Fifteenth Edition   Volume 1

CECIL
Textbook of Medicine

Edited by

PAUL B. BEESON, M.D.

Distinguished Physician, United States Veterans Administration,
Professor of Medicine, University of Washington School of Medicine

WALSH McDERMOTT, M.D.

Emeritus Professor of Public Health and Medicine, Cornell University
Medical College; Special Advisor to the President, Robert Wood Johnson Foundation

JAMES B. WYNGAARDEN, M.D.

Frederic M. Hanes Professor and Chairman,
Department of Medicine, Duke University Medical Center

W. B. SAUNDERS COMPANY · Philadelphia · London · Toronto

W. B. Saunders Company: West Washington Square
Philadelphia, PA   19105

1 St. Anne's Road
Eastbourne, East Sussex BN21 3UN, England

1 Goldthorne Avenue
Toronto, Ontario M8Z 5T9, Canada

Listed here are the latest translated editions of this book, together
with the language of the translation and the publisher.

Portuguese (14th Edition) — Editora Interamericana Ltda., Rio de Janeiro, Brazil

Serbo-Croat (11th Edition) — Medicinska Knjiga, Belgrade, Yugoslavia

Spanish (14th Edition) — Nueva Editorial Interamericana S.A. de C.V., Mexico

Single Vol: ISBN 0-7216-1663-1
Vol I: ISBN 0-7216-1664-X
Vol II: ISBN 0-7216-1666-6
Set: ISBN 0-7216-1667-4

Textbook of Medicine

Last digit is the print number: 9   8   7   6   5   4

What is a textbook? It is a putting-together of discrete pieces of information into a cohesive, meaningful pattern. In the weaving of the pattern, the editors of this Fifteenth Edition of the *Textbook of Medicine* have been mindful, as in the previous editions, of the original purposes of Russell Cecil and Robert Loeb to provide authoritative clinical guidance and a reasoned, scientific basis for the pursuit of medicine. The two ideas are complementary, for an understanding of the mechanisms of disease and its manifestations enables the physician to select appropriate diagnostic procedures and therapy. This guiding principle is underscored by introducing each major section with an overview of pathophysiology and the principles of approach to the clinical problem.

The period of time covered by the editions of this textbook extends from 1927, soon after the epochal discoveries of insulin for diabetes and the liver treatment of pernicious anemia, through an era of unprecedented productivity in biomedical research and clinical investigation; hence each succeeding edition has required substantial revision to keep pace with emerging knowledge and technology. The first edition came to about 800,000 words and had 130 contributors. The present edition runs well over 2,000,000 words and has 237 contributors. The number of individual clinical entities and syndromes has grown from about 550 in the first edition to an almost uncountable number in the current edition. For example, the subject of intestinal malabsorption, of which 41 forms are now described, was dealt with only under the term "tropical sprue" in 1927. Sickle cell anemia was given a nine-line paragraph in the first edition; there are now five chapters dealing with disorders associated with 180 different hemoglobins. The diagnostic procedures available in 1927 were relatively simple and crude (blood sugar, blood urea nitrogen, x-ray, and the use of rigid endoscopes). Modern diagnostic capabilities are, by comparison, immensely refined, including such precise aids as angiography, ultrasound, and computerized tomography, together with many new chemical determinations, some so delicate that they can measure hormone concentrations in picogram quantities.

Our therapeutic capabilities have similarly expanded. In 1927 two favorite drugs, arsenic (Fowler's solution) and potassium iodide, were each recommended for 30 to 40 different diseases. The current edition discusses the use of scores of effective and well-tested compounds, along with such high technologies as renal dialysis, parenteral nutrition, platelet transfusion, assisted respiration, and cardiac pacemakers. Surgery of the heart has revolutionized the practice of cardiology, and the replacement of joints has gained an established place in the field of rheumatology.

The flow of new ideas and new procedures continues, as reflected in this new edition. Several major Parts have been completely revised and rewritten: Respiratory Disease, Cardiovascular Diseases, Renal Diseases, Diseases of Bone, and Certain Cutaneous Diseases with Significant Systemic Manifestations. Indeed, all continuing chapters have been revised to a greater or lesser extent to fit today's situation.

Several new Parts have been added. First is one on Human Growth and Development. The remarkable lengthening in average life span that is taking place in this century calls for greater textbook emphasis on the changes that occur over time in the structure and function of the human body. Inasmuch as older patients make disproportionate demands on health services, it can be predicted that when our present medical students and house officers reach mid-career, about half their work will be in the care of people over the age of 65 years.

Another new Part—Critical Care Medicine—has been made necessary by advances both in the understanding and in the technology of supportive measures for failing respiratory, cardiac, or renal function. Coronary care units and medical intensive care units are now commonplace in general hospitals, and the specialty of critical care medicine has emerged. Inevitably, some of the matters discussed in this Part must also be mentioned in other chapters; nevertheless, it seemed desirable to bring together a general discussion of the principles of this kind of treatment in a separate Part.

Oncology is now a formal subspecialty of internal medicine, with a rapidly expanding body of knowledge from research and from clinical experience. The editors felt it appropriate, therefore, to consolidate chapters on cancer into a new Part, to give the user easier access to information, and to underscore the importance of the subject in clinical practice.

Ocular manifestations accompany many systemic diseases, and it was decided that this edition should include a Part dealing with those aspects of ophthalmology that should be part of the working knowledge of the internist or primary care physician. Special emphasis is laid on the funduscopic changes that may provide clues to the existence or progress of such conditions as lupus erythematosus, leukemia, hypertension, and hereditary disorders.

Another new Part deals with the subject of Drug-Drug Interactions. Although the detail of this subject is immense, the editors believe that certain principles which underlie such interactions can be illustrated in examples and that they would be helpful to users of the book.

Diagnostic techniques have undergone remarkable changes since the last edition; consequently much more emphasis is given to use of such procedures as fiberscopic endoscopy, ultrasound, computerized tomography, Doppler studies, nuclear imaging, and selective angiography.

This body of information is now so vast that the place

of importance of each individual piece cannot be finally judged solely by the editors; they must have expert help. For Disorders of the Nervous System and Behavior there is a separate editor, Fred Plum. In addition, nine physicians widely recognized as expert authorities in particular branches of medicine have served as Consulting Editors: Alexander Bearn (Medical Genetics), Nicholas Christy (Diseases of the Endocrine System), Philip Marsden (Protozoan and Helminthic Diseases), John Murray (Respiratory Disease), Ralph Nachman (Hematologic and Hematopoietic Diseases), Roscoe Robinson (Renal Diseases), Marvin Sleisenger (Diseases of the Digestive System), Andrew Wallace (Cardiovascular Diseases), and Sheldon Wolff (Microbial Diseases). A book is ideas made visible. This process could not have been accomplished without these consulting editors and the contributors. We are greatly indebted to them all for their selfless help.

In order to assist our users to cope with the increasing need for continuing medical education and recertification, a companion book is in preparation, to be used in self-assessment study. Its questions and answers are being devised by members of the Departments of Medicine at Duke University and the University of California, San Francisco.

To have attempted to put the essence of contemporary medicine within the covers of this textbook is an exciting and demanding adventure in which the three of us have joined as Co-Editors. For Beeson and McDermott this edition will be the last, and Wyngaarden will be joined by Lloyd H. Smith, Jr., as Co-Editor of the next edition. This change is in keeping with the book's history of orderly transition.

We cannot close without expressing our pleasure in the friendship and invaluable advice of Jack Hanley, Vice President and General Manager for Health Sciences of the W. B. Saunders Company. We wish also to thank the many other able and devoted people in the Company from whom we have learned so much. It is a special pleasure to acknowledge with gratitude the skill and untiring efforts of Dave Kilmer, Special Projects Editor at Saunders, who has so ably helped us to bring together this large assemblage of writings. Finally, we must acknowledge special indebtedness to Helen Miller, who has now been with the book for five editions, and to Patsey Sutphin, for whom this edition has been the first. Together these editorial assistants have done a splendid job not only in faultlessly handling hundreds of manuscripts and proofs, but in providing the linkage that binds contributors, publisher, consulting editors, and ourselves to the facts and ideals of medicine. Their help deserves, and has, our deepest thanks.

PAUL B. BEESON
WALSH McDERMOTT
JAMES B. WYNGAARDEN

DOSAGE NOTICE

Extraordinary efforts have been made by the authors, the editors, and the publisher of this book to ensure that dosage recommendations are precise and in agreement with the highest standards of practice.

It does happen, however, that dosage schedules are changed from time to time in the light of accumulating clinical experience and continuing laboratory studies. This is most likely to occur in the case of recently introduced products.

It is urged, therefore, that you check the package information data for the manufacturer's recommended dosage. In addition, there are some quite serious situations, each encountered only rarely, in which drug therapy must be individualized and expert judgment advises the use of a higher dosage or administration by a different route than is included in the manufacturer's recommendations. Throughout the text many such instances are indicated by a footnote.

THE EDITORS

FRANCOIS M. ABBOUD, M.D.

Shock

Professor of Medicine and Physiology; Head, Department of Medicine; and Director, Cardiovascular Center, College of Medicine, University of Iowa. Chief of Medicine, University Hospitals, Iowa City, Iowa.

ALBERT J. AGUAYO, M.D., F.R.C.P.(C.)

Mechanical Lesions of the Nerve Roots and Spinal Cord

Professor of Neurology and Neurosurgery, McGill University. Senior Physician, The Montreal General Hospital, Montreal, Quebec, Canada.

CURTIS P. ARTZ, M.D.

Electric Shock and Electric Injury

Late Distinguished University Professor and Chairman, Department of Surgery, Medical University of South Carolina. Late Chief of Surgery, Medical University Hospital, Charleston, South Carolina.

G. D. AURBACH, M.D.

Parathyroid

Chief, Metabolic Diseases Branch, National Institute of Arthritis, Metabolism, and Digestive Diseases, National Institutes of Health, Bethesda, Maryland.

K. FRANK AUSTEN, M.D.

Connective Tissue Diseases ("Collagen Diseases") Other Than Rheumatoid Arthritis: Introduction; Periarteritis Nodosa

Theodore B. Bayles Professor of Medicine, Harvard Medical School. Physician-in-Chief, Robert B. Brigham Hospital, Boston, Massachusetts.

LOUIS V. AVIOLI, M.D.

Diseases of Bone

Shoenberg Professor of Medicine, Washington University School of Medicine. Chief of Endocrinology, The Jewish Hospital of St. Louis; Attending Physician, Barnes Hospital, Jewish Hospital, and St. Louis Children's Hospital; Director, Division of Bone and Mineral Metabolism, and Director, Metabolic Bone Unit, Shriner's Hospital, St. Louis, Missouri.

ROBERT W. BALOH, M.D.

Hearing Loss

Associate Professor of Neurology, Reed Neurologic Research Center, UCLA School of Medicine. Director, Neurotology Clinic, UCLA Center for the Health Sciences, Los Angeles, California.

J. RICHARD BARINGER, M.D.

Herpes Simplex Encephalitis

Professor of Neurology and Pathology, Vice-Chairman, Department of Neurology, University of California, San Francisco. Chief, Neurology Service, Veterans Administration Hospital, San Francisco, California.

ALEXANDER G. BEARN, M.D.

Heredity; Genetic Principles: Introduction; Pedigree Analysis in Inherited Disease; Inborn Errors of Metabolism and Molecular Disease; Polygenic and Multifactorial Inheritance; Pharmacogenetics; Population Genetics; Congenital Malformations; Prevention and Management of Genetic Disease; Albinism; Wilson's Disease; The Mucopolysaccharidoses; Marfan's Syndrome; Acatalasia; Familial Dysautonomia; Laurence-Moon Syndrome; Lipoatrophic Diabetes; Lipoid Proteinosis; Werner's Syndrome

Stanton Griffis Distinguished Medical Professor and Professor of Medicine, Cornell University Medical College. Attending Physician, The New York Hospital, New York, New York.

MARGARET R. BECKLAKE, M.D., F.R.C.P.

Physical and Chemical Irritants

Professor, Department of Medicine and Department of Epidemiology and Health, McGill University. Associate of the Medical Research Council of Canada. Senior Physician, Royal Victoria Hospital, Montreal, Quebec, Canada.

PAUL B. BEESON, M.D.

On Becoming a Clinician; Granulomatous Diseases of Unproved Etiology: Introduction; Polymyalgia Rheumatica and Cranial Arteritis; Relapsing Polychondritis; Weber-Christian Disease; Fibrosing Syndromes; Eosinophilic Syndromes; Epidemic Neuromyasthenia

Distinguished Physician, United States Veterans Administration; Professor of Medicine, University of Washington, Seattle, Washington.

VICTOR S. BEHAR, M.D.

Diseases of the Myocardium: Introduction; Asymmetric Septal Hypertrophy; Familial Cardiomyopathy; Inflammatory or Infective Cardiomyopathy; Nutritional Cardiomyopathy; Cardiac Amyloidosis; Other Cardiomyopathies

Associate Professor of Medicine and Associate Director, Cardiovascular Laboratory, Duke University Medical Center, Durham, North Carolina.

JOHN E. BENNETT, M.D.

Nocardiosis; Cryptococcosis; Mucormycosis; Aspergillosis; Candidiasis

Head, Clinical Mycology Section, Laboratory of Clinical Investigation, National Institute of Allergy and Infectious Disease, Bethesda, Maryland.

ROBERT N. BERK, M.D.

Diagnostic Imaging Procedures in Gastroenterology

Professor and Chairman, Department of Radiology, University of California, San Diego School of Medicine, La Jolla. Director, Department of Radiology, University Hospital, San Diego, California.

ERNEST BEUTLER, M.D.

Galactosemia

Chairman, Department of Clinical Research, and Member, Scripps Clinic and Research Foundation, La Jolla, California.

EDWIN L. BIERMAN, M.D.

Obesity

Professor of Medicine and Head, Division of Metabolism and Endocrinology, University of Washington School of Medicine. Attending Physician, University of Washington Affiliated Hospitals, Seattle, Washington.

IRA B. BLACK, M.D.

Idiopathic Autonomic Insufficiency

Associate Professor of Neurology, Cornell University Medical College. Associate Attending Neurologist, New York Hospital, New York, New York.

LEO F. BLACK, M.D.

Cysts and Neoplasms of the Lung

Associate Professor of Medicine, Mayo Medical School. Consultant, Division of Thoracic Diseases and Internal Medicine, Mayo Clinic, Rochester, Minnesota.

DANE R. BOGGS, M.D.

The Leukopenic State

Professor of Medicine, and Chief, Division of Hematology-Oncology, University of Pittsburgh School of Medicine, Pittsburgh, Pennsylvania.

PHILIP K. BONDY, M.D.

Medical Treatment of Hormone-Dependent Cancers

Professor of Medicine, Yale University School of Medicine. Associate Chief of Staff for Research, West Haven Veterans Administration Hospital; Attending, Yale–New Haven Hospital, New Haven, Connecticut.

THOMAS H. BOTHWELL, M.D., D.Sc., F.R.C.P., F.A.C.P.(Hon.)

Hemochromatosis

Professor of Medicine, University of the Witwatersrand Medical School. Chief Physician, Johannesburg Hospital, Johannesburg, South Africa.

M. C. BRAIN, D.M., F.R.C.P., F.R.C.P.(C.)

The Anemias: Introduction; Aplastic Anemia; Sideroblastic Anemia; Myelophthisic Anemia

Professor of Medicine, McMaster University. Physician, McMaster University Medical Centre and Hamilton Civic Hospitals, Hamilton, Ontario, Canada.

LLOYD L. BRANDBORG, M.D.

Neoplastic Diseases of the Alimentary Tract: Introduction; Neoplasms of the Esophagus; Malignant Neoplasms of the Stomach; Benign Neoplasms of the Stomach

Clinical Professor of Medicine, University of California, San Francisco. Chief, Gastroenterology Section, Veterans Administration Hospital, San Francisco; Consultant, Letterman Army Medical Center, U.S. Public Health Service Hospital, San Francisco, Oakland Naval Hospital, Oakland, and David Grant Air Force Medical Center, Travis Air Force Base, California.

BARRY M. BRENNER, M.D.

Structure and Function of the Kidneys

Samuel A. Levine Professor of Medicine, Harvard Medical School. Director, Renal Division, and Physician, Peter Bent Brigham Hospital, Boston; Consultant, Veterans Administration Hospital, West Roxbury, Massachusetts.

RUBIN BRESSLER, M.D.

Drug-Drug Interactions

Professor and Head, Internal Medicine, Professor of Pharmacology, and Chief, Clinical Pharmacology, Department of Internal Medicine, University of Arizona Medical Center, Tucson, Arizona.

NEAL S. BRICKER, M.D.

The Pathophysiology of Chronic Renal Disease; Acute Renal Failure

Professor of Medicine, School of Medicine, University of California, Los Angeles. Attending Nephrologist, UCLA Hospital and Clinics, Los Angeles, California.

FRANK P. BROOKS, M.D., Sc.D.(Med.)

Diseases of the Pancreas

Professor of Medicine and Physiology, School of Medicine, University of Pennsylvania. Member, Gastrointestinal Section, Hospital of the University of Pennsylvania, Philadelphia, Pennsylvania.

ELMER B. BROWN, M.D.

Acute Hemorrhagic Anemia; Anemia Associated with Infection and Chronic Systemic Diseases; Hypochromic Anemias

Professor of Medicine and Associate Dean for Continuing Medical Education, Washington University School of Medicine. Associate Physician, Barnes Hospital, St. Louis, Missouri.

ANTHONY D. M. BRYCESON, M.D., F.R.C.P.E., D.T.M. & H.

Relapsing Fever; Tropical Phagedenic Ulcer; Leishmaniasis

Senior Lecturer, London School of Hygiene and Tropical Medicine. Consultant Physician, Hospital for Tropical Diseases, London, England.

THOMAS M. BUCHANAN, M.D.

Brucellosis

Associate Professor of Medicine, University of Washington. Head, Immunology Research Laboratory, U.S. Public Health Service Hospital, Seattle; Attending Physician in Medicine and Infectious Diseases, U.S. Public Health Service Hospital, Harborview Medical Center, and Fred Hutchison Cancer Research Center, Seattle, Washington.

BENJAMIN BURROWS, M.D.

Diseases Associated with Airways Obstruction; Abnormalities of Lung Aeration

Professor of Internal Medicine, University of Arizona College of Medicine. Director, Division of Respiratory Sciences, and Staff Physician, Arizona Health Sciences Center, Tucson, Arizona.

GEORGE F. CAHILL, Jr., M.D.

Diabetes Mellitus

Director of Research, Howard Hughes Medical Institute; Professor of Medicine, Harvard Medical School. Physician, Peter Bent Brigham Hospital, Boston, Massachusetts.

PAUL CALABRESI, M.D.

Principles of Oncologic Treatment: Irradiation, Cytotoxic Drugs, and Immunostimulatory Procedures

Professor of Internal Medicine, Brown University. Chief of Medicine, Roger Williams General Hospital, Providence, Rhode Island.

PAUL P. CARBONE, M.D.

Lymphoreticular Neoplasms: Introduction; Burkitt's Lymphoma

Professor and Chairman, Department of Human Oncology, Professor of Medicine, University of Wisconsin. Attending, University Hospitals and Middleton Veterans Administration Hospital, Madison, Wisconsin.

CHARLES C. J. CARPENTER, M.D.

Shigellosis; Cholera

Professor and Chairman, Department of Medicine, Case Western Reserve University. Physician-in-Chief, University Hospitals of Cleveland, Ohio.

HUGH CHAPLIN, Jr., M.D.

Hemoglobinuria; Transfusion Reactions

Professor of Medicine and Preventive Medicine, Washington University School of Medicine. Associate Physician, Barnes Hospital, St. Louis, Missouri.

CHARLES L. CHRISTIAN, M.D.

Diseases of the Joints

Professor of Medicine, Cornell University Medical College. Physician-in-Chief, Hospital for Special Surgery; Attending Physician, The New York Hospital, New York, New York.

NICHOLAS P. CHRISTY, M.D.

Endocrine Syndromes Associated with Cancer; Diseases of the Endocrine System: Introduction; The Anterior Pituitary

Professor of Medicine, College of Physicians and Surgeons, Columbia University. Director of Medical Service, Roosevelt Hospital; Attending Physician, Presbyterian Hospital, New York, New York.

LEIGHTON E. CLUFF, M.D.

Diseases Caused by Malleomyces; Anthrax; Listeriosis; Erysipeloid of Rosenbach

Adjunct Professor of Medicine, University of Pennsylvania School of Medicine, Philadelphia. Vice-President, Robert Wood Johnson Foundation, Princeton, New Jersey.

JAY D. COFFMAN, M.D.

Diseases of the Peripheral Vessels

Professor of Medicine, Boston University School of Medicine. Section Head, Peripheral Vascular Section, and Visiting Physician, University Hospital, Boston, Massachusetts.

C. LOCKARD CONLEY, M.D.

Hemoglobin, the Hemoglobinopathies, and the Thalassemias

Distinguished Service Professor of Medicine, Head of the Hematology Division, Department of Medicine, The Johns Hopkins University School of Medicine. Physician, The Johns Hopkins Hospital, Baltimore, Maryland.

ROBERT B. COUCH, M.D.

Mycoplasmal Diseases

Professor of Microbiology and Immunology and Medicine, Baylor College of Medicine. Attending Physician, Baylor Affiliated Hospitals: Ben Taub General Hospital, Veterans Administration Hospital, and The Methodist Hospital, Houston, Texas.

ANTHONY N. DAMATO, M.D.

Cardiac Arrhythmia

Chief, Medical Department, U.S. Public Health Service Hospital, Staten Island, New York.

JEFFERSON C. DAVIS, M.D., M.P.H.

Alterations in Atmospheric Pressure

Chief, Hyperbaric Medicine, U.S. Air Force School of Aerospace Medicine; Clinical Assistant Professor, Anesthesiology, University of Texas Health Science Center, at San Antonio; Visiting Scientist, Department of Biology, Texas A & M University.

THOMAS E. DAVIS, M.D.

Non-Hodgkin's Lymphomas

Assistant Professor of Human Oncology and Medicine, University of Wisconsin School of Medicine. Attending Physician, University Hospitals, Madison, Wisconsin.

LESLIE J. DeGROOT, M.D.

The Thyroid

Professor of Medicine, University of Chicago, Pritzker School of Medicine. Head of Endocrine Section, Billings Hospital, University of Chicago, Chicago, Illinois.

ROGER M. DES PREZ, M.D.

Tuberculosis; Extrapulmonary Tuberculosis

Professor of Medicine, Vanderbilt University Medical School. Chief, Medical Service, Veterans Administration Hospital, Nashville, Tennessee.

BERTRAM D. DINMAN, M.D., Sc.D.

Carbon Monoxide Poisoning

Adjunct Professor, Occupational Health, Graduate School of Public Health, University of Pittsburgh. Vice President, Health and Safety, Aluminum Company of America, Pittsburgh, Pennsylvania.

PHILIP R. DODGE, M.D.

Infections and Inflammatory Diseases of the Central Nervous System and Its Coverings: Introduction; Aids to Diagnosis in Intracranial and Intraspinal Inflammatory Disease; Spinal Epidural Infections; Transverse Myelitis or Myelopathy; Syphilitic Infections of the Nervous System

Professor of Pediatrics and of Neurology, Head of the Edward Mallinckrodt Department of Pediatrics, Washington University School of Medicine. Medical Director, St. Louis Children's Hospital; Pediatrician-in-Chief and Neurologist, Barnes and Affiliated Hospitals, St. Louis, Missouri.

RAPHAEL DOLIN, M.D.

Viral Gastroenteritis Caused by Norwalk-Like Agents and Rotaviruses

Head, Medical Virology Section, National Institute of Allergy and Infectious Diseases, National Institutes of Health, Bethesda, Maryland. Associate Professor of Medicine, Uniformed University of the Health Sciences.

C. T. DOLLERY, M.B., F.R.C.P.

Arterial Hypertension

Professor of Clinical Pharmacology, Royal Postgraduate Medical School. Consultant Physician, Hammersmith Hospital, London, England.

DAVID A. DRACHMAN, M.D.

Dizziness and Vertigo

Professor and Chairman, Department of Neurology, University of Massachusetts Medical Center. Attending Physician, University of Massachusetts, Worcester City Hospital, and St. Vincent Hospital, Worcester, Massachusetts.

PIERRE M. DREYFUS, M.D.

Nutritional Disorders of the Nervous System

Professor and Chairman, Department of Neurology, School of Medicine, University of California, Davis. Chief, Neurology Service, Sacramento Medical Center of the University of California, Davis, Sacramento; Consultant, U.S. Air Force Base Hospital, Travis, and Veterans Administration Hospital, Martinez, California.

PETER JAMES DYCK, M.D.

Diseases of the Peripheral Nervous System

Professor of Neurology, Mayo Medical School, Rochester, Minnesota.

DAVID L. EARNEST, M.D.

Other Diseases of the Colon, Rectum, and Anus

Associate Professor of Medicine, University of Arizona College of Medicine. Chief of Gastroenterology, University of Arizona Health Sciences Center, Tucson; Consultant, Veterans Administration Hospitals, Tucson and Phoenix, Arizona.

THEODORE C. EICKHOFF, M.D.

Colorado Tick Fever

Professor of Medicine and Head, Division of Infectious Disease, University of Colorado Medical Center, Denver, Colorado.

BRYAN T. EMMERSON, M.D., Ph.D.

Toxic Nephropathy

Professor of Medicine, University of Queensland Medical School. Physician in Charge, University Medical Unit, Princess Alexandra Hospital, Brisbane, Australia.

KARL ENGELMAN, M.D.

The Adrenal Medulla and Sympathetic Nervous System; The Carcinoid Syndrome

Associate Professor of Medicine and Pharmacology, University of Pennsylvania School of Medicine. Attending Physician, Hospital of the University of Pennsylvania, Philadelphia Veterans Administration Hospital, and Childrens Hospital of Philadelphia; Director, Clinical Research Center, Hospital of the University of Pennsylvania, Philadelphia, Pennsylvania.

ALLAN J. ERSLEV, M.D.

Polycythemia

Cardeza Research Professor of Medicine and Director, Cardeza Foundation for Hematologic Research, Thomas Jefferson University. Attending Physician, Thomas Jefferson University Hospital, Philadelphia, Pennsylvania.

ANTHONY S. FAUCI, M.D.

Wegener's Granulomatosis; Midline Granuloma; Familial Mediterranean Fever

Head, Clinical Physiology Section, Laboratory of Clinical Investigation, Deputy Clinical Director, National Institute of Allergy and Infectious Diseases, National Institutes of Health, Bethesda, Maryland.

ALVAN R. FEINSTEIN, M.D.

Science, Clinical Medicine, and the Spectrum of Disease

Professor of Medicine and Epidemiology, and Director, Robert Wood Johnson Clinical Scholar Program, Yale University School of Medicine. Attending Physician, Yale–New Haven Hospital, New Haven; Senior Biostatistician, Cooperative Studies Program Coordinating Center, West Haven Veterans Administration Hospital, West Haven, Connecticut.

F. ROBERT FEKETY, Jr., M.D.

Staphylococcal Infections

Professor of Internal Medicine, University of Michigan School of Medicine. Attending Physician and Chief, Infectious Disease Service, University Hospital, Ann Arbor, Michigan.

HARRY A. FELDMAN, M.D.

Meningococcal Disease

Professor and Chairman, Department of Preventive Medicine, State University of New York, Upstate Medical Center, Syracuse, New York.

PHILIP FELIG, M.D.

Nutritional Maintenance and Diet Therapy in Acute and Chronic Disease

C. N. H. Long Professor and Vice Chairman, Department of Medicine, and Chief, Section of Endocrinology, Yale School of Medicine. Vice Chairman, Department of Medicine and Chief of Endocrinology, Yale–New Haven Hospital, New Haven, Connecticut.

THOMAS F. FERRIS, M.D.

Renal Disease in Pregnancy

Professor and Chairman, Department of Medicine, University of Minnesota. Consultant, Veterans Administration Hospital, Minneapolis, Minnesota.

SYDNEY M. FINEGOLD, M.D.

Disease Due to Nonsporeforming Anaerobic Bacteria; Lung Abscess and Bronchiectasis

Professor of Medicine, UCLA School of Medicine. Chief, Infectious Disease Section, Wadsworth Hospital Center, Veterans Administration, Los Angeles, California.

ALFRED P. FISHMAN, M.D.

Heart Failure

William Maul Measey Professor of Medicine, University of Pennsylvania School of Medicine. Director, Cardiovascular-Pulmonary Division, Hospital of the University of Pennsylvania, Philadelphia, Pennsylvania.

ROBERT A. FISHMAN, M.D.

Intracranial Tumors and States Causing Increased Intracranial Pressure

Professor and Chairman, Department of Neurology, University of California, San Francisco. Chief, Neurology Service, University of California Hospitals, San Francisco; Attending Neurologist, San Francisco General Hospital; Consultant in Neurology, Veterans Administration Hospital, San Francisco, California.

EDMUND B. FLINK, M.D., Ph.D.

Heavy Metal Poisoning

Professor of Internal Medicine, West Virginia University Medical Center, Morgantown, West Virginia.

KATHLEEN M. FOLEY, M.D.

Neurologic Diagnostic Procedures

Assistant Professor of Neurology, Cornell University Medical College. Assistant Attending Neurologist, Memorial Sloan-Kettering Cancer Center, New York, New York.

NOBLE O. FOWLER, M.D.

Diseases of the Aorta

Professor of Medicine, University of Cincinnati College of Medicine. Director, Division of Cardiology, University of Cincinnati Medical Center; Chief Clinician, Cardiac Clinic, Cincinnati General Hospital, Cincinnati, Ohio.

DONALD S. FREDRICKSON, M.D.

Gaucher's Disease; Niemann-Pick Disease

Director, National Institutes of Health, Bethesda, Maryland.

NORBERT FREINKEL, M.D.

Hypoglycemic Disorders

Kettering Professor of Medicine; Director, Center for Endocrinology, Metabolism and Nutrition; and Chief, Section of Endocrinology, Metabolism and Nutrition; Northwestern University Medical School. Attending Physician, Northwestern Memorial Hospital; Consultant in Endocrinology and Metabolism, Veterans Administration Lakeside Hospital, Chicago, Illinois.

JOHN I. GALLIN, M.D.

The Compromised Host

Head, Bacterial Disease Section, Laboratory of Clinical Investigation, National Institute of Allergy and Infectious Disease, National Institutes of Health, Bethesda, Maryland.

KENNETH D. GARDNER, Jr., M.D.

Cystic Diseases of the Kidney

Professor of Medicine, University of New Mexico School of Medicine. Chief, Division of Renal Diseases, Bernalillo County Medical Center; Attending Nephrologist, Albuquerque Veterans Administration Hospital; Consulting Nephrologist, Presbyterian Medical Center, Albuquerque, New Mexico.

JEFFREY A. GELFAND, M.D.

Complement

Assistant Professor of Medicine, Tufts University School of Medicine. Assistant Physician, Department of Medicine, Tufts–New England Medical Center, Boston, Massachusetts.

PARK S. GERALD, M.D.

Chromosomes and Their Disorders

Professor of Pediatrics, Harvard Medical School. Chief, Clinical Genetics Division, Children's Hospital Medical Center, Boston, Massachusetts.

NORMAN GESCHWIND, M.D.

Focal Disturbances of Higher Nervous Function

James Jackson Putnam Professor of Neurology, Harvard Medical School. Neurologist-in-Chief, Beth Israel Hospital, Boston, Massachusetts.

GILBERT H. GLASER, M.D., Med.Sc.D.

The Epilepsies

Professor of Neurology and Chairman, Department of Neurology, Yale University School of Medicine. Chief of Neurology, Yale–New Haven Hospital, New Haven; Consultant in Neurology, Veterans Administration Hospital, West Haven, Connecticut.

RICHARD J. GLASSOCK, M.D.

Mechanisms of Renal Injury

Professor of Medicine, UCLA School of Medicine. Chief, Division of Nephrology and Hypertension, Los Angeles County Harbor–UCLA Medical Center, Torrance, California.

JAMES F. GLENN, M.D.

Anomalies of the Urinary Tract; Tumors of the Kidney

Professor of Urology, Duke University School of Medicine. Chief of Urology, Duke University Medical Center, Durham, North Carolina.

MARTIN GOLDBERG, M.D.

Interstitial Nephritis and Interstitial Nephropathy

Professor of Medicine, University of Pennsylvania School of Medicine. Chief, Renal-Electrolyte Section, Hospital of the University of Pennsylvania, Philadelphia, Pennsylvania.

RALPH GOLDMAN, M.D.

Aging and Geriatric Medicine

Formerly Professor of Medicine, UCLA School of Medicine. Assistant Chief Medical Director for Extended Care, Veterans Administration Central Office, Washington, D.C.

ROBERT A. GOOD, Ph.D., M.D.

The Primary Immunodeficiency Diseases

President and Director, Sloan-Kettering Institute for Cancer Research; Professor of Medicine and Pediatrics, Cornell University Medical College; Adjunct Professor, Rockefeller University, New York, New York. Attending Physician, Departments of Medicine and Pediatrics, Memorial Hospital for Cancer and Allied Diseases, New York, New York.

ROBERT A. GOODWIN, Jr., M.D.

Pulmonary Tuberculosis; Diseases Due to Mycobacteria Other Than M. tuberculosis and M. leprae

Professor of Medicine, Vanderbilt University School of Medicine. Chief, Pulmonary Disease Section, Veterans Administration Hospital, Nashville; Visiting Staff, Vanderbilt University Hospital; Consultant, St. Thomas Hospital, Nashville, Tennessee.

SHERWOOD L. GORBACH, M.D.

Typhoid Fever

Professor of Medicine and Microbiology, Tufts University

School of Medicine. Chief, Infectious Disease Service, Tufts–New England Medical Center Hospital, Boston, Massachusetts.

GARETH M. GREEN, M.D.

Infiltrative Diseases of the Lung

Professor of Environmental Health Sciences, Johns Hopkins School of Hygiene and Public Health, Baltimore, Maryland.

B. M. GREENWOOD, M.D., F.R.C.P.

African Trypanosomiasis

Senior Lecturer in Medicine, Ahmadu Bello University, Zaria, Nigeria.

MORTON I. GROSSMAN, M.D., Ph.D.

Peptic Ulcer: Pathogenesis and Pathophysiology

Professor of Medicine and Physiology, UCLA School of Medicine. Senior Medical Investigator, Veterans Administration Wadsworth Hospital Center, Los Angeles, California.

J. CAULIE GUNNELLS, Jr., M.D.

Vascular Disorders of the Kidney

Professor of Medicine, Duke University School of Medicine, Durham, North Carolina.

THORSTEIN GUTHE, M.D., M.P.H.

Nonsyphilitic Treponematoses

Former Chief Medical Officer, Venereal Diseases and Treponematoses, World Health Organization, Geneva, Switzerland. Director, Institute of Medicine, Alkem-Spigerverket, Oslo, Norway.

ROBERT J. HAGGERTY, M.D.

Common Accidental Poisoning

Roger I. Lee Professor of Health Services and Pediatrics, Harvard School of Public Health, Harvard Medical School. Senior Physician, Children's Hospital Medical Center, Boston, Massachusetts.

JAMES B. HANSHAW, M.D.

Cytomegalovirus Infections

Professor and Chairman, Department of Pediatrics, University of Massachusetts Medical School. Chief of Pediatrics, University of Massachusetts Medical Center and St. Vincent Hospital, Worcester, Massachusetts.

EDWARD D. HARRIS, Jr., M.D.

Systemic Sclerosis

Professor of Medicine, Dartmouth-Hitchcock Medical Center; Director, Arthritis Center, and Chief, Connective Tissue Disease Section. Staff Physician, Mary Hitchcock Memorial Hospital, Hanover, New Hampshire; Veterans Administration Hospital, White River Junction, Vermont.

RICHARD J. HAVEL, M.D.

Disorders of Lipid Metabolism

Professor of Medicine, University of California School of Medicine, San Francisco, California.

LEE W. HENDERSON, M.D.

Hemodialysis

Professor of Medicine in Residence, University of California, San Diego. Associate Chief of Staff for Research, Veterans Administration Hospital, San Diego; Staff Physician, University Hospital, San Diego, California.

VICTOR HERBERT, M.D., J.D.

Megaloblastic Anemias

Professor of Medicine, State University of New York, Downstate Medical Center, Brooklyn. Chief, Hematology and Nutrition Laboratory, Veterans Administration Hospital, Bronx, New York.

ALBERT HEYMAN, M.D.

Syncope; Hyperventilation

Professor of Medicine (Neurology), Duke University Medical Center, Durham, North Carolina.

HOWARD H. HIATT, M.D.

Environment

Dean, Harvard School of Public Health; Professor of Medicine, Harvard Medical School. Consultant in Medicine, Beth Israel, Peter Bent Brigham, and Children's Hospitals, Boston, Massachusetts.

JAMES F. HOLLAND, M.D.

The Acute Leukemias

Professor and Chairman, Department of Neoplastic Diseases, Mt. Sinai School of Medicine of the City University of New York. Director, Cancer Center, Mt. Sinai Hospital, New York, New York.

EDWARD W. HOOK, M.D.

Pneumococcal Pneumonia; Salmonella Infections Other Than Typhoid Fever

Henry B. Mulholland Professor of Medicine and Chairman, Department of Medicine, University of Virginia School of Medicine. Physician-in-Chief, University of Virginia Hospital, Charlottesville, Virginia.

DOROTHY M. HORSTMANN, M.D.

Mumps

Professor of Epidemiology and Pediatrics, Yale University School of Medicine. Attending, Pediatrics, Yale–New Haven Hospital, New Haven, Connecticut.

CHARLES M. HUGULEY, Jr., M.D.

The Chronic Leukemias

Professor of Medicine and Director of Cancer Center, Emory University School of Medicine. Attending Staff, Emory University Hospital and Grady Memorial Hospital, Atlanta, Georgia.

JON I. ISENBERG, M.D.

Peptic Ulcer: Diagnosis; Peptic Ulcer: Medical Therapy

Professor of Medicine, UCLA School of Medicine. Chief, Gastroenterology Section, Wadsworth Veterans Administration Hospital, Los Angeles, California.

GEORGE GEE JACKSON, M.D.

The Common Cold; Rhinoviral Respiratory Disease; Viral Pharyngitis, Laryngitis, Croup, and Bronchitis; Adenoviral Infections; Respiratory Syncytial Viral Disease; Parainfluenza Viral Diseases

Professor of Medicine, Abraham Lincoln School of Medicine; Chief, Section of Infectious Diseases. Attending Physician, University of Illinois Hospital and Veterans Administration West Side Hospital; Consultant in Infectious Diseases, Veterans Administration West Side Hospital, Chicago, Illinois.

HARRY S. JACOB, M.D.

Hemolysis Due to Intracorpuscular Abnormalities

Professor of Medicine and Chief, Section of Hematology, University of Minnesota Medical School. Attending Physician, University of Minnesota Hospitals, Minneapolis Veterans Administration Hospital, Hennepin County General Hospital, Minneapolis, and St. Paul–Ramsey General Hospital, St. Paul, Minnesota.

ERNST R. JAFFÉ, M.D.

Methemoglobinemia and Sulfhemoglobinemia

Professor of Medicine, Albert Einstein College of Medicine; Head, Division of Hematology; Senior Associate Dean; Associate Dean for Faculty. Attending Physician, Bronx Municipal Hospital Center and Hospital of the Albert Einstein College of Medicine, Bronx, New York.

D. GERAINT JAMES, M.A., M.D.(Cambridge), F.R.C.P.

Sarcoidosis

Dean and Physician, Royal Northern Hospital, London, England; Consultant Ophthalmic Physician, St. Thomas' Hospital, London. Adjunct Professor of Medicine, University of Miami, Florida. Consulting Physician, Royal Navy.

HENRY D. JANOWITZ, M.D.

Chronic Inflammatory Diseases of the Intestine

Clinical Professor of Medicine, Mount Sinai School of Medicine. Head, Division of Gastroenterology, Mount Sinai Hospital, New York, New York.

ERNEST JAWETZ, M.D., Ph.D.

Trachoma and Inclusion Conjunctivitis; Lymphogranuloma Venereum

Professor of Microbiology and Medicine, University of California Medical Center, San Francisco, California.

GRAHAM H. JEFFRIES, M.B., Ch.B. (N.Z.), D.Phil.(Oxon.)

Diseases of the Liver

Professor and Chairman, Department of Medicine, Pennsylvania State University College of Medicine. Chief, Medical Service, The Milton S. Hershey Medical Center Hospital, Hershey, Pennsylvania.

KARL M. JOHNSON, M.D.

Arthropod-Borne Viral Fevers, Viral Encephalitides and Viral Hemorrhagic Fevers: Introduction; Dengue; West Nile Fever; Fevers Caused by Group A Arboviruses; Rift Valley Fever; Sandfly Fever; Arthropod-Borne Viral Encephalitides; Viral Hemorrhagic Fevers: Introduction; Hemorrhagic Fever Caused by Dengue Viruses; Crimean Hemorrhagic Fever; Hemorrhagic Diseases Caused by Arenaviruses; African Hemorrhagic Fever; Epidemic Hemorrhagic Fever

Chief, Special Pathogens Branch, Virology Division, Bureau of Laboratories Center for Disease Control, Atlanta, Georgia.

MARIE-LOUISE JOHNSON, M.D., Ph.D.

Certain Cutaneous Diseases with Significant Systemic Manifestations

Professor of Dermatology, New York University School of Medicine. Attending, New York University Medical Center; Chief, Dermatology Service, Bellevue Hospital Center, New York, New York.

RICHARD T. JOHNSON, M.D.

Viral Infections of the Nervous System: Introduction; Viral Meningitis and Encephalitis; Herpes Zoster; Slow Infections of the Nervous System

Eisenhower Professor of Neurology and Professor of Microbiology, The Johns Hopkins University School of Medicine. Neurologist, The Johns Hopkins Hospital, Baltimore, Maryland.

THOMAS C. JONES, M.D.

Malaria; Toxoplasmosis; Pneumocystosis; Babesiosis; Trichomoniasis

Associate Professor of Medicine and Associate Professor of Public Health, Cornell University Medical College. Associate Attending Physician, The New York Hospital, New York, New York.

DESMOND G. JULIAN, M.D., F.R.C.P.

Disorders of the Coronary Arteries: Introduction; Angina Pectoris; Myocardial Infarction; Sudden Death

Professor of Cardiology, University of Newcastle-upon-Tyne. Cardiologist, Freeman Hospital, Newcastle-upon-Tyne, England.

FRED S. KANTOR, M.D.

Serum Sickness; Drug Allergy; Allergic Rhinitis; Vasomotor Rhinitis; Urticaria; Angioedema; Insect Stings

Professor of Medicine, Yale University School of Medicine; Chief, Allergy and Clinical Immunology Section, Department of Medicine. Attending Physician, Yale–New Haven Hospital, New Haven, Connecticut.

NATHAN KASE, M.D.

The Ovaries

Professor of Obstetrics and Gynecology, Yale University School of Medicine. Attending Physician, Yale–New Haven Hospital, New Haven; Consultant, Greenwich Hospital, Greenwich, Griffin Hospital, Derby, New Britain General Hospital, New Britain, St. Raphael Hospital, New Haven, Stamford Hospital, Stamford, Norwalk Hospital, Norwalk, and William W. Backus Hospital, Norwich, Connecticut. National Consultant, Department of the Air Force.

HERANT A. KATCHADOURIAN, M.D.

The Life-Cycle Perspective in Medicine; Development to Adulthood; Adulthood

Professor of Psychiatry and the Behavioral Sciences, Stanford University School of Medicine; Vice Provost and Dean of Office of Undergraduate Studies, Stanford University, Stanford, California.

DONALD KAYE, M.D.

Infective Endocarditis; Gonococcal Disease

Professor and Chairman, Department of Medicine, The Medical College of Pennsylvania. Chief of Medicine, Hospital of the Medical College of Pennsylvania; Consultant in Medicine, Veterans Administration Hospital, Philadelphia, Pennsylvania.

HUGH L. KEEGAN, Ph.D.

Arthropods as Environmental Agents of Disease; Pentastomiasis; Leeches as Agents of Disease; Snakebite; Venomous Marine Animals

Professor of Preventive Medicine, University of Mississippi School of Medicine, Jackson, Mississippi.

C. HENRY KEMPE, M.D.

Variola and Vaccinia

Professor of Pediatrics and Microbiology, University of Colorado School of Medicine. Consultant, Colorado General Hospital, Fitzsimons Army Hospital, Children's Hospital, and Veterans Administration Hospital, Denver, Colorado.

D. N. S. KERR, M.S., F.R.C.P., F.R.C.P.E.

Investigation of Renal Function; Investigation of Renal Structure and Regional Function; Chronic Renal Failure

Professor of Medicine, University of Newcastle-upon-Tyne. Consultant Physician, Royal Victoria Infirmary, Newcastle-upon-Tyne, England.

JOHN H. KERR, D.M., F.F.A., R.C.S.

Tetanus

Clinical Lecturer in Anaesthetics, University of Oxford. Consultant Anaesthetist, Oxford Area Health Authority (Teaching), Nuffield Department of Anaesthetics, Radcliffe Infirmary, Oxford, England.

SIDNEY KIBRICK, M.D., Ph.D.

Varicella

Professor of Pediatrics and Microbiology, Boston University School of Medicine. Visiting Physician for Pediatrics, Boston City Hospital, Boston, Massachusetts.

EDWIN D. KILBOURNE, M.D.

Introduction to Viral Diseases; Influenza; Measles; Rubella

Professor and Chairman, Department of Microbiology, Mount Sinai School of Medicine of the City University of New York.

PRISCILLA KINCAID-SMITH, M.D., F.R.C.P., F.R.A.C.P., D.C.P., F.R.C.P.A.

Treatment of Irreversible Renal Failure by Transplantation and Dialysis: Introduction; Renal Transplantation

Professor of Medicine, University of Melbourne. Physician-in-Charge, Department of Nephrology, Royal Melbourne Hospital, Melbourne, Australia.

S. J. KLEBANOFF, M.D., Ph.D.

Neutrophil Function; Neutrophil Dysfunction Syndromes

Professor of Medicine, University of Washington School of Medicine, Seattle, Washington.

RICHARD KNIGHT, M.B., B.Chir., M.R.C.P., Ph.D., D.T.M. and H.

Amebiasis

Senior Lecturer, Department of Tropical Medicine, Liverpool School of Tropical Medicine. Honorary Consultant Physician, (Tropical Medicine), Liverpool Area Health Authority, Liverpool, England.

HILARY KOPROWSKI, M.D.

Rabies

Wistar Professor of Research Medicine, University of Pennsylvania School of Medicine, Philadelphia, Pennsylvania.

RICHARD M. KRAUSE, M.D.

Rheumatic Fever

Director, National Institute of Allergy and Infectious Diseases, National Institutes of Health, Bethesda, Maryland.

CALVIN M. KUNIN, M.D.

Enteric Bacterial Infections; Urinary Tract Infections and Pyelonephritis

Professor of Medicine and Chairman of the Department of Medicine, Ohio State University School of Medicine, Columbus, Ohio.

HENRY G. KUNKEL, M.D.

Immune Disease: Introduction

Professor of Immunology and Medicine, Rockefeller University; Adjunct Professor of Medicine, Cornell University Medical School, New York, New York.

HAROLD P. LAMBERT, M.D., F.R.C.P.

Food Poisoning

Professor of Microbial Diseases, St. George's Hospital Medical School, London. Consultant Physician, St. George's Hospital, London, England.

MAURICE B. LANDERS, III, M.D.

Diseases of the Eye

Professor of Ophthalmology, Duke University Medical Center. Attending Ophthalmologist, Veterans Administration Hospital, Durham; Chief of Ophthalmology, Veterans Administration Hospital, Asheville, North Carolina.

DAVID H. LAW, M.D.

Gastrointestinal Bleeding

Professor of Internal Medicine (Vice Chairman), University of New Mexico School of Medicine. Chief, Medical Service, Veterans Administration Hospital, Albuquerque, New Mexico.

ALEXANDER LEAF, M.D.

Posterior Pituitary

Jackson Professor of Clinical Medicine, Harvard Medical School. Chief, Medical Services, Massachusetts General Hospital, Boston, Massachusetts.

ROBERT I. LEVY, M.D.

Prevalence and Epidemiology of Cardiovascular Disease

Director, National Heart, Lung, and Blood Institute, National Institutes of Health, Bethesda, Maryland.

HERBERT L. LEY, Jr., M.D., M.P.H.

Trench Fever; Q Fever; Bartonellosis

Medical Consultant in foods and drugs, Rockville, Maryland.

GRANT W. LIDDLE, M.D.

Adrenal Cortex

Professor and Chairman, Department of Medicine, Vanderbilt University School of Medicine. Physician-in-Chief, Vanderbilt University Hospital, Nashville, Tennessee.

PHILIP H. LIEBERMAN, M.D.

Eosinophilic Granuloma and Related Syndromes

Associate Professor of Pathology, Cornell University School of Medicine. Attending Pathologist and Chief, Surgical Pathology Service, Memorial Hospital for Cancer and Allied Diseases, New York, New York.

HAROLD I. LIEF, M.D.

Medical Aspects of Sexuality

Professor of Psychiatry, University of Pennsylvania School of Medicine. Director, Marriage Council of Philadelphia, Inc., Philadelphia, Pennsylvania.

MORTIMER B. LIPSETT, M.D.

The Testis

Director, The Clinical Center, National Institutes of Health, Bethesda, Maryland.

JOHN N. LOEB, M.D.

Mode of Action of Hormones

Associate Professor of Medicine, College of Physicians and Surgeons, Columbia University; Adjunct Associate Professor, Rockefeller University. Associate Attending Physician, Presbyterian Hospital, New York, New York.

DANIEL S. LUKAS, M.D.

Pulmonary Hypertension

Associate Professor of Medicine, Cornell University Medical College. Associate Attending Physician, The New York Hospital; Consultant, Cardiopulmonary Service, Memorial Hospital, New York, New York; Vice President of Medical Affairs, Elliot Hospital, Manchester, New Hampshire.

VANIZE MACEDO, M.D.

Chagas' Disease

Professor of Tropical Medicine, University of Brasilia. Physician, Sobradinho Hospital, Brasilia, Brazil.

ANDREW M. MARGILETH, M.D.

Cat Scratch Disease

Professor and Associate Chairman, Department of Child Health and Development, George Washington University School of Medicine; Associate Professor of Pediatrics, Howard University School of Medicine. Director, Outpatient Department, Senior Attending Staff Physician, Children's Hospital National Medical Center, Washington, D.C.

PAUL A. MARKS, M.D.

Human Carcinogenesis

Frode Jensen Professor of Medicine and of Human Genetics

and Development Director, Cancer Center, Columbia University. Attending Physician, Presbyterian Hospital, New York, New York.

PHILIP D. MARSDEN, M.D.

Protozoan and Helminthic Diseases: Introduction; Protozoan Diseases: Introduction; Trypanosomiases: Introduction; Other Protozoan Diseases: Introduction; Giardiasis; Balantidiasis; Primary Amebic Meningoencephalitis; Isosporiasis; Sarcosporidiosis; Helminthic Diseases: Introduction; The Cestodes; Hermaphroditic Flukes; The Nematodes; Disorders with Some Relation to Helminths

Professor of Tropical Medicine, University of Brasilia. Physician, Sobradinho Hospital, Brasilia, Brazil.

JOHN H. McCLEMENT, M.D.

Diseases of the Pleura, Mediastinum, Diaphragm, and Chest Wall

Professor of Medicine, New York University School of Medicine. Director, Chest Service, Bellevue Hospital, New York; Attending Physician, University Hospital, New York, New York.

WALSH McDERMOTT, M.D.

Medicine in Modern Society; Chemical Contamination of Water and Air; The Nature of Microbial Diseases; Foot-and-Mouth Disease; Bacterial Diseases: Introduction; Granuloma Inguinale; Drugs and Microbes

Emeritus Professor of Public Health and Medicine, Cornell University Medical College; Special Advisor to the President, Robert Wood Johnson Foundation, Princeton, New Jersey.

FLETCHER H. McDOWELL, M.D.

Cerebrovascular Diseases

Professor of Neurology, Cornell University Medical College. Attending Neurologist, The New York Hospital; Medical Director, Burke Rehabilitation Hospital; Consulting Neurologist, Memorial Hospital, New York, New York.

PAUL R. McHUGH, M.D.

Dementia; Psychologic Illness in Medical Practice; Psychologic Testing in Clinical Medicine

Henry Phipps Professor of Psychiatry, Department of Psychiatry, and Behavioral Science, The Johns Hopkins School of Medicine. Psychiatrist-in-Chief, The Johns Hopkins Hospital, Baltimore, Maryland.

PATRICK A. McKEE, M.D.

Thrombosis

Professor of Medicine and Assistant Professor of Biochemistry, Duke University Medical Center, Durham, North Carolina.

BYRON D. McLEES, M.D., Ph.D.

Critical Care Medicine

Chief, Department of Critical Care Medicine, Clinical Center, National Institutes of Health, Bethesda, Maryland.

JACK H. MENDELSON, M.D.

Alcohol Abuse and Alcohol-Related Illness

Professor of Psychiatry, Harvard Medical School. Director, Alcohol and Drug Abuse Research Center, McLean Hospital, Belmont, Massachusetts.

JAMES H. MEYER, M.D.

Peptic Ulcer: Complications and Surgical Treatment

Associate Professor of Medicine, University of California, Los Angeles. Chief, Division of Gastroenterology, Veterans Administration Hospital, Sepulveda, California, and UCLA/San Fernando Valley Medical Program.

ROBERT B. MILLMAN, M.D.

Drug Abuse, Dependence, and Intoxication: Introduction; The Opiates; Central Nervous System Depressants; Central Nervous System Stimulants; Cannabis; Psychedelics; Miscellaneous Inhalants

Clinical Associate Professor of Public Health, Assistant Professor of Psychiatry, Cornell University Medical College. Director, Alcohol and Drug Abuse Programs, The New York Hospital–Cornell Medical Center, New York, New York.

STANLEY R. MOHLER, M.D.

Motion Sickness and Problems of Air Travel

Professor and Vice-Chairman, Department of Community Medicine, Director of Aerospace Medicine, Wright State University School of Medicine, Dayton, Ohio.

THOMAS P. MONATH, M.D.

Yellow Fever

Director, Vector-Borne Diseases Division, Bureau of Laboratories, Center for Disease Control, Public Health Service, U.S. Department of Health, Education, and Welfare, Fort Collins, Colorado.

STEPHEN I. MORSE, M.D.

Whooping Cough

Professor and Chairman, Microbiology and Immunology, State University of New York, Downstate Medical Center, Brooklyn, New York.

ARNO G. MOTULSKY, M.D.

Genetic Counseling

Professor of Medicine and Genetics, Director, Center for Inherited Diseases, University of Washington School of Medicine. Attending Physician, University Hospital, University of Washington, Seattle, Washington.

FRANCIS P. MULDOWNEY, M.D., F.R.C.P.

Obstructive Nephropathy

Research Professor of Medicine, University College, Dublin. Physician in Charge, Metabolic and Renal Unit, St. Vincent's Hospital; Consultant Physician, Metabolic Diseases, National

Maternity Hospital; Visiting Consultant, Meath Hospital; Visiting Consultant, St. Luke's Hospital, Dublin, Ireland.

JOHN F. MURRAY, M.D.

Respiratory Disease: Introduction; Respiratory Structure and Function; Respiratory Failure

Professor of Medicine, University of California, San Francisco. Chief of the Chest Service, San Francisco General Hospital, San Francisco, California.

W. P. L. MYERS, M.D.

Cancer and Internal Medicine: An Internist's Approach to Cancer and Its Medical Manifestations; The Care of the Patient with Terminal Illness

Professor of Internal Medicine and Associate Dean, Cornell University Medical College. Vice President for Educational Affairs, Memorial Sloan-Kettering Cancer Center; Attending Physician, Memorial Hospital for Cancer and Allied Diseases and The New York Hospital; Member, Sloan-Kettering Institute for Cancer Research; Formerly Chairman, Department of Medicine, Memorial Hospital for Cancer and Allied Diseases, New York, New York.

RALPH L. NACHMAN, M.D.

Hematologic and Hematopoietic Diseases: Introduction; Hemorrhagic Disorders: Disorders of Primary Hemostasis

Professor of Medicine, Cornell University Medical College. Chief, Division of Hematology, Cornell University Medical College; Attending Physician, The New York Hospital, New York, New York.

JAMES C. NIEDERMAN, M.D.

Infectious Mononucleosis

Clinical Professor of Epidemiology and Medicine, Yale University School of Medicine. Medical Staff Member, Yale–New Haven Medical Center, New Haven, Connecticut.

THOMAS F. O'BRIEN, Jr., M.D.

Neoplasms of the Small Intestine; Neoplasms of the Large Intestine

Professor of Medicine, East Carolina School of Medicine. Chief, Gastroenterology Section, East Carolina School of Medicine; Attending Physician, Pitt County Memorial Hospital, Greenville, North Carolina.

ROBERT K. OCKNER, M.D.

Vascular Diseases of the Intestine; Diseases of the Peritoneum, Mesentery, and Omentum

Professor of Medicine, University of California School of Medicine, San Francisco. Attending Physician, University of California–Moffitt, Veterans Administration, and San Francisco General Hospitals, San Francisco, California.

ELLIOTT F. OSSERMAN, M.D.

Plasma Cell Dyscrasias

American Cancer Society Professor of Medicine, Associate

Director, Institute of Cancer Research, Columbia University College of Physicians and Surgeons. Attending Physician, Presbyterian Hospital, New York, New York.

DEMOSTHENES PAPPAGIANIS, M.D., Ph.D.

Coccidioidomycosis

Professor and Chairman, Department of Medical Microbiology, School of Medicine, University of California, Davis, California.

WILLIAM W. PARMLEY, M.D.

Circulatory Function and Control

Professor of Medicine, University of California, San Francisco, School of Medicine. Chief of Cardiology, H. C. Moffitt Hospital, San Francisco, California.

RUSSEL H. PATTERSON, Jr., M.D.

Injuries of the Head and Spine

Professor of Surgery (Neurosurgery), Cornell University Medical College. Attending Surgeon-in-Charge (Neurosurgery), The New York Hospital, New York, New York.

JOSEPH K. PERLOFF, M.D.

Congenital Heart Disease

Professor of Medicine and Pediatrics, Center for the Health Sciences, School of Medicine, University of California, Los Angeles, California.

SHELDON R. PINNELL, M.D.

Ehlers-Danlos Syndrome

Investigator, Howard Hughes Medical Institute, and Professor of Medicine (Dermatology), Duke University Medical Center, Durham, North Carolina.

FRED PLUM, M.D.

Disorders of the Nervous System and Behavior: Introduction; Consciousness and Its Disturbances: Introduction; The Pathogenesis of Stupor and Coma; Acute Drug Poisoning; The Hypothalamus and Neurologic Disorders; Headache; Acute Anterior Poliomyelitis

Professor of Neurology, Cornell University Medical College. Neurologist-in-Chief, New York Hospital, New York, New York.

JEROME B. POSNER, M.D.

Delirium and Exogenous Metabolic Brain Disease; Pain; Nonmetastatic Effects of Cancer on the Nervous System

Professor of Neurology, Cornell University Medical College. Chairman, Department of Neurology, Memorial Sloan-Kettering Cancer Center, New York, New York.

OSCAR D. RATNOFF, M.D.

Hemorrhagic Disorders: Coagulation Defects

Professor of Medicine, Case Western Reserve School of Medicine. Career Investigator of the American Heart Association; Physician, University Hospitals of Cleveland, Cleveland, Ohio.

SEYMOUR REICHLIN, M.D., Ph.D.

The Control of Anterior Pituitary Secretion; The Pineal

Professor of Medicine, Tufts University School of Medicine. Chief, Endocrine Division, and Senior Physician, New England Medical Center Hospital, Boston, Massachusetts.

HERBERT Y. REYNOLDS, M.D.

Introduction to Pneumonia; Pneumonia Due to Klebsiella pneumoniae; Legionnaires' Disease; Pneumonia and Nosocomial Respiratory Infections Caused by Aerobic Gram-Negative Bacilli

Associate Professor of Internal Medicine and Head, Pulmonary Section, Department of Internal Medicine, Yale University School of Medicine. Attending Physician, Yale–New Haven Hospital, New Haven; Pulmonary Consultant, West Haven Veterans Administration Hospital, West Haven, Connecticut.

RICHARD A. RIFKIND, M.D.

Diseases of the Spleen

Professor of Medicine and of Human Genetics and Development, Columbia University College of Physicians and Surgeons. Attending Physician and Director, Division of Hematology, Presbyterian Hospital, New York, New York.

JOHN B. ROBBINS, M.D.

Hemophilus Infections with Special Emphasis on Hemophilus influenzae Type b

Director, Division of Bacterial Products, Bureau of Biologics, Food and Drug Administration, Department of Health, Education, and Welfare, Bethesda, Maryland.

RICHARD B. ROBERTS, M.D.

Antimicrobial Therapy

Professor of Medicine and Head, Division of Infectious Diseases, Cornell University Medical College. Attending Physician, The New York Hospital, New York, New York.

ROSCOE R. ROBINSON, M.D.

The Major Renal Syndromes

Florence McAlister Professor of Medicine, Duke University School of Medicine. Director, Division of Nephrology, Duke University Medical Center, Durham, North Carolina.

HEONIR ROCHA, M.D.

Diphtheria

Professor of Medicine, Faculty of Medicine, Federal University of Bahia, Salvador-Bahia, Brazil.

ROGER N. ROSENBERG, M.D.

Inherited Degenerative Diseases

Professor of Neurology and Physiology, Chairman, Department of Neurology, The University of Texas Health Science Center, Southwestern Medical School, Dallas. Chief, Neurology Service, Parkland Memorial Hospital; Attending Neurologist, Parkland Memorial Hospital and Children's Medical Center, Dallas, Texas.

SAUL A. ROSENBERG, M.D.

Hodgkin's Disease

Professor of Medicine and Radiology, Stanford University School of Medicine. Chief, Division of Oncology, Stanford University School of Medicine, Stanford, California.

JOHN ROSS, Jr., M.D.

Acquired Valvular Heart Disease

Professor of Medicine and Head, Division of Cardiology, University of California, San Diego, School of Medicine. Attending Physician, University of California Medical Center, San Diego, California.

WENDELL F. ROSSE, M.D.

Hemolytic Disorders: Introduction; Hemolysis Due to Acquired Abnormalities

Investigator, Howard Hughes Medical Institute, and Professor of Medicine and Immunology, Duke University Medical Center. Chief, Division of Hematology–Medical Oncology, Duke University Medical Center, Durham, North Carolina.

LEWIS P. ROWLAND, M.D.

Diseases of Muscle and Neuromuscular Junction

Henry and Lucy Moses Professor and Chairman, Department of Neurology, College of Physicians and Surgeons, Columbia University. Director, Neurological Service, Neurological Institute, Presbyterian Hospital, New York, New York.

GERALD F. M. RUSSELL, M.D., F.R.C.P., F.R.C.P.Ed., F.R.C.Psych.

Anorexia Nervosa

Professor of Psychiatry, Royal Free Hospital School of Medicine, University of London. Consultant Psychiatrist, Royal Free Hospital and Friern Hospital, London, England.

DAVID C. SABISTON, Jr., M.D.

Surgical Treatment of Coronary Artery Disease

James B. Duke Professor of Surgery and Chairman of the Department of Surgery, Duke University Medical Center, Durham, North Carolina.

HERBERT A. SALTZMAN, M.D.

Therapeutic Hyperbaric Oxygen

Professor of Medicine, Duke University Medical Center, Durham, North Carolina.

JAY P. SANFORD, M.D.

Plague; Rat-Bite Fever; Leptospirosis

Professor of Medicine and Dean, Uniformed Services University School of Medicine. Attending Physician, Walter

Reed Army Medical Center, Washington, D.C., and National Naval Medical Center, Bethesda; Consultant, Clinical Center, National Institutes of Health, Bethesda, Maryland.

WILLIAM SCHAFFNER, M.D.

Psittacosis

Associate Professor of Medicine and Preventive Medicine, Vanderbilt University School of Medicine. Hospital Epidemiologist, Vanderbilt University Hospital, Nashville, Tennessee.

PHILIP S. SCHEIN, M.D.

Tumor Markers

Professor of Medicine and Pharmacology, Georgetown University School of Medicine. Assistant Director, Vincent T. Lombardi Cancer Research Center, Georgetown University Medical Center, Washington, D.C.

LABE C. SCHEINBERG, M.D.

The Demyelinating Diseases

Professor of Neurology, Albert Einstein College of Medicine of Yeshiva University. Director of Neurology and Psychiatry, St. Barnabas Hospital, Bronx, New York.

RUDI SCHMID, M.D., Ph.D.

Porphyria

Professor of Medicine, University of California, San Francisco, School of Medicine. Attending Physician and Consultant, Moffitt-University Hospital, Veterans Administration Hospital, and U.S. Army Letterman General Hospital, San Francisco, California.

ROBERT W. SCHRIER, M.D.

Other Specific Renal Diseases

Professor and Chairman, Department of Medicine, University of Colorado Medical Center, Denver, Colorado.

PETER H. SCHUR, M.D.

Systemic Lupus Erythematosus

Associate Professor of Medicine, Harvard Medical School. Physician, Robert B. Brigham Hospital, Boston, Massachusetts.

MARVIN M. SCHUSTER, M.D.

Disorders of Motility

Professor of Medicine and Assistant Professor of Psychiatry, The Johns Hopkins School of Medicine. Chief, Division of Digestive Diseases, Baltimore City Hospitals, Baltimore, Maryland.

WILLIAM B. SCHWARTZ, M.D.

Disorders of Fluid, Electrolyte, and Acid-Base Balance

Professor of Medicine, Tufts University School of Medicine. Professor of Medicine, Tufts–New England Medical Center Hospital, Boston, Massachusetts.

NEVIN S. SCRIMSHAW, Ph.D., M.D., M.P.H.

Nutrient Requirements; Assessment of Nutritional Status; Nutrition and Infection; Kwashiorkor, Marasmus, and Intermediate Forms of Protein-Calorie Malnutrition; Undernutrition, Starvation, and Hunger Edema; Deficiencies of Individual Nutrients: Vitamin Diseases

Head, Department of Nutrition and Food Science, Massachusetts Institute of Technology. Director, Clinical Research Center, Massachusetts Institute of Technology, Cambridge, Massachusetts.

CHARLES R. SCRIVER, M.D., F.R.S.C.

Hyperaminoaciduria; Branched-Chain Aminoaciduria; Hyperhistidinemia; The Hyperprolinemias and Hydroxyprolinemia; Diseases of the Urea Cycle; β-Aminoisobutyricaciduria; The Hyperglycinurias; Renal Hyperaminoacidurias; Fanconi's Syndrome; The Hyperphenylalaninemias

Professor of Biology and Pediatrics, McGill University. Director, De Belle Laboratory for Biochemical Genetics, McGill University–Montreal Children's Hospital Research Institute, Montreal, Quebec, Canada.

WILLIAM R. SHAPIRO, M.D.

Sleep and Its Disorders

Professor of Neurology, Cornell University Medical College. Attending Neurologist, Memorial Sloan-Kettering Cancer Center and The New York Hospital, New York, New York.

SOL SHERRY, M.D.

Thrombophlebitis and Phlebothrombosis; Pulmonary Embolism and Infarction

Professor and Chairman, Department of Medicine, Temple University School of Medicine. Physician-in-Chief, Temple University Hospital, Philadelphia, Pennsylvania.

J. B. SIDBURY, Jr., M.D.

Glycogen Storage Disease; Pentosuria; Fructosuria and Hereditary Fructose Intolerance

Professor, Pediatrics, Duke University Medical School; Lecturer, Pediatrics, Johns Hopkins Medical School; Professor, Child Health and Development, George Washington University School of Medicine and Health Sciences. Scientific Director, National Institute of Child Health and Human Development, National Institutes of Health, Bethesda, Maryland.

DONALD H. SILBERBERG, M.D.

Encephalitic Complications of Viral Infections and Vaccines

Professor and Vice Chairman, Department of Neurology, University of Pennsylvania School of Medicine. Neurologist, Hospital of the University of Pennsylvania, Philadelphia, Pennsylvania.

RICHARD T. SILVER, M.D.

Leukemoid Reactions; Myeloproliferative Disorders

Clinical Professor of Medicine, Cornell University Medical College. Chief, Oncology Service, Division of Hematology-Oncology, and Attending Physician, The New York Hospital, New York, New York.

MARVIN H. SLEISENGER, M.D.

Diseases of the Digestive System: Introduction; Malabsorption; Other Inflammatory Diseases of the Intestine

Professor of Medicine and Vice-Chairman, Department of Medicine, University of California, San Francisco. Chief, Medical Service, Veterans Administration Medical Center, San Francisco, California.

LLOYD H. SMITH, Jr., M.D.

Primary Hyperoxaluria; Gout; Xanthinuria; Disorders of Pyrimidine Metabolism

Professor of Medicine and Chairman, Department of Medicine, University of California, San Francisco. Chief of Medicine, Moffitt Hospital, San Francisco, California.

GORDON L. SNIDER, M.D.

Special Diagnostic Procedures in Pulmonary Disease

Professor of Medicine and Head, Pulmonary Medicine Section, Boston University School of Medicine; Lecturer, Tufts University School of Medicine. Chief, Pulmonary Medicine Section, Veterans Administration Hospital, Boston; Attending Physician, University Hospital and Boston City Hospital; Consultant Pulmonary Physician, U.S. Public Health Service Hospital, Boston, Massachusetts.

P. FREDERICK SPARLING, M.D.

Syphilis

Professor of Medicine and Bacteriology, University of North Carolina School of Medicine. Chief, Division of Infectious Diseases, Department of Internal Medicine, Memorial Hospital, Chapel Hill, North Carolina.

CHARLES J. STAHL, M.D.

Drowning

Captain, Medical Corps, United States Navy. Professor of Pathology, School of Medicine, Uniformed Services University of the Health Sciences; Professor of Pathology, School of Medicine, Georgetown University. Chairman, Department of Laboratory Medicine, National Naval Medical Center, Bethesda, Maryland; Consultant in Laboratory Medicine, Bureau of Medicine and Surgery, Washington, D.C.

GENE H. STOLLERMAN, M.D.

Streptococcal Diseases: Introduction; Group A Streptococcal Infection; Clinical Syndromes of Group A Streptococcal Infection; Treatment of Group A Streptococcal Infection and Chemoprophylaxis of Nonsuppurative Complications; Prophylaxis of Streptococcal Infection

Goodman Professor and Chairman, Department of Medicine, University of Tennessee College of Medicine. Physician-in-Chief, City of Memphis Hospital, Memphis, Tennessee.

MORTON N. SWARTZ, M.D.

Bacterial Meningitis; Parameningeal Infections

Professor of Medicine, Harvard Medical School. Physician and Chief, Infectious Disease Unit, Massachusetts General Hospital, Boston, Massachusetts.

WILLIAM C. THOMAS, Jr., M.D.

Renal Calculi

Professor, Department of Medicine, College of Medicine, University of Florida. Associate Chief of Staff for Research, Veterans Administration Hospital, Gainesville, Florida.

C. CRAIG TISHER, M.D.

Renal Changes in Other Systemic Diseases

Professor of Medicine, Associate Professor of Pathology, Duke University Medical Center, Durham, North Carolina.

H. RICHARD TYLER, M.D.

Polymyositis and Dermatomyositis

Professor of Neurology, Harvard Medical School. Head, Section of Neurology, Peter Bent Brigham Hospital; Consultant in Neurology, Children's Hospital Medical Center, Beth Israel Hospital, Robert Breck Brigham Hospital, West Roxbury Veterans Administration Hospital, and Boston Lying-In Hospital, Boston, Massachusetts.

JOHN P. UTZ, M.D.

Actinomycosis; The Mycoses: Introduction; Histoplasmosis; Blastomycosis; Paracoccidioidomycosis; Maduromycosis; Chromomycosis; Sporotrichosis

Professor of Medicine, School of Medicine, Georgetown University, Washington, D.C.

NIEL WALD, M.D.

Radiation Injury

Professor and Chairman, Department of Radiation Health, Graduate School of Public Health, and Professor of Radiology, School of Medicine, University of Pittsburgh. Active Medical Staff (Radiology) and Director, Radiation Medicine Department, Presbyterian-University Hospital, Pittsburgh; Consultant Staff, University Health Center of Pittsburgh Hospitals, Pittsburgh, and Aliquippa Hospital, Aliquippa, Pennsylvania.

ANDREW G. WALLACE, M.D.

Approach to the Patient with Cardiovascular Disease

Professor of Medicine, Duke University Medical Center. Chief, Division of Cardiology, Duke University Medical Center, Durham, North Carolina.

JOHN H. WALSH, M.D.

Peptic Ulcer: Clinical and Endocrine Aspects

Professor of Medicine, UCLA School of Medicine. Deputy Director, Center for Ulcer Research and Education, Veterans Administration Wadsworth Hospital Center, Los Angeles, California.

KENNETH S. WARREN, M.D.

Schistosomiasis

Adjunct Professor, Rockefeller University; Professor of Medicine, New York University, New York, New York.

M. F. R. WATERS, M.A., M.B., F.R.C.P., F.R.C.Path.

Leprosy

Senior Lecturer, London School of Hygiene and Tropical Medicine. Consultant Leprologist, Hospital for Tropical Diseases, London, England. Member of the Senior Scientific Staff, British Medical Research Council.

LAWRENCE W. WAY, M.D.

Diseases of the Gallbladder and Bile Ducts

Professor of Surgery, University of California School of Medicine, San Francisco. Chief of Surgery, Ft. Miley Veterans Administration Hospital, San Francisco, California.

PAUL WEBB, M.D.

Disorders Due to Heat and Cold

Principal Associate, Webb Associates, Yellow Springs, Ohio.

ROBERT E. WHALEN, M.D.

Disorders of the Pericardium; Tumors of the Heart

Professor of Medicine, Duke University Medical Center. Director, Cardiovascular Disease Service, Duke University Medical Center, Durham, North Carolina.

CHARLES L. WISSEMAN, Jr., M.S., M.D.

Rickettsial Diseases: Introduction; The Typhus Group; Rocky Mountain Spotted Fever; Tick-Borne Rickettsioses of the Eastern Hemisphere; Rickettsialpox; Scrub Typhus

Professor and Chairman, Department of Microbiology, University of Maryland School of Medicine, Baltimore, Maryland.

SHELDON M. WOLFF, M.D.

Introduction to Microbial Diseases

Endicott Professor and Chairman, Department of Medicine, Tufts University School of Medicine. Physician-in-Chief, New England Medical Center Hospital; Adjunct Professor of International Health, Fletcher School of Law and Diplomacy, Tufts University, Boston, Massachusetts.

EMANUEL WOLINSKY, M.D.

Clostridial Diseases: Introduction; Clostridial Myonecrosis; Other Clostridial Diseases; Clostridial Gastroenteritis

Professor of Medicine, Case Western Reserve University School of Medicine. Director of Microbiology and Chief of Division of Infectious Diseases, Department of Medicine, Cleveland Metropolitan General Hospital, Cleveland, Ohio.

HARVEY WOLINSKY, M.D., Ph.D.

Atherosclerosis

Professor of Medicine and Pathology, The Albert Einstein College of Medicine. Attending Physician, Bronx Municipal Hospital Center, Bronx, New York.

THEODORE E. WOODWARD, M.D.

Tularemia

Professor of Medicine and Chairman of Department of Medicine, Physician-in-Chief, University of Maryland School of Medicine and Hospital, Baltimore, Maryland.

O. M. WRONG, D.M., F.R.C.P.

Glomerular Disease: Introduction; Nephrotic Syndrome; Glomerulonephritis; Renal Involvement in Connective Tissue Diseases; Hereditary Nephritis

Professor of Medicine, University College Hospital Medical School, University of London. Consulting Physician, University College Hospital, London, England.

JAMES B. WYNGAARDEN, M.D.

Biological Science and Medical Practice; Diseases of Metabolism: Introduction; Fabry's Disease; Alcaptonuria; Cystinuria; Homocystinuria; The Lesch-Nyhan Syndrome; 2,8-Dihydroxyadenine Renal Stones; Miscellaneous Diseases of Purine Metabolism; Normal Laboratory Values of Clinical Importance

Frederic M. Hanes Professor and Chairman, Department of Medicine, Duke University Medical Center, Durham, North Carolina.

MELVIN D. YAHR, M.D.

The Extrapyramidal Disorders: Introduction; The Parkinsonian Syndrome; Essential Tremor; Senile Tremor; The Choreas; Tics; Athetosis; Dystonia Musculorum Deformans; Spasmodic Torticollis; Hemiballism

Henry P. and Georgette Goldschmidt Professor of Neurology, Chairman, Department of Neurology, Mt. Sinai School of Medicine, City University of New York. Neurologist and Chief, Mt. Sinai Hospital; Director, Neurological Service, Mt. Sinai Medical Center, New York, New York.

NATHANIEL A. YOUNG, M.D.

Enteroviral Diseases

Head, Section of Viral Oncology and Molecular Pathology, Laboratory of Pathology, National Cancer Institute; Senior Attending Physician in Infectious Diseases, Clinical Center, National Institutes of Health and National Naval Medical Center, Bethesda, Maryland.

CONTENTS

*(Detailed Table of Contents begins on the
following page)*

VOLUME 1

Part V.   Immune Disease

Part VI. Connective Tissue Diseases ("Collagen Diseases") Other Than Rheumatoid Arthritis

Part VII. Diseases of the Joints, *Charles L. Christian*

Part VIII. Granulomatous Diseases of Unproved Etiology

Part IX. Microbial Diseases

SECTION ONE. VIRAL DISEASES, 229

Viral Infections of the Respiratory Tract, 230

Viral Diseases Characterized by Cutaneous Lesions, 246

Viral Disease of Lymphoid Tissue, 264

Enteroviral Diseases, Nathaniel A. Young, 268

SECTION FOUR. CHEMOTHERAPY OF MICROBIAL DISEASE, 549

Part X. Protozoan and Helminthic Diseases

SECTION ONE. PROTOZOAN DISEASES, 566

SECTION TWO. HELMINTHIC DISEASES, 605

The Cestodes (Tapeworms), Philip D. Marsden, 606

Part XI. Disorders of the Nervous System and Behavior

SECTION ONE. CONSCIOUSNESS AND ITS DISTURBANCES, 640

SECTION TWO. FOCAL DISTURBANCES OF HIGHER NERVOUS
            FUNCTION, *Norman Geschwind*, 656

SECTION THREE. DEMENTIA, *Paul R. McHugh*, 660

SECTION TWENTY-FOUR.   DISEASES OF MUSCLE AND NEUROMUSCULAR JUNCTION, *Lewis P. Rowland*, 914

Part XII.   Respiratory Disease

Part XV. Renal Diseases

Part XVI.   Diseases of the Digestive System

SECTION ONE.   DIAGNOSTIC IMAGING PROCEDURES IN GASTROENTEROLOGY, *Robert N. Berk*, 1464

SECTION TWO.   DISORDERS OF MOTILITY, *Marvin M. Schuster*, 1475

Part XVII. Diseases of Nutrition

Part XVIII. Hematologic and Hematopoietic Diseases

SECTION ONE. THE ANEMIAS, 1714

Part XIX.   Medical Oncology

Part XX.   Diseases of Metabolism

Part XXI.   Diseases of the Endocrine System

Part XXIV.   Diseases of the Eye, *Maurice B. Landers, III*

Part XXV.   Drug-Drug Interactions, *Rubin Bressler*

Part XXVI.   Normal Laboratory Values of Clinical Importance,
James B. Wyngaarden

Index

PART I
THE NATURE OF MEDICINE

1. ON BECOMING A CLINICIAN

Paul B. Beeson

This essay is addressed to the student entering upon the study of clinical medicine. To leaf through a modern medical textbook for the first time must be a daunting experience for you. How can anyone hope to master so much scientific and technical information? The task *is* difficult, indeed impossible. Nevertheless, some encouragement should come from observing that senior medical students and young doctors on the hospital staff appear to have made a satisfactory adjustment to the challenge. Furthermore, as your acquaintance with clinical teachers grows, you will observe that although each of them has special knowledge and experience in some area of clinical medicine, they make no pretense of knowing it all. You will also find that clinicians frequently disagree, and that each of them comes to wrong conclusions from time to time. Clinical teachers must in fact appear to be very different from those under whom your preclinical work was done. Biochemists and pharmacologists have "hard" facts to propound. We, on the other hand, deal with such commodities as pain and nausea. We must accept any kind of problem. We cannot insist on working with inbred strains of people, we cannot control the environment from which they come, we know that their recollection of past events is faulty, and we cannot reduce them to subcellular fractions in order to determine what is going on. We must even question the opinions of our colleagues. We live, therefore, in an atmosphere of doubt and uncertainty, and make our decisions and take our actions on the basis of probabilities. You will have the same handicaps, and you too will make mistakes. Simply try to ensure that each mistake constitutes a learning experience which leaves you a better doctor.

Students as a rule accommodate to clinical medicine with astonishing speed. They learn by their own study and practice, by attending lectures and conferences, by observing senior people at work, and by informal discussions with fellow students and residents in ward offices, corridors, and dining rooms. Good-natured arguments facilitate the process, because debate tends to fix the information that emerges. In that connection you will find it helpful to adopt a habit of offering your point of view tentatively rather than in the form of a positive assertion.

But how should you *begin* the study of clinical medicine? I have not found it helpful (except as an editor!) to read a book like this in systematic cover-to-cover fashion. Instead, you should use it the way the mature clinician does, as a place in which information can be obtained about problems being dealt with at the time.

Inasmuch as common disorders occur commonly, this practice will in good time ensure that you will have read and thought about such frequently encountered disorders as peptic ulcer, angina pectoris, and urinary tract infection. Furthermore, although at first glance a medical text seems to be a sort of dictionary describing hundreds of unrelated entities, you will find that knowledge of one helps the study of another, because there often are dovetailing aspects or useful contrasts. I suggest that you always examine the references which accompany the discussions, and make it a practice to consult some of them. That is the kind of study doctors must carry on for themselves throughout life. Reading in connection with specific clinical problems is likely to provide knowledge that sticks.

What about the many uncommon maladies described in textbooks? The student of any age really needs only to know how to find out about them. One test of a good doctor is ability to achieve a correct diagnosis without having met the disease before.

Medical knowledge and practice are continually changing. In order to incorporate the steady flow of new information, a textbook must be extensively rewritten every few years. Let me illustrate this by citing a few examples of changes that have taken place during my own clinical career.

The third edition of this Textbook appeared in 1933, the year I graduated from medical school. It contained no mention of effective treatments for bacterial, mycobacterial, or fungal diseases; consequently, such entities as bacterial endocarditis, miliary tuberculosis, and cryptococcal meningitis were described as fatal infections with hopeless outlook. Adrenal steroids and steroid-like compounds had not been discovered. Diuretics were not available for treatment of heart failure; nor were there any drugs for control of hypertension. Anticoagulant drugs had not been introduced. The brief section entitled "Diseases of Allergy" contained nothing about lymphocytes, immune complexes, complement, or the structure of immunoglobulins. Sprue was described as an infectious disease, probably caused by *Monilia albicans*. Sydenham's chorea was thought to be due to toxins produced by an unidentified nonhemolytic streptococcus. The section on treatment of rheumatoid arthritis stated: "The most important single factor is the removal of foci of infection." The only deficiency diseases described were pellagra, beriberi, scurvy, and rickets; there was virtually no information about the nature of the responsible vitamins or of the metabolic consequences of such deficiencies. Discussions of "acidosis" and "alkalosis" were based on only one clinical chemical test — i.e., measurement of the carbon dioxide combining power of the blood. Removal of tonsils and adenoids was enthusiastically recommended: "The beneficial results of this operation are so great and so prompt that unless there is a distinct reason for its omission, it is folly to wait for spontaneous shrinking. . . ." For "falling of the stomach," recommended treatments included cacodylate of iron, strychnine in tonic doses, retention enemas of olive oil, or such surgical measures as pyloroplasty. For treatment of peptic ulcer it was mentioned that injections of nonspecific protein such as dead bacteria or milk may be followed by some success. The management of bleeding peptic ulcer called for application of an ice bag to the epigastrium; complete starvation; morphine hypodermically; and water, glucose, and soda given by rectal drip. Blood banks were unknown, and transfusion of a single unit of blood was a formidable procedure; consequently: "If the symptoms increase, transfusion of blood is advisable; in certain cases this may have to be repeated several times. When properly grouped blood cannot be quickly obtained, 10 cc of horse serum may be injected. . . ." Ulcerative colitis was covered in two brief descriptive paragraphs, which offered no suggestions as to medical or surgical treatment. Systemic lupus erythematosus, regional enteritis, and mycoplasmal pneumonia were not mentioned at all! The pathologic lesion of catarrhal jaundice (now viral hepatitis) was said to be an inflammatory swelling of the mucosa of the common bile duct. Diagnostic procedures in clinical biochemistry, endocrinology, and immunology, which now seem commonplace, had not come into use. Diagnosis by angiography, sonography, nuclear medicine, computerized tomography, and fiberscopic endoscopy were still unknown.

Nothing would be gained by a continuation of such examples; they are sufficient to illustrate the point that the conventional wisdom called clinical medicine changes rapidly. Without question, in a few decades another reader will be able to characterize much material in this edition of the Textbook as equally quaint.

The medical student should be aware, however, that exciting advances in medicine sometimes create serious new problems. Our therapy makes use of powerful drugs, all of which can do harm. Few hospital patients receive less than half a dozen different medications. In addition to intrinsic toxicity, these can interact with each other to produce unwanted effects. Part of hospital medicine today is in fact devoted to overcoming untoward effects of therapy. Knowing when to stop a certain treatment is as important as knowing when to bring it into use. There are risks, too, in many of our present invasive diagnostic procedures. In a manner of speaking, the recent scientific and technologic explosion in clinical medicine has created its own kind of pollution. One of the most important qualities needed by today's physician is ability to restrain curiosity. We should adhere to the rule that a potentially injurious diagnostic procedure should be carried out only when its possible benefit to that patient justifies the risk. A test should never be done just for the sake of "thoroughness," that is to say, before someone else suggests that it be done, or because a specialist feels it must be done to protect his or her reputation. "just in case. . . ."

Advancement in knowledge of clinical medicine is now mainly accomplished by full-time clinical scientists in medical schools and research institutes throughout the world. They concentrate on specific problems and nearly always make use of new findings and techniques developed in other biologic and physicial sciences. This kind of investigation-in-depth is essential, but requires concentration on a limited field. We have, for all time, departed from the era of clinical "giants" who were re-

garded as authorities on many aspects of internal medicine. That is why a modern textbook must be compiled from the writings of scores of contributors.

Having recognized the essential role of the specialist investigator in bringing about what are really immense advances in clinical medicine, we should give some consideration to the impact of this on trends in the practice of medicine as well as the training of future doctors. Does it follow, because we owe our advances in medical sciences to specialists, that the best medical care can only be given by specialists? Shall we say to young people now entering the profession that the age of specialization is here, and advise each of them to select a narrow field for his or her medical practice? I believe that much medical care can, and should, be the work of generalists. Diseases do not always present themselves in pure culture, and indeed the perspective of the clinical scientist can sometimes be skewed. It seems fair to say, for example, that a good general physician (now, alas, in short supply in America) can deal effectively with the great majority of episodes for which patients seek a doctor's help. When we focus on the field with which this book is concerned, it can be said with assurance that the well-trained internist is capable of dealing with most medical illnesses, including those for which hospital care is required. To do that in exemplary fashion is, however, a full-time job, which does not permit allocation of substantial portions of time and effort to research. The medical student and the house officer in a teaching hospital may need to be reminded that outside the medical school orbit much excellent medical care is provided by generalist physicians. The funds available for salaries in medical school departments go mainly to doctors who are active investigators, inasmuch as acquisition of new knowledge is a major responsibility of a university. In the setting of a teaching hospital, the clinical investigator can be a superb teacher of undergraduate and graduate medical students, and can, by combining forces with many other subspecialists in the institution, provide sophisticated medical service for patients there. This, however, is an expensive and somewhat inefficient way of offering medical care, which, although well suited to the diverse functions of a teaching institution, does not offer a realistic pattern for professional care in the outside community. In other words, specialized skill, although essential to any good system of medical care, is not needed in the proportion found among the members of medical school faculties.

Now finally, you must not only study the factual basis of clinical diagnosis and treatment, but at the same time work toward an equally difficult goal: cultivation of a proper relationship with each of your patients. This is the art of clinical practice. As Peabody described so vividly half a century ago, a hospital setting, in which you will spend the next few years, tends to be impersonal. It is easy for all of us to blend into that ambience of impersonality. More and more, people "get the bad news" during the course of a hospital stay. More and more, people must die in hospitals instead of at home. Our patients, therefore, are anxious, uncomfortable, often embarrassed, and confused by the unfamiliar surroundings. We must constantly remind ourselves of this, because successful medical care may be directly dependent on establishing an understanding and trusting relationship between ourselves and our patients. Often a good doctor scores where others have failed simply by listening to the patient and asking the right questions. Here is the way Wilfred Trotter, a great English neurosurgeon, put it:

". . . As long as medicine is an art, its chief and characteristic instrument must be human faculty. We come therefore to the very practical question of what aspects of human faculty it is necessary for the good doctor to cultivate. . . . The first to be named must always be the power of attention, of giving one's whole mind to the patient without the interposition of oneself. It sounds simple but only the very greatest doctors ever fully attain it. It is an active process and not either mere resigned listening or even politely waiting until you can interrupt. Disease often tells its secrets in a casual parenthesis. . . ."

Pickering has recently recalled an observation of Trotter at work:

". . . I asked Trotter to see a notoriously difficult patient, and marvelled how the anxious angular woman became clay in Trotter's hands. He had made it clear to her that he had listened, and that he had not only listened but had understood. I suspect that that had never happened to her before and it was for this reason that she had been, up to then, a difficult patient; that was the first time that her message had been heard. Hearing the patient's message is the *sine qua non* of a great physician. To hear that message requires first the physician's interest, second his understanding of the meaning of language, and third his sympathy and his knowledge and understanding of the circumstances of that patient's life; these again he learns best by listening to the patient."

So these are some precepts you might consider: Give each patient enough of your time. Sit down; listen; ask thoughtful questions; examine carefully; go back and do it again. Learn how to study clinical medicine, and be appropriately critical of what you read or hear. Train yourself to concentrate on each patient's problem to the exclusion of all else. Follow the example set by William Osler: "Do the kind thing and do it first."

Emerson, C. P.: Reminiscences of Sir William Osler. Internat. Assoc. Med. Museums Bull., 1926, p. 294.

Peabody, F. W.: The care of the patient. JAMA, 88:877, 1927.

Pickering, G. W.: Medicine at the crossroads: Learned profession or technological trades union? Proc. Roy. Soc. Med., 70:16, 1977.

Trotter, W.: Collected Papers. London, Oxford University Press, 1941, pp. 97–98.

2. SCIENCE, CLINICAL MEDICINE, AND THE SPECTRUM OF DISEASE

Alvan R. Feinstein

A textbook of medicine contains concepts and data for at least two distinctly different types of clinical decisions. With *explicatory** decisions, doctors choose names, causes, and mechanisms that provide intellectual explanations for the ailments observed in patients. With *interventional* decisions, doctors choose therapeutic strategies intended to prevent or to remedy the ailments. Thus, for a patient who describes his ailment as

---

*The word *explicatory* is used here to refer to diagnostic citations or pathogenetic explanations or both.

a substernal pressure provoked by exertion and relieved by rest, the doctor may make the explicatory decisions contained in such phrases as *angina pectoris, coronary artery disease,* and *myocardial ischemia.* The doctor's interventional decisions may then be expressed in recommendations about permissible physical activities, use of pharmaceutical substances, and the possible value of surgical therapy.

The explicatory decisions of clinical medicine are often regarded as its main scientific challenge. For diagnostic selections, modern technology has allowed diseases to be identified more precisely than ever before. The morphologic abnormalities that formerly could be demonstrated only at necropsy are now often revealed during life with the aid of roentgenography (including CAT scanners), biopsy, cytology, or surgical exploration; and many other ailments that cannot be depicted morphologically are identified with the aid of chemical, microbial, electrophysiologic, or other laboratory procedures. For ideas about causes and mechanisms of disease, doctors have received scientific confirmation both from the diagnostic tests performed in individual patients and from the many experimental models that have been tested during clinical investigation. The explicatory decisions thus enable doctors to apply at the bedside the major advances that laboratory research has brought to diagnostic medical science.

A doctor's interventional decisions, on the other hand, are often regarded mainly as art. The pharmaceutical, surgical, and other agents used for therapeutic intervention are highly developed from the scientific standpoint, but the decisions made about them are still often made as acts of judgment, generally unsupported by the type of scientific evidence that sustains the explicatory activities. The available evidence to prove the value of a treatment may be quantitatively defective, consisting mainly of anecdotal reports of clinical experiences that have not been thoroughly enumerated; or the evidence may seem qualitatively unappealing, depending on such "soft" data as a patient's pain, a family's anxiety, or an employer's forbearance. Even when treatments have been tested in controlled clinical trials, the results may be inconclusive because the patients under study, the investigated therapeutic regimens, or the methods of observation may differ substantially from those of customary clinical practice.

With medical activities demarcated into explicatory science and interventional art, a medical student (or a practicing clinician) often develops the belief that the purely clinical work of patient care does not present any scientific challenges. According to this belief, a clinician's principal science is contained in the "workup" that reveals diagnostic names and pathogenetic mechanisms. Once this challenge is completed, no further scientific thinking may seem necessary. After choosing a therapeutic agent according to the established diagnosis, the clinician would need only the arts of human perception and communication for telling the patient what is wrong and what is planned.

Despite popular acceptance, this demarcation of art and science in clinical work has at least three major inaccuracies. The demarcation is based on the idea that science consists only of explication, but science contains another major component: prediction. In dealing with a sick patient, a clinician is scientifically challenged not merely to explain what is wrong and how it went wrong, but also to predict what may happen and how its occurrence can be altered. To perform these predictions, a clinician must make the same type of interventional decisions with which prognosis is estimated, therapy chosen, and results evaluated. A second conceptual error arises from the belief that the choice of treatment depends almost entirely on the diagnostic citation. Although diagnosis is usually an important first step, the scientific selection and appraisal of therapy require analysis of data much more intricate than the mere identification of a disease. The most cogent information often includes symptoms, signs, and other clinical phenomena rather than a diagnostic title alone. A third misconception is the idea that important clinical phenomena cannot be expressed in "hard" scientific terms because the descriptions usually contain verbal categories rather than measured dimensions. The fallacy here is that "hard" information must be precise and reproducible, but it need not be dimensional. Some of the outstanding accomplishments of biologic science — including the work of Darwin, Virchow, and modern geneticists and electron microscopists — have been based on precise, reproducible, but nondimensional descriptions. With better standards of observation and classification, the verbal categories of "soft" clinical data could readily be improved into "hard" scientific quality.

Even when these attributes of clinical work are recognized, they may be regarded as scientifically unimportant because ordinary medical practice does not provide the experimental challenges offered by laboratory research. This belief is also inappropriate, however, because every act of clinical therapy is constructed in the same architectural sequence used for an experiment: a prepared entity is exposed to a planned maneuver and undergoes an observed response. This basic construction of an experiment can be used to outline all of a doctor's interventional decisions in clinical practice.

Despite similar challenges in the applicability of scientific methods, the "experiments" of the laboratory and bedside contain major differences in goals, reasoning, and procedures. In motive, the laboratory investigator seeks to understand how nature works and what it does; the clinician wants to change what nature has done or to thwart what it might do. In hypothesis, the laboratory investigator is innovative, wanting to test a new idea; the clinician is repetitive, wanting to reproduce the successful result achieved with the therapy used in a similar situation of the past. In cause-effect comparisons, the laboratory investigator can contrast the results of a concurrent "control group"; the clinician often relies on the "historical controls" of previous experience. In choice of data, the laboratory investigator can confine his observations only to the immediate events that seem most pertinent; the clinician must note all phenomena that can indicate a change in the patient's medical condition and way of life. These major differences in orientation require different strategies for the scientific methods used in the experiments of laboratory explication or clinical intervention, but both sets of activities offer the intellectual challenges of planning and evaluating an experiment.

In contemporary medicine, however, the methods used for acquiring and analyzing clinical data are not yet as scientifically well developed as the techniques that have been employed in laboratory research. Consequently, a doctor's explicatory decisions are often supported by excellent scientific evidence, but the in-terventional decisions are not. The purely clinical activities of contemporary medicine may thus seem more like art than science. The scientific improvement of this clinical art offers a prime target for future research, but in the meantime the reader of any compendium of clinical knowledge must deal with the state of the art in its existing form. The remainder of this essay will be concerned with certain caveats to help warn about some of the imperfections, and with a few suggestions to help resolve some of the difficulties.

One of the principal problems arises from the complex clinical spectrum associated with a disease. With increasing frequency in modern medicine, diseases are diagnostically identified as abnormalities not in a patient's clinical state (such as fever, jaundice, or chest pain), but in a paraclinical entity. The paraclinical abnormalities of disease can be diagnostically cited in such terms as morphologic structure (*coronary artery disease, carcinoma*), biochemical function (*diabetes mellitus, hyperthyroidism*), physiologic function (*atrial fibrillation, malabsorption*) or microbial invasion (*viral infection, meningococcemia*). Although the aid of modern diagnostic technology allows these paraclinical abnormalities to be diagnosed with unprecedented specificity and consistency, the principal "lesion" of each such paraclinical disease has an associated spectrum of diverse clinical manifestations that may not always occur specifically or consistently.

Some of the clinical manifestations represent the primary effects of the disease's principal abnormality, whereas other manifestations can be regarded as secondary effects or complications. In coronary artery disease, for example, angina pectoris is a primary effect and congestive heart failure is secondary. In peptic ulcer, pain is a primary effect and pyloric obstruction is secondary. Since different primary and secondary manifestations can appear alone or in various overlapping combinations, the disease in a particular patient may occur with some, all, or none of the possible clinical manifestations. For example, among patients with lung cancer, some may be wholly asymptomatic; others can have primary features, such as hemoptysis; others can have the secondary features of systemic or metastatic manifestations; and yet others may have various combinations of these primary and secondary elements. The complexity of a disease's spectrum will thus produce subsets of patients who have the same diagnosis but different clinical manifestations, and who may also differ in prognosis and therapy.

The existence of these different subsets creates important defects in any "textbook picture of disease." Since the author can seldom describe all the diverse possibilities, the "classic" textbook description is usually based on the most common or pathognomonic manifestations. The reader who expects that the disease will always occur in this classic manner may then be surprised, perplexed, or dismayed by the many occasions in which a patient appears from a less common subset. For example, in 1032 patients with lung cancer, the most common single subset consisted of 340 patients with the concurrence of pulmonic and systemic manifestations; 271 patients had pulmonic features only, and 196 had pulmonic, systemic, and metastatic manifestations; but 70 patients were wholly asymptomatic, and 34 had metastatic features only. Similarly, coronary artery disease can occur without angina pectoris in certain patients who have no symptoms or in others with manifestations only of congestive heart failure; hepatitis may first be found as advanced cirrhosis in a patient who never had jaundice.

The occurrence of an asymptomatic subset in a disease's spectrum is responsible for the frequent practice of "screening" in modern medicine. The purpose of the screening tests is to find the disease in circumstances in which it has produced no overt manifestations to arouse diagnostic suspicion. The occurrence of the many diverse subsets in a disease's spectrum is also responsible for some of the major current difficulties in evaluating prognosis and therapy. Despite similarity in diagnosis, the patients in the different subsets may have striking differences in prognosis. Thus, among a total of 1032 patients with lung cancer, the six-month survival rate was 44 per cent, but the rate ranged from 84 per cent in the localized asymptomatic subset to 14 per cent in patients who had both anatomic and symptomatic evidence of metastasis. In acute myocardial infarction, a patient with only chest pain has a much better prognosis than a patient with shock and pulmonary edema.

These natural prognostic distinctions will substantially affect the selection and appraisal of therapy. Since the "experiments" of routine clinical treatment are based on a repetitive hypothesis, a doctor chooses treatment for an individual patient by reviewing previous clinical experience, recalling the patients with similar manifestations, noting the outcomes of the therapy given to the "resemblance group," ascertaining which treatment gave the best result, and trying to reproduce that success in the current patient. To select the appropriate resemblance group, the doctor must have data for suitably demarcated subsets of patients.

Such data may not always be available. The results of previous treatment are often reported for all patients with the same disease, regardless of subsets; or the subsets distinguished in the reported results may be different from the particular one in which a subsequent patient is encountered. The absence of these details often creates difficulty in choice of treatment for an individual patient and arouses controversy in comparative evaluations of treated groups. One physician, treating diabetes mellitus with Regimen X, may have had a group of patients whose prognostic expectations were substantially different from those of another physician's patients treated with Regimen Y. One surgeon's Stage I cancer patients may be predominantly asymptomatic, whereas another surgeon's Stage I patients may have a high proportion of weight loss and fatigue. During arguments about the merits of the compared therapy, the clinicians may not realize that some of the crucial post-therapeutic differences arose not from different methods of treatment, but from prognostic differences in the subsets who constituted the treated groups.

To this complexity of clinical subsets for a single disease is added the further complexity introduced by comorbidity and demography. Since an individual patient may have more than one disease, the presence of associated ailments will create extra subsets in the spectrum of the "principal" disease, and may produce pathologic effects that alter prognosis and treatment in those subsets. The number of potential subsets for a disease becomes even larger when the cited clinical and comorbid demarcations are augmented by such demographic features as age, race, sex, and occupation.

This enormous variability of individual patients and

diseases would pose insurmountable problems in clinical decisions if each decision depended on determining a unique subset for that patient and on having adequate background information for previous experience with that subset. Fortunately, many small subsets can be combined into larger "determinant" groups for which therapeutic decisions can be based on satisfactory amounts of previous data or experience. For example, a patient with acute rheumatic fever is usually treated with salicylate if there is no clinical evidence of carditis, and with steroids if severe carditis is present. In this decision, the *no carditis* and *severe carditis* groups act as therapeutically determinant subsets, regardless of the many smaller subgroups into which the patients could be classified by virtue of demography or other clinical phenomena.

The selection of therapeutically determinant "super" subsets has traditionally been a fundamental decision in clinical judgment. The formation of the judgment may be substantially aided in the future by the availability of electronic data processing and computers for storing, augmenting, and analyzing the data of previous experience. The use of a computerized "data bank" for this type of quantification in estimating prognosis and choosing therapy offers an intriguing clinical addition to some of the other activities in which computers now receive useful medical applications. Among such activities are the calculation of complex mathematical formulas in diagnostic and therapeutic technology, the storage and display of inventories of laboratory results, the maintenance of selected components of patients' medical records, and the construction of "protocols," depicted in the flow-chart patterns of an algorithmic computer program, that provide instructions for making diagnostic or therapeutic decisions in a standard manner.

A different type of therapeutic intervention is aimed not at a disease or a determinant subset, but at a specific clinical manifestation, such as pain, constipation, or insomnia. Thus a patient may receive an antimicrobial drug for the disease pneumococcal pneumonia, but codeine for the associated symptom of pleuritic pain. Radiation or chemotherapy may be given for Hodgkin's disease, and blood transfusions for the associated weakness and anemia. For patients with acute myocardial infarction, the only treatment directed at the disease itself is bed rest. All other treatments are chosen according to the associated clinical manifestations: e.g., narcotics or analgesics for pain, diuretics or digitalis for congestive heart failure, and appropriate agents for arrhythmia.

For the many minor ailments encountered in primary medical care or family practice, a specific disease may not be diagnosed and treatment may be intended only to relieve symptoms. Encountering such ailments as an upper respiratory infection, a sprained muscle, or a gastrointestinal upset, the practitioner may decide prognostically that the ailment is self-limited and does not require more extensive diagnostic or therapeutic efforts. Another common event in general medical practice is a temporary, acute exacerbation of a chronic major ailment that has been relatively stable. In these events, which may occur in such conditions as chronic alcoholism, irritable colon syndrome, or neurotic anxiety, patients are also often treated for symptoms only.

In all the circumstances just described, the clinician's scientific challenges in interventional decisions were to determine the target(s) to be treated and to choose the best mode(s) of therapy. A different set of challenges consists of evaluating the patient's condition afterward to decide what the treatment accomplished and whether it has been successful. For this purpose, the clinician again often uses individual manifestations, rather than a disease diagnosis, as an index of accomplishment. Furthermore, the evaluation of a particular response may depend on graded subsets composed of changes in clinical manifestations. Thus the effect of treatment on congestive heart failure may be called *excellent* if both dyspnea and edema disappear; *fair* if one disappears while the other remains; and *poor* if both remain.

The data used to identify transitions in clinical state often require additional details that may not have been necessary for decisions about diagnosis, prognosis, and therapy. For example, a description of substernal chest pain provoked by exertion and relieved by rest will often suffice for a clinical diagnosis of coronary artery disease, but the evaluation of response of the angina to treatment will usually depend on further information about the angina's frequency and the associated amounts of exertion or rest. Similarly, the amount of jaundice may not be crucial for a diagnosis of hepatitis, but may be a valuable index of therapeutic response. Other examples of clinical details that are sometimes diagnostically unimportant but therapeutically valuable are the patient's weight (in treatment of edematous congestive heart failure), the size of a massive spleen (in treatment of chronic monocytic leukemia), the frequency of bowel movements (in treatment of various gastrointestinal disorders), and the frequency of urination (in treatment of cystitis or prostatitis).

The challenges of directly communicating with patients are often regarded as a nonscientific form of clinical art, mainly because the contents of the communications, which are much more complex than any of the complexities already cited, create diverse data and subsets that are even more difficult to specify. Nevertheless, many of the decisions made during these communications require the intellectual discipline used by a scientist to select suitable information, organize data, recapitulate previous experience, and evaluate responses. The discipline of scientific reasoning may not contribute to a clinician's creative insight and artful perception in dealing with the personal attributes of people, but without such reasoning the insight and perception will often be used ineffectually.

Whether a practicing doctor is involved in decisions of communication, explication, or intervention, clinical medicine will always contain and unite elements of both art and science. The complexity of people and human ailments will demand many artful judgments that cannot be expressed in scientific terms, but a scientific discipline is required for the optimal use of modern technology in identifying, explaining, preventing, or treating the ailments. To be properly adapted to its human recipients, this scientific discipline must contain suitable provision for the important personal and clinical information that is not perceived with "scientific" equipment or expressed in "scientific" dimensions. The art and science of clinical medicine are intermingled, symbiotic, and inseparable. Without the art, there can be no data for the science. Without the science, there can be no reason for the art.

3. BIOLOGICAL SCIENCE AND MEDICAL PRACTICE

James B. Wyngaarden

Every medical student and practitioner knows that the advances of clinical medicine depend in large part upon discoveries in the basic biological sciences. Much of scientific medicine derives from basic research conducted by fundamental scientists in the pursuit of truth for its own sake and eventually applied by others to medical problems. Another part stems from basic research conducted by physician-scientists with a specified clinical goal in mind—for example, the elucidation of a disease mechanism. Still other parts involve direct observations by clinical investigators or astute practitioners upon individual patients, or by epidemiologists upon populations of people. This essay is restricted to considerations of the interdependence of clinical medicine and biological science.

Most of us accept as an article of faith that applied research in the absence of basic research would sooner or later founder for the lack of a continually expanding bank of fundamental knowledge. It follows that some fraction of research in every field must always be at a basic level, conducted for its own intrinsic merit as a contribution to human understanding. Yet it is difficult to know what fraction of research should be basic and what proportion of resources should be allocated to pure science; even informed planners and policy makers are not agreed. Furthermore, it is often difficult to draw a sharp distinction betweeen pure and programmed basic science. Hypotheses, methods, and technical complexities are not qualitatively different. The same scientist may engage in both types of research, responding to different motives at one time or another.

It has been useful as an argument for support of basic science to analyze the significant antecedent discoveries that have made possible a particular practical advance. In a recent study, Comroe and Dripps chose ten major clinical innovations in cardiovascular and pulmonary medicine and traced their roots. With the help of panels of experts they concluded that over 60 per cent of the enabling discoveries were in the category of basic science, and that over 40 per cent were the result of research conducted without a particular clinical advance in mind at the time. The lags between discovery and application showed a wide range and averaged over 20 years. Often substantial development, refinement, and testing were required before the introduction of a potential new procedure or drug into clinical medicine was shown to be useful, appropriate, and safe. They concluded that some lag was essential and protective of patient and public interest.

It would not be correct, of course, to imply that all new clinical knowledge represents the final stage of a univectorial trail of development of which the seminal observations are always based in pure science. There are many positive and negative feedback loops in the process. A substantial amount of basic scientific discovery has been stimulated by clinical observations. Most of the coenzyme vitamins were recognized on the basis of human deficiency states. Most of the blood clotting factors were identified as substances present in normal blood capable of correcting a clotting defect in a patient with a hereditary bleeding condition. Many of the complex mucopolysaccharides were first identified and characterized from storage material in patients with hereditary mucopolysaccharidoses. The structure of antibodies was worked out in large part from urinary proteins of patients with multiple myeloma. Many clues to functions of the nervous system came from patients with neurologic lesions or behavioral aberrations.

However, the present bioscientific character of medical practice is a relatively recent development. Throughout most of recorded history medicine was anything but scientific, being dominated by empiricism and shackled by dogma. Diagnoses were inexact, causes of diseases poorly understood, and therapies frivolous and haphazard. Interventions by physicians consisted of bleeding, purging, cupping, administration of infusions of every known plant and of solutions of every known metal, and prescription of every possible diet — based entirely on experience, with no scientific foundation for these practices. Nor could there be such a foundation in the absence of a body of scientific biomedical knowledge.

Harbingers of change emerged slowly in the early nineteenth century, as new principles of physics and chemistry were applied to medicine. Physiologists stressed functions of organs and tissues. Its exemplars, especially Claude Bernard (1813–1878), emphasized the experimental method in establishing biological knowledge and the necessity of basing medical practice in such knowledge. Pathologists, led by Virchow (1821–1902), stressed the critical study of normal and abnormal tissues and the correlation of features of disease with precise anatomical observations. Bacteriologists, with Pasteur (1822–1895) and Koch (1843–1910) in the vanguard, began to identify the microorganisms and to implicate specific organisms in specific diseases — the anthrax bacillus in anthrax, the tubercle bacillus in consumption, the pneumococcus in lobar pneumonia, the streptococcus in puerperal fever. The groundwork for future therapies was being laid by these great Western European scientists, but there was relatively little the physician could do about most illnesses at the time. His major contributions were diagnostic, prognostic, and supportive. By correct diagnosis he could advise concerning outcome. By common-sense supportive measures he could provide comfort and maximize opportunities for recovery. But interventions were as likely as not to make things worse. The first edition of Osler's *Textbook of Medicine* in 1892 was influential for its skepticism and its therapeutic nihilism, as this outstanding physician condemned the majority of nostrums and remedies as useless, even harmful.

Slowly, specific therapies — insulin for diabetes, liver extract for pernicious anemia — or specific immunizations — diphtheria antitoxin, pneumococcic antisera — appeared. But it was not until the decade 1935–1945 that the entry of sulfonamides and penicillin into clinical medicine made a large number of previously lethal and untreatable diseases curable. It is customary to date the beginnings of modern medicine from these relatively recent events.

The language of contemporary biological science has become increasingly biochemical. The compositions of organs, tissues, cells, organelles, and membranes have been defined. The biosynthesis and catabolism of hundreds of compounds have been elucidated. The regulation of body processes has been described at progressively finer levels, and in chemical language. Pharmacologic agents are progressively understood in terms of specific loci and mechanisms of action. The expansion of new knowledge continues at a pace that is bewildering to all but experts in a given field. Current advances are particularly rapid in immunology, molecular biology, and peptide research. A beginning has been made in explaining human behavior in mechanistic terms, as more and more chemical mediators and pharmacologic modifiers are discovered.

We have entered a molecular age of basic biological science, and molecular biology is now a recognized discipline. The molecular influence pervades all the traditional disciplines underlying clinical medicine. Approximately 200 inborn errors are now understood in terms of specific missing or abnormal enzymes or other proteins. There are more than 240 known abnormal human hemoglobins, and for each of these the precise structural defect in the DNA of the mutant gene can be defined. Membrane, cytoplasmic, and nuclear receptors for hormones and drugs are exploding upon us, and old as well as new diseases are being defined in terms of receptor abnormalities — for example, type II hypercholesterolemia and nephrogenic diabetes insipidus. Recognition of opiate receptors has led to the discovery of endogenous peptides (endorphins) with analgesic activity. Their localization gives promise of further understanding of the limbic system, affective states, and addictions. Revolutionary techniques such as cell hybridization and fast-reaction measurement are reducing the gene, the cell, and even the brain to molecular terms.

Much of the recent fundamental information in science has been obtained by the process of reductionism — the exploring of details, and then details of details, until all the smallest bits of the structure, or the smallest parts of the mechanism, are exposed to scrutiny. Many of the most exciting observations of molecular biology have been made in microorganisms, which can be grown by the billions and selected for specific characteristics. Some scientists interested in mechanisms of DNA replication have even found that organisms such as *Escherichia coli* are too complex, and have switched to tiny bacterial DNA viruses whose chromosomes are about a thousandth the size of those of *E. coli*. These studies throw new light on biological mechanisms that could not at present be studied directly in eukaryotic cells.

In the biochemistry laboratory, proteins are isolated, purified, sequenced, and synthesized, their three-dimensional structure elucidated, and their active sites defined. Some of the best work has involved human proteins and has led to new understanding of clinical disorders. Islet cell tumors secrete insulin and proinsulin derived from pre-proinsulin. Lung tumors produce immunologically active parathormone-like material, resembling the C-terminal piece, or the N-terminal piece; only the latter is associated with biological activity.

The scientists responsible for our evolving understanding of biological systems know that the reductionist approach must often precede reconstitutive endeavors. Scientific progress rests on myriads of small observations, tedious measurements, and the findings of investigators asking humble, answerable questions. Instead of reaching for the whole truth, the scientist examines small, defined, and clearly separable phenomena. The pattern of science is a stepwise extension of what came before.

Critics of the bioscientific strategy of medicine have pointed out that the great advances that have dramatically reduced mortality rates consist in the improvement of the environment, the correction of malnutrition, and the control of infectious diseases through immunizations and antimicrobial agents, and that the relevant medical breakthroughs largely occurred before the prodigious expansion of federal support of biomedical science began in the early 1950's. They contend that the enormous expenditures that have made the United States pre-eminent in biomedical research have produced too little in the way of medical advance to justify their continuation, and have instead fostered the development of an extremely costly technology which has had only a minimal effect upon mortality statistics. They propose that the bioscientific strategy of medicine should be replaced by an ecological strategy for health.

These critics ignore several important realities. (1) Strategies for medicine and strategies for health are neither the same nor mutually exclusive. (2) Major advances have occurred since 1950 that have revolutionized the outlook in individual diseases or disease groups—for example, in Hodgkin's disease, acute lymphocytic leukemia of children, Parkinson's disease, and Wilson's disease. (3) Such advances have rested in most instances on a deeper and clearer understanding of underlying disease mechanisms. (4) The elucidation of a disease mechanism and the devising of rational therapy usually depend upon the application of basic scientific knowledge to a clinical problem in the laboratory or ward — for instance, the definition of pathways and rates of uric acid synthesis in gout, and the development of a xanthine oxidase inhibitor (allopurinol) for the control of hyperuricemia and hyperuricaciduria. (5) The expansion of the knowledge bank of the past quarter century justifies great optimism for the eventual control and cure of major diseases and the possible elimination of premature death from illness.

The list of human diseases for which there are as yet no definitive measures for prevention or cure is still formidable. Fresh insights into the nature of these diseases are needed. These insights can come only from continued basic research. Those who believe that there is an abundance of scientific information locked in the laboratory merely awaiting a new emphasis on human application are mistaken. Those who believe that a series of crash programs will lead to ready cures of cancer and heart, vascular, arthritic, emotional, and mental disease are misled. The essential pieces of background information are not merely awaiting assembly; most have yet to be discovered.

It is the record of recent decades that each time a major disease has come under control, through either prevention or cure, the solution has been much simpler and less costly than the half-way technologies devised during earlier stages of incomplete knowledge. Two of today's conspicuous examples of the high cost of half-way technologies are the use of the artificial kidney and renal transplantation for the treatment of chronic renal failure, and of bypass grafts for the treatment of coronary artery disease. Our lack of adequate information concerning the basic mechanisms of chronic nephritis and of atherosclerosis delays more rapid progress in prevention or cure of these conditions.

The practice of medicine is both a science and an art.

A skilled physician must have extensive medical knowledge, which is the bedrock of technical competence. In addition, he or she must have judgment, tact, decisiveness, restraint, compassion, interest, time, and other personal qualities of caring and dedication. This essay does not contend that technical competence is enough. It does contend that compassion without knowledge is insufficient. The science and the art of medicine must always be intimately linked. The student studies the science of medicine first, masters it early, and returns to it frequently. The student acquires the art of medicine — the skillful application of medical knowledge in the optimal care of the patient — more gradually and with experience.

Keeping abreast of the bioscientific, technological, and therapeutic advances of medicine has become an almost insuperable challenge for the physician. Review articles, postgraduate courses, and recertification examinations all help. But the surest way, given the realities of professional demands, is to look upon each patient as a learning experience, and to use each experience as a stimulus to self-renewal and to excellence. Internal drive will cause the student or physician to read about the condition in question and to inquire into the advances in scientific knowledge and application that have occurred since the topic was last reviewed. In this way the highest standards of personal care will be maintained. Given the pace of advance, review must occur at frequent and regular intervals. A wide range of experts must be consulted. Each edition of the *Textbook of Medicine* is a compendium of pertinent information selected and presented by experts, designed to maximize the opportunities for learning and to minimize the lag between discovery and application.

Comroe, J. H., and Dripps, R. D.: The top ten clinical advances in cardiovascular-pulmonary medicine and surgery between 1945 and 1975: How they came about. Bethesda, Md., 1977. Public Inquiries and Reports Branch, National Heart, Lung, and Blood Institute, National Institutes of Health, 1977.

Kornberg, A.: Research, the lifeline of medicine. N. Engl. J. Med., 294:1212, 1976.

Thomas, L.: Biomedical science and human health: The long-range prospect. Daedalus, 106:163, 1977.

4. MEDICINE IN MODERN SOCIETY

Walsh McDermott

Medicine is not a science but a learned profession deeply rooted in a number of sciences and charged with the obligation to apply them for man's benefit. So complex a process could hardly be reduced to a neat symmetrical design and fitted within the covers of a book. Yet this subject, the beneficial uses of medical science, is not without any design at all — it has a conceptual base on which all medical teaching and all medical books should rest. To consider this base, or certain aspects of it, seems proper at the start of a textbook of medicine. Although the book itself is addressed to medical students and graduate physicians of all ages, this essay is presented mainly for those now entering the profession.

One part of the conceptual base is set forth above in the opening sentence that ends ". . . to apply them for man's benefit." Traditionally this applying is made with compassion and in accord with a widely recognized moral and ethical code. The responsibilities of medicine are thus threefold: to generate scientific knowledge and to teach it to others; to use the knowledge for the health of an individual or a whole community; and to judge the moral and ethical propriety of each medical act that directly affects another human being. These three areas of responsibility command the efforts of individuals from a wide range of scientific disciplines and professions. The physicians who actually apply the knowledge, however, are of two sorts: those who deal through a personal encounter with one patient at a time and those who deal with people as groups.

The activities of both sorts of physicians are based on the concept that each disease entity has its own pathogenic chain — the whole series of events that determine its causation and maintenance — and that understanding this chain for a particular disease not only permits clearer recognition of its clinical manifestations, but reveals any weak links that might be exploited for prevention or therapy.

Approach to the body of knowledge organized in this way (both in books and elsewhere) is made from one of two viewpoints. The physician in public health or community medicine is constantly reaching for ways in which pathogenic chains can be broken by some continuing intervention that affects a number of people at once, e.g., to reduce the incidence of goiter by putting iodine in table salt. By contrast, physicians acting through the personal encounter system will search the same knowledge sectors and with educated discrimination will extract those elements appropriate for the solution of a problem in an individual. The viewpoints from which the knowledge is scrutinized are different, but the body of knowledge about each disease is the same. Textbooks about diseases and their pathogenic chains serve both these viewpoints and form important instruments for this process of the beneficial uses of science.

The physician who treats one patient at a time and the physician who deals with a community as a whole both exert compassion, but it is of two quite different sorts. The compassion exercised by the physician who treats individuals takes the form of a cultivated instinct to lend support and comfort to a particular fellow human being. By contrast, the "group" compassion of the public health or community physician necessarily takes the form of what the writer has previously termed "statistical compassion." By this is meant an imaginative compassion for people whom one never gets to see as individuals and, indeed, can know only as data on a graph. This compassion — the deep-seated instinct to try to help those whom one never gets to see — is a characteristic form of motivation for political leaders and other social activists, and "statistical" successes bring them major satisfactions. Such is really not the case with most physicians, who usually do not derive as much satisfaction from seeing improvement on a graph as they do from seeing improvement in an individual. *Indeed, part of the self-selection in choosing medicine as a career seems to be a self-image of a person whose professional activities are to relate directly with individuals rather than with groups.* Thus the system of public health or community medicine — based on physicians *not* seeing patients as individuals — runs contrary to most medical instincts. Yet until we have significant numbers of physicians for whom "statistical compas-

sion" is as rewarding as it is to the leaders in certain other walks of life, we will fail as a society to derive the full measure of the benefits of our medical science.

The scientific basis of medicine had been building up throughout the whole nineteenth century, but the *uses* of that science in the sense of decisively altering or preventing disease were largely accomplished through the public health or "community" physicians who dealt with people as groups. Chlorination of water supplies and the pasteurization of milk are cases in point. It was not until the discovery of insulin in 1921, and not really until the advent of the modern antimicrobial era more than 40 years ago, that the clinical physicians had much in the way of decisive therapies or preventives derived from science. Since that time most of the practical uses of biomedical science and technology have been of a nature fitted to the clinical or personal system, and, despite recent efforts, the other system has been allowed to languish. Indeed, the evolution of the highly complex and extraordinarily effective instrument that is today's university-based medical center has been almost exclusively devoted to the one system — the personal encounter system of one patient at a time.

We could tolerate this so long as what medicine had to offer was technologically simple and physicians were spread out across the whole of society much more evenly than they are now. But the coincidence of massive scientific innovation and wide social change has created a situation in which the application of medical science for man's benefit can no longer be managed by just one of the two systems — we desperately need both.

For there are two critically different populations involved, each of which is the primary responsibility of one of the systems. These two populations are the *constituency* and the *community*. The members of the constituency represent a progressively selected group, in part self-selected, and the selection is based on the presence of a medical problem, frequently one that is quite complex. Each member, in effect, has *voted* to obtain the services of a physician (or center or medical group) and has cast this vote as an individual without reference to others. The constituency is thus a collection of individuals who share in common only the fact that each has perceived a self-problem of illness or disease. It is the group known familiarly as the physician's "practice." The community, by contrast, is made up of people distinguished by the possession in common of some factor not directly related to disease. Usually, but not invariably, this common factor is a domicile located within some geographically defined boundary. In health terms, therefore, the community is a wholly unselected group, and at any one point in time many more of its members are well than are sick. *The community and the constituency thus differ strikingly in the prevalence of significant illness and disease. Because of this difference, an institutional form appropriate to meet the needs of one group would be markedly different from the form appropriate for the other.* Our challenge today is to develop such a two-type institutional form so that the needs of both groups may be equally served.

What the community needs is recognition of weakness in pathogenic chains that may be exploited in the prevention of disease. For nonpreventable disease the community needs straightforward medical care close to home, safeguarded by continuous mechanisms for identifying those who need care in the first place and mechanisms for sifting the few who need complex care from the many who do not. These few needing complex care join with a similar few from the constituency — that group of people self-selected from a much larger population base than could be satisfactorily served by a single personal encounter physician. What these properly sifted members of the constituency need is an institution that can offer a complete array of talents appropriate for the solution of any currently solvable medical problem, no matter how rarely occurring or complicated it might be. Whether for the community or for the constituency, the actual provision of the care is the responsibility of the personal encounter physician. Community medicine (or the larger public health system of which it is a part) is thus responsible *not* for the delivery of personal health services to the members of a community, but for ensuring that the community receives the proper health services of all sorts. And prominent among these are the invention of better mechanisms than we have now for both the continuous community scan of who needs care at any moment and appropriate entry points for the care of those identified. Neither of these two systems is inherently of greater social value than the other, but in the course of developing the personal encounter system to its present high point of technologic effectiveness for the individual, we have failed to mount a comparable effort for the nourishment of the other system responsible for the medical welfare of every member of the group. Without such a healthy watchdog we have allowed the personal encounter system to become unevenly distributed throughout our population. The correction of this imbalance is the critical challenge facing medicine today, and how well we meet it will determine the role of the physician in our society. For the imbalance of the two systems affects our efforts for the beneficial uses of science not only at the level of medical care for the community and the constituency, but in those even larger health matters that have to do with how the developing individual can be aided in his or her continuous interaction with the environment.

Health, like happiness, is an abstraction; it cannot be defined in exact measurable terms because its presence is so much a matter of subjective judgment. Health is a relative condition that represents the degree to which an individual can operate with effectiveness within the particular circumstances of his or her heredity and physical and cultural environment. Disease *can* be measured, and it occurs in patterns that closely reflect the major features of a particular society. The term "level of health" of a society designates which of some four or five possible patterns is present. Serious misunderstanding has arisen in recent years about the respective impacts of the two delivery systems on a society's health. Economists and other health planners have failed to recognize that there are virtually no established indicators by which to measure the impact of the personal encounter system on our nation's health. What gets measured, using the customary health indices, is the impact of the other two forces — the public health system and the life style afforded by the material culture. Each of us is under the constant influence of all three forces, and in that setting the disease pattern of the United States, including certain chronic conditions with a significant cultural linkage, has shown a steady trend toward a better level of health in recent years.

It is not possible to do justice to all these issues in this book, although some are indeed considered. For others, certain key references to the literature that has been developing in recent years are set forth below. There remain a few, however, that are so vital to the conceptual base forming the theme of this chapter that they deserve special mention.

Moral judgments must be made by the physician engaged in individual patient care, but they are to be made on his own professional acts and those of his colleagues, not on the actions of those who sought his care. Any moral judgments he might make on his patients' behavior are private matters to be kept within himself; he must not permit them to influence his own professional acts. This has long been the medical tradition, and it is important that it not be forgotten in the tumult of today's world of clashing value systems. The prospect of moral and ethical problems of an essentially new type is also now emerging before us. There is general awareness that advances in medical science are leading to various ethical conflicts that have to be faced by the personal encounter physician. What is less well recognized, however, is that this situation will also become socially serious for the nonclinical system, whether it be called public health or community medicine. Critical phenomena in human development formerly thought to represent the hand of fate are now found to be, at least in part, environmentally determined, and hence manipulable — such matters as the full expansion of an individual's intelligence or perhaps his or her degree of educability. If we develop the power to significantly influence such critical matters — and scientifically we are getting closer to it every day — we may find ourselves faced with seeking to protect the "interests" of an unborn or newborn child in the receipt of a particular intervention against the "rights" of its parents to be free from outside interference. And this question of how to ensure the best opportunity for the individual without destroying family structure in the process will not be an ethical problem to be faced by medicine in rare instances, but one that will involve whole societies. Yet we cannot run away from such questions, for it is the wise application of our science and technology, made with either form of compassion, that allows us to approach one of our major goals — that of ensuring that every child born into the world has the maximal chance to make the run through life's most productive years.

Finally, we must heed a concept of medicine that is ageless. In the life of an individual there ultimately may come a time when all the knowledge so carefully presented by the contributors to this book no longer has usefulness, yet life must go on, at least for a time. Whenever this happens, and it happens every day, it is up to each of us to follow to the fullest measure the charge laid down long ago for "the physician to become himself the treatment."

Beeson, P. B.: Some good features of the British National Health Service. Arch. Intern. Med., 133:708, 1974.

Dubos, R.: So Human an Animal. New York, Charles Scribner's Sons, 1969.

McDermott, W.: Demography, culture, and economics and the evolutionary stages of medicine. *In* Kilbourne, E. D., and Smillie, W. G. (eds.): Human Ecology and Public Health. 4th ed. New York, The Macmillan Company, 1969.

McDermott, W.: The public good and one's own. Perspect. Biol. Med., 21:167, 1978.

Morison, R. S.: Where is biology taking us? Science, 155:429, 1967.

Rogers, D. E.: The Changing Face of American Medicine. Cambridge, Mass., Ballinger Publishing Company, 1978.

PART II
HUMAN GROWTH AND DEVELOPMENT

5. HEREDITY

Alexander G. Bearn

Man is a singular creature exhibiting much genetic diversity, and able to adapt with extraordinary versatility to a wide range of environmental circumstances, some of them extreme. His genetic constitution has evolved over the last 10 to 20 million years—the period that has elapsed since we began to diverge from our nearest relative, the chimpanzee (presently vying with the gorilla for this dubious honor), who unlike man has 48 chromosomes in each diploid cell. The cranial capacity of man's immediate ancestors increased rapidly, trebling in 10 million years, although there is scant evidence that it has undergone further enlargement during the last 100,000 years. However, domestication of plants and animals as sources of food some 10,000 years ago accelerated man's cultural evolution and increased his independence from nature.

During evolution, a number of irreversible biologic steps have been taken. From the time that mammals began to evolve from amphibia and gill structures were lost, perhaps 200 million years ago, future man was condemned to a terrestrial existence. Dependence on oxygen for metabolism and life was set even earlier in the long evolutionary process.

Although man has been able to adjust to a variety of hostile environments, including ocean depths and outer space where he survives at 0 g, he has been able to do so only because his intellectual ingenuity has allowed him to equip himself with the necessary life support systems. Thus, man's present genetic constitution has established the boundary conditions for his biologic future and the cultural structures which he is able to fashion.

The revolution in biology over the past 25 years has established, in minute particulars, the sequential events that determine the structure of proteins as a result of information encoded in DNA. But the inevitability and fidelity of this information transfer have sometimes been obscured by environmental factors that influence the ultimate expression of the genetic message. In the final analysis, it is not possible to separate genes from the environment in which they act. The nature-nurture polemic is a Victorian abstraction, of no concern to modern biologists.

Despite this, it remains conventional to regard all diseases of man as due principally to either hereditary or environmental influences. The limitation of such a classification is exposed when we realize that many diseases classified as genetic can be managed by manipulating the environment rather than the abnormal gene. Restricting phenylalanine in the diet of infants with phenylketonuria is one example. Conversely, the disease scurvy, usually regarded as due to an environmental deficiency of vitamin C, could just as well be thought of as an inborn error of metabolism in which the hepatic enzyme that converts L-gluconalactone to L-ascorbic acid (present in all mammals except man, monkey, and the guinea pig) is genetically deficient.

In some diseases, such as achondroplastic dwarfism, genetic influences appear decisive and environmental factors undetectable, whereas in microbial disease and other disorders caused by exogenous environmental agents, the genetic component is considered trivial. Yet even here genetic susceptibility or resistance may play an important role. For example, human red cells which have on their surface the Duffy blood group antigen are susceptible to infection by *Plasmodium vivax* malaria. In contrast, cells which lack the Duffy factor are not subject to this infection. Many West Africans lack the Duffy marker on their cells; the parasites rarely gain entry to the red cell, and *Plasmodium vivax* malaria is rare. The uniqueness of the molecular specificity that determines the infection is evident not only from the regional absence of vivax malaria, but from the prevalence of falciparum malaria: the falciparum parasite is totally indifferent to the molecular architecture of the Duffy factor, and infection proceeds unhindered.

Thus, although in many infections the environmental agent is crucial, the importance of the genotype of the host, as in vivax malaria, should not be discounted. It seems likely that, in the past, infectious diseases were powerful selective agents, and that the ability to survive epidemic disasters was dependent at least in part on the individual's genotype (see Ch. 12).

For more than half a century, comparative studies of identical and nonidentical twins have been used to draw distinctions between hereditary and environmental influences. However, even when identical twins are reared apart, they have a shared common environment before birth, and dogmatic conclusions are treacherous.

Indeed, quantifying the balance of genetic and environmental influences in disease has been overemphasized by geneticists who have substituted algebra for biology and abstraction for reality. The greatest difficulty in sorting out the relative importance of genetic and environmental influence is encountered with common diseases. In disorders such as cancer, essential hypertension, and coronary artery disease, genetic influences are important but hard to identify in specific biochemical terms. It is occasionally possible to identify single genes that have a specific metabolic effect, such as those responsible for hypercholesterolemia and hypertriglyceridemia, but more often genetic factors are elusive.

Recently, the nature-nurture polemic, so frequently revived in sterile discussions of educability and intelligence, has been refreshingly illuminated by many fundamental studies on gene regulation. One only will be noted; evidence has now accumulated which suggests that, at any given time, as much as 80 per cent of the genetic material in the cells of higher organisms is inactive. This inactivity can be reversed by certain environmental influences. Certain steroid hormones, for example, possess the capacity to influence gene activity, and a number of these have now been shown to influence directly the synthesis of mRNA and tRNA. Indeed, the administration of estrogen to a rooster can activate genes in the rooster's liver cells so that they synthesize egg yolk proteins — proteins of more interest to the molecular biologist than to the rooster.

We can summarize by re-emphasizing that genetics is concerned with the study of hereditary variations. Most of these variations are not harmful; indeed, they confer a distinct biologic advantage by enabling the species to adapt to an ever-changing environment. When they are extreme they may be associated with clinical disease and come directly to the attention of the physician. Only by understanding the complexity of the interaction between genes and environment will the old concept of genetic diathesis be clothed in scientific reality. In the future, environmental and social change will assuredly create new diseases. Man will continue to learn more and more about his genetic constitution and, as he does, he must try to make the most of its virtues and outwit its defects.

Although the fabric of human diversity is brilliantly close-woven, it is not man's individuality that sets him apart but his awareness of it. For those who would truly understand human disease, the individuality of man's response to an ever-changing and often hostile environment is the ultimate basis of medical practice. Upon this foundation the precious and humane responsibility for the care of our patients must be built.

Bodmer, W. F., and Cavalli-Sforza, L. L.: Genetics, Evolution and Man. San Francisco, W. H. Freeman and Company, 1976.

6. ENVIRONMENT

Howard H. Hiatt

All disturbances in health reflect the interplay of environmental and genetically determined host factors. In that sense a textbook of medicine is concerned in its entirety with a consideration of man and his environment. However, the complexity of environmental factors affecting health makes it appropriate to offer a few introductory generalizations about them. Further, attention to how alteration of environmental factors can prevent or ameliorate disease is particularly urgent at this time of justifiable concern with the limitations and economic costs of therapeutic medicine.

The dimensions of man's environment are suggested when we consider that it encompasses everything that impinges on man other than the genes of the germ cell. Indeed, studies in other forms indicate that the genetic apparatus itself often includes material that was once "environment." For example, a bacterial cell may become resistant to an antimicrobial drug as a result of infection with a virus containing the information necessary for the synthesis of enzymes that inactivate the drug. Not only is the bacterium thus able to make the enzymes in question, but because viral nucleic acid may become a part of the genetic apparatus of the cell, the cell can pass on to its progeny the capacity to inactivate the drug. A related phenomenon may explain the presence of tumor viral nucleic acid in certain animal

cells. The expression of the nucleic acid in terms of tumor production may require one or more further environmental exposures — for example, to x-rays or to a chemical. This multifactorial etiology is characteristic of all diseases, and the complex interaction of causes has been likened by MacMahon and Pugh to a "web" of causation. Fortunately, effective action does not require complete unraveling of such webs — the disruption of any one thread may be sufficient to induce a favorable change in health status.

DETERMINANTS OF RESPONSE TO ENVIRONMENTAL FACTORS

It has long been recognized that many environmental substances are harmful only to individuals of a specific genetic constitution. Individuals with genetic defects in metabolic pathways may be poisoned by substances that are readily tolerated by most people. An example is the damage done by the muscle relaxant drug suxamethonium to people with abnormal forms of the enzyme pseudocholinesterase. A diet containing "normal" amounts of phenylalanine will be profoundly damaging to persons homozygous for a particular gene. People unable to convert certain dietary constituents to biologically active forms, such as those with vitamin D resistant rickets, will manifest deficiency states even when receiving the substance in amounts adequate for "normal" individuals. Such conditions are worthy of special emphasis, for although they are infrequent, they are but recognized manifestations of individual variations that are ubiquitous. Responses to drugs, chemicals, microorganisms, stress, and other environmental factors, particularly at low doses, reflect in part the genetically determined constitution of the person exposed. Differences from the "normal" in lipoprotein metabolism have already been well documented in the families of patients with complications of atherosclerosis; thus genetic predisposition probably makes the cardiovascular system of certain people more susceptible to the ravages of such known potentially harmful factors as hypertension, obesity, and too little exercise. Similarly, individual susceptibility likely explains in part why many but not all cigarette smokers develop lung cancer. Critical to preventive medicine is the development of methods for identifying people for whom specific environmental factors are hazardous, so that appropriate measures can be directed at those at risk.

Response to environmental factors is greatly affected by other environmental conditions prevailing at the time of exposure. One example is a drug the administration of which leads to altered metabolism of, and thereby to altered action of, a second drug or other chemical. Another is the effect of nutritional status on the response to infectious agents; malnutrition may explain in large part why the fatality rate from measles is so much greater in rural Guatemala than in the United States. An individual with compromised function as a result of earlier exposure to one environmental factor may be particularly prone to the effects of another; for example, people with pneumoconiosis are sensitive to carbon monoxide and those with coronary artery disease to carbon monoxide and carbon disulfide.

Timing of exposure may also be important, particularly during prenatal life. A few of the known congenital malformations and spontaneous abortions have thus far been traced to identified environmental insults, but over 80 per cent are of unknown cause. Drugs, other chemicals, viruses, bacteria, carbon monoxide, and ionizing radiation are among factors known to cause congenital malformations, but only if exposure occurs during the first trimester of pregnancy. Thalidomide, for example, given to pregnant women caused serious anomalies in their offspring. Exposure of the pregnant woman early in the sensitive period led to ear anomaly in the offspring, later to arm deformity, and later yet to leg deformity. Exposures after the first trimester produced no deformity.

Environmental factors may affect the incidence or the course of a disease, or both; the condition of the host at the time of exposure helps determine which. For example, in mice, x-rays may activate a pre-existing tumor virus, thereby producing cancer. However, even in the absence of latent oncogenic viral DNA, x-rays may themselves lead to cancer by inducing a mutation of cellular DNA. Finally, by their lethal effects on cells, x-rays may be used to destroy cancer, and thus are used therapeutically. Similarly, diethylstilbestrol will produce temporary remissions of breast cancer in some patients; however, it is also known to lead to the appearance of cancer, and some young women have developed cancer of the vagina after exposure to diethylstilbestrol during intrauterine life many years earlier. Since many environmental factors cause disease only after latent periods measured in decades, alertness and continued monitoring of potential hazards are required.

CLASSIFICATION OF ENVIRONMENTAL FACTORS

In considering the variety of environmental factors known to be harmful to health, it must be emphasized that the field is in a state of flux, and there are few broadly accepted organizing principles. Some environmental influences of major importance, particularly in developing countries, are naturally occurring. Increasingly, however, attention is focused throughout the world on the health hazards of environmental conditions created by man. Some factors are detrimental to health when present in excess, and others when deficient; many lead to problems under either circumstance. Many, and probably most, environmental factors injurious to health have yet to be identified, and new ones are constantly appearing as a result of increased population, increased affluence, and technologic advances.

A prevailing classification breaks down the principal environmental factors into chemical, physical, biologic, and social. A few examples of each follow.

CHEMICAL FACTORS. The role of chemicals in inducing human disease is variable and complicated. No chemical can be considered completely nontoxic, even though many are required in small amounts for physiologic processes. For example, the benefits of small amounts of fluoride on tooth development are now accepted. Studies of disease patterns in areas of hard and soft water supply suggest that as yet unidentified factors in water may offer some protection against atherosclerosis. Lead, arsenic, mercury, cadmium, cobalt, selenium, tin, manganese, and other metals can produce acute poisoning and may be introduced by contaminated food or water. Polychlorinated biphenyls, organochlorine, and organophosphorus insecticides may gain access via the same routes. A variety of chemicals, including silica, asbestos, lead, vinyl chloride, and many solvents, may be present in toxic amounts in the air, particularly in and near industrial plants. The exposure of workers to harmful chemicals is often reflected in higher mortality and morbidity rates in areas where certain industries are concentrated.

Over 15,000 chemicals are now in commercial production in amounts between 500 and 1 million kilograms per year, and an additional 500 are introduced annually. Some are carcinogenic, some mutagenic, some teratogenic, and some toxic in other ways. Because the long-term effects of a substance cannot be known with certainty for decades, testing for chronic as well as acute effects should be carried out before widespread human exposure is permitted. However, since it is impossible to test comprehensively all new compounds, it is particularly important to pay attention to those structurally related to other substances known to be toxic. Of crucial importance has been the recent development of short-term in vitro tests for measuring the mutagenic effects of chemicals on cultured bacterial and mammalian cells. Increasing evidence points to a close (but not perfect) correspondence between mutagenicity in cultured cells and carcinogenicity in animals. Thus the in vitro tests are now widely used as an early warning system. They have already obviated the introduction into the environment of many potentially harmful substances and have led to the withdrawal of others. In many instances in which relation between cancer and environmental exposure is well established, the specific chemicals responsible remain to be identified, as for example the carcinogenic constituents of cigarette smoke.

PHYSICAL FACTORS. Home accidents accounted for 1.3 per cent of all deaths and 4 million injuries in the United States in 1975, and automobile accidents caused 44,570 deaths and 1,800,000 injuries. Modern transportation has had detrimental effects on health in addition to the loss of life and limb caused by automobile accidents; there is evidence that one factor contributing to coronary artery disease is lack of exercise.

Excessive heat, cold, and noise are harmful, as are both nonionizing and ionizing radiation. Less than 2 per cent of our total exposure to ionizing radiation comes from occupational sources and fallout consequent to nuclear weapons testing and nuclear power development. Almost one third of our exposure is from medical diagnostic procedures, and two thirds from natural sources. However, with increasing dependence on nuclear power likely in the years ahead, this could change significantly. The effect of ionizing radiation on the gene pool is cumulative. The most important known somatic effect is carcinogenesis. Whether radiation effects contribute to mortality from causes other than cancer is uncertain.

BIOLOGIC FACTORS. Man may be exposed to pathogenic bacteria, viruses, and parasites through inspired air, ingested food and water, and skin contact. The soil is a common source of pathogenic microorganisms and parasites, and many occupations have special biologic hazards, such as anthrax and brucellosis. Many infectious agents produce both acute and chronic disease. Some virus-induced conditions, such as kuru, become manifest only after a latent period of years. Although there have been many claims and much speculation, no unequivocal evidence yet exists for a microbiologic agent as a cause of cancer in man. However, it is likely that some forms of human cancer are viral in origin. At present, the herpes viruses seem to be the best candidates.

SOCIAL FACTORS.   Social factors, including economic, psychologic, and cultural factors, all affect health. Brenner has found that there is a significant statistical relationship between unemployment and the incidence of cardiovascular disease, cirrhosis of the liver, suicide, mental illness, homicides, and the rate of imprisonment. In addition, there is evidence that schizophrenia, crime, suicide, alcoholism, and drug abuse have higher rates in impoverished and crowded areas. Infant mortality is as much as three times higher in the poverty sectors than in more affluent parts of the same cities. Knobloch and Pasamanick have shown that although black and white infants manifest no differences in developmental tests at 40 weeks of age, by three years the performance of black children is significantly behind

that of the white. Whether poverty itself, poor housing, inadequate diet, less education, a combination of these, or other factors are responsible is yet to be established. However urgent the need for more knowledge in this area, existing information is sufficient to provide strong incentive for improving conditions.

Examination of mortality data for the eighteenth, nineteenth, and early twentieth centuries reveals that some major improvements in health have resulted to a much greater extent from changes in a variety of environmental factors than from medical measures. This is particularly apparent in studies of deaths from infectious diseases in the preantimicrobial era (see accompanying figure). There is reason to believe that the improvements resulted from better nutrition, removal of hazards from the physical environment by improved water supply and sewage disposal, and a decrease in the birth rate. Other factors may also have contributed, including changes in the virulence of some of the microorganisms, notably the streptococci.

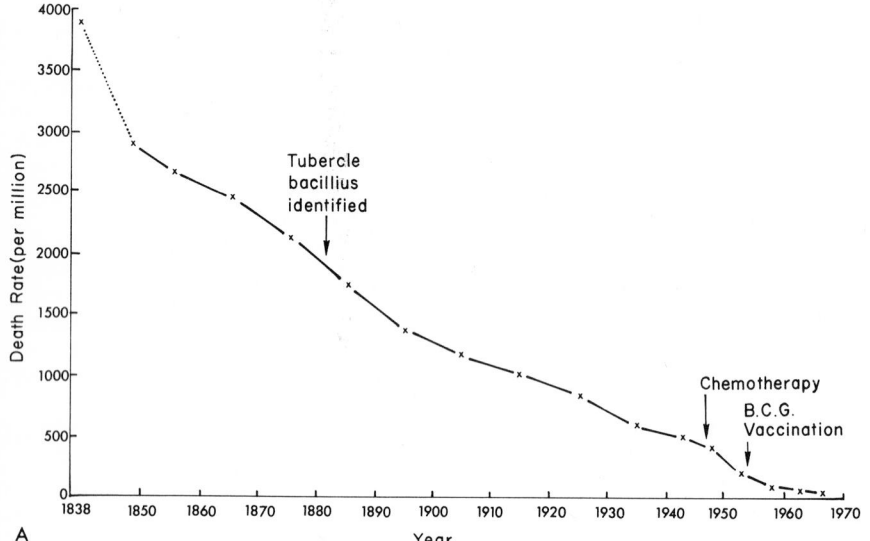

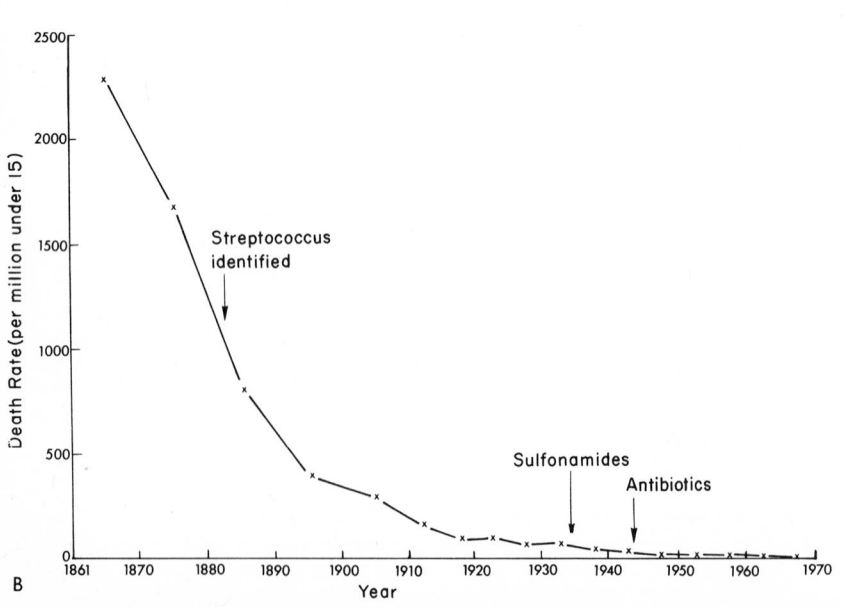

A, Respiratory tuberculosis: mean annual death rate, England and Wales. *B,* Scarlet fever: mean annual death rate of children under 15, England and Wales. (From McKeown, T., and Lowe, C. R.: An Introduction to Social Medicine. Oxford, Blackwell, 1974.)

BEHAVIORAL CHANGE

It was earlier pointed out that in order to prevent or alter an illness we do not always require an understanding of the mechanism whereby an environmental factor contributes to it, and often not even a precise identification of the specific offending factor. On the other hand, however difficult it may be to establish a cause-and-effect relationship between environmental factor and disease, it may be far more difficult to exploit such knowledge. Consider, for example, the difficulties in inducing the attitudinal and behavioral changes required to take greater advantage of the knowledge that gonorrhea is transmitted sexually and that a variety of pulmonary, cardiac, and other diseases are aggravated by cigarette smoking. One important step is, of course, behavioral change in the physician. It is unlikely that even the most enlightened patients will be appropriately moved by statistics relating cigarettes, obesity, or lack of exercise to disease if those statistics are offered by physicians who pay them no heed. Further, just as physicians who have diagnosed a condition that requires penicillin must ensure that the drug is received, so they must do everything possible to achieve the environmental and behavioral changes that they feel are dictated by their patients' health.

Much of the health benefit resulting from a recognition of responsible environmental factors and their alteration can be achieved only through action directed at population groups. Here the responsibilities of the physician include participation with other members of society in those socially acceptable actions necessary to achieve the desired ends.

CONCLUSIONS

An examination of the present state of knowledge of the relationships of environmental factors and health leads to certain conclusions. First, there is great need for careful and extensive data collection and analysis. The paucity and unreliability of available data and the complexity of the problems that confront us have led too often in this chapter and in this book to the use of such expressions as "is believed to," "may," "conflicting reports exist," and so on, and undoubtedly even more often to our overlooking associations. Better patient records and information systems are required to help correlate data concerning illness, drugs, chemicals, and physical, nutritional, social, and other environmental factors that affect health in order to alert society to dangers as early as possible. However, even these will never replace the contribution of the astute physician who regards every patient not only as a human being in need of attention and devotion, but also as one presenting a problem in need of a solution. It is relevant to recall that rubella and thalidomide were recognized as teratogens not in a research laboratory or by a computerized medical record system, but by astute clinicians in the course of their practice. (It is true, of course, that had better record systems been available at the time, the teratogenic effects might have been recognized earlier.)

The most sophisticated techniques of modern science will help demonstrate mutagenic, carcinogenic, teratogenic, and other effects of environmental factors on human cells and test organisms. Modern technology can contribute greatly needed quantification to environmental health studies. We require methods for assessing the effects of a variety of factors on human behavior and emotions and on other mental functions, although precise methodology in this area is likely to be a long way in the future. Cost-benefit studies, both medical and economic, are necessary for the physician to make enlightened decisions concerning the risks to which diagnosis and treatment inevitably expose his patient. The risk of anaphylaxis to penicillin is surely worth taking in the individual with pneumococcal pneumonia who has never had the drug previously. The risk of side effects such as thromboembolic disease from oral contraceptives now seems reasonable in the young woman seeking birth control. (Whether this will continue to be the case when all their health effects are uncovered remains uncertain.) Many other more difficult choices exist, and with the growing medical armamentarium and increasing information concerning the effects of drugs, chemicals, and procedures, many more difficult decisions are placed daily before the physician in his practice.

In recent decades there has been no improvement in over-all mortality rate from cancer.* More than 80 per cent of cases of cancer in the United States are thought to be the result, at least in part, of environmental factors. Similarly, a variety of environmental factors are known to aggravate cardiovascular disease. These and related facts make mandatory increased attention to preventive measures. The exciting implications of the application of our rapidly growing understanding of biology and chemistry to medical problems are widely recognized, and fundamental and clinical research has been and must continue to be encouraged. However, it is at least equally important that we address the present neglect of the benefits that can be achieved from available knowledge. Social and individual action could surely lead to the prevention or amelioration of many diseases, including several that are occupationally related. In this area the physician is often in a unique position to help identify problems and contribute to campaigns to alter responsible conditions.

---

*However, some changes, including a marked increase in survival of children with acute leukemia, are not reflected in the over-all data.

Brenner, H.: Estimating the Social Costs of National Economic Policy: Implications for Mental and Physical Health, and Criminal Aggression. Study prepared for the Joint Economic Committee, Congress of the U.S., October 26. Washington, D.C., U.S. Government Printing Office, 1976.

Gregg, N. M.: Congenital cataract following German measles in mother. Trans. Ophthalmol. Soc. Australia, 3:35, 1942.

Health Hazards of the Human Environment. Geneva, World Health Organization, 1972.

Knobloch, H., and Pasamanick, B.: Environmental factors affecting human development, before and after birth. Pediatrics, 26:210, 1960.

MacMahon, B., and Pugh, T. P.: Epidemiology: Principles and Methods. Boston, Little, Brown & Company, 1970.

McBride, W. G.: Thalidomide and congenital abnormalities. Lancet, 2:1358, 1961.

McKeown, T., and Lowe, C. R.: An Introduction to Social Medicine, 2nd ed. Oxford, Blackwell, 1974.

7. THE LIFE-CYCLE PERSPECTIVE IN MEDICINE

Herant A. Katchadourian

The perception of the individual in the context of the life cycle is essential for understanding patients and for dealing efficiently with their ailments and infirmities. In the seventeenth century Sir Thomas Browne wrote:

"Confound not the distinctions of thy Life which Nature hath divided, that is, Youth, Adolescence, Manhood, and old Age; nor in these divided Periods, wherein thou art in a manner Four, conceive thyself but One. Let every division be happy in its proper Virtues, nor one Vice run through all. Let each distinction have its salutary transition, and critically deliver thee from the imperfections of the former; so ordering the whole, that Prudence and Virtue may have the largest Section."

It is not merely convention that requires case histories to begin with a statement of the patient's age. Considerations related to chronologic age enter into the interpretation of the history of illness and the findings of physical examinations and laboratory tests. Since the prevalence and manifestations of illness are often age related, the fact that one is dealing with a child or an adult, an adolescent or an elderly person, significantly influences probabilistic judgments in differential diagnosis. At an even more fundamental level, the developmental phase itself determines the fact and nature of illness. Bedwetting or the presence of immature blood cells in the circulation does not carry the pathologic connotations in an infant that it would in an adult. Treatment, too, is age dependent, because the choice of procedure and dosage and even the expected outcome are significantly linked to age.

Even though a person's age is an unequivocal chronologic fact, to declare that someone is a child or an adult implies that the life span is divisible into phases and that childhood and adulthood are definable periods within it. But despite their pervasive use, terms like *child, adolescent,* or *adult* have no precise medical definition. Even more ambiguous are terms that refer to various subphases of these periods, such as *late adolescence* or *middle age.*

We take it for granted that such life phases are universal because they are biologically determined. Yet our notions about life phases are culturally defined. In spite of obvious physical differences between young and old, social differentiation is comparatively recent. Until the seventeenth century, there was no special emphasis on childhood as a separate phase of life in Western societies. In the Middle Ages, after the age of seven or so, when children could presumably look after themselves, they simply joined the world of adults, dressed like adults, and shared adult work and play. Although some went to school, there was no age grading in classrooms, and the ten- and twenty-year-olds could be taught together.

The shift away from viewing children as miniature adults began with the Reformation and the Counter Reformation in the seventeenth century. The philosophies of John Locke (1632–1704) and Jean Jacques Rousseau (1712–1778) were important early influences in shaping modern views of childhood. It was only after children had been recognized by society as a class of individuals different from adults that physicians began to make the same distinction systematically. Thus, although references to diseases of children can be found even in the most ancient of medical texts (such as the Ebers Papyrus of 1550 B.C.), medical specialization based on the age of the patient dates back only to the middle of the nineteenth century, when pediatrics began to emerge as a distinct field.

Since the turn of the century, both social and medical perspectives of the life span have tended toward further differentiation. Our modern concept of adolescence was greatly influenced by Granville Stanley Hall (1844–1924), a leading figure in American psychology and education. During the last several decades, adolescent medicine and geriatrics have become fairly well established subspecialties, even though neither of them yet qualifies for board certification. Currently there is growing interest in the specific processes and problems of adulthood itself.

Although most of the research on the life span has been done by social scientists (Goulet and Baltes; Nesselroade and Reese; Baltes and Schaie), there are now some good books by physicians in this field (Engel; Lidz). The concept of the life-cycle and life-span developmental psychology hold considerable promise for contributing to our understanding of people and how to take care of them.

The advantages to the physicians of adopting a life-cycle or life-span view can be subsumed under three general areas. First, this view extends the developmental focus beyond childhood and adolescence, so that adulthood and old age also can be seen as dynamic and changing phases of life, rather than static plateaus punctuated by periods of illness. This approach allows not only a more coherent longitudinal view of life but also a better understanding of its components over time and in a broader context. For example, sexual physiology and behavior make better sense if understood in terms of their varied manifestations at different phases of life and in relation to other significant biologic and psychosocial events occurring concurrently.

The second advantage of a life-cycle perspective is that it facilitates a multidisciplinary, integrative approach to human development and behavior. It furnishes a conceptual umbrella broad enough to incorporate a variety of views and approaches toward making cumulative sense out of the diversity of human life.

Finally, when the field of life-span developmental psychology has reached sufficient maturity, it may provide useful indices of the normative tasks and critical events that characterize the various nodal points and transitional periods of the life cycle. Such indices will help the physician assess the patient in a set of normative contexts and will facilitate more intelligent judgments in pathology. Furthermore, to the extent that such normative crises are predictable, there is allowance for anticipation and preparation to cope with them. The physician stands to gain from such knowledge not only in dealing with patients but also in the conduct of his or her own life. Although we share our patients' experiences only infrequently, in living out our own lives we are basically no different from those we set out to help.

On the other hand, the concept of the life cycle, like any other model or theory, is not a panacea. When theory becomes dogma, it entraps us into expectations that become self-fulfilling prophecies. By accepting the notion of "growing pains," we may be inclined to take lightly serious pain in a growing person. If adolescence is considered a turbulent period, then adolescents will oblige us by becoming turbulent. If middle age is expected to be a time for finding new directions, then middle-aged people may be inclined to throw away the worthwhile with the worthless in their vocational and personal lives.

Concepts like the cycle are useful at best as modest aids to our understanding the awesome complexity of human beings. Such concepts are not meant to be devices with which to wrap up life and put it in our pockets.

Aries, P.: Centuries of Childhood. New York, Knopf, 1962.

Baltes, P. B., and Schaie, K. W. (eds.): Life-Span Developmental Psychology: Personality and Socialization. New York, Academic Press, 1973.

Browne, T.: Part III, Sect. 8 of Christian Morals. In Religio Medici, Letter to a Friend, Urn-burial and Other Papers. Boston, 1878.

Engel, G. L.: Psychological Development in Health and Disease. Philadelphia, W. B. Saunders Company, 1962.

Goulet, L. R., and Baltes, P. B. (eds.): Life-Span Developmental Psychology: Research and Theory. New York, Academic Press, 1970.

Lidz, T.: The Person: His and Her Development Throughout the Life Cycle. New York, Basic Books, 1976.

Muuss, R. E.: Theories of Adolescence. New York, Random House, 1968.

Nesselroade, J. R., and Reese, H. W. (eds.): Life-Span Developmental Psychology: Methodological Issues. New York, Academic Press, 1973.

Simons, R. C., and Pardes, H.: Understanding Human Behavior in Health and Illness. Baltimore, Williams & Wilkins Company, 1977.

8. DEVELOPMENT TO ADULTHOOD

Herant A. Katchadourian

The terms "adolescent" and "adult" are both derived from the Latin "to grow" (*adolescere*): an adolescent is someone who is growing up, and an adult is someone who has grown up. Although this designation is overly simple to encompass the complex changes entailed in attaining adulthood, bodily growth and reproductive maturation are in fact among the cardinal events in this process. The period of life during which these biologic changes occur is properly referred to as "puberty," to differentiate it from the psychosocial developmental phase of "adolescence" with which it overlaps but does not coincide.

8.1. BIOLOGIC PROCESSES IN PUBERTY

The changes that constitute puberty have been classified by Marshall and Tanner as follows: (1) Acceleration and then deceleration of skeletal growth (the adolescent growth spurt). (2) Altered body composition as a result of skeletal and muscular growth, together with changes of the quantity and distribution of fat. (3) Development of the circulatory and respiratory systems, leading, particularly in boys, to increased strength and endurance. (4) The development of the gonads, reproductive organs, and secondary sex characters. (5) A combination of factors, not yet fully understood, which

modulates the activity of those nervous and endocrine elements which initiate and coordinate all these changes.

These changes result in two major biologic outcomes that have profound psychosocial repercussions. First, the child attains the physique and physiologic characteristics of the adult, including reproductive capacity. Second, most of the major adult physical sex differences become established through this process, greatly enhancing sexual dimorphism in adulthood.

These changes are virtually universal but with important differences between normal individuals in the onset, order, and rate of growth at puberty. We shall be mainly concerned here with the general patterns.

SOMATIC CHANGES. One usually becomes aware of the onset of puberty through its somatic manifestations. But these are preceded by hormonal changes, which in turn are triggered by activities in hypothalamic and other brain centers. The precise mechanisms that determine the onset of puberty are as yet unknown.

Among contemporary Western youth, the first signs of puberty become apparent at about age 10 to 11 among girls and 11 to 12 among boys (see accompanying figure). There is, however, a wide range of normal variability extending from 8½ to 13 years for girls and 9½ to 15 for boys. Most children do enter puberty within these ages (95 per cent of girls show at least one sign of puberty by age 13½); yet even at that, perfectly normal exceptions are possible at both extremes.

Puberty entails a whole host of changes, some of which are shown in the accompanying figure. Each of these events has its own schedule and range of variability. The general sequence of these events is more predictable than the ages at which they are likely to unfold. Girls enter puberty consistently earlier than boys by about two years, but here again the magnitude of discrepancy depends on what is being compared; girls grow pubic hair a year and a half earlier, but breast budding antedates testicular enlargement by six months.

It is essential to appreciate the normality of this wide range of variability during puberty. The physician must be prepared to confront adolescents of precisely the same chronologic age with dramatic differences in physical appearance, depending on whether they have entered puberty, are part way through it, or have completed the process.

Height and Weight. The pubescent growth spurt is among the more dramatic events encountered during development. Growth in stature is in progress throughout childhood. Actually, by age 10, boys have already attained 78 per cent and girls 84 per cent of their adult height. What makes the growth spurt at puberty noteworthy is mainly its rate rather than its magnitude. The height spurt typically starts at about 10½ years among girls, reaches peak velocity at 12, and ends by 14. But it may start as early as 9½ or end as late as 15 years. Among boys, the onset is usually at about 12 to 13 (or as early as 10½ and as late as 16), the peak at 14, and the end at 16 (or between 13½ and 17½). During the year of peak height velocity, a boy grows on an average of 3 to 5 inches and a girl somewhat less. This means an actual doubling in velocity of growth and approximates the rapid growth rate of the two-year-old child. Following the growth spurt, the rate of growth decelerates rapidly. Most girls at 14 years and most boys at 16 years reach 98 per cent of their ultimate adult height.

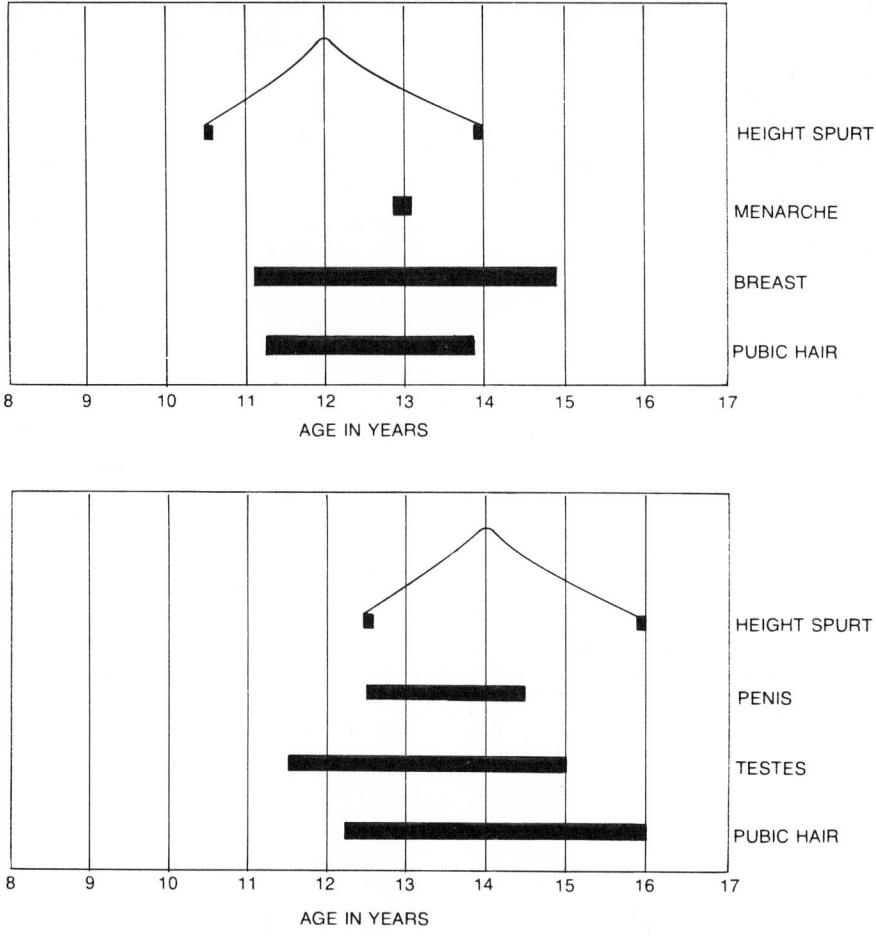

Sequence of events of puberty in girls (above) and boys (below). (From Tanner, J. M.: Sci. Am., 229:40, 1973. Copyright © 1973 by Scientific American, Inc. All rights reserved.)

Further noticeable growth in stature ceases at about 18 years in women and at 20 years in men.

Stature is determined by a host of genetic and environmental factors. It varies among children as it does among adults. During puberty further differences emerge which are transient artifacts of discrepant rates of growth. Thus an early maturing adolescent may move ahead of his peers but eventually end up no taller.

How tall a youngster will be as an adult is generally of considerable consequence to the individual and the family. Boys are usually worried about not being tall enough and girls about growing to be too tall. Physicians dealing with adolescents need to know the various normal patterns of maturation and the methods of predicting final stature by reference to skeletal age rather than chronologic age.

The gain in weight during puberty follows a similar pattern to height, but it is a more labile index of development than height. The nonskeletal growth increments are more marked than those for skeletal growth; by age 10, boys have gained only 55 per cent and girls 59 per cent of their adult weight. The factors which contribute to gain in weight are the increased size of the skeleton, muscles, and internal organs, and the amount of fat.

There is a marked sex difference between the amount and distribution of subcutaneous fat which contributes to shaping bodily contours. Infants accumulate subcutaneous fat (more in the case of females), but children gradually lose their chubbiness until shortly before puberty when they regain some of it. With the growth spurt a negative fat balance is established among boys, but not among girls, who usually enter adulthood with more body fat than males, particularly in the region of the pelvis and breasts.

Musculature and Strength. There is a marked increase in the size and strength of the musculature at puberty in both sexes but more so for males. This is the result of muscle cells becoming more numerous and larger. Among boys, the increase in number of cells is fourteen-fold; among girls, ten-fold. In females, maximum muscle cell size is reached by age 10½, whereas in males muscle cells continue to enlarge until the end of the third decade.

Body Proportions. The difference between the physique of the child and the adult is determined by variation in body proportions as well as size. During puberty body proportions undergo marked changes, and when these are in progress they may become sources of concern and distress to the adolescent who feels that he looks neither like his former childhood self nor quite like an adult. For example, legs accelerate in growth a year before the trunk, contributing to the stereotype of the gangling adolescent. Leg growth itself is not uniform; the foot accelerates first (though it stops growing soon), followed by the calf and the thigh. Similarly, hand and forearm grow ahead of the upper arm.

The adult face becomes distinctive through changes undergone during puberty. The neural pattern of growth, which also characterizes the growth of the cranium, places it ahead of other systems in the developmental schedule. Thus, throughout the growth period the size of the head becomes progressively smaller relative to the rest of the body. With the growth spurt at puberty, which affects the size of the cranium much less than the other parts of the skeleton, this trend is further exaggerated.

Other changes affect the head itself. The bones of the face grow faster than those of the cranial vault, so that at puberty the face is said to "emerge from under the skull." The profile of the adult becomes straighter, the nose and the jaw more prominent, and the lips fuller. Facial appearance is further altered by the recession of the hairline and in males by the growth of facial hair. All these changes are more marked among males.

Some sex differences in physical features are present at birth and become further exaggerated at puberty. For example, the male forearm is larger relative to height and contributes to his stronger hand grip. Other differences that emerge at puberty include the male's broader shoulders, narrower hips, and longer legs relative to trunk length.

Internal Changes. Numerous internal changes accompany the more evident manifestations of puberty. The heart, like other muscles of the body, participates in the growth spurt and its weight nearly doubles. The steady rise of systolic blood pressure throughout childhood accelerates and soon attains adult values. The concurrent decline in pulse rate is checked, and there may even be a slight increase in the resting heart rate. Blood volume, hemoglobin, and the number of red blood cells are all increased. All these changes are more marked among males.

The respiratory system undergoes similar changes. Lung size and respiratory capacity increase during puberty, whereas respiratory rate continues to decrease. These changes once again favor the male, including a greater efficiency in oxygen exchange.

The net effect of these and related physiologic alterations in puberty greatly increases the capacity for physical exertion and allows quicker recovery from its effects. Greater exercise tolerance combined with superior strength permits individuals of both sexes to vastly outperform their prepubescent selves in physical effort.

Not all changes at puberty are in the direction of growth and better performance. The lymphoid system regresses markedly. Myopic children become more so, and many new cases of myopia appear during this time.

Reproductive Maturation. The maturation of the reproductive system is the quintessential mark of puberty. It involves the accelerated growth of the internal sex organs and the external genitalia (figure). This is accompanied by the development of the so-called secondary sexual characteristics, which include the development of the female breast, the sprouting of pubic and axillary hair, the lowering pitch of the voice, and the appearance of facial hair in the male. In physiologic terms, the key events are the activation of ovulation and the menstrual cycle in females and the production of sperm and the ability to ejaculate in males. At least some prepubescent children have orgasmic capability but do not ejaculate semen prior to the development at puberty of the prostate gland, which produces most of the seminal fluid.

FEMALE REPRODUCTIVE MATURATION. Breast development is usually the first visible sign of female puberty; it starts between the ages of 8 and 13 and is completed between 13 and 18. Transient asymmetry is not unusual. Pubic hair ordinarily appears next, starting at age 11 to 12 and developing into the adult pattern by about 14; it precedes the growth of axillary hair by about a year. Breast and pubic hair growth follow predictable patterns which have been standardized and are used as indices of pubertal development.

The external genitalia become enlarged and their erotic sensitivity heightened. The internal sex organs rapidly increase in weight. Uterine musculature develops more fully, and the endometrium undergoes its elaborate cyclical changes following menarche. The vagina enlarges, with thickening of its epithelium.

Menarche does not commonly herald puberty as is sometimes erroneously assumed, but it is one of the late events. In the United States, the average age at menarche currently ranges from about 9 to 18 years (mean, 12.83). Contrary to earlier assumptions that a secular trend of decreasing ages at menarche was in progress, current data show that the age at menarche has not changed for the past three decades at least among American middle class girls.

MALE REPRODUCTIVE MATURATION. The onset of puberty in males is signaled by enlargement of the testes, which usually starts between 10 and 13½ and remains in progress until ages 14½ to 18. Pubic hair growth occurs between 12 and 16. The growth of the facial and axillary hair lags behind by two years. The first ejaculation usually occurs at 11 or 12, but mature sperm take a few more years to appear. This relative pubescent sterility in girls and boys who have otherwise matured sexually does not amount to reliable contraceptive security.

The penis begins to grow markedly about a year after testicular and pubic hair development. Deepening of the voice results from enlargement of the larynx. It is a late event in puberty and much less marked among females. Some breast enlargement may be observed in males, which eventually regresses as a rule.

NEUROENDOCRINE CONTROL OF PUBERTY. A complex set of neuroendocrine mechanisms underlies the initiation and control of puberty. They involve the interaction of hypothalamic hormones, anterior pituitary hormones (somatotropin, gonadotropins — FSH, LH) and steroid hormones from the gonads and adrenal cortex (estrogens, progestins, androgens). Other substances such as thyroid hormones and insulin also take part in these regulating mechanisms.

The nature and actions of these hormones are discussed elsewhere (see Ch. 548.2 and 549.2). The precise mechanism that initiates puberty is not known. The hypothalamus, pituitary, gonads, and body tissues have the capacity to be stimulated into adult function long before the normal ages of puberty. This means that puberty is due to the further activation of an already functional system.

The current postulate is that as the child matures, the hypothalamic receptor sites become less sensitive to inhibition by circulating low levels of steroid hormones. Consequently, under hypothalamic prompting, larger amounts of gonadotropins are produced by the pituitary, which in turn increases gonadal hormonal output. Through continuing readjustment of the equilibrium between pituitary and gonadal activities, gonadal steroids required to suppress the hypothalamus reach a level which exceeds the threshold of sensitivity of peripheral tissues to these hormones, and the physical changes of puberty are set into motion.

FACTORS AFFECTING PUBERTY. A wide range of genetic and environmental factors influence the onset and course of events in puberty. Some of these factors are well established; others are conjectural. The human pattern of puberty is the culmination of an evolutionary process starting with primates and successively carried further by monkeys, apes, and man. The current pattern of puberty in humans probably evolved with early man and has basically not changed except for relatively minor aspects such as its time of onset.

The presence of racial differences in pubertal patterns remains unsettled. The force of genetic factors is discernible in familial tendencies. Randomly chosen girls reach menarche differing on the average by 19 months; for sisters who are not twins, the difference is 13 months; for nonidentical twins, it is 10 months; for identical twins, 2.8 months.

The influence of climate is dubious; that of seasons more certain: height increases twice as fast in the spring, and growth in weight is four or five times as fast in the autumn; during spring there is a significant reduction in the incidence of menarche.

Malnutrition stunts growth and will interfere with the pubertal process. The effects are selective, as growth of sexual organs is relatively less retarded than that of other tissues. Boys are more vulnerable than girls. Differences in menarchal age in various countries and between social classes are due at least in part to nutritional factors. The effects of illness are highly variable. Most acute conditions have no lasting effect; disorders specific to the endocrine systems in question will have profound influence (see Ch. 548.2 and 548.3 and Ch. 549.2). Finally, emotional factors have considerable bearing on the developmental process, but in ways that are as yet poorly understood.

8.2. PSYCHOSOCIAL DEVELOPMENT

A comprehensive account of psychosocial aspects of normal adolescence would include psychologic reactions to the changes of puberty; emotional maturation; sexual behavior; cognitive and ideologic development; identity formation; restructuring of parental, sibling, and peer relationships; school experiences and vocational choice; participation in the youth subculture; socialization into the adult world; and so on. These events include so many complex variables and uncertainties that no concise and generally acceptable account of adolescent development is currently feasible.

We shall selectively focus here on those aspects of adolescent development that are likely to be of significance to the clinician who encounters adolescents in two contexts: first, when the issue is directly related to the process of adolescence itself and may be manifested in somatic or psychologic symptoms; and second, when some other illness, such as diabetes, occurs in an adolescent. In both cases some understanding of the normative developmental processes at work is helpful.

A central problem in adolescent psychology is whether normal adolescence is characterized by psychic turmoil. The concept that adolescence constitutes a stormy stage of life has been dominant in psychiatric thinking of the last half century (usually referred to as *Sturm und Drang*, or storm and stress). A contending view that "coming of age" need not necessarily entail turmoil has recently gained more credence through research involving adolescent populations at large rather than relying on extrapolations from clinical experience. A sensible compromise is to view adolescence as a labile period when emotional turmoil may commonly occur, without either expecting that it necessarily do so or viewing youngsters who show no such distress as pathologic.

Adolescent development is often assessed in terms of "tasks" the person must accomplish in order to successfully emerge from this stage. Beyond obvious requirements, such as the need to move toward economic self-sufficiency, the tasks that are set forth usually reflect a particular theoretical view or social value system. Some of these schemes are nevertheless quite useful for the clinician, because they provide him with a convenient framework in which to assess the young individual.

STAGES OF ADOLESCENT DEVELOPMENT. Tasks of adolescence are often subdivided as characterizing one of three subphases of adolescence. Thus, in early adolescence there is the task of psychologically integrating the ongoing somatic changes of puberty. Changes in body proportions and body image, menstruation, and enhancement of the sexual drive are among the developments that require psychologic adaptation and adjustment.

There is some reshuffling of peer groups at this time, but these remain largely monosexual. Likewise, intense outside relationships begin to form as exemplified by strong attachments and "crushes." But the home still remains the center of the youngster's life.

The adolescent makes important strides in cognitive development at this time, constituting Piaget's stage of "formal operations." Starting with age 11 to 12 and going on to 14 or 15, this process endows the adolescent with the capacity to use propositional and deductive logic. The youth can now reason abstractly, formulate hypotheses, and manipulate ideas in sophisticated adult fashion.

Similarly, Kohlberg has categorized stages of moral development that begin with "premoral" concern with avoiding punishment which is a carryover from childhood. The teenager then moves on to conventional role conformity to remain in the good graces of the family and to win approval. Only by about 16 or 17 are right and wrong understood as self-accepted moral principles.

Mid-adolescence raises the issues of dealing with family attachments and controls, revolt and conformity, participation in youth subcultures, further differentiation of gender identity, sexual experiences, and falling in love. Late adolescence is preoccupied by the task of self-definition and the identity crisis which, according to Erikson, is the phase-specific task of adolescence. The capacity for intimacy and more mature forms of love and sexual relationships characterizes adolescents approaching the threshold of adulthood.

RESTRUCTURING RELATIONSHIPS. Common social expectations require that the adolescent increasingly relate to others as an adult. This implies being less dependent and more dependable, along with a host of other expectations that are by no means consistently fulfilled by the majority of adults themselves.

The most crucial set of relationships to be redefined involves parents or other adults on whom the adolescent is economically and psychologically dependent.

Anna Freud has proposed that this detachment or emancipation from childhood ties is managed through a number of psychologic mechanisms in which the person engages without himself being quite conscious of them.

One mechanism for the adolescent to detach himself from the parents is to displace his intense feelings of attachment for them onto other people and interests. If this occurs slowly, the youngster experiences periods of moodiness and other reactions akin to those seen in mourning over a serious loss. The need to become separate may make him act seclusive or be "like a stranger" in the home. These feelings need not entirely dominate his life and may well be hidden under the continuing cordiality he maintains with his parents as well as the new and rewarding experiences he begins to develop in relating to them more like an adult.

A more abrupt expression of detachment is to run away from home. Some homes are so intolerable that this move is no less than an act of self-preservation. There are also many socially approved forms of leaving home, such as going away to boarding school or college, joining the armed forces, and so on, which may be at least in part motivated by the need to break away.

The attachment to others may take the form of friendships with peers, teachers, employers, or more distant figures such as rock stars or sports or movie figures to whom the adolescent becomes uncritically and helplessly attached as he was earlier to his parents.

A second mechanism is to reverse the feelings held toward the parents whereby love, dependence, and respect turn into various intensities of hate, revolt, and contempt. More often, positive feelings simply become tinged with ambivalence. This process is in part the result of seeing parents for who they really are and in part a means of facilitating giving them up by dwelling on their shortcomings. Since it is safer and less painful for the conflict to be shifted from the private to the public arena, the fault finding may become focused on parental substitutes, public institutions, society, and the world at large. But youth can also be critical of society on justifiable grounds quite apart from personal considerations.

Another mechanism involves the adolescent turning inward as it were and investing his own self with the intense feelings formerly reserved for parents. This would account for the narcissism and selfishness of young people, their preoccupation with their bodies, and their inflated ideas of beauty, strength, and competence. An adolescent may only indulge these thoughts in fantasies or may impose them on the world. In contrast, he may so totally lose himself in others that he thinks and acts as if he were someone else. This, too, may be indulged only in daydreams without his losing touch with reality, or it may take on pathologic expressions.

DEALING WITH DRIVES. Sexuality long antedates adolescence, yet there is a distinct upsurge in sexual interest and activity with the maturation of the reproductive system in puberty. Most societies attempt to regulate sexual behavior to widely divergent extents. So the task confronting the adolescent in this regard is socially dependent. When sexual expression in youth is frowned upon, there may be an attempt to give up the sexual impulse. When this repression is extended to all feelings of pleasure, it leads to various degrees of asceticism. The flight from sexuality may take the form of preoccupation with abstract intellectual issues or rigid and uncompromising stands toward all forms of seeming or real moral laxity.

Currently, rather than resort to such repression, many adolescents engage in various forms of sexual expression, including sexual intercourse. This confronts the physician with difficult dilemmas over such issues as contraception and abortion when he has to deal with individuals who are biologically adult but socially considered not to be so.

The expression of aggression in adolescence is a very serious social and medical problem. Violent deaths such as those resulting from accidents represent by far the leading cause of death in the second decade of life, accounting for over half of all deaths from all causes between the ages of 10 and 19. Homicide is the fifth most common cause of death among 10- to 14-year-olds. In 15- to 19-year-olds, homicide ranks second and suicide fourth.

IDENTITY FORMATION. Mainly as a result of Erikson's work, the concept of identity as the central task of adolescence has gained wide currency. Erikson's theory of psychosocial development postulates a sequence of eight phases or "ages of man." These phases derive from Freud's stages of psychosexual development, but they also go beyond them and encompass the entire life span. Each stage is defined by a phase-specific task and follows a general chronology without being linked to specific age limits.

These assignments hold true only in the sense that the phase-specific tasks reach their critical point of resolution during their respective phases. Otherwise, their solutions are prepared in previous stages and elaborated in subsequent ones.

The psychosocial transition to adulthood is accomplished during adolescence (Stage V) through the achievement of a sense of ego identity. In everyday terms, identity refers to a person's individuality, the response to the question of "Who am I?" But what Erikson means by identity is more complex. It includes a conscious sense of individual identity, an unconscious striving for a continuity of personal character, certain aspects of "ego synthesis," and the maintenance of an inner solidarity with a group's ideals and identity. The issue of identity is not settled once and for all during adolescence. What occurs at best is a clarification and reworking of earlier solutions and enough of a consolidation to provide the person with a self-sameness, even though many aspects of his personality continue to be reworked and refined in successive phases of the life cycle.

In more global terms, the criterion of attaining adulthood may be phrased in terms of achieving competence in a variety of spheres. Biologically, this means completing growth and becoming endowed with reproductive capacity. Psychologically, it requires a sufficient differentiation of the self whereby one can perceive the uniqueness of oneself in the context of other relationships. It implies the ability to recognize people for who they are and to relate to them effectively. As a minimum, it entails being able to look after oneself as well as being able to look after others in one or another context of one's choosing. It involves the capacity to help run society and be run by it.

In the final analysis, the task of becoming adult and what it means to be adult resolve into philosophical quests about the meaning and purpose of life. These are not ordinarily medical issues; yet since the physician at some level must deal with the patient as a person within a given social context, these considerations become relevant to medical practice.

Berenberg, S. R. (ed.): Puberty: Biologic and Psychosocial Components. Leider, H. E., Stenfert Kroese, B.V., 1975.

Erikson, E.: Childhood and Society. New York, Norton, 1963.

Freud, A.: Adolescence. In The Psychoanalytic Study of the Child, New York, International Universities Press, 13:255, 1958.

Grumbach, M. M., Grave, G. D., and Mayer, F. E.: Control of the Onset of Puberty. New York, John Wiley & Sons, 1974.

Heald, F. P., and Hung, W. (eds.): Adolescent Endocrinology. New York, Appleton-Century-Crofts, 1970.

Inhelder, B., and Piaget, J.: The Growth of Logical Thinking from Childhood to Adolescence. New York, Basic Books, 1958.

Kohlberg, L.: Development of moral character and ideology. In Hoffman, M. L., and Hoffman, L. W. (eds.): Review of Child Development Research, Vol. 1. New York, Russell Sage Foundation, 1964, pp. 383–433.

Marshall, W. A., and Tanner, J. M.: Puberty. In Davis, J. A., and Dobbing, J. (eds.): Scientific Foundations of Pediatrics. London, William Heinemann Medical Books, 1974.

Root, A. W.: Endocrinology of puberty: I. Normal sexual maturation. J. Pediat., 83:1, 1973.

Tanner, J. M.: Physical growth. In Mussen, P. (ed.): Carmichael's Manual of Child Psychology, Vol. I. 3rd ed. New York, John Wiley & Sons, 1970.

Zacharias, L., Rand, W. M., and Wurtman, R. J.: A prospective study of the sexual development and growth in American girls: The statistics of menarche. Obstet. Gynecol. Survey, 3:325, (Suppl.), 1976.

9. ADULTHOOD

Herant A. Katchadourian

9.1. INTRODUCTION

Unlike the pediatrician, who can turn to a vast literature on child development, physicians who deal with adults can find no comparable source of information on normative adult development. Until recently the prevailing view was that after childhood and adolescence, nothing of major consequence happened in developmental terms until toward the latter part of the normal life span, when the individual began to age. Currently gaining credence is an alternative viewpoint, whereby adulthood is seen not as a simple plateau interposed between the ascending steps of childhood and the descending steps of old age, but rather as a phase of life with its own discernible normative tasks and predictable transitions and stages. Although there is as yet no generally accepted developmental sequence for the adult years, and considerable disagreement over whether a stage theory for adulthood has any validity, knowledge accumulated in this field is of potential usefulness to the physician in understanding and treating adults.

Just as there is a great deal of normal variability in the ages at which biologic adulthood is attained, there is even more variance in the ways various cultures define an adult in psychosocial terms. Some investigators of the life cycle find it convenient nevertheless to divide the adult life span tentatively into several chronologic periods. Thus the transition to adulthood is expected to take place during the second decade of life (Katchadourian, 1977). Adulthood itself is subdivided by Levinson et al. into early adulthood, which corresponds to the age period of 20 to 40 years; middle adulthood (ages 40 to 60); and late adulthood (age 60 and older). Gerontologists divide old age into periods, such as early old age (ages 65 to 70) and advanced old age (75 years and older) (Butler).

Formidable difficulties confront investigators in this field. In order to obtain a proper time frame, for example, they must consider the interweaving of "historical time," which defines the period and hence the nature of the culture; "life time," or chronologic age of the individual; and "socially defined time," representing the age-graded expectations of appropriate behavior (Neugarten). The expectation is that during each adult developmental period a variety of biologic, psychodynamic, cultural, and social structural developmental timetables are in operation in variable degrees of synchronization. There are currently serious differences pertaining to fundamental aspects of adult developmental processes, in addition to disagreements over details, but some of the insights that are generally agreed upon will benefit the physician in his or her work.

9.2. ISSUES, CHANGES, AND STAGES

In attempting to understand the unfolding of adult life, the simplest approach is to identify those issues pertinent to adult life that are readily observable among a wide sector of the adult population. More ambitious is the attempt to delineate stages of adult development through which most individuals pass and which therefore constitute significant nodal points and predictable landmarks of adult life.

Factors within the first category are easier to identify, but because of their ubiquity and high variability they are also more difficult to systematize. Certain biologic changes become manifest more or less universally among people who live long enough. We refer to this process as "aging," but until the confounding effects of disease are eliminated, it is impossible to say whether changes in mental and physical abilities with age are due to the pathologic effects of disease or the manifestations of a normative developmental process of progressive biologic decline characteristic of all organisms. Furthermore, we have no systematic knowledge as yet as to whether these changes over time follow a discernible sequence that could conceivably be subsumed under chronologic phases or stages. Although a few physiologic events such as the menopause would seem to be notable exceptions, precisely what it is that transpires during the menopause is still far from clear.

Similarly, innumerable variables can be identified in the social realm in terms of the various adult roles individuals take on, maintain, change, or abandon. For example, a large segment of the adult population goes through divorce in addition to the sequence of courtship, marriage, parenthood, and separation from grown-up children. Similar sequences exist in vocations and other social realms. Yet the voluminous social science literature that elucidates these issues does not always help us understand how these events fit into a life-cycle perspective.

In addition to very wide cross-cultural variability in these institutions, one encounters within a given culture changes that occur over relatively short periods of time and redefine the ages at which most individuals experience these roles and what the roles signify for them. For example, Americans are getting married later and becoming parents later; from 1960 to 1976 the estimated median age at first marriage increased from 22.8 to 23.8 years for men and from 20.3 to 21.3 years for women. In 1960 there were 35 divorced persons per every 1000 people who were partners in intact marriages; by 1976 the ratio had risen to 75 per 1000. Meanwhile, women are going to work in increasingly higher proportions. The number of married women in the labor force rose from 30.5 per cent of women with husbands present in 1960 to 44.4 per cent in 1976.

Investigators have identified certain trends that are characteristic of some phases of adult life. Neugarten, for example, has described an increased tendency during middle age toward "interiority," which consists of increased emphasis upon introspection and stock-taking and conscious reappraisal of the self. Another characteristic of middle age is a change in one's perception of time. Whereas in earlier years the individual reckons time in terms of "time lived," with middle age the focus shifts to "time left to live." Although younger individuals are quite aware of their mortality, it is experienced in more personal terms during middle age and later, when a shift occurs from more abstract concern about death to a more personalized perception of its certainty and significance to one's everyday life. Additional discriminations between age groups center on attitudes toward the self and others. For instance, age-related responses have been obtained to questions such as whether marriage has been a good thing, whether parents are a cause of problems, and the possibility of changing careers (Gould).

Of various stage theories, the most widely known is Erikson's eight phases of the life cycle. In Erikson's view, the psychosocial transition to adulthood is accomplished during adolescence (Stage V) through the achievement of a sense of Identity, which in turn makes possible the establishment of a sense of Intimacy, the first phase-specific task of adulthood proper (Stage VI). Erikson defines these phase-specific tasks in terms of polar opposites of successful outcome or failure. Thus the counterpart to Intimacy is Isolation. Stage VII revolves around the issue of Generativity versus Stagnation. Using a heterosexual paradigm, Erikson sees as the central task at this phase the establishment of the next generation through the production and care of offspring, or, alternatively, through other altruistic and creative acts. The final phase of adult life confronts the task of Integrity versus Despair and Disgust. Integrity is the outcome of having taken care of things and people, originated others and generated things and ideas, and adapted to triumphs and disappointments. Because adulthood has received less attention in Erikson's work than adolescence, a great deal of Erikson's thinking about the derivatives and precursors of these adult stages of development has yet to be enunciated.

A more recent attempt to delineate stages in development comes from the work of Levinson and his associates. So far, this investigation has reported on male subjects between the ages of 18 and 45 only. Developmental phases in the lives of these men have been discerned to consist of the following: First is a transitional phase ("leaving the family") that usually stretches from the end of high school into the early twenties. During this period the young man may go through a phase of institutional living outside the home, such as in college or the military. Or, should he join the labor force, he may continue living at home but substantially outside parental control. Next is the phase of "getting into the adult world," which extends from the early twenties to the end of the twenties. During this period an initial definition of oneself as an adult is attained, and the individual fashions an initial life structure providing a link between the self and the adult world. This is a time of exploration and choice, when provisional commitments are made to an occupation. Those who resist making even tentative choices tend to develop a desperate need to settle down later on, or forfeit the chances of ever forming a reasonably satisfying life structure. Next is the "age 30 transition," a phase one passes through between the ages of 28 and 32. Like all transitional periods, this phase may be characterized by considerable turmoil, confusion, and struggle within oneself and with others, or it may simply entail a quiet reassessment of one's state and moving on.

The next period, "settling down," extends to the end of the thirties. The person now makes deeper commitments, investing more of himself in work, family, and other interests. There is a strong tendency toward maintaining order, stability, and security, while simultaneously striving to move ahead in order to "make it." In conflict with both these tendencies is the residual need to be free and unfettered. An important component of the settling-down period is "becoming one's own man," which typically is accomplished between the ages of 35 and 39 and represents the high point of early adulthood. During this phase a man has a profound need to be affirmed by society in the roles that he values most. In most instances this need involves some key event in the person's vocational career.

The "mid-life transition" ushers in another turning point, in which, irrespective of past accomplishments, the person confronts the issue of disparity between what has been gained and what one wants for himself. Major issues include the sense of bodily decline and recognition of one's mortality. There is a more acute sense of aging and further reorganization of the person's sense of gender identity. The crucial issue at mid-life is the changing relationship to the self. The mid-life transition occurs around the age of 40 and usually encompasses several years. By the mid-forties there is a period of restabilization that ushers the individual into middle adulthood.

9.3. CRISES OF ADULT LIFE

Just as a major problem in adolescent psychology is whether normal adolescence is characterized by psychic turmoil, a similar controversy involves whether certain phases of adult life have a higher potential for psychologic turbulence. Most often it is the period of mid-life that is singled out as hazardous.

Traditionally the menopause has served as an example of mid-life crisis. It represents a fairly discrete biologic event, and its psychologic repercussions have been taken to constitute a coherent entity. Physicians who treat middle-aged women could testify to having seen countless such cases. Yet what has been generally lacking is empirical research with women who go through the menopause without being seen by physicians. When examined within a broader population base, the menopause emerges as a very different entity. For instance, in one nonmedical sample studied by Neugarten, only a few of the women viewed the menopause as a major source of worry. (The women were much more concerned about getting older, developing cancer, or losing their husbands.) Although many women presumably experience the symptoms of vasomotor instability ("hot flashes") and other physiologic signs of hormonal withdrawal, the majority seem to take these events in stride without major loss of feminine identity or sexual function. Furthermore, women who have difficulty during the menopause turn out to be the same women who had difficulty with menarche, menstrual periods, and pregnancy, which would indicate that the problem is idiosyncratic, rather than related to a normative developmental crisis.

Another so-called crisis commonly assumed to affect predominantly women is related to the "empty nest" created when grown-up children leave home. A more systematic investigation reveals that the postparental stage of life is associated with a higher, rather than lower, level of life satisfaction for women. Some studies show that marital adjustment improves for both sexes during middle age, possibly because of increased companionship after the children have left home (Burr; Rollins and Feldman).

The question has been raised repeatedly whether men undergo a counterpart of the female menopause. In a literal sense, of course, they do not; but the question is more difficult to answer in the broader sense of a climacterium encompassing bodily and psychic involutional changes during the transition from middle age to old age. Unlike ovarian function, which generally ceases between the ages of 48 and 50, testicular function declines gradually in adulthood, so that the production of sperm and testosterone declines gradually over decades. Yet many of the psychologic symptoms associated with the female menopause, such as irritability and depression, seem to characterize significant numbers of middle-aged males also.

Sexual function in middle life is another common source of concern. It has long been observed that potency generally suffers with age, but age is only one factor that has a bearing on this issue, and it is by no means clear that declining potency is predominantly due to aging as such rather than illness. Without denying the possibility that a fundamental biologic process related to aging affects sexual function, one can also assume that in a large number of cases failing potency with increasing age is an artifact of psychologic factors and social expectations. It is also important to recognize the changing nature of sexual response without equating such altered responses with sexual failure. The middle-aged or older male generally requires more physical stimulation to attain erection, for example, although in his younger years psychologic arousal would often be sufficient. But once having attained an erection, an older man is likely to maintain it longer or delay ejaculation at will, thus enhancing his lasting capacity during sexual intercourse. Other changes of sexual function at the physiologic level for aging men and women have been described (Masters and Johnson). None of these alterations in sexual function can yet be linked to a particular stage or phase of adult life.

Numerous other issues critical to mid-life have been proposed in the realms of economic life, social roles, and intrapsychic processes (Butler). On reviewing the more current literature, Brim derives the following six statements that sum up theories of the male mid-life crisis and may possibly be extrapolated to women crossing the threshold of middle life:

First, the mid-life male is likely to be undergoing profound personality changes.

Second, these changes will have more than one cause.

Third, a "male mid-life crisis" will occur for some men if there are multiple, simultaneous demands for personality change; if, for instance, during the same month or year the man throws off his last illusions about great success; accepts his children for what they are; buries his father and his mother and yields to the truth of his mortality; recognizes that his sexual vigor and, indeed, interest, are declining, and even finds relief in the fact.

Fourth, these challenges may be stretched out over ten or twenty years. Some men are obsessed about their achievements, but not yet confronting the fact of death; other men are sharply disappointed in their children's personalities but not yet concerned about sexual potency. The events come sooner for some men, much later for others. There is no evidence that they are related to chronologic age in any but the most general sense — e.g., "sometime during the forties."

Fifth, there is as yet no evidence for either developmental periods or "stages" in the mid-life period, in which one event must come after another or one personality change brings another in its wake. The existence of "stages," if proved true, would be a powerful concept in studying mid-life; meanwhile, there is a danger of our using this facile scheme as a cover for loose thinking about human development, without carrying forward the necessary hard-headed analyses of the evidence.

Sixth, the "growing pains" of mid-life, like those of youth and of old age, are transitions from one comparatively steady state to another, and these changes, even when they occur in crisis dimensions, bring for many men more happiness than they found in younger days.

Brim, O. G., Jr.: Theories of the male mid-life crisis. Counseling Psychologist, 6:2, 1976.

Burr, W. R.: Satisfaction with various aspects of marriage over the life cycle: A random middle class sample, J. Marriage Family, 32:29, 1970.

Butler, R. N.: Psychiatry and psychology of the middle-aged. In Freedman, A. M., Kaplan, H. I., and Sadock, B. J. (eds.): Comprehensive Textbook of Psychiatry, Vol. 2. 2nd ed. Baltimore, Williams & Wilkins Company, 1975, pp. 2390–2404.

Erikson, E. H.: Growth and crises of the healthy personality. In Identity and the Life Cycle: Selected papers by Erik H. Erikson. Psychological Issues, 1:18, 1959.

Gould, R. L.: The phases of adult life: A study in developmental psychology. Am. J. Psychiatry, 129:521, 1972.

Katchadourian, H. A.: Biology of Adolescence. San Francisco, W. H. Freeman and Company, 1977.

Katchadourian, H. A.: Medical perspectives on adulthood. Daedalus, 105:29, 1976.

Levinson, D. J., Darrow, C. M., Klein, E. B., Levinson, M. H., and McKee, B.: Periods in the adult development of men: Ages 18 to 45. Counseling Psychologist, 6:21, 1976.

Masters, W. H., and Johnson, V. E.: Human Sexual Response. Boston, Little, Brown & Company, 1966.

Neugarten, B. L.: Adaptation and the life cycle. Counseling Psychologist, 6:16, 1976.

Rollins, B. C., and Feldman, R.: Marital satisfaction over the life cycle. J. Marriage Family, 32:20, 1970.

U. S. Bureau of Census: A statistical portrait of women in the United States. Current Population Reports, Special Studies, Series P-23, No. 50, April 1976, p. 31.

U. S. Bureau of Census: Population characteristics. Current Population Reports, Series P-20, No. 306, January 1977, pp. 1–5.

10. AGING AND GERIATRIC MEDICINE

Ralph Goldman

10.1. INTRODUCTION

Few individuals live to maturity in a world of great environmental danger. The persistence of a species requires that enough members survive and reproduce so that a balance can be established. Once this is assured, individual survival is no longer essential. In fact, post-reproductive or inefficiently reproducing individuals compete for the resources of an ecologic niche and may threaten species survival. In humans the control of infections and malnutrition, improved management of trauma, and the reduction in death associated with reproduction have produced a profound social as well as scientific revolution. Figure 1 shows changes in survival over a prolonged historical period. The magnitude of this change is exemplified by the following data: During the sixteenth century, in the city of York, England, only 45 per cent of girls survived their first year, 18 per cent reached age 20, 11 per cent reached age 40, and 3 per cent reached age 65. These data are worse than what must have been the norm for that period, but cities with similar statistics existed well into the current century. In the United States and most developed countries, more than 96 per cent of white women will now reach age 40, 82 per cent will reach age 65, and 62 per cent will reach age 75. The outlook for men is less favorable, yet 93 per cent will reach age 40 and 67 per cent will reach age 65.

The very existence of a large older population means that serious disease and injury at younger ages have decreased. Thus, although medical researchers and practitioners have been chiefly concerned with acute injuries and illnesses of younger patients, the focus of their activities must now be shifted to chronic conditions, including their acute episodes, and to a consideration of the nature and implications of the aging process itself. Since human survival no longer depends upon adequate reproduction, we have both practical and moral imperatives for the study of gerontology and the practice of geriatrics.

The word *gerontology* derives from the Greek *gerontos*, old man, and *logos*, discourse upon, and refers to the study of the aging process. The word *geriatrics* is derived from *gerontos*, and *iatros*, physician, or *iatreia*, cure, literally physician or treatment of old men. The age at which a patient becomes eligible for geriatric care is artificial and arbitrary and usually relates to a statutory criterion, such as eligibility for Social Security or the age of mandatory retirement. Geriatrics uses the knowledge of gerontology, but the latter must study the aging process, which starts much earlier in life. Aging can be said to start at conception, but for practical purposes growth and development are associated with incremental processes, whereas during maturity and senescence decremental processes predominate.

Life span refers to the longest survival for a member of a species and serves as an index of maximum potential under ideal natural conditions. *Life expectation* refers to the average length of survival from a specific age, most commonly from birth, for a given cohort. Scientific and social improvements have increased life expectancy, but have not altered life span.

Geriatrics is not limited to management of decremental disease, dementia, and death. A large portion of the practice of medicine must, by the very fact of general survival to advanced age, be with older patients not thought of as a geriatric clientele. It is necessary for the concept of geriatric care to include both ambulatory and acute, as well as chronic, disease. The role of geriatrics is to integrate the information developed by gerontology with traditional medical knowledge to increase the well-being of aging patients.

10.2. STRUCTURAL AND FUNCTIONAL CHANGES WITH AGE

A primary problem of gerontology is to identify changes which are due to age alone and to differentiate these changes, if they exist, from pathologic processes.

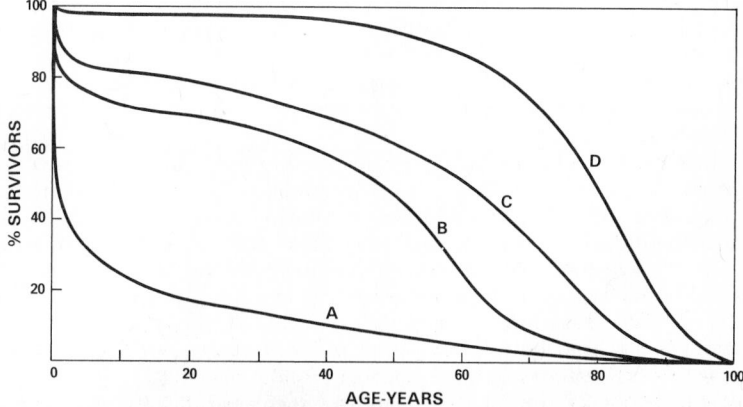

Figure 1. Cohort survival of women in different eras. A, Townswomen of York, England, sixteenth century. B, Aristocrats, England, sixteenth century. C, White women, United States, 1900. D, White women, United States, 1972.

Growth and development are universal and proceed according to an intrinsically determined pattern which can be modified by the environment within limits compatible with survival. Changes which are due to aging must also be universal. They should be unidirectional, and experience indicates that they are decremental. Although there is no a priori reason that age change should be either extrinsic or intrinsic in origin, the evidence now supports an intrinsic mechanism. The following are some of the major structural and functional changes with age which have been observed in humans and most mammals.

CELLS. Postmitotic cells, primarily muscle and nerve cells, are incapable of multiplication; they are not replaced when lost, and their number decreases with age. Mitotic cells have a limited capacity for replacement and are not immortal, as was once thought. Some cells, particularly the postmitotic cells, accumulate pigment within storage granules, and all cells show degeneration of intracellular organelles.

TISSUES. The regularity of tissue structure is lost, the individual cells enlarge, but the total number of cells decreases approximately 30 per cent. Fat deposition increases and conceals much of the loss of active cell mass. Intercellular collagen and elastin increase. The proportion of soluble collagen decreases, and there may be increased cross-linking between the long-chain collagen macromolecules. Elastin loses its discrete structure and elasticity and has an increased calcium content.

HEART. There is myocardial hypertrophy and fibrosis, and the valves become stiffer with age. The maximum cardiac rate and stroke volume, and thus the cardiac output, are progressively decreased, and the return to resting rate is prolonged. The isometric contraction and relaxation times are prolonged. Although there is a statistically valid increase in ECG intervals, there is no visually discernible abnormality in the normal pattern.

BLOOD VESSELS. The increased collagen, altered elastin, and increased calcium result in arterial rigidity with elevation of the systolic pressure, accelerated pulse wave velocity, and a loss of 10 per cent in cardiac systolic efficiency. The peripheral resistance is increased, whether due to arteriolar atrophy or spasm is not established, and the diastolic pressure is slightly elevated. The capillary basement membrane thickness increases from 700 to 1100 Angstroms between youth and old age.

EXCRETORY SYSTEM. The number of nephrons decreases 30 to 40 per cent between 25 and 85 years. The filtration rate, renal blood flow, and tubular functions are proportionately reduced, although the serum creatinine level is maintained because of reduced release from the decreasing muscle mass. The capacity for compensatory hypertrophy diminishes with age and increasingly depends upon cellular hypertrophy rather than hyperplasia.

RESPIRATORY SYSTEM. Upper respiratory infections become less frequent because of immunologic experience. The anteroposterior diameter of the chest increases and the compliance of the chest wall is decreased. The total lung capacity is unchanged, but the residual volume is doubled and the vital capacity is reduced. The maximum breathing capacity decreases about 50 per cent between the third and ninth decades. The reduced cough efficiency, decreased ciliary activity of the bronchial epithelium, and the increased dead

space enhance the potential for mechanical and infectious respiratory complications of surgery and enforced bed rest in the aged individual.

GASTROINTESTINAL SYSTEM. Hiatus hernia, atrophic gastritis, appendiceal involution, and colonic diverticulosis are increasingly common. Motility may be disorganized, and fecal incontinence is frequent in the mentally impaired. Salivary, gastric, and fasting pancreatic secretion are decreased, but after stimulation pancreatic secretion is normal. Digestion and absorption are generally adequate, although iron and calcium may be less well absorbed. The liver shows characteristic change and atrophy. There is a decreased albumin production, with a 20 per cent fall in the serum concentration. Bromsulphalein storage in hepatic cells is linearly decreased, but the secretory transport maximum is unchanged. The frequency of cholelithiasis approaches 40 per cent by the eighth decade.

ENDOCRINE SYSTEM. Blood levels of GH may be decreased and those of TSH, ACTH, and ADH are maintained. Blood levels of FSH are increased fifteen-fold and LH three-fold in postmenopausal women, whereas in men these changes are marginal. Large doses of estrogen fail to suppress FSH, and the feedback control mechanism in women is probably impaired. The serum T_4 remains normal, although the rate of turnover is decreased; T_3 is reduced 25 to 40 per cent. Responses to stress and to TSH are normal. The status of PTH is not certain, but the postmenopausal decrease in estrogen may allow an unopposed PTH effect and predispose to osteoporosis. The glucose tolerance decreases with age, and if the usual standards are used, 50 per cent of all individuals aged 70 or older would have diabetes. An adjustment in diagnostic criteria is obviously necessary. This reduced tolerance may be due to a delay in insulin release by the beta cells. Glucagon levels are unchanged. The plasma cortisol level and the circadian cycle persist, but a decreased secretion rate is matched by reduced disposal and excretion rates. The response of cortisol secretion to stress still needs clarification. The blood level and urinary excretion of aldosterone decrease 50 per cent between youth and old age, and the response to sodium depletion is reduced two thirds. The secretion of renin has a similar age-related decrease. Adrenal androgen also decreases progressively to less than one half of young adult values. Recent studies show a decrease in norepinephrine and an increase in monamine oxidase and serotonin in the brain with age. Stimulation results in a delayed but quantitatively normal increase in the excretion of epinephrine. After the menopause all female estrogen is adrenal in origin and thus decreases markedly; in males there is little age-related change. Since progesterone is a precursor of cortisol, adrenal production is probably sustained in both sexes. The production and clearance of testosterone decline, but there is no agreement that blood levels are reduced.

BLOOD. There is no decrease in the blood volume before age 80, red cell survival time is normal, and anemia is usually secondary to iron depletion. The number and distribution of leukocytes is unchanged, except for T lymphocytes, which are probably decreased. The leukocytosis of inflammation and immunoglobulin production after antigenic challenge are both decreased. Immune surveillance is markedly decreased despite an increase in total gamma globulin. Platelets may have increased adhesiveness and fibrinogen may be increased, but there is no conclusive evidence of hyper-coagulability. The erythrocyte sedimentation rate may be markedly accelerated without evidence of disease.

MUSCULOSKELETAL SYSTEM. Muscle cell loss and disorganization cause a progressive reduction in muscle strength. The poor reparative characteristics of cartilage lead to deterioration as early as the third decade, with progressive loss of joint surfaces and resultant degenerative arthritis. Throughout life there is a continuous remodeling of bone by reabsorption of interior surfaces and formation on exterior surfaces. By age 40 the reabsorption exceeds bone formation. Both the protein matrix and the bone mineral are involved, and clinical osteoporosis may result. In women 25 per cent of the bone is lost. Fractures of the vertebral body and femoral neck may result. The cumulative risk of hip fracture by age 90 approaches 25 per cent for women and 10 per cent for men.

THE INTEGUMENT. Wrinkling and sagging of the skin and graying of the hair are hallmarks of aging. The epidermis thins and contains less melanin, and cell replacement slows, resulting in delayed healing. The epidermal glands are reduced in number and function, and the skin is dry. A significant reduction in subcutaneous fat, increased collagen, and fragmented, inelastic elastin cause the observed wrinkling. The blood supply is reduced, but capillary fragility results in the common subcutaneous senile purpura. The loss of subcutaneous fat, reduction of vascularity, and slowed cell replacement contribute to the frequency and severity of decubitus ulceration. Hair distribution is subject to genetic and racial variation, but in each individual is determined by the number of active and resting hair follicles in local areas more than by follicular atrophy. Luxuriant scalp hair in youth decreases with age; facial hair appears at puberty and may persist in males, but it may appear after the menopause in Caucasian women; axillary and pubic hair appear at puberty and, in women, decrease after the menopause. Graying is due to decreased melanin production by the hair follicle. The rate of nail growth decreases 40 per cent.

NERVOUS SYSTEM. Nerve cells are postmitotic, and when lost are not replaced. The weight of the brain is essentially constant, but careful studies have shown not only a significant loss of cells, as many as 45 per cent in some cortical areas, but, more important, a loss of cellular integrity and of cellular interconnections. A consensus of several studies shows that from age 17 to age 80 years the cerebral blood flow declines from 79 to 46 ml per minute per 100 grams of brain tissue and the cerebral oxygen consumption rate decreases from 3.6 to 2.7 ml per minute per 100 grams of brain. The mean arterial pressure is constant at 90 to 100 mm Hg, but the derived cerebrovascular resistance increases from 1.3 to 2.1 mm Hg per ml blood per minute per 100 grams of brain. Patients with senile dementia cluster at the lowest levels of blood flow and oxygen utilization, but there is overlap with subjects lacking overt intellectual deterioration. Motor nerve conduction velocity decreases about 15 per cent, and sensory nerve conduction velocity may decrease 30 per cent between 20 and 95 years. Sleep levels 3 and 4 become less prominent and brief arousals more frequent with age, but total sleep time may be little affected. A reciprocal increase of monamine oxidase and decrease of norepinephrine in brain tissue may be causal to the depression and apathy so often associated with aging.

SENSORY ORGANS. Visual acuity decreases with age, primarily due to reduction in transparency of the optical portions of the system. There is also loss in the extent of the visual fields, decrease in the speed of dark adaptation, elevation in the minimal threshold of light perception, and reduction in the critical speed of flicker fusion. There is a continuous, but decelerating, formation of cells on the lens surface, which gradually lose their nuclei and become transparent. Thus the lens thickens with age and there is progressive loss of the elasticity needed to adaptively deform the lens. Between ages 42 and 45 years, previously normal individuals will need corrective glasses for near vision. Hearing decreases, particularly for high tones after age 60, especially in men. There is a decrease in the senses of taste, smell, and touch. Pain fibers appear to be intact, but clinical experience suggests that pain threshold may also be reduced.

10.3. THE GOMPERTZ CONCEPT

Benjamin Gompertz, a British actuary, proposed a concept in 1825 which did not fully arouse the interest of biologists until more than a century later. Based on data then available from Northhampton, England, he noted that at advanced ages the age-specific risk of death increased geometrically, and could be computed by the formula:

$$q_x = q_o e^{ax}$$

where q_x is the death rate at age x, q_o is the death rate at age o, and a is a constant. When age is plotted against the log of the age-specific death rate, the portion of the curve which corresponds to Gompertz's formula is essentially a straight line (Fig. 2). Thus at these ages the risk of death is determined by age, indepen-

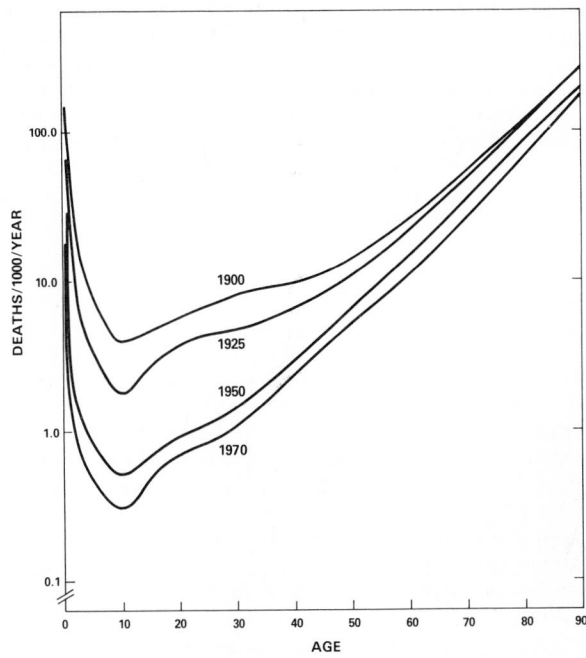

Figure 2. Mortality rates for white women, United States, 1900, 1925, 1950, and 1970.

dent of cause. The Gompertz concept has been found to be valid for all mammals.

Figure 2 shows the changes in age-specific mortality during the present century for American white women and demonstrates features which would be magnified by a longer time frame. The biggest gains have resulted from the reduction of infections and infant and maternal mortality, and in the better management of trauma. First exposures to infections occur most frequently early in life prior to the development of specific immunity. Immunization, sanitation, and antibiotics reduce the hazards of infection. The risks of childbirth are early for the infant, and in young adulthood for mothers in a society in which massive reproduction is no longer necessary. Accidents are most common as a result of the inexperience and recklessness of youth. As a result, a number of changes can be seen in the mortality risk curves. First, there is a large decrease in early mortality risk where the deviation from the Gompertz prediction is greatest. Second, the linear portion of the curve starts at an earlier age and at a lower risk level. Third, the slope of the curve is steeper. This slope defines the time required for the risk of death to double. At present the doubling time is seven years, and, if the slope remains constant, any maneuver which would eliminate 50 per cent of the causes of death (such as heart disease) would reduce the age-specific mortality by seven years. However, since the slope accelerates as the risk is reduced at lower ages, the benefits at advanced age are less prominent, and there may be a limit to the amount of reduction that can be achieved without modification of the aging process itself.

As the risk of death after maturity more closely follows the Gompertz projection, two phenomena become apparent. First, the lethality of an episode of acute disease or injury tends to parallel the Gompertz curve, suggesting that the total capability of the organism to cope with stress is decreasing with age at an accelerating rate. Second, a large number of chronic conditions, including arteriosclerosis and its manifestations, cancer, senile dementia, arthritis, diabetes, and osteoporosis, become apparent at frequencies which are less than but also parallel to the Gompertz curve. Although these conditions may manifest themselves acutely, it is clear that they are the result of progressive changes over long periods of time. These changes could result from constitutional factors, single traumas which set in motion a slow but progressive response, or multiple and continuing stimuli acting over a long period of time.

10.4. THEORIES OF AGING

The search for perpetual youth and immortality has given rise to many theories of aging, most now only of historical interest. Genetic factors are undoubtedly important, because each species has a characteristic life span, and within species there are strain differences in survival distribution. Genetic theories raise the possibility of programmed senescence or of program exhaustion. Recent knowledge of genetic mechanisms has resulted in the development of a number of error theories based on the concept that defects in protein synthesis can accumulate over time. Postmitotic cells, because of their long life, should be vulnerable particularly at the levels of transcription and translation, whereas mitotic cells should be vulnerable to somatic mutation during replication. Chromosome studies show an increase in gross abnormalities visible by light microscopy.

Another group of theories has arisen from developments in immunology. Both humoral and cellular immunocompetence decline, but autoimmune manifestations increase with age and amyloid deposits become common, particularly in the walls of blood vessels. The constant occurrence of somatic mutations could result in an ongoing immunologic response, possibly to a cell product from within a cell otherwise not distinguishable on its surface as alien, and thus free to continue producing its aberrant product. Mutation of immunocompetent cells which no longer recognize "self" would produce a graft-versus-host reaction.

In addition to the theories already noted, several others, not necessarily mutually exclusive, have attained some support. The progressive loss or impairment of postmitotic cells is a self-evident mechanism of aging. The finite limit of the reproductive capacity of mitotic cells, now very conclusively established, indicates that some limits to mortality exist on a cellular level. With age there is an accumulation of storage granules within the cellular cytoplasm, particularly lipofuscin, which may interfere with cellular functions. Quantitative increases in the amount and cross-linkage of collagen and related macromolecules have been shown for the connective tissue matrices. A similar cross-linkage of intracellular macromolecules, particularly DNA and RNA, could impair cell function. The existence of free radicals and exposure to natural radiation could produce irreversible changes in genetic and protein structures.

The accumulating evidence makes it unlikely that aging is a unitary phenomenon for which a specific therapy may be found. For the present it may be more practical to reconcile the observations of aging with certain clinical phenomena. Since aging is conceived as universal, any process which affects only a segment of the population has been considered to be a disease. However, if every individual has a potential for cancer which is held in check by immunosurveillance, the development of cancer would depend upon the level of the defense and the strength of the carcinogenetic mechanisms. Since immune competence decreases with age, cancer should occur when the defense is no longer adequate to cope with the stress. The rate of development of atherosclerosis has been linked to risk factors, particularly blood pressure, glucose tolerance, and blood lipid levels. Each increment in arterial pressure is linked with a statistical increase in mortality. Whether an individual dies of a vascular complication, cancer, or some other cause depends upon the individual vulnerability of a particular system. The risk for each potential cause of aging death and the likelihood that more than one will be present increases geometrically with age, as does the risk of death. The phenomenon of the one-horse shay, in which all parts wear out at the same moment, is just as improbable in biology as in mechanics.

The same concept could be applicable to other, nonlethal phenomena. For example, there is clear evidence that both the protein matrix and mineral content of bone decrease after the fourth decade. If this decrease were proportional in all individuals, those with the least dense bone at early maturity would be the most probable candidates for osteoporosis. There are few convincing data that therapy is effective once osteoporosis is present; it may be possible to increase maximum bone density, but this would require increased bone formation during growth. Similarly, treatment of vascular degeneration and cancer may be less effective than long-term control of appropriate risk factors. Changes in dietary patterns and effective control of blood pressure may provide future information, but the length of the human life span makes the accumulation of reliable data a prolonged process.

10.5. PSYCHOSOCIAL PROBLEMS OF THE AGED

Very few members of migratory, hunting societies lived to old age, and those few must have had unique qualities. Despite the obvious value of their wisdom, they probably were not spared if their incapacity endangered the group. The development of fixed, agricultural communities increased the security of the aged, especially after the development of property rights and rules of inheritance. Science and technology further increased the number of survivors to old age. However, the industrial revolution also broke up the family as a social and economic unit, increased social and geographic mobility, and so altered the social position of the aged that new social models have become necessary.

The popular image of the aged is negative. They are thought of as reduced in intelligence, limited in memory, rigid in concept, and uncongenial in personality. In fact, intellectual competence usually persists until quite late in life, and for a long period established knowledge and experience compensate for any slowness of learning. Even flexibility of thought is greater than was once believed. The increasing level of general education is improving the ability of the aged to adapt and to maintain interests.

Nevertheless, aging is associated with losses. There is the loss of occupation, as a source both of income and of meaningful activity. The loss of income may be more important because of reduced social leverage than lowered standard of living. Yet, with adequate income noneconomic activities can often become significant and satisfying. The loss of friends and family and separation from children become increasingly painful. The loss of vigor and attractiveness and, ultimately, the loss of health are the final reminders that the cycle is closing. Women now live eight years longer than men and are several years younger at the time of marriage. Geriatrics as a specialty must deal primarily with older women who will be widowed for an average of ten years with reduced economic resources and social contacts.

Under these conditions it is not surprising that depression is common and is often manifest as insomnia or dementia. In the latter the apparent intellectual decline is really a loss of attention created by the depression, and effective therapy can be gratifying.

In caring for aging patients, the physician must be aware of a range of problems which are less important in other age groups. First, the life experience of the patient encompasses a time period which the younger physician knows only indirectly, and the patient may be conditioned by lifetime social and ethnic considerations which also may be quite alien to him. Second, the patient may not have the economic or social resources to adhere to a prescribed regimen. Third, the patient has an increased probability of multiple problems which may be self-treated or lie in the area of another specialist. Multiple medications may be utilized with potential incompatibilities. Fourth, the patient may often be incompetent, and both the history and the therapy may suffer as a result. Fifth, the longer the survival, the more likely the loss or absence of a spouse or companion. Sixth, the need for social welfare, visiting nurse, homemaker, and related services is extensive, and when properly used can often help maintain an older patient at home as the preferred medical, social, and economic solution.

Despite the enumerated decrements associated with aging, most older individuals live remarkably active and satisfying lives. Social Security, pensions, Medicare and health insurance, and a long period of relative economic prosperity have greatly improved the economic aspects. If the individual survives, the general enfeeblement of aging is infrequently incapacitating before age 75 or 80. It is becoming usual to speak of early and late old age, since the two periods may be quite different.

It is during advanced old age that the stereotypes may be more typical. Significant senile dementia may be present in 20 per cent. Losses of hearing and vision reduce sensory input and with reduced physical mobility may aggravate the other problems of social isolation. These patients are often best managed in a home for the aged or in a skilled nursing facility if they are unable to perform the activities of daily living. It is revealing that the average age of residents in these homes is often more than 80 years.

10.6. SPECIAL PROBLEMS OF MANAGEMENT

DIET. There is little evidence that age alters the need for specific nutrients, but the total calories should be reduced to compensate for decreased metabolic activity and cell mass. Because a reduced total diet may result in an inadequate intake of vitamins and iron, a single appropriate supplement may be prescribed. No specific diet to promote longevity has yet been confirmed. The older patient will have an increased probability of need for a specific therapeutic diet, and the ability to conform to the dietary prescription must be determined.

MEDICATION. The age-related concerns of clinical pharmacology are those of drug level, receptor and effector competence, and drug toxicity. Drug levels are determined by absorption, volume of distribution, biodegradation, and excretion. Quantitatively, the 40 to 50 per cent decrease in renal function is the most important age-related factor for substances which are excreted in active form in the urine. The decrease in renal function may produce a significant increase in blood levels if dose is not adjusted. An important factor in dose level is patient compliance. Reliable information requires frequent review of all drugs taken, including over-the-counter drugs, and their amounts. Each patient should be instructed periodically to bring in all actively used drugs in their containers to determine the exact drugs taken and their amounts. This is a most instructive exercise for both patient and physician.

Recent studies have shown quantitative and qualitative changes in the receptor sites, particularly of the nervous system, heart, and muscle. The reduced number and integrity of effectors are the natural result of the changes previously described. Further information should do much to rationalize geriatric pharmacology.

Drug misadventures increase in frequency with age. The patient has had more opportunity for prior sensitization. In addition, the multiple medical problems increase the number of drugs to be administered. The frequency of pharmacologic incompatibilities and of drug-drug interactions increases geometrically with the number taken. Safe and effective drug therapy requires knowledge of the drugs used, their probable pharmacologic changes with age, tests for blood level or effect (e.g., suppression of FSH by estrogen) when possible, and close titration for effect if not. In addition, drug prescription should be selective and minimal, and the patients closely observed for untoward responses.

DECUBITUS ULCERS AND CONTRACTURES. Every attempt should be made to prevent both these complications. Frequent movement, aggressive skin care, smooth sheets, and appropriate padding are essential. Pulling, rather than lifting, a patient into the upright position may damage fragile skin by a shearing effect. Every attempt must be made to get the patient out of bed daily. When ulcers develop, care must be intensified if they are to heal. Careful enzymatic and surgical debridement, antibiotics, and occasional skin grafting are utilized when needed. Large, infected ulcers have a high mortality.

SENILE DEMENTIA. The frequency of senile dementia increases with age. The physician must rule out and treat all medical, psychologic, and social causes of decreased intellectual function and minimize their effects whenever possible. Nevertheless, true senility is a frequent reality which the family and society must be helped to accept and to manage in a positive and humane manner. In the early stages the awareness of intellectual losses may be magnified by an understandable depression which often can be minimized by social support and the proper use of mood-elevating drugs. Paranoid manifestations may also appear and also can often be controlled. The appropriate social setting may be difficult to obtain, and cooperation with a variety of social agencies is usually necessary. As with mental disease at earlier ages, the family usually has intense feelings of shame and guilt. Much support and counseling are required. Since the costs of care may be large, the family must often be reassured that there is no currently effective therapy, and that expensive searches are unnecessary and usually unwise. The development of computerized brain scanning, although rarely positive, provides a noninvasive and probably decreasingly expensive method for ruling out many potentially treatable lesions such as subdural hematomas and brain tumors.

DYING AND DEATH. Dying and death are periods of stress for the patient, family, friends, and attendants. Every attempt must be made to keep the patient comfortable. There is no excuse for a dying patient to be in pain. Analgesia, if clearly needed, as for cancer, should be prescribed on a regular schedule, and in adequate amounts. Less medicine is required to prevent than to relieve pain. The obviously dying patient should be spared unnecessary tests and procedures. Visits should be encouraged and facilitated, but governed primarily by the sense of the patient's need and desire. One of the great tragedies of modern institutional medicine is the tendency to isolate the dying patient. The family is kept at a distance, and the staff reduces interaction out of frustration and discomfort. If necessary, psychiatric consultation should be obtained, but this must be arranged with caution and sensitivity. The patient should be allowed to be dependent or hostile if it makes adjustment easier. Ideally, he should be helped to work through his own mourning reaction with its sequence of denial, anger, bargaining, depression, and final acceptance. The family and friends should also be helped through this period. The physician should always be available to his patient when needed.

10.7.   THE PHYSICIAN'S RESPONSIBILITY

Humans are mortal. Not all diseases will be cured or deaths prevented. It is only within this century that the physician's intervention has been decisive in more than occasional situations. We must not allow our newfound technical competence to separate us from our larger role as physicians. Now that our patients live out their life spans, we will more frequently be unable to cure and to prevent death. Yet, as with physicians in millenia past, we are not freed of our responsibilities to comfort, to console, to reassure, to be available. This is a responsibility which cannot be delegated; it is the essence of medical practice.

The inevitability of death and the presence of incurable disease should not lull the physician into nihilism or neglect. Most individuals are socially competent and lead active and enjoyable lives until their terminal illness. Many conditions, as with younger patients, are either self-limited or curable. Chronic disease is often subject to control, and symptoms can usually be reduced if not eliminated. Much can be done to assist the patient in maintaining independence and dignity. Most older individuals do not expect to have the capabilities of youth; nor are they afraid of death. They demand of us only that we keep them as comfortable and functional as possible, so that they can make what remains of their lives meaningful and enjoyable.

Binstock, R. H., and Shanas, E. (eds.): Handbook of Aging and the Social Sciences. New York, Van Nostrand Reinhold Company, 1976.

Birren, J. E., and Schaie, K. W. (eds.): Handbook of the Psychology of Aging. New York, Van Nostrand Reinhold Company, 1977.

Brocklehurst, J. C. (ed.): Textbook of Geriatric Medicine and Gerontology. Edinburgh and London, Churchill Livingstone, 1973.

Finch, C. E. and Havflick, L. (eds.): Handbook of the Biology of Aging. New York, Van Nostrand Reinhold Company, 1977.

Reichel, W. (ed.): Clinical Aspects of Aging. Baltimore, Williams & Wilkins Company, 1978.

Rossman, I. (ed.): Clinical Geriatrics. Philadelphia, J. B. Lippincott Company, 1971.

PART III
GENETIC PRINCIPLES

11. INTRODUCTION

Alexander G. Bearn

After Gregor Mendel established the principle of genetic transmission, Johannsen, in 1909, introduced the word *gene* to denote a unit of heredity. A structural gene is now defined, operationally, as a functional unit of inheritance situated on a chromosome and responsible for the synthesis of a specific polypeptide. It has been estimated that there are probably at least 10,000 genes in man. Since the number of well documented examples of genetic variability is of the order of 1000, it is apparent that despite the acceleration in discovery of new genetic entities 90 per cent of the human genome remains to be discovered.

MODERN GENETICS AND ITS RELATION TO INTERNAL MEDICINE. The chemical nature of the gene was unrecognized until 1944, when a soluble extract derived from pneumococci of one genotype was found to effect a stable heritable change when added to a growing culture of pneumococci of another genotype. The recognition that the transforming substance in the extract was deoxyribonucleic acid (DNA) launched the present era of molecular biology.

THE GENE AND PROTEIN SYNTHESIS. The genetic information encoded in the double-stranded DNA that determines polypeptide structure is brought to the ribosome, where the polypeptides are synthesized by a unique type of single-stranded RNA, known as messenger RNA, or mRNA. This mRNA is complementary to one of the strands of DNA, and the linear sequences in the polypeptide are precisely determined by the linear sequences of the coding units ("codons" — triplets of nucleotides coding for different amino acids) in the mRNA. These relationships are often referred to as the central dogma of molecular biology, and can be depicted schematically as shown at the bottom of this page.

The universality of this biologic truth was abruptly shaken by the discovery in 1970 that several RNA animal tumor viruses contain polymerase activity (reverse transcriptase), which used RNA as a template for the synthesis of double-stranded DNA and thus reversed the familiar direction of genetic transcription. This discovery raised the possibility that an RNA-dependent DNA polymerase might indicate the presence of an oncogenic virus which can transform normal cells into genetically stable cancer cells. Although this enzyme has now been detected in certain noncogenic viruses as well, the function of viral reverse transcriptase remains a question of central biologic importance in the problem of neoplasia.

DEOXYRIBONUCLEIC ACID (DNA). Deoxyribonucleic acid is constructed from three essential components: the five carbon sugar 2-deoxy-D-ribose; phosphoric acid, which confers on DNA its acidic properties; and nitrogenous bases. Two of the bases are purines, aden-

ine (A) and guanine (G), and two are pyrimidines, thymine (T) and cytosine (C). In 1953 Watson and Crick assembled the available physical and chemical data on DNA into a molecular model for the structure of DNA. Two polynucleotide chains are twisted together to form a double helix. The two chains are held together by hydrogen bonds between the bases which face inward forming the core, and the phosphate-sugar groups form an external helical backbone. Adenine must always pair with thymine (A-T), and guanine with cytosine (G-C). The result of this pairing leads to a precise complementary relationship between the bases on the two chains. Thus, if part of the base sequence were TTGCC, the corresponding portion of the complementary strand would read AACGG.

REPLICATION OF DNA. One of the chief attractions of the Watson-Crick model for DNA is that it contains a built-in system for self-replication. As the double helix of a parent molecule unwinds, the sequence of bases in each strand acts as a template for the synthesis of a new strand of DNA in two daughter molecules. The replication is catalyzed by the enzyme DNA polymerase and has been termed *semiconservative*, because both parental strands are conserved in the next generation, each now paired with a newly synthesized complementary partner. Recent evidence suggests that normal replication occurs in short fragments which start with an RNA primer and are then joined by a specific ligase. It is also evident that there are at least three distinct DNA polymerases, α, β, and γ. Only DNA polymerase α can initiate new DNA synthesis with an RNA primer provided by RNA polymerase. All three can function in DNA repair.

RIBONUCLEIC ACID (RNA). Ribonucleic acid differs from deoxyribonucleic acid in three important ways. (1) The sugar D-ribose replaces the 2-deoxy-D-ribose of DNA. (2) The pyrimidine base uracil (U) replaces the thymine of DNA. (3) RNA is a single-stranded polymer in contrast to double-stranded DNA.

MESSENGER RIBONUCLEIC ACID (mRNA). The genetic information encoded in the DNA of the chromosomes must be conveyed from the nucleus to the cytoplasm where the proteins are synthesized. Messenger RNA is formed by the transcription of one of the strands of DNA and is catalyzed by RNA polymerase II. The sequence of bases in mRNA is complementary to that in the corresponding uncopied strand of DNA except that uracil replaces thymine. In this way single-stranded RNA carries into the cytoplasm the genetic information originally encoded in nuclear DNA. In bacteria, mRNA has a half-life of about two minutes, and it has been calculated that during this time about 10 to 20 molecules of protein can be synthesized. In cells of higher organisms mRNAs vary in their stability over a range from minutes to many hours. For example, the half-life of globin mRNA is about 14 hours.

TRANSFER RNA (tRNA). Before amino acids are as-

$$\text{DNA (double-stranded)} \underset{}{\overset{\text{transcription}}{\rightleftharpoons}} \text{RNA (single-stranded)} \xrightarrow{\text{translation}} \text{polypeptide}$$

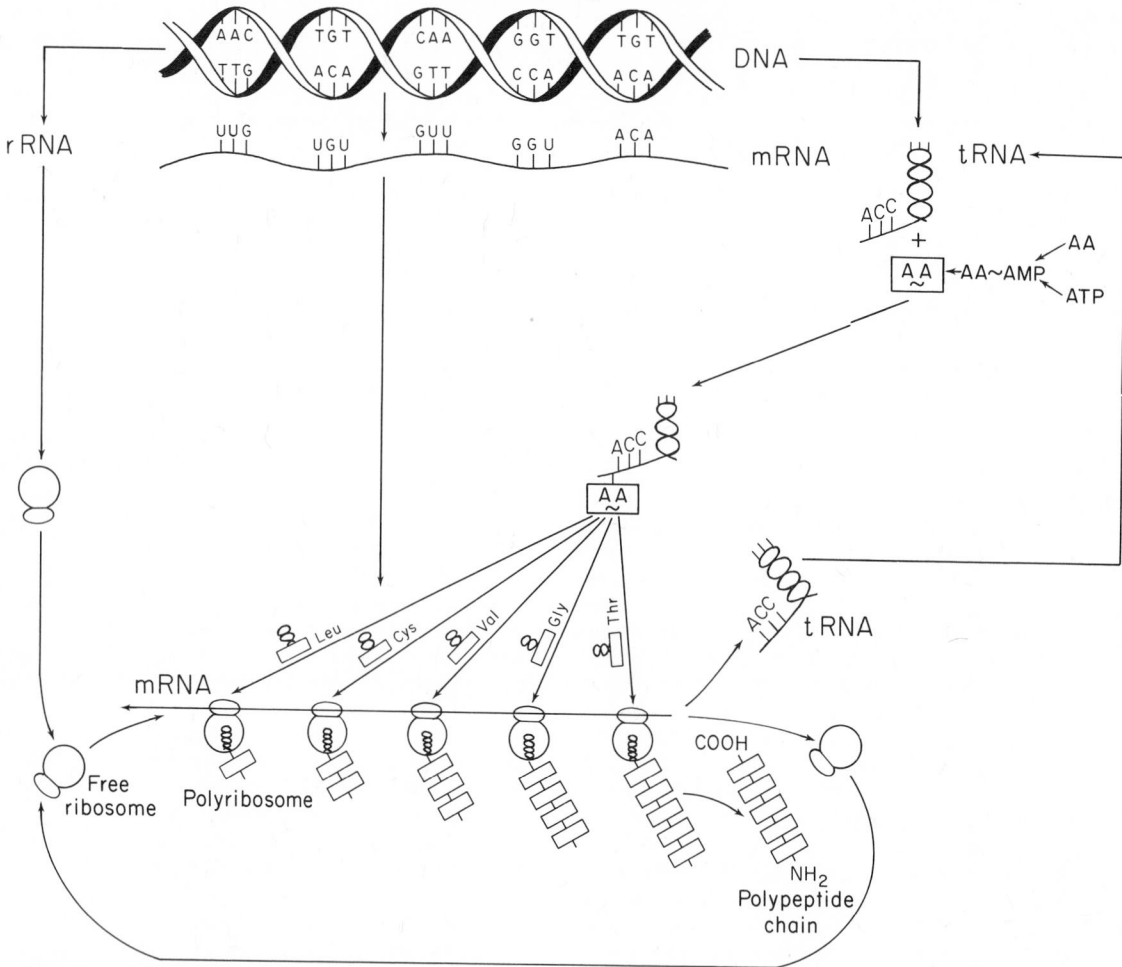

Figure 1. A schematic diagram of the genetic control of protein synthesis. A=adenine, T=thymine, G=guanine, C=cytosine, U=uracil. The codons indicated represent code words for the amino acids indicated. The messenger RNA (mRNA) moves across the ribosomes in the direction of the arrow. tRNA=transfer RNA; rRNA=ribosomal RNA. AA= amino acids.

sembled into polypeptide chains, they must first be "activated." This activation is accomplished by the enzymes known as aminoacyl-tRNA synthetases, each of which is specific for one amino acid. Such an enzyme combines ATP and an amino acid to form aminoacyladenylate, with the release of pyrophosphate. The activated amino acid is now joined to another type of RNA called transfer RNA, with the release of adenylic acid. Mammalian cells contain more than 20 different transfer RNA's, which are transcribed from DNA by RNA polymerase III. At least one transfer RNA is specific for each of the amino acids. Each transfer RNA molecule is folded into a cloverleaf pattern and has two recognition sites. One site recognizes the "activated" amino acid, whereas the second, often called the anticodon, recognizes the codon in the mRNA. Thus the fidelity of translation is assured by the specific binding of the amino acid to the appropriate tRNA catalyzed by the specific activating enzyme, and by complementary pairing of the anticodon of tRNA with the codon of the mRNA.

RIBOSOMAL RNA (rRNA). More than 80 per cent of the RNA of most cells is found in cytoplasmic particles called ribosomes. These ribosome particles represent the protein synthetic machinery of the cell and are com-

posed of about half protein and half RNA. Ribosomes from *Escherichia coli* consist of a 30 S subunit, consisting of 21 proteins and 16 S RNA, and a 50 S subunit with some 34 proteins, 5 S, and 23 S RNA. Mammalian ribosomes are somewhat larger; they have a diameter of about 200 Å and a sedimentation coefficient of 80 S and dissociate into 40 S and 60 S subunits in low concentrations of magnesium. Messenger RNA, bearing the instructions for protein synthesis, forms a complex with the smaller subunit and the initiator tRNA. The larger subunit then attaches to this complex from the functional ribosome, and the sequential assembly of amino acids into protein can now begin.

PROTEIN SYNTHESIS. Protein synthesis on the ribosome occurs in three main steps: initiation, elongation, and termination. These steps are complex and require the involvement of many protein components of the ribosome as well as rRNA.

Initiation, in bacteria, can be said to begin when the codon AUG binds $N \cdot$ formylmethionyl-tRNA to the 30 S ribosome subunit and mRNA becomes bound to the ribosomes. Thus most bacterial proteins have, as their first amino acid, N-formylmethionine. Since there are no formylated end groups in bacterial proteins, this means that the formyl group must be cleaved soon after the beginning of protein synthesis. The second codon, recognizing its specific tRNA, brings the second amino acid in sequence into alignment. A peptide bond is now formed and the messenger RNA moves along the ribosome so that the third amino acid comes into position, with further elongation of the peptide chain (Fig. 1). The messenger RNA has a distinct polarity as it moves along the ribosome, always reading from the 5′ to the 3′ end. The information that a polypeptide chain is completed and that its synthesis must be terminated is specified by a special chain-terminating codon. A ribosome takes about ten seconds to read an entire mRNA molecule of average length, and a single mRNA molecule may move over the surfaces of several ribosomes simultaneously. This explains why a cell needs relatively little mRNA to synthesize a great deal of protein. A cluster of several ribosomes all translating the same mRNA is called a polyribosome; polyribosomes synthesizing hemoglobin (a protein of molecular weight 64,500), consist, on the average, of four to six ribosomes.

CODONS. Because most proteins are composed of 20 different amino acids and because DNA has only four different nucleotide bases, it is evident that more than one base is required to prescribe for a particular amino acid. A sequence of three bases (a codon) is needed to code for each amino acid. Thus a gene with 1500 nucleotide pairs would determine the sequence of a polypeptide chain consisting of 500 amino acids. Since the four-letter code is triplet in nature, there are 64 (4 × 4 × 4) possible codons, of which 61 have been shown to code for one of the 20 amino acids. Three remaining codons, UAA, UAG, and UGA, represent signals that the polypeptide chain is completed and are called chain-terminating codons and do not code for any amino acid. Two codons serve to initiate polypeptide synthesis as well as to insert amino acids and are sometimes designated chain-initiating codons. One of the unresolved problems in eukaryotic organisms, such as man, is that they appear to possess more DNA in their genome than can be accounted for by the estimated number of unique genes. However, some genes occur

in multiple copies, and there are also stretches of noncoding DNA. The genetic code is said to be *universal* in the sense that all plant and animal species have thus far been found to use the same genetic code, and *degenerate* because certain amino acids can be specified by more than one triplet.

Certain acridine dyes, e.g., proflavine, induce mutations in bacteriophage by leading to the insertion of an extra nucleotide into the pre-existing (normal) sequence. Because of this extra nucleotide, the reading frame becomes altered distal to the point of insertion and results in a disruption of normal protein synthesis. The correct reading frame of the code can be restored by deletion of a nucleotide (or by the insertion of two extra nucleotides) distal to the insertion. This model makes the prediction that a double mutant, consisting of an insertion followed by a deletion, will result in a polypeptide chain with an altered amino acid sequence between the two mutations. If the segment of DNA between the two mutations is short, and does not code for amino acids vital for functional specificity, a protein with a normal function may still be produced. A mutation in the codon which terminates the reading of the code is referred to as a terminator mutation.

Three hemoglobin variants have been found affecting the terminating codons UAG or UAA. In each variant, the alpha chain of hemoglobin has 171 residues instead of 141. Each of these hemoglobins has an identical amino acid sequence, the alteration being at residue 141 (glutamine in Hb Constant Spring, serine in Hb Koya Dora, and lysine in Hb Icaria). The codons for each of these amino acids can be derived from UA (G or A) by a point mutation. The predicted mutation in which an amino acid–specifying codon is changed to a terminator codon has also been found. Hb McKees-Rock is a 144 residue beta chain variant which lacks the two C-terminal amino acids tyrosine and histidine, and is the result of the single step conversion of UA (C or U) tyrosine specifying codon to a terminator codon (Fig. 2).

Crossing-over between synapsing chromatids can also yield structurally abnormal proteins. In Hb Tak, for instance, misalignment and crossing-over between two

Figure 2. Hemoglobin mutants affecting terminator codons. *Key:* UCU=Serine. UCA=Serine. CAA= Glutamine. AAA=Phenylalanine. UAA=Asparagine. CAC=Histidine. UAA=Terminator. UAU=Tyrosine. AAG=Phenylalanine.

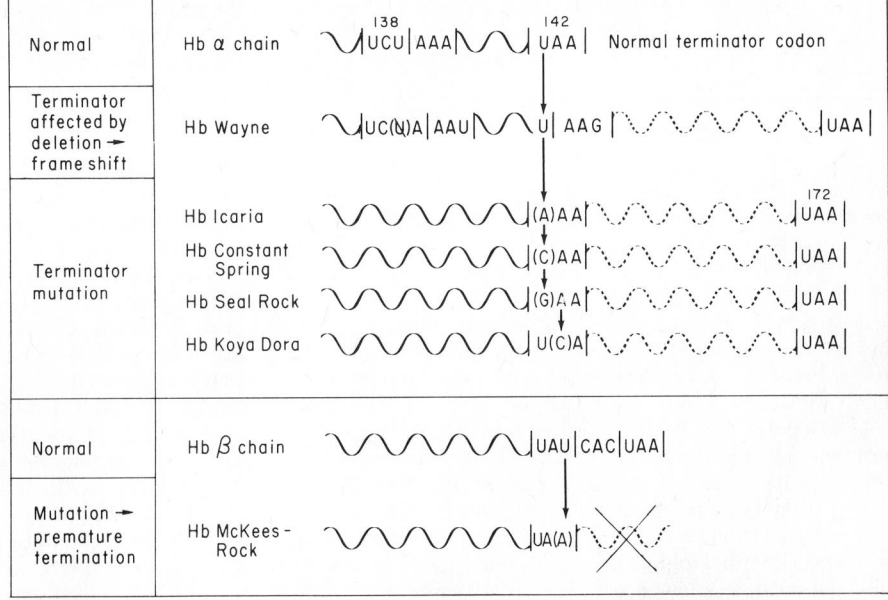

beta chains results in the insertion of two nucleotides. As a consequence, the terminating codon is not read in phase and the mRNA continues to add another 11 amino acids until the next termination codon is read at residue 157. Similar molecular rearrangements account for Hb Cranston and Hb Wayne. Hb Wayne can be derived from Hb Constant Spring by a frameshift mutation (deletion) involving the alpha 138 serine.

GENETIC REGULATORY MECHANISMS. Genetic mechanisms for the control of protein synthesis are much better understood in microorganisms than in man. The original hypothesis of Jacob and Monod postulated two classes of genes: structural genes which controlled the amino acid structure of the protein, and regulatory genes which influenced the rate of protein synthesis. Structural genes were linked together as a single functional unit, termed an operon. Thus this genetic model suggested a simple transcriptional control of protein synthesis; the amount of protein synthesis was determined by the amount of mRNA.

Direct application of this model to mammalian systems cannot be made, although the report of Ingram, in 1956, that sickle cell hemoglobin differed from normal hemoglobin in a single amino acid substitution appeared to be a neat example of a structural mutation. Since Ingram's initial observation, many structural mutants in man have been described, but whether there are regulatory mutations in man, corresponding to those seen in microorganisms, is quite unclear. Many structural mutations affect the rate of synthesis of the abnormal protein. From such observations the concept that genes controlling the structure of a protein also influence the amount of protein synthesized has gained ground, and has been termed the structure-rate hypothesis. In most instances, the mutational event leads to decreased synthesis; however, an increased enzymatic activity has been observed in G6PD Hektoen, a structural mutant in the glucose-6-phosphate dehydrogenase system, and in a pseudocholinesterase mutant, designated Cynthiana.

The molecular basis of the various forms of thalassemia (see Ch. 485.7) has become increasingly understood in recent years. Alpha thalassemia is the result of a deletion of the whole or part of the alpha-chain genes. The beta thalassemias exhibit a variety of molecular defects. Patients with classic Cooley's anemia (beta+ thal) have a reduced beta-chain mRNA synthesis; those with the less common Cooley's anemia (beta⁰ thal) have absent beta-chain mRNA, although the beta-chain genes are present (see Ch. 485.7).

In contrast to microorganisms, in which protein synthesis is controlled predominantly by genetic regulatory mechanisms, hormonal influences have a profound effect in man and other eukaryotic organisms. In certain cells, thyroxine and adrenocortical hormones influence the rate of RNA synthesis and the activity of DNA-dependent RNA polymerase. Another regulatory mechanism of protein synthesis in man involves the histones, which are closely associated with mammalian DNA. It seems likely that histones play an important role in controlling the transcription of DNA; temporary removal, or modification, of the DNA-associated histone results in an increased transcription of the DNA. When this histone modification is reversible, it provides a molecular mechanism which can adjust protein synthesis to physiologic need. Histone modification is also thought to play a key role in differentiation and development. Recent techniques for hybridizing animal cells will enable genetic regulatory mechanisms in man to be examined at the cellular level.

Watson, J. D.: Molecular Biology of the Gene. 3rd ed. New York, Benjamin, 1976.

12. PEDIGREE ANALYSIS IN INHERITED DISEASE

Alexander G. Bearn

Inspection and analysis of human pedigrees form the basis for an understanding of the application of the laws of Mendel to human disease. Analysis of a pedigree begins with the affected individual, who is referred to as the propositus, proband, or index case. Using the propositus as the point of departure, a pedigree is constructed, and the pattern of the pedigree is analyzed. It is worth emphasizing, however, that the construction of human pedigrees beyond first- and second-degree relatives is an occupation more likely to please the physician than to provide a deeper genetic understanding of the patient's disease. Human memories are notoriously untrustworthy, and great care must be exercised when very large pedigrees are compiled and recorded.

AUTOSOMAL INHERITANCE. When there are two alleles, A and a, at a locus, three possible genotypes exist, which can be represented AA, Aa, and aa. The genotypes AA and aa are called *homozygotes*; Aa is a *heterozygote*. A gene can be recognized only by the effect it produces; thus in the strictest sense it is incorrect to speak of dominant or recessive genes, but only of dominant or recessive effects. If the phenotype Aa cannot be easily distinguished from the phenotype AA, but is clearly different from aa, the effect of gene A is said to be dominant over the effect of gene a. In this circumstance there are only two phenotypes corresponding to the three genotypes AA, Aa, aa. However, the failure to detect a phenotypic difference between the genotypes AA and Aa is usually testimony to the insensitivity of the methods employed. If the gene products of A and a can both be detected in the heterozygote Aa, the genes are said to exert an effect which is *co-dominant*. It would be preferable to discard the terms "dominant" and "recessive" and instead to state whether the genes concerned are phenotypically expressed in a single or double dose; for the sake of convenience, however, the terms are often retained. Although logically indefensible, it is pragmatically useful practice to designate a trait as dominant even though the homozygote has never been observed and in fact might have quite a different phenotype.

Autosomal Dominant Traits. Autosomal genes are those genes situated on chromosomes other than the X and Y. Dominant traits are defined as those traits that are fully manifested by the presence of a gene in the heterozygous state. Thus far, approximately 750 well established autosomal dominant traits have been identified in man. (Satisfactory examples of dominant traits are those responsible for the formation of certain blood group antigens. In the ABO system, the genes controlling the formation of A and B substances are dominant over O. Thus it is not ordinarily possible to distinguish serologically AA from AO individuals, or BB from BO individuals. However, heterozygous individuals of type

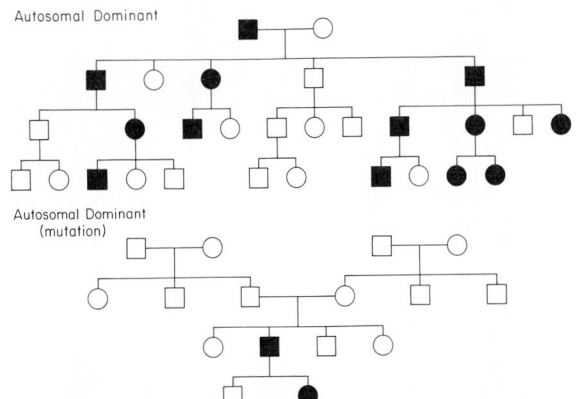

Figure 3. Pedigrees of autosomal dominant traits. In the lower pedigree the normal parents of the affected individual suggest the possibility of a new mutation. Solid symbols indicate those affected. (For details see text.)

AB can be recognized because the product of genes A and B can be detected.)

An autosomal dominant trait can be recognized in human pedigrees by its transmission from one generation to the next. Except for sporadic cases in which a fresh mutation in the germ line has arisen in either the father or the mother, and provided illegitimacy can be excluded, every affected individual has at least one affected parent and may have affected offspring and sibs (Fig. 3). The more severe the condition, the larger is the proportion of sporadic cases caused by fresh mutation. According to mendelian laws, a heterozygous affected individual married to a normal homozygote will, on the average, transmit the trait to half his offspring, both sexes being equally affected.

In contrast to recessive disorders, most dominant traits in man frequently exert only mild effects, and marked variation in the expression of the trait is the rule. In many instances the disease is not manifest until adult life. Occasionally the expression of the abnormal gene may be so weak that a generation appears to be skipped because the carrier of the abnormal gene is clinically normal. When a gene that can be clinically expressed in the heterozygous condition occurs in the homozygous state, the effect is usually more severe and may be lethal. Although examples are common in species in which experimental matings can be constructed, such examples are exceptional in man, because marriage of two clinically affected heterozygotes is rare. Possible examples include achondroplasia and the Osler-Weber-Rendu syndrome. An increased paternal age effect has been demonstrated among parents of sporadic cases of achondroplastic dwarfism, Marfan's syndrome (see Ch. 538.1), and certain other dominantly inherited disorders.

The molecular basis for the more than 750 genetically dominant diseases now known is quite obscure. It is of interest that in contrast to recessively inherited diseases in which an impairment of enzyme function is the rule, defective enzymes are only rarely found in dominant diseases. A deficiency of the inhibitor of the first component of complement, *C1-esterase inhibitor,* in hereditary angioedema and a deficiency of *uroporphyrinogen-1-synthetase* in acute intermittent porphyria are exceptions to this general rule (see Ch. 47 and 536.3). It appears that in most dominantly inherited disorders the abnormal gene determines a protein with a nonenzymatic function. In familial hypercholesterolemia the defect lies in an abnormality in the cell surface receptor that binds low density lipoprotein. Several hemolytic disorders are due to the presence of a single unstable mutant hemoglobin (see Ch. 485). The presence of one of these abnormal hemoglobin genes is sufficient to shorten the life of the red cells.

Autosomal Recessive Traits. In an autosomal recessive trait, the father and the mother of the affected individual are usually normal, as are more distant ancestors. On the average, one fourth of the brothers and sisters of the index case will be affected. If the trait is rare, an increased consanguinity will often be observed among the parents of those affected. According to mendelian laws, two normal parents, both heterozygous for a recessive trait, will produce offspring of whom, on the average, one quarter will be homozygous for the normal allele, one quarter homozygous for the abnormal allele and thus affected, and one half heterozygous for the abnormal allele, like the parents. Affected individuals usually have phenotypically normal offspring who are all carriers of the abnormal gene. If an affected individual marries an individual heterozygous for the same gene, one half of the offspring will be affected and one half will be heterozygous carriers (Fig. 4). Approximately 800 well established recessive traits have been identified in man.

Certain aspects of the segregation ratio in autosomal recessive conditions must be emphasized. Because of the small size of families and because ascertainment of the family is usually through an affected member, the mean observed proportion of affected individuals will be greater than expected. Only when the size of the sibships is large will the expected ratio of one affected to three unaffected be realized in pooled data. Thus the analysis of the expected ratio in families of various sizes requires a correction factor whose magnitude depends on the number of children in the sibship. The simplest correction is to subtract in each family the index case from the total number of affected individuals and then determine the proportion of affected children among the remaining sibs.

The disadvantage of the term "recessive" is emphasized by the increasing number of instances in which refined biochemical observations enable the recognition of the trait in the clinically normal heterozygote. Indeed, because of its importance in genetic counseling, the detection of healthy heterozygous carriers of genes that in the homozygous condition cause overt disease is

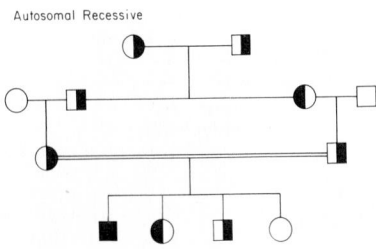

Figure 4. Pedigree of autosomal recessive trait. Note: both parents are heterozygous. One sib is affected, two are carriers, and one is normal. Double line (═══) indicates that parents are related by descent (first cousins).

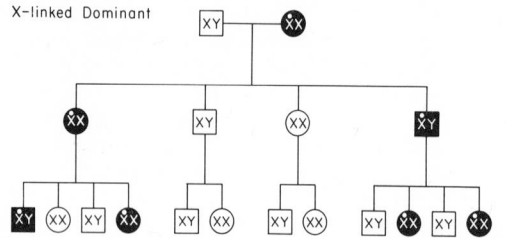

Figure 5. Pedigree of dominant X-linked trait. The X chromosome bearing the abnormal gene is designated by a small white dot.

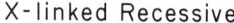

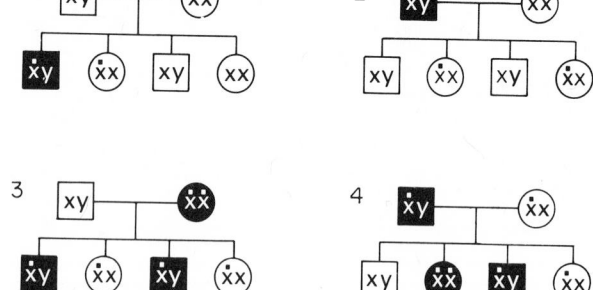

Figure 6. Pedigrees of recessive X-linked trait. The X chromosome bearing the abnormal gene is designated by a small dot. Affected individuals are indicated by solid squares (males) and circles (females). Pedigree 1 is commonly observed; pedigree 4 is rare.

becoming one of the most significant aspects of medical genetics. Detection of the sickle cell gene in black populations and the Tay-Sachs gene among Ashkenazic Jews are classic examples of the usefulness of heterozygote detection. In recent years, the biochemical detection of heterozygotes for autosomal recessive diseases has been greatly facilitated by the development of techniques to culture skin fibroblasts. Although the culturing of human fibroblasts has been relatively uninformative in dominant disorders, in approximately 25 per cent of all autosomal recessive diseases the precise biochemical defect can be detected in cultured fibroblasts derived from a simple skin biopsy.

Genetic Compounds. Heteroallelic compounds represent those conditions which are due to the inheritance of two different mutant genes derived from the same locus. Thus individuals with Hb SC disease have inherited an Hb S gene from one parent and an Hb C gene from the other. Certain unusual mucopolysaccharidoses may also represent genetic compounds (see Ch. 538.1).

X-LINKED INHERITANCE. Dominant X-Linked Traits. This mode of inheritance is uncommon. Heterozygous affected females will transmit the trait to both sexes with a frequency of 50 per cent. Affected males will transmit the trait to all their daughters, but to none of their sons (Fig. 5). This rule of X-linked dominant inheritance enables critical distinction from traits inherited in an autosomal dominant fashion, in which an affected male transmits the trait to both sons and daughters. The variability of expression of an X-linked dominant trait is less in males than in females. If the trait is uncommon, the incidence in females is roughly twice that in males. The erythrocyte antigen Xg^a and vitamin D resistant rickets (hypophosphatemic rickets) are inherited as X-linked dominant traits. Approximately 100 loci have been identified on the human X chromosome.

Recessive X-Linked Traits. Recessive X-linked traits are relatively common. On the average, half the sons of normal heterozygous females will be normal, and half will be affected. If the trait is rare, parents and relatives will be normal except for male relatives in the female line; for instance, on the average, one half of the maternal uncles will be affected. An affected male married to a normal female will have normal offspring. All their daughters will be carriers, and they, in turn, can transmit the trait to the next generation. The rare event of an affected male married to a carrier female will result in equal proportions of affected male and female offspring. The unaffected males will be genotypically normal; the unaffected females, however, will be heterozygous carriers (Fig. 6). The common red-green color blindness is inherited as an X-linked recessive trait. In the general population the frequency of affected females will be roughly the square of the frequency of affected males.

Some common mendelian disorders that are inherited in a dominant autosomal and X-linked fashion are illustrated in Table 1.

THE LYON HYPOTHESIS. Since the female bears two X chromosomes, it might have been expected that the concentration of proteins determined by genes on the X chromosome would be twice that observed in males who have only one X chromosome. Thus it might have been expected that the concentration of factor VIII (antihemophilic factor) in females would be twice that found in males. This is not the case, and the explanation is provided by a hypothesis first advanced by Mary Lyon.

TABLE 1. Some Relatively Common Mendelian Disorders

Autosomal Dominant	Autosomal Recessive	X-Linked
Familial monogenic hypercholesterolemia	Cystic fibrosis	Hemophilia A
Marfan's syndrome	Deaf mutism	Classic agammaglobulinemia (Bruton)
Adult polycystic disease	Phenylketonuria and other hereditary aminoacidurias	Pseudohypertrophic muscular dystrophy
Huntington's chorea	Wilson's disease	Glucose-6-phosphate dehydrogenase deficiency
Acute intermittent porphyria	Homocystinuria	Fabry's disease
Hereditary hemorrhagic telangiectasia	Albinism	Testicular feminization
Neurofibromatosis	Emphysema (due to alpha-1-antitrypsin deficiency)	Chronic granulomatous disease
Osteogenesis imperfecta	Friedreich's ataxia	Vitamin D resistant rickets
von Willebrand's disease		
Achondroplastic dwarfism		

In all adult female cells only one of the two X chromosomes is genetically active. Early in differentiation one of the X chromosomes becomes inactive and forms the Barr body. Inactivation is random; but once one of the two X chromosomes in any cell is inactivated, the same X chromosome remains inactive during all its subsequent cell divisions. For example, only half the X chromosomes are genetically active and synthesizing antihemophilic globulin, and thus the amount of antihemophilic globulin synthesis is approximately the same in males and females. Greater variability in expression of an X-linked trait is a natural consequence of the Lyon hypothesis. The number of cells determining a specific function at the time of inactivation is small, and thus chance alone could influence the number of such cells inactivated.

Y-LINKED INHERITANCE. If a trait is determined by a gene in the Y chromosome, it will be transmitted through the father to all his sons and none of his daughters. Thus far, the only genes that have been shown to be located in the Y chromosome are those that determine "maleness" and an antigen that influences graft rejection. (See also XYY Syndrome in Ch. 548.4.)

SEX LIMITATION. Autosomal genes that are expressed only in males may mimic sex-linkage but can be formally distinguished if affected individuals reproduce. If a gene is on an autosome, affected males can transmit the trait to their sons; if the gene is on the X chromosome, they cannot. Linkage analysis may also serve to distinguish between autosomal and X-linked genes.

MODIFICATION OF GENE EXPRESSION. The manifestation of an abnormal gene is influenced not only by its normal allele, but also by alleles at other loci, and by environment. The terms expressivity and penetrance have been employed to describe the variable manifestation of a gene. These vague words are usually best avoided unless they can be used with precision; e.g., it would be precise but cumbersome to say that the gene for Huntington's chorea is 0 per cent penetrant at the age of 10 and 95 per cent penetrant at 65. Some genetically determined traits such as those determining the blood antigens are present at birth, whereas others such as Huntington's chorea appear only in adult life. A negative correlation between the age of onset of a trait in parents and sibs suggests that the expression of a gene may be influenced by the type of normal allele present. The effect can be seen in certain dominant diseases such as the nail-patella syndrome and in the dominant form of muscular dystrophy. The concept of anticipation, which asserts that hereditary diseases tend to have a progressively earlier age of onset with successive generations, is a statistical artifact which is based on a bias of ascertainment.

CONSANGUINITY. The most common error in taking a family history is to fail to inquire about consanguinity. When confronted with a patient, particularly a child, whose disorder does not fit any clear-cut diagnosis, a history of consanguinity in the parents is often the first clue that the patient is suffering from a rare, recessively inherited disorder. In all autosomal recessive disorders the affected individual has inherited one abnormal gene from each parent. It is thus evident that an individual will be more likely to inherit the same allele from each parent if the two parents have genes inherited from a common ancestor. First cousins share, on the average, one eighth of their genes, which were derived from a common ancestor. When two first cousins marry, an offspring has, on the average, one sixteenth of the loci homozygous for a gene derived from a common ancestor. It is frequently of interest to calculate the expected frequency of first-cousin marriages among parents of those with rare autosomal recessive disorders. Providing that the frequency of the disease in the population can be estimated and the frequency of first-cousin marriages in the general population is known, the calculation can be made according to the following formula. If k is the frequency of first-cousin marriages in a rare recessive disease, then as a first approximation $k = c/16q$, where c is the frequency of first-cousin marriages in the general population and q is the frequency of the abnormal gene. The frequency of cousin marriages is variable. In some isolated populations a frequency of as high as 30 per cent has been recorded, whereas in the United States in an urban population the frequency may be as low as 0.05 per cent. Let us suppose a recessively inherited disease has a frequency in the population of 1 in 10,000 (q^2); then the frequency of the gene, which in double dose causes the disease, is 1 in 100 (q). If the frequency of consanguinity in the general population is 0.5 per cent, then k, the parental consanguinity, is 3 per cent, a six-fold increase over normal. If the disease is much rarer, 1 in 100,000, then 10 per cent of the individuals affected by the disease will have parents who are first cousins. As the frequency of c increases, the expected frequency of parents who are first cousins will also increase. In some geographically isolated populations c may reach as high as 2 per cent. If a recessively inherited disease in such an isolate has a frequency of 1 in 100,000, 40 per cent of the parents of the affected individuals will be first cousins.

It is important to realize that an increased frequency of consanguinity will not be observed if the recessive disease is common. Thus in cystic fibrosis of the pancreas, which has a frequency of approximately 1 in 2500, no increase in parental consanguinity can be detected. Although the frequency of albinism in the general population is approximately 1 per 20,000, the unexpectedly high consanguinity in the parents (k = 20 per cent) of some patients is due to the existence of more than one gene for this condition. No increase in consanguinity would be expected in dominant or X-linked traits or genetic compounds.

Although in most populations the consanguinity rate is less than 1 per cent, certain geographic and cultural isolates remain in which there is a high coefficient of inbreeding. These isolates may shelter rare genes which because of the high consanguinity rate are likely to become manifest. More than 90 per cent of patients described with the Ellis–van Creveld syndrome have been found in the Old Order Amish living in Pennsylvania, Ohio, Indiana, and Ontario. Other rare recessive diseases found within this genetic isolate include pyruvate kinase deficiency, a form of dwarfism associated with hypoplasia of the cartilage and hair, and a form of limb-girdle muscular dystrophy. It is worth remembering that, in general, the offspring of first-cousin marriages are slightly more likely to have congenital malformations, as well as mental and physical defects, than are children born to unrelated parents.

ASSOCIATION. The occurrence of two traits in the same person more often than would be expected by chance is called association. A consistent positive association between blood group A and carcinoma of the stomach, and between duodenal ulceration and blood group O, has long been recognized. Such an association may be due to many causes, and does not indicate that the genes controlling blood group antigens are on the same chromosome as those associated with the development of duodenal ulceration. If an association is found between two characters in the general population, it is important to determine whether the association persists when the two characters are examined in sibships. If geographic or social stratification is the cause of the association, the correlation will disappear. If, for example, a mixed population of Africans and Europeans is examined, a positive association between cDe Rhesus blood group (common in African populations) and dark skin color would be found. This association disappears within a sibship, but the small size of human sibships and the statistical problems associated with pooling data from different sibships make it difficult to provide a simple test.

PLEIOTROPISM. Sometimes two characters are associated because they are due to the action of a single gene. Thus clouding of the cornea and mental retardation are two traits that are associated in Hurler's syndrome. The two traits are not caused by two genes, but are due to a single gene with a so-called pleiotropic effect. When a gene causes a pleiotropic effect, the association found in the general population persists when sibships are examined. Pleiotropic effects of genes are common, and may be of clinical importance. Familial intestinal polyposis (see Ch. 426) is an early consequence of the effect of a gene that later commonly leads to carcinoma of the colon.

AUTOSOMAL LINKAGE. The site of a gene on a chromosome is termed a *locus*. Alternative forms of genes which occupy corresponding sites on homologous chromosomes are called alleles. Applied to human genetics, Mendel's law of independent assortment states that traits controlled by two or more pairs of allelic genes will be transmitted to the children of the next generation, either together or separately, by chance alone. The law holds only for genes situated on different chromosomes or at widely separated loci on the same chromosome. However, if two genes occupy closely adjacent sites on the same chromosome, they tend to segregate together and are then said to be linked. The frequency of crossing over gives an estimate of closeness of the linkage. It is important to remember that even if two genes are present on the same chromosome, they will appear unlinked if they are so widely separated that free (50 per cent) recombination between two loci can take place.

The application of somatic cell genetics as well as the development of more discriminating methods for chromosome identification has enabled the assignment of specific loci to individual autosomes. Structural loci can be assigned to all 22 autosomes. In many instances more than one genetic locus can be assigned to a particular chromosome. Chromosome 1 has 22 loci assigned, including the Rh locus.

Linkage of two genes does not cause association of the two characters in the general population unless the population is heterogeneous, as it would be in an American city, recently derived from several parts of the world. In any one sibship the two characters may be associated, in which case the genes are on the same chromosome and are said to be linked in coupling (cis configuration). If the characters are dissociated, the genes responsible are distributed on each of the two homologous chromosomes and are described as being linked in repulsion (trans configuration). A common error is to suppose that the association of two characters in the single sibship implies genetic linkage. If true linkage exists, sufficient pedigrees are collected, and the genes concerned are in equilibrium, an equal number of sibships will be found in which the two characters are not associated. If, however, the genes concerned are not in equilibrium (genetic disequilibrium), as in the case with HLA-B27 and ankylosing spondylitis, then the specific allele B27 at the HLA locus will be much more frequent in patients with the disease (see below). There are many instances of autosomal linkage in man, including the ABO blood group locus and the locus for the nail-patella syndrome; the Rh blood groups and one form of elliptocytosis; and Lutheran blood group and the secretor locus (which determines whether soluble ABO blood substances are present in saliva and other body fluids). The loci determining the β and δ chains of hemoglobin are also very closely linked (see Ch. 485.1). The development of somatic cell genetics has enabled the human chromosome map of the autosomes to be rapidly filled. One hundred fifteen genes are now assigned to the autosomes and 96 to the X chromosome. The increased information now available on the linkage of genes to specific chromosomes has been greatly enhanced by these techniques.

The linkage relationships of human genes have one important practical consequence for clinical medicine. If a mutant causing a serious inherited disease is closely linked to one causing a common trait, healthy carriers of the disease may be detected in unaffected members of the family by the presence or absence of the common trait. It would, of course, be important to know whether the two linked genes in the family under investigation were in the coupling or repulsion phase. Accurate information regarding the phase can be obtained by studying the distribution of the two traits in three generations.

THE HISTOCOMPATIBILITY LOCUS (HLA). The HLA system comprises four closely linked highly polymorphic loci on chromosome 6 (Fig. 7). These loci as ordered on the chromosome are HLA-A, HLA-C, HLA-B, and HLA-D. The A, B, and C loci are defined serologically; the D locus controls lymphocyte (LD) antigens detectable by the mixed lymphocyte test (MLD). Multiple alleles are found at each locus; HLA-A and HLA-B have more than 20 alleles, whereas at the HLA-C locus only five alleles have been identified thus far. Closely adjacent to the HLA locus are loci controlling some of the complement components. These include the genes that determine C2 and C4 deficiency and the Chido (Ch) and Rodgers (Rg) loci coding for red cell antigens. The C2 deficiency locus is particularly closely associated with DW2. Many diseases with strong associations with the HLA-B region frequently have an even stronger association with HLA-D. Since linkage of the HLA antigen to many diseases is particularly marked at the D locus, further definition of this complex area is likely to lead to information of extreme clinical importance. The immune response genes, which may serve as the T cell receptor in the mouse, have not yet been identified in man.

The association of the HLA system and disease has an unusual feature; in most disease associations such as the gene for sickle cell trait and resistance to infection with *Plasmodium falciparum*, or the Duffy blood group

HISTOCOMPATIBILITY LOCUS (Chromosome 6)

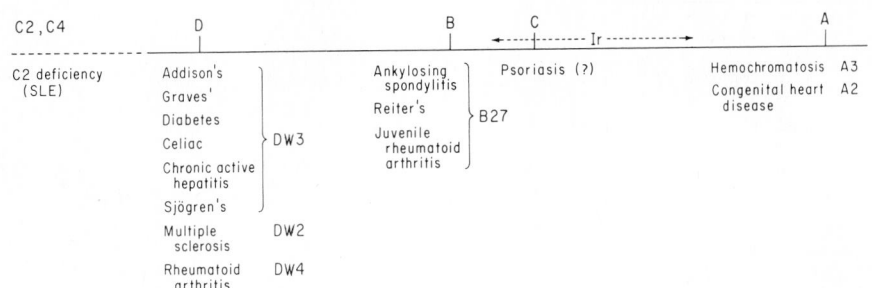

Figure 7.

and *Plasmodium vivax*, the association is with a specific disease entity. The association of specific HLA genes and disease is far ranging, and a specific HLA allele may have a significant association with several diseases.

Ankylosing Spondylitis. The frequency of the HLA-B27 allele in the white population is approximately 8 per cent. In patients with ankylosing spondylitis the frequency of B27 is over 90 per cent. In Australian aboriginals and black Africans the B27 antigen is virtually absent, and the frequency of ankylosing spondylitis in these populations is sharply reduced. In contrast, B27 occurs in 50 per cent of the adult Haida Indians of the United States, and sacroiliitis is present in 10 per cent of the adult male population. A Caucasian with the B27 antigen is approximately 100 times more likely to develop ankylosing spondylitis than one who does not possess this antigen; the increased liability in Japanese populations of B27 individuals is 300. Between 5 and 20 per cent of all individuals of both sexes, above the age of 30, with the B27 antigen have some clinical or radiologic evidence of sacroiliac joint disease.

Rheumatoid Arthritis, Sjögren's Syndrome, Reiter's Syndrome, and Multiple Sclerosis. The frequency of HLA-DW4 in patients with rheumatoid arthritis is 42 per cent compared to 16 per cent in controls, irrespective of whether the individual is positive for the rheumatoid factor. HLA-B8 is more common in patients with Sjögren's syndrome (53 per cent) than in a control population (17 per cent). Reiter's syndrome usually follows an infection of the urinary tract or bowel with *Shigella, Salmonella*, or the *Yersinia* organism. No less than 20 per cent of B27 positive individuals with *Shigella* infections will develop Reiter's syndrome. Although multiple sclerosis is strongly associated with HLA-DW2, at least 40 per cent of patients are DW2 negative.

Graves' Disease, Juvenile Diabetes, and Addison's Disease. These diseases, all of which are associated with disturbances in the immune response, are associated with an increased frequency of HLA-DW3.

Gluten Enteropathy and Chronic Active Hepatitis. The highest known disease association with the HLA system occurs in gluten enteropathy, in which 98 per cent of patients have HLA-DW3 antigen.

An association between HLA-B8 and DW3 and chronic active hepatitis has been reported, and is particularly correlated with the presence of the hepatitis associated antigen (HAA); as many as 80 per cent of the HAA positive individuals possess the B8 antigen. Recent evidence, from renal dialysis units, suggests that HLA-B8 is associated with rapid elimination of the hepatitis virus,

even though the risk of developing chronic disease is enhanced.

Mechanisms of Disease Associations. Almost all the associations of the HLA locus relate to susceptibility to disease rather than resistance. Although well over 90 per cent of patients with ankylosing spondylitis are B27 positive, no more than 20 per cent of B27 positive individuals develop the disease. Several mechanisms have been proposed to explain the association between HLA specificity and susceptibility to disease.

The immune response gene hypothesis is based on the reasonable assumption that the immune response genes (Ir gene) will map within the HLA locus in man close to the D locus, as it does in the mouse. Ir genes are dominant, as is disease susceptibility, and might cause an effect by the formation of antigen-antibody complexes or by influencing cell-mediated immunity. An alternative hypothesis suggests that the HLA gene product interacts directly with the pathogen. Certain allelic products would fail to interact with the HLA receptor on the surface of the cell, and cell-based immunity toward the virus would be affected. A third mechanism suggests that if the HLA product is molecularly similar to that of the pathogen, tolerance will obtain and the host will be unable to mount an immunologic defense.

LINKAGE DISEQUILIBRIUM. The frequency of the HLA-A1 antigen in European populations is about 0.31, and the frequency of the antigen HLA-B8, 0.21. Thus the expected frequency of individuals who possess the A1 and B8 antigens would be $(0.31 \times 0.21) = 0.065$. The observed frequency of A1+ B8+ individuals is approximately 0.17 — three times higher than expected if there were no association. The frequency of the A1 allele is 0.17 and that of B8 is 0.11. Thus the expected haplotype (a shorthand word for "haplogenotype") frequency A1, B8, if there were no association, would be $(0.17 \times 0.11) = 0.019$. In fact, the observed frequency of the A1, B8 haplotype is 0.088 — four times the expected frequency. The difference between the observed and expected frequencies is called the linkage disequilibrium $(0.088 - 0.019) = 0.069$. Thus the association between traits and linked genes, such as A1 and B, depends on the disequilibrium. Linkage disequilibrium is common among alleles on the HLA locus and accounts for the disease associations; the biologic reasons remain obscure. An interesting reason for the existence of linkage disequilibrium has been postulated. Strong selection for certain alleles at the HLA locus could have arisen in the past if catastrophic epidemic infectious disease favored the survival of individuals of a specific HLA type. Thus the HLA linkage disequilibrium we see today may represent an important relic of our evolutionary past.

Fraser, F. C., and Nora, J. J.: Genetics of Man. Philadelphia, Lea & Febiger, 1975.

McKusick, V. A.: Human Genetics. 2nd ed. Englewood Cliffs, N. J., Prentice-Hall, 1969.

Nora, J. J., and Fraser, F. C.: Medical Genetics: Principles and Practice. Philadelphia, Lea & Febiger, 1974.

Stern, C.: Principles of Human Genetics. 3rd ed. San Francisco, W. H. Freeman, 1973.

13. INBORN ERRORS OF METABOLISM AND MOLECULAR DISEASE

Alexander G. Bearn

Development of the concept of an inborn error of metabolism by Archibald Garrod in the first decade of this century was one of the most brilliant insights in the history of genetics, for it introduced the far-reaching hypothesis that the primary action of a gene is to control the synthesis of a specific enzyme. Subsequent work has fully substantiated Garrod's belief that the block in a metabolic pathway arises from an inherited deficiency of a specific enzyme. More recently the term inborn error of metabolism has been extended to include hereditary alterations in proteins that have no enzymatic functions.

The development of precise chemical methods that enable a comparison to be made between normal and genetically altered proteins led to the introduction of the term *molecular disease*, to emphasize that the difference between a normal and an affected individual might rest in the substitution of a single amino acid residue in the primary sequence of a protein molecule. Although the metabolic block may affect protein, carbohydrate, lipid, nucleic acid, porphyrin, or pigment metabolism, the *primary* defect invariably lies in the genetic specification of the synthesis of a protein.

In some inborn errors of metabolism the mutational event occurs at the active site of the enzyme. In these instances, although the enzyme will be functionally altered, the presence of cross-reacting material can be detected by immunologic methods. In other instances the mutation results in a protein which is functionally inert, and no cross-reacting material can be detected immunologically. Using the terminology of microbial genetics, the former class of mutants is frequently termed CRM (cross-reacting material) (+) and the latter CRM (−). At the pseudocholinesterase locus, for instance, 17 CRM (+) mutants and 18 CRM (−) mutants have been recognized. In the Lesch-Nyhan syndrome there is only one CRM (+) mutant; by contrast, 13 CRM (−) have been described. Even when there is no cross-reacting material detectable by immunologic methods, the protein, although no longer recognizable by antisera developed against the normal protein, may be present.

Some of the clinical conditions for which a demonstrated abnormality in a specific protein has been observed are listed in Table 2. In most of these a deficiency in a specific enzymatic activity is demonstrable, whereas in others a normal quantity of a structurally abnormal nonenzymic protein is synthesized. The classic example of a "molecular disease" affecting a nonenzyme is sickle cell anemia, in which the only difference between normal and sickle cell hemoglobin is the substitution of a valine for a glutamic acid in the β chain of hemoglobin.

It is increasingly being recognized that many of the inborn variations in metabolism are unassociated with clinical disease (Table 3). These biochemical variations represent the more conspicuous examples of the importance of human biochemical diversity. In some instances they provide a critical genetic background for the expression of an environmentally controlled disorder; in others the physiologic effect of the genetic variation is not apparent.

GENETIC HETEROGENEITY. It is becoming increasingly evident that identical or closely similar clinical syndromes may be determined by different mutant genes. In some instances, the mutations may be at different loci (nonallelic genes) (Table 4), whereas in others they occur at the same locus (allelic genes). In an individual cistron, genes may be allelic at the same codon (eualleles) or at a different codon (heteroalleles). In hemoglobins S and C the mutations occur at the same codon and are thus examples of eualleles. Hurler's and Scheie's syndromes are examples of heteroalleles, for in these instances the mutations occur at different codons but in the same cistron (see Ch. 538.1).

Even before the syndromes of recessive albinism yielded to biochemical probes, it was evident that the two clinical syndromes must be caused by genes at different loci, because it was well known that two albinos may marry and produce normally pigmented offspring. Indeed, it is a safe generalization to assume that the majority of inherited diseases presently regarded as homogeneous entities represent the clinical effects of different mutant genes.

Genetic heterogeneity can be detected at several different levels of biologic organization. Although Hurler's and Hunter's syndromes appear clinically similar, genetic heterogeneity is evident, because family studies indicate that Hurler's syndrome is controlled by a gene on an autosome, whereas in Hunter's syndrome the disease is X-linked. Similar variations exist among the spastic paraplegias: some pedigrees indicate autosomal inheritance, whereas others are clearly X-linked. Genetic heterogeneity can be demonstrated in recessive deaf mutism. Moreover, nonallelism can be definitely inferred, because marriage between deaf mutes, as with marriage between albinos, can result in normal offspring. Sometimes genetic heterogeneity can be strongly suspected from the clinical spectrum of a disease, as is the case in the various inherited mucopolysaccharidoses. When the syndromes associated with nonspherocytic anemias are examined biochemically, it is also evident that a number of different genes are involved. Heterogeneity among the X-linked hemophilias is strongly suggested as a result of functional and immunologic studies of factor VIII in different families. Heterogeneity is also evident in families exhibiting C'3 esterase deficiency. In some instances "genetic compounds" result in additional phenotypic variation. These genetic compounds arise when the individual carries two different mutant alleles. Hemoglobins S and C are controlled by euallelic genes, and individuals who have hemoglobin SC disease can thus be said to illustrate the phenotypic consequences of a genetic compound (euallelic homozygotes).

TABLE 2. Selected Inborn Errors of Metabolism

Disorder	Primary Defect	Carrier Detection	Prenatal Diagnosis
Amino acid metabolism:			
Phenylketonuria	Phenylalanine hydroxylase	+	
Albinism I	Tyrosinase		
II	?		
Tyrosinemia	p-Hydroxyphenylpyruvate oxidase (?)		
Tyrosinosis	Tyrosine transaminase		
Homocystinuria	Cystathionine synthetase	+	(+)
(a) Pyridoxine responsive			
(b) Pyridoxine unresponsive			
Cystathioninuria	γ-Cystathionase	+	(+)
Alcaptonuria	Homogentisic acid oxidase		
Maple syrup urine disease	Oxidative decarboxylase of branched chain ketoacids	+	+
Intermittent branched-chain ketoaciduria	Oxidative decarboxylase of branched chain ketoacids		(+)
Hypervalinemia	Valine transaminase		
Isovaleric acidemia	Isovaleryl-CoA-dehydrogenase		(+)
Beta-hydroxyisovaleric aciduria	Beta-methylcrotonyl-CoA-carboxylase	+	
Methylmalonic aciduria			+
(a) Vitamin B_{12} responsive	Deoxyadenosyl transferase		(+)
(b) Vitamin B_{12} unresponsive	Methylmalonyl-CoA-mutase		(+)
Hyperammonemia I	Carbamyl phosphate synthetase		
II	Ornithine transcarbamylase	+	
Citrullinemia	Argininosuccinic acid synthetase	+	(+)
Argininosuccinicaciduria	Argininosuccinase	+	(+)
Hyperargininemia	Arginase	+	
Hyperlysinemia	Lysine-ketoglutarate reductase		
Saccharopinuria	Aminoadipic semialdehyde–glutamate reductase		
Histidinemia	Histidase		
Hyperprolinemia I	Proline oxidase	+	
II	Δ'-pyrroline-5-carboxylate dehydrogenase	+	
Hydroxyprolinemia	Hydroxyproline oxidase (?)		
Ketotic hyperglycinemia	Propionyl-CoA-carboxylase	+	+
Nonketotic hyperglycinemia	Glycine decarboxylase (?)		
Hyper-beta-alaninemia	Beta-alanine-alpha-ketoglutarate amino transferase		
Carnosinemia	Carnosinase	+	
Hypersarcosinemia	Sarcosine dehydrogenase	+	
Cystinosis	?	+	+
Hartnup disease	Tubular reabsorption of monoamino-monocarboxylic acids		+
Cystinuria (three types)	Transepithelial transport of cystine and dibasic amino acids	+	
Iminoglycinuria	Transport of imino acids and glycine	+	
α-Methyl-β-hydroxybutyric acidemia	?	+	(+)
Hyperdibasic aminoaciduria	?	+	
Carbohydrate metabolism:			
Pentosuria	Xylitol dehydrogenase	+	
Fructosuria	Liver fructokinase		
Fructose intolerance	Fructose-1-phosphate aldolase		
Fructose-1,6-diphosphatase deficiency	Fructose-1,6-diphosphatase	+	
Glycogenosis I	Glucose-6-phosphatase	+	
II	Alpha-1,4-glucosidase	+	+
III	Amylo-1,6-glucosidase	+	(+)
IV	Amylo(1-4 to 1-6)-transglucosidase		(+)
V	Muscle phosphorylase		
VI	Liver phosphorylase		
VII	Muscle phosphofructokinase		
VIII	Liver phosphorylasekinase	+	
Galactosemia	Galactose-1-phosphate uridyl transferase	+	+
Galactokinase deficiency	Galactokinase	+	
Hyperoxaluria I	Alpha-ketoglutarate:glyoxalate carboligase		
II	D-Glyceric dehydrogenase		
Renal glycosuria	?		
Pyruvate decarboxylase deficiency	Pyruvate decarboxylase	+	(+)
Lactase deficiency	Lactase		
Sucrase-isomaltase deficiency	Sucrase, isomaltase		
Glucose-galactose malabsorption	?	+	
Hurler's syndrome	Alpha-L-iduronidase	+	+
Hunter's syndrome	Sulfoiduronate sulfatase	+	+
Sanfilippo's syndrome A	Heparan sulfate sulfatase	+	+
B	N-acetyl-alpha-glucosaminidase	+	(+)
Morquio's syndrome	N-acetylhexosamine-6-sulfate sulfatase	+	(+)
Scheie's syndrome	Alpha-L-iduronidase		
Maroteaux-Lamy syndrome	N-acetyl galactosamine-4-sulfatase	+	+
β-Glucuronidase deficiency	β-Glucuronidase	+	+
I-cell disease	?	+	+
Mannosidosis	Alpha-mannosidase		(+)
Fucosidosis	Alpha-1-fucosidase	+	(+)
Gaucher's disease (three types)	Glucocerebrosidase	+	+
Globoid cell leukodystrophy	Galactocerebroside beta-galactosidase	+	+
Pyruvate carboxylase deficiency	Pyruvate carboxylase		

Table continues on following page

TABLE 2. Selected Inborn Errors of Metabolism *(Continued)*

Disorder	Primary Defect	Carrier Detection	Prenatal Diagnosis
Lipid metabolism:			
Lipoprotein lipase deficiency	Low density lipoprotein receptor	+	+
Hypercholesterolemia	?		
Hypertriglyceridemia	?		
Combined hyperlipidemia	?		
Abetalipoproteinemia	Betalipoproteins		
Hypobetalipoproteinemia	Low density lipoproteins	(+)	
Tangier disease	?	+	
Norum disease	Lecithin:cholesterol acetyl transferase		
Gangliosidosis GM$_1$ (types I and II)	Beta galactosidase	+	+
Gangliosidosis GM$_2$ (Tay-Sachs)	Hexosaminidase A	+	+
Gangliosidosis GM$_2$ (Sandhoff)	Hexosaminidase A and B	+	+
Gangliosidosis GM$_2$ (juvenile, Type 3)	Hexosaminidase A	+	+
GM$_6$ (hematoside) sphingolipodystrophy	?		(+)
Fabry's disease	α-Galactosidase A	+	+
Metachromatic leukodystrophy I	Arylsulfatase A	+	+
II	Arylsulfatase A, B, C, and steroid sulfatase	+	
Lactosylceramidosis	Lactosylceramidase		
Niemann-Pick disease	Sphingomyelinase	+	+
Wolman's disease	Acid lipase	+	(+)
Cholesterylester storage disease	Acid lipase	+	(+)
Cerebrotendinous xanthomatosis	?		
Refsum's disease	Phytanic acid alpha hydroxylase	+	(+)
Ceramide lactoside lipidosis	?		(+)
Nucleic acid metabolism:			
Gout	?		
Lesch-Nyhan syndrome	Hypoxanthine-guanine phosphoribosyl transferase	+	+
Xanthinuria	Xanthine oxidase		
Xanthurenic aciduria	Kynureninase		
Orotic aciduria I	Orotidylic pyrophosphorylase and decarboxylase	+	(+)
II	Orotidylic decarboxylase		
Xeroderma pigmentosum	UV-specific endonuclease		
Porphyrin and heme metabolism:			
Erythropoietic porphyria	Uroporphyrinogen-III cosynthetase and uroporphyrinogen-I synthetase	+	(+)
Acute intermittent porphyria	Uroporphyrinogen-I synthetase	+	+
Porphyria variegata	?		
Coproporphyria	Coproporphyrin oxidase	+	
Porphyria cutanea tarda	Uroporphyrinogen decarboxylase	+	
Protoporphyria	Ferrochelatase	+	
Crigler-Najjar syndrome (two types)	Glucuronyltransferase		
Gilbert's syndrome	Bilirubin uptake		
Dubin-Johnson syndrome	Bilirubin excretion		
Erythrocyte metabolism:			
Hemolytic anemia	Pyruvate kinase	+	
	Hexokinase	+	
	Glucosephosphate isomerase	+	
	Triosephosphate isomerase	+	
	2,3-Diphosphoglyceromutase	+	
	Phosphoglycerate kinase	+	
	Glucose-6-phosphate dehydrogenase	+	(+)
	6-Phosphogluconate dehydrogenase		
	Glutathione reductase		
	Glutathione peroxidase		
	Glutathione synthetase		
Methemoglobinemia	NADH-methemoglobin reductase	+	

Table continues on opposite page.

TABLE 2.   Selected Inborn Errors of Metabolism (*Continued*)

Disorder	Primary Defect	Carrier Detection	Prenatal Diagnosis
Leukocyte metabolism:			
Myeloperoxidase deficiency	Myeloperoxidase	+	
Chronic granulomatous disease	?	+	
Chédiak-Higashi syndrome	?	+	
Abnormalities of plasma proteins:			
Analbuminemia	Albumin		
Atransferrinemia	Transferrin		
Afibrinogenemia	Fibrinogen		
Alpha$_1$-antitrypsin deficiency	Alpha$_1$-antitrypsin	+	
Acatalasemia	Catalase	+	(+)
Suxamethonium sensitivity	Pseudocholinesterase		
Hereditary angioedema	C1-inhibitor		
C1q deficiency	C1q		
C1r deficiency	C1r		
C2 deficiency	C2		
C3 deficiency	C3		
X-linked agammaglobulinemia	?		
Severe combined immunodeficiency	Adenosine deaminase (?)	+	+
Selective IgA deficiency	?		
X-linked immunodeficiency with increased IgM	?		
Hemophilia A	Factor VIII	+	
Hemophilia B	Factor IX	+	
von Willebrand's disease	?		
Hageman trait	Factor XII	+	
PTA deficiency	Factor XI	+	
Parahemophilia	Factor V	+	
Hypoprothrombinemia	Factor II	+	
Factor VII deficiency	Factor VII	+	
Factor X deficiency	Factor X	+	
Fibrin-stabilizing factor deficiency	Factor XIII	+	
Hormone and vitamin metabolism:			
Adrenogenital syndrome	21-Hydroxylase		+
	11-Hydroxylase		
	3-Beta-hydroxysteroiddehydrogenase		
	17-Hydroxylase		
	Desmolase		
Aldosterone deficiency	18-Hydroxylase		
Familial goiter	Iodide transport		
	Peroxidase		
	Iodotyrosine coupling		
	Iodotyrosine deiodinase		
	Thyroglobulin synthesis		
Renal diabetes insipidus	?	+	
Vitamin D dependent rickets	25-Hydroxycholecalciferol-1-hydroxylase		
Formiminotransferase deficiency	Formiminotransferase		
Miscellaneous:			
Cystic fibrosis	?		
Wilson's disease	?	+	
Hemochromatosis	?		
Menkes' kinky hair syndrome	Intestinal copper absorption		
Sulfite oxidase deficiency	Sulfite oxidase		
Hypophosphatasia	Alkaline phosphatase (?)	+	
Lysosomal acid phosphatase deficiency	Acid phosphatase	+	+
Renal tubular acidosis I	Gradient defect		
II	Bicarbonate wastage		
Aspartylglucosaminuria	N-aspartyl-β-glucosaminidase	+	+

(+) = Prenatal diagnosis is likely to be possible, because the enzyme defect can be detected in cell culture.

TABLE 3.   A Selection of Common Inherited Polymorphisms

Blood groups, e.g., ABO, MNS, Rh
Leukocyte groups
Platelet groups
Histocompatibility antigens (HLA)
Hemoglobin (α, β, γ, δ chains)
Myoglobin
Serum proteins:
  Albumin
  Alpha$_1$-antitrypsin
  Group-specific component (Gc)
  Haptoglobin (α, β chains)
  Ceruloplasmin
  Alpha$_2$-macroglobulin (Xm)
  Complement (C3, C4)
  Beta-lipoprotein (Ag-, Ld-, Lp-types)
  Transferrin
  Fibrinogen
  Immunoglobulins (Am, Gm, InV)
Enzymes:
  Glucose-6-phosphate dehydrogenase
  Phosphoglucomutase (PGM 1, 2, 3)
  Phosphohexoseisomerase
  Lactate dehydrogenase
  Adenine phosphoribosyl transferase
  Hypoxanthine-guanine phosphoribosyl transferase
  Peptidases (A, B, C, D, E)
  Pseudocholinesterase (E1, E2)
  Amylase
Phenylthiocarbamide testing
Beta-aminoisobutyric aciduria
Color blindness

Now that it is firmly established that genes control the specificity of particular proteins, genetic heterogeneity can also be detected by immunologic and biochemical techniques that discriminate between closely similar protein molecules. The application of these techniques to serum protein and red cell enzymes has disclosed a surprising degree of heterogeneity in normal persons. However, any estimate of genetic heterogeneity based on the application of electrophoretic techniques will be too low, because it seems that less than half the mutational events leading to a specific amino acid substitution will result in an altered net charge of the protein.

SCREENING FOR INBORN ERRORS OF METABOLISM.   The central purpose of any screening program is the detection of individuals in whom it is likely that a specific hereditary disease will develop and against which preventive or therapeutic measures are potentially available. It is important to emphasize this latter point, because screening large populations for a disease such as Duchenne muscular dystrophy, for which there is presently no treatment, is neither useful nor humane. Screening for genetic diseases can be performed at three principal phenotypic levels. In many instances the recognition of overt clinical disease represents the only phenotypic level at which the inborn error can be recognized. Thus in Huntington's chorea no biochemical abnormality has been found to be characteristic of the

TABLE 4.   Some Illustrative Examples of Genetic Diseases Showing Nonallelic Heterogeneity

Albinism
Deafness
Diabetes insipidus, neurohypophyseal type
Osteogenesis imperfecta
Pituitary dwarfism
Retinitis pigmentosa
Sanfilippo's syndrome A and B

disease, and early recognition of signs and symptoms represents the only sure means to arrive at a diagnosis. Early diagnosis of polyposis of the colon is important because of the frequency of malignant transformation. The recognition of genital abnormalities at birth in females may aid in early detection of the adrenogenital syndrome. Inborn errors can also be recognized by the presence of an abnormal metabolite in physiologic fluids. The enzymatic deficiency may lead to accumulation of the substrate for the reaction catalyzed by the normal enzyme and to a deficiency of the product. An increased level of blood galactose in galactosemia and of phenylalanine in phenylketonuria are examples in which the disturbance of the normal metabolic relationships leads to detection of disease.

Since genes control the synthesis of proteins, the most direct way of identifying an inborn error is to utilize a screening program which detects a qualitative change in the structure of the protein, e.g., electrophoretically, or by its altered enzymatic or immunologic activity. Mass screening for rare inborn errors of metabolism in the general population is expensive and time consuming, and a careful estimate of the cost of such a program must be balanced against the potential gains. For most countries the cost of extensive screening programs for genetically determined disease is prohibitive. For the moment it seems wiser to focus, with the exception of phenylketonuria, on families and populations who are particularly at risk and for whom effective therapy for the inborn errors of metabolism is available. More than 90 per cent of babies born in the United States are tested for phenylketonuria. Although the incidence of false negative tests (5 to 10 per cent) can be minimized by performing a second test after the third day of life, the practical problem of guaranteeing a second screening is insurmountable. Despite these and other difficulties, such as the devastating effect of maternal phenylketonuria on the fetus, the PKU testing program has been effective in preventing one form of mental retardation. Screening for Tay-Sachs disease among Ashkenazic Jews and sickle cell hemoglobin among black populations are examples of screening programs which, when carefully carried out, can be of undoubted benefit. Amniocentesis and the use of cultured fibroblasts to identify certain inborn errors of metabolism before birth can be expected to increase sharply in the years ahead and will increase the usefulness of screening programs.

Harris, H.: The Principles of Human Biochemical Genetics. *In* Neuberger, A., and Tatum, E. L. (eds.): Frontiers of Biology. Vol. 19. New York, American Elsevier Publishing Company, 1970.

McKusick, V. A.: Mendelian Inheritance in Man: Catalogs of Autosomal Dominant, Autosomal Recessive, and X-linked Phenotypes. 4th ed. Baltimore, The Johns Hopkins Press, 1975.

14.   POLYGENIC AND MULTIFACTORIAL INHERITANCE

Alexander G. Bearn

Traits determined by the collaboration of many genes at different loci are called polygenic, in contrast to those traits which are determined by a single gene (monogenic). Most of the differences among normal people are determined by the interaction of many ge-

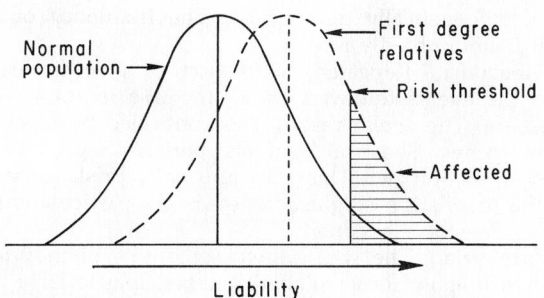

Figure 8. Diseases which conform to a polygenic multifactorial model of inheritance lead to an increased incidence of disease among the relatives of affected individuals. This increased incidence is most evident among first degree relatives.

netic and environmental factors (multifactorial inheritance).

Polygenic inheritance, in which many genes each contribute a minor effect, is best established for those traits which show continuous variation in the form of a "normal" distribution curve. Height is an example of a polygenic (and multifactorial) trait in which the extremes of the normal distribution are not considered abnormal. The degree of resemblance among relatives can be deduced from the number of genes they have in common. Dizygotic twins, however, will have 50 per cent of their genes in common, as will all sibs. Parents and children also have 50 per cent of their genes in common. Thus it would be expected that if one parent is 72 inches tall and the other 66 inches tall, all the children, on the average, would be 69 inches tall. For a variety of reasons (dominance, environment, and epistasis), the offspring are usually closer to the population average than to the average of their parents. Polygenic models have been advanced for inheritance of high blood pressure, diabetes mellitus, and rheumatoid arthritis, as well as a variety of congenital defects.

In clinical medicine polygenic and multifactorial inheritance should be suspected when the disease under consideration is "known to run in families," and when, in addition, examination of the affected and unaffected sibs in any sibship does not support inheritance in a simple dominant or recessive fashion. When this occurs, it is reasonable to suspect that within such families a large number of "risk genes" are present. "Risk genes" are of course present in the normal population, but in low frequency. If in any one individual there is a particularly large number of high "risk genes," the latent disorder becomes overt. This phenomenon is known as the "threshold effect" (Fig. 8). When examining a pedigree for a possible polygenic inheritance pattern, it is worth remembering that (1) the frequency of affected individuals is very roughly the square root of the frequency in the population, and (2) the frequency of the disease in first degree relatives will fall off in a nonlinear fashion as the relationship to the affected individual decreases; thus the frequency of cleft lip is 40 per 1000 for first degree relatives, 7 for second degree relatives, and 3 for third degree relatives. This latter fact is particularly important in genetic counseling. Thus, in distinction to monogenic traits, in which the recurrence risk in a sibship is one fourth or one half, the recurrence risk in sibs of those affected with threshold traits depends on the incidence of the trait. The elegance and complexity of the mathematical models advanced for

polygenic-multifactorial disease should not obscure the fact that each of the "risk genes" has, like any other gene, a specific biochemical consequence. Eventually, the vague concept of genetic susceptibility of polygenic inheritance must yield to the central dogma that genes control the synthesis of specific proteins each of which has a specific function.

Carter, C. O.: Genetics of common disorders. Br. Med. Bull., 25:52, 1969.

15. PHARMACOGENETICS
Alexander G. Bearn

It has long been recognized that certain people respond unusually to the administration of specific drugs. In some instances the altered reaction has an immunologic basis; in others it appears to be idiosyncratic without obvious cause; and in some the difference appears to be contingent on the genetic constitution of the host. Pharmacogenetics is concerned with those deviant responses to specific drugs that are genetically determined. The breakdown and disposal of drugs in the body are usually dependent on a series of specific gene-controlled enzymatic reactions. Mutant genes in the population that alter these reactions can result in serious clinical consequences.

INHERITED DISEASES DISCOVERED OR PRECIPITATED BY THE USE OF DRUGS. Several diseases have been disclosed or precipitated as a direct result of the administration of drugs which for their proper metabolic disposal require an intact enzyme system. In the absence of pharmacologic overload, the defective enzyme system is not stressed enough to cause clinical manifestations.

Glucose-6-Phosphate Dehydrogenase Deficiency. A severe hemolytic anemia (favism) may be produced by the ingestion of the broad bean *Vicia fava*. The anemia is due to deficiency of the X-linked enzyme glucose-6-phosphate dehydrogenase in the erythrocytes of susceptible subjects (see Glucose-6-Phosphate Dehydrogenase in Ch. 483.3). A deficiency of the enzyme is a necessary but not sufficient cause for the anemia that follows ingestion of fava beans. Additional genetic factors, presently poorly identified, are also required if the disease is to be manifest. Severe neonatal jaundice in the Mediterranean basin and Far East may occasionally be associated with glucose-6-phosphate dehydrogenase deficiency.

Persons with glucose-6-phosphate dehydrogenase deficiency are particularly susceptible to hemolytic reactions after administration of the antimalarial drug primaquine and certain other drugs, including aspirin and phenacetin. A severe hemolytic anemia may also occur during the course of acute viral hepatitis and infectious mononucleosis in individuals with deficiency of glucose-6-phosphate dehydrogenase. The mutation in the black population is characterized by a mean enzyme activity of 10 to 20 per cent of normal, and the increased susceptibility to hemolysis is restricted to the older red cells. The risk of hemolysis is significantly less than in the Mediterranean type of glucose-6-phosphate dehydrogenase deficiency in which the residual enzymatic activity is less than 5 per cent of normal and increased susceptibility to hemolysis occurs in young as well as old cells. The trait is present in about 10 per cent of blacks in the United States and may reach as high as 35 per cent in certain African and Mediterranean populations. The deficiency provides some protection against falciparum malaria and accounts for the persistence of the gene at a very high level in these populations. The relationship of glucose-6-phosphate dehydrogenase deficiency and resistance to falciparum malaria affords one of the better examples of a balanced polymorphism in which a heterozygous advantage can be clearly demonstrated.

Isoniazid. When a group of individuals is given a standard dose of the antituberculosis drug isoniazid (INH), two subpopulations can be identified. In one group the blood level of isoniazid is high and very little acetylated INH is excreted in the urine (slow inactivators), whereas in the second group the blood isoniazid is considerably lower and acetylated INH appears in the urine in large quantities (rapid inactivators). Twin studies show a similar metabolic response in monozygotic twins, whereas notable differences are apparent in dizygotic twins. Pedigree analysis indicates that the capacity to acetylate isoniazid is inherited as a simple recessive trait. The "slow inactivators" lack the liver enzyme N-acetyltransferase present in "rapid inactivators." Although it is clinically reassuring that rapid acetylators show an impairment of the antituberculosis effect of the drug, slow acetylators are more likely to encounter undesirable side effects such as peripheral neuropathy, a mischance which can be avoided if pyridoxine is administered concomitantly. It is of some clinical importance that the absence of the acetylating enzyme also makes more likely the toxic effects of the antiepileptic drug phenelzine and the antihypertensive agent hydralazine, because both these agents are acetylated by N-acetyltransferase.

The gene determining N-acetyltransferase deficiency occurs in 60 per cent of the black and white populations, but in only 10 per cent of Eskimo and Japanese populations. This polymorphism is of particular interest, because the aberrant gene has no recognizable clinical effect unless drugs which require acetylation for their metabolism are administered.

Suxamethonium (Succinylcholine). Suxamethonium is a commonly employed short-acting muscle relaxant. Its short action is due to the rapidly inactivating influence of the serum enzyme cholinesterase. Genetic variants of the enzyme are known which fail to hydrolyze suxamethonium and as a consequence cause a prolonged, but fortunately rarely fatal, apnea. This increased sensitivity to suxamethonium occurs in about 1 in 3000 patients and can be caused by a large number of different alleles at the pseudocholinesterase locus.

Hemoglobin Zürich and Other Drug-Sensitive Hemoglobins. The red cells from patients with the unstable hemoglobins (Zürich, Shepherd's Bush, and Torino) exhibit an unusual tendency to hemolysis when exposed to certain drugs. The sulfonamides are particularly offenders, but all drugs which cause hemolysis in patients with glucose-6-phosphate deficiency may be potentially harmful.

Anticoagulant Resistance. Two families have been reported in which some members are extremely resistant to warfarin and other coumarin congeners. Approximately ten times the usual dose of warfarin was needed to increase the prothrombin time to an expected level. This provides an example in which resistance to a drug is genetically determined. The frequency of the trait is undoubtedly rare.

Glaucoma. Repeated instillation of glucocorticoids into the eye is followed by an increase in intraocular pressure. The ocular response is controlled by a pair of allelic genes. Those individuals, perhaps 5 per cent of the population, who have an unusually brisk response to the instillation of glucocorticoids are particularly liable to develop glaucoma.

Porphyria. The well known sensitivity of individuals with porphyria to barbiturates, particularly the short-acting compound thiopental (thiopentone), is a classic example of a genetically determined altered response to a drug.

Malignant Hyperthermia. This is an autosomal dominantly inherited condition causing a frequently fatal hyperthermia associated with muscle rigidity that may follow the administration of anesthetic agents such as halothane, succinylcholine, or methoxyflurane. It is particularly important to inform affected individuals that half of their first-degree relatives are at a similar risk. This condition occurs in 1 out of 20,000 anesthetized patients.

Vesell, E. S.: Advances in pharmacogenetics. *In* Steinberg, A. G., and Bearn, A. G. (eds.): Progress in Medical Genetics. Vol. 9. New York, Grune & Stratton, 1973, p. 291.

16. POPULATION GENETICS
Alexander G. Bearn

GENE FREQUENCY. Although genes are expressed in individuals, it is often of interest to consider the distribution of mutant genes in the general population. The basis of population genetics is the Hardy-Weinberg law, which was formulated in a context of concern that a dominant trait would eventually displace a normal trait in the population. In particular, it arose in response to the startling assertion that because brachydactyly is a dominant trait, then "in the course of time, one would expect in the absence of counteracting factors to get three brachydactylous persons to one normal." This is quite fallacious, as the following argument will show.

If the frequency of a particular gene A is p, then its alternate allele is $(1-p)=q$; the population will consist of individuals of three genotypes: those who are homozygous AA, those who are heterozygous Aa, and those who are homozygous aa. The frequency of these genotypes in a randomly mating population will be in the proportion p^2 (AA), $2pq$ (Aa), and q^2 (aa). One important consequence of this formulation is that whatever the initial frequency of the genes A and a in the population, the proportion of the three genotypes will tend to remain constant during succeeding generations, providing that the three genotypes are equally fertile. If the mating in the population is not random or if there is unequal viability of three genotypes, the frequency calculations require considerable adjustment, and in small populations substantial changes in gene frequency may occur simply as a matter of chance.

The Hardy-Weinberg law has a very useful practical consequence. If the frequency of a recessive disease in a particular population is known, the frequency of heterozygous carriers as well as the frequency of the abnormal gene can be calculated. Thus for a recessively inherited disease aa (q^2) with a frequency of 1 per 10,000, the frequency of the gene a (q) will be the square root of 1/10,000 or 1/100. The frequency of heterozygous carriers will be $2 \times p \times q = 2 \times 99/100 \times 1/100$ or approximately 1/50. Thus for this particular inherited disease there will be 200 clinically unaffected carriers of the abnormal gene in the population for every affected individual. Cystic fibrosis of the pancreas, the most frequent recessively inherited disease in the white population, has a frequency of approximately 1 in 2500 (q^2); thus the frequency of heterozygous carriers is approximately 1 in 25 (2pq).

MUTATION AND SELECTION. A mutation is a stable heritable change in the genetic material. This change may affect a single locus, or it may consist of chromosome breakage with loss or rearrangement of the fragments. In molecular terms a point mutation can be regarded as an alteration, addition, or deletion of one of the bases of the DNA molecule. The simplest mutational event is the substitution of one nucleotide for another in the DNA sequence. Although this usually results in the substitution of one amino acid for another in the polypeptide chain (e.g., glutamic acid at position 6 of the beta polypeptide chain is replaced by valine in hemoglobin S), it is not invariable, because several different triplets can code for the same amino acid. Mutations which either insert or delete nucleotide into the genetic code usually cause more extensive substitutions in the polypeptide synthesis than single nucleotide substitutions. It will be recalled that the genetic code is read as successive triplets; an insertion or deletion will upset the regularity of the triplets, and the translation of the code into amino acids distal to the point of insertion or deletion will be altered. From what is known about the genetic code, about 75 per cent of mutations will result in a single base change, resulting in the substitution of one amino acid for another; about 20 per cent of the mutations will be synonymous, in which the base change in the codon does not change the amino acid specified; and in about 5 per cent the base triplet change will result in a nonsense triplet, leading to a chain termination and the synthesis of a polypeptide lacking a variable portion of its carboxyl terminal amino acid sequence. The effect of a mutation in a somatic cell is restricted to the life of an individual, whereas mutation in the germ line can be transmitted to future generations. The natural mutation rate can be greatly increased by x-rays, ultraviolet rays, increased temperature, and various chemical mutagens such as nitrogen mustard, ethylene sulfonate, and 5-bromouracil. Chemical mutagens are thought to achieve their effects by direct structural modification of a purine or pyrimidine base, by substitution of a base analogue for one of the normal bases, or by a frame-shift mutation.

The average spontaneous mutation rate is usually expressed as the number of mutations per locus per generation. The average spontaneous mutation rate for a number of autosomal, recessive, and X-linked traits is 3×10^{-5}. One common, often unavoidable, error in estimating mutation rates in man is the failure to recognize that indistinguishable clinical syndromes can be caused by different genes (see Genetic Heterogeneity in Ch. 13). Thus the frequencies deduced by the elegant studies of Haldane on mutation rate for hemophilia must be revised downward, because Christmas disease,

another bleeding disorder determined by a gene on the X chromosome, had not been discovered when the original calculations were made. Since heterogeneity appears to be the rule in inherited disease, all estimates of mutation rate are likely to be high. Nonhereditary conditions which mimic mutations are termed phenocopies and will also lead to overestimation of mutation rates. Spontaneous mutation rates tend to increase with advancing age. The occurrence of new mutations for chondrodystrophy is almost linearly related to paternal age. It is approximately three times more likely for a chondrodystrophic child to be born of unaffected parents if the father is 45 years of age or older than if he is 25 years old.

The frequency of most genes in the population is relatively stable. When a gene is rare and severely disadvantageous, the mutation rate is balanced by the elimination of the disadvantageous gene by natural selection. The frequency of a dominant lethal disease is twice the mutation rate; algebraically, the frequency of a dominant trait is twice the mutation rate divided by the selective disadvantage, S (S being one for a lethal). The frequency of the disadvantageous gene, however, can be stabilized at a high level if the heterozygotes are slightly favored and leave a greater number of progeny than either homozygote. The concept of *balanced polymorphism* has been defined as the existence of two or more discontinuous forms of a species in such proportion that the rarest of them cannot be maintained at its frequency in the population by recurrent mutation. As a general proposition, if the rarer of the two allelic forms occurs in a frequency that is greater than 1 per cent, the existence of balanced polymorphism should be entertained. An example of such a balanced polymorphism is the increased resistance of individuals heterozygous for sickle cell trait to falciparum malaria. Although patients with sickle cell disease (homozygotes) usually die before they can reproduce and thus cannot transmit the gene to the next generation, the incidence of the sickle cell trait may reach 40 per cent in certain West African populations. Theoretically, the high frequency of the sickle cell gene could be maintained if the heterozygote were 25 per cent more fit than the so-called normal homozygote. It has now been shown unequivocally that death from falciparum malaria is much less frequent in carriers of the sickle cell trait than in noncarriers, and thus the heterozygote does have an advantage. How much of the advantage is due to differential mortality and how much to differential fertility is uncertain, but this example serves to emphasize that the effect of genes can be assessed only in relation to a particular environment. It is, however, being slowly appreciated that the example of balanced polymorphism provided by the advantage to individuals heterozygous for the sickle cell trait may be atypical. In most instances a distinct advantage for the heterozygote cannot be demonstrated, and the possibility that certain polymorphic traits are genetically neutral is becoming increasingly discussed.

The term *genetic load* has been used to describe the total genetic disability of a population. It is composed of the *mutational load*, the load caused by recurrent mutations from a normal to a lethal or sublethal gene, and the *segregational load*, which is due to the segregation of harmful genes from favorable heterozygotes. The sickle cell gene is maintained in the population because of its heterozygous advantage, and thus contributes to the segregational load. It has been estimated that, on the average, each person has three to six genes which, if homozygous instead of heterozygous, would be lethal. The relative contribution of the segregational and mutational loads to the total load is unsettled.

Fraser, F. C., and Nora, J. J.: Genetics of Man. Philadelphia, Lea & Febiger, 1975.
Stern, C.: Principles of Human Genetics. 3rd ed. San Francisco, W. H. Freeman and Company, 1973.

17. CONGENITAL MALFORMATIONS

Alexander G. Bearn

The term congenital malformation is usually applied to important structural defects present at birth that are not caused by a birth injury. The relative importance of congenital malformation has increased as more effective control has been exercised over the environmental agents of disease. In 1900, in the United States, approximately 3.3 per cent of the total infant mortality could be ascribed to congenital malformations, whereas in 1964 congenital malformations accounted for 25 per cent of the total infant mortality. Congenital malformations are responsible for approximately 15 per cent of all deaths up to the age of 15. It has also been estimated that 7 per cent of children have a congenital malformation of consequence recognizable by the age of one year, yet only 43 per cent of such malformations are detectable at birth. In most malformations no major etiologic factor can be identified, and it must be presumed that their existence depends on complicated interactions of genetic and environmental influences or on particular genetic combinations. The frequency of many congenital malformations is compatible with a polygenic model with a threshold beyond which there is a risk of malformation. First-degree relatives (sibs and children) of an individual with a congenital malformation are at greater risk than members of the general population. This is because first-degree relatives will have a curve of distribution of high risk genes approximately halfway between the general population and those affected. The first-degree relatives of a patient with cleft lip and cleft palate are approximately 40 times more likely to develop the malformation than the population at large. The approximate frequency and sex ratio of the major malformations are shown in Table 5.

GENETIC FACTORS.   With the exception of mongolism (trisomy 21) and Turner's syndrome, relatively few congenital malformations can be ascribed to specific genes or numerical chromosomal abnormalities. Congenital hydrocephalus is occasionally inherited in an X-linked fashion. Congenital pyloric stenosis is five times more frequent in males, and harelip and cleft palate twice as common. Congenital dislocation of the hip and spina bifida are more frequent in females. Twin studies and pedigree patterns seldom provide any useful genetic information in the common malformations. The offspring of consanguineous marriages show a slight increase in the frequency of congenital malformations.

ENVIRONMENTAL FACTORS.   Contrary to popular belief, there is little direct evidence that environmental factors such as viral diseases, maternal ingestion of drugs, or maternal irradiation make a significant contribution to the *common* malformations, although each

TABLE 5.   Approximate Frequency and Sex Ratio of Common Congenital Malformations

Malformation	Frequency/1000 Births	M:F
Congenital heart disease	2.5	1:1
Pyloric stenosis	3.0 (0.5–4.0)	4:1
Talipes equinovarus	2.0	2:1
Myelomeningocele	1.5 (0.5–4.4)	1:1
Anencephaly	2.0	1:2
Down's syndrome (mongolism)	1.6	1:1
Hydrocephalus*	1.2	1:1†
Congenital dislocated hip	1.0	1:6
Cleft lip ± cleft palate	1.0	2:1
Klinefelter's syndrome	1.0	1:0

*Without spina bifida.
†Excluding X-linked recessive hydrocephalus.

of these factors materially increases the frequency of certain *specific* malformations. Recent evidence suggests that approximately 70 per cent of mothers exposed to rubella during the first trimester give birth to children with severe congenital defects, including cataracts, deafness, heart disease, and neonatal thrombocytopenic purpura.

Some evidence indicates that first-born children are more likely to have a congenital defect than later children. This is particularly true of anencephaly, congenital dislocation of the hip, talipes equinovarus, and pyloric stenosis. Striking regional differences in the incidence of congenital defects have been recognized, and have been well documented for anencephaly and spina bifida. An increased frequency of congenital dislocation of the hip in Lapps and certain American Indians is well recognized. An inexplicable but marked seasonal variation in the incidence of certain malformations has also been reported. It has been estimated that nearly one third of the pregnancies complicated by hydramnios result in congenital malformations.

The risk that a congenital malformation will recur with subsequent pregnancies depends on the specific abnormality and its cause. For the three most common neurologic malformations, anencephaly, hydrocephalus, and spina bifida, the recurrence rate in subsequent children is approximately 4 per cent after the first malformation, but much higher after two malformations. If it is recalled that the recurrence rate for a simple recessively inherited disease is 25 per cent, the role of genetic factors in congenital malformation can be put in perspective.

DRUG-INDUCED EMBRYOPATHY.   Fetal malformations may be regarded as the consequence of developmental asynchrony, and are likely to follow environmental insults during the first three months of fetal life. There is growing evidence that errors in embryonic development are particularly likely to arise between the sixth and eighth weeks. It is therefore clearly prudent to minimize frivolous medication during the first three months of pregnancy. The importance of the drugs as possible etiologic agents in congenital malformations has been emphasized, and perhaps overemphasized, by the thalidomide tragedy. Indeed, it is virtually impossible to specify a drug that will *not* result in an increased frequency of congenital malformations when administered to a sufficiently large panel of different laboratory animals. To assume that a drug that causes a congenital malformation in one species will necessarily cause one in man is as misguided as to assume that if a drug is harmless in animals, it will be harmless in man. It is certainly worth emphasizing that had thalidomide merely increased the frequency of a common malformation, such as cleft lip or cleft palate, rather than the strikingly tragic malformation of phocomelia ("seal extremities"), the causal association might still be unrecognized. During the two- to three-year period during which thalidomide (alpha-phthalimidoglutarimide) was freely available, approximately 7000 infants throughout the world were born with thalidomide-induced deformities.

Although convincing evidence of teratogenicity can be claimed only for thalidomide, steroid hormones, and folate antagonists, suspicion has fallen on alcohol, anticonvulsants, which may act by causing folate deficiency, warfarin, and an operating room environment (generally assumed to be related to anesthetic gases). Lysergic acid diethylamide (LSD) is mischievously and dangerously toxic, but whether it causes congenital malformations remains unproved.

Warkany, J.: Congenital Malformations. Chicago, Year Book Medical Publishers, 1971.

18. CHROMOSOMES AND THEIR DISORDERS

Park Gerald

18.1. INTRODUCTION

Modern human cytogenetics began in 1956, when Tjio and Levan employed techniques that had been created for use with other organisms to demonstrate the presence of 46 chromosomes (23 pairs) in cultured human fibroblasts. The field became of major medical importance with the observation in 1959 that an additional chromosome was present in patients with Down's syndrome (mongolism). It was soon thereafter brought to clinical maturity when simple means were discovered for obtaining chromosome preparations with cultured leukocytes from peripheral blood.

Modern cytogenetics entered its second and present period of growth with the introduction of a fluorescent stain which permitted identification of each of the 22 pairs of non-sex chromosomes (autosomes) as well as the 2 sex chromosomes (XX in the female and XY in the male). Additional staining procedures have since been developed which provide further evidence for the uniqueness of each chromosome pair and even of individual regions within chromosomes.

FREQUENCY OF CHROMOSOMAL ABNORMALITIES. Chromosomal abnormalities occur with greatly different frequencies at various times in life. The highest frequency and the greatest variety are found among spontaneous abortuses, 30 to 40 per cent of whom have a major chromosomal defect. Among liveborn infants, about 6 per 1000 have a chromosomal defect sufficiently severe to cause disability at some time in their lives. About half of these abnormalities involve the autosomes, whereas the remainder are sex chromosomal disorders. Among adults in the general population, the abnormalities are largely confined to the sex chromosomal disorders.

There are clinically definable subgroups within these population segments that have an increased risk for a chromosomal disorder. Infants with multiple congenital defects, for example, have a 5 to 10 per cent probability of possessing a major autosomal abnormality. The occurrence in a family of individuals with a similar group of congenital malformations is often the result of an inheritable chromosomal disorder. Such families may also have an increased number of spontaneous abortions. Sex chromosomal disorders occur with increased frequency among infertile males and among women with primary amenorrhea. They are also found to be unusually frequent among males incarcerated in penal institutions.

PREPARATION OF CELLS FOR CHROMOSOMAL ANALYSIS. The chromosomes in the nondividing (interphase) cell are so extended and intertwined that they cannot be individually distinguished. During cell division (mitosis), however, they become greatly condensed and are then visible as separate entities. Dividing cells can be arrested in that phase of mitosis (metaphase) at which the chromosomes are most contracted by treatment with colchicine. By the use of colchicine and by swelling the cells in hypotonic solution to increase the separation of the chromosomes, preparations can be produced in which each chromosome is clearly visible.

Dividing cells can be obtained directly from bone marrow or by culturing a small piece of skin. The procedure required for obtaining either of these specimens, however, is unpleasant for the patient. In addition, skin cells must be cultured for several weeks before a sufficient number of dividing cells is present. Fortunately, the normally nondividing leukocyte from peripheral blood can be stimulated to divide when exposed to phytohemagglutinin (PHA). PHA appears to act only on lymphocytes (specifically, the so-called T cell). Stimulated lymphocytes undergo a transient wave of mitoses that reaches a peak in three to four days. By a combination of PHA, colchicine, and hypotonic treatments, suitable chromosome preparations can be obtained from a few drops of capillary blood.

In view of the simplicity of the procedure, most chromosomal analyses are now carried out with peripheral blood specimens. Bone marrow cells may nonetheless be used in the study of diseases, such as myelogenous leukemia, which are confined to these cells. Skin cells may be examined when a difference between the skin cell and lymphocyte chromosome complement is suspected, or when blood samples cannot be obtained, as in abortuses.

AMNIOCENTESIS. The amniotic fluid comprises a special source of fetal cells which has attained great practical importance in recent years. Ten to 20 ml of fluid can be withdrawn with apparent safety as early as the fourteenth to fifteenth week of gestation. The amniotic cells may be examined directly for sex determination by staining for the Barr body (sex chromatin mass) or for the F body, as will be described later. More commonly, they are cultured and the dividing cells are treated to obtain metaphase preparations by the methods previously mentioned. Amniotic cells are unusual in that tetraploid cells (cells with two complete chromosomal complements) occur with significant frequency even when the fetus is cytologically normal. This may indicate that amniotic cells may arise in part from the fetal membranes and may not be totally representative of the fetus proper. Chromosomal examination of the fetus may alter in the future if procedures to obtain

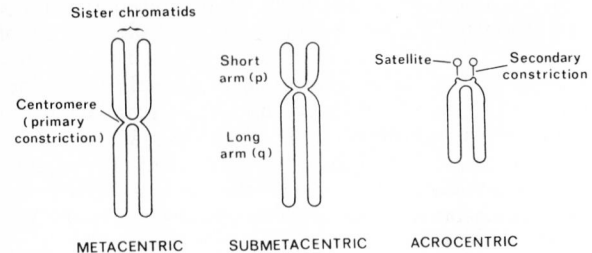

Figure 1. Schematic representation of human metaphase chromosomes and the terms commonly used to describe their gross morphologic features.

fetal blood or skin biopsies through an amnioscope can be simplified.

Amniocentesis for chromosomal analysis can be con-

sidered for those pregnancies in which the risk of a chromosomally abnormal fetus is thought to be significantly greater than the risk of damage to the fetus from the amniocentesis procedure itself (see Ch. 20).

METHODS OF CHROMOSOME IDENTIFICATION. The chromosomes present in metaphase have replicated but have not yet longitudinally divided, as would have occurred if mitosis had proceeded further. The unseparated parts are known as *sister chromatids*, or *chromatids*, and remain attached together at the centromere (Fig. 1). This leads to an X-like or inverted V configuration. The portions of a chromatid extending above and below the centromere are the chromosome arms. Chromosomes are described as metacentric, submetacentric, or acrocentric, according to the position of the centromere (Fig. 1). The acrocentric chromosomes usually possess a small amount of chromosomal material, called a satel-

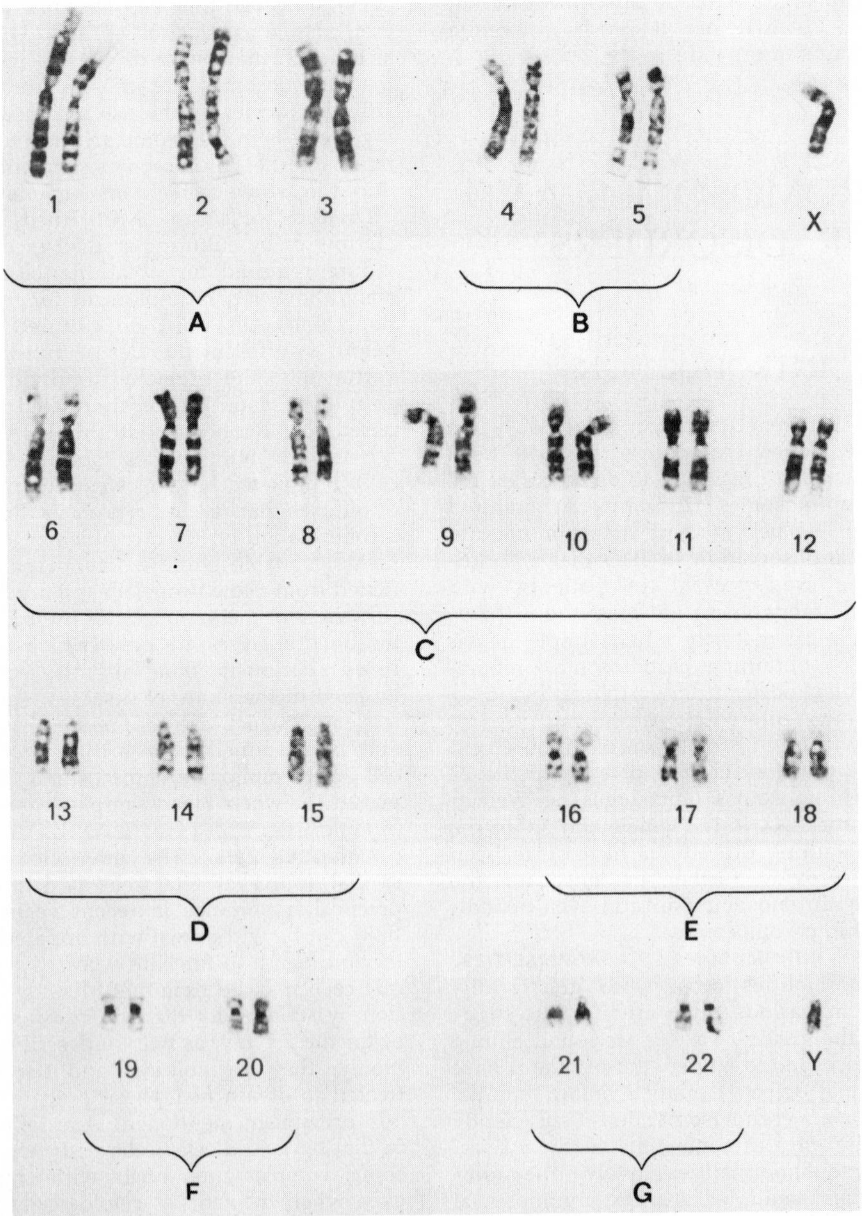

Figure 2. Karyotype of a normal male cell stained by the trypsin-Giemsa banding technique. Each chromosome pair can be identified and is given a specific number. The group designation (A, B, C, etc.), used before identification of individual chromosomes was possible, is also shown. The X chromosome in that system was classified in the C group, and the Y was frequently included in the G group. (Constructed from a karyotype kindly provided by Dr. K. Hirschhorn.)

lite, connected to the short arm by a constricted region (the secondary constriction). Secondary constrictions are also found near the centromere on the long arms of chromosomes 1, 9, and 16.

When conventional stains are used, the chromosomes display no longitudinal features other than the centromere and secondary constrictions (Fig. 1). When certain fluorescent stains, such as quinacrine mustard, are applied directly or when Giemsa stain is used after various pretreatments (e.g., trypsin, urea, heat), the chromosomes display a characteristic banded appearance (Fig. 2). The location and morphology of the individual bands in each chromosome are sufficiently constant that a system of nomenclature for each band has been devised (Fig. 3). This is becoming of great importance, because it is now possible to associate a particular gene with a particular band by such techniques as somatic cell hybridization.

The chromosomes from a single metaphase are customarily arranged in a standardized format, known as a *karyotype* (Fig. 2). Conventionally, the chromosomes are arranged in pairs and are ordered on the basis of decreasing length. Since the chromosome pairs could not be individually identified when the first karyotypes were prepared, chromosomes with similar morphology were originally classified into groups (A to G). Now that each pair can be recognized, the autosomes are numbered from 1 to 22, and the sex chromosomes are identified as X and Y (Fig. 2).

NOMENCLATURE FOR CHROMOSOMAL ABNORMALITIES. In the shorthand notation now generally used to describe the chromosome complement of an individual, the number of chromosomes is specified first, followed by the listing of the sex chromosomes. In this notation the normal female karyotype is 46,XX and the normal male is 46,XY. Any deviations from the normal karyotype are written after the sex chromosome listing. An individual autosome is referred to by number, its upper (shorter) arm by p and its lower arm by q. A plus or a minus sign written *after* the p or q indicates an increase (+) or decrease (−) in length of the arm. When written before a designated chromosome, the sign indicates that the chromosome is extra (+) or missing (−). (Examples: 46,XY, 18q− describes a male with 46 chromosomes, including one chromosome 18 whose long arm is diminished in length; 47,XX,+21 describes a female with 47 chromosomes, including an extra chromosome 21 in addition to the 46 chromosomes of the normal karyotype.)

THE BARR BODY AND THE F BODY. Despite the detail revealed by the various banding techniques, most are unable to distinguish between the two X chromosomes of the normal female. It is known that only one X chromosome is active in any cell; each X chromosome in excess of one condenses to form a sex chromatin mass (Barr body) visible at the periphery of the nucleus. The number of X chromosomes may be indirectly determined by examination of buccal mucosal cells for the number of Barr bodies.

Condensed, inactive X chromosomes are also delayed in the timing of their DNA synthesis, relative to the active X chromosome. The late-replicating X chromosome can be identified by autoradiography using tritiated thymidine, or by the incorporation into DNA of 5-bromodeoxyuridine (BUDR) in place of thymidine followed by staining with a dye that differentiates between BUDR and thymidine (the Hoechst-BUDR technique).

In over 99 per cent of males, the distal part of the long arm of the Y chromosome fluoresces brilliantly after staining with quinacrine. The intensity is sufficiently great that this region can be seen as a spot of fluorescence, the F body, in the interphase nucleus. Y-bearing cells can thereby be recognized in cells from blood, hair follicles, and tissue sections, and even in sperm.

POLYMORPHIC VARIATIONS IN THE HUMAN KARYOTYPE. In addition to those alterations in the karyotype which are directly or potentially associated with disease, some variations are known which are apparently without consequence to the individual who possesses them or to his progeny. These polymorphic variations, as they are called, may represent changes in the DNA sequence of the chromosomal region concerned. They are transmitted to progeny as part of the chromosome which contains them. The more commonly recognized variations of this type occur in the length of the short arms of the acrocentric chromosomes, the size of their satellites, the length of the fluorescent segment in the long arm of the Y, and the length of the secondary constrictions of 1, 9, and 16.

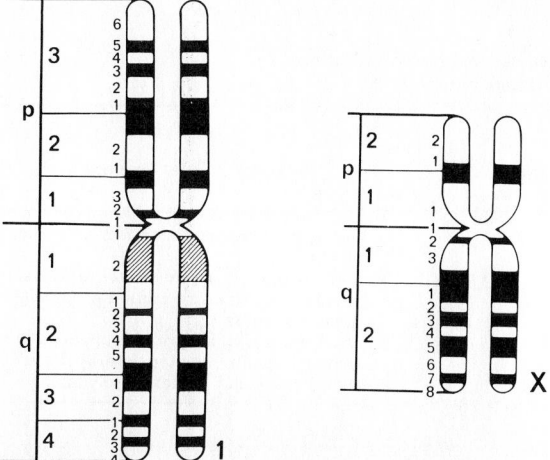

Figure 3. Schematic representation of human chromosomes 1 and X, showing their standardized banding patterns. A numbering system for the individual bands was adopted at the Paris conference (1971) on Standardization in Human Cytogenetics (Birth Defects Original Article Series, 8:1, 1972). The Rh blood group locus is in chromosome 1 near band 34 on the short arm. The loci for the following enzymes have been tentatively localized to the long arm of the X: phosphoglycerate kinase, hypoxanthine-guanine phosphoribosyl transferase, and glucose-6-phosphate dehydrogenase.

18.2.   MEIOTIC AND MITOTIC NONDISJUNCTION

MEIOTIC NONDISJUNCTION. Since gametes (sperm or ova) contain only half as much genetic material as a somatic cell, the behavior of the chromosomes during their formation is obviously a unique process, to which the term meiosis is applied. Of the many steps involved in meiosis, those of concern here are only the steps that lead to a reduction in the chromosome number from 46 in the precursor cell to 23 in the ga-

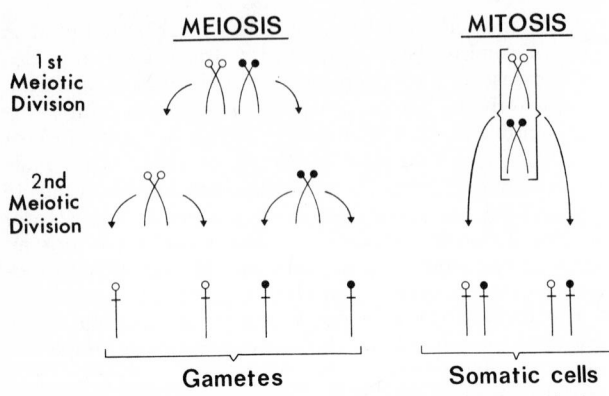

Figure 4. Schematic representation of the behavior during meiosis of a single pair of acrocentric chromosomes, contrasted with their behavior during mitosis. The round bodies on the short arms represent the satellites which are characteristically present on acrocentric chromosomes.

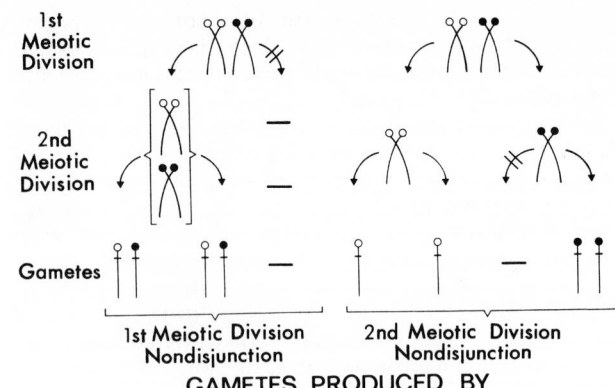

GAMETES PRODUCED BY NONDISJUNCTION

Figure 5. Production of gametes with an altered number of chromosomes by the two types of meiotic nondisjunction. When polymorphic variation in the satellites of acrocentric chromosomes occurs, a distinction may be made between first and second meiotic nondisjunction of these chromosomes.

mete. Meiosis consists of two successive stages of divisions (Fig. 4). During first meiotic division, each replicated chromosome pairs with its identical partner. Next, each member of a pair enters one of the two new daughter cells formed. During second meiotic division, sister chromatids separate at the centromere, analogous to their behavior in mitosis, and the two new chromosomes enter the two daughter cells produced at this stage (Fig. 4). Of the four cells formed from a gonadal precursor cell, each contains one chromosome from every autosomal pair and one sex chromosome (either an X or Y). (In the formation of the female sex cell, only one of the four cells becomes a functional ovum. In the male, all four cells become spermatozoa.)

Maintenance of the normal chromosome number in the gametes requires the separation of the paired chromosomes at first meiotic division and the separation of sister chromatids at second meiotic division. The failure to disjoin properly (nondisjunction) at either first or

second meiotic division will produce gametes with abnormal numbers of chromosomes (Fig. 5). This will result in formation of an individual with an abnormal number of chromosomes in each cell. By using marker genes or polymorphic variations (Fig. 5), it is sometimes possible to identify the parent in whom the nondisjunction occurred and even to distinguish between first and second meiotic division nondisjunction. It is now known that nondisjunction can occur during gametogenesis in either the male or the female and during either first or second meiotic division. Some types of meiotic errors, however, are more likely to be associated with certain kinds of chromosomal abnormalities than with others (see below).

MITOTIC NONDISJUNCTION. Mitosis resembles second meiotic division in that sister chromatids become separated, with one of the two newly formed chromosomes

Clinical and Cytogenetic Characteristics of Common Syndromes Associated with Change in Chromosome Number

Autosomal Abnormalities	Common Name	Approximate Frequency among Liveborn Infants	Mechanism of Origin	Major Clinical Findings
47, +21	Trisomy-21 or Down's syndrome	1:1000	Frequently maternal first meiotic division nondisjunction	Mental retardation, abnormal brain development (microgyria), characteristic facies, marked hypotonia
47, +18	Trisomy 18 or Edwards' syndrome	1:11,000	Meiotic nondisjunction	Mental retardation, severe failure to thrive, periarticular limitation of motion of distal interphalangeal joints
47, +13	Trisomy 13 or Patau's syndrome	1:15,000	Meiotic nondisjunction	Mental retardation, abnormal brain development (arrhinencephaly), cleft palate (and cleft lip), ocular colobomata, postaxial polydactyly
Sex Chromosomal Abnormalities				
45, X (45, XO)	Turner's syndrome	1:6000	Maternal (22%) or paternal (78%) meiotic nondisjunction	Short stature, failure of secondary sexual development, pterygium colli, neonatal edema of hands and feet
47, XXX	Triple X syndrome	1:2000	Possibly maternal meiotic nondisjunction	Usually clinically normal; may be mentally retarded and deficient in secondary sexual development
47, XXY	Klinefelter's syndrome	1:2000	Maternal (61%) or paternal (39%) meiotic nondisjunction	Mild increase in stature, micro-orchidism, infertility, gynecomastia, behavioral changes
47, XYY	XYY syndrome	1:2000	Paternal second meiotic division nondisjunction	Significantly increased stature, behavioral changes

going to each of the daughter cells. Failure of separation (mitotic nondisjunction) of the chromatids may occur and lead to creation of two cell lines, one with 47 chromosomes and one with 45 chromosomes. If mitotic nondisjunction occurs at the first cleavage division of the zygote (the cell formed by union of ovum and sperm), an individual with two cell lines (if both cell lines are viable), neither of which is normal in karyotype, will result. If mitotic nondisjunction occurs subsequent to the first cleavage division, a third and normal cell line will be present.

Individuals with two or more chromosomally distinct cell types are referred to as mosaics. Mosaicism usually results from mitotic nondisjunction or anaphase lag loss. In the latter, sister chromatids separate properly at mitosis, but one of the newly formed chromosomes fails to be incorporated in a daughter cell. This leads to creation of a new cell line with one chromosome less than the main cell line.

18.3. CHANGES IN CHROMOSOME NUMBER

Chromosomal abnormalities limited to a change in chromosome number are usually the consequence of nondisjunctional errors. This abnormality is much more common than the group of disorders which result from change in chromosomal structure. The presence of an additional autosome (trisomy) occurs with reasonable frequency, whereas the absence of an autosome is almost never found among liveborn individuals.

A change in the number of sex chromosomes is less deleterious than a change in the number of autosomes. Individuals with as many as three extra sex chromosomes are able to survive, although they are usually mentally defective and congenitally malformed. Individuals with a single sex chromosome (one X chromosome) are, surprisingly, only moderately affected. Individuals with only Y chromosomes, that is, without any X chromosome, have never been found.

The clinical features associated with the more frequently encountered changes in chromosome number are given in the accompanying table. Each type of chromosomal aberration is associated with a relatively characteristic group of clinical findings. It is therefore highly probable that the clinical findings associated with each chromosomal aberration are at least in part determined by the specific genes present on the chromosome involved.

18.4. CHANGES IN CHROMOSOMAL STRUCTURE

CHROMOSOMAL BREAKAGE. Changes in chromosomal structure are largely the consequence of chromosomal breakage. The constancy of the human karyotype from cell to cell and from individual to individual conceals the true frequency with which the continuity of the genetic material is interrupted. In most instances, a break in a chromosome is quickly repaired, with restoration of the normal chromosome structure and without harmful consequences. The exceptions to this are of two kinds and include, on the one hand, the produc-

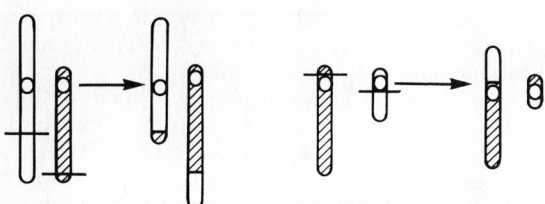

A. Reciprocal Translocation   B. Reciprocal Translocation, Centric Fusion Type

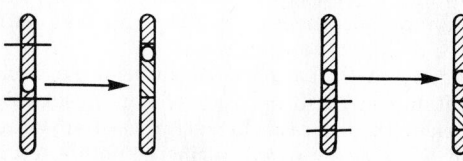

C. Inversion (Pericentric)   D. Inversion (Paracentric)

Figure 6. Schematic representation of the mechanisms underlying some types of chromosomal rearrangements. The horizontal lines represent the points of chromosomal breakage and reunion. The chromosomes are depicted as having single chromatids (i.e., they are unreplicated). It is not known, however, whether rearrangements usually occur before or after replication.

tion of chromosomal rearrangements and, on the other hand, diseases characterized by the presence of unrepaired chromosomal breaks.

CHROMOSOMAL REARRANGEMENTS; RECIPROCAL TRANSLOCATIONS. If two or more chromosomal breaks occur simultaneously in the same cell, the repair process occasionally may unite the chromosomal fragments incorrectly, with production of a chromosomal rearrangement (Fig. 6). One of the most common rearrangements encountered is that which is produced by an exchange of terminal chromosomal segments between two different chromosomes, with formation of a reciprocal translocation (Fig. 6A). A reciprocal translocation occurring between two acrocentrics, with the chromosomal breakpoints in each being located very near to the centromere, is given the special name of *centric fusion translocation* (Fig. 6B). The two most common rearrangements observed in man are centric fusions between chromosomes 14 and 21 and between chromosomes 13 and 14. The minute chromosome produced during a centric fusion translocation (Fig. 6B) is usually lost so that a cell with only 45 chromosomes results. The minute chromosome appears to have little essential genetic material, because its loss has no effect on the cell or the individual.

The types of rearrangement illustrated in Figure 6 apparently produce no change in the amount of genetic material in the cells in which they occur. Such rearrangements are described as *balanced rearrangements,* and the individuals who possess them are carriers of the balanced rearrangement.

TRANSMISSION OF A RECIPROCAL TRANSLOCATION. When meiosis occurs in a reciprocal translocation carrier, the translocated chromosomes will pair with each other, as well as with their untranslocated partners. Separation of the individual members of this pairing group is often quite abnormal, with any one, two, three, or four chromosomes of the group being incorporated in a single gamete. Since gross amounts of genetic imbalance are poorly tolerated, only a few of the possible abnormal types of progeny will be liveborn. The remaining abnormal types may appear as abortuses or may not be detected at all (because the embryo expires before implantation).

The variety of liveborn progeny expected depends dramatically upon the specific reciprocal translocation. A carrier of a centric fusion translocation between chromosomes 14 and 21, for example, will produce equal numbers of children with the balanced rearrangement and children who are chromosomally normal. A smaller number will have the genetic equivalent of an extra chromosome 21 (and have Down's syndrome), the only type of abnormal progeny produced by this rearrangement able to survive until birth.

Individuals with balanced or unbalanced reciprocal translocation may also be born of chromosomally normal parents. In this case the reciprocal translocation is assumed to have originated during gametogenesis.

Occasionally, a somatic cell may develop a chromosomal rearrangement which may then be passed on to its cellular descendants. This has been observed particularly in some forms of leukemia and in some solid tumors. Chronic myelogenous leukemia, for example, is characterized by a rearrangement (probably a reciprocal translocation) occurring in the leukemic cell which involves chromosome 22 and another autosome, usually chromosome 9. One chromosome 22 in this case has the appearance of a 22q− and is referred to as the Philadelphia chromosome (Ph[1]) (see Ch. 498.1).

CHROMOSOMAL REARRANGEMENTS; DELETIONS. A chromosome may undergo breakage so that an interstitial or a terminal segment of one arm is lost. These abnormalities are known as *chromosomal deletions*. In general they are sporadic, because the abnormality is not present in the ancestors of the affected individual. The loss of genetic material leads to production of multiple congenital malformations if an autosome is involved or to abnormal sexual development if a sex chromosome is affected. The most commonly encountered autosomal chromosomal deletion syndromes have the karyotypes 46,XX or XY,5p− (the cri du chat syndrome) and 46,XX or XY, 18q−.

DISEASES ASSOCIATED WITH UNREPAIRED CHROMOSOMAL BREAKS. There are three diseases (Bloom's syndrome, Fanconi's anemia, and ataxia telangiectasia) now known in which unrepaired chromosomal breakage commonly occurs with several times the frequency observed in normal individuals. Each of these diseases is inherited as an autosomal recessive condition. In addition to the unrepaired breaks, other cytogenetic abnormalities are present with an abnormally high frequency. These include chromosomal rearrangements, deletions, "fusion figures," and *endoreduplication* (in Fanconi's anemia). The fusion figures appear to result from a break in a single chromatid in each of two chromosomes, followed by union of the ends from nonsister chromatids. Endoreduplication is a different type of cytogenetic abnormality and results when two cycles of chromosomal replication occur without an intervening cell division — each metaphase chromosome possesses four juxtaposed sister chromatids instead of the normal two. Although chromosomal breaks and rearrangements as well as fusion figures are perhaps likely consequences of an abnormality in the DNA repair process, it is not yet possible to visualize a rational connection of this with endoreduplication.

Clinically, these three syndromes are also associated with congenital malformations and a predisposition to malignancy. This latter may also be the consequence of an alteration in a DNA repair process. By a modification of the Hoechst-BUDR technique, sister chromatids can be differentially stained. This permits the demonstration of the exchange of chromosomal segments between sister chromatids (sister chromatid exchanges). Sister chromatid exchanges (SCE) occur with considerable frequency in cells exposed to certain DNA-damaging agents, which suggests that they may be the result of repair of DNA. In Bloom's syndrome, SCE occur with *increased* frequency even without known exposure to DNA damaging agents, whereas in Fanconi's anemia SCE occur with unusually *low* frequency after such exposure.

de Grouchy, J., and Turleau, C.: Clinical Atlas of Human Chromosomes. New York, John Wiley & Sons, 1977.

Ford, E. H. R.: Human Chromosomes. New York, Academic Press, 1973.

Latt, S. A.: Optical studies of metaphase chromosome organization. Ann. Rev. Biophysics Bioengineering, 5:1, 1976.

Levine, H.: Clinical Cytogenetics. Boston, Little, Brown & Company, 1971.

Yunis, J. J.: New Chromosomal Syndromes. New York, Academic Press, 1977.

19. PREVENTION AND MANAGEMENT OF GENETIC DISEASE

Alexander G. Bearn

The cardinal principles underlying the prevention and management of disease are similar, whether the disease is determined primarily by environmental agents or by genetic influences; in both instances accurate diagnosis is a prerequisite. Treatment of the patient with inherited disease must not depend exclusively on alleviation of the metabolic defect; symptomatic treatment is often of the greatest value, and the need for sympathetic handling of a patient with a disease that is inherited, and which may be transmitted to subsequent generations, is paramount.

Although in this chapter considerable emphasis is placed on specific, individually rare, genetic syndromes, it must be realized that the magnitude of the genetic component in the causation of all disease must be assessed if control and treatment of the disease are to be optimal. Indeed, it has been a tragic misconception, too long held, that in contrast to disease caused by environmental agents, there is no effective prevention or treatment for inherited diseases. This misguided view is quickly drained of validity when it is remembered that the expression of a disease process requires the interaction of environmental and genetic influences. Realization that 20 per cent of the hyperlipidemic survivors of a myocardial infarct occurring under the age of 60 suffer from a monogenic inherited hyperlipidemic disorder suggests that it is prudent to investigate the first-degree relatives of such individuals to ascertain those particularly at risk. Moreover, an understanding of the genetic aspects of such common diseases as obesity, hypertension, and emphysema is necessary for a comprehensive approach to prevention and management. Furthermore, an awareness of genetic influences in the metabolism of many drugs will increase the effectiveness of a physician confronted with a variety of puzzling clinical syndromes.

In the balance of this chapter attention is drawn, in particular, to those specific modalities of treatment which can be applied to inherited disease, and which stem from an understanding of the nature of the primary molecular defect. Therapeutic manipulation of the cellular environment in which the gene must display its nature is an approach more tractable and less perilous than direct interference with the genetic material itself.

RESTRICTION OF SUBSTRATE. General dietary restriction is often an effective way to reduce the excessive substrate that accumulates behind an inherited metabolic block. A general reduction in protein intake will improve the clinical manifestations of a number of rare inherited diseases affecting the urea cycle, including argininosuccinicaciduria, citrullinemia, and hyperammonemia. In some rather more common diseases, such as phenylketonuria and galactosemia, specific dietary restrictions are needed. The elimination of phenylalanine from the diet of phenylketonuric infants, if instituted before two years of age, is increasingly recognized as effective therapy. Similarly, elimination of galactose in the neonatal period for patients with galactosemia has resulted in an increased mental alertness, as well as the prevention of cataracts in those individuals who have a recessively inherited galactokinase deficiency. Defective oxidation of phytanic acid is the specific inherited defect in Refsum's disease; dietary restriction of this lipid will significantly ameliorate the symptoms of this disorder.

REPLACEMENT OF THE BIOLOGICALLY ACTIVE END-PRODUCT. An inherited enzymatic defect will lead not only to an accumulation of the substrate on which the enzyme normally acts but also to a decrease in the end-product. When the end-product is of key biologic importance, simple replacement will overcome the consequences of the metabolic block. Many instances of familial goiter associated with a deficiency of a specific enzyme can be effectively prevented by the administration of thyroid hormone. Human growth hormone is effective treatment for the recessively inherited form of pituitary dwarfism, and the ill effects of X-linked diabetes insipidus can be prevented by supplying antidiuretic hormone. Oroticaciduria, in which there is an inherited deficiency of enzymes that transform orotic acid to uridine, can be circumvented by providing the uridine-starved cells with an increase in the uridine of the diet. Dietary phosphorus will overcome the excessive urinary loss of phosphate in X-linked hypophosphatemic rickets, and administration of dietary copper will effectively combat the inherited copper deficiency of Menkes' syndrome.

REMOVAL OF THE ACCUMULATION OF SUBSTRATE. In some hereditary diseases the accumulation of a "toxic product" may be responsible for the manifestations of the disease, and removal of the excess material may reverse the phenotypic consequences of the abnormal gene. Removal of the increased tissue copper in Wilson's disease by penicillamine is a particularly striking example of the effectiveness of this form of treatment. Similarly, removal of iron in hemochromatosis by phlebotomy is another example of therapy designed to remove accumulated toxic material.

AMPLIFICATION OF ENZYMATIC ACTIVITY. Active efforts are being directed toward increasing the residual enzymatic activity that is usually present in patients with autosomal recessively inherited diseases. The administration of barbiturates, for example, to patients with the Crigler-Najjar syndrome has been found to increase the activity of the enzyme glucuronyl transferase, and simultaneously to decrease the serum bilirubin level.

Many biologically important enzymes require essential cofactors for their activity. In some inborn errors of metabolism the mutational event affects the ability of the enzyme to combine with cofactor. Pyridoxine (vitamin B_6) is a cofactor for the enzyme cystathionine synthetase. In more than half the patients with homocystinuria, in whom there is a decrease in activity of this enzyme, the defect can be overcome by administration of large doses of pyridoxine (500 mg per day). Similarly, the metabolic ketoacidosis of some patients with methylmalonic aciduria can be overcome by the administration of pharmacologic doses of the cofactor vitamin B_{12}.

ENZYME REPLACEMENT. Direct replacement of the missing enzyme (or nonenzymatic protein) is an attractive and direct approach to the treatment of recessively inherited disease, and although there are a number of substantial obstacles to this simple concept, progress is being made. It should be emphasized, however, that to be effective the enzyme not only must retain its biologic activity when administered to the patient but must also gain access to the organs and cellular organelles in which excessive substrate has accumulated. Moreover, since the infused enzyme will have a finite half-life, continuous administration or gradual release from an implanted "depot store" must be achieved. Enzyme infusions have been attempted in the mucopolysaccharidoses, in which their therapeutic effect is still unproved, and in metachromatic leukodystrophy, in which the effect is rather more promising.

MODIFYING MUTANT PROTEIN. Although modification of hemoglobin by carbamylation of valine at position 6 in the beta polypeptide chain of hemoglobin S by cyanate has a profound antisickling effect in vitro, severe toxic reactions, such as peripheral neuropathy, sharply limit its clinical usefulness. This approach to the modification of mutant proteins, however, holds much promise for the future.

SURGICAL TREATMENT. Numerous examples of the application of surgery to the treatment of inherited disease could be cited. This is particularly likely to be effective in diseases transmitted in a mendelian dominant fashion. The prevention of neoplastic transformation in polyposis of the colon and the removal of the spleen in hereditary spherocytosis are examples of inherited diseases in which surgery can play an important therapeutic role. It should not be overlooked that surgery is a quick and permanent cure for polydactyly as well as for certain other dominantly inherited defects.

Allotransplantation of the organ in which the deficient enzyme is normally synthesized has been attempted in a variety of inherited diseases. Renal transplantation has been performed in patients with Fabry's disease and in cystinosis. In Fabry's disease renal transplantation appears to ameliorate the manifestations; in cystinosis allotransplantation is effective in overcoming uremic nephropathy but does not affect the disease itself. Although in general the results are encouraging, considerably more work will be needed before organ transplantation can be recommended as a routine therapeutic measure in any inborn error of metabolism. Bone marrow transplantation is presently the only effective therapy in patients with severe combined immunodeficiency disease.

20. GENETIC COUNSELING
Arno G. Motulsky

Genetic counseling includes a range of medical, genetic, and communication activities. Diagnosis of the underlying disease is followed by assessing the risks of genetic recurrence and providing information concerning these risks to the patient, to parents, or to other family members as may be required. Ideal genetic counseling should allow the individual or family to understand the full medical and genetic facts; the natural history of the disease, including its variability from patient to patient; the available modes of management; and the potential personal, economic, psychologic, and social burdens. All possible reproductive options and their advantages and disadvantages should be explained. The patient or the family should be helped to choose the most appropriate course of action considering the genetic risks, the family needs, and the ethical and religious standards of the family. Alleviation of guilt will frequently be required. Since genetic factors play an etiologic role in many different diseases, genetic counseling has become an important component of patient management. If there is a significant risk that a given disease will recur in future children, physicians should provide or arrange for genetic counseling even if the patient or parents do not specifically request such advice. Occasionally it may be appropriate to give firm and directive advice. More generally, genetic counseling should be nondirective and should provide the necessary information to allow a couple to make their own decision regarding future reproduction. The physician in his role of genetic counselor should not force his values on those who seek his advice.

DIAGNOSIS. Accurate diagnosis is a prerequisite for genetic counseling. Similar-appearing diseases may be inherited by different modes of transmission (heterogeneity) or may not be genetic at all. Apparently identical genetic diseases caused by different gene mutations may be of variable severity and carry a different burden ranging from trivial symptoms to extensive suffering. Accurate diagnosis requires a carefully obtained family history, which is best denoted by conventional pedigree symbols. Information about relatives regarding age, onset of a given disease, health status, and cause of death is obtained. Knowledge of the ethnic origin of the family may be helpful in considering certain genetic diseases; Tay-Sachs disease is common in Jews of European origin, and cystic fibrosis is rare in blacks. Advanced maternal age is a predisposing factor to chromosomal errors such as Down's and Klinefelter's syndromes. Advanced paternal age may be found when new mutations for autosomal dominant diseases such as Marfan's disease or achondroplasia are suspected. Historic data on the immediate family are more accurate than information regarding more remote relatives. Occasionally physicians' and hospital records have to

be obtained for documentation of suspected diseases. Genetic diseases manifesting anomalies of stature or a characteristic physiognomy can sometimes be recognized in photographs of family members. If the parents are related, or if both the father's and mother's ancestors originated from a restricted rural area, autosomal recessive inheritance should be considered as the possible cause for an obscure disease. The mode of inheritance together with the clinical and laboratory findings of a given patient may be helpful in defining various subtypes of clinically similar-appearing genetic disorders such as Hurler's (autosomal recessive) and Hunter's (X-linked recessive) diseases, or Marfan's disease (autosomal dominant) and homocystinuria (autosomal recessive). Diagnosis and appropriate counseling for the majority of genetic diseases require knowledge of the clinical and genetic features of the disease rather than special "genetic tests." Suitable cytogenetic and enzymatic tests should be available in the investigation of some conditions. Some patients with complex birth defects or mental retardation and many patients with gonadal and other sexual abnormalities have various cytogenetic aberrations. Most of the patients owe their abnormal karyotype to isolated events, and their parents have normal chromosomes. Cytogenetic family investigations are therefore only rarely indicated. Four to 8 per cent of couples with repeated spontaneous abortions have chromosomal translocations carried in a balanced state by one of the parents. Chromosomal analysis using banding techniques is indicated in such situations.

RECURRENCE RISKS. If a disease is transmitted by a mendelian or monogenic pattern, recurrence risks can be well defined (Table 1). Lack of clinical manifestation (diminished penetrance), variable expression, or late onset is particularly frequent in autosomal dominant disorders. In addition to the information that a given gene will be transmitted with a certain probability, the actual recurrence risk of the clinical symptomatology and the risk for severe manifestations associated with that gene must be communicated to the patient. Thus, although the risk for coronary heart diseases among patients with familial hypercholesterolemia is high, about one half of men and women by the age of 50 years and 60 years, respectively, will not exhibit clinical manifestations of coronary heart disease. About 5 per cent of all men with myocardial infarction aged 60 or below carry the gene for familial hypercholesterolemia. Some genetic diseases transmitted by an autosomal dominant mechanism, such as polycystic kidneys and Huntington's chorea, usually only express themselves clinically in the middle aged. The risk for unaffected offspring of patients, which is 50 per cent at birth, becomes progressively less as a person remains unaffected beyond the age at which these diseases first manifest. Curves plotting the age of onset can be used to quantitate these risks more precisely. McKusick's catalogue of mendelian disorders gives helpful short descriptions and literature citations for the known mendelian genetic diseases. Many human genes have been assigned to their specific chromosomal location in recent years. It will be occasionally possible to detect the affected gene carriers for a disease by studying the segregation of closely linked marker genes in families in which variants for the marker gene exist (e.g., G6PD variants and hemophilia on the X chromosome; HLA genes,

TABLE 1. Risks for Rare Mendelian Disorders in Families

Mode of Inheritance	First Degree Relatives at Risk	Risk	Other Relatives at Risk	Risk
Autosomal dominant	Sibs, parents, children (both sexes)	50%	Uncles, aunts, nephews, nieces	25%
			First cousins	12.5%
Autosomal recessive	Sibs (both sexes)	25%	Uncles, aunts, nephews, nieces, cousins	Negligible
	Children	Negligible*		
X-linked recessive	Brothers	50%†	Maternal uncle	50%†
	Sisters (carriers)	25%†	Maternal aunt (carrier)	50%†
			Maternal male cousin	25%†
			Maternal female cousin (carrier)	25%†

*Risks for children of patients affected with common autosomal recessive diseases depend upon gene frequency (highest risk [2%] for sickle cell anemia [0.08×0.25]).

†Risks are negligible when the disease in an affected patient is caused by a new mutation. Recent work suggests that the proportion of new mutations may be much less than the expected 33 per cent in X-linked lethal diseases.

PGM_3, glyoxalase, and a type of spinocerebellar ataxia on chromosome 6; secretor gene and myotonic dystrophy on a yet unassigned chromosome).

Genetic counseling in the multifactorial conditions (birth defects, common diseases of middle life, major psychoses) lacks the precision possible with counseling involving mendelian genes, as the number of genes and their relative contributions are usually unknown. Empiric risk figures based on the frequency of recurrence of the disease in many affected families are utilized for such counseling. The recurrence risks for sibs and children of patients affected with birth defects and malformations usually range between 3 and 5 per cent. Recurrence risks in first degree relatives (sibs, parents, children) for the more common multifactorial diseases of middle life such as hypertension, schizophrenia, and the affective disorders are in the range of 10 to 15 per cent. These risks increase when several immediate relatives are affected.

Recurrence risks for diabetes mellitus are often requested by families. These figures have been particularly difficult to estimate because of the heterogeneity of the condition. Extensive current work on the genetics of juvenile and late onset diabetes should provide better data in the near future. The risk of juvenile diabetes if there is one affected child and normal parents ranges around 10 per cent. The risk becomes lower with late age onset of diabetes in the affected patients and higher when several relatives are affected.

Risk assessment requires recognition of the occasional monogenic variant in a given common disease by careful consideration of the family history and possible differentiating clinical and laboratory features. For instance, about 1 per cent of men with gout carry the X-linked gene for HGPRT deficiency. The transmission of chromosomal aberrations, such as translocations, does not usually follow mendelian principles, and counseling must be based on empirically derived risk figures.

Absolute recurrence risks are more meaningful to a family than relative risks. A 1000-fold increase in recurrence risk for a certain disease in a family as compared with the general population appears frightening. However, for a condition which occurs in 1 of 100,000 births, a 1000-fold increase means that the absolute or actual risk of recurrence is only 1 per cent — a rather low risk. In mendelian diseases the recurrence risk is fixed (e.g., 25 per cent for autosomal recessive disease), whether several or no affected children preceded. Chance has no memory! In multifactorial diseases, if two or more first degree relatives are affected in a given family, more disease-producing genes are operative in

that sibship, and the risk for future offspring becomes higher.

COMMUNICATION. The meaning of genetic risks must be conveyed in terms understandable to patients. Qualitative terms such as "high" for 50 per cent risks, "substantial" for 25 per cent risks, and "low" for risks of 5 per cent or less may be helpful for optimal communication. The probability that approximately 3 per cent of all children of normal couples will develop serious birth defects, genetic disease, or mental retardation should be communicated as a measure against which the additional risks can be gauged. It is useful to discuss the concept of the total burden of the disease with the family. Some conditions may be very severe but invariably fatal in early life. The burden of such a disease would be less than one of somewhat later onset but associated with chronic crippling disease and prolonged suffering such as the Duchenne type of muscular dystrophy and others.

Once the significance of the recurrence risk and the contributions of heredity to the disorder have been considered, reproductive alternatives which are meaningful within the social, emotional, and religious framework of the particular family must be discussed. Since the issues under discussion may be complex and prove emotionally difficult for the patient and family or both, comprehension may not be optimal in a single interview. It has proved useful to have several sessions and to provide a written summary of the advice given, using lay language as much as possible. Since the full process of good communication can be time consuming, professionals known as "genetic associates" have been trained through programs in several colleges and universities in recent years. Such individuals have become useful for optimal communication with patients and families with genetic diseases in collaboration with medical geneticists who provide the medical and genetic expertise.

HETEROZYGOTE DETECTION. Heterozygote detection is particularly important in sisters of males affected with X-linked recessive diseases such as hemophilia and Duchenne type muscular dystrophy, because regardless of their husband's genetic constitution, there is a 50 per cent risk that the sons of female carriers will be affected. In contrast, autosomal recessive disease becomes evident only when *both* parents are carriers, and a heterozygote sib of an affected patient must mate with another heterozygote for the disease to occur. The chance that an unrelated mate will be a carrier is usually quite low. Specialized laboratory tests for carrier detection (such as creatine phosphokinase enzyme

TABLE 2.   Genetic Diseases—Carrier Detection* Advisable for Reproductive Decisions

Disorder	Mode of Inheritance	Method of Carrier Diagnosis	Preventive Measures in Carriers	Population Affected
Duchenne muscular dystrophy	X-linked	CPK level	Amniocentesis for male sex	All
Hemophilia	X-linked	AHG level and AHG cross-reactive material	Amniocentesis for male sex	All
Lesch-Nyhan syndrome	X-linked	HGPRT assay	Amniocentesis—HGPRT assay	All
Translocation Down's syndrome	Empirical recurrence risks apply	Chromosomal tests for balanced carrier	Amniocentesis—chromosomal study	All
Sickle cell anemia	Autosomal recessive	Hemoglobin electrophoresis	Genetic counseling	Blacks
β-Thalassemia major	Autosomal recessive	Red cell abnormalities, Hb A$_2$ increased	Genetic counseling	Mediterranean and tropical populations
Tay-Sachs disease	Autosomal recessive	Hexosaminidase A assay	Amniocentesis—hexosaminidase assay	Ashkenazic Jews

*Limited to translocation Down's syndrome, X-linked, and *frequent* autosomal recessive diseases. Detection of carriers for many rare inborn errors associated with enzyme deficiency is possible, but the risk for normal sibs of affected patients to have affected offspring is very small, because the frequency of the carrier state for such inborn errors is very low in the population.

assays in Duchenne muscular dystrophy and combined assay of antihemophilic globulin clotting and antigenic activity for hemophilia A) may be helpful but must be carefully standardized on normal subjects and known heterozygotes before applying them for individual carrier identification. Detection of carriers is relatively simple and accurate in the hemoglobinopathies, and an increasing number of heterozygote states for various enzyme deficiencies such as Tay-Sachs disease can be recognized. The significance of identical laboratory test results may differ, depending upon the a priori probability of the tested person being a carrier if there is overlap in laboratory values between "low" normals and "high" carriers. Tests which may be excellent for carrier detection in families may give too many "false positives" in screening studies of an extended kindred or particularly in the general population, in which the probability that the tested subject is a carrier is low. Heterozygote detection for cystic fibrosis — the most common recessive disease in the general American population — is not yet available. Some conditions for which carrier detection tests should be done are listed in Table 2.

REPRODUCTIVE OPTIONS.   Various data suggest that couples who sought genetic counseling have had fewer children if the genetic risk was more than 10 per cent

and the burden of the disease is great. If a couple decides that the risks for further reproduction are too high, several options besides contraception should be discussed. Adoption is becoming less practicable because fewer babies are available. Sterilization of either husband or wife may be considered, but it must be emphasized that this is an irreversible procedure. Thus sterilization is undesirable for prevention of autosomal recessive conditions, because remarriage after possible divorce or death could eliminate the genetic risks almost entirely. Artificial insemination by a donor other than the husband may be acceptable to rare couples to prevent autosomal recessive disease or autosomal dominant disease contributed by the husband.

INTRAUTERINE DIAGNOSIS.   Amniocentesis performed during the fourteenth to sixteenth week of pregnancy allows the diagnosis of genetic disease in fetuses. When performed by a trained gynecologist, the procedure has proved safe to mother and fetus. During amniocentesis amniotic fluid containing cells of fetal origin is aspirated transabdominally. After a 10- to 20-day period of cell culture, chromosomes can be visualized to ascertain fetal sex and to detect various chromosomal aberrations. Many enzyme deficiencies can be detected by suitable assays. An increased level of α-fetoprotein in amniotic fluid is frequently observed in spina bifida

TABLE 3.   Treatable and Preventable Adult Genetic Diseases with Autosomal Dominant Inheritance for Which Search in Family Members of Affected Patients Is Mandatory

Disorder	Method of Diagnosis	Treatment	Advantages of Early Diagnosis and Treatment
Hemochromatosis*	Liver biopsy most reliable	Venesection	Prevents liver, heart, and pancreatic disease
Hereditary spherocytosis	Incubated osmotic fragility test	Splenectomy	Prevents anemia and gallstones; protects against splenic rupture
Hereditary polyposis	Colonoscopy	Colectomy	Prevents colonic cancer
Gardner's syndrome	Colonoscopy—benign cysts, lipomas, fibromas on physical examination	Colectomy	Prevents colonic cancer
Familial hyperparathyroidism	Serum calcium, phosphorus, parathyroid hormone	Surgery	Prevents renal damage and other complications of hypercalcemia
Multiple endocrine adenomatosis	Serum calcium, phosphorus, blood sugar, gastrointestinal, skull x-ray, GI series	Surgery	Prevents complications of hyperparathyroidism, hypoglycemia, peptic ulcer, metastatic cancer
Medullary thyroid carcinoma–pheochromocytoma syndromes	Calcitonin, measurement of blood pressure	Surgery	Prevents thyroid carcinoma and complications of hypertension
Familial hypercholesterolemia	Serum cholesterol, LDL receptor	Diet, drugs?	Prevents premature coronary heart disease(?)

*Mode of genetic transmission may be autosomal recessive.

and other neural tube malformations. Amniocentesis is therefore indicated to rule out the following conditions: (1) chromosomal aberrations such as Down's syndrome, (2) detection of male fetuses who have a 50 per cent risk of being affected with serious X-linked diseases, (3) inborn errors of metabolism which can be detected by amniotic cell enzyme assay, and (4) spina bifida and anencephaly. Intrauterine diagnosis of the thalassemias and sickle cell anemia is possible in specialized laboratories following aspiration of fetal blood by placental puncture or fetoscopy and analysis of hemoglobin synthesis. Most amniocenteses are performed in pregnant women over 35 years of age who have a significant chance of carrying babies with Down's syndrome or in women who had a previous child with that disorder. In both situations the recurrence risk for the defect is approximately 1 per cent; this risk becomes significantly higher if either parent is a D/G translocation carrier for Down's syndrome (5 per cent for male carriers and 20 per cent for female carriers).

Intrauterine diagnosis provides a definite diagnosis and replaces statistical likelihood with certainty. Parents may select abortion if the fetus is affected, and, with monitoring of future pregnancies by amniocentesis, may be assured of unaffected children.

DETECTION OF GENETIC DISEASE IN RELATIVES. Optimal genetic counseling in some diseases should include the testing of relatives at risk (Table 3). In some conditions the detection of latent disease in sibs and other relatives, if followed by suitable therapy, may be lifesaving. A sib of a patient with Wilson's disease (autosomal recessive) has a 25 per cent chance of being affected but may be too young to exhibit overt symptoms. Sibs of patients with hereditary polyposis of the colon or Gardner's syndrome (autosomal dominant) have a 50 per cent chance of being affected and therefore carry the certain risk of developing malignant transformation of one of the many polyps. In general, vigorous attempts should be made to examine relatives, using appropriate tests, when a genetic condition causes serious preventable or treatable disease. A case can also be made for early detection of diseases such as polycystic kidneys (autosomal dominant) in family members to allow those who are affected better reproductive decisions, choice of life style and appropriate occupations, and better preparation for ultimate renal transplantation or dialysis. Possible carriers for serious X-linked diseases (such as hemophilia and Duchenne muscular dystrophy) and for chromosomal carrier status (such as Down's syndrome associated with translocation) should be sought in families for prevention by intrauterine diagnosis.

GENETIC SCREENING. Genetic counseling has usually been retrospective and has followed the advent of a sick child or relative. In prospective counseling, advice is given before a sick person is born. Such an approach is possible for common autosomal recessive diseases such as sickle cell anemia, thalassemia major, and Tay-Sachs disease in populations with high frequencies of these genes. Eight per cent of the American black population are carriers of the sickling gene, and 4 per cent of the American Jewish population of European extraction are carriers of the Tay-Sachs gene. Mass screening for heterozygote detection followed by suitable genetic counseling has been frequently carried out.

Identification of the sickle cell trait before reproduction permits the prevention of sickle cell anemia if carriers refrain from mating with each other or if those already married have no children. Such programs raise many ethical and social problems, and it is doubtful whether mating and reproductive choices which are logical from the points of view of medicine, genetics, and public health would actually be made. Unfortunately, some sickling screening programs have been established without adequate counseling. Occasionally the mistaken notion has been promoted that the sickle cell trait represents a mild form of sickle cell disease. Needless anxiety and occupational discrimination against sickle cell trait carriers have resulted. Screening programs for Tay-Sachs disease have been more successful. Intrauterine detection of this condition is readily possible on amniotic fluid cells and does not require aspiration of fetal blood. Mass screening for the genetic hyperlipidemias remains a research procedure until better methods for identifying the genetic hyperlipidemias have been developed and effective means of preventing coronary heart disease by drugs and diet have been demonstrated.

With the present tendency for couples to have smaller families, there is greater concern that children should be healthy, and thus genetic counseling will become more important. The principles of genetic counseling are simple and should be mastered by every physician. Although referral to a medical genetics clinic in a medical center is necessary for complex genetic problems, increased education in the principles of human genetics will enable genetic counseling to be undertaken by primary care physicians in many instances.

Fuhrmann, W., and Vogel, F.: Genetic Counseling. 2d ed. New York, Springer-Verlag, 1976.

Lubs, H. A., and de la Cruz, F. (eds.): Genetic Counseling. New York, Raven Press, 1977.

McKusick, V. A.: Mendelian Inheritance in Man. 4th ed. Baltimore, The Johns Hopkins Press, 1975.

Milunsky, A.: The Prevention of Genetic Disease and Mental Retardation. Philadelphia, W. B. Saunders Company, 1975.

Nora, J. J., and Fraser, F. C.: Medical Genetics: Principles and Practice. Philadelphia, Lea & Febiger, 1974.

PART IV
ENVIRONMENTAL FACTORS IN DISEASE

21. CHEMICAL CONTAMINATION OF WATER AND AIR

Walsh McDermott

Chemical contamination may occur in one's own special environment, or it may occur in the environment we share with our community, that is to say, our environment at large. Both types of contamination stem in large measure from our skill in manipulating chemicals. Public attention is largely focused on the air and water "at large," but from the standpoint of health it is probably one's own special environment that is of the greater importance. There are two reasons for this: (1) The introduction of potentially harmful chemicals occurs more often in the workplace, in the home, or in an enclosed vehicle than in the environment at large. (2) In the enclosed environments much higher concentrations of toxic materials can occur and persist, and malfunctions may develop in apparatus designed for their control. More and more, all of us are spending most of our time in a controlled environment. Dr. Lawrence Hinkle conducted a Cornell diary-questionnaire type of survey of more than 1000 men employed in a wide range of occupations in the northeastern United States; it was revealed that from October to April for most of these men the amount of time spent outside buildings, homes, and vehicles during the average working day was *less than one hour*. Although such an umbrella of artificial environment has not yet covered all portions of our population, there is no reason to doubt that something closely approximating it will eventually happen. What it does is to provide an avenue through which essentially harmless amounts of chemicals in air or water can be greatly concentrated and, in effect, sharply focused on an individual or small group. Shortly after the conclusion of an Independence Day celebration in Philadelphia, 600 "running" automobiles were backed up at the pay-as-you-leave toll collectors in a three-level underground parking lot. An outside humidity of 70 per cent prevented the ventilators from exhausting the emissions adequately. As a consequence, a traffic jam that on an unroofed parkway would have been regarded as no more than one of life's daily urban annoyances made some 150 persons ill with vomiting and other symptoms, 61 of whom received outpatient hospital care. In this case the nature of the problem was clear. But one need not force the imagination far to think of how subtle could be the early effects of undetected breaks in environmental control such as the malfunctioning of pressurized cabins in commercial aircraft or of air-cooling systems. Today's physician, aware that for a large portion of the year the patient may be spending only one hour a day in an uncontrolled environment, must determine the significant environmental facts of the other 23 hours in considerable detail. To rail against the technology that makes this necessary is not logical, because much of it — properly functioning air-cooling systems, for example — is unquestionably a positive influence for health. A severe heat wave in the United States can temporarily double the death rate — a loss of life well exceeding that of the recorded air pollution disasters. At present we may conclude that some form of technologic control would appear here to stay, and by its very existence such a "special" environment forms a potential funnel for otherwise harmless contamination to become menacing.

Contamination of air or water at the workplace presents a somewhat different sort of problem. As our skill in manipulating chemicals continues, new chemical threats are inadvertently introduced into small clusters of people in the workplace environment. Once a particular chemical can be identified as a threat to health, its dangers can be neutralized in some way, or its use in the process or the product can be abandoned. It is the initial identification that may be quite difficult, for the health damage produced by a particular chemical may take the form of a well known disease entity — asthma or primary carcinoma of the liver, to mention two actual examples. Because the disease is well characterized and known to occur in many geographic areas, there seems little sense in suspecting that it might be related to some identifiable element in the environment. Thus to detect a correlation between one or only a few instances of a well known disease and some one of the many chemicals in a particular "occupational" environment is obviously difficult. Yet the feat must be accomplished early; otherwise, conceivably large numbers of people might be seriously harmed. By no means all of the threat to health comes from newly synthesized chemicals or the breakdown of sophisticated means for their control. When technology is at fault, it is not usually *because* it is modern and sophisticated, but rather because elementary provisions for heating and ventilating are either deficient or absent altogether, and dangerous makeshifts are substituted.

A constant vigilance and a keen epidemiologic sensitivity must be a prominent part of the skill of clinicians engaged in occupational medicine. In a sense these are the pioneers of the outermost frontier of the subject of environmental contamination. Likewise, the physician not engaged in occupational medicine should be quick to consult the medical staff of his patient's workplace when some disease arises in a setting that might be viewed as representing something of a surprise.

Some of the more common chemical offenders are discussed in the chapters that follow and in Ch. 348. But the chemical nature of occupational environments is ever changing. For comprehensive coverage the practitioner or student must consult the periodical literature or textbooks in occupational medicine.

For the physician one feature characterizes these two main forms of health threat from ambient chemicals. Although there may be a considerable delay in coming to suspect the environment as culprit, once this happens the actual proof of the environmental causation and the other medical decisions follow traditional medical logic. By contrast, in the third threat, that from the environment at large, both the nature of the threat and the decisions thus made necessary are highly abstract.

Like so many problems in medicine today, the one presented by chemical contamination of our air and water is only partly medical. The effects of contaminants on an individual would be medical; yet the forces that expose the individual to the contaminants would be technologic, economic, or cultural. As modulation of these forces requires social action on a broad scale, the physician's role has to be chiefly one of educator and counselor for those of his patients who are concerned citizen activists and for the public authorities. But the physician is frequently "a concerned citizen" too. It is imperative, therefore, that while serving as counselor or educator he be able to distinguish between his advice given as a physician based on scientific and professional evidence relating to *human health*, and his advice given as a concerned citizen — albeit one with a fairly broad background in biology.

The crux of the matter is that with a very few exceptions (see below) the risks to health posed by chemical contamination of our air and water are not tangible disease realities of the sort with which the physician is accustomed to deal. Instead the fact that there are health risks at all is an intellectual judgment based mainly on biologic analogies rather than on evidence established by direct medical observations. For example, it is believed that a considerable portion of human cancers are related to some factors in the environment (see Ch. 523). The evidence for this is that there are considerable variations in the incidence of particular cancers at the same time in various places in the world and in the same place at various times, and this can be observed in situations in which it is reasonable to discount an important genetic influence. So far only four substances (tobacco, alcohol, asbestos, and betel nuts) have been convincingly incriminated as environmental factors. Except for tobacco, the groups are associated with only a small portion of the total cancers discovered each year, and all more closely resemble the contaminations of "special" environments such as the workplace rather than the environment at large. Whether contamination of our air or water at large could facilitate development of cancer cannot yet be judged. The charge that fluoridation could do so has been convincingly disproved by Doll.

In traditional medical analyses and decisions, the physician is well schooled in weighing offsetting risks. Almost invariably, however, he is dealing with risks, all of which loom for the immediate future of his patient. In weighing chemical threats from the environment, however, he must frequently offset health gains that are clear and immediate against health risks that are far off and theoretical, and indeed might become a problem only for some future generation.

A splendid example of such offsetting threats may be seen in the chemical contamination of our streams and lakes, some of which serve as community water supplies. The availability of this water made it possible to build the United States as an urbanized society, but to do so required the development of a technology whereby the water could be decontaminated of its threats to health. These threats were all actual disease-producing agents. Because they were living organisms they had the property of death and dissolution, and a highly effective technology was based on these biologic properties. For the past 50 years or so, however, on an increasing scale, we have been contaminating the water not only with our microbes but with the direct or indirect products of our chemical industry. Whereas our microbes are biodegradable, many of these chemicals are not; indeed some are not simplified at all, either by biologic degradation or by any other process of decay. Technologic solutions for this part of the problem are to be expected in the form of substituting more readily degradable pesticides and detergents. The over-all problem, however, cannot be solved purely through technologic means. For the chemical contamination, like that by man's microbes, is part of his aura and is derived from his presence and way of life. To change the aura significantly would require major changes in the way of life; yet it is only the microbial part of his aura that can be clearly incriminated as producers of disease.

Microbes, however, can contribute to the process by more ways than one. The methylation of inorganic mercury in large bodies of water appears to take place through microbial action. This microbial process is of the greatest importance; it converts a form of mercury of rather low toxicity for man into one that is quite dangerous, because, unlike inorganic mercury, methyl mercury is readily absorbed and distributed throughout the tissues of man. Strictly speaking, the *demonstrable* dangerous contamination is in the food chain, i.e., the fish; but as fish cannot methylate inorganic mercury, it is clearly a contaminant of the water. Indeed two outbreaks in Japan (the Minamata Bay and River and the Agono River) of serious disease from methyl mercury acquired through this *microbe to water to fish to man* route represent one of the few solid examples of human disease from chemical contamination of a large body of water.

The many offsetting factors that must be weighed in a judgment on the health risks of chemical contamination of water in general are well illustrated by the story of chlorophenothane (DDT). Indeed the DDT situation may be regarded as a fine prototype of the whole problem. As a pesticide this chlorinated hydrocarbon has been marvelously effective in enhancing agricultural productivity; unfortunately it is relatively stable chemically over a wide range of conditions and thus persists for long periods in the environment. Here it produces a number of unsought ecologic effects. These include critically harmful disturbances of the calcium metabolism of predatory birds; interference with various forms of marine life; and persistence in the food chain whereby it can accumulate in the tissues of a number of organisms, including man. All these effects are reason enough for insisting on strict controls on the use of DDT and on an intensive effort to develop less stable but comparably effective substitutes. Moreover, the property of accumulation in human tissue is obviously disquieting from the standpoint of human health. Thus far, however, there is no evidence that this accumulation has led to recognizable disease in humans. The World Health Organization in a 20-year experiment involving more than 200,000 DDT spraymen has received no reports of toxic effect except from accidental swallowing, and even that caused no deaths. No adverse effects were observed in a clinical study of chronic low-grade exposure in which a group of volunteers received daily for 18 months a dosage 200 times the estimated usual exposure from food (Hayes, W. S., et al., 1956).

The physician must offset the theoretic risk that these accumulations might ultimately lead to human disease against the demonstrable health gains from controlling some of the world's major diseases such as malaria (or filariasis) and those caused by arboviruses and rickettsia. At the present time, despite the presence, particularly in Central America, of mosquitoes physiologically resistant to the insecticide, there is no wholly satisfactory substitute for DDT in disease control. Faced with this choice between the clear and present danger of vector-borne diseases and the theoretic risk that tissue accumulation of low concentrations of DDT might lead to disease a few decades hence, the physician has no choice but to opt for continued use of DDT under proper control. Yet in making this choice — and the DDT situation can be viewed as the prototype of many more — he must be keenly aware of the critical nature of the factors it was *not* possible to include in the decision.

For to say that low-grade continued exposure to DDT has produced no recognizable disease in man is not to say that it exerts no *physiologic effects*. On the contrary, it is a potent inducer of the microsomal enzyme system of the liver. As this system plays a critical role in the metabolism of drugs and other chemicals introduced to the body from the outside, it serves as a major protective mechanism against chemical threats from the environment, and hence consideration of its workings is appropriate.

The activity of the microsomal enzyme system is minimal at birth and in early life but increases steadily throughout adulthood. It is inducible; and the buildup of enzymatic capability as the individual grows older is thought to be a reflection of increasing experience with chemicals from the environment acting as inducers. Activity of the system induced by one chemical may also be effective on another. Consequently when more than one drug (or adventitious chemical) are being taken into the body simultaneously, the metabolic disposition of one of the drugs can be significantly altered by the presence and inducing capabilities of the other drug or adventitious chemical. Such "cross-over" effects have obvious implications for multiple drug therapies and conceivably might also attain significance when one of the chemical compounds was an environmental contaminant. The only endogenous materials metabolized via the hepatic microsomal system are the steroid hormones, and their hydroxylation can be considerably enhanced when the system is induced. In theory, therefore, it could be imagined that the presence of DDT with its known potency as an inducer of the hepatic microsomal system could lead to an increased demand for the synthesis of some hormone. There is no evidence that such a DDT phenomenon with steroid hormones actually occurs. But the postulated phenomenon can serve as an imaginary example of how an adventitious chemical in the environment could alter the course of bodily metabolic activities *through an adaptive hepatic system that is known to exist.*

The question arises whether the decades-long stimulation of such an adaptive mechanism in an individual carries with it a risk to the total organism or whether, on balance, such continued stimulation is a good thing. In general, the many bodily systems that work toward homeostasis are regarded as normal processes whose continued operation is not harmful in itself. But some of these systems require the synthesis of protein, and this requires an allocative process involving protein precursors. In effect, therefore, as emphasized by V. R. Potter, there is a "physiologic cost" involved in each of these adaptive enzymatic processes in the sense that one is accomplished at some cost to all possible others. When the "triggering" of the system comes chiefly from the external environment, as in the hepatic microsomal system, the long-continued engagement with a wealth of chemical stimuli conceivably might result in "physiologic costs" that would be harmful to the organism. This could be so; conversely, as our knowledge advances, the notion may prove to have been ridiculously naïve. Our current state of knowledge simply does not permit judgment of the question at this time. It is really the fact that we are dealing with so many "unknowns" that serves to temper any tendency to complacency based on the present absence of detectable disease resulting from chemical contamination of our water at large. For any situation in which a variety of chemicals pass through a series of living systems that at some stage may include the human body is bound to be not only complex but a situation that is continuously subject to change. It is this fact — that the door is wide open for trouble rather than that trouble has already occurred — that characterizes our present situation with respect to possible adverse effects on health from chemical contaminants of our water.

One expressed fear about pesticides in the water also concerns contamination of the air, specifically that the world's newly released oxygen content might be undergoing subtle reduction. Approximately 60 per cent of the world's newly released oxygen each year comes from the activity of oceanic plant life which it was feared might be harmed by the pesticide pollution of the oceans. However, careful studies of Machta and Hughes have revealed that there has been no change in the world atmosphere's content of oxygen in the 60-year period from 1910 to 1970. Their "negative" data can now serve as a baseline for monitoring this question throughout the future. Fears of reduction in the global oxygen supply from combustion on land can be set completely to rest by examining the quantitative aspects of the question.

With respect to chemical contamination of the air, the challenge to the physician is the same as with water — namely, he must learn to distinguish at any one point in time between what are presently demonstrable health hazards and what are *current stimuli* that conceivably might be generating health effects to be recognized only several decades later. In broad terms, two distinct types of widespread chemical contamination exist: a "London type," composed principally of sulfur compounds from burning coal or certain grades of oil; and a "Los Angeles type," composed mainly of petroleum products introduced into the atmosphere principally from automobiles, and consisting chiefly of carbon monoxide, carbon dioxide, oxides of nitrogen, lead, and unburned or partially oxidized hydrocarbons. None of these chemicals are present in concentrations sufficiently high in themselves to produce toxicity in man. In the Los Angeles type of contamination the visible and palpable "smog" is a result of *sunlight* acting on certain of these discharged chemicals to produce more reactive chemicals, whereas in London it frequently results from *fog* physically trapping the sulfur compounds from the coal. Both types exist in both countries, but in the United States it is the hydrocarbon type that is our basic problem. It is overlaid in certain localities by the sulfur type, for the use of coal varies considerably from region to region. It is highly probable that with both types, one of the important end-results — irritation of certain body and plant cells — is much the same.

In terms of presently demonstrable effects on health, the evidence is conflicting as to whether this irritation is definitely harmful to persons who have sustained damage to their cardiovascular or bronchopulmonary systems, notably that apparently enlarging number of patients with chronic obstructive pulmonary disease (see Ch. 344.1). One may presume that it is, but thus far it has not really been possible to demonstrate it in a convincing fashion. Nevertheless, although he must act mainly on a priori reasoning, the physician would seem to be on solid ground when he attempts to protect his patients with damaged lungs or bronchi from the aggravating effects of chemically polluted urban air. Sometimes this can be accomplished by emigration, sometimes by window fans with filters. Often, however, particularly among urban poverty groups, it cannot be accomplished at all. For these unfortunates, and indeed for the majority of those with chronic pulmonary disease in all socioeconomic groups, protection, if it is to come, will have to come from the community efforts now in progress in many localities to reduce chemical contamination of the air.

It must be appreciated that virtually the entire "health case" for the need to reduce the chemical contamination of the air rests on the protection of this population with damaged cardiopulmonary systems. For no convincing case has yet been assembled to the effect that chronic obstructive pulmonary disease with its frequent cardiac sequels can be *initiated* by continued exposure to the chemical contamination of urban air. This is not to say there is no medical case at all for continued efforts to minimize contamination of the air for the sake of the far larger population with undamaged bronchopulmonary structures. On the contrary, such a case does exist. The physician must recognize clearly, however, that the case for action to protect the population at large is of quite a different nature from that for action to protect those already damaged. For those damaged the evidence is of a conventional medical sort — i.e., it is based on systematic clinical, laboratory, and epidemiologic observations. For the population at large, however, the case is not derived from actual scientific observations. On the contrary, *as in the case of chemical contamination of the water*, the argument for decontaminating the air can be no more than an intellectual judgment based mainly on biologic analogies.

There is one difference between the problems with air and with water. As mentioned previously, at present there is no recognized disease of unknown pathogenesis that seems to have any relationship to widespread chemical contamination of water. By contrast, in the disease complex of bronchitis and emphysema (chronic obstructive pulmonary disease), there *is* a commonly occurring disease grouping of unknown pathogenesis that starts in early middle age; it appears to be aggravated by chemicals in the air, and hence might also be *initiated* by them. But to demonstrate convincingly that such a causative relationship exists is a difficult task that has not yet been accomplished despite careful and intensive studies of laboratory animals and man. The epidemiologic problems involved have to do with the great difficulties in separating for analysis the various factors of conceivable relevance such as cigarette smoking and degree of exposure to particular chemicals in the air. After the first five years of planned long-term studies in the Netherlands (Van Der Lende et al., Vlagtwedde/Vlaardingen), it was not possible to demonstrate that residence in areas of high air pollution was associated with abnormalities in pulmonary function. The factor of age seemed to produce a far greater decrease of pulmonary function than smoking or living in a polluted area. Conceivably the *impact* of the chemicals that lead ultimately to disease might be something that occurs relatively early in life. Studies in young children in the United Kingdom suggest that continued exposure to high levels of pollution increases the risk of serious respiratory disease in children (Colley and Reid, 1970).

But the major problem is how to study what are in effect "water dripping on stone" effects. The chemicals now contaminating the air, taken singly or collectively, are not present in quantities that produce detectable bronchopulmonary damage in the short run. Thus if the "current stimuli" represented by these chemicals play a significant role in the pathogenesis of such a major disease grouping as chronic obstructive pulmonary disease, the effects presumably would take the form of steady but individually minute episodes of damage that ultimately fail to heal completely and emerge to significance only when accumulated over decades. Questions of this type — i.e., 30- to 40-year effects in humans — are far more difficult to answer than questions of the role of environmental contaminants on plant life or other elements of the nonhuman ecology.

To be sure, the physician in his role of public educator and counselor should support well organized efforts to develop the new methods and the new institutional arrangements for the research needed for the productive study of these medical questions of this essentially new type. But he should also not fail to stress that because of the very nature of these questions as they apply to *human health*, it seems highly unlikely that answers concerning air pollution as an initiator of disease will be forthcoming in the near future. Whatever action is to be taken, therefore, must be based on the medical information that is available now.

From the standpoint of health, therefore, we are left with the following dilemma. On the one hand, most of the actions necessary to abolish air pollution as a potential danger to health are costly and likely to prove quite disruptive to the economy and the whole style of life. To campaign for these actions in the name of health without a convincing scientific case that the evils to be corrected represent a widespread danger to health might be unwise. On the other hand, if, a few decades hence, it were shown convincingly that long-continued chemical contamination of the air *of the present sort* did have the property of initiating chronic obstructive pulmonary disease, the proportion of the population of any industrialized country that would by then have been irreversibly affected would be large indeed.

There seems to be no obvious solution for this dilemma so long as the major case for minimizing air pollution is viewed as being primarily a "health matter" and health is considered principally in terms of detectable disease. But there are more subtle aspects to health than definable disease, including even definable mental disease. There is the whole spirit involved in one's response to one's environment. The intense love of their city shown by so many Leningraders when it was under siege in World War II is a case in point. These are not the kinds of phenomena that lend themselves readily to comparative weighing in the scale against the major economic factors that might be disrupted in "air reform." Nevertheless, they deserve attention too.

What it comes down to is that, except for those already afflicted with cardiopulmonary disease, the present chemical pollution of urban air is not really a health problem in the orthodox sense; it is a widespread *social* evil that is quite unacceptable on a number of counts, of which the possible health effects are only one (Dubos). Viewed in this way it becomes the physician's role to characterize continuously what is known or seems highly probable about the health aspects of the matter. Included should be encouragement of attempts to develop more sensitive methods for the essentially permanent monitoring of the possible effects of long-continued chemical stimuli. The physician presents this knowledge not as a determining reason in itself for air control, but as only one portion of a total argument for cleansing this part of our external environment. Once the medical contribution can be regarded as but one contribution to a much larger total effort, the physician can escape from the trap of seeming to be minimizing the significances of a particular form of contamination of the air on the grounds that it is not a *known* danger to health. For the physician to operate in such a cooperative professional-social role is not new; most of the impressive early twentieth century accomplishments of medicine in extending life expectancy from birth were made in exactly this way.

Bend, J. R., and Hook, G. E. R.: Hepatic and extrahepatic mixed-function oxidases. *In* Handbook of Physiology, Section 9: Reactions to Environmental Agents. Bethesda, Md., American Physiological Society, 1977.

Carter, L. J.: Asbestos: Trouble in the air from Maryland rock quarry. Science, 197:347, 1977.

Doll, R., and Kinlen, L.: Fluoridation of water and cancer mortality in the U.S.A. Lancet, 1:1300, 1977.

Dubos, R.: Reason Awake! Science for Man. New York, Columbia University Press, 1970.

Hack, J. T.: Letter to the editor. Science, 197:1232, 1977.

Hinkle, L. E.: Hudson Basin Project, Task Group Reports, No. 9, Human Health. New York, The Rockefeller Foundation, June 1974. (Library of Congress Catalog Card No. 76–6700 38.)

Machta, L., and Hughes, E.: Atmospheric oxygen in 1967 to 1970. Science, 168: 1582, 1970.

The New York Times, July 6, 1977.

Royal College of Physicians: Air Pollution and Health. London, Pitman Medical and Scientific Publishing Company, Ltd., 1970.

Summary Report: Drinking Water and Health. Safe Drinking Water Committee, Advisory Center on Toxicology; Assembly of Life Sciences, National Research Council (Safe Drinking Water Committee), 1977. 98 pp. (Available from the Office of Public Affairs, U.S. Environmental Protection Agency, Washington, D.C. 20460).

Van Der Lende, R., et al.: Epidemiological study of the correlation between air pollution and the prevalence of airway diseases. So. Ned. Tijdschr. Geneeskd. 119:577, 1975.

22. FOOD POISONING

Harold P. Lambert

22.1. INTRODUCTION

Food may cause illness in three ways. The most common varieties are produced by *contamination with microorganisms or their products.* Although the gastrointestinal tract is an important mode of entry for many viral, bacterial, and parasitic agents of disease, the term "food poisoning" is conventionally restricted to two main types of syndromes: various forms of acute gastroenteritis caused by bacteria or their products in food; and neurologic syndromes such as botulism or paralytic shellfish poisoning caused by the toxic products of microorganisms. Second, food may be *contaminated by poisonous chemicals.* Examples include heavy metal poisoning by mercury, antimony, cadmium, arsenic, or zinc; poisoning by simple salts such as sodium fluoride or potassium chlorate; and poisoning by organic compounds such as insecticides and orthotricresyl phosphate. Third, *poisonous plants or animals may be eaten in error.* The material may be inherently poisonous, as are some species of mushroom and many other plants; or it may have become secondarily poisonous by incorporating a substance toxic to man during its own food cycle, as in certain forms of shellfish and fish poisoning.

22.2. BACTERIAL FOOD POISONING

The infectious type of bacterial food poisoning requires the ingestion of living organisms, albeit often in very large numbers, and their subsequent multiplication in the gastrointestinal tract. The most important example of this type of illness is *Salmonella* gastroenteritis, which is dealt with in Ch. 153. *Shigella* species may give rise to very similar syndromes, but these are not conventionally classified as episodes of food poisoning, although water- or food-borne outbreaks of *Shigella* infection do sometimes occur. In the toxin type of bacterial food poisoning, such as that associated with staphylococci, the illness is caused by toxin formed in food before its ingestion, and does not depend on the ingestion of living organisms. Although a generally useful concept, the distinction between the "infection" and "toxin" types of food poisoning has become less rigid than formerly with the demonstration and partial identification of a number of enterotoxins produced by bacterial gut pathogens, including those which produce disease only when ingested as living organisms.

STAPHYLOCOCCAL FOOD POISONING

ETIOLOGY AND EPIDEMIOLOGY. This common form of food poisoning is caused by the multiplication of an enterotoxin-forming strain of *Staphylococcus* in the food before ingestion. Contamination of food with staphylococci is extremely common, because the organism can be grown from the hands of about 50 per cent of people. Heavy growth may often be obtained from apparently noninfected minor cracks and cuts on the skin. Most outbreaks are caused by meat or confectionery contaminated by staphylococci of human origin, but about 10 per cent of them are milk borne, and the organism is then usually of bovine origin. The conditions needed to cause food poisoning of this type are contamination of a suitable food — most foods will support the growth of staphylococci — and a period of some hours after preparation during which the organisms are able to multiply. This may occur during a period of slow cooling after cooking or if food is held at ambient temperature in a warm climate after preparation. Later reheating or even boiling will not then prevent illness, because this is caused by preformed, heat-stable toxin and not by the ingestion of living staphylococci.

PATHOGENESIS. Detailed study of staphylococcal enterotoxin has been hindered by many technical difficulties. Strains which form enterotoxin are almost always coagulase positive, but enterotoxin production is otherwise not related to any easily measurable metabolic activities. Moreover, study of the toxin has hitherto been limited by lack of a satisfactory animal model; most workers use intraperitoneal injection of toxin in kittens as the test system. Some progress has been made in recent years, notably the differentiation of at least four and possibly five antigenic types. Enterotoxin B has been isolated in relatively pure form by Bergdoll and his colleagues. The types are antigenically specific and do not cross-react, but one staphylococcal strain may produce more than one type. The toxin, like the crude extracts, is relatively heat resistant and resistant to trypsin. Its precise mode of action is still in dispute, but experiments in monkeys suggest that this so-called enterotoxin probably has its primary site of action in the central nervous system, and that vomiting is a centrally induced response.

CLINICAL MANIFESTATIONS AND TREATMENT. The period between ingestion and illness is short, one to six hours, occasionally a little longer, and the illness is characterized by abdominal cramping pain with violent and often repeated retching and vomiting. Diarrhea is variable; it may be profuse, mild, or absent entirely. Although often violent, staphylococcal food poisoning is short lived, usually subsiding in six or eight hours and rarely lasting as long as 24 hours. It may occasionally threaten life in patients who are old or suffering from other serious disease. The patient is often recovering when first seen by a doctor, but may require an intramuscular injection of prochlorperazine, 12.5 mg, or metoclopramide, 10 mg, to control vomiting. Patients with evidence of serious depletion of extracellular fluid may require intravenous treatment using isotonic sodium chloride with added potassium.

PREVENTION. Careful training of food handlers in personal hygiene and immediate refrigeration of foods not due for immediate consumption are the most important preventive measures. Enterotoxin is not produced at ordinary domestic refrigerator temperatures. Foods should not be left to cool slowly, especially in large containers, and should be taken from the refrigerator and reheated, if this is required, immediately before serving.

Epidemiologic work on outbreaks of staphylococcal food poisoning involves standard methods of bacteriophage typing in identifying the source of the responsible strain. Since, however, terminal heating may kill the organisms in food without inactivating enterotoxin, staphylococci may not be grown from food under suspicion. Animal assays for the detection of enterotoxin are now being replaced by serologic methods. Precipitin techniques such as double gel diffusion and immunoelectrophoresis require preliminary extraction and concentration of the material, but more rapid and direct methods for detection of enterotoxin based on radioimmunoassay and reverse passive hemagglutination are being developed.

CLOSTRIDIAL FOOD POISONING

ETIOLOGY. *Clostridium perfringens* type A is responsible for about one third of the reported cases of food poisoning both in the United States and in Great Britain. It occurs in fairly large outbreaks, with an average of 35 affected people in each episode. The organism is ubiquitous. Strains can be isolated from the feces of man and of most domestic and farm animals, and samples of raw meat may often be contaminated with this organism. It has also been found in flies, soil, and dirt from kitchens. The conditions necessary for an outbreak are well defined. A meat or poultry dish, in the form of either a stew or a solid preparation such as a joint, pie, or mince, is cooked at a temperature not higher than 100° C, allowing the spores to survive. During a period of slow cooling the spores germinate, this process being provoked by "heat shock"; rapid multiplication of vegetative forms is encouraged by the rich medium and the low oxidation-reduction potential after cooking. These conditions are especially likely to apply with a large bulk of food, in which slow cooling and anaerobic conditions are likely to occur. Food eaten cold or merely warmed before serving may then cause an outbreak of food poisoning.

PATHOGENESIS. Human volunteer experiments indicate that ingestion of living organisms is necessary for the production of this form of food poisoning, and the responsible strain may often be found in large numbers in the feces of affected patients. Strains of *Cl. perfringens* type A which cause food poisoning do not differ from other strains in any way easily identifiable by routine methods, although outbreaks in Britain have most commonly been caused by strains with heat-resistant spores. The pathogenesis of the disease has yet to be defined in detail. It was believed for some time that phosphoryl choline, an end product of the action of alpha toxin (= lecithinase-phospholipase-C) was responsible for the outpouring of fluid into the bowel, but this substance has no effect in experimental systems and is probably inactive in the bowel. Recently, however, partial purification has been achieved of an antigenic heat-labile toxin, different from the other known toxins of *Cl. perfringens*, which causes accumulation of fluid in isolated loops of rabbit ileum. The toxin is a heat-labile, nondiffusible protein, antigenic and different from other known toxins produced by *Cl. perfringens*.

CLINICAL MANIFESTATIONS. The incubation period is 8 to 12 hours after ingestion of the infected food, occasionally as little as 6 or as long as 24 hours. The main features are diarrhea and griping abdominal pain. The feces are liquid but do not contain blood or mucus. A small proportion of patients suffer from nausea and vomiting. The illness is usually not severe, lasts less than 24 hours, and is unaccompanied by systemic disturbance or fever. A few deaths have been recorded in old or infirm patients.

Drug treatment is rarely necessary, but in longer attacks a kaolin mixture may be given, and patients with severe abdominal pain may need an analgesic.

PREVENTION. Preferably food should be served immediately after cooking. If it has to be kept, it should be rapidly cooled and held at a safe temperature. Cooked meat should be kept always either cold, below 5° C, or hot, over 60° C. Careful techniques of food hygiene are especially important in institutions in which large amounts of meat or poultry are cooked.

ENTERITIS NECROTICANS
(Pig-Bel)

Outbreaks of severe intestinal disease have been associated with ingestion of Cl. perfringens type C. A large outbreak was reported from Germany in 1948, and a similar syndrome known as pig-bel has more recently been described from parts of New Guinea in which pig feasts have an important economic and social function. The syndrome is characterized by severe abdominal pain, bloody diarrhea, and vomiting. Operation or autopsy reveals a severe hemorrhagic jejunitis and ileitis. Some patients die and some recover after resection of strangulated, perforated, and necrotic bowel. Others may pass through the acute phase to develop chronic small bowel obstruction and malabsorption, and some recover completely.

VIBRIO PARAHAEMOLYTICUS FOOD POISONING

V. parahaemolyticus is a halophilic marine vibrio long recognized as an inhabitant of coastal waters of Japan and as a cause of gastroenteritis associated with sea foods. More recently it has been found in American and British coastal sea waters. Techniques for its isolation and differentiation from nonpathogenic marine vibrios are now well established. In particular, pathogenic strains exhibit a specific in vitro hemolytic reaction.

In Japan gastroenteritis of this type is confined to the summer months. It is the most common cause of infective food poisoning in Japan, accounting for 59 per cent of 22,000 cases of identifiable cause in 1963. V. parahaemolyticus causes an infectious type of gastroenteritis and is associated with ingestion of raw fish or shellfish. Outbreaks in Japan have been associated with semi-dried young sardines, and especially with sushi, a food composed of cooked rice, raw fish, and shellfish. The organism, as well as episodes of food poisoning caused by its ingestion, has now been identified in many parts of the world, including the Atlantic, Pacific, and Gulf coasts of the United States, other parts of the Pacific, the United Kingdom, and Australia.

Incubation periods varying from a few hours to four days have been recorded, but the most frequent interval between ingestion and infection is 12 to 24 hours. The chief clinical features are severe diarrhea accompanied by cramping abdominal pain, nausea, and vomiting. Many patients also exhibit systemic symptoms of fever, chills, and headache. Less commonly the organism causes a dysenteric form of illness with fever and bloody diarrhea. The illness lasts for one to five days, and recovery appears to be complete. As with staphylococcal and clostridial food poisoning, the disease is rarely fatal, but old and debilitated patients may be at special risk. The role of antibiotics in treatment is uncertain, but tetracycline should be given to patients who are seriously ill.

BACILLUS CEREUS FOOD POISONING

Bacillus cereus is an aerobic, spore-bearing, gram-positive bacillus of wide natural distribution, and several outbreaks of food poisoning have been associated with high counts of the organism in the responsible food. Contamination has been traced to corn flour, rice, and other dried foods. In large outbreaks in Norway affecting as many as 600 people, the incubation period was 12 hours, and the main features were watery diarrhea, abdominal pain, and nausea lasting about 12 hours. More recently, fried or boiled rice in restaurants has been incriminated. Large quantities of rice are prepared and kept at warm kitchen temperatures for many hours, small portions being refried for a few minutes as orders are placed. In one such episode the rice contained 450×10^6 organisms per gram. The incubation period has been as short as 15 minutes to 3 hours when large inocula such as these are ingested. The pathogenesis of this form of food poisoning is not precisely established, but some strains of B. cereus cause accumulation of fluid in the rabbit ileal loop test, increased permeability in rabbit skin, and a necrotic reaction after intradermal injection in guinea pigs.

OTHER FORMS OF BACTERIAL FOOD POISONING

Many outbreaks cannot be assigned to one of the specific pathogens generally accepted as a cause of food poisoning, but many other bacteria have been implicated at one time or another as possible causes of acute gastrointestinal illness. The evidence is often inconclusive and is frequently based on high counts of the presumptive pathogen in samples of food which may have been kept at room temperature for long periods before reaching the laboratory, or on the isolation from patients' stools of organisms which form part of the normal fecal flora. Volunteer studies have often proved equivocal. With these reservations, it seems likely that diarrhea and vomiting may occasionally be caused by a considerable variety of bacteria, if circumstances have allowed their multiplication to high enough concentrations before ingestion. The genera most often implicated have been the enterococci (group D streptococci) and various members of the Enterobacteriaceae, notably E. coli, Proteus, Providencia, Pseudomonas, and Citrobacter. A remarkable and special example is the contamination of fermented coconut press cake (bongkrek), a common food in Central Java, by a species of Pseudomonas. The toxin produced causes hypoglycemia which is often fatal.

22.3. BOTULISM

ETIOLOGY. Botulism is a life-threatening illness characterized by muscle paralysis and variable gastrointestinal symptoms. It is caused by absorption from the gastrointestinal tract of ingested toxin produced by *Clostridium botulinum*. Botulism resulting from wound infection by this organism has also been recorded several times.

INCIDENCE. The unexpectedness of outbreaks of botulism, the dramatic and frightening nature of the illness, and its high mortality have attracted much attention from both laymen and doctors, but botulism is in fact an uncommon disease. From 1899 to 1969 there were 659 outbreaks in the United States, with 1696 cases and 959 deaths. The years 1970 to 1973 saw 30 outbreaks, in which 21 of the 91 patients died. Outbreaks have also been recorded in many other countries, especially in Canada, Japan, Western Europe, Scandinavia, and the U.S.S.R.

EPIDEMIOLOGY. The six strains of *Cl. botulinum* cause disease in man and in a variety of animals. Human disease is caused by types A, B, and E and occasionally by type F. Toxins produced by the different types are antigenically distinct. *Cl. botulinum*, a spore-bearing anaerobic bacillus, is widely distributed in nature. The organism has been identified in many parts of the world, in cultivated and virgin soils, in a variety of marine environments, and in many animals and animal products. The distribution of types varies in different areas, so that type A botulism is more common than type B in the United States, especially in the Western states, whereas in Europe this order is reversed. In recent years type E has superseded both types A and B in frequency. Type E organisms are especially but not exclusively associated with the aquatic environment in northern latitudes, being found in the sea bed of coastal and lake waters and in the intestinal tract of fish. However, types A and B may also be associated with a marine source.

PATHOGENESIS. Contamination of fresh food by spores of *Cl. botulinum* does not cause botulism. The spores must have germinated and toxin must have been produced by the vegetative organisms. Spores are destroyed at a temperature of 121° C or greater, as used in commercial canning processes, but can usually survive a temperature of 100° C. Type E spores are relatively heat sensitive, but smoking and light cooking may not kill them, so that food processed in these ways or preserved in the raw state may act as a vehicle of the disease. Another factor predisposing to type E botulism is the production of toxin by this organism at temperatures as low as 5° C. The cooking or preserving process is conducive to the germination of spores and, by reason of the lowered redox potential, to multiplication of the vegetative forms. Multiplication is inhibited in acid media, and botulism is rarely associated with food of pH below 4.5. All types of botulinum toxin are heat labile, and botulism could be entirely prevented by terminal heating for 20 minutes at 80° C or for 10 minutes at 90° C.

The types of food associated with botulism as a result of these contributory factors vary, with local food customs, from country to country. In the United States home-preserved vegetables constitute the most frequent source, followed by preserved fruit and fish products.

Meat and meat products are more commonly responsible in Europe. Preserved fish is the chief source of botulism in Japan, Scandinavia, and the U.S.S.R. Although most outbreaks are associated with domestic methods of preparing and preserving foods, outbreaks from commercially prepared foods also occur. Recent sources have included canned tuna fish, canned vichyssoise, and vacuum-packed smoked fish.

Ingested toxin is rapidly absorbed from the gastrointestinal tract. Toxemia may be demonstrated for periods of up to ten days or even three weeks, and it is possible that toxin continues to be formed in and absorbed from the bowel for some days after ingestion. Type E toxin is potentiated by proteolytic enzymes, including trypsin, and this phenomenon has been invoked as a mechanism which contributes to the pathogenicity of this type. Botulinum toxin is active in extremely low doses, nanogram quantities of pure toxin being lethal to mice. It prevents conduction in peripheral nerves by a presynaptic block, thus preventing release of acetylcholine without direct action on the acetylcholine release mechanism. Anticholinesterase drugs do not affect its action.

INFANT BOTULISM. This recently recognized syndrome is of special interest, since it is caused by production of toxin within the bowel lumen. Forty-two cases were described in the United States in 1977.

CLINICAL MANIFESTATIONS. Illness usually begins between 12 and 36 hours after ingesting the toxin-containing food. The first manifestations are often gastrointestinal, especially in type E disease, with nausea, vomiting, abdominal pain, and distention. Other common early symptoms are weakness, unsteadiness, and dryness of the mouth and throat. Neurologic symptoms may accompany the early gastrointestinal illness or may follow at an interval of 12 to 72 hours. Early features are blurring of vision, dysphagia, dysarthria, and weakness of a variety of muscles. Weakness spreads as the disease advances, affecting especially the respiratory system, the external ocular muscles, and muscles of the neck and proximal limb groups. Cherington, reviewing ten years' experience with botulism, found pupillary abnormalities uncommon, being present in only 2 of 14 patients. Retention of urine is common. Deep tendon reflexes are preserved. The patient remains mentally clear, and fever is not observed except as a terminal event. Paralysis may continue for many days or weeks. An occasional patient with mild disease shows myasthenic features with a response to injection of edrophonium chloride. Defects of cardiac conduction have occasionally been noted.

The chief causes of death are respiratory or bulbar paralysis or both, along with the infective complications resulting from these paralyses. Wound botulism usually follows severe injuries of the type associated with other anaerobic infections. The incubation period is 4 to 14 days, but the illness is otherwise identical with botulism caused by ingestion of toxin.

DIAGNOSIS. The illness is easily recognized if a group of patients, known to have eaten food of a type associated with botulism, present with characteristic symptoms. By contrast, diagnosis of the individual patient, in whom there may be no suspicion that the illness is a form of food poisoning, has often proved extremely difficult. The gastrointestinal features may be so severe as to stimulate intestinal obstruction, and the epigastric pain may be mistaken for that of myocardial infarction. The dry and sometimes painful throat may suggest various forms of acute pharyngitis, and the combination of sore throat and neurologic disease can cause confusion with diphtheria. The neurologic illness has been mistaken for acute polyneuritis (Guillain-Barré syndrome), encephalitis, a stroke, or myasthenia gravis. The dry mouth and fixed dilated pupils suggest atropine poisoning, as is produced by *Datura stramonium* (jimson weed). Paralytic poisoning caused by shellfish or by puffer fish (see below) is accompanied by prominent sensory symptoms not found in botulism. Electromyography is of some value, showing diminished response to a single stimulus but facilitation of action potentials with paired or repeated nerve stimulation. The changes thus resemble those found in the Eaton-Lambert syndrome.

Circulating toxin may sometimes be detected in the patient's blood or feces, even long after onset of the disease. It is detected by intraperitoneal injection in mice, controls simultaneously receiving antiserum of the different types. Suspected food is also tested for toxin in the same way, and the organism is sought by anaerobic culture.

TREATMENT. Since the greatest risk of botulism is respiratory failure, treatment is dominated by the prevention and management of this complication. Bulbar paralysis is treated by early tracheostomy, employing a cuffed endotracheal tube. Coincident or supervening respiratory muscle paralysis indicates the need for artificial ventilation applied through the tracheostomy. Specific antitoxin is probably effective in reducing the mortality of type E botulism. Although there is no such evidence in other forms of botulism, the high mortality of the disease and the difficulty of obtaining statistically valid data justify the use of antitoxin in all forms of the disease. Antitoxin should be given irrespective of the duration of illness when the diagnosis is made, because toxin may be present in the blood for many days. Unless the type of botulism is definitely known, multivalent antitoxin should be administered, because the type cannot be reliably inferred from the food source. After a preliminary test for hypersensitivity to horse serum, two vials of trivalent antitoxin (each containing 7500 IU type A, 5500 IU type B, and 8500 IU type E antitoxin) are administered by intravenous injection, and this is repeated in two to four hours. For botulism of known type, preparations containing A and B antitoxin or E antitoxin alone are available, as is a small stock of monovalent F antitoxin.

Guanidine, which enhances acetylcholine release, has been claimed as a useful adjunct in treatment. Both clinical and electromyographic improvement were observed in a number of patients who received guanidine by nasogastric tube in a dose of 15 to 50 mg per kilogram per day; unfortunately, it is less effective on respiratory than on ocular or limb weakness.

Since it is uncertain whether the long duration of toxemia in botulism is attributable to continued absorption from the bowel, gastric aspiration and colonic washouts are also used in treatment. A solution of sodium bicarbonate may be left in the stomach to promote breakdown of toxin.

PROGNOSIS. The over-all mortality of botulism is high, 60 to 70 per cent for type A, 10 to 30 per cent for type B, and 30 to 50 per cent for type E. Patients with type E botulism tend to die more quickly than those affected by other types, usually within three days of onset. Improved management of respiratory failure should lower the death rate, especially because patients who survive the stage of severe paralysis can recover completely.

SPECIAL NOTE. For assistance in suspected botulism, or for supplies of antiserum, in the United States, telephone the Center for Disease Control: 404-633-3311 (days) or 404-633-2176 (nights, weekends, and holidays).

22.4. POISONOUS PLANTS AND ANIMALS

PARALYTIC SHELLFISH POISONING

Shellfish may act as the vehicle of transmission of many pathogens, for example, infective hepatitis, *Vibrio parahaemolyticus* gastroenteritis, and diarrhea and vomiting of unknown cause. Ingestion may also give rise to an acute neurologic syndrome caused by the transmission to man of a neurotoxin acquired by shellfish from plankton on which they feed. Outbreaks are especially likely to follow a sudden increase in the population of dinoflagellate protozoa, the "red tide." The main responsible species in the Pacific Ocean is *Gonyaulax catanella*, which produces the paralytic poison *saxitoxin*, first isolated from the Alaskan butterclam *Saxidomus giganteus*. The toxin of *G. tamarensis*, responsible for outbreaks on Atlantic coasts, produces the same pharmacologic effects, although it may not be identical with saxitoxin. The toxins are water-soluble, heat-stable compounds, rapidly absorbed from the gastrointestinal tract and active in vitro at concentrations of 1 to 10 μg per milliliter. They act on vertebrate nerve fibers and on skeletal muscle fibers, abolishing action potentials by preventing depolarization. Their study has proved of great value in elucidating mechanisms of nerve conduction.

CLINICAL MANIFESTATIONS. Symptoms may begin as soon as 20 minutes after ingestion, with paresthesias of the hands and mouth, weakness of the limbs, and a floating feeling. Other common features are ataxia, headache, and vomiting, whereas in severe cases bulbar and respiratory paralysis supervene and may cause death. Mortality rates between 5 and 18 per cent have been reported in various outbreaks, but the illness is less likely to be severe if water used in cooking the shellfish has been discarded. Treatment is that of respiratory paralysis. No specific treatment is available, but patients are likely to recover if they survive the first 12 hours of the illness. The toxin of *Gymnodinium breve*, a flagellate producing red tides off the Florida coast, causes upper respiratory tract and ocular irritation in people living near the affected beaches.

A different form of paralytic shellfish poisoning is associated with ingestion of red whelk, *Neptunea antiqua*. This is caused by tetramine (tetramethylammonium hydroxide) which is produced in the salivary glands of this mollusk and causes curare-like effects on muscle.

FISH POISONING

A number of different mechanisms are involved in fish poisoning. Some species are inherently poisonous; the toxins of other species are acquired from organisms on which they feed; yet another form of fish poisoning is caused by breakdown products of bacterial action.

CIGUATERA POISONING. This can be acquired from a large number of species, about 300 in all, whose common characteristic is the narrow range of reef or coastal tropical waters which they inhabit. The toxin is thought to originate in blue-green algae consumed by herbivorous fish which are in turn the prey of carnivorous species. The toxin accumulates in the tissues and is excreted very slowly. Poisoning of this type is difficult to prevent, because the toxin is stable to heat, cold, and drying, and the taste and smell of the fish are unaffected. Symptoms commonly begin several hours after ingestion, but may be almost immediate. Nausea and vomiting are followed by paresthesias of the face, mouth, and limbs, dizziness, ataxia, muscular weakness, and severe muscle pain. The patient may die from respiratory paralysis during the first day, and in nonfatal cases the neuritic symptoms may persist for many weeks. No immunity is gained by an attack; indeed, a second episode of poisoning may be more severe.

TETRAODON POISONING. Many puffer fish found in the Pacific, Atlantic, and Indian Oceans are inherently toxic. The neurotoxin contained in their viscera (tetrodotoxin) is identical with that formerly known as tarichatoxin, found in the Californian newt *Taricha torosa* and some South American frogs. Its mode of action is similar to that of saxitoxin, and this is reflected in the syndrome of tetraodon poisoning which bears clear resemblances to paralytic shellfish poisoning (see above). Symptoms begin soon after ingestion and include paresthesias, dizziness, ataxia, and paralysis, often together with diarrhea, vomiting, and abdominal pain. The patient may die of respiratory paralysis.

SCOMBROID POISONING. Some species of the mackerel family, such as tuna and bonito, are susceptible to decomposition by *Proteus morganii*. Toxic products result from the breakdown of histidine normally contained in fish flesh. Within a few minutes of ingesting contaminated fish, the patient develops nausea, vomiting, headache, epigastric pain, dysphagia, dryness of the mouth, and severe urticaria. The illness usually lasts less than 24 hours.

OTHER FISH POISONS. Neurologic symptoms may follow ingestion of several other types of fish. Some of the toxins responsible are probably acquired from dinoflagellates, as in paralytic shellfish poisoning, but the source of other neurotoxins is still uncertain. In addition to these forms of fish poisoning, some species of the Gempylid group such as castor oil fish and snake mackerel contain a purgative oil, whereas the roe of some freshwater fish is toxic during the reproductive period, causing acute gastrointestinal symptoms with headache and fever.

MUSHROOM POISONING

In poisoning by muscarine-containing species such as *Amanita muscaria* (fly agaric) and *Amanita pantherina*, symptoms begin two or three hours after ingestion and consist of abdominal cramping, sweating, salivation, miosis, and bradycardia. Poisoning by these species is rarely fatal. By contrast, death-cup poisoning, by *Amanita phalloides* and *Amanita verna*, carries a mortality of 30 to 50 per cent or more. Two groups of toxins are contained in these mushrooms. Cyclic heptapeptides known as *phallotoxins* cause the violent symptoms of abdominal pain, vomiting, and diarrhea which begin 6 to 15 hours after ingestion. Symptoms then remit for about 48 hours. During this time tests of liver function become abnormal, and signs of hepatic and renal failure then develop, often accompanied by confusion, coma, and paralysis of the extremities. Small doses may lead to renal tubular necrosis without hepatic damage, but usually both organs are affected. This phase of the illness is probably caused by cyclic octapeptides known as *amatoxins*.

No specific treatment is available, but the stomach should be emptied by induced vomiting or gastric lavage, and atropine administered if muscarinic effects — that is, sweating, salivation, and colic — are observed. Otherwise, the general principles of management in acute hepatic and renal failure should be observed. For example, peritoneal dialysis or hemodialysis may be necessary in renal failure, and modern methods of managing acute hepatic failure may help to reduce the high mortality.

A number of pharmacologic agents have been shown to mitigate the effects of alpha-amanitin (the principal amatoxin of *A. phalloides*) in experimental systems, but their effect in human mushroom poisoning is not known.

TOXICANTS FOUND NATURALLY IN FOODS

Some substances found naturally in food cause forms of damage not usually thought of as food poisoning, partly because their effects are chronic rather than acute, and partly because the pathogenic role of many possible food toxicants is still uncertain. The mycotoxins have aroused special recent interest, but many other substances in food may be involved in the causation of chronic disease.

Antithyroid compounds in plants, mainly *Brassica* species, are thought to account for 4 per cent of the world incidence of goiter.

Cyanogenic glycosides, found especially in cassava or lima beans may be a causal agent of chronic cyanide poisoning. Tropical ataxic myelopathy and toxic amblyopia have been ascribed to this cause in several areas of high cassava consumption, but these syndromes are also found in other areas in which no such dietary factor can be invoked.

Lathyrism, a slowly progressive spastic paraplegia, is associated with the ingestion of pulse made from the seeds of *Lathyrus sativus* and other related species, which grow under adverse conditions and may become a staple diet in times of food shortage in Eritrea, parts of India, and Algeria. The toxic factor in the seeds is thought to be aminopropiononitrile.

MYCOTOXINS. Ergotism (see Ch. 368.2) is the most familiar of the illnesses caused by mold contamination of food. More recently, many other mycotoxins have been identified and their possible roles assessed in human and animal disease. Aflatoxins, products of *Aspergillus flavus* and allied species, were identified in the early 1960's after huge losses in turkey flocks, followed by outbreaks among ducks, pheasants, pigs, and calves, had been ascribed to contaminated peanut meal. In experimental animals, aflatoxin B1 causes liver necrosis, bile duct proliferation, and cirrhosis, whereas chronic or repeated administration leads to hepatocellular and cholangiocarcinoma. A probable role for this toxin in human disease is suggested by the association, established in Thailand and in several parts of Africa, between dietary intake of aflatoxin and the incidence of hepatic carcinoma.

Another group of mycotoxins, the trichothecenes, derived from *Fusarium* and other genera which cause spoilage of cereal grains, are now thought to have been responsible for alimentary toxic aleukia, widespread in the U.S.S.R. when conditions of war or famine compelled consumption of moldy grain. The main features were a hemorrhagic tendency, fever, leukopenia, agranulocytosis, and resulting sepsis.

Mycotoxins also have an indirect influence on human health by the depletion of livestock caused by moldy feed.

POISONING BY FLOWERING PLANTS

An immense number of plant species may contain constituents toxic to man, and only a few of the more common and important forms of plant poisoning can be considered here.

The first examples are all members of the family of *solanaceous plants*, in which toxic species are especially well represented.

Atropa belladonna (deadly nightshade) poisoning is caused by ingestion of the prominent black berries, which contain a number of alkaloids of the belladonna group. The symptoms and signs are those of atropine poisoning: dry mouth, dry skin, blurring of vision, dilated pupils, tachycardia and excitement, hallucinations, and delirium followed by coma — "hot as a hare, blind as a bat, dry as a bone, red as a beet, and mad as a hen."

Datura stramonium (thorn apple, jimson weed) also contains stramonium alkaloids, as do other species of this genus, and they may cause poisoning by ingestion of their seeds, of extracts of leaves, and even of nectar. Clinical manifestations are generally similar to those of atropine poisoning. Seeds may be ingested as a form of drug abuse, and the high dose thus received has led to alarming but fortunately transient syndromes characterized by hallucinations, hyperthermia, decerebrate posturing, hyperreflexia with extensor plantar responses, and electroencephalographic abnormalities.

Other familiar members of the Solanaceae are *Solanum americanum* and *S. nigrum* (common nightshade, black nightshade), *S. dulcamara* (woody nightshade, bittersweet), *Hyoscyamus niger* (henbane), and the potato plant, of which the green parts and tuber sprouts may be poisonous. Plants of this group contain a mixture of the stramonium alkaloids and of solanine, itself a mixture of alkaloids.

No specific treatment is available for these forms of poisoning. Peripheral effects caused by atropine can be antagonized by pilocarpine, but this does not affect its cerebral actions. Vomiting should be induced or the stomach emptied by gastric lavage.

The family Umbelliferae also includes many toxic species, in addition to familiar food species such as carrot, parsnip, and celery. *Conium maculatum* (hemlock), a common weed which looks somewhat like wild parsnip, contains several toxic alkaloids causing nausea and vomiting, progressive weakness, respiratory paralysis, and convulsions. Various species of *Cicuta*, the water hemlocks, are also toxic, the root containing cicutoxin, an unsaturated alcohol. Ingestion is followed by vomiting, salivation, delirium, convulsions, and paralysis. Effects similar to hemlock poisoning may result from ingestion of laburnum (family Papilionaceae), which contains the toxic alkaloid cytisine.

Some forms of poisoning are not confined to a particular plant family. Digitalis-like effects, for example, may be produced by oleander and lily-of-the-valley as well as by the foxglove.

The forms of plant poisoning discussed so far affect organs remote from the gastrointestinal tract. A number of plant products cause gastrointestinal symptoms, ranging from burning of the mouth and throat, through severe gastroenteritis (e.g., spurge laurel berries, roots and stems of pokeweed), to the hemorrhagic gastroenteritis which follows ingestion of seeds of the castor bean and certain other species.

22.5. CHEMICAL FOOD POISONING

Various forms of metallic poisoning are discussed in Ch. 24 and 379. Occasionally patients react idiosyncratically to a normal constituent of food, or to a food additive or preservative. The headache and hypertension induced by certain foods in patients receiving monoamine oxidase inhibitors are attributable to their natural tyramine content. The two examples which follow illustrate peculiar reactions to additives in food.

CHINESE RESTAURANT SYNDROME. A few people develop dramatic symptoms 10 to 20 minutes after eating some kind of Chinese food. These include tingling and burning in the back of the neck, radiating to the upper back, arms, and front of the chest. Some of them experience throbbing pain in the temples and infraorbital region. The symptoms fluctuate in severity and usually last for 45 minutes to 2 hours. The cause of this syndrome has been much disputed, but is probably the monosodium glutamate used in seasoning certain Chinese foods.

HOT DOG HEADACHE. A patient experienced several hours of bitemporal headache and facial flushing, starting within 30 minutes of eating certain kinds of cured meat. His symptoms were shown to be caused by sodium nitrite used in the curing process.

Arnon, S. S., Midura, T. F., Clay, S. A., Wood, R. M., and Chin J.: Infant botulism: Epidemiological, clinical and laboratory aspects. JAMA, 237:1946, 1977.

Barker, W. H., and Gangarosa, E. J.: Food poisoning due to *Vibrio parahaemolyticus*. Ann. Rev. Med., 25:75, 1974.

Blankenship, J. E.: Tetrodotoxin; from poison to powerful tool. Perspectives Biol. Med., 19:509, 1976.

Cherington, M.: Botulism, 10 years' experience. Arch. Neurol., 30:432, 1974.

Committee on Food Protection: Toxicants Occurring Naturally in Foods. 2nd ed. Washington, D.C., National Academy of Sciences Publication No. 73.8988, 1973, p. 346.

Crowther, J. S., and Holbrook, R.: Trends in methods for detecting food poisoning toxins produced by *Cl. botulinum* and *Staph. aureus*.

In Skinner, F. A., and Carr, J. G. (eds.): Microbiology in Agriculture Fisheries and Food. New York, Academic Press, 1976, p. 215.

Dadisman, T. A., Nelson, R., Molenda, J. R., and Garber, H. J.: *Vibrio parahaemolyticus* in Maryland. 1. Clinical and epidemiological aspects. Am. J. Epidemiol., 96:414, 1972.

Earampamoorthy, S., and Koff, R. S.: Health hazards of bivalve-mollusk ingestion. Ann. Intern. Med., 83:107, 1975.

Evans, M. H.: Mechanism of saxitoxin and tetrodotoxin poisoning. Br. Med. Bull., 25:263, 1969.

Hardin, J. W., and Arena, J. M.: Human Poisoning from Native and Cultivated Plants. 2nd ed. Durham, N. C., Duke University Press, 1973.

Hughes, J. M., Horwitz, M. A., Merson, M. H., Barker, W. H., Jr., and Gangarosa, E. J.: Foodborne disease outbreaks of chemical etiology in the U.S., 1970–74. Am. J. Epidemiol., 105:233, 1977.

Koenig, M. G., Drutz, D. J., Mushlin, A. I., Schaffner, W., and Rogers, D. E.: Type B botulism in man. Am. J. Med., 42:208, 1967.

Koenig, M. G., Spickard, A., Cardella, M. A., and Rogers, D. E.: Clinical and laboratory observations on type E botulism in man. Medicine, 43:517, 1962.

Lampe, K. F.: Systemic plant poisoning in children. Pediatrics, 54:347, 1974.

Loewenstein, M.: Epidemiology of *Cl. perfringens* food poisoning. N. Engl. J. Med., 286:1026, 1972.

Merson, M. H., and Dowell, V. R.: Epidemiologic clinical and laboratory aspects of wound botulism. N. Engl. J. Med., 289:1005, 1973.

Merson, M. H., Hughes, J. M., Dowell, V. R., Taylor, A., Barker, W. H., and Gangarosa, E. J.: Current trends in botulism in the United States. JAMA, 229:1305, 1974.

Mikolich, J. R., Paulson, G. W., and Cross, C. J.: Acute anticholinergic syndrome due to jimson seed ingestion. Ann. Intern. Med., 83:321, 1975.

Murrell, T. G. C., Roth, L., Egerton, J., Samels, J., and Walker, P. D.: Pig-bel; enteritis necroticans. Lancet, 1:217, 1966.

Nakamura, M., and Schulze, J. A.: *Clostridium perfringens* food poisoning. Ann. Rev. Microbiol., 23:359, 1970.

Portnoy, B. L., Goepfert, J. M., and Harmon, S. M.: An outbreak of *Bacillus cereus* food poisoning resulting from contaminated vegetable sprouts. Am. J. Epidemiol., 103:589, 1976.

Strong, F. M.: Toxicants occurring naturally in foods. Nutr. Rev., 32:225, 1974.

Symposium: Food, is it safe? Medlock, J. M. (ed.). Postgrad. Med. J., 50:593, 1974.

Wogan, G. N.: Mycotoxins. Ann. Rev. Pharmacol., 15:437, 1975.

Zen-Yoji, H., Sakai, S., Terayama, T., Kudo, Y., Ito, T., Benoki, M., and Nagasaki, M.: Epidemiology, enteropathogenicity and classification of *Vibrio parahaemolyticus*. J. Infect. Dis., 115:436, 1965.

23. COMMON ACCIDENTAL POISONING

Robert J. Haggerty

DEFINITION. The term "accidental poisoning" is usually limited to clinical illness that results from the introduction of exogenous chemicals into the body. These chemicals may be medications in excessive dose, other chemicals not intended for human metabolism, or biologic products, both plant and animal. The term, however, generally excludes disease produced by toxic products of microorganisms. An accident is (1) an observable tissue or biochemical injury that is (2) unplanned. This definition is too restrictive for accidental poisoning, for in many instances the physician is called upon to treat patients who have only ingested a poison but do not yet have any observable symptoms or signs of tissue or biochemical injury. Also, although most poisonings are unplanned in children, the same tissue or biochemical damage occurs when a chemical is introduced for homicidal or suicidal intent in adolescents and adults.

ETIOLOGY. Accidental poisoning is best understood

TABLE 1. Mortality: Agents Responsible for Accidental Poison Deaths in the United States, 1975*

	Less Than 5 Years of Age		Total All Ages
Medications: Total	65		3132
Salicylates and analgesics		24	1275
Sedatives and hypnotics		3	594
Psychotherapeutic drugs		11	178
Systemic and hematologic		6	61
Other		21	1024
Other substances:			
Total	49		1562
Alcohol		1	391
Petroleum and solvents		21	54
Pesticides		6	30
Heavy metals		2	13
Corrosives		4	16
Other		15	1058
Total poison deaths	114		4694

*From the National Center for Health Statistics, HRA, HEW; Reported in The National Clearinghouse for Poison Control Centers Bulletin, April, 1977.

as a problem of multiple causes — the interaction of an agent (the poison) with a host (the patient) in a particular environment. The major agents and the number of accidental poisoning deaths caused by each are listed in Table 1. In nonfatal accidental poisoning the agents responsible are quite different from those in fatal cases. The most common agents responsible for nonfatal accidental poisoning are listed in Table 2, together with the number of such accidents in different age groups. Strictly speaking, these are the etiologic agents, but to understand why a particular poisoning occurs requires knowledge of the interaction of the agent, environment, and host; this is discussed under Pathogenesis.

The route of entry of the poison (agent) is most often oral for solids and liquids, but may occasionally be by absorption through skin, rectum, or lung, or by parenteral injection.

INCIDENCE. Over 4500 accidental poison fatalities occur each year in the United States. Less than 5 per cent of these fatalities occur in children, but nearly two thirds of all accidental but nonfatal poisonings occur in preschool children. Not so evident from Table 2 is the second peak in the late teens and early twenties owing to suicide attempts. In children there are from 300 to 1000 nonfatal poison ingestions for each poison fatality. Some estimates place the total number of nonfatal poisonings as high as 300,000 to 500,000 per year in children in the United States. It is the most common medical, i.e., nonsurgical, emergency seen in preschool children. In one study, 12 per cent of all two-year-old children had experienced an accidental poisoning within the previous year. In addition to differences in the agents responsible for fatal as compared with nonfatal poisoning, the agents responsible for accidental poisoning vary considerably in their frequency between children and adults. Salicylates are the most common agent involved in children, whereas barbiturates are more common in adults. A multitude of household products (such as cleansers, solvents, and insecticides) are potentially poisonous and are available in the American home. They are more likely to be the cause of childhood than of adult poisonings.

TABLE 2. Most Common Agents Responsible for Accidental Poisoning Reported to the National Clearinghouse for Poison Information Centers, 1973

	Total All Ages	5 Years	5–14	15–24	25–44	45 and Over
Medicines	82,904	45,919	5144	15,662	12,001	4178
Internal*	73,086	37,428	4660	15,397	11,799	3802
Aspirin*	9182	6576	691	1347	453	115
Other*	63,904	30,852	3969	14,050	11,346	3687
External*	9818	8491	484	265	202	376
Cleaning and polishing agents	18,598	16,478	874	493	409	344
Petroleum products	5695	4381	505	508	243	58
Cosmetics	9167	8697	266	88	57	59
Pesticides	6414	5079	517	307	342	169
Gases and vapor	886	121	144	213	255	153
Plants	7719	6210	874	487	100	48
Turpentine, paints, etc.	6947	5937	446	300	182	82
Miscellaneous	11,290	8122	1650	718	496	304
Unknown	2140	732	206	618	405	179
Total	307,750	185,023	20,430	50,453	38,290	13,554

*These Totals are included in Medicines.

EPIDEMIOLOGY. There are more epidemiologic data available on the role of the agent in causing accidental poisoning than on the host and environmental factors, and very few data on the complex interrelations of these three factors in causing accidental poisoning (Wehrle et al.). Most of the available information is of the retrospective epidemiologic type for accidental poisoning in children. It documents incidence by age (peak childhood age one to four years), sex (males more than females, except for the poison suicides of the late teens and early twenties), socioeconomic class (no difference), season (no overall significant variation, although there are some special variations such as medications that are more frequent in the winter and pesticides in the summer), hour of day (peak in mid-morning), geographical area (lye and petroleum distillates more common in the South), and place where poisoning occurred (kitchen, bedroom, and bathroom are most common). Death *rate* for all age groups from accidental poisoning has remained steady for the past two decades at about 1 per 100,000 for all age groups. There has been a significant decrease in both the *actual number* of deaths in children under five years of age from accidental poisoning (from 422 in 1958 to 114 in 1975) and in the *rate* (from 2.5 per 100,000 in 1958 to under 1.0 in 1975. At the same time, poison fatalities in all ages rose from 3000 in 1969 to over 4500 in 1975. The most dramatic drop has occurred in aspirin poisoning. Over 20,000 total aspirin ingestions were reported to the National Clearinghouse in 1965 and only about 8000 in 1972, whereas the number of all ingestions reported actually increased. The reasons for the decline in children are probably multiple, but are likely to be from public and professional education, better therapy, safety enclosures for dispensing medicines (Schertz et al.), and limitation of the number of tablets in children's aspirin (1¼ grains) to 36 per bottle.

Since poisonous agents such as aspirin are available in nearly every home, the very real question is why more children are not poisoned when one considers the ubiquity of potentially poisonous agents.

Some children seem peculiarly susceptible to accidental poisoning (Sobel and Margolis). A child with a history of one poisoning episode is nine times as likely to have a second episode in the following year than is a child from a matched control group. Poisoned as compared to nonpoisoned control children appear to have different personalities. They are more impulsive and overactive and are likely to strike back when disciplined, to have more disturbed relationships with their parents, and to have other behavior problems. Their social environment is also different, for their parents are more likely to have marital problems, to be suffering acute illness at the time of the ingestion, or to show a more distant and tense family relationship. Whether this knowledge can lead to identification of the high-risk group before poisoning occurs and whether one can change the incidence of poisoning in this high-risk group are not known; prevention by alteration of social and environmental therapy has never been documented.

Among adults, suicide and homicide by poisoning obviously present a very different epidemiologic picture. Unlike immunization for infectious diseases, no one method of control can be expected to be effective for all types of poisoning.

PREVENTION. Prevention of accidental poisoning, in spite of these negative statements about its effectiveness, should be attempted by many groups, including physicians. Better labeling of household products and prescriptions is of importance, but it should be remembered that children of the age most often poisoned cannot read. Parents should store such medications in safe places, but locked medicine cabinets are of little practical use because they are usually left unlocked when in use. Physicians treating adults should especially warn grandparents that the digitalis, quinidine, or other potent drugs they are receiving are toxic to small children and are often taken by the child from the grandmother's pocketbook. When prescribing analgesics, especially aspirin, for an acute illness in adults, the physician should warn that those are poisonous to children and should prescribe only the minimal amounts needed for an illness. All prescriptions should be dispensed in safety cap enclosures. New laws also require household cleansers to be dispensed in safety cap containers and should be effective. A common scenario of an accidental poisoning starts with a mother with an influenzal syndrome who may have aspirin prescribed; she falls asleep, and her two-year-old child ingests a fatal amount of aspirin left on the bedside table. Other acute family crises, social as well as medical, also seem to be factors in the pathogenesis of childhood poisoning (Meyer et al.). The physician who cares for such adult crises may be the most effective person to prevent childhood accidental poisonings by seeing that adequate supervision of children is arranged when parents are sick or upset.

Most poisonings in adults are the result of suicide attempts, and of course prevention is aimed at recognition of the person at risk.

Community aspects of poison prevention include public education concerning the hazards of poisons. The Consumer Product Act of 1970 and the Commission Coordinating Safety Packaging Regulations require special labeling of hazardous substances and the listing of toxic ingredients on the label. This important step is but one of many that have been taken by the community in an effort to reduce the frequency of accidental poisoning.

National Poison Prevention Week during the third week in March serves as a focal point for health education programs. But to have any chance of success, such measures should be carried out throughout the year. The rapid development of poison information centers since the first one was formed in Chicago in 1953 to the now more than 500 in the United States is another important community action. The National Clearinghouse for Poison Information Centers of the Public Health Service coordinates activities of the local centers and is a valuable repository of information, both for treatment of poisoned patients and for preventive programs. Several poison information centers now have on-line computer terminals to the National Center for rapid access to information on the ingredients of new products. In addition, many centers now have microfiche systems to facilitate retrieval and standardize treatment. These systems have as many as 200,000 trade-name items indexed and easily accessible. The Association of Poison Control Centers, a voluntary national group, has produced educational material designed to prevent poisonings, has established standards for operation of poison control centers, including an approved list of antidotes, their indications, and doses, and has promoted scientific study of poisonings. The American Academy of Clinical Toxicology and its Board in Clinical Toxicology serve as the academic organization for poison center personnel. These organizations have stimulated research in accidental poisoning. It seems clear that these multiple approaches to prevention of poisoning need to be continued, but there is a need to critically evaluate their effectiveness and to add imaginative new programs aimed at prevention.

DIAGNOSIS. Diagnosis of accidental poisoning is made from (1) the label on the poison container, (2) the characteristic signs and symptoms in the patient, and (3) chemical analyses, in that order of importance. In most cases of acute poisoning, especially in children, there is no problem in determining that ingestion of a poison has occurred. The patient is often observed to ingest the poison or is found with the empty container. Here the problem is only to determine the chemical ingredients of the compound ingested, how much was taken, and what toxicity is to be expected. On the other hand, unlabeled prescriptions or trade-name household products (of which there are estimated to be over 250,000 potentially poisonous ones available in American homes) may present a serious problem in identification of the precise chemical involved. Poison information centers are especially equipped to deal with this aspect of diagnosis, for they keep on file trade names of potentially poisonous products and their ingredients.

Most operate 24 hours a day and are listed in the telephone book. Information on management will also be provided by these centers. Of great use to the physician in diagnosis of poisoning, as well as in therapy, is a book (Gleason et al.) which contains a section with over 17,000 trade-name household products, their ingredients, toxicity, symptoms, and treatment.

When the label is missing, identification of the poison may be aided by knowing that certain ingredients are common to household products used for the same specific purpose; e.g., most solvent cleansers contain ketones or hydrocarbons. Federal labeling legislation, which requires most hazardous household chemicals to bear a label that plainly lists ingredients, has helped in diagnosis. *The label on the container is the single most useful diagnostic bit of information in accidental poisoning.*

When the patient has not been observed to ingest a poison, the problem of diagnosis may be great. Although some poisons produce pathognomonic signs or symptoms, most do not. Almost any acute disease may be simulated, and the range of symptoms and signs that may result is so vast that one can only advise that any symptoms or signs of unknown cause must be suspected of being due to poisoning until proved otherwise. Lists of such symptoms and signs with the various poisons that can produce them are available in standard toxicology texts.

Toxicologic analysis of body fluids or of the ingested substance itself plays a numerically small but important and increasing role in the diagnosis of accidental poisoning. In those instances in which analysis is useful, it is usually much easier to analyze the remains in the container from which the poison came than to analyze body fluids in which great dilution of the poison has occurred. Recent development of chemical analyses by mass spectrometry and gas-liquid chromatography now allows toxic screens for a wide variety of poisons from small amounts of blood. Commercial laboratories provide qualitative analyses for sedatives, narcotics, psychotropics, heavy metals and pesticides, which have made diagnoses much more specific in a period as short as a few hours.

Once the poison that was ingested has been identified, there remains the problem of determining its potential for harm to the patient. This depends on the amount ingested and the toxicity of the agent. The amount can sometimes be estimated by observers who may have seen the patient ingest the poison and by the amount remaining in the container. The toxicity of a particular poison can be assessed by reference to known data on LD_{50} and minimal lethal dose. A table has been prepared that is most useful in then estimating the degree of risk to the patient (Table 3).

TABLE 3. Toxicity Rating*

Rating	Probable Lethal Dose	
	mg/kg	For 70 kg Man
6 – Super toxic	<5	A taste <7 drops
5 – Extremely toxic	5–50	7 drops to 1 tsp
4 – Very toxic	50–500	1 tsp to 1 oz
3 – Moderately toxic	500 mg–5 grams	1 oz to 1 pint
2 – Slightly toxic	5–15 grams	1 pint to 1 quart
1 – Practically nontoxic	>15 grams	>1 quart

*From Gleason, M., Gosselin, R., Hodge, H., and Smith, R.: Clinical Toxicology of Commercial Products. 4th ed. Baltimore, Williams & Wilkins Company, 1973.

TREATMENT. A common mistake in the therapy of acute poisoning is to search for a specific antidote, of which there are very few, and to delay general therapy, which may be very effective and which is all that is available for the majority of poisonings.

General principles of therapy are (1) elimination of the poison from the body, (2) inactivation of the poison, and (3) supportive measures.

Elimination of the Poison. INDUCED EMESIS. One of the most common poison problems brought to the physician is that of a child or adult who has just ingested a potential poison but is still asymptomatic. The most important part of therapy is removal of the poison from the stomach before significant absorption can occur. It is now clear that gastric lavage, the time-honored method for removal of gastric contents, is much *less* effective than induced vomiting because the stomach normally traps large quantities of material in several pouches inaccessible to the lavage tube. The most effective way to induce vomiting is to administer a large dose of syrup of ipecac (15 ml for a child one to four years old, 30 to 45 ml for adults), followed by a repeat dose if no vomiting occurs within 20 minutes (Robertson). This dose is considerably larger than is recommended in older texts, but it has been found safe and much more rapidly effective than smaller doses. Many physicians now prescribe a 1-ounce bottle of syrup of ipecac when children reach age one in order that parents will have it on hand in case of need. Vomiting is more complete if the patient drinks several ounces of fluid three to five minutes after administration of the syrup of ipecac. Mechanical induction of vomiting by gagging, although having the merit of speed, is so often not effective that it is not the first choice of methods. Parenteral administration of apomorphine has not proved to be useful. Vomiting should be induced even if several hours have elapsed after ingestion, for many poisons remain for long periods in the stomach when ingested in large quantities. Other methods of inducing vomiting such as use of a solution of powdered mustard or soap suds are not very effective.

CAUTIONS REGARDING INDUCED EMESIS. The only contraindications to induced emesis in the treatment of accidental poisoning are in patients who have ingested caustics (e.g., lyes, acids), strychnine, and hydrocarbons, and in the comatose patient. With any cause of altered consciousness, gag reflex may be altered sufficiently to increase the risk of aspiration. Ipecac does work even with ingestion of antiemetics and tranquilizers with antiemetic properties (Verhulst and Thoman). Whether one should remove hydrocarbons by careful gastric lavage is still a disputed point. A collaborative study suggests that it may be of slight advantage, and emesis is less safe and less effective than lavage. Saturated salt and sodium bicarbonate solutions should not be used as emetics.

GASTRIC LAVAGE. Even though less effective than emesis, gastric lavage is indicated for comatose poisoned patients to remove the poison from the stomach with less risk of aspiration than with emesis. A large-bore gastric lavage tube should usually be employed, and the stomach should be irrigated with copious amounts of water or physiologic saline. Aspiration can be prevented by having the patient lie on his side with the head slightly lower than the body. Sodium bicarbonate should not be used because it increases absorption of many poisons (salicylates) and causes large amounts of carbon dioxide to be released in the stomach, increasing the risk of aspiration.

OTHER METHODS OF POISON REMOVAL. No data are available on the *effectiveness of catharsis* or *colonic irrigations*. Most do not use cathartics today unless activated charcoal is also used, for ipecac will cause catharsis and there is often diarrhea produced by the original poison.

Exchange transfusion has proved useful for removal of some poisons when plasma protein binding makes any form of dialysis less effective, i.e., with boric acid and some barbiturates.

Peritoneal dialysis and hemodialysis are effective means of removing many poisons. For preschool children, and even for many adults, peritoneal dialysis (Etteldorf et al.) is preferred because proper equipment and an experienced team for hemodialysis are less available. Use of commercially prepared solutions that contain properly balanced electrolytes and albumin, together with simple multiple-holed polyethylene tubing for insertion into the peritoneal cavity, provides a relatively convenient and simple technique. In certain adult patients in whom renal failure from the poisoning is the major problem, e.g., ethylene glycol poisoning, or for whom prolonged dialysis is needed, hemodialysis has proved very useful.

The kidney is the most effective organ for removal of many poisons. If renal function was normal prior to the poisoning, this route of excretion should be facilitated by adequate fluids, usually intravenously, and in some situations by the use of *osmotic diuretics*, such as mannitol (Cirksens et al.). In salicylate poisoning renal excretion is enhanced as much as twentyfold by making the pH of the urine alkaline with sodium bicarbonate. Acid diuresis with ammonium chloride for amphetamines and phencyclidine also increases excretion of these weak bases. For patients who are seriously ill, several of these routes of elimination of the poison should be used simultaneously, i.e., gastric lavage, enhancement of urinary excretion, and peritoneal dialysis.

Inactivation of the Poison. A time-honored agent designed to inactivate many poisons has been the "universal antidote" made of two parts charcoal, one part tannic acid, and one part magnesium oxide. This mixture is of no value, but there are new data to support the use of specially prepared activated charcoal to absorb poisons in the intestinal tract. Five to 6 teaspoonfuls of such charcoal (not burnt toast) mixed in a glass of water should be swallowed or administered by gastric tube and then, after absorption has occurred, within 30 minutes, removed from the stomach, followed by saline cathartics to remove the absorbed poisons (Corby and Decker). Neutralization of ingested acids or alkalis is probably of little value, because the tissue necrosis that results from such poisons occurs almost immediately upon contact. The use of demulcents, such as olive oil or milk, makes the patient who has ingested an irritant poison more comfortable but probably does little else and should be avoided if the poison is fat-soluble.

Supportive Measures. More lives are likely to be saved by careful, early, symptomatic treatment of complications such as peripheral vascular collapse, respiratory obstruction, urinary retention, fluid imbalance, and central nervous system excitement or depression than by frantic and usually unsuccessful search for specific antidotes. All these complications are treated by the standard methods that are used when they are due to other causes.

Poisonings for Which Specific Antidotes Exist. *Cyanide poisoning* produces death within minutes. Specific antidotes are available, but unless poisoning occurs in a laboratory there is rarely time to administer them. The antidotes are sodium nitrite injected intravenously (6 to 8 ml per square meter of body surface of a 3 per cent solution at a rate of 2.5 to 5 ml per minute), which produces methemoglobinemia, followed by sodium thiosulfate intravenously (50 ml of a 25 per cent solution). Amyl nitrite inhalation may be of value immediately while the sodium nitrite is being prepared.

Heavy metal poisoning can be successfully treated by various chelating agents — BAL, EDTA, or penicillamine (Ch. 24 and 379).

Iron salts produce acute gastroenteritis, shock, liver necrosis, and, frequently, death. As few as 10 tablets of the usual size (0.3 gram) may be fatal. The specific antidote, desferrioxamine, is useful intravenously to bind absorbed iron (2.0 grams in 5 per cent of levulose solution intravenously, dose 90 mg per kilogram); 140 mg of desferrioxamine can bind about 1 gram of ferrous sulfate — 200 mg of iron. It is contraindicated orally, for it probably enhances absorption. Fluid replacement, including blood plasma, should be used for shock.

Morphine and other opium derivatives can be successfully antagonized by naloxone HCl (adult dose 0.4 mg), repeated up to three times at three-minute intervals. If no improvement occurs, another cause of symptoms should be suspected. Since the action of the antagonist lasts only one to two hours and that of morphine for six or more hours, repeat doses may be needed after two hours (see Ch. 244).

Phosphate ester insecticides such as parathion are powerful anticholinesterases. In addition to peripheral parasympathetic stimulation they produce voluntary muscle paralysis, the most serious being to the muscles of respiration. Red cell cholinesterase is a valuable laboratory test to make the diagnosis and to follow therapy. Atropine in very large doses of 1 mg subcutaneously for a child, 2 to 3 mg for an adult, every 15 to 60 minutes until symptoms subside will antagonize these peripheral parasympathomimetic toxic effects. 2-Pyridine aldoxime methiodide (PAM), a cholinesterase regenerator, is dramatically effective in relieving skeletal muscle paralysis (1 gram intravenously over a five- to ten-minute period and repeated as a slow intravenous drip as needed for respiratory paralysis). Atropine is used first. PAM is not used alone. Airway obstruction must be treated by aspiration, positioning, and occasionally tracheostomy.

Treatment of Specific Common Poisons. A few words should be said about general management of the most common poisonings, but reference to standard texts is necessary for details of treatment of these as well as for the many poisonings that cannot be discussed here.

Amphetamine poisoning is common from an overdose of reducing pills or pep pills. After removal from the stomach, chlorpromazine should be administered in full dose to counteract mania and delirium. Barbiturates should not be used because the late-stage depression that occurs with amphetamines may be compounded.

Atropine poisoning may be produced by overdose or accidental ingestion of the drug or by accidental ingestion of one of several plants, such as the jimson weed. Symptoms include those of parasympathetic blocking, intense erythema, fever, and delirium. Antihistamines and many psychotropic drugs also have anticholinergic action plus central nervous system depression. Physostigmine is a very useful diagnostic agent (dose 0.5 mg for child under five, 1 to 2 mg for child over 10, given slowly intravenously over two to three minutes). It counters both central and peripheral actions.

DDT and other chlorinated hydrocarbon insecticides are relatively uncommon causes of acute poisoning, for fatal doses in man are in the range of 250 mg per kilogram, and this amount is difficult to ingest. Central nervous system stimulation and convulsions are the most serious symptoms. Treatment is entirely symptomatic.

Hydrocarbon ingestion, especially of gasoline and kerosene, produces a severe pneumonia due mainly to direct aspiration into the lung rather than to bloodstream transport to the lungs. Most of the aspiration probably occurs during the initial swallow, but some may also occur during subsequent vomiting. If large amounts have been ingested or the hydrocarbon is a vehicle for some other toxin (i.e., insecticide), removal by emesis is preferable to leaving in the stomach. Controversy still surrounds this recommendation. For the more volatile hydrocarbons, such as charcoal lighter fluid from which central nervous system depression can occur, most now agree it should be removed by emesis. For the low volatile waxes, there is no need to remove.

Probably the only effective therapy for the patient with severe pneumonia is oxygen. Although adrenocortical steroids and prophylactic antimicrobials have been used, there is little evidence that they are the crucial element in successful therapy of this poisoning. Again, lighter fluid is the exception, and adrenal steroids do seem useful for pneumonia caused by this agent.

Carbon tetrachloride produces prompt central nervous system depression and abdominal pain. Early death is due to depression of vasomotor and respiratory centers and convulsions. If the patient survives this, he may develop renal and hepatic necrosis. The management at this stage is the same as for other causes of failure of these organs.

Methyl alcohol can cause severe metabolic acidosis and blindness with a fatal dose from as little as 2 ounces. Treatment includes emesis, ethyl alcohol to inhibit the metabolic oxidation of methanol (whiskey, 30 ml every three to four hours for adults), and sodium bicarbonate intravenously for the metabolic acidosis.

Lye and other caustics produce severe, deep burns of the esophagus that may perforate or may later cause esophageal stenosis. Initial pain, airway obstruction, and shock are treated symptomatically. Early esophagoscopy, to determine whether burns have occurred, is followed by cortisone if burns are found. After several days for healing to progress, careful dilatation of the esophagus can be begun. Management should be a team effort with the esophagoscopist.

Salicylate poisoning is the single most common cause of poisoning in children. Emesis should always be carried out if the patient is awake, even though several hours have elapsed after ingestion. Salicylates produce an initial respiratory alkalosis that is transient in children but less so in adults, followed by severe metabolic acidosis, dehydration, and loss of body potassium. With severe poisoning several routes of elimination may have to be used, i.e., by increasing urinary excretion and by peritoneal dialysis. Initial hydration should be vigorous to initiate brisk diuresis, and the fluids should include sodium bicarbonate, 2 mEq per kilogram given over one hour. Once diuresis has begun, potassium salts, approximately 35 mEq per liter of fluid, should be added to the solution. Monitoring of serum pH and electrolytes and adjustment of fluid and electrolyte administration appropriately are important for optimal therapy. Milder degrees of poisoning can usually be treated with alkali and intravenous fluids alone. Other symptoms, such as respiratory depression or convulsions, are treated symptomatically.

Cirksens, W. J., Bastian, R. C., Malloy, J. P., and Barry, K. G.: Use of mannitol in exogenous and endogenous intoxications. N. Engl. J. Med., 270:161, 1964.

Corby, D. G., and Decker, W. J.: Management of acute poisoning with activated charcoal. Pediatrics, 54:324, 1974.

Etteldorf, J. N., Dobbins, W. T., Summitt, R. L., Rainwater, W. T., and Fischer, R. L.: Intermittent peritoneal dialysis using 5 per cent albumin in the treatment of salicylate intoxication in children. J. Pediat., 58:226, 1961.

Gleason, M., Gosselin, R., Hodge, H., and Smith, R.: Clinical Toxicology of Commercial Products. 4th ed. Baltimore, Williams & Wilkins Company, 1973.

Meyer, R. J., Roelofs, H. A., Bluestone, J., and Redmond, S.: Accidental injury to the preschool child. J. Pediat., 63:95, 1963.

Robertson, W. O.: Syrup of ipecac — a slow or fast emetic? Am. J. Dis. Child., 103:136, 1962.

Rumack, B.: Anticholinergic poisoning: Treatment with physostigmine. Pediatrics, 52:449, 1973.

Schertz, R. G., Latham, G. H., and Stracener, D. E.: Child-resistant containers can prevent poisonings. Pediatrics, 43:84, 1969.

Sobel, R., and Margolis, J. A.: Repetitive poisoning in children: A psychosocial study. Pediatrics, 35:641, 1965.

Verhulst, H. L., and Thoman, M. E.: Ipecac syrup in antiemetic ingestion. JAMA, 196:433, 1966.

Wehrle, P. F., DeFreest, L., Penhollow, J., and Harris, V. G.: The epidemiology of accidental poisoning in an urban population. III. Pediatrics, 27:614, 1961.

24. HEAVY METAL POISONING

Edmund B. Flink

24.1. INTRODUCTION

Many features of poisoning by the heavy metals are similar. The important metals from the standpoint of toxicology are arsenic, lead, mercury, antimony, cadmium, and thallium. The toxic and lethal doses of each metal are small. Antimony, arsenic, lead, mercury, and thallium all have effects on enzymes of the body. Antimony, arsenic, and mercury poison sulfhydryl groups. Mercuric ions even in fairly dilute solutions denature proteins and cause protein precipitation. Thallium and cadmium have recently assumed importance industrially.

Other metals may be toxic also. *Beryllium* intoxication is discussed in Ch. 348.6, and *bismuth, copper, gold, iron, silver, and uranium* intoxications are discussed in Ch. 379. *Barium* ions cause epigastric pain, nausea, vomiting, diarrhea, chills, cramps, muscle contractions, convulsions, hypertension, tachyarrhythmia, and cardiac arrest.

Sodium sulfate or magnesium sulfate should be given immediately to precipitate the barium as sulfate. *Cobalt* was added to beer from 1957 to 1967. Ingestion of large volumes of this beer caused serious and often fatal myocardiopathy. Cobalt has been eliminated as an additive. *Manganese* poisoning occurs in mining and smelting of manganese ores. Damage to the basal ganglia of the brain occurs with attendant Parkinson-like symptoms. When symptoms begin, removal from exposure is mandatory. Proper ventilation of mines and processing plants will prevent intoxication.

Browning, E.: Toxicity of Industrial Metals. New York, Appleton-Century-Crofts, 1969.

Goodman, L. S., and Gilman, A.: Pharmacological Basis of Therapeutics. 5th ed. New York, The Macmillan Company, 1975.

Lee, D. H. K.: Metallic Contaminants and Human Health. New York, Academic Press, 1972.

Vallee, B. L., and Ulmer, D. D.: Biochemical effects of mercury, cadmium, and lead. Ann. Rev. Biochem., 41:91, 1972.

24.2. ARSENIC POISONING

EXPOSURE. Many household and garden pesticides contain arsenous oxide, copper acetoarsenite (Paris green), or calcium or lead arsenate. Drugs that contain arsenic include sodium cacodylate, Fowler's solution, and the arsphenamines (now obsolete). Fowler's solution continues to be used in treatment of asthma in certain regions. Fruits sprayed with insecticides may contain enough arsenic to be toxic. Bootlegged whiskey has occasionally been contaminated with arsenicals. Arsenic trioxide (As_2O_3) or white arsenic has been a favorite for homicidal purposes. Accidental ingestion of arsenic-containing poison continues to be an important source of exposure, especially for children.

Although toxic exposure occurs in a variety of industries, only a few cases are reported. Poisoning does occur among agricultural workers using insecticide spray or dust. Arsine (AsH_3) is a very serious industrial hazard. It is produced accidentally by the exposure of nascent hydrogen to arsenic trioxide.

Arsenic is stored in liver, nervous system, nails, hair, and other viscera and can be detected in them after excretion in urine has ceased. A single dose requires 10 to 70 days for excretion, so accumulation is possible from small daily doses.

The minimal lethal dose of arsenic trioxide (As_2O_3) is 60 to 180 mg, but there is a great variability in susceptibility. The lethal dose of arsine is smaller than this.

MANIFESTATIONS. *Acute poisoning* may be overwhelming and may produce shock and death within 20 minutes to 48 hours. Ingestion of smaller doses causes vomiting, diarrhea, abdominal pain, and muscle cramps, but does not cause corrosion of mucous membranes. If the victim survives acute poisoning, he may recover without sequelae, or he may develop symptoms of chronic poisoning.

Intravascular hemolysis and renal damage are characteristic of arsenic poisoning, so hemoglobinuria, nausea, vomiting, and abdominal pain develop within six hours after exposure. This initial illness may be quickly fatal, or recovery may begin in a few days. Instances of chronic arsine poisoning have been reported.

Chronic poisoning results from repeated ingestion of small doses. This is the usual method for homicide.

Weight loss, diarrhea or constipation, nausea, anorexia, fatigue, drowsiness, peripheral neuropathy, headache, confusion, pigmentation and scaling of the skin, hyperkeratoses of palms and soles, and transverse white lines of all fingernails (Mee's lines) are the important symptoms and signs. Hyperkeratoses may go on to malignant changes in the form of multiple basal cell cancers (Bowen's disease). Perforation of the nasal septum is common. Myocardiopathy induced by arsenic may be fatal.

Hematologic findings of chronic arsenic poisoning include anemia, leukopenia, thrombocytopenia, basophilic stippling, and disturbed erythropoiesis, and myelopoiesis.

DIAGNOSIS. The diagnosis can be established by determining arsenic in the urine. Normal persons excrete an average of 0.015 mg per day, with a range of 0.005 to 0.04 mg. Most patients with manifestations of arsenic poisoning excrete more than 0.1 mg per day.

As in lead poisoning, urine coproporphyrin III excretion is increased markedly, but delta amino levulinic acid is not increased in experimental arsenic poisoning in rabbits and probably not in human intoxication.

Hair and nails store arsenic, so analysis of arsenic content may be of diagnostic value, particularly after removal of the patient from exposure. Hair and nail samples must be very carefully washed to exclude adhering dust and extraneous material. Normal values have ranged from 0.025 to 0.088 mg per 100 grams of hair. Over 0.1 mg per 100 grams is abnormal.

TREATMENT. When a poison has been ingested, immediate induction of emesis or gastric lavage is of prime importance. Dimercaprol or 2,3-dimercaptopropanol (BAL) should be given immediately. The initial intramuscular dose of BAL is 2.5 to 3.0 mg per kilogram of body weight, followed by the same dose every four hours for six doses. For very severe poisoning, the initial dose should be 5.0 mg per kilogram, followed by 2.5 mg per kilogram, as indicated above, with additional doses at 6- to 12-hour intervals for six doses, depending on the status of the patient. BAL has not proved to be effective in arsine poisoning or in chronic poisoning, probably because the damage has already occurred. Removal from exposure in chronic poisoning is mandatory and usually suffices.

Severe anemia must be treated by transfusion. Treatment of acute renal insufficiency requires the same considerations as that resulting from a variety of causes.

PREVENTION. Proper storage and labeling of poisons in general should prevent accidental poisoning of children. Avoiding direct contact with insect sprays and wearing appropriate masks when using dusting powders will control this industrial exposure.

Heyman, A., Pfeiffer, J. B., Jr., Willet, R. W., and Taylor, H. M.: Peripheral neuropathy caused by arsenical intoxication: A study of 41 cases with observation of the effects of BAL. N. Engl. J. Med., 254:401, 1956.

Kyle, R. A., and Pease, G. L.: Hematologic aspects of arsenic intoxication. N. Engl. J. Med., 273:18, 1965.

Vallee, B. L., Ulmer, D. D., and Wacker, W. E. C.: Arsenic toxicology and biochemistry. AMA Arch. Industr. Health 21:132, 1960.

24.3. LEAD POISONING

ETIOLOGY. Exposure to lead in the home is chiefly by ingestion of white lead paint scales by children (pica), from new water systems in which white lead has been used in joints of pipes, by ingestion of soluble lead salts in foods, wines, and distilled liquors, by use of pewter dishes and earthenware dishes with a glass glaze, and by use of tetraethyl lead gasoline for cleaning purposes. Drinking of "moonshine" whiskey distilled by use of an auto radiator as a condenser has resulted in epidemics of acute lead poisoning and constitutes an important cause of lead poisoning of adults.

Ingestion of lead paint scales by young children in areas of poor and old housing constitutes the greatest problem in the United States today. In New York City 4000 cases of lead poisoning were found in 1970 and 1971 because of increased interest and availability of appropriate tests. The incidence in children is greatest in summer months and reaches a peak at the age of one to three years. Black children are at greatest risk. Siblings of children with lead intoxication should be examined also, because about a third of them have been found to have serious exposure.

Lead is dissolved and absorbed from the gastrointestinal tract, deposited in the liver, and then released into the systemic circulation. About 10 per cent of ingested lead is absorbed. The respiratory tract epithelium absorbs lead fumes or may propel particles into the pharynx, where they are swallowed. Thirty to 50 per cent of lead in air is absorbed. Tetraethyl lead and related compounds may be absorbed through the skin. Soluble lead salts, such as lead acetate or lead carbonate, are readily absorbed and can cause acute poisoning when ingested.

There are many industrial uses of lead and, therefore, many opportunities for exposure. In recent years the industrial consumption of lead in the United States has averaged about 1,110,000 tons a year. The industries using or producing lead are petroleum, mining and smelting, storage battery manufacture, printing, paint and pigment, ceramic and glass, construction (mainly plumbing and insulation), ammunition, wrecking and salvage (acetylene torch and electric arc volatilizing lead paints and alloys), battery reclaiming, and brass polishing. Any procedure that produces lead vapor, mist, or dust exposes workers to inhalation and absorption of lead from respiratory tract epithelium. A new source is paint dust generated during restoring old houses with old lead paint.

The lead-using trades have set up standards and checking procedures that have controlled industrial hazards well. Smoking and eating are restricted to uncontaminated areas. Washing hands and changing clothes before eating and leaving work are the most important personal preventive measures. The gasoline industry has rigid standards for tetraethyl lead workers, but exposure to dangerous amounts still occurs when there is a break in procedure. Cleaning and repairing large storage tanks pose a particular hazard.

PATHOLOGY. In chronic poisoning no gross or microscopic lesions are pathognomonic of lead poisoning. Lead is stored in an inert form in bone and is not harmful except when mobilized. Most of the remaining lead is found in the bone marrow, blood, liver, and kidneys. An increased amount of lead in tissues indicates exposure but not necessarily toxicity. Absence of an increased concentration of lead in tissues practically excludes lead poisoning.

In the encephalopathic type, small perivascular hemorrhages, necrosis of cells, and serous exudate around blood vessels may be found anywhere in the brain. In children with acute poisoning, nuclear inclusions are found in liver cells and renal tubular cells. Occasionally inclusions are found in renal tubule cells of lead workers. In Australia chronic lead exposure from the dust of white lead paint has been incriminated as a common cause of chronic renal failure in young adults.

CLINICAL MANIFESTATIONS. Lead poisoning is usually divided into acute and chronic forms. Although "chronic poisoning" correctly describes prolonged exposure, manifestations often are acute. It is convenient for descriptive purposes to divide symptomatology into an alimentary form, a neuromuscular form, and an encephalopathic form.

Anemia and attendant pallor and weakness are present in most patients with chronic exposure. *Insomnia, headache, dizziness,* and *irritability* are common symptoms without evidence of more serious encephalopathic disturbances. In a patient with poor oral hygiene, lead sulfide is deposited along the gingival margin of some or all teeth and produces a blue-black *"lead line."* *Stippling of the retina* adjacent to the optic disc has been described as an early sign in lead poisoning. Chronic renal failure results from chronic lead intoxication. *Saturnine gout* is particularly common in lead poisoning from "moonshine" whiskey. The renal clearance of uric acid decreases.

Alimentary Form. *Painter's* or *lead colic* is the most common feature and is the result of spasm of the bowel. Constipation is a natural consequence, and nausea, vomiting, and weight loss are common. Colic is intermittent and often severe enough to double the patient up. Between attacks there is merely a sense of pressure. Absence of tenderness differentiates the condition from appendicitis or other causes of peritoneal inflammation. Relief actually may be produced by pressure on the abdomen. Colic is not invariably present.

Neuromuscular Form. Extensor muscles of the upper extremities are more often paralyzed than flexors or lower extremity muscles. *Wrist drop* is a common and characteristic example. Muscle soreness and stiffness or hypertonus precede and accompany paralysis. The absence of sensory disturbance is important in differentiating this from other forms of peripheral neuropathy. Paralysis is confined to a functional muscle group and is not determined by the distribution of an entire motor nerve. Atrophy may occur after longstanding paralysis and may result in incomplete recovery of muscle function after termination of exposure (see Ch. 335 to 337).

Encephalopathic Form. At present this occurs primarily in children. The diagnosis is not suspected until a large amount of lead has been ingested. Because of the good safeguards in industry now, it rarely occurs in adults and then only after massive exposure to lead fumes or tetraethyl lead in a salvage operation, in cleaning large gasoline storage tanks, or in accidental breaks in techniques. Tetraethyl lead is lipid-soluble, so that exposure results almost exclusively in the encephalopathic form.

The presenting manifestations include *convulsions, aphasia, cortical blindness, mania, delirium,* or *coma.* There may be a history of antecedent behavioral changes such as irritability, insomnia, restlessness, loss of memory, hallucinations, and confusion. In fact, a toxic encephalopathy much like Korsakoff's psychosis may occur in adults.

Children may suddenly become very ill. Increased intracranial pressure may occur and is manifested by projectile vomiting, lethargy, convulsions, and coma. In very young children fontanelles bulge. The optic discs may not reflect increased pressure when the process is very acute in onset. Scattered neurologic findings indicate cerebral and cerebellar abnormalities. Blindness and deafness may occur and persist.

LABORATORY FINDINGS. The hematologic findings depend on the action of lead on hemoglobin synthesis. Lead interferes with enzymes ALA synthetase, ALA dehydrase, and heme synthetase. ALA dehydrase is uniformly low with increased burden of lead. A level of more than 600 IU per 100 ml excludes lead poisoning. ALA and coproporphyrin III accumulate and are excreted in the urine in excessive amounts, and protoporphyrin accumulates in erythrocytes as a result of the blocks in synthetic process. Normally 2 mg of ALA or less is excreted per 24 hours. Lead poisoning results in a 20- to 200-fold increase in excretion of ALA. ALA excretion is a sensitive indicator of lead intoxication. Normally 60 to 280 μg of coproporphyrin is excreted per 24 hours.

In lead poisoning free erythrocyte protoporphyrin (FEPP) ranges from 300 to 3000 μg per 100 ml (normal 15 to 60) and free erythrocyte coproporphyrin (FECP) ranges from 1 to 20 μg per 100 ml (normal 0 to 2). It is noteworthy that iron deficiency anemia and thalassemia result in FEPP values that overlap those of lead poisoning, but the range is not quite as great. If a fresh wet film of blood of a patient with lead poisoning is examined under ultraviolet light, 75 to 100 per cent of the erythrocytes have a red fluorescence. This fluorescence is the result of increased FEPP.

Lead poisoning and *hereditary acute intermittent porphyria* have manifestations that are similar. Both are characterized by colicky abdominal pain, mental symptoms, and paralysis. Acute intermittent porphyria regularly has a great increase in porphobilinogen excretion and uroporphyrin excretion, but lead poisoning usually does not result in excessive excretion of either substance.

Normochromic microcytic anemia, decreased red cell life span, decreased osmotic fragility, but increased mechanical fragility are found. Acute hemolytic anemia with hemoglobinemia, hemoglobinuria, and renal damage occur occasionally in acute poisoning. Death from shock may occur in two to three days. *Basophilic stippling* is nonspecific, is rarely found in tetraethyl lead intoxication, is seldom found in acute poisoning of children, and cannot be relied on for screening purposes. Nevertheless, it frequently furnishes the initial clue for clinical recognition of chronic lead poisoning.

Aminoaciduria, renal glycosuria, fructosuria, hyperphosphaturia, citraturia, and decreased uric acid clearance result from changes in the epithelium of the proximal convoluted tubules. These changes are like those in Fanconi's syndrome. Other toxins also cause these manifestations. The changes are usually reversible.

DIAGNOSIS. In children, particularly, the normal blood level is low. If the higher range is used with the upper limit of some 0.06 mg per 100 grams, children with serious acute poisoning will have normal levels (see accompanying table). In adults the upper limits of

Normal and Abnormal Values in Exposure to Lead

	Adults		
	Normal Industrial Exposure	"Safe" Industrial Exposure	Dangerous Industrial Exposure
Urine mg per liter	Range: 0.00 to 0.06 Mean: 0.03	0.01 to 0.15 0.08	0.08 to 0.4 0.2
Blood mg per 100 grams	Range: 0.01 to 0.05 Mean: 0.03	0.01 to 0.07 0.06	0.07 to 0.2 0.09
Feces mg per specimen	0.25	0.6 to 1.0	1.1+

	Children	
	Normal Range	Poisoning
Blood mg per 100 grams	British series 0 to 0.04	0.04 to 0.4
	American series 0.03 to 0.04	0.06+

normal coincide with the mean of "safe" exposure. Unfortunately, analytical precision is poor, often with poor agreement between laboratories.

A diagnosis of tetraethyl lead intoxication is made on the basis of history of exposure. Urine lead determination is the most valuable test. Blood values may be normal, but ALA dehydrase is low. ALA in urine is a poor indicator of tetraethyl lead poisoning.

Because of the medicolegal implications, it is important to be certain that there is evidence of increased lead excretion. Detection of an earlier exposure may be accomplished by the use of 25 mg per kilogram or a maximum of 1.0 gram of calcium disodium edetate (CaEDTA) in 5 per cent glucose solution intravenously. Striking augmentation of lead excretion to over 1.0 mg per day usually occurs. This proves previous exposure but not intoxication. There are three stages of lead poisoning: increased absorption, physiologic poisoning, and clinical poisoning.

Collection of samples for analysis must be done with great care to avoid contamination. Pyrex bottles or polyethylene flasks should be rinsed with nitric acid and distilled water. Urine and stool specimens should be passed directly into acid-cleaned containers. Tissues should be placed directly in acid-cleaned containers.

Blood now can be collected in special vacutainer 20 ml tubes (Becton, Dickinson Company) with pure gum rubber stoppers. These tubes have been chemically cleaned for lead analyses. The needle is a straight stainless steel tube. Duplicate samples are desirable.

Lead determinations on blood and urine can now be performed quickly and accurately, using an atomic absorption spectrophotometer. All state and many large city departments of health have such facilities available.

TREATMENT. Cessation of exposure is of prime importance. A saline cathartic should be given to rid the gut of any unabsorbed lead before chelation of lead is attempted, especially in the encephalopathic form in children.

Colic may be controlled temporarily by intravenous infusion of 1.0 gram of calcium gluconate. The infusion may be repeated as needed.

Fluid intake should be high unless there is increased intracranial pressure. Electrolyte concentrations should be determined and corrected if abnormal.

Chelation with CaEDTA is now the initial treatment of choice. For moderately severe intoxication of chil-

dren, 50 mg per kilogram is given per 24 hours by deep intramuscular injection in three divided doses for three to five days. For adults, 2 grams per day of CaEDTA is given in 5 per cent glucose solution continuously intravenously for five days. The minimal rest period between courses is two days but the rest period should preferably be 10 to 14 days. Urine should be collected, and an aliquot of the pooled sample should be analyzed for lead. For more severe intoxication, 2,3-dimercaptopropanol (BAL) should be given as the initial medication—4 mg per kilogram per dose intramuscularly in children and 2.5 mg per kilogram per dose intramuscularly in adults. Subsequently, BAL is given simultaneously intramuscularly, but in different sites, with 12.5 mg CaEDTA per kilogram per dose intramuscularly in children and 8.0 mg CaEDTA per kilogram per dose intramuscularly in adults every four hours for five days. In encephalopathy, the course may be extended to seven days if no improvement has occurred by the fourth day. Nephropathy has rarely been reported from therapy. When symptoms are severe, treatment should not be delayed for results of lead analysis but should be started immediately on the basis of clinical diagnosis. The use of oral CaEDTA or D-penicillamine in workers exposed to lead is not effective prophylactically and may be dangerous.

D-Penicillamine not only chelates lead but also supplies sulfhydryl groups. A dose of 30 mg per kilogram up to a total of 2.0 grams per day in four divided doses given orally is satisfactory. It is particularly useful to follow the initial CaEDTA therapy. It has the additional advantages that it can be given orally continuously, and that it is much less toxic than CaEDTA. For moderate lead intoxication, penicillamine is the agent of choice. Successful treatment with CaEDTA or penicillamine results in a return of ALA and coproporphyrin excretion to normal. Erythrocyte protoporphyrin declines very slowly after successful treatment.

The most serious manifestation is lead encephalopathy, which requires prompt and skillful treatment. Increased intracranial pressure may occur suddenly and must be treated vigorously. Infusion of urea solution in a dose of 100 mg per kilogram to 1000 mg per kilogram as 30 per cent urea in 10 per cent glucose solution or of mannitol solution (20 per cent) in a dose of 7 to 10 ml per kilogram can alleviate increased pressure effectively, but the benefit may last only a day or two, and repetition may be necessary. Dexamethasone sodium phosphate in a dose of 10 mg intravenously initially followed by 4 to 6 mg intramuscularly every four to six hours in adults is an effective alternative. Craniotomy may even be required for relief of pressure.

Physiotherapy is important for patients with neuropathy. Splinting to support the weak extremity prevents overstretching of muscles; otherwise, permanent disability can follow.

PROGNOSIS. In the gastrointestinal form the outlook is good for complete recovery after adequate treatment and prevention of re-exposure. Recovery from paralysis is usually complete even after many months of paralysis.

Encephalopathy is very serious. It causes a mortality rate of 25 per cent or more, and often leaves mental retardation and various permanent neurologic lesions in those who survive. In adults permanent blindness, extraocular muscle paralysis, or other lesions may result. The acute form caused by tetraethyl lead either is fatal or is followed by complete recovery. There is great urgency in treatment of this form. One cannot wait to get results of lead analysis before starting treatment.

Albahary, C.: Lead and hemopoiesis. Am. J. Med., 52:367, 1972.
Ball, G. V., and Sorensen, L. B.: Pathogenesis of hyperuricemia in saturnine gout. N. Engl. Med., 280:1199, 1969.
Beattie, A. D., Moore, M. R., and Goldberg, A.: Tetraethyl-lead poisoning, Lancet, 2:12, 1972.
Browder, A. A., Joselow, M. M., and Louria, D. B.: The problem of lead poisoning. Medicine, 52:121, 1972.
Chisholm, J. J.: Treatment of lead poisoning. Mod. Treatment, 8:593, 1971.
Feldman, F., Lichtman, H. C., Oransky, S., Ana, E. S., Reiser, L., and Malemud, C. J.: Serum delta aminolevulinic acid in plumbism. J. Pediat., 74:917, 1969.
Guinee, V. F.: Lead poisoning. Am. J. Med., 52:283, 1972.

24.4. MERCURY POISONING

ETIOLOGY. Acute mercury poisoning results from accidental or intentional ingestion of soluble mercuric salts such as mercuric chloride ($HgCl_2$, corrosive sublimate) and is characterized by very serious corrosive effects on the entire gastrointestinal tract and serious renal tubular cell damage.

Mercury is a liquid and is highly volatile at room temperature. In 1957 over 4 million pounds of mercury were used in the United States. It is used widely in medical research and clinical pathology laboratories, as well as in the manufacture of scientific instruments, electric meters, mercury vapor lamps, amalgams with copper, tin, silver or gold, in solders, and in the production of organic mercurial compounds. Mining cinnabar (HgS), refining mercury from it, and cleaning mercury distilling apparatus involve substantial hazards. Photoengraving, bronzing, and the production of certain paint colors such as vermilion and antifouling agents for hulls of ships all use mercury compounds.

As little as 0.1 gram of $HgCl_2$ may cause poisoning, but fatal doses are usually in excess of 1.0 gram. It is caustic and produces cell destruction by protein precipitation on direct contact. In more dilute solutions, such as concentrations effected by absorption from the intestinal tract after ingestion of a toxic dose, its effect is primarily due to selective affinity for sulfhydryl (-SH) groups of proteins, especially of enzymes. This property is counteracted by dimercaprol.

Chronic mercury poisoning results from inhalation of mercury vapor or ingestion of small amounts of mercuric nitrate or other salts, and is characterized by mental symptoms and stomatitis.

Alkyl mercury compounds (ethyl and methyl mercury) have become an important environmental problem. Alkyl mercury compounds are more readily absorbed than inorganic mercury or compounds. The compounds are soluble in organic solvents, and the covalent carbon-mercury bond is not degraded by biologic processes. Methyl mercury particularly is found in tuna and swordfish taken from waters heavily contaminated with mercury. Epidemics have occurred in Minamata and Niigata, Japan, and in several countries where seed grain treated with alkyl mercury compounds (as antifungal agents) has been diverted into food. Nearly complete intestinal absorption occurs; the liver excretes most of it into the intestine, resulting in continuous enterohepatic circulation. Methyl mercury passes the placental barrier very well and accumulates in the fetus with resultant cerebral palsy and mental retardation of the child.

ACUTE POISONING

See Ch. 379.

CHRONIC POISONING

CLINICAL MANIFESTATIONS. Stomatitis. Excessive salivation and a metallic taste are common. A blue line develops along the gingival margin. Gums become hypertrophied, bleed easily, and are sore. The teeth become loose.

Erethism. The term "erethism" is applied to the psychic disturbance characterized by irritability, shyness, and deterioration of family and social activities, suggesting hyperthyroidism. Since felt hat makers formerly used mercury salts in the manufacturing process and often became "mad," these symptoms gave rise to the phrase "mad as a hatter."

Tremors. Tremors of the eyelids, lips, tongue, fingers and extremities are characteristic of chronic poisoning. Coarse jerky movements and gross incoordination interfere with fine movements such as writing and eating. Atrophy of the cerebellar cortex and, to a lesser extent, of the cerebral cortex occurs. Microscopic changes occur in the granular layer of the cerebellum, ganglion cells, and posterior columns.

Nephrotic Syndrome. Contact with ammoniated mercury and other compounds has caused proteinuria and frank nephrotic syndrome. Removal from exposure is mandatory, so a careful history of medicinal or occupational exposure is needed.

Hypersensitivity. Hypersensitivity reactions to mercurial diuretic agents include asthma, urticaria, exfoliative dermatitis, and sudden death. Fatal accidents can be prevented by avoiding intravenous injections. Death is usually due to ventricular fibrillation.

Hypersensitivity to calomel (HgCl) results from longterm ingestion of HgCl. Hypersensitivity to ammoniated mercury or other compounds results from topical application. Fever, morbilliform rash, leukopenia, eosinophilia, and enlargement of the spleen and lymph nodes characterize this condition. Mercury fulminate used in percussion caps and detonators may cause dermatitis of exposed parts, with pruritus, papules, vesicles, and pustules.

Acrodynia or "Pink Disease." This disorder of infants and young children is characterized by irritability, insomnia, stomatitis, loss of teeth, hypertension, erythema of fingers, toes, nose, cheeks, and buttocks, and even acral gangrene. Fever, leukocytosis, and albuminuria occur. In 1948 Warkany and Hubbard suggested that sensitivity to mercury might be the cause, and that hypothesis is now fairly generally accepted. The diagnosis is established by finding excretion of more than 0.1 mg of mercury per day in the urine. An organic mercury compound, phenyl mercuric propionate, has been incorporated into house paint to prevent growth of mold. This paint has been incriminated as a source of toxic exposure.

ORGANIC MERCURY INTOXICATION

Ethyl and methyl mercury compounds have an affinity for the central nervous system and produce fatigue, headache, loss of memory, apathy, emotional instability, paresthesia, generalized ataxia, deafness, dysarthria, progressive visual deterioration, dysphagia, and, occasionally, coma and death. Changes in the central nervous system similar to the lesions of chronic mercury poisoning are found.

DIAGNOSIS. Industrial exposure and characteristic symptoms usually make recognition of chronic mercury poisoning relatively straightforward, but, in the absence of known exposure, the diagnosis may be elusive. Patients with chronic mercury poisoning excrete in excess of 0.3 mg of Hg per liter of urine. Normal values range from 0.0001 to 0.001 mg per liter. An excretion of 0.1 mg per liter is considered evidence of toxic exposure. In instances of exposure to metallic mercury for more than five years, a brown reflex from the anterior lens capsule can be seen by slit lamp. Some observers consider it an early sign of mercury poisoning. Albuminuria and hematuria are common findings in chronic poisoning.

TREATMENT. Removal of the patient from all possible exposure is of paramount importance. The use of BAL in chronic poisoning has not been established as effective treatment. However, n-acetyl-DL-penicillamine, in a dose of 500 mg four times a day, increases mercury excretion and has been used successfully in therapy of chronic mercury poisoning and acrodynia. This treatment is ineffective in methyl mercury poisoning, but promising results have been obtained here, using ion-absorbing resin to interrupt the enterohepatic circulation of mercury.

PROGNOSIS. Recovery is slow even after removal from exposure. Patients with advanced intoxication fare poorly. Only 15 per cent of the more severely involved patients recovered completely in one series. Signs of cerebellar and cerebral damage persisted and prevented return to normal activities.

PREVENTION. Removal of $HgCl_2$, calomel, and mercury ointments from the market would eliminate acute poisoning and many instances of chronic poisoning. Good safe substitutes are available for each compound. Elimination of mercuric nitrate from the felt-processing industry has already occurred. Mercury salts for fingerprinting by police departments have been replaced by barium, zinc, or bismuth. Silver has replaced mercury in the manufacture of mirrors. Stopping discharge of all mercury-containing waste will eventually stop methyl mercury contamination of fish. This has been clearly demonstrated in Sweden.

Mercury-containing paints should have a warning label "For Outside Use Only." Mercury cannot be replaced in many electrical apparatuses and scientific instruments. Proper exhaust ventilation, scrupulous avoidance of any exposed metallic mercury, and good personal hygiene are necessary precautions. The maximal allowable concentration of Hg has been set at 0.1 mg per cubic meter of air. Medical supervision is necessary wherever potential exposure exists. Neurologic signs and especially visual field changes, tremor, ataxia, and dysarthria are serious danger signals.

Amin-Zaki, L., Majeed, M. A., Clarkson, T. W., and Greenwood, M. R.: Methyl mercury poisoning in Iraqi children: Clinical observations over two years. Br. Med. J., 1:613, 1978.

Battigelli, M. C.: Mercury toxicity from industrial exposure. A critical review of the literature. J. Occup. Med., 2:337, 1960.

Hirschman, S. Z., Feingold, M., and Boylen, G.: Mercury in house paint as a cause of acrodynia. N. Engl. J. Med., 269:889, 1963.

Joselow, M. M., Louria, D. B., and Browder, A.: Mercurialism. Environmental and occupational aspects. Ann. Intern. Med., 76:119, 1972.

24.5. ANTIMONY POISONING

Antimony and potassium tartrate (tartar emetic) is used for emetic purposes, and other organic antimony compounds are used in treatment of schistosomiasis, filariasis, and certain fungal infections. Antimony is encountered in metallurgic processes, mining and smelting, and in rubber manufacturing, but industrial poisoning is rare. Finely divided antimony is more toxic than compounds of antimony. Trivalent antimony combines with sulfhydryl groups of enzymes. The symptoms of acute poisoning are similar to those of acute arsenic poisoning. Vomiting is a prominent symptom. Dimercaprol (BAL) is an effective agent for treatment of antimony poisoning, and the regimen is like that for arsenic and mercury. Dermatitis and conjunctivitis occur from exposure to dust in the smelting process. Stibine (SbH_3) is more volatile than arsine and is very toxic also. It attacks the central nervous system and causes acute hemolysis. Death occurs when there is a 0.01 per cent concentration in the air. The chemical process of formation and the effects are like those of arsine.

24.6. CADMIUM POISONING

Cadmium sulfide is associated with zinc minerals and particularly with zinc sulfide. Cadmium exposure can occur in the manufacture of alloys, vapor lamps, and storage batteries, grinding and polishing alloys, cadmium plating, welding, zinc ore smelting, and glass blowing. Inhalation of cadmium fumes results in pulmonary edema, followed in two to three days by proliferative interstitial pneumonia. Various degrees of permanent lung damage and fibrosis occur. Cadmium can be inhaled in fatal concentrations without enough discomfort to warn the worker. The inhalation of fumes with cadmium produces dryness of throat, cough, headache, vomiting, sensation of constriction in the chest, severe dyspnea, and prostration. There is no effective treatment except symptomatic treatment of pulmonary edema. Pulmonary emphysema is the principal effect of industrial exposure. Cadmium is known to be carcinogenic. It has been implicated in the pathogenesis of hypertension, but this is not established.

Foods prepared and stored in cadmium-plated containers may be contaminated sufficiently to cause poisoning. Cadmium ingestion usually does not produce fatal poisoning, but causes rather violent gastrointestinal symptoms, with sudden onset 20 to 30 minutes after eating.

Chronic poisoning from food occurs particularly in Japan. There, a great deal of mining of cadmium, lead, and zinc sulfide, as well as zinc and cadmium smelters, contaminates the streams. Water is used for irrigation of rice fields, so rice is contaminated. Chronic cadmium poisoning is endemic in these areas. A disease called "itai-itai byo" or "ouch-ouch" disease is due to severe osteomalacia which causes pain. It primarily affects women 40 to 70 years old. A Fanconi-like renal dysfunction occurs with proteinuria (largely globulins), phosphaturia, and glucosuria. This leads to typical severe osteomalacia with kyphosis, pseudofractures, and waddling gait. Osteomalacia occurs only in Japan, but the renal lesion occurs in chronic cadmium poisoning in both men and women elsewhere. Vitamin D in large doses sometimes affords relief of pain. A number of deaths have occurred, primarily from severe osteomalacia.

Friberg, L., Piscator, M., Nordberg, G. F., and Kjellström, T.: Cadmium in the Environment. 2nd ed. Cleveland, C.R.C. Press, 1974.

24.7.   THALLIUM POISONING

Thallium sulfate (Tl_2SO_4) is an extremely toxic cumulative poison (lethal dose 0.2 to 1.0 gram). It has a mild metallic taste. Thallium is absorbed from the gut and from the intact skin. It has had wide use as a rodent, ant, and cockroach poison. Because of serious and frequent accidental and deliberate (homicidal) toxicity, the U.S. Department of Agriculture banned thallium formulations for household use in 1965. Unfortunately, some of it can still be found on shelves in homes and stores.

Alopecia is a very important and unique sign. *Accumulation in nervous tissue* accounts for critical symptoms which include ataxia, choreiform movements, vomiting, constipation, restlessness, delirium with hallucinations and delusions, and, finally, coma. Blindness, loss of other special senses, facial paralysis, paresthesias, and peripheral neuropathy occur. Central lobular necrosis of the liver and renal damage also occur. Liver radiopacity increases in some patients. Urinary excretion of 10 mg per day or more indicates serious poisoning.

Various therapeutic trials, including dithiocarb, dithizone, BAL, and KCl, have been used but either have failed to bring improvement or may even be dangerous because of mobilization of thallium and redistribution to the brain. Gastric lavage should be done immediately after diagnosis up to four hours after exposure. Prussian blue (potassium ferric hexacyanoferrate II) is an excellent chelator of thallium by exchange of potassium for thallium. Prussian blue is not absorbed from the gut and is nontoxic. The recommended dose of colloidal solution is 250 mg per kilogram per day in two to four divided doses. A vigorous laxative such as castor oil is necessary for the first day or two. After this an osmotic agent such as 50 ml of 15 per cent mannitol solution will suffice. Therapy should continue until thallium excretion is less than 0.5 mg per 24 hours.

Barbier, F.: Treatment of thallium poisoning. Lancet, 2:965, 1974.
Huff, J. E.: Special communication: Thallium poisoning. Clin. Toxicol., 5:89, 1972.
Kamerbeck, H. H., Rauws, A. G., TenHam, M., and VanHeijst, A. N. P.: Prussian blue therapy of thallotoxicosis. Acta Med. Scand., 189:321, 1971.

25.   CARBON MONOXIDE POISONING

Bertram D. Dinman

DEFINITION. Carbon monoxide, a product of incomplete combustion of carbonaceous materials, is an odorless, colorless gas; its density is slightly less than air. The gas is commonly produced by the internal combustion engine, poorly vented heating devices, or gas refrigerators. Certain industrial operations such as those associated with blast furnaces and coke ovens, foundry cupolas, petroleum refineries, and underground mines also present risks of serious carbon monoxide intoxication. Less severe but potential exposures may exist in automobile repair shops, among traffic policemen, or in arc welding. Frank intoxication caused by vehicular exhausts is usually due to impaired integrity of exhaust systems and/or the automobile body. Poisoning associated with engine operation for in-car heating purposes occurs only with such defects or when the motor is run in confined spaces, e.g., deep snowdrifts, garages. Natural gas has replaced manufactured gas in the United States; since the former is free of carbon monoxide, illuminating gas per se no longer presents any risk of injury. However, carbon monoxide may be produced by the incomplete combustion of natural gas in faulty heating or other gas-burning apparatus. The most common human exposure to carbon monoxide is associated with smoking. Chronic cigarette smokers develop 3 to 8 per cent carboxyhemoglobin (COHb) concentrations. Although the foregoing exogenous sources of carbon monoxide have long been recognized, the phenomenon of endogenous carbon monoxide production is now well established; as a result of cleavage of the α-methylene bridge in the heme portion of hemoglobin, 0.3 to 1.0 ml per hour is normally produced. This leads to a normal blood COHb concentration of 0.5 to 0.8 per cent.

In contrast to the preceding anthropogenic sources of carbon monoxide, it has been estimated that approximately 3 to 25 times as much carbon monoxide is formed by natural processes. These sources of carbon monoxide are derived from atmospheric oxidation of biochemically produced methane, various free-floating components of the oceanic biomass, photo-oxidation of plant-produced terpenes, volcanic activity, and forest fires.

PATHOGENESIS. Since carbon monoxide usually exists in a gaseous form, the only significant portal of entry is via the respiratory tract. The gas diffuses across the alveolar membrane in amounts proportional to the pressure gradient for carbon monoxide between alveolar air and blood. The rate of uptake is directly proportional to the respiratory rate, duration of exposure, and carbon monoxide concentration in air. The high affinity of carbon monoxide for hemoglobin (218 times greater than that of oxygen) is responsible for its primary pathologic effect, i.e., reduction of erythrocytic oxygen-carrying capacity. As a result, all signs, symptoms, and pathologic alterations are those of tissue hypoxia. In addition to reducing blood oxygen tension, carbon monoxide in association with hemoglobin (i.e., carboxyhemoglobin) impedes that pigment's discharge of oxygen at the capillary bed. Thus capillary oxygen tensions must be decreased lower than normal in order to dissociate oxygen from the erythrocyte to the tissues. This impairment of oxygen dissociation is expressed by a shift in the oxyhemoglobin curve to the left. Such effects are further complicated in that respiratory chemoreceptors respond only to decreased blood oxygen tension; since this is not decreased (i.e., there is simply a decrease in blood oxygen content), physiologic compensatory mechanisms are not brought into play.

Aside from the formation of carboxyhemoglobin and the resultant hypoxia, there is little evidence that carbon monoxide has any significant direct effect upon tissue except at high carboxyhemoglobin concentrations.

PATHOLOGY. Carboxyhemoglobin is characteristically cherry red in color. Accordingly, the tissues and skin of poisoned individuals always grossly present a characteristic pink color when blood levels of carboxyhemoglobin exceed 30 per cent concentration levels. (Rarely, severely poisoned individuals may not manifest this change at autopsy; this results from reduction of COHb below the 30 per cent level owing to therapeutically induced respiratory clearance prior to death.) The skin may present areas of vesiculation and ulceration at pressure points. Ischemic necrosis of the cardiac papillary muscles and renal tubular degeneration may be noted. Although animal experiments suggest that repeated carbon monoxide exposures may accelerate the development of coronary atherosclerosis, the design of these experiments makes extrapolation of the results to humans difficult. Although the brain of patients dying of acute intoxication (i.e., within the first 24 hours) is congested, pink, and edematous, under these conditions this organ does not usually demonstrate specific, localized degenerative lesions. However, those surviving this acute episode can later develop diffuse degenerative changes prominently involving the cerebral cortex, globus pallidus, cerebellum, and basal ganglia. It is frequently stated that carbon monoxide–induced lesions have a predilection for certain locations in the brain, e.g., basal ganglia, hippocampal region, but in fact a consistent pattern of brain localization is not evident.

CLINICAL MANIFESTATIONS. This disease is characteristically an acute poisoning. Although chronic forms of carbon monoxide intoxication have been claimed to exist, they are not adequately documented. Repeated episodes of mild acute poisoning can occur without cumulative effects.

The clinical picture of carbon monoxide poisoning is closely correlated with the blood concentration of carboxyhemoglobin. Although levels of less than 10 per cent COHb are said to produce no clinical effects, subtle changes of central nervous system function have been consistently demonstrated at the 5 to 20 per cent COHb level (e.g., increased visual threshold, impaired higher cognate function). In addition, precipitation of anginal episodes has been noted in patients with coronary artery disease during exercise with COHb levels of 3 to 5 per cent.

Although frontal, bandlike headaches may be experienced in the 10 to 20 per cent COHb range, more commonly these occur at the upper reaches of this range. In the 20 to 30 per cent COHb range the headaches become more severe. Dyspnea on exertion may be the only other manifestation. At the 30 to 40 per cent COHb levels, headaches become very severe, and are associated with nausea and vomiting, weakness, dizziness, dimness of vision, and possibly collapse. At the 40 to 50 per cent COHb level, ataxia, syncope, and collapse may be observed, in addition to tachycardia and tachypnea. As blood levels of 50 to 60 per cent COHb supervene, there may be coma associated with intermittent convulsions, and Cheyne-Stokes respiration may develop. In the 60 to 70 per cent COHb range, coma deepens, intermittent convulsions occur, and there is clinical shock. Death may terminate such exposures, although profound shock, respiratory and cardiovascular failure, and death have been reported to be delayed until 70 to 80 per cent COHb concentrations are attained. In severe cases, leukocytosis, proteinuria, glycosuria, hematuria, and cylindruria are usually demonstrated, in addition to temperature elevation of 39° C or more.

In contrast to the relatively high levels of carboxyhemoglobin required to produce the foregoing clinical symptoms in otherwise healthy individuals, special susceptibilities among other segments of the population are becoming more clearly defined. Individuals with symptomatic arteriosclerotic heart disease experience a more rapid onset of anginal symptoms when exercised at carboxyhemoglobin levels of 2.5 per cent. Likewise, fetal carboxyhemoglobin levels are 10 to 15 per cent greater than the maternal concentration at steady-state conditions. This enhanced exposure potential for the fetus is further aggravated by the relatively slower rate of elimination of carbon monoxide by the fetus than by the mother. Aside from a decreased birth weight similar to that seen in altitude-induced hypoxia, the clinical implications of these observations as regards carbon monoxide effects on the fetus are not clear.

DIAGNOSIS. Diagnosis is established by quantitative determination of blood carboxyhemoglobin concentration; analysis of alveolar air for carbon monoxide correlates well with blood COHb. The method of Coburn, utilizing a nondispersive infrared meter, is highly accurate; the hydrogen flame–ionization detector equipped gas chromatograph provides the highest level of sensitivity. Although spectrophotometry has long been used, its sensitivity and specificity are less than with more modern techniques.

The cherry-red skin and mucous membrane coloration are highly characteristic of carbon monoxide poisoning. However, it is not readily detected until a 30 to 35 per cent COHb concentration is attained.

TREATMENT. The patient must be immediately removed from the contaminated environment. In mild cases clearance of carbon monoxide from the blood is spontaneously accomplished if respiration is sustained. Fresh air and absolute rest are sufficient in such cases; attempts at exertion of any type within four to six hours can cause a rapid recrudescence of signs and symptoms. In the event of unconsciousness — no matter how transient — hospital management and emergency treatment are indicated. Respiration must be sustained by whatever method is available — i.e., artificial respiration, intermittent positive pressure breathing apparatus. Regardless of the level of COHb initially found, normal air breathing will result in 50 per cent clearance of blood carbon monoxide in about 250 to 300 minutes; 100 per cent oxygen inhalation will achieve a similar reduction of carbon monoxide loading in 35 to 80 minutes, and oxygen at three atmospheres of pressure results in the same clearance in about 25 minutes. The use of a 95 per cent oxygen–5 per cent carbon dioxide mixture hastens oxygenation, largely owing to the Bohr shift.

Persistence of coma and the presence of shock require the usual supportive treatments. Induction of hypothermia may help prevent irreversible brain damage.

PROGNOSIS. Patients who do not become comatose usually recover without permanent sequelae. Persistence of hyperthermia, shock, or acute hypoxia-induced clinical laboratory signs for two days after intoxication holds a grave prognosis. Among those who survive such severe intoxication, a small proportion will demonstrate residual changes — e.g., major seizures, dysphasia, parkinsonism or varying degrees of hyperkinesia, mental impairment. Such severely affected patients usually manifest such signs within one week of the acute episode. However, in approximately half of these severe cases there may be apparent recovery followed by relapse after a latent period of one to three weeks. In either case, if recovery is to supervene, it should be expected within two years of the acute episode.

Carbon Monoxide, Report of the Committee on Carbon Monoxide, Committee on Medical and Biological Effects of Environmental Pollutants. Washington, D.C., National Research Council–National Academy of Sciences, 1977.

Coburn, R. F. (ed.): Biological effects of carbon monoxide. Ann. N.Y. Acad. Sci., 174:430, 1970.

Haldane, J.: The action of carbonic oxide in man. J. Physiol., 18:430, 1895.

Meigs, J. W.: Acute carbon monoxide poisoning. An analysis of one hundred five cases. AMA Arch. Indust. Hyg. Occup. Med., 6:344, 1952.

Peterson, J. E., and Stewart, R. D.: The post-exposure relationship of carbon monoxide in blood and expired air. Arch. Environ. Health, 21:165, 1970.

Richardson, J. C., Chambers, R. A., and Heywood, P. M.: Encephalopathy of anoxia and hypoglycemia. Arch. Neurol., 1:178, 1959.

Shillito, F. H., Drinker, C. K., and Shaughnessey, T. J.: The problem of nervous and mental sequelae in carbon monoxide poisoning. JAMA, 106:669, 1936.

26. DISORDERS DUE TO HEAT AND COLD

Paul Webb

26.1. INTRODUCTION

When thermoregulation fails or is overwhelmed, life-threatening disorders develop from severe heat stress or cold stress. Profound hypothermia is the result of serious loss of body heat, whereas a major accumulation of body heat produces heat stroke. Both conditions require prompt and vigorous treatment. There are other, less serious disorders from heat exposure, in which heat is not stored in large quantity; these are the more common and more easily managed heat syncope and heat exhaustion. Cold and heat can cause local tissue injury, of course, as in frostbite, immersion foot (see Ch. 368.3), and burns, but this chapter deals only with the general disorders.

26.2. HEAT STROKE

A medical emergency, heat stroke is easily diagnosed when it is expected. Thus when military men begin

training in hot climates or when seamen work in the engine rooms and galleys of ships in tropical waters, heat casualties are common, and some of them may be heat stroke. In young, healthy men who have been working hard in heat, unconsciousness, high body temperature, strong rapid pulse, and hot flushed skin are presumptive evidence of heat stroke in the absence of another obvious diagnosis such as head injury or massive infection. But in older people who have not been exerting themselves in hot work places, the diagnosis of heat stroke is not so obvious. Deaths from "excessive heat and insolation" in the United States range from 1 to 12 per 100,000 in people over 65, and many cases are missed or not reported. Heat deaths in the elderly are presumably similar in mechanism to classic heat stroke.

Prodromal symptoms, which may not be notable, include faintness, dizziness, staggering, headache, and nausea. There is a clear history of heat exposure or of heavy exertion in heat. Classically the patient in heat stroke is unconscious, although any degree of impairment of the central nervous system may present initially, from lethargy, confusion, or irrational agitation, to coma and convulsions. The body temperature is high, 40° C or higher measured in the rectum; but if the patient is not seen immediately, and if even simple measures have been started to relieve heat stress and to start cooling, the body temperature may be lower. The pulse is strong, and its rate is usually 140 or higher. Blood pressure measurement will show a normal or elevated systolic pressure and a lowered diastolic pressure. However, in the late and severe stage of the disorder, blood pressure is low as the circulation fails. The skin is flushed, and sweating may be present, or — a bad sign — reduced or absent. Heat stroke is easily distinguishable from heat syncope or heat exhaustion, with their mildly elevated body temperatures, transient disturbances of consciousness, and mild circulatory signs. Heat stroke results from excessive heat storage, with high cardiac output, cutaneous vasodilation, and low peripheral resistance. Cessation of sweating and circulatory failure are late signs. There is evidence that the heart failure is right-sided, with low resistance in the systemic circulation and high resistance in the pulmonary circulation.

One should not always expect to see all the signs of heat stroke in an elderly person whose circulatory function is not what it used to be, and in whom there may be some pre-existing infectious disease. The diagnosis should be thought of if body temperature stays high and circulation is failing. Heat deaths during heat waves typically increase one or two days after the heat wave begins, and continue for one or two days after it is over. Predisposing factors are age, obesity, lack of acclimatization, and preceding infection or gastrointestinal upset.

The greater the heat storage and the longer it has been present, the worse the prognosis. Damage is done by general cellular degeneration and widespread hemorrhages, especially those in the central nervous system, kidneys, and liver. Laboratory findings in severe cases include reduced blood coagulation, low prothrombin, and low platelet count; low urine volume, high specific gravity, albumin, and renal casts; elevated blood urea; hemoconcentration; low serum potassium and normal to high serum chloride; changes in liver function; elevation of serum enzymes; and a hyperdynamic circulatory pattern unless circulatory failure has already developed.

Treatment of heat stroke should begin at once. Its aim is to lower body temperature and to support the circulation. Effective cooling methods, in ascending order of effectiveness, are wet towels and a strong fan in a cool dry room; icebags over much of the body; water-cooled sheets such as are used to induce hypothermia; and a tub bath of cold water. The higher the body temperature, the more aggressive the cooling technique should be. Sedation may be needed to control the patient, who may struggle or who may begin to convulse. A tranquilizing cocktail of pethidine, chlorpromazine, and phenergan may be used to prevent both convulsions and shivering, or simpler means of calming a person may suffice. Cooling should be continued until the rectal temperature goes below 38° C. After the initial lowering of body temperature, continued temperature monitoring is vital, for strong cooling may produce an after-drop of temperature, and somewhat later, patients will often start to store heat again despite being in a thermally comfortable environment.

Shock must be treated with fluid replacement and possibly isoproterenol. Fluid therapy should be started judiciously, with the amount and electrolyte content guided by laboratory findings. Other supportive measures are begun when problems are identified, e.g., platelet transfusions or renal dialysis.

Ellis, F. P.: Mortality from heat illness and heat-aggravated illness in the United States. Environ. Res., 5:1, 1972.

O'Donnell, T. F., Jr., and Clowes, George H. A., Jr.: The circulatory abnormalities of heat stroke. N. Engl. J. Med., 287:734, 1972.

Shibolet, S., Coll, R., Gilat, T., and Sohar, E.: Heatstroke: Its clinical picture and mechanism in 36 cases. Quart. J. Med., 36:525, 1967.

26.3. HEAT SYNCOPE

A person who becomes dizzy or suddenly tired after exercising in the heat may abruptly faint. As soon as he is recumbent, and especially if he is removed from direct exposure to heat, he recovers. In contrast to the patient with heat stroke, the person with heat syncope has a cool, sweaty, pale skin; his pulse is weak and either mildly elevated — 100 to 120 beats per minute — or slow, as in vasovagal syncope. His blood pressure falls just before fainting, and recovers quickly when he lies down or sits with head lowered.

Lack of acclimatization and lack of training for the exercise undertaken predispose to heat syncope. Cutaneous vasodilation and blood pooling in the erect position contribute to the hypotension. Treatment is a matter of allowing the person to rest, cool down a little, and drink some extra liquid.

26.4. HEAT EXHAUSTION

Taking much longer to develop than heat syncope (often several days), heat exhaustion results from loss of fluid or loss of fluid and salt. The symptoms of prolonged water depletion are thirst, fatigue, giddiness, elevated body temperature, oliguria, and finally delirium. The water depletion results from sweating and inadequate replacement by drinking, whether voluntary or involuntary. Voluntary dehydration in heat — the failure to replace water loss even though water is available — is common, but most people catch up at the end of the day when they get out of the heat. In the tropics it is sometimes not possible to cool off at night or keep up with water replenishment. This causes problems for the non-native dweller especially.

When both water and salt become depleted, muscle cramps are added to the picture of fatigue, nausea, and giddiness. The urine chloride will be low to absent, and serum chlorides reduced.

Heat exhaustion is treated by rest in bed away from heat, and restoration of body water, or water and electrolytes. Cool liquids should be given by mouth, up to 6 or 8 liters the first day. If body temperature does not return to normal spontaneously, alcohol sponging or wet towels and a fan may be used. If the patient cannot drink, intravenous therapy should be started. Continuation of fluid and electrolyte replacement should be guided by laboratory analyses.

Prevention of heat exhaustion is a matter of ensuring an adequate fluid intake, which means enough to replace losses from sweating. These losses can be as high as 6 to 8 liters per day in men working hard in hot dry conditions. People who are not yet acclimatized to heat need supplemental salt, because their sweat contains more electrolyte than that of the acclimatized. A daily intake of 15 to 25 grams of NaCl is recommended for newcomers to hot environments; about 10 grams of this can be consumed with a meat-containing diet. The additional 5 to 15 grams is best taken in the form of salted fruit drinks and enteric-coated salt tablets. But if water and fluids are in short supply, salt tablets should not be used. The routine use of salt tablets in hot situations is no longer encouraged except possibly for people who have little experience, and then only during the first days of becoming acclimatized.

Leithead, C. S., and Lind, A. R.: Heat Stress and Heat Disorders. Philadelphia, F. A. Davis Company, 1964.

26.5. HYPOTHERMIA

When the rectal temperature is below 35° C, hypothermia is said to be present. This major loss of body heat occurs in hikers and climbers exposed to cold, in elderly people who live alone in meagerly heated homes, in people who have been drinking heavily and have fallen asleep out of doors, in accident victims, and in people accidentally immersed in cold water. In profound hypothermia people are often assumed to be dead, for their vital signs are so depressed as to be missed even by trained observers. If only a clinical mercury thermometer is available, it will fail to register low enough to point to the diagnosis.

Estimates of the frequency of hypothermia vary widely, but the incidence is possibly higher than anyone suspects. In England it has been shown that elderly people are often forced to tolerate being chronically depleted of body heat, and the same may well be true in the United States for isolated old people. This would seem to be an ideal initial condition from which to develop hypothermia. Added hunger, fatigue, or minor injury could increase the heat depletion by rendering such people helpless. Drugs such as chlorpromazine may also contribute to it.

A person in profound hypothermia is in coma and cold to the touch. The skin is pale, usually grayish in color; the neck and extremities resist bending. No peripheral pulse can be found, breathing appears to be absent, and pupillary reflexes are absent. If a low-reading thermometer can be found, the rectal temperature will show 30° C or lower. Less profound hypothermia differs in degree; there will be some signs of consciousness, reaction to pain, a detectable if slow pulse, and flexible joints.

Additional findings are hypotension; cardiac irregularities on the EKG, typically atrial fibrillation and a J wave associated with the QRS complex; low pH in the blood from metabolic acidosis, especially in patients whose hypothermia was preceded by exhaustion and prolonged shivering; low blood CO_2 content; and high blood glucose.

Rewarming is the first order of business, and a decision must be made about passive or active rewarming and, if active, whether by external or core first means. A person who is still somewhat conscious, who has a reasonable heart rhythm, and whose rectal temperature is between 31 and 35° C is probably best handled by rewarming in a warm room or in a bed with blankets. If a person is acutely hypothermic from cold water immersion, the preferred approach is immersion in a warm tub bath the temperature of which is kept at 40 to 42° C. Inhalation rewarming is suitably employed by rescue personnel, since the equipment needed is a portable source of oxygen or air and a device for heating and humidifying the gas to be delivered at 45° C. It is a decided advantage to begin treatment at once, before the patient is transported to a building with a bathtub. A person with slowly developed hypothermia, in whom fatigue, injury, or old age has produced a poor condition beyond the hypothermia, should probably be warmed actively but less aggressively, e.g., with a heating blanket kept at 37° C. Rewarming the core first may be undertaken for profound hypothermia, for there is grave danger of ventricular fibrillation at heart temperatures from 27 to 30° C. The core-warming method avoids the early return of cold blood from the arms, legs, and skin, which commonly causes an unwanted after-drop in central temperature during external rewarming. But the methods of core-warming first are not simple ones; warm peritoneal dialysis and an extracorporeal blood circuit with a heater are examples.

Other than a determined approach to restoring body heat, the management of hypothermia should be as conservative as circumstances warrant, i.e., trauma or infection must be heeded. Respiratory support, for example, should include intubation or tracheostomy only if absolutely necessary. These procedures affect an already irritable heart. Cardiac irregularities should be watched rather than treated; if arrest occurs, it should be treated by external cardiac massage, and use of a defibrillator for ventricular fibrillation. Fluid therapy should be guided by laboratory findings rather than by some predetermined rule; thus one should combat acidosis or hypokalemia specifically if present.

Anderson, S., Herbring, B. G., and Widman, B.: Accidental profound hypothermia. Br. J. Anaesth., 42:653, 1970.
Collis, M. L., Steinman, A. M., and Chaney, R. D.: Accidental hypothermia: An experimental study of practical rewarming methods. Aviat. Space Environ. Med. 48:625, 1977.
Fernandez, J. P., O'Rourke, R. A., and Ewy, G. A.: Rapid active external rewarming in accidental hypothermia. JAMA, 212:153, 1970.
Fox, R. H., Woodward, P. M., Exton-Smith, A. N., Green, M. F., Donnison, D. V., and Wicks, M. H.: Body temperatures in the elderly: A national study of physiological, social, and environmental conditions. Br. Med. J., 62:200, 1973.
Patton, J. F., and Doolittle, W. H.: Core rewarming by peritoneal dialysis following induced hypothermia in the dog. J. Appl. Physiol., 33:800, 1972.
Zingg, W.: The management of accidental hypothermia. Can. Med. Assoc. J., 96:214, 1967.

27. RADIATION INJURY
Niel Wald

DEFINITION. Radiation energy from sources of ionizing radiation which interacts with human cells, tissues, and organs produces a variety of clinical manifestations, depending on the magnitude and duration of radiation exposure and on the size and function(s) of the body area irradiated. The source of the radiation energy absorbed may be external, such as an x-ray machine, or it may be internal contamination from a radioactive isotope inhaled, ingested, injected, or absorbed through the skin or a wound.

Clinical manifestations of radiation energy absorption may be acute, with or without late sequelae, or they may be delayed and chronic. The acute manifestations include the acute radiation syndrome which typically follows whole body radiation exposure; local tissue or organ injury with little or no systemic manifestations after partial body exposure; and growth and developmental disturbances after exposure of the fetus. The clinical effects of intermittent or constant low level radiation exposure from external or internal sources may present as chronic progressive impairment of certain tissues or organs, or solely as the relatively late appearance of one or another of the long-term sequelae of radiation exposure, such as cancer and leukemia. In addition, any of these forms of exposure which impinge on the gonads may produce germ cell changes or mutations which can cause sequelae in subsequent progeny.

Tissue injury may be produced by cellular interactions with radiations of any part of the electromagnetic spectrum, including the output of the sun, lasers, or microwave equipment. Some of these, such as x-rays, gamma rays, and neutrons, are capable of penetration, and can produce internal tissue damage. Other radiations, such as alpha rays and low energy beta rays, have a very limited range in tissue and are only injurious when given off within the body by incorporated radioactive isotopes. The radiations *emitted* by ionizing radiation sources are quantitated in roentgens (r) of exposure, whereas the radiation energy *absorbed* by the tissues exposed is quantitated in rads. The same absorbed dose delivered at different rates will produce very different effects.

ETIOLOGY. Typical radiation injury is caused by exposure to *ionizing radiations*. Since the recognition of man-made radiation by Roentgen in 1895 and of natural radioactivity by Becquerel the following year, occupational and medical exposures have been the most usual sources of radiation injury, although the use of nuclear weapons in World War II produced a major addition in clinical cases. Injury from external sources occurred among the early x-ray workers, the employees of the nuclear weapons project, and the subsequent nuclear energy research and industrial organizations. In addition, unavoidable injury has been produced in some radiation therapy patients through exposure of normal tissues adjacent to the lesion under treatment.

Internal radionuclide exposure resulted in injury to employees of the radium watch dial painting industry in the 1920s. More recently, fallout from nuclear weapon tests has produced some internal radionuclide deposition in the general public. In the medical patient population, the uses of radium as a therapeutic agent and thorium as a diagnostic x-ray contrast medium have resulted in clinical sequelae decades after administration. Also, there have been instances of diagnostic and therapeutic radioisotope misadministration producing acute injury and occasionally causing death.

INCIDENCE AND PREVALENCE. The frequency with which radiation injury occurs is closely related to the availability of sources for radiation exposure and the understanding and care with which they are maintained and used. The largest potential source of radiation casualties is the military use of *nuclear weapons*. The Joint Commission for the Investigation of the Effects of the Atomic Bomb in Japan estimated the incidence of radiation injury in Hiroshima to be about 40 per cent and in Nagasaki about 50 per cent in the injured survivors. In Hiroshima about 30 per cent of the deaths in those who survived longer than one day were ascribed to radiation injury either alone or combined with blast and/or burn damage. In the survivor study population of 82,244, 141 cases of leukemia developed between 1950 and 1972. It is probable that the modern nuclear weapon effects would exceed these results. In nuclear weapon tests, some 300 people have inadvertently been exposed to local high levels of radioactive fallout, with resultant clinical manifestations in about 25 per cent.

Early peacetime uses of radioactivity led to an initial high incidence of injury. Within seven years of the demonstration of x-irradiation by Roentgen in 1895, some 200 cases of x-ray injury had been reported. After recognition of the hazard, radiation protection standards were developed internationally. There has been a marked reduction in this type of injury, although hand injuries still occur occasionally in industrial radiographers and the users of x-ray diffraction and other analytic equipment in research and development laboratories.

The discovery of natural radioactivity by Becquerel in 1896 led to the purification of radium by the Curies in 1911 and its use in medicine and industry. About 5000 watch dial painters, industrial chemists, and medical patients were involved. In 2500 of these, in whom medical information was compiled by A. M. Brues at Argonne National Laboratory through 1975, there were 408 malignant tumors, with the excess over the expected frequency involving bone and the air cavities of the head. The development of manmade radioactive material during and after World War II led to a nuclear industry population of several hundred thousand workers, but only 97 cases of clinical radiation injury had developed by 1969. Although data collection concerning medical misadministrations of radioactive isotopes designed for diagnostic and therapeutic purposes has not been systematic, several deaths and a number of injuries are known to have occurred in the very large American patient population, estimated at over 8 million annually, receiving these materials.

EPIDEMIOLOGY. The manifestations of acute or of late radiation injury are not produced solely by irradiation. It is therefore essential to utilize epidemiologic methodology in order to establish the relationship of the etiologic agent to the clinical symptomatology. Two most helpful features have been the temporal relationship of the exposure to the development of clinical effects and the quantitative dose-response relationship.

The etiologic role of radiation in the clinical syndrome of *acute* radiation injury has been shown in epidemiologic studies of the Japanese atomic bomb survivors, the Marshall Islanders and Japanese fishermen exposed to fallout from a nuclear weapon test, several groups of radiation therapy patients, and the workers involved in various industrial radiation accidents. Epidemiologic studies relating *late* radiation effects such as neoplastic diseases and life-shortening to radiation exposure have dealt with radiologists and other physicians, the Japanese population under long-term follow-up by the Atomic Bomb Casualty Commission and its successor since 1975, the Radiation Effects Research Foundation, the radium watch dial painters, therapeutically x-irradiated patients (particularly those receiving thymic irradiation in infancy), patients receiving radioactive iodine therapy, and nuclear industry employees.

PATHOGENESIS. The basic pathology begins with the interaction of the radiation with tissue within the first second of exposure. The radiation energy in photons or particles penetrating the protoplasm may interact at the atomic level to produce ion pairs. These ions combine radiochemically with cell water, producing free radicals such as H and OH which further react to produce such forms as H_2O_2 and HO_2. These, in turn, may interact with critical molecules of the cell protoplasm such as nucleic acids or enzymes. If the dose is high and interactions are numerous, the cell may be killed directly by the radiation. At lower doses, the ability of the cell to divide may be impaired permanently or temporarily. If the DNA is involved, sublethal damage of this molecule may result in reproduction of the alteration (i.e., mutation) in daughter and descendant cells. Direct cell killing begins with exposures of one or more thousands of rads, in general, although some cells such as lymphocytes and spermatogonia are affected at much lower doses. Those cells which are rapidly dividing and differentiating are most vulnerable. Mitotic arrest occurs after several hundreds of rads and is characterized by continuing function of the existing cells but no new divisions. The continuing synthesis of proteins and enzymes, despite an irreversibly impaired mitotic apparatus, leads to "giant cells" which die after several weeks because their excessive size interferes with nutrition and metabolism. At doses of about 100 rads or more, mitotic delay results from temporary impairment of the mitotic mechanism. At still lower doses transient chromosomal "stickiness" is seen, presumably caused by denaturation of the DNA-histone molecules. Also, beginning at exposures as low as a few rads, are chromosome aberrations, i.e., breaks, deletions, gaps, and abnormal forms such as ring and dicentric chromosomes.

The effects of these cellular abnormalities on the various organs depend on the rate of proliferation of new cells required. In high turnover tissues such as the blood-forming tissue and the gastrointestinal tract, the relatively short life span of the predominant cells leads to rapid depletion before the onset of mitotic recovery and new cell production. In the period of mitotic inhibition of the blood-forming tissue, for example, the consequent depletion of mature cells results in increased probability of infection and hemorrhage. The resultant pathologic manifestations are nonspecific, although the inflammatory changes accompanying infection are deficient in polymorphonuclear cells.

In tissues which have little or no continuous proliferation, such as the liver or brain, this type of radiation injury is not apparent; however, functional impairment may be detected by appropriate means. In very slow turnover tissues, such as the lens of the eye or the thyroid gland, the manifestations of acute radiation effects may require months to years before becoming evident. Also, the small arterioles damaged by local radiation injury may show a compensatory increase in cell production, leading to endothelial thickening, obliterative endarteritis, and extensive fibrosis over a prolonged period of time.

Chromosomal abnormalities produced in injured cells may be reproduced and perpetuated for decades. A long-lived component of the lymphoid cells may even carry the original radiation damage for many years before dividing. Clones of cells with the same specific chromosome abnormality may develop over a period of years as well.

CLINICAL MANIFESTATIONS. Clinical manifestations of radiation injury can be subdivided into three major forms: the acute radiation syndrome, acute local radiation injury, and delayed effects. External penetrating irradiation, as well as external and internal radionuclide contamination and local traumatic injury with radionuclide contamination, may produce these manifestations.

Acute Radiation Syndrome. This syndrome is seen typically after exposure of most or all of the body to external sources of penetrating ionizing radiation, although high doses of ^{32}P, ^{131}I, and ^{198}Au have also evoked it. It appears in three major forms, in ascending severity of injury. These are the hematologic, the gastrointestinal, and the central nervous system–cardiovascular forms. Four discernible clinical stages can be recognized, particularly when the severity of injury allows for ultimate survival. These are the initial or prodromal stage which subsides into a latent stage, followed by a stage of manifest or overt illness, and a recovery stage. The duration of each stage is inversely related to the severity of injury.

Typical manifestations of the *hematologic form* are seen after an exposure in the midlethal range (about 300 rads without treatment). Prodromal anorexia, nausea, and possibly vomiting may commence within several hours and generally subside within 48 hours. Transient waves of skin erythema and conjunctivitis may be observed over the same period or longer. The patient may be asymptomatic after the prodromal stage for one to three weeks. Then the increasing inadequacy of the body's defenses against infection and hemorrhage becomes manifest, with development of fever, oropharyngeal lesions, abscesses, petechiae, purpura, and bleeding from body orifices. Other findings include scalp pain and epilation in the third postexposure week, and recurrent anorexia and nausea accompanied by weakness, fatigue, weight loss, and emaciation. Gradual recovery ensues, beginning about the fifth to sixth week after exposure and may require several months.

The earliest laboratory finding is lymphopenia, reaching absolute lymphocyte levels below 1000 per cubic millimeter within the first 48 postexposure hours. The

reticulocytes may disappear in the same time period. A gradual fall in granulocyte counts begins during the first two weeks, reaches a plateau, or even shows an abortive rise, followed by a steep fall to a low point at about 30 days postexposure. The platelet count nadir occurs at the same time, after a more continuous fall. If the individual survives, an abrupt increase in all the cell lines mentioned, except the lymphocytes, will occur within the next week and they will rapidly reach normal levels. An initial increase in granulocyte count in the first 24 hours may occur on the basis of a nonspecific "alarm reaction," and should not mislead one to exclude radiation injury on this basis. Blood biochemical analyses may show nonspecific indicators of major cell and tissue damage such as creatinuria, increased excretion of DNA breakdown products such as beta-aminoisobutyric acid, deoxycytidine, and various other amino acids. Serum enzyme measurements such as LDH, SGOT, and SGPT may be elevated, and an early transient slight hyperbilirubinemia observed. Within 24 hours chromosome breakage and abnormal forms can be seen in peripheral blood cytogenetic preparations, with the frequency related to the magnitude of the radiation exposure.

The *gastrointestinal form* is associated with anorexia, nausea, vomiting, and diarrhea within the first few hours after exposure. These may be of sufficient severity to require active treatment but usually subside within 48 hours. A latent period follows which may last only a few days to a week before there is a major recurrence of all the gastrointestinal symptoms as well as those of infection and hemorrhage as described above. These patients generally die with a fulminating enterocolitis before the full appearance of epilation and other slower developing radiation sequelae.

Laboratory abnormalities in the gastrointestinal form of radiation injury are similar to those of the hematologic form but occur more promptly and with greater magnitude. In addition, the hematocrit may be increased as a result of hemoconcentration caused by fluid loss, which, with hypoglycemia and electrolyte imbalance, results from the loss of a functional intestinal mucosal lining.

In the *central nervous system and cardiovascular form*, immediate nausea, projectile vomiting, and explosive diarrhea are characteristic. These may be accompanied by disorientation, hyperesthesia, ataxia, sweating, prostration, and shock. There may be some improvement after several hours, but alternations develop between evidences of central nervous system hyperexcitability, including convulsions, and CNS depression, such as somnolence and coma. This is accompanied by hypotension which becomes irreversible, as does oliguria, leading to a fatal outcome in 24 to 48 hours.

Laboratory observations in the central nervous system and cardiovascular form of acute radiation injury show marked telescoping of the previously described injury syndromes with abnormalities occurring sooner and with greater severity. Complete lymphopenia and an initial granulocyte level of 30,- to 40,000 may be present within the next few hours. Prompt chromosome examination may show marked increase in aberrations, but as the circulating lymphocytes disappear, it may become difficult to find dividing cells. The biochemical evidences of tissue damage are much more striking in this form of the syndrome. In addition, biochemical evidences of azotemia secondary to hypotension become prominent.

Local Radiation Injury. Localized radiation injury may occur with acute and/or chronic clinical manifestations, depending on the total dose and dose rate at which the exposure takes place.

The early changes result in three major clinical findings: erythema, epilation, and transepidermal injury. *Erythema* comparable to a mild sunburn or a thermal burn of the first degree may appear on exposure to more than 200 to 300 rads. A transient first wave may be present within hours after exposure, associated with hyperesthesia, burning, or itching. The major redness appears two or three weeks later, the interval depending on the dose. In the lower dose range no further changes other than tanning may occur, and medical care is not necessary. A counterpart to this reaction has been described in the conjunctiva and in the anterior chamber of the eye, with inflammatory changes observed promptly after exposure.

Epilation, or loss of hair, may occur after exposure to any form of radiation, beginning with exposures to the skin of about 300 rads. It generally does not become apparent until the third week after exposure. Associated skin or scalp tenderness may occur one or two days preceding the actual hair loss. With doses greater than about 500 rads, epilation may be complete. If the exposure is much greater than 600 rads, hair may not regrow.

Transepidermal injury (dry or wet dermatitis) is comparable to a thermal second-degree burn with erythema, blistering, and pain. Confluent bullae may develop in about one and one-half to three weeks, depending on dose (usually exceeding 1000 rads). These may rupture, leaving open, weeping lesions vulnerable to infection.

With higher doses, probably on the order of 5000 rads, a more serious version of transepidermal injury occurs, in which the lesion resembles a third-degree burn. Pain occurs promptly and is intense. The raw areas may be very slow in healing, or may not heal until surgical resection and skin grafting are performed. Epilation is permanent.

Still higher doses may produce immediate tissue damage to structures below the skin. Such injuries, which have occurred in the abdominal wall, male genitalia, and extremities, are irreversible, requiring surgical excision and further reconstructive management.

Delayed Effects. Delayed effects of radiation exposure are of two varieties: those finally appearing in organs whose cells received the radiation exposure and are relatively slow in responding; and those late effects occurring in organs and tissues in which descendent cells ultimately express the initial radiation injury after a latent period which may be many years in duration. The first type of delayed effect can be seen in the male gonad, for example. Doses as low as 15 rads will produce *impairment in fertility* owing to moderate oligospermia beginning about 50 days after the exposure. Azoospermia will occur with doses of more than 200 to 300 rads for a period of roughly one to two years. Doses of 500 to 600 rads may produce permanent sterility in male or female survivors.

The lens of the eye is another late-responding tissue, with opacities appearing in the posterior subcapsular region in months to several years after exposures of about 200 rads or more. *Cataracts* of the posterior lens may develop in the majority of patients who receive more than 600 rads. The gradual development of *hypothyroidism* several years after exposure of several hundred rads is another example of delayed response. *Skin changes* constitute another late response to either acute injury or repeated low level radiation exposure. There may be loss of the detailed finger-ridge pattern and hair, abnormalities of the fingernails, and dryness of the skin. Localized hyperkeratosis may be seen, as well as breakdown of previously healed but atrophic skin, and, ultimately, neoplastic skin changes may develop in such areas.

In the *fetus* the clinical manifestations will depend largely on its age and the magnitude of exposure. If the exposure takes place in the first one to two weeks, resorption of the conceptus is probable. Between the second and sixth weeks, the effect will be on the particular organs under development at the time. Further along in gestation, there will be more subtle generalized effects ultimately expressed as deficits in growth and development, including microcephaly and mental retardation.

The most common *late effects* of radiation exposure are *neoplastic diseases*. The earliest to appear are the acute leukemias and chronic granulocytic leukemia, with a peak incidence of approximately four to seven years after the radiation exposure. Chronic lymphocytic leukemia is not increased by radiation exposure. Other neoplasms whose induction appears significantly increased by radiation exposure include cancer of the thyroid and salivary glands, lung, bone, and female breast tissues. Internally deposited radionuclides have been associated particularly with malignant neoplasms of bone and reticuloendothelial tissues such as liver, spleen, and lymph nodes. Radium deposition has involved the mastoid bones and those surrounding the paranasal sinuses in particular, whereas internally administered thorium dioxide has produced an increase of hemangiosarcomas of the liver. In addition, a generalized increase in incidence of all forms of cancer has been documented in the Japanese atomic bomb survivors. *Shortening of life expectancy* through somewhat earlier death from all causes has been demonstrated in the radiologist population but not yet in the Japanese A-bomb survivors.

DIAGNOSIS. Acute Radiation Syndrome. The manifestations of acute radiation injury are not unique to this causative agent. Therefore the diagnosis rests on the history and the evolving clinical pattern defined by time of onset and duration of the clinical signs, symptoms, and laboratory abnormalities, particularly the hematologic changes.

In the absence of an adequate history of radiation exposure, the diagnosis may be elusive. The various manifestations may suggest a wide range of conditions. Prodromes suggest psychoneurosis, food poisoning, or gastrointestinal viral infection; symptoms in the period of manifest illness may mimic aplastic anemia, leukemia, infectious gastroenteritis, typhoid fever, and even mumps (for radiation parotitis). When a radiation exposure history is elicited, hematologic and cytogenetic examinations may be used as well as physical dosimetry data obtained by personnel monitoring equipment, if any, and by reconstruction of the exposure situation, in order to obtain confirmatory and quantitative information concerning the potential severity of the injury.

However, it must be kept clearly in mind that the evolving clinical pattern is the final diagnostic criterion for the recognition and management of this form of injury.

Local Injury. Local radiation injury, particularly as it appears on the upper extremities, is often confused with thermal and chemical burns. Differentiating features are absence of waves of erythema in the latter as well as the more severe prolonged pain and slower healing associated with radiation. Recurrent tissue breakdown after healing is also suggestive of radiation injury as opposed to the other possibilities.

Delayed Effects. No clinical characteristics of the late effects of radiation exposure are unique to this etiologic agent.

Radionuclide Contamination. Radionuclides deposited on the surface of the skin may be absorbed, inhaled, or ingested into the body where they may act to produce delayed effects. In order to prevent such sequelae, the recognition of their presence is essential even though no immediate clinical manifestations are present. Such diagnostic procedures must involve close collaboration between the physician and the health physicist, the professional trained to recognize and quantitate radiation exposure in order to prevent deleterious effects of radiation. Radioactivity surveys of the suspected individual with appropriate radiation detection equipment should be carried out. It is most important to collect all urinary and fecal excretions in separate containers until sufficient data of the nature and magnitude of contamination are obtained. Some radionuclides such as radon may be sought in breath samples. An early postexposure blood sample should also be collected and preserved for radionuclide analysis. Finally, it may be necessary to carry out chest or whole body low-level radiation counting in an appropriate facility, i.e., a so-called "whole body counter."

If a traumatic wound is present, radionuclide contamination may be sought by measuring radioactivity of swabs used in cleaning the wound as well as by surveying over the surface with appropriate detectors. If the wound is the sole contaminated area, excreta samples will show whether the contaminant has been absorbed into the body and therefore is sufficiently soluble for circulation and translocation to sites remote from the wound.

TREATMENT. Acute Radiation Syndrome. The treatment of acute radiation syndrome is based on an understanding of its pathophysiology. The prodromal symptoms in the acute radiation syndrome are self-limited, but sedatives and antiemetics may be used if needed. Throughout the syndrome it is important to reduce anxiety by keeping the patient informed about the nature of his injury, the expected transient health impairment, and its anticipated duration and treatment. The prolonged weakness associated with this syndrome even during convalescence may be in some measure secondary to the prolonged anxiety and fear of the unknown often associated with radiation injury.

In the *hematologic form*, the inhibition of mitosis responsible for the overt illness is self-limited. Thus management is directed toward maintenance of the patient through the period in which his defenses against infection and hemorrhage are deficient. This is best achieved by conservative means. The threat of exogenous bacterial and viral infection is reduced by strict reverse isolation of the patient with maintenance of a clean environment by use of a laminar air flow or "life-island" methods. Attendant personnel must be screened for potential pathogens and treated prophylactically if necessary.

Prophylactic oral antimicrobial drugs to clear pathogenic bacterial and fungal organisms from the gastrointestinal tract have been used when the total granulocyte level falls below 1000 per cubic millimeter. Various blood elements may be given to replace deficiencies when needed. Donors should be limited in number and tissue typed to minimize systemic reactions to and inefficacy of transfused cells. Red cells are needed only if significant bleeding has occurred. Fresh platelets should be available for use if significant hemorrhage develops. Their use has been advocated even in the absence of bleeding when the platelet count falls below 10,000 per cubic millimeter. If available in concentrated form, normal granulocytes may be administered in the face of overt infection during the granulocytopenic phase. If not available, in the presence of a clearly life-threatening infection the use of the much greater numbers of granulocytes of patients with chronic granulocytic leukemia has been suggested, because they are capable of phagocytosis. On recovery, it is assumed that the patient's immune system will rid the body of such donor cells.

In the situation in which both biologic and dosimetric indicators suggest the high probability of a fatal outcome, bone marrow transplantation may be warranted. Because such marrow requires about two weeks to correct the deficit in circulating blood cells, such a decision should not be delayed much beyond the first postexposure week. The hazards of a graft reaction by the host if his radiation-induced immunosuppression is not sufficient, and of "graft versus host" reaction if it is too long lasting, define the narrow boundaries within which therapeutic benefit may be expected. The availability of an identical twin or a very close matching relative on tissue compatibility testing will also influence the decision. The transplantation procedures developed by Thomas et al. for managing leukemic patients after therapeutic whole body irradiation are helpful in accidental radiation injury patients also.

Management of the *gastrointestinal form* of acute radiation syndrome has not been successful thus far in the few human occurrences. Animal studies by Bond and Cronkite suggest that the vigorous and early utilization of adequate anti-infection agents, blood components, nutrients, electrolytes, and fluid may influence mortality favorably.

In the few human instances of the *central nervous system–cardiovascular form*, the progressive hypotension has not been improved by the administration of pressor agents, and the fluid administration involved has augmented the congestive heart failure which has ensued.

Local Radiation Injury. The treatment of local radiation injury is generally similar to that of thermal burns of the same severity. This includes the maintenance of asepsis, eventual removal of devitalized tissue to the degree necessary, and the use of skin grafting to cover nonhealing ulcerations. An additional feature in management is very careful and prolonged observation for possible early neoplastic changes of the skin.

Delayed Effects. Clinical management of the delayed effects of radiation exposure does not differ in any way from the management of similar pathologic conditions not caused by radiation.

Radionuclide Contamination. In the event of an accident in which radionuclide contamination is likely, only urgent first aid should be given and the patient evacuated from the site. Contaminated skin and wounds should be washed promptly, and all excreta collected.

Useful preparations for skin decontamination include soap and water, surgical and laundry detergents, and oxidizing agents. These should be accompanied by brushing and rinsing, with care taken not to abrade the skin.

Contamination of the eyes, nose, and mouth is treated initially with copious water washing as soon as possible. Isotonic irrigants may be substituted as soon as available.

For definitive wound care, the usual surgical principles apply, with modifications only in the aseptic procedures and debridement in order to avoid introduction of skin contamination into the wound. Prior to surgical treatment it may also be desirable to give intravenous diethylenetriaminepentaacetic acid (DTPA), a chelating agent available from the U.S. Department of Energy for investigational use, to minimize the retention of any contaminant which may get into circulation during surgery.

If radioactivity measurements of excreta and of the whole body suggest a residual body burden of a larger quantity than seems acceptable on the basis of medical and health physics judgment, various treatments may be used to minimize the absorption and enhance the excretion of the radionuclide.

To minimize respiratory absorption, the use of irritants, expectorants, and pulmonary lavage is under current investigation. Inhalation of DTPA aerosol mist is also currently being tested for transuranic isotope contamination.

To minimize gastrointestinal absorption, the simplest measure is to accelerate excretion with a mild laxative. For strontium-90, sodium alginate and aluminum hydroxide gel have been used orally to prevent uptake from the gut. For cesium-137, Prussian blue (ferric ferrocyanide) does the same. To promote excretion of nuclides already within the body and to reduce deposition in target organs, such as bone, a variety of agents are available. For plutonium, americium, yttrium, lanthanum, and fission products, intravenously administered chelating agents are useful, DTPA being the most effective. For strontium, the combination of high calcium intake and acidification of the blood with ammonium chloride has effectively reduced bone absorption.

PROGNOSIS. Acute Radiation Syndrome. The estimated short-term radiation exposure which would be lethal for 50 per cent of an untreated human population in 60 days ($LD_{50/60}$) is about 300 rads mean midline absorbed dose. This exposure would be expected to produce the hematologic form of the acute radiation syndrome, with half the exposed population dying within 60 days. However, an accidentally irradiated worker survived an estimated 600 rads absorbed whole body dose, with postexposure treatment, including isogeneic marrow transplantation, by Wald, Thomas, and coworkers, despite tissue damage severe enough to necessitate subsequent amputation of all four extremities. Also, Thomas et al. and others have used pre- and postexposure treatment, including isogeneic marrow, in over 100 acutely ill leukemic patients receiving 1000 rads of whole body exposure with about 20 per cent early post-treatment fatalities.

Thus it appears that successful management of the hematologic form of acute radiation injury is possible under good therapeutic circumstances. It has therefore been suggested by Wald and Watson that active supportive treatment can raise the LD_{50} to over 500 rads and heroic therapy, such as bone marrow transplantation, to over 1000 rads in accidentally exposed individuals. Clearly, such prognostic optimism would not apply to the large-scale population exposure situation such as occurred in Hiroshima and Nagasaki. Furthermore, even the best clinical management has not yet succeeded in allowing the survival of those few individuals who accidentally have received exposures resulting in major gastrointestinal or central nervous system–cardiovascular damage.

Local Radiation Injury. The outlook for good recovery from local radiation injury depends in part on the adequacy of management of the acute changes, including the removal of devitalized tissue and the prevention of secondary infection. However, the main determinant of the ultimate outcome will be the severity of injury to the underlying blood vessels.

Delayed Effects. The likelihood of a radiation-exposed individual's developing a late effect of the exposure is increased in some relation to the magnitude of the exposure. Since most radiation exposure above the natural background is due to human activities and therefore presumably controllable, increasing recent effort has been given to quantitative risk assessment for radiation carcinogenesis to facilitate better benefit-risk judgments. In 1977, both the United Nations Scientific Committee on the Effects of Atomic Radiation (UNSCEAR) and the International Commission on Radiological Protection (ICRP) reviewed human epidemiologic data and published risk approximations for radiation-induced cancer in various tissues. Although the risk estimates cannot be determined with great accuracy, it is possible, in some instances in which mutually consistent epidemiologic data are obtainable from several different sources, to classify different tissues into groups with different degrees of sensitivity to induction of malignancies by radiation. It is important to note that most of the information is derived from exposures of 100 rads or more of x- or gamma radiation at high dose rates, and therefore may represent overestimates when extrapolated to exposures of a few rads or less delivered at very low dose rates, such as received by the occupationally exposed radiation worker population.

The approximate risk of induction of radiation cancer in various tissues estimated by UNSCEAR can be summarized in terms of the number of cases expected per million persons so exposed per rad of absorbed radiation exposure. In descending order of sensitivity, with the approximate number of cases per million per rad given in parentheses following each tissue, they include thyroid (100); female breast (100); lung (25 to 50); leukemia (20 to 50); stomach, liver, large intestine, brain, and salivary glands (10 to 15); and bone, esophagus, small intestine, urinary bladder, pancreas, rectum, lymphatic tissues, and mucosa of cranial sinuses (2 to 5). It must be recognized that these estimates are very broad generalizations and that for each tissue there are differing effects of such factors as sex and age at exposure, in addition to the kind of radiation, dose, and dose rate. For example, the pediatric population is more sensitive to thyroid cancer induction, female breast cancer is induced primarily by exposure during the early reproductive period, and lung cancer is highest in males exposed at over 35 years of age. Also, the induction of cancer in the fetus is distinctly elevated, estimated roughly as 200 to 250 cases per million per rad.

The duration of the period at risk also varies with different tissues. The mean interval between exposure and leukemia development is in the region of 10 years, for example, whereas the other malignancies typically appear in an exposed population with a mean of 25 years of latency. In a population exposure, the earlier appearing leukemia may serve as an indicator for the eventual total of all fatal malignancies, which ultimately may occur in four to six times as many individuals as developed leukemia alone.

The prognosis for the various delayed effects of radiation exposure is similar to that of the same pathology in the absence of such exposure. For this reason many of the radiation-induced cancers would be expected to respond to treatment. The ICRP therefore derived maximum risk rates for fatalities from radiation-induced cancers. In descending order of risk, with approximate numbers of fatal cases per million exposed per rad in parentheses, they are female breast (50), leukemia (20), lung (20), thyroid (5), bone (5), and all other organs together (50).

Prevention. Since the foregoing discussion has indicated that there are no specific methods of reversing the course of events initiated by radiation exposure, the best measure against radiation injury is prevention. The largest *potential* source of radiation exposure to the general population is the nuclear weapon. It is therefore essential that all measures be taken to minimize the possibility of any human population receiving such an exposure again. Another potential source of population exposure, the widespread and increasing utilization of nuclear energy as a source of electric power generation, has been controlled successfully thus far.

The largest *actual* source of population exposure consists of users of radiation in the healing arts. It is evident that such usage of ionizing radiation has produced untold benefit to the same population. Nevertheless, it is incumbent on the users of medical radiation sources to minimize the exposures needed to obtain the necessary diagnostic information. This requires not only optimal operation of existing equipment by current techniques but also a continuing research and development effort to improve the efficiency of such equipment to allow reduction of exposure while obtaining the necessary biomedical information. Adequate specialized education of all users of radiation sources in the philosophy and methods of radiation protection is another factor in the preventive approach to radiation injury.

Andrews, G. A., Balish, E., Edwards, C. L., Kniseley, R. M., and Lushbaugh, C. C.: Possibilities for Improved Treatment of Persons Exposed in Radiation Accidents. In Handling of Radiation Accidents. Vienna, International Atomic Energy Agency, 1969, p. 119.

Basic Radiation Protection Criteria. NCRP Report No. 39, Washington, D.C., National Council on Radiation Protection and Measurements, 1971.

Cleary, S. F. Biological effects of microwave and radiofrequency radiation. In Straub, C. P. (ed.): Critical Reviews in Environmental Control, Vol. 7, Issue 2. Cleveland, CRC Press, 1977, p. 121.

Dalrymple, G. V., et al.: Medical Radiation Biology. Philadelphia, W. B. Saunders Company, 1973.

Management of Persons Contaminated with Radionuclides. NCRP Report

in preparation. Washington, D.C., National Council on Radiation Protection and Measurements, 1979.

Medical Radiation Exposure of Pregnant and Potentially Pregnant Women. NCRP Report No. 54. Washington, D.C., National Council on Radiation Protection and Measurements, 1977.

Norwood, W. D.: Health Protection of Radiation Workers. Springfield, Ill., Charles C Thomas, 1975.

Radiation Protection. ICRP Publication 26, Recommendations of the International Commission on Radiological Protection. New York, Pergamon Press, 1977.

Robinson, D. W.: Surgical problems in the excision and repair of radiated tissue. Plastic Reconstruct. Surg., 55:41, 1975.

Rubin, P., and Casarett, G. W.: Clinical Radiation Pathology. Philadelphia, W. B. Saunders Company, 1968.

Sources and Effects of Ionizing Radiation. United Nations Scientific Committee on the Effects of Atomic Radiation. 1977 report to the General Assembly, with annexes. New York, United Nations, 1977.

Stannard, J. N.: Toxicology of radionuclides. Ann. Rev. Pharmacol., 13:325, 1973.

The Effects on Populations of Exposure to Low Levels of Ionizing Radiation. Report of the Advisory Committee on the Biological Effects of Ionizing Radiations. Washington, National Academy of Sciences — National Research Council, 1972.

Thomas, E. D., et al.: Bone marrow transplantation. N. Engl. J. Med., 292:832, 985, 1975.

Wald, N.: Radiation injury and its management. In Wang, Y. (ed.): Handbook of Radioactive Nuclides. Part IX. Cleveland, The Chemical Rubber Co., 1969, p. 837.

Wald, N., and Watson, J. A.: Medical modification of human acute radiation injury. In Proceedings, IVth Congress. Paris, International Radiation Protection Association, 1977, p. 1183.

28.   ELECTRIC SHOCK AND ELECTRIC INJURY

*Curtis P. Artz**

Electric shock and electric injury occur when the current of electricity passes through the body. Kouwenhoven pointed out six factors that determine the effects of electricity on the body. These are type of circuit, voltage, resistance offered by the body, value of the current, pathway of the current, and duration of the contact. Direct current does not produce the same contraction of muscles that is found with alternating current.

In high voltage injury there is greater cause for respiratory arrest, because of the very severe muscular contraction. High voltage currents also cause a greater amount of tissue damage. If the victim of an electric shock retains consciousness during and after the contact, there is often a ringing in the ears and partial deafness for a time. In addition there may be visual disorders such as flashes and brilliant luminous spots. If there is a prolonged period of apnea, the neurologic manifestations of anoxia may be present.

The resistance to electric current in tissue varies in order from the greatest to the least as follows: bone, fat, tendon, skin, muscle, blood, nerve. Thin skin is less resistant, of course, than thick skin. After an electric current has penetrated the skin, it passes rapidly through the body along the lines of least resistance — that is, through the tissue fluids and along blood vessels, where it may cause degeneration of vessel walls and formation of thrombi. If the resistance of the skin is low at the time it interrupts the electric current, the current passes readily into the body. It is generally believed that the greater the skin resistance, the more severe the local burn; similarly, the less the resistance, the greater the systemic effect of the current.

The pathway of the current through the body is important. If it passes through vital organs such as the heart and the brain, the resulting injury is greater. It is always difficult, however, to tell from the cutaneous injury the exact pathway the current has taken. The difference in the susceptibility of the heart to electrical injury at different times in its contraction cycle also seems important. The longer the duration of contact, the greater the amount of damage.

INCIDENCE. There are about 1000 accidental deaths due to electric current in the United States each year. About 90 per cent of these occur in males. The highest fatality rate is experienced by men in the age range of 20 to 34. More than two fifths of the fatalities occur from June through August. Approximately two thirds of all fatal injuries from electric current occur on the job, and more than one fourth occur on home premises.

PATHOGENESIS. The wounds of electric injury are extremely variable because there are such differences in type and intensity of current, tissues through which the current passes, and degree of contact. Injuries associated with electricity may be divided into three types: true electric injury, arc burn, and flame burn.

True electric injury is caused by the passage of electric current through the skin. The entry wound is charred and depressed, whereas the exit wound is dry and gives the appearance that the electric current exploded as it made its exit. The extensive underlying tissue damage is evidenced by intense swelling. The cause of this damage is most likely due to the heat generated by the passage of the current through the tissues. The current follows blood vessels, and thrombosis even at some distance from the original injury is common. A limb that appears viable soon after an electric accident may in a few days become ischemic and finally gangrenous. Parts of the media of vessels may be weakened by cellular disintegration, and if thrombosis does not occur there may be serious hemorrhage. The death of muscle is usually very uneven. Sometimes there is a palpable pulse in the large arteries of an extremity but the nutrient artery to a muscle bundle is completely occluded.

This deeper destruction has led to the concept that electric injuries are more like crush injury than like a burn (see accompanying figure). Thermal burns usually destroy only the skin and subcutaneous tissue, whereas electric injury is deeper and frequently associated with muscle destruction.

Arc burns are produced by current coursing externally to the body from the contact point to the ground. Burns that follow the leaping of an electric arc from the conductor to the skin are mainly associated with high tension current. They are usually severe because an electric arc has a temperature of approximately 2500° C.

Flame burns result from ignition of clothing by electrical sparks or arcing.

CLINICAL MANIFESTATIONS. Tetanic contraction of muscles is common and sometimes causes fractures and dislocations. Delayed effect of electric injury includes the development of cataracts. However, the severe effects of electric injury are damage to the skin, subcutaneous tissue, and muscles. Most common is true electric injury accompanied by flame burns.

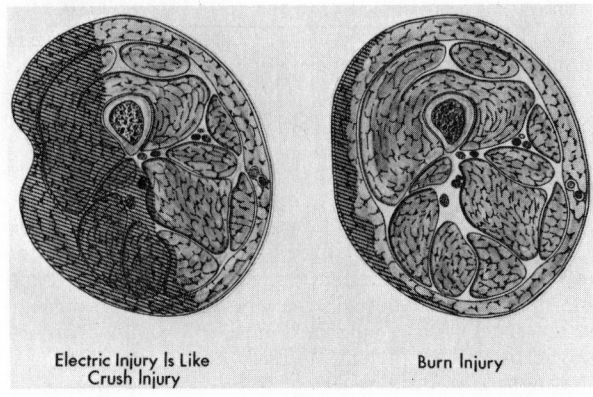

Electric injury is more like crush injury than like a burn. The damage is deep and frequently involves muscle.

Vascular Injuries. Delayed hemorrhage from large blood vessels is a threat when there is an area of extensive necrosis over the vessels. Rupture of major vessels distant from the areas of tissue necrosis may also occur. Progressive loss of blood supply to muscles may account for the fibrosis that is not uncommonly observed.

Spinal Cord Injury. Spinal cord injuries are more frequently encountered than is generally recognized, because many of these lesions are incomplete and are not associated with either vertebral fractures or the apparent path of the current. The clinical signs often are those of spastic paresis, and the patients may have little or no sensory deficit accompanying the motor changes. Such injury is difficult to diagnose, and the lesions are not suspected until ambulation provides evidence of neuromuscular imbalance.

Cardiopulmonary Injury. Anoxia and ventricular fibrillation are the principal causes of immediate death. Acute pulmonary complications are limited to pleural damage resulting in effusion and lobular pneumonitis directly adjacent to the contact point. Taylor reported electrocardiographic changes in patients who showed right bundle branch block, ectopic focus arrhythmias, or supraventricular tachycardia. There may be some longlasting cardiovascular effects, including disturbance of rhythm consisting essentially of disturbances in atrioventricular and intraventricular conduction, clinically and electrocardiographically established manifestations of acute coronary insufficiency, and subjective disturbances such as precordial pains and palpitations. Baxter reported that tachycardia and minor S-T segment alterations frequently persist for several weeks after electric injury.

Renal Effects. Renal damage is not uncommon. Most likely it is caused by a combination of the initial severe shock, direct electric current damage to the kidneys, and abnormal protein breakdown products from damaged muscles. Acute tubular necrosis is a recognized complication.

Abdominal Injury. Submucosal hemorrhages scattered throughout the gastrointestinal tract are not infrequently seen at autopsy after electric injury. This is probably because of the direct effect of the current. A most distressing diagnostic problem occurs in electric injuries to the abdomen. It is difficult to determine whether or not intra-abdominal injury is present. Too often abdominal symptoms are ascribed to nonspecific paralytic ileus. One must beware of making a diagnosis of paralytic ileus associated with electric injury and forgetting that intestinal damage as a result of the current may be present.

TREATMENT. An electric shock victim should be freed from contact with the current as quickly as possible. The rescuer must make sure that he is well insulated. If the victim is not breathing, artificial respiration must be started immediately. If the heart is not beating, there is probably ventricular fibrillation, and cardiac massage should be given until the patient can be moved to a facility where defibrillation is possible.

A most important aspect of initial resuscitation is replacement of isotonic fluid that has been rapidly lost into the area of injury. When there is true electric damage to muscle as well as to skin and subcutaneous tissue, large volumes of fluid are required. Since the injury is similar to crush injury, the principles associated with replacement therapy after crush injury are applicable. This means large quantities of lactated Ringer's solution, mannitol, and sodium bicarbonate. In extensive damage when the initial fluid therapy does not produce a clear urine, 25 grams of mannitol should be given intravenously. It should be followed by 12.5 grams per hour until the reddish brown urine clears or six doses are given. Sodium bicarbonate should be given to ensure alkalinization of the urine.

Wound Care. Management of the local wound is difficult because of the various types of injury. If the injury is small, such as is seen from low voltage current, the area should be treated with local antibacterial ointments and allowed to slough and heal.

High voltage injuries must be treated more aggressively. A surgeon should make sure that there is no underlying muscle damage. This can usually be ascertained by incising one or two areas and looking at the muscle. If there is dead muscle, the patient should be taken to the operating room as soon as his general physical condition permits, and all the dead skin, subcutaneous tissue, and muscle should be excised. Sometimes this requires amputation. In extensive injury to the extremities, fasciotomy and muscle debridement are usually accomplished at the first operation. Because of the progressive nature of the lesion, additional excision and debridement of muscle may be necessary. When there has been appreciable surface injury without deep destruction, the primary problem of management is the treatment of the entry and exit wound. Usually these are managed in the same way as a thermal burn. Associated thermal injury is treated by the application of a local antibacterial agent, and the wounds are closed by skin grafts after all the dead tissue has been removed.

Artz, C. P.: Changing concepts of electrical injury. Am. J. Surg., 128:699, 1974.

Baxter, C. R.: Present concepts in the management of major electrical injuries. Surg. Clin. North Am., 50:1401, 1970.

Kouwenhoven, W. B.: Effect of electricity on the human body. Elec. Engineering, 68:199, 1949.

Statistical Bulletin. New York, Metropolitan Life Insurance Company, May 1968.

Taylor, P. H., Pugsley, L. Q., and Vogel, E. H., Jr.: The intriguing electrical burn. J. Trauma, 2:309, 1962.

29.   MOTION SICKNESS AND PROBLEMS OF AIR TRAVEL

Stanley R. Mohler

29.1.   MOTION SICKNESS

DEFINITION. Motion sickness is the most likely reason for nausea experienced during travel on a pitching, rolling, and/or yawing conveyance, these three motions often interacting. The travel may be of any mode: air, land, sea, or space. Even riding a camel can cause motion sickness. The nausea that develops is often preceded by a feeling of fatigue, and may progress to retching and vomiting. Commonly, the skin becomes clammy and the victim prefers to withdraw from the presence of others. Vertigo (dizziness and disorientation) may be experienced, and nystagmus can often be observed (the slow motion opposite to the imposed angular acceleration, the quick return in the direction of the motion). When nystagmus occurs, some associated blurring of vision may be a major complaint.

ETIOLOGY. Repeated angular acceleration stimulations of the three semicircular canals in each ear, especially when visual contact with the actual outside horizon is lost, cause conflicting sensations of orientation. The afferent nerve signals sent to the brain centers from the body's entire motion- and position-detecting senses (semicircular canals for angular accelerations, saccule and utricle for linear accelerations, and the proprioceptive system for the gravity "downward" acceleration) are involved. The proprioceptive system contains the subcutaneous pressure and kinesthetic senses. It sends signals to the brain on the body responses to experiencing accelerations and segment position changes. When the brain can no longer resolve or ignore the aforementioned varieties of afferent signals, confusion and dismay often result. This may lead to fatigue, anxiety and adrenergic "fear" response, sweating, pallor, tachycardia, and, ultimately, nausea and vomiting.

The air traveler most often encounters motion sickness in the 0.1- to 0.7-Hz frequency range of linear acceleration. From one third to one half of airline passengers suffer motion sickness to various degrees when the linear acceleration levels (primarily in the vertical parameter) are in the range of 0.2 to 0.4 g root mean square. This is in the "moderately heavy" to "very heavy" turbulence range as described by pilots. About one in ten of the passengers of jet aircraft can be expected to experience an advanced degree of motion sickness in these frequency ranges.

In addition to the aforementioned linear acceleration aspect, the three semicircular canals in each ear detect angular accelerations at levels as low as 2.5 degrees per second^2 for a one-second period. At higher rotation rates, less time is required to detect motion. When one set of the three sets of canals (posterior, superior, lateral) is equilibrated to a constant angular velocity (for example, a constant rate turn) and the head is tilted, another set of canals receives stimulation. The canal endolymph must dissipate the angular momentum when moving to or from a given plane of rotation, producing canal sensor stimulations that the brain cannot resolve in regard to actual motion cues, giving the Coriolis effect (an uncomfortable disorientation feeling of movement different from the actual motion). At 0.6 degrees per second, the Coriolis effect can be detected. At 240 times this angular velocity, respiratory movements alone can cause the Coriolis symptoms.

It has been found that anxiety can lower the threshold for the onset of motion sickness. In addition, some persons are prone to experiencing motion sickness from childhood. No specific reason why these persons are susceptible has been found. In some cases, a labile emotional state has been implicated, as has a rigid, compulsive personality in others. However, more studies on these points are needed before positive statements can be made. The key role of the vestibular system in causing motion sickness is shown by the virtual absence of motion sickness in persons who have lost their left and right vestibular organs because of disease or surgery, or who suffered a congenital loss of these systems.

DIAGNOSIS. The progressive onset of sleepiness, fatigue, nausea, and/or vertigo, during air travel, is the prime symptom that aids in diagnosing motion sickness. This is especially so if the past history reveals prior occurrences in a given individual. The degree of the severity of the illness is usually associated directly with the degree of turbulence and maneuvering experienced. The progression of the symptoms to a state of frank vomiting is common. The signs include a clammy skin and, often, some degree of nystagmus.

The differential diagnosis must include (1) food poisoning (an occasional problem from meals served through airline caterers is staphylococcal food poisoning, often causing symptoms similar to severe motion sickness), (2) acute alcohol ingestion toxicity, (3) gastritis caused by intrinsic pathology (for example, peptic ulcer), and (4) shock. In repeated progressively severe instances of motion sickness involving a given individual, the possibility of increased intracranial pressure or some form of cranial tumor exists.

TREATMENT, PROGNOSIS, AND PREVENTION. The treatment of motion sickness is most effective when given one to two hours prior to exposure to accelerations. Reassurance is a useful aid for many travelers. Habituation of the vestibular system to accelerations usually occurs in the veteran traveler, markedly decreasing the times of motion sickness.

The following drugs have been found useful in treating motion sickness (*adult doses*):

1. Promethazine (Phenergan), 25 mg twice a day. (Note: When 25 mg ephedrine sulfate is also given simultaneously, a much more effective antimotion sickness effect results.)
2. Scopolamine (hyoscine), 1.2 mg.
3. Dimenhydrinate (Dramamine), 50 mg.
4. Cyclizine (Marezine), 50 mg.
5. Meclizine (Bonine), 50 mg.

In the 1960's, scopolamine and d-amphetamine were found to counteract motion sickness in an effective manner; but with the current trend away from prescribing amphetamines, this combination is not recommended in the routine practice of medicine.

It is quite possible that a strong placebo effect is operating in the case of drugs 4 and 5 above.

Since motion sickness is aggravated by the odors of vomitus, susceptible persons should move from its proximity. The motion-sick person should lie back and remain still, and may find that a cool damp cloth over the forehead provides comfort. The prognosis for the motion-sick person is excellent, because upon completion of the exposure to motions, recovery is usually rapid, taking place in a matter of minutes, and seldom exceeding a few hours. Prevention of motion sickness includes avoidance by susceptible persons of the types of accelerations that induce the syndrome. When this is not possible, the use of any one of the drugs given above should ameliorate or prevent motion sickness, especially if taken prior to the exposure to accelerations. It is emphasized that these drugs should not be taken by air crew members or others who must operate vehicles or machinery, because there are side effects that temporarily can impair higher mental functions and produce diminished alertness.

Gillingham, K. K.: A Primer on Vestibular Function, Spatial Disorientation, and Motion Sickness. USAF School of Aerospace Medicine, Brooks Air Force Base, Texas, Rev. 4-66, June 1966.

Graybiel, A., and Knepton, J.: Direction-specific adaptation effects acquired in a slow rotation room. Aerosp. Med., 43:1179, 1972.

Graybiel, A., Wood, C. O., Knepton, J., Hoche, J. P., and Perkins, G. F.: Human Bioassay of Antimotion Sickness Drugs. Naval Aerospace Medical Research Laboratory Report 1215, April 1975.

Lentz, J. M., and Collins, W. E.: Motion sickness susceptibility and related behavioral characteristics in men and women. Aviat. Space Environ. Med., 48:316, 1977.

von Gierke, H. E., and Clarke, N. P.: Effects of vibration and buffeting on man. In Randel, H. W. (ed.): Aerospace Medicine. Baltimore, Williams & Wilkins Company, 1971, p. 198.

Waite, R. E., and DeLucchi, M. R.: Labyrinthine and proprioceptive aspects of aerospace medicine. In Randel, H. W. (ed.): Aerospace Medicine. Baltimore, Williams & Wilkins Company, 1971, p. 254.

29.2. PROBLEMS OF AIR TRAVEL

GENERAL. U. S. airlines carried 232,100,000 passengers in 1977, many passengers characterized by extremes of age and physical status (Civil Aeronautics Board figure). Old age, infancy, and pregnancy do not alone preclude air travel. Complications accompanying these states may preclude safe travel, as may specific illnesses or conditions at any age. Persons in precarious health should be transported by air ambulance, although in individual instances safe travel may be possible if a trained health professional is along. Of course, serious contagions would preclude air travel in view of the risk to other passengers.

Passengers with specific chronic medical problems should have appropriate medications with them when traveling by air. It is very unlikely that a well provisioned medical kit will be available on a U. S. airline aircraft, as most U. S. airlines do not furnish this service at present (many non–U. S. airlines do). Therefore the diabetic, for example, should have extra insulin in his carry-on luggage, the cardiac patient should have appropriate medication along, and persons with other medical requirements should have available the appropriate drugs and equipment. Possible en route delays of several hours and even the possibility of diversions of the aircraft to another city should be considered in estimating the type and amount of medical items to carry. Possible delays in receipt of checked luggage make it wise to have all medicines in the carry-on luggage.

In addition to the above, a time factor should be included with reference to time zone changes and the relative time of taking medicine. When a diabetic travels west (lengthening the day by the number of time zones covered), a mild degree of hyperglycemia is preferable to risking hypoglycemia, and therefore the next *insulin injection* may be postponed until the local time of destination. However, when traveling several time zones to the east, resulting in a shortened day, the local destination time cannot be observed immediately for the next injection, as this would likely produce hypoglycemia. The injection may be postponed for the number of hours equivalent to the time zones crossed, or the dosage may be halved or otherwise diminished on the first day.

Persons with severe *emphysema* may arrange through the airline for airline-provided carry-on oxygen. This will assist the individual to have an adequate tracheal oxygen for the duration of the trip. Cabin altitudes may reach a maximum of about 8000 feet (2438.4 meters) equivalent altitude at the highest cruising flight altitude of the aircraft. Some advance planning to assure adequate oxygen availability in the departure and arrival terminals is also necessary. Certain other medical problems, including asthma and epilepsy, may require special medication, and this should be carried by the patient. Complicated pregnancies and advanced pregnancies are additional problems that can result in on-board flight emergencies. In all these instances, the advice of the patient's physician must be obtained, and the circumstances of the flight must be balanced against the medical condition and the purpose of the flight. In addition, the airline medical department (if the airline has one) can be consulted.

Handicapped persons with *paraplegia, blindness, deafness,* and other static problems may travel upon the advice of their physician and the airline. In some cases, an accompanying assistant will be required. Accommodation in the passenger cabin for the guide dog of a blind person can also be arranged. A major consideration in transport of the handicapped is the problem of using the toilet. If the passenger cannot tend to this alone, an accompanying attendant will be necessary, as the flight attendants do not undertake this type of care as part of their routine duties.

Persons who have upper respiratory infections with *sinusitis* or *otitis media* may experience severe discomfort as the passenger cabin repressurizes on the descent phase of flight. It is best to avoid air travel when these conditions exist, but if the problem is encountered, nasal inhalers can be of assistance in opening passageways. For aerotitis media, the Valsalva maneuver conducted with a closed mouth and nose will often open the eustachian tube and ventilate the middle ear. During the postflight period, an otolaryngologist should be consulted if symptoms persist.

Certain other potential problems preclude safe passenger flight. The few weeks following a myocardial infarction and the period of one or two weeks following abdominal or cranial surgery are generally not times for flight. In no case should flight be undertaken if there is any significant amount of trapped gas in any part of the body. A *pneumothorax* precludes safe flight.

A common bother to passengers with lower leg circulatory problems is that of *swelling of the feet and ankles* during the protracted time of sitting on long flights. This problem is due to venous stasis and can be serious from the standpoint of phlebothrombosis. Walking about the aisle during periods free from turbulence (and when the seat belt sign is off) helps diminish lower body venous stasis.

Prior to undertaking flight, crew members and passengers should allow 12 to 24 hours following *scuba diving,* depending on the depths to which the dive was carried. In the case of very deep dives, 36 hours should be allowed. If insufficient time elapses, the nitrogen stored in the fat tissue during the dive can evolve and cause the bends or chokes. Should these occur, rapid transport to a hyperbaric pressure facility is necessary for relief of symptoms and prevention of possible permanent injury (preferably by land if the distance is short; if by air, destination ground level cabin pressure should be maintained).

TIME ZONE EFFECTS, "JET LAG." A medical problem that is bothersome to air travelers undertaking lengthy flights that cover several time zones has been identified. The syndrome has been referred to by many terms, including circadian rhythm desynchronosis, transmeridian dysrhythmia, and "jet lag." The symptoms include a diminished degree of alertness, a feeling of considerable fatigue, and insomnia during nighttime hours, and may also include constipation and irritability. In addition, executives may find it difficult to solve complex problems, and athletes may find their performance markedly poorer, during the first day or two upon arrival at the destination.

The "jet lag" syndrome occurs most strongly during the two- to three-day period following east-west or west-east travel across time zones, at which time the individual is displaced geographically from the origin of the trip, although physiologically the individual is adapted to the time of the origin. If the displacement is in an easterly direction, the relative day-night cycle will be markedly shortened, and persons generally find displacement to the east to be the most fatiguing experience.

In the easterly direction, the individual is "driven" by the relatively shorter time for sleep in relation to associates. If the traveler has traversed five time zones to the east, the effective day at the destination is shortened by five hours. If he or she has flown all night, the low quality sleep acquired in the sitting position (good quality sleep necessitates a horizontal position in order that the pull of gravity along the long axis of the body be neutralized), leads to additional fatigue. It is noted that in order for refreshing stage four level sleep (the deepest sleep stage) to be achieved, the person must sleep in the horizontal position. Flights in the westerly direction lead to a stretched-out day and result in a prolonged wakeful period. This additional wakefulness is fatiguing, but is offset somewhat by the relatively longer time for sleep. Although flying to the west is not as fatiguing as flying to the east, the total time for readaptation is longer for westerly flights.

A rule of thumb for estimating readaptation following time zone dislocation is that the circadian rhythms of the body take approximately one day for each time zone (15 degrees of longitude) traversed. Serious psychophysiologic effects do not begin until three or more time zones are covered. There are wide differences in individual susceptibility to experiencing symptoms in this syndrome, and there are also wide variations in individual recovery. With increasing age, there is a general tendency for more difficulty in adapting to any time zone displacement. Recommendations for minimizing time zone displacement effects on circadian rhythms include recognizing the phenomenon, minimizing the amount of rich food and alcoholic beverages consumed during the transmeridian flights, and allowing one to two days of free rest period following arrival at the destination before engaging in complex or competitive activities. A short-acting barbiturate may be prescribed to assist sleep upon arrival at the destination should the wakeful portion of the circadian cycle be inhibiting the need for sleep.

SICKLE CELL ANEMIA. There are more than 100 identified inherited types of hemoglobinopathies that contain deletions or substitutions of certain amino acids in the alpha or beta chain of the heme moiety of hemoglobin A. Hemoglobin S is one of these hemoglobinopathies. The presence alone of the hemoglobin S genotype, sickle cell trait, does not result in any symptoms for the carrier. This genotype is detected only by laboratory tests.

The individual with hemoglobin S is most susceptible to sickling crises in the homozygous state. Crises may also occur in the heterozygous state if certain abnormal types of hemoglobin are associated with hemoglobin S. Examples are hemoglobins C, D (Los Angeles), and O (Arab). The individual with the homozygous hemoglobin S condition and the person with the combination of hemoglobin S and one or another of the various abnormal hemoglobins constitute phenotypes that experience sickle cell disease. The sickling crises of this disease occur in vivo when blood oxygen tension falls below 60 mm Hg. The total number of sickled cells depends in part upon the types of hemoglobin associated with the S type. The sickled cells can no longer pass through capillaries, and produce a cycle of vascular infarctions. It has been demonstrated that hemoglobins A and F confer resistance to sickling by the S hemoglobin. The combination of hemoglobin A and S hemoglobins does not sickle in vitro until the oxygen tension falls to about 10 mm Hg.

The hemoglobin AS genotype can be viewed as an incomplete dominance, in that although there are no sickling crises, hyposthenuria can usually be demonstrated, possibly the result of a slight tendency toward sickling in the kidneys. In World War II, 7 per cent of black pilots had the sickle cell trait. None showed any clinical manifestations of the genotype, in spite of arduous missions, including high altitude flight. There is evidence, however, that the AS genotype in some cases can have a fatal original crisis in extreme degrees of severe hypoxia. More study of this possibility must be done before definitive information is available.

In view of the aforementioned aspects concerning sickle cell anemia, the following conclusions can be made:

1. Persons with the sickle trait alone will experience no problems in air travel.

2. Persons with sickle hemoglobin in association with other abnormal hemoglobins may have sickling crises during air travel, especially if they have had a history of sickling.

3. Persons with homozygous sickle hemoglobin are very prone to hypoxic sickling crises and should avoid air travel unless absolutely necessary.

If air travel is unavoidable in categories 2 and 3 above, prophylactic oxygen should be considered, based on the past history of the individual. This must be available for the entire flight. To assure adequate kidney blood circulation with no stasis, good hydration during flight should be assured. If the cabin is to exceed an equivalent altitude of 8000 feet (2438.4 meters), the use of oxygen is essential.

Carruthers, M., Arguelles, A. E., and Mosovich, A.: Man in transit: Biochemical and physiological changes during intercontinental flights. Lancet, 1:977, 1976.

Klein, K. E., Wegmann, H. M., and Hunt, B. I.: Desynchronization of body temperature and performance circadian rhythm as a result of outgoing and homecoming transmeridian flights. Aerosp. Med., 43:119, 1972.

McKenzie, J. M.: The Aeromedical Significance of Sickle-Cell Trait: A Review. Office of Aviation Medicine Report, FAA-AM-76-15, Federal Aviation Administration, U.S.A., 1976.

Mohler, S. R.: Physiologic index as an aid in developing airline pilot scheduling patterns. Aviat. Space Environ. Med., 47:238, 1976.

Siegel, P. V., Gerathewohl, S. J., and Mohler, S. R.: Time zone effects. Science, 164:1249, 1969.

30. ALTERATIONS IN ATMOSPHERIC PRESSURE

Jefferson C. Davis

30.1. INTRODUCTION

Exposure to decreased barometric pressure in flight or to barometric pressure greater than sea level in diving presents unique pathophysiologic and therapeutic implications. In the past, medical care of workers in these environments was largely the province of flight surgeons and diving medical officers. In recent years, however, there has been rapid growth in air travel and in excursions to mountainous regions on vacation or business by the general public — often by ambulatory patients with significant medical problems. Participation in scuba (self contained underwater breathing apparatus) diving by people of all ages, in inland lakes as well as coastal waters, has expanded underwater medicine from the limited realm of the caisson worker and the commercial or military diver to include patients seen in any medical practice. Further, therapeutic use of intermittent high dose oxygen inhalation in hyperbaric or high pressure chambers (hyperbaric oxygen) has gained acceptance as an adjunct in clostridial myonecrosis and cellulitis and in carbon monoxide poisoning, as well as the promotion of healing in certain ischemic, hypoxic wounds. In order to understand the specific medical problems encountered, a brief review of the environments is necessary.

PHYSICS OF ENVIRONMENTAL PRESSURE. The weight of atmospheric air and water, at any point on or above the surface of the earth or beneath the surface of the water, can be expressed in various units of pressure. On ascent to altitude, we are passing through the blanket of air which extends from sea level to approximately 430 miles altitude, where the atmosphere is so thin that no molecular collisions occur. The atmosphere weighs 14.7 pounds per square inch, or 760 mm Hg (760 torr), at sea level. The pressure change for a given ascent is much greater at lower altitudes. For example, ascent from sea level to 3048 meters (10,000 feet) gives a pressure reduction of 237 mm Hg, from 760 mm Hg to 523 mm Hg; but the same 3048-meter altitude change, from 9146 meters (30,000 feet) to 12,192 meters (40,000 feet), gives a pressure reduction of only 85 mm Hg, from 226 mm Hg to 141 mm Hg. Contrast this pressure reduction to the linear pressure change at depth, in which each foot of sea water weighs 0.445 pound per square inch; thus, 14.7 ÷ 0.445 = 33 feet of sea water, or 10 meters. The barometric pressure (P_B) at this depth can be stated in terms of gauge pressure (that in excess of sea-level pressure) or, more conveniently, as absolute pressure (the total of sea-level atmospheric pressure plus the water pressure). Pressure can be expressed in various units; most commonly used are mm Hg, feet of sea water (FSW), meters of sea water, or atmospheres absolute (ATA). Further descent to depth gives linear pressure changes, so that at 20 meters (66 FSW), the total pressure is 3 ATA or 2280 mm Hg. Barometric pressure at any altitude is available from standard altitude charts, and pressure at any depth can be easily derived; but for clarification and because certain pressures are key in the physiologic principles to follow, selected altitudes and depths are provided in Table 1.

The earth's atmosphere is composed of a mixture of gases — including nitrogen (78.98 per cent), oxygen (20.95 per cent), argon (0.93 per cent), and carbon dioxide (0.03 per cent) — with varying amounts of water vapor and other inert rare gases, totaling 760 mm Hg at sea level according to Dalton's law ($P_B = P_{N_2} + P_{O_2} + P_{others}$). For physiologic considerations, the atmospheric composition is usually considered to consist of 21 per cent oxygen and 79 per cent nitrogen, with the rare gases being included with the inert nitrogen. For practical purposes, these percentages remain constant through the range of pressure changes, so it is the partial pressures (P_{O_2}) of gases in the mixture which change. For example, at sea level, P_{O_2} = 160 mm Hg

TABLE 1. Representative Alterations in Barometric Pressure

Altitude/depth	Absolute Pressure (mm Hg)	Absolute Pressure Atmospheres (ATA)	Absolute Pressure (PSIA)
15,200 meters (50,000 feet)	87	0.11	1.7
13,106 meters (43,000 feet)	122	0.16	2.4
5486 meters (18,000 feet)	380	0.50	7.3
3048 meters (10,000 feet)	523	0.67	10.1
Sea level	760	1.0	14.7
10 meters (33 FSW)*	1520	2.0	29.4
20 meters (66 FSW)	2280	3.0	44.1
30 meters (99 FSW)	3040	4.0	58.8
40 meters (132 FSW)	3800	5.0	73.5
50 meters (165 FSW)	4560	6.0	88.2

*FSW = Feet of sea water; 32.8 FSW = 10 meters.

(760 × 0.21), P_{N_2} = 600 mm Hg (760 × 0.79); at an altitude of 3048 meters (10,000 feet), P_{O_2} = 110 mm Hg (523 × 0.21), P_{N_2} = 413 mm Hg (523 × 0.79); and with air compressed to equal the water pressure at 20 meters (66 FSW), P_{O_2} = 479 mm Hg (2280 × 0.21), P_{N_2} = 1801 mm Hg (2280 × 0.79).

The medical problems created by changes in atmospheric pressure may be grouped into direct and indirect effects. The former result from mechanical forces created when pressure differentials develop across the walls of air-containing spaces within the body or upon its surface. Indirect effects result from alterations in partial pressures of the individual gases of the atmosphere.

Davis, J. C., and Hunt, T. K. (eds.): Hyperbaric Oxygen Therapy. Bethesda, Md., Undersea Medical Society, Inc., 1977.
Strughold, H.: The earth's atmosphere and aviation. *In* Randel, H. W. (ed.): Aerospace Medicine. Baltimore, Williams & Wilkins Company, 1971, pp. 22–34.

30.2. DIRECT EFFECTS OF CHANGES IN ATMOSPHERIC PRESSURE

Gases respond to pressure changes in accordance with Boyle's law ($P_1V_1 = P_2V_2$). Their volume varies inversely and their density, or molecular concentration, directly as the absolute pressure. The fluids and solids of the human body, being incompressible, transmit pressure freely and thus assume the pressure exerted upon the body's surface. Any alteration in pressure on the surface of the body is reflected almost instantly by an identical pressure change in body tissues and within air-containing spaces of the body. Gas pressures within the middle ears, paranasal sinuses, respiratory tract, and gastrointestinal tract can be maintained equal to external pressure only by appropriate adjustments either of the number of molecules of gas within the space or of the volume of the space. No medical difficulties arise as long as air can pass freely between such spaces and the environment. If additional air cannot enter such a space to increase its pressure during descent, a relative vacuum is created, the lining of the walls becomes hyperemic and swollen, and serum or blood may move in to eradicate the pressure differential. Conversely, during ascent with declining environmental pressure, expansion of gas volume in the fixed volume cavity produces increasing pressure. Unless air can be vented from the space, an increasing pressure gradient creates a distending force against the walls.

Pockets of air against various surfaces of the body may be produced by such factors as goggles, tight-fitting hoods, ear plugs, or wrinkles in diving suits.

CLINICAL MANIFESTATIONS. The most common direct or mechanical effect of descent from altitude, or from sea level to depth, is *barotitis media*. Because of the flutter valve effect produced by the nasopharyngeal end of the eustachian tube, equalization of middle ear pressure is usually automatic on ascent to altitude or to the surface from depth; but on descent — unless active measures (yawning, swallowing, or the modified Valsalva maneuver) are taken to open the tube — a relative vacuum is created in the middle ear. Surprisingly little pressure imbalance (60 to 100 mm Hg) produces pain as the tympanic membrane is retracted, followed by hyperemia and hemorrhage into the membrane; finally, the tympanic membrane perforates, or blood is drawn into the middle ear to equalize the pressure imbalance. Flying or diving with an upper respiratory infection may make equalization impossible and predisposes to this injury. *Barosinusitis* is less common, but the mechanisms are similar and pain can be quite intense. Barosinusitis can occur on ascent if edematous mucosa, a polyp, or mucus prevents escape of air from the sinus cavity to equalize pressure.

Prevention of these common problems is best achieved by teaching the diver not only to use techniques for pressure equalization but also to avoid pressure changes when acute coryza or allergic rhinitis restricts the eustachian tube or paranasal sinus orifices. During descent in diving, attempts to equalize middle ear pressure by a very forcible Valsalva maneuver result in elevated cerebrospinal fluid pressure. This hydrostatic pressure, transmitted by perilymph to the round window at the same time a relative vacuum exists in the middle ear, can result in *round window rupture*. The manifestations are sudden, severe vertigo, tinnitus, and persistent deafness in the affected ear. It is important to refer such a diver to an otolaryngologist immediately, so that evaluation and surgical repair can be performed.

The most serious direct effects of pressure, leading to important medical emergencies, involve the lungs. Reference to Table 1 clarifies important points. *First,* direct effects on the lungs are rare in altitude exposure, because breath-holding would have to be sustained over a long period of time during normal .ascent or descent to realize sufficient pressure changes. An exception would be in the event of catastrophic aircraft cabin decompression; but here, also, breath-holding before and during the decompression would be required. The weight of water produces great pressure changes with small depth changes. *Second,* in diving, the greatest volume changes in gases trapped in body cavities occur at shallow depths. Ascent from 4 ATA (99 FSW) to 2 ATA (33 FSW) results in an attempt to double the volume of gas which, in a fixed volume cavity, means a doubling of pressure according to Boyle's law. At shallower depths, however, the same pressure-volume change occurs with ascent from only 2 ATA (33 FSW) to the surface. This very important concept has accounted for severe *pulmonary overpressure accidents* among scuba divers who breath-held from as little as 2.2 to 3.1 meters (7 to 10 feet) of water depth.

In order to understand the direct effects of pressure change on the lung, as well as some of the indirect changes (to be discussed in Ch. 30.3), a brief description of diving modes must be introduced. (The concept of pressurized aircraft cabins has already been presented in Ch. 29.2, and will not be repeated.) The breath-holding diver carries no supplemental breathing gas supply underwater, and his depth is limited by his breath-holding time, physical stamina, and lung volume. During descent, lung volume will decrease according to Boyle's law; and, when reduced to less than residual volume, a "lung squeeze" can result in pulmonary edema and hemorrhage. Compressed gas diving (e.g., air, nitrogen-oxygen, helium-oxygen) supplies breathing gas to the diver through regulators designed to match water pressure at any depth, either from the surface by means of hoses or by compressed air or mixed breathing gas carried in high-pressure cylinders by the diver (scuba). While the lung squeeze of the breath-holding diver is avoided, the major risks to the supplied diver are on decompression.

After breathing compressed gas at pressure equal to water pressure at depth, gas must be released from the lungs by normal breathing — or, in the event of loss of gas supply at depth, by slow exhalation during ascent. Failure to do so results in intrapulmonary gas expansion, increased intra-alveolar pressure, and introduction of extra-alveolar gas (pulmonary overpressure accidents). Lung tissue distal to a poorly communicating diseased bronchial passage may be similarly damaged, even if the diver vents his excess air during ascent. The air traveler with such bronchopulmonary disease, or one who happens to be holding his breath, may be similarly injured during a sudden loss of cabin pressure at high altitude. The result may be arterial gas (air) embolism, mediastinal and subcutaneous emphysema, and/or pneumothorax. The latter two manifestations are recognized by physical and radiographic examination, and can be managed by conventional measures. In diving, a gas embolism has been reported during ascents of as little as 2.2 meters (7 FSW), and is said to be exceeded in frequency only by drowning as a cause of accidental death among divers.

Knowledge of the character of the dive, including depth, duration, air supply, and patterns of descent and ascent in relation to symptoms, often simplifies the problem of diagnosing lung injury in divers. Frothy, bloody sputum may be produced in either thoracic squeeze or lung overpressure. The overriding clinical manifestations in arterial gas embolism result from arterial gas bubbles embolizing the brain. There is sudden onset of unconsciousness, focal or generalized seizure activity, visual field loss or blindness, weakness, paralysis, and hypesthesia or confusion. The diver with these manifestations must be presumed to have gas embolism or decompression sickness.

TREATMENT. Either gas embolism or decompression sickness requires treatment by recompression at the earliest possible moment. Transport to a recompression chamber should be by the fastest method available. An aircraft used for transportation must have cabin pressure kept at or near sea-level equivalent — or, if unpressurized, flown not more than a few hundred feet above sea level. Cardiopulmonary resuscitation and bicarbonate administration may be required, because many of these casualties are also near-drowning victims. Oxygen should be administered as well as intravenous solutions, such as dextran and normal saline. Positioning the suspected gas embolism patient in the Trendelenburg position, and on the left side, seems to be of benefit.

Bond, G. F.: Arterial gas embolism. *In* Davis, J. C., and Hunt, T. K. (eds.): Hyperbaric Oxygen Therapy. Bethesda, Md., Undersea Medical Society, Inc., 1977, pp. 141–152.

30.3. INDIRECT EFFECTS OF CHANGES IN ATMOSPHERIC PRESSURE

Gases in contact with liquids dissolve in direct proportion to their partial pressures and their solubility coefficients. Gases enter and leave the body in response to gradients of partial pressure between blood and alveolar gases. Gradients of partial pressure likewise determine the movement of gases within body fluids. Alterations in respiratory gas composition (caused by the reduced barometric pressure at altitude) and the high partial pressures of inspired gases (from compressed gas sources in diving) present a series of significant hazards.

HYPOXIA

Without supplemental oxygen, the physiologic effects of the reduced atmospheric partial pressure of oxygen (Po_2) at altitude are described as hypoxic hypoxia. Other factors which lead to tissue hypoxia can coexist and be additive. Thus a patient whose oxygen transport capacity is impaired by anemia or carbon monoxide bound hemoglobin ("hypemic hypoxia"), or whose tissue oxygen utilization is impaired by cyanide or ethanol ("histotoxic hypoxia"), will be more susceptible to hypoxia at altitude. A special potentiating factor in aviation is stagnant hypoxia in an aviator exposed to high head-to-foot acceleration forces, as in recovering from an aircraft dive. The increased weight of the column of blood reduces cerebral perfusion with resultant cerebral hypoxia. Although these factors can be important contributors to hypoxia in aviation, this discussion will center on hypoxia caused by reduction in Po_2 at the decreased barometric pressures at altitude.

Inspired air is humidified in the respiratory tract, rapidly equilibrating with the 47 mm Hg vapor pressure of water at body temperature. Alveolar Pco_2 of about 40 mm Hg and water vapor of 47 mm Hg are roughly constant at any altitude, so that alveolar partial pressure of oxygen (Pa_{O_2}) can be approximated for any altitude by use of the simplified alveolar gas equation, assuming a respiratory quotient of 1:

$$Pa_{O_2} = Fi_{O_2} (P_B - Pa_{H_2O}) - Pa_{CO_2}$$
in which Fi_{O_2} = fraction of inspired O_2
P_B = barometric pressure

For example, at 3048 meters (10,000 feet), breathing air:

$$Pa_{O_2} = 0.21 (523 - 47) - 40$$
$$Pa_{O_2} = 60 \text{ mm Hg}$$

Or, at 5846 meters (18,000 feet), breathing air:

$$Pa_{O_2} = 0.21 (380 - 47) - 40$$
$$Pa_{O_2} = 30 \text{ mm Hg}$$

Alveolar Po_2 rapidly equilibrates with arterial Po_2 at the alveolar-capillary interface in healthy people, and hemoglobin is saturated according to the alveolar Po_2. The shape of the oxygen-hemoglobin dissociation curve is of great importance at altitude, with the "knee" of the curve at Po_2 of 60 mm Hg, with a fairly flat slope above this point so that a drop from the normal 100 mm Hg Pa_{O_2} at sea level to 60 mm Hg at 3048 meters (10,000 feet) causes a drop in arterial oxygen saturation of only 10 ml of oxygen per 100 ml of blood. Above this altitude, however, even small drops in Pa_{O_2} result in large decreases in arterial saturation along the steep slope of

the curve. Thus, except for a decrement in night vision at about 1220 meters (4000 feet) to 1829 meters (6000 feet), there are no significant effects of hypoxia in healthy people below 3048 meters (10,000 feet). In general, pressurized aircraft cabins are maintained well below that equivalent air pressure, so no supplemental oxygen is required. Nevertheless, patients with reduced cardiac reserve may have difficulty tolerating even this small drop in arterial oxygen saturation, and require supplemental oxygen during flight.

MANIFESTATIONS. Table 2 summarizes the major manifestations of altitude hypoxia with corresponding Pa_{O_2} breathing ambient air.

The time required for the onset of symptoms in Table 2 differs from person to person, depending on age, fitness, acclimatization, and individual variation. At higher altitudes, the progression of symptoms to the point of inability to perform useful functions (time of useful consciousness, or TUC) is quite rapid and within a narrower range of individual variation. For example, the TUC at 9146 meters (30,000 feet) is about 90 seconds, and at 13,106 meters (43,000 feet) is about 15 seconds.

PREVENTION. The use of pressurized cabins, which allows man to stay safely within the physiologically comfortable zone below 3048 meters (10,000 feet), is the main preventive factor in modern aviation. The percentage of supplemental oxygen required to maintain an alveolar Po_2 no less than the 3048 meters (10,000 feet) equivalent at an altitude can be derived by varying the Fi_{O_2} in the simplified alveolar gas equation. For example, at 12,192 meters (40,000 feet), where the barometric pressure is 141 mm Hg and Pa_{CO_2} is somewhat lower due to hyperventilation:

$$Pa_{O_2} = 1.0 (141 - 47) - 35$$
$$Pa_{O_2} = 59 \text{ mm Hg}$$

This example is equivalent to breathing air at 3048 meters (10,000 feet) and is the maximum altitude at which 100 per cent oxygen breathing is adequate to prevent hypoxia. At higher altitudes, positive pressure breathing and, finally, pressure suits are required.

TABLE 2.   Responses to Hypoxic Hypoxia

Altitude		Alveolar Po_2 (mm Hg)
3048 meters (10,000 feet)	Impairment of recent memory, judgment, and ability to perform complex calculations; increased heart rate and pulmonary ventilation	60
3658 meters (12,000 feet)	Dyspnea, impaired ability to perform complex tasks, headache, nausea, decreased visual acuity	52
4573 meters (15,000 feet)	Decrease in auditory acuity, constriction of visual fields, impaired judgment, irritability; exercise can lead to unconsciousness	46
5486 meters (18,000 feet)	Decrements in personality and intellect; threshold for loss of consciousness in resting unacclimatized individuals after several hours' exposure	40
6096 meters (20,000 feet)	Handwriting illegible in conscious subjects	33
6706 meters (22,000 feet) and above	Almost all individuals unconscious after sufficient exposure time	30

Holmstrom, F. M. G.: Hypoxia. *In* Randel, H. W. (ed.): Aerospace Medicine. Baltimore, Williams & Wilkins Company, 1971, pp. 56–85.

ACUTE MOUNTAIN SICKNESS

This is a clinical syndrome observed in unacclimatized persons, usually within a few hours after rapid exposure to high altitude. Individual tolerance varies widely. Some people experience symptoms at altitudes as low as 2134 to 2439 meters (7000 to 8000 feet), although others tolerate altitudes of 4267 meters (14,000 feet) with minimal symptoms. There appears to be no way to predict unusual susceptibility; but rapid ascent, physical exertion, and poor physical condition increase the likelihood. Initial symptoms are usually mild to incapacitating headache, exertional dyspnea, malaise, and weakness. Insomnia, anorexia, nausea, vomiting, diarrhea, and abdominal pain may occur. Mental capacity and judgment may be impaired. Inability to sleep is a common problem. Cyanosis of the lips and nail beds, Cheyne-Stokes breathing, and tachycardia are usually present. These manifestations usually subside gradually over a period of several days, but may recur at higher altitudes. In some instances, the symptoms are severe and unrelieved except by oxygen or descent to a lower altitude. Gradual ascent with periodic halts of several days to allow acclimatization will prevent or reduce the severity of symptoms. Acetazolamide, given in dosages of 250 mg every eight hours prior to and during exposure to altitude, has been reported to reduce the frequency and severity of symptoms. The mechanism of its effect is not clear; but increased ventilation and alveolar oxygen tension, decreased carbon dioxide tension and serum bicarbonate, and absence of alkalosis were observed in treated subjects. Furosemide, 80 mg every 12 hours, has produced relief of symptoms and signs usually within 48 hours, apparently in association with the induced diuresis.

Forward, S. A., Landowne, M., Follansbee, J. N., and Hansen, J. E.: Effect of acetazolamide on acute mountain sickness. N. Engl. J. Med., 279:839, 1968.

Singh, I., Khanna, P. K., Srivastava, M. C., Lal, M., Roy, S. B., and Subramanyam, C. S. V.: Acute mountain sickness. N. Engl. J. Med., 280:175, 1969.

HIGH ALTITUDE PULMONARY EDEMA

Acute pulmonary edema is an uncommon but serious and sometimes fatal complication of rapid exposure to altitudes above 2744 meters (9000 feet). Hypoxia is considered the primary etiologic agent. Many earlier fatal cases were erroneously diagnosed as pneumonia. Most susceptible appear to be young, unacclimatized persons and acclimatized residents who have sojourned at lower altitudes for a few days or weeks. Recurrences are common in those who have experienced an attack. Rapid ascent and heavy physical exertion increase susceptibility.

Autopsy findings have included wet lungs congested with serosanguineous edema fluid. Bronchiolar and alveolar edema with hyaline membranes, resembling those seen in hyaline membrane disease of the newborn, over the internal walls of alveoli, alveolar sacs, and alveolar ducts have been characteristic findings.

Dilatation of preterminal arterioles and thrombosis of septal capillaries and of small and medium-sized pulmonary arteries have also been observed. The exact pathogenic mechanism is conjectural. A comparative increase in capillary pressure is thought to be responsible for the alveolar edema. In a few cases, pulmonary artery pressure has been elevated, and electrocardiograms have suggested acute right ventricular overloading. The hyaline membrane formation, not a characteristic finding in death caused by simple hypoxia, has not been explained; but a deficient pulmonary fibrinolysis system has been postulated.

Symptoms usually appear 6 to 36 hours after exposure to altitude and may be preceded by acute mountain sickness. Exertional dyspnea, weakness, malaise, and a persistent, dry, irritating cough are the characteristic initial symptoms. Later, noisy respiration, rales, cyanosis, orthopnea, and hemoptysis develop. Unless continuous oxygen therapy is carried out or the patient descends to a lower altitude, these symptoms progress, and death occurs. Gradual acclimatization and avoidance of undue physical exertion during the early period of exposure to altitude are important preventive measures.

CHRONIC MOUNTAIN SICKNESS
(Monge's Disease)

Chronic mountain sickness is a clinical syndrome that occurs in residents at high altitudes, usually over 4267 meters (14,000 feet), characterized by loss of tolerance to hypoxia in a previously acclimatized person. The cause is not known, but associated are increased polycythemia, decreased pulmonary ventilation, increased Pco_2, lowered arterial saturation, and impaired sensitivity of the respiratory center as compared with asymptomatic residents at high altitude. Hemoglobin and hematocrit may be increased to as much as 25 grams per 100 ml and 80 per cent, as compared with 21 grams and 60 per cent in native residents. Hyperplasia and hyperactivity of marrow erythroid cells and pulmonary hypertension are greater than in the healthy residents.

The clinical manifestations are similar to those of polycythemia vera. They include marked cyanosis, dyspnea, cough, palpitations, headache, giddiness, muscular weakness, pain in the extremities, sensory and motor changes, and episodic stupor. The condition can be cured only by returning the patients to a lower altitude or to sea level.

Monge also described a less severe form of chronic mountain sickness in mountain residents that he called subacute mountain sickness. Many of the symptoms resemble those of acute mountain sickness, but they persist unless the patient descends to sea level or receives oxygen. The marked cyanosis and alveolar hypoventilation of chronic mountain sickness do not occur, and the laboratory findings are like those in asymptomatic natives.

Hultgren, H. N., and Grover, R. F.: Circulatory adaptation to high altitude. Ann. Rev. Med., 19:119, 1968.

Lenfant, C., and Sullivan, K.: Adaptation to high altitude. N. Engl. J. Med., 284:1298, 1971.

Weihe, W. H. (ed.): Physiological Effects of High Altitude. New York, The Macmillan Company, 1964.

DECOMPRESSION SICKNESS

Decompression sickness refers to the plethora of clinical manifestations first described in the middle 1800's among caisson workers who were decompressed to sea level after working in compressed air to keep water and mud out of tunnel construction (hence the previous term, "caisson disease"). Military, commercial, and, more recently, sport diving brought emphasis to studies of this complex disorder to determine safe decompression schedules and treatment of casualties. Since the 1930's, it has been recognized that decompression from sea level to altitude can produce the same disorder, and, since 1960, treatment of altitude decompression sickness persisting at ground level has been compression to greater than sea-level pressure in chambers, as has been the treatment of divers and caisson workers for decades.

PATHOPHYSIOLOGY. A brief description of diving techniques has already been given in Ch. 30.1. The compressed gas respired at increased atmospheric pressure must be a mixture of oxygen and an inert gas diluent to prevent oxygen toxicity. This inert gas is usually nitrogen for shallow depths and helium at greater depths to prevent the narcotic effects of nitrogen at high partial pressures. Here we will deal only with compressed air, which is the respiratory gas in question for cases encountered by most physicians, for deep helium oxygen diving represents a specialized area of commercial and military and scientific diving usually covered by fully trained diving medical officers.

When compressed air is breathed underwater, to balance the hydrostatic pressure of water on the thoracic wall, or from the environment of a compressed air pressurized chamber (hyperbaric chamber, compression chamber), the alveolar partial pressure of nitrogen (P_{N_2}) rises according to barometric pressure. For example, at 50 meters (165 FSW), the barometric pressure is 4560 mm Hg and the inspired P_{N_2} is $0.79 \times 4560 = 3602$ mm Hg. Allowing for water vapor, carbon dioxide, and oxygen ($P_{O_2} = 0.21 \times 4560 = 948$ mm Hg), the alveolar P_{N_2} approximates 3525 mm Hg. According to Henry's law (the amount of gas in solution varies directly with the partial pressure of gas in contact with the solution), there is rapid diffusion of the inert nitrogen across the alveolar-capillary membrane to physical solution in plasma. Upon reaching the tissues, the high P_{N_2} dissolved in arterial blood is diffused into tissues at a rate dependent on the perfusion rate of various tissues. The total nitrogen uptake by a given tissue is determined by its composition, with lipid-rich tissues taking on larger amounts of nitrogen. The body's uptake of nitrogen can thus be seen as a complex of uptake curves which results in variable loading of different tissues, increasing with time of exposure to the elevated pressure until full equilibration is achieved at approximately 24 hours (saturation). Upon decompression from the high pressure environment to lower pressures and finally to sea level, the reverse set of gradients is established for off-loading of inert gas from tissues, to venous blood, to the lung. Inert gas will stay in solution in tissues and blood within strictly defined pressure reductions; but if critical limits are exceeded, it comes out of solution into the gas phase as bubbles in blood and tissues. The limits of safe decompression are beyond the scope of this text, and represent the goal of extensive research still ongoing after more than 70 years of work. Once formed, bubbles in tissues and blood cause a series of pathophysiologic events which can culminate in permanent paralysis or death. Local tissue distortion by bubbles may cause pain, and circulating venous gas emboli may produce congestive infarction of the spinal cord or gas pulmonary embolism. At the blood-bubble interface, platelet aggregation has been seen; and, with platelet damage, there is release of vasoactive substances — such as serotonin and epinephrine — complicating the picture with vasoconstriction, and alteration of the platelet membrane makes phospholipid (platelet factor 3) available and accelerates clotting. Further, untreated, bubble-induced tissue ischemia and hypoxia result in loss of capillary integrity with resultant edema and hemoconcentration. Therapy today is directed toward this entire spectrum of events.

The sea-level dweller is in equilibrium (saturated) with the nitrogen partial pressure in the atmosphere. Upon rapid exposure to decreased barometric pressure at altitude, a series of events comparable to those described above can occur with evolution of nitrogen bubbles. Because of the relatively higher proportion of CO_2 and water vapor at altitude, these gases diffuse into bubbles and play a larger role than in diving. The precise critical altitude for bubble formation has not been defined; but, of clinical importance, the lowest documented case of altitude decompression sickness occurred at 5640 meters (18,500 feet). The incidence rises sharply with increasing altitude and with time at altitude. Most patients recover upon recompression to sea level; but for those who do not, emergency treatment in a compression chamber is required to resolve bubbles which persist at sea level because of growth while at altitude. Exposure to altitude following diving can produce bubbles at much lower altitudes. Cases of decompression sickness have been seen at as little as 1220 meters (4000 feet) after safe decompression from diving.

CLINICAL MANIFESTATIONS. The onset of symptoms and signs of decompression sickness tends to be gradual and progressive, beginning minutes to hours after an inciting dive or exposure to altitude. With certain exceptions which will be noted, the manifestations resulting from both environments are the same and can be divided into Type I (minor manifestations) and Type II (serious manifestations), as summarized in Table 3. A late manifestation is the so-called dysbaric osteonecrosis of divers and caisson workers. The exact cause of this aseptic necrosis of bone in divers is still unclear, as is its relationship to untreated previous episodes of decompression sickness. The scope of this chapter does not allow a review of the monumental research in this area.

PREVENTION AND TREATMENT. All the varied manifestations of decompression sickness usually respond rapidly to early and adequate treatment by compression. Descent from altitude produces sufficient recompression to abolish the early manifestations, but merely retards the appearance of the more slowly developing serious forms of decompression sickness. In such cases, widespread bubble formation has presumably already occurred, and descent is entirely analogous to inadequate compression therapy during which symptoms subside only temporarily.

Divers can prevent decompression sickness by knowing and following established limits for depth and time

TABLE 3. Clinical Manifestations of Decompression Sickness

Diagnosis	Symptoms and Signs
Type I (minor)	
Bends	Mild to severe, deep, "boring" pain; single or multiple joints; aggravated by exercise; may be relieved by local pressure; local lymphedema may be present
Cutaneous	Pruritus, described by the diver as "the itches or creeps"; usually clears spontaneously in minutes; mottled or marbled skin lesion with a pale and cyanotic appearance; may accompany serious manifestations
Type II (serious)	
Pulmonary ("chokes")	Substernal pain, dyspnea, nonproductive cough, cyanosis
Neurologic	1. Spinal cord (diving chiefly): Any level may be affected, but most commonly lower thoracic and upper lumbar; low back and girdling abdominal pain, hypesthesia, weakness below that level; loss of anal sphincter tone and urinary bladder control; can result in permanent paraplegia 2. Brain (altitude chiefly): Diffuse, confusing, and poorly localized; range from blurred vision, visual field defects, spotty hypesthesia, weakness, paralysis, dysphasia, headache, vertigo, to focal or generalized seizures
Shock	Poorly responsive to fluid replacement without concurrent compression chamber treatment; may be accompanied by chokes, neurologic manifestations, and mottling of skin

at depth. Adequate denitrogenation, by breathing 100 per cent oxygen prior to and during ascent, is an effective preventive measure in fliers. Fliers who have experienced decompression symptoms during a flight should delay return to even relatively low altitudes for at least 72 hours, because the expansion of bubbles still present in tissues may cause a rapid recurrence of more serious symptoms. The hazard of exposure to altitudes as low as 1220 meters (4000 feet), even after safe depth-time dives, should be recognized.

Adequate compression performed at the earliest possible time is the specific therapy for decompression sickness. Every physician should be aware of the hyperbaric chamber closest to his city. All other measures are adjunctive. Those reported to be beneficial include 100 per cent oxygen by mask, dextran and standard replacement fluids to correct hypovolemia, and injectable steroids—such as dexamethasone, 10 mg intravenously initially, with diminishing doses every six hours.

Beckman, E. L., and Elliott, D. H. (eds.): Dysbarism — Related Osteonecrosis: Proceedings of a Symposium on Dysbaric Osteonecrosis. Superintendent of Documents, U. S. Government Printing Office, 1974.

Elliott, D. H., and Hallenbeck, J. M.: The pathophysiology of decompression sickness. *In* Bennett, P. B., and Elliott, D. H. (eds.): The Physiology and Medicine of Diving and Compressed Air Work. Baltimore, Williams & Wilkins Company, 1975, pp. 435–455.

Fryer, D. I.: Subatmospheric Decompression Sickness in Man. Slough, England, Technivision Services (Library of Congress Catalog Card No. 69–19960), 1969.

Kidd, D. J., and Elliott, D. H.: Decompression disorders in divers. *In* Bennett, P. B., and Elliott, D. H. (eds.): The Physiology and Medicine of Diving and Compressed Air Work. Baltimore, Williams & Wilkins Company, 1975, pp. 471–495.

OXYGEN TOXICITY

Aside from the well-known pulmonary oxygen toxicity which occurs with prolonged inhalation of elevated partial pressure of oxygen even at sea level, oxygen-enriched breathing media in diving introduce a unique problem. One hundred per cent oxygen breathing while under pressure, to speed nitrogen elimination and shorten decompression time, was introduced by the Royal Navy and the U. S. Navy during the early 1930's. It was quickly recognized that 100 per cent oxygen breathing at high barometric pressure produced a series of central nervous system events leading to a major seizure. There was a latent period before onset, markedly shortened at deeper than 20 meters (66 FSW). The onset was hastened by exercise while breathing oxygen at depth, and by breathing oxygen in the water. Systematic studies of safe oxygen time-pressure limits have been completed. Modern oxygen decompression, hyperbaric oxygen therapy (HBO) of decompression sickness, clostridial myonecrosis, carbon monoxide poisoning, and other accepted indications stay well within these limits.

Behnke, A. R., Johnson, F. S., Poppen, J. R., and Motley, E. P.: The effect of oxygen on man at pressures from 1 to 4 atmospheres. Am. J. Physiol., 110:565, 1934–35.

Clark, J. M., and Lambertsen, C. J.: Pulmonary oxygen toxicity: A review. Pharmacol. Rev., 23:37, 1971.

Donald, K. W.: Oxygen poisoning in man. Br. Med. J., 1:667, 1947.

NITROGEN NARCOSIS

It has long been recognized that breathing the high partial pressures of nitrogen in compressed air leads to behavioral and performance decrements. This effect, which is noticeable at 4 ATA or 30 meters (99 FSW) in most people, increases progressively at depth. The symptoms are euphoria, poor judgment, and impaired ability to concentrate. These symptoms can become quite serious when critical decisions need to be made during a dive. The symptoms do not occur if helium is used to replace nitrogen as the inert gas in a breathing mixture.

31. THERAPEUTIC HYPERBARIC OXYGEN

Herbert A. Saltzman

Therapeutic application of hyperbaric oxygen is clearly beneficial in only a limited number of human illnesses. Although the full domain of clinical usefulness has yet to be determined, reasonable guidelines have been established. This review of basic principles, associated hazards, and clinical investigational experience is intended to help the reader distinguish between appropriate usage of hyperbaric oxygen, as currently understood, and costly exploitation in situations in which it is of no proved value.

DEFINITION, RATIONALE. The term hyperbaric oxygen is applied to the breathing of 100 per cent oxygen at greater than normal atmospheric pressures. This is achieved in special environmental chambers containing pressurized gas and at the same time providing technologic support for patient care. Hyperbaric oxygen provides a means for overcoming the barrier to increased oxygen transport imposed by the limited solubility of oxygen. Even though only 0.3 ml of oxygen dissolves in 100 ml of blood equilibrated at a Po_2 of 100 mm Hg, physically dissolved oxygen can be increased to almost 6 ml per 100 ml at an atmospheric pressure of 3 atmospheres absolute (ATA). Under these circumstances the Po_2 in blood will approach 2000 mm Hg. Increased oxygen concentrations have been thought to be clinically useful for the following reasons: (1) Function of hypoxic vital organs can be maintained or restored despite reduced perfusion of blood. This concept presumes satisfactory maintenance of other metabolic requirements. (2) There may be a specific desirable pharmacologic action of hyperbaric oxygen. The best example is the bactericidal effect, as employed in the treatment of clostridial myonecrosis. (3) In special circumstances wherein bubbles of gas form in tissues, removal can be expedited dramatically by treatment with hyperbaric oxygen. The increased pressure reduces bubble size, and the washout of dissolved inert gas from surrounding tissues yields a much larger and more favorable gradient for diffusion of inert gas molecules out of the bubble.

HAZARDS AND OTHER PROBLEMS. The major biologic limitations to therapeutic use of hyperbaric oxygen are (1) inability to deliver oxygen to a critical tissue if perfusion is interrupted or severely reduced by vascular disease, and (2) toxic consequences of excessive exposure. Severe and lethal pulmonary damage can be incurred in progressively shorter intervals as the inspired pressure of oxygen increases. Neurologic toxicity may occur, usually in the form of convulsions, at oxygen pressures greater than 2.5 ATA. These manifestations of toxicity are readily avoided by limiting the magnitude and duration of the exposure. Exposures of 90 minutes at an oxygen pressure of 3 ATA and longer treatments at 2 ATA have been widely employed and are very well tolerated. Intermittent exposures to hyperbaric oxygen profoundly constrain therapeutic expectations, however, as limited tissue reserves of oxygen are consumed within a few minutes. Thus sustained correction of hypoxia requires continuous treatment in the absence of other favorable biologic changes.

There are several technical problems associated with application of hyperbaric oxygen. Fire and explosive decompression are inherent risks. Exposed patients and personnel have been maimed or killed in hyperbaric chamber accidents. There are substantial costs incurred in maintaining a large hyperbaric facility. The substitution of small hyperbaric units capable of containing only a single patient, although more economical, compounds problems of adequate nursing support.

The decision to treat a patient with hyperbaric oxygen should be made after determining that alternative approaches fail to offer comparable dividends of efficacy, safety, and cost effectiveness. For example, although hyperbaric oxygen has been demonstrated to prevent or correct dangerous arrhythmias associated with myocardial ischemia, treatment with appropriate pharmacologic agents in a coronary care unit is clearly preferable.

CLINICAL EXPERIENCE. There are a small number of medical problems in which theoretical considerations, experimentation, and clinical experience justify confident employment of therapeutic hyperbaric oxygen.

Acute carbon monoxide poisoning causes profound hypoxia because hemoglobin combines with carbon monoxide preferentially, blocking oxygen transport to tissues. Concentrations of carboxyhemoglobin above 30 per cent adversely affect release of oxygen from oxyhe-

moglobin as well. The clinical consequences of cytochrome interactions with carbon monoxide are less well understood. Prompt treatment with hyperbaric oxygen at 2.5 ATA, for one hour, will greatly accelerate elimination of carbon monoxide from blood, while at the same time improving delivery of oxygen to the central nervous system. At the end of the treatment carboxyhemoglobin levels are generally below 10 per cent, and prompt recovery can be anticipated if irreversible brain damage has not already occurred.

Acute cyanide poisoning leads to profound tissue hypoxia because of blocked cytochrome function within cells. Ordinarily the process evolves so rapidly that death occurs before treatment can be implemented. Successful resuscitation with hyperbaric oxygen has been accomplished, however.

Smoke inhalation may lead to unconsciousness. Commonly carbon monoxide poisoning is the major underlying cause. Less commonly, cyanide poisoning is a significant factor. These presumptions merit prompt treatment with hyperbaric oxygen, if it is available.

In unusual circumstances of *exceptional blood loss* wherein the ensuing anemia cannot be corrected with sufficient rapidity, acute cardiorespiratory embarrassment may occur. An example is fulminant hemolytic anemia. Treatment with hyperbaric oxygen will improve oxygen transport sufficiently to avert cardiovascular decompensation, at least temporarily. The value of hyperbaric therapy in this setting is limited to unusual circumstances wherein direct blood replacement cannot be accomplished immediately.

Clostridial myonecrosis is a complex, rapidly progressive illness. Loss of limb and death are common. Adjunct therapy with hyperbaric oxygen has been shown to alter the clinical course favorably with a decrease in morbidity and increase in limb salvage. Most therapists administer five to seven treatments at 8- to 12-hour intervals. Each exposure lasts two hours, including 90 minutes at the maximum pressure of 3 ATA.

Decompression sickness is generally attributed to the formation of inert gas bubbles in tissues and blood. Brief exposures to hyperbaric oxygen have been dramatically effective in reversing the clinical manifestations of decompression sickness in most victims. There are well developed protocols of alternating exposures to oxygen and air at specified times and pressures. Experience has demonstrated these treatment schedules to be generally free of toxicity, and relief is prompt.

Air embolism, whether precipitated during ascent in the water or during open heart surgery or dialysis, generally causes a massive acute central nervous system deficit. Currently, the preferred treatment is immediate exposure to 6 ATA of air, facilitating reduction of the intravascular gas volume. Oxygen and air are breathed sequentially during decompression. Prompt improvement and recovery generally ensue if treatment is implemented within a few minutes. This requirement is readily achieved in specialized centers training personnel for rapid ascent in the ocean. In the usual hospital setting, practical considerations prevent immediate treatment and results are less satisfactory.

There are several additional illnesses in which the rationale, experimental evidence, and clinical experience are more limited but in which sufficiently promising results have been reported to justify employment of hyperbaric oxygen. *Osteoradionecrosis* is an uncommon affliction in which dissolution of bone, usually the mandible, occurs after radiation therapy. In many such patients intractable pain, sequestration of bone, and infection cause profound disability. Ultimately mandibulectomy may be necessary. Adjunct therapy with hyperbaric oxygen over an extended interval of 40 or more days, using two-hour treatments at 2 ATA, has been associated with dramatic relief of pain and healing in most patients so treated. Comparable observations have been reported for *refractory osteomyelitis*, a condition in which there are many similarities. *Meleney's ulcers* are uncommon, chronic debilitating skin lesions associated with a mixed bacterial infection. These seem to respond well to combined topical and inhalational treatment with hyperbaric oxygen. Although most *skin grafts* are accomplished successfully in modern practice, viability may be compromised by impairment of the blood supply and infection. In these circumstances some groups have reported enhanced survival of grafts after a series of intermittent two-hour treatments with hyperbaric oxygen. The need for this is rare, however. *Thermal burns* represent another acute and complex illness in which reduced complications of infection, more rapid healing, and shorter periods of hospitalization have been reported after use of hyperbaric oxygen as adjunct therapy. Benefit has been reported for the following conditions as well: actinomycosis, acute peripheral arterial insufficiency, *Bacteroides* infections, crush injuries, acute cerebral edema, acute traumatic head and spinal cord injury, intestinal obstruction, early osteomyelitis, radionecrosis of soft tissue, acute central renal artery insufficiency, retinopathy, as an adjunct to surgical restoration of continuity for a severed limb, chronic skin ulcers secondary to arterial insufficiency, and stasis ulcers. The role of hyperbaric oxygen in practical clinical management of these and other conditions is under continuing investigation.

The dramatic character of hyperbaric facilities has generated great interest among patients with unresolved chronic medical problems, and unfortunately this has led to exploitation. Hyperbaric oxygen has no proved merit in the treatment of "aging" or of such entities as wrinkles and impotence. These claims are properly rejected by responsible physicians.

Brown, I. W., Jr., and Cox, B. G.: Proceedings of the Third International Conference on Hyperbaric Medicine. Washington, D.C., National Academy of Sciences, 1966.

Davis, J. C., and Hunt, T. K.: Hyperbaric Oxygen Therapy. Bethesda, Md., Undersea Medical Society, Inc., 1978.

Hart, G.: Osteoradionecrosis. *In* Trapp, W. G., Bannister, E. W., Davison, A. J., and Trapp, P. A. (eds.): Fifth International Hyperbaric Congress Proceedings. Burnaby, Canada, Simon Fraser University, 1974, p. 845.

Holland, J. A., Hill, G. B., Wolfe, W. G., Osterhout, S., Saltzman, H. A., and Brown, I. W.: Experimental and clinical experience with hyperbaric oxygen in the treatment of clostridial myonecrosis. Surgery, 77:75, 1975.

Kindwall, E. P.: Carbon monoxide poisoning treated with hyperbaric oxygen. Resp. Ther., 5:29, 1975.

Slack, W. K., Thomas, D. A., and Perrins, D.: Hyperbaric oxygenation in chronic osteomyelitis. Lancet, 1:1093, 1965.

Wada, J., and Iwa, T.: Proceedings of the Fourth International Congress on Hyperbaric Medicine. Baltimore, Williams & Wilkins Company, 1970.

32. DROWNING

Charles J. Stahl

DEFINITION. Drowning is a pathologic condition, terminating in death, which may result from the complex biochemical, respiratory, and cardiovascular changes that follow the aspiration of fluid during immersion, or — less commonly — from asphyxia associated with obstruction of the airway. The term near-drowning implies survival after immersion, with or without aspiration of fluid, but delayed deaths of these survivors may occur several hours or several days later.

ETIOLOGY. Accidents account for most drownings. The victims are often children or other persons who have not learned to swim. Less frequently, it may result from suicide or homicide. The circumstances for accidental drowning may include the following: (1) disasters such as floods, tidal waves, shipwrecks, and vehicular accidents; (2) hazardous environmental conditions or careless acts while engaged in fishing, aquatic sport, or occupational activities; (3) impaired ability to swim because of pre-existing illness, intoxication, exhaustion, or exposure to cold water; and (4) unintentional falls into water.

INCIDENCE AND PREVALENCE. Over 8000 deaths by drowning and approximately the same number of near-drownings occur annually in the United States. This is the third most common type of accidental death. The majority of the victims are young men under 25 years of age. Several million Americans engage in the sport of underwater swimming, using either self-contained underwater breathing apparatus (scuba) or snorkel. When underwater accidents are considered alone, drowning is the most common cause of death. It occurs more frequently than deaths from barotrauma, including air embolism and decompression sickness, discussed in Ch. 30.2 and 30.3. A study by Goldhahn of fatalities among underwater swimmers using self-contained underwater breathing apparatus (scuba) indicates the need for more thorough investigation and evaluation of these cases.

PATHOGENESIS. Survivors of near-drowning have provided some knowledge of the sequence of events. The victim usually experiences panic at the time of immersion and struggles to reach the surface, unless previously incapacitated by alcohol, drugs, or injury. Breath-holding is common and persists until accumulation of carbon dioxide stimulates the respiratory center. When the victim can no longer restrain the urge to breathe, high pulmonary carbon dioxide and low pulmonary and arterial oxygen tensions are present. Gasping may result in aspiration of water or other liquid. In about 10 per cent of fatal cases, however, it is believed that the victims do not aspirate fluid, but die from asphyxia during reflex laryngospasm or breath-holding. Swallowing of water, vomiting, and coughing may occur. Convulsions precede death in some cases.

The pathophysiologic changes in drowning were poorly understood until the studies with experimental animals reported by Swann and Spafford (1951). They demonstrated that the hemodynamic and biochemical changes during drowning of dogs are affected by the type of fluid encountered. When drowning occurs in *fresh water*, rapid absorption of hypotonic water from the lungs into the circulation results in hypervolemia, hemodilution, and hemolysis. Serum electrolytes are decreased, except for potassium, which increases be-

The opinions and assertions contained herein are those of the author, and are not to be construed as official or as necessarily reflecting the views of the Department of the Navy or the Naval service at large.

cause of hemolysis. The altered ratio between sodium and potassium, as well as anoxia, may cause ventricular fibrillation in dogs. The mechanism for drowning in *sea water*, however, is probably different. As the result of the aspiration of sea water, salts pass into the circulation and fluids diffuse into alveoli. Serum electrolytes, particularly chloride and magnesium, increase markedly. Hypovolemia, hemoconcentration, and hypoproteinemia, as well as pulmonary edema, occur.

Studies of drowning and near-drowning in laboratory animals by Modell indicate that the biochemical and cardiovascular changes are dependent not only upon the tonicity of fluid but also upon the quantity of fluid aspirated. Sea water, volume for volume, is twice as lethal as fresh water, and causes more profound changes in serum electrolytes. The serum electrolytes of animals that survived aspiration of either fresh water or sea water quickly returned to normal concentrations. These studies confirm prior observations by Fuller (1963) that life-threatening changes in electrolytes may not occur in human victims of drowning. After near-drowning with aspiration of water by dogs, the most significant changes include hypoxemia, hypercarbia, and acidosis. Pulmonary edema and decreased pulmonary compliance are evident. Fresh water alters or destroys the normal surface-tension properties of *pulmonary surfactant*. Sea water only partially removes surfactant. The pathophysiologic effects are alveolar collapse, uneven ventilation, pulmonary edema, and hypoxemia. At least 20 ml of fresh water per pound of body weight must be aspirated by dogs to cause changes in electrolytes or ventricular fibrillation.

Although the pathophysiologic mechanisms seem less well understood and may differ from experimental findings, clinical evaluations of near-drowning victims indicate that fluid and electrolyte balance are restored rapidly. The majority of human drowning victims aspirate 10 ml of fluid or less per pound of body weight. Hemodilution has not been demonstrated, and hemolysis is uncommon. The changes in serum electrolytes and blood volume are often transient and depend upon the quantity and tonicity of fluid aspirated. Nonspecific electrocardiographic changes occur as the result of hypoxia. Ventricular fibrillation is uncommon in human victims. The initial effect of the aspirated fluid on the alveolar membranes and pulmonary surfactant results in collapse of alveoli, decreased compliance, and shunting of blood through nonventilated alveoli. Subsequently, hypoxia also occurs from the diffusion deficit resulting from pulmonary edema or pneumonia. The hypoxia caused by near-drowning with aspiration in human victims is manifested by arterial hypoxemia and metabolic acidosis. Retrospective clinical studies by Modell and his associates of patients who survived near-drowning show that the chance for survival is greater when the patient is alert upon admission, the initial chest roentgenograms and arterial oxygen tension are normal, and the ratio of arterial oxygen tension to the fractional concentration of oxygen in the inspired gas exceeds 150 mm Hg. Neither serum electrolyte, hematocrit, nor hemoglobin concentrations were useful predictive values of survival or threat to life. Vigorous resuscitative efforts are indicated for all near-drowning victims, as neurologic sequelae are less common than previously believed.

The pathologic findings of drowning are often non-specific. White or bloody foam, usually seen in the mouth, nose, and tracheobronchial tree, may not be evident after attempts at resuscitation. The skin of the palms and soles is often wrinkled and pale. These changes are consistent with prolonged immersion, but are not pathognomonic of drowning. Lacerations or incised wounds of skin, without evidence of vital reaction, reflect the effects of tides, collision of the body with underwater obstacles, and postmortem injuries inflicted by sharp objects such as motorboat propellers. Mutilation of a body by aquatic animals is common, particularly about the soft tissues of the face.

The lungs are heavy and edematous. In children, however, the lungs are often pink and distended with entrapped air. Pressure on the cut surfaces of the lungs yields variable degrees of frothy fluid. Foreign material from the aquatic environment, as well as vomitus, is often seen in the mouth, upper airway, and tracheobronchial tree. Depending on the postmortem interval, the pleural cavities contain variable quantities of straw-colored to dark watery fluid, which is a transudate from the edematous lungs. A relatively dry appearance of the lungs, attributed in some cases to death by reflex laryngospasm and closure of the glottis, may also result from agonal absorption and elimination of water from the lungs after cessation of respiration. Water may be found in paranasal sinuses, and hemorrhagic fluid is frequently observed in the middle ear and mastoid air cells. The latter finding is not specific for drowning, as it is also seen in other asphyxial deaths. Diatoms are microscopic unicellular or colonial algae containing silica. The significance of diatoms in the diagnosis of drowning is controversial. They may offer evidence of the aspiration of water when the same types of diatoms are demonstrated not only in the lungs but also in the water in which the body was found. After prolonged immersion in water, the changes of decomposition and the effects of aquatic life obscure the usual anatomic findings, but the pleural spaces may contain unusual amounts of sanguineous, watery fluid. The microscopic findings in the lungs may include pulmonary edema, focal intra-alveolar hemorrhage, disruption of alveoli, and demonstration of diatoms.

In laboratory animals (rats), Reidbord and Spitz (1966) observed differences in the ultrastructural changes of lungs in drownings in fresh water from those in sea water. With sea water, cellular swelling and vacuolation, as well as discontinuity of alveolar lining cells, were noted. After drowning in fresh water, the lungs of rats showed endothelial destruction, mitochondrial swelling, and cellular disruption. Histochemical changes were also reported by Spitz (1969). An acute perivasculitis, consisting mainly of neutrophils, was seen in the lungs of rats after drowning in sea water. Similar changes, but to a lesser extent, were seen in fresh-water drowning. The distribution and amount of peroxidase-positive granules in the histologic sections parallel the density of the neutrophilic infiltration around vessels. These experimental studies may serve as the basis for a distinction between drowning in sea water and drowning in fresh water.

Numerous chemical and physical tests have been applied to the diagnosis of drowning. They include tests for concentrations of chloride or magnesium in whole blood, plasma, or serum; specific gravity of plasma; refractive index, electrical conductivity, and osmolarity of blood. None of them is entirely reliable, and all require considerable judgment in interpretation. There is yet no specific laboratory test for the diagnosis of drowning.

CLINICAL MANIFESTATIONS. The victim of drowning usually experiences breath-holding and a substernal burning sensation. Loss of consciousness and aspiration of fluid may occur. Most victims have a violent struggle prior to loss of consciousness, but a few people show passive behavior. After rescue, the patient is usually unconscious, flaccid, cold, and cyanotic. Respirations are absent, and the pulse is imperceptible. If the patient is conscious, tinnitus and visual abnormalities are often reported. Frothy fluid may be seen in the nose and mouth, and examination of the chest may disclose signs of pulmonary edema. If a significant amount of water has been swallowed, nausea and vomiting may occur and gastric distention may be evident. Nonspecific electrocardiographic changes are related to the effects of hypoxia. Cardiac arrhythmias such as ventricular fibrillation, as reported for animals, are uncommon in man. Evidence of arterial hypoxemia and metabolic acidosis is provided by studies of gas and pH in blood. Serum electrolyte changes are usually transient and depend on the quantity and tonicity of fluid aspirated. The postimmersion period is sometimes complicated by pneumonia, hemoglobinuria, acute tubular necrosis, or brain damage from prolonged cerebral anoxia.

DIAGNOSIS. When the patient is a victim of near-drowning, other physical causes for disability should be considered, including injury to the cervical cord from a dive into shallow water. In the differential diagnosis of near-drowning, other causes for aquatic accidents, especially air embolism and decompression sickness, must be considered. These untoward effects of barotrauma (see Ch. 30.2 and 30.3) are usually associated with underwater swimming, diving, or the use of self-contained underwater breathing apparatus (scuba). Recognition and differentiation from near-drowning are extremely important, as recompression, the appropriate method of treatment, may bring dramatic and lifesaving results.

The diagnosis of near-drowning is usually not difficult after the circumstances are known. Diagnostic studies include chest films, electrocardiograms, electroencephalogram, central venous pressure, serial determinations of arterial gas and pH, and appropriate laboratory tests, including hematocrit, hemoglobin, leukocyte count, serum electrolytes, and serum protein determinations. Respiratory complications, particularly pneumonia, are invariably present when fever, leukocytosis, pulmonary infiltrate on chest x-ray films, and decreased arterial oxygen tension are evident.

When the body of a dead person is found immersed in water, the diagnosis of drowning alone requires exclusion of other possible causes for death. A careful appraisal of the circumstances of death and of findings from pathologic and toxicologic studies and from postmortem chemical and physical tests is required. The role of a pre-existing illness, such as heart disease, as a precipitating factor in drowning depends on demonstration of pathologic features of the disease, as well as careful correlation with the circumstances and consideration of the hazards in the environment occupied by the victim immediately before the fatal incident. In some cases of suicide, particularly in bathtubs, if a concentration of a drug sufficient to cause coma is found in the blood, the investigator should suspect that the victim ingested a lethal dose of the drug, then went into coma, and drowned subsequently. Failure to find evidence of injury, intoxication, or pre-existing disease, as well as evidence that the person was alive during the period of immersion, favors the presumption that death was caused by drowning.

TREATMENT. Prompt rescue, first aid, and resuscitation offer the best chance for survival of drowning victims. The airway is cleared of any obstructions, and dentures are removed. Resuscitation by artificial ventilation is continued until oxygen is available, spontaneous breathing occurs, or signs of death are evident. If a heart beat or carotid pulse is not detectable, closed-chest cardiac massage, as well as artificial ventilation, is required. As soon as it is available, 100 per cent oxygen, with or without intermittent positive pressure, is administered continuously en route to a hospital. Survival depends not only upon the emergency care but also the prior health of the victim, the duration of immersion, and the amount of water aspirated.

Since there are both immediate and delayed effects of near-drowning, admission to a hospital for intensive pulmonary care is indicated. If the patient is alert, has normal chest roentgenograms and arterial oxygen tension upon admission, and survives the first 24 hours, he is likely to recover. Reoxygenation should be started, followed by aspiration of the airway and suction of the stomach. Tracheostomy is rarely necessary, but abnormalities of either blood gases or chest films may indicate the need for endotracheal intubation. After insertion of an endotracheal tube, 100 per cent oxygen is given with positive end-expiratory pressure and intermittent mechanical ventilation. Subsequently, the concentration of inspired oxygen is decreased to maintain the highest arterial oxygen tension without compromising the cardiac output. The administration of sodium bicarbonate solution intravenously in a dose of 0.3 to 0.4 mEq per pound of body weight is recommended upon admission to the hospital, for a significant number of near-drowning victims have metabolic acidosis associated with hypoxia. Based on serial determinations of gases and pH in the arterial blood, arterial hypoxemia and acid-base concentrations are corrected by effective ventilation, oxygenation, buffers, or bicarbonate. Respiratory stimulants are contraindicated. As indicated, bronchodilators, diuretics, digitalization, or transfusion of whole blood, plasma, or packed red cells are given. The need for antimicrobial drugs is determined by clinical signs and roentgenographic changes, as well as by culture of tracheal secretions. Although the role of steroids in the treatment of near-drowning is uncertain, the intravenous administration of methylprednisolone sodium succinate, 5 mg per kilogram per 24 hours divided into six equal doses, has been proposed. Intensive care is continued as long as necessary to correct hypoxemia and acidosis. As the patient improves, oxygen is given by catheter or mask and reduced in concentration to 40 per cent.

PREVENTION. Continuing education programs for the public, as well as for physicians, are required to prevent drowning. Instruction in swimming, water safety, rescue, lifesaving techniques, and cardiopulmonary resuscitation is indicated for persons of all ages. Physicians have a responsibility to their communities not only to assist in the training of paramedical personnel, such as emergency medical technicians, but also to carefully evaluate prospective swimmers and divers. Rescue units and hospitals with emergency facilities should be equipped for cardiopulmonary resuscitation and intensive pulmonary care, respectively. Fear of brain damage should not deter vigorous lifesaving efforts. Siebke (1975) has reported the survival of a patient, without neurologic deficit, who was immersed for 40 minutes. The retrospective study by Modell of 81 patients who survived near-drowning revealed that only two patients had neurologic sequelae. Among 54 children, apparently dead at the time of rescue who survived near-drowning, Pearn reported that over 95 per cent recovered without neurologic abnormalities.

Bradley, M. E.: Near-drowning: Pathophysiology and treatment. *In* Strauss, R. H. (ed.): Diving Medicine. New York, Grune & Stratton, 1976, pp. 317–327.

Bucklin, R.: Drowning: A review of the physiological, experimental, and pathological findings. *In* Wecht, C. H. (ed.): Legal Medicine Annual, 1972. New York, Appleton-Century-Crofts, 1972, pp. 93–104.

den Otter, G.: Low-pressure aspiration of fresh water and sea water in the non-anoxic dog. An experimental study on the pathophysiology of drowning. Forensic Sci., 2:305, 1973.

Edmonds, C., and Thomas, R. L.: Medical aspects of diving. Part 2. Med. J. Aust., 2:1256, 1972.

Goldhahn, R. T.: SCUBA diving deaths: A review and approach for the pathologist. *In* Wecht, C. H. (ed.): Legal Medicine Annual, 1976. New York, Appleton-Century-Crofts, 1977, pp. 109–132.

Modell, J. H.: The Pathophysiology and Treatment of Drowning and Near-Drowning. Springfield, Ill., Charles C Thomas, 1971.

Modell, J. H., Graves, S. A., and Ketover, A.: Clinical course of 91 consecutive near-drowning victims. Chest, 70:231, 1976.

Pearn, J.: Neurological and psychometric studies in children surviving freshwater immersion accidents. Lancet, 1:7, 1977.

Sladen, A., and Zauder, H. L.: Methylprednisolone therapy for pulmonary edema following near drowning. JAMA, 215: 1793, 1971.

The Committee on Allied Health: Water hazards. *In* Emergency Care and Transportation of the Sick and Injured. 2nd ed., revised. Chicago, American Academy of Orthopaedic Surgeons, 1977, pp. 330–332.

Wayne, K. S.: Positive end-expiratory pressure (PEEP) ventilation. A review of mechanisms and actions. JAMA, 236:1394, 1976.

33. ARTHROPODS AS ENVIRONMENTAL AGENTS OF DISEASE

Hugh L. Keegan

33.1. INTRODUCTION

The arthropods are invertebrates characterized as a group by bilateral symmetry, chitinous exoskeleton, jointed appendages, and a single body cavity — the hemocele — which contains the internal organs and a fluid, the hemolymph. Members of several of the classes of phylum Arthropoda are of medical importance. These include class Insecta (the insects — e.g., flies, lice, fleas); class Chilopoda (the centipedes); class Arachnida (spiders, scorpions, ticks, mites); and class Crustacea (crabs, lobsters, water fleas). The pentastomids or tongue worms were formerly considered as a class in phylum Arthropoda but the consensus at present is that these wormlike parasites represent a separate phylum.

From a medical viewpoint arthropods are of primary importance as vectors of disease. Transmission of pathogens is of two types: (1) *biological transmission*, in which the arthropod is essential for transmission of the disease; and (2) *mechanical transmission*, when a disease-producing agent, which may be acquired in a variety of ways, is transmitted to man by the bite of an arthropod or through contamination of food or water by the feces or bodies of the arthropods. The first of these, biologic transmission, is of far greater importance than the second. Examples are malaria, epidemic typhus, plague, and the various forms of leishmaniasis and trypanosomiasis. The true importance of mechanical transmission has yet to be evaluated. Although many types of disease-producing organisms may survive and multiply in insects and other arthropods in the laboratory and have been found in such arthropods in nature, it is difficult to assess the importance of the arthropod in transmission of an agent which also might be acquired in food or water or by personal contact. Some arthropods, particularly the crustaceans, indirectly affect man's health by serving as intermediate hosts for helminths which parasitize man. Examples of such organisms would be the lung fluke, *Paragonimus westermani*, and the broad fish tapeworm, *Diphyllobothrium latum*.

As the diseases transmitted to man by arthropods are discussed in detail elsewhere in this textbook, the present chapters will deal only with illness and death produced directly by arthropods. Although bites by many insects and other arthropods not usually regarded as venomous may produce painful reactions in some individuals, the discussion presented here will deal primarily with *entomophobia*, an abnormal or unreasonable fear of insects and other "bugs"; *dermatosis*, skin irritation caused by bites of flies, lice, fleas, ticks, mites, and bedbugs; *myiasis*, infestation by fly larvae (maggots); injury to sense organs, caused by entry of insects or other arthropods into the eyes or ears; *allergenic effects*, caused by contact with some arthropods, or by inhalation of scales or fragments of skins of insects or by sensitization to arthropod venoms, particularly those of wasps, bees, and ants; and finally, *envenomation*, injection of venom by bites, stings, or spines, or by deposition of blister-producing secretions on the skin. This latter group would include illness produced by the Hymenoptera (wasps, bees, and ants); the Arachnida (ticks, scorpions, and spiders); the Chilopoda and Myriapoda (centipedes and millipedes); and the blister beetles of order Coleoptera.

33.2. PEDICULOSIS

Species of lice which cause pediculosis in man are the body louse, *Pediculus humanus humanus*; the head louse, *Pediculus humanus capitis*; and the pubic or crab louse, *Phthirus pubis*. These obligatory, ectoparasitic, bloodsucking insects are of medical importance as irritating pests. The body louse may serve as a vector of epidemic typhus, trench fever, and louse-borne relapsing fever. Although the head louse can harbor disease agents in the laboratory, it is not thought to be a vector in nature. The pubic louse is not known to transmit disease.

Head and body lice are similar in appearance and in

life cycles. Adult female head lice are 3 to 4 mm in length; the males are slightly smaller. Both are larger than female and male body lice. These lice are dorso-ventrally flattened, have a soft but tough skin, and are a dirty white to gray color. The legs are short and terminate in hook-like grasping organs which enable the parasite to cling firmly to hair and fibers of clothing.

After fertilization, a female body louse lays her eggs either on fibers of the clothing of the host (underclothing primarily) or on body hairs. In normal circumstances about 70 per cent of the eggs are fastened to clothing fibers. When an egg is deposited, it is "cemented" in place with a secretion which quickly hardens and renders the egg almost impossible to remove by bathing. The eggs, oval and grayish white, hatch in about a week. The nymphs which emerge are similar to the adults except in size. They molt three times before achieving maturity in eight to nine days. The total cycle from egg to egg under favorable conditions may require only 16 days.

Both immature and adult lice feed on blood. While feeding they may excrete dark red feces onto the skin. Lice are totally dependent upon the host and die in a week or less unless they can get a blood meal. They are also quite susceptible to either low or high temperatures. For this reason lice will often leave a patient and will also depart from a corpse as the body temperature lowers. This has been linked to the spread of louse-borne diseases during epidemics.

The head louse is so called because it inhabits only the head hair, particularly on the nape of the neck and behind the ears. It is not known to occur on eyebrows or lashes. Head louse infestations rarely occur in black people.

The crab louse has the same general life cycle as the head and body lice but differs in appearance and habits. The body is almost circular instead of elongate, and the lice in all stages are much slower in movement than head and body lice. As the name implies, these lice usually infest the pubic and perianal regions but may also be found on eyelashes, hair of the face, the axillae, and body hair, but seldom on head hairs (on the scalp). Adults live about a month. During this period they produce about three nits a day. Of 200 adult crab lice removed from a host, only one survived as long as 24 hours. Because of the usual mode of transmission of crab lice, the physician should consider the possibility of venereal disease in the louse-infested patient.

Head and body louse infestation is generally transmitted under conditions of crowding and poor sanitation. Skin-to-skin contact, infested clothing and bedding, and even upholstered furniture are common sources. The use of common clothing, hair brushes, and towels in family situations and close contact among playmates in schools may be important factors. Crab louse infestation is usually acquired during coitus, but parasites may also be picked up from infested bedding, clothing, or even latrine seats.

Although a characteristic irritant roseate papular dermatitis and continuous scratching by the patient are good indications of louse infestation, diagnosis is easily achieved by direct examination for active forms and nits. In suspected head louse infestations a search for parasites should be made on the nape of the neck and behind the ears. In doing this the hair should be parted with applicator sticks. Usually the nits and active forms are visible to the naked eye, but a hand lens and flashlight may help. In active infestations the nits are found attached to hair shafts about 6 to 7 mm from the scalp. In "old" infestations the nits are found on hair shafts at greater distances from the scalp. The examiner should take care to avoid infestation. Surgical gloves and wooden applicator sticks should be used, and subsequently both should be discarded.

Physical effects of louse infestation are intense itching and consequent scratching, which result in secondary infections, particularly impetigo in children. Psychologic effects are common among persons who regard louse infestation as a sign of social inferiority. With the partial exception of crab louse infestations, in which coitus is a primary factor in transmission, most louse infestations are acquired under circumstances beyond control of the individual.

Control of louse infestations is accomplished through a combination of effective treatment of the individual; disinfestation of clothing, bed linen, towels, and other items which may be of common use; and administrative measures designed to keep infested persons and their clothing from contact with others. This is of particular importance in schools and other institutions where large numbers of persons are in close contact.

During World War II several effective louse powders were developed and used in many areas to prevent or control outbreaks of epidemic typhus and other louse-borne diseases. In reaction to the developing of resistance to insecticides by lice, such powders, which at first contained DDT as the active ingredient, were later composed of formulations containing pyrethrins, lindane, dieldrin, and malathion. Because of governmental restrictions, only three of these compounds — pyrethrins, lindane, and malathion — are found in pediculicide formulations at present. Pediculicides, some of which may not be dispensed without prescription, which are currently registered with the Environmental Protection Agency, are in dust, shampoo, lotion, and cream foundations. Most contain lindane as the active ingredient. Others contain pyrethrins (in company with piperonyl butoxide), isobornyl thiocyanoacetate, carbaryl, tetrahydronaphthalene, malathion, and benzyl benzoate. Treatment should be conducted according to directions on the labels. It is probably desirable to repeat the treatment in ten days to kill newly hatched lice which may not have been affected by the original effort.

In addition to treatment of the individual, clothing, bed linen, and personal items such as hair brushes which might be in common use should be disinfested. Such items should be machine washed or dry cleaned if necessary. Combs and hair brushes should be soaked for an hour in 2 per cent Lysol solution or heated in water to a temperature of about 66° C for five to ten minutes. Freezing in a household refrigerator for about 30 minutes should also kill the parasites.

One of the most emotion-laden problems which can confront a school administrator or public health official is large-scale head louse infestation. Successful handling of such situations requires tact, knowledge, and effective organization. Control of head louse infestations depends upon prompt case finding, proper administrative handling of each case, effective treatment, and prevention of spread of the infestations. This should include examination of all students for head louse infestation as a part of routine physical examination at the beginning of each school year, administrative handling of each case to ensure that the parents understand need for treatment and will carry out such treatment, and prevention of transmission by proper assignment of lockers, wall hooks, or other methods to ensure that garments of students are not in contact. School officials should be trained in diagnosis of pediculosis, and cooperation of public officials is essential if programs are to succeed. Education of both parents and students as to the nature of the problem is of the utmost importance.

Ackerman, A. B.: Crabs — the resurgence of *Phthirus pubis*. N. Engl. J. Med., 278:950, 1968.

Buxton, P. A.: Louse: An Account of the Lice Which Infect Man, Their Medical Importance and Control. London, Edward Arnold, Ltd., 1939.

Controlling Head Lice. Atlanta, U.S. Department of Health, Education, and Welfare/Public Health Service, Center for Disease Control, 1975.

Gordon, R. M., and Lavoipierre, M. M. J.: Entomology for Students of Medicine. Oxford, Blackwell Scientific Publications, 1962.

33.3.   FLEA-BITE

The fleas, members of the insect order Siphonaptera, are small, laterally compressed, wingless, blood-sucking ectoparasites which feed on a variety of avian and mammalian hosts, including man. They are of medical importance primarily because they may transmit plague and endemic (murine) typhus and cause irritating dermatitis by their bites. These insects vary in length from 1 to 8 mm. In order to deposit eggs a female must obtain a blood meal. The eggs, which are oval and pearly white or yellowish, are deposited in nests on the host or in crevices in floors, under rugs, or between cushions on overstuffed furniture upon which dogs and cats have been lying. During her lifetime a female will deposit as many as 300 to 500 eggs in small batches of up to a dozen at a time. The eggs hatch in from a few days to a few weeks. Temperature seems to be an important factor in this process. The legless, maggot-like larvae which emerge from the eggs are quite active and move about in the nest of the host, feeding on organic debris or on partially digested blood which has passed through the alimentary tract of the adults. Under optimal conditions the larvae reach maximum size in a few weeks, but this may be prolonged due to low temperature or humidity and when adequate food is not available. When conditions are favorable, the larvae spin cocoons in which the adults will develop. The duration of life in the cocoon is extremely variable. Adults may emerge in a week or so, or the process may be delayed for several months. Although temperature and humidity are undoubtedly important factors, it is believed that vibration is of particular importance; hence the sudden appearance of large numbers of fleas in a day or so after occupancy of homes which have been vacant for some time but in which dogs and cats had previously been kept.

Most fleas spend only a portion of their lives on the host, although a few embed themselves in the integument where they remain until death. The majority feed several times a day. In so doing much of the blood ingested passes through the gut and is excreted in a semidigested condition. Fleas are attracted to a host by body warmth, vibration of the substrate, CO_2 in the breath, and perhaps odor and movement of the host. Although some species are fairly host specific, when the usual host is not available almost any warm-blooded food source is acceptable. It is in these situations that man becomes a target. Fleas live as adults for several months. In general, feeding activity is increased by rise in temperature. A major factor in spread of plague is the tendency of fleas to abandon bodies of dead animals. This has led to the practice of directing control efforts first at the flea population, then at the rodent reservoirs of disease.

Aside from the plague vectors, the most important flea parasitic on man is *Tunga penetrans*, the "jigger flea" or "chigoe." This species, which is widely distributed in Central and South America and in tropical Africa is unique in habit in that the fertilized female burrows into the skin where her presence leads to intense itching, scratching, and often severe secondary infection. As with other fleas, both males and females are blood suckers. The male leaves the host after obtaining a blood meal, but the female burrows into the skin where it is soft, commonly between the toes or around the nail beds. When the posterior end of the body is almost level with the skin surface, the female ceases to burrow and stays in position as the ova develop. During this period the abdomen swells to a diameter of 6 mm or more in about a week. Egg laying then commences, and during the following week or ten days from 150 to 200 eggs are extruded and fall to the ground. The depleted female then shrivels and dies in situ. In severe infestations extensive secondary infections, including gangrene, often occur. It is recommended that the gravid female be extracted with a needle point and that suitable antibiotics be given for prevention or control of infection. A related species, *Echidnophaga gallinacea*, a parasite of chickens, other birds, and mammals, is occasionally a problem and may cause irritating dermatitis.

The most frequent complaints concerning fleas come from those moving into quarters formerly occupied by persons with dogs or cats as pets. When the normal blood source is available, fleas will usually not bother humans; but when the reverse is true, the first person entering a flea-infested room will quickly find the lower portions of the legs dotted with fleas which rapidly converge on the target. In such cases a residual insecticidal spray should be effective in reducing the nuisance. A repeat treatment may be necessary as additional fleas emerge from their cocoons.

Gordon, R. M., and Lavoipierre, M. M. J.: Entomology for Students of Medicine. Oxford, Blackwell Scientific Publications, 1962.

33.4.   SCABIES

Scabies, also known as "the itch," "seven-year itch," and sarcoptic acariasis, is an infectious disease of the skin caused by the itch mite, *Sarcoptes scabiei*. The disease, which has been associated with wars, social upheaval, and poverty, seems to appear in epidemic cycles at 12- to 15-year intervals. Although it is most common in groups in which frequent bathing is not usual, scabies is no respecter of social or economic status. The sole requirement for infestation is contact. Close body contact, often through sexual intercourse and by sleeping with infested persons or even shaking hands, is the usual means of transmission of the parasite from one host to another. Clothing and bed linen may also be involved in the spread of the disease. Frequently, outbreaks occur in schools or other institutions where persons live in close proximity, and it is usual for all members of the family to develop infestations. *Sarcoptes scabiei* also causes sarcoptic mange in dogs, horses, and other domestic animals. Although mites found on such hosts are structurally identical with those parasitizing man, they differ physiologically and cause only transient, atypical dermatitis in humans.

As with other acarina (ticks and mites), adults of *S. scabiei* possess four pairs of legs, and immature stages have only three pairs. The adult female is usually about 350 μ long and 250 μ wide. The smaller male measures 250 by 170 μ. In the female the first two pairs of legs terminate in suckers and the last two end in long setae. The male possesses terminal suckers on the fourth pair of legs. The dorsum in both sexes bears backwardly directed spines.

There are four stages in the life cycle: egg, larva, nymph, and adult. The adult female remains in a molting pouch in the skin until she is fertilized by the male. She then extends the molting pouch into a tunnel and commences egg laying. The burrow is always superficial and never extends below the stratum corneum. Females usually extend the length of the burrow 2 or 3 mm in a 24-hour period, working chiefly at night. It has been shown that warmth provided by bed clothing or a hot shower or bath stimulates mite activity. As the female burrows, she deposits eggs. There is some difference of opinion as to whether this commences within hours after fertilization or after a four- to five-day delay. There is also some question as to the numbers of eggs produced and frequency of deposition. Some authorities believe that the female will deposit four to five eggs daily for about a month. Others are of the opinion that the eggs are deposited at two- to three-day intervals for about two months. It is agreed that the eggs, which measure about 150 by 100 μ, hatch in four to five days. The six-legged larvae which emerge from the eggs leave the tunnel, wander about the skin, and then burrow into the skin to construct almost invisible molting pouches. In these pouches males molt once and females molt twice to become nymphs, then adults. The adult male emerges from the molting pouch and wanders about over the skin surface in search of females. The adult female remains in the molting pouch until found and fertilized by the male. She then extends the molting pouch into a tunnel and commences egg laying. The cycle from egg to egg-laying female takes from 10 to 14 days. The female lives in the host for at least a month and has been known to survive off the host for ten days. It has been reported that less than 10 per cent of the eggs mature into adult mites.

Although in theory the only certain method of diagnosis of scabies is by demonstration of the parasite, the presence of papules, vesicles, and tiny serpentine burrows associated with a history of itching is adequate for diagnostic purposes. In fair-skinned persons the burrows, under magnification, may have a "peppered" appearance owing to accumulation of fecal pellets. At one end of the tunnel a tiny, pearl-shaped object, dark at one extremity, may be found. The pearl-shaped structure is the adult female, and the dark object is her mouth-parts. The parasite may be easily removed from the burrow with the point of a needle.

The burrows may vary in length from a few millimeters to several centimeters. They are usually located in areas where the skin is thin and wrinkled. Favorite spots seem to be skin between the fingers, the anterior surfaces of the wrists, the feet, the extensor surface of the elbows, the axillae, the belt line, the thighs and external genitalia in men, and under the breasts, the nipples, the abdomen, and lower portions of the buttocks in women. Itching is particularly intense at night when the mites are most active. Secondary infection by scratching is not uncommon and may also serve to reinoculate mites in new areas. Sensitization to the presence of *S. scabiei* may result in a follicular, papular eruption widely distributed over areas where mite burrows are absent. This rash seldom appears until about a month after a primary infestation, and until its appearance the patient may be unaware of his infestation. The severe itching which accompanies this rash may also lead to scratching and secondary infection. Occasionally, particularly in invalids or other persons not able to care for themselves, large numbers of mites may develop under serous crusts. This condition is commonly called "Norwegian scabies" or crusted itch.

In view of the discomfort produced by scabies infestation, it seems odd that the number of burrows and adult females parasitizing a person is usually about 10 to 15, although more than 100 may be occasionally present.

Control of scabies, particularly in schools and institutions, should be based on a program involving education, case-finding, proper treatment of individuals, and adequate laundering of underclothing and bedding. Treatment of scabies usually involves use of creams or lotions containing 1 per cent lindane, 10 per cent crotamiton, benzyl benzoate, or tetraethylthiuram monosulfide. It is generally agreed that these medications should be applied to the entire body below the chin. The medication is washed off the following day. An additional one or even two treatments may be required at seven- to ten-day intervals. One authority has urged caution to avoid overtreatment, as, even when all parasites have been killed, itching may sometimes persist for several days. Because of the long incubation period during which transmission may occur, treatment of all family members and others in close contact with the patient should be considered. Students found to be infested should be removed from school until properly treated.

Gordon, R. M., and Lavoipierre, M. M. J.: Entomology for Students of Medicine. Oxford, Blackwell Scientific Publications, 1962.
Herridge, C. F.: Norweigan scabies (crusted scabies). Br. Med. J., 1:223, 1963.
Mellanby, K.: Scabies. Middlesex, England, E. W. Classey, Ltd., 1972.
Thomsett, L. R.: Mite infestations of man contracted from dogs and cats. Br. Med. J., 2:93, 1968.

33.5. MYIASIS

Myiasis is the term for infestation of a living animal by fly larvae (maggots). Larvae of some species of flies are obligatory parasites; others are facultative in that they may develop in carrion, feces, or even vegetable debris as well as in living animals. Although some flies are fairly specific in host choice, man is not the sole host for any of the flies which cause myiasis. Several of the species which parasitize man are normally found in domestic or wild animals, and many others are accidental parasites.

Classification of myiasis is based on the portion of the body affected as well as on the symptoms produced; hence such terms as cutaneous myiasis, gastrointestinal myiasis, ophthalmomyiasis, furuncular myiasis, and creeping myiasis are encountered. The important medical problems involved are recognition of the infestation and prompt removal of maggots.

Gastrointestinal myiasis may be caused by flies of many species whose eggs or early stage larvae are accidentally ingested. One species often encountered is the rat-tailed maggot, the larva of *Eristalis tenax*. This type of myiasis may result in nausea, sharp pain, vomiting, diarrhea, and occasionally hemorrhage from the anus. *Genitourinary myiasis*, caused by several of the smaller diptera, may result from migration of maggots from the alimentary tract or from deposition of fly eggs near the genitals. Symptoms reported have been albuminuria, dysuria, hematuria, and pyuria. *Cutaneous myiasis*, including *furuncular myiasis* and *creeping myiasis*, is caused by several obligatory parasites. One of these, *Auchmeromyia luteola*, a species found only in tropical Africa, is unique in that the larva has a feeding habit similar to that of a bedbug. During the daytime it hides in crevices in the walls or floor, emerging only at night to feed on sleeping persons. *Dermatobia hominis*, the human botfly, a species widely distributed in neotropical portions of the Americas, does not directly approach the host animal but lays its eggs on mosquitoes and occasionally on ticks. When these blood-sucking arthropods contact a warm-blooded host, the eggs quickly hatch and the larvae penetrate the skin where they produce furuncular lesions as they grow. Although at first there is no pain at the invasion site, a serous exudate accompanied by swelling and severe pain may follow. The larvae may be removed by pressure, by application of petroleum jelly to the lesion (to block the spiracles through which the maggot breathes), or by surgical removal. The latter is preceded by local anesthetization to quiet the larvae as well as to relieve pain of the host.

Larvae of the botfly *Gasterophilus intestinalis*, normally a parasite of horses, may occasionally parasitize man, causing *creeping myiasis*. This is characterized by raised, reddish, serpentine lines on the skin. A larva may advance 1 to 2 cm daily, moving mainly at night. The larva is located just ahead of the inflammatory line, and because of its superficial location in the corneum it may be easily removed surgically. Another botfly, *Hypoderma lineatum*, the cattle grub, has frequently been reported as a parasite of man. As the larvae move through the subcutaneous tissues of this "unfamiliar" host, they may produce indefinite reddish lines on the skin or local painful swellings. During the infestation, which may last for months, the patient may experience severe discomfort and even temporary paralysis of limbs which have been invaded by the parasite. The most serious danger is that the maggots may enter an eye, where they have been found in both chambers. Conjunctival myiasis caused by larvae of *Oestrus ovis*, a parasite of sheep and goats, has been reported from many areas of the world. In the United States cases have frequently been reported in California.

Infestation of man by larvae of *Cochliomyia hominivorax*, the primary screw-worm, may result in serious illness. In nature these flies deposit their eggs adjacent to open wounds on cattle and other animals. The eggs quickly hatch, and, after entering the wound, the maggots burrow beneath the skin where they cause extensive tissue destruction. Infestations in man are usually nasal or aural. In such instances the flies are apparently attracted by purulent discharge. The growing larvae may cause severe local trauma and may also wander and eventually reach the brain. Removal of the larvae manually or by irrigation should be accomplished as quickly as possible, for, as the larvae mature and approach pupation, the tendency to migrate increases and so does the danger to the host.

A number of species of blue bottle, green bottle, and flesh flies which normally deposit their eggs on carrion will sometimes parasitize man if they are attracted to an open sore or to a discharge from the nose, eye, or ear. Eggs of some of these may also be swallowed along with food and give rise to gastrointestinal myiasis.

Baumhover, A. H.: Eradication of the screw worm fly: An agent of myiasis. JAMA, 196:240, 1966.

Gunther, S.: Furuncular Tambu fly myiasis of man in Gabon, Equatorial Africa. J. Trop. Med. Hyg., 70:169, 1967.

James, M. T.: The flies that cause myiasis in man. U.S. Department of Agriculture, Misc. Publ. No. 631, 1947.

Zumpt, F.: Myiasis in Man and Animals of the Old World. London, Butterworth and Company Ltd., 1965.

33.6.   ALLERGY TO ARTHROPOD PRODUCTS

Many arthropods which in most persons may cause only minor annoyance by their bites may stimulate severe allergic responses in some individuals. Others, which do not bite, may also cause similar effects by contact. Inhalant allergic response is of particular importance. Among the arthropods associated with this syndrome are spiders, ticks, mites, mayflies, caddis flies, lacewing flies, and aphids. In order for an arthropod to be of importance as an excitant of allergic symptoms, it must appear in large numbers and be widely distributed, particles from its body must be windborne at some stage in the life cycle, and the particles must be sufficiently buoyant to be carried considerable distances. Good examples are the mayflies and caddis flies. Both of these spend part of the life cycle in the water as larvae. They emerge from the water, molt, and become winged adults. The molted "skins" are light, fragile, and easily fragmented. These readily become airborne and are important causes of inhalant allergic response in areas surrounding lakes where these insects breed. In some persons, inhalation of scales and body fragments of houseflies, beetles, moths, and cockroaches may evoke allergic response.

Clinical effects may include rhinitis, expiratory wheezing, dyspnea, and a constricted feeling in the chest. Diagnosis is dependent not only on symptomatology but also on a consideration of the seasonal nature of attacks, and on a lack of response to treatment for other allergens such as pollens, molds, and housedust. Treatment consists of hyposensitization, oral bronchodilators and use of epinephrine for dyspnea and cyanosis.

TROMBICULID MITES

These mites, which include chiggers, red bugs, and harvest mites, have a wide geographic distribution; they parasitize man, other mammals, birds, amphibians, and reptiles. In most areas they are known primarily as causes of irritating dermatitis, but in Japan, portions of Central and Southeast Asia, and Australasia some are vectors of scrub typhus (tsutsugamushi disease). There is circumstantial evidence that they may be involved in the epidemiology of epidemic hemorrhagic fevers on the Asian mainland.

As with the other acarids, chiggers have four stages in the life cycle: egg, larva, nymph, and adult. Unlike the ticks, trombiculid mites are parasitic only in the larval stage. The tiny (150 by 300 μ), pale yellow or white larvae do *not* burrow into the skin but attach only while feeding. This process may require from a few hours to three or four days. The salivary secretions of the chigger dissolve the tissues adjacent to the inserted mouth-parts, so that a "feeding tube" or stylosome is formed. The actual food ingested is usually not blood but lymph and liquefied skin tissue.

Some persons develop intensely irritating dermatitis as a result of chigger attachment. Scratching may also lead to secondary infection. Although area control of chiggers in camping grounds has been achieved with DDT, dieldrin, and other insecticides (most of which are now banned by the Environmental Protection Agency), the only practical measure at present is prevention of chigger attachment by spraying clothing with insect repellent, especially with a product containing dimethylphthalate.

Baker, E. W., Evans, T. M., Gould, D. J., Hull, W. B., and Keegan, H. L.: A Manual of Parasitic Mites of Medical or Economic Importance, New York, National Pest Control Association, Inc., 1956.

Frazier, C. A.: Insect Allergy: Allergic and Toxic Reactions to Insects and Other Arthropods. St. Louis, Warren H. Green, 1969.

33.7. STINGS BY BEES, WASPS, HORNETS, AND ANTS

Except for vectors of disease agents, members of the order Hymenoptera are of far greater medical importance than all the other groups of phylum Arthropoda combined. In many regions they are also more frequent causes of illness and death than the venomous snakes, fishes, and marine invertebrates.

The stinging apparatus of the hymenopterans has been described as the "hypodermic syringe" of the arthropod world and as the most sophisticated of the invertebrate devices for envenomation. The stinging apparatus is located in the posterior part of the abdomen, between the rectum and ovaries in females, and shares a common orifice with these structures. In most species there is an "acid" and a "basic" gland associated with the stinging apparatus, but there is some disagreement as to whether the secretion of the latter is an active component of the venom. The length of the stinger varies according to species. The depth of insertion of the stinger of the honeybee is generally only 2 or 3 mm. The amount of venom injected varies from 0.2 to 0.5 mg. Although the stinger of the honeybee is lost in the act of stinging (remaining in the recipient), this is not true of other stinging hymenoptera, which may sting repeatedly at intervals of only a few seconds. Some ants may bite and sting simultaneously; indeed, some cannot sting if they are unable to engage their mandibles.

Venom composition varies greatly among the hymenopterans. Because venoms of even closely related species may possess different allergens, generalizations which might be expected to lead to more effective treatment are not warranted. At least eight toxic fractions have been identified in bee venom. Although the effects of bee sting result from the combined action of these fractions, one component, melittin, is largely responsible for the local and general toxicity. Hyaluronidase, present in bee venom, is also found in venoms of other stinging hymenopterans. Bee venom also contains histamine and, in addition, causes release of histamine in tissues by the decarboxylation of histidine. The venom contains no cholinesterase, but may contain several basic protein components, several amino acids, and at least two enzymes.

Aside from the painful local reaction following stings by bees, wasps, hornets, or ants, more serious reactions, which may lead to the death of the victim, can occur in four circumstances: (1) *Massive envenomation by a large number of stings.* Although death has been reported after a person has received only 30 to 60 bee stings, it is the consensus that ordinarily at least 400 stings are necessary to cause death in an adult. Even single stings by some of the larger hymenopterans may produce grave illness. There have been reports of death of not only man but also water buffalo and even elephants following stings by the giant bee, *Apis dorsalis.* (2) *Particular localization of the sting.* Stings on the head have been known to cause central nervous system symptoms, and stings on the throat may produce edema of the glottis. (3) *Intravascular injection of venom.* Although this is extremely rare, it has been reported. (4) *Hypersensitivity.* In hypersensitive persons even a single sting may lead to death from anaphylactic shock or laryngeal edema.

In the majority of envenomations by a hymenopteran, the initial reaction is acute local pain followed within a few minutes by local swelling and itching. The area affected shows a small, clear, round central zone surrounded by a red halo. In the case of a honeybee sting, the stinger is found in the clear zone, often still moving spasmodically. This local reaction usually subsides after a few hours. More serious effects occur when the victim is hypersensitive to the venom. In such instances onset of symptoms is rapid, usually reaching a maximum within 30 minutes or less following the sting. Location of the sting in sensitized persons may affect the outcome. In a series of 53 persons who suffered anaphylactic shock following bee sting, 5 of 20 who were stung on the head died; 1 person stung on the arm died, but all others who were stung on the neck, trunk, and legs survived. In sensitized individuals the sting may be quickly followed by abnormal swelling, massive urticaria, and shock. There is often slight fever and sometimes diarrhea and polyuria. There may also be a hot flush over the entire body, severe dyspnea, wheezing and coughing, generalized trembling, and coma.

Effects of stings by fire ants vary somewhat from those caused by bees or wasps. Although the immediate reaction is an intense, burning sensation (hence the name "fire ant"), this sensation subsides within a short time and a wheal appears at the site of venom injection. A few hours later a superficial vesicle containing a clear fluid appears. After 24 hours, the fluid becomes purulent as a result of the necrotizing properties of the venom. The pustules are sterile and may persist as long as a week if they are not broken. During this time the fluid is absorbed, leaving a crust and, in many instances, scar tissue. Occasionally a person may have systemic reactions, including nausea and vomiting, dizziness, excessive perspiration, cyanosis, asthma, and other symptoms typical of severe allergic reaction.

It is recommended that all persons showing systemic reaction to hymenopteran stings undergo a hyposensitization program involving immunizing injections with whole-body, aqueous extracts of insects to whose venoms they are sensitive. In such a program a maintenance level is first achieved, and then for a three-year period the interval between injections is gradually increased — i.e., once a month during the first year, once every two months during the second year, and up to once every three months during the third year. Thereafter maintenance doses as tolerated, equal to the antigenicity of one or more average stings of the responsible insects, are given. It has been found that the RAST procedure (radioallergosorbent procedure) is an accurate method of documenting IgE-mediated allergic sensitivity to stinging insects. In one study involving 109 sera of persons who had immediate systemic allergic reactions following insect stings, it was found that the majority contained IgE antibodies to either yellow jacket or hornet venoms. Some sera had positive RAST reactions to two or three venoms, but others had only single venom-specific IgE antibodies. Of 24 patients who had large local reactions only, the sera of 13 contained venom IgE antibodies. Immune therapy for a three-year period seems to provide a high degree of protection for most patients. In one large series it was found that 5 per cent of the patients did not reach a complete protection level during treatment and that an additional 5 per cent had a decrease in protection after treatment was stopped.

For evident severe envenomation, epinephrine hydrochloride (0.5 ml or more of a 1:1000 solution intramuscularly or part of the dose intravenously) should be given. This should be followed by an injectable antihistamine. One hundred mg of hydrocortisone should then be injected intravenously. A sensitized person should carry several sublingual tablets of isoproterenol (15 mg for adults, 10 mg for children) and several uncoated antihistamine tablets on the person at all times. If a sting occurs, the patient should swallow the antihistamine tablet and place the isoproterenol tablet under the tongue. The parents or spouse of a sensitized person should know to inject epinephrine and should keep several ampules of 1:1000 epinephrine hydrochloride on hand at all times.

Beard, R. L.: Insect Toxins and Venoms. Ann. Rev. Entomol, Vol. 8. Palo Alto, Calif., Annual Reviews, Inc., 1963.
Brown, L. L.: Fire ant allergy. South. Med. J., 65:273, 1972.
Frazier, C. A.: Insect Allergy: Allergic and Toxic Reactions to Insects and Other Arthropods. St. Louis, Warren H. Green, 1969.
Frazier, C. A.: Biting insect survey: A statistical report. Ann. Allerg. 32:200, 1974.
Lello, E. D.: Bee venom: Glands, intoxication, accidents. Mem. Inst. Butantan Simp. Internac., 33:821, 1966.
Michener, C. D.: The Brazilian Bee Problem. Ann. Rev. Entomol., Vol. 20. Palo Alto, Calif., Annual Reviews, Inc., 1975.

Mueller, H. L., Schmid, W. H., and Rubinstein, R.: Stinging insect hypersensitivity: A 20 year study of immunologic treatment. Pediatrics, 55:530, 1975.
Reisman, R. E.: Stinging insect allergy treatment failures. J. Allerg. Clin. Immunol., 52:257, 1973.
Reisman, R. E., Wypych, J., and Arbesman, C. E.: Stinging insect allergy: Detection and clinical significance of venom IgE antibodies. J. Allerg. Clin. Immunol., 56:443, 1975.

33.8. BLISTER BEETLES

Beetles of many species throughout the world qualify for the title "blister beetle." Effects of contact with these insects may vary from a vesicular dermatitis to frank blisters which may be 50 mm or more in length. Accidents occur when contact is made with beetles in vegetation or when beetles, attracted by light, enter unscreened buildings. When a beetle is brushed off the skin or crushed, a vesicant secretion deposited on the skin produces painful irritation within a few minutes. The blisters and surrounding areas are painful, but the most severe reactions occur when the secretions enter the eyes. In the tropics "whip-lash dermatitis," due to species of genus *Paederus*, is common. "Spanish fly," the supposed aphrodisiac, is actually cantharidin, secreted by beetles in the Mediterranean area. This substance, a powerful renal irritant, has frequently been misused with disastrous effects.

Treatment of dermatitis caused by blister beetles is symptomatic. As might be expected, in patients in whom large blisters are formed, prevention of secondary infection is important. In addition to antibiotics, topical and systemic administration of steroids has been reported as effective.

Armstrong, R. K., and Winfield, J. L.: *Paederus fuscipes* dermatitis. An epidemic on Okinawa. Am. J. Trop. Med. Hyg., 18:147, 1969.
Fain, A.: Toxic action of rove beetles (Coleoptera, Staphylinidae). Mem. Inst. Butantan Simp. Internac., 33:835, 1966.

33.9. SPIDER BITE

Spiders are arachnids of the order Araneida, which is divided into two suborders, the mygalomorphs of suborder Orthognatha, and the true spiders of suborder Labidognatha. The former, commonly known as "tarantulas" or bird spiders, are distinguished from the true spiders in that their jaws or chelicerae are anterior in position on the cephalothorax, are parallel, and operate vertically in a stabbing motion. In the true spiders the jaws are ventrally located and operate from side to side as pincers. Spiders differ from the ticks and mites in that the body is distinctly divided into an anterior cephalothorax and a posterior abdomen, connected by a narrow pedicle. Spiders possess four pairs of legs in all stages of development.

With very few exceptions, spiders secrete venom which is used for killing prey. Although most spiders will bite under some circumstances, less than 100 of the approximately 30,000 species which have been described have been reported as causes of spider bite in man. Still fewer can be considered as of true medical importance. Although the large, hairy mygalomorphs inspire fear, bites by members of the group are rare. Only two species of genus *Atrax* in Australia and species of genus *Harpactirella* in South Africa have consistently been reported as causing envenomation in man.

Several of the mygalomorphs in Central and South America have been shown to possess venom potent against laboratory animals, but most apparently seldom bite man. Indeed, New World mygalomorphs seem to rely for protection more on urticating hairs on the dorsal surface of the abdomen than on their chelicerae. When disturbed, these spiders will vigorously rub their hind legs over the abdomen, releasing a cloud of tiny hairs. Upon contact with the eyes, nasal mucosa, or skin these may cause intense but transitory irritation. It is possible, of course, that some of the large mygalomorphs possess venom which could be lethal for man. Fortunately, lack of contact with forest-dwelling species and the mild temperament characteristic of many species leave the question open for speculation.

Although bites by many of the true spiders have been reported, the majority of cases of even moderately severe envenomation have been caused by the black widow spiders of genus *Latrodectus* in both the Old and New Worlds; the brown spiders of genus *Loxosceles* in North and South America; the "wandering spiders" of genus *Phoneutria* in South America; the wolf spiders of genus *Lycosa*, particularly in South America; and several species of genus *Chiracanthium* in both the Old and New Worlds.

Bites by the black widow spider *Latrodectus mactans* and other members of the genus, may at first go unnoticed, marked only by two tiny puncture marks and some slight local redness. However, in a matter of a few minutes to a few hours, severe muscular pains commence, usually accompanied by a feeling of pressure on the chest. Abdominal rigidity is also characteristic. Nausea, vomiting, profuse perspiration, intestinal spasms, shock, and visual difficulty may occur. Electrocardiographic changes have been reported, as has evidence of hepatic involvement. Treatment is both symptomatic and specific. Muscle relaxants of various types have been used. Although intravenous administration of 10 per cent calcium gluconate has been used for this purpose in the past, other muscle relaxants such as mephenesin (Tolserol) and orphenadrine citrate (Norflex) have been reported to be more effective. A specific antivenin produced by Merck Sharp & Dohme (Lyovac) is highly effective in neutralizing effects of envenomation. Apparently venoms of the various species of *Latrodectus* are antigenically similar to the extent that an antivenin produced with venom of one of the species will neutralize venoms of all other spiders of the genus.

Effects of bites by *Loxosceles reclusa*, the species of genus *Loxosceles* most widely distributed in the United States, and by other members of the genus are similar. First symptoms usually appear two to three hours after the bite as mild to severe pain. In many patients, a transient erythema at the site of envenomation is quickly followed by formation of a blister surrounded by concentric areas of ischemia and erythema. This combination, termed the "bull's eye" by some, has often been used as a criterion for separation of *Loxosceles* bites from those by other spiders. Unfortunately, however, the classic picture does not always appear. Usually, within 24 hours the color of the lesion changes from red to violaceous or black. Following collapse of the blister, local necrosis occurs, leaving a persistent, slowly growing ulcer which, showing a gravitational

spread, may attain a diameter of up to 20 cm or more and cause extensive damage to skin and subcutaneous tissues. Healing may require weeks or even months. In addition to the local reaction, systemic involvement and secondary infection often follow the bite. Fever, chills, edema, nausea, vomiting, and joint pain, together with a generalized morbilliform and petechial eruption, may occur within 24 to 48 hours after envenomation. It has been suggested that the longlasting lesions following bites by *L. reclusa* may be due to stimulation of an autodestructive reaction in the host by a venom component. Rarely severe and sometimes fatal intravascular hemolysis may occur. In nearly all fatal cases, hemolytic anemia, thrombocytopenia, hemoglobinuria, and renal failure have been preterminal complications. Although this syndrome has occurred in adults, it is usually found in children 24 to 48 hours after envenomation.

An antivenin for treatment of loxoscelism in South America is produced at the Instituto Butantan in São Paulo, Brazil. Since no such product is available in the United States, management of envenomation by *L. reclusa* and related species which occur in the western states has been basically symptomatic. There have been recommendations for and against use of steroids, antihistamines, heparin, phentolamine methanesulfonate, and low molecular weight dextran. There seems to be consensus on the effectiveness of early excision of the cutaneous ulcerations. This, according to several reports, relieves pain, stops spread of the ulcer, helps control secondary infection, and prevents systemic manifestations. Antibiotics are routinely used for control of secondary infection.

In the event of intravascular hemolysis, blood replacement (particularly in the form of packed cells) may be needed. Peritoneal dialysis has been used with success in treatment of severe visceral arachnidism and renal shutdown. Hemodialysis and exchange transfusion are sometimes necessary.

House-infesting species of genus *Phoneutria* in Brazil and other areas in South America are both active and aggressive. Bites by these spiders are followed by intense pain, vertigo, visual difficulties, trembling, convulsions, hypothermia, tachycardia, urine retention, and profuse sweating. Wolf spiders of genus *Lycosa* found in the same geographic areas also enter houses and will usually bite upon contact. Effects of envenomation by these spiders may be painful, but are usually restricted to the area surrounding the bite. Treatment of envenomation by species of both these genera is based upon prompt administration of antivenin. A bivalent antivenin, effective against species of both genera and monovalent antivenins, one against species of *Phoneutria*, the other against venoms of the wolf spiders, are produced at the Instituto Butantan.

Arnold, R. E.: Brown recluse spider bites: Five cases with a review of the literature. JACEP, 5:262, 1976.

Berger, R. S.: A critical look at therapy for the brown recluse spider bite. Arch. Dermatol., 107:298, 1973.

Bücherl, W.: Spiders. In Bücherl, W., and Buckley, E. E. (eds.): Venomous Animals and Their Venoms, Vol. III. New York, Academic Press, 1971, p. 197.

Russell, F. E., Wainschel, J., and Gertsch, W. J.: Bites of spiders and other arthropods. In Conn, H. F. (ed.): Current Therapy 1973. Philadelphia, W. B. Saunders Company, 1973, p. 868.

Taylor, E. H., and Denny, W. F.: Hemolysis, renal failure and death presumed secondary to bite of brown recluse spider. South. Med. J., 59:1209, 1966.

33.10. SCORPION STING

In many areas of the world scorpion sting is a public health problem of some magnitude. Areas particularly affected are Africa, the Middle East, India, Mexico, the West Indies (particularly Trinidad), Central America, and South America (particularly Brazil and Argentina). One dangerously venomous species, *Centruroides sculpturatus,* is found in the southwestern United States. Although several hundred scorpion species have been described, published reports indicate that stings by only about 50 of these can cause serious illness and death in man.

Scorpions are arachnids with four pairs of legs and two main body divisions, the anterior cephalothorax and the posterior abdomen. The latter is further divided into a broad preabdomen and a narrow, tail-like postabdomen. This terminates in the telson, a structure which is vesicular in shape and possesses a sharp, hollow stinger. On either side of the stinger near its tip is a tiny pore which serves as an outlet for venom secreted by each of the two venom glands contained in the telson. At the anterior end of the scorpion are the conspicuous, pincer-like pedipalps which are used for seizing prey.

Scorpions produce living young and may require a year or more to reach maturity. Food consists of insects and arthropods of suitable size. These arachnids are nocturnal. During the daytime they remain hidden, and they emerge only at night to feed. Many scorpions hide under rocks, under loose tree bark, or in and around the habitations of man where they can be found in lumber piles, in crevices in walls, among clothing, behind furniture, and in any situation offering shelter and darkness. Every year thousands of accidents and many deaths are caused by contact with house-infesting species which will sting immediately if touched.

Immediate, sharp pain at the site of venom injection is a common feature of all scorpion stings; subsequent developments allow division of these accidents into two categories. In the first of these, symptoms are local and usually transitory, persisting for a few minutes or hours to a day or so. The second category includes those cases showing the systemic involvement characteristic of severe envenomation. There are no hard and fast guidelines for separation of scorpion species into "harmless" and "dangerous" groups. Some genera such as *Centruroides* and *Tityus* of the Western Hemisphere contain dangerously venomous species along with others whose stings produce relatively mild effects. Size and appearance alone are definitely *not* criteria for judgment of the medical importance of a scorpion.

Moderate local edema, which may be discolored, is frequently seen in cases of the milder type of scorpion envenomation. Regional lymph node enlargement, local itching and paresthesia, fever, nausea, and vomiting may occur. Swollen eyelids and "thick tongue," which are sometimes seen, may indicate an allergic response to the venom. In most cases of mild envenomation all signs and symptoms subside within 24 hours.

Because scorpion venoms vary greatly not only in chemical composition but also in their effects on man, it is impossible to give a simple clinical picture of scorpion sting. In various areas of the world where dangerous scorpions occur, a wide variety of characteristics of severe scorpion envenomation have been described. Some of these are anxiety and/or agitation; excessive salivation and perspiration; hyper- or hypotension; cold clammy skin; irregular pulse; unstable temperature; involuntary micturition and/or defecation; pulmonary edema; respiratory difficulties, ranging from irregular movements to respiratory paralysis; muscle tone increases, ranging from twitching and contractures in abdomen, limbs, and pharynx to convulsions, syncope, delirium, mental cloudiness, hemiplegia, shock, blurred vision, blindness, oliguria, polyuria, and hematuria; hyperglycemia; glycosuria, myocarditis; VMA elevation; and SGOT elevation.

Some authorities have felt that death from scorpion sting is always due to respiratory failure; others are of the opinion that peripheral vascular failure and myocarditis are important causes of death. In such cases the view is that cardiovascular manifestations are related to the level of circulating catecholamines elicited by the direct effect of scorpion venom on the sympathetic nervous system. Although the convulsions so frequently seen in severe scorpion envenomation may be due to direct action of the toxin on the brain, in some instances they may be the result of ventricular tachycardia.

Onset of symptoms other than local pain vary from a few minutes to as long as 24 hours following the sting. The interval between the sting and death may vary from several minutes to 30 hours. The physician should be on the alert for the sudden reappearance of symptoms after the patient seems to be on the road to recovery. Respiratory difficulties are characteristic of such relapses. Mortality rate from scorpion sting is much higher among children than adults. In a series of cases in Trinidad, the mortality rate from scorpion sting was 25 per cent among children under five years of age but only 0.25 per cent in adults. Similar data are available for stings by *Tityus serrulatus* in Brazil.

It is generally agreed that administration of a potent antivenin is the most effective treatment for scorpion sting. Various measures have been advocated for use in instances when antivenin is not available and as adjuncts to serotherapy. In mild cases no medical treatment is required, although a cube of ice over the site of the sting will reduce pain. In serious envenomation both oxygen and positive pressure breathing assistance may be needed. Atropine has been recommended as a parasympatholytic drug, and sodium phenobarbital given by the intravenous route has been helpful when convulsions occur. In the treatment of scorpion sting in the United States, morphine and meperidine are contraindicated, as these drugs have a synergistic effect with venom of the only dangerous North American species, *Centruroides sculpturatus.* An authority on scorpion sting in the Old World has stated that barbiturates, too, are contraindicated, as they have an inhibitory effect on the bulbar respiratory centers. Intravenous injections of calcium gluconate have proved helpful in relief of muscle spasms. In some areas such as India, where dangerously venomous scorpions occur and no antivenins are available, treatment is purely symptomatic. Unfortunately, scorpion venoms differ greatly in antigenicity, and antivenins produced with them are usually not paraspecific in action. This means that in each area where severe envenomation by scorpions might occur, an antivenin produced with indigenous species must be used in treatment. At present there is no commercial production of scorpion antivenin in the United States. Although antivenins produced in Mexico for treatment of stings by Mexican species of *Centruroides* are effective in neutralization of effects of envenomation by *Centruroides sculpturatus* of the southwestern United States, importation and distribution of these products are, at present, illegal. An antivenin produced at the Antivenom Production Laboratory of Arizona State University against venom of *C. sculpturatus* is distributed free throughout the state of Arizona only. Although there are many published reports of studies to characterize scorpion venoms, none of these, at least to date, has resulted in increased effectiveness of treatment of envenomation.

Efforts to eliminate scorpion sting as a medical problem have included destruction of scorpions with pesticides, mechanical barriers to prevent entry of scorpions into buildings, general policing of yards around homes to remove litter which might harbor scorpions, and common sense measures to be followed by campers or others who might be living outdoors in areas where scorpions occur.

Bücherl, W.: Classification, biology, and venom extraction of scorpions. *In* Bücherl, W., and Buckley, E. E. (eds.): Venomous Animals and Their Venoms, Vol. III. New York, Academic Press, 1971, p. 317.

Ennik, F.: A short review of scorpion biology, management of stings, and control. Calif. Vector Views, 19:69, 1972.

Gueron, M., and Yaron, R.: Cardiovascular manifestations of severe scorpion sting. Chest, 57:156, 1970.

Reddy, C. R. R. M., Suvarkakum, G., Devi, C. C., and Reddy, C. N.: Pathology of scorpion venom poisoning. J. Trop. Med. Hyg., 75:98, 1972.

Stahnke, H. L.: Some aspects of scorpion behavior. Bull. South. Calif. Acad. Sci., 65:65, 1966.

Wainshel, J., Russell, F. E., and Gertsch, W. S.: Bites of spiders and other arthropods. *In* Conn., H. F. (ed.): Current Therapy 1974. Philadelphia, W. B. Saunders Company, 1974, p. 865.

Whittemore, F. W., Keegan, H. L., and Borowitz, J. L.: Studies of scorpion antivenins. 1. Paraspecificity. Bull. WHO, 25:185, 1961.

33.11. CENTIPEDES AND MILLIPEDES

The centipedes (order Chilopoda) and the millipedes (order Diplopoda) are superficially alike in that they are wormlike in form and possess several pairs of legs; however, the millipedes possess two pairs of legs on each body segment.

The body of a centipede is composed of a series of similar segments, each of which bears a pair of legs. The head bears one pair of long antennae and associated mouth-parts. The segment immediately behind the head possesses a pair of maxillipeds or "claws," which are used in capturing prey and for defense. At the tip of each of these claws is an orifice through which venom is extruded when the centipede bites. The number of leg pairs present varies from 15 to over 100. Although most centipedes are small, some, particularly in the tropics, may reach a length of over 25 cm. Many of the species of genus *Scolopendra* are striking in appearance, with black or blue-black bodies and orange legs.

All centipedes are carnivorous and move about at night in search of food. This habit brings them in contact with man with resulting accidents, as most centipedes will bite immediately if touched. Centipede bite may be intensely painful, and the bite of at least one

species, found in Malaysia, has been compared in severity to a bite by a pit viper. In experiments with a large centipede of genus *Scolopendra* found in Texas, a single bite killed a laboratory mouse in about 30 seconds. In spite of this and the severe local pain caused by centipede bite, effects are usually transitory and there seem to have been no verifiable human deaths from this cause. Treatment is entirely symptomatic.

Unlike the centipedes, the millipedes are vegetarians. They do not bite when touched, but may squirt an irritating secretion from pores on the sides of the body. This substance may cause transitory dermatitis, or severe irritation if it reaches the eyes. Again, treatment is symptomatic.

Bücherl, W.: Venomous chilopods or centipedes. *In* Bücherl, W., and Buckley, E. E. (eds.): Venomous Animals and Their Venoms, Vol. III. New York, Academic Press, 1971, p. 169.

Keegan, H. L.: Centipedes and millipedes as pests in tropical areas. *In* Venomous and Poisonous Animals and Noxious Plants of the Pacific Region. Oxford, Pergamon Press, 1963, p. 161.

33.12. TICK PARALYSIS

Tick paralysis is a progressive, ascending flaccid paralysis of man and domestic and wild animals, caused by a toxin secreted by attached adult female (usually) hard ticks during engorgement. Although several species of ticks have been incriminated in various regions of the world, cases in man in the United States have resulted from attachment by ticks of only two species: *Dermacentor andersoni*, the Rocky Mountain wood tick, and *D. variabilis*, the American dog tick. It is believed that the toxin responsible for this condition is secreted only after the tick has been attached and feeding for one or more days.

Onset of the condition may be marked by restlessness, irritability, and numbness or tingling of the extremities, lips, throat, and face. Difficulty in walking is soon followed by inability to stand. Swallowing may become difficult or impossible. Within a day or two paralysis of the limb and trunk muscles and bulbar involvement may lead to dysphagia, slurred speech, and impaired vision. Death may result from respiratory failure or aspiration pneumonia. During the illness leukocyte and erythrocyte counts and spinal fluid, hemoglobin, and urine levels are usually normal. The temperature is only slightly elevated.

In a recent typical case, a three-year-old girl awakened unable to walk, and fell. Her parents noted extreme weakness of the legs and lack of balance. The child was examined by a physician, but except for a bruise on the leg nothing unusual was noted. On the following day the child was still weak and unable to stand. On the third day of illness, there was still no sign of improvement. However, later the same day the child's mother noted a lump on the occipital area of the scalp and found a tick. A physician removed the blood-engorged tick, and the child recovered uneventfully within a day. The tick was a female specimen of *D. andersoni*. It was thought that the tick had been acquired three weeks previously when the family had been on a camping trip.

Unless paralysis is too far advanced, rapid and complete recovery occurs within a few hours or days after removal of the tick. In most cases ticks have been found concealed in the hair and, since their bite is painless, have not been noticed. In the past, tick paralysis was sometimes confused with poliomyelitis. In polyneuritis, myelitis, syringomyelia, and spinal cord tumor, sensory loss is usually present. Sensory signs are rare in tick paralysis.

Diagnosis of tick paralysis may be delayed because the condition is not often seen. From 1960 through 1974, only 13 cases were reported from Oregon, Washington, Oklahoma, Arkansas, Mississippi, North Carolina, and Virginia. During the same period cases were reported from ten other states. Most cases of tick paralysis have been among children and adolescents. Death rates in various series of cases have ranged from 10 to 12 per cent. Deaths have generally been due to respiratory paralysis.

In Australia a canine anti-tick serum has been produced which will protect dogs from paralysis caused by attachment of *Ixodes holocyclus*. In other areas prevention lies in the use of personal protective measures. Anyone going into woods or other areas which might be tick infested should wear protective clothing — i.e., trousers tucked into boots, shirts tucked into belts, and sleeves buttoned. In addition, and of greater importance, insect repellent should be sprayed or rubbed into clothing, particularly the lower portions of trouser legs. As frequently as possible, anyone in an area where ticks are numerous should search for attached ticks. In removing these the fingers should not come into direct contact with them. Using gloves, a leaf, paper, or forceps the ticks should be removed by a gentle and then a stronger pull. Insect repellent, mineral oil, and even a heated needle or knife blade have been used for this purpose.

Gregson, J.D.: Tick Paralysis — an Appraisal of Natural and Experimental Data. Ottawa, Canadian Department of Agriculture Monograph No. 9, 1973.
Kaire, G. H.: Isolation of tick paralysis toxin from *Ixodes holocyclus*. Toxicon, 4:91, 1966.
Nelson, B. C.: Tick paralysis in a dog caused by *Ixodes pacificus*. Calif. Vector Views, 20:80, 1973.
Stanbury, J. B., and Huyck, J. H.: Tick paralysis: A critical review. Medicine, 24:219, 1945.

33.13. ALLERGY TO HOUSE-DUST MITES

Since 1964, when mites of genus *Dermatophagoides* were first shown to be important allergenic components of house dust, a veritable flood of papers by investigators throughout the world has appeared on the subject. Although 15 species of the genus have been described, much of the research concerning these arachnids has centered on two widely distributed species, *D. pteronyssinus* and *D. farinae*. It has been found in the laboratory that females of these species require an average of 30 days to develop from the egg to the adult stage. Various types of culture media have been used to rear these mites. These have included dog food, house dust, gelatin, dry hair, yeast, and skin scales. Even though mites may be present in large numbers in a home, they may not be noticed because of their small size (less than 500 μ in length) and pale color. In homes, species of the genus have been collected not only from house dust but also from overstuffed furniture, carpets, pillows, and bedding. Both temperature and humidity affect the abundance of mites. Low temperature and low humidity have adverse effects on mite development.

The allergic responses of man to house-dust mites do not differ from those evoked by contact with mite-free house dust. An examination of literature which has appeared in the past several years has revealed the same general symptoms reported from the many countries in which these mites occur. One problem has been the proper evaluation of epidemiologic data. It has been shown that there may be considerable variations in mite populations found in homes of dust-sensitive and non-dust-sensitive persons. In some localities mites are lacking from most dust samples. An additional difficulty is that house dust usually contains a variety of allergens. Recent development of commercially available pure extracts of house-dust mites has been of aid in diagnosis. Use of a vaccine prepared from cultures of *D. farinae* has shown promise in hyposensitization of asthmatic children. In addition to the techniques commonly used for protection of hypersensitive persons from contact with house dust, use of insecticides, vacuuming of infested rooms, and environmental measures involving manipulation of temperature and humidity have been suggested for mite control. However, none of these methods has been thoroughly evaluated in a field situation. In laboratory studies it has been found that cultures of *D. farinae* have been eliminated by predatory mites of two species.

Bernecker, C.: The antigenicity of house dust and mites. Acta Allerg., 25:392, 1970.
Kawai, T., March, E., Naey, S. M., and Norman, P. S.: The significance of *Dermatophagoides* allergens in house dust allergy in the Baltimore area: Assay by leukocyte histamine release. J. Allerg. 47:95, 1971.
Keh, B.: The common house dust mites of the genus *Dermatophagoides* (Acarina: Oyroglyphidae). Calif. Vector Views, 20:37, 1973.
Morita, Y., Miyamoto, T., Horiuchi, Y., Oshima, S., Katsuhata, A., and Kawai, S.: Further studies in allergenic identity between house dust and the house dust mites. Ann. Allerg., 35:362, 1975.
Wharton, G. W., and Brody, A. R.: Colloquium: The entomology of house-dust allergy. Proc. North Cent. Br. Ent. Soc. Am., 26:57, 1971.

33.14. DERMATITIS CAUSED BY CATERPILLARS AND MOTHS

In many regions, moth caterpillars as well as adult moths are of seasonal medical interest because of the irritating dermatitis, pain, and systemic manifestations produced when they contact the skin of man. These effects are caused by venom contained in the sharp hairs and spines borne singly or in clusters on the body of the caterpillar. When adult moths are involved, it is because some of these hairs adhered to the insect when it emerged from the cocoon.

Structurally, the irritating hairs and spines range from those which act in a purely mechanical manner, analogous to glass wool fibers, to complicated types resembling the "hypodermic syringe" of the hymenopterans. In many species the urticating spines are hollow and lined with venom-secreting glandular epithelium. Upon slight contact the tip of the spine breaks off and its contents pour into the skin. It has been suggested that the toxic effects, in some cases, are a result of the chemical composition of the spine rather than the venomous secretions per se. Efforts to chemically characterize lepidopteran venoms have not, as yet, met with great success. Histamine has been found in venoms of several species. Irritating, water-soluble proteolytic enzyme components have been isolated from extracts of setae of others.

Species of several genera may produce dermatitis in man. Principal offenders in the United States are the puss-caterpillar, the larva of *Megalopyge opercularis;* and the saddle-back caterpillar, the larva of *Sibine stimulea.* In East and Southeast Asia dermatitis and other symptoms have been caused by a number of species. Both caterpillars and adult moths have been involved. It has been reported that on the Japanese island of Honshu about 250,000 cases of dermatitis result yearly from contact with adults and caterpillars of *Euproctis flava,* the Oriental tussock moth. Many other species cause both dermatitis and other symptoms in man.

Symptoms following contact with urticating species may be restricted to mere reddening of the skin, itching, and mild dermatitis, but may also include sudden burning pain, swelling, lymphangitis, numbness, papule-like eruptions, blistering, urticaria, and such systemic manifestations as nausea, vomiting, and shock. Persons who have contacted the puss-caterpillar often describe the sensation as one of "through-and-through" severe pain. Appearance of large numbers of caterpillars with resulting painful contacts has caused temporary closing of schools in some areas. In one instance a military maneuver had to be cancelled when about a third of the men in a battalion acquired painful dermatitis after a one-night bivouac in a pine grove. In this episode the cause of illness was contact with empty cocoons which littered the forest floor.

Treatment of caterpillar sting is symptomatic. No antisera or other products for direct action against the venom have been developed. Codeine, morphine sulfate, and meperidine have been used in treatment with varying results. Aspirin is usually not effective in relief of pain. It has been reported that 10 ml of a 10 per cent solution of calcium gluconate given intravenously provides quick relief from the intense pain caused by the puss-caterpillar. In event of severe urticaria, administration of epinephrine has proved effective. Ice packs are sometimes helpful. Antihistamines have not been of noticeable value in therapy.

Note: In addition to their role in urticarial dermatitis, adult moths in several countries in Southeast Asia have been reported to cause severe conjunctivitis when they feed on ocular secretions. These insects may be in a state of transition from a phytophagous to a hematophagous role.

Beard, R. L.: Insect toxins and venoms. Ann. Rev. Entomol., Vol. 8. Palo Alto, Calif., Annual Reviews, Inc., 1963.

Keegan, H. L.: Caterpillars and moths as public health problems. *In* Keegan, H. L., and Macfarlane, W. V. (eds): Venomous and Poisonous Animals and Noxious Plants of the Pacific Region. Oxford, Pergamon Press, 1963, p. 161.

McGovern, J. P., Barkin, G. B., McElhenney, T. R., and Wende, R.: *Megalopyge opercularis.* Observations on its life history, of its sting in man, and report of an epidemic. JAMA, 175:1155, 1961.

Pesce, H., and Delgado, A.: Poisoning from adult moths and caterpillars. *In* Bücherl, W., and Buckley, E. E. (eds.): Venomous Animals and Their Venoms, Vol. III. New York, Academic Press, 1971, p. 119.

Sakai, M., and Toshioka, S.: References of the irritating lepidoptera of Japan. Jap. J. San. Zool., 7:107, 1956.

Zaias, N., Ioannides, G., and Taplin, D.: Dermatitis from contact with moths (genus *Hylesia*). JAMA, 207:525, 1969.

34. PENTASTOMIASIS

(Porocephaliasis, Linguatuliasis)

Hugh L. Keegan

The pentastomids are endoparasitic invertebrates which, in spite of a worm-like appearance, are not helminths but probably constitute a separate phylum. As adults most pentastomids parasitize reptiles, especially snakes, although a few utilize birds and carnivorous mammals as definitive hosts. Immature stages have been found in all orders of vertebrates, including man. Of the approximately 70 species of pentastomids, only six have been shown to infest man. Over 90 per cent of reported infestations have been due to two species: *Armillifer armillatus,* a species which in the adult stage is found in pythons and some vipers in tropical Africa, and *Linguatula serrata,* a widely distributed parasite utilizing dogs, wolves, and other carnivores as definitive hosts, and herbivores such as goats and sheep as intermediate hosts. Human infestation occurs either by ingestion of eggs of the parasite or by eating tissues of the definitive host which contain infective stage larvae.

In the first type of infestation, usually caused by *Armillifer armillatus,* eggs of the parasite are ingested in food or water or when a definitive host is being handled or skinned. In such cases the primary larvae which emerge from the ingested eggs bore through the intestinal wall and migrate to various parts of the body where they may encyst and continue development. In addition to the inflammatory response elicited by these larvae, the increase in size during growth (probably over 1000-fold) can produce severe pressure effects, especially if cysts are adjacent to passages such as bile ducts and bronchi, or are within the central nervous system. In a series of 32 autopsied patients in Africa, cysts were found in the liver, intestinal wall, mesentery, mesenteric ganglia, parietal peritoneum (renal and splenic), greater omentum, and lung.

Encysted larvae are ordinarily well tolerated. The majority of infestations are found on autopsy or as a result of x-ray examination. However, in some instances, cysts have been so numerous as to cause intestinal obstruction or to compress bile ducts or bronchi. In a few cases they have been found in the conjunctiva or floating free in the anterior chamber of the eye.

Infestation with *Linguatula serrata* is particularly common in the Middle East and North Africa, where it results from eating raw or insufficiently cooked sheep or goat liver containing the infective third stage larvae. Ingested larvae migrate from the stomach to the throat and nasopharynx where they attach to the tonsils or nasopharyngeal membrane and produce symptoms in a matter of hours. These may include pain and itching in the throat, paroxysmal coughing and sneezing, lacrimal and nasal discharge, hoarseness, dysphagia, and vomiting. Occasionally hemoptysis and temporary loss of hearing occur. There may be enlargement of the submaxillary and cervical lymph nodes. Death caused by asphyxiation resulting from edematous swelling of the tonsillar region has been reported. Fortunately these parasites do not grow to maturity in man, and the infestations are self-limiting within a week or two. This type of illness is known in the Middle East as halzoun and in the Sudan as the marrara syndrome. Similar clinical effects may be produced by nasal leeches which occur in the same geographic region.

In asymptomatic infestations the encysted parasites are found at autopsy or during x-ray examinations. The crescent-shaped, calcified cysts may be confused with other encysted parasites such as tapeworm larvae (the sparganum stage) and arthropod parasites which may penetrate living tissue (the flea, *Tunga penetrans*, and fly larvae).

Burns Cox, C. M., Prathap, K., Clark, E., and Gillman, R.: Porocephaliasis in Western Malaysia. Trans. R. Soc. Trop. Med. Hyg., 63:409, 1969.

Fain, A.: Pentastomida of snakes — their parasitological role in man and animals. Mem. Inst. Butantan Simp. Internac., 33:167, 1966.

Hopps, H. C., Keegan, H. L., Price, D. L., and Self, J. T.: Pentastomiasis. In Marcial-Rojas, R. A. (ed.): Pathology of Protozoal and Helminthic Diseases. Baltimore, Williams & Wilkins Company, 1971, p. 970.

Lindner, R. R.: Retrospective x-ray survey for porocephalosis. J. Trop. Med. Hyg., 68:155, 1965.

Prathap, K., Lau, K. S., and Bolton, J. M.: Pentastomiasis: A common finding at autopsy among Malaysian aborigines. Am. J. Trop. Med. Hyg., 18:20, 1969.

Schacher, J. F., Saab, S., Germanos, R., and Boustany, N.: The aetiology of halzoun in Lebanon: Recovery of *Linguatula serrata* nymphs from two patients. Trans. R. Soc. Trop. Med. Hyg., 63:854, 1969.

35.   LEECHES AS AGENTS OF DISEASE (Hirudiniasis)

Hugh L. Keegan

Leeches are classified as members of the class Hirudinea of the phylum Annelida. A leech is dorsoventrally flattened, possesses a ventral sucker at either end of the body, and is divided by transverse furrows into a series of annuli. The buccal cavity is located at the rear of the cavity of the oral sucker. Within the buccal cavity are three, rarely two, "jaws." These are muscular ridges, usually armed with a double or single row of tiny teeth. When a leech attaches to a host, the jaws are protruded and the teeth quickly cut through the skin as the jaws are moved in a rocking fashion. Feeding may require a half hour or more, and during this time ingested blood may increase the weight of the leech several-fold. Leeches feed infrequently and may live for months without a blood meal following a single engorgement. The shape of the leech may change considerably as the animal lengthens, contracts, or becomes distended with blood.

Blood-sucking leeches of importance to man include aquatic (freshwater) species of the genera *Hirudo*, the medicinal leeches; *Poicilobdella*, the buffalo leeches; the nasal leeches of genera *Dinobdella* and *Limnatis*; and several species of land leeches of genus *Haemadipsa*. With the exception of the nasopharyngeal leeches of genus *Limnatis*, which occur in Africa and the Middle East, the leeches of medical importance are widely distributed throughout the Pacific region, particularly on the mainland of Central and Southeast Asia and on the islands of Malaysia and Melanesia.

Initially at least, the feeding response of aquatic

leeches is stimulated by disturbance of the water. After swimming toward and contacting a suitable host, the leech will attach with the anterior sucker and quickly (usually in less than one minute) cut through the skin and commence feeding. With the majority of species the bite is painless and the person bitten is unaware of the attachment unless the leech is seen.

Land leeches are found in shaded areas on damp ground or in vegetation. Some species may ascend bushes to a height of 1 or 2 meters. Species of *Haemadipsa* are often numerous along game or cattle trails. Even a shadow passing over a leech will evoke the feeding response. The leech will "stand up" on its posterior sucker and then unerringly move toward the host in inchworm fashion. Upon contact it will quickly attach to unprotected skin, or, if boots, socks, and trousers are worn, will quickly surmount these obstacles. Almost any opening, even eyelets of shoes, offers entrance to a hungry leech.

The nasal leeches usually enter the nares or mouth of the host when the animal or man is drinking, although infestations have been reported in man and guard dogs moving through wet vegetation. Although adult land leeches are rarely greater than 50 to 60 mm in length, extended specimens of several of the buffalo leeches and of the nasal leech *Dinobdella* may exceed 200 mm.

Although leeches are annoying pests in areas where they occur, they do not transmit disease agents to man. Their medical importance lies in the repugnance which many persons feel for them; the loss of blood ingested by the leeches during feeding and the often prolonged frank bleeding or oozing of blood from the bite; the two- or three-day period of intense itching at the site of each attachment; the possibility of infection; and, of greater importance, the entry of leeches into the eye, nose, anus, or urethra.

Attachment of leeches to buccal mucosa or to the pharynx or the larynx produces a variety of symptoms. These may include breaking through one or both nostrils, nosebleeds, and hemoptysis. Hoarseness and vomiting of blood are common in such infestations. In some areas, particularly among children, hemorrhage from leech infestation may be so severe as to cause anemia leading to death. Several techniques have been used for removal of leeches from the nasopharynx. In some cases a steady pull on the specimen with forceps has been successful. In others it may be necessary to narcotize the leech before it can be removed. In one case a 1:1000 solution of epinephrine hydrochloride sprayed into the nose was effective. A spray of 5 per cent cocaine hydrochloride has also been used successfully. In cases of urethral or vaginal involvement, a strong salt solution has caused the leeches to detach. The rather drastic technique of gripping the leech with a hemostat and pressing a burning cigarette end held against it in another hemostat has been used in the removal of leeches from the nostril, buccal wall, and tonsillar fossa.

Some protection against both aquatic and land leeches is afforded by clothing, particularly if full-length trousers and field or hunting boots are worn and trouser bottoms are tucked into sock tops. However, in areas heavily infested with land leeches, use of repellent on clothing and exposed skin is essential if leech bites are to be avoided. There are no commercially produced leech repellents. The ordinary insect repellents applied to the clothing and particularly to the boots and lower portions of trouser legs are fairly effective. However, since the active ingredients in most of these are water soluble, reapplications every three to four hours or more frequently during the period of exposure are necessary if the wearer is moving through wet vegetation, is caught in heavy rain, or wades through swamps.

Cameron, A.: Haematemesis from leeches. Br. Med. J., 2:679, 1950.

Chin, T. M.: A further note on leech infestation of man. J. Parasitol., 35:215, 1949.

Keegan, H. L., Radke, M. G., and Murphy, D. A.: Nasal leech infestation in man. Am. J. Trop. Med. Hyg., 19:1029, 1970.

Keegan, H. L., Toshioka, S., and Suzuki, H.: Blood sucking Asian leeches of families Hirudidae and Haemadipsidae. Special report, 406th Medical Laboratory, U.S. Army Medical Command, Japan, 1969.

36. SNAKEBITE

Hugh L. Keegan

Although snakebite, as a cause of morbidity and mortality, is of less public health importance than hypersensitivity to hymenopteran venoms on a worldwide basis, or to scorpion stings or spider bites in many areas, snakebite remains one of the most dramatic and feared accidents to affect man. As a result of a WHO survey conducted in 1954, it was estimated that between 30,000 and 40,000 persons die from snakebite each year. Since only a small percentage of snakebites result in fatalities, it seems likely that at least 500,000 persons are bitten yearly by venomous snakes. Most deaths occur in tropical Asia and Africa where venomous snakes are numerous and where adequate medical care is often unavailable.

The venomous snakes are classified in five families: (1) Elapidae (cobras, kraits, mambas, coral snakes, and all the venomous snakes of Australia and New Guinea); (2) Viperidae (Russell's viper and related species of the genera *Vipera, Bitis, Echis,* and *Cerastes* in the Old World); (3) Crotalidae (the pit vipers: rattlesnakes, copperheads, moccasins, the fer-de-lance, the bushmaster, many species of genus *Bothrops* in the New World, and related species in East and Southeast Asia); (4) Hydrophidae (the sea snake); and (5) Colubridae (most members of the family are nonvenomous, but some, such as *Dispholidus typus,* the boomslang of South Africa, the mangrove snakes of Southeast Asia, and several species in the New World, possess venom glands and fangs which are located in the rear of the upper jaws). Although references concerning snake morphology and classification are given at the end of this discussion, the precise identification of a snake species is seldom of practical importance to a clinician. Because usually less than five or six species occur in a single area and because bites by closely related species generally produce similar results and respond to polyvalent antivenins, the physician should be concerned primarily with accurate diagnosis and effective treatment.

The simplistic notion that snake venoms can handily be characterized as either neurotoxic or hemotoxic has long since been dispelled. It is now known that venoms previously thought to be solely hemorrhagic in action may contain neurotoxic fractions and that cobra venoms, once known only as neurotoxins, possess necrotizing elements. Nevertheless, the clinical picture presented by snakebite, at least in a given geographic area, is fairly consistent. Symptoms following snakebite and severity of the illness vary according to the size and species of the snake involved, the location of the bite, and the size and physical condition of the person bitten. However, it should be realized that a bite by a venomous snake does *not* always result in envenomation. Indeed, surveys in the United States and elsewhere have shown that in many instances a bite by even a large, dangerously venomous snake will result in no envenomation or only minimal effects.

Probably the most helpful early diagnostic sign of envenomation by a viper or pit viper is the appearance of local swelling which commences often within a few minutes of the bite. This swelling progresses rapidly in severe cases and is often accompanied by ecchymosis. Pain, which usually occurs immediately, varies in intensity even in severe cases and is not a reliable criterion for judgment of the degree of envenomation. Following the initial signs and symptoms, nausea, vomiting, bleeding from the fang punctures, bleb formation, visual difficulties, and shock may occur. Later in the course of the illness, severe necrosis is frequently seen. Other signs seen in envenomation by vipers are hemoptysis, bleeding from the gums, hematemesis, and hematuria. Renal shutdown and hepatic and cardiovascular changes may also occur, and convulsions are common, particularly in children. Although death may occur within less than an hour following the bite, most deaths from snakebite occur after a matter of hours or even days. In severely bitten patients there is likely to be massive extravasation of blood into the tissues so that an entire extremity may become deep purple or black. This, coupled with massive edema, results in oozing of blood and lymph through the skin and sometimes tearing of the skin. If the bite was on an upper extremity, this process may extend onto the chest wall.

Recovery is usually prolonged over a period of weeks or months. A 56-year-old man who was bitten on the dorsum of the hand by an Eastern diamondback rattlesnake continued to have swelling in the hand a year later, and the use of his index finger was markedly restricted.

Because of the great variation in severity of effects after viper bite, grading systems have been set up to categorize the degree of illness. One such system is as follows: *Grade I*: Minimal; puncture marks are present, but little or no local swelling or discoloration and no systemic effects. *Grades II, III, and IV:* Moderate, severe, and very severe, respectively; cases in which systemic effects are evident soon after the bite range from moderate to very severe in intensity.

Although in the past the venoms of cobras, coral snakes, kraits, and their allies were generally described as neurotoxins, it is now well documented that venoms of the snakes of family Elapidae vary greatly in their effects on man. Pain, lacking after bites by some species, may be prominent in other cases. Swelling and necrosis are important features of envenomation by some of the cobras, and venoms of some Australian elapids contain both neurotoxins and coagulant fractions, whereas others contain anticoagulants. Blurring of vision, ptosis, slurred speech, dysphagia, often severe abdominal pain, and excessive salivation and sweating early in the illness may be followed by respiratory failure requiring immediate tracheostomy and mechanical respiratory assistance.

Onset of symptoms after bites by elapids may commence less than an hour after the bite, or may be delayed for several hours. It is generally considered that the sooner the signs and symptoms commence, the more severe the case. In bites by the North American coral snake, euphoria, which may be delayed in onset until several hours after the bite, is one of the first symptoms of envenomation. This is quickly followed by drowsiness, ptosis, strabismus, double vision, excessive salivation, weakness, confusion, vomiting, and hematuria. In severe cases respiratory paralysis soon occurs. It has been reported that death from coral snake envenomation usually occurs within 24 hours of the bite.

The first symptom of envenomation after a bite by a sea snake is myalgia, which may appear as early as 30 minutes following the bite. This may cause only moderate discomfort at first, but within an hour or two discomfort may greatly increase in intensity, producing severe pain on passive movements of arm, thigh, leg, and trunk muscles. Appearance of myoglobinuria within an hour or two of a bite is evidence of severe envenomation. In such cases respiratory failure may follow in a few hours. Other evidences of severe envenomation are ptosis, weakness of external eye muscles, dilatation of pupils with sluggish light reaction, and leukocytosis exceeding 20,000.

There has always been a certain amount of disagreement over first aid for snakebite, particularly as to what recommendations should be given to persons with little or no medical training. It seems to be the consensus at present that an *untrained individual* can best help a snakebite victim in the following ways: (1) Within practical limits, immobilizing the bitten part in a position below the heart (most persons are bitten on the limbs). (2) Positioning of an improvised, lightly constricting tourniquet closer to the heart than the bite. If the bite is on the leg or arm, the tourniquet should be applied above the knee or elbow respectively, where a single bone is present. The tourniquet should be moved ahead of the swelling if it progresses up the limb. (3) Obtaining assistance from the nearest medical source, or, preferably, taking the patient to a treatment facility without delay. In addition to the measures listed above, *a person with some paramedical training* may wish to carry out incision and suction *if the patient is seen less than an hour after the bite has occurred* and unavoidable delay in obtaining specific care seems likely. If this is done, an incision about 12 mm in length, and just through the skin, should be made parallel to the long axis of the limb, and through each fang mark. Either oral suction or mechanical suction with a snakebite kit can then be instituted. Although some feel that this procedure is effective if properly carried out by a trained, cool-headed individual, it is generally agreed that it is virtually a waste of time if it is started more than an hour following the bite. In the absence of a physician, and when faced with probable delay in obtaining definitive medical help, a *trained* person can administer antivenin in the field if the patient appears to be seriously ill. This should be given intravenously only after tests for hypersensitivity to horse serum have been conducted. Materials and instructions for such tests are included in each package of antivenin. If the patient is sensitive to

horse serum, administration of antivenin in the field should be used only in a situation of extreme emergency.

Use of adequate amounts of specific antivenin is of basic importance in management of snakebite in the hospital. Symptomatic measures needed will vary according to the species of snake involved and the severity of illness but may include blood transfusion, maintenance of electrolyte balance, antibiotic therapy, and use of corticosteroids for treatment of allergic response to antivenin. Oxygen may be required for treatment of shock and respiratory failure, and, because of the latter, mechanical respiratory assistance should be at hand. Antitetanus prophylaxis is important. Those who have not been previously immunized should be given a prophylactic dose of tetanus immune globulin intramuscularly. The usual dose is 250 units. Previously immunized persons who have not had a booster injection within six months of the snakebite should be given 0.5 ml of fluid tetanus toxoid intramuscularly.

In pit viper and viper bites, it is highly important that a bitten limb be immobilized in the position of function during early hospitalization. Active and passive exercise to prevent contracture should be commenced as soon as the patient's condition permits. The necrotizing action of some venoms may increase swelling and tensions in the deep fascia to the extent that blood flow may be impaired and further tissue death likely. In such instances careful surgical intervention to allow drainage and reduce tensions may be necessary in order to save the function of a hand or foot.

Except for administration of antivenin, treatment of coral snake bite is symptomatic. Because of the delayed onset of symptoms in even severe cases, it is imperative that coral snake antivenin (produced by Wyeth Laboratories) be given intravenously immediately if it is certain that the patient was bitten by a coral snake. As respiratory failure is a prominent feature of severe envenomation by coral snakes, plans should be made for tracheostomy and availability of mechanical respiratory assistance.

Although antivenin remains the single most important factor in treatment of snakebite, none of the products available has reached the goal for potency recommended by WHO years ago — i.e., that 1 ampule of antivenin be sufficiently potent to neutralize the maximum amount of venom which could be injected in a bite by a snake of the species whose bites it was designed to treat. Up to 150 ml or more of antivenin may be required for treatment of seriously ill patients. Because of widespread sensitivity to horse serum and resulting anaphylaxis if antivenin is given in treatment, this problem can be of primary importance. Although use of animals other than equines for antivenin production has been suggested, latest information is that all antivenins now available either from governmental or commercial sources are prepared by immunizing horses. Although physicians have varied in their view toward administration of antivenin, many believe that it should be withheld in cases of obvious minimal envenomation or when it is known that the snake species involved is not dangerously venomous. Of course the size, age, and general physical condition of the patient must be taken into consideration in reaching a decision.

Although there has been much improvement in antivenin potency and in preparation of effective polyvalent antivenins in recent years, development in this field has not kept up with advances in knowledge of the biochemistry and pharmacology of venoms. It is to be hoped that much of this new knowledge can soon be translated into more effective treatment.

Bücherl, W., Buckley, E. E., and Deulofeu, V. (eds.): Venomous Animals and Their Venoms, Vol. I. New York, Academic Press, 1968.

Bücherl, W., and Buckley, E. E. (eds.): Venomous Animals and Their Venoms, Vol. II. New York, Academic Press, 1971.

Glass, T. G., Jr.: Early debridement in pit viper bites. JAMA, 235:2513, 1976.

Greenwood, B. M., Warrell, D. A., Davidson, N. McD., and Ormerod, L. D.: Immunodiagnosis of snake bite. Br. Med. J., 4:743, 1974.

Harris, A. R. C., Hurst, P. E., and Saker, B. M.: Renal failure after snake bite. Med. J. Aust., 2:409, 1976.

Minton, S. A. (ed.): Snake Venoms and Envenomation. New York, Marcel Dekker, Inc., 1971.

Ohsaka, A., Hayashi, K., and Sawai, Y.: Animal, Plant, and Microbial Toxins. New York, Plenum Press, 1976.

Reid, H. A.: Epidemiology of sea-snake bites. J. Trop. Med. Hyg., 78:106, 1975.

Reid, H. A.: Antivenom in sea-snake bite poisoning. Lancet, 1:622, 1975.

37. VENOMOUS MARINE ANIMALS

Hugh L. Keegan

Envenomation by marine animals of several phyla has been of increasing importance in recent years because of widespread interest in scuba diving, shell collecting, and water sports in general. Although accidents have been more numerous in warmer waters, venomous species are ubiquitous to the extent that a knowledge of locally occurring animals is of importance to both the hobbyist and the physician. As descriptions adequate for recognition of the many species of medical importance are beyond the scope of this work, references for that purpose are given at the end of this discussion.

COELENTERATES (JELLYFISH, CORALS, SEA ANEMONES). Skin contact with many of the coelenterates, particularly the jellyfish, may result in severe pain, allergic reactions, and even death. Most accounts of severe reactions have come from tropical regions, but dangerous species also occur in regions with temperate climates.

Phylum Coelenterata has been divided into three classes: *Class I*, Hydrozoa. The most important of the orders of this class, from a medical viewpoint, is the order Siphonophora, which consists of free-swimming or floating colonies composed of both feeding and reproductive individuals attached to a stem or disk. The upper end of the colony may be a balloon-like float. *Physalia*, the Portuguese man-of-war, is the most dangerous of the Siphonophora. The tentacles dangling from the float may exceed 30 meters in length. *Class II*, Scyphozoa, the "true" jellyfish, which are solitary, not colonial, individuals. These are free-swimming forms which vary considerably in size and in toxicity for man. The best known genera are *Carybdea*, *Dactylometra*, and *Chiropsalmus*. Because of the intensity of their stings, these are known in some areas as "sea wasps" or "fire medusae." *Class III*, Anthozoa. This class includes the sea anemones and corals.

Except for cuts from contact with coral, injury to man from coelenterates is caused by nematocysts, small intracellular structures present on the tentacles of all coelenterates. Each nematocyst consists of a capsule containing a hollow, coiled, intraverted thread. These are discharged to the exterior by eversion. Some types may penetrate the skin of man, injecting a toxic substance. The nature of the toxins found in the nematocysts of the many species of coelenterates is largely unknown. The cause of discharge of the nematocysts seems to be a selective reaction to mechanical and perhaps chemical stimuli.

Symptoms following contact with venomous coelenterates vary considerably. Contact is often followed immediately by intense, burning pain. If the species is one with long tentacles, lines of contact often appear as purplish, swollen wheals. These may disappear in a few hours or in some cases vesiculate. Systemic effects, sometimes absent, may appear a few minutes after contact, or may be delayed for as much as an hour. These effects frequently include muscle spasm, particularly in the abdomen, back, and diaphragm. The patient often has great difficulty in breathing and may be nauseated. Profuse lacrimation and nasal and bronchial secretion are usual. Cardiac weakness, generalized muscular weakness, anxiety, swelling, particularly of the extremities, profuse perspiration, erythema, elevated temperature, vertigo, rapid pulse, mental confusion, and moderate dilation of the pupils may occur. Some authorities believe that the chief danger from jellyfish sting is that the victim might drown because of cramps and respiratory muscle spasm. In one series of six cases from North Queensland which ended fatally, none of the victims survived more than ten minutes after being stung. The signs were those of anaphylactic shock. In these and similar cases there was no wheal at the point of contact, and in some cases there was a delay of a half hour or more before appearance of systemic effects.

For the most part, treatment of coelenterate sting has been symptomatic. Tentacles which have adhered to the skin should be removed as soon as possible, preferably after the nematocysts have been inactivated by application of alcohol. If this is not available, bath towels, clothing, or even sand may be used. Intravenous calcium gluconate has been found to be helpful in relieving muscle spasms. Codeine, morphine, sodium phenobarbital, epinephrine, diphenylhydramine, and atropine have been used in therapy with varying success. Artificial respiration and use of oxygen may be necessary if respiration is depressed. Norepinephrine has been used to combat cardiac failure. An antivenin for treatment of stings by the sea wasp *Chiropsalmus fleckeri*, a dangerous jellyfish found in Australian waters, is produced at the Commonwealth Serum Laboratories, Melbourne, Australia.

MOLLUSCS. The most important of the marine molluscs to affect man are the cone shells. These are large, attractively colored, carnivorous snails which are widely distributed, although the species which are dangerous to man are most often found in the western and southwestern Pacific from Japan to Australia. Though perhaps 200 species of these have been described, only about 15 have been reported as causing envenomation in man. The painful, sometimes fatal sting is inflicted with a hollow, needle-like tooth which is rapidly extruded through the opening in the shell. The venom injected in this way ordinarily serves to kill small fishes and marine invertebrates which are food for cone shells. The snails, of course, do not attack man. Almost without exception, persons stung by cone shells have been shell collectors or have been gathering snails for bait. In other words, only persons who have actually been handling shells have been stung.

The victim is always aware that he has been stung. The sting has been described as a very small puncture mark and, as might be expected, usually on the hand. The sequence of symptoms following the sting varies. In some cases sharp, burning pain commences immediately. In others, pain is absent and the initial symptom is a feeling of numbness, which extends rapidly up the arm. Rapidly developing flaccid paralysis, difficulty in speech, and blurred vision occur in severe cases. Dysphagia and a feeling of constriction of the chest are common. Death, when it occurs, is due to respiratory paralysis.

Treatment is entirely symptomatic. Support of respiration is essential in severe cases. In nonfatal cases on record, most symptoms had disappeared within 24 hours. In fatal cases, death occurred in less than 12 hours, usually in 6 or less.

ECHINODERMS (STARFISHES, SEA URCHINS, SEA CUCUMBERS, AND SEA LILIES). These animals are radially symmetrical and possess structures known as tube feet, which serve as tentacles or as organs of locomotion. The sea urchins are globular, cushion-shaped, or discoidal relatives of the starfish. Unlike the former, they do not possess arms but move by tube feet or with the aid of long, movable spines. Both starfishes and sea urchins possess pedicellariae, sets of two or three spines arranged to function as pincers. There are several types of pedicellariae, some of which bear venom glands in each "jaw."

Of all the echinoderms, the sea urchins are of greatest medical importance because of wounds and envenomation which may result from penetration of spines or attachment of venom-containing pedicellariae to the skin. Throughout the Far East sea urchins are numerous in shallow, coastal waters, and are often found among coral reefs or ledges or in the intertidal shore zone. Spines of some species may be over 30 cm in length. All are sharp, brittle, and easily fragmented so that particles may remain in punctures caused by them. Most accidents occur when persons wade in infested waters with bare feet. In addition to the problem of envenomation, infection may occur when deep penetration by the spines has taken place. Symptoms resulting from attachment to the finger of pedicellariae of sea urchins in Japanese waters have included instant severe pain, fainting, difficulty of respiration, paralysis of lips, tongue, and eyelids, and relaxation of muscles of the limbs. Generalized muscular paralysis and respiratory distress have led to death in some cases.

Treatment is symptomatic. Precautionary measures against injury from starfishes and sea urchins should include wearing of shoes while wading in infested areas and use of forceps if specimens with needle-like spines are collected.

VENOMOUS FISHES. Painful and sometimes fatal stings are caused by contact with venom-bearing spines of many species of fishes in both temperate and tropical waters. These spines, which are grooved, and may be serrated, are usually located in the dorsal, pectoral, or pelvic fins, but may be present in other areas, including the top of the head and the cheek. Venom-secreting tissue lines the grooves of the spines, and sac-like venom glands may be located at the base of each grooved spine. Often an integumentary sheath may enclose the spines, particularly those of the dorsal fin. Pressure on the spine by the hand or foot of a person forces back the sheath and venom flows along the groove into the wound. These sharp, sturdy spines can easily penetrate a glove or soft-soled shoe, and even slight penetration can result in agonizing pain.

Although many fishes possess venom-bearing spines, the groups of greatest medical importance are the stingrays, catfishes, weeverfishes, stargazers, scorpion fishes, and toadfishes. *Stingrays* are flat, disk- or kite-shaped animals which possess a long tail armed with one or more barbed spines. These fishes habitually lie partially buried on the bottom in shallow water and are a serious menace to waders. Several species of bottom-dwelling *catfishes* possess serrated, venom-bearing spines on dorsal and pectoral fins. The family Scorpaenidae includes several genera with extremely dangerous species. Among these are the *scorpion fishes* of genera *Scorpaenopsis*, *Scorpaena*, and *Dactylopterus*; members of genus *Pterois*, often known as zebra fishes, lion fishes, or butterfly cod; and the *stonefishes* of genus *Synanceja*.

Stingray injuries occur when the animals are stepped upon or grazed by persons wading or diving. When this happens the animal lashes out with its tail, producing deep punctures or lacerations. The injury plus effects of the venom causes immediate excruciating pain, which may be localized or radiating. The area surrounding the puncture is at first blanched, later hyperemic and edematous. Shock, muscular twitching, convulsions, irregular respiration, and cardiac arrhythmia indicates severe envenomation.

Stonefishes are grotesque in appearance and often bear a close resemblance to weed-covered rocks or pieces of bottom debris. They are extremely difficult to detect, as they lie half-buried in bottom mud or sand or among rocks. Unlike most fishes, they do not swim away when approached, but usually lie motionless unless touched. Some species possess as many as 13 venom-bearing spines in the dorsal fin. As with stings by the other venomous fishes, immediate pain is a first symptom following contact. This may be followed by edema, paralysis, and loss of sensation in the injured limb. General effects may include syncope, impairment of all sensations, and coma. Dyspnea and general weakness may last for several months following a sting. Deaths from stings by *Synanceja verrucosa* have been reported.

SCORPION FISHES AND LION FISHES (ALSO KNOWN AS ZEBRA FISHES AND BUTTERFLY FISHES). Like stonefishes, many of these animals greatly resemble their surroundings, and are bottom-dwelling, lethargic species. Perhaps the most dangerous of these is *Scorpaenopsis diabolus*, a species widely distributed from Japan southward through Indonesia and Oceania. When disturbed, this and related species turn to face the intruding object, then flip over the pectoral fins to display their brilliantly colored undersurfaces. If further molested, the fishes spread their operculae and "butt" the offending object. Lion fishes also do not show a tendency to flee but will rotate the body to bring the tips of venomous spines in the dorsal fin directly in the path of an approaching object. Symptoms produced are similar to those caused by stonefish envenomation.

Immediate, agonizing pain has been described as characteristic of stings by *marine catfishes*. Later, tissue necrosis may occur and may be so severe as to result in loss of a limb. Deaths from catfish stings have been reported.

Treatment of venomous stings by marine fishes should be directed toward achievement of three objectives: (1) alleviation of pain, (2) combating effects of the venom, and (3) prevention of secondary infection. In injuries of this type, the prompt cleansing of the wound by irrigation with cold salt water, followed by soaking of the injured limb in hot water for 30 minutes to an hour is recommended. Infiltration of the wound area with analgesics followed by debridement, and further cleansing may be necessary if tips of spines have broken off in the tissue. The wound should be protected with an antiseptic and a sterile dressing. Tetanus prophylaxis is advised. Treatment for shock may be necessary. This should be directed toward maintenance of cardiovascular tone and prevention of further complications.

The only specific remedy for fish sting is an antiven-in produced at the Commonwealth Serum Laboratories, Melbourne, Australia, for treatment of envenomation by the stonefish, *Synanceja trachynis*. This product may be expected to have some effect in treatment of sting by related species. In the brochure containing the antivenin it is recommended that the severe pain which follows stonefish sting can usually be relieved by infiltration of the wound with emetine hydrochloride solution (65 mg per milliliter).

Cleland, J.B., and Southcott, R. V.: Injuries to Man from Marine Invertebrates in the Australian Region. National Health and Medical Research Council, Special Report Series No. 12, Commonwealth of Australia, Canberra A.C.T., 1965.

Halstead, B. W.: Poisonous and Venomous Marine Animals of the World (3 vols.). Washington, D.C., U. S. Government Printing Office, 1965–1970.

Halstead, B. W.: Venomous fishes. In Bücherl, W., and Buckley, E. E. (eds.): Venomous Animals and Their Venoms, Vol. II. New York, Academic Press, 1971, p. 587.

McMichael, D. F.: Molluscs — classification, distribution, venom apparatus and venoms, symptomatology of stings. *In* Bücherl, W., and Buckley, E. E. (eds.): Venomous Animals and Their Venoms, Vol. III. New York, Academic Press, 1971, p. 373.

Southcott, R. V.: Coelenterates of medical importance. *In* Keegan, H. L., and Macfarlane, W. V. (eds.): Venomous and Poisonous Animals and Noxious Plants of the Pacific Region. A symposium volume from Proceedings of the 10th Pacific Science Congress. Oxford, Pergamon Press, 1963, p. 41.

PART V
IMMUNE DISEASE

38. INTRODUCTION

Henry G. Kunkel

Immunology represents one of the most rapidly expanding areas of biology, and many new techniques for the study of alterations in disease have become available recently. This is particularly true at the cellular level, and much has been learned of the lymphocyte which is clearly the key cell involved in both cellular and humoral immunity. The concept of two major types of lymphocytes, T cells (thymus derived) and B cells (bone marrow derived), is firmly established. Alterations in level and defects in these cells are now recognizable.

Immunologic alterations, both at the cellular level and with respect to immunoglobulins (Igs) and antibodies, have been found in a wide variety of different diseases. However, in many instances it has proved uniquely difficult to pinpoint the abnormality as primary in the disease etiology. It is well recognized that similar changes can occur secondarily, particularly as a result of certain viral infections. In some diseases the significance of the immunologic alterations is clear, as for example in the allergic disorders, in thyroiditis, and in certain types of immune deficiency. In other diseases, such as systemic lupus erythematosus (SLE), Graves' disease, acquired hemolytic anemia, and pemphigus, immunologic alterations are present which appear to be involved in the disease process, but their origin and relative significance remain less clear. Finally, there are diseases such as rheumatoid arthritis, ulcerative colitis, and pernicious anemia in which the evidence for an immunologic disorder remains very tentative. Interest has centered in particular on the challenging question of autoimmunity and its possible pathogenic role in many of these disorders. One difficulty which has hampered investigators stems from the gradual realization that the occurrence of autoantibodies is by no means a rare phenomenon limited to specific diseases. Many normal persons appear to possess such antibodies. Some autoantibodies appear to be without harmful effects, and the possibility exists, at least in certain instances, that they may be of benefit.

Examples of widely prevalent autoantibodies that in most situations appear to be without harmful effects are immunoconglutinin or antibody to complement, the anti–gamma globulins frequently termed rheumatoid factors, and the antinuclear antibodies of many different types. All of these have been found in the serum of normal persons as well as in those with a wide variety of microbial diseases. Evidence has been obtained, however, that under certain conditions harmful effects can be produced by certain types of antinuclear and anti–gamma globulin antibodies. Characteristics such as concentration in serum, exact specificity (particularly toward antigens encountered in the serum), and physical properties such as solubility appear to govern this question.

One immunologic mechanism of tissue injury that is coming increasingly to the fore is the direct effect of antigen-antibody complexes from the circulation. This is particularly true of renal injury. Such a process appears to be involved in a number of diseases in which renal injury is manifest such as systemic lupus erythematosus and glomerulonephritis. The antigen reacting with antibody to form complexes may come from external sources such as streptococci and administered drugs, or it may come from autologous tissue breakdown products. The injury from such complexes is not limited to the kidney, a particularly sensitive target organ, but may also involve the blood vessels as a potential mechanism of vasculitis. Platelet damage represents a well documented example; complexes of drugs such as quinidine and its antibody in sensitive individuals adhere to platelets and bring about their destruction.

Considerable interest is currently centered on the important role of suppressor T cells and their special function in the regulation of immune responses. Increased suppressor cell activity appears to be involved in certain cases of immune deficiency in a situation in which B cell differentiation into antibody secreting plasma cells is inhibited. Decreased suppressor cell activity, on the other hand, may be important in the immunologic hyper-reactivity of patients with systemic lupus erythematosus and their proclivity to develop autoantibodies.

Another immunologic mechanism of disease that has come forward recently is the blockade of physiologically significant receptors by specific antibodies. Such a mechanism is well documented in myasthenia gravis and also appears involved in certain types of insulin resistance. Such a mechanism may well be more broadly significant in disease.

TYPES OF ANTIBODIES AND THEIR PROPERTIES

Five major classes of human antibodies have been characterized: IgG, IgM, IgA, IgD, and IgE. In addition, the IgG class has been divided into four subclasses which differ markedly in biologic properties: IgG1, IgG2, IgG3, and IgG4. The concentration in serum and some of the special properties of these classes and subclasses are shown in the accompanying table. All these proteins migrate in the gamma-beta area by electrophoresis, with IgG4, IgA, IgD, and IgE showing the most rapid mobility at pH 8.6. They have been determined quantitatively primarily through the use of specific antisera in radial immune diffusion assays. The five major classes are very distinct antigenically, and specific antisera are readily obtained. The four subclasses of IgG show marked cross-reactions, and it is primarily because of this distinction that they have been termed subclasses.

It is now apparent that all Igs and antibodies consist of two major polypeptide chains, the heavy or H chain and the light or L chain. Both the H and L chains have

126

Biologic Properties of Human Immunoglobulins

	IgG1	IgG2	IgG3	IgG4	IgA	IgM	IgD	IgE
Concentration mg/ml*	9.4	3.2	1.0	0.6	1.9	0.5	0.03	0.0003
Placental transfer	+	+	+	+	0	0	0	0
Complement fixation†	+	±	+	0	0	+	0	0
PCA‡ reactivity	+	0	+	+	0	0	0	0
P-K§ reactivity	0	0	0	0	0	0	0	+
Lymphocyte receptors¶	±	±	0	0	+	+	+	0
Macrophage binding	+	0	+	0	0	0	0	−

*Mean values in adult whites.
†Classic complement pathway.
‡Passive cutaneous anaphylaxis.
§Prausnitz-Küstner.
¶Ig receptors for antigen on the membranes of B lymphocytes.

a variable and a constant area. The variable portions are directly involved in the antibody combining site. The constant areas of the heavy chains differ among the classes and subclasses and are responsible for the different biologic properties shown in the table. Figure 1 illustrates the basic Ig chain structure, showing the variable and constant areas as they apply to IgG1 immunoglobulins. There are two L-H chain pairs which make up the two antigen combining sites of this type of molecule. Enzymatic splitting of the molecule has proved of great utility in the study of the various properties of antibodies. Papain produces an Fab and an Fc fragment, and each of these is readily isolated. Most of the properties of the different classes and subclasses shown in the table are based on structural differences in the Fc part of the molecule.

As shown in Figure 1, the common IgG globulin is made up of a single four-chain unit. In the case of IgM or 19S Ig as it is sometimes called, a similar four-chain monomeric unit is further polymerized into a macroglobulin consisting of five such units linked by disulfide bonds. The IgA globulin is more variable and sometimes consists of a simple four-chain 7S molecule and in other instances is polymerized to various larger sizes. Less is known about the IgD type, but this also appears to be a 7S protein made of two light and two heavy chains. The proteins of the IgE class also consist of two light and two heavy chains. However, longer heavy chains are present, making the four-chain molecule somewhat larger. These classes differ from each other in carbohydrate content, which plays an important role in solubility differences. They also differ in their ability to cross the placenta, an important property with regard to maternal-infant antibody relationships. The IgM and the IgA show little or no placental passage, in marked contrast to IgG globulin, which in cord blood reaches similar levels to those in maternal serum. A very significant special property of IgA antibodies is their occurrence as the dominant antibody in all external secretions. Saliva, tears, intestinal secretions, colostrum, and other body fluids contain primarily IgA antibodies.

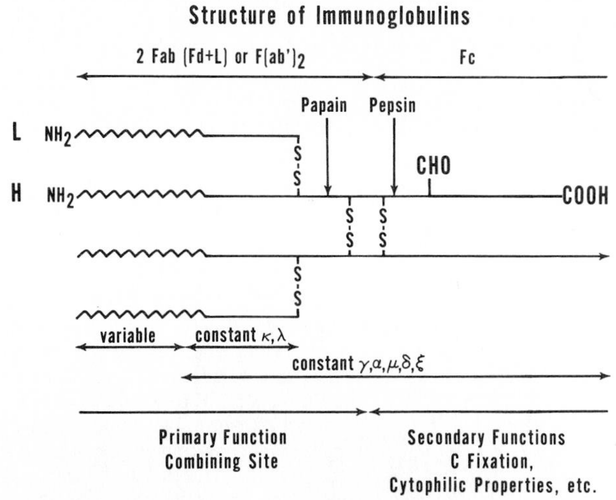

Recently it has been demonstrated that IgD is of special significance on the membrane of B type lymphocytes. It appears that IgD and IgM act as the primary receptors for antigen on the lymphocyte surface.

The total amino acid sequence is now available for a number of Igs and it is clear that marked differences occur in the variable areas of the heavy and light chains, particularly in special regions which have been termed the hypervariable areas. These amino acid substitutions account for the specific combining properties of individual antibodies for antigen. The genetic mechanism by which the huge diversity of antibody molecules is produced with amino acid differences in the hypervariable areas remains unknown. The germ line theory proposes that there are sufficient DNA units in the genome to code for all the different antibodies. The somatic theory, on the other hand, considers a variety of different mechanisms arising during cell development and involving somatic mutations from a very limited number of DNA units.

Antibodies with autospecificity have been found that belong in each of the main classes of Igs, with the possible exception of IgE. Most of the diverse antibodies encountered in the sera of SLE patients are of the IgG type, which goes along with the usual marked elevation in the total serum IgG globulin. A few, however, have been described that fall into the IgM and IgA class, particularly among the antinuclear antibodies. The rheumatoid factors as well as the majority of other anti-

Structure of Immunoglobulins

Figure 1. Diagrammatic illustration of the basic structure of the Ig molecule. There are two L chains and two H chains linked by disulfide bonds; the amino terminal ends of the chains are on the left and the carboxy terminal ends at the right. The undulating lines represent the variable portions of both the H and L chains. The sites of cleavage by papain and pepsin to give Fab and Fc fragments are indicated. The Greek letters refer to the kappa and lambda light chains and the heavy chains of the various Ig classes. The position of a carbohydrate side chain (CHO) is shown.

gamma globulins are primarily IgM macroglobulins. Most of the cryoglobulins are macroglobulins; this is also true of the cold agglutinins. Decreased solubility in the cold is a general characteristic of the antibodies of high molecular weight. It is known that these antibodies are also very sensitive to sulfhydryl compounds such as cysteine and penicillamine, which act on the disulfide bonds responsible for their polymeric structure. Attempts have been made to utilize this effect for therapeutic purposes, particularly for the cold agglutinin disease, but with limited success thus far. The antibodies of high molecular weight usually fix complement very effectively and as a result produce severe cellular injury when cells are involved as antigens. Many such antibodies are involved in hemolytic reactions of erythrocytes. In other instances the specific properties of macroglobulin antibodies make them more benign. The IgG–anti-IgG complexes found in rheumatoid arthritis sera are readily soluble under most conditions, permitting them to circulate at high concentrations with surprisingly few harmful effects. However, some of the IgG–anti-IgG complexes have been shown to have very harmful effects. This is particularly true in the disorder known as mixed cryoglobulin disease in which severe kidney disease is frequently found.

The skin-sensitizing antibodies or reagins that appear to be responsible for most of the harmful effects in the allergic diseases have many unique properties. The most striking of these is the persistence in the skin for periods of weeks after transfer to normal persons. The demonstration that these properties are characteristics of antibodies of the IgE class has been a significant recent development in immunology. Quantitatively this is a very minor class, representing only approximately 0.05 per cent of the total immunoglobulins of the serum. However, it has become clear that it is specifically involved in histamine release from leukocytes and other cells. The finding of several myeloma proteins of the IgE type has aided greatly in our understanding of the specific characteristics of proteins of this class. Their molecular weight is somewhat higher than IgG proteins and their sedimentation rate is approximately 8S. They are rich in carbohydrate and do not fix complement. It is of particular interest that IgE forming cells are concentrated in the mucosal system of the nose and respiratory tract as well as the regional lymph nodes, raising the possibility that locally formed IgE may be involved in respiratory allergy. Other types of

antibodies to allergens are also found in the sera of sensitive patients that do not have the unique skin-sensitizing properties and rapidly diffuse away from the site of the injection. These antibodies, which have been termed blocking antibodies, appear to be typical IgG globulins, in contrast to the reagins. They also combine with antigen and may prevent a reaction with the skin-sensitizing antibody.

LYMPHOCYTES AND OTHER IMMUNOLOGICALLY SIGNIFICANT CELLS

Two major classes of lymphocytes are now well documented which differ strikingly in their biologic properties. The B cell is distinguished by the presence of readily detected immunoglobulin receptors for antigen on its surface. Stimulation by antigen as well as certain mitogens cause it to differentiate into a plasma cell which is the primary antibody-producing cell. The T cell, on the other hand, plays a number of very different roles and appears to be much more heterogeneous. At least some of the T cells have specific receptors for antigen on the membrane surface; the nature of these receptors, which are not ordinary Ig, remains one of the challenging questions of immunology today. After stimulation by antigen and certain mitogens such as phytohemagglutinin and concanavallin A, individual members of T cell populations enlarge to blast cells that do not produce antibody but produce a wide variety of factors and mediators that are significant in many immunologic processes. One type, which has been termed helper factor or allogeneic factor, has a significant effect on B cells and their differentiation into antibody-producing cells. Another type, produced by suppressor T cells, has an opposing regulatory function with resulting suppression of B cell activity. Figure 2 illustrates diagrammatically some of the current concepts of these interrelationships, especially involving T cell regulation of B cell differentiation. Another important functional T cell product is the cytotoxic T cell, which specifically attaches to and destroys target cells such as tumor cells in certain instances. These cells, along with a variety of mediators produced by different T blasts, also are involved in other cellular immune reactions such as graft rejection.

A wide variety of other mediators have been described which are released by activated lymphocytes.

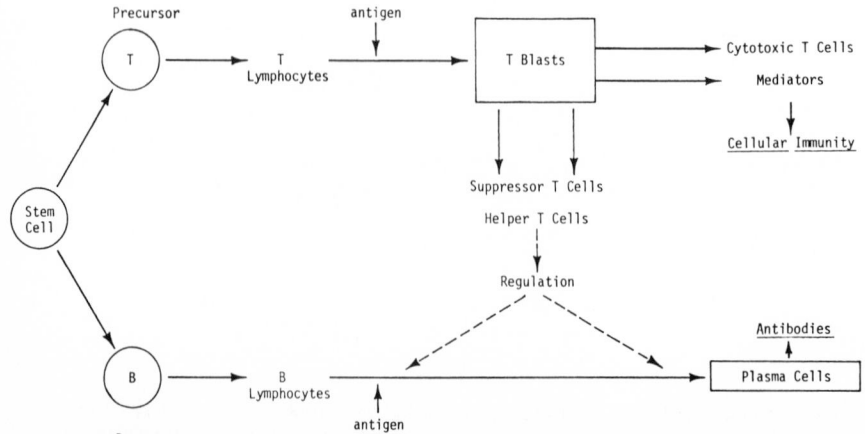

Figure 2. Diagrammatic representation of the development of immunologically active lymphoid cells of the T and B cell types from a common stem cell. Terminal differentiation of B cells to plasma cells producing antibodies and of T cells to T blasts responsible for different aspects of cellular immunity is shown. The regulating effects of T cells and their suppressor and helper functions on antibody production are also illustrated. The significant position of the macrophage in these processes is omitted.

None of these have been isolated, and it is not clear that they all represent different substances. The best known of these is "transfer factor," which is a low molecular weight dialyzable constituent that appears to transfer delayed hypersensitivity to specific antigens from a positive individual to a negative one; sensitivity to tuberculin, to diphtheria toxoid, and to coccidioidin represent three examples out of many that have been studied. Special interest has centered on "transfer factor" because of its potential value in therapy. Patients with various fungal infections, those with immune deficiency disorders, and even cancer patients have been injected with concentrated material prepared from donor lymphocytes in an attempt to produce a cellular immunity that may aid the immune response of these patients. Evidence has been obtained of therapeutic value for "transfer factor," but the final word on its usefulness is not in.

Migration inhibition factor (MIF) is another mediator released by T cells which has been widely studied. It is released in response to antigen and inhibits the migration of macrophages. This is usually measured by determining the diameter of the ring of macrophages moving out of the end of a capillary tube. It has become a widely used assay for the determination of cellular immunity to specific antigens. Other mediators include interferon, lymphotoxin, chemotactin, and skin reactive factor.

The macrophage clearly plays a key role in cellular immunologic reactions. Many aspects of this role remain poorly understood, but it is evident that a number of mediators described above affect the macrophage directly and increase its activity against bacterial or other targets. Evidence is available for the release of a variety of enzymes from macrophages after stimulation. In addition, the macrophage has been shown to play an important role in the interaction of antigen with T cells. Some workers view this as a presentation of antigen which otherwise would not activate the T cell.

Another cell type which appears to have broad significance is the K or killer cell. This cell appears to hold a high affinity for antibody and acts in conjunction with antibody to attack target cells, the so-called antibody mediated lympholysis. At present it is not known whether this is a special type of T cell or whether it represents a third type of lymphocyte. In the past it was confused with the classic cytotoxic T cell. However, it is very different and only acquires target specificity through the antibody with which it functions.

CHARACTERISTICS AND ESTIMATION OF B AND T LYMPHOCYTES

A number of different methods have been developed for differentiating B and T lymphocytes, and some of these provide quantitative results which are of use in assessing these immunologic parameters in diseased individuals. The most characteristic aspect of the B cell is the surface Ig which can be detected readily by a variety of techniques. The most widely used of these is the fluorescent antibody method in which anti-Ig antiserum that is fluorescent is used to stain the Ig on the living cell. Figure 3 illustrates the dot-like staining ob-

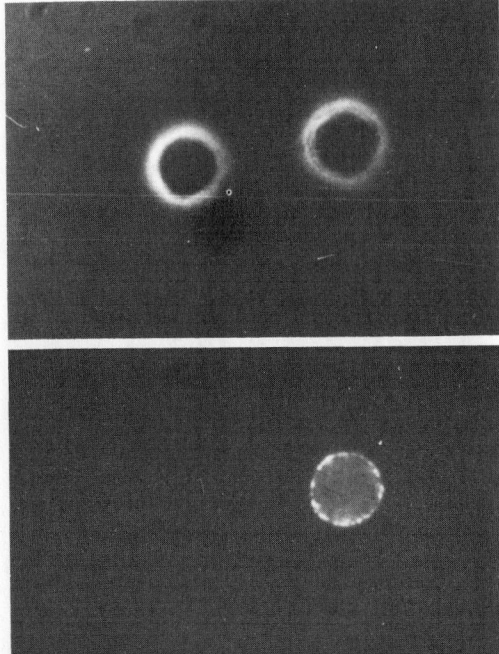

Figure 3. Surface Ig staining by the fluorescent antibody technique of a B type lymphocyte (lower frame). The upper frame shows two lymphocytes by phase contrast microscopy. One lymphocyte of the T type fails to show any Ig.

tained with such an antiserum on the surface of a B cell, whereas a T cell in the same field is entirely negative. This procedure reveals positive staining for Ig on approximately 10 per cent of normal peripheral blood lymphocytes. The Ig is primarily IgM and IgD and has been shown to be synthesized by the B cells. There are, however, numerous pitfalls in this method. The fluorescent antibodies may bind to other cells with Fc receptors, giving falsely high results. Antibodies to T cells may also interfere. These problems usually can be eliminated through the use of fluorescent antibodies in the F(ab')₂ form and through the use of short-term cultures.

Another method for determining B cells stems from the presence of a receptor for the third component of complement which is not found on T cells. Red cells that are coated with antibody and complement form rosettes around B cells, and the number of such rosettes is readily quantitated. A third procedure utilizes the B cell characteristic of reacting with the Fc portion of IgG immunoglobulins. This is a weak interaction, and stable binding occurs only when the Ig is aggregated or is in the form of an immune complex. Large aggregates of IgG are readily visualized by a variety of methods attached to B cells specifically. Other cells than B cells, however, carry the Fc receptor and to some degree the complement receptor, and falsely high values are obtained by these procedures unless these interfering cells are removed. Recently, a new antigen termed Ia has proved extremely useful for determining B cells; rabbit antisera to this component are widely available.

The T lymphocyte in the human can be detected by its selective binding of sheep red blood cells to give rosettes. This is a simple and accurate quantitative method that has come into wide use. The explanation for this useful binding procedure remains obscure. Both thymocytes and peripheral blood T cells give the rosettes. Approximately 85 per cent of blood lymphocytes are positive. Specific antisera that are T cell specific are also available and can be utilized in fluorescent antibody studies or cytotoxic assays to quantitate the T cell population. Results with the antisera usually give a lower percentage figure for blood lymphocytes than is obtained with the rosetting procedure. Specific mitogen stimulation of T cells is also used as an assay of T cell competence. Phytohemagglutinin and concanavalin A are the primary mitogens for this purpose, and the T cell response is measured by determination of the blast cells produced or through the incorporation of tritium labeled thymidine. The advantage of the mitogen procedures is that the functional competence of T cells is determined, rather than just an enumeration of T cells. The disadvantages lie in the difficulty in quantitation and the influence of other cells such as the macrophage in the response.

The *mixed lymphocyte culture* (MLC) reaction is also used as an assay of T cell function. This is usually carried out in a unidirectional system with a known stimulating lymphocyte population that is treated with mitomycin C. The latter reagent prevents these cells from responding but preserves their stimulating potential. The response is measured by the uptake of tritiated thymidine, and cells from different patients can be analyzed in terms of their response. The primary use of the MLC reaction, however, is in histocompatibility testing prior to grafting, in which compatibility is detected through an absence of any response, which is determined primarily by the MLC genes. These appear to differ from the classic HLA genes that are separate but closely linked. Because of the difficulties of the MLC test systems, the different phenotypes are only partially recognized. However, Ia antisera, obtained from pregnancy sera, are rapidly becoming available for a typing system that reflects MLC differences. One of the key developments in experimental immunology has been the delineation of immune response or *Ir* genes which are closely linked to the histocompatibility systems. The genes controlling the Ia (Ir associated) system and the MLC reactions relate closely to the Ir genes as defined in laboratory animals.

Alterations in the level and functional capacity of T and B lymphocytes have been found in a wide variety of diseases. The most striking findings are in the immune deficiency disorders (see Ch. 40.1 to 40.10), and analyses of the lymphocytes that are present are providing new insight into the basic defects. The delineation of a role of excess suppressor cells in certain individuals with immune deficiency represents one of the important developments. In Graves' disease and thyroiditis an increase in T cells and a fall in B cells have been demonstrated clearly. Alterations in Hodgkin's disease, leprosy, cancer, and connective tissue disease have been described. However, these studies are only beginning, and their significance remains to be determined. It is of special interest that the leukemic lymphocytes in the vast majority of cases of chronic lymphatic leukemia are of the B cell type. In acute lymphatic leukemia the picture is more complex. Approximately one third of the cases represent a proliferation of T cells. The remaining cases show a different and interesting new cell type that is not readily classifiable in the T or B category.

DELAYED TYPE OF HYPERSENSITIVITY

Delayed type of hypersensitivity is clearly a reaction of T cells which have been stimulated by antigen to react against targets such as infectious agents, grafts, and tumors. Antibody is not involved in this phenomenon, and disagreement exists among immunologists concerning the role of macrophages. The term "delayed type of hypersensitivity" arose from the delayed skin response of sensitive subjects to antigen; the reaction does not begin for several hours and reaches a maximum after two or three days. The term "cellular immunity" has also been used, although, as mentioned above, some types of cellular immunity also involve antibodies. Two major types of delayed hypersensitivity have been most widely studied: that induced by infection, and the other, termed contact sensitivity, resulting from exposure to a variety of substances ranging from oily resins of plants to simple chemicals employed for domestic, industrial, and medical purposes. Delayed hypersensitivity to autologous antigens has been difficult to demonstrate in humans, although it can be produced in laboratory animals by immunization with autologous antigens.

Delayed-type hypersensitivity is more strikingly evident in certain specific infections such as tuberculosis, brucellosis, lymphogranuloma venereum, mumps, vaccinia, and some fungal infections. Skin tests that depend on this type of cellular immunity have been utilized in these diseases. Tuberculin reactions have been extensively studied in humans and laboratory animals as a model for the delayed type of hypersensitivity. The skin reactivity to tuberculin can be transferred to normal recipients by means of cells from lymphoid tissue, peritoneal exudate, and peripheral blood. In laboratory animals viable cells are required, but in humans the supernatant fluid of disrupted leukocytes can transfer the reactivity. "Transfer factor," mentioned above in the discussion of mediators, represents the active principle involved.

GRAFT VERSUS HOST REACTION. Another probable manifestation of delayed-type hypersensitivity, or at least cellular immunity, is the graft versus host reaction. This has sometimes been termed "homologous disease." Initially it was largely a disorder of laboratory animals that are able to accept foreign bone marrow or lymphoid cells because they have been irradiated or otherwise treated so that these cells are not rejected. More recently it has been encountered frequently in humans who have received certain grafts, particularly bone marrow. The foreign cells react against various antigens in the host animal, resulting in a variety of clinical manifestations. The skin lesions are most characteristic: edema, erythema, and ulceration, followed by thickening, scaling, and loss of hair. Lesions of the joints and of the heart are also observed and these have aroused considerable interest because of certain similarities to those observed in some of the connective tissue disorders. Hemolytic anemia with a positive Coombs reaction has also been described. The possibility has been raised that in certain human diseases immunologically active cells react against the host in a fashion similar to that of the transferred cells in the laboratory animal experiments. The origin of such cells has been ascribed to some type of failure of tolerance mechanisms or to an alteration of host cells through somatic mutation.

SENSITIVITY TO FOREIGN ANTIGENS

Direct sensitivity to foreign antigens, the most common type of potentially injurious immunologic reaction in man, is usually a result of antigenic stimulation by foreign protein or polysaccharide antigens. These may gain entrance to the body through parenteral, oral, respiratory, or other routes. The classic example is serum sickness, usually resulting from the administration of horse or rabbit immune serum. An Arthus reaction is initiated through the direct union of antigen and antibody in the tissue spaces. Precipitates in and around small blood vessels cause secondary damage to cells, or, when antigen is in excess, soluble complexes are formed that may deposit in certain sensitive organs in the blood vessel walls and cause local inflammatory reactions.

In most of the human allergies such as hay fever and food allergy the exact mode of sensitization to external antigens is not directly apparent. Numerous factors such as heredity, intestinal absorption, respiratory secretion, and even emotional state appear involved. In such sensitive or atopic individuals the reaction to foreign antigens is more commonly of the anaphylactic type. Here the binding of antibody to tissue cells appears to play an important role. Local anaphylaxis results from the association or passive absorption of antibodies to local sites that come in contact with antigen. Not all antibodies have this property, and the IgE class is primarily involved. The antigen in turn reacts with the antibody and alters these cells, which then cause the release of histamine and other pharmacologic mediators into the tissue fluid and circulation. In the skin this gives rise to the wheal and erythema at the site of antigen introduction, as in ordinary prick and scratch diagnostic tests. Hay fever and allergic asthma are local manifestations of such reactions. Extensive urticaria may also represent an expression of local cutaneous anaphylaxis.

The antigens involved in these local allergic reactions are a very diversified group. A number have been isolated and partially characterized. The major allergen of *ragweed pollen* has been found to be a protein of approximately 37,000 molecular weight and represents a very small portion of the extractable solids of the pollen. The biologic activity of the isolated material is very high; as little as 10^{-12} grams causes a positive intracutaneous wheal and erythema reaction in sensitive individuals. A highly active protein has also been isolated from the *timothy hay pollen*. Low molecular weight nonprotein allergens have also been isolated. The best example of these is chloragenic acid, which is the active material from castor beans. Just how this is effective is not clear, but the general hypothesis is that it acts as a hapten and combines with body proteins to become a complete antigen. Similar sensitivity to a wide variety of chemicals, particularly those belonging to the group of nitrogenous aromatic substances, has been observed.

The *drug reactions* represent an analogous type of sensitivity that may become manifest in an extremely variable manner. There is a growing awareness of the possibility that sensitivity to unknown foreign materials may play a role in a variety of diseases that at present remain obscure or have been classified as possibly autoimmune in nature. Particular insight into a variety of mechanisms of immunologic cell injury has been gained from the study of the sensitization caused by drugs, particularly quinidine. In some persons thrombocytopenic purpura is the result of such sensitivity; in others it is a hemolytic anemia. It now appears that this effect is primarily the fortuitous result of the physical characteristics of the antibody produced. If the antibody is of low molecular weight, it forms a type of antigen-antibody complex with quinidine that has a particular predilection for platelets; if it is of high molecular weight, complexes are formed on union with the drug that affect primarily the erythrocytes. Complement is also intimately involved in the different effects. This system illustrates the vagaries involved in the selective action against individual target organs and may be of importance in consideration of disorders of unknown origin such as idiopathic thrombocytopenic purpura and "autoimmune" hemolytic anemia. The possibility of involvement of unknown foreign antigens, particularly haptens, is not excluded.

It has become increasingly evident that many antigens gain entrance into the body via the intestinal tract through the consumption of *food*. This has been demonstrated best for bovine milk proteins, and antibodies to a wide variety of these proteins have been found in the serum of many children and some adults. Clear precipitin reactions between bovine protein fractions and these human sera are readily observed. Usually, apparently, no ill effects result from these antibodies despite the fact that some bovine products that remain antigenic continue to gain entrance into the circulation. However, this is only one example of an antibody response to food products; many others must exist that may have important implications in, for example, certain of the intestinal disorders of unknown origin such as ulcerative colitis.

A somewhat different but very important type of reaction to foreign antigens is that produced by maternal-infant incompatibility in which the foreign antigen is introduced from the fetus. *Hemolytic disease of the newborn* is the outstanding example in which the mother produces antibodies that cause destruction of the erythrocytes in the fetus or newborn. The incompatibility leading to such effects may involve Rh antigens or those of the ABO system. Analogous phenomena have been described for leukocytes and platelets. Cytolytic or cytotoxic reactions occur in which complement is usually but not always necessary to effect the cellular damage. Many other antigens are probably involved in similar maternal-infant incompatibility, but the extent to which they lead to disease is not clear at present. One outstanding example that has become manifest recently is that for genetic types of gamma globulin. A high percentage of infants who lack the genetic gamma globulin character of the mother develop antibodies. These usually appear at approximately the sixth month after delivery and may remain throughout the life of the individual. Antibodies to IgA globulins appear to have special significance with regard to transfusion reactions. Most of these appear in individuals who lack all IgA in their serum and probably arise either through maternal immunization or through the administration of blood products.

Another indirect type of reaction to foreign antigens involves antigenic cross-reactions between such antigens and autologous tissues. In this situation an immune response is stimulated by a foreign antigen such as a bacterium, but since a constituent of the organism is antigenically similar to a constituent of the host the immune reaction damages the host tissue. Such cross-reactions have been identified, but the exact role of this mechanism in disease remains to be determined; the possibility exists that presumed autoimmune reactions may be initiated in certain instances by such foreign stimuli. Evidence has been obtained that material from the cell wall of hemolytic streptococci is related antigenically to human cardiac myofibers and the smooth muscle of blood vessel walls. This finding has led to the hypothesis that the cardiac damage of rheumatic fever thus results secondarily from the immune response to the streptococcal infection that preceded it.

SENSITIVITY TO AUTOLOGOUS ANTIGENS

It has become amply clear that many persons develop immunologic reactivity against autologous tissue antigens, but the mechanism by which this sensitivity arises remains obscure. In some instances it may be through the reaction to an unknown foreign organism that contains antigens, particularly polysaccharides, that cross-react with similar polysaccharides in the body tissues. In other instances it may arise through tissue breakdown with release of antigens into the circulation that are ordinarily buried and not subject to the usual tolerance mechanisms. Recent studies in laboratory animals indicate that autologous proteins such as gamma globulin readily become antigenic through slight alteration of the molecule. Antibodies are produced to new determinants not ordinarily exposed but, in addition, as immunization continues, additional antibodies may be produced that involve the native configuration of the protein and will react directly.

One of the best examples of autosensitization in human disease is that found in thyroiditis. There are many features that remain poorly understood, but the evidence is overwhelming that the various degrees of lymphadenoid change in the thyroid gland, particularly in Hashimoto's disease, involve some type of immune reaction against antigens in the thyroid gland. The fact that similar lesions can be produced in laboratory animals by immunization with autologous thyroid antigens lends strong support to such a view. Even in laboratory animals it remains unclear whether some type of cytotoxic antibody or a cellular autoimmunity plays the dominant role in the tissue injury.

In Goodpasture's disease antibodies reactive with autologous antigens of basement membranes have been demonstrated. These react primarily with renal and pulmonary tissues and have been eluted from these diseased organs obtained at autopsy. Clear evidence of a pathogenic role of the basement membrane antibodies in the renal disease of these patients has been obtained. The antibodies eluted from the human kidneys produce glomerulonephritis in monkeys after infusion. The evidence for a role in the pulmonary disease of these patients is more indirect. It has been demonstrated that antibodies eluted from the lung fix to renal glomerular basement membrane, and antibodies eluted from the kidney fix to pulmonary membranes. The origin of these antibodies remains obscure. Similar antibodies also appear to be involved in a few cases of idiopathic glomerulonephritis.

In many blood diseases antibodies occur in the serum that react with autologous cells and in some instances clearly produce disease. The cold agglutinin syndrome is perhaps the clearest from the standpoint of the effect of the abnormal antibody in producing erythrocyte destruction. Anemia, jaundice, and hemoglobinuria can all be traced directly to the action of the cold agglutinin. An "idiopathic" type of the syndrome and one associated with histiocytic lymphoma and lymphocytic lymphoma frequently show IgM bands that represent the cold agglutinin. These relate closely to the bands in Waldenström's macroglobulinemia and probably do not arise as a result of antigenic stimulation. Another type of disease that is usually of shorter duration follows viral or mycoplasmal pneumonia. Paroxysmal cold hemoglobinuria of the Donath-Landsteiner type is closely related and usually is associated with prenatal syphilis, although many nonsyphilitic cases have been reported. The much more common idiopathic, acquired hemolytic anemia of the warm antibody type presents a more obscure picture. Here the relationship of the erythrocyte damage to a variety of red blood cell antibodies is much more tentative. Only in a minority of cases can the antibodies be shown to have a definite specificity. In these instances it is directed against an Rh antigen, usually anti-e. Few clues are available concerning the origin of these gamma globulins that react with autologous erythrocytes.

Idiopathic thrombocytopenic purpura is another disease in which circulating antibodies react with autologous cells — in this case platelets — and cause disease through the resulting cellular injury. These antibodies have proved surprisingly difficult to detect by conventional immunologic methods, but it is now clear that they are present. The role of leukocyte autoagglutinins as a cause of leukopenia has proved even more difficult to assess. Many of the antibodies reported by early workers have been shown to result from transfusions given to these patients, with the production of isoantibodies. However, recent work indicates that autoagglutinins do occur and are responsible for some cases of leukopenia.

Systemic lupus erythematosus (SLE) is probably associated with a greater variety of antibodies with autospecificity than any other condition. The best known of these are the antinuclear antibodies, certain of which are responsible for the LE cell phenomenon. Special interest has centered on the DNA antibodies because of evidence for an association with disease activity. Antibodies to native double-stranded DNA as well as antibodies specific for the single-stranded form are found in the sera of these patients. Recently antibodies to double-stranded RNA have been detected. It has become evident that antibodies to a wide spectrum of polynucleotides are uniquely present in this disease. Numerous additional antibodies to protein and carbohydrate antigens extracted from the cytoplasm as well as the nucleus of human cells have been described. Some of these appear to be responsible for various secondary manifestations of the disease as, for example, hemolytic anemia. This is associated with a positive Coombs test, suggesting the occurrence of antibodies to autologous erythrocytes. Idiopathic thrombocytopenic purpura, probably involving antiplatelet antibodies, also occurs in these patients. Abnormalities involving blood coagulation have been of special interest to investigators; antibodies to specific clotting factors appear to be involved. The origin of these many antibodies as well as others not discussed remains obscure. Some of them appear to represent a marked elevation of antibodies found at low levels in normal persons, which is compatible with the concept that in SLE a general hyperreactivity of the immune system exists. The new concept that this situation might result from a deficiency of suppressor T cells has received some experimental support. The high prevalence in females and the familial trend of the disease have not as yet been fitted into the immunologic concepts. Recent work with various strains of mice, particularly the New Zealand NZB strain, has shown that manifestations of a disease with many features resembling SLE occur in a high proportion of the animals. Most striking are the renal disease and the hemolytic anemia. This experimental model shows a marked similarity to the human disease, and the unique antibodies to double-stranded DNA and RNA are present. Studies in these mice have suggested a significant role for secondary viral infections in potentiating various disease manifestations. Whether this also applies to the human disease remains to be proved.

The possibility has been considered that a large number of other diseases in which the cause is unknown may have as their origin some type of autoimmune mechanism. This is particularly true of *rheumatoid arthritis,* primarily because it is associated with uniquely high incidence and levels of an unusual group of antibodies called rheumatoid factors. These have been clearly demonstrated to be antibodies to gamma globulin and are capable of reacting with autologous gamma globulin. No evidence is available to suggest that the rheumatoid factors play a direct role in the arthritis; however, many workers think they may be indicative of an as yet undefined immunologic reaction. The fact that they are produced at least in part in the synovial tissue of the joints from local accumulation of plasma cells adds some weight to this concept. On the other hand, it has also become clear that the rheumatoid factors could develop as a response to some type of foreign organism. Antibodies to the organism after reaction with the particulate antigen or fragment thereof would form secondary anti–gamma globulins to these antigen-antibody complexes. This possibility has been strengthened by the experimental production of anti–gamma globulins in rabbits after injection of coliform organisms, as well as their appearance in human sera after various types of infection. In bacterial endocarditis, for example, the rheumatoid factors disappear after elimination of the organism with antimicrobial therapy. Similar attempts with such therapy in rheumatoid arthritis patients is without effect on the rheumatoid factors. The accumulated evidence indicates that there must be some profound immunologic stimulus present in the rheumatoid arthritis patient to sustain the rheumatoid factors at the extreme levels often observed and for the prolonged periods in which they are present. The nature of this stimulus remains unknown.

Another disorder showing profound immunologic abnormalities associated with arthritis similar to that in rheumatoid arthritis is *Sjögren's syndrome.* It also has been considered a possible connecting link between rheumatoid arthritis and SLE. Extreme elevation of gamma globulin similar to that found in SLE patients is observed along with many similar antinuclear and anticytoplasmic antibodies. In addition, the vast majority of these patients have rheumatoid factors, often at extreme levels. Serologically they show the findings of both rheumatoid arthritis and SLE. The lesions observed in the lacrimal, salivary, and other glands of patients with Sjögren's syndrome are highly suggestive of a local immunologic reaction. They closely resemble those observed in the thyroid gland in chronic thyroiditis, in which an immunologic alteration has been more evident.

The immunologic aspects of *pernicious anemia* are of considerable interest. Antibodies to intrinsic factor have been demonstrated in a large number of cases, and antibodies to the parietal cells of the gastric mucosa are frequently found. These have been revealed by a variety of classic immunologic procedures. In addition, the intrinsic factor antibody inhibits labeled B_{12} absorption in tests in vivo. Many of the antibodies appear to be autoantibodies and are found in untreated cases; others appear to represent antibodies to hog intrinsic factor as a result of therapy. A direct role in the pathogenesis of the disease has not been established, but they at least are important in certain therapeutic considerations.

It has been known for a number of years that the serum of patients with *myasthenia gravis* contains a number of unusual antibodies directed to muscle constituents. The idea that this disease might be autoimmune in nature was widely held. Recently, however, definitive evidence on this score has come forward. The surprising finding was made that injection of the acetylcholine receptor of the electric eel into rats as well as other species produced specific antibodies to the receptor and a myasthenia syndrome. This also has now been done with acetylcholine receptor from mammals and the disease transferred by antibody. In addition a large amount of evidence has accumulated indicating that patients with myasthenia gravis have similar antibodies that relate to disease exacerbations. It thus appears that a specific antibody that reacts with the receptor and blocks its function causes the disease manifestations.

Antibodies with autospecificity of various types have been found in a variety of other diseases. In ulcerative colitis, antibodies to colon tissue and cellular immunity to colon cells have been described. Patients with liver disease show a wide variety of antibodies to autologous cell constituents. Antibodies reactive with mitochondria are of special interest because of their specific occurrence in primary biliary cirrhosis. They are of diagnostic value, but a pathogenic role remains to be demonstrated. Pancreas antibodies have been described in patients with pancreatitis, and adrenal antibodies in patients with Addison's disease. In all these instances the major possibility that these represent antibodies secondary to tissue breakdown in the disease has not been excluded. As stressed earlier, autoantibodies are far more common than had previously been thought, and any assessment of an injurious role in a specific disease is extremely difficult.

IMMUNE COMPLEX DISEASE

When artificially made antigen-antibody complexes are injected into laboratory animals, they are deposited in a number of organs with resultant tissue injury. By far the most sensitive organ is the kidney, and acute and chronic renal disease has been produced in a number of species by this procedure. The complexes are trapped in the glomeruli and form lumpy deposits along the glomerular basement membrane. These have distinct histologic characteristics by electron microscopy and by fluorescent antibody staining techniques. In human glomerulonephritis similar deposits are frequently observed when these same procedures are utilized. In systemic lupus erythematosus such deposits in the glomeruli are particularly striking, and a large accumulation of additional evidence for antigen-antibody complex mediated renal injury is available.

Extensive studies in a number of different laboratories have demonstrated that DNA–anti-DNA complexes represent one type involved in SLE. Antibodies to DNA aroused considerable interest when they were first described in SLE approximately 17 years ago. However, they were relegated to the position of scientific curiosities, and it has only been recently that their harmful potential has been realized. Antibodies to double-stranded DNA have special significance because double-stranded DNA antigens can appear in the circulation as a result of tissue breakdown; antigen-antibody complexes are formed with fixation of complement and deposition in the most vulnerable organ, the kidney. Elution of antibody from isolated glomeruli of diseased kidneys has proved to be a very effective technique for the detection of antibodies deposited in the kidney. DNA antibody has been found in such eluates at specific concentrations as high as 1000 times those in the serum. DNA antigen has also been demonstrated in the granular deposits observed in the glomeruli. Other, more indirect evidence such as the close clinical relationship among the appearance of DNA antibodies, serum complement depression, and exacerbations of disease has also aided in establishing the significance of the DNA system. Other immune complex systems also have been demonstrated in certain of these patients, including IgG–anti-IgG, SDNA–anti-SDNA, and ribonucleoprotein–anti-ribonucleoprotein. Their exact role, as well as that of other undetermined complexes relative to the native DNA system, remains to be established. SLE, has clearly become the prototype of immune complex renal disease.

Another type of renal disease in which evidence for immune complexes is rapidly accumulating is that associated with various types of drugs. Some of these may present a picture very analogous to that of serum sickness; in others, chronic drug administration may lead to a slowly progressive glomerulonephritis. The latter situation is well illustrated in the case of penicillamine. Numerous instances of nephritis have been reported after long-term administration of this material for the treatment of cystinuria, Wilson's disease, or rheumatoid arthritis. Granular deposits of gamma globulin and complement, along the glomerular basement membrane are readily visualized in fluorescent antibody studies which closely resemble those produced in experimental animals by injection of complexes.

The presence of granular and "lumpy" deposits of gamma globulin and complement detected by fluorescent antibody techniques may be well visualized in renal biopsy specimens and have been found in a variety of different conditions such as malaria, bacterial endocarditis, and thyroiditis. Cases of chronic glomerulonephritis of unknown cause frequently show such a pattern. However, supporting evidence for specific antigen-antibody complexes is as yet unavailable for most of these. In poststreptococcal nephritis similar characteristics of complex-induced nephritis are present, and suggestive evidence for streptococcal antigens in the deposits has been obtained.

Eluates obtained from glomeruli isolated at autopsy from kidneys of patients who had subacute and chronic glomerulonephritis have in a number of instances shown high concentrations of gamma globulin. This appears to represent specific antibody, but its nature remains a mystery. The search is on in a number of laboratories for specific antigens that might react with such gamma globulin. Particular attention is being paid to various human viruses, because recent work in laboratory animals has demonstrated complexes of virus and antibody in the kidneys of mice. The task is a difficult one, however, and human tissue antigens, bacterial antigens, and even unknown drugs may be equally reasonable candidates. The possibility also seems likely that multiple antigen-antibody systems are involved in the different cases of idiopathic glomerulonephritis.

Another type of antigen-antibody complex that appears to be involved in some types of renal disease is that composed of IgG globulin and anti-IgG globulin. Such complexes are widely distributed in human sera and reach unusual levels in rheumatoid arthritis. Usually these are quite soluble, but in some patients they precipitate out in the cold as mixed cryoglobulins. Patients with such mixed cryoglobulins show a rather ill-defined clinical syndrome, but renal lesions are common. The components of such complexes along with complement have been identified in the glomeruli of these patients.

Evidence has been obtained that injury to circulating cells, particularly platelets, may be mediated by antigen-antibody complexes. A number of drug-induced thrombocytopenias fall into this category. Particular interest is currently centered on similar mechanisms in the joint inflammation of SLE and rheumatoid arthritis. Gamma globulin complexes are well known in the latter, and high concentrations have been observed in joint fluid, in which they appear to be involved in local complement depletion. Much work remains before a direct cause-and-effect relationship can be established. Lack of an adequate experimental model similar to those available for immunologic renal injury has hampered progress in this field. The recent introduction of a variety of sensitive methods for the detection of immune complexes in serum should facilitate progress in this area. One result that already is clearly of interest is the frequent detection of immune complexes in cancer patients, offering new approaches for the difficult area of human tumor immunology.

Benacerraf, B. (ed.): Immunogenetics and Immunodeficiency. London, MTP, 1975.

Dixon, F. J., and Kunkel, H. G. (eds.): Advances in Immunology, Vols. 23 and 24. New York, Academic Press, 1976.

Fudenberg, H. H., Stites, D. P., Caldwell, J. L., and Wells, J. V. (eds.): Basic and Clinical Immunology. California, Lange Medical Publications, 1976.

Möller, G. (ed.): Autoimmunity and Self-Nonself Discrimination. Transplantat. Rev. 31:1, 1976.

39. COMPLEMENT

Jeffrey A. Gelfand

GENERAL CONSIDERATIONS

The complement system is composed of a series of circulating inactive precursor proteins which, upon activation, mediate and amplify inflammatory and host defense reactions. Observations in the late 1800's led to the description by Pfeiffer and Bordet of a serum factor that would lyse cholera vibrios in combination with a specific heat-stable immune factor (antibody). This lytic factor was inactivated by heating to 56°C, and lytic activity was restored by the addition of nonimmune, fresh serum. Ehrlich and Morganroth hypothesized that antibody was necessary for the binding of the lytic factor, which they called *complement*. It is now known that this "factor," complement, is in reality a cascade of sequentially activated proteins following two major pathways of activation which merge to form a final common pathway that produces the majority of biologic effects. There have now been identified at least 15 major component proteins, as well as 5 inhibitor proteins which modulate complement reactions. Furthermore, one of these sequences, the alternative pathway, appears to function in the absence of specific antibody. This pathway contains its own primitive recognition system, being directly activated by such foreign, non-mammalian structures as repetitive polysaccharides and lipopolysaccharides. It appears to function as an "early warning system," being triggered to a variable degree by bacteria and fungi. Earlier work focused on the ability of complement to lyse antibody-sensitized erythrocytes. It is now apparent that cell lysis is not the only biologic function of complement. Opsonization, blood-stream clearance, the release of neutrophils from the bone marrow, chemotaxis of leukocytes, virus neutralization, antigen processing, histamine release, smooth muscle contraction, increased vascular permeability, and blood clotting may all be produced or enhanced by complement activation. These functions can serve to protect the host, or to produce host tissue damage. Human complement has even been identified as a necessary factor for the successful penetration and parasitization of human erythrocytes by a pathogenic protozoan, *Babesia rhodhaini*, which causes babesiosis (see Ch. 199). Finally, complement-mediated lysis of coronaviruses, virus-transformed cells, and other tumor cells may be important in immune surveillance against malignancy.

COMPLEMENT ACTIVATION. Complement activation is characterized by the conversion, in sequential fashion, of circulating precursor proteins into active ones. Some components undergo conformational changes, whereas others undergo limited proteolytic cleavage. Such changes in turn either render the component enzymatically active or complex it to a structure. A smaller fragment may be split off in the process, usually with phlogistic properties.

The classic complement pathway was the first elucidated. The components were numbered, in order of discovery, C1 to C9. Unfortunately, this did not turn out to completely correspond to the reaction sequence, hence some confusion. Components of the more recently described alternative pathway or properdin pathway are now, by convention, given capital letters (factor B

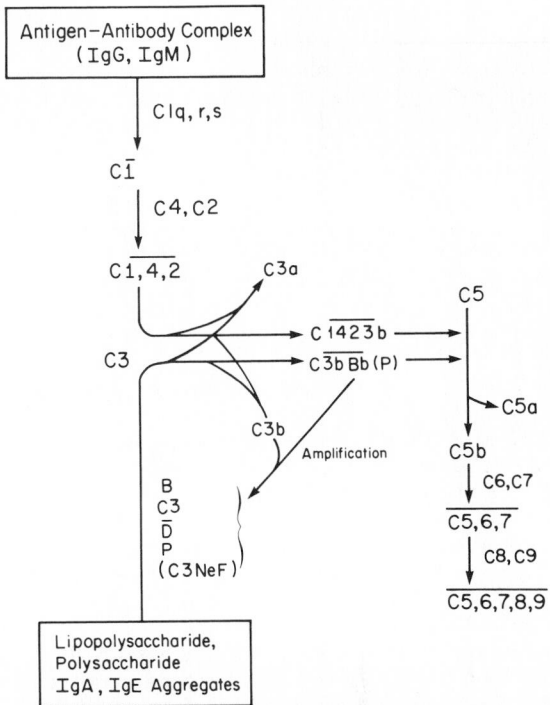

The pathways of complement activation.

or B, properdin or P). Activation of a component is indicated by a bar ($\overline{B}$ or $\overline{C1}$). Cleavage products are usually given the letter "a" for smaller, fluid phase products, whereas larger, complex-bound products are designated "b" (e.g., C5a, C5b, Bb). Further cleavage products may be termed "d," "e," and so on. An exception is C2, in which the complex-bound larger fragment is termed C2a. The pathways of activation are shown in the accompanying figure.

THE CLASSIC PATHWAY. Activation of the classic pathway occurs in the presence of antigen antibody complexes. IgG1, IgG2, IgG3, and IgM antibodies activate the classic pathway; IgA, IgD, and IgE do not.

Biologic Functions of Complement Components and Cleavage Products*

C1	Aggregates with antigen antibody complexes; combines directly with some viruses
C4b	Virus neutralization; binds to receptors on cells
C2 fragment	Kinin-like activity
C3b	Opsonic fragment; receptors for this fragment identified in neutrophils, monocytes, B lymphocytes, eosinophils, erythrocytes, renal glomeruli; cooperates in antigen processing, lymphocyte transformation
C3 fragment	Release of neutrophils from bone marrow
C3a	Anaphylatoxin (histamine release from mast cells, smooth muscle contraction, increased capillary permeability); chemotactic factor†
C5a	Anaphylatoxin (histamine release from mast cells, smooth muscle contraction, capillary permeability); chemotactic factor
C5b67	Chemotactic factor; may attach to unsensitized cells
C8	Incomplete membrane lesion, "slow leak"
C9	Complete membrane lesion, "fast leak"

*Adapted from Frank, M. M., and Atkinson, J. P.: Complement in clinical medicine. Disease-a-Month, January 1975.

†The role of C3a as a chemotactic factor is not certain.

Usually two IgG molecules fixed to antigen and in close proximity are required for C1 activation, whereas the pentameric IgM molecule does not require such a "doublet." This results in much more efficient complement activation by IgM. If one considers membrane-associated antigens on an erythrocyte, it would obviously take both spatially close antigenic sites and enough antibody to array two IgG molecules together in order to produce complement fixation with IgG.

Recent evidence suggests that C-reactive protein (CRP) can function analogously to immunoglobulin to activate the classic pathway. CRP is an acute phase serum reactant present in trace amounts in normal serum that can bind to the C-polysaccharide of the pneumococcus or other charged surfaces, and then bind and activate C1.

C1 circulates as a trimolecular complex of C1q, C1r, and C1s whose association is calcium dependent. C1q attaches to the Fc region of the antigen-bound antibody molecule, and undergoes a conformational change. This activates sequentially C1r and C1s. Activated C1 ($C\bar{1}$) has enzymatic activity (as an esterase), and proteolytically cleaves its substrates, C4 and C2, thereby creating a new cell-membrane associated complex $C\bar{1}, \bar{4}, \bar{2}$. The C42 moiety of this complex has proteolytic activity, and is termed the C3 convertase. C3 convertase splits C3 into C3a, with anaphylatoxin and possible chemotactic properties, and C3b which may be cell bound or released into the fluid phase. The bound C3b associated with the C3 convertase now becomes an enzyme that cleaves C5, termed C5 convertase. C5 is cleaved into C5b, which attaches to the cell membrane and begins the "membrane attack" sequence. C5a is released into the surrounding medium, where it effects potent chemotactic and anaphylatoxin activity. C5b binds C6 and C7, forming $C\overline{5b67}$, which can dissociate from the cell membrane. It is a chemotactic factor itself, and can attach to unsensitized cells. Cell bound $C\overline{5b67}$ will bind C8 and C9. The C5-9 complex produces holes in the cell membrane, presumably by disrupting the lipid bilayer. Exactly how this lesion is produced is not yet completely agreed upon, but it appears that $C\overline{5-8}$ opens a small channel only intermittently, whereas $C\overline{5-9}$ permanently opens a larger channel in the cell membrane, ultimately producing osmotic lysis of the cell target cell.

THE ALTERNATIVE PATHWAY. In 1954, a series of observations by Pillemer, Lepow, and associates led to the formulation of the existence of an antibody-independent system of complement activation. This was termed the properdin system, from the Latin *perdere* (to destroy). It represented a novel concept in theories of nonspecific host resistance to infection, as well as a radical departure from prevailing dogma about the requirement for specific antibody to activate complement. Although some of the details of what is now termed the alternative pathway are still unsettled, it is clear that the basic hypothesis of Pillemer is correct. Polysaccharides and lipopolysaccharides of bacteria and fungi, aggregated IgA, IgE, IgG, and even radiographic contrast media and renal dialyzer cellophane have been demonstrated to activate complement by this pathway. In the presence of these and possibly other initiating factor(s), factor $\bar{D}$, factor B, and C3b can form an alternative pathway C3 convertase, $C\overline{3bBb}$, which is stabilized by properdin (P). C3b produced by this convertase or the C42 convertase can continue to act as an

autocatalyst producing more C3 convertase with subsequent C3-C9 activation and its biologic effects. This is termed the "amplification loop." An IgG autoantibody with anti-$C\overline{3bBb}$ specificity, termed C3 nephritic factor (C3NeF), has been found in some patients with membranoproliferative glomerulonephritis and in patients with partial lipodystrophy. This factor stabilizes $C\overline{3bBb}$ in a manner analogous to P, thereby promoting complement consumption. It does not appear to be present in normal sera.

The interrelatedness of the two pathways can be appreciated when one considers that (1) C3b generated in the classic pathway can be "recruited" to enter the alternative pathway amplification loop; (2) C1 activation in animals congenitally deficient in C4 (and hence classic pathway activity) activates the alternative pathway; (3) antibody appears to increase the efficiency of alternative pathway activation; and (4) although the classic pathway is generally considered antibody dependent, recent reports indicate that viral nucleic acids can directly activate C1 and subsequent classic pathway components, in the absence of antibody. The activation of C1 by CRP bound to the C-polysaccharide of pneumococci is an additional example of antibody independent classic pathway activation.

MODULATION AND CONTROL OF COMPLEMENT ACTIVATION. Complement activation is regulated physiologically by the decay of unstable intermediates (i.e, $C\overline{3bBb}$), the formation of unstable binding sites on the molecule (the binding of C3b to the cell surface), and the function of inhibitor proteins. There are currently at least five. C1 inhibitor (C1INH) inhibits the activated C1, an esterolytic enzyme. Deficiency in the amount of function of this inhibitor can be inherited or acquired, the former producing hereditary angioedema, the latter a similar acquired syndrome.

There is an inhibitor of C3b and the alternative pathway, C3b inactivator (C3bINA). This protein proteolytically degrades C3b into biologically less active subcomponents. It also inhibits the activity of C4b. Deficiency of C3bINA results in unchecked alternative pathway activation via the amplification loop, with resultant C3 consumption and the biologic consequences of C3 depletion. There is an additional inhibitory protein directed against C3b, the C3b inactivator accelerator (A-C3bINA, or β-1H globulin, for its electrophoretic mobility). This protein binds to C3b of the alternative pathway convertase, displacing properdin factor B. It does not affect immune adherence.

A C6 inactivator (C6 INA) has been demonstrated. Its physiologic significance is unknown. Finally, the anaphylatoxins C3a and C5a are inactivated by a carboxypeptidase, anaphylatoxin inhibitor (AI).

BIOLOGIC FUNCTION OF COMPLEMENT. Complement may be critical in facilitating or mediating host defense and inflammatory reactions. Complement activation by either the classic or alternative pathways results in the formation of C3a and C5a, which have potent anaphylatoxin and chemotactic factor activity (the latter activity of C3a is controversial). Chemotactic factor directs the migration of leukocytes into the site of infection or inflammation. The anaphylatoxin activity increases local capillary permeability, permitting egress of yet more antibody and complement into the site. The next contribution of complement is to phagocytosis. Complement was identified in the 1930's as an opsonin, a serum factor facilitating phagocytosis. Initial descriptions noted the requirement for antibody, but the properdin system of Pillemer suggested an antibody-independent opsonic system.

The dramatic discovery in the late 1960's of the existence of receptors on leukocytes for immunoglobulin and complement has enabled a more integrated view of humoral, phagocytic, and cell-mediated immune mechanisms. *Immune adherence*, the adherence of complement-sensitized particles to receptors on primate erythrocytes, had been described earlier, but its biologic function was unknown. It is now known that receptors for C3b, the major opsonic fragment, exist on neutrophils, monocytes and macrophages, eosinophils, B lymphocytes, and erythrocytes. Receptors for other complement fragments have been described; the significance of these is as yet unknown. It now appears that receptors provide a specific "latching" mechanism that enables the cell to contact and hold on to a specific opsonic particle. These receptors could help clear the bloodstream of complement (or immunoglobulin) sensitized microbes, immune complexes, or even host erythrocytes (as in autoimmune hemolytic anemia). Phagocytosis is facilitated, and antigen processing by macrophages is thus enhanced. An additional provocative discovery was provided by the demonstration of receptors for complement (C3b) in the human renal glomerulus. Pathologic studies revealed an inverse correlation between the degree of C3b deposition in specimens and the ability to demonstrate C3b receptors, suggesting that these receptors were "occupied" in the pathologic samples with C3 deposition. The possibility that these receptors are involved in the pathogenesis of some forms of glomerulonephritis is obvious, although highly speculative at present.

In addition to phagocytosis, complement may play a role in host defense by enhancing virus neutralization by antibody or, independently of antibody, by the alternative pathway. Complement-mediated bacterial lysis had been thought to be relatively unimportant until the recent discovery of gonococcal sepsis associated with deficiency of C6 or C8. This suggested at least some role for bacterial lysis in host defense.

As previously noted, complement may play a role in immune surveillance against malignancy. Alternative pathway lysis of lymphoma cells, and classic pathway lysis of tumor cells have been described.

The functions of complement may also produce host damage. The direct effects of opsonic, anaphylatoxin, and lytic activities, plus those produced by chemotactic factor–attracted leukocytes, may cause tissue inflammation and destruction.

The clearance of erythrocytes in autoimmune hemolytic anemia, lysis of paroxysmal nocturnal hemoglobinuria cells (PNH-cells), various forms of glomerulonephritis (e.g., systemic lupus erythematosus, poststreptococcal, membranoproliferative), joint disease (lupus, rheumatoid, gout) and perhaps septic shock involve complement-mediated damage. The reader is directed to the appropriate chapters of this text and several excellent reviews for details.

INTERACTIONS WITH OTHER SYSTEMS. The complement system interacts with the coagulation, fibrinolytic, and kinin systems. Plasmin can activate C1 and cleave C3b from C3, thereby enabling C3b to enter the amplification loop of the alternative pathway. C1 inhibitor (C1INH) blocks the effects of activated Hageman factor in initiating both coagulation and fibrinolysis, as well as directly inhibiting factor XI and plasmin. C1INH also blocks the effects of kallikrein kinin generation.

GENETICS AND METABOLISM. Recent evidence suggests that the genes controlling synthesis of C2, C4, C8, and properdin factor B are on chromosome 6, closely linked to the major histocompatibility complex (HLA) and to a region regulating lymphocyte responsiveness. The remaining complement loci are on other chromosomes or have not yet been identified.

The sites of synthesis of various components have been investigated. Current evidence suggests that C1 synthesis takes place primarily in intestinal epithelium, although even macrophages and fibroblasts have been reported to produce C1 in vitro. The liver appears to be the major synthetic site for C3, C6, C9, and C1 inhibitor. C2, C4, and C5 appear to be produced by macrophages.

The metabolism of complement has been studied, and those components investigated have a high turnover, in the range of 1 to 2.5 percent of the plasma pool per hour. C2 and C4 production by macrophages can be increased by exposing these cells to killed pneumococci, and C3 synthesis is increased by challenge with bacterial endotoxin. There is evidence to suggest that alternative pathway activation of C3 in membranoproliferative glomerulonephritis may result in decreased synthesis of C3. Finally, there may be hormonal modulation of the production of some complement components and their inhibitors. Evidence suggests that C4 levels in mice and C1INH levels in humans may be increased by androgens.

COMPLEMENT TESTS. The clinical assays for complement either involve a determination of the amount of antigenic (complement) protein present in serum or fluid or measure the ability of that fluid to support a complement-mediated function. An example of the latter is the total hemolytic complement titer, or CH_{50}, which measures the ability of a fluid to produce lysis of sensitized sheep erythrocytes. All nine components (C1 to C9) must be present to support lysis. Decreases in individual components affect the resultant titer to a variable degree — a 70 per cent fall in the C4 level may barely affect the CH_{50}, for example. The individual components may also be tested in lytic assays, as well as immunoprecipitation tests. Care must be taken in the handling of samples. Functional titers may fall, whereas C3 antigen levels may actually rise in "aged" serum. Finally, immunofluorescence may be used to detect the involvement of complement in reactions in tissue.

COMPLEMENT AND DISEASE

HEREDITARY COMPLEMENT DEFICIENCY DISEASES. Homozygous complement deficiencies are fortunately relatively rare. Homozygous C2 deficiency is the most common of these, and has an incidence of approximately 1:10,000. Several generalizations can be made regarding hereditary deficiency states. Deficiencies of C1, C4, and C2 may be associated with connective tissue disease syndromes, most notably an "SLE-related syndrome" described by Agnello and others. Components of this syndrome may include vasculitic rash, arthritis, and glomerulonephritis. Antibodies to single-stranded DNA, rheumatoid factor, and a positive C1q precipitin test may be present in these patients. C3 deficiency may result in recurrent severe pyogenic infections, whereas deficiency of terminal components C5-C8 may result in increased susceptibility to infection, particularly with *Neisseria gonorrhoeae* and *meningitidis*. This is presumably due to defective bacteriolysis.

Deficiency of C3b inactivator (C3bINA) has already been mentioned. In the absence of C3bINA activity, C3b autocatalytically continues to activate the alternative pathway "amplification loop," and C3 deficiency occurs, with attendant susceptibility to infection. Inherited C$\overline{1}$ inhibitor deficiency, caused by either decreased synthesis or synthesis of an inactive inhibitor protein, produces hereditary angioedema (HAE). HAE is manifested by recurrent episodes of swelling of the face, extremities, abdominal viscera, or airway, the last of which may produce asphyxiation (see Ch. 47). Uninhibited C$\overline{1}$ results in consumption of C4 and C2. C2 cleavage produces a fragment with kinin-like activity. Androgens have been used successfully to increase C1INH levels, with therapeutic success.

There are no known inherited deficiencies of alternative pathway components. C3bINA deficiency depletes this pathway. C3 nephritic factor (C3NeF), an IgG anti-C3bBb antibody, occurs in association with membranoproliferative glomerulonephritis and partial lipodystrophy. Alternative pathway activation and decreased C3 levels are seen. Finally, patients with sickle cell disease have been shown to have defective alternative pathway–mediated opsonization. Evidence suggests that these patients are deficient in factor B. The cause for this association with hemoglobin SS is unknown.

ACQUIRED ABNORMALITIES. The involvement of complement in many inflammatory and host defense reactions will predictably result in a variety of serum patterns of complement activation. Furthermore, complement levels have been determined in cerebrospinal, joint, pleural, pericardial, and even subcutaneous fluids. However, several generalizations can be made. In diseases involving circulating immune complexes, C1, C4, C3, and the CH$_{50}$ may be lowered. These levels may fall before the actual clinical exacerbation which occurs, for example, in systemic lupus erythematosus (SLE) and serum sickness. Joint fluid may reflect the same pattern, and levels of C1, C4, C3 and the CH$_{50}$ are diminished in SLE and rheumatoid arthritis (although serum levels are normal in the latter).

Alternative pathway activation has been noted in a variety of situations, notably gram-negative sepsis, in which it may participate in the shock syndrome, and membranoproliferative glomerulonephritis.

It is important to stress that the determination of complement levels either antigenically or functionally yields a result which represents the vectorial sum of the processes of synthesis and consumption. Either or both may be involved in a given pathologic state, and "complement levels," whether normal or abnormal, must be interpreted with caution.

Agnello, V.: Complement deficiency states. Medicine 57:1, 1978.
Alper, C. A., and Rosen, F. S.: Clinical applications of complement assays. Adv. Intern. Med., 20:61, 1975.
Cameron, J. S., Vick, R. M., Ogg, C. S., Seymour, W. M., Chantler, C., and Turner, D. R.: Plasma C3 and C4 concentrations in management of glomerulonephritis. Br. Med. J., 3:668, 1973.
Colten, H. R.: Biosynthesis of complement. Adv. Immunol., 22:67, 1976.
Frank, M. M., and Atkinson, J.P.: Complement in clinical medicine. Disease-a-Month, January, 1975.
Gelfand, M. C., Shin, M. L., Nagle, R. B., Green, I., and Frank, M. M.: The glomerular complement receptor in immunologically mediated renal glomerular injury. N. Engl. J. Med., 295:10, 1976.
Gigli, I.: Control mechanisms of the classical and alternate complement sequences. Transplant. Proc., 6:9, 1974.
Ruddy, S., Carpenter, C. B., Chin, K. W., Knostman, J. N., Soter, N. complement metabolism: An analysis of 144 studies. Medicine, 54:165, 1975.

40. THE PRIMARY IMMUNODEFICIENCY DISEASES

Robert A. Good

40.1. INTRODUCTION

Knowledge of the lymphoid cells, their functions, and their organization into two separate major immunity systems has advanced rapidly in recent years. Current views are summarized in Table 1. Understanding of the immunity functions has derived in considerable measure from study of the primary immunodeficiencies of man. In turn, new knowledge and understanding of the relation of structure to function in the lymphoid system have made possible better definition of the several primary immunodeficiencies. A continuing interplay between clinical analyses and advancing basic understanding of immunity and the immunologic apparatus represents a fine model of how progress in medicine can proceed most rapidly to the maximal benefit of humanity. Consequently, study of the primary immunodeficiencies has had importance to medicine in recent years far beyond the numerical frequency of patients who suffer from these relatively infrequent diseases.

In Table 2 is a listing of those diseases currently recognized by a WHO expert panel as the major primary

TABLE 1. The Cellular Basis of Immune Responses

T cell system:			
Thymus-dependent T lymphocytes*	$\xrightarrow{\text{+PHA or Con-A†}}$	Blast cells	
	$\longrightarrow$	Killer cells (e.g., graft rejection)	Cell-mediated immunity
	$\xrightarrow{\text{+antigen}}$	Soluble lymphocyte factors	
B cell system:			
Thymus-independent, "bursa-equivalent" B lymphocytes	$\xrightarrow{\text{+antigen}}$	Plasma cell line	Humoral antibody synthesis

*There is evidence that T cells plus antigen can cooperate with B cells to produce antibody.
†Phytohemagglutinin or concanavallin.

TABLE 2

Type	B Cells (a)*	B Cells (b)†	T Cells	X-linked	Autosomal Recessive	Other§
X-linked agammaglobulinemia	X	(X)‡		X		
Thymic hypoplasia			X			X
Severe combined immunodeficiency	X	(X)	X	X	X	X
With dysostosis	X	?	X		X	
With adenosine deaminase deficiency	X		X		X	
With generalized hematopoietic hypoplasia	X		X		X	
Selective Ig deficiency						
IgA	?	X	(X)			X
Others		?				X
X-linked immunodeficiencies with increased IgM		X		X		
Immunodeficiency with ataxia telangiectasia		X	X		X?	
Immunodeficiency with thrombocytopenia and eczema (Wiskott-Aldrich syndrome)			X	X		
Immunodeficiency with thymoma	X*		X			X
Immunodeficiency with normo- or hypergammaglobulinemia	X	X	(X)			X
Transient hypogammaglobulinemia of infancy		X				X
Varied immunodeficiencies (largely unclassified and common)	X	X	(X)		(X)	X

*Absent or very low.
†Easily detectable or increased.
‡Some cases with circulation B-lymphocytes without detectable surface Ig have been found.
§Implies multifactorial or unknown genetic basis or no genetic basis.

immunodeficiencies of man. Included in Table 2, as well, is an effort to analyze each of the diseases in terms of its genetic basis and in terms of the types of cells primarily involved in the deficiency. Such an analysis must be recognized as ephemeral because of the rapidity of development of our knowledge and because rapid changes in understanding continue. Nevertheless, for the present these several diseases can be usefully viewed in light of this classification.

40.2. X-LINKED INFANTILE AGAMMAGLOBULINEMIA

Soon after Bruton initially described agammaglobulinemia in an eight-year-old boy, groups of patients, including multiple cases in several families, were studied in Boston, Minneapolis, and New York. From these studies, one form of agammaglobulinemia could be clearly established as being of sex-linked nature. This form has been called the Bruton type of agammaglobulinemia in recognition of the monumental contribution of the pediatrician who discovered the first of the pri-

mary immunodeficiencies and associated diseases with absence of gamma globulin in the blood. Bruton's discovery launched a period in which immunology has been maximally influenced by the "experiments of nature" represented by the several forms of primary immunodeficiency.

X-linked agammaglobulinemia is a disease in which fully developed B lymphocytes and plasma cells are absent from blood and bloodforming tissues. Production of immunoglobulins and synthesis and secretion of antibodies are grossly deficient or lacking altogether. Figure 1 represents a characteristic immunoelectrophoretic pattern comparing normal with agammaglobulinemic patients. Figure 2 compares an antigen-stimulated lymph node from a normal person (A) and a stimulated node from an eight-year-old aggamaglobulinemic child (B). Absence of germinal centers and absence of plasma cells characterize the node of the agammaglobulinemic patient. Plasma cells are not found anywhere in the body. Even the lamina propria of the intestinal tract and exudates of chronic inflammatory processes such as bronchiectasis are devoid of plasma cells in these patients.

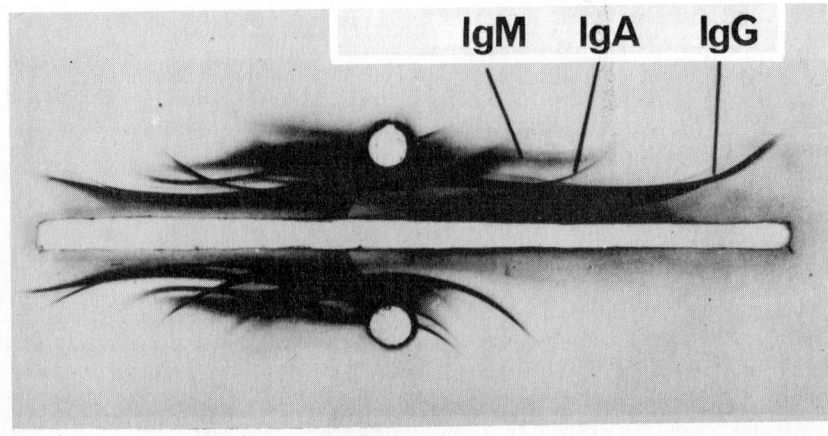

Figure 1. Normal immunoelectrophoretic pattern (above) compared with immunoelectrophoretic pattern from a patient with X-linked infantile agammaglobulinemia. Note absence of demonstrable IgM, IgA, and IgG on the immunoelectrophoretic pattern.

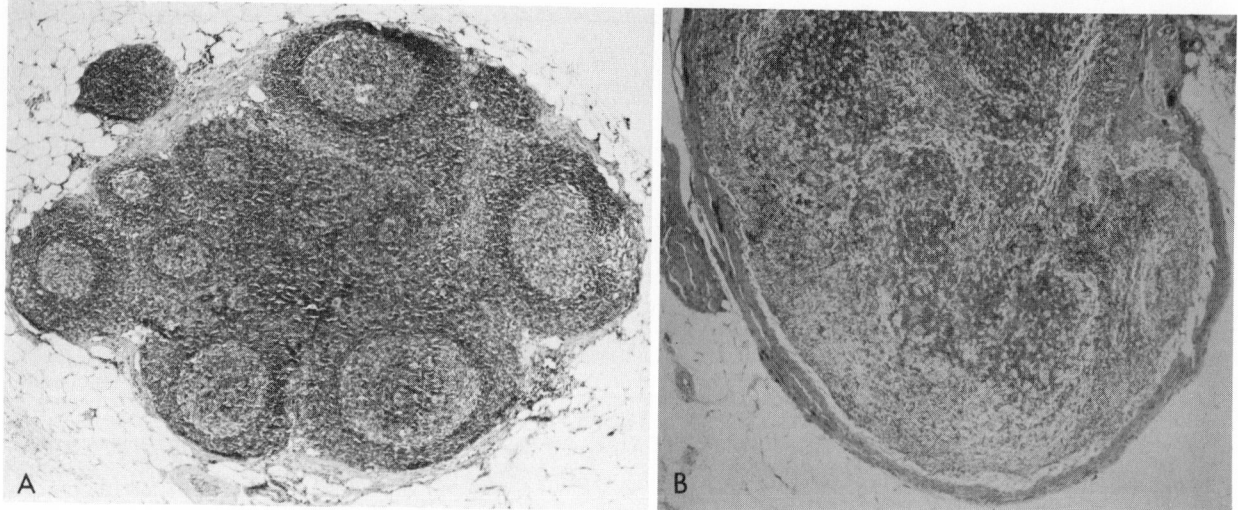

Figure 2. Comparison of normal lymph node (*A*) and lymph node of patient with X-linked infantile agammaglobulinemia (*B*) after antigenic stimulation. Note abundant germinal center formation in the normal node and absence of germinal centers in the stimulated node from the agammaglobulinemic patient.

Clinically, children with X-linked agammaglobulinemia are normal at birth, but during the second half of the first year of life they begin to have infections with the encapsulated, virulent pathogens such as pneumococci, *Hemophilus influenzae*, and *Pseudomonas aeruginosa*. Infections in these children usually respond well to appropriate drug therapy; but because of lack of humoral immunity, resistance to these infections is minimal. Untreated, the bacterial infections spread rapidly, and recurrent episodes of pneumonia, otitis, sinusitis, dermatitis, meningitis, and osteomyelitis are characteristic. By contrast, these patients seem able to resist well many other infections such as tuberculosis, histoplasmosis, and fungal and viral infections. Herpes, vaccinia, chickenpox, measles, paralytic poliomyelitis, and hepatitis, however, are unusually frequent in these children. Leukemia may also occur with inordinate frequency.

Even though immunoglobulins are virtually absent in serum and antibody synthesis is minimal or absent altogether, cell-mediated immunities, including delayed and contact allergies, are normal. Skin allograft rejection occurs with nearly normal vigor. Specific delayed allergic reactions can be transferred from the agammaglobulinemic child to an immunologically normal person, using large numbers of peripheral blood lymphocytes. Modern techniques for studying the peripheral blood lymphocytes reveal that X-linked agammaglobulinemia may be heterogeneous. The majority of patients with this disease are completely lacking B lymphocytes, as defined by the presence of readily demonstrable immunoglobulins at the cell surface. Recently, an early stage of B lymphocytes featured by cytoplasmic Ig but no surface Ig has been described in the bone marrow of patients with this disease. This interesting evidence that an early stage of B lymphocytes is present in the bone marrow needs confirmation because of its fundamental significance. In these patients T cells are somewhat increased in number, and one finds in the blood a third population of lymphocytes whose origin and exact nature are not absolutely clear. The latter may possess receptors for the third component of complement and also receptors for the Fc portion of the IgG molecule.

Diagnosis is established by analysis of the immunoelectrophoretic pattern of serum and by quantitation of each of the several immunoglobulins, using the Manchini radioimmunodiffusion or other suitable immunochemical analyses. IgM, IgA, IgD, and IgE are regularly absent, and IgG is absent or present in extremely low concentrations, 100- to 1000-fold less than that of normal persons.

Treatment involves early detection and intensive and specific treatment of the bacterial infections, as well as prophylaxis using gamma globulin concentrates injected intramuscularly at frequent intervals. Injections of 0.6 ml per kilogram of 16 per cent gamma globulin solution given intramuscularly every two weeks is a good regimen with which to start prophylactic management. Exudative enteropathy is a common complication and is often due to infestation with *Giardia lamblia*. This infection and the exudative enteropathy can be treated specifically with metronidazole. The usual immunizations may be given, although no antibodies will be formed. Although vaccinia has been tolerated, it is recommended that no live virus vaccines be used in any patient with primary or secondary immunodeficiency disease.

40.3. DiGEORGE'S SYNDROME

Counterpart to patients with X-linked agammaglobulinemia are those born without a thymus who as a consequence lack T lymphocytes in their blood and tissues. Such patients also frequently have no parathyroids. Their ears are often of abnormal appearance, and they have a characteristic facies with prominent forehead and bowed mouth. Frequently, they also have abnormalities of the first portions of the great vessels and the outflow tract from the heart. Absence of thymus is not always complete. Absence of thymic shadow on chest roentgenograms and absence of T lymphocytes and T lymphocyte functions on immunologic analysis are characteristic. The stimulated lymph nodes show well developed far cortical areas, and in some cases germinal centers are present. In other cases, germinal centers have been deficient. In all instances, the thymic dependent lymphoid areas are very grossly depleted. Plasma cells are present and may be present in normal numbers in the lymphoid tissues. The number of B lymphocytes in the blood and lymphoid tissues is usually increased. Absence of thymus and T lymphocytes may be incomplete. Treatment of the endocrinopathy requires appropriate use of vitamin D and sterol therapy to raise serum calcium level. The immunodeficiency has now been repeatedly treated successfully, using transplantation of thymus obtained from allogeneic embryos. This form of treatment has in several instances seemed to correct completely the deficiency of T lymphocytes and the defects of immunologic functions. With the appearance and increase of T lymphocytes, B lymphocytes decrease in number. Failure of thymus and T cell development of nude mice represents an autosomal recessive defect that seems to be an experimental counterpart of DiGeorge's syndrome. The cause of the human disease is unclear, and a genetic basis has not yet been established for this rare disease in man. Selective deficiency of thymus and T lymphocyte development without the associated hypoparathyroidism or great vessel anomalies has been called Nezelof's syndrome. This disease has also apparently been treated successfully by allotransplantation of fetal thymus.

40.4. SEVERE COMBINED IMMUNODEFICIENCIES
(SCID, Swiss Type Immunodeficiency)

Several different genetically determined primary immunodeficiency diseases in which both T and B lymphocyte systems fail to develop normally have now been described. Each of these diseases is genetically determined. Forms with either autosomal recessive or X-linked inheritance have been defined. Infants with each of these distinct forms of severe combined immunodeficiency disease have very gross deficiencies of both T and B immunity systems. Lymphocyte numbers, generally under 1000 per cubic millimeter, are low, but these cells are usually not absent from blood. Both T and B lymphocytes are either missing or very much reduced. Levels of all classes of immunoglobulin are low.

The thymus, lymph nodes, and spleen are small and poorly developed. Indeed, these lymphoid organs are often almost completely devoid of lymphoid cells. Antibody production and development of cell-mediated immunities are extremely deficient or absent, and lymphocytes fail to respond to phytomitogens such as phytohemagglutinin, concanavalin A, and pokewood mitogen in vitro. In some of these children, responses of blood leukocytes to stimulation with allogeneic cells have been noted.

If these patients are not treated, they regularly succumb early in life to any of many different forms of infection, i.e. *Pneumocystis carinii*, cytomegalovirus, other viruses, fungi, or low- or high-grade bacterial pathogens. Live virus immunization often leads to lethal infections. Attempts to help these children, or children with DiGeorge's syndrome, by blood transfusion often leads to death from fulminating graft-versus-host disease, because these patients cannot defend themselves against the immunologically competent lymphocytes invariably present in whole blood. If blood or blood products must be given, they should be given only after irradiation of well oxygenated blood with 1500 to 3000 r or after freezing and centrifugation.

Since both B and T immunity systems are lacking in these children, attempts have been made to correct the immunodeficiency by transplantation of bone marrow. In more than 50 instances, marrow transplantation from an appropriately matched sibling donor has made possible apparently complete restoration of both T and B immunity systems in these children. Whenever definitive markers have been available, it has been possible to establish that the new immunity systems in such marrow-reconstituted children have been derived from the bone marrow cells of the donor. For successful marrow transplantation, a sibling donor selected by HLA tissue typing and mixed leukocyte culture matching has generally been necessary.

More recently, however, in absence of a matched sibling, a satisfactory matching of a kinship donor by mixed leukocyte reaction with an SCID child has permitted reconstitution of immunity function by bone marrow transplantation. Techniques have been developed which promise sufficient matching, even among unrelated persons, to permit reconstitution of the two missing immunity systems in such patients by marrow transplantation with a donor selected from the general population. In one such instance, correction of the immunodeficiency has been successful. Fetal liver transplantation, using livers from fetuses of less than 12 weeks' gestation, has also been used to correct the cellular deficiencies in this disease. Recently, treatment of a few patients with severe combined immunodeficiency by cultured human thymus transplantation has been reported. Definitive diagnosis and immunologic reconstitution of the rare children with this disease are highly technical undertakings that should be done only by those who specialize in this therapeutic approach.

40.5. SEVERE COMBINED IMMUNODEFICIENCIES WITH ADENOSINE DEAMINASE DEFICIENCY

An autosomal recessive, genetically determined disease similar to the severe combined immunodeficiency disorders described above has recently been found to be associated with absence of the enzyme adenosine deaminase (ADA) in red blood cells, lymphoid cells, and other cells of the body. Patients lacking nucleoside phosphorylase or inosine phosphorylase who have severe combined immunodeficiency (SCID) have also been described. Clinical manifestations, immunodeficiencies, cellular defects, and susceptibility to infection in this disease are all similar to those occurring in the X-linked and autosomal recessive forms of SCID in which ADA is normal, except that, quantitatively, the functional and cellular defects seem more variable.

Approximately 15 per cent of all patients with SCID lack the enzymes ADAse, nucleoside phosphorylase, or inosine phosphorylase. In the patients with SCID and adenosine deaminase deficiency, however, some lymphoid tissue development does occur, and the thymus contains Hassall's corpuscles and has characteristics of an involuted rather than an underdeveloped thymus. Patients with ADA deficiency and SCID have repeatedly been reconstituted by marrow transplantation.

The relationship between ADA deficiency and this form of SCID is not yet clear, but it is of great interest that three forms of SCID can now be associated with an inherited inability to produce an enzyme. Whether the immunodeficiencies are due to some toxic product consequent to the enzyme deficiency or whether the enzymes are essential for some crucial step in development of the lymphoid cells remains to be determined. When the immunodeficiency associated with ADA deficiency is corrected by marrow transplantation, the lymphoid cells possess normal amounts of adenosine deaminase, but the red cells continue to lack the enzyme completely. In one instance, administration of the normal enzyme in the form of red blood cells from a normal donor has led to remission of the disease. In this patient the disease and lymphoid abnormality reappeared when the ADA-carrying red blood cells were lost.

40.6. THYMOMA WITH IMMUNODEFICIENCY

More than 50 patients have been studied in which broadly based immunodeficiency, thymoma, and hypogammaglobulinemia have been associated. The first such case provoked the extensive laboratory inquiry which established the major role played by the thymus in developmental immunobiology. Both cellular and humoral immunity functions and both T and B cell numbers are deficient in such patients. They are susceptible to a broad range of bacterial, viral, and fungal infections. In one such infection encountered by Siegal et al., normal serum possessed a factor that permitted the patient's lymphoid cells to develop in vitro into B lymphocytes with readily demonstrable surface immunoglobulin. This factor was absent from the blood or serum of the patient with the thymoma-agammaglobulinemia syndrome. Red cell aplasia or hypoplasia may sometimes be associated. Some patients with the thymoma-agammaglobulinemia syndrome appear to lack both the marrow lymphoid cell precursor of the B cell line, B lymphocytes, and plasma cells. Removal of the thymus tumor, which is composed primarily of nonlymphoid, spindle-shaped stromal epithelial cells, does not correct the immunodeficiency. The bone marrow of several of these patients has been studied and found not to contain the B cell precursor lymphocyte that appears to be present in the bone marrow in Bruton's agammaglobulinemia.

40.7. COMMON VARIABLE IMMUNODEFICIENCY

Among the most frequent forms of primary immunodeficiency diseases is that presently called the common variable immunodeficiency. This rather cumbersome term is used as temporary nomenclature for what may indeed be several different diseases. However, in this form the immunodeficiency is variable from time to time in the same patient and from patient to patient in the same family. Inheritance may be autosomal recessive or autosomal dominant. In still other patients the disease is sporadic, and because of its onset later in life has been thought to be acquired. The initial agammaglobulinemic patient described by Bruton probably would now be classified with this group.

Immunodeficiency in these patients is associated with decreased concentration of all or several immunoglobulins. Antibody production is feeble, and even cell-mediated immunity responses may be decreased. Pneumonia, sinusitis, otitis media, gastrointestinal infection and malfunction, and *Giardia lamblia* infestation are common concomitants. A wide variety of autoimmune phenomena and autoimmune diseases have been frequently encountered. Pernicious anemia, histamine-fast achlorhydria, and gastric cancer occur with high frequency early in life in patients with this syndrome.

The occurrence in these patients of much autoimmunity, autoimmune disease, e.g., Coombs-positive hemolytic anemia, autoimmune thrombocytopenic purpura, pernicious anemia, and many collagen-vascular or mesenchymal diseases, including rheumatoid arthritis and vasculitis, has represented a set of fascinating but perplexing relationships. Sprue-like syndrome with or without giardiasis is frequent.

Diagnosis is made by history of frequent and persisting infections, immunoelectrophoretic pattern, and quantitation of each of the immunoglobulin classes by radial immunodiffusion. Enumeration of T and B lymphocytes is of interest because, in spite of deficiencies in producing immunoglobulins, most of these patients have normal or only slightly reduced numbers of B lymphocytes in the circulating blood. Plasma cells are deficient in the lymphoid tissue in direct proportion to the deficits of antibody production and immunoglobulin levels. In patients possessing normal or increased amounts of IgM who have low levels of IgG and IgA, lymph nodes, spleen, and intestinal lymphatic tissue may be grossly enlarged. Germinal centers may be extraordinarily hypertrophied, suggesting the erroneous diagnosis of follicular lymphoma. Waldmann discovered that some patients with the common variable immunodeficiency have lymphocytes which suppress differentiation of B lymphocytes to plasma cells that synthesize and secrete Ig. Whether these suppressor cells are responsible for the pathogenesis of hypogammaglobulinemia, as proposed, has not yet been established. At present writing the best indications are that in a few instances these suppressor cells are pathogenetically crucial, but in most instances they are not. It is of interest that such suppressor cells have also been seen in patients with Bruton-type agammaglobulinemia, in which it seems unlikely that they are responsible for the immunodeficiency.

Treatment, as in other forms of primary immunodeficiency, involves early recognition and specific antimicrobial therapy of the frequent bacterial infections. Careful diagnosis and specific treatment of *Giardia lamblia* and fungal infections are also important. Prophylactic administration of gamma globulin concentrates in very large doses, 0.6 ml per kilogram every three to four weeks, is helpful in reducing the frequency of infections in some patients. However, in these patients even more than in patients with Bruton's X-linked infantile agammaglobulinemia, prophylaxis with currently available preparations of gamma globulin is often inadequate. More satisfactory prophylaxis has sometimes been achieved using frequent infusions of plasma from carefully selected donors free of history of hepatitis and free of both Australia antigen and antibody to Au antigen. The latter precaution is extremely important, because chronic progressive hepatitis has been an especially difficult and sometimes lethal consequence of administration of blood products to these patients. What is needed are adequate preparations of gamma globulin concentrates that are suitable for intravenous administration.

In addition to the more specific forms of therapy, prophylactic regimens such as those introduced by Mathews for the ideal pulmonary toilet in patients with cystic fibrosis are helpful. Postural and positional pulmonic drainage, breathing exercises, and inhalation therapy have all been helpful in treating and apparently in preventing pulmonary disease in these patients. The autoimmune diseases should be treated as they are in persons of greater immunologic vigor, but with cognizance of the fact that the patients are immunologically compromised and that large doses of adrenal steroids, immunosuppressive agents, and splenectomy can further debilitate the bodily defense.

40.8. ISOLATED ABSENCE OF IMMUNOGLOBULINS — SELECTIVE DEFICIENCY OF IgA

Selected absence of any of the immunoglobulin classes or subclasses can occur, and such selective deficiencies have already been described for several, e.g., selective absence of IgG2. However, none of the other immunoglobulins are so frequently lacking from blood as is IgA. The frequency of selective absence of IgA ranges from 1:700 to 1:3000, according to studies of blood bank donors from several parts of the world. Many patients lacking IgA seem to be quite healthy, but a high proportion have severe atopy, autoimmune phenomena, and autoimmune diseases. Respiratory disease is frequent, especially in those patients who possess IgE. Gastrointestinal disease is also frequent, and severe progressive sprue has been reported. Soothill and his associates have observed that classic atopy caused by production of antibody of IgE class occurs with particular frequency when the IgA system is slow to develop. One possible basis for the increased frequency of autoimmune phenomena and disease with deficiency of IgA is that the dimeric form of IgA antibodies is transferred across the epithelial barrier onto the gut surface from the site of production in the lamina propria of the gastrointestinal tract. This local antibody system normally provides a barrier to absorption of foreign proteins and other antigens. Consequently, when the local immunity system is lacking or is deficient, antigens that are cross-reactive with host constituents can be absorbed and provide excessive stimulation of the remaining systemic immunity systems. This stimulation leads to production of antibodies and immune cells that in some instances cross-react with host constituents, producing autoimmune phenomena and autoimmune disease. In keeping with this view, patients lacking IgA frequently develop antibodies to IgA, serum proteins of the bovidae, and many other antigens in food and flora in amounts far in excess of those produced by normal persons. Most patients who fail to produce IgA antibody have in their circulation at least normal numbers of B lymphocytes that produce and have at their surface IgA molecules. For reasons currently poorly understood, these cells do not differentiate to IgA-secreting plasma cells. If these cells could be induced to develop to B cells capable of secreting IgA, these patients might be much improved. Wu et al., using pokeweed mitogen, and Waldmann et al., using blast forms of putative T lymphocytes obtained from patients with Sézary's syndrome (presumably T-cell leukemia), have induced such differentiation of these IgA-producing B lymphocytes to IgA-secreting plasma cells. Some patients who fail to secrete IgA have circulating lymphocytes that inhibit differentiation of IgA secreting plasma cells. It has not been established whether these class-specific suppressor lymphocytes are of pathogenetic significance in IgA deficiency.

40.9. IMMUNODEFICIENCY DISEASES WITH ATAXIA TELANGIECTASIA AND WISKOTT-ALDRICH SYNDROME

Immunodeficiency diseases also accompany the Wiskott-Aldrich and ataxia telangiectasia syndromes. The former is a disorder of X-linked inheritance that is featured by a clinical triad, including eczema, thrombocytopenic purpura, and increased susceptibility to infection. The immunodeficiency in this syndrome is accompanied by low levels of IgM. These patients form antibody poorly to certain antigens, especially polysaccharide and small protein antigens, and show a progressive deficiency of T cell numbers and functions. The basic genetic fault is unknown, but the patients frequently succumb to infection with any of several viruses, bacteria, or fungi. Nearly 10 per cent of patients with the Wiskott-Aldrich syndrome die of cancer. Usually, but not always, the cancer takes the form of lymphoreticular sarcoma. Bleeding, especially accompanying infection, and intracranial bleeding are also frequent causes of death in these children. Treatment has generally been unsatisfactory, but platelet transfusions and plasma infusions from selected donors have been helpful in some instances. This disease has now been successfully treated by immunosuppression with alkylating agents and/or total body irradiation followed by bone marrow transplantation.

Patients with ataxia telangiectasia (see Ch. 284.5) reflect a familial and autosomal recessive, genetically determined clinical triad of progressive cerebellar ataxia, cutaneous telangiectases, and immunodeficiency. In this disease the thymus fails to develop normally and retains an embryonic appearance. T lymphocytes and T cell functions are regularly grossly deficient, and some 70 to 80 per cent of the patients lack IgA. IgE also is frequently absent from the circulation in both ataxia patients and healthy family members. These patients are troubled with frequent sinopulmonary infections, which seem to be related to the deficiency of IgA but not clearly to the deficiency of IgE.

More than 15 per cent of the patients with ataxia telangiectasia thus far studied have developed malignancies. The malignancies reported are predominantly reticulum cell sarcomas, lymphosarcomas, leukemias, and gastrointestinal cancers. Waldmann found that alpha-fetoprotein is present in inordinately high concentration in a majority of patients with ataxia telangiectasia. Chromosomal abnormalities, especially involving chromosome number 14, have been described, and this disease has been classified with the chromosomal instability syndromes along with Fanconi's anemia and Bloom's syndrome. How the immunodeficiency and chromosomal instability are related is not certain at present, but it seems likely that both the great susceptibility to certain forms of cancer in these patients and the immunodeficiency syndrome are in some way a function of the chromosomal dysmetabolism. Patients with Wiskott-Aldrich syndrome, who suffer from hematologic abnormality, profound immunodeficiency, and great susceptibility to certain malignancies, may also have a chromosomal instability at the base of all the disorders which make up the disease complex.

40.10.   OTHER PRIMARY IMMUNODEFICIENCIES

Many other forms of immunodeficiency have been discovered in recent years, and the diseases and syndromes associated with them are only now being clarified. For example, selective deficiencies of the components of the complement system are associated with serious immunodeficiency in very high frequency. These deficiencies render the patients susceptible to infection, collagen-vascular diseases, overwhelming pneumonia, or skin and bowel infections, depending on which complement component is lacking. Ongoing studies will define these associations more clearly. Some of the complement components such as C2 and C4 and factor B of the alternative pathway are clearly linked in their inheritance to the major histocompatibility region (MHR) of chromosome 6. The immunodeficiencies associated with deficiencies of these components are thus linked as well to the MHR. Hereditary angioedema is a complement component deficiency inherited as an autosomal dominant trait that is associated with absence or abnormality of the inhibitor of the C1 esterase normally present in plasma. The sometimes life-threatening attacks of edema can be aborted by giving normal plasma. Recently, prevention has become possible by treating the patients with anabolic steroids related to testosterone. Such treatment appears to induce the production of normal C1 esterase inhibition by the liver. Untreated patients with C1 esterase deficiency may develop lupus erythematosus or chronic progressive renal disease.

Patients with genetically determined deficiency of C2, which is transmitted as an autosomal recessive trait, besides showing increased susceptibility to infection, frequently develop arthritis, anaphylactoid purpura, lupus erythematosus, or other mesenchymal vascular diseases. The basis for the association of the complement component immunodeficiencies to these as yet poorly understood mesenchymal diseases is not clear but may suggest that infection, probably with a virus, underlies all of them. Similarly, inherited deficiencies of the C1r, C1s, C4, and C5 components of complement predispose to both infection and mesenchymal vascular diseases. C1r deficiency has been corrected by renal transplantation, apparently because the kidney contains cells that produce C1r. Leiner's syndrome has been associated by Miller with an abnormality of C5, and patients with this disorder have been successfully treated by regular injection of normal plasma. Deficiencies of C3 have been associated with inordinate susceptibility to many different kinds of infection and deficiencies of C6 and C7 with increased susceptibility to infections with gram-negative pathogens.

It seems fair to predict that deficiencies of each of the specific proteins involved in the defenses of the body will occur and that diseases will be associated with these deficiencies. Such deficiencies will include deficiencies of each immunoglobulin class or subclass and deficiencies of the essential lymphokines produced by lymphocytes, complement components, and cellular or humoral components of the major effector processes. The latter already include diseases in which malfunction or deficiencies of development of granulocytes occur, as in congenital neutropenia or chronic granulomatous disease. Deficiencies or abnormal function of monocytes or other cells and molecular elements involved in bodily defense are being defined. Each disease will represent an experiment of nature capable of teaching us a new lesson about how the immunity system functions. Each will require treatment, which will be made possible by the advancing knowledge of immunity functions and their organization and development. It is thus to be anticipated that the constructive interplay between clinic and laboratory will continue to produce new knowledge and to test our advancing understanding of the immunologic systems in the bodily defense. Two good illustrations of this developing new knowledge are the chronic septic granulomatous disease of childhood (CGD) and Chédiak-Higashi anomaly. In the former, increased susceptibility to infection with catalase positive microorganisms may be associated with either complete absence of glucose phosphate dehydrogenase or absence of glutathione reductase. Both these disorders are inherited as autosomal recessive traits. The most frequent form of CGD is an X-linked recessive form in which failure to generate the oxidative burst culminating in production of H_2O_2 and bacterial singlet oxygen $'O_2$, superoxide O_2^-, and OH^- radicals has been demonstrated. This disease is associated with absence on leukocytes of the antigen Kx that is associated with production of red blood cell antigens of the Kell system. In still another form of chronic granulomatous disease of childhood, the disease is inherited as an autosomal recessive trait, but no enzyme defect has been identified to date. Any of these immunodeficiency diseases should be correctable by treatment with cyclophosphamide or total body irradiation plus bone marrow transplantation. Recently, a report of major improvement in a patient with CGD, using this approach to therapy, has been presented.

The Chédiak-Higashi anomaly is an abnormality of cellular development in which leukocytes as well as many other bodily cells possess gigantic single membrane-bound particles. The leukocytes in these patients perform poorly in chemotaxis and phagocytosis, probably accounting for the increased susceptibility to infection with which these patients are troubled. Persons with the Chédiak-Higashi abnormality develop malignancies of the lymphoid and lymphoreticular system in very high frequency. These malignancies have been classified as non-Hodgkin's lymphomas, Hodgkin's disease, and reticulum cell sarcomas. The leukocytes of patients with Chédiak-Higashi syndrome have been shown to lack microtubular structure, very likely accounting for their poor performance in chemotactic responses. In most exciting recent research, it has been shown that the microtubular abnormality and functional deficiencies can be corrected by treatment of the cells in vitro with ascorbic acid. In addition, treatment of patients with this disease with ascorbic acid corrects both the deficiency of microtubules in their leukocytes and monocytes and the functional defects of their leukocytes revealed in analyses of chemotaxis and phagocytosis. Further, this dramatic new therapy appears to improve their ability to defind themselves against infection. Whether this treatment will also improve their ability to defend themselves against cancer is still enigmatic, but it is a question that is most intriguing and the answer is urgently awaited.

Because of the multiplicity of cells, proteins, peptides, developmental processes, interactions of systems, biologic amplifications, and complex effector processes that are normally involved in the defense of the body against external and internal invaders, the primary immunodeficiency diseases, once thought to be infrequent or rare diseases, turn out to be quite frequent. Indeed, in the aggregate they are about as frequent as the combination of leukemias, lymphomas, and Hodgkin's disease. Study of these diseases has aided the analysis of deficiencies in immunologic function, which are often called secondary immunodeficiencies. This is important because the secondary immunodeficiencies, being associated with nutritional deprivation, aging, viral, bacterial, and fungal infection, myelomas, leukemias, lymphomas, Hodgkin's disease, sarcomas, carcinomas, infestations, and even endocrine disturbances, represent the most frequent serious diseases of man. Understanding of these defects and development of means to correct them promise to represent truly major therapeutic advances.

Alexander, J. W., and Good, R. A. (eds): Fundamentals of Clinical Immunology. Philadelphia, W. B. Saunders Company, 1977.

Bach, F. H., and Good, R. A. (eds.): Clinical Immunobiology, Vols. 1, 2, 3. New York, Academic Press, 1972, 1974, 1976.

Bergsma, D., Good, R. A., and Finstad, J. (eds.): Immunodeficiency in Man and Animals. Sunderland, Mass., Sinauer Associates, Inc., 1975. (Birth Defects: Original Article Series, Vol. XI, No. 1, 1975.)

Boder, E., and Sedgwick, R. P.: Ataxia-telangiectasia. In Goldensohn, E., and Appel, S. (eds.): Cellular and Molecular Bases of Neurological Disease. Philadelphia, Lea & Febiger, 1973.

Bruton, O. C.: Agammaglobulinemia. Pediatrics, 9:722, 1952.

Cooper, M. D., Faulk, W. P., Fundenberg, H. H., Good, R. A., Hitzig, W., Kunkel, H. G., Roitt, I. M., Rosen, F. S., Seligmann, M., Soothill, J. R., and Wedgwood, R. H.: Meeting Report, Primary Immunodeficiency in Man. Second International Workshop of the WHO Committee. Clin. Immunol. Immunopathol., 2:416, 1974.

Day, N. K., and Good, R. A. (eds.): Biological Amplification Systems in Immunology. New York, Plenum Press, 1977. (Comprehensive Immunology, Vol. 2.)

DiGeorge, A. M.: Congenital absence of the thymus and its immunological consequences. In Bergsma, D., and Good, R. A. (eds.): Immunologic Deficiency Diseases in Man. New York, The National Foundation Press, 1968, pp. 116-121. (Birth Defects: Original Article Series Vol. IV, No. 1, 1968.)

Dupont, B., Anderson, V., Ernst, P., Faber, V., Good, R. A., Hansen, G. S., Henriksen, K., Juhl, F., Killmann, S. A., Koch, C., Müller-Berat, N., Park, B. H., Svejgaard, A., Thomsen, M., and Wiik, A.: Immunological reconstruction in severe combined immunodeficiency with HL-A incompatible bone marrow graft. Donor selection by mixed lymphocyte culture. Transplant. Proc., 5:905, 1973.

Gelfand, J. A., Sherins, R. J., Alling, D. W., and Frank, M. M.: Treatment of hereditary angioedema with danazol. Reversal of clinical and biochemical abnormalities. N. Engl. J. Med., 295:1444, 1976.

Gell, P. G. H., Coombs, R. R. A., and Lachmann, F. J. (eds.): Clinical Aspects of Immunology. 3rd ed. Oxford, Blackwell Scientific Publications, Ltd., 1975.

Golub, E. S.: The Cellular Basis of the Immune Response. Sunderland, Mass., Sinauer Associates, 1977.

Good, R. A.: Studies on agammaglobulinemia. II. Failure of plasma cell formation in bone marrow and lymph nodes of patients with agammaglobulinemia. J. Lab. Clin. Med., 46:167, 1955.

Good, R. A.: Morphological basis of the immune response and hypersensitivity. In Felton, H., et al.: Host-Parasite Relationships in Living Cells. Springfield, Ill., Charles C Thomas, 1957, pp. 68-160.

Good, R. A.: Immunodeficiency in developmental perspective. Harvey Lect., 67:1, 1973.

Good, R. A., and Zak, S. J.: Disturbances in gamma globulin synthesis as experiments of nature. Pediatrics, 18:109, 1956.

Janeway, C. A., and Rosen, F. S.: The gamma globulins. IV. Therapeutic uses of gamma globulin. N. Engl. J. Med., 275:826, 1966.

Lawton, A. R., Wu, L. Y. F., and Cooper, M. D.: The cellular basis of IgA deficiency in humans. In Mestecky, J., and Lawton, A. R., III (eds.): International Symposium on the Immunoglobulin A System, Birmingham, Ala., 1973. New York, Plenum Press, 1974, pp. 373-380. (Advances in Experimental Medicine and Biology, Vol. 45.)

Siegal, F. P., and Good, R. A.: Human lymphocyte differentiation markers and their application to immune deficiency and lymphoproliferative diseases. Clin. Haematol., 6:355, 1977.

Soothill, J. F.: Interactions in immunodeficiency. In Bergsma, D., Good, R. A., and Finstad, J. (eds.): Immunodeficiency in Man and Animals. Sunderland, Mass., Sinauer Associates, Inc., 1975, pp. 50-52. (Birth Defects: Original Article Series, Vol. XI, No. 1, 1975.)

Waldmann, T. A., Broder, S., Durm, M., and Blackman, M.: Regulation of synthesis of immunoglobulins. In Bianchi, R., Mariani, G., and McFarlane, A. S. (eds.): Plasma Protein Turnover. Baltimore, University Park Press, 1976, pp. 265-275.

Waldmann, T. A., Durm, M., Broder, S., Blackman, M., Blaese, M., and Strober, W.: Role of suppressor T cells in pathogenesis of common variable hypogammaglobulinemia. Lancet, 2:609, 1974.

Waldmann, T. A., Broder, S., Krakauer, R., MacDermott, R. P., Durm, M., Goldman, C., and Meade, B.: The role of suppressor cells in the pathogenesis of common variable hypogammaglobulinemia and the immunodeficiency associated with multiple myeloma. Fed. Proc., 35:2067, 1976.

Walker, W. A., Isselbacher, K. J., and Bloch, K. G.: Intestinal uptake of macromolecules: Effect of oral immunization. Science, 177:608, 1972.

41. THE COMPROMISED HOST

John I. Gallin

COMPONENTS OF THE HOST DEFENSES. The host defenses comprise complex and interrelated systems which are outlined in Table 1. Familiarity with these systems provides a basis for the diagnosis and management of patients with compromised defenses.

Physical Barriers. Intact skin and mucous membranes prevent microbial invasion. The skin is a complex organ, consisting of several cell types which, in addition to providing a physical barrier, produce numerous antimicrobial agents such as lactic acid, ammonia, urea, and free fatty acids. These protect the host from superficial challenges. The mucous membrane secretions, which trap inhaled microorganisms, contain soluble factors such as immunoglobulin A, lactoferrin, lysozyme, and α_1-antitrypsin, which have antibacterial activity. Proper function of the nasal and respiratory passage cilia facilitates microbial clearance. In addition, host defenses require normal anatomy of the respiratory, genitourinary, and gastrointestinal symptoms.

Inflammatory Response. The circulating phagocytes (neutrophils, monocytes, eosinophils, and basophils) are the central components of the inflammatory response. The phagocytes are manufactured and undergo maturation in the bone marrow, and upon appropriate

TABLE 1. The Host Defenses

Physical barriers
   Skin
   Mucous membranes
Inflammatory response
   Circulating phagocytes
   Humoral mediators
Reticuloendothelial system
   Fixed phagocytes
Immune response
   T cells (cell-mediated immunity, delayed hypersensitivity)
   B cells (antibody responses)
   Other mediators (i.e., lymphotoxin)

stimulation are delivered to the bloodstream where they circulate and are distributed to local tissue sites. Recruitment of phagocytic leukocytes from the bloodstream involves a complex process called diapedesis or emigration. The initial step of this process is not completely understood but seems to require phagocyte aggregation and adherence to the endothelium. The phagocytic cells migrate between the endothelial cells as they migrate to tissue sites. The availability of the potential space between endothelial cells through which phagocytes migrate is modulated by local tissue products of the complement cascade (the anaphylatoxins, or small molecular weight cleavage products of the third and fifth complement components, C3a and C5a) and the potent vasodilator bradykinin produced by activation of the fibrinolytic and kinin generating systems. The complement cascade and the fibrinolytic and kinin generating systems are activated by microbial products such as endotoxin and a variety of substances secreted by leukocytes, platelets, and fibroblasts. Locomotion of phagocytes requires cell adherence to their substratum, deformability, machinery for random locomotion, and the ability to sense a gradient of a chemical signal (chemotactic factor) and convert random locomotion (kinesis) to directed locomotion (chemotaxis). The locomotory apparatus includes an intact actin and myosin system for movement and an intact microtubule system to stabilize the cell during locomotion and organize the intracellular granules, which are secreted extracellularly during locomotion and appear to be important modulators of the inflammatory process.

The chemotactic factors are humoral mediators and include products from activation of complement (C5a) and activation of the kinin generating system (kallikrein), from neutrophils, macrophages, lymphocytes (lymphokines), and fibroblasts (collagen), as well as oxidation products of certain fatty acids. Some chemotactic factors are highly preferential for particular cell types (i.e., histamine and other mast cell products are preferential for eosinophils, whereas an alveolar macrophage product is preferential for neutrophils). After recruitment, microorganisms that have been rendered palatable by proper opsonization by complement products and immunoglobulins adhere to the phagocyte membrane and then are ingested, killed, and digested. These events require complex biochemical and biophysical events with specific mechanisms for elimination of different classes of microorganisms (see Ch. 493).

Reticuloendothelial System. The reticuloendothelial system is the major system for the clearance of circulating microorganisms from the bloodstream. The main components of the system are the fixed phagocytes, consisting of splenic macrophages, alveolar macrophages, Kupffer cells, lymph node macrophages, and microglial cells in the brain. Many or perhaps all of these macrophages are derived from circulating monocytes which migrate from the bloodstream into tissues, where they differentiate into the fixed macrophages.

The Immune Response. The T and B lymphocytes are the main components of the immune response. T lymphocytes are the functional cells of cell-mediated immunity or delayed hypersensitivity. Mature B cells, or plasma cells, produce antibodies and are the cells of humoral immunity. The thymus gland controls the maturation of the T lymphocytes; factors controlling B cell maturation in humans are not known.

Upon appropriate signal, lymphocytes are released from the bone marrow into the circulation, where they are distributed throughout the body. The mechanism of mobilizing lymphocytes to tissue sites from the circulation is poorly understood but may involve chemotaxis and/or the process of emperipolesis. Emperipolesis is the transport of cells through, rather than between, endothelial cells. At tissue sites lymphocytes perform their specific tasks. The T lymphocytes are believed to be critical in eliminating such pathogens as *Mycobacterium tuberculosis, Histoplasma capsulatum, Candida albicans,* and certain viruses. The B cells respond to antigens (which may first have to be processed by macrophages) by synthesis of the immunoglobulins (antibodies), which have important roles in complement activation, virus neutralization, and opsonization. (For a detailed review of the various components of the immune response, see Ch. 38.)

ETIOLOGY. A host may be compromised as a consequence of extrinsic (environmental) factors or abnormalities of the intrinsic components of the host defense system. Extrinsic factors include conditions that increase the infectious challenges and factors which directly impair host defenses. Examples of the former are overcrowded living conditions, as in military recruit camps where outbreaks of infectious (meningococcal) meningitis are well known; exposure to pathogenic microorganisms from sexual activity; or occupational conditions or hospitalizations with exposure to contaminated equipment used in certain diagnostic or therapeutic procedures. Other extrinsic factors associated with compromised host defenses include protein-calorie malnutrition, thermal injury, alcoholism, irradiation, and depletion of or interference with function of cells involved in host defense by iatrogenic means. Host defense defects can also result from a number of inherited and congenital disorders, as well as from acquired defects associated with numerous diseases. The particular type of infection will depend on the nature of the fundamental defect.

PATHOGENESIS AND PATHOLOGY. Pathologic models in support of predicted abnormalities of host defenses are well described for certain components of the defense system. Other examples are emerging as we understand what parameters are important to assess. Examples related to infection from penetration of the skin are obvious and include penetrating trauma and severe burns.

Mucous membrane secretions are abnormally viscid in cystic fibrosis and mucous plug formation, and obstruction with subsequent pneumonia can result. Mucociliary movement is abnormal in Kartagener's syndrome (situs inversus, chronic sinusitis, and bronchiectasis), and there is evidence that this is related to absence of a particular cilial subunit (dynein arms). Mucous secretion and cilial integrity may also be damaged by decreases in temperature and humidity, exposure to inhalants such as cigarette smoke and atmospheric pollutants, supplemental oxygen, endotracheal tubes, and thermal injury. Infection by certain respiratory viruses (i.e., influenza) and *Mycoplasma pneumoniae* can damage the mucociliary system, resulting in increased susceptibility to bronchitis and pneumonia. Recurrent bacterial pneumonias result from anatomic derangement of bronchi by obstruction from neoplasm, foreign objects, mucous plugs, or local collapse secondary to bronchiectasis and from chronic aspiration.

Gastrointestinal "blind loops" following certain surgical procedures result in overgrowth with coliform bacteria which consume vitamin B_{12} or folic acid and thereby contribute to neutropenic states. Genitourinary tract infections with gram-negative bacteria are associated with congenital and acquired abnormalities such as congenital ureteral abnormalities, urethral stricture, urethral changes following pregnancy, and urethral obstruction from stones, prostatic hypertrophy, and prostatic carcinoma.

Other anatomic defects increasing susceptibility to infection include damaged heart valves following endocarditis or rheumatic fever. Aortic aneurysms can be infected with salmonellae (particularly *Salmonella choleraesuis*), staphylococci, and streptococci. Peripheral vascular disease of diabetes mellitus is associated with infection of the distal phalanges of the toes. Foreign objects, including prosthetic devices, sutures, gauze, and intravenous or Foley catheters, interfere with normal anatomic integrity and are subject to microbial colonization and subsequent microbial dissemination.

Patients who have had splenectomy are at increased risk for *Streptococcus pneumoniae* infection, especially infants and young children. The precise basis for this is not known, but decreased clearance of bacteria is thought to be important. Children with sickle cell hemoglobinopathies without autosplenectomy, as well as patients with hemoglobinopathies from a variety of causes, are susceptible to *Salmonella, Streptococcus pneumoniae,* and *Bartonella* infection. The host defect in the hemoglobinopathies may relate to splenic dysfunction, but abnormal alternative complement pathway function and impaired phagocytosis and killing of the indicated organisms by leukocytes have been described. Splenic dysfunction is also seen in splenomegaly from a variety of causes, including passive congestion, certain collagen-vascular diseases (systemic lupus erythematosus and Felty's syndrome), and lymphomas. These examples of splenic dysfunction are associated with neutropenia from neutrophil trapping and destruction in the spleen.

A number of other conditions predispose to compromised defenses. During viral influenza there is increased susceptibility to *Streptococcus pneumoniae* and staphylococcal pneumonia. The mechanism for this is poorly understood, but impaired mucociliary function, neutropenia, and adverse effects of the virus on phagocytic cell function have been implicated. Neoplasms, malnutrition, diabetes mellitus, and effects of a variety of pharmacologic agents, especially corticosteroids and myelosuppressive agents, compromise host defenses by affecting the production, distribution, and function of leukocytes. Prolonged use of antimicrobial drugs increases susceptibility to infection with microorganisms which colonize the host, particularly *Staphylococcus aureus,* resistant gram-negative bacilli such as *Pseudomonas, Serratia,* and the gram-negative coccobacillus *Mima-Herellea,* as well as fungi *(Candida).*

Leukopenias. Perhaps the best evidence for a role of leukocytes in host defenses is the severe infections associated with leukopenias. Leukopenia exists when the peripheral white blood count is below 4000 per cubic millimeter. Although all leukocytes may be depressed, most commonly there are depressed granulocytes (neutrophils). In general, when the granulocyte count is below 500 to 1000 cells per cubic millimeter, patients are at increased risk of infection, and when there are fewer than 200 cells per cubic millimeter the inflammatory response is essentially absent and severe infection is the rule. Lymphopenia exists when the number of lymphocytes is below 1400 per cubic millimeter in children and 1000 per cubic millimeter in adults. The complete absence of leukocytes is not compatible with life in a normal environment. The particular type of infection associated with leukopenia depends upon which leukocyte population is depressed. Absence of thymus-dependent lymphocytes or T cells as in thymus aplasia (DiGeorge's syndrome) or thymus hypoplasia (Nezelof's syndrome) is associated with severe defects of cell-mediated immunity (see Ch. 40.3). Absent B lymphocytes (Bruton's X-linked agammaglobulinemia) is associated with a severe abnormality of humoral mediated immunity (see Ch. 40.2). Combined T and B cell lymphopenia (see Ch. 40.4) has a particularly poor prognosis.

The causes of leukopenias are multiple and are related to depressed marrow production (idiopathic, drug-induced, leukemias, tumor invasion of the bone marrow, and nutritional deficiencies), peripheral destruction (immune mechanisms, splenic trapping), or peripheral pooling with overwhelming bacterial infection. Leukopenia is seen following infection with bacteria (typhoid, paratyphoid fever, tuberculosis, brucellosis), viruses (influenza, measles, infectious mononucleosis, rubella), rickettsiae, and protozoa (malaria, kala-azar). (For a complete review of the leukopenias, see Ch. 495.)

Leukocyte Dysfunction. The leukocyte dysfunction syndromes also demonstrate the primary importance of leukocytes in host defenses. Patients with T cell dysfunction include those with mucocutaneous candidiasis and nucleoside phosphorylase deficiency. Combined T and B cell dysfunction are seen in adenosine deaminase deficiency and the Wiskott-Aldrich syndrome (see Ch. 40). Other patients with neutrophil dysfunctions attributable to abnormal adherence, chemotaxis, degranulation, and bactericidal activity are reviewed in Ch. 494. Defects of the humoral components of the inflammatory response include abnormalities of mediators. These include deficiencies of certain complement components (C3 and C5) with abnormal anaphylatoxin, opsonin, and chemotactic factor production. Inhibitors acting on the chemotactic factors have been described in patients with Hodgkin's disease, sarcoidosis, alcoholism, and cirrhosis. Patients deficient in the late complement components (C6 and C7) have increased susceptibility to *Neisseria* infections.

CLINICAL MANIFESTATIONS. The clinical history can be very important when evaluating a patient suspected of having a host defense defect. The type, frequency, duration, and location of infections, the intensity of the inflammatory reaction, and associated illnesses or clinical problems such as allergies or atopic dermatitis, as well as the family history, are important and are summarized in Table 2.

Leukopenias. The clinical manifestations of leukopenia without infection are minimal, or those of the underlying disease. With acute drug-induced leukopenia, chills, fever, and prostration may be the initial manifestations and may be attributed to invasion by bacteria. However, these symptoms may occur within an hour of administering a drug which results in a hapten-antibody type reaction, such as with aminopyrine, and may relate to release of endogenous pyrogens from immune lysis of leukocytes. The initial symptoms may transiently disappear, to be followed by recurrent fever,

TABLE 2. Infections in Patients with Host Defense Defects

Host Defect	Clinical Examples	Clinical Manifestation of Infections	Infectious Agents
Inflammatory response			
Neutropenia	Aplastic anemia Agranulocytosis Leukemias	Pneumonia; ulcers of skin, oral cavity, rectum, and vagina; fever; depressed inflammatory response	Gram-negative bacilli (especially *E. coli, Pseudomonas* sp., *Klebsiella, Staph. aureus*), fungi (*Candida, Aspergillus*), *Pneumocystis carinii*
Chemotaxis	Chédiak-Higashi syndrome	Subcutaneous abscesses	*Staph. aureus, Strep. pyogenes*
	Job's syndrome and variants	"Cold" abscesses, bronchitis, otitis, pneumonia, bronchiectasis	*Staph. aureus, Strep. pneumoniae, H. influenzae, E. coli, Klebsiella*
	Newborns	Bacteremia	Gram-negative bacilli
	Protein-calorie malnutrition; others (see text)	Bacteremia	Gram-negative bacilli
Phagocytosis			
Cellular defect	Systemic lupus erythematosus, megaloblastic anemia, chronic myelocytic leukemia	Otitis, bacteremia, pneumonias, meningitis	Encapsulated bacteria
Opsonin deficiency			
C3 deficiency	Inherited or acquired (i.e., systemic lupus erythematosus)	Otitis, bacteremia, pneumonia, meningitis	*Pseudomonas, Proteus, Staph. aureus, Strep. pneumoniae*
C5 dysfunction	Leiner's syndrome of newborn infants	Generalized seborrheic dermatitis, severe diarrhea, local and systemic infections	Gram-negative bacilli
Alternative complement pathway	Sickle cell disease	Pneumonia, osteomyelitis	*Salmonella, Strep. pneumoniae*
Bactericidal activity	Chronic granulomatous disease	Recurrent infection of lymph nodes, skin, lung, liver, bone, and other tissues	Catalase (+) microorganisms (*Staphylococcus, Klebsiella, E. coli, Serratia marcescens, Pseudomonas, Proteus, Salmonella, Candida, Aspergillus, Nocardia*)
Immune response			
T cells			
Deficiency	Thymic aplasia (DiGeorge's syndrome) and thymic hypoplasia (Nezelof's syndrome)	Otitis, pneumonia	Tuberculosis, *Listeria*, BCGosis, leprosy, *Candida*, cryptococci, aspergillosis, *Pneumocystis*, toxoplasmosis, *Strongyloides*, herpes simplex, herpes zoster, cytomegalovirus, measles
Dysfunction	Mucocutaneous candidasis	Candida of mucous membranes or oral cavity, esophagus, vagina, nailbeds	*Candida albicans*
	Purine nucleoside phosphorylase deficiency	Chronic pneumonias, diarrhea, candidiasis	Fungal and viral infections
B cells	Bruton's X-linked agammaglobulinemia	Sinusitis, otitis, dermatitis, pneumonia, meningitis, osteomyelitis	*Strep. pneumoniae, H. influenzae, Pseudomonas* sp.
	Dysgammaglobulinemias, agammaglobulinemia, multiple myeloma, chronic lymphocytic leukemias	Bacteremia, pneumonias, sinusitis	Fulminant hepatitis, poliomyelitis, measles, chickenpox
	IgA deficiency and nodular lymphoid hyperplasia of the intestine	Diarrhea, malabsorption	*Giardia lamblia*
Mixed T and B cells	Common variable hypogammaglobulinemia (may be due to excess T suppressor cells inhibiting B cells)	Sinusitis, bronchitis, pneumonia, bacteremia	High and low grade bacterial pathogens, *Pneumocystis*, cytomegalovirus
	Ataxia telangiectasia (decreased IgA and IgE)	Sinusitis, bronchitis, pneumonia	*Strep. pneumoniae, H. influenzae, rubella, Giardia lamblia*
	Wiskott-Aldrich syndrome (defective antibody response to polysaccharides, decreased IgE, IgM, abnormal monocyte chemotaxis)	Otitis, pneumonia	Infections seen in T and B cell dysfunction
	Severe combined immunodeficiency, adenosine deaminase deficiency	Severe infection involving multiple sites	Infections seen in T and B cell dysfunction
Mixed defects	Hodgkin's disease and lymphoma (lymphocytopenia, delayed hypersensitivity, abnormal monocyte chemotaxis)	Pneumonia, bacteremia, hepatitis	Tuberculosis, histoplasmosis, *Salmonella, Listeria, Pneumocystis*, cytomegalovirus, herpes zoster, herpes simplex, *Cryptococcus, Candida*, aspergillosis
	Diabetes mellitus (abnormal chemotaxis, phagocytosis, compromised neurovascular supply)	Cellulitis, urinary tract infections	*Staphylococcus aureus*, gram-negative *Candida*, mucormycosis
	Uremia (chemotactic defect, depressed, delayed hypersensitivity, lymphopenia)	Bacteremia, pneumonia, urinary tract infection	*Staph. aureus, E. coli, Klebsiella, Pseudomonas*

TABLE 2. Infections in Patients with Host Defense Defects *(Continued)*

Host Defect	Clinical Examples	Clinical Manifestation of Infections	Infectious Agents
	Burns (chemotactic defect, necrosis)	Cellulitis, bacteremia, pneumonia	*Staphylococcus, Strep. pyogenes, Pseudomonas* sp., *Candida*, herpes simplex
	Cystic fibrosis (mucociliary dysfunction)	Bronchitis, pneumonia	*Staph. aureus, Pseudomonas*
	Splenectomy	Pneumonia and osteomyelitis	*Streptococcus pneumoniae, Salmonella*
Iatrogenic	Foreign body (intravenous catheters, prosthetic devices)	Bacteremia, local abscesses	*Staph. aureus*, gram-negative bacilli, *Candida*
	Antibiotics	Bacteremia	*Staph. aureus*, gram-negative bacilli (*Serratia, Pseudomonas, Mima-Herellea) Candida*
	Corticosteroid therapy (depressed delayed hypersensitivity, neutrophil margination and adherence)	Bacteremia, pneumonia	*Candida, Pneumocystis, Staph. aureus*, gram-negative bacilli, others

chills, headaches, and frequently ulceration of the oropharynx and sometimes the rectum and vagina. These ulcerations are called aphthous ulcers and may be the initial clinical manifestation of neutropenia. The ulcers often have a gray membrane, but frank pus is absent. Patients receiving cytotoxic drug therapy get similar ulcers, independent of neutropenia, which may be difficult to distinguish from aphthous ulcers. Following or concomitant with this stage there are usually symptoms of local bacterial invasion. Frequently bacterial invasion is overwhelming without impressive clinical manifestations because of lack of an inflammatory reaction. Minimal skin lesions characterized by local erythema and tenderness or minimal roentgenographic findings often are the only indications of overwhelming infection with gram-negative bacilli. Careful and frequent inspection of the patient is thus required. With agranulocytosis, regional lymph nodes become enlarged. In the absence of aggressive therapy or spontaneous remission, death from overwhelming infection (usually gram-negative bacilli) ensues. If remission of the agranulocytosis occurs, immature granulocytes appear in the circulation before mature cells.

Patients with severe neutropenia also have an increased incidence of *Pneumocystis carinii* and cytomegalovirus infection as well as infection with the systemic mycoses, including candidiasis, invasive aspergillosis, and mucormycosis. Systemic candidiasis, defined as tissue invasion and not just colonization of superficial surfaces, is the most common mycosis in the neutropenic patient. Prolonged drug therapy for a bacterial infection predisposes to candidiasis and especially *C. albicans* because of normally occurring local colonization. The presence of thrush in the mouth, vagina, or skin indicates candidiasis in these patients, and indwelling catheters may serve as a portal of entry. In systemic candidiasis symptoms are usually confined to the distal esophagus or the bladder, with rare local symptoms in the lung, liver, spleen, or kidney. Symptomatic lesions in the distal esophagus in compromised hosts are usually indicative of candidiasis and are characterized by dysphagia, odynophagia, pyrosis, retrosternal pain, and gastrointestinal bleeding. On x-ray irregular scalloping of the esophageal lining is manifest. Aspergillosis (penetration of hyphae into tissues) is an infection seen in neutropenic patients who are also on corticosteroid therapy; mucormycosis is also seen in

this setting, especially in patients with diabetes mellitus. Invasion with aspergillosis almost invariably involves the lung, causing symptoms suggesting pneumonia or pulmonary emboli. Pulmonary mucormycosis is almost indistinguishable from aspergillosis.

Disorders of the Inflammatory Response. Patients with defective phagocyte chemotaxis present with minimal physical findings or findings characteristic of their underlying disease. The signs and symptoms of the infection are delayed because too few phagocytes arrive too late. Patients with defective leukocyte chemotaxis frequently have severe periodontal disease and dermatologic abnormalities, and these patients have frequent sinopulmonary infections with recurrent otitis media, bronchitis, and pneumonia. *Staphylococcus aureus* is the most frequent infectious agent, but *Streptococcus pneumoniae* and *Hemophilus influenzae* are also common. Perhaps the most common syndrome in which defective neutrophil and monocyte chemotaxis is the predominant host defect occurs in patients with eczematous and pustular dermatitis, markedly elevated IgE, recurrent "cold" staphylococcal skin infections, and recurrent bronchitis and pneumonias with subsequent bronchiectasis (Job's syndrome and its variants). The severity of the atopic dermatitis correlates with the severity of the chemotactic defect. These patients frequently have subcutaneous and lymph node abscesses requiring surgical drainage, and their facies have a characteristic broad nasal bridge. Many patients are in the teenage years at the time of evaluation for host defense defects, and few patients over 30 years of age have been noted. Usually these patients have had recurrent pneumonias since early childhood, and many have thoracotomy scars from lobectomy for the severe bronchiectasis. Some of these patients also have T cell dysfunction and mucocutaneous candidiasis. This syndrome appears to be familial in some cases. Similar clinical spectrums with high IgE and a chemotactic defect are seen in patients with incontinentia pigmenti and an unusual type of ichthyosis.

Defective neutrophil and monocyte chemotaxis and delayed degranulation of neutrophils are also noted in patients with the Chédiak-Higashi syndrome, a rare disease with autosomal recessive inheritance characterized by partial oculocutaneous albinism, nystagmus, neutropenia, recurrent cutaneous infections (particularly with *Staphylococcus aureus*), and giant lysosomes in all cells containing lysosomes. These patients usually have multiple subcutaneous scars from the recurrent infections.

An impressive list of diseases with chemotactic defects and recurrent infections has emerged in recent years and includes the following: diabetes mellitus, leukemias, malignancies (melanoma and breast carcinoma), rheumatoid arthritis, Felty's syndrome, systemic lupus erythematosus in some patients, thermal injury, bone marrow transplantation (associated with graft versus host disease and administration of antithymocyte globulin), congenital ichthyosis with *Trichophyton rubrum* infection, hypogammaglobulinemia, α-mannosidase deficiency, chronic renal failure (especially if the patient is on chronic hemodialysis), severe protein-calorie malnutrition, and severe bacterial infections and viral influenza. In most of these studies the mechanism for the chemotactic defect has not been delineated, and it is not clear whether the chemotactic defect is a cause or effect of the recurrent infections. However, a few well documented case reports of patients with severe pyogenic infections and defective leukocyte locomotion attributable to actin dysfunction or abnormal microtubule assembly clearly illustrate the importance of leukocyte chemotaxis in the host defense system.

Other phagocyte disorders include deficient phagocytosis related to abnormal opsonins as in sickle cell disease, dysfunction of the fifth complement component (Leiner's syndrome), and congenital deficiency of certain complement components (C3 and C5) or immunoglobulins. Clinical manifestations of these deficiencies are recurrent otitis media, bronchitis, pneumonia, and sepsis with encapsulated bacteria. These deficiencies, as well as those with abnormal killing of bacteria, as in chronic granulomatous disease in which there is defective hydrogen peroxide generation and recurrent severe infections of the skin, lymph nodes, lung, liver, and bone with catalase-positive microorganisms such as *Staphylococcus aureus*, enteric bacilli, *Candida*, *Aspergillus*, and *Nocardia*, are reviewed in Ch. 494.

Immune Dysfunctions. Patients with T cell abnormalities have recurrent infections from intracellular bacteria such as *M. tuberculosis*, leprosy, BCGosis, *Listeria*, and *Candida*. These patients also become infected with other fungi (cryptococcosis and aspergillosis), protozoa (*Pneumocystis carinii*, toxoplasmosis, and *Strongyloides*), and viruses (herpes simplex, herpes zoster, varicella, cytomegalovirus, and measles). The clinical presentation of these patients is discussed in Ch. 40.

In other patients the number of T cells is normal, but there is abnormal effector cell response to antigenic stimulation. Delayed skin responses to *Candida* and other naturally occurring antigens is absent, and lymphocytes from many of the patients do not respond to in vitro stimulation with antigens, especially *Candida*, by producing lymphokines or by replication. A well defined group of patients with T cell dysfunction have mucocutaneous candidiasis with *Candida albicans* infection restricted to the skin, nails, and mucous membranes. Another small group of patients deficient in purine nucleoside phosphorylase have T cell dysfunction with recurrent viral and fungal infections.

The prototype disease for B cell deficiency is Bruton's X-linked agammaglobulinemia with absent fully developed B cells and grossly deficient synthesis and secretion of antibody. These patients are subject to infection with encapsulated virulent pathogens such as *Strepto-*

coccus pneumoniae, Hemophilus influenzae, and *Pseudomonas aeruginosa.* Untreated, these infections spread rapidly, and patients have sinorespiratory infections with recurrent pneumonias and otitis media, as well as osteomyelitis, dermatitis, and meningitis. The patients usually respond to appropriate antimicrobial drugs, probably because of normal phagocyte and T cell function. Infections caused by intracellular microorganisms such as *M. tuberculosis, Histoplasma* and fungi are relatively infrequent.

Diseases with combined deficiencies of T and B cells are associated with severe infections. Such patients usually succumb early in life to many different forms of infection, including *Pneumocystis carinii*, cytomegalovirus, other viruses, and bacterial pathogens of high and low grade virulence.

DIAGNOSIS. Initial evaluation of patients with recurrent infections requires a thorough history. For example, a history of contact dermatitis (poison ivy) helps eliminate T cell dysfunction, whereas a history of mucocutaneous candidiasis suggests a T cell abnormality. Aphthous ulcers may be early signs of severe neutropenia. Staphylococcal skin infections and recurrent pneumonias suggest a chemotactic defect, and a history of recurrent infections with catalase positive microorganisms suggests chronic granulomatous disease.

Tests useful in the laboratory evaluation of compromised hosts are summarized in Table 3. Initial laboratory screening studies can be very informative. A white blood count and differential count will serve as a screen for the leukopenias. The morphology of the white cell can be particularly helpful. For example, multilobed nuclei are seen in polymorphonuclear leukocytes in vitamin B_{12} or folate deficiency, and when considering the Chédiak-Higashi syndrome the characteristic giant lysosomes can be seen. An excellent screening test used to diagnose chronic granulomatous disease is the ability of granulocytes to reduce nitroblue tetrazolium dye. This test, which is available in most medical centers, reflects leukocyte oxidative metabolism and is markedly abnormal in chronic granulomatous disease and a few related disorders of phagocyte function (see Ch. 494). Quantitative immunoglobulins assess B cell function, and in the presence of borderline hypogammaglobulinemia the capacity of patients to produce specific antibodies after immunization is important. Most hospital laboratories can measure typhoid H and O agglutinins before and after immunization with standard vaccines, and antibodies to common viruses are also usually available. T cell function can be screened by delayed hypersensitivity skin testing to common antigens (PPD, *Candida*, mumps, streptokinase, and streptodornase). A chest x-ray will help in evaluation of the thymus gland and may reveal evidence for recurrent pneumonias or bronchiectasis. Total hemolytic complement (CH_{50}) and C3 are available in many laboratories, although studies of individual complement components can be obtained only in a few research centers.

More specific studies are often necessary to define host defense defects. In addition to a bone marrow aspirate, marrow reserves can be evaluated with etiocholanolone. The inflammatory response can be estimated in vivo with a Rebuck skin window, which assesses the ability of leukocytes to accumulate at a superficial abrasion and to stick to a glass coverslip. More precise characterization of the cellular and humoral components of the inflammatory response re-

TABLE 3. Diagnostic Tests Used in the Evaluation of Host Defense Defects

Host Defense	Test
Bone marrow production	Peripheral white blood count*
	Marrow aspirate*
	Bone marrow reserve test†
Inflammatory response	Rebuck skin window*,†
	Leukocyte function
	Adherence*†
	Chemotactic response*,†
	Phagocytosis‡
	Degranulation‡
	Bactericidal activity*,†
	Nitroblue tetrazolium dye reduction (NBT test)*,†
	Hexosemonophosphate shunt activity‡
	Leukocyte glucose-6-phosphate dehydrogenase and myeloperoxidase‡
	Chemotactic and opsonic activity of serum*,†
	Complement levels (CH$_{50}$,* C3*,†)
Immune response	
T cell system (cellular immunity)	Delayed hypersensitivity skin tests to common antigens*
	Sensitization to dinitrochlorobenzene‡
	Chest x-ray to assess thymus gland*
	Quantitation of T cells†
	T cell rosettes
	Specific membrane markers
	Lymphocyte transformation studies†
	Nonspecific mitogens (pokeweed, concanavallin A)
	Specific antigens (PPD, mumps, streptokinase-streptodornase, Candida albicans)
	Lymphokine production‡
	Chemotactic lymphokines
	Macrophage migration inhibitory factor
B cell system (humoral immunity)	Quantitative immunoglobulins*
	Immunoglobulin subclasses‡
	Kinetics of antibody synthesis following primary and secondary immunization‡
	Antibodies to common viruses†
	Specific antibody response after immunization* (typhoid H and O agglutinins)

*Screening tests.
†Generally available at major medical centers.
‡Available only in specialized laboratories.

quire in vitro studies. Leukocyte adherence is measured by the ability of cells to stick to nylon wool. Locomotion can be qualitatively evaluated by looking at cells moving on glass slides and can be quantitated by measuring cell migration into different kinds of filter paper. Chemotactic factors are assessed by their ability to attract normal leukocytes. These studies of the inflammatory response are generally available in medical centers, as are studies for the quantitation of leukocyte phagocytosis and killing of bacteria. Studies of leukocyte hexose monophosphate shunt activity, leukocyte actin and myosin, or microtubule function are presently restricted to a few clinical research laboratories.

In-depth studies of the immune system include quantitation of T and B cells (and their subpopulations), using specific membrane markers. B cell function can be evaluated by the kinetics of antibody synthesis following primary and secondary immunization. Measurement of immunoglobulin G subclasses is also available. T cell function can be further characterized in vivo by monitoring the delayed hypersensitivity response after contact sensitization with dinitrochlorobenzene. T cell functional correlates to delayed hypersensitivity can be assessed in vitro by measuring

proliferative responses (tritium incorporation) to nonspecific stimuli such as mitogens (phytohemagglutinin, pokeweed mitogen, and concanavallin A) or specific stimuli such as antigens (PPD, mumps, streptokinase-streptodornase, or Candida albicans). Quantitation of the release of lymphokines (i.e., migration inhibitory factor or chemotactic lymphokines) are generally available in medical centers. Other specific tests of T cell function are available only in highly specialized laboratories.

Particularly puzzling patients with no demonstrable defect of host defenses should raise one's suspicion of the possibility of a psychologic disorder with self-inflicted lesions. Psychologic problems can be very serious, with patients inoculating fecal material subcutaneously or performing other manipulations that can manifest as severe abscesses or unexplained fevers; many of these patients are medical or paramedical professionals. Continual culture of fecal flora from wounds and localization of infections to conveniently reached areas (such as the left side of the body in right-handed individuals) should lead one to suspect psychologic problems.

MANAGEMENT. General Considerations. Management of the compromised host is based in part on the specific problems. Risk from environmental factors such as crowded living conditions, contaminated hospital respirators, or intravenous lines must be rigidly controlled. Intravenous lines should be used only when necessary; metal (scalp vein) devices should be used whenever possible, as microbial colonization with these is less than with plastic catheters. Similarly, all catheters, especially Foley catheters, should be used as little as possible, and they should be changed regularly. Antimicrobial agents should be carefully selected and used as briefly and with as much microbial specificity as possible.

Certain procedures are associated with bacteremia or local spread of infection, and compromised hosts undergoing these procedures may be at increased risk. In particular, dental manipulation, bronchoscopy, certain gastrointestinal studies (gastroscopy, jejunal biopsy, liver biopsy, sigmoidoscopy, barium enema, retrograde cholangiogams), urinary tract manipulations (catheterization, cystoscopy, retrograde pyelogram), angiograms (cardiac catheterization), orthopedic surgery, and, on rare occasions, bone marrow aspiration have been associated with bacteremia. In severely compromised hosts, administration of appropriate antimicrobials (depending on the expected bacteremia) prior to and for several hours after the procedure may prevent development of disseminated foci of infection.

Considerable controversy exists regarding the necessity for isolating patients with compromised defenses. Obviously judgment is required as to which patients require isolation. Patients with severely compromised defenses (such as patients with agranulocytosis plus corticosteroid therapy) may benefit by isolation from hospital personnel, as may those with draining staphylococcal wounds or herpes zoster. However, isolation is disruptive to hospital routine and should not be continued any longer than required. Hospital personnel with minor infections, including herpes simplex "cold sores," should not be restricted. Use of laminar flow isolation facilities may provide some benefit in selected situations; however, the availability of such units is limited to a few institutions.

Leukopenias. The compromised host with leukopenia, and in particular granulocytopenia, poses a particularly difficult management problem. This is especially true if immunosuppressive drugs such as corticosteroids are being used concurrently. If there is any possibility of an environmental or drug-induced leukopenia, the etiologic agent should be eliminated. When infections occur, inflammatory manifestations are markedly diminished or absent, and careful and frequent examination of the patient for subtle findings of infection is required. Surveillance cultures of the oral cavity, stool, and open wounds, as well as culture of withdrawn catheter tips, can be particularly helpful in the selection of initial antimicrobials when these patients become infected. Mycotic infections can be a particular problem in these patients. Heavy colonization with *Candida* (thrush of the mouth, esophagus, or vagina) should be treated with a topical antifungal agent such as mycostatin (Nystatin). Patients with urinary tract colonization with *Candida,* as judged by pseudohyphae in the urine, who have no fever or other evidence of infection, and in whom a Foley catheter is required, may benefit from bladder irrigation for several days with amphotericin B (50 μg per milliliter). If a bladder catheter is not in place, oral 5-fluorocytosine should be considered, especially if the clinical situation is not urgent and renal function is normal. With severe candidiasis, intravenous amphotericin B should be used. Patients with compromised defenses with transient candidemia that is thought to be related to contaminated intravenous lines may benefit from a short course of intravenous amphotericin B to try to prevent the establishment of disseminated foci. Fungemia in patients with malignancies and compromised defenses, especially lymphoreticular or hematopoietic malignancies, is frequently associated with disseminated fungal infection, and in these patients early use of amphotericin, sometimes prior to microbiologic confirmation, should be considered.

The use of bone marrow transplantation to reconstitute patients with agranulocytosis and other immunodeficiencies is attractive but still under investigation and at present is restricted to only a few medical centers. Use of leukocyte transfusions to transiently correct leukopenias may prove to be beneficial. Initial studies using leukocyte transfusions are encouraging, but methods for collection and storage of leukocytes and techniques for the prevention of antileukocyte antibody formation in recipients remain particular problems.

Disorders of the Inflammatory Response. Management of patients with neutrophil dysfunction syndromes requires aggressive therapy of particular infections with careful selection of antimicrobial drugs. Aggressive use of antimicrobials and early surgical drainage of abscesses in some patients (i.e., with chronic granulomatous disease) is appropriate. Long-term chemoprophylaxis has not been established as beneficial, although it may help in selected situations; chemoprophylaxis prior to procedures commonly associated with bacteremia is appropriate. Plasma transfusions may be particularly useful in infants with Leiner's syndrome (C5 dysfunction).

Manipulation of leukocyte function with pharmacologic agents may be an important future approach to management of patients with leukocyte dysfunction. Ascorbic acid has improved granulocyte function in a few patients with the Chédiak-Higashi syndrome, although this has not been seen in every patient. Several patients with the syndrome of elevated IgE, recurrent bacterial infections, atopic dermatitis, and a leukocyte chemotactic defect showed improvement of the chemotactic defect after oral levamisole. Similarly, a monocyte chemotactic defect in patients with acute influenza was also corrected by levamisole. Clinical trials with these agents have not yet been completed. It is hoped that therapeutic manipulation of inflammatory components of the host defenses will emerge as important tools in the management of these patients.

Disorders of the Immune Response. Patients with IgG immunoglobulin deficiency with recurrent bacterial infections usually benefit from replacement therapy with human gamma globulin. Maintenance of plasma IgG around 200 mg per milliliter is reported to decrease severe infections, although sinusitis, bronchitis, and otitis may persist. Intramuscular injection of IgG (100 mg per kilogram) at monthly intervals is usually adequate. Globulin injection is beneficial only in patients deficient in immunoglobulin G. An alternative therapy is infusion of fresh plasma, 10 to 20 ml per kilogram, at intervals of three to four weeks. The advantage of this is that, in addition to replacing IgG, it replaces IgM and IgA, although the IgA never enters the secretory pools. The disadvantage is the risk of transmitting hepatitis. Despite gamma globulin, repeated infections and progression of pulmonary fibrosis and bronchiectasis may persist.

Treatment of patients with T cell deficiencies is largely a research procedure. Some patients have responded to fetal thymus graft with increased numbers of T cells and improved T cell function. Other patients have responded to immune reconstitution with transfer factor therapy. Transfer factor is prepared from dialysates of leukocyte extracts and was first shown by Lawrence in 1954 to have the potential for immune reconstitution. In some patients, when the candidiasis is first cleared with a short course of intravenous amphotericin, remissions have been sustained with transfer factor therapy. Transfer factor has also been used with variable success in the reconstitution of defective cell-mediated immune responses in the Wiskott-Aldrich syndrome, in severe combined immunodeficiency, and in patients who have coccidioidomycosis, tuberculosis, or leprosy. With the recent availability of highly purified preparations of the biologically active components in transfer factor, more defined benefits of this agent should emerge. At present, therapeutic use of transfer factor should be considered investigational and its use restricted to investigators actively evaluating its therapeutic potential.

Babior, B. M.: Oxygen-dependent microbial killing by phagocytes. N. Engl. J. Med., 298:659, 721, 1978.

Cooper, M. D., and Seligman, M.: B and T lymphocytes in immunodeficiency and lymphoproliferative disorders. *In* Loor, F., and Roelants, G. E. (eds.): B and T Cells in Immune Recognition. London, John Wiley & Sons, Ltd., 1977, pp. 377–406.

Fauci, A. S.: Mechanisms of host defense. *In* Current Concepts. The Upjohn Company, 1978.

Frank, M. M., and Atkinson, J. P.: Complement in clinical medicine. Disease-a-Month, January 1975.

Gallin, J. I., and Quie, P. G. (eds): Leukocyte Chemotaxis: Methods, Physiology and Clinical Implications. New York, Raven Press, 1978.

Kirkpatrick, C. H., and Gallin, J. I.: Treatment of infectious and neoplastic diseases with transfer factor. Oncology, 29:46, 1974.

Lichtman, M. A. (ed.): Granulocyte and monocyte abnormalities. Clin. Haematol., 4:483, 1975.

Quie, P. G.: Infections due to neutrophil malfunction. Medicine, 52:411, 1973.

Wanner, A.: Clinical aspects of mucociliary transport. Am. Rev. Respir. Dis., 116:73, 1977.

Young, R. C., Bennett, J. E., Geelhoed, G. W., and Levine, A. S.: Fungemia with compromised host resistance. Ann. Intern. Med., 80:605, 1974.

42. SERUM SICKNESS

Fred S. Kantor

DEFINITION. Serum sickness is a disease characterized by fever, arthralgia, skin eruptions, and edema which appears after injection of a foreign serum or serum proteins and is dependent upon an immune response of the patient to the injected serum. Hypersensitivity reactions to a variety of drugs may produce an identical illness.

ETIOLOGY. With the advent of antimicrobial therapy, the use of serum for the treatment of microbial diseases has declined markedly; the most common cause for "serum sickness" at present is not serum itself but exogenously administered drugs, particularly the antimicrobials. Serum therapy is still used primarily for the neutralization of bacterial toxins such as tetanus and botulinus toxins and also in the form of rabies antiserum.

The incidence and severity of the disease are clearly related to the type of serum preparation as well as to the amount administered. Of patients given prophylactic tetanus antitoxin prepared in horses, approximately 2 to 5 per cent will develop symptoms of serum sickness. The figure is considerably higher for those patients receiving equine rabies antiserum; approximately 16 per cent of these patients develop serum sickness. In general, there is an increasing incidence and severity through childhood, adolescence, and adulthood. Reactions in children are quite mild, lasting from one to four days, whereas in patients over the age of 15, the disease is more frequent and more severe.

Different methods of production of various equine antisera may have a profound effect upon the serum sickness liability of the product. Most tetanus antitoxin preparations involve a peptic digestion which does not impair antitoxic properties while hydrolyzing many of the proteins present in the serum. In contrast, antirabies antiserum is not subjected to peptic digestion because of the great loss of antibody encountered with the enzymatic treatment. The most important factor concerned with the development of serum sickness is the total amount of serum administered. Recommended doses of tetanus antitoxin and rabies antisera vary considerably from time to time; from 5 to 10 ml of tetanus antitoxin may produce serum sickness in 5 to 10 per cent of patients, whereas 80 ml will almost always result in illness. Age and dose relationships in serum sickness resulting from drugs are not as clear cut as with serum or serum proteins. In most cases the drug by itself is not capable of inducing the disease and must combine with a protein of the patient to form a complete antigen or immunogen. In such a situation the genetic potential of the patient of forming complete antigens and producing antibodies to them must be considered in addition to the patient's age and the dose and duration of the drug given.

MECHANISM. The essential basis of serum sickness is antigen-antibody interaction. A blood level of circulating foreign protein can be measured in patients shortly after beginning serum treatment. In the early stages the administered protein is catabolized in a manner similar to that seen in the animal from which it came. This is the latent period and usually lasts from four to ten days, during which time the patient develops an immune response that is evidenced by the appearance of antibody directed against the injected protein. As soon as antibody appears, it combines with circulating foreign protein antigen to form soluble complexes. These complexes have a varied fate, depending upon their nature and the ratio of antigen to antibody in the complex. Experimental studies, in the rabbit primarily, have shown a deposition of antigen-antibody complexes beneath the endothelium of blood vessels and within the basement membrane of these vessels. Complexes containing antibodies of the IgM or the IgG classes may initiate fixation and activation of the complement sequence. With localization of complement-containing complexes in the walls of blood vessels, polymorphonuclear leukocytes are attracted to the site and appear to injure the vessel by release of potent enzymes found in their lysosomal granules. The vascular injury mediated by complement and polymorphonuclear leukocytes may lead to thrombosis and hemorrhage, typified by the petechial or ecchymotic rash attendant on serum sickness.

Another manifestation of the interaction of antigen and antibody is the release of potent vasoactive materials such as histamine, serotonin, bradykinin, and slow-reacting substance (SRSA), all of which lead to vasodilatation and leakage of protein and fluid from the vascular space into the tissues, resulting in edema. The disease varies from species to species in laboratory animals. As most of the work has been done in the rabbit, it is pertinent to note that the renal disease, which is a frequent and important aspect of immune complex disease in the rabbit, is often nonexistent or a very mild component in the usual human patient.

Continuation of disease is dependent upon a continual supply of antigen. Removal by the reticuloendothelial system of the immune complexes is signified by a rise in serum antibody directed against the foreign proteins, and reduction of symptoms and signs of illness. Unless the foreign proteins are readministered, the disease is self-limited. During convalescence and for long periods thereafter, antibodies against the foreign proteins are readily demonstrable in the patient's serum. Readministration of foreign antigen promptly leads to formation of immune complexes and clinical manifestations of disease, which continue until antigen is entirely removed from the circulation.

CLINICAL MANIFESTATIONS. The onset of disease is often heralded by itching and discomfort, frequently at the site of serum injection. Fully developed serum sickness is a miserable disease. The unfortunate patient lies on his side in bed with a swollen, distorted face, often resulting in closure of both eyes so that he cannot see, with a skin itching all over and often covered with an urticarial or erythematous rash. He is reluctant to scratch his skin because of the pain in all his muscles and joints upon movement, and so he lies quietly in bed suffering from headache, itching, and joint pain. Especially frightening and discomforting is the appearance of neurologic manifestations which may result in weakness of an extremity or a sensory deficit, or occasionally an isolated facial palsy. Compounding the patient's difficulties may be abdominal pain, nausea, and vomiting. Upon examination a generalized lymphadenopathy may be palpated, especially prominent in the regions draining the site of injection of the serum. At that site there may be a local rash with erythema and either urticaria or tenderness, and this may provide a potent clue for the physician as to the nature of the illness. Occasionally, auscultation of the chest reveals a cardiac arrhythmia or a pericardial friction rub. The spleen is usually not palpable. A common manifestation is fever of 38.3 to 39°C, and, in addition to the subjective complaints of joint pain, the patient may manifest objective arthritis with swelling, redness, and accumulation of fluid in joints. The skin may show a petechial or purpuric rash in addition to the more common urticarial eruption.

LABORATORY STUDIES. Examination of the blood may reveal a mild leukocytosis, and circulating plasma cells have been observed. The sedimentation rate is usually normal or only slightly elevated. Eosinophilia occurs, but is relatively uncommon. The urine may show slight proteinuria, a few red cells, and occasionally a few casts; but there are rarely significant evidences of renal impairment. Examination of the patient's serum proteins reveals circulating horse gamma globulins and macroglobulins present early in the disease, and predominantly anti-horse IgA globulin antibodies late in the disease and during convalescence. The development of antibodies to horse alpha-2-macroglobulin in the sera of patients recovering from serum sickness suggests that this component of the equine serum which lacks any antibody value could be deleted in manufacture without impairing the antitoxic benefits of the serum. Serum complement levels are reduced for variable periods during the disease and then return to normal.

TREATMENT AND PROGNOSIS. Very mild symptoms of pruritus and skin rash may be controlled by an antihistamine, such as brompheniramine, 4 mg given every four hours. Epinephrine and sympathomimetic amines have been recommended in the past for the treatment of the urticaria of serum sickness, and salicylates for the treatment of joint pains. However, for all but the mildest symptoms, adrenocortical steroids in the form of prednisone can be given with great safety and efficacy, and the patient need not suffer with less effective medications. As this is a self-limited disease with a natural course of one to three weeks, the usual hazards of steroid therapy are not realized before treatment is stopped. A treatment course of 40 mg per day for four or five days may be sufficient, even for quite severe disease. Symptomatic improvement appears often within hours of the onset of steroid therapy and sometimes is remarkable within 24 hours.

PREVENTION. Tetanus antitoxin and rabies antiserum prepared from human sera are now commercially available in many parts of the world. If a human serum can be obtained, there is no reason to choose horse serum. When equine sera must be used in treatment, patients should be carefully questioned concerning prior exposure and for allergic symptoms to other horse products, such as horse dander or horsehair, as found in horse-

hair mattresses. All patients, regardless of history, should be skin tested by production of a minimal wheal (0.01 to 0.02 ml) of a 1:10 dilution of the serum to be used. After 15 to 20 minutes the skin site is examined for an urticarial wheal, and in its absence treatment may be instituted. If the patient is allergic and the necessity for serum treatment is great, desensitization may be attempted by repeatedly injecting small amounts of serum beginning in dilutions of 1:100 and doubling the tolerated amount about every 15 or 20 minutes until the appropriate dose is achieved. Such treatment is hazardous because of possible anaphylaxis, and the indications for it should be scrutinized carefully.

In patients who have developed serum sickness after tetanus antitoxin, active immunization should be begun during the patient's convalescence from serum sickness. It is generally advisable to immunize against tetanus all individuals who are seen by the physician in connection with unrelated allergic disease and found to be sensitive to horse dander or horse products. The immunization can be accomplished by use of tetanus toxoid.

Occasionally, in the course of serum therapy *an acute anaphylactic reaction* occurs, consisting of sudden vascular collapse, severe pruritus of the face, hands, and feet, often accompanied by bronchospasm and incontinence of stool and urine. Such events must be treated promptly *with epinephrine and not adrenocortical steroids.* A tourniquet should be placed proximal to the injection site of the drug or serum, and 0.2 ml of epinephrine injected into the site of injection which will slow absorption from the site. An additional 0.3 to 0.5 ml of 1:1000 aqueous solution of epinephrine should be given subcutaneously above the tourniquet if the patient has an effective blood pressure. In the absence of adequate blood pressure, the epinephrine must be given intravenously notwithstanding the hazard of production of cardiac arrhythmia, because the drug will not be absorbed from the periphery. After epinephrine administration, diphenhydramine (Benadryl), 50 mg, should be given orally or intramuscularly. The outcome of anaphylactic reactions is usually decided in the first few minutes; rapid restoration of blood pressure with prompt treatment is an excellent prognostic sign. Fatalities are few but tend to occur when the possibility of anaphylaxis is not considered *prior* to the administration of serum or drugs so that effective measures are delayed.

Kunkel, H. G. (Chairman): Symposium on immune complex and disease. J. Exp. Med., 134:1s, 1971.
Moroz, L. A., Comerford, T. A., and Guttman, R. D.: Mixed IgG-IgA cryoglobulinemia in human serum sickness. Int. Arch. Allergy Appl. Immunol., 48:756, 1975.
Vaughan, J. H., Barnett, E. V., and Leadley, P. J.: Serum sickness: Evidence in man of antigen-antibody complexes and free light chains in the circulation during the acute reaction. Ann. Intern. Med., 67:596, 1967.
von Pirquet, C., and Schick, B.: Serum Sickness. Baltimore. Williams & Wilkins Company, 1951.

43. DRUG ALLERGY

Fred S. Kantor

The value of therapeutic agents should constantly be weighed against their potential liability. Hypersensitivity reactions must be distinguished from two other untoward effects of drugs. The first is that of intolerance, in which the usual undesirable toxic effects occur at dosages of the drug well below that expected in a normal population. An example of this type of reaction includes visual disturbances and alterations in cardiac rhythm with very small doses of digitalis. The second form of drug reaction to be distinguished from hypersensitivity is that of idiosyncrasy. Whereas intolerance is a quantitative difference, idiosyncrasy is qualitative and is based upon a biochemical alteration in the way the patient handles the drug. Such a reaction does not depend on prior exposure to the drug, is not dose dependent, and does not resemble the other pharmacologic manifestations of the drug. An example of idiosyncrasy is the hemolytic anemia produced in patients with glucose-6-phosphate dehydrogenase deficiency when treated with primaquine. Altered reactivity (von Pirquet combined these two words to produce the word "allergy") on the part of the patient always follows prior exposure, even though this may not be apparent, and its mechanism is related to the hypersensitive state as reflected by delayed hypersensitivity or antibody production.

INCIDENCE. Any drug may produce a hypersensitivity reaction, but some drugs have a much higher liability in this regard than do others. Digitalis and tetracycline have a low liability in producing allergic drug reactions, even though reports of documented cases have appeared. On the other hand, several of the antimicrobials, notably novobiocin, and certain antiinflammatory agents, such as phenylbutazone, may have a high incidence of drug reaction. In addition to the variations produced by different drugs, equal liability is not shared by all patients for development of drug reactions to a single drug, such as penicillin. Patients with a history of allergic disease or previous drug reactions, as well as patients with certain inflammatory diseases such as lupus erythematosus, are generally thought to be more prone to the development of new drug allergies.

PATHOGENESIS. Certain therapeutic agents such as insulin are complex protein molecules which are known to be immunogenic. The majority of drugs represent classes of simple chemicals which require complexing with a tissue or serum protein of the patient in order to form an antigenic or immunogenic molecule. Drugs which are highly reactive chemicals usually are the most frequent sensitizers, and conversely the more inert members of the drug armamentarium are of less allergenic potential. Sensitization by means of a simple chemical involves the formation of covalent bonds with host protein which forms a hapten-carrier conjugate. Antibodies and hypersensitivity are directed against the hapten or the hapten and a closely adjacent portion of the carrier molecule, but never to the carrier protein itself. To form a hapten-protein conjugate, the administered drug may have to undergo considerable chemical rearrangement. This may occur during the metabolism of the drug, producing an antigenic determinant which is different from the administered drug. The necessity of chemical rearrangement of the drug to form the allergenic hapten-protein complex shows the difficulty of testing in vitro for drug allergy, because before testing it is necessary to know what the antigenic determinant is.

Drug allergy has been investigated with respect to the antigenic determinant in only a limited number of cases. One of the most recent and extensive investigations has been in the case of penicillin and a derivative, the penicilloyl determinant. This has been labeled the major determinant, and as many as three — and perhaps many more — as yet undescribed chemical rearrangements may account for minor determinants, all of which can produce sensitization in given individuals and produce allergic symptoms upon administration of the drug. It should be borne in mind that not all drug immunization implies drug allergy. A good example of this is that all patients recently treated with penicillin will have developed antibodies directed against the penicilloyl determinant.

Hypersensitive reactions have been divided into *delayed hypersensitivity* and two varieties of immediate hypersensitivity: *wheal-and-flare* and *Arthus reactivity*. Serum sickness, which is discussed in Ch. 42, is an excellent example of an immediate type of hypersensitivity involving complement-fixing antibody and producing reactions of the so-called "Arthus" type.

The other type of immediate hypersensitivity, i.e., wheal-and-flare, is manifested in two major, clinically recognizable situations, urticaria and anaphylaxis. In these cases, the interaction of the drug-protein conjugate with IgE antibodies leads to release of active mediators resulting in vasodilatation and smooth muscle contraction. In this form of reaction, the hapten-protein conjugate and its respective antibody do not enter into the pathogenesis of the reaction but merely cause the release of the vasoactive material which produces the clinical effects. The last type of well-recognized mechanism is that of cellular or delayed hypersensitivity. In this form of immunity, circulating antibody is not important, and the interaction of the drug-protein conjugate is with sensitized cells, causing a release of a variety of biologically active materials which lead to perivascular accumulation of mononuclear cells and the development of induration. The best example of delayed hypersensitivity induced by drugs is skin sensitization resulting from direct contact with a variety of medications. Paradoxically, antihistamines, which have been incorporated into a variety of topical preparations for treatment of itching, burning, or allergic skin conditions, are themselves skin-sensitizing, and by combining with skin proteins form potent sensitizing agents which lead to delayed hypersensitivity and the development of the typical skin lesions of contact sensitivity. A combination of reaction types is often present in typical drug allergy, but one or another of the reaction types usually predominates and treatment is most efficacious when directed against this reaction type.

CLINICAL MANIFESTATIONS. Fever may develop immediately after administration of a drug or, more commonly, may increase in a stepwise fashion after the seventh or eighth day of administration. The fever may show a sustained or remittent course and is usually low-grade in the range of 37.8 to 39°C, although hectic fevers are often observed, accompanied by constitutional symptoms. In general, the patient appears less ill than would be anticipated from the height of the fever. A drug reaction may mimic the septic picture entirely, but it usually pursues a more indolent course. Cessation of fever within a day or two of discontinuing the offending drug is to be expected. In some cases of fever alone, and if the drug reaction involves other organ systems, such as the skin and the joints, it may take several days, up to a week, for the symptoms to slowly subside. Penicillin, diphenylhydantoin (Dilantin), and barbiturates are frequent causes of drug fever.

Skin Rash. Skin rash as a manifestation of drug allergy may take several forms. A maculopapular, very fine rash appearing in the softer skin of the axillary line and on the extensor surfaces of the extremities and along the trunk may be unnoticed by the patient. Usually, *urticarial rashes* are reported because they are accompanied by pruritus. Persistent administration of an offending drug causing maculopapular eruptions may lead to confluent erythroderma and subsequent exfoliative dermatitis. Similarly, a rash may progress to an eczematous eruption with weeping papulovesicular lesions and ill-defined patches of erythema and edema, accompanied by intense pruritus. Erythema multiforme–like eruptions may be produced by a variety of drugs and are characterized by the formation of sharply circumscribed lesions that are usually symmetrical in distribution. The individual lesions seem to spread peripherally and clear centrally to form an annular pattern with secondary and tertiary rings evolving into a "target" or "iris" lesion.

Symmetrical lesions of the lower extremities closely resembling typical erythema nodosum may also be caused by drugs, including sulfones, penicillin, and iodides. The term "fixed eruption" is used to describe an erythematous and sharply defined lesion which recurs at the same site and in the same form upon re-exposure to the same drug. Withdrawal of the drug usually leads to healing, but hyperpigmentation of the area involved may remain. Photosensitivity reactions characterized by erythema, edema, and mild scaling are sharply limited to areas exposed to light, and a clue to the examiner may be provided by the V-shaped area at the neckline, usually at the site where the collar leaves the skin exposed to light and it becomes involved. Sulfonamides and thiazide derivatives are examples known to engender photoallergic reactions.

Other Organ Systems. Drug allergy is often manifested by reactions involving the hematopoietic system. Sedormid, a once popular sedative, resulted in thrombocytopenic purpura, which was shown to depend upon the presence of drug, a serum factor demonstrated to be antibody, and the presence of platelets. Several other drugs, such as quinine and quinidine, thiouracil, and the anticonvulsant hydantoin group, have been implicated as causes of thrombocytopenic purpura. Hemolytic anemia and agranulocytosis are also common adverse reactions ascribed to drugs. Sulfonamides and thiouracil have caused both types of reaction, but aminopyrine and phenylbutazone produced mainly agranulocytosis. Care should be taken in the interpretation of allergic causality of pathologic events leading to agranulocytosis or hemolytic anemia. One of the outstanding examples of a purported allergic hemolytic anemia was that induced by the fava bean. It was later shown that the presence of an enzyme defect in the red cells of these patients resulted in their shorter life span when exposed to drug and that sensitization in the immunologic sense was not required. Aplastic anemia, involving all the formed elements of the blood, is occasionally associated with drug administration; in particular it is described with chloramphenicol, gold, and the sulfonamides.

Gastrointestinal symptoms are common adverse reactions to the administration of therapeutic agents, but the mechanism of action is rarely allergic in nature. The kidney is involved in periarteritis nodosa caused by drugs. In this disease, antimicrobial drugs, notably the sulfonamides, have been frequently implicated. Interstitial nephritis has been described with the penicillinase-resistant penicillin preparation methicillin in association with hematuria, rash, and marked eosinophilia.

The lupus erythematosus syndrome has been described following ingestion of certain drugs, particularly hydralazine, procainamide, and the hydantoin derivatives. The severity of the syndrome induced by drug ingestion may vary from only a serologic manifestation, such as a positive lupus test, to the full-blown picture of fever, arthritis, polyserositis, and hematologic manifestations. Pulmonary infiltration and eosinophilia (PIE syndrome), peripheral neuritis, and hemorrhagic encephalitis have all been ascribed to allergic drug reactions, and probably represent varieties of allergic vascular injury resident in the particular organs involved. Liver damage has been attributed to treatment with heavy metals, thorazine, and sulfonamides; the evidence supporting the allergic basis of these reactions is meager. In recent times, the introduction of halothane, a potent, widely used anesthetic agent, has led to a series of symptoms, primarily involving liver dysfunction, which in some patients strongly suggest an allergic basis.

Generalized Anaphylaxis. Generalized anaphylaxis as a manifestation of drug allergy is a clinical catastrophe with which the physician must be prepared to deal promptly. The condition is usually initiated by an injected drug, although an orally administered tablet has been reported to produce a fatal reaction. Frequently the initial symptoms are generalized pruritus, particularly on the soles of the feet and the palms of the hands, and the general development of a hyperemia of the skin, particularly about the ears, so that the individual often looks as though he had acquired a recent sunburn. Angioedema may cause distortion of the face, swelling of the eyelids, and rapid loss of effective plasma volume, leading to vascular collapse and shock. The risk of developing an anaphylactic reaction, particularly to penicillin, is enhanced by the patient's having had a prior, less serious reaction, such as a maculopapular rash.

DIAGNOSIS. Discontinuance and challenge are still the best diagnostic means available to the physician, although challenge is often inadvisable because of the danger to the patient. Certainly in cases of anaphylactic reactions or urticarial eruptions, the challenge to the patient subsequent to the subsidence of the symptoms is not warranted and is extremely dangerous. However, in drug fever, when that condition appears alone, a fractional dose may be administered after the fever subsides to further identify the cause. Unfortunately, laboratory tests have been very disappointing. The basophil degranulation test, lymphocyte stimulation test, skin window technique, and others have been reported with some success from isolated laboratories, but in general they have been found to be difficult to reproduce and have not come into general use. The necessary information concerning the intermediary metabolites of each drug and the development of specific antigenic determinants is not available for the majority of drugs which cause allergic reactions. Until this information is known, laboratory tests are not likely to be useful. The leukocyte count may be high or low, and therefore not useful; eosinophilia is not a regular occurrence.

TREATMENT AND PROPHYLAXIS. Subsidence of allergic reactions to drugs usually occurs promptly after discontinuance of the drug, often within one or two days, but in many instances prolongation of symptoms for several days and, indeed, in some instances for several weeks and months, is well recognized. Many of our foodstuffs are contaminated with medications: Chickens are fattened with estrogenic hormones, hogs are fed antimicrobials, and cows, when suffering from mastitis, may be treated with large doses of penicillin which appears in the milk. When strongly suspecting a drug hypersensitivity which fails to subside after cessation of the drug, inadvertent environmental drug administration should be carefully investigated. In general, treatment of the drug reaction should be directed against the altered physiology. In the reactions involving vasoactive substances, the use of a direct vasoconstrictor such as epinephrine may be lifesaving and should be used first, instead of the more glamorous, but less effective, group of adrenocortical steroids. The latter group of agents are very useful in the treatment of the Arthus type of immediate hypersensitivity as manifested by serum sickness and polyarteritis, as well as in many forms of delayed hypersensitivity. Epinephrine should be given in dosages of 0.5 to 1 ml of 1:1000 dilution of aqueous epinephrine, given subcutaneously. Antihistaminics such as diphenhydramine (Benadryl, 50 mg) or brompheniramine (Dimetane, 4 mg) may be administered orally or parenterally, but the intravenous use of diphenhydramine is to be avoided because serious adverse reactions to this medication have occurred. Drug reactions are self-limited diseases, and the use of steroids in these diseases is most efficacious and generally does not impose the usual liabilities of steroid therapy. Accordingly, therapy may be instituted with full doses of prednisone, 40 to 60 mg a day, and 40 mg a day may be given for three or four days, dropped to 20 mg a day for an additional several days, and discontinued without a long tapering regimen.

Demis, D. J.: Allergy and drug sensitivity of skin. Ann. Rev. Pharmacol., 9:457, 1969.

Levine, B. B.: Immunochemical mechanisms of drug allergy. Ann. Rev. Med., 17:23, 1966.

Neely, C. L., and Kraus, A. P.: Mechanisms of drug induced hemolytic anemia. Adv. Intern. Med. 18:59, 1972.

Parker, C. W.: Drug allergy. N. Engl. J. Med., 292:511, 732, 957, 1975.

44. ALLERGIC RHINITIS

(Hay Fever)

Fred S. Kantor

DEFINITION. Hay fever is the common name applied to allergic rhinitis which recurs each year at a specific season — usually spring or fall. It is characterized by rhinorrhea, sneezing, itching of the eyes, nose, ears, and palate, and edema of the nasal mucous membranes. Nonseasonal allergens, such as feathers and animal danders, may produce year-round disease called perennial allergic rhinitis; vasomotor rhinitis is a "wastebasket" term which designates perennial rhinitis without an identifiable allergic basis.

ETIOLOGY AND EPIDEMIOLOGY. Susceptible persons exposed each year to airborne pollen of many varieties of plants, particularly trees, grasses, and weeds, develop a "wheal and flare" type of immediate hypersensitivity to protein components of the pollen grains called allergens. The exact heritable basis of hay fever is still unclear, but clustering of a variety of diseases which involve "wheal and flare" hypersensitivity in certain individuals, and in families, strongly supports the view that such a basis exists. The evidence suggests that sensitivity to a particular allergen, such as ragweed, may be dependent upon transmission of a specific immune response gene and therefore might be predictable in an individual before development of the disease.

Drab, colorless plants, unattractive to birds and bees, must depend upon the wind for pollination and release of huge amounts of airborne pollen. In contrast, colorful blossoms and odoriferous plants generally release smaller amounts of heavier, stickier pollen which is not widely disseminated. "Rose fever," a form of allergic rhinitis prevalent in early summer, is a misnomer; while roses are visually in full bloom, it is the pollen from grasses such as timothy, June, and orchard grass which produces the disease.

Ragweed and grass pollen are the most common causes of allergic rhinitis in the United States. Ragweed abounds in the midwestern states, and is prevalent in the eastern and southeastern part of the country. West of the Rocky Mountains and in the dry Southwest, very little ragweed appears. Each area has a distinctive potentially sensitizing flora, and sufferers fleeing from one part of the country to another are often disappointed when symptoms rapidly reappear in their new location. In the northern United States early spring hay fever (April and May) is usually due to tree pollen; the grasses pollinate and produce symptoms in early summer (June and early July) and the ragweed in late summer and early fall. Spores of ubiquitous molds are present throughout the year but increase in numbers at different times because of increased mold growth on decaying vegetation. Spores of *Hormodendrum* peak in number in July, whereas spores of *Alternaria* increase in the fall, overlapping the ragweed season, and may be the basis of an erroneous diagnosis of ragweed hay fever.

The trees are a varied and an important group; ash, beech, birch, cedar, hickory, maple, oak, sycamore, and poplar all produce important windborne pollen, whereas the less antigenic pollens of the firs and pines are not usual sources of disease. Each species of tree produces an antigenically distinct pollen with a relatively short period of pollination lasting two to four weeks. Hypersensitivity to multiple species of trees with overlapping pollinating periods, and to grasses, molds, and ragweed, may blur the seasonal aspects of the patient's problem and suggest a perennial allergic rhinitis. Unlike the trees, grasses such as timothy, fescue, orchard, redtop, and June (Kentucky bluegrass) share important antigenic determinants and in the extreme South and West may produce year-round symptoms. A careful account of seasonal variations in symptoms coupled with a knowledge of the flora of the patient's locality and the pollinating periods of the indigenous plants is vital to the specific diagnosis and management of this group of diseases. In the British Isles and the European continent, trees and grasses are important causes of pollinosis; allergic travelers would do well to check the season of their proposed trip. Europe has little or no ragweed, so American sufferers may doubly enjoy a late summer European vacation.

Pollen grains are about 20 to 40 μ in diameter, and each species has a distinctive appearance. By collecting grains on a glass slide with a simple timed exposure or with more sophisticated air-sampling devices, pollens may be identified and enumerated. The severity of symptoms of an allergic population will vary with the pollen numbers in an approximate way, but the use of daily radio broadcast pollen numbers as a diagnostic or predictive aid is of little value. The "counts" are derived from samples obtained the previous day, and at different locations and altitudes. Often the patient will ask why he doesn't feel better (or worse) because of the low (or high) pollen count!

Allergic rhinitis may be caused by any inhaled antigen; those often implicated, in addition to plant pollen, are house dust, feathers, fungus spores, and animal danders. Food allergy is often suggested as a basis for inhalant symptoms, but manifestations in the skin such as urticaria or angioedema (see Ch. 46 and 47) are the rule, and the respiratory tract is an unlikely target organ for this type of hypersensitivity.

PATHOGENESIS. Sensitization may occur at any time of life but usually occurs in childhood or adolescence. It is curious that an adult may become sensitized to a pollen to which he has been exposed each previous year of his life; this suggests that factors other than genetic proclivity and exposure are necessary. When pollens impinge upon the nasal mucous membrane, they release a variety of protein antigens called allergens which initiate the immune response. The major allergens of grasses and ragweed have been partially purified and are low molecular weight proteins of relatively low antigenicity. This means that for a given amount of antigen, the immune response in terms of amount and avidity of antibody produced is small. The important point is that this type of antigen in low doses tends to elicit an unusual response characterized by production of reaginic antibody, which is largely or completely of the IgE class. Such antibodies are present in nanogram quantities in serum, and "fix" to the surface of cells so that passive administration will sensitize a particular skin site for weeks. Because of this quality, reaginic antibodies are sometimes called homocytotropic. Contact with the specific allergen will cause "sensitized" cells to release potent vasoactive substances, largely histamine and slow reacting substance of anaphylaxis (SRS-A). These materials cause capillary vasodilatation with leakage of fluid and colloid into the tissues leading to the major symptoms of allergic disease.

Although the symptoms produced by inhalation of pollen are localized to the mucosa with which it comes in contact, the sensitization is systemic. When peripheral leukocytes of sensitive individuals are exposed to allergen in vitro, they release histamine. This reaction affords a rapid measurement of sensitivity, usually expressed in terms of amount of allergen necessary to produce release of 50 per cent of the cellular histamine. It also provides an objective measurement of the efficacy and mechanism of treatment. Production of IgE antibody is not limited to allergic individuals; normal subjects or laboratory animals will develop this class of antibody response after subcutaneous injection of allergens. The presence of extracts of roundworms such as *Ascaris* facilitates production of IgE antibody in an unknown way. Similarly, the nasal route of allergen exposure in an allergic individual facilitates development of IgE antibody. Nonimmunologic factors also play a role in producing what may be called the "inertia" of allergic disease; patients who are well tend to remain well, whereas those who are sick tend to remain sick. Nonspecific irritants of all sorts can cause incapacitating sneezing and rhinorrhea in a patient suffering from allergic rhinitis; these might be tolerated without a sniffle at another time of year. Upper respiratory infections, particularly sinusitis, occur more frequently in the allergic patient owing to edema and obstruction of normal drainage. Similarly, the normal effects of emotional states upon the nasal mucosa are often exaggerated in the allergic patient.

CLINICAL MANIFESTATIONS. The abrupt onset of morning sneezing, usually in paroxysms of several sneezes in rapid succession, accompanied by rhinorrhea and itchiness of eyes, palate, and pharynx, is characteristic of allergic rhinitis. Symptoms recur each year at approximately the same time, corresponding to the appearance of the offending pollen in the air. Increased exposure will intensify symptoms: dry, windy days, riding in an open car, and working in a garden are frequently reported to worsen the symptoms. A hay fever sufferer notes that the morning and evening hours are the worst, with a relatively better period during the midday. Mucosal congestion and edema often lead to total blockage of the airway, necessitating mouth breathing. The conjunctivae are red and weepy, and the lids and periorbital tissues may be puffy.

Hay fever is not often accompanied by temperature elevations, and the name is therefore misleading. Fever should alert one to the common complications; sinusitis, otitis, or mastoiditis. Cough, wheezing and dyspnea are frequent companions of allergic rhinitis. Because pollen grains are too large to affect the terminal bronchioles, it was thought that the allergic reaction in the upper respiratory tract could trigger lower airway obstruction, but recent studies indicate that pollen fragments small enough to reach the bronchioles are present in the inspired air.

DIAGNOSIS. Early in the course, the differentiation of allergic rhinitis from that caused by irritants or infections is difficult, but in retrospect the patient will usually remember similar but milder symptoms at the same time in previous years. The seasonal history is the most important of all clues to correct diagnosis. Allergic rhinitis may be differentiated from viral upper respiratory infections by the presence of pruritus of eyes, nose, and pharynx and by the absence of fever, sore throat, and malaise. The nasal mucous membranes appear swollen, pale, and boggy in allergic rhinitis, and red and "angry" in viral infections; but inflammation secondary to sneezing and frequent blowing to clear the nose may blur these differences. Nasal secretions may be obtained by asking the patient to blow his nose into a piece of ordinary wax paper; smears stained with Wright's or Giemsa stains show an abundance of eosinophils in allergic rhinitis, whereas in infectious rhinitis smears reveal polymorphonuclear leukocytes.

Environmental allergens other than pollen are more

difficult to diagnose as the basis of allergic rhinitis, but a careful history will often elicit them. Inquiry should be made into the home: How old is it? What is the heating system? What are the floor, wall, and window coverings? What types of pillows, mattresses, quilts, and comforters are used by the patient and by his or her spouse? Frequently the nonallergic marriage partner will sleep on a feather pillow not five inches from the allergic one sleeping on a nonallergenic pillow. The question of what makes symptoms worse or better has a special significance in the allergic history. Often patients can specify a place or activity associated with symptoms which when avoided keeps them symptom-free.

Skin Tests. Since sensitization is systemic, the allergic individual reacts whenever contact with allergen occurs. Injection of minute quantities of allergens into the skin produces a wheal in 10 to 15 minutes in individuals with reaginic antibodies. Unfortunately, the presence of a positive skin test does not prove that the patient's symptoms are related to the allergen provoking the skin response. Often allergic individuals will have multiple positive skin reactions, such as to ragweed and grass allergen, but express symptoms in only one season and not the other. Skin tests are performed as either scratch tests or intradermal injections. Sets of skin test allergens are readily available and are often used indiscriminately. The patient may be tested with 200 to 300 skin tests with confusing results and erroneous diagnoses. A limited number of tests, 10 to 20, including house dust, common animal danders, feathers, common molds, and pollen, should suffice in all but the most difficult cases.

If skin tests are not diagnostic, why do them? They are often helpful in confirming a suspicion based on the history. The degree of skin reactivity in the untreated patient bears an approximate relationship to the degree of sensitivity and the amount of specific IgE antibody. Occasionally a positive skin test will point to a new direction of inquiry; e.g., a positive test to horse dander led to the finding that the patient was sleeping on a mattress with horse hair. Finally, when a decision is made to hyposensitize with allergen injections (see below), the degree of skin test reactivity provides guidance for a starting dosage.

Allergenic materials for testing and treatment are made by extraction of the solid allergen in a neutral buffer; usually a weight-to-volume ratio is employed, such as 1 gram of defatted ragweed pollen extracted with 100 ml of buffer producing 1:100 allergenic extract. In recent years, Kjeldahl analysis has led to standardization of extracts in protein nitrogen units (PNU) per milliliter. One PNU is equal to 10^{-8} gram N.

This "scientific"-sounding quantity may mislead the user, because only a small fraction of the extract contains the allergenic proteins and all the nitrogen is measured. Until the content of specific allergens is assayable, it is likely that the crude weight per volume or PNU per milliliter standard will be used. Extracts prepared in the same manner at different times may have wide variation in the amount of active allergen per milliliter. It is essential to be careful when using a new extract.

Intradermal tests are more sensitive than scratch tests but carry a greater likelihood of causing a constitutional reaction in a highly sensitive individual. Reactions are read after 10 to 15 minutes. A slight but definite wheal is considered 1+; a moderate reaction (wheal 6 to 10 mm) without pseudopods is read as 2+; a wheal of 10 to 15 mm with pseudopod formation is read as 3+; and wheals larger than 15 mm with a wide flare are read as 4+.

The initial intracutaneous tests with pollens should be made with solutions of antigen containing no more than 10 protein nitrogen units per milliliter, and not more than five to ten tests should be done at any one time. A minimal wheal (0.01 to 0.02 ml) is produced in the skin with a 27 needle attached to a tuberculin syringe. If little or no reaction is obtained, subsequent tests may be made with solutions containing 100 units and then 1000 units per milliliter. Reactions less than 2+ at 1000 PNU per milliliter are of doubtful significance in the untreated patient, whereas strongly positive reactions at 10 PNU per milliliter are almost always associated with symptomatic disease. The interpretation of positive reactions must be made in relation to the prevalence of the antigen in the area and the patient's history.

Circulating γE antibodies directed against a specific allergen can be evaluated by the radioallergosorbent (RAST) test. In this instance a *purified* allergen is adsorbed to an inert particle. The patient's serum is added, and the coated particles are washed. If the serum contained specific γE antibodies, they form complexes with the antigen on the particles and are measured by adding radiolabeled anti-γE antibodies. The promise of a simple in vitro test for diagnosis of allergic rhinitis is not yet fulfilled by the RAST test and, when applied, it is used in conjunction with, not instead of, skin tests.

TREATMENT. Treatment is directed toward avoiding the allergen, modifying the state of hypersensitivity, and ameliorating the symptoms. By far the most effective means is strict avoidance of the offending allergen. When this is due to an increased sensitivity to an animal dander such as that of horse or cat, merely identifying the cause will help greatly in avoidance. Often patients will "hide" their pets from the physician's inquiry because they have a strong suspicion of the offender but hope that something else will be found. Effective filtration of the air within the patient's house is now possible with a variety of electrostatic and barrier-type filters. Dust control and attention to bedding and furniture filling will be rewarding in selected cases.

Treatment with repeated injections of specific allergens has been in vogue for 70 years, and several studies have confirmed the efficacy of this mode of therapy and given insight to its mechanism. Preseasonal, coseasonal, and perennial administration of allergens all have their proponents, but perennial administration avoids the necessity of building up the dosage each year and results in the same number of patient visits. Increasing amounts of allergen are injected subcutaneously once or twice weekly, starting with a dose shown to be tolerated by skin tests. The goals of hyposensitization are two: production of a nonreaginic (blocking) antibody which can effectively compete with reaginic antibody for allergen, and reduction of the amount of reaginic antibody produced (tolerance induction), thereby decreasing cellular sensitivity to allergen. Addition of serum from a treated individual to sensitized leukocytes in vitro may increase by 100-fold the amounts of allergen necessary for 50 per cent histamine release from these leukocytes.

The increment of allergen injected at each visit is determined by the patient's skin reaction to the previous injection. If redness and swelling exceed the size of a 50-cent piece, the dose should be repeated or lowered until it is better tolerated. Often an increase in sensitivity occurs early in treatment; this may lead to a worsening in symptoms if it coincides with the patient's season. Usually patients are treated for two or more years after maximal benefit has been achieved, at which time hyposensitization is stopped. A proportion of patients will maintain their improvement, whereas, in many, a slow return of symptoms during the following year or 18 months is common. Patients should always be advised to remain in the office for 30 minutes after the injection, because the allergen may provoke a constitutional reaction. This is often heralded by reddening of the conjunctivae, nasal swelling, red ears and nose, and a feeling of faintness. Tourniquets should be applied above the injection sites and 0.2 to 0.5 ml of aqueous epinephrine 1:1000 injected above the tourniquet. Such reactions are uncommon. They are usually easily managed in the office or clinic; but if the patient leaves the office immediately after an allergen injection, the reaction at best will be very frightening and might possibly be fatal.

A variety of repository preparations, including alum-precipitated allergens, have generated interest because of a putative ability to administer more allergen in fewer injections with less likelihood of systemic reactions. The efficacy and safety of these preparations are still to be determined.

Symptomatic Treatment. Antihistamines are often helpful in ameliorating symptoms of allergic rhinitis. In general they are only partially effective, and patients complain of the soporific side effects. Brompheniramine (Dimetane) and chlorpheniramine (Chlor-Trimeton) are both available in 4 mg tablets and in long-acting preparations containing 8 or 12 mg. Both these preparations seem to have less soporific effects than Benadryl, which should be used only at bedtime. Response to these drugs is often quite variable in different patients, and several preparations should be tried if results are poor or side effects great. Dexamethasone (Decadron), administered locally by a special nasal spray inhaler, delivers 0.1 mg per spray, and it is often efficacious. Its use once on each side twice a day is often all that is necessary during a short pollen season. The local effect without systemic liability makes this therapy attractive. Systemic steroids are very effective but are used rarely because of their considerable side effects. A short course of four to five days of 30 mg per day of prednisone will help a new patient over the worst symptoms before other measures become effective or the peak of the season passes.

A variety of sympathomimetic drugs, such as Neo-Synephrine, 0.5 per cent, phenylephrine, 0.25 per cent, or Privine, 0.1 per cent, have been used intranasally to shrink the nasal mucosa, but the effects are short-lived and all cause a "rebound" swelling of the nasal mucosa which may be a self-propagating disease. These drugs are not recommended in allergic rhinitis. For relief of allergic conjunctivitis accompanying pollinosis, eye drops containing epinephrine (0.025 per cent), or dexamethasone (0.1 per cent drops) may be used for a brief period with excellent relief. Prolonged use of steroid eye drops is not recommended because of corneal thinning and cataract formation.

Ishizaka, T., and Ishizaka, K.: Biology of immunoglobulin E. Molecular basis of reaginic hypersensitivity. Prog. Allergy, 19:60, 1975.

Lichtenstein, L. M.: Allergic responses to airborne allergens and insect venoms. Fed. Proc., 36:1727, 1977.

Lieberman, P., and Patterson, R.: Immunotherapy for atopic diseases. Adv. Intern. Med. 19:391, 1974.

Norman, P.S.: Specific therapy in allergy: Pro (with reservations). Med. Clin. North Am., 58:111, 1974.

45. VASOMOTOR RHINITIS

Fred S. Kantor

Vasomotor rhinitis is a vague term describing chronic rhinitis without an allergic basis. It is indistinguishable from allergic rhinitis except for chronicity, absence of geographic or seasonal influences, and prevalence of coexistent nasal polyps. Frequently the patient has sought the use of sympathomimetic drugs administered as nose drugs such as Neo-Synephrine or Privine. The problem is compounded by the recurrent rebound rhinitis produced by these agents. Often they are the sole propagating cause of rhinitis which was once allergic or viral in origin, but which has become chronic through the use of these drugs.

The causes of vasomotor rhinitis have been ascribed to bacterial and food allergies, but documentation of these agents is meager and the mechanism is really unknown. Occasionally, a patient with allergies to a variety of ubiquitous substances may present without a clear-cut seasonal environmental history because of the overlapping allergens. These patients may recall a time when their symptoms were seasonal, and skin tests may be helpful in sorting out the problem. In general, however, the bulk of patients with perennial rhinitis at home or away, in summer and winter, will not yield a definite etiologic agent.

Treatment is symptomatic. If nose drops or sprays have been abused, it is useful to discontinue these agents on one side only for a few days and then on the other side so that the patient can breathe through the treated side while the other is recovering from the rebound effects of the drug. Antihistaminics such as brompheniramine (Dimetane), 4 mg every four hours, are sometimes helpful but rarely very successful. Some patients are helped by a nasal dexamethasone spray (Turbinaire) once on each side twice a day. This may produce relief without administering an effective systemic dose and thereby avoid the undesirable side effects.

46. URTICARIA

Fred S. Kantor

DEFINITION. Urticaria, or hives, is an eruption of the skin characterized by elevated, erythematous, sharply demarcated wheals, usually intensively pruritic, lasting hours to days but often recurrent for weeks and sometimes years.

ETIOLOGY AND PATHOGENESIS. The characteristic lesion is produced by capillary dilation in the dermis, leading to loss of fluid into the tissues. Swollen collagen bundles, widening of the dermal papillae, and flattening of the rete pegs are seen microscopically. It is useful to divide the causes into immunologic, paraimmunologic, and nonimmunologic categories.

By far the most common *immunologic cause* of acute hives is food allergy. In this circumstance, vasoactive mediators such as histamine, kinins, and slow-reacting substance of anaphylaxis (SRS-A) are released from mast cells, basophils, and other tissues, producing capillary dilation. The release of mediators is typically due to interaction of antigen with circulating, or fixed, reaginic antibody, usually of the IgE variety. This antibody can be passively transferred by the serum of an affected individual to the skin of a volunteer. A wheal is produced at the transfer site upon ingestion of the offending food antigen. This is the classic Prausnitz-Küstner (PK) reaction. Reactions of IgE antibody with antigen are not complement dependent and produce no vascular necrosis. Complement-dependent IgG-antigen interactions may also cause mediator release by cytotoxic action on mediator-containing cells. These reactions may be produced by antibodies directed against cell antigens, such as isohemagglutinins, and may also be due to antibodies directed against foreign antigens in which the antigen or the complex is passively affixed to the cell surface. The urticaria of serum sickness (see Ch. 42) is such an example. The most frequent route of antigen presentation in the production of acute urticaria is oral ingestion. Inhalation uncommonly produces hives, and occasionally contact with allergen on the skin may suffice. People sensitive to animal dander often report that contact with the fur or saliva of the animal may cause hives; patients allergic to bees may develop hives of the lips and mouth upon contact with honey.

The *"paraimmunologic" causes* are likely to involve similar mechanisms to those of the first category, but the relationship of the antigens and antibodies involved is less apparent. Infection with viruses, bacteria, and fungi may present with hives; hepatitis is a common example. Intestinal parasites, particularly the roundworms, are often associated with hives and eosinophilia. Bites of common insects such as mosquitoes, bedbugs, lice, and other biting insects may produce not only local manifestations but generalized urticaria. Neoplastic diseases, particularly lymphomas of the Hodgkin's variety, and the myeloproliferative diseases are commonly associated with hives. Finally, in the paraimmunologic category are the diseases in which immune complexes have been demonostrated and are thought to play an important etiologic role. In this group, hives are most often associated with systemic lupus erythematosus and dermatomyositis, and the palpable purpura of leukocytoclastic angiitis (Henoch-Schönlein purpura) may first appear as urticaria and then become purpuric.

The nonimmunologic causes of urticaria include physical stimuli such as cold, heat, actinic energy (solar urticaria), and pressure. Cold urticaria may be a familial or sporadic disease in which areas exposed to cold develop urticarial wheals. In about 50 per cent of the sporadic cases, a factor in serum is capable of "sensitizing" normal skin so that a wheal develops when an ice cube is applied to the site. Cold urticaria may be symptomatic of an underlying systemic disease; multiple myeloma, cryoglobulinemia, and syphilis have been reported. The mediators responsible for cold urticaria are presumed to be similar to those released by allergic reactions, but the mechanism of release remains unclear.

Solar urticaria is produced by two spectra of actinic rays of 3100 to 3700Å and 4000 to 5000Å in wavelength. Marked sun exposure in a sensitive individual has led to generalized vascular collapse. Urticaria to sunlight can be passively transferred by serum from individuals who are sensitive to the lower spectrum. The mechanism of mediator release is unknown but, unlike cold urticaria, treatment with drugs and barrier creams is quite effective (see below).

Certain drugs and chemical compounds have the capacity to cause mast cell degranulation directly, resulting in mediator release without an antigen-antibody reaction. Surface-active materials such as saponin, highly negatively charged molecules like polylysines, and many drugs share this property. Common drug examples are morphine, quinine, polymyxin B, curare, decholin, hydralazine, and meperidine. Nonimmunologic release of histamine may be the basis of many "drug reactions" which have failed to yield immunologic mechanisms such as the rare reaction to radiographic contrast agents which are iodinated organic compounds. Indeed, the warm "glow" produced by good brandy is probably more a factor of mediator release than alcohol content, as any ethanol sampler can attest.

A special form of urticaria which consists of small, almost papular, wheals surrounded by a large axon flare is called cholinergic urticaria. Affected individuals will produce a similar eruption when injected with small amounts of mecholyl or acetylcholine. The mechanisms are obscure, but clearly emotional stress, exposure to heat, such as a warm bath, or exercise may bring out the eruption.

Urticaria pigmentosa, or systemic mastocytosis, is due to infiltration of the skin by mast cells; it is believed to be a true neoplasm of very slow growth in which the chemical manifestations are much more distressing to the patient than the invasive ones. Areas of infiltration are marked by freckle-like hyperpigmentation which, upon stroking, will produce a typical linear bumpy wheal, because the skin between the accumulation of mast cells does not urticate.

Chronic urticaria implies recurrent lesions for a period of six weeks or more. The clear causal relationship of certain foods to acute urticaria has led to the assumption that the chronic form is due to an extended exposure to an unidentified allergen or urticator. Investigation of such patients yields a single causal factor in very few, and the bulk of these patients defy elucidation of a specific etiologic factor. Many writers have emphasized psychologic factors in chronic urticaria, but these are difficult to assess.

CLINICAL MANIFESTATIONS. Typically, the wheal is 1 to 5 cm in diameter, often irregular, with a blanched center ("target" lesion) and surrounding erythema. The individual lesions are evanescent, often fading within hours. Successive crops appear for the duration of the disease. The lesions tend to appear at pressure points — e.g., the belt line, the brassiere straps, or the garters. Rarely are the soles and palms affected; but when they are, the patient may complain of difficulty in walking. Pruritus is common and sometimes so severe that the patient cannot wait to get home and fling off his or her clothes. When urticaria is due to a single exposure to a food or drug, it usually appears within minutes. An ingestant taken more than 24 to 48 hours before onset is rarely the cause. Occasionally summation of two allergic stimuli may be responsible; e.g., some patients may eat frozen strawberries in winter with impunity, but during the pollen season the same strawberries will cause hives.

TREATMENT. Acute or sporadic urticaria usually responds well to antihistaminics such as brompheniramine (Dimetane), 4 mg every four hours, or tripelennamine (Pyribenzamine) 50 mg every four hours. Long-acting preparations, containing 8 and 12 mg of brompheniramine respectively, are available and may be used in a twice-a-day regimen as opposed to giving 4 mg every four hours. If the patient is in acute distress, 0.3 ml of 1:1000 epinephrine subcutaneously will often provide relief until the antihistaminic effect is apparent. In severe or unresponsive cases of sporadic urticaria, four days of prednisone, 40 mg per day may be necessary and very helpful.

In chronic urticaria the cause is rarely evident and therefore hard to remove. Most patients have been treated with antihistaminics without benefit. The use of a rigid elimination diet may not only remove hidden allergens, but more likely may also remove foods such as spices which are direct releasers of histamine. In addition to the elimination diet, liberal doses of brompheniramine (Dimetane), 8 mg every four hours, and hydroxyzine, 10 to 25 mg three times a day, are helpful. After a period of relief, cautious reduction of the drug regimen and addition of selective foods in groups, such as eggs, milk, and milk products, one at a time every three to four days, will often result in cessation of symptoms. The result is frequently a grateful patient on a full diet; the doctor, however, remains perplexed. Recently attention has been drawn to a proportion (about 1:7) of patients with chronic urticaria in whom this is a manifestation of vasculitis. This should be suspected in patients with chronic urticaria associated with hypocomplementemia, arthralgia, elevation of erythrocyte sedimentation rate, or serum globulins.

Cold urticaria is often refractory to treatment with all the agents mentioned above, and often the patient has to adjust his life style to avoid the cold. In contrast, solar urticaria is readily treated with barrier creams that filter out the actinic energy of the appropriate wave length. Hydroxychloroquine (Plaquenil), 200 mg, once daily or even twice a week, may protect a sensitive person who anticipates sun exposure.

Mathison, D. A., Arroyave, C. M., Bhat, K. N., Hurewitz, D. J., and Marnell, D. J.: Hypocomplementemia in chronic idiopathic urticaria. Ann. Intern. Med., 86:534, 1977.

Matthews, K. P.: A current review of urticaria. Med. Clin. North Am., 58:185, 1974.

47. ANGIOEDEMA

(Angioneurotic Edema)

Fred S. Kantor

DEFINITION. Angioedema is characterized by painless swelling in the subcutaneous tissues or submucosa, usually occurring about the face (eyes, lips, tongue), but any part of the body may be involved. Two types are now well recognized: sporadic, transient angioedema, related to giant urticaria but involving deeper vessels, caused primarily by food allergy; and hereditary angioedema, which is transmitted as an autosomal dominant trait and is marked by severe deficiency in function of an inhibitor to the activated first component of complement — C'1 esterase.

ETIOLOGY. The causes of the sporadic type are the same as in urticaria (see Ch. 46) and most frequently involve food allergy, although occasionally an inhalant or contactant may be incriminated. In some, emotional factors can trigger an attack. A definite relationship between aspirin ingestion and angioedema has been documented in some individuals. Often asthma and nasal polyps are also associated. Evidence does not favor an immunologic basis for this syndrome, and the mechanism is unknown; the recently reported effect of aspirin upon prostaglandins may provide an important lead.

The lesion of the familial variety is indistinguishable from the sporadic type but is not related to hypersensitivity. Serum from affected persons who are heterozygotes (the trait is dominant) has very low inhibitor activity between attacks and often none measurable during the attack. In a variant of the disease the inhibitor is present but in an inactive form. Deficiency of the inhibitor is due to impaired synthesis, because catabolic rates in affected patients are normal.

PATHOGENESIS. Sporadic angioedema may be thought of as a variant of giant urticaria, with dilation of subcutaneous instead of cutaneous vessels and leakage of fluid and colloid into the tissues. It is generally believed that interaction of ingested allergens with reaginic antibody causes release of vasoactive mediators, including histamine, slow-reacting substance of anaphylaxis (SRS-A), and, possibly, bradykinins. Because the affected capillaries are deep, redness and intradermal swelling are not features. Respiratory and gastrointestinal symptoms occur rarely; the latter should raise a strong suspicion of hereditary angioedema, because abdominal pain is a common feature of the familial disease.

The relationship of the deficiency of C'1 esterase inhibitor to the attacks of angioedema is a complicated one. Attacks are associated with the presence of active C'1, depletion of its natural substrates which are C'4 and C'2, and elevation of bradykinin levels. In addition to inhibiting C'1 esterase activity, the inhibitor is known to inhibit kallikrein and plasmin. Kallikrein converts a serum alpha globulin to bradykinin; plasmin is a broad tryptic-like enzyme which digests fibrin, may cleave C'3 to produce anaphylatoxin (a vasoactive mediator), and may digest Hageman factor into active fragments which can convert prekallikrein to kallikrein. C'1 esterase inhibitor also reduces the capacity of active Hageman factor or its fragments to convert prekallikrein to kallikrein and to convert plasminogen proactivator to the active form. To sum up: the C'1 esterase inhibitor acts at several places, and its deficiency favors the formation of vasoactive mediators from the complement sequence (C'2a, C'3a) and indirectly from the formation of active plasmin and kallikrein.

CLINICAL MANIFESTATIONS. The lesion is a tense, rounded, nonpitting swelling several centimeters in diameter which may last two or three days. In addition to the face, the hands, feet, and genitalia are often affected. In the familial form, laryngeal edema accounts for death in 30 per cent of the patients. Severe abdominal pain, vomiting, and the appearance of an acute intra-abdominal condition are common in the familial type and are important differentiating features from the sporadic variety. During abdominal attacks a characteristic pattern of bowel wall edema can sometimes be demonstrated in x-rays of the gastrointestinal tract. Attacks may be initiated after minor trauma such as tooth extraction, supporting the relationship to the clotting mechanism and the role of Hageman factor activation.

DIAGNOSIS. The sudden appearance of profound swelling without trauma or underlying infection is strongly suggestive of angioedema. Accompanying urticaria or a history of food allergy is helpful, but an inapparent insect bite can sometimes cause swelling of the eyelid or lip and must be considered. The familial form often presents with abdominal complaints accompanying the subcutaneous swelling, and laryngeal edema is also frequently noted. Symptoms of hereditary angioedema may rarely first appear in adult life, and the presence of active C'1 esterase inhibitor should be confirmed in any case involving laryngeal edema or abdominal complaints.

PROGNOSIS. The sporadic variety tends to recur either because all the causative factors are not identified, or, more likely, because the patient "cheats" and samples a forbidden food. The hereditary form of the disease is often fatal in early life, although not before reproductive age.

TREATMENT. Like urticaria, sporadic angioedema is treated with epinephrine, 0.3 to 0.5 ml, 1:1000, or an aqueous solution containing crystalline epinephrine 1:200 (Sus-Phrine), 0.6 to 0.8 ml, given in conjunction with antihistamines. Brompheniramine (Dimetane), 4 mg, tripelennamine (Pyribenzamine), 50 mg, or diphenhydramine (Benadryl), 50 mg, may be given every four hours. (Long-acting preparations, containing 8 and 12 mg of brompheniramine respectively, are available and may be used in a twice-a-day regimen as opposed to giving 4 mg every four hours.) Resolution is slow, because resorption of tissue fluid is required. Prednisone, 40 mg per day, may be given for three to four days in severe or prolonged cases. The patient should be carefully questioned about activities within the 12- to 24-hour period preceding the onset, with special reference to items passing the lips such as food, chewing gum, toothpaste, or aspirin. Usually the patient knows the culprit.

In the hereditary form of disease the aforementioned measures are useless. Poor responses to epinephrine, antihistamine, and corticosteroids are well documented. Highly encouraging results have been produced by treatment with androgen derivatives such as methyltestosterone and danazol, which not only prevent attacks of edema and abdominal pain but also cause a reversal of the biochemical defect. Danazol, 200 mg three times daily, is associated with rapid reappearance of the functional form of the serum C'1 esterase inhibitor and virtual absence of clinical attacks without virilizing side effects.

Gelfand, J. A., Sherino, R. J., Alling, D. W., and Frank, M. M.: Treatment of hereditary angioedema with danazol. Reversal of clinical and biochemical abnormalities. N. Engl. J. Med., 295:1444, 1976.

Ruddy, S., Gigli, I., and Austen, K. F.: The complement system of man. N. Engl. J. Med., 287:489, 1972.

48. INSECT STINGS

Fred S. Kantor

Allergy to antigens contained in the venom of the Hymenoptera insects (bee, wasp, hornet, yellow jacket) may produce a fatal reaction when an otherwise healthy victim is stung. Often a history is obtained of a previous sting which produced local swelling more extensive and longlasting than usual. The patient may rapidly develop shock with or without respiratory difficulty, urticaria, or angioedema, and prompt treatment is vital. If the site of the sting is known, and on an extremity, a tourniquet should be placed above the site to delay further absorption of venom. Epinephrine, 1:1000, 0.3 to 0.5 ml, should be given subcutaneously. If the patient is in shock, the intravenous route must be used, despite the hazard of arrhythmia, to ensure absorption of the drug. Bees have barbed stingers and leave the stinger and venom sac at the site. These should be removed with a forceps or scraped off with the edge of a fingernail so that the venom remaining in the venom sac is not injected through the stinger into the patient. Antihistaminics and steroids are given as adjuncts to epinephrine as described in Ch. 47.

After the acute episode is controlled and before leaving, the patient should be given an emergency kit which contains two tourniquets (stings may be multiple), forceps, or an eyebrow tweezer, a syringe for epinephrine injection (1 ml, 1:1000), and antihistamine tablets. If restung, the patient is instructed to place the tourniquet above the site, take one antihistaminic tablet (diphenhydramine [Benadryl], 50 mg), and prepare the epinephrine syringe while obtaining help from others. Muscular activity enhances the rate of absorption of venom; the patient should be urged to walk, not run, toward help. Since a generalized reaction may lead to temporary skin-test refractoriness, the patient is urged to return in three weeks for testing and hyposensitization treatment. Venom rather than allergenic extracts of the whole insect's body are more efficacious for diagnostic testing and hyposensitization treatment. Until venom extracts are freely available for treatment, the physician should keep in mind and explain to the patient that the efficacy of whole body extracts is in question; they may be used until such time as venom is available.

Lichtenstein, L. M., Valentine, M. D., and Sobotka, A. K.: A case for venom treatment in anaphylactic sensitivity to hymenoptera sting. N. Engl. J. Med., 290:122, 1974.

Zeleznick, L .D., Hunt, K. J., Sobotka, A. K., Valentine, M. D., Tippet, M. M. S., and Lichtenstein, L. M.: Diagnosis of hymenoptera hypersensitivity by skin testing with hymenoptera venoms. J. Allergy Clin. Immunol., 59:2, 1977.

PART VI

CONNECTIVE TISSUE DISEASES ("COLLAGEN DISEASES") OTHER THAN RHEUMATOID ARTHRITIS

49. INTRODUCTION

K. Frank Austen

The connective tissue ("collagen") diseases or systemic rheumatic diseases are a group of clinicopathologic entities considered together because of common or overlapping clinical and histologic features. The term "collagen diseases" was introduced by Klemperer for such reasons and not because of any conviction about a common etiology. Each of the major entities within this grouping has prominent nonspecific constitutional manifestations coupled with patterns of organ involvement which determine the clinical designation, i.e., rheumatoid arthritis, rheumatic fever, systemic lupus erythematosus, scleroderma, dermatomyositis, and periarteritis nodosa (polyarteritis nodosa). Except for rheumatic fever (see Ch. 130), these entities are considered in this Part and in Part VII. The common histologic features of the group are widespread inflammatory damage to connective tissues and blood vessels, at times associated with deposition of fibrinoid material. Fibrinoid refers to an amorphous material, mainly fibrin, staining deeply eosinophilic with hematoxylin and eosin, which is deposited along connective tissue fibers and within vessel walls, and most probably represents a nonspecific response of connective tissue to injury. Clinical findings which have been invoked to support a common grouping include cardinal features of more than one entity in the same patient; transitions between one entity and another within the same patient; possible familial aggregation; and serologic abnormalities which may predominate in one entity but have an appreciable incidence in others.

Progressive systemic sclerosis (scleroderma), polymyositis alone or with cutaneous manifestations (dermatomyositis), and systemic lupus erythematosus (SLE) have distinct clinicopathologic and/or serologic features. By contrast, periarteritis nodosa has neither a characteristic morphologic, biochemical, or immunochemical abnormalty nor a clinical presentation that is easily distinguished from systemic necrotizing angiitis of other types, including those which may be associated with any of the other connective tissue diseases. It seems pertinent, therefore, to review historically the problem of necrotizing angiitis and to include an operational classification based almost entirely upon clinical considerations. A discussion of the structure and function of the structural proteins, collagen and elastin, and the proteoglycan of the connective tissue matrix or ground substance is presented first.

CONNECTIVE TISSUE

Connective tissues are composed of various combinations of collagen, elastin, proteoglycans, and other less well characterized glycoproteins. The unique proportions and distribution of these individual components give different organs of connective tissue their particular qualities. The proteoglycans and the specific arrangement of collagen fibers at various layers give cartilage its smooth, translucent quality and its toughness with elasticity; in contrast, bone has a lesser amount of proteoglycans and a rigid structure related to mineralization within and around collagen fibers. The lens of the eye is transparent because of the precise orthogonal planes in which collagen fibrils are laid down. Skin and blood vessels are rich in elastin, which confers upon these tissues a capacity for distensibility. Basement membrane, a specialized form of collagen and glycoprotein, separates epithelium and endothelium from their environment in multiple tissues. Only in very rare diseases is a primary abnormality of the connective tissue responsible for symptoms or pathology. However, in all forms of arthritis or vasculitis the connective tissues are the site in which inflammation occurs. Although playing a passive, secondary role in pathophysiology, it is damage to connective tissue that results in the signs and symptoms of disease.

Collagen is synthesized by all mesenchymal cells and by some epithelial tissue as well. There are at least four genetic types of collagen distinguished by small but constant variations in amino acid composition: Type I collagen is found exclusively in bone, dentin, and tendon and is mixed in with other types of collagen in most other tissues; Type II collagen predominates in articular cartilage; Type III collagen (which contains an interchain disulfide bond within the helical portion of the molecule) is present in largest proportion relative to other types in skin and blood vessels; Type IV collagen, less well characterized, is an important component of basement membranes. Each collagen molecule has a biosynthetic precursor, or procollagen, which contains nonhelical peptide sequences at both NH_2^- and COOH-terminal ends of the molecule. After procollagen has been hydroxylated (hydroxyproline from proline and hydroxylysine from lysine) and glycosylated, it is released from the cell. The nonhelical ends of the molecules are cleaved off, and the collagen molecules aggregate with others to form fibrils. Each collagen molecule is formed of three α chains, each approximately 1010 amino acids in length, coiled about each other in a complex triple helical arrangement. It is this helical structure which confers upon the collagen stability, rigidity, and resistance to proteases.

This precise register of individual molecules in fibril form gives the 640 to 700 Å periodicity on electron microscopy characteristic of collagen fibrils. After fibril formation an additional change in primary structure of the molecule occurs to give cross-linking within and between different molecules. ε-Amino groups on lysine and hydroxylysine are oxidized to aldehydes. These reactive groups condense with other aldehydes or form a Schiff base with amino groups to create cross-links. These cross-links give stability through insolubility and resistance of fibrils to collagenolytic enzymes.

Recently synthesized collagen has a more rapid turnover than mature collagen. Since hydroxyproline is present only in collagen and elastin, and since collagen is the most abundant protein in the body, the excretion of urinary hydroxyproline serves as a rough index of collagen turnover. Collagen is degraded by collagenases present in mesenchymal tissues, certain epithelial tissues, and polymorphonuclear leukocytes; collagenases cleave through one site on each collagen triple helix. The reaction products uncoil, are thermally denatured at body temperature, and become immediately susceptible to multiple tissue proteases. In rheumatoid arthritis and certain skin and bone diseases, proliferation of cells which synthesize collagenase may result in excessive destruction of collagen.

Developmental abnormalities in the complicated sequence of collagen biosynthesis lead to expression of a number of diseases. For example, insufficient production of Type I collagen is found in some cases of *osteogenesis imperfecta*. Post-translational abnormalities include inadequate hydroxylation of lysine and proline in *scurvy*, inadequate hydroxylation of lysine in certain tissues in *Ehlers-Danlos* syndrome Type VI, insufficient procollagen conversion to collagen in Ehlers-Danlos *Type VII*, and inhibition of cross-link formation among collagen molecules in *homocystinuria* by the reactive sulfhydryl group in homocysteine.

Proteoglycans have a role in connective tissue not unlike that of cement in reinforced concrete. The proteoglycans are formed of subunits of disaccharides linked together (termed glycosaminoglycan chains) and joined to a protein core. In articular cartilage this core is a protein with a length of 20,000 to 50,000 Å. The disaccharide chains, many of which are sulfated, have a length of 15,000 to 36,000 Å. Each proteoglycan monomer (core protein plus disaccharide chains) is joined with others to form large aggregates with hyaluronic acid chains stabilized by a link glycoprotein. The physiologic implications of this macromolecular organization are probably related to the excluded volume effect; that is, in connective tissue, they control by virtue of size and domain the passage of other molecules to and from cells. The large net negative charge among proteoglycans serves to impart to tissues containing them in high concentration (e.g., cartilage) a resistance to compressive force. In the polysaccharide (glycosaminoglycan) component of proteoglycans one of the hexose residues of each disaccharide group is a hexosamine, and the other is a hexuronic acid moiety. Proteoglycans are synthesized by mesenchymal tissues by a complicated process involving assembly of the polysaccharide units, sulfation, and covalent linkage to the protein core.

Proteoglycans have a more rapid turnover than collagen and are degraded primarily by acid hydrolases found in lysosomes, such as cathepsin C and B. Factors such as vitamin A which destabilize lysosomal membranes can result in generalized depletion of proteoglycans from many connective tissues. Proteoglycan destruction is accentuated by an inflammatory response in the connective tissue.

Elastin has covalent cross-links, desmosine and isodesmosine, which are similar to cross-links in collagen and are formed from condensation of lysine residues on different parts of the same chain or other elastin polypeptides. Unlike collagen, which is a rigid rod, elastin is an amorphous random coil aggregate linked by these cross-links; this structure assures its return to an original configuration after it is distorted and gives rise to its elastic properties. Elastin fibers have two components: the amorphous elastin polypeptides containing a great quantity of nonpolar amino acids, and the glycoprotein microfibrils which may act as a template for amorphous elastin production. A proelastin has been described which, like procollagen, must have a COOH-terminal registration peptide cleaved away before insoluble elastic fibers can be formed.

HISTORICAL REVIEW OF ANGIITIS

The term *necrotizing angiitis* or *vasculitis* designates disorders in which there is segmental inflammation with fibrinoid necrosis of the blood vessels. Criteria that allow the definition of clinical syndromes include the gross and histologic appearance of the vascular lesions, the caliber of the affected blood vessels, the frequency of involvement of specific organs, and the absence or presence of hematologic and serologic abnormalities. Inasmuch as necrotizing angiitis is segmental and spotty in distribution, involvement of internal organs is generally not appreciated unless a partial or complete occlusion substantially compromises function. In contrast, this process is recognized visually in the skin without or with local or systemic symptoms.

The term *periarteritis nodosa* was aptly introduced by Kussmaul and Maier in 1866 to designate a morbid process manifested by numerous nodules along muscular-type arteries. Infiltration of the media with polymorphonuclear leukocytes and to a lesser extent eosinophils, plasma cells, and lymphocytes, disruption of the internal elastic lamina, fibrinoid necrosis, and extension to the adventitia and intima are characteristic. Proliferation of the intima leads to partial or total occlusion, and segmental scarring of the entire wall is responsible for the visible and/or palpable aneurysms. It is characteristic of the lesions to be in all stages of evolution from acute to healed. Additional characteristic features of periarteritis nodosa are the sparing of capillaries and veins except for involvement by spread from contiguous arteries, and the absence of involvement of pulmonary arteries despite the location of nodules in the bronchial arteries.

In 1923 Ophüls reported a patient with a periarteritis

nodosa–like illness with the additional features of pulmonary vessel lesions, extensive involvement of small arteries and veins, granulomatous vascular and extravascular reactions, and an intense eosinophilic infiltration of vascular and pulmonary parenchymal lesions. The granulomas often included an eosinophilic core of altered collagen and necrotic eosinophils surrounded by radially arranged macrophages, lymphocytes, plasma cells, and varying numbers of polymorphonuclear leukocytes, both neutrophilic and eosinophilic. A detailed study of similar patients in 1951 by Churg and Strauss emphasized the striking clinical feature of severe progressive asthma with peripheral eosinophilia followed by fever, and prompted these authors to term this entity *allergic angiitis and granulomatosis*. Rose and Spencer (1957) also appreciated these unique clinicopathologic features but preferred the term *polyarteritis with pulmonary involvement* to distinguish this group from classic polyarteritis.

In 1926 von Glahn and Pappenheimer considered that the *arteritis of rheumatic fever* could be distinguished from periarteritis nodosa by the absence of arterial thrombosis (or eosinophils), involvement of small arteries, and minimal fibrinoid necrosis. In the heart, Aschoff bodies represent a key extravascular histologic finding, although the clinical manifestations are predominantly related to rheumatic carditis.

Still another type of necrotizing vascular lesion, originally believed to be limited to the cranial arteries and characterized by the presence of multinucleated giant cells, was recognized by Horton, Magath, and Brown in 1934 and established as a clinical entity by Kilbourne and Wolff in 1946. The process usually involves the innermost layer of the media with predominantly a lymphocyte infiltration, the presence of multinucleated giant cells, fragmentation of the internal elastic lamina, and associated fibrinoid necrosis. The infiltration may extend to involve the adventitia and the intima, leading to intimal thickening with subsequent thrombosis. This entity, *giant cell arteritis*, can be predominantly local — presenting as cranial, especially temporal, or aortic arch (Takayasu's) arteritis — or it may be systemic. The syndrome of polymyalgia rheumatica seems to be associated with a local or systemic form of giant cell arteritis with or without arterial occlusion.

Necrotizing vascular lesions associated with the administration of horse antiserum and the development of clinical serum sickness were described by Clark and Kaplan in 1937. Rich observed similar lesions (1942) which he considered to be periarteritis nodosa not only in cases of serum sickness but also in circumstances of sulfonamide hypersensitivity. However, the more recent and prevailing view proposed by Zeek in 1952 is that hypersensitivity to drugs and serum, termed *hypersensitivity angiitis*, is distinguishable from periarteritis nodosa. Hypersensitivity angiitis involves small arteries, arterioles, and venules in a process of fibrinoid necrosis, occurring in the subendothelial ground substance and extending from the intima to involve the entire vessel wall; the accompanying cellular reaction is pleomorphic with polymorphonuclear neutrophil leukocyte predominance frequently including eosinophils. Hypersensitivity angiitis often involves the pulmonary system and is characterized by virtually all lesions of an episode being at a similar evolutionary stage.

Wegener's granulomatosis is distinguished from allergic granulomatosis and angiitis as defined by Churg and Strauss. Wegener in 1936 described a disease characterized by necrotizing granulomatous lesions of the upper and lower respiratory tract, generalized focal necrotizing lesions of both arteries and veins, and a glomerulitis typified by fibrin thrombi, focal necrosis of tufts, and on occasion a granulomatous reaction. This complex is somewhat similar to allergic granulomatosis and angiitis, but is is noteworthy that Wegener's granulomatosis is not associated with progressive asthma and prominent peripheral eosinophilia and does not exhibit a prominence of eosinophils in the necrotizing lesions. Thus it seems reasonable to list this entity separately; lethal midline granuloma may be a related condition or a local variant. (See Ch. 68.) More recently, variants of Wegener's granulomatosis have been recognized in which the granulomatous reactions are predominantly lymphoid- and sarcoid-like, respectively.

OPERATIONAL CLASSIFICATION OF NECROTIZING ANGIITIS

Necrotizing angiitis is a convenient generic term for the entire group of syndromes in which vascular lesions, arterial or venous or both, may involve all three layers of the vessel wall with fibrinoid necrosis and various cellular infiltrates (see accompanying table). Zeek recognized five major syndromes in this group: periarteritis nodosa, allergic angiitis and granulomatosis, rheumatic fever, giant cell arteritis, and hypersensitivity angiitis. With some modification this tabulation continues to be operationally useful. The limitations of this classification, however, are becoming increasingly apparent with the demonstration of involvement of vessels of various sizes in the same clinical process.

Rheumatic fever can be placed under a category broadened to include those collagen diseases in which necrotizing vascular lesions are present but are not the most prominent aspect of the entity, i.e., rheumatoid arthritis, scleroderma, dermatomyositis, polymyositis,

---

Necrotizing Angiitis

Periarteritis nodosa (polyarteritis nodosa)
Allergic angiitis and granulomatosis of Churg and Strauss
  ("polyarteritis nodosa with pulmonary involvement")
Connective tissue disease ("collagen disease"), associated with
  Rheumatoid arthritis
  Scleroderma
  Poly- and dermatomyositis
  Rheumatic fever
  Erythema nodosum
  Sjögren's syndrome
Giant cell arteritis
Hypersensitivity angiitis
  Drug reaction
  Henoch-Schönlein purpura
  Systemic lupus erythematosus, rheumatoid arthritis, Sjögren's
    syndrome
  Mixed cryoglobulinemia
  Nodular vasculitis
  Hypergammaglobulinemic purpura
  C2 deficiency with vasculitis
  Australian antigenemia with vasculitis
  Subacute bacterial endocarditis and other infections
  Lymphoproliferative disorders
  Erythema elevatum diutinum
Wegener's granulomatosis and variants

Sjögren's syndrome, and erythema nodosum. The situation in rheumatoid arthritis is particularly instructive in that necrotizing angiitis presents with three syndromes: polyarteritis nodosa resulting from involvement of medium-sized muscular arteries; peripheral neuropathy, digital gangrene, and cutaneous ulcers secondary to disease of small arteries; and palpable purpura as a manifestation of cutaneous necrotizing venulitis.

The category of hypersensitivity angiitis is particularly diverse and contains a variety of clinical entities distinguishable on the basis of precipitating events (drugs, hepatitis B antigenemia, subacute bacterial endocarditis, and *Mycobacterium leprae* infection), serologic abnormalities (cryoglobulinemia, hypergammaglobulinemic purpura, homozygous C2 deficiency), underlying diseases (rheumatoid arthritis, systemic lupus erythematosus, Sjögren's syndrome, lymphoproliferative disorders), and characteristic clinical presentations (Henoch-Schönlein purpura, nodular vasculitis with its lower extremity distribution and predilection for females, and erythema elevatum diutinum appearing as erythematous plaques over articular surfaces).

The problems of any effort at classification are highlighted by the vasculitis associated with Australian antigenemia and designated periarteritis nodosa by some. The clinical manifestations of urticaria, arthralgia, fever, eosinophilia, and azotemia; the pathologic findings of fibrinoid necrotizing lesions of arterioles in liver and muscle and venules in skin with deposition of immunoglobulin, viral antigen, and complement; and the serologic presence of circulating immune complexes with hypocomplementemia are entirely consistent with hypersensitivity angiitis. The demonstration of abnormalities of the medium-sized muscular arteries by angiography emphasizes the continuum of lesions characteristic of periarteritis nodosa to hypersensitivity angiitis under these etiologic circumstances. In one study only a single patient out of nine with vasculitis and hepatitis B antigenemia presented the classic manifestations of polyarteritis nodosa alone, prompting the observers to propose the generic term generalized necrotizing vasculitis for this group.

An operational classification is nonetheless a justified interim measure because there are associated implications as to prognosis, treatment, and etiology. A classification based on etiology and pathogenetic mechanisms is a further goal. The fibrinoid in the lesions of systemic lupus erythematosus contains protein residues of nuclear origin, acid mucopolysaccharides derived from altered ground substance, and fibrinogen (or derivatives), immunoglobulins, and complement proteins. These findings are interpreted to mean the presence of immune complexes, consisting of nuclear antigen and antibody, complement fixation, and secondary deposition of fibrinogen and alteration of ground substance. In vasculitis associated with Australian antigenemia, immune complexes with specific antigen have been isolated from the plasma and recognized in tissues along with complement by immunofluorescent studies. Whereas in systemic lupus erythematosus, vasculitis with Australian antigenemia, and mixed cryoglobulinemia the specificity of the antibodies contributing to or responsible for the clinicopathologic manifestations of the disease is known, such is not the case for most of the other entities shown in the table. Studies of 1-μm-thick sections stained with Giemsa's reagent have allowed the recognition of two cellular patterns in the skin of patients with cutaneous hypersensitivity angiitis. In individuals with serum hypocomplementemia the cellular infiltrate contains predominately neutrophils, whereas lymphocytes and activated lymphocytes are the predominant cells in the normocomplementemic group. Although the pathologic findings could represent different stages of a single process, transition from one to the other type of pathology in individual patients has not yet been reported, and the processes could reflect different host responses. Immunoglobulins and complement have been observed in the glomerular and cutaneous lesions of Henoch-Schönlein purpura, in the vascular lesions of rheumatoid arthritis and of periarteritis nodosa, and in the granulomatous response of allergic angiitis and granulomatosis (often with fibrinogen), but not in Wegener's granulomatosis. Such proteins could deposit nonspecifically owing to trapping, transudation or exudation, or because of aggregation of gamma globulin. It is also true, however, that deposition of immune complexes may be underestimated because of their rapid clearance. Studies should be directed toward determining the specificity of the deposited immunoglobulins. Arguments to favor specific deposition could be based on demonstration of antigen in the lesion, recognition of the antibody specificity following elution, and demonstration that the predominant L chain type or H chain subgroup in the deposit is different from the ratio observed in the circulation. Each of these criteria has been met with regard to the lesions of systemic lupus erythematosus.

Christian, C. L., and Sergent, J. S.: Vasculitis syndromes: Clinical and experimental models. Am. J. Med., 61:385, 1976.

Churg, J., and Strauss, L.: Allergic granulomatosis, allergic angiitis, and periarteritis nodosa. Am. J. Pathol., 27:277, 1951.

Frohnert, P. P., and Sheps, S. G.: Long-term follow-up study of periarteritis nodosa. Am. J. Med., 43:8, 1967.

Glass, D., Soter, N. A., and Schur, P. H.: Rheumatoid vasculitis. Arthritis Rheum., 19:950, 1976.

Gocke, D. J., Morgan, C., Lockshin, J., Hsu, K., Bombardieri, S., and Christian, C. L.: Association between polyarteritis and Australian antigen. Lancet, 2:1149, 1970.

Grant, M. E., and Prockop, D. J.: The biosynthesis of collagen. N. Engl. J. Med., 286:194, 242, 291, 1972.

Harris, E. D., Evanson, J. M., Dibona, D. R., and Krane, S. M.: Collagenase and rheumatoid arthritis. Arthritis Rheum., 13:83, 1970.

Kilbourne, E. D., and Wolff, H. G.: Cranial arteritis: Critical evaluation of syndrome of "temporal arteritis," with report of a case. Ann. Intern. Med., 24:1, 1946.

Klemperer, P.: The concept of collagen disease in medicine. Am. Rev. Respir. Dis., 83:331, 1961.

Kussmaul, A., and Maier, R.: Über eine bisher nicht beschreibene eigenthümlich Arterienerkankung (Periarteritis nodosa), die mit Morbus Brightii and rapid fortschreitender allgemeiner Muskellähmung einhergeht. Deutsch. Arch. Klin. Med., 1:484, 1866.

Liebow, A. A.: Pulmonary angiitis and granulomatosis. Am. Rev. Respir. Dis., 108:1, 1973.

Silbert, J. E.: Biosynthesis of muco-polysaccharides and proteinpolysaccharides. In Perez-Tamayo, R., and Rojkind, M. (eds.): Molecular Pathology of Connective Tissues. New York, Marcel Dekker, Inc., 1973.

Soter, N. A., Mihm, M. C., Gigli, I., Dvorak, H. F., and Austen, K. F.: Two distinct cellular patterns in cutaneous necrotizing angiitis. J. Invest. Dermat., 66:344, 1976.

Wegener, F.: Über generalisierte, septische Gefässerkrankungen. Verh. Deutsch. Ges. Path., 29:202, 1936.

Wolff, S. M., Fauci, A. S., Horn, R. G., and Dale, D. C.: Wegener's granulomatosis. Ann. Intern. Med., 81:513, 1974.

Zeek, P. M.: Periarteritis nodosa: A critical review. Am. J. Clin. Pathol., 22:777, 1952.

50. SYSTEMIC SCLEROSIS

(Scleroderma)

Edward D. Harris, Jr.

GENERAL CONSIDERATIONS. *Scleroderma* is a disease involving blood vessels and connective tissue. The clinical picture is dominated by symptoms of vascular insufficiency caused by abnormalities in small arterioles and capillaries, and by progressive fibrosis in multiple organs. Most patients have involvement predominantly of the arms and hands with Raynaud's phenomenon and acrosclerosis. The face and upper chest may be affected as well, but it is interesting that the legs and feet are involved less often, and it is rare that diffuse involvement of the entire skin is seen. Associated with the cutaneous manifestations are dysfunctions of certain viscera, particularly the esophagus, lungs, and kidneys.

Localized scleroderma, a term which includes morphea and linear scleroderma, involves the skin exclusively.

The diagnosis of systemic sclerosis is made most often in patients between the ages of 35 and 55. Between three and five new cases per million population appear each year. Only 8 per cent of cases begin in the first two decades of life. The disease is three times more common in females than in males. There is some evidence that black women have a poorer prognosis than white women, and males a poorer prognosis than females.

PATHOGENESIS AND PATHOLOGY. Pathogenesis. Data are accumulating to indicate that abnormalities in the vascular system are primarily involved in the pathogenesis of this disease. Raynaud's phenomenon with its characteristic blanching and pain followed by suffusion is a very common initial complaint in systemic sclerosis. Patients with Raynaud's phenomenon have been shown to have significantly decreased cutaneous fingertip blood flow compared with that of normal controls when both are cooled to 18° C. In clinically unaffected muscle tissue, patients with scleroderma have been shown to have loss of 80 per cent of the normal amount of capillaries; those remaining capillaries have a diameter increased over normal, swollen endothelial cells, and reduplication of the basement membrane. Surface microvessels of the nail fold in systemic sclerosis are decreased in number, dilated, and tortuous. Digital arteriograms in patients with Raynaud's syndrome and scleroderma often have shown obstruction of the proper digital arteries, and plethysmography has demonstrated decreased amplitude of reflection of the pulse. There may be a common factor of altered vascular reactivity in the development of Raynaud's phenomenon, depressed sensitivity to cholinergic agonists of the lower esophageal sphincter, pulmonary hypertension, and reduced renal cortical blood flow — all abnormalities associated with systemic sclerosis.

Studies of the proliferative lesion of scleroderma (the appearance of excessive and inappropriate collagen deposition) have revealed no significant abnormality of physical properties, amino acid analyses, cross-linking, or solubility of collagen. Areas of rapid new collagen synthesis may have a higher ratio than normal of Type III to Type I collagen.

Numerous studies have indicated that there is an increased rate of collagen synthesis in scleroderma. Increased activity of protocollagen proline hydroxylase has been found in skin biopsies from scleroderma. Medium from cultures in vitro of some scleroderma skin fibroblasts has been found to contain significantly more collagen than does medium from control cells.

Association of fibrosis with the carcinoid syndrome has generated interest in study of amine metabolism. Some patients with scleroderma have been reported to have a decreased monamine oxidase activity in plasma, although measurements of plasma catecholamine concentrations and urinary catecholamine excretion patterns have been normal.

Interest has expanded in the possible involvement of the cellular immune system in pathogenesis of scleroderma. Lymphokines (e.g., soluble products of activated lymphocytes and monocytes) which stimulate collagen production by fibroblasts and which are chemotactic for dermal fibroblasts have been defined. Mononuclear cells from scleroderma patients produce a factor chemotactic for human monocytes when cultured in the presence of collagen.

Immunoglobulin and complement have been selectively localized in vascular lesions of the kidneys of patients with scleroderma, and antinuclear antibodies have been eluted from renal tissue, suggesting, but not proving, a role for immune complexes in pathogenesis of acute renal failure in this disease.

Pathology. The result of systemic involvement in scleroderma is sclerosis. Early findings in the *skin* in active scleroderma have revealed edema, plasma cell and/or lymphocyte infiltrates around eccrine sweat glands, loss of capillaries, and endothelial proliferation. Larger vessels may show fibromucinous accumulations in the intima. The *reticular dermis* is usually thickened. It may have a normal collagen-bundle pattern or may show broad, homogeneous, acellular deposits of collagen with indistinct bundle patterns. Other findings include atrophy of the rete pegs of the epidermis, atrophy of the hair follicles and sweat glands, perivascular lymphocytic infiltration, and hyalinization of arterioles. The subcutaneous tissue is replaced by thick collagen bundles which bind the dermis to deeper structures. Pathologic changes in the musculoskeletal system include acute and chronic inflammation in the *synovium* with no pannus formation but with more sclerosis than is found in rheumatoid synovium with an equivalent inflammatory response. Fibrin deposits are laid down around *tendons*, and in *muscles* there are a variety of abnormalities, the most common being fibrosis of the perimysium and epimysium, scattered cellular infiltrates, and atrophy and necrosis of muscle fibers similar to that seen in polymyositis.

In the internal organs, microvascular abnormalities (see Pathogenesis), mild inflammation, and edema in connective tissue are followed by increased deposition of fibrous tissue in both appropriate and inappropriate loci. This leads to distortion of the architecture of the tissues affected. In the *lungs,* a relatively low-grade interstitial pneumonitis is followed by interstitial fibrosis, most marked in lower lobes. After this, cyst formation and bronchiectasis may develop. Arteriolar thickening (concentric intimal proliferation or medial hypertrophy) is seen, particularly in those patients with clinical evidence of pulmonary hypertension. In the gastrointestinal tract, the *esophagus* is frequently involved with muscle atrophy and fibrosis. Lesions secondary to reflux of gastric contents are present in 20 per cent. Fibrosis around Brunner's glands in the submucosa of the *duodenum* occurs and can be recognized on specimens obtained by peroral biopsy. Involvement of the *small bowel* begins with patchy subserosal fibrosis and may progress to almost complete replacement of smooth muscle with fibrous tissue and marked thickening of the serosa. The small bowel may develop multiple sacculations, presumably at sites of weakness in the continuity of the wall. Dilation, muscle atrophy, and fibrosis are seen in the *colon;* the fibrosis is irregular, leading to the characteristic sacculations and diverticula. The *heart* is frequently enlarged and may be the only organ weighing more than predicted for the subject's body weight. Small patches of interstitial myocardial fibrosis are commonly found. In very severe cases, as much as 60 per cent of cardiac muscle is replaced by dense, relatively acellular and avascular fibrous tissue. Endocardial or valvular thickening is unusual and is rarely of hemodynamic significance. Fibrinous pericarditis is found quite often, even in the absence of uremia. *Kidneys* in scleroderma are normal in size when renal involvement has not been present clinically. In patients dying with uremia they may be small and frequently have small cortical infarcts. Histologically, fibromucinous intimal proliferation in the interlobular arteries, fibrinoid necrosis of small arteries and arterioles (including the glomerular tufts), and thickening of the basement membrane (the "wire-loop" lesion) may all be present. These changes are similar to those seen in kidneys from patients with malignant hypertension and occasionally may be present in the absence of renal failure or severe hypertension.

CLINICAL MANIFESTATIONS AND DIAGNOSES. The disease usually begins insidiously. Raynaud's phenomenon, vague weakness, weight loss, diffuse stiffness and aching, polyarticular arthritis, and diffuse edema of the hands are the most common initial symptoms. If the illness progresses, it generally does so slowly, and is marked by characteristic organ system changes. Rarely, rapid progression to severe cutaneous and visceral involvement may occur in less than six months.

Cutaneous System. The patient with classic, well-developed acrosclerosis presents with taut, thickened, or edematous skin bound tightly to subcutaneous tissues in the hands and fingers. Feet and toes are involved less often than hands, forearms, and neck. Normal skin folds at the knuckles disappear. Chronic recurrent painful ulcerations at the ends of the digits develop, and the fingers themselves may shorten through progressive resorption of the terminal phalanges. Joints become immobilized from tight encasement in thickened skin as well as from contractures of muscles and tendons and palmar fascia. Telangiectasia, increased or decreased pigmentation, and subcutaneous calcification are common. Hair becomes thin, and the skin of the face appears smooth and waxy. The skin around the mouth may constrict, restricting lip movement and preventing adequate dental hygiene. The normal sweating mechanism is often impaired; the involved skin feels leathery and dry and may scale and itch. The CREST syndrome (calcinosis, Raynaud's phenomenon, esophageal hypomotility, sclerodactyly, and telangiectasia) and the Thibierge-Weissenbach syndrome (diffuse deposition of insoluble calcium phosphates in subcutaneous tissue in the presence of acrosclerosis) are variants of the cutaneous expression of systemic sclerosis.

Musculoskeletal System. Almost half the patients with systemic sclerosis present with joint pain or develop it during the first year of their illness. Small joints are involved more often than large ones. Joint deformity and immobility in systemic sclerosis do not result from an invasive, erosive synovitis as in rheumatoid arthritis, but are the result of encasement as subcutaneous tissue is replaced by bundles of collagen. Muscle wasting is often severe in areas such as the hands, in which joint mobility is impaired by progressive tightening of the overlying skin.

Gastrointestinal Tract. Of the internal organ systems, the gastrointestinal tract is the one most often involved in systemic sclerosis. *Oral* symptoms include xerostomia and a progressive decrease in the size of the mouth. Sjögren's syndrome is seen often, and the frequency of its association with systemic sclerosis is probably underestimated. Symptoms referable to the *esophagus,* ranging from simple dysphagia to heartburn, nausea, and substernal fullness, are found in 45 to 60 per cent of cases. The dysphagia is related to absence of coordinated peristalsis, followed by loss of amplitude of esophageal body waves and incompetence of the lower esophageal sphincter. If reflex esophagitis becomes a persistent complication, stricture may develop. There is a very frequent association of Raynaud's phenomenon and decreased esophageal peristalsis, although this association is not limited to patients with scleroderma. Vomiting, abdominal distention, and pain or diarrhea may indicate involvement of the *small intestine.* As in the esophagus, motility of the small bowel is decreased, and there may be malabsorption secondary to intraluminal stagnation with concomitant bacterial overgrowth. Functional bowel complaints secondary to pathologic changes in the *colon* are common. Disease of both large and small bowel may produce a clinical picture identical to paralytic ileus with incomplete obstruction at any level. Pneumatosis cystoides intestinalis (air-filled cysts in the mesentery which may rupture, causing peritonitis) is a rare but striking complication of scleroderma bowel disease.

An association between primary biliary cirrhosis and scleroderma with CREST syndrome is now recognized.

Heart and Lungs. Dyspnea is the most common cardiorespiratory symptom in systemic sclerosis and is present in more than 50 per cent of patients. Fine, dry crackles at the bases of the lung are the first abnormality found on physical examination. In some patients, progression to respiratory insufficiency and death from hypoxemia is related to progressive pulmonary fibrosis. The earliest abnormality of pulmonary function is a decrease in pulmonary diffusion capacity. Those exposed in their occupation to silicate dust have a predilection to develop this form of the disease. Restriction of chest wall expansion by dermal fibrosis around the thorax rarely affects respiratory function. A few patients with severe cystic and fibrotic changes in the lungs have developed multifocal alveolar cell carcinomas.

Signs of elevated pulmonary vascular resistance may develop independent of parenchymal changes in the lungs and lead to cor pulmonale and congestive heart failure.

Replacement of myocardium with fibrous tissue on a primary basis ("scleroderma heart disease") is an occasional cause of heart failure. In addition, impaired cardiac function can be attributed to right ventricular failure secondary to pulmonary hypertension.

Kidneys. The sudden development of malignant hypertension resistant to therapy and uremia progressing rapidly to death is a dreaded complication of systemic sclerosis. Most patients have had skin changes before development of abnormal renal function. Renal arteriograms reveal narrowed interlobular arteries and afferent arterioles with focal or generalized loss of the cortical nephrogram. It is rare for patients with this complication to survive longer than four months unless nephrectomy and hemodialysis and/or transplantation are carried out.

Nervous System. Involvement of the nervous system is rare. Facial pain, questionably related to a trigeminal neuropathy, is seen in occasional patients and may be disabling. Significant reduction in mean conduction velocity of peripheral nerves has been reported.

LABORATORY FINDINGS. The erythrocyte sedimentation rate is elevated in most patients with systemic sclerosis, and a mild anemia of chronic disease may be present. In addition, iron deficiency anemia may result from bleeding from esophagitis, and vitamin B_{12} and/or folic acid deficiency from overgrowth of organisms in an atonic bowel. Hemolysis is unusual, although microangiopathic hemolytic anemia has been described in scleroderma (presumably related to fragmentation of erythrocytes from contact with diseased blood vessels and/or intravascular fibrin). A number of serologic abnormalities link systemic sclerosis to other connective tissue diseases. Mild hypergammaglobulinemia is present in 30 to 50 per cent of patients, rheumatoid factor in 25 to 35 per cent, antinuclear antibodies (often with a speckled or a nucleolar pattern) in sera of 30 to 40 per cent, and LE cells in less than 10 per cent of patients. There has been no correlation found between antinuclear antibody patterns and the course and activity of disease. DNA-binding activity in serum is absent.

The electrocardiogram shows nonspecific abnormalities in almost 50 per cent of patients. The pattern of conduction defects with very low voltage is seen only in those uncommon patients with marked myocardial replacement by fibrous tissue. Echocardiogram in these cases will reveal reduced ventricular wall motion. This technique is also useful in documenting small pericardial effusions. In general the electromyogram is normal; most patients have polyphasic waves of normal duration and size. Denervation potentials are seen only rarely.

Roentgenography. Roentgenograms are important for diagnosis and follow-up evaluation. The findings of soft tissue atrophy, subcutaneous calcinosis, and resorption of the tufts of the terminal phalanges without loss of apparent joint spaces between phalanges are virtually pathognomonic of systemic sclerosis when seen on hand films. The periodontal membrane is occasionally thickened. Upper gastrointestinal films reveal a dilated, atonic esophagus in about 60 per cent of patients. Small bowel studies may demonstrate segmental atony, dilation, and sacculation in the duodenum and jejunum. Linear or cystic pneumatosis (air in the wall of the gut) is occasionally seen in flat plates of the abdomen of patients with severe small bowel involvement. Barium studies of the colon reveal wide-mouth, asym-

metrical diverticula in 20 to 40 per cent of patients; progression to a dilated, atonic megacolon rarely occurs. In patients with pulmonary involvement, chest roentgenograms reveal a diffuse reticular pattern with a honeycomb appearance in the lower lung fields. Serial films may document progression to a picture of dense interstitial fibrosis amid radiolucent cystic areas.

DIFFERENTIAL DIAGNOSIS. When systemic sclerosis presents as persistent symmetrical polyarthritis involving the hands without previous skin changes, it may be impossible to differentiate it from rheumatoid arthritis or systemic lupus erythematosus, or, if the overlying skin becomes edematous or red, dermatomyositis. In fact, "overlap" syndromes combining clinical or serologic manifestations of several of these entities are being described with increasing frequency, and one should avoid hasty classification of any clinical picture that is consistent with more than one of the connective tissue diseases.

Diseases or pathologic findings associated with Raynaud's phenomenon which must be differentiated from scleroderma include occupational trauma; anatomic lesions, e.g., scalenus anticus syndrome and cervical ribs; vasomotor syndromes resulting in disuse atrophy, e.g., Sudek's atrophy or the shoulder-hand syndrome; peripheral vascular arteriosclerosis; heavy metal or ergot poisoning; and hematologic abnormalities, e.g., polycythemia vera, paroxysmal cold hemoglobinuria, and presence of cold agglutinins or cryoproteinemia.

The atrophic changes in the skin in systemic sclerosis must be differentiated from those seen in Werner's syndrome, progeria (Hutchinson-Gilford syndrome), chronic hypostatic edema or myxedema, lichen sclerosus et atrophicus, porphyria cutanea tarda, and/or scleredema. Unlike systemic sclerosis, Werner's syndrome affects the feet more severely than the hands, and has associated with it a high-pitched voice, growth abnormalities, and premature cataracts, arteriosclerosis, and diabetes. Sclerodermatous changes have been reported in skin of patients with progeria, but the dwarf-like stature, characteristic facies, and premature death from coronary insufficiency set this syndrome apart. Porphyria cutanea tarda may have skin changes simulating scleroderma but can be differentiated on the basis of urinary or fecal porphyrin excretion. Scleredema (scleredema adultorum of Buschke) is a brawny edema which appears abruptly, involves skin of the neck and chest initially, and is characterized pathologically by the presence of a material resembling acid mucopolysaccharide diffusely interspersed among collagen bundles in the dermis. This is a self-limited process, perhaps related to a previous bacterial infection, and has a good prognosis. The cutaneous telangiectasia of scleroderma resembles Osler-Weber-Rendu disease (hereditary telangiectasia). Scleroderma-like reactions have been described in chronic graft-versus-host reactions in patients given renal allografts.

Involvement of viscera in systemic sclerosis can mimic many other illnesses. The abnormalities in pulmonary function and the roentgenographic findings seen are similar to those found in idiopathic pulmonary fibrosis (Hamman-Rich syndrome) and the pulmonary fibrosis of rheumatoid arthritis or advanced sarcoidosis. Scleroderma heart disease must be differentiated from infiltrative cardiomyopathies as well as fibrosis from diffuse coronary artery disease. The dysphagia of scleroderma is completely nonspecific, and disease of the bowel rarely can simulate sprue or any of the malabsorption syndromes, partial intestinal obstruction, or megacolon. Workers in vinyl chloride polymerization plants have an increased incidence of microvascular abnormalities, and some have scleroderma-like skin lesions or acro-osteolysis. The mechanism of this industrial disease is not known.

COURSE UNTREATED. The course of systemic sclerosis is variable. Those patients with primary acrosclerosis and decreased esophageal motility may have slowly progressive disease with no significant increased probability of early death. Others, particularly patients with pulmonary, cardiac, or renal involvement, may progress rapidly to early death. Renal failure is the cause of death of scleroderma in 20 to 40 per cent of patients. Recent data obtained using life-table methods suggest that there is a 50 to 70 per cent five-year survival. Chances for survival are worse if the patient is a black male, diagnosed over the age of 40 years, with cutaneous lesions of the trunk, pulmonary involvement, and an abnormal electrocardiogram or blood urea nitrogen greater than 40 mg per 100 ml.

TREATMENT. Patients with acrosclerosis can lead productive and useful lives. The most important goal in therapy is to preserve function in and prevent injury to the hands. Vocational and/or climatic change may be indicated. Hand care must be stressed, including instructions for active and passive exercises that the patient may do himself several times each day in order to prevent further deformity. Early signs of local infection in fingertips must be treated immediately before they progress to large ulcerations. Psychologic support can be of great value in helping a patient adjust to the discomfort and apparently inexorable progression of his disease.

Because so little is known about the underlying defect in scleroderma or its pathogenesis, no specific treatment is available. The one possible exception to this is the use of broad-spectrum antimicrobials (e.g., tetracycline, 0.25 gram twice a day, or erythromycin, 0.5 gram every day) in treatment of malabsorption associated with bacterial overgrowth in the upper small intestine. If esophageal motility is decreased, antacid therapy is used liberally to prevent secondary esophagitis and stricture. Surgical reconstruction of the esophagogastric junction has been effective in management of symptomatic reflux in selected patients. If stricture develops, bougienage will be needed. Salicylates in pharmacologic doses may decrease clinical signs of inflammation, e.g., elevated sedimentation rates, joint pain, and erythema, which is present in most patients at some time in the course of their disease.

Corticosteroids are ineffective in the treatment of systemic sclerosis; neither the vascular lesions nor the fibrosis are improved by their use. However, there is a subgroup of patients with an overlap syndrome called "mixed connective tissue disease" who present with a variety of symptoms, including Raynaud's phenomenon, arthritis, and skin changes consistent with scleroderma, but with features (including LE cells, leukopenia, inflammatory myositis, and lymphadenopathy) of other connective tissue diseases as well. Many of this group will have high titers of antinuclear antibody in a "speckled" pattern directed against an extractable nuclear antigen, a ribonucleoprotein distinct from Sm antigen. In general, this group of patients does not develop renal disease and responds to corticosteroid therapy.

Use of intra-arterial reserpine* has been advocated to decrease the frequency of Raynaud's phenomenon and potentiate healing of ulcers. Given intra-arterially (0.5 to 1.0 mg), benefit without side effects has often been prolonged. A decrease in finger vasoconstriction in response to cooling in patients with scleroderma given reserpine in the ipsilateral brachial artery has been documented. The placebo effect of this type of procedure and potential hazards of intra-arterial reserpine must be continually evaluated. Phenoxybenzamine (Dibenzyline, 20 to 100 mg per day) is an effective α-adrenergic blocking agent. The principal side effect of this class of drugs is postural hypotension. It may help relieve symptoms of Raynaud's phenomenon.

Potassium p-aminobenzoate, griseofulvin, vitamin E (1200 to 2000 IU per day), ethylenediaminetetraacetic acid, 6-aminocaproic acid infusions, and dimethyl sulfoxide applications have been employed by a number of investigators without firm proof of efficacy. D-Penicillamine,* capable of cleaving newly formed labile intermolecular cross-links of collagen in vitro, can inhibit the synthesis of collagen by active sclerodermatous skin. In doses of 750 to 1500 mg per day it may be effective in slowing progression of skin disease, although beneficial results have not been reported for visceral involvement and the toxicity of D-penicillamine is great. Pilot studies of immunosuppressive therapy are being evaluated; initial results show no clear-cut role for these drugs in systemic sclerosis. Colchicine (less than 1.5 mg per day), after initial promise, has not been proved effective in diminishing sclerosis.

Initial results in a few cases in which "scleroderma kidneys" were removed and hemodialysis and/or renal transplantation carried out have demonstrated that life of good quality can be prolonged by these aggressive approaches. Recurrence of vascular lesions in allografts has been described. To be effective, hemodialysis must be carried out relatively early in the accelerated, progressive renal failure, preferably while serum creatinine values are less than 6 to 8 mg per deciliter.

D'Angelo, W. A., Fries, J. F., Masi, A. T., and Shulman, L. E.: Pathologic observations in systemic sclerosis (scleroderma). Am. J. Med., 46:428, 1969.

Rodnan, G. P.: Progressive systemic sclerosis (scleroderma) and calcinosis. In Hollander, J. L., and McCarty, D. J. (eds.): Arthritis and Allied Conditions. 8th ed. Philadelphia, Lea & Febiger, 1972.

---

*Investigational drug for this use.

51. POLYMYOSITIS AND DERMATOMYOSITIS

H. Richard Tyler

GENERAL CONSIDERATIONS. The disorder termed polymyositis refers to an illness first described by Wagner in 1863 in which muscle weakness is the principal clinical feature. Inflammatory, degenerative, and regenerative changes can be seen in the muscles. When skin changes occur and are prominent, the cases are referred to as dermatomyositis. This subgroup was first delineated by Unverricht in 1887. The muscular lesions of dermatomyositis, however, are identical to those seen in polymyositis. Because of the dramatic skin lesions, dermatomyositis was more widely recognized. Appreciation that muscular syndromes are more common than dermatomyositis resulted from the increased use of muscle biopsy and the clinical awareness that an insidious onset and absence of muscle pain are common. If there are changes indicative of nerve damage, the term neuromyositis is occasionally used. Some authors prefer the nonspecific and noncommittal term polymyopathy and identify as separate entities only those cases whose specific cause is known. Others reserve the term polymyositis for cases with evidence of inflammatory changes in muscles. Until the cause of the majority of the cases is more clearly identified, one has to accept the need to re-evaluate nomenclature periodically. All these disorders form a large spectrum which ranges from the very acute cases with myoglobinuria to the very chronic localized disorders that mimic muscular dystrophy.

The incidence of the disease has been estimated between 0.1 and 0.6 per 100,000 population per year, with a prevalence of 6.3 per 100,000. As a cause of acute or subacute muscle weakness in an adult, polymyositis is much more common than muscular dystrophy.

The disease can appear at any age, but it is most common between the ages of 40 and 60. Females are affected about twice as frequently as males. In most instances, no precipitating cause is obvious, but some cases have followed a viral-like illness or the use of antimicrobial drugs. Virus-like particles have been noted in muscle in some cases. Their role in relation to the disease has not been defined. Hypersensitivity has been implicated by some because of the association with malignancy, the frequent relation to a previous infection, and the association with symptoms common to the other collagen diseases.

If one excludes obvious cases of collagen disease and childhood dermatomyositis, more than 10 to 15 per cent of cases are associated with malignancy. If one considers only cases above age 50, then the frequency of malignancy may double. It is important to recognize that the carcinoma may present up to three to five years after the onset of the polymyositis syndrome. The relationship between the two entities is not clear.

About 20 per cent of cases of polymyositis and dermatomyositis occur in the course of one of the other connective tissue disorders. This association favors females by 9:1.

In most instances, it is not possible to establish a definite etiology. Specific infections (such as toxoplasmosis) may cause a polymyositis, but in most cases there is no evidence of an infectious cause. It has not been possible to demonstrate antimuscle antibodies in these patients. The presence of antimyosin antibody and other antibodies in some patients is nonspecific, as it is also found in patients with muscular dystrophy and neuronal atrophy. It has been possible to produce a myositis in guinea pigs similar to human polymyositis by use of muscle plus Freund's adjuvant. In tissue culture preparations of rat skeletal muscle, "sensitized" lymph node cells from animals previously injected with muscle plus adjuvants destroyed the muscle cells when added to the culture, whereas unsensitized lymph node cells did not. The significance of these experiments for human disease remains uncertain.

The presence of particles resembling virus seen in electron microscope studies in a number of patients has raised the question of an altered reaction to a viral disease as a cause of some forms of polymyositis.

Lymphocytes or their products from affected patients have cytotoxic activity toward cells in 79 per cent of cases in one series, suggesting a cell-mediated immune response to muscle antigen. Intramuscular vascular deposits of immunoglobulin and C3 have been demonstrated, especially in the childhood form of dermatomyositis.

PATHOLOGY. Muscle biopsy may show inflammatory cells around vessels and in the interstitium frequently associated with individual muscle fiber necrosis. These necrotic muscle fibers are frequently in various stages of being phagocytized. Attempts at regeneration characterized by basophilic fibers having prominent sarcolemmal nuclei are usually impressive. It should be emphasized that histologic findings vary greatly in the same muscle and between different muscles so that sampling is important. The muscle tissue from the more chronic cases often shows surprisingly little change under the light microscope. This may consist of smaller muscle fibers, which vary significantly in cross-section diameter, associated with proliferation of sarcolemmal nuclei. In the polymyositis associated with Sjögren's syndrome, the muscle may be heavily infiltrated with plasma cells and lymphocytes. In the few studies utilizing the electron microscope, changes such as thickened basilar membranes, myofibrillary degeneration and, rarely, virus particles were seen. These studies have not contributed any new insight into the disease.

In the childhood form of dermatomyositis, there is intense perivascular inflammation with active arteritis and phlebitis. There is often occlusion of vessels with fibrin thrombi and infarction of muscles, nerves, and viscus (Banker and Victor). Other forms of more limited or less intense polymyositic syndromes in children have pathologic changes similar to those previously described.

The three useful laboratory tests, serum enzyme determinations, electromyography, and muscle biopsy, are not always abnormal. Any one or even two may yield normal findings in a particular case. In one series, electromyography was abnormal in 89 per cent and muscle biopsy was confirmatory in 63 per cent. Serum enzyme activities are usually elevated except in some slowly progressive or chronic cases.

CLINICAL MANIFESTATIONS AND DIAGNOSIS. The patient usually first notes the insidious development of *weakness in proximal muscles*. The weakness is more common at the hips than in the shoulders. Some weakness in the flexors of the neck is almost always present. Muscle discomfort or tenderness is common but can be completely absent. When present, it is more common in the shoulders, back, and arms than in the thighs. Muscular wasting is a late sign, and when it occurs it is usually in proximal muscles such as the quadriceps. The weakness is out of proportion to the loss of muscle bulk. Reflexes are depressed in proportion to muscle weakness.

The development and the rate of progression of the weakness may show great variations from patient to patient, and even in the same patient at different stages of the illness. Weakness can progress until the patient becomes bedridden, but this is unusual. Contracture of muscles may develop quickly.

A *skin rash* may or may not be present. It usually takes the form of an erythema over the face, shoulders, and arms. It can mimic erythema nodosum, eczema, or éxfoliating dermatitis, or can manifest itself by thickened, brawny, edematous skin. On occasion, the skin lesions appear primarily in areas exposed to sunlight. Erythematous, slightly raised lesions occur over bony prominences, i.e., elbows, knuckles, knees, and medial malleoli. These lesions often become scaly and atrophic. Hyperemia around the nail beds is not uncommon. In childhood forms a violaceous suffusion of the upper eyelids, called a "heliotrope" rash, is diagnostic of this disorder. This may also be seen in adults.

Dysphagia, secondary to weakness of pharyngeal muscle and hypotonicity of the upper part of the esophagus, is frequent. About one third of the patients have arthralgias, Raynaud's phenomenon, or both. Other visceral manifestations are rare. Many patients have a tachycardia. Electrocardiograms may show nonspecific T wave changes. Interstitial fibrosis and pericarditis have been noted on histologic examination. A transitory pneumonitis has also been reported. Transitional cases with some features suggesting scleroderma have occasionally demonstrated severe gastrointestinal symptoms with malabsorption, severe myopathy, and only slight skin changes. If the muscle weakness comes on acutely with such muscle necrosis, myoglobinuria will occur. This can result in acute renal failure. Polymyositis may also be seen with Sjögren's syndrome.

The *childhood form of dermatomyositis* may be much more pernicious. It starts out with skin changes, anorexia, and fatigue. Weakness, stiffness, and pain in muscles customarily follow. Low-grade fever, dysphagia, contractures, and calcinosis usually develop. A perforated viscus or mediastinitis is often the immediate cause of death.

COURSE UNTREATED. The condition can progress to severe disability and death, but most patients either improve spontaneously or proceed to a chronic phase. In earlier series, including patients primarily recognized as having dermatomyositis, case fatality rates of 50 per cent were common. In a later series of adult patients with polymyositis, it was noted that about two thirds were alive after ten years. About 50 per cent of these had complete recoveries, and the rest had some degree of residual disability. Many of the patients in this series had received some steroid therapy.

In a survey by Sheard in which adult cases were accumulated from the literature, tumors were present in nearly 20 per cent, or five times the expected incidence. When polymyositis develops in an adult male, a greater than 50 per cent chance exists that a tumor will be discovered. In another series described by Shy, it was noted that when polymyositis appeared after the age of 50 a *cancer* was found in 71 per cent of males and 24 per cent of females. The muscular weakness may precede the detection of the tumor by two or three years despite diligent search, and in this series all nine males above 50 who were followed for three years or more had an associated neoplasm. In the male, the usual carcinoma is in the lung, stomach, intestine, or prostate; and in the female, in the ovary, uterus, or breast.

Childhood dermatomyositis appears to be a very specific subgroup of polymyositic disorders. It is severely disabling and is associated with a very high fatality rate.

LABORATORY FINDINGS. The sedimentation rate is usually elevated, and there may be mild leukocytosis, especially in the acute cases. A number of enzymes which derive from muscle are usually elevated in serum. Creatine phosphokinase and aldolase are the most specific, but lactic dehydrogenase and transaminase (SGOT) are usually elevated also. Serum protein changes occur in about 50 per cent of the patients. These most commonly consist of elevations of the $\alpha2$ and γ globulins. Rheumatoid factors are positive in 10 to 50 per cent, depending on the series. About 5 per cent will have LE cells. Myoglobinuria is transient and is found only with acute and severe muscular degeneration.

In patients with dysphagia, the roentgenograms often reveal pooling of barium in the vallecular and pyriform sinuses. Hypomotility of the esophagus is present in about one third of the cases. The roentgenograms frequently reveal no abnormalities except the rare deposition of subcutaneous calcification in the childhood form of the disease. Electrocardiograms often show minor abnormalities.

Electromyography is almost always abnormal in the clinically affected muscles. There is excessive irritability of muscle when the needle is initially inserted. The motor units (which are made up of many muscle fibers supplied by a single nerve) often show a loss of amplitude, indicating a reduction in the number of functioning muscle fibers in each motor unit. The mean duration of the units is often shortened. Polyphasic discharges are common, indicating a loss of individual muscle fibers of the unit. Positive denervation waves of 20 to 50 msec and fibrillary potentials are seen, indicating some denervation or separation of a portion of the muscle from its afferent nerve supply. Repetitive discharges of pseudomyotonic firing are not uncommon. When the changes indicating denervation are prominent, the term "neuromyositis" has been used. The electromyogram is useful in indicating which muscles to biopsy. The site of biopsy should be selected to ensure that a proper sampling of abnormal muscle is being taken. It should not be taken at the site of previous electromyographic needle insertion.

DIFFERENTIAL DIAGNOSIS. The major causes of weakness, which must be differentiated from polymyositis, are those due to muscular dystrophy and disorders of the peripheral and central nervous system. Muscular dystrophy is usually a familial disorder which is longstanding and can often be traced to childhood. The involvement of proximal muscles and neck flexor weakness would be unusual in most adult forms of muscular dystrophy. In myotonic dystrophy, the only dystrophy which often demonstrates neck flexor weakness, there is a distal weakness of muscles in the extremities. There are also cataracts and myotonia to percussion. Fascioscapulohumeral muscular dystrophy and other proximal dystrophies usually spare neck flexors. All the dystrophies are characterized by family history, significant muscle wasting, and weakness; the deep tendon reflex loss is usually early and prominent. In polymyositis, reflexes are often relatively spared until severe weakness occurs. In some cases it may be impossible to distinguish a dystrophy from polymyositis. The family history may be difficult to verify, and the biopsy in chronic cases may not be characteristic. A few cases of familial polymyositis have been reported.

The weakness in peripheral neuritis tends to be distal, and careful examination usually enables one to find mild sensory loss, autonomic dysfunction, and distal areflexia. Weakness from spinal cord disease has characteristic reflex changes, such as extensor plantar responses and hyperreflexia. Occasionally, motor neuron disease (the primary muscular atrophy variant) presents as a myopathic disorder. Muscle biopsy and EMG usually distinguish between the two conditions. On occasion a subacute variety of Guillain-Barré disease can cause proximal weakness. Elevation of cerebrospinal fluid protein is helpful in establishing this entity and is not seen in polymyositis.

Of the muscular syndromes, the metabolic myopathies most closely mimic the distribution of muscle weakness and the weakness seen with polymyositis. Chronic thyroid myopathy is characterized by its involvement of proximal muscles with significant loss of muscle bulk. The reflexes are usually quite brisk. Although there are no distinctive features, the clinical signs of thyrotoxicosis and the presence of clinical tests to support hyperthyroidism usually make it easy to distinguish this group. The most common myopathy seen today is probably the one induced by excess or chronic use of corticotropin or steroids. This is especially true of the fluorinated steroids. It is identical to that seen with hyperadrenocorticism. The weakness is primarily proximal, most often involving the pelvic girdle. Early wasting of the quadriceps muscle is especially prominent. Pain and discomfort are unusual. Reflexes usually persist, and severe disabling syndromes are unusual. Muscle biopsy tends to show surprisingly little change, and then only very scattered and in single muscle fibers. These changes are usually much less than one would anticipate from the clinical status of the patients.

Since steroids are often used in the treatment of a number of clinical syndromes, it may be very difficult to establish whether progressive weakness is due to the underlying disease or the steroid treatment. Often one will have to either decrease the steroid dose sharply or increase it significantly to make such judgments. If pain is a significant problem, one must be cautious about the clinical evaluation of weakness or its disappearance with the use of high doses of steroids.

Hyperparathyroidism and hyperinsulinism have rarely been associated with syndromes of muscular weakness and must be separated from idiopathic polymyositis primarily by the associated laboratory findings. Muscle weakness is often associated with osteomalacia.

There are a number of parasitic diseases such as trichinosis and toxoplasmosis which should be considered in acute or subacute syndromes, especially when generalized symptoms and eosinophilia are noted. These are fully discussed elsewhere in this text.

Polymyalgia rheumatica is characteristically associated with significant muscular discomfort and a high sedimentation rate. Changes in serum enzymes or muscle biopsy are usually not present to any significant degree. There are noticeable short-term and even daily fluctuations of symptoms. Significant objective weakness is not common, although complaints of pain and fatigue and feelings of muscular weakness are often voiced by the patient. Although the findings in some are related to those seen with temporal arteritis, the findings in others are very similar to those of some patients seen with epidemic neuromyasthenia.

A newly described syndrome, *diffuse fasciitis associated with eosinophilia*, is easy to confuse with dermatomyositis. The biopsy specimen usually demonstrates pathology primarily in a thickened fascia rather than skin or muscle. The presence of eosinophilia in blood and bone marrow is a laboratory clue to the diagnosis.

Clinically, skin is often bound to the underlying tissue and contractions occur very easily. The cause of the syndrome is not clear. It appears to respond to steroids.

TREATMENT. The physician's obvious goal is to eradicate the active disease process, if possible, and improve the functional capacity of the patient. In almost all cases prolonged management and long-term follow-up will be necessary. Often the chronic nature and the severe disability caused by the illness make it essential for the physician to play an active role as a counselor and friend.

Many of these patients achieve significant symptomatic improvement of muscle function when treated with corticotropin, steroids, or salicylates. The use of immunosuppressive medication has been promising in a few cases. Methotrexate* has been used, especially in dermatomyositis. The disorder is rarely "cured," however, and relapses are common, especially if steroids are abruptly withdrawn. Patients may require medication for many years. The initial dose of corticotropin or steroids should be high (60 to 80 mg of prednisone) and tapered over months. It is useful to monitor serum enzymes during this period, as they often give an early indication of the patient's likely course. Relapses are common when steroids are withdrawn in the first two years, but less frequent if treatment lasts at least three years. When possible, steroids should be used on an alternate-day basis to decrease side effects. When steroid-treated and presteroid series of patients are compared in terms of long-range follow-up, as by Rose and Walton, the group receiving steroid treatment has fared better. Patients with some of the adult forms usually do well. Those with the childhood forms of dermatomyositis usually do not respond satisfactorily to steroids alone.

Banker, B. Q.: Dermatomyositis of childhood. J. Neuropathol. Exp. Neurol., 34:1, 1975.

Bohan, A., Peter, J. B., Bourman, R. L., and Pearson, C. M.: A computer-assisted analysis of 153 patients with polymyositis and dermatomyositis. Medicine, 56:255, 1977.

DeVere, R., and Bradley, W. G.: Polymyositis: Its presentation, morbidity and mortality. Brain, 98:637, 1975.

Pearson, C. M.: Polymyositis. In Milhorat, A. T. (ed.): Explanatory Concepts in Muscular Dystrophy and Related Disorders. Amsterdam, Excerpta Medica Foundation, 1967.

Schulman, L. E.: Diffuse fasciitis with eosinophilia: A new syndrome. Trans. Assoc. Am. Physicians, 88:70, 1975.

Shy, G. M.: The late onset myopathy. World Neurol., 3:149, 1962.

Walton, J. N.: Disorders of Voluntary Muscle. 3rd ed. London, J. A. Churchill, Ltd., 1974.

Walton, J. N., and Adams, R. D.: Polymyositis. Edinburgh, Livingstone, Ltd., 1958.

---

*Investigational drug for this use.

52. SYSTEMIC LUPUS ERYTHEMATOSUS

Peter H. Schur

GENERAL CONSIDERATIONS. Systemic lupus erythematosus (SLE) is a chronic, inflammatory disease of unknown cause affecting skin, joints, kidneys, nervous system, serous membranes, and often other organs of the body. The classic facial "butterfly rash" facilitates diagnosis, although the rash need not be present. The clinical course may be fulminant or indolent, but generally is characterized by periods of remissions and relapses. Patients with SLE develop distinct immunologic abnormalities, especially antinuclear antibodies. A diagnosis of SLE has frequently been confirmed by the finding of these antibodies, especially antibodies to DNA.

Lupus, which is Latin for wolf, has been used since about 1230 to describe cutaneous conditions which resemble the malar erythema of a wolf. Numerous publications in the nineteenth century by, among others, Bateman, Biett, Hebra, and Kaposi, described what we know now as lupus of the skin. In 1851, Cazenave first used the term "lupus erythemateux." Kaposi, in 1872, noted the systemic involvement in lupus, and in 1875 noted that the rash resembled a butterfly. Osler described the systemic complications of lupus and noted that they could occur in the absence of skin disease. The clinical recognition of SLE has changed greatly since Hargraves first described the LE cell test in 1948 and since the development of the immunofluorescent antinuclear factor test by Friou in 1957.

INCIDENCE AND ETIOLOGY. SLE is not a rare disorder. The prevalence rate is approximately 1 per 1000 population. The disease appears to occur more frequently in blacks than in whites and is rare among Asians. It occurs five to ten times more frequently among females than males and has been diagnosed in patients ranging from 2 to 97 years old. However, the majority of patients are first discovered to have SLE while in their third and fourth decades of life.

The cause of SLE remains unknown. Exposure to sunlight or ultraviolet radiation, viz., sunlamps, often leads to the prompt appearance of the facial butterfly rash or a rash on other exposed skin surfaces. Many other factors, including infections, surgery, and certain drugs, have been shown to be associated with exacerbations of SLE. Recent attention has focused on procainamide, hydralazine, hydantoins, and other drugs which may precipitate a lupus-like illness.

In view of the preponderance of the disease in females, endocrine factors have been thought to influence the development of SLE. The disease tends to remit during the last two trimesters of pregnancy and to relapse post partum. Inhibitors of ovulation may cause an exacerbation of SLE.

Genetic factors may influence the development of SLE in susceptible individuals. Much evidence supports this hypothesis. The high incidence of SLE among females might be considered an X-chromosome-related factor. Connective tissue disorders, including SLE, dysgammaglobulinemia, and autoimmune phenomena are observed frequently among relatives of many patients with SLE. There is a high concordance rate of SLE in twins. Immune deficiency, particularly of IgA and the second component of complement (C2), is noted with increased frequency among SLE patients. Additional evidence for a genetic role in SLE comes from studies in certain strains of inbred mice and dogs. NZB and NZW (New Zealand black and New Zealand white) mice develop an illness which includes hemolytic anemia, renal disease, and immunologic abnormalities, and is similar to human SLE. The F_1 hybrid generation, especially the females, develops the illness more frequently, at an earlier age, and with a much higher incidence of autoimmune phenomena.

Lupus erythematosus is characterized particularly by autoimmune phenomena. Patients develop antibodies to many of their own cells, cell constituents, and proteins. The origin of these autoantibodies is as obscure as is the cause of SLE. However, they do appear to represent a loss of tolerance to self antigens. Mice of the NZB strain have been found to lose their tolerance for foreign antigens much more rapidly than do other mice, possibly owing to a suppressor T cell defect.

A possible viral cause for SLE has also been proposed. Loss of tolerance may be influenced by viral infections. Structures resembling viral nucleocapsids — but shown not to be viruses — have been found much more frequently in endothelial cells in SLE patients than in normal persons. Antibody titers to certain viruses are elevated in SLE sera, but no one virus has been implicated. The presence, in many SLE patients, of antibodies to double-stranded RNA suggests reaction to an RNA virus (infection). "C" type RNA virus particles have been found in NZB mice; other viruses, including DNA and RNA viruses, can provoke the development of autoantibodies and nephritis in NZB mice. Cell-free filtrates, presumably containing a virus, have been prepared from spleens of dogs with lupus. These filtrates, when injected into normal dogs and mice, induce the formation of antinuclear antibodies; they also activate latent leukemia viruses in mice.

These data suggest that an abnormal immune response in genetically predisposed SLE patients may alter the delicate balance between immunity and tolerance and result in the development of antibodies to intracellular contents released during chronic viral infection or to new antigens to cells which result from viral infection or transformation.

PATHOGENESIS AND PATHOLOGY. Some of the manifestations of SLE appear to result from the deposition of antigen-antibody complexes in tissues. In laboratory animals, when immune complexes are formed in the circulation, serum complement levels falls and nephritis develops. In patients with SLE, especially in those with anti-DNA antibodies, a fall in complement levels is often associated with the development of nephritis. In addition, some patients with serum antibodies to DNA develop fever and nephritis as the antibody disappears and is replaced by free DNA, a sequence which presumably represents immune complex formation and deposition, followed by antigen excess. Furthermore, some sera from SLE patients with nephritis, when treated with deoxyribonuclease, have a rise in anti-DNA antibody levels. This fact suggests that DNA has been bound in vivo to the antibody as an immune complex. Also, cryoglobulins, which may represent immune complexes, have been isolated from SLE patients and shown on occasion to contain DNA and high specific activity antibodies against DNA. Immunoglobulins (especially IgG), complement components, and antigens (viz., DNA) have been detected in a granular and lumpy distribution along the renal glomerular basement membrane. After elution of the gamma globulin from the glomeruli, it has been possible to demonstrate that it consists primarily of antinuclear antibodies, including antibodies to DNA. Similar immune complexes have been demonstrated at the dermal-epidermal junction of lupus skin lesions, in nonlesional skin, and in the choroid plexus. It is hypothesized that, as the complement system is activated during immune complex formation and deposition, chemotactic factors are released and that damage to normal cells and extracellular tissue is caused both by activated terminal sequences of complement and by lysosomal enzymes released by polymorphonuclear leukocytes during phagocytosis.

The pathologic changes of SLE, even in clinically involved organs, are often minor when examined by routine histologic methods. Fibrinoid, an eosinophilic amorphous material, is commonly deposited along tissue fibers and in blood vessels. Fibrin and serum proteins (including immunoglobulins, complement, and DNA) have been detected in fibrinoid and possibly represent deposits of immune complexes. Synovium and serous membranes, including pleura and pericardium, may be edematous and contain deposits of fibrinoid. Vasculitis can involve venules, arterioles, and occasionally arteries. Hematoxylin bodies are rounded, hematoxylin-stained masses, roughly the size of nuclei, and are found in areas of inflammation. They are believed to represent in vivo LE bodies analogous to the cytoplasmic inclusions in LE cells.

Biopsies of skin lesions may show acute inflammation with liquefaction, degeneration of the basal layer with vacuolization of basal cells, edema of the dermis, and fibrinoid necrosis in the dermis and local blood vessels with cell infiltration. In chronic lesions, hyperkeratosis with follicular plugging is seen.

The spleen is the site of "onion skin lesions," which are characterized by concentric perivascular fibrosis around central and penicilliary arteries.

Libman-Sacks verrucous nonbacterial endocarditis consists of nonbacterial vegetations on the heart valves or chordae tendineae. Fibrinoid is deposited in the superficial connective tissue with infiltration of neutrophils, lymphocytes, and histiocytes. The myocardium may be involved by vasculitis.

Renal lesions are highly variable, from mild to severe. The mildest form of renal lesion consists of deposits of immunoglobulin and complement in the mesangium or along the glomerular basement membrane without any other observable histologic abnormality. The most common renal lesion is glomerulitis with minimal focal increase of cellularity, thickening of the capillary basement membrane, and fibrinoid change. In glomerulonephritis, these lesions are more generalized and severe and are usually a mixture of proliferative and membranous changes with hypercellularity of endothelial, mesangial, epithelial, and inflammatory cells, capsular inflammation leading to crescent formation, and focal thickening of the basement membrane. Some kidneys are found to have only a diffuse membranous glomerulonephritis with few cells but considerable thickening of the basement membrane. Basement membrane thickening, when associated with fibrinoid changes, results in the so-called "wire loop" lesions. There may also be hyaline thrombi in glomeruli, focal necrosis, and, occasionally, hematoxylin bodies and sclerosis in healed lesions. Tubular degenerative changes are common.

CLINICAL MANIFESTATIONS. The characteristic picture of a patient with well-advanced lupus is one of a young woman with fever, weight loss, arthralgia, a butterfly rash, pleural effusion, and nephritis. With better methods of detection (the antinuclear antibody tests), much larger groups of patients with less obvious and more varied symptoms and signs are being recognized. Most patients complain of some fatigue, arthralgia, rashes, and fever. When specific organs are involved, other symptoms may develop: pleurisy, pericarditis, edema, dyspnea and cough, Raynaud's phenomenon, bleeding, and purpura or seizures. The disease is now considered a chronic illness with periods of remission and activity.

TABLE 1. Frequency of Clinical Symptoms in Systemic Lupus Erythematosus*

	Per Cent
Weight loss	62
Fever	83
Arthralgia, arthritis	90
Skin	74
Butterfly rash	42
Photosensitivity	30
Mucous membrane lesions	12
Alopecia	27
Raynaud's phenomenon	17
Purpura	15
Urticaria	8
Renal	53
Nephrosis	18
Gastrointestinal	38
Pulmonary	47
Pleurisy	45
Effusion	24
Pneumonia	29
Cardiac	46
Pericarditis	27
Murmurs	23
EKG changes	39
Lymphadenopathy	46
Splenomegaly	15
Hepatomegaly	25
Central nervous system	32
Psychosis	15
Convulsions	15
Cytoid bodies	11

*Adapted from Dubois, E. L.: Lupus Erythematosus, New York, McGraw-Hill Book Company, 1966; Estes, D., and Christian, C. L.: Medicine, 50:85, 1971; and Fernandez-Herlihy, L.: Lahey Clinic Found. Bull., 21:49, 1972.

Musculoskeletal System. Most patients complain of pain in their joints (arthralgia) at some time. Commonly the fingers, hands, wrists, knees, ankles, and elbows are affected. Arthritis, i.e., inflammation, of joints is observed less frequently than is arthralgia. Although slight deformities at the metacarpophalangeal and proximal interphalangeal joints may occur, major joint swelling with synovial thickening, flexion deformities with subluxations, and deviation are uncommon. It is unusual for joint narrowing or cystic changes such as those seen in rheumatoid arthritis to be found on radiologic examination. The appearance of deformities or erosions on x-ray suggests a diagnosis of an overlap syndrome (rheumatoid arthritis–lupus). Muscle pain is a frequent complaint and is accompanied, occasionally, by proximal muscle atrophy. The bones are rarely affected, but an increased prevalence of aseptic necrosis of the femoral head or condyle has been noted, especially in those patients receiving corticosteroid therapy.

Mucocutaneous Manifestations. The classic "butterfly rash" is seen in less than half the patients with SLE. There may be only a blush and swelling or a scaly erythematous maculopapular rash on both cheeks and the bridge of the nose after exposure to the sun. This may clear spontaneously, only to recur. Other skin areas, particularly those exposed to the sun, may be involved. The lesions are called "discoid" when they scale, are associated with follicular plugging, and heal with atrophy, scarring (telangiectasia), hyperpigmentation, or hypopigmentation (vitiligo). Involvement may also occur on the forehead, pinna, and scalp, resulting in alopecia. Patchy hair loss is frequent and usually reversible, but discoid lupus with scarring can lead to permanent partial baldness. In these days of well-fitted hairpieces, alopecia is often undetected on cursory examination. Periungual erythema and telangiectasia are found in about 10 per cent of patients with SLE. Small ulcerations signifying an underlying vasculitis often develop on the fingertips and may progress to gangrene. Raynaud's phenomenon may occur in both fingers and toes. Painless ulcers are seen on the buccal mucosa, hard and soft palate, nose, and gums. Purpura and ecchymoses may reflect an underlying blood platelet and clotting problem, renal insufficiency, the side effects of corticosteroids, or vasculitis. Urticaria and angioedema may be present.

Renal Disease. Kidney involvement is found in about half of SLE patients and usually occurs within two years of the onset of symptoms. Acute nephritis or the nephrotic syndrome may be the presenting manifestation of SLE. The most common abnormality is a mild glomerulitis which is associated with minimal proteinuria or hematuria, or both. This lesion generally responds well to therapy initially, but may recur in mild form or as even more severe renal involvement. Acute lupus glomerulonephritis occurs less often and is associated with varying degrees of pyuria, hematuria, proteinuria, fluid retention, edema, hypertension, and azotemia. The nephrotic syndrome is associated with variable proteinuria, with fluid retention, and frequently with normal serum cholesterol levels. The finding of pyuria with fever in patients with SLE, especially in patients receiving corticosteroids, may reflect a urinary tract infection rather than lupus nephritis.

Most patients recover well from attacks of acute nephritis, with loss of edema and azotemia, but usually some proteinuria and decreased glomerular filtration rate (GFR) persist. Patients have recurrences, and some develop chronic glomerulonephritis with hypertension and proteinuria.

Cardiovascular Manifestations. The endocardium, myocardium, and pericardium are involved in nearly half the patients with SLE. Although electrocardiographic changes, such as nonspecific ST, T wave changes, are not uncommon, clinical myocarditis is seen less frequently. Myocarditis should be suspected when tachycardia is disproportionate to either fever or anemia. Cardiomegaly with congestive failure is rare. Precordial chest pain may be caused by either pleurisy or pericarditis. Careful, frequent auscultation may be rewarded by discovery of a pericardial friction rub. Tamponade or constrictive pericarditis is rare. Libman-Sacks or nonbacterial verrucous endocarditis usually occurs on the mitral valve and is recognized by murmurs which cannot be explained by fever or anemia; but generally this is a postmortem diagnosis. Bacterial endocarditis may develop on a previously damaged valve, especially in patients receiving corticosteroids. Recurrent thrombophlebitis may be the first manifestation of SLE. Occlusion of major arteries occurs rarely. Equally rare is pulmonary hypertension.

Pulmonary Involvement. Pleuritic pain is a common complaint and is often the first clue to the diagnosis of SLE. It is generally accompanied by a friction rub and a variable amount of fluid accumulation, but the effusions are often painless. There may be pulmonary infiltrates which are quite difficult to distinguish from those due to infections. The x-ray examination shows bilateral patchy infiltrations which may shift from lobe to lobe. The involvement can progress to atelectasis and to marked pulmonary insufficiency and cyanosis. Most pulmonary symptoms respond well to intensive corticosteroid therapy; but infections must be carefully considered as a cause of the infiltrate.

Neurologic and Psychologic Manifestations. Many patients have read in a dictionary or have heard that SLE is invariably a fatal illness; this understandably leads to great anxiety. Similarly the patient may be told that he or she has arthritis, which leads to ungrounded fears of disabling deformities. These natural fears and anxieties of a chronic illness are not to be confused with organic neurologic disturbances. The latter manifest themselves as behavioral disturbances, including hyperirritability, confusion, hallucinations, obsessional and paranoid reactions, and frank organic psychosis. The psychosis of SLE may easily be confused with, and in fact is difficult to differentiate from, a steroid-induced psychosis; other symptoms and signs of active SLE usually accompany the organic disease. The EEG is often abnormal in SLE with CNS involvement, but brain scans are usually normal. Organic brain damage most commonly manifests itself as convulsions, which occur in at least 15 per cent of patients. Other less frequent neurologic findings include peripheral neuropathy, hemiparesis, motor aphasia, ptosis, diplopia, and nystagmus.

"Cotton wool spots" are fluffy white exudates in the innermost layers of the retina, which may progress to cytoid bodies. They are usually present with other signs of active SLE, and are generally reversible.

Gastrointestinal Manifestations. Anorexia, nausea, vomiting, and abdominal pain are common. The cause is obscure, but may be from peritonitis, enteritis, pancreatitis, or a paralytic ileus. Diarrhea and hematochezia have been noted. The liver is often found to be enlarged because of chronic passive congestion, but this is usually transitory. Liver biopsy may be normal or show fatty infiltration and/or fibrosis.

These manifestations in SLE should not be confused with *lupoid hepatitis*, which is a condition primarily of young women with chronic active hepatitis leading to chronic liver disease and failure. Nephritis is said not to occur. Patients have high levels of gamma globulins, LE cells, and antinuclear antibodies; serum complement levels remain normal or elevated.

Lymph Nodes and Spleen. Lymph nodes, characteristically, are enlarged in SLE but are not tender. The enlarged nodes have been mistaken for lymphoma. Splenomegaly, considered very common years ago, is seen now in about 15 per cent of patients.

Menses and Pregnancy. Menses are frequently irregular or heavy, or both. In patients with circulating anticoagulants, bleeding may be profound. Although pregnancy carries some increased risk of miscarriage in the first trimester, most SLE patients without renal disease do well through term. It should be noted, however, that there is a considerable risk of postpartum exacerbation of the disease.

COURSE UNTREATED. Until recent years the natural course of untreated SLE was considered to be bleak. The average patient was considered to have but a few months or, at best, a few years to live. Since 1948, this situation has changed for the better. The reason for this improvement lies in the recognition of many cases of mild lupus through the development of very sensitive diagnostic tests (antinuclear antibodies), as well as in the development of improved forms of therapy. The

TABLE 2.   Laboratory Abnormalities in SLE*

	Per Cent
Anemia	71
Leukopenia	56
Thrombocytopenia	11
Hemolytic anemia	8
Circulating anticoagulant	2
Rheumatoid factor	19
Biologic false-positive test for syphilis	15
Hypoalbuminemia	50
Hyperglobulinemia	37
LE cell	82
Antinuclear antibodies	96
Anti-double-stranded DNA	50
Anti-single-stranded DNA	62
Anti-double-stranded RNA	51
Anti-nucleoprotein	45
Anti-"Sm"	24
Anti-RNP	46
Hypocomplementemia	66
CH50	66
C4	64
C3	52

*Adapted from Dubois, E. L.: Lupus Erythematosus, New York, McGraw-Hill Book Company, 1966; Estes, D., and Christian, C. L.: Medicine, 50:85, 1971; and Fernandez-Herlihy, L.: Lahey Clinic Found. Bull., 21:49, 1972.

disease in most patients is characterized by periods of remissions and relapses, which may be protracted or brief. The same individuals usually have recurrences of the same symptoms they had previously, such as arthritis, pleurisy, nephritis, or rashes. However, variable symptoms and signs may develop years apart. If nephritis develops, it generally does so early in the course.

The prognosis for patients seems to improve each year, but mortality rates remain high during the first year after diagnosis. Whereas in 1956, patients were given only a 50 per cent chance of surviving four years, today they have a better than 90 per cent chance to survive at least ten years. Prognosis still remains somewhat poorer for patients with diffuse proliferative glomerulonephritis or with central nervous system involvement. Patients with only skin involvement have an excellent prognosis but a 15 per cent chance of eventually developing (mild) SLE.

LABORATORY FINDINGS. Hematologic. Anemia occurs in many patients with SLE and is generally mild, normochromic, or normocytic. Anemia may also be due to infection, renal insufficiency, or bleeding. Autoagglutination of red blood cells may be observed. The Coombs test result is frequently positive, but severe hemolytic anemia is uncommon. Leukopenia occurs in about one half the patients. The differential cell count is usually normal, although mononuclear cells may be more suppressed than neutrophils. Complicating infections generally result in a rise of the white blood cell count either into the normal or elevated range. Corticosteroid therapy also causes leukocytosis. Thrombocytopenia, with or without purpura, may precede other manifestations of SLE by years or may disappear, leaving other manifestations of the disease. A circulating anticoagulant has been noted by some investigators in as many as 25 per cent of patients with SLE. This anticoagulant, either as antibody to factor VIII or, more commonly, as an inhibitor to the formation of "prothrombinase," results in prolonged clotting and pro-

thrombin times and may be associated with mild or, rarely, severe hemorrhages.

Renal. Renal dysfunction occurs in over half the patients. Most patients have only some impairment of concentrating ability, a few red and/or white blood cells in the urine, and perhaps some proteinuria (< 0.5 gram per day). Active nephritis is defined when there is hematuria (> 5 rc per hpf), pyuria (> 5 wc per hpf), erythrocyte casts, increasing proteinuria, or a decreasing glomerular filtration rate. Hematuria and pyuria are rarely seen in lupus nephritis in remission.

Plasma Proteins. The erythrocyte sedimentation rate is often elevated. Serum albumin levels are low, especially in the nephrotic syndrome. Gamma globulin levels which are elevated in many patients may be low in nephrotics. Cryoglobulins, consisting of immunoglobulins and complement components, have been noted frequently, especially in patients with renal disease.

Abnormal Immunologic Reactions. Biologic false-positive test results (BFP) for syphilis have been noted in about 15 per cent of the patients with SLE, especially in those with circulating anticoagulants. The BFP may be the first laboratory clue to the diagnosis of SLE and may precede symptoms by years. Rheumatoid factors have been found in some patients with SLE, even in the absence of clinical rheumatoid arthritis.

Most characteristic of SLE are the large number of autoantibodies which react with cells and their nuclear and cytoplasmic constituents. Historically of greatest significance is the LE cell phenomenon. The LE cell is formed in vitro as follows: some leukocytes are traumatized and release nucleoprotein (DNA-histone); the nucleoprotein reacts with an IgG antibody; and the complex is phagocytized by the remaining viable leukocytes. The LE cell consists of a leukocyte with a large purple-red homogeneous globulin inclusion body which compresses the nucleus against the cell membrane, leaving only a thin rim of cytoplasm. Because LE cells are not always present in patients with SLE, more sensitive tests have been developed for the detection of various antinuclear antibodies (ANA). An immunofluorescent (IF) technique, employing rodent liver or kidney as the source of nuclei, detects ANA in over 99 per cent of SLE patients. The antibodies are usually of the IgG or IgM class. Circulating DNA and other antigens may rarely block the detection of the ANA. With this immunofluorescent technique, different patterns of nuclear fluorescence reflect antibodies to different nuclear structures. The "homogeneous" or "diffuse" pattern reflects antibodies to nucleoprotein. The "peripheral," "rim," or "shaggy" pattern reflects primarily antibodies to DNA. The speckled pattern reflects antibodies to a group of nuclear proteins (ENA, extractable nuclear antigen), including "Sm" and ribonucleoprotein (RNP). A nucleolar pattern has also been observed and appears to represent antibodies to a nuclear RNA.

Antibodies to some antigens, especially to DNA, may also be detected by other methods, including diffusion in agar, complement fixation, agglutination, and radioimmunoassays. The titers of antibodies to DNA and, to some extent, to nucleoprotein tend to be higher during periods of clinical activity, especially of active nephritis, than during clinical remissions.

Complement levels are depressed in most patients with SLE at some time during their illness, especially when disease activity is present. Markedly depressed complement levels are seen primarily in patients with

TABLE 3. Autoantibodies in SLE

Antinuclear	Nucleoprotein
	DNA
	Histone
	Sm
	RNA
	Ribonucleoprotein
	Residue
Anticytoplasmic	Mitochondria
	Lysosomes
	Microsomes
	Ribosomes
	Cytoplasmic sap glycoprotein ("Ro")
	RNA protein
Anti-RNA	Ribosomal RNA
	Double-stranded RNA (? viral)
	Single-stranded RNA
Anticell	Red cell
	White blood cell
	Platelet
Anticlotting factors	
Antithyroid	
Rheumatoid factor	
Biologic false-positive test for syphilis	

active lupus nephritis. The low levels reflect in vivo activation and fixation of complement components by circulating immune complexes. Serial determination of whole complement levels (CH50) or of individual complement components (especially C4 and C3) may be useful in following and managing patients with SLE. SLE has also been seen in some patients with congenital deficiency of complement components, particularly C2.

DIAGNOSIS. The diagnosis of SLE can be made if any four or more of the following manifestations are present, serially or simultaneously, during any interval of observation: butterfly rash, discoid lupus, Raynaud's phenomenon, alopecia, photosensitive rash, oral or nasopharyngeal ulceration, arthritis without deformity, LE cells, chronic biologic false positive test result (BFP) for syphilis, profuse proteinuria, cellular casts, pleuritis or pericarditis, psychosis and/or convulsions, or hemolytic anemia, leukopenia, or thrombocytopenia. SLE should also be suspected — especially in young females — with unexplained fever, purpura, easy bruising, diffuse adenopathy, hepatosplenomegaly, peripheral neuropathy, endocarditis, myocarditis, interstitial pneumonitis, peritonitis, or aseptic meningitis.

Patients are frequently first diagnosed as having rheumatoid arthritis, rheumatic fever (especially children), glomerulonephritis, tuberculosis, scleroderma, vasculitis, idiopathic thrombocytopenic purpura, lymphoma, anemia, or neutropenia. The LE cell is most specific for SLE, if rheumatoid arthritis, lupoid hepatitis, or drug reactions can be excluded. Although the LE cell test is quite often negative, the antinuclear antibody test result is positive in virtually all patients with SLE. Antinuclear antibodies have also been detected in 68 per cent of patients with Sjögren's syndrome, 40 to 75 per cent of patients with scleroderma, especially the speckled pattern, 16 per cent of patients with juvenile rheumatoid arthritis, and 25 to 50 per cent of patients with rheumatoid arthritis, especially the homogeneous pattern. However, antinuclear antibodies tend to be present in higher titers in patients with SLE than in those with other disorders. Antibodies to double-stranded DNA and to an RNA-ase resistant acidic nuclear protein, termed Sm antigen by some, are highly diagnostic of SLE. Antibodies to single-stranded DNA, nucleoprotein (NP), and RNP (an RNA-ase sensitive nuclear antigen) are frequently found in patients with SLE and RA; antibodies to RNP are frequently found in patients with scleroderma.

Some patients have clinical features of SLE, scleroderma, and dermatomyositis. The term *mixed connective tissue disease* (MCTD) has been applied to these patients, as they appear to have a unique combination of clinical and laboratory findings. Some authorities, however, maintain that MCTD represents a subgroup of SLE or scleroderma. MCTD is characterized by diffuse polyarthritis and polyarthralgias, myositis, Raynaud's phenomenon, swollen hands, abnormal esophageal motility, and decreased pulmonary diffusing capacity. These patients often have severe pulmonary disease, rarely have nephritis or CNS disease, and usually respond to treatment with steroids. The serologic abnormalities seen in MCTD include a positive ANA test result with a speckled pattern and a high titer of anti-ENA (extractable nuclear antigen) antibodies, particularly to RNP. Patients with MCTD may have low levels of anti-DNA-antibodies, but most do not.

DRUG-INDUCED LUPUS. Drugs that induce lupus can be divided into two categories: drugs that induce lupus in many individuals, and drugs associated with exacerbations of SLE. In the former group are hydrazides (hydralazine, isoniazid), anticonvulsants (Dilantin), and procainamide. Over 50 per cent of subjects taking procainamide develop antinuclear antibodies, including antibodies to RNP and single-stranded DNA; about 25 per cent develop symptoms and signs of lupus. Arthralgia, pleurisy with effusion, fever, and weight loss are common features, but renal disease, hypocomplementemia, and antibodies to double-stranded DNA are not seen. Symptoms generally clear in a few weeks after discontinuation of the drug, even though antinuclear antibodies persist for months. Antinuclear antibodies appear less frequently in subjects taking hydralazine. Patients with the hydralazine lupus syndrome may have arthritis, dermatitis, serositis, leukopenia, antinuclear antibodies, and anti-DNA antibodies, but rarely have renal or central nervous system disease. Symptoms usually stop after cessation of the drug. Patients with hydralazine lupus are slow acetylators of the drug. These studies suggest that certain subjects may have a genetic predisposition for developing drug lupus. Other drugs, including penicillin, sulfonamides, and oral contraceptives, are associated with exacerbations of SLE, and rarely cause lupus-like symptoms or antinuclear antibodies in other subjects.

THERAPY AND MANAGEMENT. As there are no specific remedies for the treatment of the underlying processes of SLE, the main goals of management must be limited to the treatment of acute relapses and prevention of exacerbations. Certain measures are helpful in prevention of relapses. Sunlight, ultraviolet radiation, blood transfusions, penicillin, and sulfonamides should be avoided when possible. Surgery or infections may lead to a relapse and may require more aggressive concurrent management of the lupus. In the long-term management of this illness, both patient and physician must learn to recognize those symptoms and signs that herald relapses. Although these symptoms may involve fever and arthralgia in some patients, they may appear as hair loss, mucosal ulcers, pleurisy, weight loss, or simply fatigue in others. Before frank clinical symptoms develop, many patients will develop abnormal laboratory tests such as a reduced level of hemoglobin or serum complement or a reduced white blood cell or platelet count; an abnormal urinalysis or creatinine clearance; or a rising titer of anti-DNA antibodies.

Many of the patients seen in the hospital by physicians or students have severe but not life-threatening disease. By contrast, many of the patients seen in the office have much milder disease. The patient fearing the unknown or having heard the worst must be reassured that a majority of patients have mild to moderate disease and that with proper management many of the more serious complications can now be controlled.

Active disease should be treated aggressively to prevent permanent tissue injury. The general measures to be taken include rest when the disease is active, sunscreens, and physical therapy for muscle weakness and deformities. For those patients on moderate to high dosages of corticosteroids, salt restriction and diuretics may be of benefit. Drugs used for the treatment of SLE include topical steroids, salicylates, antimalarials, corticosteroids, and immunosuppressives. The use of corticosteroids is indicated in most patients with SLE and has improved survival. Dosage should be individualized according to the activity of the disease and side effects. *Immunosuppressives* are best used according to the guidelines of Schwartz and Gowans, whose indications are life-threatening or seriously crippling disease; presence of reversible lesions; failure to respond to conventional therapy or intolerable side effects; no active infection; no hematologic contraindication; meticulous follow-up; and objective evaluation.

The acute erythematous maculopapular rash responds well to the avoidance of sunlight, local application of corticosteroid cream, and the systemic introduction of antimalarials such as hydroxychloroquine. Systemic corticosteroids are rarely warranted. The chronic lesion, or discoid lupus, responds to these same measures to a variable degree. Severe, extensive lesions have been treated with large doses of antimalarials when all else has failed. However, the patient should be cautioned about the relative risks of retinal damage when taking large doses of antimalarials. Arthralgia and arthritis respond well to rest, physical therapy, splinting, salicylates, and antimalarials. Steroids should not be needed.

Fever often responds to rest and salicylates. Antimalarials may be beneficial. Persistent fever not responsive to these measures usually coincides with other signs of activity and responds to moderate doses of corticosteroids. Infections must be excluded.

Pericarditis and pleurisy respond well to rest and corticosteroids. Pericardial fluid, if present in moderate amounts, is best removed. Myocarditis should be treated with moderate doses of steroids, fluid restriction, and careful administration of digitalis.

Hemolytic anemia and thrombocytopenia need not be treated unless symptomatic. They generally respond well to steroids. If not, immunosuppressives or a splenectomy may be necessary.

Involvement of the central nervous system responds poorly to treatment. Organic psychosis, in addition, may be difficult to differentiate from a steroid-induced psychosis. Because of the risk of permanent brain damage, large doses of steroids (2 to 3 mg of prednisone per kilogram of body weight per day) are recommended until maximal improvement is achieved, at which time the dosage of steroids is gradually tapered. Immunosuppressives may be helpful.

Mild focal glomerulitis with minimal urinary abnormalities may respond on occasion to bed rest; however, these patients generally require systemic corticosteroid therapy, 0.5 to 1 mg of prednisone per kilogram of body weight per day. Those patients with focal or diffuse proliferative glomerulonephritis generally require higher doses, 1 to 3 mg per kilogram, depending on the severity of the renal impairment. Patients unresponsive to these regimens may benefit from immunosuppressives. Medication is maintained until hematuria clears and serum complement levels return toward normal; this usually occurs within about three weeks. The LE cells, proteinuria, elevated sedimentation rate, and high titers of antinuclear antibodies may persist. The prednisone dosage is then tapered slowly — 10 mg every five days. Complete blood counts, urinalyses, serum creatinine levels, and serum complement levels are checked regularly to detect relapses; relapses usually respond either to maintaining the dosage at that level or increasing it by 5 to 10 mg of prednisone per day. Many patients can be maintained at a dosage of 5 to 10 mg per day; some can tolerate steroids on alternate days; a few can discontinue steroids and remain asymptomatic. Continued careful monitoring and early treatment of slight relapses may avoid more severe exacerbations.

Patients with chronic membranous glomerulonephritis and nephrotic syndrome respond less well to corticosteroids or immunosuppressives. Some, usually those with normal complement levels, may have fixed proteinuria.

Dubois, E. L., and Tuffanelli, D. L.: Clinical manifestations of systemic lupus erythematosus. JAMA, 190:104, 1964.
Estes, D., and Christian, C. L.: The natural history of systemic lupus erythematosus by prospective analysis. Medicine, 50:85, 1971.
Harvey, A. M., Shulman, L. E., Tumulty, A., Conley, C. L., and Schoenrich, E. H.: Systemic lupus erythematosus: Review of the literature and clinical analysis of 138 cases. Medicine, 33:291, 1954.
Rothfield, N. F., and March, C. H.: Lupus erythematosus. In Fitzpatrick, T. B., Arndt, K. A., Clark, W. H., Eisen, A. Z., Van Scott, E. J., and Vaughan, J. H. (eds.): Dermatology in Internal Medicine. New York, McGraw-Hill Book Company, 1971, pp. 1493–1518.
Schur, P. H., and Sandson, J.: Immunological factors and clinical activity in lupus erythematosus. N. Engl. J. Med., 278:533, 1968.

53. PERIARTERITIS NODOSA

(Polyarteritis Nodosa)

K. Frank Austen

DEFINITION. Kussmaul and Maier introduced the term periarteritis nodosa in 1866 to designate a morbid process manifested by numerous grossly visible or palpable nodules along the course of medium-sized muscular arteries. The lesions are segmental in distribution, have a predilection for the crotch of bifurcations and branchings, and involve all but the pulmonary arteries. The clinical manifestations are disparate and polymorphic, and result from partial or complete arterial occlusion, hemorrhage, and glomerulitis. In view of the necrotizing nature of the process, involving the entire arterial wall, Ferrari in 1903 suggested the alternative name of polyarteritis acuta nodosa.

The incidence, age distribution, and male-to-female ratio of periarteritis nodosa are difficult to determine because a diagnostic serologic procedure is lacking, and the spotty distribution of lesions makes biopsy uncertain. Nonetheless, the condition has been reported to occur from infancy to old age, with a peak incidence in the fifth and sixth decades of life, and the male to female ratio has been estimated at from 2 to 3:1.

Generalized necrotizing angiitis in association with hepatitis B antigenemia was first reported in 1970, and by 1976 the literature contained approximately 50 such cases. The incidence of hepatitis B antigenemia has been as high as one third in patients with generalized necrotizing angiitis, a generic term introduced to indicate that these patients have disease extending from the medium-sized muscular arteries to the venules. Serous otitis media and amphetamine abuse are major associated events in the hepatitis B negative group with generalized necrotizing angiitis. On clinical grounds no criteria have been identified to distinguish between the hepatitis B positive and negative patients except that all positive hepatitis B antigenemia patients had abnormal liver chemistries. These were, however, occasionally minimal and then not different from those of the hepatitis B negative group.

PATHOLOGY. The lesions of polyarteritis involve arteries of medium and small caliber, especially at bifurcations and branchings. The segmental process involves the media, with edema, fibrinous exudation, fibrinoid necrosis, and infiltration of polymorphonuclear neutrophils and varying numbers of eosinophils, and extends to the adventitia and intima. Thrombosis and infarction or hemorrhage occur at this stage. Subsequently, the regions of fibrinoid necrosis are replaced by cellular granulation tissue, and the intima proliferates. Finally the involved segment is replaced by scar tissue with associated intimal thickening and periarterial fibrosis. These changes produce partial occlusion, thrombosis and infarction, and palpable or visible aneurysms with occasional rupture.

The glomerulitis is characterized by capillary microthrombi, focal fibrinoid necrosis, polymorphonuclear neutrophil infiltration, and capsular proliferation. With progression, the necrotizing feature of the glomerulitis is less apparent, and the process is difficult to distinguish from glomerulonephritis of other causes.

CLINICAL MANIFESTATIONS AND DIAGNOSIS. The widespread distribution of the arterial lesions produces diverse clinical manifestations, which reflect the particular organ systems in which the arterial supply has been impaired. In addition, no study including a large number of living patients has or even can limit its patient population to those with classic periarteritis as defined by Kussmaul and Maier. The available studies are likely to include an admixture of patients with allergic angiitis and granulomatosis and hypersensitivity angiitis (see Ch. 49). Among the early general symptoms and signs of periarteritis nodosa are tachycardia, fever, weight loss, and pain in viscera and/or the musculoskeletal system so that the differential diagnosis is of fever of unknown origin. Striking and specific presenting signs may relate to abdominal pain, acute glomerulitis, polyneuritis, or myocardial infarction. Pulmonary manifestations, especially intractable bronchial asthma, would indicate allergic angiitis and granulomatosis rather than classic polyarteritis nodosa.

Renal. Renal involvement in two forms, renal polyarteritis and a glomerulitis, may occur separately or together. Renal polyarteritis was the most common lesion in the postmortem studies of Rose and Spencer (see accompanying table), and in the comparable analysis performed at the Armed Forces Institute of Pathology by Mowrey (1954). Manifestations of the renal involvement include intermittent proteinuria and microscopic hematuria with occasional hyaline and granular casts. The glomerulitis is manifested by marked microscopic and even macroscopic hematuria, proteinuria, cellular casts, and progressive renal failure; survival of the acute phase is followed by progressive hypertension. It is no longer the prevailing view that hypertension precedes or occurs in the initial phase of periarteritis nodosa, but rather that it reflects healing renal polyarteritis, progressive glomerulitis, or both. Such renal involvement is the cause of death in about two thirds of patients with classic periarteritis nodosa and about one third of those with allergic angiitis and granulomatosis.

Gastrointestinal. Characteristic arterial lesions are commonly found in one or more abdominal viscera. The principal manifestation is pain, especially in the umbilical region or right upper quadrant; anorexia, nausea, and vomiting are less prominent. Impaired arterial supply to the bowel can produce mucosal ulceration, perforation, or infarction with melena or bloody diarrhea. Involvement of appendix, gallbladder, or pancreas can stimulate appendicitis, cholecystitis, or hemorrhagic pancreatitis. Liver involvement can range from hepatomegaly with or without jaundice to the signs of extensive hepatic necrosis. Splenomegaly is uncommon. There has been no consistent relationship between the development of necrotizing angiitis and the appearance of liver disease in patients with hepatitis B antigenemia. Some of the observed combinations include necrotizing angiitis as the initial clinical finding, superimposed upon chronic active hepatitis, or appearing simultaneously with an acute hepatitis. Death in this group can occur from liver failure but is more commonly due to the generalized necrotizing angiitis.

Incidence of Necrotizing Angiitis in Various Organs at Necropsy*

	Polyarteritis Nodosa (Classic)	Allergic Angiitis and Granulomatosis ("Polyarteritis with Pulmonary Involvement")
	Per Cent	*Per Cent*
Lungs (pulmonary arteries)	0	47
Heart	35	60
Kidneys: Glomerulitis	30	57
Renal polyarteritis	65	60
Stomach and intestines	30	40
Liver	54	37
Pancreas	39	17
Spleen	35	43
Brain	4	3
Periadrenal connective tissue	41	40
Voluntary muscle	20	33

*Reproduced in modified form from Rose and Spencer: Quart. J. Med., 26:43, 1957. There were 54 cases in the periarteritis group and 30 with the diagnosis of allergic angiitis and granulomatosis.

Central and Peripheral Nervous System.   Neurologic manifestations are generally late occurrences in the course of periarteritis nodosa, and their particular presentation reflects the specific brain area compromised. Headache, convulsive seizures, papillitis, and retinal hemorrhages and exudates occur with or without localizing signs referable to the cerebrum, cerebellum, or brainstem; meningeal irritation may occur as a result of subarachnoid hemorrhage. Multineuritis multiplex, that is, involvement of several or even many individual nerves at the same or different times, is a common finding and is attributed to arteritis of the vasa nervorum. The peripheral neuropathy is usually asymmetrical with both sensory and motor distribution. The former can be extremely painful, but the latter, with attendant muscular degeneration, has on occasion been so severe as to dominate the clinical presentation.

Articular and Muscular.   Arthralgia and myalgia are frequent in polyarteritis nodosa. Arthralgia is migratory, generally without swelling, and apparently due to small localized arterial lesions rather than extensive synovitis. The interpretation of those rare instances of synovitis with deformity and arterial changes of periarteritis nodosa is difficult, but it seems preferable to consider such cases as rheumatoid arthritis. Muscle pain or weakness reflects either direct involvement of the arterial supply or a peripheral neuropathy from involvement of the vasa nervorum.

Cardiac.   Polyarteritis of the coronary arteries and their branches has a frequency approaching that of renal polyarteritis, and heart failure is responsible for or contributes to death in one sixth to one half of the cases. An infantile form of periarteritis nodosa, affecting children mainly under 10 months of age, is manifested primarily by involvement of the coronary arteries. The clinical manifestations of cardiac involvement are those of partial or complete arterial occlusion as modified by the superimposition of renal hypertension and an appreciable incidence of acute pericarditis without effusion. Whereas the combination of infarction and hypertension commonly leads to left-sided failure, an occasional patient with allergic angiitis and granulomatosis will present with predominantly right-sided decompensation.

Genitourinary.   Involvement of the ovaries, testes, and epididymis is frequent, though usually asymptomatic. Mucosal ulceration in the bladder can occasionally precipitate gross hematuria with dysuria.

Cutaneous.   Cutaneous involvement of some form is believed to occur in over 25 per cent of those affected with periarteritis nodosa. The acute cutaneous manifestations of periarteritis nodosa include polymorphic exanthemata—purpuric, urticarial, and multiform in character—and severe subcutaneous hemorrhage, resulting from necrotizing arteritis, with secondary gangrene. Ulcerations and a persistent livedo reticularis are associated with the more chronic stage of the disease. A most characteristic but uncommon finding is cutaneous and subcutaneous nodules; these occur at any time in the disease course. The nodules tend to group, appear in crops, are usually movable, may regress in days or persist for months, range in size from a pea to a walnut, and may cause the overlying skin to become reddened or to ulcerate.

Allergic Angiitis and Granulomatosis ("Polyarteritis with Pulmonary Involvement").   Pulmonary lesions are absent in classic polyarteritis nodosa but almost always precede the onset of polyarteritic lesions in other organs in the process termed allergic granulomatosis and angiitis by Churg and Strauss. Such patients typically present with bronchitis, bronchial asthma, or the findings of pneumonia. The asthma is intractable and associated with a marked peripheral eosinophilia. The pneumonic episodes are transient or progressive and can include hemoptysis or pleuritic pain. The appearance and superimposition of polyarteritis nodosa in other organs is followed by a rapid deterioration, respiratory involvement accounting for half the deaths.

COURSE UNTREATED.   The course of periarteritis nodosa is progressive with destruction of vital organs. Intermittent acute episodes resulting from thrombosis of vital or nonvital structures are prominent. Death is most frequently attributed to renal involvement in cases of classic periarteritis nodosa and to pulmonary lesions in those cases classified as allergic angiitis with granulomatosis. Cardiac failure caused by a combination of infarction and renal hypertension is an additional frequent cause of death in both groups, and acute vascular accidents in the gastrointestinal tract or central nervous system account for much of the remaining mortality. In the retrospective postmortem study of Rose and Spencer, the five-year survival rate was about 10 per cent in classic periarteritis nodosa, and about 25 per cent in allergic angiitis and granulomatosis if onset was dated from the start of respiratory symptoms. The more recent report of the British Medical Research Council in 1960 placed the 54 month's survival rate in polyarteritis nodosa at nearly 50 per cent. A similar survival rate attributed to early steroid treatment has been noted in a Mayo Clinic series in which pulmonary involvement did not appear to influence the prognosis. Rare patients with polyarteritis limited to nonvital sites have been reported to experience an unusually long course or even a lasting remission. The entire issue of prognosis will be influenced by the criteria for entry into a series until the entity of periarteritis is more definitively separated from the more favorable grouping of hypersensitivity angiitis.

LABORATORY FINDINGS.   Leukocytosis, predominantly polymorphonuclear, is apparent in over 75 per cent of the cases of periarteritis nodosa or allergic angiitis and granulomatosis, eosinophilia often being marked in the latter group. The association of hepatitis B antigenemia with generalized necrotizing angiitis may be as high as one third of the cases, but probably this figure will prove to be smaller as experience widens. Hypocomplementemia, which has not been observed in classic periarteritis nodosa, has been present in patients with generalized necrotizing angiitis with or without hepatitis B antigenemia. The erythrocyte sedimentation rate is customarily elevated with or without some increase of the globulins. Abnormalities in the urine sediment, especially hematuria and proteinuria, reflect renal involvement. Abnormalities of the electrocardiogram and electroencephalogram are those expected on the basis of arterial occlusive disease or those secondary to the metabolic disturbances of uremia. Lesions apparent on chest roentgenograms are the rule in patients with allergic angiitis and granulomatosis. The findings range from transient or progressive infiltration to consolidation, cavitation, or scarring; upper and lower lobes are involved with equal frequency. As none of these findings is specific, antemortem diagnosis of polyarteritis depends upon biopsy. Since the arterial involvement is segmental and spotty in distribution, it is advisable to obtain tissue from a symptomatic site, and it is essential to section completely the entire specimen. A deep, open surgical biopsy, including subcutaneous tissue and underlying muscle, should be obtained whenever possible from a skeletal muscle exhibiting pain and tenderness. Involvement of the epididymis and testes is sufficiently common to make this a useful biopsy site, if palpation reveals the typical nodularity of segmental vascular lesions. Needle and surgical biopsies of internal organs with clinical involvement, such as liver or kidney, are gaining in favor. As an alternative or additional procedure, arteriography of several organs to detect aneurysms of medium-sized muscular arteries may be helpful.

DIFFERENTIAL DIAGNOSIS. The differential diagnosis of classic periarteritis nodosa includes all those conditions associated with necrotizing angiitis (see Ch. 49). The absence of pulmonary lesions distinguishes classic periarteritis nodosa from allergic angiitis and granulomatosis. Similarly, the relative absence of venular involvement, with or without hepatitis B antigenemia, may separate classic periarteritis nodosa from the more common generalized necrotizing angiitis. The hypocomplementemia in some patients with generalized necrotizing angiitis is more reminiscent of certain patients with hypersensitivity angiitis than of periarteritis nodosa. The other connective tissue diseases are recognized by their clinical characteristics even when necrotizing arteritis becomes prominent. For example, cases of rheumatoid arthritis with ulcerating cutaneous lesions and peripheral neuropathy often exhibit prominent rheumatoid nodules and a high titer of rheumatoid factor. Giant cell arteritis, in its limited form, cranial (especially temporal) or aortic arch (Takayasu's) arteritis, or in its disseminated state lacks the glomerulitis, peripheral neuropathy, and cutaneous manifestations notable in periarteritis nodosa. The drug-induced hypersensitivity angiitis group may be difficult to separate on purely clinical grounds, although the history of antecedent drug administration, the frequency of pulmonary involvement, infrequency of gastrointestinal manifestations, and absence of nodules along arteries are useful points. The clinical presentation in Henoch-Schönlein purpura, mostly in children and with a relatively good prognosis, is distinctive. The combination of progressive nephritis and pulmonary hemorrhage seen in Goodpasture's syndrome is unlike polyarteritis nodosa. The findings in the immunoglobulins which accompany active systemic lupus erythematosus or mixed cryoglobulinemia are distinctive; in addition, in the presence of active renal disease both entities manifest a reduced serum complement level not observed in periarteritis nodosa. Necrotizing vasculitis with or without renal disease in C2 deficiency, hypergammaglobulinemic purpura, and other syndromes listed under hypersensitivity angiitis (see Ch. 49) are differentiated by the unique features responsible for designating the entity.

The key morphologic differences between periarteritis nodosa and other causes of necrotizing angiitis are noted in Ch. 49 and include the absence of extravascular granulomas, sparing of the pulmonary arteries, failure of venous involvement except by contiguous spread, and predilection for medium-sized arteries. For allergic angiitis and granulomatosis the striking granulomatous response excludes all but Wegener's granulomatosis. The prominence of bronchial asthma, peripheral eosinophilia, and the usual absence of necrotizing lesions in the upper respiratory tract permit a tentative clinical distinction between allergic angiitis and granulomatosis (termed by some polyarteritis nodosa with pulmonary involvement) and Wegener's granulomatosis. Additional entities to be considered in the differential diagnosis are certain microbial and occlusive diseases with diverse manifestations, notably chronic meningococcemia, subacute infective endocarditis, trichinosis, certain rickettsial diseases, leptospirosis, and syphilis. A few vascular occlusive diseases, including Degos' disease and thrombotic thrombocytopenic purpura, must also be considered. Necrotizing papulosis of Degos, with its occlusive arterial lesions of the skin, gastrointestinal tract, and brain, is best characterized by the cutaneous manifestations. These lesions typically involve the trunk and extremities, begin as pink to gray papules, undergo central umbilication, and persist for variable periods with depressed (porcelain-like) centers covered with a removable scale and surrounded by a red elevated margin. The absence of both thrombocytopenia and intravascular hemolysis distinguishes periarteritis nodosa from thrombotic thrombocytopenic purpura. Additional points of help in the differential diagnosis of periarteritis nodosa in general are the rarity of Raynaud's phenomenon, the absence of the nephrotic syndrome, and the lack of lymphadenopathy.

TREATMENT. The therapy of periarteritis nodosa and allergic angiitis and granulomatosis is clearly unsatisfactory. Nonetheless, such patients can remain ambulatory and professionally active for periods of months to years after the clinical onset of the disease. The commonly employed anti-inflammatory agents such as salicylates or phenylbutazone have little or no clear effect, and thus corticosteroids have been employed most widely. Large doses, in the range of 40 to 60 mg of prednisone per day, afford symptomatic relief and apparently do improve the one-year survival statistics. On the other hand, the study by the Medical Research Council of England did not reveal a better 54 months' survival period in a steroid-treated group as compared with a control series, whereas early steroid treatment was considered efficacious in the Mayo Clinic series. The capacity of steroids in giant cell arteritis and of cyclophosphamide in Wegener's granulomatosis to produce convincing clinical responses and, apparently, even extended remissions has prompted an increased utilization of such agents in the treatment of other forms of necrotizing agiitis. Cytotoxic agents, generally accompanied by steroids, are certainly justified in the management of patients with periarteritis nodosa, generalized necrotizing angiitis, and allergic angiitis and granulomatosis.

Churg, J., and Strauss, L.: Allergic granulomatosis, allergic angiitis, and periarteritis nodosa. Am. J. Pathol., 27:277, 1951.

Collagen Diseases and Hypersensitivity Panel: Report to Medical Research Council. Br. Med. J., 1:1399, 1960.

Fink, C. W.: Polyarteritis and other diseases with necrotizing vasculitis in children. Arthritis Rheum., 20:378, 1977 (suppl.).

Gocke, D. J., Hsu, K., Morgan, C., Bombardieri, S., Lockshin, M., and Christian, C. L.: Association betwen polyarteritis and Australia antigen. Lancet, 2:1149, 1970.

Mowrey, F. H., and Lundberg, R. A.: The clinical manifestations of essential polyangitis (periarteritis nodosa) with emphasis on the hepatic manifestations. Ann. Intern. Med., 40:1145, 1954.

Reza, M. J., Dornfeld, L., Goldberg, L. S., Bluestone, R., and Pearson, C. M.: Wegener's granulomatosis. Long-term follow-up of patients treated with cyclophosphamide. Arthritis Rheum., 18:501, 1975.

Rose, G. A., and Spencer, H.: Polyarteritis nodosa. Quart. J. Med., 26:43, 1957.

Sergent, J. S., Lockshin, M. D., Christian, C. L., and Gocke, D. J.: Vasculitis with hepatitis B antigenemia. Long-term observations in nine patients. Medicine, 55:1, 1976.

Trepo, G. C., and Thivolet, J.: Antigene Australien, hépatite à virus et périartérite nouveuse. Presse Méd., 78:1575, 1970.

PART VII

DISEASES OF THE JOINTS

Charles L. Christian

54. INTRODUCTION

Although the terms "arthritis" and "rheumatism" have similar connotations, the former is restrictive, denoting inflammatory disease of joints. "Rheumatism" embraces a wide variety of illnesses that affect components of the musculoskeletal system: joints, muscles, ligaments, tendons, and bursae. Rheumatic syndromes can be classified as either inflammatory or degenerative, but the pathologic processes are sometimes less distinct than the nomenclature implies. A joint damaged by inflammatory disease is more vulnerable to degenerative influences, and syndromes that appear to be primarily degenerative in nature may be associated with the cardinal signs of inflammation. Musculoskeletal pain and stiffness, although characteristic of rheu-matic syndromes, can be significant manifestations of virtually every disease of man. Errors in diagnosis and management result from uncritical elicitation of the medical history, physical signs, and, probably most frequently, from unbalanced interpretations of laboratory data. Hyperuricemia, rheumatoid factors, and antinuclear factors are not disease specific; and radiographic evidence of degenerative joint disease does not constitute proof that pain in an extremity is due to that process.

The accompanying classification of rheumatic disease (table), condensed and somewhat amended from the American Rheumatism Association's recommended (tentative) nomenclature, indicates the diversity of illnesses that can cause manifestations of rheumatic disease.

Rheumatic Disease—Classification

1. Polyarthritis of unknown etiology:
   a. Rheumatoid arthritis
   b. Juvenile rheumatoid arthritis
   c. Ankylosing spondylitis
   d. Psoriatic arthritis
   e. Reiter's syndrome
   f. Others
2. "Connective tissue" disorders (acquired):
   a. Systemic lupus erythematosus
   b. Progressive systemic sclerosis (scleroderma)
   c. Polymyositis and dermatomyositis
   d. Necrotizing arteritis and other forms of vasculitis
3. Rheumatic fever
4. Degenerative joint disease (osteoarthritis):
   a. Primary
   b. Secondary
5. Nonarticular rheumatism:
   a. Fibrositis
   b. Intervertebral disc and low back syndromes
   c. Myositis and myalgia
   d. Tendinitis and peritendinitis (bursitis)
6. Diseases with which arthritis is frequently associated:
   a. Sarcoidosis
   b. Relapsing polychondritis
   c. Schönlein-Henoch purpura
   d. Ulcerative colitis
   e. Regional enteritis
   f. Whipple's disease
   g. Sjögren's syndrome
   h. Familial Mediterranean fever
   i. Others
7. Arthritis associated with known infectious agents:
   a. Bacterial
   b. Rickettsial
   c. Viral
   d. Fungal

   e. Parasitic
8. Traumatic and/or neurogenic disorders:
   a. Traumatic arthritis (the result of direct trauma)
   b. Neuropathic arthropathy (Charcot joints)
   c. Shoulder-hand syndrome
   d. Mechanical derangement of joints
   e. Others
9. Arthritis associated with known or strongly suspected biochemical or endocrine abnormalities:
   a. Gout
   b. Chondrocalcinosis articularis ("pseudogout")
   c. Alcaptonuria (ochronosis)
   d. Hemophilia
   e. Sickle cell disease and other hemoglobinopathies
   f. Agammaglobulinemia (hypogammaglobulinemia)
   g. Gaucher's disease
   h. Hyperparathyroidism
   i. Acromegaly
   j. Hypothyroidism
   k. Scurvy
   l. Hyperlipoproteinemia type II (xanthoma tuberosum and tendinosum)
   m. Hemochromatosis
   n. Others
10. Neoplasms
11. Allergy and drug reactions
12. Miscellaneous disorders:
    a. Pigmented villonodular synovitis and tenosynovitis
    b. Behçet's syndrome
    c. Erythema nodosum
    d. Avascular necrosis of bone
    e. Juvenile osteochondritis
    f. Erythema multiforme (Stevens-Johnson syndrome)
    g. Hypertrophic osteoarthropathy
    h. Multicentric reticulohistiocytosis

55. ARTHRITIS ASSOCIATED WITH KNOWN INFECTIOUS AGENTS

55.1. BACTERIAL ARTHRITIS

The great majority of cases of bacterial arthritis result from hematogenous spread of infections. Much less frequently, bacterial infection may result from joint aspiration or injection or by spread from contiguous osteomyelitis. In adults, gram-positive cocci (*Staphylococcus aureus, Streptococcus pyogenes, Diplococcus pneumoniae*) and *Neisseria gonorrhoeae* account for most cases. (Other areas of this text contain more detailed accounts of the problems and management of sepsis caused by specific bacterial organisms. The emphasis here is on principles of diagnosis and management that are common to all types of bacterial arthritis.)

Certain organisms appear to exhibit a tropism for joints: *N. gonorrhoeae, N. meningitidis, Hemophilus influenzae,* and *Streptobacillus moniliformis.* Host factors associated with debilitating chronic disease, rheumatoid arthritis, sickle cell anemia, hypogammaglobulinemia, and immunosuppressive therapy increase the risk of bacterial arthritis. A problem of increasing frequency is the development of low-grade infection complicating prosthetic joint placement. The recognition of infection may be delayed many months after joint replacement. Organisms of low virulence, especially *Staphylococcus albus,* predominate.

CLINICAL MANIFESTATIONS. Although inflammatory signs in a single joint should heighten one's suspicion of bacterial sepsis, the disease may be polyarticular, a pattern that predominates with gonococcal arthritis. Rigor and high temperature, common manifestations of bacterial arthritis, are rare in rheumatoid arthritis and other types of noninfectious joint disease. Inflammatory signs tend to be marked; but in the presence of debilitating disease or treatment with adrenocorticosteroids or immunosuppressive agents, pain, swelling, and erythema may be masked. In patients with chronic rheumatoid arthritis, a preponderance of inflammatory disease in one or a limited number of joints should arouse suspicion of complicating bacterial arthritis.

DIAGNOSIS. Since accurate diagnosis and effective management depend on isolation and characterization of the microbe, the highest priority is to be given to careful and complete bacteriologic studies. Although synovial fluid leukocyte counts in excess of 50,000 per cubic millimeter and reduced synovial fluid glucose content are common manifestations, no level of either is diagnostic of infection. Stained smears of joint fluid may demonstrate bacterial forms in the absence of a positive culture, especially when there has been chemotherapy. Synovial fluid and blood for microbiologic studies should be delivered without delay to the laboratory, preferably by someone involved in the patient's management. In addition to routine aerobic and anaerobic cultures, special media are needed for the isolation of *N. gonorrhoeae.* Obviously bacteriologic studies of other materials, such as sputum, urine, and cervical exudate, may help to identify the organism causing arthritis.

Radiographic signs indicating loss of articular cartilage or erosion of bone are uncommon during the first week of disease.

MANAGEMENT. Success in management, as in diagnosis, rests with identification of the pathogen. The selection of appropriate antimicrobial agents and recommendations regarding dose and duration of therapy are covered in other areas of this text (see Ch. 190). It should be remembered that bacterial arthritis is usually a part of systemic sepsis and that the involvement of the synovial bursae behaves like a closed space infection. Since there is adequate transport of the commonly employed antimicrobial agents from blood to joint fluid, there are rarely if ever indications for intra-articular therapy. When response to therapy is inadequate, measurement of bactericidal levels of drugs in synovial fluid may be indicated.

The decision whether to drain the joint bursae is influenced by the character of the exudate. When there is gross suppuration, and fluid cannot be easily aspirated with a large-bore needle, surgical incision and drainage are usually performed. When fluid can be aspirated with a needle and syringe, this is the preferred method for periodic decompression. The frequency of aspiration depends upon the extent and rate of reaccumulation. Gross joint destruction and the presence of contiguous osteomyelitis are indications for surgical drainage.

Physical therapy is inappropriate during the acute phase of bacterial arthritis. Maintenance of rest may be facilitated by removable splints. The rate at which gentle passive exercises can be graded into active motion should be tailored to each patient. Even in the absence of structural damage of weight-bearing joints, activity should not be resumed until signs of acute inflammation have subsided. The prognosis for full recovery is good when effective therapy is initiated within a week of the onset.

Gonococcal Arthritis. Gonococcal infection is discussed in Ch. 139. Because of its frequency and characteristic manifestations, this form of bacterial arthritis deserves emphasis. It is most common in females and homosexual males whose primary infections, because they are often asymptomatic, are untreated. The manifestations vary, but the most common pattern is migratory polyarthritis associated with tenosynovitis (especially in the hand and foot), followed by a "settling" in one or two joints. Shaking chills often precede or accompany the synovitis. Erythematous skin lesions, which may be macular, vesicular, or pustular (often with a necrotic center), are common in gonococcemia. The same clinical pattern can be associated with *N. meningitidis* and *H. influenzae* infections, although the latter is rare in adults.

Tuberculous Arthritis. The general decline in the frequency of tuberculosis is reflected in the relative rarity of tuberculous bone and joint disease. During the past few decades tuberculous arthritis has been predominantly an adult disease with evidence of pulmonary or disseminated disease frequently lacking. It is usually manifest in a single joint, most commonly hip, knee, or wrist, but any articulation may be affected, and occasionally two or more may be involved. Tuberculous *spondylitis* (Pott's disease), predominantly a disease of children, has dramatically decreased in western countries.

Signs of acute inflammation are usually absent. Tuberculous arthritis is most commonly confused with monoarticular rheumatoid arthritis. The ultimate differentiation, in a tuberculin-positive subject, often requires synovial biopsy and subsequent histologic and bacteriologic studies. Modern chemotherapy (see Ch. 168.14) has made surgical procedures (drainage, synovectomy, or fusion) unnecessary except in a rare patient with severe joint destruction.

55.2. VIRAL ARTHRITIS

Prevailing theories regarding the pathogenesis of rheumatoid arthritis, systemic lupus erythematosus, and related syndromes implicate atypical microbial infection. Although evidence supporting such speculations is indirect, there are well-defined, common viral infections associated with polyarthritis, notably rubella and viral hepatitis. Other viral syndromes associated with arthritis include mumps, infectious mononucleosis, and several arborvirus infections. Polyarthritis resembling acute rheumatic fever or acute rheumatoid arthritis occurs in approximately one third of women with natural or vaccine *rubella* infection. Lower frequencies of this complication are seen in men and children. Rubella arthritis usually follows the onset, or the fading phase, of the characteristic rash. The virus has been isolated from affected joints. The duration of joint inflammation varies from a few days to two weeks, rarely longer. There has been no documentation of chronic arthritis resulting from rubella infection. The management of pain and stiffness, which may be severe, should require nothing more than salicylate therapy.

Transient polyarthritis—more commonly polyarthralgia—is a significant prodromal manifestation of viral *hepatitis*. As with rubella, the pattern of arthritis resembles that of acute rheumatoid arthritis. It is frequently associated with fever and an urticarial skin eruption. These antedate the signs and symptoms of hepatitis by a few days to a few weeks, and have generally receded by the time icterus is apparent. Persistent polyarthritis has not been observed as a complication of viral hepatitis, although a small percentage of individuals with chronic active hepatitis have mild chronic or recurrent synovitis. The role that hepatitis B (Australia) antigen plays in the pathogenesis of the arthritis is not known, but certain manifestations, i.e., depressed serum complement and urticarial rash, are consistent with the hypothesis that immune complexes may be involved. Treatment is symptomatic.

55.3. OTHER FORMS OF INFECTIOUS ARTHRITIS

SYPHILITIC ARTHRITIS. Syphilis is discussed in Ch. 171. Syphilitic arthritis, in its various forms, is now rare. A mild chronic synovitis, usually of the knees, may occur at about the age of puberty in patients with prenatal syphilis *(Clutton's joints)*. Earlier skeletal manifestation of prenatal syphilis are related to periostitis and osteochondritis. Rheumatic manifestations have been attributed to secondary syphilis, but these, along with gummatous involvement of bones and joints, have more historical than current importance. The most common rheumatic expression of syphilis, neuropathic arthropathy or Charcot joint, is reviewed in Ch. 60.

MYCOTIC ARTHRITIS. Any of the invasive *mycoses* such as histoplasmosis, coccidioidomycosis, blastomycosis, and actinomycosis can affect joints, usually by extension from adjacent bone. Their manifestations generally resemble those of tuberculosis. Coccidioidomycosis can also cause the joint inflammation of erythema nodosum (see Ch. 179).

LYME ARTHRITIS. See Ch. 60.

Alpert, E., Isselbacher, K. J., and Schur, P. H.: The pathogenesis of arthritis associated with viral hepatitis: Complement component studies. N. Engl. J. Med., 285:185, 1971.

Davidson, P. T., and Horowitz, I.: Skeletal tuberculosis: A review with patient presentations and discussion. Am. J. Med., 48:77, 1970.

Keiser, H., et al.: Clinical forms of gonococcal arthritis. N. Engl. J. Med., 279:234, 1968.

Schmid, F. R.: Principles of diagnosis and treatment of infectious arthritis. *In* Hollander, J. L., and McCarty, D. J., Jr. (eds.): Arthritis and Allied Conditions. 8th ed. Philadelphia, Lea & Febiger, 1972.

Sharp, J. T.: Gonococcal arthritis. *In* Hollander, J. L., and McCarty, D. J., Jr. (eds.): Arthritis and Allied Conditions. 8th ed. Philadelphia, Lea & Febiger, 1972.

Smith, J. W., and Sanford, J. P.: Viral arthritis. Ann. Intern. Med., 67:651, 1967.

56. RHEUMATOID ARTHRITIS

DEFINITION. In 1858 Sir Alfred Garrod introduced the term rheumatoid arthritis for a syndrome which he recognized as distinct from gout and acute rheumatic fever. With only minor exceptions (Garrod included Heberden's nodes as features of rheumatoid arthritis) his description matches the modern definition. The American Rheumatism Association's criteria for "classical, definite, probable and possible rheumatoid arthritis" have led to more consistent reporting in clinical studies, but the diagnosis still rests mainly on exclusion of other causes of synovitis.

Rheumatoid arthritis is a systemic disease of unknown cause. The frequency of extra-articular manifestations justifies the concept of "rheumatoid disease," but in the majority of patients clinical and pathologic findings and disability are the result of chronic inflammation of synovial membranes. There is striking heterogeneity among patients regarding mode of onset, pattern of joint involvement, frequency of extra-articular manifestations, and clinical course. There is a tendency for symmetrical involvement of hands, wrists, and feet. Spontaneous remissions and exacerbations are characteristic. Ten to 20 per cent of patients have complete remissions, whereas the remainder have sustained fluctuating activity. Joint injury results from formation of chronic granulation tissue (pannus), products of proliferative and exudative synovitis; this is capable of altering articular and periarticular structures.

INCIDENCE AND EPIDEMIOLOGY. The frequency of rheumatoid arthritis, based on limited population surveys in Europe and North America, is in the range of 1 to 3 per cent. It is two to three times more common in females. The onset is most frequent in the fourth and fifth decades of life, but it may occur at any age. There are no consistent trends relating prevalence to geography, climate, or culture. The apparent relative rarity in tropical climates may reflect the age of indigenous populations and the level of available medical care. Multiple family members in selected kindreds may be affected; but in general, familial patterns (even in monozygotic twins) are not striking. An increased frequency of a histocompatibility antigen (HLA-DW$_4$) has been observed in rheumatoid arthritis subjects.

PATHOLOGY. The pathologic elements of chronic synovitis include exudation, cellular infiltration, and the proliferation of granulation tissue. Although polymorphonuclear leukocytes predominate in synovial fluid, the principal infiltrating cells in synovial membranes are lymphocytes. These are often arranged in nodular aggregates, occasionally as true lymphoid follicles with germinal centers. Rarely, the majority of infiltrating cells are plasmacytes. Multinucleated giant cells may be seen. None of the aforementioned histologic features are diagnostic of rheumatoid arthritis.

Pannus, presumably by its content of hydrolytic enzymes, is capable of eroding articular cartilage, subchondral bone, ligaments, and tendons. Products of exudation in synovial fluid may also contribute to cartilage injury. The variable pattern of joint disability (subluxation, loss of motion, or ankylosis) relates to destructive processes in articular and periarticular structures.

Extra-articular manifestations, although clinically evident in a minority of patients, may give rise to widespread pathologic features of rheumatoid arthritis. Many of these appear to result from focal perivascular inflammation. Ten to 20 per cent of patients with rheumatoid arthritis form *subcutaneous or periosteal nodules* over pressure or friction points. The histologic appearance of nodules (central areas of necrosis surrounded by palisading connective tissue cells and an envelope of granulation tissue) is characteristic. In rare instances, the same granulomatous process can occur in multiple organs. More commonly (probably in the range of 50 per cent of cases) there is a mild perivascular infiltration of mononuclear cells in *muscle and peripheral nerves.* An uncommon but significant complication of the disease is the development of diffuse *necrotizing arteritis* with visceral involvement indistinguishable from polyarteritis nodosa. Milder forms of vasculitis, manifested by peripheral neuropathy and *chronic skin ulcers* of the lower extremities, are much more frequent. In such patients chronic inflammation of the sclera is common.

Cardiac pathology is less evident clinically than it is histologically. At necropsy, between one third and one half of rheumatoid patients have evidence of pericarditis (usually healed). Granulomatous lesions resembling rheumatoid nodules rarely may be found in the epicardium, myocardium, valves, and proximal aorta.

Pulmonary lesions, although infrequent, are significant expressions of rheumatoid disease. They include (1) chronic *pleural effusion,* (2) *Caplan's syndrome* (exaggerated pulmonary nodule formation in rheumatoid patients exposed to silica dust), (3) involvement with *granulomatous lesions resembling rheumatoid nodules,* and (4) *interstitial fibrosis.*

The most common patterns of neurologic involvement are peripheral neuropathy and nerve root irritation or myelopathy secondary to vertebral involvement (especially at C1-C2).

PATHOGENESIS. The role of *inflammation* in the production of articular, periarticular, and extra-articular injury is evident. A variety of lysosomal enzymes, neutral proteases, and synovial collagenase are capable of hy-drolyzing constituents of connective tissue, and the role of such enzymes in the induction of tissue injury seems explicit. A more basic question, however, is: What initiates and perpetuates the inflammatory response? In this regard, immunologic theories predominate.

Immunologic Features. Synovial tissue in rheumatoid arthritis often displays histologic features characteristic of lymphoid organs, with prominent collections of lymphocytes and plasma cells (sometimes in the form of germinal centers). Immunoglobulin synthesis has been demonstrated in rheumatoid synovial tissue by immunohistologic and tissue culture studies. There is evidence for a role of immune complexes in the induction of inflammation. Synovial fluid exudate cells and synovial lining cells contain deposits of immunoglobulin and complement. Complement levels in synovial fluid are reduced in a pattern consistent with immune activation, and complexes of immunoglobulins are detectable in joint fluid. Detailed characterization of these has not been accomplished, but in part they consist of rheumatoid factors.

Rheumatoid Factors. Rheumatoid factors are autoantibodies reactive with the Fc portion of IgG. Anti–gamma globulin activities are associated with the three major classes of immunoglobulins (IgM, IgG, and IgA), but, because of the enhanced agglutinating property of IgM antibodies, standard tests measure predominantly IgM rheumatoid factors. Rheumatoid factors form soluble complexes with their antigen (IgG). The complexes of IgM rheumatoid factor with IgG have a sedimentation coefficient of approximately 22S, whereas the complexes formed with IgG rheumatoid factors are very heterogeneous, sedimenting in the "intermediate" range between IgG and IgM. These intermediate complexes, which comprise at least part of the complexes measurable in rheumatoid synovial fluid, are capable of reacting with IgM rheumatoid factors to form insoluble aggregates. It is postulated that such complexes in joint fluid, perhaps augmented by their reactivity with IgM rheumatoid factor, activate complement-dependent mediators of inflammation and promote phagocytosis and subsequent release of hydrolytic enzymes. Although this hypothesis is attractive, there are a variety of reasons why one cannot assign an exclusive and primary role to rheumatoid factors in the induction of rheumatoid synovitis. On the basis of current evidence, it is more likely that rheumatoid factors are products of the host response to a more primary event. The nature of this postulated primary event is still unknown, but there is renewed interest in an old concept that microbial disease may underlie the development of rheumatoid arthritis.

Infectious Agents. A number of clinical and pathologic features of rheumatoid arthritis are mimicked by animal models of disease where microbial causes are explicit — in particular, chronic arthritis in swine induced by species of *Mycoplasma* and by *Erysipelothrix insidiosa.* An interesting aspect of these experimental models is that by the time chronic disease has developed, the inducing microorganism is often not demonstrable. By analogy, if the microbial hypothesis for rheumatoid disease is correct, the generally negative results of efforts to recover microorganisms may thus be explained. Although speculation regarding an infectious cause of rheumatoid disease has been augmented by modern concepts of viral persistence and by studies of animal models, direct evidence in its support is lacking. There have been periodic reports of the isolation of *Mycoplasma* and bacterial forms and of demonstrations that rheumatoid synovial cells are resistant to infection by exogenous viruses, but these observations still lack confirmation.

CLINICAL MANIFESTATIONS. **Mode of Onset.** Usually, rheumatoid arthritis has an insidious onset, often beginning with poorly localized arching and stiffness. These early symptoms may be attributed to "grippe," and the subsequent evolution of frank synovitis may be sufficiently slow that the patient does not seek medical attention for many weeks. A variety of "precipitating" factors have been entertained (trauma, environmental change, infections, and psychologic stress), but none of these is constant in the antecedent history. Most patiens manifest symmetrical polyarthritis early in the course of their disease, but a significant number (approximately one third) will have inflammation limited to one or two joints. Occasionally limited expressions of the disease, i.e., monarthritis or even tenosynovitis, may persist for many weeks or months. In contrast to the gradual onset of disease that characterizes the majority, the onset is precipitous in some patients, almost to the hour of a given day.

Symptoms. *Pain,* the dominant symptom, corresponds to the pattern and intensity of joint involvement, whereas *stiffness* is more generalized and is characteristically maximal after periods of physical inactivity. *Morning stiffness* is an almost invariable feature; its intensity and duration can guide one in assessment of disease activity.

The majority of patients experience *constitutional symptoms* such as weakness, increased fatigability, and diminished appetite. Temperature elevation in excess of 38° C is uncommon. Higher temperatures should prompt search for superimposed infection, but occasionally temperatures as high as 40° C have no other explanation than active rheumatoid arthritis. Many patients complain of coldness and hypesthesias and paresthesias in the hands and feet (in the absence of signs of nerve entrapment).

Physical Signs. The physical signs of rheumatoid arthritis vary enormously according to anatomic patterns, severity, and stage of disease. The "classic" articular and extra-articular expressions are features of *chronic* rheumatoid arthritis.

GENERAL EXAMINATION. Observations of gait and performance of simple tasks, such as removal of clothing, may reveal evidence of stiffness or specific anatomic patterns of disease. Many, but not all, patients appear chronically ill and undernourished. Generalized lymphadenopathy and splenomegaly are features in some subjects (approximately 10 per cent); rarely this picture is so striking that it mimics lymphomatous disease. Dependent edema not attributable to other causes is an infrequent but significant feature. Easy bruising and increased fragility of skin are common in patients with chronic disease; both are amplified by corticosteroid therapy. Nodules are most commonly found in subcutaneous tissue, but they can occur within the dermis and periosteum. Nodules are characteristically localized over points of pressure or friction, most commonly the extensor surfaces of the proximal forearms. In a bedridden patient they may be found over the posterior aspects of the head, trunk, and spine.

SKELETAL MANIFESTATIONS. The invariable signs of swelling, tenderness, and pain on motion in early cases

may seem poorly localized to joints. A common mode of onset, with symmetrical involvement of the distal upper extremities, is diffuse swelling of the hands and wrists. More discrete enlargement of articulations (Fig. 1) may not appear for weeks or months. Warmth is usually evident, especially over the large joints such as the knee, but skin erythema is infrequent. Swelling reflects varying degrees of synovial thickening and proliferation and increased volume of synovial fluid. From palpation and ballottement, the examiner can usually estimate the relative roles of effusion and synovial proliferation.

The characteristic deformities of joints which are products of sustained chronic disease are attributable to a variety of events: loss of articular cartilage, destruction or weakening of ligaments, tendons, and capsular structures, muscle imbalance, and the physical force associated with use of the affected joints (Fig. 2). In addition, there are biologic variations which in some patients favor joint subluxation and instability and in other patients result in bony or fibrous ankylosis.

Muscle atrophy of the affected extremities may be evident within weeks of onset of rheumatoid arthritis. Whether this relates to primary myopathic change or disuse is moot, but rarely an overt myopathy, indistinguishable from polymyositis, may be a feature of the disease.

Extensions or rupture of synovial bursae beyond the confines of joint capsules can result in features of special importance to the internist. The most common example of this is the communication of joints of the wrists with the tenosynovium of the finger extensors. Popliteal cysts associated with knee synovitis may rupture into the calf and produce an inflammatory reaction that very closely resembles deep vein thrombophlebitis. The sudden onset of this complication, often associated with forceful flexion of the knee, and the intense inflammation help distinguish it from phlebitis, but this differentiation is best accomplished by arthrography. Rarely, extensions from hip synovitis may result in the formation of pelvic or inguinal masses.

EXTRA-ARTICULAR MANIFESTATIONS. Many of the features of rheumatoid arthritis that are associated with diffuse vasculitis have been discussed previously under

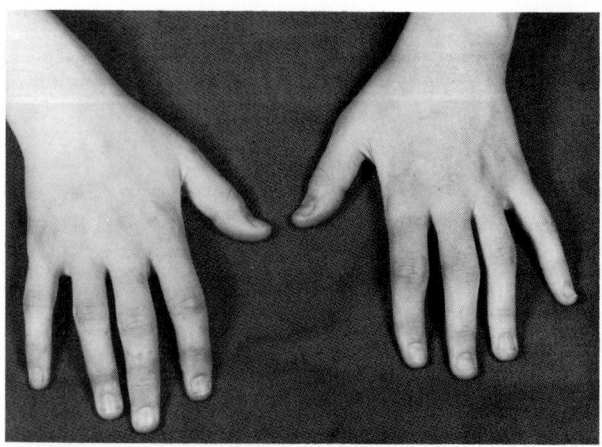

Figure 1. Early rheumatoid arthritis manifest as symmetrical swelling and slight flexion deformities of proximal interphalangeal joints of the hands. Roentgenograms were normal except for evidence of soft tissue swelling.

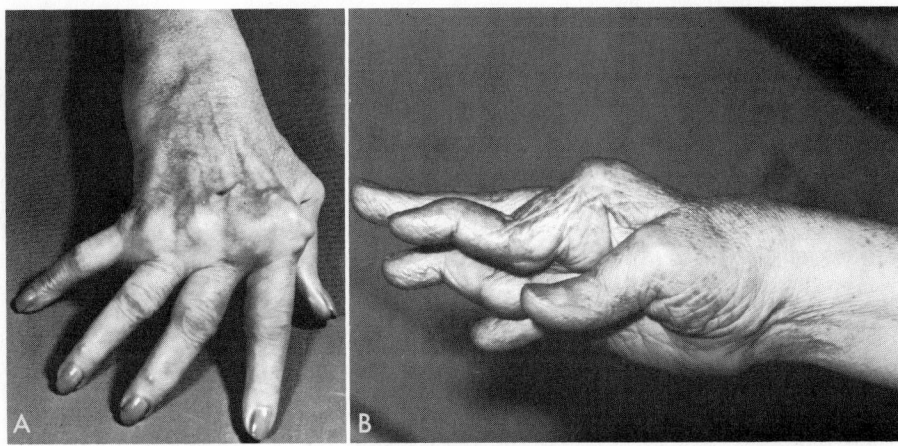

Figure 2. Hand deformities characteristic of chronic rheumatoid arthritis. *A,* Subluxation of metacarpophalangeal joints with ulnar deviation of digits. *B,* Hyperextension ("swan neck") deformities of proximal interphalangeal joints.

Pathology. The clinical expressions of vasculitis (neuropathy, chronic skin ulcers, digital gangrene, and rarely visceral arteritis) and the clinical patterns associated with disseminated granulomata (heart, lung, sclera, and dura mater) are invariably features of chronic "classic" disease and are rarely encountered in patients who lack the rheumatoid factor.

For reasons unknown, pulmonary involvement (pleural effusion, granulomatous pneumonitis, and diffuse interstitial fibrosis) is more common in males. Cavitating pulmonary nodules occasionally result in pneumothorax or chronic bronchopleural fistulas. The glucose content of rheumatoid pleural effusions is frequently less than 10 mg per 100 ml.

There are usually no problems in interpretation of neurologic signs related to peripheral neuropathy, nerve entrapment (median nerve involvement at the wrist is common), and radiculopathy. In contrast, the insidious progression of muscle weakness secondary to myelopathy from C1-C2 subluxation can mistakenly be attributed to "arthritis" and associated constitutional symptoms.

Other extra-articular manifestations of rheumatoid arthritis include amyloidosis, keratoconjunctivitis sicca, and Felty's syndrome.

CLINICAL COURSE AND PROGNOSIS. Statistics regarding the natural history of rheumatoid arthritis are based on studies in large rheumatic disease units where patients are not representative of the entire population of rheumatoid arthritics, i.e., they tend to be patients with more severe and sustained disease. Patients with more remitting patterns of disease are less apt to be entered into prognostic studies. However, even the published figures allow one to present a reasonably optimistic outlook to the patient. After 10 to 15 years of disease, over 50 per cent of patients remain fully employed and only about 10 per cent are completely incapacitated. Ten to 20 per cent of patients have virtually complete remissions; the course followed by the remainder is extremely varied. The average patient with episodic exacerbations and partial remissions will experience gradual progression of deformity and disability. The minority, with sustained disease activity and only slight remissions, may become completely disabled within a few years of onset. The *features associated with a poor prognosis,* in a statistical sense are (1) classic pattern of disease (symmetrical polyarthritis with subcutaneous nodules and high titers of rheumatoid factor), (2)

sustained disease of more than one year's duration, (3) onset below age 30, and (4) extra-articular manifestations of rheumatoid arthritis.

ROENTGENOGRAPHIC FINDINGS. Early in the disease roentgenograms of affected joints are usually negative except for evidence of soft tissue swelling and joint effusion. Osteoporosis, especially in juxta-articular locations, may be evident within weeks of onset of disease. Loss of articular cartilage, shown by reduction in the apparent "joint space," and bone erosions are rarely evident before several months of sustained disease. Subluxations, dislocations, and bony ankylosis, if they occur, are still later phenomena. Diffuse osteoporosis is common with chronic disease and is heightened with adrenocorticosteroid therapy. The frequency of avascular osteonecrosis, especially of the femoral heads, is also increased with such therapy.

LABORATORY FINDINGS. Mild *anemia,* similar to that associated with chronic infection, is common in rheumatoid arthritis. Serum levels of both iron and iron-binding protein are frequently depressed. Anemia is usually normocytic and normochromic, but if there is accompanying iron deficiency, the erythrocytes may be slightly hypochromic and microcytic. Leukocytosis, eosinophilia, and thrombocytosis are occasional laboratory features. (See Ch. 57.1 for discussion of neutropenia associated with Felty's syndrome.)

The *erythrocyte sedimentation rate* (ESR) is increased above the normal range is virtually all patients with active rheumatoid arthritis. There are a variety of other "acute phase reactants" in the serum which reflect inflammatory activity, but none of them match the simplicity of the ESR or exceed its sensitivity.

Rheumatoid *synovial fluid* is usually turbid with reduced viscosity, increased protein content, and slight reduction of glucose levels relative to the blood. Leukocyte counts (predominantly polymorphonuclear cells) vary between a few thousand and more than 50,000 cells per cubic millimeter. Cells containing inclusions are common, but these may be seen in other types of exudative synovitis. Complement in synovial fluid, relative to protein content, is commonly reduced, a finding usually associated with positive test results for rheumatoid factors.

There are no tests that are specific for rheumatoid arthritis, although the term "rheumatoid factors" has been applied to autoantibodies reactive with IgG (see Pathogenesis above). A variety of test systems are available, but more laboratories utilize the *latex fixation test,* in which polystyrene latex particles coated with IgG are agglutinated by rheumatoid factors. Less commonly applied systems include the *bentonite flocculation test* and a variety of *hemagglutination tests* employing erythrocytes coated with immunoglobulins. The latex fixation test result is positive (1:80 titer or higher) in approximately 70 per cent of rheumatoid subjects. Although test results are positive in less than 5 per cent of healthy control subjects, the rheumatoid factor is associated with other connective tissue syndromes, liver disease, and a variety of infectious diseases such as bacterial endocarditis, tuberculosis, syphilis, and leprosy. The frequency of positive test results for rheumatoid factor in the general population increases with age.

DIFFERENTIAL DIAGNOSIS. General. Differential considerations are numerous and vary according to the pattern of disease. There is seldom confusion in identifying "classic" rheumatoid arthritis, but symmetrical involvement of hand and wrist joints can be a feature of other syndromes (see below). Differentiation is more difficult and complex in patients with early acute polyarthritis or in those with arthritis limited to one or a few joints.

Chronic Polyarthritis. The most common form of chronic arthropathy, degenerative joint disease, is usually quite distinct from rheumatoid arthritis. Minimal inflammatory signs, absence of constitutional symptoms, ESR determinations in the range of normal, and the characteristic radiographic findings usually serve to identify degenerative joint disease. A clinical pattern of degenerative joint disease which has been termed "primary generalized osteoarthritis" (see Ch. 61) may be mistaken for rheumatoid arthritis, especially when there is symmetrical enlargement of interphalangeal joints in the hands. *Bouchard's nodes,* the bony enlargement of proximal interphalangeal joints of the hand (see Fig. 4B) are rather frequently misinterpreted as signs of rheumatoid arthritis.

Gout and *chondrocalcinosis* (see Ch. 535.1 and 60, respectively) may mimic chronic rheumatoid arthritis. The most definitive basis for their identification is polarized light microscopy of synovial fluid.

Other connective tissue syndromes such as *systemic lupus erythematosus* (SLE) and *progressive systemic sclerosis* are infrequently associated with chronic deforming joint change. Their differentiation from rheumatoid arthritis is based on characteristic multisystemic patterns of disease. Certain serologic features of SLE, especially hypocomplementemia and the antibodies to native deoxyribonucleic acid, are rare in rheumatoid arthritis. A few patients, with mixed clinical and laboratory features of two or more syndromes, defy classification.

The majority of patients with arthritis and *psoriasis* are indistinguishable from patients in the spectrum of rheumatoid arthritis. The designation psoriatic arthritis as a separate entity is in part arbitrary, but certain clinical and laboratory features of psoriatic arthritis (see Ch. 58.3) aid in its differentiation from rheumatoid arthritis.

Rheumatic manifestations of a wide variety of systemic diseases, including sarcoidosis, ulcerative colitis, regional enteritis, Whipple's disease, amyloidosis, acromegaly, chronic infection, and malignancies, can resemble rheumatoid arthritis. This list emphasizes the importance of exclusions in formulating a diagnosis of rheumatoid arthritis.

Acute Polyarthritis. The range of differential considerations for acute polyarthritis includes those listed above plus a variety of disorders that rarely if ever result in chronic joint disease. The most frequent set of diagnostic considerations for acute polyarthritis includes rheumatoid arthritis, acute rheumatic fever, infection, and drug hypersensitivity. Acute arthritis associated with chills and fever should be considered infectious until proved otherwise. The presence of carditis, evidence of recent streptococcal infection, fever, and prompt response to salicylate therapy contribute to the recognition of acute rheumatic fever. Important differentiating features of gonococcal arthritis are prominent tenosynovitis, the cutaneous manifestations, and, most important, isolation of the bacteria from blood or joint fluid. The common viral infections that can resemble acute rheumatoid arthritis are rubella and viral hepatitis. There are other remitting forms of polyarthritis in which viral causes are suspected but not established. A careful clinical history and the recognition of other allergic phenomena will help in the identification of drug hypersensitivity.

Monarthritis or Oligoarthritis. All the conditions listed above under Acute and Chronic Polyarthritis are appropriate to the differential diagnosis of arthritis affecting one or a limited number of joints; but when the pattern of joint involvement is restricted, the most important differential consideration is infection. A complete medical evaluation, including chest x-ray, tuberculin tests, and appropriate microbial studies, is indicated. When there is continued suspicion of bacterial or mycobacterial infection, synovial biopsy may be required.

MANAGEMENT. Basic Principles. In the management of rheumatoid arthritis, the physician should keep the following facts in mind: (1) in most patients the disease is chronic; (2) spontaneous remissions occur in almost all patients; (3) the majority of subjects can continue to lead active lives with varying degrees of restrictions; and (4) complications of drug therapy, most notably adrenocorticosteroids, can cause greater morbidity than the underlying disease.

The patient and the doctor must be educated not to expect and seek a short-term solution. The physician can present a reasonably optimistic prognosis, based on knowledge of the natural history of rheumatoid arthritis, and can assure the patient that there are conservative means of ameliorating symptoms and minimizing disability.

There are no specific dietary recommendations; rather, the general nutritional status of the patient and associated medical conditions influence diet selection. Weight reduction, in obese patients, should have high priority. Providing that the diet is well balanced, there are no indications for vitamin supplementation. The anemia of rheumatoid arthritis does not respond to hematinic therapy except to the extent that iron deficiency may be a complicating feature. Rarely the anemia may be so severe as to require transfusion.

Psychologic depression is a common consequence of chronic rheumatoid arthritis. From the physician, the patient needs sympathetic understanding of his problems and a willingness to help solve them. When depression is severe, these efforts may be facilitated by the use of antidepressive medication. If anxiety, restlessness, and insomnia are complicating features, the use of mild sedatives or tranquilizers may be indicated.

A basic program that is applicable to all patients includes (1) rest, (2) employment of salicylates for the relief of pain and suppression of inflammation, and (3) maintenance of joint function by physical measures. Some but not all patients will be candidates for medicinal therapy other than salicylates and/or orthopedic surgical procedures.

REST. Patients and physicians alike tend to be confused by the apparently conflicting goals of rest and exercise. They are not mutually exclusive (see Physical Measures below). It is clear that physical work, applied to an affected extremity, will intensify the synovitis of rheumatoid arthritis. The specific prescription of rest will vary according to the severity and pattern of involvement, but all patients should be directed to respect their symptoms of pain and fatigue and to restrict physical activities to the essentials. Any way that occupational duties can be modified to lighten the work load should be tried, and daytime rest periods are important. Occasionally when symptoms are very severe, hospitalization for attainment of more complete rest is indicated.

EMPLOYMENT OF SALICYLATES. All students of rheumatoid arthritis agree that salicylate therapy is part of the basic management. The majority of patients can tolerate acetylsalicylic acid in doses of 3.6 grams daily or more, if the physician is persistent in his recommendations. When gastrointestinal symptoms complicate therapy, ingestion of the drug with meals or the use of enteric-coated or buffered products may be helpful. When doses of acetylsalicylic acid in the range of 3.6 grams daily are tolerated but rheumatic symptoms are poorly controlled, gradual increase in the dose is warranted. It is too often concluded, on the basis of inadequate trials, that "aspirin was not effective." Measurement of blood salicylate levels is appropriate when there is a question of toxicity or absorption.

PHYSICAL MEASURES. The choice of various heat modalities (warm pool, tank, bath, shower, diathermy, or ultrasound) depends primarily on the areas affected and the availability of services. Diathermy and ultrasound treatments are contraindicated in patients with metal implants. A warm pool permitting exercise under water is optimal for the patient with very severe symptoms, but for most individuals a hot bath or shower will suffice. Morning stiffness and pain will be minimized by ingestion of salicylates followed by a hot bath.

The *goals of an exercise program* are (1) maintenance of motion of affected joints, and (2) prevention of muscle atrophy. Both of these can be achieved without submitting inflamed joints to the task of work. An active exercise program for the lower extremities can maintain motion and strength without heavy weight bearing, allowing the right combination of rest and exercise. The rate of progression from gentle passive exercises, required for the most symptomatic patient, to a more active program will vary according to the pattern of involvement and the response to therapy. In order that the patient avoid assuming a passive dependent role, it is crucial that emphasis be placed on what he or she can do independent of supervision. The average doctor is not sufficiently trained in physical medicine to write detailed prescriptions, but he should be very specific in what his goals are when referring the patient to a physical medicine service. Furthermore, he should review the program periodically with the patient and reinforce its importance in the total management. It is a moot point whether forceful active exercises are appropriate for the distal upper extremities; evidence suggests that heavy work will aggravate hand and wrist

deformities. For a patient with acutely inflamed joints, removable splints to achieve rest are helpful, but there are no convincing demonstrations that such devices prevent development of chronic hand deformities.

The role of orthopedic surgery in the management of rheumatoid arthritis is discussed subsequently in this chapter.

Other Antirheumatic Therapy. For the patient whose response to salicylate therapy has not been adequate, several other anti-inflammatory agents can be employed. These include indomethacin, phenylbutazone (and oxyphenbutazone), antimalarial drugs (chloroquine and hydroxychloroquine), gold compounds, and several compounds (propionic acid derivatives and tolmetin) marketed in the United States after 1975 (see below). The adrenocorticosteroid drugs are the most potent anti-inflammatory medications available, but their value, for reasons stated below, is limited. Unfortunately all medications employed for the treatment of rheumatoid arthritis, except gold compounds, have in common the property of promoting peptic ulceration.

Among those who specialize in the management of rheumatic disease, there is no uniformity of habit regarding the employment of agents listed above, although the majority, at some time, will institute gold therapy for the patient with sustained rheumatoid arthritis. Codeine and related analgesics may be required on a temporary basis, but their chronic use should be discouraged.

Phenylbutazone is a reasonably potent anti-inflammatory agent, but there is limited enthusiasm for its use in long-term management of rheumatoid disease. In doses of 200 to 300 mg daily, this drug may be helpful in the treatment of intermittent exacerbations. The incidence of serious toxicity (exfoliative dermatitis and hematologic complications) is low but a source of concern. The occasional patient who is helped by long-term therapy should be under close medical supervision and should have periodic blood counts.

Indomethacin, although chemically unrelated to other analgesic and anti-inflammatory drugs, has a pattern of efficacy similar to that of phenylbutazone. Both are more effective in gout and ankylosing spondylitis than in rheumatoid arthritis. In the dose range of 50 to 200 mg per day, a few patients will experience sufficient benefit to warrant its continuation. Gastrointestinal symptoms and vascular headaches are common side effects, but serious complications are rare. Concomitant aspirin therapy appears to diminish gastrointestinal absorption of indomethacin.

Several *propionic acid derivative* drugs are available for treatment of rheumatoid arthritis, and others are under study. All these compounds have anti-inflammatory, antipyretic, and analgesic properties. Ibuprofen (1200 to 1600 mg daily), naproxen (500 to 750 mg daily), and fenoprofen (2400 mg daily) impart symptomatic control roughly equivalent to that achieved with acetylsalicylic acid in the dose range of 3.6 grams daily. Gastrointestinal intolerance appears to be less frequent than with salicylates.

Tolmetin (1200 mg daily) has a spectrum and level of efficacy similar to indomethacin, a chemically related drug.

Antimalarial compounds such as chloroquine and hydroxychloroquine have moderate anti-inflammatory activity in the treatment of rheumatoid arthritis. Because of the occasional association of irreversible retinopathy, the use of antimalarials has sharply declined.

Although soluble *gold compounds* have been employed in the treatment of rheumatoid arthritis since the 1930s, their mode of action is not known. There is no evidence that they have anti-inflammatory activity; rather, clinical impressions suggest that, in some unknown way, they increase the likelihood of remission. The level of enthusiasm for chrysotherapy varies considerably among rheumatic disease specialists. Some advocate such treatment within weeks of onset of disease; others reserve it for patients who have had sustained disease for several months or more in spite of more conservative therapy. There is a cumulative effect of gold compound administration. Sensitive assays can detect trace amounts many months after discontinuation of therapy. Gold is excreted primarily in the urine. The most common complications are dermatitis and stomatitis. Renal damage, manifested by proteinuria and microscopic hematuria, and hematologic dyscrasias (thrombocytopenia and granulocytopenia) are rare but significant complications of chrysotherapy.

The preparations employed are sodium aurothiomalate (Myochrysine) and aurothioglucose (Solganal). Both are administered by deep intramuscular injection at weekly intervals. It is common practice to use small doses (10 to 25 mg) for the first two or three injections, followed by 50 mg at weekly intervals thereafter. Complete blood count and urinalysis should be obtained prior to each injection for several weeks and every few weeks after that as long as therapy is continued. If there is any sign from these tests or from clinical assessment (pruritic rash or stomatitis) of gold toxicity, therapy should be interrupted. If unequivocal evidence of gold toxicity develops, such as severe stomatitis or exfoliative dermatitis or renal or hematologic complications, treatment should not be resumed. In the case of mild, transient skin reactions, it is common practice to reinstitute the medication at reduced levels after the rash has cleared. Experience indicates that remissions, if they occur on gold therapy, will occur during the course of 20 weekly injections (approximately 1 gram total dose). In the absence of improvement during this course, there is no point in continuing therapy. For the patient experiencing a remission, it is recommended that maintenance therapy be continued (50 mg at three- to four-week intervals). The decision as to maintenance therapy in patients who experience only partial remission is more difficult.

Mild gold-induced dermatitis may persist for several weeks or more, but usually requires no therapy other than topical corticosteroids. The most common presentation consists of several scattered, well-circumscribed pruritic lesions associated with mild scaling. The discomfort associated with severe dermatitis may warrant a course of systemic corticosteroid therapy (10 to 20 mg of prednisone daily) or the use of BAL (dimercaprol). Hematologic complications, most commonly thrombocytopenia, are also indications for dimercaprol therapy. Dimercaprol, 2.5 mg per kilogram of body weight, is given every four hours for two days, followed by the same dose twice daily for approximately a week. An alternative means of promoting gold excretion is the employment of penicillamine,* although there is less clinical experience to recommend it.

Adrenocorticosteroid Therapy. SYSTEMIC THERAPY. Since the early therapeutic trials of cortisone in 1949, several related compounds with potent anti-inflammatory activity have been introduced. These include prednisone, prednisolone, triamcinolone, methylprednisolone, dexamethasone, betamethasone, and paramethasone. Electrolyte and water-retaining properties, associated with cortisone and hydroxycortisone therapy, are minimal with the newer drugs, but the more serious side effects are common to all adrenocorticosteroid preparations (see below). The approximate milligram equivalent of the various drugs that yield comparable pharmacologic effects are cortisone (25 mg), hydrocortisone (20 mg), prednisone (5 mg), triamcinolone (4 mg), methylprednisolone (4 mg), dexamethasone (0.75 mg), betamethasone (0.6 mg), and paramethasone (2 mg).

Because of frequent and potentially life-threatening complications of adrenocorticosteroid therapy, it should not be employed in the management of rheumatoid arthritis until there has been a sustained trial of more conservative therapy. In general, the more experienced the physician is in the management of rheumatoid disease, the more reluctant he is to begin adrenocorticosteroid therapy. The following facts should be pondered before initiating such treatment: (1) adrenocorticosteroid drugs suppress inflammation, but they do not correct or change the underlying process; (2) small doses, in the range of 5 to 10 mg of prednisone, often provide only partial and temporary gains; (3) over periods of months or years, there is a tendency for the dose to increase; (4) once instituted, it is very difficult to discontinue therapy; and (5) the morbidity and mortality associated with long-term adrenocorticosteroid therapy often exceed those of the underlying disease.

In the light of these facts, it is difficult to summarize indications for adrenocorticosteroid therapy of rheumatoid arthritis. If a conservative effort, employing less toxic drugs and physical measures, fails to check progressive disability and if the alternative to adrenocorticosteroid therapy seems to be chronic invalidism, such treatment may be indicated. In such cases the daily dose should not exceed 10 mg of prednisone or its equivalent; as little as 5 to 7.5 mg in divided doses may provide some benefit. Although pituitary-adrenal unresponsiveness and other complications of therapy are minimized by alternate-day or single daily dose regimens, most patients with rheumatoid arthritis do not tolerate such programs. Occasionally, sustained disease may be less severe but may compromise the occupational activity of a wage earner or mother of a household. A small dose (5 or 7.5 mg daily of prednisone or equivalent) may allow continuation of employment, but the physician and patient should make the decision deliberately and with full realization of the toxic potential of such therapy.

COMPLICATIONS OF ADRENOCORTICOSTEROID THERAPY. The frequency and severity of *osteoporosis*, a feature of rheumatoid disease regardless of therapy, are increased by adrenocorticosteroid treatment. Compression fractures of vertebral bodies are common. (Detailed discussions of the management of osteoporosis are presented in Ch. 557.) There are theoretic bases for employment of high calcium intake, vitamin D, fluorides, and anabolic steroids, but their efficacy in preventing or reversing osteoporosis is uncertain. Another frequent skeletal complication of adrenocorticosteroid therapy is *avascular osteonecrosis*, most commonly affecting the femoral head.

Although most antirheumatic drugs are associated with *peptic ulceration*, the frequency of this complication is probably highest in patients treated with adrenocorticosteroids. The problem is sometimes compounded, because the signs and symptoms of perforation and peritonitis may be masked by therapy.

Decreased host resistance to acquired or reactivated

---

*Investigational drug for this use.

infections is a well-documented feature of adrenocortico-steroid therapy. It is common practice to institute isoniazid prophylaxis in tuberculin-positive patients receiving steroid therapy.

Aggravation of latent or overt diabetes mellitus and psychic disturbances ranging from mild euphoria to frank psychosis are infrequent with the doses of adrenocortico-steroids used in the treatment of rheumatoid arthritis.

Any patient receiving daily adrenocorticosteroid therapy must be assumed to have an *inadequate pituitary adrenal response* to stress. With intercurrent illnesses, or with surgery, the dose should be increased and the patient observed closely for signs of adrenal insufficiency. The same precautions apply to those whose treatment has been discontinued up to two years prior to the stressful illness. The value of intermittent corticotropin therapy in the amelioration of pituitary adrenal unresponsiveness is unproved.

INTRA-ARTICULAR ADRENOCORTICOSTEROID THERAPY. Several adrenocorticosteroid preparations suitable for intra-articular therapy will temporarily suppress signs and symptoms of synovitis. This mode of therapy is helpful for a patient whose disability relates primarily to disease in one or two joints. With rigorous antiseptic technique, the risk of infection is low. If there is any question of antecedent infection at the time of arthrocentesis, intra-articular steroids should not be administered. The usefulness of intra-articular therapy is dependent upon the duration of symptomatic benefit. Because of clinical suspicions and experimental evidence that steroid compounds are deleterious to articular cartilage, most physicians will not inject a joint more frequently than every four to six weeks.

Immunosuppressive (Cytotoxic) Therapy. Several drugs initially developed for cancer chemotherapy have been applied in the treatment of rheumatoid arthritis. The categories of compounds include alkylating agents, purine and pyrimidine antagonists, and folic acid analogues. There is no basis for concluding that one compound is superior to another in immunosuppressive and anti-inflammatory properties, but the best data with regard to the treatment of rheumatoid arthritis derive from a controlled study of cyclophosphamide therapy. Patients receiving up to 150 mg daily of cyclophosphamide sustained significantly fewer new bone erosions over the period of study. In spite of these observations, the use of immunosuppressive agents is to be viewed as experimental therapy. Acute toxicity, especially myelosuppression, is potentially fatal and, as well, there is concern that immunosuppressive therapy may foster the emergence of primary malignant tumors.

Other Experimental Drugs. *Penicillamine,* in a well-controlled study in England, had moderate efficacy in the suppression of severe chronic rheumatoid arthritis and resulted in reductions of rheumatoid factor titers. As an antirheumatic agent, penicillamine remains in the experimental category, primarily because of potentially serious toxicity (agranulocytosis and nephropathy).

Orthopedic Surgery. Orthopedic surgeons are playing an increasingly important role in the management of rheumatoid arthritis. The value of reconstructive surgery in the rehabilitation of selected subjects is well established. Techniques of arthroplasty and prosthetic joint replacement have improved dramatically during the past decade. The rationale for synovectomy is sound, i.e., the removal of chronic pannus and its destructive potential, but proof of its efficacy is lacking. Disease frequently recurs in regenerated synovium, but the intensity of recurrent inflammation tends to be less. On the basis of current experience, synovectomy is probably warranted for patients with sustained (several months or more) proliferative synovitis affecting knee, hand, and wrist joints.

Cooperating Clinics Committee of the American Rheumatism Association: A controlled trial of cyclophosphamide in rheumatoid arthritis. N. Engl. J. Med., 283:883, 1970.

Duthie, J. R. R., et al.: Course and prognosis in rheumatoid arthritis. Ann. Rheum. Dis., 23:193, 1964.

Freyberg, R. H., Ziff, M., and Baum, J.: Gold therapy for rheumatoid arthritis. In Hollander, J. L., and McCarty, D. J., Jr. (eds.): Arthritis and Allied Conditions. 8th ed. Philadelphia, Lea & Febiger, 1972.

Hollingsworth, J. W.: Local and Systemic Complications of Rheumatoid Arthritis. Philadelphia, W. B. Saunders Company, 1968.

Ruddy, S., and Austen, K. F.: The complement system in rheumatoid synovitis: I. An analysis of complement activities in rheumatoid synovial fluids. Arthritis Rheum., 13:713, 1970.

Short, C. L., Bauer, W., and Reynolds, W. E.: Rheumatoid Arthritis. Cambridge, Harvard University Press, 1957.

Winchester, R. J., Agnello, V., and Kunkel, H. G.: Gamma globulin complexes in synovial fluids of patients with rheumatoid arthritis: Partial characterization and relationship to lowered complement levels. Clin. Exp. Immunol., 6:689, 1970.

Zvaifler, N. J.: The immunopathology of joint inflammation in rheumatoid arthritis. In Dixon, F. J., and Kunkel, H. G. (eds.): Advances in Immunology. Vol. 16. New York, Academic Press, 1972.

57. VARIANTS OF RHEUMATOID DISEASE

57.1. FELTY'S SYNDROME

Splenomegaly is observed in approximately 5 per cent of patients with rheumatoid arthritis. Felty originally described a syndrome consisting of rheumatoid arthritis, splenomegaly, and neutropenia. Anemia and thrombocytopenia are occasional features. This syndrome is most common in older individuals who have had longstanding chronic rheumatoid disease. Other extra-articular manifestations of rheumatoid disease such as rheumatoid nodules, chronic skin ulcers, and keratoconjunctivitis sicca are common. Rheumatoid factor test results are invariably positive, and antinuclear phenomena are more common than in uncomplicated rheumatoid arthritis. The indications for splenectomy are influenced primarily by the frequency and severity of infectious complications. Most patients experience hematologic remissions after splenectomy, but relapses occur in many of them.

57.2. SJÖGREN'S SYNDROME

In 1933 Sjögren called attention to the combination of rheumatoid arthritis, keratoconjunctivitis sicca, and xerostomia. The characteristic ocular and oral mucous membrane involvement may occur in the absence of rheumatic disease. In addition to its association with rheumatoid arthritis, it can be a manifestation of other connective tissue syndromes such as systemic lupus erythematosus, progressive systemic sclerosis, and polymyositis. The sicca complex is clinically manifest in approximately 10 to 15 per cent of patients with rheumatoid arthritis, but pathologic expressions, such as lymphoid infiltration of the minor salivary glands in the lip, are much more frequent. The diagnosis is most reliably established by lip biopsy. More than 90 per cent of affected patients are women, and most have had longstanding chronic arthritis. The frequency of a histocompatibility antigen (HLA-DW$_3$) in patients with sicca syndrome, in the absence of rheumatoid arthritis, was 84 per cent. (The frequency in control subjects was 24 per cent.)

The symptoms related to salivary insufficiency include difficulty with chewing and swallowing, dental caries, and ulcerations of the buccal mucous membranes. Dryness may also involve the upper respiratory tract, larynx, and tracheobronchial tree. In common with Felty's syndrome, patients with Sjögren's syndrome frequently manifest extra-articular features attributed to vasculitis. A small but significant number of patients with Sjögren's syndrome have developed reticulum cell sarcoma or a more benign lymphoproliferative disorder termed "pseudolymphoma." Because lymphomatous complications have occurred primarily in patients with a history of irradiation for parotid gland enlargement, this mode of therapy has been discouraged.

Rheumatoid factor test results are positive in the majority of patients, and antinuclear and a variety of other autoimmune reactants are associated with Sjögren's syndrome.

The treatment is symptomatic. Artificial tears of 0.5 per cent methylcellulose are helpful. Adrenocorticosteroid or immunosuppressive drugs are restricted to those patients with severe disability or life-threatening complications.

Barnes, C. G., Turnbull, A. L., and Vernon-Roberts, B.: Felty's syndrome: A clinical and pathological survey of 21 patients and their response to treatment. Ann. Rheum. Dis., 30:359, 1971.

Shearn, M. A.: Sjögren's Syndrome. Philadelphia, W. B. Saunders Company, 1971.

Whaley, K., Williamson, J., Chisholm, D. M., et al.: Sjögren's syndrome. I. Sicca components. Quart. J. Med., 42:279, 1973.

58. OTHER FORMS OF POLYARTHRITIS OF UNKNOWN ETIOLOGY

58.1. ANKYLOSING SPONDYLITIS

(Marie-Strümpell Spondylitis, von Bechterew's Syndrome, Rheumatoid Spondylitis)

In this syndrome there is prominent involvement of spinal articulations, sacroiliac joints, and paravertebral soft tissues. Because one third to one half of patients with ankylosing spondylitis manifest synovitis in peripheral joints (especially hips and shoulders), the syndrome was formerly viewed as a variant of rheumatoid arthritis. However, several features of ankylosing spondylitis are distinct from those of rheumatoid arthritis: (1) prominent ligamentous calcification and ossification with a tendency to bony ankylosis; (2) male preponderance; (3) impressive evidence of genetic transmission in selected kindreds; (4) symptomatic benefit with medications, notably phenylbutazone and indomethacin, that are minimally effective in rheumatoid arthritis; (5) absence of rheumatoid factor and rheumatoid nodules; and (6) the association of certain extra-articular manifestations such as iridocyclitis and aortitis.

ETIOLOGY. The cause of ankylosing spondylitis is unknown. The disease has been found to be 30 times more prevalent among the relatives of spondylitic patients than among relatives of controls. The striking association of ankylosing spondylitis with the histocompatibility antigen HLA-B27 has provided insight into the genetic transmission of the syndrome and, additionally, has helped define a group of spondylitic disorders. This category includes Reiter's syndrome, a subset of juvenile rheumatoid arthritis, psoriatic spondylitis, and inflammatory bowel disease that exhibits spinal involvement. The manner in which this histocompatibility antigen influences pathogenesis is unknown. Infectious causes have long been suspected but never established.

INCIDENCE AND PREVALENCE. Ankylosing spondylitis is a common cause of back pain in young men. The male-to-female ratio is approximately 8:1. In an English survey, the incidence of ankylosing spondylitis was 1 in 2000 among the population at large.

PATHOLOGY. On the basis of symptoms and early radiographic findings, the disease appears to begin in the sacroiliac joints, with subsequent involvement of zygapophyseal and costovertebral articulations, interspinous ligaments, and paravertebral tissues. The characteristic immobility of the spinal column results from bony ankylosis of zygapophyseal joints and ossification of paravertebral structures. Syndesmophytes, the bony bridges which unite adjacent vertebral bodies, form in the outer lamellae of the anulus fibrosus and adjacent connective tissue fibers. The pathologic character of synovial inflammation is not distinct from that of rheumatoid arthritis. Aortic involvement resembling syphilitic aortitis can result in aortic insufficiency. Iridocyclitis occurs in approximately 25 per cent of patients. The incidence of amyloidosis complicating ankylosing spondylitis is approximately 5 per cent. Rarely, a pattern of pulmonary fibrosis, sometimes associated with cavitation, has been described.

CLINICAL MANIFESTATIONS. In the majority of cases the onset of ankylosing spondylitis, usually in the second or third decade of life, is insidious. The initial symptoms are usually low back pain and stiffness; rarely, the first symptoms may relate to involvement of hip, shoulder, or peripheral joints. Symptoms may be sufficiently mild that the patient seeks no medical attention for months. At the other extreme, there may be debilitating pain at the outset, associated with fever, severe fatigue, and weight loss. In most patients, however, constitutional symptoms are not prominent. Pain and stiffness, which are maximal after periods of inactivity, often interrupt sleep in the early morning hours. Radicular and sciatic patterns of pain are common. The pattern and rate of spinal ankylosis are varied. The majority of patients experience gradual cephalad progression of spinal immobility, but the disease may remain confined to the sacroiliac joints and lumbar segments. The development of the poker back type of spinal deformity usually evolves gradually over a period of ten years or more. The majority of patients remain fully employed. Hip involvement, the most common cause of occupational disability, is now amenable to prosthetic surgery.

Physical signs are limited in the early stages of disease. Sacroiliac joint involvement may be evident from palpation of these joints or from orthopedic maneuvers which produce sacroiliac joint movement. Paravertebral muscle spasm and tenderness are common. Physical signs associated with the chronic phase of ankylosing spondylitis relate primarily to spinal immobility. The most accurate estimate of lumbar flexion is accomplished by comparing midline measurements from the sacrum to T-12 in flexion and extension. The normal difference in these two measurements is approximately 3 inches. The presence and progression of costovertebral joint involvement can be documented by measurements of chest expansion.

The most important extra-articular manifestations of ankylosing spondylitis are *iridocyclitis*, occurring in approximately one quarter of patients, and aortitis. The frequency of *aortic insufficiency* has been as high as 4 per cent in some series. *Cardiac conduction disturbances*, most frequently first degree A-V block, occur in about 10 per cent of cases. *Cauda equina involvement*, a rare but significant complication of longstanding spondylitis, is manifest as urinary or rectal sphincter incompetence and pain and sensory loss in the sacral distribution.

ROENTGENOGRAPHIC FINDINGS. Characteristic roentgenographic findings of ankylosing spondylitis involve the following structures: sacroiliac joints, zygapophyseal articulations, vertebral bodies, and paravertebral soft tissues. Changes in the sacroiliac joints are the earliest and most consistent findings. The margins of subchondral bone are blurred, followed by subchondral sclerosis and bony erosions. Progressive narrowing of the interosseous joint space and sacroiliac fusion develop slowly over a period of years. Sclerotic and erosive changes in zygapophyseal and costovertebral articulations are common but less readily demonstrated by x-ray. Alterations in vertebral bodies, loss of anterior concavity, and anterior marginal erosions are features of longstanding disease. Calcification and ossification of the anulus fibrosus and adjacent paravertebral ligaments give rise to the characteristic syndesmophytes that gradually bridge adjacent vertebral bodies. In advanced cases this results in the so-called *bamboo spine*. In addition to sacroiliac joints, other cartilaginous articulations such as the symphysis pubis and sternomanubrial joints may be involved. There is a tendency for ossification of ligaments and tendon insertions. Roentgenographic changes in the hips and shoulders, less commonly in more peripheral joints, are not distinct from those of rheumatoid arthritis, although the incidence of bony ankylosis of the hips is greater in ankylosing spondylitis.

The full set of roentgenographic findings, described above, is a product of many years of progressive disease. In a minority of patients with ankylosing spondylitis, the disease appears to go into remission after involvement of restricted segments of the spine.

DIAGNOSIS. Ankylosing spondylitis should be suspected in anyone, particularly a young male, with persistent or recurrent low back pain and stiffness or recurrent sciatic pain. Although associated phenomena such as elevation of erythrocyte sedimentation rate, thoracic girdle pain, arthritis in the lower limbs, and iridocyclitis will enhance the suspicion, early diagnosis should not be excluded on the basis of normal roentgenograms, because several months or, rarely, a few years may elapse before development of roentgenographic changes. Although degenerative joint disease can result in back pain and loss of spinal motion, this is a problem of later decades of life, and the roentgenographic features are distinct from ankylosing spondylitis. Joint disease identical to ankylosing spondylitis can be a feature of *ulcerative colitis, regional enteritis, Reiter's syndrome*, and *psoriasis*.

TREATMENT. The highest priority goal in the management of ankylosing spondylitis is the maintenance of a functional posture. It is doubtful that any medication will prevent ankylosis of those spinal segments involved, but the suppression of pain and inflammation is essential before an appropriate physical medicine program can be instituted.

Indomethacin and phenylbutazone are usually more effective than other antirheumatic agents in the control of pain and stiffness, but an initial trial on salicylate therapy (3.6 to 4.5 grams daily) is recommended. For those patients who do not experience sufficient relief of symptoms with salicylates, indomethacin in doses of 100 to 150 mg daily or phenylbutazone (100 to 300 mg daily) is indicated. With control of symptoms, the dose of either indomethacin or phenylbutazone should be gradually reduced to the lowest level that will maintain improvement. With continuous use of phenylbutazone, the risk of hematologic complications should be kept in mind and periodic blood counts obtained. Adrenocorticosteroid therapy is rarely indicated for ankylosing spondylitis. If all other efforts to control progressive disability fail, such therapy may be indicated, as outlined under rheumatoid arthritis (see Ch. 56). Systemic adrenocorticosteroid therapy may be required for the control of iridocyclitis. Although roentgen therapy, directed at areas of involvement, is effective in control of symptoms, this mode of treatment is not recommended because of the demonstrations of chromosomal injury and an observed incidence of leukemia that is ten times greater in patients so treated than in the general population.

For the management of ankylosing spondylitis, emphasis should be given to the institution and maintenance of an exercise program. In order that flexion deformity of the spine be avoided, the patient should sleep on a very firm mattress, preferably without a pillow. There should be a twice daily performance of exercise directed at the maintenance of erect posture, strengthening of paraspinal muscles, and promotion of chest cage motion. A hot bath or shower will often facilitate exercise activity. If physical medicine measures fail to check the progression of flexion deformity, back splints or braces may be tried. In carefully selected individuals with advanced flexion deformity, spinal osteotomy can improve posture, but this is associated with significant risk of neurologic complications. For the patient with severe hip involvement, the most frequent cause of major disability, prosthetic hip replacement offers dramatic relief.

58.2. JUVENILE RHEUMATOID ARTHRITIS

Although the definition of juvenile rheumatoid arthritis is somewhat arbitrary (onset of disease under age 16), there are clinical features which tend to distinguish it from rheumatoid arthritis in adults. These include high fever, transient morbilliform rash, leukocytosis, uveitis, local growth disturbances, low frequencies of rheumatoid factor and subcutaneous nodules, and a higher incidence of monarticular disease than is observed in adults.

The discussions of etiology, pathogenesis, and pathology of rheumatoid arthritis (see Ch. 56) are relevant to juvenile rheumatoid arthritis except for speculations regarding a pathogenic role of rheumatoid factors.

In approximately 20 per cent of children with juvenile rheumatoid arthritis, the onset is acute and fulminating and is associated with systemic manifestations such as fever, rash, pericarditis, and splenomegaly (*Still's disease*). Occasionally these features may persist for several weeks before synovitis is evident. (A similar systemic pattern of disease has been observed, rarely, in adults.) In approximately half of patients, the onset is polyarticular, resembling rheumatoid arthritis in adults. In one third of juvenile rheumatoid arthritis patients, the onset is monoarticular. Several clinical subsets of juvenile rheumatoid arthritis have been recognized. One of these is pauciarticular (involvement of a few joints) in young girls, associated with positive antinuclear test results and chronic irridocyclitis. Boys with the pauciarticular pattern of disease have a high frequency of HLA-B27 and may manifest acute iridocyclitis. The latter group of patients appears to represent the juvenile form of ankylosing spondylitis. Abnormal skeletal growth adjacent to inflamed joints results from varied degrees of accelerated local growth and premature closure of epiphyseal plates.

Leukocytosis in the range of 15,000 to 25,000 is common. Serologic evidence of recent streptococcal infection is found in a third to a half of subjects, adding to the problem of differentiation from acute rheumatic fever. No more than 10 per cent of sera are positive in the commonly employed tests for rheumatoid factor. The frequency of antinuclear antibody is higher than in adults with rheumatoid arthritis. This is especially so in children with iridocyclitis.

Distinctive roentgenographic findings include local growth disturbances (noted above), abnormal periosteal bone accretion, and prominent involvement of cervical zygapophyseal joints.

Differential considerations vary according to the pattern of juvenile rheumatoid arthritis. The systemic form of disease resembles certain infectious syndromes. Recognition of the characteristic morbilliform rash, if it is present, is important in diagnosis. The polyarticular onset of disease, when accompanied by high fever and signs of carditis, is easily confused with acute rheumatic fever. Features of juvenile rheumatoid arthritis that may aid in this distinction are frequent onset of disease under age 5, nonmigratory pattern of polyarthritis, cervical spine involvement, marked leukocytosis, and rash. The immediate suppressive effect of salicylate therapy is less striking in juvenile rheumatoid arthritis than it is in rheumatic fever.

Fifty per cent or more of patients with juvenile rheumatoid arthritis experience complete remissions. The serious consequences of extra-articular involvement relate to carditis, chronic iridocyclitis, and amyloidosis.

Principles of management outlined for rheumatoid arthritis (see Ch. 56) apply to children with chronic arthritis. Contractures and restricted motion of articulations are more common in children than in adults. The patient's parents must be given important roles in the maintenance of a physical medicine program. Aspirin

in the range of 90 to 130 mg per kilogram daily is the treatment of choice. Early in the course of the disease, adrenocorticosteroid therapy should be reserved for patients with severe systemic manifestations, such as carditis, that do not respond to salicylate therapy. Periodic ophthalmologic consultation, at approximately six-month intervals, is recommended, since iridocyclitis may be asymptomatic and missed by casual examination. Because of the threat of blindness from sustained iridocyclitis, systemic adrenocorticosteroid therapy may be indicated if this complication is severe and fails to respond to local treatment. In addition to the usual complications and limitations of adrenocorticosteroid therapy, growth retardation, a natural feature of the disease, is augmented by such treatment. The indications for the employment of gold therapy and doses are similar to those presented for rheumatoid arthritis (see Ch. 56).

58.3.   PSORIATIC ARTHRITIS

The recognition that psoriatic arthritis is a disease entity, as opposed to the coincidental occurrence of two common diseases, i.e., rheumatoid arthritis and psoriasis, is relatively recent. Based on population surveys, approximately 5 per cent of patients with cutaneous psoriasis have chronic arthritis. One quarter to one third of such patients manifest rheumatoid nodules or positive tests for rheumatoid factor, and probably represent cases of coexistence of two diseases. Patients with psoriasis and chronic arthritis are clinically heterogeneous, but some of them manifest sufficiently characteristic features to justify the term psoriatic arthritis.

Several clinical subtypes of psoriatic arthritis are recognized. The most common pattern is of a scattered asymmetrical involvement of interphalangeal joints of the hands and feet, frequently manifest as "sausage digits" (Fig. 3). Much less common, but recognized by all as "classic psoriatic arthritis" is the exclusive involvement of distal interphalangeal joints. In approximately one quarter of patients with psoriasis there is a symmetrical pattern of arthritis indistinguishable, apart from negative serology, from rheumatoid arthritis. In this group, there is a tendency for severe osteolytic involvement with resorption of bone and telescoping of digits (arthritis mutilans). Approximately 5 per cent of patients with psoriasis and arthritis manifest features identical to those of ankylosing spondylitis, although the roentgenographic character of syndesmophytes tends to differentiate the two syndromes. This pattern of disease has a striking association with the histocompatibility antigen HLA-B27.

It is important to recognize that there may be asynchronous onset of cutaneous involvement and arthritis and that a patient with typical psoriatic arthritis may have minimal or hidden cutaneous involvement. Psoriatic nail involvement occurs in over 80 per cent of patients with psoriatic arthritis, in contrast to only a 30 per cent incidence in patients with uncomplicated psoriasis. Typical psoriatic arthritis, especially spondylitis, may evolve after recurrent attacks of Reiter's syndrome.

The unique clinical patterns of psoriatic arthritis such as bone resorption, asymmetric involvement of interphalangeal joints, and spondylitis are represented in roentgenographic findings. An increased incidence of hyperuricemia in psoriatic patients probably reflects the

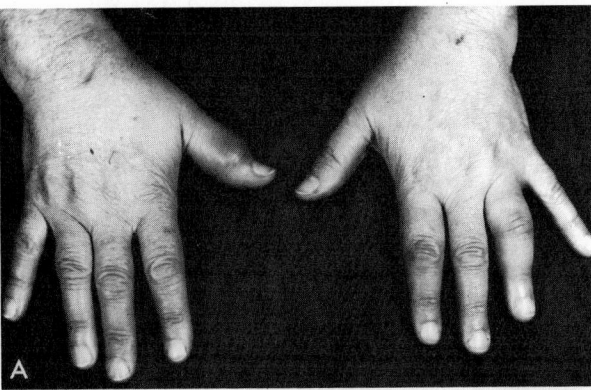
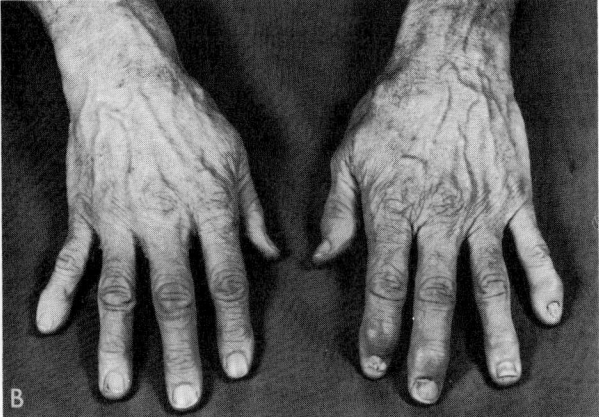

Figure 3. Common patterns of psoriatic arthritis in the hands. *A,* Asymmetrical enlargement of interphalangeal joints of right thumb and left ring finger. *B,* "Classic" involvement of distal interphalangeal joints and nails of digits two, three, and five of left hand.

increased metabolism of skin. Other than the absence of rheumatoid factor in patients with psoriatic arthritis, there are no immunologic, biochemical, or pathologic distinctions from rheumatoid arthritis.

Principles of management of psoriatic arthritis do not differ from those of rheumatoid arthritis. Antimalarial drugs are contraindicated, because they have been observed to provoke exfoliative dermatitis in psoriatic subjects. Reliance should be placed on a basic regimen of salicylates and physical therapy. Adrenocorticosteroid drugs should be employed only as a last resort. For the patient with very severe psoriatic arthritis, immunosuppressive therapy, in spite of its experimental status and considerable toxicity, is probably more appropriate than adrenocorticosteroid therapy.

For patients with severe psoriatic arthropathy that is not responsive to conventional antirheumatic therapy, methotrexate, in regimens that have proved efficacious for cutaneous psoriasis, may be employed. Intravenous or oral administration of methotrexate in doses of 10 to 25 mg once weekly (maximal dose, 50 mg per week) is usually successful in suppressing cutaneous and articular manifestations of psoriasis. A commonly employed oral regimen consists of a series of three doses (2.5 to 10 mg each) administered at 12-hour intervals each week. Close surveillance for evidence of myelosuppression is required. In addition, evidence for hepatotoxicity should be sought by periodic laboratory analyses.

58.4. REITER'S SYNDROME

Although the association of arthritis, urethritis, and conjunctivitis was recorded early in the nineteenth century, this triad of clinical manifestations bears the name of the German physician who, in 1916, described a patient with nongonococcal urethritis, conjunctivitis, and arthritis after an episode of diarrhea. Other common manifestations of the syndrome include fever, oral and genital mucous membrane lesions, cutaneous keratosis, and iritis. Most patients are young males; it is rare in women regardless of age.

ETIOLOGY. The cause of Reiter's syndrome is unknown, but most attention has focused on infectious causes. Venereal transmission seems apparent in many cases; in others the onset of Reiter's syndrome follows diarrheal illness. In several large epidemics of bacillary dysentery, a small percentage of patients have developed typical Reiter's syndrome, including genitourinary tract involvement. Mycoplasmal and chlamydial species are suspect as etiologic agents. The significance of sporadic isolation of such organisms from synovial fluid or synovial tissue is unknown. The frequency of HLA-B27 in Reiter's syndrome is close to that of ankylosing spondylitis.

CLINICAL AND LABORATORY MANIFESTATIONS. All the clinical features of Reiter's syndrome may appear simultaneously, but more commonly genitourinary or gastrointestinal symptoms precede the onset of ocular or rheumatic features by several days or a few weeks. Occasionally the classic pattern evolves slowly over weeks or months after the appearance of a single manifestation. Polyarthritis is frequently asymmetrical with predilection for involvement of articulations of the lower extremities, but the pattern of joint involvement can be varied. The majority of patients experience complete remissions within weeks or a few months of onset. A minority (range of 10 per cent) manifest persistence of synovitis in articulations of the extremities or spine and will have disability that parallels that of sustained rheumatoid arthritis or ankylosing spondylitis. Rarely, the clinical picture of chronic or recurrent Reiter's syndrome evolves into typical psoriatic arthritis.

There are no distinctive laboratory features. Peripheral blood leukocytosis is common. Properties of synovial fluid are similar to acute rheumatoid arthritis, although complement levels in joint fluid are invariably high. Roentgenographic abnormalities, equivalent to those associated with rheumatoid arthritis, are found in those patients with sustained synovitis. Periostitis, adjacent to involved joints, is a common but not distinctive feature of Reiter's syndrome.

The most common diagnostic alternative to Reiter's syndrome is *gonococcal arthritis.* The past literature is confusing because of the failure to distinguish these two syndromes and to recognize that gonococcal infection may be coincident to Reiter's syndrome. In a minority of patients, typical mucocutaneous lesions, particularly balanitis circinata and keratoderma blennorrhagica, leave no question regarding diagnosis, but the failure to isolate *N. gonorrhoeae* and the resistance of the manifestations to antimicrobial therapy are the main bases for differentiating Reiter's syndrome from gonococcal arthritis.

TREATMENT. The management of Reiter's syndrome is similar to that of rheumatoid arthritis. If salicylate therapy in the range of 3.6 to 4.5 grams daily fails to suppress synovitis or constitutional symptoms, phenyl-butazone or indomethacin (both in the range of 100 to 200 mg daily) may be beneficial. There is no experience to recommend gold therapy. There are a few reports describing remissions of very severe disease coincident to treatment with immunosuppressive agents; but in the light of their immediate and long-term toxicity, such therapy is considered experimental.

58.5. PALINDROMIC RHEUMATISM

This term has been applied to a recurring pattern of polyarthritis which results in no permanent joint deformity. The syndrome resembles gout in its acute onset and marked inflammatory signs. Rapid subsidence of signs and symptoms occurs within hours or a few days of onset. The frequency of episodes and the anatomic areas affected are variable, but for individual subjects the pattern of recurrent disease tends to be constant.

Since recurrent polyarthritis can be a feature of many rheumatic syndromes, the term palindromic rheumatism, if it is used at all, requires rigorous exclusion of other causes of synovitis. A significant number of patients, the majority in some series, with palindromic rheumatism eventually manifest typical features of rheumatoid arthritis. Systemic and constitutional symptoms are generally lacking. Since the brief episodes terminate spontaneously, there is no uniformity of opinion regarding response to therapy.

58.6. INTERMITTENT HYDRARTHROSIS

This term has been applied to the pattern of recurrent joint effusions, usually the knees, in which other inflammatory signs are minimal. The interval between episodes varies from one to a few weeks. In most reports of intermittent hydrarthrosis, there has been female preponderance. Occasionally recurrences correlate with menstruation. The diagnosis of intermittent hydrarthrosis, like palindromic rheumatism, should be restricted to individuals who have been followed long enough to exclude other causes of recurrent synovitis. A significant number of patients will eventually manifest chronic synovitis consistent with rheumatoid arthritis. When discomfort and restricted motion are attributable to joint space distention, simple arthrocentesis may be beneficial; there is no agreement regarding the efficacy of medicinal therapy in suppressing or preventing attacks.

Ansell, B. M., and Bywaters, E. G. L.: Rheumatoid arthritis (Still's disease). Pediat. Clin. North Am., 10:921, 1963.
Brewerton, D. A.: HLA-B27 and the inheritance of susceptibility to rheumatic disease. Arthritis Rheum., 19:656, 1976.
Calabro, J. J., and Marchesano, J. M.: The early natural history of juvenile rheumatoid arthritis. A ten year follow-up of 100 cases. Med. Clin. North Am., 52:569, 1968.
Kinsella, T. D., MacDonald, F. R., and Johnson, L. G.: Ankylosing spondylitis: A late re-evaluation of 92 cases. Can. Med. Assoc. J., 95:1, 1966.
Moll, J. M. H., and Wright, V.: Psoriatic arthritis. Semin. Arthritis Rheum., 3:55, 1973.
Ogryzlo, M. A.: Ankylosing spondylitis. In Hollander, J. L., and McCarty, D. J., Jr. (eds.): Arthritis and Allied Conditions. 8th ed. Philadelphia, Lea & Febiger, 1972.
Sharp, J. T.: Reiter's syndrome, In Hollander, J. L., and McCarty, D. J., Jr. (eds.): Arthritis and Allied Conditions. 8th ed. Philadelphia, Lea & Febiger, 1972.
Williams, M. H., et al.: Palindromic rheumatism: Clinical and immunological studies. Ann. Rheum. Dis., 30:375, 1971.

59. DISEASES WITH WHICH ARTHRITIS IS FREQUENTLY ASSOCIATED

Arthritis may be a significant feature of all of the syndromes listed in this chapter. Discussion here is brief and is limited to rheumatic manifestations of the various disorders. More detailed considerations will be found elsewhere in the chapters devoted to those diseases.

INFLAMMATORY BOWEL DISEASE

The reported incidence of arthritis complicating *ulcerative colitis* and *regional enteritis* (Crohn's disease) has varied, but it is generally in the range of 10 per cent. The most common rheumatic pattern is an asymmetric polyarthritis involving a few joints. In the majority of patients the disease is intermittent and results in minimal joint damage. The frequency and severity of arthritis are generally higher in those subjects with sustained and extensive bowel involvement, but occasionally rheumatic manifestations will antedate the recognition of enteric disease. *Erythema nodosum* and *uveitis* are three to four times more common in patients with enteritis and arthritis than in patients without rheumatic manifestations. In contrast to the generally benign character of rheumatic complications of enteritis, a small number (approximately 10 per cent of those with arthritis) experience a pattern of disease and disability equivalent to rheumatoid arthritis.

The incidence of *spondylitis*, which is indistinguishable from ankylosing spondylitis, in patients with ulcerative colitis and regional enteritis has varied between 2 and 6 per cent. This represents at least a twenty-fold increase in the frequency of spondylitis over that in the general population. Clinical, laboratory, or roentgenographic findings do not distinguish spondylitis complicating enteritis from ankylosing spondylitis unassociated with bowel disease, except that male predominance in the former is less striking and the incidence of HLA-B27 in subjects with enteropathic spondylitis, although increased relative to controls, is not as high as it is in ankylosing spondylitis.

There are no special recommendations regarding the management of arthritis associated with enteritis: the general principles outlined for the treatment of rheumatoid arthritis and ankylosing spondylitis (see Ch. 56 and 58.1) are appropriate. The main management effort is directed at the intestinal disease. Remissions of arthritis frequently follow surgical resection of diseased bowel, but rheumatic complications rarely affect the decision regarding surgical therapy.

Postinfectious arthritis complicating *Salmonella* and *Yersinia* enteritis shares with Reiter's syndrome and the spondylitis disorders a high association with HLA-B27.

WHIPPLE'S DISEASE

This is a rare syndrome, probably bacterial in cause, characterized by diarrhea, malabsorption, fever, anemia, increased skin pigmentation, and migratory polyarthralgia or polyarthritis. Permanent joint damage is rare.

FAMILIAL MEDITERRANEAN FEVER

Musculoskeletal pain occurs in approximately 7 per cent of patients with this heritable disease. The arthritis is usually monoarticular or limited to a few joints; most commonly involved are knees, ankles, hips, or shoulders. Severe pain and tenderness are out of proportion to other modest signs of inflammation. Arthritis, like other manifestations of this syndrome, is usually recurrent, but permanent damage to joints is rare. None of the anti-inflammatory medications have been found to be effective in the treatment of this form of arthritis. Management is limited to analgesics and local physical measures.

SARCOIDOSIS

The most common rheumatic manifestation of sarcoidosis is a transient acute polyarthritis associated with erythema nodosum and hilar adenopathy. Lower extremity joints are primarily involved. At times it is difficult to be certain whether inflammatory symptoms and signs reflect true synovitis or the cellulitis of erythema nodosum. Recovery is uniform. Most patients can be managed with salicylates but, if pain and disability are severe, a course of adrenocorticosteroid therapy may be indicated. Much less common than the acute rheumatic syndrome is chronic granulomatous synovitis that clinically resembles rheumatoid arthritis.

HYPOGAMMAGLOBULINEMIA

A mild polyarthritis, rarely deforming in character, has been observed in as many as one third of patients with congenital and acquired hypogammaglobulinemia. The pattern of joint disease resembles that of rheumatoid arthritis, although other connective tissue syndromes such as systemic lupus erythematosus, systemic sclerosis, and dermatomyositis have been associated with immune deficiency states. A variety of autoimmune phenomena and connective tissue syndromes have been observed in patients lacking IgA, the most common selective deficiency. Regression of arthritis frequently follows institution of gamma globulin therapy.

POLYCHONDRITIS

Relapsing polychondritis is a rare disorder characterized by inflammation and destruction of cartilage. In the majority of patients there is intermittent involvement of cartilage in ears, nose, trachea, pharynx, costochondral junctions, and peripheral joints. With subsidence of inflammation there may be collapse and deforming change of the ears, nose, and laryngotracheal structures. The pattern of joint involvement is usually that of recurrent polyarthritis associated with minimal residual deformity. Other manifestations include fever, iritis, episcleritis, cataracts, deafness, and aortic insufficiency. Aortic involvement, occurring in 14 per cent of reported cases, and involvement of cartilaginous structures of the respiratory tract are the two life-threatening complications of polychondritis. Pathologic studies demonstrate varying degrees of inflammation and loss of cartilage matrix. The cause is unknown. Adrenocorticosteroid therapy has been employed for life-threatening manifestations, but the generally remittent character of the disease makes it uncertain whether any mode of therapy changes its natural history. Aortic involvement has necessitated prosthetic valve replacement in a few reported patients.

BEHÇET'S SYNDROME

This syndrome was initially described as a triad (recurrent aphthous stomatitis, genital ulcerations, and iritis), but other manifestations are common: pyoderma, erythema nodosum, erythema multiforme, thrombophlebitis, and polyarthritis. Central nervous system involvement, in a minority of patients, may be fatal. Intermittent or chronic polyarthritis is usually limited to one or a few joints and rarely results in significant deformity. There is a strong suspicion that viral infection underlies the development of Behçet's syndrome, but attempts at microbial isolation have been equivocal or negative. Adrenocorticosteroid therapy is indicated if iritis is severe or if there are neurologic manifestations.

HEMOCHROMATOSIS

Joint involvement has been observed in as many as half of patients with idiopathic hemochromatosis. Joint swelling with bony enlargement is particularly common in the small joints of the hands, but other joints may be affected. The clinical and roentgenographic features resemble degenerative joint disease more than rheumatoid arthritis. There is narrowing of the joint space with subchondral erosions and sclerosis. Roentgenographic evidence of chondrocalcinosis is present in a third or more of patients with arthropathy and may account, via crystal-induced synovitis (see Chondrocalcinosis and Pseudogout in Ch. 60), for occasional acute inflammatory manifestations. The management of arthropathy is similar to that described for degenerative joint disease.

ACROMEGALY

The majority of patients with acromegaly develop an atypical form of degenerative joint disease. Increased levels of growth hormone result in hypertrophy of articular cartilage, subchondral bone, and periarticular tissues. Hypermobility of joints, a common manifestation, may contribute to degenerative change. The fingers and knees are most frequently affected. Radiographic features demonstrating overgrowth of bone are pathognomonic. Median nerve entrapment secondary to wrist synovitis is common.

HYPERPARATHYROIDISM

Patients with hyperparathyroidism are subject to a variety of associated rheumatic disorders which may occur singly or in combination. These include (1) hyperuricemia and gouty arthritis, (2) chondrocalcinosis with episodes of calcium pyrophosphate dihydrate crystal–induced synovitis, and (3) degenerative joint disease resulting from deformation of atrophic subchondral bone. Rheumatic symptoms, particularly those associated with chondrocalcinosis (see Chondrocalcinosis and Pseudogout in Ch. 60) may be the first manifestations of hyperparathyroidism.

SICKLE CELL DISEASE AND RELATED HEMOGLOBINOPATHIES

Severe polyarthralgia is a frequent manifestation of the crises of sickle cell disease. Occasionally pain is accompanied by transient joint effusion or other evidence of inflammation. The most common rheumatic symptoms result from avascular osteonecrosis of the femoral head, less commonly of other bony structures. This complication is also associated with sickle cell trait, hemoglobin C disease, SC disease, and sickle cell–thalassemia. In children, periostitis may result in transient diffuse swelling of the hands and feet. Sickle cell disease is associated with an increased incidence of bacterial arthritis and osteomyelitis, especially those caused by gram-negative organisms.

Bluestone, R., et al.: Acromegalic arthropathy. Ann. Rheum. Dis., 30:243, 1971.
Bywaters, E. G. L., Dixon, A. St. J., and Scott, J. T.: Joint lesions of hyperparathyroidism. Ann. Rheum. Dis., 22:171, 1963.
Ferguson, R. H.: Enteropathic arthritis. In Hollander, J. L., and McCarty, D. J., Jr. (eds.): Arthritis and Allied Conditions. 8th ed. Philadelphia, Lea & Febiger, 1972.
Hamilton, E., et al.: The arthropathy of idiopathic haemochromatosis. Quart. J. Med., 37:171, 1968.
McAdam, L. P., O'Hanlan, M. A., Bluestone, R., and Pearson, C. M.: Relapsing polychondritis: Prospective study of 23 patients and a review of the literature. Medicine, 55:193, 1976.
McEwen, C.: Arthritis accompanying ulcerative colitis. Clin. Orthop., 59:9, 1968.
McEwen, C., et al.: Ankylosing spondylitis and spondylitis accompanying ulcerative colitis, regional enteritis, psoriasis and Reiter's disease. A comparative study. Arthritis Rheum., 14:29, 1971.
O'Duffy, J. D., Carnery, J. A., and Deodhar, S.: Behçet's disease: A report of ten cases, three with new manifestations. Ann. Intern. Med., 75:561, 1971.
Spilberg, I., Siltzbach, L. E., and McEwen, C.: The arthritis of sarcoidosis. Arthritis Rheum., 12:126, 1969.

60. MISCELLANEOUS FORMS OF ARTHRITIS

NEUROPATHIC JOINT DISEASE (CHARCOT JOINTS)

This chronic progressive degenerative arthropathy is a complication of a variety of neurologic disorders. Impairment of proprioceptive and pain sensation deprives the affected joint of the normal protective reactions when exposed to forces of weight bearing and motion. Although any neuropathic process which impairs sensory innervation may underlie neuropathic joint disease, syphilitic tabes dorsalis, in spite of its declining frequency, and diabetic neuropathy are the most common associated conditions. Syringomyelia, myelomeningocele, and congenital indifference to pain are less frequent neurologic bases for neuropathic arthropathy. The distribution of joints affected correlates with the pattern of neuropathy. In tabes dorsalis, the knees, hips, ankles, and vertebrae are frequently involved. In diabetic neuropathy, destructive changes are limited to the distal lower extremities, and in syringomyelia the shoulder and elbow joints are most commonly affected.

Although pain is generally present, discomfort tends to be disproportionately mild relative to signs of joint destruction. Clinical, pathologic, and roentgenographic features of chronic neuropathic joint disease reflect severe degrees of destruction and disorganization of affected joints. In the early cases, the differentiation from other causes of joint derangement depends upon the demonstration of sensory neuropathy.

Management includes immobilization of affected joints and restriction of weight-bearing activities with crutches, splints, and braces. Surgical arthrodesis, although frequently unsuccessful, is indicated in selected subjects. Depending on the anatomic pattern and extent of involvement, the application of prosthetic devices after amputation may improve function.

HEMARTHROSIS

Recurrent or chronic hemarthrosis is the most common manifestation of a group of heritable disorders of blood coagulation (see Ch. 520). Hemarthrosis can be a complication of anticoagulant therapy or trauma in an otherwise normal subject.

In hemophilia, joint bleeding usually begins before the age of five and tends to recur repeatedly during childhood in response to minor injury. The most commonly affected joints are the knees, elbows, and ankles, but any articulation may be involved.

Acute hemarthrosis usually results in marked local inflammatory signs and symptoms which recede within a few days. Approximately half the patients with hemophilia develop chronic deformities in one or more joints. Some of them suffer a chronic progressive synovitis, restricted to one or a few joints, which clinically and roentgenographically resembles rheumatoid arthritis. There may be marked synovial membrane hyperplasia, destruction of articular cartilage, and erosions of subchondral bone. This chronic progressive pattern probably results from a low level of continuous or intermittent bleeding into affected joints. Joint fluid, in the chronic cases, usually contains blood and very high levels of leukocyte-derived proteases. Other musculoskeletal manifestations of hemophilia result from bleeding into muscle and bone. The resolution of large hematomas may cause formation of chronic cysts.

The first principle in management is to prevent trauma, a goal not easily achieved in children. Acute hemarthrosis should be managed by immobilization, analgesic therapy, and the administration of plasma products which contain the appropriate coagulation factor. In the choice of analgesics, it is probably wise to exclude salicylates and other drugs which alter platelet function. If there is marked distention of the joint bursae, aspiration can be accomplished after the defect in coagulation has been corrected. When pain and acute inflammation have subsided, an exercise program directed at restoration of motion should be instituted. For the patient with chronic deforming joint disease, the availability of potent plasma products has permitted application of certain surgical procedures such as synovectomy and arthroplasty.

HENOCH-SCHÖNLEIN PURPURA

Nondeforming polyarthritis, most frequently affecting knees and ankles, is a common mainfestation of this syndrome, other features being nonthrombocytopenic purpura, abdominal pain, and glomerulonephritis. The syndrome is rare in adults.

MULTICENTRIC RETICULOHISTIOCYTOSIS
(Lipoid Dermatoarthritis)

This rare disorder usually begins in the middle decades of life and affects females three times more than males. It is characterized by the development of multiple histiocytic nodules in the skin and mucous membranes and severe polyarthritis which may simulate rheumatoid arthritis. The firm reddish-brown or yellow papular nodules are most commonly found on hands, forearms, head, neck, and chest. Mutilating joint destruction, especially in the distal interphalangeal joints, occurs in approximately half the patients with this syndrome. Diagnosis is by demonstration of histiocytes and multinucleated giant cells, containing PAS-positive material, in skin or synovium. Similar infiltrates have been observed in other organs. A few reports of apparent benefit from adrenocorticosteroid or immunosuppressive therapy are difficult to interpret because of the tendency for spontaneous remissions.

HYPERTROPHIC OSTEOARTHROPATHY

This term refers to a syndrome which includes clubbing of fingers and toes, periostitis with new osseous formation at the ends of long bones, arthritis, and signs of autonomic disorders such as flushing, blanching, and profuse sweating. The syndrome occurs with a wide variety of underlying disease states. Less commonly there are hereditary and idiopathic (*pachydermoperiostosis*) forms of disease. The fully expressed pattern is usually associated with intrathoracic disease: lung carcinoma, lung abscess, empyema, bronchiectasis, chronic interstitial penumonitis, or tuberculosis. Clubbing, usually without periostitis, may be seen with cyanotic heart disease, bacterial endocarditis, biliary cirrhosis, ulcerative colitis, regional enteritis, and thyroid disease.

The distal ends of metacarpals, metatarsals, and long bones of the forearms and legs are most frequently affected. There are inflammatory changes of periosteum, synovial membranes, and periarticular structures. The periosteum is "lifted" by the deposition of new bone matrix and subsequent mineralization. Clubbing results from edema, cellular infiltration, and connective tissue proliferation of the nailbeds.

The production of a humoral substance that mediates increased vascularity and/or connective tissue proliferation has long been suspected as the pathogenic factor in hypertrophic osteoarthropathy, but no such factor has been convincingly demonstrated. Evidence that neural factors are involved derives from observations of striking resolution of signs and symptoms after denervation of the hilum or vagotomy on the same side as the thoracic lesion. Regression of osteoarthropathy has also been observed after resection of pulmonary neoplasms.

Pain, tenderness, and enlargement of the distal portions of extremities may be accompanied by acute polyarthritis that resembles rheumatoid arthritis. The differentiation of the acute polyarthritis syndrome is aided by the recognition of clubbing and roentgenographic evidence of periostitis and intrathoracic disease.

Aside from therapy directed at the associated illness, there is no effective treatment of hypertrophic osteoarthropathy. Symptomatic benefit may be obtained from salicylates, other analgesics, or adrenocorticosteroids.

CHONDROCALCINOSIS AND PSEUDOGOUT

Chondrocalcinosis is defined as the presence of calcium-containing salts in cartilaginous structures of one or more joints. These salts include calcium pyrophosphate, calcium hydroxyapatite, and calcium orthophosphate. The term pseudogout refers to the acute and/or chronic synovitis associated with the appearance of calcium pyrophosphate dihydrate crystals in joint fluid.

There is a tendency to chondrocalcinosis in patients with hyperparathyroidism, alcaptonuria, hemochromatosis, Wilson's disease, and acromegaly, and perhaps with gout as well. There appears to be a significant association of diabetes mellitus with pseudogout, and a familial pattern of chondrocalcinosis has been described. Pseudogout, like true gout, appears to be an expression of crystal-induced synovitis.

The incidence of chondrocalcinosis increases with age. Several clinical patterns have been recognized. The most common is of a progressive arthritis of large joints, especially the knee and hip. This is usually indistinguishable from degenerative joint disease, although superimposed acute inflammatory episodes are common. The intermittent acute pattern of synovitis, which resembles gout, is less common. In a small percentage of patients there is a sustained progressive synovitis that resembles rheumatoid arthritis. Since many patients with calcification of articular cartilage manifest no rheumatic signs or symptoms, the terms chondrocalcinosis and pseudogout are not synonymous.

Attacks of *pseudogout* are usually monarticular; less commonly two or more joints may be involved simultaneously. The knee is the most frequently affected joint. The diagnosis rests on roentgenographic criteria, but proof requires the demonstration of calcium pyrophosphate dihydrate crystals under polarized light microscopy. These cystals usually have rod or rhomboid shapes and show weak positive birefringence.

Roentgenographic evidence of calcification of articular fibrocartilage may be found in many structures, including menisci, intervertebral discs, and symphysis pubis. Since punctate and linear radiodensities may be more evident in asymptomatic joints, suspicion of pseudogout should direct a survey of more than the affected articulation.

The metabolic basis for crystal deposition in chondrocalcinosis is not known. There are speculations regarding inhibition or deficiency of pyrophosphatases in cartilage, synovial tissue, or joint fluid.

Aspiration of an acutely swollen joint is often sufficient therapy in itself. If inflammatory signs are marked, aspiration may be followed by intra-articular adrenocorticosteroid therapy or the oral administration of phenylbutazone.

LYME ARTHRITIS

This inflammatory arthropathy was recognized because of an unusual geographic clustering of cases in three contiguous communities in eastern Connecticut. The syndrome is usually characterized by brief, recurrent episodes of asymmetric swelling and pain in large joints. The suspicion that the disease is transmitted by an arthropod vector was strengthened by recognizing an associated dermatologic lesion, erythema chronicum migrans, previously attributed to arthropod bites. In a prospective study during 1976, the peak onset of characteristic skin lesions was in June and July, and the majority experienced onset of arthritis during the months of July to September. Lyme arthritis followed the onset of skin lesion by four weeks (median), but this interval was highly variable, up to 22 weeks. Most patients had recurrent episodes of arthritis, but permanent joint deformity was not observed.

Symptoms and signs suggestive of aseptic meningitis were observed frequently. Two patients out of 27 studied prospectively had lymphocytic meningitis, and two had unilateral Bell's palsy.

Microbiologic and serologic studies seeking evidence of infection with bacteria, mycoplasmas, viruses, and a variety of agents that are transmitted by ticks were all negative.

Spontaneous variations in the natural course of the illness have made therapeutic evaluations difficult. Salicylate therapy has been recommended for symptomatic treatment of rheumatic symptoms. When visceral manifestations or severe systemic symptoms are present, corticosteroid therapy may be indicated.

SYNOVIAL TUMORS

Pigmented villonodular synovitis is the most commonly applied term for a syndrome characterized by villous or nodular growths affecting synovial linings of joints, bursae, or tendons, and a characteristic histopathological picture, i.e., presence of inflammatory granulomas containing hemosiderin and cholesterol crystals and multinucleated giant cells. There is dispute as to whether this condition should be classified as a form of synovitis or as a true neoplasm. Joint involvement is usually monoarticular. The knee is most frequently affected, less commonly the hip, elbow, ankle, or foot. Synovial fluid is usually hemorrhagic or xanthochromic. The inflammatory mass frequently invades cartilage, subchondral bone, and periarticular structures. Pigmented villonodular synovitis may affect extra-articular bursae and tendon sheaths or may occur as a localized tumor in only part of a joint. The treatment of choice is synovectomy. Recurrence is uncommon.

Synovial chondromatosis is an uncommon disorder characterized by the presence of multiple foci of cartilage metaplasia in synovial membranes. Bits of me-taplastic growths frequently detach and grow as loose bodies in the joint cavity and ultimately become ossified. In the latter state, this condition is referred to as synovial osteochondromatosis. The knee is most commonly affected; the disease is rarely polyarticular. Symptoms include pain, swelling, limitation in motion, and intermittent locking of the affected joint. The treatment is surgical synovectomy.

A variety of benign tumors (lipoma, chondroma, hemangioma, and xanthoma) may affect joints.

Primary malignant tumors are rare. Synovioma is a highly malignant fibroblastic sarcoma which probably originates in periarticular structures. This usually occurs in late childhood or early adult years. The recommended therapy is wide excision (frequently requiring amputation), regional lymph node dissection, and irradiation. With the most aggressive management the five-year "cure" rate is usually less than 50 per cent. Synovial chondrosarcoma is a rare neoplasm that may simulate synovial chondromatosis. Radical excision or amputation is the treatment of choice.

Barrow, M. V., and Holubar, K.: Multicentric reticulohistiocytosis. Medicine, 48:287, 1969.

Eichenholz, S. M.: Charcot Joints. Springfield, Ill., Charles C Thomas, 1966.

Howell, D. S.: Hypertrophic osteoarthropathy. *In* Hollander, J. L., and McCarty, D. J., Jr. (eds.): Arthritis and Allied Conditions 8th ed. Philadelphia, Lea & Febiger, 1972.

McCarty, D. J., Kohn, N. N., and Fares, J. S.: The significance of calcium phosphate crystals in synovial fluid of arthritic patients: The pseudogout syndrome: Clinical aspect. Ann. Intern. Med., 56:711, 1962.

Moskowitz, R. W., and Katz, D.: Chondrocalcinosis and chondrocalsynovitis (pseudogout syndrome): Analysis of 24 cases. Am. J. Med., 43:322, 1967.

Steere, A. C., Malawista, S. E., Harding, J. A., Ruddy, S., Askenase, P. W., and Andiman, W. A.: Erythema chronicum migrans and Lyme arthritis. The enlarging spectrum. Ann. Intern. Med., 86:685, 1977.

61. DEGENERATIVE JOINT DISEASE

(Osteoarthritis)

Early degeneration of articular cartilage probably begins in all subjects by the end of the second decade of life. In the pathologic sense, degenerative joint disease is a "normal" response to aging. If the incidence of degenerative joint disease is estimated by minimal roentgenographic criteria, approximately 90 per cent of the population by the age 40 is affected. Although only a small proportion of those with abnormal roentgenograms are symptomatic, degenerative joint disease is the most common cause of chronic disability.

Degenerative joint disease is sometimes classified as primary and secondary. The latter denotes the acceleration or augmentation of wear by abnormal stresses associated with injuries, obesity, and mechanical joint disturbances. Primary degenerative joint disease, in which there is no abnormal wear or forces, is probably influenced by one or more biochemical abnormalities that impair cartilage metabolism.

PATHOLOGY. The earliest lesions of degenerative joint disease are microscopic alterations of articular cartilage. These include diminution of metachromatic material, decreased numbers of chondrocytes, fatty degeneration, alteration of collagen fibrils, and surface irregularities. Later morphologic changes include localized softening of the cartilage with surface flaking and fibrillations. Abrasion of fibrillated cartilage results in progressive loss of cartilaginous surfacing and exposure of subchondral bone.

Subsequent to ulcerations of cartilage, new bone formation occurs at the margin of articular cartilage. These marginal osteophytes are represented in roentgenograms as the characteristic "spurs." Other osseous changes include cysts of varying size beneath the joint surface and remodeling of subchondral bone.

Changes in synovial membranes, including fibrosis, hypertrophy, and occasionally synovitis, appear to be secondary to events affecting articular cartilage. Rarely the pathologic features of inflammation mimic those of rheumatoid arthritis.

ETIOLOGY AND PATHOGENESIS. Accepting the likely premise that primary changes in articular cartilage underlie the development of degenerative joint disease, etiologic considerations may relate to the reparative processes of cartilage. In response to injury, the metabolic activity of chondrocytes increases, but their capacity to replicate and form new matrix is limited. Secondary degenerative joint disease occurs when the forces of wear and tear exceed the restricted capacity for repair. When degenerative joint disease develops (frequently in familial patterns) in the absence of abnormal stresses, it is presumed that accelerated degeneration results from one or more biochemical abnormalities affecting cartilage metabolism. Chemical studies of degenerative cartilage have revealed several abnormalities: decreased water and chondromucoprotein contents and alterations in the profile of glycosaminoglycans. Some of these changes could be mediated by the action of lysosomal hydrolases, but the nature of the presumed biochemical defect in degenerative cartilage remains unknown.

Conditions which alter mechanical properties of joints or which affect the osseous support of articular cartilage are numerous. They include obesity, trauma, hypermobility of joints, neuropathy, acromegaly, Paget's disease of bone, hyperparathyroidism, and alterations of articular or periarticular structures by inflammatory joint disease.

CLINICAL PATTERNS OF DEGENERATIVE JOINT DISEASE. Pain is the dominant symptom of degenerative joint disease but, as noted earlier, disease which is roentgenographically moderate to severe may be asymptomatic. Pain is aggravated by joint motion or weight bearing. Transient stiffness after periods of inactivity is common. Loss of articular cartilage and osseous hypertrophy result in bony enlargement and malalignment of joints and crepitation on motion. Mild tenderness to palpation and effusions are common, but other inflammatory signs are usually absent.

The present discussion of clinical manifestations of degenerative joint disease is developed largely on anatomic lines, since signs and symptoms reflect regional patterns of involvement.

The Hand. *Heberden's nodes* are bony protuberances at the dorsal margins of distal interphalangeal joints. Early Heberden's nodes have a soft cystic consistency and may be associated with prominent inflammatory signs. The chronic stage of Heberden's nodes, characterized by bony enlargement and angular deformities (Fig. 4A), is usually minimally symptomatic. Heredity

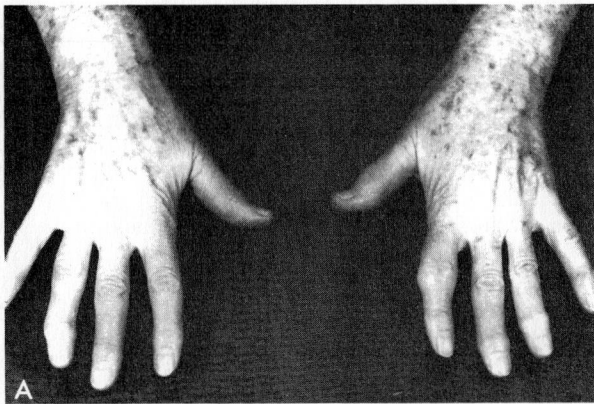
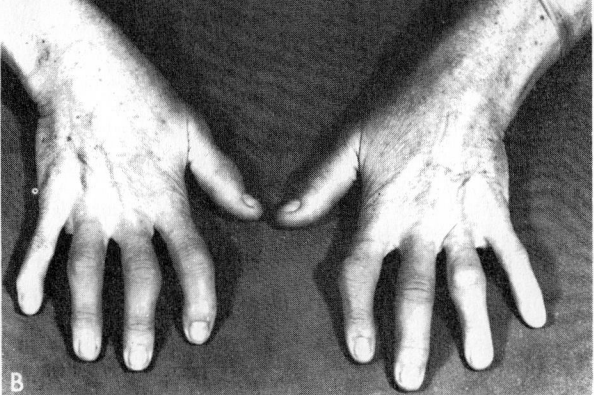

Figure 4. Hand deformities of degenerative joint disease. *A*, Bony enlargement of distal interphalangeal joints (Heberden's nodes) and similar change in one proximal interphalangeal joint (Bouchard's node). *B*, Symmetrical degenerative changes in proximal interphalangeal joints (Bouchard's nodes), a pattern that is frequently mistaken for rheumatoid arthritis.

and sex are prominently involved in the development of Heberden's nodes. They are much more common in women. On the basis of family studies, it has been postulated that a single autosomal gene is involved which is dominant in females and recessive in males.

Patients with Heberden's nodes frequently show degenerative changes in other joints of the hands. The misinterpretation of proximal interphalangeal joint involvement (Bouchard's nodes) as rheumatoid arthritis is a common error (Fig. 4B). Metacarpophalangeal joint involvement is rare. Pain on the radial side of the wrist caused by degenerative disease in the first carpometacarpal joint is a frequent manifestation.

Coxarthrosis (Malum Coxae Senilis). Symptoms of *primary degenerative hip disease* usually appear in the later decades of life, but in as many as half the cases there is evidence of antecedent hip disease such as congenital dysplasia, slipped capital femoral epiphysis, or Legg-Calvé-Perthes disease. In addition, a variety of acquired disorders such as rheumatoid arthritis and avascular necrosis of the femoral head may lead to degenerative hip disease. Groin pain on motion or weight bearing is the dominant symptom, and this is often referred to the medial aspect of the thigh or knee. Over a period of months to a few years, the majority of patients become seriously disabled because of pain and restricted motion.

Degenerative Disease of the Knee. Involvement of the knees is the most common source of major disability in degenerative joint disease. Although mild synovitis and effusion may be present, joint enlargement primarily reflects bone proliferation. Crepitation on motion is a consistent finding. Degenerative changes are usually more prominent in the medial compartment of the knee, leading to varus deformity.

An early manifestation of degenerative change in the patellofemoral joint is termed *chondromalacia patellae*. This syndrome of knee pain and mild effusion, usually associated with trauma, is seen predominantly in young adults.

Vertebral Degenerative Joint Disease, Including Herniated Disc Syndromes. Two sets of articulations are present at all levels of the spinal column: the intervertebral discs and the posterior zygapophyseal joints. In addition to these, the cervical spine (between C2 and C7) has articulations between the lateral aspects of adjacent vertebral bodies, usually referred to as *joints of Luschka*. Degenerative changes in joints of Luschka are the most common cause of pain in the cervical area. In lumbar levels degeneration and herniation of the nucleus pulposus of intervertebral discs are usually the bases for symptoms.

CERVICAL SPINE. The close proximity of cervical nerve roots to the joints of Luschka makes them vulnerable to irritation or compression from any derangement in or about the joints. Since the greatest amount of stress in the cervical spine occurs at C4-C5 and C5-C6 levels, degenerative changes in the intervertebral discs and joints of Luschka are most common there. Osteophytic spurs at the margins of joints of Luschka may impinge upon nerve roots as they leave the intervertebral foramina. The pattern of pain and neurologic findings varies according to the level involved: pain is frequently in the supraclavicular and upper trapezius regions but can be referred into the occiput and more distal upper extremity. Discomfort is aggravated by motion of the neck, particularly rotation and lateral bending.

If there is degeneration of the intervertebral discs in the cervical spine, the joints of Luschka provide a barrier against lateral herniation of the nucleus pulposus. The protrusion and subsequent osteophytic reaction may therefore encroach directly on the spinal cord rather than nerve roots. The progression of the resulting cervical myelopathy may be insidious and painless.

LUMBAR SPINE. Symptoms of degenerative disease of the lumbar spine are nearly always attributable to involvement of intervertebral discs. Protrusion or extrusion of degenerated discs is directed posterolaterally, impinging upon nerve roots or the cauda equina. Although any of the lumbar discs can herniate, this most commonly occurs at L4-L5 and L5-S1. Patients with herniated lumbar discs frequently have a history of mild or recurrent backache prior to development of more acute discomfort. Pain radiates distally into one or the other lower extremity and is aggravated by spinal movement, particularly bending to the side of the pain. There is usually marked paravertebral tenderness and aggravation of pain by straight leg raising. Loss or suppression of the ankle jerk and sensory deficit in the lateral border and sole of the foot and toes suggest L5-S1 root compression. No reflex change, sensory deficit in the lateral leg and mediodorsal aspect of the foot, and weakness of the toe extensors suggest L4-L5 root compression.

Primary Generalized Hypertrophic Osteoarthri- tis.* This is more a concept than a disease: it describes a polyarticular pattern associated with somewhat more inflammatory reaction than is customary with degenerative joint disease. There is usually involvement of the hands, including Heberden's and Bouchard's nodes, along with changes in the first carpometacarpal joints. Women in the middle years of life are most commonly affected, and a familial pattern is prominent. A closely related syndrome of degenerative joint disease has been termed *erosive osteoarthritis*.

LABORATORY FINDINGS. There are no specific laboratory abnormalities of degenerative joint disease. The erythrocyte sedimentation rate is usually normal. Synovial fluid is clear and exhibits high viscosity and normal mucin clot test. Leukocyte counts in synovial fluid vary in the range of 200 to 2000 per cubic millimeter. Fragments of cartilage are frequently identified in the fluid.

ROENTGENOGRAPHIC FEATURES. Osteophyte formation at the margins of affected joints is the basis for the most striking roentgenographic feature of degenerative joint disease, but earlier and more common findings, resulting from destruction of articular cartilage, are narrowing of the interosseous joint space and subchondral bone sclerosis. Radiolucent cysts, varying in size from a few millimeters to several centimeters, may be seen in periarticular bone.

Degeneration of cervical and lumbar discs results in interspace narrowing. Exostoses at the margins of vertebral bodies may coalesce with adjacent osteophytes, causing fusion at one or more levels. Roentgenographic documentation of intervertebral herniation requires contrast myelography. Disc degeneration is best observed by anteroposterior and lateral roentgenograms. For visualization of osteophytes encroaching on foramina, especially important in the cervical spine, oblique projections are required.

DIFFERENTIAL DIAGNOSIS. In their typical expressions, degenerative joint disease and rheumatoid arthritis are easily distinguished. The latter is usually associated with evidence of systemic disease, prominent signs of joint inflammation, and the characteristic symmetrical pattern of disease affecting the hands and wrists. When a patient presents with signs of mild inflammation in one or two weight-bearing joints of the lower extremities, the differentiation between these two syndromes is more difficult. In that setting a normal erythrocyte sedimentation rate, negative rheumatoid factor test result, and minimal abnormalities in synovial fluid support the diagnosis of degenerative joint disease. No test singly or in combination can be viewed as diagnostic; even the roentgenographic demonstration of marginal osteophytes may be a secondary change in rheumatoid arthritis. In the most experienced hands, there is a small percentage of patients in whom the diagnosis remains indeterminate.

A common diagnostic error is the interpretation of degenerative changes in proximal interphalangeal joints of the hands as evidence of rheumatoid arthritis (Fig. 4B). The deformities that characterize Heberden's and Bouchard's nodes may be marked, but this pattern of degenerative joint disease is not associated with prominent signs of inflammation, and the metacarpophalangeal joints and wrist joints are rarely or never affected.

Important aspects of differential diagnosis involve the recognition of syndromes in which secondary development of degenerative joint disease may occur. These include hemochromatosis, neuropathy, chondrocalcinosis, alcaptonuria, hypermobility of joints (including the Ehlers-Danlos syndrome), mechanical derangements of joints, and a variety of metabolic disorders that affect the support of articular cartilage by subchondral bone.

There should never be confusion in the differentiation of degenerative joint disease of the vertebral column from ankylosing spondylitis. Patients with the latter are almost invariably young men, and the roentgenographic features are distinct from those associated with degenerative joint disease.

TREATMENT. The management of degenerative joint disease is highly varied, depending upon anatomic patterns and the degree of joint deformity. An optimistic forecast is appropriate for most individuals. Patients should understand that disability can be minimized even though there is no specific remedy. The common statement that "nothing can be done for your kind of arthritis" is a false cliché.

Drugs. No medication has been shown to retard the development or progression of degenerative joint disease. The requirement for analgesic drugs is varied; many patients have so little pain that they require no medicinal therapy. Aspirin in moderate dosage (0.6 gram three to five times a day) is usually helpful for the patient with pain. Sustained salicylate therapy is superior to intermittent or erratic dosage. A common problem in degenerative joint disease, regardless of anatomic location, is the occurrence of intermittent episodes of increased pain which tend to subside spontaneously. For these recurrent episodes, phenylbutazone (100 to 300 mg daily) or indomethacin (75 to 150 mg daily) may be beneficial. Continuous use of drugs other than salicylates is rarely indicated in degenerative joint disease. Some patients with disabling hip pain, however, experience sufficient relief of symptoms with phenylbutazone or indomethacin to warrant maintenance therapy. It is common practice to prescribe muscle relaxants, such as diazepam or carisoprodol, for pain and muscle spasm of vertebral disease, but objective assessment of their efficacy is lacking.

Physical Measures. There are two general goals in the design of a physical medicine program for degenerative joint disease: minimizing the forces of work and weight bearing that apply to affected joints, and maintenance of normal joint alignment and motion. The patient with hip or knee disease should be instructed to avoid unnecessary walking or stair climbing. This recommendation is not inconsistent with the performance of an exercise program (in nonweight-bearing attitude) which can maintain muscle power and joint motion. Quadriceps isometric exercise for degenerative joint disease of the knees is particularly important. There is a powerful rationale for weight reduction for the obese patient with involvement of the spine or lower extremities. The use of a cane or a crutch can reduce forces of weight bearing applied to a symptomatic hip or knee by as much as 50 per cent. In selected patients with an unstable knee, fitting of a brace may be beneficial.

Certain physical measures are selectively relevant to degenerative joint disease of the spine. Patients need to learn to live with the altered mechanics of their spine. With cervical involvement, hyperextension and hyperflexion should be avoided. The patient should sleep supine with no more than one pillow. Most, but not all, patients with cervical radicular pain will be helped by intermittent traction. If this is beneficial, there are in-

expensive devices for applying intermittent cervical traction at home. When symptoms are acute, wearing a cervical collar will restrict movement and minimize pain.

The patient with symptomatic degenerative disease of the lumbar spine should sleep on a hard mattress and avoid bending and lifting activities. A program of graded postural exercises is important when pain has subsided. External support provided by a lumbosacral corset will frequently minimize mild chronic symptoms. When lumbar disc herniation results in severe pain or nerve deficit, hospitalization is usually indicated. The majority of such patients will experience a remission of symptoms within a two- to three-week period. Consideration of surgical therapy is appropriate for those patients who fail to respond to conservative management.

Surgical Management. The main anatomic areas affected by degenerative joint disease that are amenable to orthopedic surgical therapy are the hip, the knee, and the vertebral column. Several surgical procedures are appropriate for the patient with debilitating hip pain. These include arthrodesis (if the disease is unilateral), mold arthroplasty, osteotomy, and total joint replacement. In most centers, the last is the preferred procedure. Operative procedures for the knee with degenerative joint disease include debridement, osteotomy, and a variety of prosthetic arthroplasties. If there is reasonable preservation of motion and stability of the malaligned knee, tibial or femoral osteotomy is frequently beneficial. When there is a serious disability attributable to malalignment and instability of the knee, one or another prosthetic procedure may be indicated. However, the successes, to date, of knee joint replacement have not been as predictable as have comparable procedures for the hip.

Virtually all orthopedic surgeons agree that surgical procedures for degenerative disease of the spine are appropriate *only* after there has been a systematic and sustained trial of conservative management. If radicular pain is relentless or if there are increasing neurologic deficits from nerve root involvement or myelopathy, surgical correction is warranted.

Armstrong, J. R.: Lumbar disc lesions. 3rd ed. Baltimore, Williams & Wilkins Company, 1965.

Friedenberg, Z. B., and Miller, W. T.: Degenerative disc disease of the cervical spine J. Bone Joint Surg., 45A:1171, 1963.

Kellgren, J. H., Lawrence, J. S., and Bier, F.: Genetic factors in generalized osteo-arthritis. Ann. Rheum. Dis., 22:237, 1969.

Mankin, H. J.: Biochemical and metabolic aspects of osteoarthritis. Orthop. Clin. North Am., 2:19, 1971.

Sokoloff, L.: The Biology of Degenerative Joint Disease. Chicago, University of Chicago Press, 1969.

62. THE PAINFUL SHOULDER

Because shoulder pain is frequent and due to diverse mechanisms, this subject deserves special attention. Of prime importance is recognition that pain in the shoulder may be referred from disease affecting cervical, intrathoracic, and diaphragmatic areas. Shoulder motion is affected by the action of muscles through a "joint complex" consisting of independent articulations — glenohumeral, acromioclavicular, and sternoclavicular, as well as the scapulothoracic surface relationship. In addition, shoulder function requires movement of gliding surfaces of periarticular structures — the musculotendinous cuff, the subdeltoid bursa, and the long head of the biceps. Any of the syndromes associated with synovitis may be responsible for shoulder pain. The primary concern in this chapter is a group of painful disorders which affect the periarticular soft tissues of the shoulder.

CALCIFIC TENDINITIS AND BURSITIS

The most common cause of shoulder pain results from degeneration of the supraspinatus and infraspinatus tendons. Approximately 3 per cent of people in their middle years have calcific deposits in these rotator tendons. Although the majority of such subjects have few or no symptoms, a significant percentage develop pain because of inflammation of the parietal surface of the overlying subdeltoid bursa. An inflammatory exudate containing calcareous matter may rupture into this bursa. The symptoms may be acute, subacute, or chronic. The acute syndrome is characterized by sudden onset of pain in the shoulder area, often with radiation into the neck and proximal arm. Any motion of the shoulder girdle elicits pain. There is frequently exquisite local tenderness over the anterior and anterolateral aspect of the shoulder joint. Night pain is a prominent feature. Roentgenographic studies usually demonstrate linear calcific deposits in the involved tendon or a more diffuse calcific pattern in the subdeltoid bursa. In most instances acute symptoms abate after a few days, but in a minority subacute discomfort persists for weeks.

The treatment is influenced by the severity and duration of symptoms. Anti-inflammatory agents, such as phenylbutazone or indomethacin, and analgesics are usually sufficient to control acute symptoms. In most patients there is a spontaneous remission of pain and a disappearance of calcific deposits. When the symptoms are very acute, aspiration of calcified material and injection of adrenocorticosteroid preparation may give prompt relief. The prospects of more chronic disability can be minimized by the institution of an active exercise program as soon as the level of discomfort permits. If the patient is not making progress toward regaining normal shoulder motion with a home exercise program, supervised therapy in a physical medicine department is important. A small percentage of patients with refractory pain and persistent roentgenographic findings may require surgical exploration for removal of calcific deposits.

BICIPITAL TENDINITIS

The long head of the biceps originates from the superior surface of the glenoid. It emerges from the glenohumeral bursa to lie in the bicipital groove of the humerus where it is covered by a synovial sheath. The shoulder pain of bicipital tendinitis frequently radiates along the biceps to the forearm, and is aggravated by abduction and internal rotation. Tenderness over the bicipital groove and accentuation of pain with resisted supination of the forearm, with the elbow flexed at 90 degrees, aid in the recognition of bicipital tendinitis. The management is similar to that described for calcific

tendinitis: local injection of adrenocorticosteroid preparations, systemic anti-inflammatory agents, and an exercise program. In refractory cases, surgical exploration with tendon transfer usually yields good results.

ROTATOR CUFF TEARS

The same degenerative changes that underlie the development of shoulder tendinitis can weaken the musculotendinous rotator cuff and predispose it to rupture. In most patients with this problem, there is acute onset of shoulder pain after trauma or performance of strenuous work. If the tear is complete, the patient is unable to abduct the arm, but it can be held in abduction, once elevated to 90 degrees, by the action of the deltoid muscle. With incomplete tears, the patient has only mild pain and moderate weakness. The diagnosis of rotator cuff tears can best be established by contrast arthrography. With complete rupture of the supraspinatus tendon, surgical repair is usually warranted. In patients with partial tears, partial immobilization followed by an exercise program is appropriate.

THE SHOULDER-HAND SYNDROME
(Reflex Neurovascular Dystrophy)

This is a poorly understood disorder characterized by pain and stiffness in the shoulder, together with pain, swelling, and vasomotor phenomena in the hand. Involvement of the distal upper extremity is frequently followed by dystrophic change that resembles *Sudeck's atrophy.* The syndrome is presumed to result from reflex sympathetic stimulation analogous to that proposed for causalgia. It principally affects patients above the age of 50 and is often associated with acute illness such as myocardial infarction, trauma to the distal upper extremity, cerebrovascular accident, or pulmonary disease. The significance of associated degenerative change in the cervical spine is uncertain, because of its high frequency in the population at risk. When the disease is bilateral, the differentiation from acute rheumatoid arthritis may be difficult. Joint symptoms appear to result from periarticular involvement, but synovial biopsies, in a few cases, have disclosed mild histologic abnormalities: edema, proliferation, and disarray of synovial lining cells. There is marked variability in intensity and duration of acute symptoms and extent of dystrophic change. In a small percentage of patients the end result is "frozen shoulder" and dystrophic changes in the hands that resemble those of systemic sclerosis.

There is probably no condition for which aggressive physical therapy is more important than for the shoulder-hand syndrome. An active exercise program, facilitated by analgesic medication, should be instituted as soon as possible. When refractory pain impedes progress in the physical medicine program, a trial of systemic corticosteroid therapy (10 to 20 mg per day of prednisone or equivalent) or stellate ganglion block is warranted.

FROZEN SHOULDER

A minority of patients with any of the shoulder conditions discussed above develop chronic restriction of motion of the glenohumeral joint. When there is no apparent relationship of frozen shoulder to other shoulder disease, such as tendinitis or rotator cuff injury, the condition is sometimes termed *adhesive capsulitis*. This condition may be clincially indistinct from the shoulder-hand syndrome. Pain is generally less severe and less well localized relative to other conditions causing shoulder pain. The most important aspect of management of frozen shoulder is prevention. Early attention to the underlying cause of shoulder pain and the institution of an effective exercise program are nearly always successful in combating the progression of shoulder immobility. Management of the chronic frozen shoulder is much more difficult. Manipulation under general anesthesia followed by intensive physical therapy may be indicated when patients are not helped by conservative management.

DePalma, A. F., and Kruper, J. S.: Long-term study of shoulder joints afflicted with and treated for calcific tendinitis. Clin. Orthop., 20:61, 1961.

Kozin, F., McCarty, D. J., Sims, J., and Genant, H.: The reflex sympathetic dystrophy syndrome. 1. Clinical and histological studies: Evidence for bilaterality, response to corticosteroids and articular involvement. Am. J. Med., 60:321, 1976.

Steinbrocker, O.: The painful shoulder. *In* Hollander, J. L., and McCarty, D. J., Jr. (eds.): Arthritis and Allied Conditions. 8th ed. Philadelphia, Lea & Febiger, 1972.

63. NONARTICULAR RHEUMATISM

This term designates a group of painful disorders resulting from involvement of tendons, bursae, and other periarticular structures. Conditions causing shoulder pain are considered separately in Ch. 62.

BURSITIS

Bursae are closed synovial sacs located at sites of friction between skin, ligaments, tendons, muscles, and bones. Trauma is the most common cause of bursitis, but almost any illness characterized by joint synovitis may be associated with involvement of the lining of bursae. Bursae commonly involved include the following: subdeltoid, trochanteric, olecranon, and prepatellar. Septic or gouty bursitis can be documented by appropriate studies of aspirated fluid. Protection of an inflamed bursa from friction and trauma is the most important aspect of treatment, but moderate doses of salicylates, phenylbutazone, or indomethacin may be helpful. Local injection with an adrenocorticosteroid preparation is indicated if symptoms are severe or refractory to other treatments.

TENOSYNOVITIS

Tendon sheaths, like bursae, have synovial linings and can be involved by any process capable of inducing joint synovitis. Tenosynovitis in the hand or foot is a frequent manifestation of gonococcemia. Calcific tendinitis, a common source of shoulder pain (see Ch. 62), may be associated with marked inflammatory signs resembling acute gout. Focal thickening of the tendon sheath and adjacent tendon can result in "locking or

triggering" phenomena. This problem, termed stenosing tenovaginitis, is common in the flexor tendons of the fingers. Involvement of the abductor pollicis longus and extensor pollicis brevis tendons of the thumb (*de Quervain's syndrome*) results in pain and tenderness at the radial aspect of the wrist. There are no generalizations regarding management, since tenosynovitis may be a manifestation of various disease states, including rheumatoid arthritis and other connective tissue syndromes, infection, gout, and hypercholesterolemia. The common form of tenosynovitis, unassociated with systemic disease, will often subside with rest. If symptoms are severe or recurrent, local injections of adrenocorticosteroid preparations are usually effective. Surgical excision of the affected tendon sheath is indicated for those patients with persistent disability.

TENNIS ELBOW
(Epicondylitis)

This common condition is characterized by pain over the lateral aspect of the elbow. Tenderness is localized in the area of the common extensor insertion in the region of the lateral epicondyle. The problem, most common in middle-aged males, is related to sports or occupations that involve repetitive wrist extension or pronation-supination. Pain is accentuated by resisted wrist extension. If symptoms fail to respond to rest, injection of local adrenocorticosteroid preparations is usually successful. For the rare patient with persistent disability, surgical therapy may be needed.

CARPAL TUNNEL SYNDROME

This problem results from entrapment of the median nerve as it passes deep to the transverse carpal ligament of the wrist. Inflammation of the adjacent flexor tendon sheaths, the most common basis for median nerve entrapment, may be a feature of rheumatoid arthritis; but in most patients the tenosynovitis is localized and unassociated with systemic disease. The majority of patients are middle-aged women. The most consistent symptoms are dysesthesia, paresthesia, and hypesthesia in the middle three digits of the hand. Referred pain in the more proximal upper extremity is common. Symptoms are usually intermittent, occurring most frequently during the night. Forced flexion of the wrist or nerve compression locally may induce the characteristic symptoms. In a minority of patients, there is progressive wasting of the muscles of the thenar eminence. Conservative management consists of fitting a removable dorsal splint to hold the wrist in slight extension and the local injection of an adrenocorticosteroid preparation. Surgical release of the transverse carpal ligament is indicated for patients with persistent disability.

TIETZE'S SYNDROME

This mysterious benign disorder is characterized by painful enlargement of the upper costal cartilages. It is usually unilateral and limited to a single costochondral juncture. Occasionally the manubriosternal and sternoclavicular joints are affected. The disease may be recurrent, but remission is the rule. Some patients are concerned that they have cardiac disease; reassurance alone may be sufficient management. If discomfort is severe or recurrent, analgesics, heat, or local infiltration (adrenocorticosteroid or local anesthetic agents) may be beneficial.

FIBROSITIS

This term has been applied to a poorly defined symptom complex which is characterized by pain and stiffness in varying areas, most commonly in the neck, shoulder girdle, and posterior aspect of the trunk. Physical signs except for questionable nodules or thickening of the deep fasciae are lacking, and laboratory and roentgenographic studies are negative. The term fibrositis is based on vague hypothesis and common usage rather than on anatomic abnormalities. Localized areas of tenderness, commonly in the paravertebral areas medial to the scapula, have been termed "trigger points." The syndrome usually begins in the middle years of life. Because the majority of patients appear tense and anxious and have no recognizable objective basis for symptoms, the syndrome is often considered psychogenic. Since pain and stiffness can be manifestations of a variety of musculoskeletal, neurologic, and systemic disorders, the diagnosis of fibrositis requires the exclusion of more defined illnesses. The patient and his physician tend to share an unhappy experience in efforts to control symptoms. The results of strong reassurance that serious disease is lacking are variable, as are the results of therapy with salicylates, sedatives, tranquilizers, and muscle relaxants. Temporary relief is occasionally achieved by injection of local anesthetic into tender points or by chilling the overlying skin with ethyl chloride.

Levey, G. S., and Calabro, J. J.: Tietze's syndrome: Report of two cases and review of the literature. Arthritis Rheum., 5:261, 1962.

Phalen, G. S.: The carpal tunnel syndrome: Seventeen years' experience in diagnosis and treatment of 654 hands. J. Bone Joint Surg., 48A:211, 1966.

Swannell, A. J., Underwood, F. A., and Dixon, A. St. J.: Periarticular calcific deposits mimicking acute arthritis. Ann. Rheum. Dis., 29:380, 1970.

PART VIII

GRANULOMATOUS DISEASES OF UNPROVED ETIOLOGY

64. INTRODUCTION

Paul B. Beeson

The chapters to follow include a variety of rather uncommon and difficult-to-classify syndromes. These are characterized by long and fluctuating clinical courses, and the affected tissues show the picture of chronic inflammation, usually with formation of granulomas. Sarcoidosis is the most common and best known. The others are comparatively rare, and their natures and classifications are subject to controversy. For the purpose of textbook exposition, the best recognized clinical forms have been described as separate diseases. It should be noted, however, that there are shades of similarity and that each of these is thought by some students to be merely a variant expression of one of the other processes, e.g., panniculitis and retroperitoneal fibrosis. Some could well have been discussed with the diseases of connective tissue, as in fact they were in former editions. In the present state of knowledge — ignorance is more accurate—the editors have elected to place the descriptions of these syndromes under a heading with a noncommittal title.

65. SARCOIDOSIS

D. Geraint James

DEFINITION. Sarcoidosis is a multisystem granulomatous disorder of unknown cause most commonly affecting young adults and presenting most frequently with bilateral hilar lymphadenopathy, pulmonary infiltration, and skin or eye lesions. The diagnosis is established most securely when clinicoradiographic findings are supported by histologic evidence of widespread noncaseating epithelioid cell granulomas in more than one organ or by a positive Kveim-Siltzbach skin test. Immunologic features are depression of delayed-type hypersensitivity suggesting impaired cell-mediated immunity and raised or abnormal serum immunoglobulins suggesting lymphoproliferation. There may also be hypercalciuria with or without hypercalcemia. The course and prognosis correlate with the mode of onset: an acute onset with erythema nodosum usually heralds a self-limiting course and spontaneous resolution, whereas an insidious onset may be followed by relentless progressive fibrosis. Corticosteroids relieve symptoms and suppress inflammation and granuloma formation.

ETIOLOGY. The cause remains unknown. We do not know whether sarcoidosis is one disease or due to many contributing factors.

Infection. The various organisms claimed to be responsible for sarcoidosis have included human and anonymous mycobacteria, *Mycobacterium leprae,* fungi, viruses, and protozoa. Many organisms provoke a nonspecific granulomatous reaction, but this should not be misconstrued as multisystem sarcoidosis. Helminths provoke such reactions in the liver and central nervous system; anonymous mycobacteria cause swimming pool and fish tank granulomas, and *M. leprae* produces confusingly similar granulomas. Formerly, sarcoidosis was thought to be due to the human tubercle bacillus, but there are many important points differentiating sarcoidosis from tuberculosis.

Claims for a causal virus are longstanding, and at different times mumps, influenza, parainfluenza, Newcastle agent, and measles virus particles have been isolated.

There has been speculation concerning a transmissible agent from human sarcoid tissue into foot pads of mice, but similar changes occur with control nonsarcoid lymph node tissue. Attempts to demonstrate viruses by tissue culture of sarcoid lymph nodes have been unsuccessful.

High titers of antibodies to several viruses have been noted in sarcoidosis. This should not be misconstrued as indicative of a viral cause of sarcoidosis but rather as a reflection of lymphoproliferation by overactive B cells.

Genetic Factors. The occasional occurrence of familial sarcoidosis suggests a recessive mode of inheritance. We have observed 16 families, in whom 33 persons had sarcoidosis. The group comprised 11 brother-sister, 4 mother-offspring, and 1 uncle-niece relationships, and it was also noted once in husband and wife. The clinical, radiographic, and other features of the disorder are similar in familial and sporadic sarcoidosis, but the course of one sister was considerably worse than that of her brother, suggesting adverse hormonal factors. Four of these families were from the West Indies, suggesting a racial predisposition to familial sarcoidosis. Turiaf has also noted a greater incidence in French West Indians from Martinique; he finds familial sarcoidosis in 1 per cent of white Europeans but in 8 per cent of Martinicans living in Paris.

HLA Antigens. We have studied different clinical features individually. HLA-B8 (which was present in 27 per cent of controls) was found in 8 out of 13 with erythema nodosum alone (p < 0.015), 9 out of 11 with erythema nodosum and arthritis (p < 0.002), and 8 out of 9 with arthritis alone (p < 0.002). Thus B8 was present in 71 per cent of all patients with erythema nodosum and in 85 per cent with arthritis. It appears that there may be inherited susceptibility to arthritis and erythema nodosum in sarcoidosis, with B8 as a genetic marker for both disorders.

Allergy.   Inhalation of pine pollen and peanut dust, clay-eating, and chewing pine pitch have all been incriminated as contributory regional factors in different areas.

Chemicals.   Beryllium and zirconium are known to produce sarcoid granulomas in the sensitized individual, but other elements do not seem to be granulomagenic. Exhaustive skin testing with metals and other inorganic elements in sarcoidosis and controls has not revealed any peculiar hypersensitivity to chemicals. Skin tests for sarcoidosis, beryllium disease, zirconium hypersensitivity, and leprosy are very similar in that a sarcoid granuloma is present at the injection site one month after inoculation. Each skin test is individually specific for its own disorder, and there is no overlap.

Autoimmune Disorder.   Sarcoidosis does not satisfactorily fulfill the criteria of an autoimmune disorder. There is one pattern of sarcoidosis that could conceivably fit — namely, erythema nodosum with hilar adenopathy, a syndrome which may be associated with a circulating immune complex; and these immune complexes have been shown to be present in sarcoidosis.

IMMUNOLOGY. Impaired Cellular Immunity.   Depression of delayed-type hypersensitivity is reflected by T-cell anergy in vivo and in vitro (Fig. 1). Skin tests using tuberculin, fungal and viral antigens, and dinitrochlorobenzene are negative far more frequently than in control subjects. Sarcoid lymphocytes show diminished response to phytohemagglutinin (PHA). Quantitative tests for T cells are still crude and so results vary, but most reports indicate a reduction of the T cell subpopulation in the peripheral blood. It is likely that the number of peripheral blood sarcoid lymphocytes is most confusing and illusory to assess, for the plasma in which they are bathed may contain factors influencing

their behavior. With improved methods for assessing T cells, efforts should be directed to their enumeration within target organs and in sarcoid tissue, away from interfering T-cell antibodies.

Serum Inhibitors.   Old theories of serum anticutins and procutins in sarcoidosis have been re-evaluated now that new techniques of lymphocyte morphology suggest that serum inhibitors are responsible for depression of cell-mediated immunity in sarcoidosis. Depending on the stimulus received, regulator T cells may suppress or amplify the immune response, producing lymphokines which affect the function of other T cells. In support of this concept is evidence of increased migration inhibition factors in sarcoid lymphocytes. When sarcoid serum has been removed, there is a return to normal function of these lymphocytes. Macrophages are active secretory cells which release potent enzymes perpetuating inflammation leading to granuloma formation, disturbing the traffic of re-circulating lymphocytes, and adding to this depression of cell-mediated immunity. This depression has been overcome by transfer factor both in vitro and in vivo, by blocking or otherwise overcoming serum inhibitors emanating from suppressor T cells. Levamisole may act similarly in overcoming depression of delayed-type hypersensitivity in vitro and in treatment.

Lymphoproliferation.   Whereas there is cutaneous anergy and impaired cellular immunity, the reverse holds for humoral immunity. There is vigorous B cell activity with raised immunoglobulin levels; increased circulating antibody titers to Epstein-Barr virus, herpes simplex, rubella, measles, and parainfluenza viruses, and chlamydiae; increased antibody responses to mismatched blood; and occasional false-positive Wassermann reactions.

Circulating Immune Complexes.   Various techniques have been employed to detect circulating immune complexes. They are most evident at the stage of erythema nodosum, iritis, polyarthralgia, and bilateral hilar lymphadenopathy in which C3 activation products have been found within the first six weeks. During this early stage of acute sarcoidosis, there is activation of the complement system due to circulating immune complexes. These tests for circulating complexes subside as the acute skin lesions disappear. At present, all tests for circulating complexes are crude, and it is necessary to use a battery of different techniques. When they are detectable, the sedimentation rate is very high, so this remains the cheapest bedside indicator of these complexes.

PATHOGENESIS.   An antigenic insult, whether by an infective agent or by chemical or even vegetable matter, is met by a reticuloendothelial response in which both thymus-derived (T) cells and plasma (B) cells participate. The T cells are transformed, possibly by undergoing antigenic alteration on their cell surface, and become depleted. Serum inhibitors may block T cell function. Depletion may be due not only to T cell transformation but also to T cell interaction against transformed T cells. Depletion results in depression of delayed-type cutaneous and lymphocyte transformation tests. At the same time there is vigorous B cell proliferation, recognizable by an increase in circulating immunoglobulins. This phase of expansive lymphoproliferation with T cell eclipse is represented histologically by granuloma formation in many organ systems. During this same phase, circulating immune complexes may be

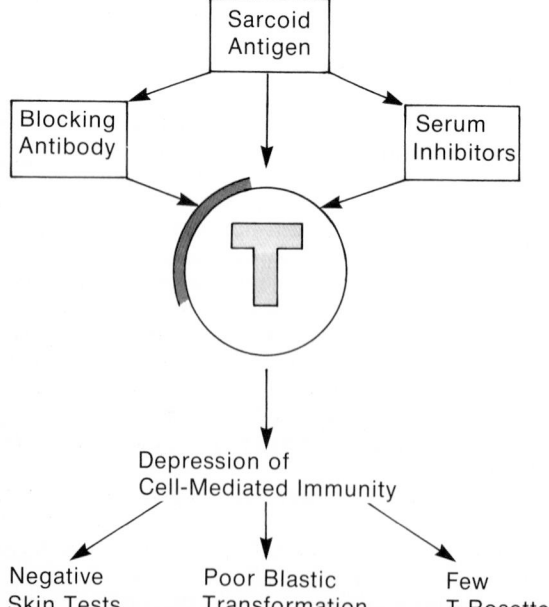

Figure 1.   Depression of cell-mediated immunity is reflected by T cell anergy in bedside skin tests and in the laboratory.

responsible for such clinical phenomena as erythema nodosum and uveitis. The antigenic insult is probably airborne, for bilateral hilar lymphadenopathy is such a frequent mode of onset. The more acute the onset and the more active the reticuloendothelial response, the more likely will there be spontaneous remission with full restoration of T cell function. If this does not occur spontaneously, then it may be induced by corticosteroids, which may overcome T cell eclipse and restore normal T cell function.

The antigen responsible for lymphoproliferation, T cell transformation, and granuloma formation almost certainly resides in Kveim-Siltzbach antigen used in the sarcoidosis skin test. There is undoubtedly a complex interrelationship between the featureless null cell, the depressed T cell, and the B cell overactivity. Serum blocking factors may coat T cells so that they look like N cells and fail to produce the necessary lymphokines which recruit more T cells. T cell anergy means lack of suppressor control, thereby allowing B cell overactivity. It remains to be seen whether thymosin, levamisole, and BCG vaccine will transform N to T cells to correct the situation and whether therapeutic injections of transfer factor will recruit other T cells to repair the defect in cell-mediated immunity.

PATHOLOGY. High turnover granulomas are characterized by epithelioid and giant cells as seen in sarcoidosis, tuberculosis, Crohn's disease, and primary biliary cirrhosis. Epithelioid cells are large mononuclear cells about 20 μ in diameter with round or oval nuclei and are derived from macrophages. They are poorly phagocytic but highly secretory, and they indicate the constant arrival of macrophages into the granuloma pool. Giant cells up to 300 μ in diameter, containing as many as 30 nuclei, are usually arranged peripherally. They are also derived by fusion of macrophages, which are constantly arriving, dividing, and aging. Within these epithelioid and giant cells may be found three types of inclusion bodies — Schaumann, asteroid, and residual bodies — all of which are nonspecific endproducts of the active metabolism and secretion which has taken place.

The sarcoid granuloma is surrounded by a peripheral rim of lymphocytes and contains macrophages, epithelioid and giant cells, and also T and B cells. Also within the granuloma are the various immunoglobulins which can be identified by immunofluorescence. As the lesion ages, reticulin fibers ramify between the epithelioid cells, which thicken and eventually become converted into collagen. The granuloma loses its outline and becomes a solid amorphous eosinophilic mass of hyaline material (Fig. 2).

So much for the morphology of the granuloma; what of its function? Macrophages are active secretory cells able to release a variety of potent enzymes, including lysozyme, glucuronidase, and angiotensin-converting enzyme. The last-named is useful for confirming the diagnosis of sarcoidosis (see Diagnosis).

EPIDEMIOLOGY. Sarcoidosis is worldwide in distribution, but is most frequently recognized in sophisticated communities with adequate diagnostic facilities. Mass chest roentgenography reveals an overall prevalence of 20 per 100,000 population, rising to a figure of 120 per 100,000 for Irishmen and 200 per 100,000 for Irishwomen in London. Although the overall prevalence is similar in men and women, it is twice as common in women of childbearing age. In the United States it is ten times more prevalent in blacks than in whites, regardless of birthplace or residence. This fact immediately raises the question of its frequency in the black population of Africa and the Caribbean. There is fresh information from South Africa indicating that sarcoidosis is ten times more frequent in the Bantu than in the white population — in fact, just as in the United States. It also afflicts the blacks in the same fashion, with gross skin lesions — including lupus pernio, papules, nodules, plaques in sites of old injury, and nail dystrophies — and a high frequency of intrathoracic involvement, bone cysts, and chronic uveitis. Of particular epidemiologic interest in the South African survey is that some of the patients had been in a leprosy institution. The diagnosis of sarcoidosis was entertained when patients had failed to improve on antileprotic, antituberculous, and antisyphilitic treatment. The South African Bantu is emerging from a scourge of tuberculosis, and sarcoidosis may follow in its wake.

Latent sarcoidosis will be found if sought in the right places. These include areas where tuberculosis has been eradicated; follow-up teams responsible for the eradication of tuberculosis should also look for sarcoidosis. It would be of interest to know the incidence of sarcoidosis in the Caribbean. Sarcoidosis is extremely common in the West Indian population in Britain and in Martinicans living in France, but is there the same preponderance in their home environments? It is possible that sarcoidosis bobs to the surface not only in the wake of tuberculosis but also after the eradication of leprosy.

CLINICAL MANIFESTATIONS. A recent worldwide re-

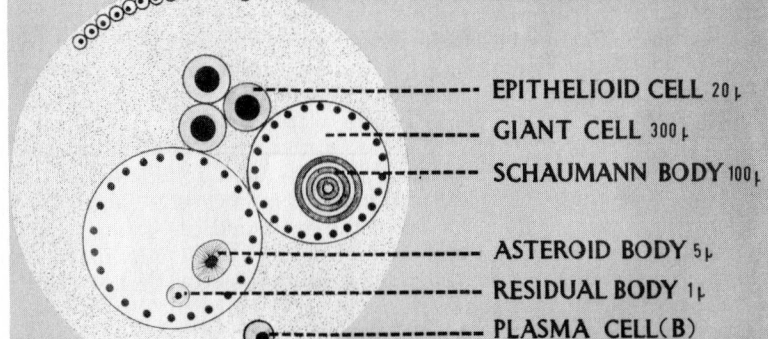

Figure 2. Features of a granuloma.

LYMPHOCYTE (T)
EPITHELIOID CELL 20 μ
GIANT CELL 300 μ
SCHAUMANN BODY 100 μ
ASTEROID BODY 5 μ
RESIDUAL BODY 1 μ
PLASMA CELL (B)

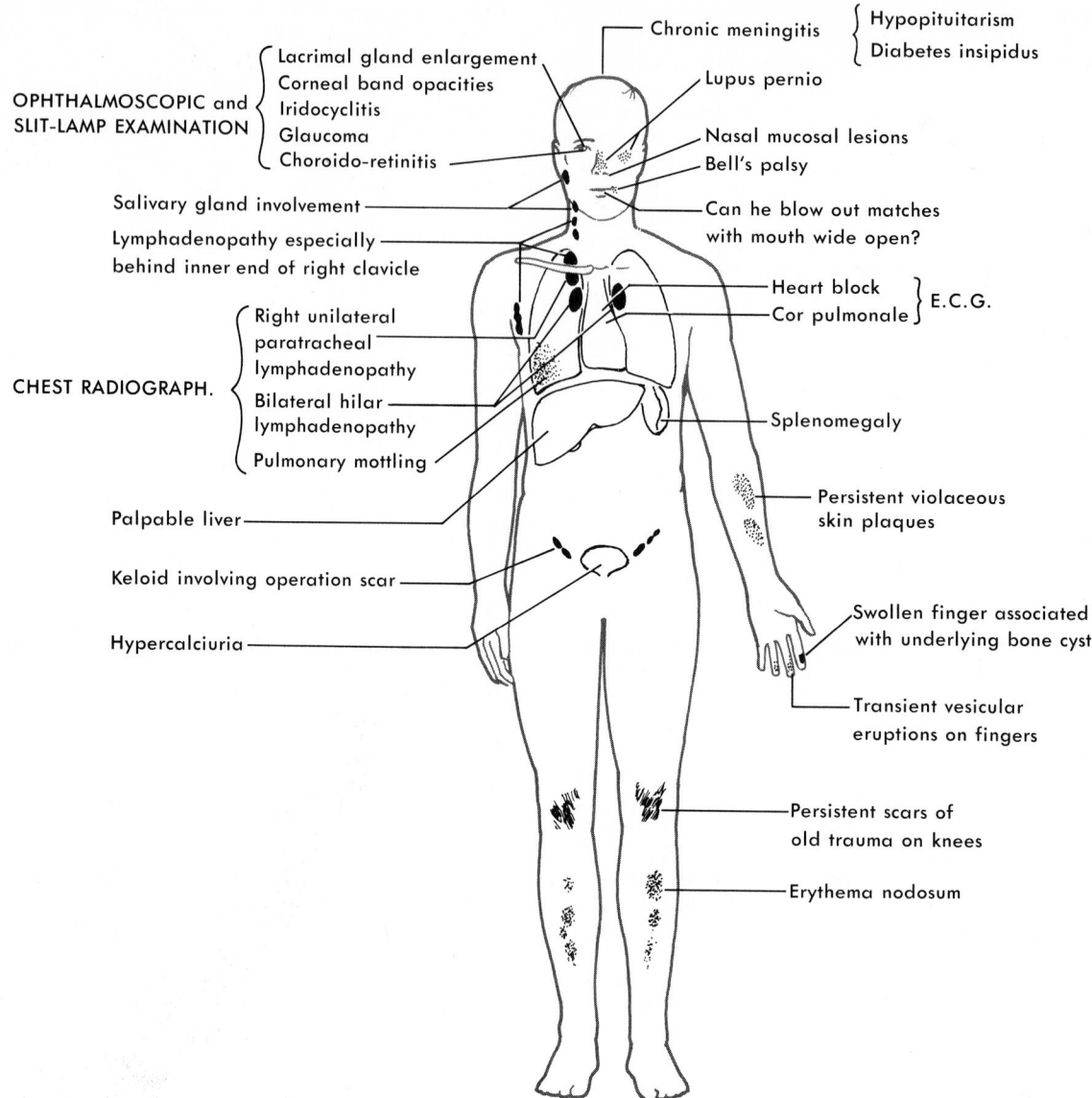

Figure 3. Clinical examination of a patient with suspected sarcoidosis.

view compares series of sarcoidosis in 11 cities. It comprises 3676 patients, 2082 (57 per cent) of whom were female and 2504 (68 per cent) of whom presented under 40 years of age (Table 1). The three common presentations were intrathoracic, dermatologic, and ophthalmic. An abnormal chest radiograph was the single most frequent presentation in 1475 patients (40 per cent), and another 783 (21 per cent) had respiratory symptoms. Seven hundred and thirty patients (20 per cent) presented with skin lesions; ocular lesions were observed in 539 (15 per cent).

Physical examination of the patient must be thorough (Fig. 3). It is incomplete unless accompanied by a chest radiograph, slit lamp examination of the eyes, and estimation of the 24-hour urinary calcium output. Multisystem involvement is a characteristic feature of sarcoidosis, with intrathoracic involvement in nine tenths of patients, ocular and skin involvement each occurring in about one quarter, and, depending on the series and country, erythema nodosum in up to one third of pa-

tients. Involvement of other tissues includes lymphadenopathy and splenomegaly in 28 per cent, neurosarcoidosis or salivary gland enlargement in 4 per cent, and bone cysts in about 3 per cent of patients (Table 1).

Sarcoidosis of the Upper Respiratory Tract. Sarcoidosis of the upper respiratory tract involves the nose, nasopharyngeal mucosa, and larynx. It is frequently associated with lupus pernio and may, in fact, precede and herald the onset of lupus pernio, a fact which is of practical clinical importance. It is a chronic manifestation occurring seven times more frequently in women and usually in the third decade, just as lupus pernio almost always occurs much more commonly in women in the fourth and fifth decades of life. A clinically significant point is that sarcoidosis may present to the nose and throat surgeon, who may perform a submucous resection for relief of nasal symptoms, with disastrous results including nasal septal perforation and progressive destruction of bone and cartilaginous septum.

Intrathoracic Sarcoidosis. Although only three fifths

TABLE 1. Data of a Worldwide Review of 3676 Patients with Sarcoidosis Followed in 11 Cities*

Features	Number of Patients	Per Cent
Total	3676	100
Women	2082	57
Age at presentation under 40 years	2504	68
Intrathoracic	3224	88
Lymph nodes and spleen	1031	28
Erythema nodosum	640	17
Other skin lesions	324	9
Ocular lesions	539	15
Parotid enlargement	160	4
Nervous system	134	4
Bones	109	3
Skin tests		
Positive Kveim-Siltzbach	1714/2189	78
Negative tuberculin	2093/3268	64
Hyperglobulinemia	808/1832	44
Hypercalcemia	200/1760	11
Treated with corticosteroids	1738	47
Mortality due to		
Sarcoidosis	84	2.2
Other causes	54	1.4

*London, New York, Paris, Los Angeles, Tokyo, Reading, Lisbon, Edinburgh, Novi Sad, Naples, Geneva. (From James, D. G., et al.: Ann. N.Y. Acad. Sci., 278:32, 1976.)

of patients have a respiratory presentation, a chest x-ray abnormality is evident at the onset in almost all patients; in the worldwide survey an abnormality was evident in 3377 (92 per cent) (Table 2).

STAGE 0. A clear chest radiograph in the presence of multisystem sarcoidosis was most unusual, occurring in only 277 patients (8 per cent).

STAGE 1. Bilateral hilar lymphadenopathy was noted in 1865 patients (51 per cent). Thus it was seen overall in half the series. Eventual resolution of this stage was noted in 65 per cent of the series overall.

STAGE 2. Hilar lymphadenopathy associated with pulmonary infiltration was the mode of presentation in 1066 (29 per cent). Chest x-ray resolution occurred in 49 per cent of these patients.

STAGE 3. It is unusual for the late stage of pulmonary infiltration with fibrosis to be a mode of presentation, and the overall resolution rate was only 20 per cent.

COURSE. When bilateral hilar lymphadenopathy alone is the initial chest x-ray appearance, the outcome is quite good, with clearance occurring in 65 per cent. When it is accompanied by erythema nodosum, the outcome is particularly favorable. Steroids are not usually necessary in these circumstances. The course of Stage 2 involvement is less favorable, and steroids are indicated to prevent progression to fibrosis. The course of Stage 3 involvement is poor, and steroids are mainly useful for relief of symptoms.

Skin Lesions. *Erythema nodosum* occurred in 640 patients (17 per cent). The incidence is higher in Britain and Scandinavia than elsewhere. It is infrequent in the black and the Asian.

Other skin lesions, including lupus pernio, maculo-papular rashes, plaques, subcutaneous nodules, and scars, occurred in 324 patients (9 per cent) of the worldwide survey. Skin disease is almost always but one manifestation of multisystem involvement, in which there is also intrathoracic disease (in nine tenths of patients), uveitis, peripheral lymphadenopathy, parotid gland enlargement, neuropathy, and bone cysts.

Ocular Lesions. If slit lamp examination is routine, uveitis is seen in one fourth of patients with sarcoidosis; however, sarcoidosis is responsible for only about 7 per cent of instances of uveitis. Ocular sarcoidosis comprises anterior and posterior uveitis, conjunctival lesions, keratoconjunctivitis, scleral plaques, retinal vasculitis, papilledema, and secondary glaucoma and cataract formation. There are certain well-defined ocular syndromes. *Heerfordt's or Waldenström's syndrome* consists of uveitis, parotid gland enlargement, fever, and, commonly, seventh cranial nerve palsy. Other components include bizarre neurologic manifestations, hyperalgesia, papilledema, meningism, and spinal fluid pleocytosis. *Löfgren's syndrome* comprises erythema nodosum, bilateral hilar lymphadenopathy and acute iritis. *Sjögren-like syndrome* consists of keratoconjunctivitis sicca with or without parotid and lacrimal gland enlargement, mimicking Sjögren's syndrome but without the arthritis which is a feature of the latter. *Chronic uveitis, lupus pernio, bone cysts, and pulmonary fibrosis* make up another well-defined syndrome.

Neurosarcoidosis. This occurs in about 4 to 7 per cent of patients with sarcoidosis. Facial palsy is the most frequent presentation either alone or with other cranial nerve palsies or with papilledema. Other features include peripheral neuropathy, myopathy, meningitis, space-occupying brain lesions, epilepsy, cerebellar ataxia, hypopituitarism, and diabetes insipidus. Neurosarcoidosis has a mortality of 10 per cent, which is twice the overall mortality of sarcoidosis. The response to corticosteroids is more likely to occur in younger patients with an explosive onset of meningitis with erythema nodosum than in those with a space-occupying intracranial mass with chronic skin lesions, chronic uveitis, or pulmonary fibrosis.

Heart. Myocardial sarcoidosis is difficult to recognize clinically. It should be considered if a patient with florid multisystem sarcoidosis develops bundle branch block, arrhythmias, congestive cardiac failure, pericarditis, or clinical evidence of cardiomyopathy. Sudden death without previous evidence of a heart lesion may occur, particularly in patients over 40 years of age. Macroscopic changes are most evident in the posterior part of the ventricular septum. Microscopy discloses granulomas or fibrous tissue or both.

Bone Cysts. Sarcoidosis of bone is most frequent in hands or feet, but rarely it involves temporal or frontal bone or the hard palate. It is associated with soft tissue swelling, joint stiffness, and pain. Involvement of other

TABLE 2. Intrathoracic Disease in a Worldwide Review of 3654 Patients with Sarcoidosis

Features	Patients	
	Number	Per Cent
Total series	3654	100
Stage at presentation:		
0	277	8
1	1865	51
2	1066	29
3	446	12
Resolution of chest roentgerams:		
Stage 1	1865	65
2	1066	49
3	446	20

systems includes lungs (in 77 per cent), lupus pernio and eyes (50 per cent), lymph nodes (32 per cent), parotids (23 per cent), liver (18 per cent), and spleen (14 per cent). There is no correlation between bone involvement and abnormal calcium metabolism. Three radiologic types of bone lesions are recognized:

PERMEATIVE. There is progressive cortical "tunneling" with remodeling of trabecular and cortical architecture.

LYTIC. Punched-out cysts are associated with pressure narrowing of the shaft, pathologic fractures, and residual cavities.

DESTRUCTIVE. Rapid destructive change may cause secondary joint surface involvement, and this may be followed by a periosteal reaction.

Pregnancy. Sarcoidosis is not a contraindication to pregnancy. In fact patients improve and are able to discontinue steroid therapy from the second trimester onward. Chest radiography is unnecessary until six months after delivery, which is the most likely time for recurrence. Excessive vitamin D intake during pregnancy must be avoided; it should be checked by determination of serum calcium level.

Childhood. In the Royal Northern Hospital, we have observed sarcoidosis in only one child under ten years of age, although we commonly see sarcoid granulomatous reactions which are mistakenly called sarcoidosis. Sarcoidosis should not be considered until the several other causes of granulomatous disorders — helminth infestation, mycobacterial infections, and chronic granulomatous disease of childhood — are excluded. We have noted sarcoidosis in 25 of 537 patients under 20 years of age (5 per cent). The main problem in management is that steroids are contraindicated in the growing child. Alternative treatments include corticotropin, oxyphenbutazone, indomethacin, and chloroquine.

DIAGNOSIS. Histology. The diagnosis is most secure when consistent clinical and radiographic findings are supported by histologic evidence of sarcoid tissue. The one without the other is commonly misconstrued. The clinical manifestations alone mimic many other disorders; conversely, histology of sarcoid granulomas alone is widely nonspecific. If there are skin lesions or peripheral lymphadenopathy, then biopsy will yield sarcoid tissue. *Fiberoptic bronchoscopy* with flexible forceps biopsy yields bronchial or lung tissue in four fifths of patients with intrathoracic disease. It is always positive in the early stage of hilar adenopathy and is least likely to be positive in those with pulmonary fibrosis.

Aspiration Liver Biopsy. This is invaluable for obtaining histologic confirmation, but it is important to establish the precise cause of the granuloma.

The histology of hepatic granulomas is similar, irrespective of the cause, so the cause is determined by collateral evidence. In Klatskin's series of 565 patients with epithelioid granulomas found on liver biopsy, the most common causes were sarcoidosis in 217 (38 per cent), underlying liver disease in 174 (31 per cent), tuberculosis in 70 (12 per cent), and schistosomiasis in 19 (3 per cent). These figures are very similar to those of our London survey, in which, of 138 patients with liver granulomas, 75 were found to have sarcoidosis (54 per cent), 26 had primary biliary cirrhosis (19 per cent), 23 had miscellaneous recognizable disorders (17 per cent), and 14 were undiagnosed (10 per cent). Ova are readily recognizable in schistosomiasis when one is alert to the possibility, but acid-fast bacilli are demonstrable in only one tenth of patients with tuberculosis. The Kveim-Siltzbach test is of considerable value, for it is positive in about 70 per cent of patients with sarcoidosis but negative in patients with hepatic granulomas due to other causes. Likewise, the antimitochondrial antibody test is almost always positive in primary biliary cirrhosis but rarely positive in other disorders.

Kveim-Siltzbach Skin Test. This is a simple, specific outpatient skin test using human sarcoid tissue. It was found to be positive in four fifths of patients with sarcoidosis in a recent worldwide survey (Table 1). It is particularly helpful in delineating multisystem sarcoidosis from the numerous other granulomatous disorders which mimic sarcoidosis. Kveim-Siltzbach antigen is a saline suspension of human sarcoid tissue prepared from the spleen of a patient suffering from active sarcoidosis. The antigen, 0.15 ml, is injected intradermally very superficially into the flexor surface of the forearm, and the inoculation site is observed for the development of a visible and palpable nodule during the ensuing six weeks. Any palpable nodule is examined by biopsy, usually one month after the injection, using a Hayes-Martin drill. This core of tissue is serially sectioned for evidence of sarcoid tissue or of a foreign body giant-cell reaction; this decision is made blind, i.e., without knowledge of the clinical picture. A Kveim-Siltzbach test is reported as positive if the intradermally injected antigen produces a nodule in the course of three to six weeks and if this nodule shows evidence of sarcoid tissue, as distinct from a foreign body giant-cell reaction.

KMIF Test. Efforts are being made to develop in vitro Kveim tests by investigating the response of peripheral lymphocytes from patients with sarcoidosis and controls to stimulation by Kveim-Siltzbach antigen, using guinea pig macrophages as the indicator cells. The technique is termed the Kveim-induced macrophage inhibition factor (KMIF) test. Sarcoid lymphocytes, when stimulated in vitro with sarcoid material, produce a macrophage inhibition factor with a migration index of less than 0.8 in three fourths of subjects. Steroids make the KMIF test negative, as they do the skin test.

Serum Angiotensin–Converting Enzyme (SACE). Assay of serum ACE is useful for confirming the diagnosis of active sarcoidosis. It is elevated in the majority of patients with active disease, but normal levels are observed in burnt-out sarcoidosis, in those receiving steroids, and in lymphoma, leukemia, and other granulomatous disorders. Reduced values have been noted in asthma, emphysema, cystic fibrosis, lung cancer, and tuberculosis. It is likely that elevated serum ACE levels reflect enzyme secretory activity by epithelioid cells of the sarcoid granuloma.

Tuberculin Reaction. The tuberculin skin test was negative at a dilution of 100 units or its equivalent in two thirds of patients in the world survey. It reflects depression of delayed type hypersensitivity and incompetent T cells. With steroid therapy or with cure there is a tendency for the tuberculin reaction to revert to the sensitivity noted before the onset of sarcoidosis.

Physiology. Two useful practical tests of lung function are the single-breath diffusing capacity and the vital capacity. In the earliest stages of bilateral hilar lymphadenopathy (Stage 1) there may be reduction in the diffusing capacity and also in arterial oxygen tension. With radiographic evidence of pulmonary involvement, there is also reduction of vital capacity, airway resistance, maximum midexpiratory flow, and arterial oxygen tension on exercise. As might be anticipated, physiologic impairment correlates well with radiographic staging of pulmonary sarcoidosis. The worse the pretreatment impairment, the greater the temporary improvement in pulmonary function with steroids.

Unlike progressive systemic sclerosis and diffuse interstitial fibrosis, sarcoidosis rarely damages the pulmonary capillary bed even in the late fibrotic stage, so membrane diffusing capacity and pulmonary capillary blood volume provide prognostic information.

BIOCHEMISTRY. Hydroxyprolinuria. This is a feature of active sarcoidosis. It is not observed in chronic fibrotic burnt-out sarcoidosis, so hydroxyprolinuria neatly distinguishes acute exudative from chronic fibrotic sarcoidosis.

Calcium Metabolism. Hypercalcemia and hypercalciuria are such well-recognized components of sarcoidosis that they have been written into the definition of the disorder; despite this, the precise mechanism of the abnormal calcium metabolism is ill understood. In the world survey of sarcoidosis, hypercalcemia was noted in 200 of 1760 patients (11 per cent) examined in various centers. In a personal series of 75 patients with histologically confirmed sarcoidosis in whom simultaneous serum and 24-hour urine calcium levels were determined, calcium was raised in the serum or urine in 37 (49 per cent), in serum and urine in 10 (13 per cent), in urine only in 27 (36 per cent), and never in the serum alone. Three lessons were learned from this study: (1) The natural history of the calcium derangement follows that of sarcoidosis in other systems. It is transient and self-limiting in acute sarcoidosis and may indeed be missed if not sought early enough. Persistent hypercalciuria, when it occurs, is associated with persistent sarcoidosis. (2) Hypercalciuria is much more frequent than hypercalcemia. Urinalysis is the more sensitive method for detecting abnormal calcium metabolism, but unfortunately it is also the more cumbersome. We did not observe hypercalcemia in the absence of hypercalciuria. (3) Abnormal calcium metabolism is one feature of a multisystem disorder in which intrathoracic abnormalities were noted in 91 per cent, peripheral lymphadenopathy in 24 per cent, skin lesions in 21 per cent, and uveitis in 15 per cent of patients.

Uric Acid Levels. Hyperuricemia reflects renal failure in sarcoidosis; there is no particular association between it and bone and joint involvement. Its importance lies in the differential diagnosis of a patient with hyperuricemia and punched-out bone cysts resembling gout. The sarcoidosis profile under these circumstances will be that of a patient with chronic fibrotic sarcoidosis, raised blood urea nitrogen levels, probably intrathoracic changes, hypercalciuria, and possible chronic uveitis and skin lesions. These features are as a rule sufficiently distinctive for differentiation from gout.

Serum Immunoglobulins. We observed abnormal immunoglobulin levels in 57 of 71 patients (80 per cent) with sarcoidosis; IgG was increased in 40 (56 per cent), IgA in 19 (27 per cent) and IgM in 9 (13 per cent). IgG was increased in half of the white and two thirds of the West Indian patients. IgA was equally distributed between the two races, but IgM levels were elevated in one third of the white and two thirds of the West Indian patients. There was no significant difference when immunoglobulin levels were compared in acute and chronic sarcoidosis groups. Abnormal IgG levels bore no special correlation with organ systems involved. There was no significant correlation between serum immunoglobulin levels and changes in chest roentgenograms, Kveim-Siltzbach tests, depression of delayed-type hypersensitivity, and hypercalcemia.

SERUM IgD. IgD is less likely to be detected in the serum of sarcoidosis patients and more likely in tuberculosis. High levels of IgD occur predominantly in older patients with tuberculosis, whereas depression of IgD occurs in middle-aged patients with sarcoidosis; the age dependence of IgD seems highly significant. Elevated levels of serum IgM in patients with sarcoidosis may represent a compensatory change associated with low levels of serum IgD.

SERUM IgE. Although there is considerable overlap, significantly higher levels seem to occur in sarcoidosis compared with tuberculosis and control groups.

DIFFERENTIAL DIAGNOSIS. There are numerous unrelated granulomatous disorders. The chest physician must distinguish sarcoidosis from tuberculosis and extrinsic allergic alveolitis; the gastroenterologist, from Crohn's enteritis and primary biliary cirrhosis; the ophthalmologist, from other causes of uveitis; and the general physician, from Hodgkin's disease. Sarcoidosis is a multisystem disorder, so it should be considered when the patient is seen to attend many different outpatient clinics, particularly respiratory, ophthalmic, and dermatologic. The quickest ways of distinguishing active sarcoidosis are the Kveim-Siltzbach skin test, which is negative in all other granulomatous disorders, and the elevated serum angiotensin-converting enzyme.

COURSE AND PROGNOSIS. There are two distinct forms of sarcoidosis, acute and chronic, with clear-cut differences in onset, natural history, course, prognosis, and response to treatment (Table 3).

Acute Sarcoidosis. There is an abrupt explosive onset most common in patients 30 years or younger. Involvement of skin, eyes, and lymph nodes is acute and eruptive, and the histology is that of exudative sarcoid tissue rich in epithelioid and giant cells. In this phase of the disorder there is a positive Kveim-Siltzbach test, hydroxyprolinuria, raised serum angiotensin-converting enzyme, and abnormal calcium metabolism. Spontaneous remission rate is high, and prognosis is good.

Transient flitting polyarthralgia commonly precedes or accompanies erythema nodosum, probably reflecting a circulating immune complex at this phase of the disorder. If the process is particularly acute and exudative with considerable prostaglandin production into the joint or eye, an effusion or severe uveitis will develop. Bone cysts and persistent polyarthritis do not occur in this form of the disease.

Chronic Sarcoidosis. There is an insidious, ill-recognized onset and a persistent unrelenting course in all tissue systems, predominantly seen in patients aged 40 years and over. The histology is that of chronic fibrotic hyaline fibrosis with little evidence of mononuclear, epithelioid, and giant cells. Hydroxyproline excretion and serum angiotensin-converting enzyme levels are both normal. the Kveim-Siltzbach test is like-

TABLE 3. Features Differentiating Acute from Chronic Sarcoidosis

Features	Acute (Transient)	Chronic (Persistent)
Age (years)	< 30	> 40
Onset	Abrupt	Insidious
Chest x-ray	Bilateral hilar lymphadenopathy	Pulmonary mottling
Eyes	Acute iritis, conjunctivitis, conjunctival nodules	Keratoconjunctivitis, chronic uveitis, glaucoma, cataract
Skin	Erythema nodosum, maculopapular rash, vesicular eruption	Lupus pernio, plaques, scars, keloids
Parotitis, Lymphadenopathy, Splenomegaly, Bell's palsy	Usually transient	Rarely permanent
Bone cysts	No	Yes
Histology	Epithelioid and giant cells	Hyaline fibrosis
Lung biopsy	Positive	Negative
Calcium metabolism	Hypercalcemia, hypercalciuria	Nephrocalcinosis
Urinary hydroxyproline	Increased	Normal
Serum angiotensin-converting enzyme	Increased	Normal
Kveim-Siltzbach test	Positive	May be negative
Spontaneous remission	Frequent	Rare
Steroid therapy	Abortive effect	Symptomatic relief
Alternative drugs	Oxyphenbutazone	Chloroquine, potassium para-amino-benzoate
Recurrence after steroid therapy	Rare	Frequent
Prognosis	Good	Poor

ly to be negative, and calcium metabolism is unremarkable; all these parameters point to lack of activity in this chronic fibrotic form of sarcoidosis (see Table 3).

It is in this form that bone cysts are noted, with overlying soft tissue swelling, joint involvement, persistent painful polyarthritis, and deformities.

Treatment is directed toward symptomatic relief only. The prognosis is poor, for the mortality is significantly increased because of lung failure, cor pulmonale and cardiac failure, and nephrocalcinosis with renal failure.

COMPLICATIONS. Pulmonary fibrosis may be followed by cor pulmonale and both respiratory and cardiac failure. Abnormal calcium metabolism may lead to nephrocalcinosis and renal failure. Chronic uveitis may be complicated by secondary glaucoma and cataract formation with failure of vision. Corticosteroid eyedrops may cause a rise in intraocular pressure, which contributes to glaucoma, and prolonged oral steroids may contribute to posterior cortical cataract formation. Myocardial sarcoidosis may be a cause of sudden death.

The overall mortality is 3.6 per cent (2.2 per cent directly caused by sarcoidosis and 1.4 per cent resulting from unrelated causes).

TREATMENT. Corticosteroids are the sheet anchor of treatment; they are particularly indicated for uveitis, worsening chest roentgenogram, breathlessness, persistent hypercalciuria, disfiguring skin lesions, myocardial and neurologic involvement, involvement of salivary and lacrimal glands, and hypersplenism.

There are alternative treatments when steroids are contraindicated or have proved ineffective; the choice depends on the form of disease, i.e., acute or chronic sarcoidosis. Oxyphenbutazone controls acute exudative sarcoidosis, whereas chloroquine and potassium para-aminobenzoate are indicated for chronic fibrotic sarcoidosis. Azathioprine may be considered for its temporary steroid-sparing effect, when otherwise massive doses of steroids would be necessary. Persistent hypercalciuria may require a low calcium diet and drugs which chelate with calcium in the intestine, sodium phytate, and inorganic phosphate.

Studies are now being made to see whether levamisole can repair defective cellular immunity with benefit.

Certain treatments, formerly popular but now contraindicated, include radiotherapy, calciferol, and antituberculous drugs.

James, D. G., Neville, E., Siltzbach, L. E., Turiaf, J., et al.: A worldwide review of sarcoidosis. Ann. N.Y. Acad. Sci., 278:321, 1976.

James, D. G., Neville, E., and Walker, A. N.: Immunology of sarcoidosis. Am. J. Med., 59:388, 1975.

Lieberman, J.: Serum angiotensin-converting enzyme in sarcoidosis. Am. J. Med., 59:365, 1975.

Sharma, O. P., Neville, E., Walker, A. N., and James, D. G.: Familial sarcoidosis: A possible genetic influence. Ann. N.Y. Acad. Sci., 278:386, 1976.

Siltzbach L. E. (ed.): Seventh International Conference on sarcoidosis and other granulomatous disorders. Ann. N.Y. Acad. Sci., 278:1, 1976.

66. POLYMYALGIA RHEUMATICA AND CRANIAL ARTERITIS

(Temporal Arteritis, Giant Cell Arteritis, Polymyalgia Arteritica)

Paul B. Beeson

66.1. INTRODUCTION

The two clinical syndromes of cranial arteritis and polymyalgia rheumatica are described together, because they are often associated and because of the probability that they represent different expressions of one process. The age distribution of patients is almost unique, and the diseases seem to follow similar courses. Most persons affected are more than 60 years of age; occurrence before age 50 is exceedingly rare. These disorders are very rare in Oriental peoples, and appear to be unknown in blacks or American Indians. The distribution of HL–A haplotypes is not remarkable. Although symptoms may come on quite abruptly and may cause serious incapacity for a time, the natural tendency is toward gradual improvement, with complete subsidence after a period of several months to several years. The remarkable age incidence and self-limited course must figure prominently in any attempt to determine the nature of these disorders. A possibility to be considered is delayed recrudescence of an infection acquired early in life, as with varicella and herpes zoster or louse-borne typhus and Brill's disease.

66.2. POLYMYALGIA RHEUMATICA

Polymyalgia rheumatica is a distinctive kind of muscular rheumatism in old people, more frequent in women than in men. It is characterized by pain and stiffness in the neck, shoulders, and back, and sometimes in the pelvic girdle. Tenderness and true muscle weakness are usually lacking. The stiffness may be particularly troublesome in the morning so that patients are barely able to get out of bed. There may be headache or painful areas over the cranium. Systemic manifestations aside from occasional low-grade pyrexia are not prominent. The patients have a vague sense of malaise simply described as "feeling rotten." Unfortunately these people are too often dismissed with the assumption that symptoms are caused by degenerative processes about which little or nothing can be done.

The distinctive laboratory finding is marked elevation of the erythrocyte sedimentation rate, i.e., more than 80 mm by the Westergren method. Mild anemia is not uncommon, and some hematologists are reporting cases of unexplained anemia in old people which, like the muscular symptoms, respond promptly to steroid therapy. Other laboratory tests are of little help. Muscle biopsy generally reveals no significant inflammatory change even when the tissue is taken from areas which seem to be the site of much pain and stiffness. Blood enzymes which sometimes become elevated in other disorders of muscle are normal in this disease. There may be slight elevation of the alpha 2 globulin. Electromyographic findings are normal. Hepatic dysfunction may be reflected by moderately elevated blood alkaline phosphatase. A possible element of autoimmunity is indicated by the observation that lymphocyte transformation occurs in the presence of muscle tissue, especially during acute phases of the symptoms. The affected muscles do not atrophy.

Because of the frequent association of polymyalgia rheumatica with cranial arteritis, and especially because cranial arteritis may cause sudden blindness, some experienced clinicians believe that biopsy of a temporal artery should be carried out in all patients with polymyalgia rheumatica. When this has been done as a routine procedure, the artery has shown the characteristic changes in more than half the cases, regardless of clinical manifestations of arteritis. Others regard this as unnecessary because a trial of steroid therapy, which would be appropriate for cranial arteritis as well as for polymyalgia, will be carried out in any event. Visual disturbances are known to occur in this disorder, but their incidence is far lower than in patients with the clinical picture of cranial arteritis.

In the differential diagnosis, rheumatoid arthritis and degenerative joint disease may present problems; however, careful questioning and examination will show that polymyalgia is a disease of muscles, not joints. Various neoplastic diseases, including multiple myeloma, have to be considered in the differential diagnosis. Similarly the collagen diseases, especially polymyositis, may resemble polymyalgia rheumatica.

Therapy with adrenal steroids is remarkably effective, usually bringing about prompt amelioration of symptoms. It should be begun with a moderately large dose, e.g., 40 to 60 mg of prednisone daily for the first week, with gradual reduction over the next few weeks to a maintenance dose of 7 to 12 mg daily for a long time.

Some experienced observers recommend at least two years of this low-dose therapy for all patients. In one large study it was found that treatment had to be maintained for at least five years in 84 per cent of cases. There are cases on record in which the symptoms have persisted for as long as ten years. Usually, by occasional trials of reduced dosage and by following the sedimentation rate, the physician can determine when to terminate steroid therapy.

Coomes, E. N., Ellis, R. M., and Kay, A. G.: A prospective study of 102 patients with the polymyalgia rheumatica syndrome. Rheumatol. Rehab., 15:270, 1976.

Esiri, M. M., MacLennan, I. C. M., and Hazleman, B. L.: Lymphocyte sensitivity to skeletal muscle in patients with polymyositis and other disorders. Clin. Exp. Immunol., 14:25, 1973.

Hamrin, B.: Polymyalgia arteritica. Acta Med. Scand., Suppl. 533, pp. 1–131, 1972.

Von Knorring, J., and Wasastjerna, C.: Liver involvement in polymyalgia rheumatica. Scand. J. Rheumatol., 5:197, 1976.

66.3. CRANIAL ARTERITIS

This entity, like polymyalgia rheumatica, occurs only in people past middle age. In a substantial proportion of cases, symptoms resembling those of polymyalgia rheumatica are present weeks or months before the onset of the severe headache which characterizes cranial arteritis. Occasionally the only clinical presentation is that of fever of unexplained origin. The distinctive feature is a granulomatous arteritis, affecting large and medium-sized arteries of the upper part of the body, especially the temporal vessels. Histologic study reveals intimal thickening, and lymphocytic infiltration of the media and adventitia. In the media there are usually numerous giant cells, of the Langhans type. Eosinophils are not conspicuous. "Skip" areas do occur, and it is advantageous to make several sections of the vessel segment chosen for biopsy.

Cranial arteritis often has an abrupt onset, with severe pain usually in one temple but sometimes in the occipital area, face, jaw, or side of the neck. This may be associated with exquisite hyperesthesia so that the patient dislikes touching the scalp, combing the hair, or washing. The pain may have a throbbing character. Pain in the tongue, blanching of the tongue, and even gangrene of the tongue have been described in this disorder, doubtless ascribable to involvement of lingual arteries. Peripheral neuropathy with both sensory and motor components has also been described. The temporal artery may be tender, thickened, and nodular; conversely it may be pulseless and impalpable. The erythrocyte sedimentation rate is elevated, and there may be a substantial fever and polymorphonuclear leukocytosis.

The most feared complication of cranial arteritis is impairment of vision. It usually develops within three months of onset of other manifestations, and can be the first sign of the disease. This may consist of blindness in one or both eyes. The pattern of involvement may be uniocular, resulting from disease of the ophthalmic artery, or occipital, resulting from disease of the vertebral artery. Visual symptoms can also be caused by weakness of extraocular muscles. A precise estimate of the frequency of this complication cannot be made, because patients with visual symptoms receive special medical attention. Some articles state that visual impairment occurs in 50 per cent of cases, but this may be too high. The danger is real, and it is generally agreed that all patients with active cranial arteritis should receive steroid treatment, especially to prevent visual loss. There is also suggestive evidence that patients with cranial arteritis are at special risk of certain other vascular accidents, including brainstem strokes and coronary occlusion.

Although it cannot be doubted that the arteries most often affected are branches of the external carotid (accounting for the use of such names as cranial arteritis and temporal arteritis), it should be recognized that other arteries may also be the site of giant cell arteritis. Autopsy has disclosed arteritis in the aorta and even in the hepatic and renal vessels. Instances of aortic aneurysm thought to be due to giant cell arteritis are on record. These may result from an associated pathologic process described under a variety of names such as medial aortopathy.

Steroid therapy should be given according to the plan outlined for polymyalgia rheumatica.

Cullen, J. F., and Coleiro, J. A.: Review. Ophthalmic complications of giant cell arteritis. Surv. Ophthalmol., 20:247, 1976.

Ghose, M. K., Shensa, S., and Lerner, P. I.: Arteritis of the aged (giant cell arteritis) and fever of unexplained origin. Am. J. Med., 60:429, 1976.

Klein, R. G., Campbell, R. J., Hunder, G. G., and Carney, J. A.: Skip lesions in temporal arteritis. Mayo Clin. Proc., 51:504, 1976.

Swinson, D. R., Goodwill, C. J., and Talbot, I. C.: Giant cell arteritis presenting as subclavian occlusion. A report of two cases. Postgrad. Med. J., 52:525, 1976.

Wilkinson, I. M. S., and Russell, R. W. R.: Arteries of the head and neck in giant cell arteritis. Arch. Neurol., 27:378, 1972.

67. RELAPSING POLYCHONDRITIS

Paul B. Beeson

This is a rare but clinically distinctive disease characterized by inflammation and degeneration of cartilaginous structures. It occurs in persons of all ages, but most often in early and middle adult life. The sexes are about equally susceptible. Most of the reported cases have been in whites, but the disease has been observed in a few blacks and Orientals. The course is usually one of many years, with unpredictable fluctuations.

The pathologic lesion is primarily a loss of the mucopolysaccharide matrix in the affected cartilage. During acute flare-ups, neutrophil infiltration of the superficial portions of the cartilage is found; later, however, the inflammatory reaction is granulomatous in character, with predominance of lymphocytes; the end result is fibrosis.

The cause is unknown. Papain will cause similar changes in animals, and some metabolic disorder could be responsible. The prevailing conjecture is that the disorder has an immunologic basis. Both humoral and cellular reactions with cartilaginous antigens have been said to be demonstrable in patients with the disorder; perhaps the clearest evidence is lymphocyte transformation and macrophage migration inhibition by the cells of affected patients in reactions with purified cartilage matrix. It is also noteworthy that other "autoimmune" diseases have been present in about one third of the reported cases of relapsing polychondritis.

The most common site of inflammation is the carti-laginous structures of the ear. The lobe of the ear is spared, but the pinna becomes red or violaceous, tender, and swollen. Another common site of disease is the nasal septum, which, especially if subjected to ill-advised submucous resection, can cause a saddle-nose deformity resembling that seen in syphilis. Hoarseness may result from laryngeal injury, and life-threatening respiratory obstruction can be caused by degeneration of the cartilaginous rings of the trachea and bronchi. The cartilages of joints may be affected, so that monarthritis or polyarthritis may be prominent manifestations. The arthritis rarely progresses to bony destruction, and is not associated with subcutaneous nodules or rheumatoid factor in the blood. The sclera may become inflamed, and severe degeneration can lead to blindness. Involvement of inner ear structures or the eustachian tubes may cause deafness, tinnitus, or vertigo.

Other sites of damage, with potentially serious effects, are the aortic valve ring and the media of the aorta. Aortic incompetence and aortic aneurysms (either in the thorax or the abdomen) are found in approximately 10 per cent of patients. The "floppy mitral valve syndrome" has also been observed to develop during the course of this disease.

Standard clinical laboratory tests are unhelpful, except that the erythrocyte sedimentation rate is a useful index of activity.

Steroid therapy has been the main form of treatment and tends to damp down the intensity of the inflammatory manifestations. It may have to be continued over long periods of time, the dose being adjusted to the intensity of the symptoms. Immunosuppressive drugs have also been tried. Recently a few reports of dramatic "cure" of the disease by the use of dapsone (100 mg twice daily), have appeared; this treatment deserves further trial in view of its simplicity and small risk of toxicity. Surgery may be required for aortic valve incompetence or aortic aneurysm.

The course is unpredictable. Some patients have died as a result of respiratory or cardiovascular disease, many have continued to have low-grade and variable activity for years, and some have appeared to go into complete remission.

Arkin, C. R., and Masi, A. T.: Relapsing polychondritis: Review of current status and case report. Sem. Arth. Rheumatism, 5:41, 1975.

Barranco, V. P., Minor, D. B., and Solomon, H.: Treatment of relapsing polychondritis with dapsone. Arch. Dermatol., 112:1286, 1976.

Cipriano, P. R., et al.: Multiple aortic aneurysms in relapsing polychondritis. Am. J. Cardiol., 37:1097, 1976.

McAdam, L. P., et al.: Relapsing polychondritis: Prospective study of 23 patients and a review of the literature. Medicine, 55:193, 1976.

68. WEGENER'S GRANULOMATOSIS

Anthony S. Fauci

DEFINITION. Wegener's granulomatosis is characterized by the classic clinicopathologic features of necrotizing granulomatous vasculitis involving the upper and lower respiratory tracts, glomerulonephritis, and variable degrees of systemic, small vessel vasculitis.

ETIOLOGY. The cause is unknown, although it is generally considered to represent an aberrant hypersensitivity reaction to an unknown antigen. There have been no associations with allergic diatheses, geographic location, travel, or domestic or occupational exposure.

INCIDENCE AND PREVALENCE. Although an uncommon disease, Wegener's granulomatosis is no longer thought of as being extremely rare, as it is now recognized earlier and more frequently in clinical practice. The male:female ratio is approximately 3:2. The disease can be seen in any age group from infancy to old age. The peak incidence is in the fourth and fifth decades.

PATHOLOGY AND PATHOGENESIS. The characteristic histopathologic features of this disease are necrotizing vasculitis of small arteries and veins together with granuloma formation.

The upper airway disease most often is manifested by involvement of the paranasal sinuses and nasopharynx with necrotizing granuloma, with or without demonstrable vasculitis. Pansinusitis with erosion of adjacent bone may occur, as well as nasal septal perforation and saddle nose deformity.

Almost all patients have lung involvement (see Ch. 346.4). The infiltrates may take any form, but are usually multiple, bilateral, and nodular, with a tendency to cavitate.

Histopathologically, the renal lesion begins as a focal and segmental necrotizing glomerulitis which may lead to rapidly progressive glomerulonephritis and renal failure.

In addition to these classic features, virtually any organ can be involved with granuloma, vasculitis, or both.

The immunopathogenesis of the disease remains an enigma. Circulating immune complexes and immune complex–like renal deposits have been demonstrated in some patients. In contradistinction, the extensive granuloma formation in various organs is suggestive of delayed type hypersensitivity or cellular immune mechanisms. It is possible that there is an overlap of more than one type of immunologic mechanism, or that there is a granulomatous response to a particular type of immune complex in this disease.

CLINICAL MANIFESTATIONS. Wegener's granulomatosis is truly a multisystem disease manifesting a variety of signs and symptoms. However, in most patients the upper airway and, less frequently, the pulmonary symptoms dominate the presenting clinical picture.

Patients usually complain of severe upper respiratory symptoms and signs such as paranasal sinus pain, drainage, and purulent or bloody nasal discharge. Nasal mucosal ulceration and septal perforation may occur, as well as the classic saddle nose deformity. Serous otitis media commonly results from eustachian tube blockage, and variable degrees of hearing impairment may occur.

Eye involvement is seen at some time in up to 60 per cent of patients and may range from mild conjunctivitis to severe episcleritis, granulomatous sclerouveitis, ciliary vessel vasculitis, and proptosis.

Pulmonary manifestations may include cough, hemoptysis, chest discomfort, and shortness of breath. However, it is not uncommon that asymptomatic pulmonary infiltrates are discovered on chest x-ray during workup for other problems.

Nonspecific symptoms such as weakness, malaise, arthralgia, anorexia, and weight loss are common. Fever may result from the underlying disease, but often reflects secondary infection in paranasal sinuses.

Skin disease resulting from vasculitis with or without granuloma is seen in more than 40 per cent of patients.

Heart involvement is infrequent and usually appears as pericarditis or coronary vasculitis. Nervous system involvement, seen in up to 20 per cent of patients, may be exhibited in the form of cranial neuritis, mononeuritis multiplex, or cerebral vasculitis and/or granuloma.

Renal disease usually determines the course and ultimate outcome of generalized Wegener's granulomatosis. Proteinuria with variable degrees of hematuria, red blood cell casts, and other sediment abnormalities may indicate smoldering disease activity. However, once renal function abnormalities appear, evidence of rapidly progressive glomerulonephritis usually ensues, leading to renal failure if appropriate therapy is not instituted. A limited form of Wegener's granulomatosis without renal involvement has been described. However, it most likely constitutes part of the spectrum of the generalized disease.

There are no diagnostic laboratory findings in this disease. The erythrocyte sedimentation rate is invariably markedly elevated. Mild anemia and leukocytosis may be seen, but eosinophilia is not characteristic. Mildly elevated bentonite flocculation titers for rheumatoid factor are common, as is mild hypergammaglobulinemia, particularly of IgA.

DIAGNOSIS. Clinically, the diagnosis can be strongly suspected when the classic picture of upper and lower airway disease together with evidence of renal involvement is present. It is confirmed by the histopathologic demonstration of necrotizing granulomatous vasculitis in appropriate tissues such as nasal or sinus mucosa. The pulmonary infiltrates are the source of tissue with the highest diagnostic yield. Percutaneous renal biopsy is extremely important in documenting glomerulonephritis, particularly in early disease or when the diagnosis is unclear by other parameters.

Recognition of the classic clinicopathologic complex of Wegener's granulomatosis should make differentiation from other similar disorders relatively easy. However, differential diagnosis should include other vasculitides, connective tissue diseases, infectious and noninfectious granulomatous diseases, and tumors of the upper airway or lung. Goodpasture's syndrome is differentiated by the demonstration of antiglomerular basement membrane antibody. Idiopathic midline granuloma (see Ch. 69) is a localized destructive disease which mutilates the upper airway and facial tissues. Wegener's granulomatosis does not erode through facial tissue, and idiopathic midline granuloma does not include lung or renal disease. Of particular interest in the differential diagnosis is a disease called *lymphomatoid granulomatosis.* It involves predominantly lungs, skin, central nervous system, and kidney. It is clearly different from Wegener's granulomatosis. The vasculitis is really an invasion and destruction of vessels by atypical lymphocytoid and plasmacytoid cells resembling a lymphoma; the renal disease is not a glomerulonephritis but a nodular infiltration of the kidney by these bizarre lymphoid cells; and upper airway disease is quite uncommon.

TREATMENT AND PROGNOSIS. The treatment of choice in this disease is cytotoxic agents, and of the cytotoxic agents, cyclophosphamide is clearly the most effective. It should be given in daily oral doses of 1 to 2 mg per kilogram per day. In initiation of treatment in fulminant cases, the drug may be given intravenously in doses of 4 to 5 mg per kilogram per day for a few days, with subsequent change to the lower oral dosage regimen. It is important to emphasize that therapeutic response can usually be induced and maintained without causing severe leukopenia. Leukocyte counts should be closely monitored during therapy, and dosages of cyclophosphamide should be adjusted to maintain the leukocyte count above 3000 per cubic millimeter and the neutrophil count no less than 1000 to 1500 per cubic millimeter in order to avoid risk of infection. In patients who cannot tolerate cyclophosphamide, azathioprine in similar doses may be used.

Corticosteroids can be used initially, together with cyclophosphamide if disease activity is fulminant. Prednisone, 60 mg per day for a brief period of time, is recommended until the cyclophosphamide becomes effective (usually within 14 days). The prednisone should then be converted to an alternate day regimen, tapered, and discontinued. Serious eye involvement is a medical emergency and constitutes one of the only absolute indications for a limited course of corticosteroids. Other situations in which courses of adjunctive corticosteroids may be used are with serosal disease such as pericarditis or with central nervous system vasculitis.

The disease was formally universally fatal, usually within months after onset of renal disease. With cyclophosphamide use, the prognosis is quite good, and long-term remissions are induced in a high percentage of patients. Several patients have maintained remission for years following discontinuation of cyclophosphamide. It is recommended that the drug be continued for at least 1 year following induction of complete remission.

Carrington, C. B., and Liebow, A. A.: Limited forms of angiitis and granulomatosis of Wegener's type. Am. J. Med., 41:497, 1966.

Fauci, A. S.: Granulomatous vasculitides: Distinct but related. Ann. Intern. Med., 87:782, 1977.

Fauci, A. S., and Wolff, S. M.: Wegener's granulomatosis: Studies in eighteen patients and a review of the literature. Medicine, 52:535, 1973.

Liebow, A. A., Carrington, C. R. B., and Friedman, P. J.: Lymphomatoid granulomatosis. Hum. Pathol., 3:457, 1972.

Reza, M. J., Dornfeld, L., Goldberg, L. S., Bluestone, R., and Pearson, C. M.: Wegener's granulomatosis. Long-term followup of patients treated with cyclophosphamide. Arthritis Rheum., 18:501, 1975.

Wolff, S. M., Fauci, A. S., Horn, R. G., and Dale, D. C.: Wegener's granulomatosis. Ann. Intern. Med., 81:513, 1974.

69. MIDLINE GRANULOMA

Anthony S. Fauci

DEFINITION. Midline granuloma is a relentlessly progressive, localized destructive process that predominantly involves the nose, paranasal sinuses, and palate, with erosion through contiguous structures such as the orbit and face. It destroys soft tissue, cartilage, and bone, and is characterized by nonspecific acute and chronic inflammation and necrosis with or without granuloma formation. It is an uncommon disease which was first described in 1897 by McBride.

ETIOLOGY. The cause of midline granuloma is unknown. Since the disease is characterized by a granulomatous inflammatory reaction suggestive of a hypersensitivity or immunologically mediated phenomenon, it has been hypothesized that this represents a localized hypersensitivity response to an unidentified antigen. Under certain circumstances the tissues of the upper airways can respond very intensely to the presence of an antigenic stimulation. It is this hyperreactivity to an

unknown stimulus which leads to the inflammatory reaction and subsequent tissue destruction characteristic of this disease. Although some patients report histories of allergic rhinitis and chronic sinusitis, there is no evidence of these conditions being predisposing factors in this disease. Biopsy materials have been cultured for various microorganisms, and no etiologic connections have been found. Certain upper airway tumors can result in inflammatory and granulomatous responses which likewise can cause necrosis and destruction of tissue. The inflammatory response is often so intense that the underlying histopathology of the neoplasm can be masked and the process closely resembles midline granuloma. However, it is clear that true midline granuloma is a distinct entity in which no identifiable cause of the localized destructive inflammatory process can be found despite multiple deep biopsies, long term followup, and even postmortem examination. This entity should appropriately be referred to as idiopathic midline granuloma, as opposed to the inflammatory and even granulomatous responses associated with upper airway neoplasms.

PATHOLOGY. The typical histopathologic features are nonspecific acute and chronic inflammation with necrosis. The tissue is infiltrated with neutrophils, monocytes, lymphocytes, plasma cells, and, in some cases, eosinophils. Although true granuloma formation with or without typical Langhans giant cells are considered the hallmark of the disease, this may not be present in every case and is often masked by the fulminant inflammation and necrosis. Thrombosis of small vessels, perivascular cellular infiltration, and secondary involvement of vessels resulting from the inflammatory process may occur, but true primary vasculitis is rarely seen. If neoplastic cells are identified, the process obviously can no longer be considered idiopathic midline granuloma. Secondary pyogenic infection of the involved tissue with its added inflammatory response is frequently found to a greater or lesser degree.

CLINICAL MANIFESTATIONS. The disease can occur in all age groups, but most patients are in the fifth and sixth decades. It is slightly more common in women than men and occurs in all races.

The clinical presentation can vary from patient to patient, but in most cases symptoms can first be related to the nose and paranasal sinuses with rhinorrhea and nasal stuffiness. Symptoms persist and intensify, often followed by purulent nasal discharge resulting from superimposed infection. Nonhealing ulcerations of the nasal mucosa occur, and perforation of the nasal septum is frequently seen. Some patients present with disease in the oral cavity either alone or concomitant with nasal and paranasal sinus involvement. This usually occurs as ulcerations of the buccal mucosa, gums, or hard and soft palate. Some patients have presented with relatively painless perforation of the palate noted by the regurgitation of food or saliva into the nasal cavity. Occasionally, patients initially complain of symptoms related to the eye. The disease may be relatively indolent or fulminant, but it is always progressive. Relentless destruction of soft tissue, cartilage, and bone occur. Erosion of paranasal sinus walls occur, with spread into contiguous structures such as the orbit with subsequent eye involvement. Destruction of the soft and hard palate, the nasal septum, and even the entire nose occurs. If left untreated, the destructive process erodes through the skin of the face, resulting in dramatic mutilation of facial structures. This understandably leads to severe psychologic difficulties in some patients. The necrotic tissue as well as the paranasal sinus cavities frequently becomes infected, usually with *Staphylococcus aureus*, and this compounds the systemic symptoms of anorexia and malaise. The necrotic tissue can be quite malodorous, although the patients themselves frequently lose their sense of smell early in the course of the destructive process. It is of interest that local lymphadenopathy rarely occurs, and that when present it is suggestive of an underlying malignancy.

There are no characteristic laboratory findings except those related to the inflammatory process such as leukocytosis, elevated erythrocyte sedimentation rate, mild anemia of chronic disease, and hyperglobulinemia. Roentgenographic studies reveal pansinusitis with destruction of various cartilaginous and bony structures of the upper airways. The disease remains localized, and laboratory abnormalities related to other organ systems should prompt one to investigate other possible causes.

Although the disease may wax and wane in its progression, if left untreated, it is uniformly fatal. It has been reported that surgical procedures in the involved areas can lead to rapid acceleration of the disease, although, following appropriate treatment, debridement of necrotic areas may be beneficial to healing. Death usually occurs from secondary systemic infection or from inanition. Other causes of death are erosion into a major blood vessel with exsanguination or erosion into the central nervous system and subsequent meningitis.

DIAGNOSIS. The diagnosis of midline granuloma is made by the characteristic histopathologic findings in biopsies of the involved tissues together with the characteristic clinical presentation, but, most important, after other diseases with similar clinicopathologic findings have been ruled out.

Midline granuloma is sometimes confused with Wegener's granulomatosis. They are clearly distinct entities. Wegener's granulomatosis is a systemic disease characterized by necrotizing granulomatous vasculitis of the upper and lower respiratory tracts with glomerulonephritis (in the generalized form). Midline granuloma rarely manifests true primary vasculitis in the lesions and by definition is a localized disease without pulmonary or renal involvement. Furthermore, the destructive qualities of the upper airway lesions are different. Wegener's granulomatosis rarely or never causes palatal perforation and does not erode through facial tissues.

The greatest difficulty in differential diagnosis arises in distinguishing true idiopathic midline granuloma from neoplasms of the upper airways, particularly midline malignant reticulosis and certain lymphomas. Since these neoplasms can elicit destructive granulomatous reactions similar to those of midline granuloma, their true malignant histopathology can be masked by the intense inflammatory reaction. Careful search for disseminated malignancy as well as complete examination of multiple adequate biopsy specimens often reveals the neoplastic nature of these other disorders while confirming the true idiopathic nature of true cases of midline granuloma.

Other diseases which must be ruled out by appropriate cultures, special stains of tissue specimens, and/or other diagnostic laboratory tests are infectious diseases such as tuberculosis, syphilis, lepromatous leprosy, histoplasmosis, blastomycosis, coccidioidomycosis, mucocutaneous leishmaniasis, and rhinoscleroma (caused by a *Klebsiella* species). Also included in the differential diagnosis is pseudotumor of the orbit.

TREATMENT. Surgical excision of the involved tissues has been attempted, only to result in continued progression and, in some cases, acceleration of the disease. Corticosteroid therapy likewise is ineffective and can cause worsening if infection is present. Cytotoxic agents have been used with reports of variable results, most of which were ultimately failures, or the diseases being treated were misdiagnosed as midline granuloma and were in reality midline neoplasms or Wegener's granulomatosis.

The treatment of choice clearly is local radiation therapy. It has been reported that low dose irradiation of 1000 rads or less induced remissions. However, relapses are common after such low doses, whereas high dose (5000 rads) radiotherapy to the involved areas has been shown to result in a high percentage of remissions.

PROGNOSIS. If left untreated, the disease is uniformly fatal. Since the use of high dose local radiotherapy, the prognosis for survival is excellent, with greater than 70 per cent remission rate and even cures after more than 10 years of follow-up. Hence the disease should no longer be referred to as "lethal" midline granuloma. It should be pointed out that high dose radiotherapy to this area is associated in some cases with serious complications and side effects. However, the risk is outweighed by the fatal alternative. The mutilation and disfigurement which result from far advanced disease are often a source of great psychologic difficulty now that survival is feasible. In this regard, reconstructive plastic surgery, as well as placement of prostheses, has resulted in dramatic functional and cosmetic improvements in patients in remission.

Blatt, I. M., Seltzer, H. S., Rubin, P., Furstenberg, A. C., Maxwell, J. H., and Schull, W. J.: Fatal granulomatosis of the respiratory tract (lethal midline granuloma — Wegener's granulomatosis). Arch. Otolaryngol., 70:7907, 1959.

Fauci, A. S., Johnson, R. E., and Wolff, S. M.: Radiation therapy of midline granuloma. Ann. Intern. Med., 84:140, 1976.

Fauci, A. S., and Wolff, S. M.: Wegener's granulomatosis: Studies in eighteen patients and a review of the literature. Medicine, 52:535, 1973.

Fechner, R. E., and Lamppin, D. W.: Midline malignant reticulosis. A clinicopathologic entity. Arch. Otolaryngol., 95:467, 1972.

Friedmann, I.: Midline granuloma. Proc. Roy. Soc. Med., 57:289, 1964.

Stewart, J. P.: Progressive lethal granulomatous ulceration of the nose. J. Laryngol., 48:657, 1933.

Walton, E. W.: Reticuloendothelial sarcoma arising in the nose and palate (granuloma gangrenescens). J. Clin. Pathol., 13:279, 1960.

70. WEBER-CHRISTIAN DISEASE

(Relapsing Febrile Nodular Nonsuppurative Panniculitis, Panniculitis)

Paul B. Beeson

In this chapter several unusual syndromes are described which may or may not be variants of the same disease. The feature shared by all is the occurrence of localized inflammatory lesions in adipose tissue.

The term *Weber-Christian disease* is usually applied to a clinical syndrome in which the principal involvement is in the panniculus adiposus. Young or middle-aged women are affected more frequently than men with this form of the disease. It is characterized by development of multiple tender nodules in the subcutaneous fat, from 5 mm to 10 cm in diameter. The lesions are located principally on the thighs and trunk and in the breasts. They are tender, and there may be some reddening of the skin. Occasionally necrosis of the skin leads to sinus formation with discharge of an oily liquid. The course is usually indolent; crops of lesions develop from time to time over periods of months or years. When the inflammation subsides, there often remains an area of loss of subcutaneous tissue which causes dimpling of skin. Systemic manifestations are usually mild, but may include malaise, low-grade fever, leukocytosis, and eosinophilia. Enlargement of the liver and spleen is reported in some cases. The illness may grumble along for months or several years and then cease.

A more serious expression of this pathologic process has been termed *systemic Weber-Christian disease*. Here there is widespread inflammation affecting not only the panniculus adiposus but also similar tissue within the abdominal and thoracic cavities. There may be parenchymatous inflammation, affecting thoracic or abdominal organs, including lungs, pericardium, pleura, bowel, spleen, kidneys, and adrenal glands. At least a dozen cases are recorded in which this form of disease has led to death.

The terms *mesenteric panniculitis* and *mesenteric lipodystrophy* have been applied to an obscure disease characterized by inflammation of the mesenteric fat. This has been encountered mainly in males, and reports of the syndrome have appeared principally in surgical journals. Symptoms include recurrent episodes of fever, abdominal pain, nausea, vomiting, and malaise. At operation the mesentery is found to be thickened, with red or yellow patches, and biopsy reveals the characteristic panniculitis or simply infiltration with lipid-laden macrophages, which may be indistinguishable from the histology of "Weber-Christian disease." Several writers have suggested that these forms of inflammation in the retroperitoneal adipose tissue may represent the initial lesion in at least some cases of retroperitoneal fibrosis. An association between some of the panniculitis syndromes and alpha$_1$-antitrypsin deficiency has been observed (Rubinstein et al., 1977). In a series of 54 cases from the Mayo Clinic, 8, or 15 per cent, were associated with malignant lymphoma. This seems more than coincidence.

An important differential diagnostic point arises in distinction of the fatty lesions in the syndromes described here from the syndromes associated with pancreatitis or acinar cell carcinoma of the pancreas. In these there may develop crops of discrete areas of inflammation in the subcutaneous fat, as well as in the fatty tissues of the body cavities, resulting from liberation of excessive quantities of pancreatic lipase. Undoubtedly this has led to confusion with other forms of lipodystrophy, such as the Weber-Christian syndrome or mesenteric panniculitis. Despite some statements to the contrary, it seems unlikely that the histologic changes found in various stages of these groups of conditions are sufficiently distinctive to permit differentiation on histologic grounds alone. In the pancreatic-

associated lesions elevation of blood lipase may provide the best clue.

Classically the pathologic findings in Weber-Christian disease are said to progress through three stages. In the early, symptomatic period, in which inflamed nodules are present, there is degeneration of fat cells, with a predominantly neutrophil infiltrate. The next stage shows a substitution of histiocytes and mononuclear cells for the neutrophils, and the histiocytes have a foamy appearance owing to ingested fat. In the third, atrophic stage fibrosis with lymphocytic cells is characteristic.

There is no specific therapy. It is difficult to evaluate any treatment because of the unpredictable remissions that characterize these diseases. Considerable relief of symptoms by use of large doses of steroids has been reported, but in other instances this has not proved helpful. Antimicrobial drugs should not be given. The use of immunosuppressive or cytotoxic agents could be considered, especially when there is evidence of systemic extension of the panniculitis, and benefit from treatment with cyclophosphamide has been reported. Other agents for which beneficial effects have been claimed include chloroquine (250 mg twice daily for one to three weeks), and thalidomide (100 mg twice daily for three or more weeks). Thalidomide is contraindicated in women of childbearing age.

Eravelly, J., and Waters, M. F. R.: Thalidomide in Weber-Christian disease. Lancet, 1:251, 1977.

Hallahan, J. D., and Klein, T.: Relapsing febrile nodular nonsuppurative panniculitis (Weber-Christian disease); review of literature and report of case. Ann. Intern. Med., 34:1179, 1951.

Kipfer, R. E., Moertel, C. G., and Dahlin, D. C.: Mesenteric lipodystrophy. Ann. Intern. Med., 80:582, 1974.

Lever, W. F., and Schaumburg-Lever, G.: Inflammatory diseases of the subcutaneous fat. In Histopathology of the Skin. 5th ed. Philadelphia, J. B. Lippincott Company, 1975, pp. 231–238.

Milner, R. D. G., and Mitchinson, M. J.: Systemic Weber-Christian disease. J. Clin. Pathol., 18:150, 1965.

Moore, S.: Syndromes resulting from dissemination of pancreatic enzymes. J. Rheumatol., 2:5, 1975.

Tannenbaum, H., Anderson, L. G., and Schur, P. H.: Association of polyarthritis, subcutaneous nodules, and pancreatic disease. J. Rheumatol., 2:14, 1975.

71. FIBROSING SYNDROMES

(Multifocal Fibrosclerosis)

Paul B. Beeson

71.1. INTRODUCTION

In rare instances the delicate fibrous areolar tissue in a certain anatomic region becomes the site of a chronic low-grade inflammatory process, leading to deposition of dense sclerotic plaques, which may obstruct or limit the movement of adjacent viscera. When the process is in the active phase, there are characteristic findings of chronic or granulomatous inflammation, featured by mononuclear cell infiltration and occasional giant cells. In the end-stages the pathologic lesion is simply that of scar tissue, so that by the time this process causes clinical manifestations there may be little evidence of the initial inflammatory reaction. As a general rule the process tends to originate in the midline, around the great vessels, and then to spread laterally. At the periphery of the lesion there appears to be an inflammation of fatty tissue; this is gradually converted to a dense fibrous mat, with little or no sign of inflammation. In at least some cases there is an accompanying vasculitis: a granulomatous inflammation in the walls of small and medium-sized veins. In most cases a clue to the inciting mechanism is lacking; hence the frequent use of the term "idiopathic" in describing the various syndromes. Indubitably this pattern of response may follow different kinds of injury. For example, there is an association between therapy with methysergide and some cases of retroperitoneal fibrosis, and the suggestion has been made that fibrosing mediastinitis can occur as a sequel to infection with *Histoplasma capsulatum*. In a number of instances the disease has developed concurrently with a neoplastic process such as reticulum cell sarcoma or carcinoid tumor.

Although most of these syndromes have been described as separate entities, depending on the clinical manifestations and the interests of the writers who have reported them, it should be emphasized that several anatomic areas may become affected in one person. For example, retroperitoneal fibrosis and sclerosing mediastinitis may be present at the same time. Even more interesting is the report by Comings and his associates of two brothers, offspring of a consanguineous marriage, who exhibited varying combinations of retroperitoneal fibrosis, mediastinal fibrosis, sclerosing cholangitis, Riedel's thyroiditis, and pseudotumor of the orbit. This remarkable constellation of syndromes in two siblings brings up the possibility of a genetic predisposition to disease of this character, but of course does not exclude other precipitating factors, e.g., common exposure to some chemical. The former possibility is given support by the recent description of an association between the occurrence of fibrosing syndromes and alpha$_1$-antitrypsin deficiency.

Alpert, L. I., and Jindrak, K.: Idiopathic retroperitoneal fibrosis and sclerosing cholangitis associated with a reticulum cell sarcoma. Gastroenterology, 62:111, 1972.

Comings, D. E., Skubi, K. B., Van Eyes, J., and Motulsky, A. G.: Familial multifocal sclerosis. Ann. Intern. Med., 66:884, 1967.

Meyer, S., and Hausman, R.: Occlusive phlebitis in multifocal fibrosclerosis. Am. J. Clin. Pathol., 65:274, 1976.

Palmer, P. E., Wolfe, H. J., and Kostas, C-I.: Multisystem fibrosis in alpha$_1$-antitrypsin deficiency. Lancet, 1:22, 1978.

Salmon, H. W.: Combined mediastinal and retroperitoneal fibrosis. Thorax, 23:158, 1968.

71.2. RETROPERITONEAL FIBROSIS
(Periureteral Fibrosis)

In retroperitoneal fibrosis the process usually begins over the promontory of the sacrum and extends laterally across the ureters and up as high as the level of the second or third lumbar vertebra. Less commonly the lesion develops in other extraperitoneal areas, for example, contiguous with the kidneys, duodenum, descending colon, or urinary bladder.

In some cases there has been an associated vasculitis in the skin and subcutaneous tissues, manifested by the formation of nodules, erythematous discolorations, and ulcerations. Similarly, inflammatory changes in small vessels at the sites of the sclerosis have been noted.

The occurrence of retroperitoneal fibrosis in patients taking methysergide for migraine has been reported with greater frequency than could be due to chance, i.e., 12 per cent of all cases reviewed by Koep and Zuidema. These authors also reported an association with some kind of neoplastic disease in 8 per cent of cases.

The disorder is about twice as common in males, and the peak age incidence is in the fifth and sixth decades. The manifestations are variable, depending on the anatomic location of the process. Pain is the most common symptom; it is vague, tends to be located in the low back, and may be accompanied by symptoms referable to the gastrointestinal tract. The patient is likely to lose weight and have low-grade fever. There may be some anemia and elevation of the erythrocyte sedimentation rate. Although the ureter is the structure most often affected, symptoms referable to the urinary tract are uncommon until obstructive uropathy has led to azotemia and other clinical manifestations of renal insufficiency. The fibrosing process may surround the inferior vena cava, but signs of obstruction of that vessel are uncommon; this contrasts with mediastinal fibrosis, in which the most common expression is superior caval obstruction.

Diagnosis of retroperitoneal fibrosis is difficult because of the lack of localizing manifestations. It is most often suggested by the findings at intravenous pyelography: displacement of the ureters toward the midline and evidence of obstruction, usually at the level of the pelvic brim. One or both ureters may be affected. Recent experience indicates that diagnosis by use of ultrasound may become very helpful. In rare instances a mass can be palpated in the pelvis or on the posterior abdominal wall. Once the presence of a mass has been disclosed, the main problem in differential diagnosis lies in distinguishing retroperitoneal fibrosis from retroperitoneal tumor, and, as already mentioned, retroperitoneal fibrosis can develop in response to various kinds of neoplastic disease. For that reason it is advised that multiple deep biopsies should be made at the time of laparotomy.

Surgical treatment, if employed before there has been severe renal damage, is often highly successful. Inasmuch as the fibrosing process is seldom invasive, the constricted organ can usually be freed by blunt dissection so that normal movement or flow is restored. Relief of ureteral obstruction is usually achieved simply by dissecting this structure free of its fibrous encasement and bringing it out on the anterior surface of the sclerotic mass. Occasionally, however, the obstruction recurs months or years after such treatment. The claim has been made that prolonged steroid therapy may be helpful, but the evidence for this is unconvincing, and prompt surgical relief should usually be attempted. Nevertheless, many people who have had experience with this disease recommend that steroid treatment be employed as an adjunct to surgical measures. When the inferior vena cava is obstructed, surgical relief is technically difficult and risky; here it may be preferable to temporize, in the hope that development of collateral pathways may alleviate the circulatory block.

The long-term outlook is fairly good if the disease is recognized and if its obstructive consequences can be treated suitably by surgical means. Prolonged observations of some successfully treated patients indicate that the disease tends to run its course and subside so that the life expectancy may not be shortened. Most deaths have been caused by renal failure.

Catino, D., Torack, R. M., and Hagstrom, J. W. C.: Idiopathic retroperitoneal fibrosis: Histochemical evidence for lateral spread of the
   process from the midline. J. Urol., 98:191, 1967.
Koep, L., and Zuidema, G. D.: The clinical significance of retroperitoneal fibrosis. Surgery, 81:250, 1977.
Ochsner, M. G., Brannan, W., Pond, H. S., and Goodlet, J. S., Jr.:
   Medical therapy in idiopathic retroperitoneal fibrosis. J. Urol.,
   114:700, 1975.
Usher, S. M., Brendler, H., and Ciavarra, V. A.: Retroperitoneal fibrosis secondary to metastatic neoplasm. Urology, 9:191, 1977.

71.3.   MEDIASTINAL FIBROSIS

Taut bundles of collagenous tissue form in the superior and anterior mediastinum with impingement on
the aorta, trachea, and pericardium, but the predominant manifestations are those caused by obstruction of
the superior vena cava: puffy, suffused appearance of
the face and conjunctivae; nonpitting edema of the
face, neck, and upper extremities; and distended veins
in the neck and upper extremities. The main task in
differential diagnosis is to distinguish this relatively
benign condition from obstruction caused by tumor.
Roentgenographic examination of the chest may reveal
little or no abnormality, but angiographic studies will
show the obstruction of the superior vena cava and its
large tributaries. Thoracotomy may be required for histologic diagnosis.

As already mentioned, histoplasmosis, and possibly
tuberculosis too, may be a cause of mediastinal fibrosis; therefore these should be considered, and a trial of
appropriate chemotherapy may be justified.

Some patients with this syndrome have shown gradual improvement over months or years, presumably because of development of collateral circulation. Attempts
to remove the fibrosing tissues from the large veins are
technically difficult and hazardous.

Goodwin, R. A., Nickell, J. A., and Dez Prez, R. M.: Mediastinal fibro-
   sis complicating healed primary histoplasmosis and tuberculosis.
   Medicine, 51:227, 1972.
Schowengerdt, C. G., Suyemoto, R., and Main, F. B.: Granulomatous
   and fibrous mediastinitis: A review and analysis of 180 cases. J.
   Thorac. Cardiovasc. Surg., 57:365, 1969.

71.4.   SCLEROSING CHOLANGITIS

A diffuse fibrous sheath sometimes envelops the
common bile duct, hepatic ducts, and gallbladder. The
clinical manifestation is usually that of insidious onset
of jaundice, although there may be some discomfort in
the right upper quadrant. Liver function tests give results compatible with extrahepatic biliary tract obstruction. The course is prolonged, with gradually deepening jaundice. Death may ensue after many months, and
the findings may be those of biliary cirrhosis.

This clinical syndrome may be associated with inflammatory bowel disease (see Ch. 413 and 414), and in
that situation progression to the clinical picture of biliary cirrhosis is rare.

Sclerosing cholangitis may also be associated with
other forms of multicentric fibrosclerosis, e.g., retroperitoneal fibrosis, Riedel's thyroiditis. Cholangiography, by either the oral or intravenous route, usually
fails to show the lesion, and even percutaneous transhepatic cholangiography may be technically difficult.
On the other hand, endoscopic retrograde cholangio-

graphy may be highly successful in demonstrating the
ductal lesion.

The diagnosis is most often accomplished by laparotomy and biopsy. The latter may be needed to distinguish this disease from a sclerosing bile duct carcinoma.

Treatment is unsatisfactory. Steroids seldom help.
Prolonged biliary tract drainage by T-tube may sometimes be useful.

Danzi, J. T., Makipour, H., and Farmer, R. G.: Primary sclerosing cholangitis. A report of nine cases and clinical review. Am. J. Gastroenterol., 65:109, 1976.
Ruskin, R. B., Katon, R. M., Bilboa, M. K., and Smith, F.: Evaluation
   of sclerosing cholangitis by endoscopic retrograde cholangiopan-
   creatography. Arch. Intern. Med., 136:232, 1976.

71.5.   FIBROSCLEROSIS IN OTHER ORGANS

Riedel's thyroiditis is a rare form of fibrotic disease affecting the structures in the anterior part of the neck
(see Ch. 546.3). This differs from Hashimoto's thyroiditis
in being equally common in males and females and in
the tendency of the fibrotic process to involve not only
the thyroid but also its neighboring structures.

Peyronie's disease is a sclerotic induration of the cor-
pora cavernosa of the penis. This disease has been encountered in association with sclerosing processes in
other parts of the body.

Pseudotumor of the orbit causes unilateral exophthalmos and is likely to be confused with tumor. It has
been seen in association with Riedel's thyroiditis, as
well as in other fibrosclerosing syndromes.

Früh, D., Jaeger, W., and Käfer, O.: Orbital involvement in retroperitoneal fibrosis (Morbus Ormond). Mod. Probl. Ophthalmol.,
   14:651, 1975.

71.6.   PRACTOLOL PERITONITIS

An unusual fibrotic syndrome has been observed in
more than 50 patients treated with the β-adrenergic
blocking drug practolol. This drug closely resembles
propranolol in chemical structure, but the risk of fibrotic reaction in the peritoneum is far smaller, perhaps
nonexistent, with propranolol. Nevertheless, there is a
little suggestive evidence that less severe disease may
develop from prolonged use of propranolol.

Practolol peritonitis seldom manifests itself in less
than 12 months after beginning treatment. Some cases
have developed as long as a year after cessation of the
therapy. It consists of a thick fibrous encasement of the
small intestine, and the symptoms are those of subacute obstruction. It has usually been possible to relieve
the symptoms by surgery, with blunt dissection to peel
away the fibrous tissue. Some improvement can be anticipated in time simply by avoidance of further treatment.

This condition seems somewhat like the retroperitoneal fibrosis that is encountered in some patients who
have taken methysergide for migraine relief.

Marshall, A. J., et al.: Practolol peritonitis. A study of 16 cases and a
   survey of small bowel function in patients taking β-adrenergic
   blockers. Quart. J. Med., 46:135, 1977.

72. EOSINOPHILIC SYNDROMES

Paul B. Beeson

72.1. INTRODUCTION

Many diseases characterized by eosinophilia are dealt with in other parts of this book, e.g., parasitic infestations, common allergic disorders, drug reactions, and skin diseases. This chapter contains a brief characterization of the cell and its behavior, with emphasis on the general pattern of diseases in which eosinophilia may or may not occur.

Although classed as a granulocyte because of certain morphologic and other similarities to the neutrophil, the eosinophil possesses some properties quite distinct from those of the neutrophil. For instance, eosinophils tend to disappear from the circulation after adrenal corticosteroids have been administered; neutrophils usually increase in number. By the same token, in acute inflammation, neutrophils predominate, locally and in the blood, whereas eosinophils recede from both areas. Conversely, in granulomatous inflammatory processes, in which neutrophils are inconspicuous, there may be both local and systemic eosinophilia. (It is partly for this reason that eosinophil behavior is dealt with in this part of the book.)

A major difference from the neutrophil is found in the fact that eosinophils behave like constituents of the immunologic apparatus. They congregate around certain kinds of antigen, especially in reactions involving immunoglobulin E. The eosinophil response becomes enhanced with repeated or continuous antigenic challenge, indicating the property of immunologic "memory." The response, which is mediated by T lymphocytes, can be ablated by administration of immunosuppressive agents, in a pattern remarkably similar to that characteristic of antibody production.

The eosinophil contains comparatively large quantities of certain enzymes, such as arylsulfatase, phospholipase, and histaminase. These are probably capable of interacting with pharmacologically active products of mast cells and basophils. It is therefore quite plausible to assume that one function of the eosinophil is to modulate the consequences of IgE-mediated allergic reactions in which mast cell and basophil products such as histamine are liberated. The eosinophil granule, when studied by electron microscopy, exhibits a crystalline substance which has been shown to be a protein, strongly basic in reaction, and undoubtedly capable of interacting with many humoral substances.

The weight of present evidence then indicates that the function(s) of the eosinophil lie mainly in interactions with endogenous products, such as those of the mast cell, and that it is comparatively unimportant in defense against bacteria, viruses, and protozoa. Whether it affords some protection against infestations by metazoan parasites is a field of active study at present.

72.2. EOSINOPHILIC PULMONARY SYNDROMES

It is notable that peripheral eosinophilia may be seen in association with many kinds of pulmonary disease. Possible factors in this include the presence of mast cells in lung tissue, the opportunity for repeated antigenic challenge by inhaled materials, and the frequency of granulomatous inflammation in pulmonary tissue. Some eosinophilic pulmonary syndromes are described in detail in Ch. 346.2. These include *Löffler's syndrome,* a benign illness usually lasting less than a month, characterized by transient pulmonary infiltrations, low fever, and peripheral eosinophilia. Some cases are undoubtedly manifestations of parasitic infestations, in which circulating parasites lodge in the lungs; however, a similar clinical picture can be observed in some drug sensitivity reactions. Steroid treatment usually causes prompt clearing and amelioration of symptoms.

An illness bearing some resemblance to Löffler's syndrome, but of longer duration and greater severity, has been called *pulmonary infiltration with eosinophilia,* or *PIE syndrome.* In this there can be marked disability, with high fever, cough, and shortness of breath persisting for months or a few years. Steroid therapy often controls the symptoms, but the disease tends to relapse when the treatment is terminated.

Tropical pulmonary eosinophilia is seen mainly in India, Southeast Asia, and the Pacific islands. The disease is characterized by fever, pulmonary infiltrates, and symptoms of asthma. As to etiology, present evidence points to filarial parasites for which man is not a natural host. Parasitemia cannot be demonstrated, but lung biopsies have revealed the presence of structures resembling filaria. The patients show antibodies to filaria and usually improve rapidly on treatment with the antifilarial drug diethylcarbamazine.

In addition to these, there are many other uncommon forms of pneumonia in which the inflammatory exudate contains eosinophils and there may or may not be blood eosinophilia. The cause of these is uncertain, and their response to steroid therapy is variable.

72.3. EOSINOPHILIC SYNDROMES AFFECTING OTHER ORGAN SYSTEMS

LÖFFLER'S EOSINOPHILIC ENDOMYOCARDITIS. This disorder is seen almost exclusively in males. It can lead to heart failure and is characterized by formation of mural thrombi, thickening of the endocardium on either side of the heart, and myocardial degeneration beneath the affected endocardium. This condition appears to be caused by presence of excessive amounts of some product of eosinophils. It can develop as a complication of any state in which there is high and prolonged blood eosinophilia, i.e., an absolute count higher than 2000 per cubic millimeter for longer than 12 months. It has been reported in association with eosinophilic leukemoid reactions, eosinophilic leukemia, eosinophilia in patients with solid tumors, and the so-called hypereosinophilic syndrome.

EOSINOPHILIC LEUKEMIA. Eosinophilic leukemia is a rare occurrence. Its existence has been disputed, but there are now on record a number of fatal illnesses characterized by the presence of immature eosinophils in the blood and marrow, blastic crises, thrombocytopenia, and anemia. In some of these, other markers of leukemia have been noted, including the Philadelphia chromosome and high levels of serum B_{12}.

HYPEREOSINOPHILIC SYNDROME. The hypereosinophilic syndrome is a name given to a disease exhibiting a myeloproliferative picture, with leukocytosis, eosinophilia, hepatomegaly, and splenomegaly. Most cases do not progress to a picture of eosinophilic leukemia, in that the eosinophils in blood appear to be mature, and that death does not result from blastic crises, thrombocytopenia, or anemia. Death may be due to heart failure, with the typical finding of Löffler's eosinophilic endomyocarditis. Another characteristic feature is high incidence of lesions in the central nervous system, not obviously caused by vascular disease. It is of interest that about 90 per cent of patients with this syndrome are males. It has recently been reported that a favorable clinical response can be obtained by treatment with hydroxyurea, whereas steroids and cyclophosphamide have had little effect.

EOSINOPHILIC COLLAGEN DISEASE. European clinicians have described a multisystem disease, with clinical features resembling dermatomyositis, in which there is marked eosinophilia. Chief complaints may be pains in the muscles and joints. The kidneys are seldom or never affected. This disease is considered by other writers simply to be a form of the hypereosinophilic syndrome described above.

EOSINOPHILIC GASTROENTERITIS. See Ch. 408.

72.4. DISEASES IN WHICH EOSINOPHILIA OCCURS OCCASIONALLY

NEOPLASTIC DISORDERS. Peripheral eosinophilia is encountered in a small proportion of patients with *carcinoma or sarcoma*, under 5 per cent. It is more likely to be present late in the disease when there has been extensive metastatic spread. Of the lymphomas, *Hodgkin's disease* is the principal form in which eosinophilia may be present. When present, it is usually just at the level of clinical recognition, but in occasional cases massive eosinophil leukemoid reaction has been observed. In the lymphoma-like syndrome called *immunoblastic lymphadenopathy*, about a third of the reported patients have had peripheral eosinophilia. Of unusual interest is a dermatologic tumor usually located in the tissues of the face or scalp, described under the term *angiolymphoid hyperplasia with eosinophilia*. The mechanism of eosinophilia associated with this small, usually nonmalignant tumor is of unusual interest.

RADIATION-RELATED EOSINOPHILIA. It has been reported that about 40 per cent of patients being treated for intra-abdominal neoplasm exhibit eosinophilia during the first few weeks after therapy has been begun.

RHEUMATOID ARTHRITIS. Perhaps 10 to 12 per cent of patients with rheumatoid arthritis may show a detectable peripheral eosinophilia at some time over the long course of their disease. In addition, in occasional cases, usually those of long standing with nodules and pleuropulmonary involvement, a substantial peripheral eosinophilia may be present.

IMMUNE DEFICIENCY SYNDROMES. Mild eosinophilia is often noted in the various kinds of immune deficiency syndromes observed in pediatric clinics. These include disorders of lymphocyte function as well as those in which there is defective neutrophil function. In any of the immune deficiency syndromes a fairly marked rise in eosinophils can accompany pneumocystis pulmonary infections.

CONGENITAL DEFECTS. Eosinophilia has been described in a significant proportion of patients with congenital heart disease, usually in forms featured by stenotic lesions. In the syndrome of thrombocytopenia with absent radius eosinophilia is frequently present.

INFLAMMATORY BOWEL DISEASE. Eosinophils are sometimes conspicuous in the inflammatory lesions of chronic ulcerative colitis, and a slight elevation of the blood eosinophils is occasionally seen in this disease. It is also reported by some observers that eosinophilia may be present during symptomatic phases of Crohn's disease and that this may be a helpful guide in the differential diagnosis between Crohn's disease and acute appendicitis.

PANCREATIC DISEASES. There is a distinctive clinical syndrome associated with acinar cell carcinoma of the pancreas, consisting of polyarthritis, areas of panniculitis in the subcutaneous fat, and blood eosinophilia. The panniculitis and arthritis are thought to be caused by pancreatic lipase affecting the subcutaneous fat or periarticular fatty tissue. There are also case reports describing symptoms similar to those just described for acinar cell carcinoma, occurring two to six weeks after acute pancreatitis.

CHRONIC ACTIVE HEPATITIS. Although not emphasized in standard clinical descriptions, reviews of reported cases of chronic active hepatitis mention eosinophilia in excess of 5 per cent in about one third of patients.

PERNICIOUS ANEMIA. Before there was a specific treatment of this disease, it was said that about one third of patients with pernicious anemia would exhibit eosinophilia at some time in the course of the disease.

ADDISON'S DISEASE. The assumption seems to have been made that Addison's disease may be characterized by eosinophilia. This must, however, be a rare event inasmuch as several fairly large series of cases of Addison's disease have not shown an elevation of the eosinophils.

SARCOIDOSIS. Prior to 1960, most reported series of cases of sarcoidosis indicated that eosinophilia was a clinical feature in an appreciable proportion of cases. Current writings about the disease deny eosinophilia as a feature. This unexplained change may be evidence to support the assumption that sarcoidosis is simply a pattern of response to a variety of environmental influences, and presumably the forms of the disease now prevalent do not seem to be those in which an eosinophil response is characteristic.

Beeson, P. B., and Bass, D. A.: The Eosinophil. Philadelphia, W. B. Saunders Company, 1977.

PART IX
MICROBIAL DISEASES

73. THE NATURE OF MICROBIAL DISEASES

Walsh McDermott

Microbial diseases are all those produced by a transmissible agent capable of multiplication in living tissue and sufficiently small in its individual units to be visible only by light or electron microscopy. One might question whether a useful purpose is served by including under the one label such diverse entities as diseases produced by protozoa and those caused by the smallest viruses. Certainly at one level of analysis a grouping of this sort is not particularly useful. For this reason, protozoa have been removed from the present Part and, with the helminths, form one of their own (Part X); general discussions of the rest of the microbial diseases have been placed with the individual subdivisions, such as viral or bacterial diseases. But there is a larger sense in which all these diseases are usefully regarded as a single group separate from and unlike all other diseases. For the nonmicrobial diseases, except for those resulting from undernutrition, are essentially individual, private affairs which, if uncontrolled, represent personal tragedies but seldom have wide public impact. By contrast, a society unable to employ contemporary technology to manage its microbial diseases is condemned to misery; infant and childhood deaths are a commonplace, pregnancy is virtually a permanent way of life for all women from their mid-teens to their mid-forties, and back-breaking toil is the lot of most people. To gain understanding of microbial disease in a scientific and technologic sense is thus an essential prerequisite to the building and maintenance of a modern society.

With that understanding of microbial disease is an appreciation of the tremendous adaptive plasticity of microbes — their great capacity for *change* both in themselves and in the conditions of their parasitism. This ability to adapt to change means that the microbial world is an enduring potential source of new diseases. It also means that there is no real prospect for a world free from microbial diseases, either those of man or of the plants and other animals. Thus if we are to continue our long record of successes in meeting microbial challenges to man, there can be no letup in our search for greater knowledge of the subject at the bedside, in the field, and in the laboratory. Our brilliant successes in the prevention and treatment of so many microbial diseases have not been founded on the extermination of the microbe. They have all been based on making the environment outside or within the human host a place in which the microbe cannot flourish to its full capacity. To exploit some weak link in the pathogenic chain in this way requires exact scientific and clinical knowledge. The incapacitation of the microbe thus affected may or may not jeopardize its survival as a species. Paleontology has taught us that species or genera

have disappeared from this planet. Our systematic study of microbes is not yet of sufficient age to document such extinction of a disease-producing microbe, but there is no reason to doubt that it could occur. There is considerable reason to doubt, however, that it can be produced by the purposeful actions of man. A far greater body of knowledge would be necessary than is now available to produce such purposeful extinction of a microbial species. This is so not only because of microbial adaptability, but also because we have so little ability to identify and successfully interrupt *all* significant ecologic relationships involved. The story of the malaria eradication campaign (see Ch. 193) is a case in point. Whether the situation with smallpox will be any different remains to be seen. In the writer's judgment, it seems most unlikely. "Final victories" in the form of microbial extinction are not to be expected, but neither are they necessary or particularly desirable. Our existing conceptual base and pluralism of practical approaches have yielded an array of triumphs that make our current management of microbial disease one of the finest chapters in the whole history of science for man's benefit. To a considerable extent, however, these practical cures and preventives rely upon the change in hygienic habits in and around the home that come with, or are made possible by, improved socioeconomic status. What is needed now is not only a continued effort in the same direction but also a new massive effort of a different sort. This new effort should be devoted to reviewing those major microbial diseases for which we already have effective technologies, with the object of developing new and quite different methods suitable for wide application in economically underdeveloped regions.

Dubos, R. J.: Man Adapting. New Haven, Yale University Press, 1965, pp. 369–399.

McDermott, W.: Microbial Persistence. Harvey Lecture, Series 63, 1967–1968. New York, Academic Press.

Morrison, R. S.: The concept of eradication and public education. The Pharos, 23:3, 1963.

74. INTRODUCTION TO MICROBIAL DISEASES

Sheldon M. Wolff

Many remarkable advances have been made in our understanding of the pathogenesis, prevention, and therapy of a variety of microbial diseases. Nonetheless, infectious diseases are still the most common problems in ambulatory patients encountered by physicians in the United States, and this group of diseases continues to be the major cause of morbidity and mortality in the world. Despite the commonly held concept that important infectious diseases have been brought into check, there continue to be ominous signs that some are not as well controlled as many have hoped or expected. For example, the emergence of penicillin-resistant pneumococci could have major consequences. Conversely, the recent demonstration of the utility of polyvalent anti-pneumococcal vaccines may prove to be much more timely and important than originally considered (see Ch. 121). The continued eruption of cholera outbreaks in certain parts of the world must create apprehension because many had assumed that pandemics of this ancient illness were part of our historic past. Even the optimistic heralding of the eradication of smallpox may be premature. Aside from the problems concerning well-described illnesses, we continue to be confronted by the appearance of previously unrecognized diseases. A conspicuous example is legionnaires' disease (see Ch. 123).

Considerable progress continues to be made regarding the etiology and therapeutic approach to microbial diseases. For example, we are beginning to amass information pertaining to the causative agents of certain forms of viral gastroenteritis (see Ch. 104). The recognition and isolation of these agents will certainly lead to rapid improvement in our ability to diagnose and, ideally, to prevent and treat these common debilitating illnesses. The enormous increase in our knowledge of the etiology of both hepatitis A and B in the past ten years has already improved our ability to categorize, to diagnose, to prevent, and to alter the severity of these viral diseases. The development of vaccines for these conditions promises to be a fruitful outcome of this exciting research. The development of chemotherapeutic agents active in viral diseases, although not yet extensively applied, has provided some exciting advances; notably, adenine arabinoside has proved effective in the treatment of the dreaded encephalitic complication of herpes simplex infection.

Despite the development of new technology (such as laminar flow rooms) and the availability of blood products (including leukocytes for replacement therapy), opportunistic infections in susceptible hosts continue to be among the most serious problems facing medicine (see Ch. 124). In fact, these life-threatening infections will undoubtedly become far more frequent as chemotherapeutic and immunosuppressive therapy finds wider clinical use. We are thus facing a major problem, for all these patients are hospitalized and the majority require treatment in intensive care units. The expense of caring for such patients is great.

Microbial diseases provided the original models for early studies in immunology. In the past two decades, we have witnessed an extraordinary increase in the understanding of immunologic processes. This wealth of knowledge has continued to provide new information concerning the pathogenesis, prevention, and recovery from microbial diseases. The role of thymus-derived (T) lymphocytes in cell-mediated immunity, of bone marrow–derived (B) lymphocytes in humoral immunity, of the alternative complement pathway in the clearing of bacteria from the bloodstream, and of secretory immunoglobulins in defense against certain viral respiratory infections are only a few examples of the importance of this newly acquired information to our understanding of infectious diseases (see Ch. 38 to 40). In addition to this information, the rapidly expanding body of knowledge concerning the inflammatory response and cell functions such as chemotaxis, phagocytosis, and microbicidal activities has greatly improved our understanding of normal and abnormal host defenses. By virtue of these new data, many previously unrecognized syn-

dromes have been described, and effective therapeutic approaches to several acquired and inherited defects have been formulated. Some new chapters and other extensively rewritten chapters attest to this profusion of knowledge.

All this new knowledge, in one way or another, represents change — change in our understanding of disease, change in our interventional skills, and change in the character and appearance of the very diseases themselves. The physician must keep up with these changes. One thing that helps in so doing is the unchanging nature of the logic involved in the approach to the patient whose illness may be a consequence of microbial disease. To outline precisely how to question and examine such a patient does not fit the scope of this chapter. Yet there are at least two questions that must be attacked and deserve mention here. The first is whether the process is indeed microbial in origin. Merely to ask the question may be enough to highlight the fact that the pneumonia is really an infarct or that the typhoid is really Hodgkin's disease. To see the major manifestation of a well-known microbial disease with no collateral evidences of infection should raise this question. At other times, in approaching the question every scrap of evidence must be carefully sifted, e.g., a high percentage of immature neutrophils within a normal total leukocyte count. On still other occasions the physician must examine the less quantifiable subtleties, such as the belief that patients with infection are generally sicker than those with the same degree of fever from other causes.

More often than not, however, the fact of infection will be clear. Indeed, the overwhelming majority of patients with microbial diseases will have self-limited and benign conditions. There will be some, however, who will have acute symptoms, and their condition could rapidly deteriorate. Such patients require immediate attention. This brings us to the answer to the second of the two major questions, namely, which of the infections conceivably present could kill this patient within the next 12 to 24 hours, and which of them could be so innocent-appearing at this stage. Most often the physician must rely on clinical knowledge and experience. Time may not permit the luxury of extensive and time-consuming laboratory examinations; yet certain key decisions must be made on how to best protect the patient until it is clear precisely what is present and to what extent steps should be taken to isolate the patient, examine contacts, and possibly start chemoprophylaxis of such contacts. Always in the forefront of the physician's thinking must be the need to ensure that proper diagnostic specimens are obtained just before whatever interventions are made.

One example of how this may be done is encountered in bacteremia due to gram-negative rods. Knowing something of the epidemiology, microbiology, and pathophysiology of this condition can sometimes be of crucial importance in the outcome of the patient's illness. If a patient with leukemia undergoing intensive chemotherapy suddenly develops chills and fever in the absence of any localizing physical findings, we must be prepared to act rapidly. Although this patient may have a localized infection, it is most likely that a generalized infection with bacteremia is present. It is useful to know that most gram-negative rod bacteremias are due to *Escherichia coli* but that in the leukemic patient *Pseudomonas aeruginosa* is the most common offender. Furthermore, it helps in deciding to institute therapy empirically to know that the mortality rate from bacteremia with this organism is higher than with other bacteria. In addition, patients with underlying rapidly fatal illnesses, such as acute leukemia, have the highest death rate from such infections. We should also realize that the risk of acquiring such an infection is greatest when the peripheral granulocyte count falls below 500 per cubic millimeter and, conversely, the replacement of granulocytes in such patients increases survival. Of crucial importance is the choice of the antimicrobial therapy to be employed early, as we cannot wait for the results of blood culture. Knowing these facts, such patients should clearly receive an aminoglycoside. Since these infections are often nosocomial, it is very helpful to know the drug-susceptibility patterns of the organisms being isolated in the hospital. Furthermore, in the granulocytopenic patients it would appear that the administration of carbenicillin with the aminoglycoside will improve the chance of survival. Needless to say, such patients may develop bacteremic shock, and, if this occurs, both monitoring and supportive measures must be instituted.

The advances of the past 30 years in prevention and care of microbial diseases are remarkable. The benefits to society of these endeavors are immeasurable. However, much remains to be done, and the study of microbial diseases should not only provide physicians with enormous pride in what their profession has accomplished, but also present the inquisitive with many still-to-be-solved riddles of immense importance.

Section One   VIRAL DISEASES

75.   INTRODUCTION TO VIRAL DISEASES

Edwin D. Kilbourne

The thread that binds together such differing diseases as influenza, mumps, smallpox, and yellow fever for common consideration in this section is the tenuous one of viral etiology. All are the result of infection with viruses, and all viruses share in common submicroscopic size and complete and intimate dependence on the cells of the host that they infect. Yet these tiny packages of protein-coated nucleic acid are as different as the diseases discussed in these pages. They vary in size from the 30 mμ RNA-containing particle of yellow fever virus to the 250 mμ antigenically complex particle of smallpox virus, with its DNA core. The relation of design and function of viruses is now being appreciated. Certain myxoviruses, including the influenza and parainfluenza viruses, possess a potent neuraminidase that probably abets their release from the mucin-coated cells of the respiratory tract. The myxoviruses are fragile and unstable in the environment, whereas the enteroviruses, including poliovirus, can pass unscathed through the barrier of gastric acidity in their journey to the target cells of the small intestine.

Neither structural nor chemical similarity of viruses, however, is any sure guide to the diseases that they may cause. Mumps and parainfluenza viruses are indistinguishable by electron microscopy and even share antigens in common, but one invades the salivary glands, pancreas, or meninges, whereas the other produces mild upper respiratory tract infection or infantile croup. Nor does viral dissimilarity predict dissimilar disease. The structurally amorphous, genetically plastic RNA virus of influenza and the geometrically precise DNA-bearing adenovirus, with its potential for latency, both evoke clinical syndromes that may be difficult to differentiate.

With this caution in mind about the great dissimilarities among viruses and their associated diseases, the common features of viral infections can be considered as useful generalizations.

Most viral infections occur in childhood, at which time any of the 200 obligate human viruses ordinarily produce acute but benign disease or no disease at all. However, the unborn child may be peculiarly vulnerable to the effects of rubella, and the newborn — if unprotected by maternal antibody — may be severely damaged by infection with the ordinarily innocuous virus of herpes simplex. With the exception of the neonatal period, the severity of disease associated with primary or initial viral infections increases with the age of the patient. Poliomyelitis is more frequent and more severe in adult infection; varicella pneumonia is essentially limited to adults; the postpuberal complications of mumps are notorious; and jaundice occurs more frequently in older than in younger patients with infectious hepatitis. It is necessary to emphasize the evidence for greater potential susceptibility of the adult because it may *appear* that the adult is less vulnerable to viral disease, protected as he is by a legacy of immunity to many viruses from his childhood experience with them. This fact of age-related susceptibility is increasingly important as the epidemiologic patterns of viral infections change with changes in man's environment and with the introduction of new vaccines. If a vaccine induces impermanent immunity so that infection is merely postponed, the consequences might be disastrous.

Although firm and enduring immunity attended by persisting humoral antibody follows most viral infections, it is unlikely that antibody formation per se is the essential mechanism of recovery. Interferon, a nonspecific and nontoxic product of virus-infected cells, is more closely related temporally to the decline of virus in tissues and to recovery from infection, but its role in the self-termination of viral infections is still conjectural. Experimental evidence that corticosteroid hormones are inhibitory to interferon synthesis may explain the deleterious effect of these hormones or of stress on certain viral infections of man — notably on the extension of recurrent herpes simplex keratitis or on varicella in children already receiving steroid therapy.

The enduring immunity of viral infections has few exceptions. The frequency of common colds is now explicable as the result of multiple infections with multiple antigenically unrelated viruses; the seemingly transient immunity of influenza reflects the changing nature of the virus itself. For most viral infections there is no indication whether protracted immunity is maintained by recurrent subclinical infection or by persistence of the virus in the host. With a few — varicella-zoster, herpes simplex, and cytomegalic inclusion disease — all associated with herpesviruses which replicate in the cell nucleus, viral genomes undoubtedly persist throughout life in the tissues, integrated in host cell DNA, and may be reactivated there to produce recurrent disease in the partially immune host. In the growing number of patients who are immunologically crippled with cancer or subjected to chemical immunosuppression for transplantation surgery, such reactivations may occur as new and sometimes terminal diseases. Other "new" viral diseases (Lassa fever, Marburg disease) have emerged recently as the result of altered relationships of man and the animal carriers of the causative viruses.

Evidence is increasing that viruses are involved in a variety of mammalian cancers and also in chronic diseases of the central nervous system. In man, the association of the herpes-like Epstein-Barr virus (EBV) with Burkitt's lymphoma and cancer of the retropharyngeal space is striking, although an etiologic relationship has not been proved. The human papilloma virus (associated with the common wart) is a member of a group of mammalian viruses — the papovaviruses — two of which have been shown to be capable of genetic integration with the host cell chromosome in the manner of lysogenic bacteriophages. One such virus (JC) has been isolated from patients with progressive multifocal leukoencephalopathy (see Ch. 310.5).

The recent direct demonstration of a measles-like virus in patients with subacute sclerosing panencephalitis suggests the awesome potential of common agents of acute infection.

In contrast to the bacterial diseases of man, the viral diseases are relatively insusceptible at present to chemotherapy, but the efficient immunity of natural viral infection can be duplicated with vaccines. The coat proteins of all viruses are antigenic, and it is reasonable to conclude that vaccines could be made for all viruses that can be cultivated in the laboratory. The great number of viral pathogens limits the feasibility of this approach, however, as does our uncertain knowledge of the ultimate potential of these viruses for good or evil. The vaccine itself may be a two-edged sword: if a living virus, it may be contaminated with alien viruses or nucleic acid, or may retain virulence expressed only in certain individuals; if inactivated, it may be poorly antigenic. At its best, however, the vaccine may be the ultimate weapon if eradication of the virus can be effected by substitution in the community of vaccine virus for wild type. A trend in this direction is evident with poliomyelitis.

The intractability of viral infections to chemotherapy is a corollary of the intimacy of virus-host association. To the extent that the viral parasite subverts the host's cellular machinery to its own synthesis, it cannot be interrupted without compromising the host as well. But the presence of novel virus-coded enzymes in infected but not in normal cells suggests the possibility of employing highly selective antimetabolites specifically directed against virus synthesis. Indeed, this effect has already been realized in vitro, and in man limited success in arresting the progression of herpes simplex encephalitis has been achieved even with an antimetabolite not specific for the virus.

Man may never be free of viruses, but it is hoped that he may gradually replace the plagues of the past with more peaceful coexistence in the future.

VIRAL INFECTIONS
OF THE RESPIRATORY TRACT

76. THE COMMON COLD

(Acute Coryza)

George Gee Jackson

DEFINITION. The common cold is a symptom complex caused by viral infection of the upper respiratory passages. Most precisely, the term applies to afebrile, acute coryza of viral origin. In the broadest sense, the common cold refers to any undifferentiated upper respiratory infection. The terms rhinitis, pharyngitis, laryngitis, and "chest cold" are sometimes used to designate the principal anatomic site of infection. The main differences between the common cold and other viral or bacterial respiratory infections are the absence of fever, the nonexudative inflammation, and the relatively mild constitutional symptoms and signs.

ETIOLOGY. Many viruses can cause the common cold. No single strain of virus accounts for more than a

TABLE 1. Viruses Associated with the Common Cold

Virus Class	Frequent	Infrequent
Picornaviruses	Rhinoviruses (numerous serotypes)	Enteroviruses (a few of many serotypes) Coxsackievirus A21, 24 (others) Coxsackievirus B3, 4, 5
Paramyxoviruses	Parainfluenza 1, 2, 3 Respiratory syncytial (RS)	Parainfluenza 4 Measles Mumps
Myxoviruses Coronaviruses Reoviruses Adenoviruses	Influenza A, B	Influenza C >2 types Type 1 Types 1, 2, 5, 6 3, 4, 7, 14, 21

small proportion of the illnesses. Isolates have been made from about 70 per cent of acute coryzal illnesses in young adults and about 35 per cent of common colds in children. Among the viruses, rhinoviruses comprise the largest single etiologic group. The viruses listed in

Table 1 show the taxonomic groups that have been etiologically related to the common cold according to their frequency in most investigations. (The coxsackie- and echoviruses listed therein are also considered separately in Ch. 90 to 98.)

The increasing ability to recover viruses and better serologic means for the diagnosis of viral infections have shown that 5 to 10 per cent of common colds are associated with more than one virus, and definite evidence of simultaneous dual infection is not rare. The causative agents of some of the infections have not been revealed by tissue culture methods currently in use. Certain of the more labile or fastidious viruses have been grown only in unusual cultures of human cell strains or in organ cultures of human embryonic trachea. Other viruses can be shown only by the transmission of illness to volunteers. More than 90 antigenically different strains of rhinoviruses are known to cause the common cold syndrome. Many different types of viruses that can cause mild respiratory illnesses in man may be prevalent in the population at any one time.

EPIDEMIOLOGY. The common cold is spread by direct person-to-person contact and by self-inoculation from hands that have become contaminated with infectious virus. Under conditions of household association, 10 per cent of adults acquired the disease from an index case. From studies in volunteers, it was shown that some persons became infected and shed virus without having symptoms. This occurs in about one third of rhinovirus colds, two thirds of coronavirus infections, and a variable number of infections with other viruses.

It is a common observation that an increase in the frequency of colds occurs in the winter. Sometimes this has been correlated with sharp changes in the temperature, humidity, or pollution of the air, but the popular belief that cold weather causes common colds cannot be substantiated from epidemiologic observations in the Arctic or tropics or from studies in volunteers. Exposure of volunteer subjects to cold did not activate latent respiratory viruses. The reason for the apparent relation between the season and common colds remains unclear. In the United States, it is usual to observe three waves of common colds per year. One occurs in the autumn a few weeks after the opening of schools, another in midwinter, and a third wave in the spring. The separate epidemics have usually been shown to be due to different viruses, each of which may have its own seasonal epidemiology.

The *incidence* of common colds is related to age and environment. Preschool children have an average of six to twelve respiratory illnesses per year, most of which are common colds. Parents with young children have approximately six viral respiratory illnesses per year, and other adults have two to three per year. Statistics gathered by the United States Public Health Service show that in the winter quarter of the year at least one half of all persons acquire a common cold; 20 per cent of persons have a similar illness in the summer quarter.

The *prevalence* of common colds is approximately 15 per cent of persons per week during the winter months. Surveillance of a group of student nurses during one winter revealed that individuals had common cold symptoms on 10 per cent of the days. Among industrial employees in the United States, common colds account for one half of all absences and one quarter of the total time lost. Similarly, acute respiratory illness is highly prevalent among military forces, especially recruits, and is a major cause of disability. In a recent National Health Interview Survey, the common cold caused 116.2 days of restricted activity per 100 persons per year, or 1.16 days per individual each year.

PATHOLOGY. The pathologic changes in the mucous membranes of the respiratory passages are edema, hyperemia, transudation, and exudation. The severity of the cytopathic effect is related to the type and virulence of the infecting virus and the extent of infection. Picornaviruses (rhinoviruses and enteroviruses) have been observed to cause more metaplasia and degeneration in smears of exfoliated cells from the nasal turbinates than the myxoviruses. This generalization does not hold for infections of the lower respiratory tract. During the acute phase of infection, protein components of the respiratory secretions are altered, and serum proteins become more abundant. Abnormal soluble substances of cellular origin also can be found. The secretion is rich in glycoprotein. Repair is relatively rapid and, insofar as is known, occurs without residual pathologic damage. Recently, however, inquiry has been made regarding the role of repeated viral respiratory infections in the pathogenesis of later degenerative diseases, such as bronchitis and emphysema.

Viral infection induces swelling and some exudation, but it causes no significant change in the bacterial flora of the nasopharynx. When the inflammatory changes are of sufficient magnitude, channels connecting the paranasal sinuses and middle ear to the airway become obstructed. Suppuration can develop from secondary bacterial growth under these conditions.

MECHANISMS OF INFECTION AND IMMUNITY. Viruses from infected persons are airborne in droplet spray that is emitted during respiration, talking, sneezing, and coughing. Particles in the size range of 5 to 50 μ are probably the most infectious. Transmission can also be made by hand contact with virus acquired from contaminated surfaces. The nasopharynx and conjunctiva are the portals of infection. The incubation period is short, usually one to four days. Proliferation of virus can often be demonstrated within 24 hours after the infection of volunteers. Virus shedding usually precedes the onset of symptoms by one to two days, and the peak excretion occurs a few days later, during the symptomatic phase of the illness. Virus excretion decreases after several days, and symptoms decrease concomitantly. Later studies from the same person as well as attempts to recover viruses from well persons indicate that the carrier state after infection is transient, and asymptomatic chronic carriers are rare. Rhinoviruses have not been recovered from more than 1 to 2 per cent of well persons in populations where colds are occurring.

Host susceptibility or resistance to infection is determined primarily by the immunologic status resulting from recent previous infection with the same or related viruses. Some physiologic functions, such as menses and fatigue, and constitutional factors, such as an allergic diathesis and vasomotor rhinitis, are secondary determinants of host susceptibility. Emotional distress and overconcern with personal health increase symptoms, whereas stoical and ascetic personality traits decrease overt susceptibility. In controlled studies, chilling did not increase the susceptibility of volunteers to infection nor did ventilation with frigid air.

The nasal secretion is the first barrier against infection of the epithelial cells of the respiratory tract. In addition to the mechanical movement of mucus, the secretion contains glycoprotein inhibitors for some myxoviruses that can compete with cell receptors for the virus. Because virus union with inhibitors is reversible whereas cellular infection is not, these inhibitors probably do no more than delay and decrease the multiplicity of infection. Specific gamma globulins of low molecular weight, principally IgA and IgG, also are contained in nasal secretion. The former is primarily the result of local antibody production and plays an important role in immunity from prior infection. The activity of IgG is related to, but poorly correlated with, the height of specific antibody in the plasma. In one study, the gradient between nasal and serum antibody was 1 to 30. During the early stages of infection, before symptoms have begun, there is an easily demonstrable increase of globulins in nasal washings.

Infection with some respiratory viruses stimulates the local production of a protein or proteins referred to as interferon. Noninfected cells exposed to interferon are protected against viral infection. The mechanism offers an attractive thesis for the termination of infection and repair of the mucosa before specific antibody is formed.

A response in serum-neutralizing antibody against the infecting virus is not always sufficiently prompt or of great enough magnitude to permit diagnosis of the causative role of a virus in the infection. Specific immunity against illness from reinfection with the same strain of virus, however, is readily demonstrable in volunteers. This clinical immunity is apparent for a period of about two years after infection. Asymptomatic infections are not entirely prevented. Reinfection in the presence of serum antibody usually results in a modified illness. The specificity of the antibody and its concentration at the site of infection on the surface of the mucosa appear to be critical factors. Although serum antibody reduces infection and illness, it is possible for infection of the respiratory mucosa to occur. In such cases, the acute inflammatory response can be exaggerated, presumably as a result of the local antigen-antibody reaction or hypersensitivity of the persons resulting from earlier infection.

CLINICAL MANIFESTATIONS. The common cold is in large part a subjective symptomatic diagnosis. The major symptoms for any individual tend to be repetitive, but they differ appreciably from person to person. Some persons have only "head colds," whereas others complain regularly of pharyngitis or cough as characteristic principal symptoms of their colds. The occurrence of symptoms that 100 young adults described as characteristic of a naturally acquired common cold is shown in Table 2.

The same symptoms occur in volunteers challenged with an infectious virus, and their time of occurrence and duration have been observed. Sneezing, headache, and malaise are the initial symptoms, followed by chilly sensations, sore throat, rhinorrhea, and nasal congestion. The chilly sensations may be associated with some lowering of oral temperature that is sometimes interpreted as the initiating cause in natural colds. Fever of any significant degree is absent. The constitutional symptoms are transient, lasting only one or two days. There is sometimes a lull for a day between the early symptoms and the development of characteristic nasopharyngeal symptoms of a full-blown cold. The dry or sore throat tends to recede as the cold progresses.

TABLE 2. The Syndrome of the Common Cold

Symptoms	Frequency
Severe:	
Nasal discharge	100
Nasal obstruction	99
Moderate:	
Sore or dry throat	96
Malaise	81
Postnasal discharge	79
Headache	78
Cough	76
Mild:	
Sneezing	97
Feverishness	49
Chilliness	43
Burning eyes and mucous membranes	28
Muscle aching	22

Nasal discharge is the hallmark of the common cold. At the onset, the secretion is clear, watery, and often profuse. Later, secretions thicken, become mucopurulent, yellow-green, and tenacious. Nasal obstruction is at first an intermittent symptom associated with an exaggeration of the rhythmic physiologic turgescence of the nasal turbinates. Later, the turbinates become swollen and boggy, encroaching on the nasal lumen, which contains increased secretions. These symptoms ordinarily run their course within a week. As the illness progresses, cough may appear as an increasingly prominent symptom, and persists for one to two weeks. It may be dry or productive of a variable amount of mucoid sputum.

Physical signs are limited to the nasopharynx, the surrounding sinuses, and middle ears. Usually, mild hyperemia, congestion, or both, are all that can be seen, and the deviation from normal may be insufficient to recognize as pathologic.

Hematologic changes have been observed in volunteers when the initial blood values and the time sequence of infection were known. Mild leukopenia with relative lymphocytosis is the initial response, followed after a day or two by a slight leukocytosis with some increase in polymorphonuclear leukocytes. A fall in the hematocrit and rise in the erythrocyte sedimentation rate can also occur. Although the aforementioned changes can be related to the infection in volunteers, their deviation from normal is not great enough to be useful in isolated cases.

Complications of a cold are usually bacterial in origin. They are infrequent and consist of suppuration in the nasopharynx and its contiguous passages. Serous effusion, however, may appear in the middle ear and perhaps in the sinuses. A recrudescence of symptoms, perhaps with fever, localized swellings and/or pus, and leukocytosis may be signs of a bacterial complication.

DIAGNOSIS. The diagnosis of a common cold is made on the basis of history and symptoms. At the peak of the illness, signs of the infection also are apparent. Examination is important for the recognition or exclusion of illnesses of more severe nature that patients may be prone to designate as a cold. The differential diagnosis includes prodromes of other infections and vascular, allergic, and neoplastic processes in the nose, pharynx, sinuses, or ears. Other serious diseases, such as bacterial endocarditis, tuberculosis, bronchitis, bronchiectasis, and lung abscess, have been called "chest colds" because of lack of characteristic symptoms and incomplete examination of the patient by a physician.

The diagnosis of common cold therefore should be avoided as a designation for a broad category of respiratory symptoms of diverse causes.

The clinical symptoms do not permit discrimination with regard to the specific viral cause of a cold. The overlap in the symptoms produced by infection with any one of many viruses that cause the common cold is so great as to preclude more than a judgment regarding the general group of viruses to which the etiologic agent might belong. Under the controlled conditions of studies in volunteers, different viruses cause appreciably different syndromes. For each, the clinical manifestations are also related to the dose, size of particle inhaled, and modifications by host factors. The diagnosis of the specific viral cause of a common cold is based on laboratory procedures. Virus isolation and/or the demonstration of a specific antibody rise in paired sera drawn several days apart are the methods most readily available. As a routine, specific viral diagnosis is not practical. It is recommended for academic reasons and in practice to determine the cause of local epidemics or to assist in the diagnosis of severe illnesses. Also, the differentiation of mycoplasmal and secondary bacterial pneumonias is essential for proper treatment.

TREATMENT AND PREVENTION. In considering treatment and prevention of the common cold, the following factors that have been discussed must be kept in mind: (1) The number of antigenically distinct viruses that cause the common cold is large. (2) Except for the time and economic loss, the infection is benign and the duration of severe symptoms is brief. (3) Viral infection does not significantly change the bacterial flora of the nasopharynx, and bacterial complications are infrequent. (4) Infection initiates production of interferon and antibodies that naturally limit the infection. (5) Specific immunity to illness with the same virus exists for one to two years after infection. (6) Reinfection can occur in the presence of antibody in the plasma.

At present there are no antimicrobial drugs of practical effectiveness in man against the viruses responsible for the common cold except for amantadine in influenza A. The use of antimicrobial drugs is thus not recommended. Carefully controlled trials with unlicensed drugs in volunteers indicate that effective chemoprophylaxis against the common cold is possible. The development of such products could initiate a more optimistic position regarding drug treatment. Suppurative complications are caused by obstruction more often than by the virulence of local bacteria. Purulent otitis or sinusitis should be treated with an appropriate antimicrobial. Group A streptococci, pneumococci, and *H. influenzae* are commonly associated with such complications and will usually respond to adequate doses of penicillin or, in the case of Group A streptococci, to erythromycin. Routine use of chemoprophylaxis selects drug-resistant strains and does not eliminate the development of suppurative complications with such strains; it is not advisable.

Supportive treatment is desirable and helpful. Additional rest in bed, warm clothing, and prevention of chilling increase the patient's comfort. If ventilatory insufficiency, stridor, and anoxemia that may accompany a cold are present, steam inhalation, a decongestant, a bronchodilator, or an expectorant may be indicated. Postural changes can help in the drainage of secretions and the raising of sputum. Because of the diverse causes and syndromes, there is no one regimen to be recommended. Aspirin in a dose of 0.6 gram for an adult or 10 mg per kilogram of body weight for children can reduce headache and malaise. However, it increases virus shedding and should generally be avoided. Oral phenylpropanolamine hydrochloride (15 to 50 mg), inhalation of hexamine vapor, or nose drops with 0.5 per cent ephedrine or phenylephrine shrink the vascular bed of the mucosa and provide temporary nasal decongestion. Nose drops in any oily vehicle should be avoided, and potent vasoconstrictors with transient action and physiologic rebound, such as epinephrine, are not desirable. Increased fluids or hard candy lozenges may be adequate for control of coughing. Cough syrups, such as elixir of terpin hydrate with codeine (64 mg per 30 ml), are more effective if necessary. Antihistamines have no effect on the common cold, except that a person prone to severe inhalant allergy may experience some reduction in the volume of nasal secretion. Large doses of vitamin C (ascorbic acid) have no significant protective effect against viral infections causing the common cold and no appreciable inhibitory effect on rhinoviral colds. Excessive amounts which have been recommended are rapidly excreted in the urine and can cause urinary symptoms owing to the increased acidity of the urine. The numerous compounded remedies, including those with vitamins, bioflavonoids, quinine, alkalinizers, multiple analgesics, antihistamines, decongestants, and tranquilizers, are developed for sales profit in a large market of uninformed and uncritical people. Their widespread and repeated use invariably leads to a few cases of hematologic disorders, eruptive or exfoliative dermatitis, and anaphylaxis or other severe idiosyncratic reactions.

Prevention of common colds by quarantine or isolation of cases is without effect because of the number of infected but asymptomatic persons and because virus excretion usually precedes the symptoms. The hygienic collection and disposal of respiratory secretions to reduce dissemination should be encouraged as common courtesy. Interruption of the airborne phase of transmission by increasing space, higher rates of air ventilation, alterations in temperature and humidity, vaporization of disinfectants, and ultraviolet irradiation of overhead air all have been given trials without clearly significant results.

Vaccines for protection against the common cold are not available. Former "cold vaccines" were bacterial suspensions and have no basis for effectiveness. The large number of antigenically distinct viruses augurs numerous difficulties in the production of an effective vaccine. Nevertheless, promising vaccines are being developed for specific groups of viruses.

Anderson, T. W., Reid, D. B. W., and Beaton, G. H.: Vitamin C and the common cold: A double-blind trial. Can. Med. Ass. J., 107:503, 1972.

Davis, D. J.: Measurements of the prevalence of viral infections. J. Infect. Dis., 133 Suppl.: A3–5, 1976.

Hendley, J. O., Wenzel, R. P., and Gwaltney, J. M.: Transmission of rhinovirus colds by self-inoculation. N. Engl. J. Med., 288:1361, 1973.

Jackson, G. G., Dowling, H. F., Anderson, T. O., Riff, L., Saporta, J., and Turck, M.: Susceptibility and immunity to common upper respiratory viral infections — the common cold. Ann. Intern. Med., 53:719, 1960.

Johnson, K. M., et al.: Role of enteroviruses in respiratory diseases. Am. Rev. Respir. Dis., 88:240, 1963.

Kaye, H. S., and Dowdle, W. R.: Seroepidemiologic survey of coronavirus (strain 229E) infections in a population of children. Am. J. Epidemiol., 101:238, 1975.

Lidwell, O. M., Morgan, R. W., and Williams, R. E. O.:The epidemiology of the common cold. IV. The effect of weather. J. Hyg. (Camb.), 63:427, 1965.

Monto, A. S., and Cavallaro, J. J.: The Tecumseh study of respiratory illness. II. Patterns of occurrence of infection with respiratory pathogens, 1965–1969. Am. J. Epidemiol., 94:280, 1971.

Tyrrell, D. A. J.: Common Colds and Related Diseases. Baltimore, Williams & Wilkins Company, 1965.

77. RHINOVIRAL RESPIRATORY DISEASE

George Gee Jackson

ETIOLOGY. For many decades, attempts were made to isolate the common cold virus. On some occasions, propagation of infectious material was accomplished for a brief period, but the viruses could not be sustained. In 1954, the virus known as 2060 and the closely related JH strain were isolated from adults with acute coryza. These viruses were believed to be enteroviruses and were designated echovirus 28. Soon thereafter, several different workers isolated similar viruses that were designated in the early literature as Salisbury agents, ERC viruses, entero-like viruses, coryzaviruses, muriviruses, and unclassified common cold viruses. Because of common biologic properties, these are all designated now as rhinoviruses. More than 90 different serotypes of rhinoviruses have been recovered from infected persons. They comprise a subclass in the family of picornaviruses, which also includes the coxsackie-, polio-, entero- and echoviruses. These are all small viruses (10 to 30 mμ) of the ribonucleic acid (RNA) type that are not inactivated by ether. The acid lability (pH 3) of rhinoviruses is probably the reason for their absence from the intestine, and is the major property that distinguishes them from enteroviruses. Rhinoviruses characteristically grow best in tissue cultures held at a reduced temperature (33° C) similar to that found in the nose of man.

EPIDEMIOLOGY. It is likely that rhinoviruses infect persons in all countries and climates. Nearly all adults have evidence of earlier infection with several different serotypes of rhinoviruses. Similar viruses have been recovered from cattle, but the transfer of infection from animals to man has not been shown. In human infections, some serotypes may occur annually, or commonly in different areas and at different times. Over the years since the methods for isolating rhinoviruses were developed, there has been a drift toward newer (higher numbered) types with fewer isolates of the serotypes that occurred earlier. Infections with rhinoviruses characteristically occur in the fall (September, October) and spring (April, May) as epidemiologic waves of acute respiratory illness; they also are the cause of a large proportion of summer colds. About 15 per cent of a young adult population will have neutralizing antibody against any one serotype. In persons with colds, one third of adults and 10 to 15 per cent of children have had rhinovirus recovered from the nasal secretion. However, children are the best transmitters of the disease. Rhinoviruses have been recovered in 1 to 3 per cent of well adults observed during epidemic disease. Infection is believed to occur by the airborne route, but transmission can also occur by hand transfer from contaminated surfaces.

CLINICAL MANIFESTATIONS AND DIAGNOSIS. Rhinovirus infections begin with headache, malaise, chilliness, a dry, scratchy sore throat, and burning nasal membranes and eyes. Nasal discharge and obstruction of the upper air passages rapidly become the dominant symptoms. Cough is a variable and later symptom. Fever is absent or of slight degree and transient. No pharyngeal exudate is observed, but cervical adenopathy can occur. In children, rhinoviruses sometimes cause croup or lower respiratory tract disease, and viremia has been found. Adults occasionally develop symptoms of lower respiratory disease, and sensitive tests of bronchial clearance are abnormal even if lower respiratory symptoms are minimal or absent. In persons prone to asthma, wheezing is common. Also, rhinovirus infections have been observed to be associated with exacerbations of chronic bronchitis. The incubation period is one to three days, and the course of illness is about one week. Rhinovirus appears in the nasal secretion a day or two before the onset of nasal symptoms, and is shed during the period of illness; persistent virus shedding for 10 to 20 days is common. The pathologic findings and pathogenesis are described in Ch. 76. A rise in neutralizing antibody in the convalescent serum occurs in only about one half of the infections.

TREATMENT. There is no specific treatment directed against propagation of the rhinovirus. Supportive measures are those given under treatment of the common cold. Quarantine is not necessary. Interferon produced by rhinovirus infection may be a principal factor in the amelioration of the disease. Pretreatment of volunteers by topical administration of high doses of interferon obtained from human leukocytes or with an interferon inducer was shown to reduce infection and illness. This is attractive, because interferon inhibits rhinoviruses without regard to serotype, but such treatment is not yet practical. In other studies, vitamin C (ascorbic acid) in doses of 3 grams per day by mouth failed to prevent infection and illness. No vaccine is available, but experimental vaccines have been effective against a single type of rhinovirus. The large number of distinct serotypes is discouraging to the prospects of developing an effective vaccine, but some strains produce heterotypic responses. Immunity to reinfection is quite specific and probably lasts only several months to two years after most infections, although detectable serum antibody may persist longer.

Beem, M.: Rhinovirus infections in nursery school children. J. Pediat., 74:818, 1969.

Blair, H. T., Greenberg, S. B., Stevens, P. M., Bilinos, P. A., and Couch, R. B.: Effects of rhinovirus infection on pulmonary function of healthy human volunteers. Am. Rev. Respir. Dis., 114:95, 1976.

Fox, J. P., Cooney, M. K., and Hall, C. E.: The Seattle virus watch. V. Epidemiologic observations of rhinovirus infections, 1965–1969, in families with young children. Am. J. Epidemiol., 101:122, 1975.

George, R. B., and Mogabgab, W. J.: Atypical pneumonia in young men with rhinovirus infections. Ann. Intern. Med., 71:1073, 1969.

Jackson, G. G., and Muldoon, R. L.: Viruses causing common respiratory infections in man. Rhinoviruses. J. Infect. Dis., 127:328, 1973.

Stanley, E. D., Jackson, G. G., Panusarn, C., Rubenis, M., and Dirda, V.: Increased virus shedding with aspirin treatment of rhinovirus infection. JAMA, 231:1248, 1975.

Stenhouse, A. C.: Rhinovirus infection in acute exacerbations of chronic bronchitis: A controlled prospective study. Br. Med. J., 3:461, 1967.

Urquhart, G. E. D., Path, M. R. C., and Stott, E. J.: Rhinoviraemia. Br. Med. J., 2:28, 1970.

78. VIRAL PHARYNGITIS, LARYNGITIS, CROUP, AND BRONCHITIS

George Gee Jackson

The same viruses that cause the common cold also cause other syndromes of respiratory illness. Pharyngitis, laryngitis, croup, or bronchitis may be even more characteristic of infection with some of the viruses than acute afebrile coryza. This clinical classification of the illnesses according to the anatomic site of predominant symptoms is the principal (although unreliable) way the physician has of differentiating diseases of different etiology. The mildest infections are those limited to the upper respiratory tract. As progressively more caudal sites are involved, the infections become more severe and cause more constitutional symptoms. *Acute rhinitis* (the common cold) and *nonexudative pharyngitis* nearly always occur without fever, whereas *exudative viral pharyngitis* is a febrile illness; type A coxsackieviruses are common causes of primary viral pharyngitis with exudate or ulcers, and herpes simplex virus can cause the syndrome. When adenovirus is the cause, *conjunctivitis* is very likely to be a prominent part of the syndrome. With viral pharyngitis the inflammation may extend into the eustachian tubes and cause *primary or secondary otitis media* and *sinusitis*. The lymphoid hyperplasia can include cervical adenitis. *Croup* is a distinctive clinical syndrome resulting from involvement of the larynx with resultant edema and stridor. It is a relatively common manifestation of respiratory viral infec-

tion in children. The classes of viruses most often causing croup are the myxoviruses and parainfluenza viruses. Bronchitis, bronchiolitis, and bronchopneumonia are severe manifestations of viral respiratory infection. They cause fever, respiratory difficulties, and symptoms that often require hospitalization of the patient. The course may be quite abrupt, including sudden unexpected death. More commonly it is acute but benign. Viral infections of the lower respiratory tract can mimic whooping cough or induce asthma or an exacerbation of chronic bronchitis. Similar nonviral infections of the lower respiratory tract with chlamydiae or mycoplasmas must be differentiated for proper therapy. The occurrence of these different clinical syndromes resulting from infection with some of the viruses responsible for the common respiratory infections is indicated in Table 3. Further details about the illnesses and their management are given in the discussions of the specific viruses.

The spectrum of diseases is caused not only by the fact that these viruses are relatively nonspecific in the clinical syndrome produced, but also because manifestations of infection are strongly influenced by age and season. Infants and children have a smaller airway and relative hypertrophy of lymphoid tissue. In them, croup and bronchitis are common symptoms of infections with the same viruses that may cause only coryza or undifferential upper respiratory infection in adults. Constitutional host factors such as allergies and proneness to asthma, bronchitis, or otitis are important determinants of the disease manifestations; sex and race and/or the socioeconomic level of the patient influence the incidence of infection and thereby, to some extent, the syndrome. The principal factor in the amelioration

TABLE 3. Spectrum of Clinical Syndromes Caused by Different Respiratory Viruses

Virus	Coryza	Pharyngitis	Croup	Bronchitis (Bronchiolitis)	Pneumonia or Systemic Disease
Influenza A, B	++		+++	++	++++
Influenza C	++			+	
Parainfluenza 1	+++	++	++++	+	
Parainfluenza 2	+		++++		
Parainfluenza 3	+++	++	+++		+++
Parainfluenza 4	+++	+			
Respiratory syncytial	+++		++	++++	+
Coronavirus	+++	+		+	
Reovirus 1	+				
Coxsackievirus					
A2, 3, 4, 6, 8, 10	+	++++	+		++
A21, 24	+++	+			
Coxsackievirus B2, 3, 4, 5	+	+	+	+	+++
Echovirus 7, 8, 11, 15, 19, 20 (others)	++	++	+		++
Rhinoviruses	++++	+	++		
Adenovirus 1, 2, 5	+	++			+
Adenovirus 3, 4, 7, 14, 21	++	++++		+	+
Herpes simplex		+++			
Nonvirus (filterable)					
Mycoplasmas		+			++++
Chlamydiae				+++	+

TABLE 4. Mechanisms that Contribute to the High Prevalence of Viral Respiratory Infection

Biologic Basis	Examples of Mechanism
New types of virus by mutation of recombination	Influenza A, B
Multiple serotypes simultaneously present	Rhinoviruses
Virus shedding before recognition of disease (and asymptomatic infections)	Influenza Parainfluenza Rhinoviruses
Latent infection with reactivation of virus	Herpes Adenoviruses 1, 2, 5, 6
Inconsistent antibody response to infection	Rhinoviruses Paramyxoviruses
Reinfection in presence of circulating antibody	Respiratory syncytial Parainfluenza 1, 3
Transient immunity after infection or vaccine	Rhinoviruses Influenza
Lasting immunity to disease but recurrent epidemics	Adenoviruses 4, 7 Measles

of viral respiratory illnesses is exerted by the preinfection immunologic status of the host owing to previous infections or vaccines.

FACTORS RELATED TO THE MANIFESTATIONS AND PREVALENCE OF VIRAL RESPIRATORY INFECTIONS

The initial infection with a virus may be resolved without establishing solid immunity to reinfection, or if immunity is established, it may be transient. The capacity of many of the respiratory viruses to cause reinfection has now been established. Reinfection in a partially immune host causes different illnesses from the initial infection. Usually the disease is milder on successive reinfections, but the dose of virus, manner of infection, season, presence of dual infection, and other factors may be of more importance. Sometimes, reinfection in the presence of antibody appears to increase the tissue response and exaggerate the symptoms.

In order for a viral infection to maintain a high prevalence of infection, one or more of several conditions is required. Some of these are virologic; others are epidemiologic or immunologic, as exemplified in Table 4. All these mechanisms are found in the case of one or another of the different viruses that cause common respiratory infections. The result is that we experience a continual endemic and cyclic epidemics of viral respiratory disease, with a large number of viruses infecting various sites of the respiratory tree and producing different anatomically designated clinical syndromes. The level of disease is exaggerated by new types of viruses or new exposures of susceptible hosts and is moderated by a progressive buildup of herd immunity developed by aging, naturally acquired infections, and vaccines. Likewise, the clinical syndrome is affected by these viral, epidemiologic, and host conditions. An appreciation of these factors is essential to the understanding of the problem of viral respiratory infections, their treatment, and control.

Beem, M. O., and Saxon, E. M.: Respiratory-tract colonization and a distinctive pneumonia syndrome in infants infected with chlamydia trachomatis. N. Engl. J. Med., 296:306, 1977.
Eadie, M. B., Stott, E. J., and Grist, N. R.: Virological studies in chronic bronchitis. Br. Med. J., 2:671, 1966.
Ferris, J. A. J., Aherne, W. A., Locke, W. S., McQuillin, J., and Gardner, P. S.: Sudden and unexpected deaths in infants: Histology and virology. Br. Med. J., 2:439, 1973.
Foy, H. M., Cooney, M. K., and Maletzky, A. J.: Incidence and etiology of pneumonia, croup, and bronchiolitis in preschool children belonging to a prepaid medical care group over a four-year period. Am. J. Epidemiol., 97:80, 1973.
Glezen, W. P., and Denny, F. W.: Epidemiology of acute lower respiratory disease in children. N. Engl. J. Med., 288:498, 1973.
Glezen, W. P., Fernald, G. W., and Lohr, J. A.: Acute respiratory disease of university students with special reference to the etiologic role of herpesvirus hominis. Am. J. Epidemiol., 101:111, 1975.
Minor, T. E., Dick, E. C., Baker, J. W., Ouellette, J. J., Cohen, M., and Reed, C. E.: Rhinovirus and influenza Type A infections as precipitants of asthma. Am. Rev. Respir. Dis., 113:149, 1976.

79. ADENOVIRAL INFECTIONS

George Gee Jackson

DEFINITION AND ETIOLOGY. The adenoviruses comprise a distinct group of viruses of the deoxyribose nucleic acid variety. The viral particle has a coat (capsid) consisting of 252 capsomeres arranged in an icosohedron, which is a structure with 20 equilateral triangular faces; it is 60 to 90 nm in size. Most of the capsomeres (240) are six sided, called hexons; the other 12, at the junctions of the triangles, are five sided, called pentons. The hexons have a common group-specific antigen characteristic of all adenoviruses. Each type has specific hexon and penton antigens. There are more than 31 specific serotypes among the strains of human origin. Only a few of them cause infections of the respiratory tract. The common types involved are 1, 2, 3, 4, 5, and 7. Types 14 and 21 also have caused acute respiratory illness. Type 8 is the principal cause of epidemic keratoconjunctivitis.

Some early isolates were recovered from surgically removed adenoids grown as tissue culture explants. These were reported as adenoidal degenerative or AD agents. The first strains from respiratory illnesses were designated RI agents. A later name, used briefly, was adenoidal-pharyngeal-conjunctival or APC agents. All the strains are now included under the term adenoviruses.

EPIDEMIOLOGY. Adenoviruses types 1, 2, and 5 infect virtually all persons early in childhood. They have been associated with febrile pharyngitis, with lower respiratory disease (sometimes fatal), and with gastrointestinal symptoms in infants. In older children and adolescents, adenoviruses, predominantly types 3 and 7 in the United States and 3, 4, 7, 14, and 21 in Europe, cause about 5 per cent of the viral respiratory illnesses. The incidence among college students may be as great as 8 per cent. At military recruit camps, infection with adenovirus types 4 and 7 is highly prevalent. It is often the predominant cause of respiratory illness, and 70 to 80 per cent of all incoming recruits become infected. Among civilian adults, adenoviruses cause only 1 to 3 per cent of respiratory illness.

Adenoviruses occur in all parts of the world. Man is the principal reservoir of infection. Many species of animals also are infected with adenoviruses, but these are of different serotypes, and cross-infection between man and animals either does not occur or is rare. Transmission is by person-to-person contact. The incubation period is three to eight days. In some investigations among civilians, respiratory infection occurred only with close or prolonged contact. However, as noted above, military inductees often become infected with adenoviruses 4 or 7 in the first few weeks of training. The syndrome called acute respiratory disease (ARD) has the highest incidence in the autumn and winter. Asymptomatic enteric infections are common. Conjunctivitis may be highly contagious and transferred by household items in common use, such as towels. Swimming pools have been an effective vehicle for the transmission of adenoviral conjunctivitis and of the disease pharyngoconjunctival fever.

PATHOGENIC MECHANISMS. During the acute infection and for a period of one to three weeks, virus is excreted in the respiratory secretions or in those of the eye, or in both. A high proportion of infected persons have virus in the stool, which may be a source for the spread of infection. Viruria also has been observed during the acute respiratory illness. Adenoviruses replicate in the nucleus of the cell and, when the concentration is high, form crystals of virus. The nuclear chromatin becomes clumped, and the cells may undergo lysis. A most remarkable aspect of adenoviral infections with types 1, 2, 3, and 5 is the capacity of the virus to persist as a latent infection in lymphoid tissue for years after the initial infection. Fifty to 90 per cent of surgically removed adenoids yield adenovirus of one of these types when cultured under conditions that will unmask latent virus. Whether this provides a source for infection of others or any harm to the host is unknown.

Some of the adenoviruses are capable of producing tumors when injected into newborn hamsters. Among the respiratory strains, some isolates of type 7 and type 3 have been oncogenic in baby hamsters. These studies on the tumorigenicity of adenoviruses also have shown the capacity of adenoviruses to combine within the same envelope (capsid) the oncogenic genome of some other tumor-producing viruses of DNA type, specifically the simian virus, SV-40. Thus under defined experimental conditions, adenoviruses can be oncogenic in their own right or act as a carrier for oncogenic material. There is no evidence that these properties give the virus any oncogenic capacity in man, but the phenomena are of basic biologic importance.

Some adrenoviruses have an associated smaller virus (AAV). It is a defective DNA virus which can multiply only in the presence of adenoviruses. The significance of AAV in the pathogenesis of adenoviral infections is not known.

CLINICAL MANIFESTATIONS AND DIFFERENTIAL DIAGNOSIS. Different clinical syndromes produced by adenoviral infections in older children and adults are characteristic. Fever and pharyngitis are the hallmarks; catarrhal otitis occurs frequently, cervical adenopathy is common, conjunctivitis may be present, and a few patients develop pneumonia. The syndromes have been given descriptive names, as follows: (1) acute febrile pharyngitis, (2) nonstreptococcal exudative pharyngitis, (3) acute respiratory disease of recruits, (4) pharyngoconjunctival fever, and (5) adenoviral pneumonia. Any single type of virus among those that cause natural respiratory infections in man can produce the entire spectrum of these clinical manifestations and also the common cold. The age of the patient and the route of inoculation are important. In newborn infants, giant cell pneumonia, myocarditis, and encephalitis have been described. In young children, mesenteric adenitis

and intussusception have been reported. Infection with adenovirus types 1, 2, 5, and 6 may occur in the preschool child without any overt illness, whereas type 7 causes severe illness in this age group, with 5 per cent fatality. The former types infect nearly all children, but type 7 infections are infrequent. The common adenoviruses have been associated in a possible interrelated role with *H. pertussis* in whooping cough. Type 11 has been found as a cause of acute hemorrhagic cystitis in children (girls).

Conjunctivitis, when present, is an acute follicular lesion, often unilateral, with marked erythema, suffusion, and narrowing of the palpebral fissure. Keratoconjunctivitis, caused by adenovirus type 8, is a serious infection of the eye with corneal infiltrates; it rarely occurs in pharyngoconjunctival fever. Pharyngeal exudate, if present, is more likely to appear on the pharyngeal wall than as follicular tonsillitis. Cervical lymph nodes are enlarged and firm but less tender than with streptococcal infections. A macular rash that is difficult to distinguish from rubella has been described in a few cases. The leukocyte count is normal or slightly elevated. A prompt antibody response usually accompanies the infection. It can be measured in the serum by complement fixation or virus neutralization tests.

TREATMENT AND PREVENTION. Treatment is supportive and with few exceptions recovery occurs without sequelae, excluding those of type 8 keratoconjunctivitis. Immunity to reinfection is demonstrable, but second infections have been observed with types 1, 2, 3, and 5. These types cause latent infections, and it is possible that later episodes represent an activation or recrudescence of the latent infection. Reinfection, if it occurs, usually causes mild illness.

Vaccine administration can elicit protective antibody and effectively prevent specific adenovirus infections. Live, enteric-coated, oral adrenovirus vaccines of types 4 and 7 have been extensively evaluated in military recruits at stations where the incidence of infection and disease is high. Given prophylactically, the vaccine stimulates antibody, prevents specific adenovirus illness, and reduces pharyngeal infection after natural exposure by about two thirds. In epidemic situations mass immunization with live virus vaccine promptly interrupts the epidemic. Use of the vaccine is not recommended for civilians because of the low incidence and sporadic occurrence of infection with adenovirus types 4 and 7 among them.

No adenovirus vaccines are available commercially.

Becroft, D. M.: Bronchiolitis obliterans, bronchiectasis, and other sequelae of adenovirus type 21 infection in young children. J. Clin. Pathol., 24:72, 1971.

Bell, J. A., Rowe, W. T., Engler, J. I., Parrott, R. H., and Huebner, R. J.: Pharyngoconjunctival fever. Epidemiological studies of a recently recognized disease entity. JAMA, 157:1083, 1955.

Brandt, C. D., Kim, H. W., Jeffries, B. C., Pyles, G., Christmas, E. E., Reid, J. L., Chanock, R. M., and Parrott, R. H.: Infections in 18,000 infants and children in a controlled study of respiratory tract disease. II. Variation in adenovirus infections by year and season. Am. J. Epidemiol., 95:218, 1972.

Chanock, R. S.: Impact of adenoviruses in human disease. Prev. Med., 3:466, 1974.

Chou, S. M., Roos, R., Burrell, R., and Gutman, L.: Subacute focal adenovirus encephalitis. J. Neuropath. Exp. Neurol., 32:34, 1973.

Dudding, B. A., Top, F. H., Jr., Winter, P. E., Buescher, E. L., Lamson, T. H., and Leibovitz, A.: Acute respiratory disease in military trainees. The adenovirus surveillance program, 1966–1971. Am. J. Epidemiol., 97:187, 1973.

Fox, J. P., Brandt, C. D., Wasserman, F. E., Hall, C. E., Spigland, L., Kogon, A., and Elveback, L. R.: The virus watch program: A continuing surveillance of viral infections in metropolitan New York families. VI. Observations of adenovirus infections: Virus excretion patterns, antibody response, efficiency of surveillance, patterns of infection, and relation to illness. Am. J. Epidemiol., 89:25, 1969.

Jackson, G. G., and Muldoon, R. L.: Viruses causing common respiratory infections in man. Adenoviruses. J. Infect. Dis., 127:328, 1973.

Klenk, E. L., Gaultney, J. V., and Bass, J. W.: Bacteriologically proved pertussis and adenovirus infection. Possible association. Am. J. Dis. Child., 124:203, 1972.

Levy, J. L., Jr.: Etiology of "idiopathic" intussusception in infants. South. Med. J., 63:642, 1970.

Pereira, M.: Adenovirus infections. Postgrad. Med. J., 49:798, 1973.

80. RESPIRATORY SYNCYTIAL VIRAL DISEASE

George Gee Jackson

DEFINITION AND ETIOLOGY. Infection with respiratory syncytial virus (RS) causes epidemic acute respiratory disease. The illnesses are rather acute in onset and may be mild or severe. Since its recognition in 1956 as an infection of man, RS has produced regular epidemics of influenza-like respiratory disease.

Respiratory syncytial virus is a paramyxovirus that resembles influenza and parainfluenza viruses in its structure and many biologic characteristics. It is serologically distinct from them, does not agglutinate erythrocytes as they do, and does not cause lesions in eggs or common laboratory animals. The virus was first isolated from chimpanzees and was designated chimpanzee coryza agent (CCA). The name respiratory syncytial virus is descriptive of the cytopathic effect of the virus in infected tissue cultures. Only one type of the virus is known; some isolates have shown minor differences when tested against specific immune serum, but these appear clinically insignificant with regard to man.

EPIDEMIOLOGY. Respiratory syncytial virus has been recovered on different continents, suggesting that it has worldwide distribution. The epidemiologic pattern of infection lies somewhere between the epidemicity of influenza A and the endemicity of the parainfluenza viruses. Usually there are sharp, well defined limits to each epidemic. In the interepidemic period, the virus is detected much less frequently, but RS virus has been isolated from illnesses in every month of the year. Epidemics recur at intervals of 8 to 16 months. These have appeared simultaneously in geographically widely separated locations. During an epidemic, a large proportion of the population may experience infection, even persons who have had prior infection and have residual serum antibody. The pattern of the epidemic spread is characteristic of airborne or direct contact transmission. The incubation period is three to seven days.

The high prevalence of infection is indicated by the fact that 70 per cent of infants at birth have appreciable amounts of maternal antibody against RS virus. During the first few months of life this declines, and between 3 and 12 months about 35 per cent develop antibody as a result of natural infection. By five years of age, 95 per cent of children have been infected. The incidence of infection with RS virus varies because of its epidemicity, but it makes a significant contribution in the production of serious respiratory diseases of children. Among hospitalized pediatric cases, RS infection has been found to be etiologic in 10 to 20 per cent. In this respect, it ranks ahead of the parainfluenza viruses or adenoviruses and is also more prevalent than influenza as a cause of hospitalization in the first year of life. RS virus is the single most frequent clinical infection causing lower respiratory illness and is a major cause of death in this age group. Among adults, the incidence is less well documented because of the milder nature of the disease, but an increase in hospital admission of adults with lower respiratory disease occurs during periods of RS virus infection.

PATHOGENESIS. Infection causes inflammation of the respiratory mucosa with a tendency for necrotizing bronchiolitis, bronchiolar obstruction, focal atelectasis, and patchy pneumonia. Among people who become infected, 80 to 90 per cent are clinically ill. Infants and adults with chronic bronchopulmonary disease are especially at risk of fatal or severe illness. Ventilatory insufficiency, sometimes severe enough to cause elevation of the arterial Pco_2 as high as 60 to 70 mm Hg, can occur in infected infants. Bacterial pneumonia can be a complication. The annual epidemiologic recurrences of disease, the reisolation of virus from the same children in successive years, and investigations in adult volunteers have all emphasized the importance of reinfections with respiratory syncytial virus. The pathogenesis of the reinfections does not depend on antigenic differences among strains. Clinical investigations show convincingly that the presence of serum neutralizing antibody against the challenge strain does not prevent reinfection or illness. Neutralizing antibody (IgA) appears in the nasal secretion after infection and is protective but not persistent. The high prevalence and importance of RS virus in the causation of respiratory disease appears to reside in this capacity to produce reinfections with clinical symptoms.

CLINICAL MANIFESTATIONS. Fever and bronchiolitis are the characteristics of infection in children. Rhinitis and pharyngitis are usually present. Otitis may occur. In one study, pneumonia was shown roentgenographically in more than two thirds of the cases. Croup may develop, but it is relatively infrequent. The average maximal temperature is 39° C, but in individual patients it may reach 40.5° C. Ordinarily, fever lasts for three days. Dyspnea, cough, and wheezing are obvious symptoms. Tachypnea, rhonchi, and crepitant rales are present on examination. A few of the patients are cyanotic. The leukocyte count is elevated to between 10,000 and 20,000 per cubic millimeter in many cases. This clinical syndrome cannot be distinguished with certainty from epidemic influenza. Ordinarily, there is more rhinitis, and the onset is less abrupt. A fatality rate of 2.5 per cent has been estimated for hospitalized patients. Sudden death of infants and young children in their cribs at home after mild respiratory symptoms has been suspected by epidemiologic association to be of RS etiology.

In about two thirds of the documented cases there is a less severe syndrome, which has been diagnosed in outpatient clinics. These patients have fever, but they have fewer constitutional symptoms than those who are hospitalized. Rhinitis and pharyngitis are relatively more prominent. Cough is frequent, but rales and rhonchi are scarce.

Among adults with prechallenge antibody, the clinical manifestation of infection is acute coryza. However, age and antibody are independent factors in the prevention of severe disease. Serum antibody per se affords little protection. An analysis of proved cases in adults admitted to a hospital in one study indicated that persons with chronic bronchitis (one half of the cases studied) had an acute exacerbation of bronchitis; in one fourth of them infection caused bronchopneumonia, and in one fourth it produced the influenza syndrome with severe constitutional symptoms. Thus the entire spectrum of viral respiratory illness is produced in adults by RS virus.

DIAGNOSIS. The suspicion of RS virus infection is based upon clinical and epidemiologic observations. The diagnosis can be made by virus isolation from the respiratory secretions or by serologic tests. Respiratory syncytial virus is recovered by the inoculation of secretions into cultures of a human epithelial cell line or diploid cell strain. The specimens should be inoculated directly into susceptible cell layers, owing to the loss of virus infectivity by freezing and thawing specimens. Under these conditions virus identification can be made within a few days. The use of specific immunofluorescent antibody to recognize viral antigens in nasopharyngeal secretions has been recommended for rapid diagnosis.

Serodiagnosis can be made by either complement-fixation (CF) or neutralization tests, using paired sera collected as early as possible after the onset of illness and again after two to three weeks. A fourfold or greater rise in the serum antibody titer is regarded as diagnostic of infection.

TREATMENT AND PREVENTION. Careful assessment of respiratory competence, close observation, and supportive care are important, especially in children, in view of the relative severity of the involvement of the lower respiratory tract. Anticipation of the possible need for tracheostomy (to reduce respiratory dead air space and assist in the removal of secretions) and mechanical assistance with ventilation in occasional patients is wise. Antimicrobial drugs have no effect on the RS virus or on the outcome of the usual infection. Isolation of the patient from other susceptible contacts should be done during hospitalization. Nosocomial spread to susceptible contacts is common (30 to 50 per cent) and includes both the patients and the attending staff. However, the spread of infection in the community is not controlled by isolation procedures.

The annual occurrence of epidemic infection and the clear demonstration of reinfections, often with equally severe sequential episodes, might suggest that immunoprophylaxis would have little effect on the infection. On the other hand, the mildness and lower frequency of infections in adults are circumstantial support for the development of immunity. The antigens of the RS virus are labile and poorly antigenic. Use of investigational inactivated vaccine that produced nonprotective levels of serum antibody augmented the clinical severity and fatality of subsequent infection. Similarly, the high fatality among infected infants in the first few months of life, when maternal antibody is demonstrable, suggests that passively acquired antibody may have a paradoxical aggravating effect. Attenuated, temperature-sensitive mutants that can be given as live virus vaccines into the respiratory passages are being developed. Perhaps the larger amount of viral antigen and repeated doses that can be given in this way will induce protection.

Beem, M.: Repeated infections with respiratory syncytial virus. J. Immunol., 98:1115, 1967.

Berglund, B.: Respiratory syncytial virus infections in families. A study of family members of children hospitalized for acute respiratory disease. Acta. Paediat. Scand., 56:395, 1967.

Fransen, H., Sterner, G., Forsgren, M., Heige, Z., Wolontis, S., Svedmyr, A., and Tunevall, G.: Acute lower respiratory illness in elderly patients with respiratory syncytial virus infection. Acta Med. Scand., 182:323, 1967.

Gardner, P. S.: Respiratory syncytial virus infections. Postgrad. Med. J., 49:788, 1973.

Hall, C. B., Geiman, J. M., Biggar, R., Kotok, D. I., Hogan, P. M., and Douglas, R. G.: Respiratory syncytial virus infections within families. N. Engl. J. Med., 294:414, 1976.

Monto, A. S., Bryan, R. E., and Rhodes, L. M.: The Tecumseh study of respiratory illness. VII. Further observations on the occurrence of respiratory syncytial virus and mycoplasma pneumoniae infections. Am. J. Epidemiol., 100:458, 1974.

Parrott, R. H., Kim, H. W., Brandt, C. D., and Chanock, R. M.: Respiratory syncytial virus in infants and children. Prev. Med., 3:473, 1974.

Sommerville, R. G.: Respiratory syncytial virus in acute exacerbations of chronic bronchitis. Lancet, 2:1247, 1963.

Urquhart, G. E., and Gibson, A. A. M.: RSV infections and infant deaths. Br. Med. J., 3:110, 1970.

81.   PARAINFLUENZA VIRAL DISEASES

(Croup)

George Gee Jackson

DEFINITION. Infection with parainfluenza viruses is a common and recurrent cause of respiratory illness. Croup is a prominent syndrome in children, but the spectrum of illness varies from the common cold to pneumonia and systemic illness.

ETIOLOGY. Parainfluenza viruses are members of the family of paramyxoviruses. In structure they closely resemble influenza virus but differ from it serologically and in some biologic respects. Four distinct types of parainfluenza viruses are recognized that cause infections in man. They are closely related to one another and have some characteristics in common with mumps, measles, and respiratory syncytial virus. Types 2 and 4 differ somewhat from types 1 and 3 in the clinical illnesses produced and in their epidemiology.

Parainfluenza viruses were first designated as hemadsorption or HA viruses, owing to their property of causing erythrocytes to absorb and stick to infected cells in tissue cultures. Type 2 was recovered from cases of croup and initially was called the "croup-associated" or CA virus. A strain of parainfluenza type 1, the Sendai virus, was first isolated in mice and called influenza D. Mice and other rodents were then recognized to have natural infection with parainfluenza viruses. The Sendai and other animal strains of parainfluenza type 1 have slight serologic differences from strains of human origin. A simian myxovirus (SV-5) is commonly found in monkey kidney tissue cultures, occasionally in eggs and other tissues. It resembles parainfluenza type 2; virus isolates from cattle with shipping fever (SF-4) were found to be parainfluenza type 3.

EPIDEMIOLOGY. Few, if any, persons escape infection and reinfection with the different types of parainfluenza viruses. Most children develop antibody from infection with parainfluenza type 3 before the age of four years. By the time they enter school, 70 per cent of children have antibody against more than one type. Among older children and adults, nasopharyngeal reinfection with types 1 and 3 is common regardless of the presence of serum antibody. Reinfection with parainfluenza viruses accounts for an appreciable proportion of common colds and upper respiratory illnesses in adults. The annual rates of infection are inversely related to age with preschool children, principally those of ages two to five years, being highest at 80 to 95 per cent per year. The over-all rates are 30 to 45 infections per 100 persons per year. This accounts for about 5 per cent of all respiratory infections in children.

Parainfluenza types 1 and 3 are endemic and cause illness in all seasons of the year. A study in Glasgow, Scotland, indicated that infections in the autumn were usually type 1 and those in the summer type 3. The former tended to have a biennial epidemic cycle, occurring predominantly in even-numbered years. Parainfluenza type 2 may be reciprocal with type 1 in its times of occurrence. Type 3 is a more infectious virus, has annual endemicity, and is associated with a wide spectrum of respiratory infections, including viral pneumonia. Similar results have been obtained from most surveys. All types can cause epidemics of respiratory disease in the winter season. Together, the parainfluenza viruses cause about 40 per cent of all cases of croup. A greater proportion of infections with types 1 and 2 cause croup, but because of its greater prevalence and transmissibility, type 3 may be a more frequent cause of the croup syndrome. Type 3 virus spreads easily from person to person. It infects virtually all contacts who have no antibody and reinfects many persons with a demonstrable level of antibody in the serum. Type 1 virus does not spread as efficiently as type 3, but is nevertheless highly transmissible. Type 2 infection has been less prevalent and more episodic in its occurrence than either type 1 or type 3 and infects older children. Infections caused by type 4 have been entirely sporadic and infrequently recognized.

Although many animal species have a high incidence of infection with the parainfluenza viruses, spread to man from these sources has not been well established.

CLINICAL MANIFESTATIONS. The clinical syndrome of croup in children is the most common characteristic of infection with parainfluenza viruses. Involvement of the trachea and bronchi also increases the amount of mucous secretions, which can become inspissated and cause additional respiratory obstruction. Type 3 infections may be symptomatically more severe and cause more lower respiratory tract disease. Although croup is the most distinctive syndrome, parainfluenza virus infections cause rhinitis or pharyngitis more than twice as often as croup, and bronchitis, bronchiolitis, or pneumonia at least as frequently as croup. Over-all, croup is a symptom in fewer than 10 per cent of infections.

The initial infection with parainfluenza viruses produces more severe disease than reinfection and produces fever of 39 to 40° C in about three fourths of the cases. Among older children and adolescents only about two thirds of infections are symptomatic. Among adults, parainfluenza viruses cause mostly upper respiratory tract disease, predominantly the common cold or afebrile coryza. About one third of patients with reinfection will have fever, but many will be asymptomatic. In dual viral infections, a parainfluenza virus has been recognized as a common member of the pair with a resultant increase in the severity of the symptoms. Extrarespiratory manifestations are occasionally associated with parainfluenza infections, usually type 3. Associations that are presumed etiologic are myocardi-

tis, pericarditis, polyarthritis, meningoencephalitis, and rash.

DIAGNOSIS. Clinical differentiation of the type of parainfluenza viral infection and even the differentiation from other viral infections of the respiratory tract cannot be made with confidence. The virus can be isolated from nasopharyngeal secretions during the illness and for a brief period thereafter. This is the most certain and may be the only way to identify the specific type of parainfluenza virus involved. However, the sampling methods used are still relatively insensitive, and culture-negative infections are quite common. Serologic responses are often heterotypic owing to the nearly universal infection of persons with type 3 early in life and the common infection with types 1, 2, and mumps viruses. A rise in antibody against one of these viruses does not permit confidence in a strain-specific diagnosis.

TREATMENT. The treatment is supportive, as described for the common cold. The croup syndrome may be very acute, and cause respiratory insufficiency requiring urgent and decisive management. A comfortably warm, draft-free environment with high humidity (steam) is recommended for reducing laryngeal stridor. Maintenance of an adequate airway is essential. Antimicrobial drugs are usually contraindicated. Inactivated virus vaccines have been produced for types 1, 2, and 3, and their antigenicity has been shown, but their effectiveness in the prevention of natural infection has not been convincing.

Buchan, K. A., Marten, K. W., and Kennedy, D. H.: Aetiology and epidemiology of viral croup in Glasgow, 1966–72. J. Hyg. (Camb.), 73:143, 1974.

Cooney, M. K., Fox, J. P., and Hall, C. E.: The Seattle virus watch. VI. Observations of infections with and illness due to parainfluenza, mumps and respiratory syncytial viruses and *Mycoplasma pneumoniae.* Am. J. Epidemiol., 101:532, 1975.

Herrmann, E. C., Jr., and Hable, K. A.: Experiences in laboratory diagnosis of parainfluenza viruses in routine medical practice. Mayo Clin. Proc., 45:177, 1970.

Jackson, G. G., and Muldoon, R. L.: Viruses causing common respiratory infections in man. Enteroviruses and paramyxoviruses. J. Infect. Dis., 128:387, 1973.

Loda, F. A., and Glezen, W. P.: Parainfluenza virus infections. Prev. Med., 3:481, 1974.

Monto, A. S.: The Tecumseh study of respiratory illnesses. V. Patterns of infection with the parainfluenzaviruses. Am. J. Epidemiol., 97:338, 1973.

Starke, J. E., Heath, R. B., and Curwen, M. P.: Infections with influenza and parainfluenza viruses in chronic bronchitis. Thorax, 20:124, 1965.

Wenzel, R. P., McCormick, D. P., and Beam, W. E.: Parainfluenza pneumonia in adults. JAMA, 221:294, 1972.

82.   INFLUENZA

Edwin D. Kilbourne

DEFINITION. Influenza is an acute, contagious disease that is usually attended by fever and prostration and is ordinarily benign in outcome. The headache, myalgia, and asthenia that characterize the disease are severe out of proportion to the symptoms originating from involvement of the respiratory tract — the primary and principal site of infection with the causative virus.

HISTORY. Epidemics of respiratory disease similar to modern influenza have been recorded through the centuries. Since the year 1510 there have been 31 pandemics described. The calamitous nature of these epidemics may have led to the naming of the disease by the Italians as an "influenza" or influence of the heavenly bodies or perhaps as an "influenza di freddo" (influence of the cold).

In 1933 the isolation of a virus in ferrets by Smith, Andrewes, and Laidlaw established the specific infectious etiology of the disease, and led rapidly to accurate definition of its epidemiology and clinical variations. The virus isolated in 1933 is now known as influenza A virus.

A second type of virus was isolated independently in 1940 by Francis and by Magill (influenza B virus). In 1950 influenza C was isolated from a patient in nonepidemic circumstances by Taylor, and later was shown by Francis and his associates to be the cause of epidemic disease.

Five pandemics of influenza have been recorded in the twentieth century (1900, 1918, 1946, 1957, and 1968). Of these, the pandemic of 1918 was most severe, accounting for at least 20 million deaths. Effective inactivated viral vaccines were introduced in the 1940's, but had never been employed in mass prophylaxis until 1976, when immunization of 50 million Americans was carried out in anticipation of a pandemic of swine influenza that never materialized.

ETIOLOGY. Influenza is a consequence of infection with certain *myxoviruses* that have common physical, chemical, and biologic properties. These viruses comprise three groups (A, B, and C), which are completely unrelated antigenically, do not induce cross-immunity to one another, and have different epidemiologic characteristics. Four major subgroups of influenza A viruses associated with human disease have been identified since discovery of the virus in 1933, each having replaced the other in chronologic succession. Serologic studies defined a virus that first appeared in swine in 1918 (HswN1) as the probable cause of the notorious human pandemic of that year. Influenza A virus subtypes are defined on the basis of antigenic analysis of their two outermost proteins. These biologically active glycoproteins (hemagglutinin [H] and neuraminidase [N]) are the primary determinants of immunity and mutate independently, as was clearly evident in the replacement of H2N2 by H3N2 (Hong Kong) virus in 1968 (see accompanying table). The hemagglutinin (H) is responsible for binding the virus to the cell; antibody to this protein therefore neutralizes the virus and is the major determinant of immunity. The viral neuraminidase (N) is instrumental in release of virus from cells; antineuraminidase antibody is not neutralizing, but limits viral replication and therefore the course of infection. As external spike-like projections from the viral envelope, H and N are in immediate contact with host antibody during infection and therefore are under selective pressure (see Epidemiology). Beneath these "spikes" the virus particle is bounded by a lipid bilayer derived from the host cell (Fig. 1). Just beneath the lipid layer the core of the particle is surrounded by

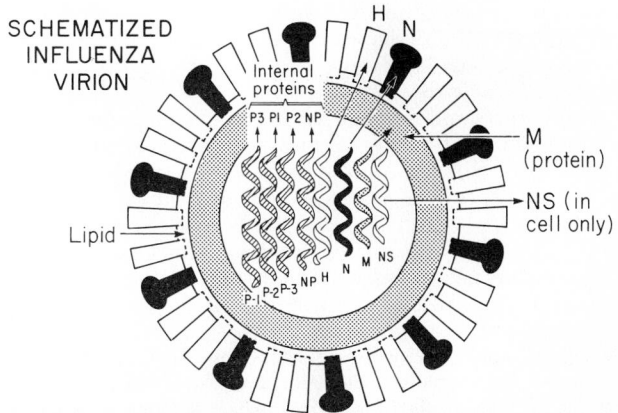

Figure 1. Schematic representation of influenza virion, indicating the eight viral genes and their polypeptide products. The relative sizes of the RNA genes are only approximate, and the structural details of their relationship to one another and to the internal proteins P1–P3 and NP are not known. (From Kilbourne, E. D.: The Harvey Lectures, series 73. New York, Academic Press, 1977–78.)

the M or membrane protein. The nucleoprotein (NP) occurs in helical form in association with the viral RNA. The internal M, NP, and three P proteins (of undefined location and function) are common to all influenza A viruses and do not differ significantly in antigenic nature from one subtype to the other. Type-specific A, B, or C categorization of virus thus depends on serologic reactions (usually complement-fixation) mediated by these internal antigens.

The viral genome within comprises eight segments of RNA (totaling 3.9×10^6 daltons) capable of reassortment during infection to provide an unusually high frequency of genetic recombination. Isolated viral RNA(s) is not infectious, because it does not constitute the message. Virus-coded transcriptase is necessary for viral replication. Thus the RNA segments code for monocistronic messages for each of the seven virion proteins and for a nonstructural protein detectable only in the host cell.

Influenza B and C viruses have been less thoroughly studied, but appear to be structurally similar to influenza A viruses. Little antigenic variation of influenza C virus has been remarked, and antigenic variation of influenza B virus has been of lesser magnitude than that observed with influenza A.

The influenza viruses are of medium size (approximately 850 Å in diameter), and by conventional electron microscopy they appear spherical or filamentous in form, with spike-like projections.

EPIDEMIOLOGY. The arbitrary designation of the three types of influenza virus as A, B, and C coincides fortuitously with their relative rank as causes of severe epidemic disease. Influenza B and C viruses have been associated chiefly with sporadic epidemics in children and young adults, notably in school or other institutional populations. Most adults carry antibodies to these viruses, probably as the result of recurrent subclinical infection. There is no evidence that pandemics of influenza B or C have occurred.

Discussions of influenza are usually concerned with the influenza A viruses, for these are the important and apparently more mutable viruses that cause widespread

Influenza Pandemics: Relation to Major Antigenic Change in Causative Viruses*

Pandemic, Year	Virus Isolation	Viral Antigens	Magnitude of Change	Pandemic	Severity†
1918	1930‡	Hsw1N1	...	Yes	Unequaled
1929	1933‡	H0N1	Moderate	?	Moderate
1946	Yes	H1N1	Moderate	Yes	Slight
1957	Yes	H2N2	Great	Yes	Great
1968	Yes	H3N2	Partial	Yes	Moderate

*From Kilbourne, E. D.: JAMA, 237:1225, 1977.

†Estimate based on excess mortality.

‡Year of isolation of probable agent. Virus not isolated in pandemic year.

epidemic and pandemic disease. The complicated and still puzzling epidemiology of influenza A is most conveniently considered by separate discussions of the *pandemic, epidemic,* and *endemic* infections — all attributable to the same virus under different conditions.

Pandemic Influenza. Pandemic or worldwide infection with influenza A viruses has occurred five times in the present century. Viruses isolated in the pandemics of 1946, 1957, and 1968 have proved to be antigenically very different with respect to their hemagglutinin antigens. The severity of pandemics can be roughly related to the magnitude of change in hemagglutinin and neuraminidase antigens (see table).

When such major antigenic changes in the virus occur — perhaps as a reciprocal of high immunity in the general population — the mutation may be so extreme that acquired immunity in the population to previously existing influenza A viruses is inadequate to prevent infection or disease initiated by the new virus, which replaces the older virus completely. Under these conditions, people of all ages and in all places are susceptible to influenza, and a worldwide epidemic or pandemic may ensue (Fig. 2). In 1976, the emergence of human infection with swine influenza virus at Fort Dix, New Jersey, was unusual in that a major epidemic did *not* follow, despite antigenic novelty of the virus. The replacement of the H3N2 subtype with the returning H1N1 ("Russian") subtype of the early 1950's appears to be in prospect.

The source of the markedly different strains of virus that suddenly appear to initiate pandemics is unknown. Direct mutation from the antecedent virus seems unlikely in view of the magnitude of change in H and N antigens. Therefore recombination in nature of human and animal influenza A viruses has been proposed to explain the recurrent decennial introduction of apparently novel viruses into the human population.

The incubation period of influenza is only 24 to 48 hours, so that, once progressive spread begins, the impact on the community is sudden and devastating. Both the incidence and the severity of illness are highly variable and are influenced by age, pregnancy, and preexisting chronic disease and by such environmental factors as crowding and season of the year. Morbidity is usually first noted among schoolchildren, then in young adults, and finally in older, less active, and presumably less exposed members of the community. Infection of the aged is more frequently followed by bacterial pneumonia. As a consequence, a "second wave" of increased community mortality may coincide with the delayed appearance of influenza in this age group — *at a time when influenza is no longer apparent in the community* by the usual criterion of absenteeism from school or industry.

Specific immunity to influenza develops rapidly after infection, but it may decline within one or two years so that recurrence of infection and disease from the same antigenic type of virus may occur *under conditions of heavy exposure* as in military barracks or boarding schools. On the other hand, the steady decline in community morbidity after the initial pandemic wave obviously points to the acquisition of immunity of some durability by most of the population.

Interpandemic "Epidemic" Influenza. Influenza occurs in its characteristic acute epidemics in the early months of the year in the north temperate zone. In a particular community the epidemic usually comes and goes within a month, rising to a peak in 12 to 14 days, and subsiding almost as rapidly. Although the case fatality rate is less than 1 per cent, the presence of influenza may be detected by a sudden increase in unspecified total mortality in the community. This mortality occurs at both extremes of age, and is occasioned principally by the bacterial pneumonias that may complicate influenza in the very young and very old.

Epidemics of influenza A have been demonstrated to occur every year since discovery of the virus, but communities are usually spared recurrence for two or more years after an epidemic.

After a pandemic, the frequency and extent of epidemics gradually abate with the development of population immunity to the new virus. Minor antigenic variations of the virus may be detected during this time, but at least a decade seems to be required for change sufficient to establish a truly "new" subtype (Fig. 2).

Endemic Influenza. The interepidemic survival of influenza virus has long been a puzzle in view of the fragility of the virus and its apparently obligate restriction to human hosts. It has become increasingly clear,

INFLUENZA PANDEMICS OF THE PAST CENTURY
(Major antigenic variations)

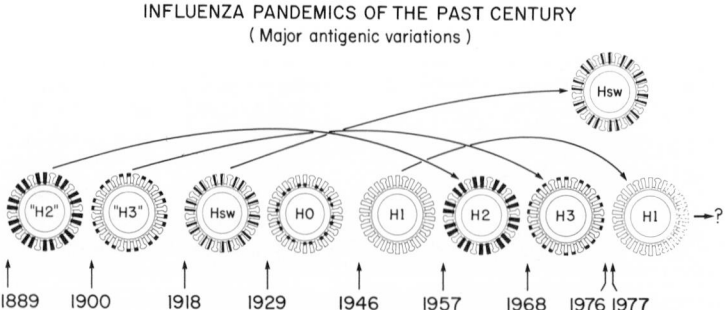

Figure 2. Schematic representation of periods of prevalence of major hemagglutinin subtypes of influenza A viruses. The year of introduction of the "new" subtypes is indicated by arrows. The designations H0, H1, and so on refer to hemagglutinin subtype of the viruses without reference to their neuraminidase antigens. Subtypes Hsw, H0, and H1 are more closely related antigenically than they are to H2 or H3. Identification of viral subtypes prior to 1933 (marking the first isolation of a human influenza virus) is inferential on the basis of studies of human antibodies. The abortive appearance of Hsw in 1976 is shown. The future prevalence of H1 is conjectural. (From Kilbourne, E. D.: The Harvey Lectures, series 73. New York, Academic Press, 1977–1978.)

however, that influenza virus infections may occur continuously within the population, either as sporadic instances of disease that are not recognized as influenza or as clinically inapparent infections. As more and more members of the population develop immunity, infections without disease become more and more frequent and serve to maintain the virus in the community. Such infections are recognized by serologic studies.

PATHOLOGY AND PATHOGENESIS. The primary lesion of influenza is a necrosis of the ciliated epithelium of the respiratory tract. In the uncomplicated infection epithelial damage is probably confined to the upper and middle portion of the respiratory tract, the trachea being the most strikingly involved. Early in infection the necrotic ciliated cells are desquamated, leaving intact the basal cell layer. On about the fifth day of illness regeneration begins in the basal layer with the development of undifferentiated "transitional" epithelium, which may simulate metaplasia. After two weeks ciliated cells may again be seen.

When influenza is complicated by bacterial pneumonia, the pathologic findings are variable and depend on the nature of the secondary invader. However, *primary influenza virus pneumonia* presents a characteristic picture. The lungs are dark red, heavy, and edematous. The trachea and bronchi contain bloody fluid, and the mucosa is hyperemic. Microscopy shows ciliated epithelium to have been lost from the trachea, bronchi, and bronchioles, but evidence of epithelial regeneration may be seen. In the submucosa, focal hemorrhage, edema, and slight leukocytic infiltration may occur. Capillary thrombosis with focal leukocytic exudate has been described. The alveolar spaces contain neutrophilic and mononuclear cells admixed with fibrin and edema fluid. Intra-alveolar hemorrhage is common in the lower lobes. The alveolar septa may be thickened, and acellular hyaline membranes may line alveolar ducts and alveoli.

Pathologic changes attributable to influenza occur only rarely outside the respiratory tract. There are no physiologic or biochemical changes in the patient that are pathognomonic of influenza. Although "leukopenia" is often stated to be characteristic, total leukocytic counts in the uncomplicated disease may vary from 2000 to 14,000 cells per cubic millimeter, and are usually in the normal range. However, *lymphocytopenia* is commonly detectable, especially in the first four days of illness. The erythrocyte sedimentation rate may be moderately elevated or normal. No characteristic changes occur in the bacterial flora of the respiratory tract.

The Complicated Disease. In primary influenza virus pneumonia, *leukocytosis* is the rule, even in the absence of bacterial pathogens, although the erythrocyte sedimentation rate may not be elevated. *Serum glutamic oxaloacetic transaminase concentrations* are elevated in proportion to the severity of pulmonary involvement and may exceed 60 units per milliliter. *Oxyhemoglobin saturation* is reduced to 46 to 85 per cent. *Partial pressure of CO_2* is elevated, and the *pH of arterial blood* is lowered. The *proteinuria* and elevated *blood urea nitrogen* concentrations that may be noted are the results of fever and dehydration and do not reflect primary renal damage. No notable changes in *serum electrolytes* or in *blood clotting* occur.

CLINICAL MANIFESTATIONS. Infection with influenza virus may be asymptomatic, may be attended only by slight fever, or may result in the "typical" prostrating disease that identifies epidemics. This disease is remarkably constant in its expression from year to year, and the uncomplicated case of pandemic influenza does not differ from the "three-day fever" of nonpandemic outbreaks. The higher fatality rates associated with the 1918 pandemic were usually attributable to secondary bacterial pneumonia. Significant variations in the disease caused by any of the A or B subtypes of virus have not occurred. Influenza C appears to be a less severe disease, but it has not yet received adequate study.

Patients with influenza almost invariably *cough*, although this symptom may not be bothersome or even noted by the patient. The cough is brief and spasmodic, and usually not productive of sputum. Other symptoms related to the destruction of respiratory epithelium are *substernal burning pain* (from the trachea), *dryness or soreness of the throat,* and *nasal obstruction and discharge.* Neither sore throat nor evidence of rhinitis is particularly prominent in influenza. Slight *pharyngeal injection* may be noted. *Epistaxis* is rare, but is valuable diagnostically when it occurs. *Conjunctival burning and injection* are common.

In 5 to 10 per cent of patients with uncomplicated disease, crepitant or musical *rales, roughened breath sounds,* or *pleural friction rub* may be detected. Such signs rarely persist for more than one or two days. *Chest pain* may accompany the friction rub, or more often is substernal and referable to the trachea.

The prostrating effects of influenza are associated with *fever, chilly sensations* (seldom with rigors), *headache,* and *myalgia. Fever* usually exceeds 38° C. and may reach 41° C. It is usually abrupt in its onset and decline and lasts for only two to five days in the absence of complications. *Headache* is often frontal and is of the throbbing sort associated with fever; its severity is proportional to the degree of fever. *Extraocular myalgia* is a characteristic but not universal complaint that may be elicited only by examination. *Myalgia* may be generalized or confined to the back or lower extremities. *Gastrointestinal symptoms* are uncommon, and occur more often in patients with pre-existing gastrointestinal disease.

In sum, the picture of uncomplicated influenza is that of a patient with flushed face and reddened eyes who lies flat in bed and coughs occasionally with a dry spasmodic cough. He moves about fitfully, complaining of headache or backache. By contrast, the rare patient with influenza virus pneumonia (see below) sits erect, is extremely anxious and agitated, gasps for breath, and manifests *cyanosis* of the lips and nailbeds.

COURSE AND COMPLICATIONS. In both pandemic and epidemic influenza the disease, although acute and prostrating, is brief, so that it is uncommon for any symptom to last beyond seven to ten days, and fever usually subsides earlier (Fig. 3). A protracted *postinfluenzal asthenia* has been emphasized in some reports. It is not clear to what extent secondary bacterial infections or psychogenic factors contribute to the state. Nevertheless, the alerting of the patient to the possibility may save some apprehension during the convalescent period. *Encephalitis* and *myocarditis* have been described infrequently as complications of influenza, and have rarely been well documented or associated with virus isolation from the brain or heart.

The important and potentially lethal complications of

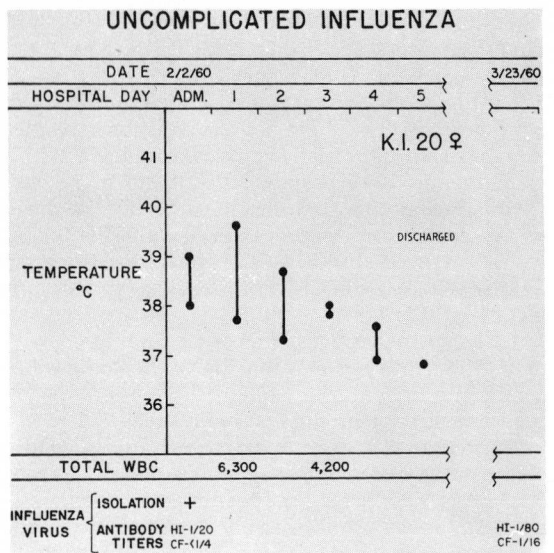

Figure 3. (From Kaye, D., et al.: Am. Rev. Respir. Dis., 85:9, 1962.)

influenza derive from infection of the lung, either with the influenza virus itself or with bacterial pathogens. The pulmonary complications of influenza may be considered as (1) *primary influenza virus pneumonia*, (2) *combined influenza virus and bacterial pneumonia*, and (3) *influenza complicated by secondary bacterial pneumonia*. All three types of complication are more frequent in patients with pre-existing cardiac or pulmonary disease or in women late in pregnancy. The aged, in whom apparent or inapparent chronic disease is more frequent, are also understandably more vulnerable to pulmonary complications of influenza. Neurologic complications have been temporally associated with influenza, as

with other respiratory viral infections. Evidence for a clear-cut causative role of the virus in such sequelae is lacking. Recently, Reye's syndrome in children (see Ch. 309.4) has occurred with increased frequency after influenza epidemics, especially influenza B.

Primary Influenza Virus Pneumonia. Primary influenza virus pneumonia is a severe disease that is usually fatal. Within 24 hours of the onset of typical symptoms of influenza, the patient experiences high fever (39.5 to 40° C), a cough productive of bloody sputum, and profound dyspnea and anxiety. Cyanosis is notable, and poor air exchange is indicated by the generalized pulmonary findings, which include suppression of breath sounds, expiratory wheezing, and diffuse, moist rales. Signs of consolidation are absent. Chest roentgenograms disclose diffuse bilateral nodular infiltrates that radiate outward from the hilum, sparing the lung periphery.

The patient almost always dies within five to ten days of the onset of illness after a course characterized by unremitting fever, progressive pulmonary involvement, and terminal vascular collapse (Fig. 4). Antibacterial drugs, oxygen, bronchodilators, and corticosteroids are usually unavailing.

Pathogenic bacteria are not recoverable from the sputum, blood, or lung during life or post mortem, and influenza virus is demonstrable in high concentrations in the lung.

Primary influenza virus pneumonia ordinarily is restricted to patients with pre-existing cardiac or pulmonary disease or pregnancy. Still more specifically, the victim usually has rheumatic cardiovascular disease and mitral stenosis. The predilection of this complication for the patient with mitral stenosis suggests that hemodynamic factors such as pulmonary hypertension are more important in its pathogenesis than general debility or the absence of specific immune mechanisms.

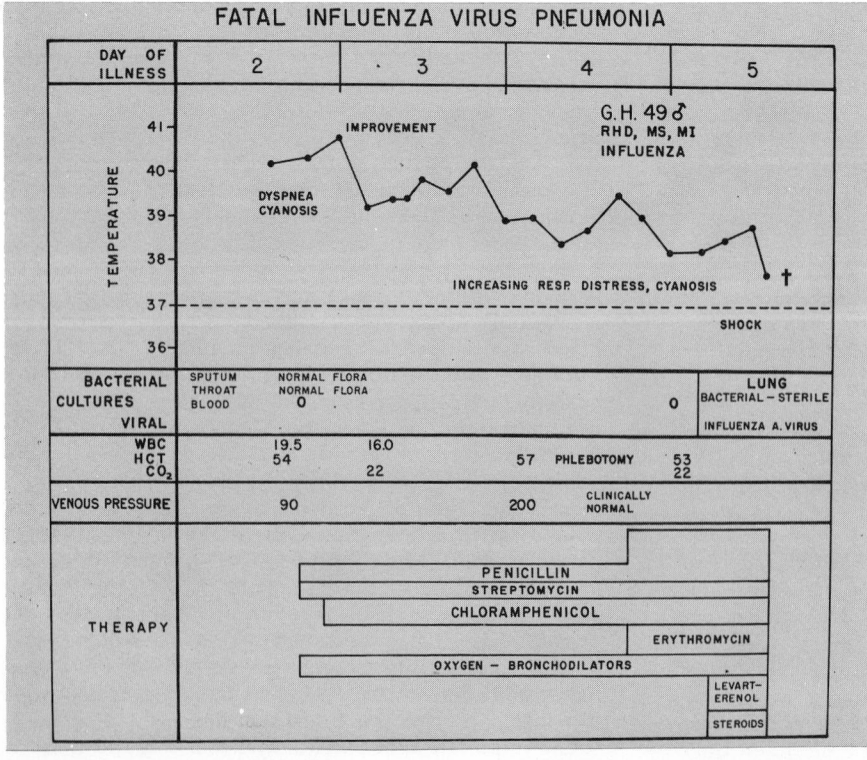

Figure 4. (From Kaye, D., et al.: Am. Rev. Respir. Dis. 85:9, 1962.)

There appears to be a graded spectrum of severity of the disease caused by influenza virus, so that, intermediate between the uncomplicated case with transient rales and the fatal virus pneumonia, occasional instances of "mild segmental influenza virus pneumonia" have been described.

Combined Influenza Virus and Bacterial Pneumonia. In patients with primary influenza virus pneumonia, infection with bacterial pathogens may supervene. In such patients the characteristic and dramatic onset of the virus pneumonia may be attended or closely followed by such symptoms of bacterial pneumonia as *productive cough, shaking chills,* or *pleuritic pain.* Signs of focal consolidation may be engrafted upon the diffuse pulmonary findings of the viral infection. Pneumococcus, *Staphylococcus, Hemophilus influenzae,* or, more rarely, group A streptococci may be demonstrated by culture of lung, blood, or sputum. In 1957–1958, pneumococcus and *Staphylococcus* were the most frequent bacterial invaders.

The host setting and course of the combined infection are basically the same as in the pneumonia associated with influenza virus infection alone.

Influenza Complicated by Secondary Bacterial Pneumonia. Bacterial pneumonia, characterized by focal consolidation, may occur after influenza in previously healthy persons as well as in the ill and infirm. This complication is further distinguished from influenza virus pneumonia by (1) the lag between influenzal symptoms and the appearance of pneumonia, sometimes with brief interval of freedom from symptoms; (2) the presence of focal and not diffuse pulmonary involvement; and (3) the absence of influenza virus in throat washings, but the presence of bacterial pathogens in the sputum. This "late" type of pulmonary complication is by far the most common.

DIAGNOSIS. In the context of an epidemic, influenza may easily be distinguished from other acute respiratory diseases, although diagnosis of the isolated case may be difficult. In its typical form influenza is characterized by relatively high fever, which sets it apart from the syndrome of the *common cold.* With the common cold, nasal symptoms predominate, but they are usually minor in influenza. *Adenoviral infections* are the most difficult to distinguish from influenza, but, in general, fever and prostration are less, onset is less sudden, and sore throat and laryngitis are more prominent in adenoviral disease. One of the clinical forms of respiratory syncytial viral disease may closely mimic influenza. The aching, febrile, minor illnesses associated with infection by various arbo- or enteroviruses may also simulate influenza but are notably unattended by cough, although sore throat may occur. In *streptococcal pharyngitis,* the greater frequency of vomiting, the predominance of sore throat, and the occurrence of cervical adenitis and leukocytosis are helpful in differential diagnosis. *Primary atypical pneumonia* is usually distinguishable clinically from influenza virus pneumonia by its more gradual onset, purulent sputum, and indolent, ordinarily benign course.

The *definitive diagnosis* of influenza depends upon isolation of the virus from throat washings or sputum and the demonstration of an increase in specific humoral antibodies. Viral isolation is most successful in the first two to three days of illness and is best accomplished by the intra-amniotic inoculation of chick embryos. Primary cultures of mammalian cells may also be used but are less satisfactory. If virus grows to high enough titer on the first passage, isolation and identification of the agent may be accomplished within 48 to 72 hours of inoculation of the specimen. Fluorescent antibody staining of exfoliated nasal epithelial cells, although infrequently used, can be applied as a quick and specific diagnostic test.

Antibody may be detected in the patient's serum by neutralization, hemagglutination-inhibition, or complement-fixation tests as early as eight to nine days after the onset of illness, but maximal response is evident only after 14 days. The diagnosis cannot be made with a single serum specimen because of the prevalence of antibody in the population; rather an *increase* in antibody titer of fourfold or more must be demonstrated by the study of two or more serum specimens obtained early in illness and in convalescence.

PROGNOSIS. The prognosis is ordinarily favorable in this brief and self-limited disease. However, the severity of the disease is a reciprocal of host susceptibility, and the outcome may be fatal in those with prior cardiac or pulmonary disease. The prognosis is also influenced by the prevalence of potential respiratory bacterial invaders in the community and the prospects for their control.

TREATMENT. There is no specific treatment for influenza. The general measures used in the symptomatic treatment of other infections are useful, including especially aspirin (0.3 to 0.6 gram) for the headache, malaise, and myalgia, and codeine sulfate (0.016 to 0.064 gram) for irritability, cough, and substernal pain. Diet may be regulated by the patient with the warning that high fat foods are not well tolerated. Fluids should be given in abundance.

Routine antibacterial prophylaxis is unnecessary and inadvisable, but may be considered for those with chronic disease with the view of forestalling the sequel of pneumococcal pneumonia. In this case, full therapeutic doses of penicillin should be given.

Treatment of primary influenza viral pneumonia is highly unsatisfactory, but oxygen therapy with positive pressure breathing devices has shown some promise.

PREVENTION. Influenza may be prevented by the parenteral injection of vaccines of influenza viruses that have been produced in the chick embryo and rendered noninfective (inactivated) by formalin or ultraviolet irradiation. The duration of protection usually does not exceed one year under conditions of epidemic exposure. Present vaccines are principally *bivalent* in that they contain the contemporary influenza A virus component and also lesser amounts of influenza B antigen. These newer vaccines have been purified by density gradient centrifugation or chromatography and are far less toxic than preparations of the past. So-called "split virus" vaccines contain antigens of the disrupted virus. They are of low reactogenicity, but may be less immunogenic than vaccines made from whole virus.

In experimental field trials amantadine hydrochloride has had a chemoprophylactic effect in influenza, as evidenced by lower infection rates and less severe illness in subjects who received the drug shortly before exposure to the infection. After infection, antibody titers were lower in drug-treated subjects, presumably reflecting a decreased antigenic stimulation from reduced viral replication. The drug is presumed to act by inhibiting virus penetration and not intracellularly on virus replication. Some evidence suggests that amantadine may have a slight therapeutic effect if given soon after the initiation of infection. Central nervous system toxicity may limit the usefulness of this compound in older people.

Because protection provided by inactivated influenza vaccine is transient, immunization of the general population is not usually indicated.

The objectives of vaccination differ in epidemic and pandemic years. In both situations, the prevention of *mortality* in the elderly and chronically ill is a major goal. In interpandemic periods, efforts to reduce morbidity have been restricted to those essential to the maintenance of community services or those particularly liable to epidemic disease such as military recruits and boarding school students. However, the wholesale morbidity associated with pandemics justifies consideration of mass immunoprophylaxis prior to or early in the course of such epidemics. An unanticipated increased risk of acquiring the Guillain-Barré syndrome

was associated with the administration of almost 50,000,000 doses of swine influenza vaccine in 1976. It is not yet clear whether or not the enhanced risk is specifically related to influenza vaccine, or whether it might also be observed following mass administration of other antigens followed by similar prospective surveillance of the immunized population. Live virus vaccines offer promise of longer immunity, but have not yet been licensed in the United States.

Douglas, J. G., Jr.: Influenza in man. *In* Kilbourne, E. D. (ed.): The Influenza Viruses and Influenza. New York, Academic Press, 1975, p. 395.

Kilbourne, E. D.: Influenza pandemics in perspective. JAMA, 237:1225, 1977.

Louria, D. B., Blumenfeld, H. L., Ellis, J. T., Kilbourne, E. D., and Rogers, D. E.: Studies on influenza in the pandemic of 1957–1958. II. Pulmonary complications of influenza. J. Clin. Invest., 38:213, 1959.

Smith, W., Andrewes, C. H., and Laidlaw, P. P.: A virus obtained from influenzal patients. Lancet, 2:66, 1933.

VIRAL DISEASES
CHARACTERIZED BY CUTANEOUS LESIONS

83. MEASLES

(Morbilli, Rubeola)

Edwin D. Kilbourne

DEFINITION.   Measles is an extremely contagious, febrile disease of high morbidity characterized by rash and catarrhal inflammation of the eyes and respiratory tract. It is principally a benign disease of children, but may afflict with equal frequency persons of any age not previously immunized by infection or vaccination.

ETIOLOGY.   Measles is caused by a medium-sized RNA paramyxovirus approximately 1400 Å in diameter. The virus is of a single antigenic type and resembles other paramyxoviruses (e.g., parainfluenza and mumps viruses) in structure and biologic activity, except that it lacks a neuraminidase. Thus measles virus is an enveloped, lipid-containing virus that is released from the infected cell by budding evagination. The virus bears external spikes that contain a hemagglutinin capable of agglutinating erythrocytes of certain primates. Hemolytic and fusing activity is carried by another viral protein. In contrast to the genome of influenza viruses, the RNA is not segmented and high frequency genetic recombination of the virus does not occur. Antigenic variation of the virus has not been noted. Measles virus is antigenically and biologically related to the viruses of canine distemper and bovine rinderpest.

Measles virus replicates most readily in primary cultures of human embryonic tissue or primate kidney cells. However, adaptation of virus to a variety of primary or continuous mammalian and avian cell cultures has been achieved. (Vaccine viruses are propagated in chick embryo cells.)

Subhuman primates have long been known to be susceptible to measles; recently, propagation of the virus in the brains of mice, hamsters, and ferrets has been achieved, demonstrating its neurotropic potential.

EPIDEMIOLOGY.   Measles is a disease of cosmopolitan distribution, endemic in all but isolated populations. It may occur at any time of the year, but most outbreaks are in the late winter and early spring, with a peak at the end of April. The disease recurs in epidemic cycles at two- to three-year intervals in most civilized communities that have been studied. This epidemic periodicity is best explained as a result of the introduction of new susceptibles into the population by birth or ingress from other areas. When the proportion of nonimmunes reaches a certain crucial concentration (45 to 50 per cent), disease and coincident dissemination of virus may occur to produce an epidemic. It is likely that virus is introduced from sources external to the involved population, probably by incoming susceptibles. Isolated communities such as the Faröe Islands (Panum) are infrequently attacked by measles, at which times manifest illness appears in virtually all persons not previously infected. In Greenland, a country not known to have been invaded previously by the disease, an epidemic resulted in overt measles in 99.9 per cent of the indigenous population (Christiansen et al.).

Throughout most of the world, measles is a disease of children; most adults possess acquired immunity. Beyond the age of ten more than 90 per cent of the population have specific antibody. Although the peak attack rate coincides with the beginning of school (age six) in technologically advanced societies, it occurs between the ages of two and three in most developing countries. A recent trend of adolescent infection in the United States may have resulted from widespread but incomplete immunization that allows unimmunized children to escape infection until later as opportunity for natural infection has declined. Morbidity and mortality rates do not appear to be influenced by sex or race. Case fatality rates are highest in children less than five years of age, and are also relatively high in the aged. Congenital infection has occurred.

There is no evidence that the virus may vary in virulence in nature. The oft-cited and notorious virulence of the disease in primitive, isolated, or crowded populations may be explained as a corollary of (1) more prevalent infection of feeble and aged adults, (2) poor environmental conditions, (3) inadequate medical care, and (4) secondary bacterial infections. A strikingly increased mortality rate is observed in areas such as West Africa in which protein-calorie malnutrition is prevalent. Because measles virus per se rarely induces fatal disease, it is evident that fatalities attributable to measles may vary in incidence according to the prevalence of bacterial pathogens and the resistance of the population to their presence.

Communicability. Measles is one of the most contagious of infections. Demonstration of virus in nasopharyngeal secretions is in accord with epidemiologic evidence that infection is disseminated and acquired by the respiratory tract. Close physical proximity or direct person-to-person contact is the usual requisite for infection.

Immunity. An unmodified attack of measles is usually followed by lifelong immunity. This observation is in accord with the observed persistence of both complement-fixing and neutralizing antibodies after infection and the relatively high titer of antibodies present even in older persons. The mechanism of persistent immunity after measles is undefined. Although persistence of infective virus after infection seems not to occur, the internal nucleocapsid of measles virus or a closely related variant is demonstrable years after infection in the brain and peripheral lymph nodes of those rare individuals afflicted with subacute sclerosing panencephalitis (SSPE) (see Ch. 310.4). Thus the potential for viral persistence exists, and in those afflicted with SSPE, antibody levels to measles virus are higher than in those who have experienced uncomplicated measles.

A more likely explanation for the persistent immunity in measles is the maintenance of such immunity by subclinical exogenous reinfection. Careful studies of isolated or closed populations after administration of live virus vaccine have demonstrated a more rapid decline of antibody titer than in populations in which measles virus is circulating. Anamnestic antibody response in the absence of disease has been shown in immune contacts of patients with measles. Thus achievement of eradication of the virus may be compromised as vaccination (see below) is more and more effective in curtailing the circulation of the wild virus; then the booster immunization provided by natural reinfection will become inoperative, and repeated vaccination in the same subject may be required. Passively transferred maternal antibody protects the young infant from measles but also reduces the possibility of effective immunization by live virus vaccines at that age.

PATHOLOGY AND PHYSIOLOGIC RESPONSES. Pathologic changes in fatal measles usually represent the compound effect of viral and secondary bacterial infection. Pneumonia is almost invariably present; it is most frequently interstitial, but may produce purulent exudate within the alveoli. More representative are changes of the uncomplicated viral disease within the tonsillar, nasopharyngeal, and appendiceal tissue removed during the prodrome. These changes consist of subepithelial round cell infiltration and the presence of multinucleated giant cells. The latter are so characteristic that skilled pathologists have predicted the development of rash from their presence in surgical specimens. Similar cells are commonly observed in tissue cultures infected with measles virus. Cytoplasmic and nuclear inclusions may be seen in epithelial cells. The lesions clinically apparent as Koplik's spots derive from inflammatory mononuclear cell infiltration of buccal submucous glands and necrosis of focal vesicular lesions of the mucosa. Rash is the result of proliferation of capillary endothelial cells in the corium and the coincident exudation of serum, and occasionally erythrocytes, into the epidermis. Viral microtubular aggregates are found in the endothelium of dermal capillaries, but not in the epidermal layer. Therefore the rash may represent an Arthus reaction elicited by viral antigen within dermal capillaries. The contribution to disease and recovery of cytotoxic immunospecific lymphocytosis is under study.

No consistent or characteristic physiologic aberrations are observed with measles. The transient hemoconcentration and albuminuria found with other febrile diseases may occur. A normal total leukocyte count or leukopenia is observed throughout the febrile period. Initially, the leukopenia is occasioned by a decline in lymphocytes on the first day of fever; subsequently, granulocytopenia ensues as well. It has been demonstrated that measles virus replicates in lymphoid tissues (spleen, thymus, lymph nodes), can multiply in vitro in peripheral blood T and B lymphocytes and monocytes, and can be isolated from blood leukocytes during the course of the disease. The incubation period is characterized by neutrophilia, and convalescence by a relative lymphocytosis. Measles virus has been isolated from the leukocytic fraction of blood, and is propagable in suspensions of leukocytes in vitro. A false-positive serologic test for syphilis may be observed.

Immunosuppressive Effects of Measles. It has long been known that cell-mediated immunity is impaired during measles. There is transient suppression of the tuberculin reaction (observed also with measles vaccines), improvement in eczema and allergic asthma, delay in wound healing, and the induction of remissions in leukemia, Hodgkin's disease, Burkitt's lymphoma, and lipoid nephrosis. Actual infection of activated lymphocytes may explain the depression of cell-mediated immunity during the acute disease. In severe disease, the magnitude of depression of the total lymphocytes has been positively correlated with a lessened chance of recovery.

CLINICAL MANIFESTATIONS. After an incubation period that averages 11 days, measles becomes clinically manifest with symptoms of fever, malaise, myalgia, and headache. Within hours *ocular symptoms* of photophobia and burning pain are evidenced by conjunctival injection, tearing, and exudate in the conjunctival sac. Concomitantly, or soon thereafter, *catarrhal inflammation of the respiratory tract* is manifested by sneezing, coughing, and nasal discharge. Less commonly, hoarseness and aphonia may reflect laryngeal involvement. In this prodromal stage of one to four days' duration, petechial lesions of the palate and pharynx or tiny white spots on the buccal mucosa *(Koplik's spots)* may herald the appearance of skin rash. The white lesions described by Koplik characteristically occur lateral to the molar teeth, and typically are mounted on red areolae of injected mucosa, which may coalesce to form a diffuse red background. Not invariably present, they constitute a valuable, if not pathognomonic, diagnostic sign. The enanthem may involve other mucous membranes such as the vaginal lining. It may "overlap" the subsequent appearance of the cutaneous rash by one to

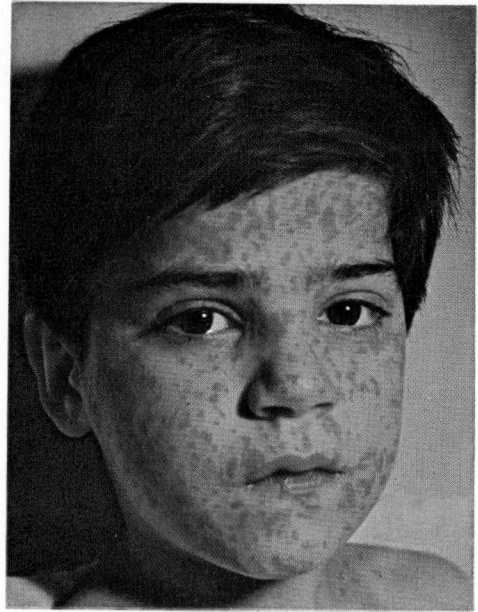

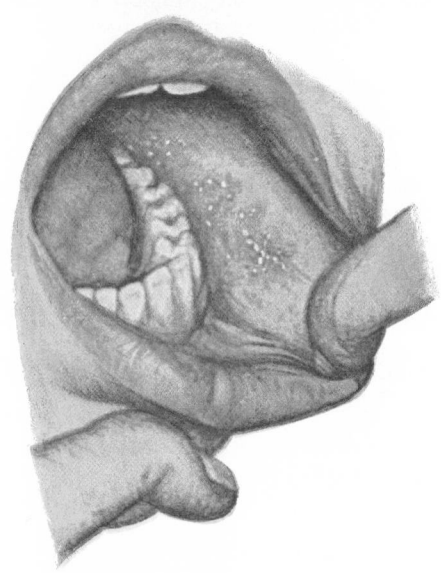

Upper: Early measles eruption. (Reproduction from Therapeutic Notes, by Courtesy of Parke, Davis & Company.) *Lower:* Koplik's spots in measles (Hecker, Trumpp, and Abt).

three days. Rarely, a transient, erythematous exanthema may occur in the prodromal period.

The *rash* of measles follows the prodromal symptoms by two to four days, occasionally as late as seven days. It first appears behind the ears or on the face as a blotchy erythema, spreads downward to cover the trunk, and finally is manifest on the extremities. The hands and feet may escape involvement. Initially, the eruption consists of discrete, reddish-brown macules that blanch with pressure. Subsequently, these lesions become slightly elevated, tend to coalesce, and may develop a hemorrhagic, nonblanching component. Rash is sometimes very extensive in children with protein-calorie malnutrition, and skin lesions associated with kwashiorkor may develop at the site of the exanthem. The rash fades in the order of its appearance; its disap-

pearance about five days after onset is attended by a fine, powdery desquamation that spares the hands and feet. At its maximum the exanthema usually marks the termination of malaise and fever in the uncomplicated illness.

The *fever* of measles is commonly of the typhoidal, progressively rising type, and falls by lysis. It persists for about six days, and frequently reaches 39.5° C. In the adult, fever may follow rather than antedate the catarrhal symptoms. Throughout the febrile period, productive *cough* and auscultatory evidence of bronchiolitis may be evident. These manifestations may persist after defervescence, and cough is often the last symptom to disappear. It is probable that bronchopulmonary symptomatology is an integral part of the primary viral infection; roentgenographic evidence of pulmonary involvement is frequently seen in the uncomplicated disease in the absence of leukocytosis and obvious bacterial infection.

COMPLICATIONS. It is difficult to distinguish between those complications directly attributable to the virus of measles and those resulting from secondary bacterial infections. The persistence or recurrence of fever and the occurrence of leukocytosis are presumptive evidence of the usual bacterial sequelae of *otitis media* or *pneumonia.* The pneumonia resembles other forms of viral pneumonia and is often caused solely by a specific reaction to the measles virus. Superimposed bacterial infection is common, however, and accounts for most of the severe or fatal cases. Pneumococcus, *Streptococcus hemolyticus, Staphylococcus aureus,* and *Hemophilus influenzae* are the usual secondary invaders. The incidence of bacterial complications is increased by crowding, debility, and the prevalence of bacterial pathogens in the population. Bacterially engendered sequelae may be unduly frequent in crowded contagious disease hospitals.

Serious complications directly related to the measles virus are rare. *Laryngitis* of sufficient severity to embarrass respiration has been observed, and may warrant tracheostomy. *Electrocardiographic abnormalities* may be found in as many as 30 per cent of children, but clinical evidence of cardiac disease is meager in such cases. *Abdominal pain* or *diarrhea* may be related to invasion of lymphoid tissue of the appendix or Peyer's patches. These symptoms may lead to unnecessary surgery before the appearance of the typical rash. The frequency of stomatitis and gastrointestinal symptoms is greater in malnourished children in tropical areas and may reflect coincident bacterial and parasitic infection.

Encephalomyelitis. A rare (0.1 per cent) but serious consequence of measles is a demyelinating encephalomyelitis that may appear from 1 to 14 days after the onset of infection. This complication is associated with a recurrence of fever, and headache, vomiting, and stiff neck. Stupor and convulsions occasionally follow. Localizing neurologic symptoms may or may not be present. Death ensues in about 10 per cent of patients; about half of survivors suffer permanent residuals of varying severity. Measles virus has been recovered from the brain of a patient with fatal measles "postinfectious" encephalitis six weeks after onset of measles. Recently, abnormal electroencephalograms were recorded in 51 per cent of children with measles *without evidence of encephalitis.* In some of the children the abnormal encephalographic findings were persistent. As noted above, the presence of virus has been demonstrated in patients with subacute sclerosing panencephalitis.

Other late sequelae of measles are thrombocytopenic purpura and exacerbation or activation of pre-existing pulmonary tuberculosis. The late complication of subacute sclerosing panencephalitis (see Immunity, above) is discussed in Ch. 310.4.

Giant-Cell Pneumonia. In children with severe disease involving the reticuloendothelial system (especially leukemia), measles virus may induce an interstitial pneumonia characterized by giant cells and intracellular inclusion bodies. The disease is usually fatal; if the patient survives, persistence of virus and poor antibody formation are evident in convalescence. The pneumonia may occur in the absence of rash so that its etiologic relation to measles may be unsuspected.

Measles Modified by Vaccine or Antibody Administration. Attenuation of the natural disease by antibody prophylaxis may result in an illness of lessened severity comparable with the milder infection of the maternally immunized newborn. Fever alone may be observed, but some degree of exanthema is usually apparent. Koplik's spots may not appear. In general, the course is truncated and relatively uncomplicated. Similar attenuated disease may occur in children partially immunized with inactivated viral vaccine.

Unfavorably Modified Measles—A New Disease. After administration of inactivated measles vaccine (no longer in general use), infection of vaccinees with either live measles vaccine or wild-type natural measles virus led to the development of a new syndrome characterized by dermal hypersensitivity to measles virus and an atypical (petechial, vesicular, or urticarial) rash atypical in distribution. In some cases pulmonary complications occurred. The mechanism of this reaction is unknown, but it may be a manifestation of delayed hypersensitivity to the viral proteins engendered by alum-precipitated inactivated viral vaccine. No such sequelae have followed primary immunization with live virus vaccine. Failure of inactivated vaccine to protect may be related to the absence of the hemolysin antigen of the viral envelope.

DIAGNOSIS. The experienced layman can diagnose typical measles. The querulous, bleary-eyed child, his face blotched and his nose crusted with exudate, presents a characteristic, if miserable, picture as he breathes open-mouthed between paroxysms of sneezing and coughing. The severity of the catarrhal symptoms distinguishes the disease from other eruptive fevers. In the prodromal period the diagnosis should be suggested by (1) fever higher than that of the usual common cold, (2) known measles in the community, and (3) Koplik's spots on the buccal mucosa.

Differential diagnosis (see accompanying table) includes consideration of rubella, scarlet fever, exanthema subitum, infectious mononucleosis, secondary syphilis, drug eruptions, and infection with certain coxsackie- and echoviruses. Of value in excluding these possibilities are the milder course and pinker rash of rubella, the sore throat and leukocytosis of scarlet fever, and serologic tests for infectious mononucleosis and syphilis. The rash of exanthema subitum does not appear until the termination of fever. Fever, enanthema, and catarrh are uncommon with the cutaneous manifestations of drug hypersensitivity.

Specific Diagnosis. Specific diagnosis depends on the isolation of measles virus from throat washings, blood, or urine by inoculation of various types of tissue culture with materials obtained during the first five days of illness. Increase in specific antibody may be detected as early as the first or second day of rash by the complement-fixation test. Antibody is also demonstrable by neutralization and hemagglutination-inhibition procedures. The latter is generally employed for serologic surveys and is correlated with susceptibility to infection.

Presumptive diagnosis may be made if giant cells are detected in stained smears of nasal exudate in the pre-eruptive period.

PROGNOSIS. Uncomplicated measles is rarely fatal, and complete recovery from the disease is the rule. Fatalities are almost always the result of secondary streptococcal or pneumococcal pneumonia, occurring principally in children below the age of five who become infected after the dissipation of passive neonatal immunity. Mortality in economically underdeveloped countries may be 250 times that observed in the United States or northern Europe. Case fatality rates are also high in elderly and tuberculous patients. Congestive cardiac failure is a common cause of death in patients over 50 years old.

Antimicrobial drugs effective against the usual secondary invaders have reduced the case fatality rate of measles sharply. The incidence of otitis media and pneumonia may be lowered by the prophylactic use of penicillin or a tetracycline early in illness.

Encephalitis occurs as frequently in mild as in severe measles (i.e., about one in a thousand cases). However, the incidence of neurologic sequelae after administration of attenuated live virus vaccine is only one in a million.

TREATMENT. There is no specific treatment for measles.

Symptomatic Therapy. In the absence of complications, bed rest is the essence of treatment in this usually benign, self-limited disease. Codeine sulfate (0.015 to

A Guide to the Differential Diagnosis of Measles

	Conjunctivitis	Rhinitis	Sore Throat	Enanthem	Leukocytosis	Specific Laboratory Tests Available
Measles	++	+	0	+	0	+
Rubella	±	±	±	±	0	+
Exanthema subitum	±	±	0	0	0	0
Enterovirus infection	0	±	±	0	±	+
Scarlet fever	±	±	++	0	+	+
Infectious mononucleosis	0	0	+	0	±	+
Drug rash	0	0	0	0	0	0

0 Not usually present; no test available.
± Variable in occurrence.
+ Present; test available.
++ Present and severe.

0.06 gram) is useful in the amelioration of headache and myalgia and is effective in the management of cough. Aspirin (0.3 to 0.6 gram) may be employed for its analgesic and antipyretic actions. Diet should be unrestricted. Bright light is not an ocular hazard, but photophobia may require darkening of the patient's room.

Antimicrobial Prophylaxis. The course of uncomplicated measles is not influenced by antimicrobial therapy. In common practice the incidence of serious bacterial infections is not sufficient to justify the routine prophylactic use of antimicrobials. Certain special circumstances may warrant full therapeutic dosage with penicillin or the tetracyclines in anticipation of the potentially fatal sequelae of pneumococcal or betahemolytic streptococcal infections. These circumstances include treatment of the chronically ill, the very young, or the aged, and the treatment of patients under crowded conditions that foster the increase and dissemination of pathogenic bacteria, as may occur in contagious disease hospitals. If careful observation of the patient is possible, rational therapy is based on the prompt recognition and etiologic definition of complications, followed by initiation of the appropriate antimicrobial drug in proper dosage.

PREVENTION. Vaccination. Highly effective vaccines are available for the prevention of measles. Most are derived from the Edmonston strain of measles virus isolated in the laboratory of Dr. John Enders. This strain, although it proved very effective in early trials as a live virus vaccine, produced febrile and other reactions (attenuated measles) with such high frequency that it has been supplanted by *"further attenuated" (live virus) vaccines* that are almost as effective as the original vaccine in inducing immunity. These live virus vaccines produce immunity by infection, and therefore need be given only as a single injection. They induce antibody response of somewhat lesser magnitude than that following natural infection. In children over one year of age, seroconversion after vaccination is 90 to 97 per cent. Although a gradual fall in antibody titer occurs in the absence of exposure to wild type virus (see Epidemiology: Immunity), serum antibody is demonstrable in most individuals 8 to 15 years after a single administration of vaccine. The occasional failure of live virus vaccine to protect has recently been related to vaccination at less than 12 months of age, at which time maternal antibody may inhibit replication of the vaccine virus. It is now recommended that measles immunization be deferred until after 15 months of age in technologically advanced countries in which infantile infection is uncommon. Reimmunization is not harmful and is recommended for those who have received vaccine before 13 to 15 months of age.

Contraindications to live virus vaccine include pregnancy, leukemia and other systemic malignant diseases, active tuberculosis, and administration of resistance-depressing drugs such as corticosteroids and antimetabolites.

Inactivated vaccine produces impermanent immunity and unfavorably alters response to later infection. It therefore is no longer recommended (see Complications, above).

Eradication of measles through administration of live virus vaccines is a scientifically reasonable possibility. The introduction of immunization in the United States in 1963 has led to a decrease in annual incidence of from about 500,000 to 35,000 cases per year. However, subsequent resurgence of disease is undoubtedly attributable to underutilization of vaccine in susceptible groups, particularly populations in impoverished circumstances. The reinstitution of Federal funds for measles vaccine in 1971 reversed the upward trend of disease in the following year.

Christiansen, P. E., et al.: An epidemic of measles in southern Greenland, 1951. Acta Med. Scand., 144:313, 430, 450, 1952–53.

Enders, J. F., Katz, S. L., Milovanovic, M. V., and Holloway, A.: Studies on an attenuated measles-virus vaccine. I. Development and preparation of the vaccine: Technics for assay of effects of vaccination. N. Engl. J. Med., 263:153, 1960.

Kimura, A., Tosaka, K., and Nakao, T.: Measles rash. I. Light and electron microscopic study of skin eruptions. Arch. Virol., 47:295, 1975.

Koplik, H.: The diagnosis of the invasion of measles from a study of the exanthema as it appears on the buccal mucous membrane. Arch. Pediat., 13:918, 1896.

Panum, P. L.: Observations Made During the Epidemic of Measles on the Faröe Islands. Delta Omega Society, 1940.

Tyler, H. R.: Neurological complications of rubeola (measles). Medicine, 36:147, 1957.

Yeager, A. S., Davis, J. H., Ross, L. A., and Harvey, B.: Measles immunization. Successes and failures. JAMA, 237:347, 1977.

84.   RUBELLA

(German Measles)

Edwin D. Kilbourne

DEFINITION. Rubella is an acute, benign, contagious disease of children and young adults. The cardinal manifestations of the illness are a pale pink rash and posterior cervical lymphadenitis. Paradoxically, this mild disease is one of the few viral infections convincingly associated with the genesis of fetal abnormalities. When infection is acquired in utero, it often results in generalized disease of the infant and protracted excretion of virus after birth. Accordingly, recognition and prevention of the disease are matters of far-reaching consequence.

ETIOLOGY. Rubella virus is a small, spherical RNA virus with a mean diameter of 550 to 600 Å. The particle is ether sensitive — an attribute of lipid-containing enveloped viruses. The virus develops by budding from marginal and intracytoplasmic membranes. On the basis of its structure and chemical characteristics, the virus has been classified as a separate genus (*Rubivirus*) of the togaviruses. Unlike other togaviruses, there is no evidence of its transmission by arthropods. The virus is clearly unrelated to the virus of measles.

The virus agglutinates the erythrocytes of newly hatched chicks — a characteristic that permits measurement of both virus and antibody. Rubella virus replicates with the production of cytopathic effects in a number of commonly employed cell culture systems, including African green monkey and human diploid cells. Virus replication and production of embryopathic effects similar to those in humans have been experimentally induced in rats.

EPIDEMIOLOGY. Precise information on the incidence of rubella is not available, but 82 to 90 per cent of young adults have specific hemagglutination-inhibiting (HI) antibodies against the virus. The mildness and brevity of clinical signs of rubella may confound the diagnosis and reporting of many instances of infection.

Studies of the experimental disease lend support to prior clinical evidence that infection may occur without rash, and indicate a further diagnostic pitfall. It can be said, however, that the disease is seen on every continent, may occur in epidemic form, and has its highest incidence in the early spring. The disease is less frequently acquired in childhood than measles, as is attested by serologic studies and by the fact that rubella is more common than measles in young adults. The higher incidence of infection in younger age groups in institutional outbreaks argues against a greater susceptibility of the adult. Prior to the introduction of rubella vaccination in the United States in 1969, the highest attack rates were observed in infants and children of less than nine years of age. Since 1972, a relative (but not absolute) increase in the number of cases in adolescents and young adults has occurred. It is probable that rubella is spread by the respiratory route by close and sustained personal contact. The usual infection is contagious during the period of prodromal symptoms and for as long as seven days after the appearance of rash. However, it is now recognized that the infant with congenitally acquired infection may excrete virus for months after birth and is contagious during this time. The epidemiologic implications of this fact — first established in the large epidemic of 1963–1964 — are yet to be determined. There is evidence that the newborn may be unusually contagious, and that although he may have no obvious stigmata of infection, yet he may be shedding virus. The relative contribution of children and young adults to the spread of infection is under debate. However, herd immunity is of little consequence in curtailing infection.

Immunity is lasting. HI antibodies have been demonstrated 30 years after initial infection. Authenticated second attacks are rare, and require serologic documentation because of the nebulous nature of the clinical syndrome. *Subclinical* reinfection demonstrated by increase in IgG serum antibody has been documented with increasing frequency as better serologic methods and increased surveillance have become available. Reinfection occurs most commonly in crowded populations in which the density of infection and probably of spread are high. It is important to note that most such reinfections are not associated with viremia and thus probably pose little threat in pregnant women. As in many other infections, IgM response serves to distinguish primary from reinfection. Presumably, as in measles, inapparent infections may boost immunity throughout life. Immunity that follows artificial immunization with live virus vaccine is of a lesser degree. (See Prevention, below.)

PATHOLOGY. Death from uncomplicated postnatally acquired rubella is unknown. Histologic changes characteristic of the disease have not been demonstrated. The onset of disease is attended by leukopenia resulting from a decrease in both lymphocytes and neutrophils. Rubella infection causes temporary suppression of response of lymphocytes to mitogens. After five days, absolute lymphocytosis is manifest. The total leukocyte count is normal at the tenth day.

Congenital Rubella. Necropsies of fetal and infantile victims of maternal infection have shown a variety of embryonal defects related to developmental arrest involving all three germ layers. Those defects most consistently associated with maternal rubella are microcephaly, cataract, patency of the ductus arteriosus, and defects of the interventricular septum. However, recent studies have revealed a wide spectrum of tissue damage in association with virologically proved disease of varying severity. In some infants hepatic and renal degeneration and myocardial necrosis without inflammation have been noted, whereas in others thrombocytopenia and purpura may be the sole abnormality. It has been proposed that the generalized visceral involvement and characteristic residua of the disease may result from a sequence of platelet damage, intravascular coagulation, and thrombosis. Another theory holds that the smaller size of the rubella-infected infant and some abnormalities may reflect inhibition of multiplication of embryonic cells by the virus.

CLINICAL MANIFESTATIONS. Postnatally Acquired Rubella. Fourteen to 21 days after exposure to the infection, the onset of rubella is evidenced by symptoms variable in their occurrence and severity. Cough, sore throat, and coryza may initiate the illness, but are often absent; headache, malaise, and myalgia may precede the eruption, especially in young adults. Commonly, fever and obvious enlargement of posterior cervical nodes antedate the appearance of the rash. Fever, when present, rarely exceeds 38° C and seldom persists beyond 48 hours. Injection of the bulbar conjunctivae may be noted. Palpable, tender, and occasionally visible lymphadenopathy involves postauricular and suboccipital nodes with sufficient frequency to be an important diagnostic sign. Generalized peripheral lymphadenitis, and, more rarely, splenomegaly, may occur.

The exanthema of rubella is usually apparent within 24 hours of the first symptoms as a faint macular erythema that first involves the face and neck. Characterized by its brevity and evanescence, it spreads rapidly to the trunk and extremities, sometimes leaving one site even as it appears at the next. The pink macules that constitute the rash blanch with pressure and rarely stain the skin. Rubella virus has been isolated from the skin lesions. Diffuse erythema on the second day of rash may closely simulate scarlet fever. The eruption has vanished by the third day. Rubella may occur without rash. An enanthema has been described that is inconstant in form and occurrence, and lacks the premonitory significance of the Koplik spots of measles. The lesions consist of red macules that usually involve the soft palate.

COMPLICATIONS. Recovery is almost always prompt and uneventful, although relapse occurs with greater frequency than in most viral diseases (5 to 8 per cent). Secondary bacterial infections rarely occur. Rare complications are arthralgia, neuritis, gingivitis, thrombocytopenic purpura, and increased capillary fragility. Heart block has been described. A *meningoencephalitis* of short duration may occur one to six days after the appearance of rash. Its incidence is estimated at 1 in 6000 cases, and it is fatal in approximately 20 per cent of those afflicted. Rubella encephalopathy is not associated with demyelinization (in contrast to other postviral encephalitides). Survivors may have electroencephalographic abnormalities, but intellectual function seems to be preserved.

Congenital Rubella. The fortuitous coincidence of the development of cell culture systems for the isolation of rubella virus and the occurrence of a global epidemic of rubella (in 1963–1964) demonstrated that the classic ocular and cardiac "teratogenic" effects of rubella are but isolated manifestations of a continuing and persisting fetal infection. It is now clear that congenital transplacental infection of the fetus occurs as a consequence of maternal infection (which may or may not be clinically evident), usually in the first trimester of pregnancy. Virus is demonstrable in placental and fetal tissues obtained by therapeutic abortion at that time. If pregnancy is not interrupted (and spontaneous abortion is uncommon), fetal infection persists, and upon delivery of the infant, virus is recoverable from the throat, urine, feces, conjunctivae, bone marrow, and cerebrospinal fluid of the living infant and from most organs at autopsy. About 10 to 15 per cent of infants born to mothers infected in the first trimester of pregnancy have stigmata of infection readily recognizable in the first year of life. These include *cardiac lesions, cataracts, glaucoma, microphthalmia,* and *esophageal atresia.* Most infants in whom virus is detectable do not have evidence of disease at birth or may simply have a lower than normal birth weight. In others, disease of intermediate severity occurs. Most prominent of these manifestations is *thrombocytopenic purpura,* which disappears soon after birth. *Hepatosplenomegaly* may persist for months. Other signs include *corneal clouding, fullness of the fontanels, lesions of the long bones,* and *electroencephalographic abnormalities.* A chronic erythematous rash associated with the presence of rubella virus in the skin has been reported in some patients. Recently, a progressive panencephalitis simulating subacute sclerosing panencephalitis has been observed in the second decade following congenital infection.

A striking finding has been the persistence of virus in the pharynx, gastrointestinal tract, and cerebrospinal fluid for as long as one year after birth (9 per cent). Infective virus was present in a congenital cataract after three years, and in the urine of a victim of congenital rubella 29 years after her birth. This evidence of continuing viral synthesis occurs coincidentally with circulating antibody (initially of maternal origin) and originally suggested a form of "immunologic tolerance" to the virus. However, it has been shown that the character of the antibody changes during the first year from IgG (presumably maternal) to IgM, indicating a primary response of the infant to the persisting viral antigen. Studies of older infants and children with stigmata of congenital rubella show them to be free of demonstrable virus and to possess the IgG immunoglobulins that characteristically persist after other viral infections. The defect in host response that is responsible for viral persistence has not yet been defined.

DIAGNOSIS. Rubella may be diagnosed clinically with assurance only during an epidemic. It may be difficult to distinguish from mild or modified measles, infectious mononucleosis, or scarlet fever. Distinction from measles may be made on the basis of pinker, nonstaining rash, the milder course, and the lesser catarrh of rubella. Sore throat is a more prominent complaint in scarlet fever; the course of infectious mononucleosis is often more protracted, and splenomegaly is more frequent than in rubella. Specific diagnosis of rubella is made by isolation of the virus in any of several cell culture systems, or by demonstration of neutralizing, hemagglutination-inhibiting, or complement-fixing antibody response during infection. The high incidence of dermatoglyphic abnormalities (50 per cent) and increased percentage of chromosome breaks described in patients following congenital rubella may prove to have diagnostic value when studied further.

PROGNOSIS. Complete recovery from postnatally acquired rubella is almost invariable. The rare deaths attributable to rubella follow the infrequent complication of meningoencephalitis. Infection in pregnancy constitutes a hazard to the fetus but not to the mother.

TREATMENT. There is no specific treatment for the disease. Few patients suffer discomfort severe enough to warrant symptomatic medication. Headache and myalgia may be controlled by aspirin; bed rest is advisable for the duration of the fever.

PREVENTION. Passive Immunization. *Administration of gamma globulin to the pregnant woman may only mask her symptoms of infection yet not protect the fetus from viral invasion.* Its use may thus only obscure the picture and confound decision about the need for therapeutic abortion. Hence the practice seems inadvisable unless continuation of pregnancy is elected.

Active Immunization. Rubella may be prevented in children and adults by the parenteral administration of attenuated live virus vaccines produced in cell cultures. Seroconversion rates after immunization are approximately 95 per cent. As with other live virus vaccines, serum antibody titers are lower than those that follow natural infection. However, antibody persists for at least eight years after vaccination, but the permanence of vaccine-induced immunity must still be established by further observation. Natural infection of individuals immunized with vaccine is not uncommon, although such infection is usually asymptomatic. In children, vaccination is attended by little or no reaction; but in women, rash, malaise, arthralgia, and mild, acute arthritis occur frequently, the incidence being directly related to age. For this reason, and in order to induce "herd immunity" to depress circulation of the virus, it is currently recommended in the United States that immunization be carried out principally in childhood. However, since the epidemic threshold—at least in semiclosed populations—is low (between 4.7 and 8.4 per cent), containment of the disease by childhood immunization has proved difficult. A high level of vaccine-induced immunity in elementary school children (83 per cent) failed to prevent the spread of rubella in one community. Despite the higher reaction rates in adults, it seems advisable to immunize adolescent girls or women of childbearing age for whose unborn children rubella may have tragic consequences. Of this population, only seronegative nonpregnant individuals should be immunized, and contraception (when appropriate) should be carried out for at least three months after vaccination. The inadvertent administration of vaccine to pregnant women has demonstrated that attenuated vaccine viruses can infect the fetus and thus have the *potential* for teratogenesis, although the risk is very low. The use of vaccine in the United States apparently has prevented a large epidemic of rubella expected in the early 1970's and has reduced the reported annual occurrence from 57,686 cases in 1969 to 16,343 in 1975.

Cooper, L. Z.: Rubella: A preventable cause of birth defects. *In* Bergsma, D. (ed.): Birth Defects: Original Article Series, Vol. IV, No. 7, Intrauterine Infections. The National Foundation, December, 1968, pp. 23–35.

Gregg, N. M.: Congenital cataract following German measles in the mother. Trans. Ophthal. Soc. Austral., 3:35, 1941.

Hayden, G. F., Modlin, J. F., and Witte, J. J.: Current status of rubella in the United States, 1969–1975. J. Infect. Dis., 135:337, 1977.

Proceedings of the International Conference on Rubella Immunization. Am. J. Dis. Child., 118, July 1969.

EXANTHEMS ASSOCIATED WITH ENTEROVIRAL INFECTIONS

See Ch. 95.

85. VARICELLA
(Chickenpox)
Sidney Kibrick

DEFINITION. Varicella is an acute infectious disease, characterized by a generalized vesicular eruption which appears in crops over several days. It is generally mild in children but may be severe in adults, newborns, and immunologically compromised patients.

Herpes zoster (shingles) is due to the same virus but is manifested by a localized eruption and primarily affects adults. It is thought to represent reactivation of a latent varicella virus in individuals with waning immunity to this agent (see Ch. 305).

ETIOLOGY. The agent responsible for these disorders is the varicella-zoster virus (V-Z virus), a member of the herpesvirus group. Weller isolated etiologic agents from both diseases in 1953 and subsequently established their similarity. Only one serotype is recognized. The virion, which is about 200 nm in diameter, has a DNA core, an icosahedral capsid, and a lipid-containing envelope. Man is the only known natural host. The virus is quite labile and loses its infectivity quickly (probably within hours) in the external environment. Complement-fixing antigens have been demonstrated in vesicle fluid and in cultures of the virus. When propagated in susceptible cells, V-Z virus produces a focal cytopathogenic effect similar to that induced in vivo, with multinucleated giant cells and intranuclear inclusions.

EPIDEMIOLOGY. The disease is spread by airborne droplets and by direct contact with infected lesions. It may also be spread from person to person by a third individual (i.e., by indirect contact) within a limited time and distance, as on a hospital ward. Varicella is communicable from one day before onset of the rash until all the vesicles have crusted — five or six days after the rash appears in the average case, somewhat longer in more severe cases. The prodrome and early stages of eruption represent the periods of greatest communicability.

Although V-Z virus may be spread by respiratory secretions, it has rarely been possible to isolate this agent from nasal or pharyngeal secretions. By contrast, infectious virus is easily recovered from vesicle fluid, and the communicability of this disease coincides with the period when virus can be recovered from the skin lesions.

Incidence and Prevalence. Varicella is primarily a disease of childhood. In temperate zones it is most common between two and eight years, with a peak on beginning school. Cases occur throughout the year but predominate in winter and spring. Inapparent infections are rare. Newborns of mothers who have had the disease are protected by maternal antibodies for up to about six months, but the degree of protection varies. Varicella is one of the most contagious of infectious diseases. Susceptible children exposed to cases in the same household had a secondary attack rate of 87 per cent. Histories of this disease in adults are often unreliable; in one study only 8 per cent of adults with supposedly negative histories acquired varicella from household contacts. Individuals with varicella usually develop lifelong immunity (but may subsequently develop zoster). Varicella may also be acquired by susceptible persons following close exposure to zoster; the attack rate has been estimated at about 15 per cent or less, however, which is considerably lower than that following similar exposure to varicella.

PATHOGENESIS AND PATHOLOGY. It is assumed but not proved that the virus enters and initially replicates in the respiratory tract. This is followed by a viremia which disseminates virus throughout the body. Focal lesions then appear in the skin and occasionally in the viscera and enlarge by virus spread from infected to contiguous cells. The occurrence of the lesions in crops is consistent with an intermittent viremia. With appearance of circulating antibody (about one to four days after onset of the rash) the viremia ceases and symptoms begin to subside.

The histopathology of the skin lesions in varicella, herpes zoster, and herpes simplex is identical. The initial skin changes occur in the endothelium of capillaries in the corium. Cells in the basal and prickle layers undergo ballooning degeneration, and edema fluid quickly accumulates, elevating the stratum corneum to form a clear vesicle containing large amounts of infective virus. The adjacent infected cells develop nuclear changes with margination of chromatin and appearance of an eosinophilic inclusion in each nucleus. In addition, multinucleated giant cells containing such inclusions begin to form at the edges and base of the lesions. As the vesicles begin to dry, they become cloudy with accumulated inflammatory cells and desquamated epidermal cells, and the viral content declines. Finally the lesions crust, the epithelial cells at their base regenerate, and the crusts are shed. In fatal cases, areas of focal necrosis associated with cells showing characteristic intranuclear inclusions may be found throughout the respiratory tract, kidneys, adrenals, liver, and other organs.

The pathologic changes associated with varicella encephalitis are nonspecific and are similar to those seen in the other viral postinfectious encephalitides (see Ch. 309).

CLINICAL MANIFESTATIONS. After an incubation period of 14 to 16 days (range, 10 to 23 days), the disease is usually manifested in young children by low-grade fever, malaise, and rash. In older patients, the eruption may be preceded by a one- or two-day prodrome consisting of fever and constitutional signs such as malaise, myalgia, and headache. The lesions, which first appear on the trunk and scalp, begin as small red macules and progress rapidly over 12 to 24 hours through stages to papules, vesicles, pustules, and crust formation. Pruritus is associated with the vesicular stage and may be quite marked. The vesicles are thin walled, superficial, and surrounded by prominent red areolae, which fade as the lesions dry. The crusts may fall off in a week or persist for several weeks, especially in lesions that become secondarily infected. Underlying areas generally heal completely over weeks to months; occasionally a pit or scar may persist.

The exanthem appears in successive crops over a

one- to six-day period. Thus, as the disease progresses, a characteristic feature is the presence of lesions in various stages of development in the same anatomic area. Those in the final crop may regress after reaching the maculopapular stage.

The varicella rash has a centripetal distribution, being most abundant on the trunk and face and relatively sparse on the extremities. It is usually increased, however, in areas of irritated, damaged, or inflamed skin.

Vesicles may also occur on the mucous membranes, especially in the mouth. Other sites which may be involved include the vaginal mucosa, conjunctiva, and pharynx. Lesions on mucous membranes break down to form shallow, generally painful ulcers, which heal without crusting.

Fever parallels the severity of the rash and persists while new lesions continue to appear. Prolongation or recurrence of fever is associated either with bacterial superinfection or with some other complication of the disease. As with many other viral infections, varicella is usually more severe in adults than in children, with higher fever, more marked rash, and more frequent complications.

About 16 to 33 per cent of adults, and uncommonly children, develop clinical or radiologic evidence of pneumonitis during their disease. Chest films show diffuse nodular densities throughout both lung fields with a tendency to concentrate at the bases and hilum. The changes subside quickly in mild cases but may persist for several months in severe cases, lagging behind clinical recovery. In some patients, fibrotic scars remain and gradually calcify over several years, resembling the radiologic changes in healed miliary tuberculosis.

Encephalitis may occur with both mild and severe cases of varicella and is responsible for 90 per cent of the neurologic complications of this disease. Its incidence is estimated at less than one per 1000 cases. The manifestations are similar to those associated with measles or vaccinial encephalitis and may be quite severe with coma, seizures, appreciable mortality, and permanent sequelae. In about one third of patients with encephalitis, especially in children, cerebellar dysfunction with ataxia is the most prominent feature, and such patients generally do well, recovering completely within one to three weeks (see Ch. 305).

Patients who are susceptible to varicella and who have leukemia, lymphoma, or congenital or acquired immunodeficiency or are on immunosuppressive medication represent a high risk group. Newborns whose mothers have developed varicella within the four days before delivery also fall into this category, presumably because they have received no maternal antibodies against this disease. In such high risk patients, varicella is generally more severe; pneumonia, disseminated visceral disease, secondary bacterial infection, central nervous system involvement, and hemorrhagic phenomena are more common, and mortality is significantly increased.

Additional manifestations which have been noted in varicella include *bullous rash, hepatitis, carditis, nephritis, orchitis, and arthritis.* About 10 per cent of cases of Reye's syndrome (acute encephalopathy and fatty degeneration of the viscera) have been associated with an immediately preceding varicella (see Ch. 309.4).

Maternal infection with V-Z virus during the first four months of pregnancy has been reported to result occasionally in a syndrome of severe congenital malformation with hypoplasia of body parts, neurologic deficits, and ocular lesions. The incidence of such cases is not known.

DIAGNOSIS. The typical case of varicella can be easily recognized on the basis of its characteristic clinical features. A history of exposure within the preceding several weeks is helpful. The demonstration of multinucleated giant cells in Wright- or Giemsa-stained scrapings of young vesicles (Tzanck smear) or in biopsies of affected tissues establishes the lesions as due to either V-Z or herpes simplex virus. Further differentiation between varicella, herpes zoster, and herpes simplex can then generally be made on the basis of associated clinical findings. Intranuclear inclusions, although also a feature of infection with these viruses, are best seen with stains which utilize acid fixatives such as Bouin's or Zenker's solution.

Viral isolation and/or serologic tests are generally necessary only to confirm unusual cases. The virus can be readily isolated from vesicle fluid and identified in appropriate tissue cultures, or the presence of viral antigen can be confirmed by immunofluorescence. The demonstration of a rising titer of complement-fixing antibodies to V-Z antigen is also useful but must be interpreted with care, as this virus shares some antigenic components with herpes simplex virus. Complement-fixing antibodies decline rapidly and may not be detectable after 6 to 12 months. Neutralizing antibodies persist, but their determination is technically difficult.

Other entities with a generalized vesicular eruption include smallpox, eczema vaccinatum, eczema herpeticum, rickettsialpox, disease due to certain coxsackieviruses, and some allergic rashes. None of these meet the criteria for diagnosis of varicella, and their differentiation from this disorder should present little difficulty.

TREATMENT. There is no specific therapy for varicella. Treatment is symptomatic and directed at relief of local discomfort and control of secondary infection. Supportive measures include aspirin for high fever and constitutional symptoms and lukewarm starch baths, calamine lotion, and/or antihistamines for pruritus. Nails should be kept clean and short to minimize skin infection from scratching. Patients with varicella pneumonia or encephalitis may need ventilatory support and attention to hydration, electrolyte balance, and nutrition. Bacterial or fungal superinfection may be important in the compromised host. There is no evidence that either prophylactic antimicrobial drugs or corticosteroids are of value in this disease. Patients who develop varicella while on immunosuppressive doses of steroids should have the dose of such medication reduced to one to one and a half times physiologic levels (0.7 to 1.0 mg of cortisone per kilogram per day or its equivalent) as rapidly as is consistent with safety, and should be maintained at this level until the disease has subsided. Patients receiving other immunosuppressive therapy should also have the dose of their medication reduced. There is no evidence that passive immunization may modify the disease in such patients.

PREVENTION. Human immune serum globulin in large doses, given to normal children within three days of exposure to varicella, does not prevent but will attenuate the disease. Zoster immune globulin (ZIG), prepared from convalescent zoster serum, is more potent and can prevent varicella under such circumstances. The ZIG does not prevent this disease in susceptible high risk children, but reduces both morbidity and mortality in this group if given within three days of exposure. *Information regarding the availability of ZIG for pediatric patients who meet high risk criteria and for high risk newborns may be obtained from the Division of Clinical Microbiology, Sidney Farber Cancer Institute, 44 Binney Street, Boston, Mass. Telephone: 617-732-3121.* Former ZIG consultants and officials from the CDC Immunological Division are available for consultation regarding alternative modes. Telephone: 404-633-311 (days) or 404-633-2176 (nights, weekends, or holidays). Exposed patients on immunosuppressive therapy should not only receive ZIG but also have the dose of their medication reduced until the risk of varicella is past.

An experimental live virus vaccine is currently being tested. Preliminary results are reported as promising.

Brunell, P. A., and Gershon, A. A.: Passive immunization against varicella-zoster infections and other modes of therapy. J. Infect. Dis., 127:415, 1973.

Cimons, I. M., Lacher, M. J., LaMonte, C. S., Levitt, L., Cady, B., and Beattie, E. J., Jr.: Treatment of varicella pneumonia. JAMA, 206:372, 1968.

Feldman, S., Hughes, W. T., and Daniel, C. B.: Varicella in children with cancer: Seventy-seven cases. Pediatrics, 56:388, 1975.

Kempe, C. H., and Gershon, A. A.: Varicella vaccine at the crossroads. Pediatrics, 60:930, 1977.

Weller, T. H.: Varicella-zoster virus. *In* Lennette, E. H. (ed.): Diagnostic Procedures for Viral and Rickettsial Infections. New York, American Public Health Association, 1969, pp. 733–754.

Williamson, A. P.: The varicella-zoster virus in the etiology of severe congenital defects. A survey of eleven reported instances. Clin. Pediat., 14:553, 1975.

86.   VARIOLA AND VACCINIA

C. Henry Kempe

86.1.   INTRODUCTION AND HISTORY

Immunization against the dread disease of smallpox was, until recently, perhaps the most widely applied immunization procedure. Over the past 150 years it has demonstrated its effectiveness beyond question. The vaccinia virus (*Poxvirus officinale*), which is in effect a laboratory strain carried for many generations in a variety of laboratory animals, differs from the newly isolated virus of cowpox (*Poxvirus bovis*), which was originally employed by Jenner (1798) and some of his fellow physicians for the immunization of man against the smallpox virus (*Poxvirus variolae*).

Smallpox was described in detail by Rhazes in the tenth century, and had been described previously by Galen in the second century. Spread from Asia to Europe and North Africa occurred in the Middle Ages, and the disease was prevalent in the sixteenth century. At approximately the same time, the disease was introduced into the West Indies by African slaves and from there into Mexico and South America. The best studied epidemics are those in the eighteenth century in England, when over 90 per cent of the cases occurred in children under ten years of age and when smallpox accounted for one third of all deaths in children. Smallpox occurred in epidemic form less frequently in North America until 1752, when over 30 per cent of the inhabitants of Boston, Massachusetts, were affected and the mortality rate was over 30 per cent (Creighton, 1894). In 1721, deliberate inoculation of smallpox (variolation) as protection against the natural disease was introduced in England from Turkey. It consisted of the inoculation of pustular material by puncturing the skin. This resulted in a febrile disease after an eight-day incubation and a general eruption on the ninth day. The mortality rate from this procedure was 1 to 2 per cent, and it is stated that 17 of 897 inoculated persons died from the disease (Woodville, 1796). Needless to say, modified infection did give rise to highly virulent natural disease in susceptible contacts. In 1738 variolation was successfully used in Charleston, South Carolina, with material that had been allowed to dry. With better care of the patients, the death rate was somewhat reduced. It was thought to be about one or two out of 500, whereas the mortality from the naturally acquired smallpox was 10 to 20 per cent. Variolation was replaced by inoculation of cowpox afer widespread acceptance of Jenner's studies published in 1798. Whether Jenner should be regarded as the originator of vaccination is not certain, but he did play a decisive role in popularizing this method of protection against smallpox, and variolation was outlawed in England in 1840.

86.2.   VARIOLA
(Smallpox)

ETIOLOGY.   Smallpox virus is readily visible with any microscope equipped with darkfield illumination or by phase contrast microscopy. With electron microscopy, the smallpox virus resembles elementary bodies of vaccinia virus. The elementary bodies are small, brick-shaped structures with a diameter of about 200 mμ. They can be demonstrated by direct examination of smears of early skin lesions. The virus is very resistant to drying, and living virus can be demonstrated in scabs kept at room temperature for over three years. Virulent virus has survived on clothing of patients, and has caused the disease in laundry workers who were not protected.

ERADICATION PROGRAM.   In 1967, when an intensified eradication program was begun, there were 42 countries reporting a total of 131,000 cases of smallpox. As it is likely that only about 1 per cent of cases were actually reported, it is estimated that 10 to 15 million cases occurred in 1967 in 30 countries that had endemic smallpox and in 12 others that experienced importations. In contrast, in 1972, 19 countries reported 65,000 cases at a time when reporting had been vastly improved.

By 1977 only one country — Somalia — had endemic smallpox. Five cases occurred in Kenya as a result of importation.

In South America, Brazil was the last country to become smallpox free. Now, after 450 years, smallpox has been eliminated from the Western Hemisphere. Variola major was last seen on the subcontinent of Asia in 1975, whereas variola minor (alastrim) occurred in 1977 in Somalia.

EPIDEMIOLOGY.   The only natural reservoir of smallpox is thought to be the patient suffering from the disease. The patient is not infective until the third day of the clinical disease, that is, one day before the maculo-papular phase of the skin eruption is noted. Contacts may be allowed at large until they actually become ill, because patients are not infective during the early pre-eruptive febrile disease.

Intensive efforts are currently being made to determine a possible nonhuman host; among the possibilities are a nonhuman primate or a rodent. The surprising and significant animal reservoirs of yellow fever and malaria, which have materially affected the eradication campaign for those two diseases, have, understandably, also been of concern to those working in the field of smallpox.

Between 1970 and 1977, 28 cases of infection occurred in humans in areas of Africa which had been free of smallpox for two years or more. Only 2 of the 28 patients had been vaccinated. No human source of infection was discovered, but none of over 100 unvaccinated close contacts subsequently contracted the disease. Virus was isolated and appeared indistinguishable from monkeypox virus isolated among outbreaks in captive monkeys, but there was no illness among monkeys in the area (Ladnyr, 1973). Therefore, although it is possible that monkeypox can cause a clinical illness resembling smallpox in man, its infectivity appears to be low.

PATHOLOGY AND PATHOGENESIS.   It is likely that the site of entry of the smallpox virus is the respiratory tract and, possibly, the eye. In the 12-day incubation period the virus probably multiplies in the regional lymphoid tissues. In the unmodified case, a massive viremia occurs at the onset of the fever, and continues during the first two or three days of the pre-eruptive phase. In this way the virus localizes in the mucous membranes and in the skin as well as in the internal tissues. After the virus disappears from the blood and the skin eruption appears, the patient feels better and the temperature tends to decrease. Antibodies are noted in the blood as early as the fourth day of the disease. The virus multiplies in the epithelial cells of the skin while relatively protected from the action of circulating antibody so that cell destruction continues for some time. When pustulation occurs, the temperature tends to rise again, probably because of the absorption of the toxic products of cell necrosis. It is of interest that patients become infectious on the third day of the disease, probably because saliva has been contaminated through the early mucosal lesions noted in the pharynx and mouth. Skin lesions become infective after the superficial cornified layer has been disrupted. Scabs remain infectious throughout the illness and until their separation during the third to fourth week of illness. The pitting is generally confined to the face and is due to destruction of sebaceous glands followed by organization and subsequent shrinking of granulation tissue and fibrosis. In cases of hemorrhagic smallpox numerous blood cells are present in the corium. Cytoplasmic inclusions are characteristic of infection with the vaccinia-variola group of viruses. Inclusion bodies can be shown best in epithelial cells, particularly of the involved skin and mucous membranes. Skin scrapings stained with hematoxylin and eosin show the inclusion to be round or oval homogeneous masses, either basophilic or acidophilic, located in the cytoplasm fairly close to the nucleus. The appearance of the inclusion bodies varies with the stage of infection but also with the method of fixation and staining, and this suggests that they consist of masses of elementary bodies. Intranuclear inclusions have also been described, but these are not invariably seen. With antimicrobial therapy, pathologic changes from bacteri-

al complications are not found, and bacterial cultures, in this situation, are usually sterile.

CLINICAL MANIFESTATIONS.   The incubation period of smallpox is generally 12 days. The illness begins with severe malaise and high fever lasting for four to six days. There is intense prostration, and the clinical impression is often that of dengue. Severe headache, photophobia, and, occasionally, vomiting are noted. A small number of patients show a prodromal or "toxemic" rash, most easily noted in the groins, the axillae, and the flanks. On the fourth day the focal rash occurs, the fever diminishes slightly, and the patient feels better, just at a time when the first macular skin lesions begin to form. The focal rash usually occurs first on the mucosa of the mouth and pharynx, the face, or the forearms, and it then spreads to the trunk and legs. *A feature of variola is the fact that lesions in any one area are all at the same stage of development, whereas in varicella they are in all stages.* The initial rash is macular and quickly becomes papular. Within two days the papules have developed into vesicles, and these, within a few hours, become cloudy and pustular. On the eighth or ninth day from the beginning of the rash, drying and crusting begin. From three to four weeks from the onset of the disease, scabs have generally fallen off, leaving pigment-free skin. Subsequently, scarring or pitting develops. The eruption is characteristically more severe on the face and the distal parts of the arms and legs, and less severe over the trunk and abdomen. The groins and axillae may be entirely spared. This centrifugal distribution is distinct from the characteristic rash of varicella, which tends to be centripetal. Lesions are often found on the palms of the hands and the soles of the feet, a situation uncommonly seen in varicella of childhood, although these parts may be involved in the adult form. Varicella may also cause osteomyelitis and arthritis. Fever generally recurs during the pustular stage, but the temperature returns to normal as the lesions become encrusted. The characteristic pustular lesions of smallpox are round, raised, and tense, with a tendency to central depression as they begin to dry out. Clinical classification of disease from the mildest form (variola sine eruptione) to modified, to confluent, to malignant confluent, to hemorrhagic indicates degrees of severity of smallpox influenced in part by age, state of immunity, and state of hormonal balance. It is of great interest that women within a short time of term, either before or after delivery, tend to have a much more severe disease than those not pregnant.

In cases modified by vaccination or transplacental immunity in the first few months of life, the rash may be scant and the evolution of lesions may be very quick. Regardless of how mild an index case of smallpox may be, the susceptible infected contacts suffer unmodified disease, and overlooked mild cases are sometimes the cause of severe epidemics. Permanent scarring may result even in the absence of purulent infection of lesions with secondary bacterial pathogens (staphylococci and streptococci) in patients who have deep lesions and serious disease.

In previous years, the bacterial complications were incriminated as the principal cause of death, particularly after the pustular phase had commenced. It is now known that the mortality rate is chiefly related to the amount of virus present in the blood during the viremic phase that occurs in the first two days of the disease before any eruption is noted. It has been shown that if the amount of virus in the blood is so great that the whole blood of the patient in the viremic pre-eruptive phase can be used as the antigen in the complement-fixation test, the patient will almost surely die, although death may be delayed for nine or ten days. Patients who die in the first week of the illness often show evidence of heart failure and terminal pneumonia. Even in the absence of any antimicrobial therapy, the lungs are often sterile, indicating that the pneumonia is caused by the smallpox virus itself. The majority of deaths occur, however, in the pustular stage toward the end of the second week of the disease. Occasionally an encephalitis has been described that is indistinguishable from that associated with measles, varicella, or smallpox vaccination and tends to occur between the eighth and sixteenth days of disease.

INFECTION IN UTERO. No congenital anomalies have been described in infants of mothers infected with smallpox, but abortion is common because of the frequent bleeding that occurs during the toxemic phase. Infection of the fetus in utero may occur during the viremic phase in the mother; if this occurs near the end of the pregnancy, the child will show clinical disease within a few days after birth. Infection has also been shown to occur at the time of birth if the disease is still active in the mother. There are two reports of smallpox in babies infected in utero a few days before birth, although the mothers showed no signs of the disease (Bancroft, 1904; Lynch, 1932).

VARIOLA MINOR. In the twentieth century, a milder clinical form of smallpox became prevalent in the Western Hemisphere. It was recognized in Brazil in 1910, when a widespread outbreak of this mild form of the disease was recorded with a mortality of only 1 per cent. To this mild type of smallpox, the name alastrim — variola minor — was given. Similar mild forms of the disease were recognized in Africa.

The vast majority of epidemics seen in this century in North America and Europe have been due to variola minor. Thus there were 12,000 cases in 1927 in England and Wales and over 48,000 cases in 1930 in the United States. In the 1930's with the widespread application of smallpox vaccination in infancy, smallpox began to decrease in the United States. An important factor in this decrease was the better preservation of smallpox vaccine with the wider availability of refrigerators. It is likely that more potent vaccines and widespread improvement of health services also contributed to the decline in the number of cases. The two types of disease (variola major and variola minor) appeared to be distinct with a markedly different mortality for the two. At present there would appear to be no evidence that an outbreak of alastrim gives rise to cases of classic variola major, although the two types may produce coexistent separate outbreaks, as they apparently did in Detroit in 1924.

There is complete cross-protection for these two infections as there is from vaccinia. The clinical picture is similar in the prodromal or pre-eruptive phase to that of variola major, but hemorrhagic and toxic cases are almost never seen. The lesions tend to be more superficial and develop more rapidly; the total illness is shorter than in classic variola major. There may be no secondary fever during the pustular stage.

DIFFERENTIAL DIAGNOSIS. Smallpox is easily diagnosed, particularly during an epidemic period. More difficult to diagnose is the first and unsuspected case in those countries where smallpox is not endemic. This is particularly true if the first case is hemorrhagic. In this situation meningococcemia, a bleeding diathesis as part of a blood dyscrasia, or typhus may be the suspected diagnosis. Very mild smallpox, modified by previous vaccination or alastrim, may be thought to be varicella, a drug eruption, or erythema multiforme. Except after known exposure, the clinical diagnosis cannot be made with certainty during the febrile phase, because the picture is indistinguishable from that of dengue, enteroviral infections, and other febrile diseases. In the eruptive phase, the most useful clinical points to remember are (1) the centrifugal distribution of lesions; (2) the fact that in a given area all the lesions are at the same stage of development; (3) the presence of a severe, febrile, three-day pre-eruptive disease; and, on occasion, (4) a known contact at least 12 days previously.

LABORATORY TESTS. Laboratory diagnostic procedures are of great value in quickly establishing the diagnosis of smallpox in the first case that appears in a community. These consist of (1) electron microscopic demonstration of viral particles in stained smears of vesicular fluid, (2) serologic or fluorescent demonstration of viral antigen in materials from cutaneous lesions, (3) isolation of virus from such materials, and (4) detection of antibodies in the serum early in the eruptive phase. The results of such tests are particularly helpful in differentiating variola from varicella and the hemorrhagic forms of the disease from other conditions (see Ch. 85). A detailed description of these procedures may be found in the reference by Downie and Kempe.

TREATMENT. No specific treatment for smallpox is currently available, although a number of promising antiviral drugs are under study. Penicillin and broad-spectrum antimicrobials have been used in the prevention and treatment of bacterial complications. There is suggestive clinical evidence that secondary late bacterial complications, including pneumonia and staphylococcal involvement of skin and bones, are decreased by the use of antimicrobial therapy. But even with such therapy the mortality rates have not been reduced below 25 per cent in most outbreaks of variola major. Good nursing care and maintenance of fluid and electrolyte balance are essential. Convalescent smallpox serum and vaccinia-immune gamma globulin have been used in the treatment of severe cases without any evidence of success.

PREVENTION OF SMALLPOX. Management of Recently Exposed Persons. The use of vaccinia-immune gamma globulin (see below) has been successful in the prophylaxis of smallpox and has reduced the incidence after known contact fourfold in control trials (Kempe et al., 1956, 1961). The results among methisazone-treated* groups have been variable (Bauer et al., 1963, 1969; Do-Valle et al., 1965; Rao et al., 1969; Heiner et al., 1971). In Heiner's study only the vaccinated contacts showed a significant reduction in attack rates (twofold), and no difference in mortality or severity was noted between tested and placebo groups.

---

*Manufactured by Burroughs Wellcome. Available in England; not available commercially in the United States.

Community Control. There is no evidence that we owe our freedom from smallpox in the United States to routine vaccination. Compulsory routine vaccination was discontinued in Great Britain in the late 1950's, and 90 per cent of the population has either never been vaccinated or not vaccinated in the past ten years. Since 1969 there have been 12 smallpox importations into England, but the experience with secondary cases, deaths, and generations of cases until control has been no different in that country than in Germany, which has a far higher level of immunity in its population. Public health policy in the United States has long held that high immunity levels are vital. This has been thoroughly discredited, because importations have caused repeated outbreaks even though as many as 90 per cent of the population in an area were vaccinated. Individuals who have not had a recent successful vaccination can be infected and may have a difficult-to-diagnose case. They can, nevertheless, transmit the infection in its most virulent form. In 1973, this has been shown again in the case of the English laboratory worker who had a greatly modified case of smallpox but still was able to transmit the infection in a fatal form to two contacts. There has been no smallpox in the United States since 1949, because we have been fortunate in not having the virus introduced rather than because our population is adequately protected. If variola major had been introduced, secondary cases would have resulted. However, their number would have depended on early versus late diagnosis, prompt versus delayed vaccination of contacts, isolation of cases, surveillance of contacts and isolation of any who developed fever during the 14 days following exposure, careful case finding, as well as on the presence of a high level of immunity in our hospital staff personnel.

In 1964, because of the persistent concern with the number of serious complications of smallpox vaccination, the writer recommended the discontinuation of nonselective routine vaccination of American children. *Selective* vaccination as a general policy was endorsed in 1971 by all major public health and professional groups, except for the American Medical Association. Vaccination is now limited to (1) travelers to endemic areas, and (2) contacts of those with proved cases of smallpox. The global eradication programs have been successful in eradicating variola major. Until alastrim has also been eradicated, however, it will be necessary to remain constantly alert that foreign quarantine procedures and selected traveler surveillance are maintained at a high level, and that adequate measures are taken, from both the clinical and laboratory points of view, in making the proper diagnosis at the earliest possible time.

With currently available techniques, an importation of smallpox and the development of some secondary cases in an unprotected population will, even with failures in early diagnosis, not result in any greater number of deaths than have occurred in the past 40 years from universal infant vaccination itself.

Control of Infected Persons, Contacts, and Environment. All cases should be reported to the local health authority, and patients should be isolated in a hospital until all crusts have disappeared. All oral, nasal, fecal, and urinary discharges and articles associated with patients should be disinfected by burning, high-pressure steam, or boiling. All contacts at home, place of work, or elsewhere should be vaccinated or revaccinated with a potent product and kept under daily surveillance for 16 days from the time of last contact. Any fever during surveillance calls for prompt isolation until smallpox can be excluded. The patient's source case should be sought assiduously. Adults with chickenpox or patients with hemorrhagic or pustular lesions of the skin need careful review for possible errors in diagnosis.

Epidemic Measures. In an epidemic the measures to be taken are as follows: (1) All smallpox patients and suspects should be isolated in hospital until they are no longer infectious. (2) All contacts should be carefully listed, vaccinated, and kept under surveillance for 16 days. (3) A public statement of the situation should be made by all available methods, and all possible contacts should be urged to be vaccinated. Potent vaccine should be provided and arrangements made for early vaccination of inner-ring and outer-ring contacts. (4) The use of vaccinia immune gamma globulin for close household contacts should further decrease the number of secondary cases. (5) Mass immunization of the entire population of a community or larger area is an emergency measure to be used only when an outbreak has given evidence of uncontrolled spread.

International Measures. The World Health Organization and countries adjacent to the one in which an outbreak occurs should be notified by telegram of the existence of any cases of smallpox. At all times, the measures applicable to ships, aircraft, and land transport arriving from smallpox areas should be enforced, as specified in International Health Regulations. It should be noted that evidence of protection by successful vaccination or revaccination (within a period of three years) is a widely enforced requirement for entry to the United States for *travelers from endemic countries but no others.*

Vaccination vs. Chemoprophylaxis. Vaccination remains the best method of prevention for any individual likely to be exposed through travel in the smallpox-endemic regions. To be fully effective, successful revaccination every three years is recommended.

Upon exposure to a case of smallpox, vaccination and revaccination should be supplemented by vaccinia-immune gamma globulin. Vaccination after exposure is effective if done promptly but may not prevent disease. It should be done in any case, however, because in an epidemic situation subsequent repeat exposures may occur. The use of vaccinia-immune gamma globulin markedly reduces clinical incidence and severity when used in full doses of 10 ml intramuscularly once for adults and 5 ml intramuscularly once for children under 12 years. Vaccinia-immune globulin and methisazone* can and should both be given, when available, for a limited number of known close contacts.

WHO and health agencies of member countries in which there is endemic smallpox depend on vaccination alone and concentrate on the elimination of specific smallpox foci. One attempt is to break the transmission chain rather than to rely on mass vaccination campaigns, which had been the accepted method in the attempts at eradication in the past. It was shown that, particularly in Africa and Asia, it is much more efficient and economical to try to interrupt transmission at a time of low seasonal incidence of smallpox. Current strategy consists of an attempt to contain outbreaks of

---

*Manufactured by Burroughs Wellcome. Available in England; not available commercially in the United States.

smallpox by the early detection and containment of cases so as to reduce smallpox incidence as quickly as possible, rather than the institution of mass vaccination.

In an outbreak in central Java in 1969, when more than 95 per cent of the 23,000,000 inhabitants in the province bore vaccination scars, almost 1700 cases of smallpox nevertheless occurred, 85 per cent of them developing in persons who had never been successfully vaccinated. In other words, in a population in which only 5 per cent had not been successfully vaccinated, continued transmission was readily possible — definite evidence that "herd immunity" does not work. The incredible success obtained in West and Central Africa, Indonesia, Ethiopia, and the Indian subcontinent is entirely due to this change of strategy based on early detection of outbreaks and the establishment of trained teams to investigate and contain them. Case finding requires a reporting network which had to be developed. The use of freeze-dried potent vaccine replaced liquid vaccine in all WHO programs. A very useful tool for case finding is the WHO photo recognition card often given to schoolchildren, who proved to be one of the most fruitful sources of information in remote villages in Asia and Africa. The schoolchild through recognition cards, visits to the principal markets which are held every week in different locations, and searching out through walking from village to village and house to house are the bases for case finding which lead to case identification and subsequent vaccination.

86.3.   VACCINIA
(Vaccination)

Smallpox vaccine commonly in use is prepared from the vaccinia lesions on the skin of inoculated calves or sheep or from the allantoic membranes of chick embryos. All currently used smallpox vaccine contains infective virus, and all successful vaccinations are deliberately induced mild viral infections. The mortality in smallpox patients successfully vaccinated many years before is less than in the unvaccinated. There is no question that regular revaccination induces a high degree of immunity even with very massive exposure to the disease.

RECOMMENDED PROGRAM FOR VACCINATION IN THE UNITED STATES

We can look forward to the time when the present eradication program will have eliminated smallpox as a threat to man. At that time, vaccination will no longer be necessary, and jennerian vaccinations will then be a matter of only historic importance. Until this is achieved, however, smallpox vaccination will continue to be necessary for those travelers to endemic areas as well as those in the armed forces.

CONTRAINDICATIONS TO VACCINATION. Primary *routine* vaccination is no longer performed on North American infants, but even *selective* vaccination is contraindicated in infant patients who fail to thrive; in persons with dysgammaglobulinemia or blood dyscrasias; in those with eczema or other dermatitides; in the presence of radiation or other immunosuppressant therapy; in those exposed to infectious diseases; or in unvaccin-

ated siblings of children with eczema. If exposure is likely, elective vaccination of the eczematous child *should* be performed, because the incidence of eczema vaccinatum in this situation is only 1 in 150 and the mortality is zero. Vaccination or revaccination is absolutely contraindicated for adult patients with neoplastic diseases, including Hodgkin's disease, lymphomas, and other conditions involving the prolonged use of corticosteroids, nitrogen mustard, or radiation therapy.

When travel outside the limits of the United States to nonendemic areas is contemplated, vaccination is no longer required for re-entry into the United States. At most, telephonic health surveillance for 14 days after re-entry to the United States may be required. This is much to be preferred to life-threatening disease from vaccination. Vaccination has not been carried out by the Quarantine Service when the patient's physician has presented written evidence that the procedure should not be performed. If such a person must travel to an endemic area, the use of vaccinia-immune gamma globulin should be considered so as to provide temporary protection and to act as a substitute for the use of vaccination with live vaccinia virus.

RECOMMENDED VACCINATION TECHNIQUES. To minimize the risk of unnecessary complications, the following practices are recommended:

Age for Primary Vaccination. In nonendemic areas, primary vaccination is not routinely done. There are no conclusive data indicating the exact period when complication rates are minimal. The presence of some transplacental maternal immunity, provided that the mother has been vaccinated, may be desirable in modifying the primary vaccination reaction, and vaccination may be carried out in the first months of life. Vaccination of newborn infants has been done without complications (Kempe et al., 1952). However, in such cases in endemic areas, revaccination should be performed after an interval of six months. If primary vaccination is delayed for several months, children who are at increased risk, such as those suffering from the Swiss type of agammaglobulinemia, will have been readily identified by their clinical course and will therefore not become casualties of smallpox vaccination. The 1966 experience in the United States fails to show a higher risk of postvaccinial encephalitis for the two-to-ten age group (Neff et al., 1968), but some European authors have stressed that the first years of life may be a safer period. The case mortality for encephalitis is certainly highest among the youngest children (Berger, 1964; Coneybeare, 1948; Muller, 1946; Neff, 1968).

Site for Vaccination. Primary vaccination and revaccination are best performed on the outer aspects of the upper arm, over the insertion of the deltoid muscle, or behind the midline. Reactions are less likely to be severe on the upper arm than on the lower extremity or other parts of the body. With proper technique, resultant scars are small and unobtrusive.

Preparation of the Vaccination Site. With a clean skin, the best preparation is none at all. The use of chemical skin cleansers may leave a residue that contains virus-inactivating material, and vigorous physical cleansing of the site may create minute abrasions that then can become sites of secondary vaccinia eruptions, with resultant involvement of a comparatively large skin area.

Vaccination Technique. Regardless of age, primary vaccination should be performed with no more than two or three pressures with the side of a bifurcated needle. These pressure points should be as close together as possible, and should be made only at one site. With the highly potent vaccines currently in use, more numerous pressure points are not necessary and certainly should not be utilized for a nonimmune person. When children or adults are to be revaccinated after a lapse of more than five years, the same small number of pressure points should be used. For revaccination within a five-year period of those persons known to have had major reaction, the full complement of 30 strokes can safely be used (Leake, 1946).

VACCINATION REACTION. The description of the reactions after vaccination or revaccination should follow the criteria recommended by the Expert Committee on Smallpox of the World Health Organization. A successful primary vaccination is one that on examination after seven to ten days presents a typical jennerian vesicle. If this is not present, vaccination must be repeated with fresh vaccine and a few more pressures of the bifurcated needle. The successful revaccination is one that on examination one week (six to ten days) later shows a vesicular or pustular lesion *or* an area of definite palpable induration and congestion surrounding a central lesion; this lesion may be a scab or an ulcer. These reactions are termed *major reactions;* all others should be called *equivocal reactions.*

A major reaction indicates virus multiplication with consequent development of immunity. An equivocal reaction may merely represent an allergic response, which could be elicited by inactive vaccine or poor technique in someone who has been sensitized by earlier vaccination; or the equivocal reaction may result from sufficient immunity to prevent virus multiplication. Since the allergic response cannot be readily differentiated from the one caused by true immunity, another vaccination should be performed, using a different lot of vaccine if there is a possibility that the first was of weak potency, and the procedure should be completed with an additional number of pressures. The site should be examined one week later; if the result is again equivocal, revaccination should be repeated, using a full 30 pressures as recommended by Leake. For the sake of expediency, an equivocal reaction to revaccination with a minimal number of insertions may be followed by vaccination at two sites, not less than 2 inches apart, using known potent vaccine. This method will make a third return unnecessary in almost all instances.

To sum up: Successful smallpox vaccination consists of the production of a major reaction. When potent vaccine and good technique are used, repeated inability to produce a major reaction can be assumed to be due to solid immunity from previous immunization.

FREQUENCY OF VACCINATION. Revaccination is essential to reinforce the immunity conferred by previous vaccination. This not only maintains a high level of immunity against smallpox but also minimizes the risk of complications on revaccination. To maintain adequate immunity against smallpox, revaccination should be carried out at approximately three-year intervals.

COMPLICATIONS OF VACCINATION

With the abandonment of universal routine vaccination of infants in 1971, complications in the United States have markedly decreased. Life-threatening complications of primary vaccination include eczema vaccinatum, postvaccinial encephalitis, and vaccinia gangrenosa (progressive vaccinia). The principal danger after revaccination is vaccinia gangrenosa, a condition in which the impairment of the patient's immune mechanism permits the continuing multiplication of the vaccinia virus. Vaccinia gangrenosa is seen in seemingly normal subjects, as well as in those suffering from dysgammaglobulinemia, Hodgkin's disease, leukemia, blood dyscrasias, and other conditions in which corticosteroid therapy or ionized irradiation has been administered therapeutically. The presence of these conditions is an absolute contraindication to vaccination.

Human vaccinia-immune globulin has been shown to be effective in the prevention and treatment of eczema vaccinatum and has also been used extensively in the treatment of other complications, in which it also produces a significant reduction in mortality. Vaccinia-immune globulin reduces the incidence of postvaccinial encephalitis. In the Royal Netherland Army, 53,630 of 106,174 recruits received hyperimmune vaccinia-immune gamma globulin, and the remaining 52,544 recruits received a placebo. In the group treated with gamma globulin, 3 cases of postvaccinial encephalitis occurred in contrast to 13 cases in the control group. There was one fatality in each group. Gamma globulin failed to have an effect on the severity and duration of the encephalitis produced by the vaccination, and it was not effective in treatment. There is evidence that transplacental maternal immunity is also effective in modifying the course of primary vaccination; significant reactions are rarely reported in very young infants whose mothers have been vaccinated in the past. In cases of vaccinia gangrenosa, the use of vaccinia-immune globulin appears to be of value. Adequate early treatment of the complications of smallpox vaccination can materially reduce the morbidity and mortality. Through the Center for Disease Control in Atlanta, Georgia, a group of experts is available for telephone consultation (day: 404-633-3311; night: 404-633-2176). When such consultation is used in conjunction with vaccinia-immune globulin, effective diagnostic and therapeutic aids are available for all.

Bauer, D. J., St. Vincent, L., Kempe, C. H., Young, P. A., and Downie, A. W.: Prophylaxis of smallpox with methisazone. Am. J. Epidemiol., 90:130, 1969.

Downie, A. W., and Kempe, C. H.: Variola and vaccinia viruses. *In* Lenette, E. H. (ed.): Diagnostic Procedures for Viral and Rickettsial Diseases. New York, American Public Health Association, 1969, Chapter 25.

DoValle, L. A. R., DeMelo, P. R., DeSalles Gomes, L. F., and Proenca, L. M.: Methisazone in prevention of variola minor among contacts. Lancet, 2:976, 1965.

Heiner, G. G., et al.: Field trials of methisazone as a prophylactic agent against smallpox. Am. J. Epidemiol., 94:435, 1971.

Kempe, C. H.: Smallpox: Recent developments in selective vaccination and eradication. Am. J. Trop. Med. Hyg., 23:775, 1974.

Kempe, C. H., et al.: The use of vaccinia hyperimmune gamma globulin in the prophylaxis of smallpox. Bull. WHO, 25:41, 1961.

Kempe, C. H., et al.: Smallpox vaccination of eczema patients with a strain of attenuated live vaccinia (CVI-78). Pediatrics, 42:980, 1968.

Meiklejohn, G.: Maxwell Finland Lecture. Smallpox: Is the end in sight? J. Infect. Dis., 133:347, 1976.

Neff, J. M.: Complications of smallpox vaccination: I. National Survey in the United States, 1963. N. Engl. J. Med., 276:125, 1967.

Rao, A. R., et al.: Chemoprophylaxis and chemotherapy in variola major: I. An Assessment of CG 662 and Marboran in prophylaxis of contacts of variola major. Indian J. Med. Res., 57:477, 1969.

WHO Expert Committee on Smallpox: Second Report, Publication 393. World Health Organization Technical Report Series. Geneva, World Health Organization, 1968.

For more detailed lists of references see the following:

Dixon, C. W.: Smallpox. London, J. & A. Churchill, Ltd., 1962.

Downie, A. W.: Smallpox. *In* Horsfall, F. L., Jr., and Tamm, I. (eds.): Viral and Rickettsial Infections of Man. 4th ed. Philadelphia, J. B. Lippincott Company, 1965.

87. FOOT-AND-MOUTH DISEASE

(Aphthous Fever)

Walsh McDermott

Foot-and-mouth disease is a viral infection of animals, chiefly cattle, which occurs in man only with great rarity. Infection, when it does occur in man, presumably results from direct contact with the agent either in the laboratory or from handling the tissues or body fluids of infected animals. The disease in man is characterized by a short incubation period followed by the appearance of a febrile illness with vesicular lesions of palms, soles, and sometimes the oropharyngeal mucosa. Neurologic involvement has not been reported, and the disease is self-limited. It may occur in a totally asymptomatic form. The disease is unrelated to hand-foot-and-mouth disease caused by certain coxsackie-viruses, notably A16 (see Ch. 95). There is no treatment of established value; the tetracycline drugs have yielded inconclusive results in the treatment of laboratory animals. Prevention of the disease in man has not been extensively studied, for man generally has a high degree of resistance to the infection. Spread among cattle is presumably by the airborne route. An effective vaccine for use in cattle has been developed. As in influenza, however, there are many types and subtypes of foot-and-mouth (FMD) virus, and it is believed that for optimal effectiveness the homologous viral strain, i.e., the "epidemic" strain, should be present in the vaccine.

Annotations: Spread of foot-and-mouth disease. Lancet, 2:580, 1969.

Flaum, A.: Foot-and-mouth disease in man. Acta Pathol. Microbiol. Scand., 16:197, 1939.

Hyslop, N. St. G.: Transmission of the virus of foot-and-mouth disease between animals and man. Bull. WHO 46:577, 1973.

88. MUMPS

Dorothy M. Horstmann

DEFINITION. Mumps is an acute contagious viral infection, most commonly manifested by nonsuppurative swelling of the parotid glands. Other salivary glands, the testes, pancreas, and central nervous system are among the various organs that may also be involved.

HISTORICAL NOTE. Hippocrates described mumps and its association with orchitis in the fifth century B.C. Because of its characteristic manifestations, the disease was one of the earliest to be recognized as a clinical entity. A classic description was written by Hamilton (1790), who stressed the importance of orchitis as a complication. He also noted that central nervous system signs sometimes accompany the parotitis, but it was early in the twentieth century before clinicians recognized meningoencephalitis as a relatively frequent manifestation. In 1940 Wesselhoeft called attention to the occurrence of oophoritis and pancreatitis, and later others reported involvement of many organs and tissues. Not until 1934 did Johnson and Goodpasture prove the viral etiology of mumps by reproducing the disease in monkeys inoculated with filtrates of infective human saliva. The virus was adapted to growth in hens' eggs in 1945 by Habel, and by Levens and Enders, who demonstrated its hemagglutinating properties. Enders and his associates also described the appearance of dermal hypersensitivity and of complement-fixing (CF) antibodies after mumps. The availability of a skin test and of serologic tools allowed the demonstration that infection with mumps virus can occur without parotitis and not infrequently without any signs at all. Immunization with a killed virus vaccine was tried in the 1950's with limited success. In 1966 Bunyak and Hilleman developed a highly effective live attenuated mumps virus vaccine, prepared in chick embryo tissue culture, which is currently widely used.

ETIOLOGY. Mumps is an RNA virus, a member of the myxovirus family that includes the influenza and parainfluenza viruses. These agents all have the property of agglutinating chicken, human, and certain other erythrocytes. In nature mumps virus infects only man; in experimental infections it induces parotitis in monkeys and meningoencephalitis in hamsters and mice. The virus multiplies in embryonated chick embryos and in a variety of tissue culture cells. For primary isolation (usually from saliva), eggs or preferably cell cultures derived from monkeys or humans are used. In tissue cultures the presence of the virus is recognized either by the appearance of cytopathic changes or by means of the hemadsorption test, which depends on the ability of the virus-infected cells to adsorb guinea pig erythrocytes. Mumps virus is associated with soluble (S) and viral (V) antigens. Antibodies to the S antigen (complement fixing) appear one week after onset; those to the V antigen are delayed and develop after two to three weeks. Only antibodies to the V antigen appear to be protective; they are measured by neutralization, CF, hemagglutination-inhibition, and indirect immunofluorescence tests. A positive skin test indicative of delayed hypersensitivity develops in persons who have been naturally infected or have received mumps vaccine.

EPIDEMIOLOGY. Mumps is a common disease, endemic all over the world. It occurs throughout the year, but there is a seasonal incidence with a regular increase in cases in winter and spring, sometimes reaching epidemic levels. In the United States approximately 20,000 cases were reported in 1977, a marked reduction from the 88,000 median for the five years beginning in 1968 when the vaccine was introduced. Under-reporting is the rule, however, not more than 1 in 10 cases being recorded. The disease incidence is the same in both sexes, but males are more prone to develop central nervous system complications. Most cases occur between the ages of 5 and 15 years; young adults are sometimes susceptible, as evidenced by epidemics in military camps and schools. A far larger number of adults acquire mumps than either measles or chickenpox. There have been scattered case reports suggesting that mumps during pregnancy may have adverse effects on the fetus, but prospective investigations have not revealed differences in rates of abortion, stillbirths, or congenital anomalies in infected and matched control study groups.

The only known reservoir of infection is man. *Transmission* is by direct contact, air-suspended droplets, or fomites contaminated with saliva. The virus is present in saliva from two to seven days before to as long as nine days after parotid swelling appears, but contagiousness is greatest around the time of onset.

Although it is a common disease, only about half the adult population in the United States give a positive history, in contrast to more than 90 per cent for measles. The difference is due in part to the high rate (approximately 30 per cent) of inapparent mumps infections. Asymptomatic infections are particularly common in children under five years old. One experience with mumps virus — whether symptomatic or silent — appears to confer lifelong immunity.

PATHOGENESIS AND PATHOLOGY. The widespread involvement of glandular and other tissues in the body indicates that mumps is a systemic infection. The virus enters and multiplies first in the upper respiratory tract; it then invades the bloodstream, and localizes in the salivary as well as other glands and in the central nervous system. The parotids are one of many target organs, the greater frequency with which they are involved being simply a reflection of greater sensitivity.

Limited observations on pathologic specimens indicate that the reaction in the parotid gland is a nonspecific inflammatory one, which is not extensive. The testes and pancreas also demonstrate inflammatory and degenerative changes. In the rare cases of encephalitis, two types of central nervous system lesions are seen — those resulting from direct viral invasion producing primary encephalitic disease, and the demyelination characteristic of postinfectious encephalitis. Mumps virus has been shown to cause aqueductal stenosis and hydrocephalus in hamsters and mice; the same lesions have been reported as very rare sequelae of mumps encephalitis in man.

CLINICAL MANIFESTATIONS. The incubation period is 14 to 21 days, usually 18. In most cases, pain and swelling in the parotid region are the first signs of the disease, although occasionally in adults pain in the testicle may be the initial symptom. Rarely, meningitis appears first, followed later by parotitis. In more severe cases, there is often a prodromal period, sometimes lasting as long as two or three days, with fever, malaise, headache, chills, sore throat, earache, and tenderness along the region of the parotid ducts.

Parotid swelling is first observed below the ear, usually obliterating the hollow between the mastoid process and the ascending ramus of the lower jaw. The gland increases in size over a two- to three-day period, but there is great variation in the degree of swelling; in mild cases it may be scarcely apparent, but in severe ones the associated edema may eventually spread superiorly to the eyes, posteriorly to the mastoid region, and inferiorly below the chin and over the anterior aspect of the neck. For the first two days, unilateral involvement is the rule, but eventually both glands are affected in about 70 per cent of cases. The skin over the swollen parotids is not usually reddened, but is tense and tender on pressure. Not infrequently the submaxillary and sublingual glands are also affected. Involvement of the sublingual glands can result in swelling of the tongue, with attendant painful swallowing. Presternal pitting edema is also occasionally present, apparently because of obstruction of the lymphatics by the enlarged salivary glands.

The patient seldom suffers severe pain except on movement of the jaws, e.g., in talking or chewing. If Stensen's duct becomes partially occluded as the gland swells, there is sharp pain on taking food or an acid drink, which stimulates the secretory mechanism. Because this occurs only with partial occlusion of the duct, it is not a constant sign. The papillae at the opening of Stensen's or Wharton's duct may be reddened, but this also is inconstant.

Constitutional symptoms vary greatly and may be virtually absent. They are especially mild in children, but tend to be more severe in adults, in whom the incidence of extraparotid lesions is higher. Fever varies with the extent of involvement, ranging between 38 and 39.5° C in full-blown, uncomplicated cases, but going as high as 40.5 and 41° C if orchitis, meningoencephalitis, or both develop.

The duration of parotid swelling and fever is dependent upon the extent and severity of the process. Usually the temperature is normal within five days, and swelling has disappeared by seven to ten days. A peculiar tendency to relapse with recurrence of parotid swelling has been noted in buglers, horn players, and others whose occupations involve similar exertion.

Neurologic Manifestations. The incidence of *aseptic meningitis* varies widely in different epidemics, but can be as high as 25 per cent. Serial examination of the cerebrospinal fluid indicates that the cell count is elevated in approximately one half of all cases of mumps. Clinically evident neurologic involvements may occur preceding, simultaneously with, or after parotitis. It affects males three times more commonly than females, and may be the only manifestation of the infection. The clinical picture of headache, fever, stiff neck, and lethargy is similar to that in other forms of viral meningitis, but the cerebrospinal fluid findings may differ in several respects. Thus cell counts tend to be higher; 500 to 1000 cells, predominantly lymphocytes, are common, and occasionally even several thousand are present. The pleocytosis in mumps is also more prolonged, and may persist for several weeks. Glucose levels below 40 mg per 100 ml have recently been reported in up to 10 per cent of cases. The protein levels are moderately elevated. *Encephalitis,* whether resulting from direct attack by the virus or occurring as postinfectious encephalitis, is rare, but in the United States mumps is the most common cause of encephalitis for which an etiology is established.

Other rare neurologic complications include permanent nerve deafness, either unilateral or bilateral; labyrinthitis; polyneuritis, sometimes affecting the facial or trigeminal nerves; disturbances in accommodation; optic neuritis, iritis, and iridocyclitis; and possibly hydrocephalus.

Orchitis. Orchitis is rare before puberty. After puberty, its incidence varies, but it usually develops in about 25 per cent of cases; there is considerable variation in different epidemics. Testicular involvement is most often unilateral, but may be bilateral, one following the other by one to nine days. The onset is commonly between the fifth and tenth days of illness, as the parotid swelling is subsiding. In mild cases there may be nothing more than discomfort, with tenderness and slight fever. In others, onset is abrupt, with a chill, fever to 40° C or higher, nausea, vomiting, sweats, backache, prostration, and severe testicular pain. Swelling of the testicle may be moderate, or the gland may rapidly reach three to four times normal size, in which case it is excessively hard, tender, and so painful that even 0.030 gram of morphine is not always effective. Epididymitis frequently accompanies orchitis; the spermatic cord may also be involved, and occasionally the prostate.

In mild cases the testicle may be normal in four days, although in the most severe, it may require three or four weeks before all evidence of inflammation has disappeared. Some degree of atrophy, apparently caused by pressure necrosis, occurs in about a third to a half of all cases of orchitis, *but in most instances it is unilateral. Even when both testes are involved, the distribution of the inflammatory reaction and loss of functional tissue are apt to be spotty, and seldom result in sterility.*

Oophoritis. Oophoritis occurs occasionally in adult females, but it may be more frequent than suspected, as mild forms are difficult to recognize. High fever, chills, lower quadrant or back pain, and palpable ovarian enlargement have been described. Sterility resulting from mumps oophoritis is virtually unknown.

Pancreatitis. In the severe form there is sudden onset of epigastric pain and tenderness, vomiting, chills, fever, and prostration. This picture, which is rare, lasts three to seven days and is followed by complete recovery. Mild forms with only abdominal pain and discomfort are thought to be more common but are difficult to diagnose.

Diabetes mellitus has been occasionally reported as a sequela of mumps, leading to the hypothesis that there is a causal relationship between the virus and juvenile onset diabetes. Recent epidemiologic studies have not provided evidence to support this concept. The solution of the problem awaits further prospective investigation.

Other Organs. More rarely, other glands or organs are involved, particularly in adults. The following have been reported as complications of mumps: prostatitis, bartholinitis, and mastitis (in both males and females); involvement of the thyroid, thymus, and lacrimal glands; splenomegaly; and hepatitis. Transient abnormalities of renal function occur frequently, but persistent nephritis is unusual, although fatal cases have been reported. Polyarthritis, occurring ten days to two weeks after onset, is a rare complication. Myocarditis, accompanied by precordial pain or heart block, has been described. Serial electrocardiograms on patients with mumps have revealed some abnormality in as high as 15 per cent, although very few patients show clinical evidence of myocarditis. Several authors have suggested that endocardial fibroelastosis is a result of intrauterine infection with mumps virus. The evidence for this is conflicting, and the issue remains unresolved.

DIAGNOSIS. Sudden onset of parotitis in a previously healthy patient with a negative history of mumps presents no diagnostic problem. Another cause of parotid swelling is suppurative parotitis, an acute bacterial infection in which there is marked tenderness, the skin over the gland is red and hot, and pus can often be expressed from the duct. Salivary calculi obstructing the duct can give rise to recurrent parotitis. Chronic enlargement of the gland occurs with tumors, Mikulicz's disease, and uveoparotid fever of sarcoidosis. Preauricular and anterior cervical lymphadenopathy may simulate parotid involvement.

Mumps infection in the absence of parotitis is often difficult to recognize. Orchitis can be due in rare instances to infection with other viruses such as coxsackievirus B, echoviruses, and lymphocytic choriomeningitis virus. A variety of viral agents cause aseptic meningitis or meningoencephalitis that cannot be distinguished clinically from central nervous system involvement caused by mumps. In such situations specific laboratory tests are necessary to establish the etiology. Mumps virus can be isolated from saliva, urine, and, in meningitis, from the cerebrospinal fluid. More commonly, confirmation of the diagnosis is based on the demonstration of a significant rise in antibody titer when acute and convalescent serum samples are tested. If only a single convalescent specimen is available, the presence of a high titer is suggestive of recent infection. The *skin test* is of no value in diagnosis, because dermal hypersensitivity usually does not develop until three to four weeks after onset; it is less reliable than serologic tests in determining immune status.

Routine laboratory tests frequently indicate a relative lymphocytosis in uncomplicated parotitis; with orchitis, pancreatitis, or aseptic meningitis, the total leukocyte count often reaches 15,00 to 20,000, with a high percentage of polymorphonuclear cells. The blood amylase is usually elevated as a result of parotitis and is therefore not a reliable indication of pancreatic involvement.

PROGNOSIS. Complete recovery is the rule, and death is extremely rare. Fatalities have been associated with encephalitis, myocarditis, and nephritis. Permanent residua are also very uncommon; they include bilateral testicular atrophy (see above) and nerve deafness.

TREATMENT. Bed rest and symptomatic therapy are all that can be offered. For parotid pain, aspirin or codeine is effective. Some patients find an ice bag applied to the parotid region comforting, but others prefer heat. The headache associated with meningitis may be relieved by lumbar puncture. If orchitis is mild, no special treatment is required; if severe, meperidine (Demerol) (0.05 to 0.1 gram) or morphine (0.01 to 0.015 gram) may be necessary to control the pain. Local support and provision of warmth by means of a nest of absorbent cotton are more effective than an ice bag to the scrotum. Corticosteroids relieve the pain but do not appear to alter the duration of illness, nor do they protect against the subsequent development of atrophy. They are not indicated in mild cases, but in severe ones hydrocortisone, 10 mg per kilogram per day, may be given for three to four days.

PREVENTION. A live attenuated mumps virus vaccine, grown in tissue cultures of chick embryo cells, was licensed in 1968. It induces an inapparent infection which is noncommunicable. To date, more than 30 million persons have been immunized in the United States. The vaccine is available as a monovalent preparation or combined with measles and rubella vaccines. It is given subcutaneously, causes virtually no clinical reaction, and induces antibody conversions in more than 90 per cent of susceptibles. The serum titers are lower than those that follow natural infection, but they have persisted satisfactorily for the seven-and-one-half-year period over which antibodies have been tested. Vaccinees have been shown to be resistant to mumps when subsequently exposed to siblings with the disease.

The vaccine may be given to persons of any age over 12 months; it is not recommended for infants under one year because of the possible presence of residual maternal antibody which interferes with the development of active immunity. If the combined measles-mumps-rubella vaccine is used, it should not be given before 15 months of age, because the immune responses to measles antigen are often inadequate in younger infants. Immunization against mumps is recommended particularly for boys approaching puberty who give no history of the disease. If the vaccine is given after exposure, it is unlikely that it will protect. However, it may be given under these circumstances so that if contact infection failed to develop in a susceptible subject who was exposed, he will be protected when he next meets the virus.

Mumps vaccine should not be given to persons with allergy to egg proteins or to neomycin. It is contraindicated for those with any disease that results in compromised immune mechanisms and for patients on immunosuppressive therapy. Since the vaccine contains live virus, it should not be given during pregnancy.

Passive Immunization.   Standard gamma globulin is ineffective; mumps hyperimmune globulin given after exposure is of questionable value in preventing parotitis, orchitis, or meningoencephalitis.

Beard, C. M., Benson, R. C., Kelalis, P. P., Elveback, L., and Kurland, L. T.: The incidence and outcome of mumps orchitis in Rochester, Minn., 1935–1974. Mayo Clin. Proc., 52:3, 1977.

Feldman, H. A.: Mumps. In Evans, A. S. (ed.): Viral Infections of Humans. New York, Plenum Publishing Corp., 1976, pp. 317–336.

Levitt, L. P., Rich, T. A., Kinde, S. W., Lewis, A. L., Gates, E. H., and Bond, J. O.: Central nervous system mumps. A review of 64 cases. Neurology, 20:829, 1970.

Reed, D., Brown, G., Merrick, R., Sever, J., and Feltz, E.: A mumps epidemic on St. George Island, Alaska. JAMA, 199:967, 1967.

Sultz, H. A., Hart, B. A., Zielezny, M., and Schlesinger, E. R.: Is mumps virus an etiologic factor in juvenile diabetes mellitus? J. Pediat., 86:654, 1975.

Weibel, R. E., Buynak, E. B., McLean, A. A., and Hilleman, M. R.: Persistence of antibody after administration of monovalent and combined live attenuated measles, mumps and rubella virus vaccines. Pediatrics, 61:5, 1978.

Wilfert, C. M.: Mumps meningoencephalitis with low cerebrospinal-fluid glucose, prolonged pleocytosis and elevation of protein. N. Engl. J. Med., 280:855, 1969.

VIRAL DISEASE OF LYMPHOID TISSUE

89.   INFECTIOUS MONONUCLEOSIS

James C. Niederman

DEFINITION.   Infectious mononucleosis is an acute infectious disease caused by Epstein-Barr virus (EBV). The infection is common in children, and the disease occurs frequently among adolescents and young adults. Identifying clinical features include fever, sore throat, lymphadenopathy, absolute lymphocytosis with an increased number of atypical lymphocytes, and the development of transient heterophil and persistent EBV antibody responses.

HISTORY.   In 1889, Emil Pfeiffer described Drüsenfieber (glandular fever), characterized by fever, mild sore throat, adenopathy, and enlargement of liver and spleen in severe cases. Sprunt and Evans named the disease "infectious mononucleosis" in 1920 and called attention to implicative hematologic changes. A detailed description of the distinct mononuclear leukocytes was made by Downey and McKinlay in 1923. Paul and Bunnell established the association between mononucleosis and heterophil antibody in 1932, and shortly thereafter Davidsohn and Walker developed guinea pig kidney and beef cell absorption techniques for increasing the specificity of this antibody determination. EBV was reported as the causal agent of infectious mononucleosis in 1968 by Henle, Henle, and Diehl; and by Niederman, McCollum, Henle, and Henle.

ETIOLOGY.   EBV, a member of the herpes group, was first recognized in electron microscopic studies of cell lines of Burkitt's lymphoma biopsies grown in tissue culture. This agent has been demonstrated in cultures of peripheral blood leukocytes from patients both during acute infectious mononucleosis and for years thereafter. In prospective clinical investigations, it has been shown that specific EBV antibodies are regularly absent before the onset of mononucleosis and develop during disease. IgG antibodies to EBV viral capsid antigen, measured by immunofluorescence techniques, are present early in clinical disease and persist for many years; in contrast, EBV-specific IgM antibodies disappear several months after acute illness.

Both heterophil and EBV antibodies develop in squirrel monkeys inoculated repeatedly with EBV autochthonous lymphoblasts. Infection of gibbons by direct pharyngeal injection of the virus has resulted in production of EBV antibodies and exudative tonsillitis. A spectrum of responses ranging from inapparent infection to lymphoid hyperplasia and malignant lymphoma has been observed in cotton-top marmosets following EBV inoculation. Atypical lymphocytes and heterophil antibody have not been demonstrated in experimentally infected marmosets; however, the EBV genome has been detected directly in tumor cell DNA by molecular hybridization techniques.

Inadvertent transmission of EBV to antibody-negative humans by blood transfusion has been associated with the development of EBV antibody and occasionally with the development of heterophil positive clinical infectious mononucleosis. EBV has been regularly demonstrated in the oropharynx of patients with infectious mononucleosis and is present in more than 80 per cent of patients during early disease; shedding persists for months and perhaps years after infection. Recent studies indicate that EBV is located extracellularly in oral fluids and suggest the existence of a cell in the oropharynx in which the full cycle of viral maturation occurs, including envelopment and release.

EPIDEMIOLOGY.   Infectious mononucleosis and EBV infections occur worldwide. Antibody to this virus has been demonstrated in every population thus far studied, and the age at which infection is acquired is related to economic factors and hygienic conditions. Infection occurs early in life in economically underdeveloped countries and is usually subclinical or inapparent. In areas where exposure and infection are delayed until older childhood and young adult life, EBV infections are more often expressed as clinical infectious mononucleosis. Occurrence of the disease among young adults, especially in the 15- to 25-year age group, is the most characteristic epidemiologic feature.

No annual or seasonal variations have been observed in the general population. However, in college students periods of high frequency occur in early fall and spring. Among college-age susceptibles, the rate of EBV infections per year is approximately 12 per cent. Measurements of clinical:subclinical cases suggest a ratio of 1:2 to 1:3 in this age group.

Seroepidemiologic studies utilizing EBV-specific IgG antibody markers have regularly indicated that absence of antibody correlates with susceptibility to infectious mononucleosis and its presence with immunity. Prospective studies of over 5000 children and young adults have now been reported in various parts of the world to support this relationship. Antibody to EBV developed in 29 per cent of subjects previously negative to antibody who were observed over periods of four to eight years; the clinical attack rate was 2 per cent per year among these susceptibles.

EBV infections occur in all ethnic groups, and population surveys have indicated no differences in antibody prevalence rates by sex. Clinical infectious mononucleosis is also equally frequent in both sexes; in adolescence, females appear to develop the disease somewhat earlier than males. High EBV antibody prevalence rates among young children in economically underdeveloped countries suggest that the virus spreads rapidly under conditions of crowding and close interpersonal contact to infect almost all susceptibles.

PATHOLOGY AND PATHOGENESIS. Gross pathologic changes in this disease are confined almost exclusively to lymphoid tissues; lymphadenopathy, nasopharyngeal lymphoid hyperplasia, and splenomegaly are outstanding features. Widespread focal and perivascular aggregates of mononuclear cells develop throughout the body. Nonspecific hyperplastic changes occur in lymph nodes without infiltration of the capsule or surrounding tissues; atypical lymphocytes found in peripheral blood are also present in nodal tissues. Nonlymphoid organs, including liver, heart, lungs, central nervous system, and kidneys, are infiltrated, and these focal lesions may be associated with functional abnormalities. Hyperplasia and occasionally small granulomatous lesions have been described in bone marrow particle sections.

Recent observations that EBV is regularly present in saliva shed light on the pathogenesis of this infection. Prolonged excretion of small amounts of infectious virus into the oropharynx accounts for the moderate contagiousness of this virus and the difficulty in demonstrating case-to-case transmission. EBV is also found in throat washings of 15 to 20 per cent of healthy antibody-positive persons without a past history of infectious mononucleosis, indicating that oropharyngeal shedding is common among those who have experienced inapparent EBV infections. Demonstration of the extracellular location of EBV in the saliva elucidates some of the epidemiologic features of infectious mononucleosis. High rates of transmission of this agent in preschool children and young adults can be explained by the greater degree of salivary exchange characteristic of these age groups in comparison with others. The regular finding of EBV in saliva and buccal fluids collected from the orifices of Stensen's ducts points to the salivary glands as a probable major site of virus production. However, the specificity of the producer cell is unknown; it could be ductal or glandular epithelium, oropharyngeal and nasopharyngeal epithelium, or specialized lymphoid cells.

CLINICAL MANIFESTATIONS. Studies of contact infections have suggested an incubation period of 30 to 50 days in the adult. Clinical mononucleosis associated with production of both heterophil and EBV antibodies has developed five weeks after blood transfusion in several patients. Young children appear to have a shorter incubation period of 4 to 14 days, but existing information is scant on this point.

During a prodromal period of four to five days, mild symptoms, including malaise, fatigue, and headache, are frequent. Initial clinical symptoms are extremely variable in severity, but include fever, sore throat, and cervical lymphadenopathy in more than 80 per cent of cases. In adults, fever in the range of 38.3 to 39.4° C may persist for seven to ten days, and elevations to 40.5° C occur in some cases. Conversely, children experience little or no fever with this infection.

Sore throat develops during the first week of disease and is the most common clinical feature of infectious mononucleosis. Inflammation and edema of pharyngeal tissues are present, and an exudative tonsillitis with a thick, gray-white exudate occurs in approximately 50 per cent of patients and persists for seven to ten days. During early disease, the uvula and palatal arch have a gelatinous appearance. At the end of the first week of disease, petechiae are observed near the border of the hard and soft palates in about one third of patients. This palatal enanthem, consisting of crops of 5 to 20 circumscribed red petechiae, is highly suggestive, but not pathognomonic, of mononucleosis.

Lymph node enlargement is a hallmark of infectious mononucleosis. Anterior and posterior cervical nodes are commonly involved, and generalized adenopathy, including axillary, epitrochlear, mediastinal, and inguinal nodes, may develop during the course of disease. The lymph nodes, usually 5 to 25 mm in diameter, may be enlarged singly or in clusters; they are firm, tense, discrete, and distinctly tender on palpation. Lymphadenopathy gradually subsides over a period of several weeks, depending on the degree and extent of involvement.

Splenomegaly develops in approximately 50 per cent of patients. Commonly, the enlarged spleen extends several centimeters below the costal margin, and enlargement is greatest during the second and third weeks of illness.

Although hepatomegaly is demonstrable in only 10 per cent of patients, liver function tests, especially serum transaminase values, are abnormal for several weeks in most cases. Frank jaundice develops in 4 to 5 per cent of patients and occurs most commonly during the first two weeks of illness; it is probably caused by hepatocellular damage, is usually mild, and is rarely associated with acholic stools.

During early disease, about 10 per cent of patients manifest a transient, faint, erythematous, or maculopapular rash on the trunk and proximal extremities. This eruption often resembles rubella, but may be scarlatiniform, urticarial, or hemorrhagic in appearance. Bilateral supraorbital edema may also be a transient early clinical finding.

Less than 1 per cent of patients, usually in the adult age group, have symptoms referable to the central nervous system. In general, neurologic manifestations depend on the anatomic site and extent of involvement; these include aseptic meningitis, Bell's palsy, encephalitis, transverse myelitis, and the Guillain-Barré syndrome. Most patients experience complete recovery; however, a small number of fatalities have been reported in association with encephalopathy and severe paralysis.

A sharp increase of peripheral blood lymphocytes, including atypical lymphocytes, occurs at the end of the first week or ten days of illness. An increase of circulating B (bone marrow–derived) lymphocytes precedes that of T (thymus-derived) lymphocytes. Transient depression of cell-mediated immune responses exists during early disease; however, decreased lymphocyte responsiveness to a variety of antigens and mitogens usually returns to normal in three to six weeks.

DIAGNOSIS. Infectious mononucleosis is diagnosed on the basis of (1) clinical manifestations, (2) characteristic blood picture, and (3) elevated titers of heterophil and EBV antibodies.

The clinical features of this disease include fever, sore throat, lymphadenopathy, and splenomegaly. An absolute increase in the number of lymphocytes and atypical lymphocytes is an essential hematologic finding. Fifty to 60 per cent of peripheral blood leukocytes are of the lymphocyte series at some stage of the disease. Early in the first week of symptoms, there may be leukopenia, but often leukocytosis with a predominance of lymphocytes is present. During the second and third weeks the total count may rise to 20,000 and may occasionally range as high as 50,000 per cubic millimeter. Atypical lymphocytes usually represent more than 10 per cent of leukocytes during disease; also known as Downey cells, these lymphocytes vary in size, shape, and staining quality with round, indented, or lobulated nuclei and basophilic, vacuolated cytoplasm. Morphologically identical cells have been observed in other diseases, including viral hepatitis, rubella, rubeola, cytomegalovirus infections, mumps, and a variety of other infectious, immunologic, and lymphoproliferative disorders. However, in these conditions, unlike mononucleosis, the percentage of atypical lymphocytes is usually less than 10 per cent. Anemia is rare in infectious mononucleosis, and the platelet count is normal in the absence of complicating thrombocytopenia.

During the course of disease, patients develop elevated titers of sheep cell agglutinins (heterophil antibodies) in the serum. These agglutinins are often present during the first week of illness, but their appearance may be delayed. In one study of 166 mononucleosis patients, the heterophil antibody test was positive in 38 per cent of cases during the first week of disease, in 60 per cent during the second week, and in 80 per cent during the third week. Elevated heterophil titers usually persist for three to six months and occasionally longer. In general, the higher the antibody titer during acute illness, the longer it persists in convalescence. Adults usually have higher heterophil antibody levels than children.

The presence of sheep cell agglutinins is not specific for infectious mononucleosis; these occur in serum sickness, hepatitis, Hodgkin's disease, rubella, and leukemia; low titers may also be found in normal persons. However, sheep cell agglutinin titers are generally higher in infectious mononucleosis than in other conditions. Qualitative tests for heterophil antibodies have now been introduced, using formalin-treated horse erythrocytes, ox red blood cells, or enzyme-treated and untreated sheep erythrocytes; a titer above 1:128 is considered significant in many laboratories.

Absorption tests utilizing guinea pig kidney and beef red cells provide specific differentiation: (1) Infectious mononucleosis heterophil antibodies are removed by beef red blood cells, but not by guinea pig kidney; (2) heterophil antibodies present in normal serum are absorbed by guinea pig kidney, but not by beef erythrocytes; and (3) heterophil antibodies in patients with serum sickness are absorbed by both antigens. The sheep or horse red cell agglutination test after serum absorption with guinea pig kidney is widely used; a level of 1:40 or higher after absorption is considered diagnostic, and a rising titer indicates recent infection. The most sensitive determination is the absorbed horse cell test; elevated titers may persist over a year after onset. The beef hemolysin test is highly specific, but detectable antibody disappears several months after clinical illness.

Specific EBV antibody responses are absent before mononucleosis and appear during the course of disease. These are assayed in a number of ways: (1) immunofluorescence techniques which demonstrate viral capsid, early, membrane, and nuclear antigens; (2) complement fixation; (3) immunodiffusion; (4) enzyme-linked immunosorbent assay (ELISA); and (5) neutralization. The most widely used clinical antibody test is the indirect immunofluorescence technique demonstrating viral capsid antigen (VCA); titers of 1:80 to 1:320 occur during early illness, and significant antibody rises develop in 15 to 20 per cent of cases. Rarely, the appearance of both EBV and heterophil antibodies is delayed for several weeks after onset of clinical symptoms. EBV-specific IgM antibody is present in serum samples collected one to three weeks after onset of mononucleosis and, like heterophil antibody, usually disappears within three to six months; EBV-specific IgM antibody has also been found in mononucleosis cases in which heterophil antibodies have not been demonstrated. The time relationships between clinical features, hematologic findings, virus shedding from the oropharynx, EBV antibody titers, and heterophil antibody levels after guinea pig kidney absorption in a typical case of infectious mononucleosis are shown in the accompanying figure.

DIFFERENTIAL DIAGNOSIS. Infectious mononucleosis resembles a number of other disorders associated with fever, exudative tonsillitis, lymphadenopathy, and splenomegaly. Early after onset, it may be confused with other forms of febrile pharyngotonsillitis, such as streptococcal or viral pharyngitis and tonsillitis, diphtheria, and Vincent's angina. Differentiation depends on throat culture results, prompt response to penicillin in the case of streptococcal infection, and the development of characteristic hematologic and serologic features of infectious mononucleosis.

Blood dyscrasias, particularly leukemia, may be mistaken for mononucleosis. Laboratory studies, including demonstration of many immature leukocytes in peripheral blood and bone marrow, an associated anemia, severe thrombocytopenia, and absence of heterophil antibody distinguish these diseases.

Rubella is characterized by a two- to four-day prodromal stage associated with fever, malaise, and lymphadenopathy prior to appearance of the rash. A distinguishing feature of the rubella exanthem is its

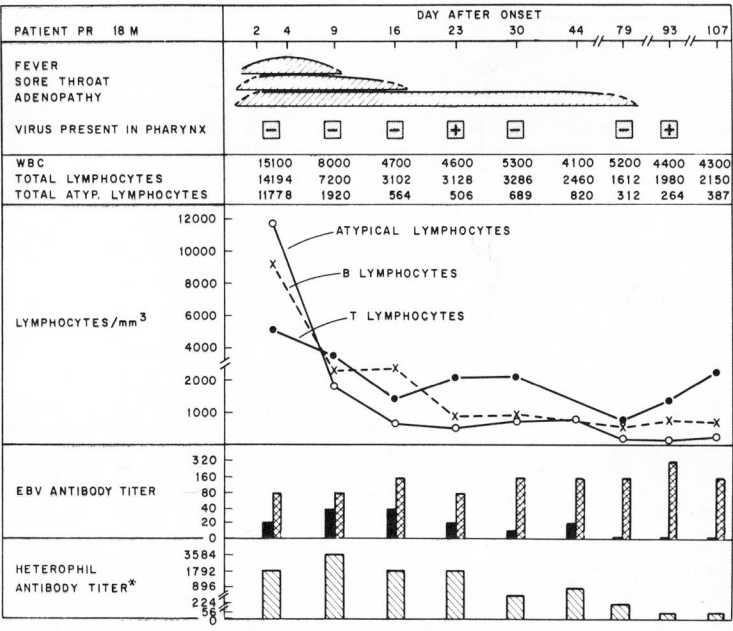

PATIENT PR 18 M	2	4	9	16	23	30	44	79	93	107
FEVER										
SORE THROAT										
ADENOPATHY										
VIRUS PRESENT IN PHARYNX		−	−	−	+	−		−	+	
WBC	15100	8000	4700	4600	5300	4100	5200	4400	4300	
TOTAL LYMPHOCYTES	14194	7200	3102	3128	3286	2460	1612	1980	2150	
TOTAL ATYP. LYMPHOCYTES	11778	1920	564	506	689	820	312	264	387	

Sequence of clinical features, atypical lymphocytosis, EBV and heterophil antibody titers, and oropharyngeal virus shedding in a typical case of infectious mononucleosis.

*AFTER ABSORPTION   ■ EBV–IgM TITER   ▨ ANTI–VCA (IgG) TITER

regular presence on the face, whereas the less florid rash of mononucleosis is prominent on the trunk and usually spares the face. The presence of large numbers of atypical lymphocytes, EBV, and heterophil antibodies indicates infectious mononucleosis. Isolation of rubella virus from the pharynx and demonstration of a rise of rubella antibody titer confirm this diagnosis.

Cytomegalovirus mononucleosis usually involves an older age group than infectious mononucleosis and is characterized by fever, splenomegaly, hepatic involvement, and atypical lymphocytes. Pharyngitis and cervical adenopathy are not features of this infection; cases may be sporadic or may follow multiple blood transfusions. Cytomegalovirus can be isolated from urine, and a rise in specific complement-fixing antibody demonstrated.

Acquired toxoplasmosis infection is associated with fever, generalized lymphadenopathy, lymphocytosis, and splenomegaly. Differentiation from infectious mononucleosis is based on isolation of *Toxoplasma gondii* and on heterophil agglutination and dye test antibody determinations.

Aseptic meningitis may be the initial diagnosis in a patient having infectious mononucleosis with central nervous system signs and symptoms. Serologic tests are required for differentiation from other forms of viral meningitis.

Infectious lymphocytosis is a benign disease of obscure etiology in children, characterized by upper respiratory tract symptoms and occasionally by abdominal pain and signs of central nervous system involvement. Leukocytosis develops and small mature lymphocytes account for 60 to 90 per cent of the white blood cell differential; this blood picture may persist for several weeks or months. Heterophil antibody is not present, and an associated rise in EBV antibody level has not been demonstrated.

TREATMENT. Therapy of uncomplicated infectious mononucleosis is chiefly symptomatic and supportive. Antimicrobial agents are not effective and do not influence the course of infection. During the acute febrile stage of disease, bed rest is advisable. Salicylates are usually sufficient to control headache and sore throat; in severe cases, codeine or meperidine (Demerol) may be necessary. Gargling and throat irrigations with normal saline solutions provide symptomatic relief of pharyngitis and stomatitis.

In cases associated with severe toxic pharyngotonsillitis in which airway encroachment secondary to oropharyngeal edema is apparent, corticosteroids are useful to induce a prompt anti-inflammatory effect. A seven- to ten-day course of prednisone may be used, starting with 40 to 60 mg the first day and decreasing this amount 5 mg daily thereafter. Full doses of steroids should be utilized in the management of other complications, including (1) airway obstruction in which a tracheostomy may also be necessary, (2) neurologic sequelae, (3) thrombocytopenic purpura and hemolytic anemia, and (4) myocarditis and pericarditis.

Corticosteroid therapy is not recommended for treatment of usual cases of infectious mononucleosis. A well controlled study of steroid therapy in uncomplicated mononucleosis patients demonstrated a decrease in duration of fever to 1.4 days in steroid-treated patients, as compared with 5.6 days in matched control patients.

Splenic rupture, usually associated with severe abdominal pain, necessitates emergency surgery; transfusions, treatment for shock, and immediate splenectomy are required.

PROGNOSIS. In general, most cases of infectious mononucleosis are mild or moderately severe; after acute symptoms subside, patients usually recover uneventfully and return to normal activities within four to six weeks. In rare instances, symptoms persist for several months, and laboratory abnormalities, including liver function tests, are slow to resolve.

Severe hepatitis and toxic encephalopathy were recently reported in a fatal case of infectious mononucleosis and Reye's syndrome in a six-year-old child. Fulminating   lymphoproliferative   disease   following infectious mononucleosis has been described in several members of the same family, suggesting a genetically determined immune defect resulting in inability to contain an EBV infection.

Carter, R. L., and Penman, H. G.: Infectious Mononucleosis. Oxford, Blackwell Scientific Publications, Ltd., 1969.
Evans, A. S., Niederman, J. C., and McCollum, R. W.: Seroepidemiologic studies of infectious mononucleosis with EB virus. N. Engl. J. Med., 279:1121, 1968.
Henle, G., Henle, W., and Diehl, V.: Relation of Burkitt's tumor associated herpes-type virus to infectious mononucleosis. Proc. Natl. Acad. Sci. U.S.A., 59:94, 1968.
Joint Investigation by University Health Physicians and P.H.L.S. Laboratories: Infectious mononucleosis and its relationship to EB virus antibody. Br. Med. J., 4:643, 1971.
Niederman, J. C., Miller, G., Pearson, H. A., Pagano, J. S., and Dowaliby, J. M.: Infectious mononucleosis: EB virus shedding in saliva and the oropharynx. N. Engl. J. Med., 294:1355, 1976.

ENTEROVIRAL DISEASES

Nathaniel A. Young

90. INTRODUCTION

The picornavirus (*pico*, small; *rna*, nucleic acid type) family consists of two genera which commonly infect man: (1) the genus *Enterovirus*, found primarily in the gut, and (2) the genus *Rhinovirus*, whose members inhabit the respiratory tract and are the most important etiologic agents of the common cold (see Ch. 77). In addition there are picornaviruses whose natural hosts are other mammals, for example, foot-and-mouth disease virus of cattle and cardioviruses of rodents. Picornaviruses have common morphologic and biophysical properties, such as size of 20 to 30 nm, RNA genome, four structural polypeptides, and resistance to organic solvents. Human enteroviruses moreover share related nucleotide sequences. Historically, enteroviruses have been further subdivided into *polioviruses, group A and B coxsackieviruses,* and *echoviruses.* Sixty-three distinct immunotypes (species) were classified, based on differences in host range and antigenic relationships (67 immunotypes were originally recognized, but redundancies in numbering and changes in classification have reduced this figure to 63). Several enteroviruses had properties which straddled these arbitrary groupings. Because of this problem, newly discovered enteroviruses are no longer subclassified as coxsackieviruses A or B or echoviruses, but are simply numbered serially, beginning with enterovirus 68. Despite these difficulties, the older classification with its vast literature is clinically useful and has been retained for the original 63 immunotypes (Table 1).

DISTINCTIVE FEATURES OF NONPOLIO ENTEROVIRUSES

COXSACKIEVIRUSES. In contrast to polioviruses, which are readily isolated in susceptible primate cell cultures and are pathogenic only for primates, coxsackieviruses produce disease in suckling mice. Named for the village of Coxsackie in New York state, they were first recovered in 1948 from the feces of children who may have also suffered from paralytic poliomyelitis. Several related but immunologically distinct types were further categorized as *group A coxsackieviruses* when the histopathologic lesions induced in mice consisted of *generalized* myositis of skeletal muscle accompanied by flaccid paralysis. In contrast, *group B coxsackieviruses* produced *focal* myositis and widespread lesions of the central nervous system, myocardium, pancreas, and brown fat accompanied by spastic paralysis. Group B coxsackieviruses can be propagated readily in susceptible cell cultures as well as in mice, whereas most group A coxsackieviruses do not produce cytopathic effects in cultured primate cells. At present 23 immunotypes of group A and 6 of group B are recognized.

ECHOVIRUSES. These viruses were first isolated from feces of healthy children shortly after the discovery of coxsackieviruses. Unlike coxsackieviruses, they produce cytopathic effects in primate cell cultures and are nonpathogenic for mice. They differ from polioviruses immunologically and in their failure to produce disease in monkeys. Because at first no disease state in any host could be attributed to these "orphan" viruses, they

TABLE 1. Human Picornaviruses

Virus	Number of Immunotypes	Cytopathic Effect or Pathogenicity for		
		Cell Cultures	Suckling Mice	Primates
I. Enteroviruses				
A. Polioviruses	3	++	−	++
B. Coxsackieviruses A	23*	±†	++	−
C. Coxsackieviruses B	6	++	++	−
D. Echoviruses	30‡	++§	−	−
E. Enteroviruses	4	++	Variable; no longer used in classification	
II. Rhinoviruses (see Ch. 77)				

*Coxsackieviruses A1–A24; coxsackievirus A23 has been reclassified as echovirus 9.
†Most immunotypes of coxsackievirus A are not readily isolated in cell cultures, but exceptions exist.
‡Echoviruses 1–34; echoviruses 1 and 8 are identical; echovirus 10 has been reclassified as reovirus 1, and echovirus 28 as rhinovirus 1A; echovirus 34 is a variant of coxsackievirus A24.
§Except echovirus 21.

TABLE 2. Clinical Spectrum of Infection with Nonpolio Enteroviruses*

	Coxsackieviruses Group A	Coxsackieviruses Group B	Echoviruses	Enteroviruses
Illness associated with many enteroviruses	Asymptomatic infection Febrile illness with or without respiratory symptoms Aseptic meningitis (1, 2, 4–7, 9, 10, 14, 16, 22, 24) Paralysis (4, 7, 9) or encephalitis	Asymptomatic infection Febrile illness with or without respiratory symptoms Aseptic meningitis (1–6) Paralysis (1–5) or encephalitis	Asymptomatic infection Febrile illness with or without respiratory symptoms Aseptic meningitis (all except 24, 26, 27, 29, 32) Paralysis (1, 2, 4, 6, 7, 9, 11, 16, 18, 30) or encephalitis	Asymptomatic infection Febrile illness with or without respiratory symptoms (68) Aseptic meningitis (71) Paralysis (70)
Illness more characteristic of particular groups or immunotypes	Herpangina (2–6, 8, 10, 22) Hand-foot-and-mouth disease (5, 10, 16) Lymphonodular pharyngitis (10) Exanthem (9)	Pleurodynia (1–5) Pericarditis (1–5) Myocarditis (1–5) Orchitis Hepatitis Generalized disease of newborn	Exanthem (especially 9, 16 but also 1–8, 11, 14, 18, 19, 25, 30, 32) Neonatal "sepsis" Neonatal diarrhea (14, 18)	Acute hemorrhagic conjunctivitis (70)
Etiologic role undefined or uncertain	Diarrhea Hemolytic-uremic syndrome Chronic myopathy Guillain-Barré syndrome	Diarrhea Endocarditis Chronic cardiomyopathy Diabetes mellitus Hemolytic-uremic syndrome Mononucleosis-like syndrome	Diarrhea Reye's syndrome	

*The most commonly implicated immunotypes are designated in parentheses.

were named echoviruses (enteric cytopathic human orphan). Currently 30 immunotypes are recognized.

NEWER ENTEROVIRUSES. The four most recent additions, enteroviruses 68–71, have been given serial numbers because of difficulties in assigning them definitively to the older categories based on host range. Their pathogenicity for mice is inconstant even among different strains of a single immunotype. All can be isolated and propagated in cell cultures.

GENERAL ASPECTS OF NONPOLIO ENTEROVIRAL INFECTIONS

EPIDEMIOLOGY. Coxsackieviruses, echoviruses, and probably most of the newer enteroviruses are distributed worldwide. There is marked seasonal variation in their prevalence in temperate climates, most infections occurring in the summer and early autumn. Enteroviral illness is distinctly unlikely during the winter. In tropical climates, however, enteroviral infections commonly occur throughout the year. Usually only one or two immunotypes are prevalent in any city each year, and these may vary from one community to another. Virus replicates briefly in the oropharynx and for longer periods in the lower intestinal tract and is shed from these sites. Enteroviruses can regularly be isolated from urban sewage. Transmission is predominantly fecal-oral, and hence enteroviral infections tend to be associated with unsanitary environments, crowding, and low socioeconomic status. Marked clustering of infections in families is observed. When one family member is infected, secondary attack rates among susceptibles (i.e., those lacking type-specific immunity) are approximately 92 per cent for polioviruses, 75 per cent for coxsackieviruses, and less than 50 per cent for echoviruses. Virus is disseminated most efficiently by children less than two years old.

INFECTION AND ILLNESS. Approximately 50 to 80 per cent of enteroviral infections are asymptomatic, and many of the remainder are characterized by undifferen-

tiated febrile illnesses lasting a few days, often accompanied by symptoms of upper respiratory tract infection. These illnesses may be caused by virtually any enterovirus immunotype and are clinically indistinguishable from infection by many other viral agents. In addition, enteroviruses have been established as the etiologic agents of a number of distinct, specifically recognizable clinical syndromes (Table 2), which may occur sporadically or in epidemics. Some of these syndromes are highly associated with a particular enterovirus group (e.g., herpangina with group A coxsackieviruses and myopericarditis with group B coxsackieviruses). Nevertheless the clinical diseases produced are not entirely specific; occasionally immunotypes from different groups may produce the same syndromes (e.g., herpangina caused by coxsackievirus B5 or carditis produced by an echovirus). Conversely, during a single epidemic one immunotype of group B coxsackievirus may cause pleurodynia, aseptic meningitis, or pericarditis in different individuals; or different strains of a single immunotype of echovirus may be associated with a high incidence of exanthem one summer but little or no exanthem in a different locality the following summer. The factors responsible for this diversity of manifestations are poorly understood.

LABORATORY DIAGNOSIS. The evidence establishing enteroviruses as the cause of specific disease syndromes has usually come from epidemics in which evidence of infection in patients with each syndrome is compared with matched controls. Establishing the etiologic role of an enterovirus in individual cases, however, is more difficult. Isolation of an enterovirus from throat secretions or feces, even when accompanied by a rising titer of type-specific antibodies, is not definitive etiologic proof of temporally associated illness because of the likelihood of intercurrent subclinical infection and prolonged (up to three months) fecal excretion of virus. On the other hand, if specimens are not collected until late in the course of illness, the intestine may be the only site from which virus is still being shed; under these circumstances fecal isolation of virus, although not definitive etiologic proof, may afford the only diagnostic clue. Isolation of virus from cerebrospinal fluid, vesicle fluid, pericardial fluid, or myocardium (as dictated by the clinical syndrome) provides convincing evidence of etiology. Measurement of type-specific neutralizing antibodies in serum is the most useful serodiagnostic test. Paired acute and convalescent sera, preferably separated by at least two weeks, are necessary, because the presence of antibodies even at high, stationary titers does not reliably distinguish recent infection from infection in the remote past. Serology has limited usefulness in the diagnosis of nonpolio enteroviral infections unless a virus has been isolated from the same patient. Without virus isolation it would be necessary, in the case of aseptic meningitis, to perform neutralization tests with more than 60 different enterovirus immunotypes. Requests to the laboratory for "viral antibody screens" are to be deplored, because it is generally feasible only to measure titers of antibody against the patient's own isolate or against one or two viruses known to be prevalent in the community at that time. A possible exception is in the case of myocarditis or pericarditis, in which measurement of antibodies against five immunotypes (coxsackieviruses B1–5) would detect the vast majority of these illnesses caused by enteroviruses.

PREVENTION AND TREATMENT. Specific chemotherapeutic agents are not available for enteroviral infections. Sanitation measures such as handwashing and containment of infectious excreta, particularly feces, should be practiced. Vaccines for nonpolio enteroviruses have not been developed, because permanent sequelae and death are rare and the immunologic diversity of the agents makes this approach unfeasible.

Kibrick, S.: Current status of Coxsackie and ECHO viruses in human disease. Prog. Med. Virol., 6:27, 1964.
Melnick, J. L.: Enteroviruses. In Evans, A. S. (ed.): Viral Infections of Humans. New York, Plenum Medical Book Company, 1976, p. 163.

POLIOMYELITIS AND ASEPTIC MENINGITIS DUE TO OTHER ENTEROVIRUSES

The most important enteroviral infections are poliomyelitis (see Ch. 307) and aseptic meningitis caused by coxsackieviruses and echoviruses, which are presented together with other causes of this syndrome (see Ch. 303).

91. PARALYSIS AND OTHER NEUROLOGIC COMPLICATIONS OF NONPOLIO ENTEROVIRAL INFECTIONS

Flaccid motor paralysis caused by enteroviruses other than polioviruses is extremely rare, but many coxsackieviruses and echoviruses have been incriminated in sporadic cases. The most commonly implicated immunotype, coxsackievirus A7, has been responsible for small outbreaks of paralytic disease in Scotland and the U.S.S.R. In general, paralytic disease caused by these viruses is transient or milder than that caused by polioviruses. A poliomyelitis-like syndrome, primarily occurring in adults, has been recognized increasingly as a complication of acute hemorrhagic conjunctivitis (see Ch. 96), which it generally follows by two to three weeks. Confirmation of the etiologic role of enterovirus 70 in this disease has been difficult, because titers of neutralizing antibodies are often maximal by the time paralysis occurs, and virus has not been recovered from the central nervous system.

Focal or generalized encephalitis accompanied by spastic paralysis may be seen in infants infected with coxsackieviruses and echoviruses. Coxsackievirus A9 has caused hemiconvulsions and hemiplegia followed by a chronic seizure disorder and porencephalic cyst. In other patients delirium, coma, cerebellar ataxia, and choreiform movements have occurred during infection with nonpolio enteroviruses.

Transverse myelitis and the Guillain-Barré syndrome have also been noted during enteroviral infections. Rarely virus has been recovered from the cerebrospinal fluid, but in most instances a firm etiologic relationship has not been established.

Grist, N. R., and Bell, E. J.: Enteroviral etiology of the paralytic poliomyelitis syndrome. Arch. Environ. Health, 21:382, 1970.
Kibrick, S.: Current status of Coxsackie and ECHO viruses in human disease. Prog. Med. Virol., 6:27, 1964.
Kono, R., Miyamura, K., Tajiri, E., Sasagawa, A., Phuapradit, P., Roongwithu, N., Vejjajiva, A., Jayavasu, C., Thongcharoen, P., Wasi, C., and Rodprassert, P.: Virological and serological studies of neurological complications of acute hemorrhagic conjunctivitis in Thailand. J. Infect. Dis., 135:706, 1977.

92.   HERPANGINA

DEFINITION. Herpangina (*herpes,* vesicular eruption; *angina,* quinsy, or inflammation of the throat) is an infectious disease characterized by fever, sore throat, and a painful vesicular enanthem typically located on the anterior pillars of the tonsils and the soft palate.

ETIOLOGY. Group A coxsackieviruses (types 1–6, 8, 10, 16, and 22) are responsible for the great majority of cases. Uncommonly, other enteroviruses have been incriminated (coxsackieviruses B1–5 and echoviruses 3, 6, 9, 17, 25, and 30).

EPIDEMIOLOGY. Herpangina occurs predominantly in children during the summer months. Sporadic cases may occur, but most reports emphasize community outbreaks. Often multiple children within the same family are afflicted at intervals of two to five days; however, inapparent infections among contacts are more common.

CLINICAL MANIFESTATIONS. The illness begins with sudden fever of 37.7 to 40° C accompanied by sore throat and dysphagia, usually lasting two to three days. The pharynx and fauces are red but with little or no exudate. Headache and abdominal pain, occasionally accompanied by vomiting, may occur. The hallmark of the disease is the presence of vesicular lesions of the fauces. These begin as punctate macules which progress, over a period of 24 hours, to 2- to 4-mm gray papules and eventually to vesicles surrounded by an erythematous halo. They are located on the soft palate, especially on the free-hanging margin between the tonsils and the uvula, or on the anterior tonsillar pillar. Less commonly they are encountered on the buccal mucosa, posterior pharynx, or hard palate. The lesions are painful, but not exquisitely so, and are never numerous; two to six is usual, rarely a dozen. Late in the illness the vesicles ulcerate. Lesions generally persist two to three days after fever has subsided and are gone by one week. *Acute lymphonodular pharyngitis* is a variant of the syndrome in which the lesions having the characteristic distribution consist of tiny nodules of packed lymphocytes which do not vesiculate or ulcerate.

DIAGNOSIS. Herpangina is a disease of the posterior oral cavity. In contrast, the vesicular enanthems of primary herpetic gingivostomatitis and hand-foot-and-mouth disease involve the front of the mouth, particularly the anterior buccal mucosa and tongue or inner aspect of the lips. Moreover, primary herpes simplex infection typically is associated with prominent gingivitis, cervical lymphadenitis, greater systemic toxicity, and sometimes *exudative* tonsillitis and pharyngitis. Vesicles of the extremities are characteristic of hand-foot-and-mouth disease but are not seen in herpangina.

LABORATORY DIAGNOSIS. The white blood cell count and differential count in herpangina are normal. Virus may be isolated from throat secretions and feces.

TREATMENT AND PROGNOSIS. Children with herpangina are rarely very ill and recover without specific therapy in a few days. Antimicrobial drugs are ineffective and are not indicated. Parotitis has been reported as a complication but is not well documented.

Huebner, R. J., Cole, R. M., Beeman, E. A., Bell, J. A., and Peers, J. H.: Herpangina. Etiologic studies of a specific infectious disease. JAMA, 145:628, 1951.

Keuth, U., Esser, I., Wilhelmi, J., and Wilhelmi, I.: Die "herpangina" Epidemie 1967-68 (ECHO 30-6-3); Bericht über 590 klinisch beobachtete Fälle im Säuglings und Kindesalter. Dtsch. Med. Wochenschr., 94:1959, 1969.

Zahorsky, J.: Herpangina (a specific infectious disease). Arch. Pediat., 41:181, 1924.

93. EPIDEMIC PLEURODYNIA

(Bornholm Disease, Epidemic Myalgia, Devil's Grip, Sylvest's Disease)

DEFINITION. Epidemic pleurodynia (*pleura*, rib or side; *odyne*, pain) is an acute, febrile infectious disease characterized by sudden, sharp, spasmodic, often relapsing pain in the intercostal region of the chest or abdomen.

ETIOLOGY. The overwhelming majority of cases of epidemic pleurodynia are caused by group B coxsackieviruses. Outbreaks of illness consistent with pleurodynia have also been associated with echovirus 1 and sporadic cases with coxsackieviruses (types A4, 6, and 10) and echoviruses (types 1, 6, 9, and 19).

EPIDEMIOLOGY. Epidemic pleurodynia is predominantly a disease of children 5 to 15 years of age and their parents. The mean age is greater than that seen in aseptic meningitis caused by enteroviruses. Three fourths of patients are less than 30 years old. Males and females are attacked equally. Although Daae in 1872 described an epidemic involving 346 people in a Norwegian community of 1950 inhabitants, it was not until 1933 that Sylvest published his classic monograph describing the disease on the Danish island of Bornholm. Since then outbreaks have been recognized in many parts of the world. In different epidemics, from one third to two thirds of the cases have been in one member of a household, but multiple cases in a single family commonly occur either simultaneously or in rapid succession at intervals of two to five days. Unlike outbreaks of enteroviral aseptic meningitis, which are seen in urban areas during most summers, intervals of many years often elapse between epidemics of pleurodynia.

PATHOGENESIS AND PATHOLOGY. Despite its name, pleurodynia almost certainly results from infection of skeletal muscle rather than serosal surfaces. This is supported by the presence of palpable muscle tenderness at the site of symptoms in many cases. Although a pleural friction rub has been noted in up to 10 per cent of cases in some epidemics, this feature has been totally absent in other outbreaks, and even small pleural effusions are rare. Patients with abdominal pain have muscle spasm, but at laparotomy even localized peritonitis is absent. Neither isolation of group B coxsackieviruses from intercostal or other skeletal muscles nor histopathologic examination of these tissues has been reported in clear-cut cases of epidemic pleurodynia.

CLINICAL MANIFESTATIONS. Although about one quarter of cases of epidemic pleurodynia may have a prodome of a "head cold," headache, anorexia, or myalgia, the typical illness is ushered in by the onset of *spasmodic* pain typically occurring over the lower rib cage or upper abdomen. The pain varies from a mild "stitch" in the side to severe crushing, constricting, or band-like pain, which in adults may closely simulate the pain of myocardial ischemia. It is frequently described as smothering, stabbing, knife-life, catching, or vise-like, but it is the spasmodic nature of the pain which is nearly universal and is its hallmark. During each paroxysm lasting several hours or more, the patient is tachypneic, with visible splinting of the chest or abdominal muscles, and appears acutely ill. Auscultation of the chest reveals no signs of pneumonia. Paroxysms are separated by intervals of several hours, during which the patient may look entirely well. The pain, which the patient localizes with a vague area covered by a hand rather than a finger, is aggravated by breathing, coughing, turning over in bed, or in fact any motion. Adults typically complain of chest pain, which is usually unilateral, less often bilateral or subxiphoid. Young children more commonly have abdominal pain. In the Birmingham epidemic of 1951, 81 per cent of children had abdominal pain, 9 per cent had chest pain, and 11 per cent had both. In the Oxford epidemic of the same year, 9 per cent of patients experienced pain in neither the chest nor the abdomen, but instead in the neck or limbs; in these patients the diagnosis was made only by epidemiologic association with other family members. Abdominal pain is more common in the epigastrium or hypochondrium than around the umbilicus or right lower quadrant. Whatever the localization, thoracic or abdominal, the individual patient generally experiences severe pain in only one or two areas of the body. Localized tenderness to pressure occurs in about one quarter of cases, occasionally accompanied by palpable or visible muscle swelling or hyperesthesia of the overlying skin.

In addition to pain there is fever of 37.8 to 39.5° C, occasionally with profuse diaphoresis. Fever occurs simultaneously with pain and is diminished or absent during intervals between paroxysms. Headache, sore throat, nausea, and vomiting may occur, and mild cervical lymphadenopathy may be present.

The illness generally lasts one to four days, but in 20 per cent of patients paroxysms may persist up to two weeks. These recrudescent paroxysms usually occur a few days after the initial attack and are shorter in duration. However, as many as 10 per cent of individuals may re-experience symptoms one or more months after complete freedom from pain. The patient recognizes these late relapses as the same disease, often identical in all respects except duration to the original attack.

Laboratory tests typically reveal no abnormalities, although about 25 per cent of patients have a white blood cell count less than 5000 per cubic millimeter on the third or fourth day of illness. Assays of muscle enzymes in serum have not been reported.

COMPLICATIONS. Most patients recover uneventfully. The two most common complications are aseptic meningitis (3 to 7 per cent), occurring 4 to 35 days after onset of pleurodynia; and orchitis (less than 5 per cent of postpubertal males), which often occurs late in the illness and may be followed by testicular atrophy. Pericarditis is rare.

DIFFERENTIAL DIAGNOSIS. In a summer epidemic, the diagnosis is not difficult in children or young adults with characteristic spasmodic pain in the chest or upper abdomen, aggravated by breathing, in the absence of signs of pneumonia. However, in the Birmingham epidemic as many children were admitted to surgical wards as to medical wards, and 9 of 49 of the former were subjected to laparotomy before the diagnosis of epidemic pleurodynia was made. The protean character of the illness can mimic chest diseases such as pneumonia, pulmonary infarction, coronary insufficiency, and the pre-eruptive phase of zoster; and abdominal diseases such as appendicitis, pancreatitis, acute cholecystitis, and perforated peptic ulcer. The absence of auscultatory findings in the chest and negative roentgenograms are helpful in excluding pneumonia, as is the spasmodic and relapsing character of the pain. With abdominal pain and muscle spasm, signs of peritoneal irritation are lacking, but in some cases it may be difficult to exclude an abdominal catastrophe.

LABORATORY DIAGNOSIS. Early in the illness, group B coxsackieviruses may be recovered from throat washings and feces, and rising titers of type-specific neutralizing antibodies can be detected in paired acute and convalescent sera. Virus has also been isolated from a testicular biopsy in a case complicated by orchitis.

PROGNOSIS AND TREATMENT. Patients with pleurodynia may appear to be extremely ill, even in extremis. However, despite the tendency for relapses, eventual recovery is invariably complete. Profound asthenia occasionally persists for months after the illness. There is no specific treatment, but salicylates or narcotic analgesics may be required for relief of pain.

Finn, J. J., Jr., Weller, T. H., and Morgan, H. R.: Epidemic pleurodyn-
ia: Clinical and etiologic studies based on one hundred and fourteen cases. Arch. Intern. Med., 83:305, 1949.
Huebner, R. J., Risser, J. A., Bell, J. A., Beeman, E. A., Beigelman, P. M., and Strong, J. C.: Epidemic pleurodynia in Texas. A study of 22 cases. N. Engl. J. Med., 248:267, 2953.
Pickles, W. N.: Sylvest's disease (Bornholm disease). N. Engl. J. Med., 250:1033, 1954.
Warin, J. F., Davies, J. B. M., Sanders, F. K., and Vizoso, A. D.: Oxford epidemic of Bornholm disease. Br. Med. J., 1:1345, 1953.

94. PERICARDITIS AND MYOCARDITIS CAUSED BY ENTEROVIRUSES

Heart disease caused by enteroviruses in neonates is quite different from illness produced in older children and adults. In neonates the virus principally attacks the myocardium and the disease is fulminant, often fatal, with involvement of other organ systems. In contrast, in older children and adults, pericarditis usually predominates over myocarditis, and the illness is generally much milder.

ETIOLOGY. Group B coxsackieviruses, types 1 to 5, cause a substantial majority of cases of pericarditis and myocarditis attributable to enteroviruses. Group A coxsackieviruses (types 1, 4, 9, and 16) and echoviruses (types 1, 3, 6–9, 19, and 22) have also been implicated in a few cases. The proportion of acute infections of the heart contributed by group B coxsackieviruses is unknown, but the best available studies suggest that they are responsible for only 13 per cent of cases of otherwise idiopathic acute pericarditis (range, 3 to 44 per cent) and 33 per cent of myocarditis. The causes of the remainder are largely unknown.

EPIDEMIOLOGY. That coxsackieviruses can infect the heart was first recognized following catastrophic outbreaks of myocarditis in newborn nurseries in South Africa and Rhodesia during the early 1950's. In recent years only sporadic cases have been reported in neonates. Infection in nurseries is presumably nosocomial, transmitted by the fecal-oral route. Neonatal myocarditis may also be acquired during birth or in utero, in which case there is frequently a history of maternal illness consistent with cosackievirus infection in the two weeks preceding delivery. In older children and adults, even during epidemics of coxsackievirus infection, cases of pericarditis and myocarditis are sporadic, because involvement of the heart is an uncommon manifestation of infection. Only 3.5 per cent of group B coxsackievirus infections in 1966 to 1970 as reported by the World Health Organization had predominantly cardiac manifestations. Because of selective reporting of more serious illnesses, even 3.5 per cent is undoubtedly an overestimate.

PATHOGENESIS AND PATHOLOGY. Coxsackieviruses and echoviruses have been isolated many times early in the illness or at autopsy from myocardium and pericardial fluid. Histologically there is focal muscle necrosis and inflammation with polymorphonuclear or round cells. These findings point to direct viral invasion of tissues as the factor responsible for the lesions. However, in laboratory animals myocardial inflammation and necrosis persist long after viral replication has ceased, and T lymphocyte function in mice appears to be necessary for both inflammation and a lethal outcome. An immunologic basis for myocardial injury is therefore suggested. Recrudescences of pericarditis reminiscent of Dressler's syndrome (see Ch. 365.2) also suggest the possibility of immunologically mediated disease.

CLINICAL MANIFESTATIONS. **Myocarditis of the Newborn.** The disease usually begins in the first week of life but occasionally up to three weeks or beyond. Typically the onset is abrupt. In one third of cases the illness is biphasic with one to three days of fever, anorexia, coryza, or loose stools followed by apparent recovery for one to seven days before the second phase begins. Circulatory failure then evolves rapidly over a period of a day or two. Only 70 per cent of infants are febrile during this phase. Most exhibit tachycardia (200 beats per minute or more), cardiomegaly, transitory systolic murmurs, and electrocardiographic changes of myocardial injury. In severely affected infants, respiratory distress, cyanosis, and the gray ashen pallor of circulatory collapse may follow, and progressive myocardial failure leads to edema, abdominal distention, and hepatomegaly. Myocarditis in fatal cases is often accompanied by disseminated viral infection involving other organs, particularly the central nervous system and the liver. In these infants liver enlargement and jaundice may reflect the combined effects of congestive heart failure and hepatocellular necrosis. Although most affected neonates are drowsy or stuporous, the presence of convulsions, bulging fontanelles, and cerebrospinal fluid pleocytosis is indicative of viral infection of the central nervous system. In fatal cases the interval from onset of illness to death is usually two to seven days, but a fulminant course with death in less than 24 hours is sometimes seen. The electrocardiogram is not of prognostic value during the acute phase. In survivors defervescence in approximately one week is accompanied by rapid improvement in cardiac function.

Myopericarditis of Older Children and Adults. Although the manifestations of coxsackievirus heart disease in older children and adults are predominantly those of pericarditis, the illness is more properly termed myopericarditis because involvement of the subepicardial myocardium is present in virtually all cases. A history of preceding upper respiratory infection is frequent. Fever, precordial pain, and a pericardial friction rub (often transient) are noted in 70 to 90 per cent of cases. Except for the common complaints of myalgia and arthralgia, noted in about 50 per cent, the symptoms and signs do not differ notably from acute serofibrinous pericarditis of other causes (see Ch. 365.2). Chest roentgenograms reveal enlargement of the cardiac silhouette in 40 to 75 per cent of patients, more commonly caused by pericardial effusion than cardiac dilatation. Pleural effusions, especially left sided, are seen in 20 to 50 per cent. The electrocardiogram is abnormal in all cases. In addition to S-T and T wave changes characteristic of pericarditis, Q waves and conduction disturbances, often accompanied by serum myocardial enzyme elevations, point to the existence of more severe myocardial involvement in occasional patients. Perhaps 10 to 15 per cent present initially with fever, gallop rhythm, and signs of severe congestive heart failure. The disease in these cases resembles myocarditis of other causes (see Ch. 366.4). Occasionally coxsackievirus myopericarditis is accompanied by aseptic meningitis; pleurodynia is rare.

LABORATORY ASPECTS. Most patients have a normal white blood cell count, but in nearly half there is a polymorphonuclear leukocytosis. Proof of enteroviral cause is made by isolation of virus from pericardial fluid or myocardium, but these specimens are not often available. Strong circumstantial evidence exists when virus is isolated from throat secretions or feces accompanied by a rising titer of type-specific neutralizing antibodies in serum. These specimens should be submitted for diagnosis whenever possible, but it is sometimes difficult to demonstrate seroconversion because many patients with coxsackievirus myopericarditis already have high, stable antibody titers within a few days of onset of illness. When no virus is isolated but a high, stable antibody titer to a group B coxsackievirus is present, the demonstration that these antibodies are of the IgM class is evidence of recent infection.

DIFFERENTIAL DIAGNOSIS. Coxsackievirus myocarditis of the newborn may resemble bacterial sepsis or pneumonia. When the liver and central nervous system are involved, the illness must be distinguished from neonatal herpes simplex without cutaneous lesions as well as from other viral infections. Although congenital heart disease may resemble neonatal myocarditis, fever or hypothermia and the nature of the electrocardiographic changes are helpful features pointing toward an infective etiology. The differential diagnosis in older individuals with pericarditis and myocarditis is found in Ch. 365.2 and 366.4.

PROGNOSIS. Although early reports indicated that coxsackievirus neonatal myocarditis was a highly lethal disease, accumulated experience now suggests that the mortality is considerably less than 50 per cent. There are few data on long-term follow-up of surviving infants. Most older children and adults recover uneventfully. In 11 of 12 adults with myocarditis caused by coxsackievirus B5, electrocardiographic abnormalities returned to normal by seven months, but the remaining subject had persistent T wave abnormalities. However, in another series 5 of 22 patients appeared to have permanent heart damage manifested by chronic congestive heart failure. The possible contribution of coxsackieviruses to chronic cardiomyopathy following unrecognized infection is unknown.

TREATMENT AND COMPLICATIONS. There is no specific treatment for the viral infection. During the acute illness pericardial pain, effusions, arrhythmias, and heart failure are managed as in patients having these disorders from other causes. Exercise and treatment with corticosteroids adversely affect the outcome of coxsackievirus myocarditis in laboratory animals. For these reasons bed rest is recommended and corticosteroids are not, although neither benefit nor harm has been clearly apparent in the few cases of steroid-treated disease in man. Constrictive pericarditis has been reported as a very rare sequel of coxsackievirus infection.

Grist, N. R., and Bell, E. J.: A six-year study of coxsackievirus B infections in heart disease. J. Hyg. (Camb.), 73:165, 1974.

Helin, M., Savola, J., and Lapinleimu, K.: Cardiac manifestations during a coxsackie B5 epidemic. Br. Med. J., 2:97, 1968.

Kibrick, S.: Current status of Coxsackie and ECHO viruses in human disease. Prog. Med. Virol., 6:27, 1964.

Koontz, C. H., and Ray, C. G.: The role of Coxsackie group B virus infections in sporadic myopericarditis. Am. Heart J., 82:750, 1971.

Sainani, G. S., Krompotic, E., and Slodki, S. J.: Adult heart disease due to the Coxsackie virus B infection. Medicine, 47:133, 1968.

95. EXANTHEMS CAUSED BY ENTEROVIRUSES

A variety of exanthems, occasionally associated with enanthems, are caused by coxsackieviruses, echoviruses, and the newer enteroviruses. In some patients they occur with aseptic meningitis, whereas in others they are associated with otherwise undifferentiated febrile summer illnesses. All occur more commonly in children than in adults with the same infection. The importance of these rashes is the clue they provide to the existence of enteroviral illness in the community, as well as their potential confusion with other childhood exanthems such as the rashes of meningococcemia, rubella, roseola infantum, varicella, and herpes simplex virus infections. The pathogenesis of enteroviral exanthems is poorly understood. In hand-foot-and-mouth disease, virus can be isolated from vesicle fluid, and the lesions are probably directly caused by hematogenously disseminated virus. Whether the maculopapular exanthems are also caused by direct viral invasion of the skin or are immunologically mediated is unknown. Whatever the mechanism, rashes may be caused by many different enteroviruses, and the type of rash elicited is with few exceptions not specific for a particular immunotype. Some, however, are distinctive:

HAND-FOOT-AND-MOUTH DISEASE
(Vesicular Stomatitis with Exanthem)

Most cases of this syndrome are caused by coxsackievirus A16, less commonly by A5 or A10, and rarely by coxsackievirus B2 or B5 or enterovirus 69. This disease is characterized by vesicular or mixed papulovesicular lesions on the dorsum, palms, or soles of the hands and feet, accompanied by vesicles or ulcers in the mouth. Children less than five years old account for 70 to 90 per cent of cases. Typically they refuse to eat and complain of a sore mouth. Oral lesions are present in nearly every case, but cutaneous lesions are seen in only about 70 per cent. The cutaneous lesions may occur in crops resembling varicella, but in hand-foot-and-mouth disease the lesions are far less numerous, do not pustulate or form scabs, and occur on the distal extremities rather than on the trunk. Vesicles are occasionally seen on the buttocks. Oral lesions are usually ulcerated and occur on the lips, tongue, anterior buccal mucosa, or hard palate, thus differentiating them from herpangina, in which the lesions occur more posteriorly. The lesions in the mouth may also resemble those of primary herpes simplex viral infection, but children with herpes generally appear more toxic, have gingivitis and prominent cervical lymphadenitis, and lack vesicles on the extremities. Patients with hand-foot-and-mouth disease do not appear very sick, and the lesions almost always disappear in less than one week.

RUBELLIFORM EXANTHEMS

A rubelliform rash caused by echovirus 9 is by far the most common enteroviral exanthem. In some epi-demics as many as 50 to 70 per cent of children infected with this agent have had rash. Less commonly, indistinguishable exanthems have been associated with many other echovirus immunotypes, as well as coxsackieviruses A and B and enterovirus 71. The rash is typically maculopapular and involves the face in all cases, the neck and chest in three quarters, and the extremities in about half. It does not itch or desquamate. Fever characteristically occurs simultaneously with the rash. Unlike rubella, posterior cervical and postauricular lymphadenopathy is not prominent. The rash of echovirus 9 or coxsackievirus A9 may have a petechial component or may be exclusively petechial and is then easily confused with meningococcemia, especially when accompanied by signs of meningeal irritation. Occasionally the rash becomes confluent or produces large, blotchy violaceous lesions, particularly on the face. Both rash and fever usually clear in three to seven days.

ROSEOLA-LIKE EXANTHEMS

Most commonly caused by echovirus 16 ("the Boston exanthem"), this illness begins with fever of 38 to 39.5° C which lasts for 24 to 48 hours. The rash, consisting of salmon pink macules on the head and trunk, which appear only as the fever is declining or shortly after defervescence, lasts one to five days. This temporal sequence has also been noted with echoviruses 11 and 25 and coxsackieviruses B1 and B5.

Adler, J. L., Mostow, S. R., Mellin, H., Janney, J. H., and Mehsen Joseph, J.: Epidemiologic investigation of hand, foot, and mouth disease. Am. J. Dis. Child., 120:309, 1970.

Horstmann, D. M.: Viral exanthems and enanthems. Pediatrics, 41:867, 1968.

Lerner, A. M.: Exanthems caused by coxsackievirus, echovirus, and reovirus infections. In Demis, D. J., Dobson, R. L., and McGuire, J. M. (eds.): Clinical Dermatology, Vol. 3, unit 14-19. New York, Harper & Row Co., 1976, pp. 1-22.

Neva, F. A., Feemster, R. F., and Gorbach, I. J.: Clinical and epidemiological features of an unusual epidemic exanthem: JAMA, 155:544, 1954.

Sabin, A. B., Krumbiegel, E. R., and Wigand, R.: ECHO type 9 virus disease. J. Dis. Child., 96:197, 1958.

96. ACUTE HEMORRHAGIC CONJUNCTIVITIS

DEFINITION. Acute hemorrhagic conjunctivitis is a contagious disease occurring in explosive epidemics in Africa, the Indian subcontinent, and the Far East. It is characterized by conjunctival injection, tearing, and subconjunctival hemorrhages.

ETIOLOGY. A great majority of cases are caused by enterovirus 70. The disease has also been caused by coxsackievirus A24 or has occurred in mixed epidemics with adenovirus 11, which produces clinically indistinguishable disease.

EPIDEMIOLOGY. Acute hemorrhagic conjunctivitis emerged as an apparently new disease in West Africa in 1969 and appeared almost simultaneously in Vietnam and Indonesia. Since then the disease has spread to North Africa, the Indian subcontinent, and most of the

Far East. In the United Kingdom and the U.S.S.R., it appeared briefly in 1971 as circumscribed outbreaks of iatrogenic infection in eye clinics after introduction from abroad. Epidemics have continued in much of Africa and Asia in subsequent years. Secondary attack rates in families are high. Attack rates for clinical disease are greatest in young adults, whereas asymptomatic infection is more common in infants and children. Antibody surveys of sera collected prior to 1969 in affected countries reveal no clear evidence even in the elderly of previous infection with enterovirus 70, but following the epidemic as many as 40 to 50 per cent of the population had neutralizing antibodies. Neither clinical disease nor evidence of previous infection has been detected in the Western Hemisphere. Available evidence suggests that the disease is transmitted from hand to eye or by fomites, such as towels.

CLINICAL MANIFESTATIONS. Following an incubation period of 12 to 72 hours, the illness begins with sudden periorbital edema, severe pain, photophobia, blurred vision, lacrimation, and conjunctival suffusion. Disease typically begins in one eye but rapidly spreads to the other. Subconjunctival hemorrhages, present in 45 per cent of cases, may be small or massive and are the most distinctive feature of the infection. A scant purulent exudate is seen in 16 per cent. Punctate epithelial keratitis is frequent but transient. Conjunctival follicles and preauricular lymphadenopathy may be present. Systemic symptoms are variously reported as absent, or low-grade fever, malaise, headache, and symptoms of upper respiratory infection occur. Recovery is usually noticeable by the second or third day and is complete by ten days.

COMPLICATIONS. Discharge from the eye may become purulent when secondary bacterial infection supervenes. The most serious complication is the rare occurrence of a poliomyelitis-like motor paralysis (see Ch. 91).

LABORATORY DIAGNOSIS. Enterovirus 70 can be recovered from conjunctival swabs, but apparently cannot regularly be isolated from the intestinal tract during the acute stage of the illness. Rising antibody titers can be demonstrated in paired acute and convalescent sera.

TREATMENT AND PREVENTION. Treatment of conjunctivitis is symptomatic. Antimicrobial agents are not indicated unless there is secondary bacterial infection. Careful handwashing and use of separate towels are indicated to prevent contagion.

Acute hemorrhagic conjunctivitis. Lancet, 1:86, 1973.

Hierholzer, J. C., Hilliard, K. A., and Esposito, J. J.: Serosurvey for "acute hemorrhagic conjunctivitis" virus (enterovirus 70) antibodies in the southeastern United States, with review of the literature and some epidemiologic implications. Am. J. Epidemiol., 102:533, 1975.

Kono, R., Sasagawa, A., Ishii, K., Sugiura, S., Ochi, M., Matsumiya, H., Uchida, Y., Kameyama, K., Kaneko, M., and Sakurai, N.: Pandemic of new type of conjunctivitis. Lancet, 1:1191, 1972.

97. DIARRHEA ASSOCIATED WITH COXSACKIE- AND ECHOVIRUSES

Perhaps because of their name, enteroviruses are frequently cited as causes of epidemic or sporadic gastroenteritis and diarrhea. The preponderance of evidence, however, suggests that other viral and bacterial agents are far more important causes of these illnesses. Echovirus 18 and possibly other echoviruses have clearly been implicated in epidemic diarrhea of the newborn, but the role of enteroviruses in sporadic diarrhea, especially in older children and adults, is less certain. The consensus of several studies with well-matched controls is that there is a variable, usually small excess of enteroviral infections in children with diarrhea. Subsequent to these studies, rotaviruses and Norwalk-like agents (see Ch. 104), as well as toxigenic *Escherichia coli*, have emerged as major causes of gastroenteritis or diarrhea in children and adults. In light of this new knowledge, additional epidemiologic studies are needed before the contribution of enteroviruses in diarrheal illness can be assessed, but their role appears to be minor.

98. RESPIRATORY ILLNESS DUE TO ENTEROVIRUSES

Undifferentiated febrile illnesses with or without respiratory symptoms ("summer grippe") are far more common manifestations of enteroviral infections than the more specific syndromes usually associated with them. Although possibly all enteroviruses may be associated with respiratory disease, such illnesses are characteristic of certain immunotypes. Coxsackievirus A21 has been responsible for outbreaks of pharyngitis and "common cold syndrome" in military recruits as well as for sporadic cases in civilians. Less commonly it has produced influenza-like disease or atypical pneumonia. Many echoviruses, but especially echovirus 11, can cause common colds. Group B coxsackieviruses and enterovirus 68 have been associated in children 2 to 15 years old with pharyngitis, tracheobronchitis, bronchiolitis, and pneumonia. The respiratory illnesses produced by enteroviruses are not clinically distinguishable from similar disease caused by rhinoviruses, parainfluenza viruses, and other respiratory viruses.

ARTHROPOD-BORNE VIRAL FEVERS, VIRAL ENCEPHALITIDES, AND VIRAL HEMORRHAGIC FEVERS
(Arboviruses and Arenaviruses)

99.   INTRODUCTION

Karl M. Johnson

Arthropod-borne viruses (arboviruses) are defined on an epidemiologic basis. Thus any virus is an arbovirus if it actually multiplies in one or more arthropods and if it is biologically transmitted to vertebrates with sufficient frequency by arthropods to make this an important means of virus survival. More than 300 distinguishable agents have been tentatively so classified. Many have similar physical and chemical properties and could reasonably be placed within families on this basis as well; others have fundamental properties relating them to animal virus groups not generally associated with recognized arthropod transmission.

Immunologic properties are currently used to cluster individual arboviruses. Viruses having such relationships are included in groups that historically began with A, B, and C; thereafter, the name of the first virus to be discovered was used to designate the group. Originally virus names were derived from antecedent diseases, e.g., yellow fever, dengue, and equine encephalitides. Later, geography in combination with disease syndrome was favored, providing names such as St. Louis encephalitis and Colorado tick fever. Finally, there are many geographically named arboviruses for which no clinical syndromes have been defined, either because they rarely infect man or because they have not been associated with morbidity of dramatic proportions.

About 90 arboviruses are known to infect man, and most of these have been shown to produce illness. With rare exceptions, such as dengue and urban yellow fever, these are zoonoses in which man is an accidental host of no apparent importance in the fundamental natural history of the virus.

Clinical syndromes produced by arboviruses share the common properties of fever and myalgia accompanied by viremia. Beyond that, classification is inevitably arbitrary, because the same virus can induce a wide variety of patterns in different patients, and different viruses have been linked to remarkably similar syndromes. Emphasis is given here to the often infrequent but spectacular severe diseases some of the agents evoke. Thus individual descriptions are placed in one of the following groups: (1) *fevers of a relatively undifferentiated type,* with or without rashes, usually benign; (2) *encephalitides,* often severe and with significant case fatality rates; and (3) *hemorrhagic fevers,* also frequently severe and fatal.

The largest number of viruses have been associated exclusively with milder, undifferentiated disease. The majority of these are encountered most commonly in tropical and semitropical countries (see table in Ch. 100.3). The classic clinical prototype is *dengue.* Those to be described represent but a small sample. Of these, *chikungunya, Mayaro, O'nyong-nyong,* and *Ross River*

are group A viruses, *dengue* and *West Nile* belong to group B, and the remainder are unclassified or are in the *sandfly fever* group. Although each gained entry to this book because of its proved epidemic disease potential for man, clinical differentiation even during epidemics is generally difficult; epidemiologic and laboratory methods are more important. When more than one such virus is simultaneously endemic, the latter techniques are essential.

All arboviruses conspicuously associated with encephalitis and hemorrhagic fever are included. In the case of the latter syndrome, all but one of the viruses belong to antigenic group B. Yellow fever is listed among the hemorrhagic fevers because many cases do not display the "classic" picture of jaundice, but manifest gastrointestinal hemorrhage (black vomit), epistaxis, and melena with fatal shock and thus fit this description better than either of the other two arbovirus clinical syndromes. Arenavirus-caused hemorrhagic fevers, although not arthropod borne, are described here because of their clinical similarity to those induced by arboviruses and because they are zoonotic infections.

It should be emphasized that all these viruses frequently provoke only mild clinically undifferentiated infections. Thus specific virologic diagnostic tests are of fundamental importance in sporadic infections as well as during epidemics. Specific diagnosis of all arboviral disease depends upon isolation of virus and/or detection of a homologous antiviral immune response. In many parts of the world malaria is first sought in acute febrile disease with or without neurologic manifestations. The findings of such parasites, however, may not solve the problem; it should be remembered that either a simultaneous arbovirus infection or a drug-resistant parasite may account for the lack of response to supposed specific chemotherapy.

Virus isolation, together with an antibody rise to that agent between acute and convalescent phase sera from the patient, provides nearly incontrovertible evidence for an etiologic association between virus and disease. Blood is the best source of virus for all the diseases here described except for Venezuelan equine encephalitis which may be gotten from pharyngeal swabs at least as readily. *Such specimens should be obtained on the very first day the patient is seen,* because viremia rarely persists for long into the encephalitic period. Since antibodies are often present at the end of the first week of symptoms, it is important to obtain the acute phase serum specimen for serologic diagnosis at this time. A convalescent serum obtained 10 to 30 days after onset will usually reveal an increase in specific antibodies when measured by the complement-fixation (CF), hemagglutination-inhibition (HI), or neutralization test. No more than 10 ml of blood need be obtained for any of these specimens unless special studies are contemplated. Materials for virus isolation should be kept chilled, or frozen at temperatures of at least −60° C if shipment for testing involves great distances.

Berge, T. O. (ed.): International Catalogue of Arboviruses. 2nd ed. Department of Health, Education, and Welfare Publication 75–8301. Washington, D.C., U. S. Government Printing Office, 1975.

Hammon, W. McD., and Sather, G. E.: Isolation and identification of arthropod-borne-viruses. *In* Lennette, E. H., and Schmidt, J. J. (eds.): Diagnostic Procedures for Virus and Rickettsial Diseases. 4th ed. New York, American Public Health Association, 1969, pp. 227–280.

100. UNDIFFERENTIATED FEVERS

100.1. DENGUE

Karl M. Johnson

DEFINITION. Dengue is an acute, febrile, self-limited infectious disease caused by an *Aedes* mosquito-borne dengue virus. Malaise, prostration, and pain of muscles and joints are characteristic, accompanied by lymphadenopathy, leukopenia, and one or two episodes of exanthem. Typically an illness of about one week is followed by one or more weeks of depression and weakness.

ETIOLOGY. Four distinct immunologic subtypes of dengue virus have been recovered from patients. These agents produce partial cross-immunity such that a primary infection will protect against another subtype only for a few months, although homologous immunity is of long duration.

EPIDEMIOLOGY. Man and certain *Aedes* mosquitoes are the essential links in the recognized natural virus cycle. Size of human populations and ecologic factors affecting the mosquito vector and multiplication of virus in that host are of prime importance. Thus the disease has occurred in all continents and many islands, but only in "summer-like" temperatures where there are large numbers of *Aedes aegypti*, *Aedes albopictus*, or *Aedes scutellaris* mosquitoes. Since infection is usually clinically apparent in adults and frequently inapparent in children, various combinations of human and *Aedes* ecology may produce nearly silent continuous endemic infection, repeated seasonal epidemics, or massive outbreaks affecting populations previously free of dengue for many years.

Viremia adequate for mosquito infection is present just prior to and for the first three days of illness. An infected mosquito requires eight to twelve days to become infective at warm temperatures. Such a mosquito is infective for life and may transmit the virus to one or more susceptible persons on whom it feeds or probes. The incubation period in man is five to six days.

Aedes aegypti, by far the most important vector, breeds, rests, and feeds in or near human habitations. It is primarily attracted to man, biting in daylight and twilight. These attributes make it an ideal virus vector and explain why dengue is principally an urban disease. In rural areas other *Aedes* species such as *A. albopictus* may transmit infection, but their habits and relatively sparse human populations render explosive epidemics uncommon.

No extrahuman virus reservoir has been conclusively documented, but there is suggestive evidence that monkeys and forest mosquitoes may be capable of virus maintenance.

PATHOLOGY. Since dengue is rarely if ever fatal, the only information available is that from biopsy of the skin rash. Such lesions consist of endothelial swelling, perivascular edema, and mononuclear infiltration of small vessels. Petechiae are characterized by extravasation of blood without significant inflammatory reaction.

CLINICAL MANIFESTATIONS. Dengue in adults is typically sudden in onset with rising temperature and only minor chilliness, headache, and fatigue. By the second day temperature is frequently 40° C, headache with ocular or retrobulbar pain is severe, and the patient complains of back pain, generalized myalgia, and aching joints. During this interval there is a diffuse blushing of the face and upper trunk, sometimes accompanied by a fleeting *erythematous macular* or *pinpoint rash* of the limbs. General lymphadenopathy is usually apparent, but hepato- or splenomegaly is rare. The leukocyte count at this stage is apt to be essentially normal.

At about the third to fifth day a *maculopapular* or *scarlatiniform rash* appears, beginning on the trunk and spreading in centripetal fashion. This generally lasts at least three days, becomes itchy as it fades, but rarely desquamates. The fever is generally of five to seven days' duration, sometimes with a fall at about the fourth day, giving a saddleback curve. The second bout of fever is often more severe, accompanied by relative or absolute bradycardia and by leukopenia. Monocytes, lymphocytes, and segmented leukocytes all decrease in absolute numbers, although there may be an absolute increase in immature polymorphonuclear cells. A few small petechiae may appear, especially on the lower extremities.

Dengue in young children is definitely a milder disease; recent longitudinal population studies in cities of endemic virus activity confirm an impression formed down the years by the paucity of description of pediatric cases during epidemics. Clinical manifestations may also vary with infecting subtype. Halstead retrospectively documented that volunteer studies done nearly 50 years ago in the Philippines employed subtype 1 and 4 viruses, the disease associated with the latter being milder and less "classic" than that caused by the former.

DIAGNOSIS. During sharp epidemics occurring in places where ecologic factors are compatible, clinical diagnosis of many cases of average severity will usually be correct. But several other arboviruses as well as rubella may be the cause. Thus laboratory confirmation of a *few* cases during an epidemic and of *every* case when the pattern is sporadic is important. Travel history during the previous ten days is essential whenever dealing with a suspect case in areas where the disease is rare.

Virus may be isolated from blood or serum of patients early in the course of illness by inoculation of suckling mice, *Aedes* mosquitoes, or cell cultures. Serologic diagnosis is also possible, using acute and convalescent (two weeks) sera, but is frequently complicated by previous infection with one or more viruses of arbovirus group B. A laboratory competent to execute and interpret tests for a number of different arboviruses is required.

TREATMENT AND PROGNOSIS. There is no specific therapy. Bed rest is indicated, as well as the usual supportive measures to maintain fluid and electrolyte balance and alleviate discomfort. Secondary bacterial infection is uncommon but should be anticipated and appropriately treated. Except in severely debilitated persons, the prognosis is uniformly excellent. Final recovery is complete, although temporary depression and lassitude are common during convalescence, and patients should not be rushed back to normal occupations.

PREVENTION. Vaccines for dengue viruses are not generally available, although experimental work on the problem continues. Individual protection is difficult, because mosquito attacks occur during daytime, and continuous use of repellent is not practical. Community protection is possible through effective control or eradication of the *Aedes* vector. Patients should be protected from mosquitoes during the first five days of illness in order to prevent further virus transmission, and space-spraying of buildings frequented by patients should be done to eliminate mosquitoes possibly infected prior to the diagnosis of the disease.

100.2. WEST NILE FEVER

Karl M. Johnson

DEFINITION. West Nile fever is an acute febrile mosquito-borne illness marked by headache, lymphadenopathy, and a macular skin eruption. It is generally self-limited, although rare cases of mortality caused by encephalitis occur in aged persons. The disease is caused by a group B arbovirus.

ETIOLOGY. West Nile virus is a small ribonucleic acid–containing virus belonging to an antigenic complex within the B group of arboviruses, which includes *Japanese B, Murray Valley*, and *St. Louis encephalitis* viruses, as well as *Ilheus* virus. Immunologic relationships are shared to a somewhat lesser degree with *yellow fever* and *dengue* viruses. Immunologic cross-protection is readily demonstrable experimentally among members of this antigenic complex. Despite the fact that such closely related viruses are frequently distributed geographically in a discontinuous manner, reflecting a long process of evolutionary segregation, West Nile and Japanese B viruses have been repeatedly recovered from the same mosquitoes in the same localities in southern India.

EPIDEMIOLOGY. Millions of people have been infected with West Nile virus, which is endemic in many parts of Africa, the Middle East, Southwest Asia, and southern Europe. Continuous human migration into Israel over the past 30 years has resulted in repeated epidemics among adults. Elsewhere the disease is mainly an affliction of children. Annual summer epidemics are correlated with seasonal peaks in populations of culicine mosquitoes. In Egypt and Israel, *Culex univittatus* is the principal epidemic vector. Much lower levels of virus transmission occur in winter when the suspected vector is *Culex pipiens*.

In ecologic terms, West Nile virus is one of the least evolved arboviruses. In addition to mosquitoes, it multiplies in, and can be experimentally transmitted by, the bite of various species of hard and soft ticks. It has been recovered from *Argas* and *Hyalomma* ticks in nature. Although the primary natural virus cycle appears

to comprise mosquitoes and wild birds, virus or antibody has been detected in rodents, camels, cattle, horses, and monkeys.

The incubation period in man is about three to six days. Most infections are clinically apparent. A number of documented laboratory infections suggest that the agent also can be transmitted by the respiratory route.

CLINICAL MANIFESTATIONS. Sudden onset of fever, lasting three to six days, is accompanied by photophobia, myalgia, and chilling. Nausea and vomiting may occur early in the febrile period. A saddleback fever curve is seen in a minority of patients, and there is usually a definite leukopenia with absolute reduction of polymorphonuclear cells by the third day of illness. At about this time a fine *maculopapular* rash is observed on the trunk and occasionally on the extremities. It is more common in children than in adults, is *nonirritating*, and fades rapidly without desquamation. Lymphadenopathy is often demonstrable at the time the patient is first seen.

Although mild meningismus is demonstrable in a minority of patients and may be accompanied by increased cells and protein in the cerebrospinal fluid, clinical encephalitis is not a feature of West Nile infection except in a handful of very old patients. Pathologic studies were not done in the few fatal cases reported. Convalescence is generally uneventful, although older patients may complain of generalized weakness for several weeks. No permanent sequelae have ever been observed.

DIAGNOSIS. Clinically this disease is so similar to dengue that laboratory diagnosis is essential in all cases. Virus isolation is by far the best hope, and blood specimens obtained as late as the fourth symptomatic day yield a reasonably high percentage of strains when inoculated into suckling mice or the yolk sacs of embryonated eggs. Serologic diagnosis may also be attempted with the usual paired serum samples, but previous infection with related group B arboviruses, including 17D live yellow fever vaccine, may render interpretation of results extremely difficult beyond the confirmation that infection was due to a mosquito-borne member of this large antigenic group.

TREATMENT AND PREVENTION. Management of patients is completely symptomatic. Complications are unusual, and the only reason to keep patients under observation after the rash has faded is to ensure the collection of appropriate diagnostic specimens in situations in which knowledge of the specific cause of illness may have public health implications.

Although there is an impression that prior infection with related group B viruses may lessen the symptomatology of West Nile fever, this has not been rigorously established. Inactivated or attenuated West Nile virus has been used in combination with other group B agents in experimental attempts to produce broad-spectrum immunity to this virus group. Such vaccines are not ready for general use. Thus mosquito control and individual protective measures against mosquito bite represent the only available means of prevention of this infection. Since the main epidemic mosquito vectors are not concentrated around human dwellings and since infection rarely causes severe human disease, expensive systematic mosquito control efforts have not often been mounted.

100.3. FEVERS CAUSED BY GROUP A ARBOVIRUSES: CHIKUNGUNYA, O'NYONG-NYONG, MAYARO, AND ROSS RIVER

Karl M. Johnson

DEFINITION. Chikungunya, O'nyong-nyong, Mayaro, and Ross River fevers are acute nonfatal diseases caused by an antigenically related, geographically dispersed complex of group A arboviruses. Maculopapular rashes and arthralgia are common features of these infections, which occur in Africa, Southeast Asia, tropical America, and Australia.

EPIDEMIOLOGY. Each of these viruses has caused epidemic disease in human populations. Perhaps the most dramatic was that due to O'nyong-nyong in East Africa from 1959 to 1962, when an estimated two million persons of all ages were affected. The important mosquito vectors of each disease are listed in the accompanying table. Chikungunya virus is often transmitted by *Aedes aegypti*; because of the rash and minor hemorrhagic phenomena associated with infection, this agent has at times been considered responsible for cases of hemorrhagic fever during outbreaks basically caused by dengue virus infection. O'nyong-nyong virus is the only known arbovirus transmitted principally by anopheline mosquitoes. Sylvan maintenance cycles involving arboreal mosquitoes and monkeys have been postulated for Mayaro and chikungunya viruses. Epidemic behavior of these agents is far from understood. Irregularly occurring outbreaks during warm rainy months are the rule. There is strong circumstantial evidence that chikungunya virus has moved steadily eastward into Asia from Africa during the last 25 years, employing a simple cycle composed of man and *Aedes aegypti* mosquitoes. The incubation periods of these agents in man vary from about 2 to 12 days. Clinical attack rates are high in relation to those for infection, with the exceptions of Ross River and Mayaro viruses, which induce mild or inapparent infection in children.

CLINICAL MANIFESTATIONS. Onset is typically abrupt, and arthralgias or rashes are more likely to be the chief complaints than are headache and fever. Fever is usually mild, and is virtually absent with Ross River virus. Chikungunya virus frequently induces a saddle-back fever curve, but the second episode, in contrast to dengue, is usually less severe. Arthralgias may or may not be symmetrical in distribution and usually involve terminal joints most severely. The maculopapular rashes are generally irritating, distributed over the trunk and extensor surfaces of the extremities, and may appear early or late in the course of the first week of symptoms. Leukopenia is a common feature of these diseases, and cervical lymphadenitis is frequently reported in cases caused by O'nyong-nyong and Ross River viruses.

DIAGNOSIS. All these viruses except Ross River can be recovered readily from the blood of patients during the initial three days of illness. Standard serologic techniques are highly reliable in making specific diagnosis, provided a second serum specimen is obtained 10 to 14 days after onset of symptoms. Differentiation of O'nyong-nyong and chikungunya viruses in East Africa may present problems. Malaria, rubella, enterovirus infection, and other nonviral causes of acute arthralgia must be considered in the differential diagnosis of individual cases.

TREATMENT AND PROGNOSIS. Treatment is symptomatic, and prognosis is uniformly excellent, although polyarthritis may persist or recur over an interval of several weeks to months. Corticosteroid therapy is contraindicated for joint pain in adults, at least until the

Etiologic and Epidemiologic Features of Undifferentiated Arbovirus Fevers

Fever	Virus	Vector(s)	Vertebrate Host(s)	Geographic Distribution	Human Epidemiologic Features
Dengue	Group B (4 types)	*Aedes aegypti*	Man	Tropics and subtropics; Old and New World	Varies from continuous endemic to repeated epidemic pattern based on human-*Aedes* population cycles
West Nile	Group B	*Culex* mosquitoes *Argas, Hyalomma* ticks	Wild birds	Mediterranean basin, Middle East, Soviet Union, Southwest Asia	Continuously endemic (tropics) to annually epidemic in Mediterranean climates
O'nyong-nyong	Group A	*Anopheles funestus, Anopheles gambiae*	Man	East Africa	Singular massive epidemic; malaria control may affect pattern
Chikungunya	Group A	*Aedes aegypti, A. africanus, Culex* mosquitoes	Man, monkeys?	Africa, Southern Asia, Philippines	Basically similar to dengue
Mayaro	Group A	*Haemagogus, Psorophora* mosquitoes	Monkeys, marsupials	Northern South America and Central America	Endemic, forest-associated infection; localized outbreaks during forest destruction
Ross River	Group A	*Culex, Aedes* mosquitoes	Wild mouse	Eastern Australia	Endemic infection in subtropical north; summer-fall epidemics farther south
Rift Valley	Ungrouped	*Aedes, Culex* mosquitoes	Large wild and domestic animals	East and South Africa	Sporadic rainy season transmission to man; mainly contact infections during livestock epizootics
Colorado tick	Bluetongue group	*Dermacentor andersoni* tick	Ground squirrels, chipmunks	Rocky Mountains of North America	Sporadic and focal summer infections during recreational and occupational activity
Sandfly	Phlebotomus fever group (20 types)	*Phlebotomus, Lutzomyia* sandflies	Man, monkeys, small wild mammals	Mediterranean basin, eastward to southern Asia; forests of tropical America	Annual seasonal transmission to children; epidemic whenever large numbers of susceptible adults introduced; forest-associated infections in American tropics

third week, when hormonal antibodies have appeared. Children possibly infected with chikungunya virus in areas where *Aedes aegypti* and dengue viruses are endemic should be hospitalized, because it is impossible to differentiate this disease from the prodrome of the dengue shock syndrome.

100.4.   COLORADO TICK FEVER

Theodore C. Eickhoff

DEFINITION.   Colorado tick fever is an acute, benign, tick-transmitted viral infection that occurs throughout the Rocky Mountain area, and is characterized by headache, back pain, a biphasic febrile course lasting about one week, and leukopenia.

ETIOLOGY.   Colorado tick fever virus is a member of the arbovirus group, in that it is transmitted to humans by the bite of the hard-shelled woodtick, *Dermacentor andersoni*. Human cases appear to be limited to the combined geographic distribution of the vector and the major mammalian reservoirs, ground squirrels and chipmunks. The virus, however, appears to be unrelated to other members of the arbovirus group. It is a double-stranded RNA virus (diplornavirus) that measures 35 to 50 nm in diameter, with a lipoprotein, hence ether-sensitive, outer coat.

EPIDEMIOLOGY.   The disease occurs during the spring and summer months, when tick exposure in the mountains is common. Disease activity appears to follow springtime in the mountains, for cases occur at lower altitudes during April and May and at higher altitudes during June and July, presumably reflecting the slower emergence of ticks at higher altitudes. Most patients give a history of having found attached ticks, but others will not be aware of the tick attachment and bite, even though they may have seen ticks on their body or clothing. Cases may occasionally be encountered in other areas of the country as a result of travel outside the endemic area during the incubation period, or from accidental transportation of infected adult ticks in clothing or bedding.

The virus has been recovered from as many as 14 per cent of *Dermacentor andersoni* collected in endemic areas. Replication of the virus within these ticks has been documented. It is not clear whether the virus is passed transovarially within the vector species. The reservoir of the disease probably resides in numerous small mammals, particularly golden-mantled ground squirrels and chipmunks, which have a prolonged viremia and infect nymphal ticks. Overwintering may thus occur in either nymphal ticks or hibernating small mammals. Adult ticks then transmit the virus to other small animals, humans being accidental hosts.

Incidence and Prevalence.   The disease has been reported from most states in the Rocky Mountain West and from western Canadian provinces, but the largest number of cases have generally been reported in Colorado. Several hundred cases are diagnosed annually in the endemic area, but it is likely that this represents but a small fraction of the total. Mild or wholly subclinical infections do occur, but their frequency has not been systemically evaluated.

The virus has been isolated from other species of ticks and from numerous species of small mammals, suggesting at least the possibility that the disease may occur over a wider geographic area than is presently appreciated.

PATHOGENESIS.   There is no unusual local reaction at the site of the tick bite inoculation, and the site of initial localization and replication of the virus is unknown. The onset of symptoms occurs three to seven days after tick exposure. Viremia can be demonstrated at the time of onset of fever, persisting not only during the febrile illness itself, but, remarkably, in red blood cells long after the virus has disappeared from serum and neutralizing antibody has appeared. The virus can be demonstrated within erythrocytes by fluorescent antibody staining for up to 120 days, and has been grown from washed erythrocytes 100 days after the original infection.

Few pathologic data in man are available, because only one fatal case has been recorded. In laboratory animals, the heart, lungs, spleen, bone marrow, and lymph nodes are important sites of viral replication. Occasional patients have clinical evidence of central nervous system or meningeal involvement, and Colorado tick fever virus has been recovered from cerebrospinal fluid.

CLINICAL MANIFESTATIONS.   The disease begins abruptly, with chilly sensations, fever of 38 to 40° C, myalgias most prominent in the back and legs, headache, retro-orbital pain, and photophobia. Malaise and nausea may occur, but vomiting is uncommon. Physical findings during the first two to three days of illness are nonspecific. The patient may be flushed, with conjunctival and pharyngeal erythema. Lymphadenopathy is not prominent, although mild splenomegaly is sometimes present. Rashes have been reported in up to 12 per cent of patients, commonly macular or maculopapular and distributed over the entire body, sometimes petechial and involving primarily the extremities. Tachycardia is in proportion to the temperature elevation.

In approximately half the cases, a distinctly biphasic illness occurs, the so-called "saddleback" fever. Symptoms abate after two to three days, temperature becomes normal or nearly so, and the patient feels relatively well for one or two days, only to suffer an abrupt return of fever, headache, and back pain, often more intense than in the first phase. The second phase lasts two to four days and then subsides, leaving the patient with weakness and lassitude that disappear entirely during the succeeding week or two. Some patients do not exhibit the typical biphasic course and experience only one bout of fever, or have a typical illness but with a third phase of fever, or have a single prolonged febrile illness lasting five to eight days.

Evidence of central nervous system involvement has been seen in a few patients, invariably children. The presenting findings have been those of aseptic meningitis with nuchal rigidity and mononuclear pleocytosis or encephalitis with a depressed sensorium or stupor. Hemorrhagic manifestations have been described in a few children with encephalitis.

Laboratory findings very early in the illness are generally not helpful, but leukopenia is usually present by the third day of illness, and becomes even more pronounced during the second phase, reaching levels as low as 2000 per cubic millimeter. The most striking decrease is in the granulocyte series, with a relative lymphocytosis, and there is frequently an accompanying thrombocytopenia. Atypical, vacuolated lymphocytes are frequently observed. Bone marrow examination reveals a maturation arrest in the granulocyte series. The white blood cell count returns to normal during convalescence.

DIAGNOSIS. At the clinical level, the diagnosis should be suspected in any person with a history of tick exposure in the endemic area three to seven days prior to the onset of a febrile illness. Findings during the first phase, however, cannot be differentiated from those of many other acute febrile illnesses. A brief symptom-free interval followed by a second febrile illness should strongly suggest the diagnosis of Colorado tick fever. Profound leukopenia is usually present by that time, and lends support to the diagnosis.

The diagnosis is confirmed by isolation of the virus from serum or whole blood, via inoculation of suckling mice. More rapid diagnosis is possible by direct immunofluorescent staining of virus in the patient's erythrocytes. A diagnostic rise in both neutralizing and complement-fixing antibodies can generally be detected by examination of acute and convalescent sera.

The differential diagnosis can be troublesome, inasmuch as Rocky Mountain spotted fever is transmitted in the tick fever endemic area by the same vector, *Dermacentor andersoni*. Parodoxically, Rocky Mountain spotted fever has become an unusual disease in the Rocky Mountain area, and is outnumbered by Colorado tick fever in the state of Colorado by 20-fold. Nevertheless, differential diagnosis may be impossible early in the course of disease before the characteristic rash of Rocky Mountain spotted fever becomes apparent. A relatively symptom-free interval after two or three days would be most unusual in Rocky Mountain spotted fever, and strongly favors the diagnosis of Colorado tick fever.

TREATMENT. Therapy is entirely supportive, there being no specific therapy. Salicylates may be necessary to minimize headache and myalgias, but are neither required nor advisable in most patients.

PROGNOSIS. The disease is almost invariably benign, and the prognosis is excellent. Severe illness, complicated by central nervous system involvement, is rarely seen in children. The immunity derived is long-lasting.

PREVENTION. Both inactivated and live attenuated vaccines have been studied, but the modest number of cases and the benign nature of the disease suggest little need for active immunization.

The most effective means of preventing the disease is the use of protective clothing or repellents by people outdoors in endemic areas during the spring and summer months, together with frequent body inspection and prompt removal of ticks. Transfusion-associated disease can be prevented by exclusion of convalescent donors for a minimum of six months.

100.5. RIFT VALLEY FEVER

Karl M. Johnson

DEFINITION. Rift Valley fever is a febrile illness of short duration characterized by headache, myalgia, prostration, photophobia, and leukopenia. It is the only such arbovirus infection accompanied by significant complications which are ocular. The virus is mosquito borne, enzootic in wild game animals, epizootic in domestic livestock, and restricted geographically to East and South Africa.

ETIOLOGY. Rift Valley virus is a 30 to 50 nm, ribonucleic acid–containing arbovirus antigenically unrelated to any other known agent. Historically it was the second disease-producing, mosquito-borne virus ever described, the first being yellow fever.

EPIDEMIOLOGY. The virus was initially recovered from sheep in East Africa. Subsequent investigations showed that infection was common among large wild mammals of the region, and that virus was naturally present in a variety of mosquito species of the genera *Aedes, Culex,* and *Erethmapodites,* many of which are now known to feed primarily on wild game. After seasonal rains which lead to high mosquito populations, the virus spills over from this wild cycle, causing epizootics with high mortality in sheep, cattle, and even fowl. The agent is pantropic in these animals, the most striking lesion being a severe necrotizing hepatitis, reminiscent of yellow fever in man.

Human infection can be acquired in at least two ways: by mosquito bite, which is usually associated with big-game hunting or with ranching activity, and by direct or aerosol contact with the virus through the handling of tissues of affected livestock, or working with the agent in the laboratory. More human disease has been associated with the "handling" mechanism than with mosquito transmission. This virus is so infectious to man, and of such potential economic hazard to the livestock industry, that it is now prohibited to bring it into the United States, even for experimental purposes.

CLINICAL MANIFESTATIONS. After an incubation period of three to six days, onset of symptoms is usually abrupt, with fever, photophobia, and severe generalized headache. There may be severe prostration, myalgia, nausea, and vomiting. Epigastric pain is a frequent complaint. Temperature oscillates between 38 and 40° C, is often "saddleback" in evolution, and may persist up to one week. Leukopenia is common, as is a relative bradycardia. Skin eruptions are almost never observed, although minor hemorrhages in skin and from mucous membranes are infrequently present. Several cases of frank hemorrhagic fever have been documented. Convalescence is usually, although not always, uneventful.

COMPLICATIONS. These consist of a *central serous retinopathy* with an associated *central scotoma*. The fundus shows exudates involving the macula that may be secondary to thrombosis of vessels. Whether such lesions represent direct viral damage or result from an immunopathologic reaction to infection is not known. The exudates usually shrink and disappear over the course of several weeks, but in a minority of patients *retinal detachment* has ensued.

DIAGNOSIS. This is above all a disease of place and of particular human activity. A history is more valuable than any other procedure. Blood obtained during the first three days of illness almost always contains virus which is lethal when inoculated into mice. Serologic diagnosis of this infection is also definitive, because interpretation of antibody responses in paired sera is never compromised by heterologous reactions with any other agent.

TREATMENT AND PREVENTION. Management of the illness, as for other arthropod-borne fevers, is symptomatic. Serial examination for retinal complications should be done, and continued rest is indicated for persons in whom such lesions occur. Since the ocular complications appear to have an acute episodic rather than a subacute or chronic allergic pathogenesis, corticosteroids are of no benefit in their management.

Prevention of infection is principally through individual anti-mosquito measures. A live attenuated vaccine has been used in animals and man in South Africa, but this has more recently been replaced for human use among persons at high risk of infection, such as veterinarians, by a formalin-killed preparation which appears to confer complete clinical protection for at least two years.

100.6. SANDFLY FEVER

Karl M. Johnson

DEFINITION. Sandfly fever is a self-limited viral disease consisting of fever, headache, and myalgia. Leukopenia and conjunctival injection are characteristic. It occurs during the warm season in the littoral of the Mediterranean Sea and eastward through Asia Minor, Pakistan, and northern India. Sporadic cases have been recognized in tropical America.

ETIOLOGY. Although the classic syndrome in the Old World is caused by two antigenically related viruses, Sicilian and Neapolitan, recent ecologic studies in various parts of the world have led to the recovery of at least 20 distinct but related agents from phlebotomine sandflies. These are now referred to as members of the phlebotomus fever group of arboviruses. Many can be isolated in suckling mice or hamsters, but cell cultures, especially an African green monkey continuous cell-line (Vero), appear to be uniformly susceptible to infection with cytopathic effect.

EPIDEMIOLOGY. The vector of classic sandfly fever is *Phlebotomus papatasii,* and the only known vertebrate host is man. The fly has a very short flight range, stays close to ground level, and breeds best during warm dry periods in small collections of organic debris beneath stones, in masonry cracks, and in other protected sites. It has a short life span, probably not more than three weeks, but because of its small size it can readily penetrate the usual barriers of screens or netting which exclude mosquitoes. Serial man-fly transmission probably accounts for much of the virus activity during the season of peak fly populations, but transovarial transmission by the vector appears to be an important mechanism for long-term virus survival in view of the repeated recovery of virus in nature from nonbiting male sandflies.

Although antibodies have been found in forest-dwelling rodents and especially arboreal mammals in tropical America, equivalent isolation rates of some serotypes from male and female flies strongly suggest that the transovarial mechanism is a basic biologic adaptation for maintenance of viruses of this antigenic group.

Human disease patterns are determined by geographic and ecologic distribution of vector and virus. In highly endemic areas most infections occur during childhood and are rarely recognized in epidemic form. Epidemics in such regions are generally the result of introduction of large numbers of susceptible adults, such as during wars and national immigration.

PATHOGENESIS. Since there are no fatalities, the pathology of this disease in man in unknown. Experimental studies in man, however, disclosed that after intracutaneous inoculation the incubation period is three to six days. Viremia is brief, usually being confined to the day prior to and that of the onset of symptoms. Postinfection immunity is type specific and is clinically complete for at least two years. It may be lifelong.

CLINICAL MANIFESTATIONS. Inapparent infection during experimental studies was rare. Onset is sudden, and peak fever is usually attained in the first 24 hours, subsiding after two to four days. It is accompanied by headache, myalgia, photophobia and ocular pain, and definite conjunctival injection. There may be erythema, but not a true eruption, over the face and upper trunk. Constipation and diarrhea sometimes occur. Bradycardia is not a feature of this disease, although the typical viral leukopenia is common. Cerebrospinal fluid remains normal. A few patients experience a second bout of fever and symptoms during the second week of evolution, but convalescence is otherwise uneventful and complete.

DIAGNOSIS, TREATMENT, AND PREVENTION. Epidemiologic history represents the best clue to diagnosis. Virus isolation and serologic procedures may be carried out but serve principally to exclude other possible causes such as dengue and influenza. Management of patients is purely symptomatic. No vaccine is generally available, but DDT and other insecticides have proved highly effective in control of the classic *Phlebotomus* vector.

Undifferentiated Fevers Exclusive of Colorado Tick Fever

Anderson, C. R., Downs, W. G., Wattley, G. H., Akin, N. W., and Reese, A. A.: Mayaro virus: A new human disease agent. II. Isolation from blood of patients in Trinidad, B.W.I. Am. J. Trop. Med. Hyg., 6:1012, 1957.

Barnett, H. C., and Suyemoto, W.: Field studies on sandfly fever and kala-azar in Pakistan, in Iran, and in Baltistan (Little Tibet). Trans. N.Y. Acad. Sci., Sec. II, 23:609, 1961.

Charris, B. J., Doherty, R. L., Fraser, J. R. E., French, E. L., and Muirden, K. D.: Epidemic polyarthritis: A cytological, virological and immunochemical study. Aust. N.Z. J. Med., 5:450, 1975.

Clarke, J. A., Marshall, I. D., and Gard, G.: Annually recurrent epidemic polyarthritis and Ross River virus activity in a coastal area of New South Wales. I. Occurrence of the disease. Am. J. Trop. Med. Hyg., 22:543, 1973.

Doherty, R. L., Barrett, E. J., Gorman, B. M., and Whitehead, R. H.: Epidemic polyarthritis in Eastern Australia, 1959–1970. Med. J. Aust., 1:5, 1971.

Halstead, S. B., Nimmannitya, S., and Margiotta, M. R.: Dengue and chikungunya virus infection in man in Thailand, 1962–1964: II. Observations on disease in outpatients. Am. J. Trop. Med. Hyg., 18:972, 1969.

Hotta, S.: Twenty years of laboratory experience with dengue virus. I. Epidemiology — past and present. In Sanders, M., and Lennette, E. H. (eds.): Applied Virology. Sheboygan, Wisc., Ellis Corporation, 1965, pp. 228–256.

Robinson, M. C.: An epidemic of virus disease in Southern province, Tanganyika Territory in 1952–1953. I. Clinical features. Trans. R. Soc. Trop. Med. Hyg., 49:28, 1955.

Sabin, A. B., Philip, C. B., and Paul, J. R.: Phlebotomus (pappataci or sandfly) fever. A disease of military importance. Summary of existing knowledge and preliminary report of original investigations. JAMA, 125:603, 693, 1944.

Schrire, L.: Macular changes in Rift Valley Fever. S. Afr. Med. J., 25:926, 1951.

Shore, H.: O'nyong-nyong fever: An epidemic disease in East Africa. III. Some clinical and epidemiological observations in the Northern province of Uganda. Trans. R. Soc. Trop. Med. Hyg., 55:361, 1961.

Spigland, I., Jasinska-Klingberg, W., Hofshi, E., and Goldblum, N.: Clinical and laboratory observations in an outbreak of West Nile fever in Israel. Harefuah, 54:275, 1958.

Taylor, R. M., Work, T. H., Hurlbut, H. S., and Rizk, F.: A study of the ecology of West Nile virus in Egypt. Am. J. Trop. Med. Hyg., 5:579, 1956.

Tesh, R.B., Chaniotis, B.N., Peralta, P. H., and Johnson, K. M.: Ecology of viruses isolated from Panamanian phlebotomine sandflies. Am. J. Trop. Med. Hyg., 23:258, 1974.

Weiss, K. E.: Rift Valley fever. A review. Bull. Epizoot. Dis. Afr., 5:431, 1957.

Wisseman, C. L., Jr.: The ecology of dengue. In May, J. M. (ed.): Studies in Disease Ecology. New York, Hafner Publishing Company, 1961, Chap. 2, p. 15.

Colorado Tick Fever

Eklund, C. M., Kohls, G. M., and Brennan, J. J.: Distribution of Colorado tick fever and virus-carrying ticks. JAMA, 157:335, 1955.

Emmons, R. W., Oshiro, L. S., Johnson, H. N., and Lennette, E. H.: Intraerythrocytic location of Colorado tick fever virus. J. Gen. Virol., 17:185, 1972.

Florio, L., Stewart, M. O., and Mugrage, E. R.: The etiology of Colorado tick fever. J. Exp. Med., 83:1, 1946.

Silver, H. K., Meiklejohn, G., and Kempe, C. H.: Colorado tick fever. Am. J. Dis. Child., 101:30, 1961.

Spruance, S. L., and Bailey, A.: Colorado tick fever. Arch. Intern. Med., 131:288, 1973.

101. ARTHROPOD-BORNE VIRAL ENCEPHALITIDES

Karl M. Johnson

101.1. INTRODUCTION

The arthropod-borne viral encephalitides comprise a group of clinically similar diseases induced by a variety of small viruses containing ribonucleic acid. Although infection usually occurs through the bite of an infectious arthropod, some of the agents are also transmitted by contact through mucous membranes, by aerosol, and by ingestion. In general, arthropods become infectious only after an extrinsic incubation period of one week or longer, which may be modified further by environmental temperature. Once infectious, however, such vectors remain so for long periods, in many cases for life. Encephalitis is usually an infrequent manifestation of human infection, but the agents to be considered all cause this dramatic and life-threatening syndrome with sufficient frequency that the term has been included as an integral part of viral nomenclature. This presentation is designed to provide the physician with the key clues necessary to aid him in sorting the variables involved in diagnosis and prognosis of infection, and to suggest areas in which ignorance rather than understanding characterizes the state of knowledge concerning these diseases and their clinical management. Because of the very real public health significance attached to the occurrence of even a single case of some of the encephalitides, the importance of specific diagnosis of arboviral encephalitis cannot be overstressed.

It is possible to subdivide these diseases in a variety of ways. They are distributed nearly worldwide, occurring in both temperate and tropical climates; they are caused by different viruses, some of which are antigenically related; they are transmitted by mosquitoes or ticks; they cause central nervous system (CNS) disease predominantly in adults or in children; and they may or may not clinically affect domestic livestock.

PATHOGENESIS AND PATHOLOGY OF ARBOVIRAL ENCE-
PHALITIS. After deposition in the skin, virus may multiply locally and spread via lymphatics to cells of the reticuloendothelial system localized in lymph nodes, small vessels, and other organs such as spleen. In vitro studies suggest that macrophages are inherently susceptible to virus replication but that lymphocytes are resistant unless "blast transformed." Release of virus from such cells leads to viremia and widespread dissemination to other organs. Clinical symptoms and pathologic changes in many of these organs suggest that vascular endothelial cells are regularly damaged, but no direct or indirect visualization of virus in such cells in man has yet been achieved.

Although myocarditis, focal hepatic necrosis, and damage to lungs and kidneys may occur, the hallmark of these agents is their ability to induce damage to the brain. Despite some variation from virus to virus, a basic similarity exists in the gross and microscopic pathology of arbovirus-induced encephalitis. Brains are minimally edematous grossly with occasional small hemorrhages. Microscopic edema and hyperemia are present in the leptomeninges and cortex. There are small hemorrhages in many parts of the brain, sometimes with small arteriolar thrombi. Most striking of all are conspicuous collections of mononuclear, occasionally polymorphonuclear leukocytes around small vessels, the so-called "perivascular cuffs." Neuronal lesions are often focal and reveal nuclei and cytoplasm in various states of degeneration. Microglial and polymorphonuclear accumulations often present a picture of focal nodules. These lesions are most common in the gray matter, midbrain, basal nuclei, brainstem, and cerebellum, although some of the viruses induce destruction of anterior horn cells of the upper spinal cord.

Leukocytes and modest increases in protein concentration in cerebrospinal fluid are almost always seen. Although polymorphonuclear cells may be slightly more numerous early in the course of disease, there is always an evolution to a pleocytosis. It is of interest also that clinical encephalitis is almost always marked by a moderate leukocytosis rather than the leukopenia so characteristic of undifferentiated and primary hemorrhagic fevers produced by arboviruses.

A central question is how much of the CNS damage produced by these arboviruses is due to direct virus-induced destruction of neurons and how much may be the result of immunologically mediated injury to small vessels and/or neurons. In most instances virus is difficult to recover at autopsy from the brain, and it is not readily obtained from cerebrospinal fluid either. This has been explained in the past on the basis that antiviral antibodies are usually present at death in fatal encephalitis such that in vivo or in vitro neutralization obscures the real sequence of events. Although some neuronal destruction almost certainly occurs, the clinical course in the majority of patients who make rapid and nearly complete recovery and the pathognomonic *mononuclear* perivascular cuffs strongly point to an immune-induced inflammatory lesion as a major contributor to disease. What is wanted are new investigations of general and local immunologic reactions in patients with these diseases. The problem is of more than theoretical interest, because an elucidation of pathogenesis might well lead to a rationale for employment of therapeutic measures which present wisdom must continue to regard as potentially more harmful than helpful.

CLINICAL MANIFESTATIONS. The shifting, protean neurologic manifestations seen in arbovirus encephalitis suggest a mixture of permanent neuronal damage and temporary central dysfunction secondary to intermittent anoxia and edema. This pattern accounts also for the observed wide range of convalescent behavior and permanent sequelae.

The temperature course is frequently bizarre, indicating an anoxic effect on central thermoregulatory function. Indeed, persistent high fever is the most ominous clinical sign, and *external artificial control of temperature may be the most important measure available* for the management of the severely ill patient.

Although statistically significant differences in the frequency of specific neurologic symptoms and signs of encephalitis caused by individual arboviruses are slowly emerging, it remains evident that the range provoked by each agent is quite broad. Symptomatology in the individual patient rarely provides assurance as to the specific etiologic agent. Unexplained differences in patterns correlated with human age, however, are sometimes striking. Thus death caused by St. Louis encephalitis virus (SLE) is almost invariably restricted to the elderly, as though the vascular reserves available to cope with an acute inflammatory anoxia were compromised. By contrast, CNS disease and death caused by Venezuelan equine encephalitis virus (VEE) are observed almost exclusively in children. Major upper motor neuron destruction leading to permanent paralysis is largely attributable to Japanese B and Russian spring-summer encephalitis viruses. Sophisticated clinical investigation of all these diseases is nearly nonexistent. More work such as that of the Southwestern University Group in Dallas, who measured cerebral blood flow and certain hormonal functions in patients with St. Louis encephalitis virus, is urgently needed.

DIFFERENTIAL DIAGNOSIS. The most common disease clinically indistinguishable from arbovirus encephalitis is that caused by *herpes simplex* virus. Previous clinical herpetic infection and the fact that this disease occurs throughout the year may offer clues to its recognition (see Ch. 304).

Enteroviruses and *leptospira* may produce disease which mimics arboviral encephalitis, and the seasonal pattern is often coincident. Indeed mixed arboviral and enteroviral epidemics are not infrequently recognized.

Meningitis and rarely encephalitis caused by *mumps* virus may also be confused with that caused by arboviruses (see Ch. 88).

Postinfectious or *postvaccinal* encephalitis after measles, rubella, or varicella infection or inoculation with rabies or vaccinia vaccines must always be considered in such cases. History is the key to these diagnoses (see Ch. 83 to 86 and Ch. 309.3).

Rabies and *lymphocytic choriomeningitis* viruses can also resemble arboviral encephalitis. History of animal bite usually establishes the former diagnosis, but the latter must usually be separated by viral diagnostic procedures.

An assortment of acute febrile encephalopathies marked by hypoglycemia, diarrhea, convulsions, and coma, with or without visceral pathologic changes, has been described. These syndromes of undetermined etiology generally do not induce significant cerebrospinal fluid pleocytosis, nor do they display the marked central inflammatory changes so typical of arbovirus infection.

Bacterial and *fungal meningitides* can usually be distinguished by reduced sugar, high protein, and a mixture of cells, as well as by presence of stainable organisms in cerebrospinal fluid. Not uncommonly, however, incompletely treated bacterial meningitis may present a real diagnostic challenge.

Tumors and *abscesses* are usually separable by strong localization of neurologic signs, by absence of high fever unless septicemia is present, and by suitable tests to document abnormal space-filling lesions. *Toxic encephalopathies* must be thought of. History and chemical determinations are the best aids to establishment of such diagnoses.

It should thus be apparent that competent microbiologic diagnostic facilities are essential to establishing the specific diagnosis, and that such competence must extend beyond the arboviruses per se.

101.2.   WESTERN EQUINE ENCEPHALITIS

ETIOLOGY. Western equine encephalitis (WEE) virus was the first such agent to be recovered from equines and humans. Isolated from an encephalitic horse in 1930 by Meyer, this agent represents the prototype for arboviruses immunologically collected into group A by Casals. The agent produces inapparent infection, mild febrile illness, or clinical encephalitis in both equines and humans.

EPIDEMIOLOGY. This virus, as well as its immunologic relative, Venezuelan equine encephalitis (VEE), is restricted to the Western Hemisphere. Eastern equine encephalitis (EEE), another group A agent of the New World, recently has been found to occur in Europe. Virologic and serologic studies have disclosed seasonal mosquito-bird activity cycles in many areas of the United States and Canada and in parts of southern and eastern South America as well. It is not present in tropical Middle America. In North America clinical infection of man has been recognized in the Mississippi drainage basin, the Great Plains, and the valleys between the western mountains. In most of these regions the mosquito vector is *Culex tarsalis,* and a variety of small birds appear to provide the principal blood virus source for mosquito infection. Equines and humans are frequently infected, as disclosed by population surveys for specific antibodies, but do not develop viremia of sufficient concentration to serve as hosts for further amplification of the basic cycle. Seasonal temperature fluctuations play a decisive role in disease transmission, exerting effects on mosquito population, on virus incubation period in mosquitoes, and on migratory behavior of birds. Thus WEE is a disease of summer and early fall.

Experimental work has shown that WEE virus may persist during winter in hibernating snakes and claims for such a mechanism in nature have been made but are as yet not generally accepted as valid. Human attack rates are highest in young adult males and in infants less than one year old. This pattern is due to the strong geographic localization of WEE virus and to the fact that agricultural irrigation projects vastly increase the breeding habitat available for *Culex tarsalis.* Incubation period of infection in man is generally five to ten days. Mortality among patients with encephalitis may reach 10 per cent.

CLINICAL MANIFESTATIONS. A two- to four-day pro- drome of fever, headache, and myalgia commonly pre- cedes the appearance of CNS signs in children; adults more often experience abrupt onset of stiff neck and drowsiness with fever and muscle aching. Clinically, CNS disease is almost always more severe in children, who, in addition to the hallmark signs of disorienta- tion, somnolence, and coma, often suffer convulsions, abnormal reflexes, and flaccid or spastic paralyses. Fever lasts for a week or more, but rarely for two, and ranges from 39 to 40°C. Higher temperatures are prog- nostically ominous and should be reduced by external means.

Clinical improvement at the end of the febrile period is often dramatic in adults, most of whom make un- eventful recoveries without residual motor or psycho- logic residua. Children, especially the very young, are not so fortunate; more than half of them are left with permanent damage, producing mental retardation, emotional instability, or spastic paralyses.

Although leukopenia may be present early in the course of illness, a mild leukocytosis with polymorpho- nuclear cells predominating is more common. Cerebro- spinal fluid is clear, contains normal sugar concentra- tion but moderately increased protein, and nearly always shows a mild pleocytosis.

DIAGNOSIS. Encephalitic signs occurring in both children and adults during summer should immediately raise suspicion of an arboviral causation. The major dif- ferential is similar disease caused by enteroviruses. Specific laboratory diagnosis is required in both in- stances.

Although WEE virus has been recovered on occasion from brain tissue of patients dying during the first week of disease, isolation of the agent from blood or cerebrospinal fluid is difficult even during the initial three days of symptoms. Specific diagnosis thus de- pends on demonstration of increasing anti-WEE anti- body titers in sequentially collected sera. A specimen should be obtained and frozen as part of the initial ex- amination of the patient, because such antibodies often appear during the first week of symptoms. The second serum can be taken 10 to 14 days later. Although single convalescent sera are of limited usefulness in areas where WEE infection is common, detection of specific antibodies of the IgM class is good evidence for very recent infection. This test is of proved utility in cases occurring among infants who have residual IgG from their immune mothers.

TREATMENT. Control of high fever and maintenance of water and electrolyte balance are the essential meas- ures in management of patients. When necessary, re- duction of fever should be by use of external chilling techniques rather than by use of analgesics such as as- pirin. Continuous care should be taken to see that a patient's airway and normal respiratory function are maintained.

Convalescence is usually prolonged and should never be forced. Children should be thoroughly examined at intervals up to a year after acute encephalitis in order to detect those who may require psychiatric or special educational and motor therapy.

PREVENTION. During epizootics or epidemics the prime objective is to prevent mosquitoes from biting babies. Houses should be screened; cribs, bassinets, and carriages should be covered by fine mesh netting.

Transmission of WEE virus can also occur in utero; thus *pregnant women* should be especially protected against mosquito attack by restricting outdoor activity, by using repellents, and by use of residual and knock- down insecticides within and near their homes.

Community-wide organized control programs to re- duce mosquito populations are important in areas where repeated epidemics have occurred. Based on combinations of insecticide and management of irriga- tion water, the value of such measures has been docu- mented in California, Colorado, and Texas.

Epizootics of WEE in equines frequently precede human epidemics. An effective formalin-killed chick embryo virus vaccine is now used to protect horses, thus reducing the "sentinel" value of this species as a warning of an impending epidemic. The vaccine is not licensed for use in human medicine.

101.3. EASTERN EQUINE ENCEPHALITIS

ETIOLOGY. Eastern equine encephalitis (EEE) virus is a group A arbovirus which produces severe encepha- litis and death in a high proportion of equine and human infections. It was first isolated in 1933 by Ten Broeck and Merrill and has been shown to be the most common cause of summertime epizootic-epidemic arbo- viral encephalitis in the eastern United States. Most outbreaks have occurred along the seaboard from northern Florida to Canada. Sporadic disease outbreaks also have been documented in some of the Caribbean islands during the fall. An antigenically distinguishable EEE virus variant is present in Middle and parts of South America. To date this variant has been associated with acute neurologic disease in equines but only rare- ly in man.

EPIDEMIOLOGY. Basic elements in the natural cycle of EEE virus in North America are the mosquito *Culex melanura* and a large number of species of small wild birds. Although reminiscent of WEE epidemiology, that of EEE differs significantly owing to the fact that *Culex melanura* distribution is strongly localized to a series of coastal fresh water hardwood swamps. Virus activity in these swamps occurs each summer, commencing later as one moves from south to north. Two possible mech- anisms may account for this seasonal chain: either the virus overwinters in each swamp by infection of verte- brates (hibernating turtles as well as contact infections among rodents have been proposed), or the *Culex*-bird cycle is maintained through the winter in the most southerly swamps where frost is unusual. In the latter case spring migration of birds could provide the means for reintroduction of virus into northern swamps each year. Southward fall bird migration definitely seems to account for the Caribbean outbreaks because EEE- infected migrants have been detected in the southern United States and on the islands, and virus strains re- covered during these autumnal epizootic epidemics were identified antigenically as North American rather than South American in origin.

Epizootics in equines and in exotic gallinaceous birds such as pheasants, chukar partridges, and Pekin ducks usually precede by one to three weeks the appearance of human encephalitis. Evidence has accumulated indicating that accessory mosquito vectors such as the salt-marsh *Aedes sollicitans* and the widely dispersed *Aedes vexans* may be important in transmission of virus to these abnormal hosts. As with WEE virus, equines and humans are of no or very limited significance as hosts for further mosquito infection. Disease patterns observed in game-bird farms strongly suggest, moreover, that direct contact infection is important in the epizootics which at times devastate these exotic species.

Although EEE infection of wild birds is usually not symptomatic, the reverse is true for horses and humans. More than half of equine infections are clinically overt, and mortality among such animals may approach 90 per cent. Serologic surveys among human populations resident very close to the fresh-water swamps have revealed individuals with specific antibodies and no history or stigmata of encephalitis. Nevertheless, it is probable that clinical encephalitis occurs in a high proportion of human North American EEE infections. Mortality among hospitalized patients runs to 50 per cent or higher, and many survivors have residual neurologic dysfunction regardless of age.

CLINICAL MANIFESTATIONS.   The incubation period is assumed to be about seven to ten days, after which there is sudden onset of high fever, headache, conjunctivitis, nausea, and vomiting. This pattern, particularly common in adults, progresses rapidly from drowsiness to delirium and coma. There is stiff neck and irritability, at times accompanied by positive Kernig's sign, absent or hyperactive reflexes, and muscle spasticity in the extremities, often asymmetrical. Patients, if conscious, may be unable to speak or swallow. Excessive salivation is common. The disease terminates fatally within the first two weeks, usually within seven days, or shifting signs of deep CNS involvement may continue for several weeks, the patient gradually returning to consciousness. Serial neurologic examination usually discloses which centers and nerve supplies have sustained permanent damage.

Polymorphonuclear leukocytosis which can reach 50,000 cells per cubic millimeter is characteristic. During the first days of disease the CSF, usually under considerable pressure, also contains such cells in numbers up to 1000. Protein is elevated; as illness progresses, the cells become predominantly mononuclear.

A diphasic pattern of illness is often seen in children. After a day or two of fever, headache, and gastrointestinal upset, followed by two or three days of clinical improvement, there is fulminating onset of high fever, vomiting, delirium, convulsions, and coma. There may be intermittent or persistent opisthotonos, generalized rigidity, and localized paralyses. Circulatory stasis or mechanical obstruction leads to clinical cyanosis, especially in the very young.

Convalescence is slow, and during this time neurologic residua become apparent. There may be permanent damage to cranial nerves, as to those regulating muscle function of one or more extremities. Mental or emotional deterioration, or both, may be so severe as to require permanent institutional care.

DIAGNOSIS.   Although EEE virus can be isolated from the brains of persons who die during the first week of illness, little success attends attempts to recover the agent from blood or CSF specimens during the acute illness. Sera taken during the first seven days of disease may contain neutralizing and hemagglutination-inhibiting antibodies for EEE virus. If so, the diagnosis is likely, because such substances are rarely found in the general population. A second serum obtained at about 14 days usually shows rising titers of specific antibodies.

TREATMENT.   There is no specific chemotherapy, and there is no evidence that passively administered anti-EEE antibodies alter the course of clinically apparent disease. Thus management is that of any desperately ill patient: careful control of fluid and electrolyte balance, constant maintenance of a patient's airway, and external treatment of direct life-threatening hyperthermia. Secondary bacterial infections, if they occur, generally appear after the most acute primary phase of disease, and are those attendant to mechanical maintenance of respiratory and urinary function, physical inactivity, and bed sores. Physiotherapy to minimize paralytic contractures should begin after the febrile period.

PREVENTION.   The principles are similar to those for WEE infection. There is a killed virus vaccine for equine, but not human, use. Since the ecology of EEE virus is centered in natural rather than man-modified habitats, organized mosquito-control efforts directed specifically at annual disease prevention are not economically feasible. Insecticides, however, are of some value both near residences and in accessible areas of mosquito-virus activity whenever a human epidemic exists or is threatened by the appearance of an epizootic.

Convalescent human plasma has been used to prevent disease after inadvertent direct exposure to EEE virus in laboratory workers. It is of unproved value and appears to be of no help unless given within 24 hours of the accident.

101.4.   VENEZUELAN EQUINE ENCEPHALITIS

ETIOLOGY.   Venezuelan equine encephalitis (VEE) virus is a group A arbovirus which causes fatal CNS disease in equines and an acute influenza-like syndrome in humans. During large epidemics cases of encephalitis are seen in young children, but the incidence of neurologic signs in this age group rarely exceeds 1 to 3 per cent of infections.

First isolated from horses by Kubes and Rios during a 1938 epizootic in Venezuela, the virus was not associated with human disease until several years later. Investigation of arbovirus ecology in tropical America during the past three decades has resulted in the recognition of several antigenic subtypes of VEE virus which differ in pathogenicity for equines and possibly humans and which have distinct cycles of maintenance and transmission. Taken together, VEE viruses have killed more equines and produced more human illness in the Western Hemisphere than any other arbovirus.

EPIDEMIOLOGY.   Enzootic VEE virus cycles have been carefully studied in Trinidad, Colombia, Panama, Brazil, Mexico, and the United States (Florida Everglades). Virus activity was always focal, localized to shaded fresh-water swamps or to slow-moving bodies of water where floating water lettuce plants, *Pistia*, were common. The vector mosquitoes in each instance were members of the taxonomically complex subgenus *Culex melanoconion*. Small rodents, or in some cases water birds, are the principal vertebrate hosts. These animals develop high levels of virus in blood without significant mortality. Humans resident near or entering such enzootic foci suffer overt clinical infection, because the mosquito vectors are opportunistic rather than highly specialized blood feeders.

For some time it was thought that such enzootic foci were the sources for the periodic equine-human VEE outbreaks that swept large parts of Venezuela, Colombia, Ecuador, and Peru. But antigenic analysis of virus strains from all countries where VEE occurs together with experimental studies in horses has disclosed that enzootic VEE viruses were never involved in epizootics. Such strains, although capable of infecting and inducing cross-immunity, produced no encephalitis or sufficient viremia to infect mosquitoes when inoculated into equines. In contrast, antigenically distinct epizootic virus strains are highly pathogenic for equines, and induce truly dramatic viremias in them. Many genera and species of mosquitoes are thus infected and capable of further transmission of virus to equines, humans, and other vertebrates. Unlike the related WEE and EEE viruses, then, the equine is the single major host responsible for amplification and dissemination of the classic VEE strains. At present no mechanism has been discovered to account for interepizootic maintenance of such viruses in nature. Epizootics of VEE typically take place in rural tropical regions characterized by climates having a pronounced dry season. Cattle raising is the dominant land use, and outbreaks most often occur after the advent of the rainy season. Although human-mosquito transmission chains are possible, the timing of human disease one to two weeks after appearance of equine encephalitis suggests that epidemic VEE in man is mainly a spillover from the fulminant equine-mosquito cycle. At times nearly all equines and large fractions of rural human populations are infected during such outbreaks. Many thousands of human infections, most of them clinically apparent, can thus occur in a few weeks.

All subtypes of VEE virus are highly infectious for humans and other vertebrates when administered via the respiratory route. Thus many laboratory infections have been recorded.

CLINICAL MANIFESTATIONS. Onset of illness is typically abrupt, patients frequently reporting the exact time of appearance of severe headache, chills, fever, and explosive vomiting and diarrhea. These symptoms ensue two to four days after infectious mosquito bite but can occur within 24 hours after exposure to highly infectious aerosols. Conjunctival injection and mild sore throat are present early in the clinical course, and myalgia is usually intense. Fever often reaches 40° C. In general the first day of symptoms is the worst, and the fever curve shows daily evening peaks which regress to normal after three to five days. Mild somnolence is common, but severe neurologic signs are seen in only a small percentage of cases, nearly always among children. Individual cases may thus be readily confused with influenza, acute infectious or toxic gastroenteritis, or leptospirosis.

During the first day of illness blood leukocytes are usually normal or slightly increased in numbers, with a strong shift toward polymorphonuclear dominance and a conspicuous eosinopenia. There follows a definite leukopenia, and by the fourth or fifth day a relative lymphocytosis is usual. Normal total and differential values are re-established by about the tenth day.

Nuchal stiffness is unusual, and the CSF generally shows no cells or a very mild pleocytosis with normal protein. Children exhibiting more serious neurologic signs, including abnormal reflexes, spastic paralyses, convulsions, and coma, usually experience a biphasic febrile course with the second fever elevation associated with CNS signs. Epilepsy, paralyses, tremors, hallucinations, and emotional instability may persist as permanent sequelae of infection in children, and occasional cases of residual epilepsy and intention tremors have been cited among adults.

Most fatalities occur in children under five years of age. Autopsies revealed gross and histologic changes similar to those seen with other arboviruses causing encephalitis, but in addition were noteworthy for the presence of scattered gross focal hemorrhages in brain, heart, and lungs.

DIAGNOSIS. Since clinical presentation of VEE infection is rarely overtly encephalitic, the diagnosis will be missed unless it is considered in a patient with high fever, respiratory symptoms, and gastrointestinal upset who resides in or has recently visited either an enzootic focus or an epizootic area of tropical America. Virus can be recovered with ease, however, from either blood or throat swab specimens taken during the initial 72 hours of symptoms. Since patients are potentially infectious for humans and mosquitoes during this phase, the importance of establishing the cause is obvious. Paired serum samples obtained early in illness and about ten days later will reliably reveal rising levels of specific anti-VEE antibodies.

TREATMENT. There is no specific treatment. Analgesics and external chilling may be required to control hyperthermia. Life-threatening fluid and electrolyte imbalance may result from vomiting and diarrhea in children and must be alertly detected and corrected. Patients frequently complain of lassitude and inability to concentrate mentally for one to four weeks after fever has subsided, but convalescence is otherwise usually uneventful.

PROPHYLAXIS. Formalin-inactivated vaccines have been used to protect equines in South America for 30 years. The potency of these products is borderline at best, and the frequent persistence of live VEE virus in them may well have been the cause of subsequent major epizootics. An experimental live attenuated vaccine, strain TC-83, has been used with success in immunizing laboratory personnel at high risk of aerosol infection. This vaccine, which produces febrile reactions in up to 20 per cent of adult recipients, has not been tested in children or pregnant women. It has been associated with birth defects when inoculated into pregnant rhesus monkeys and seems unlikely ever to be generally safe for human protection.

Nevertheless, this vaccine is the single most important tool available for interdiction of human VEE epidemics. Most mosquitoes acquire virus from equines, and it has been shown that mass vaccination of equines prevents further viremic infection of these animals within three days. Once horse infections cease, transmission to man generally comes to an end within a short interval as infected mosquitoes die. Insecticides are useful in killing infected mosquitoes when temporally combined with equine vaccination.

Since patients are potentially infectious, precautions should be taken to prevent them from mosquito bite. Although medical personnel attending patients are potentially at risk of acquiring the disease by aerosol, the infrequent occurrence of significant coughing during VEE infection may explain the absence of well-documented instances of such transmission.

101.5. CALIFORNIA ENCEPHALITIS

DEFINITION. California encephalitis is an acute CNS disease which occurs during summer in many areas of the United States and is caused by one or more antigenically related viruses of the California arbovirus complex.

ETIOLOGY. The original virus strain of this antigenic complex was recovered from *Aedes dorsalis* and *Culex tarsalis* mosquitoes in the San Joaquin Valley of California in the 1940s. Serologic studies showed this agent to be associated with a few cases of childhood encephalitis previously thought clinically to be caused by WEE or St. Louis encephalitis viruses.

In 1960 the La Crosse strain was recovered from the brain of a six-year-old child who died of encephalitis. Although very few other isolates have been made from man, antigens prepared from the La Crosse agent have been used in recent years to document many cases of acute CNS disease in different regions of the United States.

At least six antigenically related California arboviruses have been recovered from a variety of mosquitoes and wild vertebrates in the United States. Related agents are known from tropical America, Europe, Africa, and Asia. One variant is annually active in the far north of western Canada and Alaska.

EPIDEMIOLOGY. Frequent epidemics of California encephalitis have been documented in Wisconsin, Indiana, Minnesota, and Ohio, and sporadic cases are on record from North Carolina and Florida. It is probable that the disease occurs over a much wider area of the midwestern and southern United States but is not diagnosed because specific serologic tests are not generally employed and because cases often appear sporadically in a large number of small rural communities.

The La Crosse virus is transmitted principally by tree-hole breeding mosquitoes of the genus *Aedes*. Small mammals such as rabbits, chipmunks, and squirrels provide sources of virus for new mosquito infection, but the basic mechanism of virus maintenance is probably transovarial transmission of virus through the various life stages of the mosquito. This behavior was recently proved for *Aedes triseriatus*, the first known instance of insect maintenance of a mosquito-borne arbovirus.

More than 90 per cent of human cases of encephalitis occur in persons 15 years old or under. Males are more often affected than females, probably because exposure to the virus is most frequently related to the outdoor recreational pursuits of camping, fishing, or hunting in woodlands where infected day-biting *Aedes* mosquitoes are present. Although mortality from California encephalitis has not been established, it is low, not exceeding 5 per cent. Serologic studies also show that human infection with these viruses is far more common than clinical encephalitis.

CLINICAL MANIFESTATIONS. Although not accurately known, the incubation period is probably between five and ten days. Onset of symptoms is typically insidious, with mild fever and headache for several days. As these symptoms increase, the headache usually becomes frontal, and the complaints are sometimes ascribed by patient or relatives to a minor traumatic incident. Mental confusion may or may not precede the sudden occurrence of convulsions, which may be the only overt sign of CNS disease on admission to hospital. Coma may supervene, and meningeal signs are occasionally seen, but shifting deep neurologic signs such as paralyses and reflex changes are rarely observed.

Mild to severe leukocytosis is characteristic of the acute stage of illness, counts sometimes reaching 30,000 per cubic millimeter. Cerebrospinal fluid is clear under moderate pressure and contains up to several hundred leukocytes, predominantly polymorphonuclear early, becoming mononuclear as illness progresses.

Fever generally subsides by lysis after a course of less than two weeks. Motor and sensory neurologic sequelae have not been observed, but emotional and learning dysfunction has been noted in children several months after physical convalescence is complete.

DIAGNOSIS. The differential diagnosis of importance is that between viral encephalitis and post-traumatic *subdural hematoma*. Favoring the former are season of occurrence, history of forest exposure, the presence of leukocytosis, a clear cerebrospinal fluid, and the absence of localizing neurologic signs.

Specific diagnosis of California encephalitis must be made serologically, no isolate having yet been obtained from blood or excretions of acutely ill patients. Thus a fourfold or greater increase in CF, HI, or neutralizing antibodies between acute and early convalescent serum specimens provides the only confirmation of etiology.

TREATMENT AND PROPHYLAXIS. Management of patients is completely symptomatic. Hyperthermia and respiratory failure, although unusual, are the dangerous signs that must be detected and corrected without delay. No vaccine is available, nor has any experimental work been reported in this direction. Mosquito control is virtually impossible on a large scale because of the specialized breeding habits of the vector species. Protective clothing, nets, and repellents are the only effective measures available to individuals entering the woodlands where infected mosquitoes are present.

101.6. ST. LOUIS ENCEPHALITIS

DEFINITION. St. Louis encephalitis (SLE) was the first recognized and is the most important arboviral encephalitis in the United States. It occurs sporadically and in major outbreaks during late summer and fall, afflicting rural populations in the West and urban-suburban communities elsewhere in the nation.

ETIOLOGY. St. Louis encephalitis virus is a group B arbovirus, most closely related antigenically to Japanese B and Murray Valley encephalitis viruses. It occurs only in the Western Hemisphere. A closely related virus, Rocio, was recently associated with a major epidemic of encephalitis in southern Brazil.

EPIDEMIOLOGY. The causative virus was first recovered from fatal cases during a major outbreak of encephalitis in St. Louis in 1933. Since that time sporadic cases and outbreaks of varying intensity have occurred in rural Washington and California, and in suburban and urban areas of Florida, Texas, Illinois, the lower Ohio and Mississippi Valleys, Pennsylvania, and New Jersey. Presence of virus is indicated by antibodies and/or isolation of virus strains from wildlife in Mexico, Central America, South America, and several Caribbean islands.

The basic virus cycle leading to human outbreaks involves birds and certain *Culex* mosquitoes. Although the possible mechanisms for virus survival during winter are not precisely known, they include reintroduction by northward migrating birds, recrudescent infection in nonmigratory birds, persistence of infected adult mosquitoes, and persistent infection in hibernating bats. The principal mosquito vector in the western United States is *Culex tarsalis*, especially abundant in irrigated agricultural areas. The vectors of urban-suburban epidemics elsewhere in the country are *C. pipiens*, *C. quinquefasciatus*, and *C. nigripalpus*. The virus has been recovered from many different mosquitoes in tropical America, many of them strongly arboreal in activity pattern, but it is not clear which are the most important in ecologic terms.

Although the distribution of SLE virus in the United States overlaps to a considerable degree with that of both EEE and WEE viruses, two important epidemiologic features distinguish the former from the latter group A viruses. First, although all three agents "spill over" from birds to horses, only EEE and WEE cause equine disease. Second, because the extrinsic incubation period in the mosquito is longer for SLE than for the equine viruses, St. Louis encephalitis always occurs later in the summer and is not found as far north as the group A encephalitides.

CLINICAL MANIFESTATIONS. Acute disease probably occurs in no more than 1 to 2 per cent of St. Louis encephalitis virus infections. Usually the course is benign, comprising a few days of fever and pronounced headache followed by complete recovery. More severe disease is occasionally seen in young children and occurs in a substantial number of adults more than 40 years of age. After an incubation period variously estimated at up to two weeks, there is acute onset of fever and altered sensorium. Convulsions are more common in children than in adults. The most common neurologic signs are stiff neck, tremors of the hands and face, dysdiadochokinesia, and nystagmus. Cranial nerve abnormalities are found in about 20 per cent of cases. Myalgia, photophobia, and conjunctival suffusion are common, and acute urinary symptoms with unexplained mild pyuria and increased blood urea nitrogen concentration occur in nearly one fourth of patients.

White blood cell counts are usually normal to moderately elevated, and increased numbers of immature polymorphonuclear leukocytes may be found early in the course. Although an occasional patient has no cells in the cerebrospinal fluid on admission to hospital, all eventually show a pleocytosis, the total number of leukocytes rarely exceeding 500. Although some polymorphonuclear cells may be present at the beginning, later examinations reveal only lymphocytes. Cerebrospinal fluid protein is typically increased, but rarely exceeds 100 mg per 100 ml.

DIAGNOSIS. Given appropriate season and place, the differential diagnosis of St. Louis encephalitis virus infection centers on other arboviruses and enteroviral meningitis in children and on *acute cerebrovascular accidents* in the elderly. An infectious cause may not even be considered in the latter group until a cluster of cases demands explanation. The virus itself has never been recovered from blood or cerebrospinal fluid of patients, and only rarely from brains of persons who die during the first week of illness. Specific diagnosis is thus dependent upon serologic testing of paired sera. The most practical technique is that of complement fixation, although the neutralization test provides the most definitive result if the early acute specimen is recovered before significant levels of antibody have been produced.

TREATMENT AND PROGNOSIS. Treatment is purely symptomatic. Persistent fever above 40° C is an ominous sign and should be vigorously combated. About 10 to 25 per cent of adults with acute encephalitis die, most of them from complications of underlying diseases. Such deaths generally occur after the first 10 days of illness when most of the neurologic manifestations have subsided. Hyponatremia is a frequent problem in management of the acute phase of disease, and in some cases has been ascribed to a partial persistent elaboration of antidiuretic hormone. Convalescence is often quite prolonged, and long-term examination of patients reveals frequent persistence of personality changes and emotional disturbance. Motor deficits are uncommon.

PREVENTION. There is no specific vaccine. Surveillance of seasonal mosquito-avian activity patterns of the virus in endemic regions is valuable as a guide to the timing of measures designed to reduce populations of vector mosquitoes. Emergency use of insecticides against adult mosquitoes during urban-suburban epidemics is probably of considerable help in reducing morbidity.

101.7. JAPANESE B ENCEPHALITIS

DEFINITION. Japanese B encephalitis is a severe arbovirus disease which occurs in eastern Asia. Summer-fall outbreaks occur in Siberia, Korea, Japan, Taiwan, and other Pacific islands. Continuous endemic virus transmission has been proved or is suspected in Southeast Asia, the Philippines, and East Indies.

ETIOLOGY. The causative agent is a group of B arbovirus closely related antigenically to St. Louis, Murray Valley, and West Nile viruses. Unlike these agents, however, Japanese B virus is pathogenic for certain monkeys and equines, and has been shown to induce abortion or stillbirth in pregnant sows, a fact of major economic significance to the porcine industry of Japan and Taiwan.

EPIDEMIOLOGY. The basic cycle of infection in both temperate and tropical areas is mosquito-vertebrate-mosquito. In temperate areas the primary vector is *Culex tritaeniorhyncus*, and the important vertebrate hosts are herons, egrets, and pigs. Virus is detected in a given locale annually, first in mosquitoes in July, and then in birds and pigs within a few weeks. Epidemics of encephalitis occur later, in August and September, and by November virus has apparently disappeared. Winter survival has not been elucidated. Epidemics tend to be larger in alternate years for reasons not clearly understood.

In tropical areas virus transmission is less strongly seasonal, and although the basic cycle is similar to that of temperate zones, other vectors such as *C. gelidus* in Malaysia, Thailand, and Vietnam and *C. annulirostris* on Guam are important. Regardless of area, the ratio of inapparent to disease-associated infections in man is very high. Annual infection rates in children may reach 10 per cent, but only 1 in 300 to 500 infections results in clinical disease. This ratio apparently declines with increasing age, one case of encephalitis occurring per 25 infections in United States troops.

CLINICAL MANIFESTATIONS. Japanese B infection is similar to that of St. Louis encephalitis virus in the high frequency of inapparent infection or mild illness, in onset, and in the signs or symptoms of central nervous system disease. But urinary tract symptoms and signs are less common, and the over-all severity of neurologic disease is more severe in Japanese B infections. Children commonly evidence paralysis of the face or extremities. Adults tend toward bilateral paresis without sensory changes. Sensorial changes, spastic rigidity, cerebellar signs, and coma are frequent in adults. The fever usually peaks four or five days after onset, then slowly subsides. Relative bradycardia is often seen, accompanied by a modest transient leukocytosis. Cerebrospinal fluid pressure is often increased moderately, and pleocytosis and increased protein are invariably present.

DIAGNOSIS. Although epidemiologic considerations may strongly suggest it, specific diagnosis requires a variety of virologic procedures. Isolation of virus from blood has been reported but is uncommonly achieved. Virus or, more often, fluorescent antigen can sometimes be demonstrated in brain tissue of fatal cases. Serologic diagnosis offers the best possibility of establishing the cause, but in many areas of Southeast Asia and India this is often confounded by the prior presence of antibodies to other related group B viruses. In Japan, where fewer such problems exist, it has been shown that primary infection induces early IgM antibodies reactive in neutralization and HI tests only, whereas IgG antibodies reactive in CF test are detectable eight or more days after onset of disease. Depending on the timing of serum specimens, diagnosis may thus require use of any or all three procedures. Detection of specific IgM HI antibodies has increased by precision of diagnosis in areas where related group B viruses are endemic.

TREATMENT AND PROGNOSIS. Intensive supportive care is mandatory and is all that is available. Artificial control of hyperthermia is frequently required. Anticonvulsant drugs may be needed, although prognosis in such cases is generally poor. The mortality rate varies from about 30 per cent for those under 20 years of age to nearly 80 per cent in older persons. Severity of clinical disease is directly correlated with quantitative antibody response. It has also been shown that early appearance of IgG antibodies was more common in persons who had received one dose of inactivated vaccine or who were more than 50 years old. Correlation of disease severity with early IgG immune response has not yet been reported.

Permanent sequelae are most common in children under age ten, severe residual damage generally being reserved for the very young. These changes run the gamut of upper motor paralyses, cerebellar syndromes, personality changes, and mental deterioration frequently requiring permanent institutional care.

PREVENTION. Formolized vaccine has been widely used in Japan and, providing that two or more doses are given, is credited with significant protection. A live attenuated vaccine has been tried in pigs in an effort to prevent annual amplification of the natural virus cycle; but although individual animals can be thus protected, the suppression of vaccine virus replication by passively acquired antibodies and the rapid turnover of this economically exploited species in Japan effectively preclude large-scale use of this measure. Specific vector control is not practical either, although modernization of rice culture techniques with attendant increased use of insecticides has apparently reduced peak mosquito vector populations in both Japan and South Korea, and is credited with significant reduction in epidemic disease transmission in recent years.

101.8.   MURRAY VALLEY ENCEPHALITIS

Murray Valley encephalitis is similar to Japanese B encephalitis in pathogenesis and clinical features, and is caused by a very closely related virus. Diagnosis requires laboratory studies similar to those for other group B encephalitides.

The disease almost certainly was recognized in 1917–18 when an epidemic of 134 cases, then called *Australian X disease*, occurred in the Murray and Darling River valleys of Victoria and New South Wales. Virus strains isolated at the time were lost. Sporadic cases occurred during the next three decades, but the present designation was established during an outbreak of some 40 cases in 1951, more than a third of them fatal. This time the virus was recovered and completely characterized. Many inapparent human infections were detected. Endemic infection is maintained in a bird-mosquito cycle in Northern Australia and New Guinea, and it has been postulated that the virus is intermittently brought south by migratory birds, where an amplifying cycle involving domestic fowl, water birds, and *Culex annulirostris* mosquitoes produces epidemic disease, most commonly among children. Another epidemic in 1974 confirmed and extended these basic observations.

101.9.   TICK-BORNE GROUP B ARBOVIRUS DISEASES: RUSSIAN SPRING-SUMMER ENCEPHALITIS, LOUPING ILL, KYASANUR FOREST DISEASE, OMSK HEMORRHAGIC FEVER

DEFINITION. The tick-borne complex of group B arboviruses cause mild to severe febrile illness with frequent neurologic abnormalities and in two instances (Kyasanur Forest disease [KFD] and Omsk hemorrhagic fever [OHF]) acute hemorrhagic manifestations. These agents are distributed throughout Eurasia (KFD, OHF, Russian spring-summer encephalitis [RSSE]) and Great Britain (louping ill). Powassan virus occurs in Canada and the northern United States but has so far caused only a few recognized cases of human disease.

ETIOLOGY. The group B tick-borne arboviruses constitute an antigenic complex readily distinguishable from most mosquito-borne group B agents, and separable into several closely related subtypes. With the exception of RSSE and OHF, which overlap geographically, these viruses are found in distinct regions of the world. Suckling mice and a variety of cell cultures have proved most satisfactory for virus isolation, and a complete range of serologic techniques is available for differential classification. Hemorrhagic pneumonia is induced in muskrats by inoculation of OHF virus, encephalitis with occasional hemorrhagic diathesis follows administration of KFD virus to langur and bonnet monkeys, and varying clinical encephalitis occurs upon intracerebral inoculation of monkeys, sheep, and goats with the remaining members of the complex.

EPIDEMIOLOGY. The viruses persist in discrete geographic foci by interchange between wild and domestic vertebrates and ixodid ticks, principally of the genera *Ixodes, Dermacentor,* and *Haemaphysalis.*

Many vertebrates, including rodents, birds, bats, sheep, goats, and cattle, experience clinically silent viremic infection. The capacity of the tick vectors to transmit virus transovarially has been experimentally documented, thus providing a fundamental mechanism for winter survival of some of the viruses. Persistent infection of hibernating species such as bats and hedgehogs has also been demonstrated. In the case of OHF and KFD viruses, respectively, viremia and overt fatal infection occur naturally in muskrats and monkeys, and major epizootics among these animals often precede or accompany outbreaks in man.

In addition to tick transmission, RSSE infection in man may be acquired through *raw milk* of infected goats and sheep. Tick-transmitted infection may result from factors affecting residence, occupation, or recreation. Residents of rural forested areas, particularly agricultural, veterinary, and forest workers, are at highest risk. Seasonal disease patterns reflect temperature-dependent tick activity, with peaks ranging from late spring to autumn, depending on the tick and the geographic locality. Some of the agents can also apparently infect man by the respiratory route, as evidenced by winter outbreaks among trappers and skinners of muskrats (OHF) and by aerosol-associated laboratory infections (OHF, KFD).

CLINICAL MANIFESTATIONS AND PATHOLOGY. Onset is typically abrupt after an incubation period of 3 to 12 days. The pattern is frequently diphasic except for OHF, the initial phase consisting of fever, headache, myalgia, gastrointestinal disturbances, and, in KFD, mild to moderate hemorrhages from the nose and intestines. Leukopenia is common during this phase, which lasts five to ten days.

The second phase usually begins with high fever and severe headache. Louping ill is usually mild to moderate in over-all severity, but RSSE infection tends to be progressively more severe from Europe to Far Eastern Asia. Although serous meningitis is the most common form over-all, infection in the easternmost part of the Soviet Union is frequently grossly encephalomyelitic, with transient or permanent flaccid paralysis, nystagmus, deafness, and somnolence. Bulbospinal disease is the most serious, resulting in neck and shoulder paralysis or even death. The second phase of KFD also is predominantly neurologic, although severity is usually

moderate. Moderate leukocytosis and cerebrospinal fluid pleocytosis and elevated protein are characteristic of this phase. The latter abnormalities have been shown to persist in louping ill for weeks after apparent clinical recovery.

Pathologically the lesions produced by these viruses are generally similar to those observed with other arbovirus encephalitides or hemorrhagic fevers (inflammatory vasculitis in brain or focal capillary hemorrhages without inflammation). But not infrequently RSSE virus produces neuronal damage in the cervical cord reminiscent of poliomyelitis, and the viruses of OHF and KFD induce a focal hemorrhagic bronchopneumonia with occasional necrotic foci in the liver and gastrointestinal tract.

DIAGNOSIS AND TREATMENT. Specific diagnosis, in contrast to disease caused by most mosquito-borne encephalitides, can often be made by isolation of the virus from blood during the initial febrile phase, or from brain in rapidly fatal infection. Serologic diagnosis is even more reliable, although access to all three common techniques is necessary to establish the cause in some instances. With the exception of RSSE-OHF, anamnestic responses to infection with related agents are usually not a problem. Treatment is symptomatic. Blood loss in OHF and KFD is rarely sufficient to warrant transfusion.

PROGNOSIS AND PREVENTION. Louping ill virus infection has not caused fatalities or permanent neurologic sequelae. Far eastern RSSE, in contrast, has a fatality rate of more than 15 per cent and leaves many survivors with permanent paralysis of an arm or the shoulder girdle. Soviet workers also claim that 3 to 5 per cent of paralytic patients follow a chronic progressive course that develops into clonic spasms, epilepsy, and death. Strong indirect evidence for chronic virus persistence in the brain of one patient during a period of 14 years with final deterioration and death has been obtained by Japanese workers. Fatality rates do not exceed 5 per cent for KFD and OHF and there are no permanent sequelae associated with these diseases.

Soviet workers have administered formolized mouse brain RSSE vaccine to thousands of persons with reported good results. Work proceeds in that country on a live attenuated vaccine. Otherwise, protection is largely individual against tick bite, consisting of adequate clothing and insect repellents. Aerial spraying of insecticides has been tried on a large scale for tick control in parts of Russia but has been abandoned as too expensive.

Bennett, N. M.: Murray Valley encephalitis, 1974: Clinical features. Med. J. Aust., 2:446, 1976.

Blaskovic, D., and Nosek, J.: The ecological approach to the study of tick-borne encephalitis, In Melnick, J. L. (ed.): Progress in Medical Virology. Vol. 14. Basel and New York, S. Karger, 1972, pp. 275–320.

Feemster, R. F.: Equine encephalitis in Massachusetts. N. Engl. J. Med., 257:701, 1957.

Grabow, J. D., Mathews, C. G., Chun, R. W. M., and Thompson, W. H.: The electroencephalogram and clinical sequelae of California arbovirus encephalitis. Neurology, 19:394, 1969.

Hart, K. L., Keen, D., and Belle, E. A.: An outbreak of eastern equine encephalomyelitis in Jamaica, West Indies. I. Description of human cases. Am. J. Trop. Med. Hyg., 13:331, 1964.

Hilty, M. D., Haynes, R. E., Azimi, P. H., and Cramblett, H. G.: California encephalitis in children. Am. J. Dis. Child., 124:530, 1972.

Johnson, K. M., and Martin, D. H.: Venezuelan equine encephalitis. In Brandly, C. A., and Cornelius, C. E. (eds.): Advances in Veterinary

Science and Comparative Medicine. Vol. 18. New York, Academic Press, 1974, pp. 79–115.

Leon, C. A., Jaramillo, R., Martinez, S., ·Fernandez, F., Tellez, H., Lasso, B., and Guzman, R. de: Sequelae of Venezuelan equine encephalitis in humans: A four-year follow-up. Int. J. Epidemiol., 4:131, 1975.

Lincoln, A. F., and Sivertson, S. E.: Acute phase of Japanese B encephalitis. Two hundred and one cases in American soldiers, Korea, 1950. JAMA, 150:268, 1952.

Matthews, C. G., Chun, R. W. M., Grabow, J. D., and Thompson, W. H.: Psychological sequelae in children following California arbovirus encephalitis. Neurology, 18:1023, 1968.

Parkin, W. E., Hammon, W. McD., and Sather, G. W.: Review of current epidemiological literature on viruses of the California arbovirus group. Am. J. Trop. Med. Hyg., 21:964, 1972.

Quick, D. T., Thompson, J. M., and Bond, J. O.: The 1962 epidemic of St. Louis encephalitis in Florida. IV. Clinical features of cases occurring in the Tampa Bay area. Am. J. Epidemiol., 81:415, 1965.

Venezuelan Encephalitis: Washington, D.C., Pan-American Health Organization Publication Number 243, 1972, pp. 416.

Wallis, R. C.: Recent advances in research on the eastern encephalitis virus. Yale J. Biol. Med., 37:413, 1965.

Weaver, O. M., Haymaker, W., Pieper, S., and Kirland, R.: Sequelae of the arthropod-borne encephalitides. V. Japanese encephalitis. Neurology, 8:887, 1958.

Webb, H. E., and Rao, L.: Kyasanur Forest disease: A general clinical study in which some cases with neurological complications were observed. Trans. R. Soc. Trop. Hyg., 55:284, 1961.

White, M. G., Carter, N. W., et al.: Pathophysiology of epidemic St. Louis encephalitis. Ann. Intern. Med., 71:691, 1969.

102. VIRAL HEMORRHAGIC FEVERS

102.1. INTRODUCTION

Karl M. Johnson

The viral hemorrhagic fevers form a group of acute diseases in which bleeding is a prominent clinical manifestation. These diseases occur in different parts of the world, are caused by ribonucleic acid–containing viruses, and may be transmitted to man by mosquitoes, by ticks, or by direct contact with excreta of virus-infected rodents (see accompanying table). Despite its longstanding fame as a cause of acute hepatocellular necrosis, *yellow fever* is included under this heading because of its recognized ability to induce gastrointestinal hemorrhage and a shock syndrome similar to that seen with other viruses of the group.

After a variable period of a few days to one to three weeks, during which virus multiplies in lymphoid cells and produces a viremia, hemorrhagic fever patients experience fever, myalgia, and other nonspecific symptoms. Bleeding ensues, generally near the end of the febrile period, and although usually not sufficient per se to account for it, such hemorrhage is the harbinger of a clinical crisis dominated by hypovolemic shock. In at least two instances, epidemic hemorrhagic fever and dengue hemorrhagic fever, there is evidence that shock is caused by a widespread capillary vascular lesion in which plasma protein escapes the circulation much faster than erythrocytes. Thrombocytopenia and deficits in various circulating hemostatic factors are frequently present, but it is not clear whether they are etiologically related to this condition.

How the hemorrhagic syndrome is produced thus remains a mystery. No evidence for a direct virus-induced lesion of capillary endothelium has been ob-

tained to date. Disseminated intravascular coagulation (DIC) has been shown in a few instances and postulated in others. But even assuming that DIC occurs, we have no clear idea about the vital pathophysiologic triggers for this chain reaction. Certain facts suggest, however, that altered immunologic function may be important in the pathogenesis of hemorrhagic fever. First, the pathology of such viral disease, unlike that associated with arboviral encephalitis, is characterized by the absence of inflammatory tissue reaction. Second, the high evidence of secondary bacterial infections and the delay of specific humoral antibody response observed in arenavirus-caused disease and Crimean hemorrhagic fever implies a direct suppression of B-cell lymphocyte function. Finally, there is the possibility that antigen-antibody complexes may be important in the genesis of some of these conditions. Available data include long incubation period, leukocytosis, and acute, reversible renal insufficiency in epidemic hemorrhagic fever; the temporal association between hemorrhagic disease and secondary dengue virus infection together with reduction of circulating complement components is even more suggestive. As for the arboviral encephalitides, elucidation of the operative variables is important. Clinical management of disease and vaccine development appear to offer more hope of averting fatal infection than does interruption of the nonhuman natural virus cycles.

102.2. YELLOW FEVER

Thomas P. Monath

DEFINITION. Yellow fever is an acute mosquito-borne viral infection characterized, in its severe form, by fever, jaundice, hemorrhage, and albuminuria. The disease is endemic-epidemic in tropical regions of the Americas and Africa, where it remains a major public health problem, but it does not occur in Asia.

ETIOLOGY. Yellow fever virus is the prototype of the flavivirus taxonomic group which is composed of a variety of other medically important, antigenically related viruses, including several which also cause hemorrhagic fevers (dengue, Omsk hemorrhagic fever, and Kyasanur Forest disease). Yellow fever virus (and other flaviviruses) are spherical, enveloped, RNA-containing particles of approximately 38 mμ in size; virions develop by budding from intracytoplasmic membranes of infected cells and accumulate in cisternae of the endoplasmic reticulum. Since the virus shares antigenic determinants with many other flaviviruses, some of which are common in the yellow fever endemic zone, serologic responses to infection are often nonspecific or difficult to interpret. Strains of yellow fever virus from Africa and South America are distinguishable in special serologic tests; strain variation in virulence markers for laboratory animals also occurs. However, no clear geographic differences have been shown in the clinical features of the human disease. Yellow fever virus is pathogenic for a variety of cell cultures, newborn mice, adult mice (when injected intracerebrally), and some monkey species. Rhesus monkeys have been used as an experimental model of the human disease.

EPIDEMIOLOGY. Two epidemiologic forms of yellow fever are classically distinguished on the basis of dif-

Viral Hemorrhagic Fevers: Etiologic and Epidemiologic Considerations

	Causative Agent	Vector(s)	Vertebrate Host(s)	Geographical Distribution	Epidemiologic Features of Involvement of Man	Control	Remarks
Yellow fever (urban)	YF virus—a group B arbovirus	*Aedes aegypti* in cities	Man	Human populations (usually urban) in tropics of South and Central America and Africa	Person-to-person passage by *Aedes aegypti*	*Aedes aegypti* control; vaccination	Sylvan YF can spread to cities
Yellow fever (sylvan)	YF virus—a group B arbovirus	*Haemagogus* mosquitoes in New World; *Aedes* species in Africa	Monkeys of several genera and species	Forests and jungles of South and Central American and West, Central, and East Africa	Man infected by exposure in jungle (i.e., woodcutters, hunters, etc.)	Vaccination	Human cases sporadic and unpredictable; disease often a "silent" endemic in forests
Dengue hemorrhagic fever	Dengue viruses of four types; group B arboviruses	*Aedes aegypti*	Man (involvement of other primates has been postulated)	Tropical and subtropical cities of Southeast Asia and Philippines	Small children usually involved in cities where *Aedes aegypti* densities are high	*Aedes aegypti* control; mosquito repellent, screens, etc.	Disease may represent an immunologic over-response to a sequential infection with a different dengue strain
Omsk hemorrhagic fever	Two distinguishable subtypes of HF virus	Ticks of genus *Dermacentor*	Small rodents and muskrats	Omsk region of USSR; northern Roumania	People exposed in fields and wooded lands.	Tick repellents and protective clothing	
Kyasanur forest disease	KFD virus—a group B arbovirus	Ticks of several species in genus *Haemaphysalis*	Monkeys (rhesus and langur) and small rodents and birds	Mysore State, India	People exposed in fields and wooded lands	Tick control; tick repellents and protective clothing	Monkey mortality signals epidemic activity
Argentine hemorrhagic fever	Junin virus, an arenavirus LCM-related	None proved; mites suspected	Small rodents: *Akodon; Calomys laucha, musculinus*	Argentina: NW of Buenos Aires extending west to Province of Cordoba	Field workers at harvest time are particularly at risk	Rodent control in fields	Infected rodents contaminate environment with urine
Bolivian hemorrhagic fever	Machupo virus, an arenavirus LCM-related	None recognized	Small rodent, *Calomys callosus*	Beni Province of Bolivia	Residents of small, rodent-infested villages and homes; 1971 nosocomial outbreak in Cochabamba, Bolivia	Rodent control in villages; full isolation in hospital patient care	High mortality in man
Lassa fever	Lassa virus, an arenavirus LCM-related	None required	Small rodent; *Mastomys natalensis*	West Africa: Nigeria, Liberia, Sierra Leone	Residents of small rodent-infested villages; dramatic nosocomial outbreaks	None known; possibly rodent control	High mortality in man
Crimean hemorrhagic fever	CHF-Congo virus; an ungrouped arbovirus	Ticks of several genera	Larger domestic animals implicated; also African hedgehog	Southern USSR, Bulgaria, East and West Africa	Cowhands and field workers in USSR; nosocomial outbreaks reported	Tick control relating to livestock; full isolation in patient care	Human disease important in USSR; importance to man in Africa not known
Korean hemorrhagic fever (hemor. nephroso-nephritis)	Not known; virus suspected	Not known	Possibly small mammals	Korea; northern Eurasia to and including Scandinavia	Rural or sylvan exposure (military, forest occupations, farmers)	None	A baffling epidemiologic and clinical entity

ferent mosquito vectors and vertebrate hosts involved in the cycle of virus transmission. These forms are clinically and pathoanatomically identical. In the *urban* form, yellow fever virus is passed from a viremic person to another, nonimmune individual by the agency of the peridomestic mosquito, *Aedes aegypti*. As with other arboviruses, a period of extrinsic incubation in the vector is required before virus can be transmitted; this interval (6 to 30 days in *Ae. aegypti*) is temperature dependent. *Jungle* (or sylvan) yellow fever is a zoonotic infection, incidentally acquired through the bite of one of a variety of forest mosquito vector species, which maintains the virus in a monkey-mosquito-monkey cycle. The epidemiology and epizootiology of the disease in the Americas and in Africa differ and must be considered separately. Despite years of intensive study,

many aspects of the ecology of yellow fever remain poorly understood.

Between 50 and 300 cases of *jungle yellow fever* are recognized annually in South America. The virus is active primarily in Brazil, Peru, Bolivia, and Colombia in forested and sparsely populated areas under limited cultivation, drained by tributaries of the Amazon, Orinoco, and Magdalena Rivers. Human cases reach a peak during the rainy months (in most areas, December through March). Human cases are often sporadic, but small epidemics (involving 20 to 50 cases) are not uncommon. In the past, large outbreaks have been associated with monkey epizootics which appear at 5- to 40-year intervals and spread through natural corridors into forested areas, such as Central America, normally outside the enzootic zone. In the forest canopy, the virus circulates in a primary cycle involving monkeys and marmosets and mosquitoes of the genus *Haemagogus*. The exact location of virus activity in the vast tropical forests of South America is difficult or impossible to ascertain at any point in time, and indeed the virus is constantly moving, thus assuring a supply of susceptible hosts adequate for maintenance of the cycle. Presence of the virus is, however, sometimes evident on the basis of monkey deaths, because some New World species succumb to the infection. Humans may accidentally acquire the disease during vocational activities, such as woodcutting, which bring them into contact with *Haemagogus* mosquitoes. Dramatic outbreaks have occurred when groups of unvaccinated laborers have penetrated jungle areas. Mosquito species of the drought-resistant genus *Sabethes* play a secondary role in the yellow fever cycle but may be important in maintaining transmission over the dry season.

In the Americas, *urban yellow fever* has not occurred since 1954 (in Trinidad), largely because of the eradication of *Aedes aegypti* mosquitoes from population centers of South America. Nonetheless, some *aegypti*-infested areas of northern South America remain in juxtaposition to the jungle cycle, and the risk of a viremic individual traveling to receptive regions of the Caribbean and southern United States is recognized. The recent occurrence of dengue epidemics in the Caribbean is prima facie evidence that this region is receptive to yellow fever.

The situation in Africa is considerably more complex. Relatively few sporadic cases are recognized annually, but this reflects under-reporting and inadequate surveillance and diagnostic facilities. Large epidemics, which occur at irregular intervals in areas of West, Central, and East Africa between 0 and 15 degrees N, have involved as many as 100,000 cases, with 30,000 deaths. Epidemics sustained by the peridomestic *Ae. aegypti* vector have occurred in both the urban and rural environments of West Africa. Epidemic yellow fever in the savannah and forest-savannah transition areas of West Africa has been transmitted by nondomestic *Aedes* species, including *luteocephalus* and *africanus*, with man acting as the probable intermediate host. Jungle yellow fever (transmission from monkey to man by wild *Aedes*) may occur but has not been documented in West Africa, where forested areas and nonhuman primate populations are now quite restricted. Enzootic transmission has nonetheless been documented in monkeys and wild *Aedes* (*africanus* and other species) inhabiting riverine forests.

In the more extensive forests of Central and East Africa, a jungle cycle analogous to that in the Americas operates, with *Aedes africanus* as the principal vector. Sporadic cases and epidemics in persons entering the forest or living at the forest fringe have resulted from exposure to this mosquito. In some areas, another vector, *Ae. simpsoni*, links the jungle cycle with human populations and has been responsible for intensive interhuman transmission.

All races are equally susceptible to yellow fever infection. The disease produced in native populations of Africa is thought to be milder than in whites, but this is probably a reflection of background immunity and cross-protection by related endemic flaviviruses; some outbreaks of yellow fever involving Africans have been severe, with high death rates. Nonimmune persons of all ages and both sexes are equally susceptible. The age and sex distribution is, however, determined by the rate of natural immunization in endemic areas, by vaccination campaign policies, and by occupational exposures. Adult males employed in woodcutting or agricultural pursuits are primarily affected by jungle yellow fever.

PATHOLOGY AND PATHOGENESIS. Gross pathologic lesions are relatively few; signs include icterus; hemorrhages or petechiae of the mucous membranes, stomach, duodenum, renal capsule, and urinary bladder; and small amounts of pleural and peritoneal fluid. Histopathologic changes of the liver may be characteristic, but even experienced pathologists may not be able to make an unequivocal diagnosis in atypical cases. Conditions with which yellow fever has been confused on the basis of liver pathology include Lassa fever, African (Marburg-Ebola virus) hemorrhagic fever, viral hepatitis, and leptospirosis. The typical yellow fever lesion is marked by cloudy swelling, then by coagulative necrosis of hepatocytes in the midzone of the liver lobule, sparing cells bordering the central vein. The centrilobular trabeculae show a degree of disorganization. Eosinophilic degeneration of hepatocytes results in the formation of *Councilman bodies;* intranuclear eosinophilic granular inclusions (Torres bodies) have also been described. Multi- and microvacuolar fatty change is nearly always present, especially after the eighth day of illness. An inflammatory response is absent or limited to a mild interstitial histiocytic infiltration late in the disease. The reticulin framework is preserved. Characteristic changes have been seen in biopsy specimens taken as early as the third day of illness; interpretation of biopsy or necropsy material obtained after the tenth day is often difficult. Histopathologic changes in other organs are variable and less specific. Renal glomerular changes are relatively insignificant compared to acute tubular necrosis and fatty metamorphosis, which may be marked. The myocardial fibers show moderate cloudy swelling, degeneration, and fatty infiltration. Lymphocytic elements in the spleen and nodes are depleted, and large mononuclear or histiocytic cells accumulate in the splenic follicles. The brain may show edema and petechial hemorrhages.

The *pathologic physiology* of yellow fever is poorly understood. Direct viral injury to the cells of major target organs, such as the liver, kidney, and heart, undoubtedly underlie the pathogenic process and may be mediated by activation of intracellular lysozymes. Immunopathologic mechanisms are also suspected but not proved. Hepatic coma has not been clinically or electroencephalographically defined, and the role of hepatic failure in the disease is uncertain. Some patients have prominent signs of acute renal failure, and deaths have been attributed to uremia. It is not known whether acute tubular necrosis is due to direct viral injury or is secondary to hemodynamic causes or hepatocellular necrosis. Deaths (especially late in the disease) have occurred because of cardiac failure or arrhythmia, but are rare. Hemorrhage undoubtedly exacerbates hypotension and oliguria and may precipitate vascular collapse and death, but it is usually minor and must be considered only a contributory problem; rhesus monkeys die in a fashion similar to humans, with little or no overt hemorrhagic manifestations. Evidence for disseminated intravascular coagulation as the basis for the hemorrhagic diathesis is conflicting. Acid-base and electrolyte imbalances have been poorly defined. At present, the complex pathophysiologic interrelationships of yellow fever cannot be specified, and directions for specific therapeutic interventions are consequently undetermined.

CLINICAL MANIFESTATIONS. Yellow fever infection produces a clinical spectrum varying from very mild, nonspecific, febrile illness to a malignant, sometimes fatal form with pathognomonic features. The precise frequency with which the various clinical forms occur is uncertain; however, it is clear that abortive infections are the rule and that the classic symptoms of severe yellow fever are found in only 10 to 20 per cent of cases. The incubation period (interval between bite of infected mosquito and onset of symptoms) is generally three to six days.

The typical or mild case will not be suspected or clinically diagnosed except in the setting of an epidemic. In its mildest form it is characterized by sudden onset of fever and headache, without other symptoms, lasting 48 hours or less. In other patients, the fever is higher, the headache more distressing, and the illness accompanied by a grippe-like syndrome with nausea, myalgia, slight albuminuria, and bradycardia in relation to the presence of fever (Faget's sign). The illness lasts several days, with uneventful recovery.

The severe forms of yellow fever begin abruptly with fever to 40° C, chills or chilliness, severe headache, and generalized myalgia often most acute in the lower back. The patient appears distressed and anxious, the conjunctiva congested, the face and neck flushed, the tongue reddened at the tip and edges, the breath foul smelling. Anorexia, nausea, vomiting, and constipation are present, and minor gingival hemorrhages or epistaxis may occur. Despite a persistent or rising temperature, the pulse may fall. This syndrome, persisting for approximately three days, corresponds to the "period of infection," during which yellow fever virus is present in the blood. It may be followed by a "period of remission," with partial or complete defervescence and mitigation of symptoms, usually lasting several to 24 hours. The fever and systemic symptoms then reappear with more *frequent vomiting, epigastric pain, prostration,* and the *appearance of jaundice* ("period of intoxication"). Viremia is generally absent, and antibodies appear during this phase. Hematemesis, coffee grounds or black (vomito negro), is a characteristic and frightening sign. It may be accompanied or followed by other hemorrhagic manifestations, including melena, metrorrhagia, petechiae, ecchymoses, and diffuse oozing from the mucous membranes. Dehydration resulting from vomiting and increased insensible losses is frequent. Renal damage is evidenced by the sudden appearance of albuminuria, which may rapidly increase, and by diminishing urine output. The pulse remains dissociated from fever, but may weaken as the blood and pulse pressures decrease. The patient recovers either rapidly after a period of intoxication of three to four days or over a protracted course of up to two weeks. Fatalities (occurring in up to 50 per cent of severe yellow fever cases) generally occur on the seventh to tenth day of illness, and are preceded by increasing albuminuria, hemorrhages, rising pulse, hypotension, oliguria, and azotemia. Hypothermia, a severe agitated delirium, intractable hiccup, stupor, and coma are terminal signs.

In individual cases hepatic, renal, or myocardial involvement predominates, with clinical signs of relatively pure hepatitis, acute renal failure, or hypotension and hypokinetic heart failure. Pre-eminent central nervous system involvement, producing meningoencephalitic signs, has also been described. Atypical, fulminant cases occur, with death on the second or third day in the absence of hepatic or renal signs.

Physical findings during the period of intoxication include scleral and dermal icterus, hemorrhagic manifestations, epigastric (rarely hepatic) tenderness without organomegaly, and the changes already noted in vital signs.

The convalescent stage is sometimes prolonged, with profound asthenia lasting one to two weeks. Late death, occurring at the end of convalescence or even weeks after complete recovery from the acute illness, is a rare but well documented phenomenon attributed to yellow fever myocardial damage, cardiac arrhythmia, or failure. Suppurative parotitis (resulting from dehydration) and secondary bacterial pneumonia are recognized complications.

CLINICAL LABORATORY FINDINGS. Leukopenia (neutropenia) occurs most often during the early phase of illness; the white blood count is, however, often normal or elevated. Prolongation of the clotting, prothrombin, and partial thromboplastin times is marked in cases with jaundice. The platelet count is usually normal, but may be decreased. The total and conjugated serum bilirubin rise together and may reach levels of 15 to 20 mg per deciliter in severe cases. Serum glutamic-oxaloacetic transaminase and serum glutamic pyruvic transaminase levels are markedly elevated in all icteric (but inconstantly and to lower levels in anicteric) patients, with peak values between days 5 and 10 of the illness, and return to normal by days 10 to 20. The alkaline phosphatase is generally normal, but other tests reflecting liver function (serum proteins, thymol turbidity, cholesterol) may be abnormal. In patients with severe hepatic damage, hypoglycemia has been occasionally noted.

During the period of infection, the urine may contain a small amount of albumin, which then increases suddenly on the fourth or fifth day, reaching levels of 3 to 5 (rarely as high as 40) grams per liter. The urine may coagulate in patients with massive proteinuria. The urine contains bile; the cell sediment may be abnormal but is not diagnostically helpful. The cerebrospinal fluid is clear, without cells, but it is often under increased pressure, and contains a mildly raised concentration of protein. ST-T wave electrocardiographic abnormalities have been described.

DIAGNOSIS. In endemic areas, recognition and diagnosis of a case are of great importance because it may indicate the presence of an epidemic and stimulate preventive or control measures. Because the incubation period is sufficiently long to permit an infected person to travel a long distance, the diagnosis should be suspected in all patients with fever and jaundice coming from tropical America or Africa. Specific diagnosis depends upon histopathologic study, isolation of the virus, or demonstration of a specific antibody response. The hemorrhagic diathesis renders liver biopsy hazardous, and pathologic diagnosis is thus a postmortem procedure. The virus is most readily isolated (by inoculation of mice or cell cultures) from serum obtained during the first three or four days of illness (period of infection), but it may be recovered from serum up to the twelfth day and occasionally from liver at death.

Serologic methods useful in the diagnosis of yellow

fever include hemagglutination-inhibition (HI), complement-fixation (CF), neutralization (N), and radioimmunoassay tests. The HI and N antibodies appear within a week of onset; the CF antibodies appear later. Paired, acute, and convalescent phase specimens are required to establish the diagnosis by rise in antibody titer. Cross-reactions with other flaviviruses and the high prevalence of background immunity to flaviviruses in tropical populations make serodiagnosis difficult in many cases.

Virus isolation and serologic tests are applicable to the diagnosis of all clinical forms of yellow fever and are the only means available of establishing the cause of abortive and mild infections.

DIFFERENTIAL DIAGNOSIS. Mild yellow fever cannot be clinically distinguished from a wide array of other infections. In the presence of jaundice and the other signs of severe yellow fever, conditions that must be differentiated include viral hepatitis, falciparum malaria, spirochetal infections (tick-borne relapsing fever and Weil's disease), Rift Valley fever, typhoid, Q fever, typhus, and surgical, drug-induced, and toxic causes. Other diseases (usually without jaundice) that may be confused with yellow fever include Lassa, African (Marburg-Ebola virus), Bolivian, and Argentine hemorrhagic fevers.

PROGNOSIS. Up to 50 per cent of patients with severe forms of yellow fever die; it should be recognized that patients in most reported series have been cared for under primitive conditions. The fatality rate of *all* patients with clinical illness is much lower (2 to 5 per cent). The prognosis should be guarded for the patient who, after a brief remission, enters a clear period of intoxication with rising fever, jaundice, and albuminuria. Certain clinical and laboratory features appear to correlate with a poor prognosis. These include early onset of bilirubinemia and albuminuria rising to high levels; prolongation of the prothrombin time beyond 25 per cent of normal; a rising and weakening pulse during the period of intoxication; and the appearance of coma, hypothermia, and intractable hiccup.

Relapses have not been described. The possibility of late death from myocardial or renal injury must be considered.

TREATMENT. No specific therapy exists at present. Complete bed rest, supportive care, and close monitoring of vital functions are essential. During the stage of infection, mild sedatives, analgesics, and antiemetics may be indicated, and attention should be given to fluid and electrolyte balance. Aspirin is contraindicated because of the bleeding diathesis. General and specific supportive measures are of critical importance during the period of intoxication if vomiting is severe, if hemorrhage appears, or if hypertension, hypokinetic heart failure, oliguria, azotemia, and electrolyte and acid-base imbalance become evident. In theory, these consequences of severe yellow fever might be lessened by intensive counter-regulation. Heroic measures (hyperalimentation, exchange blood transfusion) aimed at improving hepatic and neurologic function have been tried in experimentally infected rhesus monkeys, but without success.

Secondary bacterial infections or concurrent infections (in particular, malaria) should be treated by the usual appropriate means.

Return to activity should be gradual.

PREVENTION AND CONTROL. The patient with yellow fever should be isolated from possible contact with mosquitoes under netting or in a screened room.

Yellow fever 17D is one of the safest live, attenuated vaccines available and provides effective, longlasting immunity. For purposes of international certification, vaccination is considered valid for 10 years, but immunity has been documented to last 19 years and may be lifelong. Since yellow fever exists as a silent enzoosis over wide areas of the tropics and appears in epidemic form with little warning and without early recognition, vaccination of travelers is imperative. Immunity can be demonstrated within 10 days after vaccination. Mild vaccine reactions occur rarely, and serious complications have been exceedingly uncommon. No untoward consequences for the fetus have been recorded; but on theoretical grounds, pregnant women should not be vaccinated unless the risk of acquiring yellow fever is considered great. The vaccine is prepared in chicken embryos and should be used with caution in persons hypersensitive to egg proteins. The 17D vaccine available in the United States is presently contaminated with avian leukosis virus, but follow-up studies have not correlated this contaminant with any known human disease. Leukosis-free vaccine is commercially available in England and is under development in the United States. The French neurotropic viral vaccine is no longer produced or used anywhere in the world.

In the event of an epidemic, the disease may be controlled by mass vaccination and the use of insecticides to reduce infected vector populations.

102.3. HEMORRHAGIC FEVER CAUSED BY DENGUE VIRUSES

Karl M. Johnson

DEFINITION. These hemorrhagic fevers of Southeast Asia and India are acute, infectious, urban, mosquito-borne diseases caused by dengue viruses. Endoepidemic in pattern, dengue hemorrhagic fever is clinically defined as a dengue disease that worsens two or more days after onset, and is characterized by hypoproteinemia and one or more hemostatic abnormalities such as thrombocytopenia, prolonged bleeding time, or elevated prothrombin time. The dengue shock syndrome consists of hemorrhagic fever plus shock (hypotension or a pulse pressure of 20 mm Hg or less) and hemoconcentration (hematocrit at least 20 per cent greater than convalescent value). Chikungunya virus infections fulfilling these criteria are rarely encountered.

ETIOLOGY. All evidence suggests that these diseases are caused by each of the four recognized dengue virus subtypes. How they produce such disease is still not clear. A current hypothesis is that severe dengue disease is produced by an immunologic reaction that occurs in some individuals experiencing a second dengue infection. However, hemorrhagic fever has been unequivocally caused by primary dengue infection.

EPIDEMIOLOGY. These hemorrhagic fevers were first seen in epidemic proportions in Manila and Bangkok (1954) and in Singapore (1960). Other outbreaks have been reported from Malaysia, South Vietnam, India, Indonesia, and Oceania. In Bangkok age-specific rates in children have reached 7 to 8 per 1000. In most outbreaks cases occur only in children, principally below the age of 8 years; otherwise, the epidemiology of infection leading to dengue hemorrhagic fever is basically similar to that associated with ordinary dengue fever; outbreaks occur during the rainy season in large urban centers where *Aedes aegypti* is well established. Halstead has proposed that dengue hemorrhagic fever is an immune disease, brought on usually by a second (but not a third) dengue virus infection in a previously sensitized host. The syndromes have not been observed in many places where dengue is or has been prevalent, including the New World and many parts of Southeast Asia, Australasia, and Oceania.

PATHOLOGY. Autopsy data are scant. The chief abnormalities include generalized vascular congestion and dilatation with edema and multiple focal hemorrhages in most organs, mild to moderate pleural effusion and ascites, mononuclear cell infiltration of interstitial tissues and alveolar walls of lungs, focal myocardial congestion, and a decrease in mature lymphocytes with proliferation of mononuclear forms in the germinal centers of lymph follicles.

Necrosis is unusual, and no specific damage of the blood vessels has been observed. Perivascular infiltration by mononuclear cells is common, but there is no evidence for significant vasculitis or for platelet or thrombin thrombosis of vessel walls. About one third of cases show evidence of globulin on endothelial surfaces and the walls of arterioles. The bone marrow often shows maturation arrest of megakaryocytes, and sometimes there is marked generalized cellular hypoplasia with rapid restoration to normal after emergence from shock.

Pathologic change in the liver, although generally inconspicuous, consists of focal lesions and varies greatly in degree of severity. These lesions are of particular interest, because occasionally Councilman bodies and other changes characteristic of yellow fever are observed.

PATHOGENESIS OR MECHANISM OF DISEASE. The pathogenesis is as yet poorly understood. The vascular congestion, dilatation, and increased permeability lead to the extensive edema and hemorrhage observed in the gastrointestinal tract, the skin, and other tissues. The cause of these vascular changes is unknown, but they result in loss of plasma volume and associated electrolyte disturbances. Platelet deficiency probably plays a role in the hemorrhages. Bleeding time is usually prolonged, prothrombin times are somewhat prolonged, clot retraction is poor, and the blood fibrinogen is slightly reduced. None of these changes is very profound. The circulatory collapse and shock observed appear to be far in excess of what might be expected from the extent of loss of edema fluid and blood. The adrenal changes suggest exhaustion of steroid reserve. Death in some cases has been accompanied by severe hyperkalemia.

CLINICAL MANIFESTATIONS. The onset is that of a dengue infection, usually abrupt, with fever. Nausea and vomiting are common. The throat appears injected, and there may be a dry cough. About the second or third day petechiae appear, usually first on the face or distal portions of the extremities but sparing the axillae and chest. The tourniquet test may be conspicuously positive before petechiae appear. Purpura and large ecchymoses as well as other manifestations of bleeding tendency are occasionally prominent. There may be severe abdominal pain and tenderness. About the third or fourth day, vomiting may produce copious coffee-

ground material. Melena also is not uncommon, but gross bleeding from the intestines is rare. Shock is likely to occur in severe cases about the fourth day, and this critical state lasts about 12 to 24 hours. At this time the temperature falls to normal, the blood pressure and pulse pressure are low or unmeasurable, and the limbs are cool and present a purple or brownish mottled appearance. Perspiration is frequently profuse. The face and hands appear edematous. Restlessness and apprehension are conspicuous as the patient enters shock. This state of shock is entirely out of proportion to the apparent loss of blood. Thrombocytopenia is noted during this period, and bleeding time is prolonged. Leukocytes remain at approximately normal levels, but are elevated in number in serious cases more frequently than they are depressed. The total and differential leukocyte counts are not those observed in dengue. Although the numbers of both immature and mature polymorphonuclear cells are decreased, there is an increase in lymphocytes and sometimes in monocytes.

DIAGNOSIS. Hemorrhagic fever begins as an extension of a classic dengue infection, and the early dengue syndrome intergrades into the milder and atypical manifestations of the later hemorrhagic syndrome. The diagnosis in a febrile child acutely ill for only two or three days is rendered highly probable by the presentation of petechiae, purpuric lesions, and unusual ecchymosis of the skin with most prominent distribution on the extremities and face, together with melena, thrombocytopenia, and a relatively normal leukocyte count. In a milder case or at an earlier stage, the tourniquet test may be of great assistance in detecting unusual capillary fragility. The rapid development of circulatory collapse and shock during the fourth to sixth day, associated with the aforementioned findings, differentiates this from most other exanthematous diseases. Meningococcemia and the Waterhouse-Friderichsen syndrome need careful consideration. Thrombocytopenic purpura can be expected to have an entirely different onset and is usually not associated with fever. Laboratory methods available for diagnosis are those described for dengue fever.

TREATMENT. There is no specific therapy, but case fatality rates can be greatly reduced by skillful management directed toward combating shock. Close monitoring of pulse, respiration, and blood pressure during the course of treatment is essential for at least 48 hours, because shock can occur and recur. Oxygen should be administered if there is cyanosis or labored breathing. Hypovolemia should be treated by administration of lactated Ringer's solution or 5 per cent glucose in normal saline, on the basis of 20 ml per kilogram of body weight, administered rapidly. In profound or unresponsive shock, plasma or a plasma expander (dextran in normal saline) can be given at the rate of 20 ml per kilogram of body weight. When signs improve, 5 per cent glucose in normal saline or in lactated Ringer's solution should be given at the rate of 10 ml per kilogram per hour, and continued until vital signs are normal. Acidosis should be corrected with sodium bicarbonate as necessary.

Whole blood should be given only if blood loss is known to be large. Administration of whole blood to a patient with elevated hematocrit may result in heart failure. Paraldehyde or chloral hydrate may be required for children who are markedly agitated. Salicylates administered during the febrile period may cause bleeding and acidosis, and they should not be given to febrile patients during a hemorrhagic fever outbreak. Pressor amines, alpha-adrenergic blocking agents, and steroids have not been demonstrated to be of value in treatment.

PROGNOSIS. Death is almost always associated with shock, and rarely occurs after the sixth day of illness. Case fatality rates among hospitalized patients have ranged from 5 to 50 per cent, depending to a large extent upon the condition of patients on admission and the facilities available for treatment. Careful management should be able to save all but the 5 or 10 per cent of patients admitted in a moribund state. Residual effects have not been observed, and, in contrast to primary dengue, recovery is usually prompt and complete seven to ten days after onset. Mental depression is seldom observed.

PREVENTION. The control of this hemorrhagic fever is the same as that for dengue, and consists of mosquito control or protection from mosquito bites and isolation of the patient from mosquitoes. No vaccine is available, and if the immunologic theory of causation is confirmed, vaccines as presently conceived would be specifically contraindicated.

102.4.   CRIMEAN HEMORRHAGIC FEVER

Karl M. Johnson

DEFINITION. Crimean hemorrhagic fever (CHF) is an acute febrile disease, often marked by severe hemorrhage and high mortality, occurring in the Soviet Union, Bulgaria, and Pakistan.

ETIOLOGY. The CHF agent is an arbovirus first isolated from human blood specimens in 1967. It is pathogenic for suckling mice and grows in several types of cultured cells. This virus is indistinguishable from Congo virus of Africa in CF and neutralization tests. Strains from Eurasia and Africa are thus referred to as CHF-Congo virus.

EPIDEMIOLOGY. CHF-Congo virus is naturally transmitted by several species of hard ticks belonging to the genera *Hyalomma, Rhipicephalus, Amblyomma,* and *Boophilus.* Active foci of infection with transmission to man exist in the lower Don and Volga river basins, in the Central Asian republics of Kazakstan and Uzbekistan of the Soviet Union, and in Pakistan. Few human cases have been recognized in Africa. The disease occurs most frequently among adults who are heavily exposed to ticks while working among cattle. Cases begin to appear in April and reach a peak during summer months. Proved or presumed vertebrate hosts for the virus include cattle, goats, hares, rooks, and hedgehogs. Transovarial tick transmission is suspected but not yet proved. Nosocomial human infections have occurred repeatedly in Central Asia, suggesting transmission by aerosol. The incubation period is estimated at about one week.

CLINICAL MANIFESTATIONS. Onset is typically abrupt with high, unremitting fever, chills, headache, and myalgia. There may be hyperemia of the upper trunk and neck, conjunctival effusion, vomiting, and diarrhea. Hepatomegaly is noted in about half the cases; splenomegaly is uncommon. Pronounced panleukopenia is almost invariably present, as is thrombocytopenia.

Bleeding begins on about the fourth day of illness. Petechiae appear in the oral mucosa and skin, at times presenting as frank *purpura hemorrhagica*. Nose, gums, and intestinal tract are the most common sites of bleeding, and in this disease above all other viral hemorrhagic fevers, blood loss per se may be life threatening. Stiff neck, hyperexcitability, or coma occurs in about 10 per cent of cases and these are grave prognostic signs. The cerebrospinal fluid, however, contains no leukocytes or increased protein. There may be proteinuria and microscopic hematuria, but renal function is rarely compromised. The fever and bleeding generally resolve by lysis at about the eighth day. Hypovolemic shock with a paradoxical rising hematocrit may appear just prior to the end of fever and is the most common cause of death.

DIAGNOSIS. Virus can be easily obtained from blood of patients during the first few days of illness. Specific CF and neutralizing antibodies appear in the sera of most patients 30 to 60 days after onset of symptoms.

TREATMENT AND PROGNOSIS. Therapy is symptomatic. Management of fluid, electrolyte, and erythrocyte balance forms the continuous clinical challenge. Shock is a grave problem and should be anticipated and treated as outlined in Ch. 102.5 and 356. Whole blood transfusion may be necessary. Intercurrent bacterial infection is very common, especially pneumonia. Mortality in the Soviet Union ranges from 20 to 50 per cent. Patients surviving the acute illness generally recover completely, albeit quite slowly. Several instances of mono- or polyneuritis persisting for several months have been recorded.

PREVENTION. There is no vaccine yet available; thus avoidance of the disease in endemic foci depends on personal measures designed to prevent tick bites. Several nosocomial infections have occurred in the Soviet Union and Pakistan. Thus strict isolation of patients and use of protective clothing and respirators by medical personnel are indicated.

102.5.   HEMORRHAGIC DISEASES CAUSED BY ARENAVIRUSES: ARGENTINE AND BOLIVIAN HEMORRHAGIC FEVERS AND LASSA FEVER*

Karl M. Johnson

DEFINITION. Argentine and Bolivian hemorrhagic fevers and Lassa fever are acute diseases caused respectively by Junin, Machupo, and Lassa viruses. Clinically, the diseases share the common features of fever, severe myalgia, leukopenia, hemorrhagic manifestations, shock, and (excluding Lassa fever) neurologic abnormalities.

ETIOLOGY. The three viruses are serologically and morphologically related, and related to lymphocytic choriomeningitis virus, in a grouping designated as arenaviruses.

GEOGRAPHICAL DISTRIBUTION, INCIDENCE, AND PREVALENCE. Argentine hemorrhagic fever is localized to the provinces of Córdoba and Junin in northern Argentina,

---

*The author wishes to express his thanks to Dr. Wilbur G. Downs for his considerable assistance in the preparation of this chapter, particularly with reference to the material on Lassa fever.

where several hundred to several thousand cases occur annually, principally in agricultural field hands, in the harvest months. Bolivian hemorrhagic fever has been reported only from Beni province of Bolivia, between the rivers Mamore and Branco, with the exception of a hospital outbreak in Cochabamba, Bolivia, in 1971, traceable to contact with a person from Beni province. Infections are seen in inhabitants of certain of the small towns, as well as in rural populations. Lassa fever has been reported from Nigeria, Liberia, and Sierra Leone, and hospital outbreaks account for most of the cases reported. Case fatality rates are estimates in the usual absence of prompt and specific diagnosis, but may be as high as 50 per cent in hospitalized cases of Lassa, and 10 to 20 per cent for the South American diseases.

EPIDEMIOLOGY AND PROBABLE MODE OF TRANSMISSION. The viruses have been isolated from wild rodents: Junin, most commonly from *Calomys musculinus*, *Calomys laucha*, and also *Akodon arenicola*; Machupo, from *Calomys callosus*; and Lassa, from *Mastomys natalensis*. An attractive current hypothesis is that infection is acquired by direct human contact (ingestion, inhalation, or entrance through mucous membranes or skin breaks) with virus-containing rodent excreta. For all three agents, persistent infection in rodents has been demonstrated, with viremia readily detectable for months. A similar pattern of chronic virus infection in rodents has been described for lymphocytic choriomeningitis virus.

PATHOLOGY. Few cases have received full study. Findings include irregularly focal diapedesis and capillary hemorrhage without much evidence of inflammatory reaction. Gross hemorrhages may be seen in the mucosa of the stomach and intestines and in the brain. Pulmonary infection, probably intercurrent, is frequently seen. Focal liver necrosis is prominent in Lassa fever.

CLINICAL MANIFESTATIONS. Although as many as half of all etiologically confirmed cases appear as acute undifferentiated fevers, the findings and clinical course of "full-blown" Argentine and Bolivian infections are so nearly identical as to justify joint description. The same holds for Lassa fever. Onset is usually gradual, with increasing fever, headache, diffuse myalgia, and anorexia. By the third day the temperature may be 39.5 to 40.5° C, with severe myalgia, particularly in the lumbar regions (or legs in Lassa fever). Conjunctival injection is present, a flush involving the upper trunk and face is frequently observed, and there may be a relative bradycardia. Beginning about the fourth day, scattered fine petechiae may appear on the face and neck, about the pectoral girdle, and/or in the buccal mucosa or palate. Aphthous ulcers of the oral mucosa and exudative pharyngitis have been a noteworthy feature of Lassa infections. The Rumpel-Leede test is frequently positive. Frank hemorrhages from one or more sites, including the stomach, intestines, nose, gums, and uterus, accompanied by microscopic hematuria, may occur. Hemorrhagic phenomena are not a common feature of Lassa infections. Although hemorrhage per se is rarely the precipitating cause, a hypotensive crisis frequently develops between the sixth and eighth days, coincident with a rapid return of temperature to normal after five or more days of sustained fever. Patients surviving this stress for 48 hours generally make slow but complete recovery.

Perhaps a fifth of the patients with the Bolivian or Argentine disease develop neurologic signs. These are quite characteristic, and begin on about the fifth or sixth day with a fine intention tremor of the tongue. This may become so severe as to render speech unintelligible and to preclude oral ingestion of solid or even liquid food. If so, gross intention tremors of the extremities usually appear, occasionally accompanied by an intermittent nystagmus. Such patients often become delirious, and may experience generalized clonic and tonic convulsions. The cerebrospinal fluid appears normal, however, and contains neither leukocytes nor virus. Convalescence is marked by weakness and signs of autonomic nervous system lability such as postural hypotension, spontaneous flushing and blanching of the skin, and episodes of diaphoresis.

In addition to delirium and occasional coma, 5 to 10 per cent of Lassa fever patients suffer significant permanent damage to one or both eighth cranial nerves. Some Lassa fever patients have shown electrocardiographic evidence of myocardial involvement.

Transient loss of scalp hair and typical Beau's lines in the nails, particularly those of the fingers, are observed in a majority of cases several weeks after subsidence of the high, sustained fever. Many patients are not able to resume full activity for at least one month after illness.

Leukopenia is almost invariably present, and cell counts may be as low as 1000 per cubic millimeter by the fourth or fifth day. All elements are reduced nearly equally, and there is often a mild to moderate thrombocytopenia during the first week. Usually the peripheral blood picture returns to normal rapidly after defervescence, although there may be transient relative lymphocytosis and mild anemia. During the latter portion of the febrile period, progressive increase in hematocrit similar to, but usually milder than, that of hemorrhagic nephrosonephritis (q.v.) is frequently observed. At about the same time, moderate proteinuria is common, although renal function is rarely compromised seriously, and frank azotemia and hyperkalemia are almost never present.

DIAGNOSIS. The presence of high fever, severe myalgia, and leukopenia should arouse immediate suspicion of viral hemorrhagic fever within the known endemic areas of its occurrence. Potential intimate contact with wild rodents in a rural or semirural setting serves to strengthen the likelihood of this diagnosis. Since these findings and all others described cannot be relied upon to differentiate the disease clinically from other infections such as yellow fever, typhoid and paratyphoid fevers, typhus, malaria, and leptospirosis, specific identification of cases depends upon laboratory confirmation. Virus can sometimes be isolated from blood, throat washing, and urine during the febrile period. At autopsy splenic tissue almost always yields the agent. Serologic detection of infection is a reliable method if paired acute and convalescent serums are employed. Both group-reacting complement-fixing antibodies and virus type-specific neutralizing antibodies appear in three to four weeks and reach peak values in seven to ten weeks after the onset of illness. Fluorescent antibodies appear in Lassa infections as early as seven days after the onset of symptoms.

These three agents have been responsible for several fatal laboratory infections, and work with the viruses should be carried out only with strictest precautionary measures, and complete isolation from other laboratory activities, in special high-risk laboratories.

TREATMENT. In the absence of any specific therapy,

successful treatment presents an acute challenge in the science and art of physiologic management. Patients require complete rest and maximal comfort. Mild sedatives and analgesics should be judiciously used. Careful measurement of fluid intake and output is mandatory. The electrolyte balance should be checked regularly; marked underhydration and overhydration are to be avoided, because these conditions appear to compromise the patient's ability to weather the hypotensive crisis. Daily hematocrit determinations and examinations of urine for protein are the most valuable tests for anticipating and managing this problem. Frequent measurement of blood pressure is also important, because many patients enter the shock phase with persistent relative bradycardia and warm, dry skin. Raising the foot of the bed may suffice to stabilize the pressure at levels adequate to preserve vital urinary output. If not, careful administration of human plasma or concentrated albumin (not whole blood) is indicated. In one instance of a Lassa infection, administration of plasma from a recovered patient appeared to be effective. Great care should be exercised in administering plasma or other fluids intravenously during shock, because intractable pulmonary edema is readily induced. Complications, particularly bacterial infections, should be anticipated and promptly treated. Convalescence should never be hurried.

PROGNOSIS. Although the case mortality may exceed 20 per cent, there is no single finding early in the disease that aids prognosis in the individual case. In general, the very young and the very old, as well as those who do not receive medical attention prior to the sixth day of disease, are subject to the highest risk. The onset of severe shock and neurologic abnormalities are both ominous prognostic signs, and at least half the patients exhibiting these signs succumb. The prognosis in Lassa fever is even poorer in diagnosed cases.

PREVENTION. Effective elimination of intimate human contact with certain wild rodents represents the only proved method for prevention of disease. This may be achieved by maintaining sound standards of personal and environmental hygiene. Campaigns to eliminate rodents, repair buildings, and clean rubbish near dwellings are highly successful when the disease is acquired mainly from peridomestic animals. There is insufficient evidence at present to warrant recommendation of systematic measures to control attacks by any potential arthropod vector.

Hospital outbreaks involving medical staff have provided most of the Lassa fever cases to date. A hospital outbreak of Machupo virus has occurred in Cochabamba, Bolivia. Such outbreaks can be extremely dangerous to personnel and demoralizing to hospital operation.

102.6. AFRICAN HEMORRHAGIC FEVER

(Marburg Disease)

Karl M. Johnson

DEFINITION. African hemorrhagic fever is an acute, highly fatal disease characterized by fever, prostration, rash, proteinuria, major hemorrhagic manifestations, pancreatitis, and hepatitis.

HISTORY. The disease was first described in Germany in 1967 and named Marburg disease. It was acquired through contact with green monkeys, *Cercopithecus aethiops,* imported from Uganda. Secondary nosocomial cases occurred. Three further cases occurred in South Africa in 1975, with origin postulated in Rhodesia. Major outbreaks with several hundreds of cases occurred in Sudan and Zaire in 1976.

ETIOLOGY. This syndrome is caused by morphologically identical viruses, Marburg and Ebola, which are immunologically distinct. These agents probably contain RNA, are about 100 nm in diameter, and have a helical capsid, but vary extremely in length. Particles as long as $14\mu m$ have been found.

EPIDEMIOLOGY. The ecology of Marburg and Ebola viruses is presently unknown. No evidence for Marburg infection was detected in green monkeys captured in Uganda subsequent to the original outbreak. The source of the index infection in Rhodesia and of the Ebola outbreaks in Sudan and Zaire remains a mystery. Transmission is person-to-person, associated with close contact with patients. In Zaire contaminated needles were the source of many infections. Incubation period is about one week.

PATHOLOGY. These viruses attack the lymphoreticular system, the liver, and possibly the pancreas. Prominent hepatocellular necrosis without inflammatory reaction is a hallmark of infection. Large eosinophilic inclusions are found in liver cells, but the over-all pattern of destruction is diffuse, rather than strongly midzonal as in yellow fever.

CLINICAL MANIFESTATIONS AND PATHOLOGIC PHYSIOLOGY. Onset is typically insidious with headache and progressive fever. There is severe myalgia, and often vomiting and/or diarrhea occur. About the fourth day of illness sore throat and abdominal pain appear, and a day or so later many patients develop a fine maculopapular rash over the trunk and back which spreads to the limbs and may fade in two or three days. Bleeding, principally gastrointestinal, begins on the fifth to seventh days and is associated with rapid decompensation, ending in shock and death. Leukopenia, thrombocytopenia, and proteinuria are almost invariably present. There are extreme elevations of plasma transaminases and of amylase. In the few cases studied, definitive evidence for disseminated intravascular coagulation was found.

DIAGNOSIS. High persistent viremia is the basis for establishment of the diagnosis in acute cases. Virus is recovered by inoculation of blood into Vero cell cultures or guinea pigs which undergo a febrile infection. No attempt at virus isolation should be made except in a specially protected facility. Immunofluorescent antibodies appear during the second week after onset and persist for several years. This method is more sensitive than the complement-fixation technique, which also has been used.

PROGNOSIS AND TREATMENT. With sophisticated medical management, mortality in Marburg infection is 25 to 30 per cent. Ebola virus infections treated in rural hospitals were 50 to 90 per cent fatal, the worst prognosis of any viral disease other than rabies. In addition to intensive supportive care, which should include continuous nasogastric aspiration to combat pancreatitis, two other forms of active intervention may be of value: continuous intravenous heparin therapy for intravascular coagulation, and *early* administration of plasma containing virus-specific antibodies.

PREVENTION. The secondary attack rate in African hemorrhagic fever rarely exceeds 10 per cent. Transmission can be interrupted by scrupulous isolation of patients, careful disposal of virus-contaminated excreta and fomites, and the use of protective clothing and full-face respirators by medical personnel.

102.7. EPIDEMIC HEMORRHAGIC FEVER: HEMORRHAGIC NEPHROSONEPHRITIS

Karl M. Johnson

DEFINITION. Epidemic hemorrhagic fever is an acute disease that occurs in northeastern Asia and, in milder form, in northern European U.S.S.R., Scandinavia, Czechoslovakia, Rumania, and Bulgaria. It is characterized by fever, prostration, vomiting, proteinuria, hemorrhagic manifestations, shock, and renal failure.

HISTORY. The disease was first described in the far east of the Soviet Union in the 1930's, with suggestive history as far back as 1913. An epidemic in United Nations troops in Korea, beginning in 1951, attracted much attention.

ETIOLOGY. The disease is caused by a filterable agent first recovered from the striped field mouse, *Apodemus agrarius*, in Korea. Strains also have been recovered from patients.

EPIDEMIOLOGY. The disease is rural, characterized by isolated cases widely separated in place. Environmental exposure in forests or fields near forests is invariably noted. Person-to-person transmission does not occur. Soviet workers believe that the disease is transmitted directly from asymptomatically infected rodents to man by means of virus-contaminated rodent excreta. Some outbreaks in Europe have coincided with population "explosions" of the redbacked vole (*Clethrionomys glareolus*), involving invasion by rodents of fields, barns, and even houses.

PATHOLOGY. Profound, protein-rich retroperitoneal edema is characteristic of early death in shock, but not of later deaths. Changes in various organs apparently have a similar pathogenesis and consist of widespread, often focal, congestion and hemorrhage, sometimes accompanied by necrosis, without significant inflammatory response. The "pathognomonic" lesion is found in the kidneys, which appear swollen and, when incised, exhibit extreme hemorrhagic congestion sharply localized to the medulla. Gross congestion or hemorrhage derived from dilated, congested small blood vessels is also found frequently in the right atrium, the pituitary, and the stomach, and less often in intestines, adrenals, lungs, and central nervous system. Liver and spleen are usually not grossly involved. Petechial hemorrhages may occur in the skin, heart, adrenals, brain, and serous surfaces.

CLINICAL MANIFESTATIONS AND PATHOLOGIC PHYSIOLOGY. The following description is based on the minority of patients (about 20 per cent) who exhibit the more severe form of disease, which can be divided into five clinical phases. All patients, however, have fever, proteinuria, and isohyposthenuria.

The febrile phase lasts three to eight days and is characterized by fever, malaise, a flush over the face and neck, and injection of the eyes and palate. Toward the end of this period, petechiae occur, blood platelets decrease, traces of protein appear in the urine, and the hematocrit begins to rise.

The hypotensive phase develops suddenly during defervescence and lasts one to three days. Shock is insidious with warm dry extremities and initially no increase in pulse rate. The dominant feature is a reduction in effective blood volume owing to a loss of plasma from the vascular system. Hematocrit values may reach 70 per cent, and erythrocytes are sequestered in dilated capillaries. Nausea and vomiting are common, as are back and abdominal pain, the latter having occasioned ill-advised exploratory laparotomy in misdiagnosed cases. Heavy proteinuria and oliguria progressing to acute renal failure occur during this interval. Capillary hemorrhages are most prominent at this time also, and blood leukocytes, earlier normal or reduced, now show a leukemoid reaction.

The oliguric phase begins as the sequestered plasma returns to the vascular system and the hematocrit falls. Deaths during this three- to five-day interval are due to pulmonary edema, hyperkalemia, and shock secondary to dehydration or secondary pulmonary infections. Some patients become hypertensive and display a reactive hypervolemic syndrome that responds to phlebotomy. Biochemical abnormalities associated with renal failure appear at this time.

The diuretic phase, lasting for days or weeks, usually initiates clinical recovery but is fraught with problems in clinical management. Diuresis of 3 to 8 liters daily and isohyposthenuria lead to an extremely brittle situation with respect to hemodynamics and salt balance. Hypokalemia and hypernatremia can be problems. Shock may occur, and bacterial pulmonary infections are common. Nearly a third of all deaths occur during this phase.

Convalescence requires three to twelve weeks and is marked by gradual return of appetite, strength, and urinary concentrating ability.

DIAGNOSIS. Specific diagnosis is made by immunofluorescent technique, using lung sections from *Apodemus* rodents as source of antigen. Most patients already have low titers of antibody in acute phase sera, but diagnostic increases in titer regularly occur by the end of the second week of symptoms. The antibodies persist at least ten years. Retrospective serodiagnosis has now been confirmed in patients from the Soviet Union, Finland, and Japan, as well as Korea. Asymptomatic infections are unusual, but mild clinically apparent cases have been documented.

PROGNOSIS AND TREATMENT. Because antimicrobial drugs, convalescent serum, hormones, and other agents are entirely ineffective, the management of hemorrhagic fever must be supportive and based on an understanding of its physiologic and biochemical characteristics and on frequent clinical observations. Adequate sedation with barbiturates or opiates is frequently required for restlessness. Contrary to the practice in other febrile diseases, fluid intake must be limited because any excess will simply leak out of damaged capillaries and increase edema and symptoms. When intravenous fluid is required, it usually should be 10 per cent dextrose in water, and must be given very slowly. If shock fails to respond to simple measures such as shock blocks, then concentrated (salt-poor) human serum albumin to restore plasma volume may be required. Treatment in the oliguric phase is that of acute renal failure, with careful control of electrolytes and particular attention to hyperkalemia. If oliguria persists, hemodialysis or peritoneal dialysis is indicated. Soviet workers have so treated 60 severe cases and report only three deaths. The chief problem of the diuretic phase is one of careful matching of fluid and electrolyte intake against the brisk urinary output, so as to avoid excessive dehydration and shock, on the one hand, and hypervolemia and pulmonary edema, on the other. Electrolyte abnormalities are still a problem, especially potassium deficiency. Overall mortality under optimal conditions seldom surpasses 5 per cent.

PREVENTION. Preventive measures are based on the assumption that the disease is transmitted by rodents with or without the aid of an associated arthropod vector. Vigorous rodent control measures, as well as dipping of clothing in acaricidal solutions and the individual use of insect repellents, are recommended in endemic areas during seasonal periods of disease activity.

Barnes, W. J. S., and Rosen, L.: Fatal hemorrhagic disease and shock associated with primary dengue infection on a Pacific island. Am. J. Trop. Med. Hyg., 23:495, 1974.

Bokisch, V. A., Top, F. H., Jr., Russell, R. K., Dixon, F. J., and Muller-Eberhard, H. J.: The potential pathogenic role of complement in dengue hemorrhagic shock syndrome. N. Engl. J. Med., 289:996, 1973.

Casals, J., Henderson, B. E., Hoogstraal, H., Johnson, K. M., and Shelokov, A.: A review of Soviet viral hemorrhagic fevers, 1969. J. Infect. Dis., 122:437, 1970.

Groot, H., and Bahia Ribiero, R.: Neutralizing and hemagglutination-inhibiting antibodies to yellow fever 17 years after vaccination with 17D vaccine. Bull. WHO, 27:699, 1962.

Halstead, S. B., et al.: Observations related to pathogenesis of dengue hemorrhagic fever. Yale J. Biol. Med., 42:261, 1970.

International symposium on arenaviral infections of public health importance. Bull. WHO, 52:381, 1975.

Johnson, K. M., Halstead, S. B., and Cohen, S. N.: Hemorrhagic fevers of Southeast Asia and South America: A comparative appraisal. In Melnick, J. L. (ed.): Progress in Medical Virology, Vol. 9. Basel/New York, S. Karger, 1967, pp. 105–158.

Johnson, K. M., Webb, P. A., Lange, J. V., and Murphy, F. A.: Isolation and partial characterization of a new virus causing haemorrhagic fever in Zaire. Lancet, 1:569, 1977.

Lee, H. W., Lee, P. W., and Johnson, K. M.: Isolation of the etiologic agent of Korean hemorrhagic fever. J. Infect. Dis., 137:298, 1978.

Mertens, P. E., Patton, R., Baum, J. J., and Monath, T. P.: Clinical presentation of Lassa fever cases during the hospital epidemic at Zorzar, Liberia, March–April 1972. Am. J. Trop. Med. Hyg., 22:780, 1973.

Pantheir, R.: Yellow fever: In Debré, R., and Celers, J. (eds.): Clinicial Virology. Philadelphia, W. B. Saunders Company, 1970, pp. 299–315.

Sabattini, M., and Maiztegui, J. I.: Fiebre hemorrágica argentina. Medicina (Buenos Aires), 30: Suppl. 1, 111, 1970.

Simpson, D. I. H., Knight, E. M., et al.: Congo virus: A hitherto undescribed virus occurring in Africa. Part I. Human isolation — clinical notes. East Afr. Med. J., 44:87, 1967.

Smorodintsev, A. A., Kazbintsev, L. I., and Chudakov, V. G.: Virus Hemorrhagic Fevers (Y. Halperin, translator). Washington, D.C., Office of Technical Services, U.S. Department of Commerce, 1964.

Stode, G. K.: Yellow Fever. New York, McGraw-Hill Book Company, 1951.

Symposium on Epidemic Hemorrhagic Fever. Am. J. Med., 16:617, 1954.

Viral haemorrhagic fever. Weekly Epidemiol. Rec. WHO, 52:177, 1977.

WHO Expert Committee on Yellow Fever, Third Report. WHO Tech. Rep. Ser. No. 479, 1971.

VIRAL DISEASES CHARACTERIZED BY PROTRACTED, RECURRENT, OR LATENT INFECTION

These diseases are discussed in detail in Ch. 310.

VIRAL DISEASES (PRESUMPTIVE)

103. CAT SCRATCH DISEASE

(Benign Nonbacterial Regional Lymphadenitis, Inoculation Lymphoreticulosis)

Andrew M. Margileth

DEFINITION. Cat scratch disease is a benign, self-limited disease characterized by tender regional lymphadenopathy and frequently preceded by a primary skin lesion following cat contact or scratches, or both. The disease is being recognized more frequently in both children and adults. Persistence of the adenopathy for several months in a generally healthy patient with gradual spontaneous resolution of the enlarged bubo is its natural course.

ETIOLOGY. Since 1967, when Warwick reviewed the etiologic investigations in cat scratch disease, little information regarding etiology has been published. A number of studies, including those of the writer and his associates, have not demonstrated any instance of complicity of fungi or bacteria, including rickettsiae or mycobacteria. It is presumed therefore that the etiologic agent is probably a virus. Particles that could represent viral particles have been detected (Kalter, 1970) in the cell cytoplasm of biopsied human lymph nodes. It appears that during acute illness patients with cat scratch disease have a transient state of lymphocyte unresponsiveness similar to that of patients with a variety of illnesses caused by viruses and mycoplasmas.

EPIDEMIOLOGY. Since the initial description by Debré (1950), more than 1500 patients with cat scratch disease have been reported in about 600 articles. An estimated 2000 unreported cases occur annually in the United States, primarily in children. The true incidence is unknown, because the number of reported cases varies greatly depending on the interest of the physician and the availability of the skin test antigen. The disease is worldwide, occurring in all races and apparently equally in both sexes. In temperate zones, most cases have occurred during fall and winter. Seasonal variation is minimal in warmer climates. Several epidemics in the same house or geographic locality have been recorded.

TRANSMISSION AND COMMUNICABILITY. The mode of transmission is presumably by direct contact, as the bubo usually follows a scratch, bite, or lick from a young cat. Cat contact occurs in 90 per cent of patients. The disease has also been thought to have developed through dog bite or scratch and, rarely, following a scratch from a thorn, wood splinter, or fish bone. An inoculation site may be detected in 55 to 96 per cent of patients. The disease has been transmitted experimentally to man, monkeys, baboons, and Hartley guinea pigs. There is no evidence that the disease can be transmitted from human to human. Regional lymphadenopathy was produced in each species following an intradermal injection of material aspirated from suppurative lymph nodes of human patients. Attempts to isolate virus from cat saliva or claws have been unsuccessful. The healthy cat — often a kitten — apparently acts as a mechanical vector for the infective agent, for skin tests with CS antigen on the implicated cats have been nonreactive. The writer's studies in family outbreaks have shown that the family cat usually transmits the causative agent no longer than two to three weeks.

PATHOGENESIS AND PATHOLOGY. No serologic test is available to measure antibodies to the causative agent. Fortunately, the cat scratch skin test is reliable and has a high degree of specificity; the reaction is a delayed hypersensitivity type. A positive reaction is usually detected at the time the clinical diagnosis is suspected; however, conversion may be delayed up to four weeks thereafter. Cutaneous reactivity lasts up to ten years. Second attacks have not been reported. A recurrence in the nodes originally involved has been observed, but is quite rare.

Biopsied lymph nodes may show distinct yet nonspecific stages, depending upon the interval between the time of onset and the time of biopsy. The early lesions reveal a reticulum cell hyperplasia followed by necrotizing granulomas, occasionally with giant cells, then multiple microabscesses, and, weeks to months later, frank abscess formation. Consequently, a presumptive histopathologic diagnosis of tularemia, brucellosis, tuberculosis, or sarcoidosis might be considered. Rarely a biopsy made early before suppuration has appeared has shown histologic changes, including reticulum cell hyperplasia and granulomas, which have been confused with those of Hodgkin's disease.

CLINICAL MANIFESTATIONS. The patient usually is not ill in spite of impressive lymphadenopathy; however, malaise, fever, and influenza-like symptoms may be present. Three to ten days elapse from the time of the scratch or contact until a primary skin papule or pustule forms. It may exhibit one or more erythematous papules. Rarely unilateral conjunctival granulomas occur. An inoculation site (a scratch or a primary lesion, or both) may be detected in more than half the patients, de-

pending upon the thoroughness of the examination and the duration of the bubo when first seen. Most primary lesions persist for one to three weeks; lesions rarely persist for seven weeks. The primary lesion usually heals without scar formation. Regional lymphadenopathy usually develops about two weeks after the scratch (observed range, 3 to 50 days). Lymphangitis has not been observed. Tender nodes, present in 80 per cent of patients for the first one or two weeks, are commonly found in the head, neck, or axilla. Epitrochlear, inguinal, femoral, or popliteal areas are involved less frequently. Multiple site involvement has occurred in about 10 to 20 per cent of cases in the writer's experience. Node size varies from 1 to 5 cm in the majority of cases. Enlargement persists for two to four months; lymphadenopathy rarely lasts for 6 to 24 months. Macroscopic node suppuration occurs in about one tenth of patients seen in office practice and in about one quarter of those admitted to hospitals.

No clinical signs other than lymphadenopathy occurred in approximately half of our 413 patients observed at various times throughout a 19-year period. In about one third of similar reported cases, patients had fever (38.3 to 41.2° C) lasting for 5 to 9 (1 to 30) days; 32 per cent of our 413 patients had malaise or an influenza-like syndrome lasting about 4 (1 to 21) days. Splenomegaly occurred in 16 per cent of the last 100 patients. Exanthems, i.e., maculopapular, petechial, or erythema nodosum or multiforme types, have been reported in 4 per cent of affected patients. The rash usually lasted 4 to 9 (3 to 14) days.

Unusual clinical manifestations reported include the oculoglandular syndrome of Parinaud (40 cases), presenting as an ocular granuloma or conjunctivitis with parotid area swelling caused by preauricular lymphadenopathy; encephalitis (41); thrombocytopenic purpura (7); osteomyelitis (4); and primary atypical pneumonia (4). In any patient with an ocular granuloma or conjunctivitis and parotid area swelling (preauricular lymphadenopathy), cat scratch disease should always be considered.

Children with central nervous system involvement may develop encephalopathy, meningitis, radiculitis, polyneuritis, or myelitis with paraplegia. Onset of neu-

TABLE 1.   Clinical Features in 100 Patients with Cat Scratch Adenopathy and a Positive Skin Test (April 1975 to July 1977)

Category	Percentage of Patients
Animal contact	
Cat	88
Dog	9
None	3
Animal scratch	
Cat	72
Dog	3
None	23
Primary lesion	
Skin papule or pustule	53
Eye granuloma	3
Symptoms and signs	
None	66
Fever (38.3–42.1° C)	26
Malaise	17
Splenomegaly	16
Sore throat	7
Headache	5
Parotid swelling	2

TABLE 2. Cat Scratch Lymphadenopathy in 100 Patients—Clinical Characteristics of Involved Nodes and Duration of Adenopathy (April 1975 to July 1977)

Adenopathy (N = 100)	Per Cent	Size (cm) (N = 100)	Per Cent
Single node	46	1.0 to <3.0	46
Multiple nodes	54	3.0 to <5.0	39
Multiple sites	23	≥5.0	15
Tender nodes	81		
Suppuration	10		

Location (N = 120)	Per Cent	Duration (N = 100)	Per Cent
Head: total (N = 29)	24	Prior to diagnosis	
Submandibular	21	2 to <4 weeks	56
Preauricular	3	1 to <2 months	20
Neck: total (N = 44)	37	2 to <4 months	17
Posterior	20	4 to <6 months	4
Anterior	10	6 to <12 months	3
Supraclavicular	7	Regression (months, <1.0 cm)	
Extremities: total (N = 47)	39	1 to <2	24
Axillary	27	2 to <6	62
Epitrochlear	6	6 to <12	8
Inguinal	4	12 to <24	4
Femoral	2	≥24	1

rologic symptoms is sudden, usually with fever, and occurs within one to six weeks of the onset of adenopathy. Major symptoms and signs found in 41 cases of neurologic involvement were as follows: coma or convulsions in two thirds, neurologic abnormalities, noted above, in 25 per cent, and lethargy and/or confusion in one sixth. In 12 of 22 patients (55 per cent) with neurologic involvement, cerebrospinal fluid pleocytosis, elevated protein, or both were detected. Electroencephalograms were abnormal in most patients. Severe manifestations have lasted for one to two weeks, with gradual recovery to normal status in one to six months in most patients.

Recovery from thrombocytopenic purpura, osteomyelitis, pneumonitis, and Parinaud's syndrome has been complete.

DIAGNOSIS. Regional lymphadenopathy developing two weeks after cat contact and/or scratches, and especially if a primary inoculation papule or pustule followed the scratch, suggests a diagnosis of cat scratch disease. Three of the four following manifestations would confirm the diagnosis in a typical case, whereas all four would be necessary in an atypical case: (1) a history of animal (usually cat) contact or presence of a scratch or a primary dermal or eye lesion; (2) aspiration of sterile pus from the node (a presumptive diagnostic test) or negative laboratory studies excluding other etiologic possibilities; (3) a positive skin test to cat scratch antigen (5 per cent false positives occur; use of only one antigen may give a false negative result in 10 to 20 per cent of patients); (4) node biopsy revealing histopathology consistent with cat scratch disease.

If a negative skin test is found to one or two different cat scratch antigens applied simultaneously and again four weeks later, and if other studies are negative, a biopsy must be considered to rule out a benign tumor or lymphoma. The presence of tenderness favors cat scratch or a pyogenic or mycobacterial adenopathy rather than a neoplasm.

Skin Tests. A skin test using cat scratch antigen is positive in 90 per cent of patients who are clinically suspected of having cat scratch disease and have had cat scratches and/or contact. A negative skin test often occurs if the duration of illness is less than three or four weeks, and about 10 per cent of patients with typical cat scratch disease will have negative skin tests with one or two different antigens. The positive reaction consists of a wheal or papule with 5 mm or more of induration, with or without erythema, occurring 48 to 72 hours after intradermal inoculation of 0.1 ml of antigen. Induration may persist for five to six days or longer. A positive test may be obtained for years (10 to 28) after the initial episode and hence does not necessarily indicate concurrent disease. False positive reactions have been reported in veterinarians (12 to 29 per cent), healthy persons (4 to 5 per cent), and family contacts; the over-all incidence is 5 per cent. Thus the limit of confidence for a positive reaction is about 95 per cent. If the reaction is negative at four-week intervals, the disease can be excluded with reasonable certainty, especially if two different antigens are used. Repeated skin testing with CS antigen in the same patients has not produced positive reactions. Skin tests with PPD-S and atypical PPD mycobacterium antigens have been rarely positive in patients with cat scratch disease; six patients with the disease had positive reactions to PPD Battey out of 413 patients tested. Dog contact and/or scratches were noted with greater frequency (8 per cent) in this period (1975 to 1977) than in the Margileth 1968 and 1971 studies.

Since CS antigen is not available commercially, all aspirated pus from affected nodes should be saved to prepare test antigen. This subject is treated in greater detail elsewhere (Margileth, 1968, 1971).

Laboratory Data. Laboratory tests are not diagnostic, but eosinophilia has been reported. At the onset the number of polymorphonuclear cells may be increased with a mild leukocytosis. A sedimentation rate, usually elevated during the first few weeks of adenopathy, suggests an inflammatory lymphadenitis, and is recommended.

DIFFERENTIAL DIAGNOSIS. Cat scratch disease should be considered in all patients with persistent lymphadenopathy (over three weeks), because it is the most common cause of chronic regional lymphadenitis in children or adolescents. The presence of an inoculation (dermal or ocular) lesion would strongly suggest cat scratch disease. Other, less common causes are sporotrichosis, primary syphilis, lymphogranuloma venereum, typical or atypical tuberculosis, other bacterial adenitis, tularemia, brucellosis, histoplasmosis, coccidioidomycosis, sarcoidosis, toxoplasmosis, infectious mononucleosis, and benign or malignant tumors. In atypical forms of cat scratch disease, one must consider benign recurrent parotid lymphosialadenopathy, Parinaud's oculoglandular disease, encephalitis, pneumonia, thrombocytopenic purpura, erythema nodosum, and osteomyelitis, as well as fluctuant lymphadenopathy simulating cystic hygroma or a thyroglossal duct cyst. If CS skin tests are negative, as well as appropriate cultures and serologic and other skin tests, a node biopsy will usually determine the cause.

TREATMENT. In the majority of patients the disease is self-limited. The best therapy is reassurance that the adenopathy is benign and in most cases will subside spontaneously within two or three months. Thus management consists of reassurance with appropriate follow-up examination, analgesics for pain, and aspiration if suppuration occurs. Lack of response to antimicrobials is the rule; if cat scratch disease is suspected, antimicrobial drugs are not recommended. In the child whose node suppurates, needle aspiration on an ambulatory basis is preferred to incision and drainage. Aspiration is performed, usually without local anesthesia. After washing with Betadine cleanser, a needle (18 or 20 gauge) is inserted through normal skin at the base of the mass in order to avoid a chronic sinus tract in the event that a tuberculous lesion is present. Aspiration provides material for skin test antigen, relieves painful adenopathy, and usually allows the patient to become symptom free within 24 to 48 hours. If fluid recurs, reaspiration may be necessary. Application of moist soaks to the primary lesion may facilitate drainage and shorten the duration of lymphadenopathy. The efficacy of steroid therapy in cat scratch disease is questionable, and it is not recommended. Excisional biopsy of the node may be necessary in selected patients because of persistent pain or for diagnostic purposes. Spontaneous drainage occurred in 6 per cent of our last 100 patients.

PROGNOSIS. The prognosis is excellent; lymphadenopathy usually regresses spontaneously in two to three months. One attack appears to confer lifelong immunity. Complications and sequelae are almost nonexistent and have not been seen or reported in typical cases. In France in one patient with encephalopathy, death apparently occurred during treatment of continued seizures with hypothermia. Rare patients have been reported to have had chronic adenopathy for two years; we have observed one such case in an adult in our most recent series. Only two patients have had a recurrence of the same adenopathy after a three-year period of well-being.

PREVENTION. Because of increasing numbers of household pets (50 million cats in the United States), cat scratch disease will be difficult to prevent. Disposal of the suspect cat is not recommended, because the cat involved is invariably well. Four to 9 per cent of family members scratched by the same cat may develop cat scratch disease. The patient with the disease does not require isolation or quarantine, as there is no evidence of disease spread from man to man. Active or passive protection is not available.

Altman, R. P., and Margileth, A. M.: Cervical lymphadenopathy from atypical mycobacteria — diagnosis and surgical treatment. J. Pediat. Surg., 10:419, 1975.

Margileth, A. M.: Cat-scratch disease in 65 patients: Evaluation of cat scratch skin test antigen in 109 subjects. Clin. Proc. Child. Hosp. D.C., 27:213, 1971.

Margileth, A. M., London, W. T., and Sever, J. L.: Cat scratch disease virus? Negative viral studies in mammals. Submitted for publication.

Warwick, W. J.: The cat-scratch syndrome; many diseases or one disease? Prog. Med. Virol., 9:256, 1967.

104. VIRAL GASTROENTERITIS CAUSED BY NORWALK-LIKE AGENTS AND ROTAVIRUSES

(Acute Infectious Nonbacterial Gastroenteritis, Epidemic Diarrhea, Winter Vomiting Disease)

Raphael Dolin

DEFINITION. The term "nonbacterial gastroenteritis," along with the descriptive phrases listed above, has referred to a group of acute, common, self-limited illnesses characterized chiefly by vomiting and/or diarrhea. An infectious cause for these diseases had been previously suspected, but it has been only recently that specific viral agents which cause at least a portion of such illnesses have been detected.

ETIOLOGY. Two groups of viral agents which induce acute gastroenteritis have been described. The first is the Norwalk-like agents, generally named after the location of the outbreak from which they have been derived (Norwalk, Hawaii, Montgomery County, "W," and Ditchling agents). These agents have not been cultivated in vitro and have been only partly characterized. They are small (26 to 27 nm in diameter), nonenveloped viral agents found in the stools of acutely ill patients. The biophysical properties of the best studied of these, the Norwalk agent, resemble those of parvoviruses. They have, thus, also been referred to as "parvovirus-like" agents. Among the Norwalk-like agents, at least three antigenic types have been detected thus far.

The second group, described in 1973, is the rotaviruses, also referred to earlier as "duovirus" or "reovirus-like" agents, which have been tentatively classified within the family of Reoviridae of mammalian viruses. They are 66 to 70 nm in diameter, contain double-stranded RNA, and have a characteristic double shell appearance. Although strain differences have not been fully analyzed, human rotaviruses appear to be of at least two antigenic types. Human rotaviruses can only be grown with difficulty in vitro, but can be detected directly in stool by a variety of techniques (see below).

It is of interest that other, previously described groups of viruses which infect the gastrointestinal tract (e.g., enteroviruses) do not appear to be major causes of acute gastroenteritis (see Ch. 97).

EPIDEMIOLOGY. Little is known about the specific epidemiology of the Norwalk-like agents because of the lack of suitable detection methods. Naturally occurring illnesses from which these agents have been derived appear to be exceedingly common and widespread and involve all age groups. Illness occurs most frequently between September and March in the Northern Hemisphere, and can present in distinct outbreaks with explosive patterns of spread.

Rotaviruses, on the other hand, have a well described epidemiologic pattern. Rotavirus-induced gastroenteritis occurs most frequently between 6 and 24 months of age, and occasionally up to 4 years of age. Disease also occurs in neonates. Illness in older children and adults is apparently unusual, although reinfection is common. Fifty-two to 90 per cent of individuals above two years of age have serum antibody against rotavirus. Rotavirus infections are seen primarily during the winter months in both Northern and Southern Hemispheres. Cases occur both sporadically and in distinct outbreaks during that time. Rotavirus infections have accounted for 42 to 55 per cent of hospitalized cases of gastroenteritis among infants and young children in studies carried out throughout the world.

PATHOGENESIS. *Acute infection with Norwalk and Hawaii agents* results in reversible histopathologic lesions which primarily involve the upper jejunum, with relative sparing of the stomach and rectum. The jejunal mucosa remains intact, but there is marked blunting of villi and shortening of microvilli. The lamina propria is infiltrated with both polymorphonuclear and mononuclear cells. Acute illness is also accompanied by malabsorption of d-xylose and fat. *Rotavirus infections* induce a similar pathology in the duodenum and jejunum, although inflammatory changes can on occasion be seen in the stomach and rectum.

The characteristics of immunity to infection with Norwalk-like agents and rotaviruses are not well defined. Such immunity does not correlate closely with serum antibody levels, and, in the case of the Norwalk agent, appears to wane after one to two years.

CLINICAL MANIFESTATIONS. *Illness induced by the Norwalk-like agents* consists of nausea, abdominal cramps, vomiting, and/or diarrhea, often accompanied by headache and myalgias. Onset of illness is often abrupt, and although both vomiting and diarrhea usually occur, either can be present alone. Low-grade fever ($< 38.9°$ C) can be found in approximately 50 to 60 per cent of patients. Incubation period for illness is generally from 18 to 48 hours, and disease manifestations last from 48 to 72 hours. Disease remits spontaneously and without known sequelae.

Rotavirus infections have clinical features which are similar to those described for the Norwalk-like agents. Incubation periods range from 24 hours to 96 hours, and among hospitalized children illness lasts for five to eight days. Even among hospitalized children, illness appears to be generally mild, although occasionally more severe and rarely fatal cases have been reported. Rotaviruses appear to be one of the causes of infantile diarrhea, which is a source of significant morbidity and mortality in economically underdeveloped countries.

DIAGNOSIS. Laboratory Tests. Norwalk-like agents, and antibody directed against them, currently can be detected only by immune electron microscopy, a spe-

cialized technique not suited for routine or large-scale investigations. Norwalk agent is found in stools during the first four to five days of illness, and serum antibody rises are noted two to six weeks later. Rotaviruses are easily detected in stools by a variety of techniques, including complement fixation (CF), immunofluorescence, and conventional electron microscopy. Virus can be found in stools for up to eight days and occasionally longer after onset of illness, and serum antibody (CF) rises are seen by two weeks after illness.

Clinical Diagnosis. Clinical diagnosis of infection with Norwalk-like agents or rotaviruses can be suspected on the basis of epidemiologic information (age, time of year, secondary cases). Although illness is generally milder than that observed with several bacterial pathogens, individual virus-induced cases cannot be differentiated from other causes of acute gastroenteritis on clinical grounds alone. Fecal leukocytes are absent in Norwalk-induced disease, and are usually absent in rotavirus infections, which may prove helpful for early differentiation from *Shigella* or *Salmonella* enteritis (see Ch. 153 and 155).

TREATMENT. Acute viral gastroenteritis is generally a benign, self-limited illness which requires no specific therapy. In severe cases, particularly in the very young, fluid replacement may be necessary, which can be generally provided in the form of clear liquids by mouth. In severe fluid loss, intravenous fluid and electrolyte replacement should be administered promptly. Occasionally, symptomatic treatment of headache or nausea may be required, and restriction of activity during acute illness according to the patient's own symptoms would appear to be prudent. Administration of inhibitors of intestinal motility may be considered in severe diarrhea, but their effect on these illnesses has not been studied.

PREVENTION. There are currently no available methods for prevention or control of these diseases, which represent major public health problems. In addition to the Norwalk-like agents and the rotaviruses, it is likely that other agents which induce acute gastroenteritis will be found in future studies.

Appleton, A. Z., Buckley, M., Thom, B. T., Colton, J. L., and Henderson, S.: Virus-like particles in winter vomiting disease. Lancet, 1:409, 1977.

Bishop, R. F., Davidson, G. P., Holmes, I. H., and Ruck, B. J.: Virus particles in epithelial cells of duodenal mucosa from children with acute nonbacterial gastroenteritis. Lancet, 2:1281, 1973.

Dolin, R., Blacklow, N. R., DuPont, H., Buscho, R. F., Wyatt, R. G., Kasel, J. A., Hornick, R., and Chanock, R. M.: Biological properties of Norwalk agent of acute infectious nonbacterial gastroenteritis. Proc. Soc. Exp. Biol. Med., 140:578, 1972.

Dolin, R., Levy, A. G., Wyatt, R. G., Thornhill, T. S., and Gardner, J. D.: Viral gastroenteritis induced by the Hawaii agent: Jejunal histopathology and serologic response. Am. J. Med., 59:761, 1975.

Flewett, T. H., Davies, H., Bryden, A. S., and Robertson, M. J.: Acute gastroenteritis associated with reovirus-like particles. J. Clin. Path., 27:608, 1974.

Kapikian, A. Z., Kim, H. W., Wyatt, R. G., Cline, W. L., Arrobio, J. O., Brandt, C. O., Rodriguez, W. J., Sack, D. A., Chanock, R. M., and Parrot, R. H.: Human reovirus-like agent as the major pathogen associated with winter gastroenteritis in hospitalized infants and young children. N. Engl. J. Med., 294:965, 1976.

Kapikian, A. Z., Wyatt, R. G., Dolin, R., Thornhill, T. S., Kalica, A. R., and Chanock, R. M.: Visualization of a 27 nm particle associated with acute infectious nonbacterial gastroenteritis. J. Virol., 10:1075, 1972.

Middleton, P. J., Szymanski, M. T., Abbott, G. D., Bortolussi, R., and Hamilton, J. R.: Orbivirus acute gastroenteritis of infancy. Lancet, 1:1241, 1974.

105. EPIDEMIC NEUROMYASTHENIA
(Iceland Disease, Benign Myalgic Encephalomyelitis)
Paul B. Beeson

Between 1934 and 1960, several epidemics were reported of symptoms resembling those of poliomyelitis. The acute phase was often followed by a prolonged period of disability, with headache, muscular weakness, fatigue, and mood depression.

Most outbreaks have occurred in summer, and about half of those reported have involved hospital personnel, especially student nurses. In all instances the attack rate has been much higher in women. Sporadic cases have been reported, but the diagnosis is difficult in the absence of an epidemic.

Severe generalized headache is nearly always a prominent complaint at the onset, and frequently there are pain and stiffness of the neck. Generalized tenderness of the muscles is common, and they frequently exhibit a characteristic of rapid fatigue and loss of motor power on repeated contraction. In perhaps 40 per cent of affected persons, areas of muscle weakness or paralysis appear during the first two weeks. These may be in the trunk or the extremities, and the pattern of involvement often changes from day to day. Cranial nerve signs, bladder dysfunction, and paresthesia may also be noted. In most cases complete recovery of neurologic function occurs within four to eight weeks, but relapses and exacerbations are common during the next few months.

Fever is inconspicuous or absent. The cerebrospinal fluid is usually normal, and routine tests of blood and urine reveal nothing of significance.

A striking feature of this illness is the prolonged period of disability after subsidence of the acute phase. Particularly troublesome are the behavioral manifestations of irritability and mood depression, which together with easy fatigue may interfere with normal living for months and even years after the acute episode. In this stage the subject may present a picture of hysteria or of simple neurasthenia.

Deaths have not been reported; therefore nothing is known of the pathology.

Extensive laboratory investigations failed to yield evidence of participation of any known pathogenic microorganism; nevertheless, the presumption had seemed warranted that it was an infectious disease. However, McEvedy and Beard have cast doubt on the likelihood of an infectious etiology. They carefully reviewed the reports of 15 recorded outbreaks, with special attention to the well-documented epidemic among nurses at the Royal Free Hospital, London. They suggest alternatively that these epidemics represented psychosocial phenomena: either mass hysteria among the subjects or altered medical perception. Their analysis and argument are persuasive, and the apparent lessening of the disease coincident with control of poliomyelitis further strengthens the case that some of the epidemics were indeed examples of mass hysteria.

Acheson, E. D.: The clinical syndrome variously called benign myalgic encephalomyelitis, Iceland disease and epidemic neuromyasthenia. Am. J. Med., 26:569, 1959.

Dillon, M. J., Marshall, W. C., Dudgeon, J. A., and Steigman, A. J.: Epidemic neuromyasthenia: Outbreak among nurses at a children's hospital. Br. Med. J., 1:301, 1974.

McEvedy, C. P., and Beard, A. W.: Concept of benign myalgic encephalomyelitis. Br. Med. J., 1:11, 1970.

Section Two   BACTERIAL DISEASES

106. INTRODUCTION
Walsh McDermott

In recent decades the term "bacterial diseases" has undergone considerable expansion for several reasons: (1) Certain organisms, the rickettsiae, the chlamydiae, and, for all practical purposes, the mycoplasmas, are now considered to be bacteria; (2) new organisms causing new conditions such as legionnaires' disease get discovered; and (3) there have been significant changes in the relation to man of bacterial species long known as "harmless." The first of these changes is of little consequence to most readers, for it is essentially a question of semantics. The second change likewise presents no real problems, for the emergence of recognizable entities such as legionnaires' disease does not happen every day, and, when they are recognized, their description can be easily included in an additional chapter. It is the third change — the continuing alteration in our relation to our own, or the "community," bacterial flora — that continues to significantly expand what the physician should know. As so much of this changing relationship in bacterial disease is a consequence of our increasing capability to intervene, its degree of prominence is a crude indicator of the state of the health services available. Thus it is that for the past few decades the problems presented by bacterial and mycotic disease have presented themselves in two different forms, depending largely upon the nature of the society.

In the economically underdeveloped parts of the world, the individual diseases have presented in classic form, each occupying its traditional niche in the overall pattern. By contrast, in nations with highly developed health services, the familiar bacterial diseases have by no means disappeared, but their menace has been largely nullified by vaccines and by prompt and appropriate antimicrobial therapy. For example, one hears that lobar pneumonia "has largely disappeared." In actuality, it *has* become much less prominent, not because its major cause, pneumococcal infection, is any less frequent, but because with prompt chemotherapy the early pneumonic lesion is halted in its progress well short of the confines of the lobe. It is the same old pneumonia, but it is no longer "lobar." Expressed differently, without any change in the annual incidence of pneumococcal infection or disease, the annual incidence of *serious problems* from this cause has substantially diminished. Ideally they will be diminished still further by the appropriate use of the vaccine. In place of such clinical problems there are now essentially new menaces in the serious systemic disease produced by *E. coli, Proteus* species, *Pseudomonas, Candida,* and other microbes that were formerly regarded as basically harmless inhabitants of man. The diseases produced by staphylococci and tubercle bacilli can likewise be regarded as being partially of this sort, in that the microbes can subsist harmlessly in the tissues for considerable periods between eruptions as destructive disease. In effect these new clinical patterns represent *endogenous microbial disease* — clinical entities that appear almost exclusively in people with some temporary or sustained lowering of local or general defenses. Because of the resulting changes in the tissue environment, disease-producing microbes are evoked from the dormant or latent state. Generally speaking, these changes in the internal milieu represent a direct or indirect consequence of our modern therapies. They are the unsought-for effects of practical therapeutic gains that in themselves represent great scientific achievements. And because weakened hosts and powerful therapies tend to be congregated in hospitals, such infections are particularly prominent there — the so-called "nosocomial infections." The practices involved include the use of corticosteroids and immunosuppressants; the suppression of customary microbial flora by drugs, thus compromising the protection to the host afforded by *bacterial interference;* surgical procedures, e.g., subtotal gastrectomy or splenectomy that can reduce previously acquired host resistance; and the longer survival of many patients despite protracted, severe, and ultimately fatal illness. Sometimes, as elucidated in the studies by Pierce and Sanford, it is the equipment that is at fault.

The striking change in a large university center in just the first two decades of the "antibiotic era" may be seen from Rogers' study published in 1959 (see accompanying table). *Over-all* infections were either the major or a significant contributory cause of death in 28 per cent of patients hospitalized in 1938, in contrast to only 14 per cent of those hospitalized in 1958. In terms of the number of persons involved, therefore, great progress has been made. The nature of today's problem could be foreseen, however, by the observation that in 1938 most of the "28 per cent" *were admitted* to the hospital with infection; less than 10 per cent of the infections were hospital associated. Only 20 years later, when much of the current technology was available, over *half* of the "14 per cent" with serious infections had acquired them after having been admitted to the hospital for a nonmicrobial — usually life-threatening — disease problem.

Changing Pattern of Life-Threatening Microbial Disease at Necropsy (%) of 200 Consecutive Admissions in Each Period

Etiology	Year of Study	
	1938–1940	1957–1958
Pneumococci, streptococci, tubercle bacilli	20	2
Staphylococci	8	8
Gram-negative bacilli (aerobic)	4	11
Mycotic	1	4
"Hospital-associated infections"	7	54

The increasing ability to alter man's internal environment has had the effect that virtually no microbial species today can be considered nonpathogenic, for in appropriate circumstances virtually any can give rise to disease. All these mechanisms unleash what are, in effect, "new" microbial disease. There are other "new" diseases that may have been similarly unleashed or may have merely become easier to recognize by virtue of the selectivity of drug action. The separation of "atypical" pneumonia from bacterial pneumonia by the introduction of sulfonamide back in the 1930's and the importance of "atypical" mycobacteria as disease agents once antituberculous therapy was introduced are cases in point. What is happening was biologically predictable, and the changing nature of the situation may be expected to continue.

To be capable of staying with this change, the physician must know considerably more about the behavior of microbes, as they cause disease and are exposed to drugs with an otherwise normal or a compromised host, than he had to master only one or two decades ago. This knowledge is of two sorts: certain concepts and principles related to the microbe-drug-host interactions, and a body of knowledge sufficient to permit him to make microbiologically relevant diagnoses on clinical grounds. Knowledge of the latter sort is presented in the individual chapters that follow. For discussion of host defenses, see Ch. 41 and 119; for their behavior during administration of immunosuppressive drugs, the reader is referred to Ch. 38, 40, and 527. Endogenous microbial disease itself is discussed in Ch. 124, whereas the concepts and principles related to microbe-drug-host interactions are considered in Ch. 189 and 190.

McDermott, W.: Inapparent Infection. The Dyer Lecture. Public Health Rep., 74:485, 1959.

National Nosocomial Infections Study — United States, 1975-1976. MMWR, Vol. 26, No. 46, November 18, 1977.

Pierce, A. K., and Sanford, J. P.: Bacterial contamination of aerosols. Arch. Intern. Med., 131:156, 1973.

Rogers, D., et al.: Infections in the altered host. *In* Year Book of Medicine, 1978, Chicago, Year Book Medical Publishers.

Rogers, D. E.: The changing pattern of life-threatening microbial disease. N. Engl. J. Med., 261:677, 1959.

RICKETTSIAL DISEASES

107. INTRODUCTION

Charles L. Wisseman, Jr.

The diseases commonly referred to as the rickettsial diseases of man consist of several clinical entities, usually acute, self-limited fevers, caused by bacteria of the family Rickettsiaceae. They fall naturally into the typhus-like diseases (typhus groups, spotted fever group, and scrub typhus group), Q fever, and trench fever. The typhus-like diseases are caused by organisms of the genus *Rickettsia;* Q fever by *Coxiella burnetii;* and trench fever by *Rochalimaea quintana. Bartonella bacilliformis,* the cause of bartonellosis, belonging to the family Bartonellaceae, is included here for convenience because it is the only other member of the order Rickettsiales known to cause human disease and because there are certain selected superficial similarities (facultative intracellular parasite, arthropod transmission).

Organisms of the *Rickettsia, Coxiella,* and *Rochalimaea* genera, although very different in many respects, are very small bacteria (the former concept of intermediate between bacteria and viruses is no longer tenable) with a gram-negative bacterium-like cell wall, bacterial type internal structure (typical prokaryotic DNA arrangement with a genome size roughly equivalent to that of *Neisseria;* ribosomes), often a slime layer or microcapsule, and a substantially similar independent metabolic activity. Organisms of the genus *Rickettsia* and *Coxiella burnetii* are obligate intracellular parasites, i.e., they are known to date to grow only within eukaryotic host cells. *Rochalimaea quintana* can be grown on cell-free medium and grows extracellularly in the louse gut, but *may* be a facultative intracellular parasite in man. All organisms of the genus *Rickettsia* have the capacity to penetrate directly through the host cell plasma membrane into the cytoplasm, can cause host cell lysis from without, and multiply by binary fission free in the host cell cytoplasm not surrounded by a vacuolar membrane. Different species vary in their capacity to interact with other host cell membranes. Thus members of the spotted fever group can penetrate into the host cell nucleus, and these, as well as *R. mooseri,* can escape through the plasma membrane without requiring complete host cell destruction as does *R. prowazekii. Coxiella burnetii,* on the other hand, does not actively penetrate into host cells, is probably taken in by endocytosis, and grows within a membrane bound vacuole. These differences in action on host cell membranes are probably related to differences in disease patterns (host response) and immune mechanisms. Active penetration of host cells appears to be correlated with mouse lethal toxic action and hemolytic properties. On the other hand, members of the genus *Rickettsia* which have been studied and *Coxiella burnetii* have endotoxins similar in physiologic action to those of gram-negative bacilli.

All rickettsioses are transmitted by arthropod vectors, although Q fever is usually acquired from domestic animals. Many years ago, McGaw proposed an epidemiologically useful classification of rickettsial diseases based on arthropod vector — viz., louse-borne, flea-borne, tick-borne, and mite-borne. With the exception of louse-borne typhus and trench fevers, in which man is the key vertebrate host and reservoir, all the rickettsioses are zoonoses, existing in a natural cycle involving arthropods (vectors and in some cases reservoirs) and vertebrate (usually mammalian) hosts. In these, man acquires the disease by accidentally intruding into the natural cycle and is a "dead-end" host not sustaining the infection cycle. The reservoir mechanism varies considerably among the rickettsioses. The nonsterile immunity in the vertebrate host, with persisting infection and potential or proved capacity for recrudescence, appears to be important in louse-borne typhus and trench fever, in which the main reservoir is man, and in murine typhus in the rat. In these three infections, the vector (the human body louse in the first two and fleas in the last) does not transmit the organism transovarially to the next generation, and, in the case of louse-borne typhus, the infection in the louse vector is almost invariably fatal to the louse in a week or two. On the other hand, in the case of tick-, mite- and chigger-borne rickettsioses, the organism is efficiently transmitted transovarially to succeeding generations, a process which probably constitutes the main reservoir mechanism, whereas the vertebrate infection possibly only serves an amplifying role in some instances. *Coxiella burnetii,* possibly originally tick-borne, is sustained

TABLE 1.   Selected Biologic Properties of Rickettsiae

	DNA %GC	Slime Layer or Micro-capsule	Endo-toxin Action	Host Cell Membrane Actions			Replication Site			
				Mode of Entry into Host Cells*	Mouse Lethal Toxin	Hemo-lysin	Cytoplasm		Nucleus	Type‡ in CE Cells
							Free†	Vacuole		
Typhus group										
R. prowazekii	28–30	+	+	Active	+	+	+	0	0	1
R. mooseri	28–30	+	+	Active	+	+	+	0	0	2
R. canada	28–30	?	?	Active	+	?	+	0	+	?
Spotted fever group	32–33	+	?	Active	+	?	+	0	+	2
Scrub typhus group	?	Probably	?	Active	+	?	+	0	0	?
Coxiella burnetii	42.9	+	+	Passive	0	0	0	+	0	?
Rochalimaea quintana	38.8	?	?	?Passive	0	0	?	?	?	?

*Active = active penetration; passive = endocytosis by host cell.

†Free = free in cytoplasm with no surrounding vacuolar membrane.

‡Type 1 growth cycle = rickettsiae are retained within host cell until it breaks down. Type 2 growth cycle = in early stages, rickettsiae escape through plasma membrane without apparent host cell damage; rapidly spreading type of infection.

TABLE 2. Summary of Some Epidemiologic Features of Selected Rickettsial Diseases of Man

Disease	Organism	Natural Cycle		Usual Mode of Transmission to Man	Common Occupational or Environmental Association	Geographic Distribution
		Arthropod Vector	Reservoir/ Mammalian Host			
Typhus group						
Murine typhus	*Rickettsia mooseri* (*R. typhi*)	Flea	Rodents	Infected flea feces into broken skin or aerosol to mucous membranes	Rat-infested premises (shops, warehouses, grain elevators)	Scattered foci, worldwide
Epidemic typhus	*R. prowazekii*	Body louse	Man*	Infected crushed louse or feces into broken skin or aerosol to mucous membranes	Lousy human population with louse transfer	Worldwide
Brill's disease	*R. prowazekii*	Recrudescence months to years after primary attack of louse-borne typhus			Unknown; ?stress	Worldwide
Spotted fever group (selected examples)						
Rocky Mountain spotted fever	*R. rickettsii*	Ixodid ticks	Ticks, small mammals	Tick bite, mechanical transfer to mucous membranes, ?airborne	Tick-infested terrain, houses, dogs	Western Hemisphere
Boutonneuse fever	*R. conorii*	Ixodid ticks	Ticks, rodents, dogs	Tick bite	Tick-infested terrain, houses, dogs	Mediterranean, littoral, Africa, ?Indian subcontinent
Rickettsialpox	*R. akari*	Mouse mite	Mite, mice	Mouse mite bite	Unique mouse- and mite-infested premises (incinerators)	United States, U.S.S.R., Korea, ?Central Africa
Scrub typhus						
Tsutsugamushi disease	*R. tsutsugamushi* (multiple serotypes)	Chigger	Chigger, ?rodents	Chigger bite	Chigger-infested terrain; secondary scrub, grass airfields, golf courses	Asia, Australia, New Guinea, Pacific islands
Q fever†	*Coxiella burnetii*	?Ticks	Ticks, mammals	Inhalation of dried airborne infective material; ?tick bite	Domestic animals or products, dairies, lambing pens, slaughterhouses	Worldwide
Trench fever†	*Rochalimaea quintana*	Body louse	Man	Infected crushed louse or feces into broken skin; ?aerosol to mucous membranes	Lousy human population with louse transfer	Africa, Mexico, ?South America, ?Eastern Europe

*Recent isolations of putative *R. prowazekii* from flying squirrels in the eastern United States have not been evaluated as reservoirs for human infection. Previous claims of involvement of domestic animals are now largely discounted.

†Though *C. burnetii* and *R. quintana* are not strictly "rickettsiae" and Q fever and trench fever differ clinically from the others, they are conventionally considered with the rickettsiae.

by vertical passage in its vertebrate host (e.g., sheep, cattle) by virtue of its capacity to multiply to phenomenal levels in placental tissues and to be excreted in milk.

Thus, although they are commonly lumped together under the "rickettsial diseases of man," and possessing some points in common, it is apparent that there are major differences in the biologic properties of the organisms involved, in their interactions with host cells, and in their natural infection cycles and reservoir mechanisms. It is likely that organisms of diverse origin have acquired certain similar properties related to cell parasitism through a process of convergent evolution and that within groups diversification has occurred through divergent evolution. However, some similarities in cell tropism and the restricted ways in which man responds to injury have conspired to produce a group of clinical entities with many to few common features.

PATHOGENESIS, PATHOLOGY, IMMUNITY. Since the human diseases caused by members of the genus *Rickettsia* share many common features, although there are sufficient differences in detail to yield distinct clinical entities, it is convenient to consider here pathogenesis and immunity in a generalized framework.

The route of infection is frequently through the skin, injected through the vector mouth parts in the case of tick-, mite-, and chigger-borne rickettsioses and by contamination of broken skin by infected louse or flea feces in the case of louse-borne typhus and murine typhus, respectively. Airborne rickettsiae in dried louse or flea feces may initiate airborne infection through the respiratory tract or conjunctiva. Aerosols of all rickettsiae are highly infectious via the respiratory tract.

Some local proliferation undoubtedly occurs at the inoculation site with all *Rickettsia* species. In some (e.g., scrub typhus, rickettsialpox, fièvre boutonneuse), a visible lesion (the *eschar*) develops at the inoculation site during the incubation period. The route or routes of dissemination of the infection from the inoculation site are not precisely known. However, regional lymphadenopathy (e.g., in scrub typhus) suggests lymphatic spread on the one hand, whereas on the other hand demonstration of rickettsiae in endothelial cells of small blood vessels at the inoculation site opens the possibility of hematogenous dissemination.

Some dissemination to, and proliferation in, distant sites must take place during the incubation period, but the organs or tissues involved have not been identified in man. Patent rickettsemia probably appears only late in the incubation period, e.g., only a few hours prior to the onset of clinical disease in volunteers infected with *R. tsutsugamushi,* is regularly present at onset, and persists throughout the febrile period of disease despite the appearance of humoral antibodies by the end of the first week of disease. It is unknown if this early wave of patent rickettsemia is fed and sustained by, or is responsible for, initiating the characteristic widespread infection of endothelial cells in small blood vessels. *Nevertheless, disseminated focal infection of the small blood vessels (capillaries, arterioles, and venules) of the skin, and, to a lesser but significant extent, in other organs such as brain, lung, heart, and kidneys, is the single most important known pathophysiologic feature of these diseases.* At focal points in the small blood vessels, rickettsiae infect, multiply in, and damage endothelial cells with cell necrosis, hypertrophy, and proliferation. Infection is limited to the endothelial cells in typhus and scrub typhus infections but may extend to all layers in Rocky Mountain spotted fever, causing necrosis of the media. At the sites of endothelial damage, platelet-fibrin thrombi tend to form, which, along with endothelial hypertrophy and proliferation, partially or completely occlude the vascular lumen. At these sites of infection and vascular damage there develops the typical perivascular inflammatory response, with polymorphonuclear and monocytic cells early and macrophages, lymphocytes, and occasional plasma cells later, coinciding approximately temporally with antibody response, suggesting the possibility of superimposition of a vascular immunopathologic component. This sequence suggests that perhaps a typical rickettsial infection evolves through an *early phase,* in which vascular damage is primarily the direct result of rickettsial infection, and a *late phase,* in which additional vascular damage is produced by immunologic mechanisms. The latter is unproved, but is consistent with the fact that in typhus and scrub typhus infections patients appear more "toxic" in this late phase and show greater vascular instability, and most deaths occur in the period *after* antibodies are demonstrable. On the other hand, the greater severity of vascular lesions, frequent early deaths, and often little perivascular cellular response and early unresponsiveness to antirickettsial therapy in early fatal cases of Rocky Mountain spotted fever suggest that direct rickettsia-induced vascular damage alone can initiate irreversible pathophysiologic changes.

The disseminated vascular lesions can account for many of the clinical and pathophysiologic abnormalities seen in these infections, viz., rash, edema and increased extravascular fluid space, hypotension, and gangrene (in louse-borne typhus and Rocky Mountain spotted fever), as well as the clotting abnormalities (up to disseminated intravascular clotting) which have been recognized recently to some extent in several rickettsial diseases but which are seen more regularly and in such a severe form in Rocky Mountain spotted fever that they may be a major problem contributing to death. The classic typhus nodules in the brain, most frequent in the midbrain and nuclear areas, are of the same vascular origin and help explain the mental changes and cranial nerve deficits. In Rocky Mountain spotted fever, discrete microinfarcts may occur in the central nervous system with persisting electroencephalographic changes. The heart often shows, in addition to the typical perivascular lesions, some edema, a diffuse mononuclear infiltrate of unknown origin, and a minor amount of muscle necrosis. Nonspecific electrocardiographic changes are common. Despite the dramatic histologic appearance of the heart, limited studies during World War II suggested that cardiac function was not impaired. This matter should be reinvestigated by modern methods. Typical perivascular lesions occur in the portal areas of the liver, along with nonspecific focal areas of fatty degeneration in hepatocytes. However, the origin of abnormal transaminase blood levels remains unknown. The kidneys also show focal interstitial vascular lesions and lesions involving a few nephrons. The characteristic oliguria and azotemia of typhus have been attributed in the past to prerenal causes, e.g., hypotension, tissue catabolism, but the occurrence of rickettsial antigen in the urine early, followed by its disappearance with antibody response, suggests that transient immune complex disease should be sought by modern methods. The lung shows a variable degree of interstitial type pneumonitis, on histologic examination and by x-ray, regardless of route of infection. Cough is a common early clinical manifestation, but physical signs are scant.

Immunity to the infecting rickettsial strain following recovery from infection tends to be solid and longlasting but of a nonsterile type, i.e., the rickettsiae are not entirely eradicated and may remain "latent" for at least many months to many years. The bases for immunity are not yet completely understood, although rapid advances are now being made in this field. An antibody response is detectable around the end of the first week of disease, but this does not cause an immediate control of rickettsemia. Cell-mediated immunity also develops, but the kinetics of its evolution in man have not yet been clearly documented. Laboratory studies suggest that both antibody-mediated and cell-mediated mechanisms contribute to immunity. Moreover, studies of murine typhus infection in guinea pigs showed a temporal correlation between the development of an immune response as measured by serum antibodies and the development of the typical mononuclear perivascular lesions, leaving open the possibility of a late immunopathologic component.

GENERAL CLINICAL CONSIDERATIONS. In classic form, the typhus-like rickettsial diseases (typhus group, spotted fever group, and scrub typhus group) display many common clinical features which may vary in degree and in detail, e.g., fever, headache, cough, prostration, rash, altered mental state, hypotension, normal to low white blood count. *Especially at the onset,* however, the signs and symptoms are those common to many acute infectious diseases, differential clinical diagnosis is difficult, and specific laboratory diagnostic methods are limited. Sometimes an early sign, such as an eschar, which is variable even in the rickettsioses in which it occurs, is helpful. Later, rash, hypotension, changes in mental state, and the like may give clues. But rickettsioses vary in severity, and not all cases are classic. Moreover, in many areas, other infectious diseases exist which are confusing clinically, especially in that early period when the correct choice of chemotherapy may be lifesaving (as with Rocky Mountain spotted fever, meningococcemia, or cerebral malaria). Hence, one must be acutely sensitive to the different possibilities in one's area of practice and must devise a kind of strategy for the diagnosis and management, sometimes empirically on the basis of probabilities, of a rickettsia-like disease, using all available bits of epidemiologic, clinical, and laboratory information. Simple observation of the patient for the development of diagnostic clinical or laboratory features is a hazardous practice. In the United States, the single major factor contributory to the continuing 5 to 10 per cent mortality in Rocky Mountain spotted fever is delay in institution of specific chemotherapy. Listed below are some practical considerations which have emerged from analysis of experiences of others and from the author's personal experience in several parts of the world.

The history of potential exposure (occupation, travel, recreational activities in wilderness areas), as well as of tick bite, is extremely important in alerting the physician to the possibility of a rickettsial disease. Modern air travel makes it possible to return from any part of the world within the incubation period of a rickettsial disease, e.g., scrub typhus and Kenya tick typhus in travelers returning to the United States.

In a given area, certain diseases commonly cause difficult clinical differential diagnostic problems. For example, in the United States, the two diseases most commonly confused with Rocky Mountain spotted fever are measles and meningococcemia. In central and east Africa, two diseases which cause major differential diagnostic problems with louse-borne typhus are cerebral falciparum malaria and typhoid fever. Milder cases of typhus may be indistinguishable clinically from influenza.

The most sophisticated modern laboratory diagnostic aids can sometimes help distinguish within hours between measles, meningococcemia, and Rocky Mountain spotted fever. Blood smears for malaria should be routine where malaria and rickettsial diseases coexist. Typhoid can be detected by cultures. (Only *early* diagnostic measures are stressed here. It is no victory to make a retrospective diagnosis!) Outside the United States and Europe, however, laboratory facilities may be unavailable, and an empirical therapeutic approach is often successful. For example, when it is not possible to distinguish between malaria, typhus, and typhoid, a combination of chloramphenicol and chloroquine often gives a satisfactory clinical response; or a "typhus suspect" not responding in 48 hours to a tetracycline drug can often be treated successfully with chloramphenicol.

Finally, outside the United States, a patient with a rickettsial infection may have another concurrent infection, e.g., typhus plus relapsing fever or trench fever; or typhus or scrub typhus plus malaria, bacterial pneumonia, or dysentery. These must also be diagnosed and treated specifically.

LABORATORY DIAGNOSIS. Methods for retrospective diagnoses (isolation of organism and serologic response) of rickettsial infections are reasonably well developed, although not universally available, and methods for specific diagnosis in the acute phase of disease, when crucial decisions about specific chemotherapy must be made, are generally unsatisfactory but are improving. The following paragraphs have been written specifically for the practicing physician, beginning with methods applicable to the early, acute phase and proceeding to more specific methods which sometimes tend to be only confirmatory or retrospective.

Exclusion of Diseases Which Present Common Differential Diagnostic Problems in a Given Locality. Examples include malaria smear, skin lesion smear for meningococci, demonstration of measles antigen in respiratory epithelial cells by fluorescence microscopy, and cultures for typhoid and other enteric fevers.

Direct Demonstration of Rickettsiae in Tissues or Rickettsial Antigens in Urine in Acute Phase of Dis-ease. Attempts to demonstrate rickettsiae directly in tissues or cells of patients and to demonstrate rickettsial antigens in body fluids, such as urine, have been explored for many years with variable degrees of success, although none is yet available for routine diagnosis.

DIRECT MICROSCOPIC DEMONSTRATION OF RICKETTSIAE IN TISSUES. For diagnostic purposes, rickettsiae have been demonstrated in endothelial cells of skin biopsies, blood leukocytes (with or without a short period of in vitro incubation), and bone marrow smears in typhus and spotted fever infections of man or animals. The use of fluorescein-conjugated antisera permits identification of the organisms, specific at least to group. Refinement and standardization of these methods promise to yield practical routine methods for the early specific diagnosis of rickettsial infections and should be pursued vigorously. A different application of the general method is the direct demonstration by fluorescent antibody staining of *R. rickettsii* in attached ticks removed from a person (see Prevention and Control in Ch. 109).

DEMONSTRATION OF RICKETTSIAL ANTIGENS IN ACUTE PHASE URINE. Although theoretically feasible, demonstrable in certain experimental infections in animals, and sporadically reported in human disease, reliable demonstration of rickettsial antigens in acute phase urine has been fraught with difficulty. Application of modern immunologic methods (e.g., immunodiffusion, counterimmunoelectrophoresis, radioimmunoassay, enzyme-linked immunosorbent assay [ELISA] may improve sensitivity, specificity, and reliability and deserves concerted effort.

Isolation of Rickettsiae. The isolation of rickettsiae from the blood or tissues of a patient is hazardous, requires special laboratory facilities and trained personnel, usually does not yield results in time to influence patient management, and hence, was not encouraged as a routine procedure in the past. However, methods are improving, and moreover it is now urgent to change this position because serologic retrospective diagnoses are ill equipped to identify new species or variants of rickettsiae. A growing diversity of rickettsial agents (e.g., the flying squirrel agent and *R. canada* in the typhus group, new members of the spotted fever group) is being recognized in the United States and elsewhere, whose importance as causes of human disease remains unknown; this is partly because conventional serologic tests for retrospective diagnosis are largely *group* specific, might not recognize variants at the species level, and would not detect infections with totally new agents (e.g., the agent of "Kawasaki disease"). Isolation and characterization of the agent are the keystones of identification of new diseases.

Although isolation and identification of rickettsial agents are usually beyond the competence of the ordinary hospital laboratory, mechanisms do exist for accomplishing this. In the United States, properly collected and preserved (frozen at $-70°$ C or lower) specimens can be sent through state health departments to the Center for Disease Control in Atlanta, Georgia, where specially trained personnel and special facilities exist to handle and characterize such agents. Moreover, the World Health Organization has established in this country and abroad a series of reference laboratories which are also capable of handling such agents.

Serologic Diagnosis. Serologic methods remain the mainstay of routine laboratory diagnosis of rickettsial infections and for epidemiologic purposes. However,

TABLE 3. Some Clinical Features of Selected Rickettsial Diseases

Disease	Usual Incubation Period (Days)	Rash				Usual Duration of Disease* (Days)	Usual Severity†	Fever After Chemotherapy (Hours)
		Eschar	Onset, Day of Disease	Distribution	Type			
Typhus group Murine typhus	12 (8–16)	None	5–7	Trunk → extremities	Macular, maculopapular	12 (8–16)	Moderate	48–72
Epidemic typhus	12 (10–14)	None	5–7	Trunk → extremities	Macular, maculopapular, petechial	14 (10–18)	Severe	48–72
Brill's disease	—	None		Trunk → extremities	Macular	7–11	Relatively mild	48–72
Spotted fever group Rocky Mountain spotted fever	7 (3–12)	None	3–5	Extremities → trunk, face	Macular, maculopapular, petechial	16 (10–20)	Severe	72
Boutonneuse fever	5–7	Often present	3–4	Trunk, extremities, face, palms, soles	Macular, maculopapular, petechial	10 (7–14)	Moderate	—
Rickettsialpox	?9–17	Often present	1–3	Trunk → face, extremities	Papular vesicular	7 (3–11)	Relatively mild	—
Scrub typhus (tsutsugamushi disease)	1–12 (9–18)	Often present	4–6	Trunk → extremities	Macular, maculopapular	14 (10–20)	Mild to severe	24–36
Q fever	10–19	None		None		6 (2–21)	Relatively‡ mild	48 (occasionally slow)

*Untreated disease.
†Severity can vary greatly.
‡Occasional chronic infections occur (e.g., hepatitis, endocarditis).

since an antibody response rarely occurs with any of the rickettsioses before the end of the first week of disease, and since a rise in antibody titer is more or less essential to a solid diagnosis, convincing serologic diagnosis may become available only *after* the critical point has been passed with respect to lifesaving decisions about chemotherapy. At present, serologic tests consist of (1) nonspecific (Weil-Felix) tests generally available to hospital laboratories through commercially produced antigens (a part of the "febrile agglutinin" package) and (2) more specific tests, generally available at State Health Departments, the CDC, and the WHO reference laboratories.

WEIL-FELIX REACTION. Based upon unique sharing of polysaccharide antigens between certain *Proteus* strains and some rickettsiae, this agglutination test performed with suspensions of rough *Proteus* OX-2, OX-19, and OX-K strains has an historical aura and the advantage of simplicity, ready availability of antigens, and sensitivity to early antibody response.

Proteus agglutinins tend to appear early (toward the end of the first week), attain peak titers between three and four weeks after onset, and then rapidly decline. The Weil-Felix test is not positive in all rickettsial infections, is variable in recrudescent typhus (Brill-Zinsser disease), will not distinguish between typhus and spotted fever group infections, is not positive in all scrub typhus infections (about 70 per cent positive in primary infections and fewer in second infections), and may yield "false positive" results in *Proteus* infections, relapsing fever, and leptospirosis. Nevertheless, properly applied and interpreted along with other information,

the test can be useful. Until more specific tests are generally available to physicians within a time frame useful for patient management, the Weil-Felix test, despite its deficiencies, will not die.

COMPLEMENT FIXATION (CF) TEST. For most of the rickettsioses, except for the scrub typhus group, the CF test remains the standard of serodiagnosis and seroepidemiology. With group ("soluble") antigens, sera can be screened for evidence of infection with any member of the typhus or spotted fever group and with the "specific" rickettsial body antigens; the offending organism can often be identified by titer differences, depending in part on the time of specimen collection, previous exposure to related organisms, and the like. By comparing titers obtained with low and high antigen doses or before and after treatment with ethanethiol or 2-mercaptoethanol, some information can be obtained on the presence of IgM and IgG antibodies. In a single serum specimen, such information allows one to judge if antibodies present are the result of recent or remote infection or to differentiate between primary louse-borne typhus (early IgM response) and recrudescent typhus (Brill-Zinsser disease) (secondary early IgG response). In the case of Q fever, persisting high titers with Phase I antigen suggest chronic infection (e.g., hepatitis, endocarditis).

There are some pitfalls. Spotted fever group antigens tend to be anticomplementary and are often unsatisfactory. Moreover, discrimination between infections of man caused by different members of the spotted fever group is not entirely satisfactory. Some cross-reactions may occur between typhus and spotted fever group in-

TABLE 4. Some Typical Serologic Responses in Rickettsial Infections of Man*

Rickettsial Infection	Well-Felix Test†					Complement Fixation				Agglutination				Indirect Fluorescent Antibody Test‡			
	Agglutination with Proteus Strain			Kinetics		Specificity		Kinetics		Specificity		Kinetics		Specificity		Kinetics	
	OX-19	OX-2	OX-K	Day First Positive	Persistence	Group	Species or Strain	Day First Positive	Persistence	Group	Species or Strain	Day First Positive	Persistence	Group	Species or Strain	Day First Positive	Persistence
Typhus group	+++	+	0	5–9	Short	++	++	7–10	Long	++	+	5–7	Unknown	++	+	?	?
Brill-Zinsser disease	Variable, often negative			—	—	++	+	4–5	Long	++	+	Unknown	Unknown	++	Unknown	?	?
Spotted fever group	+++	+	0	5–12	Short	++§	+§	8–14	Long	++	+	Unknown	Unknown	++	+	?	?
		+++		5–12	Short												
Rickettsialpox	0	0	0	—	—	++§	+§	8–14	Long					++	++	?	?
Scrub typhus group	0	0	0–+++	10–14	Short	+	++	10–14	Unknown	++	+	Unknown	Unknown	++	+	?	?
Q fever	0	0	0	—	—	Single serotype				Test not available / Single serotype				Single serotype		?	?
Phase I antigen								8–14	Inter-mediate¶			10–14	Inter-mediate			?	?
Phase II antigen												5–8				?	?

*Variations of microbial or host origin, early chemotherapy, etc., may alter "typical" responses.

†"False positives" may occur—viz., Proteus infections, relapsing fever, leptospirosis. "Significant" titer in single specimen is ≥ 1:160.

‡Experience is sufficient to establish utility in diagnosis but insufficient to establish precise patterns.

§Complement fixation test is of limited use in spotted fever group infections because antigens tend to be anticomplementary.

¶Phase I complement fixation antibodies ordinarily tend to be low and transient but may persist in high titer in chronic infections (e.g., hepatitis, endocarditis).

fections. Prior experience with a related organism may result in higher titers to that organism than to the current infecting agent. Thus, as with all serologic tests, interpretation requires care and knowledge of potential problems.

AGGLUTINATION TESTS. Agglutination tests with highly purified rickettsial suspensions are receiving increasing attention because they are simple to perform, are unaffected by anticomplementary factors in serum or antigen, are highly sensitive, and usually detect antibodies somewhat earlier in disease than does the CF test. Persistence of antibodies has not yet been thoroughly documented. Group specificity is good. Species specificity appears to be fair among the spotted fever group, but some problems have been encountered in distinguishing between murine and epidemic typhus infections of man (as opposed to high specificity in rodents). This test requires large amounts of antigen compared with the CF test. However, the original tube test has now been largely replaced with a highly satisfactory microtiter adaptation (MA test). (*Note:* The agglutination tests referred to here are not to be confused with the Giroud type of microscopic agglutination test, which is performed with relatively crude antigens and which is often unreliable).

INDIRECT FLUORESCENT ANTIBODY TESTS (IFA). IFA tests are undergoing rapid development for diagnostic and epidemiologic purposes. They are sensitive and useful with anticomplementary sera or blood collected on filter paper. IFA tests may be positive when blocking factors interfere with CF or MA tests. They can be made group specific. Methods for improved species differentiation are under study. IgG, IgM, and IgA antibody titers can be determined directly. Kinetics of antibody response have not yet been clearly defined. The IFA test is currently the most sensitive and reliable test available for the diagnosis of scrub typhus.

OTHER TESTS. Toxin neutralization tests, passive hemagglutination tests, and radioimmune precipitation tests have special uses. New tests, such as the ELISA type test, are under development and evaluation.

TREATMENT OF RICKETTSIAL DISEASES. The general principles of therapy are similar for all the common rickettsial diseases. Optimal management includes (1) specific antimicrobial therapy directed against the offending rickettsial agent; (2) supportive measures to correct physiologic abnormalities; (3) good nursing care to prevent serious complications; and (4) prompt, appropriate therapy of complications. In mild cases, patients treated early may require little more than the specific antimicrobial therapy. Vigorous supportive measures and good nursing may be lifesaving in severe cases.

Clinical Classification. A clinical classification system for efficient management of patients evolved during a large epidemic of louse-borne typhus fever is also useful in the sporadic, individual case of any of the rickettsioses. Thus the patient is evaluated immediately on admission according to duration and general severity of disease, neurologic involvement (coma, delirium, lucid state but inability to swallow), physiologic derangements (hypotension, shock, renal impairment, clotting derangement), state of nutrition and hydration, and presence or absence of complications. For practical management purposes, patients can then be classified as (1) mild or severe, (2) cooperative or uncooperative, and (3) uncomplicated or complicated. Even moderately severe but uncomplicated rickettsial infection in a cooperative patient is usually simple to manage with orally administered antibiotics, fluids, and nutriments. The uncooperative patient or the patient with complications requires added measures. Management is greatly simplified if the uncooperative patient can be brought quickly to the stage at which oral medications and fluids are possible (see below).

Antirickettsial Therapy. *Prompt adequate antirickettsial therapy is the single most important factor in shortening the disease, reducing mortality, and speeding convalescence.* In cooperative uncomplicated cases this may be the only medication required.

Antimicrobial drugs of the tetracycline series are the drugs of choice for the treatment of all rickettsial diseases. Although also highly effective, chloramphenicol is not recommended, unless tetracyclines cannot be used, because of the occasional complication of aplastic anemia. These drugs shorten the course of disease dramatically and reduce fatality rates virtually to zero except in neglected, complicated, or fulminating cases. The patient often begins to respond by 24 hours and is afebrile in one to four days, usually two to three days, depending on the specific rickettsia and the stage of disease at the time therapy is begun.

Penicillin, streptomycin, and sulfonamides are clinically ineffective. Practical concentrations of a wide range of aminoglycosides, semisynthetic penicillins, and cephalosporins do not inhibit *R. prowazekii* growth in vitro in cell cultures. *Note: Except for chloramphenicol, none of the drugs (ampicillin, amoxycillin, cotrimoxazole) used for the treatment of typhoid fever, a serious differential diagnostic problem in some areas, gives clinical and/or in vitro evidence of effectiveness in typhus fever. Whether or not this applies to the other rickettsioses remains to be determined.*

Tetracycline HCl is given orally in a total daily dose of 25 to 50 mg per kilogram of body weight. Two grams per day in divided doses at 4- to 6- or even 12-hour intervals usually suffices for adult patients. Chloramphenicol is given orally in amounts of 50 and 75 mg per kilogram of body weight per day for adults and children, respectively, usually in divided doses at 4- to 6- or even 12-hour intervals. (*Caution:* Doses larger than 25 mg per kilogram of body weight may be severely toxic for *newborn infants.*) Intravenous tetracycline is given in a dosage of 0.5 gram every 6 to 12 hours, to a maximum of 2 grams per day for adults. Although likely to cause pain or local reaction, up to 0.5 gram of the intramuscular tetracycline preparation can be given, if necessary, every 12 hours for a day or two until the patient can take the oral preparation. Chloramphenicol succinate, appropriately diluted, is given intravenously to adults in a dose of 1.0 gram every 8 to 12 hours. Parenteral therapy should be replaced with oral therapy as soon as the patient can swallow. When parenteral preparations are unavailable or intravenous drip therapy is impractical, oral preparations suspended in fluid may be administered by stomach tube.

Since neither tetracycline HCl nor chloramphenicol is rickettsicidal under ordinary circumstances, and since neither eradicates the organism from the body, ultimate freedom from clinical relapse (i.e., "cure") is probably dependent on an adequate immune response by the patient. Duration of therapy is dependent on the pharmacology of the particular drug employed; the susceptibility of the organism to, and rate of recovery from, the inhibitory effects of the drug employed, which may vary from one species of organism to another; and the stage of the disease at the time therapy is begun. Although not necessarily the minimal effective regimen, a practical conservative guide to duration of tetracycline or chloramphenicol therapy is to administer the drug until the patient has been afebrile for 48 hours and for an additional period until the total time elapsed from onset of disease is 12 to 14 days. Relapses respond to re-treatment with the same drug. The usual precautions are observed for administering antimicrobials, e.g., adjustment of dosage to compensate for problems of immaturity in infants and of renal or hepatic dysfunction of rickettsial or other origin, staining of developing teeth, changes in microbial flora and superinfection, pregnancy, drug susceptibilities, or blood dyscrasias.

The introduction of new lipotropic tetracycline derivatives which produce prolonged high blood and tissue levels after a single dose (viz., doxycycline and minocycline) has literally revolutionized the management of louse-borne typhus and perhaps scrub typhus. A *single* 100-mg dose of doxycycline will *cure* most adults, and a *single* 50-mg dose will cure most children, with only an occasional transient relapse which does not require additional therapy. A single 200-mg dose is rarely followed by relapse. Under extreme circumstances, single-dose doxycycline therapy, requiring only a single contact between patient and medical personnel, has been applied successfully on an outpatient basis. Unless in extremis from typhus or suffering from some unrelated disease, almost all patients will survive whether "hospitalized," at home, or transiently disoriented in the bush. Single-dose doxycycline is currently the treatment of choice for louse-borne typhus. Comparable results have been obtained with minocycline, but, because of its tendency to cause otitic complications, it is not recommended as a first choice drug.

Experience with single-dose doxycycline treatment of other rickettsioses is limited. However, some substantial evidence indicates that a single 200-mg dose of doxycycline will cure scrub typhus, with some transient recrudescences. On the other hand, very limited and uncontrolled observations suggest that a single dose will not suffice for the treatment of murine typhus or Rocky Mountain spotted fever, although a daily dose of 100 to 200 mg on a schedule described for tetracycline HCl is effective.

Antimicrobial Resistance. Antimicrobial resistance has not yet been encountered in naturally occurring rickettsial disease. However, in the laboratory, *R. prowazekii* strains have been selected that are resistant to erythromycin, chloramphenicol, penicillin, and certain other inhibitors. Moreover, it has been shown that therapeutic doses of antirickettsial drugs produce blood levels which transiently inhibit the growth of *R. prowazekii* in the louse gut, thereby creating potentially selective conditions. Since not all treated typhus patients are in fact effectively deloused, the possibility exists for the selection of antimicrobial-resistant strains of *R. prowazekii* which might emerge in either current epidemics or future epidemics through recrudescence of infection by antimicrobial-resistant strains.

Steroids. Although not rigorously controlled, studies have shown that corticosteroids given in conjunction with antimicrobial drugs may cause rapid defervescence, dramatic reversal of neurologic impairment (coma, difficulty in swallowing), and an apparent improvement in the general well-being of the patient without adversely affecting the infectious process. A comatose typhus patient given steroid therapy in the evening may be sitting up on the side of the bed in the morning, conversing with his fellow patients and able to take medication and fluids by mouth. Similar effects may be seen in patients unable to swallow. More limited observations with scrub typhus and Rocky Mountain spotted fever have shown similar apparently beneficial effects, although of course reversal of intravascular clotting in Rocky Mountain spotted fever will not be effected. This has been accomplished by giving 100 mg of hydrocortisone intravenously and 200 to 300 mg of cortisone acetate intramuscularly in addition to 500 mg of tetracycline intramuscularly upon admission. (*Falciparum malaria must be excluded by blood smear in patients at risk to both diseases.*) Often within 24 hours a typhus patient is able to swallow the final dose of antibiotic (100 mg of doxycycline), to take oral fluids, to attend to elimination, and to move spontaneously to reduce the chances of developing pressure necroses or thrombophlebitis. Usually no more therapy of any kind, antimicrobial or steroid, is required, and nutrition presents no problem. This therapy is reserved for seriously ill or "uncooperative" patients.

Fluid and Electrolyte Balance. Oral fluids sufficient to ensure a daily urine output of at least 1500 ml suffice for the conscious, cooperative patient. The comatose patient will require parenteral fluids to maintain an adequate urine output. Fluids should be given slowly so as not to tax the potentially labile cardiovascular system. Excess electrolytes contribute to the general edema and to cardiac load when the fluid re-enters the vascular compartment. Urine output, the presence of oliguria, and laboratory determinations will serve as guides to the proper volume and proportion of electrolytes, glucose and water.

Hepatic and Renal Systems. The cause of the disturbed liver (abnormal tests, rarely jaundice) and kidney (azotemia, albuminuria, oliguria) functions remains controversial, but these abnormalities are usually transient and disappear with convalescence. Hence management, if required, is guided by identification of the specific abnormalities present through appropriate tests and by the presence of other complicating abnormalities.

Cardiovascular System, Including Blood. The most prominent manifestations of the typhus, scrub typhus, and spotted fever groups of rickettsial diseases can be attributed to abnormalities of the cardiovascular system. Indeed, hypotension is common, and peripheral vascular collapse, frequently in the second week of disease, is a leading cause of death and has been difficult to manage. Its cause is only incompletely understood. However, the widespread focal lesions of the small vessels are assumed to be contributory to increased vascular permeability and collapse and may also account for some of the clotting abnormalities (thrombocytopenia, disseminated intravascular clotting as a result of endothelial damage, and defective synthesis from liver impairment) which have recently been recognized in certain rickettsioses. This in turn would help explain certain complications — hemorrhage, vascular occlusion (gangrene, hemiplegia, others), and thrombophlebitis — and would suggest more rational approaches to their prevention and management, especially when specifically identified by appropriate laboratory tests.

Accordingly, whole blood and plasma should be avoided. Albumin may be used to combat hypoproteinemia. Red cells are preferred to correct significant anemia. Heparin has been described as treatment for rickettsia-associated intravascular clotting, but others have failed to detect benefit in the intravascular clotting accompanying Rocky Mountain spotted fever.

The management of peripheral vascular collapse is empirical and largely of unproved benefit: (1) oxygen; (2) judicious use of salt-poor concentrated albumin as a plasma expander and to reduce edema; (3) vasopressor drugs, e.g., levarterenol bitartrate (Levophed); and (4) corticosteroids such as hydrocortisone.

Pulmonary edema and congestive heart failure, resulting from excessive intake of salt and water or from rapid resorption of edema fluid with vascular healing, are treated with digitalis. No guidelines are available for the use of diuretics, but if their use is contemplated, consideration should be given to the state of renal function.

Massive intravascular hemolysis, described in glucose-6-phosphate dehydrogenase–deficient subjects with murine or scrub typhus, has been managed successfully with peritoneal dialysis.

Other Complications. Bacterial pneumonia, still frequent in epidemic typhus, or other bacterial infections are treated with appropriate antimicrobial agents according to the causative organisms and their sensitivity patterns. Gangrene, decubitus ulcers, and thrombophlebitis are treated by the usual surgical and medical methods. Unless caused by a large destructive process (hemorrhage or thrombosis of a large vessel), neurologic abnormalities usually resolve with convalescence, although personality changes and deafness have been known to persist in some patients for months.

Nursing Care. Patients may be irrational or agitated and may injure themselves or even attempt self-destruction. Close observation and restraint may be required. Comatose patients should be turned frequently to prevent pressure necrosis, thrombophlebitis, and hypostatic pneumonia. Special skin care and protection of bony prominences may be desirable in view of the vascular damage associated with the disease. Good oral hygiene reduces the chances of suppurative parotitis.

Special Considerations. Although classic Q fever often responds promptly to chemotherapy with tetracycline drugs or chloramphenicol as outlined above, the response in some cases is slower and less dramatic. Treatment of chronic infection is less satisfactory. Chemotherapy of *C. burnetii* endocarditis is especially unsatisfactory, probably due to the fact that most antirickettsial drugs are only rickettsiostatic. There has been very limited success with combined chemotherapy administered over a period of many months. However, surgical replacement of the affected heart valve has been somewhat more successful.

Trench fever has been reported to respond to tetracycline drugs, but no information is available concerning the effects of brief chemotherapy on the persistence of the organism in the blood or on subsequent relapse rates.

General

Horsfall, F. L., Jr., and Tamm, I. (eds.): Viral and Rickettsial Infections of Man. 4th ed. Philadelphia, J. B. Lippincott Company, 1965.
Moulton, F. R. (ed.): Symposium on Rickettsial Diseases (Dec., 1946, Boston). Washington, D.C., American Association for the Advancement of Science, 1948.
Topping, N. H., et al.: Studies of typhus fever. National Institute of Health Bull. No. 183, 1945.

Weiss, E.: Growth and physiology of rickettsiae. Bacteriol. Rev., 37:259, 1973.
Wisseman, C. L., Jr.: Some biological properties of rickettsiae pathogenic for man. Zentralbl. Bakteriol. [Orig.] 206:299, 1968.
Wisseman, C. L. Jr. (ed.): Symposium on the spotted fever group of rickettsiae (Commission on Rickettsial Diseases, Armed Forces Epidemiological Board). Walter Reed Army Institute of Research Medical Science, Publication no. 7. Washington, D.C., Government Printing Office, 1960.
Zdrodovskii, P. F., and Golinevich, H. M.: The Rickettsial Diseases. New York, Pergamon Press, Inc., 1960.

Laboratory Diagnosis

DeShazo, R. D., Boyce, J. R., Osterman, J. V., and Stephenson, E. H.: Early diagnosis of Rocky Mountain spotted fever. Use of primary monocyte culture technique. JAMA, 235:1353, 1976.
Elisberg, B. L., and Bozeman, F. L.: Serologic diagnosis of rickettsial diseases by indirect immunofluorescence. Arch. Inst. Pasteur Tunis, 43:193, 1966.
Elisberg, B. L., and Bozeman, F. M.: Rickettsiae. In Lennette, E. H., and Schmidt, N. J. (eds.): Diagnostic Procedures for Viral and Rickettsial Infections. 4th ed. New York, American Public Health Association, 1969, pp. 826–868.
Fiset, P., Ormsbee, R. A., Silberman, R., Peacock, M., and Spielman, S. H.: A microagglutination technique for detection and measurement of rickettsial antibodies. Acta Virol. (Praha), 13:60, 1969.
Murphy, J. R., Wisseman, C. L., Jr., and Snyder, L. B.: Plaque assay for *Rickettsia mooseri* in tissue samples. Proc. Soc. Exp. Biol. Med., 153:151, 1976.
Murray, E. S., O'Connor, J. M., and Gaon, J. A.: Differentiation of 19S and 7S complement-fixing antibodies in primary versus recrudescent typhus by either ethanethiol or heat. Proc. Soc. Exp. Biol. Med., 119:291, 1965.
Ormsbee, R., Peacock, M., Casper, E., Plorde, J., Gabre-Kirdan, T., and Wright, L.: Serologic diagnosis of epidemic typhus fever. Am. J. Epidemiol., 105:261, 1977.
Philip, R. N., Casper, E. A., MacCormack, J. N., Sexton, D. J., Thomas, L. A., Anacker, R. L., Burgdorfer, W., and Vick, S.: A comparison of serologic methods for diagnosis of Rocky Mountain spotted fever. Am. J. Epidemiol., 105:56, 1977.
Robinson, D. M., Brown, G., Gan, E., and Huxsoll, D. L.: Adaptation of a microimmunofluorescence test to the study of human *Rickettsia tsutsugamushi* antibody. Am. J. Trop. Med. Hyg., 25:900, 1976.
Woodward, T. E., Pederson, C. E., Jr., Oster, C. N., Bagley, L. R., Romberger, J., and Snyder, M. J.: Prompt confirmation of Rocky Mountain spotted fever: Identification of rickettsiae in skin tissues. J. Infect. Dis., 134:297, 1976.

Clinicopathologic

Allen, A. C., and Spitz, S.: A comparative study of the pathology of scrub typhus and other rickettsial diseases. Am. J. Pathol., 21:603, 1945.
National Research Council Committee on Pathology: Pathology of epidemic typhus. Arch. Pathol., 56:397, 512, 1953.
Whelton, A., Donadio, J. V., Jr., and Elisberg, B. L.: Acute renal failure complicating rickettsial infections in glucose-6-phosphate dehydrogenase–deficient individuals. Ann. Intern. Med., 69:323, 1968.
Wolbach, S. B., Todd, J. L., and Palfrey, F. W.: The Etiology and Pathology of Typhus. Cambridge, Harvard University Press, 1922.
Wright, L. J., Barker, L. F., Mickenberg, I. D., and Wolff, S. M.: Laboratory-acquired typhus fevers. Ann. Intern. Med., 69:731, 1968.
Zarafonetis, C. J. D.: The typhus fevers. In Coates, J. B., and Havens, W. P. (eds.): Medical Department, United States Army. Internal Medicine in World War II. Vol. II, Infectious Diseases. Washington, D.C., Office of the Surgeon General, Department of the Army, 1963, pp. 143–223.
See Ch. 109 for selected references on coagulation abnormalities.

Chemotherapy/Treatment

Fabrikant, I. B., El Batawi, Y., and Wisseman, C. L., Jr.: Cortisone action at different stages of experimental *Rickettsia mooseri* infection in mice. Arch. Inst. Pasteur Tunis, 43:205, 1966 (review of corticosteroids).
Ley, H. L., Jr., and Smadel, J. E.: Antibiotic therapy of rickettsial diseases. Antibiot. Chemother., 4:792, 1954.
Sheehy, T. W., Hazlett, D., and Turk, R. E.: Scrub typhus: A comparison of chloramphenicol and tetracycline and its treatment. Arch. Intern. Med., 132:77, 1973.
Wisseman, C. L., Jr., et al.: Antibodies and clinical relapse of murine typhus fever following early chemotherapy. Ann. Intern. Med., 57:743, 1962.
Woodward, T. E.: Therapy of the rickettsial diseases with a discussion of chemoprophylaxis. Arch. Inst. Pasteur Tunis, 36:507, 1959.

108. THE TYPHUS GROUP

Charles L. Wisseman, Jr.

Three clinical and epidemiologic entities comprise the established diseases of the typhus group: (1) primary louse-borne epidemic typhus (*Rickettsia prowazekii*); (2) its recrudescent form, Brill-Zinsser disease (*R. prowazekii*); and (3) flea-borne murine typhus (*R. mooseri* [*R. typhi*]). These diseases are similar clinically and pathologically but differ in intensity of certain symptoms and signs, severity, and case fatality rate. This conventional listing of typhus group diseases has been complicated in the United States in recent years by (1) the isolation of a new species, *R. canada*, from ticks in Canada and its implication on serologic grounds as the possible cause of a Rocky Mountain spotted fever–like disease in Georgia; (2) the isolation of *R. prowazekii*–like rickettsiae from flying squirrels in the eastern United States and the growing suspicion of the occurrence of sporadic non–*R. mooseri* typhus cases in southern states; and (3) the strong one-way serologic cross-reactions between *R. canada* and *R. prowazekii*. Much more information, especially isolation and characterization of the agents from human cases, is needed for clarification.

108.1. EPIDEMIC LOUSE-BORNE TYPHUS FEVER

(Many Synonyms: Classic, Historic, European Typhus; Jail, War, Camp, Ship Fever; Fleckfieber [German]; Typhus Exanthématique [French]; Tifus Exantemático, Tabardillo [Spanish]; Dermotypho [Italian])

HISTORY. Typhus fever is one of the great epidemic diseases of mankind. It is best known in its epidemic form, which tends to emerge in association with wars, famines, and other forms of human misfortunes. Although it is probably ancient on an historical time scale and has been suggested as a possible cause of the plague of Athens in 430 B.C., the first reasonably accurate medical description of typhus is generally attributed to Fracastorius in 1546. In the ensuing four centuries it has changed the course of history, often being more decisive in military campaigns than the battles themselves, as Zinsser has recounted in his *Rats, Lice and History*. Typhus fever was an important factor in World War I and during the subsequent famine and sociopolitical unrest in Russia and eastern Europe between 1918 and 1922, when an estimated 30,000,000 cases of typhus with 3,000,000 deaths occurred. During World War II, millions of cases occurred in North Africa, Italy, Nazi prison camps, eastern Europe, and even Soviet Central Asia. At present, only sporadic cases are encountered in eastern Europe. The disease resurges from time to time in Afghanistan, probably occurs in the Himalaya Mountains, is epidemic to endemoepidemic in Central Africa and Ethiopia, and causes sporadic outbreaks in southern Africa. Typhus has a long history, dating from the Spanish conquistadores, in Mexico, Central America, and the Andean countries of South America, where it remains highly endemic with occasional sharp village outbreaks.

It was not until 1837 that Gerhard in Philadelphia clearly differentiated typhus from typhoid fever on clinical and pathologic grounds. Typhoid fever is still called *typhus abdominalis* in Europe, and the distinction between typhus and typhoid still poses practical problems of differential clinical diagnosis.

Louse transmission of typhus was demonstrated by Nicolle, Compte, and Consiel in 1909; da Rocha-Lima described the organism in the gut of the body louse and named it *Rickettsia prowazekii*. The classic work of Wolbach, Todd, and Palfrey (1922) clearly associated the clinical, pathologic, and etiologic aspects of typhus.

DEFINITION. Classic typhus fever is an acute infectious disease transmitted by the human body louse (*Pediculus humanus humanus*) and characterized clinically by sudden onset, sustained high fever of about two weeks' duration, a macular rash, and altered mental state.

ETIOLOGY (see Ch. 107). *Rickettsia prowazekii* is a small pleomorphic bacterium, ranging from coccobacillary to filamentous, with distinct tinctorial properties. Outer layers of the envelope possess group as well as specific antigens. No evidence has been obtained for significant variations in antigenic composition or virulence for man in strains from different areas, but attenuation has been observed as a laboratory phenomenon.

TRANSMISSION AND EPIDEMIOLOGY. The natural infection cycle is restricted to man and the human body louse (*Pediculus humanus humanus*), although the organism can also grow in the head louse (*Pediculus humanus capitis*). The louse acquires the rickettsia by feeding on the blood of a typhus patient during the rickettsemic phase. The organism multiplies in, and destroys, cells of the louse midgut, achieving numbers greater than 10^8 organisms per louse and causing death of the louse in one to two weeks. Large numbers of rickettsiae are excreted in the feces. The organism is not transmitted by bite. Instead, crushed infective lice or louse feces contaminate bite sites or other breaks in the skin, or airborne infective louse feces gain access through the respiratory tract.

The louse regularly dies of *R. prowazekii* infection, does not transmit the organism transovarially to the next generation, and is not a reservoir of typhus. Putative domestic animal reservoirs have largely been discounted as laboratory artifacts, but the role of the flying squirrel in the eastern United States has not yet been evaluated. Man, through the phenomenon of persisting infection and subsequent recrudescence (see Ch. 108.2) remains the most likely candidate for the major interepidemic reservoir.

One major key to epidemic typhus is the body louse vector. Typhus can occur anywhere when living conditions and political, socioeconomic, environmental, and cultural factors predispose to lousiness and the transfer of lice among people. These are currently supplied in mountainous parts of the Northern and Southern Hemispheres, as well as equatorial regions, in deserts (Sahara, Arabian deserts) where heavy clothing is worn continuously, and in tropical regions among nearly naked populations whose waistbands or arm and leg ornaments provide harborage for lice.

Depending upon many factors, louse-borne typhus can occur as a truly sharp epidemic disease, as a prolonged endemoepidemic disease (as in Ethiopia today), or as a highly endemic infection with sporadic, often unrecognized infections in young age groups but with sporadic sharp village outbreaks involving all age groups (as in Andean countries today).

PATHOLOGY. The general pathology and pathophysiologic features are described in Ch. 107.

CLINICAL MANIFESTATIONS AND COURSE. The following description applies to untreated full-blown classic typhus fever in adults. The incubation period usually is from 8 to 12 days but may be as short as 6 days or as long as 15 days. The disease may be divided into the prodromal, early, and late phases (see Pathogenesis in Ch. 107).

Prodromes of vague malaise and headache are not uncommon. The early phase is usually ushered in by the abrupt onset of fever, severe headache, myalgia of the back and legs, and chills or chilly sensations. The headache is intense and intractable, and persists day and night. Over the first two or three days the temperature attains a level of about 39 to 41° C, where it remains with only slight fluctuations until death or recovery. The skin is usually hot and dry. The face is flushed or dusky; the conjunctivae are suffused; photophobia is frequent. Deafness, tinnitus, and sometimes vertigo are prominent features. The mental state is dull. Weakness and prostration may be mild early, but after two or three days may become profound. Unproductive cough with sparse physical findings occurs in about two thirds of the cases. Nausea, vomiting, and diarrhea occur but are uncommon. Constipation is usually present.

The characteristic rash appears between the fourth and seventh days and ushers in the late phase of disease. In some instances, it is preceded by a diffuse, transient erythema. The lesions first appear on the trunk and axillary folds and spread to the extremities, sparing the face, palms, and soles, except in very severely ill patients. At first the lesions are pinkish red macules which blanch on pressure. The evolution of the rash depends on the severity of the illness. In mild cases it may fade completely in one or two days; in cases of moderate severity, it may become maculopapular, and may become hemorrhagic, changing to reddish brown and lasting for one to two weeks before fading; in very severe cases the lesions may be exceedingly numerous, almost confluent, quickly becoming hemorrhagic or even purpuric. The rash may be absent in 5 to 10 per cent of cases. With experience and proper lighting, it may be seen without too much difficulty in dark-skinned persons.

At first the pulse rate is slow in relation to the temperature, but by the end of the first week it becomes rapid (110 to 140), weak, and frequently undulating or irregular. The blood pressure is usually low, sometimes with a systolic pressure below 80 mm Hg, and there may be brief episodes of severe hypotension. Cyanosis may be present.

The mental state progresses from dullness to stupor, or occasionally to coma. The stupor may be interrupted by brief periods of delirium, excitement, or vigorous activity. Cranial nerves are selectively and variably involved (deafness, dysphagia, dysphonia). Coarse tremors may appear. Incontinence of urine and feces is encountered in moderately or severely ill patients.

Oliguria, proteinuria, and azotemia are common. Jaundice is rare, but elevations in serum transaminases may appear early. The white blood count may show a leukopenia early. In the second and third weeks of the disease it is normal or only slightly elevated unless complications ensue. Eosinophils are absent or rare in the early stages of typhus. Anemia may develop in the second or third week.

Death from typhus usually occurs between the ninth and eighteenth days of illness. The terminal period is usually characterized by a profound stupor, peripheral vascular collapse, and severe renal failure. When recovery is the outcome, the temperature begins to decline after 14 to 18 days and reaches a normal level by rapid lysis in two to four days. The mental and physical state of the patient improves strikingly as the temperature falls, but strength returns more slowly (two to three months).

Secondary bacterial bronchopneumonia, otitis media, and parotitis are common in untreated patients. Thrombosis may affect the large arteries with serious results (e.g., hemiplegia). Thrombosis of small vessels in the skin may lead to gangrene, particularly of the toes, fingers, or ear lobes. Necrosis of the skin may occur over the bony prominences, especially over the sacrum or greater trochanter.

Severity of disease and case fatality rate increase with age, being less severe and often uncharacteristic in younger children and increasing rapidly in those over the age of 40 years. In persons who contract typhus after having received killed typhus vaccine, the disease is greatly modified — with headache, fever of a few days' duration, and a transient rash but rare complications and negligible mortality.

PROGNOSIS. Depending on host factors, such as age, stress, nutritional state, other concurrent diseases, and perhaps the past typhus history of the population, case fatality rate in untreated typhus may range from 10 per cent or less to 60 per cent. Deep coma and severe hypotension and tachycardia associated with falling body temperature are signs of poor prognosis. Even such cases, however, often respond dramatically to appropriate chemotherapy and supportive measures. Appropriate treatment reduces the mortality rate in ordinary severe typhus fever virtually to zero.

TREATMENT. Treatment is described in Ch. 107. A single 200-mg oral dose of the long-acting tetracycline, doxycycline, is the treatment of choice under ordinary circumstances.

PREVENTION AND CONTROL. Infected lice and louse feces on a typhus patient present a special hazard to all nonimmune contacts, including physicians and attendants among whom infection is a common occupational hazard. Decontamination and delousing of the typhus patient and his clothing (including blankets and hats) are performed immediately upon hospitalization. Clothing and bedding are best decontaminated by heat, because this will kill the lice as well as the rickettsiae. After the patient is decontaminated and deloused, isolation and quarantine are not necessary.

Control of louse-borne typhus currently depends heavily upon control of the louse vector. When simple hygienic measures (e.g., bathing and laundering of clothes) cannot be followed, application of insecticide dusts (10 per cent DDT, 1 per cent malathion, 1 per cent lindane, or newer carbamates, depending upon local louse-resistance patterns) to fully clothed persons is very effective for reducing louse populations and controlling disease in acute outbreaks. Insecticides alone are less effective for long-term louse control in areas where conditions conducive to lousiness persist and where louse strains resistant to insecticides can be, and are, selected. The older methods of subjecting clothes and bedding to heat or fumigants (e.g., methyl bromide) are effective but cumbersome. It is possible but unproved that repellent-treated clothing (e.g., M-1960, diethyltoluamide) would reduce the chances of louse acquisition.

Vaccines composed of killed *R. prowazekii* are available, have been used extensively, definitely reduce the duration, severity, and mortality in vaccinated persons who acquire clinical typhus, and probably reduce the incidence of disease, although there are no quantitative controlled studies to assess accurately the degree of protection afforded. The attenuated E strain of *R. prowazekii*, when used experimentally as a living vaccine, has demonstrated substantial protection. The attenuated, immunizing infection occasionally is clinically overt, resembling an extremely modified typhus infection not requiring therapy. This vaccine is not yet generally available.

108.2. BRILL-ZINSSER DISEASE
(Recrudescent Typhus)

HISTORY. In 1898 in New York, Nathan Brill reported a relatively mild typhus-like disease in immigrants from eastern Europe in the absence of body lice. Similar febrile illnesses were subsequently encountered in other cities in the eastern United States and were commonly referred to as Brill's disease. Then, in 1912, Anderson and Goldberger established the relationship between Brill's disease and typhus, and in 1931 murine typhus was recognized as a distinct entity. On the basis of an epidemiologic study, Zinsser in 1934 postulated that Brill's disease was in fact the late recrudescence of a latent infection following primary louse-borne typhus. This appeared to be confirmed, and the epidemiologic significance underlined in 1953, when Murray and Snyder infected body lice by allowing them to feed on Brill-Zinsser disease patients and then demonstrated that the organism was indistinguishable from fully virulent *R. prowazekii*.

DEFINITION. Brill-Zinsser disease is a recrudescence of typhus months to years after primary infection and clinically resembles a mild form of primary typhus.

ETIOLOGY. The etiologic agent is unmodified, fully virulent *R. prowazekii* that has persisted in tissues of the patient since his primary attack of typhus.

INTEREPIDEMIC SURVIVAL AND EPIDEMIOLOGIC CONSIDERATIONS. The nonsterile immunity and long persisting "latent" *R. prowazekii* infection that follows primary typhus constitutes, through rickettsemic recrudescence months to years later, the interepidemic reservoir for typhus and the mechanism by which the rickettsia is again made available to the louse vector. Neither the factors that precipitate recrudescence nor the precise rate of recrudescence among typhus convalescents is known. The efficiency with which lice become infected with *R. prowazekii* is apparently less during feeding upon Brill-Zinsser disease patients than upon primary typhus patients. Nevertheless, typhus outbreaks are known to have originated from Brill-Zinsser disease patients. This mechanism probably also plays a role in sustaining endemicity.

PATHOLOGY. The basic vascular lesions are similar to those of primary typhus.

CLINICAL MANIFESTATIONS AND COURSE. Recrudescent typhus is similar to primary typhus except that the fever is on the average lower and of shorter duration, the rash is less intense and often absent, and the case fatality rate is low. Nevertheless, it can be a serious and debilitating disease. Whether or not subclinical recrudescences occur is unknown.

DIAGNOSIS. The occurrence of a typhus-like disease of more than a few days' duration, with or without rash, in a patient who has no other stigmata of other bacterial infection and who has a history of previous primary typhus or residence in a typhus-endemic area should be considered as a potential candidate for Brill-Zinsser disease. In the laboratory, the organism can be demonstrated in vascular endothelial cells by skin biopsy. The Weil-Felix test is frequently negative. However, the diagnosis of *R. prowazekii* infection can be made with specific rickettsial serologic tests, and recrudescent typhus can be differentiated from primary typhus by the rapid appearance of dominantly IgG antibodies (secondary type of antibody response), as opposed to a somewhat slower antibody response, initially with a prominent IgM component, in primary typhus.

PROGNOSIS. Uncomplicated, untreated Brill-Zinsser disease has a low case fatality rate which should be reduced virtually to zero with specific antirickettsial treatment.

TREATMENT. Treatment is the same as for primary louse-borne typhus, as outlined in Ch. 107.

PREVENTION AND CONTROL. Prevention of primary louse-borne typhus infection is the only known reliable method for preventing Brill-Zinsser disease. None of the currently available antirickettsial chemotherapeutic agents are known to eradicate *R. prowazekii* from the infected person; hence, adequate antimicrobial therapy of primary louse-borne typhus probably will not prevent later recrudescence of infection. Since the factors leading to recrudescence are unknown, no specific manipulations of the host can be recommended. It is unknown, for example, if periodic vaccination of persons with a past history of primary louse-borne typhus will reduce the incidence of recrudescence. Prompt delousing of a patient with Brill-Zinsser disease will prevent the patient from becoming a source of primary louse-borne typhus infections in contacts.

108.3. MURINE OR FLEA-BORNE TYPHUS FEVER

HISTORY. In 1926, Maxcy's studies suggested a flea, mite, or tick vector and a rodent reservoir of the sporadic cases of typhus in the southeastern United States. In 1928 Mooser reported the distinctive characteristics of the microorganism; he suggested the term "murine typhus." In 1931, Dyer, Rumreich, and Badger obtained rickettsiae from rats in Baltimore, and in the same year Mooser, Castaneda, and Zinsser isolated a similar strain from the brains of rats in Mexico City. It was established that the infection is kept alive in a rat reservoir, is picked up from the rats by fleas, and is transferred by the flea vector to man. From rat to rat the infection can pass by both rat fleas and the rat louse, *Polyplax spinulosa*. Murine typhus was promptly found to be distributed all over the world, often existing in the same places where classic epidemic typhus fever occurs.

DEFINITION. Murine typhus fever is an acute, infectious disease communicable from rodent hosts to man sporadically by means of the rat flea (*Xenopsylla cheopis*). The disease is similar clinically to classic epidemic typhus except that it is much milder.

ETIOLOGY. The causative organism, *Rickettsia mooseri (R. typhi)*, is similar to *R. prowazekii* in ultrastructure, metabolism, guanine and cytosine content of DNA, and staining characteristics and shares group antigens with *R. prowazekii* and *R. canada,* but it differs in specific antigens and host range. Significant cross-immunity between *R. mooseri* and *R. prowazekii* is produced by infection but not by killed vaccines.

TRANSMISSION AND EPIDEMIOLOGY. Murine typhus is not communicable from man to man. It is a zoonosis maintained in nature in a cycle involving rats and certain other small mammals as amplifying hosts and reservoirs and fleas and rat lice as vectors. In the rat flea (*Xenopsylla cheopis*) and perhaps other fleas infected by feeding upon rickettsemic rats, the organism grows in cells of the gut without killing the flea and is shed in the feces for the life of the flea. There is no transovarial transmission. It is transmitted to man, not by bite of the flea, but rather by contamination of broken skin with infective feces or by inhalation of dried infective feces.

Murine typhus is widely distributed over the world in the areas penetrated by *Rattus rattus* and *Rattus norvegicus* and where the vector fleas coexist. In some areas under appropriate conditions there may be spillover of *R. mooseri* from *Rattus* into other spatially closely associated small mammals and to man. Seasonal incidence of human infections appears to correlate with the periods of abundance of vector fleas, which in the United States is in the summer months. Rats are commensal animals closely associated with buildings or structures containing food (such as warehouses, markets, grain elevators, and godowns). Hence, acquisition of murine typhus by man is often associated with certain places and occupations.

PATHOLOGY. Although because of the low death rate few postmortem studies have been made, it is assumed that the lesions in man, as is the case in experimental infection of laboratory animals, are similar to those in louse-borne typhus.

CLINICAL MANIFESTATIONS AND COURSE. The incubation period of murine typhus lasts from 6 to 14 days. The symptoms are similar to those of louse-borne typhus, the principal differences being that murine typhus is a milder and shorter disease, the rash is less extensive and persists for shorter periods, there are fewer complications, and the case fatality rate is lower.

Although murine typhus is often referred to as mild, and truly mild cases do occur, this is mildness *relative* to louse-borne typhus. On an absolute scale, however, it can be severe and debilitating and may require two to three months for convalescence in untreated patients.

DIAGNOSIS. Clinical Diagnosis. The diagnosis of murine typhus may be suspected when a patient has sustained fever of several days' duration accompanied by headache, generalized aches and pains, and a macular or maculopapular rash appearing on the trunk on the fifth or sixth day after onset of fever. The patient with murine typhus may give a history of activities that have brought him into contact with places where rats are numerous. However, there is often no definite recollection of a flea bite. It is impossible on clinical evidence alone to distinguish an ordinary case of murine typhus from a case of Brill-Zinsser disease or a mild case of louse-borne typhus.

Laboratory Diagnosis. Diagnosis can often be made by specific rickettsial serologic tests or by isolation of the agent. (See Laboratory Diagnosis in Ch. 107.)

PROGNOSIS. The case fatality rate is usually less than 5 per cent in untreated patients and is virtually zero with rapid convalescence in uncomplicated murine typhus treated with appropriate antirickettsial drugs.

TREATMENT. Treatment follows the guidelines given in Ch. 107 with respect to the multiple dose antimicrobial regimen.

PREVENTION AND CONTROL. Individual preventive measures include avoiding endemic foci where rats and their fleas abound (e.g., warehouses, storage areas, grain elevators) or wearing repellent-treated clothing to prevent acquisition of fleas. A killed vaccine has been produced, but is unevaluated and is not now available.

General control measures are directed at reducing rat and flea populations. Among others, these include rat-proof construction and prevention of access of rats to food materials; reduction of rat populations by poison baits (e.g., warfarin, alphanaphthylthiourea), trapping, or poison gases into burrows; and reduction of the flea population through application of appropriate insecticides (such as DDT) to rat runs. When contemplating a rodent control program, it is important to plan insecticide application for flea control prior to, or simultaneously with, the rodent control measures to prevent increased exposure of man to fleas seeking alternative hosts.

Fox, J. P., Montoya, J. A., Jordan, M. D., Cornojo Ubillus, J. R., Garcia, J. L., Estrada, M. A., and Gelfand, H. M.: Immunization of man against epidemic typhus by infection with avirulent *Rickettsia prowazekii* (strain E). Arch. Inst. Pasteur Tunis, 36:449, 1959.

Gaon, J. A., and Murray, E. S.: The natural history of recrudescent typhus (Brill-Zinsser disease) in Bosnia. Bull. WHO, 35:133, 1966.

Hoeprich, P. D. (ed.): Infectious Diseases. New York, Harper & Row, 1972.

MacArthur, W. P.: The Athenian plague: A medical note. Classical Quarterly, 4:171, 1954.

Miller, E. S., and Beeson, P. B.: Murine typhus fever. Medicine, 25:1, 1946.

Murray, E. S., and Snyder, J. C.: Brill-Zinsser disease: The interepidemic reservoir of epidemic louse-borne typhus fever. Proceedings, Sixth International Congress of Microbiology, Rome; 4, Section 11, 31-44, 1953.

Price, W. H., et. al.: Ecologic studies of the interepidemic survival of louse-borne epidemic typhus fever. Am. J. Hyg., 67:154 1958.

Proceedings of the International Symposium on the Control of Lice and Louse-borne Diseases, Washington, D.C., December 4-6, 1972. Pan American Health Organization Scientific Publication No. 263, 1973.

Smadel, J. E.: Status of the rickettsioses in the United States. Ann. Intern. Med., 51:421, 1959.

Snyder, J. C.: The typhus fevers. *In* Horsfall, F. L., Jr., and Tamm, I. (eds.): Viral and Rickettsial Infections of Man. 4th ed. Philadelphia, J. B. Lippincott Company, 1965, Chapter 50.

Stuart, B. M., and Pullen, R. L.: Endemic (murine) typhus fever: Clinical observations of 180 cases. Ann. Intern. Med., 23:520, 1945.

Wisseman, C. L., Jr.: Problems of rickettsial diseases and vaccines: Desirable developments. Proceedings of the International Conference on the Application of Vaccines against Viral Rickettsial and Bacterial Diseases of Man, Washington, D.C., 14-18 Dec. 1970. Pan American Health Organization Scientific Publication No. 226, 1971, pp. 289-303.

Wisseman, C. L., Jr.: Concepts of louse-borne typhus control in developing countries: The use of the living attenuated E strain typhus vaccine in epidemic and endemic situations. *In* Kohn, A., and Klingberg, M. A. (eds.): Immunity in Viral and Rickettsial Diseases. New York, Plenum Publishing Co., 1972, pp. 97-130.

Wolbach, S. B., Todd, J. L., and Palfrey, F. W.: The Etiology and Pathology of Typhus. Cambridge, Mass., Harvard University Press, 1922.

Zdrodovskii, P. F., and Golinevich, H. M.: The Rickettsial Diseases. New York, Pergamon Press, 1960.

Zinsser, H.: Rats, Lice, and History. Boston, Little, Brown and Company, 1935.

109. ROCKY MOUNTAIN SPOTTED FEVER

(Spotted Fever, Tick Typhus [England], Fiebre Manchada [Mexico], Fiebre Petequial [Colombia], Febre Maculosa, São Paulo Typhus [Brazil])

Charles L. Wisseman, Jr.

DEFINITION. Rocky Mountain spotted fever is a mild to severe acute infectious disease of the Western Hemisphere caused by *Rickettsia rickettsii* and transmitted to man by several species of ticks. The disease is characterized by sudden onset with chills and headache, by fever of about two to three weeks' duration, and by a rash on the extremities and trunk beginning about the fourth day of disease.

ETIOLOGY. The disease is caused by *Rickettsia rickettsii*, the prototype species of the spotted fever group of rickettsiae with which it shares group antigens but from which it can be differentiated by more specific tests (see Ch. 107). It differs from the typhus and scrub typhus group organisms in its capacity to grow in the nucleus as well as the cytoplasm of host cells (see Ch. 107). Both mild and highly virulent strains coexist in many parts of the United States. Although several other species of the spotted fever group have been isolated from ticks in the United States (*R. parkeri, R. montana,* other recent isolates), to date only typical *R. rickettsii* has been isolated from infections of man. More intensive efforts to isolate and characterize rickettsiae from patients is needed to clarify the role, if any, of these other spotted fever group agents as causes of human disease.

DISTRIBUTION AND INCIDENCE. Although originally encountered in Rocky Mountain states (Montana and Idaho), Rocky Mountain spotted fever has been recognized in at least 46 states and is actually more prevalent in the south Atlantic states than in the west. In the eastern United States it extends from Cape Cod and some adjacent islands, through a focus on Long Island, to Florida, with almost half the cases in the United States occurring in Maryland, Virginia, North Carolina, and Georgia. The number of cases per year in the United States has risen steadily over the past several years to more than 700 in 1976. The reasons for this increase are not fully understood, but many include abundance of ticks, extension of suburbs into tick-infested rural areas, and increased recreational activities in wilderness areas. Rocky Mountain spotted fever has also been recognized in several provinces of Canada, Mexico, Central America (Panama, Costa Rica) and South America (Colombia, Brazil).

TRANSMISSION AND EPIDEMIOLOGY. Rocky Mountain spotted fever is a zoonosis maintained in a natural cycle between certain tick species and small (rodents, rabbits) and perhaps larger mammals. The ticks not only serve as vectors but also have an important reservoir function, because the infected female tick efficiently transmits the rickettsia transovarially to its progeny. Mammalian hosts probably serve more as an amplifying mechanism for infection of new ticks than they do as true reservoirs. Man, a dead-end host for *R. rickettsii,* becomes infected when he intrudes into this zoonotic cycle (as for recreational or occupational reasons) and is bitten by an infected tick. However, dogs can bring infected ticks into human dwellings.

Although multiple tick species (both hard and soft varieties) are known to become naturally infected and may play a role in transmission among animals, the main tick vectors for man are hard (Ixodid) ticks: the wood tick, *Dermacentor andersoni,* in the western United States; the dog tick, *Dermacentor variabilis,* in the eastern United States; *Amblyomma americanum* in Texas and Oklahoma; the brown dog tick, *Rhipicephalus sanguineus,* in northern Mexico (and introduced into the United States); and *Amblyomma cajennense* in Brazil and Colombia.

PATHOLOGY. The pathology of Rocky Mountain spotted fever conforms in general to the description in Ch. 107. Of special note is the fact that the vasculitis in Rocky Mountain spotted fever is not limited to the endothelium and is more severe than in typhus or scrub typhus, causing more pronounced thrombotic occlusion and necrosis of the muscular layers. Microinfarcts are seen with some frequency in the central nervous system.

CLINICAL MANIFESTATIONS AND COURSE. A history of tick bite can be elicited in the majority of, but not all, patients. Variation in incubation period (2 to 14, average 7 days) and severity of disease are seen in Rocky Mountain spotted fever, with a tendency for an inverse relationship between the two. Very severe disease often is preceded by a short (two- to five-day) incubation period. Prodromes, when present, consist of anorexia, irritability, malaise, feverishness, and chilly sensations. Attacks may be so mild that the patient remains ambulatory, or so severe that death may occur within three to six days of onset. The more typical infections are sudden in onset, with severe headache, chills, fever, prostration, myalgia (especially of the back and legs), nausea with occasional vomiting, conjunctival injections, and photophobia. There may be abdominal muscular pain, tenderness of muscles on palpation, and arthralgia.

Body temperature reaches 39 to 40° C in the first two days, is sustained at elevated levels for about 2 weeks, and declines by slow lysis over three or four days. Hyperthermia in the range of 41° C is a serious sign. Body temperature falling to near or below normal levels in the face of severe hypotension and tachycardia carries a grave prognosis.

The characteristic rash appears on about the fourth day (two to six days), first about the wrists and ankles, and then extends rapidly over all or most of the body, including palms, soles, face, and, occasionally, the mucous membranes of the mouth and throat. At first, the lesions are pink macules, 2 to 5 mm in diameter, which blanch on pressure. In two or three days, they become fixed, darker red, or purplish, maculopapular, and, about the fourth day, petechial. Hemorrhagic lesions may coalesce. The rash begins to disappear as the fever subsides but often remains as pigmented spots for weeks.

Early in the disease the pulse is full, regular, and elevated in proportion to fever. Later, it becomes more rapid and feeble, and some degree of hypotension develops. The electrocardiogram may show minor S-T deflections and prolonged P-R intervals. In some cases, hypotension may attain shock levels, and gangrene of fingers, toes, ears, nose, or genitalia may develop. Thrombosis of larger vessels may lead to loss of a portion of a limb or hemiplegia. The skin may become necrotic over body prominences. Hemorrhage from the nose, gastrointestinal tract, or kidney may occur. In recent years, disturbances in clotting mechanisms have been observed. Platelet counts are frequently low. Varying degrees of disseminated intravascular coagulation have been observed.

Central nervous system involvement is manifest by restlessness, insomnia, delirium, stupor, and, in severe cases, coma. Convulsions, muscular rigidity, tremors, and athetoid movements may occur. Cranial nerve involvement is variable. Transient deafness is common, but peripheral neuritis is uncommon. Electroencephalographic changes may persist for many months. Incontinence of urine and feces may be present in severe cases.

The liver may be enlarged and serum albumin depressed, but jaundice is not common. Oliguria and some azotemia are common in severe cases. Anuria and marked azotemia may be seen in critically ill patients. Complicating secondary bacterial infections (bronchopneumonia, otitis media, parotitis) occur but are uncommon.

Defervescence is usually by slow lysis. Convalescence may take weeks to months. Death, when it occurs in the nonfulminant variety, usually occurs late in the second week of disease (range about 9 to 18 days after onset).

DIAGNOSIS. An acute febrile illness with or without rash, in a person with a history of tick-bite, exposure to ticks (either in a tick-infested rural or suburban area or contact with a tick-infested dog), or, equally important, recreational or occupational activities which might have brought the patient into a potentially tick-infested area, should alert the physician to the possibility of Rocky Mountain spotted fever. Although other diseases, especially those with rash, may present transient early differential diagnostic problems, the two diseases which have consistently caused the greatest confusion are measles and meningococcemia. The most promising laboratory diagnostic method for providing a specific diagnosis early enough in the disease to permit effective specific therapeutic intervention is the demonstration by the fluorescent antibody technique of spotted fever group rickettsiae in skin biopsies. Isolation attempts, which are encouraged, and serologic diagnostic methods (see Laboratory Diagnosis in Ch. 107) are useful and important but rarely yield results in time for most efficient management.

PROGNOSIS. Although mild cases occur, the rapid, severe course in some patients makes it imperative to regard any suspected case of Rocky Mountain spotted fever essentially as a medical emergency. In untreated cases, the over-all case fatality rate was about 20 per cent, with areas of low ($\leqslant$ 10 per cent) and high ($\geqslant$60 per cent) rates. Prognosis depends on severity of infection, host factors (such as age, presence of other disease), and *the time after onset at which specific antirickettsial chemotherapy is started.* Even with effective antirickettsial drugs available, the case fatality rate has remained at 5 to 10 per cent. Analysis of fatal cases in recent years has shown that the single most important factor was *delay in institution of antirickettsial therapy,*

whatever the reason. With the time between onset and death as short as three to six days, the critical period when antimicrobial therapy can influence the outcome may be very short indeed and does not leave much latitude for correcting errors in clinical diagnosis.

TREATMENT. Prompt administration of a tetracycline antibiotic or chloramphenicol (see Treatment of Rickettsial Diseases in Ch. 107) is the single most important specific therapeutic measure. However, apparently serious physiologic derangements follow rapidly on the tissue damage produced by the rickettsial infection. Once initiated, these physiologic derangements do not respond directly to antimicrobial therapy and may require vigorous supportive measures and attempts at specific intervention. Shock and the consequences of disseminated intravascular clotting have been particularly resistant to correction in severe cases.

PREVENTION AND CONTROL. Individual preventive measures are directed primarily at prevention of tick bite. The chances of ticks attaching should be minimized by (1) avoiding places especially likely to harbor ticks (e.g., brush where livestock and game take refuge); (2) wearing boots and protective clothing designed to exclude ticks (preferably impregnated with a tick repellent, such as N-N-butylacetanilide); and (3) carefully inspecting the *entire* body once or twice daily to remove all ticks. Ticks usually crawl about on the body or in the clothing for some time prior to attaching. Thus frequent inspection usually discloses ticks before they attach. Moreover, since the chance of transmission of Rocky Mountain spotted fever appears to be a function of the duration of attachment, early removal of an attached tick probably reduces the chances of infection. Ticks should be removed (from man or dogs) with a pair of forceps, exerting gentle steady traction so that the mouth parts are released intact from the skin. Most other commonly recommended methods of tick removal are less satisfactory. Contact between tick and fingers should be avoided, because rickettsiae in tick feces or body fluids may enter a break in the skin or be transferred to mucous membranes and initiate infection.

For families living in tick-infested areas, an especially effective preventive measure is for parents to establish the routine of examining themselves and their children for ticks every evening at bath time during the tick season, and to teach the children to examine themselves as soon as they are old enough. In the author's own family, over the years this practice has detected many ticks, all still unattached.

The Rocky Mountain Laboratory of the United States Public Health Service has recently begun a service through state health departments to examine individual ticks for *R. rickettsii* (the "hemolymph" test). It is best practice today to place a person from whom a positive tick has been removed under close observation, recording morning and evening temperatures for two weeks, and instituting full antirickettsial chemotherapy only, but promptly, when a significant rise in temperature first appears. Attempts at chemoprophylaxis are likely only to delay onset of disease.

The current commercial killed *R. rickettsii* vaccine is of dubious value, and its manufacture may be discontinued. In a human vaccination-challenge study, it failed to protect against disease when minimal human infectious challenge doses were given intradermally, although the incubation period was lengthened. On the other hand, an uncontrolled retrospective study of potentially exposed laboratory personnel suggested protection against airborne infections. An experimental killed vaccine which may have greater potency has been developed but is not yet generally available.

Area control of ticks is still very difficult and is usually considered impractical. Ticks are unusually resistant to most insecticides. Yet, some measure of control may be achieved in time on small plots of ground, such as suburban lots, by intensive acaricidal treatment, the clearing of underbrush, intensive gardening or cultivation, and a reduction of the wild animal population. Changes in land use may affect tick populations. Some progress is being made toward identifying the specific habitat alterations that affect tick populations.

Atkin, M. D., Strauss, H. S., and Fisher, G. U.: A case report of "Cape Cod" Rocky Mountain spotted fever with multipe coagulation disturbances. Pediatrics, 36:627, 1965.

Graybill, J. R., Hawiger, J., and Des Prez, R. M.: Complement and coagulation in Rocky Mountain spotted fever. South. Med. J., 66:410, 1973.

Hand, W. L., Miller, J. B., Reinarz, J. A., and Sanford, J. P.: Rocky Mountain spotted fever. A vascular disease. Arch. Intern. Med., 125:879, 1970.

Harrell, G. T.: Rocky Mountain spotted fever. Medicine, 28:333, 1949.

Hattwick, M. A. W., O'Brien, R. J., and Hanson, B. F.: Rocky Mountain spotted fever: Epidemiology of an increasing problem. Ann. Intern. Med., 84:732, 1976.

Haynes, R. E., Sanders, D. Y., and Cramblett, H. G.: Rocky Mountain spotted fever in children. J. Pediat. 76:685, 1970.

Kurnick, J. E., Malinow, S. H. and Snyderman, M. C.: Disseminated intravascular coagulation in Rocky Mountain spotted fever. South. Med. J., 67:623, 1974.

Lackman, D. B., Bell, E. J., Stoenner, H. G., and Pickens, E. G.: The Rocky Mountain spotted fever group of rickettsias. Health Lab. Sci., 2:135, 1965.

Lennette, E. H.: Rocky Mountain spotted fever (editorial). N. Engl. J. Med., 297:884, 1977.

Miller, J. Q., and Price, T. R.: The nervous system in Rocky Mountain spotted fever. Neurology, 22:561, 1972.

Oster, C. N., Burke, D. S., Kenyon, R. H., Ascher, M. D., Harber, P., and Pedersen, C. E., Jr.: Laboratory-acquired Rocky Mountain spotted fever. N. Engl. J. Med., 297:859, 1977.

Ricketts, H. T.: Contributions to Medical Science by Howard Taylor Ricketts, 1870–1910. Chicago, University of Chicago Press, 1911, p. 278.

Sexton, D. J., Banks, P. M., Weig, S., and Roe, C. R.: Late appearance of skin rash and abnormal serum enzymes in Rocky Mountain spotted fever. J. Pediat., 87:580, 1975.

Wisseman, C. L., Jr. (ed.): Symposium on the Spotted Fever Group of Rickettsiae. Medical Science Publication No. 7, Walter Reed Army Institute of Research. Washington, D.C., U.S. Government Printing Office, 1960.

Woodward, T. E., and Jackson, E. B.: Spotted fever rickettsiae. In Horsfall, F. L., Jr., and Tamm, I. (eds.): Viral and Rickettsial Infections of Man. 4th ed. Philadelphia, J. B. Lippincott Company, 1965, p. 1095.

110. TICK-BORNE RICKETTSIOSES OF THE EASTERN HEMISPHERE*

Charles L. Wisseman, Jr.

DEFINITION. Three diseases, caused by three different members of the spotted fever group of rickettsiae, are currently the best recognized tick-borne rickettsioses of the Eastern Hemisphere and occur over distinct broad geographic areas: (1) African tick typhus (*R. conorii*), (2) North Asian tick-borne rickettsiosis (*R. sibirica*), and (3) Queensland tick typhus (*R. australis*). Each is a zoonosis, with man an accidental, dead-end host, and is transmitted by the bite of one or more species of ixodid ticks. The three diseases, mild to moderate in severity, closely resemble one another with a short (average five- to seven-day) incubation period, a primary lesion (eschar, tache noire), a fever of a few days' to two weeks' duration, and a maculopapular to almost nodular rash which appears three to five days after onset.

As might be expected with a microorganism that shows distinct tendencies for geographic variants distributed over extensive and divergent land masses with enormous faunal variation, several lines of evidence, especially in the past few years, suggested that the tick-borne rickettsioses of the Eastern Hemisphere are probably more complex than is implied by the generally accepted classification given above. For example, a spotted fever group rickettsia, apparently distinct from *R. sibirica* and *R. conorii,* has been isolated from ticks in Slovakia. Two different, possibly new species of spotted fever group rickettsiae, probably not *R. conorii,* have been isolated from ticks from dogs and hedgehogs in Israel, and one of these was also isolated from a patient with clinical tick typhus. Moreover, some cases of tick typhus in this area differ from classic boutonneuse fever (*R. conorii*) by the absence of a primary lesion and possibly more fatalities. Early descriptions of "Indian tick typhus" suggested the possibility of more than one entity. The only strain of "Indian tick typhus" rickettsiae studied by modern methods and found to be identical with, or very similar to, *R. conorii* was isolated from a tick taken from a dog near the dwelling of a patient with Indian tick typhus in Kashmir. However, more recently multiple spotted fever group rickettsiae have been isolated from ticks in Pakistan, viz., *R. conorii*-like, *R. sibirica*-like, and one or two probable new species. Thus clinical tick typhus in south Asia may have multiple causes. Occasional human cases of tick typhus, with eschar, have been recognized in southeast Asia, viz., Indochina and Malaysia. Such infections are probably often misdiagnosed as scrub typhus. Serologic evidence has been presented for widespread spotted fever group rickettsial infection among small mammals in Malaysia. However, the rickettsial agent or agents responsible for the human and small mammal infections have not been isolated and identified. Only a single strain of spotted fever group rickettsiae, probably a new species, has been isolated from ticks in Thailand. Much work remains to be done to clarify the problem of the rickettsioses of the Eastern Hemisphere. It is especially important to isolate and fully characterize the rickettsiae from patients with tick typhus in order that the agents most commonly associated with human disease can be identified.

For lack of more comprehensive knowledge, the descriptions below are confined to the three established rickettsioses.

*My former colleague and author of this chapter in the previous edition of this book, Dr. Herbert Ley, left this chapter essentially unchanged from that originally written by our mutual mentor, friend, and colleague, Dr. Joseph E. Smadel, who masterfully and concisely unified concepts in a difficult area on the basis of the best information available at the time. Some of this chapter has been retained in its original form with minor editorial changes because it is difficult to improve upon excellence. Newer information, however, of the kind that Dr. Smadel would have strongly fostered, has reintroduced certain complexities and uncertainties, reflected primarily in the paragraphs on Definition and on History, Etiology, Distribution, and Epidemiology. I look forward to the time when sufficient information is available to permit a second generation of unification and simplification. CLW Jr.

HISTORY, ETIOLOGY, DISTRIBUTION, AND EPIDEMIOLOGY. *Boutonneuse fever* was first recognized in 1910 in Tunisia by Conor and Bruch. During the next several decades similar diseases were recognized in other parts of Africa, in parts of Europe and the Middle East adjacent to the Mediterranian, Black and Caspian Seas, and in India where they were often given local names — e.g., Marseille fever, Indian tick typhus, Kenya tick typhus, South African tick typhus. Subsequent application of modern rickettsiologic methods led to the conclusion that all of these were in reality infection by *R. conorii* or closely related spotted fever group rickettsiae and could be classified under a single entity, African tick typhus. This probably is correct to a large degree. However, the serologic methods employed have limitations and cannot readily discriminate between infections caused by a new species and those caused by other members of this serologically cross-reactive group unless that new agent is included in the battery of specific antigens. The recent findings (see above) of a multiplicity of established and probable new species of spotted fever group rickettsiae along with *R. conorii* in some of the areas of presumed African tick typhus (*R. conorii*) distribution (e.g., Europe, Israel, India) suggest that considerable work must yet be done to clarify the question of distribution and nature of "African tick typhus." In the Mediterranean littoral, the main vector of fièvre boutonneuse is the dog tick, *Rhipicephalus sanguineus,* and the disease is often acquired in and around human habitations, i.e., a domesticated or urban pattern. In other areas, the causative agent of the local disease is transmitted by ticks which are parasitic on wild animals, and hence the disease is acquired in rural areas, e.g., certain stretches of the South African veldt.

North Asian tick-borne rickettsiosis (Siberian tick typhus), now known to be caused by *R. sibirica,* was first recognized as a clinical entity distinct from the other rickettsioses of the U.S.S.R. in the mid to late 1930's. It has since been found distributed from European Russia through Siberia to the Soviet Far East and, more recently, possibly to the Indo-Pakistan subcontinent. Several species of ixodid ticks have been implicated as vectors in different geographic regions. Its acquisition is characteristically in a sylvan or rural setting.

Queensland tick typhus is usually acquired in rural areas heavily infested with the tick, *Ixodes holocyclus,* and a history of tick bite and an eschar are common. The agent, *R. australis,* however, has only been isolated from the blood of patients. Antibodies have been detected in the blood of some small marsupials and a rat, suggesting a natural sylvan small animal–tick cycle.

PATHOLOGY. In fatal cases, which are few and usually limited to the aged and debilitated, the findings are similar to those in Rocky Mountain spotted fever except for the presence of the tache noire, the black button–like necrotic primary lesion that is generally found on the surface areas of the body ordinarily covered by clothing. The basic pathologic changes are found in the small blood vessels (see Ch. 107).

SYMPTOMS, LABORATORY FINDINGS, AND DIAGNOSIS. The three tick-borne rickettsioses that occur in different parts of the Eastern Hemisphere resemble one another closely. After an incubation period of about five to seven days, the disease begins with fever, headache, malaise, myalgia, and conjunctival injection. The primary lesion, which is present in most cases at the onset of fever, consists of a small ulcer 2 to 5 mm in diameter with a black center and a red areola; the regional lymph nodes are enlarged. The generalized erythematous maculopapular rash appears about the fourth day and quickly involves most of the body, including the palms and soles and often the face. In severe cases the rash becomes hemorrhagic. Fever abates during the second week. The prognosis is good except in the aged and debilitated. Complications and sequelae are unusual.

North Asian tick-borne rickettsiosis has been the subject of considerable laboratory and clinical observation by Soviet investigators. Mild hypotension, electrocardiographic changes, a reversal of the A/G ratio in serum (depressed albumin, early increased alpha globulins, followed by increase in gamma globulins), and abnormal liver function tests are noteworthy.

The laboratory findings of greatest importance are those derived from the serologic tests with Weil-Felix and rickettsial antigens (see Ch. 107). Agglutinins against *Proteus* OX-19 develop during the second week, and complement-fixing antibodies appear shortly thereafter.

Diagnosis is established by the clinical picture, including the tache noire, the geographic location, and positive serologic reactions. In the differential diagnosis the typhus fevers, meningococcal infections, and measles must be considered.

TREATMENT. Adequate information is available to indicate that treatment with the broad-spectrum antimicrobial drugs is as effective in patients with African tick typhus and North Asian tick-borne rickettsiosis as in those with other rickettsioses (see Ch. 107 for details of therapy). Presumably, these measures are also applicable to the other tick-borne rickettsioses of the Eastern Hemisphere. All the newly recognized strains display in vitro susceptibility to tetracyclines of the same order as *R. rickettsii* and presumably would respond to similar therapeutic regimens (see Ch. 107).

PROPHYLAXIS. Prevention of human disease is based on avoiding the bites of infected ticks. In Ch. 109 details are set forth regarding personal prophylaxis, including the use of protective clothing, chemical insect repellents, and reduction of tick population by measures involved in terrain control. Experimental vaccines prepared from formalin-treated yolk sac tissue infected with some of the three established Eastern Hemisphere rickettsiae under discussion are effective in animals, but commercial vaccines for human use are not available.

Bozeman, F. M., Humphries, J. W., Campbell, J. M., and O'Hara, P. L.: Laboratory studies of the spotted fever group of rickettsiae. *In* Wisseman, C. L., Jr. (ed.): Symposium on the Spotted Fever Group of Rickettsiae. Medical Science Publication No. 7, Walter Reed Army Institute of Research. Washington, D.C., U. S. Government Printing Office, 1960, p. 7.

Goldwasser, R. A., Klingberg, M. A., Klingberg, W., Steiman, Y., and Swartz, T. A.: Laboratory and epidemiological studies of rickettsial spotted fever in Israel. *In* Frontiers of Internal Medicine, Proceedings of 12th International Congress of Internal Medicine, Tel Aviv, 1974. Basel, Karger, 1975, pp. 270–275.

Hoogstraal, H.: Ticks in relation to human disease caused by *Rickettsia* species. Ann. Rev. Entomol., 12:377, 1967.

Lyskovtsev, M. M.: Tickborne rickettsiosis. Translation from the Russian in Miscellaneous Publications of the Entomological Society of America, 6:41, 1968.

Rehaček, I., Palonová, A., Zupancìková, M., Urvolgyi, J., Kovácová, E., Járábek, L., and Brezina, R.: Study of rickettsioses in Slovakia. I. *Coxiella burnetii* and rickettsiae of the spotted fever (SF) group in

ticks and serological surveys in animals and humans in certain selected localities in the Lucenec and V. Krtis districts. J. Hyg. Epidemiol. Microbiol. Immunol., 19:105, 1975.

Robertson, R. G., and Wisseman, C. L., Jr.: Tick-borne rickettsiae of
the spotted fever group in West Pakistan. II. Serological classification of isolates from West Pakistan and Thailand: Evidence for two
new species. Am. J. Epidemiol., 97:55, 1973.

Woodward, T. E., and Jackson, E. B.: Spotted fever rickettsiae. In Horsfall, F. L., Jr., and Tamm, I. (eds.): Viral and Rickettsial Infections
of Man. 4th ed. Philadelphia, J. B. Lippincott Company, 1965, p.
1095.

Zdrodovskii, P. I., and Golinevich, H. M.: The Rickettsial Diseases,
New York, Pergamon Press, 1960, p. 191.

111.　RICKETTSIALPOX

Charles L. Wisseman, Jr.

DEFINITION. Rickettsialpox is a mite-borne rickettsial
disease, mild and self-limited, which is characterized
by an initial eschar-like lesion and a fever of a week's
duration accompanied by headache, backache, and a
generalized papulovesicular rash.

ETIOLOGY. Rickettsialpox is caused by *Rickettsia
akari*, a member of the spotted fever group on the basis
of shared group antigens but with unique specfic antigens and certain biologic properties.

DISTRIBUTION AND INCIDENCE. The disease has been
reported from certain cities in the United States (New
York, Boston, West Haven, Ct., Philadelphia, Pittsburgh, and Cleveland) and from the U.S.S.R. In the
first three years after the disease was described in 1946,
about 500 cases were reported in the United States,
mostly from New York, but the number reported has
since decreased markedly. Although the reasons for the
decrease are not clearly established, it may be due to
under-reporting of disease or to control measures.

TRANSMISSION AND EPIDEMIOLOGY. Although detailed information is sparse, it is clear that rickettsialpox is a zoonosis which can involve house mice (*Mus
musculus*) and mouse mites (*Allodermanyssus sanguineus*). *R. akari* has also been isolated from rats in the
U.S.S.R. and from voles (small field "mice") in Korea.
It is unknown if the basic natural cycle involves field
rodents and their ectoparasites with occasional spillover
into the mouse-mite cycle or if the latter is in fact the
basic sustaining cycle. Regardless, in the United States
the mouse-mite cycle, greatly amplified and concentrated in discrete foci artificially created by, and frequented
by, man himself (e.g., improperly fired apartment
house incinerators), was responsible for bringing *R.
akari* and man into effective contact with one another.
The usually large mite population, which infested the
walls and floors of the incinerator rooms, had access to
people entering the foci with a frequency not usually
encountered under natural circumstances. Transmission
is presumably by bite of the mite. Simple control measures directed at the mice and mites have virtually eliminated the human disease.

PATHOLOGY. As no fatal cases have been encountered, studies of the pathology of rickettsialpox have
been limited to an examination of skin biopsies. Histologically, the eschar of rickettsialpox resembles the eschars of scrub typhus and boutonneuse fever. The skin

lesions composing the rash show a typical perivascular
infiltration by mononuclear cells. Later, necrosis of the
superficial epithelium leads to intraepidermal vesicle
formation.

CLINICAL MANIFESTATIONS AND COURSE. The incubation period varies from about ten days to three weeks.
An initial lesion (the eschar) appears at the site of the
mite bite about a week before onset of fever in about
90 per cent of the cases, gradually enlarging and progressing from a papular lesion through vesicle formation, finally to form a dark encrusted lesion 0.5 to 1.5
cm in diameter. The onset of an intermittent fever is
sudden and is accompanied by chills or chilly sensations, drenching sweats, headache, anorexia, and photophobia. The temperature ranges from about 38 to
40° C, lasts for about a week, is accompanied by headache, lassitude, and myalgia, and then gradually subsides. A sparse eruption appears on the trunk, extremities, and mucous membranes between the first and
fourth days of fever, beginning as discrete maculopapular lesions and evolving into a vesiculopapular rash.
The vesicles are firm, are sometimes surrounded by erythema, and, on drying, form a dark crust that falls off
without leaving a scar.

DIAGNOSIS.　Clinical Diagnosis. The clinical characteristics of the disease are so distinctive that in most
patients a presumptive diagnosis may be made on clinical grounds. Chickenpox in adults poses the most difficult diagnostic problem. Important points in differentiation are as follows: the vesicles in rickettsialpox are
seen to arise from the center of discrete papules; the
lesions tend to appear at the same time instead of in
crops; on the average, the number of lesions is fewer
than in chickenpox; and there often is an initial lesion
at the site of the mite bite. In smallpox, the lesions
progress on to pustulation.

Laboratory Diagnosis. Laboratory diagnosis depends on isolation of the agent and on serologic response measured by rickettsial group and specific antigens. The Weil-Felix test is negative (see Ch. 107).

PROGNOSIS. Even without specific therapy, the
course of the disease is benign, the prognosis excellent,
and death unusual.

TREATMENT. Response to tetracycline drugs, given
as outlined in Ch. 107, is rapid without relapse.

PREVENTION AND CONTROL. The transient emergence
of rickettsialpox from a silent zoonosis to a human disease problem was an artifact of urban living, and its
apparent disappearance is probably a result of minor
changes in human behavior. The prevention and control of rickettsialpox depend on rodent and mite control
by (1) the elimination of mice and mouse harborages,
which should include proper care and firing of incinerators in dwellings, and (2) the application of residual
acaricides to walls and other mite-infested areas. No
vaccines have been developed.

Dolgopol, V. B.: Histologic changes in rickettsialpox. Am. J. Pathol.,
24:119, 1948.

Greenberg, M., Pelliteri, O., Klein, I. F., and Huebner, R. J.: Rickettsialpox — a newly recognized rickettsial disease. II. Clinical observations. JAMA, 133:901, 1947.

Lackman, D. B.: A review of information on rickettsialpox in the United States. Clin. Pediat. 2:296, 1963.

Roueché, B.: The alerting of Mr. Pomerantz. In Roueché, B.: Eleven
Blue Men. Boston, Little, Brown & Company, 1954, p. 48.

112. SCRUB TYPHUS (Chigger-Borne Rickettsiosis; Many Local Names: Tsutsugamushi Disease, Japanese River or Flood Fever, Mite-Borne Typhus, Tropical Typhus, Rural Typhus, Mossman Fever, Others)

Charles L. Wisseman, Jr.

DEFINITION. Scrub typhus is an acute, febrile, typhus-like disease of rural Asia transmitted by the bite of larval trombiculid mites (chiggers). The site of infection is often marked by an eschar accompanied by regional lymphadenitis.

ETIOLOGY. The disease is caused by infection with *Rickettsia tsutsugamushi* (*R. orientalis*). The organism, although an obligate intracellular parasite multiplying free in host cell cytoplasm, differs substantially from other members of the genus *Rickettsia* in ultrastructure, tinctorial properties, and certain biologic features, holds no known antigens in common with them, but shares an antigen with *Proteus* OX-K. Multiple serotypes exist which produce substantial homologous immunity but only transient cross-immunity in man. Virulence of strain for mice and man varies from low to very high.

DISTRIBUTION AND INCIDENCE. Scrub typhus is widely distributed in eastern and southern Asia and the islands of the western and southern Pacific. It is known as far north as the island of Hokkaido in Japan and the Primorye region of asiatic U.S.S.R., as far south as the northern tip of Australia, and as far west as Pakistan and Tadzhikistan. Endemic infection is unknown in the New World, Europe, and Western Asia; but cases imported during the incubation period following infection in an endemic area have been recognized in the United States.

Because of a general lack of diagnostic and medical facilities in endemic areas, scrub typhus is best known from its occurrence in substantial numbers when large groups of nonimmune persons enter an endemic area, such as in military operations, road building, land clearing, and certain agricultural settings such as rubber plantations. It is an important military disease, e.g., in World War II, Vietnam, the Indo-Pakistan war, and current campaigns against "insurgents" in Burma and Thailand. Application of modern epidemiologic and laboratory methods is currently revealing, as expected, that scrub typhus is a major cause of febrile disease in rural populations indigenous to endemic areas and thus promises to emerge as one of the major causes of febrile disease in Asia.

TRANSMISSION AND EPIDEMIOLOGY. Scrub typhus is a zoonosis whose main constant elements constitute a tetrad: (1) *R. tsutsugamushi*; (2) chiggers of the *Leptotrombidium deliense* group; (3) wild rats, especially of the subgenus *Rattus*; and (4) transitional vegetation. Man, not essential to maintenance of the infection cycle, is a dead-end host and acquires the disease when he intrudes into an endemic focus. The characteristic epidemiologic features of chigger-borne typhus, such as a marked focal distribution of cases and sudden outbreaks among field personnel, are explained by attributes of the vector chiggers. In temperate zones, most vector chiggers are active at some time during the warm months. On the Izu islands of Japan, *Leptotrombidium scutellare* transmits the disease in the winter. In tropical and subtropical regions, the disease may be more prevalent at one time of the year than another, depending on rainfall, flooding, and other factors. Chigger-borne rickettsiosis is transmitted by the bite of the infected larval mite. Since the chigger is the only parasitic stage of the mite and usually feeds only once, if infected, it must have acquired the organism transovarially from its mother. Naturally infected chiggers presumably constitute the main reservoirs of *R. tsutsugamushi* in nature. Chiggers of the *Leptotrombidium deliense* group are the main vectors to man and perhaps to other hosts as well; *L. deliense*, *L. akamushi*, *L. fletcheri*, *L. arenicola*, *L. pallidum*, *L. pavlovskyi*, and *L. scutellare* are known vectors. Infections also occur in areas where none of the known vectors is present. *Rickettsia tsutsugamushi*–infected chiggers often occur in very circumscribed foci or "islands." Rats, particularly wild rats of the subgenus *Rattus*, serve as prime hosts of *Leptotrombidium* throughout their native ranges. Other small mammals (e.g., field mice, voles, shrews) often serve as secondary hosts.

The rickettsiosis exists in a wide variety of habitats, ranging from semideserts to alpine meadows and subarctic scree in the Himalayas, and from disturbed rain forest to seashores. Some kind of transitional or secondary vegetation is characteristic of all terrain where outbreaks occur, and is present in some form in all known foci of chigger-borne rickettsiosis, even if only as fringe habitat along streams in deep forest. All known foci are characterized by changing environmental conditions, whether induced by man (e.g., clearing of forest) or by nature, either suddenly (e.g., landslides) or cyclically (tidal zones, spring floods, glacial runoff).

PATHOLOGY. The pathologic features of scrub typhus conform generally to those described in Ch. 107. Of special note in scrub typhus is the primary local ulcer with regional and, later, generalized lymphadenopathy. Vascular thrombosis is less frequent than in epidemic typhus and Rocky Mountain spotted fever, but inflammatory lesions of larger arteries are more common.

CLINICAL MANIFESTATIONS AND COURSE. The spectrum of clinical severity of untreated scrub typhus ranges from inapparent or mild to severe or mortal, with mortality rates varying from 0 to more than 30 per cent in different places and outbreaks. The following description pertains to a classic, relatively severe untreated case of scrub typhus.

The bite of the infecting chigger, which may be on any part of the body, is usually unnoticed; but in roughly 60 to 70 per cent of the primary infections and substantially fewer in second infections, a small painless papule develops during the 6- to 18-day (usually 9-

to 12-day) incubation period. It enlarges, undergoes central necrosis, and crusts to form the eschar or primary lesion which is well developed at the onset of disease. The regional lymph nodes are enlarged and tender. Prodromes of headache, malaise, anorexia, and weakness may occur. The onset is usually acute. The fever rises progressively during the first few days, sometimes accompanied by chills after about the third day, to 39.5 to 40.5° C, accompanied by severe headache, ocular pain, conjunctival injection, anorexia, generalized aches, malaise, apathy, and cough. Interstitial pneumonitis is common. The pulse remains relatively slow. Toward the end of the first week, a macular rash, later sometimes papular, often appears, first on the trunk and then on the extremities. About this time there is generalized lymphadenopathy, soft splenic enlargement, and sometimes hepatomegaly.

During the second week of disease, the temperature remains elevated and signs of complex multiple organ system involvement appear. Apathy may give way to more pronounced signs of meningoencephalitis: delirium and restlessness, stupor, coma, convulsions, muscular weakness, hyperesthesias, and coarse intention tremors. Cranial nerves are selectively involved: varying degrees of nerve deafness and papilledema and congestion of retinal vessels are common; dysarthria and dysphagia are less frequent. Signs of diffuse and focal myocarditis may appear: soft first heart sound, systolic murmurs, ectopic beats, occasional cardiac enlargement, transient gallop rhythm, and minor abnormalities of the electrocardiogram (prolonged P-R interval, inverted T waves). Classic congestive failure is rare, but varying degrees of circulatory failure may appear: increasing pulse rate, falling blood pressure (commonly below 100 mm Hg systolic), rapid shallow respirations, cyanosis, sweating, and cold clammy skin. Gangrene is rare, but edema may be overt in severe cases. Clinical evidence for renal insufficiency is often absent, but oliguria or anuria occur in some. Spontaneous diuresis is fairly common late in the febrile course or in early convalescence.

In untreated cases, defervescence is by lysis usually after about 10 to 14 days (21 or more days in severe cases). Convalescence is prolonged. However, in nonfatal cases, all abnormalities appear to be completely reversible, although some, such as cardiovascular instability, personality changes, and deafness, may occasionally persist for weeks to months. Long-term (ten years or more) follow-up of United States servicemen who survived scrub typhus in World War II failed to reveal any significant residua.

An early leukopenia (1000 to 5000 white blood cells per cubic millimeter) gives way to slightly depressed or normal total white blood counts, which may become somewhat elevated late in the disease. Total serum proteins are usually normal or low, but the albumin-globulin (A/G) ratio is often reversed. Occasional clotting disturbances have been reported recently, including disseminated intravascular clotting syndrome. Jaundice is rare, but serum transaminase enzyme levels may be elevated. Albuminuria is common. Isosthenuria, oliguria, and azotemia may occur.

DIAGNOSIS. A typhus-like illness with a history of possible exposure in endemic areas and an eschar (in only about 40 to 70 per cent) with regional lymphadenitis should alert the physician to the possibility of scrub typhus. Differential diagnosis may be difficult in some endemic regions where the clinical picture may suggest other rickettsial infections (especially tick-borne typhus, which may also have an eschar) and other nonrickettsial infections (see General Clinical Considerations in Ch. 107). The Weil-Felix test with *Proteus* OX-K, not positive in all cases, is useful because of general availability. The indirect fluorescent antibody test is currently the serodiagnostic method of choice (see Laboratory Diagnosis in Ch. 107). Isolation can be accomplished by inoculating blood or tissue homogenates intraperitoneally into white mice.

PROGNOSIS. Untreated, the mortality ranges from essentially zero to over 30 per cent in different foci. Prompt antibiotic therapy reduces mortality virtually to zero.

TREATMENT. Tetracycline drugs, given as recommended in Ch. 107, and appropriate supportive measures are recommended treatment. A single dose of doxycycline may prove to be adequate for treatment.

PREVENTION AND CONTROL. Effective killed vaccines have not yet been developed to prevent scrub typhus. Transient cross-immunity among serotypes and more persistent homologous immunity can be induced by intentional infection with a virulent strain, followed by carefully timed chemoprophylaxis which permits subclinical immunizing infection, but this procedure is useful only under limited circumstances. Practical chemoprophylaxis with a long-acting tetracycline (doxycycline) is theoretically feasible and is currently under investigation. But practically, at this time, preventive measures against scrub typhus are directed primarily against the chigger vector. Mite-infested terrain should be avoided whenever possible. Individual prophylaxis against attack by larval mites consists of wearing protective clothing, impregnated with a mite repellent (benzyl benzoate, M-1960), and applying diethyltoluamide to exposed skin areas. The vector population in and around camp sites in endemic zones can be reduced (1) by treating the area intensively with acaricides (e.g., dieldrin), (2) possibly by reducing the rodent population through intensive poison bait campaigns, and (3) by destroying vegetation (bulldozing, power oil burners, herbicides). However, appropriate and relevant environmental, medical, and ecologic considerations must temper decisions on the use of persisting acaricides and herbicides.

Brown, G. W., Robinson, D. M., and Huxsoll, D. L.: Scrub typhus: A common cause of illness in indigenous populations. Trans. R. Soc. Trop. Med. Hyg., 70:444, 1976.

Deller, J. J., Jr., and Russell, P. K.: An analysis of fevers of unknown origin in American Soldiers in Vietnam. Ann. Intern. Med., 66:1129, 1967.

Ley, H. L., Jr., et al.: Immunization against scrub typhus. IV. Living Karp vaccine and chemoprophylaxis in volunteers. Am. J. Hyg., 56:303, 1952.

Smadel, J. E.: Influence of antibiotics on immunologic responses in scrub typhus. Am. J. Med., 17:246, 1954.

Smadel, J. E., and Elisberg, B. L.: Scrub typhus rickettsia. *In* Horsfall, F. L., Jr., and Tamm, I. (eds.): Viral and Rickettsial Infections of Man. 4th ed. Philadelphia, J. B. Lippincott Company, 1965, p. 1130.

Tamiya, T. (ed.): Recent Advances in Studies of Tsutsugamushi Disease in Japan. Tokyo, Medical Culture Inc., 1962.

Traub, R., and Wisseman, C. L., Jr.: Ecological considerations in scrub typhus. III. Methods of area control. Bull. WHO, 39:231, 1968.

Traub, R., and Wisseman, C. L., Jr.: The ecology of chigger-borne rickettsioses (scrub typhus) (review article). J. Med. Entomol., 11:237, 1974.

113. TRENCH FEVER
(Five-Day or Quintana Fever, Shin Bone Fever, Volhynian Fever)

Herbert L. Ley, Jr.

DEFINITION. Trench fever is a self-limited louse-borne rickettsial disease characterized by intermittent fever, generalized aches and pains, negligible mortality, and multiple relapses.

ETIOLOGY AND EPIDEMIOLOGY. The disease is caused by *Rochalimaea quintana*, a rickettsial agent that grows extracellularly in the louse intestine and is excreted in louse feces. Transmission takes place by rubbing louse feces into skin abrasions or into the bite wound left by the louse. The incubation period of the disease may vary from 5 to 38 days, but is usually two to four weeks. The disease was a major military problem during World War I, when an estimated 1,000,000 cases occurred in western Europe. It was not seen in epidemic form again until World War II when 80,000 cases were reported in eastern Europe. Recent studies have demonstrated the disease in endemic form in Mexico. During epidemics man is clearly the principal reservoir. He may also be the major long-term reservoir because the disease agent has been isolated from asymptomatic patients years after their initial infection.

PATHOLOGY AND CLINICAL MANIFESTATIONS. Because the disease has a negligible mortality, information on the histopathologic changes is limited. Biopsy studies reveal only perivascular inflammation, principally in the form of lymphocytic infiltrations. The presenting symptoms of the disease are recurrent fever, severe weakness, headache, dizziness, back and leg pains (particularly in the shins), and photophobia. Physical and laboratory examinations are not remarkable except for slight enlargement of the spleen and liver, areas of cutaneous tenderness distributed over the body, and a moderate leukocytosis. A transient rash of erythematous macules or papules occurs in about 70 per cent of patients. The patient's fever may rise as high as 40.5° C in an irregular fashion with intervals of nearly normal temperature between peaks of fever. The fever may last for only four or five days in the more fortunate patients. In others, the initial pyrexia may be followed after five or six days of normal temperature by one to eight relapses of fever similar to the initial episode. In still other patients, the initial fever may decline, shading into relapses without a true afebrile period, producing a "saddleback" or "typhoidal" fever curve.

DIAGNOSIS. The most important fact supporting the diagnosis of trench fever is a history of contact with lice within the incubation period of the disease. Xenodiagnosis — the feeding of clean uninfected lice on a patient suspected of having the disease — is a useful diagnostic aid. The lice are examined a week after feeding on the patient for the presence of rickettsiae in the lumen of the gut. The technique of cultivation of *R. quintana* on blood agar containing 10 per cent of fresh blood has also been used diagnostically. Recently developed serologic tests appear promising in the diagnosis of the disease. The differential diagnosis of the disease should include leptospirosis, dengue, malaria, relapsing fever, and the typhus fevers.

TREATMENT AND PROGNOSIS. Although the tetracyclines and other antimicrobials may be expected to be as effective in the treatment of trench fever as in the treatment of the other rickettsial diseases, in the absence of epidemics of trench fever no reliable information about their efficacy is available. Because the disease has a negligible mortality, the long-term prognosis is excellent. Even without treatment the majority of patients are able to return to full activity within one to two months after onset, although a few continue to experience recurrences of the symptoms of infection for months or years.

PREVENTION. The only practicable method of control of trench fever is the elimination of the louse vector of the disease by dusting clothing with residual insecticides. Ten per cent DDT powders proved highly effective for louse control during the World War II period, but the development of DDT resistance in lice in many parts of the world has forced the use of 1 per cent lindane or 1 per cent malathion powders. For additional comments on louse control, see Ch. 108.

Trench Fever: Report of Commission on Trench Fever. American Red Cross Medical Research Committee. London, Oxford University Press, 1918.

Varela, G., Vinson, J. W., and Molina-Pasquel, C.: Trench fever. II. Propagation of *Rickettsia quintana* on cell-free medium from the blood of two patients. Am. J. Trop. Med., 18:708, 1969.

Vinson, J. W., Varela, G., and Molina-Pasquel, C.: Trench fever. III. Induction of clinical disease in volunteers inoculated with *Rickettsia quintana* propagated on blood agar. Am. J. Trop. Med., 18:713, 1969.

Warren, J.: Trench fever rickettsia. *In* Horsfall, F. L., Jr., and Tamm, I. (eds.): Viral and Rickettsial Infections of Man. 4th ed. Philadelphia, J. B. Lippincott Company, p. 1161.

114. Q FEVER

Herbert L. Ley, Jr.

DEFINITION. Q fever is a self-limited rickettsial infection characterized by fever, headache, and constitutional symptoms, associated, in approximately half the patients, with a pneumonitis. It is unique among the rickettsial diseases of man in that human infection is most commonly acquired by inhalation of the agent rather than by contact with an arthropod vector.

ETIOLOGY. The disease is caused by *Coxiella burnetii*, a rickettsial agent having the general biologic characteristics of this class of microorganisms by possessing, in addition, a resistance to desiccation and to exposure in the dusts and soils that is unique among the rickettsiae. The organism may be propagated in embryonated eggs and in mice, hamsters, and guinea pigs, and has frequently infected laboratory personnel engaged in isolation studies on clinical material. Both patients and animals develop agglutinating and complement-fixing antibodies for the agent. On the other hand, *C. burnetii*, unlike most of the other rickettsiae, does not stimulate the production of Weil-Felix *Proteus* agglutinins in man.

EPIDEMIOLOGY. Incidence and Distribution. The true incidence of the disease in the human population is impossible to determine because the majority of infections are undiagnosed. Isolated serologic surveys have revealed that many persons exposed to infection in sheep and cattle ranches, abattoirs, meat packing plants, or wool processing plants present serologic evidence of past infection. More detailed investigation of animals and arthropods on a worldwide basis has shown *C. burnetii* to be ubiquitous in distribution except for the countries of Denmark, Finland, Ireland, the Netherlands, Norway, and Sweden. In the United States the disease, first recognized in the states of Montana and California, is now recognized as prevalent in most of the states in which sheep and cattle are produced. Small numbers of cases have been reported for most of the remaining states.

Transmission. The epidemiology of the disease is complex because it involves two major patterns of transmission. The first pattern, described in Australia, is a disease cycle in wild animals with transmission of the agent from animal to animal by a tick vector. Although the species of animal and arthropod vary from country to country, such a cycle has been demonstrated in Australia in two forms, bandicoot-tick-cattle and kangaroo-tick-sheep. In both these cycles the agent can be transmitted indefinitely as an inapparent infection in the wild reservoir (bandicoot and kangaroo) by ticks, but it may also be transmitted laterally by arthropod to a domestic animal in close contact with man. In these and similar cycles recognized in other parts of the world, *C. burnetii*, like the other rickettsial agents of human disease, is vector-transmitted.

However, Q fever patients rarely give a history of tick bite. Human infection with the agent has now been shown to occur almost exclusively by a second transmission pattern capable of sustaining itself independently of the wild animal cycle. The reservoirs of infection in the second pattern are animals domesticated by man, principally cattle, sheep, and goats, in which *C. burnetii* produces only an inapparent or mild infection. In sheep, Q fever organisms are excreted in very large numbers in placental tissue, and to a lesser degree in birth fluids, milk, and feces. In the cow, and probably the goat, excretion occurs mainly through the placenta and milk. *With all infected animals, the period of parturition is associated with the formation of a primary infectious aerosol, easily demonstrated by air-sampling studies.* Such aerosols infect other cattle in the herd and also the human population in direct contact with the animals. Further, because contaminated clothing, wool, hides, bedding, and soil may be the source of secondary aerosols, *the infections may be transmitted via these vehicles at considerable distances from the infected cattle;* in certain circumstances these distances are measurable in miles. The unique resistance of *C. burnetii* to prolonged exposure in nature contributes to the spread of the agent by such infectious microenvironments. Within California, where the local epidemiology of the disease has been studied in great detail, sheep are the major reservoir for human infection in the northern part of the state and cattle in the southern part. In the latter area milk may be a vehicle of infection if consumed raw. Although the pulmonary route is the most important portal of access of the agent to man, the transmission of the rickettsia from man to man by this method is rare, despite the occurrence of an infectious pneumonitis in some patients. Studies in Egypt, where the disease is endemic, have demonstrated that Q fever can be transmitted to the human fetus in utero without producing clinical signs of infection in the infant at birth.

PATHOLOGY. Because the mortality rate is low, postmortem studies have been limited. In those patients having a pneumonitis, the histopathology is similar to that seen in the viral pneumonias and psittacosis. Recent studies in patients have directed attention to hepatic pathology during the acute phase of the disease, demonstrable both in biochemical abnormalities of liver function (elevated cephalin-cholesterol flocculation, alkaline phosphatase, and thymol turbidity tests) and in histologic abnormalities in biopsy specimens (focal inflammation and granulomas). Q fever endocarditis, producing valvular vegetations from which rickettsiae may be isolated, has also been described. There is increasing evidence that Q fever can occasionally also cause myocarditis and paroxysmal ventricular tachycardia.

CLINICAL MANIFESTATIONS. After an incubation period of 9 to 20 days after respiratory exposure, most patients complain of an abrupt onset of fever, headache, muscle pains, and severe malaise. The temperature may rise as high as 40° C and remain elevated, with considerable fluctuation, for one to three weeks. Occasionally, patients may suffer a prolonged fever of several months' duration. In contrast to the other rickettsial infections, there is no rash. In approximately half the patients there is roentgenographic evidence of pneumonitis, manifested clinically as a slight, nonproductive cough developing in the second week of fever.

DIAGNOSIS. Q fever should always be suspected in a patient having a febrile illness for which no obvious cause can be found. If the patient's occupation brings him into contact with sheep, cattle, or goats, or byproducts such as wool or hides, particular care should be exercised to exclude Q fever from consideration. The presence of Q fever should be suspected in any patient in whom the differential diagnosis includes viral pneumonia, psittacosis, primary atypical pneumonia, pulmonary mycotic disease, or comparable infections. Furthermore, recent data would also support consideration of Q fever in the differential diagnoses of endocarditis and of hepatitis with or without jaundice.

Diagnostic laboratory studies usually must be limited to serologic studies because of the extensive history of accidentally acquired laboratory infections resulting from attempts at isolation. Either complement-fixation or agglutination tests may be employed, and with either test a fourfold or greater rise in titer of antibody may be expected to occur between the first and fourth weeks of illness. Recent reports have emphasized the importance of both strain and phase variation in the selection of antigens for diagnostic use.

TREATMENT AND PROGNOSIS. The tetracyclines or chloramphenicol are both effective in treatment of acute infections with *C. burnetii*, but because of the nature of chloramphenicol toxicity, the tetracyclines are definitely to be preferred. The dosage of antimicrobial given should be the same as that for epidemic typhus or Rocky Mountain spotted fever. The mortality is low (1 per cent or less), even in untreated patients, and is lower still in those treated with antimicrobial drugs. Therapy should be continued for approximately one week even though the patient usually becomes afebrile within 48 hours. Patients occasionally may experience relapses after treatment, and when this complication occurs additional drug therapy should be administered. No clinical data are available concerning the effectiveness of the lipotrophic tetracycline derivatives in the treatment of Q fever. Prognosis is less favorable for the rare patient in whom Q fever endocarditis develops. In some of these patients the disease has been reported to have been unresponsive to antimicrobial therapy, although favorable results have been reported in one patient treated with co-trimoxazole.

PREVENTION. Experimental lots of yolk-sac vaccines have been effective in prevention of clinical disease in volunteers experimentally infected via the respiratory route. Because this vaccine is not commercially available, control measures are limited to minimizing exposure to the agent. In particular, milk from cattle, sheep, and goats in endemic areas should be pasteurized or boiled before use. Because rickettsiae are excreted in the sputum and urine of patients, these materials should be disinfected by autoclaving to prevent secondary infection in hospitals.

Barraclough, D., and Papert, A. J.: Q fever presenting with paroxysmal ventricular tachycardia. Br. Med. J., 2:423, 1975.

Editorial: Chronic Q fever or Q fever endocarditis. Lancet, 1:1171, 1976.

Fiset, P., Wisseman, C. L., and el Batawi, Y.: Immunologic evidence of human fetal infection with Coxiella burnetii. Am. J. Epidemiol., 101:65, 1975.

Freeman, R., and Hodson, M. E.: Q fever endocarditis with trimethoprim and sulfamethoxazole. Br. Med. J., 1:419, 1972.

Ormsbee, R. A.: Q fever rickettsia. In Horsfall, F. L., Jr., and Tamm, I. (eds.): Viral and Rickettsial Infections of Man. 4th ed. Philadelphia, J. B. Lippincott Company, 1965, p. 1144.

Powell, O. W.: Liver involvement in "Q" fever. Aust. Ann. Med., 10:52, 1961.

Sheridan, P., MacCaig, J. N., and Hart, R. J. C.: Myocarditis complicating Q fever. Br. Med. J., 2:155, 1974.

Tigertt, W. D., and Benenson, A. S.: Studies on Q fever in man. Trans. Assoc. Am. Physicians, 69:98, 1956.

115. BARTONELLOSIS
(Carrión's Disease, Oroya Fever, Verruga Peruana)

Herbert L. Ley, Jr.

DEFINITION. Bartonellosis is an insect-borne microbial disease limited to South America. It is characterized by two distinctive clinical stages. The first of these (Oroya fever) presents a severe febrile infection associated with a marked anemia, bone and joint pains, bacteremia, and an appreciable mortality. The second stage (verruga peruana) is more benign and is distinguished by the appearance of a generalized eruption of hemangiomatous papules and nodules.

ETIOLOGY. The disease is caused by *Bartonella bacilliformis*, a small gram-negative pleomorphic bacillus that may be cultivated readily in enriched bacteriologic media. The disease is transmitted to man by the bite of sandflies of the genus *Phlebotomus*, with development of the characteristic symptoms of Oroya fever after an incubation period of two weeks to three months.

EPIDEMIOLOGY. Although a number of epidemics of the disease have been reported, it is more commonly seen as sporadic cases among populations of Peru, Colombia, and Ecuador, and is restricted within these countries to those who live at altitudes of 1500 to 9000 feet on both slopes of the Andes. In general, the distribution of the disease coincides with the ecologic zones supporting populations of *Phlebotomus*.

In Peru the disease is transmitted by *Phlebotomus verrugarum*, a night-biting sandfly. The biting habits of the vectors in the other countries are similar, although the species of *Phlebotomus* involved in transmission in the other areas are not conclusively identified. The

principal reservoir of the disease appears to be man; no additional animal reservoirs have as yet been implicated in nature. Reports of cultivation of the agent from apparently healthy persons suggest that as much as 10 per cent of infections may be subclinical. Persons convalescent from the disease are known to have a low-level bacteremia for months or years, providing frequent opportunities for infection of the disease vector.

PATHOLOGY AND PHYSIOLOGIC RESPONSES. In the Oroya fever stage of illness the causative organism may be found in peripheral blood smears stained with Giemsa or Wright's stain as well as in the reticuloendothelial cells of the viscera and lymphatics. In the blood the parasite is found both free in the plasma and adhering to the erythrocytes. The parasitization of the erythrocytes causes an increased mechanical fragility and also an increased sequestration of the cells in the spleen and the liver. A hypochromic and macrocytic anemia develops rapidly during the febrile period, erythrocyte counts decreasing within a period of only a few days to levels of one million to two million cells per cubic millimeter. The bone marrow is hyperplastic, with an abundance of nucleated erythrocytes. The pathologic findings secondary to the anemia are present in the verruga stage of infection. The histopathology of the skin lesions is that of dilation of the capillaries and proliferation of the vascular endothelial cells that may be shown to contain the causative agent.

CLINICAL MANIFESTATIONS. The presenting symptoms of patients with Oroya fever are intermittent high fever, painful muscles and joints, tender enlarged lymph nodes, and the systemic symptoms and prostration of a severe anemia. These symptoms may persist from several weeks to several months in untreated patients, half of whom may die within the first three weeks of fever. If the patient survives, gradual convalescence is punctuated, after a few days to a month, by the appearance of the cutaneous lesions of the second phase of the disease. The verrugae may persist for a month to a year in untreated persons, but mortality is negligible. Occasional patients may experience only the fever and anemia without the skin manifestations or only the cutaneous lesions without the initial fever. Although these two aspects of the infection were once thought to be different diseases, there is no doubt that both syndromes are manifestations of infection with the same organism. The current interpretation that the skin lesions are an expression of developing immunity in the patient is supported by the observation that second attacks of the disease are exceedingly rare even in highly endemic areas and that the attacks are almost always caused by verruga rather than by Oroya fever.

DIAGNOSIS. In endemic areas the diagnosis can usually be made on the basis of clinical findings. In the acute stage of Oroya fever both blood smears and blood culture usually reveal the presence of the agent. As the patient progresses toward the verruga stage of infection, or with treatment, the organism becomes more difficult to demonstrate.

TREATMENT AND PROGNOSIS. The prognosis in the untreated patient depends upon both the nature and the severity of his infection. Mortality in the Oroya fever phase of the disease may exceed 50 per cent, particularly when the infection is complicated by concurrent attacks of malaria, amebiasis, tuberculosis, salmonellosis, or other diseases. The disease responds well to treatment with penicillin, streptomycin, and the tetracyclines. Chloramphenicol is favored by many South American clinicians because of the frequency of concurrent salmonella infections, but the risks of its potentially more serious toxicity must be weighed against the fact that the other drugs mentioned are therapeutically effective. In general, as in the rickettsial infections, the tetracyclines are the preferred form of antimicrobial therapy for bartonellosis. When the broad-spectrum antimicrobials have been used, oral doses of 1 to 2 grams per day have been used for a period of a week or more with excellent results. Patients become afebrile in 24 to 48 hours, and, if they receive transfusions, recover strength rapidly. Although the mortality of the verruga stage of infection is less than 5 per cent, antimicrobial therapy is desirable to hasten the disappearance of the skin lesions.

PREVENTION. Control measures are directed principally against the *Phlebotomus* vector. Because the insect is a night feeder and moves by a series of short "hops" between surfaces, the application of a residual insecticide to the exterior and interior of doorways, windows, and other avenues of entry to human habitation is effective. Where insecticide application is impracticable, bed nets or insect repellents provide significant protection. Control of breeding of the vector is difficult, but may be undertaken when it is otherwise impossible to prevent contact of the vector with man. No protective vaccine is available. Patients need not be isolated in hospital wards if the vector is absent because the disease is not transmitted by person-to-person contact.

Goldstein, E.: Bartonellosis. *In* Hoeprich, P. D. (ed.): Infectious Diseases. Hagerstown, Md., Harper & Row, 1972, p. 1159.
Reynafarje, C., and Ramos, J.: The hemolytic anemia of human bartonellosis. Blood, 17:562, 1961.
Weinman, D.: The Bartonella Group. *In:* Dubos, R. J., and Hirsch, J. G. (eds.): Bacterial and Mycotic Infections of Man. 4th ed. Philadelphia, J. B. Lippincott Company, 1965, p. 775.

DISEASES CAUSED BY CHLAMYDIAE

116. TRACHOMA AND INCLUSION CONJUNCTIVITIS

Ernest Jawetz

DEFINITION. Trachoma and "inclusion conjunctivitis" are chronic infectious diseases of the eye and genital tract, caused by closely related microorganisms and exhibiting overlapping spectra of clinical manifestations and epidemiologic patterns. These range from mild and self-limited to severe and blinding eye disease and a spectrum of involvement of the genital tract.

ETIOLOGY. The agents of *trachoma and inclusion conjunctivitis* are members of the psittacosis–lymphogranuloma venereum–trachoma group. Formerly these agents were considered viruses; now they are called *chlamydiae*. They are nonmotile, gram-negative, obligate intracellular parasites which multiply in the cytoplasm of their host cells by a distinctive developmental cycle. Chlamydiae differ from viruses in many important respects: they possess both RNA and DNA; they multiply by binary fission; they possess bacterial types of cell walls and ribosomes; they produce a variety of metabolically active enzymes; and their growth can be inhibited by several antibacterial drugs. It is probable that chlamydiae are closely related to gram-negative bacteria, but lack some significant mechanism for the production of metabolic energy so that they are restricted to an intracellular existence.

Chlamydiae fall into two distinct species: *C. psittaci* and *C. trachomatis*. The latter can infect epithelial cells of conjunctiva, cornea, urethra, and cervix of man and monkey, but does not replicate in most other tissues of the body. The infective particle ("elementary body") is a sphere with a diameter of 250 nanometers (millimicrons) and stains purple with Giemsa's or red with Macchiavello's stain. The infective particle is taken into the host cell by phagocytosis and, after replication, results in the development of an inclusion body. This is an oval or crescent-shaped mass of "elementary bodies" embedded in a matrix of glycogen, lying in the cytoplasm of an epithelial cell often adjacent to the nucleus. Inclusion bodies can be stained brightly with specific immunofluorescence.

Chlamydiae can be grown in the yolk sac of embryonated eggs and, by special techniques, in cell culture. The growth of chlamydiae is markedly inhibited by tetracyclines, erythromycins, and chloramphenicol, but not by aminoglycosides. Therefore aminoglycosides can be used to suppress bacterial contaminants in clinical specimens and to aid in isolation of chlamydiae in the laboratory.

All chlamydiae share a heat-stable group antigen. These are lipopolysaccharides detectable by complement-fixation tests. In addition, species- and type-specific antigens have been detected in the cell wall. Infected persons may develop antibodies to both types of antigens in serum and tears. By immunofluorescence tests specific antigens and antibodies can be identified. Thus genital chlamydial isolates usually fall within certain antigenic groups (D to K), whereas ocular isolates from endemic trachoma areas usually fall within other groups (A, B, C). At least 12 specific antigenic groups have been identified to date. There exist cross-reactions between the specific antigens of the chlamydiae of lymphogranuloma venereum and of trachoma and inclusion conjunctivitis. The immunologic labels are the only laboratory characteristics which differentiate different chlamydiae.

Chlamydiae can persist in man for years, with or without symptoms and signs of infection. Subclinical infection in the eye can be activated by trauma, corticosteroids, and bacterial superinfection. The development of scarring and blindness in some endemic trachoma regions is attributable to a large extent to recurrent bacterial infections of the eye, especially with *Hemophilus* or *Neisseria*.

EPIDEMIOLOGY. Since antiquity, trachomatous infection was recognized in the Mediterranean basin and in the Orient. Today, trachomatous eye disease is very prevalent in Africa and Asia. It has been estimated that up to 400 million persons may have eye infections with chlamydiae, and up to 20 million may be economically blinded as a result. Trachoma flourishes in areas that are hot and dry, and that have a shortage of available water and poor hygienic customs. In such areas endemic levels are high, and initial infection commonly occurs in early childhood. In certain parts of the world, e.g., in North Africa, virtually the entire population is infected with chlamydiae before reaching adulthood. The high prevalence of bacterial superinfection in such populations undoubtedly contributes to the severity of eye disease and to its causing widespread blindness. In parts of the United States, e.g., Indian reservations of the Southwest, endemic chlamydial infection is relatively common, but it rarely leads to major visual impairment, perhaps because bacterial superinfection is infrequent. Throughout the world sporadic cases of ocular chlamydial infection occur, often with a clinical picture resembling trachoma. It is probable that some of these originate in genital infections rather than in contact with ocular trachoma.

Active cases of ocular chlamydial infection shed the infective agent in desquamated conjunctival cells, conjunctival exudate, or tears. The infectious agent may be transmitted by fingers, fomites, and perhaps flies. Patients with early active infection probably shed more infective chlamydiae and thus are more infectious for contacts than are those with chronic infection. However, even patients with longstanding scarred eye disease, and without signs of current activity, may shed chlamydiae and thus serve as a source of infection.

These comments concern ocular chlamydial infection, particularly typical endemic trachoma. *Typical inclusion conjunctivitis* has a radically different epidemiologic pattern. Inclusion conjunctivitis is fundamentally an infection of the adult human genital tract, transmitted as a venereal disease. In the female the chlamydiae grow mainly in the transitional epithelium of the cervix. These cells may contain typical inclusions, and occasionally a mild cervicitis is present. In the male, genital infection may produce nongonococcal *urethritis*, as the chlamydial agent replicates in urethral epithelium. In both sexes, adult genital tract infection and proctitis are often asymptomatic. Adults may transfer genital secretions to their own or other eyes by fingers, by fomites, and — occasionally — in swimming pools. The infection may pass from the cervix of the infected mother to the eye of her newborn during passage through the birth canal. The newborn infant may then develop eye disease between 5 and 14 days after birth.

The epidemiologic patterns described for typical trachoma and typical inclusion conjunctivitis may be mixed. Thus the genital tract of women in endemic trachoma regions may harbor chlamydiae and these may produce either inclusion conjunctivitis or clinically typical trachoma in the offspring. Genital isolates from adults in nonendemic areas may, upon inoculation into the eye, give rise to disease resembling either inclusion conjunctivitis or trachoma.

PATHOLOGY AND PATHOGENESIS. *Chlamydia trachomatis* invades mainly the epithelium of the conjunctiva, cervix, and urethra. The earliest sign of infection is the appearance of inclusion bodies within epithelial cells and neutrophil infiltration of the epithelium of mucous membranes. Subepithelial infiltration with plasma cells and lymphocytes and the development of lymphoid follicles then follow. In the cornea, epithelial keratitis is often accompanied by the formation of subepithelial opacities. Blood vessels from the limbus, accompanied by fibroblasts, may invade the cornea to form a pannus. Progression of the inflammatory process leads to necrosis and scar formation in the conjunctiva. In classic trachoma, these changes occur more markedly in the upper half of the conjunctival sac and cornea; in inclusion conjunctivitis, more markedly in the lower conjunctiva. Inflammatory changes, lymphoid infiltration, necrosis, and scar formation have also been observed in chlamydial infection of cervix and urethra.

Classic inclusion conjunctivitis of the newborn is an *acute purulent conjunctivitis*; in the adult it is a *follicular conjunctivitis*. However, all pathologic changes from limited follicular conjunctivitis to full-blown "trachoma" with scars and pannus may follow inoculation of genital isolates into the adult eye.

Classic, chronic, severe trachoma in hyperendemic areas progresses to marked lid deformation and loss of vision. As a result of cellular infiltration and scarring near the lid margins, the tarsal plate is bowed and the lid margins inverted (entropion), and some eyelashes turn inward (trichiasis), rubbing against the cornea with each lid movement, and aggravating corneal opacification. The scarring may destroy tear function, with resulting keratinization of corneal epithelium.

Chlamydiae exhibit a pronounced tendency to persist in infected tissues for years even in the absence of signs of active disease, and this predisposes to relapses and to chronicity.

CLINICAL MANIFESTATIONS. In experimental human infection with *Chlamydia trachomatis* the incubation period is from two to seven days. *Inclusion conjunctivitis* of the newborn usually begins between the fifth and fourteenth days of life (whereas gonococcal ophthalmia usually begins two days after birth). The incubation period of naturally occurring trachoma is uncertain because the onset is often insidious, particularly in children. Early symptoms of chlamydial infection are those of irritation, lacrimation, and mucopurulent discharge. The earliest physical signs are conjunctival hyperemia, mucopurulent discharge, papillary hypertrophy in infants, and follicular hypertrophy in adults. Newborns may develop pneumonitis.

Typical *trachoma* in children and adults begins as a follicular conjunctivitis, most noticeable in the conjunctiva of the upper lid and the tarsal plate. There are epithelial keratitis and subepithelial corneal infiltration, followed by gradual corneal vascularization from the upper limbus downward. This evolves into a dense fibrovascular pannus extending over part, or all, of the cornea, grossly impairing vision. Linear or stellate scars appear on the conjunctiva. Progressive scarring of the subepithelial tissues leads to deformation of the tarsal plate, resulting in entropion, trichiasis, and further corneal damage. These changes often follow secondary bacterial infection, which may also produce corneal ulceration and accelerate loss of vision. Typically there are no systemic symptoms or signs of infection, and the eye is the sole involved organ.

Typical *inclusion conjunctivitis* of the newborn presents as an acute purulent conjunctivitis with papillary hypertrophy but little involvement of the cornea. Over a period of weeks or months this tends to regress spontaneously and to heal with little scarring. In the adult, inclusion conjunctivitis is an acute mucopurulent conjunctivitis, often accompanied by preauricular adenopathy. Follicular hypertrophy is most noticeable in the conjunctiva of the lower lid, and tends to persist for weeks or months, occasionally accompanied by epithelial keratitis and subepithelial corneal infiltrates. Some adults with chronic inclusion conjunctivitis develop pannus and a few scars of conjunctiva and cornea.

Adult genital chlamydial infection usually precedes the eye involvement. Adult *cervicitis* and *urethritis* either are asymptomatic or produce only slight discharge and discomfort. This nongonococcal urethritis forms a substantial portion of the acute urethritis in the male seen in venereal disease clinics (see Ch. 139).

All intermediate stages between minimal self-limited inclusion conjunctivitis and typical progressive trachoma can occur as a result of infection with chlamydiae agents of either ocular or genital origin. The typical, severe trachoma that leads to blindness and is seen in hyperendemic areas occurs probably as a result of long-standing infection with many relapses of chlamydial activity, hypersensitivity reactions, and repeated bacterial superinfections. Conversely, the self-limited inclusion conjunctivitis of the newborn may be characteristic of a first infection, without hypersensitivity reaction, and without bacterial complications in an immunologically immature host. The basis for different clinical patterns of mild or severe disease seen in different areas of the world is not clearly understood.

DIAGNOSIS. The traditional criteria for the diagnosis of trachoma are the triad of follicular hypertrophy, most prominent on the upper tarsal conjunctiva, pannus, and conjunctival scars. The last two signs may be detected only by biomicroscopic examination (slit lamp).

The diagnosis of inclusion conjunctivitis rests on finding typical inclusions in a purulent conjunctivitis of the newborn or in a follicular conjunctivitis of the adult. There should be only minimal vascular invasion of the cornea. Examination of the adult genital tract may reveal cervicitis and urethritis with moderate discharge and inclusions in epithelial cells. Proctitis may be present.

Among laboratory tests for chlamydial infections, the demonstration of typical intracytoplasmic inclusions in conjunctival or genital epithelial cells is most widely used. Specific immunofluorescent stain is more sensitive than Giemsa stain. Polymorphonuclear leukocytes are often prominent in scrapings that contain chlamydial inclusions. Isolation of chlamydiae in embryonated eggs or in specially treated cell cultures remains a specialized laboratory procedure. Serologic tests can support the diagnosis only if a rise in complement-fixing or immunofluorescence antibodies occurs during acute disease.

DIFFERENTIAL DIAGNOSIS. In differential diagnosis of ocular chlamydial infections, adenovirus infections, herpetic keratoconjunctivitis, folliculosis of children, chronic follicular conjunctivitis (Axenfeld type), reactions to allergens and irritating chemicals, and certain bacterial infections must be considered. Some of these entities may coexist with chlamydial infections, and repeated competent ophthalmologic examinations and elaborate laboratory assistance may be required to establish a correct diagnosis. The demonstration of morphologically typical chlamydial inclusions by immunofluorescent or Giemsa stain is most helpful when combined with efforts to isolate viruses or bacteria of possible etiologic significance.

The differential diagnosis between ocular trachoma and oculogenital inclusion conjunctivitis requires epidemiologic considerations, clinical and laboratory examination of the genital tract, and a "typing" of the isolate by immunofluorescent tests. The eye lesions of trachoma and of oculogenital inclusion conjunctivitis in the adult cannot be distinguished. The most important differential diagnosis of inclusion conjunctivitis of the newborn is chemical or bacterial conjunctivitis.

TREATMENT AND PROGNOSIS. Chlamydiae are susceptible to several antibacterial drugs. Tetracyclines and sulfonamides have been most widely used in treatment. Tetracycline suspensions or ointments can cling to the conjunctiva for prolonged effect. Ophthalmic topical tetracycline preparations have been administered in various dosage schedules for several months in chronic endemic trachoma. In inclusion conjunctivitis of the newborn, there is a strong natural tendency toward healing. The administration of topical tetracycline two to four times daily for three weeks further accelerates healing.

Oral tetracycline hydrochloride, 1 to 2 grams in three divided daily doses, or doxycycline, 2.5 to 4.0 mg per kilogram in a single daily dose, or oral trisulfapyrimidines, 4 grams daily in divided doses for five to six weeks, can suppress signs of activity in chronic trachoma of adults. However, these treatment regimens often fail to eradicate the infectious agent. By contrast, in acute chlamydial infections these oral drug regimens alone, or combined with topical tetracycline, may result in permanent cure. This applies to acute infections of either the eye or the genital tract.

In areas of hyperendemic trachoma, mass treatment must be applied to early infection of children and must be repeated at intervals in order to control chlamydial infection before scarring occurs. Repeated courses of drug treatment are probably beneficial by reducing the reservoir of infection, by temporarily suppressing microbial and clinical activity in the patient, and by controlling bacteral superinfection. Even one monthly dose of 300 mg of doxycycline provides clinical benefit by converting severe to mild eye disease and preventing visual impairment.

Drug therapy has no influence on established scars or pannus. Surgical correction is required in serious entropion or trichiasis. Topical corticosteroids and caustics have no place in therapy.

PREVENTION. Endemic trachoma is favored by ignorance, poverty, and cultural patterns that oppose hygienic improvement and medical treatment. In addition, the sheer lack of water available for washing seems to be important.

The most potent preventive measures include efforts to increase the total supply of water, simple cleanliness such as frequent hand washing, avoidance of common towel or common eye pencil, and measures to reduce flies. It is also important to detect mild, early infection in young children in endemic areas and to apply effective drug treatment repeatedly. This prevents the blinding progression of the disease, and probably reduces the infective reservoir. Detection and treatment of adults who already suffer visual impairment can probably reduce the source of infection for children. Entire family groups or communities should be treated simultaneously.

Prevention of genital chlamydial infections requires the control of sexual promiscuity, early diagnosis and effective treatment of cases and sexual contacts, and prolonged follow-up to establish that the genital or ocular infection is not relapsing. Effective treatment of pregnant women with genital chlamydial infection can prevent inclusion conjunctivitis in the newborn. The usual instillations into the eye of the newborn (silver nitrate or penicillin) do not prevent inclusion conjunctivitis. A newborn baby with inclusion conjunctivitis should be isolated to prevent spread to others.

Experimental vaccines against chlamydial infections have failed to protect against infection or against progression of disease.

Natural infection engenders only minimal protection against reinfection. The most that could be expected of artificial immunization is an attenuation of the disease resulting from infection. The best current hope for control of chlamydial infections rests on a combination of public health measures and drug treatment.

Dunlop, E. M. C., Jones, B. R., Darougar, S., and Treharne, J. D.: Chlamydia and non-specific urethritis. Br. Med. J., 2:575, 1973.

Grayston, J. T., and Wang S. P.: New knowledge of chlamydiae and the diseases they cause. J. Infect. Dis., 132:87, 1975.

Holmes, K. K., Handsfield, H. H., Wang, S. P., Wentworth, B. B., Turck, M., Anderson, J. B., and Alexander, R. E.: Etiology of non-gonococcal urethritis. N. Engl. J. Med., 292:1199, 1975.

Jawetz, E.: Chemotherapy of chlamydial infections. In Garattini, S., Goldin, A., Hawking, F., and Kopin, I. J. (eds.): Advances in Pharmacology and Chemotherapy. Vol. 7. New York, Academic Press, 1969, pp. 253–282.

Jawetz, E., Hanna, L., Dawson, C., Wood, R., and Briones, O.: Subclinical infections with TRIC agents. Am. J. Ophthal., 63:1413, 1967.

Jones, B. R., and Darougar, S.: Communicable ophthalmia: The blinding scourge of the Middle East. Br. J. Ophthalmol., 60:492, 1976.

Moulder, J. W.: The relation of the psittacosis group (chlamydiae) to bacteria and viruses. Ann. Rev. Microbiol., 20:107, 1966.

Richmond, S. J., and Sparling, P. F.: Genital chlamydial infections. Am. J. Epidemiol., 103:438, 1976.

117. LYMPHOGRANULOMA VENEREUM

Ernest Jawetz

DEFINITION. Lymphogranuloma venereum (LGV) is an acute and chronic venereal disease with prominent systemic manifestations, caused by a chlamydial agent closely related to trachoma and inclusion conjunctivitis agents. LGV produces early genital lesions followed by enlargement and suppuration of regional lymph nodes and a variety of febrile systemic manifestations. Late results are prominent inguinal draining sinuses in men and fibrosing proctitis and rectal strictures in women and homosexual males.

ETIOLOGY. The chlamydiae of LGV are members of the species and share the characteristics of *C. trachomatis*, including the formation of compact intracytoplasmic inclusions with a glycogen matrix, inhibition of growth by sulfonamides, and antigenic features. All LGV chlamydiae carry the chlamydial group reactive antigen. Specific antigens have been defined by immunofluorescence, thus permitting classification of LGV isolates into three specific antigenic types. These antigens cross-react with type-specific antigens of other *C. trachomatis*. LGV chlamydiae differ from ocular isolates in growing more readily in cell cultures and in several animal tissues.

EPIDEMIOLOGY. LGV is transmitted almost exclusively by sexual contact. The genital tract and rectum of chronically infected persons serve as reservoirs of infection. The highest incidence of the disease has been reported from subtropical and tropical areas, but the in-

fection occurs all over the world. Definitive serologic surveys of LGV infection by appropriate specific methods have not been performed.

PATHOGENESIS AND PATHOLOGY. A primary vesicular or ulcerative lesion develops at the site of inoculation one to four weeks after infection. The chlamydiae spread rapidly to regional lymph nodes which become enlarged and inflamed. From the penis or vulva the spread is mainly to inguinal and iliac nodes. From the vagina or rectum the spread is mainly to perirectal and pelvic nodes. The involved nodes become matted and suppurate and may discharge pus through multiple sinus tracts.

During the stage of early, active lymphadenitis, the chlamydiae may become widely disseminated by the bloodstream and may reach various organs, including the central nervous system. In the late, chronic stages of infection, fibrosis, obstruction, and strictures develop. Lymphatic obstruction may lead to elephantiasis of external genitalia (penis, scrotum, vulva). Chronic proctitis may lead to progressive rectal strictures, with obstruction of the bowel lumen and fistula formation.

The histologic appearance of involved lymph nodes shows acute and chronic inflammation, suppuration, and fibrosis, but is not specific or diagnostic of LGV.

CLINICAL MANIFESTATIONS. Several days to several weeks after exposure, a small, evanescent papule or vesicle develops on any part of the external genitalia, anus, or rectum. The lesion may ulcerate, but usually — especially in women — it remains unnoticed and heals in a few days. Soon thereafter the regional lymph nodes enlarge and tend to become matted and often painful. In males, inguinal nodes are most commonly involved both above and below Poupart's ligament, and the overlying skin often turns purplish as the nodes suppurate and eventually discharge pus through multiple sinus tracts. In females, the perirectal nodes are prominently involved with proctitis and bloody mucopurulent anal discharge. This is also seen in homosexual males.

During the stage of active lymphadenitis, there are often marked systemic symptoms, including fever, headaches, meningismus, conjunctivitis, skin rashes, nausea and vomiting, and arthralgias. Rarely is there meningitis, arthritis, or pericarditis. Unless effective antimicrobial therapy is instituted at that stage, the chronic inflammatory process progresses to fibrosis, lymphatic obstruction, and rectal strictures. The lymphatic obstruction may lead to elephantiasis of the penis, scrotum, or vulva. The chronic proctitis of women or homosexual males may lead to progressive rectal strictures, rectosigmoid obstruction, and fistula formation.

DIAGNOSIS. LGV must be considered in every case of enlarged, matted, tender inguinal lymph nodes, active proctitis, draining inguinal or perianal fistulas, and rectal strictures. It must be distinguished from inguinal adenopathy of any cause, including pyogenic infection of lower extremities, plague, tularemia, chancroid, granuloma inguinale, syphilis, and inflammatory or neoplastic lesions of the rectum. A clinical impression of LGV can be supported by the demonstration of the chlamydiae, a skin test, or a meaningful serologic response, but histologic appearance of biopsied tissue is not specific.

Material from fluctuant suppurating nodes may be obtained by aspiration or biopsy. When inoculated into x-irradiated cell cultures, into embryonated eggs, or, by intracerebral injection, into mice, LGV chlamydiae can sometimes be isolated. Only rarely can chlamydial inclusions be seen in stained smears of such material.

The skin test (Frei test) consists of the intradermal injection of LGV antigens, prepared in embryonated eggs, and a suitable control of egg material. The test is considered positive if an indurated area or papule — at least 6 mm larger than the control site — develops in 48 hours. Reactivity to chlamydial group antigen develops within three to eight weeks after LGV infection and may remain positive for life. This delayed hypersensitivity reaction may be positive after *any* chlamydial infection. A negative skin test cannot exclude LGV infection. Skin tests with commercial antigens are sometimes negative even when LGV chlamydiae are isolated from pus, or when the serologic response unequivocally proves a chlamydial infection. Thus the Frei test is of only limited value in the diagnosis of suspected LGV infection. Early antimicrobial drug treatment may interfere with the development of a positive skin test and antibody response.

The complement-fixation (CF) test with heat-stable group reactive antigen is at present the most generally available test for LGV and other systemic chlamydial infections. In the presence of inguinal adenopathy or proctitis, a rise of antibody titer in sera taken two to three weeks apart strongly supports the diagnosis of LGV. In untreated LGV patients, the CF titer is often 1:64 or more, and such a high titer in a single serum from a patient with a compatible clinical picture also supports the diagnosis. With effective treatment the titer declines. Persisting high antibody titers suggest chronic persistent infection. Indirect immunofluorescence tests for antibodies to LGV antigens are as sensitive as and more specific than CF tests but are not generally available.

Other abnormal laboratory findings are less helpful. The white blood cell count is often elevated during lymph node suppuration or proctitis, sometimes with a relative monocytosis. Total serum proteins may be elevated with a reversed albumin-globulin ratio. Gamma globulin, cryoglobulin, rheumatoid factor, and IgM are sometimes significantly increased in serum.

TREATMENT. The growth of LGV chlamydiae can be inhibited by sulfonamides, tetracyclines, and some other antimicrobials. Full systemic doses of a soluble sulfonamide (e.g., trisulfapyrimidines USP, 6 to 8 grams on day one with 4 grams daily thereafter) or of a tetracycline (e.g., tetracycline HCl, 2 to 3 grams daily) are administered for three to four weeks as early in the course of LGV infection as possible. LGV acquired since 1967 in Southeast Asia has responded more regularly to tetracycline than to sulfonamides. In some patients, two or three courses of treatment are required. Supportive therapy consists of bed rest, compresses to inflamed areas, analgesics, and aspiration of fluctuant sites. Treatment is guided by the subsiding of constitutional symptoms and of lymph node swelling, closure of fistulas, and resolution of proctitis. If the infection is eradicated, the serum antibody titer drops markedly over a period of six to eight months.

PROGNOSIS. Although the acute illness in early LGV is usually self-limited, the chronic complications resulting from lymphatic blockade or rectal stricture are debilitating and often require surgical correction. It is important therefore to prevent these late complications by early diagnosis and prolonged or repeated treatment. Death from LGV uncomplicated by bacterial superinfection is very rare. There may be an increased incidence of anorectal carcinoma in persons with anorectal chronic LGV.

PREVENTION. Since LGV is generally acquired as a venereal disease, all measures applicable to the prevention of venereal diseases are pertinent. No active immunization is available.

Abrams, A. J.: Lymphogranuloma venereum. JAMA, 205:59, 1968.
Jawetz, E.: Chemotherapy of chlamydial infections. Adv. Pharmacol. Chemother., 7:235, 1969.
Schachter, J., Smith, D. E., Dawson, C. R., Anderson, W. R., Deller, J. J., Hoke, A. W., Smart, W. H., and Meyer, K. F.: Lymphogranuloma venereum. Comparison of the Frei test, complement fixation test, and isolation of the agent. J. Infect. Dis., 120:372, 1969.
Sowmini, C. N., Gopalan, K. N., and Chandrasekhara Roa, G.: Minocycline in the treatment of lymphogranuloma venereum. J. Am. Ven. Dis. Assoc., 2:19, 1976.
Thorsteinsson, S. B., Musher, D. M., Min, K. W., and Gyorkey, F.: Lymphogranuloma venereum, a cause of cervical lymphadenopathy. JAMA, 235:1882, 1976.

118.   PSITTACOSIS
(Ornithosis, Parrot Fever)
William Schaffner

DEFINITION. Psittacosis is a specific infection of birds produced by the obligate intracellular bacteria, *Chlamydia psittaci*. When transmitted to man, this agent can produce asymptomatic infection, a transient influenza-like illness, or serious pneumonic disease characterized by high fever, headache, cough, myalgia, pulmonary infiltrates, and a significant mortality. Because many species of birds other than the order Psittaciformes transmit psittacosis, *ornithosis* has been suggested as a more accurate title. Usage has made psittacosis the accepted term for the human disease.

HISTORY. In 1879, Ritter, a Swiss physician, described seven cases of an unusual pneumonia that occurred after contact with tropical birds. Morange, in 1894, established the parrot as a vector and termed the disease *psittacosis* after the Greek *psittakos* (the parrot). During 1929–1930 a serious epidemic of pneumonia occurred in Europe and America after shipments of infected South American parrots. This epidemic led to clearer recognition of psittacosis as a human disease. The etiologic agent was demonstrated to be a filterable agent by Bedson, Western, and Simpson in 1930. Subsequent studies have shown that over 90 species of birds can harbor the agent, and its worldwide distribution has been documented. Reported cases in the United States have declined since 1960, probably as a consequence of requiring tetracycline treatment of imported psittacine birds.

ETIOLOGY. *C. psittaci* is an obligate intracellular parasite. It is morphologically and serologically related to lymphogranuloma venereum, to trachoma, and to a number of mammalian agents that produce pneumonitis, meningoencephalitis, and abortion in their native hosts but that do not produce human disease. Because of their large size (250 to 400 mμ), possession of both RNA and DNA, a demonstrable cell wall containing muramic acid, division by binary fission, and their susceptibility to chemotherapeutic agents known to inhibit bacterial enzyme systems, these agents have recently been reclassified as specialized bacteria. Parrots and parakeets are common carriers and until recently represented the major source of human infection. With better control of psittacine disease in aviaries, other birds now contribute more human infections, and cases have resulted from contact with turkeys, pigeons, ducks, chickens, pheasants, finches, and other fowl. Although individuals of both sexes and all ages are susceptible, overt clinical infections in children are uncommon. Persons working with birds are at greatest risk of infection, and there is an increased incidence of psittacosis in pet shop employees, pigeon handlers, and poultry workers, especially in turkey processing plants. There is no risk associated with eating poultry products.

The agent is present in the blood, tissue, feathers, and discharges of infected birds. It is hardy and can withstand drying. Although the avian disease can be fatal, infected birds frequently show only minimal evidence of illness, such as ruffled feathers, lethargy, and failure to eat. Birds having active infections are most likely to transmit the disease, but asymptomatic carriers are common, and birds that recover can shed transmissible agent for many months. In general, human psittacosis acquired from psittacine birds or turkeys has been more severe than that acquired from pigeons, ducks, chickens, or pheasants. Bird ectoparasites can harbor the agent and may serve as a source of reinfection for domestic flocks. Antimicrobials incorporated in bird foodstuffs may not eradicate psittacosis from infected parrots or parakeets but can render them less infectious for man.

Psittacosis is generally acquired by the respiratory route through inhalation of infected dried bird excreta, more rarely by handling the feathers and the tissues of infected birds. On rare occasion the disease may be acquired through an open lesion or the bite of a bird. Mouth-to-beak intimacies have led to infection in man. Small epidemics have been attributed to aerosols of dust laden with dried excreta. Cases have been reported after only brief exposure to birds. There is some evidence that the incubation period may be shortened by a large inoculum. Person-to-person transmission of psittacosis, although rare, has been documented. These cases of "human" strain psittacosis have been severe, with high mortality.

PATHOLOGY. In birds, the principal sites of disease are the liver, spleen, and pericardium. In man, the lung is most commonly involved. The psittacosis agent generally gains access to the human body via the respiratory route, and then rapidly enters the blood and reaches the reticuloendothelial cells of the liver and spleen. After replication in these sites, invasion of the lung is by hematogenous spread. The agent can be isolated from the blood and sputum during the first two weeks of illness, and has been found in the spleen in fatal cases. The mature pulmonary lesion is a lobular pneumonitis. The process is initiated by inflammation and progressive edema of the alveolar cells. Exudation is often accompanied by small hemorrhages, accounting for clinical hemoptysis. Polymorphonuclear leukocytes appear early in the process. Later inflammatory exudates show lymphocytes and large numbers of mononuclear leukocytes within the alveoli and interstitial spaces. The mucosa of the trachea and bronchi generally remains intact but is edematous and invaded with mononuclear cells. Thick, gelatinous plugs of mucus may fill major and minor bronchi and account for the severe cyanosis and progressive anoxia seen in fatal cases. Foci of necrosis may occur in more severely affected areas of

the lung and are sometimes associated with capillary thrombi. The process is generally most severe in dependent bronchopulmonary segments. Vasculitis and thrombosis may account for many findings. Large monocytes and macrophages containing cytoplasmic inclusion bodies, which may represent the agent (LCL bodies), are characteristic of psittacosis infection. Hyperplasia and monocytic infiltration of pulmonary and hilar lymph nodes and splenic enlargement with occasional areas of focal necrosis may occur. Rarely the liver may show intralobular focal necrosis and swollen Kupffer cells containing the psittacosis elementary bodies. Changes in the myocardium, heart valves, pericardium, meninges, brain, adrenals, and kidneys have been reported.

CLINICAL MANIFESTATIONS. Wide variations can occur in the clinical picture. The incubation period ranges from 7 to 15 days but may occasionally be longer. Asymptomatic infection or mild influenza-like infections probably are the rule. Moderate or severe infections, although less frequent, are more commonly diagnosed. The onset of illness may be insidious, but it often starts with chills and a fever that rises slowly from initial levels of 38 or 39 to 39.5 to 40.5° C during the first week of illness. As with some other instances of intracellular infection, the pulse may be slow relative to the height of the fever. Headache is severe. Malaise, anorexia, severe myalgias, particularly in the neck and back, and arthralgias are common. Cough is generally prominent but may be delayed until late in the first week. Small amounts of mucoid sputum with occasional blood streaking are the rule, and pleuritic pain is rare. Changes in mentation are often seen. Delirium or stupor may occur in severe cases toward the end of the first week, and is usually associated with severe pulmonary involvement, cyanosis, and other evidences of anoxia. Other neurologic manifestations are uncommon. Nausea and vomiting are frequent. Epistaxis may occur early in the course of the illness. A macular rash (Horder's spots) resembling that seen in typhoid has occasionally been described. Jaundice and progressive nitrogen retention have been reported in severe cases. Severe dyspnea, tachypnea, tachycardia, cyanosis, jaundice, delirium, and stupor are all poor prognostic signs.

The physical findings of pneumonia are often sparse. Chest roentgenograms often reveal evidence of infiltrates not detected at the bedside. Examination may reveal only fever, painful muscle groups, an elevated respiratory rate, and a relative bradycardia. Fine, crepitant rales may be heard in localized areas over the lungs. Frank percussion or auscultatory changes suggestive of true consolidation are less common. Pleurisy with effusion can occur but is unusual. Mild hepatomegaly is frequent. A palpable spleen has been noted in a substantial number of patients. Splenomegaly in a patient with undiagnosed acute pneumonitis should raise the consideration of psittacosis. An erythematous pharynx may be noted. In rare instances there may be signs of pericarditis or myocarditis. In prolonged, severe illness, thrombophlebitis and pulmonary infarction have been reported as late complications.

Patients with mild cases may recover in seven to eight days. More severe infections may last 12 to 21 days without specific treatment. Fever is ordinarily sustained or remittent, and when accompanied by bradycardia, resembles the fever seen in untreated typhoid infections. Defervescence is generally slow, and a prolonged convalescence is common. Relapses have been reported even after appropriate treatment. Complicating bacterial infections are rare. Second attacks have been described. Recently, British physicians have reported occasional cases of endocarditis caused by *C. psittaci* in patients with sterile blood cultures.

LABORATORY FINDINGS. Simple laboratory studies are not helpful in establishing a diagnosis. The leukocyte count is usually normal, but leukopenia or low-grade leukocytosis ranging to over 20,000 cells per cubic millimeter may occur. The erythrocyte sedimentation rate is generally elevated. Proteinuria is common during the febrile period. Chest roentgenograms generally show soft patchy infiltrates radiating outward from the hilum, which tend to be more prominent in dependent lobes or segments. Occasionally diffuse miliary, nodular, or frank lobar distribution of infiltrates is seen.

A specific diagnosis can be made only by isolation of the agent or by serologic studies. The agent is present in the blood and sputum during the first two to three weeks, but isolation is hazardous, and should not be attempted except in special laboratories. Diagnosis is generally made by a fourfold rise in complement-fixing antibodies against a heat-stable group antigen prepared from psittacosis agent grown in eggs. Paired acute and convalescent sera should always be tested. A significant change in antibody titers is generally present by the twelfth to fourteenth day of disease; the titers are usually maximal by 30 days, then slowly disappear. Treatment can delay or suppress antibody response. A serum complement-fixation titer of 1:16 during the acute illness is presumptive evidence of psittacosis. There is considerable cross-reaction between antigens prepared from psittacosis and lymphogranuloma venereum agents. False positive complement-fixation tests may occur with Q fever or brucellosis. Cutaneous hypersensitivity to the Frei antigen may develop during psittacosis.

DIFFERENTIAL DIAGNOSIS. Specific diagnosis of psittacosis is of extreme importance because of its potential severity (reported case fatality rates show a wide range but have attained 40 per cent), its response to antimicrobials, and the public health significance of psittacosis infection. All cases should be reported to the local health department. The syndrome of viral pneumonia accompanied by protracted high fever, unusually severe headache, and relative bradycardia should suggest psittacosis. Often a history of contact with birds is the only clue to diagnosis and may be elicited only by repeated questioning of the patient and family. When pneumonic symptoms are prominent, psittacosis must be differentiated from viral pneumonias, mycoplasmal pneumonia, influenza, Q fever, tularemia, tuberculosis, fungal infection, and bacterial pneumonia distal to an obstructed bronchus. If pneumonic symptoms are not prominent, psittacosis can be confused with other systemic febrile illnesses such as typhoid fever, brucellosis, infectious mononucleosis, infectious hepatitis, miliary tuberculosis, or the viral meningoencephalitides.

TREATMENT. The tetracyclines are the drugs of choice, and early diagnosis and initiation of treatment may be lifesaving. After institution of therapy with 2 to 3 grams daily, both fever and symptoms are generally controlled within 48 to 72 hours, although the response may be indolent. Although the disease apparently responds to penicillin in doses above 2 million units daily, tetracycline remains the drug of choice. Treatment should be continued for at least 10 days after defervescence to prevent relapse. The high fever and progressive anoxia secondary to extensive pulmonary involvement in severe cases may require appropriate measures directed at these problems.

Harding, H. B.: The bacteria-like chlamydiae of ornithosis and the diseases they cause. CRC Crit. Rev. Clin. Lab. Sci., 1:451, 1970.
Meyer, K. F.: The ecology of psittacosis and ornithosis. Medicine, 21:175, 1942.
Schaffner, W., Drutz, D. J., Duncan, G. W., and Koenig, M. G.: The clinical spectrum of endemic psittacosis. Arch. Intern. Med., 119:433, 1967.
Ward, C., and Ward, A. M.: Acquired valvular heart-disease in patients who keep pet birds. Lancet, 2:734, 1974.

PNEUMONIA

119. INTRODUCTION TO PNEUMONIA

Herbert Y. Reynolds

Pneumonia is a general term denoting a group of clinically manifest diseases that result from microbial infection of lung parenchyma. It is a commonly encountered disease and, in one form or another, continues to be a leading cause of death in the United States. Histologically, the pneumonias represent an inflammatory reaction in the interstitium of alveoli and an accumulation of exudate in alveolar lumina. Consolidation and a degree of nonfunction may occur in affected lung tissue. With successful inactivation of the infecting agent, resolution occurs and normal lung structure is usually restored. Exceptions to the complete healing phase occur in certain necrotizing pneumonias, those caused by staphylococcal or gram-negative bacteria, after which lung scars or fibrosis may develop.

For the physician to discover that a pneumonia, i.e., an intrapulmonary process of some sort, is present in an adult patient is no very difficult feat; neither is that knowledge particularly helpful unless two further steps can be taken. These are detection of evidence that the disease is indeed microbial in origin and not an infarct or neoplasm, and identification of the specific microbe or kind of microbe that is involved. Every aspect of management — the choice of treatment, the complications to be watched for, and the hour-by-hour prognosis — depends on the nature of this information. To obtain it *accurately and in proper time* requires the physician to be wholly familiar with the various ways in which each one of the microbial pneumonias expresses itself. Some of these — for example, plague pneumonia — he may never see. Yet he must know at least enough about plague pneumonia so that he could avert its terrible consequences for others should he ever encounter a case. Other forms of pneumonia encountered relatively rarely arise as complications of some familiar microbial disease such as measles or tuberculosis or streptococcal disease. Occasionally, well-known viruses such as influenza or chickenpox cause pneumonia, or the physician may be asked to see a patient with psittacosis. In the compromised host, necrotizing pneumonias caused by *Pseudomonas* and other gram-negative bacilli are commonplace. Most of the time, in an adult patient the physician is dealing with *mycoplasmal pneumonia* or with *one of three bacterial* pneumonias, pneumococcal, staphylococcal, or some other form of necrotizing pneumonia in an obviously altered host. This narrowing of the probabilities does not really lighten the seriousness of making the correct choice. The most effective treatment for pneumococcal pneumonia is utterly without value in *Klebsiella* pneumonia; a choice of therapy based on a diagnosis of mycoplasmal pneumonia when the patient actually has staphylococcal pneumonia could result in a fatality.

Mycoplasmal, pneumococcal, certain other primary bacterial pneumonias, and the necrotizing (frequently nosocomial) pneumonias are considered in Ch. 120 to 124. Because staphylococcal pneumonia is so closely related to influenza, it is discussed under influenza (see Ch. 82), as well as under staphylococcal disease (see Ch. 134). The pneumonias caused by viruses, rickettsiae, certain fungal species, i.e., *Histoplasma*, coccidioidomycosis, and *Aspergillus*) and other taxonomically less well defined species, such as *Pneumocystis carinii*, are considered in the individual chapters dealing with those infections.

Many microbial agents can infect the lungs and cause pneumonia, but bacteria do so most frequently. Although a common disease, bacterial pneumonia is a relatively rare occurrence in normal people, considering the burden of microorganisms in the ambient air and our frequent exposure to infectious respiratory droplets and secretions from sneezing and coughing fellow humans. This attests to the effectiveness of the lung host defense system. This defense system consists of a complex interrelationship of anatomic barriers and cleansing mechanisms present in the nasopharynx and upper airways and between local cellular and humoral factors operant in the terminal air-exchange units (alveoli). This might be described as the "natural defense system" of the respiratory tract. With respect to infectious agents, normal lungs are kept sterile beyond the first bronchial divisions.

Microorganisms reach lung tissue in several ways: (1) by direct inhalation of infectious particles from ambient air or by aspiration of secretions from the mouth and nasopharynx; (2) by deposition in lung vasculature following hematogenous spread from another site; and (3) by exogenous penetration of lung tissue. The last-named route includes trauma as well as iatrogenic inoculation of lung tissue with bacteria during chest surgery or from other kinds of diagnostic or therapeutic procedures, e.g., bronchoscopy. The inhalation-aspiration route is by far the most important. Also important are the size and configuration of inhaled particles and droplets which determine the site or level of deposition in the respiratory tract. For example, approximately 90 per cent of particles between 5 and 10 μ in diameter impact at some point along the trachea or in major bronchi, whereas those between 0.5 and 3 μ in size may escape filtration and be deposited in terminal air spaces or leave the body via expired air. Because many bacteria are in this small size range, they frequently plumb the airways to the alveoli. Of importance in pneumonia are the forces that can become operative to keep them there. Factors influencing the location of viral particles in the lungs are not so clear. Common to both viruses and mycoplasmas is their injury of the ciliary epithelium lining the trachea and lower respiratory tract. Such injury, caused in particular by viral infections, is a well-recognized predisposing factor to bacterial superinfection frequently with staphylococci. After viral infections, bacteria may not be cleared normally from the lower airways owing to damage in the ciliary clearing action of the respiratory epithelium. Subsequent stasis of mucus and respiratory secretions may inhibit phagocytosis and allows for bacterial multiplication; breaks in the lining surface permit submucosal penetration of bacteria. Pneumonia is a common aftermath.

In the upper respiratory tract and large airways, a combination of mechanisms excludes particulate material: (1) anatomic barriers such as the epiglottis, (2) frequent branching of the pulmonary tree (to affect aerodynamic filtration of inspired air), (3) mucociliary clearance of particulates which impact on the mucosa, (4) acute bronchial constriction, and (5) the cough response. When infectious agents, bacteria in particular, elude the physical or mechanical defenses described above and are deposited in the terminal airways and alveoli, another group of host factors takes over. These include phospholipid surfactant and proteins (immunoglobulins and complement factors) in the alveolar lining material and phagocytic cells, i.e., alveolar macrophages and polymorphonuclear neutrophils (PMN's). Anatomically, lung structure changes at the level of respiratory bronchioles and the terminal units (alveolar ducts and alveoli), in that ciliated epithelium and mucus-secreting cells (goblet cells and mucus glands), are no longer present. Therefore, mucociliary clearance does not exist, nor does coughing effectively clear material from the alveoli. Thus microbial clearance and removal of other antigenic material from alveoli are dependent entirely on cellular and humoral factors. Functionally, this portion of the airways from respiratory bronchioles to alveoli might be considered the lower respiratory tract.

If a bacterium of critical size is deposited in an alveolus (in the absence of edema fluid of either circulatory or inflammatory origin), the microbe may encounter at least three substances which conceivably might inactivate it, exclusive of its eventual inactivation by phagocytosis. First, surfactant, secreted by Type II pneumocytes, may have antibacterial activity against staphylococci and rough colony strains of some gram-negative rod bacteria. Second, immunoglobulins, principally of the IgG class and, in lesser concentration, monomeric and secretory forms of IgA, may have specific opsonic antibody activity for the bacterium. Although IgE is present and is considered to be a secretory immunoglobulin, no participation in the opsonic process has been identified for this immunoglobulin class. Third, complement components, especially properdin Factor B, might interact with the bacterium and trigger the alternative complement pathway. One or all of these possibilities described can prepare the bacterium for ingestion by an alveolar macrophage, or the activated complement sequence can lyse it directly. Although alveolar macrophages avidly phagocytose some inert particles, they ingest viable bacteria with considerably less enthusiasm. Coating or opsonizing the organisms will enhance phagocytosis approximately tenfold. However, immunoglobulin G appears to be the only substance capable of increasing alveolar macrophage phagocytosis. There is suggestive evidence that complement can function to enhance or amplify the process. Once phagocytosis has occurred, the alveolar macrophage can inactivate susceptible organisms. Intracellular killing proceeds but at an often slower rate than that measured in PMN's and along less well studied metabolic pathways. Whereas PMN's may kill ingested bacteria with one or a combination of four antimicrobial systems (H_2O_2, superoxide anion [O_2^-], myeloperoxidase, or halide anion), the process is less certain in alveolar macrophages.

Following containment of bacteria, the fate of alveolar macrophages is not certain. They are long-lived tissue cells which can survive at least several months and presumably are capable of handling repeated bacterial and other microbial challenges. Because they are mobile cells, they can migrate to other alveoli through the "pores of Kohn" or move to more proximal areas of the respiratory tract and get aboard the mucociliary escalator for elimination from the lungs. In addition, macrophages gain entry into lung lymphatics and can be carried to regional lymph nodes. This exit gives access to systemic lymphoid tissue and is important in initiating cellular immune responses. Undoubtedly, macrophages are instrumental in degrading antigenic material and presenting it to appropriate lymphocytes in these nodes.

Alveolar macrophages can usually inactivate microorganisms, and host defense surveillance is successful. Under this happy circumstance, clinical disease and pneumonitis never develop. However, if a sufficiently large bacterial inoculum reaches the lower respiratory tract, or if particularly virulent microorganisms are inhaled, the macrophage system can be overwhelmed. In such a situation, the lung parenchyma mounts an extensive inflammatory response that may be perceived as clinical illness. A chest roentgenogram usually reveals an infiltrate. The development of the inflammatory response and hence pneumonia is a deliberate and controlled reaction in the lungs. The ingredients of initiation, amplification, and, finally, suppression are present which make this sequence likely and will be reviewed.

The alveolar macrophage is the only resident phagocyte normally present in the alveoli. It is the bona fide first line of cellular defense on the airside of the lower respiratory tract. However, reserve phagocytic cells, the PMN's, are close by but located in the intravascular compartment. A plentiful supply of PMN's resides in the network of lung capillaries and by estimation may account for up to 30 per cent of the body's pool of marginated PMN's. Even though PMN's are in close proximity to alveolar spaces, they are nonetheless separated by several planes of tissue—capillary endothelium, interstitial space, and alveolar epithelium. Therefore granulocyte movement into the alveoli must be an orderly reaction initiated from the alveolar side. This is termed directed migration or chemotaxis. At least two mechanisms for chemotactic activity exist which can set in motion the inflammatory response in the alveoli: direct generation of chemotactic factors by microorganisms entering the alveoli, and release of chemotactic factors from alveolar macrophages following phagocytosis which might amplify the response. *The first* is best explained with the example of gram-negative rod bacteria

known to contain lipopolysaccharide substances termed endotoxins. Some complement components, particularly Factor B, are present in small amounts in brochoalveolar fluids as sampled by lavage of normal human lungs. Bacterial endotoxin can activate directly the alternative complement pathway, leading to the formation of fragments known to be potent stimulators of PMN chemotaxis, namely C5a and possibly C3a. Furthermore, endotoxin has the potential to convert Hageman factor, also a constituent of bronchoalveolar fluids, to an activated state which can subsequently initiate several pathways: coagulation, fibrinolysis, and kinin generation. In the fibrinolysis sequence, the enzyme plasminogen activator has chemotactic activity for PMN's and for mononuclear cells. In the kinin system, the enzyme kallikrein is chemotactic, and bradykinin is capable of increasing vascular permeability and may account for the accumulation of fluid and other humoral substances in alveoli that accompany pneumonia. Kinin activation is probably a nonspecific and nonimmune reaction (see Ch. 41). *The second mechanism* seems more specific and emanates from the alveolar macrophage itself. In vitro and in vivo studies with macrophages from monkeys and guinea pigs have shown that following phagocytosis of opsonized bacteria, a chemotactic factor is synthesized and secreted which will selectively attract PMN's. Such a factor is of small molecular weight (<5000 daltons), heat labile, and unaffected by antisera to complement components C3a and C5a, which neutralize their respective activities. Although this factor was identified first in macrophages of monkey and guinea pig origin, it has now been found in human cells as well. This mechanism would permit alveolar macrophages to recruit secondary phagocytes, PMN's, to help contain unruly bacteria in the alveoli. Once PMN's and other components of edema fluid have filled alveolar spaces, an exudative inflammatory reaction exists in lung parenchyma and pathologically pneumonitis is present. Ultimately lung tissues become consolidated.

Because of the inflammatory reaction, another quite significant mechanism of host defense — surface phagocytosis — assumes importance in pneumonia caused by well-encapsulated organisms. This phenomenon is of particular importance in patients who receive antimicrobial therapy early in the course of their disease. The reader should consult Ch. 121 for a presentation of this aspect of the subject.

After pneumonia has developed and pending successful containment of the infection, resolution and healing phases eventually occur. At present, however, little is known about the processes that turn off or limit the acute inflammatory reaction of pneumonia and initiate recovery. As in other disease situations, defects in immunoregulation of this part of host immunity are being explored (see Ch. 41). Serum-derived chemotactic factor inactivator can inhibit immune-complex deposition in animal lung tissue and modify the ensuing inflammatory response. The identification of such inhibitors and the potential for manipulating them is a part of lung immunophysiology that is still in its infancy.

A number of patients with *recurrent bacterial pneumonia* as a major clinical problem have been found to be deficient in either granulocyte or mononuclear cell chemotaxis or both. Inability to mobilize phagocytes to the alveoli in response to an inoculum of bacteria may be a fundamental defect (see Ch. 41).

As indicated above, in most persons with pneumonia, the physician's opportunity for error comes not from overlooking altogether that respiratory disease is present, but from either falsely minimizing its importance ("a little bronchitis") or from lightheartedly mislabeling a quite serious *nonmicrobial* condition, such as pulmonary infarction, as "a viral pneumonia." The physician's two immediate assignments — to establish that a pneumonic process is present and to amass evidence that it is most probably microbial in origin — are met by sharp awareness of what it is that is being sought and the prompt use of the relevant clinical and the readily available and simple laboratory techniques. A urine examination, for example, might reveal that a young, previously well adult with a slight cough, sudden rigor, left-sided midback pain, and a temperature of 39.5° C had an acute infection of the urinary tract. Young adults often have the classic symptoms which can be readily pinpointed to the lower respiratory tract, whereas infants and the elderly may have so few respiratory symptoms as to cause concern that infection may be arising from another organ system. Elderly or severely ill patients may have an unimpressive amount of cough, scant sputum production, and little evidence of respiratory symptoms. Only after excluding infection systematically in other organ systems, such as the previously cited urinary tract, does the respiratory tract receive greater consideration. The onset of fever and agitation or altered mentation frequently ushers in an acquired or nosocomial lung infection in a hospitalized or immunocompromised patient (see Ch. 124). Obviously, a high index of suspicion is sometimes needed plus confirming evidence from the physical examination and other laboratory aids.

Once the nature of respiratory illness is determined, other problems come to mind which should be weighed appropriately. Will the patient require hospitalization versus outpatient management? Does the patient have any obvious risk factors or underlying illnesses which make him or her susceptible to a specific bacterial infection? Are there any special epidemiologic considerations, and — of special importance — are any other members of the immediate family ill? Is this a recurrent pneumonia? What other peculiar problems of the patient may complicate medical management, such as drug allergies, compromised renal or liver function, poor superficial arm veins which prevent easy intravenous access, and so on? Obviously, some of the considerations are not relevant for every case. The points for emphasis, however, are the use of a mental check list to cover most facets of the patient's presentation and initiation of an orderly plan for the management of the particular respiratory infection.

Three principles of patient management bear repeating and deserve emphasis: (1) obtain all the necessary specimens for appropriate bacteriologic cultures before antimicrobial therapy is begun so that there is a reasonable chance for laboratory recovery of the organism; (2) ensure that the drug therapy is as specific as one's certainty of the etiologic agent allows, yet sufficiently broad — temporarily at least — to cover the common yet unsuspected microorganisms as well; and (3) tailor or change the antimicrobial coverage in several days when the results of the cultures are available. A few days of a broad-spectrum antimicrobial coverage will usually not cause superinfections or selection of the drug-resistant bacteria, as long as the physician wisely discontinues unnecessary drugs and appropriately narrows the antimicrobial spectrum as soon as possible.

It is of great importance to recognize that, if the chemotherapy of pneumonia is to be maximally effective, the correct drug or drug combination must be chosen quickly so that it can be given before irreversible changes have occurred. Yet to do this may be quite difficult, because periods of 24 hours or more are frequently necessary before laboratory techniques can reveal the particular microbe involved. Consequently, almost invariably the initial therapy must be chosen on the basis of the skillful interpretation of essentially *clinical* phenomena and must be heavily weighted toward protecting the patient against the most dangerous of the conceivable diagnoses in that particular set of circumstances. It is likewise of importance to make periodic (at least daily) reviews of the situation and to be quick to discontinue unneeded drugs once the identity of the microbe is known. For a discussion of this question, the reader is referred to Ch. 189.

Since the adequate examination and culture of respiratory secretions is so necessary for the rational treatment of pneumonia, the physician should be vigorous in his attempt to get adequate specimens. If the patient is not producing sputum, an attempt to induce secretions by nebulization of ultrasonic water particles is reasonable. Such particles (which may vary in size between 0.8 and 10 μ in diameter) serve as an irritant and stimulate most subjects to cough. Attempts to obtain lung secretions by passing a small rubber catheter through the nose or mouth — the red snake — rarely get beyond the vocal cords of an alert patient and should be recognized to accomplish little more than to greatly distress an already sick patient in order to obtain a sample of oropharyngeal fluids.

Within a few days of the start of therapy, the great majority of patients with a primary pneumonia can be assigned to one of three categories: a convincing bacteriologic diagnosis has been established by culture of the sputum, blood, or pleural fluid; absolute diagnostic proof is lacking but the patient is clearly recovering with antimicrobial therapy; or the patient is clearly recovering but without wholly convincing evidence that the pneumonia was bacterial in origin. There remains a fourth group, which is quite small. This consists of patients with impressive evidence of microbial pneumonia yet no real indication as to its cause. An appreciable number of these cases turn out to be fungal infections or caused by opportunistic organisms.

For this quite small group of pneumonias, the physician is justified in using various invasive methods to obtain material for microbiologic diagnosis, because to do so would be very much in the interests of the patient. This situation clearly differs from that obtaining in the usual patient with primary pneumonia, in whom such invasive procedures are seldom necessary. The nonprimary — the so-called nosocomial — pneumonias present a situation of their own. With them (see Ch. 124) the patient is usually suffering from at least one serious underlying disease, and the identity of the microbe causing the pneumonia can be considerably more difficult to establish than is the case with the primary pneumonias. At times, therefore, it seems proper on balance to use invasive procedures to establish the microbial agent in a nosocomial pneumonia. The point for emphasis, however, is that, as in primary pneumonia, the instances in which it is appropriate to do this are rare. Because such instances do occur, however, in the interest of completeness, the various techniques are set forth here:

Percutaneous transtracheal aspiration is a direct approach which eliminates much of the contaminating oral, microbial flora. The aspirate, performed through a plastic catheter (No. 14 or 16 size) and needle inserted through the cricothyroid membrane into the airway lumen, is obtained after a small injection of saline which makes the patient cough. If the head of the supine patient is placed below the level of the trachea and major bronchi, liquid injected through the transtracheal catheter may gravitate toward the larynx and possibly accumulate in the oropharynx. Under this circumstance, the patient may inhale oropharyngeal contents during coughing episodes which ensue. Thus transtracheal specimens can become contaminated with mouth flora and yield confusing results if shortcomings in the procedure are not recognized. Although this procedure is generally safe, occasionally some hazard accompanies it such as air leak, leading to subcutaneous or mediastinal emphysema, cardiac arrhythmia, or tracheal bleeding. The physician should use the procedure when indicated, with due caution and awareness of its complications. Anaerobic cultures should be planted as well as routine aerobic ones when a tracheal aspirate is obtained.

The availability of *fiberoptic bronchoscopy* with bronchial lavage and brushing provides another approach to lower respiratory secretions. The risk of bronchoscopy is small even in patients with extensive pneumonia; the administration of supplemental oxygen during the procedure is usually indicated. Often a direct view of the affected lung anatomy, particularly if a loss of volume in the lung lobe accompanies the infection, may provide evidence of an endobronchial obstruction. Removal of secretions or a mucus plug could make the procedure therapeutic as well as diagnostic.

Usually, the lavage fluid or brush culture will contain the offending pathogen; however, microbial cultures from the bronchoscopy specimens also contain contaminating flora from the nasopharynx. Interpretation of culture results is often confusing, and deciding what the predominant organism is may be difficult. To date, no one has perfected a completely reliable way to collect bronchoscopy lavage specimens to avoid this contamination. Several suggestions may improve specificity of the culture results somewhat. By using an area sampling technique to obtain oropharyngeal fluid and a nasal swab for nasal secretions, the nasopharynx can be cultured just prior to bronchoscopy. Then mouth organisms can be transiently suppressed by having the patient rinse the mouth and gargle with an antiseptic solution. Subsequent passage of the bronchoscope through an oropharyngeal tube or an endotracheal tube may reduce contamination even more. Final comparison between the oropharyngeal and nasal culture results and those obtained from lavage specimens may reveal differences that will be helpful in diagnosis. Quantitative bacterial cultures will not add much useful information in this setting and therefore are not recommended. Furthermore, if the patient has chronic bronchitis, for example, and already has colonization of the upper respiratory tract and tracheobronchial tree with *Streptococcus pneumoniae* or *Hemophilus* species, it is virtually impossible to localize or delimit the source of these bacteria in a meaningful way.

Direct examination and culture of affected lung tissue is often indicated. Physicians who care for adult patients with pneumonia generally do not think in terms of needle aspiration of lung tissue. Pediatricians, on the other hand, confronted with undiagnosed pneumonias in infants, feel more comforatble with the procedure and use it frequently. Precise indications for a needle aspirate in an adult cannot be formulated unequivocally; however, a localized, peripheral infiltrate which is "well situated" may lend itself to a needle approach with relatively small risk of complication. Spreading microorganisms along the needle track or soiling the pleural surface is always a consideration, but in actual practice it seems to occur rarely. A small pneumothorax may complicate a needle aspiration, but the frequency of this occurrence depends somewhat on the

type and size of the needle used. Often the factor of most significance is the skill and experience of the physician doing the procedure; this usually dictates the frequency and success with which needle aspiration is used within a particular hospital or medical community. The need to do a *small open thoracotomy* to obtain lung tissue is often easier to agree upon. This approach gives the best piece of tissue and is tolerated surprisingly well by even the sickest patient. Generally thoracic surgeons are extremely skillful in managing this situation. Open lung biopsy is often necessary in the immunocompromised patient with an advancing, undiagnosed, pulmonary infiltrate and pneumonia. However, two failings often are observed with the procedure. Medical personnel procrastinate and wait too long to get the biopsy, thus delaying appropriate antimicrobial therapy, or they do not coordinate the handling of the tissue with the microbiologist and pathologist to ensure optimal analysis. A brief presurgical consultation with all the principals is most helpful. The pathologist can often suggest the best area of lung to biopsy, and having the microbiology laboratory prepared can ensure that the most appropriate cultures are quickly planted.

Each of the procedures, as noted above, carries with it some risk of producing a potentially serious complication in a patient who may be already quite sick. The use of any of these procedures should be carefully limited to those relatively rare situations in which the additional knowledge to be obtained could be of significant benefit to the patient.

Antimicrobial therapy — plus appropriate support with fluids, antipyretic drugs, oxygen, suction or postural drainage, and the other modalities employed to treat serious lung infection — remains the cornerstone of medical management. Intelligent use of antimicrobial drugs is not easy, and frequent reappraisal of their choice and patient response must be practiced. The perennial problem of emerging microbial resistance remains; therefore proper selection and use of new antimicrobials to meet the need require the continual education and attention of medical personnel. Although current drug use will be addressed in succeeding chapters, new patterns of microbial resistance must be carefully sought. Without constantly maintaining such vigilance, our accepted therapies could rapidly become obsolete.

Bartlett, J. G., Rosenblatt, J. E., and Finegold, S. M.: Percutaneous transtracheal aspiration in the diagnosis of anaerobic pulmonary infection. Ann. Intern. Med., 79:535, 1973.

Green, G. M., Jakab, G. J., Low, R. B., and Davis, G. S.: Defense mechanisms of respiratory membrane. Am. Rev. Respir. Dis., 115:479, 1977.

Haas, H., Morris, J. F., Samson, S., Kilbourn, J. P., and Kim, P. J.: Bacterial flora of the respiratory tract in chronic brochitis: Comparison of transtracheal fiberbronchoscopic and oropharyngeal sampling methods. Am. Rev. Respir. Dis., 116:41, 1977.

Hahn, H. H., and Beaty, H. N.: Transtracheal aspiration in the evaluation of patients with pneumonia. Ann. Intern. Med., 72:183, 1970.

Johanson, W. G., Pierce, A. K., and Sanford, J. P.: Area sampling technique for quantitative pharyngeal cultures. J. Appl. Microbiol., 18:276, 1969.

Kaltreider, H. B.: Expression of immune mechanisms in the lung. Am. Rev. Respir. Dis., 113:347, 1976.

Kazmierowski, J. A., Aduan, R. P., and Reynolds, H. Y.: Pulmonary host defense: Coordinated interaction of mechanical, cellular and humoral immune systems of the lung. Bull. Europ. Physiopath. Resp., 13:103, 1977.

Kazmierowski, J. A., Gallin, J. I., and Reynolds, H. Y.: Mechanisms for the inflammatory response in primate lungs: Demonstration and partial characterization of an alveolar macrophage–derived chemotactic factor with preferential activity for the polymorphonuclear leukocytes. J. Clin. Invest., 59:273, 1977.

Newhouse, M., Sanchis, J., and Bienenstock, J.: Lung defense mechanisms (medical progress). N. Engl. J. Med., 295:990, 1045, 1976.

Reynolds, H. Y., Atkinson, J. P., Newball, H. H., and Frank, M. M.:

Receptors for immunoglobulin and complement on human alveolar macrophages. J. Immunol., 114:1813, 1975.

Reynolds, H. Y., Kazmierowski, J. A., and Newball, H. H.: Specificity of opsonic antibodies to enhance phagocytosis of *Pseudomonas aeruginosa* by human alveolar macrophages. J. Clin. Invest., 56:376, 1975.

Reynolds, H. Y., and Newball, H. H.: Fluid and cellular milieu of the human respiratory tract. *In* Kirkpatrick, C. H., and Reynolds, H. Y. (eds.): Immunologic and Infectious Reactions in the Lung. New York, Marcel Dekker, Inc., 1976, p. 3.

Robertson, J., Caldwell, J. R., Castle, J. R., and Waldman, R. H.: Evidence for the presence of components of the alternate (properdin) pathway of complement activation in respiratory secretions. J. Immunol., 117:900, 1976.

The Human Mycoplasmas

Species	Usual Site of Occurrence
M. pneumoniae	Respiratory tract
M. salivarium	Oropharynx
M. orale 1	Oropharynx
M. orale 2	Oropharynx
M. orale 3	Oropharynx
M. fermentans	Oropharynx and genital tract (rarely detected)
M. hominis	Genital tract
Ureaplasma urealyticum (T-mycoplasmas)	Genital tract

120. MYCOPLASMAL DISEASES

Robert B. Couch

120.1.   INTRODUCTION

The mycoplasmas (formerly called pleuropneumonia-like organisms, PPLO) are the smallest free-living organisms. Recent classification places them in the class Mollicutes, which is divided into two distinct families, Mycoplasmataceae and Acholeplasmataceae, and three genera, *Mycoplasma* (>40 species), *Acholeplasma* (five species), and *Ureaplasma* (one species). These organisms share a number of properties with bacteria, e.g., growth outside the host cell, susceptibility to antimicrobial drugs, generation of metabolic energy, reproduction by binary fission, and possession of both RNA and DNA. In contrast to bacteria, they do not possess a cell wall or the ability to synthesize cell wall precursors. The mycoplasmas are commonly confused with L-forms of bacteria, because L-forms also lack a cell wall and their colonial morphology resembles that of mycoplasmas. However, L-forms are related to their bacterial parents and are unrelated to the mycoplasmas.

Members of the genus *Mycoplasma* cause a variety of diseases in lower animals. These include sinusitis, pneumonia, arteritis, arthritis, and neurologic disease. Because of these varied pathologic states in animals, it has been proposed that many inflammatory diseases of man of unknown etiology are caused by mycoplasmas. In this regard, extensive efforts to incriminate mycoplasmas in the etiology of rheumatoid arthritis have thus far been inconclusive. At present, eight species of human mycoplasmas have been identified. Only one species, *Mycoplasma pneumoniae*, has been clearly shown to produce disease in man, and the disease is essentially limited to the respiratory tract. Two species are commonly cultured from the genitourinary tract; their role in disease there is not wholly clear, but probably at times they are the primary causative agent of disease. The other known species appear to be commensals. Nevertheless, because of the variety of animal diseases described, it would be surprising if some other human diseases are not caused by mycoplasmas.

The eight species of human mycoplasmas and their usual anatomic site of occurrence are shown in the accompanying table. *M. pneumoniae* is a significant cause of acute respiratory disease, including pneumonia. *M. salivarium* and *M. orale* 1 are common inhabitants of the oropharynx, particularly if oral hygiene is poor. *M.* *orale* 2 and 3 are uncommon inhabitants of the oropharynx, and *M. fermentans* has on rare occasions been recovered from the oropharynx and genital tract. None of the latter five species have been shown to cause human disease. *M. hominis* and the T-mycoplasmas (so called because of the "tiny" colonies produced on agar medium) have been collectively called the genital mycoplasmas (see Ch. 120.3).

120.2.   PNEUMONIA AND OTHER RESPIRATORY DISEASES CAUSED BY M. PNEUMONIAE

DEFINITION.   Pneumonia is the most severe manifestation of respiratory infection with *Mycoplasma pneumoniae*. Bronchitis, pharyngitis, and asymptomatic infections are frequently seen, particularly in young children; pneumonia occurs predominantly among older children and young adults. The disease responds to treatment with the tetracyclines and erythromycins.

HISTORY.   A pneumonia that was unlike lobar pneumonia of *Diplococcus pneumoniae* was recognized in the 1930's. Extensive bacteriologic studies failed to reveal a specific etiology in many of these cases, and Dingle and Finland in 1942 applied the term primary atypical pneumonia to this group of nonbacterial pneumonias. In 1943 the discovery that cold hemagglutinins developed in the sera of many of the patients provided a useful diagnostic test. During World War II the Armed Forces Commission on Acute Respiratory Disease described many of the clinical and epidemiologic characteristics of an atypical pneumonia, retrospectively identified by serologic tests as caused by infection with *M. pneumoniae*.

The causative agent was first isolated by Eaton in cotton rats, and subsequently was shown to infect hamsters and chicken embryos. It is filterable and for this reason was considered to be a virus for many years. In 1957, Liu reported an immunofluorescent test for antibody, using sections of infected chicken embryo bronchi for antigen, and Chanock in 1961 reported that the organism was the cause of most cases of pneumonia associated with the development of cold hemagglutinins. Subsequent to these studies and the demonstration that the organism was a *Mycoplasma,* it was given the name *Mycoplasma pneumoniae.*

ETIOLOGY.   *Mycoplasma pneumoniae* can readily be distinguished from the seven other known human species of *Mycoplasma*. The organism is about 200 nm in size. It will grow aerobically or anaerobically on artificial media, but the medium must be enriched with 20 per cent horse serum and yeast extract. On solid medium, the small granular colonies grow embedded in the surface of the agar, and are best detected by microscopic examination. Tentative identification procedures utilize the fact that *M. pneumoniae* ferments glucose, exhibits hemadsorption, hemolyzes guinea pig and sheep red blood cells, and is resistant to methylene blue. Final identification requires serologic procedures.

Analysis of the lipids of *M. pneumoniae* has partially explained some of the serologic responses noted in this infection. The protective antigen appears to be a glycolipid contained in the membrane of the organism. A phospholipid which reacts with some Wassermann-positive sera has been identified, and cross-reactions with glycolipids of *Streptococcus* MG and the I antigen of human erythrocytes probably account for these occasional serologic responses. The anti-tissue antibodies noted in this infection may have a similar explanation.

EPIDEMIOLOGY. *M. pneumoniae* infection is endemic in large populations, but numerous localized outbreaks have occurred in schools and military populations. There is no periodicity such as occurs with influenza and no seasonal prevalence as with bacterial and viral respiratory illnesses.

The basic epidemiologic unit is the family, where the infection is often introduced by five- to nine-year-old schoolchildren. Infection spreads slowly but will ultimately involve 80 to 90 per cent of family members who are not immune. Though most common in young schoolage children, the very young, adolescents, and young adults frequently acquire the infection. It is uncommon after age 50, but may occur at any age.

Roentgenographic evidence of pneumonia occurs in 30 to 50 per cent of infected family members, but studies in the military have suggested that less than 10 per cent of infections result in pneumonia. Recent reports suggest that infection may be more common in infants and preschool children than was formerly thought, but pneumonia is uncommon. Thus an age relationship to the likelihood of occurrence of pneumonia exists, but the reasons for this are not clear.

PATHOGENESIS. *M. pneumoniae* is a primary pathogen of the respiratory tract that is spread by close and frequent contact between infected and susceptible persons. The organism can be recovered from sputum and throat swab specimens two to three days prior to onset of illness. Thereafter, the concentration of organisms in secretions rises to the time of occurrence of illness and remains high for four to six days. After illness subsides, the agent may persist in respiratory secretions for several weeks in a considerable percentage of cases, and positive cultures frequently occur after antimicrobial treatment.

The organism grows on the ciliated border and between respiratory epithelial cells. All evidence indicates that it does not invade lung parenchyma. It has been suggested that the peroxide produced by the organism might produce cell damage; more recently it has been suggested that the illness may be a result of hypersensitivity to the organism or one or more of its products as a result of prior mild or asymptomatic infection.

Resistance to infection has been shown to correlate with presence and magnitude of serum antibody. Antibody is detectable in respiratory secretions, and recent data suggest that resistance more closely correlates with this antibody than with serum antibody. The association between antibody and resistance probably accounts for prevalence of the infection in younger age groups, as most adults have higher levels of serum antibody. Nevertheless, reinfection may occur at any age and be accompanied by pneumonia.

PATHOLOGY. From the limited studies available, it is apparent that a great variety of pathologic findings may occur in pneumonia, including patchy or confluent bronchopneumonia, interstitial pneumonia, and lobar pneumonia. Pleuritis with a small pleural effusion may be present, but significant pleural effusion is rare. Macroscopic examination usually reveals patchy areas of lung infiltration and inflamed bronchial and bronchiolar lumina containing mucoid and occasionally purulent exudate. Microscopic sections reveal mononuclear peribronchial and peribronchiolar infiltrates with edema and mononuclear cell infiltration of neighboring alveolar septa. Mucosal cell lining of respiratory passages usually remains intact, and polymorphonuclear cell infiltration is prominent only if necrosis and sloughing of the mucosal cell lining occur. Pathology in other organs of the body has been described for a few patients with evidence of *M. pneumoniae* infection and death as a result of severe hemolysis, encephalitis, myocarditis, or pancreatitis. A predominance of mononuclear cells with edema and sometimes intravascular thrombosis and necrosis characterizes the pathology of involved organs.

CLINICAL MANIFESTATIONS. Infection may be manifested by pneumonia, tracheobronchitis, pharyngitis, or myringitis. Pneumonia is the most serious and best described syndrome. The incubation period to onset of illness is about three weeks, most cases occurring in 15 to 25 days.

Pneumonia. The onset of pneumonia is usually insidious, with malaise and headache as prominent symptoms. For a period of two to three days these symptoms increase in severity, and feverishness, myalgias, and sore throat may also occur. Cough is usually not prominent until two to three days after onset of illness. It is either nonproductive or productive of small amounts of mucoid sputum that occasionally contain flecks of blood. *Despite the delayed appearance of cough, it becomes the dominant respiratory symptom in mycoplasmal pneumonia, and its absence or the occurrence of only mild cough makes a clinical diagnosis questionable.* In some cases cough occurs early, and patients may exhibit the paroxysms, substernal discomfort, and tracheal tenderness characteristic of acute tracheobronchitis. Headache is commonly reported as the most distressing symptom in an adult. Ear discomfort, owing to myringitis, mild nasal symptoms, and prominent sore throat may also occur, especially in the younger age groups. Substernal or diffuse chest discomfort on inspiration is common, but typical pleuritic pain is rare. Arthralgias, anorexia, nausea, and vomiting may also be reported.

Patients usually do not appear seriously ill. Tachypnea, dyspnea, and cyanosis are rare and are not seen unless pulmonary involvement is extensive or other disease is present. Fever is present in virtually all cases of pneumonia; it varies between 37.7 and >40° C, although it is usually under 39° C.

Physical examination usually reveals mild nasal obstruction and discharge and mild to moderate injection of the posterior pharynx. Mild injection of the tympanic membranes is commonly seen, and about 15 per cent of patients will exhibit frank myringitis, some of whom will develop blebs or bullae. Hemorrhage into the blebs or bullae is common, and these patients usually complain of severe ear pain. Tender cervical lymphadenopathy is a common finding, particularly when pharyngitis is also present.

Findings on chest examination may be minimal, and

roentgenographic findings that seem out of proportion to physical findings frequently occur. Auscultation of the chest may reveal rhonchi and wheezes over the involved area of the lung owing to mucus in large bronchi and bronchioles, and fine to medium moist rales may also be heard. In the occasional patient with more extensive disease, signs of consolidation may be detected.

Tracheobronchitis. Tracheobronchitis alone may occur from infection with *M. pneumoniae* and is more common than pneumonia. The onset and clinical picture are little different from that described for pneumonia, and a significant proportion of cases clinically diagnosed as tracheobronchitis will exhibit infiltration when x-rays are obtained. The cases in which the chest x-rays are normal tend to be less severe.

Pharyngitis. Pharyngitis frequently accompanies the tracheobronchitis and pneumonia caused by *M. pneumoniae;* however, pharyngitis alone may also occur. The onset and constitutional manifestations are similar to those described for pneumonia, but sore throat appears early and persists as the predominant symptom. Mild nasal symptoms and some cough may also occur. Pharyngeal examination may reveal a diffusely erythematous pharynx with or without pharyngeal and tonsillar exudate, or only mild pharyngeal congestion may be present. Tender cervical lymph nodes frequently accompany pharyngitis.

Ear Disease. Myringitis, occasionally accompanied by blebs or bullae, is most commonly seen in association with disease of the respiratory tract; however, it has also been reported as an isolated disease occurrence. Such patients complain of ear pain which on occasion may be severe.

ROENTGENOGRAPHIC FINDINGS. No roentgenographic changes can be considered typical of mycoplasmal pneumonia. Infiltrates are usually unilateral, confined to a lower lobe, and more prominent near the hilum. Frequently a single segment is involved, but on occasion the infiltrate may be extensive and lobar or may involve more than one lobe. Small pleural effusions are not uncommon.

LABORATORY FINDINGS. In pneumonia and the other mycoplasmal respiratory diseases, the leukocyte counts are usually within normal limits and rarely exceed 10,000 to 15,000 per cubic millimeter. Differential counts usually reveal slight neutrophilia with counts of 60 to 85 per cent neutrophils. During the period of acute illness lymphopenia may be seen. The erythrocyte sedimentation rate is usually elevated. Urinalysis reveals normal findings except for occasional albuminuria, which may be attributed to fever. Gram stain of sputum may reveal neutrophils without a predominant bacterium, and culture of sputum usually reveals normal flora.

COURSE AND COMPLICATIONS. The clinical course is variable and is best described for pneumonia. Illness on occasion may be severe, but very few deaths from pneumonia have occurred. Fever is variable in duration, lasting from three days to two weeks. Fever usually subsides by lysis, and when this occurs, slow but progressive improvement in the cough, malaise, and lethargy ensues. However, symptoms may persist for three to six weeks. Roentgenographic abnormalities frequently persist for two to four weeks.

Recent reports of hospitalized patients with evidence of *M. pneumoniae* infection have emphasized the severe manifestations the pneumonia may exhibit and the occurrence of a variety of nonrespiratory complications. An accurate estimation of the incidence of these various complications is not available, but they are uncommon. The most common pulmonary *complication* is relapse soon after clinical recovery, and disease may involve the same or a different lobe of the lung. Patients with severe bilateral pneumonia, marked pleural effusions, lung abscess, pneumatoceles, and residual pleural abnormality have also been reported. Clinically apparent intravascular hemolysis in association with demonstrable cold hemagglutinins occurs in a small percentage of patients. Such patients usually exhibit cold hemagglutinin titers of 1:500 or greater and also have demonstrable hemagglutinins at room temperature. Hemolysis usually occurs when fever subsides or chilling of peripheral tissues occurs.

M. pneumoniae has been associated with nervous system and cutaneous disease, although respiratory disease is also usually present. Patients with nervous system disease have had psychosis, meningitis, meningoencephalitis, neuropathy, or cerebellar ataxia. Variable numbers and types of cells have been noted in the cerebrospinal fluid, although mononuclear cells are prominent. Skin manifestations have included urticaria, vesicular eruptions, maculopapular eruptions, erythema multiforme, and erythema nodosum, although many patients were simultaneously receiving drugs, so that causation is not certain. A reported association with Stevens-Johnson syndrome is perhaps of special significance, as these cases are frequently preceded by respiratory symptoms and accompanied by pneumonia. Evidence of *M. pneumoniae* infection should be sought in such cases.

Bronchiectasis, pericarditis, myocarditis, Guillain-Barré syndrome, arthritis, hepatitis, pancreatitis, and thrombocytopenic purpura have also been reported as complications of *M. pneumoniae* infection.

DIAGNOSIS. Early diagnosis can be made only by clinical means. The presence of marked headache, lassitude, myalgias, definite nasopharyngeal findings, and nonproductive cough suggests nonbacterial pneumonia. Absence of the usual features of bacterial pneumonia, such as sudden onset, shaking chills, pleuritic pain, and purulent or bloody sputum, offers important support for the diagnosis. Other causes of pulmonary infiltration such as tuberculosis, mycotic infection, pulmonary infarction, and malignancy must be considered.

Among the causes of nonbacterial pneumonia that may mimic mycoplasmal pneumonia are psittacosis and Q fever, for which an exposure history should be sought, and adenoviral and influenzal pneumonias, which are usually more acute in onset and occur primarily during recognizable epidemics. If the age of the patient is 5 to 30 years and other similar cases have occurred in a family, diagnosis is more certain, but the only clinical finding that makes mycoplasmal pneumonia almost a certain diagnosis is the additional presence of myringitis with a bleb or bulla on the tympanic membrane.

Isolation of *M. pneumoniae* may be accomplished from sputum or throat swab specimens. Either enriched solid or special liquid medium may be used, although identifiable isolations are not usually detected for at least five days after inoculation, and 14 to 21 days of incubation may be required.

The cold hemagglutinin test is generally available and

useful. Sera of about 50 per cent of patients with *M. pneumoniae* pneumonia will develop a rise in titer of this autoantibody which agglutinates human red blood cells when reacted in the cold (4° C). It is more likely to occur in more severely ill patients, and usually appears toward the end of the first week or the beginning of the second week of illness. *Serum for this test should be separated from red blood cells before refrigeration.* Positive direct Coombs test and an occasional false positive serologic test for syphilis may occur.

A variety of serologic procedures have been described for detecting rise in specific serum antibody titer to *M. pneumoniae* between acute and convalescent sera. Complement fixation is the most available procedure and will demonstrate a rise in titer in 75 to 80 per cent of cases. Growth inhibition and mycoplasmacidal antibody assays are more sensitive but they require experience with cultivation techniques which is not widely available.

TREATMENT. Tetracycline and its derivatives and erythromycin have been shown to hasten the disappearance of fever, rales, and cough in treated cases of pneumonia. Since definitive diagnosis is not possible within the first few days after onset of illness, decisions regarding administration of antimicrobials must be made on clinical grounds. Patients presumed to have mycoplasmal pneumonia should receive tetracycline or its equivalent in doses of 0.25 gram every six hours. Erythromycin in doses of 0.5 gram every eight hours appears to be an acceptable alternative. Incomplete relief of cough, occasional relapse, and continued shedding of the organism frequently follow six- to eight-day courses of treatment with these antimicrobials. It is possible that continuing treatment for two to three weeks will provide more complete recovery, and therefore this duration of treatment is recommended. The additional use of antipyretics, antitussives, intermittent positive pressure breathing, oxygen, and the like is determined by individual needs.

It is recommended that all patients with bullous myringitis be treated with erythromycin or tetracycline for 10 to 14 days. Treatment of patients with pharyngitis and tracheobronchitis on a routine basis is not recommended unless the organism has been isolated, because these illnesses are indistinguishable by clinical techniques from the great majority of acute respiratory illnesses caused by viruses. However, if protracted illness occurs and *M. pneumoniae* has been isolated, the antimicrobials listed above may be used. An effect of antimicrobial therapy on the nonrespiratory complications of *M. pneumoniae* infections has not been shown; indeed, the occasional occurrence of these complications during adequate antimicrobial therapy raises questions regarding the role of the organism in their causation.

PREVENTION. No established method is presently available to prevent *M. pneumoniae* infection. Patients in the acute stage of pneumonia should probably be isolated and attempts made in the home to prevent close contact with ill individuals. There is no vaccine currently available.

Chanock, R.: *Mycoplasma* infections of man. N. Engl. J. Med., 272:1257, 1965.

Couch, R.: *Mycoplasma pneumoniae. In* Knight, V. (ed.): Viral and Mycoplasmal Infections of the Respiratory Tract. Philadelphia. Lea & Febiger, 1973, pp. 217–235.

Hayflick, L. (ed.): The Mycoplasmatales and the L-phase of Bacteria. New York, Appleton-Century-Crofts, 1969.

Mufson, M., Manko, M., Kingston, J., and Chanock, R.: Eaton agent pneumonia: Clinical features. J.A.M.A, 178:369, 1961.

Murray, H., Masur, H., Senterfit, L., and Roberts, R.: The protean manifestations of *Mycoplasma pneumoniae* infection in adults. Am. J. Med., 58:229, 1975.

120.3. MYCOPLASMAS IN GENITOURINARY DISEASE

ETIOLOGY. *Mycoplasma hominis* and *Ureaplasma urealyticum* (T-mycoplasmas) may cause genitourinary disease. *M. hominis* typically produces colonies on agar with the often-described "fried-egg" appearance. Colonies are usually 200 to 300 μ in diameter and are best visualized by microscopy. This colony size contrasts to that of the T-mycoplasmas, which is 10 to 30 μ in diameter. On agar medium *M. hominis* grows well under aerobic conditions, whereas T-mycoplasmas grow best anaerobically. Both grow well in broth, and tentative identification procedures employ the preferential metabolism of arginine by *M. hominis* and the fact that T-mycoplasmas possess a urease system and grow best in an acidic medium. The T-mycoplasmas are antigenically heterogeneous, and the number and significance of types or subtypes has not yet been delineated. A recent report suggests that *M. hominis* is also antigenically heterogeneous.

EPIDEMIOLOGY. The genital mycoplasmas may be recovered from the distal urethra of both the male and female and the vulva, vagina, and cervix of the latter. Presumably because of intimate association with mucosal surfaces, specimens that contain epithelial cells are superior to urine or secretion specimens for isolation tests.

Infants may become colonized with genital mycoplasmas at birth, presumably acquiring them from the birth canal. The frequency of recovery of organisms decreases for the first year or two of life, and most individuals then remain free of genital mycoplasmas until puberty. Mycoplasmas then reappear, and frequencies are directly proportional to extent of sexual activity and promiscuity, suggesting the possibility of infection being acquired venereally.

Despite the fact that genital mycoplasmas are commonly recovered from the urogenital tract, disease is uncommon. This suggests a low order of pathogenicity for these organisms.

CLINICAL MANIFESTATIONS. **Nonspecific Urethritis.** The syndrome of dysuria, urgency, and frequency of urination with urethral discharge and without evidence of gonococcal infection has been called nonspecific or nongonococcal urethritis. A negative urine culture for bacteria and absence of prostatitis if the patient is a male are essential supportive findings. Patients with postgonococcal urethritis in which the gonococcus disappears but symptoms of urethritis remain are also included in this category of patients. The urethritis may be caused by a T-mycoplasma but apparently not by *M. hominis* (chlamydiae are the most likely alternative to T-mycoplasmas) (see Ch. 139).

Pelvic Inflammatory Disease. Patients with lower abdominal pain and fever who exhibit tenderness on movement of the cervix and in the adnexal areas are usually designated as having pelvic inflammatory disease. In most instances acute or subacute salpingitis is present, although tubo-ovarian abscesses or pelvic abscesses elsewhere may present similar findings. *M. hominis* may cause the disease in many of these cases.

Cervicitis and vaginitis as separate disease entities may occasionally be caused by *M. hominis,* although the data are inconclusive in this regard.

Mycoplasmal Disease in Pregnancy. Both *M. hominis* and the T-mycoplasmas have been recovered from the uterus, amnion, and fetus. Infection is more likely to occur with *M. hominis* than with T-mycoplasmas and to occur during therapeutic or spontaneous abortion, or when premature rupture of the membranes has occurred. Blood cultures are occasionally positive, and such patients exhibit fever and serum antibody responses. The frequency and significance of mycoplasmal infection of the uterus and products of conception are uncertain, but it seems probable that *M. hominis* is responsible for some cases of spontaneous abortion and puerperal infection. Infertility, infant low birth weight, and fetal death have been attributed to mycoplasma infection, but a causative relationship has not been established.

Postpartum fever in patients with normal pregnancy and delivery may occasionally be caused by invasion of the bloodstream with *M. hominis* or T-mycoplasma. The frequency of such cases attributable to mycoplasmas is apparently low.

TREATMENT. All mycoplasmas are susceptible to the tetracyclines. *M. hominis* is susceptible to lincomycin and resistant to erythromycin, whereas the converse is true for the T-mycoplasmas. Patients with nonspecific urethritis should receive tetracycline or its equivalent in doses of 0.25 gram every six hours for five to seven days. Although T-mycoplasmas are also susceptible to erythromycin, results of treatment have been somewhat better with tetracycline. Failure to respond may be attributable to resistance of the infecting strain to tetracycline, a recently reported finding of uncertain frequency. When erythromycin is used for therapy of nonspecific urethritis, patients should receive 0.5 gram every eight hours for five to seven days. Relapse and/or reinfection occurs in about 20 per cent of patients within three months. Second courses of the drug are frequently beneficial, but the sexual contacts of such patients should be examined for T-mycoplasmas. Unexplained recurrent nonspecific urethritis is an indication for urologic evaluation for structural abnormality of the urethra.

Since pelvic inflammatory disease may be caused by gonococci, *M. hominis,* and perhaps other bacteria, and since the site of disease is not accessible for obtaining culture specimens, antimicrobial therapy directed toward the specific cause is often not possible. In nonhospitalized patients tetracycline has been reported to be effective treatment. In most instances of postpartum fever associated with mycoplasmas, spontaneous cure without specific antimycoplasmal therapy occurs. Patients considered as candidates for treatment should receive tetracycline in doses noted above.

McCormack, W. M., Braun, P., Lee, Y. H., Klein, J. O., and Kass, E. H.: The genital mycoplasmas. N. Engl. J. Med., 288:78, 1973.

121. PNEUMOCOCCAL PNEUMONIA

Edward W. Hook

DEFINITION. Pneumococcal pneumonia is an acute bacterial infection of the lungs caused by *Streptococcus pneumoniae* (the pneumococcus) and characterized clinically by an abrupt onset, rigor, fever, chest pain, cough, and bloody sputum. Bacterial pneumonia occurring in otherwise healthy persons is usually caused by the pneumococcus.

BACTERIOLOGY AND IMMUNOLOGY. The somatic portion of the lancet-shaped pneumococcal cell is gram positive. In its virulent form (smooth, S), the pneumococcus has an outer capsule consisting of a high molecular weight polysaccharide polymer that is specific for each serologic type. In addition to the type-specific capsular antigen, there is a species-specific carbohydrate in the cell wall, known as the "C" substance. The capsule of pneumococcus acts as an armor against phagocytic cells and thus contributes significantly to the pathogenicity of the organism. Pneumococcal variants having no capsules (rough, R strains) are essentially avirulent. Antibody to the type-specific carbohydrate promotes phagocytosis by combining with the highly polymerized polysaccharide of the capsular gel. The pneumococcus also produces hyaluronidase, a hemolysin that causes greenish discoloration around colonies on blood agar, and autolytic enzymes that, when activated, render the organism gram negative and eventually cause its dissolution.

Pneumococci grow rapidly on a variety of bacteriologic media. Blood agar and beef infusion broth containing 0.5 per cent dextrose and 5 per cent blood or serum are the media most commonly used. On blood agar virulent strains form circular, glistening, dome-shaped colonies that are alpha hemolytic. Because of the great quantity of capsular polysaccharide formed by type 3 pneumococcus, its colonies are more mucoid and usually much larger than those of other types. Unlike other alpha-hemolytic streptococci, the pneumococcus is soluble in bile, sodium deoxycholate, and other surface-active agents, is highly sensitive to ethyl hydrocuprein chloride (optochin), and, with a few exceptions, is mouse virulent.

The extraordinary virulence of pneumococci for mice may be made use of in isolating the organisms from sputum. The technique usually used consists in injecting intraperitoneally 0.5 ml of sputum previously emulsified by having been drawn repeatedly into a tuberculin syringe. When virulent pneumococci are present, the mouse usually dies within 48 hours, and a pure culture of the organism can be isolated from the heart's blood. Since other bacteria in the sputum do not ordinarily produce fatal infections in mice, the animal serves as a convenient and highly sensitive differential "culture medium" for the isolation of pneumococci.

At least 85 different serologic types of pneumococci have been identified by agglutination tests with specific antiserums or by the quellung test. The latter is based upon the fact that when pneumococci come in contact with homologous capsular antibody, a capsular precipitin reaction and swelling occur, rendering the capsule easily visible under the microscope.

Specific polysaccharide, which has diffused away from the bacteria, can often be identified in the sputum, blood, or urine of patients with pneumococcal pneumonia. The lungs of patients with extensive pneumonia may contain up to 2 grams of capsular polysaccharide. The detection of these bacterial antigens in clinical specimens by counterimmunoelectrophoresis is gaining acceptance as a sensitive method for the rapid (e.g., two hours) diagnosis of infection.

Anticapsular antibody usually appears in the blood of patients with pneumococcal pneumonia between the fifth and tenth days of the disease. In some untreated patients, its appearance coincides with recovery; in others no such relation is demonstrable. The development of measurable type-specific antibody is delayed in patients with antigenemia detectable by counterimmunoelectrophoresis.

EPIDEMIOLOGY. Pneumococcal pneumonia may occur at any season, but it is most common during the winter and early spring, when viral respiratory infections are most prevalent.

The types of pneumococci that most commonly cause pneumonia in adults in the United States are types 1, 3, 4, 6, 7, 8, 12, 14, 18, and 19. Together, these ten types account for about three quarters of all cases. The most common types encountered in childhood pneumonias are 1, 6, 14, 19, and 23.

Pneumococci, particularly of the higher types, are frequently present in the respiratory tracts of normal subjects. Ordinarily the prevalence of carriers of highly pathogenic types is relatively low, except for type 3, which is a common inhabitant of the normal pharynx. Nevertheless, there is evidence that normal carriers play a more important role in the dissemination of infective types than do patients ill with pneumonia. Occasionally, in relatively closed communities, high carrier rates of pathogenic types are encountered. In such circumstances the occurrence of widespread viral disease of the respiratory tract may result in an epidemic of pneumococcal pneumonia. Except for these rare epidemics, most of which occur in hospitals or custodial institutions, the disease is sporadic.

PATHOGENESIS AND PATHOLOGY. The lung is the only major viscus of the body exposed to air. As the atmosphere, particularly in congested places, contains many pathogenic bacteria, it is remarkable that pneumonia is not more common. The failure of normal subjects to acquire acute bacterial pneumonia as an airborne infection is due to efficient defense barriers of the lower respiratory tract. These barriers include (1) the epiglottal reflex, which prevents aspiration of infected secretions; (2) the sticky mucus that lines the bronchial tree and to which airborne organisms adhere; (3) the cilia of the respiratory epithelium, which keep the mucus moving constantly toward the pharynx at the rate of 1 to 3 cm per hour; (4) the cough reflex, which serves to propel mucus or foreign bodies out of the lower tract; (5) the lymphatics that drain the terminal bronchi and bronchioles; (6) phagocytic cells, especially alveolar macrophages that are ever present in the normal alveoli; and (7) opsonins and specific antibody. In addition, the alveoli themselves are relatively dry and thus offer a poor medium for growth of bacteria that succeed in reaching them. Acute bacterial pneumonia results only when the defense barriers of the normal respiratory tract fail (see Ch. 119).

The thesis that bacterial pneumonia usually results from aspiration of infected secretions from the upper respiratory tract is strongly supported by both experimental and clinical observations. Rats infected with pneumococci in the nasopharynx regularly exhibit pulmonary lesions only when subjected to experimental procedures involving chilling of the body, anesthesia,

administration of morphine, or alcoholic intoxication, all of which are predisposing factors in human pneumonia and have been shown in laboratory animals to slow the epiglottal reflex and thus to facilitate aspiration. Experimental pneumonia can best be produced by intrabronchial inoculation of organisms suspended in mixtures of gastric mucin or starch having viscosities similar to that of mucus. Viral infection of the upper respiratory tract in man usually precedes the onset of acute bacterial pneumonia by several days. Not only is the volume of secretion from the nasopharynx greater than normal during viral infections such as the common cold, but also the number of pathogenic microorganisms in the secretions is significantly increased. Thus the stage is set for aspiration of infected mucus. That such aspiration often occurs at the onset of pneumonia in man is suggested by the usual sites of initial involvement of the lung. The earliest lesions of bacterial pneumonia usually appear in those parts of the lungs into which aspirated fluid is most likely to drain. Whereas most airborne bacteria are caught on the sticky surfaces of the bronchial tree and never reach the alveoli, organisms contained in thin nasopharyngeal secretions are readily carried into the alveoli by the liquid mucus. The latter, like Lipiodol, cannot all be ejected by ciliary action, and much of it penetrates to the farthest reaches of the bronchial tree, where it establishes the initial focus of infection.

Other factors known to predispose patients to acute bacterial pneumonia include exposure to noxious gases and anesthetics, cardiac failure, influenza viral infection of the lungs, and trauma to the thorax. A feature common to all these conditions is the accumulation of fluid in the alveoli. Harford (1950) has shown that the dry lungs of normal mice are able to rid themselves of large numbers of inspired bacteria, whereas lungs containing fluid are readily infected. This observation suggests that pulmonary edema, by providing a suitable culture medium for the bacteria, may facilitate the establishment of active infection within the alveoli. Influenza also causes destruction of the ciliated columnar epithelial cells lining the tracheobronchial tree, thus interfering with function of cilia. In addition, influenza virus also apparently inhibits phagocytosis.

Pneumococcal pneumonia may also occur as a complication of bronchogenic carcinoma, chronic pulmonary disease, such as bronchiectasis or lung abscess, or any process that produces obstruction of a bronchus.

Splenectomy carries an increased risk of severe bacteremic infections which are predominantly although not exclusively pneumococcal in etiology. The clinical course is often fulminant, frequently associated with evidence of diffuse intravascular coagulation and a high mortality rate. Although it appears that even healthy adults with post-traumatic splenectomies show increased susceptibility, the risk is greatest in infants and young children, in patients with underlying diseases which compromise reticuloendothelial function, and during the early postsplenectomy years. The mechanism of this relationship is unknown, but it appears that the spleen is important in removing encapsulated bacteria in the absence of antibody.

Persons with sickle cell anemia and other sickle hemoglobinopathies are especially vulnerable to severe pneumococcal infections, especially meningitis. The pneumococcus, not *Hemophilus influenzae*, is the most common cause of bacteremia and meningitis in children with sickle cell anemia. The factors accounting for this relationship are probably multiple and include deficiency of heat-labile opsonins which is secondary to a defect in the function of the alternative complement pathway (see Ch. 39), functional asplenia in some instances and actual splenic atrophy in others, and impaired phagocytic and killing capacity of reticuloendothelial cells.

In patients with severe pneumococcal infection with bacteremia and pneumonia or extrapulmonary sites of infection in cerebrospinal, pleural, or peritoneal fluids, the frequency of some other underlying disease exceeds 50 per cent. The incidence of pneumococcal pneumonia is increased in patients with hypogammaglobulinemia or multiple myeloma.

Early Lesion. Once the infection has gained a foothold within the alveoli, the lesion evolves in a characteristic manner. The first response of the lung to bacterial invasion is an outpouring of edema fluid into the alveoli which serves to "float" organisms into new alveoli through the pores of Kohn and terminal bronchioles. Centrifugal spread of infection occurs. After the outpouring of edema fluid, polymorphonuclear leukocytes and some erythrocytes accumulate in the infected alveoli, first in small numbers but later in such quantities as to fill each alveolus and thus render the area completely consolidated. Once the infected alveoli become crowded with leukocytes, phagocytosis of bacteria takes place, and the invading organisms are destroyed. Macrophages appear in the exudate, and resolution begins only after most of the organisms have been ingested.

Spreading Lesion. Three stages in the inflammatory reaction account for the distinguishing histologic features of the spreading pneumonic lesion. In the outermost portion there appears an "edema zone" in which the alveoli are filled with serous fluid containing only bacteria. Inside the edema zone a second zone may be identified in which there are signs of early consolidation with leukocytes in most of the alveoli. Here phagocytosis is often noted. Still more centrally a third transition to a "zone of advanced consolidation" is noted where the alveoli are packed with cells and where beginning resolution may be evident.

All stages of inflammation can be found in a spreading lesion. In the most recently invaded areas at the periphery, edema and hemorrhage predominate, causing "red hepatization," whereas in the older, more central parts of the lesion, dense consolidation with leukocytes accounts for the characteristic color of "gray hepatization."

Pneumococcal pneumonia may involve a lobe or segment of the lung, or lesions may be patchy in distribution and concentrated particularly about the bronchi. Bronchopneumonia is especially common in infants, the elderly, and persons with other lung diseases such as chronic obstructive pulmonary disease. Because a clear-cut distinction between pneumococcal bronchopneumonia and lobar pneumonia cannot always be made even by the pathologist, and because management for the two conditions is the same, it is rarely important for the clinician to differentiate them. The etiology rather than the anatomy of the lesion determines therapy.

Interlobar Spread. The spread of the pneumonic process may be stopped by the pleural boundaries of the lobe. Often, however, the infection spreads to other lobes of the lungs by flow of infected edema fluid from bronchi of the involved lung into the bronchial tree of a new lobe.

Bacteremia. Bacteremia is common during the course of pneumococcal pneumonia, particularly when the infection is fulminating. The fact that organisms appear in the thoracic duct in experimental pneumonia before they appear in the systemic circulation suggests that the bacteria reach the bloodstream via the lymphatics. Blood cultures are positive in 20 to 30 per cent of patients with pneumococcal pneumonia. The prevalence of bacteremia increases with age, and is more common with type 2 pneumonia and less common with type 3 pneumonia than with other pneumococcal types.

Invasion of Pleura and Pericardium. The exact mechanism whereby pneumococci invade the pleura or pericardium is not known. As the lymphatics at the periphery of the lung drain outward toward the pleura, it is possible that the pleural invasion results from lymphangitic spread. When infection of a pleural or pericardial cavity occurs, there results an outpouring of serous fluid followed by the deposit of fibrin. Leukocytes accumulate in the infected cavity, and, if infection persists, a purulent focus results. The pus in such cavities is at first thin but later becomes thick and stringy as a result not only of fibrin formation but also of the presence of deoxyribonucleic acid derived from the nuclei of disintegrating leukocytes. Finally, the thick fibrinous pus becomes walled off, forming loculated foci of chronic suppuration.

Similar purulent foci may occur in the meninges, peritoneum, or joints, as a result of hematogenous spread. Acute vegetations on the endocardium of the heart valves are sometimes encountered. Children with nephrotic syndrome are more prone to pneumococcal peritonitis than normal children. Pneumococcal peritonitis also occurs as a complication of hepatic cirrhosis with ascites.

Mechanism of Recovery. Surface Phagocytosis. Owing to the antiphagocytic properties of their capsules, fully encapsulated, virulent pneumococci are resistant to phagocytosis when suspended in a fluid medium devoid of opsonins. In the presence of relatively immovable cellular surfaces, however, as in the alveoli, leukocytes are able to trap the encapsulated organisms and ingest them without the aid of opsonizing antibody.

Heat-Labile Opsonins. Leukocytes in vivo are also assisted, right from the start of infection, by heat-labile opsonins that are present in normal plasma. These opsonins, which gain access to acute inflammatory exudates, are immunologically polyspecific, i.e., they act on all sorts of bacteria, in contrast to the monospecific anticapsular antibody that is eventually generated. In nonimmune individuals the majority of serum opsonizing activity for pneumococci results from alternative pathway activation of C3 and C5 and fixation of the cleavage products C3b and C5b to the surface of the organism.

Anticapsular Opsonins. Most patients with pneumococcal pneumonia who survive long enough eventually generate an excess of monospecific anticapsular antibody. The process usually takes five to ten days. These newly formed immunoglobulins not only agglutinate the pneumococci in the edema zone of the lesion and thereby inhibit their spread, but also act as potent accessory opsonins and further increase the efficiency of phagocytosis.

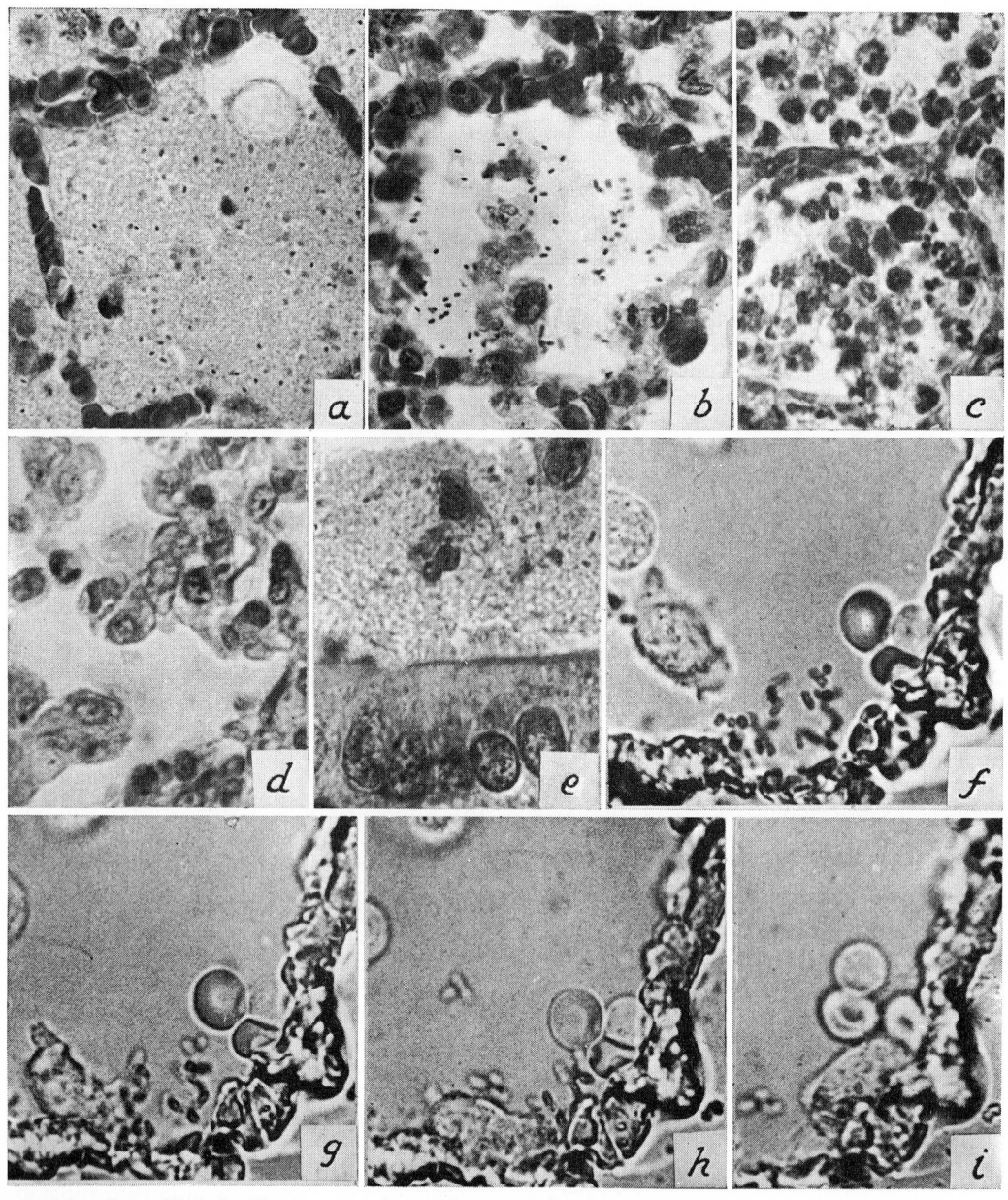

a, Pneumococci in edema-filled alveoli at margin of spreading pneumonic lesion (×800).

b, Beginning stage of polymorphonuclear exudation in zone of early consolidation. Note leukocytes in alveolar capillaries, some in process of diapedesis (×800).

c, Leukocyte exudate (still predominantly polymorphonuclear) in inner zone of advanced consolidation. Pneumococci have been phagocytized and destroyed (×800).

d, Alveolar macrophage reaction characteristic of late stage of resolution (×800).

e, Pneumococci in edema fluid contained within lumen of a large bronchus. Such infected bronchial fluid causes spread of pneumonia to other lobes of the lungs (×1250).

f–i, Surface phagocytosis of encapsulated microorganisms in formalin-fixed rat lung (×1250). Bacteria shown in these photomicrographs are klebsiellae, but same results have been obtained with pneumococci.

f, Polymorphonuclear leukocyte is seen approaching bacteria near alveolar wall. Time 12:30.

g, Leukocyte has reached alveolar wall and is about to trap organisms against the tissue surface. Time 12:31.

h, Cell has trapped some of the encapsulated bacteria against the wall and is in the process of phagocytizing them. Time 12:32.

i, Having ingested several of the organisms, the leukocyte is moving up the alveolar wall. Time 12:35.

(Photomicrographs from studies on experimental pneumonia. W. B. Wood et al.: J. Exp. Med., Vol. 73; and Smith and Wood: *ibid.*, Vol. 86.)

MACROPHAGE REACTION. The exact role of the "macrophage reaction" in the recovery process is not entirely clear. Because the appearance of macrophages in the alveolar exudate coincides in general with the disappearance of organisms from the lesion, it has long been assumed that these large mononuclear phagocytes take an active part in destroying the bacteria, and in the final analysis tip the scales in favor of the cellular defenses of the host. Studies relating to experimental lymphadenitis cast some doubt upon this assumption. The "macrophage reaction" in a regional lymph node draining an area of active infection can be artificially initiated at any stage of the nodal inflammation by merely cutting the afferent lymph vessels bringing bacteria to the node. Thus it appears that macrophages accumulate in the exudate only when the active stimulus of direct bacterial invasion has been eliminated. If this interpretation is correct, the polymorphonuclear leukocytes may be looked upon as the "shock troops" that play the major role in controlling the infection, whereas the macrophages serve primarily to remove the particulate debris from the resolving exudate and thus promote clearing of the lesion.

RESOLUTION. One of the most remarkable features of pneumococcal pneumonia is the completeness with which it resolves. Even when several lobes are completely consolidated, recovery usually results in restoration of the entire pulmonary parenchyma to its normal state within a few weeks. Not all the processes that take part in this dramatic resolution have been identified, but they include (1) the action of cytolytic enzymes upon disintegrating leukocytes; (2) transport of cells from the lesion via lymphatics; and (3) phagocytosis and digestion of cellular debris by macrophages. The rarity with which tissue necrosis occurs in pneumococcal pneumonia, despite the violence of the inflammatory response, appears to account for the completeness of the healing. Occasionally recovery proceeds more slowly than usual and leads to "delayed resolution." The factors responsible for delaying the removal of exudate from the lesion in such cases are not known. In rare instances, as the result of irreversible damage to the pulmonary parenchyma, resolution fails to take place altogether, and the lesion becomes the site of intense fibroblastic activity that leads to permanent scarring or "organized pneumonia."

Infection with type 3 pneumococcus may occasionally lead to pulmonary necrosis and abscess formation. This pneumococcus has a large capsule that interferes with phagocytosis and accounts, at least in part, for its extraordinary pathogenicity.

SUPPURATIVE EXTRAPULMONARY FOCI. Suppurative pneumococcal lesions, which occur in such extrapulmonary sites as the pleura, pericardium, meninges, joints, mastoids, or accessory sinuses, resolve much less readily, even with intensive chemotherapy, than does uncomplicated pneumococcal pneumonia. In such areas of suppuration, phagocytosis appears to be relatively inefficient, because trapping of bacteria by leukocytes in the exudate is inefficient and many of the leukocytes in the exudate are not viable. Although a drug like penicillin may reach the organisms in a purulent focus, it may not destroy them, because pneumococci do not multiply rapidly in pus of long standing, and "resting" bacteria are not susceptible to the bactericidal action of penicillin. In fact, suppurative pneumococcal lesions may respond satisfactorily only when chemo-

therapy is combined with some form of drainage that removes the bulk of the necrotic exudate.

CLINICAL MANIFESTATIONS. Symptoms. Victims of pneumococcal pneumonia are often seriously ill when first seen. The degree of prostration may be such that an adequate history can be obtained only from the family. The story of a mild nasopharyngitis preceding by several days the onset of major symptoms is frequently elicited. The first distressing symptom is usually a shaking chill, lasting for several minutes to a half hour. More than 80 per cent of patients with pneumococcal pneumonia experience one or more chills during the earliest stages of the disease. The initial rigor is often so violent as to cause the bed to shake and the patient's teeth to chatter. It is followed in about one case in three by vomiting. The initial chill usually coincides with bacterial invasion of the lung and marks the onset of fever. Several chills may occur at the start of pneumococcal pneumonia, but repeated attacks of rigor late in the disease suggest an extrapulmonary complication such as empyema, pneumonia caused by some other bacterium, or administration of antipyretics.

CHEST PAIN. In approximately 70 per cent of cases, severe chest pain occurs at the onset and may even precede the rigor. The pain, which is "stabbing" in character and exaggerated by cough and respiration, is caused by inflammation of the pleura resulting from the characteristically peripheral location of the initial lesion. There may be local tenderness in the chest wall at the site of the pleurisy. When the diaphragmatic surfaces of the pleura are affected, the pain may be referred either to the corresponding side of the lower chest wall and upper abdomen or to the shoulder. The patient may gain some relief from the knifelike pain by lying on the affected side on a firm surface, thereby splinting that half of the thorax.

COUGH. A cough may be absent at the onset, but usually is a prominent symptom during the course of the disease. Stimulation of the cough reflex results from irritation of the lower respiratory tract and from accumulation of mucus and exudate within the bronchial tree. Approximately 75 per cent of patients raise diffusely bloody or "rusty" sputum in contrast to "blood-streaked" sputum. The thorough mixing of the blood appears to be due to the fact that bleeding occurs directly into the alveolar exudate and thus constitutes an integral part of the inflammatory response to the infection. When the sputum is particularly sticky or jelly-like, type 3 pneumococcus or *Klebsiella* should be suspected, because both these organisms produce an inordinate amount of capsular polysaccharide that causes the exudate to be highly viscous.

FEVER AND TOXEMIA. Constant features of the disease are fever and toxemia, with the temperature usually ranging between 39.5 and 41° C. During the febrile period complaints of malaise, anorexia, weakness, myalgia, and general prostration are extremely common. Pneumococcal pneumonia may occasionally progress with great rapidity, and the general condition of the patient may deteriorate alarmingly within a few hours.

Physical Signs. Patients with well-established pneumococcal pneumonia appear acutely ill. There is moderate to severe respiratory distress. The nostrils dilate with each inspiration. Paroxysms of hacking cough, often productive of bloody or rusty sputum, occur during the examination. The chest pain, which is usually unilateral, may be so severe as to interfere with the patient's breathing and coughing; in these circumstances grunting expiration results. The location of the pain indicates immediately the approximate site of at least part of the lesion. The patient occasionally appears apprehensive and may even be delirious.

The temperature, pulse rate, and respiratory rate are usually elevated by the time the patient seeks the aid of a physician. The temperature should be taken by rectum, because oral measurement with the subject breathing rapidly through the mouth is likely to be inaccurate. The pulse pressure is characteristically widened, as in any high fever.

The skin is usually hot and moist, with beads of perspiration visible on the face and forehead. Cold extremities may indicate impending shock. Herpetic blisters are frequently noted about the mouth. The lips, mucous membranes, and nail beds are often cyanotic as a result of blood passing through poorly aerated lung. The cyanosis may be exaggerated by lowered respiratory exchange associated with rapid shallow breathing, often resulting from pleural pain. Icterus of the sclerae should be carefully looked for because of the prognostic significance of overt jaundice in pneumonia.

The ears should always be examined with an otoscope to exclude the presence of active otitis. Tenderness over a mastoid process or over an accessory nasal sinus should also be noted. The presence of exudate in the pharynx or over the tonsils suggests the possibility of streptococcal or adenoviral pneumonia. Definite nuchal rigidity may indicate pneumococcal meningitis, a serious complication of pneumonia. The neck veins must be carefully examined to detect the presence of increased venous pressure caused by complicating congestive heart failure. Deviation of the trachea constitutes an important sign of either atelectasis (toward the involved side) or pleural effusion (away from the involved side).

EXAMINATION OF THE CHEST. Diminished respiratory excursion or a slight inspiratory lag of one side of the chest often reveals the side of the principal lesion. A localized area of tenderness in the chest wall, noted during percussion, may be one of the earliest signs of pleural invasion. Careful percussion and auscultation do not always reveal signs of consolidation. In early cases, particularly, there may be no conclusive physical signs. Lesions at a distance from the chest wall are difficult to outline by percussion. When consolidation is extensive, the typical findings of dullness to percussion, bronchial or tubular breath sounds, and fine crackling rales are easily elicited, except in the presence of complicating bronchial obstruction or extensive pleural effusion. A coarse "leathery" friction rub is frequently audible in the region of consolidation.

Examination of the heart may be difficult because of loud respiratory sounds. An apical systolic murmur is frequently heard during high fever and is often of no significance. Diastolic murmurs, on the other hand, arising from either the mitral or aortic valve, are usually indicative of underlying organic heart disease or complicating pneumococcal endocarditis. A pericardial friction rub often constitutes the first sign of spread of the pneumococcal infection to the pericardial cavity. Ventricular premature contractions are not uncommon in the presence of any moderate or severe infection.

ABDOMINAL DISTENTION. Distention of the abdomen is frequently encountered. When tympany is noted in the left axilla and left upper quadrant, acute gastrectasia should be suspected. Occasionally, the examiner will note rigidity and even tenderness in one or both upper quadrants of the abdomen, suggesting a subdiaphragmatic lesion. This sign is usually due to referred pain resulting from involvement of the parietal pleura over the outer part of the diaphragm.

Digital examination of the rectum may be postponed if the patient is acutely ill, but in women a sufficiently complete pelvic examination should be performed to exclude the possibility of an infected abortion, which may lead to metastatic bacterial pneumonia. The neurologic examination is rarely abnormal in pneumococcal pneumonia except in the presence of meningitis or brain abscess.

LABORATORY FINDINGS. As in most acute bacterial infections, the total leukocyte count in pneumococcal pneumonia is elevated, and there is a "shift to the left" in the differential count. The number of leukocytes in the peripheral blood during the active infection usually ranges from 10,000 to 25,000 per cubic millimeter; counts above 40,000 are occasionally encountered. Leukopenia (with a "shift to the left") is observed in fulminating pneumococcal infections, particularly in the presence of bacteremia and in alcoholics.

Although the presence and location of the pulmonary lesion can usually be determined by physical examination, confirmatory roentgenographic evidence is often helpful. Both posteroanterior and lateral views of the chest should be taken. Pneumococcal infection of the lungs usually begins in the right middle lobe or in one of the lower lobes. The pulmonary process is limited to a single lobe in the majority of patients. In fact, it is not unusual for the process to be limited to a single pulmonary segment. In the series of Austrian and Gold, collected since the introduction of antimicrobial drugs, fewer than one third of the patients with pneumococcal pneumonia and bacteremia had more than a single lobe involved. Bulging interlobar fissure may be observed occasionally in pneumococcal pneumonia, although it is much more characteristic of Friedländer's pneumonia.

Whenever the diagnosis of pneumococcal pneumonia is suspected, the patient's blood should be cultured. Anaerobic as well as aerobic cultures are recommended to aid detection of pneumonia caused by a microbe other than pneumococcus. A blood culture positive for pneumococci provides important information regarding both etiology and prognosis.

Pneumococci are usually present in sputum, nasopharynx, and material aspirated from the trachea. Sputum for smear and culture may be difficult to obtain, but this usually can be accomplished by urging the patient to cough, or a paroxysm of cough can be induced by passing a nasal catheter into the trachea. If a sputum specimen cannot be obtained, a nasopharyngeal culture should be collected, because there is a high positive correlation between specific pneumococci isolated from cultures of the nasopharynx and from the sputum of patients with pneumococcal pneumonia. Transtracheal aspiration or lung puncture is not indicated for the diagnosis of bacterial pneumonia in the usual patient.

The sputum in pneumococcal pneumonia shows large numbers of gram-positive, lancet-shaped diplococci in association with polymorphonuclear leukocytes. Gram-positive cocci which are not pneumococci are frequently observed in sputum smears and account for the poor correlation of results of studies to identify pneumococci on Gram-stained sputum smears and on sputum cultures. Omniserum, a pool of antibody against 84 of the known 85 pneumococcal types, can be used for definitive identification of pneumococci in sputum. The results of the quellung reaction with omniserum correlate with the results of cultures in about 90 per cent of cases. Because the carrier rate of pneumococci in the general population may be quite high, positive identification of pneumococci in sputum or nasopharynx does not establish a definitive diagnosis of pneumococcal pneumonia.

The technique of counterimmunoelectrophoresis for detection of specific polysaccharides in sputum, blood, or body fluids can be helpful in establishing definitive diagnosis, even in patients who have received antimicrobial therapy. Capsular antigens persist in secretions or fluids rendered sterile by antimicrobial drugs. Antigen can be detected in the sputum of the majority of patients with pneumococcal pneumonia, but positive results may also be obtained in patients with bronchitis without pneumonia. Circulating polysaccharide can be detected in the blood of at least one half of patients with pneumococcal bacteremia but much less often in the absence of demonstrable bacteremia. The concentration of polysaccharide in the circulation declines progressively during antimicrobial therapy, but circulating antigen remains detectable in two thirds of the patients with antigenemia for two weeks or longer.

Other laboratory examinations that may be of value in the management of the patient include hematocrit, blood electrolyte, and urea determinations.

CLINICAL COURSE. During the course of the disease the patient should be examined carefully once a day. More frequent physical examinations may unduly exhaust an acutely ill subject. The common complications of pneumococcal pneumonia should be specifically looked for during each examination, particularly when fever persists.

Defervescence. The fever of untreated pneumococcal pneumonia either may terminate abruptly by "crisis" five to ten days after onset or may gradually subside by lysis. When effective antibacterial therapy is used, a dramatic crisis may occur within 24 hours, or the fever may persist for several days. Physical signs in the chest may also change, coarse sticky rales of resolution replacing the fine crepitant rales and tubular breath sounds of consolidation. Complete clearing of the pulmonary lesion may occur within a few days, but usually the auscultatory signs of resolution persist for a week or more after defervescence. If resolution is not complete within 21 days, it is arbitrarily classified as delayed. The promptness of defervescence and the speed of resolution are in general inversely proportional to the age and extent of the lesion at the time treatment is begun. There is a high incidence of protracted illness and delayed resolution of pulmonary infiltrates in patients with polysaccharide antigenemia which persists for more than three weeks.

Crisis marking the start of recovery must be differentiated from the "pseudocrisis" occasionally noted at the onset of shock or at the time of interlobar spread of the infection. Although the temperature may fall precipitously during a pseudocrisis, the pulse rate remains elevated, and the patient's general condition fails to improve.

Relapse. Relapse may occur in pneumococcal pneumonia when chemotherapy is discontinued too soon. If fever, tachycardia, and other signs of active infection recur while the patient is still receiving penicillin therapy, it may usually be assumed that a previously unrecognized purulent complication of the pneumococcal infection (such as empyema) exists, that a drug-resistant secondary invader has gained a foothold in the lung, that hypersensitivity of the patient to penicillin has caused the development of drug fever, or that the diagnosis of pneumococcal pneumonia is incorrect.

COMPLICATIONS. Pleural Effusion. The most common specific complication of pneumococcal pneumonia is pleurisy with effusion. In somewhat less than 10 per cent of cases, fluid can be demonstrated in the pleural cavity by either physical or roentgenographic examination. Such effusions are usually small, and, when sterile, are rarely of significance. They result from inflammation of the pleura overlying the lesion in the lung. Occasionally they may be of sufficient volume to cause respiratory embarrassment and necessitate thoracentesis. Whenever pleural effusion is detected in a patient who has failed to respond promptly to treatment, a thoracentesis should be performed to determine whether the fluid is infected and thus represents an early empyema.

Empyema. Empyema, though less common than sterile pleural effusion, is far more serious. Before the advent of chemotherapy, the incidence of this complication was approximately 5 per cent. With the use of penicillin, empyema is much less common (less than 2 per cent). Its presence is indicated by continued fever (often irregular), persistent leukocytosis, and signs of pleural effusion. Localized tenderness is frequently noted in the chest wall overlying the site of the lesion. The exudate in the pleural cavity may become loculated by thick, fibrinous adhesions. When the lesion is confined to an interlobar fissure or is located in the thoracic "gutter" adjacent to the spine, it may be detectable only by roentgenographic methods. Repeated exploratory thoracenteses, done preferably with the help of fluoroscopy, may be required to prove the presence of empyema. Its detection is of the greatest importance, because, once discovered, it is amenable to proper therapy, whereas, if left untreated, it may eventually drain exteriorly through the chest wall (empyema necessitatis) or rupture into a bronchus and cause a bronchopleural fistula. Rarely, empyema heals spontaneously, causing calcification of the pleura.

Meningitis and Endocarditis. Two serious complications of pneumococcal pneumonia that are often associated with one another are endocarditis and meningitis. Pneumococci usually localize on the aortic valve, producing aortic insufficiency. The development of pneumococcal endocarditis is rare at present. Equally serious is *pneumococcal meningitis* resulting from blood-borne metastasis to the meninges. About 20 per cent of cases of pneumococcal meningitis develop secondary to pneumococcal infection of the lung. The meningitis is characterized by the presence in the pia-arachnoid of a heavily infected exudate, which may cause subarachnoid block or may lead to localized subarachnoid abscesses. Unless vigorous therapy is instituted promptly, the prognosis is hopeless. Even when treatment is intensive, the patient may fail to recover, or may sustain permanent damage to the brain.

Pericarditis. Like the other complications of pneumococcal pneumonia, pericarditis has also become relatively rare since the introduction of potent antimicrobial drugs. When the pericardium is invaded, the patient usually experiences precordial pain, and a leathery friction rub may be heard over the heart. Pericardial effusion usually results, causing a "dampening" of the heart sounds. If the fluid is sterile, the condition is benign, unless so large a volume accumulates as to cause cardiac tamponade. Empyema of the pericardium, on the other hand, is a serious complication requiring prompt and vigorous treatment. Pericardiocentesis is mandatory to establish the diagnosis of purulent pericarditis.

Other Specific Complications. Still rarer specific complications include peritonitis and pyogenic arthritis. Occasionally the pulmonary lesion of pneumococcal pneumonia fails to resolve even after many weeks, and finally is replaced by fibrous tissue.

Nonspecific Complications. *Acute dilatation of the stomach* (gastrectasia) and *paralytic ileus* occur particularly in patients suffering from anoxia and severe toxemia and give rise to gaseous distention of the abdomen (tympanites) that causes discomfort and often increases respiratory embarrassment. *Shock*, likewise, is a complication of severe toxemia and indicates a serious prognosis. *Congestive heart failure* occurs frequently as a complication of severe pneumonia in patients with underlying heart disease. As congestive heart failure is an important predisposing factor in bacterial pneumonia, it is not surprising that they are often associated, and obviously both must be treated. The diagnosis of congestive heart failure in the presence of pneumonia may at times be difficult, but it should be considered in any patient with abnormal distention of neck veins, peripheral edema, an enlarged tender liver, and elevated venous pressure. Pulmonary signs of congestion are difficult to interpret in patients with pneumonia.

Jaundice, the pathogenesis of which is controversial, may be related to lysis of erythrocytes in pneumonic lesions, depressed liver function resulting from anoxia, or focal hepatic necrosis consequent to the pneumococcal infection. Pneumococcal pneumonia may also precipitate hemolysis and jaundice in persons with glucose-6-phosphate dehydrogenase deficiency. The presence of prominent icterus usually indicates a poor prognosis, and may be associated with chronic liver disease, e.g., cirrhosis. As in any bedridden patient, *phlebothrombosis* may occur during pneumonia. Its early presence should suggest the possibility that the pulmonary lesion is due to infarction of the lung rather than to primary pneumonia. *Herpes labialis* occurs in at least 10 per cent of patients with pneumococcal pneumonia.

DIFFERENTIAL DIAGNOSIS. Pneumonia resulting from organisms other than pneumococcus may at times be difficult to differentiate from pneumococcal pneumonia. Only by bacteriologic study of the sputum can pneumonia caused by *Klebsiella pneumoniae* (Friedländer's bacillus), *Staphylococcus aureus*, or *group A Streptococcus* be identified. *Tuberculous pneumonia* rarely causes the acute prostration characteristic of coccal infection. *Mycoplasmal pneumonia* and other infections of the lungs, such as psittacosis and Q fever, do not often cause shaking chills, diffusely bloody sputum, severe pleural pain, or a marked leukocytosis, although they may at times be confused with acute bacterial pneumonia. *Tularemic pneumonia, legionnaires' disease*, and pneumonia caused by *H. influenzae*, especially common in young children, must also be considered. When the diagnosis

is in doubt, repeated examinations of the sputum should be made, using both the Gram and "acid-fast" stains.

The most important noninfectious processes that must be differentiated from pneumococcal pneumonia are pulmonary infarction and atelectasis. *Pulmonary infarction* may be exceedingly difficult to differentiate from pneumonia. The dyspnea, pleural pain, hemoptysis, fever, physical signs of pulmonary consolidation, roentgenographic findings, and leukocytosis are all in keeping with an acute infection of the lungs. Frequently, however, the initial symptom is intense pleural pain of sudden onset; shaking chills rarely occur; there is no preceding history of respiratory infection; the fever is usually not high; frank hemoptysis is common; pulmonary signs, when present, appear early; and the total leukocyte count rarely reaches 20,000 per cubic millimeter. Moreover, although the chest signs develop rapidly in pneumococcal pneumonia, they appear right away with a pulmonary infarct. Combination ventilation-perfusion radionuclide scanning reveals similar defects in pneumonia and pulmonary infarction. Perfusion defects without corresponding ventilation defects are evidence for pulmonary embolism; such perfusion defects in association with a matched ventilation-perfusion defect in the area of a pulmonary infiltrate suggest pulmonary infarction as the cause of the infiltrate.

When a pulmonary infarct becomes infected, as sometimes happens, differentiation from primary bacterial pneumonia may be extremely difficult. Although in such cases the patients should receive antimicrobial treatment as in pneumonia, recognition of the infarction is of importance because of the need for anticoagulant therapy.

Pulmonary atelectasis, resulting from bronchial obstruction, not only may simulate pneumonia but often leads to serious infection of the lung if the bronchial obstruction is not relieved. Aspiration of mucus during or after surgical anesthesia is a common cause of atelectasis. Dyspnea, cough, chest pain, splinting of one side of the thorax, dullness to percussion, and suppressed breath sounds may all suggest primary pneumonia. Fever and leukocytosis also are noted when infection is present. As pulmonary atelectasis may be relieved by forced coughing and postural drainage or, if necessary, by bronchoscopy, it is important to differentiate it from primary pneumonia. Occasionally, sufficient shift of the mediastinum occurs to make the diagnosis obvious. Collapse of a segment of the lung may also result from chronic bronchial obstruction caused by neoplasms, such as bronchogenic carcinoma, or by an aortic aneurysm.

Subdiaphragmatic infection may be confused with pneumonia. Subdiaphragmatic abscess, liver abscess, or other infections in the upper abdomen may extend to the diaphragm and produce local inflammation, small collections of pleural fluid, chest pain, and atelectasis secondary to decreased respiratory excursions. Conversely, pneumococcal pneumonia may simulate intra-abdominal disease. Pleurisy may result in pain referred to the abdomen so as to suggest acute appendicitis or cholecystitis.

Even when the diagnosis of pneumococcal pneumonia is established beyond doubt, the possibility of a second underlying lesion of the lung must be borne in mind. Chronic obstructive pulmonary disease or lung abscess may lead to repeated attacks of bacterial pneumonia and often becomes evident only after the pneumonic consolidation has resolved. Bronchogenic carcinoma or any lesion partially obstructing a bronchus may lead to recurrent pneumonia of the same pulmonary segment.

TREATMENT. The treatment of pneumococcal pneumonia may best be discussed under three headings: (1) antibacterial therapy, (2) supportive measures, and (3) the treatment of complications. Before the advent of effective antibacterial therapy, supportive treatment was of the greatest importance. The introduction, first, of antipneumococcal serum and, later, of sulfonamides, penicillin, and the other antimicrobial drugs has so altered the management of pneumococcal pneumonia that today supportive treatment is rarely crucial, and serious complications are only occasionally encountered.

Antibacterial Therapy. PENICILLIN. Penicillin is at present the drug of choice in the treatment of pneumococcal pneumonia. The vast majority of strains of the pneumococcus isolated in the United States and most other areas of the world are susceptible to penicillin, and most are inhibited in broth by concentrations of less than 0.02 μg per milliliter. However, a number of reports have appeared since 1967 which describe the isolation of pneumococci relatively resistant to penicillin G in Australia, New Guinea, England, Canada, and the United States. The minimal inhibitory concentration of benzylpenicillin for these strains is 0.1 to 2.0 μg per milliliter, although most strains isolated in the United States are inhibited by 0.2 to 0.4 μg per milliliter. Some of these strains have shown relative resistance to the penicillinase-resistant penicillins and cephalosporins, but most have been fully susceptible to antimicrobials other than benzylpenicillin.

The emergence of these relatively resistant strains of pneumococci in a number of different areas of the world has not altered our present over-all approach to the therapy of pneumococcal pneumonia. The dose of penicillin usually utilized in therapy of pneumonia is sufficient to inhibit or kill these strains. However, several reports of delayed response or failure of penicillin therapy of pneumococcal meningitis caused by these strains of "intermediate sensitivity" have been reported. Clinicians should consider the possibility that delay in response to therapy of pneumococcal infection, especially at sites where high concentrations of penicillin may be difficult to achieve, could be related to relative resistance of the infecting organism to penicillin.

A recent development in South Africa regarding the susceptibility of pneumococci to antimicrobials is of great potential importance. In May 1977, pneumococci highly resistant to multiple antimicrobial agents were isolated from pediatric patients and staff of several hospitals in Durban and Johannesburg, South Africa. These organisms are highly resistant to benzylpenicillin, penicillinase-resistant penicillins, ampicillin, cephalothin, erythromycin, clindamycin, tetracycline, and chloramphenicol, but are sensitive to rifampin, vancomycin, bacitracin, and fusidic acid. These organisms spread readily among patients in the hospital and, in addition to producing an asymptomatic carrier state, have also caused pneumonia, bacteremia, and meningitis unresponsive to conventional therapy. Physicians should be alert to the spread or emergence of these organisms in other areas of the world.

The effectiveness of antimicrobial treatment is due in part to the natural resistance of the host, which accounts for the destruction of a large proportion of the invading bacteria. Host resistance, which results primarily from the activity of phagocytic cells in the lung, when combined with the bacteriostatic and bactericidal effects of drug therapy, controls promptly all but the most malignant pneumonia. Even with no treatment at all, approximately seven of every ten patients with pneumococcal pneumonia eventually recover, but some will have experienced a very severe illness before recovery has occurred.

Antipneumococcal therapy should be initiated promptly, therefore, in order to halt the spread of the infection both locally and through the bloodstream. An effective method is to give aqueous procaine penicillin G intramuscularly in a dose of 300,000 units at 12-hour intervals. Some authorities recommend the administration of aqueous penicillin G by the intramuscular route in doses of 300,000 units several times during the first 24-hour period of observation in addition to the procaine penicillin. In the presence of shock, penicillin G should be given intravenously. Treatment should be maintained for at least one week or until the temperature has been normal for 72 hours; if treatment is discontinued too soon, relapse may occur.

Penicillin may also be given by mouth. However, in a serious infection such as pneumococcal pneumonia, it is inadvisable to rely on oral penicillin therapy in acutely ill patients. Parenteral therapy throughout provides the greatest margin of safety. If parenteral therapy is not feasible or advisable throughout the period of treatment, procaine penicillin G can be given parenterally initially and penicillin V can then be given orally after defervescence. When oral penicillin V is used, it should be given in a dosage of at least 250 mg every six hours.

Response to penicillin therapy is often dramatic. Bacteremia, when present at the start of treatment, clears within a few hours. A crisis, characterized by rapid defervescence and a striking subsidence of symptoms, occurs in less than 48 hours in approximately half the patients. The others experience a more gradual recovery, the temperature falling by lysis over a period of four to seven days. Frequently a secondary rise in temperature occurs after the crisis. This elevation is usually low-grade and subsides spontaneously within a few hours, or at most a few days.

When a patient's pneumonia fails to respond satisfactorily to penicillin therapy, four possible explanations should be considered: (1) that the patient is suffering from a serious complication such as empyema, endocarditis, meningitis, or pulmonary suppuration (possibly secondary to bronchogenic carcinoma); (2) that the primary infection is of nonpneumococcal origin and is due to an agent that is resistant to the action of penicillin, e.g., a penicillin-resistant strain of *Staphylococcus* or *Klebsiella*; (3) that drug fever has developed as a result of penicillin hypersensitivity; or (4) that the diagnosis of microbial pneumonia is incorrect and some other condition accounts for the fever and pulmonary lesions. Occasionally, patients will respond initially to treatment only to have unmistakable signs of persistent pneumonia subsequently develop in spite of continued therapy. This sequence of events is usually due to the presence of a mixed infection, the initial response to treatment resulting from control of penicillin-susceptible organisms, and the relapse occurring as a result of persistence of a penicillin-resistant species.

Re-examination of the sputum and modification of the antimicrobial therapy are immediately indicated. Patients with underlying chronic pulmonary disease are particularly prone to such mixed infections.

Persons giving a history of having had a penicillin reaction in the past should not be treated with penicillin.

OTHER ANTIMICROBIAL DRUGS. Cephalothin or cefazolin can be used as effective alternatives to penicillin for parenteral therapy in patients hypersensitive to penicillin. Patients hypersensitive to penicillin sometimes show cross-sensitivity to cephalosporins; a cutaneous scratch test with the cephalosporin to be used should probably be performed in these patients to determine whether the drug can be used as an alternative to penicillin. Cephalothin should be administered in doses of 1 gram every four hours by the intramuscular or intravenous route, and cefazolin should be given in doses of 0.5 gram every six hours. Cephalosporins should not be used in therapy of pneumococcal meningitis. Erythromycin in doses of 250 mg every six hours by the oral route is also adequate for treatment of patients with a history of penicillin allergy, provided they are not severely ill. Resistance of pneumococci to erythromycin has been reported but is quite rare. Methicillin, cloxacillin, and nafcillin are also effective in the treatment of pneumococcal pneumonia. Tetracyclines should not be used in treating pneumococcal infections unless the organism is known to be susceptible. The prevalence of tetracycline-resistant pneumococci has increased greatly in recent years, now exceeding 5 per cent in many areas of the world. Pneumococci are relatively resistant to gentamicin, and pneumococcal pneumonia has been shown to progress during the administration of this drug.

Supportive Treatment. Patients suffering from pneumococcal pneumonia should be kept at bed rest, and visitors to the sick room should be limited to the immediate family. Pleural pain, if mild, may be treated with codeine sulfate (30 to 60 mg) orally. A tight chest binder may relieve pain but is inadvisable because it inhibits effectiveness of cough. Hypoxemia should be treated with oxygen administered by nasal catheter or by mask. Acetylsalicylic acid should not be used, because it interferes with the utilization of the fever curve to evaluate response to therapy.

FLUID AND ELECTROLYTES. During the acute state of pneumococcal pneumonia, considerable fluid is lost from the body, chiefly through the skin as the result of high fever. Dehydration may develop rapidly and, if severe, may become a contributing factor in the development of shock. Intravenous fluids and electrolytes may be required to control dehydration. When hydration is adequate, the specific gravity of the urine should remain below 1.020. Pneumonia may occasionally lead to the syndrome of inappropriate secretion of antidiuretic hormone.

DIET. Many patients with pneumococcal pneumonia are too ill to tolerate a full diet and should receive only liquids during the height of the fever. Fruit juices, ginger ale, and soups are well tolerated. After the crisis a regular diet may be prescribed.

The patient should be kept in bed until the temperature is approximately normal and should be observed closely until the pneumonic lesion has resolved. As already emphasized, all patients should be subjected to a follow-up roentgenographic examination three to four weeks after recovery.

Treatment of Complications. SHOCK. Patients with peripheral vascular collapse (shock) resulting from severe pneumococcal pneumonia usually respond poorly to the accepted forms of antishock therapy. The prognosis is almost invariably grave when this complication develops. Oxygen therapy should be begun immediately, even if cyanosis is absent. Hemodynamic monitoring should be used as a guide for fluid replacement. The use of corticosteroids has not been demonstrated to be of value.

ABDOMINAL DISTENTION. Decompression is indicated if distention is severe. Acute gastric and ileal dilatation is best managed with the use of gastric suction; a rectal tube may be indicated if colonic distention is a problem.

DELIRIUM TREMENS. Delirium tremens may sometimes be difficult to control in patients with a history of chronic alcoholism. Restraints may be required. The safest sedative to control hyperactivity in these patients is diazepam (Valium) in a dose of 0.066 mg per kilogram every four to six hours.

EMPYEMA AND PERICARDITIS. The treatment of choice for empyema and purulent pericarditis is systemic antimicrobial therapy and surgical drainage. Injection of penicillin into the pleural or pericardial cavity is not required. Repeated needle aspirations are occasionally effective but do not provide effective drainage in most patients.

The treatment of the remaining two major complications of pneumococcal pneumonia, namely endocarditis and meningitis, is discussed in Ch. 131 and 140.

PROGNOSIS. The case fatality rate in untreated pneumococcal pneumonia ranges from 20 to 40 per cent. The widespread use of sulfonamide drugs in the late 1930's resulted in a lowering of the fatality rate among treated patients to approximately 10 per cent. Penicillin therapy has lowered the rate still further. At present approximately 95 per cent of patients with pneumococcal pneumonia recover when properly treated with penicillin.

The prognosis in pneumococcal pneumonia is influenced adversely by each of the following: (1) old age (and also infancy), (2) late treatment, (3) infection with certain types of pneumococci (particularly types 2 and 3), (4) involvement of more than one lobe of the lung, (5) leukopenia, (6) occurrence of bacteremia, (7) capsular polysaccharide detectable in blood by counterimmunoelectrophoresis, (8) jaundice, (9) the presence of complications (notably shock and meningitis), (10) pregnancy (particularly in the third trimester), (11) the presence of other disease such as heart disease or cirrhosis of the liver, and (12) alcoholic intoxication and delirium tremens. Through a consideration of these factors a rough estimate may be made of the severity of the infection in each case, and therapy may be modified accordingly.

Even with the most intensive penicillin treatment, a significant number of patients will die of pneumococcal pneumonia. A recent study, for example, has revealed that in patients destined, at the onset of illness, to die within five days (because of complicating disease, old age, etc.), penicillin therapy has little if any effect. Similarly, the case fatality rate in type 3 pneumococcal pneumonia with bacteremia still exceeds 50 per cent regardless of treatment.

PREVENTION. Because pneumococcal pneumonia is not highly contagious and usually responds promptly to early therapy, prophylaxis constitutes less of a problem than in many other infectious diseases. It is estimated that only one in every 500 persons of all ages in the United States may be expected to contract the disease in any one year.

Although pneumococcal pneumonia can undoubtedly be prevented (or at least aborted) in many patients by the intensive treatment of every upper respiratory tract infection with antimicrobial drugs, their use for this purpose should be avoided. The possible inconvenience to the patient of hypersensitivity reactions and the danger of favoring drug-resistant strains of bacteria outweigh the advantages to be gained in preventing such a relatively uncommon and readily treatable disease as pneumococcal pneumonia. Some authorities do recommend penicillin prophylaxis for children with sickle cell anemia less than three or four years of age whose circulating erythrocytes contain Howell-Jolly bodies as an indicator of splenic hypofunction.

During recent years Austrian has redirected attention to the possibility of specific immunization as a means of preventing pneumococcal infection. During World War II, MacLeod and colleagues showed in controlled experiments in man that pneumococcal polysaccharides are effective antigens, evoking the formation of antibody that persists for years and that confers type-specific immunity to pneumococcal infection. Austrian has proposed immunization of that portion of the population at greatest risk with the types of pneumococci that are most often responsible for disease. Austrian's data, reported in 1972, show that 62 per cent of 2000 cases of pneumococcal bacteremia in adults were caused by six types (1, 3, 4, 7, 8, 12), and that 70 per cent of 100 bacteremias in the pediatric age group were caused by six types (1, 6, 14, 18, 19, 23). Pneumococci of capsular types 6, 14, 19, and 23 are responsible for about 60 per cent of cases of otitis media in children. Since high risk groups can be identified and a large proportion of infections are caused by a few pneumococcal types, commercially available vaccine against those types was introduced in 1978. Vaccination is recommended for those over 2 years of age with a high risk of serious pneumococcal infection, especially patients with asplenia, sickle cell anemia, nephrotic syndrome, chronic cardiopulmonary diseases, or other deficiencies of host resistance. Whether effective immunization of certain groups by polysaccharide vaccines will be followed by an increasing occurrence of infections with other pneumococcal types is unknown but is a definite possibility.

Patient Isolation. The cross-infection rate in pneumococcal pneumonia is low, and patients receiving chemotherapy are probably not highly infectious. Isolation is not indicated in the usual patient.

Applebaum, P. C., et al.: *Streptococcus pneumoniae* responding to penicillin and chloramphenicol. Lancet, 2:995, 1977.

Austrian, R.: Current status of bacterial pneumonia with especial reference to pneumococcal infection. J. Clin. Path. (suppl.), 21:93, 1968.

Austrian, R., and Gold, J.: Pneumococcal bacteremia with especial reference to bacteremic pneumococcal pneumonia. Ann. Intern. Med., 60:759, 1964.

Austrian, R., Howie, V. M., and Ploussard, J. H.: The bacteriology of pneumococcal otitis media. Johns Hopkins Med. J., 141:104, 1977.

Blazevic, D. J., et al.: Penicillin-resistant *Streptococcus pneumoniae* — Minnesota. MMWR, 26: October 21, 1977.

Coonrod, J. D., and Drennan, D. P.: Pneumococcal pneumonia. Capsular polysaccharide antigenemia and antibody response. Ann. Intern. Med., 84:254, 1976.

Coonrod, J. D., and Rytel, M. W.: Detection of type-specific pneumococcal antigens by counterimmunoelectrophoresis. II. Etiologic diagnosis of pneumonia. J. Lab. Clin. Med., 81:778, 1973.

Jay, S. J., Johanson, W. G., Jr., and Pierce, A. K.: The radiographic resolution of *Streptococcus pneumoniae*. N. Engl. J. Med., 293:798, 1975.

Kauffman, C. A., Watanakunakorn, C., and Phair, J. P.: Pneumococcal arthritis. J. Rheumatol., 3:409, 1976.

Kauffman, C. A., Watanakunakorn, C., and Phair, J. P.: Purulent pneumonococcal pericarditis. A continuing problem in the antibiotic era. Am. J. Med., 54:743, 1973.

Lerner, A. M., and Jan Kauskas, K.: The classic bacterial pneumonias. Disease-a-Month, February 1975, pp. 1–46.

Lukems, J. N.: Hemoglobin S, the pneumococcus and the spleen. Am. J. Dis. Child., 123:6, 1972.

Spencer, R. C., and Savage, M. A.: Use of counter and rocket immunoelectrophoresis in acute respiratory infections due to *Streptococcus pneumoniae*. J. Clin. Pathol., 29:187, 1976.

Wood, W. B.: Studies of the Cellular Immunology of Acute Bacterial Infections. The Harvey Lectures, Series 47, 1951–52.

122. PNEUMONIA DUE TO KLEBSIELLA PNEUMONIAE
(Friedländer's Pneumonia)

Herbert Y. Reynolds

Klebsiella may persist in the oropharynx of normal persons, although the prevalence is low, 1 to 6 per cent. There is no tendency for contacts to acquire the organism from a carrier, and it is difficult to implant organisms in the pharynx of healthy volunteers. As is the case with a number of other bacteria, the prevalence of *Klebsiella* in pharyngeal cultures increases (up to 20 per cent) in hospitalized subjects. Pulmonary infections arise most likely from the inhalation or aspiration of organisms from the oropharynx during circumstances in which the major pulmonary antibacterial defense mechanisms are compromised, but the demarcation is often indistinct, as classic primary *Klebsiella* pneumonia occurs in patients with underlying conditions such as alcoholism, chronic obstructive airways disease (emphysema-bronchitis) or diabetes mellitus. Operationally, infections may be considered as primary if *Klebsiella* organisms are isolated from specimens obtained when the patient first seeks medical aid. The designation "secondary" is then applied to those infections that either represent superinfection of an underlying infection or are opportunistic in origin. The present chapter is concerned with the primary pneumonia and hence includes the antimicrobial therapy of *Klebsiella* pulmonary disease. The management of the so-called "secondary" *Klebsiella* bronchopulmonary infections is essentially the same as for any nosocomial pneumonia (see Ch. 124).

In patients with primary pneumonia, males predominate heavily (80 to 90 per cent) and most infections occur in middle-aged and older patients. A common coexisting disease is alcoholism (66 per cent). Both chronic bronchopulmonary disease and, to a lesser extent, diabetes mellitus appear to predispose to *Klebsiella* pneumonia.

PATHOLOGY. The outstanding characteristic of *Klebsiella* pneumonia is its destructiveness; it is a necrotizing pneumonia. In fatal cases lobar involvement most often occurs, but infection may be lobular or may be a combination of both; an upper lobe is most frequently involved. The pleural surface is covered by a fibrinous exudate, and adhesions form early. Empyema is appreciably more frequent than in pneumococcal pneumonia and probably occurs in about one fifth of cases. Microscopically, in the acute stage the alveolar walls are congested. Usually the alveoli are filled with an exudate composed of a mixture of predominantly polymorphonuclear cells. There is abscess formation in association with the necrosis of the alveolar walls. Other findings at autopsy may include extrapulmonary sites of dissemination, e.g., pericarditis or meningitis. Evidence of alcoholic hepatitis and alcoholic cirrhosis is common.

CLINICAL MANIFESTATIONS. The onset is usually sudden (90 per cent), associated with cough productive of sputum (90 per cent), pleuritic chest pain (80 per cent), and true rigors (60 per cent). Early prostration is a usual feature. Occasionally the acute onset is preceded by a nondescript upper respiratory infection and cough. Rarely, epigastric pain and vomiting are the initial symptoms. Typically the sputum is described as a nonputrid homogeneous thick mixture of blood and mucus, often brick red in color. In some patients the sputum is sufficiently thick to be expectorated with difficulty. In others it is thin, resembling currant jelly. Almost always it is either blood tinged or rusty, and frank hemoptysis may occur. On examination, the patient appears acutely ill, febrile, dyspneic, and often cyanotic. Tachycardia is present in proportion to the fever. Chest examination usually reveals signs of pulmonary consolidation. There may be loss of lung volume as manifested by decreased size and expansion of the involved hemithorax and diaphragmatic elevation. Auscultation may reveal suppressed breath sounds with few rales, despite evidence of considerable consolidation. Involvement of more than one lobe is frequent (in two thirds of patients), with a predilection for upper lobes.

LABORATORY AND ROENTGENOGRAPHIC FINDINGS. Peripheral leukocyte counts vary from marked leukopenia to leukocytosis, but leukopenia (and neutropenia) is a poor prognostic sign. In one quarter of patients the total leukocyte count may be in the normal range. On sputum culture, other gram-negative bacilli may be isolated in addition to *Klebsiella*. A mixed sputum flora containing other gram-negative bacilli such as *Pseudomonas spp.* is especially common in secondary infections. A pulmonary source is often incriminated in patients with *Klebsiella* bacteremia. This is unusual, because in other types of gram-negative bacillary bacteremia the urinary tract usually represents the major primary source, followed by the gastrointestinal tract.

The roentgenographic features are variable and include massive lobar consolidation, lobular involvement, lung abscess formation with either multiple small thin-walled or large abscess cavities, and residual parenchymal fibrosis. Bulging of a fissure, sharp advancing borders of the infiltrates, and abscess formation occur with greater frequency than in other types of pneumonia. The pneumonic infiltrate is relatively dense, but shadows of similar density are seen with other types of pneumonia. Bronchopneumonic distribution is less characteristic but can occur, and even bilateral perihilar infiltrates are reported.

COMPLICATIONS. Rapid destruction of pulmonary tissue with suppurative or residual fibrosis occurs in as many as half of the surviving patients. Necrosis may occur within 24 to 48 hours, and abscess formation may be recognized within four days. Other less common pulmonary complications include pleural effusion and pneumothorax. In the past, activation of quiescent pulmonary tuberculosis has been reported. It is believed that some of these cases actually represent a slough of localized tuberculous disease by the necrotizing *Klebsiella* pneumonia.

The course of illness is not marked by frequent extrapulmonary manifestations, but they can occur and include pericarditis, meningitis, gastroenteritis, erythematous skin rashes, and nonsuppurative polyarthritis.

PROGNOSIS AND TREATMENT. In the preantimicrobial era, the case mortality of *Klebsiella* pneumonia ranged from 51 to 97 per cent. The use of antimicrobials has markedly decreased mortality, but in some series the mortality remains nearly 50 per cent. In these series there has been a predominance of severely ill, alcoholic patients, although good results have been reported even in this group. Analysis of the mode of death frequently reveals that inadequate removal of tenacious pulmonary secretions was a significant factor. The correlation of bloodstream invasion and fatality is frequently close.

The majority of strains of *Klebsiella* are susceptible in vitro to chloramphenicol, the cephalosporins, and the aminoglycosides. The antimicrobial regimen of choice varies according to the gravity of the acute clinical situation and the extent of the underlying problem. Because the necrosis of lung tissue can occur so rapidly, it is essential that maximally effective antimicrobial therapy be started immediately. In patients with life-threatening infection, which is at least potentially always the case, a two-drug regimen of cephalothin intravenously and gentamicin intramuscularly is recommended. After several days of such therapy, if the infection is clearly well under control, the cephalothin may be discontinued. Meticulous measures directed at supportive care — maintenance of clear airways, adequate but not excessive ventilation and oxygenation, adequate fluid and electrolyte replacement, and often control of delirium tremens — are essential.

An emerging problem is the developing resistance of *Klebsiella* to gentamicin. In such a clinical situation another aminoglycoside should be chosen, and, if possible, drug-susceptibility studies should be done. Streptomycin, amikacin, and tobramycin are the principal drugs from which a choice must be made.

CHRONIC CAVITARY KLEBSIELLA DISEASE

Occasionally a patient will be seen with a chronic cavitary disease of the lung resulting from infection with *Klebsiella*. In some cases this chronic disease is a known sequel to a primary pneumonia. In other cases, there is no convincing history of such an acute process and the disease appears to have been persisting in subacute or chronic form for many months. Because of the rarity of this form of *Klebsiella* disease, its natural history has not been well characterized. It should be treated initially with the drug-pairing regimen of cephalothin and gentamicin, which can be appropriately modified as improvement occurs. The general treatment should be that for any other lung abscess, including presumably the use of surgical excision in rare cases (see Ch. 347.1).

Bloomfield, A. L.: The fate of bacteria introduced into the upper air passages. V. The Friedländer bacilli. Bull. Johns Hopkins Hosp., 31:203, 1920.

Jervey, L. P., Jr., and Hamburger, M.: The treatment of acute Friedländer's pneumonia. Arch. Intern. Med., 99:1, 1957.

Knight, L., Fraser, R. G., and Robson, H. G.: Massive pulmonary gangrene: A severe complication of Klebsiella pneumonia. Can. Med. Assoc. J., 112:196, 1975.

Manfredi, F., Daly, W. J., and Behnke, R. H.: Clinical observations of acute Friedländer's pneumonia. Ann. Intern. Med., 58:642, 1963.

Pierce, A. K., and Sanford, J. P.: Aerobic gram-negative bacillary pneumonias. Am. Rev. Respir. Dis., 110:647, 1974.

123.   LEGIONNAIRES' DISEASE

Herbert Y. Reynolds

In the late summer of 1976, a mysterious outbreak of severe respiratory illness occurred in Pennsylvania. Initially the disease developed among people who attended a State American Legion convention in Philadelphia at the end of July. Because a microbial agent was not readily identified and mortality initially appeared to be high, the outbreak received wide publicity and evoked concern that a new and virulent infection would become rampant. Public expectation was ripe for a sensational respiratory disease, for this was the year of the abortive swine influenza immunization program for the epidemic that failed to materialize. Later, when an etiologic agent was isolated from lung tissue of legionnaires' disease victims and a fluorescent antibody stain was developed, several interesting findings placed the legionnaires' disease outbreak in better perspective. It became apparent that this disease was not new, nor was the Philadelphia outbreak the first. In fact, based on serial changes in antibody titers, about 0.5 to 1.5 per cent of patients with an etiologically undiagnosed viral-like pneumonia may actually be infected with the legionnaires' agent. However, legionnaires' disease is usually a more serious infection than viral-like pneumonias. The Center for Disease Control estimates that there may be 45,000 cases annually in the United States.

The status of the disease is still in flux, and much is still not understood. Factual data about new outbreaks and recent developments in the drug susceptibilities of the putative bacterium are to be found in the daily newspapers rather than in the medical literature. As yet, the bacterium has not been classified taxonomically.

BACKGROUND. As mentioned, an outbreak of severe epidemic respiratory illness occurred chiefly among conventioneers who attended a State American Legion convention in Philadelphia between July 21 and 24, 1976. The outbreak had all the hallmarks of an infectious disease, with an onset of approximately six to eight days after the affected individual arrived at the convention in the Bellevue-Stratford Hotel. The illness, unfortunately dubbed legionnaires' disease, was not confined to participants in the American Legion convention, but included non-convention-goers as well. In one fatal case categorized as Broad Street pneumonia, the victim had been within a block of the Bellevue-Stratford but had not gone inside the hotel for three weeks prior to the convention. Other cases occurred among people who attended the Catholic Eucharistic convention during the first week in August. In total, 180 cases were recorded in Philadelphia, including 29 deaths.

Preliminary evidence indicated that neither food nor drink could be implicated as sources of the disease agent. Distribution of most cases at the headquarters hotel by room of occupancy showed no unusual pattern of occurrence. Illness in the American Legion conventioneers was associated with time spent in the hotel and clearly related to time spent in the lobby. The only other factor associated with illness was cigarette smoking. The illness was not contagious, and the hotel personnel were unaffected. Inhalation exposure to a list of toxins was entertained, especially to nickel carbonyl because nickel concentrations in lung tissues were found to be elevated. Apparently this cause and effect was not substantiated further. However, the presence of a significant pre-existing illness, such as cardiopulmonary disease, malignancy, or diabetes mellitus, was associated with a 29 per cent case-fatality ratio, compared with a 5 per cent ratio for those without. The actual number of cases of clinical disease was small compared with the several thousand legionnaires and guests who attended the convention and, for that matter, was very small when contrasted with the large number of tourists who visited Philadelphia for the Bicentennial celebration.

Approximately six months later, a presumptive etiologic agent (a gram-negative bacillus) was recovered from infected lung tissue. This bacterium provided an antigen source for an indirect immunofluorescent antibody staining test. With the availability of this assay some interesting developments occurred. First, previous outbreaks of undiagnosed pneumonia were solved. In 1965, 94 cases of unexplained pneumonia had occurred at St. Elizabeth's Hospital, a psychiatric hospital in the District of Columbia. Sixteen deaths occurred. Acute and convalescent sera were available from 14 patients, and 13 showed significant rises in antibody staining titers implicating the legionnaires' bacterium as the infecting agent. An equally baffling outbreak of respiratory illness in Pontiac, Michigan, in 1968 was also found to have been caused by the legionnaires' agent. In 1977, a number of outbreaks occurred, especially in the late summer. Clusters of cases have been found in Columbus, Ohio, Burlington, Vermont, Kingsport, Tennessee and Los Angeles, California; sporadic cases have been widely distributed across the country. In Burlington, Vermont, 32 cases of legionnaires' disease have been identified at this writing; 17 of the cases were fatal. The interesting twist to this outbreak was the development of disease in a number of patients requiring hemodialysis or renal homografting.

Clearly, this type of pneumonia is a nationwide phenomenon. The mortality rate appears to be about 15 to 20 per cent.

ETIOLOGY. The presumptive causative organism was finally isolated about six months after the index cases were discovered from lung tissues of one fatal case of legionnaires' respiratory disease and of one fatal case of "Broad Street pneumonia." Recovery of the microorganism was accomplished by inoculation of guinea pigs intraperitoneally. After a one- to two-day incubation period, the inoculated guinea pigs developed a febrile illness characterized in most animals by watery eyes and prostration. Spleen suspensions from these febrile guinea pigs were inoculated into yolk sacs of embryonated eggs from antibiotic-free chickens. The embryos died after four to six days, and microscopic smears of the yolk sacs (Gimenez stain) revealed pleomorphic gram-negative bacilli. The bacterial-like organisms proved difficult to grow on several artificial culture media but apparently did grow satisfactorily on Mueller-Hinton medium which was supplemented with 1 per cent hemoglobin and 1 per cent bacterial nutrients. Starch, iron, and cysteine seem to be essential ingredients for growth. Colonies could be detected in three to five days after inoculation with infected yolk-sac material or after transfer from other bacterial medium. Because most bacteria when inoculated into the yolk sac kill eggs in one to two days, it was thought that the organism's slow growth might imply that is was an unusual *Rickettsia.* However, the organisms were larger than *Rickettsia,* and they did not react with any standard rickettsial antigens in complement fixation tests. The organism was not acid fast.

The yolk-sac isolate is being called a bacterium on the basis of its size and morphology. The two yolk-sac isolates initially recovered appear similar. Both have been used as antigen in an indirect fluorescent antibody staining test. When both antigen preparations have been assayed with immune serum from selected patients with legionnaires' disease, comparable antibody titers have been found. Thus both yolk-sac isolates appear to be antigenically similar.

Antemortem cultures of respiratory secretions, blood, and lung tissue have not yielded growth of the organisms. However, the bacterium has been cultured from pleural fluid of at least two patients and the diagnosis substantiated. At present, the diagnosis of legionnaires' respiratory disease is usually made from fluorescent antibody staining titers in serum. Seroconversion ($\geq$4-fold titer increase) in paired sera, with one titer at least 1:128, and a typical clinical illness in the absence of an established microbial cause seem to be sufficient criteria for the diagnosis. Antibody titers are being performed by the Center for Disease Control at Atlanta and by a number of state health laboratories, as well. The availability of antibody testing will undoubtedly become more convenient in the near future. Direct fluorescent antibody technique and silver impregnation stains may be used to demonstrate organisms in tissues.

CLINICAL PRESENTATION. Many cases are clearly associated with institutions, including hospitals. Immunosuppressed hosts, particularly those receiving corticosteroids, and debilitated individuals are especially susceptible. The illness begins with headache, malaise, muscle pains, and a slight nonproductive cough; in some patients diarrhea is noted first. This rather mild illness may persist for two or three days, followed by the onset of rigors and high fever. True shaking chills occur, and fever is an impressive finding in most patients (39 to 40.5°C). The fever is usually nonremittent. Relatively slow pulse in relation to fever is common. The cough remains nonproductive or produces mucoid sputum. A chest x-ray can show either a diffuse patchy or scattered infiltrate with evidence of alveolar filling or a more discrete lobar infiltration. The total blood leukocyte count can be elevated to a range of 12,000 to 18,000 per cubic millimeter, with some left shift.

This is the extent and severity of the disease in some patients, and they gradually improve in a week or so, often without specific treatment. Other patients will progress in three to four days to a severe form of pneumonia with evidence of extensive three- to five-lobe infiltration or consolidation and marked obtundation and disorientation. The obtundation and disorientation are out of proportion to the extent of the lung involvement and hypoxia. The chest x-ray lags several days behind the fulminant respiratory and clinical picture. Some patients experience pleuritic chest pain, and hemoptysis

may occur. Shock occurs occasionally and is associated with a grave prognosis. A number of patients develop small pleural effusions; uncompromised patients seem to have larger effusions. As mentioned, cultures of pleural fluid have yielded the organism in several patients. The chest x-ray usually shows extensive air space filling and air bronchograms. However, a peculiar but distinctive x-ray pattern can be found with the disease and consists of the appearance of large fuzzy densities throughout the lung fields which almost have the appearance of widespread pulmonary metastases. Abnormal liver function tests (SGOT, alkaline phosphatase, LDH) are common, as are hyponatremia and hypophosphatemia. Renal function impairment, apparently directly attributable to the disease, may occur occasionally. Several clues which may tip one to the diagnosis of legionnaires' disease are extensive pneumonia without an obvious etiologic agent, predisposed host, nonproductive or mucoid cough, chills, high nonremitting fever, temperature-pulse dissociation, pleuritic chest pain, presence of diarrhea, myalgia, inappropriate obtundation, abnormal liver function tests, hypophosphatemia, failure of response to cephalosporins or gentamicin, and favorable response to erythromycin.

Postmortem examination of the lungs reveals an acute diffuse pattern of alveolar damage. Histopathologic changes include presence of hyaline membranes, regenerating alveolar epithelium, sparse interstitial round cell infiltrate, and intra-alveolar proteinaceous debris. Organisms may be demonstrated within macrophages or polymorphonuclear leukocytes among the intra-alveolar debris. This pattern of injury is nonspecific and may be caused by many infections and toxic agents. Focal bacterial pneumonia is often present, suggesting that a superimposed infection has occurred.

TREATMENT AND PROGNOSIS. Full supportive respiratory care is often required, including supplemental oxygen and mechanical ventilatory support with tracheostomy or endotracheal intubation. Details for pulmonary care will not be reviewed here (see Ch. 351). Prompt antimicrobial therapy is important, and erythromycin, given as 2 to 4 grams per day in divided doses intravenously, seems to be an effective drug. Antimicrobial susceptibility of the legionnaires' disease bacterium was evaluated in protection studies in embryonated hens' eggs and in vitro by agar dilution. Erythromycin was effective. Moreover, erythromycin has proved to be effective treatment in the guinea pig model of the disease. Tetracycline may also be effective. Recent information indicates that rifampin may be an effective drug as well, but its use is not advocated as a single drug regimen.

Chandler, F. W., Hicklin, M. D., and Blackmon, J. A.: Legionnaires' disease: Demonstration of the agent in tissue. N. Engl. J. Med., 297:1218, 1977.

Chen, J. R., Francisco, R. B., and Miller, T. E.: Legionnaires' disease: Nickel levels. Science, 196:906, 1977.

Fraser, D. W., et al.: Legionnaires' disease: Description of an epidemic. N. Engl. J. Med., 297:1189, 1977.

Keys, T. F.: A sporadic case of pneumonia due to legionnaires' disease. Mayo Clin. Proc., 52:657, 1977.

Legionnaires' disease. Lancet, 2:1265, 1977.

McDade, J. E., et al.: Legionnaires' disease: Isolation of a bacterium. N. Engl. J. Med., 297:1197, 1977.

124. PNEUMONIA AND NOSOCOMIAL RESPIRATORY INFECTIONS CAUSED BY AEROBIC GRAM-NEGATIVE BACILLI

(Pseudomonas, Escherichia Coli, and Serratia)

Herbert Y. Reynolds

Bacterial species that belong to the families Enterobacteriaceae and Pseudomonadaceae are considered together because of (1) similarities in the pulmonary infection they produce and (2) common circumstances in which they cause disease. Only a few of the bacteria that are frequently encountered as respiratory pathogens will be discussed individually. Others may be important in special instances, but statistically are less of a problem. Specialized texts on microbial diseases and the periodical literature can supply more detailed information about rare or unusual infections.

The family Enterobacteriaceae is composed of numerous interrelated bacilli, all of which are gram-negative, are nonsporing, grow on ordinary media, and rapidly ferment glucose. The following genera are included in the family: *Shigella, Escherichia, Salmonella, Arizona, Citrobacter, Edwardsiella, Klebsiella, Enterobacter, Serratia, Proteus, Providencia,* and *Erwinia.* The nonfermenting aerobic gram-negative bacilli are recognized with almost equal frequency. Organisms in this category include *Pseudomonas aeruginosa, P. maltophilia, P. pseudomallei, P. cepacia, P. stutzeri, Acinetobacter lwoffi* (previously *Mima polymorpha*), *Acinetobacter anitratus* (previously *Herellea vaginicola* and *Achromobacter anitratus*), *Alcaligenes spp., Achromobacter spp., Flavobacterium spp., Moraxella spp.,* and *Aeromonas hydrophilia.* Infections caused by *Pseudomonas pseudomallei* (melioidosis) are presented in Ch. 159.2.

Pulmonary infections associated with the small aerobic gram-negative bacilli belonging to the genera *Bordetella, Brucella, Hemophilus,* and *Yersinia,* as well as nonsporulating anaerobic gram-negative bacilli, e.g., *Bacteroides* and *Fusobacterium,* are discussed in the individual chapters dealing with each of these infections. Pneumonia caused by *Klebsiella* is the subject of Ch. 122.

Aerobic gram-negative bacilli are frequently the cause of respiratory infection in two groups of patients: those who develop a superinfection or acquire an infection in the hospital (nosocomial) and those who are immunocompromised. Many patients become infected with their endogenous bacterial flora. These clinical conditions are not necessarily distinct, but will be separated for convenience of discussion. For example, primary *Klebsiella* pneumonia (see Ch. 122) may be associated with a number of underlying of perhaps predisposing conditions in the patient, such as alcoholism, chronic obstructive airways disease (emphysema), and diabetes mellitus. By contrast, nosocomial, i.e., hospital-acquired, infections can occur from environmental bacteria or from an organism considered to be part of the normal bacterial flora of the gut or oropharynx.

NOSOCOMIAL PNEUMONIA

Mechanisms and Prevalence

Many common aerobic gram-negative bacteria normally inhabit the human gastrointestinal tract. Moreover, a significant number of healthy, normal people have oropharyngeal colonization with a small number of these bacteria. Certain species such as *Pseudomonas aeruginosa* can be isolated from various skin sites (hands and axillae) in some instances. Since these bacteria are part of the normal microbial flora, they rarely cause primary infection. However, an unwanted byproduct of modern medicine, which can manipulate so many facets of human physiology to salvage and restore health, is the development of iatrogenic and drug-induced infections. The magnitude of this infectious disease problem is large in terms of patient morbidity and mortality, and the financial burden to the health care system. Hospital-acquired infections developed in approximately 3.5 per cent of hospitalized patients (range, 2.6 to 5.8 per cent) reported for 1975–1976 in the National Nosocomial Infections Study of the Center for Disease Control. Urinary tract and surgical wound infections were most common, but lower respiratory tract infections were reported for 21 per cent of the infections of medical patients and 15 per cent of the infections of surgical patients. Perhaps more disturbing than the frequency of respiratory infections is the poor success generally cited for treatment and control. Serious underlying disease is usually present and, despite antimicrobial therapy, the case mortality from nosocomial pneumonia may approach 50 per cent, depending somewhat on the specific causative bacterium and the clinical setting of the patient. The statistics become even worse in patients immunocompromised by acute bone marrow failure and leukemia. In such a group reported from the National Institutes of Health, Bethesda, Maryland, deaths were caused by systemic infections in 46 per cent, in most cases from a gram-negative bacterium and/or fungal species. In the other half of the group, death was attributed to pneumonia caused most frequently by fungal species but closely followed by gram-negative rod bacteria. In the past bacterial deaths accounted for an even higher percentage. The early administration of drug combinations having a broad antibacterial spectrum in febrile, granulocytopenic cancer patients has more effectively controlled some bacterial infections. However, the emergence of drug-resistant strains of *Klebsiella pneumoniae, Pseudomonas aeruginosa,* and others to commonly used aminoglycosides (gentamicin, for example) could alter tremendously the prospects for bacterial control. Superinfection of the respiratory tract with fungi (*Aspergillus* frequently) and other opportunistic organisms (*Pneumocystis carinii*) continues to gain in importance at a time when gram-negative bacterial ones seem to be coming under better control. The therapy for fungal and other opportunistic infections is not usually started as promptly as is the rule for bacterial infections because of the persistent difficulty in obtaining an early and reliable diagnosis. Invasive procedures to obtain lung tissue for a histologic diagnosis are sometimes necessary, thus adding to the delay in instituting appropriate therapy.

Predisposing Factors

Conditions which lead to nosocomial pneumonia are well defined and are usually obvious. Susceptible patients invariably have one or a combination of the following: (1) chronic debilitating illness often requiring prolonged hospitalization; (2) prior therapy with antimicrobial drugs having a broad spectrum; (3) a breach of the airway by tracheostomy or endotracheal tube; and (4) impaired host immunity (cellular and/or humoral) owing to a primary disease or as a consequence of immunosuppressive therapy.

The hospital environment itself has been implicated as a prime source of opportunistic microorganisms, and to some extent it is. Certainly it is a good repository for some hardy drug-resistant strains; but this may vary, as with staphylococci, which may exhibit more drug resistance among community strains than hospital-associated ones. In this context, however, it is well to remember the point emphasized by Feingold (1970) that *hospitalization itself does not predispose the patient to infection; rather, the hospitalized patient is often an altered host with enhanced susceptibility to infection because of either the disease or the therapy.* For this reason the term "nosocomial," strictly defined as an infection originating in a hospital or as one which is not clinically evident or incubating at the time of hospital admission, does not differentiate the etiology and site of infection or the circumstances inducing it. Other descriptions such as iatrogenic or autogenic infection and superinfection are often more appropriate. Thus it is important to remember that these infections may not be acquired from the hospital environment or hospital personnel but may arise from the indigenous microbial flora of the patient.

Hospitalization per se is associated with some striking changes in patterns of bacterial colonization of the respiratory tract which seem significant. As mentioned, the isolation of a variety of potentially pathologic species of gram-negative rods from the oropharynx occurs in a significant percentage (18 per cent) of normal people. Other studies (Johanson et al., 1969, 1972) have reported a lower incidence of gram-negative rod recovery (2 to 12 per cent), but these did not utilize a broth culture medium, which seems to facilitate bacterial recovery. Generally the oropharynx of a normal person is not a very suitable environment for growth of aerobic gram-negative bacteria. Yet colonization developed rapidly in patients admitted to a medical intensive care unit and occurred in about 40 per cent of them within four days of admission to the unit. Such colonization of the respiratory tract apparently plays a major role in the pathogenesis of nosocomial respiratory infections. In the study by Johanson, Pierce, and Sanford, 22 of 95 patients (23 per cent) who were colonized with gram-negative bacilli developed respiratory infections with these bacteria. By comparison, only 4 of 118 patients (3.3 per cent) who were never colonized with these bacteria developed infections. There is additional evidence that susceptibility to oropharyngeal colonization of the hospitalized patient with gram-negative bacilli is related to the severity of the primary underlying disease and is therefore greatest in the moribund subject. The

precise mechanism for such colonization in the chronically or severely ill patient is unknown, but undoubtedly it is related to altered upper airway clearance mechanisms to be discussed. It is noteworthy that when pharyngeal and sputum cultures become positive for Enterobacteriaceae or Pseudomonadaceae and other pathogenic bacteria, it is likely that the respiratory tract is also colonized with these microorganisms. Such a pattern should alert one to impending respiratory infection. New techniques to assess adherence of bacteria to the patient's in vitro cultured buccal mucosa cells may prove important in selecting patients who are more susceptible to bacterial colonization. Consequently, such susceptible persons might profit from prophylactic use of a tropical antimicrobial drug in the oropharynx to prevent colonization with potential pathogens. The future will decide the usefulness of this approach.

The importance of prior antimicrobial therapy as a determinant of oropharyngeal colonization with gram-negative bacilli is not as obvious as might be expected. Several of the cited studies which recorded development of colonization in hospitalized patients failed to find strong evidence that prior or concomitant antimicrobial use was a requisite factor, although such therapy did indeed increase the occurrence of colonization (Pierce and Sanford). On the contrary, in principle, broad-spectrum antimicrobial therapy that reduces a proportion of the normal bacterial flora of the gastrointestinal tract and naso-oropharyngeal area should improve the opportunity for more drug-resistant strains to emerge. Perhaps of greater significance nowadays is the emergence of fungal strains in the wake of a bacterial void so that colonization with these opportunistic organisms presages respiratory infection.

An interruption in the continuity of the airway with a tracheostomy, for example, is often associated with bacterial colonization of the tracheobronchial tree and with recurrent respiratory infections. Obviously, important mechanical barriers which guard entry into the lungs are bypassed and microorganisms have direct access. The situation is compounded if ventilatory equipment is attached which may itself contain a source of bacteria and, in fact, forcefully aerosolize them into the airways. In the time since it was demonstrated that contaminated inhalation respiratory equipment could be the source of nosocomial pneumonia, significant improvement has occurred in the general care and handling of this equipment in many respiratory therapy programs, with the pleasing result that this form of iatrogenic infection is less frequent.

The immunocompromised patient presents a complex array of disordered host defenses, and the lungs are but one organ system at risk for infection. Predisposition to pneumonia with gram-negative bacilli occurs because a number of cellular components in the respiratory tract are either vulnerable to the direct effects of various antineoplastic chemotherapy drugs and anti-inflammatory agents, or may have been depleted because renewal from the bone marrow, for example, is inadequate. (See Ch. 41 and 527.)

Granulocytopenia is the most common abnormality in patients who have ineffective granulocytopoiesis or are receiving cytotoxic chemotherapy. This results from an inadequate systemic supply of circulating phagocytic cells; subsequently, a lack of reserve or marginated granulocytes develops in capillary storage areas. The lung capillary vasculature is but one such involved site.

The effect is to deplete the lower respiratory tract of secondary phagocytes that can be attracted to alveolar areas and to diminish the cellular inflammatory response.

Available evidence indicates that bone marrow–derived circulating monocytes are the precursors of tissue macrophages in the lungs. After the monocyte enters the pulmonary lymphoreticular system, it undergoes further development into a mature phagocytic macrophage which has a life span of several months. Alveolar macrophages obtained by lung lavage from leukemia patients who have been leukopenic (monocytopenic) for several months are functionally and morphologically normal, despite intensive chemotherapy. Such findings indicate longevity of alveolar macrophages. Moreover, some human pulmonary macrophages are capable of a slow rate of replication, which suggests that the number of lung macrophages can be maintained in part by local cell proliferation when the usual influx of cells from peripheral blood and from bone marrow is absent. Although it is difficult to demonstrate that alveolar macrophages are readily depleted in immunosuppressed subjects, in contrast to short-lived polymorphonuclear granulocytes, it is probable that subtle metabolic effects from cytotoxic drugs impair the phagocytic and bactericidal capacity of lung macrophages. This would help account for the greater susceptibility to respiratory infections in these patients. For example, it has been demonstrated that corticosteroids, experimentally, impair the release of lysosomal enzymes from macrophages and granulocytes, impede the migration of cells into inflammatory sites, diminish phagocytosis by macrophages, block the response of macrophages to migration inhibition factor produced by immune lymphocytes, and interfere with granulocyte chemotaxis (Fauci et al., 1974, 1976).

Lymphoid tissue is extensive along the airways, and its alteration could directly affect the lung's handling of antigenic substances contained in respired air. Cell-mediated immune responses could be blunted, and development might be impaired of immunoglobulin-producing lymphocytes and plasma cells which secrete local secretory antibodies onto respiratory mucosal surfaces. However, assessment of the integrity of lymphoid tissue in the lungs of normal people or the immunosuppressed is difficult, because suitable methods are lacking. Customary techniques such as skin testing or antigenic stimulation of peripheral blood lymphocytes are not necessarily representative of immunologic events occurring in vivo in lung tissue. Thus the demonstration of abnormal lymphocyte function in the respiratory tract remains a theoretic consideration. Yet certain populations of lymphocytes are sensitive to radiotherapy (T cells) and may be eliminated when various forms of irradiation therapy are given. Cytotoxic drugs such as cyclophosphamide have various effects on both major subpopulations of lymphocytes (B and T cells).

The consequence of injury to other cell-types in the lung, such as surfactant-secreting Type II alveolar epithelial cells, various mucus-producing cells, and ciliated epithelial cells, are largely conjectural, because the deleterious effects of immunosuppressive agents on these cell-types have not been established. Yet it seems plausible that drastic regimens of immunosuppressive therapy may impair the function of these cells. The cumulative effects of diminished surfactant production promoting lung atelectasis, altered mucus secretion, and reduced ciliary clearance all could contribute to stasis and accumulation of lung secretions which promote local bacterial growth and subsequent pneumonia.

Possible Future Management of Nosocomial Pneumonia

What is the future of therapy in the immunocompromised host? Without question, the cornerstone of the medical treatment for bacterial respiratory infections is antimicrobial therapy. This is likely to remain the situation in the forseeable future, and other forms of therapy will be at best adjuncts. Although the antimicrobial drugs have provided splendid therapy for many infections, the increasing prevalence of many bacteria resistant to them necessitates constant re-evaluation of drug dosages and drug combinations and the continual development of new antimicrobial agents.

As mentioned, granulocytopenia is usually present when an immunosuppressed patient develops a serious bacterial infection. The absence of granulocytes may allow bacteria to become established in lung tissue. Moreover, should bacteremia develop, death of the patient from sepsis can occur quickly. Logically, the replacement of these phagocytic cells by transfusion is a reasonable mode of therapy. A number of clinical trials using granulocyte transfusions show the usefulness of this therapy for certain patients with bacteremia. The rationale is to prevent or contain the infection with chemotherapy and granulocyte transfusion support until there is a return of indigenous bone marrow function and circulating granulocytes. Whether such therapy would prove useful in specific organ infections such as pneumonia remains to be determined.

Alveolar macrophages are not depleted in immunosuppressed patients, despite many weeks of peripheral blood leukopenia and monocytopenia which would be expected to remove precursor cells. Although lung macrophages may undergo some local cellular replication in the immunosuppressed patient, this is judged to be insufficient to maintain the quota of lung phagocytes. Despite the longevity of the macrophage, the high incidence of pulmonary infections in the immunosuppressed patient suggests that it does not function well. Conceivably the situation might be ameliorated by a stimulus such as BCG and perhaps someday by infusion of purely monocytic preparations into leukemic hosts.

The delivery of a specific antibody is generally agreed to be desirable for an immunocompromised patient. The appropriate way to give such therapy is not established and reflects persisting inadequacies in antibody technology. Questions remain about the best route of immunization, the appropriate antigens to use, and the level or quantity of circulating antibody which is protective. In the immunodeficient host, active primary or booster immunization does not reliably provide high or lasting antibody titers, and a supplemental form of passive immunization is usually necessary. Yet loss of body tissue mass from cachexia and/or thrombocytopenia limits the use of parenteral gamma globulin, making intravenous preparations in the form of hyperimmune plasma desirable. The class of immunoglobulin antibody delivered is also important. IgG would appear to be the preferable form of opsonic antibody for established lower lung infections, whereas secretory IgA agglutinating antibody might be preferable to prevent bacterial adherence and colonization in the upper respiratory tract. Currently available parenteral gamma globulin preparations and plasma will both supply IgG antibody adequately, but neither contains a suitable form of IgA (see Ch. 40.8).

Perhaps the most critical decision is selection of the appropriate antigen for immunization of the patient or the donor. In the case of pneumococcal prophylaxis, a multivalent polysaccharide vaccine containing antigens to a limited number of common clinical strains is now available (see Ch. 121). For the gram-negative bacteria, which so frequently cause pulmonary infections in immunosuppressed hosts, the selection of appropriate antigens is not so evident. The variety of infecting strains of Enterobacteriaceae is so large that a comprehensive vaccine, including even the most commonly incriminated strains, is impractical. The alternative approach is to select an antigen which will elicit an antibody that is broadly reactive with many strains and will offer protection against a large number of similar infecting bacteria. In fact, this solution has been achieved experimentally (McCabe; Young et al.) A similar approach has been taken for *Pseudomonas*. Immunization with a J_5 mutant (^{R}c glycolipid antigen) of *Escherichia coli* 0:111 induces antibody that protects against *P. aeruginosa* and Enterobacteriaceae organisms. The protein moiety of the endotoxin (OEP) from *P. aeruginosa* has been used for experimental immunization; it affords protection from *P. aeruginosa* infection regardless of the serotype of the organisms. Thus the most important factor in devising practical immunization for the immunodeficient host — the proper selection of antigens that evoke cross-reactive antibodies — is being addressed and should improve the prospects for antibody immunoprophylaxis.

PNEUMONIA CAUSED BY PSEUDOMONAS

Pseudomonas, which is a distinct genus of bacteria and is not included in the family Enterobacteriaceae, is widespread in the environment and is generally part of the usual bacterial flora of hospitals and intensive care units. *Pseudomonas* organisms are frequently carried on the skin (axillary and anogenital areas) of normal people and transiently may be part of the intestinal flora in a significant number (up to 20 per cent). Almost any alteration in normal health status, such as hospitalization or antimicrobial or immunosuppressive therapy, is associated with increased carriage of *Pseudomonas* organisms. People with cystic fibrosis usually have persistent colonization of their respiratory tract with these bacteria.

For this discussion, *Pseudomonas* respiratory infection refers to those caused by *Pseudomonas aeruginosa*, which is the most important pathogen of the genus. The reader should remember, however, that other *Pseudomonas* species can cause serious infections (*P. pseudomallei* [melioidosis] and *P. mallei* [glanders]). Moreover, other less frequently encountered species are being implicated in human infection. *P. cepacia* has the distinction of being the only one in this group of clinical pathogens that is generally not susceptible to gentamicin, hence making drug-susceptibility testing necessary for proper drug selection.

PREDISPOSING FACTORS. *Pseudomonas* rarely produces infection in a normal person but is a frequent cause of sepsis and pneumonia in the abnormal host. Currently it is the second most frequent organism isolated from patients with nosocomial pneumonia (*Klebsiella* now has assumed first place in many recent series). In the past, chronic lung or heart disease was an associated condition that apparently increased susceptibility to *Pseudomonas* pneumonia; now the presence of leukopenia (granulocytopenia) and other evidence of immunosuppressive disease or treatment is more common. *Pseudomonas* infection is likely to be an acquired or secondary pneumonia following any one of the predisposing causes already outlined. As a form of primary pneumonia, it is essentially limited to patients who are receiving inhalation therapy that incorporates reservoir nebulization. Following *Pseudomonas* bacteremia, pulmonary complications are well described, consisting of nodular areas of lung infarction with massive bacterial infiltration of arterial and venous walls. Such bacteremia produces a form of necrotizing pneumonia. This presentation may occur in illicit intravenous drug users who develop *Pseudomonas* tricuspid endocarditis.

PATHOLOGY. On microscopic section, the intra-alveolar inflammatory exudate is a mixture of polymorphonuclear leukocytic and mononuclear cells, or the cellular infiltrates may consist predominantly of mononuclear cells admixed with fragmented pyknotic nuclei of necrotic neutrophils. At a later stage, alveolar spaces are filled with a deeply basophilic granular material containing large macrophage-like cells and dense colonies of gram-negative bacilli. In the areas of an abscess there is often focal hemorrhage. The dominant microscopic lesion is that of alveolar septal necrosis. In association with these necrotizing lesions, necrosis of arterial walls and secondary thrombosis of vessels have been encountered when the *Pseudomonas* pneumonia is of bacteremic origin or associated with nebulizing therapy equipment. In primary *Pseudomonas* pneumonia, as reported by Tillotson and Lerner (1968), the vascular involvement is not a feature. *Pseudomonas cepacia* is also associated with a necrotizing granulomatous pneumonia.

CLINICAL FEATURES AND COURSE. In patients with *Pseudomonas* pneumonia, apprehension, toxicity, confusion, and progressive cyanosis are characteristic; hemoptysis is unusual. Relative bradycardia may occur. Alteration in diurnal temperature patterns, with the peak temperature in early morning, was noted by Tillotson and Lerner. The physical signs over the thorax are not characteristic. The development of empyema is common (30 to 50 per cent). Roentgenograms reveal bilateral pneumonic infiltrates, usually in the lower lobe, that are often nodular and may undergo necrosis with abscesses that may be small but are often greater than 1 cm is diameter. A pattern of interstitial infiltration may be seen. With resolution of pneumonia, areas of lung with poor expansion and residual "scarring" may be noted on follow-up chest films.

LABORATORY FINDINGS. The usual laboratory tests such as leukocyte counts are of little help, being either normal or moderately increased and often reflecting the bone marrow status of an underlying disease. Cultures of sputum are of only moderate help, because *Pseudomonas* organisms are frequently present as commensals in patients who are receiving antimicrobial therapy or in those who are critically ill. In the relatively rare situations in which it becomes necessary to establish with certainty the organism involved, specimens could be collected by the transtracheal technique. With empyema, thoracentesis with staining and culture of the fluid will help confirm the diagnosis and facilitate the selection of optimal therapy.

PROGNOSIS AND TREATMENT. Prognosis varies with the underlying condition of the patient. Case mortality rates in the range of 80 per cent are not uncommon with *Pseudomonas* pneumonia, especially if bacteremia develops. However, in recent years, the mortality seems to be distinctly less and appears to be about 35 per cent. Several important things have occurred. First, better antimicrobial drugs are available. The use of an aminoglycoside, gentamicin, and carbenicillin in combination for *Pseudomonas aeruginosa* infections has had a dramatic impact. (It should be remembered, however, that the gentamicin can be inactivated by carbenicillin when the two remain long in the same solution [see Ch. 190].) Second, medical personnel are much more aware of their role in the transmission of this ubiquitous microorganism, and appropriate changes in patient care techniques have been made. Third, meticulous cleanliness of respiratory ventilation equipment and use of disposable endotracheal or tracheostomy suctioning devices are routine. Sadly, however, microbial resistance to one or both of these mainstay antibiotics is now seen on occasion. In 1976, two other aminoglycosides became available, tobramycin and amikacin. Both are effective against many gentamicin-resistant *P. aeruginosa*. Tobramycin appears to be the drug of choice for nonresistant strains of this organism. Undoubtedly, it will be necessary to have additional antimicrobials in the future to keep ahead of the adaptable *Pseudomonas* strains.

Clinical experience and experimental results in leukopenic animal models indicate that a single aminoglycoside (i.e., gentamicin) is usually insufficient to eradicate and cure an extensive *Pseudomonas* pneumonia. Tobramycin appears no better in this situation and probably offers a measurable advantage only when a gentamicin-resistant organism is the cause. The two drugs give slightly different degrees of oto- or nephrotoxicity and other side effects which may dictate the choice of drugs in some patients. The combined use of an aminoglycoside and carbenicillin does offer an improvement in therapy and outcome. Carbenicillin, which seems an especially effective drug in leukopenic patients, should not, however, be relied upon as a single drug, because drug resistance may develop quickly in this setting. Other forms of supportive care are very essential also. Because *Pseudomonas* organisms are difficult to clear from infected lung tissue, patients will frequently relapse after drug therapy is discontinued, despite what is considered an adequate course of therapy. Re-treatment is usually necessary and should be done in conjunction with drug-susceptibility testing of the bacterium to confirm appropriate drug selection. With successful treatment, *Pseudomonas* may still reappear in the sputum, making it necessary to distinguish between relapse and persistent colonization of the respiratory tract. Changing lung infiltrates and clinical signs help to separate the two. As discussed above, current experimental work might lead to other therapies in practical form, such as passive antibody administration of anti-*Pseudomonas* gamma globulin or prophylactic immunization of high-risk patients with *Pseudomonas* lipopolysaccharide antigens. Granulocyte transfusion therapy in appropriate patients could be considered a reasonable possibility at present and does offer hope for improving current therapy.

PNEUMONIA DUE TO OTHER AEROBIC GRAM-NEGATIVE BACILLI
(E. Coli, Serratia Marcescens, and Proteus sp.)

The large number of bacterial species other than *Klebsiella pneumoniae* that belong to the families Enterobacteriaceae and Achromobacteraceae may produce pulmonary infection. In addition, in many hospitals other gram-negative organisms such as *Serratia marcescens* are being encountered, especially in hospital-associated secondary pneumonia.

Primary *E. coli* pneumonia tends to be present as a scattered pneumonic process in the lower lobes. The pulse is proportional to the temperature. Early findings include rales without consolidation. Empyema formation is less common than with *Klebsiella* or *Pseudomonas*. *E. coli* bacteremia from a urinary source more commonly results in lung infection than does that from other gram-negative bacilli.

Proteus species also produce a clinical picture similar to that of *Klebsiella* (see Ch. 122), with fever, chills, dyspnea, pleuritic chest pain, and cough productive of purulent sputum. Signs of consolidation are usual. Roentgenograms reveal dense infiltrates in the posterior segment of an upper lobe or superior segment of the right lower lobe. Progression to lung abscess or empyema is common.

Serratia infections, which are always secondary, have been associated with the clinical oddity "pseudohemoptysis" owing to a red pigment produced by some strains of *Serratia marcescens*. Other features may include abscess formation, empyema, or both.

Clinical experience with the other bacterial genera such as *Flavobacterium* and *Acinetobacter* is limited, but suggests that their clinical manifestations are similar to those of secondary *Klebsiella* infections.

The antimicrobial regimen of choice may be selected according to the physician's knowledge of the epidemiologic pattern of drug resistance to be anticipated in a given community, but should be confirmed, when possible, by tests on an individual patient's organism.

Brachman, P. S.: Nosocomial respiratory infections. Prev. Med., 3:500, 1974.

Gilardi, G. L.: Infrequently encountered *Pseudomonas* species causing infection in humans. Ann. Intern. Med., 77:211, 1972.

Johanson, W. G., Pierce, A. K., and Sanford, J. P.: Changing pharyngeal bacterial flora of the hospitalized patients. N. Engl. J. Med., 281:1137, 1969.

Johanson, W. G., Pierce, A. K., Sanford, J. P., and Thomas, G. D.: Nosocomial respiratory infections with gram-negative bacilli: The significance of colonization of the respiratory tract. Ann. Intern. Med., 77:701, 1972.

McCabe, W. R.: Immunization with R mutant of *S. minnesota*. I. Protection against challenge with heterologous gram-negative bacilli. J. Immunol., 108:601, 1972.

National Nosocomial Infections Study — United States, 1975–76. MMWR, Vol. 26, No. 46, November 18, 1977.

Pennington, J. W., Reynolds, H. Y., Wood, R. E., Robinson, R. B., and Levine, A. S.: Use of *Pseudomonas aeruginosa* vaccine in patients with acute leukemia and cystic fibrosis. Am. J. Med., 58:629, 1975.

Pierce, A. K., and Sanford, J. P.: Aerobic gram-negative bacillary pneumonias: State of the art. Am. Rev. Respir. Dis., 110:647, 1974.

Reynolds, H. Y.: Prevention and future control of hospital-associated infections commonly caused by gram-negative bacteria. Prev. Med., 3:507, 1974.

Reynolds, H. Y., Levine, A. S., Wood, R. E., Zierdt, C. H., Dale, D. C., and Pennington, J. E.: *Pseudomonas aeruginosa* infections: Persisting problems and current research to find new therapies. Ann. Intern. Med., 82:819, 1975.

Rosenthal, S., and Tager, I. B.: Prevalence of gram-negative rods in the normal pharyngeal flora. Ann. Intern. Med., 83:355, 1975.

Westwood, J. C. N., Legace, S., and Mitchell, M. D.: Hospital acquired infection: Present and future impact and need for positive action. Can. Med. Assoc. J., 110:769, 1974.

Williams, D. M., Krick, J. A., and Remington, J. S.: Pulmonary infection in the compromised host. Part 1. Am. Rev. Respir. Dis., 114:359, 1976.

Young, L. S., Stevens, P., and Ingram, J.: Functional role of antibody against "core" glycolipid of Enterobacteriaceae. J. Clin. Invest., 56:850, 1975.

STREPTOCOCCAL DISEASES

125. INTRODUCTION

Gene H. Stollerman

Streptococci constitute a large heterogeneous group of gram-positive bacteria that are very common parasites of man. Their name derives from their growth in liquid media as chains of globular bacteria. Classification of streptococci has been confusing, because a single species may cause a variety of diseases and because several kinds of streptococci can often be cultured from the same site of infection.

CLASSIFICATION

The modern classification of streptococci is based upon Lancefield's identification of the group-specific cell wall "C" carbohydrate antigens which are present in beta-hemolytic streptococci and in some nonhemolytic species as well.

GROUP A INFECTIONS. The most important human streptococcal pathogen, *Streptococcus pyogenes,* can be identified as containing group A carbohydrate with specific rabbit antiserum to the carbohydrate cell wall antigens, and thus can be distinguished from other beta-hemolytic streptococci which are also frequently isolated from the respiratory tract of man. Diseases caused by group A streptococci will be considered in detail in Ch. 126 to 130 and in Ch. 374.3. Streptococci belonging to other serogroups that are of importance to man will be mentioned briefly here.

The traditional classification of streptococci by their properties of hemolysis on the surface of blood agar plates is clinically useful. It helps to distinguish hemolytic streptococci, to which the more virulent species belong, from the alpha-hemolytic viridans streptococci ("green" streptococci), the predominant normal flora of the upper respiratory tract, and the nonhemolytic streptococci which include the enterococci, a common inhabitant of the gastrointestinal tract.

Beta-hemolytic streptococci are those that produce a completely clear zone around the colony as a result of the formation of either extracellular hemolysin, streptolysin O and streptolysin S, or both. Classification of streptococci based on the type of hemolysis they produce, however, is unsatisfactory for many reasons. Many species belonging to specific serologic groups may be nonhemolytic, such as group D. On the other hand, some enterococci belonging to the usually nonhemolytic group D may produce beta hemolysis, or some apparently nonhemolytic colonies may become alpha hemolytic upon prolonged incubation. Beta hemolysis is therefore primarily useful in the first step of the identification of group A organisms which are, with only rare exceptions, consistently hemolytic.

GROUP B INFECTIONS. The group B organisms are classically represented by the species *Streptococcus agalactiae*. They were well known for many years as the cause of bovine mastitis but produced human disease rarely. Until recently, little attention was paid to group B organisms in man, although it was known that they could colonize the vagina and genitourinary tract and were occasionally found in the upper respiratory tract as well. In fact, between 5 and 10 per cent of hemolytic streptococci isolated from man were identified in many studies as group B. In the past two decades, however, group B streptococci have been reported with increasing frequency as a cause of perinatal infections. In the preantimicrobial era, group A streptococci were the common agent of puerperal fever. Since the early 1960's, however, group B streptococci have emerged as a major cause of puerperal infection and as a cause of neonatal sepsis, with or without meningitis. These organisms have been subdivided into five serotypes — Ia, Ib, Ic, II, and III — based on their polysaccharide capsular antigens and minor protein determinants. Types Ia and III are the strains most often isolated from septic infants in the first week of life, and type III is predominantly associated with meningitis. Transplacentally acquired opsonic antibodies appear to be important as a mechanism of neonatal host defense, and considerable interest now exists in the possibility of immunizing against what is currently the most common serious neonatal bacterial infection in the United States.

The frequency with which group B streptococci are recovered from the female genital tract (and the male genitourinary tract as well) appears to be increasing, and cervicovaginal carrier rates in normal pregnant women vary from 3 to 6 per cent. In some studies, approximately one third of infants born to such carriers have contracted serious group B infections. Group B organisms also seem to be causing bacteremic complications of pyelonephritis in both men and women more often than heretofore, especially in diabetics and other compromised hosts. These infections have remained susceptible to penicillin so far.

GROUP D INFECTIONS. This group includes *Streptococcus faecalis,* often referred to as enterococcus because of the frequency with which it is found in the human gastrointestinal tract. Enterococci may also be cultured from the oropharynx and, although usually nonhemolytic, some strains can produce beta or alpha hemolysis.

S. faecalis is an exceptionally hardy organism which can resist heat (62° C for 30 minutes), grow well at room temperature, multiply in hypertonic media (6.5 per cent sodium chloride), and grow in the presence of 0.05 per cent sodium azide.

Enterococci are often isolated from the blood in bacterial endocarditis and from the urine in urinary tract obstruction. The precise role of these organisms in the pathogenesis of pyelonephritis has not been fully evaluated. They can be associated with suppurative abdominal lesions, especially after bowel surgery.

The failure of some laboratories to distinguish the enterococci from other streptococci often leads to inappropriate therapy in serious infections. These organisms may also be recovered from the respiratory tract and may be regarded mistakenly as penicillin-resistant group A streptococci. This error occurs most often during the post-treatment follow-up study of cases of group A streptococcal sore throat and may lead to needless overtreatment in an attempt to eradicate the organisms from the pharynx. Enterococci do *not* cause pharyngitis and tonsillitis.

STREPTOCOCCI OF OTHER GROUPS. Strains of groups C, E, G, H, K, and O are isolated from the respiratory tract of man but are of little clinical significance. "Human" group C strains may occasionally cause illnesses that resemble those of group A, but such infections are relatively rare. Moreover, as far as is known, only group A organisms cause rheumatic fever. Group G may occasionally cause mild infections, but these are relatively infrequent and are uncomplicated. Groups A, C, and G all elaborate in vivo antigenically similar streptolysin O, streptokinase, hyaluronidase, and erythrogenic toxin.

ALPHA-HEMOLYTIC STREPTOCOCCI ("GREEN" STREPTO-COCCI). The alpha-hemolytic streptococci are often referred to collectively as the *viridans group*. They have never been satisfactorily classified. Their colonies are surrounded by a narrow zone of incompletely hemolyzed red cells (some red cells are spared for unknown reasons). Green discoloration of the colonies occurs owing to the formation of an unidentified reductant of hemoglobin. The degree of "greening" varies with the animal source of blood and is best brought out by sheep red blood cells which differentiate most clearly beta from alpha hemolysis.

Viridans streptococci make up the predominant normal flora of the upper respiratory tract and are generally nonpathogenic except as a cause of subacute bacterial endocarditis. *Streptococcus salivarius* is one of the most commonly encountered of these species. The importance of the streptococci that colonize the oral cavity in the pathogenesis of caries is now well recognized. Species in saliva, such as *Streptococcus mutans, sanguis,* and *mitis,* have remarkable affinity for the enamel of teeth. When the diet is rich in sucrose, the bacteria produce particular long chain polysaccharides which stick to enamel. The formation of lactic acid by the adherent bacteria dissolves enamel and thus causes caries. Bacterial adherence of this kind seems to be due to surface substances with specific affinities for host cell membranes (see Ch. 126). Variations in host susceptibility to caries may be related to factors in saliva and in diet that affect bacterial adherence.

The term *nonhemolytic Streptococcus* is confusing because it is often used to include any *Streptococcus* that is not beta hemolytic, and because many nonhemolytic species (including the common *Streptococcus faecalis*) possess the same group specific cell wall antigens as certain hemolytic strains. The organisms of the nonhemolytic group are generally of low pathogenicity for man and, like alpha-hemolytic streptococci, are of concern to physicians primarily as causative agents of subacute bacterial endocarditis. They may multiply and cause inflammation in traumatized or diseased structures and wounds and in obstructed sinuses, bronchi, and urinary and biliary tracts.

ANAEROBIC STREPTOCOCCI. The varieties of streptococci considered above are facultative anaerobes. Microaerophilic streptococci which are *obligate* anaerobes do exist, however, and cause human disease. They are usually nonhemolytic and have not been systematically classified. One of the most ubiquitous genera of these is the *Peptostreptococcus,* a major component of the anaerobic intestinal flora. These organisms are found in the mouth, bowel, and female genital tract. Their virulence is low and they tend to multiply in necrotic or frankly gangrenous lesions, producing a foul odor such as may be noted in lung abscesses or intra-abdominal or intrauterine infections. They may cause very extensive necrotizing wound infections. Although most anaerobic streptococci are susceptible to antimicrobial drugs, usually penicillin, the lesions in which they are found often require adequate surgical drainage as well as chemotherapy. Peritonsillar, brain, lung, liver, and intra-abdominal abscesses resulting from mixed anaerobic bacterial infections may contain peptostreptococci. *Peptostreptococcus* is also involved in the pathogenesis of necrotizing fasciitis, producing, in synergy with aerobic streptococci or staphylococci, a fulminant, often fatal wound infection (Meleney's synergistic gangrene).

126. GROUP A STREPTOCOCCAL INFECTION

Gene H. Stollerman

HISTORY. Many of the clinical syndromes caused by group A streptococcal infection were recognized for many years before the discovery of *Streptococcus pyogenes* by Rosenbach in 1884. Thus Sydenham is often stated to have described scarlet fever, but the early accounts are inadequate and inexact. Certainly clinical recognition of scarlet fever, of tonsillitis and pharyngitis without a skin rash, of erysipelas, and of puerperal sepsis date back for many centuries before the modern era of bacteriology. Significant understanding of streptococcal infections, however, began with the discovery by Schottmüller, in 1903, that certain strains produce hemolysis on blood agar. Brown, in 1919, defined this reaction in greater detail and coined the descriptive terms that are still in use.

The streptococcal cause of scarlet fever and tonsillitis was known by 1895. The more modern work of the Dicks and of Dochez (1925) resolved the temporary issues raised concerning the possible role of other pharyngeal bacteria in scarlet fever, and Bloomfield clearly defined the streptococcal etiology of most cases of tonsillitis. The serologic classification of the organism into groups by Lancefield and into types by Lancefield and Griffith by 1935 and the introduction of the antistreptolysin O titer by Todd (1932) to identify streptococcal infection immunologically led to the modern era of the clinical bacteriology, immunology, and epidemiology of streptococcal infections and their nonsuppurative sequels, acute rheumatic fever (ARF) and acute glomerulonephritis (AGN).

The great epidemics of streptococcal disease in the armed forces in World War II supplied an enormous volume of clinical material for the clearer definition of the epidemiology of group A streptococcal disease and of the effect of penicillin therapy and prophylaxis upon the prevention of rheumatic fever and glomerulonephritis. The current era has been one of precise chemical definition of the structure and antigenic composition of *Streptococcus* and the pathophysiologic effects of the cellular and extracellular antigenic and nonantigenic products it produces. Of particular interest has been the demonstration of immunologic cross-reactivity of streptococcal products with tissues of the heart and of the skin and the demonstration of complement-fixing immune complexes in the glomeruli of patients with acute nephritis.

The recent intensive studies of group A streptococcal skin infections have clarified the roles of these organisms in impetigo and secondary pyodermas and have pointed out the difference in the serotypes that produce such infections from those that produce pharyngitis alone. Such studies have sharpened the distinction between three populations of group A streptococci: (1) those that infect the throat but not the skin and that cause acute rheumatic fever (ARF) but not acute glomerulonephritis (AGN); (2) the streptococcal pharyngeal strains that cause AGN; and (3) the pyoderma strains that primarily affect the skin but may also be found in the throat, and that cause AGN but apparently little or no ARF. The persistent enigma of the pathogenesis of ARF and of AGN continues to stimulate studies that unfold the remarkable complexity and variation of *Streptococcus pyogenes.*

PATHOGENESIS. The two most common sites of infection with streptococci in man are the nasopharynx and the skin. Most of our knowledge of the host-parasite relation is based on studies of the former, whereas streptococcal skin infection received little attention until recently. A growing interest in the role of streptococcal pyoderma in acute glomerulonephritis has led to increasing awareness of many distinctive features that set skin infections apart from those of the upper respiratory tract. In the ensuing discussion, some of these will be pointed out, and the specific clinical features of skin infections will be considered separately.

Strains of group A streptococci may vary greatly in infectivity or virulence. During epidemics of pharyngitis, most strains isolated from the throats of patients who are acutely ill contain relatively large amounts of the type-specific surface antigen, M protein. More than 70 antigenically distinct types of M protein have been differentiated so far. This substance has particular importance in the pathogenesis of group A streptococcal infection because immunity is type specific, that is, dependent upon antibody to the homologous type of M protein. Such antibodies tend to persist for many years after infection. For this reason, repeated infections with strains of different M types occur during the lifetime of most persons, but reinfection with the same M serotype is very rare unless the type-specific immune response is suppressed by penicillin therapy.

The production of large amounts of M protein is correlated with the ability of *Streptococcus* to resist phagocytosis. A hyaluronic acid capsule, which may attain very large size in some epidemic strains and produce large mucoid colonies, also contributes to the organism's resistance to phagocytosis, particularly in certain laboratory animals such as mice. Rapid passage of group A streptococci through mice usually results in increase in M protein production by group A strains and

frequently in an increased size of the capsule. Interestingly, strains that form mucoid colonies (large capsules) are rarely if every found in the skin. In the presence of homologous anti-M antibody, virulent group A streptococci are rapidly and efficiently destroyed by human blood phagocytes. This phenomenon forms the basis for the so-called bactericidal test for the presence of circulating type-specific anti-M antibody.

Despite the location of the type-specific M protein on the surface "hairs" or "fimbriae" that project from the streptococcal cell wall and the envelope of hyaluronic acid that surrounds them, the factor responsible for the *adherence* of streptococci to mucosal cells has been shown recently to be a lipoteichoic acid (LTA), a bacterial cell wall substance with high affinity for cell membranes. The same LTA is found also in other serogroups of streptococci, viridans streptococci, and staphylococci. The role of LTA in the localization of streptococcal infections and its possible role in the deposition of streptococcal antigens in various organs is currently receiving considerable attention.

It is not yet clear to what extent cross-immunity exists to strains of streptococci less virulent than those that are rich in M protein and that are highly encapsulated. Strains of group A organisms lacking both these virulence factors are readily phagocytized and destroyed by human and animal blood. It is possible that with increasing age and number of previous streptococcal infections, the human host acquires greater resistance to all but the most virulent strains of group A streptococci. This may account, in part, for the striking age incidence in the epidemiology of human group A streptococcal pharyngitis and streptococcal pyoderma. It also may account for the progressive tendency, between infancy and childhood, for nasopharyngeal inflammatory reactions to become more and more focalized and intense. Certainly, immediate and delayed skin allergy to streptococcal products becomes increasingly frequent and severe during childhood and adolescence. Indeed, the widespread incidence of immediate and delayed allergy to streptococcal products has seriously hampered the development of effective vaccines against streptococcal M protein preparations.

The portion of highly purified M protein which is not the type-specific determinant is, instead, one or more determinants common to most if not all M proteins and has been called "M-associated" or "non-type-specific M" protein. Both cellular and humoral hypersensitivity to these antigens are intense in man, and antibodies prepared to them can cross-react with streptococcal protoplast membranes and with the sarcolemma of myocardial tissues.

Recently the type-specific M determinant has been separated and purified in T24 streptococci by extraction with dilute pepsin at suboptimal pH. This purified M protein fraction has been shown to be free of cross-reactivity with other M proteins, molecularly homogeneous by amino acid sequencing, immunogenic in laboratory animals, and far less toxic in human skin than any previously studied M protein preparation. Such progress in the immunochemical definition of the type-specific determinant and its separation from the stubbornly associated cross-reactive and toxic moieties has again encouraged prospects for human immunization against group A streptococci.

Other somatic protein antigens of the streptococcal surface that are of clinical significance are the so-called

T proteins of group A streptococci. Although these play no part in virulence, they are useful antigenic markers of streptococci, particularly when the latter have dissociated to less virulent strains with the loss of their M protein marker. The T antigens include a number of immunologically distinct proteins which resist digestion by proteolytic enzymes. Antisera prepared against these antigens can identify the T type of trypsin-digested whole streptococci by a slide agglutination method. This method has proved particularly useful in identifying pyoderma streptococci (see below) which could not be serotyped with available anti-M sera because these organisms contained M proteins of hitherto unidentified types. Thus the T type pattern of a streptococcal strain is a useful marker in following its epidemiology, especially when its M protein marker is unknown or not present. There is little difficulty in M-typing the strains isolated from most outbreaks of acute streptococcal respiratory infection, but it is seldom possible to identify an M antigen in more than 50 per cent of any large and unselected collection of cultures. This is generally not due to the absence of M antigen but to the difficulty of preparing anti-M antisera to some types and the apparent large number of M proteins which still remain unidentified.

No definite biologic property has been defined for the "C"-carbohydrate group A antigen. The antigenic determinant of group A polysaccharide has been shown to be composed of repeating units of a dimer of N-acetyl glucosamine and rhamnose. Antibodies against this somatic antigen are not readily demonstrated in man by conventional antibody tests, but recent studies employing radioactive-labeled antigen have identified very persistent antibodies to group A polysaccharide in the sera of patients with rheumatic heart disease. The mucopeptide (peptidoglycan) which forms the backbone of the streptococcal cell wall cross-reacts with the structurally similar mucopeptides of many other bacteria and produces many of the same biologic reactions as the endotoxins of gram-negative bacteria.

In the course of human infections, group A organisms produce a great variety of antigenic extracellular products, such as streptolysin O, streptokinase (fibrinolysin), hyaluronidase, nicotinamide adenine dinucleotidase (NADase), several deoxyribonucleases (DNAses), and proteinases. The antibody responses to many of these substances are useful in diagnosis (see below), and some of these products undoubtedly contribute to the pathologic features of streptococcal infection. For example, the breakdown of fibrin and nucleic acids by streptokinase and the DNAases, respectively, produces the characteristic thin pus of streptococcal infections and, with hyaluronidase, may aid the organisms' rapid spread through tissues, as observed in streptococcal cellulitis and lymphagitis. The erythrogenic toxin causes the typical erythema of scarlet fever (see below). The pathogenic role of other toxins is not yet clearly understood.

A streptococcal product receiving attention recently for its possible biologic significance is a type-specific lipoprotein lipase which causes opalescence in serum. This "serum opacity reaction" (SOR) has been used to identify strains of certain M protein serotypes. SOR+ strains appear to produce less intense anti-M immune responses and seem to be rarely associated with rheumatic fever.

With the virtual disappearance of diphtheria in the United States, the group A Streptococcus is the only significant bacterial organism that commonly causes primary sore throat, that is, that can invade the normal tissues of the pharynx. Because nasal and throat carriage of these organisms is very common, virulent streptococci may be inoculated into open wounds or skin abrasions, producing rapidly spreading cellulitis and lymphangitis or erysipelas; they may contaminate the denuded postpartum endometrium to produce puerperal sepsis; they may secondarily infect the lungs to produce a streptococcal pneumonia after viral respiratory diseases such as influenza. Therefore group A streptococci have always been a major cause of sepsis and suppurative complications. In addition, certain so-called nonsuppurative complications such as rheumatic fever and glomerulonephritis may follow streptococcal infection by pathogenic mechanisms that are not yet clear. The relation of streptococcal antigens to the pathogenesis of ARF and AGN is discussed in Ch. 130 and 374.3.

EPIDEMIOLOGY. Quantitatively, upper respiratory infections, including scarlet fever, pharyngitis, and tonsillitis, are the most important forms of group A streptococcal infection. Illness in these categories occurs most frequently in children from 5 to 15 years of age, but younger and older persons are also highly susceptible to infection. The key to the understanding of the epidemiology of streptococcal infection is an appreciation of its mode of transmission. Transmission of group A streptococcal infections occurs as a result of direct contact between infected persons or healthy carriers and susceptible persons. Significant extrahuman or animal reservoirs of these organisms do not exist, although occasional outbreaks caused by contamination of an article of food, often milk, have occurred. In general, however, streptococci dissociate rapidly outside the human host, and organisms recovered from clothing, bedding, or house dust, although identifiable as group A, have been found to be noninfective when inoculated into the throats of human volunteers. Children, among whom infection is commonplace and healthy carriers are abundant, are primarily responsible for the spread of streptococcal disease. The introduction of an untreated, infected five-year-old into a family will be followed by pharyngeal infection of more than half of his siblings and a significant number of adults in the household. The spread of an M-typable, virulent strain of group A Streptococcus through a family occurs much more readily than that of non-M-typable organisms. The problem of control of hemolytic streptococcal disease is complicated by the fact that a very large proportion of infections by these organisms is either exceedingly mild or completely inapparent. Persons with this type of "subclinical" infection are fully capable of disseminating the streptococci, but will not necessarily come under the care of a physician who could apply modern chemotherapy, eradicate streptococci from the pharyngeal tissues, and eliminate the possibility of transmission of the disease.

Epidemiologic factors such as climate, season, and geography are important primarily as they affect close contact of individuals. For example, military recruit populations, particularly when mobilized in large camps in cold climates and crowded housing conditions, provide the most ideal circumstances for the rapid passage of the organism from individual to individual, and such populations give rise to some of the most severe epidemics on record. Streptococcal disease is most severe in civilian populations when poverty and poor housing promote the most crowded living conditions.

In the northern cities of the United States pharyngeal streptococcal infections vary strikingly with the season of the year. The peak incidence occurs between December and May, and only sporadic infections appear during the hot summer months. In family studies of a large metropolitan area in the northern part of the United States, it was estimated that a streptococcal infection occurs approximately once every three to four years during childhood and adolescence, and that in a middle class population in this metropolis only about 2 per cent of all respiratory illnesses that occurred were due to group A streptococcal infection.

The epidemiology of *scarlet fever* is the same as that of other group A streptococcal infections except that the strains producing the infection seem to be lysogenized by a bacteriophage that induces the production of erythrogenic toxin in a manner analogous to diphtheria organisms that produce diphtheria toxin. Thus the epidemiology of scarlet fever is essentially that of any other strain of group A *Streptococcus* that does not produce the erythrogenic toxin. This explains the mild sporadic cases of scarlet fever, the severe epidemics of streptococcal pharyngitis *without* any scarlet fever cases, and the localized outburst of scarlet fever in a single concentrated population such as a school or institution.

The epidemiology of streptococcal *pyoderma* is strikingly different from that of streptococcal pharyngitis in several respects. Seasonal occurrence of the two is quite disparate in temperate climates: pharyngitis is more common and intense in cold weather, whereas streptococcal pyoderma occurs often in the late summer and early fall. The close indoor contact during the colder months may facilitate respiratory spread, whereas increased exposure of the uncovered skin to minor trauma and insect bites may favor skin infection during the warmer months. Although, geographically, epidemic streptococcal pharyngitis is more common in temperate or cold climates and streptococcal pyoderma in hot or tropical climates, exceptions are not uncommon in both diseases.

Streptococcal pyoderma affects an even younger age group than pharyngitis, occurring most often in children of preschool age and in infants. Transmission of streptococcal pyoderma may be aided mechanically by insects, particularly flies, that are attracted to skin lesions. Poverty and filth, as well as crowding, are major predisposing factors. Patients with streptococcal pyoderma often harbor the same organisms in the throat that colonize the skin.

The Contrasting Epidemiology of Acute Rheumatic Fever and Acute Glomerulonephritis (see accompanying figure). Students of the nonsuppurative sequels of group A streptococcal infection have long been impressed with the extreme rarity with which ARF and AGN occur in the same patient at the same time, and the antecedent infection is considered, therefore, to be due to a strain that is *either* "rheumatogenic" *or* "nephritogenic," but not both. Simultaneous appearance of both sequelae has not been a feature of the reported experience of large numbers of patients with either disease in severe epidemics in which a single streptococcal strain could be identified as the cause. The route of infection also seems to differentiate rheu-

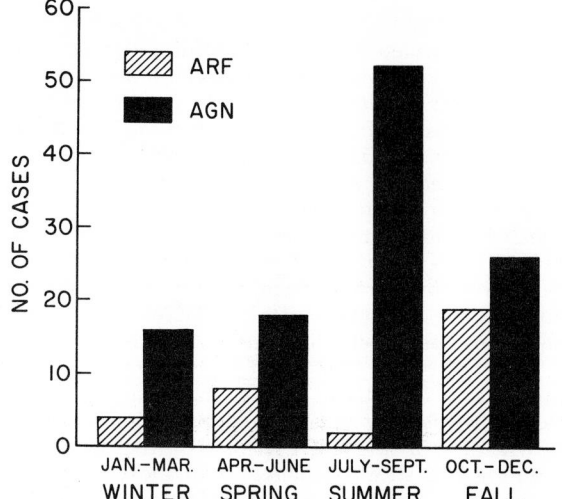

Seasonal distribution of acute rheumatic fever (ARF) and acute glomerulonephritis (AGN) admissions at City of Memphis Hospitals, September 1965–August 1968. (After Bisno, A. L., Pearce, I. A., Wall, H. P., Moody, M. D., and Stollerman, G. H.: N. Engl. J. Med., 283:561, 1970.)

matogenic from nephritogenic strains. Acute rheumatic fever seems to be almost always, if not exclusively, a complication of a pharyngeal infection. Acute glomerulonephritis occurs after *either* skin or pharyngeal infection. Although skin strains often parasitize the throat, the best known rheumatogenic pharyngeal strains do not seem to parasitize the skin.

The strains which belong to the M serotypes that have clearly caused pharyngitis followed by rheumatic fever are those commonly encountered in the throats of children in the cities of the temperate zones of the United States and western Europe and include, among others, 1, 3, 5, 6, 14, 18, 19, and 24. *All* strains containing these M antigens are not necessarily nonnephritogenic, and from time to time sporadic cases of AGN have appeared which seemed to be due to strains representing some of these serotypes (types 1, 3, and 6).

The identification of M type 12 organisms as the major pharyngeal serotype that has been associated with AGN (Rammelkamp et al., 1952) is of interest because this M serotype is one of the most common ones encountered in the throats of schoolchildren, and yet AGN does not appear consistently in populations harboring this strain. Thus not all members of a given M serotype are necessarily nephritogenic.

The recent attention to the bacteriology of skin strains of steptococci has revealed them to contain M and T proteins of types hitherto unrecognized. Since the identification of the nephritogenic type 49 (Red Lake) skin strain, a seemingly endless procession of new M types has been identified, and the number accepted by international reference laboratories now exceeds 70. Although AGN has occurred in association with most of the strains in these categories, no specific M or T antigen per se has been related to this complication.

The factors of infection determining the attack rate of rheumatic fever are also quantitative. The attack rate may vary from as low as 0.3 per cent after very mild, sporadic streptococcal infections associated with strains of low virulence to as high as 3 per cent or greater after infections with highly virulent strains of group A streptococci. The two factors that appear to have most influence on the frequency with which rheumatic fever follows a streptococcal infection are (1) the duration of convalescent carriage of the strain after the infection, and (2) the magnitude of the immunologic response associated with the infection. Thus patients with relatively feeble antistreptolysin O responses may show an attack rate of rheumatic fever of considerably less than 1 per cent, whereas those with the most vigorous streptococcal antistreptolysin O responses may suffer attack rates of rheumatic fever as high as 5 to 10 per cent. The acquisition of streptococci in the throat and their subsequent carriage *without* immunologic response has not been associated with reactivation of rheumatic fever in rheumatic subjects, nor do primary attacks of rheumatic fever occur very often without a well defined immune response. The epidemiology of rheumatic fever is therefore a reflection of the prevalence and severity of group A streptococcal pharyngitis.

127. CLINICAL SYNDROMES OF GROUP A STREPTOCOCCAL INFECTION

Gene H. Stollerman

127.1. STREPTOCOCCAL SORE THROAT

The classic syndrome described as most typical of group A streptococcal infection in older children and adults is as follows:

SYMPTOMS. There is a sudden onset of sore throat, sometimes associated with abdominal pain and nausea, especially in children, accompanied by constitutional symptoms of malaise, headache, and feverishness.

SIGNS. Redness and edema of the throat are present, particularly an *exudate* on the tonsils or tonsillar fossae; enlargement and particularly *tenderness* of the anterior cervical nodes, and fever of 38.2° C or greater. Helpful laboratory data, other than results of throat culture, include leukocytosis greater than 12,000 leukocytes per cubic millimeter.

Although this classic syndrome is, indeed, associated with group A streptococcal infection, the full clinical picture develops in a minority of patients with pharyngitis, except during epidemics. Much more common in clinical practice is the patient with some, but not all, of the aforementioned signs and symptoms. It is not unusual for mild streptococcal disease to be associated with *nonexudative* pharyngitis, and, conversely, for viral infections, particularly adenovirus and Epstein-Barr virus, to produce purulent tonsillar exudate and a syndrome indistinguishable from streptococcal tonsillitis. Hemolytic streptococci are the only common *bacterial* cause of nonexudative pharyngitis. Many viral infections may mimic this clinical state, making the study of upper respiratory infection without bacteriologic control most difficult.

Streptococcal respiratory infection is not accompanied by significant cough or by coryza. The presence of either of these manifestations should suggest a different cause. *Rhinorrhea* does occur in young children, who may develop suppurative sinusitis.

SCARLET FEVER. The disease is clinically similar in almost all respects to tonsillitis and pharyngitis caused by nonscarlatinal strains of group A streptococci. Its name, however, comes from the presence of a skin rash caused by the erythrogenic toxin produced by scarlatinal strains. The erythrogenic effect of the toxin on the skin can be neutralized by antitoxin. This is the basis of the diagnostic *Schultz-Charlton reaction.* The injection of 0.1 ml of scarlet fever antitoxin, or of 0.2 to 0.3 ml of convalescent human serum, into an area where the rash is florid will be followed by blanching around the site of injection in 8 to 12 hours. Streptococcal antitoxin is no longer readily available, and usually clinical and bacteriologic studies suffice for diagnosis.

The enanthem of scarlet fever includes a tongue that may be bright red with large papillae (raspberry tongue) or coated with the red papillae protruding (strawberry tongue). These manifestations of the disease are rarely seen in adults. The rash usually appears on the second day of the disease. It consists of a diffuse, bright scarlet erythema with many points of deeper red. The distribution is variable, but the trunk and inner aspects of the arms and thighs are most often affected. In many cases the rash is clearly seen only in the axillae and groins. The face is flushed and red, but a pale area, the *circumoral pallor,* is often seen around the mouth. The palms and soles are not erythematous. Petechiae and occasionally ecchymoses are observed, especially in severely ill patients. The application of a tourniquet to the arm for five minutes will be associated with the appearance of large numbers of petechiae distal to the obstruction in nearly all cases. This is the *Rumpel-Leede* sign; it is not specific for scarlet fever. The erythema disappears usually by the sixth to the ninth day of infection in association with the return of the temperature and the throat to normal. *Desquamation of the skin* is characteristic of scarlet fever, and it begins as a fine scaling of the face and body that is usually completed during the second week. About this time the extensive and characteristic desquamation of the palms and soles starts and continues for one to two weeks. Often the diagnosis is made retrospectively in patients who show this desquamation after a sore throat and in whom the scarlatinal rash may have been overlooked. *Eosinophilia* may be a feature of scarlet fever, especially during desquamation, and is sometimes striking (up to 20 per cent).

The course and clinical features of scarlet fever vary greatly with the severity of the disease. Many mild cases are observed in which constitutional symptoms and sore throat are minimal, fever is low grade and of short duration, and the rash is evanescent. A florid eruption is sometimes seen in persons in whom all other evidences of the disease are slight, indicating that the reaction to the erythrogenic toxin per se is not primarily responsible for the systemic manifestations of scarlet fever. Again, the situation is comparable to that in diphtheria. A mild sore throat with a strain that is a potent toxin-producer may result in a clinical picture dominated by the effects of the exotoxin. Conversely, severe pharyngeal infection may be present with a strain that is a relatively mild toxin-producer, and the clinical manifestations resulting from the toxin may be slight.

COURSE OF STREPTOCOCCAL PHARYNGITIS. The course of untreated hemolytic streptococcal pharyngitis in older children and adults is benign. Seventy-five per cent of patients are afebrile within 72 hours after onset, but sore throat, abnormal signs in the pharynx, and tender adenitis may persist for two or three days after the return of the temperature to normal. Although the whole process is shortened 24 to 48 hours by appropriate antimicrobial therapy, it is not always easy to distinguish the treated from the untreated patient. An acute pharyngitis that *fails to respond* to adequate penicillin therapy is virtually never due to group A streptococcal infection. On the other hand, the course of viral pharyngitis is often also very brief, and a spontaneous defervescence in 24 to 48 hours may mislead the clinician who has treated the patient into believing the patient has had a therapeutic response to penicillin therapy. In severe streptococcal infections, leukocytosis, when present in the acute stage, may persist in more than one half of untreated patients for a week or more, but this disappears more quickly after the institution of antimicrobial therapy. The erythrocyte sedimentation rate returns to normal in 80 per cent of patients by the third week.

Group A streptococci tend to persist in the pharynx for long periods after recovery if antimicrobial therapy has not been employed. In general, the more virulent the strain, the longer and more consistent is the duration of convalescent throat carriage. Under epidemic conditions, 80 per cent of untreated patients may carry the infecting strain for as long as four weeks. On the other hand, sporadic and mild streptococcal infections among schoolchildren studied in recent years have not been as frequently associated with such prolonged throat carriage.

Streptococcal pharyngitis in infants and small children lacks an acute and well defined onset, has *rhinorrhea* as a dominant manifestation, is rarely associated with high fever, and runs a protracted and indeterminate course. The physical signs in the throat are nondescript, and usually do not permit an accurate clinical diagnosis. Suppurative complications such as otitis media and cervical lymphadenitis occur frequently.

The change of the pharyngeal response after the first few years of life to an explosive onset with fever, sore throat, and exudative pharyngitis may be a reflection of the sharp increase in delayed hypersensitivity (cellular immunity) that appears after the first or second year of life as a result of repeated infection with different types of group A streptococci. It is noteworthy that rheumatic fever is very rare before heightened cellular and humoral immunity to the *Streptococcus* occurs, whereas acute glomerulonephritis is common.

DIAGNOSIS OF STREPTOCOCCAL PHARYNGITIS. Streptococcal tonsillitis and pharyngitis in its typical form needs to be differentiated from diphtheria, nonstreptococcal exudative pharyngitis (usually adenovirus), and infectious mononucleosis. When streptococcal infection is nonexudative, however, it cannot be differentiated (in the absence of scarlet fever) from a variety of viral agents producing an identical clinical picture. Cough, coryza, and rhinorrhea (in adults) make a nonbacterial disorder more likely. Unfortunately therefore the clinical diagnosis of the kind of streptococcal pharyngitis that now occurs most commonly as a sporadic infection

in civilian communities is usually a crude guess. It is possible, however, to *exclude* the diagnosis of streptococcal disease in considerably more than half the patients studied for sporadic pharyngitis by the use of throat cultures. The incidence of throat cultures positive for beta-hemolytic streptococci decreases progressively with age in patients with sporadic acute respiratory diseases in civilian communities. In several large cities in the northern sections of the United States, surveys have shown that less than 5 per cent of adults who had routine cultures for upper respiratory infections harbored group A streptococci in their throats. It is obvious therefore that without bacteriologic confirmation, the clinical diagnosis of viral versus streptococcal pharyngitis is quite unsatisfactory.

Before any antimicrobial therapy is administered, swabs should be passed through the mouth under direct vision, using a good light, and rubbed over the tonsils and posterior pharynx. The swab should be streaked directly, with a minimum of delay, on sheep blood agar plates of low dextrose content. After incubation overnight, the number of hemolytic streptococci present should be recorded in a roughly quantitative manner. These organisms will be very numerous in nearly all cases if they are the cause of the infection. The presence of a few does not provide convincing evidence that they are responsible for the illness, because 5 to 10 per cent of the general population are nasopharyngeal carriers of these organisms. Serologic grouping and typing of the isolated organisms are usually not necessary for routine clinical diagnosis. Because all group A streptococci are susceptible in vitro to discs containing less than 0.02 unit of bacitracin, some laboratories determine the bacitracin susceptibility of hemolytic streptococci routinely. A hemolytic *Streptococcus* resistant to such low concentrations of bacitracin is virtually never a group A *Streptococcus*. On the other hand, approximately 5 per cent of non-group A hemolytic streptococci are also susceptible to this low concentration.

Immunologic Diagnosis of Streptococcal Pharyngitis. The immunologic diagnosis of group A streptococcal infection is of no value in the treatment of the acute illness, because an antibody response will not usually be detected until 10 to 20 days after the onset of the disease. Measurement of antistreptolysin O, anti-DNAse B, antihyaluronidase, antistreptokinase, or anti-NADase is of great value in determining whether or not there has been preceding streptococcal pharyngitis in patients with possible rheumatic fever or glomerulonephritis. The presence of low titers of such antibodies during convalescence virtually excludes recent streptococcal disease except in patients who have been intensively treated early in the illness.

It should be noted that streptococcal pyoderma does not produce an equally strong immune response to all streptococcal antigens. In particular, antistreptolysin O and anti-NADase are increased relatively infrequently, whereas anti-DNAse B and antihyaluronidase, particularly the former, are better indicators of streptococcal pyoderma.

Recently, a sensitive hemagglutination test has been devised for detecting an increase in streptococcal antibodies in human serum following group A infections. The test depends on the detection of one or more extracellular antigens that adhere to the membrane of red blood cells. The extracellular substance or substances have not been clearly identified but do not appear to be any one of the aforementioned extracellular products. They have been called "streptozyme" and the hemagglutinating antibodies to them, "antistreptozyme." Although the test is not yet immunologically standardized and not yet proved to be entirely specific for group A streptococci, the frequency with which this system reflects antecedent group A streptococcal infection is very high, approaching 100 per cent in rheumatic fever and in poststreptococcal glomerulonephritis. A low antistreptozyme titer therefore in a patient with migratory polyarthritis or acute glomerulonephritis helps to exclude a streptococcal cause for either condition.

The clinician should be aware that elevated serum levels of streptococcal antibodies may persist for long periods of time after an immune response has occurred. Such elevated serum levels do not necessarily imply an unfavorable prognosis, and are not an indication for additional prolonged antimicrobial therapy.

The Value of Throat Cultures in Deciding When to Treat. There may be some difficulty in interpreting the significance of a throat culture weakly positive for hemolytic streptococci when streptococcal disease is mild and sporadic. Such a positive culture may represent the acquisition of a strain temporarily in the pharynx that does not actually invade the deeper tissues of the host, does not produce a significant immune response, and does not lead to acute rheumatic fever. Such a positive culture may also represent the convalescent carriage of an infection that occurred several weeks previously and may bear no relation to subsequent acute symptoms of viral pharyngitis from which the patient may now be suffering. The physician's problem in deciding which patient with pharyngitis to treat with antimicrobial drugs will be clarified if he obtains throat cultures routinely in all such patients whom he examines. By doing this he becomes alert to the epidemiology of the infections he encounters. A throat culture negative for beta-hemolytic streptococci will exclude a great many patients from unnecessary and promiscuous use of expensive antimicrobial drugs. In outbreaks of exudative pharyngitis, negative throat cultures in a succession of patients will immediately reveal the nonstreptococcal nature of the disease encountered. Conversely, a succession of strongly positive cultures leaves little doubt that a local outbreak of streptococcal pharyngitis is in progress.

When exudative pharyngitis is associated with a throat culture heavily seeded with beta-hemolytic streptococci, there is little argument with the general recommendation for prompt and adequate antimicrobial therapy. Moreover, when a succession of such cases is observed, the practitioner is immediately alerted to the need to culture material from the throats of asymptomatic contacts to prevent the spread of an epidemic. It is with the sporadic cases of nonexudative pharyngitis that are associated with positive throat cultures that some argument has been raised as to the need to employ intensive penicillin therapy in the regimens recommended for the prevention of rheumatic fever (see below). In some populations and under some conditions, such intensive treatment may not be necessary. At present, however, these conditions have not yet been sufficiently defined to justify broad generalizations. Until further studies define more precisely the risk of withholding or modifying chemotherapy of such infections, it is safer to err on the side of overtreatment

and thus to ensure the prevention of passage of streptococcal strains through a population. Indeed, with the assistance of the throat culture, all contacts of patients with well diagnosed exudative streptococcal pharyngitis may be studied for acquisition of potentially dangerous strains, and those identified as carriers may be treated. The consequence of such practice would undoubtedly have a profound influence on the epidemiology of streptococcal infection and therefore upon the incidence of rheumatic fever and glomerulonephritis.

COMPLICATIONS OF PHARYNGITIS. Suppurative and nonsuppurative complications may follow untreated streptococcal tonsillitis and pharyngitis.

Suppurative Complications. *Peritonsillar abscess* or *quinsy sore throat* is an interesting and infrequent complication of streptococcal tonsillitis. Its exact pathogenesis is unknown. Suppuration extends through the capsule of the palatine tonsil into the loose connective tissue of the neck. This is associated with formation of brawny edema of the affected side with movement of the tonsil toward the midline of the throat. An abscess eventually forms and drains in untreated cases, *but the pus does not regularly contain streptococci.* It is probable that the initial streptococcal infection does not cause this lesion directly, but may permit commensal organisms such as anaerobic gram-negative bacilli of the oropharynx and anaerobic nonhemolytic streptococci to gain a foothold in the affected tissues. The onset of this complication is marked by an abrupt increase in soreness and swelling of the neck, and often by increased fever and malaise. The involved tonsil and anterior pillar are greatly swollen, the cervical nodes are large and tender, and eventually a fluctuant mass may be felt in the affected area with the gloved finger. Complications of peritonsillar abscess arise when the infection extends further into the neck or leads to the development of suppurative thrombophlebitis. Peritonsillar abscess is only rarely seen today, because severe hemolytic streptococcal tonsillitis is often treated early in its course with effective antimicrobial agents.

Direct extension of hemolytic streptococci from the locus in the throat to the surrounding tissues may result in certain suppurative complications. *Paranasal sinusitis, otitis media, mastoiditis, suppurative cervical adenitis,* and *impetigo* are the most common, and will occur most frequently in untreated children less than four years old. It has been demonstrated that otitis media occurring early in the course of streptococcal respiratory infection is caused by the same serologic type that was present in the throat at the onset. A similar complication that develops after the first week is likely to be the result of a reinfection, and a different type will be recovered from the purulent exudate. Bacteremia was once observed rather frequently during the course of streptococcal respiratory infection and was often associated with metastatic lesions in the joints, bones, and elsewhere. Such cases are now almost unknown, even if antimicrobial therapy is withheld. Similarly, there has been a nearly complete disappearance of group A streptococcal meningitis. Pneumonia has always been a surprisingly uncommon complication of streptococcal upper respiratory infections. Tender cervical adenitis is regularly present and is not to be regarded as a complication unless the lymph nodes become very large and fluctuant. All the various suppurative streptococcal complications may be prevented by early and adequate antimicrobial therapy. Response to similar management is excellent if any such complications should develop in an untreated patient.

Nonsuppurative Complications. The principal non-suppurative complications of streptococcal disease, acute rheumatic fever (ARF) and acute glomerulonephritis (AGN), are discussed in Ch. 130 (ARF) and in Ch. 374.3 (AGN).

127.2.   STREPTOCOCCAL SKIN INFECTIONS

STREPTOCOCCAL PYODERMA

CLINICAL FEATURES. Aside from secondary infections of wounds or burns, group A streptococci can cause at least two kinds of skin infection, *pyoderma* and *erysipelas*. These differ markedly in clinical appearance, in epidemiology, in pathogenesis, and perhaps in the strains of streptococci causing infection. The term streptococcal pyoderma includes all kinds of streptococcal skin infections, other than erysipelas, many of which are secondary infections. The term *impetigo,* or *impetigo contagiosa,* describes what often appears to be a *primary* infection, is initially and transiently vesicular, and presents as crusted, nonscarring lesions in its later stages.

The initial lesion of streptococcal impetigo is a papule that develops rapidly into a vesicle with a small surrounding area of erythema. The vesicles are often missed clinically because of their evanescence and rapid transformation into pustules with thick, amber-colored crusts that appear to be "stuck on" the skin. Aside from occasional itching and burning, the lesions are not painful unless they become deep seated. Regional lymph nodes are commonly involved even without extensive local cellulitis. Often an apparently innocuous lesion may yield large numbers of group A streptococci in cultures taken beneath dried crusts, and such indolent-appearing lesions can produce full-blown acute glomerulonephritis. Bacteremia, which is rare in streptococcal pharyngitis, occurs more frequently with skin and wound infections, and occasionally scarlet fever has been reported. Superficial streptococcal skin infections often pursue a chronic course of weeks or months, and their onset is often difficult to establish. A deeply ulcerated form is known as *ecthyma.*

Contagiousness of streptococcal skin infections is evident from the tendency of multiple cases to occur in a family and from their tendency to occur in epidemics. The importance of antecedent skin trauma is apparent in the epidemiology of streptococcal pyoderma (see above). Its preponderance in the summer when insect bites and trauma to exposed parts of children are most common, especially in populations in which poverty results in poor hygiene, neglect, flies, and crowding, suggests the conditions for maximal opportunity of invasion of the skin by virulent strains. Because of the frequency, especially in children, of such minor skin trauma as mosquito bites, abrasions, burns, eczema, scabies, and pediculosis, it is often difficult to determine whether or not group A streptococci invade the unbroken skin. In epidemic conditions owing to particularly virulent strains, the clinical appearance of the lesions often suggests direct invasion, but it is virtually impossible to exclude minute and transient antecedent trauma.

DIAGNOSIS. The frequency with which staphylococci colonize the skin makes contamination of skin lesions with these organisms almost the rule. Cultures of lesions more clearly considered streptococcal pyoderma are frequently also associated with staphylococci, and the relative role of each organism in the etiology of impetigo has caused much confusion and controversy. Although the issue is not entirely settled, current evidence suggests that impetigo can be divided on clinical, bacteriologic, and epidemiologic grounds into two basic forms: *a bullous type,* in infants, which forms thin, varnish-like crusts and is primarily staphylococcal in origin, and *a vesicular type,* which develops thick "stuck-on" crusts and is primarily streptococcal in etiology. Whereas the classic bullous impetigo caused by staphylococci yields a pure culture of phage Type 71 organisms, the early vesicular stage of streptococcal impetigo may yield pure cultures of group A streptococci, but in the purulent and crusted stages large numbers of staphylococci may be present also. The latter are of a variety of phage types suggesting secondary colonization.

Skin cultures of pyodermas should be made after careful cleansing of the surface of the lesions with gauze soaked in sterile warm water, avoiding antiseptics, soaps, and detergents that kill or suppress the more fastidious streptococci and favor the survival of the more adaptable *Staphylococcus.* Often the removal of crusts and careful culture of the serous exudate beneath will yield large numbers of hemolytic streptococci in almost pure culture. Sheep blood agar plates incubated anaerobically or in 10 per cent CO_2 favor the growth of streptococci.

The higher numbered M and T serotypes associated with pyoderma strains of group A streptococci set them apart from the primarily pharyngeal strains, although it should be noted that throat carriage of the "skin strains" may be high in populations in which much pyoderma is present, especially during the summer months.

The weak antistreptolysin O response to pyoderma strains should be borne in mind, and anti-DNAse B, antihyaluronidase, or antistreptozyme titers should be measured when studies of the immune response to these streptococcal infections are indicated (see above), as in the diagnosis of poststreptococcal AGN.

ERYSIPELAS

This form of group A streptococcal skin infection has special characteristics and may be considered in greater detail. Erysipelas usually involves the face and head, but may affect any area of the body. Other than an occasional case of a group C strain that has been recognized, erysipelas is caused by group A streptococci. The precise way in which the bacteria are introduced into the skin in primary facial erysipelas has not been determined. Large numbers of group A streptococci are fairly constantly present among the nasopharyngeal flora of patients with early erysipelas. It may be that the primary infection is a nasopharyngitis from which the organism is transferred to the skin.

After reaching the face, the streptococci may enter

the skin through minute abrasions that are not recognizable after the disease is well established. In surgical and wound erysipelas, it is probable that streptococci are introduced into the traumatized areas from external sources, usually the nose and throat of attendants and other patients. The epidemiology of facial erysipelas differs somewhat from that of group A streptococcal infection in the affected age groups. This disease, when large numbers of cases were observed in the past, was rather common in infancy, rare between the ages of six and thirty, and predominantly a disorder of middle age. There had been no explanation for this discrepancy in age distribution.

Erysipelas usually begins as an abrupt onset of fever with a shaking chill. A history of preceding acute or subacute upper respiratory infection is obtained in about one third of adult cases and more frequently in infants. Very early in the disease a definite zone of redness and edema of the skin appears, most frequently around the birdge of the nose or around a surgical incision, traumatic wound, area of dermatitis, or the newly severed umbilical cord. Facial erysipelas is usually self-limited if no antibacterial therapy is administered. Under these circumstances, the temperature remains at a high level for four to ten days and then falls by lysis or crisis. During this interval a local process involves a large part of the face. As the lesion develops and spreads from the central focus, the skin is red, hot, edematous, and glistening. Blebs are frequently formed. The advancing edge of the lesion is sharply defined and slightly elevated. Great swelling occurs when the infection involves the eyelids.

The disease may involve one or both sides of the face, and usually remains active and spreading until the cheeks and eyelids are affected. Very often the inflammatory process does not extend over the bony prominences, and is limited to the area between the mandible, the malar eminence, and the hairline. In certain cases the ear is included, but spread to the scalp and trunk is rare except in infants.

Untreated *erysipelas of the trunk or extremities,* which usually occurs in infants or persons who have undergone surgery or have been injured, is a more malignant disease. Large areas of skin are often involved rapidly, prostration frequently occurs, and death is a common event. In this form of the disorder it is often possible to observe the characteristic recovery of the skin first affected while the process advances elsewhere. Healing of the skin requires one to two weeks after the temperature has returned to normal.

127.3. HEMOLYTIC STREPTOCOCCAL PNEUMONIA

Group A hemolytic streptococci were once responsible for 3 to 5 per cent of cases of bacterial pneumonia, but this form of disease is now rarely seen. It usually appears as a complication of influenza or other viral respiratory infection or in persons with underlying pulmonary disease. It is almost never observed as a sequel to streptococcal tonsillitis and pharyngitis or scarlet fever.

The pneumonic process is lobular in distribution in the lung. Empyema develops in 30 to 40 per cent of untreated cases. It is present early in the illness and is characterized by the formation of large amounts of thin fluid. Bacteremia is demonstrable in 10 to 15 per cent of the cases of streptococcal pneumonia. The demonstration of large numbers of hemolytic streptococci in the sputum by cultural methods, or the isolation of these organisms from the blood or pleural fluid, is required for diagnosis. (See Ch. 119 to 124.)

128. TREATMENT OF GROUP A STREPTOCOCCAL INFECTION AND CHEMOPROPHYLAXIS OF NONSUPPURATIVE COMPLICATIONS

Gene H. Stollerman

The management of the various group A streptococcal illnesses should include those general measures that are applied in all acute infections. Bed rest, light or liquid diet if pharyngeal discomfort is present and severe, and adequate but not excessive fluid intake are indicated.

Most important is the prompt institution of appropriate antimicrobial therapy, which has four goals: (1) the prompt control of the acute suppurative process in the respiratory tract or elsewhere, (2) the prevention of suppurative complications, (3) the prevention of nonsuppurative complications, and (4) the elimination of the carrier state and the prevention of transmission of the organism to others. The third and fourth goals will be fully attained only if the organism is permanently eradicated from the tissues. This can best be accomplished by the administration of penicillin. Sulfonamides are not effective either in eradicating the carrier state or in preventing an immunologic response, and thus do not prevent nonsuppurative complications. Erythromycin is an acceptable second choice to penicillin in the presence of allergy to penicillin. Tetracycline-resistant group A streptococci have been described with increasing frequency, and this drug is therefore an unreliable choice. It is essential that treatment in full doses be given over a period of at least ten days, regardless of which of the effective drugs is used.

Group A streptococci are among the most susceptible of all bacteria to the action of penicillin. The range of susceptibility for all strains of this serologic group is extremely narrow, between 0.01 and 0.04 unit per milliliter of culture. Moreover, no penicillin-resistant strains of group A streptococci have been demonstrated.

Duration of exposure to penicillin is the most important factor in therapy. Prolonged exposure to small concentrations of pencillin therefore is just as effective as a more intensive form of treatment of group A streptococcal pharyngitis. A single intramuscular injection of 600,000 units of benzathine penicillin provides blood levels that are barely detectable but that persist for about ten days; 1.2 million units results in levels that persist for at least two to four weeks or more. Such doses cure streptococcal pharyngitis, terminate carriage in the throat, and prevent rheumatic fever with optimal efficiency. Shorter-acting penicillin salts, such as aqueous procaine pencillin, must be administered still more often (usually daily for ten days) in a dose of 300,000 or 600,000 units intramuscularly to accomplish the same results. In the treatment of streptococcal pharyngitis, combinations of aqueous, procaine, and benzathine penicillin have no advantage over a single injection of benzathine penicillin G alone if a dose of at least 600,000 units or, preferably, 1.2 million units of the latter is employed.

If given orally, penicillin G must be administered in doses of 200,000 to 250,000 units four times daily for ten days. Thus, penicillinemia of about ten days' duration, regardless of the choice of preparation, is necessary to ensure the highest rates of bacteriologic cure. Sulfonamides are ineffective in preventing rheumatic fever when used to treat streptococcal pharyngitis. They do not suppress the immune response, do not terminate pharyngeal carriage of streptococci, and thus do not reduce the attack rate of subsequent rheumatic fever. They may be used, however, as continuous prophylaxis to *prevent* new infections (see below).

PREVENTION OF RHEUMATIC FEVER

Treatment of streptococcal sore throat should be started as soon as a definite diagnosis of streptococcal infection is made. It has been shown, however, that a short delay (even for several days) in initiating antimicrobial therapy while awaiting throat culture results does not significantly interfere with rheumatic fever prevention. One exception to this statement involves the patient with a history of rheumatic fever. In such a patient, the prevention of rheumatic recurrence is not always possible unless treatment is instituted at the first clinical sign of streptococcal infection. In such a patient, any delay of therapy entails the risk of reactivation of the disease. Certain features of the chemoprophylaxis of rheumatic fever are also presented in Ch. 130.

Patients with more serious streptococcal infections, such as streptococcal pneumonia, severe wound infections with sepsis, or suppurative complications of ordinary respiratory infection, should receive 600,000 units of procaine penicillin G per day intramuscularly for several days until the illness is well controlled, when a shift to a single dose of benzathine penicillin or to oral penicillin may be made. The response of extrapharyngeal suppurative complications of streptococcal infection to penicillin is good, and recovery without surgical intervention is the rule, with one exception. Sterilization of abscesses in well-established suppurative cervical adenitis is most difficult. Incision and drainage is usually required in such cases unless spontaneous rupture occurs. As in all situations of antimicrobial therapy in the presence of pus and necrosis, prolonged therapy for as long as several weeks may be required when adequate debridement is not possible. For patients allergic to penicillin, erythromycin is recommended in doses of 1 gram per day, which may be given in four divided doses for a period of ten days. Severely ill patients may receive 500 mg of erythromycin twice daily intravenously for a short time until they are able to accept the drug by month.

PREVENTION OF GLOMERULONEPHRITIS

Unlike the situation in rheumatic fever, treatment of streptococcal sore throat after the infection is well established will often fail to prevent acute glomerulonephritis. The latent period of this complication is much shorter than that of rheumatic fever. However, the spread of a nephritogenic strain through a family, school, or community can be stopped with effective antimicrobial therapy. In the case of pyoderma, the onset of the infection is not sharp and the symptoms are often not severe enough to make the patient seek treatment. Even when he does, the infection may be too well established to prevent glomerulonephritis in the patient himself. *Awareness of the presence of an index case of acute glomerulonephritis in the population he attends is therefore of great importance to the physician.* It will help him determine how promptly and vigorously he identifies, cultures, and treats patients with streptococcal infections and their contacts.

The treatment of streptococcal pyoderma has been studied far less methodically than pharyngitis and has varied widely in practice. The principles guiding the treatment of pyoderma may be somewhat different from those of pharyngitis in which prevention of rheumatic fever requires thorough eradication of group A streptococci. Unlike pharyngeal infections, topical treatment of skin infections may be adequate for mild cases of impetigo. Whether or not parenteral antimicrobial drugs are used, the removal of crusts and cleansing of the affected skin surfaces with soap seems to be an important part of the treatment of streptococcal pyoderma. In patients with extensive, persistent, or recurring impetigo, intramuscular benzathine penicillin is the treatment of choice.

Again, the decision to treat pyoderma with penicillin may depend upon, in addition to the severity of the infection, the appearance of an index case of acute glomerulonephritis in the population. In such instances, it is prudent to use an injection of benzathine penicillin G, which is the most effective measure. Where hygienic conditions are not improved, however, skin infections may recur after penicillin treatment, and it may be difficult to eradicate a nephritogenic strain from the population by penicillin therapy of infected individuals alone.

Obviously, the decision of when and how to treat a patient with a streptococcal infection, and whether or not to identify and treat his contacts, will vary with the severity of the infection, with the epidemiologic setting in which the infection occurs, and with the awareness of the presence or absence of index cases of rheumatic fever or acute glomerulonephritis in the community.

129. PROPHYLAXIS OF STREPTOCOCCAL INFECTION

Gene H. Stollerman

MASS PROPHYLAXIS. Mass prophylaxis is the term applied to the treatment of an entire population, both healthy and affected persons, to interrupt or prevent an epidemic, impending or in progress. This has been done frequently in military populations when epidemic streptococcal pharyngitis and its aftermath of rheumatic fever or glomerulonephritis have appeared. Occasionally, similar measures have been taken against local epidemics in schools or institutions. A single injection of 1.2 million units of benzathine penicillin G intramuscularly has proved extremely effective for this purpose because it (1) is therapeutic in those actually infected, (2) terminates pharyngeal carriage, and (3) protects against the acquisition of new infections for four to five weeks.

Unfortunately, no form of immunization is available. However, alert medical practitioners who will promptly detect and adequately treat streptococcal infections, a good system of public health reporting of rheumatic fever and acute glomerulonephritis, and good facilities for routine use of throat cultures should reduce extensive epidemics of streptococcal disease to a rarity. This should so alter the spread of streptococcal infections as to diminish the virulence and epidemicity of the *Streptococcus* and thereby continue the present trend in the decline of nonsuppurative complications of streptococcal disease.

Tonsillectomy has been employed prophylactically in the past, but is now known to be useless for this purpose, as it does not prevent infection by hemolytic streptococci. Subsequently acquired streptococcal respiratory illnesses may be less severe, but the frequency of occurrence of nonsuppurative complications is not reduced.

CONTINUOUS CHEMOPROPHYLAXIS. Continuous chemoprophylaxis against group A streptococci has proved to be highly effective in preventing recurrences of rheumatic fever (see below) and may be attained by one of three regimens listed here in order of their apparent efficacy and practicability:

1. Benzathine penicillin G in a single injection of 1.2 million units will provide protection for about 30 days. The disadvantages and discomfort of this regimen have to be weighed against the susceptibility to rheumatic recurrences of the individual patient. Those with rheumatic heart disease, those who have had a recent attack of rheumatic fever, and those exposed to an environment in which the incidence of streptococcal infection is frequent deserve the most effective protection. For such patients, benzathine penicillin by injection monthly is recommended.

2. Sulfonamide in daily administration by mouth of 1.0 gram of sulfadiazine or one of the other sulfapyrimidines provides satisfactory prophylaxis, but failures will occur. Toxic reactions may be observed during the first 60 days of continuous treatment. These have been rare, however, with the small doses of sulfadiazine that have been employed extensively.

3. Oral penicillin in doses of 200,000 (125 mg) units of penicillin G has been employed widely for prevention of streptococcal infections. This regimen has not been any more effective, however, than the daily dose of 1.0 gram of sulfadiazine. Indeed, 200,000 units of penicillin *twice* daily has not proved as yet to be clearly superior to the single dose. It is possible that the oral dose of penicillin may have to be increased to nearly therapeutic proportions to be more effective than sulfonamides, and this would increase further its expense and impracticability.

Baker, C. J., and Kasper, D. L.: Correlation of maternal antibody deficiency with susceptibility to neonatal group B streptococcal infection. N. Engl. J. Med., 294:752, 1976.

Beachey, E. H., and Ofek, I.: Epithelial binding of group A streptococci by lipotheichoic acid on fimbriae denuded of M protein. J. Exp. Med., 143:759, 1976.

Beachey, E. H., Stollerman, G. H., Chiang, E. Y., Chiang, T. M., Seyer, J. M., and Kang, A. H.: Purification and properties of M protein extracted from group A streptococci with pepsin: Covalent structure of the amino terminal region of type 24 M antigen. J. Exp. Med., 145:1469, 1977.

Bisno, A. L., and Ofek, I.: Serologic diagnosis of streptococcal infection: Comparison of a rapid hemagglutination technique with conventional antibody tests. Am. J. Dis. Child., 127:676, 1974.

Bisno, A. L., and Stollerman, G. H.: Streptococcal antibodies in the diagnosis of rheumatic fever. *In* Cohen, A. S. (ed.): Laboratory Diagnostic Procedure in the Rheumatic Diseases. 2nd ed. Boston, Little, Brown & Company, 1974, pp. 207–263.

Gibbons, R. J., and Van Houte, J.: Bacterial adherence in oral microbial ecology. Ann. Rev. Microbiol., 29:19, 1975.

Rammelkamp, C. H., Jr.: Epidemiology of Streptococcal Infections. Harvey Lectures, Series 51, 1955–56. New York, Academic Press, 1957, p. 113.

Rheumatic Fever Committee, American Heart Association: Prevention of Rheumatic fever. Circulation, 55:S1, 1977.

Seegal, D., and Seegal, B. C.: Facial erysipelas: A study of 281 cases treated at the Massachusetts General Hospital from 1870–1927. JAMA, 93:430, 1929.

Stollerman, G. H.: The relative rheumatogenicity of strains of group A streptococci. Mod. Concepts Cardiovasc. Dis., 44:35, 1975.

Stollerman, G. H.: Rheumatic Fever and Streptococcal Infection. New York, Grune & Stratton, 1975.

Stollerman, G. H.: Streptococcal vaccines revisited. J. Lab. Clin. Med., 91: 872, 1978.

Wannamaker, L. W.: Infections of the throat and skin. N. Engl. J. Med., 282:23, 78, 1970.

Wannamaker, L. W., and Matsen, J. M. (eds.): Streptococci and Streptococcal Diseases. New York, Academic Press, 1972.

Wood, H. F., Feinstein, A. R., Taranta, A., Epstein, J. A., and Simpson, R.: Rheumatic fever in children and adolescents. III. Comparative effectiveness of three prophylaxis regimens in preventing streptococcal infections and rheumatic recurrences. Ann. Intern. Med., 60 S5:31, 1964.

130. RHEUMATIC FEVER

Richard M. Krause

DEFINITION. Rheumatic fever is an uncommon, but by no means rare, delayed sequel of an upper respiratory tract infection caused by group A hemolytic streptococci. The pathogenesis remains obscure. Multiple focal aseptic inflammatory lesions are the basis for the acute manifestations, which may include migratory arthritis, carditis, chorea, erythema marginatum, and subcutaneous nodules, as well as a number of less prominent signs and symptoms. Recurrences of rheumatic fever are common after an untreated streptococcal infection in patients with a previous history of this disease. The acute disease is of limited duration, but the carditis may lead to permanent valvular damage. It is for this reason that extensive studies have been concerned with methods to prevent first attacks as well as recurrences of rheumatic fever. Prevention can be achieved only by the prompt detection, diagnosis, and treatment of streptococcal pharyngitis set forth in the immediately preceding chapters.

ETIOLOGY AND PATHOGENESIS. Despite the decline in recent years in the incidence of rheumatic fever, interest in the disease is unabated because of its unique relationship to streptococcal infections. All the available evidence indicates that only group A streptococcal infections of the upper respiratory tract lead to rheumatic fever. Further, the two episodes are separated by a latent period during which the signs and symptoms of either illness are commonly absent. Although streptococci may be present in the throat from the onset of pharyngitis to the onset of rheumatic fever, there is no satisfactory evidence that foci of living streptococci contribute to the occurrence of rheumatic inflammatory lesions. Thus rheumatic fever appears to be a *reaction* to the streptococcal infection, and not a continuation of the infectious process.

The epidemiologic, clinical, and laboratory evidence for the association between streptococcal infections and rheumatic fever deserves special comment. Numerous epidemiologic studies have described a temporal relationship between these two diseases. Prior to the days of penicillin, an epidemic of scarlet fever in a closed population, such as a boarding school, was followed in two to four weeks by an uncommonly high incidence of rheumatic fever. But the certain relationship between the two diseases was only established once there had been major advances in the bacteriology of streptococci. The advent of methods to delineate the antigenic structure of the group A *Streptococcus* and the immune response to the various streptococcal antigens permitted the identification of the group A *Streptococcus* as the only pathogen that causes the pharyngitis leading to rheumatic fever. The serologic methods to detect antibodies to streptococcal antigens played an especially important role in establishing this relationship. With such methods, it was possible to determine for the first time that nearly every patient with rheumatic fever had a preceding streptococcal sore throat. This was not always evident from the results of throat cultures taken at the onset of rheumatic fever. Although group A streptococci may persist in the throat during the interval between streptococcal pharyngitis and rheumatic fever, it is not uncommon for repeated cultures of the pharynx to be negative for these organisms.

The most persuasive argument in favor of a relationship between streptococcal pharyngitis and acute rheumatic fever stems from the treatment schedules that have been devised to prevent primary as well as recurrent attacks of rheumatic fever. In brief, it is clear that adequate antimicrobial therapy of streptococcal pharyngitis will prevent a subsequent attack of rheumatic fever.

Once the bacteriology of streptococcal pharyngitis was clarified, the recurrent nature of rheumatic fever was no longer a mystery. Group A streptococci are classified into more than 70 serologic types on the basis of serologically distinct M proteins. Almost all serologic types are apparently capable of causing a pharyngitis that can lead to rheumatic fever (the possible exceptions to this rule are some of the recent new types of streptococci that have been most prominently isolated from skin lesions, some of which are associated primarily with the occurrence of acute nephritis). Because immunity to streptococcal infections is M-type specific, infection with one type results in no significant protection against the many other types. Thus it is common for a child to experience several different streptococcal infections during the school years, and this, in turn, makes possible repeated attacks of rheumatic fever. A child who has had an attack of rheumatic fever retains a special susceptibility to repeated attacks in subsequent years. However, the reason for this special susceptibility remains to be explained.

Most, if not all, serologic M types of group A streptococcal infections of the pharynx can lead to rheumatic fever. Although the attack rate of rheumatic fever is as high as 3 per cent following untreated streptococcal pharyngitis during epidemics, the rate is 0.5 per cent or less following sporadic infections. Epidemiologic evidence indicates that rheumatic fever occurs only after streptococcal pharyngitis, but not in association with streptococcal skin infections, e.g., impetigo. It is conceivable that the response to the pharyngeal infection is qualitatively and quantitatively different from the response to skin infections. It is known, for example, that the antibody response to streptolysin O is more likely to be elevated after pharyngeal infections than after skin infections, whereas the antibody response to DNAse B occurs with high frequency after infection at either site. Thus it is conceivable that the special consequences of a pharyngeal infection set the stage for the occurrence of rheumatic fever.

The selective occurrence of rheumatic fever in only a few people with pharyngitis argues for the importance of host factors in addition to the infectious process in the pathogenesis of rheumatic fever. It is possible that the accumulative effects of repetitive streptococcal infections in any one individual are a factor that increases the risk. Young children under the age of three have streptococcal pharyngitis, but rheumatic fever is uncommon in this age group. Throughout the remainder of childhood repetitive streptococcal infections lead to delayed hypersensitivity to streptococcal products, but such hypersensitivity is not commonly present in children less than three years of age. It is after the age of four that rheumatic fever is most common in children. The possible importance of genetic factors in predisposition has been suggested. Although it has been observed that rheumatic fever may occur in families, no clear-cut genetic pattern has been found. In a study of monozygotic twins, less than one fifth were concordant for rheumatic fever. Unsatisfactory and inconclusive though these studies are, the selective occurrence of rheumatic fever in only a few of all those infected with streptococci suggests that predisposing factors work in conjunction with the infectious process to produce rheumatic fever, but the nature of such contributory causes has remained obscure.

Although the central role of streptococcal infections in the etiology of rheumatic fever is now established beyond question, the mechanism by which the hemolytic streptococci initiate the disease process is unknown. For convenience, evidence can be marshaled for the support of three different theories of pathogenesis. Each of these theories is less than satisfactory.

The most currently attractive hypothesis is that rheumatic fever is a consequence of an immunologic response or hypersensitivity reaction, or both, to streptococcal antigens. An immunologic mechanism is suggested by the intriguing parallel between the latent period of serum sickness and rheumatic fever. Patients who develop rheumatic fever appear to have an exaggerated antibody response to streptococcal antigens. Such patients commonly, but not always, have a higher antistreptolysin O response than those who do not develop this complication after streptococcal pharyngitis.

The arguments suggesting that autoimmunity may be

of importance in pathogenesis cannot be recorded in detail here. The occurrence of autoantibodies that react with mammalian muscle in the sera of patients with rheumatic fever in concentrations greater than in the sera of patients who do not develop this complication has been emphasized. What remain to be determined are the source of antigenic stimulus for this autoantibody and the pathologic significance of such autoantibody. Because this autoantibody cross-reacts with a streptococcal antigen, it has been argued that these antibodies are only another manifestation of the immune response to the preceding streptococcal infection. It is also possible, however, that the host's own tissues were so altered by the toxic processes at the time of infection that altered tissue antigens became the stimulus for autoantibody production. In addition to the controversy over the source of the stimulus that gives rise to these autoantibodies, there is the additional controversy over their pathologic significance. It is unknown if they participate in the genesis of the inflammatory lesions in a manner similar to the autoantibodies to nucleic acid which appear to be intimately associated with the inflammatory lesions of lupus erythematosus.

Another possible explanation for the pathogenesis of rheumatic fever is that the inflammation is a direct consequence of the deleterious effects of streptococcal toxins produced at the time of the infection. Despite the marked toxicity of certain streptococcal products, such as streptolysin O and S, there is little evidence for or against the importance of toxins in pathogenesis.

It remains to mention the possible role of persistent foci of the infecting *Streptococcus* in the pathogenesis of rheumatic fever. Aside from several earlier bacteriologic reports prior to the era of antimicrobial drugs, there is little bacteriologic evidence for a direct infection of the heart valves, the myocardium, or other organs involved in rheumatic fever. Nevertheless, because the prevention of rheumatic fever requires the successful and complete eradication of the infecting *Streptococcus* from the pharynx by drug therapy, the view lingers that persistence of the infecting *Streptococcus* in some form may be a factor in the disease process.

EPIDEMIOLOGY. It is obvious from what has been said that the epidemiology of acute rheumatic fever and the epidemiology of streptococcal pharyngitis are clearly interrelated. The incidence of the two diseases is related. Any environmental or host factor that enhances the occurrence of streptococcal pharyngitis will enhance the occurrence of rheumatic fever. Streptococcal disease is most common between the ages of five and fifteen years, with a peak incidence between six and eight years, and this is the age group with the highest attack rate of rheumatic fever. Although adults have fewer streptococcal infections than children because of acquired immunity and less exposure to streptococci, the special circumstances of military service or close association with children enhance the risk of higher attack rates for adults.

As is the case for most other respiratory diseases, the occurrence of streptococcal pharyngitis fluctuates widely with the seasons. The occurrence of acute rheumatic fever parallels such fluctuations. The peak occurrence falls in the late winter and early spring months, although not uncommonly the number of cases increases sharply for a brief period shortly after the onset of school in the early fall.

Classic epidemiologic studies indicate that rheumatic fever occurs most commonly in the temperate zones. But recent reports from Africa, India, and countries of Southeast Asia suggest that rheumatic heart disease is by no means rare in these areas. This has prompted a search for acute rheumatic fever in economically underdeveloped countries of the world. A recent clinical study in Egypt has revealed that rheumatic fever there has the same characteristics as the disease which occurs in the United States and Europe.

Socioeconomic factors such as overcrowding, either in tenement areas or in army barracks, that favor the spread of streptococcal disease also favor the occurrence of rheumatic fever. There is no evidence for differences of susceptibility because of race or sex, although chorea and mitral stenosis are more common in females, and aortic insufficiency is more common in males.

A number of factors have undoubtedly been responsible for the decline in the occurrence of rheumatic fever and rheumatic heart disease in the past several decades. Not the least of these are improvements of socioeconomic conditions and the treatment of streptococcal infections with penicillin. Certainly antimicrobial therapy has had a major impact on the prevention of recurrent attacks of rheumatic fever, and such cases have shown a precipitous decline. Less well documented is the decline in first attacks. Indeed, long-time students of the disease have commented on the persistent occurrence of first attacks in the large cities of the United States, and suggest that the over-all decline in cases stems from the prevention of recurrences as well as from the prevention of first attacks.

For the United States at large, the yearly incidence of first attacks of rheumatic fever has been estimated at about 50,000 to 100,000 children, but for a variety of reasons such estimates are unsatisfactory. The disease is not reportable in all states and, in addition, without unequivocal pathognomonic signs and symptoms that clearly establish diagnosis, the disease is both over- and underreported. Some idea of the continued occurrence of rheumatic fever in the population can be obtained by the examination of schoolchildren, college students, and military recruits for the prevalence of rheumatic heart disease. Among schoolchildren, the prevalence is between 0.7 and 1.6 per 1000. The prevalence for freshmen college students and servicemen is between 6 and 9 per 1000.

CLINICAL MANIFESTATIONS. The most striking clinical manifestations are due to arthritis, carditis, and chorea. Each sign and symptom of rheumatic fever may be either mild or severe, and the severity of each may vary independently. Thus severe carditis may be associated with minimal or no evidence of arthritis, and vice versa. Because the manifestations of rheumatic fever at first glance appear so variable, and because no single set of manifestations is typical for rheumatic fever, the Jones criteria have been devised as a guide to aid in the differential diagnosis. The signs and symptoms that comprise the Jones criteria are listed in the accompanying table. Use of these criteria for guidance in differential diagnosis will be discussed later.

Although a history of a preceding streptococcal pharyngitis is common, this infection may have been so mild as to have escaped medical attention. Indeed, a number of patients can recall no recent sore throat. The interval between the pharyngitis and the onset of rheu-

Clinical and Laboratory Manifestations of Acute Rheumatic Fever

Major Manifestations	Minor Manifestations

1. Carditis
2. Polyarthritis
3. Chorea
4. Erythema marginatum
5. Subcutaneous nodules
	1. Clinical
	  a. Previous rheumatic fever or
	    rheumatic heart disease
	  b. Arthralgia
	  c. Fever
	2. Laboratory
	  a. Acute phase reactions, elevated
	    erythrocyte sedimentation rate,
	    C-reactive protein, leukocytosis
	  b. Prolonged P-R interval

plus

Supporting evidence of preceding streptococcal infection (increased ASO or other streptococcal antibodies, positive throat culture for group A Streptococcus, recent scarlet fever)

The Jones criteria (revised) have been employed as a guide in the diagnosis of rheumatic fever, but this scheme has not received universal acceptance. The presence of two major manifestations, or of one major and two minor manifestations, indicates a high probability of the presence of rheumatic fever *if supported by evidence of a preceding streptococcal infection*. The absence of the latter should make the diagnosis doubtful, except in situations in which rheumatic fever is first discovered after a long, latent period from the antecedent infection, e.g., Sydenham's chorea or low-grade carditis.

Adapted from the recommendations of the Committee of The American Heart Association (Circulation, 32:664, 1965.)

matic fever has been termed the latent period. This is a period of one to five weeks, and during this time the patient usually appears entirely well. On some occasions, however, laboratory examination will reveal evidence of disease activity.

The onset of rheumatic fever, with characteristic signs and symptoms, is usually sudden, but it may be insidious. In the latter case, diagnosis depends on observation of the clinical course and the interpretation of laboratory data. Usually the first symptoms are fever and joint pain. Fever may be high and sustained in severe cases, but more frequently it is moderate and often low grade. Sore throat is not uncommon, even though examination reveals minimal evidence of acute inflammation. Epistaxis occurs commonly both at the onset and throughout the acute stage of the disease, and in some cases results in serious loss of blood. In children, severe abdominal pain is not uncommon, and vomiting may occur. Localization of such pain in the right lower quadrant with fleeting signs of peritoneal inflammation may suggest the diagnosis of appendicitis.

Arthritis. The arthritis in rheumatic fever may involve multiple joints, but a characteristic feature is that the inflammation occurs and subsides in the joints first affected, only to occur in others that were initially spared. This phenomenon has been termed migratory polyarthritis. The large joints of the extremities are most frequently affected, but all are potentially susceptible. Arthritis can occur in the hands, feet, or spine, or in such joints as the sternoclavicular and the temporomandibular.

The manifestations of arthritis may be either mild with vague discomfort in the joints of the extremities, or severe. Acutely inflamed and swollen joints are commonly very painful. In mild cases there may be no objective evidence of arthritis. When arthritis is severe, the skin over the joint shows local redness and heat, the joint is swollen, and fluid is obviously present within the joint cavity. Passive or active movement of the joint is extremely painful. The fluid in such cases is turbid and contains leukocytes, indicating an inflammatory reaction, but is sterile on bacteriologic culture.

Although uncommon, the arthritis may not affect multiple joints. Experienced clinicians have observed the occasional case in which arthritis may persist for prolonged periods in only one joint, with minimal evidence of arthritis in the others.

There is usually a difference between the pattern of arthritis in children and that in adults. Frank arthritis is less common in children between four and six years of age. Only mild joint pains may be noted, or merely vague localized aching in the extremities. It is this type of complaint that has been referred to in the past as "growing pains." Such symptoms and low-grade fever suggest a mild illness, but examination of the heart may reveal severe carditis. It bears repetition that rheumatic fever can occur without any evidence of joint involvement whatever.

Carditis. Palpitation and precordial chest pain or discomfort are common symptoms. If the carditis is severe, symptoms of cardiac failure may occur in addition to those of rheumatic fever. The final and definitive diagnosis of carditis depends upon the physical, roentgenographic, and electrocardiographic examinations.

The carditis may be mild or severe. In mild cases, tachycardia, persistent during sleep, may be the only sign suggesting carditis. Bradycardia has been well documented in rheumatic fever, particularly during the recovery process. In the more severe cases, generalized cardiac enlargement frequently occurs, often associated with a diffuse precordial impulse.

On auscultation, the heart sounds in the apical area may be muffled, indistinct, and of poor quality. The second sound in the pulmonic area is usually greatly accentuated in comparison with the second aortic sound. Gallop rhythm may occur, and is usually an indication of serious myocardial disease. The sounds may seem distant if precordial effusion is present, and the pericarditis may produce a to-and-fro friction rub (see Ch 365).

Cardiac murmurs may be present at the initial examination, or they may develop during the first few weeks of the illness. Several characteristic murmurs, occurring alone or in any combination, are indicative of carditis. These are a holosystolic apical murmur due to relative or actual mitral regurgitation; a diastolic murmur along the left sternal border at the third and fourth interspaces, due to relative or actual aortic regurgitation; and an apical mid-diastolic rumble often associated with mitral regurgitation during acute carditis and referred to as a Carey-Coombs murmur. As the murmurs may disappear permanently on recovery, their final significance cannot be determined except by repeated examinations during and after convalescence. Mitral stenosis and aortic stenosis are late manifestations of cardiac damage that do not develop until months or years after the initial or repeated attacks.

Disturbances of the conduction system are a common feature of rheumatic carditis. Although certain irregularities, such as second-degree heart block, can be recognized clinically, the electrocardiogram is the best method to detect all potential conduction system disturbances. One of the most commonly observed electrocardiographic changes is the prolongation of the P-R interval. In some cases, the Wenckebach phenomenon is observed. Further delay in conduction may lead to drop beats, with the occurrence of couplets and triplets. Finally, complete dissociation is indicated by an independent rhythm for both the ventricles and the atria. Atrial fibrillation is uncommon during the acute attack.

In addition to these conduction abnormalities, the electrocardiogram may show T wave changes, such as inversion of the T wave in one or more leads. When pericarditis is present, elevation of the S-T segment is observed initially. Late in the course, the configuration of the T wave stimulates that seen in coronary disease.

Although cardiac enlargement, when present, is usually detectable on physical examination, the dilatation of the various chambers of the heart is more accurately determined by roentgenography of the chest. It is not uncommon for dilatation to arise rapidly when severe myocarditis is present.

The recurrence of active rheumatic fever should be suspected in patients with chronic rheumatic heart disease when the character of the murmurs changes over a short period of time. Cardiac failure may occur, but in carditis associated with recurrent rheumatic fever in such cases poses several diagnostic problems, because the manifestations of acute rheumatic carditis are superimposed on those of chronic valvular disease. Furthermore, the status of the pre-existing heart disease is often unknown. When there is evidence of advanced valvular deformity, all final assessment of the extent of cardiac damage must await convalescence from the acute attack.

Erythema Marginatum. *Erythema marginatum* or *circinatum* of the skin is one of the characteristic manifestations of acute rheumatic fever and occurs in 10 to 20 per cent of the childhood cases. Because it comes and goes, it is frequently missed, particularly if the patients are not examined *completely*. It is a multiform type of erythema, and consists of roughly circular lesions that may be distributed over the extremities, the trunk, and sometimes the face, and that spread centrifugally, leaving a clear center. The lesions tend to coalesce so that, although individual areas are iris-like, the larger areas are serpiginous in outline. The erythema blanches on pressure and may be evanescent, disappearing and later reappearing at the same sites. The lesions are usually not elevated, although in some cases a slight papular quality may be detected. Most commonly, no discomfort is associated with the lesions. Erythema marginatum is uncommon in other diseases.

Subcutaneous Rheumatic Nodules. These lesions are one of the physical findings that lend strong support to the diagnosis of rheumatic fever, but in recent years they have occurred less commonly than was the case in the past. They are firm, insensitive nodules that occur over the bony prominences of the various joints and tendons of the extremities, the spine, and the back of the head. They are loosely attached to the underlying tissue, and the skin is freely movable over them. If the joint can be flexed without undue pain, the nodules are more readily apparent because of the tension of the skin. If nodules are numerous, they may occur in a symmetrical distribution. The nodules are more frequently encountered in the more severe cases of rheumatic fever with serious cardiac involvement.

Sydenham's Chorea. Chorea may occur in combination with other symptoms of rheumatic fever, but it is commonly seen as the sole manifestation of the disease. This phenomenon is explained by the fact that chorea tends to make its appearance late in the course of rheumatic fever. The onset may be delayed for as long as six months after the initiating streptococcal infection, although the delay is usually less than this. Patients with chorea may have had an easily recognizable preceding attack of arthritis and carditis, and, indeed, may have been hospitalized with it, only to have the chorea occur as a late manifestation at a time when all other evidence of any inflammatory process had disappeared. When the onset of chorea is delayed and the other manifestations of rheumatic fever have abated, the laboratory findings are often normal. It is not uncommon for chorea to occur in patients who can recall no earlier illness. It seems likely that such individuals had an attack of acute rheumatic fever in the recent past which was so mild that it escaped clinical detection. It is for this reason that patients with so-called "pure chorea" may develop rheumatic heart disease.

The onset of chorea is usually insidious, and the parents of the child with chorea may first note increased awkwardness and a tendency to spill food or drop objects that is attributed to carelessness. Even the appearance of involuntary purposeless movements of the extremities may be discounted as nervousness. However, with further progression of the disease, the irregular and uncontrollable movements become obvious. They may become extensive, and may involve not only the hands, feet, arms, and legs, but the tongue and facial muscles. The severity may range from no more than minimal involuntary movements observed only by close inspection, to violent, continual activity, totally incapacitating the patient and requiring protection from self-injury. In moderate cases, interference with all coordinated activity, such as writing and eating, is common. On occasion, chorea may be limited to one side of the body. The disease appears to affect females somewhat more frequently than males.

Miscellaneous Clinical Manifestations. Rheumatic pneumonitis may occur, but this is difficult to detect clinically, particularly if there is superimposed heart failure. Rheumatic pneumonia has seldom been seen in recent years, probably because the disease process itself appears to be much milder than in former times. Such few cases as do occur are in patients with severe rheumatic fever.

LABORATORY FINDINGS. Hematology. There are no characteristic abnormalities of the leukocyte differential count that are indicative of rheumatic fever. Leukocytosis is common, but not always present, with a total count from 12,000 to 24,000 per cubic millimeter. This is associated with an increase in the percentage of polymorphonuclear cells.

A moderate degree of anemia is generally seen, which is normochromic with proportional decreases in the hemoglobin concentration and the erythrocyte count. The anemia usually persists for as long as the rheumatic process is active. The most severe anemias are obviously encountered in patients who have an associated blood loss owing to epistaxis.

Urinary Findings. Some proteinuria and an increase in the number of red and white cells in the urine are common during the acute phase of the disease. However, it is seldom that these abnormalities are as great as those characteristically encountered in acute glomerulonephritis. When this is the case, simultaneous acute nephritis and rheumatic fever must be considered, but such a combination is a most uncommon event.

Evidence for a Prior Streptococcal Infection. The

most important laboratory information for establishing the diagnosis of rheumatic fever is data that substantiate the prior occurrence of streptococcal pharyngitis. The detection of group A beta-hemolytic streptococci by a throat culture is helpful in this regard, but of greater usefulness is the serologic detection of antibodies that are indicative of a previous streptococcal infection.

Because the streptococci that caused the initial infection may persist for many weeks in the pharynx in those instances in which antimicrobial therapy was not given or was inadequate, a throat culture may detect the infecting group A streptococci at the time of the onset of rheumatic fever. But such a finding is only suggestive of a preceding streptococcal pharyngitis and is not an unambiguous indication of it. This stems from the fact that 5 to 30 per cent of the healthy population may carry group A streptococci in the pharynx during the respiratory disease season. Thus the recovery of this organism from a patient may be an inadvertent finding and not indicative of a preceding streptococcal sore throat. Nevertheless, the throat culture is helpful, and should be obtained in all cases. When the patient has a negative throat culture, it is frequently possible to isolate the group A streptococci from other members of the family. Such a finding is indicative of a recent intrafamilial spread of streptococci.

The most helpful information that is indicative of a recent streptococcal infection is obtained with tests that detect serum antibodies to streptococcal antigens. The most widely employed test is the antistreptolysin O determination. As with all antibody tests, the detection of an antibody rise over a one- to three-week interval is the only unequivocal evidence for the recent occurrence of a streptococcal infection. If a patient is seen in the first few days after the onset of rheumatic fever, the antistreplysin O titer at that time may be less than the titer seen several weeks after onset of rheumatic fever. Not uncommonly, however, the titer has reached a maximal plateau so that it is not possible to detect a progressive increase in titer. When this is the case, the antistreptolysin O titer should be at least 250 units in adults and at least 333 units in children over five years of age to be acceptable as an indication of a previous streptococcal infection. Obviously, a certain proportion of the individuals in the normal population have had a recent streptococcal infection at any one time, and they will have antistreptolysin O titers similar to these.

Approximately 15 to 20 per cent of the patients with rheumatic fever and nearly all patients who exhibit only chorea have a low or borderline low antistreptolysin O titer. In such instances, it is helpful to employ another antibody test. The anti-DNAse B test is becoming widely accepted as a second antibody test, and it is a useful means to obtain additional evidence for the occurrence of a previous streptococcal infection. When both these antibody tests are used, it is possible to obtain antibody evidence for a preceding streptococcal infection in almost all cases of rheumatic fever.

One other serologic test should be mentioned because it may be used more widely in the future. It has been noted that nearly all patients with rheumatic fever have readily detectable serum autoantibodies that react with muscle tissue, including heart, whereas the concentration of these antibodies is very much less or absent in sera of patients with other rheumatic diseases. Such findings suggest that this antibody test may have clinical usefulness for the differential diagnosis of rheumatic fever.

Other Laboratory Tests. An elevated sedimentation rate and a positive C-reactive protein are present in rheumatic fever, but these findings are nonspecific indicators of inflammation, and they cannot be used to differentiate rheumatic fever from other diseases. However, a normal C-reactive protein and a normal sedimentation rate are helpful in excluding active rheumatic fever. The sedimentation rate, when properly done, is strikingly elevated in all cases of *acute* rheumatic fever, exclusive of patients with chorea, and other concomitant diseases such as sickle cell disease or fibrinogenemia. If the sedimentation rate and the C-reactive protein are normal, active rheumatic fever is unlikely in patients with mild symptoms, such as vague arthralgia and lassitude.

DIAGNOSIS AND DIFFERENTIAL DIAGNOSIS. A history of severe sore throat in the recent past, migrating polyarthritis, carditis, fever, and an elevated antistreptolysin O titer is such a classic combination of signs and symptoms that the diagnosis can seldom be questioned. But the problem is often not as straightforward as this. *Furthermore, it cannot be emphasized too strongly that there is no specific diagnostic laboratory test for rheumatic fever.*

The various major manifestations of rheumatic fever that have been described above are considered to be part of the same disease because they occur together with a frequency that far exceeds chance. Because they may occur singly or in various combinations in any individual patient, the diagnostic criteria originally proposed by Jones have been suggested as a guide to diagnosis. These criteria are listed in the table. Any combination of these criteria can occur in patients with other disorders. It is for this reason that stress is placed on supporting evidence for a preceding streptococcal infection. When this is the case, the diagnosis is weighed in favor of rheumatic fever and against the other connective tissue disorders that may mimic it. The footnote to the table should be especially noted.

The designations major and minor for the various criteria are based on the diagnostic importance of the particular findings. The major ones are more indicative of rheumatic fever than the minor. The occurrence of two major manifestations is strong presumptive evidence for rheumatic fever. Only one major manifestation and any combination of the minor suggest possible rheumatic fever. In any case, if evidence is lacking for a preceding streptococcal pharyngitis, the possibility of other diseases must be kept in mind.

In many ways the most useful purpose of the criteria is their value in reducing overdiagnosis. For example, not uncommonly, patients, after streptococcal infections, may have vague pains in the extremities, an increased sedimentation rate, and a borderline temperature elevation. Careful follow-up of such patients has not revealed the delayed occurrence of rheumatic heart disease. Therefore the diagnosis of rheumatic fever should be made with caution and only with clear evidence of one or more of the major manifestations. When the diagnosis is in doubt, because the symptoms are of such a mild nature, treatment with aspirin and steroids should be withheld until the signs and symptoms are unmistakable. Early treatment of a questionable case may so depress the disease activity that clearcut clinical signs and symptoms do not develop.

In the early stages, during the acute onset, *rheumatoid arthritis* and *systemic lupus erythematosus* may mimic rheumatic fever. Indeed, if the streptococcal antibody tests are elevated, the diagnosis may be in question unless the special diagnostic tests for the other diseases are clearly positive. Usually as time progresses, the special distinctive clinical features of rheumatoid arthritis and lupus serve to exclude the diagnosis of rheumatic fever. On occasion, at the onset, Still's disease may be confused with rheumatic fever, but again the clinical course will aid in differentiating the two.

Subacute bacterial endocarditis can occur in persons with valves previously damaged by rheumatic fever, and it often presents a clinical picture that is not readily distinguishable from a rheumatic recurrence. Vague pains in the extremities are more common than overt arthritis, but these symptoms together with fever and debility in a known rheumatic patient are sufficient to suggest a rheumatic recurrence. The difficulties are increased by the fact that in some cases it is not possible to recover the offending organism in a blood culture. The characteristic petechiae and painful septic emboli of endocarditis are helpful in differential diagnosis (see Ch. 131).

The so-called *benign idiopathic pericarditis* is not rheumatic in origin and has been observed with coxsackievirus infection. It is indistinguishable in the acute phase from those cases of rheumatic fever in which pericarditis is the major detectable manifestation. The diagnosis of idiopathic pericarditis is dependent primarily on elimination of other possibilities and on the subsequent course of the disease, which is characterized by complete recovery without residual damage. Thus the final conclusion is often reached only in retrospect, and must remain somewhat uncertain because rheumatic pericarditis with minimal involvement of the myocardium and endocardium could conceivably behave in a similar fashion.

Fever, arthritis, and positive acute phase reactants may also occur in bacterial arthritis, serum sickness, subacute bacterial endocarditis, sickle cell anemia, and acute aleukemic leukemia. In such cases in which confusion exists, only a careful assessment of the clinical course, physical examination, and laboratory findings will exclude rheumatic fever.

Persistent monarticular arthritis, without other major manifestations of rheumatic fever, is usually not due to rheumatic fever, and osteomyelitis or local injury must be considered.

THERAPY. There is no specific treatment for rheumatic fever. Therapeutic measures are devised to promote, or at least ideally not to hinder, the natural healing processes. Bed rest is always prescribed, and most students agree that it should continue until the acute manifestations of arthritis and carditis are under control. It is not at all clear that absolute bed rest without bath privileges is essential. A program for a progressive increase in recreational and occupational therapy has important psychologic value and should be an integral part of the long-term bed rest management. Schooling should not be neglected during this time. Hospital or home visit teaching programs, or both, are available in many cities, and instruction should be begun as soon as the acute manifestations of the disease are brought under control by anti-inflammatory therapy.

After the first few weeks of bed rest, gradual ambulation can be started. During the period of bed rest, the patient is permitted a number of activities in increasing amounts, such as sitting up in a chair, occupational therapy, and schoolwork. In some patients with pronounced tachycardia, as well as evidence of severe myocarditis, the period of bed rest should be prolonged.

The period of bed rest is a good time for patients of all ages to be informed about the nature of the illness and the optimistic prospects for an active, long life. The need for a continuous program to prevent streptococcal pharyngitis should be discussed in detail. It is at this time, also, that patients with more severe forms of heart disease should be advised that some curtailment of normal physical activity may be necessary during convalescence. But pessimism is not warranted. All too often, patients are left with the impression that their useful, active life is at an end. This is almost invariably not the case.

If there is no evidence of rheumatic carditis or heart disease following the termination of therapy, full physical activity can be gradually resumed. Any long-term restrictions on physical activity in patients with persistent rheumatic heart disease will depend on an assessment of valvular disease.

It is recommended that all patients with acute rheumatic fever be treated with a course of penicillin to eliminate the hemolytic *Streptococcus* from the pharynx. This is recommended even if the throat culture does not reveal group A beta-hemolytic streptococci, because these organisms may persist in areas where they remain undetected, such as the crypts of the tonsils. Parenteral penicillin is the drug of choice unless there is a history of allergy to it. Three hundred thousand units of procaine penicillin G once a day in children and twice a day in adults for ten days is an effective dose. A single dose of 1.2 million units of long-acting benzathine penicillin is preferred by many, as the one injection facilitates administration. Oral penicillin, 200,000 units four times a day, also for ten days, is acceptable therapy, but requires careful supervision in order to be sure that all doses are taken without fail. If there is a history of penicillin allergy, the drug of choice is erythromycin. The dose is 250 mg four times a day for ten days. Sulfonamide in any form should never be used. After completion of the ten-day course of penicillin or erythromycin, a continuous prophylaxis regimen should be started to prevent reinfection with group A streptococci and to reduce the risk of recurrent attacks of acute rheumatic fever (see Ch. 128). Prevention of infective endocarditis is an important aspect in the management of patients with rheumatic heart disease. This is discussed in Ch. 131.

Aspirin and Steroid Therapy. Most patients respond rapidly to either steroid or aspirin therapy. After one or two weeks, arthritis and fever have disappeared, and the acute phase reactants frequently have returned to normal, or nearly so. On occasion, neither fever nor arthritis responds to full aspirin dosage, and steroids are required to control the disease. Many, but not all, clinicians favor use of steroids in nearly all patients with carditis. It is certainly indicated in patients with severe carditis and pancarditis. Some prefer to withdraw the steroid treatment after several weeks and continue treatment by substituting aspirin. Others continue steroid therapy for the full course. The arthritis in nearly all patients responds readily to aspirin alone. The evidence remains equivocal for the beneficial effect of steroid therapy in preventing the development of permanent rheumatic heart disease, even though there is apparent clinical improvement in the acute carditis when steroids are used.

It should be stressed again that when full and adequate treatment eliminates all the clinical manifestations of the disease, including laboratory abnormalities, the underlying disease process is still continuing unabated for its natural course. If the drugs are withdrawn before the process is at an end, the disease with all its clinical manifestations will recur. Duration of therapy is discussed below.

The daily dose of aspirin is 60 mg per pound of body weight. The actual dose per day varies from 3 grams in young children to 10 grams in adults. It is preferable to give this total amount in at least six divided doses. Aspirin should be given throughout the 24-hour day, at least during the early stages of the disease. Individual variation in the efficacy of absorption or excretion of the drug and in its therapeutic effectiveness requires readjustment of the dose in many cases. The aim is to give the minimal dose that results in full control of symptoms and to avoid serious toxic side reactions because of overdosage. Studies on the concentration of salicylates in the blood have shown that optimal therapeutic effect usually requires at least 25 mg per 100 ml of serum. The optimal therapeutic range is between 25 and 35 mg per 100 ml of serum. Levels greater than the upper limit are associated with toxicity. When aspirin is given in conjunction with the prednisone, it is frequently necessary to give a daily dose of aspirin larger than that recommended above in order to achieve the therapeutic salicylate level. Furthermore, as aspirin is continued upon the withdrawal of prednisone, less aspirin is frequently required to maintain an adequate serum salicylate level.

The most common toxic manifestations of aspirin therapy are nausea, vomiting, and gastric distress. Tinnitus and partial but temporary impairment of hearing usually occur only at full therapeutic dosage. Hyperpnea frequently results from central stimulatory action in respiration and can lead to alkalosis. It is uncommon to see the more severe metabolic disturbances of acute salicylate toxicity.

In practice, nausea and vomiting are the most frequent complications that result from starting aspirin. This can be minimized if the initial daily dosage is below the optimum and then is gradually increased over a period of a few days. Attempts to achieve full and optimal salicylate levels within 24 hours often result in severe nausea and vomiting. In such cases it may be difficult to reach an effective therapeutic level of salicylate, and in such instances steroids afford an alternative therapeutic approach. The use of sodium bicarbonate to reduce gastric irritation is not recommended, as it increases the excretion of salicylate and interferes with the maintenance of an anti-inflammatory concentration of the drug in the blood. If a portion of the aspirin is given as enteric-coated pills, some degree of gastric irritation can be eliminated.

Prednisone is the recommended steroid because a low salt diet and added potassium are usually not required. There is no firm agreement on the dosage of this drug. The usual procedure is to begin with a relatively large daily dose until activity of the disease appears to be under control, and then to reduce the dosage to the minimal amount that will maintain the full effect. In the experience of many, the total daily dosage of 0.3 to 0.5 mg per pound given in divided doses is adequate to bring the signs of inflammation, including fever, rapidly under control. Almost all signs and symptoms are suppressed in two or three days. It is at this point that the daily dose may be reduced. After two or three weeks of steroid therapy, some prefer to shift to aspirin, particularly for those patients without carditis. The advantage of this is that most side effects of prolonged steroid therapy, such as the mild manifestations of Cushing's disease, are avoided. Prolonged use of steroid therapy may lead to complications, such as infections, growth retardation, gastric ulcers, and toxic psychoses.

The treatment of chorea is symptomatic. There is no evidence that either steroids or aspirin have any influence on the symptoms of chorea. The usual case lasts from two weeks to several months, but in rare instances it may persist longer. Nevertheless, almost without exception, complete recovery is the rule. Many patients show improvement when bright light, noise, and undue activity are eliminated from their bedroom. In some cases, measures must be taken to prevent self-injury from violent chorea movements, including tongue-biting. Phenobarbital and other sedatives may be helpful.

Duration of Therapy. The duration of therapy bears some relationship to the severity of the acute manifestations. The disease process in the typical mild case without carditis subsides in three to four weeks. When severe arthritis and carditis are present, the natural course lasts two to three months. Such estimates for the duration of the disease can be used to determine the termination of therapy, recognizing, however, that disease activity in the occasional case may persist for many months. Laboratory tests such as determination of the sedimentation rate and the C-reactive protein assume normal values during the course of adequate therapy. For this reason, they cannot be used to determine the duration of therapy.

Many clinicians prefer to withdraw either aspirin or steroid therapy gradually over a period of one or two weeks. After withdrawal, a clinical "rebound" is commonly seen. This may be so mild that only the acute phase reactants indicate its occurrence, but not uncommonly clinical manifestations are present. These may be mild or severe, and include fever, arthritis, and tachycardia. Usually the rebound subsides in five to ten days without use of anti-inflammatory drugs. The occurrence of positive C-reactive protein, an elevated sedimentation rate, and an elevated white count, without significant clinical manifestations, is not sufficient grounds for reinstituting therapy. But progressive clinical severity and particularly the emergence of severe carditis may require reinstitution of therapy. In such instances, it is assumed that the natural duration of the disease has yet to run its course. In practice, if therapy must be reinstated because of the emergence of carditis, the drugs are continued for another three to four weeks.

If no significant rebound occurs, ambulation should begin, and usually full activity, except vigorous exercise, may be permitted three to four weeks after the termination of therapy. If persistent rheumatic heart disease is present, the permissible level of physical activity is determined by an assessment of its severity.

PREVENTION. Prior to the days of antimicrobial drugs, measures were not available to prevent recurrences of rheumatic fever. Now properly supervised continuous chemoprophylaxis is effective in preventing these recurrences, and it should be employed for all patients with a well-documented history of rheumatic fever or unequivocal evidence of rheumatic heart disease. Prophylaxis prevents streptococcal pharyngitis and therefore the recurrences of rheumatic fever.

A detailed consideration of drug regimens for prophylaxis has been presented in Ch. 128. Intramuscular benzathine penicillin, 1.2 million units each month, is the preferred drug and route of administration. Such a route of administration does not leave open to question the degree of patient compliance, as is the case with orally administered penicillin.

The duration of antimicrobial prophylaxis should be extended through childhood. In the case of adolescents and adults, it should not be terminated as long as the patient is associated with population groups that have high attack rates of streptococcal infections, such as military recruits, schoolchildren, medical personnel, and school teachers. Because of the risk of additional valvular damage during a recurrence, *prophylaxis should be continued for life for all patients with definite rheumatic heart disease.* Contrary to popular belief, people in late middle age can have a recurrence of rheumatic fever after streptococcal pharyngitis.

Epidemiologic studies clearly indicate that streptococcal disease spreads in the home and in the school. The physician must be alert to the occurrence of streptococcal pharyngitis in the family and the school of the patient on prophylaxis. This is a potential risk to the patient, and strict compliance with the prophylaxis must be urged. If streptococcal disease occurs in the family, it should be treated with adequate antimicrobial drugs.

For a number of reasons, the prevention of first attacks of rheumatic fever is difficult to achieve. Prompt recognition and treatment of streptococcal pharyngitis is hampered in a number of cases by the fact that the symptoms are so mild that the patient does not see a physician. Not uncommonly, when the patient is seen by a doctor, the disease is misdiagnosed or the antimicrobial therapy prescribed is inadequate. For example, the tetracyclines should never be used to treat streptococcal pharyngitis, because 25 to 40 per cent of all group A streptococci are now resistant to this family of drugs.

The occasion arises when special measures are needed to control epidemics of streptococcal pharyngitis in a school or a community or in an army recruit camp. Several unexpected cases of rheumatic fever in a short period of time in a small population group should alert the physician to the possibility that there is a serious streptococcal epidemic in the community in question. Methods to curtail such epidemics have been described in Ch. 129.

PROGNOSIS. Recovery from the acute attack is the rule. Death at this stage is very rare, even in cases of severe carditis, because of the anti-inflammatory effects of steroid therapy. The disease process in mild cases of rheumatic fever without carditis usually subsides in two to four weeks, and the patient usually makes a complete recovery. When carditis is present, the disease usually persists for six weeks to three months. Patients with carditis during the acute attack may progress to valvular rheumatic heart disease. This is less common in patients without carditis, but absence of carditis during an acute attack is unfortunately not an absolute guarantee against the development of subsequent valvular deformity. Approximately one third of the rheumatic fever patients develop valvular heart disease.

Chronic disability and death owing to rheumatic heart disease are related to recurrent attacks. In former years, before antimicrobial therapy, patients who had had rheumatic fever usually suffered recurrences. Additional valvular deformity was the frequent outcome of each recurrence. As a result, a progressive severity of rheumatic heart disease was common. In current times the prognosis is more optimistic. Progressively severe valvular deformity after an initial attack, if recurrences are prevented, appears to be much less common than in former times, but this point requires further epidemiologic study. The efficacy of adequate chemoprophylaxis in the prevention of recurrences is clearly documented. In one study more than two thirds of the patients with a history of rheumatic fever who were not on prophylaxis had one or more recurrences over an eight-year follow-up period. If prophylaxis is adequately supervised and the drug is taken without fail, a recurrence is an extremely uncommon event.

Kuttner, A. G., and Mayer, F. E.: Carditis during second attacks of rheumatic fever: Its incidence in patients without clinical evidence of cardiac involvement in their initial rheumatic episode. N. Engl. J. Med., 268:1259, 1963.

Lendrum, B. L., Simon, A. J., and Mack, I.: Relation of duration of bed rest in acute rheumatic fever to heart disease present 2 to 14 years later. Pediatrics, 24:389, 1959.

Markowitz, M., and Gordis, L.: Rheumatic Fever. 2nd ed. Philadelphia, W. B. Saunders Company, 1972.

McCarty, M.: Missing links in the streptococcal chain leading to rheumatic fever: The T. Duckett Jones Memorial Lecture. Circulation, 24:488, 1964.

United Kingdom and United States Joint Report: The natural history of rheumatic fever and rheumatic heart disease: Ten-year report of a co-operative clinical trial of ACTH, cortisone, and aspirin. Circulation, 32:457, 1965.

Wood, H. F., and McCarty, M.: Laboratory aids in the diagnosis of rheumatic fever and in evaluation of disease activity. Am. J. Med., 17:768, 1954.

Zabriskie, J. B., Hsu, K. C., and Seegal, G. C.: Heart-reactive antibody associated with rheumatic fever: Characterization and diagnostic significance. Clin. Exp. Immunol., 7:147, 1970.

ENDOCARDITIS

131. INFECTIVE ENDOCARDITIS

Donald Kaye

DEFINITION

Infective endocarditis is defined as infection on the endocardium. Most commonly a heart valve is involved, but infection may be on a septal defect or mural endocardium. Infection of an arteriovenous shunt or coarctation of the aorta is more properly called endarteritis. However, the clinical syndrome of endarteritis is similar to that of endocarditis, and therefore the discussion of endocarditis relates to both endocarditis and endarteritis.

CLASSIFICATION

For many years infective endocarditis has been classified by course into acute and subacute disease. *Acute endocarditis* is most frequently caused by *Staphylococcus aureus* (and occasionally by pneumococci, group A streptococci, gonococci, or other organisms); it often occurs on a normal heart valve and results in rapid severe destruction. Metastatic foci of infection are common. Untreated, the infection will kill in days to weeks. However, the mortality rate is high even with appropriate therapy. *Subacute endocarditis* is usually caused by streptococci of the viridans group and occurs on already damaged valves, producing additional damage slowly. Metastatic foci of infection are rare, and results of treatment are good. Without therapy the infection will take six or more weeks and even up to years to kill. The correlations between infecting organism, rapidity of the course, and underlying valvular disease are not perfect. For example, endocarditis caused by streptococci of the viridans group can occasionally cause endocarditis with an acute course on a normal valve, and *S. aureus* can cause subacute disease.

Although the division of infective endocarditis into acute and subacute forms is useful, it is more important to classify by infecting organism (e.g. enterococcal endocarditis, *S. aureus* endocarditis, and so on). The identity of the organism has implications for the course (i.e. acute or subacute), but more important, has therapeutic implications for the antimicrobial regimen.

MICROBIOLOGY

Almost any species of bacteria is capable of producing infective endocarditis. However, streptococci and staphylococci account for the vast majority of cases (over 90 per cent) in which an infecting organism can be identified.

STREPTOCOCCI. In most reported series, streptococci are the causative microorganisms in 60 to 80 per cent of cases of endocarditis with demonstrated bacteremia. Viridans streptococci (most commonly *S. sanguis* and *S. mitis*) are numerically the most important of the streptococci, accounting for about 50 per cent of the cases of streptococcal endocarditis. Enterococci are the next most frequent streptococci and cause about 15 per cent of cases. The remaining streptococci, including microaerophilic and anaerobic streptococci, nonhemolytic streptococci, group A beta-hemolytic streptococci, and streptococci of other groups, are isolated in the remainder of the cases. There has been a trend during the past 30 years toward an increasing incidence of enterococcal endocarditis and a decreasing incidence of viridans streptococcal endocarditis.

Enterococci and group A beta-hemolytic streptococci can attack normal or previously damaged heart valves and may cause rapid destruction. The other streptococci are much more likely to cause endocarditis on already damaged heart valves and rarely cause rapid destruction. Enterococci also can cause abscesses, e.g., in the spleen, which are uncommon with other streptococci.

STAPHYLOCOCCI. Staphylococci are the causative microorganisms in 10 to 30 per cent of cases of infective endocarditis with positive blood cultures. *S. aureus* is isolated much more frequently than *S. epidermidis*. If patients with acute endocarditis only are considered, *S. aureus* is the causative agent in the vast majority. In patients with subacute disease, *S. epidermidis* is found more often than *S. aureus*. The incidence of staphylococcal endocarditis has risen over the past 30 years, and part of the increase is attributable to the high frequency of staphylococcal endocarditis in narcotic addicts and in patients following cardiac surgery.

S. aureus attacks either normal or previously damaged heart valves and causes rapid destruction. The course is often fulminant, leading to death from overwhelming bacteremia within days or from heart failure within weeks. Abscesses are common at multiple sites (e.g., kidneys, lungs, brain, and heart). *S. epidermidis* usually attacks abnormal heart valves without causing rapid destruction.

S. PNEUMONIAE. The pneumococcus, which was responsible for 10 per cent or more of cases of endocarditis before the advent of antimicrobial therapy, is now an uncommon cause. This organism can attack normal or previously damaged heart valves and can cause rapid destruction with a fulminant course. The coexistence of

---

Differences Between Acute and Subacute Infective Endocarditis*

	Acute	Subacute
Causative agent	Capable of primary invasion (e.g., *S. aureus*)	Normally noninvasive, usually viridans streptococcus
Pre-existing valve damage	Often not present	Usually present
Metastatic foci of infection	Common	Rare
Duration if untreated	Days to weeks	Months to one to two years
Response of infection to appropriate chemotherapy	Cure rate of 50% or less	High cure rate

*Modified from Beeson, P. B.: Infective endocarditis. *In* Beeson, P. B., and McDermott, W. (eds.): Textbook of Medicine. 14th ed. Philadelphia, W. B. Saunders Company, 1975.

endocarditis in patients with pneumococcal meningitis and pneumonia is common (up to one third of cases).

N. GONORRHOEAE. Neisseria (notably gonococcus), once a common cause of endocarditis (5 to 10 per cent of cases), now rarely causes the disease. It can attack and rapidly destroy normal or previously damaged heart valves. Gonococcal endocarditis was a common cause of endocarditis involving the right side of the heart; 25 per cent of patients with gonococcal endocarditis in the older series had right-sided involvement. About 50 per cent had double daily temperature elevations, and jaundice was common. Both these manifestations are rare in other types of endocarditis.

OTHER BACTERIA. Almost all species of bacteria are reported as occasionally causing endocarditis, including the enteric gram-negative bacilli, *Salmonella, Streptobacillus, Serratia marcescens, Bacteroides, Hemophilus, Brucella,* meningococci, *Listeria,* and even diphtheroids. Gram-negative bacilli account for less than 5 per cent of cases of endocarditis but are common causes in drug addicts and patients with prosthetic heart valves.

FUNGI. *Candida, Aspergillus,* and *Histoplasma* species are the most common causes of fungal endocarditis, with *Candida* endocarditis occurring most frequently. In addition, *Blastomyces, Cryptococcus, Mucor, Torulopsis,* and other fungi can cause endocarditis. *C. albicans* is the most common candidal organism isolated, but *C. tropicalis, C. krusei, C. parapsilosis,* and other candidal species have also caused endocarditis. *Candida-* and *Aspergillus*-induced endocarditis often occur in patients with intravascular catheters who frequently have received corticosteroids, broad-spectrum antimicrobial drugs, or cytotoxic agents. Fungal endocarditis is common in narcotic addicts (*Candida*) and in patients following cardiac surgery (*Candida* and *Aspergillus*).

The course of fungal endocarditis is usually subacute. Large friable vegetations are common and give rise to large emboli, often to the lower extremities. In patients with prosthetic cardiac valves, malfunction of the valve may occur because of the size of the vegetations. The prognosis is grave in fungal endocarditis, partly because of the relatively poor activity of the available antifungal agents and their toxicity for man, features that make their use difficult.

OTHER MICROORGANISMS. Spirochetes (e.g., *Spirillum minus*), cell wall–deficient bacteria, rickettsiae (*Coxiella burnetii*), and the psittacosis agent have all been reported as rare causes of endocarditis.

EPIDEMIOLOGY

SEX AND AGE. The proportion of males is somewhat higher than that of females in most reported series. The mean age of patients with endocarditis has increased during the past 30 years: at present, mean ages in most series range from the mid 40's to the 50's, with 50 per cent or more being 50 years or older. The mean age of males with endocarditis is about six or seven years higher than the mean age of females. Endocarditis is uncommon in children.

UNDERLYING HEART DISEASE. *Rheumatic valvular disease* is the underlying cardiac disease in about 40 to 60 per cent of patients with infective endocarditis. The mitral valve is most commonly involved. Aortic valve infection is also common. Right-sided endocarditis occurs in fewer than 10 per cent of patients with endocarditis superimposed on rheumatic heart disease and usually involves the tricuspid valve.

Congenital heart disease is the underlying lesion in about 10 per cent of patients with endocarditis. Some of the congenital lesions that predispose to endocarditis are patent ductus arteriosus, ventricular septal defect, tetralogy of Fallot, coarctation of the aorta, pulmonary stenosis, and bicuspid aortic valve. In contrast, atrial septal defects of the secundum type rarely serve as an underlying lesion in endocarditis.

Degenerative heart disease can be a predisposing cardiac lesion in endocarditis. For example, endocarditis has been reported on a calcified mitral annulus and on valves with degenerative changes. Calcific aortic stenosis resulting from degenerative aortic valve disease or a bicuspid aortic valve is being seen with increasing frequency in the elderly and can serve as an underlying lesion for endocarditis. Infective endocarditis has also been reported in patients with *hypertrophic subaortic stenosis,* the *systolic click syndrome* (mitral valve prolapse), *Marfan's syndrome,* and *syphilitic aortic valve disease.*

A new and important cardiac lesion which serves as an underlying abnormality for production of endocarditis is the *prosthetic cardiac valve.* Similarly, intravascular sutures, pacemaker wires, and Teflon-Silastic tubes serve as predisposing factors to development of endocarditis or endarteritis. Arterioarterial or arteriovenous fistulas also predispose to endocarditis.

In 20 to 40 per cent of patients with infective endocarditis, *no underlying heart disease* can be recognized. It is likely that some of these patients have underlying lesions that are difficult to recognize (e.g., degenerative heart disease, hypertrophic subaortic stenosis, systolic click syndrome). Others probably have no underlying lesions at all.

PATHOGENESIS AND PATHOLOGY

The characteristic lesions of infective endocarditis are vegetations on the valve leaflets or elsewhere on the endocardium. The disease usually arises secondary to localization of microorganisms on a sterile thrombotic vegetation. This type of sterile vegetation is termed nonbacterial thrombotic endocarditis and may form as a result of trauma to the endothelial cells (e.g., from intracardiac foreign bodies). Thrombi also may form over a subendothelial inflammatory reaction, such as in acute rheumatic fever or myocardial infarction. Vegetations commonly on the mitral and aortic valves (marantic endocarditis) are found at autopsy in patients with wasting disease, particularly from malignant tumors. Infective endocarditis has complicated sterile thrombus formation in all these circumstances.

When bacteremia occurs, the surface of the vegetation can become secondarily infected and converted to the typical vegetation of infective endocarditis. This results from deposition of platelets and fibrin over the bacteria. The vegetation then becomes a "protected site" into which phagocytic cells penetrate poorly. Although healthy valves may develop the lesions of nonbacterial thrombotic endocarditis, damaged valves appear to be much more frequently affected.

HYDRODYNAMIC FORCES. Sites of involvement suggest an important role for hydrodynamic forces. Endocarditis occurs where blood flows through a narrow orifice at a high velocity from a high- to a low-pressure chamber. Lateral pressure is lowest and the velocity of blood greatest a short distance downstream from the opening between the two chambers. A decrease in lateral pressure lowers perfusion of the intima, perhaps resulting in an area more susceptible to infection. This is the location where infective endocarditis initially develops in patients with congenital heart defects or valvular insufficiency. For example, endocarditis is found immediately distal to the constriction in coarctation of the aorta, on the pulmonary artery immediately beyond the junction with the ductus in patent ductus arteriosus, and on the right side of the defect in ventricular septal defect.

Endocarditis does not usually occur when there is only a small pressure gradient, as in artrial septal defects, or when a congenital defect is large enough practically to abolish the pressure gradient. Valvular endocarditis occurs more frequently in valvular incompetence than in pure stenosis and is characteristically on the atrial side of the incompetent mitral valve and the ventricular surface of the incompetent aortic valve. A high velocity stream of blood can produce satellite-infected lesions at distant points of impact. The reported cures of endocarditis at the sites of patent ductus arteriosus and arteriovenous fistulas with surgical ligation alone emphasize the role of hydrodynamic factors in both the initiation and maintenance of the infective process.

Experimental observations suggest that a hyperdynamic state of the cardiovascular system alone can initiate nonbacterial and subsequently infective endocarditis. Spontaneous endocarditis of the mitral and aortic valves occurs in dogs following surgical production of large arteriovenous fistulas and has been described in patients with traumatic arteriovenous fistulas and in patients undergoing hemodialysis with surgically produced arteriovenous fistulas or shunts.

INHERENT PATHOGENICITY. Microorganisms that possess little pathogenicity in other situations, e.g., alpha-hemolytic (viridans) streptococci, usually implant on heart valves deformed by pre-existing disease, although more virulent microorganisms, e.g., S. aureus and pneumococci, can implant on apparently normal valves. Infective endocarditis is found at autopsy in as high as 65 per cent of patients with S. aureus bacteremia and in one-third of patients with both pneumococcal pneumonia and meningitis.

INVASION OF CIRCULATION. Organisms must gain access to the circulation in sufficient numbers for a sufficient interval for endocarditis to result. Invasion of the bloodstream occurs in many infections. For example, transient bacteremia is found in about 30 per cent of patients with early pneumococcal pneumonia and is seen following compression of infected foci (e.g., bones, gums, tonsils, boils, prostate, diverticula, and endometrium).

BACTEREMIA. Transient bacteremia is common during traumatic procedures involving the epithelial surfaces normally laden with an indigenous bacterial flora (oropharynx, genitourinary and gastrointestinal tracts, and skin). Surgical incision of the skin, ordinarily inhabited by staphylococci and diphtheroids, is often associated with bacteremia, usually staphylococcal (either S. aureus or S. epidermidis). Bacteremia occurs in about 25 per cent of patients after toothbrushing, chewing hard candy, or use of an oral irrigation device. Streptococci of the viridans group are the most common bacteria isolated from the blood, either alone or more often mixed with other bacteria, after trauma to the tissues of the mouth. In one study, following tooth extraction, over 90 per cent of patients had mixed bacteremia, which included viridans streptococci in 74 per cent and Bacteroides melaninogenicus in 61 per cent of bacteremic patients. Many other bacterial species are occasionally isolated from blood after dental procedures (peptostreptococci, diptheroids, peptococci, staphylococci, fusobacteria, actinomyces, veillonella, bacteroides, spirillum, and vibrios). The frequency of bacteremia is related to the degree of periodontal disease and to the amount of trauma.

PORTAL OF ENTRY. Although the portal of entry for the initiating episode of bacteremia in endocarditis is often not apparent, oral cavity infection or operative or manipulative dental procedures appear to be the most common clinically apparent portals of entry, especially in endocarditis caused by viridans streptococci. Endocarditis caused by viridans streptococci has also occurred in edentulous patients in association with oral ulcers from poorly fitting dentures.

The incidence of bacteremia after sigmoidoscopy and barium enema has been reported to be about 10 per cent, with one half caused by enterococci. Similarly, bacteremia occurs in up to one third of patients after transurethral prostatic resection, cystoscopy, urethral dilatation, and urethral catheterization. The organisms are usually enterococci and gram-negative bacilli.

Endocarditis, especially enterococcal endocarditis, has developed after urinary tract surgery or instrumentation, prostatic massage or resection, delivery, abortion, pelvic infection, operative intervention or instrumentation of the female reproductive tract, and placement of a contraceptive uterine device. Instrumentation of the gastrointestinal tract has occasionally been implicated as a portal of entry for microorganisms in patients with endocarditis.

Endocarditis has also followed intravenous injection in drug addicts and has occurred with the prolonged use of plastic intravenous catheters.

MECHANISMS IN PRODUCTION OF LESIONS. The pathogenesis of the manifestations of endocarditis is both a result of the vegetations themselves, and an *immue reaction* to the infection. The vegetations may become so extensive, especially in fungal endocarditis, that the valve orifice is occluded. There may be rapid, massive destruction of tissue with consequent valvular insufficiency, especially in S. aureus endocarditis. Areas of healing may cause scar formation and consequent valvular stenosis or insufficiency. Infection may extend along the chordae tendineae or into the myocardium from the periphery of the valve, e.g., into the mitral annulus or along the sinus of Valsalva into the aortic ring, producing burrowing abscesses. Conduction abnormalities, fistulas (between a chamber of the heart and either another chamber or the pericardium or major vessels), or rupture of the chordae, a papillary muscle, or the ventricular septum may result. Valve ring abscesses with conduction abnormalities carry a grave prognostic significance.

The vegetations, containing necrotic calcified infected debris, are friable, and pieces break off and are swept into the circulation. Multiple emboli occlude the blood supply both to the heart itself and to the brain, kidney, spleen, liver, extremities, and lung (in endocarditis of the right side of the heart). Infarcts and perhaps abscesses (with *S. aureus* endocarditis) result at these sites. Septic embolization to the vasa vasorum or direct bacterial invasion of the arterial wall may result in formation of mycotic aneurysms which may rupture. Aneurysms involve medium or large arteries frequently at bifurcations. They most often develop in the cerebral arteries, abdominal aorta, sinus of Valsalva, ligated ductus arteriosus, and superior mesenteric, splenic, coronary, and pulmonary arteries. Vessels within the head are involved in about 50 per cent of the cases, vessels within the abdomen and chest in about 40 per cent, and vessels in the limbs in about 10 per cent of cases.

In addition, vasculitis on an immunologic basis is thought to contribute to the findings. Patients with infective endocarditis usually have high circulating antibody titers against the infecting microorganism. This contributes to the formation of immune complexes. Complexes composed of immunoglobulin and complement have been demonstrated in the glomeruli of patients with endocarditis and diffuse glomerulonephritis. In addition to glomerulonephritis, Roth's spots, petechiae, and Osler's nodes are thought to usually be due to allergic vasculitis. In contrast, Janeway's lesions are thought to be on an embolic basis.

Myocarditis is an important complication of endocarditis. Although its exact pathogenesis is still undetermined, present theories include ischemic damage secondary to coronary artery occlusion by emboli, damage produced by microbial toxins, myocardial invasion by organisms, or the result of immune complex deposition in blood vessels. Myocardial abscesses or myocardial infarction secondary to an arterial embolus may occur.

In addition to emboli or abscess formation, the kidneys may be involved with focal embolic glomerulitis or diffuse glomerulonephritis. The diffuse glomerulonephritis has been shown to be related to immune complex deposition, and it is likely that the focal type has the same cause. Focal glomerulitis occurs in over half of patients with subacute endocarditis. Diffuse glomerulonephritis is less common.

CLINICAL MANIFESTATIONS

In most patients with infective endocarditis, no event can be identified as the etiologic factor in the endocarditis. A history of a dental procedure can be elicited in only 15 to 20 per cent of patients with endocarditis caused by streptococci of the viridans group. About 50 per cent of patients with enterococcal endocarditis have had a preceding urologic or genital tract procedure, and about 35 per cent of patients with staphylococcal endocarditis have a history of a preceding staphylococcal infection. Symptoms of endocarditis generally start within two or three weeks of the procedure. The onset is usually gradual, with mild fever and malaise with endocarditis caused by streptococci of the viridans group and other organisms of low pathogenicity. With *S. aureus*, pneumococci and other organisms of high pathogenicity, the onset is often acute with high fever.

For purposes of orientation, it may be helpful to present prototypes of patients with the syndromes of subacute and acute bacterial endocarditis.

SUBACUTE ENDOCARDITIS. A 44-year-old white man with rheumatic heart disease was admitted to the hospital with four weeks of malaise, weakness, and anorexia without any cardiac symptoms. Erythromycin had been given from 12 to 7 days prior to admission, during which time the patient felt better. However, symptoms returned several days after stopping the drug. During the illness he had lost 10 pounds. There was no recent history of a dental procedure. Although he denied fever, a rectal temperature was found to be 38.4° C. Murmurs of mitral stenosis and mitral insufficiency were heard. There were no petechiae, but an enlarged spleen was palpated. He was started on antimicrobial therapy, and subsequently five blood cultures, taken at time of admission, were positive for viridans streptococci (*S. mitis*).

ACUTE ENDOCARDITIS. A 60-year-old female who had been in good health was admitted to the hospital with a history of sudden onset of high fever and recurrent shaking chills starting five days before and dyspnea starting on the day of admission. There was no history of heart disease. The rectal temperature was 40° C, and the blood pressure was 160/40 mm Hg. Bibasilar rales and a loud murmur of aortic insufficiency were present. There were no petechiae or splenomegaly. Although antimicrobial therapy was promptly initiated on the night of admission, she developed severe pulmonary edema, had a cardiac arrest, and died. Five of five blood cultures, taken at time of admission, were subsequently positive for *S. aureus*.

FEVER. Fever is present in almost all patients during the course of endocarditis. Most exceptions are elderly patients or patients with renal failure, congestive heart failure, or severe debility. The temperature is usually low grade (less than 39.4° C) except with acute disease.

CARDIAC MURMUR. Cardiac murmurs are almost always present except with acute endocarditis or in intravenous narcotic addicts. Those who develop endocarditis secondary to intravenous drug abuse often have vegetations on the tricuspid valve, and murmurs are frequently absent. True changes in murmurs or the appearance of a new murmur is uncommon except in acute endocarditis in which a new murmur (particularly aortic insufficiency) is a frequent occurrence. Changes in the intensities of murmurs during the course of endocarditis are often due to changes in heart rate and/or cardiac output such as occur with development of anemia and do not necessarily indicate progressive valvular damage.

SPLENOMEGALY. Splenomegaly is present in 25 to 60 per cent of reported cases of endocarditis and is most common in disease of long duration (i.e., less common in acute endocarditis).

PETECHIAE. Petechiae are present in 20 to 40 per cent of patients, most commonly in patients with more prolonged illness. Petechiae are most frequently found in the conjunctivae, palate, buccal mucosa, and extremities. Care must be taken in the interpretation of petechiae in areas of the body where they may have been induced by local trauma, such as the hard palate in patients with poorly fitting dentures or the lower conjunctival sac in women who wear eye makeup. Petechiae may also be found in elderly persons in whom there is no evidence of infection.

OTHER SIGNS. *Splinter hemorrhages* are subungual, linear, dark red streaks that may appear in endocarditis, but are also commonly the result of local trauma. What are commonly called *Roth's spots* are oval, retinal hemorrhages with a clear pale center. These are seen in less than 5 per cent of patients with endocarditis and may also occur in collagen vascular diseases and in severe anemia. *Osler's nodes* are small tender nodules most frequently found on the finger or toe pads which persist for hours to days. They are found in 10 to 25 per cent of patients with endocarditis, but also occur in other diseases such as typhoid fever and collagen vascular disease; they are uncommon in acute endocarditis. *Clubbing of the fingers* is present in some patients, usually those with longstanding disease. *Janeway's lesions* are nontender, macular, hemorrhagic areas on the palms and soles most commonly seen in acute endocarditis.

EMBOLIC EPISODES. Clinically apparent embolic episodes are recognized in about one third of patients with endocarditis and may occur early (as the first symptom) or late (after successful therapy). Splenic emboli with infarction may cause left upper quadrant pain radiating to the shoulder. Retinal emboli cause blindness, and coronary artery emboli can cause myocardial infarction. Emboli to large arteries such as the femoral or brachial arteries are often the result of fungal endocarditis with its large friable cardiac vegetations. Pulmonary emboli often occur in right-sided carditis, especially common in narcotic addicts, in whom the emboli may be the presenting symptoms. Pulmonary emboli may also be seen in endocarditis in patients with congenital heart disease with left-to-right shunts.

MYCOTIC ANEURYSMS. Mycotic aneurysms occur in about 15 per cent of patients with infective endocarditis, most commonly with less virulent organisms such as viridans streptococci. The aneurysms are most often found in the brain, where they tend to be small. Symptoms from mycotic aneurysms are usually lacking but may be those of an expanding mass until rupture occurs. These lesions can rupture at any time before, during, or even years after therapy for endocarditis.

NEUROLOGIC MANIFESTATIONS. Neurologic manifestations are present in about one third of patients with endocarditis. Major cerebral emboli occur not infrequently and usually involve the middle cerebral artery system. Mycotic aneurysms also most often involve this system. Rupture results in hemorrhage into the brain, ventricle, or subarachnoid space. Patients with endocarditis can also develop toxic encephalopathy and/or personality changes. Brain abscess and purulent meningitis are most common with *S. aureus* endocarditis.

CONGESTIVE HEART FAILURE. Congestive heart failure is a frequent complication of endocarditis and may occur at any time during the course of the disease, including long after cure. It carries a bad prognosis. Some of the factors which contribute to heart failure are valve destruction, myocarditis from vasculitis, coronary artery emboli with infarction, and myocardial abscesses.

RENAL DISEASE. Renal disease is present in most patients with infective endocarditis. Up to 50 per cent of endocarditis patients have microscopic hematuria, and proteinuria is even more common. These findings may be due to renal emboli, focal embolic glomerulitis, or diffuse glomerulonephritis. Renal insufficiency may occur in diffuse glomerulonephritis but is rare as a consequence of emboli or focal embolic glomerulitis.

SPECIAL SYNDROMES

ENTEROCOCCAL ENDOCARDITIS. Enterococci (*S. faecalis* varieties *zymogenes* and *liquefaciens*, *S. faecium*, and *S. durans*) are alpha-, beta-, or gamma-hemolytic streptococci that are normal inhabitants of the gastrointestinal tract, the anterior urethra, and occasionally the mouth of man. Enterococci may be distinguished from other streptococci by their ability to grow in media containing sodium azide, 0.1 per cent methylene blue, 40 per cent bile, or 6.5 per cent sodium chloride and to grow at 45° C. All enterococci are in Lancefield's group D, although all organisms in group D are not enterococci.

Two other group D streptococci, *S. bovis* and *S. equinus*, should be separated from the enterococci, because endocarditis caused by these two species can be treated like endocarditis caused by viridans streptococci. To separate *S. bovis* and *S. equinus* from the enterococci, biochemical tests must be performed, such as the ability to grow in 6.5 per cent sodium chloride broth. For all practical purposes *S. bovis* and *S. equinus* can be demonstrated not to be enterococci by the fact that they are highly susceptible to penicillin G (inhibited by 0.1 μg per milliliter), whereas enterococci are much more resistant.

Enterococcal endocarditis is more common in men than in women. The average age for males is near 60 years, whereas in women it is just under 40 years. This age distribution is probably closely related to the suspected portal of entry of the organism. About 50 per cent of patients give a history of genitourinary tract manipulation, trauma, or disease within three months of their admission to the hospital. For men this usually means cystoscopy, urethral catheterization, or prostatectomy, thus explaining the older age in males. For women the genitourinary factors are abortions, pregnancy, cesarean section, and urethral catheterization. Since many of these manipulations occur mainly during the childbearing years, this explains the lower age of female patients.

About one half of the patients with enterococcal endocarditis have no prior history of heart murmurs, indicating the ability of enterococci to attack normal heart valves. There is a tendency to form metastatic abscesses.

ENDOCARDITIS IN DRUG ABUSERS. Infective endocarditis is a complication of parenteral narcotic addiction. In these patients bacteremia may result from cellulitis or phlebitis at sites of injection or from drug contamination with virulent microorganisms. The skin is probably the most common source of microorganisms responsible for endocarditis in the addict. *S. aureus* is responsible for over 50 per cent of cases, and fungi (mainly *Candida*) and gram-negative bacilli (about one-third of which are *Pseudomonas* species) cause most of the remaining cases. Viridans streptococci are uncommon infecting agents in endocarditis in addicts.

Only about 20 per cent of narcotic addicts presenting with their first episode of endocarditis appear to have previously damaged heart valves. The tricuspid valve is infected in over 50 per cent of addicts, the aortic in 35 per cent and the mitral in about 30 per cent. There is a striking association of *S. aureus* endocarditis with tricuspid valve involvement; over 75 per cent with *S. aureus* infection have endocarditis on the tricuspid valve. Gram-negative bacilli also commonly involve the tricuspid valve (about 50 per cent of gram-negative bacillary cases), whereas fungi and streptococci (often enterococci) usually involve the left side of the heart.

Signs and symptoms of pulmonary emboli or pneumonia related to septic pulmonary emboli are common presentations in addicts with tricuspid valve endocarditis, and murmurs are frequently absent.

PROSTHETIC VALVE ENDOCARDITIS. The widespread use of prosthetic heart valves (and other intracardiac foreign bodies such as sutures or pacemaker wires) has created a new form of endocarditis. An intracardiac prosthesis predisposes to the development of endocarditis and makes eradication of the infection extremely difficult.

Endocarditis occurs at least two or three times more frequently after insertion of a prosthetic heart valve than after other open-heart operations and has been reported to occur in 1 to 3 per cent of patients with prosthetic valves. Endocarditis is much more likely to occur on aortic than mitral valve prostheses. The infection is usually found on the suture line.

Prosthetic valve endocarditis is usually divided into early endocarditis (onset within two months of valve replacement) and late endocarditis (onset after two months). Early endocarditis is a consequence of contamination during the surgical procedure or bacteremia in the postoperative period, whereas late endocarditis is probably related to episodes of transient bacteremia associated with dental, skin, and genitourinary tract trauma or infections.

The causative microorganisms in prosthetic valve endocarditis differ from those usually seen in other patients with endocarditis. About one third of both early and late endocarditis episodes are caused by staphylococci, with S. epidermidis occurring as a more frequent infecting organism than S. aureus. Gram-negative bacilli cause up to 25 per cent of early cases and are less common in late endocarditis. Fungi (most commonly Candida) are responsible for up to 25 per cent of early cases and are much less common in late endocarditis. Streptococci are the most frequent single causes of late endocarditis (about 40 per cent of cases) but are uncommon infecting organisms in early endocarditis. Diphtheroids have been the infecting organisms in up to 20 per cent of early cases and are less common in late endocarditis.

Early prosthetic valve endocarditis is often associated with valve dysfunction or dehiscence and a fulminant course. Although late endocarditis may have a similar clinical course, it is commonly characterized by a clinical syndrome indistinguishable from that occurring in patients without prosthetic valves. This is especially likely when the infecting organism is a streptococcus.

LABORATORY FINDINGS

Anemia is an almost constant finding in infective endocarditis except in acute cases. The anemia is usually normocytic and normochromic. Most patients with endocarditis have normal white blood cell and differential counts. However, in acute disease, leukocytosis may be present. Proteinuria, gross or microscopic hematuria, or both are present in most patients. The erythrocyte sedimentation rate is almost always elevated except in the presence of congestive heart failure. In those with severe renal complications (usually diffuse glomerulonephritis), the blood urea nitrogen or serum creatinine may be elevated.

About 50 per cent of patients with endocarditis of at least several weeks' duration have a positive serum test for rheumatoid factor. This tends to disappear with cure of endocarditis. The serum complement may be decreased, especially in patients with glomerulonephritis. Large mononuclear cells have been described in the first drop of blood obtained after massage of the ear lobe ("ear lobe histiocytes") in about 25 per cent of patients with endocarditis. These cells are found in other chronic infections such as typhoid fever and malaria.

The demonstration of serum antibodies to teichoic acid (a major cell wall antigen in S. aureus) may be helpful in suggesting the possibility of endocarditis in a patient presenting with staphylococcal bacteremia. Bacteria can be seen inside leukocytes in buffy coat preparations of blood in about 50 per cent of patients with bacterial endocarditis.

The single most important finding in patients with endocarditis is bacteremia or fungemia. Blood cultures should be obtained promptly in anyone with suspected endocarditis and should be positive in over 95 per cent of patients. The bacteremia of endocarditis is constant; if any cultures are positive, it is likely that all will be positive. Therefore there is no advantage to obtaining cultures at any particular time or level of body temperature. Culture of arterial blood or marrow offers no advantage over culture of antecubital vein blood.

In patients with subacute disease who have not received previous antimicrobial therapy, five blood cultures should be obtained over a period of 12 to 24 hours and therapy initiated. If previous therapy has been given, treatment may be expeditiously delayed in an attempt to obtain positive blood cultures. In general, in acute disease therapy should not be delayed for more than two to three hours while obtaining cultures. Proper technique of blood culture involves thorough cleansing of the skin with a bactericidal disinfectant (e.g., 70 per cent alcohol and iodine), obtaining only one culture from each venipuncture, using anaerobic as well as aerobic techniques, keeping cultures for three weeks, and making periodic blind Gram stains and subcultures. In selected patients (especially those who have received previous antimicrobial therapy), cultures in hypertonic media may be helpful in an attempt to isolate cell-wall deficient forms.

Blood cultures have usually been negative in those rare cases of endocarditis caused by *Aspergillus*, *Histoplasma*, and *Coxiella burnetii*. In fungal endocarditis, large emboli to the lower extremities are common, necessitating embolectomy. Histologic examination and culture of the embolus may be diagnostic. Serologic tests for *C. burnetii* are positive in patients with endocarditis caused by this organism. Blood cultures may be sterile in patients with *Brucella* endocarditis unless special techniques are used.

Echocardiograms, although not diagnostic, may suggest the location of a vegetation. Serial phonocardiography and cineradiography are useful in evaluating patients with prosthetic valve endocarditis for valve dysfunction or dehiscence. Disappearance of an opening or closing click suggests presence of a vegetation on the valve; this is especially likely to occur with large vegetations, as are seen in fungal endocarditis. Cineradiography of the valve will show abnormal motion if the sutures are pulling out.

DIFFERENTIAL DIAGNOSIS

The possibility of infective endocarditis should be suspected in any patient with a heart murmur and unexplained fever present for at least one week. However, many other diseases can present with these same manifestations. A definitive diagnosis can be made only in the presence of positive blood cultures. In the small percentage of patients with sterile blood cultures, the differential diagnosis can be very difficult.

Some of the clinical entities which can exactly duplicate the syndrome of infective endocarditis (including fever, murmur, and emboli) are atrial myxoma and nonbacterial thrombotic endocarditis. Acute rheumatic fever, lupus erythematosus, and sickle cell disease can also produce fever and heart murmur. Any patient with an existing heart murmur can develop fever related to another illness such as infectious mononucleosis, toxoplasmosis, multiple pulmonary emboli, miliary tuberculosis, or lymphoma. Drug fever is another important possibility. Therefore in the absence of positive blood cultures, a search must be made for other causes of fever.

Following cardiac surgery, fever may be related to bacterial infection at sites other than the prosthetic valve, to the postcardiotomy syndrome, or to a "post-pump syndrome" (e.g., cytomegalovirus infection).

TREATMENT

Principles of Therapy

In order to achieve cure of infective endocarditis, it is necessary to eradicate essentially all microorganisms from the vegetation. Unlike other infections, inhibition of growth of the microorganism is not adequate for cure, because the cellular and humoral host defense mechanisms that normally eliminate organisms from other sites are not very effective in the vegetation of endocarditis. Therefore *bactericidal drug regimens are necessary in therapy of endocarditis, and treatment must be continued for a long enough period of time to achieve sterilization of the vegetation.* In addition, sufficient concentrations of antimicrobial agents must be reached in the serum to guarantee penetration of antibacterial concentrations into the vegetation. Available evidence indicates that if peak serum concentrations are bactericidal for the infecting microorganism at a 1:8 dilution in normal serum, therapy is probably adequate. Except for unusual circumstances, the route of administration should be parenteral to guarantee adequate absorption of drugs.

Different regimens have been used in therapy of infective endocarditis. One fact that seems incontrovertible is that therapeutic regimens, including penicillins and cephalosporins (and perhaps vancomycin), give far better results than regimens in which these drugs cannot be used either because of resistance of the organisms or because of drug reactions.

Drug susceptibility tests using disks are usually not very helpful in management of patients with bacterial endocarditis; more precise determinations of bacteriostatic and bactericidal end-points by broth dilution tests are necessary. These tests are critical when infection is caused by organisms other than gram-positive cocci, treatment has failed, or drug regimens other than penicillins or cephalosporins must be used. In vitro tests are also helpful in selecting appropriate drug combinations and in determining the dilution at which the patient's serum is bactericidal for the infecting organism. Once the infecting microorganism is isolated, it should be saved for future testing (e.g., serum antibacterial activity, evaluation of different antimicrobial drugs, or comparison with a strain obtained during relapse).

Intravascular catheters are to be avoided in treatment of endocarditis, as their use increases the risk of superinfection of the vegetation. This does not seem to be a problem with intravascular needles. Anticoagulants were used at one time to reduce the size of the vegetation in conjunction with antimicrobial drugs. However, the increased risk of hemorrhage (especially intracranial) far outweighs any advantage.

Specific Antimicrobial Regimens

The initial treatment of subacute infective endocarditis while awaiting culture results should be directed at the most common infecting organism, the streptococcus. As enterococci require the most vigorous therapy, the regimen is directed against the enterococcus. However, if the course is acute, if the patient has an intracardiac foreign body, or if the patient is a parenteral drug abuser, therapy for staphylococcal endocarditis must be added. This is the principle of initially treating for the most resistant infecting organism likely to be present. However, once the infecting organism is isolated, the regimen should promptly be altered. For example, if a streptococcus highly susceptible to penicillin is isolated, there would be no need for antistaphylococcal agents, and the dose of streptomycin would be decreased or stopped to avoid ototoxicity. In the event that cultures remain sterile and culture-negative endocarditis is felt to be present, treatment for enterococcal endocarditis is continued for six weeks, provided that the response is adequate.

STREPTOCOCCI. *Streptococci inhibited by 0.1 μg per milliliter penicillin G:* (These are classified as *penicillin-susceptible* and include over 90 per cent of viridans streptococci but no enterococci.) Although penicillin alone is highly active in vitro against these strains, the combination of penicillin and streptomycin exerts a more rapid bactericidal action than does penicillin alone. Three regimens have been widely used: (1) penicillin alone for four weeks in doses of 4 to 5 million units daily, which results in a low relapse rate (e.g., 1 per cent) after therapy is stopped; (2) penicillin and streptomycin in combination for two weeks, which results in a relapse rate of about 5 per cent; and (3) penicillin plus streptomycin for two weeks with penicillin therapy extended another two weeks, which results in essentially no relapses.

The writer's preferred regimen is procaine penicillin, 1.2 million units administered intramuscularly every six hours for four weeks, plus streptomycin, 0.5 gram given intramuscularly every 12 hours for the first two weeks. If the patient prefers intravenous infusions, penicillin G can be given intravenously in doses of 10 to 20 million units each day rather than by intramuscular injections. If penicillin is contraindicated because of hypersensitivity, cephalothin or cefazolin can be given instead in doses of 2 grams every four hours or 1 to 2 grams every six hours, respectively. Cephalosporins should be administered for four weeks, together with streptomycin for the first two weeks. Patients who are hypersensitive to penicillin may also be hypersensitive to the cephalosporins. If neither penicillin nor a cephalosporin can be used, vancomycin can be given intravenously in a dose of 0.5 gram every six hours for four weeks, together with streptomycin for the first two weeks.

In these regimens, streptomycin should be discontinued if vestibular toxicity occurs and should not be used if renal insufficiency is present.

Streptococci resistant to 0.1 μg per milliliter penicillin G: (These are classified as *relatively resistant to penicillin* and include all enterococci and up to 10 per cent of viridans streptococci.) Larger doses of penicillin must be used in these patients than are used for the therapy of endocarditis caused by penicillin-susceptible streptococci. Penicillin or ampicillin alone is inadequate therapy for enterococcal endocarditis, and an aminoglycoside must be added. In vitro, streptomycin combined with penicillin provides a more rapid and more complete bactericidal effect than penicillin alone against the majority of strains of enterococci. Some strains of enterococci do not demonstrate this in vitro effect with penicillin and streptomycin but do with penicillin and gentamicin. The enterococci that demonstrate a more rapid and complete bactericidal effect in the presence of streptomycin are inhibited by 2000 μg per milliliter, and those that do not are resistant to 2000 μg per milliliter of streptomycin. Thus this simple in vitro test can help predict which strains will or will not demonstrate the penicillin-streptomycin potentiation.

The therapy recommended for *enterococcal endocarditis* is aqueous penicillin G, 20 million units daily intravenously by continuous drip for six weeks, plus streptomycin, 1 gram every 12 hours intramuscularly for the first two weeks, followed by 0.5 gram every 12 hours for the remaining four weeks. The serum antibacterial activity should be determined, and if a 1:8 dilution does not inhibit the infecting enterococcus, the dose of penicillin should be doubled.

Although it is clear that penicillin plus gentamicin is bactericidal against more strains of enterococci in vitro than penicillin plus streptomycin, there are no clinical data to suggest that penicillin plus gentamicin is superior treatment. However, some investigators advocate the use of penicillin plus gentamicin (1.0 to 1.5 mg per kilogram of body weight every eight hours) as initial therapy in enterococcal endocarditis until in vitro studies are complete. Others prefer to use penicillin plus streptomycin, because renal toxicity is a more serious problem with gentamicin than with streptomycin. Once in vitro tests are completed, penicillin plus gentamicin may be used if there is an apparent advantage of gentamicin. If relapse occurs following a course of penicillin and streptomycin, the penicillin-gentamicin combination should be tried if tests in vitro demonstrate an advantage of this combination.

Vertigo or disturbances of balance develop in 20 to 30 per cent of patients who receive streptomycin for six weeks. If ototoxicity develops, the streptomycin may be terminated at four weeks, although penicillin is continued for the full six-week course. In patients with renal insufficiency, serum levels of streptomycin should be measured and the doses of streptomycin adjusted to maintain peak serum concentrations (one hour after dosage) between 10 and 15 μg per milliliter.

In contrast to endocarditis caused by penicillin-susceptible streptococci, *cephalosporins have no place in the treatment of enterococcal endocarditis.* Enterococci are highly resistant to cephalosporins in vitro, and the clinical results have been unsatisfactory. No alternative drug has been extensively tested for efficacy in the treatment of enterococcal endocarditis. Therefore an effort should be made to use penicillin in most patients who have a history of allergy to penicillin or in patients developing minor reactions during the course of therapy. In a patient with a history of a rash to penicillin, a "desensitization" procedure should be tried. This involves a scratch test through a drop of penicillin G (100 units per milliliter). This is followed in 30 to 45 minutes by graded amounts of penicillin intradermally, beginning at 0.001 unit per 0.1 ml of test solution and continued in tenfold increments every 30 to 45 minutes; with increasing amounts, administration is changed to the subcutaneous, intramuscular, and finally intravenous route. Epinephrine and diphenhydramine should be on hand for emergency use during the procedure if needed for an anaphylactic reaction. It is important to maintain continuous intravenous administration of penicillin throughout the course of treatment. If the intravenous infusion is stopped, it may be necessary to repeat the entire "desensitization."

Patients with a history of anaphylaxis to penicillin or those who develop severe reactions can be treated with vancomycin in a dose of 0.5 gram intravenously every six hours for four to six weeks. Streptomycin combined with vancomycin provides a more rapid and complete bactericidal effect against most enterococci than vancomycin alone and probably should be included in the therapeutic program. Vancomycin is difficult to administer intravenously because of the occurrence of phlebitis. On occasion it is nephrotoxic and ototoxic. A decision to use vancomycin in therapy should be made only after careful deliberation.

Endocarditis caused by streptococci that are not inhibited by 0.1 μg per milliliter penicillin G in vitro, i.e., relatively resistant, should probably be managed in the same manner as enterococcal endocarditis. However, with these nonenterococcal, relatively resistant streptococci, a cephalosporin can often be used as substitute therapy in the penicillin-allergic patient, provided that adequate serum bactericidal activity is achieved. Obviously, in such instances, the fact that the organism is *not* an enterococcus must be clearly established (see Laboratory Findings, above).

STAPHYLOCOCCI. *S. aureus* endocarditis is frequently a fulminant disease, requiring immediate antimicrobial therapy. It should be suspected when endocarditis occurs either in narcotic addicts or after the insertion of prosthetic heart valves or in the presence of the clinical syndrome of acute endocarditis. More than 50 per cent of community-acquired and over 80 per cent of hospital-acquired *S. aureus* produce penicillinase and are therefore resistant to penicillin. Only penicillinase-resistant penicillins (nafcillin, methicillin, or oxacillin) or cephalosporins may be relied on in initial treatment of staphylococcal endocarditis. Therapy must be given for four to six weeks. The doses are 2 grams of nafcillin, methicillin, oxacillin, or cephalothin intravenously every four hours or 1 to 2 grams of cefazolin intramuscularly or intravenously every six hours. Only when staphylococci are exquisitely susceptible to penicillin G (i.e., inhibited by 0.1 μg per milliliter) can penicillin G be used and then only in high doses (e.g., 20 million units daily by continuous intravenous infusion). If a penicillin or cephalosporin cannot be used, vancomycin, 0.5 gram intravenously every six hours, is the drug of choice.

Penicillins and gentamicin have been shown to result in a more rapid bactericidal effect against *S. aureus* than penicillins alone, both in vitro and in an animal model of endocarditis. Because of the high mortality of *S. aureus* endocarditis, some investigators have recommended the use of the combination in infection in man. At present, there is no clinical evidence to suggest that the combination has any advantage over the penicillin or cephalosporin alone. Furthermore, the additional toxicity of the aminoglycoside is sufficient to warrant further investigation before recommending routine use of the combination.

Resistance of *S. aureus* to methicillin has been noted elsewhere in the world, but it is not a major problem in the United States. Methicillin-resistant strains of *S. aureus* are resistant to other penicillinase-resistant penicillins such as nafcillin or oxacillin, and to the cephalosporins as well. Endocarditis caused by methicillin-resistant *S. aureus*, although rare, requires vancomycin therapy.

S. epidermidis endocarditis, which is often associated with prosthetic valves, should initially be treated with a cephalosporin. These organisms are often resistant to penicillin G and occasionally to methicillin but usually are susceptible to the cephalosporins. *S. epidermidis* endocarditis caused by a cephalosporin-resistant strain will require therapy with vancomycin.

OTHER ORGANISMS. *Pneumococcal, gonococcal,* and *meningococcal* endocarditis should be treated with 20 million units of penicillin G intravenously daily for four weeks. However, if a case of endocarditis should occur with one of the recently described strains of gonococci that produce penicillinase, penicillin G will not be appropriate therapy, and a regimen would have to be chosen on the basis of in vitro bactericidal tests.

The therapy of endocarditis caused by *gram-negative bacilli* must consist of bactericidal antimicrobials, preferably a penicillin or cephalosporin with or without an aminoglycoside, and must be given in sufficient doses to achieve peak concentrations in the serum that are bactericidal for the infecting organism at a 1:8 dilution. Penicillin G or ampicillin (for *E. coli, Proteus mirabilis,* or *Salmonella*), cephalosporins (for *E. coli, Proteus mirabilis,* or *Klebsiella* species), and carbenicillin (for *Enterobacter* species, *Pseudomonas aeruginosa,* or *Proteus* species other than *P. mirabilis*) are the drugs most likely to be effective but must be selected on the basis of in vitro bactericidal tests. An aminoglycoside such as gentamicin is often added to achieve a greater bactericidal effect; this is particularly important in *Pseudomonas* endocarditis. The usual doses are as follows: penicillin G, 20 million units or more intravenously daily; ampicillin, 2 grams or more every four hours intramuscularly or intravenously; cephalothin, 2 grams or more every four hours intravenously; cefazolin, 1 to 2 grams every six hours intramuscularly or intravenously; carbenicillin, 500 mg per kilogram of body weight daily intravenously in divided doses every four hours; and gentamicin, 1 to 1.7 mg per kilogram intramuscularly every eight hours. The adequacy of therapy must be monitored by testing serum bactericidal activity. Therapy is continued for four to six weeks.

If the gram-negative bacillus is resistant to the penicillins and cephalosporins, either an aminoglycoside as sole therapy or bacteriostatic antimicrobials may have to be used. The results of therapy with these alternatives are usually poor. Surgical management to remove the vegetation and replace the valve may be necessary for cure.

If *other infecting bacteria* are found, the susceptibility to antimicrobial agents must be determined in vitro. If the organism is susceptible to a penicillin or cephalosporin, therapy with one of these agents in high doses plus streptomycin (unless streptomycin does not increase the bactericidal activity in vitro) should be given for four to

six weeks. Serum bactericidal activity should be monitored. If the organism is resistant to all penicillins and cephalosporins, vancomycin with (or without) streptomycin should be used if in vitro studies indicate susceptibility. If the organism is resistant to penicillins, cephalosporins, and vancomycin, therapy will probably be unsuccessful. Under these circumstances, treatment should be initiated with the bactericidal drug grouping that demonstrates the best activity in vitro; if the patient does not respond, or if relapse occurs after four to six weeks of therapy, antimicrobial therapy plus cardiac surgery to remove the vegetation and replace the valve will probably be necessary.

Results of therapy of *fungal endocarditis* have been very disappointing. Amphotericin B, the only fungicidal agent available for parenteral use, is very toxic and difficult to use. It is difficult to achieve adequate fungicidal serum levels with amphotericin without causing profound toxicity. Another agent, flucytosine, is fungistatic but may increase the fungicidal activity of amphotericin B in vitro. Amphotericin B is generally administered intravenously in a dose of 0.5 mg per kilogram daily; flucytosine is given orally in a dose of 75 to 150 mg per kilogram each day. Although some cures have been reported with antifungal therapy alone, surgical intervention with valve replacement is usually necessary to achieve a cure.

ENDOCARDITIS WITH STERILE BLOOD CULTURES. Most experts favor treating these patients as they would patients with enterococcal endocarditis. If there is no clinical response to the penicillin plus aminoglycoside regimen within three to five days, the dose of penicillin should be doubled to 40 million units daily. When the course is acute and fulminant, antistaphylococcal therapy with a penicillinase-resistant penicillin or cephalosporin should be added.

ENDOCARDITIS ON INTRACARDIAC PROSTHESES OR SUTURES. These patients probably require longer courses of therapy than patients without intravascular foreign bodies. Treatment is usually continued for at least six weeks for streptococci inhibited by 0.1 μg per milliliter of penicillin and eight weeks for all other microorganisms. With the exception of streptococcal endocarditis, results of medical therapy of prosthetic valve endocarditis have been very poor. Therefore in patients with endocarditis caused by organisms other than streptococci, valve replacement should be carefully considered.

Untoward Effects of Antimicrobial Therapy

Hypersensitivity reactions are common during therapy with penicillins. If a rash develops, therapy can be continued and antihistamines or even corticosteroids given to suppress the reaction. If the reaction is severe, requiring discontinuation of a penicillin, a cephalosporin can be tried if appropriate therapy. When neither penicillins nor cephalosporins can be used, vancomycin is the best alternative for endocarditis caused by gram-positive organisms.

The large amounts of penicillins used daily are accompanied by significant cation loads that may be of clinical significance. Twenty million units of potassium penicillin G contains approximately 34 mEq of potassium; 10 grams of nafcillin contains about 30 mEq of sodium; and 30 grams of carbenicillin contains about 141 mEq of sodium. Streptomycin, gentamicin, and vancomycin are all potentially nephrotoxic and ototoxic and must be used in reduced doses in patients with renal insufficiency; serum levels should be monitored during therapy to achieve therapeutic but nontoxic serum concentrations.

Surgery in the Management of Endocarditis

When appropriate microbicidal therapy is not available and positive blood cultures continue on therapy or relapse occurs after therapy is discontinued, removal of the vegetation and replacement of the valve with a prosthesis should be considered. The surgical repair should ideally be performed after several days or more of the best available antimicrobial therapy. The therapy should then be continued for two weeks or longer in the case of organisms that tend to produce metastatic foci. Some investigators have found it unnecessary to replace the tricuspid valve after removal. *Immediate valve replacement (even after only hours of therapy) is essential in patients developing congestive heart failure secondary to severe valvular insufficiency.* Surgery should also be strongly considered in patients with recurrent emboli despite adequate antimicrobial therapy.

Current evidence indicates that to achieve cure in fungal endocarditis, surgical intervention is almost always required in addition to treatment with antifungal agents. Because of the toxicity of antifungal agents and the complications of continued infection (e.g., large emboli), early valve resection is best.

Patients with prosthetic valve endocarditis often require valve replacement for cure. The indications for valve replacement are valve dysfunction, continuation of embolization, organisms resistant to bactericidal antimicrobials, infection with fungi, and continuing bacteremia during or relapses after an appropriate course of therapy. Surgery is most often required in early prosthetic valve endocarditis both because of the microorganisms involved (fungi and other resistant organisms) and because of valve dysfunction.

RESPONSE TO THERAPY AND PROGNOSIS

RESPONSE. Defervescence and an increased sense of well-being usually occur within several days to a week of initiation of appropriate antimicrobial therapy. Blood cultures should be obtained periodically during treatment and generally become negative within several days of onset of therapy. Lack of response of fever (at times accompanied by persistently positive blood cultures) may be associated with metastatic abscess formation (especially in *S. aureus* endocarditis).

The most common cause of persistent or recurrent fever during therapy with an appropriate drug regimen is a reaction to the antimicrobial agents, either true drug fever or inflammation at the site of administration. Another cause of febrile episodes is emboli. Superinfection of a heart valve, although rare, is especially likely when intravascular plastic catheters are used.

Weight gain, a fall in erythrocyte sedimentation rate, and disappearance of rheumatoid factor follow the fall in temperature, but may be delayed in some patients for as long as several weeks after therapy has been discontinued. Regression of clubbing occurs after many weeks. Hematuria, proteinuria, and changes in renal function tend to disappear with therapy. Splenomegaly may persist for months. Although anemia may respond within weeks, the rise in hemoglobin may be very slow and may not occur until weeks after discontinuation of therapy.

Petechiae, Osler's nodes, and emboli may occur during and for weeks after successful antimicrobial therapy. Mycotic aneurysms may regress on drug therapy or may become clinically evident by rupture weeks to months after successful therapy.

Heart failure may occur at any time during or after therapy and is a poor prognostic sign. Patients with aortic insufficiency are especially likely to develop heart failure and have a high mortality. Even with mild heart failure, aortic insufficiency may be associated with sudden death. In addition to valvular insufficiency, vegetations (especially in fungal endocarditis) may become large enough to cause obstruction of the valvular orifice.

The vast majority of relapses should be detected with blood cultures obtained one, two and four weeks after discontinuation of therapy.

PROGNOSIS. The factors that tend to make the prognosis relatively bad are (1) nonstreptococcal disease, (2) development of heart failure, (3) aortic valve involvement, (4) prosthetic valve, and (5) old age. The cure rate in streptococcal endocarditis is about 90 per cent. The failures are not due to uncontrolled infection but to death from heart failure, an embolus, rupture of a mycotic aneurysm, or renal failure. The cure rate in staphylococcal endocarditis is about 50 per cent, most deaths being due to early overwhelming infection or to heart failure. Results in endocarditis caused by fungi and gram-negative bacilli have been poor. Early cardiac surgery for heart failure or for cases refractory to antimicrobial therapy should improve these results.

Following cure of infective endocarditis, there is an increase in morbidity and mortality as compared with those in the normal population. This increase is in part related to the pre-existing underlying heart disease and in part to the consequences of the endocarditis. The mortality rate without cardiac surgery is about 5 per cent per year for the first four years and then 2 to 3 per cent annually thereafter. The prognosis is much poorer in the presence of aortic insufficiency, with only about 70 per cent alive in two years; thereafter the mortality is less than 4 per cent annually. With cardiac surgery, the survival rates should be higher.

About two thirds of the deaths are due to heart failure, with embolic phenomena, renal failure, and rupture of a mycotic aneurysm accounting for most of the remainder. The onset of heart failure can occur early in endocarditis or may be delayed for weeks, months, or even years after successful therapy. Emboli can occur months (and perhaps years) after cure of endocarditis. Mycotic aneurysms can rupture months or years after cure of infective endocarditis. Renal failure resulting from the glomerulonephritis of endocarditis is usually reversible with cure of endocarditis. About 5 to 8 per cent of patients who have been cured of one episode of endocarditis will have one or more additional episodes over a period of years.

PROPHYLAXIS OF ENDOCARDITIS

An apparent portal of entry for the infecting organism can be demonstrated in only a minority of patients with infective endocarditis. However, it seems clear that the oropharynx serves as the site of origin for most patients, with the genitourinary tract next. It is obvious that oral hygiene should be optimal in patients with underlying cardiac lesions that predispose to endocarditis, especially those who are to have prosthetic cardiac valves implanted.

Although the risk of endocarditis is small and there is no proof of efficacy, antimicrobial prophylaxis is recommended for patients with predisposing cardiac lesions who are to undergo procedures known to result in transient bacteremia. The cardiac conditions for which prophylaxis is recommended are valvular or congenital heart disease (except for uncomplicated atrial septal defect), intracardiac prostheses, and previous episode of infective endocarditis. The antimicrobial therapy is directed at the bacteria which lodge at an endocardial site and therefore is analogous to treatment of very early endocarditis.

DENTAL MANIPULATIONS AND OTHER PROCEDURES IN THE MOUTH, NOSE, OR THROAT. Prophylaxis is directed against viridans streptococci and is recommended for all procedures likely to cause gingival bleeding and for tonsillectomy and bronchoscopy. Based on data in laboratory animals, regimens likely to be effective are (1) aqueous penicillin G, 1 million units, mixed with procaine penicillin, 600,000 units, *plus* streptomycin, 1 gram, both intramuscularly 30 minutes before the procedure; (2) aqueous penicillin G, 1 million units, mixed with procaine penicillin, 600,000 units, intramuscularly 30 minutes before the procedure, followed by penicillin V, 0.5 gram orally every six hours for eight doses; (3) vancomycin, 1 gram intravenously over a 30- to 60-minute period starting 30 to 60 minutes before the procedure; or (4) penicillin V, 2 grams orally 30 minutes before the procedure and then 0.5 gram every six hours for eight doses. The penicillin-plus-streptomycin regimen is preferred for patients with prosthetic heart valves, and vancomycin should be used in the patient who is hypersensitive to penicillin. Erythromycin, 1 gram orally one and one half hours before the procedure and then 500 mg every six hours for eight doses, is probably less effective. The American Heart Association recommends continuation of therapy after penicillin plus streptomycin (penicillin V, 500 mg orally every six hours for eight doses) and after vancomycin (erythromycin, 500 mg orally every six hours for eight doses), but this additional oral treatment is probably unnecessary except in the case of a prolonged procedure.

GENITOURINARY AND GASTROINTESTINAL TRACT PROCEDURES OR SURGERY. Prophylaxis is directed against enterococci and is recommended for procedures that cause significant trauma to the genitourinary or gastrointestinal tracts (e.g., urethral catheterization, prostatic surgery, and colonic or gallbladder surgery). Regimens likely to be effective are (1) ampicillin (1 gram intramuscularly or intravenously) plus gentamicin (1.5 mg per kilogram intramuscularly or intravenously) or streptomycin (1 gram intramuscularly) 30 minutes before the procedure, and then two additional doses every eight hours for ampicillin plus gentamicin and every 12 hours for ampicillin plus streptomycin; or (2) vancomycin, 1 gram intravenously over a 30- to 60-minute period starting 30 to 60 minutes before the procedure, plus streptomycin, 1 gram intramuscularly 30 to 60 minutes before the procedure.

CARDIAC SURGERY. Prophylaxis is directed against staphylococci and consists of 2 grams of methicillin, oxacillin, nafcillin, or cephalothin intravenously every four hours starting one hour before the procedure and continuing for several days. Vancomycin in a dose of 0.5 gram intravenously every six hours can be used in patients hypersensitive to penicillins and cephalosporins. Because of an extremely low risk of endocarditis, prophylaxis is not recommended in association with cardiac catheterization.

A. H. A. Committee Report: Prevention of bacterial endocarditis. Circulation, 56:139A, 1977.
Bayer, A. S., Theofilopoulos, A. N., Eisenberg, R, Dixon, F. J., and Guze, L. B.: Circulating immune complexes in infective endocarditis. N. Engl. J. Med., 295:1500, 1976.
Dreyer, N. P., and Fields, B. N.: Heroin-associated infective endocarditis. A report of 28 cases. Am. Intern. Med., 78:699, 1973.
Duma, R. J.: Infections of Prosthetic Heart Valves and Vascular Grafts. Baltimore, University Park Press, 1977.
Kaye, D.: Infective Endocarditis. Baltimore, University Park Press, 1976.
Mandell, G. L., Kaye, D., Levison, M. E., and Hook, E. W.: Enterococcal endocarditis. An analysis of 38 patients observed at the New York Hospital–Cornell Medical Center. Arch. Intern. Med., 125:258, 1970.
Rubinstein, E., Noriega, E. R., Simberkoff, M. S., Holzman, R., and Rahal, J. J., Jr.: Fungal endocarditis: Analysis of 24 cases and review of the literature. Medicine, 54:331, 1975.
Wolfe, J. C., and Johnson, W. D., Jr.: Penicillin-sensitive streptococcal endocarditis: In vitro and clinical observations on penicillin-streptomycin therapy. Ann. Intern Med., 81:178, 1974.

STAPHYLOCOCCAL INFECTIONS

F. Robert Fekety, Jr.

132. INTRODUCTION

Staphylococci are the most common cause of suppurative skin infections of man. They also cause bacteremia and serious infections of lungs, pleura, endocardium, meninges, muscles, bones, joints, and other viscera. Staphylococcal infections became more frequent and troublesome after antimicrobial drugs were introduced. Staphylococci are ubiquitous in our environment and are constituents of our normal flora. They are resistant to some of our most useful antimicrobial drugs and increase in prevalence when these agents are used. Hospitalized patients are frequently exposed to staphylococci as well as being highly susceptible to them. Such patients are most likely to develop serious staphylococcal infections and to have difficulty in handling them. Hospital-acquired staphylococcal infections are still an important problem even though we have developed several good drugs for treating them.

BACTERIOLOGY. Staphylococci are spherical gram-positive cocci that grow well either aerobically or anaerobically on simple laboratory media. Grapelike clusters of organisms are seen in stained smears of cultures; small irregular clusters, pairs, and short chains are seen in smears of pus. When gram-positive cocci are seen *within* leukocytes, it is very likely that they are staphylococci, as other cocci are usually killed and digested soon after phagocytosis, but pathogenic staphylococci are not.

Staphylococci are the most important pathogens in

the genus *Micrococcus,* which includes many sapro-phytes. Pathogenic staphylococci are noteworthy for their metabolic and biochemical versatility. Two species can be tentatively identified by pigment production: *S. aureus* is characteristically golden yellow on agar, and *S. epidermidis* (formerly *S. albus*) is white. *S. aureus* often grows as white colonies on primary isolation; cream-colored, orange, or lemon-yellow colonies of *S. aureus* are also seen. *S. aureus* is the most important pathogenic *Staphylococcus.*

Pathogenic staphylococci can produce a variety of ex-otoxins with hemolytic, necrotizing, leukocidal, vaso-spastic, or lethal properties. They are capable of fer-menting mannitol and other sugars, and produce other possibly important substances, including lysozyme, ca-talase, enterotoxin, epidermolysin, fibrinolysin, hya-luronidase, lipase, thermonuclease, beta-lactamase, phosphatase, deoxyribonuclease, protease, and coagu-lase (a plasma-clotting substance). The pathogenetic role of these toxins and enzymes is still uncertain. Coa-gulase and thermonuclease production and mannitol fermentation correlate well with pathogenicity for man. By convention, coagulase-positive, mannitol-fermenting staphylococci are called *S. aureus.* The tube coagulase test is more reliable than the slide test, which measures bound coagulase (clumping factor).

Coagulase-negative and mannitol-negative isolates are called *S. epidermidis. S. epidermidis* does not often cause infection of man unless susceptibility is increased or there is a nidus of infected foreign material, such as an intracardiac prosthesis or an intravascular plastic catheter or shunt. These opportunistic organisms are being recognized more and more frequently as the etio-logic agents in endocarditis, bacteremia, and other serious infections, and *they can no longer be dismissed automatically as contaminants whenever they are isolated from cultures of blood or other specimens.*

Nonhemolytic, coagulase-negative staphylococci that ferment mannitol under certain conditions have been classified recently as *Staphylococcus saprophyticus.* They can also be recognized by their resistance to novobio-cin. These organisms can cause urinary tract infections, especially in young women. This is the primary reason for calling attention to them and for attempting to dis-tinguish them from *S. epidermidis,* which often is a con-taminant in urine cultures.

PATHOGENESIS. Suppuration and abscess formation are the characteristic features of staphylococcal infec-tion. When staphylococci lodge in susceptible tissues, multiply, and produce their exotoxins, an acute inflam-matory reaction ensues. Small blood vessels thrombose, and fibrin is deposited about the lesion, which be-comes avascular, necrotic, and surrounded by fibro-blasts. The tissues become hypertonic, edematous, tense, and painful. The center of the lesion gradually liquefies, forming the characteristic thick, creamy yel-low pus which is slightly acidic, hypoxic, and com-posed of dead organisms, leukocytes, and proteina-ceous substances. Further evolution of the lesion is slow even when antimicrobials are given unless it drains, after which it usually begins to heal. Antimi-crobial drugs do not affect undrained abscesses very much, (1) because the drugs may not diffuse into ab-scesses very well, (2) because they may be destroyed or inactivated there, or (3) because the organisms in ab-scesses may not be multiplying and thus are in a rela-tively insusceptible state. Granulomatous reactions are

occasionally seen at sites of chronic staphylococcal in-fections.

Very little that is conclusive has been established about the mechanisms of the pathogenicity of staphylo-cocci. Virulence probably is the result of multiple mechanisms acting together. There are obvious clinical implications for the dermonecrotic, lethal, and leuko-cidal toxins, but their true importance is unknown. Fi-brin products of coagulase activity may help wall off the lesion and protect the organism from granulocytes, but the resultant fibrin network may also enhance sur-face phagocytosis. Lipases may nullify the bactericidal action of cutaneous lipids. Capsular structures and cell wall teichoic acids may be antiphagocytic.

Some of the substances that may be important in pathogenesis have been used as antigens in experimen-tal vaccines, but immunization as a means of enhanc-ing resistance to staphylococci has met with little suc-cess. Most adults possess serum antibodies to a number of staphylococcal antigens, but high titers of these anti-bodies have not correlated well with protection from disease. The factors important in promoting phago-cytosis and intracellular killing of the organism are incompletely understood. Protein A, a component of staphylococcal cell walls, nonspecifically binds anti-staphylococcal (and other) antibodies at the Fc frag-ment instead of appropriately at the Fab fragment. This reverse attachment of immune globulins appears to ren-der them functionally ineffective, and may be the ex-planation for the observation that neither vaccination nor the disease seems to result in immunity despite the production of large amounts of antibody. In addition, there is some evidence that hypersensitivity reactions to antigenic products of the microorganism may lower local resistance to infection. Additional studies are re-quired if safe and effective vaccination against staphy-lococci is to become possible.

EPIDEMIOLOGY. Pathogenic staphylococci are nor-mally acquired by a high percentage of healthy infants within a few days or weeks of birth. They may be re-sponsible for epidemics in nurseries. Most healthy humans harbor virulent staphylococci in the anterior nares or on the skin, either occasionally or consistently. Clinical disease occurs in exposed persons or asymp-tomatic carriers when local or general resistance is de-creased or when exposure is heavy. Staphylococci are abundant in our environment and can survive in dust for long periods, but implantation of large numbers of staphylococci derived from air and other exogenous sources seems an uncommon explanation for disease. To produce skin infections experimentally in healthy persons more than a million pathogenic staphylococci must be inoculated, and no significant differences have been demonstrated between strains derived from le-sions or from healthy mucous membranes. In the pres-ence of a silk suture, the infective dose is reduced to less than 100 organisms. The evidence that certain strains of pathogenic staphylococci are especially viru-lent is inconclusive, but the epidemiologic evidence suggests that enhanced virulence may be responsible for nursery outbreaks. Factors that increase host sus-ceptibility to relatively small numbers of ordinary staphylococci seem of greatest importance in explaining the development of staphylococcal disease.

Although numerous conditions are known to predis-pose to staphylococcal infection, the mechanisms caus-ing staphylococci to become invasive are not well understood. Skin infections usually begin about hair follicles, sebaceous glands, or at sites of wounds, abrasions, or foreign bodies such as intravenous catheters. Greasy substances, oils, sunburn, and other conditions causing blockage of the ducts of cutaneous glands predispose to infection. In some cases infection results from multiplication of the organism within serous exudates, hematomas, or devitalized tissues. Burns, surgical wounds, and chronic dermatitic lesions frequently become secondarily infected with staphylococci. Diabetics seem to have an increased frequency of cutaneous staphylococcal infections, possibly because their acute defensive inflammatory responses may be delayed and deficient (especially during ketoacidosis), because of vascular disease and gangrene, and because of the frequent exposure that diabetics have to hospitals and to medical procedures that increase the risk of infection. The chronic granulomatous disease of childhood is characterized by refractory infections with catalase-positive organisms such as staphylococci, because the granulocytes of the affected individuals are unable to generate sufficient hydrogen peroxide to permit intraleukocytic bactericidal mechanisms to operate normally. Other congenital or acquired conditions associated with frequent staphylococcal infections have been described; eczema, elevated serum IgE or depressed IgM levels, and depressed leukocyte chemotaxis are often documented. Malnutrition and a variety of chronic debilitating diseases predispose to serious staphylococcal infection. In some cases this association may be attributable to treatment with antimicrobial drugs that encourage overgrowth of drug-resistant, pathogenic staphylococci. In others, it may be the consequence of therapeutic efforts or disease processes that adversely affected cellular or humoral defense mechanisms. Neoplasms, uremia, lengthy operations, and treatment with adrenal steroids and cytotoxic or immunosuppressive agents predispose to staphylococcal infection. Influenza, measles, diabetes mellitus, and cystic fibrosis predispose to staphylococcal pneumonia. Newborn infants are hypersusceptible to this organism and are subject to severe spreading skin infections and primary staphylococcal pneumonia with pneumatocele formation.

Because of their ubiquity, versatility, and resistance to antimicrobial drugs, staphylococci have become a major cause of serious infections in highly susceptible persons who tend to congregate in hospitals (see Ch. 124). Bacteriophage typing of staphylococci has contributed to understanding the modes of transmission of these infections. Man is the major source of the organism. Patients and personnel in hospitals are more commonly asymptomatic carriers of the organism than are those without hospital contact. The organism is most often found in the anterior nares, in intertriginous areas and hair, and on the hands. Carriers and infected patients readily contaminate their environment, and staphylococci can be isolated from air, dust, floors, mops, blankets, clothing, dressing carts, and other fomites. Heavily colonized or clinically infected patients tend to shed more organisms than do asymptomatic carriers. The usual habitat of *S. epidermidis* is the skin and mucous membranes of man and animals.

Studies in nurseries for the newborn have shown that transmission of the organism occurs primarily via the hands of personnel who either are carriers or have recently handled infected or colonized newborns. The spread of organisms from heavily colonized infants ("cloud-babies") via the airborne route may occur, but this seems much less frequent than transmission via hands. Postoperative wound infections are more frequent in nasal carriers of staphylococci and often appear to be attributable to strains carried by the patient prior to operation (endogenous infection). Infected patients or personnel are also important sources of strains causing wound infections (exogenous infections); the usual mechanism is contact spread via hands. Air, environment, or fomites are less common sources of the organism. All these mechanisms contribute to the perpetuation of the reservoir of staphylococci in the hospital and to the spread of organisms to personnel and highly susceptible patients, especially those treated with antimicrobial drugs.

Most authorities believe that special attention to measures such as isolation and frequent handwashing in order to prevent the spread of staphylococci is worthwhile. Infected patients can shed large numbers of bacteria into the environment and should be isolated unless the infection is at a closed site (e.g., blood, meninges). Personnel with clinical infections should not have contact with susceptible patients. The indiscriminate use of antimicrobial drugs favors the transmission and survival of drug-resistant strains. Few surgical procedures are indications for prophylactic antimicrobials, for there is little evidence that such agents are capable of preventing staphylococcal infection. Because so many persons are asymptomatic carriers of pathogenic staphylococci, it is not practical to exclude all of them from contact with susceptible persons in hospitals. Actually, healthy carriers of ordinary strains seem unlikely to acquire new and potentially more dangerous strains, which is probably an example of *bacterial interference*. However, it may be necessary during outbreaks to exclude carriers of *especially dangerous* staphylococcal strains (as demonstrated by both bacteriophage typing and clinical experience) from nurseries, delivery rooms, and operating rooms.

TREATMENT. Although antimicrobial therapy has markedly improved the prognosis in serious staphylococcal infection, it must be emphasized that surgical drainage of abscesses and removal of infected foreign bodies are not only equally important but may be the only way to achieve a cure. Patients with staphylococcal infections usually respond relatively slowly to therapy, and despite optimal treatment the mortality rate is high in persons with compromised defense mechanisms. Although antimicrobial therapy is considered in detail in Ch. 187 and 188, there are certain points that should be stressed here.

Appropriate cultures and drug susceptibility tests should always be obtained to confirm the diagnosis of serious staphylococcal disease and to guide therapy. Although many antimicrobial drugs are now available for treating these infections, the unpredictable susceptibility of the organism narrows the initial choice to only a few. Bacteriophage typing of staphylococci has contrib- Bactericidal penicillin analogues are preferred unless the patient is allergic to them. Because most isolates causing infection in the hospital and in the community are resistant to penicillin G and ampicillin, the choice should be limited to drugs that are not significantly inactivated by staphylococcal beta-lactamase. Toxic-appearing patients with serious infections are best treated parenterally. Methicillin, oxacillin, nafcillin, cephalothin, cefazolin, and cephapirin are recommended for serious infection. Used properly, they seem to produce equally good therapeutic results. Many experts still prefer methicillin, but nafcillin has become increasingly popular because it is the most active derivative and rarely causes nephritis or other serious side effects. The cephalosporins are especially useful with mixed infections because of their relatively broad spectrum. Cephaloridine should rarely be used because it is nephrotoxic when used in doses greater than 4.0 grams per day. Cefazolin is a well tolerated new cephalosporin preparation providing good serum antistaphylococcal activity, and is preferred over the other cephalosporins for intramuscular use. Cephalosporins should be avoided in treating central nervous system staphylococcal infections unless intravenous therapy is supplemented with intrathecal cephaloridine (50 mg daily).*

For oral therapy of less serious infections, cloxacillin, dicloxacillin, and the more expensive cephalexin are suitable and equally efficacious when given properly. Oxacillin and nafcillin are not recommended for oral use because their absorption is too erratic.

The penicillinase-resistant penicillin analogues are adequate for the treatment of infections caused by more susceptible organisms such as penicillin-susceptible staphylococci, pneumococci, and group A beta streptococci when the dosages commonly recommended for staphylococcal disease are used. Consequently, it is *not* necessary to add penicillin G to the regimen when these organisms are suspected of playing a role in the illness. However, many persons prefer to use both penicillin G and methicillin or nafcillin initially and to switch to the more active drug when the nature of the etiologic agent becomes clear. If the organism is susceptible to it, penicillin is preferred because it is usually the most active drug as well as the most convenient and inexpensive one to administer. Penicillin V is better than penicillin G for oral therapy of staphylococcal infections because of its better absorption.

If the patient is allergic to penicillin, all the semisynthetic penicillins should be avoided. Vancomycin (0.5 gram intravenously every six hours), clindamycin, cephalothin, cefazolin, or cephalexin are suitable substitutes, but allergic cross-reactions between penicillin and the cephalosporins have been observed. Tetracyclines, including minocycline, and chloramphenicol are less frequently employed because of drug resistance, fear of toxicity, or lack of bactericidal action.

Because there are several suitable antimicrobial agents and many different clinical situations, only general guidelines for dosage and duration of treatment can be given here. A delay in initiating appropriate therapy for these necrotizing infections is often deleterious. These infections respond slowly and often require high doses of antimicrobial drugs for long periods. Relapses are common if therapy is terminated too early, especially if the lesion has not drained or foreign bodies are not removed. It is unusual for staphylococci to become resistant to penicillin derivatives *during therapy of closed infections*, such as endocarditis. Endocarditis and other serious infections are usually treated for at least four to six weeks. In serious infections, parenteral therapy is preferred because of the desirability of ensuring high concentrations of the antimicrobial in blood and tissues. In order to maintain adequate serum antistaphylococcal activity, the interval between intravenous doses of penicillins and cephalosporins should not exceed four hours in critically ill patients; also, the drugs should not be given rapidly as an intravenous bolus in order to avoid neurotoxic reactions and the rapid renal elimination of the drug.

Although methicillin-resistant strains of *S. aureus* have been encountered frequently in Europe, they are not common in the United States. Faulty testing disks occasionally are responsible for their spurious detection. Methicillin-resistant organisms usually show resistance to other semisynthetic penicillins and cephalosporins. Resistant strains grow better at 30° than at 37°C and in high concentrations of sodium chloride. They may be recognizable only after prolonged incubation (48 hours) in the presence of methicillin or oxacillin, presumably because the isolates contain only a small proportion of resistant clones. Most laboratories do not employ these special conditions routinely. Resistant organisms seem less virulent than methicillin-susceptible staphylococci, but they have occasionally been of clinical importance. Wide misuse of the new penicillins will probably result eventually in an increase in the prevalence of these strains. Vancomycin, gentamicin, clindamycin, or a combination of kanamycin or gentamicin with cephalothin or methicillin has been recommended for treatment of infections with these organisms.

Attention has been directed to the observation that certain drugs (including methicillin, oxacillin, gentamicin, vancomycin, or cephalosporins) that are ordinarily considered bactericidal may be primarily bacteriostatic for some staphylococci. In a few instances of serious infection with such isolates, responses to treatment have been slow or unsatisfactory. In the hope of increasing the rapidity and frequency of response, there has been a growing tendency to treat serious staphylococcal sepsis with a combination of bactericidal drugs such as a penicillin and gentamicin. In vitro studies have shown a more rapid killing effect with such combinations, and experimental infections in animal models also have been controlled more rapidly with them. However, there is no proof as yet that therapeutic results in humans are better with combination therapy.

Cephalosporins, vancomycin, gentamicin, and the macrolides are the most active antimicrobials against *S. epidermidis*. These coagulase-negative organisms are often surprisingly resistant to methicillin and the other semisynthetic penicillins.

133. CUTANEOUS STAPHYLOCOCCAL INFECTIONS

133.1. FURUNCLES

A furuncle (boil) is an acute circumscribed staphylococcal abscess of the skin and subcutaneous tissues. The term folliculitis refers to pustular furuncles involving hair follicles. Folliculitis is common in persons with

---

*Intrathecal use is not mentioned in the manufacturer's package insert approved by the U.S. Food and Drug Administration. Therefore its use in these circumstances must be considered investigational.

oily skin, poor hygiene, or occupational exposure to cutting oils. Deep folliculitis of the beard area is known as *sycosis barbae*. Patients with multiple or recurrent furuncles are said to have furunculosis; otherwise normal adults commonly experience an average of five or six furuncles per year. Furunculosis is an important problem in the newborn.

Furuncles are most common on the face, neck, buttocks, thighs, perineum, breasts, and axillary skin. Most furuncles begin at the base of a hair follicle and take three to five days to evolve. Itching or pain may be the earliest symptom. As the center of the lesion becomes necrotic and hypertonic, fluid is drawn into the furuncle and it swells, thinning the overlapping erythematous skin. Spontaneous drainage usually occurs soon thereafter. A hard core of necrotic debris is sometimes extruded from the center of the abscess. Relief of pain and onset of healing are usually rapid after drainage occurs, although erythema and swelling may persist for several weeks. A furuncle may regress without draining and form a "blind boil" that is indolent and prone to exacerbation following minor local trauma.

When the sebaceous glands of the face and upper back are extensively involved with furuncles, the condition is referred to as *pustular acne vulgaris. Juvenile acne* is not caused by staphylococci, but these organisms may secondarily infect acne lesions.

Furuncles involving blocked apocrine sweat glands (*hidradenitis suppurativa*) frequently become chronic. This troublesome infection tends to spread to other local sweat glands and hair follicles and leads to interconnecting draining sinuses and extensive scarring. Lesions occur in the axillary, perianal, and genital areas. Various organisms can be responsible. Hidradenitis is difficult to cure solely with antimicrobial therapy and drainage. Excision of the involved tissues and skin grafting are frequently necessary and usually successful.

Although systemic symptoms and bacteremia are unusual with an ordinary furuncle unless the lesion is squeezed or manipulated, asymptomatic bacteremia secondary to a furuncle is probably fairly common. Furuncles are believed to be important in the pathogenesis of endocarditis, osteomyelitis, pyarthrosis, and other metastatic infections developing after hematogenous dissemination. Septic thrombophlebitis resulting from local extension of infection is another serious complication of furuncles. Lesions in the middle third of the face are especially dangerous, because they may spread intracranially via emissary veins and cause cavernous sinus thrombophlebitis.

133.2. CARBUNCLES

A carbuncle is a large furuncle or an aggregate of interconnected furuncles. Carbuncles often drain through multiple skin openings. They represent an acute suppurative inflammation of subcutaneous tissues extending between hair follicles in clefts along fibrous and adipose tissues. They occur where the skin is especially thick and tough (such as the back of the neck). Carbuncles may attain the size of lemons, and can be associated with extreme pain, chills, fever, leukocytosis, malaise, prostration, and bacteremia. They are serious and sometimes fatal infections.

133.3. IMPETIGO

Impetigo is a superficial primary pyoderma caused by group A beta streptococci, *S. aureus,* or both (see Ch. 127.2). Most common in infants and children, it begins as macules and progresses to vesicles and bullae which rupture, releasing a cloudy yellow fluid that forms crusts and reveals a weeping denuded area. The lesions may become chronic and resemble fungal infections. They are superficial, are rarely larger than 2 cm, and spread by autoinoculation. Streptococci are usually responsible for impetigo, but there is good evidence that staphylococci of bacteriophage type 71 may be involved in some cases.

133.4. THE SCALDED SKIN SYNDROME

An association of bacteriophage group II staphylococci with exfoliative dermatitis has been recognized in three distinct but related clinical entities: (1) *Generalized exfoliative dermatitis (scalded skin syndrome, pemphigus neonatorum, Ritter's disease, staphylococcal toxic epidermal necrolysis)* is severe and characterized by generalized painful erythema, formation of large flaccid bullae, a positive Nikolsky sign (epidermis is detached easily by the examining finger), and shedding of the upper epidermis in large sheets. The focus of infection may be at a distant site. The disease is usually seen in newborns but has been recognized in adults, and is often confused with pemphigus. (2) *Bullous impetigo* is a localized form of the scalded skin syndrome in which the infection occurs at the site of the lesion. (3) *Staphylococcal scarlet fever* is a mild variant of the generalized scalded skin syndrome and is clinically similar to streptococcal scarlet fever. A localized infection is the usual focus.

These three clinical variants appear to represent the spectrum of a disease process with a common etiology — the epidermolytic exotoxin produced usually by group II staphylococci (especially types 3A, 3C, 55, and 71). Antibodies to the streptococcal erythrogenic toxin do not seem to be cross-reactive. The disease has been duplicated in an experimental model. The characteristic lesion consists of intraepidermal cleavage through desmosomes of the stratum granulosum. Other forms of toxic epidermal necrolysis can be distinguished easily because they show necrosis of the entire epidermis with a deeper cleavage plane near the dermoepidermal junction. Frozen sections of peeled skin or cytologic studies of cells from the denuded base of a lesion can yield a diagnosis rapidly.

133.5. TREATMENT OF CUTANEOUS INFECTIONS

Some authorities believe that furuncles and pustules can be aborted at early stages by the administration of an antimicrobial drug or by the local application of an antiseptic such as alcohol. Once drained, small lesions require no further therapy, but they should be kept covered with a dressing or zinc oxide ointment to prevent spread of organisms. More severe lesions require both local and systemic therapy. Rest, heat, and elevation of the affected site relieve pains and hasten resolution. Warm compresses hasten maturation of the lesion, but care should be taken to prevent maceration. Incision should be delayed until frank suppuration and fluctuance are detectable, as early incision is ineffective and may promote bacteremia.

Antimicrobials should be given for large furuncles, for those on the face or neck, or for those accompanied by lymphadenitis, fever, or other systemic reaction. They should also be given if the patient has diabetes, congenital or valvular heart disease, or another underlying disease predisposing to complications, or if surgical incision is to be performed. Oral therapy with penicillin, erythromycin, or clindamycin is usually satisfactory. Therapy should be continued until signs of active inflammation have disappeared; a week is usually sufficient. Gamma globulin, adrenal steroids, and vaccines are of no proved value.

Impetigo responds rapidly to treatment with appropriate antimicrobials given systemically; topical bacitracin ointment may be adequate in mild cases.

133.6. PREVENTION OF CUTANEOUS INFECTIONS

Furuncles are difficult to prevent because the resistance of the patient usually cannot be influenced and the organism is ubiquitous. However, measures that protect the skin and minimize contact with the organism may be worthwhile. Predisposing conditions should be treated or eliminated. Skin irritants and abrasive tight clothing should be avoided. The fingernails should be kept short, and frequent handwashing should be stressed. Draining lesions should be considered highly contaminated and kept covered. Daily bathing and shampooing with antiseptic soap may be useful. Very rarely it may be possible to treat carriers with antimicrobials for several weeks or months and to eliminate the organism and thus prevent recurrences. Antimicrobial ointments (gentamicin or neomycin-bacitracin) or 2 per cent hexachlorophene cream may be applied several times daily to susceptible areas or to the anterior nares to suppress the organism. A short course of treatment with both dicloxacillin and rifampin may eradicate the organism. It is sometimes possible to get rid of a troublesome organism by intentionally inducing nasal carriage with a relatively nonpathogenic species after the more virulent staphylococcal strain has been suppressed by drug therapy (bacterial interference). The 502A strain of *S. aureus* has been employed for this purpose in patients with recurrent furunculosis. Small numbers of organisms of the 502A strain have been used to intentionally colonize the umbilicus and nares of newborn infants in order to prevent acquisition of more dangerous strains. Outbreaks in nurseries have been terminated in this way. Infections have been caused in infants and adults by strain 502A, and its use is still experimental. Staphylococcus vaccines, toxoids, and bacteriophage lysates are of no proved value in prevention, and irradiation to produce atrophy of cutaneous glands is not recommended.

134. STAPHYLOCOCCAL PNEUMONIA

Staphylococci cause less than 5 per cent of all bacterial pneumonias, except during influenza epidemics, but the disease is especially important because of its high mortality rate (up to 50 per cent) (see Ch. 119 to 124).

In so-called *primary staphylococcal pneumonia*, the organisms gain access to the lung via the tracheobronchial tree. Primary staphylococcal pneumonia is most often seen in infants; in children with cystic fibrosis or measles; in adults with influenza; or in debilitated, hospitalized persons being treated with antimicrobials, steroids, cancer chemotherapy, or immunosuppressants.

The diagnosis of primary staphylococcal pneumonia in adults with serious underlying diseases is often difficult. High remittent fever, multiple chills, cyanosis, rapidly progressive dyspnea, chest pain, and the production of thick, creamy yellow, salmon-colored, or reddish-yellow sputum should lead to the suspicion of staphylococcal pneumonia. Peripheral vascular collapse and marked signs of toxicity should also cause one to suspect the diagnosis in patients with pulmonary filtrates. Staphylococcal pneumonia developing in association with influenza or an underlying debilitating illness characteristically begins with a sudden and marked worsening of the illness, accompanied by prostration, cyanosis, tachypnea, bloody or purulent sputum, and high fever. Fever, cough, sputum production, dyspnea, and chest pain may be minimal during early stages of staphylococcal pneumonia. In infants the sudden development of pneumothorax, pneumatoceles, or empyema is characteristic. Necrosis with formation of multiple abscesses is characteristic in adults, but pneumothorax can occur, particularly in patients treated with adrenal steroids.

Hematogenous or secondary staphylococcal pneumonia is seen most frequently in narcotic addicts with endocarditis and in others with bacteremia from a focus elsewhere. Secondary staphylococcal pneumonia is characterized by multiple peripheral infiltrates that resemble embolic lesions and progress to necrosis and abscess formation, with a high frequency of pleuritic pain and empyema. Pneumothorax may occur, characteristically in young children. The signs of septicemia frequently overshadow the pulmonary disease in these patients.

The physical findings in patients with staphylococcal pneumonia are highly variable. A toxic appearance and low-grade fever may be the only detectable manifestations, particularly when the pneumonia is early and in a central location or interstitial, which is common. Patchy pneumonia with multiple small abscesses is another common presentation, and can be detected by the presence of either coarse or fine rales. Dullness to percussion is not an early sign, and signs of frank consolidation are rarely found. Pleural effusion and empyema are frequent, but the fluid is commonly loculated in interlobar fissures and may not be readily detected or aspirated.

The leukocyte count is usually elevated to between 15,000 and 25,000 per cubic millimeter. A leukocyte count greater than 15,000 in an adult with influenza should raise the question of a secondary bacterial pneumonia. The Gram-stained smear of the sputum usually shows polymorphonuclear leukocytes and large numbers of clustered gram-positive cocci. When cocci are seen within leukocytes in sputum, staphylococcal pneumonia is the presumptive diagnosis. The blood culture is *not* often positive unless the pneumonia is secondary to staphylococcal bacteremia originating at some other site.

DIFFERENTIAL DIAGNOSIS. All other forms of pneumonia must be considered. The distinction from pneumonia caused by gram-negative organisms is especially important in patients developing pneumonia in the hospital. A carefully performed Gram stain of a good sample of sputum is the keystone of choosing initial therapy, and may be helpful in interpreting subsequent culture reports. Abscess formation, salmon-colored sputum, and an appropriate host for the development of staphylococcal pneumonia are helpful clues.

As drug-resistant staphylococci frequently colonize the respiratory tract soon after the administration of antimicrobial drugs, one should not diagnose staphylococcal pneumonia solely on the basis of a sputum culture revealing rare or moderate numbers of the organism in someone under treatment for other pulmonary infections.

PROGNOSIS. Even under the best of circumstances, the case fatality rate for pneumonia is 15 to 20 per cent. Higher fatality rates are seen in very young infants and in elderly or debilitated patients. As this pneumonia is characterized by necrosis of lung parenchyma, recovery is usually slow. Improvement following the initiation of therapy is often not evident for 48 to 72 hours, and the illness usually lasts three to four weeks. Convalescence may be prolonged when empyema is present. Bronchiectasis can be a consequence of staphylococcal pneumonia.

TREATMENT. Once the diagnosis is tentatively established, vigorous parenteral antimicrobial therapy should be initiated promptly. Methicillin, oxacillin, nafcillin, cephalothin, or cefazolin, in doses of at least 1 gram every four to six hours, are preferred and equally good. The organism should be considered resistant to penicillin and ampicillin until it is demonstrated to be susceptible. If the organism is susceptible, penicillin G (20 million units intravenously per day) is the drug of choice. If the patient is allergic to penicillin, vancomycin (0.5 gram intravenously every six to eight hours) or clindamycin (600 mg four times per day) may be used. Therapy should be continued for 10 to 14 days or more after the patient shows a definite clinical response. The clinical response is usually very gradual. When empyema is present, it may be helpful to administer antimicrobial drugs directly into the pleural cavity, and proteolytic enzymes may be instilled to help thin the exudate. Because the pus is often loculated or too thick for needle aspiration, surgical drainage of empyema with a chest tube is usually required. Oxygen, bronchodilators, expectorants, fluids, and other supportive measures are important.

135. STAPHYLOCOCCAL OSTEOMYELITIS

Staphylococcus aureus is the etiologic agent in the majority of instances of *primary or hematogenous osteomyelitis*. The disease is becoming uncommon and is readily cured if treated early with appropriate antimicrobials. Bacteremia occurring from a skin infection which may be no more serious than a furuncle is the usual inciting event. *Secondary staphylococcal osteomyelitis* is usually related to penetrating trauma, surgery, or a contiguous focus of infection. It is also seen in patients with diabetes mellitus or peripheral vascular disease following local cutaneous infections.

Hematogenous staphylococcal osteomyelitis is primarily a disease of children, adolescents, and intravenous drug abusers. It is more frequent in males. It usually begins in the metaphyseal area of the diaphysis near the epiphyseal plate, and is uncommon following epiphyseal closure. The metaphysis is a weak spot in growing bones. It has a terminal blood supply subject to bacterial embolization and thrombosis. The capillary and venous networks in this area are extensive, and minor injuries may result in hematomas that afford a nidus for bacteria. Furthermore, the capillaries in this area are deficient in phagocytic lining cells. The most common sites of involvement are the lower femur, upper tibia, ankle, wrist, or hip, but any metaphyseal area can be involved. The vertebrae are more commonly involved in adults, particularly narcotic addicts. As the infectious process develops in the metaphysis, the arterial blood supply is usually compromised, because it is terminal and encased in rigid bony canals. Thromboses and vascular insufficiency develop and lead to necrosis of bone. Early radiologic signs of osteomyelitis include decalcification or rarefaction of bone due to hyperemia and injury to osteoblasts, and periosteal elevation. If the infection is untreated, a sequestrum of necrotic bone will separate in six to eight weeks. Treatment with antimicrobial drugs has practically eliminated this result. In pyogenic osteomyelitis it is characteristic for the periosteum to react to the infection by forming a layer of reparative bone (osteosclerosis) called the involucrum. Reactive bone formation is much less common in tuberculous osteomyelitis, unless the process has been going on for more than six months.

The infection tends to spread along the diaphysis or outward to the subperiosteal space, where an abscess often forms, particularly in children. From there the infection may extend and involve nearby joints. This is seen in about 10 per cent of cases, and is more frequent when the hip or shoulder bones are infected. It is uncommon for the infection to enter the joint by crossing the epiphyseal plate barrier in children, but this is not unusual in adults. In addition, sterile joint effusions are not uncommon when there is an osteomyelitic focus nearby.

If not treated early or adequately, the infection tends to become chronic, with recurrent exacerbations, formation of draining sinuses, and extensive scarring eventually requiring surgical debridement and saucerization of bone. Amyloidosis occasionally develops after long-standing osteomyelitis.

Staphylococcal infections of vertebrae and intervertebral discs are especially frequent in intravenous drug abusers. They are also seen following pelvic and urinary tract infections, but other organisms are more frequent in these settings. The patients usually complain of back pain accentuated by straining or coughing, pain radiating down the leg, or abdominal pain. Paravertebral abscesses are a frequent complication. Narrowing of the disc space, erosion of the vertebral end-plates, and bridging of the disc space by new bone formation are important radiologic findings. The condition may be mistaken for tuberculous spondylitis, but osteophytic bridging or isolated involvement of the vertebral arches or processes is unusual in tuberculosis. Acute endocarditis is an occasional complication of staphylococcal vertebral osteomyelitis.

High fever, chills, throbbing bone pain, local tenderness, muscle spasms, splinting, or limping are the early manifestations. Redness, swelling, and warmth are seen later. Bacteremia is frequent in osteomyelitis, and the patient may appear delirious and critically ill. The systemic signs and symptoms may overshadow the local manifestations. Leukocytosis and anemia are common. Rarefaction of bone is the earliest radiologic sign, but may not appear until 10 to 14 days after onset. Periosteal reaction with new bone formation is seen after the disease has been present for at least a month. Bone scans using radioactive technetium, strontium, fluorine, or gallium can localize the lesion prior to x-ray changes. They are particularly useful in drug addicts who present with fever and vague complaints referable to the lower back.

Rheumatic fever, traumatic lesions, leukemia, scurvy, pyogenic arthritis, hemoglobinopathies, Ewing's tumor, and other neoplasms should be considered in the differential diagnosis of osteomyelitis.

TREATMENT. With appropriate treatment, death from acute osteomyelitis is rare, and progression to chronic osteomyelitis is not likely. Mixed infection with other organisms, such as *Pseudomonas*, is seen fairly often. Empirical treatment without the aid of exudate or aspirated or operative specimens for culture and Gram stain is hazardous and should be avoided. Since early treatment is important, therapy directed against staphylococci should be started as soon as cultures have been obtained when this organism appears likely. Parenteral bactericidal drugs should be given initially. One of the penicillins, cephalosporins, or clindamycin is recommended. Gentamicin is useful in addicts when *Pseudomonas* as well as *Staphylococcus* is suspected. Immobilization is important for relief of pain and for clinical improvement. Some evidence of a clinical response should be noted within four days. It may be necessary to aspirate a subperiosteal abscess, or to surgically drain it. Vigorous parenteral treatment should be continued for at least four weeks. Subsequent oral therapy is not needed in most cases. Radiologic signs of the infection may never become apparent if treatment is given early. Although small sequestra usually absorb spontaneously, larger pieces of dead bone require surgical removal, especially if there is a slow or incomplete clinical response. Operative removal of foreign bodies is frequently necessary to achieve a cure in secondary osteomyelitis.

With chronic osteomyelitis, antimicrobial therapy should be given, and sequestrectomy, saucerization of infected bone, and removal of sinus tracts should be performed. Only rarely will such patients respond to drug therapy alone. Closed irrigation with antimicrobial agents is occasionally a useful adjunct to surgery.

136. STAPHYLOCOCCAL BACTEREMIA AND ENDOCARDITIS

Bacteremia may occur with any localized staphylococcal infection, but is relatively uncommon with minor postoperative wound infections and pneumonia, unless of hematogenous origin. Carbuncles, skin infections, infected intravascular shunts, catheters, and other foreign bodies, endocarditis, and osteomyelitis are the most common foci causing bacteremia. Staphylococcal bacteremia is frequent in patients with marked granulocytopenia or serious chronic debilitating diseases. It is usually associated with hectic fever, repeated shaking chills, and marked systemic toxicity. Widespread metastatic abscesses may develop in kidneys, lungs, bone, skin, brain, meninges, myocardium, and other viscera.

Bacteremia with coagulase-negative staphylococci sometimes pursues an indolent course for many weeks with remarkably few clinical manifestations. Bloodstream infections with these organisms are usually seen following ventriculoatriostomy shunting or cardiac surgery with insertion of prostheses. A proliferative and membranous glomerulonephritis and the nephrotic syndrome may be seen as a result of chronic *S. epidermidis* bacteremia in patients with infected shunts, and prompt improvement in the renal disease may follow removal of the shunt.

Endocarditis frequently complicates staphylococcal bacteremia from another site. The disease is usually of the acute, malignant, or ulcerative type with *S. aureus*, but a form indistinguishable from that caused by *S. viridans* is occasionally seen, especially when *S. epidermidis* is responsible. The illness usually has an acute onset with shaking chills, high fever, changing cardiac murmurs, cutaneous pustules and petechiae, splinter hemorrhages, metastatic abscesses, hematuria, progressive anemia, and marked leukocytosis. Thrombocytopenia and disseminated intravascular coagulation may be seen. Normal heart valves may be destroyed in just a few days. Abscess of the myocardial valve ring occurs frequently and should be suspected when arrhythmias develop.

Acute staphylococcal endocarditis in heroin addicts is often characterized by involvement of the tricuspid valve. Multiple septic pulmonary emboli and infarcts with abscess formation and empyema are the usual presenting manifestations. The classic peripheral cutaneous manifestations of endocarditis, such as splenomegaly, Osler's nodes, and splinter hemorrhages, may be lacking in right-sided endocarditis, but blood cultures are usually positive. Antibodies to staphylococcal teichoic acid are usually present, and tests for rheumatoid factor are often positive. Cerebral manifestations relative to abscess formation, embolization, meningitis, and subarachnoid hemorrhage are frequent. Panophthalmitis is occasionally a complication. A murmur from the tricuspid lesion is usually present but is often overlooked initially until pulmonary emboli call attention to its presence. Other clues to tricuspid involvement are atrial or ventricular diastolic gallops along the lower left sternal border and the external jugular vein, or a short soft systolic murmur along the lower left sternal border which is increased with inspiration (Carvallo's sign), and with the patient standing.

Acute proliferative glomerulonephritis of the immune complex type may develop during the course of staphylococcal endocarditis and is sometimes confused with an allergic reaction to drugs used in treatment.

The distinction between endocarditis and bacteremia originating from another focus may be difficult. Continuous bacteremia suggests endocarditis or other intravascular focus; intermittent bacteremia suggests an extravascular focus.

TREATMENT. Even with appropriate therapy, staphylococcal bacteremia still has a mortality rate of about 40 per cent. Patients over the age of 50 or with underlying diseases have a mortality rate of more than 60 per cent. Parenteral therapy is necessary, and the regimen must be bactericidal. Therapy for endocarditis should be continued for four to eight weeks. A clear-cut clinical response to treatment may not be seen until the end of the first week. Surgical treatment of the focus of infection is always important to consider. When the site of infection is an intravascular foreign body, the infection is rarely cured until the foreign material is removed. However, infected cardiac prostheses are not usually replaced until at least one course of intensive treatment has proved unsuccessful, because 5 to 10 per cent of these infections may be cured with medical therapy alone. Early replacement of damaged valves may be necessary if there is severe or intractable heart failure.

If there is a removable focus of infection, no evidence of heart disease or metastatic infection, no serious derangement of host defenses, no teichoic acid antibodies, and a prompt clinical response, treatment of staphylococcal bacteremia can be terminated at the end of two or three weeks. In doubtful cases in which endocarditis remains a good possibility, therapy should be given for at least four weeks.

137.   MISCELLANEOUS INFECTIONS

Staphlyococci are commonly found in *nose* or *throat* cultures, but they do not cause pharyngitis or tonsillitis, except in patients with agranulocytosis or leukemia. Their presence in healthy persons usually represents nothing more than colonization, and does not by itself justify treatment with antimicrobial therapy. Staphylococci have been recognized as a cause of cervical lymphadenitis in infants.

Staphylococcal pyarthrosis represents a diagnostic and therapeutic challenge in adults. It may occur following orthopedic surgery or in association with osteomyelitis. Infected skin ulcers or contaminated intra-articular injections or aspirations are often responsible. Rheumatoid factor may bind antistaphylococcal antibodies and contribute to lowered resistance. Joint infection should be suspected in all patients with rheumatoid arthritis who show an apparent exacerbation of joint disease with fever, pain, effusion, and leukocytosis. Chills favor the diagnosis of septic arthritis over rheumatoid disease. Joint fluid aspiration is essential for early diagnosis. Immobilization, repeated aspiration, surgical drainage when indicated, and appropriate antimicrobial drugs given for two to four weeks are the treatment.

Staphylococcal meningitis is uncommon. It is usually the result of penetrating trauma, local surgery, or bacterial endocarditis. Therapy must be vigorous. If the organism is known to be susceptible to penicillin G, 24 to 30 million units should be given daily by the intravenous route. If it is resistant to penicillin G or of unknown susceptibility, nafcillin (12 grams per day), oxacillin (12 grams per day) or methicillin (12 to 24 grams per day) may be used. Cephalosporins are not recommended unless they are supplemented with intrathecal cephaloridine* (50 mg daily).

Primary spinal epidural abscess is a neurosurgical emergency in which prompt recognition and treatment are indicated to prevent permanent spinal cord damage. It is sometimes seen in narcotic addicts in association with vertebral osteomyelitis. The process is usually acute, located dorsally in the lower thoracic or lumbar regions, and most often caused by staphylococci. Fever, localized spinal tenderness, and rigidity of the spine are followed by root pain, localized weakness, progressive paresthesias, sphincter changes, and evidence of spinal cord compression. The lumbar spinal fluid usually is under reduced pressure and shows pleocytosis, but may be normal. Myelography localizes the lesion but *is seldom necessary*. Antimicrobials are merely adjuncts to treatment, for total recovery depends on early diagnosis followed by *prompt* surgery, usually laminectomy and drainage (see Ch. 299).

Staphylococcal pericarditis usually occurs following bacteremia, often in association with osteomyelitis or endocarditis, with formation of focal myocardial abscesses and spread to the pericardium. The staphylococcus is the most frequent cause of purulent pericarditis. Treatment consists of antimicrobial therapy and pericardiocentesis, but if rapid improvement is not noted, open surgical drainage should be instituted.

Staphylococcal parotitis is seen in debilitated adults, especially those who become dehydrated and receive inadequate mouth care. Extensive edema, erythema, and tenderness are seen in the parotid area, and pus may be seen oozing from Stensen's duct. The patient usually has a high fever and disorientation. Shock and death are common. Irradiation of the gland may be a useful therapeutic adjunct, but appropriate antimicrobial therapy and supportive care are more important.

Staphylococcal (tropical) pyomyositis is a relatively common disease of indigenous residents of hot, humid tropical areas. It is occasionally seen in temperate climates, where it is usually misdiagnosed. Bacteremia resulting from minor superficial lesions is followed by abscess formation beneath the deep fascia of skeletal muscles, especially in the upper leg. Local trauma may be important in determining the site. There is diffuse swelling of the limb, but usually no fluctuance or regional adenopathy. The skin may become tense and cellulitic, but is often normal. Fever may be minimal during the first week of illness. The diagnosis is usually made at operation, when multiple abscesses are found to have coalesced and extended between muscle fasciculi and within fascial compartments. It is uncommon for osteomyelitis to coexist. Staphylococci of bacteriophage group II are usually implicated. Surgical drainage and antimicrobial drugs are efficacious.

138.   STAPHYLOCOCCAL GASTROENTERITIS AND ENTEROCOLITIS

The enterotoxins produced by staphylococci are an important cause of acute epidemic gastroenteritis or food poisoning. The toxin is formed prior to ingestion of contaminated and usually improperly refrigerated or stored food (see Ch. 22.2).

Staphylococci are normal inhabitants of the intestines, although they are not usually detected unless se-

---

*Intrathecal use is not mentioned in the manufacturer's package insert approved by the U.S. Food and Drug Administration. Therefore its use in these circumstances must be considered investigational.

lective media are used. They may increase during antimicrobial therapy, and patients may concomitantly experience mild diarrhea. Much more rarely the organisms cause acute necrotizing pseudomembranous enterocolitis. Most common following abdominal surgery, shock, or antimicrobial therapy, or in leukemia, this syndrome has a high mortality rate. Locally produced enterotoxin is thought to be responsible for the manifestations of the disease, but the pathogenesis is still uncertain. Staphylococci are implicated in only a relatively small proportion of total cases. Recent data suggest that toxigenic *Clostridium difficile* is the most important cause of the disease. Symptoms include abdominal pain, distention, ileus, fever, diarrhea, bloody stools, electrolyte depletion, dehydration, and shock. Gram stain of the stool reveals leukocytes and large numbers of cocci in sheets and clumps, and establishes the diagnosis of staphylococcal enterocolitis. Vancomycin given by *mouth* is useful in treatment. The usual dose is 0.5 gram every six hours. Parenteral therapy with another appropriate drug may also be given. Oral neomycin is no longer recommended, as many staphylococci in hospitals are resistant to it. Shock and electrolyte imbalance should be treated vigorously with appropriate fluids.

Andriole, V. T., and Lyons, R. W.: Coagulase-negative staphylococcus. Ann. N. Y. Acad. Sci., 174:533, 1970.

Banks, T., Fletcher, R., and Ali, N.: Infective endocarditis in heroin addicts. Am. J. Med., 55:444, 1973.

Barrett, F. F., McGehee, R. F., and Finland, M.: Methicillin-resistant *Staphylococcus aureus* at Boston City Hospital. N. Engl. J. Med., 279:441, 1968.

Boyle, J. D., Pearce, M. L., and Guze, L. B.: Purulent pericarditis: Review of literature and report of eleven cases. Medicine, 40:119, 1961.

Cluff, L. E., Reynolds, R. C., Page, D. L., and Breckenridge, J. C.: Staphylococcal bacteremia and altered host resistance. Ann. Intern. Med., 69:859, 1968.

Cohen, J. O. (ed.): The Staphylococci. New York, Wiley-Interscience, 1972.

Elek, S. D.: Staphylococcus Pyogenes. Edinburgh, E. and S. Livingstone, Ltd., 1959.

Elias, P. M., Fritsch, P. and Epstein, E. H.: Staphylococcal scalded skin syndrome. Arch. Dermatol., 113:207, 1977.

Fekety, F. R.: The epidemiology and prevention of staphylococcal infection. Medicine, 43:593, 1964.

Iannini, P. B., and Crossley, K.: Therapy of *Staphylococcus aureus* bacteremia associated with a removable focus of infection. Ann. Intern. Med., 84:558, 1976.

Karten, I.: Septic arthritis complicating rheumatoid arthritis. Ann. Intern. Med., 70:1147, 1969.

Keys, T. F., and Hewitt, W. L.: Endocarditis due to micrococci and *Staphylococcus epidermidis*. Arch. Intern. Med., 132:216, 1973.

Levin, M. J., Gardner, P., and Waldvogel, F. A.: "Tropical" pyomyositis. N. Engl. J. Med., 284:196, 1971.

Mailbach, H. I., Strauss, W. G., and Shinefield, H. R.: Bacterial interference: Relating to chronic furunculosis in man. Br. J. Dermatol., 81: Suppl. 1:69, 1969.

McCloskey, R. V.: Scarlet fever and necrotizing fasciitis caused by coagulase-positive hemolytic *Staphylococcus aureus*, phage type 85. Ann. Intern. Med., 78:85, 1973.

Pollack, N., Spinner, M., and Richman, R.: Hematogenous pyogenic spondylitis. N.Y. J. Med., 64:2870, 1964.

Rahal, J. J., MacMahon, H. E., and Weinstein, L.: Thrombocytopenia and symmetrical peripheral gangrene associated with staphylococcal and streptococcal bacteremia. Ann. Intern. Med., 69:35, 1968.

Shinefield, H. R., Ribble, J. C., Boris, M., and Eichenwald, H.: Bacterial interference: Its effect on nursery acquired infection with *Staphylococcus aureus*. Am. J. Dis. Child., 105:646, 1963.

Smith, D. T.: Autogenous vaccines in theory and practice. Arch. Intern. Med., 125:344, 1970.

Stickler, G. B., Shin, W. H., Burke, E. C., Holley, K. E., Miller, R. H., and Segar, W. H.: Diffuse glomerulonephritis associated with infected ventriculoatrial shunt. N. Engl. J. Med., 279:1077, 1968.

Tu, W. H., Shearn, M. A., and Lee, J. C.: Acute diffuse glomerulonephritis in acute staphylococcal endocarditis. Ann. Intern. Med., 71:335, 1969.

Tuazon, C. U., and Sheagren, J. N.: Teichoic acid antibodies in the diagnosis of serious infections with *Staphylococcus aureus*. Ann. Intern. Med., 84:543, 1976.

VanProhaska, J., Mock, F., Baker, W., and Collins, R.: Pseudomembranous (staphylococcal) enterocolitis. Surg. Gynecol. Obstet., 112:103, 1961.

Waldvogel, F. A., Medoff, G., and Swartz, M. N.: Osteomyelitis: A review of clinical features, therapeutic considerations and unusual aspects. N. Engl. J. Med., 282:198, 260, 316, 1970.

Watanakunakorn, C., Tan, J. S., and Phair, J. P.: Some salient features of *Staphylococcus aureus* endocarditis. Am. J. Med., 54:473, 1973.

Wentworth, B. B.: Bacteriophage typing of staphylococci. Bacteriol. Rev., 27:253, 1963.

Williams, D. N., Lung, M. E., and Blazevic, D. J.: Significance of urinary isolates of coagulase-negative Micrococcaceae. J. Clin. Microbiol., 3:556, 1976.

DISEASES CAUSED BY NEISSERIA

139. GONOCOCCAL DISEASE

Donald Kaye

DEFINITION. Gonorrhea is an infection of the mucous membrane of the urethra and genital tract caused by *Neisseria gonorrhoeae*. Involvement of the pharynx and anal canal is common. Infection is almost always the result of sexual contact. After invasion of mucosal sites, gonococci may spread and cause infections such as arthritis, tenosynovitis, perihepatitis, endocarditis, and meningitis.

ETIOLOGY. *N. gonorrhoeae* is a gram-negative coccus that was first described by Neisser in 1879 in exudates from patients with gonorrhea. In stained smears of exudates the organisms appear as diplococci with flattened or slightly concave adjacent sides and resemble a pair of kidney beans. A considerable portion of the organisms in exudates are within polymorphonuclear leukocytes. Gonococci grown in laboratory media assume an oval or spherical form, and single cocci and clumps of cocci may be found in addition to diplococci. *N. gonorrhoeae* can be distinguished from other *Neisseria* by its ability to ferment glucose but not maltose or sucrose.

Primary isolation of the gonococcus is difficult. The organism is fastidious in its growth requirements, and is susceptible to toxic substances that are present in many media. Blood, serum, ascitic fluid, or other agents must be added for enrichment, as growth will usually not occur on plain agar. Blood is commonly used, and the medium is heated (chocolate agar) to reduce the deleterious effect exerted by certain amino acids toxic to the gonococcus. Commercial media are available that satisfy the various growth requirements of *N. gonorrhoeae*. Most strains require an atmosphere of 2 to 10 per cent carbon dioxide. Overgrowth with other bacterica occasionally occurs in cultures of exudate from the urethra, vagina, and cervix and is frequent in cultures from the pharynx and anal canal if nonselective media are used.

Colonies of *N. gonorrhoeae* are round, gray-white, and translucent. On subculture on special media, four morphologically different colonial variants can be recognized: T_1, T_2, T_3, and T_4. T_1 and T_2 colonies are virulent, and the gonococci in the colonies are covered with tiny hairlike projections called pili. T_3 and T_4 colonies are much less virulent, and the gonococci do not have pili. Pili may be important for attachment of gonococci to mucosal cells in the pathogenesis of infection.

All *Neisseria* produce an oxidase that can be used for tentative identification of colonies of *N. gonorrhoeae* (colonies turn purple on exposure to 1 per cent para-aminodimethylaniline monohydrochloride). With cultures from the genital tract, the combination of colonies of typical morphology composed of gram-negative diplococci and a positive oxidase test is strong presumptive evidence of the presence of *N. gonorrhoeae*. However, confirmation by fermentation reactions or by fluorescent antibody techniques is necessary for definitive identification.

Thayer-Martin selective medium, containing a mixture of antimicrobials, permits growth of *N. meningitidis* and *N. gonorrhoeae* but inhibits growth of many other bacteria frequently found in specimens from urethra, cervix, vagina, anal canal, and pharynx.

EPIDEMIOLOGY.   *N. gonorrhoeae* is a parasite of man; it does not cause disease in animals in nature. Gonorrhea is almost always acquired from sexual contact. Exceptions are gonococcal conjunctivitis (which occurs primarily in infants) and vulvovaginitis. Conjunctivitis results either from passage of the infant through an infected genital tract (ophthalmia neonatorum) or from contamination after birth. Vulvovaginitis is an infection of the genital tract of infants and preadolescent girls that results from direct contact with infected adults or, rarely, can be spread by contact with towels or linens contaminated with gonococci.

Repeated attacks of gonorrhea are common; therefore individual attacks seem to confer little or no immunity. However, individual variation in susceptibility to infection has been demonstrated after inoculation of *N. gonorrhoeae* into the urethras of male volunteers. Trauma to the urethra probably increases susceptibility to gonorrhea. After an episode of acute gonorrhea, *N. gonorrhoeae* may remain in the genital tract for months. Chronic asymptomatic carriers of the gonococcus are important in the epidemiology of gonorrhea because they are difficult to detect and therefore are rarely treated. It has been common knowledge that most women with gonorrhea are relatively asymptomatic, but only recently has it been reported that as many as 10 per cent of males with gonorrhea seen in a venereal disease clinic may be asymptomatic and that up to 40 per cent of asymptomatic male contacts of women with symptomatic gonorrhea have positive urethral cultures.

There has been an increase in the reported incidence of gonococcal infections in recent years. However, the true *incidence* and *prevalence* of gonorrhea are unknown because of problems in diagnosis, antimicrobial therapy by nonmedical persons, incomplete reporting by physicians, and the presence of many undetected asymptomatic carriers. It has been estimated that over 2 million new cases of gonorrhea occur annually in the United States. The magnitude of the problem of asymp-

tomatic gonorrhea may be demonstrated by the fact that there is about a 5 per cent prevalence of asymptomatic gonorrhea in pregnant women.

Gonorrhea is a disease of the sexually active, and most cases occur in patients 15 to 24 years of age. Gonorrhea rates are higher among military personnel, migrant groups (such as itinerant laborers and seafarers), homosexuals, and prostitutes. In surveys 10 to 33 per cent of prostitutes have gonorrhea.

PATHOGENESIS AND PATHOLOGY.   In males the urethra is attacked first, resulting in purulent urethritis and involvement of the urethral glands. Direct spread of infection may result in prostatitis, epididymitis, or seminal vesiculitis (all rare conditions currently). During stages of healing, stricture formation may occur. Gonococcal proctitis in the male is almost always the result of rectal intercourse.

In the female, urethritis is mild and transient. Bartholin's and Skene's glands and glands of the cervix may become infected with or without involvement of the urethra. Contiguous spread of infection can cause acute salpingitis, which is said to occur in about 10 per cent of women with genital tract gonorrhea. Proctitis may result from contiguous spread or rectal intercourse. Gonococcal salpingitis is usually bilateral and may cause pyosalpinx and formation of a tubo-ovarian abscess. The inflammation tends to heal with fibrosis and adhesions that may produce obstruction of the fallopian tubes and sterility. Subsequent secondary infections with other microorganisms (chronic pelvic inflammatory disease) may play a major role in the destructive process. Ascent of infection to the fallopian tubes often occurs during or just after menstruation. Although endometrial infection is usual when *N. gonorrhoeae* invades the fallopian tubes, it is not serious and tends to subside promptly. The vagina does not become infected in adults, probably because of the presence of squamous epithelium with many layers of cells and the lack of glands.

Conjunctivitis is the most common manifestation of gonococcal disease in infants. It is a destructive inflammation of the eye and before the use of antimicrobial agents frequently caused blindness. Between one year of age and pubescence, gonococcal infection is rare in males but causes vulvovaginitis in females. The increased susceptibility to gonococcal infection of the immature vaginal mucous membrane in contrast to the resistance of the mucosa of adults is probably explained by the thin mucous membrane present prior to adolescence.

Gonococcal infection of the pharynx is common and results from oral-genital contact. Gonococcal pharyngeal infection has been demonstrated in up to 20 per cent of homosexual men and 20 per cent of women practicing fellatio who had gonococcal infection at any site. In 3 to 8 per cent of these patients, only pharyngeal cultures are positive for gonococci.

N. gonorrhoeae have been found to produce a protease that cleaves human IgA. This destruction of IgA may play a role in the ability of gonococci to produce infection on mucosal surfaces.

Occasionally invasion of the blood occurs and *N. gonorrhoeae* may disseminate and produce infection at distant foci. Joints are the most frequent extragenital sites of localization, but tenosynovitis, endocarditis, meningitis, skin lesions, and infection at other foci may also occur.

Dissemination of gonoccocal infection is about twice

as common in women as in men and is probably more common in homosexual males than in heterosexual males. This is probably explained by the fact that men with gonococcal urethritis are usually symptomatic (90 to 95 per cent) and therefore are treated promptly, greatly decreasing the chances of dissemination of infection. In contrast, women with gonorrhea and males with gonococcal proctitis or pharyngitis (almost always homosexuals) are usually asymptomatic and are therefore unlikely to be treated. There is also a disproportionately high incidence of men with asymptomatic urethral gonorrhea among males with disseminated gonococcal infection. The source for dissemination may be the genital tract, rectum, or pharynx. It has been estimated that dissemination of gonococcal infection occurs in up to 3 per cent of women with gonorrhea and is most prone to occur during pregnancy or during or just after menstruation. Strains of *N. gonorrhoeae* that disseminate have usually been found to be highly susceptible to penicillin G and to require arginine, hypoxanthine, and uracil for growth.

CLINICAL MANIFESTATIONS. Gonorrhea in the Male. The incubation period of gonococcal urethritis in the male is usually two to eight days. There is sudden onset of dysuria, urgency, and frequency associated with mucoid urethral discharge that rapidly becomes purulent and profuse. Gonococcal urethritis usually does not cause fever, but prostatitis, seminal vesiculitis, or epididymitis is frequently associated with fever. Acute urinary retention may result from involvement of the prostate. Rectal examination reveals tenderness of the affected organ in the presence of prostatitis or seminal vesiculitis. Epididymitis causes severe pain and tenderness of the epididymis.

Untreated gonorrhea subsides over a period of weeks, but a small amount of mucoid discharge from the urethra may continue to be found each morning for months. Urethral stricture is a common sequela of untreated urethritis, especially after recurrent attacks of gonorrhea. Epididymitis can result in sterility.

About 5 to 10 per cent of men who develop urethral infection remain asymptomatic, do not seek therapy, and become an important vector for spread of infection.

Gonorrhea in the Female. In females the disease may begin with dysuria, urgency, and frequency after an incubation period of two to eight days. However, the urethritis is frequently of short duration and often is mild or completely asymptomatic. Cervicitis gives rise to a mucopurulent discharge that varies from scant to profuse. Involvement of Skene's ducts or Bartholin's glands is common, and abscess formation may occur. Gonococci can be isolated from the anal canal in 20 to 50 per cent of women with gonorrhea, and occasionally can produce symptomatic proctitis. In 5 per cent of women with gonococcal infection only the anorectal culture contains gonoccoci. The duration of symptoms from an untreated infection that remains localized in the lower genital tract is usually no longer than a month or two. However, the patient may remain a carrier of the disease for many months.

Salpingitis is manifested by acute onset of fever and lower abdominal pain. Physical examination usually reveals lower abdominal tenderness, pain on movement of the cervix, and tenderness of the adnexa (with or without palpable masses). Subsequently pelvic inflammatory disease with pelvic pain and fever may recur and is usually caused by bacteria other than gonococci. Sterility is common.

Extragenital Gonococcal Infection. PROCTITIS. Gonococcal proctitis is usually asymptomatic but may be manifested by anal discharge, burning rectal pain, blood and pus in the stools, and pain on defecation.

PHARYNGITIS. Gonococcal infection in the oropharynx can probably cause symptomatic pharyngitis, tonsillitis, and gingivitis but is usually asymptomatic.

ARTHRITIS. Arthritis is the most common form of clinically recognized disseminated gonococcal infection; it usually occurs within one to three weeks after initial infection in the genital tract or may follow pharyngeal or rectal infection. Onset may be gradual with migratory polyarthalgias leading to frank arthritis in one or more joints, or it may be sudden with hot, swollen, and extremely painful joints. Fever and leukocytosis are usually present. Over 75 per cent of patients have polyarthritis. The joints that are most commonly involved are the knees, ankles, and wrists, but any joint may be involved, including the spine and sternoclavicular and temporomandibular joints. *Tenosynovitis*, which is rarely observed in other types of pyogenic arthritis, is common in gonococcal arthritis and most often occurs about the wrists and ankles. The skin lesions associated with gonococcal bacteremia are also frequently present.

N. gonorrhoeae can be isolated from joint fluid in only 25 to 50 per cent of cases. The fluid ranges from serous to frankly purulent, has the protein content of an exudate, and usually contains increased numbers of leukocytes that are mainly polymorphonuclear. Muscle wasting about the joint and permanent deformity may result. Some authorities have described two types of arthritis produced by the gonococcus: (1) polyarticular arthritis, usually with no or small effusions that tend to be sterile, often associated with bacteremia and skin lesions, and (2) frank pyogenic arthritis (often involving one joint from which gonococci can frequently be isolated) without bacteremia or skin lesions. The first type has been attributed by some to hypersensitivity, but it seems more likely that it represents the initial or bacteremic phase during which organisms localize in joints. Frank pyogenic arthritis may occur after a clinically apparent or inapparent bacteremic phase. Sterility of the joint fluid in patients during the bacteremic phase may be due to taking cultures early in disease, before microorganisms in the joint have sufficient time to proliferate.

GONOCOCCAL BACTEREMIA. Gonococcal bacteremia can produce a syndrome with recurrent episodes of fever, skin lesions, tenosynovitis, arthralgia or arthritis, mild to severe constitutional symptoms, and intermittently positive blood cultures. This syndrome occurs with infection in the genital tract, anal canal or pharynx, and, if untreated, can recur over a period of months or even years. The rash usually appears during the first day of symptoms and may recur with each episode of fever. The rash is found on the distal part of the extremities and consists of scanty pin-point erythematous macules that rapidly become maculopapular, vesiculopustular, and frequently hemorrhagic. Bullae can form. The mature lesion is elevated, has a dirty gray necrotic center, and is surrounded by erythema. It heals in three to four days. Gram-negative cocci can often be seen in stains of fluid from the lesions, but cultures for *N. gonorrhoeae* are usually negative. Immunofluorescent studies on the exudate from the pustules demonstrate *N. gonorrhoeae* in a high percentage of patients. Identical skin lesions may be seen in patients with meningococcemia, which can present an indistinguishable clinical sydrome.

GONOCOCCAL ENDOCARDITIS. Gonococcal endocarditis is extremely rare at present. In most patients, previously normal valves are attacked. The valves on the left side of the heart are involved most often, but valves on the right side are affected with a higher frequency than with endocarditis caused by other bacteria. A double daily temperature elevation (double quotidian) is common in patients with gonococcal endocarditis.

PERIHEPATITIS (FITZ-HUGH–CURTIS SYNDROME). Perihepatitis is a rare complication in women with gonococcal pelvic inflammatory disease and results from direct spread of gonococci from the pelvis to the upper abdomen. It is manifested by fever, upper quadrant pain (usually right upper quadrant), tenderness and spasm of the abdominal wall, and occasionally a friction rub over the liver. During the acute stage the gallbladder temporarily may not be visualized on cholecystography; this can lead to an erroneous diagnosis of cholecystitis. The patient often has a recent history of pelvic pain or vaginal discharge, and physical examination may reveal evidence of pelvic inflammatory disease. N. gonorrhoeae can frequently be demonstrated in the cervical or vaginal discharge.

The symptoms respond to antimicrobial therapy. The untreated disease subsides after one to four weeks of fever and abdominal pain, leaving "violin-string" adhesions between the anterior surface of the liver and the anterior abdominal wall. This syndrome has been reported in a male, probably caused by lymphatic or hematogenous dissemination.

DIAGNOSIS. In the male the combination of urethritis and the presence of intracellular gram-negative diplococci in smears of exudate from the urethra is strong presumptive evidence of gonorrhea. Confirmation is obtained by culture or, if available, fluorescent antibody studies. Cultures of the anal canal should be obtained in homosexual males. Urethral cultures in asymptomatic males are made by inserting a wire tipped with a calcium alginate swab into the urethra.

For routine screening, cervical cultures will detect the vast majority of females with asymptomatic gonorrhea. Gonorrhea should be suspected in any female contact of an infected male. Similarly the asymptomatic carrier state should be suspected in asymptomatic male contacts of symptomatic females or asymptomatic females detected by routine cultures. In the female with suspected gonorrhea, cultures of exudate from the cervix and anal canal should be obtained in addition to urethral cultures.

Pharyngeal cultures for N. gonorrhoeae should be obtained from homosexual males and females practicing fellatio. In all patients with suspected disseminated gonococcal infections, cultures of the pharynx and anal canal should be obtained in addition to genital tract cultures.

Gonococci die within hours if allowed to dry. Therefore exudates should be inoculated as soon as possible on Thayer-Martin medium or on a suitable transport medium for N. gonorrhoeae such as Transgrow, which is available commercially.

With use of fluorescent antibody it is frequently possible to make a definite identification of N. gonorrhoeae in exudate within one hour of obtaining a specimen.

A substantial portion of the cases of urethritis in men in the United States today are nongonococcal. A substantial portion of these are caused by Chlamydia trachomatis. Although the evidence is not conclusive, many of the remaining cases may be due to Ureaplasma urealyticum. Trichomonas vaginalis can also cause

urethritis. The urethral discharge in gonorrhea is usually profuse and yellow, whereas in nongonococcal urethritis the discharge is usually white and scanty. However, Gram stain and culture are necessary for definitive differentiation. The chlamydial form of urethritis is discussed in Ch. 116.

Salpingitis. Acute salpingitis must be differentiated from appendicitis and tubal pregnancy. The presence of bilateral tenderness in the adnexa with or without masses, a history of recent sexual intercourse followed by urethritis or vaginal discharge, and demonstration of gonococci in the cervical exudate are strongly suggestive of gonococcal salpingitis. When it is impossible to differentiate acute salpingitis from appendicitis or tubal pregnancy, the diagnosis must be established at laparoscopy or laparotomy.

Bacteria indigenous to the female genital tract (e.g., anaerobic gram-positive cocci) are also responsible for cases of acute salpingitis and for continuing infection following an episode of gonococcal salpingitis (chronic pelvic inflammatory disease). The risk of pelvic inflammatory disease seems to be increased by intrauterine devices.

Arthritis; Blood-Borne Lesions. The diagnosis of gonococcal arthritis or bacteremia with skin lesions should be suspected in a patient with the appropriate clinical syndrome, especially if there is a recent history of urethritis or vaginal discharge. Tenosynovitis is suggestive of disseminated gonococcal infection. Isolation of N. gonorrhoeae from the genital tract, rectum, or pharynx is supportive evidence, and demonstration of gonococci in skin lesions, blood, or joint fluid is confirmatory. The serum complement-fixation test for gonococci may be of aid in suggesting gonococcal arthritis, especially if titers are rising. However, this test is not generally available. Other serologic tests which look promising are currently under investigation.

When stains and cultures of joint fluid are negative for gonococci (50 to 75 per cent of cases), it is frequently difficult to differentiate gonococcal arthritis from Reiter's syndrome (nonbacterial urethritis, conjuctivitis, and arthritis) (see Ch. 58.4). The problem in differential diagnosis is compounded by the fact that patients with Reiter's syndrome may have concomitant gonococcal urethritis. Urethritis and arthritis in a female suggest gonococcal arthritis, because this disease is more common in females, whereas Reiter's syndrome is rare in females. The presence of tenosynovitis and response to antimicrobial therapy strongly imply gonococcal arthritis. Patients with Reiter's syndrome frequently have prolonged courses with recurrences, do not respond to antimicrobial therapy, and develop keratodermia blennorrhagica (a symmetrical eruption with a predilection for the soles, palms, and genitals).

Gonococcal arthritis can often be differentiated from acute rheumatic fever, rheumatoid arthritis, and gout by the absence of carditis, lack of rheumatoid factor in serum, and failure to respond to colchicine, respectively.

When N. gonorrhoeae cannot be isolated from the joint, the response to penicillin therapy is often the strongest confirmatory evidence of gonococcal arthritis.

TREATMENT AND PROGNOSIS. Prior to 1954, all gonococci were highly susceptible to penicillin, and a single injection of 300,000 units of penicillin cured almost all cases of gonorrhea. Subsequently, gonococcal strains of increased resistance to penicillin (requiring up to 2.0 μg per milliliter for inhibition) have constituted as much as 50 per cent or more of all isolates. Concomitantly there has been a striking increase in the frequency of failure of therapy with 600,000 to 2,400,000 units of penicillin, requiring larger doses for cure.

N. gonorrhoeae have also been becoming more resistant to tetracycline. The same strains of N. gonorrhoeae that are relatively resistant to penicillin also tend to have increased resistance to tetracycline and ampicillin but not to spectinomycin.

In 1976, for the first time, strains of gonococci were isolated that produced penicillinase and were therefore highly resistant to penicillin in vitro and against which penicillin was totally ineffective clinically. These gonococci also tend to be relatively resistant to tetracycline. Many of these strains seem to have originated in Southeast Asia, where they are widely disseminated. Cases have been reported from various areas (Australia, Belgium, Canada, Denmark, Hong Kong, Japan, Korea, the Netherlands, New Zealand, Norway, the Philippines, Singapore, Sweden, Switzerland, and Great Britain) and from many states within the United States. Because these strains are not yet widely disseminated within the United States, the recommendations for initial treatment of gonorrhea assume that the infecting organism is not a penicillinase producer. However, if the patient or contact has had any relationship with Southeast Asia, the infecting organism is assumed to be a penicillinase producer.

The recommendations of the Venereal Diseases Branch of the Center for Disease Control for treatment of uncomplicated gonorrhea (urethral, cervical, pharyngeal, or anal canal) or *for patients with known exposure* to gonorrhea are as follows: The regimen of choice is aqueous procaine penicillin (4.8 million units) administered intramuscularly at one visit (two sites of injection), together with 1 gram of oral probenecid just before the penicillin. An alternative regimen is 3.5 grams of oral ampicillin simultaneously with 1 gram of probenecid. When penicillin or ampicillin is contraindicated, spectinomycin, 2 grams in one intramuscular injection, or tetracycline hydrochloride orally, 1.5 grams initially, followed by 0.5 gram four times a day for four days (total 9.5 grams), can be used. If the infection is caused by a strain suspected to be a penicillinase producer, initial treatment should be with spectinomycin. However, spectinomycin should not be used indiscriminately as rare isolates of gonococci are resistant to spectinomycin and widespread use of the drug may encourage spread of these strains.

If a penicillin cannot be used in a pregnant patient because of hypersensitivity, since tetracycline is contraindicated, one of the following regimens is suggested: erythromycin, 1.5 grams orally, followed by 500 mg four times daily for a total of 9.5 grams; cefazolin, 2 grams intramuscularly, together with 1.0 gram of probenecid orally; or spectinomycin, 2 grams intramuscularly. Each of these regimens has problems: (1) the efficacy of the erythromycin regimen has not been established; (2) cefazolin should not be used in a patient with a history of anaphylaxis to pencillin because of the danger of cross-reactions; and (3) the safety of spectinomycin for the fetus has not been established.

Spectinomycin and ampicillin do not seem to be effective in eliminating N. gonorrhoeae from the pharynx. With this exception, the cure rates with these regimens in the United States before the introduction of penicillinase-producing gonococci were 97 per cent for procaine penicillin, 93 per cent for ampicillin, 96 per

cent for tetracycline, and 95 per cent for spectinomycin. Aqueous procaine penicillin and spectinomycin have the important advantage of one-visit parenteral therapy which guarantees absorption of the total course of treatment. A major advantage of the procaine penicillin regimen (although clearly more painful) is that it will cure incubating syphilis. A disadvantage of the penicillin regimen in addition to the possibility of hypersensitivity is the possibility of neurotoxicity from the procaine (procaine reaction). The advantage of the tetracycline regimen is that it will usually prevent postgonococcal urethritis in males (see below).

Urethritis should subside within two to three days after therapy. A watery urethral discharge may persist in males for weeks despite elimination of gonococci. This is frequently due to so-called postgonococcal urethritis, which is actually nongonococcal urethritis (e.g., chlamydial) acquired at the same time as the gonorrhea. Postgonococcal urethritis can usually be prevented by use of tetracycline for therapy of gonorrhea. If severe enough to require therapy, postgonococcal urethritis will usually respond to 500 mg of tetracycline four times a day for seven days; the sexual partner should be treated simultaneously to avoid reinfection.

Relapse of gonorrhea occurs most commonly during the first week after treatment. Therefore to evaluate cure, a culture should be obtained seven days after completion of therapy. In homosexual males and in females, anorectal cultures should be obtained as well as cervical cultures. If relapse occurs (and relapse is often difficult to differentiate from reinfection), the patient should be retreated with spectinomycin.

Causes of apparent failure of therapy, other than infection with gonococci resistant to penicillin, are failure to distinguish between relapse and reinfection, failure to identify nongonococcal urethritis, and possibly the presence of other penicillinase-producing bacteria at the site of infection.

Patients with gonococcal prostatitis, seminal vesiculitis, epididymitis, salpingitis, or perihepatitis should be hospitalized and treated with 20 million units of aqueous penicillin G intravenously each day. Following clear-cut improvement, therapy can be changed to 0.5 gram of ampicillin orally four times a day to complete ten days of treatment. Patients who are allergic to penicillin or who are treated as outpatients can be given 1.5 grams of tetracycline orally, followed by 0.5 gram four times a day for ten days. Outpatients can also be treated with the procaine penicillin plus probenecid or ampicillin plus probenecid regimens for uncomplicated gonorrhea, followed by 0.5 gram of ampicillin orally four times a day for ten days. Because of the possibility of polymicrobial infection in pelvic inflammatory disease, aminoglycosides (for enteric gram-negative bacilli), often along with clindamycin or chloramphenicol (for B. fragilis), are frequently added to the regimen in the severely ill patient with salpingitis.

Recent evidence indicates that gonococci that are relatively resistant to penicillin are less likely to cause bacteremia and disseminated infection, i.e., are less pathogenic. Consequently, in the treatment of disseminated infection, after several days of intravenous penicillin therapy the course can be completed with oral ampicillin. Patients with gonococcal arthritis or bacteremia with skin lesions (arthritis-dermatitis syndrome) should be treated with aqueous penicillin G, 10 million units intravenously each day for three days or until there is clear-cut improvement. Therapy can then be changed to oral ampicillin, 0.5 gram four times a day, to complete at least seven days of therapy. Other effective regimens are ampicillin, 3.5 grams orally, plus 1.0 gram probenecid, followed by 0.5 gram of ampicillin four times a day, or tetracycline, 1.5 gram orally, followed by 0.5 gram four times a day for at least seven days. In the penicillin-allergic pregnant patient (in whom tetracycline is contraindicated) erythromycin, 500 mg intravenously every six hours for at least three days, can be used.

There has been little experience with treatment of salpingitis or disseminated gonococcal infection caused by penicillinase-producing gonococci. Although not approved for repeated doses, spectinomycin intramuscularly in a dose of 2 grams every six to twelve hours for seven to ten days would probably be the most effective therapy. Other regimens that probably would be effective are cefazolin in doses of 2 grams every six hours intramuscularly or intravenously or trimethoprim-sulfamethoxazole in a dose of about 3200 mg of sulfamethoxazole and 640 mg of trimethoprim daily orally.

Response of gonococcal infections to therapy usually occurs within two to three days. However, arthritis frequently responds more slowly, and it may take seven to ten days for the patient to become afebrile.

In acute gonococcal disease in the genital tract, surgery is indicated only for drainage of abscesses. However, in the chronic state in some female patients it may become necessary to remove involved pelvic organs. In gonococcal arthritis, pus should be aspirated by needle when possible. With the exception of the hip, open drainage of the joint is rarely necessary. Injection of penicillin into the joint is not indicated. Physiotherapy should be started during the period of convalescence to promote return of function of the joint.

For gonococcal endocarditis or meningitis, 20 million units of aqueous penicillin G should be administered intravenously each day for four weeks in the case of endocarditis and for two weeks for meningitis. Chloramphenicol would probably be the agent of choice in meningitis caused by penicillinase-producing gonococci; in endocarditis, drug susceptibility tests would be necessary to select effective bactericidal therapy.

About 3 per cent of patients with gonorrhea may be in the incubation period of syphilis. The doses of procaine penicillin recommended for therapy of uncomplicated gonorrhea will cure incubating syphilis but will not cure established syphilis. Therefore serologic tests for syphilis should be performed prior to initiation of therapy in all patients treated for gonococcal infections. If the serologic test is positive, therapy for syphilis must be initiated. If the serologic test is negative, no follow-up tests are required if procaine penicillin is used to treat the gonorrhea. Ampicillin, spectinomycin, and tetracycline in the doses recommended for gonor-

rhea have not been shown to abort incubating syphilis. Therefore serologic tests for syphilis should be obtained three months after therapy for gonorrhea with these regimens.

PREVENTION. Use of a condom provides a high degree of protection for the uninfected partner. Past experience has indicated that prophylactic use of oral penicillin in a dose of 250,000 units within two to three hours after exposure markedly decreases the incidence of infection. *Sexual partners of patients with gonorrhea should be identified and treated as quickly as possible to prevent further spread of disease.*

The instillation of 1 per cent silver nitrate (Credé method) or an antimicrobial drug into the eyes of the newborn has largely eradicated gonococcal ophthalmia neonatorum.

Barr, J., and Danielsson, D.: Septic gonococcal dermatitis. Br. Med. J., 1:482, 1971.

Blankenship, R. M., Holmes, R. K., and Sanford, S. P.: Treatment of disseminated gonococcal infection. N. Engl. J. Med., 290:267, 1974.

Danielsson, D., Juhlin, L., and Mardh, P.: Genital Infections and Their Complications. Uppsala, Almqvist and Wiksell International, 1975.

Eschenbach, D. A., Buchanan, T. M., Pollock, H. M., Forsyth, P. S., Alexander, E. R., Lin., J., Wang, S., Wentworth, B. B., McCormack, W. M., and Holmes, K. K.: Polymicrobial etiology of acute pelvic inflammatory disease. N. Engl. J. Med., 293:166, 1975.

Handsfield, H. H., Lipman, T. O., Harnisch, J. P., Tronca, E., and Holmes, K. K.: Asymptomatic gonorrhea in men: Diagnosis, natural course, prevalence and significance. N. Engl. J. Med., 290:117, 1974.

Handsfield, H. H., Wiesner, P. J., and Holmes, K. K.: Treatment of the gonococcal arthritis-dermatitis syndrome. Ann. Intern. Med., 84:661, 1976.

Jaffe, H. W., Biddle, J. W., Thornsberry, C., Johnson, R. E., Kaufman, R. E., Reynolds, G. H., Wiesner, P. J., and The Cooperative Study Group: National gonorrhea therapy monitoring study: In vitro antibiotic susceptibility and its correlation with treatment results. N. Engl. J. Med., 294:5, 1976.

Kaufman, R. E., Johnson, R. E., Jaffe, H. W., Thornsberry, C., Reynolds, G. H., Wiesner, P. J., and The Cooperative Study Group: National gonorrhea therapy monitoring study: Treatment results. N. Engl. J. Med., 294:1, 1976.

McCormack, W. M., and Finland, M.: Spectinomycin. Ann. Intern. Med., 84:712, 1976.

Oriel, J. D., Reeve, P., Thomas, B. J., and Nicol, C. S.: Infection with Chlamydia group A in men with urethritis due to Neisseria gonorrhoeae. J. Infect. Dis., 131:376, 1975.

Penicillin-resistant gonorrhea: New strain spreading worldwide. Science, 194:1395, 1976.

Recommended treatment schedules for gonorrhea — 1974. Arch. Intern. Med., 135:615, 1975

Vickers, F. N., and Maloney, P. J.: Gonococcal perihepatitis. Report of three cases with comments on diagnosis and treatment. Arch. Intern. Med., 114:120, 1964.

Wiesner, P. J.: Gonococcal pharyngeal infection. Clin. Obstet. Gynecol., 18:121, 1975.

MENINGOCOCCAL DISEASE

See Ch. 141.

BACTERIAL MENINGITIS

140. BACTERIAL MENINGITIS

Morton N. Swartz

Meningitis is an inflammation of the arachnoid, the pia mater, and the intervening cerebrospinal fluid. The inflammatory process extends throughout the subarachnoid space about the brain and spinal cord, and regularly involves the ventricles. Pyogenic meningitis, considered in this chapter, is usually an acute infection due to bacteria which evoke a polymorphonuclear response in the cerebrospinal fluid (CSF). One of its major forms, that caused by meningococci, is considered in Ch. 141; less acute forms of bacterial meningitis, characterized by a mononuclear cell response in the CSF, are discussed in Ch. 168.8 and 301.

ETIOLOGY AND INCIDENCE. *Streptococcus pneumoniae, Neisseria meningitidis,* and *Hemophilus influenzae* type b are the three most common causes of pyogenic meningitis, accounting for approximately 70 per cent of cases. The relative frequencies with which the different bacterial species cause meningitis are age related (see accompanying table). In the newborn, gram-negative bacilli (most frequently *E. coli* strains containing K1 capsular antigen, but also other enteric bacilli and *Pseudomonas*) and group B streptococci are the principal causes. Beyond the first month of life and extending through childhood, *H. influenzae* and *N. meningitidis* are the most frequent causes of bacterial meningitis. In adults *S. pneumoniae* and *N. meningitidis* are responsible for most cases. Meningococcal meningitis is the only type which occurs in outbreaks; its relative frequency among the meningitides will depend on whether statistics have been gathered during an epidemic period. In about 10 per cent of patients with pyogenic meningitis the bacterial cause cannot be defined. Simultaneous mixed meningitis is rare, occurring in the setting of neonatal meningitis, penetrating head injury, or intraventricular rupture of a cerebral abscess; the isolation of anaerobes should strongly suggest the last of these.

CLINICAL SETTINGS. The clinical setting in which meningitis develops may provide a clue as to the specific bacterial cause. Meningococcal disease, including meningitis, may occur sporadically and in cyclic outbreaks; military recruits are particularly susceptible, but large urban outbreaks also occur, as in Brazil in 1971 (see Ch. 141).

Certain predisposing factors are frequently associated with the development of *pneumococcal meningitis. Acute otitis media* and *mastoiditis* occur in about 30 per cent of patients. *Pneumonia* is present in about 25 per cent of patients with pneumococcal meningitis, a much higher frequency than in meningitis caused by *H. influenzae* or *N. meningitidis. Acute pneumococcal sinusitis* is occasionally the initial focus from which infection spreads to the meninges. A significant head injury (recent or remote) has occurred in about 10 per cent of patients with pneumococcal meningitis. CSF rhinorrhea (usually caused by a defect or fracture in the cribriform plate) is present in about 5 per cent of patients with pneumococcal meningitis. Among patients with recurrent bacterial meningitis, a pneumococcal cause is found about ten times as frequently as any other. Meningitis occurring in young children with sickle cell anemia is most likely to be due to *S. pneumoniae.* A variety of defects in host defenses (primary or acquired immunoglobulin deficiencies, the asplenic state) may predispose to pneumococcal disease, particularly meningitis. Alcoholism is an underlying problem in 10 to 25 per cent of adults with pneumococcal meningitis in urban hospitals.

S. aureus meningitis is seen most commonly as a complication of a neurosurgical procedure, following penetrating skull trauma, or secondary to staphylococcal bacteremia and endocarditis. Meningitis caused by *gram-negative bacilli* is usually a nosocomial infection, occurring principally in neonatal and neurosurgical patients. Among the latter, *Klebsiella, Enterobacter,* and *Pseudomonas aeruginosa* have been the organisms most frequently involved. Bacteremic *Klebsiella* meningitis is sometimes seen in patients with diabetes mellitus. The most frequent causes of bacterial meningitis in patients with neoplastic disease are gram-negative bacilli, *Listeria monocytogenes, S. pneumoniae,* and *S. aureus.* Meningitis caused by *group A streptococci* is uncommon, but occasionally occurs following acute otitis media, mastoiditis, or sinusitis. *Clostridium perfringens* is a rare cause of meningitis usually secondary to a penetrating injury.

The age-related incidence (children under five years) of *H. influenzae* type b meningitis is so striking that the occurrence of this disease in an adult should raise the question of the presence of an underlying anatomic or immunologic defect, circumventing the usual barrier interposed by serum bactericidal mechanisms.

PATHOLOGY. The purulent exudate is distributed widely in the subarachnoid space, most abundant in the basal cisterns and about the cerebellum initially, but also extending into the sulci over the cerebrum. The exudate in pneumococcal meningitis tends to be more evident over the convexities of the brain than in the basilar region. There is no direct invasion of cerebral tissue by the infecting organism or the inflammatory exudate, but the subjacent brain becomes congested and edematous. The effectiveness of the pial barrier accounts for the fact that cerebral abscess does not complicate bacterial meningitis. Indeed, when these two processes coexist, the sequence usually has been that of

Bacterial Causes of Meningitis

	Adults (>15 years) (%)	Children (1 month to 15 years) (%)	Neonates (<1 month) (%)
S. pneumoniae	30–50	10–20	0–5
N. meningitidis	10–30	30–40	0–1
H. influenzae	1–3	35–45	0–1
Streptococci	5–10	2–4	10–25
Staphylococci	5–15	1–2	5
Listeria	5	1–2	2–10
Gram-negative bacilli	1–10	1–2	55–60

an initial abscess subsequently leaking its contents into the ventricular system, producing meningitis. Structures adjacent to the meninges may show a variety of pathologic changes secondary to bacterial meningitis. *Cortical thrombophlebitis* results from venous stasis and adjacent meningeal inflammation. Infarction of cerebral tissue may follow. *Involvement of small pial arteries* with peripheral aneurysm formation and vascular occlusion occurs occasionally in bacterial meningitis. In fulminating cases (particularly meningococcal meningitis), *cerebral edema* may be marked even though the CSF pleocytosis is only moderate. Rarely such patients develop temporal lobe and cerebellar herniation, resulting in compression of the midbrain and medulla. *Damage to cranial nerves* occurs in areas where dense exudate accumulates; the third and sixth cranial nerves are also vulnerable to damage by increased intracranial pressure. *Ventriculitis* probably occurs in most cases of bacterial meningitis; rarely this progresses to the accumulation of pus, *ventricular empyema. Hydrocephalus* can develop during meningitis from obstruction to CSF flow within the ventricular system (obstructive hydrocephalus) or extraventricularly (communicating hydrocephalus). *Subdural effusions* are sterile transudates which develop over the cerebral cortex in about 15 per cent of infants with bacterial meningitis. Rarely such effusions become infected, producing a subdural empyema. In the past the diagnosis has been made almost exclusively in infants, in whom abnormal transillumination or increasing head size can be detected. Its frequency in adults is not known. Cerebral CAT scanning techniques may provide an answer.

PATHOGENESIS. Bacteria may reach the meninges by several routes: (1) systemic bacteremia, (2) direct ingress from the upper respiratory tract or skin through an anatomic defect (e.g., skull fracture, eroding sequestrum, meningocoele), (3) passage intracranially via venules in the nasopharynx, or (4) spread from a contiguous focus of infection (infection of the paranasal sinuses, leakage of a brain abscess). Bacteremic spread to the meninges is probably the most frequent path of infection. Bacteremia is common in meningitis and suggests this route; but bacteremia also can be a consequence of meningitis as suggested by its occurrence in experimental meningitis following bacterial inoculation into the subarachnoid space of animals and by its occurrence in about 30 per cent of patients with post-traumatic pneumococcal meningitis. The primary focus initiating the bacteremia is usually in the upper respiratory tract or lung (pneumonia), but may be in the heart (endocarditis) or the gastrointestinal or urinary tracts. Once established in any part of the meninges, infection quickly extends throughout the subarachnoid space.

CLINICAL MANIFESTATIONS. History. An acute onset of fever, generalized headache, vomiting, and stiff neck is common to many types of meningitis. Although some patients develop bacterial meningitis in the absence of respiratory symptoms, the majority of patients with pyogenic meningitis of the three common causes have had an antecedent or accompanying upper respiratory tract infection, acute otitis (or mastoiditis), or pneumonia. Myalgias (particularly in meningococcal disease), backache, and generalized weakness are common symptoms. The illness usually progresses rapidly with development of confusion, obtundation, and loss of consciousness. Rarely the onset may be less acute,

with meningeal signs present for several days to a week prior to hospitalization.

General Physical Findings. Evidences of meningeal irritation (drowsiness and decreased mentation, stiff neck, positive Kernig's and Brudzinski's signs) are usually present. In certain patients the findings of meningitis may be easily overlooked; obtunded elderly patients with congestive failure or pneumonia may develop meningitis without prominent meningeal signs. Their lethargy should be investigated carefully and meningeal signs should be sought; if any doubt exists, examination of the CSF is indicated.

The presence of a petechial, purpuric, or ecchymotic rash in a patient with meningeal findings almost always indicates meningococcal infection and requires prompt treatment because of the rapidity with which this infection can progress (see Ch. 141). Rarely, extensive petechial and purpuric lesions occur in meningitis caused by *S. pneumoniae* or *H. influenzae*. Very rarely skin lesions almost indistinguishable from those of meningococcal bacteremia occur in patients with acute *S. aureus* endocarditis who also have meningeal signs and a CSF pleocytosis (secondary either to staphylococcal meningitis or to embolic cerebral infarction). Usually one or two of the lesions in such a patient are those of purulent purpura; aspiration of material reveals staphylococci on Gram stain. In the summer months viral aseptic meningitis (particularly caused by echovirus 9) may produce meningeal signs, macular and petechial skin lesions, and a CSF pleocytosis of several hundred to 1000 cells.

Neurologic Findings and Complications. *Cranial nerve abnormalities*, involving principally the third, fourth, sixth, or seventh nerves, occur in 10 to 20 per cent of patients with bacterial meningitis. These usually disappear shortly after recovery. Partial or complete sensorineural hearing loss (sometimes irreversible) occurs in about 20 per cent of patients with bacterial meningitis over the age of three years, and is not correlated with coincident otitis media. Hearing loss occurs more frequently after meningitis caused by *N. meningitidis* than after that caused by *H. influenzae* or *S. pneumoniae*.

Seizures (focal or generalized) occur during the acute phase of bacterial meningitis in 20 to 30 per cent of patients and may be due to readily reversible causes (high fever in infants; penicillin neurotoxicity when large doses are administered intravenously in the presence of renal failure) or to focal cerebral injury. Seizures can occur during the first few days, or can appear with associated focal neurologic deficits caused by cortical vein phlebitis seven to ten days after the onset of the meningitis.

Brain swelling and increased CSF pressure are associated with seizures, third nerve dysfunction, abnormal reflexes, coma, hypertension, and bradycardia. Papilledema is rare in bacterial meningitis even with high CSF pressures. Its presence should raise the possibility of some other associated or independent suppurative intracranial process (subdural empyema, brain abscess). Marked central hyperpnea sometimes occurs in patients with severe bacterial meningitis; CSF acidosis (principally caused by increased lactic acid levels) provides much of the respiratory stimulus.

Focal cerebral signs (hemiparesis, dysphasia, visual field defects) occur in about 15 per cent of patients with bacterial meningitis. They may develop during early meningitis secondary to occlusive vascular processes or some days later. It is important to distinguish lateralizing findings resulting from postictal changes (Todd's paralysis) which usually persist for no more than several hours.

Prompt treatment of bacterial meningitis usually results in rapid recovery of neurologic function. Persistent or late onset of obtundation and coma without focal findings suggests the development of brain swelling, subdural effusions (in the infant), hydrocephalus, loculated ventriculitis, or cortical thrombophlebitis. The last two are commonly associated with fever and a continuing CSF pleocytosis.

Residual neurologic damage remains in 10 to 20 per cent of patients who recover from bacterial meningitis.

LABORATORY DIAGNOSIS. Cerebrospinal Fluid Examination. Initial CSF pressure is usually moderately elevated (200 to 300 mm H_2O). Striking elevations (over 400 mm) occur in occasional patients with acute brain swelling complicating meningitis in the absence of an associated mass lesion.

GRAM-STAINED SMEAR. By the time of hospitalization, most patients with pyogenic meningitis have large numbers (at least 10^5 per milliliter) of bacteria in the cerebrospinal fluid. Careful examination of the Gram-stained smear of the spun sediment of CSF reveals the etiologic agent in 70 to 80 per cent of cases. In most instances when gram-positive diplococci (or short-chaining cocci) are observed on stained CSF smear they are pneumococci. In certain clinical settings it is important to distinguish the organism from the relatively penicillin-resistant enterococcus, which would require the addition of an aminoglycoside to penicillin in treatment. If sufficient organisms are present in the CSF, prompt identification of a pneumococcus can be made by the quellung reaction, employing pooled pneumococcal antisera. Culture of the cerebrospinal fluid reveals the etiologic agent in 80 to 90 per cent of patients with bacterial meningitis.

SPECIAL IMMUNOLOGIC AND SEROLOGIC PROCEDURES. In patients in whom the etiologic agent is not identified on Gram-stained smear of the CSF, rapid diagnosis may sometimes be made by detection of specific bacterial antigens by countercurrent immunoelectrophoresis (CIE). This technique has been employed most extensively in the rapid diagnosis of meningitis caused by H. influenzae type b, but has also been used in the diagnosis of meningococcal and pneumococcal meningitis; identification of the pathogen can be accomplished in 55 to 80 per cent of cases of meningitis resulting from these three common pathogens. Failure to detect these antigens does *not* exclude bacterial meningitis. The reliability of the test depends on the activity and specificity of the antisera employed; false-positive results may occur because of cross-reactivity of some antigens (e.g., E. coli K1 with group B meningococcus). Since the bacterial cause can be found on Gram-stained smear in most cases of bacterial meningitis, the role of CIE appears to be as an adjunct in rapid diagnosis when no organisms are observed or in providing a specific rather than a morphologic (Gram stain) diagnosis.

The limulus gelation assay for endotoxin is positive in the CSF of patients with meningitis caused by gram-negative bacteria but not in the case of meningitis caused by gram-positive organisms.

CELL COUNT. The cell count in untreated meningitis usually ranges between 100 and 10,000 per cubic millimeter, with polymorphonuclear leukocytes predominating initially (80 per cent or more) and lymphocytes appearing subsequently. Extremely high cell counts (>50,000 per cubic millimeter) may occur rarely in primary bacterial meningitis, but should also raise the possibility of intraventricular rupture of a cerebral abscess. Cell counts as low as 10 to 20 may be observed early in bacterial meningitis (particularly that caused by N. meningitidis and H. influenzae). Occasionally, in granulocytopenic patients or in the elderly with overwhelming pneumococcal meningitis, the cerebrospinal fluid may contain very few leukocytes and yet may appear grossly turbid just because of the presence of myriads of organisms. Meningitis caused by several bacterial species (M. tuberculosis, T. pallidum) characteristically produces a lymphocytic pleocytosis. Listeria monocytogenes meningitis in infants may produce a primarily lymphocytic response in the CSF; in the adult there is usually a polymorphonuclear response, but rarely lymphocytes predominate.

GLUCOSE. The CSF glucose is reduced to values of 40 mg per deciliter or below (or less than 50 to 60 per cent of the simultaneous blood level) in over 50 per cent of patients with bacterial meningitis; this finding can be very valuable in distinguishing bacterial meningitis from most viral meningitides or parameningeal infections. A normal CSF glucose does not exclude the diagnosis of bacterial meningitis. The simultaneous blood glucose level should be determined, because patients with diabetes mellitus (or who are receiving intravenous glucose infusions) will have an elevated level of glucose in the CSF, and its significance can be appreciated only on comparison with the simultaneous blood level. However, it may take 90 to 120 minutes for equilibration to occur after major shifts in the level of glucose in the circulation. The hypoglycorrhachia characteristic of pyogenic meningitis appears to be due to interference with the normal carrier-facilitated diffusion of glucose.

PROTEIN. The level of protein in the cerebrospinal fluid is usually elevated above 100 mg per deciliter, and the higher values are more commonly observed in pneumococcal meningitis. Extreme elevations, up to 1000 mg per deciliter or more, indicate impending or actual subarachnoid block secondary to the meningitis.

OTHER ABNORMALITIES IN THE CSF. Elevated levels of lactic acid occur in pyogenic meningitis. Lactic dehydrogenase levels (particularly isozymes 4 and 5 derived from granulocytes) are commonly elevated in patients with bacterial meningitis. Although the levels of lactic dehydrogenase are higher in patients with bacterial meningitis than in those with viral infections of the central nervous system, these alterations are not of help in determining the specific etiologic agent involved.

Other Laboratory Tests. BLOOD AND RESPIRATORY TRACT CULTURES. Bacteremia is demonstrable in about 80 per cent of patients with H. influenzae meningitis, 50 per cent of those with pneumococcal meningitis, and 30 to 40 per cent of those with meningococcal meningitis. Cultures of the upper respiratory tract have not proved helpful in establishing an etiologic diagnosis. Determination of serum creatinine and electrolytes is important in view of the gravity of the illness, the occurrence of specific abnormalities secondary to the meningitis (syndrome of inappropriate secretion of antidiuretic hormone), and problems in therapy in the presence of renal dysfunction (seizures and hyperkalemia with high-dose penicillin therapy). In patients with extensive petechial and purpuric skin lesions, evaluation for coagulopathy is indicated.

RADIOLOGIC STUDIES. In view of the frequency with which pyogenic meningitis is associated with primary foci of infection in the chest, nasal sinuses, or mastoid, roentgenograms of these areas should be taken at the appropriate time after institution of antimicrobial therapy. If a mass lesion (cerebral abscess, subdural empyema) is suspected by history, clinical setting, or physicial findings (papilledema), then radionuclide or CAT scans should be performed.

DIAGNOSIS. The diagnosis of bacterial meningitis is not difficult in a febrile patient with meningeal symptoms and signs developing in the setting of a predisposing illness. The diagnosis may be less obvious in the elderly, obtunded patient with pneumonia or the confused alcoholic patient in impending delirium tremens. Examination of the cerebrospinal fluid should be carried out promptly under these circumstances or whenever there is any question of meningitis.

Headache, fever, vomiting, stiff neck, and CSF pleocytosis are features of meningeal inflammation and are common to many types of meningitis (e.g., bacterial, fungal, viral) and also to some parameningeal processes. The cerebrospinal fluid findings are most helpful in distinguishing among these processes (see Ch. 298). In the patient with meningitis whose cerebrospinal fluid does not reveal the etiologic agent on examination of Gram-stained smear, particularly when the CSF glucose is normal and the polymorphonuclear pleocytosis is atypical, certain treatable processes which can mimic bacterial meningitis should be considered in differential diagnosis: (1) *Parameningeal infections.* The presence of infections (chronic ear or nasal accessory sinus infections, lung abscess) predisposing to brain abscess, epidural (cerebral or spinal) abscess, subdural empyema, or pyogenic venous sinus phlebitis should be sought. Neurologic findings may appear in the course of primary bacterial meningitis, but their presence should alert the physician to the need for close scrutiny for the presence of a space-occupying infectious process in the central nervous system. Neurologic symptoms or findings antedating the onset of meningeal symptoms should raise the question of a parameningeal infection. The isolation of an anaerobic organism should suggest the possibility of intraventricular leakage of a cerebral abscess. (2) *Bacterial endocarditis.* Bacterial meningitis may occur during bacterial endocarditis caused by pyogenic organisms such as *S. aureus* and enterococci. In subacute bacterial endocarditis sterile embolic infarctions of the brain may occur and produce meningeal signs and a CSF pleocytosis containing several hundred cells, including polymorphonuclear leukocytes. A history of dental manipulation, fever, and anorexia antedating the meningitis should be sought; careful examination for heart murmurs and peripheral stigmata of endocarditis is indicated. (3) *"Chemical" meningitis.* The clinical and CSF findings (polymorphonuclear pleocytosis and even reduced glucose level) of bacterial meningitis may be produced by chemically induced inflammation. Acute meningitis following a diagnostic lumbar puncture or spinal anesthesia may be due to bacterial (usually *Pseudomonas* species or coliform organisms) or chemical contamination of equipment or anesthetic agent. Endogenous chemical meningitis resulting from leakage into the subarachnoid space of material from an epidermoid tumor or a craniopharyngioma can produce a polymorphonuclear pleocytosis and hypoglycorrhachia. Birefringent material may be seen on polarizing microscopy of the CSF sediment.

NON-NEUROLOGIC COMPLICATIONS. Shock. When shock occurs in pyogenic meningitis it is usually a manifestation of an accompanying intense bacteremia, as in fulminant meningococcemia, rather than of the meningitis itself. Shock is the result both of the bacteremia (and possible associated endotoxemia) and of cardiac injury (myocarditis). Management is guided by the principles of septic shock therapy with appropriate modifications for myocardial failure. (See Ch. 141.)

Coagulation Disorders. Coagulopathies are frequently associated with the intense bacteremias (usually meningococcal, occasionally pneumococcal) and hypotension which can accompany meningitis. The changes may be mild such as thrombocytopenia (with or without prolongation of prothrombin and partial thromboplastin times) or more marked with clinical evidences of disseminated intravascular coagulation (see Ch. 521.5).

Septic Complications. ENDOCARDITIS. Previously, 5 to 10 per cent of patients with pneumococcal meningitis, particularly those with bacteremia and pneumonia as well, developed acute endocarditis, most commonly on the aortic valve. The incidence is currently much lower, as a result of earlier treatment of the initiating infection. The early diagnosis of simultaneous pneumococcal endocarditis in a patient with meningitis may be difficult, because treatment of meningitis may control the manifestations of endocarditis. However, in such patients, febrile relapse and a new murmur may appear shortly after completion of antimicrobial therapy for meningitis.

PYOGENIC ARTHRITIS. Septic arthritis may result from the bacteremia associated with pyogenic meningitis. Most commonly it occurs with pneumococcal meningitis, but it may complicate meningitis caused by *N. meningitidis, H. influenzae,* or *S. aureus.*

Prolonged Fever. With appropriate antimicrobial treatment of meningitis of the three most common bacterial causes, patients become afebrile within two to five days. Sometimes fever persists beyond this or recurs after an afebrile period. In the patient with persisting headache, obtundation, and cerebral findings, inadequate drug therapy or neurologic sequelae (cortical venous thrombophlebitis, ventriculitis, subdural collections) are important considerations. Re-evaluation of the cerebrospinal fluid, particularly Gram-stained smear and culture, is essential under these circumstances. Drug fever may be responsible in the patient who continues to show clinical improvement in all other respects. Metastatic infection (septic arthritis, purulent pericarditis, thoracic empyema, endocarditis) may be the cause of continuing or recurrent fever.

A syndrome consisting of fever, arthritis, and pericarditis three to six days after initiation of effective antimicrobial therapy of meningococcal meningitis occurs in about 10 per cent of patients. Synovial and pericardial fluids are characteristically serosanguineous and sterile, unlike the purulent fluid which can occur in both sites early in the course of meningococcal infection. The clinical features are reminiscent of those of serum sickness. Immunopathologic study of skin and synovial lesions implicates immune complex formation in their genesis. Pericardial effusions usually do not become hemodynamically significant, but close observation is indicated. Symptomatic relief is provided by salicylates.

RECURRENT MENINGITIS. Repeated episodes of bacterial meningitis generally indicate a host defect, either in local anatomy or in antibacterial and immunologic defenses. *S. pneumoniae* is by far the most frequent cause of recurrent meningitis. Eleven per cent of patients with pneumococcal meningitis have had more than one episode, whereas 0.5 per cent of patients with meningitis caused by other organisms have had recurrent attacks. A history of head trauma is much more frequent in patients with recurrent meningitis. Organisms may directly enter the subarachnoid space, through a defect in the cribriform plate (the most common site), via a basilar skull fracture, through an erosive sequestrum of the mastoid, through congenital dermal defects along the craniospinal axis (usually evident before adult life), or as a consequence of penetrating cranial trauma or neurosurgical procedures. The anatomic defect may produce a frank CSF leak (rhinorrhea or, less commonly, otorrhea) or may entrap a vascular cuff of meninges which might subsequently serve as a direct route for organisms to reach the meninges. CSF rhinorrhea may be intermittent, and meningitis may occur months or years after head injury.

Any patient with bacterial meningitis, particularly if meningitis is recurrent, should be evaluated carefully for any congenital or post-traumatic defects. The presence of CSF rhinorrhea should be sought at admission and subsequently (rhinorrhea may clear during active meningitis only to recur when inflammation has resolved). Demonstration of glucose in nasal secretions with glucose oxidase "sticks" (Dextrostix) suggests the presence of cerebrospinal fluid. Quantitative determination of glucose and chloride content of nasal secretions can definitively establish the presence of CSF rhinorrhea.

Recurrent pneumococcal meningitis may occur without apparent predisposing circumstances, and cryptic CSF leaks should be sought actively in such patients by polytomography of the frontal and mastoid regions and by radioisotope techniques. (Radioiodine-labeled albumin is introduced intrathecally, and pledgets of cotton placed in the nares are subsequently examined for the radionuclide.) Surgical closure of CSF fistulas should be carried out to prevent further episodes of meningitis.

In most patients with CSF otorrhea and rhinorrhea following an acute head injury, the leak ceases in one or two weeks. *Persistent rhinorrhea for more than four to six weeks is an indication for surgical repair.* Prolonged administration of penicillin will not prevent pneumococcal meningitis and may encourage infection with more drug-resistant species.

Rarely, recurrent meningitis of nonbacterial etiology may mimic bacterial meningitis. *Mollaret's meningitis* consists of repeated febrile episodes of mild meningeal symptomatology, usually without neurologic abnormalities. Initially, large "endothelial" cells may be seen in the CSF along with polymorphonuclear leukocytes, which subsequently are replaced by lymphocytes. *Behçet's syndrome,* characterized by relapsing oral and genital ulcers and ocular lesions (hypopyon), may exhibit a variety of neurologic abnormalities, including recurrent meningitis.

PROGNOSIS. The introduction of antimicrobial agents has converted bacterial meningitis from a disease that was almost always fatal to one in which the majority of patients survive without significant neurologic residua. The mortality rate for bacterial meningitis varies with the etiologic agent and the clinical circumstances. With current antimicrobial therapy the mortality rate for *H. influenzae* meningitis is below 5 per cent and that for meningococcal meningitis is about 10 per cent. The highest mortality is with pneumococcal meningitis, in which the rate is about 20 per cent. Poor prognostic factors include advanced age, presence of other foci of infection, underlying diseases (leukemia, alcoholism), coma, and delay in instituting appropriate therapy.

TREATMENT. Antimicrobial Agents. *Antimicrobial therapy should be begun promptly in this life-threatening emergency.* If the etiologic agent is observed on Gram-stained smear of the CSF sediment, specific therapy can be initiated. If the etiologic agent is not observed on smear (or not detected by counterimmunoelectrophoresis), treatment for bacterial meningitis of unknown cause should be started, aiming at the most likely possibilities based on available clinical clues (age of the patient, presence of a purpuric rash, a recent neurosurgical procedure, CSF rhinorrhea).

With the exception of chloramphenicol, the commonly employed antimicrobial agents do not readily penetrate the normal blood-brain barrier; but the passage of penicillin and other antimicrobials is enhanced in the presence of meningeal inflammation. Antimicrobial drugs should be administered intravenously throughout the treatment period; reduction in dosage as the patient improves should be avoided, because normalization of the blood-brain barrier during recovery reduces the CSF levels of drug that are achievable. Bactericidal drugs (penicillin, ampicillin) are preferred whenever possible in the treatment of meningitis caused by susceptible bacteria. Several antimicrobial drugs (cephalosporins, clindamycin) which do not provide effective levels in the cerebrospinal fluid should not be used.

MENINGITIS OF SPECIFIC BACTERIAL CAUSE. The treatment of choice for pneumococcal meningitis in the adult is penicillin (24 million units daily in divided doses every two hours) or ampicillin (12 grams daily in divided doses every two to three hours). Chloramphenicol (4 to 6 grams intravenously daily) is a suitable alternative in the patient with a major penicillin allergy. The recent emergence in South Africa of pneumococcal strains significantly resistant to most antimicrobial drugs, including penicillin and chloramphenicol, indicates a need for determining antimicrobial susceptibilities of pneumococcal isolates from cerebrospinal fluid and blood.

The treatment of meningococcal meningitis is the same as for pneumococcal meningitis (see Ch. 141).

The recent appearance of *H. influenzae* strains highly resistant to ampicillin has dictated a change in initial management of this form of meningitis. Chloramphenicol (100 mg per kilogram intravenously daily for a child; 4 grams intravenously daily for an adult), either alone or in combination with ampicillin (300 to 400 mg per kilogram intravenously per day for a child; 12 grams intravenously per day for an adult), is the preferred treatment until drug susceptibilities are determined. If the organism is proved susceptible to ampicillin, then this drug can be used alone in treatment.

Adult meningitis caused by *S. aureus* should be treated with a penicillinase-resistant penicillin (oxacillin or nafcillin in a dosage of 10 to 12 grams intravenously per day). In occasional cases, particularly when staphylococcal meningitis complicates a craniotomy, adjunctive intrathecal therapy (5000 to 10,000 units of bacitracin)* may be considered. Vancomycin (2.0 grams intravenously daily in the adult) has been used as an alternative in the penicillin-allergic patient, and adjunctive therapy with intrathecal bacitracin may be indicated.

Treatment of enterococcal meningitis in the adult involves the use of intravenous penicillin (24 million units daily) or ampicillin (12 grams daily), supplemented with parenterally administered gentamicin (3 to 5 mg per kilogram daily in divided doses every eight hours). In the patient who fails to respond promptly to parenteral therapy, adjunctive intrathecal therapy with gentamicin* (3 to 5 mg) should be considered.

Initial treatment of adults with gram-negative bacillary meningitis involves the use of chloramphenicol (4 grams intravenously daily) as well as intravenous gentamicin (5 mg per kilogram daily in divided doses every eight hours) and intrathecal gentamicin* (3 to 5 mg administered at intervals of 24 hours for the first few days). Intrathecal (or intraventricular) therapy is particularly important in patients with meningitis after neurosurgical procedures. Following identification of the specific infecting species and determination of its drug susceptibilities, alterations in antimicrobial therapy may be indicated; if the organism is *Pseudomonas aeruginosa,* parenteral and intrathecal gentamicin would be continued but carbenicillin (30 to 40 grams intravenously daily) would be substituted for chloramphenicol.

Initial treatment of meningitis when the etiologic agent cannot be identified on Gram-stained smear of cerebrospinal fluid is based on available clinical clues. *In the neonate,* a wide range of gram-positive (group B streptococci, *Listeria*) and gram-negative organisms (*E. coli, Klebsiella, H. influenzae*) may be the cause, indicating the use of combined therapy with drugs such as ampicillin and gentamicin. *In children,* therapy is directed at the three most frequent pathogens: *H. influenzae, S. pneumoniae,* and *N. meningitidis.* The appearance of ampicillin resistance among strains of *H. influenzae* has necessitated the shift from single drug therapy (ampicillin) to a two-drug approach (ampicillin-chloramphenicol or penicillin-chloramphenicol) in the treatment of meningitis of unknown cause in this age group, pending results of culture. *In adults,* therapy with ampicillin or penicillin is directed at the most common pathogens (*S. pneumoniae* and *N. meningitidis*). However, because *H. influenzae* type b infections appear to be increasing in adults, and because of the increased incidence of gram-negative bacillary meningitis in certain clinical settings, broader initial therapy may be indicated if clinical features suggest unusual organisms.

Duration of Therapy. The frequency of cerebrospinal fluid examinations depends on the clinical course, but a repeat examination should be done in 48 hours if there has not been satisfactory improvement. Meningococci are rapidly eliminated from the circulation and cerebrospinal fluid with appropriate antimicrobial therapy, which should be continued for at least five to seven days after the patient becomes afebrile. *H. influenzae* meningitis should be treated for a minimum of

ten days (at least for seven days after the patient becomes afebrile); re-examination of the CSF at that time usually shows cell counts of less than 60 (over 90 per cent mononuclear). Since pneumococcal meningitis produces a more intense inflammatory response, antimicrobial treatment should be continued for 10 to 14 days and follow-up examination of the cerebrospinal fluid should show resolution. More prolonged therapy is indicated with concomitant parameningeal infection or mastoiditis. Treatment of gram-negative bacillary meningitis with parenteral antimicrobials is prolonged, usually for a minimum of three weeks, in order to prevent relapse.

Other Aspects of Treatment. Occasional patients with acute bacterial meningitis develop marked brain swelling (CSF pressure exceeding 400 mm H_2O), which may lead to temporal lobe or cerebellar herniation following lumbar puncture. To reduce this increased pressure, an intravenous infusion of 20 per cent mannitol solution (1.5 to 2.0 grams per kilogram) is administered over 20 to 60 minutes. Continued control of increased intracranial pressure, if needed therafter, may be effected with mannitol, dexamethasone (10 mg intravenously, followed by 4 mg every six hours), or both. Brain swelling is about the only indication for the use of corticosteroids in the treatment of pyogenic meningitis; they should be employed only when the appropriate antimicrobial drugs are administered. Fluid restriction (1200 to 1500 ml daily in adults) is advisable during the first 24 to 48 hours to minimize brain swelling.

Patients with acute bacterial meningitis should receive constant nursing attention to ensure prompt recognition of seizures and to prevent aspiration. If seizures occur, they should be treated acutely with diazepam (Valium) administered slowly intravenously in a dose of 5 to 10 mg in the adult. Maintenance anticonvulsant therapy can be continued thereafter with intravenous diphenylhydantoin (Dilantin) until the medication can be administered orally. Sedation should be avoided because of the danger of respiratory depression and aspiration.

Bayer, A. S., Seidel, J. S., Yoshikawa, T. T., Anthony, B. F., and Guze, L. B.: Group D enterococcal meningitis. Arch. Intern. Med., 136:883, 1976.

Carpenter, R. R., and Petersdorf, R. G.: The clinical spectrum of bacterial meningitis. Am. J. Med., 33:262, 1962.

Chernik, N. L., Armstrong, D., and Posner, J. B.: Central nervous system infections in patients with cancer. Medicine, 52:563, 1973.

Colding, H., and Lind, I.: Counterimmunoelectrophoresis in the diagnosis of bacterial meningitis. J. Clin. Microbiol., 5:405, 1977.

Finland, M., and Barnes, M. W.: Acute bacterial meningitis at Boston City Hospital during 12 selected years, 1935–1972. J. Infect. Dis. 136:400, 1977.

Hand, W. L., and Sanford, J. P.: Posttraumatic bacterial meningitis. Ann. Intern. Med., 72:869, 1970.

Hermans, P. E., Goldstein, N. P., and Wellman, W. E.: Mollaret's meningitis and differential diagnosis of recurrent meningitis. Am. J. Med., 52:128, 1972.

Hyslop, N. E., and Swartz, M. N.: Bacterial meningitis. Postgrad. Med., 58:120, 1975.

Levin, S., Nelson, K. E., Spies, H. W., and Lepper, M. H.: Pneumococcal meningitis: The problem of the unseen cerebrospinal fluid leak. Am. J. Med. Sci., 264:319, 1972.

Mangi, R. J., Quintiliani, R., and Andriole, V. T.: Gram-negative bacillary meningitis. Am. J. Med., 59:829, 1975.

McCracken, G. H.: Rapid identification of specific etiology in meningitis. J. Pediat., 88:706, 1976.

Swartz, M. N., and Dodge, P. R.: Bacterial meningitis—a review of selected aspects. N. Engl. J. Med., 272:725, 779, 842, 898, 954, 1003, 1965.

Tugwell, P., Greenwood, B. M., and Warrell, D. A.: Pneumococcal meningitis: A clinical and laboratory study. Quart. J. Med., 45:583, 1976.

---

*Intrathecal use is not mentioned in the manufacturer's package insert approved by the U.S. Food and Drug Administration. Therefore its use in these circumstances must be considered investigational.

141. MENINGOCOCCAL DISEASE

Harry A. Feldman

DEFINITION. Meningococcal infections may affect the upper and lower respiratory tracts, blood (meningococcemia), central nervous system (meningococcal meningitis, cerebrospinal fever, spotted fever, or epidemic cerebrospinal meningitis), joints (arthritis), heart, pericardium, eyes, skin, urethra, cervix, and rectum, singly or in any combination in a given patient. First recognized in 1805 by Vieusseux in Geneva and in 1806 by Danielson and Mann in Massachusetts, *meningococcal meningitis*, the best known form, occurs sporadically and as localized or widespread epidemics.

ETIOLOGY. *Neisseria meningitidis*, a variable sized gram-negative coccus which may be seen singly or as biscuit-shaped diplococci, was established to cause meningitis by Weichselbaum in 1887. Metabolically fastidious, the organism grows best on enriched culture media at 37° C in an atmosphere of increased CO_2 concentration. Mueller-Hinton or meat infusion broths or agar containing 10 per cent of blood (rabbit, sheep, or horse) or human ascitic fluid are excellent. Chocolate agar is very good for initial isolation. The addition of vancomycin and colistin with or without nystatin (modified Thayer-Martin agar) is especially useful for isolation from throats or other areas of marked contamination. Meningococci are very susceptible to chilling or drying, so all cultures should be inoculated and incubated promptly. Since some meningococcal strains are exquisitely susceptible to sulfonamides, media inoculated with specimens from patients receiving such drugs should contain para-aminobenzoic acid (5 mg per 100 ml).

Identification of meningococci is based on morphology, Gram staining, oxidative utilization of glucose and maltose but not sucrose, and immunologic reactions. The following serogroups are recognized: A, B, C, D, X, Y, Z, 29-E, and W-135. Those which most commonly cause illness are A, B, C, and Y. Group D is exceedingly rare. The groups are identified through their specific polysaccharide antigens. A and C organisms have prominent capsules so young cultures or organisms in cerebrospinal fluid quell (capsular swelling) with specific antisera. Groups B and C have been further subdivided on the basis of protein antigens, some of which are shared. Group A strains can be subdivided similarly within the group. At present these characteristics appear to be useful for epidemiologic studies, but their role in protection remains undefined.

Lipopolysaccharides or "endotoxins" in purified form have been prepared from meningococci. These are toxic for animals and are increasingly being demonstrated to play significant roles in the pathogenesis of human disease.

EPIDEMIOLOGY. The epidemiology of meningococcal infections is complicated by the multiplicity of their serogroups. Sporadic infections may be seen almost constantly in all areas. Major epidemics are generally caused by group A organisms and seem to occur in 20- to 30-year cycles. For example, during World Wars I and II there were massive civilian and military outbreaks which persisted for several years. Groups B and C produce most cases in the intervening years. The remaining groups are usually detected in carriers and sporadic cases. Group Y is the most frequent disease producer after A, B, and C. Thus the over-all picture is that of high waves about every 20 to 30 years and lower ones in the interims. There are localized exceptions to this generalization. Detroit had a major group A epidemic in 1929, with 724 cases reported in an eight-month period and a general mortality rate of 50 per cent (no specific treatment available). In infants, however, the mortality rate was 84 per cent, and in those over 40 years, 72 per cent. Santiago, Chile, had a severe group A epidemic in 1941 to 1942 with 5885 cases; of these, 15.9 per cent were fatal (sulfonamides used).

In recent years the most devastated areas have been that portion of Africa which lies below the Sahara and north of the Equator, and Brazil. The African "meningitis belt" now averages about 10,000 cases per year with about 1200 deaths, but from 1939 to 1962 it reported 593,738 cases with 102,956 (17 per cent) deaths! In earlier outbreaks in the same area, as many as 85 per cent of cases were fatal. Here, as in South Africa, group A organisms continue to predominate. The Brazilian epidemic was centered in São Paulo but occurred in other areas as well. It began unusually as a group C epidemic in 1971, which in 1973 became a predominately group A outbreak. It began to die out in 1975 and faded drastically in 1976. The great mystery here is the unanswered question as to what conditions made it possible for two epidemics to overlap in the same general area.

Other recent epidemics, all caused by group A, have occurred in Canada, Finland, Outer Mongolia, and Morocco. Group A infections remain rare in the United States, except for a localized nidus in the "skid row" area of Seattle and, to a lesser extent, among a similar population in Anchorage.

About 60 per cent of cases occur in those less than 15 years of age. Military recruits for some unknown reason are especially vulnerable. About 80 per cent of their cases are seen within the first 90 days of service, most often in the first month. The incidence of both cases and carriers is usually higher in males. Race and color (except for those with sickle cell disease) do not seem to influence either incidence or susceptibility, but socioeconomic level does. The higher rates reported among blacks in certain urban areas probably reflect increased poverty with its concomitant crowding. The exact incubation period is often nondeterminable, but the range is probably one to ten days. There are a few instances reported in which this may have been a long as three weeks.

The portal of entry of meningococci is the upper respiratory tract, and transmission from person to person may result from direct or intimate contact, airborne droplets, or articles contaminated with fresh secretions from the respiratory tract. Mouth-to-mouth resuscitation has resulted in several cases in physicians. In one instance, nasopharyngeal carriage followed a kidney transplant from a donor who had died of unrecognized meningococcemia; in another, meningococcal pneumonia also followed a kidney transplant. Yet even during severe epidemics, the majority of clinical infections seems to be unrelated to others, so that case-to-case spread is almost impossible to trace. Posterior nasopharyngeal culture surveys during outbreaks may demonstrate carrier rates as high as 90 per cent, constantly or intermittently, without clinical evidence of disease. Although the carrier rate often is less than 5 per cent during interepidemic periods, much of the population may harbor meningococci at some time.

Until 1963, meningococci of all serogroups were highly susceptible to sulfonamides so that such drugs were exceedingly effective for both the treatment of cases and mass prophylaxis. Unfortunately, sulfonamide-resistant group B meningococci were found to be prevalent in that year. Markedly resistant group C strains were detected soon after. Recently, and perhaps even more disturbing, sulfonamide-resistant group A strains first were isolated during an epidemic in North Africa, and subsequently in the "belt" below the Sahara, South Africa, Australia, Brazil, Canada, Finland, Greece, Mongolia, Norway, and Southeast Asia. This phenomenon is now so widespread that all cases caused by organisms of *any* serogroup must be considered to be the result of sulfonamide-resistant strains unless specifically proved otherwise. The same holds for carrier strains.

The physician is often concerned with the question of whether family members or other contacts of meningococcal patients are at excessive risk from this disease. Fortunately, secondary cases are unusual, but they do occur. In the Detroit epidemic of 1929, 4 per cent of cases were in affected households. In the Santiago epidemic of 1941–1942, the over-all secondary attack rate was 2.5 per cent. Because most of these follow within ten days (many four days) of the index case, they are often considered to be co-primaries. Acceptance of this concept leads to another control approach which will be dealt with subsequently (see Prevention). Household carrier rates, on the other hand, generally are high. In several studies of families of meningococcal patients, 45 to 50 per cent were found to be carrying organisms of the same serogroup as the patient, providing some justification for the anxieties of both families and physicians over household cases. Unfortunately, these no longer can be resolved by the relatively simple procedure which was possible when sulfonamide-susceptible strains were the rule.

PATHOGENESIS AND PATHOLOGY. In meningococcemia the essential lesion is vascular, with endothelial damage, inflammation of vessel walls with necrosis and thrombosis, and focal hemorrhages into cutaneous, subcutaneous, submucosal, and synovial tissues. In rapidly extending meningococcemia the Waterhouse-Friderichsen syndrome is often present. This is usually but not necessarily accompanied by bilateral adrenal hemorrhages.

Involvement of the central nervous system is characterized by *acute purulent meningitis*, although, if suspected early, there may be only hyperemia. Some degree of encephalitis usually accompanies the meningitis. When treatment is delayed or ineffective, permanent cranial nerve damage may be anticipated.

The pathogenesis of meningococcal infections is usually initiated by the colonization of the posterior nasopharynx and adjoining structures by organisms entering through the upper respiratory passages. Symptoms and signs of an acute upper respiratory infection may result, although this is not accepted by all observers. If invasion of the bloodstream follows, this may be relatively asymptomatic in some, but in others there may be metastatic lesions in skin, meninges, joints, eyes, lungs, pericardium, urethra, and other organs and tissues. The sites and extent of these localizations determine the symptoms and signs that follow.

We are totally at a loss to explain why meningococcal infections are so limited and innocuous in some individuals and so extensive and overwhelming in others. No microbe can kill more quickly; deaths have been observed within several hours after the first symptom.

Chemical alterations reflecting the severity of the meningococcal infection may be profound. Their cause is not known, but to some degree they are endotoxic in origin and furthered by the release of various substances from damaged tissue cells. Hemorrhagic manifestations may result from direct vascular damage because of a Schwartzman-like reaction, thrombocytopenia, or both. Other changes are those found in acute sepsis: fever, dehydration, reduction in blood volume, and altered acid-base and negative nitrogen balances. In severely ill patients, cyanosis, circulatory collapse, and other signs of shock appear, probably the result of the combined actions of bacterial endotoxins and tissue anoxia. Alterations suggestive of acute adrenal insufficiency, low serum sodium, elevated potassium, low chloride, and hypoglycemia may be present and are consistent with absent or diminished cortical secretion by damaged adrenal glands. There is no evidence that adrenal insufficiency as judged by the degree of excretion of corticosteroids in fulminating infections per se occurs independently of glandular destruction.

CLINICAL MANIFESTATIONS. A sequential development of clinical manifestations of meningococcal infections can be discerned from a number of cases, but any one patient may present with symptoms and signs of advanced diffuse illness. The usual sequence consists of infection of the upper respiratory tract, bacteremia, septicemia, meningitis, and/or other metastatic localization. One stage may be dominant, giving the appearance of mild illness, grave illness, or none.

Infection of the Upper Respiratory Tract. The upper respiratory tract is the most frequent site of meningococcal infection. Most patients have no or inconsequential symptoms so that the organism is detectable only by culture of the posterior nasopharynx. Whether symptoms result from such colonization is contested by many observers, because descriptions of this stage usually have been derived from military recruits at a time when they are subject to many viral and mycoplasmal respiratory infections. On the other hand, many but not all patients with meningococcal illnesses give histories of preceding or concurrent nasopharyngitis.

Meningococcemia. Bacteremic meningococcal infections may vary from acute fulminating illnesses of a few hours' duration to indolent, chronic infections lasting days, weeks, or, rarely, months. Symptoms may be relentlessly progressive or intermittent, with relapses and recrudescences at different times.

MILD OR SUBACUTE MENINGOCOCCEMIA. The most common form of meningococcemia is that of a relatively mild, acute, or subacute infection. Prodromal symptoms are frequently absent except for those of a mild upper respiratory infection in some. Onset is usually sudden, with fever, chilliness or frank chills that may be recurrent, malaise, myalgia, and apathy. The presenting symptoms may be any combination of these, but frequently the initial complaints are those of recurrent fever, rash, arthralgia, acute mono- or polyarthritis, conjunctivitis, nausea, and vomiting. Symptoms may regress or persist if the disease progresses. Fever may be remittent and irregular with elevations to 39 or 39.5° C. The pulse rate is proportionate to the fever. Respirations are usually normal or only slightly increased except when pneumonia or pleurisy is present.

The most striking feature on physical examination is the rash, which occurs often. It appears soon after onset, is variable (the severest is petechial or purpuric), measuring from 1 or 2 mm to 1 cm or more in diameter, and is pink to reddish blue (see accompanying figure). Early in the disease there may be a generalized, mottled erythema which appears dusky in slightly cyanotic patients. Light pink macules resembling the "rose spots" of typhoid, wheals, or nodules like erythema nodosum may appear before petechiae and ecchymoses. Careful search in good daylight may be necessary to detect early lesions. Occasionally, vesicular, pustular, or bullous lesions are present. Superficial or deep ulcerations may result from petechiae, especially when coalescent. These are sometimes very extensive and ultimately may require grafting. The rash often appears first on the wrists and ankles, but any area may be involved, including the conjunctivae and the mucous membranes. Hemorrhagic lesions fade to a brown, rusty color three or four days after their appearance; if new crops appear, often after chills, a variety of skin lesions may be present at the same time. This is more likely when treatment is delayed or unsuccessful.

Other physical findings, including splenomegaly, are inconstant. Herpetic lesions of the lip are found in about 10 per cent of the cases. Unless meningismus develops, symptoms referable to the central nervous system are absent, although those resulting from metastatic localizations are usually self-evident, depending upon their site.

The firm diagnosis is established with laboratory aids. Leukocytosis up to 40,000 cells per cubic millimeter with 80 to 90 per cent neutrophils is almost always present. In overwhelming cases, leukopenia may be profound and gram-negative intracellular diplococci may be seen within leukocytes in stained smears from capillary blood, buffy coat, or skin lesions. A blood culture positive for meningococci furnishes final etiologic proof. It should be emphasized that several cultures of the blood may be necessary to detect meningococci and that growth of the organism in liquid medium may be slow. Other laboratory examinations are either normal or compatible with any febrile illness.

The subsequent course is dependent on therapy, although some patients with very mild disease recover spontaneously after several weeks or months. Any of the complications and sequelae of meningococcal infections may develop.

ACUTE FULMINATING MENINGOCOCCEMIA. This differs from the milder form in the rapidity with which it progresses and in its overwhelming character. The onset is usually abrupt and quite dramatic, with a shaking chill, severe headache, dizziness or vertigo, collapse, and unconsciousness. Patients with massive purpura, low blood pressure, rapid, quiet respiration, and overwhelming bacteremia are said to have the Waterhouse-Friderichsen syndrome. They are often clear mentally. Their extensive rash (see figure) involves skin and mucous membranes as well as internal organs such as skeletal muscle and, classically, the adrenal glands. Leukopenia is another indicator of the gravity of the patient's condition. Body temperature may be subnormal, normal, or elevated. Within a few hours there may be circulatory collapse with intravascular coagulation. Often there is a consumptive coagulopathy (see Ch. 140).

Others may have the encephalitic form, which is characterized by rapidly developing coma, rapid stertorous breathing, a petechial but not massive purpuric rash, and normal blood pressure. Some may present with a combination of encephalitis and adrenal involve-

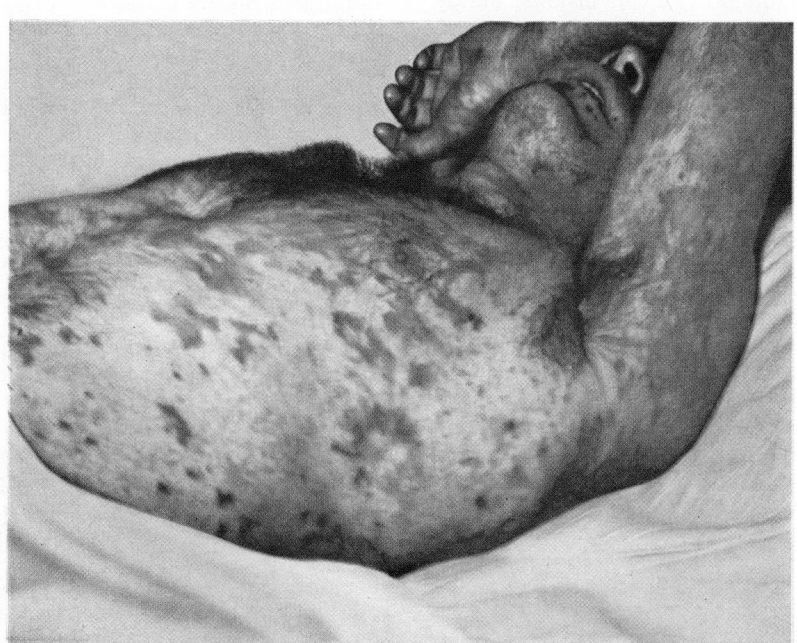

Skin lesions in fulminating meningococcemia. (Courtesy of Dr. Worth B. Daniels.)

ment with early deep coma, low blood pressure, and purpura. Occasionally, the pituitary gland, like the adrenals, is damaged by hemorrhage. These severe illnesses are often rapidly fatal. It is in the attempt to prevent or to reverse this rapid course that so much emphasis is placed upon early, intensive treatment.

CHRONIC MENINGOCOCCEMIA. Chronic meningococcemia is an uncommon form of meningococcal disease in which episodes of fever of a few days' duration recur at intervals of days, weeks, or, more rarely, months. Chills and arthralgic symptoms are frequent, but rash may be absent or evanescent. Repeated cultures of the blood may be necessary before meningococci are recovered. Failure to suspect, recognize, and treat chronic meningococcemia may result in meningitis or endocarditis.

Meningitis. Although meningitis constitutes only a relatively small percentage of the total number of meningococcal infections, it is the most characteristic and important manifestation. The onset and symptoms are often indistinguishable from those of a generalized infection; in some, meningeal involvement seems to predominate. In others, both groups of symptoms appear almost simultaneously, but there may be great variations in their intensity and severity. In addition to the signs of sepsis and the rash, patients with meningitis have evidence of inflammation of the meninges: pain in the neck and back on forward flexion of the head, stiff neck, retraction of the head or severe opisthotonos, positive Kernig's and Brudzinski's signs, hyperesthesia, hyperirritability, and exaggerated reflexes. Unequal reflexes are unusual, but may be present. Involvement of the cranial nerves, when present, may result in strabismus and deafness. The increased intracranial pressure may lead to severe headache, nausea, vomiting, dilated or irregular pupils, engorgement of the fundal veins, choking of the discs, irregular slow pulse, and moderately elevated blood pressure. Cheyne-Stokes or Biot's respiration may appear. As the disease progresses, restlessness and irritability may be followed by delirium or by generalized or jacksonian type convulsions; the patient may become greatly depressed, somnolent, and finally stuporous and comatose. The signs of meningitis in infants may be no more than refusal of feedings, vomiting or regurgitation, diarrhea, irritability, and fever. Convulsions and bulging of the fontanelles may be noted in more severely ill young infants.

LABORATORY FINDINGS IN MENINGITIS. The cerebrospinal fluid is under increased pressure and varies from clear to frankly purulent. The cell count is elevated, often to thousands per cubic millimeter, mostly neutrophils. Gram-negative intra- and extracellular diplococci can be seen in variable numbers in stained smears of the sediment. The total protein in the cerebrospinal fluid is increased, and its sugar content is usually reduced. Meningococci may be grown from the fluid by proper cultural methods. Although fluid obtained early in meningitis may have few or no cells and no reduction of its glucose content, cultures often are positive.

COURSE OF MENINGITIS. Extremely variable, the course is greatly influenced by therapy. In untreated cases the temperature is erratic, and symptoms progress to early death or to chronic meningitis with severe sequelae or delayed death.

COMPLICATIONS OF MENINGOCOCCAL INFECTIONS. The complications of the different forms of meningococcal infections include intercurrent infections, metastatic localizations, and permanent damage to the central nervous system. These may appear during the acute stage or subsequently. Intercurrent infections of the respiratory tract with other agents may occur. Bacteremic or metastatic complications include conjunctivitis, panophthalmitis, otitis, purulent mono- or polyarthritis, pneumonia, pleurisy, pericarditis, myocarditis, endocarditis, orchitis, epididymitis, jaundice, hepatorenal failure, transient albuminuria and hematuria, and adrenal hemorrhage with necrosis. Infection of the central nervous system may produce convulsions, transient or permanent paralyses, hemiplegia, neuroradiculitis, encephalitis, encephalomyelitis, altered cerebration, cranial nerve damage, cerebral thrombosis, and brain abscess. Organization of exudate in the ventricular channels and the subarachnoid space may mechanically obstruct the flow of cerebrospinal fluid, producing hydrocephalus. The accumulation of subdural fluid of high protein content, which when encapsulated resembles a subdural hematoma, is fairly frequent in infants and young children. *Recurrent meningitis* caused by meningococci or other bacteria is usually due to structural defects of bone resulting from trauma or other causes which sometimes require surgical repair. Complications resulting from therapy can be avoided or minimized, if anticipated.

Permanent sequelae may result from almost any complication; the most frequent are deafness, ocular palsies, blindness, hydrocephalus, diminished intellectual capacity, and psychoses.

DIAGNOSIS. The specific diagnosis of meningococcal disease depends primarily upon differentiation from other acute systemic infections. Final confirmation of the diagnosis requires identification of a meningococcus as the causative organism. During an epidemic, especially in a recruit military camp or a closed population, all cases of fever with abrupt onset, of prostration with or without fever, of petechial or purpuric rash, of drowsiness or coma, and of meningitis should be treated vigorously as meningococcal infections whether or not organisms are found in initial smears and cultures.

Meningococcal infections in their early stages may resemble any acute systemic infection. In sepsis caused by pyogenic organisms such as staphylococci, streptococci, or pneumococci, there may be a preceding upper respiratory infection, recurrent fever, malaise, arthralgia, and leukocytosis. A rash similar to that of severe meningococcemia and even signs of the Waterhouse-Friderichsen syndrome may be present in such cases. Final proof of cause is accomplished by isolation of the offending organisms from the blood, joint fluid, sputum, and so forth. Meningococcal infections also must be differentiated from the acute exanthems, typhus (both endemic and epidemic), typhoid and other enteric fevers, subacute bacterial endocarditis, rheumatic fever, brucellosis, and others.

Diagnosis of Meningitis. The diagnosis of meningococcal meningitis requires differentiation from meningismus, other bacterial meningitides, viral meningoencephalitis, myeloencephalitis resulting from bacterial toxins (tetanus, botulinus) or chemicals, and noninfectious illnesses such as subarachnoid or cerebral hemorrhages or thrombosis, diabetic coma, and uremia. In most cases of meningococcal meningitis, the diagnosis is readily established by the specific identification of the organism; in others the cause may not be determinable when the patient is first seen, but a number of helpful procedures can be carried out. The usual medical history should be obtained with a careful inquiry into recent localized infections, especially of the ear. Trauma to the head should be investigated, because this predisposes to secondary bacterial meningitides, more likely to be caused by *H. influenzae* or pneumococci.

Physical examination should include a thorough search for diseases of the eyes and upper respiratory passages, sinuses, and ears, and for evidence of injury to the head, in addition to careful general and neurologic examinations. A complete blood count should be made and cultures of the blood and posterior nasopharynx obtained. Any suspected localized areas of infection likewise should be cultured. Urinalysis and determinations of serum electrolytes and the blood nonprotein nitrogen may aid in the differential diagnosis and help to indicate precautions to be observed in therapy. In seriously ill, or perhaps all, patients, blood coagulation analyses should be performed to determine the presence of a consumptive coagulopathy. Bleeding from the upper gastrointestinal tract ("stress ulcers") should be suspected in the very sick, especially those in shock.

Lumbar puncture should be performed as soon as possible and before specific treatment is instituted. After determining the initial pressure, fluid should be removed slowly until the pressure is reduced to an approximately normal level. The dynamics of the cerebrospinal fluids can then be estimated by jugular compression for evidence of block or sinus thrombosis. Examination of the cerebrospinal fluid should include the following: gross appearance, total and differential cell counts, determination of sugar (compare with blood level) and protein, and cultures and examination of Gram-stained smears. If organisms are seen, they can often be identified tentatively from their appearance and precisely with proper and *potent* antisera by a positive direct quellung test if of group A or C. Where the technique is available, counterimmunoelectrophoresis can be used, often successfully even when organisms are not seen on smear.

A *presumptive diagnosis* can usually be made from the Gram-stained smear, the differential cell count, and the sugar content of the cerebrospinal fluid. Caution should be exercised in the interpretation of smears, because even experienced observers may be misled by overdecolorized or dead gram-positive diplococci or other bacteria. Final identification depends on serogrouping organisms from culture. The leukocytes are almost entirely neutrophils in purulent meningitides, except for those caused by tubercle bacilli. In the latter, as in viral infections (mumps, herpes, coxsackieviruses, echoviruses and others), mononucleated cells predominate except in their early stages. The sugar content is usually decreased in bacterial meningitis and normal or elevated in viral infections. In meningismus the fluid is usually normal. The proportion of erythrocytes to leukocytes is similar to that in whole blood in cases of subarachnoid hemorrhage. The history, other physical findings, and special laboratory tests should help to differentiate myeloencephalitides resulting from toxins or chemicals.

TREATMENT. During the past 30 years, groups A, B, C, and, less often, Y meningococci have been responsible for almost all meningococcal infections regardless of their clinical forms. Until about 1963, practically all meningococcal strains were exquisitely susceptible to the sulfonamide drugs, whether in carriers or cases. For these reasons, the sulfonamides were the agents of choice for both treatment and prophylaxis. They are still excellent, but only when specific tests have demonstrated that the patient or carrier has a sulfonamide-susceptible organism.

Since sulfonamide-resistant group A, B, C, and Y strains are now commonplace, the treatment of choice is penicillin G in massive dosage. For adults, this means 20,000,000 units per day intravenously or 1,000,000 units every two hours intramuscularly. The latter route should not be used for patients in or on the verge of shock, because of possible failure of absorption. When the 20,000,000-unit dose is used intravenously, it is best to divide it into four or more doses per day rather than to administer it by continuous drip. Doses in children should be reduced in accordance with pediatric therapeutic principles.

Ampicillin may be used as an alternative, although an occasional patient does not seem to respond adequately to this drug. Close observation of the patient's course will alert the physician to this problem should it arise. The dose should be at least 150 mg per kilogram per day for children and 10 to 12 grams per day for adults, parenterally, divided into six to eight doses.

In patients known to be truly allergic to penicillin, and ill with sulfonamide-resistant strains of meningococci, chloramphenicol is the alternative drug of choice. The use of this drug imposes precautions of its own. These can be managed but close watch should be kept on the hematopoietic system and the drug withdrawn immediately if a complication appears. Thus far, no meningococci resistant to penicillin or chloramphenicol have been identified. If the patient's organism is found to be susceptible to sulfonamide, treatment can be altered accordingly. Cephalothins and lincomycin should not be used, because therapeutic failures have followed their administration.

Patients with meningococcal disease are usually more dehydrated than they appear. Care should be taken to ensure a daily urine output of more than 1000 ml. Treatment should be continued at least until all signs and symptoms have been normal for a minimum of two days and preferably for five. It may be stopped abruptly. Relapse occurs occasionally and requires prompt treatment.

Patients with fulminating meningococcemia or meningitis, or both, should be started on therapy as soon as the diagnosis is suspected and specimens obtained without waiting for bacteriologic confirmation. Penicillin should be given by vein. (Patients allergic to penicillin are best treated with chloramphenicol.) The central venous pressure should be monitored and corrected as necessary. Disseminated intravascular coagulation, when diagnosed, should be managed as in any other disease state (see Ch. 521.5). Norepinephrine, intravenously, may be required to maintain blood pressure. Steroids are clearly required if there is evidence of adrenal collapse; such patients are managed as are those with acute adrenal insufficiency. Otherwise, there is no good evidence that steroids are of any positive value. These severely ill patients are the most likely ones to bleed from gastric lesions ("stress ulcers") which require special handling, contraindicating steroids. Intravenous infusions will be required to correct dehydration, but an excess should be avoided. Oxygen therapy should be instituted and maintained as long as cyanosis or dyspnea is present. Blood transfusions have not been shown to be of significant value in this type of circulatory failure.

Certain laboratory tests such as *hematologic examinations* should be repeated as aids in monitoring the patient's course. This is especially true for patients admitted with severe leukopenia or thrombocytopenia. Their reversal is of considerable positive prognostic significance. *Blood cultures* should be repeated if the fever persists or returns, for continued bacteremia suggests the presence of endocarditis or other metastatic localization. *Repeat lumbar punctures* are indicated if there is persistent increased intracranial pressure, failure to respond to adequate therapy, or relapse of meningitis.

Symptomatic and supportive treatment is essential for patients with meningococcal infections. Sedation should be minimal, yet sufficient to assure adequate rest but not to interfere with the assessment of the patient's course. Approximately one month of convalescence is required for complete recovery in most cases and even more for those who had severe illnesses.

The treatment of complications of meningococcal infections is primarily that of the underlying disease. Should fever or signs of meningeal irritation reappear, then the most probable causes are recurrence of infection with the meningococcus because of inadequate treatment, drug fever, or superinfection with another organism. In such circumstances, the cerebrospinal fluid and blood should be re-examined and cultured. If the meningococcal infection has relapsed, intensive treatment should be reinstituted and maintained until the patient has fully recovered.

PROGNOSIS. The prognosis in meningococcal infections has improved enormously since the sulfonamides and penicillin became available. In untreated cases of meningococcemia and meningitis, the mortality formerly varied from 20 to 90 per cent, averaging about 70 per cent. The introduction of serum therapy reduced this to about 50 per cent. With the sulfonamides, the case fatality rate was reduced to 5 to 10 per cent, depending upon age and complicating conditions. The recent recognition of sulfonamide-resistant meningococci has not altered this significantly, because cases can be treated as successfully with penicillin. Age is perhaps the most important factor in prognosis, for the greatest mortality, despite adequate therapy, occurs in those less than 2 or more than 40 years old. In the U.S. Army during World War II, the over-all mortality was slightly less than 5 per cent and, in some series, even below 1 per cent. More than 90 per cent of these cases were caused by sulfonamide-susceptible group A strains. In addition to a most favorable age distribution in the Army, the excellent physical condition of patients, early diagnosis, and the prompt institution of effective therapy were probably responsible for this remarkable recovery rate. The prognosis is still poor in fulminating cases with abrupt onset, extensive cutaneous lesions, and circulatory collapse. In spite of rapid, intensive therapy, such cases frequently terminate fatally. Relapses, recurrences, and complications have been greatly reduced by specific treatment so that the prognosis for total recovery is generally good. The most frequent permanent sequelae despite adequate treatment are deafness, cranial nerve paralyses, mental deficiency, and, less often, blindness and hydrocephalus. These are all relatively uncommon and usually result from treatment delays for whatever cause.

PREVENTION. Prophylaxis as applied to meningococcal infections during the past 30 years represented an outgrowth of the World War II experience, which indicated not only that sulfadiazine rapidly cured meningococcal disease but also that the nasopharyngeal carrier state was reversed (not true of penicillin) soon after such treatment was begun. After several successful trials in military recruits, a policy was adopted whereby small amounts of sulfadiazine were administered simultaneously to all members of recruit training centers, schools, ships, and similar groups upon the recognition of a predetermined number of cases. This resulted in an immediate reduction in carriers and a sharp decrease in cases, reflecting the interaction of a susceptible organism with an effective drug when administered to a total population at risk. Because of the fears often generated by the diagnosis of meningitis, the same sulfadiazine regimen was adopted for general use by physicians and health departments to treat family and hospital (staff) contacts of sporadic cases. But the "secondary" cases which occasionally occur in households usually begin within 96 hours or less of that of the index patient, suggesting that they may be coprimary rather than secondary. Less often, this interval may be as long as seven to ten days. It would seem then that if disease is to be prevented under such circumstances, therapeutic rather than "prophylactic" medication is needed. Unless the causative strain is known to be sulfonamide susceptible, it must be assumed to be resistant, requiring penicillin dosage in the therapeutic range. If taken orally, this will require 8 million or more units per day in young or older adults. Suitably reduced doses should be prescribed for children. Either oral or parenteral regimens for *streptococcal prophylaxis* provide *no* protection for meningococcal infections.

The recommendation for meningococcal disease is really for intervention rather than prevention. Alternatively, one can observe closely (including nasopharyngeal cultures) and treat immediately upon the appearance of any symptoms. But over-all, the risk is very low and should not induce the hysteria which so often accompanies the hospital admission or diagnosis of a case of meningococcal meningitis. The isolation of patients after 24 to 48 hours of adequate therapy is not indicated.

Although the foregoing is suitable for the immediate contact or family, it is not applicable to a population group such as in a camp, school, or mental institution. In such instances the objective is to rapidly reduce the over-all carrier level to a point at which transfer is impeded, decreasing the case rate. Again, sulfonamides are the most effective drugs for this purpose, but only when the causative organisms are susceptible. Penicillin, in contrast to sulfonamides, often fails to eliminate the carrier state, even in therapeutic doses. Rifampin (600 mg daily for five days) has been used for this purpose in military and civilian populations. Meningococcal carrier rates are reduced quite effectively by rifampin, but resistance does occur and increases with reuse. Recent experience has indicated considerable toxicity with minocycline so that it has been all but discontinued for meningococcal prophylaxis. The widespread use of rifampin in populations with high tuberculosis rates probably should be exercised with some caution because of possible increased resistance among tubercle bacilli. At no time should rifampin be used for the treatment of cases of meningococcal disease.

Vaccines. There is considerable reason for optimism regarding meningococcal vaccines. Potent group-specific polysaccharides have been prepared from meningococci of groups A, C, and Y but not yet from B. After very careful graduated trials, group C meningococcal polysaccharide vaccine, in single subcutaneous doses of 50 μg, was made routine for all American military recruits. Disease caused by this serogroup has all but been eliminated from that population. Group A polysaccharide vaccine has been found to be equally effective in a Finnish epidemic and among South African miners, and combined group A and C vaccine also was efficacious in the massive Brazilian epidemic which was caused by organisms of both serogroups. The duration of protection has not yet been established, although it would appear likely to be of long duration. Measurable responses to polysaccharide vaccines are quite different and diminished in children (especially under 18 months of age) than adults. Although group A and C polysaccharide vaccines have been licensed in the United States and elsewhere, they are not available for general use in the United States.

Artenstein, M. S., Gold, R., Zimmerly, J. G., Wyle, F. A., Schneider, H., and Harkins, C.: Prevention of meningococcal disease by group C polysaccharide vaccine. N. Engl. J. Med., 282:417, 1970.

Evans, R. W., Glick, B., Kimball, F., and Lobell, M.: Fatal intravascular consumption coagulopathy in meningococcal sepsis. Am. J. Med., 46:910, 1969.

Feldman, H. A.: *Neisseria* infections other than gonococcal. *In* Bodily, H. L., Updyke, E. L., and Mason, J. O. (eds.): Diagnostic Procedures for Bacterial, Mycotic and Parasitic Infections. 5th ed. New York, American Public Health Association, Inc., 1970.

Feldman, H. A.: Meningococcal Infections. *In* Stollerman, G. H. (ed.): Advances in Internal Medicine, Vol. 18. Chicago, Year Book Medical Publishers, 1972, pp. 117–140.

Makela, P. H., Kayhty, H., Weckstrom, P., Sivonen, A., and Renkonen, O.-V.: Effect of group-A meningococcal vaccine in army recruits in Finland. Lancet, 2:883, 1975.

142. HEMOPHILUS INFECTIONS WITH SPECIAL EMPHASIS ON HEMOPHILUS INFLUENZAE TYPE B

John B. Robbins

Pfeiffer, in 1892, identified the genus *Hemophilus* from the sputum of individuals with respiratory disease during an influenza pandemic. The requirement of the microbe for whole blood prompted his designation *Hemophilus influenzae*. Studies, especially during the influenza pandemics of 1917 and 1918, revealed that this organism was not the etiologic cause of influenza. Subsequently, other bacterial species have been designated *Hemophilus* because of similar morphology, physiology, and growth requirement for blood-enriched media (see accompanying table). All *Hemophilus* species are facultatively aerobic, nonmotile, and nonsporeforming. *H. influenzae* is the most important for its potential for serious human disease.

Clinical Differentiation of *Hemophilus* Species

Species	Normal Habitat	Growth Factor Requirement		Hemolysis
		X	V	
H. influenzae	Upper respiratory tract	+	+	−
H. parainfluenzae	Upper respiratory tract	−	+	−
H. aegyptius	Upper respiratory tract, eye	+	+	−
H. hemolyticus	Upper respiratory tract	+	+	+
H. parahemolyticus	Upper respiratory tract	−	+	+
H. ducreyi	Genital	+	−	+

ETIOLOGY. *H. influenzae* exists in the encapsulated form (opalescent colonies) with raised mucoid appearance and the uncapsulated form (flat bluish translucent colonies). On optimal media, the organisms appear as comparatively small uniform coccobacilli (1 to 1.5 by 0.3 μ). However, under less than optimal conditions, especially in body fluids, *H. influenzae* exhibits polymorphism and may be long slender filaments, often attaining a length of 20 to 30 μ. Its bipolar bodies may retain the gram-positive stain under certain conditions, and *H. influenzae* has often been mistaken for pneumococci or meningococci. *H. influenzae* requires V factor (heat labile, NAD) and X factor (hemin). These nutritive factors are the basis for differentiation among *Hemophilus* species (see table).

Occasionally, mistakes may be made by the exuberant transfer of colonies from chocolate agar (containing both growth factors) to a differential medium. In this case, the small amounts of nutrients carried over on thick swabs may be sufficient to allow other *Hemophilus* species to grow, resulting in confusion, such as has occurred between *H. parainfluenzae* and *H. influenzae*. *H. influenzae* will grow in any enriched nonselective medium. Complex mixtures, such as brain-heart infusion plus hemolyzed blood, provide the most effective medium in the author's experience. Enriched media, such as chocolate agar, lose their nutritive activity because of the factor V decay. Further, if the blood supplement is not carefully prepared (extensive heat may destroy its enriching properties), laboratories may fail to report *H. influenzae* isolates. Quality control measures, such as growing standardized *H. influenzae* strains, should be practiced. The "satellite" phenomenon is often used to accelerate the growth of *H. influenzae* on blood agar. In this technique, the formation of NAD and hemin mediated by *Staphylococcus aureus* provides a local environment that favors *Hemophilus* growth.

As defined by Pittman, there are six chemically and serologically distinct capsular polysaccharide antigens. With the use of the appropriate antisera, these capsular polysaccharides may be visualized on fresh isolates or bacteria grown under optimal conditions by a variety of techniques, including the quellung reaction and immunoprecipitation. Although the over-all chemical and physical properties of the six capsules are similar, virtually all serious human disease is caused by type b.

ECOLOGY. *H. influenzae* is usually found in the upper respiratory tract. The nonencapsulated form can be recovered from nasopharyngeal cultures of about 80 per cent of healthy individuals. In contrast, encapsulated organisms, especially type b, are found in comparatively few individuals (1 to 3 per cent) during infancy and early childhood and only rarely in healthy adults. In cases of severe systemic *H. influenzae* type b disease, case contacts, including siblings and parents, usually have positive cultures.

PATHOGENICITY AND IMMUNITY. The relation of the type b capsule to systemic disease with *H. influenzae* resembles that observed for pneumococcal and meningococcal capsular polysaccharides. The presence of the capsule inhibits effective phagocytosis. However, the mechanism by which *H. influenzae* type b invades the nasopharyngeal mucosa of only some individuals is not known. It has been suggested that toxic substances in this organism may inhibit ciliary action or that simultaneous infection with some viruses may predispose to septicemia. Pathogen-free infant rat models suggest that the escape of one organism into the blood in a nonimmune individual is sufficient to cause septicemia. When concentration of organisms in the blood reaches a critical level (approximately 10^3 per milliliter), the chance of penetrating the meninges increases considerably.

Immunity to systemic disease is mediated by serum antibodies. Serum concentrations of 0.15 to 0.2 μg of anti-type b antibodies have been shown to be protective. However, complete protection against this disease with currently available *H. influenzae* type b capsular polysaccharide vaccines in infants up to 18 months has not yet been achieved because of poor immunogenicity in this high-risk age group. Antibodies to other surface bacterial components, such as outer membrane proteins and lipopolysaccharides, may also confer protection. Their use as potential vaccines is also under study. Other host resistance mechanisms are important, as shown by the extreme susceptibility of individuals who have splenic dysfunction, such as is seen in excessive hemolytic states as sickle cell anemia or its variants, in splenectomy, or in congenital absence of the spleen. Individuals with deficient immunoglobulin synthesis, including highly specialized defects such as that of IgG 2, are extraordinarily susceptible to repeated and severe *H. influenzae* type b disease. Passive immunization of X-linked hypogammaglobulinemia patients with pooled immunoglobulin is highly effective preventive therapy.

Meningitis is the most important and frequent of serious systemic disease with *H. influenzae* type b. This organism is the leading cause of all bacterial meningitis in the United States. Other important *H. influenzae* type b diseases include epiglottitis, pyoarthrosis, and pneumonia and its complications, including empyema, osteomyelitis, and pericarditis. Occasionally, superficial and deep cellulitis in the buccal area may occur. This may be recognized by a bluish hue to the surrounding tissues and is usually accompanied by a septicemia. The over-all incidence in the United States is 4.5 per 100,000, but in children up to five years of age the incidence is 50 to 80 per 100,000. The incidence is also much higher in adults with acquired immunologic defects. In one survey, *H. influenzae* type b was found to be the most common cause of bacterial meningitis in adults in New York City. Some have suggested that the frequency of *H. influenzae* type b diseases has recently increased, but improved laboratory facilities and increasing awareness of this organism as a pathogen may have contributed to these figures. Unusually high attack rates of systemic *H. influenzae* type b diseases, including meningitis, occur in certain communities and closed populations such as day care nurseries.

DIAGNOSIS. Systemic disease with *H. influenzae* type b is most accurately diagnosed by identification of the organism in body fluids, such as the blood, cerebrospinal fluid, or pleural fluid. Care must be taken that the medium used for cultivation of the organism is fresh and can sustain *H. influenzae* growth. The use of 5 per cent carbon dioxide and high humidity environment increases the rapidity with which the organism can be identified and recovered from fluids with low concentration of organisms or in patients treated with antimicrobials.

Immunochemical identification of the capsule may be accomplished by the quellung reaction of fresh isolates and by the demonstration of the capsular material in body fluids. The use of concentrated urine samples from patients with systemic disease with *H. influenzae* type b is very productive. There are many bacterial antigens cross-reactive with the type b capsular polysaccharide, including one *E. coli* capsular type, K100; also, gram-positive bacteria containing ribitol phosphate as a component of their cell wall teichoic acid, including pneumococcus types 6B, 29, and 34, some *Bacillus* species, and *S. aureus,* could yield false-positive reactions. In addition, circulating type b antigen may be masked by host antibody. In this case, dissociation techniques for measuring type b antigen have been reported. The determination of trace and unique *H. influenzae* type b metabolites by more sophisticated techniques seems promising, but such techniques are not yet available in most centers.

Meningitis caused by *H. influenzae* type b does not present any distinctive clinical features (see Ch. 140).

Epiglottitis caused by this organism presents an acute clinical emergency in any age group. The appearance of upper respiratory obstruction associated with a clinical infection, especially with fever, pain, and no external swelling, should alert the physician to the possibility of *H. influenzae* type b epiglottitis. Direct visualization of the inflamed, cherry red epiglottis is diagnostic. In many cases, the simple maneuvering of the tongue may acutely increase the respiratory obstruction, and tracheal intubation or tracheostomy may be necessary. Thus facilities must be at hand if this acute infectious upper respiratory obstruction is suspected.

Fever of unknown origin in children is often due to *H. influenzae* type b. Such individuals respond rapidly to proper therapy without evidence of localized disease. However, complications or blood-borne infections such as meningitis and osteomyelitis may occur.

TREATMENT. Prior to the availability of effective therapeutic agents, systemic *H. influenzae* diseases, particularly meningitis and epiglottitis, had at least a 95 per cent mortality. Currently, highly effective antimicrobial drugs, including ampicillin and chloramphenicol, are available. However, the use of ampicillin has been curtailed because of the widespread emergence of beta lactamase–producing *H. influenzae* type b disease isolates. Surveillance studies in many communities indicate that at least 10 per cent of disease isolates produce this inactivating enzyme. The diagnosis of ampicillin resistance is achieved by acid liberated from penicillin or a chromogen for a cephalin derivative synthesized for penicillinase detection. Chloramphenicol, despite its bone marrow toxicity, provides a highly effective agent for the treatment of all systemic *H. influenzae* type b diseases, including meningitis and arthritis. However, some disease isolates have shown resistance to chloramphenicol and tetracycline. It is now recommended that all *systemic* diseases with

H. influenzae type b be treated with chloramphenicol until their drug resistance patterns can be determined. Ampicillin remains the drug of choice for susceptible organisms. Surveillance is necessary to assess the frequency of the drug resistance patterns.

Antimicrobial therapy for meningitis has been recommended for approximately seven to ten days (see Ch. 140). Cellular and protein levels may require more than two weeks to return to normal. In children, persistent fever with meningitis may signify localized collections of fluid. Signs of increasing intracranial pressure or localizing signs may warrant further diagnostic studies to identify such complications as subdural empyema or intracortical abscess formation. Endocarditis or pericarditis caused by *H. influenzae* type b has been treated successfully by approximately four to six weeks of therapy. The other aspects of treatment of meningitis, mentioned in Ch. 140, apply to the treatment of *H. influenzae* type b diseases at all ages.

Other H. Influenzae Diseases. Nonencapsulated *H. influenzae* organisms are frequently found in the respiratory tracts of individuals with chronic lung disease. Their pathogenic role has been incompletely defined, but it seems probable that high sputum populations of *H. influenzae* in those with chronic lung disease exert a deleterious effect. The finding of *H. influenzae* in the sputum of patients with chronic lung disease poses a therapeutic problem. Most physicians feel that when this finding is accompanied by signs of respiratory infection, antimicrobial therapy is indicated. Treatment resulting in diminution or disappearance of *H. influenzae* from the sputum of such patients often results in marked relief of symptoms such as fever, cough, and dyspnea. *H. influenzae* is often found in the exudate of infants and children with middle ear infection. In most cases, these are nonencapsulated organisms and the response to antimicrobial therapy is rapid. In about 3 to 4 per cent of cases, however, type b organisms may be isolated directly from middle ear aspirants. This finding may be accompanied by *H. influenzae* type b systemic disease, including meningitis. Accurate etiologic diagnosis of otitis media with nasopharyngeal cultures is not possible. Accordingly, in most instances, acute otitis media is treated with the antimicrobial drugs designed to combat the agents most often responsible for this infectious disease in the appropriate age group.

PREVENTION. It has been reported with increasing frequency that secondary cases of *H. influenzae* type b disease, especially meningitis, may occur under certain unusual conditions, such as day care nurseries or chronic care institutions. In this case, there have been reports of trials with various antimicrobial agents and immunization with the purified capsular polysaccharide. The latter, in its present form, prevents disease in individuals for more than two years. Various antimicrobials, including ampicillin for the treatment of drug-susceptible organisms, sulfonamides, and others, have been used without any clear definition of their effectiveness in preventing further disease in outbreak situations. It should be realized that secondary cases occur among families, especially when there are siblings of susceptible age in close contact with the affected patient. Indeed, the secondary attack rate under certain circumstances is comparable to that for meningococcal disease. Attempts at disease prevention of siblings should include antimicrobial regimens designed to treat meningitis. The morbidity (fixed central nervous deficits) remains high even after optimal therapy, and vaccine development for prevention is under active research.

Other Human Hemophilus Species. *H. influenzae* types a, c, d, e, and f, as well as *H. parainfluenzae, H. aphrophilus,* and *H. hemolyticus,* occasionally are isolated from individuals with systemic bacterial infections. There is yet no known predisposing lesion to identify the pathogenic processes involved in infection with such unusual organisms. The treatment of these *Hemophilus* infections requires no unusual therapy except for the caution that their isolation may be impeded by the use of conventional or outdated media. *H. aegyptius* is the cause of a severe form of conjunctivitis. This form of conjunctivitis may occur in epidemic form, especially in the summer among crowded communities such as those seen in summer camps. Its diagnosis can be achieved by direct smear of the purified fluid or by cultivation on appropriate media. Therapy with antimicrobials is successful. Drug resistance among these *Hemophilus* species has been reported, but its frequency is not well characterized.

H. ducreyi is the cause of chancroid. This venereal disease is characterized by a one- to two-week incubation with centrally ulcerating lesions of about 2 to 20 ml on or in the immediate genital area. There is usually painful nonindurated lymphadenopathy accompanying these lesions. Suppuration of the regional lymph nodes may make the diagnosis of simultaneous syphilis difficult. Sulfadiazine remains the treatment of choice for chancroid, but it should be realized that the symptoms of chancroid may obscure simultaneous infection with syphilis, which requires a different therapy (see Ch. 171).

Peltola, H., Kayhty, H., Sivonen, A., and Makela, P. H.: *Haemophilus influenzae* type b capsular polysaccharide vaccine in children: A double blind field study of 100,000 vaccinees 3 months to 5 years of age in Finland. Pediatrics 60:730, 1977.

Pittman, M.: Variation and type specificity in the bacterial species *Haemophilus influenzae.* J. Exp. Med., 53:471, 1931.

Robbins, J. B., and Hill, J. C. (eds.): Current status and prospects for improved and new bacterial vaccines. A symposium held at the National Institutes of Health, Bethesda, Maryland, March 29–April 1, 1976. J. Infect. Dis., *136* (suppl.), August 1977.

Robbins, J. B., Schneerson, R., Argaman, M., and Handzel, Z. T.: *Haemophilus influenzae* type b: Disease and immunity in humans. Ann. Intern. Med., 78:259, 1973.

Schneerson, R., and Robbins, J.: Induction of serum *Haemophilus influenzae* type b capsular antibodies in adult volunteers fed cross-reacting *Escherichia coli* 075:K 100:H5. N. Engl. J. Med., 292:1093, 1975.

Smith, D. H., Ingram, D. L., Smith, R. L., Gilles, F., and Bresnan, M. J.: Bacterial meningitis. A symposium. Pediatrics, 52:586, 1973.

WHOOPING COUGH

143. WHOOPING COUGH

(Pertussis)

Stephen I. Morse

DEFINITION. Whooping cough is an acute respiratory illness that classically affects infants and young children. The etiologic agent is usually *Bordetella pertussis;* occasionally *B. parapertussis* and rarely *B. bronchiseptica* produce a similar syndrome. The descriptive name derives from a distressing, prolonged inspiratory effort that follows paroxysmal coughing. Whooping cough is still responsible for a significant number of deaths in infants in areas where pertussis immunization is not practiced.

HISTORY. The disease was first recorded in the middle of the sixteenth century by Moulton and by DeBaillou. Whether whooping cough was indigenous to Europe or had been transported there in the preceding century is uncertain. Sydenham applied the name "pertussis" to any illness accompanied by violent coughing, but the term became restricted to the epidemic disease that was a well-recognized clinical entity by the middle of the eighteenth century. In 1900 Bordet and Gengou observed coccobacilli in the sputum of a child with whooping cough, but it was not until 1906 that they were able to culture the organism. Many years passed before the Bordet-Gengou bacillus was universally accepted as the etiologic agent of whooping cough was indigenous to Europe or had been trans- morphologic changes on prolonged cultivation, thereby ac- counting for the difficulties in establishing the etiologic role of the agent and the inconstant protective effect of immunizing preparations. Although the mortality rate of whooping cough in the United States began to decline in the early part of this century, the incidence in young children did not significantly decrease until after the use of prophylactic vaccines became widespread.

ETIOLOGY. When first isolated, *Bordetella pertussis* is a minute, nonmotile, weakly staining, gram-negative coccobacillus, 0.5 to 1.0 μ in length. Capsules can be demonstrated by special procedures, and bipolar meta- chromatic granules are present. The complex medium containing blood originally employed by Bordet and Gengou is still often used for cultivation. *Primary iso- lates, phase I organisms, will not grow on conventional laboratory media,* but will do so after prolonged passage. At the same time colonial morphology changes, marked pleomorphism of individual cells is evident, and there is an alteration in antigenic composition. This occurs in a series of phases, and the change from phase I to phase IV has been likened to the smooth to rough tran- sition of other microbes. Only phase I organisms are virulent, and *only phase I organisms* provide effective immunizing material.

Members of the *Bordetella* genus were formerly re- garded as species of *Hemophilus.* However, the *Borde- tella* group does not have the strict requirement for X and V growth factors, and they are antigenically dis- tinct. The addition of blood to Bordet-Gengou medium is required for the growth of phase I organisms, but the blood acts to neutralize bacterial substances, probably fatty acids, rather than to provide nutrients. Charcoal, starch, or ion exchange resins can be substituted for blood.

B. pertussis produces a heat-stable toxin (endotoxin) and a heat-labile toxin. A role of toxins in the develop- ment of disease has not been demonstrated. A hemag- glutinin has also been isolated. The capsular material does not swell in the presence of antiserum. A species agglutinogen has been recognized as well as agglutinat- ing factors that differ between strains. Serotyping is therefore a useful epidemiologic tool. The role of the interaction between the organism and phagocytes has not been defined, although the presence of antisera ap- pears to increase uptake of *B. pertussis* by leukocytes.

Remarkable biologic effects are induced in laboratory animals by the injection of killed phase I organisms. These include development of heightened sensitivity to histamine and serotonin; increased susceptibility to an- aphylaxis and to experimental allergic encephalomyeli- tis; increased antibody production, including reaginic antibody, in response to heterologous antigens; and hyperleukocytosis and hyperlymphocytosis. The factors responsible for these reactions have not been character- ized fully.

It should be emphasized that none, of the cellular components or products of *B. pertussis* have been shown to be of central importance in the pathogenesis of whooping cough.

Approximately 5 to 10 per cent of clinical whooping cough is caused by *B. parapertussis.* The animal patho- gen *B. bronchiseptica* is responsible for a very minor percentage of cases. These organisms can be differen- tiated from *B. pertussis* by appropriate further bacterio- logic or serologic procedures. It has recently been sug- gested that adenoviruses, along or in concert with *B. pertussis,* may play an etiologic role in some cases of whooping cough.

EPIDEMIOLOGY. In communities of susceptibles the family attack rate is 80 to 90 per cent, which is extreme- ly high for a bacterial disease, approaching that seen in varicella or measles. Transmission is by droplet infec- tion. Carriers of *B. pertussis* are found infrequently, and the reservoir is therefore unknown. Disease usually occurs in late winter in the northern climates and in late spring in southern zones, but there is great varia- tion.

The mortality rate from whooping cough has fallen since the turn of this century owing to improved sup- portive therapy. The incidence of whooping cough, however, did not change until after the 1940's, when immunization of young children became standard prac- tice. In the five-year periods 1926–1930, 1936–1940, 1956–1960, and 1965–1969, the fatality rate per thousand cases in the United States was 39.1, 19.4, 6.8, and 5.9 respectively. In the same time frames, the number of reported cases was 909,705; 956,262; 146,989; and 32,329, respectively. The majority of deaths, over 70 per cent, occur in children under one year of age, with the preponderance in infants under the age of six months.

Neither immunization against pertussis nor natural dis- ease provides lifelong protection. In the case of artificial immunization, an attack rate greater than 50 per cent has been reported when the interval after immuniza- tion exceeds 12 years, a rate no different from that in unimmunized individuals of the same age. Thus in the face of routine immunization, it is possible that pertussis will become primarily a disease of older children and adults.

PATHOLOGY. Interpretation of pathologic material obtained at autopsy is difficult because of the common presence of complicating respiratory infections. Lesions caused by *B. pertussis* are found principally in the bronchi and bronchioles, but changes are also seen in the nasopharynx, larynx, and trachea. Masses of bacteria are intertwined with the cilia of the columnar epithelium together with mucopurulent exudate. There is also necrosis of the midzonal and basilar epithelium with infiltration of polymorphonuclear leukocytes and macrophages. Peribronchial accumulation of lymphocytes and granulocytes produces the picture of interstitial pneumonitis. Secondary atelectasis and localized emphysema are common. The alveoli in uncomplicated whooping cough do not contain exudate.

CLINICAL MANIFESTATIONS. After an incubation period of 7 to 16 days, symptoms appear. It is customary to divide the clinical course into three stages, each of two weeks' duration, but variation is frequent, particularly in the immunized community.

Catarrhal Stage. Whooping cough begins with symptoms indistinguishable from those of a mild viral upper respiratory infection or common cold. Sneezing is frequent, the conjunctivae are injected, and a nocturnal cough appears. The temperature may be slightly elevated at this time. Infectivity is greatest during the catarrhal stage.

Paroxysmal Stage. Seven to 14 days after onset, the cough becomes more frequent, diurnal, and then paroxysmal. In a typical paroxysm there is a series of 15 to 20 short coughs of increasing intensity, and then with a deep inspiration the air is drawn into the lungs, making the "whoop." A tenacious mucus plug is usually expelled, and vomiting frequently follows the spasmodic episode. Paroxysms may occur as often as every half hour, and are accompanied by signs of increased venous pressure. The conjunctivae are deeply engorged; there is periorbital edema; and petechial hemorrhages, particularly about the forehead, as well as epistaxis are common. During the attack the infant may be cyanotic until the crowing whoop occurs. In between paroxysms the child usually feels well though justifiably apprehensive.

Physical examination of the chest is usually unremarkable, although scattered rhonchi may be heard. The chest roentgenogram sometimes reveals hilar and mediastinal nodal enlargement. The presence of fever immediately suggests the development of a secondary infectious process.

Convalescent Stage. Gradually the paroxysms become less frequent and less intense, vomiting ceases, and slow recovery ensues. Often for many months even a mild, unrelated respiratory infection will be manifested by a return of paroxysmal cough and whoop.

It is important to recognize those patients with whooping cough in whom variation from the pattern frequently occurs. In young infants the paroxysms and the whoop are often absent; instead, choking spells and apneic periods may be the major manifestations. Second attacks of whooping cough as well as disease occurring in previously immunized individuals often present simply as an upper respiratory illness or bronchitis.

Complications. Complications may be related to the primary disease or to secondary events. Alterations in acid-base balance occur as a result of metabolic alkalosis when vomiting is severe. Recurrent vomiting can also lead to malnutrition. Anoxemic manifestations are seen when ventilation is markedly impaired. Central nervous system changes can result from cerebral anoxia or hemorrhages consequent to the elevated venous pressure. Rarely, cortical degeneration occurs, but the exact pathogenesis of the encephalopathy is unknown. A serous meningitis with lymphocytosis of the cerebrospinal fluid has been described. Localized areas of emphysema and atelectasis generally return to normal after the disease has run its course, and pneumothorax and interstitial emphysema are infrequently seen.

The major cause of death in whooping cough is complicating pneumonia or bronchopneumonia caused by other bacteria or viruses. In addition, secondary bacterial otitis media occurs frequently.

DIAGNOSIS. There is little difficulty in making the clinical diagnosis of whooping cough in a patient who, after a variable period of coryzal symptoms, develops paroxysmal coughing with a terminal inspiratory whoop. Toward the end of the catarrhal stage, or early in the spasmodic phase, leukocytosis often occurs. In contrast to the leukocytosis found in most bacterial diseases, the predominating cell type is the mature small lymphocyte. Characteristically the leukocyte count ranges from 15,000 to 30,000 per cubic millimeter, and 80 per cent of the cells are small lymphocytes. However, the leukocyte count either may be normal or may reach a level greater than 100,000 per cubic millimeter. Polymorphonuclear leukocytosis suggests a secondary bacterial complication.

Difficulty in recognizing whooping cough occurs in the catarrhal stage, in abortive or mild cases, and in young infants. Epidemiologic awareness may suggest the possibility, but microbiologic identification of the organisms is required. During the early stages of whooping cough *B. pertussis* can be isolated from approximately 90 per cent of patients. By the third or fourth week of illness the organism can be recovered in only 50 per cent of cases, and in the convalescent stage it is unusual to obtain a positive culture.

Adequate specimens and appropriate media are essential if bacteriologic diagnosis is to be efficient. *Specimens are best obtained by pernasal swab rather than by the cough plate method.* A sterile cotton swab wrapped about a flexible copper wire is passed through the nares, and mucus is obtained from the posterior pharynx. The swab must not be allowed to dry out because *B. pertussis* is readily killed by desiccation. As quickly as possible the specimen is plated onto fresh Bordet-Gengou medium, to which penicillin has been added to prevent overgrowth of adventitious organisms. Incubation is at 35° C, and although the trained observer can recognize the small, bisected pearl colonies of *B. pertussis* within 48 hours, at least 72 hours of growth is usually required. Presumptive identification can be made by agglutination tests with appropriate antisera. It is virtually impossible to distinguish between *Bordetella* species on primary isolation except by serologic means.

A fluorescent antibody staining procedure that can be applied directly to clinical specimens as well as to organisms grown in culture is now in more general use.

Serologic procedures are of little help in the diagnosis of whooping cough because a rise in titer of most antibodies does not occur until at least the third week of illness.

It is difficult to distinguish abortive or mild cases of pertussis from tracheobronchitis caused by other agents except by bacteriologic means. On the other hand, paroxysmal coughing may be associated with pulmonary lesions such as allergic bronchitis, atypical pneumonia, or cystic fibrosis.

TREATMENT. Mild cases of pertussis require only supportive treatment. Specific therapy of severe whooping cough has been disappointing despite the in vitro susceptibility of *B. pertussis* to various antimicrobial agents and the protective effect of passively administered antibody in experimental disease.

Antimicrobials. A number of antimicrobial drugs have significant in vitro activity against *B. pertussis*. Agents that readily eradicate the organisms in human disease may shorten the course of the illness if given in the catarrhal or early paroxysmal stages. In the established paroxysmal stage the organisms can also be readily eliminated by antimicrobials, but the course of the illness is unaltered. Even in the paroxysmal stage the use of drugs is justified in order to render the patient noninfectious.

Erythromycin, oxytetracycline, and several other drugs are effective in eliminating organisms. Erythromycin is the drug of choice. The daily dose is 50 mg per kilogram of body weight given in four divided doses. The organism is eliminated after a few days of therapy, but because bacteriologic relapse may occur, treatment should be continued for 10 to 14 days.

Immunotherapy. Hyperimmune human gamma globulin is used in therapy of unimmunized patients, particularly small infants, but its effect is controversial. The usual dose is 1.25 or 2.5 ml intramuscularly for three successive days.

Supportive Therapy. Particularly in the young infant, supportive measures combined with careful nursing care are of paramount importance. Specific attention must be devoted to the maintenance of proper water and electrolyte balance, adequate nutrition, and sufficient oxygenation. Constant alertness for the presence of secondary infectious complications such as pneumonia is required, and appropriate therapy should be promptly instituted upon discovery.

PREVENTION. The great communicability of whooping cough, particularly during the first few weeks of illness, makes it desirable to isolate the patient for four to six weeks, or, ideally, until cultures are negative. Unfortunately, the diagnosis is usually not made until the end of the catarrhal stage, and by then spread of the disease has already occurred. Exposed susceptibles should receive erythromycin prophylaxis, and contacts under four years of age who have been previously immunized should receive a booster dose of vaccine in addition to erythromycin. Booster doses of vaccine have been used to protect adults, such as hospital staff, but side effects tend to be frequent, and erythromycin chemoprophylaxis may be preferable.

Active Immunization. The fall in incidence of whooping cough in the very young is directly related to widespread immunization with suitable, killed suspensions of *B. pertussis*. The highest risk of serious morbidity and mortality is in the young infant. Women of childbearing age generally do not have significant levels

of protective antibody in their sera, and consequently the newborn are not protected by maternal antibodies. Therefore active immunization is begun as early as is commensurate with the production of a satisfactory immune response. At present, it is recommended that the infant receive three injections of pertussis vaccine at one-month intervals beginning at 6 to 12 weeks of age. Each injection provides four NIH* units. The NIH unit-age is based upon the ability of a vaccine to protect mice against a standard intracerebral infection. The pertussis suspension is usually incorporated into a triple vaccine with alum-precipitated diphtheria and tetanus toxoids (DPT). Booster injections are given one and five years after completion of the initial course. Administration of pertussis vaccine to those over six years of age is not generally recommended because of an apparent increased incidence of untoward reactions. However, low doses have been administered to adults without incident. There is no protection against parapertussis.

As previously noted, immunization does not confer lifelong protection. Approximately 80 per cent of those vaccinated within four years of exposure will be protected, whereas 80 to 90 per cent of a matched unimmunized group with similar exposure will contract pertussis. However, as the time after immunization increases, the attack rate in both groups approaches 50 per cent.

Instances of "vaccine failure" have usually been shown to be due to the use of preparations of low potency. However, it has been suggested that a change in the dominant serotype causing disease, unrepresented in certain vaccine preparations, may be of importance. This controversial point is under study.

Local reactions as well as fever may occur after injection of pertussis vaccine. The exact incidence of the more severe complication of encephalopathy is uncertain, but both fatalities and residua have been reported. The occurrence of neurotoxicity appears to be decreasing as more refined immunizing suspensions are used, and certain soluble extracts of *B. pertussis* may prove to be effective without engendering serious side effects. Despite the small, but real, incidence of neurologic complications of pertussis immunization, the risk still seems far less than the hazards of whooping cough in the young child. Nevertheless, in infants with a personal or family history of convulsions or other neurologic disorders, pertussis immunization should be deferred, or very small doses should be cautiously administered. Care should also be exercised in the immunization of children with a family history of an allergic diathesis.

Linneman, C. C., Jr., Ramundo, N., Perlstein, P. H., Minton, S. D., Englender, G. S., McCormick, J. B., and Hayes, P. S.: Use of pertussis vaccine in an epidemic involving hospital staff. Lancet, 2:540, 1975.

Morse, S. I.: Biologically active components and properties of *Bordetella pertussis*. Adv. Appl. Microbiol., 20:9, 1976.

Nelson, K. E., Gavitt, F., Batt, M. D., Kallick, C. A., Reddi, K. T., and Levin, S.: The role of adenoviruses in the pertussis syndrome. J. Pediat. 86:335, 1975.

Olson, L. C.: Pertussis. Medicine, 54:427, 1975.

Steigman, A. J. (ed.): Report of the Committee on Infectious Diseases. 18th ed. Evanston, Ill., American Academy of Pediatrics, 1977.

*National Institutes of Health.

GRANULOMA INGUINALE

144. GRANULOMA INGUINALE

Walsh McDermott

Granuloma inguinale is an indolent granulomatous and ulcerative disease usually localized to the genitalia or perianal region and caused by a pleomorphic coccobacillus, *Donovania granulomatis*, the so-called "Donovan body." When grown on artificial medium, the presumed organism, *Calymmatobacterium granulomatis*, develops a large capsule that reacts immunologically with klebsiella capsular material. It also resembles *K. pneumoniae* in morphology. The infection appears to be customarily transmitted during coitus or other close body contact, and the degree of communicability appears to be relatively low. The lesion tends to be single, and may rarely appear on surfaces of the body other than the genitalia. Systemic infection, notably with the production of arthritis or osteomyelitis, has been reported. Usually the lesion appears on the genitalia or in the perianal area as a relatively painless nodular infiltration that soon breaks down, leaving a sharply demarcated ulcer with friable granulation tissue at the base. On histologic examination, the lesion appears well vascularized and is the site of considerable cellular infiltration, especially with polymorphonuclear leukocytes and monocytes. In appropriately stained tissue scrapings (Wright-Giemsa), the microbe *C. granulomatis* may be seen situated principally within the monocytes, although smaller numbers of extracellular microorganisms can usually be identified. The lesion spreads by direct extension, it is highly destructive to the skin and subcutaneous tissue, and secondary infection with other microorganisms is common. Rarely, if sufficiently extensive, the process may cause elephantiasis of the genitalia.

There is nothing particularly characteristic about the lesions of granuloma inguinale, and the early lesion is indistinguishable from those produced by *T. pallidum*, *H. ducreyi*, or other processes that involve the genitalia. The diagnosis can be established only by appropriate microbiologic techniques, and these should be employed whenever the physician encounters a genital lesion (or an indolent ulceration elsewhere) that is not clearly caused by some other process. Microscopy of deep scrapings or impression smears from the lesion of granuloma inguinale stained by the Wright-Giemsa method usually reveals the microbe within the monocytes. The ease with which the microorganisms, can be detected varies to some extent with the age of the lesion. In a relatively old lesion, the scrapings should be made from the depth of the lesion, and an extensive search of the smears may be necessary. The microorganisms can also be cultured in medium containing chick embryo yolk by methods originally developed by Anderson and her associates. Antigen prepared from capsular material of *C. granulomatis* has been employed in a complement-fixation reaction and in a cutaneous reaction, but these have not had wide application.

Granuloma inguinale was initially treated successfully with streptomycin and tetracycline, but this is no longer the case. Ampicillin has become the drug of choice. In all but 2 of 31 patients treated by Breschi et al. with ampicillin, the lesions healed completely. The two failures were successfully treated by a second course of ampicillin in one and by a two-week course of lincomycin following a dorsal slit in the other. Ampicillin should be given in individual doses of 500 mg orally every six hours for two weeks. With extensive lesions, the chemotherapy should be extended for one or two weeks more. In uncircumcised men, a dorsal slit may be necessary if the ulceration is beneath a partial phimosis. Lincomycin in the same dosage as recommended above for ampicillin has been used successfully in patients known to have shown allergy to penicillin, and should be employed in such circumstances.

No detailed studies are available concerning the prevention of granuloma inguinale. It seems likely, however, that thorough washing of the genitalia with soap and water immediately after sexual intercourse has a significant influence in reducing the probability of infection.

Anderson, K., Goodpasture, E. W., and DeMonbreun, W. A.: Immunologic relationship of *Donovania granulomatis* to granuloma inguinale. J. Exp. Med., 81:41, 1945.

Breschi, L. C., Goldman, G., and Shapiro, S. R.: Granuloma inguinale in Vietnam: Successful therapy with ampicillin and lincomycin. J. Am. Vener. Dis. Assoc., 1:118, 1975.

Davis, B. D., Dulbecco, R., Eisen, H. N., Ginsberg, H. S., and Wood, W. B., Jr.: Microbiology. New York, Hoeber Medical Division, Harper & Row, 1970, Chap. 36.

DIPHTHERIA

145. DIPHTHERIA

Heonir Rocha

Diphtheria is an acute infectious disease caused by a bacillus, *Corynebacterium diphtheriae*. The infection usually localizes in the pharynx, larynx, and nostrils and occasionally in the skin, and gives rise to both local and systemic signs. The latter are related to the production of a potent soluble exotoxin elaborated by the microorganisms multiplying at the site of infection.

ETIOLOGY. *Corynebacterium diphtheriae* is a gram-positive, nonsporulating, nonmotile pleomorphic bacillus, which grows best aerobically and does not form gas. In stained smears diphtheria bacilli are frequently club shaped in appearance and are arranged in palisade form. The most common media used to isolate the bacilli are Löffler's and potassium tellurite agar. By the appearance on tellurite agar and the ability to ferment starch and glycogen, three distinct types of colonies can be idenfitied: *gravis*, *mitis*, and *intermedius*. All three types can produce the same powerful toxin, which is a heat-labile polypeptide, with a molecular weight of 62,000, produced by bacterial cells infected with a lysogenic bacteriophage. In so-called avirulent diphtheria strains no parasitism with bacteriophages can be demonstrated, and the bacilli fail to produce toxin. Thus acquisition of phage leads to toxigenicity, and the amount of toxin produced depends on genetic and nutritional factors. The ability to produce toxin under laboratory conditions is not entirely related to potential for causing severe disease, because several virulent strains are poor toxin formers. Around 10 per cent of *Corynebacterium diphtheriae* isolated from clinically typical cases were nontoxigenic when tested by the Eleck-plate method or by guinea pig inoculation. It should be mentioned that nontoxigenic *Corynebacterium diphtheriae* can cause symptomatic infection in humans. Diphtheria caused by nontoxigenic strains, however, is mild and behaves as localized disease caused by toxigenic strains.

It is usually said that the *gravis* strain is more frequently associated with epidemic diphtheria; also, that the case fatality rate associated with any epidemic is determined by the proportion of cases infected with the *gravis* or *mitis* types. However, these views are not generally accepted. Although there seems to be a trend toward more severe infection with the *gravis* and *mitis* types, without question the same clinical picture can be produced by all three types.

EPIDEMIOLOGY AND IMMUNITY. Diphtheria has a world-wide distribution, its natural incidence being greatest in temperate climates. The disease occurs predominantly in poor socioeconomic conditions where inadequately immunized hosts and crowding are common. It exhibits a tendency to be most prevalent in autumn and winter but can give rise to epidemics at any time of year.

The human host is the only significant reservoir of *Corynebacterium diphtheriae,* which is transmitted directly or indirectly from one person to another. The usual habitat of *Corynebacterium diphtheriae* is the respiratory tract. The organism can multiply in the mucous membranes of the respiratory tract (pharynx or nares) of immunized hosts without giving rise to clinical disease. The transmission of diphtheria is mainly via droplets, although fomites and dust may have a minor role. Milk has been shown to be a vehicle of infection in rare instances. Duration and closeness of contact are the important factors in transmission. In some tropical areas the skin has been implicated as a major reservoir of *Corynebacterium diphtheriae* infection.

Immunity against the disease depends basically upon the existence of antitoxin in the blood of the host, which is formed in response to direct stimulation of diphtheria toxin either by artificial immunization or by clinical or subclinical infection. Infants under the age of six months are normally protected by passive immunity received through the placenta from immune mothers. Adults are usually protected by artificial immunization or subclinical infection. It has been suggested that undiagnosed cutaneous diphtheria may be the main way whereby natural immunization is acquired in tropical countries.

A relatively simple method to gain valuable information concerning a patient's immune status is to observe the local reaction after the intradermal injection of 0.1 ml of diluted, highly purified diphtheria toxin (Schick test). A positive reaction is interpreted to mean that the patient is susceptible to the disease; a negative reaction indicates that the levels of antitoxin exceed 0.03 unit per milliliter and that the host is not likely to acquire the clinical disease. It should be mentioned, however, that immunization status does not appear to reduce the likelihood of acquiring disease from nontoxigenic strains and has no discernible effect on the severity of clinical illness associated with those strains.

The maximal age incidence of diphtheria lies in the period of two to six years. The disease is an unusual occurrence in adults in endemic areas. However, recently in the United States, approximately 25 per cent of the cases occurred in persons 15 years of age or older.

PATHOGENESIS. The most serious consequences of *Corynebacterium diphtheriae* infection are the result of production and absorption of an extremely active and damaging exotoxin. The organisms multiply on epithelial cells at the infected site (usually pharynx), secreting the specific toxin which produces local signs and is absorbed, resulting in a systemic illness. The initial cytotoxic effect of the toxin is in tissues immediately adjacent to the bacterial growth, resulting in necrotic changes. As a consequence, an exudate which tends to coalesce is formed during the initial 24 to 48 hours. This fibrinous exudate contains leukocytes, necrotic epithelial cells, red blood cells, and the growing diphtheria bacillus. The exudate forms a tough membrane (so-called pseudomembrane) which is firmly attached, with a white shiny center and a gray or brownish periphery. If this membrane is forcibly removed, bleeding occurs. Occasionally it extends throughout the tracheobronchial tree, forming a cast. In the trachea and larynx, probably because of mucus production, this membrane tends to be adherent. Edema of soft tissues subjacent to the membrane may be intense. These local lesions when present in the larynx can result in encroachment of the airway with varying degrees of respiratory obstruction. Tracheal and bronchial obstruction can also result from detachment of the pseudomembrane.

From the local site of production the soluble toxin is disseminated by the blood and lymphatics and can produce degenerative changes in the heart, nervous system, and kidneys. The diphtheria toxin is regularly lethal to the affected cells. It becomes absorbed to the cell membrane, penetrates into the cell, and alters the protein synthesis by interfering with the transfer of amino acids from RNA to the growing polypeptide chain. By breaking disulfide bonds, the molecule can be split into two fragments; fragment B has no independent activity, but is required for the transport of fragment A into cells. Fragment A inactivates the EF-2 (elongation factor), which is required for translocation of polypeptidyl–transfer RNA from the acceptor to the donor site on the eukaryotic ribosome. This results in abrupt arrest of protein synthesis, presumably bringing about degeneration and death of the cell. Specific antitoxin may neutralize even adsorbed toxin, but does not prevent the chain of events once the toxin penetrates the cell.

Diphtheria infection may be localized infrequently in wounds, buccal mucosa, vagina, and conjunctiva. These extrarespiratory locations usually give rise to milder disease with much less systemic illness.

CLINICAL MANIFESTATIONS.   The incubation period of diphtheria varies from one to seven days, but is most commonly two to four days. The clinical picture depends upon the anatomic location of the lesions and the severity of the toxic process.

Faucial diphtheria is the most common clinical presentation and includes the most toxic forms. In a typical case the onset is usually sudden, with low-grade fever (37 to 38° C), malaise, and mild sore throat. The pharynx is only moderately injected, and a thick tonsillar whitish exudate is frequently seen. This exudate usually spreads from one tonsil to the other and may invade the pillars, uvula, soft palate, and pharyngeal wall. Moderate tonsillar as well as cervical lymph node enlargement is usually present.

In some cases the membrane or exudate is limited to the tonsils *(tonsillar diphtheria)*, and toxic manifestations are inconspicuous. In other cases, there is spread of the original process to the uvula, posterior pharyngeal wall, and posterior nasal mucosa *(nasopharyngeal diphtheria)*, sometimes with massive cervical lymphadenopathy (bullneck appearance) and signs of toxemia. In this clinical form the child is pale, lethargic, prostrated, restless at times, and extremely weak. The pulse is rapid and thin; heart beats become muffled; respiration is labored and frequently noisy. This state of toxemia may result in death within a few days if the condition remains untreated. Finally, in some patients the infection spreads downward to the larynx, producing a clinical picture of progressive laryngeal obstruction *(laryngeal diphtheria)*. When the larynx is involved, the first symptoms are hoarseness, dyspnea, a brassy cough, and an increasing expiratory and inspiratory stridor. In a few instances laryngeal involvement may be the first sign of infection. As the obstruction progresses, dyspnea becomes more severe, bronchial secretions accumulate, the accessory muscles of respiration come into full play, and there are supra- and infrasternal retraction at each stridulous breath. If obstruction is not relieved, the patient becomes extremely restless, anxious, and cyanotic, and the condition then merges into severe exhaustion and a comatose stage.

In some cases the infection is basically localized in the anterior nasal area *(anterior nasal diphtheria)*. Clinically it is manifested by bilateral or unilateral serous or serosanguineous discharge which erodes the skin around the nostrils and the upper lips, occasionally resulting in small crusted lesions. Small rounded ulcers, some of them covered with a whitish exudate, are usually seen in the anterior part of the nasal septum. Constitutional symptoms are lacking, and this process is chiefly important because of its epidemiologic implications. It is frequently undiagnosed in an endemic area, and may be an important source of spreading the disease.

Other parts of the body may be the site of primary or secondary diphtheric lesions, the most commonly described being the skin. *Cutaneous diphtheria* takes the form of chronic nonhealing ulcers, sometimes covered with a grayish membranous exudate. It seems probable that these ulcers, mainly described in the tropics, have a complex etiology. Treatment with antitoxin alone usually gives disappointing results. Involvement of the conjunctiva, vagina, or ear by *Corynebacterium diphtheriae* has been rarely reported. These uncommon localizations are practically always secondary to faucial infection.

DIAGNOSIS. In most instances of diphtheric oropharyngeal infection, a presumptive diagnosis must be made on clinical grounds, without awaiting laboratory confirmation, because therapy should be started at once.

The clinical manifestations which should arouse suspicion of *nasopharyngeal diphtheria* are (1) insidious onset of a painless pharyngitis associated with an exudate (usually localized or predominantly in one tonsillar area); (2) association of a faucial exudate with insidious and progressive signs of laryngeal obstruction or with a serous or serosanguineous nasal discharge; and (3) the presence of faucial exudate with marked cervical adenopathy and signs of toxicity (prostration, tachycardia, marked pallor).

For laboratory diagnosis, a swab from the suspected site (usually a pharyngeal and a nasal swab are taken) should be promptly inoculated on a Löffler slant, a tellurite plate, and a blood agar plate. Identification of the etiologic agent can be made after overnight incubation on the basis of colony formation, cellular morphology, and sometimes fermentation reactions. Immunofluorescence techniques have been tried for the rapid diagnosis of diphtheria. For reliable results the specimen has to be incubated four hours before applying the fluorescent antibody technique. Slides prepared directly from throat swabs are unsatisfactory. The fluorescent antibody technique is not of value for the identification of toxigenic strains. Tests to detect the toxigenicity of diphtheria-like organisms cultured (guinea pig skin reaction, in vitro test on agar plate or Elek-plate method, and tissue culture test) are usually performed days after therapy has been started, because they require the isolation of *Corynebacterium diphtheriae*; two to three days thereafter are necessary for correct reading.

Several conditions may be confused with diphtheria, especially during an epidemic bout. This is the case, for instance, with streptococcal pharyngitis. In this condition there is usually high fever (39 to 40° C) with frequent chills, the throat is fiery red, the exudate is thin and easily removable, and swallowing is painful. Other pharyngeal infections which may be accompanied by an exudate are adenoviral exudative pharyngitis, infectious mononucleosis, Vincent's angina, and angina of agranulocytosis. Rhinitis associated with diphtheria must be differentiated from rhinitis of simple colds and from foreign bodies in the nostrils. The distressful laryngeal manifestations of diphtheria should be differentiated from acute obstructive laryngitis, either infectious (viral, *Hemophilus*) or allergic.

COMPLICATIONS. The most important complications of diphtheria are related to the cardiovascular and nervous systems. They are most frequently associated with the severe forms of the disease.

Although electrocardiographic changes have been described in a high percentage (25 per cent) of cases of diphtheria, clinically manifest myocarditis is less common. The onset of myocarditis is often insidious, appearing in the second or third week of the infection. Characteristically, the patient exhibits a weak rising pulse with distant heart sounds and a profound weakness and lethargy. When heart failure ensues, the patient becomes dyspneic, with marked pallor and epigastric pain, and he develops cardiac enlargement and an apical diastolic gallop. The most common electrocardiographic changes are T wave flattening or inversion, bundle branch block or intraventricular block, and several types of disorders of rhythm (premature contractions and atrial fibrillation).

Diphtheria myocarditis, particularly when associated with heart block, carries an extremely poor prognosis. Despite vigorous treatment, including steroids and digitalis, the mortality rate is very high. Glucagon has also been tried but is ineffective.

Nervous system involvement is manifested by cranial nerve or peripheral nerve paralysis. The most common form of cranial nerve palsy is paralysis of the soft palate, which is suspected by the development of nasal regurgitation of fluid upon attempted swallowing. Nasal speech may be present but is frequently slight. This condition is mild, and recovery usually occurs within two weeks. Ciliary paresis and oculomotor paralysis (affecting both sides) make up the next most common form. Rarely, facial, pharyngeal, or laryngeal paralysis is observed.

Peripheral neuritis, usually affecting the limbs, may appear from about the fourth to the eighth week. It varies greatly in extent but is frequently manifested by weakness in the dorsiflexors of the feet, accompanied by decreased or absent tendon reflexes in the lower extremities. Less commonly, the upper limbs, the neck, and the trunk may be involved. The prognosis is good. Diphtheric polyneuritis has been described after cutaneous diphtheria.

It must be emphasized that recovery from the complications of diphtheria is nearly always complete insofar as can be determined by clinical examination. It has been suggested that a lowering of cardiac reserve can persist in some cases, but this assumption needs further documentation.

TREATMENT. The most important act in the treatment of diphtheria is to administer antitoxin as soon as the diphtheria is suspected on clinical grounds without awaiting laboratory confirmation. Admittedly this practice will result in the unnecessary use of antitoxin in some cases. But this is of little consequence in view of the considerable improvement in prognosis in severe forms of the disease when antitoxin is administered early and in adequate amounts.

Opinions vary as to what constitutes an efficient dose. It is usually accepted that in mild or moderate cases a dose of 30,000 to 50,000 units, injected intramuscularly, is enough. In severe cases, 60,000 to 100,000 units is the recommended dose, half of it being given by slow intravenous infusion in critically ill patients. As the antitoxin is a horse protein, precautions should be observed to avoid severe hypersensitivity reactions (anaphylaxis). It is mandatory to inquire if allergy to horse serum is known, and to perform a conjunctival or intracutaneous skin test with a 1:10 saline dilution of the antitoxin. If a positive reaction is obtained by either method, desensitization with increasing doses of antiserum is recommended. Epinephrine must be at hand before antitoxin is administered by any route.

As the *Corynebacterium diphtheriae* is susceptible to several antimicrobials, these drugs have been used routinely, in addition to antitoxin, in cases of diphtheria. Penicillin G is still the drug of choice, and is usually given as procaine penicillin, 400,000 units intramuscularly every 12 hours, for a period of 8 to 12 days. Erythromycin, also very active against the diphtheria

bacillus, is an alternative drug and is recommended in a dosage of 30 to 40 mg per kilogram of body weight for a similar period. In suspected cases, these drugs must not be administered without the antitoxin, because they may mask the infection and thus may make it impossible to establish a laboratory diagnosis.

Bed rest is essential in all patients during the acute phase of the disease; this can vary in completeness and duration, depending on the degree of toxicity and the presence of cardiac involvement. In any event, the patient's return to activity should be carefully guided by the physician. Complications such as dehydration, shock, and congestive heart failure should be promptly diagnosed and properly treated.

In cases exhibiting marked toxicity and in patients with severe laryngeal involvement and/or shock, corticosteroids (prednisone, 3 to 5 mg per kilogram of body weight per day) have been advocated along with the antitoxin and antimicrobial. Cases of laryngeal obstruction may require emergency tracheostomy and careful postoperative aspiration to avoid complications. Such patients need special nursing for safety.

Patients with diphtheria should be isolated, preferably in hospital. Before their discharge from isolation, cultures from throat and nose (or local lesion) should be taken, and at least two consecutive negative cultures should be obtained.

PREVENTION. Diphtheria may be effectively prevented by *active immunization.* The primary course of immunization should be administered within the first year of life, preferably between the third and sixth months. Of the preparations available, *fluid toxoid* and *alum-precipitated toxoid* are the most commonly used. The primary course of fluid toxoid consists of three intramuscular injections (0.5 ml, 1.0 ml, and 1.0 ml) at weekly intervals (one to three weeks). For immunization with the alum-precipitated toxoid, two 1-ml intramuscular injections administered at intervals of one to two months are enough. Despite its greater antigenic potency, the alum-precipitated toxoid also has a greater sensitizing ability, and may induce sterile local abscesses at the injection site owing to the irritating effect of the alum upon tissues. Both fluid and alum-precipitated toxoid are excellent immunizing agents, conferring immunity to at least 90 per cent of those receiving a primary course. After this immunization in infancy, one stimulating dose should be given one or two years later, and another given at the time the child enters school.

Diphtheria toxoid has been combined with immunizations against tetanus and pertussis and should be given within the first year of life. All children under six years of age who are not immunized are susceptible to diphtheria and should be actively immunized without preliminary Schick testing. In older children and adults, before immunization with toxoid, a sensitivity test should be done. The development of a local reaction within 48 hours of the intracutaneous injection of 0.1 ml of 1:10 dilution of toxoid in normal saline *(Moloney test)* is a warning that toxoid should be administered cautiously in multiple small diluted doses.

Passive immunization against diphtheria may be rapidly conferred by subcutaneous inoculation of 1500 units of diphtheria antitoxin. This procedure should be limited to persons peculiarly at risk of infection, such as nonimmunized children heavily exposed to an infected case. The protection is limited to a period of two to three weeks, and active immunization with a toxoid preparation should be started at the same time. Human diphtheria antitoxin is not yet available.

Treatment of Diphtheria Carriers. Whenever diphtheria is common, carrier rates are high. In approximately 15 to 20 per cent of cases, the cultures will remain positive for as long as one month after the disease, but they will subsequently become negative in most instances. Erythromycin in a dosage of 30 to 40 mg per kilogram of body weight has been found effective for treatment of carriers. Benzathine penicillin could be used (600,000 units for children of ages one to five years, and 1,200,000 units for older patients) only when patients cannot be relied upon to complete a seven-day course of oral therapy. Tonsillectomy and adenoidectomy have also been advocated to eliminate the carrier state.

Barksdale, L., Garmiese, L., and Horibata, K.: Virulence, toxigeny, and lysogeny in *Corynebacterium diphtheriae*. Ann. N.Y. Acad. Sci., 88:1093, 1960.

Bray, J. P., Burt, E. G., Potter, E. V., Poon-King, T., and Earle, D.: Epidemic diphtheria and skin infections in Trinidad. J. Infect. Dis., 126:34, 1972.

Collier, R. J.: Diphtheria toxin: Mode of action and structure. Bact. Rev., 39:54, 1975.

McCloskey, R. V., Eller, J. J., Green, M., Mauney, C. V., and Richards, S. E. M.: The 1970 epidemic of diphtheria in San Antonio. Ann. intern. Med., 75:495, 1971.

McCracken, A. W., and Mauney, C. V.: Identification of *Corynebacterium diphtheriae* by immunofluorescence during a diphtheria epidemic. J. Clin. Pathol., 24:641, 1971.

Naiditch, M. J., and Bower, A. A.: Diphtheria: Study of 1433 cases observed during 10-year period at Los Angeles County Hospital. Am. J. Med., 17:229, 1954.

Scheid, W.: Diphtherial paralysis. An analysis of 2292 cases of diphtheria in adults, which included 174 cases of polyneuritis. J. Nerv. Ment. Dis., 116:1095, 1952.

CLOSTRIDIAL DISEASES

146. INTRODUCTION

Emanuel Wolinsky

The clostridia are spore-forming anaerobic gram-positive bacilli that for the most part lead a saprophytic existence in nature. They may be found in large numbers in the intestinal tracts of humans and animals, and in the soil. They are capable of producing disease by virtue of their elaboration of powerful exotoxins, but special conditions must be present in the tissues to allow the organisms to germinate, proliferate, and elaborate toxins. The mere presence of clostridia in the wound or on the surface of the body is not significant. Most clostridial disease is caused by *C. perfringens*, although occasionally *C. novyi (oedematiens), septicum, sordellii (bifermentans), histolyticum,* and *fallax* may be human pathogens.

The pathologic states attributable to clostridial infection cover a wide range of severity and localization, from the relatively benign wound infection to the highly fatal gas gangrene; from transient bacteremia to life-threatening septicemia; from relatively mild food poisoning to necrotic enteritis; and from pleural empyema to purulent meningitis. The neurotoxic disease caused by *C. tetani* is discussed below, and that caused by *C. botulinum* is discussed in Ch. 22.3.

BACTERIOLOGY

All the clostridia owe their pathogenicity to the elaboration of exotoxins that have enzymatic activity. Four major toxins and eight minor ones have been described and given Greek letters. The most important of them is the alpha toxin, which is a lecithinase capable of splitting lecithin in the red cell envelope and causing severe hemolysis. Many of the species of clostridia have been separated into types according to their ability to elaborate specific exotoxins. *C. perfringens* may be divided into five or six toxigenic types; Type A elaborates more alpha toxin than any other type or species and is by far the most important variety of *Clostridium* in human disease, particularly gas gangrene.

147. CLOSTRIDIAL MYONECROSIS

(Gas Gangrene)

Emanuel Wolinsky

The clostridial gas gangrene is best called *clostridial myonecrosis* because the outstanding feature is rapidly progressive muscle necrosis with relatively little inflammatory reaction, and because other organisms can produce skin and subcutaneous gangrene, and myositis, with gas formation. The disease most often arises from traumatic or surgical wounds in which anoxic conditions prevail as a result of ischemia or crushed muscle. Battle wounds of World Wars I and II supplied plentiful case material for study; gas gangrene occurred in approximately 10 per cent of World War I wounds and in 1 per cent of those that occurred in World War II. In civilian practice the rate of gas gangrene among 188,000 major open wounds has been estimated to be 1.8 per cent. The rate of contamination or local infection of open wounds, on the other hand, amounts to 30 to 80 per cent. The soil is the usual source of the clostridia in exogenous infection, the intestine or biliary tract in autogenous infection.

PATHOGENESIS. The factors that predispose to the invasion of muscle by the bacilli with the subsequent elaboration of exotoxins are related to lack of oxygen and lowering of the oxidation-reduction potential of the tissues. These factors are (1) impaired local vascular supply owing to vessel trauma or pressure from foreign bodies, casts, or tourniquets; (2) presence of metallic bodies, clothing, or dirt in the wound; (3) presence of necrotic tissue or hemorrhage; and (4) growth of aerobic microorganisms in the wound.

Under these circumstances the bacilli can multiply anaerobically and elaborate toxins, which diffuse out and damage surrounding muscle, which in turn becomes colonized with the bacilli. Thus the disease spreads rapidly to surrounding muscles and gains momentum. The severe generalized toxemia remains poorly explained. Alpha toxin is not found in the blood, and it is postulated that a toxic factor that acts on certain vital centers or enzymes is produced by the interaction of clostridial toxin with necrotic muscle.

CLINICAL MANIFESTATIONS. The clinical picture of gas gangrene is dominated by rapidly progressive toxemia and shock. After a relatively short incubation period of one to four days the patient suddenly exhibits restlessness and anxiety; the temperature and pulse rate begin to rise and the blood pressure to fall. He is noted to be pale and sweating. The wound becomes painful and markedly swollen. Some hours later, after progression of the signs and symptoms, a thin brownish exudate begins to ooze from the wound, and a small amount of crepitus may be noted in the surrounding tissues. A bronze discoloration starts at the edge of the wound and progresses outward. Blebs filled with purplish fluid may appear. An odor characterized as "mousy" or "sickly sweet" is described by many observers. By this time the patient may be anuric and in irreversible vascular collapse. When the muscle is exposed by incision, it appears to be "cooked" or dead — it does not bleed when cut or retract when pinched. Smears from *involved muscle* show many large gram-positive rods and no other organisms, but very few pus cells. Smears and cultures from the *wound exudate* at the surface may reveal other organisms in addition to the clostridia, especially in grossly contaminated wounds. Roentgenograms reveal the presence of gas in and around muscle bundles in the form of fernlike, lacy patterns. Untreated, fully developed clostridial myonecrosis is almost always fatal.

Myonecrosis must be differentiated from clostridial and nonclostridial *crepitant cellulitis*, from *anaerobic streptococcal myonecrosis*, and from *physical* and *chemical* causes of gas in the tissues. *Clostridial cellulitis* (anaerobic cellulitis, local gas gangrene, epifascial gas gangrene, or gas-forming fasciitis) is a gas-forming infection of connective tissue mainly localized to subcutaneous areas with spread in fascial planes, but healthy muscle is not involved. It arises as a result of clostridial infection of tissue already necrotic from ischemia or trauma. The onset is gradual, and toxemia, pain, and swelling are less than in gas gangrene. A large amount of gas is distributed in the form of large bubbles along the fascial planes, but not in the muscle. Incision will show that the muscle is viable, and smears from muscle tissue away from the open wound will not reveal organisms.

Nonclostridial crepitant cellulitis is similar to clostridial cellulitis, except that the infection is associated with other organisms, usually in a mixed flora consisting of two or more of the following: aerogenic coliforms (*E. coli*, *Klebsiella*, *Enterobacter*), anaerobic streptococci, *Bacteroides*, and gamma streptococci. In many cases this mixed bacterial flora in gas-forming cellulitis includes clostridia; these cases do not appear to differ in prognosis from those in which clostridia are absent. It is not clear how often cellulitis progresses to myonecrosis, but varying degrees of muscle gangrene may be seen in patients who present with classic anaerobic cellulitis, especially of the nonclostridial variety. Thus a sharp distinction between cellulitis and myonecrosis is not always possible, although one or the other condition usually predominates.

Anaerobic streptococcal myonecrosis was described by MacLennan in infected war wounds from the Middle East in 1948, but there have been few reports since then. Other organisms, especially group A streptococci and *Staph. aureus*, were always found with the primary agent, and 3 of 19 patients had anaerobic streptococcal bacteremia.

Simple contamination of wounds with clostridia is not uncommon. The organisms, usually in association with a mixed flora, exist as saprophytes on necrotic tissue and debris and do not invade further. Clostridia may also be found in localized collections of purulent material in wounds, or in foul-smelling brownish fluid known as a "gas abscess" or a "Welch abscess." Drainage will usually suffice to bring these conditions under control.

DIAGNOSIS. The diagnosis of gas gangrene is essentially a clinical one. Upon first suspicion of the disease, dressings and casts must be removed and the wound or suspected area thoroughly inspected. Roentgenograms may help to show the fine bubbles of gas distributed in and around muscle bundles. Incision should be made into the muscle so that the characteristic appearance may be appreciated. At the same time a specimen of muscle may be examined by Gram stain of imprint slides and by anaerobic cultural techniques. Smears and cultures from the exudate around the wound surface may be misleading. Tables 1 and 2 summarize the most important findings for the differential diagnosis.

TREATMENT. Treatment must be prompt and vigorous. Most important is thorough *debridement* and *excision* of all devitalized tissue and dead muscle. Hopelessly involved extremities usually need to be amputated except perhaps under the influence of hyperbaric oxygen. It is said that if any infected muscle is left behind, it will prevent cure. General *supportive measures* should include intravenous fluids and blood, other measures to combat vascular collapse and shock, and peritoneal dialysis when necessary. *Antimicrobial* treatment is given to prevent bloodstream invasion and to suppress further spread of infection. Penicillin is the drug of choice given in large doses of 10 to 20 million units per day intravenously. A cephalosporin or clindamycin may be substituted in patients allergic to penicillin. Approximately 20 per cent of *C. perfringens* strains are resistant to tetracycline, and erythromycin is not suitable because of poor activity at low redox potential and in acidic environment. *Antitoxin* is recommended, especially during the first few hours of the disease, in the hope of neutralizing any free toxin in

TABLE 1. Classification of Histotoxic Clostridial Disease

Traumatic
  A. Wound infection (war and civilian)
    1. Simple contamination
    2. Localized (purulent or "gas abscess")
    3. Gas-forming cellulitis
    4. Myonecrosis
  B. Uterine infection (postabortion and postpartum)
  C. Burns, panophthalmitis, brain abscess, etc.

Nontraumatic
  A. Postoperative (abdominal, amputation)
  B. Postinjection
  C. Spontaneous
    1. Localized (pneumonia, empyema, cholecystitis, myonecrosis)
    2. Septicemic (malignant disease, intestinal lesion)
  D. Bacteremia without hemolysis or sepsis (from decubitus ulcer, gangrenous extremity, uterus)

TABLE 2. Gas-Forming Soft Tissue Infections

	Clostridial Myonecrosis	"Anaerobic" Cellulitis	Streptococcal Myonecrosis
Onset	Sudden	Gradual	Gradual
Toxemia	Extreme	Slight	Slight
Pain	May be severe	Slight	Gradually increasing
Swelling	Marked	Slight	Marked
Skin color	Bronze	No change	Erythematous
Exudate	Thin, brown	Thin, bloody; later purulent	Profuse, thin seropurulent
Gas	Little, in muscle	Profuse, large bubbles in fascial planes	Little, in muscle
Muscle	Dead, "cooked," healthy muscle invaded	Not involved	Initially edematous, then hemorrhagic
Bacteriology	Mixed flora from exudate or open wound; from muscle aspirate pure gram-positive rods	May be pure clostridia or mixed flora from exudate or subcutaneous tissue; no organisms in muscle aspirate	Anaerobic streptococci, along with Group A *Streptococcus*, *Staph. aureus*, etc., from exudate and muscle
Prognosis	Serious	Good	Good
Treatment	Radical surgery, penicillin, antitoxin, hyperbaric oxygen	Surgical drainage and debridement, appropriate antimicrobials	Surgical drainage and debridement, penicillin

the body fluids, although its usefulness is doubtful because the exotoxins are very rapidly bound to cells. The recommended dose is 40 thousand units of trivalent or pentavalent antitoxin intravenously at once and 20 to 40 thousand units repeated at four- to six-hour intervals. The usual precautions for horse serum must be observed. *Hyperbaric oxygen* at 3 atmospheres has been recommended by some as a dramatically successful mode of therapy that should take precedence over immediate surgical treatment and antitoxin. It is said that debridement may be deferred until systemic toxicity has been relieved and demarcation between necrotic and viable tissue is clear. In this way loss of tissue may be minimized and amputation sometimes avoided. If a suitable chamber is not available locally, it is probably unwise to delay surgical extirpation in favor of a long journey (see Ch. 31).

Treatment of "anaerobic" cellulitis and streptococcal myonecrosis need not be so radical. Usually wide excision and debridement along with supportive measures and appropriate antimicrobials will suffice. A Gram-stained smear of wound exudate and muscle aspirate will help one to decide whether penicillin alone should be given (for pure *Clostridium* or *Streptococcus*) or whether antistaphylococcal, antibacteroides, or anticoliform agents should be added or substituted. Reasonable drug regimens for mixed anaerobic cellulitis are gentamicin plus clindamycin, or chloramphenicol alone. A penicillinase-resistant penicillin or cephalosporin should be included if staphylococci are recognized.

PREVENTION. The prophylactic use of antitoxin and antimicrobials at the time of injury does not prevent gas gangrene. Careful attention to good surgical technique is most important. All devitalized tissue must be excised and vascular supply left intact. Care must be taken with tourniquets and casts to prevent undue ischemia. Plaster of Paris itself may be contaminated with clostridia.

UTERINE INFECTION

Postabortion and postpartum clostridial infections of the uterus are still important causes of serious disease in obstetrics. At least 5 per cent of women harbor clostridia in the vagina as simple contaminants. Fulminant infection usually follows criminal abortion or prolonged and difficult labor, and presents a clinical picture similar to that seen in traumatic gas gangrene. Unlike wound gas gangrene, however, uterine infection is frequently accompanied by clostridial sepsis leading to jaundice, hemolysis, hemoglobinemia, hemoglobinuria, and renal shutdown. As in wound infection, there may be various grades of clostridial involvement, from simple contamination to secondary invasion of necrotic matter in the uterus or a dead fetus to true invasion of intact uterine muscle producing myonecrosis or "physometra." Clostridial infection must be differentiated from the more slowly progressive uterine infection produced by anaerobic streptococci and *Bacteroides* which commonly leads to pelvic thrombophlebitis and septic pulmonary infarcts.

Treatment is essentially the same as that outlined above, except that a decision must be made quickly on whether to do a hysterectomy or merely to empty the uterus. Evidence of uterine perforation or necrosis will call for the more radical procedure. Antimicrobial therapy should probably include clindamycin or chloramphenicol in addition to penicillin to control *Bacteroides*.

POSTOPERATIVE GAS GANGRENE

Nontraumatic gas gangrene that follows surgical operations is probably the most common variety of the disease in civilian hospitals today. Of 42 cases of *C. perfringens* infection reported from a single hospital, 18 followed operations and 10 were secondary to trauma (Pyrtek and Bartus, 1962). Most of these infections involve the abdominal wall after biliary or intestinal surgery, or the leg or hip after amputation or correction of hip fractures, although the complication has been described after many other kinds of surgical procedures. Recent investigation in England indicated that most of these infections were sporadic and autogenous in origin, probably as a result of fecal contamination of the skin. Parker called attention to the importance of adequate preoperative sterilization of the skin with sporicidal agents and the advisability of giving prophylactic penicillin from a few hours before operation to one week after to those patients at greatest risk from postoperative clostridial infections — elderly patients who will have hip surgery or thigh amputations.

Altemeier, W. A., and Culbertson, W. R.: Acute non-clostridial crepitant cellulitis. Surg. Gynecol. Obstet., 87:206, 1948.

Ayliffe, G. A. J., and Lowbury, E. J. L.: Sources of gas gangrene in hospital. Br. Med. J., 2:333, 1969.

Darke, S. G., King, A. M., and Slack, W. K.: Gas gangrene and related infection: Classification, clinical features and aetiology, management and mortality. A report of 88 cases. Br. J. Surg., 64:104, 1977.

Holland, J. A., Hill G. B., Wolfe, W. G., Osterhout, S., Saltzman, H. A., and Brown, I. W.: Experimental and clinical experience with hyperbaric oxygen in the treatment of clostridial myonecrosis. Surgery, 77:75, 1975.

MacLennan, J. D.: The histotoxic clostridial infections of man. Bact. Rev., 26:177, 1962.

Parker, M. T.: Postoperative clostridial infections in Britain. Br. Med. J., 3:671, 1969.

Roding, B., Groenveld, P. H., and Boerema, I.: Ten years' experience in the treatment of gas gangrene in hyperbaric oxygen. Surg. Gynecol. Obstet., 134:579, 1972.

Schwartzman, J. D., Reller, L. B., and Wang, W. L.: Susceptibility of Clostridium perfringens isolated from human infections to twenty antibiotics. Antimicrob. Agents Chemother., 11:695, 1977.

VanBeek, A., Zook, E., Yaw, P., Gardner, R., Smith, R., and Glover, J. L.: Nonclostridial gas-forming infections. A collective review and report of seven cases. Arch. Surg., 108:552, 1974.

Weinstein, L., and Barza, M. A.: Gas gangrene. N. Engl. J. Med., 289:1129, 1973.

148. OTHER CLOSTRIDIAL DISEASES

Emanuel Wolinksy

SEPTICEMIA

Clostridial septicemia occurs rarely from traumatic wound gangrene, occasionally from postoperative gas gangrene, and commonly from uterine infection. In addition, nontraumatic or spontaneous clostridial septicemia has been described from such conditions as acute cholecystitis, perforated peptic ulcer, ulcerating carcinoma of the colon, acute pancreatitis, diverticulitis, appendiceal abscess, decubitus ulcer, and gangrenous limbs. Septicemia may occur in terminal cancer patients from portals of entry such as ulcerations of the respiratory or alimentary tracts. A study of 21 patients suffering from various malignant diseases who had septicemia caused by *C. septicum* has been reported. As a result of septicemia, infection may localize in the pleura, myocardium, endocardium, and meninges. Benign clostridial bacteremia without hemolysis was observed in a series of 20 patients, all of whom survived (Rathbun, 1968). Neonatal omphalitis and septicemia occur rarely.

MISCELLANEOUS FORMS

Pneumonia and empyema may be associated with clostridial infection, usually as a result of aspiration of contaminated material from the mouth or the stomach, but occasionally by way of the bloodstream. Penetrating injuries may lead to serious clostridial infections of the eye, brain, and meninges. Severe gas gangrene may result from injections into the buttock or thigh, presumably from inadequately sterilized skin. In at least one instance the organism was also isolated from cotton sponges soaked in alcohol.

Alpern, R. J., and Dowell, V. R., Jr.: Nonhistotoxic clostridial bacteremia. Am. J. Clin. Path., 55:717, 1971.

Bogdan, J. C., and Rapkin, R. H.: Clostridia infection in the newborn. Pediatrics, 58:120, 1976.

Cabrera, A., Tsukada, Y., and Pickren, J. W.: Clostridial gas gangrene and septicemia in malignant disease. Cancer, 18:800, 1965.

149. CLOSTRIDIAL GASTROENTERITIS

Emanuel Wolinsky

Clostridial food poisoning has been the second most common variety reported to the Communicable Disease Center, representing 16 per cent of the total outbreaks and 34 per cent of the cases. It is discussed in Ch. 22.2.

A similar disease, called "pig-bel," is endemic in Papua, New Guinea, and has been attributed hypothetically to lack of proteolytic activity resulting from low protein diet and trypsin inhibitors in the dietary staple, sweet potato. Without protease, the beta toxin of Type C organisms may initiate the disease.

Lawrence, G., and Walker, P. D.: Pathogenesis of enteritis necroticans in Papua, New Guinea. Lancet, 1:125, 1976.

150. TETANUS*

John H. Kerr

Tetanus, often called "lockjaw," is a disease of the nervous system characterized by intense activity of motor neurons resulting in severe muscle spasms. It is caused by an exotoxin of *Clostridium tetani*.

HISTORY. Tetanus has caught the imagination of physicians since Hippocrates, and this is probably due in part to the horrifying nature of the clinical picture in the established untreated case. The presence of the causative organism in soil was demonstrated by Nicolaier, who produced tetanus in animals by soil injections. The *Clostridium* was isolated in pure culture in 1899 by Kitasato, and in 1892 Nocard immunized horses by injections of antitoxin horse serum. Passive immunization after wounding saved many lives in World War I, and active immunization with toxoid almost eliminated tetanus in the allied armies in World War II. Curare was first suggested as having an application in the treatment of tetanus in 1811, but as curare in sufficient dosage to abolish the spasm of severe tetanus will certainly paralyze the muscles of ventilation, the large-scale use of curare had to wait almost 150 years until intermittent positive pressure ventilation (IPPV) through a cuffed tracheostomy tube was introduced into the treatment of tetanus in Denmark in 1953 (Bjørnboe et al.).

ETIOLOGY AND PATHOGENESIS. *Clostridium tetani* is a gram-positive actively motile bacillus which in its spore-bearing form has a characteristic "drumstick" appearance. Spores may develop at either end of the bacillus, giving a "dumbbell" appearance. It is a strict anaerobe, and spores will not germinate in the presence of even the smallest amount of oxygen. An oxidation-reduction potential of +0.01 volt or less at pH7 is required if germination is to take place. The *Clostridium* grows well on laboratory media at 37° C, and growth occurs slowly at 22° C. Vegetative bacilli are readily killed by antiseptics and by heat, but spores are highly resistant to antiseptics and, to a certain extent, are resistant to heat. To kill most spores, boiling for one hour is necessary, but the most resistant may require boiling for four hours. Autoclaving for ten minutes at 120° C

---

*This chapter is based on the one contributed to the previous edition by Professor A. Crampton Smith, with whom the author has worked for many years.

may, however, be relied on to sterilize contaminated objects. *Clostridium tetani* is commonly found in soil and in the feces of domestic animals and humans. Presumably by contamination with soil and feces, spores can be recovered from dust and clothing; in suitable surroundings such as dried earth, spores will survive for many years.

Clostridium tetani produces two exotoxins, tetanospasmin and tetanolysin, and of these tetanospasmin is the neurotoxin which produces the typical muscle spasm of tetanus. It is extremely potent, each milligram of crystallized toxin containing 50 to 75 million mouse-lethal doses. This extreme toxicity may be the reason why an attack of tetanus does not confer immunity, as it is postulated that the fatal dose of tetanus toxin is less than the amount required to provoke an immune response. Tetanolysin can cause hemolysis on blood agar plates, but does not seem to play any significant part in the pathologic process caused by the *Clostridium*.

There have been differences of opinion about the site of action of tetanospasmin and about the route by which it spreads, but it now seems firmly established that the toxin acts in the spinal cord and in the brainstem and that it spreads centrally along motor nerve trunks and up the spinal cord. Tetanus will follow the intravenous injection of toxin into animals, but the route by which toxin in the blood enters the nervous system is not clear. Toxin injected intramuscularly apparently spreads not only by passing up motor nerves but also by absorption into the blood, and it has been suggested that vascular spread is the more important route in generalized tetanus.

EPIDEMIOLOGY. The incidence of tetanus is difficult to establish because it is not a notifiable disease in many countries. The total world deaths each year, however, probably exceed 400,000. If the average crude fatality rate is about 45 per cent (and it may be higher), there must be nearly 1 million cases in the world every year. Tetanus is thus still a major public health problem in economically underdeveloped countries. The disease is common in warm climates and in rural areas that are highly cultivated and consequently have a large population of men and animals. Agricultural workers, in whom injuries may easily be contaminated with the *Clostridium*, are particularly at risk. *Clostridium tetani* can also be found in urban areas, but the degree of contamination is not high, and it is likely that the increased standard of living and hygiene which urbanization implies also contributes to a lower incidence of tetanus in cities. It remains a common, and usually lethal, complication of drug addiction. Further evidence of the importance of education and hygiene is the absence of neonatal tetanus in countries where obstetric hygiene is good, compared with the high incidence in countries where dung is sometimes used as a dressing for the umbilical stump.

PREVENTION OF TETANUS. Before Injury. ACTIVE IMMUNIZATION. The United States Public Health Service Advisory Committee has stated that the need for active immunization against tetanus is universal and that such immunization is the only way by which tetanus may be eliminated as an important health problem. There is little doubt that active immunization with adsorbed tetanus toxoid will convey a remarkably high degree of immunity. La Force et al. (1969) calculated that the incidence of tetanus in the under-ten age group in the United States of America was about 3.8 per 100 million. This underscores the excellent results obtained by active immunization of American and British military personnel in World War II.

In the United Kingdom, the recommended course of injections is three doses of adsorbed toxoid in a mixed vaccine, one injection at six months of age, and two others, with six to eight weeks between first and second and six months between second and third. A booster is advised at school entry and another at age 15 to 19. Thereafter, booster doses should be given at ten-year intervals. The American Academy of Pediatrics suggests three injections of toxoid no less than one month apart in infancy, a reinforcing dose about 12 months later, and a fifth or booster injection on entering school. Subsequent routine toxoid boosters should be administered at intervals of approximately ten years. Placental transfer of maternal tetanus antibodies appears to take place so that at least temporary passive immunity can be conferred on the neonate. Active immunization in pregnancy has proved to be an effective method of reducing the incidence of neonatal tetanus.

After Injury. PREVENTION OF CONTAMINATION. Simple measures that prevent contamination can contribute significantly to the prevention of tetanus, and the effect of attention to treatment of the umbilical stump on the incidence of neonatal tetanus is a good example of the effectiveness of simple hygiene. The aim of surgery in prophylaxis is to remove all dead tissue and foreign bodies from a wound. This will not only remove spore-bearing material but will also deny the spores the anaerobic conditions necessary for their growth. Tetanus occurs significantly often in patients in whom no wound is found, so that a precise definition of a "tetanus-prone" wound is difficult, although it is generally agreed that certain features increase the likelihood of tetanus. These features include an interval of more than six to eight hours between injury and treatment, heavy contamination of the wound with soil or manure, the retention of devitalized tissue or foreign bodies within the wound, and deep puncture wounds in which anaerobic conditions may occur.

Active Immunization. The protection against tetanus conferred by a full course of three injections of adsorbed toxoid lasts for at least ten years, and the reactivation provided by a booster dose of toxoid is equally long lived. Since the incidence of local reactions to toxoid is considerable, both United States and United Kingdom authorities recommend that a booster dose of toxoid is required after injury only if the patient is known, or suspected, not to have been actively immunized at all, or if more than ten years has elapsed since immunization or the most recent toxoid booster. If the wounds are of the "tetanus-prone" type described above, it is suggested that a toxoid booster be given if there has been an interval of more than five years since immunization or the most recent booster.

Passive Immunization. The use of passive immunization by means of antitoxin has probably saved many lives. The absence of a controlled trial precludes certainty, but circumstantial evidence is very strong. Experiments in laboratory animals show that antitoxin given soon after inoculation with tetanus will protect against the disease, and Bruce (1920), reviewing 1458 cases of tetanus occurring in World War I, showed that the incidence of tetanus, after prophylactic antitoxin was available in large quantities, fell from 9 per 1000 wounded to 1.4 per 1000 wounded. Other improvements in surgical care could have been contributory, but it seems likely that antitoxin was an important factor in the decrease in incidence.

Although antitoxin produced by the active immunization of horses has been widely employed since 1894, methods for the production of human tetanus antitoxin have been developed recently, and this agent is now widely available. Human tetanus immune globulin has two great advantages over equine antitetanus serum and should be employed whenever available. The first advantage is that the severe and sometimes fatal anaphylactic reactions which were relatively common after injection of horse serum are extremely rare after human antitoxin, so that it is not believed necessary to recommend a small test dose of human tetanus immune globulin before administration of the full dose. Epinephrine should, however, be available whenever either human or equine antitoxin is to be given. The second advantage is that human tetanus immune globulin shows less tendency than equine antitoxin to form the immune complexes which are excreted rapidly. An intramuscular injection of 250 units of human tetanus immune globulin maintains a blood level at or above that recommended for prophylaxis (0.01 unit per milliliter) for a period of four weeks, whereas 1500 units of equine antitoxin is required to produce a comparable but shorter-lived protection.

Tetanus antitoxin need not be given after clean, minor wounds; but if a wound with "tetanus-prone" features is present, a prophylactic dose of 250 units of human tetanus immune globulin should be administered intramuscularly unless the patient has been fully immunized against tetanus. United States recommendations are that two previous toxoid injections provide adequate immunization unless the wound is more than 24 hours old, whereas the United Kingdom recommendations suggest that tetanus antitoxin should be given unless a full course of three toxoid injections or a booster dose of toxoid has been received within ten years. If tetanus antitoxin is to be given, active immunization should be commenced immediately with an injection of adsorbed toxoid into another limb.

Chemoprophylaxis. Antimicrobial drugs can inhibit the multiplication of *Clostridium tetani* and kill the vegetative form of the organism. By killing aerobic organisms coexisting with the *Clostridium*, antimicrobial drugs can prevent multiplication by denying the *Clostridium* the conditions favorable to its growth; they have no effect, however, on tetanus toxin. Although data have been presented showing no increase in the incidence of tetanus after the substitution of chemoprophylaxis for passive immunization with equine antitetanus serum, the less toxic human antitoxin is currently recommended for tetanus prophylaxis if indicated after injury.

If human antitoxin is not available and chemoprophylaxis is to be employed, the drug chosen must be one to which the organism is susceptible and also one to which the patient is not sensitive. *Clostridium tetani* is susceptible to a variety of drugs, including penicillin, tetracycline, and erythromycin, so that it is probably not difficult to make a suitable choice for a particular patient. Smith (1964) has shown that in mice inoculated with tetanus spores, chemoprophylaxis was effective if it was started four hours after inoculation but not if started eight hours after inoculation. The time interval in humans is not established, but it is suggested that in

injuries seen later than six hours after infliction, some other form of prophylaxis should be chosen. Antimicrobial therapy must be continued for a sufficient time to ensure that tetanus spores cannot survive, and this means for at least five days.

PATHOGENESIS. If tetanus is to supervene, the *Clostridium* must be introduced into human tissue, and the disease may follow a trivial or a serious injury. In countries with good medical services, serious wounds receive effective treatment and tetanus is usually avoided. Apparently minor wounds then become a common cause of the disease, and in quite a high proportion of cases no responsible injury can be identified. The site of action and method of spread of the exotoxin have been mentioned, but it is rather surprising that no unequivocal evidence of recognizable pathologic lesions caused by tetanus has yet been forthcoming even after careful postmortem studies.

CLINICAL FEATURES AND CRITERIA OF SEVERITY IN TETANUS. The criteria of severity may be established in two ways: from the history, and from the symptoms and signs.

From the History. The severity of an attack of tetanus is related to the incubation period (the period from injury to the first sign of tetanus) and the onset period, described by Cole (1940) as the period from the first sign to the first generalized spasm. If the former is less than nine days and the latter less than 48 hours, the attack of tetanus may be expected to be severe. The length of the onset period is, in general, the more reliable guide to the expected severity of the attack.

From the Symptoms and Signs. In *the mild case*, tetanus usually presents with rigidity of muscles, and this rigidity may be severe enough to cause pain. The patient with mild tetanus may have "local tetanus," in which rigidity affects only one limb, or the patient may have mild generalized rigidity. Stiffness of the jaw muscles causes trismus, and stiffness of the facial muscles may cause a change of expression. Stiffness of the muscles of the neck and back may cause discomfort or even pain on attempted flexion of the spine.

In *the moderate case*, the patient has more severe generalized rigidity. Trismus is pronounced, the mouth can hardly be opened, and rigidity of the muscles of the face may cause the sneering "risus sardonicus." Opisthotonos may be pronounced, but more typically the stiffness of the antagonist muscles makes the patient lie "at attention" in bed, and the muscles of the back and abdomen are hard to the touch. Patients with moderate tetanus may show mild exacerbations of this generalized rigidity as "reflex spasms." These spasms may arise spontaneously or more commonly as a result of stimuli. The important difference, however, between the patient with mild and the patient with moderate tetanus is the presence or absence of dysphagia. Spasm of the pharyngeal muscles makes swallowing difficult, and the patient coughs or splutters while drinking. This will predispose to the inhalation of pharyngeal contents and is the diagnostic characteristic of the moderate case.

The patient with *a severe case* is distinguished from the patient with a moderate case by the presence of reflex spasms that may be of appalling intensity. If the spasms are untreated, opisthotonos becomes extreme and the intense muscle spasm may fracture vertebrae. Spasm of the laryngeal muscles, the diaphragm, and the intercostals prevents ventilation and cyanosis occurs. The occurrence of reflex spasms that cause cyanosis and cannot be controlled except by powerful relaxants such as curare is the characteristic feature of the severe case of tetanus.

Autonomic Disturbances. Disturbances of the autonomic nervous system occur frequently in severely affected tetanus patients and may prove fatal, particularly when the disease occurs in drug addicts. Younger patients often develop a fluctuating hypertension and increasing tachycardia after a few days of treatment, and cardiovascular responses to stimuli such as the aspiration of secretions from the respiratory tract become exaggerated so that systolic blood pressures of over 300 mm Hg are not uncommon. Patients sweat profusely, and may become extremely vasoconstricted peripherally with a sharp line of demarcation between warm and cold skin. Hyperpyrexia occurs in the absence of significant secondary infection and probably reflects the inability of the vasoconstricted patient to lose heat. High metabolic rates have been measured in spite of muscular paralysis, and the cardiac output is often disproportionately high in relation to tissue oxygen utilization, suggesting increased neurogenic drive to the heart. Raised plasma and urine catecholamine levels occur in association with these disturbances, and it seems likely that the sympathetic nervous system is grossly overactive and incoordinate. Prolonged overactivity has been followed by supraventricular tachycardia and multifocal ventricular ectopic beats, unresponsive hypotension, sudden bradycardia, and cardiac arrest.

Perhaps fortunately, patients with severe tetanus often remember little of their illness, but many recall weird and sometimes frightening dreams. Electroencephalography usually shows a sleep pattern with activation during stimulation such as tracheal aspiration.

DIAGNOSIS. The diagnosis of the established case of tetanus is all too easy, and strychnine poisoning is the only condition which is truly similar to established tetanus. Trismus may occur from dental infections, and the author has seen one case of hysterical tetanus. Overdose with or sensitivity to the phenothiazine group of drugs can be confused with tetanus, but the movements in these conditions usually include grimacing and jaw movements in which the jaw is opened widely.

CAUSES OF DEATH IN TETANUS. One of the most remarkable features of tetanus is that when patients recover, even from the most severe forms of the disease, they recover completely. It would therefore seem reasonable to study the causes of death carefully in tetanus so that by avoiding them the natural tendency of the disease toward recovery may be exploited. In a survey in Oxford, the causes of death in 20 of 110 patients were as follows: bronchopneumonia, 4; pulmonary embolus, 3; technical failure, 2; coincidental causes, 6; and no identifiable cause of death, 5.

Bronchopulmonary complications of tetanus are becoming less common now that the management of patients receiving intermittent positive pressure ventilation (IPPV) through a tracheostomy tube is better understood, and it is likely that chest complications will become still less common in the future. In general on the writer's service, pulmonary embolus is not a common cause of death in patients with other diseases treated by tracheostomy and IPPV. However, the difference in the incidence of pulmonary embolus between patients with tetanus requiring treatment with curare and IPPV and patients with other diseases similarly treated is so striking that anticoagulants are now used in patients with tetanus severe enough to merit treatment in this way. The incidence of technical failure underlines the complexity of treating the fully paralyzed patient; the coincidental causes of death apparently had nothing to do with the main disease. No identifiable cause of death could be found in five patients who had all displayed the pattern of clinical features suggestive of sympathetic overactivity.

TREATMENT. Treatment in tetanus is essentially symptomatic, but all patients with the disease should receive antimicrobial drugs and active and passive immunization, and should undergo wound excision. To allow the earliest possible detection of possibly lethal manifestations of the disease such as severe muscular or laryngeal spasms, the treatment of tetanus should be conducted in a well lighted intensive care unit rather than in isolation in a darkened side room. Treatment with penicillin (1 million units six hourly intramuscularly) or tetracycline (100 mg six hourly intramuscularly) should be commenced to ensure that all clostridia are killed. Human antitetanus immunoglobulin (3000 to 10,000 units) should be administered intravenously to produce a high blood level as early as possible. Investigations are under way in several parts of the world to assess the efficacy and dangers of administering a much smaller dose of the expensive human tetanus immunoglobulin via the intrathecal route. If a focus of infection is found, surgical debridement should be carried out shortly after administration of the antitoxin so that any toxin released into the circulation at surgery is neutralized. Because an attack of tetanus does not confer immunity, active immunization with adsorbed toxoid should be started and a full course of injections given during the recovery period.

Symptomatic Measures. Muscular Hypertonicity. The trismus and increased muscle tone of the mild case of tetanus can usually be controlled adequately with small doses of diazepam (10 mg. three to four hourly orally or parenterally). Barbiturates and chlorpromazine have also been widely and effectively employed against these symptoms.

Dysphagia and Airway Management. Trismus is a common early symptom in tetanus and is frequently accompanied by incoordination of the swallowing and laryngeal protective reflexes. Correct management of the airway is of vital importance, because laryngeal spasm may occur spontaneously or may be induced by attempts to swallow saliva or to pass a nasogastric tube. In addition, dysphagia may allow inhalation of infected material and saliva from the mouth so that atelectasis and pneumonia can follow; the latter remains a common cause of death in tetanus.

To minimize pulmonary complications, protection of the airway by intubation with a cuffed tube is advocated as soon as dysphagia is suspected. The symptom may be demonstrated as a tendency to cough and clear the throat after swallowing a mouthful of water, and, in more advanced form, as an inability to swallow saliva so that the patient drools or spits it out. Orotracheal intubation should be performed under general anesthesia and after muscle paralysis, allowing an elective tracheostomy with a cuffed tube. Meticulous pulmonary care should be instituted and maintained until normal pharyngolaryngeal function returns.

Muscle Spasms. Muscle spasms in tetanus can be

either localized or generalized and of varying severity. Sustained contraction of the muscles is exhausting, painful, and, if the respiratory muscles become involved, dangerous. When large doses of diazepam or chlorpromazine are employed in attempts to control severe spasms, oversedation may lead to hypoventilation between spasms. In this situation, and when muscle spasms themselves interfere with ventilation, therapeutic paralysis should be induced with curare and the resultant ventilatory failure treated with intermittent positive pressure ventilation. Curare is given intramuscularly or intravenously and with sufficient frequency to allow ventilation to proceed freely and to keep the patient comfortable. This method of treatment has proved most satisfactory when used early in the disease rather than after prolonged attempts to manage the patient with sedative agents. Smythe et al. have reported remarkable success in neonates with similar techniques.

Once curarization and IPPV have commenced, anxiety in the conscious but paretic patient should be minimized by frequent reassurance from the nursing staff and by mild hypnosis from diazepam or a barbiturate. Some of the most severely affected patients, however, become unresponsive and appear comatose for periods of one to three weeks during the critical phase of their illness, and in this situation sedative agents and muscle relaxants should be administered only if clearly indicated. These patients usually regain consciousness during the recovery phase and appear normal apart from amnesia. After one to four weeks of treatment, curare requirements decrease and diazepam may be reinstituted to reduce muscle stiffness during weaning from IPPV.

NUTRITION. Patients with mild tetanus may be fed orally, but once dysphagia develops a nasogastric tube should be inserted while the patient is anesthetized for tracheostomy. The considerable caloric (2500 cals per day) and fluid requirements of the tetanus patient can be satisfied effectively over the two- to four-week period of dysphagia by nasogastric feeding; since tube feedings normally contain milk, the chance of gastrointestinal bleeding is reduced. Paralytic ileus occurs fairly frequently in severe tetanus but usually responds to intermittent gastric drainage followed by the instillation of antacids and gut stimulants (e.g., metoclopramide).

FLUID BALANCE. The maintenance of a balanced fluid status in the severe tetanus patient is complicated by the considerable insensible fluid losses produced by profuse sweating and by unswallowed saliva. If reliance is placed entirely upon measured fluid input and output, fluid losses may be seriously underestimated, and dehydration may result.

Underhydration in an immobilized patient increases the possibility of deep venous thrombosis and of pulmonary embolism, and the latter has already been mentioned as a common cause of death in tetanus. Although anticoagulation started 24 hours after tracheostomy and continued until remobilization has been practiced without significant complication in several centers, protection against pulmonary embolism has not been complete, and it is likely that avoidance of dehydration is equally important.

Insensible fluid losses are best monitored by weighing the patient each day, and dehydration is avoided by measuring the specific gravity (or osmolality) of the urine regularly. Enough fluid should be given paren-terally or by nasogastric tube to produce a daily urine flow of 1.5 to 2 liters and to maintain the urine specific gravity below 1.015. Particular care must be taken to react promptly to the severe hypovolemia which may develop rapidly when overactivity of the sympathetic nervous system causes excessive sweating in association with paralytic ileus.

Cardiovascular Disturbances. In some of the tetanus patients who show severe muscular symptoms, cardiovascular changes in the form of tachycardia, hypertension, and increased responses to therapeutic maneuvers, such as tracheal aspiration, may appear after two to five days of treatment by curarization and artificial ventilation. These changes are probably produced by overactivity of the sympathetic nervous system and have been controlled successfully with adrenergic blocking agents. To reduce the tachycardia resulting from the intense sympathetic stimulation of the heart, a beta-adrenergic blocking agent such as propranolol (10 mg three to six hourly via the nasogastric tube) should be administered until the heart rate averages less than 100; if hypertension persists, an antihypertensive (e.g., bethanidine, 10 mg two to six hourly) should be added.*

Although other combinations of antiadrenergic agents might be more effective, short-acting drugs are preferred, because, particularly in drug addicts and in elderly patients, the pattern of autonomic disturbance may change very rapidly. In these groups of patients, episodes of profound hypotension and bradycardia may suddenly occur and, on occasion, lead to cardiac arrest. Provided that resuscitation is prompt, the cardiovascular status may be restored rapidly and repeatedly by measures such as tracheal aspiration and mildly painful stimuli which result in the release of endogenous catecholamines. These sudden and readily reversible episodes, during which the circulation appears unstimulated and dilated, must be contrasted with the unresponsive preterminal hypotension accompanied by tachycardia, vasoconstriction, and hyperpyrexia which has followed prolonged and unrelieved sympathetic overactivity. In view of the varying patterns of cardiovascular disturbance, continuous direct monitoring of heart rate and of arterial and central venous blood pressures has proved of considerable benefit in guiding therapy.

In summary, in a *mild case* the patient needs (1) wound excision, (2) human or equine antitoxin, (3) penicillin or another appropriate antimicrobial drug, and (4) a centrally acting relaxant and sedative drug, such as diazepam.

In the *moderate case* the patient needs in addition (5) tracheostomy and the insertion of a cuffed rubber tracheostomy tube to separate the pharynx from the trachea and to make inhalation of foreign material impossible, and (6) nasogastric tube feeding.

In the *severe case* the patient needs in addition (7) virtually complete paralysis with curare or another powerful relaxant and IPPV, (8) anticoagulant drugs, and (9), if sympathetic overactivity is present, treatment with alpha- and beta-adrenergic blockers.

PROGNOSIS. The patient with mild tetanus will almost certainly survive whether treated or not. The patient with moderate tetanus, if untreated, is at risk

---

*Bethanidine is not available in the United States; guanethidine might be substituted.

from inhalation of foreign material, and repeated episodes of this kind may lead to fatal pneumonia. The patient with moderate tetanus, if treated, should not die except from causes unrelated to the primary disease. The patient with severe tetanus who is having reflex spasms severe enough to cause cyanosis will certainly die if untreated, but even with treatment the severity of the illness and the complexity of the therapeutic regimen make the outlook uncertain. In the United Kingdom in 1967, even in the best centers, the mortality in patients with tetanus severe enough to indicate treatment with curare and IPPV varied between 10 and 40 per cent. Over-all mortality in the best hands is often still as high as 20 per cent, and at the extremes of age the mortality may be higher. It is paradoxical that in advanced countries where the immunization programs are efficient, mortality in the cases that do occur is high, not only because unimmunized patients are generally at the extremes of age, but also because patients who escape the immunization programs tend to have a poor physical status.

Adams, E. B., Laurence, D. R., and Smith, J. W. G.: Tetanus. Oxford, Blackwell Scientific Publications, 1969.

Bjørnboe, M., Ibsen, B., and Johnson, S.: Et tilfaelde af tetanus behandlet med curarisering, tracheostomi of overtryksventilation med kvaelstofforilte og ilt. Ugeskr. Laeger., 115:1535, 1953.

Fraser, D. W.: Preventing tetanus in patients with wounds. Ann. Intern. Med., 84:95, 1976.

Sanders, R. K. M., Martyn, B., Joseph, R., and Peacock, M. L.: Intrathecal antitetanus serum (horse) in the treatment of tetanus. Lancet, 1:974, 1977.

Smythe, P. M., Bowie, M. D., and Voss, T. J. V.: Treatment of tetanus neonatorum with muscle relaxants and intermittent positive pressure ventilation. Br. Med. J., 1:223, 1974.

Tsueda, K., Oliver, P. B., and Richter, R. W.: Cardiovascular manifestations of tetanus. Anesthesiology, 40:588, 1974.

ANAEROBIC BACTERIA

151. DISEASE DUE TO NONSPOREFORMING ANAEROBIC BACTERIA

Sydney M. Finegold

DEFINITION. Essentially every type of infection may be caused by nonsporeforming anaerobes. No organ or tissue of the body is immune to infection with these organisms. The majority of anaerobic infections involve two or more anaerobes, but infection with a single species of anaerobe does occur. Aerobic or facultatively anaerobic organisms may also be present in mixed infections. In mixed anaerobic infections, clostridia may be found together with nonsporeforming anaerobic bacilli and cocci. There are a number of unique features associated with certain clostridial infections, however, and it is convenient to consider these infections separately (see Ch. 146 to 150). Actinomycosis may also show distinctive clinical features; this disease (also often a mixed infection) is discussed in Ch. 163.

ETIOLOGY. The nonsporulating anaerobic bacteria are distributed widely throughout the body as indigenous flora. Numerically, they are the dominant flora on the various mucosal surfaces.

The anaerobic gram-negative bacilli and the anaerobic cocci are the major etiologic agents in anaerobic infections. They are encountered at least 15 times as frequently as clostridia. Gram-positive nonsporeforming anaerobic bacilli are encountered less commonly.

Anaerobic Gram-Negative Bacilli. The anaerobic gram-negative bacilli found in human infections belong to the genera *Bacteroides* and *Fusobacterium*, the former being encountered with much greater frequency. The *Bacteroides fragilis* group (five closely related species) is the most commonly seen of all anaerobes. It is of added importance because it is the most resistant of the anaerobes to antimicrobial compounds. The species of the *B. fragilis* group recovered most often from infections are, in order, *fragilis*, *thetaiotaomicron*, and *vulgatus*.

The *B. fragilis* group, like other gram-negative anaerobic rods, stains poorly. The staining is usually irregular. There is a variable amount of pleomorphism. Two other *Bacteroides* species seen relatively often, though rarely as single infecting agents, are *B. melaninogenicus* (coccobacilli) and *B. oralis* (morphologically similar to *B. fragilis*). *Fusobacterium nucleatum*, the fusiform bacillus, is the most frequently found of the fusobacteria. This organism is long and thin, with tapered ends; it is seen often in pairs end to end. Long filaments may also be noted. Granules (sometimes gram-positive) may be seen. *F. necrophorum*, formerly commonly encountered, is now seen much less. Other species of *Fusobacterium* seen include *F. mortiferum* and *F. varium*, the latter being relatively resistant to antimicrobials. Medically important fusobacteria other than *F. nucleatum* tend to be highly pleomorphic, with long filaments containing central swellings, large, free round bodies, and considerable irregularity of staining.

The spirochetes of the genus *Treponema*, also gram-negative anaerobes, which are part of the indigenous flora, are very likely not pathogenic, judging from experimental studies. The old terms "fusospirochetal infection" and "Vincent's infection" are therefore no longer appropriate.

Anaerobic Cocci. The anaerobic cocci include gram-positive streptococci (*Peptostreptococcus*), gram-positive cocci in pairs or masses (*Peptococcus*), and gram-negative cocci (*Veillonella, Megasphaera, Acidaminococcus*). The gram-negative cocci are not important pathogens. The anaerobic cocci are not usually pleomorphic, but many are smaller than facultative streptococci. *Veillonella* are tiny cocci in masses. As a group, anaerobic cocci are found in human disease almost as often as are the gram-negative anaerobic bacilli. The most commonly encountered species include *Peptostreptococcus anaerobius, intermedius* (this organism is actually microaerophilic), and *micros*, and *Peptococcus magnus, asaccharolyticus*, and *prevotii*.

The microaerophilic cocci and streptococci are a very poorly characterized heterogeneous group. They are best defined as organisms which tolerate reduced oxygen tension (18 per cent oxygen) — with or without added carbon dioxide. Most of these are actually facultative streptococci. These organisms are encountered in serious infections with some frequency, not uncommonly in pure culture. They are considered with the obligate anaerobes because they will often be overlooked unless good anaerobic techniques are used for transporting and culturing clinical specimens.

Gram-Positive Nonsporeforming Anaerobic Bacilli. The most commonly encountered gram-positive anaerobic nonsporeforming bacilli belong to the genus *Eubacterium*, particularly *E. lentum*, *E. alactolyticum*, and *E. limosum*. Gram-positive anaerobic bacilli in general destain readily and may appear gram-negative. *Eubacterium* strains may be filamentous. *Propionibacterium* strains, chiefly *P. acnes*, are seldom involved in infections of significance other than endocarditis (in patients with pre-existing valvular disease or artificial heart valves) or other infections related to implanted artificial prostheses. *Bifidobacterium eriksonii* is another well-established pathogen. *Actinomyces* may also be involved in infections without the distinctive clinical features of actinomycosis.

Features of Infections Due to Various Organisms. There are differences in the types of infection involving various anaerobes related to differences in their distribution in the body as normal flora. Thus the anaerobic cocci are encountered more often in oral and pulmonary infections and in female genital infections than in intra-abdominal disease. *Bacteroides fragilis*, which is the dominant member of the colonic flora, is involved in intra-abdominal infection commonly but is less frequently involved in dental infections or lung abscess. Aside from these differences, all the nonsporeforming anaerobes may be involved in any of the infections to be discussed in this chapter. Furthermore, the clinical picture is basically the same in these conditions regardless of the specific flora involved. Minor exceptions include distinctive odors related to end-products of metabolism (e.g., butyric acid produced in large amounts by *Fusobacterium* strains), the occasional formation of soft granules resembling sulfur granules by *Fusobacterium*, and the production of black color in blood-containing exudates by *B. melaninogenicus*.

Relative Importance of Various Organisms in Mixed Infections. It is difficult to determine the role of each species recovered from a mixed anaerobic infection and to assess the relative importance of the anaerobes and aerobic or facultative bacteria in mixed infections. Quantitative culture techniques may help. A small number of patients with pulmonary and intra-abdominal mixed infections of mild to moderate severity have been treated with agents active only against the anaerobes and have done well. This suggests that the anaerobes may have been the key pathogens.

EPIDEMIOLOGY. Anaerobic infections are the most frequently overlooked or misdiagnosed of all bacterial infections. Fortunately, the introduction of simplified anaerobic cultural procedures and an increased awareness of anaerobes and their importance on the part of bacteriologists and clinicians are beginning to overcome the problem.

Good data on the incidence of anaerobes in various infections are not always available. One big problem has been a tendency to overlook anaerobes in mixed cultures when one or more aerobic or facultative forms are present. Problems in specific identification have interfered with accurate determination of the involvement of particular organisms in various anaerobic infections.

There are now a number of studies supporting the view that anaerobes are common causes of infection. Some years ago Stokes (1958) found anaerobes in over 10 per cent of 4737 positive cultures of clinical specimens. Lodenkämper and Stienen (1955) detected 690 anaerobic infections in an eight-year period. Mattman et al. (1958) found anaerobic cocci in 45 per cent of 437 positive cultures from hospitalized patients. Martin (1974) isolated 10,998 anaerobes from clinical specimens in a two-year period.

A number of studies have combined good clinical and bacteriologic analysis to yield reliable information on the incidence of anaerobes in certain infections. Thus Heineman and Braude (1962) have shown that anaerobes are the dominant cause of brain abscess. Frederick and Braude (1974) noted an important role for anaerobes in chronic sinusitis. Bartlett and coworkers (1972, 1973, 1974) have established that lung abscess and aspiration pneumonia are most often due to anaerobes and that these organisms are important causes of necrotizing pneumonia and of empyema. Several groups have data to indicate that 85 to 95 per cent of cases of intra-abdominal abscess and of peritonitis involve anaerobes. Very likely well over half of all cases of pyogenic liver abscess also involve these organisms. A number of workers have documented the importance of anaerobes in a variety of obstetric and gynecologic infections. Other types of infections in which anaerobes play an important role include chronic otitis media, gingivitis and other oral infections, dental infections, bronchiectasis, other pulmonary infections, breast abscess, appendicitis, diverticulitis, abdominal and other wound infections, puerperal sepsis, ischiorectal and perirectal abscess, infected pilonidal sinuses, gas-forming cellulitis, necrotizing fasciitis, human and animal bite infections, and septic thrombophlebitis.

PATHOGENESIS OR MECHANISMS. Anaerobic bacteria basically are saprophytic members of the indigenous flora. Under certain conditions, however, they may invade and produce disease.

A simplistic definition of anaerobic bacteria would be bacteria which cannot survive in the presence of air. However, it is well known that a number of anaerobes generally regarded as fairly fastidious will tolerate 2 to 8 per cent oxygen in the atmosphere, and a number of these organisms will tolerate considerably more. Another factor determining whether or not the environment is suitable for growth of anaerobic bacteria is the oxidation-reduction potential of the medium. This is a measure of the tendency of the system to give up electrons and is usually expressed as the Eh value in millivolts. The Eh of a system is a function not only of its inherent reducing tendency but also of its hydrogen ion concentration, the Eh becoming more negative as the hydrogen ion concentration decreases.

One of the major defenses of the body against infection by anaerobes is the normal Eh (+120 mv). Lowering of the redox potential permits anaerobic growth in tissues, even those exposed to air. Lowered oxidation-reduction potential results from impaired blood supply, tissue necrosis, and growth of facultative bacteria in a wound. Thus vascular disease, epinephrine injection, cold, shock, edema, trauma, surgery, presence of a foreign body, malignancy, gas production by microorganisms, and aerobic infection all may predispose to anaerobic infection. The predisposition of diabetics to anaerobic infection is undoubtedly related at least partially to impaired blood supply and lowering of Eh. The association of malignancy (particularly of the colon, the bronchus, and the uterus) and anaerobic infection is well established; at times, anaerobic infection may be the first clue to the malignant process.

Certain toxins such as collagenase, hyaluronidase, deoxyribonuclease, and proteinases account for the virulence of some anaerobic infections.

The septic thrombophlebitis seen commonly in anaerobic infections may relate to production of heparinase by anaerobic bacteria and to acceleration of coagulation by gram-negative anaerobic rods. This lesion may lead to metastatic infection and helps account for the difficulty in eradicating anaerobic infections. Tissue destruction and abscess formation are also common manifestations of anaerobic infection.

Previous antimicrobial therapy is a not uncommon background for anaerobic infection. Preoperative "bowel preparation" with oral neomycin often results in a residual anaerobic flora, as many anaerobes tolerate even the very high concentrations achieved in the bowel lumen with such therapy. The popular combination of an aminoglycoside plus a cephalosporin (given parenterally) may lead to anaerobic superinfection, particularly with *Bacteroides fragilis*.

Conditions which predispose to infection in general (malnutrition, severe debilitating disease, corticosteroid and other immunosuppressive therapy, granulocytopenia) also facilitate anaerobic infection.

Aspiration and poor dental hygiene are common background factors in anaerobic pulmonary infection.

The unique involvement of only certain species of the *B. fragilis* group in infection is probably related to capsule formation (Kasper, 1976) and to resistance to normal serum bactericidal factors (Casciato et al., 1973). Under anaerobic conditions the granulocyte phagocytic bactericidal system may not function efficiently.

CLINICAL MANIFESTATIONS. For the most part the manifestations of anaerobic infection are those of the basic process (e.g., peritonsillar abscess, cholangitis, endometritis). Tissue necrosis, abscess formation, and septic thrombophlebitis are common with anaerobic infection, as are a foul odor and gas in tissues or in discharges.

Tonsillitis, Ludwig's Angina. Exudative tonsillitis (Vincent's angina) used to be a common anaerobic infection, usually caused by *Fusobacterium necrophorum*. The local tonsillar infection undoubtedly still occurs but is rarely recognized as an anaerobic process. The dreaded Ludwig's angina (cellulitis of the submandibular space), probably an anaerobic infection in most cases, is also uncommon now.

Bacteremia, Endocarditis. In recent years, bacteremia caused by anaerobes has dominated clinical reports on anaerobic infections. Most likely this is because anaerobes are much more likely to be present in pure culture in bacteremia than in other types of anaerobic infection, and consequently it is much easier to isolate the offending organism. On the other hand, it is clear that anaerobic bacteremia is relatively common, accounting for 10 to 15 per cent of all bacteremias. The primary sources of anaerobic bacteremia at present are the gastrointestinal and gynecologic tracts. Less common sites include infected decubitus ulcers and other wounds. Septic shock and disseminated intravascular coagulation have been described in the course of anaerobic bacteremia.

In large series of endocarditis, only 1 to 2 per cent of positive blood cultures have yielded anaerobes as a rule. As high as 15 per cent, however, were sterile in the presence of strong clinical or pathologic evidence of endocarditis. Our experience is that approximately 10 per cent of cases of endocarditis are caused by anaerobic or microaerophilic cocci. The main portals of entry for anaerobes in bacterial endocarditis are the mouth, the gastrointestinal tract, and, to a lesser extent, the genitourinary tract. The incidence of pre-existing heart disease is lower in the case of anaerobic endocarditis, and there is evidence to indicate that embolization may be more common in the case of the disease involving anaerobes.

Pleuropulmonary Infection. Anaerobic pulmonary infection is commonly overlooked. Unfortunately, even when suspected, it has often not been confirmed by proper culture of appropriate specimens. Coughed sputum culture is unsatisfactory because of the presence of anaerobes as normal upper respiratory tract flora. The clinical course of anaerobic pulmonary infection ranges from incidentally discovered infection to fulminant infection. Most patients present with a smoldering illness. The most common underlying condition is a predisposition to aspirate caused by altered consciousness or dysphagia. Important clues to anaerobic etiology are aspiration, pulmonary necrosis, indolent course, and foul-smelling sputum or pus. The principal types of anaerobic pulmonary infection are lung abscess, necrotizing pneumonia, and pneumonia without necrosis; many patients have an associated empyema.

Anaerobes are probably second only to the pneumococcus as causes of pneumonia in hospitalized patients, because aspiration pneumonia is a common event.

Intra-abdominal Infection. Anaerobes are a prime cause of peritonitis and intra-abdominal abscess and are involved in virtually all cases of complicated appendicitis or diverticulitis.

Anaerobes (especially nonsporeformers) play a relatively minor role in gallbladder infection.

Genitourinary Tract Infection. Various urinary tract infections may involve anaerobes, but these organisms are not common causes of such infection. Factors predisposing to anaerobic urinary tract infection are stones, malignancy, obstruction, and previous renal tuberculosis.

A large variety of female genital tract infections involve anaerobic bacteria. Clostridia cause the most serious female genital tract infections, but infections in this system are much more commonly produced by nonsporeforming anaerobic bacteria. Predisposing conditions include pregnancy, the puerperium (particularly with premature rupture of the membranes, prolonged labor, or postpartum hemorrhage), abortion (spontaneous or induced), malignancy, radiation, surgery, cauterization, stenosis, uterine fibroids, and old gonococcal salpingitis.

Skin, Soft Tissue, and Muscle Infection. These infections include such entities as cellulitis, pyoderma, infected cysts, infection of decubitus and other ulcers, abscesses, bacterial synergistic gangrene, chronic undermining ulcer of Meleney, necrotizing fasciitis, bite infection, noma, and tropical ulcer. Anaerobes are common infecting agents in hidradenitis suppurativa. Subcutaneous abscesses involving anaerobes are seen in narcotic addicts who are "skin-poppers."

Anaerobic (gas-forming) cellulitis is an acute soft tissue infection, seen particularly in diabetics and commonly ascribed to coliforms. Although gas-producing nonanaerobes may be involved, it is our experience that anaerobes predominate. Muscle is usually not involved, but it is essential that clostridial myositis be ruled out. This differentiation may require surgery, which, in any case, is important therapeutically.

Anaerobic streptococci may produce a myositis simulating "gas gangrene," but the infection is much less severe. Bacteroides and anaerobic cocci may be involved in a milder form of myositis known as synergistic anaerobic cellulitis, as well as in necrotizing fasciitis.

Bone and Joint Infection. Osteomyelitis caused by anaerobes is probably overlooked often. Anaerobes are relatively common in infected diabetic ulcers of the foot with bony involvement.

There are a number of well-documented cases of purulent arthritis caused by anaerobes, chiefly gram-negative bacilli. Predisposing factors include underlying joint disease and local or systemic corticosteroid therapy. Any joint may be affected, but there is a peculiar susceptibility of the sternoclavicular and sacroiliac joints.

DIAGNOSIS. Clues Suggesting Anaerobic Infection. Features indicating the likelihood of anaerobic infection include foul or putrid odor, infection located near mucosal surfaces (particularly with manipulation of the associated organs), tissue necrosis, gas in tissues or discharges, infection associated with malignancy or other tissue-destructive process, endocarditis with negative routine blood cultures, infection related to the use of aminoglycoside antimicrobials (by any route) and/or broad-spectrum penicillins or cephalosporins, septic thrombophlebitis, infection after bites, black coloration or red fluorescence under ultraviolet light of discharges or lesions (*B. melaninogenicus* infection), unique morphology on Gram stain of exudate, and failure to obtain growth on routine culture (particularly when organisms are seen on Gram stain of exudate).

Specimen Collection. The major consideration is to avoid "contaminating" a specimen with normal flora, because anaerobes are prevalent as indigenous flora.

Expectorated sputum is not suitable for anaerobic culture. Bronchoscopically obtained specimens are also not suitable, although it is possible that quantitative culture of material obtained via a sheathed fiberoptic bronchoscope may prove useful. This is not established. Transtracheal needle aspiration or direct lung puncture is the optimal method of obtaining specimens from patients with suspected anaerobic pulmonary infection, unless empyema fluid is available.

In the case of uterine infection, there is no satisfactory method for obtaining reliable bacteriologic data unless there is an accompanying bacteremia. However, quantitation of growth from carefully obtained intrauterine cultures may be of some value.

In the case of abscesses, the unbroken skin or mucosal surface is decontaminated, and pus is removed with a syringe. This is preferable to using a swab on a portion of an exposed lesion.

Voided midstream urine may contain anaerobes from the urethral flora; therefore percutaneous suprapubic bladder aspiration is necessary.

Specimen Transport. Proper transport of specimens to the laboratory is crucial for recovery of anaerobes which may be present. Since some anaerobes are tolerant to oxygen contact, a laboratory which isolates such organisms as *B. fragilis* and *C. perfringens* may not realize that it is overlooking more demanding anaerobes. Many anaerobes responsible for clinical infections do not tolerate oxygen exposure well, so that special transport methods are needed to ensure their survival. Various means for proper anaerobic transport include the following:

1. Syringe technique — eliminate all air from specimen in syringe and needle and then stick needle into a sterile rubber stopper (for transport time of 30 minutes or less).
2. Gassed-out tubes — inject specimen into butyl rubber-stopped tube which has been gassed out with oxygen-free CO_2. Commercial vials of this type are available.

TREATMENT. General Aspects. Surgical aspects of therapy are extremely important. Drainage of collections of pus and excision of necrotic tissue are commonly necessary, and in minor infections they may be all that is required. Obstructions must be relieved and tissues decompressed when this is indicated.

Anticoagulant therapy or venous ligation may be indicated in patients with septic phlebitis. Treatment of shock and disseminated intravascular coagulation, when they occur, and general supportive measures are important aspects of therapy.

Local use of hydrogen peroxide or zinc peroxide is useful. Hyperbaric oxygen therapy is not indicated in infection with nonsporeforming anaerobes.

Antimicrobial Therapy. In vitro susceptibility tests, properly performed, serve as a good guide to drug therapy of anaerobic infections. Standardized disc susceptibility tests are available for most anaerobic bacteria but are most satisfactory with organisms which have been identified. Use of a disc test without measurement of zones of inhibition, or application of standards which were developed for aerobic and facultative organisms, yields completely undependable results. Conventional tube or plate dilution tests with incubation in an anaerobic jar are reliable. Patterns of susceptibility to selected drugs are noted in the accompanying table.

Penicillin is active against most anaerobes other than *Bacteroides fragilis;* however, this organism is the anaerobe most commonly isolated from infection. Certain strains of anaerobic cocci require as much as 16.0 to 32.0 μg per milliliter for inhibition, and occasional strains of *Fusobacterium varium* are resistant to penicillin. Dosage of penicillin G should be at least 8 to 12 million units daily in the case of seriously ill adults or infection with relatively resistant strains. Ampicillin and cephaloridine are usually comparable to penicillin G, but several other penicillins and cephalosporins are less active. Some agents in these classes may be useful because very high blood levels are achieved safely or because of their resistance to beta lactamases.

Tetracycline is no longer valuable in many geographic areas, because many strains of anaerobes of all types are now resistant. Two new tetracycline derivatives, doxycycline and minocycline, are more active, but susceptibility testing is required because a number of strains of most types of anaerobes are resistant.

Lincomycin, erythromycin, and vancomycin are active against certain anaerobes; more information is needed, however, on the validity of in vitro tests with these drugs, and they are not approved by the Food and Drug Administration for use in anaerobic infections.

Susceptibility of Anaerobes to Selected Antimicrobial Agents

	Microaerophilic and Anaerobic Cocci	Bacteroides fragilis	Bacteroides melaninogenicus	Fusobacterium varium	Other Fusobacterium Species	Eubacterium
Penicillin G	+++ to ++++	+	++++*	+++*	++++	++++
Clindamycin	++ to +++	+++	+++	++	+++	++ to +++
Metronidazole†	++	+++	+++	+++	+++	++
Chloramphenicol	+++	+++	+++	+++	+++	+++

++++ Drug of choice.   ++ Moderate activity.
+++ Good activity.   + Poor or inconsistent activity.

*A few strains are resistant.
†Experimental for anaerobic infections.

Chloramphenicol is active against all anaerobes, with only rare strains resistant, and is very effective clinically. It penetrates the central nervous system well. However, because of its serious and unpredictable toxicity, it should be reserved for seriously ill patients and used only until bacteriologic data indicate that a less toxic drug would be suitable. Nevertheless, chloramphenicol is the drug of choice for serious anaerobic infection of uncertain cause. Initial dosage of chloramphenicol in such a patient should be 40 to 50 mg per kilogram of body weight daily; once the patient has shown a good response, 30 mg per kilogram per day should be adequate.

Clindamycin (7-chlorolincomycin) has broad activity against anaerobes, with only *Fusobacterium varium*, among the nonsporeformers, commonly resistant. However, a number of strains of *Clostridium* other than *C. perfringens* are not uncommonly resistant; this is also true for a number of *Peptococcus* strains and occasional strains of *B. fragilis*. Clindamycin is one of the drugs of choice for nonsporeforming anaerobic infections, except in central nervous system infections and in very serious infections in which the nature of the infecting organism and its susceptibility to clindamycin are not yet known. Colitis caused by clindamycin is an uncommon but sometimes serious complication; it is now known to be caused primarily or exclusively by *Clostridium difficile*. Oral dosage for adults is 150 to 450 mg every six hours, and parenteral dosage is 600 to 2700 mg per day (in two to four equal doses), depending on the severity of the infection. Daily doses as high as 4.8 grams have been given intravenously to critically ill patients.

Metronidazole has broad activity against anaerobic microorganisms and is consistently bactericidal versus *Bacteroides fragilis* and other anaerobes. It is very effective in anaerobic infections, but it has not yet been approved by the U.S. Food and Drug Administration for this purpose.

Although it is true that *Bacteroides fragilis* infections are more common below the diaphragm and that most anaerobes recovered from infections above the diaphragm are penicillin susceptible, there is too much overlap for practical application of this knowledge in the individual case — particularly if the patient has a serious infection. For example, *B. fragilis* is part of the infecting flora of 10 to 20 per cent of anaerobic pulmonary infections. It has also been recovered from such infections as sinusitis, mastoiditis, and brain abscess.

Therapy with antimicrobial agents in anaerobic infections must be intensive and prolonged. These infections have a considerable tendency to relapse.

PROGNOSIS. In general, infection with nonsporeforming anaerobes carries a relatively good prognosis, provided the diagnosis is suspected and confirmed early and appropriate therapy instituted promptly. To some extent, of course, the prognosis varies with the site and extent of the lesion. Brain abscess is still a very serious infection with a significant mortality (50 per cent). The over-all mortality in anaerobic pulmonary infections is 15 to 20 per cent, with a distinctly higher mortality in the case of necrotizing pneumonia (30 per cent). The mortality in liver abscess varies greatly from series to series, depending primarily on whether or not cases were discovered ante mortem and on how early they were picked up. On the whole, the mortality is in the range of 25 to 50 per cent. The mortality in sepsis caused by nonsporeforming anaerobes is 30 per cent. In patients with endocarditis caused by gram-negative anaerobic bacilli, mortality is also 30 per cent, but it is higher in cases caused by *Bacteroides fragilis* than in those caused by other, more sensitive gram-negative anaerobic bacilli. The mortality in endocarditis caused by anaerobic cocci is not significantly different from that caused by facultative streptococci. The availability of a number of effective drugs has permitted a reduction in mortality and morbidity resulting from anaerobic infection.

PREVENTION. The major principles in prophylaxis are avoidance or early correction of conditions which reduce the redox potential of the tissues and avoidance of the introduction of anaerobes from the indigenous flora into sites where they may set up infection. Discriminate use of antimicrobial drugs will minimize anaerobic superinfection.

Early appropriate therapy of anaerobic infections will prevent metastatic infection.

Precautions to minimize the possibility of aspiration will be helpful in preventing anaerobic pulmonary infection. Good surgical technique (e.g., minimal devitalization of tissue, use of closed methods of resection) will prevent postoperative anaerobic infections.

Bartlett, J., and Finegold, S. M.: Anaerobic pleuropulmonary infections. Medicine, 51:413, 1972.

Finegold, S. M.: Anaerobic Bacteria in Human Disease. New York, Academic Press, 1977.

Gorbach, S. L., and Bartlett, J. G.: Anaerobic infections. N. Engl. J. Med., 290:1177, 1237, 1289, 1974.

Ledger, W. J.: Infection in the Female. Philadelphia, Lea & Febiger, 1977.

Marcoux, J. A., Zabransky, R. J., Washington, J. A., II, Wellman, W. E., and Martin, W. J.: Bacteroides bacteremia: A review of 123 cases. Minn. Med., 53:1169, 1970.

Saksena, D. S., Block, M. A., McHenry, M. C., and Truant, J. P.: Bacteroidaceae: Anaerobic organisms encountered in surgical infections. Surgery, 63:261, 1968.

TYPHOID FEVER AND SALMONELLOSIS

152. TYPHOID FEVER

Sherwood L. Gorbach

Typhoid ("cloudy") fever is a febrile illness of prolonged duration which is marked by hectic fever, delirium, enlargement of the spleen, abdominal pain, and a variety of systemic manifestations. Although caused primarily by *Salmonella typhi*, typhoidal disease occasionally is produced by other types of salmonellae. The portal of entry is the gastrointestinal tract, but typhoid fever is not truly an intestinal disease, having more systemic symptoms than those related to the bowel. There is a mortality of 1 to 5 per cent in drug-treated patients; the causes of death are intestinal perforation, hemorrhage, and severe toxemia.

EPIDEMIOLOGY. Improvements in environmental sanitation have reduced the incidence of typhoid fever in the industrialized nations. Approximately 500 cases occur each year in the United States, with the greatest occurrence in young people. Most cases are sporadic, but are invariably related to a human carrier. The organism is essentially confined to humans, either in a disease state or as a carrier. Large-scale epidemics of typhoid occur on a regular basis, usually traced to contaminated food which may be imported from an endemic area or to contaminated water supplies. A recent epidemic in Mexico has been associated with bottled beverages.

Typhoid fever is a classic food- and water-borne pathogen. The major routes of passage are by the five F's: flies, fingers, food, feces, and fomites. *S. typhi* is extremely hardy and can survive for extended periods in polluted waters, contaminated foods, and soiled bedclothes. In earlier times, typhoid fever was considered "morbus medicorum," being capable of spread within hospitals to cause a high mortality among doctors and nurses. With effective chemotherapy and intelligent isolation procedures, intrahospital spread is extremely uncommon.

Since *S. typhi* cohabits exclusively with man, the occurrence of a single case means the presence of a carrier. An investigation by public health authorities should be instituted to determine the source and the presence of other cases. Chronic carriers, as they are discovered, are registered with the health authorities, and the microorganism is phage typed so that it can be traced in the event of an outbreak. However, the registered carriers represent only a minority of the potential reservoir, and do not take account of the "imported" cases of typhoid, which include nearly half of the acute infections in the United States.

PATHOGENESIS AND PATHOLOGY. The pathologic events of typhoid fever are initiated in the intestinal tract following oral ingestion of typhoid bacilli. The organism penetrates the small bowel mucosa, sparing the stomach, and makes its way rapidly to the lymphatics, the mesenteric nodes, and, within minutes, to the bloodstream. There is a paucity of local inflammatory findings, which explains the lack of intestinal symptoms at this stage. This sequence of events is in marked contrast to that of other forms of salmonellosis and to shigellosis in which the intestinal findings are prominent at the onset.

The organism must survive passage through the stomach, warding off the destructive action of gastric acid. Food and beverages, the classic vehicles of typhoid fever, also serve as an excellent buffer to acid. The number of bacilli ingested is a critical determinant of infection. An inoculum of 10^9 bacilli produces disease in 95 per cent of apparently healthy people, whereas 10^3 organisms rarely cause symptoms. The incubation period is inversely related to inoculum size; an inoculum of 10^9 bacilli is associated with a five-day latent period, which is extended to nine days or longer in those receiving a smaller dose.

Following the initial bacteremia, the organism is sequestered in macrophages and monocytic cells of the reticuloendothelial system. It undergoes multiplication, and re-emerges several days later in recurrent waves of bacteremia, an event which initiates the symptomatic phase of infection. Now in great numbers, the organism is spread throughout the host, infecting many organ sites. The intestinal tract may be seeded by direct bacteremic spread, as, for example, to Peyer's patches in the terminal ileum. Alternatively, the gallbladder contains a large number of bacilli, and contaminated bile is another method of infecting the gut.

Hyperplasia of the reticuloendothelial system, including lymph nodes, liver, and spleen, is characteristic of typhoid fever. The liver contains discrete, micronodular areas of necrosis, surrounded by macrophages and lymphocytes. Inflammation of the gallbladder is common, and may lead to acute cholecystitis. Patients with preexisting gallbladder disease have a penchant for becoming carriers, because the bacillus becomes intimately associated with the chronic infection and may be incorporated within the gallstones themselves. Lymphoid follicles in the gut, such as Peyer's patches, become hyperplastic, with infiltration of macrophages, lymphocytes, and red blood cells. Subsequently, a follicle may ulcerate and penetrate through the submucosa to the intestinal lumen, discharging in its wake large numbers of typhoid bacilli. As the bowel wall is progressively involved, it becomes paper-thin, and is susceptible to transmural perforation into the peritoneal cavity. This occurs most commonly in the distal ileum, 25 cm from the ileocecal sphincter. Erosion into blood vessels produces severe intestinal hemorrhage.

An analogy has been drawn between the biologic effects of endotoxin and typhoid fever. Both cause chills, fever, headache, nausea, and vomiting, as well as the laboratory findings of leukopenia and thrombocytopenia. With endotoxin, however, increasing doses produce a state of tolerance in which further administration has no effect. By contrast, typhoid fever is a relentless and sustained state of illness. Administration of viable typhoid organisms to volunteers rendered tolerant to endotoxin still produces symptoms. Thus typhoid fever cannot be explained merely as a reaction to endotoxin, although this material may play some role in the disease state.

CLINICAL MANIFESTATIONS. Typhoid fever lasts about four weeks, evolving in a manner consistent with the pathophysiologic events. Classically, the illness is described as a series of one-week stages. Although in general the illness follows such a pattern, individual cases may deviate significantly, and the illness may persist (with accompanying bacteremia) with only slight improvement for four weeks or more. The *incubation period* is generally 7 to 14 days, with wide variations on either extreme. During the *first week*, the triad of fever, headache, and abdominal pain is commonly encountered. The onset usually is insidious with a stepladder rise of fever which later becomes persistent. It is accompanied by a dull headache. The pulse is often slower than would be expected for the degree of temperature elevation. Abdominal pain is localized to the right lower quadrant in most instances, although it can be diffuse. In approximately 50 per cent of patients, there is no change in bowel habits; in fact, constipation is more common than diarrhea in children. Near the end of the first week, enlargement of the spleen is noticeable. An evanescent and rather classic rash, "rose spots," becomes manifest at this time. It is observed in approximately 70 per cent of whites, but considerably less frequently in dark-skinned persons. Rose spots are deeply red, 2- to 4-mm macules, often present in clusters, blanching on pressure; they occur most often on the upper anterior abdominal wall and lower thorax. During the *second week*, the fever becomes more continuous. The patient looks sick and withdrawn, although he may be fully responsive. In some, marked deterioration in the mental condition, lassitude, delirium, and even coma may develop. Cough is commonly present and epistaxis is not infrequent. During the *third week*, the patient's illness continues in the "typhoidal state." There may be disoriented mentation and, in some cases, extreme toxemia. In this period there may be intestinal involvement, manifested clinically by greenish "pea-soup" diarrhea and the dire complications of intestinal perforation and hemorrhage. The *fourth week* usually but not invariably brings slackening of the fever and improvement in clinical status. The patient becomes more interested in the surroundings. There is significant weight loss, anemia, and profound fatigue. Typhoid fever is among the longest and most debilitating of microbial diseases.

The clinical course is altered by many factors, such as the pathogenicity of the infecting strain, the immune and nutritional status of the host, the size of the infecting dose, and antimicrobial therapy.

COMPLICATIONS. Since the typhoid bacillus is widely disseminated through recurrent waves of bacteremia, many organ sites are involved. Pneumonia occurs in 10 per cent of patients, although cough, without radiographic findings, is encountered in approximately two thirds. Rarely there is a small pleural effusion. During the severe toxemic phase, patients may aspirate gastric contents and develop a suppurative pneumonia. Severe headache, delirium, and even coma are often noted, but suppurative disease of the brain and meninges is quite uncommon, being seen in less than 1 per cent of patients. Typhoid pyelonephritis associated with renal pain, hematuria, and pyuria is occasionally encountered. The gallbladder and liver are often involved with inflammatory changes. Acute cholecystitis can occur during the initial period of typhoid fever. Jaundice, on the basis of diffuse hepatic inflammation, has been observed in some patients. The microorganism may spread to bone, especially ribs and spine, and to the large joints. Nerve deafness, conjunctivitis, keratitis, and optic neuritis have all been seen on rare occasions.

Although the litany of organ site involvement is long, the pre-eminent complications are intestinal hemorrhage and perforation. These events are most apt to occur in the third week and during convalescence and are not closely related to the severity of the disease. However, they tend to occur in the same patient, with the bleeding serving as a warning of a possible perforation to come. Bleeding may be sudden and severe, or a slow ooze. Prior to chemotherapy, the incidence of hemorrhage was 7 to 20 per cent in various series; it is somewhat less frequent since specific treatment has been available. The ileum is the main site of bowel perforation. The onset may be sudden with signs of acute abdomen. Or there may be a leak of intraluminal contents to form an abscess in the lower quadrant or pelvis, producing a more chronic, insidious course. Approximately 3 per cent of patients with typhoid fever will experience intestinal perforation.

RELAPSE. After defervescence has occurred and the patient has apparently "ridden through the storm," there remains a potential for recurrence. The relapse generally occurs eight to ten days after cessation of drug therapy and consists of a re-enactment of the major manifestations such as fever, chills, skin rash, and bacteremia. Early chemotherapy of the initial infection may increase the potential for relapse because it prevents the development of natural immunity, an important feature in eventually controlling the organism within the host.

CARRIERS. The disappearance of typhoid bacilli from the bowel has a prolonged and unpredictable course. After six weeks, approximately 50 per cent of typhoid victims are still shedding the organism in their feces. This figure progressively declines so that after three months only 5 to 10 per cent are excreters. A chronic carrier is defined as a person with stool cultures positive for *S. typhi* at least one year following an episode of typhoid or, in some cases, positive stool cultures without a documented history of disease. The possibility of spontaneously aborting the carrier state is very unlikely after this time. Chronic carriers are more common in older age groups, in women (a 3:1 ratio of women to men), and in people with gallbladder disease. The organism usually is harbored in the gallbladder, often forming part of gallstones, and persists in a noninflammatory symbiotic relationship with the host, causing neither local inflammation nor systemic symptoms. Occasionally, the gallbladder is free of the organism, and it is apparently carried in the large bowel. In the usual case, the bile contains enormous numbers of bacilli, up to 10^9 per milliliter, and they are discharged in the feces in varying concentrations. The organisms are viable and fully infective, so the carrier may be a source of new infection.

LABORATORY FINDINGS. Many laboratory features of typhoid fever are consistent with prolonged sepsis. A normochromic, normocytic anemia persists throughout the infection; it may be made worse by intestinal blood loss or a reaction of the bone marrow to agents such as chloramphenicol. Thrombocytopenia occurs during the initial hectic period of the disease. Leukopenia is characteristic of the first week of illness, with the major depression in polymorphonuclear leukocytes.

The definitive diagnosis of typhoid fever is established by isolating the organism. During the first week, blood cultures are positive in 90 per cent of patients. As bacteremia abates during the subsequent weeks, other sites become colonized. It is not always appreciated, however, that, if the clinical illness persists essentially unimproved, the bacteremia likewise persists. As a consequence, the blood culture may be positive for several weeks or more. The blood culture thus is the primary diagnostic test. Stool cultures usually become positive in the second and third weeks when the organisms are shed from the lymphoid follicles of the intestinal wall. During the third week, urine culture yields typhoid bacilli in approximately 30 per cent of patients. Rose spots harbor the organism, and they can be sampled by small skin snips of the lesion which are cultured in nutrient broth. These are positive in two thirds of patients. A most useful source is the bone marrow, which is positive for *S. typhi* in 90 per cent of patients, even when they have received some antimicrobial therapy.

The titer of agglutinins (Widal test) against somatic (O) and flagellar (H) antigens rises during the third week of illness. An O titer of 1:80 or more in nonimmunized individuals is suggestive of typhoid fever. Higher initial titers or a fourfold rise provides stronger evidence. The H antigen is more nonspecific, and is likely to be elevated from prior immunization or infection by other enteric bacteria. There are many false-positive and occasional false-negative Widal reactions so that a diagnosis based on titer rises alone is rather tenuous.

DIAGNOSIS. In endemic regions the most perplexing diagnosis is between typhoid fever and malaria, because both diseases can cause fever, chills, splenomegaly, and neutropenia. Travelers to such areas may acquire either disease so that they present with the same diagnostic dilemma. Blood smears usually are positive in malaria, and typhoid is identified by isolating the organism in culture or, as an early clue, a positive Widal reaction. In certain parts of the world, Lassa fever or dengue is a diagnostic alternative. Other salmonellae can mimic typhoid fever. Among bacterial infections which may be confused with typhoid, tuberculosis, shigellosis, leptospirosis, and bacteremias associated with cholecystitis and pyelonephritis should be given consideration. Viral agents such as infectious mononucleosis and infectious hepatitis can present with similar symptoms. Patients having delirium or coma with normal cerebrospinal fluid may be thought to have viral encephalitis rather than typhoid fever. Rickettsial diseases may be considered, but the absence of a characteristic rash would militate against this diagnosis.

TREATMENT. Drug resistance, mediated by plasmids, can occur among typhoid bacilli. Most strains are susceptible to chloramphenicol and ampicillin, although notable epidemics with strains resistant to either of these drugs have been reported in recent years. Hence, a great effort should be made in each case to isolate the organism and to perform drug susceptibility tests. Chloramphenicol remains the standard therapy because of its proved efficacy and its high activity against most clinical isolates of typhoid bacilli. The response to therapy is remarkably constant, as defervescence regularly occurs three to five days after initiating treatment. The clinical condition improves within one to two days, with decreased toxemia and slowly declining fever. In adults, chloramphenicol should be given in a total daily dose of 3 to 4 grams, administered in four equally divided doses. Occasionally in very sick patients it may be necessary to give the drug by the intravenous route, and the same total daily dose of 3 to 4 grams should be used. Oral medication can then be given after improvement in the clinical status. Chloramphenicol is well

absorbed from the intestinal tract, but is rather poorly absorbed from intramuscular sites. Thus the intramuscular route is to be avoided. The duration of treatment is two weeks; prolongation of this treatment does not reduce the incidence of complications or carriers. Intestinal perforation and hemorrhage can occur during what is apparently successful treatment. Relapse may follow an otherwise uneventful course, and should be treated with the same drug.

Ampicillin has been recommended as alternative therapy, but it has been somewhat disappointing in comparison with chloramphenicol. The dose is 6 grams per day, intravenously, in four to six divided doses. Amoxicillin, a closely related drug, provides better absorption and increased efficacy. Several studies have shown that amoxicillin, in doses of 4 grams per day in four divided doses, has good activity, but is somewhat less effective than chloramphenicol. Co-trimoxazole has also been used in the therapy of typhoid fever, and the initial results are promising.

Corticosteroids are administered for severe toxemia and fever, and may produce a dramatic response in the patient with profound sepsis. The treatment should be given in high doses, 60 mg per day of prednisone divided in four doses, and rapidly tapered over the next three days. The wide experience with steroid treatment has failed to show any adverse effects, although the potentiality for masking intestinal perforation is still present. Thus steroids are best reserved for patients with severe toxicity.

Intestinal perforation is managed by standard surgical practices. All patients should be treated with nasogastric suction. Indications for operation are progressive peritoneal signs or localization of an abscess. Simple closure of the perforation is the treatment of choice. However, the ileum may be riddled with multiple perforations, and resection or exteriorization of the intestinal loop may be required. Intestinal perforation can lead to secondary infection with enteric bacilli, so it is advisable to initiate treatment with a broad-spectrum antimicrobial such as an aminoglycoside, in addition to continuing chloramphenicol.

Good nursing care plays a major role in the recovery from typhoid fever. The pyrexia can be managed with tepid baths and sponging. Salicylates and antipyretics should be avoided, as they cause severe sweating and may lower the blood pressure.

A chronic carrier, who has been discharging *S. typhi* for longer than one year, can be treated with antimicrobials in an attempt to eliminate the infection. One regimen which works in approximately two thirds of patients is 6 grams of ampicillin per day in four divided doses for six weeks. Reappearance of the carrier state following such treatment is generally associated with gallbladder disease. In persons with gallstones or chronic cholecystitis, cholecystectomy eliminates the carrier state in 85 per cent. This procedure, however, is recommended only for those whose profession is not compatible with the typhoid carrier state, i.e., food handlers and health care providers.

PROGNOSIS. Prior to antimicrobial therapy, the case mortality of typhoid fever was around 10 to 15 per cent. The introduction of chloramphenicol has reduced this to 1 per cent, and most patients now succumb to either perforation or hemorrhage. However, in areas of the world with poor nutrition and limited medical facilities, the mortality may be higher. Factors which influence a lethal outcome are severity of the disease at time of admission (coma is a poor prognostic sign); age, with the very young and the very old being at greatest risk; and prior infection, because a second attack, although uncommon, is less severe than the primary episode.

PROPHYLAXIS. For control of intrahospital spread, enteric precautions should be initiated; fecal, urine, and blood specimens should be disposed of by double-bag techniques and always handled with gloves. Additional precautions are unwarranted.

Typhoid vaccine affords 70 per cent protection. This relative immunity can be overcome by a large inoculum of bacilli. The most active vaccine is the acetone-dried product which is administered in two doses of 0.5 ml, subcutaneously, at four-week intervals. The phenol-inactivated product has somewhat reduced immunogenicity, but it produces less local discomfort, a problem which is prominent with the acetone-dried vaccine. There is no relationship between serum antibody levels measured against O, H, or Vi antigens and resistance to disease, relapse, or reinfection. It is apparent that the major forces of immunity act at the intestinal mucosa surface. Oral live vaccines, theoretically the most attractive approach, have not proved successful, because either they have failed to colonize the intestine or the mutated vaccine strain has reverted to a pathogen. Despite its limitations, typhoid vaccine is recommended for travelers to endemic regions; revaccination should be done every three years with a single 0.5-ml dose.

Hornick, R. B., Greisman, S. E., Woodward, T. E., DuPont, H. L., Dawkins, A. T., and Snyder, M. J.: Typhoid fever: Pathogenesis and immunologic control. N. Engl. J. Med., 283:686, 739, 1970.

Johnson, W. D., Jr., Hook, E. W., Lindsey, E., and Kaye, D.: Treatment of chronic typhoid carriers with ampicillin. Antimicrob. Agents Chemother., 3:439, 1973.

Kim, J-P., Oh, S-K., and Jarret, F.: Management of ileal perforation due to typhoid fever. Ann. Surg., 181:88, 1975.

Pillay, N., Adams, E. B., and North-Coombes, D.: Comparative trial of amoxycillin and chloramphenicol in treatment of typhoid fever in adults. Lancet, 2:333, 1975.

Snyder, M. J., Gonzalez, O., Palomino, C., Music, S. I., Hornick, R. B., Perroni, J., Woodward, W. E., Gonzalez, C., DuPont, H. L., and Woodward, T. E.: Comparative efficacy of chloramphenicol, ampicillin, and co-trimoxazole in the treatment of typhoid fever. Lancet, 2:1155, 1976.

Wicks, C. B., Holmes, G. S., and Davidson, L.: Endemic typhoid fever. Quart. J. Med., 159:341, 1971.

Woodward, T. E., and Smadel, J. E.: Management of typhoid fever and its complications. Ann. Intern. Med., 60:144, 1964.

153. SALMONELLA INFECTIONS OTHER THAN TYPHOID FEVER

Edward W. Hook

DEFINITION. The genus *Salmonella* consists of more than 1700 serotypes and variants. These organisms with a few exceptions are primary pathogens for animals that are readily transmitted to man. The outstanding exception is *S. typhi*, which is a parasite only of man and does not cause disease in lower animals in nature.

Human infection with *Salmonella* may be expressed as *acute gastroenteritis*, *enteric fever* (paratyphoid fever), *bacteremia*, or *localized metastatic infection* at almost any

site. The clinical syndromes resulting from *Salmonella* infection cannot always be sharply differentiated and sometimes overlap.

Transient *asymptomatic infection* of the intestinal tract is also common with most serotypes. A *chronic carrier state* may occur occasionally after infection with *Salmonella* other than *S. typhi*, and is characterized by prolonged excretion of the organism in feces or urine.

Typhoid fever is considered in a separate chapter (see Ch. 152) because of its historical identity, the host specificity of the pathogen, and the wealth of data on basic and clinical aspects of the disease. This separation is unrealistic to the extent that an illness closely resembling typhoid fever can result from infection with other salmonellae, and *S. typhi* can on occasion produce all the clinical syndromes described for the other *Salmonella* serotypes.

ETIOLOGY. Salmonellae are gram-negative, aerobic, nonsporing rods that grow readily on simple culture media. Presumptive identification of salmonellae involves relatively simple biochemical tests and agglutination reactions performed with group-specific antisera. The majority of strains isolated from man fall into groups A through E. Definitive identification of serotype depends on precise analysis of the somatic (O) and flagellar (H) antigens of the organism. Subdivision of certain serotypes, for example *S. typhimurium*, can be achieved by bacteriophage typing. Specific identification of all isolates is desirable, especially for epidemiologic reasons, and can be obtained through local, state, or federal health agencies.

Salmonella serotypes most frequently isolated from human infections in the United States during 1975 were, in descending order of frequency, *S. typhimurium*, *S. newport*, *S. enteritidis*, *S. heidelberg*, *S. agona*, *S. infantis*, *S. saint-paul*, *S. typhi*, *S. oranienburg*, and *S. javiana*. These ten serotypes accounted for about 70 per cent of the total *Salmonella* isolates from man during 1975. *S. typhimurium* is the serotype most frequently isolated year after year, usually accounting for 20 to 30 per cent of the total.

EPIDEMIOLOGY. Salmonellae are widespread among members of the Animal Kingdom in all parts of the world. Virtually all domestic and many wild animal species have been shown to harbor these organisms, and infection rates range from 1 per cent to more than 40 per cent. For example, in certain studies salmonellae have been isolated from 41 per cent of turkeys, 7 to 50 per cent of swine, and 24 per cent of apparently healthy cattle.

In 1975, 23,445 isolations of *Salmonella* from humans were reported in the United States. The annual incidence of reported isolations has remained approximately constant since 1963, the first full year of operation of the Salmonella Surveillance System in the United States. The true incidence of human salmonellosis is probably much higher than the number of reported cases. It is estimated that only about 1 per cent of cases are reported.

The prevalence of asymptomatic human carriers of salmonellae in the general population has been estimated to be about 0.2 per cent. The carrier state in the vast majority of these people is transient and probably represents persistence of organisms in the stools after asymptomatic or mild intestinal infection. The transient carrier state is more frequent in persons whose occupations provide opportunity for contact with *Salmonella* in foods, such as professional food processors or abattoir workers, than in the general population.

Man almost always acquires *Salmonella* infection by the oral route. Any item of food or drink can be contaminated directly or indirectly with viable bacilli from infected animals or man and can serve as a source of infection. Although the role of human carriers in the spread of salmonellosis must not be minimized, the majority of infections of man in the United States are related to the enormous reservoirs of salmonellae in lower animals.

The greatest single source of human disease is poultry products, including chickens, turkeys, ducks, and eggs. Other animal meats, especially pork, beef, and lamb, also serve as sources of infection. Salmonellae on meats or other foods contaminate utensils, tables, and other items in the processing plant, market, or kitchen, and may be transferred from these items to previously uninfected foods. A significant proportion (1 to 58 per cent) of raw meat purchased in retail markets is contaminated with salmonellae.

Eggs or egg products are common sources of *Salmonella* infection. The bacilli may be found on the external surface of the eggshell, between the shell and the shell membranes, or in yolks of eggs from hens with ovarian infection. The incidence of infection of eggs is low, but pooling of large numbers for freezing or drying increases the possibility of contamination of large quantities of materials. Prepared food mixtures containing dried eggs have been implicated many times in outbreaks of *Salmonella* infection.

Sterilization of contaminated foods is not always achieved by cooking. Viable salmonellae contaminating large birds such as turkeys, especially if the fowl is stuffed, may persist despite the baking process, and organisms in eggs occasionally survive frying, scrambling, or boiling in the shell.

The numerous byproducts of the meat-packing industry, such as bone meal, fertilizer, domestic animal food, and fish meal, often contain salmonellae and may serve as sources of infection, especially among lower animals. Finally, in considering potential sources of infection, household pets, including dogs, cats, birds, and turtles, should not be overlooked; all have been shown to harbor salmonellae.

Direct transmission from man to man without food as the intermediate source does occur. Transmission by person-to-person contact appears to be a relatively common mode of spread in hospital outbreaks, especially those occurring in nurseries or pediatric wards. For example, salmonellae may be introduced into a nursery by a newborn infected at birth from an infected mother and then spread to other babies by nursery attendants. Several nursery and hospital outbreaks have also been described in which infection appeared to be perpetuated by airborne spread of salmonellae.

S. choleraesuis bacteremia has been reported in immunologically compromised patients who received platelet transfusions from a donor with chronic intermittent bacteremia secondary to minimally symptomatic osteomyelitis.

The incidence of *Salmonella* infection shows a seasonal pattern. In the United States, the largest number of infections are reported in July through November and the smallest number in February through April. Children under two years of age have the highest incidence of infection.

PATHOLOGY. Death from *Salmonella* gastroenteritis occurs primarily in infants, the aged, and persons with underlying diseases. The intestinal mucosa is red and swollen and often shows petechial hemorrhages. The pathologic findings in paratyphoid fever are qualitatively similar to those of typhoid fever, although the involvement of Peyer's patches is less prominent and ulcerations are much less frequent. Intestinal lesions are usually absent in patients with *Salmonella* bacteremia, and the findings are similar to those of any acute generalized infection. Blood-borne salmonellae may localize in almost any organ, producing single or multiple suppurative lesions.

PATHOGENESIS. Multiplication of salmonellae in the intestinal tract is associated with invasion of mucosal cells of the small intestine, inflammation of the intestinal mucosa, and symptoms of gastroenteritis. Gastroenteritis is a true infection of the mucosa; ingestion of a large number of dead bacilli will not produce the disease. The mechanism of the production of diarrhea is unknown. However, certain salmonellae have been reported to cause ileal secretion in experimental infections by stimulating adenylate cyclase.

Salmonellae multiplying in the intestinal tract occasionally gain access to the blood, producing transient bacteremia or localized infections that can serve as sources of persistent bacteremia. The pathogenesis of enteric or paratyphoid fever is similar to that of typhoid fever.

The prevalence of salmonellae in foods for human consumption makes it almost inevitable that man come in contact with these organisms relatively frequently. The outcome of such exposures depends on many factors, especially the characteristics of the *Salmonella* serotype, the number of bacteria ingested, and the status of the host.

Almost every serotype of *Salmonella* has the capacity to produce asymptomatic infection, acute gastroenteritis, bacteremia with or without localized infection, or paratyphoid fever. However, some serotypes are much more likely to produce certain of these clinical syndromes than others. For example, *S. anatum* usually produces inapparent infection or gastroenteritis and only rarely invades the blood. In contrast, *S. choleraesuis* only occasionally produces gastroenteritis or inapparent infection but is a common cause of bacteremia or metastatic infection. Differences in pathogenicity are observed not only between serotypes but also between strains of the same serotype.

Limited information is available on the number of organisms required to produce salmonellosis in man. Experiments in volunteers suggest that a large number (approximately 10^5 to 10^6) of viable salmonellae are usually required to produce gastroenteritis in normal adults. However, several outbreaks have been described in which as few as 100 to 1000 cells were apparently responsible for illness. A transient carrier state may follow ingestion of inocula 10 or 100 times smaller than those required to produce disease.

The resistance of the host also plays a major role in determining the wide range of responses from no disease to rapidly fatal illness observed in human salmonellosis. Local factors in the stomach and intestine may be the first lines of defense. It is known that salmonellae are rapidly killed at a pH of 2, a level readily attained in the stomach, and that concomitant administration of certain antacids reduces the challenge dose of organisms required to initiate infection under experimental conditions. It has been established that major gastric surgery, including subtotal gastrectomy, gastroenterostomy, and/or vagotomy, predisposes to *Salmonella* gastroenteritis. The mechanism of this effect is unknown, but may be related to reduced bactericidal activity of gastric juice or altered intestinal flora. It has been shown in experimental *Salmonella* infections of mice that the microbial flora of the normal intestine exerts a protective action by suppressing multiplication of salmonellae. In these studies alteration of intestinal flora by antimicrobial drugs increased susceptibility to infection with S. *typhimurium* 100,000 times, and resistance was restored by re-establishing the normal enteric flora. Prior antimicrobial therapy also enhances susceptibility of man to symptomatic intestinal infection with salmonellae.

The incidence of severe *Salmonella* infections is increased in patients with certain underlying diseases. Another process, such as hepatic cirrhosis, lupus erythematosus, leukemia, lymphoma, or neoplasm, is present in one third to one half of patients with *Salmonella* bacteremia. These conditions are associated with a general depression of resistance to microbial invasion, and secondary infection is not unexpected. However, in a few diseases — acute bartonellosis, sickle cell anemia, and, perhaps, malaria — there appears to be a predisposition to infection with salmonellae that exceeds any general susceptibility to other bacterial species. The acute hemolytic phase of bartonellosis is complicated by the development of *Salmonella* bacteremia in as many as 40 per cent of cases. Patients with sickle cell anemia and other sickle hemoglobinopathies are unusually susceptible to invasion of the blood by *Salmonella*, and there is a strong tendency for localization of infection in bone. In fact, *Salmonella* species, not staphylococci, account for the vast majority of instances of osteomyelitis in patients with sickle cell anemia. Osteomyelitis is probably related to the localization of organisms in the areas of ischemia and necrosis of bone so common in sickle cell anemia; this is but one example of the striking tendency of salmonellae to localize at sites of pre-existing disease. Localization of salmonellae has been reported in vascular aneurysms, bone compressed by aortic aneurysms, hematomas, areas of infarction, and a variety of cysts and neoplasms.

CLINICAL MANIFESTATIONS. Salmonella Gastroenteritis. Symptoms of gastroenteritis develop 8 to 48 hours after ingestion of contaminated food. The relatively long incubation period represents the time required for multiplication and invasion by the organism. Nausea and vomiting are common initial manifestations and are rapidly followed by colicky abdominal pain and persistent diarrhea, occasionally with mucus or blood. Nausea and vomiting are rarely severe or protracted. An initial chill is not unusual, and fever of 38 to 39° C is common. Symptoms usually subside in two to five days, and recovery is uneventful.

Considerable variation in the severity of *Salmonella* gastroenteritis is observed, even among patients infected at the same meal. Some patients have a mild afebrile disease with a few loose stools, whereas others have high fever and 30 to 40 liquid stools per day. Severe diarrhea occasionally occurs in an afebrile patient. Abdominal pain may be intense, localized, and associated with rebound tenderness, suggesting appendicitis or some other acute intra-abdominal process. Symptoms of gastroenteritis persist in some patients for as long as two weeks. Active proctitis and colitis may occur and play a role in the tenesmus and small-volume bloody stools seen in some patients.

The leukocyte count is usually normal, and blood cultures are sterile in almost all cases. Stools of patients with diarrhea may contain large numbers of polymorphonuclear neutrophils. The causative organism can be isolated from the feces of almost all patients during the acute illness. About 50 per cent of the patients continue to have stool cultures positive for salmonellae at two weeks after onset of gastroenteritis, but only 15 per cent remain positive at the end of the fourth week. A small proportion of patients continue to excrete organisms after two months, but in most of these the cultures become negative in the next six months. The period of excretion of organisms in stool tends to be longer in infants than in older children or adults. The term "chronic enteric carrier" should be reserved for the patient shown to have persistently positive stools with the same *Salmonella* species for one or more years.

Enteric (Paratyphoid) Fever. Salmonellae other than S. *typhi* may produce an illness with all the features of typhoid fever, including prolonged sustained fever, respiratory and gastrointestinal symptoms, rose spots, leukopenia, and positive blood, stool, and urine cultures. Although paratyphoid fever may be clinically indistinguishable from typhoid fever, it is usually milder with a shorter course and a lower mortality rate. The organisms most likely to produce this syndrome are S. *paratyphi A*, S. *paratyphi B*, and S. *choleraesuis*. Paratyphoid fever is occasionally preceded by manifestations of *Salmonella* gastroenteritis.

Bacteremia. Salmonellae also produce a clinical syndrome that is characterized by chills, prolonged intermittent fever, anorexia, and weight loss. The characteristic features of typhoid or paratyphoid fever, such as rose spots, sustained fever, and leukopenia, are absent. Patients with this form of illness usually have no gastrointestinal complaints, and, indeed, stool cultures are usually negative for the causative organism despite its presence in blood. The leukocyte count is normal in most cases.

A prolonged febrile illness lasting weeks or months and characterized by weight loss, anemia, hepatosplenomegaly, and bacteremia with salmonellae, including S. *typhi*, has been described in South America and the Middle East in patients with schistosomiasis. The organisms apparently find a protected environment for multiplication within the gut of the worm. Eradication of the worms may also result in cure of the bacterial infection (see Ch. 210).

Localized Disease. Signs of localized infection appear in many cases of *Salmonella* bacteremia. Abscess formation may occur at almost any site, or bronchopneumonia, empyema, endocarditis, pericarditis, pyelonephritis, osteomyelitis, or arthritis may develop. Meningitis is a focal manifestation more common in newborns and infants than in adults. Patients with localized infections usually have striking polymorphonuclear leukocytosis as high as 20,000 to 30,000 cells per cubic millimeter of blood.

DIAGNOSIS. *Salmonella* gastroenteritis must be differentiated from other acute diarrheal diseases, especially shigellosis, invasive and enterotoxigenic *Escherichia coli* infection, staphylococcal food poisoning, and enteritis produced by *Vibrio parahaemolyticus, Yersinia enterocolitica,* and viral agents. A short incubation period, absence of fever, and prominence of nausea and vomiting are characteristic of staphylococcal food poisoning, whereas tenesmus, dysentery, and numerous fecal leukocytes suggest a diagnosis of shigellosis. However, differentiation on the basis of clinical information alone is difficult, especially in sporadic cases, and definitive diagnosis depends on isolation of the causative organism from the stool.

In patients with enteric fever, blood cultures are usually positive early in the course of the disease, and feces and urine become positive somewhat later. In patients with *Salmonella* bacteremia, the organisms can be isolated from blood, or in some cases from pus or exudate from localized infection.

Patients with salmonellosis may show during the course of illness a fourfold or greater increase in titer of agglutinins against the causative organism or closely related species. However, agglutination tests performed in the ordinary clinical laboratory are usually not helpful in diagnosis.

TREATMENT. The most important aspect of the management of patients with *Salmonella* gastroenteritis is prompt correction of dehydration and electrolyte disturbances. Diphenoxylate hydrochloride with atropine (Lomotil), paregoric, or small doses of morphine may be used to relieve abdominal cramps and diarrhea if contraindications do not exist. Some authorities feel that administration of such agents is not indicated. Inhibition of gut motility does enhance susceptibility to intestinal infection in laboratory animals. There is no convincing evidence that antimicrobial drugs, including chloramphenicol, ampicillin, or co-trimoxazole, reduce the duration of illness or the period of excretion of organisms in the stool. In fact, the period of excretion of salmonellae in the stool during convalescence after symptomatic intestinal infection is actually longer in patients who have been treated with antimicrobial drugs during the acute illness than in patients who have received no antimicrobial therapy.

In *Salmonella* bacteremia, paratyphoid fever, or localized infections of bones, joints, meninges, and other sites, chloramphenicol is the drug of choice and should be administered in divided doses of about 50 mg per kilogram per day for at least two weeks. Four to six days may be required for defervescence in favorable cases and even longer in patients with localized infection. In patients with localized infections, it may be necessary to continue antimicrobial therapy for four to six weeks, and surgical drainage of collections of pus may be required. Salmonellae persisting in tissues during chloramphenicol therapy may be responsible for relapse after the antimicrobial is discontinued. Relapse is not related to the emergence of chloramphenicol-resistant strains during therapy, and clinical response to a second or third course of therapy usually differs in no way from the first.

Ampicillin has also been shown to be effective in treating paratyphoid fever, but the response to ampicillin is slower than the response to chloramphenicol.

Ampicillin is also often effective in the treatment of other systemic *Salmonella* infections if the causative organism is susceptible to this drug. Ampicillin is preferred over chloramphenicol for patients requiring prolonged therapy. Ampicillin resistance is common among *Salmonella* serotypes. In a recent study in the United States, about 30 per cent of strains of *S. typhimurium, S. heidelberg,* and *S. newport* were found to be resistant to ampicillin. Resistance to the aminoglycosides, sulfonamides, or tetracyclines is also common, but resistance to chloramphenicol or co-trimoxazole is uncommon. Resistance is usually to multiple antimicrobials and is transferable by R-factors. Nosocomial outbreaks with serotypes resistant to ampicillin, chloramphenicol, and co-trimoxazole have been described.

Co-trimoxazole appears to be of some value in the therapy of enteric fever, but its relative position among effective antimicrobials has not been established at present.

Excretion of salmonellae in stool after clinical or subclinical infection ceases spontaneously in almost all patients; the convalescent carrier state is not an indication for antimicrobial therapy. Chronic enteric carriers of salmonellae other than *S. typhi* are managed as are typhoid carriers.

PROGNOSIS. The case fatality rate in *Salmonella* gastroenteritis rarely exceeds 1 or 2 per cent, and probably averages about 0.3 per cent. Fatalities occur almost entirely in infants, the aged, and persons with major underlying disease. The case fatality rate in the more serious systemic infections is high; it approaches 20 per cent in *S. choleraesuis* bacteremia.

PREVENTION. Every effort should be made to prevent the spread of salmonellae among the population by the excreta of patients with acute illness and convalescent or chronic carriers. Patients with acute illness should be isolated, and convalescent or chronic carriers should not be employed as food handlers and should practice strict personal hygiene.

The control of salmonellosis among animals and prevention of spread of infection to man present many problems. Progress is being made in developing methods of detection and control of salmonellosis in domestic animals and in improving hygienic conditions in food-processing and food-dispensing establishments.

Aserkoff, B., and Bennett, J. V.: Effect of therapy in acute salmonellosis on salmonellae in feces. N. Engl. J. Med., 281:636, 1969.

Bennett, I. L., Jr., and Hook, E. W.: Infectious diseases (some aspects of salmonellosis). Ann. Rev. Med., 10:1, 1959.

Center for Disease Control: Salmonella Surveillance Annual Summary, 1975. Issued September 1976, Atlanta, Georgia.

D'Aoust, J. Y., and Pivnick, H.: Small infectious doses of *Salmonella*. Lancet, 1:866, 1976.

Hornick, R. B.: *Salmonella* infections — newer perspectives of an old infection. Trans. Am. Clin. Climatol. Assoc., 85:164, 1973.

Lintz, D., Kapila, R., Pilgrim, E., Tecson, F., Dorn, R., and Louria, D.: Nosocomial *Salmonella* epidemic. Arch. Intern. Med., 136:968, 1976.

Musher, D. M., and Rubenstein, A. D.: Permanent carriers of nontyphosa salmonellae. Arch. Intern. Med., 132:869, 1973.

Neu, H. C., Cherubin, C. E., Longo, E. D., Flouton, B., and Winter, J.: Antimicrobial resistance and R-factor transfer among isolates of *Salmonella* in the northeastern United States. A comparison of human and animal isolates. J. Infect. Dis., 132:617, 1975.

Rhame, F. S., Root, R. K., MacLowry, J. D., Dadisman, T. A., and Bennett, J. V.: Salmonella septicemia from platelet transfusions. Study of an outbreak traced to a hematogenous carrier of *Salmonella choleraesuis*. Ann. Intern. Med., 78:633, 1973.

Wahab, M. F. A., Robertson, R. P., and Raasch, F. O.: Paratyphoid A fever. Ann. Intern. Med., 70:913, 1969.

OTHER BACTERIAL INFECTIONS

154. ENTERIC BACTERIAL INFECTIONS

Calvin M. Kunin

DEFINITION. The wide variety of microorganisms commonly found in the gastrointestinal tract, particularly the gram-negative, nonsporulating bacilli, have become increasingly important in clinical medicine. They are the principal organisms found in infections of the abdominal viscera, peritoneum, and urinary tract, as well as being frequent secondary invaders of the respiratory tract, burned or traumatized skin, and sites of decreased host resistance and instrumentation. Currently, they are the most frequent cause of life-threatening bacteremia. Infections with these organisms will be considered together because of their common habitat in the gut and on mucous surfaces, the similarity of epidemiologic and pathogenic characteristics, and the common approach used in diagnosis, treatment, and prevention.

BACTERIOLOGY. The gastrointestinal flora is exceedingly complex. The large intestine contains about 10^{10} to 10^{11} organisms per gram of contents. Of these, 90 to 95 per cent are obligate anaerobes. Most common are the gram-negative bacilli, *Bacteroides* and *Fusobacterium*, gram-positive bacilli, including *Bifidobacterium*, *Eubacterium*, and *Corynebacterium* species, and a wide variety of anaerobic streptococci. Other anaerobes include the gram-positive spore-forming rods of the clostridia species and gram-negative cocci, *Veillonella* (see Ch. 151). Enterococci are also present. The well-known aerobic gram-negative rods, which are members of the family Enterobacteriaceae, account for only 5 to 10 per cent of the total flora. These include the most common, *E. coli*, as well as the *Klebsiella-Enterobacter* group, *Proteus*, *Providencia*, *Edwardsiella*, *Serratia*, and, under pathologic conditions, *Salmonella* and *Shigella*. *Pseudomonas* is an entirely unrelated species, and is usually found in only small numbers in the bowel. Various yeasts are also found in lesser numbers in the normal large intestine.

Although the human gastrointestinal tract is usually considered to be colonized in the anatomic regions proximal to the cardia of the stomach and distal to the ileocecal valve, recent studies have demonstrated organisms in the jejunum and almost always in the ileum. Moderate changes in the diet do not affect the ratio of predominant bacteria in the feces, but antimicrobial therapy has a strong selective effect and is the single most important reason for the increasing emergence in human infection of these heretofore unusual organisms.

All the microorganisms of the gastrointestinal tract are potentially pathogenic under conditions of altered host resistance. The major diagnostic problem is to differentiate superficial colonization from actual tissue invasion.

ENDOTOXIN. The gram-negative bacteria of the gastrointestinal tract produce disease by invasion of tissue and by release of a pharmacologically active lipopolysaccharide from the cell wall, known as endotoxin. Endotoxins from a wide variety of unrelated species behave quite similarly, regardless of the inherent pathogenicity of the microorganism from which they are derived or their antigenic structure.

In the intact microorganism they exist as complexes of lipid, polysaccharide, and protein. The biologic activity seems to be a property of a lipid and carbohydrate portion. The cell wall of gram-negative bacteria may be roughly divided into three regions. The outermost region contains the chains of specific sugars which characterize the O-specific antigens and determine individual serotypes within a species. This is linked to a core polysaccharide which is of similar structure among related groups of bacteria. This is in turn linked through 2-keto-3-deoxyoctonate trisaccharides to the major lipid component termed lipid A. Evidence has now accumulated to indicate that all the properties of endotoxin may be accounted for by this complex lipid substance. Lipid A is a polymer containing glucosamine disaccharide units linked through pyrophosphate bridges and esterified with lauric, palmitic, and myristic acids. Perhaps the most important finding in recent years is that lipid A is immunogenic and will induce antibodies which cross-react among the gram-negative bacteria. Animal studies reveal that antibody prepared against the active component of endotoxin will protect against challenge from heterologous gram-negative bacteria; however, better protection is obtained by immunization with specific O antigens which induce opsonizing antibodies. The frequency of shock and death in patients with gram-negative bacteria appears to be lower in individuals with initially high titers of cross-reacting antibody to the Re or core lipopolysaccharide (lipid A) component. These findings hold promise for development of immunoprophylaxis and therapy.

When inoculated intravenously, the endotoxins cause fever, leukopenia, circulatory collapse, capillary hemorrhages, necrosis of tumors, and the Shwartzman phenomenon. Noteworthy is the remarkable tolerance that develops after repeated injections of endotoxin. For example, the first intravenous injection in man of as little as 0.01 ml of typhoid vaccine will give rise to a violent response, with chill and high fever; yet after 10 to 14 daily injections of increasing quantities, the subject can accept 25 ml or more without symptoms and with only a slight rise in temperature. This state of tolerance is not obviously dependent on specific antibodies; it extends to endotoxins of unrelated bacterial strains. The clinical features of gram-negative bacteremia resemble the reaction of laboratory animals or man to intravenous injection of purified endotoxic preparations, and may well represent a direct "pharmacologic" response to bacterial endotoxin. In other types of infectious process there is reason to doubt that such phenomena as fever, leukocytosis, and leukopenia are direct effects of endotoxin liberation.

The phenomenon of endotoxin tolerance may explain the remarkable tendency of the symptoms of pyelonephritis to subside spontaneously. By contrast, endotoxin tolerance is not a feature of experimental typhoid fever, but, rather, volunteers infected with this organism have been shown to be hypersensitive to its effects. Endotoxin tolerance is currently under intensive study because of the presumed important pathologic effect of this substance. The often conflicting observations on tolerance to the fever-producing property of endotoxin now appear to be due to the fact that multiple phenomena are operating simultaneously. Endotoxin is believed to be pyrogenic by inducing macrophages (monocytes, Kupffer and related cells) to release a protein, termed endogenous pyrogen. This protein is carried in the circulation to the temperature-regulating nuclei in the hypothalamus, producing an alteration in thermoregulation. Frequent, repeated doses of endotoxin are thought to exhaust the cells' capability of releasing this substance. More prolonged exposure is believed to induce antibodies which block the action of endotoxin.

ANTIBODIES. Antibodies reacting with most Enterobacteriaceae can be demonstrated in sera of normal animals and man, probably because of the continual production of antigen in the gastrointestinal tract. Gram-negative bacteria contain a wide variety of antigenic determinants. The best studied include the H or flagellar antigens which are heat-labile proteins present in motile strains. They have not been shown to be of pathogenetic significance. Some of the enteric bacteria contain K or capsular polysaccharides. They constitute the Vi antigens of *S. typhi* and are particularly prominent in *Klebsiella,* but are not confined to these groups. These surface slime layers interfere with phagocytosis and may be important in imparting virulence to encapsulated strains. They appear to account for invasiveness but not toxicity. *E. coli* K_1 capsular antigen, which is immunochemically identical to meningococcal Group B polysaccharide, appears to be the most important property of strains that are associated with neonatal meningitis. The K antigens also have been linked to invasiveness of *E. coli* in pyelonephritis. The Enterobacteriaceae share a common antigen (CA). Antibody to core lipopolysaccharide, described above, is currently thought to be the key determinant of resistance to endotoxin damage. Antibodies to the O or somatic antigens of *E. coli* have been most extensively studied. Very low titers are present in human newborns, presumably because they are mostly of the high molecular weight IgM variety, and do not readily pass the placenta. Human colostrum is rich in O antibody, but this is not absorbed during breast feeding. Colonization of the digestive tract, however, is soon accompanied by appearance of a wide variety of antibodies in serum, which contains virtually all the *E. coli* O antibodies by one year of age.

As a rule, most strains are susceptible to lysis by the combined effects of antibody and complement. Invasive strains are often found to be insusceptible to lysis in vitro. This system may be of great importance in preventing strains from invading and persisting in the blood.

TESTS FOR ENDOTOXEMIA. A remarkably sensitive test for endotoxemia has been developed, based on the finding that small amounts will cause gelation of lysates of amebocytes of the horseshoe crab. The test must be currently considered primarily as a research test, because, although it is commonly positive in gram-negative bacteremia, this is not always true, and a positive test does not correlate well with the outcome of infection. Since endotoxemia does not require living organisms, the test may be positive in the absence of detectable bacteremia.

THE ROLE OF ENTERIC BACTERIA IN PYOGENIC INFECTIONS OF THE ABDOMINAL CAVITY

The mixed flora of the intestinal tract participates in infections that originate from lesions of the bowel, such as appendicitis, cholangitis, diverticulitis, and perforation (from ulcerative colitis, ileitis, or carcinoma). These may lead to subdiaphragmatic, hepatic, and pelvic abscesses, which are frequent causes of fever of unknown origin in the patient recovering from abdominal surgery or trauma to this region. Because enteric bacteria grow luxuriantly in both aerobic and anaerobic media and therefore are likely to predominate in cultures, their relative importance tends to be exaggerated. There is good reason to believe that anaerobic bacteria — bacteroides, clostridia, and anaerobic streptococci — play important roles in this process. It should be pointed out here that a "fecal" odor of pus, though often ascribed to coliforms, is doubtless caused by associated anaerobic bacteria. Anaerobic bacteria are usually present as mixtures of two or more species. They should be suspected when there is foul pus and when organisms can be visualized microscopically but fail to grow under routine conditions.

OTHER INFECTIONS CAUSED BY THE ENTERIC BACTERIA

GASTROENTERITIS. A significant proportion of cases of gastroenteritis occurring in the neonatal period of life appear to be caused by *E. coli* as well as *Salmonella* and *Shigella.* Outbreaks of diarrhea among adults, particularly travelers abroad, have been associated with enterotoxigenic strains of *E. coli.* It was formerly thought that enteropathic *E. coli* were limited to a small number of serotypes. It is now clear that the pathogenetic properties of these strains are due to a surface factor that permits colonization and the ability to secrete one or both of two enterotoxins (a heat-labile protein resembling that of *V. cholerae* or a heat-stable toxin). These properties may be transmitted by plasmids to other *E. coli.* Thus the presence of a common serotype in an outbreak is more likely to be an epidemiologic marker than to denote virulence. Sporadic epidemics with invasive strains have been reported after ingestion of imported cheese. Certain strains of *Proteus* and *Pseudomonas* have at times also been held responsible for similar illness.

MENINGITIS AND BRAIN ABSCESS. During the first four weeks of life, purulent meningitis is frequently caused by members of the enteric group of bacteria. Such cases occur sporadically in nurseries, and may be associated with infection of any other tissue of the body (see discussion of K antigens, above). Infants with meningoceles are especially liable to enteric bacterial meningitis. In adults, such infections are rare, but may occasionally be seen as complications of gram-negative bacteremia or in association with other diseases affecting host resistance, e.g., diabetes mellitus or lymphoma (see Ch. 140). Nontraumatic brain abscess is frequently due to infection by multiple species of anaerobic organisms similar to those found in the gastrointestinal tract. The sites of origin include chronically infected ears, sinuses, lung, abdomen, and pelvis.

BACTEREMIA IN HEPATIC CIRRHOSIS. Occasionally persons with cirrhosis of the liver develop an acute febrile illness and are found to have bacteremia caused by one of the enteric organisms, usually *E. coli.* Occasionally patients with ascites develop "spontaneous" peritonitis, but in most of these cases the bacteremia comes "out of the blue" without evidence of localized sepsis anywhere. The illness is short and self-limited or responds to appropriate chemotherapy. Speculation as to its pathogenesis has included the possibility of shunting bacteria away from the filtering action of the liver, impairment of humoral or cellular defense mechanisms, or complement inactivation owing to high blood ammonia. In actuality a satisfactory explanation is lacking at present.

SURFACE INFECTION. Enteric bacteria, particularly *Proteus* and *Pseudomonas,* are commonly recovered from the surfaces of burns, varicose ulcers, decubitus ulcers, tracheostomy sites, and the like. Generally, these organisms appear to play no pathogenic role, and satisfactory healing may proceed regardless of their presence. They can at times result in fulminant gram-negative sepsis, particularly in the patient with severe burns. The exudate from the sinus of a chronic osteomyelitis or chronic otitis media often contains *Proteus* as the dominant organism. Otitis of the external auditory canal owing to *Pseudomonas* may give troublesome local symptoms, especially in swimmers.

PERIRECTAL ABSCESS. Perirectal abscess is an important complication in patients with marked granulocytopenia. Rectal examination should be carefully performed in such patients, particularly when they develop fever and perianal pain.

ABSCESSES AT SITES OF SUBCUTANEOUS INJECTIONS. Rarely, enteric bacilli cause abscesses in subcutaneous tissue at sites of hypodermic injections, notably in diabetic subjects who inject their own insulin. These are sometimes characterized by gas formation, and they thus arouse fear of more serious clostridial infection, whereas, in fact, they are usually of minor clinical importance.

METASTATIC INFECTIONS. Despite the frequency with which enteric bacteria succeed in invading the blood, metastatic localization of infection is rare. There are, however, occasional instances of such suppurative lesions as arthritis and panophthalmitis in patients with bacteremia originating in acute pyelonephritis. Of special interest in this regard is osteomyelitis of the spine. This is usually seen in men with prostatic disease, chronic cystitis, and posterior urethritis. Possibly the method of spread here is by way of septic emboli to the spine through the vertebral venous plexus.

SUPERINFECTION. Enteric bacteria frequently predominate in the bronchial secretions of patients who are chronically ill or are treated with antimicrobial agents. In most instances, this is not of significance and simply represents emergence of bacterial strains after the suppression of the primary pathogens. Transtracheal aspiration, followed by Gram stain and culture of the secretions, is a useful method to distinguish between colonization of the pharynx versus true infection of the lower respiratory tract. Pharyngeal colonization is not an indication for antimicrobial therapy unless there is clinical evidence of tissue invasion by the newly emergent organism. Primary gram-negative bacterial pneumonia often superimposed on viral influenza, however, does occur and may be exceedingly difficult to manage.

GRAM-NEGATIVE BACTEREMIA

Bacteremia caused by gram-negative bacilli has become a problem of greater relative importance since the advent of penicillin and better control of gram-positive coccal infections. Urinary tract infection accounts for about one half of all cases of blood invasion by the enteric bacteria. Other causes include surgical disease of the gastrointestinal tract, infections developing at the site of "cut-downs" and intravenous catheters, postpartum or postabortal sepsis (including the so-called "placental bacteremia"), and infection of wounds, ulcers, burns, and internal prosthetic devices such as heart valves. Sometimes there is a clearly apparent precipitating factor such as cystoscopy, surgical or obstetrical procedure, or manipulation of an infected wound.

These bacteremias have clinical characteristics closely resembling the recognized biologic effects of gram-negative bacterial endotoxins. Onset of symptoms may occur with a shaking chill and rise in temperature to 38 to 40.5° C. There is an initial leukopenia, but after 6 to 12 hours usually there is leukocytosis. An *important and highly significant accompaniment is circulatory embarrassment with lowering of the blood pressure.* This may be manifested only by some alteration in the patient's state of consciousness, and the skin may continue to feel warm, although sometimes the skin is cold and clammy. Occasionally patients slip into a shocklike state without much elevation of temperature; hence infection of this kind must always be taken into consideration in evaluation of peripheral circulatory failure. Some patients, however, do develop the syndrome of disseminated intravascular coagulation (DIC). This phenomenon is not unique to gram-negative bacteremia and may be due to such diverse causes as rickettsial and gram-positive bacterial infections. The most common findings are reduced platelet count, low factor V levels in plasma, and fibrin split products in serum. Serum complement is low only in the most seriously ill patients (see Ch. 140). With so-called "gram-negative shock" there is diminution in urine output, increase in proteinuria, and often a rise in nonprotein nitrogen of the blood. The cardiac output may be unpredictably low, normal, or elevated. Some patients show shifts in acid-base balance in the direction of metabolic acidosis, whereas others have compensatory hyperventilation. The pH of the blood, however, often remains normal. Lactic acidosis is common in severely ill patients. It is characterized by a marked anion gap with low levels of both serum bicarbonate and Pco_2. These findings are often confusing, particularly if they occur in patients with complicating problems such as pulmonary or renal insufficiency or congestive heart failure. Serum lactate levels are helpful in sorting out these factors. Much depends on the nature of the underlying disease and the renal reserve. The outlook is grave, being influenced by age, associated disease, and evidence of shock. When obvious signs of circulatory collapse are present, the fatality rate may be as high as 75 per cent.

UNIQUE FEATURES OF PSEUDOMONAS INFECTIONS

Pseudomonas infections, although often similar to those caused by other gram-negative bacteria, sometimes have unique characteristics. As already mentioned, this organism frequently appears in necrotic tissue, as in ulcers, burns, or draining sinuses. Usually such colonization is of little clinical significance, and mere removal of necrotic tissue may cause it to disappear. Nevertheless, under certain circumstances, especially in chronically debilitated persons or in patients with agranulocytosis or acute leukemia, severe sepsis may be produced by this class of bacteria. In addition to endotoxin, *Pseudomonas aeruginosa* produces several enzymes, including collagenase, proteases, elastase, and a recently described exotoxin (PA toxin) whose mode of action is similar to that of diphtheria toxin.

Pseudomonas is notoriously resistant to antimicrobial therapy; hence it tends to emerge as the dominant microorganism after eradication of other bacteria by drugs. It may then be responsible for the phenomenon of superinfection, as in the bronchopulmonary infections that may complicate prophylactic chemotherapy of chronic lung disease.

Because *Pseudomonas* commonly occurs in tap water, and because it may be resistant to antiseptics used in sterilizing instruments, it is likely to be carried into the body by such procedures as cystoscopy. Furthermore, meningitis after lumbar puncture has been associated with this organism.

Tissue invasion, most often seen in patients with leukopenia or relapse in leukemia, is characterized by necrotizing vasculitis with bacterial invasion of the walls of arteries and veins. This leads to a distinctive necrotic skin lesion (called ecthyma gangrenosum) that is found most commonly along the axillary folds or in the anogenital area, but may also develop on any part of the body. It may begin as a vesicle that later becomes necrotic. The typical lesion of ecthyma gangrenosum is a round, indurated ulcer with a black center that varies from a few millimeters to several centimeters in diameter.

TREATMENT OF ENTERIC BACTERIAL INFECTIONS

GENERAL PRINCIPLES. The major clinical problems in management of enteric bacterial infections are (1) differentiation of superficial contamination that often requires no treatment from true or potential tissue invasion, (2) early recognition and drainage of abscesses, (3) anticipation of the role of anaerobic bacteria that cannot be readily cultured, and (4) early recognition of bacteremic shock. *Many of these infections are preventable,* particularly those arising from instrumentation of the urinary tract, intravenous catheters and contaminated fluids, suction, and ventilation equipment. *Every physician must consider elimination of such sources of contamination as one of his prime responsibilities.*

GRAM-NEGATIVE BACTEREMIA. The presence of gram-negative organisms in the blood should alert the physician to search for a site of origin such as intravenous or urinary catheters and abdominal, pelvic, or perirectal abscesses. Removal of devices and drainage of abscesses should be done as soon as possible. It should be remembered that gram-negative bacteremia is more common than is usually suspected and is often transient and without complication. For example, bacteremia may occur after gastrointestinal endoscopy, urinary instrumentation, and manipulation of the bowel during surgery. These events often go undetected, or there is a single temperature rise and no further complications. Antimicrobial therapy probably plays little role in management of these transient episodes. The main problem is caused by the release of endotoxin, which is not affected by antimicrobial drugs. Judgment will therefore have to be made to determine whether there is an infected site which requires treatment.

The site of origin of the infection, the underlying illness of the patient, and prior receipt of antimicrobial agents are key determinants in planning therapy. The response to antimicrobial agents and the mortality from gram-negative bacteremia are closely related to whether the patient has rapidly fatal, ultimately fatal, or nonfatal underlying diseases. Consequently, the nature and status of the underlying disease is a major determinant in selecting appropriate treatment. The treatment must often be begun in the rapidly and ultimately fatal group before organisms are isolated and their drug susceptibility patterns are determined.

In rapidly fatal conditions (severe leukopenia, acute leukemia, extensive burns, and immunosuppressed patients), gram-negative bacteremia often occurs in hospital settings where there are organisms with multiple-drug resistance such as *Pseudomonas, Klebsiella, Serratia, Providencia,* and *Proteus.* In the febrile patient, after obtaining blood and other cultures from suspected sites of infection, therapy should be begun with an aminoglycoside (gentamicin, tobramycin, or amikacin) and either carbenicillin or ticarcillin. The addition of a parenteral or antistaphylococcal agent such as a penicillinase-resistant penicillin (methicillin, oxacillin, or nafcillin) or cephalosporin (cephalothin, cefazolin, or cephapirin) should also be considered. The choice of a specific aminoglycoside drug, such as amikacin, will depend on whether the hospital has a high frequency of endemic strains resistant to gentamicin or tobramycin. Once the organism is isolated from the blood or suspected site of infection, therapy should be altered, if needed, to the most appropriate, least toxic agent(s).

In ultimately fatal conditions (severe obstructive pulmonary disease, end-stage renal failure, obstructive uropathy, or carcinomatosis), there is usually a determinable site of infection. After obtaining blood and other cultures of the suspected site (transtracheal aspiration, urinary catheterization, thoracentesis, paracentesis, lumbar puncture, subcutaneous aspiration of an abscess) and gram-negative bacilli are seen on Gram stain in association with polymorphonuclear leukocytes, therapy should be begun. Until drug susceptibility tests are available, treatment should be started with an aminoglycoside drug as described above. Gram-negative meningitis often requires intrathecal injection of aminoglycosides. When *Klebsiella* is strongly suspected (such as in pneumonia), a cephalosporin may be added. When anaerobic organisms are suspected in the lower respiratory tract, penicillin should be added; when they are suspected in the abdomen, pelvis, or anogenital area, clindamycin or chloramphenicol should be added. Once drug susceptibility data are available, therapy may be changed to the most appropriate agent(s).

In nonfatal conditions, such as urinary tract infections, osteomyelitis, cholecystitis, or abdominal, pelvic, or wound infections in an otherwise healthy patient, therapy will depend on the urgency of the patient's condition, the most likely invasive organism, and the local pattern of drug susceptibility to common organisms, such as *E. coli.* In the acutely ill hospitalized patient, a parenteral form of an aminoglycoside or cephalosporin or ampicillin may be used. Clindamycin or chloramphenicol should be added in abdominal, pelvic, or decubitus infections when anaerobes are suspected. Acute cholecystitis is usually associated with *E. coli* and may be treated with ampicillin, tetracycline, or a cephalosporin. Acute urinary infections are most likely to respond to oral agents such as co-trimoxazole or nitrofurantoin. Alternative agents, such as ampicillin, tetracycline, nalidixic acid, a sulfonamide, or an oral cephalosporin may be used, depending on drug susceptibility tests. *Pseudomonas* infections occurring in nonfatal conditions often can be treated with an aminoglycoside antimicrobial when the organism is susceptible. Carbenicillin or ticarcillin need only be added or used when the organism is resistant to an aminoglycoside or when the patient has severe renal failure or fails to respond to other agents. Oral carbenicillin should be reserved for treatment of *Pseudomonas* urinary infections outside the hospital because of the danger of selecting resistant organisms. *Antimicrobial therapy is ineffective for more than a few days in the patient with an indwelling urinary catheter and should be reserved for acute episodes of sepsis.*

Management of bacteremic shock is complex, requiring corrective measures designed to improve cardiac function, tissue perfusion, and electrolyte imbalance, particularly acidosis. This requires monitoring of the central venous pressure by a well-placed catheter in the superior vena cava or right atrium in an attempt to achieve a pressure of about 8 to 12 cm of water, and following the dynamics of pressure changes as fluid replacement is given. Replacement fluids include blood, dextran, and saline solutions. Drugs such as dopamine may be used to increase cardiac output and improve tissue perfusion; vasopressors such as metaraminol should be used sparingly except in severe shock. High doses of corticosteroids are widely used, but their efficacy has not been established by controlled studies. Heparin may be useful in the syndrome of disseminated intravascular coagulation (see Ch. 356).

Finegold, S. M.: Anaerobic Bacteria in Human Disease. New York, Academic Press, 1977.

Fried, M. A., and Vosti, K. L.: Importance of underlying disease in patients with gram-negative bacteremia. Arch. Intern. Med., 121:418, 1968.

Mangi, R. J., Quintiliani, R., and Andriole, V. T.: Gram-negative bacillary meningitis. Am. J. Med., 59:829, 1975.

Young, L. S., Martin, W. J., Meyer, R. D., Weinstein, R. J., and Anderson, E. T.: Gram-negative rod bacteremia: Microbiologic, immunologic and therapeutic considerations. Ann. Intern. Med., 86:456, 1977.

155. SHIGELLOSIS

Charles C. J. Carpenter

DEFINITION. Shigellosis is a specific acute bacterial infection of the intestinal tract of man, with predominant involvement of the distal colon, sigmoid, and rectum, caused by bacteria of the genus *Shigella*. It most commonly presents as a clinically nonspecific diarrhea. In the more severe cases, the initial mild diarrhea is accompanied by fever and followed by true dysentery, with cramping abdominal pains, tenesmus, and frequent stools in which mucus, leukocytes, and erythrocytes are abundant.

ETIOLOGY. Shigellae (dysentery bacilli) are nonmotile, gram-negative, rod-shaped bacilli belonging to the family Enterobacteriaceae. Four species of shigellae are recognized, based on antigenic and biochemical properties: *S. dysenteriae* (Group A), *S. flexneri* (Group B), *S. boydii* (Group C), and *S. sonnei* (Group D). Among these species there are 39 serotypes, each of which is designated by the species name followed by a specific Arabic number. With the exception of *S. flexneri* 6, they do not ferment lactose. The most common species in the United States until 1965 was *S. flexneri*, but this species has now largely been replaced by *S. sonnei*. *S. sonnei* is now the most commonly reported shigella in Western Europe and Japan, as well as North America. *S. boydii* is so rarely encountered in the United States that its isolation usually indicates exposure during foreign travel. *S. dysenteriae*, the most virulent shigella, is now unusual in the more developed countries, but is currently prevalent in Central America.

EPIDEMIOLOGY. Incidence and Prevalence. Despite generally high standards of hygiene in the United States, there were over 16,000 cases of shigellosis reported to the Center for Disease Control in 1976. *S. sonnei* was the predominant etiologic agent, and the great majority of patients were children. The few cases caused by *S. dysenteriae* could generally be traced to contact with individuals from infected areas in Central America. The true incidence is undoubtedly severalfold higher than the number of reported cases.

The same general pattern of infection has been observed throughout Western Europe and Japan in the past ten years. In Eastern Europe and Russia, where the over-all incidence of shigellosis is greater, *S. flexneri* has continued to be the predominant microorganism. *S. flexneri* is also the most commonly isolated species in most of the economically underdeveloped nations of the world. *S. dysenteriae* 1 (Shiga bacillus), which has nearly disappeared as a major cause of dysentery in most parts of the world, re-emerged as a major epidemic problem throughout Central America from 1969 to 1973; imported cases of dysentery caused by the Shiga bacillus continue to be reported sporadically from the southwestern United States.

Spread of Infection. Shigellosis is found throughout the world. Although seasonal patterns vary in different regions, the incidence of shigellosis characteristically peaks in the late summer and early autumn in the United States. Man remains the only known reservoir of *Shigella* infection. During clinical illness and for a variable period (up to six weeks) following recovery, shigellae excreted in the stools may be transmitted to other persons. Although the organisms are quite sensitive to desiccation, they may survive for long periods in foods and water. Transmission most often occurs by close person-to-person contact involving contaminated hands. Children in the one- to four-year age group are at highest risk of developing shigellosis, and young males are affected more often than young females. In young adults the incidence is higher in women than in men, probably reflecting the fact that many young adult women are in close contact with ill children, either in the home or in an institutional setting. Intrafamilial spread is especially likely to occur when the initial case has occurred in a preschool child. Attack rates in affected families range from 10 to 80 per cent.

Custodial institutions, especially those caring for the retarded, are frequent settings for large epidemics. Because of the difficulty in maintaining adequate hygiene among residents in these settings, endemic shigellosis is often a nearly intractable problem. Up to 30 per cent of admissions to certain custodial institutions experience an episode of shigellosis within a year of arrival. Nursery schools and day care centers, because of the young age group and the close contact of the populations, have especially high attack rates whenever shigellae are introduced.

Since shigellae are transmitted primarily by the fecal-oral route, crowded living conditions, poor housing, poor water supply, and inadequate sewage facilities all correlate significantly with increased risk of infection. Therefore, within the United States, the urban ghetto areas and Indian reservations are settings in which incidence of shigellosis is excessively high. By the same token, rural villages in the economically underdeveloped nations are areas of high rates of shigellosis. The recent pandemic spread of S. dysenteriae 1 (Shiga bacillus) from Guatemala and El Salvador throughout Central America and Mexico was a matter of grave concern. This pandemic has, however, subsided without major spread to either South America or the United States. As has been true of pandemics in the past, the reason for the development of the 1969–1973 Central American Shiga bacillus pandemic remains obscure.

PATHOGENESIS AND PATHOPHYSIOLOGY. Although moderately resistant to acid, shigellae have less difficulty than other enteric pathogens in passing the human gastric barrier. In volunteer studies, as few as 200 ingested bacilli regularly initiate disease in 25 per cent of healthy volunteers. This contrasts strikingly with the much larger numbers of typhoid bacilli and the strikingly greater number of cholera bacilli which must be ingested to produce disease in man. During the incubation period, which is usually 36 to 72 hours, the organisms traverse the small bowel and proliferate in the lower ileum and colon. In the colon shigellae reach concentrations of 10^6 to 10^{10} organisms per gram of stool. Unlike the case with certain other enteric pathogens (V. cholerae and enterotoxigenic E. coli), epithelial cell penetration is essential to the pathogenesis of shigellosis. Multiplication of bacteria occurs within the epithelial cells of the colon, predominantly in the villi, and this is followed by an acute inflammatory response in the subjacent lamina propria. This results in destruction of the villous tips, distortion of the mucosal architecture, and the formation of superficial microabscesses. In the more severe cases, long segments of colon may be affected with a diffuse inflammatory process which,

however, remains confined to the lamina propria. The altered mucosa is friable and is covered with an exudate of polymorphonuclear leukocytes. Stool therefore contains large numbers of erythrocytes and leukocytes. Since the inflammation is superficial, bacteremia is rare and colonic perforation seldom occurs as a complication of shigellosis.

S. dysenteriae and certain strains of S. flexneri and S. sonnei produce an enterotoxin which causes secretion of isotonic fluid by the small bowel. The role of this enterotoxin in the pathogenesis of clinical shigellosis is not certain, but it has been suggested that the enterotoxin is responsible for the mild watery diarrhea which often precedes full-blown bacillary dysentery. It is possible that the enterotoxin is entirely responsible for the clinical manifestations in those mild cases characterized by only short-lived, nonbloody diarrhea.

CLINICAL MANIFESTATIONS. Shigellosis is often a biphasic disease, beginning with cramping abdominal pain and watery diarrhea, sometimes accompanied by fever (up to 40° C) and generalized myalgias. Fluid and electrolyte losses are greatest during this phase of the illness; such losses are rarely voluminous enough to be life threatening except in very young children and in the elderly. This first phase usually lasts for one to three days; in the more severely ill patients, it is followed by a second phase, which, in the absence of treatment, may last for weeks. The second phase is that of true dysentery; the character of the stool changes with a decrease in the quantity of each bowel movement and the appearance of bright red blood and mucus in the feces. During this phase, tenesmus may become a vexing feature, and anorexia and weight loss are common. Fever is not prominent during the second phase of the illness.

It is important to emphasize that many patients who are infected with shigellae, especially S. sonnei, are entirely asymptomatic, and an additional large number simply have mild cramping abdominal pain and watery diarrhea which cannot clinically be differentiated from the illnesses caused by several other microorganisms. Only the more severe cases, presenting with the classic bacillary dysentery pattern, can readily be diagnosed clinically as shigellosis. Of the Shigella strains now encountered in the United States, S. dysenteriae is the most virulent and by far the least common. S. flexneri is intermediate in both virulence and frequency, and S. sonnei, which accounts for 80 per cent of cases in the United States, presents the mildest clinical picture.

The onset of shigellosis is often more fulminant in children, who may present with unexplained high fever with or without convulsions. Neurologic symptoms and signs, including delirium, headache, nuchal rigidity, and lethargy, rarely occur in adults, but are quite common in children in the one- to four-year age group. Roughly 25 per cent of children hospitalized for shigellosis experience convulsions. The basis for the convulsions is unknown; it seems unlikely that the neurologic manifestations are caused by Shigella neurotoxin, as similar neurologic manifestations may be seen in children with salmonellosis.

DIAGNOSIS. Shigellosis should be considered in any patient with the acute onset of fever and diarrhea. Diagnosis is more likely, however, in the high-risk groups delineated above. Examination of the stool is quite useful in the diagnosis. Blood, pus, and mucus may be seen grossly in severe bacillary dysentery; even in milder forms of the disease, microscopic examination of the stool reveals numerous leukocytes and erythrocytes. The fecal leukocyte examination should be performed with a portion of liquid stool, preferably containing mucus. A drop of stool is placed on a microscopic slide and mixed thoroughly with two drops of methylene blue solution. A cover slip is placed over the mixture for microscopic examination. The presence of abundant polymorphonuclear leukocytes helps in distinguishing shigellosis from salmonellosis (in which leukocytes are present but are predominantly mononuclear) and from diarrheal syndromes caused by enterotoxigenic *E. coli* and *Vibrio cholerae* (in which fecal leukocytes are characteristically absent). The peripheral white cell count is of little diagnostic value, in that the white cell count may range from less than 3000 to more than 30,000, with a mean value in the high-normal range. Sigmoidoscopic examination characteristically reveals diffuse erythema and a friable mucosa, with shallow ulcers which are characteristically 3 to 7 mm in diameter.

Definitive diagnosis depends on isolating shigellae by use of selective media. A rectal swab, a swab of a colonic ulcer obtained by sigmoidoscopic examination, or a freshly passed stool specimen should be inoculated immediately on culture plates or into carrying media. If a delay of more than a few hours is anticipated before appropriate culture media are available, the stool should be placed in a buffered glycerol-saline solution for preservation. Since isolation rates of shigellae from freshly passed stools of patients known to have shigellosis may be as low as 67 per cent, culturing for three successive days is recommended in order to maximize the chance of isolation. Stool cultures are generally positive within 24 hours after the onset of symptoms and may remain positive for several weeks in the absence of antimicrobial therapy. Blood cultures are so rarely positive as to be of no diagnostic value.

Appropriate culture media include blood, desoxycholate, and salmonella-shigella (S-S) agars. Selected colonies suggestive of shigellae should be placed on triple sugar-iron agar and lysine-iron agar. Colonies showing an alkaline slant and acid butt without gas or hydrogen sulfide in either agar should be definitively diagnosed by agglutination with polyvalent shigella antisera. It is important to recognize that the commonly used S-S agar is inhibitory for the most virulent of the *Shigella* species, *S. dysenteriae* 1.

Definitive bacteriologic diagnosis becomes of critical importance in distinguishing the more severe and prolonged cases of shigellosis from ulcerative colitis, with which it may be confused both clinically and by sigmoidoscopic examination. Occasional patients with shigellosis have been subjected to colectomy with the mistaken diagnosis of ulcerative colitis; a positive culture for shigellae could clearly prevent such a therapeutic misadventure.

TREATMENT. The three steps in the treatment of shigellosis include correction of fluid and electrolyte balance, antimicrobial therapy, and symptomatic relief. Although voluminous diarrhea is unusual in shigellosis, fluid loss may be lethal in the very young and the very old. Fluid losses in shigellosis are qualitatively similar to those in other bacterial diarrheal diseases, and the patient should be treated with appropriate in-

travenous fluids (lactated Ringer's solution is a generally available and adequate solution) in quantities adequate to correct clinical signs of saline depletion. The requirement for intravenous fluids is generally brief, but will be lifesaving in exceptional cases.

The efficacy of antimicrobial agents in treating shigellosis has been well established. Although infections with *Shigella sonnei, flexneri,* and *boydii* are generally self-limited except in the very young and very old, appropriate antimicrobial therapy may decrease the duration of symptoms by 50 per cent and decrease the duration of excretion of shigellae (an important epidemiologic factor) by a far greater percentage. Infection by *S. dysenteriae* 1 may result in a 10 to 20 per cent mortality rate in the absence of antimicrobial therapy, and appropriate antimicrobials are therefore mandatory with this pathogen. Ampicillin is currently the drug of choice for shigellosis in the United States. It should be administered orally in four divided doses for a total of 2 grams a day to adults and 100 mg per kilogram per day to children for a five-day period. Because of the increasing frequency of plasmid-mediated antimicrobial resistance to *Shigella* infections, drug susceptibility testing is important. For patients with ampicillin-resistant isolates, tetracycline is sometimes effective. It is important to recognize that certain drugs which appear effective in vitro, especially orally administered, nonabsorbable antimicrobials such as neomycin or kanamycin, are *not* effective in vivo, and that sulfonamide resistance is so widespread as to nullify the value of these chemotherapeutic agents when used alone. However, cotrimoxazole is an alternative drug to which significant resistance has not yet been demonstrated.

Agents which decrease intestinal motility should *not* be used. Such preparations as diphenoxylate and paregoric may exacerbate symptoms, presumably by retarding intestinal clearance of the microorganisms. There is no convincing evidence that the pectin- or bismuth-containing preparations are of any positive value.

PROGNOSIS. The mortality rate in untreated shigellosis is dependent upon the infectious strain, and ranges from greater than 20 per cent in certain outbreaks of infection caused by *S. dysenteriae* 1 to less than 1 per cent in many outbreaks caused by *S. sonnei*. Even with infection caused by *S. dysenteriae* 1, the mortality rate should approach zero if appropriate fluid replacement and antimicrobial therapy are initiated early in the course of the disease.

PREVENTION. Individuals excreting shigellae, whether symptomatic or not, should be excluded from all phases of food-handling until cultures of stool specimens collected on three consecutive days, after antimicrobial therapy has been discontinued, are reported as negative. In outbreaks in custodial institutions or day care centers, strict and early separation of those with illness from those who are unaffected is mandatory. Targeted antimicrobial chemoprophylaxis in this setting has generally been disappointing. The most important control measure is scrupulous handwashing by all individuals involved in handling food.

Recognition, reporting, and investigation of epidemics in schools and institutions remain important, and reporting of shigellosis cases to health authorities should be considered mandatory.

For the traveler to countries with major *Shigella* problems, no chemoprophylactic agent is an adequate substitute for good personal hygiene and the avoidance of contaminated water, fruits, and vegetables. No effective vaccine is yet available.

DuPont, H. L., and Hornick, R. B.: Adverse effect of Lomotil therapy in shigellosis. JAMA, 226:1525, 1973.

DuPont, H. L., Hornick, R. B., Dawkins, A. T., Snyder, M. J., and Formal, S. B.: The response of man to virulent *Shigella flexneri* 2a. J. Infect. Dis., 119:296, 1969.

Haltalin, K. C., Kusmiesz, H. T., Hinton, L. V., and Nelson, J. D.: Treatment of acute diarrhea in outpatients. Am. J. Dis. Child., 124:554, 1972.

Harris, J. C., DuPont, H. L., and Hornick, R. B.: Fecal leukocytes in diarrheal illness. Ann. Intern. Med., 76:697, 1972.

Keusch, G. T., and Jacewicz, M.: The pathogenesis of *Shigella* diarrhea. VI. Toxin and antitoxin in *Shigella flexneri* and *Shigella sonnei* infections in humans. J. Infect. Dis., 135:552, 1977.

Neisman, J. B., Martin, K. I., Lewis, J. N., Friedman, C. T. H., and Gangarosa, E. J.: Impact in the United States of the Shiga dysentery pandemic of Central America and Mexico; a review of the surveillance data through 1972. J. Infect. Dis., 128:574, 1973.

Ogawa, H.: Experimental approach in studies on pathogenesis of bacillary dysentery — with special reference to the invasion of bacilli into intestinal mucosa. Acta Pathol., 20:261, 1970.

156.   CHOLERA

(Asiatic Cholera)

Charles C. J. Carpenter

DEFINITION.   Cholera is an acute specific infectious disease of man caused by *Vibrio cholerae*. All manifestations of the disease are caused by an enterotoxin elaborated by *Vibrio cholerae* which have colonized the small bowel of the susceptible individual. In its most severe form the disease is characterized by voluminous diarrhea, with rapid loss of fluid and electrolytes from the gastrointestinal tract, resulting in hypovolemic shock, metabolic acidosis, and, if untreated, death. Cholera is endemic in the Gangetic Delta of the Indian subcontinent, and has been responsible for seven major pandemics during the past 150 years.

ETIOLOGY.   In his classic study in 1857, John Snow carefully described an outbreak of cholera in London, and clearly incriminated contaminated water as the source of the disease. In 1883, Koch identified *Vibrio cholerae* as the etiologic agent of this disease by identifying this microorganism in the feces of large numbers of patients with cholera. *Vibrio cholerae* are short (0.2 to 0.4 μm by 1.5 to 4.0 μm), slightly curved, gram-negative rods and may readily be seen in the gram-stained smears of the watery excreta of patients with cholera. Vibrios grow aerobically on a variety of nutrient media at 37° C, preferentially at an alkaline pH. There are two biotypes of *Vibrio cholerae*, the "classic" and the eltor. The eltor biotype is hardier than the classic strain, persists longer in nature, and is more likely to cause a carrier state in man; the eltor biotype can be readily distinguished from the classic biotype by its resistance to polymyxin B. The distinction between the two biotypes is important for epidemiologic purposes. *Vibrio cholerae* can be differentiated from noncholera vibrios by antigenic and fermentative reactions, as well as by biologic testing.

EPIDEMIOLOGY.   Incidence and Prevalence.   For the past century and a half, cholera has remained endemic in the common delta of the Ganges and Brahmaputra

Rivers. The disease has caused seven worldwide pandemics since 1817, and the three major North American epidemics of 1832, 1848, and 1867 have shown that the potential distribution of cholera is worldwide. The period 1961 to 1976 witnessed a seventh pandemic spread of cholera from Indonesia westward through South and Central Asia to Western Europe and to the entire African continent. Serious outbreaks of cholera occurred in Israel in 1970, in Spain in 1972, in Italy in the summer of 1973, in Portugal and Guam in 1974, and in Syria in 1977. Isolated cases have been identified in travelers returning to most of the nations of Western Europe, as well as to Canada and Japan. An isolated case was identified in Port Lavaca, Texas, in 1973. Although there has been no further geographic spread of the disease in 1977, cholera appears to have become endemic in several Central and Western African nations which had been previously free of this disease for at least four decades. Fewer than 70 thousand cases of cholera were reported to the World Health Organization in 1977, representing a sharp decrease from 148,000 cases at the peak of the seventh pandemic in 1971.

Spread of Infection.   Man is the only natural host and victim of *Vibrio cholerae*. Most major epidemics of this disease have been water borne, and water plays the major role in the transmission of *Vibrio cholerae* in the endemic rural areas in the Gangetic Delta. During major pandemics, however, the direct contamination of food with infectious excreta may be important. Contaminated fresh vegetables appeared to have been a major factor in the transmission of cholera in Israel in the outbreak in 1970, and shellfish may have been a significant factor in the spread of cholera in Naples in 1973. Persons with mild or asymptomatic infections (contact carriers) may play a significant role in the dissemination of epidemic disease. The clinical case-to-infection ratio with infection by the classic *V. cholerae* biotype is about 1:6; with infection by the eltor biotype, this ratio may be as low as 1:50. A prolonged gallbladder carrier state may develop in 3 to 5 per cent of adult patients convalescing from cholera caused by the eltor biotype. The gallbladder carrier state is more common in older convalescents and has never been observed in the pediatric age group. The role of such convalescent carriers in the transmission of the disease has not been clarified. *Vibrio cholerae* does not survive well in fresh water, but may survive for long periods in sea water; this has recently been reaffirmed in association with the 1973 outbreak of cholera in Portugal.

In the cholera endemic areas of Bangladesh and West Bengal, cholera is predominantly a disease of children. Attack rates are ten times greater in the one- to five-year age group than in those over 20 years of age. When the disease spreads to previously uninvolved areas, the attack rates are initially at least as high in adults as in children. As the disease becomes endemic in new locations, as has occurred in the Philippines over the past 15 years, the endemic epidemiologic pattern develops, with the disease becoming far more common in young children than in adults.

PATHOGENESIS.   *Vibrio cholerae* causes disease when a large number of viable organisms are ingested, survive passage through the stomach, colonize the small bowel, and produce enterotoxin. The incubation period may vary from 12 hours to as long as 6 days. Because of the remarkable susceptibility of *Vibrio cholerae* to gastric acid, an enormous number of microorganisms must be ingested to cause this disease in a previously healthy individual. Volunteer studies have indicated that ingestion of even 10 billion organisms will not consistently produce clinical disease in healthy adults. If, however, gastric acid is neutralized by sodium bicarbonate, ingestion of 1 million viable organisms produces clinical disease in roughly 50 per cent of normal individuals. The individual with relative or absolute achlorhydria is therefore abnormally susceptible to cholera, and this susceptibility has been demonstrated by the very sharp increase in incidence of cholera in individuals with total or subtotal gastrectomy in the recent outbreaks of cholera in Israel and Italy.

Once vibrios have colonized the small bowel, an enterotoxin, with a molecular weight of 84,000, is produced. The binding unit of this enterotoxin combines rapidly, and apparently irreversibly, to a monosialoganglioside in the small bowel epithelial cell wall, allowing the active toxin subunit to stimulate adenyl cyclase in the intestinal epithelial cells. The resultant increase in intracellular levels of cyclic adenosine 3',5'-monophosphate leads to rapid excretion of electrolytes into the small bowel lumen. The action of the cholera toxin on the small bowel mucosa causes no visible morphologic damage to the gut mucosa, and this is reflected in the very low protein content, and the virtual absence of leukocytes, in the cholera stool.

All signs, symptoms, and metabolic derangements in cholera result directly from the rapid loss of fluid and electrolytes from the gut. All segments of the small bowel participate in the increased secretion of isotonic fluid. Precise studies have demonstrated that, in the adult, cholera stool is nearly isotonic with plasma, with sodium and chloride concentrations slightly less than those of plasma, bicarbonate concentration approximately twice that of plasma, and potassium concentration three to fives times that of plasma.

CLINICAL MANIFESTATIONS. The clinical onset of cholera is generally that of abrupt, painless, watery diarrhea. Stool volumes vary greatly, and in all epidemics there are large numbers of mild cases in which the fluid loss is not severe enough to require hospitalization. In the more severe cases, however, the initial stool volume may exceed 1500. At variable intervals after the onset of diarrhea, vomiting ensues; this is also characteristically effortless and productive of rice-watery material. In fulminant cases, severe muscle cramps, most commonly involving the gastrocnemius group, almost invariably develop. Prostration occurs at varying intervals following the onset of symptoms, in direct relationship to the magnitude of the fluid loss.

When first seen by the physician, the severely ill cholera patient presents a characteristic appearance: collapsed, cyanotic, with no palpable peripheral pulses, pinched facies, and scaphoid abdomen. The voice is very weak, high-pitched, and often nearly inaudible. Vital signs include tachycardia, varying degrees of tachypnea, hypopyrexia, and hypotension, often with no obtainable blood pressure. Heart sounds are faint or inaudible, and bowel sounds are hypoactive or entirely absent. Major alterations in mental status are not common in adults; the adult usually remains well oriented, although apathetic, even in the face of severe hypovolemic shock. As many as 10 per cent of small children, however, may have central nervous system abnormalities that range from stupor to convulsions.

Laboratory abnormalities are those which would be expected to result from a massive gastrointestinal loss of an isotonic, alkaline, virtually protein-free fluid (see accompanying table). These include increased plasma and whole blood specific gravity, elevated plasma protein, decreased plasma bicarbonate, low arterial pH, normal plasma sodium, slightly increased plasma chloride, and moderately elevated plasma potassium. Since the bicarbonate loss is proportional to stool volume, the decrease in whole blood pH is roughly proportional to the increase in plasma protein concentration at all stages of the untreated disease.

The illness may last from 12 hours to 7 days, and later clinical manifestations depend on adequacy of therapy. With adequate fluid and electrolyte repletion, recovery is remarkably rapid. If therapy is inadequate, the case mortality rate may exceed 50 per cent. The important causes of death are hypovolemic shock, uncompensated metabolic acidosis, and renal failure. When renal failure occurs, the characteristic pathologic findings are those of acute tubular necrosis secondary to prolonged hypotension.

DIAGNOSIS. The working diagnosis of cholera should be made on the basis of the clinical picture; appropriate fluid and electrolyte replacement therapy, as indicated by the physical findings, should be initiated immediately. Although a cholera-like illness may be caused by microorganisms other than *Vibrio cholerae*, most frequently by enterotoxigenic *Escherichia coli*, the resulting physiologic and metabolic abnormalities are the same, so that identical intravenous and oral electrolyte therapy may be used in all such cases.

Once appropriate therapy has been initiated, a geographic history should be obtained. The diagnosis of cholera is unlikely if the patient has not recently been in a known endemic or epidemic area. Stool examination should then be performed. Since the cholera enterotoxin causes neither inflammation nor destruction of intestinal mucosa, no leukocytes or erythrocytes are usually seen on microscopic examination of a fresh cholera stool stained with methylene blue. This dictum is, however, not absolute, as cholera may occasionally be superimposed on other acute or chronic inflammatory bowel disease. With *darkfield microscopy*, rapid tentative diagnosis can be made by direct observation of the characteristic rapid motility of the comma-shaped bacilli in fresh stool. Group- and type-specific antisera immobilize homologous strains and clearly distinguish them from other vibrios. *Fluorescent microscopy*, using fluorescein-labeled type-specific antibody, when available, also provides a rapid and accurate means of diagnosis.

Diagnostic culture techniques are relatively simple. A reliable and practical method consists of direct plating of feces on thiosulfate–citrate–bile salt–sucrose (TCBS)

Serial Blood Chemical Determinations in Cholera; Average Values in 40 Consecutive Patients

	On Admission	Four Hours	24 Hours
Sodium*	152	156	153
Chloride*	117	118	113
Potassium*	5.7	3.3	3.1
Bicarbonate*	7.4	21.0	24.5
Arterial pH	7.21	7.43	7.46
Plasma specific gravity	1.043	1.026	1.026

*Plasma electrolyte values are expressed in milliequivalents per liter of plasma H_2O.

agar. On TCBS agar typical opaque yellow colonies appear in 18 hours. Distinction between the two major serotypes, Inaba and Ogawa, requires agglutination with type-specific antisera. Identification of the eltor biotype of *Vibrio cholerae*, which is important for epidemiologic purposes, can be simply determined on the basis of the resistance of this biotype to polymyxin B.

TREATMENT. Successful therapy demands only prompt replacement of gastrointestinal losses of fluid and electrolytes. A "diarrhea treatment solution," recommended for intravenous therapy by the World Health Organization, is uniformly effective in both adult and pediatric patients; this solution may be simply prepared by adding 4 grams of sodium chloride, 6.5 grams of sodium acetate, 1 gram of potassium chloride and 10 grams of glucose to a liter of sterile distilled water. Alternatively, lactated Ringer's solution may be administered. Either of these intravenous fluid preparations should be infused intravenously and rapidly, 50 to 100 ml per minute, until a strong radial pulse has been restored. Subsequently the same fluid should be infused in quantities equal to gastrointestinal losses. If these losses cannot be measured accurately, intravenous fluid should be given at a rate sufficient to maintain a normal pulse volume and normal skin turgor. Overhydration can be avoided by careful observation of the neck veins and by auscultation of the lungs. Close observation of the patient is mandatory during the acute phase of the illness, as an adult patient can lose as much as 1 liter of isotonic fluid per hour during the first 24 hours of the disease. Inadequate or delayed restoration of electrolyte losses results in a very high incidence of acute renal insufficiency.

In children, complications are both more frequent and more severe. The most serious include stupor, coma, and convulsions (unique to pediatric patients), pulmonary edema, and cardiac arrhythmias. The central nervous system complications may be due to hypoglycemia (observed only in pediatric patients); hypernatremia resulting from the administration of isotonic fluid to the pediatric patient (who, unlike the adult patient, produces feces with a sodium concentration significantly less than that of plasma); or cerebral edema, presumably secondary to rapid fluid shifts during the administration of intravenous fluids. Pulmonary edema may result if fluids are given intravenously at too rapid a rate prior to the correction of the metabolic acidosis. Serious cardiac arrhythmias may result from potassium depletion in children, but rarely occur in adults with cholera. Each of these complications can be avoided by the careful administration of intravenous fluids that are carefully designed to replace the fecal electrolyte losses. The "diarrhea treatment solution," recommended by the World Health Organization for cholera as well as for other acute diarrheal diseases, has been used successfully to correct the acidosis, hypokalemia, and hypoglycemia without provoking hypernatremia. If lactated Ringer's solution is used in the pediatric patient, peroral supplementation of potassium and glucose is needed. The outcome in pediatric cholera should be essentially as favorable as that in the adult disease, with an over-all mortality rate of less than 1 per cent.

Peroral replacement of water and electrolytes is also remarkably effective in adults, and in children who are alert. This development of peroral therapy has greatly increased the capability to treat cholera in field conditions and thus represents a major achievement in the effort to use modern science and technology for the health problems of economically underdeveloped countries. An oral glucose-electrolyte solution (prepared by the addition of 20 grams of glucose, 3.5 grams of sodium chloride, 2.5 grams of sodium bicarbonate, and 1.5 grams of potassium chloride to 1 liter of drinking water) can be given in mild cholera cases throughout the course of illness, and is also satisfactory in more severe cases once the hypovolemic shock has been corrected by the initial rapid intravenous fluid therapy. When oral therapy is employed, about 1.5 volumes of oral solution must be given to replace each volume of stool lost. Glucose is an essential component of this solution in that the success of oral therapy in cholera depends upon enhanced intestinal absorption of sodium in the presence of intraluminal glucose.

Although adequate fluid therapy results in rapid recovery in virtually all cholera patients (table), adjunctive therapy with antimicrobials dramatically reduces the duration and volume of diarrhea and results in rapid eradication of vibrios from the feces. Tetracycline, in a total daily dose of 40 to 50 mg per kilogram of body weight divided into four equal portions and given perorally every six hours for two days, has been uniformly successful. Furazolidone and chloramphenicol are also of value, but are slightly less effective than tetracycline.

PROGNOSIS. Without treatment, mortality rates in cholera epidemics have exceeded 50 per cent. With adequate therapy, however, the mortality rate approaches zero. Largely because of the mechanical problems inherent in the administration of large amounts of fluid to small children, a mortality rate of 1 to 2 per cent still obtains in pediatric patients despite the best current therapy. A single attack of cholera confers only relatively short-lived, type-specific protection against subsequent infection by *V. cholerae*.

PREVENTION. Immunization, using two injections of standard commercial vaccine (containing 10 billion killed bacteria per milliliter), provides 60 to 80 per cent protection for three to six months to adults in cholera endemic areas. In recent field trials, immunization with toxoid proved to be no more effective than the standard whole-cell vaccine. Since immunization against cholera has not proved to be effective in altering the transmission of this disease, administration of cholera vaccine is no longer a requirement for entrance into the United States from cholera endemic areas. At present, careful hygiene provides the only certain protection against cholera.

Barua, D., and Burrows, W.: Cholera. Philadelphia, W.B. Saunders Company, 1974.

Carpenter, C. C. J., Mitra, P. P., and Sack, R. B.: Clinical studies in Asiatic cholera. Parts I-VI. Bull. Johns Hopkins Hosp., 118:165, 1966.

Holmgren, J., Lonnroth, I., Mansson, J. E., and Svennerholm, L.: Interaction of cholera toxin and membrane GM-1 ganglioside of small intestine. Proc. Natl. Acad. Sci. U.S.A., 72:2520, 1975.

Hornick, R. B., Music, S. I., Wenzel, R., Cash, R., Lebonati, J. P., Snyder, M. J., and Woodward, T. E.: The Broad Street pump revisited: Response of volunteers to ingested cholera vibrios. Bull. N.Y. Acad. Med., 47:1181, 1971.

Mahalanobis, D., Choudhuri, A. B., Bagchi, N. G., Bhattacharya, A. K., and Simpson, T. W.: Oral therapy of cholera among Bangladesh refugees. Johns Hopkins Med. J., 132:197, 1973.

Pierce, N. F., Sack, R. B., Mitra, R. C., Banwell, J. G., Brigham, K. L., Fedson, D. S., and Mondal, A.: Replacement of water and electrolyte losses in cholera by an oral glucose-electrolyte solution. Ann. Intern. Med., 70:1173, 1969.

Wallace, C. K., Anderson, P. N., Brown, T. C., Khanra, S. R., Lewis, G. W., Pierce, N. F., Sanyal, S. N., Segre, G. V., and Waldman, R. H.: Optimal antibiotic therapy in cholera. Bull. WHO, 39:239, 1968.

157. PLAGUE

Jay P. Sanford

DEFINITION. Plague is an infection caused by *Yersinia pestis* which in man usually presents in either of two major clinical patterns: acute lymphadenitis (bubonic plague) or acute severe pneumonia (pneumonic plague). Plague is primarily an infection of rodents caused by *Y. pestis* with transmission by a flea vector. Man usually acquires bubonic plague through the aberrant bite of plague-infected rodent fleas. With the occurrence of bacteremia, secondary pulmonary involvement may occur, which in turn may be followed by subsequent human-to-human respiratory transmission. In the fifteenth century, plague, which was known as the black death, assumed catastrophic proportions, killing an estimated one quarter of the population of Europe. The pathophysiology underlying the clinical features of black death appear to be multiple, but would appear to include the occurrence of profound cyanosis and disseminated intravascular coagulation with purpura and extensive symmetrical peripheral gangrene.

ETIOLOGY. *Y. pestis* is a gram-negative, nonmotile, aerobic coccobacillus which in smears from tissues or secretions stains in a bipolar "safety pin" pattern. This classic appearance is best demonstrated with Wayson's (methylene blue and carbofuchsin) or Giemsa's stain rather than with Gram's stain. The organism grows readily on most culture media, ordinary nutrient agar, blood agar, or deoxycholate agar with optimal growth at 28° C, although it will grow at temperatures of 1 to 43° C. However, growth is slow, requiring 48 hours before colonies are readily discernible. *Y. pestis* may remain viable for weeks in dry sputum or flea feces at room temperature. *Y. pestis* produces a number of antigenic components, several of which are of major importance in the pathogenesis of disease. These include a capsular antigen, which is a heat-labile protein designated as Fraction 1 (F1), and the VW antigens, which include a protein V and lipoprotein W. The F1 and VW antigens which render the organism resistant to phagocytosis are produced during growth at 37° C, but are not produced during growth at 28° C. *Y. pestis* contains an endotoxin, which may be less lethal than endotoxins extracted from Enterobacteriaceae, and exotoxins which are lethal (cardiotoxic) for the mouse and rat but against which other species appear to be resistant.

EPIDEMIOLOGY. Geographic Distribution and Prevalence. Plague is endemic in Vietnam, other parts of Indochina, India, Burma, Java, and South Central and East Africa, including Madagascar. The disease also has been reported sporadically in Egypt, Saudi Arabia, North Africa (Tunisia and Morocco), South America (Argentina, Bolivia, Brazil, Ecuador, Peru, and Venezuela), and the western and southwestern United States (Arizona, California, Colorado, New Mexico, Oregon, and Texas). In 1967, at the peak of an outbreak which subsequently declined, over 5000 cases were reported to the World Health Organization from South Vietnam. In the United States during the past ten years, an average of 7.4 cases per year (1 to 20) has been reported. In the United States since 1950, 60 per cent of cases have been in persons less than 20 years old, with a predominance of males (55 per cent). The over-all fatality-to-case ratio has been 20 per cent.

Transmission and Host Range. Plague is a natural disease of both domestic and wild rodents. Rats are the primary reservoir in urban areas. The oriental rat flea (*Xenopsylla cheopis*) becomes infected when it feeds on the blood of a bacteremic rat, which usually dies a short time after becoming bacteremic. Levels of *Y. pestis* in the rat may reach 10^7 bacilli per milliliter of blood. With the death of its host, the hungry flea seeks another host. The transmission from rat to rat by fleas is not primarily mechanical but involves biologic transmission, which is dependent upon the "blocking" of the flea proventriculus with plague bacilli. The extrinsic incubation period required for *X. cheopis* to become "blocked" varies, but on the average it requires two weeks. The ingested blood, which contains *Y. pestis*, is coagulated in the flea stomach by a coagulase produced by the organism embedding the bacilli in a matrix of fibrin. This fibrin anchor serves to retain *Y. pestis* in the proventriculus until the organ is occluded by a mass of multiplying bacilli. The "blocked" flea, which undergoes progressive desiccation, makes repeated attempts to feed; at each attempt, being unable to pass the blood meal past the blocked proventriculus, the flea regurgitates, thereby inoculating 25,000 to 100,000 bacilli into the site of the bite. It has been observed that flea-borne bubonic plague cannot exist in epidemic proportions when the mean ambient temperature is above 27.5° C. This observation seems particularly enigmatic, because the F1 and VW antigens which are antiphagocytic are not elaborated at these lower temperatures. Cavanaugh has elucidated the enigma by showing that when temperatures are elevated to about 27° C, fibrin is rapidly destroyed by a fibrinolytic factor elaborated by *Y. pestis* and a trypsin-like enzyme of the flea stomach. In the absence of the fibrin anchor, *Y. pestis* is eliminated from the stomach and proventriculus and fleas become noninfective. In the rat-flea-rat cycle, if another rodent is not available, the flea will accept a human host as a blood source; man then becomes an accidental host in the usual rat-flea-rat transmission cycle.

Epizootic plague occurs when *Y. pestis* is introduced into rodent or small mammal populations (e.g., prairie dogs) that are more highly susceptible to the lethal effects of infection than is the rat. The risk of exposure is high when man interfaces with epizootic plague. Transmission from animal hosts to man is termed zootic plague, whereas transmission from man to man is termed demic plague.

In recent years in the United States all but one case have resulted from exposure in rural or suburban settings. The principal animals involved have been ground squirrels, prairie dogs, marmots, wood rats, rabbits, and hares. Human infection from rabbits and hares usually results from direct tissue contact rather than flea bites. Carnivorous animals — including cats, dogs, and coyotes — in areas of enzootic and epizootic plague regularly show serologic evidence of infection. Recently, several human cases have been associated with handling of sick or dead dogs, coyotes, or cats. The communicability of plague pneumonia varies with the extent of cough and character of sputum, which often is thick and tenacious. Secondary cases have occurred most frequently in household contacts and medical personnel. Fortunately, no spread to contacts in the United States has been observed since 1925. The introduction of air travel requires that physicians throughout the world consider the occurrence of plague and recognize that air travel increases the danger of transmission. The index of clinical suspicion of plague outside endemic areas (e.g., the Southwest) is unfortunately low, as reflected in the occurrence of plague in a geologist who was infected in New Mexico but developed disease which was unrecognized and fatal in New England, or in a soldier who returned from Vietnam.

Y. pestis has been isolated from the throats of healthy persons who are in contact with pneumonic and presumably uncomplicated bubonic plague infections. Experimental evidence suggests that persons with plague infections of the upper respiratory tract, including asymptomatic pharyngeal "carriers" of *Y. pestis*, probably are incapable of respiratory transmission to other persons.

PATHOGENESIS. *Y. pestis* may enter the body via the blood, skin, conjunctiva, or mucous membranes of the respiratory or digestive tracts. The organisms which enter the body through the bites of fleas lack F1 and VW antigen, and hence are readily phagocytized by neutrophils and promptly killed. However, some organisms are phagocytized by mononuclear cells. Cavanaugh and associates have shown that at 37° C the organisms produce F1 and VW antigens and are able to kill the mononuclear cell. The organisms released from mononuclear cells are able to resist phagocytosis by neutrophils and reach lymph nodes. A local vesicle or pustule may form at the site of inoculation. If *Y. pestis* passes the local pustule, organisms reach lymph nodes which acutely enlarge and become embedded in a gelatinous periglandular edema. Infection may be contained at this stage, and is designated as pestis minor. If bacilli escape from the regional nodes, they pass into the bloodstream with the potential for involvement of multiple organs: lungs, spleen, meninges, and liver. In 42 patients studied by Butler and associates, 40 per cent had positive blood cultures. Endotoxemia as measured by the limulus gelation test has been demonstrated in some patients with negative blood cultures. A strong association has been demonstrated between axillary location of buboes and the development of meningitis and pneumonia.

CLINICAL MANIFESTATIONS. Bubonic plague is the more common form. The incubation period may vary from a few hours to 12 days, but is usually two to five days. The onset is abrupt, often associated with chills, and the temperature rises to 39.4 to 41.4° C. The pulse often is rapid and thready and hypotension occurs. Painful, enlarged lymph nodes appear simultaneously with or even shortly before the fever. Usually, there is no primary lesion at the site of the bite, but occasionally a primary cutaneous lesion, varying from a small vesicle with slight local lymphangitis to an eschar, may be seen. The most commonly involved lymph nodes are femoral or inguinal (50 per cent), followed by axillary (22 per cent), cervical (10 per cent), or multiple nodes (14 per cent). The nodes are usually tender and vary in size from 1 to 5 cm. The overlying skin often is smooth and reddened. In addition, headache and gastrointestinal complaints, anorexia, vomiting, and abdominal pain are common (about one fourth of patients). Restlessness, delirium, confusion, and incoordination may occur. The liver and spleen may be palpable.

Benign forms of bubonic plague, such as pestis minor with lymphadenitis, fever, headache, and prostration, may subside within a week. This is usually seen only in endemic areas. Recently, the occurrence of asymptomatic pharyngeal carriers of *Y. pestis* has been recognized.

Primary pneumonic plague has an incubation period usually lasting only two to three days, followed by the abrupt onset of high fever, chills, tachycardia, and headache, which is often severe. Initially, cough is not a prominent symptom. Within 20 to 24 hours a productive cough develops. Sputum is mucoid but rapidly shows blood specks, then uniformly becomes pink or bright red (resembling raspberry syrup) and foamy in character. There is associated tachypnea and dyspnea but no pleurisy. Signs of consolidation are rare; rales may be absent. Chest radiographs show a rapidly progressing pneumonia. Most untreated patients die one and one half to two days after onset of symptoms.

Primary septicemic plague, which usually occurs in association with the bubonic form, presents as an acute fulminant illness which may be fatal before either lymph node or pulmonary manifestations predominate. Other, less classic forms are pharyngeal plague and plague meningitis.

LABORATORY FEATURES. Hematocrit determinations have been normal or reflect other causes of anemia. Leukocyte counts are elevated in over 90 per cent of patients when initially seen. In patients with bubonic plague whose clinical conditions are stable, the usual leukocyte counts are 15,000 to 20,000 per cubic millimeter, with a marked neutrophilia. In patients who appear "septic" or who are hypotensive, leukocyte counts are usually 30,000 per cubic millimeter or higher. Peripheral blood smears will often (approximately 10 per cent) show *Y. pestis*. Patients commonly develop disseminated intravascular coagulation (86 per cent in a group of patients studied by Butler and associates), as manifested by elevated titers of fibrinogen-fibrin degradation products, thrombocytopenia, and hypofibrinogenemia, although none showed overt bleeding. Electrocardiograms have usually been normal, although STT segment depression consistent with ischemia associated with marked tachycardia may be seen. Liver function tests usually are normal, although elevations in SGOT have been seen. In patients with plague meningitis, endotoxin may be demonstrated in cerebrospinal fluid, using the limulus lysate gelation test.

DIAGNOSIS. This is based on recovery of *Y. pestis*, which may be cultured from blood (almost half of patients have positive cultures), sputum, or lymph node aspirate. Prompt smears of lymph node aspirate stained with Wayson's stain (or methylene blue) usually provide a rapid presumptive diagnosis. Surgical drainage of a bubo may disseminate organisms: hence needle aspiration is preferable. *Y. pestis* can be grown on ordinary culture media or isolated by animal inoculation. Since most pyogenic bacteria grow within 24 hours, a "negative" culture at 24 hours should raise suspicion of tularemia and plague. Serologic tests include complement fixation, passive hemagglutination, and immunofluorescent staining of a node, secretions, or tissues. Since clinical illness occurs in vaccinated individuals, a vaccine history does not exclude plague in the differential diagnosis.

Differential diagnostic considerations in the patient with buboes include tularemia, lymphogranuloma venereum, impetigo with lymphadenitis, and erysipelas, whereas such considerations in the patient with pneumonic involvement must include the spectrum of acute, viral, bacterial, fungal, and parasitologic causes. It is noteworthy that several of the patients seen in the southwestern United States have been admitted with diagnoses of incarcerated hernias.

THERAPY AND MANAGEMENT. Treatment, which should be immediate upon suspicion of plague, includes general supportive measures and specific therapy. Prompt treatment will reduce mortality to 5 per cent. In the septicemic or pneumonic forms, treatment must begin within 24 hours to afford protection. The tetracyclines, chloramphenicol, and streptomycin are highly effective against naturally transmitted forms of plague. Streptomycin, 0.5 gram intramuscularly every three hours for 48 hours, followed by 1.5 to 2.0 grams per day for seven to ten days, is preferred. Occasional (about 1 per cent) strains of *Y. pestis* encountered in Vietnam were resistant in vitro to streptomycin. These strains were susceptible in vitro to kanamycin, which has been shown to be effective. Gentamicin has not been proved to be effective and should not be relied upon as an alternative. As an alternative, tetracycline or chloramphenicol, 500 mg intravaneously every three hours for 48 hours, 4 grams per day orally for the next two days, and then 3 grams per day orally for an additional four to five days, may be used, and is preferred by some authorities. Patients with plague meningitis should receive chloramphenicol as well as streptomycin. Recent studies suggest that co-trimoxazole is effective, but the duration of fever and incidence of complications were greater than occurred in patients treated with streptomycin. Penicillins are not effective. Some authors have advised against the use of streptomycin because of possible Herxheimer reactions. Such reactions were not encountered in patients treated in Vietnam. Despite laboratory evidence of disseminated intravascular coagulation based upon extrapolation from other infections, heparin therapy would not seem indicated. Routine aseptic precautions are adequate for patients with bubonic plague. In contrast, primary or secondary plague pneumonia demands strict isolation. Response to streptomycin treatment usually is prompt, most patients becoming afebrile within the first week (median, four days). Buboes usually become nontender concomitantly with defervescence and either resolve or become smaller. Occasional nodes become fluctuant and require incision. It should be noted that positive cultures may be obtained from such nodes after seven to ten days of therapy.

PREVENTION. Prevention is based upon rodent control and use of repellents to minimize attacks by fleas. There is indirect evidence from Vietnam that the killed plague vaccine used in the United States is highly effective in preventing plague. Although vaccination against plague is not required by any country as a condition for entry and is not recommended for travelers to most countries, it is advisable for all persons traveling to the interior regions of Indochina. Immunization is also recommended for persons whose occupation brings them into frequent contact with wild rodents in plague enzootic areas.

Butler, T., Bell, W. R., Linh, N. N., Tiep, N. D., and Arnold, K.: *Yersinia pestis* infection in Vietnam. I. Clinical and hematologic aspects. J. Infect. Dis. (Suppl.), 124:5, 1974.

Butler, T., Levin, J., Linh, N. N., Chau, D. M., Adickman, M., and Arnold, K.: *Yersinia pestis* infection in Vietnam. II. Quantitative blood cultures and detection of endotoxin in cerebrospinal fluid of patients with meningitis. J. Infect. Dis., 133:493, 1976.

Cantey, J. R.: Plague in Vietnam. Clinical observations and treatment with kanamycin. Arch. Intern. Med., 133:1380, 1974.

Cavanaugh, D. C.: Specific effect of temperature upon transmission of the plague bacillus of the oriental rat flea, *Xenopsylla cheopis*. Am. J. Trop. Med. Hyg. 20:264, 1971.

Cavanaugh, D. C., and Randall, R.: The role of multiplication of *Pasteurella pestis* and mononuclear phagocytes in the pathogenesis of flea-borne plague. J. Immunol., 83:348, 159.

Pollitzer, R.: Plague. WHO Monograph No. 22, Geneva, 1954.

Reed, W. P., Palmer, D. L., Williams, R. C., and Kisch, A. L: Bubonic plague in the southwestern United States: A review of recent experience. Medicine, 49:465, 1970.

Schwade, J., and Sanford, J. P.: Hepatic granulomata due to "benign" plague imported from Vietnam: Case report. Milit. Med., 139:554, 1974.

158. TULAREMIA

Theodore E. Woodward

DEFINITION. Most cases of tularemia are characterized by the formation of a focal ulcer at the site of entry of the causative bacillus, enlargement of regional lymph nodes, and a constitutional reaction of fever, prostration, myalgia, and headache. There may be pneumonia, which is occasionally accompanied by pleurisy or a typhoid-like illness.

Francisella tularensis, the microbial agent, is transmitted to humans by insect vectors such as ticks or deer flies, by the handling or ingestion of infected animal tissues, or by inhalation of infected aerosols. The clinical diagnosis is confirmed by demonstration of bacteremia, by isolation of the bacillus from the sputum, tissue exudates, or gastric washings, and by demonstration of serum agglutinins in early convalescence.

HISTORICAL FEATURES. The knowledge of the ecology and clinical features of tularemia has been developed in the United States through the pioneering work of Francis and other Public Health Service investigators. McCoy described the disease in 1911 while studying a plaguelike illness in ground squirrels in Tulare County, California. The first clinical description and bacteriologic proof of illness is attributed to Wherry and Lamb in 1914. In a series of studies conducted in Utah and elsewhere, Francis (1928) incriminated rabbits as important animal hosts and established the transmissibility of disease by deer flies.

ETIOLOGY, SPECIFIC LABORATORY DIAGNOSIS, AND EPIDEMIOLOGY. Tularemia is caused by a pleomorphic, nonmotile, small gram-negative rod. There is only one serologic group of all *F. tularensis* isolates. However, there are two varieties recognized which vary in virulence. One variety is highly virulent for rabbit and man (Jellson type A) and is found only in North America. It ferments glycerol and has citrulline ureidase activity. The second variety is avirulent for the rabbit but causes mild tularemia in man (Jellson type B). It is found in Europe, Asia, and North America. This variety lacks glycerol-fermenting enzymes and also citrulline ureidase.

CULTURE. Blood-glucose cysteine agar is the basic medium needed for propagating the organism. All culturing and animal inoculations should be done in an appropriate contagion hood to minimize laboratory-acquired infections. The routine inoculation of animals (mice or guinea pigs) is not generally recommended because of the risk of infecting personnel and also initiating an epizootic. Organisms can be recovered from ulcers and draining regional lymph nodes during the first few weeks in patients with ulceroglandular tularemia. Patients with pneumonic disease or symptoms of a bronchitis may have organisms isolated from bronchial secretions and gastric washings. Bacteremia does occur, but few organisms are present and are difficult to isolate. Bone marrow aspirations may yield *F. tularensis.* The organisms should be identifiable within two to four days in the culture media.

Serologic Diagnosis. The conventional serum agglutination reaction is a very useful diagnostic test, because specific agglutinins appear within eight to ten days from the onset of illness. Maximal titers are reached in about four weeks. Demonstration of a rise in titer through examination of serial specimens is confirmatory evidence of infection, although single titers of 1:160 or more are usually significant. Sera from patients with brucellosis or tularemia may show cross-agglutination, although the titer is usually higher with the homologous antigen.

Cutaneous Test. Foshay described a diagnostic skin test that consists of the intradermal inoculation of a purified antigen consisting of a killed suspension of *F. tularensis.* The reaction is of the delayed tuberculin type, becoming positive in 48 hours. The test is highly specific and becomes positive during the first week of tularemia either prior to or coincident with the development of agglutinins. The test remains positive for years.

EPIDEMIOLOGY. Tularemia has been detected in many areas of the Northern Hemisphere, including Japan, Central Europe, Asian and European Russia, and Scandinavia. Man can be infected by as few as 50 organisms injected intradermally, and that number and probably fewer *F. tularensis* delivered as a small particle (<5 microns) aerosol will cause pneumonic disease. This unique infectiousness of these bacilli for man points up the need for caution when culturing or inoculating animals as well as when handling infected animals. The organisms are found in many species of animals. In North America, the cottontail rabbit is associated with many cases of ulceroglandular and typhoidal forms of tularemia. These animals will have large numbers of tularemia organisms in the liver and bloodstream. In the process of eviscerating an infected animal, there is ample opportunity for direct hand contamination as well as generation of an infectious aerosol. Tiny puncture wounds of the skin, hair follicles, or cracks around nail beds can serve as portals of entry for the initiation of ulceroglandular tularemia. Restricted sale of wild rabbits in metropolitan areas has resulted in a sharp decline of the disease.

Many cases have their origin from infected arthropods such as ticks, deer flies, or mosquitoes. In North America the ticks *Dermacentor andersoni, Dermacentor variabilis,* and the Lone Star tick are important reservoirs and vectors. Infected female ticks transmit *F. tularensis* transovarially. A primary ulcer often forms at the site of tick attachment.

Tularemia occurs in all seasons: among hunters and trappers in the fall and winter, and during the spring and summer when ticks and deer flies are active. All ages and both sexes are susceptible. Since 1967, fewer than 200 cases have been reported annually in the United States.

MECHANISM OF INFECTION AND PATHOLOGY. The disease may present in a variety of forms with two major subdivisions, depending on whether or not the initial site of entry can be visualized. In all forms there is lymph node involvement. In most instances there is a primary ulcer, variable in size, which may be located on the skin (ulceroglandular), in the eye (oculoglandular), or in the nasopharynx with necrotizing lesions. Sometimes the cutaneous lesion may be insignificant, so that the picture is that of "glandular tularemia" without an overt primary lesion. The entry also may be through the intestinal tract (enteric or typhoidal) or via the lungs (pulmonary).

After infection, *F. tularensis* reaches the blood via the lymphatics and nodes; the microbe, although phagocytized, resides intracellularly without loss of viability. Granulomatous lesions develop within the reticuloendothelial system, particularly in lymph nodes, liver, and spleen. These lesions, usually hyperplastic, bear some resemblance to tuberculosis and may caseate or form small local abscesses. The macrophage is the predominant cell type that surrounds an area of caseous necrosis. Langhans' cells are observed occasionally, and the larger lesions are liable to central abscess formation.

Pneumonia is a common development in tularemia, occurring in approximately 30 per cent of patients who acquire the disease, regardless of the type of infection. Histologically, the early lesion is edematous, and consists of fibrin and leukocytes associated with necrosis of alveolar walls. In non-necrotic areas the exudate consists of the large mononuclear type. The gross lesions resemble the pneumonia of tuberculosis, although histologically there is less epithelioid cell transformation. Tubercle-like nodules are more common in lymph nodes than in the lungs. Mediastinal nodes are involved frequently.

CLINICAL MANIFESTATIONS. The incubation period of tularemia ranges from two to ten days. Headache, fever, and toxic signs characterize all forms of the illness and are in no way dissimilar to those in other infectious illnesses. The pertinent historic and epidemiologic features are often helpful clues, and in approximately three fourths of all patients there is a primary lesion associated with adenopathy.

Ulceroglandular Tularemia. The initial lesion begins as a reddish papule, which is often undermined and more extensive than the small area of superficial induration indicates. Neighboring and draining lymph nodes are enlarged, tender, and discrete. Fluctuation of these nodes occurs later in the illness, after two or more weeks, when other acute signs may have partially abated. Such diseased nodes may subsequently require incision and drainage. The lymph nodes during the early stages are laden with *F. tularensis* and, if incised, may provoke bacteremia and toxemia. Fluctuant buboes four or more weeks old are usually sterile. Generalized lymphadenopathy occurs. Systemic signs of toxemia may be severe in ulceroglandular tularemia, although most cases are mild or moderate in severity. Pneumonia of all gradations may accompany this type of infection.

Occasionally, tularemia referred to as the glandular type may occur as generalized adenopathy and toxemia but without cutaneous lesions.

Enteric Form of Tularemia (Typhoidal or Cryptogenic). Man is not readily infected by the oral route. Aerosols consisting of large particles or the swallowing of huge numbers of tularemia bacilli will cause illness characterized by symptoms of abdominal pain, high fever, and toxicity, which can be confused with the symptoms of typhoid fever. Usually there are prominent enlarged cervical lymph nodes. This typhoidal systemic reaction may typify any of the clinical varieties of tularemia regardless of the presence of a cutaneous lesion. The term "cryptogenic" has often been used to connote the absence of an obvious portal of entry.

Pulmonary Tularemia. Lung involvement occurs in all forms of tularemia, subsequent to the bacteremia. Available evidence suggests that primary tularemic pneumonia is an entity, particularly in those persons such as laboratory workers who are exposed to infected aerosols. The incubation period varies from two to five days, depending upon the number of viable bacteria inhaled. In addition to headache, fever, malaise, and prostration, there is a nonproductive harassing cough and a sensation of substernal discomfort. Later the sputum may be mucoid or bloody and, in severely ill patients, pleural pain, dyspnea, tachycardia, and cyanosis occur.

In spite of extensive pulmonary involvement, there may be a paucity of physical signs. The early roentgenographic signs, seldom evident before the second to the fourth day of fever, consist of small irregular oval lesions with hilar adenopathy. Later in the illness, the infiltrate may be annular. True abscess formation is rare, although during resolution and convalescence, which in untreated patients or in those treated late may be prolonged, shadows suggesting abscess formation may be noted. Pleuritis with effusion is not uncommon.

Oculoglandular Tularemia. After ocular contamination there may be pain, photophobia, intense congestion, itching, lacrimation, chemosis, and a mucopurulent discharge. Small yellowish granulomatous lesions may appear on the palpebral conjunctivae or cornea and may eventually ulcerate. The preauricular and other regional lymph nodes may enlarge and ultimately suppurate. In untreated patients, serious ocular complications, including corneal perforation or optic atrophy, may ensue.

Other General Manifestations. Initially, in severely ill patients, there is a rigor followed by pyrexia that persists for a month or more. The fever may be continuously high or remittent, and defervescence is usually gradual. Hepatomegaly and splenomegaly with tenderness over the respective organs are relatively common. Toxic signs in all cases include fever, headache, myalgia, and nausea. Rashes are very uncommon; when present, they consist of localized papular lesions along the peripheral lymphatics or maculopapular body eruptions. In untreated patients or in those first given antimicrobial therapy late in the course of illness, convalescence may be prolonged with sporadic episodes of fever, weakness, muscular pains, and chronic respiratory signs.

NONSPECIFIC LABORATORY FINDINGS. The erythrocyte sedimentation rate and C-reactive protein are elevated during the active stages. In contrast, the total blood leukocyte count is usually normal or low. Occasionally there may be moderate leukocytosis. Mild albuminuria may occur at the height of illness.

DIFFERENTIAL DIAGNOSIS. Ulceroglandular tularemia is recognized readily in endemic areas. Punctate lesions with surrounding erythema at the site of prior arthropod attachment suggest *Rocky Mountain spotted fever,* particularly when associated with fever, headache, and toxic signs. The absence of a rash would favor tularemia, because patients with rickettsial disease develop a characteristic exanthem. *Meningococcemia* is recognized by its fulminant character, the typical exanthem, leuko-

cytosis, and the bacteriologic findings. Fever, toxic signs, pharyngitis, adenitis, hepatomegaly, and splenomegaly are common to tularemia and *infectious mononucleosis.* The hematologic and serologic findings are usually distinctive. *Cat scratch disease* is characterized by peripheral ulceration and regional adenopathy; a history of contact with cats, the cutaneous reaction to specific antigens, and the absence of agglutinins for *F. tularensis* are distinguishing features. *Ecthyma* and *furunculi* are similar in some respects to this form of tularemia, although lymphadenitis and systemic signs are less likely to develop.

The lesions of *sporotrichosis* are multiple, occur along the course of lymphatics, attach themselves firmly to the skin, and are freely movable.

Certain forms of tularemia may present with clinical features similar to those of psittacosis, Q fever, and mycoplasmal pneumonia. Broad-spectrum antimicrobial drugs are effective in each of these conditions. Appropriate serologic tests or viral isolation may be required to define the precise cause. Influenza with associated pneumonia is similar but does not respond to specific drugs, and its clinical course is short. Fungal diseases, such as *histoplasmosis* and *coccidioidomycosis,* may be acute and may simulate pulmonary tularemia. Consideration of the history, the epidemiologic data, and the cutaneous manifestations, as well as the bacteriologic and serologic findings, usually will permit proper identification.

The presence of unexplained pleural effusion, similar to tuberculous fibrinous pleurisy, requires differentiation. The results of cultural and serologic tests will aid in differentiation.

COMPLICATIONS. Pericarditis and meningitis are distinctive but unusual complications of tularemia. Pericardial involvement may develop by direct extension from the pulmonary lesions or lymph nodes, and is characterized by a fibrinous or fibrocaseous exudate. In untreated patients constrictive pericarditis may ensue. Tularemic meningitis is characterized by a lymphocytic pleocytosis in the cerebrospinal fluid, and was usually fatal prior to the availability of specific antimicrobial drugs. Rare instances of tularemic peritonitis, perisplenitis, osteomyelitis, and endocarditis have been reported.

TREATMENT. Specific Therapy. Tularemia is very amenable to treatment with antimicrobial drugs. Streptomycin is preferable, but the broad-spectrum antimicrobials are equally beneficial in ameliorating the active manifestations. They are less effective, however, in eradicating the organism, primarily because of their bacteriostatic mode of action. With the latter drugs, relapses are liable to occur if treatment is initiated within the first week of illness.

AMINOGLYCOSIDES. Streptomycin, when given in doses of 1.0 gram daily to adults for about one week, results in prompt recovery. Most patients are improved within 24 hours, and are afebrile within 48 hours. Relapses are uncommon with streptomycin except when insufficient drug is given during the very early stages of illness. Strains resistant to streptomycin have been induced in vitro but have not been isolated from patients with naturally acquired disease. Kanamycin and gentamicin are equally effective, but the experience with these drugs is meager, and kanamycin carries with it a greater risk of ototoxicity.

TETRACYCLINE AND CHLORAMPHENICOL TREAT-

MENT. Broad-spectrum antimicrobials are very effective in rendering the patient afebrile and free from toxicity within 48 to 72 hours. Relapses are uncommon when therapy is initiated 10 to 12 days after the onset of illness, but are frequent if it is given during the first week. *F. tularensis* does not develop resistance to chloramphenicol or tetracycline; hence, retreatment leads to prompt response.

The following dosage schedule is considered optimal: for tetracycline, an initial oral dose of 25 mg per kilogram of body weight; and for chloramphenicol, 50 mg per kilogram of body weight. Subsequent daily doses are calculated on the same basis as the initial loading dose, dividing the requirement equally and giving it at six- to eight-hour intervals. Antimicrobial therapy is continued until the patient is improved and has been afebrile for about five to seven days.

No supplementary chemotherapy is necessary with any of the aforementioned regimens. Tetracycline is preferred solely because reactions to it are potentially less serious.

General Management. An adequate diet with appropriate protein intake is advisable. Oxygen treatment is indicated for all severely ill patients with pneumonia whether or not cyanosis is present. Other supportive measures useful for treating patients with pneumonia, such as frequent turning and the performing of a tracheostomy to provide a proper airway, are indicated. Thoracentesis for removal of fluid will allay respiratory embarassment.

The local ulcer requires no special measures. During the early several weeks of illness, lymph nodes should not be manipulated unduly or incised. Later, fluctuant buboes, which are usually sterile, may require incision and drainage. Recovery ensues rapidly.

PROGNOSIS AND POSTINFECTION IMMUNITY. In untreated patients, the case fatality rate in ulceroglandular tularemia was formerly approximately 5 per cent. However, of those patients with typhoidal tularemia or with pulmonary manifestations, about 30 per cent succumbed. With the advent of streptomycin and later the broad-spectrum antimicrobials, death from tularemia has been virtually eliminated and the morbidity shortened drastically to several days after institution of treatment, even among severely ill patients.

Second attacks of tularemia with systemic complications are uncommon, because recovery from the initial episode usually confers immunity. However, it is not unusual for patients to develop primary lesions when reinfected long after the initial systemic infection. Viable *F. tularensis* may be isolated from such recurrent primary ulcers, which resemble a Koch reaction. Under these conditions, systemic manifestations are unusual.

Under test conditions in volunteers, when streptomycin is given soon after intradermal infection (before the onset of clinical illness), an attack may be aborted fully. Immunity does not develop, agglutinins fail to appear, and such subjects are prone to further infection. This phenomenon is of little practical significance, as patients are usually encountered after a week or more of active clinical illness. Partial to complete resistance to infection follows such antigenic stimulation.

CONTROL MEASURES. General. In infected areas those measures designed to repel ticks, mosquitoes, or deer flies should be employed. Gloves should be used for handling all potentially infected animals, particularly rabbits, and animals to be consumed should be cooked thoroughly. Laboratory workers exposed to infected aerosols should exercise care by wearing suitable masks and utilizing other protective devices.

Vaccination. The available killed vaccines afford only partial protection to man against tularemia. Viable attenuated preparations have been used with considerable success in the Soviet Union. The vaccine is administered intradermally and provokes a reaction similar in severity to that which follows smallpox immunization. Significant protection has been demonstrated in volunteers in the United States vaccinated with a similar viable product and who subsequently were exposed to virulent strains of *F. tularensis* by the respiratory or cutaneous routes. In those subjects who have developed clinical illness after immunization, the disease has been mild.

Foshay, L.: Tularemia. Ann. Rev. Microbiol., 4:313, 1950.

McCrumb, F. R.: Aerosol infection of man with *Pasteurella tularensis*. Bact. Rev., 25:262, 1961.

Meyer, K. F.: Pasteurella and franciscella. *In* Dubos, R., and Hirsch, J. G. (eds.): Bacterial and Mycotic Infections of Man. 4th ed. Philadelphia, J. B. Lippincott Company, 1965, Chap. 27, p. 659.

Young, L. S.: Tularemia epidemic, Vermont, 1968. Forty-seven cases linked to contact with muskrats. N. Engl. J. Med., 280:1253, 1969.

159. DISEASES CAUSED BY MALLEOMYCES

Leighton E. Cluff

159.1. GLANDERS
(Farcy)

DEFINITION. Glanders, or farcy, is an infectious disease of horses, mules, and donkeys caused by *Malleomyces mallei*. The infection is occasionally transmitted to man, and is characterized by an acute fulminant febrile illness or a chronic indolent disease with abscesses of the respiratory tract or skin. Farcy refers to the nodular abscesses observed in skin, lymphatics, and subcutaneous tissues.

ETIOLOGY. Glanders was described by Aristotle about 330 B.C., and the occurrence of the disease in horses was observed by Apeyrtos about 375 A.D. Royer's (1837) monograph on glanders in man remains the classic description of the disease. The microorganism responsible for glanders was isolated in 1882. It is a gram-negative bacillus culturable aerobically on ordinary nutrient media. It is variously called *Malleomyces mallei*, *Bacillus mallei*, or *Pfeiferella mallei*. *M. mallei* is nonmotile. It elaborates a specific antigen (mallein) upon lysis that is used as a skin test material for diagnostic purposes. The bacillus is antigenically separable from *M. pseudomallei*, which causes melioidosis. When grown on potato slices or potato infusion agar, *M. mallei* produces a brown pigment resembling that of *Pseudomonas aeruginosa*. The bacillus produces fatal infection experimentally in guinea pigs and hamsters but will not cause disease in rats, cattle, hogs, or fowl.

EPIDEMIOLOGY. Glanders has probably never been a common disease in man. It occurs almost exclusively in persons handling horses. It has been reported from all parts of the world. It has been eradicated in the United

States and the United Kingdom, but may still occur in Asia and South America.

Glanders is a communicable disease among horses, and it may occur sporadically in other animal species in contact with horses. In horses, glanders is manifested by nasal symptoms and abscesses and by cutaneous nodules or abscesses (farcy). The bacillus preferentially invades areas of abraded or injured skin. Experimental infection can be induced in animals by inhalation of the bacillus, and certain laboratory-acquired infections indicate that infection may develop in man after inhalation of the microorganism. *Unlike melioidosis, glanders can be transmitted from person to person.*

PATHOLOGY AND PATHOGENESIS. Characteristically glanders is associated with cellulitis, necrosis, abscess, and thromboses with septic embolization. Healing occurs by fibrosis, and, rarely, by calcification.

CLINICAL MANIFESTATIONS. Glanders may occur as a fulminant acute febrile disease, as a chronic indolent and relapsing disease, or as a subclinical occult infection detectable incidentally at postmortem examination or by serologic test. The two principal features of glanders are (1) nasal cellulitis and necrosis-producing septal perforation and palatal and pharyngeal ulceration; or (2) cutaneous cellulitis, vesiculation, and ulceration at the site of inoculation of the bacillus into the skin, followed by lymphangitis with nodular abscesses along the lymphatics and lymphadenopathy (farcy).

Pulmonary involvement is common in glanders, producing pneumonia, abscesses, pleural effusion, and empyema. Occasionally, in chronic indolent glanders, small nodular granulomatous lesions may be found in the lungs. Hilar lymph node enlargement is common in pulmonary glanders.

When glanders becomes disseminated, destructive polyarthritis, subcutaneous and muscular abscesses, osteomyelitis, meningitis, and pustular skin lesions, particularly over the joints and face, are seen. Prostration and stupor may develop, and are followed by death in two to three weeks.

Chronic glanders may be punctuated by recurrent acute relapses with bacteremia, often resulting in a fulminant course and death. Amyloidosis may be a complication of chronic glanders.

Fever and chills, headache, and backache are common in acute glanders. Leukopenia or a normal leukocyte count is the rule, but leukocytosis has been observed.

DIAGNOSIS. There are no pathognomonic chronic clinical features of glanders. The nodules along lymphatics resemble those seen in sporotrichosis. The respiratory lesions may be difficult to distinguish from other ulcerative infections of the nose and mouth. The cutaneous lesion often resembles streptococcal cellulitis. The multiple abscesses mimic many mycotic and staphylococcal infections and are difficult to distinguish from those of melioidosis. The acute fulminant illness may resemble typhoid fever or disseminated tuberculosis. The diagnosis of glanders can be established by combination of a history of exposure to horses, isolation of *M. mallei*, serologic tests (agglutination, complement-fixation), and skin test with sterile culture filtrate (mallein). Inoculation of infected material into guinea pigs may facilitate identification of the microorganism.

TREATMENT. There are reports of successful treatment of glanders with sulfonamides. Sulfadiazine, ad-

ministered in divided doses by mouth for a total daily dosage of 100 mg per kilogram for a three-week period, is recommended. Tetracycline, chloramphenicol, and streptomycin may be useful, but there is little clinical experience with these drugs in glanders. Because of the serious prognosis and the lack of documented experience with drug therapy, it is advisable to administer daily streptomycin (1.0 gram) or tetracycline in association with a sulfonamide until all evidences of disease have disappeared. Incision, drainage, and excision of abscesses must be done with caution, for the infection may be disseminated by such manipulation.

PROGNOSIS. Although a few patients have been cured with chemotherapy, the effect of treatment on the mortality rate is not known. *More than 90 per cent of patients with glanders will die from the disease if untreated.* However, the frequency of occurrence of occult or subclinical glanders is not known.

PREVENTION. Infected horses have been identified by skin tests with mallein and by serologic tests. Destruction of infected animals has eliminated glanders as a public health problem in the United States and most other countries.

Howe, C., and Miller, W. R.: Human glanders. Report of six cases. Ann. Intern. Med., 26:115, 1947.
Howe, C., and Miller, W. R.: The pseudomallei: A review. J. Infect. Dis., 124:598, 1971.
Mendelson, R. W.: Glanders. U.S. Armed Forces Med. J., 1:781, 1950.

159.2. MELIOIDOSIS

DEFINITION. Melioidosis is a rare disease of man caused by *Malleomyces pseudomallei*. It has been observed most frequently in Malaysia, the People's Republic of China, Burma, India, and other parts of the Far East and Southeast Asia, but has only rarely been observed in North and South America. It is a disease of wild rodents and some domesticated animals, and probably is transmitted to man by contact with diseased animals or animal excreta and possibly by contact with contaminated soil. The disease in man appears in a subclinical (detectable only by serologic tests), pulmonary, septicemic, or extrapulmonary form. The septicemic and pulmonary disease may be acute and fatal. The pulmonary and extrapulmonary infection with abscesses may be chronic and debilitating.

ETIOLOGY. Melioidosis was first identified by Whitmore and Krishnaswami (1912) in Rangoon. The disease was recognized as similar to glanders and attributable to a gram-negative bacillus resembling but differing from *Malleomyces mallei*. The microorganism causing melioidosis has been variously called *Malleomyces pseudomallei*, *Bacillus whitmori*, and *Pfeiferella whitmori*. It is a motile bacillus that grows aerobically on nutrient agar. Culturally it may resemble *Klebsiella* and *Pseudomonas aeruginosa*. *M. pseudomallei* is antigenically distinguishable from *M. mallei*. It produces fatal infection in guinea pigs, rabbits, and other laboratory animals.

EPIDEMIOLOGY. *M. pseudomallei* has been found to cause disease sporadically, endemically, and epidemically among a wide variety of animal species, including rats, rabbits, goats, hogs, dogs, cats, and horses. In addition, the bacillus has been found to be harbored by mosquitoes and fleas. Frequently, the initial manifestations of melioidosis in man are cutaneous abscesses, diarrhea, and pneumonia; therefore it is probable that the disease is transmitted by direct contact with infected animals or by ingestion or inhalation of contaminated material. All these routes of inoculation can produce the disease experimentally in animals. It is unlikely that melioidosis is ever transmitted from man to man. Infection has been observed in narcotic addicts, and in infants, or in patients with diabetes mellitus, renal or liver disease, and pregnancy as predisposing factors.

CLINICAL MANIFESTATIONS. Melioidosis may appear acutely or insidiously, and most often follows a fulminant course with septicemia or a chronic indolent course with multiple abscess formation. The incubation period of the disease is not known. The acute illness is often associated with fever, chills, cough, production of bloody and purulent sputum, diarrhea, or abdominal pain. Physical examination may reveal signs of pneumonia, empyema, lung abscess, hepatomegaly, jaundice, and splenomegaly. *A subacute or chronic illness may follow the acute disease or may develop in the absence of an acute illness.* In this situation the patient often has osteomyelitis, suppurating lymphadenopathy, subcutaneous abscesses, psoas abscess, lung abscess, pyelonephritis, or liver or spleen abscess. Bronchocutaneous and other types of fistulas may appear. Patients with this chronic illness may survive for many months, and occasionally may recover.

DIAGNOSIS. Inapparent infection has been recognized by serologic tests in 6 to 8 per cent of adult men in some parts of Southeast Asia. Only 1 per cent of adult women have been similarly infected. Melioidosis may resemble typhoid fever, malaria, mycotic infection, and occasionally acute staphylococcal septicemia or staphylococcal pneumonia. The chronic pulmonary disease most resembles tuberculosis. Melioidosis can be differentiated from these diseases only by bacteriologic identification of the bacillus from blood, sputum, urine, or pus. Hemagglutination and complement fixation tests may be useful when acute and convalescent serologic titers are compared. A single positive test may only indicate previous clinical and subclinical infection.

The leukocyte count of the peripheral blood often is normal in melioidosis, but may rise to levels of 20,000 per cubic millimeter. Urinalysis may show pyuria and hematuria.

TREATMENT AND PREVENTION. There is no available antigen for active immunization against melioidosis. Prevention of the disease is possible by controlled sanitation and improved standards of living. Patients have been successfully treated with chloramphenicol, sulfonamides, or tetracycline, given over long periods of time. The drug susceptibility of *M. pseudomallei*, however, is variable. In adults, 3 grams of tetracycline a day orally for 90 days or, alternatively, in septicemia, large doses of chloramphenicol are preferred. Surgical drainage of abscesses is essential for proper management.

Buchman, R. J., Kmiecik, J. E., and LaNove, A. M.: Extrapulmonary melioidosis. Ann. J. Surg., 125:324, 1973.
Howe, C., and Miller, W. R.: The pseudomallei: A review. J. Infect. Dis., 124:598, 1971.
Khaira, B. S., Young, W. B., and Hart, P. DeV.: Melioidosis. Br. Med. J., 1:949, 1959.
Prevatt, A. L., and Hunt, J. S.: Chronic systemic melioidosis. Review of literature. Am. J. Med., 23:810, 1957.
Spotnitz, M., Rudnitsky, A., and Rambaud, J. J.: Melioidosis pneumonitis. JAMA, 202:950, 1967.

160. ANTHRAX

Leighton E. Cluff

DEFINITION. Anthrax is an infectious disease of wild and domesticated animals caused by *Bacillus anthracis*. Occasionally it is transmitted to man. A necrotic ulcer of the skin or mucous membranes is the most common feature of the disease, but hemorrhagic mediastinitis and disseminated infection with hemorrhagic meningitis may also develop. Depending upon the most prominent feature of the disease, anthrax has been variously referred to as *malignant pustule, splenic fever, woolsorters' disease, milzbrand,* and *charbon.*

ETIOLOGY. *Bacillus anthracis* was identified in 1849 by Davaine, and was further characterized by Koch in 1877. It is a gram-positive, sporeforming, encapsulated, hemolytic, aerobic microorganism. It resembles *B. subtilis* and *B. cereus* but can be differentiated from these organisms by its virulence for laboratory animals such as the mouse and rabbit, by its lack of hemolytic activity on blood agar, and by lysis of *B. anthracis* with specific bacteriophage. In broth, the bacillus elaborates an antigen that can be used for specific immunization ("protective antigen"). The spores of *B. anthracis* are killed by boiling for ten minutes but survive for long periods of time in soil, in animal carcasses, and after aerosolization.

EPIDEMIOLOGY. Anthrax has occurred sporadically and in epidemics throughout the world. Cattle, sheep, goats, horses, and swine are most commonly found to have anthrax; outbreaks of the disease in these animals rarely occur in the United States. Although the disease has been acquired by butchering, skinning, or dissecting infected carcasses, human infection in the United States is observed almost exclusively in persons handling imported contaminated hides, wool, goat hair, or other animal products. Epidemics of anthrax occurred in cattle in Texas and in horses in the state of Washington during 1974, attributed to contaminated saddle packs containing goat hair imported from Pakistan. No human infections were known to have been contracted during these outbreaks, although cats fed carcass meat developed anthrax. Three human infections occurred in the United States in 1975–1976. The infection may be transmitted to man by direct contact, inhalation, and ingestion of infected material.

PATHOLOGY AND PATHOGENESIS. Anthrax is characterized by edema, hemorrhage, necrosis, and various degrees of inflammation. *B. anthracis* possesses a glutamyl polypeptide capsule that interferes with phagocytosis, and this contributes to its pathogenicity. The gelatinous edema of anthrax infection contains large amounts of bacterial capsular material. The serum of many animals has lytic activity against the bacillus, but this anthracidal substance seems to bear little or no relationship to natural resistance. It is probable that *B. anthracis* initiates infection in the skin only through abrasions, cuts, or other types of injury. During the course of lethal anthrax infection in laboratory animals, Smith and Keppie demonstrated a bacterial toxin in blood which is responsible for death. This lethal toxin can be neutralized by specific antitoxin.

CLINICAL MANIFESTATIONS. The skin lesion of anthrax usually begins as a small erythematous papule that becomes vesicular, necrotic, and covered with a dark crust or eschar. Intense nonpitting edema, which may not be erythematous, often surrounds and may extend a considerable distance from the eschar. Characteristically the lesion is pruritic but not very tender or hot. The skin lesion is commonly on exposed areas of hands, arms, neck, or face; and there may be mild regional lymph node enlargement. Lymphangitis is not usually observed. Constitutional symptoms and fever are frequently absent unless the skin disease is severe or the infection becomes disseminated, when high fever, prostration, and death may occur.

Infrequently anthrax may develop without a lesion, possibly after inoculation into the skin, but probably more commonly after inhalation of spores of the bacillus in contaminated air. Characteristically, this form of anthrax is severe and is associated with disseminated infection. *Hemorrhagic mediastinitis,* often without pneumonia, and *hemorrhagic meningitis* may occur. Death is common in this form of anthrax; the illness may begin abruptly, be of short duration, and terminate rapidly. Dyspnea and cyanosis are indicative of respiratory or ventilatory insufficiency. Roentgenographic examination of the chest in inhalation anthrax reveals widening of the mediastinum. Leukocytosis is ordinarily not pronounced. Pleural effusion may complicate pulmonary anthrax. Anthrax in man from ingestion of bacilli is rare.

DIAGNOSIS. Anthrax is most readily diagnosed in persons known to have been exposed to animals or animal products potentially contaminated with *B. anthracis.* Cutaneous anthrax can be differentiated from many other bacterial infections of the skin by the insignificance of regional adenopathy, lymphangitis, and cellulitis in relation to the severity of the eschar and edema. Furthermore, pruritus, lack of tenderness, and intense nonpitting edema are characteristic of anthrax. Small skin lesions, however, may be more difficult to recognize. Pulmonary anthrax can be identified by a history of occupational exposure and acute widening of the mediastinum shown by roentgenographic examination. Anthrax meningitis is confused with subarachnoid hemorrhage or cerebrovascular accident, but is usually associated with prominent signs of infection, and gram-positive bacilli can be seen in the cerebrospinal fluid.

In disseminated anthrax infection, blood cultures are often positive. Occasionally, the bacilli may be identified in the centrifugal sediment of blood treated with 3 per cent acetic acid solution and stained with Wright's stain.

In cutaneous anthrax, the bacilli can usually be cultured from the lesions, or typical encapsulated bacilli will be seen when stained with a polychrome eosin–methylene blue stain (Wright or Giemsa). Their direct cultivation on peptone agar should always be attempted. If the specimen has to be shipped, the specimen should be dried on silk threads or on a sterile glass slide. In view of the occurrence of anthrax-like bacilli on the skin, it is imperative that diagnoses be confirmed by animal inoculations, preferably in guinea pigs or mice or by specific bacteriophage lysis. In pulmonary anthrax, the bacillus has been found microscopically in the sputum and in the pleural exudate.

An agar-gel precipitin serologic test has been useful in epidemiologic studies of anthrax. This test, however, is of no value in diagnosing the acute disease.

PROGNOSIS. Cutaneous anthrax is often a self-limited disease, but dissemination of the infection and death may occur in 20 per cent of patients. A fatal outcome in cutaneous anthrax can be averted by appropriate treatment, but treatment of disseminated infection is often unsuccessful in preventing death.

TREATMENT. *B. anthracis* is susceptible to the action of penicillin, the tetracyclines, chloramphenicol, erythromycin, and streptomycin. Penicillin G should be given in total daily doses of at least 1.2 million units, starting as soon as anthrax is diagnosed or seriously suspected. The effectiveness of the tetracyclines is probably not quite so great as that of penicillin; nevertheless, they are effective in cutaneous anthrax and may be administered in a total daily dose of 2.0 grams. Therapy with penicillin or the tetracyclines should be continued for seven days. It should be emphasized that in patients with disseminated anthrax, the progressive course may be so rapid that antimicrobial drugs may not save the patient's life.

PREVENTION. Anthrax can be prevented in man by control of infected animals or animal products. Autoclaving or treatment of imported goat hair with 5.25 per cent sodium hypochlorite (Chlorox) is often impracticable, although this is the means employed to prevent infection from clothing, rugs, and other products, such as shaving brushes, made of potentially infected materials. Vaccination with "protective antigen" is effective in preventing infection in persons likely to be occupationally exposed.

Brachman, P. S.: Human anthrax in the United States. *In* Hobby, G. L. (ed.): Antimicrobial Agents and Chemotherapy. Baltimore, Williams & Wilkins Company, 1965.
Brachman, P. S., Plotkin, S. A., Bumford, F. H., and Atchison, M. M.: An epidemic of inhalation anthrax. II. Epidemiologic investigation. Am. J. Hyg., 72:6, 1960.
Gold, H.: Anthrax: Report of 117 cases. Arch. Intern. Med., 96:387, 1955.
Hughes, M. H.: Anthrax. Br. Med. J., 1:488, 1973.
Plotkin, S. A., Brachman, P. S., Utell, M., Bumford, F. H., and Atchison, M. M.: Epidemic of inhalation anthrax, first in twentieth century. I. Clinical features. Am. J. Med., 29:992, 1960.

161. LISTERIOSIS

Leighton E. Cluff

DEFINITION. Listeriosis is an infectious disease of animals and man with exceptionally protean manifestations, including meningitis, disseminated granulomas, lymphadenopathy, respiratory symptoms, and ill-defined acute febrile illness. It can produce abortion and fetal or neonatal death. The infection is caused by a gram-positive bacillus called *Listeria monocytogenes* and is worldwide in distribution.

ETIOLOGY. Infection of the human being with *Listeria monocytogenes* was identified in 1929 by Nyfeldt. The microorganism was first characterized, however, by Murray, Webb, and Swann in 1926, during an epizootic among rabbits and guinea pigs. Subsequently the microorganism has been identified as a cause of disease in fox, raccoon, goat, lemming, mouse, rat, hamster, pig, horse, cow, dog, domestic fowl and wild birds, and other animals. *L. monocytogenes* is a gram-positive, nonsporeforming, aerobic or microaerophilic, motile bacillus. It ferments a number of sugars, with formation of acid but no gas. It can be grown on nutrient agar or broth, preferably containing 1 per cent glucose, and produces beta hemolysis on blood agar. *L. monocy-*

togenes resembles *Erysipelothrix rhuziopathiae* and diphtheroids, but can be differentiated from these bacteria by its motility (best at 20 to 30° C), its specific antigenicity, and its animal pathogenicity. *Listeria* regularly — and *Erysipelothrix* occasionally — produces purulent keratoconjunctivitis in rabbits after inoculation into the conjunctival space, whereas diphtheroids do not.

EPIDEMIOLOGY. Listeriosis in man and animals has been observed throughout the world. It has been recognized more frequently in humans in recent years, but its true incidence is not known. Confusion in bacteriologic differentiation accounts largely for inadequate recognition of listeriosis. In addition, the diverse manifestations of the disease render it difficult to identify clinically.

Listeriosis may develop after inhalation, ingestion, or direct contact with contaminated food or animal products. The disease is most common in persons living in rural areas. Although infection with *Listeria* occurs in many domesticated and wild animals, there are only rare instances of epizootics or outbreaks in animals other than man. Transmission of infection from person to person probably occurs under some circumstances, notably in nursery outbreaks. Women can carry *Listeria* in the vagina, and infection may be transmitted venereally. Whether or not man can be an asymptomatic carrier of *Listeria* under other conditions is not known.

PATHOLOGY AND PATHOGENESIS. Human listeriosis is characterized by disseminated granulomas and focal necrosis or suppuration in involved tissues. Lesions may develop in liver, intestinal tract, gallbladder, skin, mucous membranes of the respiratory tract, lung, heart, spleen, lymph nodes, placenta, and brain. The fetus may be infected transplacentally through the umbilical vein, with production of septicemia. Debilitating diseases such as chronic infection and cancer predispose to the occurrence of listeriosis. Pregnancy may increase susceptibility to infection, but the disease in pregnant women may be less severe than in other persons. Administration of adrenal cortical steroids may also increase susceptibility to listeriosis. Infection also occurs in persons with no underlying disease.

CLINICAL MANIFESTATIONS. *Meningitis* is the most commonly recognized form of listeriosis in the United States. It is characterized at onset by symptoms of headache, myalgia, fever, chills, nausea, vomiting, and photophobia, followed by the development of stiff neck, stupor, convulsions, somnolence, and, finally, death. The onset may be abrupt or gradual, and the initial symptoms may be those of gastrointestinal or respiratory illness. Examination reveals manifestations of meningitis or encephalitis in varying degrees of severity. There may be pharyngitis, rhinitis, otitis media, neck rigidity, ocular palsy, and signs of depressed cerebral function. Leukocytosis is common, with granulocytosis and, occasionally, monocytosis, in the early phase of the disease. The cerebrospinal fluid, with decreased sugar, elevated protein, and cell counts of 150 to 3000 per cubic millimeter, is indistinguishable from that in many purulent meningitides. Early, the cells in the fluid may be principally granulocytes, but later there may be a predominance of mononuclear cells.

Febrile pharyngitis with cervical and generalized lymphadenopathy can be caused by *Listeria*, and may be difficult to differentiate from *infectious mononucleosis*.

Patients with this type of illness, however, may have an abrupt onset of fever, chills, headache, myalgia, conjunctivitis, macular rash, and sore throat. Lymph nodes in the neck and elsewhere may enlarge, and there may be hepatosplenomegaly. Blood leukocytes occasionally increase in number with a more or less pronounced monocytosis. The absorbed heterophil serologic test for infectious mononucleosis is negative, *Listeria* can be isolated from blood and pharynx, and there will be a rising serum agglutinin titer for *Listeria*.

Lymph node enlargement in the neck and elsewhere without respiratory symptoms may also be attributed to listeriosis. In addition, lymph node enlargement associated only with conjunctivitis may occur. Isolated acute upper respiratory illness may be attributable to listeriosis, although for obvious reasons this diagnosis is seldom established. Chronic urethritis in men has been described, and possibly may be responsible for subclinical or occult infection, demonstrable by culture of the bacillus from bone marrow.

Papular skin lesions associated with disseminated listeriosis have been seen in infants, but adults may acquire primary cutaneous infection after direct contact with infected animal tissues.

Disseminated listeriosis in infants has been reported frequently in Europe, but infrequently in the United States. The disease may arise by transplacental infection of the fetus, causing abortion, fetal death, or serious illness within several days after birth. Outbreaks of infection may develop in newborn nurseries, probably by person-to-person transmission. The disease is characterized by disseminated visceral granulomas and abscesses. When it manifests itself in infants a few weeks old, it often begins as a mild febrile illness with cough, coryza, gastrointestinal symptoms, and pneumonia. Granulomas may be formed on the posterior pharyngeal wall. Granulocytosis and occasionally mononucleosis are present. Pleural and pericardial effusions may develop. Listeriosis has been reported as a common cause of neonatal death and fetal damage in Europe.

Listeriosis in pregnancy may be subclinical or may be associated with an acute febrile illness resembling influenza and occasionally pyelonephritis; it is rarely severe. Its occurrence after the fifth month of pregnancy, however, is likely to affect the fetus seriously. A woman may become a vaginal carrier of *Listeria* and may possibly infect her infant at birth.

Disseminated listeriosis in adults has an abrupt onset with chill and fever. Meningitis can occur, as well as bacterial endocarditis. Blood cultures are usually positive, and there may be a consumptive coagulopathy. This type of listeriosis is observed most often in patients with carcinoma or debilitating disease, and its development may have been facilitated by adrenal steroid therapy.

DIAGNOSIS. There are no pathognomonic clinical features of human listeriosis. The diagnosis rests on isolation of the microorganism or rising agglutinin titers in the serum. It is likely that the recognition of listeriosis has been difficult because of the failure to differentiate *Listeria* from diphtheroid bacilli in culture. The isolation of microorganisms resembling diphtheroids from infectious material or blood should alert one to the necessity for further bacteriologic characterization.

Listeriosis may resemble influenza, miliary tuberculosis, typhoid fever, mycotic infections, and several bacterial infections with septicemia. *Infectious mononucleosis* is most often confused with listeriosis in adults, for the two diseases may be clinically alike. However, listeriosis is infrequently associated with monocytosis, it does not produce a positive absorbed heterophil serologic test, and in systemic disease the bacillus can be isolated from blood, bone marrow, urine, or upper respiratory tract.

TREATMENT. *Listeria monocytogenes* is susceptible in vitro to sulfonamides, penicillin, tetracycline, chloramphenicol, erythromycin, novobiocin, and occasionally streptomycin. Penicillin is the drug of choice, but the tetracyclines and erythromycin are also effective. Some have recommended use of the aminoglycosides, but most strains of *Listeria* are susceptible to less toxic antimicrobial drugs, and these are preferred unless in vitro resistance is demonstrated. Penicillin G should be administered in a dose of 250,000 units per kilogram of body weight each day and should be continued for about seven days after the patient with meningitis becomes afebrile. In other types of infection, treatment should be given for a period of several days, depending upon the course of the disease.

PROGNOSIS. Listeria meningitis has a fatality rate of 70 per cent in untreated patients. The fatality rate in treated patients is considerably lower. The prognosis in adults with pharyngitis and lymph node enlargement is good, whether treated or not, but meningitis may supervene. Recovery from meningitis may leave residual symptoms of central nervous system damage. Infection of the newborn is very serious; the fatality rate and the incidence of congenital defects are high. Untreated, disseminated listeriosis is usually a fatal disease.

PREVENTION. Listeriosis must be regarded as primarily a contagious disease of animals; prevention of human infection would require elimination of animal reservoirs, but this would not prevent person-to-person transmission. Pasteurization prevents transmission of the disease by contaminated milk. Animal products, including meat, should be declared unfit for consumption if the disease is found in slaughtered animals. Better recognition of the disease should clarify its epidemiology and indirectly facilitate control measures. There are no effective agents for immunization.

Gray, M. L., and Killinger, A. H.: *Listeria monocytogenes* and listeric infections. Bact. Rev., 30:309, 1966.

Hoeprich, P. D.: Infections due to *Listeria monocytogenes.* Medicine, 37:143, 1958.

Lowenstein, M. S., Fox, M. D., and Martin, S. M.: Human listeriosis in the U.S. J. Infect. Dis., 123:328, 1971.

Medoff, G., Kunz, L. J., and Weinberg, A. N.: Listeriosis in humans: An evaluation. J. Infect. Dis., 123:247, 1971.

Moore, R. M., and Zehmer, R. B.: Listeriosis in the U.S., 1971. J. Infect. Dis., 127:610, 1973.

162. ERYSIPELOID OF ROSENBACH

Leighton E. Cluff

Erysipeloid of Rosenbach is a specific infectious disease attributable to *Erysipelothrix rhuziopathia.* It occurs in man after contact with infected animals or animal products, particularly swine, cattle, sheep, fish, birds, dogs, horses, reindeer, rabbits, mink, rats, and mice. The disease in man therefore usually arises in abattoir employees, butchers, kitchen workers, those handling fish, those handling animal hides and pelts, and those working with bone or bone meal. Most infections in human beings can be related to skin injury. The causative microorganism is a gram-positive bacillus, nonsporeforming, that can be grown aerobically or anaerobically on nutrient broth containing 1 per cent glucose or upon blood agar. It produces death in laboratory animals, particularly mice, causing focal abscesses in the liver or cutaneous cellulitis. The bacillus is susceptible in vitro to tetracycline, penicillin, chloramphenicol, cephalosporins, erythromycin, and clindamycin.

Erysipeloid in man occurs seasonally, usually in summer and early fall, and is worldwide in distribution. Most commonly it is characterized by a nonsuppurative violaceous lesion of the hand or fingers that is swollen, is very slightly tender, and has a sharply defined margin rarely extending above the wrist. In contrast to streptococcal cellulitis, there are usually burning, tingling, and itching, but little pain in the involved area; rarely does the patient have systemic symptoms of fever, chills, malaise, or headache. Lymphangitis is infrequent, and when it develops it is often attributable to secondary infection with staphylococci or streptococci. The localized disease is self-limited, lasting a few days, and resolution is rapid, associated with brownish discoloration of the involved skin and rarely desquamation. A bacteriologic diagnosis can be made by culture of material aspirated or biopsied from the margin of the lesion, but isolation of the bacillus is not invariable. Ordinarily, the lesion is sufficiently distinctive to permit a clinical diagnosis when the microorganism is not cultured.

Infrequently *Erysipelothrix* infections may become disseminated, causing a diffuse involvement of skin. Rarely, bacteremia may develop, and bacterial endocarditis can occur.

Erysipeloid continues to occur frequently in exposed persons. The ubiquitousness of the bacillus has made it difficult to eradicate the disease. The ordinarily benign character of the infection, however, has made it an insignificant public health problem. Treatment of erysipeloid with penicillin in a dose of 1.2 million units of benzathine penicillin G shortens the localized illness. Disseminated infection should be treated with penicillin G in a dose of 6 to 12 million units each day for four to six weeks. Relapses of the disease have occurred in persons who are untreated or who receive inadequate treatment.

Ewing, M.: Erysipeloid. Med. J. Aust., 1:449, 1957.

Klauden, J. V.: Erysipeloid as an occupational disease. J.A.M.A., 111:1345, 1938.

Price, J. E. L., and Bennett, W. E. J.: The erysipeloid of Rosenbach. Br. Med. J., 2:1060, 1951.

Sneath, P. H. A., Abbott, J. D., and Cunliffe, A. C.: The bacteriology of erysipeloid. Br. Med. J., 2:1063, 1951.

163. ACTINOMYCOSIS

John P. Utz

DEFINITION. Actinomycosis is a chronic, systemic disease characterized by multiple indurated abscesses and sinus tracts characteristically in the face, neck, chest, and abdomen.

HISTORY. Lebert is credited with the first report, in 1857, of actinomycosis in man. Bollinger described the disease in cattle in 1876. In 1877 Harz named the causative organism *Actinomyces bovis*. In 1878 Israel clearly defined the disease in man by a summary of the clinical and pathologic characteristics observed in 38 patients. The same author in collaboration with Wolff in 1891 succeeded in growing the microorganism in anaerobic culture. In 1910 Lord observed *A. bovis* in and about carious teeth and tonsillar crypts in the mouths of otherwise normal persons.

ETIOLOGY. Actinomycosis in man is caused by *A. israelii* and in cattle by *A. bovis*, but species characteristics overlap. In the normal mouth *A. israelii* grows as a pleomorphic rod-shaped bacterium and in tissues as a granule. In draining pus, mycelial clumps measuring 1 to 2 mm in diameter and colored white to yellow have been termed "sulfur" granules. Microscopically these are composed of 0.5 to 1.0 μ filaments which stain gram-positive. On agar media under strictly anaerobic conditions, *A. israelii* grows as a white spherical or lobulated colony. Laboratory animals are generally not susceptible to experimental infection. Although long considered to be a fungus, the microbe is now classified under the bacteria, a designation that more closely fits certain of its major characteristics, including susceptibility to penicillin.

EPIDEMIOLOGY. The disease is worldwide in distribution. During the first part of the twentieth century it was viewed as being the most common of the "systemic mycoses," but the incidence has been decreasing of late. Males are affected almost twice as frequently as females, and the illness seems most common among farmers and in rural areas. Disease is produced by direct invasion of contiguous tissues by *A. israelii* commonly present in the mouth or bowel. There is virtually always concurrent infection with other anaerobic bacteria. Disease in the brain, heart valves, or extremities may be exceptional instances of hematogenous dissemination. Disease in cows, dogs, or swine has no contagious relation to that in man.

PATHOLOGY. In tissues the characteristic and classic findings are the actinomycotic granules. These are usually found in abscesses and are surrounded by polymorphonuclear leukocytes. Chronic granulomatous reactions are also seen with giant cells, especially about granules.

CLINICAL MANIFESTATIONS. Cervicofacial Form. The cervicofacial form occurs in less than half of all cases. Infection probably spreads secondarily to trauma or to carious teeth or infected tonsils. The subcutaneous tissues at the angle of the mandible and of the neck have a characteristic "woody" or indurated feeling, and the skin over these areas is reddened and may have single or multiple draining sinus tracts. Pain is seldom prominent even with osteomyelitic or periosteal lesions of bone.

Thoracic Form. This form of disease arises from aspiration into the bronchi of *A. israelii* or in a few instances from extension of disease from the esophagus to mediastinal tissues and secondarily to pleura and lung. Fever and cough are minimal early in the illness. As disease progresses to consolidation, pleurisy, and draining sinuses, prominent symptoms are weight loss, night sweats, and high fever. Rib involvement occurs occasionally, pleural effusion rarely. Pericarditis (with effusion) and multiple systemic to pulmonary artery fistulas have recently been described.

Abdominal Form. Actinomycosis of the abdomen

generally follows appendicitis, appendiceal abscess, a perforating lesion of the stomach, or a diverticulum of the large bowel. An abdominal mass is usually palpable, and may be extensive; and there may be burrowing sinus tracts, some of which may open to the skin in the inguinal or other regions. Pelvic actinomycosis can occur in patients with an intrauterine contraceptive device. Retroperitoneal and thoracic spread through the diaphragm are common.

Other Forms. Approximately 10 per cent of patients have lesions in the brain, heart valves, anorectal area, or subcutaneous tissue of the extremities. Rare instances of actinomycosis of the finger have been attributed to injury to the hand by an adversary's tooth.

DIAGNOSIS. The diagnosis of actinomycosis is supported by the finding in pus of granules that microscopically are composed of gram-positive, branching, often beaded filaments. It should be emphasized that granules may be expressed from otherwise normal tonsils and may not be found in cerebrospinal fluid in cases of central nervous system disease. The diagnosis is confirmed by the isolation of the microorganism in anaerobic culture from a lesion.

Skin test and serologic methods of confirmation are unreliable and are generally unavailable.

Cervicofacial forms of actinomycosis must be distinguished from Ludwig's angina, tuberculosis, osteomyelitis, and malignancy. The thoracic form of disease is suggestive of tuberculosis, other fungal infections, and malignancy. Abdominal actinomycosis is often suspected of being tuberculosis, malignant disease, and, occasionally, amebiasis.

TREATMENT. Penicillin, first used for actinomycosis in 1944, continues to be the best drug in treating all forms of the disease. Although most strains are inhibited in vitro by levels of 0.1 unit per milliliter, the nature of the pathologic process leads often to treatment failures and necessitates prolonged therapy. Doses of 10 to 20 million units parenterally daily for at least six weeks or until lesions have healed are recommended. In penicillin-allergic patients, alternative agents are tetracycline, clindamycin, or chloramphenicol.

Surgical resection and incision and drainage of chronically infected tissues are important adjunctive therapeutic measures.

PROGNOSIS. Prior to antimicrobial therapy, prognosis for life was poor in all forms. With penicillin therapy, the approximate recovery rates are as follows: cervicofacial, 90 per cent; abdominal, 80 per cent; and thoracic, 40 per cent.

Cope, V. Z.: Actinomycosis. London, Oxford University Press, 1938.

Lerner, P. I.: Susceptibility of pathogenic actinomycetes to antimicrobial compounds. Antimicrob. Agents Chemother., 5:302, 1974.

Slack, J. M., and Gerencser, M. A.: Actinomyces and Filamentous Bacteria. Minneapolis, Burgess, 1975.

164. NOCARDIOSIS

John E. Bennett

DEFINITION. Nocardiosis is an uncommon acute or chronic suppurative infection, most often originating in the lung, with a marked tendency to spread to brain and other organs.

HISTORY. Eppinger described the first case in 1890 and isolated the etiologic agent.

ETIOLOGY. *Nocardia asteroides* is the etiologic agent in most cases of nocardiosis. *N. brasiliensis* and *N. caviae* cause an occasional case of nocardiosis. *N. brasiliensis* more typically is responsible for mycetoma or, rarely, a lymphocutaneous disease resembling sporotrichosis. *Nocardia* species are aerobic, higher bacteria with branching hyphae less than 1 μ wide. Hyphae are weakly gram-positive and weakly acid fast. On Gram stain of pus, *Nocardia* often appear beaded and refractile. *Nocardia* grow readily at 25 or 37° C on many drug-free culture media. Colonies are initially smooth and white or cream colored, later becoming chalky with an orange or yellow hue. Growth is often apparent in the first week of incubation. Identification of an isolate as *N. asteroides, N. caviae,* or *N. brasiliensis* is a complex task, best assigned to a reference laboratory.

EPIDEMIOLOGY. *Nocardia* organisms are soil saprophytes. Portal of entry is the lung or, rarely, through trauma to the skin or gastrointestinal tract. Man-to-man transmission is unknown. Nocardiosis is infrequent but worldwide. Infection in males is two to three times as common as in females. Disease occurs at any age but is more frequent in older adults. No occupational predisposition is known. Many patients have pre-existing debilitating conditions, such as neoplasia, immunosuppressive therapy, alveolar proteinosis, or chronic granulomatous disease of childhood.

PATHOLOGY. The lung lesion is a bronchopneumonia, with a tendency to suppuration, empyema, and abscess formation. Brain lesions are poorly encapsulated abscesses, often multiple. Purulent meningitis may result from rupture of a brain abscess into the cerebrospinal fluid. Neutrophils are the most prominent inflammatory cell in all sites, but lymphocytes and plasma cells also occur. Giant cells or epithelioid cells are infrequent. Branching filaments of *Nocardia* are scattered in the lesion, with no granule formation. Hyphae are best demonstrated histologically by a tissue Gram stain, such as Brown and Brenn. An overstained Gomori methenamine silver procedure can also be used.

CLINICAL MANIFESTATIONS. Presenting symptoms usually refer to the lung, brain, or subcutaneous tissue, in that decreasing order of frequency. Pulmonary infection may be acute or of many months' duration. Symptoms include fever, cough, purulent sputum, weight loss, anorexia, fatigue, dyspnea, and chest pain. Radiologic appearance of the lung lesion is variable, but typically there are one or more areas of dense pneumonia. Lesions tend to cavitate with time. Infection sometimes extends from the lung into the chest wall, forming a subcutaneous abscess. The central nervous system is infected in 30 per cent of cases. This may be the initial or sole manifestation of the disease or may be a late complication of pulmonary nocardiosis. Clinically the neurologic disease presents as a brain abscess or purulent meningitis. Skin or subcutaneous abscesses also occur in about 30 per cent of cases, usually in the presence of pulmonary nocardiosis. Dissemination to many other organs may occur, particularly heart, kidney, spleen, and liver.

DIAGNOSIS. A refractory, suppurative pneumonitis should suggest the possibility of nocardiosis, particularly in the presence of immunosuppression, brain abscess, or skin abscesses. Sputum, bronchoscopic washings, pleural fluid, percutaneous lung aspirates, and pus aspirated from other sites should be Gram stained and cultured for *Nocardia*. Cultures of blood, bone marrow, urine, or cerebrospinal fluid are rarely positive.

Branching, gram-positive filaments on smear raise the possibility of actinomycosis or nocardiosis. *Nocardia* can usually, but not always, be distinguished from *Actinomyces* on smear by the absence of granules and weak acid-fastness of the former. Acid-fastness is best demonstrated by a modified Ziehl-Neelsen stain or in tissue by a modified Fite-Faraco stain. Use of dilute sulfuric acid rather than acid-alcohol during destaining is critical. Diagnosis of nocardiosis by culture alone is fraught with problems. *Nocardia* organisms are difficult to isolate from heavily contaminated specimens, such as sputum, and accurate culture identification of *Nocardia* requires both time and expertise.

Occasionally *Nocardia* is isolated from a specimen, usually sputum, either as a contaminant or as the cause of a mild, self-limiting disease. It is much more common, however, for subsequent developments to indicate that the *Nocardia* had been the cause of symptoms incorrectly ascribed to tuberculosis, neoplasm, or another disorder.

TREATMENT. Treatment of choice is enough sulfadiazine to give serum concentrations of 10 to 15 mg per 100 ml. Six to nine grams per day is usually required for an adult. Copious fluid intake and urine alkalinization with oral sodium bicarbonate are necessary to prevent crystalluria. After about a month, if the patient is improving, sulfadiazine dosage may be reduced to 4 to 6 grams per day, or an equivalent amount of sulfisoxazole or trisulfapyrimidines may be used instead. Therapy is usually continued at this dose for 12 to 18 months. Pus in the brain, pleura, or soft tissues should be drained. Whether or not drugs other than sulfonamides are useful is an open question. Only a few patients not receiving sulfonamides have survived. It is common practice for patients responding poorly to sulfonamides to be given an additional drug, particularly ampicillin, 150 mg per kilogram per day. Cycloserine, erythromycin, minocycline, and co-trimoxazole also have their advocates.

PROGNOSIS. Clinically apparent nocardiosis is usually fatal without treatment. With appropriate therapy, nocardiosis confined to the lung has the best prognosis (50 to 60 per cent survival) and central nervous system infection the worst (13 per cent survival). The occurrence of nocardiosis in the presence of immunosuppressive therapy portends a poor prognosis.

Frazier, A. R., Rosenow, E. C., and Roberts, G.: Nocardiosis. A review of 25 cases occurring during 24 months. Mayo Clin. Proc., 50:657, 1975.

Krick, J. A., Stinson, E. B., and Remington, J. S.: *Nocardia* infection in heart transplant patients. Ann. Intern. Med., 82:18, 1975.

Palmer, D. L., Harvey, R. L., and Wheeler, J. K.: Diagnostic and therapeutic considerations in *Nocardia asteroides* infection. Medicine, 53:391, 1974.

Young, L. S., Armstrong, D., Blevins, A., and Lieberman, P.: *Nocardia asteroides* infection complicating neoplastic disease. Am. J. Med., 50:356, 1971.

165. BRUCELLOSIS

Thomas M. Buchanan

DEFINITION. Brucellosis is an infectious disease characterized by fever, sweats, weakness, malaise, and weight loss that is transmitted to man from animals or animal products containing bacteria of the genus *Brucella*.

ETIOLOGY. *Brucella suis, Brucella abortus, Brucella me-*

litensis, and *Brucella canis* may all cause human brucellosis. Brucellae are small, nonmotile, nonsporeforming, gram-negative rods. The four species are differentiated by biochemical and serologic reactions. Hogs are generally infected with *Br. suis,* cattle with *Br. abortus,* sheep and goats with *Br. melitensis,* and dogs with *Br. canis.* However, infections of swine with *Br. abortus* or of cattle with *Br. suis* may occur, and *Brucella* infection of caribou, deer, horses, moose, cats, and chickens has been reported. Animal-to-animal transmission is usually venereal or via ingestion of infected tissue or milk. Human infection most commonly results from ingestion of infected animal tissue or milk products, or through skin wounds directly bathed in freshly killed infected animal tissues, as in abattoir workers. Human infection via inoculation of the conjunctival sac has also been documented (for example, with strain 19, an attenuated *Br. abortus* used to vaccinate cattle), and there is epidemiologic evidence to suggest rare infection via inhalation of aerosols containing *Brucella* organisms. In recent years, approximately 57 per cent of patients in the United States have been infected with *Br. suis,* 33 per cent with *Br. abortus,* and 10 per cent with *Br. melitensis* or an unidentified *Brucella* species.

EPIDEMIOLOGY. Since 1970, cases of human brucellosis in the United States have ranged from 175 to 328 per year, with 328 cases in 1975 and 271 in 1976. Worldwide, the disease is more common and closely correlates with the extent of animal brucellosis in any country. States with the highest incidence of brucellosis during the past ten years were Iowa, Virginia, Illinois, Minnesota, Nebraska, California, Tennessee, North Carolina, Georgia, Florida, Mississippi, Arkansas, and Louisiana. Texas, Oklahoma, Missouri, and Pennsylvania each reported more than 40 cases during this same period, and all states except Nevada and the District of Columbia experienced one or more cases of human brucellosis during this interval.

Brucellosis most frequently occurs in persons with high rates of exposure to *Brucella*-infected tissues, milk, or milk products. This includes slaughterhouse workers (some persons handle 3000 freshly killed hogs or 800 freshly killed cattle per day), livestock producers, veterinarians, and persons who ingest unpasteurized milk or milk products. In 1976 in the United States, brucellosis patients by occupation were packing house employees (54 per cent), livestock producers (11 per cent), veterinarians and meat inspectors (9 per cent), and farmers, students, children, and other miscellaneous categories (18 per cent). The number of organisms required to produce infection via different routes is least for penetration through broken skin; considerably more for exposure to *Brucella* organisms through the conjunctival sac or by ingestion of contaminated materials; and still more for inhalation of infected aerosols. Brucellae may remain viable in unpasteurized milk or cheese for approximately 10 or 90 days, respectively. Isolation of *Brucella* from infected meat markedly decreases over a few days with refrigeration, and particularly with the curing and smoking processes used for ham and bacon. In the abattoir setting, persons with a combination of both high accidental cut rates and considerable exposure to the blood and lymph of freshly killed animals are most likely to develop *Brucella* infections. *Brucella* infections are often controlled by the patient's immune response, and asymptomatic infections are up to ten times more common than symptomatic disease and the

clinical syndrome of brucellosis. Approximately 90 per cent of patients are immune to developing subsequent clinical brucellosis following recovery from their first infection. Therefore in populations with high exposures to potentially infected tissues (e.g., abattoir workers), most cases are seen in younger persons who have been exposed for shorter periods to potentially infected tissues and are less likely to have developed immunity. Also, brucellosis affects men more commonly than women; in 1975, brucellosis was nearly six times more frequent in men than in women.

PATHOGENESIS AND PATHOLOGY. *Brucella* organisms penetrate the epithelial cells of the human skin (i.e., hands), oropharynx, conjunctivae, or lung. In the submucosa they interact with polymorphonuclear leukocytes (PMN) and/or tissue macrophages. Many are phagocytized, and, if the inoculum is sufficient, some spread via the lymphatics to regional lymph nodes. The most common sites of lymphadenitis in brucellosis are in the axillary, cervical, and supraclavicular locations, perhaps reflecting the high frequency of the hand-wound or oropharyngeal routes of infections. If the inoculum is sufficient to overcome host immune attempts at localization of *Brucella* organisms within the lymph nodes, bacteremia follows. The usual incubation period between infection and bacteremia with associated symptoms is 10 to 11 days with a heavy inoculum, and two to three weeks with a smaller inoculum. Incubation periods as short as seven days or as long as three months have been reported. Bacteremia is usually accompanied by phagocytosis of nearly all free *Brucella* organisms within a few hours by circulating PMN. These phagocytized brucellae are further localized most commonly to the spleen, liver, and bone marrow. The patient's fever, chills, and sweats may in part result from endogenous pyrogen release from PMN that have phagocytized *Brucella* organisms. Brucellae are located with phagocytic vacuoles within PMN, and transient intracellular survival and even multiplication of *Brucella* organisms within phagocytes have been reported. In most instances, the inoculum is not large, the human host defenses prevail, granuloma formation does not occur, and the patient recovers. Similarly, even with a large inoculum, prompt (within three to four weeks of onset of symptoms) treatment of sufficient duration (four to eight weeks) results in rapid healing of the small granulomas and complete recovery. However, if the inoculum is large and the patient is not treated, small granulomas may fuse to form large granulomas that may eventually suppurate and serve as a source for recurrent bacteremia. Persistent bacteremia may lead to multiple system involvement, including most commonly infections and abscesses of the skeletal system (spine and joints), genitourinary tract (kidneys, bladder, epididymis, testes, urethra), optic nerve, lung, liver (abnormal liver function tests, jaundice), and cardiovascular system (endocarditis, myocarditis, pericarditis). *Br. suis* and *Br. melitensis* are more virulent than *Br. abortus* and more readily form abscesses.

CLINICAL MANIFESTATIONS. Over 90 per cent of patients experience chilly sensations, sweats, and fever, accompanied by weakness and general malaise. The fever ranges from 38.3 to 40° C, and approximately 70 per cent of patients experience body aches. Over half of patients with brucellosis complain of anorexia and experience weight loss, averaging 15 to 20 pounds. Nearly 45 per cent of patients complain of headaches. Cough and/or arthralgias are present in approximately 20 to 25 per cent of patients. Diarrhea, constipation, visual disturbance, eye pain, dizziness, tinnitus, or genitourinary disturbance may occur, although less frequently. The most common signs of brucellosis in addition to fever are lymphadenopathy (up to 40 per cent), splenomegaly (up to 40 per cent), hepatomegaly (up to 8 per cent), and tenderness over the spine (up to 6 per cent), with the prevalence of each sign reflecting the chronicity of infection in the patient population studied. The average number of work days lost for an abattoir worker with brucellosis varies from 30 to 50 days. One third to one half of patients experience a sudden onset of symptoms; in the remainder the onset is gradual, over several days to weeks.

Observed complications in patients with untreated and longstanding brucellosis have included pleurisy, pleural effusion, lung abscess, millet-seed pulmonary calcification, empyema, pneumonia, chronic pulmonary granuloma, spondylitis, suppurative arthritis, osteomyelitis, hydroarthrosis, epididymitis, orchitis, cystitis, pyelitis, nephritis, optic neuritis, keratitis, uveitis, retinopathy, meningitis, encephalitis, neuritis, hemolytic anemia, thrombocytopenia or pancytopenia associated with hypersplenism, cholecystitis, pericholecystic or subdiaphragmatic abscesses, chronic cutaneous ulcers, endocarditis, myocarditis, thrombophlebitis, pulmonary embolization, and cardiac rupture. Many diseases more common than brucellosis have signs and symptoms that partially or almost totally mimic brucellosis. It is therefore important to exclude other more common illnesses and to obtain objective evidence of *Brucella* infection before making a diagnosis of brucellosis. Diseases that may resemble brucellosis include influenza; infectious mononucleosis; toxoplasmosis; viral hepatitis; acute pyelonephritis; ankylosing spondylitis; thyrotoxicosis; disseminated gonococcal infection; rheumatic fever; systemic lupus erythematosus; malaria; tuberculosis; sarcoidosis; leptospirosis; typhoid fever; Hodgkin's disease; lymphoblastic and lymphocytic leukemia; myeloblastic and myelocytic leukemia; metastatic carcinoma of the lung, colon, prostate, pancreas, stomach, or liver; and thiamin deficiency. If the patient has had recent exposure to animal tissue or products potentially infected with *Brucella* organisms, the clinical suspicion of brucellosis should be increased. However, even abattoir workers experience influenza or influenza-like viral syndromes more frequently than brucellosis.

Objective findings useful for evaluation of possible brucellosis in a patient include physical signs, cultures, serologic data, and x-rays. The absence of at least intermittent fever of 38.3° C or higher makes a diagnosis of brucellosis extremely unlikely (less than 5 per cent of patients). Weight loss is present in approximately half of patients, and lymphadenopathy and splenomegaly are other common signs.

The definitive evidence of *Brucella* infection is the isolation of *Brucella* organisms from the patient. *However, culturing Brucella organisms may be dangerous to laboratory personnel. All cultures should be clearly marked "possible brucellosis" and should be processed with sterile techniques in a biohazard hood certified for handling class III infectious agents. Culturing for Brucella organisms is not recommended for hospitals and clinics without these facilities.* Early in the course of illness, particularly in association with fever and chills, the patient is likely to have *Brucella* bacteremia. Approximately 50 to 75 per cent of these patients who have not received antimicrobial drugs will yield *Brucella* organisms from their blood when one or two samples are cultured in standard blood culture bottles (containing trypticase soy broth) for one to three weeks in the presence of 5 to 10 per cent CO_2. Later in the course of the illness, bacteremia is less frequent and organisms are more likely to be isolated from infected lymph nodes, or from granulomas involving the spleen, liver, or skeletal system (most frequently, spine). During the past ten years only 15 to 20 per cent of brucellosis cases in the United States have been confirmed by culture. Most cases (80 to 85 per cent) were diagnosed serologically.

The most reliable and standardized *serologic screening test* for brucellosis is the standard tube *Brucella* agglutination test. A four-fold or greater rise in titer for sera drawn one to four weeks apart is indicative of recent exposure to *Brucella* or *Brucella*-like antigens. Separate sera should be tested on the same day, in the same laboratory, and under identical conditions to examine for seroconversion. Significant seroconversion is defined as fourfold or greater rise in titer from an initial titer of at least 40 or higher to eventual titer of 160 or higher. The titer is the reciprocal of the maximal serum dilution that produces 50 per cent or more agglutination of the *Brucella* organisms under the test conditions. Most patients develop rising agglutination titers to *Brucella* antigens within one to two weeks of illness, and approximately 80 per cent of persons have an eightfold or higher rise in their agglutinins during the acute illness. Within three weeks of illness, approximately 97 per cent of patients with brucellosis will have serologic evidence of their infection if a single serum sample is tested. With repeat testing, less than 0.7 per cent of all patients will remain seronegative (titer <160). The maximal *Brucella* agglutination titers in sera from persons with asymptomatic *Brucella* infections may reach as high as titers in patients with clinical brucellosis. It should be noted that the *Brucella* skin test, cholera vaccination, or infection with *Vibrio cholerae, Pasteurella tularensis,* or *Yersinia enterocolitica* may cause seroconversion to elevated *Brucella* agglutination titers and not represent *Brucella* infection. Provided that these "cross-reactive" causes of seroconversion are ruled out, a fourfold rise in titer of *Brucella* agglutinating antibodies is indicative of current *Brucella* infection. If such a patient has signs and symptoms compatible with brucellosis, then it is likely that the patient has a symptomatic *Brucella* infection known as brucellosis.

The standard *Brucella* agglutination test is performed as follows: (1) Serial twofold dilutions of the patient's serum are prepared in normal saline, beginning with a 1:10 dilution. (2) Antigen consisting of a standardized diluted suspension of *Brucella abortus* strain No. 1119 (available from the Department of Agriculture, National Animal Diseases Laboratory, Ames, Iowa) is added to each serum-containing well. The tubes containing antigen and serum are mixed and incubated at 37° C for 48 hours. The serum titer is the reciprocal of the maximal serum dilution that produces 50 per cent or more agglutination of the bacterial suspension. This agglutination is accomplished by divalent (IgG) or multivalent (IgM) antibodies bridging two or more *Brucella* organisms. The latticework produced forms a clump that can be seen by observing each agglutination test tube with a fluorescent light against a dark background. A titer of 160 or higher is very rare in persons with no exposure to *Brucella* organisms and is considered indicative of past or present antigenic stimulation with *Brucella* organisms or antigens "cross-reactive" with *Brucella* species. If the clinical suspicion of brucellosis is strong, the patient's serum should be tested in dilutions as high as 1:1280, because prozones — falsely negative tests for agglutination due to "blocking" IgA or nonagglutinating IgG antibodies — have been reported in titers as high as 640.

Significance of Elevated Antibody Titer. During the first one to two weeks of illness, the primary agglutinating antibody response to *Brucella* is of the IgM immunoglobulin class. Thereafter, IgG antibodies are formed in addition to IgM antibodies. Both IgG and IgM agglutinating antibodies are detected in the standard *Brucella* agglutination test. However, with early diagnosis and prompt treatment of sufficient duration, IgG agglutinating antibodies rarely persist beyond 6 to 12 months following onset of the disease. However, if the diagnosis is delayed for many months to years and no treatment is received, some patients (fewer than 15 per cent) will develop continuing *Brucella* infection with potentially serious complications. These patients will maintain elevated IgG *Brucella* agglutinins until diagnosed and treated. This information is useful to the clinician, because the *Brucella* agglutination performed in the presence of 0.05 M 2-mercaptoethanol (2-ME) recognizes only IgG agglutinating antibodies to *Brucella*. Thus in the absence of a rising agglutination titer, a single elevated 2-ME *Brucella* agglutination test titer is the most objective evidence that the patient has a current or recent infection. A titer of 160 or higher in the 2-ME test suggests either a current or recent asymptomatic infection or, if the patient is symptomatic, active infection with disease and the need for treatment. Titers of 40 to 80 in the 2-ME *Brucella* agglutination test are rarely associated with significant recent infections. In a patient with symptoms of three or more weeks' duration, a 2-ME *Brucella* agglutination titer of 20 or lower essentially eliminates the possibility that the patient's symptoms are due to brucellosis. A significant proportion of patients maintain elevated IgM agglutinating antibodies and consequently have elevated standard *Brucella* agglutination titers for many years, even after presumed complete cure of their brucellosis. In fact, standard *Brucella* agglutination titers of ≤160 are very common in completely asymptomatic abattoir workers. For this reason, the 2-ME *Brucella* agglutination test that measures only IgG agglutinating antibodies is the most useful indicator of whether the patient was cured (negative test).

The Brucella skin test is not recommended for diagnostic purposes, because it may remain positive for many years following symptomatic or asymptomatic *Brucella* infection and it may interfere with interpretation of serologic tests by causing a rise in titer of the standard tube agglutination test.

TREATMENT. The combination of streptomycin and tetracycline is superior to tetracycline alone, and tetracycline therapy should be maintained for a minimum of six weeks. These antimicrobials quickly kill *Brucella* organisms in vitro, but during brucellosis some organisms survive the antimicrobial therapy, perhaps by being located within cells, granulomas, or abscesses. The long duration of chemotherapy permits mobilization of the humoral and cellular immunity that is required for eventual complete elimination of infecting *Brucella* organisms. A regimen used successfully to treat more than 200 workers who acquired brucellosis in a midwest slaughterhouse was streptomycin, 1 gram daily intramuscularly during days 1 to 6 and 8 to 13; and tetracycline, 500 mg orally four times daily during

days 1 to 45. One of these patients developed significant complications of his brucellosis that lasted six to eight months, and none developed chronic disease (illness ≥1 year's duration) or death. Relapses occurred in approximately 2 per cent of the patients, and these responded to retreatment. Nearly all were able to return to their former work in the abattoir. Variations on the streptomycin-tetracycline regimen have been reported, e.g., substitution of another aminoglycoside, gentamicin, for the streptomycin, use of a tetracycline with prolonged action (doxycycline), or use of co-trimoxazole as a supplement. However, at present the efficacy of these alternatives to the streptomycin-tetracycline therapy is unproved, and further investigations are warranted before their value can be established. After six weeks of treatment, if the patient is without signs or symptoms of brucellosis and has evidence of decreasing agglutination titers, antimicrobial therapy may be discontinued. Relapses occur in less than 5 per cent of cases when the patient receives treatment early in the course of illness and for six weeks' duration. Relapse is more frequent when treatment is delayed or of insufficient duration. Most relapses occur within three months, and nearly all develop within ten months of completing initial therapy. Nearly all relapses rapidly respond to a repeat course of therapy.

PROGNOSIS. Brucellosis diagnosed within one month of onset of illness and treated with appropriate antimicrobial therapy for a sufficient period is a completely curable illness. Even before antimicrobial therapy was available, 85 per cent of patients recovered within three months. With chemotherapy, chronic brucellosis (illness lasting more than one year) or severe complications have become extremely rare. When either of these situations is found, it is almost invariably associated with a prolonged delay before diagnosis and/or failure to take prescribed medications. Acute brucellosis produces substantial malaise, weakness, fever, and weight loss and is frequently associated with an inability to work for one to two months, even with antimicrobial therapy. Without therapy, complications such as *Brucella* abscesses of the liver, spleen, vertebral column, heart valve, skin, meninges, lung, or bone marrow may occur; but with therapy, these complications are rare (less than 1 per cent). They almost invariably occur only in patients with continuous or intermittent fever of 38.3° C or higher and positive standard and 2-ME *Brucella* agglutination test results (titer greater than 160).

A febrile patient with chronic symptoms suggestive of a complication of brucellosis or of chronic brucellosis should be screened with a standard agglutination test. If this is positive, a 2-ME *Brucella* agglutination test should be performed. A titer of lower than 40 in the 2-ME *Brucella* agglutination test is strong evidence against chronic brucellosis or a complication of brucellosis. The absence of fever, a localized lesion, and elevated 2-ME resistant *Brucella* agglutinins essentially eliminate the possibility that the patient may have chronic brucellosis or a complication of brucellosis. When complications of brucellosis are demonstrated, they usually respond to a combination of surgical removal of the localized lesion and antimicrobial therapy. Hypersensitivity to *Brucella* antigens may occur, but in recent years it has been very unusual even among abattoir workers who are maximally exposed to potentially infected animal tissue. Therefore patients should be allowed to return to their former work, even if it means re-exposure to *Brucella* antigens, as development of hypersensitivity is unlikely. Also, immunity to reinfection follows the first *Brucella* infection in most (92 per cent) cases, and thus patients returning to work following treatment are less likely to acquire brucellosis than are previously uninfected employees. However, if symptoms resembling hypersensitivity occur, it should be determined whether small amounts of *Brucella* antigens can induce these symptoms. If so, these patients should avoid *Brucella* antigens, and this may require changing occupations.

PREVENTION. Infection with *Brucella* confers an impressive immunity. Reinfection occurs but is uncommon (fewer than 5 per cent of patients). Effective prevention of brucellosis in cattle results from a live attenuated *Brucella* vaccine. No vaccine is presently available for humans. The risk of acquiring brucellosis may be reduced by decreasing one's exposure to freshly killed animal tissue from potentially infected animals, and by drinking pasteurized milk and milk products. Slaughterhouse workers, meat inspectors, and veterinarians who occupationally examine large numbers of cattle and hogs may reduce their risk of infection by wearing protective gloves and goggles or eyeglasses and by avoiding hand or arm cuts that might provide a route of entry for *Brucella* organisms. Complete elimination of brucellosis in humans will first require elimination of *Brucella* infection in animals.

Alton, G. G., et al.: Laboratory Techniques in Brucellosis. Geneva, World Health Organization, 1975.

Buchanan, T. M., et al.: Brucellosis in the United States, 1960–1972: An abattoir-associated disease. I. Clinical features and therapy. II. Diagnostic aspects. III. Epidemiology and evidence for acquired immunity. Medicine, 53:403, 415, 427, 1974.

Morales-Otero, P.: *Brucella abortus* in Porto Rico. Porto Rico J. Public Health Trop. Med., 6:3, 1930.

Reports of the Commission for the Investigation of Mediterranean Fever. London, Harrison & Sons, Part 1 to 7, 1905–1907.

Reddin, J. L.: Significance of 7S and macroglobulin *Brucella* agglutinins in human brucellosis. N. Engl. J. Med., 275:1263, 1965.

Smith, C. C.: Treatment of human brucellosis. Scott. Med. J., 21:132, 1976.

Spink, W. W.: The Nature of Brucellosis. Minneapolis, University of Minnesota Press, 1956.

Zoonoses Surveillance, Annual Brucellosis Summaries. Atlanta, Center for Disease Control, published yearly.

DISEASES DUE TO MYCOBACTERIA

166. TUBERCULOSIS

Roger Des Prez

GENERAL CONSIDERATIONS

Tuberculosis is a chronic infection, potentially of lifelong duration, caused by two species of mycobacteria, *M. tuberculosis* and, rarely, *M. bovis*. It is almost always initiated by inhalation of infectious material, rarely by ingestion, and more rarely still by cutaneous inoculation (prosector's wart). Early in infection a silent bloodstream spread seeds the lymphatic system and other organs throughout the body, leaving foci which may cause clinical illness after long periods of latency. Tuberculosis must be differentiated on bacteriologic grounds from chronic infections caused by other species of mycobacteria.

Although paleopathologic evidence indicates that humans were infected with tuberculosis in neolithic times, the infection became epidemic with the Industrial Revolution, which produced the crowded living conditions most favorable to its spread. In the mid-nineteenth century, it is said to have accounted for one quarter of adult deaths in Europe. During that century three great strides led to an accurate conception of the disease and its cause. In 1804, Laennec published the opinion that the many different forms of tuberculosis in the lungs and elsewhere, previously regarded as different diseases, were actually different manifestations of one disease. By 1839, the term *tuberculosis* had come into use, reflecting the unifying anatomic feature of tubercle formation. In 1865, Villemin established the contagious nature of the process by infecting laboratory animals with diseased tissue. In 1882, Koch reported isolation and culture of the tubercle bacillus and successful production of disease in animals by these isolates.

The sanatorium movement, which began because of emphasis on climate in treatment, received further impetus from the demonstration of the infectious nature of the process. As a result, phthisiology became a distinct and sophisticated medical specialty but one which was separated from the mainstream of medicine. The development of diagnostic radiology led to an appreciation of the pivotal importance of cavity formation. Treatment, other than general supportive measures and bed rest, became directed almost entirely at the goal of cavity closure, utilizing methods such as pneumoperitoneum, therapeutic pneumothorax, and collapse of the chest wall by surgical measures (thoracoplasty).

By 1947, it had become established that streptomycin (SM) was a truly effective antituberculous drug, initiating the chemotherapy era. Soon after, it was shown that combination of SM with para-aminosalicylic acid (PAS) tended to prevent treatment failures associated with development of bacterial resistance to SM, establishing the principle of combined drug therapy. The availability of effective drug treatment also made it possible for the first time to resect diseased tissue, a procedure which had previously frequently resulted in spread of infection. Some form of pulmonary resection became a part of treatment of many if not most cases. This attitude persisted for some 15 years until it became clear that resection added very little to the long-term results of effective and extended drug therapy.

In 1952, isoniazid (INH) was established as an antituberculous drug of a different and higher order than SM, and tuberculosis became a medically curable illness in most cases. Since patients on treatment became rapidly noninfectious and required little bed rest or specialized therapeutic methods aimed at cavity collapse, the need for sanatoriums disappeared, and tuberculosis became, perhaps for the first time, the legitimate province of the general physician and general hospital. Treatment began to be applied not only to patients with demonstrably active cases but also to individuals in whom active disease seemed only reasonably likely to develop (chemoprophylaxis). Finally, the more meticulous bacteriologic techniques required to determine drug susceptibility of infecting strains was, more than anything else, responsible for the recognition and eventual definition of many other pathogenic mycobacteria, all of which are less susceptible to isoniazid.

BACTERIOLOGY

Mycobacteria are acid-fast, nonmotile, nonsporulating, weakly gram-positive rods classified in the order Actinomycetales. Until recently, only *M. tuberculosis*, the human tubercle bacillus, and *M. bovis* were regarded as pathogenic for man. *M. avium*, which causes tuberculosis in poultry and swine, is thought to produce human disease only rarely. Recently other mycobacteria, previously either unrecognized or regarded as saprophytes, have become recognized as human pathogens. The clinical importance of these "atypical" mycobacteria is discussed in Ch. 169.

Such distinguishing characteristics as slow growth rate, resistance to chemical disinfectants, and the ability to survive within phagocytic cells are attributed to the hydrophobic, lipid-rich (60 per cent of dry weight) mycobacterial cell wall. Its composition accounts for the typical diagnostic staining characteristics. In the Ziehl-Neelsen method, staining with carbolfuchsin is facilitated by steaming the smear. Subsequent treatment with acid-alcohol elutes carbolfuchsin from other bacteria and organic material, but "acid-fast" mycobacteria resist decoloration.

When pulmonary tuberculosis is sufficiently advanced to cause symptoms, most patients will demonstrate acid-fast bacilli in the sputum. Because it facilitates a more rapid scanning of a sputum smear, an auramine-rhodamine fluorescent stain is now commonly used. The first sputum raised in the morning is the best material to submit for culture. When sputum is not produced, respiratory secretions can be obtained by gastric aspiration or stimulated by inhalation of heated, hypertonic aerosols (10 per cent saline). The aerosol is inhaled for 15 minutes, and all sputum raised then and for a 15-minute period thereafter is collected. Gastric aspiration has been largely abandoned. The procedure, however, is effective for culture purposes when accomplished immediately upon awakening in the morning before the overnight gastric contents have passed from the stomach.

Differentiation of Clinically Important Myobacterial Species

Definitive identification of mycobacteria is usually accomplished by reference laboratories, but good species identification can be achieved by a few simple observations. Rate of growth and production of pigment were used by Runyon to classify the so-called "atypical" mycobacteria into four groups: Group I is characterized by formation of yellow colonies after brief exposure to light (photochromogens), Group II by production of yellow or orange colonies without light stimulation (scotochromogens), Group III by nonpigmented colonies, and Group IV by growth within seven days. These characteristics, together with nonsusceptibility to isoniazid, lack of production of niacin, and production of the enzyme catalase, suffice for tentative identification of those mycobacteria known to be of pathogenic importance in man. *M. tuberculosis* usually requires two or three weeks for visible growth. Colonies are rough, and no pigment is produced. It is the only species which produces a positive niacin test. Isoniazid-susceptible strains of *M. tuberculosis* produce catalase, whereas isoniazid-resistant strains are usually catalase negative. *M. bovis* resembles *M. tuberculosis* but does not produce niacin. The *photochromogenic* property of *M. kansasii* (Runyon Group I) is its most distinguishing characteristic. Growth is slow, colonies are either rough or smooth, moderate isoniazid resistance is usual, catalase production is marked, and niacin is not produced. *M. marinum* (Runyon Group I) resembles *M. kansasii* except that growth is poor at 37° C and good at room temperature. *M. avium* and *M. intracellulare* (the Battey bacillus) grow slowly, produce smooth, thin, nonpigmented colonies, are highly resistant to isoniazid, produce catalase, and do not produce niacin. They are serologically closely related and differ only in that *M. avium* grows well at 45° C and *M. intracellulare* does not. They are classified in Runyon's Group III. *Scotochromogenic mycobacteria* (Runyon Group II) produce yellow to orange pigment in the dark, grow slowly, have smooth colonies, are highly resistant to isoniazid, produce catalase, and do not produce niacin. *Rapid growers* (Runyon Group IV) produce colonies within seven days and are catalase positive, niacin negative, and very resistant to isoniazid.

EPIDEMIOLOGY

In much of the world, bovine tuberculosis remains a significant problem and infection by mouth is frequent. In Western nations, however, infection is almost always by inhalation. Most importance is attached to the dried residue of droplets aerosolized by cough, called *droplet nuclei*, which may remain suspended in air for prolonged periods and are sufficiently small to reach terminal air passages where removal is difficult and bacterial multiplication can begin. Well-studied epidemics in certain closed environments such as naval vessels and boarding schools indicate that one person with cavitary disease may "poison" the environment with droplet nuclei and infect virtually all susceptibles in the same environment, even in the temporary absence of the infectious person himself. A tuberculosis ward is probably not a place of great risk when care is taken, because persons receiving chemotherapy become rapidly noninfectious. Infected urine may rarely be contagious for young children using the same toilet facilities, owing to droplet nuclei formed from urine aerosolization. Transmission of tuberculosis by the genital route is rare. Inoculation of abraded skin by contaminated tissues at autopsy examination may produce a primary skin infection in tuberculin-negative individuals (prosector's wart). Fomites are of no importance in the spread of infection.

INCIDENCE AND PREVALENCE. The decline in tuberculosis mortality which began in the middle of the last century was probably due to improved living conditions and heightened social awareness. In the past 20 years of drug treatment, mortality has declined somewhat more rapidly but the incidence of new cases has fallen less, suggesting a residue of older individuals infected in earlier years. In the young, it is clear that the new case rate has drastically fallen in urban United States. In 1928, 53 per cent of 16-year-old schoolchildren in Philadelphia were tuberculin positive. By 1968, this had decreased to 1.4 per cent. At present, less than 10 per cent of cases of active tuberculosis represent new infections, the remainder developing in persons infected years previously, and succumbing to host-dependent factors, such as age and intercurrent illness, favoring progression of the infection. In the United States active disease is now most frequently diagnosed in nonwhite older males.

IMMUNOLOGIC RESPONSE AND PATHOLOGIC FEATURES

Tuberculosis is the prototype of infections which require cellular immune responses for control. Infection induces a rich antibody response, but what role, if any, these antibodies play in control of infection is not clear. In the first few weeks after established infection, the previously unexposed host has virtually no defense against multiplication of the infectious inoculum either at the initial site or at various metastatic foci established by lymphohematogenous dissemination. During this silent period, lymphocytes genetically coded to react with antigens of the tubercle bacillus proliferate and circulate throughout the lymphatic system. At some interval, usually three to six weeks after infection, the population of specifically reactive lymphocytes usually reaches sufficient size and dissemination to bring the infection under control. The mechanism by which this is accomplished is the elaboration, by reactive lymphocytes in contact with antigen, of a series of lymphocyte products which attract or entrap macrophages at the site of the lymphocyte-antigen interaction, stimulate them to a metabolically more active state in which their mycobactericidal activity is greatly enhanced, and cause some macrophages to differentiate into epithelioid cells and fibroblasts. This sequence of events results in a quite efficient control of infection. However, activated lymphocytes may also elaborate cytotoxic materials which in some instances, particularly when large concentrations of antigen interact with large populations of reactive lymphocytes, may cause cellular necrosis, an event of central importance in the progression of the infection. Although the details of these antigen-lymphocyte-macrophage interactions are by no means clear, *in a general sense tissue hypersensitivity, as manifested by the tuberculin reaction and by cellular necrosis, and cellular immunity, as manifested by successful containment of the infection, are parallel consequences of the appearance of a population of specifically reactive lymphocytes.*

The pathologic response to tuberculous infection is determined in large part by interaction of these two factors, the population of specifically reactive lymphocytes present in the host and the mass of antigen present in the lesion, as modified by structural characteristics of the tissue involved. Small numbers of bacilli in a host with well established lymphocyte reactivity to tuberculosis antigens induce *tubercle formation,* characterized by central multinucleated giant cells surrounded by a cluster of epithelioid cells. More peripherally, lymphocytes are seen admixed with fibroblasts and, in older lesions, fibrosis. Visible bacilli are few or absent. Lesions of this histologic character are termed *productive* and represent successful local containment of infection. When large bacterial concentrations coexist with high levels of lymphocyte reactivity, an exudate rich in fibrin and a nonspecific inflammatory reaction containing polymorphonuclear leukocytes, monocytes, and small numbers of epithelioid and giant cells results; such lesions, termed *exudative,* may progress to *caseous necrosis.* In contrast to many other infections, tissue autolysis in tuberculosis is initially incomplete. The term caseous depicts its cheesy, semisolid, or solid consistency, which appears microscopically as amorphous, homogeneous, eosinophilic material. When specific lymphocyte reactivity has waned because of age or intercurrent illness, and breakdown of a previously quiescent chronic focus leads to extensive bacteremia, the cellular response may be minimal or lacking entirely in the presence of large concentrations of multiplying bacteria in the miliary foci. This histologic picture has been termed *nonreactive tuberculosis.*

Since the histopathologic response is determined in part by local factors, quite different patterns may occur simultaneously in the same individual and even in different parts of the same lesion, some representing progression and some successful containment. In pulmonary caseous foci, for instance, the histologic response at increasing distances from the caseous center (where antigen concentration is greatest) comes more and more to resemble that associated with successful containment of infection, with tubercle formation and fibrosis predominating. It is important to emphasize that these histologic features are not diagnostic of tuberculosis and may be seen in some combination in a wide variety of other conditions.

PATHOGENESIS

The tubercle bacillus requires ready access to oxygen for growth, and even under the most favorable circum-stances cell division occurs no more frequently than every day or two, explaining the chronic character of tuberculous disease. In unfavorable circumstances it may become metabolically dormant and persist in necrotic tissue for years. Infection by inhalation requires very few bacilli contained in a particle small enough to escape the mucociliary clearance mechanism of the conducting airways and lodge in the air-exchanging portion of the lung (respiratory bronchioles, alveolar ducts, or alveoli). Bacterial multiplication proceeds with little or no reaction, spreads to regional nodes in the hilum of the lung, and thence gains access to the bloodstream. *It is important to emphasize that asymptomatic lymphohematogenous dissemination of the primary infection before the acquisition of tuberculin hypersensitivity probably occurs in all instances; it is this event which sets the stage for the development of chronic pulmonary and extrapulmonary tuberculosis at a later time.* The metastatic bacterial colonies throughout the body also multiply in unimpeded fashion prior to development of tuberculin reactivity. Circulating bacilli are most efficiently cleared from the bloodstream by reticuloendothelial organs, but bacterial multiplication is favored in those areas known to be associated with clinical tuberculosis, most importantly the apices of the lungs, and to a lesser degree the kidneys, richly vascularized skeletal areas, and lymph nodes. The fact that the lung apices provide a particularly favorable environment for metastatic foci of infection has been attributed to the high oxygen tensions in these areas, but this is conjectural.

As mentioned, the subsequent development of *tuberculin hypersensitivity* and *cellular immunity* greatly alters the balance in favor of the host. Activated macrophages reduce the bacterial population at both initial and metastatic foci, and further bacterial growth is inhibited. It is likely, however, that slowly metabolizing viable bacilli persist at most foci. When antigen concentration at the site of initial infection and in the regional lymph nodes is sufficiently large, cellular necrosis may develop and eventually calcify, producing the so-called *Ghon complex.* This roentgenographic finding, for years considered pathognomonic of tuberculosis, is now known to be caused also by certain fungi, notably histoplasmosis and coccidioidomycosis, and other mycobacteria.

FATE OF THE PRIMARY INFECTION. In most people, the infection remains quiescent after the development of tuberculin hypersensitivity and is of no further clinical significance. In an appreciable number, however, infection may evolve into clinical tuberculosis in a number of ways. In some, particularly the very young, the preallergic bacteremia (early hematogenous dissemination) may progress directly into *generalized acute hematogenous tuberculosis.* The resemblance of the resulting disseminated tubercles to millet seeds led to the designation *miliary tuberculosis.* At times it is the strategic location of miliary tubercles rather than progression of the bacteremia which is critical, particularly with respect to development of *tuberculous meningitis,* because subependymal foci in brain or spinal cord may rupture into the subarachnoid space and produce spread of the infection via the subarachnoid fluid. Meningitis may occur in the setting of obvious, progressive bloodstream infection but also may be due to a nonprogressive and otherwise asymptomatic bacteremia.

Local rather than hematogenous events may also determine the outcome. The initial focus may directly evolve into progressive pneumonia (*progressive prima-*

ry); rarely cavitation may result. Large hilar nodes may become necrotic, liquefy, discharge into the bronchial tree, and produce tuberculous pneumonia in this fashion, or, particularly in the young, often partially compress the major bronchi, producing bronchial obstruction and collapse of a pulmonary segment or lobe. When the site of the initial infection is subpleural in location, rupture into the pleural space may occur, producing the clinical picture of *serofibrinous pleurisy with effusion*. A hematogenous focus located near the pleural surface can also produce this syndrome.

Numerically, the most frequent serious sequel of the preallergic bacteremia is chronic pulmonary tuberculosis. Pulmonary sequestration of blood-borne bacteria occurs in a distribution proportional to blood flow, but conditions in the superior and posterior aspects of the lungs greatly favor bacterial multiplication. Over the years it has been a matter of controversy whether chronic apical pulmonary tuberculosis of the so-called *reinfection type* results from breakdown of latent residua seeded at the time of the initial infection (*endogenous reinfection*) or from acquisition of new infection from the environment (*exogenous reinfection*). Many authorities assume that both can occur. However, it now seems likely that exogenous reinfection is considerably less important, and that pulmonary tuberculosis is almost always a direct consequence of the primary infection, with progression (then or later) in that area caused by local factors favoring bacterial growth, whereas the initial focus, when located in the mid or lower lung fields, almost always regresses.

The time at which apical pulmonary tuberculosis appears depends on three factors: first, the period of life in which infection occurs; second, normal, age-dependent factors favoring or inhibiting growth of the apical lesion; and third, non-age-related factors altering resistance. All mortality curves from urban populations in the early part of this century, in which infection in childhood was the rule, demonstrate a peak in the first three years of life owing to the relative deficiency in cellular immunity which characterizes this period of life. In very young children, progressive hematogenous tuberculosis, particularly miliary and meningeal disease, constituted a large part of the over-all mortality. Older prepubertal children (roughly between 5 and 15), although in no way resistant to *infection*, very seldom manifested progressive *disease*. After puberty a second mortality peak was seen, which continued through the second and into the third decade and was more pronounced in females than in males. Thereafter, the death rate continued at a lower level until old age, when a third, less dramatic mortality peak was seen. At present, in countries with low prevalence, clinical tuberculosis is becoming more a disease of the elderly, particularly the older male, presumably caused in part by waning immunologic competence in old age.

As mentioned, persons infected during the disease-resistant period of childhood (roughly 5 to 15) are prone to develop clinical tuberculosis in the postpubertal and early adult period of life, presumably owing to age-dependent host factors favoring evolution of the infection. In contrast, apical pulmonary tuberculosis caused by infection after childhood most often becomes manifest within two years of initial infection. Beyond this period of maximal jeopardy, quiescent foci in the lungs and elsewhere may evolve to produce clinical disease at any time when a combination of local and systemic factors favors reactivation.

The importance of local factors in reactivation of previously quiescent foci is illustrated by development of tuberculous arthritis after joint injury, activation of pulmonary tuberculosis by destructive lung disease such as lung abscess or carcinoma, and the appearance of late hematogenous dissemination after trauma. Thus any tuberculin-positive individual is at risk to develop any form of tuberculosis, often as a result of a remote and clinically undetectable primary infection. The role of immunologic senescence or other processes altering cellular immunity needs to be emphasized; reactivation of tuberculosis becomes progressively likely as individuals become more aged.

ENDOBRONCHIAL SPREAD OF CHRONIC PULMONARY TUBERCULOSIS: THE IMPORTANCE OF CAVITY FORMATION. In contrast to the earliest stages of tuberculous infection in which lymphohematogenous dissemination is the rule, once chronic pulmonary tuberculosis has become established, further spread occurs for the most part via the bronchial tree. The cavity, which is responsible both for progression of pulmonary disease in the individual and for infection of others, has provided the environment which has nurtured the tubercle bacillus through so many centuries of coexistence with the human species. *Especially in the era prior to the availability of effective drugs, cavity formation was the pivotal event in the course of pulmonary tuberculosis, to the prevention or treatment of which most forms of therapy were directed.*

LATE HEMATOGENOUS DISSEMINATION. Foci seeded at the time of the preallergic bacteremia may, after prolonged quiescent periods, break down and liberate bacteria into the bloodstream. Chronic pulmonary foci may cause late bacteremia in this manner, but extrapulmonary and often clinically inapparent foci, particularly in lymph nodes, bones, and the urogenital system, cause most instances of miliary tuberculosis in older individuals.

THE TUBERCULIN TEST

The tuberculin test is best performed by intracutaneous injection of 0.1 ml of purified protein derivative (PPD of Seibert). Proper introduction will be indicated by a raised white area that persists for some minutes after injection. Dosage is expressed in terms of tuberculin units (1 TU is 0.00002 mg; 5 TU is 0.0001 mg; 250 TU is 0.005 mg). In children or in persons with ocular involvement, the 1 TU dose is used. In adults a 5 TU dose is employed first. *Production of visible and palpable induration over 10 mm in diameter after 48 to 72 hours is considered virtually diagnostic of infection with M. tuberculosis.* A smaller reaction is of uncertain significance, because it may be due to other mycobacterial infections. If the test is negative, retesting with 250 TU is carried out. A positive reaction to this larger (second-strength) dosage is also of uncertain significance, because it may reflect cross-reactivity. A negative reaction in a *nonfebrile, relatively well individual* in whom generalized cutaneous anergy can be ruled out by a positive skin test to candida or mumps antigen is strong evidence against tuberculosis. However, as many as 15 per cent or more of persons constitutionally ill with proved tuberculosis may fail to react to 250 TU when first tested, becoming reactive again as health returns. Associated illnesses such as Hodgkin's disease, sarcoidosis, less commonly other neoplasias, and acute infections, notably the viral exanthems, may also cause false negatives. False positives are almost always due to infections with other mycobacterial species. Repeated testing may recall sensitivity to 250 TU in remotely infected individuals in whom reactivity had waned.

FACTORS MODIFYING THE COURSE OF TUBERCULOSIS

Nutritional status, mental and physical stress, and exhaustion modify the course of tuberculosis, as is well illustrated by the peak in mortality statistics observed during the major wars in both belligerent and nonbelligerent nations. *Pregnancy, delivery, and the puerperium*, long regarded as risk periods, have probably been overemphasized. Although statistical evidence is lacking, there is little doubt that *prolonged therapy with corticosteroids* predisposes to exacerbation of tuberculosis, as does *therapy with oncolytic or immunosuppressive agents*. *Diabetes* predisposes to clinical tuberculosis, and the disease tends to be more fulminant, particularly in young, poorly controlled diabetics. *Silicosis* or *anthracosilicosis* alters host response to tuberculosis in important ways. Instances of infection with the usually nonpathogenic *M. avium* and other mycobacteria of usually decreased virulence is observed in silicotics. Once established, silicotuberculosis may produce massive conglomerate fibrosis with little potential for resolution and little response to antituberculous drugs. Moreover, conglomerate fibrosis often contains quite small bacterial populations held fast within the fibrotic masses, making bacteriologic diagnosis difficult. In times past, *sarcoidosis* was thought to predispose to the progression of tuberculosis, but this no longer appears to be the case. *Hodgkin's disease, leukemia, and other lymphatic neoplasms* are often confused with tuberculosis and may also be complicated by active tuberculosis caused presumably by the detrimental effects of these diseases on cellular immune mechanisms. *Carcinoma* and *destructive infections* such as histoplasmosis, other mycobacterial infections, and lung abscess may erode an old tuberculous focus, releasing tubercle bacilli which may or may not produce disease. Severe viral illness, notably rubella and influenza, may have detrimental effects on the course of tuberculosis. *Gastric resection*, for unknown reasons, favors the progression of previously inactive pulmonary foci, and as many as 4 to 6 per cent will develop active disease. *Pulmonary surgery* may also cause progression of quiescent pulmonary foci. The role of various types of trauma in activating latent foci has been mentioned previously.

PREVENTION OF TUBERCULOSIS

Vaccination

BCG (bacille Calmette Guérin) is a strain of *M. bovis* with attenuated virulence for man. Several large studies have produced convincing evidence that vaccination with an effective strain of BCG in high-risk groups will prevent approximately four of every five cases of active tuberculosis which otherwise would have developed. Also of benefit is the fact that vaccinated persons who do become ill develop less progressive forms of tuberculosis. Miliary and meningeal disease in young children, for instance, is rare after BCG vaccination, a major advantage, considering the gravity of these conditions in the very young. (Disseminated infection with BCG itself is so rare as to be of no importance.)

BCG vaccination programs have been carried out with substantial success in some European countries and the United Kingdom. In the United States the falling rates of infection and disease make vaccination valuable only in specialized circumstances (see below). Tuberculin positivity is induced by BCG, thus destroying the major indicator of early infection, an important consideration weighing against vaccination in areas of low prevalence; the success of isoniazid prophylaxis (see below) is another. Almost all authorities advise the use of BCG in tuberculin-negative children in areas in which 20 per cent or more of secondary schoolchildren are tuberculin positive. (Vaccination is, of course, of no use in tuberculin-positive persons.) Vaccination may also be appropriate for missionary or government personnel prior to assignment to areas of known high prevalence, in groups of health professionals with high (over 20 per cent) incidence of infection, and even in some military personnel. Vaccination of infants born to tuberculous mothers or who must live in known high-risk environments is the procedure of choice, but is compromised somewhat by the problem of keeping the infant isolated for the four- to ten-week period required for development of tuberculin hypersensitivity in response to BCG vaccination.

Chemoprophylaxis

The term chemoprophylaxis has been applied to two distinct situations: first, the treatment of tuberculin-negative individuals in the hope of preventing infection in high-risk situations; and second, treatment of tuberculin-positive persons in the hope of preventing evolution of infection into disease. In a practical sense, it means treatment with isoniazid.

Circumstances in which *infection prophylaxis* (primary prophylaxis) is indicated are few. When an infant cannot be isolated from a mother with active tuberculosis long enough to establish tuberculin hypersensitivity with BCG, isoniazid may be administered to the child until and for a few months after the mother stops discharging tubercle bacilli in the sputum under treatment. When the period of risk cannot be defined, such as in households with recalcitrant infectious patients or in geographic pockets of known high risk, it may be useful to continue therapy for two years or more, because the morbidity associated with meningitis is less in older children. Alternatively, it may be reasonable to stop chemoprophylaxis at some point for a period long enough to achieve vaccination and tuberculin conversion and then to resume therapy for another year, assuming that the conversion might be due to either vaccination or infection, and that in either case protection would result. Prophylactic treatment of tuberculin-negative household contacts of newly discovered patients with active cases, particularly children and young adults, is advised by many. Two and one-half per cent of untreated household contacts will develop active tuberculosis within the next year regardless of tuberculosis status at the time of testing.

Certain exposure to highly contaminated material, as in laboratory accidents or in mouth-to-mouth resuscitation of positive patients, may be covered with prophylactic isoniazid for a period of several months. In the latter situation, attention should be given to the possibility of isoniazid resistance if these data are available, and therapy adjusted accordingly. The status of the tuberculin test during and after treatment should be monitored.

In certain conditions, notably sarcoidosis and Hodgkin's disease, cutaneous anergy may make it impossible to determine whether or not infection has occurred, the roentgenographic and histologic abnormalities may resemble those produced by tuberculosis, and both may require corticosteroid therapy (see below). For these reasons, some persons with sarcoidosis, Hodgkin's disease, and related lymphomas are treated with isoniazid without certain knowledge whether or not infection has in fact occurred. Similarly, prolonged corticosteroid therapy in gravely ill individuals is ordinarily accompanied by isoniazid regardless of tuberculin status.

In contrast, *disease prophylaxis* (secondary prophylaxis) is a frequently employed and well established procedure. Its greatest use is in the *recent tuberculin converter*, which in point of fact represents treatment of an early and active infection. Treatment of children under five years with a positive reaction to a 5 TU dose of tuberculin is recommended without exception. This may also be the case in older persons in whom tuberculin conversion is known to be a relatively recent (within two years) event. Early studies of isoniazid prophylaxis in known recent converters demonstrated an incidence of 5 per cent active tuberculosis within the first year in the nontreated controls. Household contacts of newly discovered patients who are tuberculin positive at the time of contact study and not treated demonstrate a similar incidence of overt disease. This figure probably represents the morbidity of large infections in susceptible age groups, and it is likely that quantitatively smaller inocula in less susceptible age groups produce considerably less disease; nevertheless, the morbidity of a tuberculous infection is substantial during the first 12 to 18 months after infection, and continues to carry some risk throughout life. The protection afforded by treatment of the tuberculin converter persists for many years.

Individuals under 35 with positive (greater than 10 mm induration) reactions to 5 TU in whom prior tuberculin status is not known should in most instances receive chemoprophylaxis. Over that age, the risk of isoniazid-induced hepatitis exceeds the risk of development of active tuberculosis. Reactions requiring large (250 TU) concentrations of tuberculin to be elicited in the well population have entirely different implications and are not taken as evidence of possible recent conversion or indication for treatment.

In addition to treatment of the preclinical infection, as defined above, a number of situations known to be prejudicial to the course of tuberculous infection constitute sufficient reason for chemoprophylaxis in tuberculin-positive individuals. These include *silicosis, severe and poorly controlled diabetes, the postgastrectomy state, progressive neoplastic disease of the lung or of the myeloid or lymphatic systems* (particularly when treatment with oncolytic agents is employed), and *prolonged treatment with corticosteroids*. The occurrence of severe viral illness in a tuberculin-positive individual is regarded by some as an indication for chemoprophylaxis. Persons with an *undiagnosed pulmonary infiltrate and a positive tuberculin reaction*, in whom for one reason or another definitive diagnosis is not indicated, should be given prophylaxis, as the risk for the development of manifest active disease is approximately 1 per cent per year in such individuals. It is essential in such circumstances, however, to ensure that the period of prophylaxis does not serve to postpone appropriate diagnostic approaches for more serious diseases. Similarly, *patients with known presumably inactive tuberculosis who had received either inadequate or no chemotherapy in the past* will demonstrate a similar (approximately 1 per cent per year) rate of relapse and should receive chemoprophylaxis.

Chemoprophylaxis in adults consists of isoniazid in dosage of 300 mg once daily for a period of a year. In children, the dose is 6 to 8 mg per kilogram. The indications for the use of isoniazid in uncertain situations should be balanced against the real risk of hepatotoxicity, particularly in older persons. The incidence of *isoniazid hepatitis* is negligible in those under 20 years of age, 0.3 per cent between 20 and 35, 1.2 per cent between 35 and 50, and 2.3 per cent over 50. In older age groups women are more frequently affected than men. The symptom complex is identical to that of viral hepatitis (nausea, malaise, fever, vomiting, dark urine, and jaundice in some combination), and the histologic picture is also indistinguishable, ranging from mild hepatocellular disease to severe hepatic necrosis or chronic active hepatitis. Prolonged reactions may lead to cirrhosis. Most cases develop within the first two months of treatment, but may occur at any time. Everyone receiving isoniazid should be told of the symptoms of isoniazid hepatitis, and ideally should be seen monthly by a knowledgeable medical worker. If careful surveillance of symptoms is maintained, periodic liver function testing is probably not necessary. The great majority of fatalities have occurred in persons who continued to take isoniazid in spite of recognizable symptoms and signs of liver dysfunction. The presence of established unrelated liver disease complicates the picture. There is no evidence that liver disease predisposes to isoniazid hepatotoxicity, but its detection is more difficult in the presence of unrelated liver disease, and the consequences of hepatotoxicity might be more serious in the presence of an already damaged liver.

167. PULMONARY TUBERCULOSIS

Robert A. Goodwin, Jr.

SYMPTOMATIC PRIMARY INFECTION

The primary infection consists of a small parenchymal focus or cluster of small infiltrates with regional hilar and mediastinal lymphadenitis of varying degrees usually attended by few or no recognizable symptoms. It is more often symptomatic in infants and young children because of an age-related tendency to more extensive lymphadenitis and lymphohematogenous spread, and accordingly has traditionally been termed childhood tuberculosis. At the time of tuberculin conversion, fever and lassitude may be present; rarely *erythema nodosum* or symptomatic inflammation of the eye (*phlyctenular keratoconjunctivitis*) will develop. Hilar lymphadenitis may partially compress the major bronchi, producing a brassy cough and occasionally sputum and localized bronchial obstruction. The chest roentgenogram will often reveal hilar adenopathy, usually unilateral, and at times a small parenchymal infiltrate.

Diagnosis is based on a positive and usually strongly reactive tuberculin test. Acid-fast bacilli may occasionally be found in sputum smears, and cultures positive for *M. tuberculosis* can probably be demonstrated in most patients if obtained repeatedly. Syndromes based on hilar adenopathy, pleural effusion, and, rarely, direct progression of the initial pulmonary infiltrate may be seen.

Hilar adenopathy may compress the small and relatively flaccid bronchi in the very young, producing partial or complete bronchial obstruction and obstructive pneumonitis. Involvement of the bronchial wall and mucosa by direct extension from contiguous tuberculous lymphadenitis can seed tuberculous foci distally. Prolonged obstruction and endobronchial scarring may result in distal bronchiectasis. Occasionally a node will rupture into a bronchus, producing intense bronchitis and pneumonitis which may go into caseation. (This may also occur in the adult [see below].) *Tuberculous pleurisy and effusion* (see Ch. 350.1) is an important and not uncommon complication occurring soon after infection in both children and young adults. Although this syndrome is itself usually self-limited, two thirds of patients will subsequently develop progressive pulmonary or extrapulmonary tuberculosis; accordingly, tuberculin-positive patients with unexplained pleural effusion should be treated as having active tuberculosis unless another cause can be definitely established. The term *progressive primary* connotes direct evolution of the initial infiltrate into a pneumonic, caseous process. It differs from apical chronic pulmonary tuberculosis in that hilar adenopathy is prominent and the process most often involves the middle or lower lung fields.

Features characteristic of childhood tuberculosis may occasionally be seen in young adults, and prominent hilar adenitis may be confused with lymphoma.

TREATMENT. Children are usually given a larger dosage of isoniazid (10 to 15 mg per kilogram) than adults, because the risks of isoniazid toxicity are negligible in the young. An uncomplicated infection is usually treated with isoniazid alone except when drug resistance seems likely on epidemiologic grounds (contact with a known drug-resistant patient). Symptoms resulting from bronchial compression may be benefited by brief corticosteroid treatment (prednisone, 20 to 40 mg daily). Treatment of progressive caseous pulmonary parenchymal disease requires more than one drug.

CHRONIC PULMONARY TUBERCULOSIS

Pulmonary tuberculosis in adults is predominantly an apical parenchymal process almost always caused by evolution of hematogenous foci seeded during the preallergic phase of the initial infection. This may occur fairly promptly or after long periods of quiescence. Whether or not a latent period intervenes, these metastatic foci gain largest size and are therefore most unstable in the superior areas of the lung in which local factors favor bacterial growth.

Chronic pulmonary tuberculosis begins as a small patch of pneumonia surrounding a growing bacterial colony, most commonly in the posterior or apical segment of an upper lobe or the apical segment of a lower lobe. The inflammatory response in the sensitized host produces fibrin-rich alveolar fluid containing a mixture of inflammatory cells. Intense inflammation may progress to caseous necrosis which, while solid, is an effective mechanism of host defense, causing the death of most organisms. (Invariably, however, a few metabolically dormant organisms persist.) However, caseous foci

in upper lung zones have a marked tendency to liquefy and discharge into the bronchial tree, producing a cavity in open communication with inspired air, from which infectious secretions spread via the bronchi to other areas of the lung and to the outside environment. *Once reactivation occurs, the progressive nature of tuberculosis in the sensitized host is largely due to the combination of these factors: (1) the tendency of apical caseous foci to liquefy; (2) the access of liquefied infectious material to the bronchial tree; and (3) the aerobic nature of the organisms, resulting in huge bacterial populations within open cavities.*

Bronchogenic spread of infectious material is enhanced by coughing, which aerosolizes infectious material and then on inhalation distributes it widely throughout the lung. Sooner or later new foci of disease develop, which then may undergo caseous necrosis and then heal, or liquefy, slough, and produce another cavity. New lesions usually appear first in the segment or lobe initially involved, producing scattered, patchy disease. The apical posterior areas of the contralateral lung are quite apt to become involved. In addition to the exudative response, some associated productive tissue reaction is usually found, characterized by giant cells and epithelioid cells forming tubercles and leading eventually to fibrosis and healing. This is particularly true in the anterior and basal portions of the lung, areas which respond to continual bronchogenic seeding from apical cavities with granuloma formation, fibrosis, and scarring but very rarely become necrotic or cavitary. Almost all lesions will contain some mixture of exudative and productive tissue responses, with progression in one area and regression in another. The pace and tempo of progressive disease is highly variable in different individuals and in the same individual at different times. Intercurrent or genetic factors, vigorous hypersensitivity reactions, and large numbers of organisms favor acute and rapidly progressive reactions which may produce confluent pneumonia (*tuberculous pneumonia or phthisis florida*). At the other end of the spectrum, relatively effective immunity and low bacterial populations favor predominantly productive lesions with a greater tendency to spontaneous healing.

Mechanisms of healing are basically the same whether spontaneous or after drug treatment. The exudative component of the early infiltrate may resolve with preservation of normal lung architecture. More often it is replaced with fibrous tissue. Solid caseous foci may become encapsulated by fibrosis. An open cavity occasionally may become obstructed by granulation tissue at the bronchocavitary junction, and become inspissated and encapsulated, producing a tenuous form of healing. An open cavity probably always remains infectious except after prolonged antimicrobial therapy, which may eliminate all necrotic and infectious tissue and result in a clean fibrotic cavity wall. Regardless of the type and extent of healing, however, it is probable that dormant organisms capable of renewed growth and reactivation of disease persist in all cases.

SYMPTOMS. Small apical infiltrates may persist for months or even years in tenuous balance, undergoing minor extensions and regressions and producing no symptoms. Discovery of such cases by chest roentgenogram is a fortunate event. When the infection reaches a certain size, however, absorption of antigenic substances results in entirely nonspecific *constitutional symptoms* such as anorexia, fatigue, fever, chilliness, night sweats, and wasting. Constitutional symptoms usually begin insidiously and progress slowly. Weight loss and fatigue are more likely to lead to medical attention than is fever, usually in the afternoon, which is often unrecognized.

Symptoms resulting from local pulmonary inflammation are also variable in degree and in time of onset. *Cough* and *sputum* are the most consistent, due both to secretions draining from a cavity and to superficial bronchial mucosal and submucosal disease caused by these highly infectious secretions. Their presence indicates advanced disease. Cough may vary from mild to severe, and sputum may be scant and mucoid or copious and purulent.

Hemoptysis and *chest pain* are unpredictable symptoms which cause the patient great concern and are likely to lead to medical attention. Hemoptysis may be due to slough of a caseous lesion or bronchial ulceration. It usually is minor in degree but nevertheless connotes advanced disease. Particularly in late chronic disease, bleeding may be copious and sudden, owing to rupture of an artery within the fibrous walls of a cavity (Rasmussen's aneurysm). Exsanguination is unusual, but, particularly in extensive disease, there may be a real threat of drowning, requiring prompt positioning for drainage (prone or Trendelenburg) and avoidance of drugs which suppress cough. (Hemoptysis may also be due to an aspergilloma in an old healed cavity and so does not necessarily connote reactivation of inactive tuberculosis.) *Pleural pain* usually is due to extension of inflammation to the pleural surface with involvement of the parietal pleura without production of pleural fluid (*dry pleurisy*). Much less commonly, pleural pain will be associated with serofibrinous pleurisy with effusion (which usually occurs prior to established apical pulmonary tuberculosis), and rarely tuberculous empyema will be discovered. Rarely, medical attention is not sought until disease in other tissues bathed in highly infectious pulmonary secretions occurs, such as painful pharyngeal ulcers, hoarseness and dysphagia resulting from laryngeal involvement, tuberculous otitis media, or anal pain caused by a tuberculous perirectal abscess. Shortness of breath is common in pneumonic or extensive destructive disease.

PHYSICAL EXAMINATION. Physical findings usually underestimate the extent of involvement and may be entirely negative even with advanced disease. However, the physical examination provides some information not obtainable in any other way, such as asymmetry in respiratory excursion, contraction of the hemithorax, and deviation of the trachea. Dullness to percussion and increased tactile fremitus are usual over the side of the lesion. Dullness associated with decreased fremitus may detect pleural thickening or pleural fluid. Auscultation may reveal rales, very frequently detected only during quick inspiration following a short cough (posttussic rales). (Interestingly, rales may persist for years after disease has become inactive, presumably because of permanent distortion of small bronchi.) Tubular breath sounds and whispered pectoriloquy may be heard. Distant, hollow tubular breath sounds heard over cavities are termed *amphoric*, as they resemble sounds made by blowing across the mouth of a jar (amphora). Forced hyperventilation may detect local stenosis and obstruction of a bronchus. Scrotal examination may uncover an asymptomatic epididymal nodule. Careful funduscopic examination may reveal choroidal tubercles. Physical findings must be correlated with the chest roentgenogram. Neither is adequate without the other.

ROENTGENOLOGIC FINDINGS. The chest roentgenogram is central to diagnosis, determination of extent and character of disease, and evaluation of response to treatment. Although not diagnostic, the finding of a patchy infiltrate located in the apical posterior area is highly suggestive of tuberculosis. Cavities can usually be seen on the standard posteroanterior chest roentgenogram, but may be missed, and are much more clearly seen with planigrams. Certain histopathologic characteristics of the infiltrates can be estimated from the chest roentgenogram. Exudative lesions tend to have soft indistinct margins. Increased density suggests caseation. Productive lesions tend to be small and nodular with sharply defined margins. Scar tissue produces quite sharp margins and tends to contract. Healing exudative lesions first become smaller and less dense and then, as scarring develops, become more sharply defined. Roentgenographic stability, except for slow further contraction, is one criterion indicating achievement of quiescent or inactive status.

OTHER LABORATORY FINDINGS. A normocytic, normochromic anemia is usual and may be severe. The white blood count is usually normal; a monocytosis of 8 to 15 per cent may be seen. Prolonged and severe infections may cause hyperglobulinemia and hypoalbuminemia. Hematuria or pyuria may disclose coexisting renal tuberculosis; marked albuminuria may indicate amyloidosis. A low serum sodium is sometimes found in extensive chronic pulmonary tuberculosis, more often due to abnormal retention of water (inappropriate secretion of antidiuretic hormone) than to coexistent Addison's disease. It is important to rule out diabetes.

DIAGNOSIS. A strong presumptive diagnosis of tuberculosis may often be made on the basis of roentgenographic characteristics alone. A stained sputum smear positive for acid-fast bacteria on microscopy — a finding usual in extensive disease — will in the proper setting provide nearly conclusive evidence. It must be remembered, however, that any destructive process in the lung, particularly in the apical posterior area, may erode an inactive focus and cause appearance of acidfast bacilli in the sputum with or without development of new, active tuberculosis. A positive tuberculin test, although of great use in children, has limited diagnostic significance in older age groups. A negative reaction to 250 TU when a positive reaction to candida or mumps antigen indicates that anergy is not present is very strong but still not completely conclusive evidence against active tuberculosis. *Histologic demonstration of granulomatous disease* provides only presumptive evidence of tuberculosis, and even demonstration of acidfast bacteria is not definitive in that they may represent mycobacteria other than *M. tuberculosis*. Definitive diagnosis requires culture and speciation of the organism.

DIFFERENTIAL DIAGNOSIS. Although tuberculosis may be confused with virtually any intrathoracic condition, certain diseases are frequently considered in differential diagnosis. *Fungal disease*, particularly histoplasmosis, and disease caused by other mycobacteria can be indistinguishable from chronic cavitary or fibroid tuberculosis. (Coexistence of histoplasmosis and tuberculosis in the same individual is not rare.) *Bronchiectasis* may present with symptoms suggesting tuberculosis, and bronchiectatic and emphysematous areas surrounded by infiltrate may mimic cavitation roentgenographically. *Cavitary lung abscess* often involves the dorsal segments of the lower lobes and posterior segments of the upper lobes owing to patterns of aspiration during unconsciousness. Typically lung abscess causes little in the way of physical findings, may have a fluid level, and is not associated with patchy bronchogenic infiltrates; in contrast, physical findings are prominent over tuberculous cavities, fluid levels are rare, and patchy infiltrates elsewhere are the rule. *Acute bacterial pneumonias* may resemble florid tuberculosis in all particulars except for the sputum examination and response to antimicrobial drugs. *Neoplasm* may resemble tuberculosis, as in an isolated coin lesion, an obstructing and inconspicuous endobronchial tumor causing distal chronic inflammation, or a caviting neoplastic mass. (An irregular cavity wall suggests necrotic neoplasm.) The association between neoplasm and tuberculosis is complex: first, in that cancer may erode into and reactivate a latent tuberculous focus; second, in that saphrophytic mycobacteria may be found in association with a destructive neoplasm; and third, in that chronic scarring in a tuberculous focus may induce neoplastic degeneration. New roentgenographic progression of a previously stable, fibrotic tuberculous focus may be due to "scar cancer" rather than progressive infection.

LOWER AND MIDDLE LOBE TUBERCULOSIS IN OLDER INDIVIDUALS. As tuberculosis in young adults becomes less frequent, certain atypical presentations in older individuals are being recognized. A progressive infiltrate in the lower or mid-lung field may rarely be due to a progressive primary infection, presumably because of deficient immune mechanisms in the elderly. Also, tuberculous hilar lymph nodes from a remote infection may rupture into a bronchus, causing tuberculous pneumonia in the associated lobe or segment. For some unexplained reason, middle lobe tuberculosis is not uncommon in diabetics.

CLASSIFICATION OF PULMONARY TUBERCULOSIS. Previous classifications included the following description of the extent of disease. *Minimal:* the total area of disease, taken in the aggregate, is less than the area from the second chondrocostal junction and the fifth vertebral body to the apex of the lung on one side, and no cavity is demonstrable (planigrams usually required). *Moderately advanced:* The aggregate total area of scattered, small lesions is less than one lung field, or of dense, confluent lesions less than the equivalent of one third of one lung field. The total diameter of cavitation, if present, is less than 4 cm. *Far advanced:* Disease greater in extent than moderately advanced.

The present classification (American Thoracic Society, 1974) is as follows:

  0. No tuberculosis exposure, not infected (no history of exposure, negative tuberculin skin test).
  I. Tuberculosis exposure, no evidence of infection (history of exposure, negative tuberculin skin test).
  II. Tuberculous infection, without disease (positive tuberculin skin test, negative bacteriologic studies (if done), no roentgenographic findings compatible with tuberculosis, no symptoms due to tuberculosis). Chemotherapy status (preventive therapy), dates, if given.
  III. Tuberculosis: infected, with disease.

The current status of the patient's tuberculosis shall be described by the following characteristics:

  A. Location of disease (e.g., pulmonary, pleural, lymphatic).
  B. Bacteriologic status (microscopy and culture with dates).
  C. Chemotherapy status (give dates).

TREATMENT OF PULMONARY TUBERCULOSIS

Treatment of pulmonary tuberculosis, long the province of specialized physicians in special hospitals, now is properly the responsibility of the general internist. Although in most instances treatment is best initiated in a hospital setting, providing easier accomplishment of laboratory studies and perhaps more importantly a period in which education of the patient and the family

can be accomplished, it is perfectly acceptable in individuals who are not in poor health otherwise to initiate and complete therapy entirely in an outpatient setting. It is well established that individuals on treatment very promptly become noninfectious for others in the environment even when sputum smears and cultures remain positive. If the patient can be taught to cough into tissue and to maintain a brief period of modified separation from the rest of the family, it is probable that serious infectiousness ceases entirely with initiation of therapy, or a week or two thereafter, and even the minor risk of infectiousness within that initial period is hardly of consequence compared to the risk already undergone by those in the patient's environment prior to diagnosis. The crux of tuberculosis control is diagnosis and treatment of the patient and proper investigation and treatment of contacts (see Chemoprophylaxis in Ch. 166) and not patient isolation. It should be restated that tuberculosis is communicated by aerosolized secretions and not at all by fomites. Competent treatment requires knowledge of the antituberculosis drugs, an understanding of the principles of combined and prolonged drug therapy, and an appreciation of how cases should be followed, particularly with regard to monitoring of patient compliance and the development of drug resistance. Effective use of drugs now available should provide cure in 95 to 100 per cent of previously untreated cases. In actual practice, results are less satisfactory. In part this may reflect poor medical direction, but much more important is the often carefully obscured failure of the patient to follow his drug regimen.

THE ANTITUBERCULOSIS DRUGS. *Isoniazid* (INH) remains the keystone of original treatment of pulmonary tuberculosis. It is highly effective (bactericidal against actively metabolizing cells, bacteriostatic against metabolically dormant cells), well absorbed, distributed throughout all tissues in effective concentrations, of low toxicity, and inexpensive. Drug resistance may emerge in the presence of very large bacterial populations such as are associated with pulmonary or renal cavities, and one or more companion drugs must be added to prevent this. However, INH, in contrast to all other antituberculosis drugs, may retain some in vivo effectiveness even when in vitro studies indicate resistance, probably owing in part to a slightly decreased pathogenicity of INH-resistant strains. Accordingly, it is advisable *in all regimens not continuing rifampin* to continue administration of INH in spite of development of in vitro resistance, while adding other effective drugs. The marginal benefit of continuing INH when rifampin is added to INH-resistant infections does not at present justify the increased risk of hepatotoxicity of INH-rifampin in combination. The incidence of INH-resistant isolates from previously untreated patients has remained for some years at approximately 2 per cent in the United States and England, although in other areas this figure may be higher. Allergic reactions to INH are uncommon. Transient elevations of SGOT occur in 10 per cent of patients, and INH-related hepatitis, reversible in its early stages, occurs in less than 1 per cent. (See Chemoprophylaxis in Ch. 166.) INH depletes body pyridoxine stores and may induce peripheral neuritis, particularly in nutritionally compromised patients such as alcoholics. Pyridoxine (50 mg a day) is often given with INH and is mandatory with doses greater than 300 mg daily and in severe alcoholics. INH dosage is 5 mg per kilogram of body weight, which in most adults usually is rounded off to 300 mg in a single daily dose. Larger doses (10 to 15 mg per kilogram) may be given at cost of greater toxicity (pyridoxine always added) in extensive caseous disease and in INH-resistant infections, particularly when supporting drug therapy is weak.

Rifampin (RMP) is a new antituberculosis agent of the same order of effectiveness, low incidence of toxicity, and high degree of patient acceptance as INH. It is expensive. Its effectiveness (with companion drugs) in INH-resistant treatment failures has radically changed the prognosis in such cases from uncertain at best to favorable in the majority. Its role in initial treatment has yet to be established. Clinical evidence in studies of short-term (six- to nine-month) chemotherapy indicates that RMP plus INH is more effective than any other regimen, resulting in fewer relapses after discontinuation of therapy than is the case with any other regimen administered for this period of time. However, when therapy is continued for 18 months, as is routinely recommended although at times hard to achieve, there is no advantage to the combined use of these two most potent agents. Further, hepatotoxicity is increased by the use of INH and RMP together in comparison to regimens containing only one or the other. Finally, in contrast to INH, RMP loses all effectiveness when resistant strains emerge. At present it seems justifiable to employ both agents in treatment of cases of extraordinary gravity such as extensive miliary or caseous pulmonary tuberculosis associated with marked debility. At the time of this writing, however, it is the author's practice to reserve RMP for retreatment in the usual case of pulmonary tuberculosis when it seems likely that compliance with 18 months of drug treatment can be achieved.

RMP is excreted by the liver and should be used cautiously in the presence of liver disease. Rarely it may cause bilirubinemia, usually with larger than ordinary dosage. Thrombocytopenic purpura and a serum sickness type of reaction have been observed. These allergic phenomena are rare at conventional daily dosage but are not uncommon when larger than usual dosage and intervals greater than 24 hours are employed. Therefore use of RMP in intermittent courses is not recommended. The recommended dosage is 450 to 600 mg administered by mouth in a single daily dose given at least an hour before or after meals, as food delays absorption. At the beginning of treatment RMP colors the urine a reddish orange, a somewhat alarming finding to which the patient should be alerted.

Streptomycin (SM) is substantially less effective than INH or RMP but more effective than any other agent. It is often administered for a few months as the third drug in three-drug therapy (INH ± ethambutol + SM) of severe disease. In conjunction with INH, it offers a strong two-drug regimen for hospitalized patients. In the unusual situation in which neither INH or RMP can be used, SM in combination with two other drugs, optimally including pyrazinamide (see below), provides acceptable therapy. SM is excreted by the kidneys, and toxic levels may develop when renal function is compromised. Eighth nerve toxicity (especially the vestibular branch) is a troublesome complication, more serious in those over 50 in whom the ability to compensate for loss of vestibular function is less effective. SM is administered intramuscularly in a dose of 1 gram daily during the first few months of treatment, but may be reduced to 1 gram two or three times weekly thereafter.

*Ethambutol** (EMB) is the most useful oral companion drug for INH (replacing PAS) in original treatment cases, and, if not previously used, for RMP in retreatment (INH-resistant) cases. A tendency to induce optic neuritis (loss of visual acuity, field constriction, and loss of green color discrimination) limits dosage. An acceptable incidence of 2 per cent allows the use of 25 mg per kilogram of body weight in hospitalized patients, but 15 to 20 mg per kilogram is recommended for outpatient treatment, at which dosage the incidence of optic neuritis is negligible.

Para-aminosalicylic acid (PAS), the principal companion drug to INH for years, has now been replaced by the much less toxic EMB. PAS is difficult to take and poorly tolerated because of gastric irritation. In addition, it causes serious hypersensitivity reactions more frequently than any other antituberculosis drug. PAS is now used mainly as a companion drug in retreatment cases with limited drug options. It is usually administered as the sodium salt in a dose of 5 grams three times daily with meals or 10 grams in a single daily dose given on a full stomach.

Pyrazinamide (PZA) follows SM in antimicrobial effectiveness, but its value is limited by early development of drug resistance (as early as six weeks in an active infection). This may be offset by its use with multiple drugs, with a strong drug, or in an already fairly well controlled infection. SM plus PZA is a good combination. Hepatotoxicity is a limiting factor, with 15 per cent showing altered liver function tests and 3 per cent frank jaundice, and with reported fatal hepatitis as high as 1 per cent. The usual oral dosage is a total of 2 to 3 grams daily given in two to three divided doses.

Ethionamide (ETH) is moderately effective in retreatment cases as a companion drug with a strong agent or as one of three or more weak drugs. Patient intolerance is moderately high due to central nervous system mediated nausea. It is administered by mouth in a dose of 500 to 1000 mg daily, most often as 250 mg three times daily.

*Cycloserine** (CS) is a toxic and rather ineffective drug used in retreatment with a strong drug or as a member of a three or more drug combination. Its tendency to induce a variety of central nervous system symptoms, including convulsions, limits the dosage to 0.5 to 1.0 gram daily, the lower being of questionable effectiveness and the higher a dose that few tolerate. A regimen of 250 mg three times daily is a reasonable compromise.

*Capreomycin** (CM) is an aminoglycoside approaching SM in effectiveness, with similar dosage requirements and toxicity. There is no cross-resistance with SM and in general it can be substituted for that drug, but it is best to include it in a three-drug regimen.

*Viomycin** (VM) and *kanamycin* (KM), aminoglycosides less effective and more toxic than SM or CM, are used only in retreatment with quite limited antimicrobial drug resources. The aminoglycosides have additive toxicities, and only one can be used at a time.

COMBINED DRUG THEAPY. Drug resistance may be *primary* (in previously untreated patients) or may emerge during treatment. Although a matter of continuing concern, primary resistance is not yet a major problem in most areas. Continuing surveys in the United States and Great Britain indicate a rather stable level of 2 to 3 per cent of previously untreated infections primarily resistant to either INH or SM, and less than 1 per cent to both drugs. However, some careful studies have demonstrated a higher incidence of primary drug resistance in children in urban areas of known high prevalence.

Drug resistance emerging during treatment is a major problem recognized ever since earliest drug trials. Canetti's detailed studies provide insight into the mechanisms of this phenomenon. Naturally occurring mutants resistant to INH appear at a predictable rate of 1 per 10^5 or 10^6 bacterial cells. This is true with respect to SM and in general other antituberculosis drugs. When INH is administered alone and the bacterial population is large, drug-susceptible cells are killed or suppressed and resistant mutants may in time repopulate the site of infection. This is of little practical importance in closed (noncavitary) lesions with a low bacterial population (10^3 to 10^5 cells per gram tissue), but is extremely important in open cavitary lesions associated with huge bacterial populations. Pulmonary cavities usually contain 10^7 to 10^9 but occasionally 10^{10} or more organisms; therefore as many as 10^3 or more INH-resistant bacteria might be present from the outset, providing an ample nidus for establishment of a drug-resistant infection once the larger susceptible population is suppressed. Under these circumstances, significant numbers of resistant organisms may appear in the sputum in a few weeks, and after three to four months the major portion

---

*Conditions for safe use in children have not been established. The Editors.

*Conditions for safe use in children have not been established. The Editors.

of the bacterial population may be INH-resistant. If two effective drugs are used at the same time and organisms resistant to each are present in a ratio of 1 to 10^5 bacterial cells, then the population of organisms resistant to both would be approximately 1 in 10^{10} bacteria, making emergence of resistance unlikely. This is the basis of the principle of combined therapy in which two or more effective drugs are used, each active against organisms resistant to the other (see Ch. 189).

If in the course of treatment the development of drug resistance appears to be threatening (continued presence of significant numbers of tubercle bacilli in the sputum after three to four months), caution should be exercised in introducing a single new drug without ensuring (recent drug susceptibility studies) the presence of at least one other drug to which the organisms are known to be susceptible. When in doubt, it is best to add two new drugs in compliance with the principle of combined therapy.

PROLONGED THERAPY. The principle of prolonged therapy was also established early by the occurrence of relapse when treatment was terminated too soon because of limited supplies of drug. Such relapses were ordinarily due to organisms still susceptible to the agents administered. Since the antituberculosis drugs are bacteriostatic for dormant organisms, suppressive therapy must be continued until the slow processes of host healing mechanisms secure control of residual infection. This usually means a treatment course of at least 18 months, and in advanced disease 24 months. As discussed below, the exceptions to this rule are drug regimens containing both INH and RMP. As brief a period as nine or even six months' treatment with these have produced results comparable to 18 months' treatment with standard, INH-containing regimens, but at a cost of greater hepatotoxicity and the disadvantage of not having RMP in reserve should treatment fail.

INITIAL TREATMENT. In the initial treatment of pulmonary tuberculosis, the most generally used *all-purpose* drug regimen is *SM (two months) + INH + EMB* for 18 months (SM, 1 gram daily first two months; INH, 300 mg, and EMB, 25 mg per kilogram, first three months, then 15 mg per kilogram thereafter — all given in a single daily dose). However, a more individualized approach is recommended when feasible, taking into account first the character of the disease and then patient response in order to minimize drug toxicity by reducing drug coverage on the one hand and giving added drug support when needed on the other. Based on the character of the disease, the following drug regimens are recommended for initiation of therapy: *(1) Double therapy, INH + EMB in usual mild or moderate disease with small infiltrates and thin-walled cavities, and (2) triple therapy, SM (until sputum conversion) + INH + EMB in extensive and severe disease, particularly when large areas of caseation or thick-walled cavities are identified.*

The rate of disappearance of tubercle bacilli from the sputum is an important prognostic event during the course of drug therapy. Although there is some correlation of severity of disease and persistence of organisms in the sputum, this is not predictable, and some as yet not understood biologic relationship between host, organisms, and drugs also determines whether patients are "rapid converters" or "slow converters." Slow sputum conversion favors drug resistance and a greater tendency to relapse if drug therapy is terminated too soon. Tubercle bacilli may disappear from the sputum by smear and culture as early as one month into drug treatment even in extensive disease, but more often sputum conversion takes place between the first and third months of treatment. Beyond this point the continued presence of organisms in the sputum defines the slow converter (if lapse in drug taking can be excluded), and after four to six months of continued discharge of tubercle bacilli in the sputum drug resistance is very likely to have developed.

The better prognosis of those who show prompt sputum conversion on either the two- or three-drug regimen allows safe termination of treatment in 18 months, and, in addition, drug coverage may be reduced to INH alone during the suppressive phase of treatment beginning six months after tubercle bacilli have disappeared from the sputum. On the other hand, the continued presence of tubercle bacilli in the sputum four months or more into drug therapy (even in the absence of drug resistance) indicates the need for more prolonged and vigorous therapy. Consequently, it is recommended that drug therapy be continued for a total of 24 months and that at least two drugs (INH and EMB) be used throughout (in the triple-drug regimen SM is best continued at least until reversal of infectiousness has been demonstrated).

Because of the threat of drug resistance when tubercle bacilli persist in the sputum well beyond four months into drug therapy, drug susceptibility studies are critically important at this time. The introduction of *two new drugs* (SM + PAS or RMP + SM) is advisable in a threatening situation pending report of drug susceptibility studies. Further therapy for a total of 24 months should be based on at least two drugs to which the organism is shown to be susceptible (or to which it has not previously been exposed), including one strong drug (INH, RMP, or SM).

Ordinarily a bacteriologic diagnosis is established at least by microscopy before institution of drugs. If smears are negative on microscopy, five or six adequate sputum specimens should be submitted for culture before initiating drug therapy. In severely ill patients, drugs should be started immediately, because a few days of antituberculosis drugs will not interfere with demonstration of tubercle bacilli on sputum smear or culture. Monthly chest roentgenograms allow adequate monitoring of the active course of the disease, and three monthly intervals suffice during healing stages. After the first month and before reversal of infectiousness, it is best to obtain sputum specimens at fortnightly intervals in order to detect either disappearance of the bacilli or early evidence of drug resistance. Drug susceptibility studies for the commonly used drugs should be obtained before treatment, and again in three or four months if sputum remains positive, or at any time of bacteriologic relapse.

All patients receiving INH should be instructed regarding symptoms suggestive of hepatitis and questioned concerning these at monthly intervals (see Chemoprophylaxis in Ch. 166). Patients receiving EMB should be questioned regarding visual symptoms; if they are receiving high doses, visual acuity (Snellen chart) and green color perception should be tested regularly. Patients receiving SM should be questioned concerning hearing and vestibular function and tested regularly for high frequency loss if over 50 years of age.

In patients with marked debility and severe constitutional symptoms, *corticosteroid therapy* in relatively low doses (30 mg daily of prednisone) will usually effect prompt symptomatic improvement, decrease fever, and promptly repair serious anemia when this is present. It is usually possible to taper the dose by 2.5-mg decrements every four or five days. In the rare instance of hypoxia resulting from a diffusion defect, usually in severe miliary tuberculosis but also observed in extensive bronchogenic dissemination, a larger dosage of corticosteroids (60 to 80 mg of prednisone daily) may be necessary for a few days before quickly decreasing to 30 mg of prednisone daily and then tapering. The unusual coexistence of Addison's disease and active pulmonary tuberculosis should be borne in mind. The adverse effect of steroids on tuberculous infection can be disregarded in the presence of effective antituberculosis drug therapy.

TREATMENT OF THE NONCOMPLIANT PATIENT. Patient failure to take drugs is the most frequent and important cause of treatment failure. There are many reasons such as simple forgetfulness, the illusion of health associated with the disappearance of symptoms, and the always underestimated reluctance of almost all persons to subject themselves to any discipline for prolonged periods. Alcoholics are almost predictably noncompliant and should probably be always regarded as potentially so. It is impossible to overemphasize the importance of a suspicious attitude regarding compliance with therapy. Every physician who treats tuberculosis has often observed relapse in a patient who indignantly maintains that he has taken his drugs faithfully — only to find that the infection is still drug susceptible and that the disease promptly responds to the same drugs given under supervision.

Two treatment methods have been applied successfully to the management of tuberculosis in alcoholics and other noncompliant patients. *Short-term chemotherapy,* using INH (300 mg) plus RMP (600 mg) daily, possibly with the addition of SM (1 gram) or PZA (1 gram twice a day), or both, is given under supervision for a period of six months. This ordinarily requires hospitalization. If completed successfully, this short-term vigorous course is thought to be comparable to 18 months of standard therapy. Continued suppressive therapy with INH is recommended for another 6 to 12 months, but in this circumstance noncompliance is less important. *Intermittent chemotherapy,* usually provided by a public health clinic and usually requiring some means of bringing the patient to the clinic or the medications to the patient, has been successful throughout the world. In the United States, an initial period of intensive hospital treatment as outlined above (usually two to three months) is followed by an intermittent twice weekly drug regimen of either (1) INH, 15 mg per kilogram orally, plus EMB, 50 mg per kilogram orally,* or (2) INH, 15 mg per kilogram orally, plus SM, 25 to 30 mg per kilogram intramuscularly, given for a total of 18 months. RMP is not recommended in intermittent therapy because of the tendency to allergic reactions under these circumstances.

RETREATMENT. In most retreatment circumstances it is very important that the patient be managed in a hospital experienced with tuberculosis. Expert judgment is particularly important in drug-resistant tuberculosis in order to attain maximal effectiveness from limited drug resources. The determination of the susceptibility of the organism to all available drugs is critical to proper management.

In drug-resistant infections, RMP, if it has been held in reserve, offers an excellent chance for final successful treatment when combined with one other drug to which the organism is susceptible and under circumstances guaranteeing uninterrupted drug ingestion for at least 24 months. An infinite variety of circumstances attends each retreatment case. Some of these, along with certain principles of retreatment, are tabulated here: (1) A relapse following prompt reversal of infectiousness almost always indicates that drugs have been stopped too soon, usually by the patient. If drugs were stopped completely, most will harbor drug-susceptible strains and respond again to the initial drug regimen. (2) If lapse in treatment and relapse are followed by irregular drug ingestion, resistant organisms will probably be present. (3) A patient with tubercle bacilli in the sputum after more than four to six months of treatment is probably excreting drug-resistant organisms. (4) Under circumstances of suspected or presumed drug resistance, a two- or three-drug combination, including an unused strong drug (INH, RMP, SM) and an unused companion type drug (EMB, PZA, ETH, PAS, CS), may be added to drugs previously given while awaiting drug susceptibility studies. (5) CM can replace SM in the aforementioned regimens. VM and KM are less effective and more toxic, and their use is limited to last-resort situations. (6) SM, CM, VM, and KM have similar and additive toxicities, and no more than one should be used at the same time. (7) If only drugs of limited effectiveness remain available (ETH, CS, PAS, and either VM or KM), three or four should be used at the same time and INH also given in high dosage (15 mg per kilogram). INH-resistant strains are less pathogenic and more susceptible to the weaker drugs, and INH should therefore be given in high dosage even though drug resistance is already established.

OTHER FORMS OF TREATMENT. Bed Rest. Modified bed rest is beneficial during symptomatic disease, but its effect is insignificant compared to drugs in over-all therapy. In treatment failures resistant to all drugs, modified bed rest and continued use of INH together in time salvage many apparently hopeless cases. In retreatment cases with resistance to all but the weakest drugs, modified bed rest will improve chance of success.

Surgery. Surgery is now rarely used in the treatment of pulmonary tuberculosis. However, surgical resection may still occasionally have a place in treatment failures with residual cavities and meager drug resources or when lack of patient cooperation compromises the prospects of successful use of limited drug resources. Here experienced judgment is critically important.

DURATION OF OBSERVATION. The incidence of relapse following adequate antimicrobial therapy of tuberculosis is of such a low order that the time-honored custom of long-term or lifelong follow-up of patients with tuberculosis is no longer considered necessary by many authorities. Therefore, routine follow-up chest roentgenogram and sputum examinations after successful treatment are no longer considered important. However, exception should be made in the case of unusually extensive disease, unusually slow bacteriologic response to treatment, patients in whom there is reason to question faithfulness of drug taking, and certain high-risk patients such as diabetics.

---

*See p. vi, Dosage Notice, immediately following Preface.

168. EXTRAPULMONARY TUBERCULOSIS

Roger Des Prez

168.1. INTRODUCTION

Extrapulmonary tuberculosis falls into two groups on the basis of pathogenesis. The first comprises conditions resulting from *lymphohematogenous dissemination,* (*miliary tuberculosis, tuberculosis of bone and joints, renal tuberculosis,* most cases of *tuberculous lymphadenitis, female genital tuberculosis, peritonitis, pericarditis, meningitis,* and some instances of *pleural effusion and tuberculous laryngitis*). These illnesses may coexist with tuberculosis elsewhere or *may be isolated clinical manifestations.* The second comprises conditions which complicate pulmonary tuberculosis caused either by bronchial or gastrointestinal spread of infectious secretions (*intracanalicular spread),* or by direct contiguous invasion (pleura, pericardium, esophagus). Urogenital tuberculosis may represent a combination when a hematogenous renal focus cavitates and seeds the lower urinary tract via the ureter.

168.2. PRINCIPLES OF DRUG THERAPY

Most extrapulmonary tuberculosis responds more readily to drugs than does advanced pulmonary tuberculosis, because the bacterial populations are small. The exception is cavitary renal tuberculosis, which may contain large bacterial populations requiring combined drug therapy. In the remainder, the likelihood of drug resistance developing on therapy is negligible, and the choice of a drug regimen depends on how life threatening the illness is judged to be. Those conditions carrying a threat of early mortality (miliary and meningeal tuberculosis, and probably spondylitis and pericarditis) are treated with maximal drug therapy (isoniazid and daily streptomycin, or isoniazid and rifampin) at least until response is established, thus increasing antimicrobial potency and eliminating the small possibility of a primarily isoniazid-resistant infection. Less threatening conditions such as involvement of serous membranes, lymph nodes, the skeletal system (excluding the spine), and genital tuberculosis are treated with isoniazid and ethambutol for 18 to 24 months. Although not widely accepted, some authorities treat these conditions with isoniazid alone. As a rule, response is good. When it is not, other drugs may be added without significant loss (see Treatment in Ch. 167).

168.3. TUBERCULOSIS OF THE PLEURA

Subpleural foci established during the preallergic bacillemic phase of the primary infection may, when tuberculin hypersensitivity develops, rupture into the pleural space, evoking a brisk allergic reaction and the clinical syndrome of *primary serofibrinous pleurisy with effusion.* This occurrence, of itself usually unilateral and self-limiting, is important in identifying rather extensive initial (primary) infections which are very likely to result in progressive tuberculosis elsewhere at a later time. Unilateral or bilateral pleural effusion, occasionally with concurrent tuberculous peritonitis or pericarditis, may also result from subpleural foci established as a part of acute or subacute hematogenous (miliary) tuberculosis. Established chronic pulmonary tuberculosis more frequently causes local inflammation and visceral-parietal pleural adhesions (dry pleurisy), precluding sudden delivery of large amounts of antigenic material into the pleural cavity. However, uncommonly, serofibrinous pleurisy with effusion can complicate chronic pulmonary foci, and, rarely, rupture of a necrotic chronic focus into the pleural space may produce tuberculous empyema and bronchopleural fistula (see Ch. 350.1 for a more complete discussion).

168.4. ENDOBRONCHIAL TUBERCULOSIS

Cavitary tuberculosis inevitably produces bronchial mucosal infection in the immediate vicinity of the cavity and usually in spotty distribution elsewhere. In the days before drug therapy, such involvement at times obstructed the bronchocavitary junction or even a whole segment or lobe, with subsequent inspissation, fibrosis, and contraction, an important although tenuous healing mechanism. Superficial bronchial lesions respond promptly to chemotherapy, and now usually require little attention. However, partial degrees of bronchial cicatrization may cause nontuberculous complications such as atelectasis and obstructive pneumonitis, and rarely may produce complete obstruction of a bronchus even during the course of chemotherapy. Some degree of permanent bronchial distortion probably occurs in all moderately extensive pulmonary tuberculosis. Tuberculosis of the trachea, now rare, is an extension of florid endobronchial tuberculosis. The consequences of bronchial involvement in childhood are discussed in Ch. 167.

168.5. TUBERCULOSIS OF THE LARYNX

Prior to drug therapy, tuberculosis of the larynx was a dread late complication of extensive pulmonary tuberculosis. The onset of hoarseness, dysphagia, and perhaps pain, sometimes referred to the ear, often initiated a downhill course, with extensive bronchogenic spread throughout both lung fields from copious, thin, laryngeal secretions. This is now almost never seen, even in patients with a drug-resistant strain and highly infectious sputum. Rarely isolated tuberculous ulcers or nodules with intact mucosa, resembling carcinoma, are diagnosed either by biopsy or by association with active pulmonary tuberculosis. Laryngeal lesions are now more commonly seeded via the bloodstream, usually accompanied by hematogenous involvement of the lung as well, but rarely as a clinically isolated focus. Pain, often accentuated by swallowing, and hoarseness are prominent symptoms. Response to drug therapy is excellent and surgery usually unnecessary.

168.6. GASTROINTESTINAL TUBERCULOSIS

Gastrointestinal tuberculosis frequently complicated extensive pulmonary tuberculosis in years past, and also was caused by ingestion of contaminated milk. It is now rare, but occasionally complaints related to a gastrointestinal focus may lead to recognition of pulmonary tuberculosis; even more rarely, gastrointestinal tuberculosis presents in the absence of recognizable active pulmonary disease.

Tuberculosis of the tongue and mouth may present as painful ulcers or as a nonhealing tooth socket after dental extraction. Untreated, the process is indolently progressive, but response to chemotherapy is rapid. Extension of oropharyngeal disease via the eustachian tube may produce *tuberculosis of the middle ear and mastoid bone. Tuberculosis of the tonsil and pharyngeal lymphatic tissue* was common when bovine tuberculosis was epidemic; draining regional nodes were termed *scrofula. Tuberculosis of the esophagus* may very rarely result from penetration of an adjacent node, leading to bronchoesophageal fistula or to ulcerative or hyperplastic disease on the esophageal wall. *Tuberculosis of the stomach,* rare even when untreated pulmonary tuberculosis was common, has been described as resembling diffuse neoplastic involvement (linitis plastica type) or nonhealing ulcers, and may, if caused by extension from an adjacent lymph node focus, present as an isolated clinical manifestation. Hyperplastic or ulcerative *duodenal tuberculosis* may resemble peptic or neoplastic obstructive disease. Tuberculosis of the intestine may produce ulceration with bleeding and a tendency to perforation and fistula formation, hyperplasia with obstructive symptoms, or a combination of the two. *Tuberculosis of the small intestine* is more liable to produce perforation than disease elsewhere in the bowel. *Ileocecal tuberculosis* is the most frequently observed form of bowel involvement, presumably because of cecal pooling of infectious fecal material producing mucosal disease, occult bleeding, obstruction, or fistula formation. *Tuberculosis of the ascending and transverse colon* is much less common, and may present as a concentric, hyperplastic lesion producing obstruction. *Tuberculosis of the sigmoid colon* may resemble carcinoma, atypical ulcerative colitis, or diverticulitis. All these lesions may perforate and produce *tuberculous perirectal and pelvic abscesses and fistula in ano.* Diagnosis is now almost always an unexpected finding at surgery, but if it is established by nonsurgical means, the effects of chemotherapy should be determined. Even advanced lesions usually respond satisfactorily, but occasionally death results in spite of chemotherapy and surgery.

168.7. MILIARY TUBERCULOSIS

The term *acute miliary tuberculosis* was coined to describe the appearance of lungs and other organs from fatal cases of progressive tuberculous bacteremia in which the disseminated small tubercles suggested millet seeds. It is at present applied to the more extensive and acute form of hematogenous (bloodstream) dissemination. The hematogenous phase of the primary infection is especially liable to evolve into miliary tuberculosis in very young children and, together with the

associated meningitis, accounts for most tuberculosis deaths in this age group. In adults miliary tuberculosis may be an early sequel of the primary infection as in children, or may be due to old residua of remote infections which reactivate, undergo necrosis, and seed the circulation. A pulmonary focus may be responsible, but more frequently a previously undetected or clinically undetectable lymphatic, genitourinary, or skeletal focus is the cause. Such foci may cause multiple bacteremic episodes, and the process may be protracted, intermittent, and low grade (chronic hematogenous tuberculosis). Host factors such as debility; advanced age; intercurrent therapy with oncolytic agents, immunosuppressives, or corticosteroid hormones; malignant disease, particularly of the lymphatic and hematopoietic systems; and occasionally local injury are frequently associated with activation of latent foci.

CLINICAL FEATURES AND DIAGNOSIS. Acute Miliary Tuberculosis. In the very young, the illness is usually an acute and severe illness, with high intermittent fevers, night sweats, and occasionally rigors. Complications such as pleural effusion, peritonitis, or meningitis occur in as many as two thirds, usually developing several weeks after the onset of constitutional symptoms. A similar acute illness may occur in adults as well. The onset, although perhaps not actually abrupt, can nevertheless be dated. The patient is prostrated, frequently had a moderately severe headache, and, although conscious and oriented, usually seems to wish to be left alone. A leukopenia is present, sometimes as low as 3500 to 4000 cells per cubic millimeter, and there is a considerable increase of immature forms. Although meningeal signs may be absent, eventually meningitis appears in about two thirds of patients. However, in some, miliary tuberculosis may be covert and subtle, with weeks or months of nonspecific, slowly progressive constitutional symptoms such as weight loss, weakness, and low-grade or absent fever. This clinical picture, ascribed to small, intermittent bacteremic episodes and designated *chronic hematogenous tuberculosis,* is more common with increasing age. As in the more acute form, the initial clinical manifestation may be serous membrane involvement, meningitis, or, less commonly, disseminated lymphatic involvement. Choroidal tubercles are often absent. Splenomegaly is unusual in both acute and chronic miliary disease. In an appreciable number, particularly older individuals (see below), specific symptoms may be entirely lacking. *Accordingly, the diagnosis of miliary tuberculosis should be entertained in any wasting illness with or without fever.* Often a therapeutic trial of isoniazid will be diagnostic. Very uncommonly the tissue response to hematogenous dissemination is atypical, consisting of foci containing myriads of acid-fast organisms, nonspecific tissue necrosis, and a sparse polymorphonuclear cellular infiltrate. This histologic picture has been termed *nonreactive tuberculosis.* The usual clinical course is acute overwhelming sepsis; less commonly a more protracted fever of unknown origin is observed. Splenomegaly and a variety of hematologic disorders (see below) are the rule in patients with this histologic picture.

Diagnostic studies are usually initiated because of the appearance of a typical miliary infiltration on chest roentgenogram. However, *individuals may succumb to miliary tuberculosis before the miliary pulmonary infiltrate has become roentgenographically detectable.* The tuberculin test is of little help, because *as many as one fourth of patients with proved cases may be initially tuberculin negative,* reactivity returning when treatment results in improvement. Anemia is usual. The white blood count is usually normal or depressed initially (see below). Gastric and urine cultures, although frequently positive, are of little immediate diagnostic help. *Culture of spinal fluid may be positive without pleocytosis, protein elevation, or meningeal signs.* Evidence of associated tuberculosis is helpful but often lacking. In many, a tentative diagnosis is made when granulomatous lesions are discovered on bone marrow aspiration or liver biopsy. Culture of these tissues may be positive without histologic evidence of disease, and negative findings do not exclude the diagnosis.

Primary Hepatic Tuberculosis. Rarely miliary tuberculosis may present as fever and a pattern of hepatic functional derangement, suggesting disseminated hepatic infiltration of neoplastic or nontuberculous granulomatous origin (elevation of serum alkaline phosphatase, less elevation of serum bilirubin, and little indication of hepatocellular damage), resembling at times extrahepatic obstruction with ascending cholangitis. Diagnosis is made by liver biopsy.

Primary Splenic Tuberculosis. Even more rarely miliary tuberculosis may present as clinically isolated splenomegaly with or without the hematologic consequences of splenic enlargement (hypersplenism).

Miliary Tuberculosis and Hematologic Disease. Many hematologic illnesses may be mimicked by miliary tuberculosis (leukemoid reaction, leukopenia, thrombocytopenia, aregenerative anemia, hemolytic anemia, myelofibrosis, and even polycythemia). This is particularly the case with the histologic picture of *nonreactive tuberculosis.* The confusion is compounded by the fact that, particularly when steroid therapy has been employed, miliary tuberculosis may complicate, as well as mimic, serious hematologic illnesses. Some authorities state that miliary tuberculosis may present the clinical picture of leukemia as well. However, probably all such cases actually represent coexistent leukemia and hematogenous tuberculosis, and the hematologic abnormality is not reversed by antituberculous chemotherapy.

Electrolyte Abnormalities. A surprising number of patients with miliary tuberculosis, especially but not exclusively those complicated by meningitis, will demonstrate hyponatremia. Although the possibility of coexistent adrenal insufficiency should always be entertained, the syndrome of inappropriate secretion of antidiuretic hormone is a much more frequent cause.

TREATMENT AND PROGNOSIS. Treatment of miliary tuberculosis with regimens containing isoniazid should be successful in virtually all except those dying within the first few weeks or with serious underlying disease. The prognosis with concurrent meningitis is less favorable. Maximal drug therapy with isoniazid, 300 mg, and rifampin, 600 mg once daily, is recommended. When a good response has been established and the infecting strain is known to be isoniazid susceptible, rifampin may be discontinued. Isoniazid should be continued for a total of at least two years. (A good response to isoniazid in a therapeutic trial of unproved disease makes it unnecessary to add another drug.) Response to treatment may be dramatic or may require some weeks. Adjunctive therapy with corticosteroids is advisable in severe cases with extensive pulmonary involvement and serious hypoxemia, and also in cases with poor response resulting from severe debility. It is, of course, mandatory in the rare instance of coexistent adrenal insufficiency. Other causes for poor response to treatment, such as miliary disease caused by mycobacteria other than *M. tuberculosis,* are rare, presumably owing to the decreased virulence of these organisms.

168.8. TUBERCULOUS MENINGITIS

Tuberculous meningitis is invariably fatal when untreated and often produces incapacitating neurologic damage, particularly in the very young, even with prompt therapy. It was long regarded as primarily a children's disease, but at present one half or more of cases are observed in adults. Meningitis complicates the majority of untreated cases of miliary tuberculosis. The infection reaches the subarachnoid space by direct extension from a subjacent focus, most frequently a small, subependymal tubercle, less frequently a tuberculoma or parameningeal focus in the spine, middle ear, or elsewhere. Since the critical factor is location, extensive bacteremia merely enhances the probability of a strategically placed subependymal tubercle, but such a lesion may be also seeded during a small, transient, otherwise inapparent hematogenous phase, as in the preallergic bacteremia of the primary infection, and may remain latent for years. Once infectious material ruptures into the subarachnoid space, an allergic inflammatory response spreads infection via the spinal fluid, implanting bacilli elsewhere on the meningeal surfaces. Involvement is usually most marked at the base of the brain and may produce a grossly thickened, space-occupying exudate, causing pressure injury to adjacent cranial nerves and long tracts. Obstructed basilar foramina may cause hydrocephalus. Vascular thrombosis and ischemic brain damage may also occur.

CLINICAL FEATURES AND DIAGNOSIS. The usual case of tuberculous meningitis is an illness of one to six weeks' duration, beginning with a nonspecific febrile prodrome and followed in many with focal neurologic signs, particularly oculomotor palsies, pupillary changes, and other cranial nerve abnormalities, and then the development of meningeal signs and symptoms associated with mononuclear pleocytosis and a low sugar concentration in the cerebrospinal fluid. However, the illness may be abrupt and severe, resembling pyogenic meningitis, or subtle and chronic. In some instances defects in mentation or affect may develop with little to suggest infection. Extrameningeal tuberculosis is clinically apparent in one half and the tuberculin test is positive in three fourths, *but the absence of both does not exclude the diagnosis.* A variety of neurologic abnormalities may develop, including pupillary abnormalities, cranial nerve palsies, blindness, deafness, long tract signs, subarachnoid block, disorders of consciousness ranging from mild confusion to dementia or coma, and, as mentioned, the syndrome of inappropriate secretion of antidiuretic hormone.

An increase of cells in the cerebrospinal fluid, more than half mononuclear cells, is the rule. Cell counts are rarely over 1000 per cubic millimeter, more frequently in the 50 to 200 range, and may be as low as only a few lymphocytes. Uncommonly, in acute severe disease cerebrospinal fluid may, early on, contain predominantly polymorphonuclear leukocytes resembling pyogenic meningitis. The cerebrospinal fluid protein is almost always elevated and glucose usually depressed in comparison with simultaneously determined blood glucose. Smears of the spinal fluid sediment will reveal acid-fast bacilli on microscopy in less than 25 per cent; this return may be improved if the pellicle which forms on the top of the fluid specimen, if it is allowed to sit for several hours, is stained and examined. Culture will eventually be positive for *M. tuberculosis* in 75 per cent of cases. Of the spinal fluid abnormalities, only the degree of pressure elevation has prognostic import, higher pressures being associated with a tendency to herniation at the base of the brain. Accordingly, fluid should be removed cautiously and slowly.

TREATMENT AND PROGNOSIS.   Therapy should always include isoniazid and either rifampin or streptomycin, probably the former. Early in the course, isoniazid should be administered in larger than conventional dosage (8 to 12 mg per kilogram in the adult, and 15 to 20 mg per kilogram in children) with pyridoxine (100 mg per day). If response is favorable, these dosages may be reduced after four weeks or so. Isoniazid may be given by mouth or by intramuscular administration if oral therapy is not possible (equal total dose). Rifampin is administered as described for pulmonary tuberculosis. Intrathecal therapy is not indicated.

Bacteriologic cure should be achieved in three fourths or more, but permanent neurologic residua (weakness, paralysis, blindness, or deafness, other cranial nerve palsies, hydrocephalus, compromised intelligence, and rarely, symptoms and signs of pituitary or hypothalamic dysfunction such as precocious puberty, obesity, diabetes insipidus, and panhypopituitarism) may result in as many as 25 per cent. These are local complications of the inflammatory response, and accordingly adjunctive anti-inflammatory therapy should be advantageous. Use of *corticosteroid hormones or corticotropin* has received wide acceptance. Although evidence is conflicting, most studies reveal a slight but definite survival advantage in groups receiving adjunctive corticosteroid therapy, particularly in prevention of brainstem herniation. The response to corticosteroid therapy may be dramatic, with rapid clearing of sensorium, regression of abnormalities in the cerebrospinal fluid, defervescence, and loss of headache. Even if long-term benefits are slight, this symptomatic improvement justifies corticosteroid therapy. Prednisone (60 to 80 mg per day) is recommended in all cases of established tuberculous meningitis complicated by altered consciousness, neurologic abnormality, subarachnoid block, or spinal fluid pressures in excess of 300 ml of water. This will include most cases. The corticosteroid therapy may be tapered rapidly in the second or third week to a level of 30 mg, then decreased at a slower rate every third or fourth day, using the signs and symptoms of meningeal inflammation as a guide to dosage reduction, and usually discontinued entirely after six to eight weeks.

168.9.   TUBERCULOMAS

Tuberculomas, once the most frequent cause of intracranial mass lesions in children, are now rare. Except in cases in which meningitis develops as a result of extension to the subarachnoid space, the symptoms are those of an expanding cerebral or cerebellar mass. Diagnosis is usually made at surgery. Antimicrobial therapy

should be administered when the diagnosis is made, both in hope of some resolution and to prevent development of meningitis. In the spinal cord *epidural granulomas* may behave clinically exactly like metastatic neoplasm, causing paraplegia with no evidence of infection or spinal fluid abnormalities and diagnosed at laminectomy.

168.10.   TUBERCULOUS PERICARDITIS

The subject of pericarditis is covered in Ch. 365.2, and this discussion concerns only aspects unique to tuberculous pericarditis. The pericardium is most often contaminated by an adjacent mediastinal node, less frequently by a pulmonary focus, and rarely as a part of generalized hematogenous tuberculosis, evoking an allergic effusion which disseminates the infection over the entire pericardial surface. Associated pleural effusion is present in approximately half the patients, and peritoneal involvement may also occur, a syndrome termed *tuberculous polyserositis*. Although always associated with other tuberculosis foci, frequently pericarditis is the only clinically apparent manifestation. Prior to the era of chemotherapy, tuberculous pericarditis was fatal in 90 per cent or more of cases, with deaths caused both by progressive infection and by acute and chronic cardiovascular complications such as tamponade, constriction, restriction, and myocardial and coronary artery involvement.

Features tending to differentiate tuberculosis from other causes of pericarditis are a somewhat chronic course, less prominent pain, decreased frequency and prominence of a pericardial friction rub, and symptoms of chronic systemic infection. At times a symptom complex resembling progressive right heart failure leads to the diagnosis. Etiologic diagnosis of tuberculous pericarditis, once the anatomic process has been established, is always difficult. The tuberculin test is usually positive (over 90 per cent) but may be negative. *Pericardiocentesis* is often employed for both diagnosis and relief of tamponade. *This procedure is associated with significant morbidity and mortality and, if done, should always be preceded by unequivocal evidence of pericardial fluid.* It is not only risky, but also provides meager diagnostic information. The character of the fluid will not differentiate tuberculous disease from other causes of pericardial exudate (with the possible exception of pyogenic pericarditis). The fluid is rarely positive for acid-fast bacilli on microscopy, and culture (positive in approximately 40 per cent) requires too much time to be of immediate therapeutic assistance. It is the writer's preference to advise pericardiocentesis only for temporary relief of tamponade or to exclude the possibility of a pyogenic process when associated clinical manifestations (high remittent fever, marked leukocytosis, associated nontuberculous infection) make this uncommon process a serious consideration. Pericardiocentesis is best carried out in association with right heart catheterization and only after arrangements for prompt thoracotomy have been made, should this become necessary. When the presence of documented tuberculous disease elsewhere makes tuberculous pericarditis likely and little hemodynamic compromise is present, therapy may be initiated with isoniazid, 300 mg, and rifampin, 600 mg, in a single daily dose, and the course carefully followed. If, because of uncertain diagnosis, unfavorable hemodynamic conditions, or less than prompt improvement, this approach becomes unsatisfactory and the general condition of the patient is otherwise fairly good, we advise thoracotomy and anterior pericardial stripping. The advantages of this approach are (1) accurate diagnosis; (2) relief of tamponade and very probably prevention of some instances which would otherwise progress to constrictive or restrictive disease; (3) a favorable surgical technical situation prior to the development of chronic inflammation, scarring, and fibrosis; and (4) relief of right atrial hypertension which favors fluid retention, venous thrombosis, and pulmonary embolization. Our personal experience with patients succumbing to pulmonary embolic disease had led us to this rather prompt and decisive diagnostic and therapeutic approach.

Some authorities advise the use of corticosteroids to favor resolution of the inflammatory process. Although this is acceptable when the diagnosis is certain and the inflammatory reaction is particularly intense, in most cases therapy is initiated before mycobacterial diagnosis has been established. In these the risk of an infectious process not susceptible to antituberculous drugs, although minor, is always present.

168.11. TUBERCULOUS PERITONITIS

Tuberculous peritonitis usually results from rupture of an adjacent caseous lymph node, fallopian tube, or subserosal tubercle into the peritoneal cavity, or as a component of generalized hematogenous tuberculosis. It frequently may be the only clinical manifestation of infection. Peritoneal involvement from a bowel focus is rare. The most frequent clinical picture is the relatively abrupt onset of unexplained ascites, usually associated with some fever and abdominal discomfort. The syndromes of chronic fibroid peritonitis (doughy abdomen) and of localized abdominal tumor are rare. The process may be loculated and hyperplastic with gelatinous exudate tending to fibrosis and caseation, but much more frequently involves the entire peritoneal surface with development of clear or slightly cloudy ascites containing several hundred to several thousand mononuclear cells per milliliter. Erroneous initial diagnoses, which are almost the rule, include peritoneal carcinomatosis, unexplained ascites, fever of unknown origin, bowel obstruction, or, in unusual cases of abrupt onset, bacterial peritonitis or perforated viscus. Some fever is the rule, and the tuberculin test is most often positive. Recognition of tuberculous peritonitis in cirrhotics may be difficult, because the symptoms may resemble those of uncomplicated cirrhosis with ascites, requiring paracentesis for detection (ascitic fluid in uncomplicated cirrhosis usually contains less than 800 cells). Fever, abdominal pain, or both in the cirrhotic with ascites should raise the question of some other complicating abdominal condition, including tuberculous peritonitis.

Diagnosis may be made on the basis of clinically detectable tuberculosis in the chest or elsewhere, but frequently is the result of laparotomy or response to specific antituberculous chemotherapy. The peritoneal fluid resembles that found in tuberculous pleurisy with effusion, but is indistinguishable from that which may occur in peritoneal carcinomatosis. In acute cases the ascitic pleocytosis may be predominantly polymorphonuclear, at least early on, suggesting a pyogenic process. Acid-fast stain of the fluid sediment is rarely positive, and tubercle bacilli can be cultured in fewer than 20 per cent of cases. Needle biopsy of the parietal peritoneum (Cope or Abrams needle) will be diagnostic in most patients, but has resulted in death from occult intraperitoneal bleeding. Accordingly, if tissue is required, a limited exploratory laparotomy is safer. When the therapeutic implications of tissue diagnosis are limited to the question of whether or not to treat for tuberculosis, a trial of isoniazid is often an acceptable alternative. Multiple drug therapy, at present isoniazid and ethambutol, is advised by most authorities, but single drug therapy with isoniazid for a period of 24 months has produced completely satisfactory responses in all cases known to the writer.

168.12. TUBERCULOUS LYMPHADENITIS

Prior to the control of bovine tuberculosis, cervical tuberculous lymphadenitis or *scrofula* was commonplace due to local infection of the oropharynx and draining cervical lymphatics. This mode of acquisition of tuberculous cervical lymphadenitis is now extremely rare in areas with no bovine tuberculosis problem. In contrast, in children, cervical granulomatous lymphadenitis caused by mycobacteria other than *M. tuberculosis* and *M. bovis* is almost certainly acquired by the oral route (see Ch. 169).

The term tuberculous lymphadenitis is now used to describe superficial lymph node involvement either caused by extensive lymphatic spread from a primary pulmonary focus or as a part of a generalized lymphohematogenous dissemination. The cervical and mediastinal nodes are most frequently involved. Clinical evidence of associated tuberculosis is lacking in more than half the cases. Painless or, less frequently, painful unilateral cervical node enlargement is the usual presenting complaint, but multiple areas of lymphadenopathy may be present. The nodes may become fluctuant and drain. Systemic symptoms are frequent but may be lacking completely or so subtle as to have gone unnoticed.

Drug therapy (isoniazid and ethambutol) may produce complete resolution, but, in as many as one half in some series, response to drugs, especially when fluctuant areas are present, may be inadequate, requiring repeated aspiration or surgical excision. In some cases cervical lymphadenitis may locally progress or develop de novo while coexisting pulmonary disease is responding well to chemotherapy. This does not represent bacterial resistance to the antimicrobials but rather the fact that tuberculous nodes, especially when necrosis has taken place, may be very slow to resolve or actually enlarge even when the infection is well controlled. Prolonged rest or hospitalization is not necessary once treatment has been initiated. Careful bacteriologic investigation is mandatory in view of the frequency of granulomatous lymphadenitis caused by other mycobacteria which are more drug resistant and more frequently require surgical removal.

168.13. GENITOURINARY TUBERCULOSIS

RENAL TUBERCULOSIS

Renal tuberculosis develops from foci in the cortex seeded via the bloodstream. Although it is usually unilateral when detected, 50 per cent of cases will become bilateral in the absence of treatment, because of progression of contralateral hematogenous foci which are probably always present. The bacilli lodge in the cortex, but infection does not become progressive until it reaches the medulla (via the renal tubules), where the environment is much more favorable to bacterial multiplication. Foci in the renal papillae may cause obstruction and retrograde involvement of the obstructed segment, or may undergo necrosis, excavate, and seed the ureteral and vesical mucosa. Papillary obstruction with infection may cause segmental renal obstruction; scarring in the renal pelvis and ureters may cause obstructive hydronephrosis; and the contaminated urine may cause bladder irritability, contracture, and scarring as well as infection of the male genitalia. The interval between the initial infection and active renal tuberculosis, when this can be dated by some early manifestation such as pleural effusion, is usually quite long, often many years.

Symptoms are usually subtle and often lacking entirely even with advanced cavitary renal tuberculosis. Sterile pyuria should suggest tuberculosis, especially with frequency and dysuria, but it should be kept in mind that infection with conventional urinary pathogens may coexist with renal tuberculosis. Pyuria may be intermittent and low grade (10 WBC per high power field). Intermittent hematuria may be the only recognizable abnormality. Fever and backache are uncommon and probably late symptoms. Male genital tuberculosis (epididymitis or orchitis) is often the first clue to renal involvement. Some evidence of intrathoracic tuberculosis, usually healed but at times active, will be present in as many as one half. Hypertension and renal insufficiency, when present, are almost always due to some coexistent process other than tuberculosis.

Culture of several early morning urine specimens will yield the diagnosis in 80 per cent or more of active cases; diagnosis in the remainder is based on evidence of tuberculosis elsewhere together with pyelographic abnormality or persistent pyuria. Demonstration of acid-fast bacilli by microscopy of concentrated sediment should be regarded with suspicion, although the smega bacillus may be responsible. Intravenous pyelography, which is abnormal to some degree in two thirds or more, may provide the first evidence of disease and is necessary to assess the degree of involvement and whether or not ureteral stricture is present. However, unless calcification is present, the findings are nonspecific.

Treatment with a two-drug regimen including isoniazid for a period of at least two years will arrest the disease in most instances. Relapse is usually associated with emergence of drug resistance, and retreatment with two drugs to which the infection is susceptible is advised. Intravenous pyelograms at three-month intervals to detect and treat ureteral strictures complicating the healing process are recommended by some authorities. Very rarely obstruction with complicating pyogenic infection or pain may require partial or complete nephrectomy, but this is unnecessary in the absence of symptoms regardless of the degree of renal destruction. Hypertension is not an indication for nephrectomy.

MALE GENITAL TUBERCULOSIS

Male genital tuberculosis affects the *prostate*, the *seminal vesicles*, the *epididymides*, and more rarely the *testes*; it may be secondary to recent or remote renal tuberculosis or to lymphohematogenous spread. Most instances present as an epididymal lesion, varying from a firm, painless, small nodule to an inflamed and draining mass. Diagnosis is usually made by prostatic or epididymal biopsy. Some instances may be detected because of poor healing and fistula formation complicating prostatic or scrotal surgery; in these, diagnoses may require a therapeutic trial of isoniazid, because culture of the draining material is often unrevealing. Response to drug therapy with isoniazid and ethambutol is excellent in most patients, and surgery usually is not required except for diagnosis.

FEMALE GENITAL TUBERCULOSIS

Female pelvic tuberculosis begins as a hematogenous endosalpingeal focus. Infection may spread to the ovary, the endometrium, and, rarely, the cervix, producing an ulcerating granuloma resembling carcinoma. Local or generalized peritonitis may also develop. The most common symptoms are menstrual disorders and abdominal pain. Most patients are sterile. In a small number, pregnancy and delivery appear to activate a previously latent focus. When conception does occur, tubal disease favors ectopic pregnancy. Pelvic inflammatory disease unresponsive to antimicrobial therapy may lead to the recognition of tuberculosis. In the majority, however, local and constitutional symptoms are mild or absent. Diagnosis is made by histologic study and culture of endometrial scrapings, culture of menstrual blood, and often by exploratory laparotomy. Response to a drug regimen containing isoniazid is usually excellent, and surgery is only rarely necessary to remove large tubo-ovarian abscesses.

168.14. TUBERCULOSIS OF BONES AND JOINTS

Blood-borne tubercle bacilli tend to lodge in the anterior aspects of vertebral bodies and in the metaphyseal areas of long bones. Evolution of foci in bone may produce cystic areas of osteomyelitis without joint involvement but often erode the end plate and involve the adjacent joint space. At present, bone and joint tuberculosis is not common in the United States, but several cases are seen each year on most medical services. It remains a major problem in some other areas of the world.

TUBERCULOUS SPONDYLITIS

The most grave form of skeletal tuberculosis is *tuberculous spondylitis* or *Pott's disease*. The originating focus is usually in the anterior aspect of the vertebral body near an intervertebral disc. The developing infection may erode the cortex, destroy the intervertebral disc, and involve the adjacent vertebral body. The roentgenographic picture of rarefaction and destruction of adjacent areas of two vertebral bodies, loss of the intervening disc space, and a tendency to anterior wedging or collapse is typical of tuberculous spondylitis, but is also caused by other infectious processes. The anterior foreshortening and angulation of the spine may result in a visible and tender posterior bony prominence or gibbus. Less frequently, the infection may begin in the center or posterior aspect of the vertebral body. The thoracic, thoracolumbar, cervical, and lumbosacral areas are involved in order of decreasing frequency. More than one area may be involved with intervening normal vertebrae. Characteristically, the infection dissects anterolaterally from the vertebral body, producing a paraspinal abscess. In the thoracolumbar area, this may be seen as mediastinal widening or a pear-shaped retrocardiac density on chest roentgenogram. In the lumbar area, the psoas shadow may be lost. In the cervical area, the abscess may cause anterior displacement or even obstruction of the esophagus or trachea. Pus dissecting under the firm paraspinal ligamentous structures may result in very high pressures in the abscess and produce ischemic paralysis in the subjacent spinal cord. This high abscess pressure also may cause the pus to dissect along ligamentous planes and present as a fluctuant or firm mass in the groin, the gluteal area, or the supraclavicular space.

CLINICAL FEATURES AND DIAGNOSIS. Symptoms are usually insidious and prolonged, and may not include fever, although weight loss is common. Local back pain is frequent, and referred pain imitating renal colic or abdominal disorders occurs. Walking may be painful, and the gait may become stilted. Miliary, meningeal, or pulmonary tuberculosis may develop and dominate the picture in the untreated patient. Severe anterior angulation of the spine may eventually produce a hunchback deformity. Frequently, however, it is the development of *weakness or paralysis* of the sphincters or legs which leads to medical attention. Paralysis, now the most serious consequence of Pott's disease, may develop owing to pressure from abscess fluid, to generalized inflammatory edema, or to intrusion of bony sequestrum or granulation tissue on the anterior aspect of the cord. Paralysis resulting from angulation and displacement is unusual, as the anatomic abnormality develops slowly, but violent movement may produce sudden cord transection when spine instability is marked.

In prior years most infectious spondylitis was tuberculous. However, it is now clear that entirely similar roentgenographic and clinical pictures can be produced by several other organisms, notably staphylococci, gram-negative enterobacteria, fungi, and rarely mycobacteria other than *M. tuberculosis*. Accordingly, in the absence of strong ancillary evidence for tuberculosis, aspiration or open biopsy of the vertebral body is indicated for microbiologic diagnosis.

TREATMENT. The most important aspect of the treatment of Pott's disease is antimicrobial therapy. Usually isoniazid and streptomycin or rifampin for a period of two years or more are recommended. Some period of bed rest during the first month or two is usually recommended, but its usefulness in the uncomplicated case, except to relieve pain or in patients with marked instability of the spine, is not established. Body casting is generally not indicated except as an adjunct to surgical procedures. When paralysis develops or fails to improve on therapy, surgery is required; the procedure, whether abscess evacuation, debridement of granulation tissue, or removal of sequestra, is dictated by the findings at operation. Usually some form of spinal fusion will also be carried out. Although orthopedic opinion tends to favor prompt surgical intervention with debridement, spinal fusion, and casting, experienced internists prefer to assess the effects of drug therapy and bed rest while maintaining close surveillance of the neurologic status, and many individuals will achieve stable spines and remission of neurologic symptoms without operative intervention or casting.

TUBERCULOUS ARTHRITIS

CLINICAL FINDINGS AND DIAGNOSIS. Tuberculous arthritis involves the hips, knees, elbows, shoulders, and small joints of the hands and feet in roughly that order. The initial symptoms are pain on motion or weight bearing, usually with some swelling. The process is usually monarticular, chronic, and associated eventually with considerable muscle wasting, pain, and stiffness, although low grade and trivial symptoms may have been present for months or even years at the time of diagnosis. A history of trauma to the involved joint can frequently be obtained. In the absence of proved associated tuberculosis, diagnosis requires biopsy, histologic study, and culture. The need for verification by culture as well as histology has been emphasized by reports of cases of granulomatous arthritis caused by mycobacteria other than *M. tuberculosis* (see Ch. 169).

TREATMENT. Isoniazid and ethambutol provide effective drug therapy; isoniazid alone is adequate in most cases. Intra-articular injection of drugs is not recommended. Many and perhaps most instances of tuberculous arthritis will heal with preservation of joint function when treated with mild immobilization, bed rest until pain is gone in the case of weight-bearing joints, and chemotherapy. When progress is not entirely satisfactory, joint exploration and removal of hypertrophied and fragmented synovial granulation tissue may be required. Casting and procedures to effect joint fusion are rarely necessary and often detrimental.

OTHER FORMS OF SKELETAL TUBERCULOSIS

Cystic tuberculosis of bone (tuberculous caries or *tuberculosa multiplex cystica*) is a rare condition in which osteolytic cystic areas of long and flat bones, particularly the ribs, and occasionally the tubular bones of the hands or feet are caused by tuberculosis. *Tuberculosis of the costochondral junction* may present as a cold abscess overlying the area of involvement. *Tuberculosis of the tendon sheaths and bursae* is usually secondary to involvement of the adjacent joint bone, but may be present in the absence of bony involvement. These usually respond readily to chemotherapy, but chronic lesions may require surgical evacuation of fibrinous material referred to as rice bodies.

168.15. RARE FORMS OF TUBERCULOSIS

Ocular tuberculosis is one of the causes of *granulomatous intraocular infection. Phlyctenular keratoconjunctivitis* is a rare allergic external ocular inflammation observed in children at the time of the primary infection and characterized by small blisters (phlyctenules) at the junction of conjunctiva and cornea. *Choroidal tubercles* often provide a clue to the presence of disseminated tuberculosis. They produce no symptoms and are difficult to differentiate from other retinal exudates.

Cutaneous tuberculosis, once important but now only rarely seen, is usually grouped into two categories. The first, in which organisms are present, includes *lupus vulgaris, tuberculosis verrucosa cutis* (anatomic or prosector's wart), *scrofuloderma* (the skin changes surrounding a draining tuberculous sinus or overlying a tuberculous node), and *tuberculosis orificialis* (nodular and ulcerated lesions around the mouth or other orifice through which highly infectious material passes). These are all very responsive to isoniazid. The second group comprises the *tuberculids* (including *erythema induratum* or Bazin's disease). These reactions are thought to be allergic and comprise a variety of erythematous, papular, and ulcerative forms. Their relationship to tuberculosis is poorly understood. *Tuberculosis cutis miliaris acuta disseminata* is a rare complication of overwhelming miliary tuberculosis, usually in children.

Tuberculosis of the adrenals is important only as a now uncommon cause of adrenal insufficiency. Tuberculosis of the *thyroid, pancreas,* and *breast* may all occur and mimic other infections or neoplastic change in these organs.

American Lung Association: Preventive therapy of tuberculous infection. Am. Rev. Respir. Dis., 110:371, 1974.

Berger, H. W., and Mejia, E.: Tuberculous pleurisy. Chest, 63:88, 1973.

Black, M., Mitchell, J. R., Zimmerman, H. J., Ishak, K. G., and Epler, G. R.: Isoniazid-associated hepatitis in 114 patients. Gastroenterology, 69:289, 1975.

Brown, A. B., Gilbert, R. A., and Telinde, R. W.: Pelvic tuberculosis. Obstet. Gynecol., 2:476, 1953.

Canetti, G.: Present aspects of bacterial resistance in tuberculosis. Rev. Respir. Dis., 92:687, 1965.

Christensen, W. I.: Genitourinary tuberculosis: Review of 102 cases. Medicine, 53:377, 1974.

Davidson, P. T., and Horowitz, I.: Skeletal tuberculosis. A review with patient presentations and discussion. Am. J. Med., 48:77, 1970.

Diagnostic Standards and Classification of Tuberculosis and other Mycobacterial Diseases. 13th ed. New York, American Lung Association, 1974.

Fox, W., and Mitchison, D. A.: Short-course chemotherapy for pulmonary tuberculosis. Am. Rev. Resp. Dis., 111:325, 1975.

Gelb, A. F., Leffler, C., Brewin, A., Mascatello, V., and Lyons, H. A.: Miliary tuberculosis. Am. Rev. Respir. Dis., 108:1327, 1973.

Goyette, E. M.: The treatment of tuberculous pericarditis. Prog. Cardiovasc. Dis., 3:141, 1960.

Huhti, E., Brander, E., Paloheimo, S., and Sutinen, S.: Tuberculosis of the cervical lymph nodes: A clinical, pathological and bacteriological study. Tubercle, 56:27, 1975.

Johnston, R. F., and Wildrick, K. H.: The impact of chemotherapy on the care of patients with tuberculosis. Am. Rev. Respir. Dis., 109:636, 1974.

Kocen, R. S., and Parsons, M.: Neurological complications of tuberculosis: Some unusual manifestations. Quart. J. Med., 39:17, 1970.

Konstam, P. G., and Blesovsky, A.: The ambulant treatment of spinal tuberculosis. Br. J. Surg., 50:26, 1962.

Newman, R., Doster, B. E., Murray, F. J., and Woolpert, S. F.: Rifampin in initial treatment of pulmonary tuberculosis. A United States Public Health Service tuberculosis therapy trial. Am. Rev. Respir. Dis., 109:216, 1974.

O'Brien, J. R.: Non-reactive tuberculosis. J. Clin. Path., 7:216, 1954.

Rich, A.: The Pathogenesis of Tuberculosis. 2nd ed. Springfield, Ill., Charles C Thomas, 1951.

Singh, M. M., Bhargava, A. N., and Jain, K. P.: Tuberculous peritonitis. An evaluation of pathogenetic mechanisms, diagnostic procedures and therapeutic measures. N. Engl. J. Med., 281:1091, 1969.

Smith, D. T.: Diagnostic and prognostic significance of the quantitative tuberculin tests. Ann. Intern. Med., 67:919, 1967.

Smith, D. T.: Isoniazid prophylaxis and BCG vaccination in the control of tuberculosis. High-risk groups. Arch. Environ. Health, 23:235, 1971.

Wales, J. M., Mumtaz, H., and MacLeod, W. M.: Gastrointestinal tuberculosis. Br. J. Dis. Chest, 70:39, 1976.

169. DISEASES DUE TO MYCOBACTERIA OTHER THAN M. TUBERCULOSIS AND M. LEPRAE

Robert A. Goodwin, Jr.

The term tuberculosis traditionally refers to infection associated with *M. tuberculosis (var. hominis* and *var. bovis).* It has long been known that other mycobacterial species exist in nature, some of which cause disease in animals. For years their role in human disease was unappreciated due largely to the overwhelming prevalence of *M. tuberculosis.* When found, their significance was denied because of the notion that mycobacteria were human pathogens only if they produced disease in the guinea pig (these did not). In recent years modern culture methods and drug susceptibility studies stimulated by the chemotherapy era have identified many mycobacterial species other than *M. tuberculosis* in human disease tissue. Much of the most important bacteriologic work on these "atypical" mycobacteria has been carried out by Runyon, who classified them into four groups primarily on the basis of the presence and type of pigment production and growth rate. (See Bacteriology in Ch. 166.) Most recently most of the known human pathogens have received tentative species designations, which will be employed herein. The relationship of these to the Runyon classification is as follows: *M. kansasii* and *M. marinum* — Runyon Group I (photochromogens); *M. scrofulaceum* — Runyon Group II (scotochromogens); *M. intracellulare* (Battey bacilli), *M. avium,* and *M. xenopi* — Runyon Group III (nonpigmented species); *M. fortuitum* — Runyon Group IV (rapid growers).

Human infection with many of these opportunistic mycobacteria is found throughout most of the world. Many of the organisms involved are widespread in nature, being found particularly in the soil and in water. *M. kansasii* has been recovered from milk in Dallas and tap water in California, but its source in nature is not clear. *M. intracellulare* is readily found in soil and in house dust, and has been demonstrated in throat swabs of normal individuals. *M. avium,* also of widespread distribution, is found in chickens and other birds as well as in household mammals. *M. scrofulaceum* has been isolated from soil and water, and is frequently found in oropharyngeal secretions of healthy men. *M. fortuitum* has widespread distribution in nature, may be found in saliva of normal persons, and is probably a frequent skin contaminant. *There is no evidence of man-to-man transmission of any of these, and no source case has ever been identified in human disease.*

The diseases produced by these organisms have

roentgenologic, pathologic, and, to some extent, clinical similarities to tuberculosis, but there are distinct differences in virulence, treatment, and prognosis. The term *mycobacteriosis* has been suggested to differentiate them from tuberculosis. However, species orientation is preferable, because there are differences in organ susceptibility, treatment, and prognosis. It is convenient from a clinical standpoint to group these infections according to organ involvement. Pulmonary disease, mainly in older white men with chronic bronchitis and emphysema, is the most common clinical manifestation. Lymphadenitis in children and granulomatous skin lesions in all age groups are next in frequency. Injection abscesses are not uncommon. Rarely, disseminated disease, meningitis, renal or skeletal involvement, penetrating wound infection, and corneal ulcers following trauma are reported.

PULMONARY DISEASE

M. kansasii and *M. intracellulare* (Battey bacilli) and, less frequently, *M. avium* and *M. fortuitum* may produce a chronic granulomatous pulmonary disease in susceptible individuals, as may rarely *M. xenopi* and *M. chelonei* (subsp. chelonei) and even more rarely *M. aquae*, *M. szulgai*, *M. scrofulaceum*, and *M. simiae*.

PREVALENCE. In the United States and Europe, 1 to 5 per cent of hospital admissions for tuberculosis are due to infection with either *M. kansasii* or *M. intracellulare*. There are geographic variations, particularly in the United States. The incidence of *M. intracellulare* infections is relatively high in Georgia and northern Florida, and *M. kansasii* infection is much more frequent in the central United States. In some localities the incidence is as high as 7 to 15 per cent of hospital admissions for tuberculosis.

CLINICAL MANIFESTATIONS. Pulmonary disease caused by *M. kansasii*, *M. intracellulare*, *M. avium*, *M. fortuitum*, and other "atypical" mycobacteria primarily affects white males over the age of 45; less frequently, by roughly a factor of 1 to 10, females and blacks; and rarely or never, children. Chronic bronchitis, emphysema, bullous disease, silicosis and other pneumoconioses, and, in *M. fortuitum* infection, lipoid pneumonia and achalasia are commonly present singly or in combination, and pre-existing chronic pulmonary disease in all probability is prerequisite to colonization with these saprophytic organisms. In this and other respects these pulmonary infections are more akin to that of *H. capsulatum*, a fungus of low human pathogenicity known to colonize abnormal pulmonary spaces, than to the much more virulent *M. tuberculosis* to which they are commonly compared. The earliest stages of these infections have not been described. The later stages are characterized by the presence of multiple thin-walled cavities, inconspicuous exudative and caseous disease, slowly progressive fibrosis, and a course marked by periods of stability and regression but, in general, slow progression.

Clinical symptoms when present tend to be mild. At least 50 per cent are said to be asymptomatic, and disease is often discovered on routine chest roentgenogram. Cough with expectoration to some extent probably occurs in all and is the most common complaint when recorded. Hemoptysis is not uncommon and occurred in 30 per cent in one series. Aching chest pain is an occasional complaint. Constitutional symptoms when present are mild and nonspecific and include malaise, fatigue, mild weight loss, and occasionally feverishness. Fever when found is low grade; chills and night sweats are rare. Constitutional symptoms usually disappear on rest. Remission and spontaneous healing may occur, but usually there is gradual progression over a period of many years. The infected individual usually dies of some other cause, and in only 15 per cent or less can death be attributed to the pulmonary disease and then as a result of pulmonary insufficiency. None of these opportunistic infections are contagious, and isolation is unnecessary.

DIAGNOSIS. Diagnosis is dependent upon bacteriologic identification of the specific organisms. With the exception of *M. kansasii*, mycobacteria other than *M. tuberculosis* may be found in oropharyngeal secretions of normals; therefore diagnosis of disease required repeated demonstration of the organism in significant numbers in the presence of compatible pulmonary disease. A tuberculosis-like disease that does not respond to antimicrobial therapy or the demonstration that the infecting organisms are highly drug resistant should suggest the possibility of another mycobacterial species.

TREATMENT. Only *M. kansasii* shows significant *in vitro* susceptibility to the antituberculosis drugs, although the degree of susceptibility is not always comparable to that of *M. tuberculosis*. Although no controlled studies have been done, it appears that a regimen of streptomycin (1 gram), isoniazid (300 mg), and ethambutol (25 mg per kilogram, reduced in two or three months to 15 mg per kilogram) given daily for 18 months will result in healing in 90 to 95 per cent of cases. Rifampin (600 mg daily) is probably the most effective drug, but rifampin-containing regimens have not been shown to exhibit any superiority, and some prefer to reserve this drug for the few patients requiring retreatment. This drug does have the advantage of oral administration, and a full oral regimen of rifampin, isoniazid, and ethambutol is reasonable and practical but carries greater hazard of liver toxicity. Whether two-drug regimens are effective has not been determined. Surgery is no longer considered necessary or advisable except for the few instances of drug failures.

M. intracellulare, *M. avium*, *M. fortuitum*, and all other saprophytic mycobacteria causing pulmonary disease are highly resistant in vitro to all the antituberculosis drugs. Some may show in vitro susceptibility to rifampin at levels unattainable in treatment of human disease. In spite of demonstrated in vitro resistance, many physicians use antituberculosis drugs in various combinations, and some report improvement, particularly with combinations including three or more drugs. However, there have been no controlled studies and no firm evidence of benefit. It has long been observed that significant improvement occurs with rest therapy, although relapse usually takes place in the presence of residual cavities. Surgical resection has been successful in controlling 75 per cent of *M. intracellulare* infections, and this would probably apply to the other pulmonary mycobacterioses as well. The incidence of surgical complications in these infections of low virulence is remarkably low even without effective drug coverage. A decision for or against surgery must be individualized, taking into account pulmonary function status, the severity of symptoms, evidence of progression, and other factors. Rest therapy for several months with or without a rifampin-containing drug regimen (such as rifampin, ethambutol, and streptomycin) is recommended for significant disease without prominent cavitation, and surgical excision (if not contraindicated) for localized extensive cavitary disease.

LYMPHADENITIS

Infants and young children may respond to a primary infection with certain atypical mycobacteria with the clinical manifestations of scrofula. Reports from the United States, Europe, and Australia in recent years indicate that 75 per cent of granulomatous cervical adenitis suggestive of tuberculosis is actually caused by mycobacteria other than *M. tuberculosis. M. scrofulaceum,* a scotochromogen, *M. avium, M. intracellulare,* and, less commonly, *M. kansasii* are the responsible agents. Each of these may be the predominant cause of adenitis in certain geographic areas and not found at all in others. In the vast majority the adenitis is cervical, occasionally preauricular, and rarely inguinal, axillary, or epitrochlear. Cervical adenitis most commonly occurs in the submaxillary and submandibular areas and is almost always unilateral, in most instances representing a regional component of a primary infection. Submaxillary and submandibular involvement suggests that the buccal mucosa is the portal of entry; involvement of the preauricular node implies conjunctival infection. In the extremities the infection usually follows a puncture wound. The pathology of the lesion is similar to that of tuberculosis, as are the clinical manifestations. Enlarged, firm, and nontender single nodes or groups of nodes may appear and persist unchanged or progress to fluctuation, drainage, and sinus formation, sometimes quite rapidly. Surgical excision is usually employed for both diagnosis and treatment. Infections with *M. kansasii* may be an exception, and a trial of drug treatment is indicated (see Pulmonary Disease, above). Isoniazid treatment of granulomatous cervical adenitis is recommended prior to cultural identification because the infection may be due to *M. tuberculosis.* If antigens are available, the demonstration of skin hypersensitivity to some other mycobacterial species and a negative or smaller reaction to PPD-S (*M. tuberculosis*) is regarded as diagnostic. PPD-B (Battey) may be used for this purpose. Although recurrence may develop in an adjacent lymph node, surgical excision of grossly involved nodes is usually curative.

SUPERFICIAL SKIN DISEASE

In addition to *M. leprae* (leprosy) and *M. tuberculosis,* two other mycobacteria, *M. marinum* and *M. ulcerans,* occasionally produce skin infections. Both have temperature requirements below 37° C, accounting for limitation of infection to superficial areas of the skin. *M. marinum,* previously referred to as *M. balnei,* is a photochromogenic saprophyte first described in marine fish. It is widely distributed in nature, occurring in soil, water, and freshwater fish as well. The temperature for optimal growth is 30 to 32° C. It has been implicated in epidemics of granulomatous skin disease traced to infected swimming pools, beaches of several of the Hawaiian Islands, and, more rarely, tropical fish aquariums. The granulomas occur at the site of minor abrasions, most commonly on the elbows, but also on the knees, toes, fingers, dorsum of the feet, and bridge of the nose, appearing two to three weeks after exposure as papules or nodules which increase slowly in size and may ulcerate. A line of granulomatous nodules may follow the draining lymphatics. Spontaneous healing is to be expected after several months. Diagnosis may be established by culturing a biopsy of the lesion at 30° C. Histologically, the tissue usually suggests a tuberculosis-like granuloma, but may appear to be a nonspecific chronic inflammatory reaction. Rifampin may speed spontaneous healing.

Disease caused by *M. ulcerans* is relatively rare in most areas of the world but strangely is quite common in the Buruli district of the upper Nile in Africa. This organism has a limited temperature requirement in the range of 32 to 33° C. Disease begins as a painless nodule, usually on the extremities, which may grow rapidly and ulcerate. The ulcers (Buruli ulcers), seldom less than 5 cm in diameter and often much larger, have characteristic undermined margins. They tend to be persistent and progressively destructive. Surgical excision is curative and much simpler when the lesion is recognized in the preulcerative stages.

OTHER INFECTIONS

Several hundred cases of *injection abscesses* have been reported, mostly caused by the common saprophyte, *M. fortuitum,* but also by *M. chelonei* (subsp. *abscessus*). These have occurred mostly in adults and usually respond to incision and drainage but occasionally require excision. The same organisms, and more rarely *M. kansasii,* have occasionally caused penetrating wound infections. *M. fortuitum* infection may result in corneal ulceration following trauma.

A dozen or so usually fatal cases of *disseminated* infection have been reported in young children and more rarely in immunologically deficient adults. Many different mycobacteria have been implicated, including *M. kansasii, M. avium, M. intracellulare, M. scrofulaceum,* and *M. fortuitum.* Rare cases of multiple and single *bone and joint* lesions have been reported, mostly in children, caused by the same organisms implicated in disseminated infection with the addition of *M. triviale.* Rare cases of *meningitis* in children and adults are reported with *M. avium, M. kansasii,* and *M. fortuitum.* One case of renal infection caused by *M. kansasii* has been found. A single case of *pleural effusion* caused by *M. fortuitum* has been reported.

Bates, J. H.: A study of pulmonary disease associated with mycobacteria other than *Mycobacterium tuberculosis:* Clinical characteristics. Am. Rev. Respir. Dis., 96:1151, 1967.

Corpe, R. F.: Clinical aspects, medical and surgical, in the management of Battey-type pulmonary disease. Dis. Chest, 45:380, 1964.

Harris, G. D., Johanson, W. G., and Nicholson, D. P.: Response to chemotherapy of pulmonary infection due to *Mycobacterium kansasii.* Am. Rev. Respir. Dis., 112:31, 1975.

Lincoln, E. M., and Gilbert, L. A.: Disease in children due to mycobacteria other than *Mycobacterium tuberculosis.* Am. Rev. Respir. Dis., 105:683, 1972.

Pfuetze, K. H., and Hubble, R.: Nontuberculous mycobacterial diseases. Disease-a-Month, September 1968.

Schaefer, W. B., and Davis, C. L.: A bacteriologic and histopathologic study of skin granuloma due to *Mycobacterium balnei.* Am. Rev. Respir. Dis., 84:837, 1961.

170. LEPROSY
(Hansen's Disease)

M. F. R. Waters

DEFINITION. Leprosy is a chronic inflammatory disease of man caused by *Mycobacterium leprae*, which displays a wide clinical "spectrum" related to host ability to develop specific cell-mediated immunity (CMI). In high resistant "tuberculoid" leprosy, the localized signs are restricted to skin and nerve. Low resistant "lepromatous" leprosy is a generalized disease involving many systems, with widespread lesions of skin, peripheral nerves, upper respiratory tract, eyes, testes, and the reticuloendothelial system. Common complications include more acute, immunologically mediated, inflammatory episodes ("reactions"), secondary inflammation in the anesthetic areas which result from nerve damage, and deformity of hands, feet, and face.

ETIOLOGY AND MICROBIOLOGY. Although Hansen recognized the leprosy bacillus in 1873, as yet *M. leprae* has not been cultured in vitro. Past attempts to infect human volunteers were unsatisfactory, and successful experimental transmission was not achieved until 1960, when Shepard reported limited infection in mouse footpads. Since that date, leprosy has been one of the fastest growing points in medical research. In 1967, Rees and his colleagues obtained lepromatous leprosy in thymectomized-irradiated mice. In 1971, Kirchheimer and Storrs described lepromatous leprosy developing in a proportion of immunologically normal nine-banded armadillos inoculated with leprosy bacilli. Subsequently, the only known animal reservoir, a small focus in armadillos, was discovered in Louisiana.

M. leprae is an intracellular, rod-shaped, acid-fast organism, 1 to 7 μ long and 0.25 μ in width; morphologically it resembles *M. tuberculosis*. However, in suspensions prepared from lepromatous tissues, bacilli are frequently arranged in characteristic "cigar-bundle" groups and in larger aggregates or "globi" derived from multinucleate Virchow giant cells. The cytoplasm of many bacilli is fragmented; such bacilli are dead. The percentage of solid-staining, presumed viable bacilli is known as the morphologic index (MI). Dead organisms are only slowly broken down, and may remain in tissues for many months or years.

In normal mice, a footpad inoculum of 5000 or 10,000 bacilli yields 10^6 after about six months, but no subsequent increase occurs. During the log phase of multiplication, the generation time is 12 to 13 days, the longest of any known bacterium. In thymectomized-irradiated mice, yields of 10^9 bacilli per footpad are not uncommon and systemic spread occurs, but the generation time remains unchanged. The footpad technique has been applied to studying the effect of drugs in leprosy, the detection of drug resistance, and the immunology and pathogenesis of the disease.

M. leprae is most easily detected in patients by Wade's "scraped incision" method. After cleansing, the skin is pinched to exclude blood, and a small cut made in the skinfold some 2 to 3 mm deep. One side of the cut is then scraped with the back of the scalpel point. The tissue pulp collected on the blade is spread on a glass slide, dried, fixed, and stained by the Ziehl-Neelsen method, care being taken never to overheat the carbolfuchsin. Leprosy bacilli are very scanty in tuberculoid lesions, and are often not detected by routine methods. They become more numerous as the spectrum is crossed and are present in huge numbers in lepromatous lesions. A lepromatous patient may have more than 10^{12} bacilli in the body. The density of bacilli in smears or tissues is termed the bacterial index (BI).

A standardized, autoclaved suspension of *M. leprae* is used as a prognostic intradermal skin test, the "lepromin test," which gives an accurate assessment of specific CMI in leprosy patients; it is negative in lepromatous and positive in tuberculoid leprosy. However, the test is often positive in nonleprosy patients, including those who have never visited leprosy-endemic areas, and shows some cross-reactivity with tuberculin. Therefore it is of no diagnostic or epidemiologic value.

EPIDEMIOLOGY. Incidence and Prevalence. Although governmental returns indicate a world total of 12 million leprosy patients, many consider that 15 million is a more accurate estimate, and that 1 million new patients will arise over the next five years. The importance of leprosy lies not only in numbers but also in the chronicity of the disease, which frequently disables but now seldom kills. Therefore it makes disproportionate demands on the health services and economies of developing countries.

Leprosy occurs in almost all tropical and warm temperate regions, including Japan and Korea, and is endemic in several states of the United States. It has only recently died out in certain northern European countries and Canada. It seems to be related particularly to overcrowding, so that as living standards rise, the disease becomes less common.

Transmission. Because *M. leprae* cannot be cultured, and because there is no simple, specific immunologic test of past or present infection, epidemiologic studies have hitherto been restricted to clinical cases. These have been further hampered by the long incubation period of three or more years. Close (household) contacts of lepromatous patients may show a tenfold higher incidence of leprosy and those of tuberculoid patients a twofold higher incidence than the general population. Lepromatous patients are thought to form the main source of infection in the community.

The lepromatous dermis is full of bacilli, but these are not shed in significant numbers through the intact epidermis. However, leprosy bacilli are excreted freely in lepromatous nasal secretions, so that 24-hour yields are comparable in numbers to those of *M. tuberculosis* coughed up in cavitary pulmonary tuberculosis. Bacilli from dried nasal secretions remain viable after being kept in the dark for at least 24 hours, and thus could be largely responsible for the spread of leprosy. The possibility of insect spread is also being reinvestigated. It has been assumed that *M. leprae* gains entry through the skin or the respiratory tract.

Studies in twins and other subjects suggest that lepromatous disease is a host-determined characteristic possessed by a fixed proportion of all people. Godal (1971) has developed a specific lymphocyte transformation test (LTT) which may help to clarify the epidemiology of leprosy.

PATHOLOGY AND CLINICAL MANIFESTATIONS. Leprosy has two special features. One is the invasion by *M. leprae* of certain superficial nerves, which may become thickened and firm. The other is the wide range of clinical and histologic manifestations, reflecting the intricacies of the host-parasite relationship. Skin lesions, which are best seen in good oblique light, may occur anywhere, although rarely on the hairy scalp and perineum. Nerves of predilection, which should always be palpated, include the ulnars at and above the medial humeral epicondyle, the superficial radials and medians at the wrist, the great auriculars at the edge of the sternocleidomastoid muscle, and the lateral popliteals (common peroneal) at the neck of the fibula. Appropriate muscle weakness and wasting may occur, resulting in claw hand (ulnar and/or median), foot drop, claw toes, and facial nerve paralysis, the last-named usually incomplete but including lagophthalmos. Wrist drop is comparatively rare.

The spectrum of leprosy has been particularly well defined by Ridley and Jopling, who proposed a five-group system of classification according to certain immunologic features, principally *the cytology* of the host cells of the macrophage-histiocyte series (whether histiocytic or epithelioid), *the bacterial density*, and *the degree of infiltration by lymphocytes*. Their classification enables the majority of patients to be diagnosed accurately from the clinical features, although the intermediate "borderline" (dimorphous) groups are relatively unstable, and tend to move toward lepromatous in the absence of treatment and toward tuberculoid after institution of effective chemotherapy. The five groups are, in order across the spectrum, *tuberculoid* (TT), *borderline-tuberculoid* (BT), *borderline* (BB), *borderline-lepromatous* (BL), and *lepromatous* (LL). Their distinctive clinical manifestations are now described, and these, with their corresponding pathologic, bacteriologic, and immunologic features, are summarized in the accompanying table.

Tuberculoid (TT). The typical tuberculoid lesion is large and annular, with a sharply raised outer edge and a thin erythematous rim which slopes gradually to a hypopigmented, flattened center. In profile, it resembles a saucer the right way up. The surface is dry, hairless, and sometimes scaly, with loss of sweating and marked anesthesia. Sometimes the lesion is a plaque with a dry, pebbly surface, or a macule. The lesion is usually single — at most two or three may be present — and, frequently, running to it may be palpated a thickened cutaneous sensory nerve in which caseation may occur. Sometimes, one of the nerves of predilection in the region of the skin lesion may be enlarged; rarely the only sign is a thickened nerve. Tuberculoid leprosy appears to be related to delay in the development of adequate cell-mediated immunity, and it forms a stable group.

Borderline-Tuberculoid (BT). The skin lesions resemble those of TT leprosy, but are usually multiple, though asymmetrical, and smaller in size, or else small "satellite" lesions may be present near the periphery of larger lesions. Sharp-edged papules may also occur. Enlarged cutaneous sensory nerves are less commonly found, but frequently one or more nerves of predilection are thickened. Therefore BT leprosy is often associated with deformity of one or both hands and/or feet; a patient may present with, or later develop, a plantar ulcer in an anesthetic foot or burns or infection of anesthetic fingers. Lagophthalmos may result in exposure keratitis.

Borderline (BB). The rather numerous, though asymmetrical, skin lesions are erythematous or hyperpigmented, and vary markedly in size. They occur as papules, plaques, and most characteristically as annular

Summary of the Clinical, Histologic, Bacteriologic and Immunologic Findings of the Five Groups of the Leprosy Spectrum

	TT	BT	BB	BL	LL
Skin lesions					
Numbers	1 to 3	Very few to moderate	Moderate	Moderate to many	Very many
Symmetry	Very asymmetrical	Asymmetrical	Asymmetrical	Slightly asymmetrical	Symmetrical
Anesthesia	Very marked	Marked	Marked to moderate	Slight to nil	Nil
Nerve enlargement					
Cutaneous sensory	Common	May occur	0	0	0
Peripheral nerves*	0 or one	Common; asymmetrical	Common; asymmetrical	Moderately asymmetrical	Symmetrical
Skin histology					
Granuloma cell	Epithelioid	Epithelioid	Epithelioid	Histiocyte	Foamy histiocyte
Lymphocytes	+++	+++	+	± or ++	±†
Dermal nerves	Destroyed	Mostly destroyed	Some visible	Visible	Easily visible
Bacilli numbers (routine examination)	0	0, + or ++	+, ++ or +++	++++	+++++
Lymph nodes					
Paracortical infiltrate	Nil; immunoblasts	Sarcoid-like	Diffuse epithelioid	Diffuse histiocytes	Massive infiltrate with foamy histiocytes and Virchow cells
Germinal centers	Normal	Normal	Normal	Some hypertrophy	Gross hypertrophy
Lepromin test	+++	++	± or 0	0	0
Reactions					
ENL	0	0	0	Rare	Very common
Lepra	?	Common	Very common	Very common	(Rare)‡

*Nerves of predilection, i.e. ulnar, median, lateral popliteal, facial, great auricular, and posterior tibial.

†In LL leprosy, the peripheral blood shows an absolute decrease in T and an absolute increase in B lymphocytes.

‡Lepra reactions are occasionally seen in treated LL patients who have developed from borderline (BT, BB, or BL) in the absence of treatment.

lesions with broad rims. The outer edge is often flattish and irregular; it rises to a thick inner edge, and the anesthetic, hypopigmented center is always sharply "punched out." The profile resembles a saucer the wrong way up, except that where the cup should sit is a deep central depression. Satellite lesions are common. Moderate and widespread, though asymmetrical, enlargement of the nerves of predilection may occur with or without associated muscle weakness and wasting.

Borderline-Lepromatous (BL). The skin lesions are numerous, but are not usually bilaterally symmetrical. They consist of erythematous or hyperpigmented papules, nodules, or plaques which appear moist and succulent, and which possess normal sensation or show only mild hypoesthesia. Small, indefinite-edged, hypopigmented macules may also be present. Some nodules may be dimpled, and often one or two lesions, usually the first to appear, have punched-out, hypopigmented, anesthetic centers, indicating progression from BB leprosy. Nerves of predilection close to the latter are often markedly thickened; elsewhere they may be only slightly enlarged. Ear lobes may appear normal, or be asymmetrically (more rarely symmetrically) enlarged. The eyebrows, nasal cartilage, and eyes are unaffected. Although bacilli are very numerous in the lesions, they are often undetected in normal-looking skin.

Lepromatous (LL). Lesions show marked bilateral symmetry. Skin lesions are very numerous, with erythematous, smooth, shiny surfaces, and are neither anesthetic nor anhidrotic. Early cases may have numerous, small, hypopigmented macules with vague edges and small papules with indefinite edges; nerves may be but slightly thickened at this stage, although significant involvement of the nasal mucosa is frequently detected. With time, plaques and nodules develop, and the skin progressively thickens as lepromatous infiltrate increases; rarely, but especially in Central America, infiltrate alone occurs. The ear lobes enlarge, and the lines of the face coarsen and deepen (leonine facies). The lips often swell, and the eyebrows and eyelashes become scanty and are lost. Iritis and keratitis are common. Nasal blockage occurs, with ulceration and bloodstreaked discharge, and in time the nasal cartilage and bones may be gradually destroyed, resulting in saddle-nose deformity. Lepromatous laryngitis may cause hoarseness. Edema of the extremities may occur, lymph nodes often enlarge, and testicular involvement frequently leads to atrophy and occasionally to gynecomastia. Dermal nerve damage leads to a progressive pseudo- "glove-and-stocking" anesthesia; light touch, pain, and temperature sensation are eventually lost over most of the body except scalp and flexures, but position sense is well preserved. Very numerous bacilli are present not only in the skin, in the draining lymph nodes, and in nerves of predilection, but also in the liver, spleen, bone marrow, and blood; there are relatively few in the kidney, and the lungs, heart, and central nervous system are not clinically involved in the infection.

In some peoples, such as the Chinese, many of the lepromatous cases originate as borderline, and a small number of residual BB-type lesions may be found; otherwise the signs are consistent with LL. In treated LL patients whose disease relapses, the new lesions are usually asymmetrical initially, but otherwise retain lepromatous characteristics.

Indeterminate Leprosy. Some child contacts of adult cases develop a single (occasionally two or three) hypopigmented macule, 2 to 5 cm in diameter, which shows hypoesthesia and decreased sweating. Histologically, there is lymphocytic infiltrate around the dermal appendages and neurovascular bundles. If left untreated, about one quarter later develop leprosy which may be of any type on the spectrum.

Reactions. Erythema Nodosum Leprosum (ENL) — Lepromatous Lepra Reaction. More than 50 per cent of treated LL patients, and the occasional untreated LL or treated BL patient, suffer from episodes of erythema nodosum leprosum. Over the course of a few hours, a crop of painful erythematous papules develops, typically on the extensor surfaces of the body except the scalp. The papules last for two to three days, becoming more purple, and then gradually subside, leaving dark staining of the skin. The episodes are usually associated with fever and general malaise. They may be isolated or may occur continuously over months or years, leading, if untreated, to gross prostration, weakness, and occasionally death. In severe ENL, the papules may form sterile pustules and ulcers. A frequent complication is painful neuritis, usually of the ulnar, median or lateral popliteal nerves, and muscle weakness may increase. Lymphadenitis, iritis, and orchitis may also occur, and more rarely nephritis and large-joint arthritis. The ENL is due to immune complex formation, resulting in vasculitis and polymorphonuclear infiltrate. The antigen is probably derived from the cytoplasm of dead leprosy bacilli, and serum immunoglobulin levels are markedly elevated in LL leprosy.

Nonlepromatous Lepra Reactions. These occur very frequently in BT, BB, and BL leprosy. The leprous lesions themselves become markedly swollen, erythematous, and often scaly, and new lesions may appear. The reaction lasts for many weeks or months. Systemic upset and fever are uncommon, but neuritis may occur, and ulceration of the friable skin may lead to unsightly scarring. The reaction is often associated with change in specific CMI and therefore of a patient's leprosy classification, so that untreated patients become more lepromatous and treated patients more tuberculoid.

DIAGNOSIS AND DIFFERENTIAL DIAGNOSIS. It is essential to consider leprosy in all patients with skin or peripheral nerve lesions who have resided in endemic areas. The three most helpful findings are (1) thickening of one or more nerves, either of predilection or cutaneous sensory; nerve enlargement is found in some TT, many BT, and the great majority of BB, BL, and LL patients; (2) anesthetic skin lesions, which are found in almost all TT, BT, and BB patients, in many BL patients, and in those LL patients who have evolved from borderline; and (3) acid-fast bacilli (AFB) in skin smears, which are positive in many BT and in all untreated BB, BL, and LL patients. Smears are usually taken from both ear lobes and up to six typical skin lesions. Leprosy should be suspected when skin or nasal symptoms persist despite routine treatment; in chronic, painless, plantar ulceration; in foot drop unassociated with trauma; or in unusual presentations of arthritis and erythema nodosum. Confirmation should be obtained by skin biopsy or, in neural leprosy without skin lesions, by biopsy of a thickened sensory nerve.

Lack of anesthesia differentiates vitiligo, mycotic infections, lupus erythematosus, and psoriasis from TT and BT leprosy. Nerves are not enlarged in neurologic conditions such as syringomyelia, motor neuron disease, and Friedreich's ataxia; they are enlarged in hereditary sensory neuropathy of Dejerine and Sotta, which can be differentiated by the absence of skin lesions and of AFB and by the familial history. Dermal leishmaniasis, yaws, secondary syphilis, and neurofibromatosis may resemble LL leprosy, but there is no nerve thickening, and smears for AFB are negative.

TREATMENT. Treatment is made difficult by the excessive prejudice and outdated fear of leprosy persisting in many cultures, and by the extreme chronicity of the infection and slowness of response to treatment which is related in part to the unique generation time of *M. leprae.*

Treatment of the Infection. The drug of choice remains DDS (dapsone, 4-4'diaminodiphenyl sulfone), which is as cheap as aspirin and may be administered by mouth or parenterally. In LL and BL patients, clinical improvement is detected from about three months after starting DDS (often earlier in TT, BT, and BB leprosy), and around this time bacilli from nose and skin will no longer infect mice. The MI reaches zero by six months, but the BI takes many years to become negative. Small numbers of viable, probably dormant, bacilli have been shown to persist in a number of tissue sites, in LL patients treated continuously for at least ten years; such patients may relapse if treatment is stopped. Therefore it is recommended that DDS be given for the following minimum periods:

Indeterminate and TT	3 years
BT	5 years
BB	7 years
BL	15 years
LL	20 years or for life

Although the minimal effective dose of DDS is less than 1 mg, the recommended standard adult dose in LL and BL leprosy is 100 mg daily by mouth or 300 to 400 mg twice weekly by injection. This results in an incidence of drug resistance of only 2.5 per cent, whereas the incidence may be many times higher on lower dosage, especially if irregularly taken. Secondary (emergent) resistance to DDS has not yet been reported from the other types of leprosy (TT, BT, BB, and indeterminate), in which bacillary loads are so much lower. In these, a dosage of 50 mg DDS daily is acceptable.

Sulfone resistance has been detected 4 to 25 years after the start of treatment, sometimes long after the patient has become smear negative. New active lesions, usually asymmetrical papules and small plaques with high BI and MI, are found on a background of old, resolving, or resolved lepromatous leprosy. Bacilli from these lesions will grow in the footpads of mice treated with DDS mixed in their diet (Pettit and Rees, 1964). Clinically, resistance must be distinguished from relapse off treatment by a therapeutic trial of DDS, 400 mg given regularly twice weekly by injection. In drug-susceptible relapse, uninterrupted improvement occurs. In resistant patients, some initial improvement may occur if there is a mixed bacterial population of partially and highly resistant organisms, but the MI is unlikely to fall to 0, and further new lesions, with raised MI, will sooner or later appear.

Toxic effects of DDS include dose-related sulfhemoglobinemia and hemolytic anemia, the latter especially in glucose-6-phosphate dehydrogenase–deficient patients. Drug allergy, which occurs in one in several

hundred cases, may be serious and even fatal; three to seven weeks after starting DDS the patient develops fever, pruritus, and dermatitis, which may become exfoliative, and jaundice and psychosis sometimes occur. DDS must be stopped immediately and prednisolone given for several weeks.

To reduce the risk of DDS resistance, it is now recommended that a second antileprosy drug should be given with DDS during an initial intensive course of treatment in LL and BL leprosy for a duration of up to six months. Available drugs include rifampin, clofazimine, and ethionamide (or prothionamide). Alternative treatment is also required in sulfone allergy and in proved cases of sulfone resistance. Clofazimine (B663, Lamprene), a rimino-phenazine dye, is both antimycobacterial and, in high dosage, anti-inflammatory. It is relatively nontoxic, its chief disadvantage being that it causes a reddish-brown pigmentation of the skin which is objectionable to most light-skinned patients. In a dose of 100 mg daily, it appears clinically and bacteriologically approximately as effective as DDS. Clofazimine resistance has not yet been reported, although the drug has been given for over 14 years to sulfone-resistant patients. It is used widely in dark-skinned races, in a dose of 100 mg three times a day (a dose level that should not usually be maintained for longer than about three months) to control ENL and lepra reactions, although several weeks elapse before its full anti-inflammatory effect is produced.

Rifampin is bactericidal. It kills leprosy bacilli faster than any other drug tried hitherto, so that patients may be rendered minimal public health risks within a few days; clinical improvement is seen in about three weeks, and the MI falls to zero within six weeks. It has been used for more than a decade in the treatment of DDS-resistant leprosy, usually in combination with the second-line drug thiambutosine, or with ethionamide, with excellent results, although the BI falls no faster than with clofazimine. Dosage is 600 mg daily, and intermittent therapy is under trial. Rifampin combined with DDS is of particular value in the initial therapy of sulfone-susceptible LL leprosy, when a rapid therapeutic effect is especially desirable.

Treatment of Reactions. In mild erythema nodosum leprosum, paracetamol or aspirin may suffice. Somewhat more severe episodes often respond to two or three courses of stibophen,* 2 ml daily parenterally for five days. In severe continuous ENL,or in all episodes complicated by significant neuritis or iritis, there are three alternative regimens. Prednisone, given in addition to DDS, rapidly suppresses ENL, but in the long term severe steroid toxicity is common. Therefore steroids are best reserved for short-term cover for operations, childbirth, and similar situations. The drug thalidomide is equally effective in controlling reactions, but its use is contraindicated in women because of its teratogenic potential. The dosage is initially 200 mg twice daily; subsequently it is progressively lowered to a maintenance dose, usually of 50 to 100 mg nightly, which may be continued for years. DDS must not be discontinued. The third alternative is clofazimine in high dosage. In light-skinned males and postmenopausal females thalidomide is probably the drug of choice; in dark-skinned patients and premenopausal women clofazimine is the safest drug, provided that a rapid action is not required. *Lepra reactions* can often be con-

---

*Discontinued by manufacturer in May 1977.

trolled with paracetamol, with or without stibophen. But whenever neuritis occurs or when there is risk of skin ulceration, the signs of inflammation should be suppressed with prednisone. Although steroids may be required for some months, toxicity is rare, because the dosage is usually less than for ENL and the total duration of the reaction is shorter. In dark-skinned patients, clofazimine can be commenced with the prednisone, and the latter drug slowly withdrawn. Thalidomide is useless in this type of reaction.

Other Treatment. Patients must be educated to protect their anesthetic limbs. The healing of plantar ulcers is aided by rest and plaster splints. Reconstructive surgery and physiotherapy are valuable in the rehabilitation of deformed patients. The use of transfer factor in LL and BL leprosy is being assessed.

PROGNOSIS. Even without treatment, patients with TT leprosy and three quarters of those with "indeterminate" disease eventually cure themselves; however, the patients with BL, most BB, and many BT forms of disease tend to lose cell-mediated immunity, and their disease becomes more lepromatous. Widespread nerve damage may develop in the BT and BB groups. Patients with the LL form used to die from uncontrolled leprosy, intercurrent infection, or amyloid nephritis, and blindness was common. With correct treatment, the prognosis now is good. Death from leprosy is rare, although amyloidosis is still seen occasionally, especially in inadequately treated ENL. Patients who fail to care for anesthetic extremities may suffer from repeated trauma or infection, resulting in gradual absorption of digits, or amputation may become necessary for chronic osteomyelitis. Even with careful management, reactional neuritis may sometimes cause increased deformity, and ENL may also, if rarely, result in blindness or significant renal damage.

PREVENTION. Because *M. leprae* cannot be grown in vitro, there is no specific vaccine. The precise value of BCG in protecting against early leprosy is being further assessed. Prophylactic DDS or acedapsone (diacetyl DDS) may be justified in special local situations. Otherwise prevention rests on early diagnosis of cases, and annual examination of known contacts may be rewarding.

Committee on Experimental Chemotherapy: Experimental chemotherapy in leprosy. Bull. WHO, 53:425, 1976.

Pearson, J. M. H., Rees, R. J. W., and Waters, M. F. R.: Sulphone resistance in leprosy. A review of one hundred proven clinical cases. Lancet, 2:69, 1975.

Ridley, D. S., and Jopling, W. H.: Classification of leprosy according to immunity. A five-group system. Int. J. Lepr., 34:255, 1966.

WHO Expert Committee on Leprosy. Fifth Report. Technical Report Series 607. Geneva, World Health Organization, 1977.

TREPONEMAL DISEASES

171. SYPHILIS

P. Frederick Sparling

DEFINITION. Syphilis is a subacute to chronic infectious disease caused by the bacterium *Treponema pallidum.* It is usually acquired by sexual contact with another infected individual. Syphilis is remarkable among infectious diseases in its large variety of clinical presentations. It progresses, if untreated, through primary, secondary, and tertiary stages. The early stages (primary and secondary) are infectious. Spontaneous healing of early lesions occurs, followed by a long latent period. In about 30 per cent of untreated patients, late disease of the heart, central nervous system, or other organs ultimately develops. At one time this disease was termed "the great imitator." Although the disease is less common now than previously, it still remains a great challenge to the clinician because of its protean manifestations, and is of great interest to biologists as well because of the long and tenuous balance between the host and the invading spirochete.

ETIOLOGY. The etiology of syphilis was first discovered in 1905 by Schaudinn and Hoffman when they visualized spirochetal organisms in early infectious lesions. The causative agent of syphilis, *Treponema pallidum,* is closely related to other pathogenic spirochetes, including those causing yaws *(Treponema pertenue)* and pinta *(Treponema carateum). T. pallidum* is also related in a more distant manner to other pathogenic spirochetes, including *Leptospira* (cause of leptospirosis) and *Borrelia* (cause of relapsing fever).

T. pallidum is a thin, helical cell approximately 0.15 μ wide and 6 to 50 μ long. Ordinarily there are approximately 6 to 14 spirals. The organism is tapered on either end. It is too thin to be seen by ordinary Gram stain but can be visualized in wet mounts by darkfield microscopy (see below), or by silver stains or fluorescent antibody methods.

The organism bears considerable structural resemblance to gram-negative bacteria. A peptidoglycan cell wall is closely adherent to the cytoplasmic membrane. The exterior surface of the cell is made up of a trilaminar lipoprotein outer envelope. This is structurally similar to the outer membrane of gram-negative bacteria, but no biologically active endotoxin has been identified in *T. pallidum* or in any other pathogenic spirochete. Between the outer envelope and the cell wall are six axial fibrils. The axial fibrils are attached three at each end and overlap in the center of the organism. They are structurally and biochemically similar to flagellae, and may be in part responsible for the motility of the organism. The spiral shape of the cell is primarily determined by the peptidoglycan cell wall. Microtubular structures have been seen in the cytoplasm of many treponemes, including *T. pallidum;* treponemes are apparently the only bacteria with microtubules.

It has not been possible to culture *T. pallidum* in vitro. Motility is prolonged under microaerophilic to anaerobic conditions. *T. pallidum* was formerly considered a strict anaerobe, but recent evidence shows that it is a microaerophilic to aerophilic organism. It can be maintained by serial passage in rabbits without loss of virulence. The Nichols strain of *T. pallidum* has been maintained in the laboratory in this manner for over 50 years. Only a few strains of *T. pallidum* have been isolated in rabbits and carefully studied, and little evidence is available regarding the genetic diversity of the organism. All studied isolates have been susceptible to penicillin and are similar antigenically. Immunity to the homologous strain develops readily in rabbits, but protection is often not conferred against heterologous isolates of *T. pallidum*. The only known natural hosts for *T. pallidum* are man and certain monkeys and higher apes. A related organism, *T. paraluis-cuniculi*, is a pathogenic spirochete of rabbits.

HISTORY. A great epidemic of syphilis occurred throughout Europe in the late fifteenth century. Because of the severity of the infection it was termed the "great pox" in contrast to another prevalent infection, smallpox. Severe morbidity and sometimes death occurred during the secondary stage of syphilis at that time; in later periods secondary syphilis has usually not been so severe. The pandemic started soon after Columbus returned from the West Indies, and one school holds that the disease was imported into a nonimmune population by the returning sailors. However, there is evidence in the Old Testament and also in ancient Chinese writings of similar diseases, and there are other reasons for disbelieving the Columbian origin of syphilis. Among these are the extensive knowledge of the course of the disease and the effectiveness of mercurial therapy in writings published only a relatively few years after Columbus and his men returned. It seems more likely that syphilis was endemic in Europe, but rose to particular prominence in the late fifteenth century because of the wartime conditions which prevailed. It will probably never be possible to settle the precise point of origin of syphilis.

The disease was recognized to be sexually transmitted in the early sixteenth century. Its name is derived from the sixteenth century poem by Fracastorius about the mythical shepherd, Syphilis, who was afflicted with the disease. The major cardiovascular and neurologic complications were recognized later in the eighteenth and nineteenth centuries. Many great figures of Western civilization had syphilis of the central nervous system, with untold effects on the course of history. The disease was confused with gonorrhea for some time, in part because of experiments by the great eighteenth century physician and surgeon John Hunter. He inoculated himself with pus from a patient with gonorrhea, and subsequently (and unfortunately) developed both gonorrhea and syphilis. The latter was eventually fatal. He concluded that both infections had a single cause. A clear distinction between syphilis and gonorrhea was finally made by Ricord in the mid 1800's.

Syphilis was treated for centuries with various heavy metal preparations. Until 1910, inunctions of mercury were the mainstay of therapy which was apparently moderately effective, although extremely toxic. In 1910, Ehrlich introduced arsphenamine, the "magic bullet." This and subsequent arsenical compounds were more effective and less toxic than mercurial compounds and were revolutionary at the time. They had to be administered for periods of up to two years to be effective. Bismuth salts also were effective and were frequently used in combination with arsenicals between World War I and World War II. The final revolution occurred in 1943, when penicillin was introduced for therapy of syphilis. It was so effective and exhibited so little toxicity that many thought that this ancient disease would soon be eradicated. Although syphilis did decline rapidly in incidence after World War II, it has proved to be a resilient foe and continues to be a significant problem.

PATHOGENESIS AND HOST RESPONSE. *T. pallidum* may penetrate through normal mucosal membranes and also may penetrate through minor abrasions of epithelial surfaces. In experimental rabbit syphilis, spirochetes can be found in the lymphatic system within 30 minutes of inoculation and are found in blood shortly thereafter. There have been occasional instances in man of transfusion syphilis using blood from a donor who was in the incubation stage of his disease. Therefore it seems clear that syphilis is a generalized disease from the onset in man as well. However, the first lesions to appear are at the site of primary inoculation, presumably because of the large numbers of treponemes implanted at this site. In laboratory animals, there is an inverse relationship between numbers of treponemes inoculated and time required for development of the primary cutaneous lesion. The minimum number of treponemes required to establish infection is not known, but may be as low as one treponeme. Multiplication of organisms is very slow, with a division time in rabbits of approximately 33 hours. Similarly slow growth of treponemes in man probably accounts in part for the protracted nature of the illness, and for the relatively long incubation period of 10 to 90 days before appearance of the primary chancre (average time, 21 days).

T. pallidum is not known to produce any toxins. Although the outer membrane structurally resembles those of gram-negative bacteria, there is no biologically active endotoxin in *T. pallidum*. Hyaluronic acid has been seen in experimental lesions, and it has been postulated that the hyaluronic acid slime layer may serve to protect treponemes against host defenses. No true capsule of treponemes is known. Recent evidence shows that treponemes are capable of specific attachment to host cells, but it is not known whether attachment results in damage to host cells. Most treponemes are found in intercellular spaces, but occasional treponemes can be seen within phagocytic cells. However, there is no evidence for intracellular survival of treponemes.

The primary pathologic lesion of syphilis is a focal endarteritis. There is an increase in adventitial cells, endothelial proliferation, and presence of an inflammatory cuff around affected vessels. Lymphocytes, plasma cells, and monocytes predominate in the inflammatory lesion, and in some cases polymorphonuclear cells are seen as well. The vessel lumen is frequently obliterated. With healing there is considerable fibrosis. Treponemes may be seen in most early lesions of syphilis, and in some of the late lesions such as the meningoencephalitis of general paresis.

Granulomatous reaction is also frequently seen in secondary syphilis and in late syphilis. The granuloma is histologically nonspecific, and more than a few cases of syphilis have been incorrectly diagnosed as sarcoidosis or other granulomatous diseases. There is evidence from human inoculation studies that the pathogenesis of the gumma, which is a granulomatous lesion, involves hypersensitivity to small numbers of virulent treponemes introduced into a previously sensitized host.

Intracutaneous inoculation of patients with syphilis in various stages with partially purified antigens of *T. pallidum* showed that delayed cellular hypersensitivity developed only in late secondary syphilis but was uniformly present in latent syphilis. Recent studies have shown that there may be temporary hyporesponsiveness of lymphocytes from patients with primary and secondary syphilis to treponemal antigens; some studies have suggested that this partial inhibition of lymphocyte transformation in primary and secondary syphilis is due to a factor which appears in plasma. It is possible but not yet proved that the explanation for the unusual waxing and waning of lesions in early syphilis depends on the balance between development of effective cellular immunity and suppression of thymus-derived lymphocyte function.

The host also responds to infection with production of numerous antibodies, and in some instances circulating immune complexes may be formed. The nephrotic syndrome has been recognized occasionally in secondary syphilis, and renal biopsies from such cases have shown membranous glomerulonephritis characterized by focal subepithelial basement membrane deposits. The deposits contain both IgG and C3, and treponemal antibody.

Rarely patients may develop paroxysmal cold hemoglobinuria. This is due to production of an IgG antibody which binds to the red cell at 4° C and which, upon rewarming of the blood in the presence of complement, results in hemolysis. Thus patients may develop massive hemolysis and hemoglobinuria after cold exposure. This was formerly usually due to congenital syphilis but is now almost always due to other infections. Treatment with penicillin usually stops the attacks.

Antibodies useful in diagnosis are discussed under Serologic Tests, below.

EPIDEMIOLOGY. Syphilis, with the exception of congenital syphilis, is acquired almost exclusively by intimate contact with the infectious lesions of primary or secondary syphilis (chancre, mucous patches, condylomata lata). This is usually through sexual intercourse, including anogenital and orogenital intercourse. Health workers have sometimes been infected during unsuspecting examination of patients with infectious lesions. Infection by contact with fomites is extremely uncommon.

Syphilis is most common in large cities, and in young sexually active individuals. The highest rate in both men and women occurs at ages 20 to 24, followed by ages 25 to 29 and 15 to 19 years. Among predominantly rural areas in the United States the disease is most prevalent in the southeast.

Syphilis spares no class, race, or group, but is more prevalent in the United States among the poorly educated and economically deprived than among more economically prosperous groups. Studies of patients with repeat venereal disease, who are probably representative of syphilis patients, show increased rates of broken families and mental illness, as well as earlier age of onset of sexual activity and greater promiscuity. Increased numbers of different sexual partners and perhaps indiscriminate choice of partner increase the risk of acquiring sexually transmitted disease. Patients with primary and secondary syphilis name on the average nearly three different sexual contacts within the previous 90 days. A cornerstone of syphilis control is epidemiologic investigation of sexual contacts of patients with primary or secondary lesions, and of patients with early latent disease.

In recent years male homosexuals have apparently accounted for an increasing proportion of the total cases of infectious syphilis. The ratio of male:female cases of primary and secondary syphilis in the United States rose from 1.6:1.0 in 1965 to 2.5:1.0 in 1975. In many large cities over 50 per cent of all infectious syphilis occurs in male homosexuals. In 1975, more than half of all white males with infectious syphilis named at least one male sexual partner during the recent past. In contrast only 2 per cent of primary and secondary syphilis in females occurred in women who named a sexual contact of the same sex. Similar trends have been noted in other countries.

Another important method of case detection is routine serologic testing. Of the approximately 38 million blood specimens examined annually in the United States, approximately 1 million are reactive. Almost 14 per cent of all primary and secondary syphilis is initially detected through tracing of a reactive serology. Approximately 35 per cent of primary and secondary syphilis and 75 per cent of early latent syphilis are detected annually by either serologic screening or contact treating.

The annual incidence of syphilis has generally declined worldwide for approximately 100 years with the exception of periods of extensive war. Reported annual rates of all stages of syphilis were approximately 200 per 100,000 in the 1930's in the United States, and peaked at approximately 430 cases per 100,000 in 1943. Reported cases of infectious primary and secondary syphilis in the United States peaked in 1947 at approximately 73 cases per 100,000 population. With introduction of penicillin there was a rapid decline in primary and secondary syphilis after World War II, to annual rates of approximately 4 cases per 100,000 in 1957. This resulted in declining federal expenditure for syphilis control, however, and there was a subsequent resurgence in infectious primary and secondary syphilis in the United States, reaching peaks of over 12 cases per 100,000 in 1965 and again in 1975. Intensified epidemiologic control efforts have recently resulted in renewed decline in rates of early syphilis. Total reported cases of primary and secondary syphilis in 1976 were 23,731. Over 71,000 cases of syphilis (all types) were reported in the United States in 1976, ranking syphilis third in incidence behind gonorrhea and varicella among reported infectious diseases.

The reported figures are considerably less than the true incidence of the disease. Surveys of private physicians who treat most cases of early syphilis showed that they report less than 20 per cent of cases to public health authorities. It has therefore been estimated that over 80,000 new cases of primary and secondary syphilis occurred in the United States in 1974, and that there may currently be 360,000 untreated cases of syphilis in all stages in the United States.

Reported deaths from syphilis declined from 2434 in 1965 to 200 in 1976. Infant deaths from syphilis and first admissions for syphilitic psychoses have fallen by 98 to 99 per cent since 1940. Less than 800 total cases of congenital syphilis were reported in 1976 in the United States, of which only 170 were among infants less than one year of age. Patients with clinically manifest late syphilis, particularly gummas, are becoming less common, perhaps as a result of the effectiveness of penicillin therapy for early syphilis. However, surveys indicate that there still are significant numbers of patients with untreated cardiovascular and neurologic syphilis, especially among older age groups. There is suggestive evidence that neurosyphilis may be presenting with atypical clinical manifestations, and therefore not easily recognized.

NATURAL COURSE OF UNTREATED SYPHILIS. The incubation period from time of exposure to development of the primary lesion at the place of initial inoculation of treponemes averages approximately 21 days, but ranges from 10 to 90 days. A painless papule develops, and gradually breaks down to form a clean-based ulcer with raised indurated margins. This persists for several weeks (two to six weeks) and then heals spontaneously.

Several weeks after disappearance of the chancre the patient characteristically develops a secondary stage characterized by low grade fever, headache, malaise, generalized lymphadenopathy, and a mucocutaneous rash. There may be involvement of visceral organs. The secondary eruption may occur while the primary chancre is still healing or may occur several months after the disappearance of the chancre. The secondary lesions heal spontaneously within two to six weeks, and the infection then enters latency. Some patients may later develop relapsing lesions similar to those of the secondary stage; rarely the relapse will take the form of recurrence of the primary chancre. About one third of untreated patients eventually develop late destructive tertiary lesions involving one or more of the eyes, central nervous system, heart, or other organs. These may occur at any time from a few years after initial infection to as late as 25 years following infection.

The course of untreated syphilis has been extensively studied in two large groups of patients. In the Oslo Study (1891–1951), over 2000 untreated patients diagnosed clinically (without serologic tests or lumbar punctures) were followed for the ultimate course of the disease. None of these patients received treatment with arsenicals or other compounds. A smaller prospective study was also done in the United States among black Afro-American males in rural Alabama (the Tuskegee Study, 1932–1972). This study, which was initiated in the arsenical era because of uncertainty that the beneficial effects of treatment outweighed the toxicity of prolonged exposure to arsenical compounds, extended into the penicillin era. It has been subjected to much criticism because curative penicillin therapy was not given when it became available in the mid 1940's, although antimicrobial drugs given for other purposes may have influenced the course of the disease in some patients.

In the Oslo Study, relapsing secondary lesions developed in the first four years after infection in nearly 25 per cent of patients. Twenty-eight per cent of patients eventually developed tertiary syphilis. The most common late lesions were benign tertiary gummas of the skin, mucous membranes, and skeleton. Cardiovascular syphilis was diagnosed in slightly over 10 per cent and symptomatic neurosyphilis in 6.5 per cent of patients. Syphilis was the primary cause of death in 50 per cent of males and 8 per cent of females. Pregnancy had a beneficial effect on the disease. Among autopsied patients cardiovascular syphilis was proved in 35 per cent of men and 22 per cent of women. Serious late complications were more common in men than in women.

The Tuskegee Study showed that among men aged 25 to 50 years, death rates were 75 per cent greater in syphilitics than in appropriately matched noninfected control subjects. Cardiovascular or central nervous system syphilis was the primary cause of death in 30 per cent of syphilitic men. Among autopsied patients aortitis was found in about 50 per cent of syphilitics with a persistently positive serologic test. Central nervous system syphilis was found in only 4 per cent. There was no definite anatomic basis for some of the excess mortality among syphilitics noted in the Tuskegee Study. Thus the incidence of cardiovascular syphilis was higher but the incidence of neurological syphilis was lower in the Tuskegee Study than in the Oslo Study. On the basis of these data, plus other uncontrolled clinical observations, it has been suggested that black patients are particularly prone to development of cardio-vascular syphilis, and white patients to central nervous system syphilis, but the evidence is not definitive. The reasons for the possible racial differences are unknown.

CLINICAL MANIFESTATIONS. Primary Syphilis. The typical lesion of primary syphilis is the chancre, a painless, clean-based, indurated ulcer occurring 10 to 90 (average, 21) days after exposure to a sexual contact with infectious primary or secondary lesions. The chancre starts as a papule, but then superficial erosion occurs, resulting in the typical ulcer. The borders of the ulcer are raised, firm, and indurated. Occasionally, secondary infections change the appearance, resulting in a painful lesion. Most chancres are single, but multiple ulcers are sometimes seen, particularly when skin folds are opposed ("kissing chancres"). The untreated chancre heals in several weeks, leaving a faint scar. The chancre is usually associated with regional adenopathy, which may be either unilateral or bilateral. The regional nodes are movable, discrete, and rubbery. If the chancre occurs in the cervix or in the rectum, the affected regional iliac nodes are not palpable.

It was formerly taught that 90 per cent of chancres occurred in the genital region. Presently a much higher proportion of nongenital chancres are observed, particularly among male homosexuals, in whom chancres in or near the rectum are common. Rectal chancres may have an atypical appearance mimicking rectal fissures or other more benign lesions, and are frequently overlooked. Conversely, they have also been mistaken for malignant disease. In general it is reasonable to assume that any ulcer occurring in the genital area or, in male homosexuals, around the rectum is syphilitic until proved otherwise. Chancres may also be seen in the pharynx, on the tongue, around the lips, on the fingers, on the nipples, or in many other diverse areas. The morphology depends in part on the area of the body in which they occur and also on the host immune response. Chancres in previously infected individuals may be small and may remain papular. Chancres of the finger may appear more erosive and may be quite painful.

The *differential diagnosis* of a genital ulcer should include lesions caused by herpesvirus hominis type II. Herpetic ulcers can usually be distinguished because they are multiple, superficial, and, if seen early, vesicular. They are often painful. Herpetic ulcers, unlike syphilitic ulcers, have a positive Tzanck test—multinucleated giant cells in the base of the ulcer. The ulcers of chancroid are usually painful, often multiple, and frequently exudative and nonindurated. Lymphogranuloma venereum may produce a small papular lesion associated with a regional adenopathy. Other conditions which must be distinguished include granuloma inguinale, drug eruptions, carcinoma, superficial fungal infections, traumatic lesions, and lichen planus. Of these, the one most likely to cause difficulty is the ulcer of granuloma inguinale, which is usually redder and more granular in appearance (see Ch. 144). Final distinction in most cases is made on the basis of darkfield examination which is positive only in syphilis.

Secondary Syphilis. Approximately four to eight weeks following the appearance of the primary chancre, patients typically develop lesions of secondary syphilis. They may complain of *malaise, fever, headache, sore throat,* and other systemic symptoms. Most patients have generalized lymphadenopathy, including the epitrochlear nodes. Approximately 30 per cent of patients

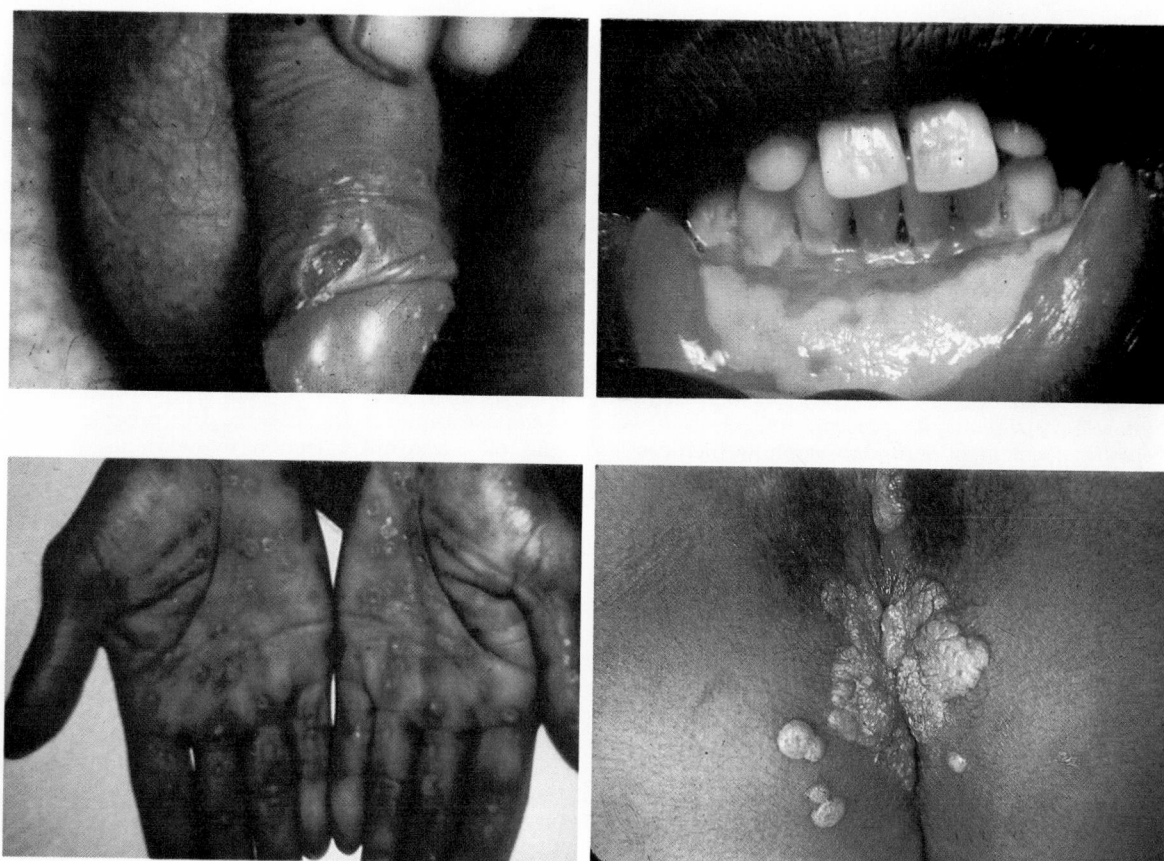

A, Primary syphilis, chancre. *B,* Secondary syphilis, mucous patch. *C,* Secondary syphilis, papulosquamous rash. *D,* Secondary syphilis, condylomata lata.

will have evidence of the healing chancre, although many patients, including male homosexuals and women, give no history of a primary lesion.

At least 80 per cent of patients with secondary syphilis have cutaneous lesions or lesions of the mucocutaneous junctions at some point in their illness. The diagnosis is usually first suspected on the basis of the cutaneous eruption. The rash is often minimally symptomatic, however, and many patients with late syphilis do not recall either primary or secondary lesions. The rashes are quite varied in their appearance, but have certain characteristic features. The lesions are usually widespread and are symmetrical in distribution. They often are pink, coppery, or dusky red, particularly the earliest macular lesions. They usually are nonpruritic, although occasional exceptions have been noted, and are almost never vesicular or bullous in adults. They are indurated except for the very earliest macular lesions and frequently have a superficial scale (papulosquamous lesions). They tend to be polymorphic and rounded, and on healing they may leave residual pigmentation or depigmentation. The lesions may be quite faint and difficult to visualize, particularly on dark-skinned individuals.

The earliest pink macular lesions are frequently seen on the margins of the ribs or the sides of the trunk with later spread to the rest of the body. The face is often spared except around the mouth. Subsequently a papular rash appears which is usually generalized but is *quite marked on the palms and soles.* These frequently are associated with a superficial scale and may be hy-

perpigmented. When the rash occurs on the face, it may be pustular, resembling acne vulgaris. On occasion the scale may be so great as to resemble psoriasis. Ulceration may occur, producing lesions resembling ecthyma. In malnourished or debilitated patients extensive destructive ulcerative lesions with a heaped-up crust may occur, the so-called rupial lesion. Lesions around the hair follicles may result in a patchy alopecia of the beard or of the scalp.

Ringed or annular lesions may occur, especially around the face, particularly on black individuals. Lesions at the angle of the mouth or the corner of the nose may have a central linear erosion (the so-called "split papule").

In warm, moist areas such as the perineum, large pale flat-topped papules may coalesce to form condylomata lata. These may also be seen in the axilla and rarely in a generalized form. They are extremely infectious. They are not to be confused with the common venereal warts (condylomata acuminata), which are small, often multiple, and more sharply raised than condylomata lata.

Other lesions of the mucous membranes are common. The palate and pharynx may be inflamed. Approximately 30 per cent of patients develop the so-called mucous patch. This is a slightly raised oval area covered by a grayish-white membrane, which when raised reveals a pink base that does not bleed. These may be seen on the genitalia, in the mouth, or on the tongue, and, like condylomata lata, are highly infectious.

Other manifestations of secondary syphilis include hepatitis, which has been reported in up to 10 per cent of patients in some series. Jaundice is rare, but an elevated alkaline phosphatase is common. Liver biopsy reveals small areas of focal necrosis and mononuclear infiltrate or periportal vasculitis. Spirochetes can often be visualized with silver stains. Periostitis with widespread lytic lesions of bone has been reported occasionally; use of bone scans appears to be a sensitive test for early syphilitic osteitis. An immune complex type of nephropathy with transient nephrotic syndrome has been rarely documented. There may be iritis or an anterior uveitis. From 10 to 30 per cent of patients have pleocytosis in the cerebrospinal fluid, but symptomatic meningitis is seen in less than 1 per cent of patients. Symptomatic gastritis may be present.

Differential diagnosis of secondary syphilis includes a large number of diseases. The cutaneous eruptions may be mimicked by pityriasis rosea, which can be differentiated by the occurrence of lesions along lines of skin cleavage and frequently by the presence of a herald patch in pityriasis rosea. Drug eruptions, acute febrile exanthems, psoriasis, lichen planus, scabies, and other diseases must also be considered in some cases. The mucous patch may superficially resemble oral candidiasis (thrush). Infectious mononucleosis may appear very similar to secondary syphilis, with sore throat, generalized adenopathy, hepatitis, and a generalized rash. Infectious hepatitis may also cause confusion. A high index of suspicion is required to make the diagnosis of syphilis in some cases. Unfortunately even classic cases with widespread, hyperpigmented, papulosquamous lesions involving the palms and the soles are not infrequently misdiagnosed in the current era. Fortunately, if the serologic tests for syphilis are obtained, they will be found to be positive in 99 per cent of patients. The condylomata lata and mucous patches contain large numbers of treponemes as seen on darkfield examination. Aspiration of lymph nodes may occasionally reveal motile *T. pallidum.* Hardly in any other disease is it of such importance as in suspected syphilis to make a careful and complete examination of the entire skin, mucous membranes, and body systems.

Relapsing Syphilis. Condylomata lata are likely to recur. The skin manifestations tend to be unilateral, the eruptions more dense, marked, with fewer lesions, and sometimes solitary. They are also more infiltrated and of somewhat longer standing, and have some characteristics that resemble the skin lesions in late syphilis. This reflects the increasing immunity with the duration of the early disease. Neurorecurrences, as well as ophthalmic and other relapsing manifestations, may occur. If the patient has been inadequately treated, relapses may be delayed.

Latent Syphilis. By definition latent syphilis is that stage in which there are no clinical signs of syphilis and the cerebrospinal fluid is normal. Latency begins with the passing of the first attack of secondary syphilis and may last for a lifetime thereafter. It is usually detected by positive specific treponemal antibody tests for syphilis. The test must be shown to be reactive on more than one occasion to rule out technical errors. Diseases known to cause occasional false-positive treponemal tests for syphilis, such as systemic lupus erythematosus, must be excluded. In addition, congenital syphilis must be excluded before the diagnosis of latent

syphilis can be made. Patients may or may not have a history of earlier primary or secondary syphilis, although such history is obviously helpful in making a firm diagnosis of latent syphilis.

Latency has been divided into two stages: *early* and *late latency.* Early latency is ordinarily considered infection of less than four years' duration, based upon evidence in the Oslo Study that mucocutaneous relapse could occur at any time during the first four years. However, more recent evidence suggests that most relapses occur in the first year, and epidemiologic evidence shows that most infectious spread of syphilis occurs during the first year of infection. *Therefore early latency in the United States is now defined as the first year after infection.* Late latent syphilis is ordinarily not infectious except for the case of the pregnant woman, who may transmit infection to her fetus after many years. Approximately 30 per cent of untreated patients with latent syphilis eventually develop late (tertiary) complications of syphilis. Since treponemal antibody tests usually remain reactive for life, it is likely that small numbers of treponemes persist throughout latency even if the patient shows no ill effects of the disease.

Late Syphilis. Late or tertiary syphilis is the destructive stage of the disease and can be crippling. It has affected many prominent figures in history, and until the advent of penicillin it was a dread complication of this infection. Late syphilitic complications are still important medical problems, but newly recognized cases of late syphilis have been declining steadily in the United States since World War II.

Late syphilis is usually very slowly progressive, although certain neurologic syndromes may have sudden onset due to endarteritis and thrombosis in the central nervous system. Late syphilis is noninfectious. Any organ of the body may be involved, but three main types of disease may be distinguished: late benign (gummatous), cardiovascular, and neurosyphilis.

LATE BENIGN SYPHILIS. Late benign syphilis or gumma was the most common complication of late syphilis in the Oslo Study. In the penicillin era gummas are quite rare. They typically develop from one to ten years after the initial infection and may involve any part of the body. Although they may be very destructive, they respond very rapidly to treatment and therefore are clinically relatively benign. Histologically the gumma is a granuloma. The histology is nonspecific and may be associated with central necrosis surrounded by epithelioid and fibroblastic cells and occasionally giant cells. There is sometimes vasculitis. *T. pallidum* is ordinarily not demonstrable by silver stains but can sometimes be recovered by inoculation of rabbits.

Clinically gummas may be solitary or multiple. They are usually asymmetrical, and are often grouped. They may start as a superficial nodule or as a deeper lesion which breaks down to form punched-out ulcers. They are ordinarily indolent and slowly progressive with curving or polycyclic borders. They are indurated on palpation. There often is central healing with an atrophic scar surrounded by hyperpigmented borders. Cutaneous gummas may resemble other chronic granulomatous ulcerative lesions caused by tuberculosis, sarcoidosis, leprosy, and other deep fungal infections. Precise histologic diagnosis may not be possible. However, the syphilitic gumma is the only such lesion to heal dramatically with penicillin therapy. Another form of gumma is papulosquamous, and may mimic psoriasis.

Gummas may also involve deep visceral organs, of which the most common are the respiratory tract, the gastrointestinal tract, and bones. In earlier centuries gummas of the nose and palate commonly resulted in septal perforations and disfiguring facial lesions. Gummas may also involve the larynx or the pulmonary parenchyma. Gumma of the stomach may masquerade as carcinoma of the stomach or lymphoma. Gummas of the liver were once the most common form of visceral syphilis, presenting often with hepatosplenomegaly and anemia, occasionally with fever and jaundice. Skeletal gummas typically produce lesions in the long bones, skull, and clavicle. A characteristic symptom is nocturnal pain. Radiologic abnormalities when present include periostitis and either lytic or sclerotic destructive osteitis.

Cardiovascular Syphilis. The primary cardiovascular complications of syphilis are aortic insufficiency and aortic aneurysm, usually of the ascending aorta. Less commonly other large arteries may be involved, and rarely involvement of the coronary ostia results in coronary insufficiency. These complications in all cases are due to obliterative endarteritis of the vasa vasorum with resultant damage to the intima and media of the great vessels. This results in dilatation of the ascending aorta and eventually in stretching of the ring of the aortic valve, producing aortic insufficiency. The valve cusps remain normal. Death may eventually result from congestive heart failure. Recently there has been some success with placing prosthetic heart valves in patients with syphilitic aortic insufficiency. Even in the present era, aneurysms are seen presenting as a pulsating mass bulging through the anterior chest wall. Occasionally syphilitic aortitis may involve the descending aorta, but this is almost always proximal to the renal arteries, unlike atherosclerotic aneurysms, which typically involve the descending aorta below the renal arteries.

The disease usually begins within five to ten years after initial infection but may not become clinically manifest until a total of 20 or 30 years after infection. Cardiovascular syphilis is thought to be more common in men than in women and possibly in blacks than in whites. Conceivably this could represent an effect of mechanical stress on a damaged aorta and the relative frequency of chronic hard physical exertion by various groups. The effects of genetic and nutritional factors on development of this and other complications of late syphilis are unclear. Cardiovascular syphilis does not occur after congenital infection — a phenomenon that remains unexplained.

Asymptomatic aortitis is best diagnosed by visualizing linear calcifications in the wall of the ascending aorta by x-ray. The signs of syphilitic aortic insufficiency are the same as for aortic insufficiency of other causes. Syphilitic aneurysms may be fusiform but are more typically saccular, and do not lead to aortic dissection. Approximately 10 to 25 per cent of patients with cardiovascular syphilis have coexistent neurosyphilis, and it is therefore mandatory to do a lumbar puncture in all patients with cardiovascular syphilis.

At present, syphilis is a relatively more common cause of aortic insufficiency among the elderly than among younger patients; this is due to the progressively decreasing incidence of new cases of late cardiovascular syphilis.

Neurosyphilis. Neurosyphilis may be divided into four groups: asymptomatic, meningovascular, tabes dorsalis, and general paresis. Division is not absolute and there may be considerable overlap between syndromes. There is limited evidence that currently occurring cases of neurosyphilis are more likely than heretofore to be variants of the classic syndromes, possibly as a result of use of antimicrobials for other diseases.

Asymptomatic Neurosyphilis. Asymptomatic neurosyphilis is diagnosed when there is a positive VDRL* in the cerebrospinal fluid (CSF) in the absence of signs and symptoms of neurologic disease. False-positive VDRL tests do not occur in CSF in the absence of a traumatic tap. The CSF usually shows an increased total protein and a lymphocytic pleocytosis, but some of these findings may be absent. If the CSF is normal two or more years after the initial infection, the patient is not likely to develop a positive CSF later. Although up to 30 per cent of patients with untreated secondary syphilis have an abnormal CSF, studies show that penicillin therapy prevents progression to late symptomatic neurosyphilis. Because of this, routine lumbar punctures for examination of CSF are not indicated in early syphilis. Unfortunately, it has become common practice to avoid lumbar punctures in later stages of syphilis as well, electing instead of treat with doses of penicillin which are thought to be effective for neurosyphilis, if present. As a result, there are few data on the present frequency and course of asymptomatic neurosyphilis.

Many laboratories perform an FTA-ABS* test on spinal fluid. Admittedly, there are published reports of positive FTA-ABS tests in the CSF of patients with otherwise normal spinal fluid, in whom there were clinical signs and symptoms compatible with neurosyphilis. However, the CSF FTA-ABS test has not been standardized, and there is some evidence that positive CSF FTA-ABS tests are the result of passive transfer of serum antibody into spinal fluid. At present no diagnosis of asymptomatic (or symptomatic) neurosyphilis should be based on the CSF FTA-ABS* test.

Meningovascular Syphilis. An acute to subacute aseptic meningitis may occur at any time after the primary stage but usually within the first year of infection. It frequently involves the base of the brain and may result in unilateral or bilateral cranial nerve palsies. In about 10 per cent of cases, the onset of meningitis coincides with the rash of secondary syphilis. The spinal fluid shows a lymphocytic pleocytosis with increased protein and usually normal glucose concentration. The CSF VDRL is nearly always positive. Rarely CSF glucose concentration is decreased. This syndrome can mimic tuberculous or fungal meningitis or nonpurulent meningitis of various causes.

In other patients, the meningeal involvement may be less prominent but there is sufficient endarteritis and perivascular inflammation to result in cerebrovascular thrombosis and infarction, with signs and symptoms typical of those of cerebrovascular accidents of any cause. This usually occurs five to ten years after the initial infection and is more common in males. There often is an associated aseptic meningitis as well. Most cerebrovascular accidents are not due to syphilitic ar-

---

*See Serologic Tests, below. Also refer to Table 1.

teritis even in patients with a positive serologic test for syphilis. However, syphilis should be considered as the cause in young patients with a history of syphilis and without other causes for cerebrovascular accidents.

A variety of other meningeal syndromes may rarely be seen, including transverse myelitis and radiculitis. A rare syndrome of meningomyelitis may involve the lateral regions of the cord, resulting in anterior horn damage and paralysis of one or more extremities.

Tabes Dorsalis. Tabes dorsalis is a slowly progressive degenerative disease involving the posterior columns and posterior roots of the spinal cord, resulting in progressive loss of peripheral reflexes, impairment of vibration and position sense, and progressive ataxia. There may be chronic destructive changes in the large joints of the affected limbs in far advanced cases (Charcot's joints). Incontinence of the bladder and impotence are common. Sudden and severe painful crises of uncertain cause are a characteristic part of the syndrome. These may involve the larynx, vagina, rectum, or other organs. Not infrequently severe sharp abdominal pains lead to exploratory surgery. Lightning pains in the extremities are severe and may require opiates for relief. These may be triggered by exposure to cold or other stresses, or may arise with no obvious precipitating cause.

The eyes are frequently involved as well. Optic atrophy is seen in 20 per cent of cases. The pupils are abnormal in 90 per cent of cases, with bilaterally small pupils which fail to constrict further in response to light but which do constrict normally to accommodation (Argyll Robertson pupils).

The cause of tabes dorsalis is unclear. Spirochetes cannot be demonstrated in the posterior column or dorsal roots.

Onset of the disease is usually delayed, often not being seen until 20 to 30 years after initial onset of infection. It is thought to be more common in whites and in males. Typical cases presenting with lightning pains, ataxia, Argyll Robertson pupils, absent deep tendon reflexes, and loss of posterior column function are easy to diagnose. Atypical cases may be more troublesome, particularly because the VDRL test in the serum is normal in as many as 30 to 40 per cent of cases, and 10 to 20 per cent of cases (even before the advent of penicillin) have normal CSF as well. The FTA-ABS test in serum is nearly always positive.

Treatment is unsatisfactory. Penicillin does not reverse the symptoms, although it does usually result in clearing of the abnormal spinal fluid. Carbamazepine in doses of 400 to 800 mg per day has been reported to be effective in treatment of the lightning pains.

Tabes dorsalis is now thought generally to be quite uncommon, although a recent survey of newly diagnosed late syphilis in Denmark in the decade 1961 to 1970 showed that in approximately 10 per cent of all persons with late syphilis and 40 per cent of all with clinical neurosyphilis there was evidence of tabes dorsalis.

General Paresis. This form of neurosyphilis is a chronic meningoencephalitis resulting in gradually progressive loss of cortical function. It typically occurs 10 to 20 years after the initial infection. Pathologically there is a perivascular and meningeal chronic inflammatory reaction with thickening of the meninges, a granular ependymitis, degeneration of the cortical parenchyma, and abundant spirochetes in the tissues.

The most devastating effect of general paresis is on the mind. This was formerly a common cause of insanity and was one of the first diseases for which a definite cause of insanity was found. With effective penicillin therapy this disease has become much less common; in the United States, first admissions to mental hospitals because of syphilitic psychosis have declined from 7694 in 1940 to 154 in 1968, the last year for which definite figures are available.

Symptomatically in its early stages general paresis results in nonspecific symptoms such as irritability, fatigability, headaches, forgetfulness, and personality changes. Later there is impaired memory, defective judgment, lack of insight, confusion, and often depression or marked elation. The patients may be delusional, and seizures are sometimes seen. There may also be loss of other cortical functions, including paralysis or aphasia.

Physical signs of the illness are primarily those of the altered mental status. Cranial nerve palsies are uncommon. Optic atrophy is rare. The complete Argyll Robertson pupil is also uncommon, but irregular or otherwise abnormal pupils are not infrequent. Peripheral reflexes are often somewhat increased.

The cerebrospinal fluid is nearly always abnormal with lymphocytic pleocytosis and increased total protein. The VDRL is nearly always reactive in both spinal fluid and serum. The disease responds well to penicillin therapy if administered early, although as many as a third of treated patients may develop progressive neurologic decline in later years. Fever therapy induced with malaria was formerly an effective adjunct to treatment with arsenicals, but has now been abandoned.

Classic general paresis is now infrequently seen in the United States, but there is increasing evidence that variant forms of paresis may be occurring in significant numbers. Nearly 4 per cent of a recent series of over 200 elderly patients with dementia or psychiatric illness, most of whom were not hospitalized, had evidence of inadequately treated or untreated syphilis. Some investigators believe that small doses of antimicrobial drugs given for other reasons may be modifying the expression of late neurologic syphilis. Further investigation is needed before clear conclusions can be drawn, but it remains reasonable to suspect syphilis as the cause of undiagnosed neurologic illness. Since the VDRL may be negative in patients with late neurologic syphilis, the FTA-ABS test on serum must be performed before syphilis can be excluded.

Congenital Syphilis. Congenital syphilis results from transplacental hematogenous spread of syphilis from the mother to the fetus. The incidence of congenital syphilis among newborns or infants under one year of age in the United States rose from 180 cases in 1957 to 422 cases in 1972, but has since declined to less than 200 cases annually. Each case of congenital syphilis represents a tragedy which possibly could have been prevented by better case reporting and by proper prenatal care. A VDRL should be obtained in all expectant mothers at the beginning and near the end of pregnancy.

It has generally been held that maternal syphilis cannot be transmitted to the fetus until the sixteenth to eighteenth week of pregnancy. However, recent data show that spirochetes can be found in abortuses of as little as nine to ten weeks' gestation. The risk of fetal infection is greatest in the early stages of untreated maternal syphilis and declines slowly thereafter, but the mother may infect her fetus during at least the first five years of her infection. Adequate treatment of the mother prior to the sixteenth week will usually prevent manifest clinical illness in the neonate. Later treatment may not prevent late sequelae of the disease in the child. Untreated maternal infection may result in stillbirth, neonatal death, prematurity, or syndromes of early or late congenital syphilis among surviving infants.

Manifestations of early congenital syphilis are often seen in the perinatal period, but may not develop until the infant has been discharged from the hospital. The disease resembles secondary syphilis of the adult except that the rash may be vesicular or bullous, which is extremely rare in adults. There often is rhinitis, hepatosplenomegaly, hemolytic anemia, jaundice, and pseudoparalysis (immobility of one or more extremities) due to painful osteochondritis. There may be thrombocytopenia and leukocytosis. The early stages of congenital syphilis must be differentiated from rubella, cytomegalovirus infection, toxoplasmosis, bacterial sepsis, and other diseases.

Late congenital syphilis is defined as congenital syphilis of more than two years' duration. The disease may remain latent with no manifest late damage. Cardiovascular alterations have not been observed in congenital syphilis. Neurologic manifestations are common, and there may be eighth nerve deafness and interstitial keratitis. The latter occurs in over 10 per cent of patients but may not be manifest until the tenth year of life or later. Periostitis may result in prominent frontal bones, depression of the bridge of the nose ("saddle nose"), poor development of the maxilla, and anterior bowing of the tibias ("saber shins"). There may be late onset arthritis of the knees (Clutton's joints). The permanent dentition may show characteristic abnormalities known as Hutchinson's teeth; the upper central incisors are widely spaced, centrally notched, and tapered in the manner of a screwdriver. The molars may show multiple poorly developed cusps (mulberry molars). Some of the late manifestations such as interstitial keratitis and Clutton's joints may be due to hypersensitivity responses, and are benefited by corticosteroids in some cases.

DIAGNOSIS. Darkfield Examination. The most definitive means of making a diagnosis is finding spirochetes of typical morphology and motility in lesions of early acquired or congenital syphilis. The darkfield examination is almost always positive in primary syphilis and in the moist mucosal lesions of secondary and congenital syphilis. It may occasionally be positive in aspirates of lymph nodes in secondary syphilis. Problems arise, however, because of false-negative examinations in primary syphilis owing to application by the patient of soaps or other toxic compounds to the lesions. A single negative examination is therefore insufficient to exclude syphilis. Patients with suspicious lesions but with an initially negative darkfield examination should be instructed to avoid washing the lesion and to return daily for two successive examinations. Confusion may also arise because of presence of spirochetes which are morphologically indistinguishable from *T. pallidum* in the mouth, particularly around the gingival margins. For lesions in these areas therefore diagnosis often depends upon clinical appearance, history, and serologic testing.

To perform the darkfield examination, the surface of the suspected ulcerative lesion should be cleaned with saline and gauze without production of bleeding. Presence of red cells in the specimen makes it difficult to visualize small numbers of *T. pallidum*. Squeezing of the lesion (with gloves on!) may help produce serous fluid, which is picked up on a glass slide, covered with a coverslip, and examined with the darkfield microscope. Living *T. pallida* demonstrate gradual motion to and fro, rotational movement around the long axis, and rather sudden 90 degree bending near the center of the organism. Since most physicians do not have the proper equipment and are not familiar with the techniques of darkfield microscopy, the state public health authorities can be called for assistance. A mail-in darkfield test, in which lesion fluid is drawn up in a capillary tube, sealed, and mailed to a state laboratory for fluorescent antibody identification of treponemes, is under investigation but not readily available.

T. pallidum may also be demonstrated in biopsies or pathologic specimens by fluorescent antibody stains or by silver stains.

Serologic Tests. Two basic types of humoral antibody are stimulated by infection with *T. pallidum*: nonspecific antibody directed against diphosphatidyl glycerol (cardiolipin), which is a normal component of many tissues; and specific treponemal antibodies. Nonspecific antibodies against cardiolipin were formerly designated "reagin," a term which should be discarded to avoid confusion with another "reagin," IgE. The kinds of tests used in syphilis are summarized in Table 1.

NONSPECIFIC TESTS. Anticardiolipin antibodies were first discovered by Wassermann in 1907, using extracts of congenitally syphilitic livers as the antigen for a complement fixation test. Subsequently it was shown that normal livers contained the same antigen as do many other tissues; the antigen for this class of test is now extracted from beef heart. As yet there is no convincing explanation for why patients infected with *T. pallidum* develop increasing titers of antibody against a normal tissue component.

The Wassermann test has now been replaced by related tests. The standard test in use today for detection of anticardiolipin antibody is the Venereal Disease Research Laboratories (VDRL) test, which is an easily quantitated slide flocculation test. Many similar tests,

TABLE 1. Serologic Tests for Syphilis

Type	Use
Nonspecific (anticardiolipin) antibodies:	
VDRL (slide flocculation)	Screening, quantitation, following response to treatment
RPR (agglutination)	Screening
Kolmer (complement fixation)	Limited
Specific treponemal antibodies:	
FTA-ABS (immunofluorescence with absorbed serum)	Confirmatory, diagnostic, not for routine screening
MHA-TP (microhemagglutination)	Similar to FTA-ABS but can be quantitated and automated
TPI (immobilization)	Most specific but not generally available

VDRL = Venereal Disease Research Laboratories test.
RPR = Rapid plasma reagin test.
FTA-ABS = Fluorescent treponemal antibody absorption test.
TPI = *Treponema pallidum* immobilization test.
MHA-TP = Microhemagglutination assay for *T. pallidum*.

including the rapid plasma reagin (RPR) test and the unheated serum reagin (USR) test, are frequently used for screening for syphilis.

The VDRL and related tests are simple, well standardized, cheap, and easy to perform and are the screening tests of choice. The VDRL is the test of choice for following response of patients to treatment. Since the VDRL detects antibody against a normal tissue component, it may be falsely positive in a significant number of patients. The relative proportion of patients with a false-positive VDRL depends on the prevalence of syphilis in the community; the lower the prevalence of syphilis, the higher the proportion of positive VDRL tests which are due to nonsyphilitic causes.

The VDRL test begins to turn positive a week or two after the onset of the chancre. In large series of patients with primary syphilis, approximately two thirds have had a positive VDRL test. Obviously then a negative VDRL test does not exclude primary syphilis, particularly if the lesion is less than two weeks old. The VDRL is positive in 99 per cent of patients with secondary syphilis, the only exceptions being patients with such high titers of antibody that they are in antibody excess; dilution of the serum will then paradoxically result in conversion of a negative test to positive. VDRL reactivity tends to diminish in later stages of the disease, and only about 70 per cent of patients with cardiovascular or neurosyphilis have a positive VDRL test.

The *quantitative titer* of the VDRL test is somewhat useful in diagnosis and quite useful in following therapeutic response. The titer is reported as the highest dilution which gives a positive response. Most patients with secondary syphilis have titers of at least 1:16. Most patients with false-positive VDRL tests have titers of less than 1:8. No single titer is in itself diagnostic. Significant rises (fourfold or greater) in paired sera, however, are strongly indicative of acute syphilis.

TREPONEMAL TESTS. There are many varieties of specific treponemal antibody tests. The first and still perhaps best test is the *Treponema pallidum* immobilization (TPI) test, which when properly performed is nearly completely specific for infection by *T. pallidum* or related pathogenic spirochetes. Unfortunately it is cumbersome and expensive and therefore is not routinely done in the United States at present. The most widely used treponemal antibody test is the fluorescent treponemal antibody absorption (FTA-ABS) test. Patient serum is absorbed with extracts of nonpathogenic cultivable treponemes to remove cross-reacting group treponemal antibody. The absorbed serum is reacted with dried *T. pallidum* on a glass slide, and specific antitreponemal antibodies are detected by subsequent addition of fluorescein-labeled anti-human gamma globulin. Other treponemal tests are based on agglutination of red cells to which *T. pallidum* antigens have been fixed. The most commonly used hemagglutination test is the microhemagglutination assay for *T. pallidum* (MHA-TP).

The precise nature of the antigens involved in these tests is not known. Characterization of the antigens of *T. pallidum* has been greatly hindered by inability to grow the organism in cell-free culture. Antibodies reactive in the various tests are found in all major immunoglobulin classes (IgG, IgM, IgA). A modification of the FTA-ABS test has been developed using fluorescein-labeled anti-human IgM (IgM FTA-ABS). The IgM FTA-ABS test is of some use in diagnosis of early congenital syphilis but is of no use in distinguishing acute disease from old infections in adults.

The FTA-ABS test is best used as a confirmatory test. It is somewhat more difficult to perform than the VDRL test and cannot be easily quantitated. It is sensitive and has a high degree of specificity, being positive in only approximately 1 per cent of normal individuals. It is positive in 85 per cent of patients with primary syphilis, 99 per cent with secondary syphilis, and in at least 95 per cent with late syphilis. It may therefore be the only test positive in patients with cardiovascular or neurologic syphilis. In late syphilis the FTA-ABS test usually remains positive for life despite adequate therapy. It (as well as the TPI and MHA-TP) is positive in other treponemal diseases such as pinta, yaws, and bejel.

The FTA-ABS test is reported in terms of relative brilliance of fluorescence, from borderline to 4+. Borderline reactivity has the same meaning as nonreactive for clinical purposes. Most laboratories report 1+ positive tests as reactive, but some studies have shown that such tests may be relatively difficult to reproduce. Occasional laboratories therefore only report as positive tests with 2+ or greater reactivity. In patients lacking historical or clinical evidence of syphilis but with a reactive FTA-ABS test, one should repeat the FTA-ABS test. Use of another treponemal test such as the MHA-TP may be helpful in certain problem cases.

The MHA-TP test is less sensitive than either the VDRL or the FTA-ABS test in primary syphilis. Its sensitivity and specificity otherwise are nearly identical to those of the FTA-ABS test, being positive in nearly all patients with secondary syphilis and in 95 per cent or more of patients with late syphilis. An automated version of the MHA-TP test is now being developed for widespread use. The reactivity of serologic tests for syphilis in various stages of disease is shown in Table 2.

False-Positive Serologic Tests for Syphilis. The VDRL or RPR test may be positive in a variety of diseases other than syphilis. A false-positive test is defined as a reproducible positive test in a patient with no clinical or historical evidence of syphilis, and whose serum FTA-ABS or MHA-TP test is negative.

"Acute" (less than six months) false-positive VDRL tests occur with low frequency in atypical pneumonia, malaria, and other bacterial or viral infections, and may occur after smallpox or other vaccinations as well. *Chronic false-positive VDRL tests* (lasting longer than six months) are relatively common in autoimmune disorders such as systemic lupus erythematosus, in narcotic addicts, in leprosy, and in aged persons. From 8 to 20 per cent of patients with systemic lupus erythematosus have been reported as having false-positive VDRL test, and the false-positive test may develop many years prior to the onset of other manifestations of the disease. A chronic false-positive VDRL test in females age

TABLE 2. Frequency of Positive Serologic Tests in Untreated Syphilis

Stage	VDRL (%)	FTA-ABS (%)	MHA-TP (%)
Primary	70	85	50-60
Secondary	99	100	100
Latent or late	70	98	98

TABLE 3. Penicillin Treatment Practice in Syphilis as Recommended by
United States Public Health Service (1976)

Indications for Syphilis Therapy†	Dosage and Administration*		
	Benzathine Penicillin G	Aqueous Benzyl Penicillin G or Procaine Penicillin G	Procaine Penicillin G in Aluminum Stearate Suspension (PAM)
Primary, secondary, and early latent syphilis (<1 year); epidemiologic treatment	Total of 2.4 million units; single IM dose of two injections of 1.2 million units in one session	Total of 4.8 million units IM in doses of 600,000 units daily for eight consecutive days	Total of 4.8 million units IM; first dose 2.4 million units and 1.2 million units at each of two subsequent injections three days apart (over nine days)
Late latent (>1 year) or when cerebrospinal fluid was not examined in "latency"; asymptomatic neurosyphilis, symptomatic neurosyphilis, cardiovascular syphilis, late benign (cutaneous, osseous, visceral gumma)	Total of 7.2 million units IM in doses of 2.4 million units at seven-day intervals, over 21 days	Total of 9 million units IM in doses of 600,000 units daily over 15 days; in selected cases of symptomatic CNS syphilis, 2 to 4 million units of aqueous (crystalline) penicillin G intravenously every four hours for at least ten days	No recommendation by USPHS; total dose of 9 million units over 15 to 21 days is effective
Congenital Early			
Up to two years of age	If CSF is normal: Total of 50,000 units per kilogram IM in a single or divided dose at one session	If CSF is abnormal: Total of 50,000 units per kilogram IM per day for ten consecutive days‡	No recommendation by USPHS
Late			
Two to 12 years, weight 32 kg (71 lb) or less	Same as for early congenital syphilis	Same as for early congenital syphilis	Same as for early congenital syphilis
Over 12 years, or over 32 kg	Same as for adult late latent syphilis	Same as for adult late latent syphilis	Same as for adult late latent syphilis

*Individual doses can be divided for injection in each buttock to minimize discomfort.
†In *pregnancy*, treatment is dependent on the stage of syphilis.
‡For aqueous penicillin, give in two divided doses per day; for procaine penicillin, give as one daily dose.

20 or younger carries a significant risk of future development of systemic lupus erythematosus, thyroiditis, or other autoimmune disorders, and such patients should be followed carefully for a considerable period of time. As many as one third of patients with narcotic addiction have a false-positive VDRL test. Over 1 per cent of patients aged 70 and 10 per cent of patients over age 80 have a low titer false-positive VDRL test. Most false-positive VDRL tests have a titer of 1:8 or less, although occasional patients with lymphoma and other diseases have been described with very high titer false-positive VDRL tests.

A positive FTA-ABS test is usually indicative of recent or past syphilis. However, there is an increased incidence of false-positive FTA-ABS tests in systemic lupus erythematosus and in other chronic diseases associated with hyperglobulinemia, including rheumatoid arthritis, biliary cirrhosis, and others. False-positive tests are of two kinds in systemic lupus erythematosus: the most common is one with a beaded pattern of fluorescence, which has been shown to be due to anti-DNA antibodies; there also may be homogeneous fluorescence of the treponeme indistinguishable from a true positive test in syphilis. Patients with systemic lupus who have a false-positive FTA-ABS test almost always have a negative VDRL test (and conversely, patients with SLE with a positive VDRL usually have a negative FTA-ABS).

Occasionally one encounters reproducible positive FTA-ABS tests in patients with no clinical or historical evidence of syphilis, and in whom there is no evidence of diseases associated with false-positive FTA-ABS tests. It may be wise to obtain cerebrospinal fluid for examination of total protein, cells, and VDRL reactivity in order to rule out neurosyphilis. If in doubt and if the patient is not allergic to penicillin, it is often wisest to treat such patients for possible syphilis.

IgM FTA-ABS Test for Congenital Syphilis. Mothers with a positive VDRL or FTA-ABS test will deliver infants with a positive VDRL and FTA-ABS test because of passive transfer of the IgG antibodies reactive in these tests. Since many infants with congenital syphilis are clinically normal at birth but develop serious symptomatic disease some weeks later, it is important to determine whether a newborn with a positive VDRL or FTA-ABS test has passively transferred maternal antibody or is actively infected. Since maternal IgM antibodies are not passively transferred to the fetus, an IgM FTA-ABS test has been developed to test for syphilis in the newborn. Unfortunately there is approximately a 35 per cent incidence of false-negative IgM FTA-ABS tests in delayed-onset congenital syphilis. There also is a false-positive rate of approximately 10 per cent. For these reasons the IgM FTA-ABS test is of limited use in diagnosis of neonatal syphilis.

If the mother has been adequately treated for syphilis during pregnancy and the infant is clinically normal at birth, one may elect to follow the infant carefully by serial examination and VDRL titers. If the positive VDRL in the infant is due to passively transferred maternal antibody, the titer of reactivity will fall markedly in the first two months of life. A rising titer indicates active disease and the need for treatment. Many physicians are unwilling to risk failure of proper follow-up of VDRL-positive but clinically normal neonates, and instead administer effective therapy immediately. The risk of penicillin allergy in neonates is very low.

TREATMENT. There have been many therapies for syphilis in the past, including mercurial, arsenical, and bismuth compounds, as well as induced fever. All of these have been replaced by penicillin because it is more effective, simple, and safe.

T. pallidum is highly susceptible to penicillin, being inhibited by less than 0.01 μg of penicillin G. Since treponemes divide slowly, and since penicillin acts only on dividing cells, it is necessary to maintain serum levels of penicillin for many days. Studies in animals and in man show that more therapy is required as the length of infection increases. Current recommendations for treatment of syphilis are summarized in Table 3.

Early (Less Than One Year) Infectious Syphilis. Early syphilis may be treated with a single injection of 2.4 million units of *benzathine penicillin G*, which provides low but effective serum levels for over two weeks. Extensive studies in the 1940's and 1950's with regimens which provided similar serum levels and duration of therapy showed that approximately 95 per cent of patients were cured by such treatment. Many of the remaining 5 per cent who had clinical or serologic evidence of relapse may actually have been reinfected. It is not necessary to examine the cerebrospinal fluid at this stage, because penicillin prevents development of later neurosyphilis. Motile treponemes disappear from primary lesions in 24 hours.

A single injection of 2.4 million units of *aqueous procaine penicillin,* which provides relatively high serum levels for a brief period, is ineffective in established early syphilis, but is curative if the disease is still in the incubating stage (e.g., in a patient who is being treated for gonorrhea and who happened to acquire syphilis simultaneously). Other regimens currently useful for gonorrhea have uncertain effects on incubating syphilis, and careful follow-up for syphilis is indicated in gonorrhea patients treated with regimens other than procaine penicillin. The incidence of incubating syphilis in gonorrhea patients is 2 per cent or more in several series.

For patients allergic to penicillin, tetracycline hydrochloride may be given in a total dose of 30 grams over 15 days, or erythromycin base may be given in a total dose of 30 grams over 15 days. Particularly careful follow-up is necessary in patients treated with drugs other than penicillin, because patients may not be fully compliant with these prolonged courses of oral therapy and these regimens have been less fully evaluated clinically. Cephaloridine or other cephalosporins may be effective but have not been well studied. Chloramphenicol is of equivocal efficacy and for this reason, as well as because of the risk of toxicity, should not be used. Spectinomycin has essentially no effect on syphilis.

Syphilis of More Than One Year's Duration. Larger doses of penicillin are needed for *neurosyphilis* (see Ch. 301) than for syphilis of less than one year's duration. In general, patients with general paresis respond better to treatment than do patients with tabes dorsalis, although patients with paresis should be expected to show residual effects of the infection. This is particularly true in advanced cases. Meningovascular syphilis usually responds well, except for residual damage to cranial nerves or cortical function resulting from ischemic infarcts. Published studies show that a total of 6.0 to 9.0 million units of penicillin G results in a satisfactory clinical response in approximately 90 per cent of patients with neurosyphilis.

Currently used benzathine penicillin regimens have received relatively little study in neurosyphilis. Benzathine penicillin G in a total dose of 7.2 million units given as 2.4 million units weekly for three successive weeks is effective in most patients. However, there are reports of patients who have failed standard penicillin therapy for neurosyphilis but who responded to intensive intravenous therapy which provided high serum levels of penicillin. Benzathine penicillin does not provide measurable levels of penicillin in the spinal fluid or aqueous humor of the eye. *Therefore in cases of symptomatic central nervous system syphilis, which is a serious disease, there is considerable rationale to treatment with* *aqueous penicillin G, 600,000 units daily for 15 days, or for intensive intravenous therapy with penicillin G (20 million units per day for at least 10 days in hospital).* Therapy of neurosyphilis not infrequently results in increased CSF pleocytosis for seven to ten days after starting treatment, and may transiently convert a normal CSF to abnormal.

Limited evidence suggests that treating *latent syphilis* with 7.2 million units total dose of benzathine penicillin is curative even if the patient has asymptomatic neurosyphilis. However, because of the possible lack of the efficacy of benzathine penicillin in some patients with central nervous system syphilis, it is desirable to examine cerebrospinal fluid in all patients with latent syphilis to exclude asymptomatic neurosyphilis. Alternatively, one may reasonably elect to perform a lumbar puncture at the conclusion of the follow-up period (two years); if the CSF is normal, the patient can be reassured that neurosyphilis will not develop.

There is no evidence that therapy with antimicrobial drugs is clinically beneficial to patients with *cardiovascular syphilis.* Nevertheless, treatment of cardiovascular syphilis is recommended in order to prevent further progression of disease and because approximately 15 per cent of patients with cardiovascular syphilis have associated neurosyphilis.

There is no evidence as to the efficacy of other antimicrobials in treatment of late syphilis. Therefore if patients are allergic to penicillin, it is mandatory that the cerebrospinal fluid be examined before therapy is undertaken. Either tetracycline, 2 grams daily for 30 days, or erythromycin, 2 grams daily for 30 days, is probably effective.

Syphilis in Pregnancy. All pregnant women should be examined with a VDRL or RPR test during pregnancy; if they are at high risk for syphilis, a second test should be obtained before delivery. Because of the risk of infection to the fetus, evaluation and treatment of the VDRL-positive patient should be done as rapidly as possible, particularly for patients first seen in the later stages of pregnancy. If a confirmatory FTA-ABS test is positive and the patient has not been treated, penicillin (or erythromycin for patients who are allergic to penicillin) should be administered in doses appropriate for early or late syphilis as outlined above. For patients who are VDRL positive but FTA-ABS negative and who have no clinical signs of syphilis, treatment may be withheld. In such patients a quantitative VDRL test and another FTA-ABS test should be repeated in four weeks. If the VDRL titer has risen by fourfold or more, or if clinical signs of syphilis have developed, the patient should be treated. If after repeat examination the diagnosis remains equivocal, the patient should be treated to prevent possible disease in the neonate. After treatment a quantitative VDRL titer should be followed monthly; if it rises fourfold, the patient should be treated a second time.

Congenital Syphilis. Proper treatment of the mother usually prevents active congenital syphilis in the neonate. However, infected infants may be clinically normal at birth, and the infant may be seronegative if the mother's infection was acquired late in pregnancy. The infant should be treated at birth if the mother had received no or inadequate treatment, or had been treated with drugs other than penicillin, or if the infant cannot be carefully followed up for several months after birth. Cerebrospinal fluid should be examined before treatment of the infant. If the cerebrospinal fluid is normal, treatment may be with a single injection of 50,000 units per kilogram of benzathine penicillin G. If the fluid is abnormal, treatment should be with aqueous penicillin G, 50,000 units per kilogram intramuscularly or intravenously daily, given in two divided doses, for a minimum of ten days. Alternatively, a single daily intramuscular injection of procaine penicillin G, 50,000 units per kilogram, may be given for ten days. These recommendations are based upon the failure of benzathine penicillin to provide adequate treponemicidal levels in spinal fluid, and on evidence that aqueous or procaine penicillin does provide adequate cerebrospinal fluid levels of penicillin.

Tetracycline should not be used to treat children of less than eight years of age. Antimicrobial agents other than penicillin are not recommended for treatment of congenital syphilis.

Follow-up Examinations. All patients with early syphilis or congenital syphilis should return for quantitative VDRL titers and clinical examination 3, 6, and 12 months after treatment. Patients with late latent syphilis should be examined also at 24 months after therapy; if cerebrospinal fluid was not examined prior to therapy, a lumbar puncture should be done prior to discharge to rule out inadequately treated asymptomatic neurosyphilis.

The quantitative VDRL titer should return to normal within 12 months after therapy of primary syphilis or 24 months after therapy of secondary syphilis. In a small percentage of patients with early syphilis, the VDRL will remain reactive in low titer for long periods of time. Chronic low titer VDRL reactivity after therapy is much more common in late syphilis and should not be viewed with alarm. A progressively rising VDRL titer after therapy (a fourfold or greater rise) is sufficient evidence for retreatment. Patients with treated early syphilis are fully susceptible to reinfection, and many clinical and serologic relapses after therapy are probably reinfections. As such they represent failures of proper epidemiologic case finding and preventive therapy of the patient's sexual contacts.

Patients with neurosyphilis should be followed with serologic tests for at least three years and with repeat examination of cerebrospinal fluid at six-month intervals. The cerebrospinal fluid pleocytosis is the first abnormality to disappear, but cell counts may not be normal for one to two years. The elevated cerebrospinal fluid protein falls more slowly, followed by the positive cerebrospinal fluid VDRL test, which may take years to become negative. Rising cerebrospinal fluid cell counts, protein, and VDRL titer obtained at follow-up are an indication for retreatment.

Epidemiologic Investigation and Treatment. All patients with syphilis should be reported to public health authorities. In the absence of an effective vaccine, control of syphilis depends on finding and treating persons with infectious lesions of primary and secondary syphilis before they can further transmit the disease, and on finding and treating persons with incubating syphilis before they have developed infectious lesions. All patients with early syphilis (less than one year) should be carefully interviewed by qualified persons to determine the nature of their recent sex contacts. Approximately 16 per cent of the named recent contacts of patients with early syphilis will be found to have active untreated syphilis on examination, and a similar proportion of

individuals named as suspects or associates will also have active syphilis. Approximately 20 per cent of cases of early syphilis seen in the United States at present are found by epidemiologic investigation of index cases with syphilis.

Most authorities, particularly in the United States, recommend treatment of sexual contacts of patients with early syphilis even if the contacts are clinically and serologically normal on examination. This is justifiable, because 30 per cent of clinically normal individuals named as contacts of persons with infectious lesions of syphilis within the previous 30 days will go on to develop syphilis if untreated. In general, preventive treatment is given to all sexual contacts of the past 90 days, although nearly all cases of syphilis in contacts will have developed within 60 days of exposure.

Jarisch-Herxheimer Reaction. Up to 60 per cent of patients with early syphilis, and a significant proportion of patients with later stages of syphilis, experience a transient febrile reaction after therapy for syphilis. This usually occurs in the first few hours after therapy, peaks at six to eight hours, and disappears within 12 to 24 hours of therapy. Temperature elevation is usually low grade, and there is often associated myalgia, headache, and malaise. The skin lesions of secondary syphilis are often exacerbated during the Herxheimer reaction, and cutaneous lesions which were not visible may become visible. It is usually of no clinical significance and may be treated with salicylates in most cases. In patients with syphilis of the coronary ostia or of the optic nerve, there is a theoretical risk that local inflammation coincident with the Herxheimer reaction could precipitate serious damage. This is the subject of much discussion in the old literature, but there is little current evidence that "local Herxheimer reactions" constitute a significant risk to the patient. Corticosteroids have been used to prevent adverse effects of the Herxheimer reaction, but there is no evidence that they are clinically beneficial (other than reducing fever) or necessary. Institution of treatment with small doses of penicillin does not prevent the Herxheimer reaction.

The pathogenesis of the Herxheimer reaction is unclear. It may be due to liberation of antigens from the spirochetes. There is evidence of activation of the complement cascade, including transient consumption of C3, C4, C6, and C7, and of transient decrease in treponemal antibodies coincident with the Herxheimer reaction. There is also evidence for endotoxemia, obtained by positive limulus amebocyte gelation tests, at the time of the Herxheimer reaction, although T. pallidum does not contain biologically active endotoxin. These seemingly contradictory observations could be explained if the reaction resulted in release of endogenous endotoxin from the gut.

Persistence of Treponemes After Treatment. Studies in man and in rabbits have shown that spiral forms may be visualized by silver stains in lymph nodes after effective treatment. Living virulent treponemes have occasionally been recovered by rabbit inoculation from lymph nodes, cerebrospinal fluid, or ocular fluids after effective treatment has been given. These documented cases of treponemal persistence are very rare, however. There are many other reports of spiral forms in various body tissues and fluids which stain with fluorescent treponemal antibodies; the significance of these is difficult to assess, as infectivity tests in rabbits were not performed in the majority of these reports. At present there is little reason to worry about persistence of virulent treponemes after therapy with penicillin, with the possible exception of central nervous system syphilis, which needs further evaluation. There is no evidence for selection of penicillin-resistant mutants of *T. pallidum* to date.

PROSPECTS FOR PREVENTION. Solid immunity develops in rabbits following prolonged infection with virulent *T. pallidum*. It has not yet been possible to passively transfer immunity in laboratory animals by either immune serum or immune lymphocytes alone, suggesting that both cellular and humoral systems are necessary for immunity. Rabbits have been effectively immunized with multiple injections of treponemes which have been rendered avirulent by irradiation or by exposure to cold. However, a very large number of injections and a large mass of treponemes are necessary to effect immunity in the laboratory animal. For this reason and since *T. pallidum* cannot yet be grown in a virulent state in cell-free medium, there is no immediate prospect for a vaccine. However, significant immunity does develop in man after prolonged infection, and it should be possible to develop an effective vaccine after successful cultivation of *T. pallidum* has been accomplished. There is reason for optimism that this may happen in the foreseeable future. For the present, control depends entirely on clinical awareness on the part of physicians, adequate reporting to public health authorities, and vigorous application of epidemiologic investigation and preventive treatment of sexual contacts.

There is a real need for better health education, starting in the schools. It is not unreasonable to educate about sexually transmitted disease as early as the sixth grade. The public needs to be reminded that condoms will help to prevent disease, and that soap and water may possibly avert an infection if used immediately after exposure. Many contraceptive foams are treponemicidal. Patients can be educated to report to a physician upon the earliest signs of disease. It is difficult to alter patterns of sexual behavior, but proper education and case reporting will help control the incidence of syphilis. Each physician bears a portion of the over-all responsibility for this task.

Bryceson, A. D. M.: Clinical pathology of the Jarisch-Herxheimer reaction. J. Infect. Dis., 133:696, 1976.

Drusin, L. M., Singer, C., Valenti, A. J., and Armstrong, D.: Infectious syphilis mimicking neoplastic disease. Arch. Intern. Med., 137:156, 1977.

Fehér, J., Somogyi, T., Timmer, M., and Józsa, L.: Early syphilitic hepatitis. Lancet, 2:896, 1975.

Fischer, A., Kristensen, J. K., and Husfelt, V.: Tertiary syphilis in Denmark 1961–1970. A description of 105 cases not previously diagnosed or specifically treated. Acta Dermatovener., 56:485, 1976.

Fulford, K. W. M., Johnson, N., Loveday, C., Storey, J., and Tedder, R. S.: Changes in anti-vascular complement and anti-treponemal antibody titres preceding the Jarisch-Herxheimer reaction in secondary syphilis. J. Clin. Exp. Immunol., 24:483, 1976.

Gamble, C. N., and Reardan, J. B.: Immunopathogenesis of syphilitic glomerulonephritis: Elution of antitreponemal antibody from glomerular immune-complex deposits. N. Engl. J. Med., 292:449, 1975.

Gjestland, T.: The Oslo study of untreated syphilis: An epidemiologic investigation of the natural course of the syphilitic infection based upon a re-study of the Boeck-Bruusgaard material. Acta Derm. Venereol., 35: Suppl. 34, 1955.

Kaufman, R. E., Olansky, D. C., and Wiesner, P. J.: The FTA-ABS (IgM) test for neonatal congenital syphilis: A critical review. J. Am. Vener. Dis. Assoc., 1:79, 1974.

Magnuson, H. J., Thomas, E. W., Olansky, S., Kaplan, B. I., De Mello, L., and Cutler, J. C.: Inoculation syphilis in human volunteers. Medicine, 35:33, 1956.

Musher, D. M., Schell, R. F., Jones, R. H., and Jones, A. M.: Lympho-

cyte transformation in syphilis: An in vitro correlate or immune suppression in vivo? Infect. Immun., 11:1261, 1975.

Prewitt, T. A.: Syphilitic aortic insufficiency. JAMA, 211:637, 1970.

Raskind, M. A., and Eisdorfer, C.: Screening for syphilis in an aged psychiatrically impaired population. West. J. Med., 125:361, 1976.

Schroeter, A. L., Turner, R. H., Lucas, J. B., and Brown, W. J.: Therapy for incubating syphilis: Effectiveness of gonorrhea treatment. JAMA, 218:711, 1971.

Sparling, P. F.: Diagnosis and treatment of syphilis. N. Engl. J. Med., 284:642, 1971.

Syphilotherapy 1976: Position papers for the current USPHS recommendations. J. Am. Vener. Dis. Assoc., 3:98, 1976.

Tramont, E. C.: Persistence of *Treponema pallidum* following penicillin G therapy: Report of two cases. JAMA, 236:2206, 1976.

Turner, T. B.: Syphilis and the treponematoses. *In* Mudd, S. (ed.): Infectious Agents and Host Reactions. Philadelphia, W. B. Saunders Company, 1970.

Wilner, E., and Brody, J. A.: Prognosis of general paresis after treatment. Lancet, 2:1370, 1968.

172. NONSYPHILITIC TREPONEMATOSES

Thorstein Guthe

172.1. YAWS

(Frambesia Tropica, Pian, Bouba, Parangi, Patek)

DEFINITION. Yaws is produced by a spirochetal microorganism, *T. pertenue*, which causes a chronic human infection, most often with onset in childhood. An initial cutaneous lesion usually appears, followed by relapsing infectious secondary nondestructive lesions of the skin, periosteum, and bones, frequently interspersed with symptom-free periods. Late manifestations include destructive and deforming lesions of skin, bones, and joints. Hyperkeratosis, notably of the soles, may develop in secondary and late yaws. There is no evidence of cardiac or nervous system involvement or of prenatal manifestations. Infected persons slowly develop relative immunity, and humoral antibodies can be detected by serologic tests reactive also in other treponematoses (syphilis, pinta).

HISTORY. Yaws probably existed in Africa from remote times. Early accounts suggest that it was brought to the West Indies with the slave trade in the sixteenth century. By the eighteenth century it had become a serious health problem of the Antilles, Central America, and South America, as well as in areas of Oceania and Southeast Asia. Savages (1778) proposed the name frambesia for the disease because of the raspberry-like appearance of its papillomatous secondary lesions. Moseley (1800) observed its clinical course, notably that yaws ends in enlarged nodes and destructive lesions. Maxwell (1839) determined its incubation period to be three to four weeks after inoculation of lesion material to humans. Castellani (1905) identified *T. pertenue* as the causative microorganism of yaws. Lambert (1923) first attempted community-wide treatment with arsenicals in the Pacific Isles. The advent of long-acting penicillin preparations and single injection therapy revolutionized case treatment and made possible important reduction of yaws by mass penicillin campaigns (World Health Organization, 1950–1970) in the tropics.

The author wishes to acknowledge the valuable advice of his colleagues Drs. J. Ridet and G. Causse, Medical Officers, Communicable Diseases Division, World Health Organization, Geneva, concerning this chapter.

ETIOLOGY. The causative agent, *T. pertenue,* is a helical cell 8 to 12 μ in length and about 0.2 μ in diameter, with several closely set spirals. It resembles *T. pallidum* (syphilis) and *T. carateum* (pinta) morphologically in dark-field illumination and structurally in electron microphotographs. *T. pertenue* has not been grown in vitro, but will survive in special media for several days without multiplication. Strains stored in glycerin remain virulent for many years at −70° C (CO_2 ice) or lower temperatures, e.g., liquid nitrogen or helium. *T. pertenue* is pathogenic for the same animal species as *T. pallidum.* The latter causes subclinical "silent" infection in the hamster, whereas *T. pertenue* causes a specific dermatitis — a procedure sometimes used to differentiate between treponemes in the laboratory (Vaisman, 1969). Pathogenic treponemes closely resembling or identical with *T. pertenue* have been isolated from wild cynomolgous African monkeys (Fribourg-Blanc et al.; Sepetjian et al., 1968).

EPIDEMIOLOGY AND PATHOGENESIS. Despite mass penicillin campaigns in recent years, yaws has remained a disease of many rural communities in the intertropical zone in Africa, the Americas, Southeast Asia, and Oceania. Areas of high prevalence of active yaws sometimes lie within a few miles of communities where the disease is rarely observed, depending on the ecologic situation, the evolutionary stage of endemicity, and the number of susceptibles at any given time. There is also a higher frequency of early yaws lesion in the rainy than in the dry season (Harding, 1947). Moreover, skin lesions are less frequent in cooler climates in mountainous tropical communities where they also become less moist and where papillomas tend to erupt in sweaty, mucocutaneous junctions and skin folds rather than involving the flat body surfaces (Ramsey, 1925). Furthermore, the occasional yaws lesions encountered after mass penicillin campaigns appear to be less extensive and less moist. In areas where no further lesions are encountered after such campaigns, continued specific seroreactivity (TPI) in a small proportion of children born after the campaigns could suggest the possibility of asymptomatic infection taking place in the new circumstances.

T. pertenue is incapable of penetrating unbroken skin. It is also unable to pass the placenta and cause congenital yaws. Transmission usually occurs through contact of skin abrasions, cuts, or lesions, e.g., trauma, injury, dermatoses, with infectious yaws lesions of another person. Indirect transmission via contaminated hands is believed to occur among children. Nursing mothers are sometimes infected directly by their infants. In addition to early infectious lesions, untreated latent yaws cases — which are liable to relapse with active lesions — form an important part of the reservoir maintaining the disease in rural communities. Humidity, moisture-holding soil, and mean annual temperatures of 27° C or more are also necessary for the spread of yaws. Moreover, transmission is favored by scant clothing, bare feet, crowded dwellings, and deficient personal hygiene. The gradual improvement of environmental and socioeconomic conditions will reduce the attack rate of yaws (Saxena and Prasad, 1963).

No true vector has been found in which *T. pertenue* actually multiplies, but it has been shown that disease can be transmitted by experimentally infected gnats. In some areas *Hippelates pallipes* may serve as mechanical carriers (Kumm and Turner, 1936). Geographic coexistence of foci of human yaws and natural treponematoses of wild cynomolgous monkeys has been observed in Africa (Baylet et al., 1970).

The age distribution of yaws depends on the rate of transmission and level of endemicity. In hyperendemic communities, e.g., the former Netherlands New Guinea (Kranendonk), the highest incidence of infectious lesions was in the two- to five-year-olds, with a seroprevalence of more than 90 per cent, pointing to an early almost complete epidemic "saturation" of the community with yaws. In areas of moderate or low endemicity the highest seroprevalence is in older age groups. For example, this has been observed among the pygmies in the Cameroons and in Zaire, where FTA/ABS seroreactivity was found to be 45 to 50 per cent in those more than 30 years of age (Pampligione and Wilkinson). After mass penicillin campaigns in areas of high endemicity, maximal seroprevalence was in the 45- to 59-year-olds, e.g., Nigeria, signaling regression of a hyperendemic situation many years ago. In the latter instance many more young individuals are susceptible to yaws in the new generation, but there are also more barriers to impede renewed spread of the infection, e.g., education, health consciousness, chemotherapy, and health services. On the other hand, the greater number of serologically nonreactive young people in the new generation have, when reaching puberty, less protective cross-immunity to infection with venereal syphilis. This, in turn, has been reported to be among the reasons for the increased incidence of syphilis noted in tropical countries in the last decade.

PATHOLOGY. A main pathologic feature of yaws is the involvement of the skin. In early lesions the epidermis is thickened. There is cell infiltration ("plasmocytoma") of the dermis, hyperplasia, edema, and the presence of many treponemes. The papillae are elongated, often with thickening of the interpapillary pegs. Proliferation of vascular endothelium and obstruction of vessels are less characteristic of yaws than of syphilis. The epithelium may show hyperkeratosis, become superficially eroded, and be covered by dried exudate. The acanthotic epidermis and the papillary proliferation give rise to a fungating, frambesiform, crust-covered lesion. Diffuse periostitis and cortical rarefaction of the long bones are common in early yaws and are more marked than in venereal syphilis. The late lesions of yaws are due to a different tissue response, and endarteritis is observed histopathologically. Late lesions include ulcerating granulomatous nodules and gumma of the skin and bones. The gumma is built of elements similar to syphilitic lesions. Late skeletal affliction is mostly characterized by periosteal proliferation, rarefaction, or destruction of multiple areas of the long bones which can lead to extensive deformities.

CLINICAL CHARACTERISTICS. At the site of entry of *T. pertenue* an initial lesion usually develops after an incubation period of three to four weeks. The implantation is facilitated by previous breaks in the skin (abrasion, injury, vaccination). The lesion is a papule situated on the legs in more than half the cases. In babies and toddlers it often appears on the buttocks or in the perineum. The papule grows into a round, broad-based granulomatous lesion ("mother yaw") covered by a serous crust from which *T. pertenue* can be recovered. The regional lymph nodes are frequently enlarged, not

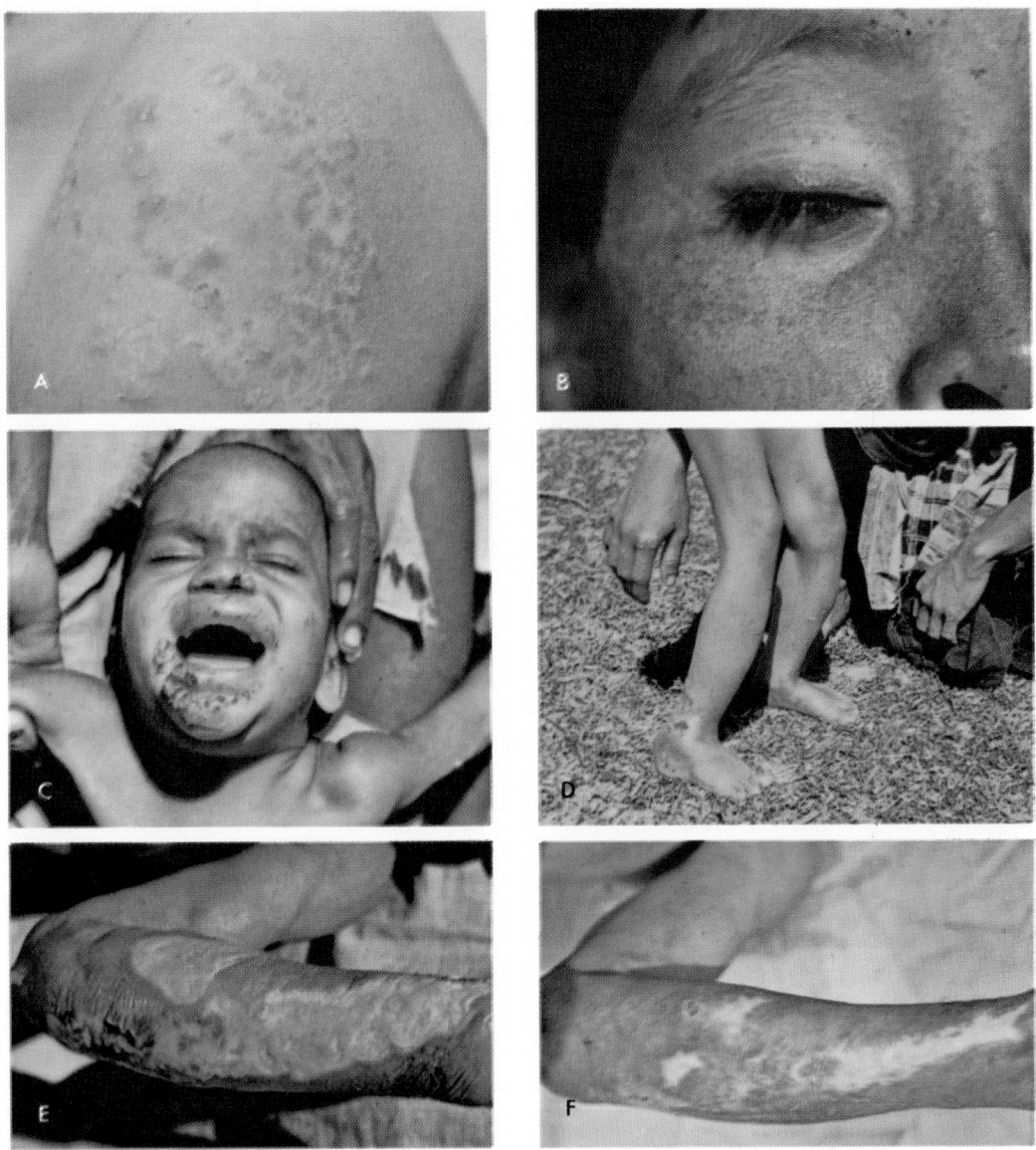

A, Initial lesions in early pinta. *B*, Late pigmented blue variety pinta. *C*, Early papillomatous yaws. *D*, Osteoperiostitis of yaws. *E*, Deep ulcerated late yaws of arm before therapy with long-acting penicillin. *F*, Same patient after treatment.

"shotty," and do not suppurate. An initial lesion will heal spontaneously within three to six months; ulcerating initial lesions require more time to heal.

As a result of early treponemia a generalized secondary eruption appears before or after the healing of the initial lesion. The most frequent and characteristic eruptions are roundish, raised, rough, granulomatous papules ("yaws" or frambesides), often covered by a brownish crust. These lesions appear anywhere on the skin, but rarely on the scalp. They sometimes show arciform arrangements. Secondary lesions may last for more than six months. A new crop may appear before the preceding lesions heal. Relapsing crops tend increasingly to become localized, e.g., to periaxillary, perianal, or circumoral areas. Sometimes the papilloma may be solitary. Plantar papules appear late, often after the generalized eruption, and are modified by a thick keratotic layer characteristic of barefoot people: a cherry-like granuloma appears in a well of cracked horny layer, frequently giving rise to painful disability ("crab yaws"). On the body, micropapular as well as various forms of macular or desquamative macular ("pian dartre") lesions may also appear. Lesions of mucous membranes are rare, but occur. Desquamatous macules can develop in the palms and notably on the soles, which are sometimes covered by a thick hyperkeratotic layer. In addition to skin eruptions in early yaws, there is superficial lymph node enlargement. In many cases there are pain and tenderness of the tibial shaft and other long bones owing to early periostitis. Such periostitis sometimes leads to saber tibia and polydactylitis. In many cases the general health of the patient appears little affected; in others there are systemic manifestations, with irregular fever, loss of appetite, and weight loss.

The secondary lesions begin to regress after several months, but relapses may occur on and off for four to five years before true latency is reached. The latter can be interrupted by late lesions of several types. (1) *Superficial ulcerations* of the skin with central healing tendency are observed, and *cutaneous and subcutaneous nodules* with ulceration and marginal healing may leave markedly dyspigmented atrophic scars, sometimes with deforming contractures. (2) *Diffuse or more localized hyperkeratosis* of the soles — less frequently of the palms — with fissuring and pitting can result in a characteristic mottled pattern, occasionally complicated by ulceration and sometimes developing more than 15 years after the infection. (3) *Osteal or periosteal gummatous lesions* of the tibia and other long bones may penetrate subcutaneous and cutaneous tissues, resulting in chronic ulcerations. These may also affect tarsal and carpal bones, the scapula, the sternum, and the skull. Affliction of palatonasal structures may lead to gangosa (rhinopharyngitis mutilans), a spectacular condition similar to that in syphilis. The osteitis and periostitis can occur both in association with generalized skin lesions and after these have receded.

Other yaws lesions are less common and include painless subcutaneous fibromatous juxta-articular nodes, paranasal egg-shaped swelling of the superior maxillary bone (goundou), chronic late macular or hyperkeratotic lesions of palmar surfaces, and volar aspects of wrists and insteps of soles, frequently followed by depigmentation.

DIAGNOSIS. Typical early yaws lesions are generally not confused clinically with other conditions. Ulcerated initial leg lesions may sometimes be mistaken for other ulcerations, e.g., tropical ulcer. Also, spirochetes found in tropical ulcers resembling *Borrelia vincentii* may be mistaken for *T. pertenue*. Facial yaws papules may look like crusted impetigo. Individual lesions may resemble those of secondary syphilis or cutaneous leishmaniasis. Demonstration of treponemes by microscopic darkfield examination of exudate from the lesion and seroreactivity in reagin and treponemal antibody tests (VDRL, FTA-ABS, TPI, TPHA) serve to distinguish yaws from other conditions except those of the treponematosis group. Differential tests using *T. pertenue* as antigen have not given uneqivocal findings (Garner et al.). Reagin tests become positive in serum about a month after the initial lesion (Li and Soebekti, 1955), and TPI titers can be very high (1:2560) in early yaws (WHO, Eastern Nigeria, 1968). Ulcerating contractures and mutilating lesions may present differential diagnostic problems in relation notably to leprosy and tuberculosis. Hyperkeratosis of the soles is often confused with other plantar conditions, mainly keratoma plantare sulcatum, plantar pitting, and tropical hyperkeratotic conditions of unknown origin (Hackett and Lowenthal).

PROGNOSIS. In infected persons the prognosis is favorable when early treatment is provided. Otherwise, periodic infectious recurrences over many years give rise to months of incapacity. An undetermined number of infected persons develop late lesions. Others go on to spontaneous clinical cure; some also become serologically nonreactive ("burnt-out yaws"). Among those developing late chronic lesions, extensive invalidism, deformities, and functional impairment often result.

TREATMENT AND CONTROL. The aim of treatment of individual patients is cure of the early disease and prevention of late manifestations. Intramuscular injection of 1.2 million units of benzathine penicillin (DBED) or 2.4 million units of PAM (procaine penicillin G in oil and 2 per cent monosterate)* in adults and half doses for children suffices to cause disappearance of early lesions and prevent relapses. The response is dramatic. The early lesions usually become darkfield-negative within 48 hours, and healing takes place within one to two weeks. Serologic titers decline, but many retain low-titer reagin seroreactivity, depending on the duration of the infection (D'Mello and Krag, 1955). Penicillin sometimes causes a Herxheimer reaction. The usual safeguards against hypersensitivity reactions to penicillin should be taken (see Ch. 43). Persons with late yaws lesions may require repeated therapy. Oxytetracycline and chloretetracycline are reported to be useful in cases of deforming osteoperiostitis, indolent gummas, or ulcerations. A minimum of two grams daily for five to ten days in adults and proportionately less for children are given. Ulcerations of late yaws may also require application of local antiseptic dressings. Deformities caused by chronic osteitis and contractures may necessitate local surgery in addition to drug therapy.

In the efforts to achieve community-wide control of yaws, the previous work of the Jamaica Yaws Commission (1936) was in recent years extended under the auspices of the World Health Organization. Since 1950, more than 210 million people in 49 countries were examined, and some 53 million treated with long-acting penicillin in large-scale control programs. The aim was

---

*Not available in United States of America.

(1) to survey entire area populations so as to control the reservoir of infection; (2) to interrupt the spread of yaws through mass treatment, rendering early cases noncontagious, preventing infectious recurrences, and aborting incubating disease; and (3) to undertake post-campaign yaws surveillance by periodic resurveys to detect and promply treat overlooked cases or new infections that might arise. Untreated early cases free of clinical symptoms between outbreaks form an important part of the reservoir of infection and contribute to maintain the disease in rural communities. Accordingly, mass treatment criteria in these campaigns were based on a certain association in the population between the occurrence of clinically active lesions and of seroprevalence owing both to such lesions and to clinically symptom-free infections (Hackett and Guthe). The criteria for mass treatment are as follows: (1) When the prevalence of active yaws cases is 10 per cent or higher (hyperendemic areas), more than 50 per cent of the population is seroreactive, and all members of the community are to be treated. (2) When there are 5 to 10 per cent of active cases (mesoendemic area), all children and their obvious contacts are treated, because most contagious cases occur in the lower age groups. (3) Where there are less than 5 per cent active cases (hypoendemic areas), solely case and contact treatment is provided. This wide use of penicillin results in rapid regression of active lesions. The prevalence thus declined within a few years from more than 20 per cent to less than 1 per cent after mass campaigns in many areas. Examples of reduction in *infectious* yaws are: in N. Nigeria from 4.2 (1954) to 0.1 per cent (1964); in W. Samoa 3 per cent (1955) to nil (1965).

Indifference must be anticipated in rural populations toward long-term surveillance after mass campaigns that resulted in "disappearance" of community-wide diseases. In the case of yaws, seroepidemiologic studies have shown continued low-level transmission with tendency to focal outbreaks ten to fifteen years after mass campaigns (Guthe). Using cardiolipin serology, 40 per cent of children in areas of Indonesia remained seroreactive four to eight years after treatment, and 13 per cent of the seroreactive children still had high seroreactivity titers. A potential for clinical relapses therefore remains. It is really not possible to drive a community disease out of existence by the use of a drug alone even if the population coverage in mass campaigns is nearly complete. Broader measures are needed, notably development of basic health services, into the functions of which the continued surveillance of communicable diseases can be integrated following mass campaigns, e.g., against yaws. (World Health Organization, 1970).

PROPHYLAXIS. Prevention of yaws depends on avoidance of minor injuries to the skin, and of shielding of open wounds and abrasions from contamination by insects. Open infectious lesions should be protected. Health eduation should aim at improvement of personal hygiene (soap) and community hygiene (water). Children with infectious lesions should be treated and excluded from school until noninfectious. Mass therapy represents an important control measure. No method of artificial immunization is available.

Fluker, J. L., and Hewitt, A. B.: Late yaws. Br. J. Vener. Dis., 46:264, 1970.
Garner, M. F., Backhouse, J. L., Daskalopoulos, G., and Walsh, J. L.: Use of *T. pertenue* in the fluorescent and immobilization tests. In-

vestigation of sera from yaws areas found reactive only in the TPHA test. Br. J. Vener. Dis., 50:264, 1974.
Guthe, T.: Clinical serological and epidemiological features of framboesia tropica (yaws) and its control in rural communities. Acta Dermatovener. (Stockholm) 49:343, 1969.
Hackett, C. J., and Guthe, T.: Some important aspects of yaws eradication. Bull. WHO, 15:869, 1956.
Hackett, C. J., and Lowenthal, L. J. A.: Differential Diagnosis of Yaws. WHO Org. Monograph Series No. 45, Geneva, 1960.
Kantor, I., et al.: Test patterns of yaws antibodies in New Zealand. Arch. Dermatol., 103:226, 1971.
Pampiglione, S., and Wilkinson, A. E.: A study of yaws among pygmies in Cameroon and Zaire, Br. J. Vener. Dis., 51:165, 1975.
Turner, L. H.: Notes on the Treponematoses with an Illustrated Account of Yaws. Kuala Lumpur, Government Press (Institute for Medical Research, Federation of Malaya, Bulletin No. 9), 1959.
Turner, T. B., and Śaunders, G. M.: Yaws in Jamaica: 1. An epidemiological study of two rural communities. Am. J. Hyg., 21:483, 1935.
World Health Organization: Bibliography on yaws 1905–1962. Geneva, 1963.
World Health Organization: Scientific Group of Treponematoses Research. WHO Techn. Rep. Ser., No. 455, 1970.

172.2.   BEJEL

(Endemic Syphilis, Nonvenereal Childhood Syphilis, Belesh, Dichuchwa, Njovera, Skerljevo)

DEFINITION. Bejel is a chronic, inflammatory childhood disease of the treponematosis group. The early disease is characterized by infectious mucocutaneous lesions and osseous manifestations resembling those of secondary syphilis. After disappearance of early lesions and an undetermined latency period, late manifestations may develop. There are skin and bone lesions similar to those of late "benign" venereal syphilis. If they occur at all, cardiovascular, nervous system, and prenatally acquired manifestations are extremely rare.

ETIOLOGY. The bejel treponeme is morphologically indistinguishable from *T. pallidum*, *T. pertenue*, and *T. carateum*. It is present in early lesions or lymph node aspirate. The organism has not been cultivated in vitro. In laboratory animals Turner and Hollander showed consistent differences in cinical reaction as compared with that of yaws and venereal syphilis treponemes. The bejel treponeme is apparently an intermediate between the two (Paris-Hamelin et al., 1968). Like other treponematoses, bejel is accompanied by antibody formation with seroreactivity in reagin, e.g., VDRL, and treponemal antibody (TPI-FTA) tests. Childhood infections with bejel protects against later infection with syphilis.

EPIDEMIOLOGY. Humans are the reservoir of bejel. Treponemes are most likely transmitted directly among children by skin-to-skin contact, or by hands moistened with treponeme-containing saliva, or indirectly via drinking flasks, the spouts of which have been demonstrated to contain treponemes (Grin). Treponeme implantation is generally facilitated by labial and oral fissures, occurring in dry climates, or by small mucosal lesions. Bejel is a household disease. In some instances 60 to 70 per cent of rural community populations have been reported to be infected. Narrow huts, crowded dwellings, unhygienic living conditions, and low socioeconomic standards favor transmission.

There are many scattered endemic centers of bejel in backward rural areas north and south of the tropics.

Bejel occurs along the Kalahari and Sahara deserts in Africa, in the countries of the Balkans and the Eastern Mediterranean region, on the Arabian peninsula, in central Asian countries, and in Australia. It prevails in arid areas in contrast to yaws, which is encountered in moist, tropical jungle regions. Bejel was first described as a disease of nomadic people, subsequently to occur in settled rural populations, e.g., among the Dogons of Mali, the Islamic descendants of Bosnia, and the Bakwenas of Botswana. Previously it was widespread in the Middle East and Europe. Bejel has not been observed in the Western Hemisphere, where pinta and yaws are the prevailing childhood treponematoses. Bejel is in regression from its higher prevalence of two to three decades ago as a result of extensive mass penicillin campaigns and some improvement of health services. In certain areas the prevalence of bejel has remained higher than that of yaws because of occurrence in nomadic tribes, on account of geographic inaccessibility of endemic foci, and inadequacy of health services (Basset, 1963). It is likely to recur when mass treatment has been incomplete. Thus in Niger infectious lesions (5 per cent) and seroreactivity (30 to 40 per cent) were found some years after a mass treatment campaign.

CLINICAL MANIFESTATIONS AND DIAGNOSIS. The experimental incubation period is approximately three weeks. Initial lesions are rarely encountered. The earliest lesions are mucous patches of the secondary type localized to the oral and faucial mucosa. "Split papules" occur at the oral angles. Local papular condylomata lata or anal, genital, or other intertriginous skin areas were observed in 25 per cent of infected children in Iraq (Guthe and Luger). Generalized secondary rashes and alopecia are relatively rare. Regional lymphadenopathy is common. Polyadenitis is rare. The early disease is followed by a latency period of undetermined duration, with seroreactivity as the sole sign of infection. Late "benign" manifestations of the skin develop in some patients. They do not differ in character from those in late venereal syphilis. Superficial tuberoulcerative skin lesions and characteristic serpiginous nodular ulcers occur. Nasopharyngeal ulcerations may occur and range from palate perforation to rhinopharyngitis mutilans as in yaws and syphilis (gangosa). Gummatous ulceration of the breast may occur in women previously infected with bejel who are suckling a child with oral lesions, a phenomenon which supports the concept that gummas may be delayed hypersensitivity reactions from repeated exposure (see Ch. 171). Juxta-articular nodes have been described in some geographic areas.

Bone lesions are the most frequent manifestations of late bejel, affecting the clavicle, the frontal bones, the tibias, and other long bones (Goldstein et al.), giving rise to swelling, tenderness, and pain. There is periosteal and endosteal proliferation, and deformities may result. Isolated cases of cardiovascular and neurologic system involvement have been described in Bosnia (Grin) and Botswana (Murray et al.). Incidental cases of prenatally acquired disease have also been reported. No case of prenatal or systemic disease was observed in several thousand examinations in a WHO project in Syria which included radiologic and cerebrospinal fluid examinations. When observed, the systemic manifestations may be due to the occurrence also of venereal syphilis in the geographic area concerned.

DIAGNOSIS. The diagnosis of early bejel is established on epidemiologic and clinical grounds. It may be confirmed by darkfield demonstration of treponemes in the lesions or in node aspirate and by serologic tests (VDRL), reactive in nearly 100 per cent of cases. Serodiagnostic tests cannot differentiate latent bejel from latent yaws or syphilis. Because late clinical lesions are similar to those of yaws and syphilis, the local epidemiologic situation is an important diagnostic consideration. As distinct from the manifestations of late prenatal syphilis, dental deformities and interstitial keratitis are not observed in bejel.

TREATMENT AND PREVENTION. Penicillin is as effective against bejel as it is against yaws, syphilis, and pinta. In the control campaigns initiated by the World Health Organization in several countries, one dose of 1.2 million units of long-acting penicillin PAM* or benzathine penicillin G (DBED) was given intramuscularly in early cases, with two further doses at three- to seven-day intervals to patients with late manifestations. Half doses are used for contacts. The longer acting benzathine penicillin is preferred in contact treatment among nomadic tribes. Rapid healing of early lesions was followed by seroreversal in a large proportion of cases. Late destructive lesions required more time. Healing with scars progressed slowly but definitely and with some reduction in reaginemia, but with little or no effect on treponemal antibody tests (TPI-FTA), as in venereal syphilis.

Seroepidemiologic studies undertaken in Bosnia, Yugoslavia, 20 years after the penicillin mass campaign — which was followed by systematic periodic surveillance over ten years — showed that childhood infection had been reduced to nil, the community seroimmunologic profiles indicating complete interruption of transmission. During this period adequate basic health services were provided, health education promoted, and general socioeconomic development took place. Bosnia remains the only example of eradication of endemic treponematoses. However, eradication of childhood infection has resulted in a population susceptible to venereal syphilis in later life. The absence of protective cross-immunity has thus created a new epidemiologic situation in which sporadic cases of the sexually transmitted treponematosis occurs.

Goldstein, M. S., Arensburg, C., and Natan, H.: Pathology of Bedouin skeletal remains from two sites in Israel. Am. J. Phys. Anthropol., 45:891, 1975.

Grin, E. I., and Guthe, T.: Evaluation of previous mass campaigns against endemic syphilis in Bosnia and Herzegovina. Br. J. Vener. Dis., 49:1, 1973.

Guthe, T., and Luger, A.: Epidemiological aspects of non-venereal "endemic" syphilis. Dermatologica, 115:248, 1957.

Hudson, E. H.: Non-venereal Syphilis. Edinburgh and London, E. & S. Livingstone, Ltd., 1958.

Turner, T. B.: Syphilis and the treponematoses. In Mudd, S. (ed.): Infectious Agents and Host Reactions. Philadelphia, W. B. Saunders Company, 1969.

Turner, T. B., and Hollander, D. H.: Biology of the Treponematoses. WHO Monograph series no. 35, Geneva, 1957.

*Not available in United States of America.

172.3. PINTA

(Mal del Pinto, Carate)

DEFINITION. Pinta is a skin infection with a chronic course. It is caused by *Treponema carateum*, giving rise to an initial lesion and a generalized secondary rash, both containing treponemes. Late skin manifestations comprise extensive dyschromic (treponeme-containing) and achromic (treponeme-free) conspicuous splotches. Antibodies are produced, detectable by serologic tests reactive also in syphilis and yaws. Organ systems are not involved, physical health is not impaired, and prenatal disease is not known.

HISTORY. Manifestations of pinta were described by Muciño (1798) and by Berecochea and Corona (1811). Frequent seroreactivity (Wassermann complement fixation test) in pinta patients led Menck (1926) to imply association with syphilis and made Herrejon (1927) assume a treponeme to be the causative microorganism. Armenteros and Triana (1938) identified *T. carateum* in Cuban pinta. Leon Blanco (1939) obtained early generalized eruptions by self-inoculation of darkfield-controlled material from lesions. In therapy Corona (1811) showed the usefulness of mercury, Maria Graz (1913) of arsenobenzoles, and Varela (1944) of penicillin.

ETIOLOGY. The etiologic agent, *T. carateum*, is a slender helical cell, 8 to 35 μ long and 0.2 to 0.3 μ wide. It has regular spirals, performs characteristic movements in microscopic darkfield examination, and is morphologically indistinguishable from the treponemes causing syphilis and yaws. *T. carateum* has not been cultivated in vitro.

EPIDEMIOLOGY. Pinta is an endemic treponematosis of large rural populations in tropical forest and valley regions of Central and South America. For example, in rural areas of Mexico the prevalence of pinta varied from 1.3 to 9 per cent (1964) of the census population. Pinta cases occasionally reported from Pacific islands, India, Indonesia, and West Africa have not been verified and may have been "pintide" yaws. Unlike yaws, pinta is not a disease of earliest childhood. Community data (Mexico) indicate age-specific prevalences of early pinta lesions to be 2.5 per cent below five years of age, 8.8 per cent between five and ten years, and 12.2 per cent between ten and fifteen years. In late life some early lesions occur also after 40 years of age.

Transmission presumably takes place by person-to-person contact and is facilitated by poor hygiene, low economic standards, and limited health services. Treponemes are present in early lesions as well as in extensive late dyschromic lesions, where they can be found up to 40 years after the infection. Pinta does not appear to be very contagious, because an infected spouse with treponeme-containing lesions may sometimes not infect a serologically nonreactive partner or other family members. Scratches and insect bites may provide portals of entry for the agent. Blanco found 63 per cent of 257 initial lesions located on the legs and dorsum of feet. Arthropods (Simuliidae, *Hippelates*, or *Ornithodorus*) have not been convincingly demonstrated

to be reservoirs of treponemes or biologic vectors, although mechanical transmission cannot be excluded.

Host-Treponeme Relationship. Laboratory animal infection has been achieved in the chimpanzee (Kuhn et al., 1968). Man is the only known natural host of *T. carateum*.

As in syphilis, two types of antibody are formed during the human infection: (1) *Reagin*, detectable by cardiolipin antigen tests (VDRL), appears two to six months after the infection. (2) *Treponemal antibody*, identified in treponemal tests (fluorescent [FTA], hemagglutinating [TPHA] and immobilizing [TPI] antibody tests), is produced notably during dyschromic late manifestations but possibly before this stage. In untreated pinta the antibodies persist for many years. Asymptomatic seroreactors in communities affected by pinta are rare or absent. Superinfection can be achieved experimentally during the early generalized erythrosquamous stage of disease, but not after establishment of dyschromic late lesions. Varying degrees of cross-immunity between pinta, syphilis, yaws, and bejel have been reported (Medina, 1965). However, knowledge of humoral and cell-mediated immunity mechanisms is lacking. The same applies to immunologic (immunopathologic) processes possibly concerned in the genesis of lesions. Related aspects are discussed in Ch. 171.

The histopathology of pinta is characterized by a perivascular infiltrate of inflammatory cells composed of lymphocytes, some plasma cells, histiocytes, and macrophages. Swollen endothelial cells show no proliferation, arterioles and capillaries are not obliterated (as is the case in syphilis), and granulomatous tuberculoid structure is not observed. In dyschromic lesions accumulation of melanin-filled chromatophores in the upper corium is characteristic, and is caused by pigment "fall-out" from the epidermis. This might be a consequence of the primary process. In achromic lesions the picture is quite different — epidermis is atrophic with flattened rete pegs, melanocytes and melanin are lacking, elastic fibers are destroyed, and there is collagenic sclerosis, which explains the porcelain whiteness of achromic lesions. The pigment changes may result from direct action of *T. carateum* on the epidermal "melanin unit" (a melanocyte with a pool of associated malpighian cells [Duchon et al., 1968]). Pinta lesions are localized to skin areas exposed to sunlight. This is unrelated to the number and distribution of melanocytes. A photosensitization process is therefore unlikely.

CLINICAL MANIFESTATIONS AND DIAGNOSIS. The incubation period in experimental pinta is 7 to 21 days. In man, the initial manifestation is a small papule developing by extension or by coalescence with satellite lesions into a scaly maculopapular lesion. There is regional lymphadenopathy. A generalized erythrosquamous rash develops three to nine months after infection, and can be of the "wandering" type. Palpable polyadenitis is not a feature of secondary pinta in contrast to secondary syphilis. One to three years after the initial lesion, sizable dyschromic macules develop. These late lesions develop from secondary pintides or independently, and pass from slate blue through violet to brown and white — the final achromic phase of the pathogenic process. The time required to pass through these stages varies for different patches in the same individual, and the coexisting colored and white skin areas present a mottled appearance. Dyschromic lesions

The author wishes to acknowledge the valuable advice of his colleague Dr. S. Christiansen, Scientific Adviser, WHO Reference Centre for Treponematoses, State Serum Institute, Copenhagen, Denmark, concerning this chapter.

are usually located on frontal skin, cheeks, ears, forearms, back of hands, and dorsum of feet, but never the scalp. Blue lesions may be punctate, but most often appear as smudges on the brow, cheeks, and side of nose, and may last for one to two years. Brown lesions last much longer, and white elements are of lifelong duration. The achromic lesions are porcelain white and exhibit a "geographic coast" appearance; the skin is not supple and has no skin lines or lanugo. A different clinical course of pinta has been described in Cuba (Pardo-Castello, 1942), where the early phase is limited to palms and soles, with hyperpigmented spots turning into keratotic elements. The hyperpigmentation extends to the backs of hands and forearms. In Cuba implication of the cardiovascular and nervous systems has also been suggested. Such systemic involvement has not been verified in other pinta-affected areas of Central and South America. For instance Mazotti (1966) found nonreactive treponemal antibody tests (TPI) in the cerebrospinal fluid of a series of advanced pinta patients in Mexico. Neither were abnormalities found in the cerebrospinal fluid of pinta patients in Venezuela (Lawton-Smith and Medina, 1971).

Early pinta may be difficult to differentiate from *neurodermatitis* (darkfield examination is decisive even if there is seroreactivity); *trichophytosis of the glabrous skin* (pinta does not have vesicles or pustules); *pityriasis alba* (early pinta is more infiltrated); *tinea versicolor* (secondary pintides are more sharply delineated and infiltrated); or *psoriasis* (on removal of scales in pinta no bleeding points appear on a smooth surface). In *late pinta* the leukoderma may closely resemble similar lesions in *syphilis* and *yaws* (scarring); *vitiligo* (supple skin in scalp and perianal areas); *chloasma* (pregnancy and disorders of female genitals); *melanosis* (telangiectasis and poikiloderma are not features of pinta); or *incontinentia pigmenti* (urticaria prior to spots in infancy, pattern of splotches different, concomitant retinal and organ disease).

LABORATORY METHODS. A diagnosis of pinta depends on microscopic darkfield demonstration of *T. carateum* in fluid from early initial and secondary generalized lesions and late dyschromic lesions, as well as on serologic reagin and treponemal antibody tests. Methodologic considerations and interpretations concerning these are related to those in syphilis.

TREATMENT. The treatment of choice is repository, long-acting penicillin, notably procaine penicillin G in oil with aluminium monostearate (PAM)* and benza-

thine penicillin G (DBED). The considerations regarding time-dose relationship, oral therapy, and alternative antimicrobial drugs in persons hypersensitive to penicillin are the same as are discussed in Ch. 171. Rein et al. obtained highly satisfactory treatment results with 2.4 to 4.8 million units of PAM in early and late pinta. Injections of 2.4 million units of the longer-acting benzathine penicillin G can be effectively applied in a single dose or two injections of 1.2 million units in each buttock in one session.

PROGNOSIS. Pinta neither endangers life nor gives rise to prenatal disease. It has little appreciable effect on general health of patients. Treatment causes treponemes to disappear rapidly from the lesions, which sometimes regress very slowly, depending on their extent. Achromic patches in which atrophy of the epidermis has occurred do not change. However, the disfigurement from pinta, notably of younger persons, is sometimes associated with psychologic misery and social ostracism. Freedom of choice of habitat, mate, and employment is curtailed.

PREVENTION. Pinta prevention consists in examination and treatment with long-acting penicillin, of all patients and their contacts, along with improvement of rural health services, hygiene, and economic standards. In the frame of the international treponematoses program of the World Health Organization (WHO) and the Pan-American Health Organization (PAHO), extensive penicillin treatment campaigns have been undertaken in rural endemic pinta areas by several national health administrations in Central and South America during the last two decades. For instance, in Mexico more than 350,000 pinta patients and contacts have been treated since 1959. Prevalence was reduced from 5.9 to 0.4 per cent in nine main states. In 1974 only 248 cases were discovered. The age pattern and the stages of the disease indicated the effectiveness of the campaign (Lopez de Nava).

Chandler, F. W., Kaufman, A. F., and Kuhn, U.S., III: The histopathology of experimental pinta in the chimpanzee. J. Invest. Dermatol., 58:103, 1972.

Lopez de Nava, G.: Eradication of pinta disease in Mexico. Activities and results. Sal. Publ. Mex., 18:383, 1976.

Mazotti, L.: Negatividad de la prueba de inmovilizaciom de treponemas (TPI) en el liquido cefalorraquideo de 10 enfermos de pinto (carate). Rev. Inst. Salubr. Enferm. Trop., 22: Nos. 1 and 2, 1962.

Rein, C. R., Kitchen, D. K., Marquez, F., and Varela, G.: Repository penicillin therapy of pinta in the Mexican peasant. J. Invest. Dermatol., 18:137, 1952.

Smith, J. L., et al.: Neuro-ophthalmological study of late yaws and pinta. II. The Caracas project. Br. J. Vener. Dis., 47:226, 1971.

*Not available in United States of America.

SPIRILLARY AND LEPTOSPIRAL DISEASES

173. RELAPSING FEVER

Anthony D. M. Bryceson

173.1. INTRODUCTION

DEFINITION. Relapsing fever is a systemic infection with spirochetes of the genus *Borrelia* that are transmitted from man to man by the body louse, *Pediculus humanus*, or by soft-backed ticks of the genus *Ornithodoros*. Many species of tick-borne borreliae that infect man are zoonotic and so have an animal reservoir. Other species are of veterinary importance.

The disease is characterized by an abrupt, severe, self-limiting infection lasting several days with one or more relapses of diminishing duration and severity. The brunt of the infection is borne by the spleen, liver, brain, and myocardium, and there may be profound disturbance of the coagulation system. Treatment may be complicated by a severe Jarisch-Herxheimer reaction.

ETIOLOGY AND PATHOGENESIS. Borreliae are helical organisms 3 to 25 μ long with 4 to 30 coils. The body of the organism is 0.2 to 0.5 μ thick. They divide transversely. Borreliae contain endotoxin-like activity, but it is not known whether they contain lipopolysaccharide. Borreliae are susceptible to drying and to most chemical disinfectants, but survive for three months in citrated blood in the refrigerator, and much longer at $-70°$ C. They do not grow readily on artificial culture medium, but do so in chick embryos. Tick-borne species may be maintained in rodents or in ticks.

Epidemic or *louse-borne relapsing fever* is caused by *B. recurrentis*. Organisms circulate in the patient's bloodstream, are taken up by the louse when it feeds, and develop in the coelomic cavity. The louse becomes infective five to eight days later and remains so throughout its few weeks of life. Infected coelomic fluid is spilled on the skin when the louse is crushed during scratching. Spirochetes can penetrate broken skin, intact mucosa, and possibly intact skin, and so infect man.

Tick-borne disease may be caused by one of a wide range of spirochetes which are more or less specific for their vector. The tick becomes infected by feeding on human blood, and is infective three to four days later when spirochetes may be found in saliva and coxal fluid, which carry the organism into the bite of the tick when it next feeds. The tick remains infective for life, which is on average two years but may be as long as 25 years. Ticks are hardy and need not feed more than once a year. In addition, the ovaries of the tick become infected and the spirochete is transmitted to larvae and nymphs, which are infective for man. Up to 100 per cent of eggs of the most efficient vector, *O. moubata*, are infected. This tick is the only reservoir of *B. duttonii*. Borreliae transmitted by other species of ticks have, in addition, another reservoir, usually a rodent, whose burrow the tick shares. In nature a wide range of animals have been found infected with borreliae capable of infecting man. Lice can transmit tick-borne borreliae, but ticks cannot transmit *B. recurrentis*.

Borreliae circulate in the blood during the febrile periods and disappear during the remissions. They produce a *relapsing* infection because of antigenic variation. Spirochetes isolated from the blood during a relapse can be shown serologically to be distinct from the previous isolate. In louse-borne disease up to eight antigenically distinct isolates have been recognized. They tend to follow a regular pattern of variation and to revert to their original identity on passage through the vector. During each febrile episode variant specific antibodies are formed which immobilize and, in the presence of complement, lyse the organism. It is not clear to what extent spontaneous remission and antigenic variation are inherent properties of borreliae or are mediated by the patient's immune response.

173.2. LOUSE-BORNE RELAPSING FEVER

(Yellow Plague, Yellow Famine Fever, Vagabond Fever, Bilious Typhoid, Recurrent Fever)

EPIDEMIOLOGY. Man is the only reservoir of infection. In times of peace and prosperity, as now, louse-borne disease is restricted to a few endemic foci where it smolders ready to break out into epidemics in times of war, the movement of refugees, famine, and the breakdown of medical services.

The most important focus is the Ethiopian highlands, where about 10,000 cases occur annually, and whence it has spread into Sudan. Other foci may be found in the high Andes, in Afghanistan, in Cambodia, and possibly in the People's Republic of China. Important characteristics of endemic foci are cold, which discourages washing, and poverty, which encourages overcrowding and movement of laborers. These conditions favor the multiplication and spread of lice. Microfoci of disease are found in jails, army camps, and orphanages. Transmission is greatest in the winter months.

Louse-borne relapsing fever is one of the classic epidemic diseases of history. In ancient times it ravaged Europe as one of the famine fevers. After World War I it killed 5 million people in Europe and hundreds of thousands in Africa. During World War II there were 1 million cases in north Africa, besides many other lesser outbreaks, and from 1945 to 1947 there were over 1 million cases in Egypt alone with a case mortality of 8 per cent. Epidemic typhus (see Ch. 108.1) has often accompanied outbreaks of louse-borne relapsing fever, and the two diseases have been confused in the past. The present state of unrest in Africa threatens the epidemic spread of this disease within and beyond that continent. Nomads, pilgrims, seasonal laborers, traders, and dealers in old clothes may spread the disease, as well as soldiers and refugees. All are susceptible to infection, but the highest incidence is in young men. Immunity after an attack lasts at least one year.

PATHOGENESIS. Severity of illness bears little relationship to density of spirochetemia, which commonly ranges between 5000 and 500,000 microorganisms per milliliter during the febrile episodes. Most tissues of the body are invaded by the spirochete. Hepatocellular damage is present in all patients, and biochemical tests of hepatic function are deranged. Hyperbilirubinemia, mainly unconjugated, is present in three quarters of patients, and the urine contains an excess of urobilinogen and frequently bile. Histologically, parenchymatous cells are degenerate, sinuses congested, and endothelial cells prominent. In the spleen spirochetes accumulate in the sinuses, and there are miliary foci of necrosis and sometimes larger infarcts which may become secondarily infected. Perisplenitis is common. Dehydration is common and renal function is impaired, over half the patients having protein or cells in their urine; blood urea nitrogen is raised in four fifths of patients. Histologic examination shows tubular damage. There is no gross electrolyte disturbance. Heart failure with pulmonary edema develops in a few patients; prolonged Q-Tc interval is present in two fifths of electrocardiograms and prolonged P-R interval in a smaller proportion. Autopsy specimens show petechial hemorrhages on the serosal surfaces and, on microscopy, interstitial myocarditis with focal myocardial necrosis. There is no defect of pulmonary ventilation, but pulmonary venous admixture may exceed 20 per cent of cardiac output and lowers arterial oxygen saturation to 85 per cent. The high metabolic rate is reflected in the tachycardia (90 to 160 beats per minute), tachypnea (20 to 70 breaths per minute), and increased cardiac output (8 to 14 liters per minute). Systemic vascular resistance is low.

Borreliae, especially the tick-borne species, are neurotropic. Cerebrospinal fluid contains a moderate excess of polymorphonuclear leukocytes, lymphocytes, and protein; meninges may be inflamed, and cranial nerve palsies occasionally develop.

Bleeding occurs in half the patients. The early petechial rash is due to clumps of circulating spirochetes impacted in capillaries and is associated with thrombocytopenia, which is present in 85 per cent of patients. Later in the infection severe bleeding is associated with hepatocellular damage, and prolonged prothrombin and partial thromboplastin times are found in half the patients. Epistaxis may be profuse and prolonged, and there may be bleeding in the brain, meninges, subdural space, gut, urinary tract, and serosal surfaces.

In most patients fibrinogen levels are elevated; but in a few who develop widespread bleeding and shock, a low fibrinogen level is accompanied by other evidence of disseminated intravascular coagulation.

CLINICAL MANIFESTATIONS. After an incubation period of 2 to 15 days, the illness starts with chills, repeated several times during the day, and high fever. Few other diseases make the patient so ill so quickly. During the first two or three days chills and fever are accompanied by profound malaise, severe headache, dizziness, and nightmares. A bitter taste, thirst, and dysphagia are followed by anorexia, nausea, and vomiting in one third of the patients. Generalized aches and pains are common, especially in muscles and lower back. Two thirds complain of upper abdominal pain and of pain on breathing and, more rarely, of pain in the left shoulder. Half the patients cough, with mucoid frothy sputum. One quarter have epistaxis.

By the third day the patient is apathetic, with glazed expression, dull or confused mind, hot forehead, and cold hands. He is shivering and breathless. The presence of epistaxis, a petechial or purpuric rash, jaundice, or tenderness over the liver or spleen strongly suggests the diagnosis. The rash is most commonly over the shoulders, sides of the trunk, and inner aspects of the arms and thighs. The incidence of physical signs varies from one outbreak to another. All patients have fever and tachycardia. Systolic blood pressure is often low, and one quarter of patients have a gallop rhythm. Respiration is rapid, but added breath sounds are rarely heard. The liver or spleen is palpable in half the patients. In addition to confusion, two fifths of patients have signs of meningism, iritis, or cranial nerve palsies. Deafness or blindness occasionally develops. Delirium and coma may follow. Half the patients have tender muscles. Abortion or miscarriage is common.

Complications from secondary bacterial infection include pneumonia, endocarditis, and diarrhea. Concomitant infections such as typhus, malaria, typhoid, and dysentery are common in epidemics.

Throughout the illness the temperature remains around 39 to 40° C; sweating is slight. After 3 to 13 days the temperature falls by crisis. This is accompanied by physiologic changes similar to, but less severe than, those which characterize the Jarisch-Herxheimer reaction after treatment (see below) and may be fatal. If he survives, the patient remains exhausted for several days.

In the untreated patient there is an afebrile remission of five to seven days, rarely longer, during which he still feels unwell; it is followed by a second attack of fever. This relapse seldom lasts more than four days. Its features are those of the first attack, although less severe and without a rash. Second and third relapses may follow, rarely more, after which the patient makes a gradual but complete recovery.

DIAGNOSIS. Diagnosis is suggested by the typical clinical picture in the appropriate environment, and is confirmed by demonstrating spirochetes in peripheral blood taken from the first or second day of the illness onward. Thick and thin films are prepared and stained with Field's stain or Leishman's stain as for the diagnosis of malaria (see Ch. 193), and examined under the oil immersion objective. In the thick film tangled clumps of spirochetes are seen, whereas in the thin film individual spirochetes lie between the erythrocytes. Platelets are scanty. During remission spirochetes are difficult or impossible to find in the blood. There is no place for serologic tests which are technically difficult and hazardous, or for the inoculation of laboratory animals. In up to 30 per cent of patients anticardiolysin antibody (detectable by VDRL tests) is present transiently, and Weil-Felix OXK or OX19 titers may be raised.

There is usually a mild normocytic normochromic anemia, moderate polymorpholeukocytosis, and marked thrombocytopenia. Biochemical evidence of hepatocellular and renal damage is usual. The cerebrospinal fluid may contain a slight excess of cells, lymphocytes more than polymorphonuclear leukocytes, and of protein.

DIFFERENTIAL DIAGNOSIS. Relapsing fever, once suspected, is easy to diagnose or exclude. Clinical differentiation is from other causes of febrile jaundice, of meningism, of abdominal or chest pain with fever, and of septicemia.

Of the causes of febrile jaundice, malaria is the most important to differentiate, as specific therapy for it may be lifesaving. Severe *Plasmodium falciparum* infections may have most of the features of relapsing fever, but the rash is absent and hemorrhage is rare; muscle tenderness is unusual. Leptospirosis has many features in common with relapsing fever; it is often an occupational hazard (see Ch. 176). Rat-bite fever, especially that caused by *Spirillum minus,* is a less severe relapsing fever, with its own epidemiologic setting. Yellow fever may be suspected on epidemiologic as well as clinical grounds and is diagnosed by animal inoculation, serologically or at autopsy. Viral hepatitis (A or B) is seldom as severe or hemorrhagic and is a diagnosis of exclusion. A sickle crisis, presenting in someone flying in from a relapsing fever area, may show fever, jaundice, and generalized pains.

TREATMENT. The objectives of treatment are to support failing organs and systems, to kill the spirochete, to mitigate the effects of the ensuing Jarisch-Herxheimer reaction, and to prevent relapse.

The patient must be put to bed until at least three days after the first dose of an antimicrobial drug. Drinking is encouraged; but if there is vomiting, intravenous rehydration with 0.18 per cent saline in 4.3 per cent dextrose may be needed. Jugular or central venous pressure should be monitored. Nursing care for the febrile debilitated patient is needed, and sometimes for restlessness, delirium, unconsciousness, convulsions, and incontinence during the reaction. Pain may be relieved by oral paracetamol (acetaminol), known as acetaminophen in the United States, 1 gram every four hours.

Borrelia recurrentis is susceptible to penicillin, erythromycin, streptomycin, tetracycline, and chloramphenicol. The faster the organism is killed, the worse the reaction. Oral medication is often vomited. A slowly released preparation of penicillin given by intramuscular injection is the best compromise. Procaine penicillin in a dose of 300,000 units clears the blood of spirochetes in eight to nine hours. Penicillin aluminium monostearate,* 600,000 units, induces a less severe reaction and is considered by some to be safer, but the blood is not cleared of spirochetes for 17 hours (Warrell et al., 1976). Intravenous tetracycline, which clears the blood in one to two hours, in dangerous because it induces the most severe reaction. In an epidemic or when diagnostic facilities are poor, a single dose of 100 mg of doxycycline by mouth has the advantage of curing louse-borne typhus as well as relapsing fever. Penicillin is not completely effective in clearing borreliae from the brain, and the relapse rate after its use is 3 per cent. Relapse is prevented by giving the patient tetracycline, 500 mg, or doxycycline, 100 mg, by mouth the following day.

Petechial hemorrhage is unimportant. Severe hemorrhage is treated by blood transfusion. Vitamin K, 20 mg, may be given, but the prothrombin time returns to normal within three days of treatment regardless. There has been little experience with use of heparin to treat disseminated intravascular coagulation in relapsing fever. Liver and kidney function return rapidly to normal after treatment, and there is seldom need for specific support. Intercurrent infection should be sought and treated, especially typhoid.

JARISCH-HERXHEIMER REACTION. As spirochetes are killed, either during the natural crisis or following an antimicrobial drug, they are phagocytosed and removed from the circulation, and the Jarisch-Herxheimer reac-

tion begins. The characteristic feature is the chill, just before which the patient becomes uncomfortable, restless, or delirious and may pass urine or stool or may vomit. The chill lasts 10 to 30 minutes. After the chill, the patient suddenly feels hot and soon breaks out into a profuse sweat, after which he feels comfortable and falls asleep exhausted. During and after the chill the temperature rises to 40 to 42° C.

The metabolic rate rises sharply and attains a peak during the chill, and the cardiac output reaches 10 liters per minute. Ventilation is stimulated to cope with the demand for oxygen, and the respiratory rate may rise above 80 breaths per minute. Despite this, arterial oxygen saturation remains low and lactic acidosis develops. Arterial blood pressure rises sharply immediately before the chill, falls abruptly after it to dangerously low levels, and remains low for at least eight hours and often for two or three days. During this period the systemic vascular resistance falls and peripheral vessels dilate. The first eight hours after the chill are critical: the cardiac output is strained to its limit, the circulatory volume is falling, death of spirochetes in the myocardium precipitates or aggravates myocarditis (in about one third of the patients treated with tetracycline), and cardiac failure may follow. There is also evidence suggesting accelerated defibrination.

It is not certain whether the reaction is due primarily to endotoxin release, massive intravascular phagocytosis, or immune complex deposition.

Management of Jarisch-Herxheimer Reaction. HYPERPYREXIA. The oral temperature is taken every 30 minutes after treatment is given. If, after the chill, the oral temperature rises above 40° C, the patient should be sponged with tepid water and fanned vigorously until the temperature falls to 38.5° C.

SHOCK. After the profuse sweating, the patient is deceptively quiet and warm, and the pulse may feel full, but the blood pressure and pulse rate should be recorded every 30 minutes. If the systolic pressure falls below 60 mm Hg, the foot of the bed is raised and oral fluids are encouraged. If this is inadequate, intravenous fluid is given, with monitoring of the central venous pressure· and listening for evidence of pulmonary edema. A peripheral vasoconstrictor drug such as metaraminol bitartrate, 10 mg by intramuscular injection, may be helpful.

MYOCARDIAL FAILURE. This responds to sitting the patient upright and giving digoxin, 1 mg intravenously, followed by 0.5 mg twice daily for a few days.

CEREBRAL EDEMA. Prolonged coma may be due to intracranial hemorrhage or to cerebral edema; mannitol, 2 grams per kilogram of body weight, may be given as 20 per cent solution intravenously.

LACTIC ACIDOSIS. Lactic acidosis may be prevented by letting the patient breathe 100 per cent oxygen during the reaction. This seems to speed convalescence, but its benefit during the reaction is uncertain.

Corticosteroids in large doses, such as hydrocortisone, 1 gram hourly, reduce fever before the reaction but do not mitigate any of the changes of the reaction.

PROGNOSIS. The case mortality of louse-borne relapsing fever has varied markedly (4 to 40 per cent) in different outbreaks, depending upon age, nutrition, underlying disease, residual immunity, variations in the virulence of the organism during an epidemic, and the availability, nature, and timing of treatment. In the

---

*No longer available in the United States.

individual case deep jaundice, coma, and shock are bad prognostic signs. Early treatment improves the prognosis, but treatment late in the attack may induce a reaction which is more severe than the natural crisis. The disease tends to kill during the first attack, or just after the crisis, rather than during the relapses.

PREVENTION. During an outbreak, anti-louse measures are instituted in the population at risk. Clothes are treated by dry heat or insecticide powder, such as carbaryl 5 per cent or malathion 5 per cent, which are superseding gammexane 1 per cent and DDT 10 per cent, to which lice are resistant in many parts of the world. Personal hygiene and cleanliness are important, and this may be helped by shaving body and head hair. Mass prophylaxis with penicillin aluminium monostearate,* 1 million units, or doxycycline, 100 mg, would seem sensible but has not been tried. Patients and their clothes should be deloused with insecticide, and medical attendants should wear gloves while performing venipuncture or handling blood samples. If blood is spilled on the skin, tetracycline, 500 mg orally, should be taken once. International Sanitary Regulations require notification of cases and may direct disinfection of persons arriving from infected areas. There is no vaccine.

173.3.   TICK-BORNE RELAPSING FEVER

(Tick Fever; Many Local Names in Endemic Areas)

EPIDEMIOLOGY. The patterns of endemic or tick-borne relapsing fever depend upon the habits of their vectors and animal reservoirs and of man's contact with the ticks. The patterns vary from place to place.

In the far western United States and Texas, ticks live in caves; in Kansas, in prairie dog burrows; in Washington state, in owl burrows; in southwest Texas, in rodent burrows. Hunters and vacationers tend to become infected. *Ornithodoros turicata* inhabits caves frequented by goats and sheep, but is becoming domesticated in Central Mexico. *O. hermsi* lives in or near cabins at high altitude where it is associated with hibernating rodents. Early summer visitors acquire the disease. *O. erraticus* inhabits a wide range of animal burrows on the Mediterranean coast, and the disease affects both settled and nomadic peoples. *O. tholozani* inhabits caves and burrows and is attracted to fowls and camels and so reaches a large human population. It travels on sheep and camels on long caravan routes.

O. moubata has the closest association with man. It is found throughout the savanna of Central, East, and South Africa but not in the deserts, forests, or mountains. It prefers to live in and near human huts in cracks and crevices in the earthen floor, but is also found in animal burrows. It emerges at nightfall to feed on the inhabitants. The disease is therefore truly endemic, and sporadic cases occur throughout the year, most commonly in children. Visitors of any age are susceptible.

PATHOGENESIS. This is essentially the same as for the louse-borne disease, but tick-borne borreliae are more neurotropic, which alters slightly the clinical pattern and increases the liability to relapse. During remissions borreliae survive principally in the brain and seem relatively resistant to antimicrobial drugs and possibly to antibodies. The infection may cross the placenta.

CLINICAL MANIFESTATIONS. In endemic areas where people are repeatedly exposed to infection, the disease is commonly mild and brief. In nonimmunes it may be severe, and in general it follows the same course as the louse-borne infection.

The duration of the febrile periods and remissions is less regular than in the louse-borne disease, and the number of relapses tends to be greater. *B. duttonii* causes the most severe infection, and in the untreated nonimmune patient ten relapses of ten days each are not uncommon. Mediterranean and Middle Eastern infections are less severe and the American ones least so.

Neurologic complications are common. Iridocyclitis occurs in up to 15 per cent of patients and presents with eye pain, ciliary injection, and dim vision. Up to 30 per cent develop other complications, including coma, convulsions, cranial nerve lesions, hemiplegia, peripheral neuritis, and transverse myelitis. Nightmares, hallucinations, and severe anxiety and depressive states may develop. Most neurologic and psychiatric changes eventually disappear. Neurologic signs may be the sole feature of a late relapse.

DIAGNOSIS. Ticks emerge at night and their bite is often painless, so there may not be a clear history of bite. Sometimes their bites give rise to a local allergic response. Spirochetemia is often scantier than in louse-borne disease. Repeated examination of blood slides may be necessary. A concentration technique that has been used successfully in animals is to examine the buffy coat of blood centrifuged in a microhematocrit tube. Alternatively, 2 ml of blood may be inoculated intraperitoneally into mice; tail blood is examined for spirochetes from the second to fourteenth days. Occasionally during a relapse, only the cerebrospinal fluid may contain spirochetes.

PROGNOSIS. The initial attack of tick-borne relapsing fever is not usually so severe as the louse-borne variety, but, untreated, the disease is far more prolonged and debilitating, and death usually occurs in one of the relapses. The mortality is in general less, being very low in the United States, Middle East, and Asia and rising to 5 per cent in Africa, but a mortality of 27 per cent has been reported from Venezuela.

TREATMENT. Some strains of tick-borne Borreliae are not susceptible to penicillin; therefore tetracycline is commonly used. The dose is 250 mg orally every six hours until the patient is afebrile. Relapse is prevented by giving 500 mg six hourly for seven days, or 2 grams weekly for four weeks. In patients who are vomiting, 250 mg of tetracycline can be given intravenously, but a severe reaction can be expected within two hours. Alternatively, an initial dose of procaine penicillin may be tried, as for the louse-borne disease.

PREVENTION. In areas where the disease is endemic and the tick is associated with houses or frequents caves, as in Africa with *O. moubata* and parts of central Asia with *O. tholozani,* an insecticide should be sprayed, preferably in an oily base, on the lower part of the walls of the huts, on their floors, and at their entrances. A suitable preparation is 3 per cent benzene hexachloride in diesoline, which keeps huts free of ticks for over two years. Powders have a much shorter effect. Travelers should sleep under mosquito nets and inspect their clothing in the morning. A light kept burning at night discourages ticks. In the long run, better housing controls the disease. In areas where the disease is sporadic and ticks live in caves or burrows,

---

*No longer available in the United States.

anti-tick measures are impracticable, and personal prophylaxis is advised. It is best to avoid entering caves or using old camp sites; second best is the use of insect repellents. Clothes may be impregnated with 5 per cent dimethylphthalate in a 2 per cent oil emulsion. Washing with 10 per cent carbol soap is also effective. Insect repellent creams may be applied to the skin. Summer cabins in the Rocky Mountains should be rodent proof, and wooden walls and floors treated with creosote. In the spring, bedding should be treated with insecticide. There is no vaccine.

Bryceson, A. D. M., Parry, E. H. O., Perine, P. L., Warrell, D. A., Vukotich, D., and Leithead, C. S.: Louse-borne relapsing fever. Quart. J. Med., 39:130, 1970.

Coffey, E., and Eveland, W. C.: Experimental relapsing fever initiated by *B. hermsi*. J. Infect. Dis. 117:28, 1967.

Felsenfeld, O.: Borrelia. Strains, Vectors, Human and Animal Borreliosis. St. Louis, W. H. Green, 1971.

Parry, E. H. O., Warrell, D. A., Perine, P. L., Vukotich, D., and Bryceson, A. D. M.: Some effects of louse-borne relapsing fever on the function of the heart. Am. J. Med., 49:472, 1970.

Perine, P. L., Krause, D. W., Awoke, S., and McDade, J. E.: Single dose doxycycline treatment of louse-borne relapsing fever and epidemic typhus. Lancet, 2:742, 1974.

Warrell, D. A., Pope, H. M., Parry, E. H. O., Perine, P. L., and Bryceson, A. D. M.: Cardiorespiratory disturbances associated with infective fever in man: Studies of Ethiopian louse-borne relapsing fever. Clin. Sci., 39:123, 1970.

174. TROPICAL PHAGEDENIC ULCER

Anthony D. M. Bryceson

DEFINITION. Tropical phagedenic ulcer is an acute specific ulcer of skin and subcutaneous tissue, associated in its early stages with infection with *Borrelia vincentii* and anaerobic bacteria of the genus *Bacteroides*. The ulcer is usually situated below the knee, has certain typical characteristics, and commonly becomes chronic.

ETIOLOGY AND PATHOGENESIS. *B. vincentii* is a loosely coiled spirochete 5 to 10 μ long; it is a common oral commensal. *Bacteroides* is a curved, cigar-shaped rod 5 to 14 μ long, often beaded when stained; it, too, is an oral commensal and is common in moist soils. Either or both of these organisms are present in the acute stage of the ulcer. They gain entry through a tiny wound in the skin. Experimentally, they will cause ulcers only in malnourished subjects or animals. Other organisms, especially cocci, may also be found in established ulcers.

EPIDEMIOLOGY. The condition is common and widespread in the tropics and rare elsewhere. It may be found in all climates and at any altitude. In some countries hot wet areas are especially affected. In parts of some countries, active ulcers have a prevalence of 2 per cent and scars of 15 per cent. It is often the most common complaint of hospital outpatients, representing up to one third of new patients, and may be the most common cause of surgical admissions.

Tropical ulcer is typically a sporadic disease, especially affecting adolescent males. It is most common in the lower socioeconomic groups. Although the patient may not appear grossly malnourished, there is a clear clinical and experimental association with malnutrition. No specific nutritional deficiency has been identified, but tropical ulcer is rare in those who eat adequate animal protein and is especially common in labor gangs, ill-

kept prisoners of war, and other physically deprived groups, among whom it can appear as an epidemic. This association with malnutrition and deprivation is also found in two other infections with the same organisms, cancrum oris and trench mouth.

PATHOGENESIS, CLINICAL MANIFESTATIONS, AND PROGNOSIS. The lesion starts at the site of a minor wound or insect bite, which the patient can usually recall. Often the site is neglected or treated with a native remedy, or sucked by mouth to clean it. A small blister appears, containing serosanguineous fluid, and ruptures, exposing an ash gray slough which has a characteristic foul smell. The ulcer spreads rapidly to involve subcutaneous tissue and often muscle and tendon down to bone. It reaches its final diameter of 1 to 40 cm in a few days. The central slough liquefies, exposing a gray-brown base. The ulcer is circular, with a raised edge and surrounding edema, and may encircle the limb. It is painful and bleeds easily. Regional lymph nodes may be enlarged and tender. The most common sites of tropical ulcers are over the bony parts of the leg at the level of, or just above, the ankle.

Histologic examination shows three layers: a superficial layer of coagulation necrosis in which organisms are abundant, a layer of granulation tissue, and a highly vascular base. The edge of the ulcer shows pseudo-epitheliomatous hyperplasia.

Fifty per cent of ulcers heal spontaneously within three months, and 80 per cent within six months.

Chronic ulcers become less painful and lose their odor. They become irregular with a rigid base and edge and are filled with pink granulation tissue. Histologically there is much surrounding fibrosis. Squamous cell carcinoma develops in 9 per cent of chronic ulcers after a period of three months to 50 years. Tetanus and gangrene are rarer complications.

DIAGNOSIS. In the acute stage the appearances and smell are typical. The specific organisms can be demonstrated in a drop of fluid aspirated from the ulcer, either by darkfield microscopy or by Gram stain or staining with 1 per cent carbolfuchsin. Histologic examination is seldom needed. It is more difficult to identify the cause of chronic ulcers. The differential diagnosis includes yaws (serology and radiology), cutaneous diphtheria (climate, culture), Buruli ulcer (undermining, acid-fast bacilli), squamous cell carcinoma and melanoma (histology), and varicose ulcers (age group, venous abnormality).

TREATMENT. In the acute stage the patient is put to bed and the limb elevated. The ulcer is dressed with sterile saline or resorcinol monoacetate (Euresol). Hydrogen peroxide may be used for a few days to help slough out. Strong antiseptics are contraindicated. Penicillin is given by intramuscular injection for seven days; procaine penicillin, 600,000 units twice daily, or penicillin aluminium monostearate,* 1,200,000 units daily, is suitable. Metronidazole, 200 mg thrice daily by mouth, is a suitable alternative to penicillin. The synergistic effect of the two drugs has not been tested.

This treatment controls the infection and cleans the ulcer. Ulcers under 5 cm in diameter should now heal satisfactorily. Ulcers over 5 cm should be grafted with split skin.

Chronic ulcers are treated initially in the same way, and are then completely excised and grafted. A walking

---

*No longer available in the United States.

plaster may then be applied, and healing is complete within three weeks.

PREVENTION. Good nutrition and physical health are the best preventives. Legs should be covered while walking in country where thorns or sharp grass may scratch them. Minor cuts and scratches should be washed and treated with local antiseptic.

Edington, G. M., and Gillies, H. M.: Tropical ulcers. *In* Pathology in the Tropics. London, Arnold, 1976, p. 726.

Lindler, R. R., and Adeniyi-Jones, C.: The effect of metronidazole on tropical ulcers. Trans. R. Soc. Trop. Med. Hyg., 62:712, 1968.

Lowenthal, L. J. A.: Tropical phagedenic ulcer: A review. *In* Lincicome, D. R. (ed.): International Review of Tropical Medicine. New York, Academic Press, 1963, p. 267.

175. RAT-BITE FEVER

Jay P. Sanford

Rat-bite fever represents two clinically somewhat similar but etiologically distinct diseases which usually follow the bite of a rat or other rodent. Streptobacillary rat-bite fever is caused by the pleomorphic gram-negative bacillus *Streptobacillus moniliformis*, whereas spirillary rat-bite fever is caused by *spirillum minus*. In the United States, streptobacillary rat-bite fever is far more common.

Rat-bite fever occurs throughout the world, with a higher incidence in urban areas where sanitation is poor and the rat population is great. In the United States, approximately half of the reported cases have occurred in children under 12 years of age. Rat-bite fever is said to follow about 10 per cent of rat bites; however, with an estimated 14,000 persons bitten by rats annually in the United States, this estimated frequency appears excessively high.

STREPTOBACILLARY RAT-BITE FEVER

EPIDEMIOLOGY. *Streptobacillus moniliformis* is found in the oropharynx of healthy rats. Although several epidemics have apparently been associated with the ingestion of raw milk, Haverhill fever, the portal of entry is usually an animal bite. Animals incriminated include rats, mice, weasels, dogs, and cats. Currently rat-bite fever represents a particular hazard to biomedical laboratory workers.

CLINICAL MANIFESTATIONS. Following a bite, the primary wound usually heals promptly. After an incubation period of 1 to 22 (usually less than 10) days, the patient abruptly develops severe chills, fever, vomiting, headache, and pains in the joints and back. The fever tends to remit in two to five days. About the third day, a morbilliform, petechial rash appears over the feet and hands in more than 90 per cent of patients. After remitting briefly, the fever recurs and is characteristically (70 per cent of patients) associated with arthralgia and arthritis. In most patients, multiple joints, especially the wrists and elbows, are involved. Untreated, the joint findings may persist for several days to several months.

Cases have been reported of patients who develop infective endocarditis caused by *Streptobacillus moniliformis*. In such instances there are usually no aspects of the history, such as that of rat bites or clinical features, to lead one to suspect *Streptobacillus moniliformis* as the etiologic agent.

LABORATORY FEATURES. Leukocyte counts may range between 6000 and 30,000 per cubic millimeter. There are no other distinctive features. False-positive serologic tests for syphilis have been reported in 25 per cent of cases.

DIAGNOSIS. Diagnosis is confirmed by culturing the organism from blood or joint fluid on ordinary nutrient media, although growth is enhanced by addition of 20 per cent horse serum to the medium and incubation under 5 to 10 per cent CO_2.

The differential diagnosis includes the following viral diseases: rubella with associated arthralgia-arthritis (however, the rash in rubella is centripetal); hepatitis B virus infection with arthralgia-arthritis, although the rash is usually urticarial; and dengue, although a diphasic febrile course is typical, a maculopapular rash appears on the third to fifth day, severe arthralgia is characteristic, and arthritis is not a feature (also, in dengue the peripheral leukocyte count usually is less than 5000 per cubic millimeter by the third to fifth day). In Africa, other arboviral causes which are associated with rash and arthritis include Chikungunya, O'nyong-nyong, and Sindbis virus; in Australia, epidemics of polyarthritis associated with rashes occur with Ross River virus. The rash of streptobacillary rat-bite fever may resemble that seen with Rocky Mountain spotted fever in character, distribution, and time of occurrence. Other bacterial diseases to be considered in the differential diagnosis include disseminated gonococcal infection, chronic meningococcemia, and leptospirosis, especially in children, in whom peripheral rash is more frequent.

THERAPY. The organisms are susceptible to penicillin, the tetracyclines, and most other antimicrobial drugs. Penicillin V (phenoxymethyl penicillin, 2.0 grams per day divided into three or four doses, or procaine penicillin, 600,000 units intramuscularly every 12 hours for 10 days, is recommended. In patients with hypersensitivity to penicillins, tetracycline, 2.0 grams per day orally divided into four doses, is an effective alternative.

PROGNOSIS AND SEQUELAE. Mortality is low except with endocarditis. Treatment will shorten the febrile course.

SPIRILLARY RAT-BITE FEVER
(Sodoku)

EPIDEMIOLOGY. *Spirillum minus* is a cause of ocular infection in rats, the organism apparently reaching the rat's mouth by way of the nasolacrimal ducts. Occasionally, the bites of cats have been incriminated.

CLINICAL MANIFESTATIONS. Following a bite, the initial wound usually heals promptly. After an incubation period of 4 to 28 (usually greater than 10) days, inflammation recurs at the primary wound site, with associated fever and regional lymphadenitis. A roseolar-urticarial rash may occur, but it is less evident than with streptobacillary rat-bite fever. Arthritis is rare. An episode lasts three to four days and then subsides. Recurrence is usual after a few days.

LABORATORY FEATURES. The leukocyte count usually is 5000 to 30,000 per cubic millimeter. False-positive serologic tests for syphilis occur in about one half of patients.

DIAGNOSIS. *Spirillum minus* has not been cultured on

artificial medium; hence diagnosis is established by demonstrating *Spirillum minus* in a darkfield preparation of exudate from an infected site or lymph node. Alternatively, inoculation of material intraperitoneally into mice and examination of the mouse blood 5 to 15 days later by Giemsa stain or darkfield microscopy may enable demonstration of the spirillum.

THERAPY. Response to treatment with penicillin or with the aminoglycoside streptomycin is prompt.

Cole, J. S., Stoll, R W., and Bulger, R. J. Rat-bite fever: Report of three cases. Ann. Intern. Med., 71:979, 1969.

Place, E. H., and Sutton, L. E.: Erythema arthriticum epidemicum (Haverhill fever). Arch. Intern. Med., 54:659, 1934.

Roughgarden, J. W.: Antimicrobial therapy of rat-bite fever. Arch Intern. Med., 116:39, 1965.

Watkins, C. G.: Rat-bite fever. J. Pediat. 28:429, 1946.

176. LEPTOSPIROSIS

Jay P. Sanford

DEFINITION. Leptospirosis is an inclusive term applied to disease caused by all leptospires regardless of specific serotype. Correlation of clinical syndromes with infection by differing serotypes indicates that a single serotype of *Leptospira* may be responsible for a variety of clinical features; likewise, a single syndrome, e.g., aseptic meningitis, may be caused by multiple serotypes of leptospires. Hence, the general term leptospirosis is preferred rather than the synonyms such as Weil's disease or Canicola fever.

ETIOLOGY. The genus *Leptospira* contains only one species, *L. interrogans,* which may be subdivided into two complexes, interrogans and biflexa. The interrogans complex includes most of the pathogenic strains, whereas the biflexa complex includes mainly saprophytic strains with no recognized hosts. Despite contrary common usage, an example of the correct designation of leptospira is as follows: pomona serogroup of *L. interrogans,* not *L. pomona.* The interrogans complex now contains about 130 serotypes arranged in 16 serogroups (the number in parentheses refers to number of serotypes within the serogroup): Icterohemorrhagiae (13), Hebdomadis (28), Autumnalis (13), Canicola (11), Australis (10), Tarassovi or Hyos (10), Pyrogenes (9), Bataviae (8), Javanica (6), Pomona (6), Ballum (3), Cynopteri (3), Celledoni (2), Grippotyphosa (2), Panama (2), and Shermani (1). At least 22 serotypes of *Leptospira* occur naturally in the United States.

EPIDEMIOLOGY. Leptospirosis, although not a common disease, has been reported from all regions of the United States. Between 1960 and 1976, 50 to 90 cases were reported annually. Occasional upswings in the number of cases have been the result of common source outbreaks.

Infection in man is incidental and is not essential to the maintenance of leptospirosis. Infection occurs in a wide range of domestic and wild animal hosts. In many species, such as opossums, skunks, raccoons, and foxes, infectivity ratios in the range of 10 to 50 per cent are not unusual. Interspecies spread of specific serotypes of leptospires between animal hosts is frequent, e.g., *pomona*, a serotype principally associated with livestock, has been demonstrated in dogs. The infection in animals may vary from inapparent illness to severe fatal disease. The carrier state may develop in many animals wherein the host may shed leptospires in its urine for months to years.

It has not been established that pathogenic leptospires are capable of multiplication outside a host. Survival in nature is governed by factors including pH of the urine, soil, or water into which they are shed and ambient temperature. Acid urine permits only limited survival; however, if the urine is neutral or alkaline and is shed into a similar moist environment which has low salinity and is not badly polluted with microorganisms or detergents, and with a temperature above 22° C, leptospires may survive for several weeks. Human infections can occur either directly by contact with urine or tissue of an infected animal or indirectly through contaminated water, soil, or vegetation. The usual portals of entry are abraded skin, particularly about the feet, and exposed mucous membranes, conjunctival, nasal, and oral. The concept that organisms can penetrate intact skin has been questioned. Although leptospires have been isolated from ticks, they appear to be unimportant in transmission.

With the ubiquitous infection of animals, leptospirosis in man can occur in all age groups, at all seasons, and in both sexes. However, it is primarily a disease of teenage children and young adults (at least 50 per cent of patients are between ages 10 and 39 years), occurs predominantly in males (75 per cent), and develops most frequently in hot weather (in the United States two thirds of infections occur from June to October). The wide spectrum of animal hosts results in both urban and rural human disease. Leptospirosis has been considered an occupational disease; however, improved methods of rat control and better standards of hygiene have reduced the incidence among occupational groups such as coal miners and sewermen. Currently only 10 per cent of patients in the United States have direct contact with animals, i.e., farmers, abattoir workers, or veterinarians. The majority of patients have incidental exposure, two thirds being children, students, or housewives. Swimming or partial immersion in contaminated water has been implicated in one fifth of patients and has accounted for most of the recognized common source outbreaks.

PATHOLOGY. In patients who have died with hepatic involvement (Weil's syndrome), renal involvement, or both, the significant gross changes include hemorrhages and bile-staining of tissues. The hemorrhages, which vary from petechial to ecchymotic, are widespread but are most prominent in skeletal muscle, kidneys, adrenals, liver, stomach, spleen, and lungs.

In skeletal muscle, focal necrotic and necrobiotic changes thought to be rather typical of leptospirosis occur. Biopsies early in the illness demonstrate swelling, vacuolation, and subsequently hyalinization. Leptospiral antigen has been demonstrated in these lesions by the fluorescent antibody technique. Healing ensues by the formation of new myofibrils with minimal fibrosis.

The renal lesion in the acute phase involves the tubules predominantly and varies from simple dilatation of distal convoluted tubules to degeneration, necrosis, and basement membrane rupture. Interstitial edema and cellular infiltrates, consisting of lymphocytes, neutrophilic leukocytes, histiocytes, and plasma cells, are uniformly present. Glomerular lesions either are absent or consist of mesangial hyperplasia and focal foot process fusion, which are interpreted as representing nonspecific changes. Microscopic alterations in the liver are not diagnostic, and correlate poorly with the degree of function impairment. The changes include frequent double nuclei and cloudy swelling of hepatocytes, disruption of liver cords, enlargement of Kupffer cells, and bile stasis in biliary canaliculi. The changes in the brain and meninges are also minimal and are not diagnostic. Microscopic evidence of myocarditis, including focal hemorrhages, interstitial edema, and focal infiltration with lymphocytes and plasma cells, has been recorded. Pulmonary findings consist of a patchy, localized hemorrhagic pneumonitis. Special staining techniques utilizing silver impregnation methods have demonstrated organisms in the lumina of renal tubules but rarely in other organs.

CLINICAL MANIFESTATIONS. General Features. The incubation period after immersion or accidental laboratory exposure has shown extremes of 2 to 26 days, the usual range being 7 to 13 days and the average, 10 days.

Leptospirosis is typically a biphasic illness. *The leptospiremic or first phase* is characterized by the presence of leptospires in the blood and cerebrospinal fluid. The onset is typically abrupt (75 to 100 per cent of patients). Initial symptoms include headache, which is usually frontal, less often retro-orbital, but occasionally may be bitemporal or occipital. Severe muscle aching occurs in most patients, the muscles of the thighs and lumbar areas being most prominently involved and often accompanied by pain on palpation. The myalgia may be accompanied by extreme cutaneous hyperesthesia (causalgia). Chills followed by high fever are prominent. The leptospiremic phase typically lasts four to nine days. Features during this interval include recurrent chills, high spiking temperature curve (usually reaching 39° C or greater), headache, and continued severe myalgia. Anorexia, nausea, vomiting, and abdominal pain are encountered in about one half of patients. Occasional patients have diarrhea (7 to 29 per cent). Pulmonary manifestations, usually either cough or chest pain, have varied in frequency of occurrence from less than 25 to 86 per cent. Hemoptysis occurs but is rare. Examination during this phase reveals an acutely ill febrile patient. A relative bradycardia may be noted. The blood pressure is usually normal in adults. In children hypertension is common. Disturbances in sensorium may be encountered in up to 25 per cent of patients. The most characteristic sign is conjunctival suffusion which usually appears on the third or fourth day. It may be lacking in some patients, but more often it is overlooked because of its benign nature. This may be associated with photophobia, but serous or purulent secretion is unusual. Less common findings (in 10 to 50 per cent of patients) may include pharyngeal injection, nuchal rigidity, lymphadenopathy, cutaneous hemorrhages, and skin rashes that are usually macular, maculopapular, or urticarial, and usually occur on the trunk. Uncommon findings (usually less than 10 per cent) are erythema nodosum, splenomegaly, hepatomegaly, or jaundice. Defervescence and improvement in symptoms coincide with the disappearance of leptospires from the blood and cerebrospinal fluid.

The second phase has been characterized as the "immune" phase and correlates with the appearance of circulating antibodies which are predominantly IgM class.

The clinical manifestations of this phase exhibit greater variability than those during the first phase After a relatively asymptomatic period of one to three days, the fever and earlier symptoms recur and meningismus may develop. The fever rarely exceeds 39° C and is usually of one to three days' duration. It is not uncommon for fever to be absent or quite transient. Even when symptoms or signs of meningeal irritation are absent, routine examination of cerebrospinal fluid after the seventh day has revealed pleocytosis in 50 to 90 per cent of patients. Less common features include iridocyclitis, optic neuritis, and other nervous system manifestations, including encephalitis, myelitis, and peripheral neuropathy.

Some clinicians recognize a third or convalescent phase, usually between the second and fourth weeks, when fever and aching may recur. The pathogenesis of this stage is poorly understood.

Leptospirosis during pregnancy may be associated with an increased risk of fetal loss.

Specific Features. WEIL'S SYNDROME. Weil's syndrome, which may be due to serotypes other than *icterohemorrhagiae*, is defined as severe leptospirosis with jaundice, usually accompanied by azotemia, hemorrhages, anemia, disturbances in consciousness, and continued fever. There is uncertainty as to the pathogenesis of the syndrome, i.e., whether it represents direct toxic damage caused by leptospires or whether it is the consequence of immune response to leptospiral antigens. The consensus favors toxic damage.

The onset and first stage are identical with the less severe forms. The distinctive features of Weil's syndrome appear from the third to the sixth day but may not reach their peak until well into the second stage. As in the other forms of leptospirosis, there is a tendency for the fever to lyse about the seventh day; however, with its recurrence it is marked and may persist for several weeks. Either renal or hepatic manifestations may predominate. Hepatic disturbances include tenderness in the right upper quadrant and hepatic enlargement, both of which are common when jaundice is present. SGOT values are rarely increased more than fivefold regardless of the degree of hyperbilirubinemia, which is predominantly conjugated (direct). The mechanism of hyperbilirubinemia appears to be an intracellular block to bilirubin excretion.

Renal manifestations consist primarily of proteinuria, pyuria, hematuria, and azotemia. Dysuria is rare. The maximal level of blood urea nitrogen is usually reached on the fifth to seventh day. Serious renal damage usually occurs in the form of acute tubular necrosis associated with oliguria. Hemorrhagic manifestations include epistaxis, hemoptysis, gastrointestinal bleeding, hemorrhage into the adrenal glands, hemorrhagic pneumonitis, and subarachnoid hemorrhage. These have been explained on the basis of capillary injury. In addition, in some patients hypoprothrombinemia and thrombocytopenia have been observed.

ASEPTIC MENINGITIS. A leptospiral cause has been incriminated in 5 to 13 per cent of patients with aseptic meningitis. The pleocytosis is not present before the immune phase, when it develops rapidly. There are usually tens to hundreds of cells, occasionally 1000 per cubic millimeter, which may be neutrophils or mononuclear cells. The cerebrospinal fluid glucose level is almost always normal, but occasional instances of lowered glucose levels have been recorded. With leptospirosis the cerebrospinal fluid protein may exceed 100 mg per 100 ml early in the course. Xanthochromic cerebrospinal fluid has been observed in the presence of jaundice. Each of the serotypes of leptospires that are pathogenic for man is probably capable of association with this syndrome. The most prevalent serotypes have been *Canicola, Icterohemorrhagiae,*and *Pomona.*

PRETIBIAL (FORT BRAGG) FEVER. An illness was observed in the summer of 1942 that had an onset identical with that of the first phase of leptospirosis. The most distinctive feature was the development of a rash on about the fourth day, characterized by 2 to 5 cm slightly raised erythematous lesions that were usually symmetrically distributed over the pretibial areas. In contrast to other leptospiral syndromes, splenomegaly occurred in 95 per cent of these patients. This outbreak, which related to exposure while swimming, was caused by the Autumnalis serogroup. Subsequently Pomona has been observed in association with rashes, which are usually truncal in distribution but have also been pretibial in location.

MYOCARDITIS. Cardiac arrhythmias, including paroxysmal atrial fibrillation, atrial flutter, and ventricular tachycardia, have been described, but are usually of little clinical significance. However, on rare occasions definite cardiac dilatation with acute left ventricular failure has been observed. Associated manifestations have included jaundice, pulmonary infiltrates, arthritis, and skin rashes. The serogroups thus far incriminated have included Icterohemorrhagiae and Pomona.

CHILDREN. Several clinical features occur in children which are not seen or are very rare in adults: acalculous cholecystitis (five of nine children in one series), pancreatitis, abdominal causalgia, peripheral desquamation of rash which may be associated with gangrene, and cardiopulmonary arrest. The features of desquamation, myocardial involvement, and hydrops of the gallbladder suggest the recently described "mucocutaneous lymph node syndrome."

LABORATORY FEATURES. Leukocyte counts vary from leukopenic levels to mild elevations in the anicteric patients. In patients with jaundice, leukocytosis as high as 70,000 per cubic millimeter may be present. However, regardless of the total leukocyte count, neutrophilia of greater than 70 per cent is very frequently encountered during the first stage.

Hemolytic substances have been demonstrated in cultures of pathogenic leptospires. In contrast to many hemolysins of bacterial origin, which are not hemolytic in vivo, the leptospiral hemolysins appear active in vivo. In patients with jaundice, anemia may be severe and is most characteristically due to intravascular hemolysis. Anemia owing to leptospirosis is unusual in anicteric patients.

Rarely thrombocytopenia sufficient in magnitude to be associated with bleeding is encountered. The erythrocyte sedimentation rate is elevated in more than one half of patients but is usually less than 50 mm per hour.

Urinalyses during the leptospiremic phase reveal a high frequency of abnormalities, including mild proteinuria, casts, and an increase in cellular elements. In anicteric infections, these abnormalities rapidly disappear after the beginning of illness. Proteinuria and abnormalities in urine sediment are usually not associated with elevations in blood urea nitrogen values. Since the

anicteric form of the disease has often gone undiagnosed, estimates of the frequency of azotemia and jaundice are probably high. Azotemia has been reported in approximately one fourth of patients. In three fourths of these patients the blood urea nitrogen is less than 100 mg per 100 ml. Azotemia is usually associated with the occurrence of jaundice. The serum bilirubin levels may reach 65 mg per 100 ml; however, in two thirds of patients the levels are less than 20 mg per 100 ml. During the first phase one half of patients have increased serum creatine phosphokinase (CPK) values. In contrast, increases are not seen in viral hepatitis. Mean transaminase values in leptospirosis approximate five times normal. A slight increase in transaminase with a definite increase in CPK suggests leptospirosis rather than viral hepatitis.

DIAGNOSIS. Diagnosis is based upon either cultural or serologic studies. The most common initial diagnostic impressions in patients with leptospirosis are meningitis, hepatitis, nephritis, "FUO," and influenza. Leptospires may be isolated quite readily during the first phase from blood and cerebrospinal fluid or during the second phase from the urine. Leptospires may be excreted in the urine for up to 11 months after the onset of illness. Whole blood should be inoculated immediately into tubes containing semisolid medium, such as Fletcher's. If culture medium is not available, leptospires reportedly will remain viable up to 11 days in blood anticoagulated with sodium oxalate. Animal inoculation (preferably of either suckling hamsters or guinea pigs) may also be used and is of particular value if specimens, e.g., urine, are contaminated. Direct examination of blood or urine by darkfield methods so frequently results in failure or misdiagnosis that it should not be employed as the only diagnostic test. Antibodies appear from the sixth to the twelfth day of illness. Four serologic tests are available: the macroscopic plate agglutination test (the easiest to perform but a relatively insensitive technique), hemolytic test (complex in performance but requiring only a single antigen), microscopic agglutination test (complex in performance but most specific), and complement-fixation test. Serologic criteria for diagnosis include a fourfold or greater rise in titer during the course. Cross-agglutination reactions between various serotypes commonly occur so that the infecting serotype often cannot be determined with certainty without isolation of leptospires.

PROGNOSIS AND SEQUELAE. Between 1966 and 1975, a case fatality ratio of 9.8 per cent has been reported in the United States. Age is the most significant host factor related to increased mortality. In a representative series, the mortality rose from 10 per cent in men less than 50 years of age to 56 per cent in those over 51 years of age. In anicteric patients, mortality is essentially unknown. With the occurrence of jaundice, mortality in various series has ranged from 15 to 40 per cent. The long-term prognosis after the acute renal lesion of leptospirosis is good. However, a few patients exhibit residual tubular dysfunction, e.g., a defect in renal concentrating ability, and a patient with permanent renal damage has been recorded.

THERAPY AND MANAGEMENT. A variety of antimicrobial drugs, including penicillin, streptomycin, the tetracycline congeners and erythromycin, have been effective in vitro and against experimental leptospiral infections. The data obtained from controlled observations in man are conflicting as to over-all efficacy. If antimicrobial drugs have any beneficial effect, they must be administered within four days, and preferably within two days, of the onset of illness. This means that the decision to start chemotherapy must be made mainly on clinical suspicion (see Ch. 189). The agents most studied have been penicillin G and the various tetracycline congeners. Turner states that large doses of penicillin G or tetracycline are beneficial. Within four to six hours after initiation of penicillin G therapy, a Jarisch-Herxheimer type reaction may occur, which suggests antileptospiral activity. There is general agreement that antimicrobials administered after the fifth day have no beneficial effect. Since diagnosis within the first five days requires a very high index of suspicion, management is primarily supportive. The clinical impression exists that early bed rest may minimize the subsequent morbidity. The presence of azotemia and jaundice requires meticulous attention to fluid and electrolyte therapy.

Alston, J. M., and Broom, J. C.: Leptospirosis in man and animals. Edinburgh and London, E. S. Livingstone, Ltd., 1958.

Edwards, G. A., and Domm, B. M.: Human leptospirosis. Medicine, 39:117, 1960.

Feigin, R. D., and Anderson, D. C.: Human leptospirosis. C.R.C. Crit. Rev. Clin. Lab. Sci., 5:413, 1975.

Heath, C. W., Jr., Alexander, A. D., and Galton, M. M.: Leptospirosis in the United States. Analysis of 483 cases in man. 1949–1961. N. Engl. J. Med., 273:857, 915, 1965.

Johnson, R. C.: The Biology of Parasitic Spirochetes. New York, Academic Press, 1976.

Johnson, W. D. Jr., Silva, I. C., and Rocha, H.: Serum creatine phosphokinase in leptospirosis. JAMA, 233:981, 1975.

Turner, L. H.: Leptospirosis. Br. Med. J., 1:537, 1973.

Wong, M. L., Kaplan, S., Dunkle, L. M., Strechenberg, B. W., and Feigin, R. D.: Leptospirosis: A childhood disease. J. Pediat., 90:532, 1977.

Section Three THE MYCOSES

177. INTRODUCTION

John P. Utz

Increased awareness by physicians, continuing improvement in cultural techniques and in their use by laboratory technicians, and the existence of a valuable (and difficult) antifungal agent, amphotericin B, have led to an increased importance of the systemic mycoses in human disease. The fact that infection occurs with fungi that are free-living forms in soil, decaying vegetation, and bird excreta poses a difficult problem of control. The deliberate impairment of immune response, e.g., to decrease host-versus-graft reactions in patients with organ transplants, has created still another setting for infection by "opportunistic" fungi.

Although the chapters that follow are devoted to the mycoses per se, it should be pointed out that fungi have other pathways through which they can produce disease. P. K. C. Austwick has well summarized these phenomena:

Fungi cause three main types of animal and human disease:

Mycoses: diseases resulting from the invasion of living tissues by the fungus.

Allergies: diseases resulting from the development of hypersensitivity to fungal antigens.

Mycotoxicoses resulting from the ingestion of toxic fungal metabolites formed in food, and *mycetisms* resulting from the ingestion of toxic fungal fruiting bodies.

There are also three indirect ways in which fungi can be involved in pathogenic processes in animals, viz., by inducing the formation of toxic substances (including estrogens) by a host plant which is then eaten by an animal; by so degrading a foodstuff that macronutrient deficiencies appear in animals feeding on it; and by forming substances such as enzymes, which, although not acting directly on metabolic processes themselves, affect the availability of growth substances to the animal, e.g., vitamins, which may lead to micronutrient deficiency.

Fungal pathogenicity thus covers a much wider range of activity than that seen in other pathogenic microorganisms, and its height of complexity may be realized when it is possible for all three types of disease to be present in one individual animal, each caused by the same species of fungus playing three different roles at one time. Infection and allergy due to *Aspergillus fumigatus* are not uncommon together in man.

Further complications arise in the existence of two types of fungal thallus morphology in vivo. Firstly, apical hyphal growth leads to spherical or disc-like colonies whose spread is by peripheral extension and by fragmentation, a process compensating for its slowness of dissemination by the provision of relatively large inocula for its extension, and so of more certainty of success. Secondly, the self-replication of single cells either as yeast cells or endosporulating spherules can more readily play a leading role in the dissemination of infection in the body, but for this the fungus is generally dependent upon phagocytosis. It may be said that, in the first instance, the fungus is essentially active, making its own way through the tissues and, in the second, passive and dependent on the bloodstream or blood cells for transport. The latter type of growth is also directly comparable to that in many bacterial and viral infections, being frequently accompanied by acute pyrexial symptoms, while the former is generally associated with a chronic inflammatory process extending sometimes over many years.

Failure to understand this fundamental difference in the behavior in vivo of fungi has led to much confusion in the classification of fungal disease, and it still remains a major problem when trying to generalize on the pathogenesis of the mycoses. The ability of fungi to adopt a wide range of vegetative morphology according to their environment is being increasingly observed, and a number of filamentous saprophytic fungi are now known to be capable of budding as yeast cells under defined experimental conditions, e.g., *Mucor rouxii* and *Aspergillus parasiticus* (Bartnicki-Garcia and Nickerson, 1962; Detroy and Ciegler, 1971). The possession of hyphae or of a unicellular state therefore bears no relationship to the classification or to the potential pathogenicity of the species.*

The systemic mycoses have important properties in common in addition to their point of origin in nature. With few exceptions, they are not contagious from animal to man or man to man, and epidemics or outbreaks arise from a common source. Infection is acquired by inhalation or, in a few instances, by traumatic implantation. The primary focus is usually the lung, and infection spreads hematogenously or, less commonly, by direct extension. The gross and microscopic appearance of infected tissue is that of a granulomatous process. The immunologic response is generally effective (reinfection is rare), and cellular and serologically mediated immune mechanisms have been demonstrated (see Ch. 38 and 40).

178. HISTOPLASMOSIS

John P. Utz

DEFINITION. Histoplasmosis is a systemic fungal disease, respiratory in origin, that spreads to the pulmonary lymphatics and by the blood to the mediastinal lymph nodes, spleen, liver, adrenals, gastrointestinal tract, kidneys, skin, central nervous system, heart, and other organs. It may be asymptomatic, acute and benign, or progressive and eventually fatal.

HISTORY. Darling in Panama in 1905 reported three fatal cases of disseminated disease, which he considered to be due to a *"plasmodium"* with a *"capsule,"* in *histiocytes* which he termed *Histoplasma capsulatum.* In a study of tissue section, da Rocha Lima concluded in 1913 that the agent was a fungus. In 1934 De Monbreun correctly identified the fungus in cultural and in laboratory animal studies. Ten years later Christie and Peterson recognized the benign form of human disease with pulmonary calcification and associated skin hypersensitivity to histoplasmin. Subsequently, Palmer showed widely varying rates of hypersensitivity according to geographic areas in this country.

ETIOLOGY. *H. capsulatum* has two morphologic forms, *yeast* and *hyphal,* dependent upon a variety of environmental factors. The yeast form seen in tissues measures 2 to 3 by 3 to 4 μ and has a clear area resulting from skrinkage of cytoplasm from the rigid cell wall. In artificial media or natural substrate the yeast form is converted readily at room temperatures to the hyphal form with the production on Sabouraud's glucose medium of a white to brown cottony mold. On microscopic examination this is composed of branched hyphae, characteristic spherical forms with spiny projections (tuberculate macroconidia) 8 to 14 μ in diameter, and smaller forms (microconidia) measuring 2 to 5 μ. Conversion of the hyphal to the yeast form occurs characteristically after inoculation into animals or less readily on enriched media at 37° C. Skin hypersensitivity, complement-fixing, and other antigens have been demonstrated. Mice and guinea pigs are susceptible to experimental infection.

EPIDEMIOLOGY. Histoplasmosis occurs with highest frequency in infancy and old age and equally in the

sexes except more often in the male in old age. It has been reported in more than 30 countries in both temperate and tropical zones. Skin hypersensitivity rates are as high as 80 to 90 per cent in some parts of the eastern and midwestern United States. Rates of skin reactivity increase rapidly with age to young adulthood and then more slowly thereafter. Man and animals are infected by inhalation of the fungus in dust. Soil from chicken houses or from areas contaminated or composted by bat or bird dung is especially rich in fungi. Massive exposure through such activities as destruction of chicken houses, exploration of caves, or community "clean-up" activities has resulted in outbreaks. Fifty per cent of dogs and cats in some areas and many species of wild animals are known to be infected. *Histoplasma duboisii,* a closely related fungus, produces in African patients a disease marked by lymphadenopathy and bone, joint, and skin involvement.

PATHOLOGY. The tissue reaction is characteristically engulfment of yeast forms by histiocytes or macrophages derived from organs of the reticuloendothelial system. Epithelioid or histiocytic granulomas are formed, with tubercle-like nodules, caseation necrosis, and calcification in the lung, lymph nodes, liver, spleen, adrenals, and other organs. The organism can best be identified in tissues by culture or by use of special stains (periodic acid–Schiff, Gridley, or Gomori methenamine silver methods). However, fungal cells may be few, crowded, and not differentiated with certainty from those of *H. duboisii, Blastomyces dermatitidis, Torulopsis glabrata,* or *Candida albicans.*

CLINICAL MANIFESTATIONS. On the basis of delayed cutaneous hypersensitivity studies, it appears that primary infection with *H. capsulatum* is usually asymptomatic or produces a respiratory illness that is not distinctive.

Primary Acute Form. The primary acute form is characterized by respiratory symptoms of cough, shortness of breath, pleuritic chest pain, hoarseness, hemoptysis, and cyanosis in that order. Associated generalized symptoms are commonly fever, chills, myalgia, malaise, and weight loss. In focal outbreaks, where there is exposure to large numbers of spores, sudden onset and pleuritic pain are common. Pleural effusion, however, is rare. The chest film may show bilateral disease with the characteristic diffuse miliary type of lesion from hematogenous seeding, or, more commonly, localized infiltrations, especially in the lower lobes. There may be hilar and peritracheal lymphadenopathy unaccompanied by other lesions. That infection is not localized to lungs alone is attested to by the frequent splenic calcification seen later and the occasional isolation of *H. capsulatum* from urine during the acute illness. In many patients lesions resolve completely, but in others calcification or fibrotic scarring persists. Calcified peribronchial nodes may compress the bronchus, leading to bronchiectasis, or may erode and result in broncholithiasis. A distinctive residue of primary infection is the solitary nodule of the lung, located just beneath the pleura, appearing roentgenographically as a "coin lesion." Mediastinal histoplasmosis with esophageal abscess or superior vena cava syndrome is being increasingly reported.

Progressive Disseminated Form. Rarely the disease progresses and resembles that form originally described by Darling. Pulmonary findings are often not prominent; illness is characterized instead by fever, enlarge-

---

*From Austwick, P. K. C.: The pathogenicity of fungi. *In* Microbial Pathogenicity in Man and Animals. Twenty-second Symposium of the Society for General Microbiology, Imperial College, London. Cambridge, England, Cambridge University Press, 1972.

ment of the liver and spleen, generalized lymphade-nopathy, weight loss, anemia, and leukopenia. One particular feature may predominate, and the illness then appears as endocarditis, pericarditis, meningitis, adrenal insufficiency, or multiple ulcerations of mouth, pharynx, larynx, stomach, or small or large bowel. Belief in *H. capsulatum* uveitis persists despite the extraordinary rarity of isolation of the fungus from any material derived from patients.

Chronic Cavitary Form.   In older adult males especially, a chronic, cavitary pulmonary disease occurs that closely simulates and is often labeled tuberculosis. This form is characterized by cough, weight loss, dyspnea, low-grade fever, chest pain, and hemoptysis. This form is most likely a reactivation of a previously quiescent primary infection.

DIAGNOSIS.   The isolation in culture and microscopic identification of the fungus establish the diagnosis. In suspected cases of acute primary disease both sputum and urine should be cultured. In the widely disseminated forms, the fungus may be cultured from blood, bone marrow, cerebrospinal fluid, ulcer swabs, urine, sputum, lymph nodes, and material from liver biopsy. Conversion of a skin test from negative to positive and a titer of the complement-fixing antibodies that rises and falls or is in excess of 1:32 only support the clinical impression. A single positive histoplasmin skin test indicates only recent or remote exposure to this or related antigen. Frequently, both skin and complement-fixation tests are negative in a patient with severe or early disease. Careful microscopic study of properly stained tissue sections may reveal characteristic fungal forms, providing additional supporting evidence for the clinical diagnosis (see Pathology).

Acute primary histoplasmosis should be considered in the differential diagnosis of any persistent febrile respiratory disease, especially those occurring after exposure to chicken or other bird excreta and in any pneumonia without appropriate bacteria in sputum. Hepatosplenomegaly, lymphadenopathy, anemia, and leukopenia of the severe disseminated form may closely simulate Hodgkin's disease and leukemia. Mucosal alterations so closely resemble cancer that repeated biopsies for tissue study have been performed, all with negative results, before cultures were done. As a general rule, histoplasmosis should be suspected in any patient with findings suggestive of tuberculosis but without supporting laboratory data.

TREATMENT.   Amphotericin B is the most active of the presently available antifungal drugs for the treatment of the disease in man. The drug is customarily given intravenously; 1.0 mg dissolved in 500 ml of a 5 per cent glucose solution is recommended as the first dose. Dosage should be increased daily by increments of 5 to 10 mg. At present there are many recommendations and no consensus as to optimal daily dosage (from 0.5 to 1.0 mg per kilogram), duration of therapy (from 6 to 14 weeks), or total dosage (from irrelevant to about 2 grams). Each infusion should be administered over at least a two-hour period and preferably longer, e.g., four to six hours. Such undesired side effects as local thrombophlebitis, fever, chills, nausea, vomiting, anorexia, rise in serum urea nitrogen, hypokalemia, and anemia may occur in approximately 80 per cent of patients but should not require abandonment of the therapy. After treatment is stopped, most indices of renal function return toward normal, but in about 80

per cent of patients on higher drug doses the values are never again the same as before treatment. Salicylates, antihistamines, and corticoids reduce the severity or frequency of such side effects of treatment as nausea, chills, and fever.

A few patients with localized disease in the lungs have been helped by surgical excision of lesions.

PROGNOSIS.   Except in localized outbreaks with inhalation of large numbers of fungi, acute primary histoplasmosis is almost always a benign illness from which the patient recovers rapidly. Therapy usually has not been administered.

Since progressive disseminated disease is fatal in 80 to 90 per cent, and the chronic cavitary form in 30 per cent of cases, chemotherapy is indicated. Approximately 80 to 90 per cent of patients with severe disease have recovered with amphotericin B treatment.

Corticoid treatment has been associated with deleterious effects in experimental infections of animals and with relapse after amphotericin B therapy in man.

Austwick, P. K. C.: The pathogenicity of fungi. *In* Microbial Pathogenicity in Man and Animals. Twenty-second Symposium of the Society for General Microbiology, Imperial College, London, April 1972. Cambridge, England, Cambridge University Press, 1972.

Butler, W. T.: Pharmacology, toxicity and therapeutic usefulness of amphotericin B. JAMA, 195:371, 1966.

Drutz, D. J., Spickard, A., Rodgers, D. E., and Koenig, M. G.: Treatment of disseminated mycotic infections: A new approach to amphotericin B treatment. Am. J. Med., 45:406, 1968.

Goodwin, R. A., Jr., and Des Prez, R. M.: Histoplasmosis. Am. Rev. Respir. Dis., 117:929, 1978.

Vanek, J., and Schwarz, J.: The gamut of histoplasmosis. Am. J. Med., 50:89, 1971.

179.   COCCIDIOIDOMYCOSIS

(Valley Fever)

Demosthenes Pappagianis

DEFINITION.   Coccidioidomycosis is a fungal infection usually acquired by the respiratory route. In most cases it is arrested in the lungs, but it may spread to virtually all organs or tissues. Chronic persistent infection may ensue. Infrequently the infection is fatal.

HISTORY.   The disease we recognize as coccidioidomycosis was first described in 1892 by Alejandro Posadas in an Argentinian man in Buenos Aires. In the infected tissues a cystlike organism thought to be a protozoan was observed. The second case was reported in 1894 by Rixford in California, the place of origin of the succeeding several hundred recognized cases. The resemblance of the organism to the protozoan *Coccidia* led to the name *Coccidioides*. Ophuls and Moffitt in 1900 recognized the causative organism as a cultivable mold in vitro. Most early recognized cases of coccidioidal infection were severe, often with widespread cutaneous and visceral lesions, and frequently fatal, but Gifford and Dickson in the early 1930's established that San Joaquin or valley fever was a mild infection caused by *Coccidioides immitis*. Introduction of amphotericin B in 1956 led to successful therapy in coccidioidal infections with an otherwise dismal outlook.

ETIOLOGY.   In the infected host, *C. immitis* exists as a spherule (sporangium), 20 to 100 μm in diameter, and reproduces by formation of few to several hundred endospores. These endospores are released and in turn enlarge to mature spherules. The filamentous septate *mycelial* form usually found in cultures and in nature produces chains of *arthrospores*. These arthrospores (about $2 \times 5 \mu m$) are readily airborne and constitute the inhaled infectious form of the organism. Confirmation of the identity of *C. immitis* requires demonstration of the spherule form of the organism in the patient or by animal inoculation, and constitutes the single best diagnostic procedure.

EPIDEMIOLOGY. Coccidioidomycosis is usually encountered in the southwestern United States (California, Arizona, New Mexico, Texas, southern portions of Nevada and Utah), Mexico, Central America, Argentina, Paraguay, Venezuela, and Colombia. These areas correspond to location of *C. immitis* in the soil. Travelers may acquire the infection during brief visits to these areas. Rarely exportation of the fungus on some product of the endemic region can lead to infection elsewhere. The true *incidence* is likely greater than the 300 to 400 cases reported per year in California, or the more than 500 per year in Arizona. Some 50 deaths per year caused by coccidioidomycosis are reported in the United States. It has been estimated that 25,000 to 35,000 new infections occur per year in California. About a fifth of those so affected will have symptomatic infections that bring them to a physician. The *prevalence* of coccidioidomycosis increases during the dry, dusty summer and fall. An occupational risk of infection exists in agricultural or other disturbers of the soil. In some endemic areas the proportion of the population which has been infected increases with time of residence and may exceed 85 per cent. *C. immitis* survives for months at -20 to $42°$ C and a pH of 4 to 9. It can be found in rodent burrows and elsewhere, persisting for years in the soil. Rodents, dogs, cattle, sheep, and other animals are also infected by inhalation of arthrospores. The infection is not spread from animals to man or from man to man (although one case of in utero infection has been reported).

Humans from a few weeks to 85 years of age have been infected. In general, infection may be milder in children. In adults, about 60 per cent of infections are asymptomatic. Of the 40 per cent with symptomatic infections, most will recover. Approximately 1 in 100 adult white males with symptoms will develop disseminated coccidioidomycosis. Filipinos and blacks have higher rates of dissemination. Adult white females less frequently develop disseminated coccidioidomycosis, perhaps associated with their greater tendency to develop the prognostically favorable erythema nodosum.

PATHOGENESIS AND PATHOLOGY. The nature of the response to infection with *C. immitis* appears related to the morphologic states of the organism and to the development of delayed hypersensitivity. Endospores appear to induce a granulocytic response, spherules a macrophagic response. Lesions may resemble closely the granulomatous lesion of tuberculosis or sarcoid, but frequently there is juxtaposed suppuration. The mixed inflammatory reaction may yield amorphous necrosis, hyalinization, fibrosis, and calcification. The contribution of delayed hypersensitivity to pathogenesis is not clear, but anergy to coccidioidin is prognostically unfavorable.

Primary infection usually presents as a pneumonitis. (Fewer than 20 cases of primary cutaneous coccidioidomycosis have been reported.) The infection is usually arrested in the pulmonary parenchyma and regional nodes. Occasionally the organisms spread lymphogenously and hematogenously to virtually any tissue (the gastrointestinal mucosa has not been involved, and the brain and the endocardium only rarely). Such dissemination usually ensues early after the primary infection, but occasionally the pulmonary lesion has cleared by the time dissemination is apparent. In about 5 to 10 per cent of patients with primary pulmonary coccidioidomycosis, a chronic cavity or granuloma will develop. Viable *C. immitis* may persist for years in such lesions, although the patient's clinical status remains favorable. Pulmonary cavities occur and recur more frequently in patients with diabetes mellitus. Prognostically more serious but less frequent is an apical chronic progressive fibrocavitary disease.

CLINICAL MANIFESTATIONS. Clinically apparent primary pulmonary coccidioidomycosis will develop in 7 to 28 days (average, 10 to 16 days) after inhalation of the spores, presenting with fever, malaise, pleuritic pain, dry cough, night sweats, anorexia, headache, and weight loss. Chest pain is common and may be severe. Early after onset of symptoms, a macular, urticarial, scarlatiniform or morbilliform rash may develop transiently. It may be seen particularly in the inguinal areas and on the palms and soles, even before coccidioidin sensitivity develops. Such a rash is seen more frequently in children.

Along with the respiratory component, "valley fever" classically includes erythema nodosum of the anterior tibia or erythema multiforme of the extensor aspects of the upper extremities, palms, and upper thorax and neck. This may be seen in about 40 per cent of adult white females and 5 per cent of adult white males who have symptomatic infections, and is accompanied by arthralgia and swelling of ankles and knees. Erythema nodosum indicates marked sensitivity to coccidioidin and is not likely to be coccidioidal in cause if the skin test is negative. Initially primary coccidioidomycosis may be bronchial or peribronchial. The chest x-ray may reveal pneumonitis resembling acute bacterial, mycoplasmal, viral, or other fungal pneumonias with lobar, lobular, or scattered patches of infiltrate. Hilar densities (parenchymal and adenopathy) and pleural effusion are common. Infrequently there is pericardial effusion. A transient cavity occasionally develops during the acute phase. Primary infection of the skin yields an ulcerative lesion and regional adenopathy. Resolution of primary pulmonary coccidioidomycosis usually occurs within several weeks, although asthenia and easy fatigability may last for several months. There may be persistent and unexplained chest pain despite recovery from the acute infection.

Dissemination of the infection to metapulmonary tissues, including the meninges, may also be recognized only after the primary pulmonary lesion has faded. The progression is sometimes difficult to discern clinically until an overt lesion of bone, skin, lymph node, or meninges is detected. It may be suspected from deterioration of the patient with persistent fever, weight loss, marked bronchomediastinal adenopathy, or mental deterioration (in meningitis), or from laboratory parameters to be discussed below.

Chronic cavities, coccidioidomas, or *bronchiectasis* may remain after apparent clearing of the primary pneumonitis, or they may be detected on routine roentgenograms years after the primary infection. Hemoptysis may be the first indication of a pulmonary cavity.

DIAGNOSIS. Awareness of the extreme variability of clinical patterns offered by coccidioidomycosis is essential. It may resemble influenza; bacterial, mycoplasmal, or other mycotic pneumonia; acute or chronic tuberculosis or histoplasmosis; or neoplasms. The hilar or bronchomediastinal adenopathy may resemble that of sarcoid or lymphomas. The chronic pulmonary cavity is characteristically thin-walled on x-ray, but may resemble a pulmonary abscess or be partially filled with fluid. Coccidioidal fibrosis or bronchiectasis may resemble that of other causes. Lesions of bones or soft tissues may resemble those of blastomycosis, tuberculosis, or other bacterial infections. The erythrocyte sedimentation rate is elevated, and there is often a moderate leukocytosis, sometimes with eosinophilia. Sustained eosinophilia is unfavorable.

Coccidioidal meningitis may resemble tuberculosis or other mycotic meningitis. Decrease in the cerebrospinal fluid (CSF) glucose is often an early significant change. Occasionally in the early stages there may be a polymorphonuclear pleocytosis, but the onset is usually more insidious and the CSF changes in cell and protein are suggestive of chronic or "aseptic" meningitis. A "paretic" colloidal gold curve often accompanies these changes.

Coccidioidomycosis is confirmed by direct demonstration of endosporulating spherules in biopsied tissue or exudates utilizing special fungal stains. *Cultures* from lesions or sputum also yield a diagnosis, provided that animal inoculation or special culture methods are used to confirm the production of spherules. The CSF should be cultured but often fails to yield C. immitis.

The time involved and hazard of working with C. immitis cultures require that appropriate skin test and serologic studies be carried out. The coccidioidin (mycelial phase antigen) skin test may become positive in three days to three weeks after onset of symptoms. (A newly developed antigen, spherulin, appears more reactive in detecting sensitivity.) A positive coccidioidin skin test means past or present infection. A negative test does not exclude a coccidioidal cause, for the test is often negative in disseminated infections or with old pulmonary lesions (cavities or coccidioidomas). The skin test should be repeated in following the course of the illness, for anergy is unfavorable. The skin test does not interfere with coccidioidal serologic studies. Precipitins (IgM) are produced early and assist in diagnosis of primary infections. These are detected by a tube test and by a latex particle agglutination test. They fade within the first few weeks but may persist in severe infections and may reappear, e.g., with a bronchopleural fistula or in reinfection via ventriculoperitoneal or ventriculoatrial shunt. Complement-fixing (CF) antibodies (IgG) appear later and may persist for many months or years after recovery. They are readily detected by immunodiffusion. The CF antibody titer rises proportional to severity (extent of involvement). Thus metapulmonary dissemination is usually reflected in an elevated titer (usually above 1:16, but this level may vary between laboratories), and declining titer indicates improvement. Pleural, joint, and cerebrospinal fluids may contain CF antibody, although usually at lower titer than in the serum. In coccidioidal meningitis the CSF infrequently is seronegative but the serum positive. The basilar meningitis may yield CF-positive cisternal and lumbar fluids even though the ventricular fluid is negative. Complement fixation by the CSF is usually diagnostic of coccidioidal meningitis, although an extradural (paravertebral) abscess can yield CF an-

tibody in the CSF. In this instance the CSF protein is elevated, with glucose and cells normal.

The CF test is positive in about 60 per cent of cases (immunodiffusion is more often positive) with chronic coccidioidal cavities, but is often negative in patients with asymptomatic coccidioidomas. Thus diagnosis of the latter often is not assisted by serologic tests. Cross-reactions occur between C. immitis, Histoplasma capsulatum, and Blastomyces dermatitidis in serologic and skin tests. Primary coccidioidal infections are sometimes accompanied by higher CF titers with Histoplasma and Blastomyces antigens. Sequential sera should yield higher homologous titers.

TREATMENT. Symptomatic therapy is indicated for primary coccidioidomycosis. Amphotericin B, the most extensively used antifungal agent, should be applied in most cases of disseminated disease, although miconazole has been effective in some cases. Occasionally, as with a small single cutaneous lesion, excision may be curative. In the absence of overt evidence of dissemination, systemic amphotericin may be administered for severe primary coccidioidal infection or when the clinical or laboratory picture indicates likelihood of dissemination. Amphotericin may be administered intravenously on alternate days, with the dose gradually raised to 1.0 mg per kilogram of body weight. The MIC in vitro of most strains of C. immitis is approximately 1 μg per milliliter. Prolonged therapy is often needed in coccidioidomycosis, increasing the risk of nephropathy, hypokalemia, anemia, phlebitis, and other side effects. Meningitis can be treated preferably by intracisternal administration of up to 1.0 mg, usually three times a week. Arachnoiditis has frequently complicated lumbar administration. The use of 10 per cent (hyperbaric) glucose with amphotericin, with the patient's head lowered, may lessen but does not eliminate arachnoiditis. Under some circumstances amphotericin may be given by the intraventricular route via the Ommaya reservoir and catheter. The total dose required must be determined by the progress of the patient. Therapy of meningitis should be continued for at least three months after the CSF becomes normal, but continued vigilance for years is required because of the possibility of relapse.

Excisional therapy may also be needed for osseous, articular, or soft tissue lesions. Pulmonary cavities, although generally benign, may be resected if complicated by progressive enlargement, rupture into the pleural space, hemorrhage, or secondary infection. Pre- and postoperative therapy with amphotericin is advisable, although some thoracic surgeons have had few complications without such coverage. Treatment of chronic pulmonary cavities or fibrocavitary disease with amphotericin B is usually without benefit. The usually benign solitary pulmonary nodule may have to be resected for differentiation from other lesions.

Immunotherapy with Lawrence's leukocyte transfer factor from coccidioidin-sensitive donors has had limited trials. This may provide an important additional therapeutic modality, particularly in anergic patients who have not responded to amphotericin or who may be at risk of recurrence of cavities, e.g., diabetics.

PROGNOSIS. Prior to amphotericin therapy, more than half the patients with disseminated infections and all with coccidioidal meningitis died. With amphotericin therapy, patients with coccidioidal meningitis have survived for 15 to 20 years, some apparently cured.

Nonmeningeal disseminated infections have also been successfully treated, although infections involving joints may be recurrent despite treatment with amphotericin B. Recovery from infection leads to resistance to reinfection (exogenous reinfection has occurred only in a very few laboratory workers). Immunosuppressive therapy of intercurrent disease such as Hodgkin's disease with accompanying cytotoxic therapy may reactivate old arrested coccidioidomycosis.

PREVENTION. A vaccine prepared from killed spherules has provided good protection of laboratory animals and has appeared safe in humans. However, it has not had a field trial in humans exposed to infection. Avoidance of exposure to the arthrospores would prevent infection, but the widespread distribution of the organism and impracticality of eradicating it from the soil make avoidance difficult in those who are occupationally tied to the soil. The use of lightweight masks or other measures to reduce inhalation of spores during overt dusty exposures is justified.

Ajello, L. (ed.): Coccidioidomycosis. Tucson, University of Arizona Press, 1967.

Ajello, L. (ed.): Coccidioidomycosis. Miami, Fla., Symposia Specialists, 1977.

Drutz, D., and Catanzaro, A.: Coccidioidomycosis. Am. Rev. Respir. Dis., 117:559, 727, 1978.

Fiese, M. J.: Coccidioidomycosis. Springfield, Ill., Charles C Thomas, 1958.

Huntington, R. W., Jr.: Coccidioidomycosis. In Baker, R. D. (ed.): Human Infection with Fungi, Actinomycetes and Algae. New York, Springer-Verlag, 1971, Chap. 6.

Smith, C. E., Saito, M. T., and Simons, S. A.: Pattern of 39,500 serologic tests in coccidioidomycosis. JAMA, 160:546, 1956.

180. BLASTOMYCOSIS

(North American)

John P. Utz

DEFINITION. Blastomycosis is a chronic systemic fungal disease, respiratory in origin, which, classically, disseminates to the skin and occasionally to subcutaneous tissue, bone, and other organs.

HISTORY. In 1894 Gilchrist and in 1898 Gilchrist and Stokes reported the first two cases and named the responsible fungus *Blastomyces dermatitidis.*

ETIOLOGY. *B. dermatitidis* is a dimorphic fungus existing in tissue as a yeastlike form (8 to 15 μ, rarely 30 μ), with a characteristic thick wall (0.5 to 0.75 μ). The yeast form reproduces by budding, and the typical bud is characterized by its large size and attachment to the parent cell by a persistent wall and a wide pore. On Sabouraud's glucose medium *B. dermatitidis* grows as a white mycelium composed of slender hyphae to which are attached, either directly or by lateral slender stalks (conidiophores), smooth spherical 2 to 10 μ forms (conidia). The perfect, sexual state, *Ajellomyces dermatitidis,* has recently been defined. Skin hypersensitivity, complement-fixing, and other antigens have been demonstrated. Mice and other laboratory animals are susceptible to experimental infection.

EPIDEMIOLOGY. Blastomycosis was at first exclusively American in distribution: Canada, Mexico, Central America, northern Latin America, and, in 98 per cent of reported cases, the United States. However, cases have now been reported from widely separated sites in Africa. The disease affects all ages, but there is a slightly higher frequency in the third and fourth decades. Men are affected six to nine times more frequently than women. Infection results from inhalation of conidia, but the saprophytic source of the fungus in nature is not known. In one reported instance, genital infection was acquired conjugally. Benign, subclinical cases have been reported, but the skin test studies do not support a high incidence of infection in certain areas similar to that of histoplasmosis and coccidioidomycosis. Common source epidemics have been reported in Big Fork, Minnesota, and Pick County, North Carolina.

PATHOLOGY. The characteristic tissue response to *B. dermatitidis* is a combination of suppuration and epithelioid and giant cell granulomas. In the lung the disease may be localized or may spread as a pneumonia. Cavitation and circumscribed, calcific nodules are rarely encountered. The skin lesions reveal characteristically pseudoepitheliomatous hyperplasia and microabscesses in which *B. dermatitidis* may be seen. In bone, subcutaneous tissue, meninges, prostate, epididymis, and other organs the histologic appearance is again a combination of suppuration and granulomas.

CLINICAL MANIFESTATIONS.   Primary Pulmonary Form. Primary pulmonary blastomycosis begins usually as a mild respiratory infection (rarely as a fulminant pneumonia) with cough, pleuritic chest pain, and, occasionally, hemoptysis. As the disease progresses, generalized symptoms of fever, night sweats, anorexia, and weight loss appear. Physical signs may not be prominent. However, there may be dullness, bronchial breath sounds, and rales characteristic of consolidation. Roentgenographically, manifestations vary from those of a consolidated lobar pneumonia to multiple infiltrations. Hilar adenopathy is common, localized nodules are less so, and cavitation is rare. Although pleural disease is common, effusion is characteristically extremely rare.

Cutaneous Form. Although cutaneous blastomycosis represents spread from a primary pulmonary infection, the presenting complaint of many patients is a cutaneous lesion, either solitary or multiple. The initial papule or pustule progresses within weeks or months into an ulcerated or warty lesion. The advancing border of this lesion is serpiginous, dusky red, or violaceous, elevated 1 to 3 mm, and has an outer edge that slopes abruptly. The base of the lesion contains small abscesses, from which characteristic budding yeast cells can be demonstrated. The central area may become crusted, or, in older lesions, may heal with a thin atrophic scar. In contrast to the skin lesion that follows accidental laboratory implantation, regional lymphadenopathy does not occur.

Other Systemic Forms. A subcutaneous form of the disease consists of single or more often multiple soft to firm nodules, palpable deep beneath the skin. These may enlarge to become bulging abscesses, but in various stages contain pus. The skin over the nodules may have a slightly reddish hue.

Osteomyelitis or periostitis of long bones or spine occurs frequently. The first manifestation of disease may be a psoas abscess. A septic arthritis may occur either alone or by extension from bone.

Genitourinary blastomycosis is frequently seen in men and is manifested by pain and swelling of the epididymis, prostate, or seminal vesicles.

There may also be involvement of the central nervous system, eye, adrenals, thyroid, and larynx. In contrast to histoplasmosis, the gastrointestinal tract is almost never involved.

DIAGNOSIS. Although skin lesions may be strongly suggestive, the diagnosis of blastomycosis is confirmed by the finding of typical budding yeast cells in direct preparations or by the culture and identification of *B. dermatitidis* from pus or lesions. When appropriate, sputum, urine, cerebrospinal fluid, bone marrow, or other biopsy and autopsy tissue should also be cultured. Skin tests are almost always negative, especially in earlier stages of the disease, and serologic procedures may show a higher titer or a positive reaction only to *Histoplasma capsulatum*.

The pulmonary form of the disease is rarely diagnosed clinically or roentgenographically and is usually thought to be tuberculosis or, less frequently, sarcoidosis, acute bacterial pneumonia, malignancy, or other fungal infections more common in the geographic area. Skin lesions are suggestive of basal cell carcinoma, tuberculosis, nodulo-ulcerative syphilid, pyoderma, or other fungal infections. Other systemic manifestations mimic those of tuberculosis or other chronic bacterial infection.

TREATMENT. Amphotericin B has been used extensively for all forms of blastomycosis. Details of administration are given in Ch. 178. Rather less drug is necessary, however, and for involvement of organs and tissues other than bones, 1 to 2 grams is usually sufficient.

2-Hydroxystilbamidine, administered intravenously, is probably less toxic than amphotericin B. It is a satisfactory alternative only in nonprogressive cutaneous disease. The usual dosage has been 225 mg per day and 8.0 grams per course of therapy.

Surgical drainage of abscesses is frequently indicated. Chemotherapy before and after surgery is advisable.

PROGNOSIS. Pulmonary infection of an inapparent or benign form occurs only rarely. Blastomycosis is, if untreated, a chronic and usually progressive disease. Cutaneous and other disseminated disease is eventually fatal in 10 to 30 per cent of cases.

Except with moribund patients chemotherapy usually effects a prompt recovery. Relapse requiring additional therapy has occurred, however, in at least 10 to 15 per cent of patients.

Lockwood, W. R., Allison, F. L., Batson, B. E., and Busey, J. F.: The treatment of North American blastomycosis: Ten years' experience. Am. Rev. Respir. Dis., 100:314, 1969.

Witorsch, P., and Utz, J. P.: North American blastomycosis. A study of 40 patients. Medicine, 47:169, 1969.

181. PARACOCCIDIOIDO-MYCOSIS

(South American Blastomycosis)

John P. Utz

DEFINITION. Paracoccidioidomycosis is a chronic systemic fungal disease, probably respiratory or gastrointestinal in origin, with dissemination to the lymph nodes, skin, lung, and other organs.

HISTORY. Lutz in 1908 first described the disease and the organism observed in tissues of a Brazilian patient. In 1909 and 1912, Splendore described more fully the characteristics of the disease and the fungus.

ETIOLOGY. The disease is caused by a dimorphic fungus, *Paracoccidioides brasiliensis*, which appears in tissues and exudates as a multiple-budding yeast 2 to 60 μ in diameter. The bud is characterized by a thin wall (0.2 to 1.0 μ) and narrow pore. At temperatures less than 30° C on Sabouraud's glucose medium, a white (later brown) membranous or wrinkled mycelium appears that microscopically is composed of branching hyphae and oval forms (conidia). Delayed cutaneous hypersensitivity and complement-fixing antigens have been demonstrated. Guinea pigs and mice can be experimentally infected.

EPIDEMIOLOGY. Except for reports of occasional immigrants to North America, the disease occurs exclusively in residents of Central and South America and is especially prevalent in Brazil. It is approximately ten times more frequent in males, and is slightly more frequent in persons 40 to 50 years of age. Manual laborers and farmers seem especially susceptible. Infection is probably acquired by the respiratory route, but a saprophytic, environmental source of fungi is not known. Disease in animals and animal-to-man or man-to-man spread are unknown. Widespread infection of a benign form has been suggested by skin test surveys.

PATHOLOGY. The histopathologic reaction to *P. brasiliensis* may be suppurative with abscess formation; in other sites it may be granulomatous with fibroblasts, macrophages, lymphocytes, caseation, and giant cells containing organisms. Lesions are seen in the mucosa of the gastrointestinal tract, lymph nodes, spleen, lungs, and liver.

CLINICAL FORMS. Primary. The primary lesion is commonly on the oral or nasal mucosa. Rarely, the conjunctival or anorectal mucosa may be involved. The earliest lesion is a papule that ulcerates and spreads to adjacent tissue.

Cutaneous Form. A variety of skin lesions may be seen, most of which progress to an ulcerative, crusted form suggestive of blastomycosis. In contrast, however, regional lymphadenopathy frequently accompanies skin lesions only in paracoccidioidomycosis. A keloidal form (Lobo's disease) of milder nature, without lymphadenopathy and caused by a different species (*Loboa loboi*) may be another type of paracoccidioidomycosis.

Lymphangitic Form. In this form there are lymphangitis and enlargement of regional lymph nodes, which suppurate and drain. Cervical and submandibular nodes are most commonly affected.

Visceral Form. The gastrointestinal tract is frequently involved as a primary site of infection. The spleen, adrenals, lungs, and liver may be affected by hematogenous spread. Bone, myocardium, and central nervous system involvement are less frequently seen.

DIAGNOSIS. The diagnosis is established by the culture and identification of *P. brasiliensis* and is only supported by positive skin and complement-fixation tests.

The disease must be differentiated from syphilis, tuberculous adenitis and skin disease, yaws, leishmaniasis, and other fungal infections.

TREATMENT. Amphotericin B (see Ch. 178) is the

drug of choice. Continuous sulfonamide therapy, still employed today, results in remission but not cure.

PROGNOSIS.   All forms of the disease are fatal if untreated. Over 90 per cent of cases are cured by amphotericin B.

Emmons, C. W., Binford, C. H., Utz, J. P., and Kwon-Chung, K. J.: Medical Mycology. 3rd ed. Philadelphia, Lea & Febiger, 1977.
Paracoccidioidomycosis. Scientific Publication No. 254. Washington, D.C., Pan American Health Organization, 1972.

182.   MADUROMYCOSIS

(Mycetoma, Madura Foot)

John P. Utz

DEFINITION.   Maduromycosis is a chronic systemic fungal disease that follows traumatic or imperceptible implantation of the skin. It is characterized by swelling, induration, suppuration, and draining sinuses of the skin, subcutaneous tissue, and bone, typically of the foot.

HISTORY.   The disease was first recognized and described in 1712 by Kaempfer in India, and was called Madura foot, after the city of that name. It has been suggested, however, that Madura foot was described by Sophocles in the hero of *Philoctetes*.

ETIOLOGY.   Many species of ten genera have been reported as etiologic agents; the most common of these have been *Madurella mycetomi*, *Nocardia brasiliensis*, and, in the United States, *Allescheria boydii*. In tissues or pus these fungi, except for *Nocardia* (see Ch. 164), are characterized by the appearance of "grains" of oval or irregular shape measuring 0.5 to 2.0 mm, and of white, red, black, or yellow color. Microscopically they are composed of 2 to 4 μ segmented, branched hyphae or round encysted forms (chlamydospores).

A. boydii grows rapidly on Sabouraud's glucose medium, forming a white (later gray or brown) cottony, aerial mycelium, which microscopically consists of thin hyphae to which are attached short or long stalks (conidiophores) bearing a single 8 to 10 by 5 to 7 μ pyriform or ovoid form (conidium). Large (50 to 200 μ) flask-shaped vessels containing asci and spores (4 to 7 μ) can be seen when material from the surface of agar is crushed and examined.

When inoculated intraperitoneally into mice, *A. boydii* is pathogenic, but progressive disease similar to that in humans has not been produced.

EPIDEMIOLOGY.   Although occasionally reported from temperate areas, the disease is seen most often in those tropical zones where few people wear shoes. The disease occurs chiefly in adults and more often in males. Most causative organisms are saprophytes of soil or plants. The disease has been reported in the dog, cow, and horse, but animal-to-man or man-to-man spread has not been reported.

PATHOLOGY.   The typical swollen foot has numerous draining sinuses communicating with abscesses of the skin, subcutaneous tissue, or bone. Drainage sites have characteristic collars of fibrous or epithelial tissues. Suppuration with epithelioid, plasma, and giant cells is intermingled with areas of fibrosis, and one or the other reaction may predominate. With Gram, hematoxylin and eosin, or periodic acid–Schiff stains, fungal cells may be seen either in pus or within macrophages or giant cells.

CLINICAL FORMS.   Although lesions have been reported on the leg, torso, hand, and face, the characteristic site of disease is the foot. The first manifestation consists of a papule, small nodule, indurated area with a vesicle, or an abscess that ruptures with sinus tract formation. Infection spreads and new nodules appear, leading to generalized swelling and distortion of the toes. Pain is infrequent, and there are few generalized symptoms. Roentgenographic examination may show lytic lesions with reaction and proliferation of the bone.

DIAGNOSIS.   Diagnosis is confirmed by the demonstration of granules in draining material, but the specific cause is dependent on isolation of the fungus in culture. Serologic and skin tests have not been developed for most of the responsible fungi. Maduromycosis must be distinguished from other fungal infections and from tuberculosis, yaws, neoplasms, and elephantiasis.

TREATMENT.   With the variety of antimicrobial agents available, each with specific activity, it is essential that definitive mycologic studies be done prior to treatment to determine the identity and, if feasible, the drug susceptibility of the causative fungus. The failure to do so in many past reports is undoubtedly a factor in the generally pessimistic attitude toward treatment and the early resort to amputation.

The drug of choice for infections caused by *Nocardia brasiliensis* is a sulfonamide (see Ch. 164), whereas for those caused by *Aspergillus,* amphotericin B is indicated (see Ch. 187). Tetracycline and diaminodiphenylsulfone have been reported to be successful in a few cases of *M. mycetomi* infections. Amphotericin B has been reported ineffective in two cases of *A. boydii* infection.

PROGNOSIS.   The disease is usually progressive and rarely self-limited.

Butz, W. C., and Ajello, L.: Black grain mycetoma. Arch. Dermatol., 104:197, 1971.
Rippon, J. W.: Medical Mycology. Philadelphia, W. B. Saunders Company, 1974.
Zeisler, E. B.: A case from Sophocles. Arch. Dermatol., 84:136, 1961.

183.   CHROMOMYCOSIS

John P. Utz

DEFINITION.   Chromomycosis is a chronic systemic fungal disease, acquired in the cutaneous form by traumatic or imperceptible implantation, and characterized by wartlike, ulcerated, crusted lesions of the skin and subcutaneous tissues.

HISTORY.   Although rare in this country, chromomycosis was first reported from Boston in 1915, separately by Lane and Medlar, and the organism responsible was named *Phialophora verrucosa* by Thaxter. Subsequently, cases caused by other genera of fungi were described by Brumpt and Carrion.

ETIOLOGY.   A number of fungi have been incriminated, but chiefly *Phialophora verrucosa*, *P. pedrosoi*, *P. compactum*, and *Cladosporium carrioni*. In tissues these fungi resemble each other and appear as single or clustered, round, thick-walled, 6 to 12 μ budding cells of a striking brown color, from which the disease draws its name. On culture, mycelia are produced that vary according to genus and species. Skin hypersensitivity and complement-fixing antigens have been demonstrated in some fungal species. Laboratory animals are susceptible to experimental infection, but the equivalent of natural disease in man is not produced.

EPIDEMIOLOGY. The disease is seen more often in adult males in the rural areas of the tropics, especially in Brazil, Puerto Rico, and Cuba. The responsible fungi are saprophytes of soil, but are found more often in decaying wood and vegetation. Infection in animals has not been reported, and animal-to-man or man-to-man spread is unknown.

PATHOLOGY. Varying degrees of hyperkeratoses, acanthosis, and pseudoepitheliomatous hyperplasia are seen. In the cutis the reaction may be granulomatous with mononuclear, epithelioid, and Langhans' giant cells. Fungal cells are seen readily with hematoxylin and eosin stains.

CLINICAL FORMS. Chromomycosis is a disease of the skin and subcutaneous tissue.

The first patient reported had lesions of the buttock. The most common site is the lower extremity. The disease appears also, in descending order of frequency, on the hand, forearm, arm, neck, and shoulders. The earliest lesion is a nodule or pustule that, over a period of weeks to months, ulcerates, drains, enlarges, dries, and becomes violaceous and wartlike. There is rarely pain, but itching is common. Lesions do not spread generally, but scratching results in autoinoculation and satellite or secondary distal lesions.

DIAGNOSIS. Although older typical skin lesions may be clinically and histologically suggestive, the diagnosis is confirmed by the culture and identification of the causative fungus.

Early lesions may be confused with blastomycosis, tuberculosis, leprosy, yaws, and syphilis.

TREATMENT. Surgical resection of early skin lesions has been the most common and efficacious therapy. Amputation has been required in a small number of cases. Most of the fungi causing chromomycosis are resistant to amphotericin B, but successful treatment has been reported in two cases when the drug was injected locally into the skin. This drug needs further trial in this disease.

PROGNOSIS. The cutaneous form of chromomycosis is chronic and compatible with long life (in one case, 40 years).

Al-Doory, Y.: Chromomycosis. Missoula, Montana, Mountain Press, 1972.

184. CRYPTOCOCCOSIS

(European Blastomycosis, Torulosis)

John E. Bennett

DEFINITION. Cryptococcosis is a systemic fungal infection, its most common and most lethal manifestation being meningoencephalitis.

HISTORY. Busse, who reported the first case in 1894, observed the fungus in tissue and isolated the causative agent. That same year Sanfelice isolated from peach juice the same fungus, naming it *Saccharomyces hominis*. The fungus received no less than 37 additional names until 1952, when Lodder and Kreger-Van Rij's monumental taxonomic study of yeast gave the fungus its current name, *Cryptococcus neoformans*. The fungus was rarely isolated from natural sources until 1955, when Emmons demonstrated that *C. neoformans* was a frequent saprophyte in weathered pigeon droppings. This lent support to the emerging concept that the disease was acquired by inhalation of fungus-laden dust. The discovery of amphotericin B, reported by Gold and co-workers in 1956, was to provide the first successful chemotherapy of cryptococcosis.

ETIOLOGY. Cryptococcosis is caused by *Cryptococcus neoformans,* a round or oval yeastlike fungus measuring 4 to 7 μ in diameter. It reproduces by budding. This fungus is unique among systemic mycoses of man in that it is highly encapsulated in tissue. The polysaccharide capsule releases into the host the soluble antigen which provides a means of serologic diagnosis. The fungus can be isolated as a smooth, creamy white colony on a variety of common laboratory media. Culture identification is by gross and microscopic appearance, biochemical reactions, and growth at 37° C.

EPIDEMIOLOGY. The disease is sporadic throughout the world, with no clear focal outbreaks in man or sharply defined areas of high endemicity. Disease occurs occasionally in warm-blooded feral and domestic animals, excluding birds. Cryptococcal mastitis may spread through dairy herds, probably by way of milking machines, and contaminate unpasteurized milk. No spread of infection from animal to man or man to man has been reported. Reservoir of infection is probably saprophytic sources in nature, such as weathered pigeon droppings. Presumed portal of entry is the lung, although this site is often clinically inapparent. The fungus is not a part of the normal flora of man or animals, although occasionally it appears to colonize a patient's damaged bronchial tree. No occupational group is known to be predisposed to cryptococcosis. Infection is uncommon before puberty and is more frequent in males. Predisposing factors include Hodgkin's disease, lymphoma, leukemia, sarcoidosis, and supraphysiologic doses of adrenal corticosteroids.

PATHOLOGY. The most frequent and characteristic abnormality on gross examination occurs in the brain, which shows basilar arachnoiditis and focal collections of small, glistening, gelatinous cysts, particularly in the cortical gray matter and basal ganglia. Microscopic examination reveals the cysts to be clumps of cryptococci, with little surrounding inflammation. A dense inflammatory response to the fungus may be noted in meninges or brain but is more characteristic of extraneural lesions. Cellular response consists of macrophages, giant cells, and lymphocytes. Necrosis is seen occasionally at the center of a dense inflammatory response, particularly in the lung. Features notable for their infrequency include polymorphonuclear leukocytes, calcification, extensive scarring, and hemorrhage.

CLINICAL MANIFESTATIONS. Meningoencephalitis. Symptoms begin with the insidious onset of headache, followed by nausea, vomiting, blurred vision, or decreased mental acuity. Less frequent symptoms include photophobia, diplopia, and gait ataxia. Gradually the patient becomes lethargic and prefers to remain undisturbed. Somnolence or irritability may appear. Fever is low grade or absent. Although no one physical finding is highly frequent or characteristic, examination may disclose papilledema, mild to moderate nuchal rigidity, cranial nerve palsies, or extensor plantar response.

Extraneural Cryptococcosis. Pulmonary cryptococcosis is the second most common clinical manifestation. Even patients with no clinically apparent pneumonitis but with cryptococcosis elsewhere in the body are often found to have a pulmonary focus on careful postmortem examination or sometimes on sputum culture. Chest symptoms and radiologic findings, when present, commonly mimic primary or metastatic carcinoma in the lung. Pleural effusions, cavitation, and hilar adenopathy are not common. Skin lesions occur in 10 per cent of patients with cryptococcosis, and bone lesions occur in about 5 per cent. Either may be the sole clinical manifestation of the infection or may be associated with disease in other organs. Skin lesions begin as asymptomatic papules, pustules, or soft subcutaneous nodules. They tend to become painful as they slowly enlarge, ulcerate, and drain glary pus. Osteolytic lesions may appear in almost any bone and present as a cold abscess. Rare clinical manifestations include prostatitis, hepatitis, endocarditis, pericarditis, renal abscess, and endophthalmitis.

DIAGNOSIS. Lumbar puncture in patients with symptomatic cryptococcal meningoencephalitis usually reveals one or more of the following abnormalities: elevated opening pressure, pleocytosis predominantly composed of mononuclear cells, increased protein concentration, and hypoglycorrhachia. A smear of cerebrospinal fluid sediment, mixed with India ink, reveals encapsulated yeast in about half the cases. The smear may be difficult to interpret and provides only a tentative, albeit useful, diagnosis. Another rapid diagnostic aid is serologic detection of cryptococcal antigen in serum and cerebrospinal fluid. With current techniques, about 90 per cent of patients with cryptococcal meningitis have detectable antigen if both sites are tested. Extraneural cryptococcosis may result in serum antigen if infection is extensive. A falling antigen titer during recovery is a favorable prognostic sign.

Final diagnosis depends upon culture or biopsy. Several milliliters of cerebrospinal fluid should be cultured for cryptococci in cases of indolent meningoencephalitis and also in every case of documented extraneural cryptococcosis, in order to detect subclinical extension to the central nervous system. The frequency of subclinical renal infection in disseminated cryptococcosis makes urine culture useful. Sputum, blood, prostatic fluid, and pus from cutaneous lesions may also yield the fungus. Biopsy may be required to diagnose cryptococcosis in the lung, skin, or bone. Histologic diagnosis can usually be made with accuracy by those experienced in this area.

THERAPY. Intravenous amphotericin B is the treatment of choice for cryptococcosis of the central nervous system. Treatment should be continued for at least four weeks after all weekly cultures become negative. 5-Fluorocytosine therapy cures some cases of cryptococcosis, but drug resistance often arises during therapy. Combination therapy, using 5-fluorocytosine and low-dose intravenous amphotericin B, is probably better than amphotericin B alone in cryptococcal meningitis, but experience is required to avoid serious toxic reactions to 5-fluorocytosine. Intrathecal amphotericin B may be a useful adjunct in patients failing an adequate trial of intravenous therapy or with such poor renal function

that reduced doses of intravenous amphotericin B are obligatory. Development of communicating or noncommunicating hydrocephalus may require neurosurgical intervention.

Intravenous amphotericin B is the usual treatment of choice for extraneural cryptococcosis. A probable exception is the patient without either hematologic malignancy or immunosuppressive therapy who, on thorough study, has infection confined to one focus in lung, skin, or bone. Surgical excision of skin or lung lesions, curettage of bone lesions, or simply prolonged observation may be warranted if the lesion is not extensive and is stable or regressing.

PROGNOSIS. Cryptococcal meningoencephalitis is invariably fatal unless treated. With currently available therapy, the case fatality rate is about 25 per cent. Patients with Hodgkin's disease, lymphoma, or leukemia or who require continued immunosuppressive therapy fare less well. Death usually results from the sequelae of coma or from brainstem compression. Despite successful therapy, patients may be left with optic atrophy, hydrocephalus, personality changes, or decreased mental acuity.

Diamond, R. D., and Bennett, J. E.: Prognostic factors in cryptococcal meningitis. Ann. Intern. Med., 80:176, 1974.
Fetter, B. F., Klintworth, G. K., and Hendry, W. S.: Mycoses of the Central Nervous System. Baltimore, Williams & Wilkins Company, 1967.
Salfelder, K.: Cryptococcosis. In Baker, R. E. (ed.): Human Infections with Fungi, Actinomycetes and Algae. New York, Springer-Verlag, 1971, pp. 383–464.

185. SPOROTRICHOSIS

John P. Utz

DEFINITION. Sporotrichosis is a chronic systemic fungal disease, acquired usually by traumatic implantation and localized to cutaneous lymphatic tissues, or rarely by the respiratory route with dissemination throughout the body.

HISTORY. From a patient at Johns Hopkins Hospital, in 1896 Schenck isolated a fungus that was identified by E. F. Smith as *Sporotrichum*; it was named *Sporotrichum schenckii* by Hektoen and Perkins in 1900. A great number of cases were seen subsequently in France, and more than 2800 cases in a single epidemic in the gold mines of South Africa.

ETIOLOGY. *Sporothrix schenckii*, a dimorphic fungus, is occasionally observed in tissues as round to cigar-shaped yeast- or bacteria-like forms. On Sabouraud's glucose medium at room temperature, a white, cottony, aerial mycelium appears that in three to seven days becomes wrinkled and changes in color from cream to black. Microscopically, branching, septate hyphae are seen, 2 μ in width, bearing directly or on lateral branches ovoid to spherical bodies (conidia) measuring 2 to 4 by 2 to 6 μ in diameter. Mice are susceptible to experimental infection. Delayed cutaneous hypersensitivity and agglutinogen antigens have been demonstrated.

EPIDEMIOLOGY. The disease is worldwide in distribution; it has appeared epidemically in South Africa and in localized outbreaks in Mexico and Florida. It is more common in men. It frequently affects laborers, farmers, and florists and is considered a true occupational disease. The fungus exists in its saprophytic form in soil, peat moss, and decaying vegetation and on thorns. In the cutaneous lymphatic forms, infection results from accidental implantation into the skin. In disseminated forms, the mode of entry is probably respiratory. Spontaneous sporotrichosis has been reported in dogs, horses, mules, cats, and other animals, and human disease has resulted from animal contact. Direct transfer from man to man is not known to occur.

PATHOLOGY. The histopathologic reaction to *S. schenckii* is varied, frequently acute and suppurative, but also subacute or chronic. In some instances granulomas are seen with epithelioid and giant cells either diffusely distributed or localized in a typical tubercle. Fungi may be seen more readily after staining with a modified Schiff-MacManus technique.

CLINICAL FORMS. Cutaneous Lymphatic Form. The earliest lesion is a pustule, papule, or nodule of the skin appearing characteristically on a finger and at a site where the patient may recall an earlier, seemingly insignificant scratch or prick. The nodule enlarges, becomes red to violaceous, and is followed by a chain of subcutaneous nodules along regional lymphatics. These are at first freely movable, but become attached to the skin, and may ulcerate and drain a thin gray to yellow pus. Streaking and pain characteristic of acute lymphangitis are not present. Generalized symptoms are rare.

Other Forms. Other forms may appear secondary to the cutaneous lymphatic lesion either by direct extension to contiguous, subcutaneous tissue, bone, and joint or by hematogenous spread to distant sites. Sometimes the original site of infection is inapparent, and the disease presents as a septic arthritis or osteomyelitis. Less frequently, there may be involvement of the eye, gastrointestinal tract, central nervous system, or skin. In disseminated disease, systemic symptoms of fever, weight loss, inanition, malaise, pain at sites of lesion, anemia, and leukocytosis are commonly present. Two forms of pulmonary disease are now recognized. The more common is chronic cavitary, resembling tuberculosis. The other is less chronic, resolves spontaneously, and is characterized by hilar lymphadenopathy with a sparing of lung parenchyma.

DIAGNOSIS. Although the diagnosis may seem readily apparent in the cutaneous lymphatic form of disease, the clinical impression is confirmed by the culture and identification of the fungus. Agglutination or complement-fixation serologic and skin tests may be helpful, but are not generally available.

Cutaneous lymphatic sporotrichosis must be distinguished from tularemia, pyoderma of bacterial origin, and other fungal infections. Disseminated disease resembles tuberculosis, staphylococcal osteomyelitis, or neoplastic disease.

TREATMENT. The cutaneous lymphatic form of disease responds slowly but progressively to the oral administration of iodides in the form of a saturated solution (1 gram per milliliter) of potassium iodide given in dosage of 4 to 5 ml three times daily. Treatment should be prolonged one to two months beyond the time of apparent healing.

Disseminated disease, especially of bone and joints, is frequently resistant to iodide therapy. Dramatic improvement has been seen in a few patients treated with amphotericin B, and for this form of disease this drug is recommended.

PROGNOSIS. Untreated cutaneous lymphatic sporotrichosis may persist for many months to years. Treated lesions respond slowly but completely. Disseminated disease is progressive and usually fatal unless treated.

Baum, G. L., Donnerberg, R. L., Stewart, D., Mulligan, W. J., and Putnam, L. R.: Pulmonary sporotrichosis. N. Engl. J. Med. 280:410, 1969.

Crout, J. E., Brewer, N. S., and Tompkins, R. B.: Sporotrichosis arthritis. Ann. Intern. Med., 86:294, 1977.

Wilson, D. E., Mann, J. J., Bennett, J. E., and Utz, J. P.: Clinical features of extracutaneous sporotrichosis. Medicine, 46:265, 1967.

186. MUCORMYCOSIS

John E. Bennett

DEFINITION. Mucormycosis is an acute, often fatal infection caused by fungi of the order Mucorales. Phycomycosis is a term which encompasses mucormycosis and several other mycoses.

HISTORY. Two cases of pulmonary mucormycosis reported by Fürbringer in 1876 were probably the first cases described with enough clarity to permit any confidence in the diagnosis. It was not until 1943 that Gregory described mucormycosis originating in nose and paranasal sinuses.

ETIOLOGY. *Rhizopus* and *Mucor* species are the principal pathogens of mucormycosis. These fungi appear in tissue as hyphae 6 to 50 μ wide, rarely septate, irregular in contour, and tending to branch at nearly right angles. Hyphae may be demonstrated histologically by staining with hematoxylin and eosin, Gomori methenamine silver, or periodic acid–Schiff. Growth at 25 or 37° C is profuse and rapidly spreading on most media. Identification of the culture is based largely on microscopic appearance. Only very specialized laboratories are competent to pursue identification beyond a tentative designation of genus.

EPIDEMIOLOGY. Mucormycosis is uncommon and sporadic around the world, usually afflicting patients with serious pre-existing disease. *Mucormycosis of the paranasal sinuses and contiguous structures occurs predominantly in patients with poorly controlled diabetes mellitus.* Pulmonary and disseminated mucormycosis also occurs occasionally in diabetics but is most prevalent in immunosuppressed patients, particularly treated leukemics. Among the varied underlying disorders present in patients with gastrointestinal mucormycosis, uremia, severe malnutrition, and diarrheal diseases seem prominent. Mucormycosis occurs at any age, with no strong predilection for race or sex. It does not spread from man to man. Disease is probably acquired by inhalation of fungal spores. Mucorales are ubiquitous in the environment, growing on decaying vegetation, dung, and foods of high sugar content.

PATHOLOGY. Necrosis is the predominant gross and microscopic finding. This is accounted for in part by the propensity of hyphae to proliferate within small and medium-sized arteries, producing thrombosis. Infarcted areas may be ischemic or hemorrhagic. Neutrophils predominate in the inflammatory response.

CLINICAL MANIFESTATIONS. Mucormycosis originating in the nose and paranasal sinuses produces a characteristic clinical entity. Initial symptoms mimic bacterial sinusitis, with low-grade fever and sinus pain. However, nasal discharge is not purulent but is thin and sometimes blood streaked. Over the next few days, infection spreads to contiguous structures. Invasion of the orbit may lead to reduced range of ocular motion, proptosis, chemosis, or blurred vision. Direct invasion of the globe or thrombosis of the ophthalmic artery may occur. Nasal turbinates or hard palate develop areas which are black, friable, and bloodless. Frontal or temporal lobes of the brain may be infected by direct extension, producing headache and deepening stupor. Invasion of the carotid artery within the cavernous sinus may cause embolization, mycotic aneurysm, or thrombosis. Without treatment, the patient usually dies in coma a few days to a few weeks from onset.

Pulmonary mucormycosis presents as a rapidly progressive dense bronchopneumonia, accompanied by high fever, toxicity, and tachypnea, but with little cough or sputum. The necrotic central portion of a lesion is sometimes expectorated, producing hyphae in sputum and a cavity on chest x-ray. Gastrointestinal lesions of mucormycosis begin as one or more shallow ulcerations in esophagus, stomach, or intestine. The ulcer tends to enlarge, deepen, and perforate the viscus. Disseminated mucormycosis may originate in nasal area, lung, or gastrointestinal tract. Sometimes no portal is evident. Hematogenous spread may involve brain or other organs. Pulmonary and disseminated mucormycosis are clinically indistinguishable from invasive aspergillosis.

DIAGNOSIS. *Cranial mucormycosis* is easily mistaken for bacterial sinusitis with cavernous sinus thrombosis. The diagnosis requires biopsy of infected mucosa in the nose or sinus. Hyphae are often abundant on histologic section or wet smear of crushed tissue. Hyphae seen in cross-section may be mistaken for yeast. Occasionally hyphae are confused with capillaries, or vice versa.

Pulmonary and disseminated infections caused by Mucorales, *Aspergillus,* and *Pseudomonas aeruginosa* have many similarities. Diagnosis of mucormycosis, like that of aspergillosis, requires biopsy. In the proper clinical setting, demonstration of broad, nonseptate hyphae in bronchial brush specimens or sputum would be strongly suggestive. Culture of biopsy specimens is certainly of interest, but isolation of a ubiquitous organism like Mucorales must be interpreted with caution. Blood cultures are very rarely positive for the fungus.

TREATMENT. Mucormycosis originating in the nose and paranasal areas should be treated by optimal regulation of diabetes mellitus, extensive surgical debridement, and intravenous amphotericin B. After debridement, sinus cavities can be irrigated daily with amphotericin B, 1 mg per milliliter. Although good guidelines for dose and duration of intravenous amphotericin B are not available, it has been customary to treat vigorously at least until disease progression halts. Treatment should probably continue for another month beyond that. Tomograms of the orbit and sinuses can be very helpful in evaluating disease progression. Carotid arteriogram may demonstrate extension to the ophthalmic artery or carotid siphon. Electroencephalogram and lumbar puncture provide late evidence of intracranial extension.

Intravenous amphotericin B is probably useful in other forms of mucormycosis, but too few patients have been treated for this question to be answered.

PROGNOSIS. A substantial number of cures have been reported recently in mucormycosis of the nose, sinus, and orbit. Prognosis is poor once central nervous

system signs appear. Other forms of mucormycosis have largely been diagnosed post mortem.

Baker, R. D.: Mucormycosis. *In* Human Infection with Fungi, Actinomycetes and Algae, New York, Springer-Verlag, 1971, pp. 832–918.

Bartrum, R. J., Watnick, M., and Herman, P. G.: Roentgenographic findings in pulmonary mucormycosis. Am. J. Roentgenol., 117:810, 1973.

Meyer, R. D., and Armstrong, D.: Mucormycosis — changing status. Crit. Rev. Clin. Lab. Sci., 4:421, 1973.

Price, D. L., Wolpow, E. R., and Richardson, E. P.: Intracranial phycomycosis: A clinicopathological and radiologic study. J. Neurol. Sci., 14:359, 1971.

187. ASPERGILLOSIS

John E. Bennett

DEFINITION. The term aspergillosis embraces a variety of diseases which have in common growth of the fungus *Aspergillus* in tissue or within air-containing spaces of the body, such as bronchus or pulmonary cavity.

HISTORY. Micheli first described the genus *Aspergillus* in 1729. The first case of aspergillosis in man was probably observed by Sluyter in 1847, although disease in birds had been reported before then. In 1856 Virchow reviewed the literature and reported four autopsied cases. Renon's classic paper of 1897 attracted attention to the disease.

ETIOLOGY. The etiologic agent *Aspergillus* is a fungus largely composed of septate hyphae about 4 μ in diameter. Sporulating structures, called conidial heads, may be seen when the fungus is growing in nature, on artificial medium, or within air-containing spaces of the body. The most frequent pathogen for man is *Aspergillus fumigatus*. However, many other species can clearly cause either invasive or noninvasive disease in man, particularly *Aspergillus flavus*. Aspergilli grow rapidly on many routine laboratory media and, because of their ubiquity, are encountered in the laboratory as airborne contaminants. Identification is by gross and microscopic appearance.

EPIDEMIOLOGY. Aspergilli are often found growing on decaying vegetation. Under proper conditions millions of spores, about 2 to 4 μ in diameter, may be released into the air. Inhalation of these spores must be a common event, but disease is infrequent. Both insects and animals may acquire aspergillosis. The disease is an economically important cause of mycotic abortion in cattle and horses. In man the disease is sporadic and worldwide, with no clear occupational predisposition. Transmission from animal to man or man to man has not been encountered.

PATHOLOGY. The fungus is capable of eliciting a wide variety of tissue responses, depending upon site and host. A ball of hyphae may be situated within an ectatic bronchus or epithelialized lung cavity and provoke little or no histologic response. During invasion of tissue in a markedly immunosuppressed host, blood vessel invasion by hyphae, thrombosis, necrosis, and hemorrhagic infarction are prominent features. In invasion of more normal tissue, a pyogenic necrotic reaction is common, but epithelioid granulomas with giant cells may be observed instead. Chronic, fibrosing, nonnecrotizing granulomatous inflammation has typically been seen in the paranasal sinus and orbit.

Inhalation of *Aspergillus* spores may provoke an allergic response without invasion of the body, but this condition will not be considered here. Certain aspergilli, given proper growth conditions, produce proteolytic enzymes or toxins. As far as is known, these substances play no important role in aspergillosis.

CLINICAL MANIFESTATIONS. Pulmonary Aspergillosis. *Aspergillus* can colonize ectatic bronchi, cysts, or cavities in the lung. Colonization is usually a sequel of a chronic inflammatory process, such as tuberculosis, bronchiectasis, histoplasmosis, or sarcoidosis. A ball of hyphae may form within an air-containing space, particularly in the upper lobes, and is termed an aspergilloma. The fungus rarely invades the wall of the cavity, cyst, or bronchus in such patients. During bacterial pneumonia, lung abscess, or empyema in a colonized patient, *Aspergillus* may appear in the inflammatory process, although its role is uncertain. In most patients it is difficult to determine clinically whether specific symptoms or signs of disease progression are due to the underlying condition or to some allergic, inflammatory, or obstructive process caused by *Aspergillus*. The most common symptoms are chronic productive cough and hemoptysis. *Aspergillus* can cause chronic pneumonia in patients with chronic granulomatous disease of childhood or, rarely, in previously healthy persons. In a few instances, acute bilateral pneumonia has occurred in normal persons, usually after a presumed massive inhalation of spores. However, the majority of patients with invasive aspergillosis now being encountered are markedly neutropenic or are receiving immunosuppressive therapy, or both. A patch of pneumonia appears and steadily becomes larger and denser. The lesion may remain focal or, at any time, may spread hematogenously to one or more sites in the lung, brain, or other organs. The lung lesion may also erode directly through the diaphragm or pericardium.

Lesions of Extrapulmonary Origin. Necrotizing lesions originating in the palate, paranasal sinuses, epiglottis, or gastrointestinal tract may occur in the immunosuppressed patient. *Aspergillus* may infect intracardiac or intravascular prostheses. Chronic granulomatous inflammation may originate in the paranasal sinuses and spread to orbit or brain. Progressive mycotic keratitis caused by *Aspergillus* may follow corneal trauma. Growth of *Aspergillus* on cerumen and detritus within the external auditory canal is termed otomycosis.

DIAGNOSIS. Culture of *Aspergillus* from sputum usually has no clinical significance. Repeated isolation of *Aspergillus* from sputum or demonstration of hyphae on sputum smear suggests endobronchial colonization. Precipitins to *Aspergillus* antigens are often demonstrable in the sera of such colonized patients. Radiologic appearance of an aspergilloma is distinctive. In the severely immunosuppressed patient, isolation of *Aspergillus* from even a single sputum should raise suspicion of possible invasive infection. Biopsy is usually required to diagnose invasive aspergillosis in lung, paranasal sinus, orbit, or brain. Histology may provide evidence of tissue invasion and permit a presumptive diagnosis of aspergillosis. For absolute confirmation and determination of species, the biopsy should be cultured. Neither serologic tests nor cultures of blood, cerebrospinal fluid, or urine are helpful in most forms of invasive aspergillosis.

TREATMENT. Surgical excision may be helpful in fungus ball of the lung or in aspergillosis of the parana-

sal sinus and orbit. Measures to improve bronchopulmonary drainage may assist the patient with endobronchial colonization. Intravenous amphotericin B is not helpful in endobronchial or endocavitary aspergillosis, but in invasive pulmonary aspergillosis a prolonged course of treatment will occasionally arrest progression. Ultimate cure of invasive pulmonary aspergillosis requires not only intravenous amphotericin B but also significant restoration of the host's defense mechanisms.

PROGNOSIS. Endobronchial or endocavitary aspergillosis rarely becomes invasive or disseminated. Although the condition is not usually the sole cause of death, it may contribute problems to an already damaged lung. Cure is infrequent in invasive aspergillosis of the lung, heart, paranasal sinus, orbit, or brain.

Green, W. R., Font, R. L., and Zimmerman, L. E.: Aspergillosis of the orbit. Arch. Ophthalmol., 82:302, 1969.
Kilman, J. W., Ahn, C., Andrews, N. C., and Klassen, K.: Surgery for pulmonary aspergillosis. J. Thorac. Cardiovasc. Surg., 57:642, 1969.
Young, R. C., Bennett, J. E., Vogel, C., Carbone, P. P., and DeVita, V. T.: Aspergillosis. Spectrum of the disease in 98 patients. Medicine, 49:147, 1970.

188. CANDIDIASIS

(Candidosis, Moniliasis, Thrush)

John E. Bennett

DEFINITION. Candidiasis is an infection of the skin, mucous membranes, or viscera caused by species of *Candida*, a yeastlike fungus. Thrush refers to candidiasis of mucous membranes, as in the mouth or vagina.

HISTORY. Thrush as a clinical entity has been appreciated for centuries, but its relationship to fungi was unknown until Langenbeck isolated the pathogen from a patient's throat in 1839. Among the many names applied to this fungus, the most significant have been *Oidium albicans* (given by Robin in 1853), *Monilia albicans* (Zopf, 1890), and *Candida albicans* (Berkhout, 1923).

ETIOLOGY. *Candida albicans* is the usual cause of candidiasis. A substantial number of cases of disseminated candidiasis have been caused by other species of *Candida*, particularly *C. tropicalis* and *C. parapsilosis*. The size and shape of *Candida* cells are variable, but most commonly the cells are oval and 4 to 6 μ in their longest axis. Growth usually appears within a few days of incubation at 25 or 37° C. Deep inoculation into certain media, such as corn meal Tween 80 agar, causes *Candida* to grow as long tubules called pseudohyphae. Individual species of *Candida* are distinguished by their ability to utilize or ferment certain sugars. For routine laboratory purposes, *C. albicans* can be identified by its ability to form chlamydospores or, in the presence of serum, to form germ tubes. *Candida* species look very similar in infected tissue, but usually can be distinguished from other fungi. *Candida* generally, but not always, grows in tissue as both budding yeast and pseudohyphae. Both tissue forms are well demonstrated by Gomori methenamine silver, periodic acid–Schiff, or tissue Gram stains.

EPIDEMIOLOGY. *C. albicans* is a frequent commensal in the human mouth, gastrointestinal tract, and vagina.

Candida is also commonly isolated from the gut of animals. Isolation of this fungus from the environment is unusual, and most of the exceptions could have represented contamination by animals or man. This leads to the presumption that the fungus is spread from man to man and animal to animal. It is usually impossible to trace this spread, because colonization is asymptomatic. A probable exception is the newborn infant, in whom colonization usually leads to oral thrush. Later in life, disease seems to occur when a previously colonized patient becomes more vulnerable to tissue invasion. A wide variety of conditions predispose to candidiasis, particularly diabetes mellitus and therapy with either broad-spectrum antimicrobials or adrenal corticosteroids. Chronic maceration predisposes to cutaneous candidiasis, as in paronychia of bartenders and housewives, intertrigo of obese patients, or diaper rash. Women in the later months of pregnancy are particularly susceptible to vulvovaginal candidiasis. Patients with acute leukemia are prone to gastrointestinal and systemic candidiasis. An important route for acquiring systemic candidiasis is through unsterile intravenous injections of narcotics or through use of plastic intravenous catheters. When the infusion through the catheter is designed to meet the patient's total caloric requirement, the risk of systemic candidiasis goes even higher.

PATHOLOGY. In mucocutaneous candidiasis, pseudohyphae and yeast tend to be confined to the epithelium. Leukocytes infiltrate the epithelium as well as the submucosa or corium. Parakeratosis is usual. Ulceration and hyphal invasion of the submucosa is a more frequent characteristic of gastrointestinal candidiasis. In systemic candidiasis, abscesses may be found in almost any organ, but kidney, brain, spleen, heart, and liver are frequent sites. Such abscesses on gross inspection may appear as small, white, firm, cheesy nodules. Histologically these foci show necrosis, leukocytes, pseudohyphae, and yeast. Giant cells are seen occasionally. In the immunosuppressed patient, inflammatory cells may be scanty or absent. Patients with plastic intravenous catheters may develop at the catheter tip an endovenous fibrin sleeve containing *Candida*. Presumably, this can continue to seed the bloodstream for several days after withdrawal of the catheter.

CLINICAL MANIFESTATIONS. The mouth is the most common site of candidiasis. *Oral thrush* is usually an acute, self-limiting disease which presents as discrete and confluent white plaques on the oral and pharyngeal mucosa. The plaque is a pseudomembrane which can be scraped off with difficulty, exposing a red base. *Candida denture stomatitis* is characterized by well-circumscribed areas of erythema and edema in the mucosa under the upper dentures. *Candida* also appears to cause chronic hyperplastic oral lesions resembling leukoplakia. All the aforementioned oral lesions tend to be asymptomatic. *Cutaneous candidiasis* can present as diaper rash, red macerated areas in large skin folds, fissuring and desquamation in interdigital areas, angular cheilitis, paronychia, balanitis, or pruritus ani. *Chronic mucocutaneous candidiasis*, also called *Candida granuloma*, is an uncommon disease, usually beginning in early childhood, in which hyperkeratotic lesions wax and wane in the skin and mucous membranes for many years. The most severe skin lesions occur on the face, scalp, and hands. Involvement of mouth, vagina, and nails is usual. Children with this disorder frequently seem to have defective function of thymus-derived lymphocytes and tend to develop hypofunction of the parathyroid, thyroid, and adrenal glands.

The most common symptom of *Candida vaginitis* is pruritus. Other frequent symptoms include discharge and burning pain, the latter being worse on urination or intercourse. Speculum examination reveals an inflamed vaginal mucosa and a thin exudate, sometimes with white curds. Within the gastrointestinal tract, the *esophagus* is the most common site of candidiasis and the only site likely to be symptomatic. Substernal burning and either pain or a sense of obstruction on swallowing may occur. Blood-borne *Candida abscesses* are usually manifest only as fever and toxicity. Hematogenous dissemination to the choroid is detected on funduscopic examination as fluffy white retinal exudates. The abscesses gradually enlarge and extend into the vitreous humor, which becomes increasingly hazy. Cells and flare may also appear in the anterior chamber. The most common symptoms are orbital or retro-orbital pain, blurring, scotoma, and opacities floating across the visual field. *Candidiasis of the endocardium* or around the edges of an intracardiac prosthesis resembles bacterial infections in these sites. *Candida meningitis* clinically mimics cryptococcosis. *Pulmonary and renal candidiasis* are usually hematogenous in origin and cause no focal symptoms. Extensive renal cortical abscesses may cause azotemia. *Candidiasis in the lining of the bladder or renal pelvis* usually appears in a diabetic patient with chronic or recurrent bacterial urinary tract infections or after instrumentation or surgery on the urinary tract. Dysuria, pyuria, and passage of pseudohyphae in the urine are frequent findings. Rarely, pseudohyphae will be found packed in a necrotic renal papilla. A sloughed papilla, largely then a ball of fungus, may obstruct a ureter.

DIAGNOSIS. Demonstration of pseudohyphae on smear with confirmation by culture is the procedure of choice for diagnosing candidiasis of epithelial surfaces. Scrapings for this purpose may be made of skin, oral mucosa, vagina, or nails. Cerebrospinal fluid and joint fluid cultures are helpful in diagnosing *Candida* meningitis or arthritis. Progression of funduscopic findings usually permits an operational diagnosis of *Candida* endophthalmitis. Esophagram and esophagoscopy can aid the diagnosis of *Candida* esophagitis. Biopsy is required to diagnose candidiasis of lung or liver. Blood cultures are very useful in diagnosing *Candida* endocarditis but are less commonly positive in other forms of systemic candidiasis. The fungus can be isolated from blood, using the same routine media employed for bacteria, but one to three weeks of incubation are often required and the bottles should be vented. Rarely, *Candida* is seen on blood smear. Skin tests with *Candida* antigens are so commonly positive in normal people that they are not useful in diagnosing candidiasis. Diagnostic interpretation of serologic tests for candidiasis remains controversial.

TREATMENT. Oral thrush is best treated by rinsing the mouth with and then swallowing nystatin suspension, 100,000 units four times daily. Painting the lesions with 1 per cent aqueous gentian violet is a messy but effective alternative. Vaginal thrush usually responds to deep insertion of a nystatin vaginal suppository once or twice daily for two weeks. Cutaneous candidiasis of macerated areas requires measures to keep the skin dry plus topical nystatin or amphotericin B. Mild symptoms of *Candida* esophagitis may respond to the patient's sucking on a nystatin suppository three or four times daily. With pronounced esophageal symptoms, a short course of intravenous amphotericin B is more beneficial. Bladder thrush may be eradicated by bladder irrigation with amphotericin B, 50 μg per milliliter. If a Foley catheter is not in place, oral 5-fluorocytosine is an alternative. Isolation of *Candida* from blood may or may not indicate the need for intravenous amphotericin B. If the patient is febrile and severely immunosuppressed, a single positive blood culture for *Candida* is generally an indication for prompt chemotherapy. All too often the patient dies before additional blood cultures are reported positive. In the patient who is not immunosuppressed, significance of candidemia depends upon the number of positive cultures and the presence or absence of a plastic intravenous catheter. Multiple positive blood cultures in the absence of such a catheter indicate the need for chemotherapy. In the presence of such a catheter, discovery of candidemia should prompt removal of the catheter and culturing of its tip. If the patient is not seriously ill and is improving, treatment may be postponed to await clinical progress and the results of subsequent blood cultures. The species of *Candida* isolated is irrelevant to the decision about therapy. Temporization is inappropriate when endocarditis, endophthalmitis, arthritis, or other hematogenous lesions are detect-

ed. Systemic candidiasis is treated with the same daily doses of intravenous amphotericin B as are used with other systemic mycoses. Adequate guidelines for judging duration of therapy are not known. There is also inadequate information to judge whether 5-fluorocytosine has a role in the treatment of systemic candidiasis.

PROGNOSIS. Most forms of mucocutaneous candidiasis are benign and respond to local treatment, although relapse is not rare. Chronic mucocutaneous candidiasis of children responds to intravenous amphotericin B, but relapse is virtually inevitable. For some reason these children rarely develop systemic candidiasis. The ability of treatment to prevent death from most forms of systemic candidiasis and to eradicate candidiasis of the urinary and gastrointestinal mucosa depends largely on the severity of the underlying condition. Candidiasis of the endocardium or around an intracardiac prosthesis is usually fatal despite treatment.

Edwards, J. E., Jr., Foos, R. Y., Montgomerie, J. Z., and Guze, L.: Ocular manifestations of *Candida* septicaemia. Review of 76 cases of haematogenous *candida* endophthalmitis. Medicine, 53:47, 1974.

Eras, P., Goldstein, M. J., and Sherlock, P.: Candida infection of the gastrointestinal tract. Medicine, 51:367, 1972.

Kirkpatrick, C. H., Rich, P. R., and Bennett, J. E.: Chronic mucocutaneous candidiasis. Ann. Intern. Med., 74:955, 1971.

Young, R. C., Bennett, J. E., Geelhoed, G., and Levine, E.: Fungemia with compromised host resistance. Ann. Intern. Med., 80:605, 1974.

Section Four CHEMOTHERAPY OF MICROBIAL DISEASE

189. DRUGS AND MICROBES

Walsh McDermott

In choosing the initial therapy for a patient with a presumed microbial disease, the physician is confronted with a formidable dilemma. On the one hand, if therapy is to be maximally effective, the correct drug or drug-pairing must be chosen quickly so that it may be administered before significant tissue damage or irreversible physiologic changes have occurred. On the other hand, if the choice is to be made quickly, it is difficult to make it exactly; for there are still only a few techniques by which the cause of an infection can be positively identified during the early hours of acute illness. Thus the physician is in the uncomfortable position of knowing that if he is to obtain the greatest advantages of antimicrobial therapy for his patient, he must make the correct choice of drugs one to five days before solid evidence of the identity of the infection will be forthcoming. An obvious way out of the dilemma would be by the introduction of rapid diagnostic methods illustrated by techniques such as the quellung test or the use of fluorescent-tagged antibody to swiftly identify organisms. However, surprisingly little effort has been devoted to developing a better, more rapid diagnostic technology. Given this situation, the physician has to rely on his *clinical* acumen and a full knowledge of all the microbial diseases that might reasonably

be expected to institute threats to his patients. In actuality, to make this choice of the initial drug regimen from evidence obtained at the bedside is not as difficult as it sounds once the physician realizes what it is that he should be trying to do. While doing it, he can also be comforted by the thought that the expert consultant must go through exactly the same exercise; for he, too, seldom has any secret diagnostic weapons, and is equally hampered by the slowness of the available diagnostic tests. Attempts should be made to differentiate, on clinical grounds, those situations or syndromes that require immediate and intensive action from those that properly may be left to unfold until precise identification becomes possible. Moreover, when a choice of therapy is made, it should be made on the basis of careful consideration of the most serious threats to the patient that are likely. The drug or drugs chosen should be the ones that do most to protect the patient overnight or for a somewhat longer interval against the reasonably likely threats, while at the same time do the least to mask the identity of other infections that might conceivably be present. Above all, once the identity of the infecting microbe *is* established, the physician should be quick to discontinue all but the scientifically relevant therapy.

An example of the exercise involved is as follows:

A young man was first seen with a high fever, a cough, and obviously excruciating pleural pain. His systolic blood pressure was 90 mm of mercury; his leukocyte count was 4000 per cubic millimeter, with a marked increase in immature neutrophils. Less than four hours previously, he had been enjoying himself at the theater, although he had had a mild respiratory infection for the preceding five or six days.

It was apparent that he had an infection, that it was progressing rapidly, and that it involved lung and pleura. What reasonable inferences could be drawn concerning the identity of the infection and hence both its relative threat to him and the appropriate choice of therapy?

At least four microbial species, pneumococcus, *Streptococcus, S. aureus,* and *Klebsiella* (Friedländer's bacillus), are capable of producing this particular situation, and faced with the individual case there is absolutely no way of differentiating one from another at the bedside. Nevertheless, the clinician knows that this syndrome occurs in such a severe fulminating form in less than 5 per cent of pneumococcal pneumonias, whereas such severity is the characteristic picture of the rapidly necrotizing pneumonias caused by staphylococci, klebsiellae, or, in some instances, streptococci. He also knows that primary staphylococcal pneumonia is extremely rare in the absence of viral influenza, but that as a complication of viral influenza it is by no means uncommon. Here his day-to-day "community epidemiologic knowledge" can stand him in good stead, for he should know whether viral influenza "is around" or has not been seen for some time; in this case, it has been "around." He likewise has discovered that his patient is a medical student, and he knows that staphylococci acquired from hospitalized patients are even more apt to be penicillinase producers than in the world at large, where, to be sure, they are by no means uncommon. He knows that primary streptococcal pneumonia of this severe type is a rarer phenomenon than primary staphylococcal pneumonia except in the middle of an outbreak of viral influenza. By contrast, *Klebsiella* pneumonia, although a not unlikely possibility in such a severe pneumonia syndrome, characteristically occurs in middle-aged weakened hosts and would be a most unlikely happening in an otherwise healthy young man.

In this situation as described, the amount of immediately useful knowledge that was produced is considerable. Armed with this knowledge, the physician who knows that he must start drug therapy right away actually has a pretty good idea of the nature of the problem. Indeed, the assembled information made it seem most likely that the patient had a primary staphylococcal pneumonia. Be that as it may, the physician knows the drug regimen he chooses must provide maximal protection against pneumococcus and *Streptococcus* (penicillin); maximal protection against *Klebsiella* (an aminoglycoside such as gentamicin or streptomycin); and maximal protection against *Staphylococcus,* including penicillinase producers (methicillin or a similar drug, along with gentamicin or streptomycin). Eighteen to 24 hours later when the identity of the infection presumably would become known, the therapy could be modified appropriately. It so happened that the cause of the illness was discovered to be a penicillinase-producing strain of *S. aureus* which was well controlled by the therapy. It should be stressed that once the microbe is identified, the physician's responsibility to modify the therapy is great. Almost invariably the patient has been receiving one or more drugs that are now known to be unnecessary, and the risks of their toxicities should be terminated promptly.

The body of knowledge from which selectivity of the sort described can be obtained is presented in the various chapters on bacterial and mycotic diseases and in Ch. 41. There are other sorts of knowledge also necessary to the clinician—knowledge about antimicrobial therapy and the drugs themselves (see Ch. 190) and information about some of the microbial mechanisms whereby the impact of drug therapy could be withstood and the microbe survive. One form of survival, viewing the microbial world as a whole, is the "new diseases" that emerge as *endogenous microbial diseases,* so-called nosocomial infections (see Ch. 124). These "new diseases" are a form of microbial survival of drug challenge, because they ensure that *some* microbes will endure. To ensure the survival of a particular microbial species and hence a particular disease, however, there are two other and quite different survival patterns, *microbial persistence* and *microbial drug resistance.* The latter phenomenon, under the name "drug-fastness," has been recognized since the early days of this century. Microbial persistence, on the other hand, was not recognized — indeed could not be recognized — until the development of penicillin, because it was only then that a powerful antimicrobial drug could be given in virtually any dosage and thus permit exclusion of the obvious possibility that the microbial survival was only a consequence of underdosage.

MICROBIAL PERSISTENCE. Microbial persistence can be defined as the phenomenon whereby a microbial strain that is susceptible to a drug in the test tube is nevertheless capable of surviving long-term exposure to that drug in the body. Persistence is thus sharply distinguished from drug resistance, which is a heritable property of a microbial strain and is demonstrable in the test tube as well as in the body. In numerical terms, microbial persistence is of the greater importance, because it is the phenomenon that is responsible for most instances of post-treatment relapse, that interferes with the effectiveness of chemoprophylaxis, and that balks attempts to use drugs for the "eradication" of microbes (see Ch. 190). Once recognized and studied, it became clear that microbial persistence—the drug-related phenomenon—was only one aspect of the larger phenomenon of latent microbial infection with its potentiality for evocation as endogenous microbial disease. As our knowledge accumulates, it is likewise beginning to appear that microbial persistence and genotypic drug resistance are veering toward each other, and may eventually come to overlap. Persistence thus serves as a link between the other two phenomena, and indeed all three may ultimately be seen to shade into each other. However, we are not yet at that point. Recognition of the present clearly visible difference among the three has been most valuable in that it has made it possible for each to be recognized, reasonably well defined, and isolated for study. For more detailed consideration of these phenomena, the reader is referred to the references at the end of this chapter. Certain aspects of microbial persistence and heritable drug resistance deserve mention at this point.

Until microbial persistence was recognized in the 1940's, the conceptual base of antimicrobial therapy was *therapia sterilisans magna* as originally conceived by Ehrlich; namely, the goal was to effect a total eradication of the infecting microbes from the host. With penicillin and the subsequently introduced drugs, it was discovered that such total eradication did not occur uniformly and predictably. In a significant number of cases of virtually any bacterial disease, drug-susceptible cells of the infecting strain could be isolated well after completion of drug therapy. At times these persisters would increase and produce clinical relapse, which was then easily treatable by the appropriate drug. At other times they would persist in the carrier state or might ultimately disappear either into latency or presumably by leaving the host altogether. Evidence was obtained that this microbial survival could not be explained by failure of drug delivery, namely, that the microbes were located in some sanctuary such as a body compartment or the center of a necrotic area where they could not be reached by the molecules of drug in the extracellular fluid; nor could the phenomoneon be explained on the basis that the drug molecules were deviated from making contact with the microbes because the inflammatory-necrotic lesion either chemically degraded the drug or wholly bound it in some way. On the contrary, convincing evidence exists that the capacity to persist is a nonheritable property of a minority of the microbial population, and it is mediated by the ability to assume a metabolic state that has been termed "drug indifference" or "physiologic" spore formation. To what extent bacterial pleomorphism, including such forms as protoplasts, plays a role in persistence is not known. Another phenomenon of penicillin survival demonstrated in vitro has been designated *tolerance* (Sabath et al.). This may represent a fifth form of drug resistance (see below); an aspect of persistence; or, most likely, another phenomenon linking the two together. Whatever may be the mechanism or mechanisms of microbial persistence, it is also clear that even though an infecting microbial population may be wholly drug susceptible in the conventional sense, actual therapy with that drug will not be uniformly or predictably *eradicative*. This is the case irrespective of whether the drug is classified as "bacteriostatic" or "bactericidal." It is this capacity of drug-susceptible bacteria to survive and outlast periods of drug administration that is responsible for most clinical relapse, failures to eliminate the carrier state, and certain failures of chemoprophylaxis. It is not generally known that Ehrlich in his late years came to perceive that *magna sterilisans* conceived as eradication was untenable. He then subtly changed the *concept* of the "sterilisans" without changing the *word*, and offered the idea that the bacteria in the tissues were in effect rendered sterile, i.e., incapable of having progeny. In the last analysis all that is added to this "latter-day Ehrlich" by the present concept of microbial persistence is the point that the sterile state is reversible.

DRUG RESISTANCE. Strictly speaking, any microbial strain that is unaffected by appropriate concentrations of a drug in vitro could be called drug resistant. In actual practice, however, the designation is reserved for the drug-resistant representatives of bacterial species that are customarily susceptible to the drug in question. *Primary resistance* refers to situations in which the infecting bacterial strain is already drug resistant at the time it initiates the infection. *Emergent resistance* refers to the emergence to predominance of a drug-resistant population during the treatment of a microbial disease that was drug susceptible when treatment was started.

All drug-susceptible bacterial species possess the capability to show emergent resistance—that is to say, to escape during therapy — to *some* drug or drugs. But *all drugs* are not associated with emergent resistance. Specifically, no instance of emergent resistance to penicillin has been observed,* and all penicillin resistance is primary. Whether drug resistance can emerge or not thus *depends not so much on the bacterial species as on the drug.* This clearly indicates that there exists a phenomenon of drug action on a microbe wherein the emergence to predominance of drug-resistant forms is a great rarity. The existence of such a phenomenon in drug action is of obvious importance in considerations

of the possible mechanisms involved in multiple drug regimens, as discussed below. Although still important, this distinction between primary and emergent resistance is diminished by virtue of the relatively abrupt appearance of pneumococci highly resistant to penicillin among patients and staff of an inpatient pediatric service in South Africa (see Ch. 121). The speed with which this situation became evident created a problem not too far removed from that facing the physician when a patient's disease responding well to antimicrobial therapy "escapes" because of emergent resistance. The issue really comes down to the precise nature of the change in the pneumococcal cell. If it is a process that can occur speedily, as with pneumococci and sulfonamide, emergent resistance presumably will occur, and the physician will have to be alert for the occurrence of either form of penicillin resistance in his patients with pneumococcal pneumonia. Conceivably, with another type of process, only primary resistance has to be feared; whether it is likely to be present or would constitute a great rarity is a judgment in which the physician would be guided by his up-to-the-minute knowledge of "community epidemiology."

Four Different Forms of Drug Resistance. The pluralistic nature of this broad phenomenon called "drug resistance" can readily be seen by examining different drugs or drug-microbe pairings. At least four distinct forms are identifiable. There is the *sulfonamide-streptomycin form*, in which the resistant bacteria maintain full pathogenic potential and are otherwise altered little, if at all, except for their loss of susceptibility to the drug. There is the *major isoniazid form*, in which certain enzymes have been lost (catalase and peroxidase), and the pathogenicity for laboratory animals, including primates, has been significantly reduced. (There is another, much less frequently encountered form of isoniazid resistance in which full pathogenicity is maintained.) There is a form characterized by *episomal or plasmid transfer*, exemplified by enteric bacteria but also by staphylococci. There is also a form seen most clearly with penicillin and staphylococci in which the critical element in producing the resistance is the *presence of a beta-lactamase*, so-called penicillinase. In some strains of staphylococci the enzyme is inducible; in other strains and species it can be constitutive. Combinations of these various forms of phenomena occur. For example, some strains of isoniazid-resistant tubercle bacilli are of the sulfonamide-streptomycin form, although these are rare; the genetic capability of staphylococci to elaborate penicillinase can be passed from one cell to another by episomal transfer, and the actual enzymatic process of synthesizing penicillinase is induced by exposure to the substrate penicillin.

Episomal transfer is an example of nonchromosomal inheritance, for bacteria not only have chromosomal genes but also have what are in effect free-floating genes that can pass from one cell to another as if they were a virus. The particles are of two sorts: *the episomes* and *the plasmid*. The difference between them is that the plasmid does not attach itself to the chromosome at any time, whereas the episome can either exist freely in the cytoplasm or at times attach itself to the chromosome. Synergism between an episomal gene and a chromosomal gene can occur. In one such experiment, two genes, one present in the episomal factor and the other in the chromosomal, each of which singly conferred resistance to streptomycin concentrations of 25 mg per

---

*The penicillin-resistant pneumococci reported from Australia (Hausman et al., 1971) were not isolated in a situation of *emergent* resistance. This also appears to have been the case with the strains isolated by Tempest et al. (1974) at the Navajo Medical Center.

milliliter, *cooperated* to yield organisms to 1000 mg per milliliter. It is believed that the synergism was acquired as a direct result of genetic recombination between the chromosome and the episomal factor. The "infection" of the strain of *E. coli* in the form of the episomal factor could be removed by treatment with an acridine dye — in effect, a form of drug therapy in vitro. The last-named observation is of considerable theoretic significance when one attempts to analyze the ways in which two-drug therapy can be more effective than the more powerful drug used alone.

Aid to the Clinician. In what way is the clinician benefited by acquaintance with this expanding body of knowledge on the multiple forms of what can only loosely be called "drug resistance"? The principal gain—and it is by no means a minor one—is that he is able to perceive that *the results of testing a microbial strain for drug susceptibility in vitro represent only one bit of information, and one that is not always relevant to the therapeutic problem presented by his patient.* The identity of the microbial species, its probable source, e.g., whether acquired in hospital or acquired from a drug-treated household contact, and the *history* of drugs received earlier in the illness and their observed effects usually represent a body of evidence of greater reliability and predictive value than drug-susceptibility tests as they are frequently performed. For example, the highly successful streptomycin-penicillin treatment of enterocococcal endocarditis would never have been instituted had the results of the streptomycin-susceptibility tests been the controlling factor. Likewise, a patient's pulmonary tuberculosis may respond well to isoniazid despite isoniazid resistance of the patient's strain when subjected to conventional drug-susceptibility tests. But this is not always the case, which merely reflects that there is obviously more than one form of isoniazid resistance. What is clear is that the clinician should be very wary of abandoning a particular drug therapy that appears to be working satisfactorily and introducing a substitute *solely* on the basis of drug-susceptibility tests. Like many laboratory procedures, drug-susceptibility tests have a place, but their results should seldom be the sole factor in determining the choice of therapy.

DRUG PAIRINGS. Consideration of the mechanisms of drug resistance leads to scrutiny of the use of two antimicrobial drugs together. One of the avowed goals of such multidrug therapy is to postpone or prevent drug resistance of the emergent type; the other is to obtain greater antimicrobial effectiveness per unit of time. Conceivably the same process could be responsible for both effects, although this is not the customary way of looking at the matter. With respect to drug resistance, the orthodox explanation dates from Ehrlich's day and is based on the notion that emergent resistance is prevented or postponed because drug A is effective against those bacterial mutants that are resistant to drug B, and vice versa. By this concept it would be possible for a two-drug regimen to affect emergent resistance without exerting an enhanced antimicrobial effectiveness per unit of time. The enhanced effectiveness phenomenon, which is seen, for example, in the penicillin-streptomycin treatment of enterococcal endocarditis, presumably would have to be explained on some other basis. The issue here is not whether, in appropriate circumstances, two-drug therapy can affect emergent resistance or increase total antimicrobial effectiveness.

The question is *how* these phenomena are brought about. If the combined drug action is exerted independently, with drug A acting on cells resistant to drug B, virtually any two-drug regimen would be expected to be effective. Contrariwise, if the respective drug actions are dependent, it would presumably represent a highly specialized phenomenon. To settle this issue would thus be a matter of considerable practical importance. Unfortunately, a reasonably complete and authoritative answer cannot be given at this time.

It can be said from the relatively few sets of observations available (see McCune et al.) that enhancement of antimicrobial effectiveness by concurrent administration of two drugs appears to be a *dependent* phenomenon, *with both drugs generally acting on the same microbial cell.* The phenomenon seems to have considerable specificity in terms of drugs and microbial species involved; hence superior drug pairings are relatively rare, and are not to be expected with just any pairing and any drug-susceptible parasite. Whether the "dependent" mechanism is also the major way by which two-drug regimens influence emergent resistance is less clear. In the writer's judgment, there is considerable reason to believe that this is indeed the case and that *when a drug pairing does exert an influence on emergent resistance, it does so by the action of both drugs on the microbes susceptible to both drugs.* Hence in large measure the action would consist of both drugs acting on the same microbial cell. As in the situation with enhancement, such effective drug pairings would represent highly specialized sets of circumstances.

The indication that drug pairings superior to the more powerful drug alone are special affairs is in agreement with the rarity with which multiple drug regimens are of demonstrated value in clinical medicine. Indeed to all intents and purposes, the examples are largely limited to infections with enterococci, tubercle bacilli, and viridans streptococci. Conceivably it might be possible to add *Pseudomonas aeruginosa* infections and the drug pairing of gentamicin and carbenicillin to the list. The problem here, as in general, is that most microbial infections do not produce *human disease* in a form that lends itself to comparative measurements of drug effectiveness, even when it is ethically permissible to do so. It is important for the physician to keep reminding himself therefore that, except for these few microbial diseases, the solid justification for the use of more than one antimicrobial drug at a time is largely limited to situations in which an etiologic diagnosis has not yet (or never) been established. Usually, as discussed above, this occurs only during the early hours of treatment, and the physician should be quick to change to single drug therapy as the situation is clarified.

NEED FOR SELECTIVITY. The day has gone by when the physician could prescribe all two or three of the available antimicrobial drugs to an acutely febrile patient and relax with the comforting thought that all that modern science could do was being done. With today's multiplicity of drugs, the emergence of "new" microbial diseases, and our considerably expanded knowledge about mechanisms of microbial survival, the physician must be highly selective in his drug choices, and hence must have mastery of a considerably greater body of clinical and laboratory-derived knowledge than was needed even a few decades ago. The physician's "comforting thought" today is of quite a different sort. It consists of the knowledge that, however difficult modern science is making things for *him* in the management of infections, it is making things ever so much better for his patients.

Applebaum, P. C., et al.: *Streptococcus pneumoniae* responding to penicillin and chloramphenicol. Lancet, 2:995, 1977.

Blazevic, D. J., et al.: Penicillin-resistant *Streptococcus pneumoniae*–Minnesota. MMWR, 26: October 21, 1977.

Davis, B. D., Dulbecco, R., Eisen, H. N., Ginsberg, H. S., Wood, W. B., Jr., and McCarty, M. (eds.): Microbiology. 2nd ed. New York, Harper & Row, 1973.

Dubos, R. J.: Man Adapting. New Haven, Yale University Press, 1965.

McCune, R. M., Feldman, F. M., and McDermott, W.: Microbial persistence. II. Characteristics of the sterile state of tubercle bacilli. J. Exp. Med., 123:469, 1966.

McDermott, W.: Microbial Persistence. Harvey Lecture Series No. 63, 1969, pp. 1–31.

McDermott, W.: Microbial drug resistance. Barnwell Lecture. Am. Rev. Respir. Dis., 102:855, 1970.

Sabath, L. D., et al.: A new type of penicillin resistance of *Staphylococcus aureus*. Lancet, 1:443, 1977.

190. ANTIMICROBIAL THERAPY

Richard B. Roberts

The announcement of the first sulfonamide in 1935 ushered in the modern era of antimicrobial therapy, an era characterized by the dramatic reduction in incidence, morbidity, and mortality of many infectious diseases. The most outstanding examples include the reduction in disease incidence or death caused by pneumococcal pneumonia, microbial endocarditis, tuberculosis, and syphilis. The impact by this class of agents on medical, public health, and economic factors related to disease states has been unparalleled in the history of drug therapy.

The abuse of these therapeutic agents, however, is alarming. In the United States, production of antimicrobial agents and the use of these drugs by physicians has steadily increased in the past two decades. Antimicrobial agents are a commonly prescribed medication in office practice (about 15 per cent of all drugs), and approximately one third of hospitalized patients receive such drugs. Surveys have suggested that two thirds of these patients receive the incorrect agent or an inappropriate dose. Indiscriminate use of these drugs may be accompanied by such complications as adverse reactions (allergic or dose related), superinfection, emergence of resistant organisms, and delay in identifying the causative organism.

Since many clinical situations dictate that antimicrobial therapy be instituted prior to identification of the specific etiologic microbe, intelligent use of these drugs requires a thorough knowledge of the suspected infectious process as well as of the changing patterns of microbial resistance. (see Ch. 189). In addition, an understanding of the physical and chemical properties of antimicrobial agents is important, because these properties determine adequate drug levels and toxicity, depending on absorption, distribution, and excretion of these drugs.

SELECTION OF ANTIMICROBIAL AGENTS

Host Determinants

AGE AND WEIGHT. The dose of an antimicrobial drug is usually calculated on the basis of body weight and, less commonly, body surface (Table 1). The route of administration, dosage, and the incidence of adverse reactions may also vary, depending on the age of the patient. For example, in the neonate and aged patient, renal function may be compromised, and the dosage of drugs excreted by the kidney should be adjusted accordingly. *Tetracycline* should not be used in pregnant women, infants, or young children, because this drug may cause enamel hypoplasia, tooth discoloration, and disturbance in bone growth. *Sulfonamides* should not be given to newborns because of possible elevated serum levels owing to abnormalities in acetylation or kernicterus owing to displacement of bilirubin from serum albumin. Similarly, the liver of premature and newborn babies produces only small amounts of glucuronyl transferase, the enzyme necessary to inactivate *chloramphenicol*. High levels of the biologically active drug may cause the "gray baby syndrome," characterized by abdominal distention, progressive pallor and cyanosis, vasomotor collapse, and death.

SITE OF INFECTION. The anatomic location of an infectious process often determines the choice of the antimicrobial and the route of its administration. Clinical studies have shown that adequate levels of most antimicrobial agents except the polymyxins are achieved in inflamed joints, making intra-articular instillation unnecessary. Antimicrobial drugs also penetrate inflamed pleura. Aminoglycosides should not be instilled into a body cavity (i.e., pleural or peritoneal), because neuromuscular blockade and respiratory paralysis may occur. Adequate drainage in addition to effective drug levels in the blood is necessary in infections associated with obstruction in the respiratory, biliary, or urinary tracts. Adequate levels of an antimicrobial agent in the cerebrospinal fluid are determined in part by the pharmacologic properties of the drug and meningeal inflammation. The penicillins, because of their low toxicity, can be given in sufficient dosage parenterally to achieve adequate levels in the cerebrospinal fluid. Chloramphenicol and sulfonamides cross the blood-brain barrier and are effective in bacterial meningitis. However, therapeutic levels of cephalothin and clindamycin in the cerebrospinal fluid are not achieved in the presence of normal or inflamed meninges, and these drugs should not be used in bacterial meningitis. Gentamicin and polymyxin B cross the blood-brain barrier poorly and should be given intrathecally as well as parenterally to patients with gram-negative bacillary meningitis.

UNDERLYING DISEASE. Serious and life-threatening infections in the compromised host present as one of the most difficult diagnostic and therapeutic challenges in medicine. A variety of microbes, including bacteria, viruses, fungi, and protozoa, infect patients who have malignant disorders or who receive immunosuppressive and cytotoxic therapy for cancer, rheumatic diseases, and renal transplantation. These patients often require antimicrobial therapy before the etiologic agent or agents are identified. Since infections in the compromised host are usually severe and are caused by a number of diverse microorganisms, an aggressive diagnostic approach, often culminating in invasive biopsy procedures, may be necessary. Initial antibacterial therapy should include a penicillinase-resistant penicillin or a cephalosporin and gentamicin. Carbenicillin is added if the clinical or laboratory findings are consistent with *Pseudomonas* bacteremia. Clindamycin should be given if anaerobic organisms, especially *Bacteroides fragilis*, are suspected. These drugs should be given in maximal doses parenterally. If the initial bacterial cultures are negative after three to five days, the patient should be re-evaluated. If diagnostic studies are negative, the drug therapy should be discontinued, because superinfection with resistant gram-negative bacilli and fungi may occur. Even with appropriate therapy, clinical response may be delayed and may ultimately depend on remission of the underlying disease or reduction of immunosuppressive therapy.

Function of the liver and kidneys may be affected by many underlying diseases. Since these are the major excretory organs for antimicrobial drugs, either many antimicrobial drugs should not be used or their dosage should be modified in the face of compromised hepatic or renal function. These precautions are discussed subsequently under the heading Excretion.

GENETIC FACTORS. The genetic background of patients may play a determinant part in the use of some antimicrobial agents. Although there may be other examples as yet unrecognized, the following known phenomena are important in determining, in part, the response to therapy as well as the risk of adverse reactions.

The rate at which isoniazid and sulfapyridine are conjugated and biologically inactivated in the liver is genetically determined. These drugs are inactivated in the liver by acetylation. Studies have shown that certain groups of patients receiving a sulfonamide or isoniazid acetylate the drug rapidly and others slowly. The rate of acetylation determines the concentration and duration of biologically active drug in the serum. Although sulfapyridine is not commonly used, salicylazosulfapyridine, which is often administered to patients with mild ulcerative colitis, is metabolized by the microbial flora of the colon to sulfapyridine and 5-aminosalicylic acid. The former metabolite is rapidly absorbed into the systemic circulation and is responsible for the adverse reactions that accompany the use of salicylazosulfapyridine.

Acute hemolytic anemia is associated with the administration of certain antimicrobial agents in patients with glucose-6-phosphate dehydrogenase deficiency. This enzyme abnormality is transmitted as a sex-linked partially dominant characteristic with full expression in homozygous males. Affected females are usually heterozygous. The antimicrobial agents that may precipitate acute hemolysis in these patients are chloramphenicol, niridazole, nitrofurantoin, primaquine, and sulfonamides. Sulfonamides may also be responsible for acute hemolysis in patients with certain hemoglobinopathies.

DRUG SUSCEPTIBILITY. One of the most important determinants in the selection of an antimicrobial agent is the susceptibility of the causative organism. It is imperative that appropriate stains and cultures of blood, secretions, cavity fluids, and the like be obtained prior to the institution of antimicrobial therapy. Once the organism has been isolated, drug-susceptibility determinations may be performed by either one of two methods: the disc (agar) *diffusion* technique, or the tube (broth) or plate (agar) *dilution* technique. The former method is routinely used in most clinical laboratories. Because of the many factors which may influence drug-susceptibility determinations, standardization of this method must take into account the growth of the organism, the inoculum size, the type and quantity of media employed, the size and concentration of drug-

impregnated discs, and the duration and environmental conditions of incubation. If these conditions are adhered to, the diameter of the area of growth inhibition about the impregnated disc distinguishes resistant from susceptible strains. In addition, precautions concerning specific bacteria or drugs must also be taken into consideration. Resistance of *Staphylococcus aureus* to methicillin is reliable only if the zones are measured within 20 hours of incubation, because methicillin deteriorates rapidly at incubating temperatures. Fastidious and slow-growing organisms such as *Bacteroides* and certain streptococci may not produce visible colonies within 24 hours, and reports of susceptibility may not be reliable. Disc susceptibility tests performed in anaerobic jars may give misleading results. Colistin and polymyxin B diffuse poorly in agar, and the drug-susceptibility results may be inaccurate. The standarized disc test is not recommended for gonococci or for *Mycobacterium tuberculosis*.

In certain clinical settings, namely patients with endocarditis and osteomyelitis, a more precise method for determining the susceptibility of an organism may be indicated. The *dilution method* — that is, twofold dilutions of the drug in broth or agar containing a standardized inoculum of the infecting organism — is the technique commonly employed in many laboratories. Results are expressed as the minimal inhibitory concentration, or MIC, which is the smallest amount of drug that will inhibit growth after 18 to 24 hours of incubation.

The serum antibacterial activity may also be determined. At a specified time after the drug is given (usually one hour after parenteral administration), serum is collected and serially diluted in a medium inoculated with the organism. A serum dilution of 1:8 or greater that inhibits the growth of the test organism is indicative of an adequate blood level for serious and life-threatening infections. Accurate serum concentrations can be determined by impregnating discs with known concentrations of a drug and other discs with serum dilutions from the patient. These discs are placed on agar previously inoculated with the organism, and zones of growth inhibition are compared after incubation. More recently, radioimmunoassay procedures have been developed for determining the serum levels of certain aminoglycosides.

Knowledge of the drug-susceptibility patterns of bacteria is important for the intelligent use of antimicrobial agents. For example, despite the common use of penicillin G, group A streptococci, pneumococci, and meningococci have remained generally susceptible to it. Methicillin-resistant *Staphylococcus aureus* strains, however, have been reported especially from Denmark and less commonly from England and the United States. These strains are also resistant to the cephalosporins. Patterns of susceptibility and resistance of gram-negative bacilli vary from hospital to hospital as well as temporally within the same institution. This phenomenon is principally due to the widespread use of antimicrobial agents active against gram-negative bacilli and the development of emergent resistance. Because of the changing patterns of susceptibility and resistance of bacteria, continuous laboratory surveillance of the incidence and susceptibility of isolates by hospital epidemiologists and clinical laboratories is extremely important. The antimicrobial susceptibilities of various microbes are discussed later in this chapter.

BACTERICIDAL AND BACTERIOSTATIC DRUGS. Bactericidal agents are drugs that kill organisms at or near the minimal inhibitory concentration. Examples of bactericidal agents include the penicillins, cephalosporins, vancomycin, aminoglycosides, and polymyxins. In general, patients with severe infections should receive bactericidal drugs. This is especially true in patients with abnormal host defense mechanisms involving antibody function, phagocyte function, or cellular immunity. Bacteriostatic drugs inhibit the growth of organisms and include erythromycin, lincomycin, clindamycin, chloramphenicol, tetracycline, and the sulfonamides. Erythromycin, lincomycin, and clindamycin may have bactericidal activity at high concentrations against certain organisms. An intact immunologic system is an important determinant in the response of patients receiving bacteriostatic drugs. In many clinical situations, such as upper respiratory tract infections, anaerobic infections, and uncomplicated urinary tract infections, bacteriostatic drugs are as effective clinically as bactericidal agents.

COMBINATION THERAPY. The administration of more than one antimicrobial agent at the same time is indicated for (1) initial therapy in a critically ill patient when the causative organism is not known, (2) polymicrobial infection in which the organisms are not susceptible to one antimicrobial agent, (3) reducing or postponing the emergence of resistance to one or both agents, such as in the therapy for tuberculosis, and (4) synergism. Synergism is best exemplified by the penicillins, the cephalosporins, vancomycin, and the aminoglycosides. In vitro studies suggest that this enhanced antimicrobial effect by bactericidal agents may be due to the inhibition of cell wall synthesis by the penicillins or vancomycin resulting in increased permeability and penetration of the aminoglycosides. The combination of penicillin or vancomycin with streptomycin or gentamicin should be used in patients with enterococcal endocarditis. Limited clinical studies suggest that carbenicillin and an aminoglycoside may be more effective than either drug alone in severe *Pseudomonas aeruginosa* infections. (For additional discussion of multiple drug therapy, see Ch. 189.)

Antagonism between two antimicrobial agents can be demonstrated in vitro. Since bactericidal drugs such as penicillin inhibit cell wall synthesis or rapidly multiplying bacteria, the simultaneous use of a bacteriostatic drug may interfere with bactericidal activity. It is uncommon, however, to detect adverse effects clinically with combined bactericidal and bacteriostatic therapy.

Absorption and Distribution

Pharmacologic properties differ markedly between classes of antimicrobial agents and between agents within the same class. Knowledge of these properties is important for the intelligent use of these drugs. Antimicrobial drugs may be administered by various routes, including topical, oral, and parenteral (intramuscular and intravenous). *Topical administration* should be restricted to special circumstances whenever possible because of possible absorption into the systemic circulation, allergic reactions, and the development of microbial resistance. Examples of appropriate local administration include severe burns, intravenous catheter sites, and purulent conjunctivitis. The *oral route* is used chiefly in initial therapy for mild to mod-

erately severe infections and for the completion of therapy in patients with severe infections. Because of the variable absorption of antimicrobial agents in the presence of gastric acidity, oral medications should be given in the fasting state, i.e., 1 to 2 hours before or after meals. *Parenteral administration* of antimicrobial drugs is indicated for severe infections that require high and sustained blood levels. Many drugs cannot be administered intramuscularly because of severe pain. These include cephalothin, vancomycin, erythromycin, chloramphenicol, and tetracycline. *Intravenous administration* is indicated in patients with severe infections or hypotension, or when appropriate levels cannot be achieved by the intramuscular route. Intravenous appliances must be changed every 24 to 48 hours to avoid thrombophlebitis and local infection with or without bacteremia. In general, medications should be diluted in 50 to 100 ml of solution and allowed to run in over a period of 15 to 30 minutes. Adverse reactions, especially associated with the aminoglycosides and polymyxins, may occur with rapid intravenous administration. Intrathecal and intra-articular therapy may be necessary in gram-negative infections. Complications associated with intrathecal administration include arachnoiditis with severe pain, paresthesias, and transient to permanent paralysis. The intrapleural or intraperitoneal administration of antimicrobial drugs is not recommended.

The distribution of a drug is a complex phenomenon and depends on many factors, including (1) molecular size, (2) electrical charge at pH 7.4, (3) lipid solubility, (4) plasma protein binding, and (5) presence of inflammation. If adequate blood levels are present, most antimicrobial agents will enter infected synovial and serous fluids. However, even in the presence of inflamed meninges, therapeutic levels of cephalothin, clindamycin, polymyxin, or gentamicin may not be achieved.

Excretion

The liver and the kidneys are the two principal excretory organs for antimicrobial agents. Renal clearance, by either glomerular filtration or tubular secretion, or both, is a major determinant of serum levels. Probenecid increases and prolongs the serum level of those antimicrobials excreted by tubular secretion (i.e., the penicillins and cephalosporins). Repeated evaluation of hepatic and renal function must be performed when antimicrobial agents are given in high doses for a prolonged period of time. Ampicillin, nafcillin, erythromycin, tetracycline, chloramphenicol, lincomycin, clindamycin, and novobiocin should be used with caution in patients with liver disease. In the face of impaired renal function, the following agents should be administered with caution, and the dosage reduced accordingly: amphotericin B, cephaloridine, colistimethate, flucytosine, methenamine mandelate, neomycin, nitrofurantoin, penicillins, polymyxin B, the aminoglycosides, sulfonamides, tetracycline, and vancomycin. Many of these agents not only are excreted largely by the kidney but also are nephrotoxic. Although the initial loading dose is the same, subsequent doses are reduced or the duration between doses is prolonged. Formulas for drug dose and interval between doses have been derived based on renal function, i.e., serum creatinine or creatinine clearance. These guidelines are useful but cannot be relied upon alone. Adjustments are best guided by repeated determinations of the serum concentration of the drug. In addition, knowledge of the dialyzability of antimicrobial agents with hemodialysis and peritoneal dialysis is necessary for the management of patients with acute and chronic renal failure.

Adverse Reactions

The administration of antimicrobial agents may be associated with toxic or allergic reactions. Adverse reactions are widely variable, as shown by the following examples: (1) local irritation at the site of administration; (2) hypersensitivity reactions; (3) dose-related hepatic, renal, and bone marrow toxicity; and (4) adverse reactions caused by the composition of the drug prepa-

ration (i.e., hyperkalemia with potassium penicillin G, fluid retention with disodium carbenicllin). The adverse reactions associated with specific antimicrobial agents are discussed below.

SPECIFIC ANTIMICROBIAL AGENTS

Antimicrobial agents may be classified as to their chemical structure, mechanism of action, antimicrobial spectrum of activity, and bactericidal versus bacteriostatic properties. Table 1 lists the common antibacterial agents with their route of administration, dosage, and mechanism of action. More detailed descriptions of the indications of each drug are included in the chapters dealing with specific organisms or infectious diseases.

TABLE 1. Antimicrobial Agents for Bacterial, Fungal, and Viral Infections

	Adult Daily Dosage (Time Interval of Divided Doses)	Route	Mechanism of Action
Adenine arabinoside		Local	Inhibition of nucleoprotein synthesis
Amantadine hydrochloride	200 mg/day	PO	Unknown
Amikacin	15 mg/kg/day (q. 8–12 hours)	IM, IV	Inhibition of protein synthesis (30S ribosomal binding)
Aminosalicylic acid	12 grams/day (t.i.d.)	PO	Replacement of para-aminobenzoic acid
Amphotericin B	1.0 mg/kg/day or every other day (total dose: 2–3 grams) or 15–50 mg/day × 10 weeks	IV	Interaction with sterols of cell membrane
Bacitracin	t.i.d.	Local	Inhibition of cell wall synthesis
Capreomycin	1 gram/day	IM	Unknown
Cephalosporins			Inhibition of cell wall synthesis
Cephalothin	4–12 grams/day (q. 4–6 hours)	IV	
Cephapirin	4–12 grams/day (q. 4–6 hours)	IM, IV	
Cephaloridine	2–4 grams/day (q. 6 hours)	IM	
Cefazolin	2–6 grams/day (q. 6–8 hours)	IM, IV	
Cephradine	2–6 grams/day (q. 4–6 hours) 1–2 grams/day (q.i.d.)	IM, IV, PO	Inhibition of cell wall synthesis
Cephalexin	1–4 grams/day (q.i.d.)	PO	
Chloramphenicol	2–4 grams/day (q. 6 hours) 1–2 grams/day (q.i.d.)	IV PO	Inhibition of protein synthesis (50S ribosomal binding)
Clindamycin	0.6–4.5 grams/day (q. 6–8 hours) 0.4–1.2 grams/day (q.i.d.)	IM, IV PO	Inhibition of protein synthesis
Co-trimoxazole (trimethoprim-sulfamethoxazole)	4 tablets/day (q. 12 hours) (1 tablet = T80 mg/S400 mg)	PO	Sequential inhibition of folic acid reduction
Cycloserine	500–750 mg/day (q. 12 hours)	PO	Inhibition of cell wall synthesis
Cytarabine	10–100 mg/square meter/day	IV	Inhibition of nucleoprotein synthesis
Erythromycins			Inhibition of protein synthesis (50S ribosomal binding)
Erythromycin ethylsuccinate	1–4 grams/day (q. 6 hours) 400 mg/day (q. 6 hours)	PO IM	
Erythromycin stearate	1–4 grams/day (q. 6 hours)	PO	
Erythromycin gluceptate	1–4 grams/day (q. 6 hours)	IV	
Erythromycin lactobionate	1–4 grams/day (q. 6 hours)	IV	
Ethambutol	15 mg/kg/day	PO	Unknown
Ethionamide	500–750 mg/day (q. 12 hours)	PO	Unknown
Flucytosine	150 mg/kg/day × 6 weeks (q. 6 hours)	PO	Inhibition of nucleoprotein synthesis (competition with cytosine)
Gentamicin	3–6 mg/kg/day (q. 8 hours) 4–6 mg/day	IV, IM IT	Inhibition of protein synthesis (30S ribosomal binding)
Idoxuridine	100 mg/kg/day	IV Local	Inhibition of nucleoprotein synthesis (competition with thymidylic acid)
Isoniazid	300 mg/day	PO	Inhibition of enzymes requiring pyridoxal as cofactor
Kanamycin	15 mg/kg/day (q. 8–12 hours) 4–8 grams/day (q. 4–6 hours)	IV, IM PO	Inhibition of protein synthesis (30S ribosomal binding)
Lincomycin	2–8 grams/day (q. 6 hours) 0.6–2.4 grams/day (q. 6–12 hours) 2 grams/day (q.i.d.)	IV IM PO	Inhibition of protein synthesis (50S ribosomal binding)
Methenamine mandelate	4–12 grams/day (q.i.d.)	PO	Unknown
Methisazone	1.5 grams/day × 2 days	PO	Inhibition of nucleoprotein synthesis
Nalidixic acid	2–4 grams/day (q.i.d.)	PO	Unknown
Neomycin	4–8 grams/day (q. 6 hours) t.i.d.	PO Local	Inhibition of protein synthesis (30S ribosomal binding)
Nitrofurans			Unknown
Nitrofurantoin	5–10 mg/kg/day (q.i.d.)	PO	
Novobiocin	2–4 grams/day (q. 6 hours) 1–2 grams/day (q. 6 hours)	PO IV	Unknown

The antituberculous drugs (isoniazid, rifampin, strep-tomycin, para-aminosalicylic acid, pyrazinamide, cap-reomycin, cycloserine, ethambutol, ethionamide, and viomycin), the antiviral drugs (adenine arabinoside, amantadine hydrochloride, cytarabine, idoxuridine, and methisazone), and the antifungal agents (ampho-tericin B, flucytosine, and nystatin) are included in Table 1 and are discussed in detail in the chapters deal-ing with the respective diseases for which they are used. Table 2 lists the antiprotozoan and antimetazoan drugs with their clinical indications, dose, route of ad-ministration, and toxicity. The following antiparasitic drugs are not approved by the Food and Drug Admin-istration for general use in the United States: antimony sodium gluconate, bithional, melarsoprol, niclosamide, niridazole, pentamidine, and suramin. These agents, however, may be easily obtained for therapy of the in-dicated diseases by calling the Parasitic Diseases

Branch of the Center for Disease Control in Atlanta, Georgia, at 404–633–3311.

PENICILLINS. Penicillinase-Sensitive Penicillins. The penicillins that are susceptible to penicillinase are penicillin G (benzyl penicillin), phenoxymethyl penicillin, amoxicillin, ampicillin, carbenicillin, and ti-carcillin. Penicillin G has three intramuscular forms which differ in the rate of absorption, thus affecting the concentration and duration of drug in serum. *Aqueous crystalline penicillin G* is well absorbed but is painful and is therefore usually given intravenously. *Procaine penicillin G* is well tolerated intramuscularly and is slowly absorbed so that injections are only necessary every six to twelve hours. *Benzathine penicillin G* is also given intramuscularly and is slowly released from the site of injection over three to four weeks. Procaine pen-icillin G and benzathine pencillin should not be admin-istered intravenously. Penicillin G is unstable in the

TABLE 1. Antimicrobial Agents for Bacterial, Fungal, and Viral Infections (*Continued*)

	Adult Daily Dosage (Time Interval of Divided Doses)	Route	Mechanism of Action
Nystatin	1.5–3 million units (t.i.d.)	PO	Interaction with sterols of cell membrane
Penicillins, penicillinase-sensitive			Inhibition of cell wall synthesis
Aqueous crystalline penicillin G	0.6–20 million units/day (q. 2–6 hours)	IV, IM	
Procaine penicillin G	600,000–4.8 million units/day (q. 6–12 hours)	IM	
Benzathine penicillin G	600,000–2.4 million units (q. 4 weeks)	IM	
Phenoxymethyl penicillin	1–4 grams/day (q.i.d.)	PO	
Penicillins with gram-negative bacillary activity			Inhibition of cell wall synthesis
Amoxicillin	0.75–1.5 grams/day (q. 8 hours)	PO	
Ampicillin	4–12 grams/day (q. 4–6 hours)	IV, IM	
	1–4 grams/day (q. 6 hours)	PO	
Carbenicillin	4–35 grams/day (q. 4 hours)	IV, IM	
	2–4 grams/day (q.i.d.)	PO	
Ticarcillin	4–20 grams/day (q. 4 hours)	IV, IM	
Penicillins, penicillinase-resistant			Inhibition of cell wall synthesis
Cloxacillin	2–4 grams/day (q. 6 hours)	PO	
Dicloxacillin	1–2 grams/day (q. 6 hours)	PO	
Methicillin	6–12 grams/day (q. 4–6 hours)	IV, IM	
Nafcillin	4–8 grams/day (q. 4–6 hours)	IV, IM	
Oxacillin	4–8 grams/day (q. 6 hours)	IV, IM	
	2–4 grams/day (q. 4–6 hours)	PO	
Polymyxins			Disruption of cell wall–membrane complex
Polymyxin B	2.5 mg/kg/day (q. 8 hours)	IV, IM	
	5.0 mg/day	IT	
Polymyxin E			
Colistimethate sodium	5.0 mg/kg/day (q. 6 hours)	IV, IM	
Colistin sulfate	5.0 mg/kg/day (q. 6 hours)	PO	
Pyrazinamide	25 to 30 mg/kg/day in 3 or 4 divided doses	PO	Unknown
Rifampin	600 mg/day	PO	Inhibition of DNA-dependent RNA polymerase
Spectinomycin	2.0 grams/day	IM	Inhibition of protein synthesis (30S ribosomal binding)
Streptomycin	1–2 grams/day (q. 12–24 hours)	IM	Inhibition of protein synthesis (30S ribosomal binding)
Sulfonamides			Competition with para-aminobenzoic acid
Sulfisoxazole	4–6 grams/day (q. 6 hours)	PO, IV	
Sulfasalazine	4–8 grams/day (q. 3–6 hours)	PO	
Tetracyclines			Inhibition of protein synthesis
Tetracycline HCl	IV: 0.5–1.0 gram/day (q. 12 hours)	IV, PO	
Chlortetracycline		IV, PO	
Oxytetracycline	PO: 1–2 grams/day (q. 6 hours)	IV, PO	
Demeclocycline	0.6–1.2 grams/day (q. 6 hours)	PO	
Methacycline	0.6–0.9 gram/day (q. 6–12 hours)	PO	
Doxycycline	0.1–0.2 gram/day (q. 12 hours)	IV, PO	
Minocycline	0.1–0.4 gram/day (q. 12 hours)	PO	
Tobramycin	3–6 mg/kg/day (q. 8 hours)	IM, IV	Inhibition of protein synthesis (30S ribosomal binding)
Vancomycin	2 grams/day (q. 6 hours)	IV	Inhibition of cell wall synthesis
Viomycin	1 gram twice weekly	IM	Inhibition of protein synthesis

Table 2. Antimicrobial Agents for Protozoan and Metazoan Infections

Protozoan Infections	Infecting Organism	Antimicrobial Agent	Adult Dose	Route	Adverse Reactions (Most Frequent Are *Italicized*)
Amebiasis Asymptomatic cyst	*Entamoeba histolytica*	Diiodohydroxyquin	650 mg t.i.d. × 3 weeks	PO	*Iodine toxicoderma*, rash, slight thyroid enlargement, nausea
Intestinal disease		Metronidazole	750 mg t.i.d. × 5–10 days	PO	*Nausea*, vomiting, diarrhea; *headache*, vertigo, insomnia, ataxia
Hepatic disease		Diiodohydroxyquin	650 mg t.i.d. × 3 weeks	PO	See above
		Metronidazole and	750 mg t.i.d. × 10 days	PO	See above
		Chloroquine	500 mg q.d. × 10 days	PO	*Vomiting, headache, pruritus*, ocular damage, convulsions, psychosis, rash; hair, nail, and mucous membrane discoloration
Giardiasis	*G. lamblia*	Quinacrine	100 mg t.i.d. × 5 days	PO	*Vomiting, vertigo, headache*; psychosis, blood dyscrasia, ocular damage, rash, hepatic necrosis
		or Metronidazole	250 mg t.i.d. × 10 days	PO	See above
Leishmaniasis Visceral	*L. donovani*	Antimony Na gluconate*	600 mg q.d. × 10 days	IM	Similar to antimony potassium tartrate but less severe
Cutaneous	*L. tropica*	Antimony Na gluconate*	600 mg q.d. × 10 days	IM	See above
Mucocutaneous	*L. brasiliensis*	Antimony Na gluconate*	600 mg q.d. × 10 days	IM	See above
Toxoplasmosis Moderate–severe illness	*T. gondii*	Pyrimethamine and	75 mg first day, then 25 mg q.d. × 4 weeks	PO	*Folic acid deficiency*, blood dyscrasia, rash, vomiting, convulsions, shock
Immunosuppressed host		Sulfadiazine plus	1 gram q.i.d. × 4 weeks	PO	*Rash*, photosensitivity, hepatic and renal toxicity, blood dyscrasia, vasculitis
Malaria	*Plasmodium vivax, malariae, ovale*	Folinic acid	6 mg q. 2 days	IM	
		Chloroquine followed by	1 gram, then 500 mg in 6 hours, then 500 mg q.d. × 2 days	PO	See above
		Primaquine	26.3 mg q.d. × 14 days	PO	*Hemolytic anemia* in G-6-PD deficient patients, neutropenia, nausea, hypertension
	P. falciparum Chloroquine-susceptible	Chloroquine	1 gram, then 500 mg in 6 hours, then 500 mg q.d. × 2 days	PO	See above
	Chloroquine-resistant	Quinine and	650 mg t.i.d. × 14 days	PO	*Cinchonism, hypotension, arrhythmias*, blood dyscrasias, photosensitivity, blindness
		Pyrimethamine plus	25 mg b.i.d. × 3 days	PO	See above
		Sulfadiazine	500 mg q.i.d. × 5 days		See above
	Comatose patient	Quinine†	600 mg/300 ml saline q. 8 hours until PO tolerated	IV	See above
Trichomoniasis	*T. vaginalis*	Metronidazole	250 mg t.i.d. × 10 days	PO	See above
Trypanosomiasis	*T. gambiense* and *T. rhodesiense*	Suramin*	1 gram on days 1, 3, 7, 14, and 21 after 100 mg test dose	IV	*Rash, pruritus, paresthesias, vomiting*, peripheral neuropathy, shock
		followed by Melarsoprol*	2.0–3.6 mg/kg q.d. for 3 days; repeat after 1 week and, if necessary, after an additional 10–21 days	IV	*Encephalopathy*, vomiting, neuropathy, rash, myocarditis, hypertension
	T. cruzi	Nifurtimox*	8 mg/kg q.d. × 120 days	PO	Nausea, dizziness, insomnia, peripheral neuropathy
Pneumocystosis	*P. carinii*	Pentamidine*	4 mg/kg/day × 12–14 days	IM	See above
		or Co-trimoxazole	20 mg/kg and 100 mg/kg q.d.	PO	See above (i.e., sulfadiazine)

*Available from Center for Disease Control (404-633-3311, Ext. 3670).

†If parenteral preparations of quinine are not available locally, they may be obtained from the Parasitic Disease Drug Service, Center for Disease Control (404-633-3311, Ext. 3670).

presence of gastric acid. *Phenoxymethyl penicillin*, although ten times less active than benzyl penicillin, is acid stable and is preferred for oral therapy. Renal clearance of the penicillins is by glomerular filtration and tubular secretion, and the simultaneous administration of probenecid will increase and prolong serum levels. However, probenecid may cause such adverse reactions as nausea, vomiting, hypersensitivity reactions (rash and fever), and rarely the nephrotic syndrome, hepatocellular injury, and aplastic anemia. Acute gout as well as the development of uric acid stones may be precipitated by probenecid. Penicillin G is active against streptococci of groups A, B, C, and G, viridans streptococci, pneumococci, nonpenicillinase-producing staphylococci, *Corynebacterium diphtheriae, Listeria monocytogenes*, anaerobic streptococci, *Fusobacterium, Clostridia*, treponemes, *Leptospira* species, *Neisseria, Pasteurella multocida*, and *Actinomyces*.

Penicillins with gram-negative bacillary activity include ampicillin and carbenicillin. *Ampicillin* differs from penicillin G only in the presence of an amino group on the side chain. This minor alteration is responsible for the difference in antimicrobial activity. Ampicillin is active against enterococci, *Hemophilus influenzae, Shigella, Salmonella, Escherichia coli*, and *Proteus mirabilis*. Indole-positive *Proteus* species (i.e., *P. rettgeri, P. morgani, P. vulgaris*) and *Pseudomonas* species are resistant. Ampicillin may be given either parenterally or orally, and the serum half-life is twice as long as that of penicillin G. *Amoxicillin*, an analogue of ampicillin and available only in oral form, has several pharmacologic advantages over ampicillin. It is more stable in the presence of gastric acid and thus better absorbed. Serum levels are higher and more prolonged than those of ampicillin. Both drugs have the same spectrum of antibacterial activity.

Carbenicillin is also similar in structure to penicillin G except for a carboxyl group on the side chain. It is active in vitro against *E. coli, Pseudomonas* species, *Proteus* species, and some strains of *Enterobacter*. The minimal inhibitory concentrations for *Pseudomonas* are very high when compared to other drug susceptibilities (i.e.,

TABLE 2. Antimicrobial Agents for Protozoan and Metazoan Infections (*Continued*)

Metazoan Infections	Infecting Organism	Antimicrobial Agent	Adult Dose	Route	Adverse Reactions (Most Frequent Are *Italicized*)
Intestinal nematodes	*Ascaris lumbricoides* (roundworm)	Pyrantel pamoate	11 mg/kg (maximum 1 gram), single dose	PO	*GI disturbance*, headache, dizziness, rash, fever
	Enterobius vermicularis (pinworm)	Pyrantel pamoate	11 mg/kg, single dose; repeat after 2 weeks	PO	
	Necator americanus (hookworm)	Mebendazole	100 mg b.i.d. × 3 days	PO	*GI disturbance*
	Ancylostoma duodenale (hookworm)	Mebendazole	100 mg b.i.d. × 3 days	PO	
	Trichuris trichiura (whipworm)	Mebendazole	100 mg b.i.d. × 3 days	PO	
	Strongyloides stercoralis	Thiabendazole	25 mg/kg b.i.d. × 2 days	PO	*Nausea, vomiting, vertigo, rash,* leukopenia, color vision disturbance, tinnitus, shock
Tissue nematodes					
Filariasis	*Wuchereria bancrofti*	Diethylcarbamazine	2 mg/kg t.i.d. × 14 days	PO	*Allergic and febrile reactions* due to worm disintegration; encephalopathy
	Loa loa	Diethylcarbamazine	2 mg/kg t.i.d. × 14 days	PO	See above
River blindness	*Onchocerca volvulus*	Diethylcarbamazine plus	2 mg/kg t.i.d. × 14 days	PO	See above
		Suramin*	1 gram per week × 5 weeks	IV	See above
Trichinosis	*Trichinella spiralis*	Thiabendazole and/or	25 mg/kg q.d. until symptoms subside	PO	See above
		Prednisone	40 mg q.d. for 3–5 days	PO	
Cestodes (tapeworms)	*Taenia saginata* (beef tapeworm)	Niclosamide*	2 grams in a single dose	PO	Nausea, abdominal pain
	Diphyllobothrium latum (fish tapeworm)	Niclosamide*	2 grams in a single dose	PO	
	Taenia solium (pork tapeworm)	Niclosamide*	2 grams in a single dose	PO	
Trematodes (flukes)					
Schistosomiasis	*S. mansoni*	Niridazole*	25 mg/kg q.d. × 5–7 days	PO	*Vomiting, diarrhea, dizziness, headache,* EKG changes, rash, insomnia, paresthesias, convulsions, psychosis, hemolysis
	S. haematobium	Niridazole*	25 mg/kg q.d. × 5–7 days	PO	See above
	S. japonicum	Niridazole*	25 mg/kg q.d. × 5–7 days	PO	See above
Paragonimiasis	*P. westermani*	Bithionol*	50 mg/kg q.o.d. × 15 doses	PO	*Photosensitivity, urticaria, abdominal pain, vomiting, and diarrhea*

*Available from Center for Disease Control (404-633-3311, Ext. 3670).

75 to 100 μg per milliliter). However, carbenicillin is a relatively nontoxic agent which can be given in doses of 30 to 40 grams per day intravenously with serum levels of 200 to 400 μg per milliliter. One half this dose is usually adequate for *E. coli, Proteus,* and *Enterobacter* infections. Carbenicillin is principally excreted by the kidneys, and very high urine levels are present after 0.5 or 1.0 gram is given parenterally (1000 μg per milliliter of urine or more). Thus a dose of 4 to 6 grams per day is adequate for uncomplicated urinary tract infections. Since *Pseudomonas aeruginosa* may develop resistance during therapy, especially if the drug is given in suboptimal doses, carbenicillin should not be used alone in patients with severe infections, cystic fibrosis, or chronic urinary tract obstruction when prolonged therapy may be indicated. In addition, superinfection, especially with *Klebsiella* species and *Serratia* species, is not uncommon. An oral form of carbenicillin, the indanyl salt of the sodium ester, is indicated only in uncomplicated urinary tract infections caused by susceptible organisms. Whereas serum levels are low after 0.5 to 1.0 gram orally, urine levels are in excess of the minimal inhibitory concentration of susceptible gram-negative bacilli.

Ticarcillin, now available for general use, is two to four times more active against *Pseudomonas aeruginosa* than carbenicillin. Otherwise, the spectrum of activity and pharmacologic properties of the two drugs are similar.

Penicillinase-Resistant Penicillins. The semisynthetic penicillins that resist penicillinase are methicillin, nafcillin, oxacillin, cloxacillin, and dicloxacillin. The principal indication for using these penicillins is infections caused by *Staphylococcus aureus* which produce penicillinase. These drugs are also active against group A streptococci and pneumococci. Cloxacillin and dicloxacillin are acid stable and are the preferred agents for oral therapy. Nafcillin is the only penicillinase-resistant penicillin excreted primarily by the liver, and the dose need not be significantly altered in patients with renal failure.

Adverse Reactions to the Penicillins. In general, severe adverse reactions to the penicillins are uncommon, and a wide range exists between therapeutic and toxic serum levels. Hypersensitivity reactions occur in 2 to 5 per cent of patients. These reactions may take two clinical forms: (1) immediate reactions, including anaphylaxis, accelerated urticaria, and angioneurotic edema; and (2) delayed reactions, which are more common and include delayed urticaria, morbilliform eruption, and serum sickness. Hypersensitivity reactions have been reported with all the penicillin derivatives. Patients allergic to one penicillin are allergic to all congeners. Drug fever is not uncommon. Coombs-positive hemolytic anemia may result from the formation of antibody to penicillin-coated red cells. This is most likely to occur when large parenteral doses are given over a long period of time. Central nervous system toxicity, characterized by myoclonus and generalized seizures, may be seen when high doses of parenteral penicillins are administered to patients especially with renal insufficiency. Hyperkalemia may be seen in patients with renal insufficiency, because the potassium salt of penicillin G has 1.6 mEq of K+ per million units. Diarrhea is common in patients receiving oral ampicillin. Skin rashes have been reported to be more common in patients with infectious mononucleosis who receive oral ampicillin. Carbenicillin must be used with caution in patients in whom sodium restriction is important, because 1 gram of carbenicillin contains 4.7 mEq of sodium. Carbenicillin may cause elevated hepatic enzymes, neutropenia, and increased clotting and prothrombin times with bleeding in patients with renal insufficiency. Methicillin and, less commonly, penicillin G have been reported to cause interstitial nephritis and reversible azotemia. Bone marrow depression with anemia and leukopenia has also been associated with methicillin therapy.

CEPHALOSPORINS. Six cephalosporins are currently marketed in the United States: cephalothin, cephapirin, cefazolin, cephaloridine, cephradine, and cephalexin. The cephalosporins are active against most organisms susceptible to the penicillins, i.e., group A streptococci, viridans streptococci, pneumococci, *Staphylococcus aureus,* and *C. diphtheriae.* Susceptible gram-negative bacilli include *Escherichia coli, Klebsiella,* and *Proteus mirabilis. Enterobacter* species, indole-positive *Proteus* strains and *Pseudomonas* species are resistant to the cephalosporins. Cephalothin, cephapirin, cefazolin, and cephaloridine are used parenterally; cephaloglycin and cephalexin, orally. *Cephalothin* is usually given intravenously, because intramuscular injections of greater than 0.5 gram are painful. Renal clearance is rapid, and the drug should be given every four hours. *Cephapirin* has antibacterial spectra and pharmacologic properties similar to cephalothin. *Cefazolin* has several pharmacologic advantages over cephalothin. Because of its low renal clearance and longer half-life, serum levels are two to three times higher and more sustained. Cefazolin may produce less thrombophlebitis than cephalothin and may be given intramuscularly. *Cephaloridine* should be given only by the parenteral route and must be avoided in patients with renal insufficiency. *Cephalexin* is acid stable and well absorbed. Urine levels are within the therapeutic range after a 0.5 to 1.0 gram oral dose. Since the excretion of the cephalosporins is by tubular secretion, serum levels may be increased and prolonged with the simultaneous administration of probenecid. Since the cephalosporins do not achieve therapeutic levels in the cerebrospinal fluid, these agents should not be used in patients with bacterial meningitis. *Cephradine* is available in both parenteral and oral forms.

At the time of this writing, two new compounds, cephamandole, a cephalosporin, and cefoxitin, a cephamycin, appear to be more resistant to the action of cephalosporinase and therefore more active than other cephalosporins against certain gram-negative bacilli.

Adverse reactions to the cephalosporins are relatively uncommon. The question of cross-allergenicity between the penicillins and the cephalosporins remains controversial. The incidence of cross-sensitization must be low, because cephalosporin compounds have been given successfully to many patients with prior penicillin reactions. However, the cephalosporins should probably not be administered to patients with a documented history of an immediate hypersensitivity reaction to pencillin. Thrombophlebitis is commonly seen with the intravenous use of large doses of cephalothin and cephapirin, and frequent changes of the intravenous site are necessary if these drugs have to be given over an extended period of time. A positive Coombs test without hemolysis may occur with large doses of cephalothin; leukopenia is rare and usually responds to discontinuing the drug. Cephaloridine is nephrotoxic, especially if the dose is greater than 4 grams per day or if patients are receiving ethacrynic acid or furosemide.

Acute tubular necrosis has also been reported in patients receiving cephalothin and gentamicin. The specific role of either drug or the combination in this complication is unknown. Nausea and vomiting may accompany the administration of the oral cephalosporins. The presence of cephalexin in the urine may give a false positive test for glucose with Benedict's solution or Clinitest tablets.

VANCOMYCIN. Vancomycin is active against penicillinase-producing *Staphylococcus aureus* and *S. epidermidis,* viridans streptococci, and enterococci. It is an important alternative drug in patients allergic to the penicillins and the cephalosporins who have severe staphylococcal infections or endocarditis caused by penicillin-resistant viridans streptococci and enterococci. Methicillin-resistant *Staphylococcus aureus* strains are usually resistant to the cephalosporins but susceptible to vancomycin. All gram-negative bacilli are resistant to this antimicrobial. Vancomycin can only be administered intravenously. Pain at the site of injection is frequent and thrombophlebitis common. Chills, fever, and urticaria may also accompany its administration. The more severe adverse reactions include reversible nephrotoxicity with albuminuria, casts, and azotemia, and ototoxicity with deafness when very high blood levels are achieved.

ERYTHROMYCIN, LINCOMYCIN, AND CLINDAMYCIN. *Erythromycin* is one of two macrolide antimicrobials. It should be classified with lincomycin and clindamycin, because all three drugs have a similar mechanism of action (inhibition of protein synthesis by binding the 50S ribosomal unit). The spectrum of activity of these drugs, with a few exceptions, is similar. Erythromycin is active against group A streptococci, pneumococci, and *Staphylococcus aureus. Mycoplasma pneumoniae* and *T. pallidum* are also susceptible to it. Erythromycin may be used in patients allergic to penicillin who have respiratory tract or soft tissue infections caused by pneumococci and group A streptococci, respectively. It may be used as the primary drug in *M. pneumoniae* infections. Erythromycin should not be used for serious *Staphylococcus aureus* infections. Local irritation at the site of parenteral administration is common, and gastrointestinal disturbance may be associated with oral therapy. Erythromycin estolate may produce reversible cholestatic hepatitis, and other preparations of erythromycin should be used. Hypersensitivity reactions, such as rash and eosinophilia, and drug fever are uncommon.

Triacetyloleandomycin is also a macrolide antimicrobial, but it is used infrequently because of adverse reactions.

Lincomycin and clindamycin (a chloro-derivative of lincomycin) are also active against group A streptococci, pneumococci, and penicillinase-producing staphylococci. Enterococci, gram-negative bacilli, and *Mycoplasma pneumoniae* are resistant. Many strains of *Staphylococcus aureus* resistant to erythromycin are also resistant to lincomycin and clindamycin. Staphylococci resistant to erythromycin but susceptible to lincomycin or clindamycin may rapidly develop resistance to the latter drugs during lincomycin-clindamycin therapy (dissociated cross-resistance). Clindamycin is well absorbed from the gastrointestinal tract and produces higher serum levels than oral lincomycin. Clindamycin is also more active against many anaerobes, especially *Bacteroides fragilis,* and has become the drug of choice in the initial therapy of severe anaerobic infections. Erythromycin crosses the blood-brain barrier, but lincomycin and clindamycin do not, and therefore the latter agents should not be used in bacterial meningitis. Gastrointestinal disturbances such as nausea, vomiting, abdominal cramps, and diarrhea occur with clindamycin and lincomycin. Pseudomembranous colitis has been observed with both drugs. Rapid intravenous administration may be associated with cardiopulmonary arrest. Reversible hepatocellular toxicity and bone marrow depression (leukopenia) have been reported after clindamycin therapy. Hypersensitivity reactions such as rash and generalized pruritus are rare.

NOVOBIOCIN. The antibacterical spectrum of novobiocin is similar to that of penicillin G and erythromycin; *Staphylococcus aureus* and pneumococci are susceptible to this antimicrobial. It is well absorbed from the gastrointestinal tract and may also be given intravenously. However, the high incidence of adverse reactions precludes the routine use of this drug, and it is rarely prescribed at present. Toxic reactions include gastrointestinal disturbances (nausea, vomiting, diarrhea, and bleeding), bone marrow depression (pancytopenia), hypersensitivity reactions (eosinophilia, rash, fever, angioedema, exudative erythema multiforme), alopecia, and yellow discoloration of the skin and sclera caused by a degradation product of the drug.

BACITRACIN. Bacitracin is a polypeptide antimicrobial agent for topical use only. *Staphylococcus aureus*, *Staphylococcus epidermidis*, enterococci, viridans streptococci, and group A streptococci are susceptible to it. Gram-negative bacilli are resistant to bacitracin. The antibiotic is stable in ointments only when it is incorporated in petrolatum. Bacitracin is indicated in open superficial skin infections such as eczema, dermal ulcers, and minor wounds infected with drug-susceptible bacteria. Purulent conjunctivitis and infected corneal ulcers may also respond to topical bacitracin when caused by similar organisms. Furunculosis, impetigo, pyoderma, and subcutaneous abscesses should not be treated with topical bacitracin alone. Adverse reactions are rarely seen with this topical drug.

AMINOGLYCOSIDES. The six drugs that belong to this class of antimicrobial agents are streptomycin, neomycin, kanamycin, gentamicin, tobramycin, and amikacin. *Streptomycin*, one of the first aminoglycosides available for parenteral administration, was widely used in the 1940's and 1950's, because *Mycobacterium tuberculosis* and gram-negative bacilli, especially *Escherichia coli*, *Klebsiella-Enterobacter* species, and *Proteus* strains were susceptible. However, with the development of other drugs for these infections and because adverse reactions, notably vestibular toxicity, are a risk, the use of intramuscular streptomycin is now limited to a few specific diseases. Most strains of enterococci are resistant to streptomycin in vitro. Nevertheless, streptomycin in combination with penicillin or vancomycin is the therapy of choice in patients with penicillin-resistant viridans streptococcal and enterococcal endocarditis. These drug combinations should also be used for prophylaxis against enterococcal bacteremia in patients with underlying congenital or valvular heart disease who have urogenital or gastrointestinal manipulation. Streptomycin has substantial activity against *M. tuberculosis*, and the indications for its use in this disease are discussed in Ch. 167. Streptomycin may also be used in the therapy of plague, tularemia, and brucellosis. *Neomycin*, also discovered in the 1940's, has limited clinical application because of nephrotoxicity and neurotoxicity. The drug is poorly absorbed from the gastrointestinal tract and is therefore useful in patients with severe hepatic disease with impending or frank coma, inhibiting bacterial growth in the intestinal tract and reducing absorption of nitrogenous compounds. Unfortunately, neomycin is widely used in topical antimicrobial preparations, many of which are available without a prescription. There is no evidence from controlled studies that neomycin is effective in healing or preventing skin infections. Indeed, topical neomycin frequently causes contact dermatitis. Injudicious use of neomycin in patients with extensive wounds or burns or instillation into body cavities may result in absorption of the drug and life-threatening adverse reactions.

Kanamycin is closely related to neomycin but is less toxic. It is active against most gram-negative bacilli, including *E. coli*, *Klebsiella-Enterobacter* species, and *Proteus* species. The drug is also active in vitro against *Shigella*, *Staphylococcus aureus*, and *M. tuberculosis*, but is not indicated for clinical use in these infections, because less toxic agents are available. *Pseudomonas aeruginosa* strains are universally resistant to kanamycin. Ampicillin plus kanamycin has been the initial therapy of choice in suspected neonatal sepsis. However, if it is known that kanamycin-resistant gram-negative organisms have been isolated from the nursery, ampicillin plus gentamicin is recommended.

Gentamicin is widely used for serious gram-negative bacillary infections. It is active against *Pseudomonas* species as well as *E. coli*, *Klebsiella-Enterobacter* species, and *Proteus* species. *Staphylococcus aureus* strains are also susceptible to gentamicin; however, less toxic antistaphylococcal agents are available, and gentamicin should not be used for this purpose. Gentamicin may be given by either the intramuscular or the intravenous route. Therapeutic levels in the cerebrospinal fluid are usually not achieved with parenteral administration, and intrathecal injections are indicated in patients with gram-negative bacillary meningitis. In patients with urinary tract infections, the urine should be alkaline for maximal antimicrobial activity. Carbenicillin when mixed with gentamicin in the same solution will inactivate the latter drug over a prolonged period of time.

Recently, two additional aminoglycosides have become available for general use. *Tobramycin* is two to six times more active against *P. aeruginosa* than gentamicin and is the drug of choice for infections caused by this microbe. The spectrum of gram-negative bacillary activity and pharmacologic properties of the two drugs are similar. *Amikacin*, despite a chemical structure similar to that of kanamycin, has excellent activity against *P. aeruginosa*. Since amikacin is a poor substrate for many of the enzymes produced by gram-negative organisms that inactivate gentamicin and tobramycin, this drug should be reserved at present for infections caused by gentamicin- and tobramycin-resistant organisms.

Adverse reactions are commonly seen with administration of the aminoglycosides. These agents are excreted principally by the kidneys and should be avoided or the dose adjusted in patients with compromised renal function. Furthermore, the therapeutic serum level often approximates the toxic level, and adverse reactions may be unavoidable in patients with life-threatening infections. Since gentamicin has such a wide spectrum of activity against aerobic gram-negative bacilli, it is often used in conjunction with a penicillinase-resistant penicillin or a cephalosporin for the initial therapy in patients with malignancies or who are on immunosuppressive or cytotoxic agents. If the infecting organism proves to be susceptible to a less toxic drug, gentamicin should be discontinued and that agent instituted for the remainder of the patient's therapy. The aminoglycosides should never be injected into body cavities or given rapidly by vein, because neuromuscular blockade with respiratory arrest may ensue. This curare-like effect may be reversed with neostigmine or calcium gluconate. All the aminoglycosides are nephrotoxic and neurotoxic. Neomycin, kanamycin, and amikacin cause auditory toxicity with deafness. Deafness is more commonly seen in patients with renal insufficiency or in patients receiving ethacrynic acid or furosemide. Streptomycin, gentamicin, and tobramycin usually cause vestibular damage which may be irreversible. Occasionally deafness may also occur. During long-term therapy, patients must be closely followed with daily tandem-walking and weekly caloric reactions and audiograms. Paresthesias, peripheral neuropathy, and optic neuritis are rarely observed. Hypersensitivity reactions have been reported with each of the aminoglycosides.

POLYMYXINS. Polymyxin B and polymyxin E are polypeptide antimicrobials that are active against *E. coli, Klebsiella-Enterobacter* species, and *Pseudomonas* species. *Proteus* species are resistant to these drugs. Polymyxin B is given parenterally and may also be administered intrathecally. The polymyxins do not cross the blood-brain barrier and must be given both parenterally and intrathecally in patients with gram-negative bacillary meningitis. Polymyxin E has two forms, parenteral colistimethate sodium and oral colistin sulfate, a nonabsorbable antimicrobial. Although active in vitro against many species of gram-negative bacilli, polymyxin is most useful in the therapy of *Pseudomonas aeruginosa* infections. Since the polymyxins are excreted by the kidneys, caution must be used when these agents are given to patients with renal insufficiency. Serious adverse reactions are dose related. Neurotoxic reactions include circumoral or fingertip paresthesias that are usually reversible. Ataxia, slurred speech, and blurred vision are uncommon. Respiratory paralysis may occur with rapid intravenous administration or in patients receiving succinylcholine and may be reversed by intravenous calcium gluconate but not neostigmine. Azotemia and impaired renal function are seen with high doses. Hypersensitivity reactions have been reported and include eosinophilia and rash.

SPECTINOMYCIN. Spectinomycin is active against *Neisseria gonorrhoeae* and has been approved only for use in uncomplicated gonorrhea. The drug does not have treponemicidal activity. It should be considered for use in patients with gonococcal urethritis and cervicitis who are allergic to penicillin, because it can be given as a single dose intramuscularly. There is no cross-resistance between spectinomycin and penicillin. Although spectinomycin inhibits protein synthesis by binding 30S ribosomal subunits (similar to the aminoglycosides), adverse reactions, except for fever and urticaria, have been uncommon to date.

CHLORAMPHENICOL. Chloramphenicol has a broad spectrum of activity against the rickettsiae, gram-positive bacteria, gram-negative bacteria, including *Salmonella* and *Shigella,* and anaerobic bacteria. The drug is well absorbed from the gastrointestinal tract. It is metabolized by the liver and can therefore be used in patients with renal insufficiency. Adequate levels in the cerebrospinal fluid are present after intravenous injection. Chloramphenicol causes bone marrow aplasia and fatal pancytopenia in 1 of every 40,000 or more courses of therapy or 1 of 25,000 to 50,000 people exposed. This severe toxic reaction is a form of hypersensitivity or idiosyncratic reaction which cannot be predicted before therapy. For this reason, chloramphenicol should be used only for certain specific, severe infections. These indications include (1) typhoid fever or other *Salmonella* infections, (2) initial therapy for *Hemophilus influenzae* meningitis, (3) as an alternative drug for penicillin G in pneumococcal and meningococcal meningitis, (4) severe anaerobic infections for which clindamycin is not effective, (5) gram-negative bacillary infections that do not respond to other antimicrobial agents, and (6) severe rickettsial infections when tetracycline is not effective.

Anemia which is dose related and not a hypersensitivity reaction may occur with prolonged use. This form of bone marrow depression is reversible and is characterized by interference with iron metabolism, with increased serum iron and saturation of iron-binding globulin, decreased reticulocyte count, and vacuolization of red cell precursors. Patients receiving chloramphenicol must have repeated complete blood counts and serum iron and saturation determinations. This type of anemia is most commonly seen in patients with liver disease or renal insufficiency and in those receiving high doses. Fatal toxicity may develop in neonates ("gray baby syndrome"). Optic neuritis and peripheral neuropathy are rarely seen with prolonged therapy. Hypersensitivity reactions have been reported.

TETRACYCLINES. The tetracyclines have a broad spectrum of activity. *Rickettsia, Chlamydia, Mycoplasma pneumoniae,* gram-positive and gram-negative bacteria, certain anaerobic organisms, and *T. pallidum* are susceptible to the tetracyclines. At present, 25 to 50 per cent of group A streptococci, 5 to 10 per cent of pneumococci, and most *Staphylococcus aureus* isolates are resistant. In addition, many aerobic gram-negative bacilli and *Bacteroides* species are also resistant. These changing susceptibility patterns since the introduction of tetracycline in the 1940's have made it necessary to restrict the use of these drugs to the following indications: (1) *Rickettsia* infections; (2) *M. pneumoniae* infections; (3) *Chlamydia* infections, including psittacosis, trachoma, lymphogranuloma venereum, and nongonococcal urethritis; (4) granuloma inguinale and chancroid; (5) alternative therapy for gonorrhea and syphilis; and (6) urinary tract infections caused by susceptible gram-negative bacilli.

Tetracycline has replaced *chlortetracycline* and *oxytetracycline* as the agent of choice. It may be given orally or intravenously, although thrombophlebitis often accompanies the latter route of administration. Tetracycline should be avoided in patients with renal insufficiency. Four long-acting tetracyclines are available: *demethylchlortetracycline, methacycline, doxycycline,* and *minocycline.* The rate of renal excretion of these agents is less and oral absorption greater than those of tetracycline, resulting in prolonged serum levels. Minor variations in the degree of antibacterial activity exist among the four preparations which are reflected in the amount of drug recommended per dose. Doxycycline does not accumulate in the serum of patients with renal insufficiency and may be advantageous when the status of renal function is unknown. However, because of the low renal clearance of both doxycycline and minocycline, their usefulness in urinary tract infections may be limited by low urinary concentrations. With few exceptions all the tetracycline compounds produce the same adverse reactions. These include gastrointestinal disturbances such as nausea, vomiting, and diarrhea, thrombophlebitis with intravenous administration, staining and hypoplasia of dental enamel and disturbed bone growth in neonates and young children, pseudotumor cerebri with bulging fontanelles and increased cerebrospinal fluid pressure in infants, and acute fatty degeneration of the liver in pregnant women and patients with renal insufficiency. Photosensitivity reactions are not infrequently seen with the long-acting tetracyclines. A variant of the Fanconi syndrome caused by toxic products may occur with administration of outdated tetracycline preparations. Superinfections with resistant gram-negative bacilli, *Staphylococcus aureus*, and *Candida* may occur with prolonged therapy.

SULFONAMIDES. For four decades, sulfonamides have been widely prescribed for a variety of clinical infections. However, their present use is limited because of resistance of gram-positive and gram-negative organisms, the availability of more active antimicrobial agents, and adverse reactions. The major indications are (1) nocardiosis; (2) suppressive therapy for paracoccidioidomycosis; (3) prophylaxis in sulfadiazine-susceptible meningococcal infections; (4) alternative prophylaxis for acute rheumatic fever in patients allergic to penicillin; (5) uncomplicated urinary tract infections caused by susceptible organisms, especially *E. coli*; (6) salicylazosulfapyridine therapy in patients with mild ulcerative colitis; (7) certain protozoal infections (toxoplasmosis, *Pneumocystis carinii*, and chloroquine-resistant *P. falciparum* malaria); and (8) when administered in combination with antifolate compounds, chronic urinary tract infections and typhoid fever.

Sulfisoxazole is well absorbed from the gastrointestinal tract and may also be administered parenterally if necessary. The drug is chiefly excreted by glomerular filtration and thus is not affected by probenecid. *Sulfamethoxazole* is a congener of sulfisoxazole, but is absorbed less and the renal excretion is delayed. The more potent *sulfadiazine*, once widely used, is less soluble and tends to cause crystalluria. The incidence of crystalluria is decreased by increasing fluid intake and maintaining an alkaline urine. The risk of precipitation of the drug in the renal tubules is appreciably increased if the sulfadiazine is administered intravenously. Long-acting sulfonamides, such as *sulfamethoxypyridazine* and *sulfadimethoxine*, although widely used in the past, have no place in clinical antimicrobial therapy because of their toxic effects. The poorly absorbed sulfonamides, *succinylsulfathiazole* and *phthalylsulfathiazole*, are principally used to decrease bacterial counts in the intestine prior to surgery. These agents are of doubtful value. *Salicylazosulfapyridine* may decrease the severity of disease in patients with mild ulcerative colitis. This effect may be due to the antibacterial action of sulfapyridine or the anti-inflammatory effect of 5-aminosalicylic acid.

Adverse reactions caused by the sulfonamides include the following: hypersensitivity reactions with fever, rash, photosensitivity, and rarely vasculitis; nephrotoxicity with crystalluria and renal tubular necrosis; kernicterus in the newborn; hepatitis (occasionally with noncaseating granuloma); agranulocytosis and aplastic anemia; and acute hemolytic anemia in patients with G-6-PD deficiency. Long-acting sulfonamides may cause Stevens-Johnson syndrome and myocarditis.

TRIMETHOPRIM-SULFAMETHOXAZOLE (CO-TRIMOXAZOLE). This drug combination sequentially inhibits the utilization of para-aminobenzoic acid by bacteria in the synthesis of folic acid. A double sequential blockage is thus produced, and relatively low concentrations of each drug are required for antimicrobial activity. At present, the drug combination (trimethoprim, 80 mg; sulfamethoxazole, 400 mg) has been approved in the United States only for chronic urinary tract infections and pneumocystis infections. Clinically trials suggest that it may be useful in patients with bronchitis, gonorrhea, and possibly typhoid fever resistant to both chloramphenicol and ampicillin. Adverse reactions are the same as those described for the sulfonamides, including the Stevens-Johnson syndrome, and those caused by trimethoprim, including nausea, vomiting, skin rashes, and macrocytic anemia resulting from folic acid deficiency. Serious nephrotoxicity has been reported in patients with diminished renal function.

NITROFURANTOIN. Nitrofurantoin is an oral antibacterial agent that is excreted in the urine by both glomerular filtration and tubular secretion. The drug is most active against *E. coli*, *Klebsiella-Enterobacter* species, and some strains of enterococci. The susceptibility of *Proteus* strains is variable, and *Pseudomonas* species are resistant. Nitrofurantoin should be used only for uncomplicated urinary tract infections or suppressive therapy in patients with chronic urinary tract infections. The drug is most active in the presence of an acid urine, and emergent resistance has not been noted. It should not be prescribed in pregnant women, because it crosses the placenta, or in patients with renal insufficiency. Adverse reactions include nausea and vomiting, hypersensitivity reactions (fever, rash, allergic pneumonitis), paresthesias which may progress to severe polyneuropathy if the drug is not discontinued, acute hemolytic anemia in patients with G-6-PD deficiency, and cholestatic hepatitis.

NALIDIXIC ACID. Nalidixic acid is also an oral antimicrobial agent used in the therapy of uncomplicated urinary tract infections. The drug is active against strains of *E. coli*, *Klebsiella-Enterobacter* species, and *Proteus* species; *Pseudomonas* species are resistant. Gram-negative bacilli may rapidly develop resistance to this agent, and repeated urine cultures with drug-susceptibility determinations should be performed during therapy. Adverse reactions include nausea, vomiting, hypersensitivity reactions (rash, eosinophilia, photosensitivity), and rarely cholestatic jaundice, blood dyscrasias, visual disturbances, toxic psychosis, and convulsive seizures. Severe headache associated with papilledema has been observed in children.

METHENAMINE MANDELATE AND HIPPURATE. These antimicrobial compounds are the salts of methenamine and mandelic acid and hippuric acid, respectively. They are well absorbed from the gastrointestinal tract and rapidly excreted in the urine. They are bactericidal in acidic urine (pH less than 5.5). An acidifying agent is necessary if the infecting organism forms ammonia. Methenamine mandelate or hippurate may be used for chronic suppression of urinary tract infections. *Escherichia coli* is susceptible to these drugs. *Proteus* species and *Pseudomonas* are usually resistant. Adverse reactions are uncommon and include epigastric pain, dysuria, crystalluria, and metabolic acidosis, especially in patients with renal insufficiency.

FAILURE OF ANTIMICROBIAL THERAPY

The failure of a patient to respond to antimicrobial therapy may be due to factors related to the host and the nature of the disease or to an error in the choice, dosage, or route of administration of the drug. The following causes are most common: (1) incorrect diagnosis; (2) impaired host defense mechanisms; (3) inadequate dose, route of administration, or distribution of drug; (4) closed space infection; (5) presence of a foreign body; (6) superinfection; and (7) microbial drug resistance.

Resistance of microorganisms to antimicrobial agents may be classified as primary (natural) or emergent (acquired) (see Ch. 189). Microorganisms acquire resistance by either mutation or episomal transfer. Mutation patterns may be multi-step, involving a number of genes, or large-step, involving one gene. The efficiency of mutation is increased in the presence of low-dose antimicrobial drug administration. Both gram-positive and gram-negative bacteria develop resistance by mutation. Recognition of episomal transfer of resistance is presently restricted to gram-negative bacilli and *Staphylococcus aureus*. The transfer of cytoplasmic DNA (R factor) requires cell-to-cell contact and is termed conjugation. The transfer of resistance may be single or multiple, and occurs most commonly in the gastrointestinal tract. It is often designated infectious drug resistance.

CHEMOPROPHYLAXIS

Antimicrobial agents are often administered to individuals who are believed to be at some increased risk of acquiring a bacterial infection.

Prophylaxis is usually successful only when a single drug is given for a specific organism. The antimicrobial drugs and their clinical indications which are considered to be of value are summarized in Table 3. Except for the use of amantadine in influenza A infection (see Ch. 82), antimicrobial prophylaxis is not effective in either viral respiratory diseases or viral exanthems. In addition, prophylaxis is not indicated in clean abdominal surgery or congestive heart failure. Unlike the therapeutic situation in which the identity of the offending microbe might be in doubt and there is urgency in selecting therapy, with chemoprophylaxis there is usually no urgency, and the microbe in question is known. Consequently, the use of antimicrobial drugs in chemoprophylaxis should be more rational than in therapy. Unfortunately, this is not always the case, and in many

TABLE 3. Recommendations for Antimicrobial Prophylaxis

Disease or Clinical Setting	Etiologic Agent	Antimicrobial Drug
Acute rheumatic fever (recurrent)	Group A streptococcus	Penicillin, erythromycin, sulfonamide
Meningococcal infections	*Neisseria meningitidis*	
	Sulfonamide-susceptible	Sulfisoxazole
	Sulfonamide-resistant	Rifampin
Microbial endocarditis		
Oral cavity instrumentation	Viridans streptococcus	Penicillin, erythromycin
Urogenital and gastrointestinal instrumentation	Enterococcus	Penicillin or vancomycin plus streptomycin
Open heart surgery	*Staphylococcus aureus* and *epidermidis*	Penicillinase-resistant penicillin, cephalosporin
Newborn nursery epidemics	Enteropathic *E. coli*	Neomycin, Colistin
	Staphylococcus aureus	Penicillinase-resistant penicillin
	Group A streptococci	Penicillin
Tuberculin reactors of certain sorts	*Mycobacterium tuberculosis*	Isoniazid
Malaria	Plasmodia	
	Chloroquine-susceptible	Chloroquine followed by primaquine
	Chloroquine-resistant (*P. falciparum*)	Pyrimethamine and sulfadoxine *or* Chloroguanide and sulfone
Ophthalmia neonatorum	*Neisseria gonorrhoeae*	Silver nitrate, penicillin
Burns		Silver sulfadiazine, silver nitrate
Bronchitis (chronic)	Pneumococcus or *Hemophilus influenzae*	Ampicillin, tetracycline

instances the prophylactic use of antimicrobial agents is unwarranted, ineffective, and often dangerous because of toxic reactions, superinfection, and emergent resistance. The matter of drug toxicity requires comment. Selection of a drug is a matter of weighing offsetting risks. It is easy to forget that a degree of drug toxicity that is acceptable when weighed against an instance of a particular disease may be unacceptable when weighed against the chance that someone *might* acquire that disease. Finally, although one must emphasize the need for caution in chemoprophylaxis, it is fitting to remember that in terms of the number of people benefited, the use of the drugs in this way represents one of the greatest achievements of modern biomedical science and technology.

Balows, A.: Current Techniques for Antibiotic Susceptibility Testing. Springfield, Ill., Charles C Thomas, 1974.

Goodman, L. S., and Gilman, A.: The Pharmacological Basis of Therapeutics. 4th ed. New York, Macmillan, 1970.

Handbook of Antimicrobial Therapy. The Medical Letter on Drugs and Therapeutics (revised ed.), 1977.

Kunin, C. M., et al.: Use of antibiotics. A brief exposition of the problem and some tentative solutions. Ann. Intern. Med., 79:555, 1973.

Lowbury, E. J. L., and Ayliffe, G. A. L.: Drug Resistance in Antimicrobial Therapy. Springfield, Ill., Charles C Thomas, 1974.

Pratt, W. B.: Chemotherapy of Infections. New York, Oxford University Press, 1977.

Weinstein, L., and Dalton, A. C.: Host determinants of response to antimicrobial agents. N. Engl. J. Med., 279:467, 1968.

PART X
PROTOZOAN AND HELMINTHIC DISEASES

191. INTRODUCTION

Philip D. Marsden

With rapid air travel, so-called parasitic infections are becoming more important in temperate climes. They have always been important in the tropics.

Parasitic disease is usually taken to imply infections caused by protozoa and helminths, although, in their relationship to the host, bacteria, viruses, and rickettsiae equally fulfill the general criteria used to describe an organism as parasitic. The reason for this nomenclature is historic; because they are bigger organisms, helminths and protozoa were discovered relatively early by medical investigators. *Ascaris* and tapeworms are dramatic enough to have been recognized in ancient times, and protozoa were seen with the first crude microscopes.

A knowledge of where the infection occurs in the world is important, and this information is included in the succeeding chapters. For example, schistosomiasis would not be considered as a cause of portal hypertension in a patient from the Indian subcontinent, and malaria caused by *Plasmodium vivax* is rare in West Africa.

For the correct diagnosis of parasitic disease the physician must be as competent at the microscope and in using the laboratory procedures to find parasites as he is at defining the clinical presentation at the bedside and interpreting it. As with other infectious diseases, a firm diagnosis rests on finding the infectious agent. Recently serologic tests have been used much more to aid diagnosis, and, interpreted wisely, they are valuable. Broadly speaking, they mean that a patient has developed antibodies of a certain type to a parasitic antigen. Rarely do they give any confirmation about the status of the parasite in the body of man in terms of numbers present or whether they are multiplying. Positive serologic findings should often be an indication for redoubling one's efforts to find the parasite.

Whether a complement fixation test, hemagglutination test, fluorescent antibody test, or gel diffusion test is positive at a significant titer must be decided in the light of known facts about the specificity of the tests.

Many of the drugs used are toxic to man but more toxic to the parasites. We know little of the mechanisms of drug action in many cases, e.g., Pentostam in leishmaniasis. With some drugs such as heavy metal containing compounds and emetine the toxic dose for man is near the therapeutic dose. Physicians should be especially careful to check their prescriptions of these drugs, especially if they are not used to prescribing them often.

The Center for Disease Control, Atlanta, Georgia, offers unique services to the physician in the United States for the management of parasitic disease. Not only is there a laboratory for diagnostic serology, but a number of rare drugs previously not available in the United States and mentioned in this book have become available through the Parasitic Disease Drug Service in the Epidemiology Program. These include drugs for the treatment of both types of human trypanosomiasis, leishmaniasis, amebiasis, pneumocystis infection, and schistosomiasis.

With regard to diagnostic serology, Dr. Irving G. Kagan has kindly provided the information on serologic tests available for parasitic diseases in the United States (see accompanying table).

Immunodiagnostic Tests for Parasitic Infections

	Complement Fixation	Precipitin	Particle Agglutination Tests				Fluorescent Antibody	ELISA
			Bentonite Flocculation	Hemagglutination	Latex Agglutination	Cholesterol Flocculation		
Trichinosis	+	+	+*	±*	+*	+*	+*	0
Echinococcosis	+	+	+*	+*	+*		+	0
Schistosomiasis	+*		±*	±*		+*	+*	0
Ascariasis/toxocariasis			+*	+*			0	±*
Filariasis	±		+*	+*	0		0	0
Cysticercosis	+	0		+*	±		0	±*
Chagas' disease	+*	±	0	+*	0		0*	0
Leishmaniasis	+			+*			0	0
Toxoplasmosis	+*			+*	0		+*	±*
Amebiasis	+*	+	±*	+*	±		±*	0
Malaria				±*			+*	0

*Tests available in the United States.
ELISA = Enzyme-linked immunosorbent assay.
0 = Under experimental investigation.
± = Used for diagnosis, but requires further evaluation for routine use.
+ = Generally accepted useful routine diagnostic test.
Adapted from data supplied by Dr. Irving Kagan, Center for Disease Control.

Section One   PROTOZOAN DISEASES

192.   INTRODUCTION

Philip D. Marsden

Malaria remains the greatest challenge in parasitic disease both in terms of prevalence (over 500 million people still live in malarious areas) and in the amount of morbidity and mortality it causes. In many tropical countries, notably Africa, malaria has a profound influence on the pattern of clinical medicine.

Trypanosomiasis is a good example of geographically restricted disease. *Trypanosoma brucei* infections are restricted to Africa because tsetse flies (*Glossina* species) are not found elsewhere. African sleeping sickness demands attention because human infections once established are so frequently fatal. Also, this same group of trypanosomes are responsible for widespread fatal disease in cattle, profoundly influencing animal husbandry. South American trypanosomiasis (Chagas' disease) is restricted to the Americas because again the great majority of reduviid bugs occur in this location. The significance of this infection as a public health problem is a matter of current concern. One estimate suggests that 7 million people are infected and 30 million exposed to the risk of infection. Permanent cardiac damage often ensues, and at the time of writing there is no cure.

Also in the family Trypanosomatidae, the genus *Leishmania* is responsible for considerable human suffering. Visceral leishmaniasis is a debilitating infection, and without treatment the terminal event is usually a secondary bacterial infection, often a pneumonia. Cutaneous and mucocutaneous leishmaniasis can be disfiguring infections. Therapy is far from satisfactory.

Amebiasis ranks fourth in this consideration, because, although bowel infections are widely prevalent, invasive disease is less common. Then come a miscellany of rarer protozoal disease entities.

The reader will appreciate that the first three groups of diseases caused by protozoa all have arthropod vectors: *Anopheles* for malaria, *Glossina* and Reduviidae for trypanosomiasis, and *Phlebotomus* for leishmaniasis. It is relevant and important for medical people to have some knowledge of these vectors. A few examples of why this is so will suffice. At the time of writing there have been a few cases of indigenous vivax malaria recognized in the United States. Epidemiologic work has revealed vector *Anopheles* in the area. Xenodiagnosis using clean Reduviidae is the best way of finding *Trypanosoma cruzi* parasites in a patient with a chronic infection, and because of this these insects are most important, as they are used in diagnostic medicine. *Phlebotomus* remains very susceptible to DDT, and spraying of this insect's habitats will result in the control of human leishmaniasis.

Another medical consideration worth emphasizing is that blood protozoa can be transmitted by blood transfusion. Particularly important in this respect are malaria and *Trypanosoma cruzi* infections. Suitable selection of donors in temperate countries is necessary to avoid this complication in nonimmune persons exposed to the risk of malaria parasites in transfused blood. *Trypanosoma cruzi* infections transmitted by blood transfusion are said to be particularly acute. It is of interest that recent advances in immunology enable us to screen blood donors for malaria with the indirect fluorescent antibody test, whereas for *Trypanosoma cruzi* the valuable complement-fixation test or an indirect fluorescent antibody test is available.

Belding, D. L.: Textbook of Parasitology. 3rd ed. New York, Appleton-Century-Crofts, Inc., 1965.

Faust, E. C., and Russell, P. F.: Clinical Parasitology. 8th ed. Philadelphia, Lea & Febiger, 1970.

Hunter, G. W., Swartzwelder, J. C. and Clyde, D. F.: Tropical Medicine. 5th ed. Philadelphia, W. B. Saunders Company, 1976.

Wilcocks, C., and Manson-Bahr, P. E. C.: Manson's Tropical Diseases. 17th ed. Baltimore, Williams & Wilkins Company, 1972.

Woodruff, A. W.: Medicine in the Tropics. New York, Longman, 1974.

193.   MALARIA

Thomas C. Jones

GENERAL CONSIDERATIONS.   Malaria is characterized by shaking chills, relapsing fever, prostration, splenomegaly, and anemia. After the initial illness, the disease may follow a chronic or relapsing course. It is caused by four species of the genus *Plasmodium* (*P. vivax, P. falciparum, P. malariae,* and *P. ovale*). The infection is maintained in nature by the feeding habits of female mosquitoes of the genus *Anopheles,* in which sporogony occurs, feeding on blood of humans, in which schizogony and gametocytogony occur. Malaria remains a common cause of morbidity and mortality in the world. Delay in diagnosis or inappropriate therapy may lead to severe complications which include coma, acute renal failure, severe anemia, pulmonary edema, or shock. Recognition of the association between malaria and hemoglobinopathies, persistent hypergammaglobulinemia, and the tropical splenomegaly syndrome has emphasized the often subtle but significant influence of malaria on populations living in endemic areas.

HISTORY.   The term malaria originated in the seventeenth century in Italy where the death of patients after intermittent or so-called Roman fevers was attributed to the bad air (mal'aria) of the marsh and swamp lands. These fevers were recognized in ancient times in China, India, and Mesopotamia, but the earliest record of quotidian, tertian, and quartan fevers was that of Hippocrates in the fifth century B.C. The Greeks and Romans were aware of the association of these fevers with marsh lands and conducted one of the earliest public health campaigns by draining the stagnant water. Cinchona bark was recognized as being effective against fevers in 1600 in Peru, after which it was widely used in Europe. Torti, in 1712, clearly distinguished the fevers that responded to cinchona from those that did not.

The protozoan was first described in the blood of a patient

by Charles Laveran in 1880, who observed the parasite in an unstained smear of fresh blood. In 1891 Romanowsky developed a technique for staining blood smears for accurate study of the erythrocytic stage of malaria. In 1897, William MacCallum observed penetration and fertilization of the female gamete, documenting that a sexual cycle occurred in malaria. The role of the mosquito as a vector in malaria was postulated by Sir Patrick Manson after he documented that filaria could develop in the mosquito. The careful studies of Sir Ronald Ross in 1898 documented that in avian malaria the protozoan developed in the stomach of infected mosquitoes and migrated to the salivary glands, from which it could infect healthy birds. Several months later Bignami, Bastianelli, and Grassi documented the transmission of malaria to man by *Anopheles* mosquitoes. Our present knowledge of the malaria cycle was completed in 1948 when Shortt, Garnham, Bray, and others confirmed the presence of the pre-erythrocytic stage in man.

A decrease in the prevalence of malaria during this century has resulted from campaigns to control mosquitoes and the widespread use of drug therapy directed against malaria. The systematic approach to mosquito control organized by Col. William Gorgas in the Canal Zone in 1906 was one of the outstanding achievements in preventive medical science. Effective insecticides were first introduced in 1939, and a number of synthetic antimalarial drugs were developed. The global program of malaria eradication was instituted during the 1950's. It has become clear recently, however, that various biologic, technical, and socioeconomic problems in some countries have required that careful methods of malaria control be substituted for attempts at eradication of the disease.

EPIDEMIOLOGY. Malaria is an endemic disease in parts of Africa, Asia, and Central and South America, where environmental factors, including temperature, humidity, and standing water, support the breeding of mosquitoes and where there is close contact between the mosquitoes and man. The disease in these areas contributes to a high infant mortality and syndromes of chronic malaria. The prevalence of malaria in endemic areas is usually determined by documenting the proportion of people with large spleens (spleen rate) or the proportion of people with blood smears positive for malaria parasites (parasite rate). It has been estimated that 100 million cases of malaria occur each year. Approximately 1 per cent of these patients die of the disease, although this figure can vary from less than 1 per cent to over 10 per cent, depending on the species of *Plasmodium* most prevalent, the level of immunity of the host, and the availability of prompt medical care.

Acute disease caused by malaria often occurs when nonimmune persons enter endemic areas. Through the centuries the most impressive effects of malaria have been recorded during time of war when large numbers of nonimmunes are placed in malarious areas. This has certainly been the major factor contributing to the incidence of malaria in American citizens in the past 35 years. The number of cases of malaria in the United States rose from less than 100 in 1960 to 4000 in 1970 as a direct result of the exposure of nonimmune military personnel to the disease in Vietnam.

Epidemics of malaria may occur when the parasite is introduced into a region with a large nonimmune population. This occurred in the Soviet Union after World War I when more than 5 million cases were reported in 1923; and in Ethiopia in 1958 when 3 million cases and 150,000 deaths caused by malaria were reported. Such epidemics are reminders of the potential threat to localities where effective malaria eradication has created a large nonimmune population but where mosquito vectors persist in large numbers. Vectors for transmission

of plasmodia, primarily *A. quadrimaculatus* and *A. freeborni*, persist in parts of the United States. In the past 25 years there have been a dozen outbreaks of malaria resulting from mosquito transmission within the United States.

Falciparum and vivax malaria are widely spread throughout the tropics and subtropics, particularly in hot, humid regions. Malariae malaria is also widespread, but it is of lower prevalence, and it tends to be less evenly distributed. Ovale malaria is primarily seen in West Africa.

During the past decade malaria has been found to be associated geographically with several other conditions, including various erythrocyte abnormalities and Burkitt's lymphoma. Patients with sickle hemoglobin have been shown to acquire falciparum malaria as frequently as those with normal hemoglobin, but their disease is less severe. The malaria parasite appears less able to divide in these abnormal erythrocytes. Other hemoglobinopathies and inherited enzyme defects, including hemoglobin C, D, E, K, O, b-thalassemia, and glucose-6-phosphate dehydrogenase deficiency, have also been shown to occur more commonly in areas endemic for malaria. These defects appear to provide a selective advantage for survival in malarious areas. Correlation of the prevalence of Burkitt's lymphoma with prevalence of malaria has led to suggestions that chronic malaria suppresses mechanisms for immunologic surveillance, leading to expression of this tumor. Some work in laboratory animals chronically infected with malaria supports this view, but the relationship needs further clarification.

The epidemiology of malaria is inseparable from the epidemiology of its mosquito vectors. Entomologists must document different and changing characteristics of the numerous species of anopheline mosquitoes, including their flying and resting habits, feeding habits, and degree of resistance to insecticides. For example, a change in mosquito living habits from domestic to sylvatic in Central America has rendered the usual technique of household DDT residual spraying less effective. Several instances have been recorded in which mosquito feeding habits changed from cattle to man, resulting in epidemic malaria.

Although the mosquito is the primary vector for malaria, direct transfer of infected erythrocytes from one individual to another by blood transfusion or syringe usage in common by addicts will cause malaria. In these cases the sexual cycle in the mosquito and the pre-erythrocytic stages of malaria in man are bypassed. In the past 20 years, over 50 cases of malaria transmitted by transfusions were reported in the United States. The American Association of Blood Banks has recommended that blood not be taken from anyone who has emigrated from an endemic area or had malaria during the preceding three years, or who has visited a malarious area during which antimalarial prophylaxis was taken in the preceding two years. Travelers to malarial areas who remained symptom free and who did not take antimalarials may donate blood after six months. An epidemic of vivax malaria (which affected 47 persons) was reported from California after the sharing of heroin injection equipment by drug addicts. In the past, malaria was transmitted intentionally by physicians as a method of causing fever in patients for treatment of neurosyphilis and other diseases. Congenitally acquired malaria probably occurs more commonly in

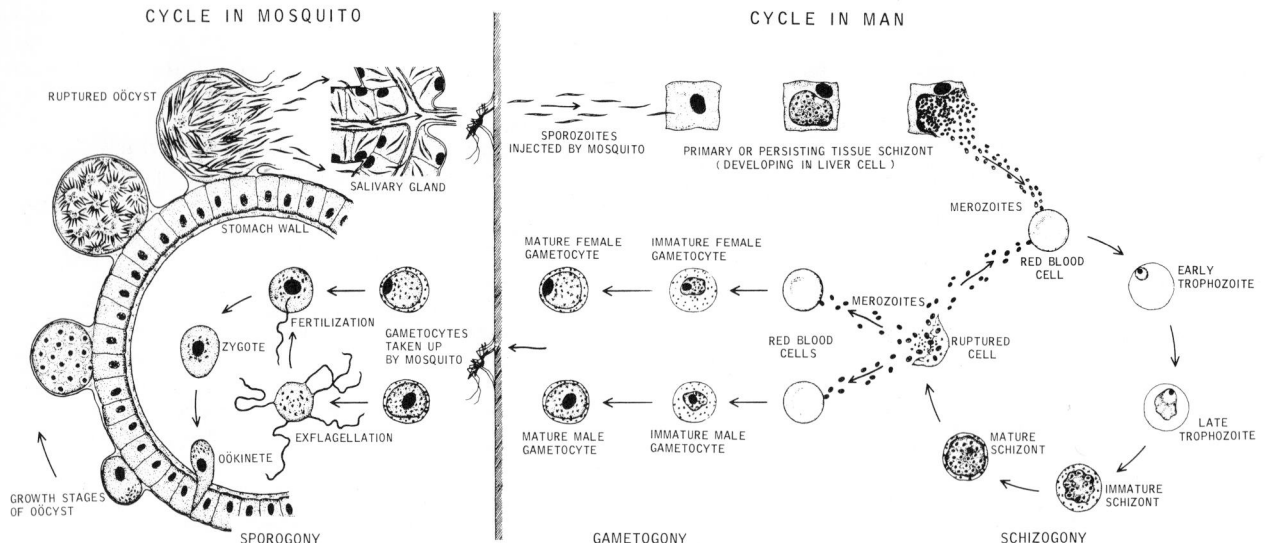

Figure 1. Life cycle of *Plasmodium* in mosquito and man. (Adapted from Alvarado, C. A., and Bruce-Chwatt, L. J.: Scientific American, Vol. 206, May, 1962. Copyright © 1962, by Scientific American, Inc. All rights reserved.)

endemic areas than has been recorded. Transmission of malaria of monkeys, *P. knowlesi* and *P. cynomolgi*, from monkey to man has been demonstrated in the laboratory and rarely documented in nature.

The major thrust against malaria has been the worldwide cooperative program of malaria eradication begun approximately 25 years ago. The program was a unified approach divided into four carefully defined phases: preparatory, attack, consolidation, and maintenance. The techniques included concentrated spraying with residual insecticides, use of antimalarial drugs, and case-detection surveys. Recently, a number of problems have challenged the completion of malaria eradication using these techniques: inadequate finances in some regions; social disorganization during war and natural disaster; resistance of mosquitoes to insecticides; and resistance of plasmodia to antimalarial drugs. Realization of these limitations has led to programs concentrating on malaria control rather than eradicaton. There has been an increased interest in malaria immunity, both to define mechanisms of natural or acquired resistance and to develop potentially useful vaccines.

THE PROTOZOAN. Over 100 different species of *Plasmodium* are capable of infecting the red blood cells of mammals, birds, and reptiles. There are several hundred species of *Anopheles* mosquitoes which can be infected by the protozoan and therefore transmit the disease. Male anopheline mosquitoes feed on nectar and therefore do not transmit the infection. The female requires products of a blood meal for egg production. Female mosquitoes vary in their feeding habits so that only 50 species participate in transmission of human malaria. During the process of feeding, the mosquito injects fluid from the salivary glands. Sporozoites may be released with the salivary fluid if the mosquito ate a blood meal two to four weeks previously which contained male and female malaria gametocytes (Fig. 1).

The sporozoites enter the circulation immediately, and a transient parasitemia occurs which lasts less than one hour. During this period the sporozoites enter hepatic parenchymal cells, initiating the *pre-erythrocytic* stage of plasmodium infection by forming a primary

hepatic schizont. The duration of this pre-erythrocytic stage is usually short in *P. falciparum* (5.5 to 7 days) and *P. vivax* (6 to 8 days) but somewhat longer in *P. ovale* (9 days) and *P. malariae* (13 to 16 days). Merozoites are then released from the hepatic cells and enter circulating erythrocytes. Occasionally, when the number of sporozoites inoculated is very low, the period from infection to onset of erythrocyte infection lasts for months or even years. In falciparum malaria the tissue phase terminates at the beginning of the *erythrocyte cycle;* in vivax and ovale malaria, the hepatic forms persist.* This species variation necessitates different therapeutic approaches in treating malaria. The species also differ in the number of merozoites released after primary hepatic schizogony: *P. falciparum,* about 40,000 from each infected cell; *P. ovale,* 15,000; *P. vivax,* 10,000; and *P. malariae,* 2000. The large number of merozoites released into the cirulation in *P. falciparum* may contribute to the high levels of parasitemia seen in this infection and perhaps to the increased frequency with which erythrocytes are observed to contain multiple organisms.

The merozoite attaches to specific receptors on the red blood cell and then enters by inducing erythrocyte endocytosis, and the organism begins to develop within a vacuole in the erythrocyte. Using Giemsa or Wright stains, the parasite is first identified with light microscopy as a characteristic "ring-form," an early *trophozoite* (Figs. 2A and 2B). The organism increases in size, partially filling the red blood cell; this is termed the late *trophozoite*. Later the nuclear material is segregated by schizogony, and the red cell becomes partially filled with the cytoplasm and the multiple nuclei of the *schizont* (Fig. 2C). The erythrocyte cycle is completed when the red blood cells rupture, releasing the merozoites formed from the schizont, which then invade other erythrocytes. This cycle takes 48 hours in *P.*

---

*The exoerythrocytic state is described in this chapter as "persistent" rather than cyclic, based on the arguments presented by Coatney et al. in the first cited reference. It is recognized that not all malariologists agree with this change in terms or the implied change in the nature of tissue schizogony and the mechanism of relapse.

falciparum, P. vivax, and *P. ovale* malaria, and 72 hours in *P. malariae* infection. Symptoms of fever and chills coincide with the release of merozoites; hence the clinical descriptions of tertian malaria (fevers on days one and three) and quartan malaria (fevers on days one and four). The number of merozoites formed during erythrocyte schizogony is helpful in species diagnosis. Examination of a mature schizont of *P. malariae* will reveal 6 to 12 developing merozoites, *P. ovale* 6 to 16, and *P. vivax* 12 to 24.

By mechanisms which remain unknown, some merozoites do not continue the cycle of schizogony but develop into female and male gametocytes (Fig. 1). These first appear in the peripheral blood several days after the onset of the erythrocytic cycle, and they may persist for weeks after schizogony has been suppressed. During the blood meal of an *Anopheles* mosquito, the gametocytes are ingested. Conditions exist in the stomach of the mosquito for the male gametocyte to form motile male gametes (exflagellation) which then fertilize the female gamete. After fertilization, the *zygote* becomes a motile *ookinete*, penetrates the stomach wall, and multiplies in an enlarging *oocyst*. Rupture of this cyst allows release of sporozoites which are distributed throughout the mosquito and accumulate in the salivary gland. The formation of sporozoites completes the process of *sporogony*, the sexual or mosquito cycle of malaria.

PATHOGENESIS AND IMMUNITY. There has been no documentation of generalized or significant host injury or response during the periods of sporozoitemia or hepatic schizogony, although antisporozoite antibodies have been demonstrated. After release of merozoites from the hepatic cells into the circulation, however, marked changes occur. Parasitized and nonparasitized red blood cells undergo alterations. In *P. falciparum* infection the erythrocytes develop electron-dense knob-like projections, take unusual shapes, and become less deformable. They also become more adhesive to vascular endothelium and more permeable to sodium, and demonstrate increased osmotic fragility. During the erythrocyte cycle, red blood cells are damaged at the time merozoites are released, leading to intravascular hemolysis and progressive anemia. Damage to vascular endothelium also occurs. B lymphocytes begin to produce immunoglobulin M and G antibodies directed against the merozoites, and excess antibody is seen in the plasma in several days. These antibodies coat merozoites, after which they do not enter uninfected red cells, and they are removed from the circulation by phagocytic cells in the bone marrow, spleen, and liver. T lymphocytes release materials which stimulate increased metabolic and phagocytic activity of macrophages. This series of events produces the clinical and pathologic changes observed in acute and chronic malaria.

In acute falciparum malaria a number of complications result from alteration of the red blood cells and the vascular endothelium. The severe anemia and the adherence of red cells to capillary endothelium decrease oxygen supply to the tissues. The anoxia causes serious functional impairment of the brain and kidneys, less commonly of the liver, myocardium, and bone marrow. In fatal cases of falciparum malaria the brain is edematous, and blood vessels are occluded by parasitized erythrocytes, and surrounded by areas of hemorrhage and necrosis. The kidney may show ischemia of the renal cortex and diffuse glomerulitis, as well as tubular necrosis. The liver may show centrilobular degeneration and necrosis. These changes in the kidney and liver are believed related more to ischemia secondary to severe anemia and hypovolemia than to vascular obstruction by erythrocytes. In patients who die in pulmonary edema unrelated to fluid overload, the cardiac and pulmonary vessels are filled with parasitized red cells. Impaired bone marrow function in man is manifested by thrombocytopenia, absence of reticulocytes, and varying degrees of leukopenia.

Accelerated intravascular coagulation can be documented in patients with malaria; that is, factors V, VII, VIII, X, fibrinogen, and platelets are decreased, prothrombin and partial thromboplastin times are prolonged, and fibrin degradation products are increased. However, disseminated intravascular coagulation is not a prominent feature at autopsy of patients who die of malaria.

During the acute attack of falciparum malaria, most patients develop vasodilation, just as in other acute febrile diseases. This results in decreased effective circulating blood volume and orthostatic hypotension. Changes secondary to this include increased aldosterone levels, increased plasma volume, hyponatremia, and reversal of the urinary sodium to potassium ratio.

Some of the clinical and pathologic features of malaria are related to the host immune response. Patients occasionally have a Coombs-positive hemolytic anemia. This may partially explain the rapid intravascular hemolysis which exceeds that attributable to the level of parasitemia alone. "Blackwater fever," the complication of falciparum malaria characterized by rapid hemolysis and acute renal failure, occurs both in patients who have received quinine and in patients who have a history of previous exposure to the *Plasmodium* and who have not received quinine. Antibody damage to red cells has been postulated in both situations. The pathologic changes seen in blackwater fever include renal ischemia and tubular necrosis. Recent evidence has suggested that the glomerulitis seen in some patients with falciparum malaria may be induced by immune complexes.

The pathologic picture in malaria of long duration is in large part that due to the immune response. Marked elevation of the serum immunoglobulins (IgG and IgM) is seen, and the liver and spleen are enlarged consistent with continued stimulation to the reticuloendothelial system. Anemia is common. A number of patients in an area hyperendemic for malaria develop marked splenomegaly (tropical splenomegaly syndrome). Parasites may not be demonstrable in peripheral blood smears, but elevated fluorescent antimalarial antibody titers are present, and the patients respond to prolonged therapy with antimalarials. Liver biopsy frequently shows hepatic sinusoidal lymphocytosis. In *P. malariae* infection of long duration, nephrotic syndrome is not uncommon. There is good evidence that this is related to immune complex injury to the glomerulus. Preliminary evidence has suggested that patients with chronic malaria have depressed cellular immune responses.

Host Resistance. Resistance to malaria involves numerous complex metabolic and immunologic factors. As mentioned previously, certain hemoglobinopathies and enzyme defects of the erythrocytes render patients less vulnerable to the severe complications of malaria. Blacks are less susceptible to *P. vivax* infection than

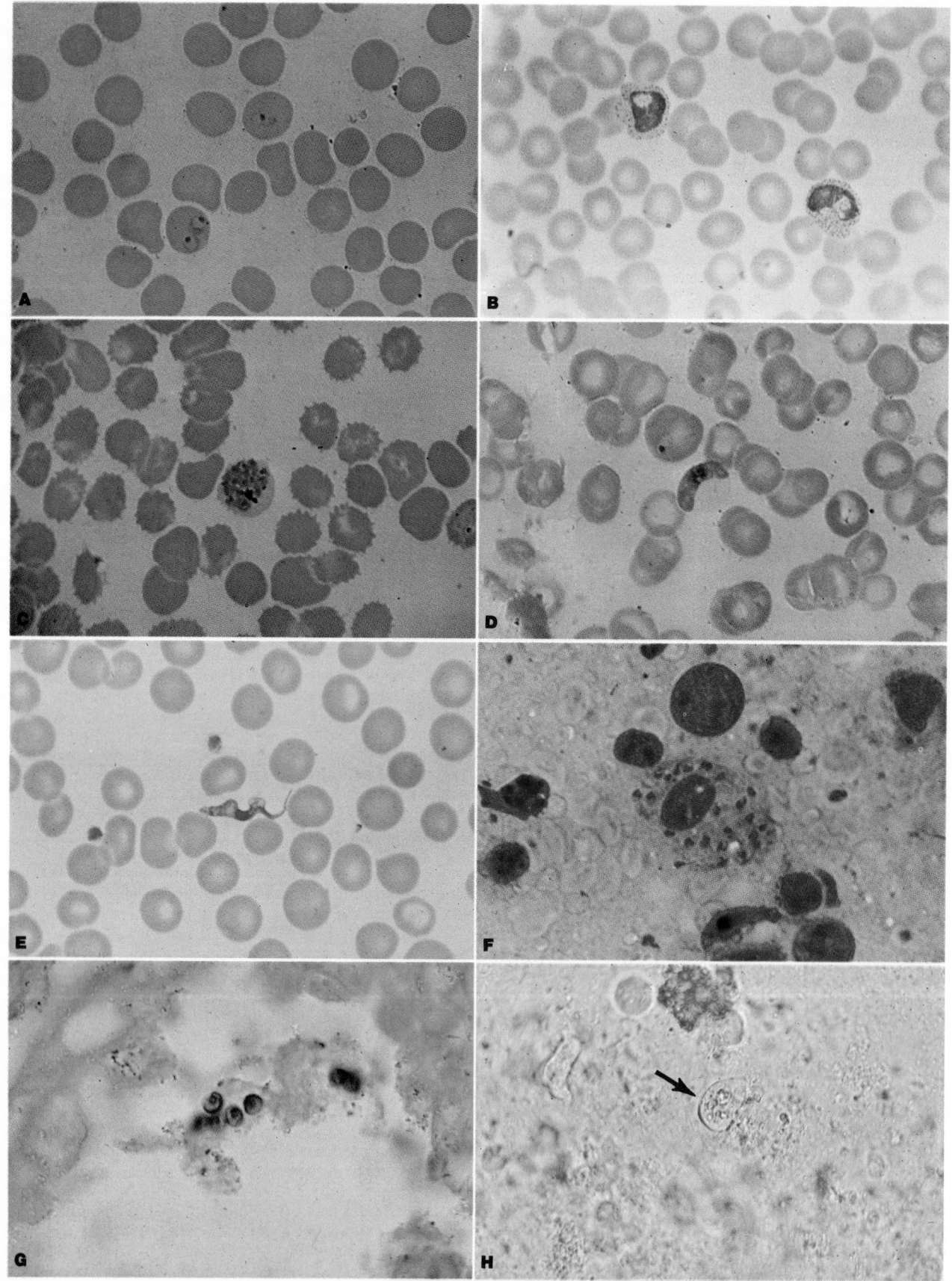

Figure 2.   *See opposite page for legend.*

whites. This has recently been shown to be associated with the absence of Duffy blood group substance in a majority of blacks. *Acquired immunity* to malaria requires both humoral and cellular defense mechanisms. Circulating antibodies are of primary importance in control of the acute infection, documented by studies in which antimalaria IgG was transferred to infected hosts and found to be protective. This protection was species specific. The role of antibody has been shown by the transfer of immunity from mother to fetus, with protection of the neonate during the period in which maternal IgG persists. Whether decreases in immunoglobulin levels contribute to relapse of malaria has not been clearly shown. The importance of cellular defense mechanisms has been suggested by the intense phagocytic activity of cells of the reticuloendothelial system during malaria infection.

CLINICAL MANIFESTATIONS. The patient with malaria experiences chills and fever, often associated with frontal headache and myalgias. In the early period of the illness the fever may be persistent for several days before developing into a synchronous periodicity, the hallmark of tertian or quartan malaria. When the typical pattern has been established, the patient has a chill, a rise in temperature to 40 to 41° C, headache, and myalgias. This is followed in several hours by diffuse sweating and a fall in temperature. In vivax and ovale malaria these paroxysms occur every 48 hours (benign tertian malaria) and in malariae malaria every 72 hours (quartan malaria). In falciparum malaria the temperature is usually persistently elevated, but it may occasionally progress to a 48-hour cycle (malignant tertian malaria). Between the paroxysms of chills and fever, the patient often feels well except for some weakness or fatigue.

The illness may occasionally begin with nonspecific symptoms such as *malaise, dry cough,* and *abdominal pain.* Most patients have *nausea* and *anorexia; vomiting* is less common. These symptoms may mislead the physician into making a diagnosis of pharyngitis, influenza, or gastroenteritis. Occasionally, the only sign of malaria is fever. In the postoperative surgical patient, fever caused by malaria is frequently confused with that caused by drug allergy. Rarely fever may be absent.

Physical examination reveals a tachycardia, and the skin is warm and flushed. *Jaundice* is not common, but occasionally it can be a prominent feature of the illness. *Hepatomegaly* is commonly found, and the liver may be moderately tender. The spleen is often palpable in acute malaria and is usually quite soft and occasionally tender. Attempts to palpate the spleen should be made carefully in view of the relative ease with which splenic rupture can occur. *Splenomegaly* is more commonly found in the early stage of vivax and ovale malaria than in falciparum malaria. Orthostatic hypotension can be documented in falciparum malaria. Lesions of herpes simplex virus may be seen.

Examination of peripheral blood after several days of illness reveals a normochromic, normocytic anemia which is usually mild, but it may be severe in prolonged infections or in those presenting with high parasitemia or acute hemolysis. The number of reticulocytes is usually normal until several days after therapy has been begun; then reticulocytosis is seen. The white blood cell count is normal or low. Monocytosis may be present, but eosinophilia is not a feature of malaria. Thrombocytopenia of a moderate degree is usually present. Serum $\alpha 1$ glycoproteins are increased, whereas $\alpha 2$ glycoproteins (containing haptoglobin) are decreased. A false-positive serologic test for syphilis (VDRL) may occur. The serum transaminases are almost always elevated to moderate degrees and total bilirubin is often elevated. This is predominantly indirect bilirubin, but occasionally increased conjugated bilirubin is seen. Severe cases of malaria may be associated with sufficient liver dysfunction to be misdiagnosed as infectious hepatitis. Tests for determining intestinal absorption have been shown to be abnormal in some malaria patients. Urinalysis reveals trace amounts of albumin and bilirubin in uncomplicated cases, and rarely marked proteinuria has been documented. In falciparum malaria hyponatremia, reversal of the urinary sodium/potassium ratio, and transient increases in serum creatinine and blood urea nitrogen can frequently be recorded.

Fever and related symptoms gradually subside over several weeks in untreated vivax, ovale, and malariae malaria. However, relapse of vivax or ovale infection may occur months or even years later. The illness at the time of relapse is usually milder and of shorter duration than the initial illness. Death caused by infection with these species is very uncommon.

Complications. In falciparum malaria high levels of parasitemia and serious complications may develop rapidly. The most important of these complications are *coma, severe hemolytic anemia, acute renal failure,* and *acute pulmonary edema.* The patient may first demonstrate confusion with increasing lethargy, and within a few hours be unconscious. Focal neurologic signs are uncommon, but hyperreflexia and Babinski signs may be seen. Examination of the cerebrospinal fluid will reveal increased pressure and increased protein, without

Figure 2. *A* to *D* show various erythrocyte forms of falciparum or vivax malaria (× 1500).

A, "Ring forms" of *Plasmodium falciparum.* Note the delicate rings and an erythrocyte containing two organisms.

B, Trophozoite of *Plasmodium vivax.* The red cell is enlarged, Schüffner's dots are seen, and the parasite is large and ameboid.

C, Schizont of *Plasmodium vivax* with at least 18 merozoite nuclei.

D, Gametocyte of *Plasmodium falciparum.* The crescent or banana shape is characteristic.

E, *Trypanosoma rhodesiense* in the peripheral blood. It has a nucleus, posterior kinetoplast, an undulating membrane, and flagellum (× 1500).

F, Spleen smear showing a cell filled with *Leishmania donovani.* The rod-shaped kinetoplast and large round nucleus appear as two adjacent red dots.

G, Methenamine silver nitrate stain of clump of *Pneumocystis* cysts. They appear as black circles against the blue background (× 800).

H, Stool sample observed by light microscopy, showing a motile *Entamoeba histolytica* moving in a straight line across the field. The ameba contains lucent vacuoles and shows a pseudopod directed to the upper right (× 500).

(*A, C, D,* and *F* are photographs taken by T. C. Jones from the Cornell Parasitology teaching slides; *B* is from the collection of H. Zaiman, originally photographed by M. Wittner; *E* and *G* were provided by R. B. Roberts; *H* is a photograph of fresh material provided by T. C. Jones.)

pleocytosis. *Massive intravascular hemolysis* may result from high levels of parasitemia, quinine therapy, drug administration to patients with glucose-6-phosphate dehydrogenase deficiency, or hypersensitivity after previous malaria infections. Hemoglobinuria, acute tubular necrosis, and renal failure may result. *Hemolysis, hemoglobinuria,* and *renal failure* make up the striking clinical picture of severe malaria known as "blackwater fever." Acute renal failure may occur in the absence of signs of intravascular hemolysis and can be detected early only by careful monitoring of the urine volume and serum creatinine or urea nitrogen levels. Acute pulmonary edema is an uncommon complication, but it may develop rapidly and be particularly refractory to therapy. Pulmonary edema may be due to excessive fluid administration, but a number of cases have been reported in which intravascular volume was normal. Patients may present with signs and symptoms of vascular collapse — so-called algid malaria. A rare complication of malaria is splenic rupture, the only complication which is probably more common in vivax than falciparum malaria. Patients who survive untreated falciparum malaria may have recurrences of symptoms for a number of months, but thereafter they remain asymptomatic.

Syndromes Associated with Chronic Malaria. Syndromes associated with chronic malaria are most likely the result of repeated exposure of immune patients to *Plasmodium* and occur predominantly in hyperendemic areas of malaria. The patients may be asymptomatic, but they have intermittently detectable parasitemia, hypergammaglobulinemia, elevated antimalaria antibody titers, anemia, and splenic enlargement. Some patients develop marked splenomegaly — the tropical splenomegaly syndrome. Patients infected with *P. malariae* may develop nephrotic syndrome (quartan nephrosis). This is most common in children. It is associated with a poor prognosis and does not respond well to corticosteroid administration.

DIAGNOSIS. The diagnosis of malaria must be suspected in every patient with fever, coma, or shock who has lived or traveled in a malarious area, has received a blood transfusion, or may be a drug addict. The only technique for confirming the clinical suspicion of malaria is the identification of plasmodia in fixed, stained blood smears. The diagnosis may be made by an alert technician during examination of a differential white count. However, it is usually only when a high suspicion of the possibility of malaria exists that the proper smears will be done and the necessary time taken to make the diagnosis.

Thin blood smears are made by placing a drop of blood on the end of a glass slide, touching the drop with another slide, and rapidly moving the edge of the second slide along the surface of the first. A thick blood smear is made by placing a drop of blood on a slide, then spreading it to fill a diameter of about 1 cm. The slides are allowed to dry. The thin blood smear is fixed in methanol and stained with Giemsa, or fixed and stained with Wright's. The thick blood smear is first dipped in water to lyse the red blood cells, then fixed and similarly stained. For the inexperienced observer the thin smear is easiest to examine and most likely to yield the diagnosis in the nonimmune patient with malaria. Careful examination of several thousand red blood cells on a properly stained smear will usually reveal the protozoan. When malaria is suspected but smears do not reveal the organism, smears should be repeated several times a day. The highest level of parasitemia is said to be demonstrable several hours *after* a chill. A thick smear can be particularly helpful for finding the characteristic gametocyte of falciparum malaria (Fig. 2D), but it may also reveal organisms when they are too infrequent to be easily identified on a thin smear.

The correct diagnosis of the species of *Plasmodium* is critical in determining therapy and prognosis in malaria. The following brief description and the photomicrographs in Figure 2 were selected to aid in differentiating *P. vivax* and *P. falciparum* in peripheral blood.

Differentiation of P. Vivax and P. Falciparum in Blood Smears. The following characteristics can be used to identify *P. falciparum*. Only the ring forms are usually seen in the peripheral blood; they are small and delicate, often with two chromatin dots (Fig. 2A). The erythrocytes containing these protozoa are not conspicuously enlarged, and red dots (Schüffner's dots) are not present. The level of parasitemia may be high (more than 5 to 10 per cent of the erythrocytes infected), and some erythrocytes may contain several parasites. Organisms may appear to be on the surface of the erythrocyte (appliqué forms). *P. vivax* ring forms are often larger than falciparum rings and in later stages appear quite pleomorphic (Fig. 2B). The infected erythrocytes are usually larger than normal, and if properly stained, Schüffner's dots can be identified. By examining blood films at various times, the maturation of *P. vivax* in the peripheral blood can be documented. The mature schizont (Fig. 2C) contains 12 to 24 chromatin dots, and the parasite cytoplasm almost fills the red blood cell. The gametocyte of *P. falciparum* is very characteristic (Fig. 2D) and should be looked for carefully since it substantiates the diagnosis. It has a crescent or banana shape, whereas the shape of *P. vivax* gametocytes is globular.

Mixed Infection. Even after one species of malaria is identified, it must be kept in mind that the patient could have a mixed infection (1 to 2 per cent of cases). Mixed infection can best be diagnosed by careful review of several thin blood films. Repeated blood films for one to two days after the start of treatment should show decreasing levels of parasitemia. If a *P. vivax* infection is diagnosed and treated with chloroquine but parasitemia is seen to be increasing, a mixed infection with chloroquine-resistant *P. falciparum* should be suspected. At present, *P. falciparum* infection acquired in Asia and parts of Central and South America is resistant to chloroquine (see below). All patients diagnosed as having *P. falciparum* should have repeated smears during therapy to ensure that the parasitemia is decreasing.

Chloroquine Susceptibility Test. A technique for documenting whether *P. falciparum* is susceptible or resistant has been developed. At the time of initial diagnosis and before therapy is instituted, a sample of the patient's blood is defibrinated and added to vials (1 ml each) containing varying concentrations of chloroquine and 5 mg of glucose per 100 ml. During 24 hours of incubation, *P. falciparum* will mature to the schizont stage in the vials containing insufficent levels of chloroquine. Chloroquine susceptibility can be calculated from these data.

Antibody Tests. Antibody tests for malaria are not useful in the diagnosis of the acute illness. The indirect fluorescent antibody and hemagglutination tests are of value in testing populations to determine the prevalence of malaria and in screening blood donors when tracing cases of transfusion-induced malaria. They have also been of help in confirming recent malaria and supporting morphologic diagnosis of malaria species.

Differential Diagnosis. The differential diagnosis of malaria is lengthy and varies, depending upon the area of the world, the dominant malaria species, and whether the disease is acute or chronic. The fever of malaria must be separated from fever caused by dengue and other arboviruses, typhus, amebiasis, typhoid, relapsing fever, heat stroke, drug allergy, influenza, bacterial pneumonias, and wound infections. Intermittent chills secondary to antipyretics may simulate the chills and fever of malaria in all these conditions. Cerebral malaria must be distinguished from viral encephalitides, drug overdose, and other causes of coma. The jaundice of malaria must be distinguished from viral hepatitis and leptospirosis. In more chronic malaria infection in which splenomegaly and anemia are prominent, one must also consider infective endocarditis, schistosomiasis, visceral leishmaniasis, and lymphoma.

THERAPY. Elimination of Parasitemia. The initial therapeutic goal in the treatment of malaria is to eliminate the erythrocytic stage of the infection, because all the acute symptoms are due to this hematogenous process. Chloroquine, a 4-aminoquinoline, is the drug of choice to accomplish this purpose. It can be given orally, or parenterally if the patient is vomiting. Chloroquine diphosphate is given orally as follows: 1 gram initially (600 mg of base), followed by 500 mg (300 mg of base) at 6 hours, 24 hours, and 48 hours after the initial dose (total dose 2.5 grams; 1.5 grams of base). Children should receive a loading dose of 17 mg per kilogram, followed by 8.5 mg per kilogram at 6, 24, and 48 hours.* Chloroquine hydrochloride is available for intramuscular or intravenous injection. It is important to note that the hydrochloride salt contains a different quantity of chloroquine base than the diphosphate salt. Chloroquine base, 300 mg, is given intramuscularly every six hours for three doses (total of 900 mg base). On the second and third days therapy may be changed to oral medication, or single intramuscular injections can be continued until a total dose of 1.5 grams chloroquine base is reached. Intravenous medication with chloroquine is seldom indicated, because the patient in shock or coma will usually be given quinine realizing the possibility of a drug-resistant infection (see below). If intravenous chloroquine is considered necessary, 300 mg of base is diluted in 300 ml of saline and given over 30 to 60 minutes. It can be given every six to eight hours, but not in excess of a total daily dose of 1000 mg of base.

The exact mechanism of action of chloroquine remains unknown. It interrupts the vacuolar digestive mechanisms of protozoa, and it binds strongly to nucleic acids. Higher concentrations of the drug are found in infected erythrocytes than in uninfected cells or plasma. This enhanced uptake of chloroquine by parasitized cells may be very important, as suggested by the observation that chloroquine-resistant strains do not enhance the concentration of chloroquine by erythrocytes. In spite of the fact that chloroquine is also concentrated in the liver, it is ineffective in inhibiting tissue schizogony. Chloroquine is absorbed rapidly from the gastrointestinal tract. Fifty per cent becomes bound to plasma proteins, and only about 10 per cent of the active compound is excreted in the urine. Most of the drug is concentrated in tissue, and degradation probably occurs in the liver. It disappears from tissue over a period of several weeks after the drug is stopped. Chloroquine is usually well tolerated, but it can cause transient headache, visual disturbances, nausea, and vomiting. At toxic levels it can cause delirium, psychotic reactions, and convulsions. Its use is not contraindicated during pregnancy for treatment of malaria. When given for prolonged periods in doses higher than that used in malaria chemoprophylaxis, punctate keratitis and retinitis have been recorded. Amodiaquine is as effective as chloroquine for treating malaria.

Drug-Resistant Plasmodia. When falciparum malaria is diagnosed, a careful history must include the country where the infection was acquired. If the illness was acquired in South America or Central America, and the level of parasitemia is greater than 2 per cent of erythrocytes, or if it was acquired in any part of Asia, regardless of the level of parasitemia, or if the source of the infection is unknown (such as in transfusion malaria) and parasitemia is high, then quinine sulfate should be used instead of chloroquine. *P. falciparum* acquired in the areas cited has been documented to show varying degrees of resistance to chloroquine.

Resistance of plasmodia to antimalarial drugs has been recognized for many years. Shortly after pyrimethamine and proguanil were introduced, strains resistant to these drugs were identified. This was not unexpected, because protozoa have been known to rapidly develop resistance to inhibitors of folate metabolism. Strains of *P. falciparum* which required higher than standard doses of quinine for inhibition were recorded many years ago. Only in the past decade, however, has the problem of drug resistance been brought to particular attention by appearance of resistance of *P. falciparum* to previously accepted therapeutic levels of chloroquine. Resistant strains apeared in several parts of the world at about the same time, unrelated to whether chloroquine had been commonly used in the area or not.

Resistance of *P. falciparum* to chloroquine has been divided, based on response in level of parasitemia after initiation of therapy: no reduction (termed RIII level of resistance), and partial reduction (termed RII). The first level of chloroquine resistance (RI), to be considered in more detail below, is one in which *patent* parasitemia is eradicated but parasitemia and clinical symptoms recur in a few days to several weeks; i.e., recrudescent malaria. At present, quinine is effective in removing patent parasitemia in these cases; however, a number of other drugs are necessary to prevent recrudescence. Careful attention to the diagnosis of chloroquine-resistant malaria is now an integral part of the management of patients with malaria (see Diagnosis).

To eradicate parasitemia in cases suspected to be caused by chloroquine-resistant strains, quinine is given orally, 650 mg every eight hours for 10 to 14 days. Quinine dihydrochloride is used intravenously in patients unable to take the drug orally. Quinine, 600 mg, is dissolved in 100 to 200 ml of 5 per cent glucose and water and administered over 30 minutes. This is repeated every eight hours. The mechanism of action of quinine against the malaria parasite is unknown. It has been shown to block protein synthetic and glycolytic pathways. It is absorbed readily from the gastrointesti-

---

*See p. vi, Dosage Notice, immediately following Preface.

nal tract, and over 70 per cent is bound to plasma proteins. Like chloroquine, it is concentrated in tissues, including erythrocytes. Only 5 per cent of administered quinine is excreted unchanged in the urine. The most common side effects of quinine are tinnitus, vertigo, nausea, and vomiting. Although these symptoms are annoying, they are not indications to discontinue medication. Since deafness and blindness have been reported due to quinine, blood levels should be checked and decreased dosage should be considered in those with signs of significant nerve toxicity. A Coombs-positive hemolytic anemia is a rare complication of quinine therapy.

Prevention of Recrudescent Falciparum Malaria. Recrudescence of falciparum malaria occurs frequently in patients whose infection was acquired in Asia, Central America, or South America. Recrudescence is due to persistence during an asymptomatic period of erythrocytic stages of *P. falciparum* at undetectable levels, followed by increased parasitemia and symptoms several days to six weeks after apparently successful control of the illness by chloroquine or quinine. This is the first level of chloroquine resistance (RI). To prevent this, several drugs have been added to the initial therapeutic program for treatment of falciparum malaria acquired in the areas previously mentioned. Most commonly, pyrimethamine is given, 50 mg orally per day for three days in combination with sulfadiazine, 1 gram every six hours for five days. A long-acting sulfonamide, e.g., sulfadoxine,* is frequently used in place of sulfadiazine. These drugs act by blocking folate metabolism at the paraminobenzoic acid and the dehydrofolate reductase steps. They can cause bone marrow suppression and allergic reactions. Difference of opinion exists over whether these drugs should be started on the first day of chloroquine or quinine therapy or several days later. We recommend that the drugs be started at the end of chloroquine treatment or on the fourth day of quinine therapy. This reduces the possibility of complicating the clinical picture by potential side effects of the drugs. Clindamycin or tetracycline has been found effective in combination with quinine against recrudescence of falciparum malaria. In cases in which recrudescence has occurred repeatedly, intravenous quinine has been used in place of oral quinine in combination with these drugs.

Gametocytes usually disappear from the peripheral blood within a few days after schizogony is interrupted, and no specific therapy is needed. Primaquine is an effective gametocidal drug and can be used in the rare patient with prolonged asymptomatic gametocytemia.

Prevention of Relapse Due to Persistent Hepatic Schizonts. Relapse of *P. vivax* and *P. ovale* malaria is caused by the persistence of hepatic schizogony.† Primaquine, an 8-aminoquinoline, is usually effective in preventing relapse (approximately 90 per cent of patients are cured). Since relapse is common in these infections, chloroquine therapy should always be followed by a course of primaquine. The adult dose is 15 mg of base daily for 14 days. Children should be given 0.25 mg per kilogram of body weight per day for 14 days. If relapse occurs after a full course of primaquine, a second 14-day period of therapy is usually successful.

The mechanism of action of primaquine is unknown, but it does appear to block glycolysis.

Primaquine can induce hemolysis in patients whose erythrocytes are deficient in glucose-6-phosphate dehydrogenase. Therefore patients should be tested for this deficiency before therapy is started, and if glucose-6-phosphate dehydrogenase deficiency is documented, red blood cell counts should be monitored carefully during treatment.

Supportive Therapy. Treatment of malaria is often accomplished with ease even in cases of falciparum malaria. However, since the course of falciparum malaria is unpredictable and complications may develop rapidly, all cases should be approached as medical emergencies. The management of a patient with malaria includes complete bed rest during the period of orthostatic hypotension. In the occasional patient with very high fever, this should be controlled by continuous antipyretic administration, sponging, and cooling. Frequent determinations of hematocrit, electrolytes, creatinine, urine volume, bilirubin, and transaminases are necessary. The level of consciousness should be carefully monitored.

The patient with falciparum malaria should receive transfusions with packed erythrocytes if severe anemia develops. The vascular volume and cardiac function should be monitored carefully by following the blood pressure, and in severe cases monitoring the central venous pressure may be necessary. Intravenous fluids should be given judiciously with full knowledge of the vascular volume, renal function, and serum electrolytes.

If cerebral malaria develops, the patient should be managed according to procedures used in the care of any comatose patient (see Ch. 219). Corticosteroids have been advocated in these cases to reduce cerebral edema. Heparin therapy should be considered in the rare patients documented to have clinically significant intravascular coagulation.

If the patient develops oliguria, a trial of furosemide or mannitol may be given. However, when acute renal failure is present, judicious administration of fluids associated with hemodialysis or peritoneal dialysis is indicated (see Ch. 372). The dose of quinine should be reduced to half in patients with renal failure, but maintained at therapeutic levels once hemo- or peritoneal dialysis is instituted.

If signs of pulmonary edema develop, standard therapeutic approaches are indicated, including digitalis preparations and methods to reduce the central venous pressure. This complication, however, has been quite refractory to treatment.

PREVENTION. An individual entering an area where malaria remains endemic must avoid contact with mosquitoes and systematically take drug prophylaxis. Use of mosquito netting, screens, insecticides, and mosquito repellents are the main mechanisms for avoiding contact with mosquitoes. The best repellent available at present is N,N-diethyltoluamide. It remains effective for up to 18 hours, a considerable advance over the odor repellents which are of value for only two or four hours.

The best means of malaria prevention is chemoprophylaxis. This is a cumbersome method, requiring intelligence, compulsiveness, and often willingness to tolerate the mild side effects of the medicaton. Travelers should check with medical officials in the area they visit for up-to-date advice on malaria chemoprophy-

---

*This ultralong-acting sulfonamide is not available in the United States, but is available in the United Kingdom.
    †See footnote, page 568.

laxis. The primary drug recommended for prophylaxis for travelers from the United States is chloroquine diphosphate or sulfate. Five hundred milligrams (300 mg of chloroquine base) is taken once a week. Children of ages 8 to 12 should receive 250 mg; ages 4 to 7, 200 mg; and ages 1 to 3, 125 mg; infants should receive 75 mg weekly. Where malaria is hyperendemic, 500 mg twice weekly has been recommended. Chloroquine should be started one to two weeks before entering the malarious area and continued for six weeks after departure from the area. Chloroquine does not prevent the hepatic infection, but simply suppresses the erythrocytic stage; *therefore the period of prophylaxis after leaving the malarious area is very important.* It is this period which travelers most often ignore and which leads to their illness several weeks after leaving the endemic area. After chloroquine prophylaxis, primaquine (15 mg of base per day) should be given for 14 days to eradicate the hepatic stages of plasmodia infections.

A single tablet containing 300 mg of chloroquine base and 45 mg of primaquine base was used for chemoprophylaxis by the U.S. military during the Vietnam war. This tablet is not recommended for use in preference to chloroquine alone. However, if primaquine is unavailable, this drug combination may be used after the traveler leaves the endemic area; it will prevent chloroquine-sensitive falciparum malaria and relapsing malaria. One tablet is taken per week for eight weeks. It is important that this combination *not* be used in the treatment of malaria, because the dose of primaquine base is at toxic levels when 1.5 grams of chloroquine base is given.

Prophylaxis When Chloroquine Resistance Is Present. Chloroquine prophylaxis may be ineffective in areas such as Asia and parts of Central and South America where chloroquine-resistant falciparum malaria is encountered. Travelers to these areas must balance their likely level of exposure to infected mosquitoes with the dangers of more vigorous chemoprophylaxis. The Center for Disease Control has recommended that travelers to these countries take chloroquine in the dose usually recommended for other areas of the world (500 mg once weekly). Chloroguanide hydrochloride (100 to 200 mg per day) is an effective alternative to chloroquine chemoprophylaxis. The travelers must be told that these drugs may not be effective, and they should seek medical care promptly if fever occurs. A drug combination which at present is completely effective in preventing chloroquine-resistant falciparum malaria is pyrimethamine, 25 mg, plus sulfadoxine,* 500 mg, taken once a week. This combination is not available in the United States, but it can be obtained in many other countries. Another effective drug combination is chloroguanide hydrochloride, 100 mg per day, plus dapsone, 25 mg daily. However, an increased risk of agranulocytosis caused by dapsone makes it less desirable as chemoprophylaxis for civilian travelers unless heavy exposure to infected mosquitoes is anticipated.

Prevention in a Community. Prevention of malaria in communities in endemic areas requires a coordinated effort directed at reducing the number of *Anophleles* mosquitoes and identifying and treating human cases of malaria. *Anopheles* are reduced in the environment by draining or filling breeding areas and by the use of larvicides. Effective campaigns against adult mosquitoes usually include spraying of all buildings with residual insecticides twice a year. DDT has been particularly effective for this purpose in the past; however, because of mosquito resistance and potential unacceptable side effects of DDT, other drugs such as hexachlorocyclohexane, dieldrin, malathion, and carbamates are now being used.

In areas endemic for malaria, use of chemoprophylactic drugs is usually reserved for children or pregnant women (to prevent congenital transmission of malaria). In some areas entire populations are treated by including the drug in the salt distribution for daily use. These approaches are used to reduce morbidity and mortality before adequate immunity is acquired. It is hoped that some form of active immunization will replace this method in the future.

Coatney, G. R., Collins, W. E., Warren, M., and Contacos, P. G.: The Primate Malarias. U.S. Department of Health, Education, and Welfare, National Institutes of Health. Washington, D.C., U.S. Government Printing Office, 1971.

Hall, A. P.: The treatment of malaria. Br. Med. J., 1:323, 1976.

Inter-American Malaria Research Symposium. Am. J. Trop. Med. Hyg., 21:613, 1972.

Jeffery, G. M.: Malaria control in the twentieth century. Am. J. Trop. Med. Hyg., 25:361, 1976.

Maegraith, B., and Fletcher, A.: The pathogenesis of mammalian malaria. Adv. Parasitol., 10:49, 1972.

Miller, L. H.: Malaria. *In* Hoeprich, P. D. (ed.): Infectious Diseases. 2nd ed. Hagerstown, Md., Harper & Row, 1977, p. 1075.

Miller, L. H., Mason, S. J., Dovorak, J. A., McGinniss, M. H., and Rothman, I. K.: Erythrocyte receptors for (*Plasmodium knowlesi*) malaria: The Duffy blood group determinants. Science, 189:561, 1975.

Neva, F. A., Sheagren, J. N., Shulman, N. R., and Canfield, C. J.: Malaria: Host-defense mechanisms and complications. Ann. Intern. Med., 73:295, 1970.

World Health Organization: Chemotherapy of Malaria and Resistance to Antimalarials. WHO Tech. Rep. Series No. 529, 1973.

194. TRYPANOSOMIASES

194.1. INTRODUCTION

Philip D. Marsden

Some differences between the four species of trypanosomes which can be found in the bloodstream of man are listed in the accompanying table. *Trypanosoma rangeli* is nonpathogenic but may be mistaken for *T. cruzi* in bug feces during xenodiagnosis. In contrast to *T. cruzi*, *T. rangeli* can be found in the hemolymph and salivary glands of reduviid bugs. In areas where the two species coexist, dissection of such bugs is necessary.

There are similarities as well as differences between Chagas' disease and African sleeping sickness. Essentially both infections have three phases. There is an initial phase of local multiplication following inoculation and a secondary phase of bloodstream dissemination with reticuloendothelial activation; together, these constitute the acute phase of Chagas' disease and first and second stages of sleeping sickness. The blood trypanosome can be found in blood films at this time.

The prolonged tertiary phase is one of organ localization and damage, involving tropisms that are still poorly understood. With the development of immunity the trypanosome is no longer visible in blood films, and

---

*This ultralong-acting sulfonamide is not available in the United States, but is available in the United Kingdom.

Some Differences Between the Human Trypanosomiases

	Trypanosoma gambiense, rhodesiense	*Trypanosoma cruzi*	*Trypanosoma rangeli*
Geographic distribution	Africa	South and Central America	Central and South America
Insect vector	*Glossina*	Reduviidae	Reduviidae
Pathogenicity for insect vector	Low	Low	High
Pathogenicity for man	High	High	Low
Method of transmission by insect	Saliva (bite)	Contamination with feces	Saliva (bite)
Site of dominant human pathology	Brain	Heart muscle, smooth muscle of gut	No pathology
Multiplying form of organism in man	Trypanomastigote	Amastigote	Trypanomastigote
Size of kinetoplast of blood trypanosome	Small	Large	Small

special diagnostic techniques are necessary to demonstrate it. Serology becomes important as a diagnostic aid. During the dissemination phase trypanosomes come in contact with all body tissues, but chronic inflammatory processes proceed principally in the cerebrum in African trypanosomiasis and in the heart and smooth muscle in Chagas' disease. In both diseases evidence of autoimmune mechanisms responsible for this pathology has begun to appear in the literature. Both diseases are notoriously difficult to treat, and to date vaccine production has been impossible. The best hope for control lies in breaking the contact between man and the infected insect vector.

Cancado, J. R.: Doenca de Chagas. Belo Horizonte. Imprensa Oficial do Estado de Minas Gerais, 1968.
D'Alessandro, A.: Biology of *Trypanosoma (Herpetosoma) rangeli*. Tejera, 1920. *In* Lumsden, W. H. R., and Evans, D. A.: Biology of the Kinetoplastida. Vol. I. London, Academic Press, 1976, pp. 327–403.
Mulligan, H. W., and Potts, W. H. (eds.): The African Trypanosomiases. London, Allen and Unwin, 1970.

194.2. AFRICAN TRYPANOSOMIASIS
(Sleeping Sickness)

B. M. Greenwood

DEFINITION AND ETIOLOGY. *Trypanosoma brucei*, the causative agent of African trypanosomiasis, is named after Sir David Bruce, who, in 1894, demonstrated that this organism caused the cattle disease nagana. Eight years later it was shown that the same trypanosome caused human sleeping sickness, a disease that occurs in two forms — West African or Gambian sleeping sickness and East African or Rhodesian sleeping sickness. Trypanosomes causing these diseases cannot be distinguished morphologically, but differentiation of strains that are pathogenic for man from those that are not is often important. In the past this has been achieved by infecting human volunteers, but safer methods are now available. Nonpathogenic strains (*T. b. brucei*) lose their infectivity for laboratory animals when incubated in human serum, whereas the two strains pathogenic for man (*T. b. gambiense* and *T. b. rhodesiense*) do not. These two strains can usually be differentiated by the electrophoretic pattern of two of their component enzymes, alanine aminotransferase and aspartate aminotransferase.

On light microscopy *T. brucei* is seen to be an elongated trypanosome with a prominent nucleus, kinetoplast, and flagellum. Its length varies from 10 to 40 μ, slender and stumpy forms being found in the patient at the same time. Electron microscopy has revealed the detailed struc-

ture of the trypanosome. It is coated with an amorphous material which contains the variant antigens which are of vital importance to its survival.

EPIDEMIOLOGY. Distribution and Prevalence of Sleeping Sickness. Sleeping sickness is restricted to tropical Africa where it has probably occurred in scattered foci for many centuries. The disease was described in the ancient kingdom of Mali in the fourteenth century, and sleeping sickness was well known to the West African slave traders. Around 1890, major epidemics broke out in the Congo basin, around Lake Victoria, and in Nigeria, perhaps because the early colonial explorers and traders carried the disease into areas where it had not previously occurred. At least half a million people died in these epidemics. In the 1930's, the disease again became very active in West Africa, 300,000 cases occurring in Nigeria alone. Since 1950, the incidence of the disease has declined, with the exception of a major outbreak in Zaire in the early 1960's which followed a breakdown in surveillance measures. Zaire still accounts for most of the 5000 to 10,000 cases of sleeping sickness reported annually. Small outbreaks still occur intermittently in nearly all West and Central African countries south of the Sahara. In East Africa the disease is most active in Tanzania and Zambia, a few cases occurring in neighboring countries. In 1968, a new focus of sleeping sickness was discovered in Ethiopia. When present in cattle, trypanosomiasis also affects human health indirectly through its role in contributing to protein malnutrition. In large areas of tropical Africa it is not possible to rear cattle because of trypanosomiasis; in other areas the infection produces sickly animals giving a poor yield of meat.

Pathway of Infection. Tsetse flies are the natural vector of African trypanosomiasis, but it is possible that the disease may occasionally be transmitted mechanically by other biting flies. Intrauterine transmission has been recorded. Infections have followed accidental inoculation with trypanosomes in the laboratory.

When a tsetse fly bites an infected host, trypanosomes are sucked into the midgut with the blood meal. Here they pass through the peritrophic membrane, migrate forward between it and the gut wall, penetrate the gut wall, and reach the salivary glands where development into new infective forms occurs. When a new host is bitten, trypanosomes pass down the proboscis with the saliva to start a new infection. Development within the fly takes two to five weeks.

Epidemiology of Gambian Sleeping Sickness. Man is the only known natural host of *T. b. gambiense*. Pigs, rodents, and other animals can be infected experimentally, but the existence of an important natural reservoir has never been established. Gambian sleeping sickness is spread mainly by two species of tsetse fly, *Glossina palpalis* and *G. tachinoides*. These flies inhabit the shaded areas alongside rivers and streams, areas where their human victims can often be found as they come to the stream for water. In some areas these flies will also rest and bite within a village. Contact between man and these species of tsetse flies is often very close, providing ideal conditions for transmission of the disease.

Epidemiology of Rhodesian Sleeping Sickness. *T. b. rhodesiense* differs from *T. b. gambiense* in being primarily a parasite of wild game, man acting only as an occasional and accidental host. Rhodesian sleeping sickness is spread by tsetse flies of the *G. morsitans* group, flies that can live in open savanna with enough vegetation to provide shade and resting places. Rhodesian sleeping sickness is an occupational disease, occurring mainly in those whose work takes them into areas of bush where wild game, especially the bushbuck, survives. Hunters, fishermen, honey-gatherers, and tourists are all at risk. This form of trypanosomiasis is usually a sporadic infection, but epidemics can occur. In the epidemic situation direct man-to-man transmission probably takes place.

PATHOLOGY. Few studies of the pathology of African trypanosomiasis have been made since the classic work of Mott published in 1906. In the early stage of the disease the lymph nodes and spleen are enlarged and infiltrated with plasma cells and macrophages. Later, lymph nodes shrink and patchy fibrosis occurs. Lymphocytic infiltration of the pericardium and myocardium may be found, especially in the Rhodesian form of the disease. Characteristic changes are found in the brain and meninges once invasion of the central nervous system has occurred. These changes are most marked in longstanding cases of Gambian sleeping sickness. The meninges are thickened and infiltrated with lymphocytes, plasma cells, and morular cells. Morular cells are large cells with an eccentric nucleus displaced by numerous cytoplasmic vesicles which contain IgM. As the disease progresses, chronic inflammatory changes extend along the perivascular spaces to produce prominent perivascular cuffing. Finally, infiltration of the brain substance with lymphocytes, plasma cells, and morular cells takes place with accompanying neuronal degeneration and microglial proliferation.

PATHOGENESIS AND IMMUNITY. The immune response of the host probably plays an important part in the pathogenesis of sleeping sickness. Stimulation of the reticuloendothelial and humoral immune systems contributes to the lymphadenopathy and splenomegaly of the early phase of the disease. Vessel damage is an important feature of the advanced stage of the infection and may be due to immune complex deposition, for patients with sleeping sickness have high levels of circulating immune complexes and have laboratory features indicating activation of the complement and kinin pathways.

T. brucei possesses surface and core antigens which both induce a humoral immune response. Little is known about the role of cell-mediated immunity in this infection. In the presence of antibody, trypanosomes are lysed or taken up by cells of the reticuloendothelial system, but successful eradication of the parasite is prevented by the phenomenon of antigenic variation. By progressive alteration of the structure of its surface antigens, the trypanosome is able to keep continually one step ahead of the host's immune response and thus to persist until the host eventually dies. The mechanism of antigenic variation is not known, but contact with antibody probably initiates the antigenic switch.

Large amounts of IgM are produced in the serum and cerebrospinal fluid of patients with sleeping sickness. Only a small proportion of this immunoglobulin is parasite-specific antibody; the rest contains antibodies with a wide variety of specificities, including autoantibodies. The mechanism of this polyclonal B lymphocyte activation is not understood and is currently being studied. Humoral and cellular immune responses are suppressed in patients with sleeping sickness, and this immunosuppression may underlie their increased susceptibility to secondary infections such as pneumonia.

CLINICAL FEATURES. Sleeping sickness passes through three pathologic and clinical phases: an initial phase in which trypanosomes are localized to the site of the tsetse fly bite; an early or systemic phase in which trypanosomes are widely distributed throughout the body; and a neurologic or advanced stage in which trypanosomes are largely restricted to the central nervous system. Rhodesian sleeping sickness is usually a much more rapidly progressive illness than Gambian sleeping sickness with less distinction between systemic and neurologic stages. However, this distinction is not an absolute one; in some outbreaks Gambian sleeping sickness has progressed rapidly, whereas occasionally Rhodesian sleeping sickness follows a more benign course.

Gambian Sleeping Sickness. Ten days after a bite by an infected tsetse fly, a small nodular lesion, a chancre, may develop at the site of the bite and persist for two to three weeks. This lesion, if it occurs, frequently passes unnoticed.

Months or even years after an infected bite, systemic invasion with trypanosomes occurs. Fever and lymphadenopathy are the main features of this early stage of the infection. Fever is usually intermittent and may be mild.

Some Contrasting Features of Gambian and Rhodesian Sleeping Sickness

	Gambian Sleeping Sickness	Rhodesian Sleeping Sickness
Causative organism	*Trypanosoma brucei gambiense*	*Trypanosoma brucei rhodesiense*
Distribution	West and Central Africa	East Africa
Source of infection	Man	Wild game (man)
Vector	*Glossina palpalis* or *tachinoides* (riverine tsetse)	*Glossina morsitans* (savanna tsetse)
Clinical features		
Lymphadenopathy	++	+
Heart failure	0	++
Neurologic	++	+
Disseminated intravascular coagulation	0	+
Diagnosis	Trypanosomes in lymph node juice or CSF	Trypanosomes in blood or CSF
Course of infection	Slow	Rapid

Lymphadenopathy may be general, but the posterior cervical nodes are nearly always involved. Enlarged nodes are firm but not usually tender. Moderate splenomegaly may occur. Urticarial rashes, erythematous rashes, and localized edema may be seen. A variety of eye lesions have been recorded, but these are rare. Electrocardiograms are often abnormal, but clinical signs of heart disease are unusual. Mild normocytic anemia and mild thrombocytopenia are common. The serum IgM level is nearly always raised.

Months or years after the first appearance of symptoms, the clinical features of the early phase of the disease regress to be replaced by new symptoms and signs indicating invasion of the nervous system. Mild behavioral and personality changes are often the first sign of central nervous system involvement. Later, more florid psychologic changes may occur with hallucinations and delusions. Headache and backache are common complaints. Drowsiness during the day, the feature from which the disease takes its name, may occur but is not invariable, and some patients are manic. If no treatment is given, the patient's level of consciousness progressively deteriorates until finally he lapses into stupor. Convulsions occasionally occur. Chorea and athetosis are the most frequently encountered localizing neurologic signs. Pyramidal tract involvement is less frequent, and cranial nerve lesions are rare. Obesity and impotence or amenorrhea probably follow from damage to the hypothalamus. Severe itching is a frequent but unexplained symptom that may lead to skin changes. The cerebrospinal fluid shows an increase in cells and protein, much of which is IgM. Most of the cells are lymphocytes, but a few plasma cells and morular cells may be seen. Trypanosomes may be present.

Rhodesian Sleeping Sickness. The clinical picture of Rhodesian sleeping sickness is similar to that described above, but on presentation the patient is usually more acutely ill than a patient with Gambian sleeping sickness, and the disease progresses more rapidly. Heart failure and jaundice occur more frequently than in Gambian sleeping sickness, but lymphadenopathy is usually less prominent. Neurologic features similar to those described above may be present, but sometimes death occurs before these have had time to develop. Anemia and thrombocytopenia are usual, and disseminated intravascular coagulation may occur. Liver function tests are often abnormal, and an abnormal electrocardiogram is usually obtained. Cerebrospinal fluid changes are the same as those described above.

DIAGNOSIS. The chancre of trypanosomiasis has no special features and is unlikely to be recognized unless there is a strong reason for suspecting trypanosomiasis. It must be differentiated from an allergic reaction to a tsetse fly bite. Trypanosomes are present in juice obtained from the lesion.

The clinical features of the early phase of sleeping sickness are similar to those of many infectious, neoplastic, and connective tissue diseases. Trypanosomiasis must be considered in the differential diagnosis of unexplained pyrexia or lymphadenopathy in any patient who has visited an endemic area. Diagnosis of Rhodesian sleeping sickness can usually be made by the demonstration of trypanosomes in a thick blood film. However, trypanosomes are rarely found in the blood of patients with Gambian sleeping sickness even when concentration, culture, or animal inoculation is used. Diagnosis is most readily made in the early stage of this form of sleeping sickness by the detection of trypanosomes in the juice obtained on puncturing an enlarged lymph node with a venipuncture needle.

Once invasion of the central nervous system has occurred, clinical diagnosis of sleeping sickness is usually not difficult. However, tragic misdiagnoses have been made in patients with predominantly psychologic features. Chorea may be so marked as to suggest Sydenham's chorea, and confusion with other extrapyramidal syndromes may occur occasionally. Diagnosis of the advanced stage of sleeping sickness is confirmed by examination of the cerebrospinal fluid. Trypanosomes can be found in most patients provided both that the cerebrospinal fluid is examined immediately after collection and that scrupulously clean glassware is used. Measurement of the cerebrospinal fluid IgM level is often of great diagnostic help in patients in whom trypanosomes cannot be found. A high cerebrospinal fluid IgM in the presence of a modest increase in total protein is a characteristic feature of sleeping sickness very rarely found in other diseases, such as tuberculous meningitis and neurovascular syphilis, with which it might be confused.

Many different serologic tests have been used to diagnose sleeping sickness; the recently developed ELISA test is especially promising. These tests have proved of great value in survey work but are of less value in the investigation of individual patients, as false-positive and false-negative reactions can occur.

TREATMENT. General Measures. Whenever possible, patients with sleeping sickness should be treated in hospital. Lumbar puncture to determine the stage of the disease must be carried out before treatment is started. If abnormalities are found (a raised cell count or protein), the patient must be treated as having a case of advanced disease, even if there are no clinical signs of central nervous system involvement. Poorly nourished patients may require dietary supplements. A search should be made for any associated infections, and these should be treated. Malaria prophylaxis should be given if malaria is endemic.

Many different drugs and dosage regimens have been used in the treatment of sleeping sickness, but few controlled trials have been undertaken and the treatment schedules currently in use were largely established empirically. All the drugs used in the treatment of sleeping sickness were developed many years ago, and all are toxic; there is still a great need for safer effective drugs.

Chemotherapy of Early Disease. Suramin is an effective treatment for early Gambian and Rhodesian sleeping sickness, but it is ineffective in advanced disease as it penetrates poorly into the cerebrospinal fluid. Suramin* is a white powder which is made up in an aqueous solution immediately before use and given intravenously in a dose of 20 mg per kilogram of body weight. Occasionally it causes vomiting and collapse, so it is customary to start with a test dose of one fifth of this amount. A course comprises five to ten injections given at two- to five-day intervals. The drug can cause renal damage; because of this, it should not be given in more than a single course and the urine should be tested for protein and casts before each injection. Mild proteinuria can be ignored; but if heavy proteinuria develops or if casts are found, treatment should be stopped. Three injections of melarsoprol (see below) is an effective alternative form of treatment which is considered by some to be the treatment of

---

*Available from the Center for Disease Control (404-633-3311, Ext. 3670).

choice. Berenil is also effective but has been less widely used.

Chemotherapy of Advanced Disease. Melarsoprol (Mel B) is the treatment of choice for both Gambian and Rhodesian sleeping sickness once involvement of the central nervous system has occurred, even though the drug is very toxic. It is possible that toxicity is reduced by a prior course of suramin, but melarsoprol should be started right away in patients who are very sick. Mel B is dispensed as a 3.6 per cent solution in polyethylene glycol. This is very irritating and is liable to produce thrombophlebitis. The full dosage of Mel B* is 3.6 mg (0.1 ml) per kilogram of body weight given intravenously up to a maximum of 5.0 ml. The following is an effective schedule of treatment for an adult: 2.5 ml on day 1 and 3, followed by 5.0 ml on day 5; rest for one to two weeks; 5.0 ml on days 8, 10, and 12; rest for a further week; and then 5.0 ml on days 15, 17 and 19 (total dose, 40.0 ml). Other schedules employ a more gradual build-up to full dosage. Treatment schedules should be kept flexible and slowed down if reactions occur. Febrile reactions are common after the first injection of Mel B, especially if suramin has not been given. Mel B can produce rashes, marrow depression, and renal damage, but its most serious side effect is an encephalopathy which occurs in about 5 per cent of patients. Encephalopathy occurs most frequently at the time of the third or fourth injection; it may develop very rapidly and is sometimes fatal. Dimercaprol (BAL) has been used to treat this complication of Mel B treatment, but its value has not been clearly established. It has been suggested that corticosteroids protect patients from Mel B encephalopathy, but no protection was demonstrated in a recent controlled trial.

Follow-up and Treatment of Relapses. The results of treatment of patients with early disease with suramin are excellent, but occasional patients subsequently develop neurologic disease and require treatment with a full course of Mel B. Regular follow-up with clinical examination and lumbar puncture is therefore necessary for at least a year after treatment.

Patients with neurologic disease also require regular follow-up, for treatment failures and relapses occasionally occur. Patients with a relapse of advanced disease should receive another full course of Mel B* (total dosage, 40.0 ml for an adult) together with nitrofurazone, for, despite the toxicity of this drug, there is an impression that patients treated with melarsoprol and nitrofurazone do better than those receiving melarsoprol alone. The adult dosage of nitrofurazone* is 0.5 gram given by mouth every six hours for five days, this course being repeated on two or three occasions. Nitrofurazone is a toxic drug causing peripheral neuropathy and hemolytic anemia, especially in those with glucose-6-phosphatase deficiency.

PROGNOSIS. Many patients with early Gambian sleeping sickness remain relatively well for months or years, and it is possible that a few recover spontaneously. Once central nervous system involvement has occurred, death is inevitable unless treatment is given. Death frequently follows a secondary infection, often pneumonia, in a stuporous and malnourished patient. Patients with Rhodesian sleeping sickness may die from heart failure.

The results of treatment of patients in the early phase of sleeping sickness are excellent, over 90 per cent making a complete recovery. However, a few patients subsequently develop central nervous system involvement and require further treatment. Mel B achieves a parasitologic "cure" in at least 90 per cent of cases of advanced disease, and many patients make a complete recovery. Unfortunately some patients are left with irreversible neurologic damage. These patients must be differentiated from those who have had a true relapse and require further treatment. About 5 per cent of patients die as a result of Mel B treatment.

An attack of sleeping sickness does not induce protective immunity, and reinfection may occur.

CONTROL AND PROPHYLAXIS. Many different approaches have been made to the control of sleeping sickness. In West Africa, survey teams have been used extensively to detect and treat asymptomatic patients early in the course of their disease, thus reducing the reservoir of infection. In East Africa, attempts have been made to reduce the reservoir of infection in wild game. Man-fly contact can be reduced by encouraging farmers to live in villages rather than in scattered hamlets. Tsetse flies can be destroyed by hand catching, trapping, or destruction of their natural habitat, but most control programs now rely on insecticides sprayed either by hand or from the air. Several large aerial spraying projects are now in progress aimed mainly at destruction of the tsetse flies responsible for cattle trypanosomiasis, but the vectors of human sleeping sickness are also being destroyed.

Pentamidine* has been successfully used as a chemoprophylactic in Gambian sleeping sickness when given by a single intramuscular injection of 4 mg per kilogram every three to six months. However, its use carries the risk of producing cryptic infections, and the drug can cause diabetes. It should therefore be used only in those who are in great danger of being infected.

The occurrence of antigenic variation has been a major obstacle to the development of a successful vaccine. However, recent progress in culture of *T. brucei* in vitro and in analysis of the detailed chemical structure of its variant antigens holds out hope for the future.

Apted, F. I. C.: Clinical manifestations and diagnosis of sleeping sickness. *In* Mulligan, H. W. (ed.): The African Trypanosomiases. London, George Allen and Unwin, 1970, p. 661.

Ford, J.: The Role of the African Trypanosomiases in African Ecology. Oxford, Clarendon Press, 1971.

Goodwin, L. G.: The African scene; mechanisms of pathogenesis in trypanosomiasis. *In* Trypanosomiasis and Leishmaniasis with Special Reference to Chagas' Disease. Ciba Foundation Symposium, 20. Amsterdam, Associated Scientific Publishers, 1974, p. 107.

Mott, F. W.: Histological observations on sleeping sickness and other trypanosome infections. Reports of the Sleeping Sickness Commission of the Royal Society, 7:3, 1906.

Vickerman, K.: Antigenic variation in African trypanosomes. *In* Parasites in the Immunised Host: Mechanisms of Survival. Ciba Foundation Symposium, 25. Amsterdam, Associated Scientific Publishers, 1974, p. 53.

194.3. CHAGAS' DISEASE
(American Trypanosomiasis)

Vanize Macedo

DEFINITION. Chagas' disease, an infection caused by *Trypanosoma cruzi* and named after its Brazilian discoverer, Carlos Chagas, is found only in the Western Hemisphere. A distinction must be made between in-

---

*Available from the Center for Disease Control (404-633-3311, Ext. 3670).

*Available from the Center for Disease Control (404-633-3311, Ext. 3670).

fection and disease. The majority of infected patients develop no signs of clinically detectable disease. Chagas himself described the two main disease forms occurring years after the initial infection: a chronic cardiomyopathy often with intracardiac conduction defects, and dilatation of the esophagus or colon (the mega syndromes).

ETIOLOGY. The trypanomastigote is visible in peripheral blood films of man and the multitude of naturally or experimentally infected animals studied in the early or acute phase of the disease. It is polymorphic, 15 to 25 μ long, and has a large subterminal kinetoplast. The proportion of narrow, broad, and intermediate forms appears to vary with the strain. Multiplication takes place only in an amastigote phase in host cells. The trypanomastigote penetrates a host cell (frequently a cardiac or smooth muscle cell), rounds up, and commences to replicate by binary fission every 12 hours. The time of rupture of this host cell will depend on its size. The amastigotes change into trypanomastigotes, which are released to circulate in the peripheral blood and penetrate new cells. Experimentally, myotropic, neurotropic, and reticulotropic strains have been identified, and it is possible that different strains of *T. cruzi* are responsible for geographic variations in the human disease. After a period of weeks, the host immune response suppresses the trypanomastigote parasitemia to subpatent levels. Small numbers continue to circulate for years.

EVOLUTIONARY CYCLE. The insect vector of *T. cruzi* is a hemipteran, a reduviid bug of the subfamily Triatominae, of which about 100 species have been described. They are obligate blood suckers and withdraw a large blood meal rapidly by directly tapping a subcutaneous capillary with their stylet mouth parts. The great majority of these are sylvatic and maintain cycles among wild animals. Such bugs are found from within 200 miles of New York to the south of Argentina. For reasons that are unclear, a small number of species have become highly domesticated, and those cohabiting with man are the transmitters of Chagas' disease. The most important species in this respect are *Triatoma infestans*, *Panstrongylus megistus*, and *Rhodnius prolixus*.

T. cruzi probably originated as a parasite of these insects which remain extraordinarily susceptible to infection with the protozoan. All stages of the bug are easily infected after ingestion of blood from an infected mammalian host, even one in which circulating trypanosomes cannot be detected by any other means. *T. cruzi* undergoes a complex cycle of morphogenesis as it passes down the intestines of the bug. Infective trypanomastigotes can be found in the rectum after 20 to 30 days, and these will penetrate cells to replicate and initiate the infection in mammalian hosts.

EPIDEMIOLOGY. Transmission is usually at night, when the bugs are active. They feed mainly on the face and arms, the uncovered parts of sleeping man. As they engorge with blood, the rise in intra-abdominal pressure promotes defecation, and the trypanomastigotes in the feces can penetrate mucous membranes or small skin abrasions. The three main species of transmitting bugs all tend to defecate soon after feeding.

Congenital transmission and infection by blood transfusion can occur. More rarely, transmisson may occur as a result of a laboratory accident. There exists the possibility of contamination by the digestive tract.

Chagas' disease has been described in all the countries of South America and Central America with the exception of Guyana and Surinam. In Mexico it is rare. Two autochthonous acute cases have been reported in Texas. The high standard of housing and the discrete nature of the sylvatic cycles makes transmission to man a very rare event in North America. Chagas' disease is a serious public health problem in South America, principally in Argentina, Brazil, Chile, Uruguay, and Venezuela. There are geographic differences in the disease; for example, cardiomyopathy is rare in Chile, and the mega syndromes are unknown in Venezuela. From some countries (e.g., Bolivia) there is little information on the status of Chagas' disease.

It is estimated that the prevalence of trypanosomiasis may reach 20 per cent in the rural zones of the countries where it is endemic. Socioeconomic conditions are bad in these areas and dwellings are of poor construction with mud and sticks, building materials which favor bug colonization. Chagas' disease is intimately linked with economic underdevelopment.

The medicosocial importance of the disease has not been determined, and we do not know for certain the role American trypanosomiasis plays in the economy of countries where it is endemic. Cardiopathy is the most important form of the disease, causing a significant mortality and inability to work in the most productive phase of life. Many employers in Brazil will not hire a worker with positive serology.

PATHOGENESIS. The local tissue inflammation promoted by rupture of nests of amastigotes of *T. cruzi* was the first interpretation of the pathology of the disease. This view explains the alterations that occur in the acute phase but not all those that occur in the chronic phase. In this phase amastigotes are rarely found. Early workers introduced theories of allergic or hypersensitivity reactions to hypothetical toxins of *T. cruzi* to explain the chronic inflammation in the absence of a parasite. A neurotoxin was said to be responsible for degeneration of parasympathetic ganglia. Although such denervation goes far to explain the genesis of the mega syndromes, it is only one factor in the development of cardiac disease.

There is evidence suggesting that an autoimmune process is at work in the chronic cardiomyopathy of Chagas' disease. Santos, Buch, and Teixeira have demonstrated that sensitized lymphocytes from rabbits chronically infected with *T. cruzi* are cytotoxic to normal cardiac cells. Cossio and colleagues have identified circulating autoantibodies to heart tissue in patients with chronic cardiomyopathy.

The importance of strains of the parasite or reinfection in the pathogenesis of Chagas' disease is still not clear.

PATHOLOGY. In the acute phase the infection is generalized, and amastigotes of *T. cruzi* can be found in cells of the reticuloendothelial system. Initially reticular cells are parasitized, and in a short time smooth and striated muscle cells, including cardiac muscle, glial and nerve cells, and fat cells are invaded.

The inoculation lesion shows inflammation with infiltration of lymphocytes and plasma cells and fibroblastic proliferation. The heart is enlarged and flabby, with predominance of dilatation over hypertrophy. Hemorrhagic foci may be seen on the endocardium. Microscopically there is diffuse edema, both intestinal and interfibrillar congestion, and the presence of amastigotes in the cardiac fibers. The cardiac fibers show hyaline necrosis and degeneration (lesions of Margarino Torres). In the central nervous system there is mononuclear infiltration of the leptomeninges, congestive perivascular inflammation, and hemorrhage with glial proliferation and neurophagia. Amastigotes may be encountered in the cells of the central nervous system.

In the chronic cardiac form the heart is enlarged with both hypertrophy and dilatation so that the apex is formed by the terminations of both ventricles. The epicardium is congested, and there may be a small pericardial effusion. There are no organic valvular lesions. The thinned myocardium of the apex may distend to form an apical aneurysm, a characteristic lesion of Chagas' disease. Mural thrombosis is frequent on the endocardium, particularly in the right atrium and the apex of the left ventricle. Thrombosis at the apex is an important finding in Chagas' myocarditis. These intracardiac thrombi are the source of emboli principally to the lungs, kidneys, cerebrum, and spleen. There is chronic passive congestion of the organs.

Microscopy demonstrates an intense diffuse myocarditis with focal areas of cellular infiltration containing mononuclear cells, lymphocytes, and plasma cells. There is hypertrophy of the cardiac fibers with small areas of focal necrosis, hemorrhage, and granular degeneration. A variable degree of fibrosis is associated with edema and vascular dilatation and congestion. Tissue amastigotes are rarely seen in chronic cases.

Andrade has shown that these inflammatory changes directly involve the conducting system of the heart, particularly the sinoatrial node, the interior third of the atrioventricular node, the right half of the main bundle, the right bundle branch, and the anterior ramification of the left bundle branch. He established a good correlation between the electrocardiogram in life and these pathologic changes.

In the indeterminate form of Chagas' disease, active myocarditis with granuloma formation and neuronal destruction of Auerbach's plexus has been found, but in lesser degree than established cardiomyopathy. In megaesophagus and megacolon the organ is dilated with focal myositis associated with a diminution in the number of nerve cells in Auerbach's plexus.

In the congenital form a chronic placentitis with ischemia of the chorionic villi occurs. Edema and a histiocytic inflammatory infiltrate are present with small foci of necrosis in these villi. Amastigotes are visible in the cytoplasm of macrophages.

CLINICAL PRESENTATION. Chagas' disease has an acute and chronic phase. It is noteworthy that in endemic areas discrepancies exist between the prevalence of the chronic phase and the small number of cases diagnosed as acute disease.

Acute Phase. In areas endemic for Chagas' disease, the acute phase is diagnosed in about 1 per cent of patients. Probably in the majority of individuals the initial phase of the infection is inapparent. Seventy per cent of patients in this phase are children under ten years of age. Acute Chagas' disease is rare in adults.

The incubation period is 4 to 12 days. The signs at the portal of entry often call the attention of the physician to the possible diagnosis of the disease. Romaña's sign is present in half the patients in the acute phase. This is a unilateral, bipalpebral, firm, violaceous edema, frequently with conjunctivitis and enlargement of the preauricular gland. An inoculation chagoma may occur in exposed areas, such as the face or arms, where

the bug has an opportunity of biting. This also is characterized by erythema and infiltrative tumefaction of the skin with satellite ganglion reaction, which, when it disappears, leaves hyperpigmentation. It is found in 25 per cent of patients in the acute phase. A minority of patients do not present signs of a portal of entry.

The disease is characterized by prolonged fever, asthenia, enlargement of lymphatic glands, edema of the face and legs, and hepatosplenomegaly. Tachycardia is frequently present even in the absence of temperature. This is a sign of myocarditis which is benign in the majority of cases and only diagnosed on electrocardiogram.

The signs of the acute phase disappear in two to four months. The so-called schizotrypanides are skin rashes that rarely occur in the acute phase. They may take the form of erythematous indurated plaques or may be morbilliform or urticarial in type, suggesting an allergic nature. Meningoencephalitis is also a rare complication, often occurring in children under one year of age and usually fatal. Clinical evidence of encephalitis may be complicated by convulsions.

Congenital Disease. Since this is rarely diagnosed, its prevalence in endemic areas cannot be estimated. Such newborns are underweight and afebrile, and have hepatosplenomegaly and often edema. Petechiae, bruising, and frank hemorrhage may be noted. Meningoencephalitis may produce convulsions and tremors of the face and limbs. If jaundice is present, it disappears in the third week. Metastatic chagomas have been described, with skin infiltration, infection, and even necrosis.

The Chronic Phase. INDETERMINATE FORM. After the acute phase, individuals can stay for many years or all their lives in a latent or indeterminate phase. These subjects do not have clinical, radiologic, or electrocardiographic signs. In endemic areas, approximately half of those infected show this form. It is probable that this number will diminish as more sophisticated methods for detecting disease are developed.

CARDIAC FORM. This is the most important clinical form of the chronic phase, and its prevalence can reach 30 per cent of individuals in an endemic area. The majority of patients have no cardiac symptoms or signs but only electrocardiographic evidence of disease.

Palpitations, usually the result of extrasystoles, are a frequent initial symptom. They may be accompanied by dizziness and precordial pain. Right-sided ventricular failure predominates, and dyspnea is infrequent.

Physical examination shows an irregular pulse and distant heart sounds, fixed splitting of the pulmonary second sound, gallop rhythm, and a functional regurgitant murmur in the mitral area. In advanced cases, tricuspid regurgitation can occur and cyanosis is present. Thromboembolic phenomena are very frequent and may precede symptoms of cardiac insufficiency. Total atrioventricular block is rare but is frequently accompanied by Stokes-Adams attacks.

DIGESTIVE FORM. The digestive form is characterized by dilatation and alteration in motility of the esophagus or colon. Rarely the stomach or small intestine shows similar changes.

In megaesophagus the principal symptom is longstanding dysphagia, which begins with difficulty with solid food and progresses until the patient can swallow only soft foods with the aid of frequent sips of water. In advanced cases, patients have pain on swallowing, regurgitation, and pyrosis with a sensation of suffocation. Hiccup, sialorrhea, and nocturnal cough are associated symptoms. Hypersalivation is accompanied by parotid gland enlargement. Marked weight loss is present, and aspiration pneumonias may occur in advanced cases.

Megacolon is evidenced by retention of feces and gas and often progresses to fecaloma formation. Volvulus and intestinal obstruction are frequent complications. The majority of cases of megacolon are associated with megaesophagus. Half of the patients with digestive forms of Chagas' disease have abnormal electrocardiograms.

OTHER CLINICAL FORMS. Rare complications are megaureter, megabladder, megagallbladder, and bronchiectasis. The forms of central nervous system involvement in chronic infection, described by Chagas himself, are still debatable. The denervation process has been implicated in the dysfunction of various exocrine and endocrine glands.

DIAGNOSIS. Acute Phase. The acute phase is usually diagnosed by finding the trypanomastigote in the peripheral blood on direct examination of thick films. This is the best criterion for diagnosing the acute phase. Should this fail, simple concentration methods are usually positive, such as examination of the leukocyte cream after centrifugation or allowing the blood to clot and examining the supernatant (Strout's method). Biopsy of the calf muscle shows myositis and frequently nests of amastigotes.

The *xenodiagnostic test* is often positive before 30 days owing to the high number of circulating trypanosomes. Similarly, cultures (NNN) and subinoculation of mice recover the organism. The serologic reactions, usually positive in this early stage, are precipitins and agglutinins. There is a raised IgM. The complement fixation test becomes positive four to six weeks after infection. The indirect immunofluorescent test becomes positive earlier than the hemagglutination and complement fixation tests. The white cell count shows leukocytosis caused by an intense lymphocytosis with atypical lymphocytes. The erythrocyte sedimentation rate is increased, as are the mucoproteins. Heterophil antibodies may appear in the serum, and the Paul Bunnell reaction may be positive. Protein electrophoresis reveals a slight hypoalbuminemia with a rise in gamma and alpha 2 globulins. The transaminases are slightly elevated. The electrocardiogram may show sinus tachycardia, low voltage complexes, first degree atrioventricular block, increased QT space, primary alterations in ventricular repolarization, and sometimes subepicardial ischemia. Alterations in cardiac rhythm are rare at this stage and a bad prognostic sign.

On x-ray examination, there may be enlargement of the cardiac shadow, which may be transitory. At times such enlargement is due to a pericardial effusion. Marked cardiomegaly indicates a bad prognosis.

Chronic Phase. Evidence of infection is established mainly by serologic tests such as complement fixation, hemagglutination, and immunofluorescence. Xenodiagnosis, using 40 bugs, will isolate an organism in about 50 per cent of cases. In the indeterminate phase, only these investigations will be positive.

A chest x-ray may be normal, but frequently a degree of cardiomegaly is seen progressing to marked global enlargement of the heart. The electrocardiogram is valuable, as conduction defects are common. In the endemic area of São Felipe, Brazil, the following abnormalities were present in a frequency of 15 to 20 per cent: complete right bundle branch block with anterior hemiblock, ventricular extrasystoles, first degree atrioventricular block, and alterations in ventricular repolarization. Total atrioventricular block or complete left bundle branch block occurred in only 0.2 per cent. There may be evidence of septal fibrosis. Digestive tract involvement is revealed by radiologic studies in a patient with a suggestive history. Both the esophagus and colon are dilated, with abnormal peristalsis and evidence of retained food residues.

Rezende has proposed the following classification of megaesophagus based on radiologic findings:

Group I — The caliber of the esophagus is normal, but there is slow transit and retention of barium.

Group II — The caliber of the esophagus is slightly or moderately enlarged with marked retention of contrast. Tertiary waves are present.

Group III — The esophagus is greatly enlarged and hypotonic with marked barium retention.

Group IV—Dolichomegaesophagus occurs, with massive retention capacity, atonia, and doubling of the esophagus on top of the diaphragm.

DIFFERENTIAL DIAGNOSIS. Romaña's sign must be distinguished from conjunctivitis, orbital cellulitis, cavernous sinus thrombosis, insect bites, and trauma, all of which produce unilateral orbital edema. Clinically the acute phase may resemble typhoid fever, infectious mononucleosis, kala-azar, brucellosis, toxoplasmosis, and acute glomerulonephritis. Other types of acute myocarditis must be considered.

Congenital infections must be distinguished from syphilis, toxoplasmosis, and cytomegalic inclusion disease.

Chronic cardiomyopathy involves a differential diagnosis from the cardiomyopathies associated with alcohol, pregnancy, idiopathic cardiomyopathy, endomyocardial fibrosis, and ischemic heart disease. The absence of organic valvular lesions usually permits a distinction from rheumatic valvular disease. Carcinoma of the esophagus may mimic megaesophagus. The presence of positive serology and electrocardiographic changes assist in the differential diagnosis from megaesophagus and megacolon not caused by Chagas' disease.

EVOLUTION AND PROGNOSIS. Chagas' cardiomyopathy is variable in its course and of uncertain prognosis. In the acute phase only 10 per cent of patients die of myocarditis or acute meningoencephalitis. The latter condition usually occurs in children under one year of age. The indeterminate phase can last a lifetime. The factors influencing the evolution of the disease are not clear. There is some evidence that reinfections could play a role in an endemic area. The strain of parasite and the host's response to it could be important. Cardiomyopathy begins in the second to fifth decade. Heart failure in these age groups leads to death one to five years after its initial appearance. The prognosis is poor if cardiac failure appears before 30 years of age.

A longitudinal study in São Felipe, Brazil, showed that each year the disease made a detectable progression in 5.5 per cent of patients. The mortality was 0.7 per cent per year. The principal cause of death was cardiac failure in 58.3 per cent. Sudden death from conduction defects occurred in 37.5 per cent. The following electrocardiographic changes were associated with a 50 per cent mortality in five years: total atrioventricular block, atrial fibrillation, left bundle branch block, multifocal extrasystoles, and septal fibrosis.

TREATMENT. Two drugs appear to kill circulating trypanosomes and may have value in the specific treatment of Chagas' disease. These are nifurtimox, a nitrofuran derivative (Bayer 2502 [Lampit]), and benznidazole, a nitroimidazole RO7–1051 Rochagan).

Nifurtimox* is used in a dose of 8 mg per kilogram of body weight per day for a period of 120 days. With regard to eradicating parasitemia, it has given good results in patients in the acute and chronic phases in Chile, Argentina, and southern Brazil. In other areas of Brazil, such as Bahia, Goiás, and Minas Gerais, the results have been less satisfactory, only 40 per cent of individuals being uniformly negative on repeated xenodiagnosis after treatment. Experiments in animals infected with different strains of *T. cruzi* demonstrated different susceptibilities to nifurtimox. This reinforces the hypothesis that different strains of *T. cruzi* may be responsible for these variations in response to treatment. Benznidazole* is used in a dose of 5 mg per kilogram per day for 60 days and also eradicates parasitemia in a proportion of patients. Both these drugs have serious side effects and should be used only under direct medical supervision. The side effects include polyneuritis, dizziness, loss of weight, nausea, and insomnia. With use of benznidazole, exfoliative dermatitis and thrombocytopenic purpura have also been seen.

It is not known how important such specific treatment is in arresting the disease. If parasitemia is an important factor in the evolution of the disease, then certainly the acute phase should be treated. In the acute phase, both serologic tests and xenodiagnosis may remain negative after treatment. In the chronic phase, those in whom xenodiagnosis becomes negative remain positive serologically. It is still not clear whether such treatment is of value in the chronic phase.

When chronic myocarditis is associated with heart failure, the treatment is symptomatic. Digitalis must be used with care because of sensitivity of the damaged cardiac fiber, and the response is poor in relation to other cardiomyopathies. Extrasystoles, the most frequent arrhythmia, may be helped by procainamide. In ventricular tachycardia, procainamide and lidocaine are the drugs indicated. Beta-adrenergic blocking agents are dangerous in acute arrhythmias in Chagas' myocarditis, as they may produce bradycardia and shock. Deaths have been reported after the use of propranolol. In Stokes-Adams crises, isopropyl norepinephrine is useful. In patients with total atrioventricular block and a normal or slightly enlarged heart, implantation of the pacemaker is indicated. When there is marked cardiac enlargement, this measure carries a poor prognosis, because either the weak cardiac muscle cannot support the new rhythm or an intramural clot may become dislodged.

Initially megaesophagus is treated by balloon dilatation; in more advanced cases cardiotomy is often successful. Operations consisting of excision of the aperistaltic esophagus and replacement with a segment of colon or small intestine have been developed. In megacolon evacuation of a fecaloma may be an emergency procedure. It has to be carried out with care, for rupture of the colon and septicemia can follow the procedure. Resection of the aperistaltic segment may relieve persistent constipation.

PROPHYLAXIS. Since transmission usually occurs in a domestic setting in poor-quality housing, Chagas' disease is a direct reflection of poverty. The important prophylactic measures in the control of Chagas' disease are better housing, public health education, and application of insecticides in the house and its environs. Benzene hexachloride (BHC), the insecticide of choice, is applied in a suspension of 500 mg of the gamma isomer per square meter every six months.

In blood banks in endemic areas of Chagas' disease, 1:4000 gentian violet is added to stored blood 24 hours before use in order to kill the trypanosomes. To date no results that can be applied to humans have been obtained with immunoprotection for Chagas' disease.

American Trypanosomiasis Research. PAHO Scientific Publication 318, 1975.

Andrade, Z., and Andrade, S. G.: Chagas' disease (American trypanosomiasis). *In* Marcial-Rojas, R. A. (ed.): Pathology of Protozoal and Helminthic Disease. Baltimore, Williams & Wilkins Company, 1971.

Chagas, C.: Processos patojênicos da tripanosomiase americana. Memórias do Instituto Oswaldo Cruz, 8:5, 1916.

Köberle, F.: Patologia y anatomía patológica de la enfermedad de Chagas. Bol. Sanit. Panam., 51:404, 1961.

Laranja, F. S., Dias, E., Nóbrega, G., and Miranda, A.: Chagas' disease — a clinical epidemiologic and pathologic study. Circulation, 14:1035, 1956.

Prata, A., Andrade, Z., and Guimarães, A.: Chagas' heart disease. *In* Shaper, A. G., Hutt, M. S. R., and Fejfar, Z. (eds.): Cardiovascular Disease in the Tropics. London, British Medical Association, 1974.

Romaña, C.: Enfermedad de Chagas. Buenos Aires, Lopez Liberos, 1963.

World Health Organization: Chagas' Disease: Report of a Study Group. Technical Report Series No. 202, 1960.

195. LEISHMANIASIS

Anthony D. M. Bryceson

195.1. INTRODUCTION

DEFINITION. Leishmaniasis is an infection with parasites of the genus *Leishmania*. It is usually a zoonosis transmitted by phlebotomine sandflies between wild or peridomestic animals, especially rodents or canines. Man is infected when he interrupts the natural cycle.

In man the infection is either visceral or cutaneous. Visceral leishmaniasis is a severe chronic infection of the reticuloendothelial system, characterized by fever, chills, weight loss, splenomegaly, leukopenia, anemia, and a high natural mortality. It is caused by *L. donovani*. Cutaneous leishmaniasis is characterized by single or several chronic sores which usually heal spontaneously. In parts of South and Central America, severely mutilating metastatic lesions of the mouth and nose are seen. Cutaneous leishmaniasis is caused by *L. tropica* in the Old World, and by members of the *L. mexicana* and *L. brasiliensis* groups in the New World.

ETIOLOGY. *Leishmania* exist in two forms, one in the vertebrate host, including man, and the other in the sandfly and in artificial culture. In the vertebrate host the parasite is in the amastigote (Leishman-Donovan body) stage, so called because it has no free flagellum.

---

*Available from Center for Disease Control (404-633-3311, Ext. 3670).

It is a round or oval body 2 to 3 μ across, containing a nucleus and a smaller kinetoplast which stain respectively red and purple with Giemsa, Wright's or Leishman's stain, and stand out against the pale blue cytoplasm. *Leishmania* are strict intracellular parasites and are found in macrophages in which they multiply by binary fission. Heavily parasitized host cells rupture, and fresh cells are invaded. Sandflies become infected when they feed on an infected person or animal and take up parasites from blood or skin. In the sandfly the parasite is in the promastigote (leptomonad) stage, so called because of the anterior origin of its flagellum. Promastigotes are supple, highly motile, spindle-shaped organisms, 15 to 25 μ long and 1.5 to 3.5 μ broad. Promastigotes are found in the hindgut or midgut of the sandfly, where they divide and whence they migrate forward into the pharynx and buccal cavity, rendering the sandfly infective. The cycle of development in the sandfly takes about seven days. Once inoculated into man, the promastigote rapidly penetrates macrophages, flagellum first, and transforms into an amastigote.

Biochemical taxonomy of *Leishmania* (isoenzymes, DNA analysis) has proved a valuable adjunct to the traditional epidemiologic and serologic methods of species differentiation.

IMMUNOLOGY. The patterns of disease in man are partly determined by the species of parasite (tropism for skin or viscera, differences in immunogenicity and allergenicity) and partly by man's response to the parasite. Resistance to *Leishmania* depends upon the development of specific cell-mediated immunity. The capacity of individuals to mount such a response varies, and consequently leishmaniasis presents a spectrum of disease in the same way that leprosy does. At one end of the spectrum lie visceral leishmaniasis and diffuse cutaneous leishmaniasis, characterized by abundance of parasites, absence of lymphocytes in lesions, insensitivity to leishmanin, and poor prognosis. At the other end lie the self-healing sores, with relatively scanty parasites, marked lymphocytic infiltration, and leishmanin sensitivity. Accompanying cell-mediated immunity is delayed hypersensitivity to numerous parasite antigens, which causes the destructive pathology of leishmanial ulcers, especially in the chronic conditions of mucocutaneous leishmaniasis (see below) and leishmaniasis recidiva (see below) in which the normal balance between immunity and hypersensitivity has been lost. The mechanisms underlying these abnormal immune responses are not understood.

Antibody, which is produced in large quantities in visceral leishmaniasis, is not protective, and it has been suggested that it may even contribute to the pathogenesis of hemolytic anemia, nephritis, and amyloidosis. Healing is usually accompanied by long-lasting immunity to the particular species of *Leishmania* involved, but not to other species.

Leishmanin (Montenegro) Test. Leishmanin is a suspension of 10^6 promastigotes in 1 ml of 0.5 per cent phenol saline. The test is performed by injecting 0.1 ml intradermally into the volar surface of the forearm. A palpable nodule, 5 mm or more in diameter after 48 to 72 hours, is considered positive. The test is an index of delayed hypersensitivity, but not necessarily of immunity to *Leishmania*. It is not species specific. It is used to map out the extent of past infection in a community and may be of help in diagnosis in individual patients.

195.2.   VISCERAL LEISHMANIASIS
(Kala-Azar, Ponos)

EPIDEMIOLOGY. It has been suggested that the zoonotic origin of *L. donovani* was among jackals in the steppes of Central Asia, where sporadic cases of visceral leishmaniasis are still sometimes seen among nomads and in settlers in the outskirts of rapidly expanding towns. From here the disease spread and developed three distinct epidemiologic patterns.

Visceral Leishmaniasis with a Canine Reservoir. This is the pattern in a belt which stretches from Portugal to Peking between latitudes 30 and 48 degrees North, the most important areas being the Mediterranean littoral, including North Africa, the shores of the Caspian Sea, central Soviet Asia, and northeast China. The main vectors are *Phlebotomus perniciosus* and *P. ariasi* in Western Europe, *P. major* in Eastern Europe, *P. papatasii* in the Middle East, and *P. chinensis* in China. In the Mediterranean and Chinese foci, the host-parasite relationship is relatively stable, and the disease is most common among children between one and four years of age. For this reason the parasite is sometimes called *L. infantum*, although adults in areas into which the disease has newly been introduced or visitors of any age are highly susceptible. Domestic dogs and foxes are the reservoir.

Portuguese and Spanish settlers possibly introduced *L. donovani*, also called *L. chagasi*, into the New World and initiated a zoonosis among foxes and dogs, although man may still be an occasional reservoir. The likely vector is *Lutzomyia longipalpis*. Visceral leishmaniasis is epidemic in northeast Brazil and sporadic in Amazonia, northern Argentina, and Paraguay and extends up through Venezuela and Colombia as far as Guatemala and Mexico. In Brazil male children are most commonly affected.

Visceral Leishmaniasis with a Rodent Vector. This is the pattern in Africa south of the Sahara from Lake Chad in the west to Somalia in the east, sparing the highlands of Ethiopia. The apparent absence of the disease in West Africa and south of the equator is unexplained. In the Sudan the zoonosis is between the Nile rat (*Arvicanthus niloticus*) and *P. orientalis* on the flood plains of the Nile and its tributaries. Visceral leishmaniasis is found among nomads who occupy temporary villages in riverine acacia woodland and migrant workers from adjoining countries.

In Kenya the disease is associated with termite hills where the vector *P. martini* rests and around which village men gather in the evenings. The reservoir is probably the gerbil *Tatara vicina*. The disease is usually sporadic, but epidemics have occurred. Males are affected four times as often as females, and the disease is most common in teenagers.

Visceral Leishmaniasis with a Human Reservoir. This is true epidemic kala-azar and is the pattern of the disease in northeast India, Bangladesh, Assam, and Burma. Classically the disease spreads along the Brahmaputra valley every 20 years or so. Transmission is by the highly anthropophilic, domestic sandfly *P. argentipes*. Often, many cases are found to have originated from one house. The age and sex pattern is the same as in Africa. Man is the only reservoir, and *P. argentipes* is readily infected from blood or from the lesions of post-kala-azar dermal leishmaniasis. The disease virtually disappeared over large areas as a result of DDT spraying for malaria control, but returned in epidemic form in Bihar in 1975.

FACTORS AFFECTING TRANSMISSION. Opportunities for contact with infected sandflies largely determine the pattern of disease in a given area. This is modified by the level of immunity of the population or individual. An attack of visceral leishmaniasis confers lifelong immunity, which determines the periodicity of epidemics. Subclinical infections with *L. donovani* or possibly even lizard and rodent species of *Leishmania* affect the pattern of spread in Africa and around the Mediterranean.

PATHOLOGY. The organs most severely affected are the spleen, liver, bone marrow, lymph nodes, intestines, and skin. The patient suffers from hyperplasia within and damage to these organs and from effects secondary to splenomegaly, reticuloendothelial blockage, and chronic parasitemia. Histologically the disease is characterized by massive proliferation of parasitized macrophages with little or no lymphocytic response. In Africa and Central Asia a cutaneous nodule or leishmanioma commonly develops at the site of parasite inoculation. Parasites multiply within histiocytes which may become the focus of a tuberculoid granuloma that heals spontaneously, and the infection proceeds no further. In the majority of cases, however, after a period of months, the infection disseminates.

The spleen is grossly enlarged, smooth, and firm and the capsule thick. The pulp is friable and infarcts are usual. There is massive hyperplasia of reticuloendothelial cells which are heavily parasitized. In the liver, Kupffer cells are hyperplastic and contain parasites. Occasionally parenchymal cells are parasitized. In chronic untreated cases there is parenchymal cell degeneration which may be followed after several years by fibrosis and even cirrhosis with clinical and biochemical evidence of hepatic dysfunction.

The bone marrow is heavily infiltrated with parasitized macrophages. Erythropoiesis and granulopoiesis are normal in the early stages of the disease, but may be depressed later. The peripheral blood shows anemia and leukopenia. The anemia is probably due to increased plasma volume, sequestration of erythrocytes in the spleen, and hemolysis. Leukopenia is due to splenic pooling and is said to predispose the patient to secondary infections. Lymph nodes and lymphoid tissue of the nasopharynx and gut are enlarged and contain many parasitized cells.

Kidneys may show cloudy swelling of tubular cells. Immunoglobulin and complement are deposited in the glomerular basement membrane. In fatal cases hyaline thickening of the glomerular mesangium has been found, and in chronic cases amyloidosis can develop. The skin, although normal in appearance, contains many intracellular parasites. In *post-kala-azar dermal leishmaniasis* there is variable infiltration with lymphocytes, histiocytes, and parasites.

In visceral leishmaniasis there is an enormous overproduction of IgG, only a small fraction of which is specific antibody. Some of it is autoantibody.

CLINICAL FEATURES. The incubation period is normally two to six months, but may be as short as ten days or as long as nine years. The onset is usually insidious, especially in indigenous peoples who may feel well and have a good appetite despite daily bouts of fever; however, in those who are poorly nourished and have several underlying parasitic infections, the disease may then progress rapidly. In Africa a primary cutaneous nodule may be noticed for a few months before there are any systemic symptoms. The earliest symptom is fever. This is usually gradual in onset and accompanied by sweats, often without preceding chills. Alternatively, the onset is sudden with high fever and chills. This is common in Americans and Europeans who have contracted the disease while visiting an endemic area. Associated with fever there may be dizziness, weakness, and weight loss. Other common early symptoms include cough, diarrhea, pain, or discomfort in the left hypochondrium and symptoms of complicating secondary infections.

The important physical findings are fever, splenomegaly, lymphadenopathy, and skin changes. Fever at first is often inconstant, with apyrexial periods of several days or weeks. In over 80 per cent of cases, however, the fever eventually develops a characteristic pattern with twice daily elevations reaching 38 to 40° C, and may then undulate as in brucellosis. In the most acute cases fever and toxemia may be the only signs. Splenic enlargement is not necessarily rapidly progressive, nor does the size of the spleen correlate with the duration of the disease. In many instances, however, it reaches the right iliac fossa. It is firm and not tender unless there has been a recent subcapsular infarct. The liver enlarges more slowly and becomes palpable in about 20 per cent of cases and is likewise firm and not tender. Generalized lymphadenopathy is common in patients from Mediterranean countries, Africa, or China. Various changes have been reported in the skin. Classically there is hyperpigmentation of hands, feet, and abdomen. This may be missed in black Africans; in lighter-skinned Indians it looks gray or black (kala-azar means black sickness). In Africans warty eruptions or ulcers of the skin and oronasal lesions are occasionally seen (Abdalla et al, 1975).

COURSE AND COMPLICATIONS. As the disease progresses, anemia becomes clinically apparent. There may be bleeding from the nose or gums. In longstanding cases jaundice and signs of hypoalbuminemia may develop, namely, brittle hair, opaque nails, subcutaneous edema and ascites. Finally, after a course which may run for a few months or for five years, the patient becomes emaciated and exhausted. Intercurrent infections are the cause of death in 90 per cent of fatal cases. The most common are cancrum oris, pneumonia, pulmonary tuberculosis, bacillary dysentery, amebic dysentery, and, in Africa, brucellosis. Massive gastrointestinal hemorrhage accounts for another 1 to 2 per cent.

Post-Kala-Azar Dermal Leishmaniasis. About 20 per cent of Indian patients develop a rash one to two years after treatment or spontaneous recovery. The lesions develop slowly and may last for several, even 20, years. In Africa the rash develops in 2 per cent of cases, usually during treatment, and does not persist. It commonly starts as hypopigmented or erythematous macules on the face and sometimes on the arms, legs, and trunk. On the face the rash gradually becomes papular or nodular, especially on the forehead, cheeks, and earlobes, and closely resembles lepromatous leprosy. In 25 per cent of cases the lesions resolve spontaneously.

DIAGNOSIS AND LABORATORY FINDINGS. The diagnosis must be suspected in any person living in, or having visited, an endemic area who has a prolonged fever. The diagnosis is likely in the presence of splenomegaly, granulocytopenia, anemia, and hyperglobulinemia and is made by isolation of the parasite or by characteristic immunologic changes.

ISOLATION OF PARASITE. This is best done by needle aspiration of bone marrow, spleen, liver, lymph nodes, or blood. Material obtained is:

1. Used to make a thin film on a glass microscope slide, stained, and examined under oil immersion for amastigotes, which must be distinguished from platelets. Parasitized macrophages usually rupture on smearing and free parasites must be looked for (see Fig. 2F, Ch. 193). Bone marrow aspiration is the procedure of choice. However, splenic puncture is safe so long as the tip of the spleen is well below the costal margin and the prothrombin and bleeding times are normal. A hypodermic needle on a syringe is inserted into the spleen, allowed to rest a moment, and withdrawn without suction. Organisms are seen in about 90 per cent of splenic aspirates and rather less often from other tissues. Buffy coat preparations show parasites in over 90 per cent of cases in India, but in only about 1 per cent in Africa.

2. Inoculated onto NNN (Novy-MacNeal-Nicolle) medium overlaid with balanced salt solution, containing streptomycin and penicillin (but not amphotericin). Cultures are kept in the dark at 22 to 25° C (not at 37° C), and every three to four days a drop of fluid is taken and examined wet for promastigotes. If after four weeks no parasites are seen, the fluid overlay is reinoculated onto a fresh NNN slope. Culture greatly improves the chances of making a diagnosis.

3. Inoculated intraperitoneally into hamsters, which are susceptible to a single amastigote. Though sensitive, this method is slow and seldom valuable.

IMMUNOLOGIC TESTS. Antileishmanial antibodies can be demonstrated by indirect immunofluorescence of promastigotes in over 90 per cent of cases and by precipitation in gel in 95 per cent. Cross-reactions with *Trypanosoma cruzi* antibodies can be absorbed out. Complement fixation is positive in 65 per cent, but if the older antigen made from Kedrowsky's bacillus is used, reactions may be expected in some patients with mycobacterial disease. Serum obtained by eluting blood dried onto filter paper in the field can be used satisfactorily in all these techniques. The leishmanin test is *negative* in cases of active visceral leishmaniasis, but becomes positive after recovery, being most intense after one to two years, after which it fades slowly.

Total serum proteins are raised up to and over 10 grams per 100 ml. This increase is due almost entirely to the IgG fraction of gamma globulin. On immunoelectrophoresis the IgG pattern is characteristically skewed. In some cases IgM is also slightly increased, but this is said to be transient and to revert rapidly to normal on treatment. In advanced cases serum albumin levels fall. This disturbed globulin pattern underlies the older diagnostic aldehyde test which is also positive in other diseases with a grossly disturbed globulin pattern.

LABORATORY FINDINGS. The principal laboratory findings have to do with the blood and with the plasma proteins.

Blood Changes. Leukopenia is the most characteristic finding. The total count is below 2000 cells per cubic millimeter in 75 per cent of cases. There are an absolute neutropenia and eosinopenia and a relative lymphocytosis and monocytosis. Agranulocytosis occasionally develops. Anemia is slower in onset but becomes severe. It is normocytic and normochromic unless complicated by bleeding or deficiency states. There is often a mild reticulocytosis, and erythrocyte half-life is reduced. Thrombocytopenia is usual and progresses with the disease. Early on, tests of clotting are normal but later

the prothrombin, partial thromboplastin, bleeding, and clotting times are prolonged. There are no characteristic findings in the urine.

DIFFERENTIAL DIAGNOSIS. In Europeans, Americans, and others who are not immune, malaria must be excluded by examination of thick and thin blood films. In immunes, the presence of malarial parasites in the blood film does not exclude the additional diagnosis of leishmaniasis. In many parts of the tropics where malaria and schistosomiasis are endemic, a palpable spleen is commonplace and is usually unrelated to a recent febrile illness. Diseases which can be confused with visceral leishmaniasis include aleukemic leukemia and lymphomas, tropical splenomegaly syndrome (serum IgM, liver biopsy), cirrhosis of the liver with portal hypertension and hypersplenism, miliary tuberculosis, histoplasmosis, acute schistosomiasis, brucellosis, typhoid, and other septicemias, including bacterial endocarditis.

PROGNOSIS. Studies of an epidemic of visceral leishmaniasis in Italy suggest that subclinical infection is four times as common as classic kala-azar (Pampiglione et al., 1974, 1975). Untreated, 75 to 90 per cent of patients with established disease die. Treated, in all early cases, patients should recover. The mortality of late or severe disease in malnourished patients treated under difficult conditions can be over 25 per cent. Bad prognostic signs include extreme emaciation and toxemia, agranulocytosis, and the absence of the lymphocytosis which usually appears during treatment.

TREATMENT. **Chemotherapy.** Pentavalent antimony is the drug of choice, and, of the available preparations, sodium stibogluconate* (Sb) (Pentostam, Solustibostam) is probably the best. This is marketed as a solution containing 100 mg Sb per milliliter. The dose is 0.1 to 0.2 ml per kilogram of body weight daily by intravenous or intramuscular injection, not exceeding 10 ml per dose. In India six injections are usually adequate, but elsewhere 30 are considered necessary. Alternative preparations include the following: (1) Meglumine antimoniate (Glucantime, 30 mg per ml), 0.4 ml per kilogram of body weight daily for 14 days. (2) Ethyl stibamine (Neostibosan), which must be freshly prepared as a 5 per cent solution. The adult dose is 0.1 gram the first day, 0.2 gram the second day, and 0.3 gram daily thereafter for 8 to 16 doses by intravenous injection. (3) Urea stibamine, 100 to 200 mg intravenously on alternate days for 15 doses. Side effects of pentavalent antimony are cumulative but rare. They are nausea, vomiting, urticaria, bradycardia, and electrocardiographic changes. The response to antimonial treatment varies in kala-azar from different parts of the world. It is excellent in India and Brazil but less satisfactory in patients from East Africa or the Mediterranean. The choice then lies between two toxic drugs, pentamidine isethionate* (Lomidine, 40 mg per milliliter) and amphotericin B (Fungizone). The dose of pentamidine is 0.1 ml per kilogram of body weight by intramuscular injection every three to four days for ten doses, or less frequently if side effects develop. If the drug is accidentally injected intravenously, the patient will collapse, but recovers quickly if the feet are raised. Cumulative side effects include fatigue, anorexia, nausea, abdominal pain and, in 2 per cent of cases, prolonged hypoglycemia. Ten per cent of patients develop diabetes whose onset is not related to

---

*Available from Center for Disease Control (404-633-3311, Ext. 3670).

the duration of treatment. If this drug has to be used, a glucose tolerance test should be performed weekly. Amphotericin B is given by slow intravenous infusion in 5 per cent dextrose in a dose of 1 mg per kilogram of body weight on alternate days to a total of 2 grams for a 50-kg adult. Side effects include rigors, thrombophlebitis, nausea, vomiting, fatigue, anemia, and uremia. This drug is more difficult to administer than pentamidine but is preferable.

Supportive Treatment. Bed rest, good nursing care, oral hygiene, an adequate fluid intake, and sufficient food are all desirable. Complicating infections must be sought and treated. Anemia responds as the patient recovers, but if severe, and especially if there is bleeding, blood transfusion should be given. Deficiencies of iron, folate, and other vitamins need treating.

Response to Treatment. Little improvement may be seen until the course of treatment is nearly over. The patient then continues to improve steadily. Lymphocytosis and reticulocytosis develop. No criterion of cure has been established. The patient should be seen monthly for six months and at a year. At each visit blood is cultured for *Leishmania*, spleen size is measured, and hemoglobin and serum IgG estimated. Complement-fixing antibody should not be detectable after six months. The spleen does not always become impalpable, and may indicate that cirrhosis has developed.

Relapses and Post-Kala-Azar Dermal Leishmaniasis. These usually respond to a further course or courses of antimony. If not, one of the other drugs may be used. One month should elapse before repeating a course. Rarely, if repeated courses of drugs fail to eliminate the parasite, the spleen remains huge, and the patient suffers from hypersplenism, splenectomy may be indicated. It must be followed by a course of chemotherapy, and in malarial areas by antimalarial prophylaxis for life.

PREVENTION. On a mass scale the detailed epidemiology of the local disease must be known. This will enable reservoir control (destruction of stray dogs, early detection and treatment of cases) and vector control (insecticide spraying in the right places) to be carried out, and people may be able to avoid contact with infected flies, e.g., Kenyan termite hills. In some areas insecticide spraying against malarial mosquitoes reduced or eliminated kala-azar. Personal prophylaxis depends on wearing protective clothing in the evenings, the use of insect repellents, and sleeping under fine mesh netting.

195.3. CUTANEOUS LEISHMANIASIS OF THE OLD WORLD

(Oriental Sore)

EPIDEMIOLOGY. The innumerable names of this disease (Delhi or Bagdad boil, Biskra button, Aleppo evil, bouton de Crete, little sister) testify to its extent and familiarity throughout the Mediterranean basin, the Near and Middle East, and parts of India. Four epidemiologic situations are recognized.

"Rural" leishmaniasis throughout these areas is caused by the subspecies *L. tropica major*. The disease is a zoonosis among the desert gerbils (*Rhombomys opimus*) and is transmitted to man by *Phlebotomus papatasii*. Where village settlements are close to gerbil colonies, up to 100 per cent of the population become infected, usually in early childhood. Travelers, hunters, and soldiers also get the disease. In "urban" leishmaniasis, the parasite *L. tropica minor* is adapted to dogs and to man, either of whom can act as reservoirs. *P. sergenti* is the main vector. This disease was the scourge of Middle Eastern cities; every adult inhabitant bore the scar, and few visitors were spared.

In Africa two distinct zoonoses exist. In West Africa the situation is "rural." Human cases are uncommon and sporadic. The vector and reservoir are not definitely established, but rodents and dogs are probably involved. In Ethiopia and Kenya the disease is confined to the highlands, where the reservoir is the rock hyrax (*Procavia*). The vector is *P. longipes*, which bites villagers at night in their houses. The parasite has recently been designated *L. aethiopica.*

PATHOLOGY. At the site of inoculation there is a massive infiltration with monocytes and histiocytes which take up the parasites and support their growth. The lesion then becomes surrounded by or mixed with lymphocytes and a few plasma cells. Macrophages develop into epithelioid cells, and parasites diminish. In later cases loose tubercles composed of loosely packed cells may develop. The overlying dermis ulcerates. The epidermis shows hyperkeratosis, acanthosis, pseudoepitheliomatous hyperplasia, intraepidermal necrosis, and ulceration. Healing is accompanied by fibrosis and is followed by lifelong immunity. Second infections are seen in only about 2 per 1000 cases, and then often in association with a generalized depression of immunity.

If cell-mediated immunity fails to develop, the patient gets diffuse cutaneous leishmaniasis, the disease spreading to other parts of the skin. Histologic study shows masses of heavily parasitized macrophages with little or no lymphocytic infiltration or epidermal change. The leishmanin test is negative.

In leishmaniasis recidiva, failure to heal is associated with exquisite delayed hypersensitivity, extreme chronicity, a tuberculoid histology with epithelioid giant cells but without caseation, and scanty or undetectable parasites.

CLINICAL MANIFESTATIONS. The earliest lesion is a small erythematous papule, appearing two to eight weeks after the sandfly bite. It may itch slightly. The typical "urban" sore grows slowly into a nodule 1 to 2 cm across, and after a period of weeks or months forms a central crust under which is a shallow ulcer. The edge of the lesion is characteristically studded with small satellite papules. The sore usually remains in this state for a few more months and then heals gradually, leaving a depressed mottled scar. The whole process takes from three months to two years. The most common site is the face, followed by the arms and legs. There may be one or several sores. Immunity after healing is usually lifelong, but second infections may develop in old age or in patients taking corticosteroid drugs. About 1 per cent of urban sores develop *leishmaniasis recidiva (lupoid leishmaniasis)*. The ulcer fails to heal completely, scarring centrally but spreading peripherally, or heals and recrudesces at the edge of the scar. The lesion lasts for many years and resembles cutaneous tuberculosis.

There are many variants of the typical pattern of Oriental sore. "Rural" sores are commonly multiple, rapid

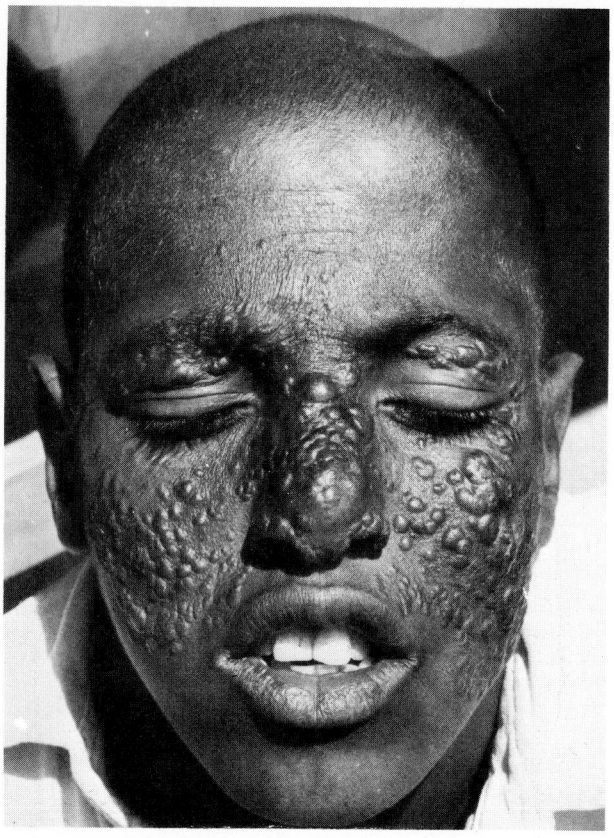

Early diffuse cutaneous leishmaniasis in an Ethiopian. Post-kala-azar dermal leishmaniasis may also look like this.

in evolution, and more florid, and produce more scarring. Ethiopian lesions are solitary, facial, milder, and slower in evolution, although lesions affecting the mucocutaneous border of the nose are extremely chronic and disfiguring.

Ethiopia and Kenya are the only Old World countries where *diffuse cutaneous leishmaniasis* is found. It is a rare condition, occurring in perhaps 1 in 100,000 cases. The primary nodule does not ulcerate, but after a period of months or years starts to spread locally, and

the disease disseminates to other parts of the skin, notably on the face and the extensor surfaces of the limbs, producing infiltrative and nodular lesions which may resemble lepromatous leprosy and do not heal spontaneously. The viscera are not involved, and the patient feels well.

DIAGNOSIS. Leishmaniasis must be suspected as the cause of any chronic nodule or ulcer in a person living in or having recently visited an endemic area. Typical sores are diagnosable on sight. Diagnosis is confirmed by finding parasites in stained slit skin smears taken from a nonulcerated part of the lesion. The slit must reach the dermis, and the smears must contain tissue juice, not blood or pus. If unsuccessful, the crust is removed, the ulcer cleaned of all debris, and smears made of tissue scraped from the base of the ulcer. These methods are simpler and more likely to show parasites than is histology. In healing lesions and lupoid leishmaniasis, parasites are scanty and culture of juice or biopsy tissue may be necessary.

The leishmanin test becomes positive as the lesion ulcerates and is of diagnostic value in patients who do not live in endemic areas; it also may help to distinguish lupoid leishmaniasis from cutaneous tuberculosis, late syphilis, and fungal granulomas, which may be histologically similar.

There are no characteristic blood changes, and antibodies are difficult to demonstrate by usual techniques.

TREATMENT. Treatment remains unsatisfactory, but, as almost all cases heal spontaneously, the systemic use of toxic drugs is seldom justified. Fortunately most cases respond to a course of pentavalent antimony* Failure to respond is usually due to inadequate dosage or duration of treatment. Local infiltration with 0.5 ml 2 per cent berberine sulfate or 15 per cent mepacrine is often effective. Indolent sores may respond to heating to 50° C by coned infrared rays, to curettage and skin grafting, or to intralesional injections of corticosteroids combined with a course of antimony. Secondary infection is treated with the customary antimicrobial drugs.

PREVENTION. Detailed epidemiologic knowledge has permitted attacks on the reservoir in Central Asia and in Middle Eastern cities, where demolition of mud

---

*Available from Center for Disease Control (404-633-3311, Ext. 3670).

Cutaneous Leishmaniasis of the New World: Epidemiology

Parasite	Vector to Man	Reservoir	Geography	Human Disease
L. mexicana mexicana	*Lutzomyia olmeca*	Numerous rodents	Yucatan, Central America	"Chicle ulcer, bay sore" in forest workers; single skin lesions, healing in six months; diffuse cutaneous leishmaniasis
L. mexicana amazonensis	*Lutzomyia flaviscutellata*	Numerous rodents	Brazil, Trinidad; ?= *L. pifanoi*, Venezuela	Rare, single skin lesions; diffuse cutaneous leishmaniasis
L. brasiliensis brasiliensis	*Psychodopygus wellcomei*, *Lutzomyia spp.*	Uncertain	All Amazon forests, esp. Brazil	"Espundia"; single or few large persistent destructive skin ulcers; oronasal metastases common
L. brasiliensis guyanensis	*Lutzomyia anduzei*	Unknown	Guyanas, into Brazil, Venezuela	"Forest yaws, pian bois"; multiple, widespread, deep skin ulcers, with nodular lymphatic metastases; ? oronasal metastases
L. brasiliensis panamensis	*Lutzomyia trapidoi*, *Psychodopygus panamensis*, and others	Rodents, sloths, dogs	Panama	Single or few deep skin ulcers with nodular lymphatic metastases; ? oronasal metastases
L. peruviana	*Lutzomyia verrucarum*, ? *Lutzomyia peruensis*	Dogs	Peru, west slopes of Andes to 3000 meters	"Uta"; single or few skin lesions, healing in one year

buildings and antimalarial spraying have reduced the number of sandflies. Immunization with live, virulent organisms is practiced on a mass scale in Russia and traditionally in the Middle East (see R. A. Neal, 1968).

195.4. CUTANEOUS LEISHMANIASIS OF THE NEW WORLD

(Including American Mucocutaneous Leishmaniasis or Espundia)

EPIDEMIOLOGY AND PARASITOLOGY. Cutaneous leishmaniasis is endemic in Central and South America as far south as the Parana Estuary in the east and the Peruvian Andes in the west. In this extensive and varied terrain many different zoonoses exist, each associated with its own reservoirs and vectors and a particular pattern of human disease. Two main groups of parasites are now distinguished, those of *L. mexicana* and of *L. brasiliensis.* The former, which grows easily in NNN medium and in the hamster, is responsible for most of the cutaneous leishmaniasis in Central America and a little in Brazil. The latter, which grows poorly in NNN medium and in the hamster, is responsible for most of the disease in South America, including mucocutaneous leishmaniasis. Epidemiologic details are summarized in the accompanying table.

Cutaneous leishmaniasis presents a formidable obstacle to the development of the Central and South American forests, in large areas of which transmission of the infection is extremely high. This is particularly true in Brazil, where many workers on the trans-Amazonian highway become infected and run the risk of developing mutilating oronasal metastatic lesions. Amerindians, on the other hand, commonly develop transient mild infections so that by the age of 40 years up to 100 per cent are sensitive to leishmanin. They rarely develop mucocutaneous lesions.

PATHOLOGY. The pathology of cutaneous lesions is similar to that of Oriental sore. Metastatic lesions of *L. brasiliensis* arise in the mucosa of the nose and mouth and show at first a typical leishmanial granuloma with numerous parasites, which later become scanty, and can be seen also in cells in cartilage, which is rapidly invaded and destroyed. There is vasculitis with edema, necrosis, and fibrosis.

CLINICAL MANIFESTATIONS. Cutaneous lesions develop and heal in the same way as Oriental sores, but tend to be less nodular and more ulcerative and destructive. Lesions of *L. mexicana* on the pinna may last for many years and slowly destroy the cartilage. Regional variations are given in the table.

In espundia, from 2 per cent (Panama) to 80 per cent (Paraguay) of primary cutaneous sores are followed after a period ranging from a few days to 25 years by metastatic lesions of the nose or mouth, most commonly on the mucocutaneous borders, but sometimes on the palate or larynx and rarely on the conjunctiva or external genitalia. Nasal obstruction is the most common early symptom. These lesions may arise many years after the primary lesion has healed. At first there is crusting or polyp formation, and then ulceration and perforation of the septum. Alternatively, large protruding granulomas of the nose and lips develop. The lesion heals slowly, if at all, after many years. Scarring

may constrict the nose or mouth, producing gross deformity and making eating difficult. Secondary sepsis is common and increases the patient's debility.

Diffuse cutaneous leishmaniasis is a rare disease described mainly from Venezuela and northern Brazil. Its clinical features are the same as in Ethiopia.

DIAGNOSIS. The approach to diagnosis is set forth in Ch. 195.2 and 195.3. In late cases of espundia it may be impossible to isolate the parasite, but geographic history, clinical pattern, and leishmanin sensitivity make the diagnosis likely. Antibodies are detectable by immunofluorescence in over 90 per cent of patients with cutaneous or oronasal lesions, and disappear when the disease has been successfully treated. Blastomycosis is added to the list of differential diagnoses.

TREATMENT. The milder varieties of solitary sores seldom need treatment, unless they are disfiguring. If there is any suspicion that a sore has been caused by *L. brasiliensis,* it must be treated by a course of pentavalent antimony (see Ch. 195.2). Established oronasal lesions frequently do not respond to antimony, or are liable to relapse. Amphotericin B (see Ch. 195.2) is then the drug of choice. Diffuse cutaneous leishmaniasis responds initially to antimony, but becomes resistant in relapse. Amphotericin B should then be tried.

PREVENTION. Prevention in South America is difficult. Intensity of transmission in the forest and lack of detailed epidemiologic information make mass prophylaxis a hopeless approach at the moment. People who are obliged to enter the forest could attempt to follow a regimen of the application of insect repellents every few hours and of sleeping under a fine mesh netting, but admittedly both these procedures can produce considerable discomfort.

Chance, M. L., Peters, W., and Shchory, L.: Biochemical taxonomy of *Leishmania.* Ann. Trop. Med. Parasit., *68*:307, 317, 1974.

Lainson, R., and Shaw, J. J.: Leishmaniasis of the New World: Taxonomic problems. Br. Med. Bull, 28:44, 1972.

Manson-Bahr, P. E. C., and Winslow, D. J.: Cutaneous leishmaniasis. *In* Marcial-Rojas, R. A. (ed.): Pathology of Rickettsial and Helminthic Diseases. Baltimore, Williams & Wilkins Company, 1971, p. 97.

Marsden, P. D., and Nonata, R. R.: Mucocutaneous leishmaniasis: A review of clinical aspects. Rev. Soc. Bras. Med. Trop., 9:309, 1975.

Most, H., and Lavietes, R. H.: Kala-azar in American military personnel. Medicine, 26:221, 1947.

Symposium on leishmaniasis. Bull. WHO, 44:477, 1971.

Turk, J. L., and Bryceson, A. D. M.: Immunological phenomena in leprosy and related diseases. Adv. Immunol., 13:209, 1971.

Walton, B. C., Brooks, W. H., and Arjona, I.: Serodiagnosis of American leishmaniasis by indirect fluorescent antibody test. Am. J. Trop. Med. Hyg., 21:296, 1972.

Wilcocks, C., and Manson-Bahr, P. E. C. (eds.): Manson's Tropical Diseases. 17th ed. Baltimore, Williams & Wilkins Company, 1972.

Winslow, D. J.: Visceral leishmaniasis. *In* Marcial-Rojas, R. A. (ed.): Pathology of Rickettsial and Helminthic Diseases. Baltimore, Williams & Wilkins Company, 1971, p. 86.

196. AMEBIASIS

Richard Knight

DEFINITION. Amebiasis is caused by infection with *Entamoeba histolytica.* This species normally lives as a commensal within the large bowel lumen, where it may persist for several years. Symptoms of the disease may be produced if there is bowel wall invasion or subsequent blood-borne spread to the liver.

ETIOLOGY. Noninvasive trophozoites of *E. histolytica* measure 10 to 20 μ in diameter and live adjacent to the mucosa of the proximal colon, where they feed upon bacteria and exfoliated epithelial cells. They multiply by binary fission every eight hours; some of them round up, eliminate their cytoplasmic inclusions, and secrete a rigid cell wall to become uninucleate spherical cysts (10 to 16 μ in diameter); immature cysts contain a large glycogen vacuole. The cysts mature either within the bowel lumen or outside the body. Most mature cysts have four nuclei resulting from two nuclear divisions, and cigar-shaped chromatoid bars that constitute a ribosome store. When these mature cysts are ingested, they undergo one additional nuclear division. The cyst wall is destroyed in the small intestine, releasing eight motile uninucleate amebae or trophozoites.

Invasive *E. histolytica* are larger than noninvasive forms, up to 50 μ, and move much more actively by unidirectional pseudopodial movement. They contain ingested erythrocytes — hence the term hematophagous — and few or no bacteria.

Freshly isolated strains of *E. histolytica* behave differently when inoculated intracecally into weanling rats, those from patients with dysentery often being the most pathogenic. Strain virulence is relatively unstable and in culture often decreases quite rapidly, although it may usually be restored by animal passage. A few strains have been isolated that differ from *E. histolytica* antigenically and by their ability to grow at room temperature and in hypotonic media. These atypical or *E. histolytica*–like amebae are probably never pathogenic; *all other strains of E. histolytica are potentially virulent.*

EPIDEMIOLOGY. About 10 per cent of the world's population harbor *E. histolytica*. In the United States the prevalence is 2 to 5 per cent, in some tropical countries over 40 per cent. Poverty and poor sanitation encourage infection. Cysts may survive a month in water but are killed by drying. Rats, dogs, and certain monkeys are sometimes infected, but almost all human infections are from cysts passed by human carriers. *Encystment does not occur outside the body,* so patients passing only trophozoites in their stools are not infectious. Food is the most common vehicle of transmission; it may be contaminated by infected food handlers or flies. Direct contamination with human feces used as fertilizer is most common with salad vegetables. Direct fecal spread is important among children or the mentally handicapped in institutions, where infection rates may be very high.

Water-borne infection occurs, occasionally in epidemic form, as in the famous Chicago epidemic in which there were 1400 known cases and more than 100 deaths. Epidemics are probably not often recognized because the incubation period is so variable and many infections asymptomatic. Cysts may appear in the stool as early as four days after infection. The rate of spontaneous loss of infection is perhaps 15 per cent per year, so persons coming to temperate countries from the tropics may remain infected for five years or more. In countries where there is continuous transmission, prevalence rates remain stable from year to year. In certain parts of the world, such as Mexico, parts of South America, the West Coast of Africa, Natal, and Southeast Asia, invasive disease is especially common. The incidence of disease does not necessarily correlate with the prevalence of infection.

PATHOGENESIS AND PATHOLOGY. Commensal trophozoites thrive adjacent to the colonic mucosa where the oxygen tension is moderately low and the pH between 6.0 and 6.5. Host tissues are damaged only by direct contact with amebae, when membrane-bound cytolytic enzymes are released from dendritic plasmalemmal processes. The relatively anoxic and acid conditions of cell necrosis favor further penetration of amebae into the tissues. Although some amebic bowel lesions are secondarily infected, the role of intestinal bacteria in pathogenesis is still uncertain. They may act mainly by creating a milieu suitable for amebic growth.

Amebic ulceration is most common in the cecum and rectosigmoid, but may affect any part of the large bowel, appendix, and terminal ileum. The initial lesions are small, discrete superficial mucosal erosions which may then extend more deeply through the muscularis mucosae and spread laterally, producing ulcers that are flask shaped in cross-section. Lesions may coalesce, causing extensive mucosal loss. Blood vessel involvement usually results in local thrombosis. Penetration may extend through the muscle coats, causing *peritonitis,* the most dangerous complication of intestinal amebiasis. Microscopically, tissue necrosis is the main change; amebae occur throughout the lesion, but particularly at the advancing edge, and even beyond into healthy tissue. In tissue sections, amebae may appear shrunken and be surrounded by a clear space. They stain rather indistinctly with ordinary hematoxylin and eosin but stand out clearly as bright red bodies with periodic acid–Schiff stain; iron hematoxylin staining is necessary to show the nuclear structure clearly. The lymphocytic inflammatory response is slight or moderate; some neutrophils are also present, especially if there is secondary bacterial infection.

Ulcers heal rapidly after treatment, and persistent scarring is uncommon. Sometimes localized bowel lesions show a more vigorous host response, with edema and a marked inflammatory reaction producing an amebic granuloma or ameboma. These are most common in the cecum and rectosigmoid and may be multiple.

Although strain virulence may influence the probability of tissue invasion, host factors are also important. Women in late pregnancy and the puerperium are especially susceptible, as are patients on cytotoxic or corticosteroid therapy. Colonic cancers may be secondarily invaded by *E. histolytica. Trichuris trichiura* infections and intestinal schistosomiasis may also encourage invasion. The low protein diets of developing countries may enhance susceptibility, especially in children.

Hepatic Involvement. In many patients with invasive intestinal disease, amebae probably reach the liver via the portal vein, but most are destroyed. Hepatomegaly is frequent in acute amebic dysentery because of products of colonic tissue destruction or bacteria reaching the liver. Established amebic infection of the liver usually causes progressive cytolytic lesions that extend in all directions, with trophozoites proliferating near the advancing edge. Perhaps these lesions begin at the sites of venous embolism or thrombosis. Secondary bacterial infection is rare, and the content of such a "liver abscess" is necrotic liquefied liver tissue. The abscess is sharply demarcated from surrounding liver, which shows edema, hyperemia, and a narrow zone of lymphocytic and polymorphonuclear infiltration; a fibroblastic reaction occurs in longstanding lesions. Most liver abscesses are solitary and occur long after any clinically evident bowel ulceration; but both solitary and the rarer multiple abscesses may develop during or shortly after a bout of dysentery. The term *amebic hepatitis* has been used by clinicians, but there is no pathologic basis for a diffuse lesion of this kind. In adults, 80 to 90 per cent of amebic liver abscesses occur in men, but before puberty both sexes are similarly affected. No other host factors have been definitely identified, although pre-existing liver disease and alcoholism may be relevant. Most complications of liver abscess are due to direct spread to adjacent structures.

Antibody Response. Tissue invasion provokes a humoral antibody response, mainly IgG, and a skin sensitivity to injected amebic antigen. It is not known whether this response has any protective function. Using sensitive techniques, antibodies can be detected in 25 per cent or more of apparently healthy carriers, suggesting that mild self-limiting bowel invasion is more common than has been supposed.

CLINICAL MANIFESTATIONS. Intestinal Amebiasis. Most persons with *E. histolytica* in the stool have no symptoms, and many will remain symptomless carriers for the whole duration of their infection. Invasive bowel disease begins most commonly between one and six months after infection but sometimes much later, especially in an immunologically compromised host.

The disease spectrum is wide, and the clinical picture depends on the severity and extent of bowel wall involvement. Most commonly, ulceration is localized and not severe enough to produce dysentery. The patient complains of colicky pains in the right or left iliac fossa, flatulence, and an altered bowel habit, often with some diarrhea. A little blood or mucus may be noted in the stool; there is little constitutional upset. The cecum or sigmoid colon may be tender or feel abnormal on palpation. Symptoms may persist intermittently for months thereafter, and spontaneous cure is not uncommon.

Widespread colonic or rectosigmoid ulceration produces amebic dysentery with frequent bloody stools. Dysentery may begin abruptly, but often follows a varied period of the milder colonic symptoms noted above. Initially, many patients remain ambulant, but later, fever, colicky abdominal pains, and tenesmus appear. The illness is usually less acute than bacillary dysentery and dehydration less evident. There may be colonic tenderness and some hepatomegaly. The stool is often offensive and contains some fecal matter; much of the blood present is altered unless there is rectal ulceration. Sigmoidoscopic appearances are not pathognomonic, but the procedure is useful for initial assessment and follow-up; scrapings should be examined immediately for hematophagous trophozoites. In the rare fulminating form of the disease, toxic megacolon occurs with progressive abdominal distention, vomiting, dehydration, and electrolyte loss; some very ill patients have relatively few bowel actions. Sigmoidoscopy and barium enema examination should not be carried out in patients with severe dysentery; when the diagnosis is in doubt, a limited endoscopy may be justified.

Amebomas may present as a tender abdominal mass, sometimes with fever and constitutional upset. Partial bowel obstruction may occur, especially when the lesion is annular. The appendix may be affected primarily, or secondarily by a cecal lesion. This may resemble simple appendicitis, except that pain begins in the right iliac fossa, and guarding and rigidity are slight unless perforation has occurred.

COMPLICATIONS. A grossly diseased and atonic large bowel may perforate at several points. Absent bowel sounds with relatively little pain, rigidity, or tenderness should suggest this very dangerous possibility. Free gas in the peritoneum confirms it. Less commonly, when perforation is localized, classic signs of peritonitis are produced. Local perforation can also lead to pericolic abscess or retroperitoneal fecal cellulitis. *Fibrous strictures* of the colon rarely follow amebic dysentery or amebomas, but may require surgical relief. Serious hemorrhage is uncommon, but can be life threatening. Amebic ulceration or an ameboma may rarely initiate a cecocolic intussusception. Irritable bowel syndrome may follow amebic colitis and persist for several months. Much rarer is the syndrome of postdysenteric colitis which can continue for several years despite eradication of the amebic infection. It is distinct from simple ulcerative colitis and is associated with very high amebic antibody titers; endoscopy shows a reddened edematous mucosa, sometimes with superficial erosions. Barium enema examination will exclude the rare possibility of internal fistulas.

Cutaneous amebiasis takes the form of deep, painful, and rapidly spreading ulceration. The most common sites are the perianal area, perineum, laparotomy incisions, and colostomy stomas. Rarely, the uterine cervix is affected, giving lesions that may resemble carcinoma. Penile lesions may follow anal coitus.

Hepatic Amebiasis. About half of all patients with liver abscess have a history suggestive of amebic dysentery between a week and many years previously. Solitary lesions are most common in the upper part of the right lobe; multiple lesions are often associated with coexistent dysentery. The illness begins insidiously with fever, sweating, and pain in the liver region. If the diaphragm is involved, there may be right pleuritic or shoulder pain. Most patients present within a few weeks of onset; as the disease progresses, weight loss and anemia develop. *Those developing the condition in temperate countries after returning from the tropics rarely have bowel symptoms.* Hepatomegaly is always present, but if enlargement is mainly upward, it may not be very evident on abdominal palpation. Left lobe lesions are palpable as an epigastric mass. Liver tenderness is mainly localized to the site of the lesion, and, in suspected cases, all the lower right intercostal spaces should be carefully palpated. Pain on heavy percussion or compression of the liver is not a very specific sign, because many types of liver and chest disease will be painful with these procedures. Crepitations and signs of lung consolidation or pleural fluid in the lower right chest are quite common. Jaundice occurs only when lesions are very large or numerous. The blood sedimentation rate is raised, and normally there is polymorphonuclear leukocytosis and some normocytic normochromic anemia. Levels of serum transaminase and alkaline phosphatase are variable and of little diagnostic value. *The most suggestive roentgenographic finding* is an immobile, raised, or bulging right hemidiaphragm; lung or pleural involvement may also be visible. Liver scans help considerably to show the site, size, and number of lesions present; radioisotope scans are probably most useful, but ultrasound and computerized axial tomography may also be helpful.

COMPLICATIONS. Rupture through the diaphragm can produce amebic lung abscess or empyema and sometimes a bronchohepatic fistula so that the patient coughs up amebic pus. Extension to the body surface may lead to sinus formation and cutaneous lesions. Amebic peritonitis follows rupture into the peritoneum, and the primary source may be evident only at laparotomy. The gut, stomach, vena cava, spleen, and right kidney can also be involved by direct spread. A dangerous complication of left lobe lesions is *amebic pericarditis;* urgent aspiration may be necessary to relieve tamponade, and fibrous constrictive pericarditis is a rare late sequel. More than 100 cases of *amebic brain abscess* have been reported. All have been associated with liver abscess and, so far, all patients have died. This condition should not be confused with primary amebic meningoencephalitis caused by free-living amebae (*Naegleria*). Hematogenous lesions also occasionally occur in the lung and perhaps elsewhere.

DIFFERENTIAL DIAGNOSIS.   Intestinal Amebiasis. Amebic dysentery may resemble bacillary dysentery, nonspecific ulcerative colitis, intestinal salmonellosis, and, more rarely, heavy infection with intestinal schistosomiasis or *Trichuris trichiura.* Patients with nondysenteric colitis are often suspected of having irritable bowel syndrome, and blood in the stool may be attributed to hemorrhoids. Diverticulitis, carcinoma, and Crohn's disease of the colon may require exclusion by barium enema and sigmoidoscopy. *The finding of E. histolytica should not delay the search for another disease, especially because amebic ulceration may be superimposed upon a carcinoma.* Amebomas may mimic neoplastic, infective, and granulomatous conditions of the large bowel, including lymphogranuloma venereum when the rectum is involved. The interpretation of therapeutic trials with tissue amebicides may be difficult, and the delay can make a tumor inoperable.

Hepatic Amebiasis. In the differential diagnosis of hepatic amebiasis, it is necessary to exclude primary and secondary neoplasms of the liver, subphrenic abscess, and pyogenic liver abscesses, including those caused by migrating *Ascaris* worms. Other conditions to be considered are hydatid cyst, the painful or tender hepatomegaly of viral or alcoholic hepatitis, and various pleural or lung lesions of the right lower chest. Liver scans and amebic serology have made *diagnostic needle aspiration* less often necessary, but the finding of relatively odorless brownish or pink material with no bacteria on Gram staining is almost pathognomonic. An 8-cm pleural aspiration needle 1.5 to 2.0 mm in diameter connected to a large syringe via a three-way tap is normally used. When there is no definite clinical evidence as to the site of the lesion, the eighth or ninth right intercostal space should be explored in the midaxillary line.

LABORATORY   DIAGNOSIS.   Microscopy and Culture. The finding of hematophagous trophozoites in fresh stools or material obtained at endoscopy confirms the presence of invasive colonic amebiasis. Symptomless carriers and those with mild ulceration of the proximal colon pass only cysts in their stools. Liver abscess patients pass cysts or, less commonly, hematophagous trophozoites; sometimes, however, no bowel infection can be demonstrated.

Hematophagous trophozoites should be sought in temporary wet mounts of dysenteric stools, bowel wall scrapings, material from suspected skin lesions, and in the last portion of pus obtained at liver aspiration. If necessary, the material should be diluted with buffered saline (ideally, pH 6.8). In nondysenteric stools, flecks

of mucus or pus should be looked for and examined. Trophozoites remain active and recognizable for about 30 minutes above 18° C (see Fig. 2, Ch. 193). If delay will inevitably be longer than this, the specimen should be kept cool as activity is restored, even after several hours at 4° C. If necessary, amebae may be preserved in polyvinyl alcohol and identified after staining with Heidenhain's iron hematoxylin or Gomori's trichrome stain; alternatively, a smear may be fixed in Schaudinn's fixative and stained later. In wet mounts, the definitive identification of nonhematophagous *E. histolytica* is not possible, and even in stained preparations, it is not easy; for this reason purged stool specimens are of no help unless hematophagous amebae are obtained. On the other hand, *E. histolytica* cysts can be readily recognized in wet mounts, using dilute Lugol's iodine to define nuclear and chromatoid morphology. Cyst concentration techniques using formol ether sedimentation or zinc sulfate flotation give a diagnostic sensitivity of about 70 per cent per specimen compared with 30 per cent without concentration. Examination of concentrates from stools obtained on three separate days is normally sufficient to exclude an intraluminal amebic infection. Cysts in stool may be preserved in 10 per cent formalin, but this reduces the effectiveness of concentration procedures. Besides *E. histolytica,* three nonpathogenic species of *Entamoeba* may infect man; they are never hematophagous and may be recognized by their cystic stages.

E. hartmanni is closely related to *E. histolytica* but is smaller, the peripheral nuclear chromatin is more clumped, and the quadrinucleate cysts are less than 10 μ in diameter (mean, 8 μ). *E. coli* is another common commensal, whose sluggish trophozoites (20 to 30 μ) have coarse granular endoplasm. The karyosome is eccentric and the peripheral chromatin coarser than that of *E. histolytica.* Mature cysts (12 to 20 μ) have eight nuclei and thin-pointed chromatoids. *E. polecki* is primarily a pig parasite and is rare in man except in parts of New Guinea where pigs and man live in close association. The mature cyst has only one nucleus and resembles an immature *E. histolytica* cyst.

Cultivation of *E. histolytica* from fresh stool is not difficult with appropriate media, and is sometimes helpful in confirming the diagnosis. Stained preparations of isolates must be made for accurate identification. If amebic liver pus is to be cultured, the medium should be preconditioned with *Escherichia coli.*

Serologic Tests. The most sensitive tests for the detection of amebic antibodies are indirect hemagglutination, indirect immunofluorescence, and counterimmunoelectrophoresis. Latex agglutination and gel diffusion precipitation tests are also used. Over 90 per cent of patients with liver abscess normally have positive serologic tests, compared with 60 to 80 per cent of those with invasive intestinal disease. Results must be interpreted with caution, as antibody may persist for several years, and in endemic areas some asymptomatic carriers and noninfected persons will have positive reactions. However, negative serologic tests are quite strong evidence against a diagnosis of liver abscess. Serologic tests are also valuable in suspected amebomas and other localized colonic lesions beyond the reach of sigmoidoscopy.

TREATMENT.   Clinical Pharmacology. TISSUE AMEBICIDES.   Metronidazole (Flagyl) is a potent and safe oral ambicide that is rapidly absorbed by the small bowel to reach all tissues. It is also useful in the treatment of intraluminal infections, because some is excreted in the bile in modified form and some directly into the colon. A five- or eight-day course of 750 or 800 mg thrice daily is effective in all forms of invasive amebiasis. Paradoxically, higher doses are required to eliminate a bowel infection than to destroy all tissue-invading amebae. Side effects very rarely necessitate stopping treatment; they include dizziness, nausea, abdominal pain, a metallic taste in the mouth, brownish discoloration of the urine, and a confusional state if alcohol is taken. The effectiveness of metronidazole has greatly simplified the chemotherapy of amebiasis, but its action is slightly less rapid than that of emetine, and a few treatment failures have been reported. A parenteral preparation of metronidazole has recently become available and may find a place in the treatment of amebic peritonitis.

Intramuscular emetine hydrochloride and the synthetic compound dehydroemetine dihydrochloride* are the most rapidly acting tissue amebicides, but both are toxic and cumulative. Emetine is given in a dose of 1 mg per kilogram of body weight daily (maximum, 60 mg daily) for up to ten days. *Serious cardiotoxicity* is suggested by hypotension, dyspnea, precordial pain, tachycardia, and palpitations, but is unusual until at least six doses have been given. Electrocardiographic changes include T wave inversion, prolongation of P-R interval, widening of the QRS complex, and arrhythmias. Less serious side effects are weakness, nausea, and vomiting, local myositis at the site of injection, and, rarely, a more generalized myositis. A course of treatment should not exceed ten days and should not be repeated without an interval of at least two weeks. Complete bed rest is essential. The drug should not be given to patients with cardiovascular disease, and is not generally recommended for pregnant women or for children. Dehydroemetine is excreted more rapidly in the urine than emetine, and a daily dose of 1.25 mg per kilogram of body weight (maximum, 90 mg daily) is necessary; it is probably less cardiotoxic.

The only indication for chloroquine is hepatic amebiasis, because the drug is concentrated by, and accumulates within, the liver. The usual regimen for adults consists of 150 mg base twice daily for three weeks. Some toxicity may occur with this regimen, including T wave changes on the electrocardiogram. *Patients being treated for invasive intestinal amebiasis with drugs other than emetine or metronidazole should be given a two-week course of chloroquine to prevent the development of hepatic lesions.*

LUMINAL AMEBICIDES. Tetracycline can be very useful in some patients with invasive intestinal disease; it acts upon bacteria within the lesions, but also has some direct amebicidal activity. Tetracycline is used in situations when a parenteral drug is needed, and when metronidazole or emetine is contraindicated or not available. It should not be used for long-term treatment (four weeks or more) in those under the age of puberty. If the drug is used alone, parasitic cure is uncommon, and there may be clinical relapse. For adults, the dosage is 250 or 500 mg every six hours for five to ten days.

Numerous substances have been used to eliminate the bowel infection in symptomless carriers and in patients with invasive disease who are not given metro-nidazole. The most effective are diiodohydroxyquin, diloxanide furoate (Furamide),* and paromomycin (Humatin). The adverse effects of diiodohydroxyquin are mild diarrhea, pruritus ani, rashes, and rarely iodism. The related compound clioquinol (iodochlorohydroxyquin) has been incriminated as a rare cause of myelo-optic neuropathy.

Management. INTESTINAL AMEBIASIS. Amebic dysentery and nondysenteric colitis should be treated with emetine, metronidazole, or tetracycline, depending upon drug availability and contraindications. If emetine is given, only a three- to six-day course is normally required to control the acute phase of the disease. It should be combined with or followed by metronidazole or tetracycline with chloroquine. Tetracycline should probably be given to all patients with severe dysentery. Amebic peritonitis should be treated medically with gastric suction and intravenous fluid and electrolytes, together with emetine and parenteral tetracycline. If the diagnosis is made at laparotomy, surgical repair may be difficult because the bowel wall is so friable. Amebomas may be successfully treated with a full course of metronidazole or a ten-day course of emetine. In all forms of intestinal disease, if metronidazole is not used, a luminally active drug must also be given to eradicate the infection.

In countries where transmission rates are low, such as the United States and Western Europe, it is generally recommended that all detected symptomless infections should be treated to prevent later invasive disease or transmission to others. Suitable regimens for adults are diiodohydroxyquin, 650 mg thrice daily for 21 days; entamide furoate, 500 mg thrice daily for 10 days; or paromomycin, 500 mg thrice daily for seven days. Alternatively, a full course of metronidazole can be given, particularly if there is suspicion of tissue invasion or concurrent infection with *Giardia lamblia*.

HEPATIC AMEBIASIS. Liver abscess may be successfully treated with a ten-day course of emetine plus chloroquine for three weeks and a luminal amebicide. Alternatively, a five- or eight-day course of metronidazole may be used; 400 or 500 mg thrice daily will cure the liver lesion, but 750 or 800 mg should be given to eliminate the coexistent gut infection which must be assumed to be present. Being better tolerated, metronidazole will usually be the treatment of choice; however, unless the lesion is drained, resolution may be slower with this drug, and a few therapeutic failures have been reported.

Aspiration of the liver is sometimes necessary for therapeutic purposes as well as for diagnosis. Consequently, if it is at all possible, the patient with liver abscess should be treated in association with a surgeon. This is easily accomplished in a large metropolitan center. By contrast, in a remote rural area it may be necessary for the physician to perform needle aspiration. However, if drainage of the abscess is necessary and satisfactory facilities are available, it is preferable that this procedure, whether by needle or through laparotomy, be conducted as a surgical procedure. There is some risk of spreading the infection within the peritoneal cavity, but this is greatly lessened by preaspiration chemotherapy.

The indications for surgical drainage are as follows: (1) when aspiration is strongly indicated on clinical

---

*Available from Center for Disease Control (404-633-3311, Ext. 3670).

*Available from Center for Disease Control (404-633-3311, Ext. 3670).

grounds, but attempts by percutaneous route have failed to locate or adequately drain the lesion; (2) when the lesion continues to refill despite chemotherapy and several percutaneous aspirations; and (3) in the presence of left lobe lesions when not superficial or when the diagnosis is uncertain. An indwelling soft rubber drain is rarely required after surgical drainage; if used, it must be connected to a sterile underwater seal and removed early.

The principal indications for percutaneous aspiration are: (1) very large lesions and those in the left lobe, especially when there is clinical or radiologic evidence that rupture is imminent; (2) after rupture, if this has occurred into the pleural cavity or pericardium (these also must be aspirated); and (3) poor clinical response after five days of medical treatment. Sometimes the procedure may have to be repeated two or three times. The principal complications are hemorrhage and introduction of bacterial infection; the latter is suggested if the aspirate changes color, becomes very liquid or offensive, or contains gas. Bleeding is less common than might be expected, because in liver abscess the right hemidiaphragm rarely moves with respiration.

Amebic lung lesions will respond to treatment given for the associated liver lesion. Cutaneous lesions respond to either emetine or metronidazole.

PROGNOSIS. Despite a normally rapid response to treatment, invasive intestinal disease may relapse if the infection is not eliminated. Host factors may be relevant in some persons, including perhaps those with mild nonspecific colitis. If symptoms recur, care must be taken to exclude other colonic disease. There is so far no evidence of drug resistance by any strain of *E. histolytica*. Amebic peritonitis, especially when there are multiple gut perforations, carries a grave prognosis; but permanent sequelae after any form of amebic colitis are rare. Hepatic scanning suggests that filling defects normally disappear within two or four months after treatment of liver abscess. Failure to aspirate large lesions adequately may lead to clinical relapse or much slower resolution. Healing occurs with little scar formation, but if the lesion was secondarily infected, bizarre hepatic calcification may be seen years afterward. Published reports of unselected patients suggest that a 10 per cent mortality is not unusual in liver abscess, but the prognosis can be much better with early diagnosis and adequate treatment.

After successful treatment for amebiasis, there is no reason why a person from a temperate country should not return to the tropics.

PREVENTION. Chlorination of water supplies does not destroy *E. histolytica* cysts, but proper filtration is effective. A weak solution of iodine is a more potent cysticide than chlorine. Salads and vegetables may be soaked in vinegar or potassium permanganate solution; these are procedures of doubtful benefit, and for some they render the food inedible. A solution of sodium hypochlorite has been found useful. Visitors to the tropics should avoid purchasing food from street vendors and from premises where flies are evident. Fruit that can be skinned should be safe. Boiling water for five minutes kills cysts. Members of domestic staffs involved in food handling should have their stools examined.

Intermittent mass chemotherapy with entamide furoate and metronidazole has been successfully attempted in Mexico and elsewhere where invasive disease is common; it may also be useful in mental institutions in temperate countries. *Personal chemoprophylaxis* by visitors to the tropics is not recommended, and it is better for such persons to avoid eating uncooked foods and to have their stools examined on return.

Amoebiasis: Report of a WHO Expert Committee. WHO Technical Report Series No. 421, 1–52, 1969.

Barbour, G. L., and Juniper, K., Jr.: A clinical comparison of amebic and pyogenic abscess of the liver. Am. J. Med., 53:323, 1972.

Biagi–F., F., and Beltran, H. F.: The challenge of amoebiasis: Understanding pathogenic mechanisms. Int. Rev. Trop. Med., 3:219, 1969.

Elsdon-Dew, R.: The epidemiology of amoebiasis. Adv. Parasitol., 6:1, 1968.

Krogstad, D. J., et al.: Amebiasis: Epidemiologic studies in the United States, 1971–1974. Ann. Intern. Med., 88:89, 1978.

Powell, S. J.: New developments in the therapy of amoebiasis. Gut, 11:967, 1970.

Sepulveda, B., and Diamond, L. S.: Amebiasis. Instituto Mexicano del Seguro Social, Mexico, 1976.

Wilmot, A. J.: Clinical Amoebiasis. Oxford, Blackwell, 1962.

197.   TOXOPLASMOSIS

Thomas C. Jones

GENERAL CONSIDERATIONS. Toxoplasmosis is a common infection of mammals and birds which occasionally results in protean disease. It is caused by the protozoan *Toxoplasma gondii*. In man, tissue parasitism during the proliferative phase may occur without signs or symptoms; it may lead to a transient illness characterized by lymphadenopathy, fever, and fatigue; or it may cause extensive damage to the brain, eyes, muscle, heart, liver, or lungs. Severe manifestations of the disease most commonly occur when a fetus is infected (congenital toxoplasmosis) or when infection occurs in patients with impaired immunity. Chronic infection may lead to a recurrent inflammatory process usually recognized by progressive ocular damage. When members of the cat family ingest *Toxoplasma* organisms, infection of epithelial cells in the intestinal tract results in production of oocysts which, when excreted, provide an important means by which the infection is transmitted in nature. Viable organisms within cysts in muscles and brain of infected animals provide a continued source of infection to carnivores.

HISTORY. In 1907 *Toxoplasma gondii* was recognized as a distinct protozoan and named by Nicolle and Manceaux. The first human case of congenital infection was recorded in 1923 by Janku in Prague, and in 1938 Wolf, Cowen, and Paige described the first cases from which the parasite was isolated. Toxoplasmosis in adults was first described by Pinkerton and Henderson in 1941. Eye damage caused by *Toxoplasma* in adults was first suggested by Frenkel and confirmed after observations made by Wilder in 1952. The present realization that 500 million humans are infected with the protozoan evolved from the extensive epidemiologic studies of Feldman, Desmonts, Thalhammer, and Jacobs, and from the recognition by Siim and others of the varied, often mild clinical patterns of acquired infection. In 1967, Hutchison first suggested that the cat played a role in the life cycle of *Toxoplasma gondii*, a cycle which was subsequently delineated in 1970.

THE PROTOZOAN. When mammals or birds ingest either infective oocysts or cysts in muscle or brain of other animals, an *intermediate* or asexual cycle of *Toxoplasma* infection is initiated. This consists of an obligate intracellular *proliferative stage* and a *cyst* stage. In the proliferative stage, *trophozoites*, which are ovoid or arc shaped, 3 to 4 μ in diameter, 6 to 7 μ in length, enter host cells by endocytosis and then divide by endodyogeny; two daughter cells are formed within each parent. Division continues until the host cell ruptures, releasing organisms which in turn infect adjacent cells. As the host develops immunity, parasite proliferation gradually slows, and a firm wall (cyst) forms around the organism allowing the *Toxoplasma* to persist for years in this cyst stage.

When *cats* ingest cysts or oocysts of *Toxoplasma gondii*, however, an addition process can occur, i.e., the *definitive* or sexual cycle initiated within the cat's intestinal epithelial cells. Parasites released from cysts or oocysts penetrate the epithelial cells where they first enter a proliferative stage and then mature by gametogony into *macro-* or *microgametocytes*. A *zygote*, formed by union of the gametocytes, matures in one to four days into an infective *oocyst*. The mature infective oocyst is oblong, 9 by 13 μ, and it contains two *sporocysts*, each of which contains four *sporozoites*. Oocysts are excreted by the cat for one to three weeks, beginning three to five days after ingestion of the *Toxoplasma*-containing tissue. Cats generally also acquire a systemic infection (intermediate cycle) at the time of first exposure to *Toxoplasma*, just as other mammals do. They occasionally repeat the sexual cycle after reinfection, although the period of oocyst shedding may be shorter.

EPIDEMIOLOGY. *Toxoplasma gondii* infects almost all mammals and birds. The usual life cycle in nature is among cats, small mammals, and birds, but man has intruded on this cycle with his taste for uncooked meats and his close association with cats. In some areas, such as Tahiti and the Easter Islands, the prevalence of *Toxoplasma* infection is near 100 per cent. In most parts of the world the prevalence ranges between 20 and 60 per cent of the population. Only in very dry areas, such as Arizona, and in very cold areas, such as northern Alaska, are low prevalence rates found. A few small islands in the Pacific, where cats have never been introduced, have remained free of toxoplasmosis.

The means by which the parasite is transmitted varies from one area to another: in one, oocyst ingestion seems more likely; in another, cyst ingestion. For instance, the very high rates in certain parts of the tropics are believed to be due to close contact with cat feces. In these areas infection is often acquired in childhood. The oocysts are resistant to drying and to a wide range of temperatures, and may remain infectious in moist soil for a year. Ingestion of oocysts is made more likely by the demonstration that cockroaches and flies can disseminate them to various exposed foods. In the United States the population appears to acquire the infection more commonly by ingesting uncooked infected meat. The infection is acquired at a rate of 1 per cent of the population per year of life from age 15 to age 50. Mutton and pork have been found to be more frequently infected than beef. Rarely, transmission of infection has followed accidental inoculation of trophozoites by laboratory workers, organ transplantation, and leukocyte transfusion from immunosuppressed donors. Blood transfusions from healthy donors have not been shown to be a means of transmitting toxoplasmosis.

Transplacental Transmission. Transplacental transmission in humans occurs only at the time of parasitemia, during the acute infection. The frequency of this secondary form of transmission therefore follows the frequency of acquisition of infection during childbearing years. In the United States and Europe 0.5 to 1.0 per cent of women have been demonstrated to have rising or very high antibody titers to *Toxoplasma* during pregnancy. Forty per cent of these adult infections are transmitted to the fetus. This may result in abortion or stillbirth, or an infant with clinical signs of toxoplasmosis (one third to one half of infected infants). Alternatively, infected infants may be completely asymptomatic but may show an antibody response to *Toxoplasma* antigens as evidence of transplacental infection. These infected asymptomatic infants are believed to make up a population which later in life may show signs of recurrent retinochoroiditis. There is no significant relationship in humans between chronic *Toxoplasma* infection and either recurrent abortion or prematurity.

PATHOGENESIS AND IMMUNITY. Multiplication of *Toxoplasma* organisms within cells causes little obvious disturbance to host cell function until the dividing parasites cause the cell to rupture. Adjacent cells are then infected, resulting in progressive tissue necrosis and an acute inflammatory response (edema and infiltration with mononuclear cells and a few polymorphonuclear leukocytes). Organisms are disseminated hematogenously throughout the body. New sites of necrosis and inflammation are initiated, particularly in myocardium and skeletal muscle. In those patients who develop severe generalized toxoplasmosis significant encephalitis, myocarditis, myositis, pneumonitis, hepatitis, and skin rash have been documented.

Generalized lymph node enlargement, along with other signs of systemic infection such as fever and malaise, develops one to two weeks after ingestion of infectious tissue. These lymph nodes show histocytic hyperplasia rather than follicular hyperplasia, giving the hematoxylin-eosin–stained section a rather typical appearance of containing predominantly eosin reactive cells. The architecture of the lymph node is preserved. Necrosis and giant cells are not seen, and only rarely can groups of *Toxoplasma* organisms be identified. Occasionally, even in relatively mild infections, myositis or myocarditis can be demonstrated.

Associated with the development of marked lymphoreticular activity, both humoral and cellular immunity can be demonstrated. Antibodies against various *Toxoplasma* antigens can be demonstrated in the peripheral blood. Later *Toxoplasma* antigen induces lymphocyte proliferation and lymphokine production, and mononuclear cells no longer support division of intracellular *Toxoplasma*. The acute infection resolves, but *Toxoplasma* organisms remain viable within cysts in the infected tissue for the lifetime of the host.

Congenital Infection; Immunologic Deficiency. Although the healthy adult usually deals effectively with the *Toxoplasma* infection, the immunologically deficient patient does not. The best example of this is the pathologic changes of congenital toxoplasmosis. The infected placenta may show areas of necrosis, inflammatory cells, and parasites, more frequently on the fetal than on the maternal side of the placenta. The fetal brain shows necrosis, glial cell proliferation, and perivascular lymphocytic infiltration. *Toxoplasma* can be identified in these lesions. High ventricular fluid protein, aqueductal obstruction, and hydrocephalus are often seen. If the infant survives several months, calcification of these areas occurs. Necrotic lesions in the retina are also seen. Organisms can be isolated from numerous organs of the body, but extensive inflammation is most often identified as pneumonitis, myocarditis, hepatitis, and splenitis.

About half the infections which occur in utero are caused by a sufficiently low number of organisms or are of low enough virulence that infection is manifest only by the appearance of humoral and cellular immune responses. Cysts develop and persist in brain, retina, and cardiac and skeletal muscle. Rupture of these cysts, many years later, can lead to transient episodes of inflammatory response and scarring. These inflammatory lesions are usually well localized, but in the retina they lead to significant organ impairment. The enucleated eye may show areas of necrosis in the retina often associated with proliferating *Toxoplasma* organisms, as well as a granulomatous inflammation of the choroid and sclera. The eye damage is the result of proliferation of organisms released at the time of cyst rupture which invade other cells, combined with damage caused by the vigorous hypersensitivity reaction.

In the patients with abnormal or suppressed immune responses, primary infection or cyst rupture may lead to symptomatic myositis, myocarditis, retinochoroiditis, or encephalitis.

CLINICAL MANIFESTATIONS. Manifestations of toxoplasmosis can be divided into four clinical patterns: acquired disease in otherwise healthy individuals, congenital infection, retinochoroiditis, and disease in the altered host.

Acquired Toxoplasmosis. Patients with acquired toxoplasmosis usually present with lymphadenopathy (90 per cent), fever (40 per cent), or malaise (40 per cent). Lymph node enlargement may be the only sign, and since cervical lymph node enlargement is particularly common, the patient may seek medical attention only because of concern about a neck mass. The nodes are usually nontender and rubbery in consistency. Generalized lymphadenopathy occurs in over half the cases, and transient splenomegaly has been recorded in approximately one third. The fever is usually low grade, but occasionally it may be high and of prolonged duration. Fatigue is often rather marked and may be associated with generalized muscle discomfort. Less commonly recorded signs or symptoms have included sore throat, headache, and a maculopapular rash. The pharynx is usually hyperemic; exudative pharyngitis is not seen. Specific organ involvement in this form of the disease includes myocardium (rarely pericardium), skeletal muscle, brain, rarely liver, and skin. When such organ involvement occurs, the abnormalities in organ function may dominate the clinical picture. Retinochoroiditis in association with the acute acquired disease is unusual.

The course of the illness is quite variable. Occasionally fever, malaise, and specific organ involvement are marked and the illness prolonged. More commonly, fever lasts only a few days or weeks, although fatigue and lymphadenopathy may persist for several months. Lymph nodes will occasionally fluctuate in size during the recovery period.

Laboratory tests usually reveal a normal total leukocyte count with a slight monocytosis or lymphocytosis. Atypical lymphocytes may be described, but they are usually not present in large numbers. Hematocrit and hemoglobin are usually normal; however, a Coombs-negative hemolytic anemia has occasionally been reported. Serum transaminases are usually normal, but early in the illness they may be slightly elevated (less than 100 U). The Paul-Bunnell test for heterophil antibodies is negative. The electrocardiogram may show ST and T wave abnormalities in cases in which myocarditis is prominent. The chest film is usually normal; hilar adenopathy is very rare. Lymph node biopsy shows histocytic hyperplasia. Antibodies against *Toxoplasma* antigens are present in high or rising titers.

Congenital Toxoplasmosis. Cases of congenital toxoplasmosis may be manifested as micro-ophthalmia, microcephaly, seizures, retardation, hepatosplenomegaly, pneumonitis, rash, and fever. If aqueduct of Sylvius obstruction has occurred, hydrocephalus will be prominent. Occasionally, signs may not be obvious at birth, but they may progress during the first months of life. Cerebral calcification may be seen after several months. The infant will show progressive signs of failure to thrive, followed by death. Cases of congenital toxoplasmosis may be mild, demonstrating only mental retardation, a seizure disorder, or retinochoroiditis. Laboratory tests reflect the severity of the specific organ involved. *Toxoplasma* antibody titers are elevated and will show a persistent or rising titer as maternal antibody disappears.

Toxoplasmic Retinochoroiditis. This form of toxoplasmosis is usually a late sequela of otherwise asymptomatic congenital infection, though infection of the eye during adult acquired illness has been recorded. Symptoms are usually first noted in the second or third decade of life. Patients have recurrent episodes of ocular pain and decreased vision associated with progressive loss of vision. The lesion is retinal, with an associated posterior uveitis. *Toxoplasma* infection probably does not cause an isolated anterior uveitis. Systemic signs of *Toxoplasma* infection are not usually present. *Toxoplasma* antibody titers are frequently low and tend not to change.

Toxoplasmosis in the Altered Host. Toxoplasmosis may present as a disseminated disease in patients with neoplasms of the lymphatic system, particularly Hodgkin's disease, or in patients being treated with immunosuppressive drugs. The clinical manifestations of the systemic disease are variable. Fever, encephalitis, myositis, hepatosplenomegaly, or myocarditis may occur. Pneumonitis has been described rarely in this setting. Lymphadenopathy may or may not be present. The primary difficulty is in separating the numerous other causes of these signs or symptoms from those caused by toxoplasmosis. At present one clinical pattern seems dominant, that is, progressive signs of encephalitis (confusion, headache, coma). In a patient with altered cellular immunity, these signs should lead to a consideration of and probably treatment for toxoplasmosis. If untreated, this illness is almost always progressive and fatal. *Toxoplasma* antibody titers are usually elevated; but changing titers are often not seen.

DIAGNOSIS. The diagnosis of toxoplasmosis rests on the presence of changing or elevated titers of antitoxoplasma antibodies and on isolation of the parasite from infected tissue. The antibody tests available include the indirect fluorescent antibody test (IFA), the Sabin-Feldman dye test, and a complement fixation test. The IFA and dye test show high antitoxoplasma antibody titers usually from the time of earliest symptoms (one to two weeks after infection). A titer of 1:1024 or higher, or evidence of a rising titer, is suggestive of active infection. The high titers will decrease during the subsequent months and after two to four years reach low levels (1:16 to 1:256) for the lifetime of the individual. An IgM-IFA test has been developed which demonstrates immunofluorescence of IgM-coated organisms at titers of patient serum greater than 1:20 during the first few months after infection. An indirect hemagglutination test is available; however, the rise in antibody titer is too slow to be helpful clinically.

The complement fixation test becomes positive later than the dye test, three to six weeks after infection, when symptoms are often present. Thus one is often able to see a changing titer over several weeks by using this test in a patient whose dye test is elevated. A significant complement fixation test is a titer of 1:8 or greater or a fourfold increase in titer. This test usually becomes negative within a few years after infection. In conjunction with the dye test it can help separate those patients with persistently high dye test antibody titers from those with recent infection. This may help in deciding if symptoms which began weeks or a few months previously are due to recent *Toxoplasma* infection or, in an asymptomatic pregnant female, whether the infection was recently acquired. Treatment may transiently decrease complement fixing antibody titers.

In congenital toxoplasmosis the contribution of transferred maternal IgG antitoxoplasma antibody must be excluded. This is done by performing several tests over the first few months; if positive titers are due to maternal antibody, the titer will fall about 50 per cent per month over four to six months. If the infant had been infected, the titer would remain stable, dip transiently, or increase. One may also test for IgM antitoxoplasma antibodies by using an IFA test to determine if the observed antibodies are fetal or maternal in origin. Since IgM antibodies do not cross the placenta, their presence indicates fetal antibody synthesis. In some infected infants this test may be falsely negative.

The diagnosis of *Toxoplasma* retinochoroiditis by serologic means is difficult. Since the infection is chronic, dye test and IFA titers are usually positive in low titer, and complement fixing antibodies are absent. The diagnosis of toxoplasmic retinochoroiditis may be suggested by finding higher antibody titers in the anterior chamber fluid than in the serum, or by isolating the organism at the time of enucleation. A negative dye test or IFA excludes *Toxoplasma* as the cause of retinochoroiditis.

The use of serologic tests in the immunodeficient patient to determine "activity" of the infection has also been difficult. Some patients with repeatedly low antibody titers have demonstrated a sudden rise in titer associated with a moribund state and death; however, at autopsy, disseminated toxoplasmosis could not be implicated as a factor contributing to death. Elevated antibody titers, plus progressive encephalitis, should be sufficient to warrant antitoxoplasma therapy in an immunodeficient patient. Evidence of the organism on biopsy of organs such as muscle, kidney, lung, and liver should also be an indication for therapy in these patients.

The diagnosis of toxoplasmosis can be substantiated by isolation of the organism. Biopsy material (particularly lymph node or muscle), tissue at the time of autopsy, or blood, sputum, or cerebrospinal fluid can be inoculated intraperitoneally into *Toxoplasma*-free laboratory animals. Smears of peritoneal fluid can be made at seven to ten days, stained by Giemsa technique, and examined for the protozoa. If the smear is negative, the peritoneal fluid should be injected intraperitoneally into another animal. If the infected animals survive for three weeks, they are sacrificed and their brains examined for *Toxoplasma* cysts and their serum for *Toxoplasma* antibody. Isolation of *Toxoplasma* organisms from human tissue should be correlated with histopathology of the tissue and antibody titers.

The differential diagnosis in a patient with lymphadenopathy and fever usually rests between lymphoma and infectious mononucleosis, although numerous infections, such as tuberculosis, brucellosis, tularemia, cat scratch disease, and certain systemic viral and rickettsial illnesses, must be considered. Toxoplasmosis can be distinguished from infectious mononucleosis by absence of marked atypical lymphocytosis and heterophil antibodies and normal or nearly normal hepatic transaminases; and from lymphoma by absence of anemia, hilar adenopathy, and a lymph node biopsy which shows histocytic hyperplasia rather than neoplastic cells. The other numerous causes of lymphadenopathy and fever must be excluded by appropriate serologic and skin tests, biopsy, and cultures. *Toxoplasma* encephalitis may resemble the localized necrosis of herpes infection.

Congenital toxoplasmosis must be distinguished from cytomegalovirus infection. Microcephaly is more common in cytomegalovirus infection than in toxoplasmosis. Ventricular fluid protein content is often higher in toxoplasmosis than in cytomegalovirus infection. Bacterial and fungal meningoencephalitis must be excluded by appropriate cultures. Viral encephalitis, particularly the rubella syndrome, must be considered. Congenital malformations are unusual in toxoplasmosis.

Toxoplasmic retinochoroiditis must be distinguished from cytomegalovirus, herpes, tuberculosis, histoplasmosis, and sarcoidosis by appearance of the retinal lesion and appropriate serologic and skin tests.

TREATMENT. A combination of pyrimethamine (Daraprim) and sulfadiazine has been shown to be effective in controlling *Toxoplasma* during the proliferative stage. There is no known therapy for eradicating organisms in the cyst stage. Pyrimethamine is given orally, 75 mg the first day, followed by 25 mg per day for one month. Infants are given 1 mg per kilogram per day for the first three days, and then 0.5 mg per kilogram per day thereafter. An intramuscular preparation is not commercially available. Sulfadiazine is given orally, 4 grams daily in divided doses for one month. Infants can be given 100 mg per kilogram per day. Sufficient fluid intake to maintain good urine flow should be assured during sulfadiazine therapy. Whether the drug combination co-trimoxazole will be a useful, less toxic agent in treating toxoplasmosis requires further study. Other sulfonamides such as the triple sulfonamides can be substituted for sulfadiazine; however, sulfisoxazole (Gantrisin) has been found ineffective. Other drugs such as spiramycin, clindamycin, and sulfones are less effective than the aforementioned drugs. Since pyrimethamine and sulfonamide inhibit folate synthesis, folinic acid (leucovorin), 6 mg per day, should be used in conjunction with the aforementioned therapy to prevent potential bone marrow toxicity. Platelet counts and white blood cell counts should be performed twice weekly during therapy.

Study of the effectiveness of these drugs in acquired human toxoplasmosis has been limited by the marked variability and spontaneous improvement without therapy. However, in some cases there has been evidence that this treatment shortens the period of fever and malaise, although lymphadenopathy may persist. It has therefore been recommended that only patients with fever, myalgias, or malaise be considered for therapy. Asymptomatic adults should be considered for treatment (1) after accidental laboratory infection and (2) when a pregnant female demonstrates serologic evidence of recent infection, only after appropriate consultations and considerations have led to a rejection of therapeutic abortion and have weighed potential fetal damage from the drugs. There is no adequate evidence to recommend treating dye-test-positive women who wish to become pregnant or who abort habitually, or in treating asymptomatic women after delivery of a congenitally damaged infant.

Congenital toxoplasmosis should be treated whether asymptomatic or symptomatic, because the proliferative stage may continue for several months before adequate immunity has developed to control the infection. Treatment will not be effective when given late in the course of the disease or when severe central nervous system damage has already occurred.

In toxoplasmic retinochoroiditis, the primary therapy should be directed at controlling the hypersensitivity response with corticosteroids. Pyrimethamine and sulfadiazine should be used in conjunction with this therapy to prevent dissemination of infection and to limit local damage caused by proliferating organisms.

In patients with altered immunity and toxoplasmosis, good therapeutic response to this drug combination has been recorded. Fever has been controlled, and evidence of progressive encephalitis has been reversed. In these patients long-term therapy has to be considered because appropriate immunologic responses do not occur, making relapse of the disease likely.

PREVENTION. Toxoplasmosis is commonly transmitted by consumption of undercooked meat or *Toxoplasma* oocysts. Thus, dye-test-negative pregnant women or patients with depressed cellular immunity should avoid both these sources of infection. Meat should be cooked at a temperature in excess of 60° C for at least 15 minutes. Susceptible individuals should avoid soil or sand boxes where cats may defecate, because oocysts may survive in these places for months. If cats are kept in the house, they should not be fed raw meat or allowed access to wild rodents or birds. Baseline antibody testing should be done in patients who are to receive immunosuppressive drugs, who have lymphatic malignancies, or who are to act as organ or leukocyte donors.

Beverley, J. K. A.: Toxoplasmosis. Br. Med. J., 2:475, 1973.

Feldman, H. A.: Toxoplasmosis. N. Engl. J. Med., 279:1370, 1431, 1968.

Frenkel, J. K.: Toxoplasma in and around us. Bio. Science, 26:343, 1973.

Frenkel, J. K.: Toxoplasmosis. *In* Marcial-Rojas, R. D. (ed.): Pathology of Protozoal and Helminthic Diseases. Baltimore, Williams & Wilkins Company, 1971, p. 254.

Kean, B. H.: Clinical toxoplasmosis — 50 years. Trans. R. Soc. Trop. Med. Hyg., 66:549, 1972.

Remington, J. S.: Toxoplasmosis — recent developments. Ann. Rev. Med., 21:201, 1970.

Ruskin, J., and Remington, J. S.: Toxoplasmosis in the compromised host. Ann. Intern. Med., 84:193, 1976.

Wallace, G. D.: The role of the cat in the natural history of *Toxoplasma gondii*. Am. J. Trop. Med. Hyg., 22:313, 1973.

198. PNEUMOCYSTOSIS

Thomas C. Jones

Pneumocystosis is an acute pulmonary disease characterized by fever, tachypnea, dyspnea, and cyanosis which occurs in immunodeficient patients and malnourished or premature infants. It is caused by species of the genus *Pneumocystis*, organisms of uncertain classification, but probably protozoa. The organisms cause asymptomatic infection in healthy mammalian hosts and are seen extracellularly in the pulmonary alveoli.

HISTORY. In 1909 Carlos Chagas described what he thought was a stage of sporogony of *Trypanosoma cruzi* occurring in the lungs of experimentally infected guinea pigs. The next year Carini observed the same forms in rats infected with *T. lewisi*. In 1912 Delanoe and Delanoe recognized that the "cyst of Carini" was not part of the life cycle of trypanosomes, but was a different organism. The first reports of such an organism in humans appeared in 1938 when Ammich and Beneke independently described them in the lungs of infants dying during the first year of life. Epidemics of the disease in institutionalized children were subsequently described throughout Europe. In 1953 Vanek, Jirovec, and Lukes recognized the relationship between *Pneumocystis* and the pathologic entity interstitial plasma cell pneumonia. Reports of pneumocystosis have increased since that time, associated with the increased use of corticosteroids and antimetabolites as therapy in malignant disease or in patients undergoing organ transplantation, and with the increased life span of patients with congenital immunodeficient syndromes.

ORGANISM. The life cycle of *Pneumocystis* is unknown. At present, one can only postulate that the life cycle in lungs of infected mammals includes an extracystic body or trophozoite which changes to a cyst followed by the development of oval bodies (sporozoites) within the cyst. These are then released to initiate another cycle. A trophozoite-to-trophozoite cycle may also occur. Both cyst and trophozoite stages of the organism are found in exudate within the alveoli. The cyst is the form commonly demonstrated in clinical specimens. It is 5 to 6 μ in diameter, and its outer wall stains well with methenamine silver nitrate (see Fig. 2G, Ch. 193), Gram-Weigert stains or periodic acid–Schiff reagents. Using Giemsa stain, the sporozoites (1 to 2 μ in diameter) can be recognized within the cyst and are usually eight in number. After release from the cyst, the organisms are termed trophozoites. They move freely about the alveoli, and gradually undergo changes, including loss of internal structure, appearance of villous microprojections on the outer membrane, and development of an unusual trilaminar membrane, characteristics which identify it as a new cyst.

EPIDEMIOLOGY. *Pneumocystis* species are widely distributed, affecting rodents, rabbits, sheep, dogs, and other mammals, in addition to humans. It is unlikely that animals serve as a reservoir for infection of humans, since organisms of different mammals appear to be host specific. Evidence at present best supports the thesis that infection is transmitted by the respiratory route by droplet spray. In a few cases congenital infection has been considered the most likely route of infection. The disease is principally one of immunodeficient subjects.

Epidemiologic data suggest that the organism is quite infectious, that infection is usually asymptomatic, and that apparently healthy, infected individuals can transmit the disease to immunodeficient patients. This is supported by observations in animals that healthy rats and rabbits when caged communally acquire the infection, and when the animals are rendered immunodeficient by corticosteroid administration, disease may be manifest. It is supported in humans by the increased prevalence of antibodies to *Pneumocystis* in personnel working in medical institutions (7 to 15 per cent), the epidemics of disease in the institutionalized infants, and the sporadic clusters of cases in hospitalized immunodeficient patients.

Disease that follows recent infection or reactivation of latent infection has been seen most commonly in patients with hypogammaglobulinemia of immunoglobulins G or M, in malnourished infants in the second to fourth months of life (when passively transferred maternal antibodies first reach low levels), or in patients receiving corticosteroids or antimetabolites. A few patients not on immunosuppressive drugs and with normal immunoglobulin levels and a few patients with isolated defects in cellular immunity have acquired the disease. Organisms reach high numbers in the lungs of infected persons showing clinical disease, and it is likely that these patients can more readily spread the disease than asymptomatic carriers.

PATHOLOGY AND PATHOGENESIS. When conditions exist in the alveoli for the multiplication of *Pneumocystis*, an inflammatory response is elicited which includes transudation of fluid into the alveoli and thickening of alveolar interstitial spaces. The alveoli become filled with foamy, proteinaceous material in which trophozoite nuclei are found along with clumps of the *Pneumocystis* cysts. The interstitial spaces have been noted to contain predominantly plasma cells and alveolar epithelial cells when pathologic material was studied in malnourished or premature infants; hence the origin of the pathologic description, interstitial plasma cell pneumonia. However, in the immunodeficient child or adult, this pattern is not seen. The inflammatory response in these patients has been described as primarily lymphocytes, macrophages, and occasionally eosinophils. Polymorphonuclear leukocytes are not seen. The lung is usually diffusely involved with this process, although localized disease has occasionally been described. The lung is firm and rubbery in consistency. Other organisms, such as cytomegalovirus or bacteria, are frequently found in association with *Pneumocystis*. Less commonly, *Pneumocystis* is found in lungs which also contain mycobacteria, fungi, or toxoplasma. Rarely, pneumocystis may become generalized, involving lymph nodes, spleen, and bone marrow.

CLINICAL MANIFESTATIONS. The major symptoms of pneumocystosis are tachypnea and a nonproductive cough. These symptoms often develop insidiously over a period of several weeks and may be associated with fever, dyspnea, and cyanosis. It has been noted that these symptoms may first appear during the period when corticosteroids are being withdrawn. The disease may also present with an abrupt onset (over two to three days) of high, spiking fever, cough, dyspnea, and cyanosis, with the patient reaching a moribund state within a few days. Most of the patients presenting with this rapid course have been on continuous high doses of corticosteroids. In the United States at present the disease which presents with an abrupt onset may be more common than the more insidious onset characteristic of the illness seen in institutionalized infants in Europe. After renal, bone marrow, or cardiac transplantation, pneumocystosis is an important cause of pneumonia occurring three to four months later.

On physical examination the patient shows signs of respiratory distress (tachypnea and dyspnea) associated with fever and cyanosis. Auscultation of the lungs may reveal no abnormalities, although scattered rales and rhonchi may be heard.

There are no diagnostic laboratory tests. *The white blood cell count* may reflect the underlying disease of the patient or other complications, but leukocytosis may be seen. Significant eosinophilia has occasionally been reported, particularly in children with humoral immune deficiency. *The blood gases* will usually indicate hyperventilation and decreased oxygen saturation even while the patient is on continuous oxygen, consistent with an alveolar capillary block syndrome. Some have reported associated mild respiratory acidosis. *The chest radiograph* usually shows diffuse mixed alveolar and interstitial pneumonitis. This appears as a granular haziness beginning in the hilar region, which progresses to a frank alveolar pattern with air bronchograms. Atypical features such as asymmetrical involvement, segmental infiltrates, and pleural effusions occur in up to half the cases.

Course. In immunodeficient patients the course of pneumocystosis will usually be one of progressive deterioration unless improvement occurs in the underlying immune defect. Increasing pulmonary consolidation, cyanosis, and death are the natural history of the disease. After institution of specific therapy against pneumocystis, improvement begins in five to ten days. The roentgenographic findings may become transiently worse after institution of therapy, but will then show gradual improvement over one to three weeks. Some have suggested that pneumocystosis of long duration may lead to interstitial fibrosis or emphysema. This has been difficult to document in view of the many factors leading to pulmonary changes in these patients.

DIAGNOSIS. Once the suspicion of pneumocystosis is raised by the clinical setting of immune deficiency and progressive pulmonary symptoms, pulmonary secretions should be examined by methenamine silver, Gram-Weigert, or Giemsa stains. If these examinations are negative, the patient should be considered for lung biopsy. Most centers now recommend transbronchial or open lung biopsy rather than percutaneous needle biopsy, because the latter provides no visualization of the lung and a greater risk of lung collapse or bleeding. Biopsy is required to distinguish pneumocystosis from drug-induced interstitial fibrosis, cytomegalovirus infection, *Aspergillus* or other fungi, unusual forms of bacterial bronchopneumonia, toxoplasmosis, or leukemic infiltration. Impression smears of the biopsy specimen at the time of surgery can be fixed in methanol and stained with Giemsa, methenamine silver, or Gram-Weigert stains and carefully examined for the presence of *Pneumocystis* cysts. Specimens are also preserved for bacterial and fungal cultures. If the biopsy must be delayed, or if surgery is believed to be contraindicated for other reasons, then a therapeutic trial with specific drugs against *Pneumocystis* should be instituted. Immunofluorescent antibody tests are now being evaluated. However, they show significantly elevated titers in only about 30 per cent of cases of pneumocystosis. Although measurement of antibody response using fluorescent antibody techniques is relatively insensitive, it appears to be specific. Thus a change in titer from negative to positive adds support to the diagnosis, whereas the absence of such a change does not exclude it.

TREATMENT.   Therapy for pneumocystosis, if started early in the disease, has proved to be quite successful. During the past decade pentamidine isethionate has been used. This has reduced mortality from *Pneumocystis* infection from near 100 per cent to below 50 per cent and considerably lower in some circumstances. The drug is made rapidly available by calling the Parasitic Disease Drug Service, U.S. Public Health Service (404–633–3311). The patient is given 4 mg per kilogram per day intramuscularly for 12 to 14 days. The mechanism of action of the drug remains unknown, but it does cause megaloblastic cell changes, inhibits incorporation of nucleotides into DNA and RNA, and inhibits oxidative phosphorylation. Folinic acid therapy can be used in patients who develop signs of folate deficiency without interfering with action of the drug against the organism. Pentamidine may also cause hypoglycemia, hyperglycemia, and nephrotoxicity. When given intravenously, hypotension can occur. The possibility that pentamidine causes pulmonary interstitial fibrosis has been raised by studies in animals. Because of these observed and potential toxic effects, another drug combination, co-trimoxazole, the fixed combination of trimethoprim and sulfamethoxazole, has been tested for treatment of pneumocystosis. Although there have been fewer patients treated with this combination than with pentamidine, it appears to be effective and less toxic. This drug combination interferes with the synthesis of folinic acid. For treatment of adults, 20 mg per kilogram per day of trimethoprim and 100 mg per kilogram per day of sulfamethoxazole, divided into four doses, can be given by mouth. An intravenous preparation is available as an investigational drug from the manufacturer. Since inadequate levels of the drug have been documented in the serum of critically ill patients after oral therapy, serum concentrations should be checked. If levels of trimethoprim are less than 4.6 μg per milliliter, parenteral therapy should be used.

Because of the relationship between the occurrence of pneumocystosis and hypogammaglobulinemia, gamma globulin administration has been recommended. However, commercially available gamma globulin has proved to be of little value when given alone for treatment of pneumocystosis. In general, attempts should be made to reduce the dose of corticosteroids when signs of pneumocystosis appear; however, in some patients whose respiratory symptoms developed during tapering of corticosteroids, a transient *increase* in the dose of these drugs while pneumocystosis therapy is started should be considered. Supportive measures such as oxygen therapy, assisted ventilation, and careful fluid and electrolyte balance are important parts of the management.

PREVENTION.   In order to interrupt spread of *Pneumocystis* infection, a great deal must be learned about its life cycle. Since the diseased patient may be able to spread the organism to other patients, healthy person-

nel, and relatives, appropriate respiratory precautions should be considered when the diagnosis is suspected. Attention to preventing contact between susceptible patients and diseased patients in open wards and in clinics may reduce the spread of the disease. For certain highly susceptible patient populations, prophylactic treatment with co-trimoxazole has been found to be beneficial. The disease will be better controlled when the relationships between certain types of immune deficiency or corticosteroids and rapid proliferation of the organism are better understood.

Burke, B. A., and Good, R. A.: *Pneumocystis carinii* infection. Medicine, 52:23, 1973.

Norman, L., and Kagan, I. G.: Some observations on the serology of *Pneumocystis carinii* infections in the United States. Infect. Immun., 8:317, 1973.

Robbins, J. B., DeVita, V. T., and Dutz, W.: Symposium on *Pneumocystis carinii* Infection. National Cancer Institute Monograph 43. U.S. Department of Health, Education and Welfare, October 1976.

Rosen, P., Armstrong, D., and Ramos, C.: *Pneumocystis carinii* pneumonia. A clinicopathologic study of twenty patients with neoplastic diseases. Am. J. Med., 53:428, 1972.

Walzer, P. D., Perl, D. P., Krogstad, D. J., Rawson, P. G., and Schultz, M. G.: *Pneumocystis carinii* pneumonia in the United States. Epidemiologic, diagnostic, and clinical features. Ann. Intern. Med., 80:83, 1974.

199.   BABESIOSIS

(Babesiasis, Piroplasmosis)

Thomas C. Jones

Babesiosis is an acute febrile illness characterized by myalgias, fatigue, and hemolytic anemia caused by species of the intraerythrocytic protozoa, *Babesia*, transmitted by infected ticks. Animal infection with *Babesia* has long been recognized; however, significant transmission of disease to man has been documented only recently. In asplenic patients the disease is likely to be serious and may be fatal.

HISTORY.   Babès, in 1888, identified the organism in the peripheral blood of cattle with anemia and fever. Smith and Kilborne in 1893 observed a similar organism as the cause of Texas cattle fever, described it as a protozoan, and documented the role of the tick as vector — the first demonstration that arthropods could transmit protozoan diseases. In 1904, Wilson and Chowning described blood smears from several patients in Montana which looked like piroplasmosis of cattle; they termed the organism *Piroplasma hominis*. These cases were identified in the midst of another tick-borne disease, Rocky Mountain spotted fever, and were therefore considered to be examples of this rickettsial disease. In retrospect, these cases may have been the first descriptions of babesiosis in man. Svkrabalo reported in 1957 a fatal case of babesiosis presenting with fever, anemia, and hemoglobinuria in a splenectomized man. Twenty additional cases have been identified in the past decade, 16 of which have occurred on Nantucket and Martha's Vineyard islands and on the tip of Long Island.

ORGANISM.   *Babesia* is a protozoan with asexual multiplication (shizogony) occurring in mammalian erythrocytes and a sexual cycle (sporogony) in the tick. The organism is introduced during the bite of the tick, when sporozoites in salivary glands enter the bloodstream and invade erythrocytes. In the erythrocyte stained with Romanowsky stains, organisms are 2 to 3 μ in diameter with blue-staining, irregularly shaped cytoplasm and a red nucleus. They may appear as ring, binucleate, or quadrinucleate forms. *Babesia* does not produce pigment within the red cell, a feature clearly distinguishing it from *Plasmodium*. A period of prolonged parasitemia occurs. When a tick ingests parasitized red blood cells, the sexual cycle occurs in the digestive tract of the tick with formation of zygotes and ookinetes. A systemic infection of the tick allows transmission of the organism at the time of its next blood meal as well as infection of the tick eggs, leading to vertical transmission to larvae, another source of mammalian infection. Congenital transmission of infection in ticks complicates the epidemiology by allowing long periods of tick infection in the absence of contact with mammalian blood cells.

PATHOLOGY AND IMMUNITY. Babesiosis leads to red cell destruction (hemolytic anemia, hyperbilirubinemia, hemoglobinuria, splenic enlargement) and capillary obstruction associated with parasitized red blood cells (leading to tissue anoxia). In those patients who have been autopsied, findings have included generalized hyperemia and hemorrhage. The liver revealed parasitized red cells, many within phagocytic cells, but no pigment deposition as seen in malaria. The kidneys showed the changes of tubular nephrosis consistent with intravascular hemolysis and hemoglobin damage. In animals a proliferative glomerulitis has been demonstrated and glomerular deposits of IgG and C3 documented.

A delicate balance between progressive infection and host immune response leads to prolonged parasitemia with variable signs of tissue injury. The severe illness which has been described in humans without spleens (three of four patients died) and the documented severe illness in experimentally splenectomized animals gives strong support for the role of this organ in the immune response to *Babesia*.

Hamsters infected with *B. microti* of human origin demonstrated excess antibody in the serum by two weeks after infection, which reached a peak titer of 1:1280 by eight weeks. In these animals, parasitemia persisted until the sixth week. Marked splenic enlargement occurred during this period. Parasitemia recurred in hamsters splenectomized three to four months after infection. In infected animals *B. microti* have been shown to undergo degenerative changes within the red cells. This observation and cross-immunity between *Babesia* and *Plasmodium* suggest that an immunologically nonspecific substance could be important in the immune response. Antibody may contribute to control of the infection by agglutination or opsonization of organisms and by inhibiting the entry of *Babesia* into red cells.

EPIDEMIOLOGY. A number of species of Babesia have been described. These have been characterized as host specific: *B. bigemina* and *B. bovis* in cattle, *B. ovis* in sheep, *B. canis* in dogs, *B. equi* in horses, and *B. microti* in rodents. It is now clear both from cross-species animal infections and the emergence of disease in humans that these zoonoses can infect and cause disease in more than one animal species. Infection in splenectomized man has been due to *B. bovis* acquired from ticks feeding on cattle and one case possibly due to *B. equi*. The disease in man on Nantucket island has been caused by the rodent species, *B. microti*, and has led to illness in immunologically normal humans.

Infection with *B. microti* in those exposed to infected ticks is probably frequent. On Nantucket island, of 133 persons with a history of tick bite, 10 had significant antibody titers against *B. microti* (>1:64) consistent with recent infection. Infection of rodents with *B. microti* has been recognized in many parts of the world for decades. Recent studies on Nantucket confirmed a very high rate of parasitemia (82 per cent) in field and white-footed mice. The deer tick, *Ixodes scapularis*, has

become abundant in the past few decades and has replaced the rodent tick, *Ixodes muris*, as the dominant tick. This change in the ecology of ticks may have contributed to the emergence of infection in man. A change in the organism itself rendering it more adaptable to infection in man is possible, but comparative studies have not been done.

CLINICAL MANIFESTATIONS. The clinical manifestations of babesiosis are undoubtedly quite varied. The following description is based on detailed observations on only a few patients. The first signs of illness have occurred one to six weeks after a tick bite, although only a few patients have recalled such a bite. There may be absence of a history of tick bite because the small tick larvae may go unnoticed.

The first symptoms include fatigue, general malaise, and anorexia, followed in a few days by fever. The fever may be high (40° C), and drenching sweats, chills, myalgias, and arthralgias may accompany it. Nausea and vomiting may occur. Several of the patients have had symptoms of depression, emotional lability, and transient hyperesthesias. The illness may be sudden in onset or quite indolent and prolonged, lasting a month before diagnosis. On physical examination, splenomegaly has been noted in two of eight patients. No rash or lymphadenopathy has been recorded. In the fatal cases in asplenic patients, signs of massive hemolysis (pallor, icterus, and dark urine), prostration, dehydration, and renal insufficiency were most prominent.

Patients demonstrate a low hemoglobin and a moderate reticulocytosis. Leukocyte counts are normal, but some patients have thrombocytopenia. Urinalysis usually shows proteinuria. Liver function tests may be slightly abnormal. Peripheral blood smears show 1 to 10 per cent of erythrocytes infected with *Babesia* organisms.

DIAGNOSIS. The diagnosis of babesiosis should be suspected in any patient with fever and unexplained hemolytic anemia. This should be considered particularly if the laboratory reports identify malaria parasite on smear. Diagnosis can usually be made by observing the nonpigmented organisms in erythrocytes on thick and thin peripheral blood smears. In suspected cases in which the smear is equivocal, inoculation of laboratory rodents will allow confirmation of the diagnosis. The Center for Disease Control has developed a serologic test using *B. microti* antigen which appears specific and which will be helpful in both clinical diagnosis and epidemiology.

THERAPY. Treatment with chloroquine phosphate, 1500 mg initially, followed by 500 mg daily or every other day until symptoms subside and parasitemia decreases, has been recommended. Parasitemia may continue for many weeks even while the patient is on therapy. Malaise and fatigue may also persist for several weeks. Pentamidine, 4 mg per kilogram per day, may be more effective and should be used in severely ill patients. Supportive therapy for acute renal failure with dialysis and for anemia with blood transfusion may be necessary in severe cases.

PREVENTION. No chemoprophylaxis is available. Avoiding tick-infested areas will decrease likelihood of acquiring the disease. Removal of ticks present on the skin, use of clothing impregnated with tick repellents, and use of insecticide sprays all have value in limiting transmission of tick-borne diseases. Patients who have had splenectomy should avoid occupations and vacations which might bring them in contact with infected ticks.

Anderson, A. E., Cassaday, P. B., and Healy, G. R.: Babesiosis in man. Am. J. Clin. Pathol. 62:612, 1974.

Annable, C. R., and Ward, P. A.: Immunopathology of the renal complications of babesiosis. J. Immunol., 112:1, 1974.

Healy, G. R., Spielman A., and Gleason, N.: Human babesiosis: Reservoir of infection on Nantucket island. Science, 192:479, 1976.

Ruebush, T. K., II, Cassaday, P. B., Marsh, J. H., Lisker, S. A., Voorhees, D. B., Mahoney, E. B., and Healy, G. R.: Human babesiosis on Nantucket island. Ann. Intern. Med., 86:6, 1977.

Svkrabalo, Z.: Babesiosis (piroplasmosis). In Marcial-Rojas, R. A. (ed.): Pathology of Protozoal and Helminthic Diseases. Baltimore, Williams & Wilkins Company, 1971, p. 225.

200. OTHER PROTOZOAN DISEASES

200.1. INTRODUCTION

Philip D. Marsden

Apart from *Entamoeba histolytica*, at least four genera and seven species of amebae have been established as living in man. Common stool amebae are *Entamoeba coli*, *Endolimax nana*, and *Iodamoeba bütschlii*. They are nonpathogenic, but such protozoa have a double importance. First, they must be distinguished from the pathogenic *E. histolytica* by the available clear morphologic criteria. Second, they provide an index of fecal contamination. If any stool protozoan is encountered, it is wise to examine a further specimen, for, because of the variable appearance of protozoa in the stool, the second specimen may reveal a pathogen. *Dientamoeba fragilis* has a delicate ameba form without a cystic stage. Some clinicians believe it is a cause of mild diarrhea, but the evidence is not convincing.

Several flagellates are also found in the stool, among them the nonpathogenic *Trichomonas hominis* and *Chilomastix mesnili*. Information on the differential diagnosis of these intestinal protozoa can be found in texts of parasitology. Here we will consider briefly the clinical significance of six pathogenic types of protozoa: *Giardia lamblia* and *Trichomonas vaginalis* (both flagellates), *Balantidium coli* (a ciliate), *Naegleria* and *Acanthamoeba* (amebae), and *Isospora* and *Sarcocystis* (sporozoa).

Knight, R.: Giardiasis, isosporiasis, and balantidiasis. Clin. Gastroenterol., 7:31, 1978.

200.2. GIARDIASIS

Philip D. Marsden

Abdominal pain, distention and flatulence, and recurrent diarrhea may be associated with *Giardia lamblia* infection, especially in children. Inhabiting the duodenum and upper jejunum, the parasite is a pear-shaped flagellate, anteriorly broad and rounded and tapering to a point not unlike a tennis racket. It is convex dorsally with a ventral attachment disc. There are sets of identical structures on either side of the median line. When stained, there are two nuclei, four pairs of flagella, and a parabasal body. In fresh stool this trophozoite is actively motile with an irregular characteristic progression. It reproduces by longitudinal binary fission.

The thick-walled cysts are 10 to 14 μ by 6 to 10 μ and have two to four nuclei with curved rods or axostyles. In some infections several million cysts per gram of feces may be passed. Only in patients with very rapid bowel transit times do trophozoites appear in the stool, although they may be found in duodenal samples obtained by duodenal aspiration, biopsy, or, preferably, Beal's string test. Cultivation of *Giardia* in vitro has been achieved but is not a practical diagnostic procedure.

The infective cysts are transmitted in food and drink, and the infection is cosmopolitan. The great majority of patients are asymptomatic, but there is no doubt that heavy infections are associated with symptoms. There is an association between symptomatic giardiasis and the immunodeficiency syndrome of nonselective variable hypogammaglobulinemia. Diarrhea is the most common symptom, and the stools are pale and contain mucus. *Giardia* is in fact a cause of steatorrhea, and patients have abnormal fat balances and D-xylose tests which return to normal after successful treatment. The hypothesis that this malabsorption is the result of a mechanical barrier produced by large numbers of parasites attached to the microvillar surface is attractive, but effects on digestive enzyme activity and microvillar function are possible. Villous flattening with inflammatory infiltration has been demonstrated.

Diarrhea may alternate with constipation, and apart from these symptoms epigastric pain resembling a peptic ulcer may be a disabling symptom. Anorexia, meat intolerance, and loss of weight may occur. Although *Giardia* may be found in the gallbladder, the evidence that it is responsible for cholecystitis is unsatisfactory. Giardiasis must be distinguished from other causes of malabsorption and peptic ulcer.

Giardiasis, symptomatic or not, should always be treated. Two drugs are equally effective. Metronidazole (Flagyl), 250 or 400 mg three times a day for five to ten days, has few side effects. Good cure rates have been obtained with single doses of 2 grams. It is the drug of choice for children and when *Giardia* coexists with *Entamoeba histolytica*. Quinacrine hydrochloride (Atabrine, mepacrine), in an *adult* dose of 100 mg three times a day after food for seven days, is an established therapy, but the drug has a bitter taste, and nausea and vomiting may result. It may also stain the skin yellow, but psychosis does not occur at this dosage level. Both drugs have about an 80 per cent cure rate, and in the event of failure of one drug the other can be tried. The follow-up procedures are similar to those in amebiasis.

Hoskins, L. C., Winawer, S. J., Broitman, S. A., Gottlieb, L. S., and Zamchek, N.: Clinical giardiasis and intestinal malabsorption. Gastroenterology, 53:265, 1967.

Yardley, J. H., Takano, J., and Hendrix, T. B.: Epithelial and other mucosal lesions of the jejunum in giardiasis: Jejunal biopsy studies. Bull. Hopkins Hosp., 115:389, 1964.

200.3. TRICHOMONIASIS

Thomas C. Jones

Another group of lumen-dwelling protozoa with flagella are the trichomonads. Three species of the genus *Trichomonas* frequently inhabit man: *Trichomonas hominis*, *Trichomonas tenax*, and *Trichomonas vaginalis*. Only the last-named is considered pathogenic.

T. vaginalis is a pear-shaped, colorless, single-celled

organism 10 to 20 μ in size with two pairs of anterior flagella, an eccentrically located nucleus, an undulating membrane, and a structure termed an axostyle leading to a posterior flagellum. The flagella and undulating membrane move the organism rapidly through exudative material in a jerky, rotating manner. Its survival on mucosal surfaces is dependent on certain environmental conditions. For instance, activity of the organism decreases rapidly at a pH below 5.

The organism can persist in endocervical or uethral glands without causing symptoms, or it can induce inflammation on the mucosal surfaces of the vagina, urethra, urinary bladder, or prostate. The inflamed area takes on a characteristic "strawberry-like" appearance owing to vasodilation. Exudate filled with polymorphonuclear leukocytes and mononuclear cells covers the surface. *Trichomonas* infection can make interpretation of cervical Papanicolaou smears more difficult, but there is no evidence that infection contributes to carcinoma of the cervix.

Patients usually present with symptoms of vaginal itching or burning and a yellow blood-tinged discharge. These symptoms are more commonly associated with menstruation. If the urethra is involved, symptoms of dysuria and a mild urethral discharge are seen. Approximately 20 per cent of females with documented *Trichomonas* infection are asymptomatic.

Diagnosis is made by observing the motile organisms in fresh specimens of vaginal discharge. A drop of warm saline containing methylene blue is mixed with the exudate and examined immediately, using low-power microscopy. *T. vaginalis* can also be cultured. Nitroimidazoles, such as metronidazole, provide effective therapy. One gram of metronidazole should be given in a single dose to both sexual partners. If this is ineffective, the more traditional therapy of 250 mg three times daily for ten days can be used. Because of potential drug side effects, only patients documented to have *Trichomonas* vaginitis and their sexual partners should be treated. Failure to treat both partners results in reinfection, so-called "Ping-Pong" vaginitis. The infection is usually acquired by sexual intercourse. It can be transmitted to infants at the time of birth, and may survive on nonmucosal surfaces for a sufficient time to be spread in places such as mental institutions where personal hygiene is poor. In severely immunocompromised patients, trichomonads have been identified in pleural and cerebrospinal fluids consistent with communication between these sites and mucosal surfaces.

Dykers, J. R.: Single dose metronidazole for trichomonal vaginitis: A follow-up. N. Engl. J. Med., 295:395, 1976.
Trussell, R. E.: Trichomonas Vaginalis and Trichomoniasis. Springfield, Ill., Charles C Thomas, 1947.

200.4. BALANTIDIASIS

Philip D. Marsden

Balantidium coli is the largest protozoan of man, measuring 50 to 70 μ in length by 30 to 60 μ in width. It infects the colon of man and may produce diarrhea and dysentery. When viewed under the low power of the microscope in a saline smear of stool, the grayish-green trophozoite can be seen gliding across the field powered by spiral longitudinal rows of cilia. There is a large oval macronucleus and a smaller micronu-

cleus. A cytostome or mouth ingests organic matter that circulates as food vacuoles. Erythrophagocytosis has been observed. Reproduction is by binary fission or conjugation. A resistant cyst form is passed in formed stools, and this is the infective form. *Cosmopolitan in distribution, it is a rare infection of man although common in pigs.* When man and pig share shelter, human infections are common, and this accounts for the high incidence of human infection in parts of New Guinea (20 per cent) and Peru. *B. coli* of man can be transmitted to monkeys, cats, guinea pigs, and rats, but the importance of these animals as reservoirs is minor. Handling pigs in slaughterhouses may be an occupational risk.

This ciliate can be a tissue invader, and similar factors to those mentioned for *E. histolytica* may well determine this behavior. Proteolytic secretions produce necrosis and ulceration of the mucosa. Columns of balantidia may be seen lying in the submucosa. Secondary infection with bacteria results in an accompanying inflammatory reaction. The ulcers are often quite large and deep, with a broad, indurated base. A liver abscess with *B. coli* in situ has been described, and balantidia have been found in the lung and heart in isolated cases.

Less than one fifth of infected persons have symptoms. Severe infections are associated with diarrhea and the passage of blood and mucus in the stools. Constitutional symptoms of fever, nausea, vomiting, and asthenia are described. Examination of fresh stools reveals the trophozoite or cyst. Culture of the stools on media similar to those used for amebiasis may reveal an infection when conventional microscopy has failed; in symptomatic patients this is usually not necessary. Balantidiasis must be differentiated from amebic dysentery and ulcerative colitis. Although arsenical preparations have been used in the past, oxytetracycline is the drug of choice in an adult dose of 500 mg five times a day for ten days. Paromomycin (Humatin) is also effective. The value of metronidazole is still uncertain. Spontaneous recovery has been noted. The infection may be fatal if bowel perforation occurs.

Arean, V. M., and Koppisch, E.: Balantidiasis: A review and report of cases. Am. J. Path., 32:1089, 1956.
Garcia Laverde, A., and De Bonilla, L.: Clinical trials with metronidazole in human balantidiasis. Am. J. Trop. Med. Hyg., 24:781, 1975.
Van der Hoeven, J. A., and Rijpstra, A. C.: Intestinal parasites in the central mountain district of Netherlands, New Guinea. An important focus of *Balantidium coli*. Docum. Med. Geog. Trop., 9:225, 1957.

200.5. PRIMARY AMEBIC MENINGOENCEPHALITIS

Philip D. Marsden

Recently it has been realized that *free-living amebae* are capable of producing severe brain lesions in man. Several species are implicated, but *Naegleria gruberi* had been the species usually identified when cultures are made. They can be cultured on plain agar plates with *Aerobacter aerogenes* as a nutrient source, but we need to know more about their cultural requirements. The *Naegleria* amebae possess the capacity to transform in culture from ameboid trophozoites to highly mobile flagellates. Another organism, *Acanthamoeba castellani*, was among the first to be recognized. An ameba 6 to 8 μ long, with foamy cytoplasm, a nucleus of 2 μ, and a 1 μ darkly staining central karyosome, it is present as a commensal in human mouths and throats and was shown to be pathogenic for mice and monkeys before the first cases were reported in man. An initial report from Australia in 1965 described a rapidly progressive meningitis that proved fatal. Early symptoms in the first two days or so are fever, severe frontal headache, defects of olfactory sense, lethargy, sore throat, and obstructed nostrils. By the third day vomiting and impaired consciousness may be present, progressing to deepening coma and death on the fourth day. At postmortem, destruction of the inferior surface of the frontal lobes and olfactory bulbs was seen, associated with a purulent exudate. Histologic examination revealed columns of amebae extending into the brain substance, especially via the perivascular spaces.

This clinical entity has now been reported from several parts of the United States (Florida, Virginia, Texas) and from Great Britain and Czechoslovakia. It is usually found in children and young people, and is invariably fatal. It appears to be acquired by swimming, diving, or water skiing in lakes known to contain large numbers of free-living amebae. Pressure changes under water probably force the amebae through the cribriform plate. *Naegleria* has repeatedly been found in the cerebrospinal fluid of man. The CSF also shows an increased protein level, decreased sugar, neutrophils, and red cells, but is bacteriologically sterile. Most of the patients to date have died, usually because the diagnosis has been missed.

Emetine, arsenicals, sulfonamides, tetracyclines, and metronidazole have been used without success. Amphotericin B therapy has resulted in recovery of a patient in whom *Naegleria* organisms were recovered from the CSF, and in vitro studies show that therapeutic concentrations are amebicidal. In one fatal case *Naegleria gruberi* was recovered from the lungs, liver, spleen and heart blood, as well as from the central nervous system. In patients with persistent eye inflammation *Acanthamoeba polyphaga* has been isolated. Since such free-living amebae are ubiquitous, doubtless reports from other countries will appear in the future

Carter, R. F.: Primary amoebic meningo-encephalitis. Trans. Roy. Soc. Trop. Med. Hyg., 66:193, 1972.
Culbertson, C. G.: Pathogenic acanthamoeba (Hartmannella). Am. J. Clin. Path., 35:195, 1961.
Dumar, R. J., Helwig, W. B., and Martinez, A. J.: Meningoencephalitis and brain abscess due to a free-living amoeba. Ann. Interno. Med., 88:468, 1978.
Duma, R. J., Rosenblum, W. I., McGehee, R. F., Jones, M. M., and Clifford, N. E.: Primary amoebic meningoencephalitis caused by Naegleria. Ann. Intern. Med., 74:923, 1971.
Visvesvaka, G. S., Jones, D. B., and Robinson, N. M.: Isolation, identification and biological characterization of Acanthamoeba polyphaga from a human eye. Am. J. Trop. Med. Hyg., 24:784, 1975.

200.6. ISOSPORIASIS
(Coccidiosis)

Philip D. Marsden

Isospora have alternate asexual and sexual generation in the same host, and the nature of the cycle is not dis-

similar to plasmodia in the forms produced. There is probably only one human species, *Isospora belli*, which parasitizes the small intestinal epithelium. The cycles of schizogony and gametogony have now been described in small bowel mucosal biopsies from symptomatic patients, and it has been suggested that this organism causes a malabsorption syndrome. Until recently the case for the pathogenicity of *Isospora* rested mainly on laboratory infections that resulted in diarrhea lasting about three weeks, accompanied by the passage of the diagnostic form of the parasite in the stool. This is a thick-walled oocyst 25 to 35 μ × 12 to 16 μ in size. Both ends are rounded, and one is contracted to form a neck. This stage is the zygote. Further development in two to four days results in the formation of two sporoblasts, which mature into oval sporocysts. Each sporocyst ultimately contains four sporozoites. These oocysts are very resistant to physical and chemical insult and will readily sporulate in potassium dichromate. Many instances of spurious parasitemia have been reported in man when oocysts of various animals and fish coccidia have passed unchanged through the bowel to appear in the stool and pose a diagnostic problem. The mild persistent diarrhea during the active phase of the infection is usually accompanied only by nausea and abdominal discomfort. In a report cited below, the patients had severe diarrhea and steatorrhea unresponsive to therapy, and three died.

Brandborg, L. L., Golberg, S. B., and Breidenbach, W. C.: Human coccidiosis — a possible cause of malabsorption. The life cycle in small bowel mucosal biopsies as a diagnostic feature. N. Engl. J. Med., 283:1306, 1970.
Smitskamp, H., and Oey-Muller, E.: Geographical distribution and clinical significance of human coccidiosis. Trop. Geogr. Med., 18:133, 1966.

200.7. SARCOSPORIDIOSIS

Philip D. Marsden

The genus *Sarcocystis*, like *Isospora, Toxoplasma,* and *Plasmodium,* belongs to the subphylum Sporozoa, parasites which show alterations of generations, one sexual (sporogony) and the other asexual (schizogony). Unlike *Isospora,* however, in *Sarcocystis* these two cycles occur in different hosts. The parasite previously designated *Isospora hominis* has been renamed *Sarcocystis hominis* because sporocysts appear in the stools of man following the ingestion of sarcocysts in uncooked beef or pork. Man also acts as an intermediate host for *Sarcocystis lindemanni* which may cause polymyositis sometimes associated with eosinophilia. Both these parasites are rarely reported, but their true prevalence in man is unknown.

Jeffrey, H. C.: Sarcosporidiosis in man. Trans. Roy. Soc. Trop. Med. Hyg., 68:17, 1974.
Rommel, M., and Heydorn, A. O.: Beiträge zum Lebenszyklus der Sarkosporidien. III. Isospora hominis (Raillet and Lucet, 1891) Wenyon, 1923, eine Dauerform der Sarkosporidien des Rindes und des Schweins. Berl. Münch. Tieraerztl. Wochenschr., 85:143, 1972.

Section Two HELMINTHIC DISEASES

201. INTRODUCTION

Philip D. Marsden

Compared to protozoans, helminths are very large organisms with a complex cellular structure. As they feed on host tissue, their metabolism results in various protein secretions and excretions; and because they themselves largely consist of complex protein, it is not surprising that invasion of the body by worms is frequently associated with an eosinophilic response. Thus, in the invasive stage of schistosomes, hookworm, ascaris, and similar parasites, an eosinophilia is usual. Yet when these worms have matured and settled at their site of election, eosinophilia often is not found. It might be argued in the case of intestinal nematodes that this is because they are in the gut and in a strict sense outside the body, but because the phenomenon also occurs with schistosomiasis and tissue filariae this is too facile an explanation. At present the mechanisms and course of eosinophilia produced in a host in response to a foreign protein are not clearly understood (Beeson and Bass).

With regard to immunology, understandably, complex helminths produce complex crude antigens of low specificity. At the moment, with a few exceptions, group-specific reactions with antigens for schistosomes, hermaphroditic flukes, nematodes, and cestodes are all that are available using tests such as complement fixation or indirect hemagglutination. Skin tests on the whole are much less satisfactory than those based on serology. Many of these helminths are recognized by the presence of characteristic progeny in the form of either eggs in the stools, sputum, or urine, or larvae in the tissues.

The concept of the over-all population or load of worms is important in human disease, as *the parasitic load* is one of the factors determining the extent of pathology (another would be the host response). Today many helminthic infections can be quantitated, and these methods will be mentioned under diagnosis. Another important aspect of worm infections is their relatively long life. Many flukes live for decades after the infection has been acquired, and similarly many filarial species are long lived. This illustrates the importance of obtaining a very detailed history of the patient's move-

TABLE 1. Prevalence of Common Helminth Infections in Man*

Parasite	Source of Infection	Approximate Locality	Estimated Incidence in U.S. and Canada	Estimated World Incidence
Trematodes (flukes):				
Schistosoma japonicum	Water through skin	Far East	—	46,000,000
Schistosoma haematobium	Water through skin	Africa, Middle East	—	39,200,000
Schistosoma mansoni	Water through skin	Africa, South America, Caribbean	—	29,200,000
Clonorchis sinensis	Fish	Far East	—	19,000,000
Opisthorchis felineus	Fish	Far East	—	1,100,000
Paragonimus westermani	Crabs, crayfish	Africa, South America	—	3,200,000
Fasciolopsis buski	Water nuts	Far East	—	10,000,000
Cestodes (tapeworms):				
Diphyllobothrium latum	Fish	Around Arctic Circle, N. Europe, Russia, America	†	10,400,000
Taenia saginata	Beef	Cosmopolitan	10,000	38,900,000
Taenia solium	Pork	Cosmopolitan	†	2,500,000
Echinococcus granulosus	Dog feces	Cosmopolitan	†	†
Nematodes (roundworms):				
Intestinal nematodes				
Strongyloides stercoralis	Human feces	Cosmopolitan	400,000	34,900,000
Hookworm	Human feces	Cosmopolitan	1,800,000	456,800,000
Ascaris lumbricoides	Human feces	Cosmopolitan	3,000,000	644,400,000
Trichuris trichiura	Human feces	Cosmopolitan	400,000	355,100,000
Enterobius vermicularis	Human feces	Cosmopolitan	18,000,000	208,800,000
Tissue nematodes				
Trichinella spiralis	Pork	Cosmopolitan	21,100,000	27,800,000
Wuchereria bancrofti and *Brugia malayi*	Mosquitoes	Africa, South America, South Asia	—	189,000,000
Loa loa	*Chrysops*	Equatorial Africa	—	13,000,000
Dipetalonema perstans	*Culicoides*	Africa, South America	—	27,000,000
Mansonella ozzardi	*Culicoides*	South America	—	7,000,000
Onchocerca volvulus	*Simulium*	Equatorial Africa, Central America	—	19,800,000
Dracunculus medinensis	*Cyclops*	Middle East, India, Africa	—	48,300,000

*Based on data culculated by N. R. Stoll (J. Parasit., 33:1, 1947). Since the world population has subsequently increased by more than 50 per cent, all the figures given can be regarded as extremely conservative. For instance, it is said that 180 million people in the world are infected with one of the three species of schistosomes that infect humans.

†Represents less than 100,000 infections.

ments around the world, because a visit to an endemic area 20 years ago may be connected with a current clinical problem.

It must be remembered that there are a large number of helminths that rarely infect man, and many cannot be included in this book. For information on these a standard textbook on parasitology (see references in Ch. 192) should be consulted. An important topical point is that we are now beginning to realize that for every worm adapted to man there are many others which gain access to man's tissues but fail to mature because they are natural parasites of other mammals or birds. These may cause very puzzling clinical problems. An increasing proportion of unexplained eosinophilia encountered in clinical practice is being explained on a basis of invasion of the body by a worm that will not mature in man because he is not the definitive host.

By a simple classification, worms may be separated into trematodes or flukes, cestodes or tapeworms, and nematodes or roundworms. A check list adapted from H. W. Brown's table in the twelfth edition of this text is given here in Table 1, together with information on the source of infection and the main areas of occurrence in the world. The most important helminthic infections in terms of disease in man and incidence are schistosomiasis, hookworm, and filariasis.

Beeson, P. B., and Bass, D. A.: The Eosinophil. Philadelphia, W. B. Saunders Company, 1977.
Marcial Rojas, R. A. (ed.): Pathology of Protozoal and Helminthic Diseases with Clinical Correlations. Baltimore, Williams & Wilkins Company, 1971.
Marsden, P. D. (ed.): Intestinal Parasites. Clinics in Gastroenterology, Vol. 7, No. 1. Philadelphia, W. B. Saunders Company, 1978.
Muller, R.: Worms and Disease. London, Heinemann, 1975.

THE CESTODES
(Tapeworms)

Philip D. Marsden

202. INTRODUCTION

The cestodes are endoparasitic flatworms, the hermaphroditic adults of which are flat and ribbonlike and inhabit the intestinal tract of vertebrates. *Taenia* species and the fish tapeworm may have a life of 25 to 30 years if left alone. The larval forms may require more than one intermediate host and develop in the tissues of vertebrates, and in some instances invertebrates. Most adult tapeworms consist of a scolex or head equipped for attachment with suckers, hooks, or grooves and a strobila or tapelike chain of progressively developing segments or proglottides. The neck is the site of segment generation, and mature segments are complete hermaphroditic units with both sets of sex organs. There is no digestive system, food being absorbed directly through the cuticle. There are longitudinal primitive excretory systems and a nervous system. In gravid segments the uterus is loaded with eggs, and these pass out of the bowel either in the segment or free in the stool. The delicate outer membrane of the eggs is often lost, but the thick-walled inner membrane contains a form infective for the intermediate host.

When eggs are ingested by the appropriate intermediate host, larvae (termed oncospheres) are released which are capable of penetrating the intestinal mucosa. The method by which the larvae develop into encysted forms differs among the cestodes and leads to different clinical patterns. Oncospheres in *Taenia solium* each

develop into a small (0.5 to 1.0 cm) fluid-filled structure containing a single inverted "head." These are called *cysticerci*, or bladder worms, and many such larvae distributed in various organs cause the disease cysticercosis. The oncospheres in *Hymenolepis nana* penetrate only into the intestinal mucosa. They develop similarly to those just described; however, fluid is usually not present in the larva, and hence it is termed a *cysticercoid*. In the case of *Echinococcus granulosus*, usually only one oncosphere is able to develop (unilocular) within the intermediate host. However, this larva develops an internal germinating membrane capable of producing an entire population of daughter and granddaughter cysts within the primary cyst. This cyst is called an *echinococcal* or *hydatid* cyst. It continues to enlarge as the population of scolices within increases and will commonly reach a diameter of 20 to 30 cm after many years.

The clinical pattern of disease reflects these various methods of development; the cysticercoid of *H. nana* presents as intestinal irritation; the cysticercus of *T. solium* leads to multiple small lesions, often in the brain, causing seizure disorders; the *Echinococcus* produces a single large space-occupying lesion which often because of its size interferes with liver, lung, or cardiac function.

In the following chapters, we will deal with only the six most common of the 30 or more species of tapeworm which have been found in man. These are listed in Table 2. They will be discussed in the order cited in

TABLE 2. Common Important Tapeworms

Official Name	Intermediate Host(s)	Stage in Man
Diphyllobothrium latum	Water fleas, freshwater fish	Adult worm
Taenia saginata	Cattle (beef)	Adult worm
Taenia solium	Pigs (pork)	Adult worm and larval stage
Hymenolepis nana	Man	Adult worm and larval stage
Echinococcus granulosus	Man, sheep, cattle	Larval stage
Echinococcus multilocularis	Man, sheep, cattle	Larval stage

the table: first those in which man is the definitive host, then those in which he serves as both definitive and intermediate host, and finally those in which only the larval stage can develop in man.

Jones, T. C.: Cestodes. Clin. Gastroenterol., 7:105, 1978.

203. DIPHYLLOBOTHRIUM LATUM
(The Fish Tapeworm)

Infection with the fish tapeworm is most common in temperate areas such as Scandinavia and around the Baltic Sea. It also occurs in Canada and in the northern United States, notably Alaska. Central Europe is an endemic focus. In the tropics relatively few reports have appeared from the Philippines, Madagascar, Botswana, Uganda, and Chile. A human parasite, *Diphyllobothrium pacificum*, has been described from Peru. The adult is the largest tapeworm of man, reaching 10 meters and having 4000 segments. (The spatulate head has two deep sucking grooves for attachment to the wall of the ileum.) The gravid segment disintegrates, and operculated ova are passed in the feces.

From the egg a ciliated embryo is eaten by a freshwater flea (*Cyclops* or *Diaptomus* species) in which it develops to a *procercoid*. When the infected flea is swallowed by freshwater fish, e.g., salmon, pike, further development takes place in the muscles of the fish to the *plerocercoid*, the form infective to man. The plerocercoid on being liberated into the small intestine grows to an adult in three to six weeks. Although the adult worm causes no pathologic lesion, there is a very important complication to this infection, namely a megaloblastic anemia. This appears to be due to the avidity of the worm for vitamin B_{12}. Forty-four per cent of a single dose of Co^{60} labeled vitamin B_{12} has been absorbed by a worm, the radioactivity being concentrated in the proximal growing part. Also, the nearer the worm is to the jejunum, the greater the chance of developing megaloblastic anemia. It is not clear why the worm needs so much vitamin B_{12}. The worm also appears to require folic acid in the same way. Thus the full range of neurologic symptoms of subacute combined degeneration of the cord may appear, particularly in severe cases of multiple parasitism. Peripheral neuritis appears very early in the parasitism, and recently optic atrophy has been reported.

The *diagnosis* is made by direct examination of the stools, because the eggs are present in very large numbers. Yellowish-brown and operculated, they have to be distinguished from fluke eggs such as *Paragonimus*, but the large number in the stool favors the diagnosis of fish tapeworm even to the uninitiated. The operculum is actually less conspicuous in *Diphyllobothrium*, and there is a small knob at the anopercular end (mean size, 70 by 45 μ). Because the treatment for the tapeworms of this group and of the *Taenia* genus is the same, they are considered together later.

Prophylaxis is readily accomplished by thoroughly cooking fish before consumption. Freezing of fish for 48 hours at $-10°$ C will also prevent infection. The infection is not uncommon in New York among Jewish housewives who make their own gefilte fish and sample it in the process.

SPARGANOSIS

This condition requires mention here, because it is the name of an infection caused by the migrating larvae or spargana of several species of tapeworm related to *D. latum* but requiring final hosts other than man. It presents as a migrating subcutaneous painful swelling suggesting a cellulitis. Marked eosinophilia is usually present. The eye may be involved with orbital swelling or even actual penetration of the globe. In China this results from applying infected frogs on poultices to the eye. Biopsy reveals inflammatory tissue reactions and an immature cestode, many of which are quite impossible to identify. *Diphyllobothrium mansonoides (Spirometra mansonoides)* is a common offender. So-called *Sparganum proliferum* is unknown in the adult stage, but may distribute thousands of larvae throughout the body, and in contrast to other forms carries a poorer prognosis. This type of infection is rare, but occurs in many tropical countries, diagnosis being made by finding the plerocercoid larvae in tissues.

Bjorkenheim, G.: Neurological changes in pernicious tapeworm anemia. Acta Med. Scand., 140 (Supplement): 260, 1971.
Swartzwelder, J. C., Beaver, P. C., and Hood, M. W.: Sparganosis in the southern United States. Am. J. Trop. Med. Hyg., 13:43, 1964.
Vik, R.: The genus *Diphyllobothrium*. Exp. Parasitol., 15:361, 1964.
Von Bowsdorff, B.: Diphyllobothriasis in man. New York, Academic Press, 1977.

204. TAENIA SAGINATA
(The Beef Tapeworm)

The beef tapeworm has a cosmopolitan distribution, being particularly common in the Middle East, Kenya, and Ethiopia. In the last-named country many people habitually take a monthly purge of herbs to get rid of an impressive length of worm, but rarely get rid of the head. Beef tapeworm is also common in parts of South America, Mexico, and Russia. In all these countries it is acquired by eating undercooked or raw beef — a delicacy in Ethiopia. It is doubtful whether *T. saginata* causes any symptoms, although epigastric pain, appetite disturbances, and general malaise have been ascribed to the presence of the worm. It is possible that multiple worms may be associated with symptoms. Very rarely the worm may block the pancreatic or cystic duct or appendix, producing acute inflammation (16 such cases have been reported). The 5- to 10-meter adult worm has four suckers on the head to attach it to the wall of the small intestine. The gravid segments are usually recognized in the stool but, being muscular, they can traverse the anal sphincter and appear in the underclothing. They contain more than 12 uterine branches, which distinguish them from *T. solium*, although recently some doubt has been cast on the reliability of this criterion. Characteristic *Taenia* eggs may be found in the stool or on the anal margin. When the eggs are swallowed by cattle, llamas, or buffaloes, the hatched embryos gain the skeletal muscles by the bloodstream after bowel penetration and develop into the encysted bladder-like larval forms or cysticerci which are infective for man.

Man is the only definitive host in which the adult worm can develop. The larval cysticercus form has been reported only three times in man, so host specificity seems to be strict. Treatment will be discussed later; prevention consists in not ingesting beef containing cysticerci.

Pawloski, Z., and Schultz, M. G.: Taeniasis and cysticercosis (*Taenia saginata*). Adv. Parasitol., 10:269, 1972.

205. TAENIA SOLIUM
(The Pork Tapeworm Causing Human Cysticercosis Due to Cysticercus Cellulosae)

In contrast to *T. saginata*, both larval and adult forms of this species can develop in man. Again this worm is cosmopolitan in distribution although relatively rare in North America and western Europe; cysticercosis is the most common identifiable cause of epilepsy in the Durban African population and is a serious disease because of the frequency of brain involvement. It is common in Mexico and parts of Central and South America. Man, again the only definitive host of importance, acquires the infection by eating undercooked measly pork containing cysticerci. Pigs and wild boars are the usual intermediate hosts.

The adult worm usually causes no symptoms in the small intestine. For attachment the head has four suckers and two rows of hooklets on a prominent rostellum. It is smaller than *T. saginata* (2 to 4 meters). Its segments are more delicate than *T. saginata* and there are usually less than twelve branches to the uterus in the gravid segment. The eggs are indistinguishable from *T. saginata*, both being approximately 35 μ, thick-walled, brown, and containing an embryonic oncosphere with six hooklets. In *T. solium* infection, however, these eggs are infective to man, but must pass through the stomach and undergo tryptic digestion before hatching occurs. The usual way in which man is infected with eggs is by external autoinfection, transferring eggs from the anus to the mouth or to food fecally contaminated by a carrier of the worm. Internal autoinfection by regurgitating segments of the worm into the stomach is a theoretic possibility, but has not been recorded.

Once free from the egg in the intestine, the oncosphere penetrates the intestinal wall with its hooklets and, as in the pig, settles in the body tissues. The invaded organs in order of frequency are subcutaneous tissue, brain, eye, muscles, heart, liver, lung, and peritoneum. The cysticercus matures in four months to an ellipsoidal translucent cyst, 10 to 20 by 5 to 10 mm, with an opaque invaginated scolex with suckers and hooks. It is gradually surrounded by a thick fibrous capsule and may live for years. Death is frequently associated with calcification. Some authors distinguish *Cysticercus cellulosae*, in which a scolex is present, from *Cysticercus racemosus;* the latter is a degenerate cyst in which the scolex is absent.

The invasive phase may be associated with fever, headache, muscle pain, and high eosinophilia. Usually years after this stage more serious symptoms occur owing to brain involvement, with the onset of epilepsy, personality changes, signs of raised intracranial pressure, or long tract signs. In every patient with epilepsy of late onset coming from an endemic area, especially if eosinophilia is present, this possibility should be excluded by (1) taking a detailed history, especially in relation to a past history of tapeworm infection; the stool should be examined for *Taenia* eggs and segments, because rarely the worm may still be in situ; (2) having a full physical examination, especially for subcutaneous nodules containing cysticerci; biopsy will establish the diagnosis; (3) taking roentgenograms of the skull, buttocks, and thighs for calcified cysticerci which have a characteristic size and shape; and (4) performing either a complement-fixation test or an indirect hemagglutination test, using antigen from lyophilized pig cysticerci. The cerebrospinal fluid may be under increased pressure, show an excess of eosinophils, and demonstrate a positive complement fixation test. More rarely the globe of the eye is involved, as well as the heart and skeletal muscle. A cysticercus may be visible on the tongue. Sometimes the cysticerci become secondarily infected. In the brain, inflammation around them may produce internal hydrocephalus. Although the adult worm can be eradicated easily, there is no medical treatment for *Cysticercus cellulosae* save palliative anticonvulsants. Mebendazole has been shown to kill cysticerci in mice. Rarely surgical intervention may be necessary in cases of raised intracranial pressure. Again prophylaxis rests on avoiding opportunities of eating infected meat and the inspection and thorough cooking of pork.

Campbell, W. C., and Blair, L. S.: Prevention and cure of hepatic cysticercosis in mice. J. Parisitol., 60:1049, 1974.
Marquez-Monter, H.: Cysticercosis. *In* Marcial Rojas, R. A., (ed.): Pathology of Protozoal and Helminthic Diseases. Baltimore, Williams & Wilkins Company, 1971.
Powell, S. J., Procter, E. M., Wilmot, A. J., and McLeod, I. N., Cysticercosis and epilepsy in Africans: A clinical and serological study. Ann. Trop. Med. Parasitol., 60:152, 1966.

206. TREATMENT OF INFECTIONS WITH ADULTS OF THE FISH, BEEF, AND PORK TAPEWORM

Niclosamide (hydroxychlorobenzamide, Yomesan)* is safe, effective, and easy to administer. When the patient wakes in the morning, two tablets of 0.5 gram each are chewed thoroughly and swallowed with a little water. The same procedure is repeated one hour later. No fasting or purgation is necessary, and children receive a proportionately smaller dose. Alternatively, paromomycin can be used in the adult. The dosage for niclosamide and for paromomycin is the same: 1 gram every four hours, for a total of 4 grams. The worm disintegrates so that unfortunately the head cannot be sought as proof of cure. For this reason follow-up at six months is desirable.

Quinacrine hydrochloride (Atabrine, mepacrine) is indicated in cases in which the aforementioned therapy had been unsuccessful. The rationale is that a single comparatively large dose of this drug causes the worm

---

*Available from Center for Disease Control (404-633-3311, Ext. 3670).

to release its hold and it can then be voided. The most successful technique for adults is as follows: Admit the patient to hospital and give only fluids for 36 to 48 hours. Then pass a tube into the duodenum and, with the patient resting quietly, inject 1 gram of quinacrine hydrochloride down the tube in 40 ml of water, using a 20-ml syringe. Half an hour later a saline purge is injected down the tube, and all feces saved for the next 24 hours. Long lengths of the worm stained yellow with the drug are passed, and the head should be identified. If the head is not dislodged, the worm will regenerate in two to three months, and segments will reappear in the stools. The duodenal tube reduces the chances of vomiting the drug. If the head of the worm is found, one can usually reassure the patient that the worm is eliminated unless it is a rare case of multiple infection. It must be remembered that feces from patients harboring *T. solium* are an infectious risk. The patient should scrub his hands after defecation and pass his feces into disinfectant.

Keeling, J. E. W.: The chemotherapy of cestode infections. *In* Goldin, A., Hawking, F., and Schnitzer, R. J. (eds.): Advances in Chemotherapy. New York, Academic Press, 1968, Vol. 3, pp. 109–152.

207. HYMENOLEPIS NANA (Dwarf Tapeworm)

H. nana is less important as a cause of symptomatic disease than the other tapeworms described here. However, since it is spread directly by contact with contaminated stool, the infection can reach epidemic proportions in institutions where fecal-oral exposure is difficult to control, such as in mental hospitals or schools for young children. In one study of children in a school for the mentally retarded (Willowbrook, New York), almost 8 per cent were found to be infected.

Clinical manifestations of this infection include anorexia, diarrhea, and abdominal pain secondary to irritation of the intestinal mucosa. In addition, systemic signs and symptoms such as headache, dizziness, and occasionally seizures are not infrequent. The treatment of choice is hydroxychlorobenzamide (niclosamide),* 2 grams daily for three days, followed a week later by a second course of therapy. This treatment schedule has been developed because relapse occurred when shorter courses of therapy were used. Relapse is thought to occur for two reasons: first, the chlorobenzamide is effective only against the adult; and second, the cysticercoid stage may persist in the mucosa for several weeks before developing into an adult.

Yoeli, M., Most, H., Hammond, J., and Scheinesson, G. P.: Parasitic infections in a closed community. Results of a 10-year survey in Willowbrook State School. Trans. R. Soc. Trop. Med. Hyg., 66:764, 1972.

208. ECHINOCOCCOSIS (Hydatid Disease)

There are two species of the genus *Echinococcus* which infect man, *Echinococcus granulosus* and *Echinococcus multilocularis*. They are the most important ces-

---

*Available from Center for Disease Control (404-633-3311, Ext. 3670).

todes producing serious disease in man because of the size and location of their larval form, the hydatid cyst. Man is only one of a number of intermediate hosts, other important ones being sheep, cattle, and deer. The definitive hosts for these very small adult tapeworms are canines such as dogs, wolves, jackals, and foxes.

Hydatid disease is cosmopolitan because infected stock have been distributed all over the world for breeding purposes. The incidence of human infection is low in many countries, but where the triad of man, dog, and sheep or cattle is common, hydatid disease is relatively frequent. Examples are countries such as Australia, Argentina, Chile, Kenya, New Zealand, and the United Kingdom (Wales). It has been reported from 15 states in the United States. A distinct variant, *E. granulosus var. canadensis*, is present in Alaska and is also found in Canada.

Human infection follows ingestion of the eggs excreted by infected dogs. The adult tapeworm measures only 2.5 to 9.2 mm and has a head with hooklets and suckers, a growing neck, and only three segments: immature, sexually mature, and gravid. Heavy infections of dogs are common, but the worm lives for only about six months in the upper jejunum. The eggs produced are indistinguishable from *Taenia* eggs and like them produce an oncosphere with six hooklets. On reaching the intestine of the intermediate host such as man, they pass through the intestinal wall and circulate in the blood and can develop in any body tissue. It may take 20 to 30 years before the slowly growing hydatid cyst causes symptoms. Often they remain small (less than 10 cm), but they may grow as large as the human head. The host parasite factors determining growth are not clearly understood, but growth is variable from 0.25 to 1 cm a year. The structure of a developed hydatid cyst is complex. Briefly, it really consists of a whole colony of infective larval forms, for inside the laminated, defined cyst wall is a germinal layer that is constantly budding off new infective individuals. The cyst is filled with fluid, and second and third generation cysts containing thousands of infective forms or scolices are suspended in this fluid. There is little wonder that when a dog eats an infected sheep's liver he acquires many adult *Echinococcus* organisms.

When the infective embryo or oncosphere passes into the portal circulation of man, it is first held up in the liver where more than half (58 per cent) of those that survive develop. Many are destroyed by phagocytic cells. The next tissue filter is the lungs, where 27 per cent lodge. Finally, 15 per cent escape into the general circulation to involve the abdominal cavity, muscle, kidney, spleen, bone, heart, and brain.

ECHINOCOCCUS GRANULOSUS

Echinococcus granulosus is the common species; there are several types of cysts, as follows: (1) The classic unilocular cyst is usually fertile and surrounded by a false capsule of host tissue fibrosis. Rupture of such a cyst will cause dissemination of daughter cysts with secondary hydatids. (2) Alveolar hydatids have a reticulated irregular outline resulting from uneven growth of the germinal membrane. They resemble those of *E. multilocularis*, but there is no metastatic growth. This cyst usually occurs in the liver and is difficult to remove. It is often sterile, and its contents degenerate. (3) Osseous hydatid. The nature of bone does not permit a host or parasite capsule to form. Daughter cysts form in the bone medulla, erode the cortex, and produce a pathologic fracture. If they escape from the bone, the cysts grow in their normal spherical shape with the usual capsules in the extraosseous tissues.

Clinically, the hydatid cysts may produce signs of a space-occupying lesion in relation to the organ in which they occur. In the liver abdominal pain and vomiting may be presenting symptoms, a mass being visible or palpable. Usually the cysts are too tense to show fluctuation. In the lung they are usually detected on routine chest films as spherical, well-defined shadows. They are more common in the right lung, and rarely are associated with cough and hemoptysis. Those of the brain are indistinguishable from a cerebral tumor. In the kidney, hematuria or loin pain may be the first sign, whereas hydatid cyst of bone may present as a pathologic fracture.

The *complications* of hydatid disease are important. The most serious is rupture and dissemination of further infective larvae. Patients with suspected hydatid disease should always be gently palpated — a leaking cyst may present as anaphylactic shock with an urticarial rash and high eosinophilia. The cyst may become secondarily infected with bacteria and present similarly to a liver or lung abscess.

A suggestive tumor in a patient from an endemic area demands the following investigations. An eosinophilia may be present. Plain roentgenograms may show calcification in the cyst wall, although this does not mean that the cyst is not infective. An isotope scan of the liver reveals the extent of the tumor, but gives no clue as to its nature. In the chest film the round, uniformly dense shadow is suggestive. A skin test using cyst air in the cyst means communication with a bronchus and possibly secondary infection. A skin test using cyst fluid is positive in the majority of patients, but it has been shown that the reaction depends on the concentration (nitrogen content) of protein in the fluid injected. A cross-reaction occurs in patients with schistosomiasis. Until there is universal acceptance of a standard skin test antigen, a negative result is meaningless. Hydatid complement-fixation tests, hemagglutination tests, and bentonite flocculation tests are all practicable and are helpful. A scolex antigen is probably the best (Bull. WHO, 1968). Rarely cyst fragments, such as scolices, may be found in the sputum or urine. It must be recalled that one in five patients has multiple cysts, so that if a cyst is located in one site, especially if it is not the liver, there may be others. *A liver scan should be done in every patient with an extrahepatic cyst. Diagnostic aspiration is never indicated because of the risk of rupture.* In the liver and lung, carcinoma and abscess are often difficult differential diagnoses.

It should be emphasized that many hydatid cysts never get very large (5 to 10 cm) and never cause symptoms. Until recently there was no medical treatment for human hydatidosis. Now limited studies suggest that fluoromebendazole in an oral adult dose of 2 grams daily for six months to a year may kill the organism. The suggestion that specific antibodies and immune complexes are useful in assessing treatment requires confirmation. Surgery is indicated only in cysts that are enlarging, producing pressure symptoms, or developing complications. The physician should consult a surgeon who has experience with this problem. If possible the cyst should be removed entirely. To prevent spillage and dissemination, the cyst is usually aspirated at operation after packing off the site; 20 ml of fluid is withdrawn, and an equal quantity of 1 per cent iodine or 30 per cent sodium chloride is introduced to kill the scolices. Injection of a 1 per cent aqueous solution of iodine in a volume amounting to one twentieth of the whole cyst volume is lethal to scolices within one minute. Anaphylactic reactions resulting from spillage during operation may require corticosteroids.

E. granulosus var. *canadensis* is common in Alaska and Canada where it has a sylvatic cycle in deer and wolves. It produces smaller and more delicate cysts in man than the classic *E. granulosus;* the latter are more frequent in the lung, are usually asymptomatic, and almost never cause serious complications so that the distinction is important.

ECHINOCOCCUS MULTILOCULARIS

The medical importance of distinguishing between these two species is that *Echinococcus multilocularis* does not produce large single cysts with endogenous growth and well-defined fibrous tissue encapsulation but rather an aggregate of innumerable small cysts that multiply by exogenous budding to produce the so-called alveolar or malignant hydatid. More than 90 per cent occur in liver, which is progressively honeycombed by a multitude of small cysts. They may become confluent and even metastasize like a malignancy. Intrahepatic or portal hypertension develops with splenomegaly, and biliary obstruction may produce icterus. The hepatic infection may be difficult to differentiate from a malignancy. As surgical techniques improve, this infection may become an indication for a total liver transplant. This species of cestode occurs in south central Europe, Russia, and Alaska. Rarely cases have occurred in Australia, England, and Argentina.

Prevention of infection with both these species entails elimination of the infection from dogs by worming with arecoline hydrobromide regularly and preventing their eating infected offal. Contamination of the hands, food, and drink with dog feces should be avoided.

Arana Iniguez, R.: Hydatid echinococcosis of the nervous system. *In* Spillane, J. D. (ed.): Tropical Neurology. New York, Oxford University Press, 1973, p. 408.

Bouree, P., and Molimard, R.: Treatment of trichinococcosis. Br. Med. J., 1:307, 1978.

Danis, M., Brücker, G., Gentilini, M., et al.: Treatment of hepatic hydatid disease. Br. Med. J., 2:1356, 1977.

Dew, H. R.: Hydatid Disease. Sydney, Australian Publishing Co., Ltd., 1928.

Echinococcosis. Bull. WHO, 39: No. 1, 1968.

Jalayer, T., and Askavi, I.: A study of the effect of aqueous iodine on hydatid cysts in vitro and in vivo. Ann. Trop. Med. Parasitol., 60:169, 1966.

Katz, A. M., and Pan, C.: *Echinococcus* disease in the United States. Am. J. Med., 25:759, 1958.

Wilson, J. F., Diddams, A. C., and Rausch, R. L.: Cystic hydatid disease in Alaska. A review of 101 cases of *Echinococcus granulosus* infection. Am. Rev. Respir. Dis., 98:1, 1967.

209.   OTHER TAPEWORMS

Two other species of adult tapeworms that parasitize the human intestine are usually mentioned; but in comparison with those discussed above, they are of little importance in human disease. The rat tapeworm *Hymenolepis diminuta* is acquired by swallowing insects carrying the *Taenia* eggs from rats. *Dipylidium caninum* is the common tapeworm of cats and dogs throughout the world, and is transmitted by their fleas to children handling the pets. The gravid proglottids are shaped like melon seeds and may be seen in the stool. For these parasites niclosamide or paromomycin can be used.*

Coenurus infections of man, like hydatid, take the

form of cystlike larvae in the tissue; 64 cases have been recorded to date. Infection in temperate regions is probably due to the larval cyst *Multiceps multiceps* (a dog tapeworm) and usually occurs in the central nervous system. Similar cysts are found in the brain of sheep, producing a fatal disease known as gid, which is characterized by somnolence, loss of weight, visual disturbance, and ataxia. In Africa *Taenia brauni* seems to be responsible for similar "hydatid-like" cysts in the subcutaneous tissues of man.

---

*Available from Center for Disease Control (404-633-3311, Ext. 3670).

Templeton, A. C.: Anatomical and geographical location of human *Coenurus* infection. Trop. Geogr. Med., 23:105, 1971.

DISEASES CAUSED BY TREMATODES
(Flukes)

210. SCHISTOSOMIASIS
(Bilharziasis)

Kenneth S. Warren

DEFINITION. Schistosomiasis, a chronic infection of more than 200,000,000 people in Asia, Africa, the Caribbean region, and South America, is caused by three different worm species, *Schistosoma mansoni*, *S. japonicum*, and *S. haematobium*. Infection occurs during immersion in fresh water containing schistosome cercariae. These larval forms penetrate the skin and migrate via the lungs and liver to the final habitat of the half-inch-long adult worms: the veins of the intestines and urinary bladder. The worms themselves do not multiply within man, but produce large numbers of eggs, many of which remain in the body, damaging primarily the intestines, liver, and urinary tract. Eggs that are excreted in the urine and feces and that reach fresh water hatch into ciliated miracidia. These organisms penetrate into snails, multiply, and develop into cercariae, the infective form for man.

ETIOLOGY. Although the cercariae of many different schistosome species penetrate human skin, there are three major species that complete their life cycles in man and are thus capable of causing systemic disease: *Schistosoma mansoni*, *japonicum*, and *haematobium*. The life cycles of these schistosomes are essentially similar, all being digenetic trematodes alternating a sexual phase of reproduction in man (definitive host) with an asexual reproductive phase in snails (intermediate host). Nevertheless, at each phase of the life cycle there are differences among the species that play crucial roles in the epidemiology, pathogenesis, and clinical picture of the disease.

The adult worms or schistosomes are members of the class Trematoda of the phylum Platyhelminthes or flatworms. The male worms (10 to 20 × 0.5 to 1 mm) have cleft bodies within which the longer and thinner females reside, *S. japonicum* being the largest of the three species. The worms may live in man for as long as 30 years, but recent evidence suggests that their mean life span is five to ten years. The habitats of the adult *S. mansoni*, *japonicum*, and *haematobium* worms are, re-

spectively, the veins of the large intestine, small intestine, and urinary bladder.

The worms absorb metabolites through both their intestines and integument. Their energy processes depend on anaerobic catabolism of carbohydrates; the schistosomes utilize an amount of glucose equivalent to one fifth of their dry body weight each hour and convert 80 per cent of it to lactic acid. In addition, the ingestion of red blood cells appears to be of nutritional significance, as the worms contain a proteolytic enzyme that breaks down globin; the remaining insoluble hematin-like pigment is regurgitated because the schistosome intestine terminates blindly. The rapid metabolic rate of these worms may in part be related to their continual output of large numbers of eggs, estimated at 1400 to 3000 per day for *S. japonicum* and one tenth that number for *S. mansoni*. The eggs of the last-named species are released singly, whereas those of the other two species are deposited in large aggregates. They embryonate over a period of six days and increase in size, reaching a mean of 66 by 155 μ for *S. mansoni*, 60 by 143 μ for *S. haematobium*, and 67 by 89 μ for *S. japonicum*. The shape of the eggs is distinctive, *S. mansoni* being ellipsoidal and having a lateral spine; *S. haematobium*, also ellipsoidal but with a terminal spine; and *S. japonicum*, spheroidal with a tiny knob. The eggs remain viable for approximately 21 days after laying, during which time they must pass out of the body if their life cycle is to be completed. Passage from the blood vessels through the tissues and into the lumen of the excretory organs is apparently facilitated by enzymatic secretions of the eggs plus muscular movements of the gut or bladder. A large proportion of the eggs, however, either remain in the intestinal and vesical tissues or break free in the bloodstream and are carried into the liver and lungs.

The eggs that pass out of the body in feces or urine and reach fresh water hatch rapidly into free-swimming ciliated miracidia. The miracidia of *S. mansoni* are negatively geotropic and positively phototropic, although those of *S. haematobium* appear to be the opposite. Their average life span is about six hours. If during this time a snail is encountered, the organisms may penetrate it, and if it is of the genus *Biomphalaria* for *S. mansoni*, *Bulinus* for *S. haematobium*, or *Oncomelania* for

S. japonicum, the organism can complete its life cycle. The former two snail genera are aquatic, the latter amphibious. The miracidium remains close to the site of penetration, developing into a mother sporocyst. After about ten days daughter sporocysts begin to migrate into the digestive gland of the snail, and at about five weeks from the inception of the process cercariae produced from the daughter sporocysts begin to be shed by the snail. Maximal stimulus for shedding of *S. mansoni* and *haematobium* cercariae is provided by light, but darkness seems to favor the output of *S. japonicum* cercariae. The average daily output of *S. mansoni* and *S. haematobium* cercariae is about 700, but that of *S. japonicum* cercariae is only about two. These organisms may live for two to three days under ideal conditions, but their infectivity is lost by 20 hours; under field conditions both their life span and their infectivity are usually greatly reduced. The fork-tailed schistosome cercariae are about 125 to 200 μ in length by 50 to 75 μ in width. *S. mansoni* and *haematobium* cercariae alternate periods of rest, during which they sink slowly, with periods of movement, during which they rise toward the surface of the water. In contrast, *S. japonicum* cercariae attach themselves to the surface film where they tend to remain at rest. When cercariae encounter mammalian skin, they attach themselves with suckers, and by mechanical means, aided by enzymatic secretions, the heads penetrate, leaving the tails behind. This process occurs during immersion in water or while the skin remains moist (drying kills the organism), and takes four to ten minutes for *S. mansoni,* but only a few seconds to three minutes for *S. japonicum.*

As the worms do not multiply in the mammalian host, each cercaria that penetrates the skin can develop into only one worm. Many cercariae die in the skin, however, and in the best of experimental hosts only about 60 per cent of the *S. mansoni* organisms reach maturity. Within a few hours to days the schistosomula (the cercariae are completely changed both biochemically and physiologically immediately after penetration) migrate to the lungs by either the bloodstream or lymphatics. After a few days in the pulmonary vessels the schistosomula migrate to the liver, largely by the bloodstream. This phase takes ten to twelve days for *S. mansoni,* a somewhat shorter period for *S. japonicum,* and a longer one for *S. haematobium.* Once in the intrahepatic portal venules the worms rapidly reach maturity, mate, and move against the blood flow to their final habitats. Egg output is detectable at five to six weeks for *S. japonicum,* seven to eight weeks for *S. mansoni,* and ten to twelve weeks for *S. haematobium.*

EPIDEMIOLOGY. Initial infection in schistosomiasis usually occurs in childhood, and reinfection may continue as long as there is contact with fresh water. It must be remembered that the worms do not multiply in the human body, that complete immunity apparently does not occur, and that the worms may live for decades. Under these circumstances the incidence of schistosomiasis in endemic areas is low and occurs principally in children, but the prevalence of the disease may build up to massive proportions.

The worldwide prevalence of schistosomiasis is now estimated at over 200,000,000 cases. It is known to be endemic in 71 countries that have a total population of 1,362,635,000.

In Africa, *S. haematobium* and *S. mansoni* are widespread. Only the former species occurs in Tunisia, Algeria, Morocco, Mauritania, Guinea-Bissau, Niger, the Congo Republic (Brazzaville), Somalia, and the island of Mauritius. Both species are found in all other countries, including the Malagasy Republic. Sixty per cent of Africans live in areas where exposure to schistosomes is possible, and 40 per cent of these (about 75,000,000 people) are infected.

In Southwest Asia, *S. haematobium* is endemic in Aden, Saudi Arabia, Yemen, Israel, Iraq, Iran, Syria, Turkey, and Lebanon. *S. mansoni* occurs in the first four of these countries, and is particularly prevalent in Yemen, where half the 3,500,000 population are thought to be infected. The highest prevalence rate for *S. haematobium* occurs in Iraq, where 20 per cent of the exposed population of 5,000,000 are infected. Of the 87,003,000 population of Southwest Asia an estimated 10,745,000 are exposed to infection.

In the Orient, *S. japonicum* occurs in China, Japan, the Philippines, and the Celebes. The prevalence in China was estimated at 32,000,000, but it is reported that this number has been substantially reduced by a recent massive control campaign. Schistosomiasis is under control in Japan, but seems to be spreading in the Philippines. Small foci of schistosomiasis japonica have recently been discovered in Thailand and Laos. Of the 868,531,000 population of Southeast Asia, 337,051,500 are estimated to be exposed. A small focus of *S. haematobium* infection was found in India, in Maharashtra State, but it is now believed that transmission there has ceased.

In endemic areas of the New World (population 98,339,000) where only *S. mansoni* is found, 18,199,750 people are estimated to be exposed. Brazil has the largest number of cases, estimated at 8,000,000, and the infection seems to be spreading. Schistosomiasis also occurs in Venezuela, where it is apparently on the wane, and in Surinam. It is endemic in the following Caribbean islands: Puerto Rico, Vieques, Dominican Republic, Antigua, Guadeloupe, Martinique, and St. Lucia. The parasite has not been found in any of the Central American countries.

The one tiny focus of schistosomiasis in Europe, *S. haematobium* in southern Portugal, has now been eliminated.

The life cycle of schistosomiasis will become established only in areas where there is a susceptible snail species. Thus the infection is prevalent on the West Indian island of St. Lucia, although St. Vincent, 30 miles away, is completely free of the parasite. There are 1,450,000 Puerto Ricans now living on the mainland of the United States, and 100,000 immigrants from other areas endemic for schistosomiasis entering this country each year, but the presence of susceptible snails in the continental United States has not been established. Prevalence rates within endemic areas may be exceedingly variable, ranging from close to 100 per cent in some localities to almost none in others. This is governed by the interaction of multiple local ecologic factors relating to both the snail and human populations. Another important factor in the epidemiology of schistosomiasis is the variation in geographic strains of the species; for example, *S. japonicum* on Formosa is highly infective to domestic and wild animals but not to man, and *S. mansoni* in Africa south of the Sahara appears to be relatively avirulent.

Animal reservoirs are undoubtedly of significance in maintaining the life cycle of *S. japonicum* — in particular, cows and dogs. Natural *S. mansoni* infections have been found in rodents, baboons, insectivores, and dogs in Africa, but it is generally believed that animal reservoirs do not play a significant role in the life cycle of this species. *S. haematobium* is rarely encountered in animals.

Although *transmission patterns* differ among the three species of schistosomes, *there is little question that for each species agricultural development, particularly irrigation, may lead to a marked increase in the prevalence of schistosomiasis.* A major epidemic occurred in Egypt after the construction of the low Aswan dam, and in Rhodesia after development of large scale irrigation schemes.

In regard to morbidity and mortality, precise demographic figures are not available, particularly because schistosomiasis is such an insidious disease. The few investigations of morbidity now available show little or no effect of schistosomiasis on educational attainment or work capacity. Most studies suggest, however, that disease and death in schistosomiasis are correlated with intensity of infection. As the worms do not multiply in man, the number of parasites in a given individual is related to the degree of water contact and perhaps the occurrence of partial immunity. Under these conditions, schistosomes have an overdispersed distribution in which most members of the host population bear low worm burdens. As far as has been determined, little or no morbidity occurs in the large majority of the population carrying infections of low intensity. Though the proportion of heavily infected individuals is small, when this figure is multiplied against the vast number of people with schistosomiasis, it becomes obvious that this helminthic infection constitutes a major medical problem. In addition, there is no question that in all its forms schistosomiasis is potentially lethal — Katayama fever in *S. japonicum* infections, portal hypertension with hematemesis in both schistosomiasis japonica and mansoni, uremia in *S. haematobium* infection, and cor pulmonale in all three. Schistosomiasis may also potentiate the development of other diseases such as hepatitis, hepatoma, cirrhosis, and cancer of the urinary bladder.

PATHOGENESIS AND CLINICAL MANIFESTATIONS. Basic to an understanding of the disease processes in schistosomiasis are these facts: the schistosomes do not multiply in man; complete immunity does not follow initial infection; repeated infections usually occur; the worms are relatively long lived; most individuals have low worm burdens, but large numbers of worms may accumulate; and a large proportion of schistosome eggs are not excreted but remain within the body. Disease is correlated with the intensity of infection and is related not only to the presence of the various stages of the schistosomes in the body tissues and their secretions and excretions, but to the inflammatory responses of the host as well.

Clinically, three distinct syndromes occur at different stages of schistosome infection. Within one day of cercarial penetration, swimmer's itch, a pruritic papular rash, may appear. Several weeks later Katayama fever, a self-limited but possibly fatal illness resembling serum sickness, may develop. Finally, after many years, during which the infection may be either asymptomatic or associated with relatively mild intestinal or urinary tract symptoms, fibrosis of the liver may result in the signs and symptoms of portal hypertension in schistosomiasis mansoni and japonica; fibrosis of the ureters and bladder in schistosomiasis haematobia may result in changes associated with urinary tract obstruction.

Schistosome Dermatitis. Schistosomiasis begins with penetration of the skin by cercariae. These organisms are not discriminating and will penetrate the skin of most animals whether they are susceptible or insusceptible, living or dead. When nonhuman schistosomes, those that complete their life cycle in animals or birds, enter the skin of man, they die. Even in highly susceptible experimental hosts many *S. mansoni* cercariae die in the skin and perhaps in the lung; in the hamster almost 40 per cent are lost in this manner. In the highest primate thus far studied, the chimpanzee, 4 to 8 per cent of *S. mansoni* cercariae, 14 to 40 per cent of *S. haematobium* cercariae, and 1 to 48 per cent of *S. japonicum* cercariae were recovered as adult schistosomes. In most laboratory animals the recovery rate for *S. japonicum* is higher than that for the other two species.

The death of cercariae in the skin leads to the development of a pruritic papular rash known as swimmer's itch. This syndrome occurs in its most severe form after exposure to animal schistosomes, and has been shown to be a sensitization phenomenon, rarely occurring on primary exposure. Papules appear in sensitized persons at 5 to 15 hours, and there is massive round cell invasion of the dermis and epidermis, suggesting a delayed hypersensitivity response. Swimmer's itch has been demonstrated in infected patients experimentally reexposed to *S. mansoni* and *S. haematobium* cercariae. A mild form of swimmer's itch appears to occur in patients exposed to *S. japonicum* cercariae, but the rice paddy dermatitis of the Far East is caused mainly by avian schistosomes.

Katayama Fever. The next clinical phase of schistosomiasis begins 20 to 60 days after exposure and has been known in Japan as Katayama fever since the mid-nineteenth century. This syndrome occurs most frequently and is most severe in *S. japonicum* infections; in schistosomiasis mansoni it is usually found only in patients with very heavy initial infection; it is rarely if ever seen in schistosomiasis haematobia. In addition to fever, the patient suffers from chills, sweating, anorexia, headache, diarrhea, and cough. Hepatosplenomegaly is frequent, and generalized lymphadenopathy and urticaria are often seen. Eosinophilia occurs in most cases, averaging about 40 per cent. The fever may last for several weeks; when it subsides the other signs and symptoms also disappear. Death may occur in the Katayama fever stage of schistosomiasis japonica, but rarely does so in *S. mansoni* infection. At autopsy, massive infection is almost invariably found, with large numbers of eggs in the liver and intestines; 1608 worm pairs were demonstrated at autopsy in a Brazilian child. Katayama fever, which usually appears on initial infection, begins at about the time of onset of egg-laying by the worms; thus large amounts of antigen are suddenly added to moderate levels of cross-reacting antibody formed in response to the developing worms. It is possible, therefore, that this serum sickness–like syndrome may be a form of immune-complex disease.

Chronic Schistosomiasis. A correlation between the number of worms and the development and extent of chronic disease (except for patients with advanced liver fibrosis) was recently demonstrated by techniques quantitating human worm burdens at surgery and at autopsy. Heavy worm burdens were apparently a prerequisite for the development of severe disease, whereas light infections appeared to be of little consequence pathologically. *Thus patients with few worms may never show any signs or symptoms related to schistosome infection.*

It is said that patients with chronic schistosomiasis mansoni or japonica may complain of fatigue, abdominal pain, and intermittent diarrhea or dysentery. Although this may be true in selected hospital populations, recent controlled field studies have revealed few such signs and symptoms, even in heavily infected individuals. On sigmoidoscopy, particularly in Egypt, granulomatous nodules or polyps may be observed. In *S. haematobium* infection, terminal hematuria, and, occasionally, dysuria and frequency are found. Mild chronic blood loss has been measured by radioisotope labeling in both *S. mansoni* and *S. haematobium* infections, but anemia is not usually seen in areas where there is normal iron intake. All the aforementioned signs and symptoms are related to the passage of eggs through the mucosa of the intestine and the urinary bladder.

Many eggs do not, however, leave the body; in laboratory animals less than half of them are excreted. Over a period of 20 years, for each *S. mansoni* worm pair producing eggs at a rate of 300 per day, at least 1,000,000 eggs will remain in the body. This figure can be multiplied by 10 for each *S. japonicum* worm pair.

In *S. mansoni* and *S. japonicum* infections, some of the eggs remain in the intestinal walls, but many of them enter the circulation and are carried into the liver. In schistosomiasis haematobia many eggs remain in the tissues of the bladder and adjacent organs, but some (usually too few to cause significant disease) enter the lungs via the inferior vena cava as well as the liver via the portal system. *Granulomatous inflammation* develops around the eggs trapped in the tissues; in the case of *S. mansoni* this has been demonstrated to be an immunologic response of the delayed hypersensitivity type. Both the eggs and the reactions to them are being constantly resorbed, but if large numbers of eggs gather together, the fibrosis subsequent to inflammation may remain. In schistosomiasis mansoni and japonica this leads to hepatic portal fibrosis, and in schistosomiasis haematobia, to fibrosis of the ureters and bladder.

Hepatosplenic Schistosomiasis. As the liver parenchyma is relatively unharmed by the pathologic processes involved in hepatic schistosomiasis japonica and mansoni, the clinical consequences of the disease relate primarily to granulomatous inflammation and portal fibrosis. Pathophysiologically this results in an intrahepatic block to portal blood flow and the development of portal hypertension and portal-systemic collateral circulation. The lesion is presinusoidal; thus intrasplenic and portal pressures are markedly elevated, whereas wedged hepatic vein pressure is normal. Total liver blood flow tends to remain within normal limits owing to a compensatory increase in arterial flow.

Clinically, the earliest sign of significant liver involvement is hepatomegaly. With progression, the spleen enlarges and becomes firm in consistency. Eventually it may extend to well below the umbilicus. At this point the patient tends to be in good general health, but may consult a physician because of a dragging feeling in the left upper abdominal quadrant.

The other major factor bringing the patient to the physician is a sudden hematemesis because of bleeding esophageal varices. Such an episode may not reappear for many years or may recur at fairly frequent intervals. The consequences of hematemesis in schistosomiasis are very different from those in cirrhosis of the liver: the blood ammonia concentration tends to remain normal, hepatic coma rarely occurs, and mortality is very low, being primarily due to exsanguination. This is consistent with relatively normal liver function. Jaundice is almost never seen in uncomplicated schistosomiasis, and the levels of both conjugated and unconjugated bilirubin are usually normal. Serum albumin concentration is normal or only slightly decreased, and globulin is somewhat elevated. As a consequence, ascites and edema are rarely encountered. Even sulfobromophthalein retention is often normal in these patients. Stigmata of chronic liver disease such as palmar erythema, spider angiomas, altered hair distribution, and gynecomastia are rare. Patients may suffer multiple severe hematemeses; but aside from temporary changes, liver function tends to remain relatively normal.

In spite of moderate chronic and occasional severe acute intestinal blood loss, a significant degree of anemia rarely occurs in uncomplicated schistosomiasis. The white blood count is usually within normal limits, but there is a moderate eosinophilia. Splenomegaly, however, may result in hypersplenism, the patient developing leukopenia, thrombocytopenia, and anemia with decreased red blood cell life span.

Patients with decompensated hepatic disease characterized by liver parenchymal malfunction and all the physical stigmata of this state, including jaundice and ascites, are seen in localities in which schistosomiasis is endemic. This is particularly common in the case of schistosomiasis japonica, and may, perhaps, be related to overwhelming embolization of the liver with the large numbers of eggs produced by this parasite. Pathologists have stated, however, that *it has not been possible to prove the transformation of advanced schistosomal fibrosis into true cirrhosis.* In Egypt it has been suggested that patients with schistosomiasis might concomitantly have other forms of liver disease. Finally, it must be recognized that all those infected with *S. mansoni* and *S. japonicum* perforce have some degree of liver involvement, and that the effect of malnutrition, hepatotoxins, and hepatitis may be potentiated; such interrelationships have been demonstrated in laboratory animals.

Pulmonary Schistosomiasis. Pulmonary schistosomiasis, which in its most severe state is characterized by signs and symptoms of cor pulmonale, is a complication of hepatosplenic schistosomiasis. Portal-systemic collateral circulation enables the eggs to bypass the liver, and they are trapped in the pulmonary capillary bed. Arteritis with angiomatoid formation occurs, and there is obstruction to pulmonary blood flow. Pulmonary hypertension is found in every case, but cardiac output usually remains within the normal range. Arterial oxygen saturation is usually normal, and cyanosis is rare. The lungs are often involved in schistosomiasis haematobia because of the passage of eggs from the vesical plexuses into the inferior vena cava, but egg embolization appears to be relatively light, and significant disease is uncommon.

Urinary Tract Schistosomiasis. Severe urinary tract disease may occur in both the early and late phases of *S. haematobium* infection. Initially there may be ureteral obstruction owing to florid granulomatous inflammatory reactions to the eggs in both the ureters and the bladder; these lesions appear to be highly reversible after antischistosomal therapy. Later in the course of the disease irreversible fibrosis may supervene. Bladder fibrosis and calcification lead to frequency and dysuria. On cystoscopy, so-called sandy patches may be seen on the bladder walls; these are made up of large numbers of schistosome eggs. The disease may progress through hydronephrosis, secondary infection, and finally uremia. An association between cancer of the bladder and urinary schistosomiasis has been demonstrated.

In the past decade there has been a growing impression among Brazilian clinicians and pathologists that there is an increased frequency of renal disease in patients with schistosomiasis mansoni. Initially proteinuria was noted in patients with hepatosplenic schistosomiasis, and then, at autopsy, the renal glomeruli of similar patients were found to have pathologic changes. This was followed by ultrastructural and immunocytochemical studies which revealed electron-dense deposits in the glomerular basement membranes which contained immunoglobulins. Similar deposits have been observed in laboratory animals. It should be pointed out, however, that specific schistosomal antigen has not been demonstrated as yet, and comparable lesions have been found in the kidneys of patients with cirrhosis of the liver.

Central Nervous System Schistosomiasis. Schistosomiasis of the central nervous system, although relatively rare, is an important complication of the infection. *S. japonicum* usually involves the brain, whereas *S. mansoni* and *S. haematobium* tend to affect the spinal cord. Schistosomiasis japonica is reputed to be one of the important causes of focal epilepsy in the Far East. The disease may also present as a space-occupying lesion or occasionally as a generalized encephalitis. Cerebral schistosomiasis japonica may appear at any time in the course of infection from the first three weeks on. At autopsy the lesions almost always consist of large collections of eggs in the venous circulatory system, suggesting the presence of adult worms, although they have never been found. *S. mansoni* and *S. haematobium* in the spinal cord may be associated with a transverse myelitis-like syndrome; at surgery or autopsy large granulomas made up of eggs are usually found.

The development of chronic salmonellosis has been described in schistosomiasis in both man and laboratory animals. In the latter, schistosomiasis has also been associated with increased severity of viral hepatitis and intestinal amebiasis.

DIAGNOSIS. When schistosomiasis is considered as a diagnosis in nonendemic areas, the first question that should be asked is: "Where have you been?" It must then be determined whether there was contact with fresh water, whether transient pruritus was observed soon thereafter, and if there was a febrile episode several weeks later. For schistosomiasis mansoni and japonica, abdominal symptoms and signs might be considered, and for *S. haematobium* infection, terminal hematuria, dysuria, and frequency are important. The presence of eosinophilia is a useful sign of schistosome infection. A wide variety of serologic tests (e.g., complement-fixation, flocculation, fluorescent antibody,

and circumoval precipitin) and a skin test of the immediate type are available. *These immunologic methods, which are all based on detection of circulating antibody, essentially have no place in the diagnosis of the individual case,* as cross-reactions with other parasitic infections providing false-positive results are relatively common; false-negative reactions also occur.

Definitive diagnosis can be made only by finding schistosome eggs in the excreta (feces or urine) or in a biopsy specimen — usually rectal. Eggs may not be present in the early stages of acute schistosomiasis. Schistosome eggs are relatively large, and are easy to identify because of their distinctive shape. Direct fecal smear is too insensitive, but techniques which provide both concentration and quantitation of eggs in the feces have been developed. This is important, because correlations between egg output and intensity of infection have been made. The Kato thick smear technique is a simple and highly effective method for fecal egg counting. A small portion of stool (schistosome eggs are distributed randomly in feces) is passed through 105-mesh stainless steel bolting cloth (W. S. Tyler Co., Cleveland, Ohio) and 50 mg is added to a tared glass slide and covered with a cellophane cover slip (no. 124PD, E. I. DuPont de Nemours, Inc., Film Department, Wilmington, Delaware) impregnated with 50 per cent glycerin. The slides are inverted and pressed onto a bed of filter paper, turned face up, and left for a period of at least 48 hours during which the fecal matter clears. Although the embryo within the egg also clears, the characteristic shape of the egg shell can be easily seen. After counting all the eggs in the sample, multiplication by 20 provides the number of eggs per gram of feces.

Rectal biopsy is a highly efficient method for the diagnosis of *S. mansoni* and *japonicum* infection, and will often help detect *S. haematobium* eggs. Through a proctoscope, snips are taken from the valves of Houston (8 to 10 cm from the anus), pressed between glass slides, and examined immediately under a microscope. Sometimes only opaque dead eggs are observed, suggesting a burnt-out or successfully treated infection. Liver biopsy has been suggested as a means of diagnosis, but will only rarely detect an infection not revealed by the aforementioned methods.

For the diagnosis of schistosomiasis haematobia, urine is collected at midday, because a diurnal variation in egg output has been demonstrated. The urine specimen is centrifuged and the sediment examined. For quantitative data a 10 ml aliquot of urine collected between 1100 and 1300 hours is passed through a Nuclepore Filter (13 mm in diameter with a pore size of 10 μm) held in a PT-013 chamber (Nuclepore Corp., Pleasanton, California). The filter is removed, placed face down on a microscope slide, and examined immediately at $\times$ 40 magnification, and the terminal-spined eggs are counted. *S. mansoni* eggs are occasionally found in urine.

For determining the severity of intestinal disease, sigmoidoscopy and barium enema are of value. The extent of liver disease may be estimated by liver biopsy, barium swallow, esophagoscopy, and especially splenoportography with measurement of intrasplenic pressure. In schistosomiasis haematobia, cystoscopy and intravenous pyelography are useful techniques.

TREATMENT. Antischistosomal treatment should never be instituted without proof of infection by the demonstration of living eggs in excreta or biopsy specimens, except in the rare case of suspected schistosomiasis of the central nervous system. A positive serologic or skin test does not provide a definitive diagnosis. Complete cure is not necessary and indeed is not always desirable in schistosomiasis (particularly in endemic areas where reinfection may occur), because disease is related to intensity of infection, surviving worms do not multiply, and immunity may be premunitive, i.e., dependent on the presence of living organisms. The recent use of quantitative egg counts has shown that in cases in which cure is not achieved by the full course of treatment with an established drug, egg output is usually reduced by over 90 per cent. Thus striving for cure by increasing the drug dosage or repeating the course of treatment is rarely necessary and, because of the toxicity of the antischistosomal drugs, may actually be harmful.

None of the drugs now available for human use have any effect on the schistosomes during their early migratory phases in the body (the first three to six weeks), thus rendering it difficult to treat Katayama fever; steroids have been used to suppress the clinical manifestations during this stage of the infection. The three schistosome species vary considerably in their response to drugs, *S. haematobium* being the most susceptible and *S. japonicum* the most resistant. Under these circumstances it is generally stated that it is still necessary to treat schistosomiasis japonica with the highly toxic antimony potassium tartrate (tartar emetic). In a 1972 report of a World Health Organization consultant group, however, it was noted that the cure rates in *S. japonicum* infections with tartar emetic, stibocaptate (Astiban), and niridazole (Ambilhar), respectively, ranged between 40 and 75, 40 and 75, and 40 and 70 per cent. Thus it can be recommended that those infected with any of the three species of human schistosomes be treated with niridazole or stibocaptate, the latter when there are signs or symptoms of liver or cerebral disease. Both these drugs may be obtained from the Parasitic Disease Drug Service of the Center for Disease Control, Atlanta, Georgia 30333. Particularly in the case of *S. mansoni* infections, it would not be unreasonable to withhold treatment with these drugs in asymptomatic individuals with very low egg counts.

Niridazole is administered orally in two divided doses totaling 25 mg per kilogram of body weight daily, for a period of five to seven days. Vomiting, diarrhea, cramps, and dizziness may occur. Side effects are greatly exacerbated in patients with signs and symptoms of liver or cerebral disease. Under these circumstances stibocaptate can be substituted; this antimony compound is administered intramuscularly in a dose of 8 mg per kilogram once per week for five weeks. Antimony compounds are cardiotoxic; stibocaptate is also associated with anorexia, vomiting, abdominal pain, headache, and pain at the site of injection. Recently good success has been reported in treating human *Schistosoma mansoni* infections in Brazil with a new drug, oxamniquine. Relatively nontoxic, it is given in a single oral dose for adults of 15 mg per kilogram of body weight. Further research will establish the importance of this compound.

Utilizing a combination of surgery and a single dose of antischistosomal drug, many of the worms can be sieved out of the bloodstream. Although such extracorporeal hemofiltration is a valuable research tool, it should never be used as a form of treatment.

In general, the surgical treatment of schistosomiasis should be approached with caution. Many of the apparently irreversible lesions of urinary tract schistosomiasis will resolve completely after antischistosomal treatment, particularly in young patients. Cerebral schistosomiasis japonica is frequently cured or markedly ameliorated by drug therapy. Finally, prophylactic portacaval shunts should never be performed in hepatosplenic schistosomiasis, because hematemesis is not invariable and is unpredictable in onset, and, when it occurs, mortality is low. If the creation of shunt by surgery is necessitated by repeated bleeding episodes, splenorenal anastomosis is preferable to portacaval shunt because of a much lower incidence of chronic portal systemic encephalopathy. Prior to shunting, however, antischistosomal therapy is necessary to prevent prolonged passage of eggs into the lungs which may lead to the development of cor pulmonale.

PROGNOSIS. The prognosis is usually good. Many patients with schistosomiasis never have symptoms or signs of disease, or have only relatively mild ones. Epidemiologically, both the infection and the disease reach their peak in early adult life and decline with age. Disregarding the factor of death among heavily infected patients, this may be due to decreased exposure to infection, gradual death of the worms, slow development of immunity, and diminution in the inflammatory response to the parasite and its products.

The early stages of hepatic or urinary tract disease appear to be reversible after antischistosomal therapy. Although late disease seems relatively irreversible, progression may be halted and gradual improvement may follow drug therapy. In hepatosplenic schistosomiasis the prognosis in patients suffering a hematemesis is far better than in those with cirrhosis, because the former do not tend to go into hepatic coma. Patients with cerebral schistosomiasis japonica may show remarkable improvement after antischistosome therapy.

PREVENTION. On the individual level, schistosomiasis may be prevented by avoidance of contaminated waters. If this is not possible, boots should be worn; if contaminated water reaches the skin, rapid drying or rubbing with alcohol will prevent infection. Storage of water for several days will ensure the death of cercariae, as will the boiling of drinking water. Sea water is safe for swimming, although the mouths of rivers and streams should be avoided; chlorination of swimming pools will prevent infection. Repellents are of no great value, and vaccines or prophylactic drugs are not available.

There are three approaches to the control of schistosomiasis on a mass basis: (1) destruction of the snail intermediate host, (2) prevention of snail infection by the treatment of human infection and the construction of privies, and (3) elimination of contact with contaminated water by the provision of safe water supplies. Destruction of the snail is primarily based on the use of molluscicides such as the various copper salts, sodium pentachlorophenate, Bayluscide, and n-trityl-morpholone. Molluscicides, however, are quickly inactivated by sunlight and adsorption to mud and organic matter; they pass rapidly through running water or are diluted in vast bodies of still water, and they often destroy other aquatic fauna and flora. Also, although molluscicides may appear to be highly effective, only a few surviving snails can rapidly repopulate an area. Many biologic control measures have been advocated, including the use of nonsusceptible snail species which may compete for miracidia, food, and space; snail-eating fish and ducks; and snail pathogens. None of these measures has shown outstanding promise. The snails that transmit *S. japonicum* are amphibious and are frequently found along the banks of water courses; their eradication can necessitate the use of earth-moving equipment and flame throwers. When the snails are "buried" in this way, as in the campaigns in the People's Republic of China, it appears to reduce the infectivity of the environment.

An attempt to break the life cycle at the stage of transmission from man to the snail has been hampered by the lack of practical mass therapy. The recent development of effective oral drugs and of a single-dose intramuscular drug offers great promise for the future. An important adjunct to this approach is the construction of privies. Breaking the cycle at the stage of transmission from the snail to man can be accomplished by the provision of safe water supplies for washing and recreational purposes.

Control measures based on the destruction of snails are an end in themselves, and in addition may be inimical to the environment. In contrast, mass antischistosomal treatment coupled with the construction of privies or the provision of safe water supplies should contribute greatly to the general health of the population.

Arap Siongok, T. K., Mahmoud, A. A. F., Ouma, J. H., Warren, K. S., Muller, A. S., Handa, A. K., and Houser, H. B.: Morbidity in schistosomiasis mansoni in relation to intensity of infection: Study of a community in Machakos, Kenya. Am. J. Trop. Med. Hyg., 25:273, 1976.

Cheever, A. W., Kamel, I. A., Elwi, A. M., Mosimann, J. E., and Danner, R.: *Schistosoma mansoni* and *S. haematobium* infections in Egypt: II. Quantitative parasitological findings at necropsy. Am. J. Trop. Med. Hyg., 26:702, 1977.

Clark, W. D., Cox, P. M., Jr., Ratner, L. H., and Correa-Coronas, R.: Acute schistosomiasis mansoni in 10 boys. An outbreak in Caguas, Puerto Rico. Ann. Intern. Med., 73:379, 1970.

Lehman, J. S., Jr., Farid, Z., Smith, J. H., Bassily, S., and El-Masry, N. A.: Urinary schistosomiasis in Egypt: Clinical, radiological, bacteriological and parasitological correlations. Trans. R. Soc. Trop. Med. Hyg., 67:384, 1973.

Warren, K. S.: Regulation of the prevalence and intensity of schistosomiasis in man. Immunology or ecology? J. Infect. Dis., 127:595, 1973.

Warren, K. S.: Schistosomiasis: A multiplicity of immunopathology. J. Invest. Dermatol., 67:464, 1976.

Warren, K. S., Rebouças, G., and Baptista, A. G.: Ammonia metabolism and hepatic coma in hepatosplenic schistosomiasis. Patients studied before and after portacaval shunt. Ann. Intern. Med., 62:1113, 1965.

WHO Reports on Schistosomicidal Drugs. II. Report of a WHO consultant group on the comparative evaluation of new schistosomicidal drugs for use in treatment campaigns. Bol. Of. Sanit. Panam. (English), 6:89, 1972.

211. HERMAPHRODITIC FLUKES

Philip D. Marsden

211.1. INTRODUCTION

The hermaphroditic flukes, unlike *Schistosoma* flukes, have both sets of sex organs in the same worm, and frequently self-fertilization occurs. These flukes are flat leaflike worms with oral and ventral suckers. They have a complex life cycle. The egg hatches to produce a motile ciliated *miracidium*, which penetrates the soft tissue of a snail and undergoes a cycle of development similar to that in schistosomiasis. *Cercariae* are produced by the snail after a few weeks, but unlike schistosomes these cercariae encyst in a second intermediate host, either fish, crab, or plant. These encysted cercariae or *metacercariae* are a relatively resistant form which can survive adverse conditions. If the metacercaria is then ingested by man, it hatches to produce an immature fluke which migrates through the body tissues to gain its site of final development. This varies with the species concerned, being the liver for *Clonorchis* and *Fasciola*, the lung for *Paragonimus*, and the intestine for *Fasciolopsis buski*. None of these trematodes are principally human parasites, and they show different degrees of adaptation to man.

Initial invasion is often accompanied by eosinophilia, but it takes a month or longer before the characteristic eggs are produced. All the eggs have an operculum or lid through which the miracidia escape, unlike *Schistosoma* eggs. Some of these flukes live for a long time, producing progressive damage in the tissues of the host. When searching for the ova of trematodes in the biliary tree, duodenal aspiration may be more rewarding than stool examination. Therapy, especially in the hepatic hermaphroditic trematodes, is unsatisfactory.

Skah, S. K. K.: Digenetic trematodes. Clin. Gastroenterol., 7:87, 1978.

211.2. HEPATIC HERMAPHRODITIC FLUKES

CLONORCHIASIS (CLONORCHIS SINENSIS). Man is infected by eating the flesh of undercooked or raw freshwater fish in which the metacercariae are encysted. More than 40 species of fish, mainly of the carp and salmon (cyprinoid) group, have been found to harbor metacercariae. The natural definitive hosts other than man are fish-eating mammals, including cats, dogs, mink, and rats. Widespread in the Far East, the main endemic areas of human infection are Japan, Korea, China, and Vietnam. As the flukes live for decades (20 to 30 years) in the biliary tree, immigrants from Asia have been found infested in many countries. A portion of the Chinese in New York and San Francisco are infected. Infections recorded in Hawaiians are attributed to imports of infected frozen, dried, or pickled fish from Japan.

It appears that most of the larval flukes ascend the biliary tree directly from the duodenum, but some may pass via the portal circulation to the liver. They mature in the bile ducts, and the grayish-brown adults, measuring 10 to 20 mm by 2 to 4 mm, move sluggishly around by means of their suckers in the distal biliary passages. They feed on secretions from the mucosa of the bile duct and possibly also on cellular elements. Occasionally they gain access to the gallbladder and pancreatic ducts. In effect they cause a chronic cholangitis with inflammation of the biliary tree, proliferation of the biliary epithelium, and progressive portal fibrosis. The severity of these changes depends upon the load of flukes.

After ingesting the metacercariae, the patient may present with epigastric pain, malaise, and tender hepatomegaly. An eosinophilia is usually present in the early stages, but no eggs can be found until about one month has passed and the flukes have matured. Light infections are often asymptomatic, but a firm liver edge is often discovered within the costal margin on routine examination. In an Asian, this finding should prompt a careful search for ova in the stool. In heavy infections (10,000 to 20,000 flukes), more serious sequelae occur. The marked portal fibrosis may be associated with signs of portal hypertension. Extension of the fibrosis into the liver parenchyma may be associated with liver cell death and fatty change. Jaundice is more likely to be associated with biliary obstruction owing to a mass of flukes or stone formation. Cholangiocarcinoma is a late complication of severe clonorchiasis, a metaplastic change occurring in the irritated biliary epithelium. In Hong Kong there is a high incidence in males after the fourth decade, the adenocarcinomas showing varying degrees of differentiation. Suppurative cholangitis and chronic pancreatitis are other complications.

The diagnosis is made by finding the eggs in the stool. Unfortunately they are not characteristic and can be easily confused with a number of other trematodes producing small, similar eggs (Heterophyes, Opisthorchis, Metagonimus). The eggs average 29 by 16 μ; they are light brown and ovoid. There is a definite shoulder in the shell wall near the operculum and a boss at the anopercular end.

The invasive stage must be distinguished from that of other fluke infections, visceral larval migrans, and hepatic amebiasis. The last-named condition is not associated with eosinophilia. The late stages may resemble cirrhosis and uncomplicated cholecystitis. Hypoglycemic coma can also be a manifestation of a hepatocellular carcinoma. In the elderly, repeated nonparasitic cholangitis is sometimes a difficult diagnosis to establish in patients with pyrexia of unknown origin.

Treatment and Prevention. Most investigators agree that the drugs available for treating this infection are often ineffective and disappointing. In those patients who have no symptoms, no treatment is advised. Prolonged chloroquine therapy is chiefly suppressive; however, it is still the drug of choice. Chloroquine diphosphate in a dose of 300 mg base (two 250 mg tablets) three times a day for three to six weeks is a standard course. Some workers have increased this dose or used it for periods of up to a year. Various percentages of cures are claimed, but it depends on the criteria used and especially on what stool concentration technique is employed and how frequently. At the higher dosage levels the more severe side effects of chloroquine toxicity may be seen, namely, corneal deposits and retinopathy, central nervous system changes (a parkinsonian-like syndrome), dyspigmentation, cardiac arrhythmias, and peripheral myopathy and neuropathy. The compound hexachloroparaxylol proved effective, but alarming toxicity tests in studies in laboratory animals have resulted in its withdrawal. Biliary obstruction may require surgical relief, and at surgery as many flukes as possible should be removed from the biliary tree. Prevention of this infection relates to the competent cooking of freshwater fish.

OPISTHORCHIASIS (OPISTHORCHIS VIVERRINI AND FELINEUS). Opisthorchis felineus is prevalent in the Philippines, India, Japan, and Vietnam, as well as in the U.S.S.R. and parts of Eastern Europe, whereas Opisthorchis viverrini is common in north Thailand and Laos.

The life cycles of these flukes are similar to that of Clonorchis sinensis and are completed in about four months under favorable conditions. Snails are infected by fecal contaminants of water from infected persons or animal reservoirs, e.g., cats. In northeast Thailand 90 per cent of people more than ten years of age are infected with O. viverrini, and 3.5 million in the whole country. With all infections of this type, as might be expected, the incidence rises with age. The source of infection is a popular dish of raw fish, rice, vegetables, and spices.

The pathologic findings are similar to those in Clonorchis sinensis, although stone formation is said to be unusual. Cholangiocarcinoma has also been reported to be associated with this infection. The eggs are indistinguishable from Clonorchis. This emphasizes the importance of a geographic history, for the only other way of distinguishing the parasite would be by examination of the adult flukes. Percutaneous transhepatic cholangiography may reveal radiologic changes such as a single cystic cavity or mulberry-like dilatation of the intrahepatic bile ducts.

DICROCOELIASIS. Dicrocoelium dendriticum is acquired by eating ants in which the metacercariae have developed following ingestion by the ant of slime balls containing cercariae secreted by the snail. Infections are generally uncommon, but occur in Europe and Asia and around the Mediterranean basin. Being light infections, their main importance is for the physician to recognize the small, fully embryonated thick-shelled eggs (40 μ by 25 μ) for what they are. Spurious parasitism, in which nonhuman species ingested in liver pass through the bowel unchanged, is well documented.

FASCIOLIASIS (FASCIOLA HEPATICA). This is also a biliary fluke, but it is less well adapted to man than is Clonorchis sinensis. It is a common parasite of sheep, producing marked liver damage. Worldwide in distribution in sheep, it is prevalent in low wet pastures where suitable species of snails are indigenous. The metacercariae encyst on plants, and man is infected mainly as a result of eating wild watercress and other plants gathered in these pastures. Human infections are more common where such salad is favored, e.g., Europe, Cuba, and Chile. In England outbreaks are associated with particularly wet summers.

The adult fluke is large, 2 to 3 cm in length by 0.8 to 1.3 cm in breadth, and may occlude the common bile duct. Indeed, many human infections have been first recognized at surgery for biliary obstruction. Again an invasive stage of fever, eosinophilia, and hepatomegaly is associated with larval flukes moving through the liver substance to gain the biliary tract, for the larval flukes produced from the metacercariae in the jejunum pass across the peritoneal cavity to pierce Glisson's capsule and move through the liver substance. Far fewer flukes than Clonorchis are found in man, but again hyperplasia, necrosis, and cystic dilation of the biliary tract, accompanied by leukocytic infiltration and eventually periportal fibrosis, can ensue if the load of flukes is heavy enough. The differential diagnosis is similar to that of clonorchiasis.

The diagnosis depends on finding large yellowish operculate eggs 130 to 150 μ in length in the feces or aspirated bile. Liver should be excluded from the patient's diet in areas where raw liver is eaten, because eggs in such livers will pass through the intestinal tract unchanged. A complement-fixation test using an extract of the adult fluke as antigen is a useful diagnostic aid, especially in infections in which the flukes are ectopic. A hemagglutination test has also been developed.

Unlike the other hepatic hermaphroditic flukes. *Fasciola hepatica* and the closely allied *Fasciola gigantica* are occasionally found in sites other than the liver. This could be related to man's being a relatively poor host species. Thus a migrating subcutaneous swelling associated with intense eosinophilia may contain such an immature fluke, and there are records of occurrences in many sites, including the brain.

A further oddity associated with *Fasciola hepatica* infection is the parasitization of the pharynx by young post-metacercarial flukes which are acquired by eating raw liver in which the young flukes are actively migrating. This occurs in Lebanon, where such raw sheep and goat livers are eaten; the patient complains of intense inflammation of the back of the throat. This syndrome of parasitic pharyngitis, known as halzoun, can also be produced by a leech or a pentosomid (a worm-like arthropod).

Bithionol,* a drug used for *Paragonimus,* has replaced emetine and chloroquine for initial therapy. It is given in an oral dose of 30 to 50 mg per kilogram on alternate days for 10 to 15 doses.

Ectopic flukes are removed surgically.

Clonorchiasis

Hou, P. C.: The relationship between primary carcinoma of the liver and infestation with *Clonorchis sinensis*. J. Pathol., 72:239, 1956.
Komiya, L.: Clonorchis and clonorchiasis. *In* Dawes, B. (ed.): Advances in Parasitology. London, Academic Press, 1966, Vol. 4, pp. 53–106.
Viranuvatti, V., and Stitnimankam, T.: Liver fluke infection and infestation in South East Asia. *In* Popper, H., and Schaffner, F. (eds.): Progress in Liver Disease, Vol. 4. New York, Grune & Stratton, 1972, pp. 537–547.
Weng, H. C., Chung, H. L., Ho, L. Y., and Hou, T. C.: Studies in *Clonorchis sinensis* in the past 10 years. Chin. Med. J. (Peking), 80:441, 1960.

Opisthorchiasis

Harinasuta, C.: Opisthorchiasis in Thailand: A review. *In* Harinasuta, C. (ed.): Proceedings of the Fourth Southeast Asian Seminar on Parasitology and Tropical Medicine: Schistosomiasis and Other Snail-Transmitted Helminthiases. Manila, 1969, pp. 177–199.

Fascioliasis

Hardman, E. W., Jones, R. L. H., and Davies, A. H.: Fascioliasis — a large outbreak. Br. Med. J., 3:502, 1970.
Khalil, G. M., and Schacher, J. F.: *Linguatula serrata* in relation to halzoun and the Marrara syndrome. Am. J. Trop. Med., 14:736, 1965.
Neghume, A., and Ossandan, M.: Ectopic and hepatic fascioliasis. Am. J. Trop. Med., 23:545, 1943.
Pantelouris, E. M.: The Common Liver Fluke. Oxford, Pergamon Press, 1964.

211.3. LUNG HERMAPHRODITIC FLUKES

(Paragonimiasis)

Although *Paragonimus westermani* is the most common species of this group infecting man, recently a number of other human pathogens have been recognized in the genus *Paragonimus,* which to date numbers more than 31 species. These include *P. africanus* found in Nigeria, the Cameroons, and the Congo, and two new Chinese flukes, *P. skrjabini* and *P. heterotremus. P. westermani* is widely distributed in the Far East, occur-

ring as an important human infection in China, Japan, Vietnam, Korea, Formosa, the Philippines, and Thailand. Species also occur in South America in Peru, Colombia, Ecuador, and Venezuela.

Paragonimiasis is a chronic lung infection of man caused by this group of flukes, the adults living in cystic spaces in the lung. Reddish-brown plump oval flukes, they resemble in size a coffee bean (0.8 to 1.6 cm long by 0.4 to 0.8 cm wide). They are covered with little spines and live singly or in pairs in the lung parenchyma, feeding on host exudates. They live five to six years usually. Oval yellowish-brown operculated ova (85 μ by 35 μ) are coughed up in thick, blood-stained sputum. These hatch to produce a miracidium which invades specific snails. The cercariae subsequently produced by these snails encyst as metacercariae in the muscles and viscera of freshwater crabs. Man acquires the infection by eating the crabs raw or partly cooked. The larval flukes released from the metacercariae usually migrate to the lung via the peritoneal cavity, penetrating the diaphragm, but may mature in the abdomen or brain.

For many species man is not the definitive host, felines being preferred. For instance, other hosts apart from man for *P. westermani* are cats, tigers, leopards, mink, badgers, dogs, lions, and rats. *P. westermani* was discovered by Westerman in 1877 in a tiger in the Amsterdam zoo.

PATHOGENESIS AND PATHOLOGY. The larval fluke tunnels into the lung at the periphery. There is an inflammatory reaction around it with many eosinophils. Later it forms a cystic space with a fibrous tissue wall. These cysts usually communicate with a bronchus and often become secondarily infected with abscess formation. Death of the fluke is often followed by calcification. Ova may be reaspirated, with an eosinophilic inflammatory response and the formation of small lung granulomas.

Although the target organ for *Paragonimus* is the lung, it must be realized that often adults go astray, and if the invading species is one less adapted to man, this is more liable to happen. Thus a characteristic feature of *P. skrjabini* infection is migrating subcutaneous nodules that contain active flukes. Such granulomas in the subcutaneous tissue may require excision as in fascioliasis.

In the brain the temporal and occipital lobes are occasionally the site of an eosinophilic granuloma containing flukes and, in a few cases, ova. A transverse myelitis is known. Flukes in the peritoneal cavity produce adhesions and abscesses, and ulceration of the intestine occurs with ova in the stool. Adult and mature flukes have been found in many other organs, including intestine, spermatic cord, testis and scrotum, vagina, and muscles.

CLINICAL MANIFESTATIONS. Lung infections are encountered with symptoms of persistent hemoptysis, breathlessness on exertion, pleural pain, and recurrent pulmonary infections. The condition is known as endemic hemoptysis. Clubbing of the fingers is common, and persistent rales may be heard over the affected lung segments as in nonparasitic bronchiectasis. A lung abscess may be present. Pneumothorax, pleural effusion, and empyema are rarer complications. Chest films early in the disease show infiltrations, but later dense nodular opacities or ring shadows indicate the site of the cysts. Pleural adhesions and calcification are late

*Available from Center for Disease Control (404-633-3311, Ext. 3670).

signs. Coexistent pulmonary tuberculosis occurs in some patients. There are rarely more than 20 parasites in the lungs.

It has been estimated that there were 5000 cases of cerebral paragonimiasis in South Korea in January 1968. Cerebral paragonimiasis may present signs of a space-occupying lesion with epilepsy and paresis of varying degrees. Ophthalmic signs are optic atrophy associated with papilledema or direct involvement with the inflammatory process. The cerebrospinal fluid shows a raised protein, and eosinophils are present. There may be calcifications present on skull roentgenograms; pneumoencephalography may show the site of a pseudotumor. Abdominal paragonimiasis is a difficult condition to diagnose, but an abdominal mass in a patient with lung disease should raise this suspicion.

DIAGNOSIS. This rests mainly on finding ova in the sputum. One third of patients also have ova in the stools because of swallowed sputum or a coincidental intestinal lesion. Complement-fixation tests are useful, and positive results correlate closely with an active infection. Yokogawa has treated patients on this basis alone. The intradermal test remains positive for a long while after active infection and is not a reliable guide. Work goes on defining the antigenic structure of the parasite. The extent to which the *Paragonimus* antigen cross-reacts with other flukes is not clear.

Pulmonary paragonimiasis may resemble bronchiectasis, lung abscess, bronchial carcinoma, or — most important of all — pulmonary tuberculosis. Cerebral paragonimiasis mimics other space-occupying lesions but especially other helminths in the brain. These include *Fasciola*, *Schistosoma japonicum*, *Angiostrongylus cantonensis*, and hydatid.

PROGNOSIS. Fatalities are rare, and lung lesions resolve spontaneously in five to ten years. Cerebral involvement may be associated with persistent epilepsy. Two per cent of the cases of lung paragonimiasis are complicated by pulmonary tuberculosis.

TREATMENT. Bithionol* (Actamer, Biton) is 2,2'-thiobis(4,6-dichlorophenol) and is given orally in a dose of 30 to 50 mg per kilogram of body weight on alternate days for 10 to 15 doses. Skin reactions and gastrointestinal irritation are rarely severe enough to interrupt treatment. Results are far superior to those obtained with chloroquine or emetine drugs used in the past. Granulomas containing *Paragonimus* adults and ova may require surgical removal from the skin, testis, abdominal organs, or brain.

PREVENTION. It might be thought that it would be a simple matter to dissuade people from eating raw, fresh salted, pickled, or imperfectly cooked crabs and crayfish, but such local delicacies are not easily relinquished. Drunken crab, a favorite dish, involves immersing live crabs in alcohol prior to consumption. In Korea and West Africa, fresh crab juice is used as a home remedy in the treatment of measles.

Chang, H. T., Wang, C. W., Yü, C. F., Hsü, C. F., and Fang, J. C.: Paragonimiasis, a clinical study of 200 adult cases. Chin. Med. J., 77:3, 1958.

Grados, O. B., Cuba, C. C., Morales, F. N., and Mazabel, T. C.: Epidemiologia de la paragonimiasis en el Peru. Arch. Peruanos Pat. Clin., 26:33, 1972.

Miyazaki, I.: Lung Flukes in the Western Hemisphere. Tokyo, Overseas Technical Cooperation Agency, 1972.

Nwokolo, C.: Endemic paragonimiasis in Eastern Nigeria. Clinical fea-

tures and epidemiology of the recent outbreak following the Nigerian Civil War. Trop. Geogr. Med., 24:138, 1972.

Yokogawa, M.: Paragonimus and paragonimiasis. In Dawes, B. (ed.): Advances in Parasitology. London, Academic Press, 1969, Vol. 7, pp. 375–387.

Yokogawa, S., Cort, W. W., and Yokogawa, M.: Paragonimus and paragonimiasis. Exp. Parasitol., 10:81, 139, 1960.

Yokogawa, M., Okawa, T., Tsuji, M., Iwasaki, M., and Shigeyasu, M.: Chemotherapy of paragonimiasis with bithionol. III. The follow-up studies for 1 year after treatment with bithionol. Jap. J. Parasit., 11:103, 1962.

211.4.   INTESTINAL HERMAPHRODITIC FLUKES

FASCIOLOPSIASIS
(Fasciolopsis Buski)

Fasciolopsis buski is a large fleshy fluke, 3 cm long and 1.2 cm wide. It is found mainly in China but also in India, Indonesia, Thailand, Malaya, and Taiwan, normally as an intestinal parasite of pigs. The eggs are passed in the feces, and miracidia are released to penetrate a snail. The cercariae subsequently produced encyst as metacercariae on edible water plants called water caltrop or water chestnuts. The tubers and fruits of these plants are eaten fresh and raw from July to September and as they are peeled with the teeth, people are easily infected. The ponds are often fertilized with night soil or contaminated by pigs.

Most infections are asymptomatic, but foci of inflammation may occur at the site of attachment of the worms in the small intestine. In heavy infections abdominal pain may simulate a peptic ulcer, and there may be alternating diarrhea and constipation. A recent investigation does not suggest that malabsorption occurs. Intestinal stasis, ulceration, and even obstruction have occurred. Several thousand worms may be harbored by the patient, and in severe cases, especially in children, edema of the face and trunk has been described. The mechanism of this edema may be complex, as anemia and hypoproteinemia from blood loss in the bowel are possible. Definite allergic edemas do not appear to be reported in the literature, but there is a variable eosinophilia with heavy loads. Ascites and death from exhaustion are rare.

DIAGNOSIS. Diagnosis depends on finding the characteristic eggs in the stool. These are large, 130 to 140 μ by 80 to 85 μ, yellowish, and rather similar to *Fasciola* but with a smaller operculum. Occasionally an adult fluke may be vomited or passed in the stool. Facial edema may raise the question of differentiating fasciolopsiasis from trichinosis or the nephrotic syndrome.

THERAPY. The old cheap anthelmintics are effective, such as tetrachloroethylene* in a dose of 0.1 ml per kilogram body weight or hexylresorcinol in an adult dose of 1 gram. Since these are difficult to obtain now, piperazine (see Ch. 213.8) or bephenium hydroxynaphthoate (5-gram oral dose for adults) can be used. Not all flukes may be eradicated, but the therapy can be repeated after a few days. Prevention entails cooking the offending plants, eradicating snails with molluscicides, and preventing fecal contamination of ponds.

---

*Available from Center for Disease Control (404-633-3311, Ext. 3670).

*Not available in the United States except as a veterinarian product, Nema worm caps.

OTHER INTESTINAL HERMAPHRODITIC FLUKES

Two very small intestinal flukes—*Heterophyes heterophyes* and *Metagonimus yokogawai*—deserve mention. The former is found in Egypt, Tunisia, South China, India, and the Philippines, and the latter occurs in the Far East and Indonesia. Both are acquired by eating raw or inadequately cooked fish that contain the respective metacercariae. The adult flukes, 2 to 3 mm long, are attached to the mucosa of the small intestine and are alleged to produce superficial inflammation and ulceration. Usually they are not present in sufficient numbers to produce symptoms. Very rarely eggs may gain access to the circulation and be found in internal organs. Usually they are passed in the stool and closely resemble *Clonorchis* eggs, which is perhaps their main importance. Both species can be treated with tetrachloroethylene as used for hookworm. Many species of the genus *Echinostoma* can also infect man in the Far East, but again rarely produce symptoms. Their eggs resemble those of *Fasciola* but are smaller. *Gastrodiscoides hominis* is a fascinating fluke with a large ventral sucker. Like the others, it can produce diarrhea. It occurs in Assam, Indochina, India, and Malaysia. In Canada the eggs of *Metorchis conjunctus* are occasionally found in the stools of man.

Barlow, C. H.: The life cycle of the human intestinal fluke *Fasciolopsis buski* (Lankester). Amer. J. Hyg., Monograph 4, 1925.

Cross, J. H.: Fasciolopsiasis in South East Asia and the Far East: A review. *In* Harinasuta, C. (ed.): Proceedings of the Fourth Southeast Asian Seminar on Parasitology and Tropical Medicine: Schistosomiasis and Other Snail-Transmitted Helminthiases. Manila, 1969, pp. 177–199.

Plaut, A. G., Kampanort-Sanyakorn, C., and Manning, G. S.: A clinical study of *Fasciolopsis buski* in Thailand. Trans. Roy. Soc. Trop. Med. Hyg., 63:470, 1969.

THE NEMATODES
(Roundworms)

Philip D. Marsden

212. INTRODUCTION

Roundworms have an intestinal tract and a large body cavity bordered by a complex cuticle and containing the reproductive, nervous, and excretory systems. They have elongated, cylindrical, bilaterally symmetrical, smooth, nonsegmented, translucent, flesh-colored bodies, often filiform, with a pointed posterior and rounded anterior end. The Nematoda constitute the second largest class in the Animal Kingdom, with 500,000 species. Many are free living. They are unisexual, and the female is usually bigger than the male. There is a great variation in size among the common species infecting man. For example, in the intestinal nematodes a female *Ascaris* may reach 18 cm whereas a female *Strongyloides* is smaller than 1 mm. Their bodies are muscular and require high carbohydrate reserves.

The common nematodes infecting man can be roughly divided into the *intestinal nematodes,* of which the common ones in order of importance are hookworms, *Ascaris, Strongyloides, Trichuris,* and *Oxyuris,* and the *tissue nematodes.* The latter group includes *Trichinella* and the various filarial worms. Heyneman has suggested that the life cycles of the intestinal nematodes of man can be shown to demonstrate an increasing dependence upon the host and a decrease in the proportion of metabolically active time in the free-living stages if they are arranged in a certain sequence. This sequence reflects different degrees of adaption by the parasite to the host and is presented in Table 1.

Rhabditis, a free-living nematode which rarely infects man, is but one step away from the relatively common *Strongyloides stercoralis. Strongyloides* represents the first stage in parasitic adaption. Hookworms are obligate parasites with no free-living stage. Both these nematodes and *Ascaris* have a phase of lung migration by immature larvae in the host, the explanation of which is not known. *Ascaris, Trichuris,* and *Enterobius* have progressively shorter oval maturation times. *Trichinella spiralis* is viviparous; the intestinal phase is transient, and the larvae persist in the host muscle.

Although the adult *Trichinella* organisms are intestinal nematodes, from a clinical viewpoint trichinosis can be considered as a tissue parasite infection, as it is the larvae that produce the disease syndrome. The final break from the free-living state is illustrated by the filariae, in which the adult worms live in the host tissue, specific arthropods serving as the intermediate hosts. Whether filariae evolved from insect parasites or arose by adaption of intestinal parasites to insects after ingestion of eggs by coprophagic insects is a matter for speculation.

As in schistosomiasis, the number of worms present in the host determines the clinical manifestations, and many mild infections are asymptomatic. Quantitative techniques to determine adult worm load are commonly used in some nematode infections. Among the intestinal nematodes, *Strongyloides* and *Oxyuris* infections

TABLE 1. Sequence for Common Human Intestinal Nematodes (Heyneman)

Species	Details of Life Cycle
Strongyloides stercoralis	Most primitive since parasitism is irregular and exists in free-living adult stage in soil
Necator americanus *Ancylostoma duodenale*	Regular parasitism; no free-living adults, only larvae in soil
Ascaris lumbricoides	All hatched larval stages as well as adults in host; only eggs in soil
Trichuris trichiura	Similar to *Ascaris,* but newly hatched larvae do not migrate through host's body; all development confined to the intestine
Enterobius vermicularis	Eggs infective shortly after being laid; soil phase for eggs rarely involved
Trichinella spiralis	No eggs laid; larvae hatch within female, are deposited in mucosa, which they penetrate, and migrate via blood stream to encyst in tissues

cannot be quantitated owing to the variability in excretion of progeny. *Ascaris* produces so many eggs that quantitative techniques are usually not worthwhile, but hookworms and *Trichuris* eggs can be quantitated by a stool-dilution technique. For example, in Stoll's method 3 grams of stool is emulsified in 42 ml of water in a special flask. Tenth normal sodium hydroxide may be used to soften hard feces. Glass beads and shaking after standing produces a uniform fine emulsion; 0.15 ml volume of this is pipetted onto a glass slide, and all the eggs counted in this volume are equivalent to 0.01 gram of feces. Knowing the number of eggs per gram of stool, the total volume of stool, the egg output per female worm, and the usual sex ratio of the species population, it is possible to calculate the approximate worm load. The Kato technique has gained popularity as a quick quantitative method. All the eggs are counted in 50 mg of stool cleared under a glycerin-soaked cellophane cover slip. Tissue helminths can also be quantitated in terms of larval output by expressing results in *Trichinella spiralis* infections as the number of larvae per gram of skeletal muscle or the number of microfilariae per milliliter of blood at a certain time of day. *Onchocerca* infections are likewise expressed as number of microfilariae per milligram of skin.

Multiple infections with intestinal nematodes often occur, especially in the tropics (for example, *Ascaris*, hookworm, and *Trichuris* in conjunction). Broad-spectrum anthelmintics have been developed to facilitate single dose oral treatment. Notable among these are the benzimidazoles, of which thiabendazole was the first broad-spectrum drug; the latest, mebendazole, shows great promise, although it is expensive.

Another important feature of nematode infections is the frequency with which infections with nonhuman parasites are encountered as abortive infections, with larvae only rarely maturing to adults, thus suggesting helminths in a process of adaption into man. A number of such parasites will be mentioned in the text that follows, including the genera *Oesophagostomum, Toxocara, Anasakis, Angiostrongylus, Dirofilaria,* and others of clinical importance.

Heyneman's sequence is followed in the present discussion of the nematodes, although it is important to point out that, in terms of human suffering, hookworm and Bancroftian filariasis are by far the most serious infections.

Beaver, P. C.: The nature of visceral larva migrans. J. Parasitol., 55:3, 1969.

Davis, A.: Drug Treatment of Intestinal Helminthiases. Geneva, World Health Organization, 1973.

Heyneman, D.: The life cycle of the nematodes parasitic in man: An evolutionary sequence. Med. J. Malaya, 20:249, 1966.

Knight, R., Schultz, M. G., Hoskins, D. W., and Marsden, P. D.: Intestinal parasites, a progress report. Gut, 14:145, 1973.

Stevens, D. P.: Quantitative techniques. Clin. Gastroenterol., 7:231, 1978.

213. INTESTINAL NEMATODES

213.1. STRONGYLOIDIASIS
(Cochin-China Diarrhea)

DEFINITION. Strongyloidiasis is an infection of the small intestine with the invasive small nematode *Strongyloides stercoralis*. Most infections are asymptomatic, but a few can be life threatening; because of this, treatment is always necessary.

ETIOLOGY AND TRANSMISSION. The parasitic female worm is small (2.2 mm long) and lives in the mucosa of the intestinal villi. The parasitic male has rarely been observed, and experimental work suggests that parthenogenesis is the rule. The eggs produced by the female hatch rapidly, producing larvae in the small intestine, and these may reinvade the bowel mucosa before being voided in the feces (internal autoinfection). On the other hand, they may invade immediately after voiding via the perianal skin (external autoinfection). Other larvae become infective within hours of contact with the soil, and invasion of a fresh host occurs via the skin. Alternatively, voided larvae may develop into *free-living adults in the soil.* These adults produce further generations of infective larvae in the soil. These alternative cycles make the life history of *Strongyloides* the most difficult one to grasp.

After skin penetration, the infective larvae undergo the same curious migration as hookworms via the venous system to the lungs (in 24 to 48 hours). Autoinfective forms may take a peritoneal or lymphatic route to the same site. From the lungs the developing larvae ascend the trachea, drop down into the stomach, and mature in the small intestine. Because of the frequency of autoinfection this nematode is self-perpetuating, and infections can last for 30 to 40 years. Man is the only common host, although primates and dogs can be experimentally infected.

DISTRIBUTION. The parasite is cosmopolitan, but it is more frequent in the tropics. Local habitats where warmth, moisture, and lack of sanitation favor the free-living existence are endemic sites. Curiously enough, in nearly all populations, however, the infection seems to be sporadic and an incidence comparable with that seen in hookworm infection is not encountered. This infection, like all intestinal parasitic infections, has been reported in high incidence from some mental institutions. Resistance to reinfection has been suggested by animal studies.

PATHOLOGY AND PATHOGENESIS. The adult female worms burrow through the intestinal submucosa above the muscularis mucosae, depositing eggs as they go. They cause a chronic inflammatory cell infiltrate with many eosinophils. The rapidly hatching larvae are responsible for most of the pathologic findings, and their powers of penetration are such they can be distributed widely throughout the body. For reasons not clearly understood, the whole process may be accelerated (the so-called hyperinfective syndrome). Debility on the part of the host, malnutrition, or corticoid administration favors the development of this syndrome. Obviously prolonged bowel transit time would increase the possibility of internal autoinfection. Inflammation of the small bowel may be so intense as to cause malabsorption, thickening, and edema visible roentgenographically. The mesenteric lymph nodes enlarge, and ulceration and necrosis of the mucosa may occur. The lungs and liver may also show abscess formation, and fatty changes in the liver may indicate primary or secondary malnutrition. In recent years several series of fatal cases have been described from the West Indies, Brazil, and Africa. Acute small bowel obstruction has been described, as well as *E. coli* bacteremia with meningitis, the latter perhaps arising from bacteria being introduced from the bowel on migrating larvae. The gut may be invaded at any level by larvae, and gastric and colonic involvement are well documented. Rarely larvae are found in other abdominal organs. Involvement of the kidney, heart, and endocrine glands is described.

CLINICAL MANIFESTATIONS. Dermal invasion, either as a result of primary exposure or by external autoinfection, may be characterized by linear, erythematous, urticarial wheals, which are the sites of migrating larvae. Particularly common around the buttocks, they may occur anywhere, and are often recognized for what they are, as they are relatively fast moving. It is a form of cutaneous larva migrans (see Ch. 213.4). Lung invasion may be associated with signs of bronchospasm or pneumonia. These may be short-lived or recurrent if several waves of larvae arrive in the lung. Hemoptysis is not uncommon as the larvae burst through the pulmonary alveoli. They may be found in the sputum, and there is usually a marked eosinophilia. Bowel involvement may give rise to a variety of clinical manifestations, but again it must be stressed that many light infections are asymptomatic. The most common gastrointestinal symptom is epigastric pain, which is often to the right of the midline, constant, and of a dull, aching character, mimicking peptic ulcer. Tenderness may be present on abdominal palpation over the duodenum. In heavy infections diarrhea is common; it may not be just the result of inflammation but may also reflect the coexistent malabsorption. Upper abdominal pain and vomiting from the involved upper gut are frequent, but intestinal obstruction is rare. Marked large bowel involvement may resemble ulcerative colitis. In the hyperinfective syndrome an eosinophilia is often present and death may result from disseminated inflammatory lesions, often with superimposed bacterial infection.

DIAGNOSIS. Strongyloidiasis must always be thought of in patients with unexplained eosinophilia. The high eosinophilia is probably associated with recurrent larval invasion. The diagnosis is made by finding the larvae in the stool, preferably by using a concentration technique. Unfortunately there are a number of difficulties. In warm climates fresh stool should be examined, as hookworm larvae hatch quickly from the eggs; they can be differentiated, but only by an expert. The excretion of larvae in strongyloidiasis is intermittent, and multiple stool specimens should be examined. The Baermann funnel technique, filter paper culture technique, and Beal's string test have facilitated diagnosis. Sometimes larvae are demonstrated in the duodenal aspirate or sputum when other techniques have failed. Jejunal biopsy may show larvae and adult parasites in section in the mucosa. The filarial complement-fixation test is often positive and of diagnositc help in difficult cases. Barium studies may show thickening and deformities of the small bowel owing to inflammatory edema.

TREATMENT. As so little is known about the conditions governing development of serious infections, all patients should be treated with thiabendazole, 25 mg per kilogram twice daily for three days. The tablets should be chewed; they have an orange taste. Common side effects are nausea, vomiting, and vertigo. It is said not to kill larvae or eggs, so treatment may have to be repeated. Rarely cases are resistant to repeated thiabendazole therapy. Recently cambendazole, a related compound, has been used with success. Assessment of parasitologic cure requires repeated stool examinations using special techniques. The eosinophilia should fall within eight weeks. The prognosis is good in otherwise healthy subjects, but may be poor in the exceptional circumstances described above. Prophylaxis involves avoiding unsanitary conditions when infection is likely. Strongyloides of nutria and raccoons have caused transient creeping eruptions (cutaneous larva migrans) in Louisiana trappers. The position of *Strongyloides fulleburni* as a human pathogen is unclear at this time.

Bras, G., Richards, R. C., Irvine, R. A., Milner, P. F. A., and Ragbeer, M. M. S.: Infection with *Strongyloides stercoralis* in Jamaica. Lancet, 2:1257, 1964.

Carvalho Filho, E.: Strongyloidiasis. Clin. Gastroenterol., 7:179, 1978.

Rodrigues, L. D., Martirani, J., Cabeca, M., Soares, W., and Brandao, J. A.: Cambendazol: Nova antihelmitico na terapeutica da estrongiloidiase. Rev. Inst. Med. Trop. São Paulo, 19:57, 1977.

Stemmerman, G. N.: Strongyloidiasis in migrants. Pathological and clinical considerations. Gastroenterology, 53:59, 1967.

Tanaka, H.: Experimental and epidemiological strongyloidiasis of Amaini Oshima Island. Jap. J. Exp. Med., 28:159, 1958.

213.2. CAPILLARIASIS

Until recently the genus *Capillaria* appeared to infect man so rarely that it would not have merited inclusion in a general work of this kind. The most common form, *Capillaria hepatica* (less than 20 cases reported), was recognized by finding *Trichuris*-like eggs encapsulated in the liver. Species of the genus had also been reported in the lungs and skin of man.

Recently, however, a new parasite of man *Capillaria philippinensis*, has been described from the northern Philippines, where more than 1000 cases and 100 deaths have been confirmed. Patients with intestinal capillariasis have colicky abdominal pain, chronic diarrhea, muscle wasting, and edema, which may lead to debility and death in four months. Clinical studies have shown the presence of a severe protein-losing enteropathy in these patients with malabsorption of fats and sugars.

A tiny nematode (3 to 4 mm by 0.03 to 0.04 mm), *C. philippinensis* is confined to the small intestine, particularly the jejunum. The eggs detected in the stool are similar to *Trichuris trichiura* (to which the *Capillaria* are closely related) but are smaller, are more oval, and have less prominent bipolar plugs. There is evidence that hatching may occur in the small intestine, and tissue invasion of the bowel similar to strongyloidiasis has been noted at postmortem examination. The mode of transmission of the disease is not fully worked out, but three species of fish have been found to contain infective larvae. It is still uncertain whether interhuman transmission occurs.

Intravenous feeding is necessary in severe cases. Mebendazole is the treatment of choice in an oral dose of 100 to 400 mg per day for 10 to 30 days.

Cross, J. H., Banzon, T., Clarke, M. D., Basaca Servilla, V., Watten, R. H., and Dizon, J. J.: Studies on the experimental transmission of *Capillaria philippinensis* in monkeys. Trans. R. Soc. Trop. Med. Hyg., 66:819, 1972.

Singson, C. N., Banzon, T. C., and Cross, J. H.: Mebendazole in the treatment of intestinal capillariasis. Am. J. Trop. Med. Hyg., 24:932, 1975.

Watten, R. H., Beckner, W. M., Cross, J. H., Gunning, J. J., and Jarmillo, J.: Clinical studies of *Capillaria philippinensis*. Trans. Roy. Soc. Trop. Med. Hyg., 66:828, 1972.

213.3. HOOKWORM DISEASE
(Ancylostomiasis, Miner's Anemia)

DEFINITION. The two common hookworms of man, *Ancylostoma duodenale* and *Necator americanus,* attach themselves to the small bowel by their buccal capsules and suck blood, thereby causing chronic blood loss. Depending on their number and the iron stores of the host, a variable degree of anemia often results. A distinction is made between hookworm infection when the load is too light to produce symptoms and hookworm disease.

PATHOGENIC CHAIN. Etiology. The human hookworms measure about 1 cm in length, the female being slightly longer than the male, which is recognizable by an expanded posterior end, the copulating bursa. *A. duodenale* is larger than *Necator americanus,* and the two species are differentiated most easily by the fact that *A. duodenale* has two pairs of teeth in its buccal capsule, whereas *N. americanus* has a pair of cutting plates only. The eggs of the two species are indistinguishable and are passed in the feces. In warm moist soil the larva hatches within 48 hours. The rhabditiform larva has a free-living cycle in the soil, feeding on bacteria, during which time it molts twice. The filariform larvae resulting from the second molt are the infected stage for man and can survive several months in favorable conditions. They tend to migrate up grass stems or gain any elevation up to 3 feet, and on coming into contact with the skin of man, quickly penetrate it, enter the bloodstream, and are transported to the lungs. Like *Strongyloides,* there they leave the vascular system and emerge into the alveoli, migrate up the bronchi and trachea, and down the esophagus to reach the small intestine where maturity is attained. In contrast to *N. americanus,* with *Ancylostoma duodenale* a duodenal infection is easily acquired in the mucosa of the upper intestinal tract, and the migrating larvae in the body tissues can remain dormant for nine months before completing development. Usually eggs appear in the stool five or more weeks after invasion, and the adults live one to nine years. A dog hookworm, *Ancylostoma ceylonicum,* has been described as an occasional human pathogen in the Orient.

Epidemiology. Over 400 million people have hookworm infections, but in the majority the worm load is small. *Ancylostoma duodenale* is the Old World hookworm, being prevalent in Europe, North Africa, and the Middle and Far East. *Necator americanus* is found more in the New World and tropical Africa. During the past 30 years both parasites have become widely distributed, and rigid geographic demarcations are not possible.

The survival of larvae is favored by a damp sandy soil, high in humus content at a temperature of 24 to 32° C. Promiscuous defecation and the absence of shoes are the chief factors responsible for infections. Such conditions occur in mines as well as on the surface of the ground. Urban people tend to have less hookworm than agricultural rural workers at locations where night soil is often used as fertilizer. Infection can be acquired by ingesting or handling contaminated vegetables. Coffee, banana, sugar cane, rice, and sweet potato fields are ideal for the growth and development of larvae. Often one locality is used as a communal latrine in the area, and people reinfect themselves by visiting these sites again and again. *The distinction between hookworm infection and hookworm disease is important.* Methods of estimating the intensity of the infection show that in endemic areas most patients have few worms and no significant anemia. Those who have hookworm anemia have more worms, and these heavy infections could be the result of repeated exposure or a failure of immunity on the part of the host. With canine hookworm, small repeated infections give almost complete immunity. Antibodies have been demonstrated in sera of infected patients, but this degree of immunity to reinfection seen in the dog does not seem to occur.

Pathology and Pathogenesis. Inflammatory cell infiltration is seen at the site of penetration of the hookworm larvae, and in the lungs small hemorrhages occur with eosinophilic and leukocytic infiltration. An eosinophilia is present during the invasive phase. The main feature of the established disease is the active sucking of blood by the worms. They create a negative pressure in the buccal capsule and suck in a piece of mucosa which acts as both an anchorage and a source of blood. It is still not clear what hookworms abstract from the blood. Vital preparations in vitro show red cells being vigorously expelled from the posterior end. *Ancylostoma* sucks between 0.16 and 0.34 ml of blood per day and *Necator,* 0.03 to 0.05. The development of anemia depends upon three factors: the iron content of the diet, the state of the iron reserves, and the intensity and duration of infection.

When iron intake is high, a heavy worm load is needed to produce a significant anemia. Up to 60 per cent of the iron from the hemoglobin extracted by the hookworm is reabsorbed in the intestine. At open operation small punctate hemorrhagic spots are encountered at the site of attachment. In addition to anemia, hypoalbuminemia occurs owing to a combination of blood loss and a low rate of albumin synthesis, possibly associated with anoxia affecting liver cell function. Malabsorption is said to occur in a few cases with partial villous atrophy and chronic inflammatory cell infiltration of the lamina propria.

CLINICAL MANIFESTATIONS. The site of skin penetration by the larvae is associated with pruritus and the development of an erythematous papular eruption (ground itch) which may last several days or even longer, depending on the host's immune response. Within a week after penetration the patient may have a transient asthmatic attack, but this is not as commonly seen as in invasive ascariasis.

Established hookworm disease is associated with general symptoms of anemia, weakness, fatigue, dyspnea, palpitation, and mental and physical retardation. Pica may be noted. On examination the skin and mucus membrane are pale. Peripheral edema is due possibly to a variety of factors, namely, hypoalbuminemia, a rise of capillary venous pressure, and tissue anoxia. In severe cases there is evidence of congestive cardiac failure. The pulse is rapid with a high pulse pressure. On auscultation of the enlarged heart, a third heart sound and an ejection type of systolic murmur are commonly heard; regurgitant systolic and even diastolic murmurs may occur and disappear when the anemia is corrected. For this reason it is very unwise to diagnose a valvular lesion clinically in such anemic patients until that anemia has been corrected. The hemoglobin may be very low (2 grams per 100 ml) and the patient still ambulant.

The patient may complain of upper abdominal pain, and radiologic changes suggestive of a duodenitis have been reported.

DIAGNOSIS AND DIFFERENTIAL DIAGNOSIS. Stool microscopy, either by a direct smear or by a concentration technique, reveals hookworm ova. Quantitation of the egg excretion enables the physician to decide whether the patient has a significant worm load. This is done by diluting a known volume of stool and counting a sample (Stoll technique) or by using a Kato thick smear, which must be read promptly or else the eggs will clear beyond recognition. Hookworm ova are 60 to 70 μ long by 35 to 40 μ wide and have a characteristic morphology with a clear shell and developing embryo inside. They must be distinguished, however, from both *Trichostrongylus* and *Ternidens deminutus,* both of which have larger eggs. Test tube cultivation of ova and differentiation of the resultant larvae are of value in doubtful cases. A skin test using an extract of *Necator americanus* larvae of standard nitrogen content has proved useful in screening a hookworm-infected population. Fluorescent antibody, complement-fixation, and hemagglutination tests have been developed but have little clinical application.

The anemia of hookworm disease is a classic iron deficiency anemia with a low hemoglobin, mean corpuscular hemoglobin concentration and serum iron, and a high iron-binding capacity. On the film the red cells are microcytic and hypochromic. Folic acid deficiency may sometimes be superimposed on macrocytosis. The serum albumin is low, and liver function tests may be abnormal. In the edematous patient there may be confusion with kwashiorkor, wet beriberi, or the nephrotic syndrome. The anemia has to be differentiated from other iron deficiency anemias.

TREATMENT. Tetrachloroethylene* and bephenium hydroxynaphthoate (see previous edition) are being replaced by newer less toxic drugs. Mebendazole in an oral dose of 100 mg twice a day for three days can be used for adults and children over two years of age. Pyrantel pamoate or embonate in a single oral dose of 11 mg per kilogram of body weight (maximum dose, 1 gram) is also accompanied by few side effects and is effective. These drugs also act on coexistent *Ascaris* infections. Both drugs will remove a large number of worms at the first dose, but to get rid of the last 5 to 10 per cent is often very difficult. In many areas total eradication may not be desirable or necessary.

The anemia responds well to ferrous sulfate, 200 or 300 mg three times daily. Occasionally the hemoglobin is so low, or there is an associated acute infection, that the patient presents in extremis owing to heart failure. Pregnancy may also precipitate acute heart failure. Intraperitoneal blood transfusion or exchange transfusions have been lifesaving. The prognosis is good in most cases. It is wise to delay treating the hookworm infection until the hemoglobin is above 50 per cent after oral iron. Without treatment of the worm infection, the anemia will relapse when iron therapy is discontinued. *Prevention* involves the sanitary disposal of human excreta and the prevention of soil pollution. The wearing of shoes cuts down the opportunities for infection.

---

*Available in the United States only as a veterinarian product, Nema worm caps.

Banwell, J. G., and Shad, G. A.: Hookworm. Clin. Gastroenterol., 7:129, 1978.
Gilles, H. M., Williams, E. J. W., and Ball, P. A. J.: Hookworm infection and anemia. Quart. J. Med., 33:1, 1964.
Roche, M., and Layrisse, M.: Nature and causes of hookworm anemia. Am. J. Trop. Med., 15:1031, 1966.
Stoll, N. R.: On endemic hookworm, where do we stand to-day? Exp. Parasitol., 12:241, 1962.
Stoll, N. R.: For hookworm diagnosis is finding one egg enough? Ann. N.Y. Acad. Sci., 98:712, 1962.

213.4. CUTANEOUS LARVA MIGRANS
(Creeping Eruption)

Cutaneous larva migrans is considered at this point because its most common cause is *Ancylostoma braziliense,* although it may be produced by a variety of other helminths. It is characterized by an erythematous, serpiginous, intracutaneous track or burrow, the anterior end of which is observed to migrate at the rate of 1 to 2 cm per day. There is often intense irritation, and secondary infection may result from scratching. This migration is due to the infective larva of *A. braziliense* (the cat and dog hookworm), which does not visceralize in man but wanders around in the skin. This migration may last for 2 to 50 weeks before the larva dies. Rarely some larvae reach the lungs, causing high eosinophilia and patchy pulmonary infiltration.

Patients are often infected by lying on beaches contaminated by dog or cat feces. The feet, legs, and hands are the most common sites, and the appearance of the lesion is usually diagnostic. It is virtually impossible to remove the larva from the skin.

Ancylostoma braziliense is found in the southern United States, Central America, the Caribbean, and tropical South America, as well as in tropical Africa and parts of the Far East, especially the Malay peninsula. There have been several reports of the worm maturing in the gut of man and eggs appearing in the feces, so there is not an absolute host specificity. Two other dog hookworms, *Uncinaria stenocephala* and *Ancylostoma caninum,* can produce similar lesions. Occasionally the ground itch of the two common human hookworms may persist and resemble creeping eruption in immune subjects.

The larva migrans track of *Strongyloides stercoralis* tends to be a short line, erythematous and rapidly moving (larva currens). Rodent *Strongyloides* may produce similar lesions but no mature worms. A form of myiasis with the horse botfly maggot (*Gasterophilus*) can produce a larger deeper migrating form of cutaneous larva migrans.

TREATMENT. Thiabendazole by mouth, 25 mg per kilogram per day for two days, is usually effective. If not, the dose can be doubled and repeated. Alternatively, the advancing end of the burrow can be treated with topical thiabendazole sprinkled on elastoplast or in a cream containing 15 per cent thiabendazole powder in a hydrosoluble base. This drug has completely superseded the other, more unsatisfactory treatments such as ethyl chloride spray and Hetrazan.

Battistini, F.: Treatment of creeping eruption with topical thiabendazole. Tex. Rep. Biol. Med., 27 (Supplement 2):645, 1969.
Beaver, P. C.: Larva migrans. Exp. Parasitol., 5:587, 1956.
Stone, O. J.: Systemic and topical thiabendazole for creeping eruption. Tex. Rep. Biol. Med., 27 (Supplement 2):659, 1969.

213.5. TRICHOSTRONGYLIASIS

The adult worms of the genus *Trichostrongylus* are much smaller than hookworms, being under 100 mm long. They lie embedded in the mucosa of the duodenum and jejunum, where they suck a small quantity of blood. Eight species have been reported in man. Infections are most frequent in the Far East, especially in Japan, China, Korea, and Indonesia. High infection rates have been reported in Iran and south and western Asia. Worm loads in man are usually light and asymptomatic. Infection is acquired by ingesting salad contaminated with infective third-stage larvae. The importance of *Trichostrongylus* lies in the fact that the egg is frequently mistaken for hookworm. These "hookworm eggs" appear to persist after therapy and are termed drug resistant. Frequently, these so-called drug-resistant hookworms turn out to be *Trichostrongylus*. The eggs of *Trichostrongylus* are larger and more sharply pointed at one end and have more advanced embryonation than hookworm ova. They are from 73 to 94 μ in length and 40 to 50 μ in width. Larvae recovered from fecal culture of the ova can also be distinguished from hookworm. Treatment is seldom needed, but pyrantel pamoate or thiabendazole is effective in the majority of cases.

Ghadirian, E., and Arfaa, F): Present status of *Trichostrongylus* in Iran. Am. J. Trop. Med. Hyg., 24:935, 1975.

Marcial Rojas, R. A.: Trichostrongyliasis. *In* Marcial Rojas, R. A. (ed.): Pathology of Protozoal and Helminthic Disease with Clinical Correlation. Baltimore, Williams & Wilkins Company, 1971, p. 753.

Wolfe, M. S.: Oxyuris, trichostrongylus and trichuris. Clin. Gastroenterol., 7:201, 1978.

213.6. GNATHOSTOMIASIS

Although *Gnathostoma* species are more closely related to *Ascaris*, this group is mentioned at this point because it also presents as *creeping eruptions* or, more commonly, as *migratory swelling in the subcutaneous tissues*. More than 100 human infections with the immature stages of *Gnathostoma spinigerum* have been reported from the Far East, particularly Thailand. Normally a parasite of wild felines, dogs, and foxes, *Gnathostoma* infects man when he eats the larvae in undercooked fish (fermented fish is a Thai delicacy). The larva causes a migratory swelling, often in the subcutaneous tissues, associated with an intense eosinophilia. Occasionally the larva comes to the skin surface and resembles cutaneous larva migrans, but the area of involvement is larger. Sometimes the larva burrows deep into the internal tissues and may lodge in the gut wall or elsewhere and produce an abscess. Indeed, secondary infection frequently occurs. Brain involvement in fatal cases with eosinophilic meningitis has been reported. Eye involvement with iritis and orbital cellulitis is also described. If the worm does not reach the body surface, the symptoms can persist for months. Some recommend extraction of the worm, but Hetrazan has been said to be useful. There is insufficient experience with thiabendazole thus far to permit a definite statement of its value, but its trial seems reasonable.

Miyazaki, I.: On the genus *Gnathostoma* and human gnathostomiasis with special reference to Japan. Exp. Parasitol., 9:338, 1960.

213.7. OESOPHAGOSTOMIASIS

Oesophagostomiasis is more closely related to hookworm and *Strongyloides* than to *Gnathostoma*, but like *Gnathostoma* it may rarely form a tumor in the human gut wall. Again, man is not the definitive host. The infection is often carried by pet monkeys, and the clinical picture is usually one of intestinal obstruction. Bacterial infection of the tumor nodule is common. Surgical excision of the tumor shows it to contain worms of *Oesophagostomum* species.

Anthony, P. P., and McAdam, I. W. J.: Helminthic pseudotumours of the bowel: Thirty-four cases of helminthoma. Gut, 13:8, 1972.

213.8. ASCARIASIS

DEFINITION. Ascariasis is infection with *Ascaris lumbricoides*, the large roundworm of man. The adults mature in the small intestine and can produce disease by intestinal obstruction or migration. The passage of larvae through the lungs may result in pneumonitis.

ETIOLOGY. *Ascaris* is a large whitish nematode; the female (20 to 35 cm) is larger than the male (15 to 30 cm), which often has a curly tail. The vulva of the female is situated ventrally at the junction of the anterior and middle thirds of the worm. Frequent copulation is necessary to ensure the continuous production of fertile eggs. A female worm has a reproductive capacity of 26 to 27 million eggs and a daily output of 200,000. The life span of the adult worms is relatively short (12 to 24 months). They are not attached to the wall of the jejunum, but bridge themselves across the lumen and by their muscle tone maintain themselves against the fecal stream. In a largely anaerobic environment they obtain nourishment from the semidigested food of the host and possibly from epithelial cells of the intestinal mucosa. The high protein and vitamin content of the parasite suggests that they deprive the host of nutrients.

The brownish eggs with a thick shell and albuminous coat become infective ten days after being passed in the stool. Fertile and infertile eggs have a different morphology. On ingestion of infective eggs by man, the larvae hatch in the small intestine, and, penetrating its wall, are carried by the blood and lymphatic system to the lungs. It has been suggested that this migration is necessitated by the need for oxygen, which is not available in the intestine, at this stage of the life cycle. Here, like hookworm and *Strongyloides*, the larvae migrate up the respiratory passages to the epiglottis and down to the esophagus. A new generation of eggs appears in the feces approximately two months after the ingestion of embryonated eggs.

EPIDEMIOLOGY. Although cosmopolitan, this worm is most abundant in the tropics, where sanitation is poor. One in every four people in the world is infected with *Ascaris lumbricoides*. The eggs are killed by direct sunlight and temperatures above 45° C; nevertheless, under optimal conditions they may remain viable for ten years. The eggs pass unchanged through the intestine of animals with the possible exception of the pig. The pig *Ascaris*, *Ascaris suum*, is morphologically identical to the human *Ascaris*, and there is some evidence that cross-infections can occur. The susceptibility to infection is greatest in childhood, reaching a peak at puberty, and transmission is by fecal contamination of food and drink. Circulating antibodies appear to play some role in host immunity.

PATHOLOGY AND CLINICAL MANIFESTATIONS. Light infections of a dozen or so worms often pass unnoticed, especially in adults. During the phase of larval migration, especially if many eggs have been ingested, respiratory symptoms may appear 4 to 16 days after infection. The pulmonary migration of larvae is associated with fever, cough, occasionally hemoptysis, and either crepitations or more rarely the signs of consolidation on auscultation of the chest. The sputum contains larvae and eosinophils, and there is a high blood eosinophilia. Sections of the lungs at this stage would show larvae in the bronchioles with patchy infiltration of alveoli with polymorphs and eosinophil leukocytes. Aberrant larvae may lodge in the liver, producing granulomatous lesions and hepatomegaly. More rarely such larvae, which fail to re-enter the circulation, are found in other abdominal organs.

When adult worms are present in the intestine, the established infection is often associated with occasional colicky abdominal pain and some abdominal distention. These adults may produce complications by mechanical effects within the gastrointestinal tract, or by wandering outside it, or more rarely by producing allergic manifestations in a sensitized host.

Heavy loads of worms may particularly be associated with intestinal obstruction, intussusception, volvulus, appendicitis, and hernial strangulation. A bolus of *Ascaris* may be a common cause of intestinal obstruction in childhood in an endemic area. Before undertaking bowel surgery, an *Ascaris* infection should always be excluded, because these worms are difficult to control once the bowel is opened, and considerable peritoneal soiling may result. Migration of adult worms may occur spontaneously or as a result of some stimulus such as fever or tetrachloroethylene. The *Ascaris* adults may perforate a suture line or cause a bile or pancreatic duct obstruction. Occasionally they migrate into the stomach and are vomited up, or pass down into the large bowel and out with the stool. Adult worms have been described issuing from umbilical fistulas, and even from the nose or ear. Obstruction of the bile duct is associated with cholangitis, and eggs may be deposited in the liver. *A. lumbricoides* has been said by some to be second only to *E. histolytica* in producing liver abscesses. Blockage of the pancreatic duct results in acute pancreatitis. Once the adult worm has left the bowel, it often dies, releasing foreign protein that may produce a reaction in a sensitized host. These reactions range from facial edema and giant urticaria to acute local necrosis and anaphylaxis. Laboratory personnel who work with *Ascaris* invariably become sensitized to the worms. Young pigs infected with *Ascaris* do not gain weight normally, and it is possible that heavy loads of human *Ascaris* may affect children similarly, as the worms will consume much food in the actively growing phase.

DIAGNOSIS. Examination of the feces reveals the characteristic ova. Usually in view of the number of ova produced, they can be found in ordinary direct smear. Although fertilized eggs are easy to recognize, unfertilized eggs assume bizarre shapes and may be mistaken for debris. Rarely one encounters infections of immature worms or only male worms. Sometimes an infection is diagnosed in barium meal examination, as the barium can be seen in the *Ascaris* gut. Although many serologic tests have been developed for *Ascaris*, including complement-fixation, hemagglutination, and gel diffusion, they are seldom used for diagnostic purposes.

TREATMENT. Although piperazine is still widely used, it is being replaced by new, less toxic drugs such as levamisole, pyrantel, and mebendazole. Levamisole is given in a single oral dose of 15 mg for adults and 5 mg per kilogram for children. Pyrantel embonate is also given in a single oral dose 11 mg per kilogram of body weight (maximum dose, 1 gram). The dose of mebendazole is the same as that given for hookworm (see Ch. 213.3). Piperazine salts act by blocking the neuromuscular junctions of the worm. The paralyzed worm can no longer bridge itself across the intestinal lumen and is carried along in the fecal stream and passed in the stool. Piperazine citrate is given in a dose of 75 mg per kilogram to a maximal single dose of 4 grams. This will clear 75 per cent of patients of their worms, but the dose can be repeated the following day with safety. No special preparation or purgation is necessary. Neurotoxic effects from piperazine have been reported in patients with renal failure who cannot excrete the drug. Being a cheap drug, piperazine is still widely used in the tropics. In multiple intestinal helminthic infections, *Ascaris* should always be treated first.

When examining stools for ova after therapy, it must be remembered that eggs may be passed in the stool for up to a week after the worms have been eradicated owing to the delay in the colonic circulation of feces.

The following regimen is suggested to deal with *intestinal obstruction* caused by *Ascaris*. Initially conservative treatment with nasogastric suction, intravenous fluids, and piperazine therapy should be tried for 48 hours. If no improvement follows, at laparotomy it is often possible to manipulate the bolus of worms into the large bowel through the terminal ileum. Only if this is not possible should enterotomy and worm extraction be performed.

PREVENTION. This consists of disposal of human excreta in sanitary privies and toilets. Children must be taught to use these facilities and avoid contamination of food with ova.

Blumenthal, D. S., and Schultz, M. G.: Incidence of intestinal obstruction in children infected with *Ascaris lumbricoides*. Am. J. Trop. Med. Hyg., 24:801, 1975.

Chang, C. C., and Han, C. T.: Biliary ascariasis in childhood. A clinical analysis of 788 cases. Chin. Med. J. (Peking), 85:167, 1966.

Gelpi, A. P., and Mustafa, A.: Seasonal pneumonitis with eosinophilia: A study of larval ascariasis in Saudi Arabia. Am. J. Trop. Med. Hyg., 16:646, 1967.

Lejkina, E. S.: Research in *Ascaris* immunity and immunodiagnosis. Bull. WHO, 32:699, 1965.

Pawlowski, Z. S.: Ascariasis. Clin. Gastroenterol., 7:157, 1978.

Piggott, J., Hansbarger, E. A., and Neafie, R. G.: Human ascariasis. Am. J. Clin. Path., 53:223, 1970.

The Control of Ascariasis. World Health Organization Technical Report, Series No. 379, 1967.

213.9. TOXOCARIASIS
(Visceral Larva Migrans)

Toxocariasis is an accidental human infection with the cat and dog *Ascaris* (*Toxocara cati* and *Toxocara canis*). The eggs of these species are infective two to three weeks after being passed, and if ingested by man the second stage larvae emerge. These penetrate the intestinal wall and reach the liver. The majority remain in the liver but others migrate to other organs, particularly the brain and the eye. Rarely they complete their cycle of development in man and produce adult worms in the bowel. Children are particularly susceptible because of more frequent soiling of the fingers and habits of playing with puppies, in which the incidence of infection is very high. Initially reported from the southern United States, these parasites are common in dogs and cats in many parts of the world. Although many reports have come from North America and Europe, it is likely that this syndrome also occurs in other parts of the world.

The migrating larvae produce "eosinophilic trails" and tissue inflammation in the affected organ. Usually a granuloma forms with epithelial cells, fibroblasts, lymphocytes, plasma cells, and occasional giant cells. A fibrous capsule eventually encloses the larva, which may remain alive for months. The granulomas can be seen macroscopically as small grayish-white spots. Such granulomas have been found in the lungs, eyes, brain, heart, kidney, and striated muscle.

The most common clinical form is that of a patient with a mild fever and tender hepatomegaly. Routine investigation reveals a marked eosinophilia (50 to 60 per cent), and further questioning often brings to light a history of contact with dogs. These signs and symptoms may persist for 18 months. The serum globulins may be elevated and anti-γ globulins are found. Another clinical form is as an *endophthalmitis* with a space-occupying granuloma visibly distorting the contour of the retina on funduscopy. In the past such granulomas were often mistaken for retinoblastomas, and the eye was removed. Several such series of "retinoblastomas" have been examined, and many of the tumors were found to consist of granulomas containing *Toxocara* larvae. Many mild infections are asymptomatic.

The syndrome of tender hepatomegaly and eosinophilia must be distinguished from invasive schistosomiasis or fascioliasis. A variety of nematodes can produce visceral larva migrans in special circumstances, among them *Ascaris lumbricoides, Necator americanus,* and *Strongyloides stercoralis.* Other nonhuman nematodes such as *Gnathostoma, Capillaria,* and *Dirofilaria* may be involved in granuloma formation in the liver. Sarcoidosis and periarteritis nodosa may mimic this disease. Blind liver biopsy is seldom helpful, but where facilities exist, direct visualization of surface granulomas of the liver with a peritoneoscope may enable biopsy of a granuloma to be made. A definitive diagnosis can often be made by examination of this granuloma. A diagnosis of second-stage *Toxocara* larva can be made on a section at mid-gut level, showing a maximal width of 12 to 20 μ and lateral alae. A variety of serologic tests are available but lack specificity, as they cross-react with other helminthic infections. However, in areas where such infections are rarely encountered, a fluorescent antibody test or an indirect hemagglutination test may be helpful.

TREATMENT. Diethylcarbamazine (see Bancroftian Filariasis in Ch. 214.3) has been used and does kill some larvae in the tissues of infected mice. A resolution of symptoms has followed the use of thiabendazole in one case in a dose of 25 mg per kilogram twice daily for seven days. The prognosis is good if the source of infection is removed by treating the dog with piperazine. Care must be taken to worm pets regularly, especially puppies, if they are in contact with children.

Huntley, C. C., Costas, M. C., Williams, R. C., Lyerly, A. D., and Watson, R. G.: Anti-γ-globulin factors in visceral larva migrans. JAMA, 197:552, 1966.
Kagan, I. G.: The serological diagnosis of visceral larva migrans. Clin. Pediat. (Phila), 7:508, 1968.
Mok, C. H.: Visceral larva migrans: A discussion based on a review of the literature. Clin. Pediat. (Phila.), 7:565, 1968.
Nelson, J. D., McConnell, T. H., and Moore, D. V.: Thiabendazole therapy of visceral larva migrans: A case report. Am. J. Trop. Med. Hyg., 15:903, 1966.
Woodruff, A. W.: Toxocariasis. Br. Med. J., 3:663, 1970.

213.10.   ANISAKIASIS

Although the full life cycle is still unknown, it appears that man is occasionally infected by the ascarid *Anisakis marina,* which has its larval stages in herrings. The adult worms develop in marine mammals such as seals, dolphins, porpoises, and whales. Man is infected by eating raw or undercooked herrings, and infection has occurred where such food is considered a delicacy, namely, northeastern Europe (particularly the Netherlands) and Japan. The larvae appear to burrow into the wall of the stomach or small bowel to produce an eosinophilic granulomatous mass that may be mistaken for a malignancy. Perforation of the bowel wall has been reported, as has stenosis following granuloma formation. Usually the correct diagnosis is not made until the specimen is examined after surgical resection. Government regulations in the Netherlands require that all raw herring be frozen at $-20°$ C for 24 hours to kill the larvae. This has practically abolished the disease.

Van Thiel, P. H.: The present state of anisakiasis and its causative worms. Trop. Geog. Med., 28:73, 1976.
Yokogawa, M., and Yoshimura, H.: Clinicopathologic studies on larval anisakiasis in Japan. Am. J. Trop. Med. Hyg., 16:723, 1967.

213.11.   TRICHURIASIS
(Whipworm Infection, Trichocephaliasis)

In trichuriasis, the adult worms are shaped like a whip. The long anterior threadlike portion of the worm consists of a cellular esophagus buried deep into the submucosa of the colon, making it difficult to dislodge. These adults are pinkish-gray and are 30 to 50 mm long. The male is distinguished from the female by its coiled caudal extremity. The female produces 5000 to 10,000 eggs per day. The eggs are 50 to 55 μ long, golden brown with prominent characteristic bipolar plugs. Under favorable conditions they become infective in three to five weeks, and when ingested by man the first stage larva hatches in the small intestine and spends three to ten days in the intestinal villi. Then it passes down to the large bowel where it matures in 30 to 90 days. The adult worms live for three to five years.

Of worldwide distribution, trichuriasis is most frequently encountered in the tropics. Often in a particular endemic locality, the infestation has a patchy distribution because of dense shade, heavy rainfall, and the clay soils that hold water as well as fecal pollution, thus facilitating transmission. In the United States, whipworm infection is found in the southern Appalachians and southwestern Louisiana; it is not infrequent in Puerto Rico.

The great majority of infections are asymptomatic; only heavy loads of worms cause clinical illness. The worms are distributed throughout the colon and rectum, and heavy infections may be associated with colic and diarrhea with blood. *Trichuris trichiura* abstracts 0.005 ml of blood per worm from the host each day. In children in precarious iron balance a load of over 800 worms may be associated with an iron deficiency anemia. Up to 5000 worms have been recovered from heavily infected children. In such infections rectal prolapse may complicate the diarrhea, and the appearance of the congested mucosa associated with the whitish bodies of the worms has been described as the "coconut cake" rectum. Early infections may be associated with a mild blood eosinophilia. *Trichuris* has been implicated as a predisposing factor to acute amebic dysentery by causing an initial breach of the mucosa, this suggestion being based on finding a higher incidence of *Trichuris* in patients with acute bowel amebiasis than is normal for the area. *Trichuris* is often associated with other helminthic and protozoal infections. Appendicitis and peritonitis with the presence of worms in the peritoneal cavity have been described.

Diagnosis is made by finding the eggs in the feces, either on direct smear or by concentration methods. In the rare *Trichuris* dysentery the eggs may appear in aggregates in the mucoid stools, together with eosinophils and Charcot-Leyden crystals. Egg counts below 10,000 per gram are unlikely to be associated with symptoms.

Treatment should be confined to heavily infected individuals presenting with symptoms and to those employed as food handlers, nurses, and so forth. Mebendazole, in an oral dose of 100 mg twice a day for three days, gave a cure rate of 64.3 per cent in one trial. It is well tolerated and has a direct ovicidal effect. A second or even a third course can be given. Thiabendazole in a similar dose to that used in *Strongyloides* (25 mg per kilogram of body weight twice daily for two days) eradicates the infection in one third of cases, and the course can be repeated after one week.

Boon, W. H., and Hoh, K. K.: Severe whipworm infection in children. Singapore Med. J., 2:34, 1966.

Franz, K. H., Schneider, W. J., and Pohlman, M. H.: Clinical trials with thiabendazole against intestinal nematodes infecting humans. Am. J. Trop. Med. Hyg., 14:383, 1965.

Jung, R. C., and Jelliffe, D. B.: The clinical picture and treatment of whipworm infection. West Afr. Med. J., 1:11, 1952.

Layrisse, M., Aparideo, L., Martinez Torres, C., and Roche, M.: Blood loss due to infection with *Trichuris trichiura*. Am. J. Trop. Med. Hyg., 16:613, 1967.

Sargent, R. G., Savoury, A. M., Mina, A., and Lee, P. R.: A clinical evaluation of mebendazole in the treatment of trichuriasis. Am. J. Trop. Med. Hyg., 23:375, 1974.

Wagner, E. D., and Chavarria, A. P.: In vivo effects of a new anthelmintic, mebendazole (R 17,635), on the eggs of *Trichuris trichiura* and hookworm. Am. J. Trop. Med. Hyg., 23:151, 1974.

213.12. ENTEROBIASIS

(Oxyuriasis, Pinworm or Seatworm Infection)

Infestation with the pinworm, *Enterobius vermicularis*, is not limited to rural communities and the poor as with many intestinal nematodes, but occurs also in urban communities. Reportedly worldwide in distribution, it appears to be rarer in the tropics. Children are more commonly infected than adults.

The adult female worm is 8 to 13 mm long, and the male, which is rarely seen, 2 to 5 mm. Both live in the cecum and adjacent large and small bowel. The females migrate at night to the anal orifice, where they deposit their eggs. Within a few hours larvae develop in the eggs, which are then infectious and on ingestion hatch in the duodenum and migrate to the large bowel where they mature in 15 to 28 days. The ova can be transferred from the anal margin to the mouth by contamination of the hands, and ova lodge under the nails after scratching of the anal margin. The eggs also become widely disseminated in the environment, notable in bedclothes and dust samples. It has been suggested that hatching of larvae on the anal margin may result in the colon's being colonized from below as a form of autoinfection. Fortunately the eggs are relatively susceptible to drying, and in a warm dry environment survive only a few days.

Usually pinworm infestation is harmless and is often asymptomatic. Pruritus ani is the chief complaint caused by the migrating female worms. Numerous other symptoms have been described, including enuresis, irritability, and insomnia, which may result from the pruritus. Less convincing reported manifestations are abdominal pain, teeth grinding, nausea, and weight loss.

Rarely the female worm may penetrate into the mucosa of the bowel, where it has been a primary cause of appendicitis. Occasionally female worms migrate into the vagina, causing an intense vulvitis. Prostatitis is a rare complication in the male, and secondary ischiorectal abscesses may follow perianal eczema. Granulomas may form around worms that enter tissues, and such granulomas have been described in the uterus, fallopian tubes, and peritoneum, presumably associated with migration of worms up the female genital tract. A rare case not reported in the literature occurred in a mentally deficient child who developed pulmonary eosinophilic granulomas owing to massive inhalation of *Enterobius* eggs present in the dust of the mental institution.

The best method for finding *Enterobius* eggs is by means of the sealing tape (Scotch tape) swab. A piece of Scotch tape 2 inches long is folded, sticky side out, over the end of a wooden tongue depressor and pressed firmly against the perianal region. The tape is then stuck to the slide, acting as a coverslip, and the specimen is scanned for the typical eggs, which are 50 to 60 μ in length, are flattened on one side, and contain a developing embryo. The patient can be given six such swabs, and he does the examination every morning for six mornings on rising and before taking a bath. All can then be examined at the laboratory. Adult worms are rarely observed in feces or on the perianal skin, or seen with the sigmoidoscope. All members of the family should be examined in view of the frequency with which whole families are infected. The eosinophil count is rarely elevated in this infection.

Single-dose treatment is practical with either mebendazole, a 100-mg tablet for all ages, or pyrantel pamoate, 1 ml per 5 kilograms of body weight to a maximal dose of 15 ml. Pyrvinium pamoate, in a dose of 5 mg per kilogram, should be repeated after two weeks.

This drug turns the stool red, and may occasionally be associated with vomiting, diarrhea, and skin rashes. The methods of transmission should be explained to the patient, and care of personal hygiene (short nails, frequent baths, and clean underclothes) instituted before treatment. Follow-up tape swabs are necessary. There is a tendency for some patients to become overanxious about this infection, occasionally with the development of a "worm neurosis." They should be strongly reassured.

Chandrasoma, P. T., and Mendis, K. M.: Enterobius vermicularis in ectopic sites. Am. J. Trop. Med. Hyg., 26:644, 1977.

Cram, E. B.: Studies on oxyuriasis, xxviii. Summary and conclusions. Am. J. Dis. Child., 65:46, 1943.

Most, H., Gellin, G. A., Yager, R., Aron, B., Friedlander, M., and Quarfordt, S.: Enterobius (pinworm infection): A study of 951 Puerto Rican and 315 non-Puerto Rican children in New York City. Am. J. Trop. Med. Hyg., 12:65, 1963.

214.   TISSUE NEMATODES

214.1.   TRICHINOSIS*

(Trichiniasis, Trichinellosis)

DEFINITION AND ETIOLOGY. Trichinosis is a self-limited infection of the intestine (by the adult parasite) and of the striated muscle (by the larvae) produced by a small nematode, *Trichinella spiralis*. The same animal host thus acts as both the final and the intermediate host, harboring the adults temporarily and the encysted larvae for long periods. When infected meat containing larvae is ingested, these larvae are released into the upper small intestine by the action of digestive juices. They become adult in five to seven days, the males and females mate, and the fertile female begins to deposit larvae into the mucosa. These larvae pass into the circulation through the hepatic and pulmonary filters, and are carried to all parts of the body. They burrow into the muscles and encyst and complete their development in striated muscle. In other tissues such as the myocardium, brain, and eye, the larvae disintegrate and are absorbed. Among the muscles heavily parasitized are the diaphragmatic, masseteric, intercostal, laryngeal, extraocular, nuchal, pectoral, deltoid, gluteus, biceps, and gastrocnemius. A total of 1500 larvae are liberated by each female worm, usually in four to eight weeks but up to 16 weeks, after which the females die.

Larvae attain a size of 0.4 by 0.025 mm in a cyst in the muscle by the thirty-fifth day. The capsule is complete in three months, and calcification occurs within six months to two years. Recent evidence suggests that there may be strain differences in relation to host susceptibility. The parasite is chiefly found in man, hogs, rats, bears, foxes, walruses, dogs, and cats, but any carnivorous or omnivorous animal may be infected.

EPIDEMIOLOGY. Generally of worldwide distribution, the parasite has not been reported from the islands of the Pacific, Brazil, or Australia. It occurs more frequently in the Northern Hemisphere than in the tropics. It is common in Europe and the United States. Fatal cases have recently been described from Kenya and Chile. It is rare east of the Suez Canal. In the United States there has been a marked reduction in the incidence of the infection, owing to laws requiring the cooking of garbage fed to hogs, storage of meat at low temperature, and education of the public resulting in thorough cooking of pork.

Until quite recently, trichinosis was relatively common in New York City, as pork was being obtained from garbage-fed hogs in New Jersey. However, hog-rearing in this way has substantially declined. Pigs become infected by eating infected meat and occasionally infected rats. Rats are infected in the same way. One of the main methods of transmission is in sausages, wursts, or hamburgers in which the beef is diluted (or actually contaminated in mechanical grinders) with a little pork. Infections from bear and walrus meat have been reported. The low incidence in the tropics is probably due to the fact that meat of any kind is a luxury to many people. Hindus, Jews, and Moslems eschew pork, and the Chinese cook it very well.

PATHOLOGY AND PATHOGENESIS. Three to four days after invasion of the muscle, the fiber becomes edematous, loses its cross striations, and undergoes basophilic degeneration. The nuclei increase in number and size, and there is interstitial inflammation around the muscle with a chronic inflammatory cell infiltrate. The severity of the disease depends on the adult worm load, the age of the patient, and the degree of host resistance as well as the numbers of organs involved.

In the heart a focal interstitial myocarditis may occur. Acute nonsuppurative meningitis may be associated with larvae in the cerebrospinal fluid. Larvae may cause lesions in the choroid and retina. Catarrhal enteritis, pulmonary edema, and pneumonia may occur in the early stages of the disease.

CLINICAL MANIFESTATIONS. The cardinal features of trichinosis are fever, orbital edema, myalgia, and eosinophilia. Only a small percentage of infected patients have sufficient parasites, however, to produce such clinically recognizable disease. The clinical picture can be divided into distinct stages in a symptomatic infection. First, there is the stage of adult maturation during the first weeks after infection associated with transient gastrointestinal symptoms. From the seventh to the fourteenth day larviposition begins, and muscle penetration commences. This is usually associated with an irregular persistent fever (37.8 to 40.5° C), urticarial rash, and occasionally respiratory symptoms in the form of cough and bronchospasm. Muscle pains become prominent and unusual, but the characteristic physical signs are bilateral orbital edema and subungual and subconjunctival hemorrhages. A severe infection may result in death four to eight weeks after infection from toxemia, secondary pneumonia, myocardial failure, or trichinous encephalitis. Severe muscle involvement may render breathing, masticating, swallowing, or locomotion painful. An eosinophilia beginning seven days after the infection may rise to very high levels (70 per cent) and persist for months. Serum transaminases are also elevated in the invasive stage.

DIAGNOSIS AND DIFFERENTIAL DIAGNOSIS. Although the rising eosinophilia together with a suggestive clinical picture leads one to suspect this diagnosis, it is proved by finding the larvae in a muscle biopsy. This should be done in the fourth week of infection when a small piece of

---

*The present chapter is based on the article on trichinosis prepared by Dr. Harold W. Brown for the twelfth edition of this book. Little new clinical information has developed in the interval; what has appeared has been incorporated in the basic article.   P.D.M.

muscle is removed from the deltoid or gastrocnemius. Crushed between two microscope slides and examined under the low-power objective of the microscope, the living coiled larvae can be seen. In light infections when the direct examination is negative, the biopsy specimen can be incubated overnight in an acid-pepsin mixture and the centrifuged deposit examined for larvae.

Calcified cysts and calcified larvae represent older infections, as calcification usually takes 18 months, but the larva may live inside the calcified cyst for many years. Calcified cysts appear as tiny white spots in fresh muscle, but are too small to be detected radiologically.

A variety of serologic tests are available. The bentonite flocculation test is as sensitive as the complement-fixation test and much easier to perform. It is usually positive four weeks after infection, but may be present earlier. A change from a negative to a positive test during the illness is significant. The indirect fluorescent antibody test detects some infections at an earlier stage. Few other parasitic infections are associated with such persistent fever or generalized muscular aches and tender muscles. Polymyositis of nonparasitic cause may present like this and be associated with eosinophilia. Periarteritis nodosa may also mimic trichinosis.

TREATMENT. Congestive cardiac failure should be searched for and, if present, should be treated. Mild analgesics can be given for the muscle pain. Anti-inflammatory steroids (prednisone, dexamethasone) relieve fever, edema, and muscle pain in severe acute cases but are said not to affect the adult worms' fecundity or the number of larvae settling in the muscle. In patients with central nervous system involvement this effect of steroids is dramatic.

Thiabendazole, in a dose of 25 mg per kilogram of body weight for five to seven days, has also produced a marked resolution of the symptoms of fever and muscle pain, but living larvae have still been recovered on muscle biopsy after much larger courses of the drug. In severe infections the use of corticosteroids and thiabendazole may be lifesaving, but when the parasite load is not considerable, the prognosis is good even without treatment.

PREVENTION. The ultimate prevention of trichinosis is dependent on its elimination in hogs, and the incidence in these animals can be greatly reduced by heat-sterilizing garbage. Freezing meat at −32° C for a few hours (or −15 to −30° C for several weeks) kills larvae, as does gamma radiation of the meat. Pigs fed on a diet containing 0.1 per cent thiabendazole fail to incubate *T. spiralis* on challenge. Routine meat inspection does not detect the infection, and serologic and skin tests on pigs have not been helpful in detecting infected animals. The chief safeguard at present is the thorough cooking of pork at 60° C for 30 minutes for each pound of meat.

Gould, S. E.: Trichinosis in Man and Animals. Springfield, Ill., Charles C Thomas, 1970.
Hennekeuser, M. H., Pabst, K., Poeplau, W., and Gerok, W.: Thiabendazole for the treatment of trichinosis in humans. Tex. Rep. Biol. Med., 27 (Supplement 2):581, 1969.
Kim, C. W.: Trichinellosis. New York, Intext Educational Publishers, 1974.
Maynard, J. E., and Kagan, I. G.: Trichinosis (serology). Practitioner, 191:622, 1963.
Moser, R. H.: Trichinosis from Bismarck to polar bears. JAMA, 228:735, 1974.
Proceedings of the International Commission in Trichinellosis: No. VI. Wiad, Parazyt., 14:127, 1968.
Zimmerman, W. J., Steele, J. H., and Kagan, I. G.: The changing status of trichiniasis in the U.S. population. Public Health Rep., 83:957, 1968.

214.2. ANGIOSTRONGYLIASIS

ANGIOSTRONGYLUS CANTONENSIS. Eosinophilic meningoencephalitis, a syndrome caused by *Angiostrongylus cantonensis* (the rat lung worm), was first recognized in New Caledonia in 1950, and has since been reported from Hawaii, Tahiti, other Pacific Islands, Indonesia, and Thailand. The human disease has only been reported from the Far East and the Pacific to date, although infected rats have been found in Madagascar, Mauritius, Ceylon, and Sarawak.

The life cycle was described by workers in Australia in 1955 before the importance of the worm as a human pathogen was known. A delicate filiform nematode, 17 to 25 mm in length, the adult lives in the lungs of rats, and the eggs are coughed up, swallowed, and pass out in the feces as first-stage larvae. Further development occurs in slugs and snails to the third-stage infective larvae. These larvae are ingested by man either while in this intermediate host or after they have been shed by it onto some other article of food, e.g., lettuce. Crabs and freshwater prawns have also been found to be infected with these metastrongyloid larvae, but probably act as paratenic hosts. The dispersal of the giant African land snail *Achatina fulica* may have assisted the spread of the infection. When infective larvae are ingested by the rat, they migrate to the brain and reach young adulthood in four weeks. They then migrate to the pulmonary arteries and after two more weeks start laying eggs. Unfortunately if man accidentally ingests these infective larvae, they migrate to the brain (as in the rat), and there produce the clinical picture of a meningoencephalitis associated with fever, signs of cerebral irritation, mental deficit, and varying degrees of loss of consciousness. Mild blood eosinophilia is present, and lumbar puncture reveals a fluid under increased pressure with increased protein and many eosinophils (from 100 to 3000 per cubic millimeter). Occasionally patients present with a facial nerve lesion or complaints of diplopia and paresthesia. A complement-fixation test using an extract of adult worms as antigen has been developed. The illness usually persists for some weeks or months and then the patient recovers spontaneously.

Young adult worms have been found in the brain and cerebrospinal fluid of man, and experimental infection of monkeys produces a similar syndrome. The pathology of the brain in fatal cases is one of focal areas of softening, the meninges and subarachnoid space being infiltrated with plasma cells, lymphocytes, eosinophils, and neutrophils. There is perivascular cuffing with chronic inflammatory cells in the brain substance. Careful sectioning of the brain is necessary to find the 0.16 to 8 mm nematodes.

This condition must be differentiated from a variety of other parasitic infections involving the central nervous system. In Thailand cerebral gnathostomiasis and *Angiostrongylus* infections occur. Cerebral paragonimiasis could be an important differential diagnosis in parts of the Far East. In other situations the syndrome of eosinophilic meningitis could be produced by cysticercosis, hydatid, schistosomiasis, fascioliasis, trichinosis, and possibly strongyloidiasis. Refinements of serologic diagnostic techniques will help in this sometimes difficult clinical problem.

The author has been able to trace no references to treatment with thiabendazole, although this would seem to be the drug to try. Prevention entails education regarding dangerous foods such as raw crabs and prawns and undercooked snails, and making sure that lettuce is free of slugs and snails. Freezing of crustaceans and molluscs at −15° C for 12 hours has been found to be effective in destroying the infective larvae of *A. cantonensis*.

MORERASTRONGYLUS COSTARICENSIS. Human disease caused by this parasite has been described from Costa Rica where 130 cases have been studied. The worm also occurs in Honduras and Panama. Patients, usually children, present with right iliac fossa pain, fever, and blood eosinophilia, and often an abdominal mass is palpable. At operation an eosinophilic granulomatous cecal pseudo-tumor is found to contain adult worms and eggs.

The intermediate host is a slug, *Vaginulus (Sarasinula) plebius,* and the definitive host is the cotton rat *Sigmodon hispidus.* Infected slugs contaminate lettuce leaves with infective third-stage larvae, and man acquires the disease by ingesting the slug itself on contaminated salad. In the rodent host — and probably in man — the cycle occurs in the abdominal cavity. The third and fourth larval molts occur in lymph vessels. After three months the young adults move to radicles of the mesenteric arteries, mate, mature, and oviposit. Arteritis and thrombosis may be followed by macro- or microinfarcts of the gut, with ulceration and necrosis of the gut wall. Fistulization or generalized peritonitis may ensue. Neither larvae nor eggs are usually detected in the stools of man.

In *Morerastrongylus costaricensis* infection of man, sexually mature adult worms develop, and as such this species is better adapted to man than *Angiostrongylus cantonensis.*

Alicata, J. E.: Present status of *Angiostrongylus cantonensis* infection in man and animals in the tropics. J. Trop. Med. Hyg., 72:53, 1969.
Mackerras, M. T., and Sanders, D. F.: The life history of the rat lungworm *Angiostrongylus cantonensis* (Chen) (Nematoda; Metastrongylidae). Aust. J. Zool., 3:1, 1955.
Morera, P.: Life cycle and redescription of *Angiostrongylus costaricensis* (Morera and Cespedes 1971). Am. J. Trop. Med. Hyg., 22:613, 1973.
Schollhaminer, G., Aubry, P., and Rigaud, J. L.: Quelques réflexions sur la méningite à éosinophiles a Tahiti. Étude clinique et biologique de 165 observations, à propos d'un cas atypique. Bull. Soc. Pathol. Exot., 59:341, 1966.

214.3.   FILARIASIS

GENERAL CONSIDERATIONS

To talk of filariasis as such is to use a general term like anemia, for there are seven types of nematodes found in man belonging to the superfamily Filarioidea, as well as one member of the superfamily Dracunculoidea (the guinea worm), which is usually included in a consideration of this group. Of these Filarioidea, the embryos or microfilariae are found in the blood in five and in the subcutaneous tissues in two species. The adults are viviparous, and the blood microfilariae demonstrate a periodicity in the peripheral blood, depending on the species. They may remain ensheathed in their elongated egg shell or have no sheath. These microfilariae are distinguished on their criteria as well as on the pattern of distribution of nuclei seen in stained specimens in their tails. Giemsa stain can be used, but better results of sheath staining are obtained with Delafield's hematoxylin or Mayer's acid hemalum.

In Table 2 the various species are listed and the characteristics of their microfilariae are shown. The adult worms live for many years, whereas blood microfilariae have a life of three to six months. After being bitten by an infected arthropod it may take 1 year to 18 months before microfilariae are present in the peripheral blood, a long prepatent period. The controlling mechanism for periodicity has never been satisfactorily explained for many of these human species. However, Hawking's work suggests that at least two circadian rhythms are involved, one mechanism within the microfilariae themselves, and the other some physiological tide in the host (body temperature for certain animal species). This periodicity fits the habits of the insect vector; for instance, the *Loa* insect vector flies by day, but most bancrofti infections are transmitted nocturnally. The geographic distribution of these species is of particular importance, because in some it is markedly restricted. For instance *Loa loa* is a filarid of Equatorial Africa, and *Mansonella ozzardi* is found only in South America.

Not all the species listed are significantly pathogenic. Few symptoms have been ascribed to *Mansonella ozzardi* infections, and the case for the pathogenicity of *D. perstans* is very shaky. Two of these filarial infections are notable in terms of their importance in man. These are the *Wuchereria-Brugia complex,* which produces bancroftian filariasis with lymphatic obstruction and elephantiasis, and *onchocerciasis,* which is a common cause of blindness in endemic areas. Multiple infections occur in endemic areas; for instance, in parts of West Africa a patient may be seen infected with *Loa loa,* bancrofti, perstans, and onchocerciasis.

This final group of the most modified nematodes will be considered in the order in which they are listed in Table 2, except that the guinea worm will be considered first. Dirofilariasis and pulmonary tropical eosinophilia will then be reviewed.

TABLE 2.   Common Filarioidea of Man as Distinguished by Characteristics of Microfilariae

	Periodicity of Microfilariae	Sheathed or Unsheathed	Tail Morphology
Microfilariae in blood:			
Wuchereria bancrofti	Majority nocturnal	Sheathed	Nuclei not to tip of tail
Brugia malayi	Majority nocturnal	Sheathed	Two distinct nuclei in tail tip
Loa loa	Diurnal	Sheathed	Nuclei to tip of tail
Mansonella ozzardi	Nonperiodic	Not sheathed	Nuclei not to tip of tail
Dipetalonema perstans	Nocturnally subperiodic	Not sheathed	Nuclei to tip of tail
Microfilariae in subcutaneous tissues:			
Onchocerca volvulus	Nonperiodic	Not sheathed	Nuclei not to tip of tail
Dipetalonema streptocerca	Nonperiodic	Not sheathed	Nuclei to tip of tail, which is crooked

Hawking, F.: Advances in filariasis. Trans. R. Soc. Trop. Med. Hyg., 59:9, 1965.

Hawking, F., Moore, P., Gammage, K., and Worms, M. J.: Periodicity of microfilariae. XII. The effect of variations in host body temperature on the cycle of *Loa loa, Monnigofilaria setariosa. Dirofilaria immitis*, and other filariae. Trans. R. Soc. Trop. Med. Hyg., 61:674, 1967.

Sasa, M.: Human Filariasis. Baltimore, University Park Press, 1976.

Muller, R.: Dracunculus and dracunculiasis. *In* Dawes, B. (ed.): Advances in Parasitology, Vol. 9, New York, Academic Press, 1973, p. 73.

Pardanani, D. S., Trivedi, V. D., Joshi, L. G., Daulatram, J., and Nandi, J. S.: Metronidazole (Flagyl) in dracunculiasis: A double blind study. Ann. Trop. Med. Parasitol., 71:45, 1977.

Raffier, G.: Efficacy of thiabendazole in the treatment of dracunculiasis. Texas Rep. Biol. Med., 27(Supplement 2):601, 1969.

DRACONTIASIS
(Guinea Worm)

Infection with the guinea worm (*Dracunculus medinensis*) usually presents as a skin ulceration at the site of emergence of the female adult worm. Man is probably the only reservoir, although monkeys and dogs can be experimentally infected. Human infections are widespread in the tropics, occurring in local distribution in West Africa and the Nile Valley, the Middle East, India and Pakistan, the Caribbean Islands, and Guyana. Infection occurs on ingesting infected water fleas (*Cyclops*) present in drinking water from shallow wells or ponds. The infective larvae in the *Cyclops* penetrate the intestinal walls and mature in the loose connective tissue under the skin, especially that of legs and feet. The male worm is small and dies after copulation. The female requires a year to become gravid, and then measures up to a meter long and is 2 mm in diameter. When ready to discharge larvae, she approaches the skin surface, and a blister is produced by secretion of a toxic substance from the anterior end of the worm. The blister breaks down to form an ulcer a few centimeters across, and the anterior end of the worm protrudes into this ulcer. On contact with water the head of the worm ruptures, and the uterus periodically discharges the tightly coiled larvae infective to the water flea. Secondary infection of the ulcer with resultant cellulitis is common. Generalized allergic symptoms may occur prior to the blister formation or when surgical removal of the worm is attempted. Multiple infections are common. The lesion is usually on the lower leg, but may occur on the genitalia, buttocks, or upper limbs. In water carriers lesions have been observed on the back, suggesting that the worm is positively hydrotropic. Alternatively, the mature female may never reach the surface of the body and may be absorbed or calcify in the tissue. The radiologic appearance is pathognomonic because the worm is so large. If a gravid worm dies in situ or is broken during extraction, cellulitis and secondary infection often occur. This may give rise to contractures. Also *Clostridium tetani* may contaminate the wound and tetanus may result. Rarely the adult worm involves serous cavities, the extradural space, or joints. Guinea worm arthritis appears to be due to the presence of the adult worm or larvae in the joint. A microscopic diagnosis can be made by finding embryos in the exudate from the guinea worm ulcer after exposure to a few drops of water.

Gradually winding the worm out of the ulcer by turning it on a stick a few centimeters a day is still common practice. Surgical extraction is also practiced. Metronidazole (Flagyl) in an adult dose of 400 mg three times a day for 10 to 20 days rapidly reduces symptoms. Thiabendazole is also effective. Prevention involves constructing water sources that cannot be contaminated and killing *Cyclops* by chlorination or boiling water to be used for drinking.

BANCROFTIAN FILARIASIS

ETIOLOGY. Bancroftian filariasis is caused by the filarial worm *Wuchereria bancrofti*. The adult worms reside in the lymphatic system and produce recurrent lymphangitis with fibrosis and obstruction. The infection is transmitted by culicine and anopheline mosquitoes.

The threadlike adult worms are 4 to 10 cm long and live for decades. The female worm is viviparous, producing microfilariae 130 to 320 μ long which are found in the peripheral blood; in some forms this occurs only at night, whereas during the day the microfilariae are in the lungs. If ingested by a suitable mosquito, these microfilariae develop in the thoracic muscles of the insect and are present in the mouth parts after two weeks. They enter the skin through the puncture wound when the mosquito next feeds, and, finding their way to the lymphatics of the host, the males and females mate and mature. More than a year after infection microfilariae appear in the peripheral blood.

EPIDEMIOLOGY. Man is the only definitive host of this common type of filariasis. Periodic bancroftian filariasis is found throughout tropical Africa and North Africa, as well as in the tropical coastal borders of Asia and Queensland. It is endemic in the West Indies and the northern countries of South America. In the northern Pacific bancroftian filariasis exhibits nocturnal periodicity, but in the Pacific Islands east of 160 degrees of longitude (including New Caledonia, Fiji, Samoa, the Ellis and Cook Islands, Society Islands, and the Marquesas) the microfilariae are nonperiodic, being present in the peripheral blood throughout the 24-hour period. The term *W. bancrofti var. pacifica* has been applied to this strain.

PATHOLOGY. The severity of the lesions probably depends on the adult worm load and their site of development and the susceptibility of the host. Light infections are often asymptomatic, and microfilariae are detected on incidental blood examinations. Maturing adults in the lymphatics are associated with endothelial thickening, fibrin deposition, and infiltration with eosinophils, histiocytes, and lymphocytes. Giant cells occur. Fibrotic and inflammatory changes tend to obstruct the lymphatics, and this process is exacerbated by death of the worms, which may calcify. There is reactive hyperplasia in the lymph nodes, and small granulomas are seen. An eosinophilic endophlebitis of the small veins is present in the lymph nodes. The testicles and epididymis often show similar changes with evidence of chronic inflammation. Worms may not be present at the site of inflammation. Secretions of the worm, especially after molting, are thought to be responsible for some of these changes. As lymphatic obstruction becomes more extensive, chronic edema develops in the infected areas. Recently lymphedema has been produced in laboratory animals with longstanding brugia infections.

CLINICAL MANIFESTATIONS. Attacks of fever, headache, and lymphadenopathy sometimes associated with urticarial rashes are known as filarial fever and occur in the acute phase of the disease. Often, however, no history of this early phase can be obtained. Epididymitis may occur as a lone lesion. Lymphatics most affected are those of the inguinal region, upper arms, and spermatic cord. Chronic lymphadenopathy is often the only sign of infection for years. Retrograde lymphangitis may be noted. In a small proportion of infected individuals, with increasing lymphatic obstruction over the years, all degrees of chronic edema occur, affecting especially the lower limbs and scrotum. Initially the edema is pitting, but as organization of collagen occurs in the edematous subcutaneous tissues, it becomes nonpitting. Eventually the giant limbs of elephantiasis are produced. The skin over the affected part, at first smooth, later becomes scaly and is fissured at the points where the fascia is attached to the skin. Hyperkeratosis produces warts and nodules. Varicose nodes in the groin are the result of lymphatic dilatation and may lead to scrotal lymphedema. Infection may supervene in any of these lesions with formation of a chronic discharging sinus. Chronic inflammatory disease of the testicle and epididymis with or without hydrocele occurs.

Chyluria may be renal or vesical in origin, depending on the level at which the lymph varix communicates with the urinary tract. Cystoscopy and intravenous or retrograde pyelography help to establish the site of communication.

DIAGNOSIS. In the early stages and when lymphadenopathy only is present, microfilariae are usually present in night blood films. Although the motile microfilariae are easily seen in fresh films, staining is necessary for identification. Microfilariae may be absent in the late stage; thus they were found in only 4 per cent of patients with elephantiasis, and 30 per cent of patients with hydrocele had microfilariae in one series. Concentration techniques are available for microfilariae, and they may be found in the chylous urine or hydrocele fluid. A millipore filtration concentration technique has shown that small numbers of microfilariae are circulating during the day in periodic infections. Eosinophilia is not a constant finding. The filarial complement-fixation test and skin test, although only group specific, are useful in suggesting a filarial cause for a lymphedema. Lymphangiograms reveal the extent of the lymphatic obstruction and may be a useful preoperative measure. It is rarely justified to remove an enlarged lymph node to find the adults because this still further prejudices the lymphatic circulation. In an endemic area surgeons frequently encounter adult worms when operating on the groin.

The differential diagnosis depends on the type of clinical syndrome. Lymphadenopathy caused by other infections and neoplasms must be considered. Elephantiasis may be associated with congenital defects of the lymphatic drainage as well as tuberculous inguinal lymphadenitis. Tuberculosis, *Schistosoma haematobium,* and gonorrhea produce epididymitis, and relatively few hydroceles are filarial. Lymphatic obstruction caused by many other agents may produce lymphedema and chyluria.

TREATMENT. Diethylcarbamazine (Banocide, Hetrazan) is believed to kill a large proportion of adults as well as microfilariae. It is usually given in an oral dose of 6 mg per kilogram, in three divided doses after meals. This dose is then given for 14 days. Reactions are mild in comparison with those seen in onchocerciasis, but fever, nausea and vomiting, and skin rashes may occur as with any drug. The arsenical Mel W and the antimonial Astiban (sodium dimercaptosuccinate) kill adult filariae, but are too toxic for general use. All patients with microfilaremia should receive an adequate course of treatment.

The management of lymphedema depends on its severity. Mild degrees are best treated with elevation of the foot of the bed and an elastic stocking. Careful instructions regarding foot care should be given, as ascending streptococcal cellulitis is common in the edematous tissues and further prejudices the lymphatic circulation. Some workers believe the *Streptococcus* to be more important in producing lymphangitis than the worms themselves. Any foot sepsis requires early and vigorous treatment with antimicrobial drugs. Tinea infections should be eradicated. Banocide therapy is often given in elephantiasis on the ground that it may prevent further lymphatic damage, but clinical improvement is seldom observed.

A variety of surgical operations have been devised to remove the edematous subcutaneous tissue from the leg, scrotum, and breasts. Success depends on the type of operation and the skill of the surgeon. In scrotal elephantiasis care must be taken to preserve the testicles. Hydroceles can be treated by the injection of sclerosing agents. Chyluria of bladder origin can be terminated by fulgurating the leaking bladder lymphatics. Renal chyluria is best left alone, although in the past kidneys have been wrapped in cellophane with the subsequent production of renal hypertension.

PREVENTION. Diethylcarbamazine, 3 mg per kilogram per month for 12 to 18 months, has been effective in mass treatment for preventive purposes. Residual DDT or dieldrin is effective against many of the mosquito vectors, and systematic destruction of mosquito-breeding sites has also met with success. Biologic control of mosquito vectors is receiving intensive field trials, but thus far they have not resulted in methods for mass application.

MALAYAN FILARIASIS

A disease similar to bancroftian filariasis is produced by a closely related filarial worm, *Brugia malayi.* The sheathed microfilariae of this species have two distinct caudal nuclei. Transmitted by *Mansonoides* mosquitoes, it is the only filarial infection of man in Malaya and Borneo, whereas in India, Ceylon, and tropical China it coexists with *W. bancrofti. Brugia malayi* is responsible for only mild lymphedema in man, usually below the knee, with enlargement of the popliteal and femoral nodes. In contrast to bancroftian filariasis, the microfilaremia rates in the Malayan form are quite high in children younger than five years. In this infection, also, there are two types of organisms, one with nocturnal periodicity, and another subperiodic form. The latter is found in many animals (primates, carnivores, and rodents) and is a true zoonosis.

Galindo, L., Von Lichtenberg, F., and Baldison, C.: Bancroftian filariasis in Puerto Rico: Infection pattern and tissue lesions. Am. J. Trop. Med., 11:739, 1962.

Nelson, G. S.: The pathology of filarial infections. Helminth. Abst., 35:Pt. 4, 311, 1966.

Schacher, J. F., and Sahyoun, P. F.: A chronological study of the histopathology of filarial disease in cats and dogs caused by *Brugia phangi* (Buckley and Edeson, 1956). Trans. R. Soc. Trop. Med. Hyg., 61:234, 1967.

Turner, L. H.: Studies on filariasis in Malaya: the clinical features of filariasis due to *Wuchereria malayi*. Trans. R. Soc. Trop. Med. Hyg., 53:154, 1959.

Wilson, T.: Filariasis in Malaya — A general review. Trans. R. Soc. Trop. Med. Hyg., 55:107, 1961.

LOIASIS

Loa loa infection is characterized by the appearance of transient swellings mainly on the limbs; these are thought to be the site of the migrating adult worms in the subcutaneous tissue. Occasionally a worm will traverse the conjunctiva of the eye.

The male adult worm is 30 mm long and the female 70 mm. They live for many years, and gain access to the body through the proboscis of biting flies (deer flies of the genus *Chrysops*). These worms appear to be in a state of continuous migration in the subcutaneous tissues of the body. It is not clearly understood how the sexes locate each other, but they meet and mate, and the female produces microfilariae that appear in the blood during the day and are infective to the insect vector.

Man is the only reservoir host, with the possible exception of monkeys. Human loiasis is restricted to Africa, mainly the West Coast. It occurs from Sierra Leone to the Cameroons and extends into the heart of Africa in the region of the Congo basin.

CLINICAL MANIFESTATIONS. The main clinical manifestation is the repeated occurrence of hot erythematous swellings (5 to 10 cm or more) called Calabar swellings after the endemic area of Calabar. These occur in the upper limbs particularly, are painful, and subside in a few days. They are associated with the presence of an adult worm. A similar swelling occurs around the eye when the adult worm crosses the eye beneath the conjunctivae. The patient notices the worm in his line of vision ("like a submarine, doctor") and it is worth inquiring for such a history. Calabar swellings seem to occur more frequently in the extremities. Why this is so is not known. Routine roentgenography in endemic areas often reveals calcified dead worms lying between the metacarpals. Rarely, neurologic symptoms may be associated with the infection if the Calabar swelling involves a peripheral nerve. Also the parasite has been found in the cerebrospinal fluid associated with a meningoencephalitis.

DIAGNOSIS. The initial diagnosis is usually based on a history of Calabar swellings in a patient coming from an endemic area. Examination of the daytime blood reveals sheathed microfilariae with a characteristic distribution of caudal nuclei. In early loiasis, microfilariae may not be detected even by concentration techniques. Very high eosinophil counts are encountered at this stage (50 to 70 per cent). A positive filarial complement-fixation test is usually present. Occasionally the adult worm can be extracted as it crosses the eye.

TREATMENT. Diethylcarbamazine (Hetrazan) kills both adults and microfilariae. One course of 6 mg per kilogram of body weight for 14 days is all that is necessary. Reactions are rare.

Woodruff, A. W.: Loiasis, In Fairley, N. H., Woodruff, A. W., and Walters, J. H. (eds.): Recent Advances in Tropical Medicine. London, J. & A. Churchill, Ltd., 1961, pp. 178–194.

MANSONELLA OZZARDI

Mansonella ozzardi is found only in the New World, occurring in South America and certain foci in the Caribbean. *Culicoides* midges are the vectors in Trinidad; in Brazil, *Simulium amazonicum* has been implicated. The adult worms are embedded in visceral adipose tissue. Although they are usually regarded as nonpathogenic, fever, headache, lymphadenitis, and erythematous irritant skin rashes have been reported in association with their presence. Cold extremities, the result of peripheral vasoconstriction caused by a postulated filarial toxin, have been reported. The microfilariae show no particular periodicity and are about twice the size of perstans and have a different caudal morphology. A recent survey, cited below, showed that of 810 Colombian Indians, 96.2 per cent harbored microfilariae of *Mansonella ozzardi*. Diethylcarbamazine (Hetrazan) is ineffective.

Marinkelle, C. J., and German, E.: Mansonelliasis in the Comisaría del Vaupes of Colombia. Trop. Geog. Med., 22:101, 1970.

Undiano, C.: Importance and present-day concepts of the pathogenicity of *Mansonella* infections. Fev. Fac. Cienc. Med. Univ. Cordoba, 24:183, 1966.

DIPETALONEMA PERSTANS

Filariasis caused by *Dipetalonema perstans* has an extensive distribution in Equatorial Africa, the Caribbean, and South America, where it sometimes overlaps with *Mansonella ozzardi*. The adult worms are found in association with the serous cavities of the body, usually behind the limiting membrane. They may be seen at postmortem examination moving behind the peritoneum or pleura. The small (100 μ) unsheathed microfilariae are found in the blood throughout the 24 hours, but there is a peak in the peripheral blood population at night. A *Culicoides* species, a small balck midge, is responsible for transmission.

The vast majority of patients exhibiting microfilaremia have no symptoms, but there have been recent reports of clinical symptoms associated with this infection. These reports include fever, Calabar swellings, arthritis, and upper abdominal pain associated with hepatomegaly. A high eosinophilia is often present in cases with scanty embryos, and such a finding in a patient from an endemic area should prompt a careful search for these. Diethylcarbamazine (Hetrazan) has little effect on the adults or on the microfilariae.

Wiseman, R. A.: *Acanthocheilonema perstans*: A cause of significant eosinophilia in the tropics. Comments on its pathogenicity. Trans. R. Soc. Trop. Med. Hyg., 61:667, 1967.

ONCHOCERCIASIS
(River Blindness)

River blindness is a form of cutaneous filariasis caused by infection with *Onchocerca volvulus* and is characterized by skin irritation, corneal opacities, and skin nodules.

ETIOLOGY. The threadlike adult worms lie tangled together in fibrous nodules in the subcutaneous tissues or fascial planes. Microfilariae produced by the females become widely distributed in the surrounding skin. Female black flies (buffalo gnats) of the genus *Simulium* ingest these larvae while taking a blood meal. After development in the fly for one week, the larvae are infective for man and are deposited when the fly next bites. They take more than a year to mature, mate, and produce microfilariae. Adult worms live 7 to 15 years.

EPIDEMIOLOGY. Human onchocerciasis is found on the West Coast of Africa from Sierra Leone to the Congo and in the east from the Sudan to Nyasaland. It also occurs in Guatemala, Mexico, Eastern Venezuela, Northern Brazil, and Surinam. *Simulium* larvae and pupae are usually found in rapidly running highly oxygenated water. Small insects (3 mm long), the flies bite low on the legs in Africa, but more around the head in Central America, which may account for the high incidence of nodules on the head in the latter locality. In East Africa *Simulium naevi* larvae and pupae evaded detection for many years until they were found on the shells of fresh-water crabs.

PATHOGENESIS AND PATHOLOGY. An initial inflammatory reaction around the adult worm is followed by a foreign body granulomatous reaction and fibrous capsule formation. The nodules are literally the graveyards of the adult worms, for these eventually die and degenerate, sometimes with secondary abscess formation. The microfilariae in the surrounding subcutaneous tissues produce a low-grade inflammatory reaction with lymphocytes, plasma cells, and eosinophils. Thickening of the epidermis and dermis owing to fibrosis eventually occurs, with destruction of elastic fibers and sometimes reduction in pigmentation.

Microfilariae migrate into the tissues of the eye to produce important inflammatory lesions which may result in blindness. Punctate keratitis is associated with death of microfilariae in the cornea, and such multiple corneal opacities may result in permanent corneal scarring. A low-grade iritis and iridocyclitis result in pupillary distortion and even occlusion. Choroidoretinitis also occurs.

CLINICAL MANIFESTATIONS. Any patient who has a persistent irritating skin rash or visual disturbances and has been in one of the endemic areas may have onchocerciasis. More rarely, the presenting complaint takes the form of deep-seated muscular pains. The early skin lesions consist of an erythematous papular irritant rash. In heavy infections definite thickening and hyperkeratosis of the skin occur (craw-craw or crocodile skin). Rarer late complications are depigmentation and pendulous bags in the groins containing sclerosed lymph nodes.

Nodules vary much in size from a few centimeters to as big as a tennis ball. They are frequently detected over bony prominences such as the greater trochanter, the iliac crest, the olecranons, ribs, and occiput. Often the adult worms are located deep in the fascial planes, and no nodules are palpable. To detect the small milky dots of punctate keratitis near the limbus the eyes should be examined with a strong pencil torch, the beam directed obliquely across the cornea. Signs of iritis may be present. With a slit lamp, microfilariae may be visible in the aqueous humor. Funduscopic examination may reveal the much rarer posterior segment lesion.

DIAGNOSIS. Skin shavings are used to demonstrate microfilariae. Thin sections of the superficial skin are removed with a razor blade, mounted in saline, teased out, and examined. Many motile microfilariae emerge from those snips within an hour after they have been made. Blood contamination can be avoided if the shavings are superficial, and this is important if there is coexistent blood microfilaremia. If there is a definite site of skin irritation, shavings should be taken from this area. In lightly infected patients multiple shavings may be necessary to detect microfilariae, and quite often they are not found. The reaction to a test dose of 50 mg of diethylcarbamazine (Mazzotti's test) in the form of an exacerbation of the itching rash is suggestive, as are an eosinophilia and a positive filarial complement-fixation test. In up to 35 per cent of cases microfilariae can be found in the urine.

Scabies and superficial mycoses are the most common irritant skin rashes of the tropics and are important differential diagnoses. Although an infection with no mortality, the recurrent irritation of onchocerciasis can be most distressing. Severe ocular lesions may induce total blindness, and this is the blinding filarid.

TREATMENT. When practicable, all nodules should be excised; this simple measure will reduce the load of adult worms. Suramin* is effective in killing adult worms and is more suitable for mass treatment programs. The side effects and method of administration of this drug are mentioned under African Trypanosomiasis (see Ch. 194.2), which should be consulted before its use. A suitable course for onchocerciasis is 1 gram weekly for six weeks. As the drug is nephrotoxic, treatment should be stopped if more than 30 mg per 100 ml of protein appears in the urine.

Diethylcarbamazine is effective in killing microfilariae but does not kill the adult worms. In sensitized individuals, reactions occur when the microfilariae die in the tissues. Skin irritation becomes more intense, and there may be edema of the skin with fever, headache, and malaise. More serious is acute inflammation of the eye which may prejudice sight. As these reactions are dose related, it is usual to start therapy with a small dose of the drug (0.25 mg per kilogram) and increase gradually to a maximum dose of 6 mg per kilogram of body weight per day for three weeks. Eye reactions can be controlled with 1 per cent cortisone acetate eye drops and the general reactions controlled with antihistamines and, in severe cases, with systemic steroids.

PREVENTION. *Simulium* larvae and pupae are very sensitive to small concentrations of DDT in the river water (less than 1 part per million), and this has been the most effective form of control of the insect vector. Personal prophylaxis is possible to a limited extent by avoiding places where biting *Simulium* are numerous.

---

*Available from Center for Disease Control (404-633-3311, Ext. 3670).

Buck, A. A. (ed.): Onchocerciasis. Symptomatology, Pathology, and Diagnosis. Geneva, World Health Organization, 1974.

Duke, B. O. L.: Onchocerciasis. Br. Med. J., 4:301, 1968.

Nelson, D. S.: Onchocerciasis. In Dawes, B. (ed.): Advances in Parasitology. Volume 8. New York, Academic Press, 1970, p. 173.

Onchocerciasis in the Western Hemisphere. PAHO Sc. Pub. No. 298. Washington, D.C., 1974.

WHO Expert Committee on Onchocerciasis. World Health Organization Technical Report Series No. 335, 1–92, 1966.

STREPTOCERCIASIS

Dipetalonema streptocerca is carried by midges of the genus *Culicoides*. It occurs in Central Africa, particularly in the Congo and neighboring countries. The adult worms are found in the region of the shoulder girdle, and the microfilariae produced in the skin cause a reddish brown irritant rash which may be associated with some degree of edema. Skin shavings reveal the unsheathed microfilariae with the crooked tails and the nuclei going down to the tip. Treatment with diethylcarbamazine is effective.

Meyers, W. M., Connor, D. H., Harman, L. E., Fleshman, K., Moris, R. and Neafie, R. G.: Human streptocerciasis: A clinicopathologic study of 40 Africans (Zairans), including identification of the adult filaria. Am. J. Trop. Med. Hyg., 21:528, 1972.

DIROFILARIASIS

Several dirofilariae have been reported to occasionally cause symptoms in man, particularly in the United States. Such infections have also been reported from the Mediterranean basin, South America, and Africa. In Louisiana and Texas a subcutaneous filarid of raccoons (*Dirofilaria tenuis*) occasionally invades man, but does not mature. It produces a painful subcutaneous nodule, consisting of an eosinophilic inflammatory reaction around the worm; this may be a granuloma or may be located in a lymph node. This diagnosis is usually made after biopsy. Mosquitoes transmit the infection.

Other species found in man include *D. conjunctivae*, *D. repens*, and *D. immitis*. Adult worms have been detected in the heart and great vessels and in the eye. They have also caused infarcts in the lung and "coin" lesions at the hila which may be mistaken for a bronchial carcinoma and excised before the nature is known. In sections the worm is seen in cross-section in the center of an infarcted area infiltrated with eosinophils.

Beaver, P. C., and Orihel, T. C.: Human infection with filariae of animals in the United States. Am. J. Trop. Med. Hyg., 14:1010, 1965.

Beskin, C. A., Colvin, S. H., Jr., and Beaver, P. C.: Pulmonary dirofilariasis, cause of a pulmonary nodular disease. JAMA, 198:665, 1966.

POSSIBLE HUMAN MENINGONEMIASIS

Orihel has pointed out that microfilariae recovered from patients with neurologic disorders in Rhodesia and thought to be *Dipetalonema perstans* more closely resemble *Meningonema peruzzii*. The adults of this species inhabit the leptomeninges of the brainstem in African monkeys.

Orihel, T. C.: Cerebral filariasis in Rhodesia — a zoonotic infection. Am. J. Trop. Med. Hyg., 22:596, 1973.

PULMONARY TROPICAL EOSINOPHILIA
(Eosinophilic Lung, Weingarten's Syndrome)

Since the early part of this century Indian physicians have recognized a syndrome of paroxysmal cough and nocturnal bronchospasm associated with high eosinophilia, and have called it pulmonary tropical eosinophilia. Low fever, dyspnea, and malaise may be accompanying symptoms. The absolute eosinophil count is above 3000 per cubic millimeter, and may reach very high levels. Chest films may show increased reticulation, prominence of bronchovascular markings, or diffuse miliary mottling of the lung fields. In Ball's series of 1000 cases the great majority were Indian; the condition is much more common among Indians in Singapore. It is now generally accepted that this syndrome is caused by occult filarial infections. The evidence that this is so can be listed as follows: (1) Patients have a consistently high titer of filarial complement-fixing antibodies in the absence of evidence of microfilariae in the blood. (2) There is a clinical, hematologic, and serologic response to therapy with the antifilarial drug diethylcarbamazine. (3) The syndrome has been produced in a volunteer by inoculation of *Brugia malayi* infective larvae and *Brugia pahangi* (a feline filaria). (4) Microfilariae have been demonstrated in lung granulomas in such cases by several groups of workers.

It is possible that eosinophilic lung results from an alteration in host immunity to the filarial parasite, giving rise to allergic phenomena manifested by persistent hypereosinophilia and pulmonary symptoms. What is not yet settled is the precise identification of the parasite. It is likely that several species of filaria of the genera *Wuchereria* and *Brugia*, some human, some animal, may be involved, depending on the locality in which the syndrome occurs. The high incidence in Indians is noteworthy and may suggest a genetic predisposition in certain racial groups. The course of diethylcarbamazide recommended is similar to that for bancroftian filariasis. Often the symptoms get temporarily worse after starting the drug, but invariably they resolve, and a second course of the drug or the use of carbarsone as an alternative is seldom necessary.

The question of occult filariasis has been reviewed, and it has been pointed out that in many instances it has not been possible to identify the helminth responsible because of the difficulty of interpreting the microfilariae in tissue sections even if they are found. Quite apart from the well defined clinical entity of pulmonary tropical eosinophilia there are patients presenting with signs of reticuloendothelial activation (enlarged lymph nodes, hepatosplenomegaly) and eosinophilia for which it is difficult to find a cause.

Ball, J. D.: Tropical pulmonary eosinophilia. Trans. R. Soc. Trop. Med. Hyg., 44:237, 1950.

Donohugh, D. L.: Tropical eosinophilia, an etiologic enquiry. N. Engl. J. Med., 269:1357, 1963.

Danaraj, T. J., Pacheco, G., Shanmugaratnam, K., and Beaver, P. C.: The etiology and pathology of eosinophilic lung (tropical eosinophilia). Am. J. Trop. Med. Hyg., 15:183, 1966.

Islam, N.: Tropical eosinophilia. East Pakistan, Islam A. Chittagong, 1964.

Lie Kian, J., and Shandosham, A. A.: The pathology of clinical filariasis due to *Wuchereria bancrofti* and *Brugia malayi* and a discussion of occult filariasis. In Shandosham, A. A., and Zaman, V. (eds.): Proceedings of Seminar on Filariasis and Immunology of Parasitic Infections, and Laboratory Meeting. Kuala Lumpur, Malaysia, Rajiv Printers, 1969, p. 125.

DISORDERS WITH SOME RELATION TO HELMINTHS

Philip D. Marsden

215. EOSINOPHILIA IN RELATION TO HELMINTHIC INFECTIONS

Hypereosinophilic states are considered elsewhere in this book, and conditions such as periarteritis nodosa, eosinophilic leukemia, and allergic diseases are discussed in the appropriate chapters. However, the author believes that a number of the cases of unexplained eosinophilia seen today in diagnostic units will in time be explained on the basis of helminthic infections, and it is worthwhile making one or two general points in relation to such infections.

As can be seen from the preceding chapters, almost all helminthic infections in contrast to protozoal infections are at some time or other associated with eosinophilia. In terms of the parasites for which man is the definitive host, the eosinophilia often coincides with the invasive phase of a trematode, cestode, or nematode infection, and the diagnosis may not be apparent until several weeks or months later when the adults begin to produce progeny. For this reason patients with obscure eosinophilia should always be kept under observation, and stool or tissue specimens examined after an interval. Some parasites are notorious in presenting a problem of eosinophilia for diagnosis, notably *Strongyloides* and *Trichinella* infections. After effective treatment of helminthic infections, particularly those in close contact with body tissues, there is often a pronounced rise in circulating eosinophils.

Perhaps more interesting is the clinical situation in which a patient has a significant human helminth load and yet little or no expected eosinophilia in the absence of cortisone therapy. Recent work suggesting that sensitized lymphocytes play an important role in the genesis of eosinophilia may throw some light on this problem.

Eosinophilia is a prominent feature of infections with nonhuman helminths, e.g., *Angiostrongylus*, and situations in which there is an abnormal host response, e.g., pulmonary tropical eosinophilia. It appears that a small number of nonhuman helminths passing through man's tissues may engender marked eosinophilia and even hypergammaglobulinemia, e.g., toxocariasis, gnatho-

stomiasis. To find the helminths responsible is impossible in many patients, and when found they may be very difficult to identify. Our elucidation of this clinical problem appears to rest on the elaboration of more specific and sensitive serologic tests, and the techniques of indirect hemagglutination, gel diffusion, indirect fluorescent antibody tests, and similar procedures are useful here to detect host response to helminthic antigens. However, much difficult work will be needed to characterize these complex antigens.

Finally, in a clinical consideration of this problem, common things occur commonly. A survey of a series of patients with occult eosinophilia in a large teaching hospital in New York City revealed a few cases of strongyloidiasis, but eosinophilia was most frequently one of the signs of a reaction to drug therapy.

Beeson, P. B., and Bass, D. A.: The Esoinophil. Philadelphia, W. B. Saunders Company, 1977.

216. TROPICAL PYOMYOSITIS

This is a condition of a large deep-seated abscess, single or multiple, occurring in any voluntary muscle. Strange lumps for diagnosis in the tropics sometimes turn out to be deep-seated abscesses. By far the most frequent organism isolated is *Staphylococcus aureus*. Histologically there are areas of focal muscle necrosis with inflammatory cell infiltration. The regional lymph nodes are rarely affected, and there may be no fever or leukocytosis in the peripheral blood. The cause is unknown. Subcutaneous helminthic infection, particularly filaria, and sickle cell disease have been suggested as predisposing conditions, but as yet there is no convincing evidence to this effect. Treatment consists of antimicrobial therapy (initially with penicillin) and surgical drainage.

Elebute, E. A.: Pyomyositis. *In* Schwartz, S. I., Adesola, A. O., Elebute, E. A., and Rob, C. G. (eds.): Tropical Surgery, New York, McGraw-Hill Book Company, 1971.

Marcus, R. T., and Foster, W. D.: Observations on the clinical features, aetiology and geographical distribution of pyomyositis in East Africa. East Afr. Med. J., 45:167, 1968.

Tropical myositis. Lancet, 1:862, 1978.

PART XI
DISORDERS OF THE NERVOUS SYSTEM AND BEHAVIOR

217. INTRODUCTION

Fred Plum

The scientific revolution has begun to invade if not yet fully conquer the fields of neurology and psychiatry. The 12 years that have elapsed since I first had the privilege of writing this introductory chapter have spawned pharmacologic treatments for depression and mania, the knowledge of the infectious nature of Creutzfeldt-Jakob disease, the realization that slow or latent viral infections can cause neurologic disease, a specific and rational treatment for parkinsonism, the awareness that myasthenia gravis is an immunologic disorder and can be treated as such, and much of our understanding of how the hypothalamus specifically regulates the pituitary gland. Since the last edition of this textbook appeared, medicine has learned that man's nervous system not only contains specific receptors to which opiates bind to produce their extraordinary effects, but that brain-made endogenous peptides, the enkephalins or endorphins, attach to these natural sites to modify intrinsic sensations and behavior. Also since the last edition, computerized transaxial (CT) scanning has transformed diagnostic neurology, seemingly making obsolete many of the physician's traditional slow and imprecise approaches to the patient.

The aforementioned discoveries have meant marvelous advances in clinical care. Unfortunately, however, new diagnostic machines and new drugs to treat symptoms can sometimes leave untouched many of the complex, human needs of patients, and this can be especially true of individuals with neurologic complaints. The neurologic and psychiatric patient, perhaps more than most, requires a physician who not only sees a symptom or disease but looks beyond that to see who is sick and asks why.

Most diseases express themselves, sooner or later, through nervous system symptoms, and this fact sometimes makes neurology complicated and also places limitations on the information to be gained from the diagnostic machines that neurologists use. Pain, sensory loss, weakness, disturbed thinking, and impaired mood or alertness can reflect a systemic disorder as often as a primary neurologic illness. Perhaps even more frequently, such symptoms derive from man's faulty adjustment to his environment. Unless they specifically remind themselves to do otherwise, physicians educated to respond predominantly to the diagnostic accuracies of blood tests, CT scans, contrast radiographs, electrical nerve and muscle studies, and electroencephalographic tracings may overlook the fact that none of these tests or machines can detect most of the miseries which bring most patients to seek the help of their doctors. Most patients consult physicians because they are afraid — afraid of pain, of cancer, of heart disease, of losing their memories and minds, of humiliation, of loneliness — ultimately, of death. It takes clinical experience and wisdom to separate symptoms born of these fears from complaints which arise from a diseased structure or function. The descriptions and approaches included in Part XI attempt to give the physician a framework for making that separation in patients with neurologic problems.

A word of reassurance may be in order about how to approach the patient with a neurologic complaint or a suspected neurologic lesion. If one is logical, systematic and thorough, the seeming complexities of such patients will be found rapidly to become analyzable. The most reliable approach to neurologic patients lies in the full, thorough, and educated application of clinical method, emphasizing neither the laboratory nor the bedside examination at the expense of the other. A recent analysis of diagnostic accuracy in medical illnesses indicates that a careful history provides 80 per cent of diagnoses and that the laboratory adds no more than another 10 per cent. Obviously, the history, physical examination, and laboratory all offer important confirmations of each other. But all evidence still indicates that a careful history contributes the largest share of neurologic diagnosis even when all the new technical diagnostic procedures are fully utilized. Accurate diagnosis in neurology still depends mainly on the thorough understanding of the pathologic physiology of signs and symptoms.

Part XI is organized in two main categories. The first considers the more general functions of the nervous system: how it is organized, how it handles certain normal activities, and how it expresses psychologic and somatic symptoms in response to either real or symbolic threat or injury. The second takes the more traditional approach, and discusses neurologic diseases according to anatomic and causative categories. Heavy emphasis is placed on the mechanism of disease and, when known, the biochemistry of its treatment.

As the following chapters regrettably illustrate, many neurologic and neuromuscular diseases still lack satisfactory specific treament. Yet this shortcoming should not becloud the principle that much of the practice of medicine directs itself at protecting or recouping brain function, sometimes at the necessary, temporary expense of other organs. Man's brain makes him human.

Damage it and life loses its meaning in direct proportion, no matter what other physiologic benefits may accrue in the process. The brain cannot be regenerated, repaired, or homotransplanted. It accumulates no metabolic debts and, unless supplied continuously by an effective circulation carrying large amounts of oxygen and glucose, it digests itself irreparably. One cannot "let the brain go" while solving other medical problems. If an elderly man with severe anemia suffers an ischemic stroke while awaiting accurate blood studies, there is no satisfaction later in a correct hematologic diagnosis. If an adolescent girl suffers permanent dementia from hypoglycemia while having her diabetes regulated, the perfect control of glycosuria seems hardly worth it. To maintain the integrity of the nervous system remains the first goal in therapeutics.

Section One CONSCIOUSNESS AND ITS DISTURBANCES

218. INTRODUCTION

Fred Plum

From the medical standpoint, consciousness includes two interdependent but separate functions, namely, wakefulness and psychologically recognizable mental activity. Dementia, apathy, amnesia, and aphasia are conditions in which the content of consciousness is reduced but, as long as enough appropriate responses remain in other behavioral functions, consciousness is considered to be preserved. Obtundation and drowsiness describe states of impaired alertness or wakefulness, often with an excessive tendency to sleep. Stupor is a state wherein subjects arouse when vigorously stimulated, but immediately sink back again as soon as external stimuli are withdrawn. Coma is complete unresponsiveness with eyes closed and no evidence of psychologically appropriate responses to stimulation.

The present physiologic concept of consciousness is that it depends upon a close functional interaction between the intact cerebral hemispheres and the central gray matter of the upper brainstem. The hemispheres contribute most of the specific components of consciousness, including language, memory, intellect, and learned responses to sensory stimuli. But in order for the cerebrum to function, the organism must be aroused or activated by more caudally placed mechanisms that reside in the thalamus, hypothalamus, midbrain, and upper pons. An important component of this arousal mechanism is located within what Magoun and his colleagues called the ascending reticular activating system; other brainstem systems also influence cerebral cortical activity and the state of consciousness.

The relation of the cerebral cortex to consciousness is more quantitative than qualitative: All hemispheric lesions undoubtedly reduce, at least to some degree, the content of man's consciousness, and the total loss of the cortex causes at least several weeks of coma even if the brainstem is intact. Between the extremes of an injury so small that it is clinically almost undetectable and so large that it causes coma lies a continuum along which the size of the lesion and the impairment of mind, memory, wit, and personality are roughly proportional.

219. THE PATHOGENESIS OF STUPOR AND COMA

Fred Plum

As noted in Ch. 218, consciousness depends on the integrity of the sum of the physiologic activity of the two cerebral hemispheres and an activating system located in the central core of the upper brainstem. It follows that to produce an alteration of consciousness, a disease or dysfunction must damage or depress either the two hemispheres or the brainstem core or both. A potentially bewildering series of individual maladies can have one or both of these effects, as may be seen in the accompanying table. However, if one examines the mechanisms by which neurologic diseases cause coma, all these maladies fall into three categories that can be distinguished by their signs and symptoms: (1) supratentorial mass lesions, (2) subtentorial compressive or destructive lesions, and (3) metabolic brain diseases.

The Common Causes of Stupor and Coma

Supratentorial lesions (causing upper brainstem dysfunction)
  Cerebral hemorrhage
  Large cerebral infarction
  Subdural hematoma
  Epidural hematoma
  Brain tumor
  Brain abscess (rare)

Subtentorial lesions (compressing or destroying the reticular formation)
  Pontine or cerebellar hemorrhage
  Infarction
  Tumor
  Cerebellar abscess

Metabolic and diffuse lesions (see also Table 1 in Ch. 220)
  Anoxia or ischemia
  Hypoglycemia
  Nutritional deficiency
  Endogenous organ failure or deficiency
  Ionic and electrolyte disorders
  Exogenous poison
  Infections
    Meningitis
    Encephalitis
  Concussion and postictal states

SUPRATENTORIAL MASS LESIONS

Supratentorial masses are rarely so large that they produce coma by directly destroying or replacing the cerebral hemispheres. Rather, they interfere with consciousness because they shift and squeeze the contents of the supratentorial compartment and, in so doing, compress the diencephalon. The expanding process can originate anywhere in the hemisphere and ultimately produce this reaction because the fibrous tentorium and the bones of the base of the skull resist movement except toward the tentorial opening. As a result, when supratentorial masses demand room for expansion, the diencephalic tectum and adjacent midbrain are likely to be compressed, and the diencephalon may be displaced downward through the tentorial notch (transtentorial herniation).

How do supratentorial masses progress so that these reactions occur? The brain has certain common responses to injury, including edema, vascular dilatation, and the invasion of leukocytes and proliferation of glial cells. The intensity, tempo, and exact contribution of each of these responses varies according to the nature of the original lesion and the rate at which it appears, but each shares in the brain's defenses against neoplasms, infections, infarcts, and irritants. Thus the original lesion gradually enlarges and, ripple-like, tends to impair structures ever more remote from itself in the inexpansible intracranial cavity. The remote effects are due partly to edema spreading away from the edges of the primary lesion and partly to an actual shift of the brain within the skull, compressing normal tissues and blood vessels against rigid structures such as the falx cerebri and the tentorium. At this stage, clinical signs of increased intracranial pressure are common and imply that an intracranial lesion is already exerting generalized deleterious effects.

The clinical picture of supratentorial mass lesions producing stupor or coma has several distinctive features. If a history is available, localizing symptoms such as frontal headache, focal seizures, or other changes consistent with hemispheric disease will usually be found to have preceded unconsciousness. Physically, most patients demonstrate a combination of *focal* hemispheral signs, e.g., sensorimotor defect, aphasia, and visual field defect, reflecting the site of the original pathologic process, plus *diffuse* signs of supratentorial dysfunction, indicating that the lesion is exerting remote effects on the opposite hemisphere and the deep diencephalon. An important negative finding is that, unless the patient is in the terminal stages of illness, no evidence of direct subtentorial brainstem dysfunction can be found: pupillary and oculovestibular reflexes remain intact. As a supratentorial lesion progresses, the neurologic signs and symptoms evolve in a characteristic, orderly, rostral-caudal pattern. The more rostrally located neurologic functions first disappear, followed by more caudal impairment, first in the diencephalon and then down the brainstem almost as if the structures were being progressively transected from above downward, each plane of function being removed almost completely before the next is impaired.

The aforementioned description needs amplification to be complete. Some supratentorial masses begin and enlarge in neurologically silent areas such as the frontal lobes or the subdural space and lack a focal signature. Lesions of this type may be revealed only when the patient develops signs of diffuse forebrain dysfunction plus, perhaps, headache and evidence of increased intracranial pressure.

Stupor or coma with supratentorial lesions is ominous because it implies that the deeply located upper brainstem is already compressed or distorted and that the much more serious complication of herniation of the forebrain downward into the tentorial notch is about to occur. Such herniation begins either with direct downward displacement of the diencephalon (central herniation) or with the uncus of the temporal lobe squeezing into the tentorial notch and against the midbrain (uncal herniation). Either way, if the hernia develops fully, it usually impacts itself upon the midbrain and nearly always results in permanent brain damage or death. A characteristic constellation of symptoms heralds each of these patterns of transtentorial herniation. With impending *central* herniation, stupor becomes gradually deeper, and the subjects sigh, yawn, or develop periodic respirations. The pupils shrink to 1 to 2 mm in diameter, but retain their light reflexes. Oculovestibular reflexes are brisk, and the extremities stiffen into bilateral rigidity or spasticity, combined with extensor plantar responses. With *uncal* herniation, signs are in many ways similar to the above except that as the uncus slides over the tentorial edge, it often compresses the third nerve ahead of it, even before the diencephalon is squeezed. The result is that the pupil on the side of the herniation begins to dilate more than its fellow. Eventually, the pupil dilates widely and becomes light-fixed, and the patient becomes stuporous. Shortly afterward, oculomotor functions of the third nerve are usually impaired, and the involved eye turns outward. If the herniating process continues, the opposite third nerve becomes involved as well, and then the brainstem. To initiate effective treatment one must recognize the process before this advanced stage and halt it with osmotic decompressing agents or surgical treatment. Otherwise, when conditions progress this far, few subjects recover without substantial, permanent neurologic injury.

SUBTENTORIAL MASS OR DESTRUCTIVE LESIONS

These conditions cause stupor or coma if they destroy or compress the centrally located activating systems in the brainstem anywhere above approximately the midpons. Expanding lesions of the posterior fossa have the same effect if they compress the midbrain upward. Compression against the medulla oblongata with an ensuing cerebellar pressure cone produces stiff neck, along with respiratory and cardiac irregularities, but does not directly cause loss of consciousness.

The characteristic clinical feature of subtentorial destruction or compression causing coma is the presence of restricted and usually asymmetrical signs of focal brainstem dysfunction, which frequently can be anatomically pinpointed to a single locus by the clinical findings. Seldom do the signs indicate complete brainstem transection. This restricted, discrete localization is unlike metabolic lesions causing coma in which the signs commonly indicate incomplete dysfunction at several different levels of the brain, and also is unlike the secondary brainstem dysfunction and coma that follow supratentorial herniation, in which *all* function at any given level tends to be lost as the process progresses from rostral to caudal along the neuraxis.

Purely compressive lesions of the posterior fossa rarely cause coma until late in their course when the patient is near death. The pathologic process involved is usually a hemorrhage, abscess, or tumor of the cerebellum or fourth ventricle. As a result, occipital headache, nystagmus, diplopia, nausea, vomiting, cranial nerve signs, and ataxia usually precede unconsciousness. Important points in distinguishing both destructive and compressive posterior fossa lesions from metabolic depression of the brainstem are that in metabolic depression oculovestibular responses are generally preserved until the advanced stages, and pupillary light reflexes are nearly always preserved. By contrast, structural brainstem lesions causing coma always disrupt the oculovestibular responses, and those involving the midbrain also interrupt the pupillary reflexes.

METABOLIC DEPRESSION OF THE BRAIN CAUSING COMA

Primary metabolic encephalopathies are intrinsic to the neuron, the glial cell, or the white matter, respectively. They often produce dementia, but rarely cause coma except terminally. *Secondary* metabolic encephalopathies are those in which brain function is disrupted either because the brain is not supplied with a required substance, e.g., thiamine, oxygen, or glucose, or because it is poisoned by an ingested or endogenous toxin, e.g., depressant drugs or the products of uremia. The secondary metabolic encephalopathies are frequent causes of delirium as well as of stupor and coma; their relationship to the normal metabolism of the brain is discussed in detail in Ch. 220.

Experimental evidence conflicts as to whether most metabolic agents causing coma depress mainly the brainstem reticular formation or the cerebral cortex. Clinically, most patients with metabolic encephalopathy appear to suffer depression of the forebrain more than of the brainstem. The remarkable finding with most metabolic encephalopathies, however, is the uneven degree to which they affect different parts of the brain without regard for simple anatomic levels. Thus metabolic encephalopathy characteristically depresses certain susceptible functions at several different brain levels, but at the same time spares other functions that emanate from identical levels. For example, nearly all metabolic poisons spare the pupillary light reflex so that reactive pupils persist into the deepest stages of metabolic coma until asphyxia intervenes. (Poisoning with glutethimide or parasympathomimetics provides the only exception to this rule, both drugs blocking the light reflex in large, coma-causing doses.) Most of the metabolic encephalopathies cause delirium before stupor or coma, and many of them are accompanied in their early stages by asterixis, a flapping irregular tremor of the outstretched hands, or by random myoclonic muscle twitches. Although the metabolic encephalopathies occasionally produce asymmetrical motor signs, they more characteristically impair body movement symmetrically, and they never impair central sensory pathways except as an accompaniment to the over-all depression of the sensorium.

To epitomize, diseases causing stupor or coma fall into three categories:

1. Supratentorial mass lesions present with asymmetrical neurologic signs of hemispheral dysfunction combined with evidence of intact subtentorial brainstem function. As supratentorial lesions evolve, the signs indicate progressive rostral-caudal neurologic deterioration, almost as if the brain were being serially sectioned from top to bottom.

2. Subtentorial compressive and destructive lesions present from the outset with either cranial nerve abnormalities or other focal brainstem signs, including pupillary and oculovestibular reflex abnormalities. Long tract motor signs are usually present and asymmetrical.

3. Metabolic brain diseases present a picture of either diffuse cortical depression or, more often, of impaired function in both the hemispheres and the brainstem accompanied by retained pupillary light reflexes. The multifocal distribution of metabolic encephalopathy is usually symmetrical and not accompanied by sensory impairments.

APPROACH TO THE PATIENT IN STUPOR OR COMA

The physician must ensure that the brain and other vital organs receive no further injury while he obtains whatever history, examinations, and laboratory data are required. Before anything else he must provide a free and open airway and determine that the subject is breathing deeply enough to oxygenate his lungs and eliminate carbon dioxide. Next, the heart and blood pressure should be examined, and possible sources of bleeding checked to be certain that cardiac output and blood volume are sufficient to supply the metabolic needs of the brain and kidney. In all patients in coma an intravenous infusion or central venous pressure line should be started, using a large-bore needle. Blood samples for typing and cross-matching, as well as for other appropriate laboratory determinations, can be obtained at this time. Whenever the cause of coma is doubtful, and particularly when the clinical signs suggest a metabolic disorder, blood should be taken for sugar determination, and then 50 ml of 50 per cent glucose given intravenously. Hypoglycemic encephalopathy can take many forms, some of which mimic other diseases. If glucose is given promptly, no further cerebral damage occurs while the doctor awaits definitive laboratory diagnosis. Intravenous sugar harms nothing if the coma has another cause.

Beyond these immediate, lifesaving measures, it requires considerable restraint to approach a patient in a coma methodically, for the urge to act without delay is understandably strong but potentially dangerous. Inquiry into both the past medical history and the circumstances under which the patient lost consciousness generally discloses more of diagnostic value than any other maneuver. Is there any suggestion that head trauma could have occurred recently? Has there been renal, hepatic, or myocardial disease? Could a seizure have preceded the present unconsciousness? Has the subject been taking insulin? Have there been recent changes in mood, behavior, or neurologic function to suggest an evolving intracranial process? Was the subject "blue," depressed, or moody, and did he have access to depressant drugs? Is he a "spree" drinker? These and other questions must be covered comprehensively with relatives, past physicians, friends, police, or ambulance personnel.

One must perform both a meticulous neurologic examination and a thoughtful physical review of every body system, because disease in remote organs often causes or accentuates dysfunction in the brain.

Fever implies infection, inflammation, or neoplasm. On the other hand, hypothermia (30 to 36° C) in a patient not severely exposed to cold suggests depressant drug poisoning, hypoglycemia, or severe lower brainstem injury, as by infarction. Hypertension may be the cause of hypertensive encephalopathy or the underlying cause of cerebral hemorrhage. Conversely, an elevated blood pressure can be a symptom of subarachnoid hemorrhage in a subject not previously hypertensive. Hypotension in a supine patient implies low blood volume (hemorrhagic or traumatic shock; severe nutritional and fluid depletion), low cardiac output (myocardial infarction), or low peripheral resistance (depressant drug poisoning). Tachycardia (over 160 per minute) can mean that unconsciousness is the result of lowered cardiac output from a supraventricular cardiac arrhythmia. Bradycardia suggests heart block and the Adams-Stokes syndrome or a myocardial infarct.

The pattern and depth of respiration are often informative in evaluating both neurologic function and acid-base balance, so much so that the evaluation of breathing is discussed more fully in Ch. 220.

The skin should be searched for petechiae (thrombocytopenic or nonthrombocytopenic purpura, meningococcemia, and bacterial endocarditis), bruises, evidence of nutritional deficiency, icterus, angiomatous spiders, and the bright pinkness of carbon monoxide poisoning. Fleshy or clubbed fingertips suggest carcinoma of the lung, or, less often, lung abscess or congenital heart disease (with brain embolism or abscess). A meticulous examination of the optic fundi is imperative but should be completed without cycloplegics, the use of which destroys the potential diagnostic value of pupillary reactions in coma. In the fundus oculi, the pathologic changes of many diseases causing coma can be viewed directly: increased intracranial pressure, hypertensive vascular disease, diabetes, blood dyscrasia, tuberculosis, sarcoidosis, bacterial endocarditis, cryptococcosis, collagen vascular disease, and even subarachnoid hemorrhage producing subhyaloid bleeding.

Chest examination has two potentially rewarding findings: cardiac murmurs suggest bacterial endocarditis with consequent focal, embolic encephalitis; the wheezes and obstructive sounds of the pulmonary cripple suggest CO_2 retention causing narcosis. In the abdominal examination, the presence of masses suggesting polycystic kidneys increases the chances that subarachnoid hemorrhage has occurred, whereas liver enlargement (hepatic coma is common with hepatomas) or splenic enlargement (both blood dyscrasias and infectious mononucleosis can cause encephalitis-like illnesses) can provide valuable leads.

During the neurologic examination, certain potentially informative steps are sometimes overlooked. The skull should always be palpated and inspected meticulously. Edema of the scalp commonly overlies fresh fracture lines, and basal skull fractures predispose to blood pigment stains behind the ear (Battle's sign) and about the orbit (raccoon eyes). Blood also may escape from basal fractures into the ear canals, the middle ears, or the nostrils. The skull should be percussed, because focal or unilateral skull tenderness, manifested by grimacing or withdrawal in a stuporous subject, often overlies an intracranial mass lesion. The neck should be tested carefully: stiff neck can reflect meningitis, cerebellar tonsillar herniation, or, occasionally, simply skeletal muscle spasticity. The stiff neck of acute bacterial meningitis is rarely equivocal; that of impending herniation is commonly less severe and lacks accompanying signs of infection or a prominent Kernig sign. It usually requires several hours or a day or more for stiff neck to develop after subarachnoid bleeding.

It is useful to watch the unconscious patient for a time, observing whether or not the extremities move equally and whether tremor, myoclonus, or single or repetitive seizures involve any part of the body. Status epilepticus with focal continuous epilepsy is not uncommon, but is often overlooked.

Laboratory Examination of the Patient in Coma

Patients should be subjected to a skull roentgenogram (looking for fracture lines, densities, and pineal shifts), a blood count and smear, and a urinalysis. When the clinical findings are consistent with metabolic encephalopathy but the cause is uncertain, the blood glucose and serum sodium, potassium, and bicarbonate should be obtained promptly. Knowledge of the arterial pH greatly helps diagnosis in metabolic coma (see Table 3 in Ch. 220).

When to do a lumbar puncture is always a serious question. All physicians are aware that in patients with increased intracranial pressure the procedure sometimes induces fatal herniation of the brain through the tentorium or foramen magnum. For this reason, lumbar puncture is best avoided if the physician strongly suspects his patient of having an expanding intracranial mass, particularly in the posterior fossa. Such forbearance is particularly advisable when CT scanning is immediately available. There are certain treatable diseases such as meningitis, however, that can be diagnosed only by lumbar puncture, and many others in which the procedure yields valuable preliminary diagnostic information. When the advice of neurologic specialists is unavailable, the doctor has no choice but to proceed with lumbar puncture if the diagnosis is in doubt and he believes the procedure has a reasonable chance of offering valuable information. Certain steps minimize the risk. One is to use a small (No. 20), sharp needle. Another is to fill the manometer with saline and attach it to the needle before releasing fluid, a technique that prevents sudden subarachnoid pressure shifts. Jugular manometrics should *never* be performed, for they offer little useful data and increase the risk of impacting potential intracranial herniations.

Magoun, H. W.: The Waking Brain. 2nd ed. Springfield, Ill., Charles C Thomas, 1963.

Plum, F., and Posner, J. B.: The Diagnosis of Stupor and Coma. 2nd ed. Philadelphia, F. A. Davis Company, 1972.

220. DELIRIUM AND EXOGENOUS METABOLIC BRAIN DISEASE

Jerome B. Posner

INTRODUCTION

There are few situations in clinical medicine that confuse and distress the physician so much as when he confronts a patient whose state of consciousness is rapidly deteriorating. The physician's task in such a situation is both enormous and exacting. First he must decide which of three major categories of disease is responsible for the patient's condition: (1) structural brain disease (e.g., brain tumors, subdural hematomas, cerebral infarctions); (2) "functional" brain disease (e.g., schizophrenia, manic-depressive psychosis); or (3) metabolic brain disease or delirium (see definitions below). If the patient's disorder falls into one of the first two categories (discussed elsewhere in this book), the physician can obtain help from highly skilled specialists in those areas (neurologists, neurosurgeons, or psychiatrists). If the patient's behavioral change is due to metabolic brain disease, the general physician must then determine himself which of a bewildering variety of metabolic defects is responsible (Table 1) and must rapidly begin treatment to assure that the metabolic defect does not produce irreversible brain damage. While he is carrying out these exacting tasks, he is often impeded by the fact that the patient is noisy, obstre-

---

TABLE 1.   Causes of Metabolic Brain Disease

I. Deprivation of oxygen, substrate, or metabolic cofactors
  *A. Hypoxia (interference with oxygen supply to the entire brain—cerebral blood flow normal)
    1. Decreased oxygen tension and content of blood
        Pulmonary disease
        Alveolar hypoventilation
        Decreased atmospheric oxygen tension
    2. Decreased oxygen content of blood—normal tension
        Anemia
        Carbon monoxide poisoning
        Methemoglobinemia
  *B. Ischemia (diffuse or widespread multifocal interference with blood supply to brain)
    1. Decreased cerebral blood flow resulting from decreased cardiac output
        Stokes-Adams syndrome, cardiac arrest, cardiac arrhythmias
        Myocardial infarction
        Congestive heart failure
        Aortic stenosis
        Pulmonary embolus
    2. Decreased cerebral blood flow resulting from decreased peripheral resistance in systemic circulation
        Syncope: orthostatic, vasovagal
        Carotid sinus hypersensitivity
        Low blood volume
    3. Decreased cerebral blood flow due to generalized increase in cerebrovascular resistance
        Hyperventilation syndrome
        Increased blood viscosity (polycythemia), cryo- and macroglobinemia
    4. Decreased local cerebral blood flow due to widespread small vessel occlusion
        Disseminated intravascular coagulation
        Systemic lupus erythematosus
        Subacute bacterial endocarditis
        Cardiopulmonary bypass
    5. Alterations of blood flow due to failure of autoregulation
        Hypertensive encephalopathy
  *C. Hypoglycemia
        Resulting from exogenous insulin
        Spontaneous (endogenous insulin, liver disease, etc.)
    D. Cofactor deficiency
        Thiamin (Wernicke's encephalopathy)
        Niacin
        Pyridoxine
        B_{12}
        Folate

II. Diseases of organs other than brain
  *A. Diseases of nonendocrine organs
        Liver (hepatic coma)
        Kidney (uremic coma)
        Lung (CO_2 narcosis)
  *B. Hyper- and/or hypofunction of endocrine organs
        Pituitary

Thyroid (myxedema-thyrotoxicosis)
Parathyroid (hyper- and hypoparathyroidism)
Adrenal (Addison's disease, Cushing's disease, pheochromocytoma)
Pancreas (diabetes, hypoglycemia)
  C. Other systemic diseases
        Diabetes
        Cancer
        Porphyria
        Sepsis
        Fever

III. Exogenous poisons
  *A. Sedative drugs
    B. Acid poisons or poisons with acidic breakdown products
        Paraldehyde
        Methyl alcohol
        Ethylene glycol
    C. Other enzyme inhibitors
        Heavy metals
        Organic phosphates
        Cyanide
        Salicylates
    D. Psychotropic drugs
        Tricyclic antidepressants and anticholinergic drugs
        Amphetamines
        Lithium
        Phenothiazines
        LSD-mescaline
        Monoamine oxidase inhibitors
    E. Others
        Penicillin
        Anticonvulsants
        Steroids
        Cardiac glycosides

IV. Diseases producing toxins or enzyme inhibition in CNS
    A. Meningitis
    B. Encephalitis
    C. Subarachnoid hemorrhage

V. Abnormalities of fluid, ionic or acid-base environment of CNS
    A. Water and sodium (hyper- and hyponatremia) (hypo- and hyperosmolality)
    B. Acidosis (metabolic and respiratory)
    C. Alkalosis (metabolic and respiratory)
    D. Magnesium (hyper- and hypomagnesemia)
    E. Calcium (hyper- and hypocalcemia)
    F. ? Trace metal deficiency or excess

VI. Miscellaneous diseases of unknown cause
    A. Seizures and postictal states
  *B. "Postoperative" delirium
    C. Concussion
  *D. "Sensory deprivation"
    E. Drug withdrawal states

---

*Alone or in combination, the most common causes of delirium seen on medical or surgical wards.

perous, and uncooperative, and by his own knowledge that appropriate treatment is essential and inappropriate treatment (e.g., injudicious use of sedative drugs in patients with incipient respiratory failure) potentially deleterious or even fatal. To deal with metabolic brain disease, the physician must understand some pathophysiologic aspects of cerebral metabolism and must undertake a systematic and thorough physical and laboratory examination of the patient.

DEFINITIONS

Metabolic encephalopathy is a term applied to the behavioral changes which result from diffuse or widespread multifocal failure of cerebral metabolism. When the cerebral disorder arises from an intrinsic failure of neuronal or glial metabolism, it is referred to as *primary or endogenous encephalopathy*. The primary disorders usually begin insidiously, progress inexorably, and produce a clinical picture of dementia, as discussed in Ch. 226 to 231. When the encephalopathy results from interference with brain metabolism by extracerebral disease, it is called *secondary or exogenous metabolic encephalopathy*. The secondary encephalopathies usually begin acutely or subacutely and often subside with time and/or treatment. They produce a clinical picture in which confusion, thinking errors, behavioral abnormalities, disorders of consciousness, and abnormal motor activity predominate. The causes of secondary metabolic encephalopathy are as many and varied as the illnesses that disturb body chemistry. Some causes of metabolic encephalopathy are listed in Table 1.

In some instances, the distinction, both clinically and pathophysiologically, between primary and secondary metabolic encephalopathies is blurred. For example, both vitamin B_{12} deficiency and hypothyroidism interfere with brain metabolism, causing an exogenous metabolic encephalopathy. The usual clinical findings in these disorders, however, resemble dementia (see definition below) rather than delirium, although on occasion either can produce a subacute delirium. The brain dysfunction is reversible by appropriate treatment in each of these disorders, and in this respect both resemble exogenous encephalopathy rather than endogenous encephalopathy. On the other hand, some primary disorders of the central nervous system, such as encephalitis, meningitis, concussion, and seizure disorders, appear acutely, are reversible with appropriate treatment, and clinically resemble delirium rather than dementia. For this reason, these disorders are grouped with the secondary metabolic encephalopathies in Table 1.

Metabolic brain disease is common and often misdiagnosed. When mild, it produces intellectual dullness, social indifference, and vague perplexity easily mistaken by observers for psychogenic depression or simply low intelligence. More severe encephalopathy elicits either a florid picture of tremulous agitation, rich and frightening hallucinations, and periods of seemingly complete loss of contact with the environment, or a more quiet, withdrawn, akinetic state which may fade into stupor or coma. The former, often called *delirium* or *toxic psychosis*, may be confused with a functional psychosis, and the latter, often called *acute* or *subacute confusional state*, is likely to be mistaken for structural brain disease. Although certain specific systemic disorders characteristically cause one or another of the aforementioned syndromes, each can occur with any of the metabolic brain diseases; thus the terms "delirium," "toxic psychosis," and "confusional state" are used interchangeably in this chapter to describe the wakeful stage of metabolic encephalopathy. A patient who is drowsy but can be coaxed to respond to verbal stimuli is *obtunded*. When he no longer responds to verbal stimuli but responds appropriately to noxious cutaneous stimuli, he is *stuporous*. If he does not respond appropriately to noxious stimuli, he is *comatose*.

The term *dementia* is used operationally to describe an irreversible loss of memory and cognitive functions, usually insidious in onset, irreversible, and often, but not always, due to intrinsic disease of the brain. Demented patients usually do not have the clouding of consciousness associated with delirium. However, an insidiously developing, quiet delirium may be clinically indistinguishable from the early stages of dementia.

SOME PATHOPHYSIOLOGIC ASPECTS OF METABOLIC BRAIN DISEASE

Pathologic changes in metabolic brain disease depend upon the nature and severity of the illness. The brains of some patients delirious during life are entirely normal at postmortem examination. In some cases, however, at least microscopic pathologic changes can be identified if the process causing delirium has lasted for some hours or days prior to death. The pathologic changes, if present, are bilateral, symmetrical, and usually diffusely or multifocally distributed in the cerebral hemispheres. Lesions may be present in the neurons, the glial cells, or the white matter, depending on the nature of the primary illness.

Perhaps the most common pathologic cerebral changes are observed after anoxia, ischemia, or hypoglycemia. The mildest abnormalities are visible only microscopically and consist of "microvacuoles" in neuronal cytoplasm of neocortex and hippocampus. The microvacuoles are swollen mitochondria, and this change is probably reversible. With more severe insults there is dissolution of the Nissl granules (particles of ribonucleic acid) and generalized pallor of staining. Finally, the nuclei shrink and become hyperchromatic, and irregular basophilic rings and granules appear in the swollen cytoplasm. These changes are not reversible. After severe and prolonged insults, all neurons in the cerebral cortex may disappear, and the third layer of the cortex may completely degenerate so that the naked eye detects a thin line of spongy necrosis (laminar necrosis). Anoxic changes also affect the basal ganglia to cause grossly visible focal necrosis of the globus pallidus. Occasionally, there may be diffuse demyelination of the subcortical white matter. Characteristically, the brainstem and spinal cord are spared unless the process has been overwhelmingly severe.

A nonspecific but common pathologic change in patients who have died with uremia, hyponatremia, diabetic coma, or CO_2 narcosis is cerebral swelling, recognized grossly by flattened gyri, narrowed sulci, and small ventricles. Microscopically, large perivascular and perineuronal spaces attest to the presence of edema.

Unusual glial cells with ballooned, lobulated nuclei are found in the cortex and basal ganglia of patients who die in hepatic coma, and are relatively specific for this disorder. Widespread perivascular "cuffs" of lymphocytes or polymorphonuclear leukocytes indicate an inflammatory lesion of the brain and meninges from viral or bacterial invasion.

In most cases of metabolic brain disease, the cerebral oxygen uptake declines in rough proportion to the degree of brain dysfunction observed clinically. So far, we understand in only a few instances how systemic illnesses interfere with cerebral metabolism, but these few serve as models to suggest the possible mechanisms for the others. The following material outlines some of our knowledge of normal and abnormal cerebral metabolism.

GLUCOSE. Glucose is the brain's only substrate under physiologic conditions, and is transferred across the blood-brain barrier by facilitated transport. Other substances can serve as substrates of brain in extraordinary circumstances (e.g., ketone bodies during starvation). Under normal circumstances, each 100 grams of brain utilizes about 31 μmol (5.5 mg) of glucose per minute, which represents almost the body's entire basal glucose consumption. Under aerobic conditions, 85 per cent of brain glucose uptake is oxidized to form CO_2, water, and energy; the remainder is probably accounted for by production of lactate, pyruvate, and other intermediates of glucose metabolism, and by synthesis of some chemicals. Under anaerobic conditions, lactic acid is the end product of glucose metabolism, but the energy so produced is insufficient to maintain neuronal function. There are about 2 grams of reserve glucose (as such and as glycogen) in the brain, an amount that allows the brain of a hypoglycemic patient to survive (although not to function at a normal metabolic rate) for about 90 minutes without suffering irreversible damage. The blood glucose concentration at which cerebral metabolism fails and clinical symptoms develop is variable from patient to patient, but, in general, levels below 30 mg per 100 ml cause confusion, and below 10 to 15 mg per 100 ml, coma.

OXYGEN. Oxygen, the other substance vital for normal cerebral function, is not stored by the brain, and a few seconds of anoxia is sufficient to cause coma. After a variable period of time, usually minutes, both hypoxia and ischemia cause irreversible neuronal damage. The normal brain consumes about 156 μmol (3.5 ml) of oxygen per 100 grams per minute and produces an equal amount of carbon dioxide (R.Q. = 1). Cerebral oxygen consumption represents about 20 per cent of the total body oxygen consumption at rest and is remarkably constant in normal man, whether awake or sleeping. However, significant deviations in oxygen consumption occur with brain dysfunction. For example, seizures increase the brain's demand for oxygen and usually are associated with an increased cerebral blood flow and oxygen uptake. Sedative drugs decrease the brain's metabolic demands; an overdose is usually associated with decreased blood flow and oxygen uptake. Clinically, delirium usually accompanies oxygen uptakes below 2.5 ml and when the uptake falls below 2.0 ml per 100 grams per minute, most patients are unconscious. The degree of hypoxia necessary to cause clinical symptoms depends not only on the blood oxygen tension but also on hemoglobin concentration, cerebral blood flow, and serum pH. In general, Pa_{O_2} values below 50 mm Hg cause delirium, and below 25 mm Hg, coma.

Blood brings both glucose and oxygen to the brain. Under resting conditions, each 100 grams of the brain receives 55 ml of blood each minute; the total brain blood flow of 800 ml per minute is about 15 per cent of the cardiac output. If the flow falls, the brain compensates by extracting more oxygen and more glucose from the blood it receives. Increased extraction of oxygen maintains normal metabolism in the face of a decreased cerebral blood flow up to the point where so much oxygen has been extracted that the oxygen tension of the brain's venous blood falls to about 20 mm of mercury (a level at which hemoglobin is about 35 per cent saturated). At this point, which is reached when cerebral blood flow falls to about half of normal, the oxygen tension is too low to maintain normal metabolism, and the patient loses consciousness. With hemoglobin concentrations below about 8 grams per 100 ml, cerebral blood flow must increase to assure an adequate oxygen supply. Profound anemia thus becomes a potential contributor to cerebral hypoxia.

OTHER SUBSTANCES. In addition to glucose and oxygen, the brain requires other substances (e.g., enzymes, vitamins, amino acids, electrolytes) to maintain metabolism, synthesize transmitter substances, preserve cellular structure, and maintain membrane potentials. Abnormalities of any of these essential substances lead to metabolic brain disease. The unique function of nervous tissue is to transmit electrical impulses, both within cells and by synaptic transmission between cells. The integrity of intracellular transmission depends not only on energy from oxidative metabolism (to maintain the sodium pump) but also on finely controlled intra- and extracellular electrolyte balance. Thus, for example, alterations of extracellular sodium, an ion necessary for propagation of the action potential, produce behavioral changes and delirium. Lithium, a cation with properties similar to both sodium and potassium, changes behavior in manic patients and, in overdose, can lead to severe delirium and coma. The integrity of intercellular transmission is regulated by the synthesis, release, re-uptake, and breakdown of transmitter substances and by maintenance of postsynaptic transmitter receptor sites. Several substances have been identified as putative transmitters in the nervous system, including norepinephrine, dopamine, serotonin, acetylcholine, and amino acids, especially glycine, gamma-aminobutyric acid, and glutamic acid. Most psychotropic drugs are believed to exert their behavioral effects by altering the activity of biogenic amines in the central nervous system, and in overdose most of these drugs produce delirium and sometimes coma. By the same token, severe alterations in amino acid metabolism lead to delirium. Interference with transmitter function may occur when the synthesis, breakdown, or release of the transmitter is inhibited, or when a foreign substance having a structure similar to the transmitter competes for sites on the postsynaptic receptor. Such a "false transmitter" may be the mechanism by which hallucinogenic drugs act, and may also be responsible for the production of "hepatic coma." However, despite these considerations, in no instance is the exact mechanism of delirium in either electrolyte or putative transmitter abnormalities clearly understood.

The biochemical common denominator of metabolic brain disease is decreased oxygen uptake: Is there an anatomic common denominator? Two concepts have arisen delineating a principal locus of metabolic brain disease. One is that the neurons of the cerebral cortex are affected first and, as the process becomes more severe, subcortical structures are affected from the rostral end downward, the phylogenetically oldest and most caudal structures resisting most strongly. This view is supported by the pathologic distribution of cerebral anoxic and hypoglycemic changes and by physiologic studies of hypoglycemic animals in which abnormal electrical activity was recorded from the cortex before it appeared in the hypothalamus.

The second concept is that the neurons of the brainstem reticular formation are the most susceptible to metabolic change and, at least at first, the cortical neurons cease to function only because they lose their reticular stimulation. This concept is supported by physiologic experiments on animals, demonstrating that moderate degrees of hypoxia, hypoglycemia, anesthesia, and cyanide poisoning all block electrical conduction through the reticular formation before they block the ability of cortical neurons to receive messages via other afferent pathways (the lemniscal system).

Neither of these experimental concepts fully explains the several human disease states in which metabolic lesions clinically affect several different levels of the neuraxis simultaneously, with the major locus of early dysfunction differing not only from patient to patient but sometimes from one attack to the next in the same patient. This phenomenon is exemplified by the varied picture of hypoglycemia: Some patients first suffer loss of consciousness and have bilaterally synchronous slow waves in the EEG, suggesting an initial reticular involvement. Others first experience restricted cerebral motor or sensory signs unaccompanied by either EEG abnormalities or impaired consciousness. Still other patients convulse with one attack of hypoglycemia but suffer only quiet coma in the next. It appears that in the clinical situation, regional factors such as blood flow and energy requirements must vary from moment to moment to predispose first one part of the brain and then another to metabolic insult.

CLINICAL FEATURES OF METABOLIC BRAIN DISEASE

The purpose of the physical and laboratory examination in a patient with suspected metabolic brain disease is twofold: first, to determine if the observed changes in consciousness are due to metabolic brain disease (i.e., to rule out structural brain disease or psychiatric dysfunction); and second, to determine exactly the type of metabolic defect causing the delirium. In general, evaluation of the state of consciousness, motor activity, and autonomic activity, as detailed below, helps to answer the first question, whereas the general physical examination, examination of ventilation, and laboratory examination (the latter two detailed below) help to answer the second question. It cannot, however, be overemphasized that, despite the difficulties of examining a delirious patient, a thorough and systematic general physical, neurologic, and laboratory examination *must* be undertaken if a definitive diagnosis is to be established and definitive treatment to be applied. Some principles of the examination are outlined in Table 2.

STATE OF CONSCIOUSNESS AND MENTAL CONTENT. Mental changes are the earliest and most subtle sign of metabolic brain disease. Restlessness or lethargy, emotional lability, insomnia or drowsiness, and vivid nightmares may appear before other mental changes. Patients often appear fearful and anxious, or depressed, and may express the fear that they are "going crazy." They may be restless, irritable, and easily distracted. Conversely, they may lie quietly or sleep when left alone, and rarely read or tend to the world around them. With more severe metabolic disturbances, patients become drowsy and finally stuporous or comatose. The particular affect that prevails in patients with metabolic encephalopathy depends partly on the nature of the illness and partly on the rapidity of its development; previous personality often has surprisingly little influence. Thus, barbiturate- or alcohol-withdrawal syndromes, acute liver necrosis, and porphyria often cause an agitated delirium, whereas uremia, pulmonary encephalopathy, and anoxia usually produce a more quiet illness. Rapidly developing metabolic abnormalities are more likely to produce agitated delirium than those that develop more slowly.

Disturbances in cognition appear along with altered alertness and awareness and are characterized by difficulties with immediate recall and the ability to abstract. Normal subjects readily recall and repeat 6 or 7 digits forward and 5 or 6 backward and can identify the common denominator between such pairs as an apple and an orange or a fly and a tree, but delirious patients cannot. However, innate intelligence and education also determine cognitive abilities and, unless the physician has examined the patient previously, it is difficult to attribute mild disturbances to a metabolic defect. An early sign of delirium, although usually not as early a sign as altered alertness and cognition, is impairment of memory and orientation. Loss of memory for recent events is a hallmark of metabolic and other organic brain disease and is tested by asking the patient about the names of his doctors, some important current events, and his recent activities. Orientation to place

TABLE 2. Physical Examination of Patients with Suspected Metabolic Brain Disease

History (from relatives or friends)
    Previous medical illnesses (diabetes, uremia, heart disease)
    Previous psychiatric history
    Access to drugs (sedative, psychotropic drugs)
    Recent complaints (headache, depression)

General physical examination
    Evidence of trauma
    Evidence of chronic or acute systemic illness
    Ventilation

Neurologic examination
    Mental status
        Affect (agitated, depressed, apathetic)
        Alertness (delirium, obtundation, stupor, coma)
        Memory (recent events, recall of objects)
        Orientation (time, place, person)
        Perceptual abnormalities (illusions, delusions, hallucinations)
        Psychomotor activity
    Motor examination
        Focal weakness
        Tremor
        Asterixis
        Myoclonus
        Seizures
    Autonomic examination
        Pupillary size and responses
        Temperature
        Heart rate and rhythm
        Diaphoresis

and time should be specifically tested by asking the date and year, the day of the week, and the present location. Orientation for time, particularly the year, is lost early in patients with delirium and orientation for place a little later.

Perceptual errors, e.g., mistaking the physician for an old friend or family member, illusions, and hallucinations are common accompaniments of delirium. They frighten and agitate some patients, but are quietly tolerated by others. The nature of the illusions and hallucinations seems to reflect the individual's personality, and often the same hallucinations accompany separate episodes of delirium. A quiet, withdrawn patient must be specifically asked about hallucinations, because he often fails either to volunteer the information or to behave as if he were hallucinating. Hallucinations of metabolic origin are usually visual, contrasting with those of schizophrenia, which are usually auditory.

Fluctuations of the mental status are common in metabolic encephalopathy. Patients may be totally out of contact one moment and lucid the next. Lucid intervals appear unpredictably and last for minutes or hours. Some of the fluctuation is environmentally related. Thus delirious patients characteristically become more disoriented at night, in unfamiliar surroundings, and in situations in which restraints and background noise and unfamiliar activity replace familiar sensory stimuli. One study demonstrated a significantly higher incidence of postoperative delirium in patients treated in a windowless intensive care unit than in those treated in a similar one with windows.

MOTOR ACTIVITY. Tremor, asterixis, and multifocal myoclonus are characteristic of metabolic brain disease, and the specificity of the latter two makes them the most important physical signs that distinguish metabolic encephalopathy from psychiatric illness or from structural brain disease.

The *tremor* of delirious patients is coarse and irregular at a rate of about eight to ten per second. It is usually absent at complete rest. It is best seen in the fingers of the outstretched hands. It is less specific than asterixis and multifocal myoclonus, and may be seen in patients with psychiatric disease as well as systemic illness not associated with delirium.

Asterixis is an abnormal, involuntary jerking movement elicited in the hands by asking patients to dorsiflex the wrist and spread the extended fingers. In its mildest form there are irregular random lateral jerking movements of the fingers at the metacarpal phalangeal joints. With fully developed asterixis there is sudden palmar flexion of the fingers at the metacarpal phalangeal joint and of the wrist. The movements are asynchronous in the two hands and are nonrhythmic. They occur every 2 to 30 seconds, recover quickly, and cannot be controlled by the patient, even when he is aware of their presence. Asterixis may also involve the feet and tongue. In the obtunded patient the same movement can sometimes be evoked by passively dorsiflexing the wrist or the ankles. Bilateral asterixis almost universally accompanies metabolic encephalopathy at some stage of the illness. It is absent in patients with psychiatric disorders unless they are taking large amounts of drugs, and is encountered rarely, and then unilaterally, in patients with gross structural brain disease such as decompensating subdural hematomas or deep hemispheral infarcts, especially involving the basal ganglia.

Multifocal myoclonus consists of sudden nonrhythmic, nonpatterned gross muscle contractions in a resting person. The movements are most common in the face and shoulders but occur anywhere in the body. Multifocal myoclonus can often be elicited, if not present at rest, by passive movements of the shoulder and upper arm. It occurs in a later and more severe stage of metabolic illness than does asterixis, and may physiologically represent a more intense and widespread manifestation of that abnormal movement. Multifocal myoclonus makes its most frequent appearance in uremia, hypercarbic-anoxic encephalopathy, and penicillin overdose, but can occur in virtually all metabolic encephalopathies.

Psychomotor activity ranges from extreme hyperactivity to total immobility. Delirious patients may be unwilling or unable to stay in bed, pacing the halls, in constant movement, with outbursts of aggressiveness which may culminate in attacks on others. With more severe delirium, there may be groping movements, picking at the bedclothes, and constant tossing and turning. Such patients may fall out of bed and injure themselves. Increased psychomotor activity is typically observed in acute deliria such as delirium tremens and drug withdrawal states. More commonly, delirium is manifested by reduced activity, with the patient lethargic, drowsy, and generally bradykinetic. The same patient may run the gamut from psychomotor overactivity to reduced activity during the course of the same delirium. *Speech* is often abnormal. Patients with increased psychomotor behavior often speak rapidly, with a muttering or slurred speech which, because of its speed, is incomprehensible. Patients with reduced psychomotor activity may speak slowly, monotonously, and so softly as not to be clearly heard.

Seizures, weakness, and *hyperactive stretch reflexes* frequently accompany severe metabolic brain disease. The seizures are usually generalized, and the motor abnormalities are usually symmetrical. Focal paresis and focal seizures are by no means rare, however, especially with anoxia, hypoglycemia, or hyperosmolality. Signs of focal disturbance make it more difficult to distinguish between metabolic and structural brain disease. However, in metabolic brain disease the focal signs are usually mild and fleeting, and they are accompanied by more widespread neurologic dysfunction than occurs with gross structural disease.

AUTONOMIC ACTIVITY. *Pupillary light reactions are always preserved in metabolic coma with the few exceptions to be mentioned, and absence of the pupillary light reaction strongly suggests a structural lesion.* The exceptions are glutethimide intoxication, which may produce mid-position or slightly dilated fixed pupils; anticholinergic drug administration, which produces fixed, dilated pupils; and exposure to severe anoxia, or asphyxia, which produces fixed dilated pupils and, if sustained, probably implies irreversible brain damage. The pupils, whatever their size and reaction to light, are usually symmetrical in patients comatose from metabolic brain disease, but often asymmetrical in patients comatose from structural brain disease.

Hypothermia is common in delirious patients with myxedema, hypoglycemia, and barbiturate intoxication. Hyperthermia with profuse perspiration and tachycardia accompanies most agitated deliria and is especially common with delirium tremens. Hyperthermia without perspiration suggests anticholinergic drug ingestion or infection. Hyperthermia also marks salicylate and occasionally phenothiazine overdosage.

VENTILATION. The clinical features of delirium that have been described are common to many metabolic disorders and aid little in the differential diagnosis of specific types of metabolic coma. Ventilation is an exception. A rapid evaluation of the patient's ventilatory status, coupled with an estimate of blood acid-base balance, frequently narrows the range of possible causes of metabolic coma. A careful clinical examination of the respiratory rate and depth usually allows the physician to estimate whether his patient is hyperventilating, eupneic, or hypoventilating. Caution must be exercised in evaluating patients with severe emphysema whose respiratory effort is increased and who may be tachypneic but nevertheless hypoventilating because of ineffective lungs. Caution must also be used in evaluating patients poisoned with depressant drugs who appear to be hypoventilating but are actually eupneic because their metabolic needs are so low. Unexplained abnormalities in the respiratory pattern demand rapid determination of blood gas and acid-base status. A delirious and clinically *hyperventilating* adult with a low serum pH probably has diabetic ketosis, uremia, lactic acidosis, or poisoning with an acidic product. Severe metabolic acidosis, if not treated, is rapidly lethal. Uremia, diabetes, and Addison's disease can be treated specifically (see Ch. 371, 531.1, and 547.3), and the others often respond to prompt and urgent treatment of the acidosis by infusion of bicarbonate. If, however, the serum pH is elevated in the delirious and hyperventilating adult, pulmonary disease, cardiac disease, hepatic coma, or neurogenic hyperventilation are the probable causes. Pneumonia is probably the most common cause of mild respiratory alkalosis in unconscious patients; the others can be evaluated by appropriate laboratory tests. When the serum pH is elevated and the bicarbonate is between 10 and 15 mEq per liter (mixed respiratory alkalosis and metabolic acidosis), sepsis, especially with gram-negative organisms, salicylism (which causes acidosis in children, alkalosis in adults), and severe hepatic coma are the probable causes.

A similar analysis can be applied to *hypoventilating* patients. In these, the severe problems are depressant drug poisoning, which produces a low serum pH with a normal bicarbonate, and chronic pulmonary failure, which produces a low serum pH and usually a high serum bicarbonate. (The serum bicarbonate level indicates the duration of hypoventilation.) Both situations demand ventilatory support.

ELECTROENCEPHALOGRAM (EEG). The EEG is useful in evaluating patients with metabolic brain disease because it is usually slower than in normal subjects and because it is symmetrical. The slowing indicates that there is neural dysfunction, and the bilateral symmetry suggests a diffuse process. The degree of slowing roughly parallels the severity of the encephalopathy. Patients with agitated deliria are often exceptions in that such patients, particularly those suffering from drug withdrawal, may have rapid rather than slow EEG's. Normal 8 to 13 Hz activity, however, is usually absent. The normal EEG has a basic frequency of 8 to 13 Hz. In metabolic disease, bilateral, synchronous, paroxysmal bursts of 1 to 3 Hz activity are frequently superimposed upon a background of mildly slow 5 to 7 Hz activity. A normal EEG is incompatible with severe delirium. An EEG with focal or unilateral slow activity strongly suggests a structural and not a metabolic brain disorder.

OTHER LABORATORY TESTS. The causes of metabolic coma are legion, and a final diagnosis usually depends on extensive laboratory tests. The tests which should be performed immediately to establish the presence of life-threatening metabolic defects are listed in Table 3, along with those whose results are not available immediately but should be done as soon as possible if the diagnosis is unclear.

DIAGNOSIS OF METABOLIC ENCEPHALOPATHY

The physician should consider metabolic encephalopathy as the possible diagnosis for every patient whose thinking, behavior, or state of consciousness has recently become disordered. The diagnosis requires, first, that one establish that metabolic encephalopathy rather than psychiatric disease, a structural brain lesion, or dementia is causing the abnormal behavior and, second, that one identify the specific metabolic illness responsible.

Psychiatric disease is distinguished in the awake patient by examination of the mental status and motor function. Psychotic patients are oriented and usually have normal cognitive function if one can enlist their cooperation. Delirious patients are disoriented and confused. Some patients with psychogenic amnesia claim to be confused about who they are as well as to the place and time; patients with metabolic brain disorders always know who they are. Hallucinations in psychiatric illness are usually auditory; in metabolic illness they are usually visual. Recent memory and cognitive abilities are generally preserved in psychiatric patients but are lost early in patients with metabolic illness. Tremor plagues anxious patients, and occasionally generalized seizures wrack those with catatonic schizophrenia, but asterixis and multifocal myoclonus are never present in psychiatric disease. Asterixis, if carefully searched for, is present in most patients with metabolic brain disease. Rarely, a patient with "hysterical coma" will present a diagnostic problem. Such patients are quietly unresponsive, and all their limbs are flaccid, but they often strongly resist passive eye opening. If the diagnosis is doubtful, irrigating the tympanum with 50 ml of cold water is informative; this procedure produces

TABLE 3.   Laboratory Evaluation of Metabolic Brain Disease

Test	Reason for Test
Immediate:	
Glucose	Hypoglycemia, hyperosmolar coma
Na^+	Osmolar abnormalities
Ca^{++}	Hyper- or hypocalcemia
BUN	Uremia
pH, Pco_2	Acidosis, alkalosis
Po_2	Hypoxia
Lumbar puncture	Infection, hemorrhage
Later:	
Liver function tests	Hepatic coma
Sedative drug levels	Overdose
Blood and CSF culture	Sepsis, encephalitis, meningitis
Full electrolytes, including Mg^{++}	Electrolyte imbalance
Coagulation profile	Intravascular coagulation
EEG	

physiologic nystagmus in the patient with "hysterical coma," but only tonic eye deviation in the comatose patient with metabolic disease. The EEG in "hysterical coma" shows a normal awake record; it is always abnormal in metabolic coma. The EEG is less helpful in distinguishing agitated delirium from affective psychosis. The EEG in patients with an agitated delirium (e.g., alcohol withdrawal) is often not slow but instead marked by low voltage fast activity with no normal 8 to 13 Hz waves, a pattern seen at times in normal or psychotic patients.

Supratentorial mass lesions that encroach on the diencephalon produce diffuse brain dysfunction (see Ch. 219). However, supratentorial lesions produce focal motor and/or sensory signs early in the illness, often before mental changes, and these focal signs either persist or grow worse. Hemiparesis or hemisensory defects, although occasionally present in metabolic disease, are usually mild, often fleeting, and generally appear only after consciousness is lost. Late in the course of mass lesions, when transtentorial herniation has impaired midbrain function, bilateral decorticate or decerebrate rigidity usually replaces unilateral motor signs. These motor signs of midbrain dysfunction may also be present in metabolic coma, but in metabolic coma the pupillary light reflexes are retained, thereby ruling out a structural lesion. The EEG of a patient with a supratentorial mass lesion is usually slow either focally in one area or laterally over one hemisphere; that of a patient with metabolic brain disease, even when focal neurologic abnormalities are present, is usually symmetrically slow. Computerized transaxial tomography (CT scanning) (see Ch. 267) is the best single laboratory test to identify mass lesions in the brain and should be performed whenever the cause of an encephalopathy is in doubt.

Subtentorial structural lesions are distinguished from metabolic brain disease by the presence in the former of signs of cranial nerve and focal brainstem dysfunction. In patients with subtentorial lesions causing changes in consciousness, the pupils are almost always abnormal, either because pontine and medullary sympathetic pathways are involved or because the third nerve nuclei or fibers are destroyed. Both pupillary light reflexes and the ciliospinal reflex (pupillary dilatation to noxious cutaneous stimuli) are preserved in metabolic disease. Dysconjugate eye movements are common with subtentorial lesions, rare with metabolic disease. Unilateral facial weakness involving both the brow and lower face, unilateral facial anesthesia, absent caloric responses to one side, or eye deviation toward a paralyzed arm and leg all suggest a subtentorial lesion and are against the diagnosis of metabolic disease.

Dementia is the expression of irreversible metabolic brain disease in which the primary metabolic error usually resides in the brain rather than affects the brain secondarily. For this reason, the incipient signs of dementia can resemble delirium, and distinction may sometimes be difficult. In general, dementia begins gradually, whereas delirium begins either acutely or subacutely. Recent memory loss, cognitive difficulties, and disorientation to place occur early in dementia and precede any change in consciousness, whereas lethargy, apathy, decreased awareness, and disorientation in time are early marks of delirium. Tremor, asterixis, and myoclonus are rare in dementia (except myoclonus in Creutzfeldt-Jakob disease). Mild or moderate dementia

reduces the brain's defenses against metabolic insults, and thus it is common for a fully reversible delirium to complicate mild systemic illnesses in demented patients. In these cases only treatment of the systemic disorders will separate the delirious component from the dementia (see Ch. 226 to 231).

DIFFERENTIAL DIAGNOSIS. Delirium means that a metabolic illness is so advanced that it not only threatens brain function but may threaten life itself unless promptly diagnosed and reversed by treatment. Since the neurologic manifestations of the various metabolic encephalopathies are often similar, specific diagnosis by physical examination is often impossible, so some systematic approach to the problem is needed.

In Table 1 are listed all of the common and many of the less frequent causes of metabolic brain disease. Those marked with an asterisk either alone or in combination account for most of the delirium encountered on general medical wards. The table is designed as a checklist; the specific symptoms, signs, and management of each of the systemic disorders causing delirium can be found elsewhere in this book. Table 3 lists the laboratory tests most helpful in achieving a definitive diagnosis.

When the cause of delirium is unclear, the first conditions to consider are *hypoxia, hypoglycemia,* and *metabolic acidosis.* Unless promptly treated, all three are potentially rapidly lethal, and the first two very quickly damage the brain irreversibly.

Certain physical signs, such as respiratory abnormalities, convulsions, and fever, suggest specific diagnoses. The examination of respiration aids in the diagnosis of pulmonary encephalopathy, sedative drug poisoning, "gram-negative sepsis," and hepatic coma. Often an early clue to the diagnosis of hepatic coma is the presence of respiratory alkalosis, which then prompts liver function tests or a blood ammonia determination to support the diagnosis. *Generalized convulsions* occur in many metabolic brain disorders, especially with hypoxia and hypoglycemia. Repeated seizures are dangerous since they create the risk of brain damage and should be treated even before their cause is clear. If hypoxia and hypoglycemia are not the cause, repeated seizures suggest sedative drug withdrawal, uremia, hyponatremia, hypocalcemia, or penicillin encephalopathy.

Agitated delirium accompanied by fever prompts immediate consideration of intracranial infection. Often the patient with meningitis is so combative that nuchal rigidity cannot be adequately assessed, and only lumbar puncture confirms the diagnosis. A lumbar puncture should be performed on any patient who is delirious without obvious cause and who lacks evidence of chronically increased intracranial pressure (e.g., papilledema, history of chronic progressive headache and/or focal neurologic signs). If one suspects that a mass lesion is the cause of delirium, a CT scan should be performed before lumbar puncture. Encephalitis and subarachnoid hemorrhage often present initially with delirium accompanied by little or no fever and no nuchal rigidity, and may not be diagnosed unless the cerebrospinal fluid is examined. In any delirious patient with nystagmus or ocular palsies, thiamin deficiency encephalopathy (see Ch. 285 to 287) should be immediately considered, because if this condition is untreated, cardiovascular collapse and death may follow.

Once the dangerous and potentially lethal illnesses detailed above are excluded, there is time to consider the many other causes of metabolic brain disease and to make the tests appropriate to their diagnosis. In most cases, a single cause for delirium is not found. Instead, the patient has multiple metabolic defects, no one of which is sufficient to produce delirium, but the sum total of which in a susceptible patient is responsible. A common example is an *elderly* patient with mild *congestive heart failure, anemia,* and *hypoxia* being given *sedative drugs* for agitation and diuretics which have caused an electrolyte imbalance. The dismay caused by the multiplicity of diagnostic possibilities is partially offset when the physician makes the happy therapeutic discovery that treatment of any one of the metabolic disorders may substantially improve his patient's delirium.

PROGNOSIS AND TREATMENT OF METABOLIC BRAIN DISEASE

Metabolic brain disease can be definitively treated only by correcting the systemic disorder responsible for the delirium, and the effectiveness of this correction, in turn, determines the prognosis of the delirium. With the exception of severe hypoxia, hypoglycemia, or thiamin deficiency, all of which can cause neuronal death, delirium clears as the systemic disorder causing it improves. Often, however, the encephalopathy improves much more slowly than the systemic illness so that severe encephalopathy may persist four to five days or more after the systemic disorder has been fully reversed. Such a delay need not portend an unfavorable outcome, and vigorous efforts to prevent infections and other complications of delirium and coma are indicated during this period, for full recovery of cerebral function still is possible.

Certain general therapeutic measures apply to all delirious patients (Table 4). An adequate *airway* and *oxygenation* of the blood must be assured. For stuporous or comatose patients, this may require an endotracheal tube or tracheostomy. *Blood volume, cardiac output,* and *blood pressure* must be maintained at near normal levels to assure adequate cerebral blood flow. If the cause of coma is not known, a blood glucose should be obtained; but even before the results are reported, intravenous glucose (50 ml of 50 per cent solution) should be given to assure that hypoglycemia will not cause irreversible brain damage. Abnormalities of *acid-base balance* and of *electrolyte balance* should be corrected. Correction should be carried out over several hours, because too rapid correction often leads to other metabolic abnormalities. Infection should be treated and fever lowered. If the diagnosis is unclear and narcotic overdose is a potential cause of the patient's delirium, a diagnostic test of naloxone should be considered. How-

ever, it must be remembered that naloxone will cause acute withdrawal symptoms in patients tolerant to narcotics and may reverse narcotic encephalopathy but wear off before the narcotics are fully metabolized.

The awake, delirious patient should be kept in a quiet room, away from the unfamiliar noises and bustle of the general ward. The room should be well lighted, especially at night, because darkness accentuates disorientation and hallucinations. Physicians and nurses can reassure the patient by introducing themselves at each contact and quietly apprising him of his whereabouts. All procedures must be carefully and often repetitively explained before they are done. Drugs not essential for treatment of the patient's systemic illness should be withdrawn. This applies particularly to sedatives, narcotics, and tranquilizers, all of which commonly cause or accentuate delirium; it also applies to extensive use of diuretics, antihypertensive drugs, anticonvulsants, and even digitalis, medications that are less widely recognized to cause or accentuate delirium. If the patient is agitated and hyperactive, small doses of diazepam, starting with 5 mg orally and increasing as necessary, can be given to quiet him but not to render him unresponsive.

Careful attention is required to other systemic disorders that, although not of themselves sufficiently severe to cause delirium, may increase an already present encephalopathy. Oxygen should be given to mildly hypoxic patients, and transfusions should be administered to those with significant anemia. Mild electrolyte disorders such as hypokalemia and hyponatremia are diagnosed by periodic serum electrolyte determinations and are corrected by appropriate fluid control. Such measures often improve a patient's delirium considerably, even if the primary cause cannot be treated. Fluid losses should be routinely measured and replaced parenterally if the patient is not eating. Vital signs and the state of consciousness must be checked frequently to ensure that sudden worsening does not go undetected.

Jacobs, J. W., Bernhard, M. R., Delgado, A., and Strain, J. J.: Screening for organic mental syndromes in the medically ill. Ann. Intern. Med., 86:40, 1977.

Metabolic and deficiency diseases of the nervous system, Part II. *In* Vinken, P. J., and Bruyn, G. W. (eds.): Handbook of Clinical Neurology, Vol. 28. Amsterdam, Elsevier North-Holland Biomedical Press, 1976.

Plum, F., and Posner, J. B.: The Diagnosis of Stupor and Coma. 2nd ed. Philadelphia, F. A. Davis Company, 1972.

Sokoloff, L.: Circulation and energy metabolism of the brain. *In* Siegel, G. J., Albers, R. W., Katzman, R., and Agranoff, B. W. (eds.): Basic Neurochemistry. 2nd ed. Boston, Little, Brown & Company, 1976, Chap. 19, pp. 388–413.

221. SLEEP AND ITS DISORDERS

William R. Shapiro

The average adult sleeps 7½ to 8 hours out of every 24. Despite the fact that a third of life is spent sleeping, little is understood of its function. Sleep is an active state. Cerebral metabolism diminishes hardly at all during sleep, and although sleeping individuals often appear quiescent, they are known to go through a series of contortion-like movements as many as 20 times in the course of a given night. Twenty-five per cent of the

---

TABLE 4. Immediate Treatment of Metabolic Brain Disease

1. Assure oxygenation
2. Maintain circulation
3. Give glucose
4. Restore acid-base balance
5. Treat infection
6. Control body temperature
7. Stop seizures
8. Consider naloxone

night is spent dreaming, and a large body of literature, both scientific and mythological, has been devoted to explaining dreams. Sleep is essential, but studies in man and animals do not, as was once thought, indicate that sleep deprivation produces permanent physiologic damage in adults, although temporary neurologic and psychologic changes can be demonstrated. Recently neuroendocrinologic research has shown that some hormonal secretions have cyclic rhythms which may relate to sleep. Growth hormone output is increased during the early hours, and prolactin output increases during the morning hours of sleep. Disturbances of sleep represent a major source of distress to patients and a cause for the consumption of enormous quantities of sleep-related medications.

PHYSIOLOGY AND PHARMACOLOGY OF SLEEP

Studies from several sources have identified sleep not merely as a cessation of contact with the environment, but also as an active state in which cerebral metabolism does not diminish and in which several active processes can be identified. Two sleep states can be defined. One, called slow wave (SW) sleep, consists of gradual slowing of the electroencephalographic (EEG) rhythms, with increasing amplitude and synchronization through four stages from mild drowsiness (stage 1) to profound somnolence (stage 4). A second sleep state, called rapid eye movement (REM) sleep, is characterized by EEG activity which is low voltage, fast, and desynchronized and is associated with, respectively, rapid eye movements (hence its name), profound hypotonicity of the skeletal muscles with an associated low voltage electromyogram, and absent reflexes. Other phasic components identifiable in REM sleep include abrupt changes in respiration, pupil diameter, blood pressure, and pulse rate, muscle twitching, and penile erection. In electrical recordings abrupt spike activity in the pons and geniculate and occipital cortex (PGO waves) are detected. The two sleep states characteristically cycle during normal sleep. SW sleep occurs early, with the subject progressing through the four stages and returning back toward stage 2 in the course of the first 90 to 100 minutes. This is followed by REM sleep lasting 15 to 20 minutes, after which the subject returns again to SW sleep. REM sleep gradually occurs more often during the night, but on average makes up about 25 per cent of adult sleep time. Much of dreaming occurs during REM sleep, and subjects awakened during this state have described vivid, colorful, frequently uninhibited dreams. Dreaming of a more prosaic nature occurs also during SW sleep, but it tends to be related more to the subject's daily activities than does the imaginative introspective dreaming of REM sleep. The cycling between SW sleep and REM sleep varies with age, there being a greater proportion of REM sleep in infants and young children than in adults. There is evidence that human beings have a specific biologic need for a certain minimum of REM sleep as well as total sleep, and humans deprived of REM sleep experience a rebound in which extra REM sleep periods occur.

The mechanism by which sleep-wake cycles occur has been an active area of investigation. It has been determined that the brainstem contains structures iden-

tifiable both anatomically and neuropharmacologically which can cycle sleep-wake patterns in the absence of cerebral connections. On the other hand, it is possible to sever the connections between brainstem and cerebrum in animals and still demonstrate sleep-wake cycles in the cerebral cortex by EEG. Although inconsistencies still exist in the experimental evidence, a working model of the sleep-wake cycle system can be constructed which is based primarily on Jouvet's work with the decerebrate cat. In Jouvet's model, sleeping-waking cycles are regulated by two antagonistic ascending monoaminergic systems that operate tonically. One system involves serotonin (5-hydroxytryptamine) containing neurons lying primarily in the raphe nuclei that are important in inducing SW sleep and priming REM sleep. The other includes catecholaminergic neurons (mostly noradrenergic) and acetylcholinergic neurons occupying the nucleus locus ceruleus and nucleus locus subceruleus that appear to induce cortical arousal and the waking state and also subserve elements of REM sleep. It is possible to isolate regions of these nuclei that specifically mediate the components of the REM state.

DISORDERS OF SLEEP

There are three major disorders of sleep. *Insomnia* means too little sleep; *hypersomnia*, an excess of sleep, usually during the day. *Disturbed sleep* occurs during otherwise normal sleep and includes enuresis, sleepwalking, and night terrors.

When considering the diagnosis of a sleep disorder, it is important to bear in mind the variable nature of sleep. Some individuals require more than eight hours of sleep, whereas a few get along well on three or four. Women usually sleep longer than men. Children require more sleep than young adults, and less sleep is needed with advancing age. In most people a few nocturnal awakenings normally occur; they become of medical concern only when they increase in number or duration so much that they substantially reduce total sleep time. Similarly, many individuals normally nap during the day; hypersomnia implies excessive somnolence, especially an increase over the subject's usual level.

Insomnia

According to Kales, insomnia is the sleep disturbance most frequently treated by the general physician. It may consist of difficulty of falling asleep, difficulty in staying asleep, too early awakenings, or a combination of these. Insomnia may be a symptom associated with medical disorders. Chronic pain may produce difficulty in sleeping throughout the night. Pulmonary insufficiency may cause frequent nocturnal awakenings. Insomnia may accompany acute infectious illness and is common in Sydenham's chorea and in bulbar poliomyelitis. More often no specific medical disorder is present and the complaint is treated symptomatically, usually by hypnotic medications. It is estimated that 7 to 10 per cent of the population uses hypnotics, including alcohol, minor tranquilizers, and nonprescription sleeping medications. Psychologic factors probably contribute to insomnia in most such patients. In direct testing, over three fourths of insomniacs evaluated on the Minnesota Multiphasic Personality Inventory (MMPI) showed high scores on the depression scale. At least one MMPI scale was abnormal in 85 per cent of insomniac patients. Further, many chronic insomniacs are described as tense, complaining individuals who are oversensitive to minor discomforts and unable to relax easily. The advent of sleep laboratory research has disclosed that the degree of sleeplessness is frequently overestimated by patients. The Sleep Disorders Clinic at Stanford University found that compared with laboratory recordings of 122 drug-free subjects who complained of chronic insomnia, most subjects consistently underestimated the amount of time they slept and overestimated the latency in falling asleep. On the other hand, most patients had more arousals during the night than they reported. *Drug treatment does not alleviate insomnia for more than a few days.* In direct sleep laboratory studies, Kales found that compared to drug-free insomniacs, those chronically habituated to hypnotics have more awakenings during the night, less stage 3 and 4 SW sleep, the same degree of prolonged sleep latency, and a marked reduction in REM sleep. If patients attempt to reduce hypnotic medications abruptly, there is profound REM rebound with excessive dreaming and increased insomnia. Patients continue to take hypnotics, and may increase the dose, because of the REM rebound. The problem of chronic use of sleeping medications is complicated by the patients' failure to recognize the psychologic components of their insomnia, denying depression and focusing on the somatic complaint of poor sleep.

It is apparent that the evaluation of chronic insomnia requires special attention to the patient's psychologic needs. Since psychologic testing indicates that the majority of patients with chronic insomnia are depressed, the physician must inquire into associated symptoms of depression, including poor appetite, early awakenings, sadness, crying spells, significant weight loss, changing bowel habits, and personal loss. If the physician determines that the patient's major problem is depression, referral for psychotherapy may be indicated.

Treatment of chronic insomnia depends on the results of evaluation: specific medical disorders should be treated directly. Symptomatic treatment of the insomnia requires attention to general measures and specific pharmacologic considerations. Helpful measures in the general treatment of chronic insomnia include reduction of stimulant drugs, i.e., caffeine or amphetamines, regulation of bedtime and wake time, elimination of daytime naps, relaxation exercises, and recommendation for moderate daily exercise. Some persons simply need the reassurance that they require less sleep than others.

Pharmacologic therapy for insomnia requires an awareness that many drugs affect sleep. Some are designed specifically to induce or ward off sleep. Others not designed to alter sleep do so as a side effect. For example, L-dopa, used to treat Parkinson's disease, and exogenous corticosteroid hormones regularly produce insomnia. Drug effect depends on host circumstances and previous exposure. Many sedative drugs under certain circumstances actually produce excitement; barbiturates given to elderly patients may cause an agitated

confusion. Conversely, amphetamine and methylphenidate, both stimulants, can quiet hyperactive children. Chronic administration of both sedative and analeptic drugs can rapidly lead to tolerance; abrupt withdrawal can lead to profound physiologic disturbance. The following points should be observed when prescribing such drugs. Barbiturates lead to tolerance within two weeks. They then become ineffective after a short while, and, because they profoundly depress REM sleep as tolerance develops, there is marked REM rebound and restlessness on withdrawal. Benzodiazepines are similar to barbiturates, although Kales has reported that flurazepam does not lose its effectiveness in two weeks. Less REM rebound is reported following cessation of benzodiazepines than occurs with barbiturates. Tricyclic antidepressants and monoamine oxidase (MAO) inhibitors reduce REM sleep during chronic therapy; REM rebound occurs after drug withdrawal. Amphetamines tend to decrease REM sleep, but withdrawal effects have not been studied. Variable effects on sleep have been produced by analgesics and alcohol and by antipsychotic agents. In part the effects depend on the subjects; normal healthy volunteers differ more in their response to single doses of opiates than do subjects addicted to such compounds.

Pharmacologic therapy for insomnia should be limited, whenever possible, to occasional use of sleeping medications for acute episodes. Most hypnotics may be used safely for up to three days; typical bedtime doses are secobarbital, 100 mg; pentobarbital, 100 mg; and chloral hydrate, 1 gram. Glutethimide has been reported as a cause for suicide in a sufficient number of patients to suggest replacement by another hypnotic. Chronic use of hypnotics does not relieve insomnia. If therapy must extend for more than a few days, flurazepam is the drug of choice because it surpresses REM sleep less than barbiturates and does not produce tolerance after two weeks. Flurazepam, 15 mg, is administered at bedtime to be increased after a week to 30 mg if sleep is not improved. For drug-withdrawal insomnia and hypnotic drug dependency, very slow drug withdrawal is recommended to avoid REM rebound. The therapeutic dose should be reduced no more frequently than once every five or six days, and the patient must be informed that increased dreaming, vivid dreams, and even nightmares may occur. Insomnia often improves after withdrawal. Because of the REM rebound special care must be taken in withdrawing hypnotics too quickly from those patients who suffer from coronary artery disease or duodenal ulcer, as both of these conditions are potentially made worse by excessive REM sleep.

Hypersomnia

NARCOLEPSY. Narcolepsy is a chronic disorder characterized by irresistable episodes of sleep occurring from a few to many times a day, between which the patient may be alert or drowsy. Narcolepsy may be accompanied by cataplexy, sleep paralysis, and/or hypnagogic hallucinations. *Cataplexy* is a sudden decrease or loss of muscle tone that may be generalized or confined to individual muscles. When mild, cataplexy consists of a sense of weakness, a tendency to drop things, or of having one lower limb give way; when severe, the patient may fall in a heap. Such attacks generally last less than a minute and occur from one to 12 to 25 times in 24-hour period. They may be precipitated by heightened emotional tone — e.g., laughter or anger — but when severe they occur spontaneously or with any kind of movement. *Sleep paralysis*, like cataplexy, is also characterized by the inability to move but occurs when the patient is either falling asleep or just coming out of a sleep spell. *Hypnagogic hallucinations* are vivid, visual, or auditory dreamlike states which occur while dozing or while being aroused. They are so vivid that patients may act out the dream state on awakening and are surprised to discover that they have been dreaming. These four symptoms constitute the narcoleptic tetrad. Twenty-five per cent of narcoleptic patients have sleep attacks only, whereas 70 per cent have both narcolepsy and cataplexy. Approximately 12 per cent of patients experience all four symptoms. The incidence in men and women is approximately equal. A family history is present in half the patients. Although the disease commonly begins in the teens and twenties, the diagnosis is frequently delayed for five to eight years because neither the patient nor the physician recognizes the nature of the attacks.

The pathogenesis of narcolepsy is unknown, but two theories have been proposed. Yoss and Daly suggested that narcolepsy represents one end of a continuous spectrum from full wakefulness to deep sleep. Narcoleptic patients are thought to have a genetically determined greater incidence of otherwise normal drowsiness (reduced vigilance), and the degree of such sleepiness can be determined by pupillographic studies. The second theory was advanced after the two different sleep states, SW and REM, were recognized. In most normal subjects an interval of an hour to an hour and a half elapses between falling asleep and the first appearance of REM sleep in the EEG tracing. In the patients with narcolepsy, especially those with cataplexy, the sleep syndrome may begin abruptly with a period of REM sleep. Narcoleptic patients without cataplexy may have non-REM onset sleep attacks. The thesis that narcolepsy-cataplexy is associated with REM onset sleep patterns explains cataplexy as the sudden loss of motor tone that occurs with REM. Hypnagogic hallucinations represent the dream component of the REM state, and sleep paralysis is also associated with loss of motor tone occurring during sleep. Amphetamines inhibit both SW sleep and REM sleep but only to a moderate degree, whereas tricyclic antidepressants profoundly inhibit REM sleep but do not influence SW sleep and have no effect on the sleep attacks of narcolepsy. It is the REM inhibiting property of the antidepressants which makes them effective in treating cataplexy. They appear to suppress the tonic components of REM sleep, apparently by action on brainstem structures responsible for inhibition of muscle activity and reflexia. It is likely that the narcoleptic disorder involves both the REM and SW systems, because methysergide is mildly effective against narcoleptic sleep attacks, suggesting an effect on the SW serotonergic system.

Narcolepsy is distinguished from other causes of hypersomnia, for example, structural brain lesions, because the latter occur more acutely and with greater severity. Narcoleptic patients are easily aroused, whereas patients with structural lesions causing lethargy become progressively unarousable and have associated respiratory, cranial nerve, and motor signs. In structural brain disease there is usually impaired cognition. Narcolepsy dates to early life with a stable course over many years. Late onset hypersomnia may occur in sleep apnea or other syndromes associated with hypoventilation (see below). Occasionally narcolepsy itself may be associated with sleep apnea.

Treatment of narcolepsy is difficult, both because it requires stimulants whose side effects are difficult to control and because it requires a regulated, almost rigid life style usually unacceptable to young patients. Dextroamphetamine sulfate in the form of sustained release capsules or tablets at doses of 15 to 50 mg per day is generally effective against the sleep attacks, especially in the first years of use. Tolerance develops, however, and the drug becomes less effective. Methylphenidate has the advantage that tolerance develops more slowly than with the amphetamines, and it has a reduced excitatory potential. Methylphenidate is used in doses up to 200 mg per day but must be administered on an empty stomach. It is the drug of choice in narcoleptic patients who are also hypertensive. Unfortunately methlyphenidate does not prevent cataplexy, and the amphetamines are only minimally effective. The tricyclic antidepressants, including imipramine and desmethylimipramine, are effective in moderately high doses, but the most effective drug to treat cataplexy is clomipramine. Clomipramine may be used in doses of 25 to 75 mg a day according to the number and severity of cataplectic attacks. A troublesome side effect of the tricyclic antidepressants is the tendency to produce impotence in men. They also exaggerate the natural tendency of narcoleptic patients to overeat and increase the difficulty in controlling weight. Monoamine oxidase inhibitors and L-dopa have been used to treat narcolepsy, but their side effects preclude general use. Although narcolepsy is a benign disorder, its course may be gradually progressive, the patient becoming refractory to therapy. Whether this constitutes progression of the disease or increasing tolerance to the medication produced by weight gain or other factors is not known.

SLEEP APNEA. The specific association of hypersomnia and chronic alveolar hypoventilation in the presence of extreme obesity, polycythemia, and excessive appetite is called the pickwickian syndrome. Cessation of respiration while sleeping was first described in patients with severe bulbar poliomyelitis. A similar disorder may follow surgery of the high spinal cord or brainstem in which patients become apneic upon falling asleep. This is called "Ondine's curse," a literary illusion to the revenge that Ondine, a river nymph, takes upon a deceitful mortal who jilted her; the curse requires him to attend consciously to his autonomic functions, and when he falls asleep he stops breathing and dies. More common than any of these is the disorder characterized by hypersomnia with obstructive periodic apneas during sleep, so-called *sleep apnea*.

The patient with sleep apnea usually presents with excessive daytime sleepiness of subacute or chronic duration. A history is obtained from family members that the patient snores loudly and excessively through the night. The spouse may report that the patient's sleep is often disturbed by sudden starts and violent arm swings which sometimes produce injury and occasionally necessitate separation of sleeping arrangements. A minority of the patients have known narcolepsy. Constitutionally, sleep apnea patients often complain of morning headaches, are frequently hypertensive, and may have cardiac arrhythmias. Most patients with sleep apnea are obese middle-aged men, but a few have the severe obesity and hypercapnia of the pickwickian patients, and the syndrome can occur in nonobese individuals, women, and children. It may also be related to the sudden infant death syndrome. Nocturnal sleep recordings in these patients are characterized by up to hundreds of episodes of apnea with abrupt awakenings. The Po_2 falls during apnea, the Pco_2 rises, and both are reversed as the patient awakens and takes four or five breaths. The cycle repeats as the patient lapses into sleep. Apnea occurs during both REM and SW sleep but has been observed to be more specifically associated with REM sleep. Three types were initially described: a central apnea, in which there was cessation of diaphragmatic excursions; upper airway apnea, characterized by obstruction to airflow past the oral pharynx but with persistent diaphragm movement; and a mixed apnea, defined by cessation of air flow and absent respiratory effort early in the episode, followed by unsuccessful attempts at respiration later in the episode. It is now recognized that most patients have intermittent upper airway obstruction as the cause of their apnea. The pathogenesis of sleep apnea remains obscure. Functional obstruction in the oral pharynx seems to be caused by recurrent closure of the upper pharyngeal wall and posterior movement of the tongue. There is secondary downward movement of the soft palate and hypopharyngeal closure from abortive thoracic and diaphragmatic respiratory movements. The questions of the cause of the upper pharyngeal collapse and the pathogenesis of the daytime somnolence remain to be explained.

Sleep apnea sometimes responds to vigorous weight reduction. Otherwise, treatment of sleep apnea secondary to upper airway obstruction is tracheostomy, although weight reduction and tricyclic antidepressants may reduce daytime somnolence. The presence of associated cardiovascular abnormalities requires that the patient be treated promptly. Following tracheostomy, most patients improve remarkably, the daytime somnolence disappears, nocturnal sleep is uninterrupted, and constitutional symptoms, including hypertension and the arrhythmias, usually improve.

OTHER CAUSES OF HYPERSOMNIA. With the recent rise in amphetamine abuse, occasional patients are seen with hypersomnolence secondary to amphetamine addiction or abrupt withdrawal. Tolerance and dependency paradoxically increase daytime sleepiness; the diagnosis depends on the history of chronic use of stimulant medication. A rare condition of recurrent hypersomnia combined with excessive eating is sometimes observed in adolescent males and is known as the *Kleine-Levin syndrome.* The cause is unknown, but the attacks last several days to a week or more, during which the patient eats voraciously and often develops disturbed behavior. Intervals of months to years of normal behavior separate the attacks. There is no treatment, and the attacks tend to disappear as the patient reaches adulthood.

Disturbed Sleep

Somnambulism or sleepwalking has been reported to occur in 15 per cent of children at least once between ages 5 and 12. Most reports describe aimless wandering usually without falls. Somnambulism may occur in isolation or in association with *enuresis.* The latter, bedwetting at night with daytime continence, occurs in 10 per cent of children between ages 4 and 14 and is more common in boys. Its cause is thought to be functional, but only rarely does it indicate severe psychopathology. Both sleepwalking and enuresis occur during stages 3 and 4 of SW sleep. Both tend to disappear with age. They should be treated with reassurance. Enuresis has been reported to respond to tricyclic antidepressants.

Night terrors (pavor nocturnus) also occur in children, usually associated with stage 3 and 4 of SW sleep. The child suddenly awakens, intensely afraid, with tachypnea and tachycardia. The attack lasts only minutes and is rarely recalled in the morning. Most children grow out of the episodes. Night terrors can be distinguished from nightmares, in that the latter are less intense, tend to occur during the dreaming of REM sleep, and are usually remembered.

Physiology and Pharmacology

Petre-Quadens, O., and Schlag, J. D. (eds.): Basic Sleep Mechanisms. New York, Academic Press, 1974.
Williams, R. L., and Karaccen, I.: Pharmacology of Sleep. New York, Wiley, 1976.

Insomnia

Carskadon, M. A., Dement, W. C., Mitler, M. M., Guilleminault, C., Zarcove, V. P., and Spiegel, R.: Self-reports versus sleep laboratory findings in 122 drug-free subjects with complaints of chronic insomnia. Am. J. Psychiat., 133:1382, 1976.
Kales, A., and Kales, J. D.: Sleep disorders. Recent findings in the diagnosis and treatment of disturbed sleep. N. Engl. J. Med., 290:487, 1974.
Regestein, Q. R.: Treating insomnia: A practical guide for managing chronic sleeplessness, circa 1975. Compr. Psychiatry, 17:517, 1976.

Hypersomnia

Guilleminault, C., and Dement, W. C.: 235 cases of excessive daytime sleepiness. J. Neurol. Sci., 31:13, 1977.
Guilleminault, C., Dement, W. C., and Passouant, P. (eds.): Narcolepsy. Advances in Sleep Research, Vol. 3. New York, Spectrum, 1976.
Guilleminault, C., Elridge, F. L., Tilkian, A., Simmons, F. B., and Dement, W. C.: Sleep apnea syndrome due to upper airway obstruction. A review of 25 cases. Arch. Intern. Med., 137:296, 1977.
Parkes, J. D.: The sleepy patient. Lancet, 1:990, 1977.

Section Two FOCAL DISTURBANCES OF HIGHER NERVOUS FUNCTION

Norman Geschwind

222. LANGUAGE, APHASIA, AND RELATED DISORDERS

Language is one of the most striking biologic attributes of man. Recent evidence suggesting that some potential for language exists in chimpanzees may open up new possibilities for investigation of the neurologic foundations of linguistic behavior. At present, however, nearly all our knowledge of the neural substrate of language is based on man. Detailed postmortem studies of well-described patients have provided the majority of the information, but useful data have been accumulated from patients with other types of disorders and from studies of the effects of stimulation of the brain during operations.

A striking feature of the human brain is dominance, i.e., the superiority of one hemisphere in the performance of certain functions. Dominance is not known definitely to exist in any mammal other than man. There is, however, left-brain dominance for singing in birds. About 93 per cent of people are right-handed, and at least 99 per cent of right handers have left hemisphere dominance for speech.

The situation is more complex and less well defined in the non-right-handed, i.e., the left handers and those with varying degrees of ambidexterity. Such patients become aphasic as a result of a lesion in *either* hemisphere, although left hemisphere lesions generally produce more lasting disability. A third group, *pathologic left handers*, who have suffered early childhood injury to the left hemisphere, are usually right-brained for speech.

The cause of dominance was in dispute for many years. We now know that the temporal speech region on the left is generally larger than the corresponding area on the right. The nondominant side is, however, endowed genetically with the capacity to develop language. Thus if the dominant hemisphere is damaged before age nine, there is nearly always excellent recovery of language over a period of months or even years, although the over-all degree of mental development is slowed. Spontaneous recovery from aphasia also occurs in later life but less frequently. Dominance in the intact human can be studied by two recently developed techniques. The *Wada test* consists of the injection of sodium amytal into the internal carotid artery. This causes a hemiplegia on the side opposite the injection, but aphasia results only from injection on the dominant side, especially in non-right-handed patients. Another technique, the *Kimura test*, is that of dichotic listening, in which different words are simultaneously presented to the two ears. Normal individuals tend to report first the words presented to the ear opposite the dominant hemisphere.

223. APHASIA

The aphasias may be defined as disorders of language secondary to lesions of the brain. In most cases there is disorder of the output of speech. In the experience of the author, aphasia in spoken speech is invariably accompanied by similar abnormalities in writing. Aphasia in spoken language is of two major types: (1) *Nonfluent aphasia,* in which few words are produced slowly and with great effort, and sounds are incorrectly articulated. Production of grammatical words is relatively more affected so that sentences tend to be ungrammatical, e.g., "Weather sunny." (2) *Fluent aphasia,* in the more extreme forms of which the patient produces runs of well-articulated speech, which has the rhythm and melody of normal language and a basically normal grammatical structure, but which tends to convey little information, e.g., "I was at the other one and then I was at this one," a fluent aphasic's circumlocutory manner of explaining that he was in another hospital previously. The speech of these patients usually contains many incorrect words, called *paraphasias. Literal* (or phonemic) *paraphasias* are substitutions of well-articulated but incorrect sounds, e.g., "spoot" for "spoon," and *verbal paraphasias* are incorrect usages of words, e.g., "knife" for "fork," or "department" for "hospital."

The terms *expressive* and *receptive* aphasia should be avoided, as they have been used with different meanings in the literature. Thus some authors use expressive aphasia to describe only the nonfluent forms, whereas others use it to describe both nonfluent and fluent forms. Receptive aphasia has been used to describe pure word deafness by some; others use it for the full syndrome of Wernicke's aphasia, in which all modalities of language are affected.

In differential diagnosis, one must be wary of describing *mutism* as aphasia, because even severe aphasics are usually not mute. Causes of mutism are (1) uncooperativeness; (2) psychiatric disorders, e.g., severe depression or schizophrenia; (3) widespread disorders of brain, such as trauma, subarachnoid hemorrhage, or metabolic disorders; (4) lesions of mesencephalic and pontine tegmentum; and (5) bilateral lesions of the cranial nerves serving the speech organs, their nuclei, or their supranuclear pathways.

Dysarthria should not be confused with aphasia. Dysarthric speech is incorrectly articulated, but, if transcribed, shows correct grammar and word usage. A helpful clue is that if a patient who is mute or has completely unintelligible speech can produce fully normal language (not just his own name) in writing or on a typewriter, he is almost certainly not aphasic.

A common error is to misdiagnose a fluent aphasia as *schizophrenic word-salad.* Several clues help to make the differential diagnosis. Fluent aphasia is much more common than schizophrenic word-salad. The schizophrenic speech disorder ususally develops in chronic "back ward" schizophrenics. By contrast, fluent aphasia may come on abruptly as the result of a stroke in a previously well person. Finally, fluent aphasia from vascular disease usually occurs in older people, whereas schizophrenia almost always is manifest before the age of 30.

APHASIC SYNDROMES AND THEIR LOCALIZATIONS. *Broca's aphasia* is the result of a lesion of Broca's area, i.e., the portion of the frontal lobe just anterior to the face, lip, tongue, and mouth area of the motor cortex. This produces a nonfluent aphasia, and writing is also involved. Repetition is impaired. The patient's greatest difficulty in repetition is with phrases consisting of small "grammatical" words (e.g., "If he were here I would go there") rather than with long words. Comprehension of language is intact. There is nearly always a right hemiplegia. *Wernicke's aphasia* results from a lesion of Wernicke's area, the posterior portion of the superior temporal gyrus. The aphasia is typically fluent. Written language is equally impaired. Comprehension of spoken and written language is severely impaired. Repetition of spoken language is poor. There is usually no hemiplegia, and other elementary neurologic signs are usually lacking. *Conduction aphasia* results from a lesion of the parietal operculum, i.e., the region lying above the sylvian fissure. There is fluent aphasia involving speech and writing, with severely impaired repetition but intact comprehension. Elementary neurologic signs are usually absent, with the occasional exception of cortical sensory loss on the opposite side. Some patients with Wernicke's area lesions may recover comprehension and are therefore left with the same syndrome. *Anomic aphasia* is characterized by fluent aphasia in speech and impairment of written language, but with intact comprehension and repetition. The components of Gerstmann's syndrome (discussed in Ch. 224) are often present. In this syndrome the lesion, if focal, is at the region of the parietotemporal junction, but a similar sydrome is produced in nonfocal widespread disease of the brain, such as is caused by metabolic disease or by large masses with raised intracranial pressure regardless of their location. It is also the most common form of aphasia in patients with closed head injury. Anomic aphasia may also be seen in the recovery stage from almost any other form of aphasia. Thus, in contrast to Broca's, Wernicke's, and conduction aphasia, anomic aphasia is much more difficult to localize.

These four syndromes are the most common, and although overlapping forms are common, relatively pure forms are not rare. Certain other syndromes are much less common.

Isolation of the speech area is caused by a large lesion involving the cortex and underlying white matter in a C-shaped configuration that spares Broca's area, Wernicke's area, and their interconnections, but destroys the cortex and underlying white matter that surround the speech region. These patients either may show little spontaneous speech or may have fluent abnormal speech. The most striking characteristic of this disorder is that, despite an almost total lack of comprehension, the patient can repeat well without dysarthria. This lesion is usually the result of anoxia or of carotid insufficiency. *Alexia without agraphia* is a syndrome in which the patient speaks and writes normally but cannot comprehend written language. The lesion, almost always the result of infarction in the distribution of the left posterior cerebral artery, consists of destruction of the left visual cortex and the splenium, i.e., the posterior portion, of the corpus callosum. In *alexia with agraphia* the patient can neither write nor comprehend written language, but other language functions are normal. Other components of Gerstmann's syndrome (see Ch. 224) may be present. The lesion involves a portion of the left angular gyrus. A right visual field defect may occur if the lesion extends deeply into the white matter but is often absent. *Pure word-deafness* described a syndrome in which there is dense incomprehension of language in the presence of intact hearing, although other language functions are intact. Two types of lesion produce this; either a single lesion lying subcortically in the posterior temporal lobe or bilateral lesions of the middle portion of the first temporal gyrus. *Pure agraphia* is extremely rare as the result of any focal lesion, but is common in patients with confusional states of toxic, metabolic, or traumatic orgin.

Aphemia is an uncommon syndrome in which the patient has speech which is slow, effortful and dysarthric, but without significant disorder of grammar or word choice. The patient's written language is essentially normal. A right hemiplegia is often present at the onset but usually disappears. Aphemic patients usually improve markedly, but it may take up to three years. It is likely that this syndrome results from small lesions in Broca's area, whereas larger lesions produce the typical Broca's aphasia with a right hemiplegia.

Aphasic syndromes in children are more difficult to localize. Mutism is more common in childhood aphasia. Fluent aphasia occurs very rarely in childhood even with lesions that usually lead to fluent forms in adults. Older adults are more likely than younger adults to have grossly fluent aphasias.

Aphasias in left handers have some special properties. Left handers appear to become aphasic with lesions in either hemisphere, although those occurring after right hemisphere lesions are more likely to be transient. Most permanent severe aphasias in left handers result from left-sided lesions. Comprehenshion difficulty is less common in left handers, and apraxia (see below) is also less common as an accompaniment of aphasia. Recovery is better not only in left handers but also, according to Luria, in right handers with left-handed parents, siblings, or children.

At present the evidence is that most *recovery in adult aphasics* takes place spontaneously. Although speech therapy has not been proved to produce major changes, it can be very useful in mobilizing the patient's residual language capacities for most effective communication.

224. OTHER DISORDERS OF THE HIGHER FUNCTIONS

APRAXIA. Apraxia is the inability to perform a learned act in response to a stimulus which would normally elicit it, and which cannot be accounted for by weakness, incoordination, reflex change, sensory loss, incomprehension, inattention, or uncooperativeness. Three lesions may produce apraxia. With lesions of the corpus callosum there will be apraxia of the left side of the body, but not of the right or of the face. Patients with Broca's aphasia (who usually have a right hemiplegia) will show apraxia that is usually most marked in the face and is also often present in the left limbs. With lesions in the left parietal operculum, producing a conduction aphasia, there is usually apraxia in the face (where it is most marked) and in the limbs of both sides of the body. In all forms of apraxia, axial movements, i.e., movements in which the muscles of the trunk or neck are involved, e.g., "stand up," "sit down," "turn around," and movement of eye-closing and eye-opening as well as movements of the eyes (e.g., "look up") are preserved. In all forms of apraxia the defect is most marked to verbal command (although the patient comprehends), usually somewhat less marked on imitation of the examiner, and least marked in the handling of objects, although in some patients even this latter category is impaired.

AGNOSIA. Agnosia is a failure of recognition of complex stimuli in the face of preserved elementary perception. The most common form is visual agnosia, in which there are usually bilateral posterior occipital lobe lesions. The agnosias are less well understood than the aphasias or apraxias.

CALLOSAL SYNDROMES. These were first brilliantly described by Hugo Liepmann in the early 1900's, but have been rediscovered only in recent years. In some cases of anterior cerebral artery occlusion there is infarction of the anterior four fifths of the corpus callosum. The patient will carry out verbal commands with the right hand but not the left. He will name objects held (concealed from vision) in the right hand but not the left. He can, however, with the left hand draw or select from a group of objects the one previously held in the left hand. He manifests, in brief, inability to transfer information between the two hemispheres. Involvement of the splenium of the corpus callosum plays a role in alexia without agraphia (see Ch. 223).

GERSTMANN'S SYNDROME. This consists of agraphia, right-left disorientation, acalculia (difficulty in carrying out calculations), and finger agnosia (inability to name fingers or to identify them). The patient almost invariably also shows constructional disorder, i.e., a difficulty in drawing or copying designs, especially three-dimensional ones. When all the components of this syndrome are present, the lesion almost invariably lies in the left posterior parietal region. It should, however, be kept in mind that a single component has little localizing value.

RIGHT HEMISPHERE SYNDROMES. Lesions of the right parietal region produce constructional difficulty that is more severe on the average than that produced from any other site. It should be recalled, however, that constructional difficulty is common with left hemisphere lesions. Patients with right hemisphere lesions may also show a dressing disorder manifested by great difficulty in putting on clothes. Milder degrees of the difficulty may be brought out by such maneuvers as putting one sleeve of the bathrobe inside out; the patient may be unable to get the bathrobe on properly.

A striking feature of acute lesions of the right hemisphere is *anosognosia*, i.e., a tendency to deny or neglect disability or, when admitting its presence, to be unconcerned with it. It is a common experience that the patient with an acute left hemiplegia will show this type of behavior, although by contrast the patient with an acute right hemiplegia will, even if aphasic, usually show appropriate awareness of disability and will be depressed. These disorders in right hemisphere lesions are always accompanied by a curious mental state, in which the patient shows apathy, poor attention, and often jocularity. These states (and the accompanying unconcern with illness) are usually transient, but are sometimes permanent in cases of large right parietal lesions. These curious mental states probably reflect the fact that the right hemisphere has a special role in many aspects of subjective emotional response and emotional expression.

Not all patients who deny illness suffer from right hemisphere disease. Weinstein has shown that a patient with any disability may deny illness if he is sufficiently obtunded. Thus a patient may deny blindness resulting even from disease of the eyes if he develops a confusional state from metabolic disorder or drugs.

225. MEMORY

Memory describes the processes by which past experience is stored and retrieved. Disorders of memory include *anterograde amnesia*, i.e., the failure to store new memories, or *retrograde amnesia*, i.e., disorders of storage or retrieval of memories laid down in the past.

Certain separable stages in memory storage have become clear from clinical observation. There is a stage of *immediate* memory, which is the ability to retain material presented as long as attention is not distracted. This is examined by such tests as digit span, i.e., the ability to repeat a series of digits spoken by the examiner. Most normal persons can immediately repeat a series of seven such digits. The next step is *transfer* to the long-term memory store. The first step in this is *intermediate memory* storage, and the later step is called *remote memory*. The reason for separating these steps will become clear when we discuss the clinical syndromes.

ANATOMY OF MEMORY

Memories are probably held in short-term store simply by continuation of nervous activity. The transfer to the long-term store probably involves some molecular change either in nerve membrane or in intracellular organelles. The neural structures most involved appear to lie in the limbic system, especially the hippocampal region, mammillary bodies, and, according to some authors, the dorsomedial nuclei of the thalamus (Victor et al.). The intactness of these structures appears to be important, in some as yet undefined way, in the transfer of memories from the intermediate to the long-term stores. The memories are probably not laid down in these limbic structures, because their destruction does not lead to loss of remote memories. They must therefore act on the structures which are the sites of storage. The limbic structures are also important, as will be seen below, in retrieval from the intermediate store.

CLINICAL DISORDERS OF MEMORY

Memory disorder may be evidence in widespread disorder of the brain such as may be produced by drugs or metabolic disorders. On the other hand, memory may be relatively or dramatically spared in many of the dementias. Thus memory is much less impaired than such functions as calculation and abstraction in general paresis. By contrast, in Alzheimer's disease, in which involvement of hippocampus is prominent, memory disorder is a salient feature of the initial states in most but not all cases. In Pick's disease, which is much less common, memory is frequently spared.

Disease processes predominantly affecting the hippocampal-mammillary system will produce significant memory disorder with little or no effect on other intellectual functions. This clinical state is called *Korsakoff's syndrome*. When caused by thiamin deficiency, the most striking lesions are in the mammillary bodies. The hippocampus may be involved in Alzheimer's disease, head injury, or tumors. Disease of the posterior cerebral artery may cause infarction of the hippocampus. Herpes simplex encephalitis has a predilection for all the structures of the limbic system. Occasional cases of severe memory loss have been reported after bilateral removal of the medial temporal structures surgically.

In order to produce a permanent memory deficit, bilateral lesions of the mammillo-hippocampal system are required. However, a unilateral lesion of the *left* hippocampus will produce a transient memory disorder, which may last as long as three months (Geschwind and Fusillo).

The memory disorder that sometimes follows head injury illustrates well the different states of the memory process outlined above. A patient who shows this disorder, let us say a week after the episode, may exhibit the following picture. He will be alert, awake, and cooperative and may, on a standard I.Q. test, score in a normal or even superior range. In addition his immediate memory, as shown, for example, by digit span, will be normal. By contrast he shows an anterograde amnesia, i.e., an inability to learn new material. He also shows a retrograde amnesia extending back from 3 to 20 years. More remote memories, in particular most of what was learned before the age of 12, are usually but not invariably much better preserved. Over the next two or three months the condition improves. The ability to learn new material reappears (but the patient will have a permanent gap in his memory for the period in which he lacked this ability). The retrograde amnesia gradually shrinks until it reaches its permanent form, with a duration of seconds to minutes. The long retrograde amnesia must therefore have been a disorder of retrieval rather than storage. It thus appears that the integrity of the limbic structures is necessary for the retrieval from intermediate but not remote memory. In cases of persistent Korsakoff's syndrome, such as occur frequently with other forms of disorders that produce permanent bilateral limbic system damage, the retrograde amnesia does not improve significantly.

A prominent feature of many but not all cases of Korsakoff's syndrome, especially in the early stages, is *confabulation*, i.e., the tendency of the patient to invent fanciful replies to questions whose answers he does not know. Confabulation usually becomes less marked with the passage of time. Some patients with Korsakoff's syndrome show distinct improvement, although not to normal, over periods of months or even several years.

Functional amnesia occurs in hysteria (usually in young people) or in older patients who are depressed. A similar clinical picture seen in malingerers is usually easy to recognize. The patient may show either a highly selective memory disorder, e.g., denying that he is married, although all other recent and remote facts are preserved, or a global disorder, e.g., professing total amnesia for all events of his life. Failure of a patient without aphasia to state his own name is invariably not organic in orgin. Another common syndrome is the fugue state in which the patient denies any memory of his activities for a period of time ranging from hours to weeks, during which his external activities appeared normal or during which he disappeared and traveled extensively. Although some short-lasting fugue states may occasionally be the result of temporal lobe epilepsy, the author's experience has been that these are nearly all functional in origin.

Kral, on the basis of study of several hundred aging subjects, has pointed out that the finding of true Korsakoff's syndrome leads to a poor prognosis for psychologic function and survival. He has distinguished another syndrome of *benign forgetfulness* with onset usually in middle life. Patients with this disorder have difficulty remembering specific details, especially proper names, although they recognize the correct answer, and on other occasions recall the same data without difficulty. These patients are very embarrassed by these failures to recall. The senile Korsakoff patient is more likely to forget recent events in more global fashion, often fails to recognize the correct data, and is often unconcerned. The benign disorder tends to remain delimited over many years, and is compatible with the highest levels of professional activity. It is more common in men, whereas senile dementia is more common in women.

In some patients *mid-life depression* is associated with distinct memory impairment. When this is the presenting symptom the correct diagnosis may be overlooked. When the depression is successfully treated, the memory disorder clears.

Recovery from memory disorder: Post-traumatic Korsakoff's syndromes typically improve, as pointed out above. A seemingly permanent metabolic amnestic syndrome also may improve slowly over many years. There is no evidence that any therapy is effective in treating memory disorders, but active research is now going on in this field.

Geschwind, N.: Disconnexion syndromes in animals and man. Brain, 88:237, 585, 1965.

Geschwind, N.: The organization of language and the brain. Science, 170:940, 1970.

Geschwind, N., and Fusillo, M.: Color-naming defects in association with alexia. Arch. Neurol., 15:137, 1966.

Kral, V. A.: Senescent forgetfulness: Benign and malignant. Can. Med. Assoc. J., 86:257, 1962.

Victor, M., Adams, R. D., and Collins, G. H.: The Wernicke-Korsakoff Syndrome. Philadelphia, F. A. Davis Company, 1971.

Zangwill, O. L.: Cerebral Dominance and Its Relation to Psychological Function. Springfield, Ill., Charles C Thomas, 1960.

Section Three   DEMENTIA

Paul R. McHugh

226.   INTRODUCTION

GENERAL CONSIDERATIONS. Dementia means deterioration in intellectual capacity. The condition is distinguished from mental retardation, in which subnormal intellectual ability has been lifelong and may or may not be caused by brain injury; and from aphasia and Korsakoff's psychosis, in which specific intellectual skills (language and memory, respectively) have deteriorated without a proportional disturbance in other cognitive functions.

Dementia is a clinical entity. Any pathologic process affecting the cerebral hemispheres can lead to an impairment in intellectual capacity. The extent of the brain injury and not its location or the nature of the neuropathology determines its severity. Treatment and prognosis, however, depend on the nature of the pathologic process. Some pathologies and the dementias they produce are relentlessly progressive. Others are curable. Therefore the diagnostic task consists of two steps: first, the recognition of dementia; and second, the identification of the cerebral pathology producing it. The first step requires skill in the assessment of mental function; the second, an appreciation of the clinical features, course, and diagnostic laboratory data that characterize various cerebral pathologies.

CLINICAL MANIFESTATIONS.   The earliest symptoms of dementia can pass almost unrecognized. They appear as disturbances in the patient's capacities for problem solving, grasp of situation, and agility of thought. He may carry out his daily routines at home and at work adequately, but he becomes less efficient and may fail in tasks that are demanding or require his special skills. The changes may be hard to distinguish from fatigue or boredom. The appreciation of their importance will depend on how well the examiner knows the patient and on how much the patient's livelihood depends upon mental capacity. Thus relatives and fellow workers usually notice a change before doctors can be sure of it; and professional, managerial, or skilled workers are more quickly brought for help than are individuals with unskilled occupations.

As a dementia progresses, however, the disability will be obvious to all because its symptoms are defects in basic mental functions. Memory failure is often the first definite symptom. The patient becomes forgetful particularly of the events of the day, overlooks appointments, fails to remember conversations, or forgets the purpose of his errands.

Other symptoms reflect the patient's bewilderment in the face of complexity. He becomes lost in attempting to find his way in the city. He fails to understand a conversation, particularly if several people are involved, as at a meeting. He cannot follow directions that involve a series of steps.

Language presents special difficulties. He is unable to use words with facility and pertinence, but depends on clichés and habitual forms of expression. His conversation becomes rambling and repetitious, his letters long and vague, his directions to others involved and obscure. Defining a word or a proverb for his examining physician is very difficult because he is unable to call up the meaning of abstract words and concepts.

At this stage in a dementing illness, habit often sustains the patient's social behavior. He can for example take part in superficial, polite conversation giving appropriate replies. But if a mental status examination is carried beyond casual interchange to test memory, orientation, or grasp of situation, this façade of customary manners and speech cannot hide the deficits in mental capacity.

The demented patient often suffers from emotional disturbances. Sudden outbursts of emotion, taking the form of anger, tears, or aggressiveness, may occur when the patient is attempting a task that is beyond his present mental skill. These *catastrophic reactions* are usually of short duration, but their repeated appearance may be a prominent feature of the illness almost from its onset.

More sustained and chronic emotional disorders, such as depression and anxiety, are also seen in dementing illness for reasons that are not immediately obvious. They may represent a response of a patient who comprehends his growing difficulties but may also represent injury to central nervous system mechanisms mediating emotional expression.

A symptom seen in some dementing patients and easily confused with depression is a progressive apathy or mental inertia. This may be just a loss of sparkle or liveliness of character, but progresses to involve initiative and physical energy. Such apathy can result in much poorer performance in daily affairs than can be explained at first by the cognitive disabilities, but worsens as the dementia progresses and can reach such a state of unresponsiveness that the patient is inaccessible to examination.

Finally, if the dementing disorder is relentlessly progressive, the patient will lose all his mental powers. He loses his remote memories, now failing to recognize his closest relatives. He cannot care for any of his physical needs. He becomes bedridden, unaware of his situation, and dependent, and soon dies of intercurrent infection or malnutrition.

DIAGNOSIS.   It is not difficult to recognize advanced intellectual impairment. More taxing is the recognition of intellectual impairment when it is slight and potentially reversible. The tests of cognitive function that are part of the neurologic examination of every patient are intended to accomplish this, but they must be interpreted with care.

It is customary to test (1) orientation to time, place, and person; (2) language skills, by naming common objects and comprehending commands; (3) fund of knowledge, such as the names of some capital cities and of presidents; (4) recent memory, by setting three objects to be remembered for 5, 10, and 30 minutes; (5) attention span, by asking for a serial subtraction of 7 from 100 or any other arithmetic task that requires "carrying over"; (6) abstract reasoning power, by asking for definitions of proverbs or the similarity of words such as apple-orange, ear-eye, poem-statue; and (7) constructional capacity, by asking the patient to draw simple objects such as a clock or to copy an abstract design.

As a means of scoring cognitive impairment and following its progress, the Mini-Mental Status of Folstein et al. has proved useful. It employs several of these standard clinical tests to derive a quantitative assessment that is sensitive, reliable, and brief enough to be part of every bedside examination.

The results of these tests must be interpreted in the light of other knowledge about the patient. If the patient was a gifted professional person whose family has noted a decline in his judgment and an increasing forgetfulness, the discovery that he cannot hold three words in mind for five minutes and that he interprets proverbs clumsily provides some evidence that he is suffering from a disturbance to his intellectual power. On the other hand, if the patient was not a person with intellectual achievements in the past and has received a poor education, difficulties in proverb interpretation or fund of knowledge are less likely to represent brain disease. Although it is possible to find all the intellectual functions disturbed in dementia, the tests for recent memory, for attention, and for constructional capacity are most useful. Deficiencies here are easy to document; these functions are affected early in the course of many brain diseases, and they are little dependent on education. Also, tests for recent memory are useful in differentiating a patient with mental retardation from an individual of limited intelligence who is developing a brain disease, since memory function is intact in the mildly retarded individual.

It is important to differentiate Korsakoff's syndrome and aphasia. The patient with Korsakoff's syndrome will fail the test of recent memory. He will be disoriented to time and place, but he will be able to name objects, obey commands, and accomplish tasks of abstract reasoning and drawing if he can hold the question in mind. His disorder is in memory. The rest of his intellectual function is relatively spared. The aphasic patient will have severe problems in naming objects and comprehending words. But if this difficulty can be surmounted, it will be evident that language is specifically disturbed, and other mental functions such as memory, orientation, and constructional capacity are relatively intact.

It is sometimes useful to supplement the bedside tests of mental function with standardized examination of intellectual skills. The Wechsler Adult Intelligence Scale as described in Ch. 236 is most often employed.

DIAGNOSTIC ISSUES IN DEMENTIA. As mentioned previously, the symptoms of dementia appear with an injury to the cerebral hemispheres, and are not specific for a particular pathology. It is the course of their development, the associated neurologic signs, and the laboratory findings that permit diagnosis of the pathologic entities producing the dementia.

Since the same symptoms can be produced by curable, reversible pathology as by incurable and progressive disorders, the first diagnostic consideration should reflect a search for the treatable pathologic entities. All the following conditions represent potentially treatable disorders that should be considered and excluded in every patient: general paresis, myxedema, intracranial mass lesions such as tumors, hematomas and abscesses, hepatolenticular degeneration (Wilson's disease), avitaminosis B (particularly niacin deficiency [pellagra] and

B_{12} deficiency), occult hydrocephalus, and a depressive illness in advanced age. Many of these conditions can be diagnosed by evidence derived from the clinical examination; others demand clinical laboratory studies. A group of laboratory tests are required in the diagnostic evaluation. As a routine, all patients should have a lumbar puncture to measure intracerebral pressure and to obtain a sample of cerebrospinal fluid for analysis. Cell count, protein content, and a test for the antisyphilis antibodies will be needed in cerebrospinal fluid. Blood serologic examination for syphilis, analysis for protein-bound iodine, and serum B_{12} analysis are also indicated. An electroencephalogram may reveal a local lesion or a severe generalized slowing of the rhythms characteristic of delirium. Skull roentgenograms can also reveal a local lesion. The recently developed brain CT scan (see Ch. 267) has become the radiographic procedure of choice in the diagnosis of dementia, providing information that can be critical in the diagnosis of many different cerebral pathologies.

The onset and course of a dementing disorder must be carefully analyzed when considering the likely pathologic entities. Was the onset abrupt or insidious, was the subsequent course a gradual and relentless loss of mental faculties, or was it a series of sudden losses producing a steplike decline? Did it require months or only a few weeks to develop? Different pathologic entities produce different clinical histories in these respects.

Thus the typical dementia produced by arteriosclerotic disease of the brain (*multi-infarct dementia*) will take the course of occlusive vascular infarctions. The mental decline will come with "strokes." It will be a steplike decline with each step sudden in onset, varying in extent, intermittent and unpredictable in timing, and usually associated with some motor-sensory deficits on neurologic examination. The dementia of the degenerative disorders such as Alzheimer's disease appears insidiously rather than suddenly, progresses slowly but steadily rather than irregularly and intermittently, and is free of motor-sensory features until the condition is advanced. The dementia of general paresis or pellagra tends to be subacute and steadily progressive.

An occasional elderly patient with a depressive illness will present with a dementia syndrome quite responsive to treatment of his depression. The course of such depressions is helpful in diagnosis, since, in contrast to Alzheimer's disease, the dementia appears and progresses in a subacute fashion (days to a few weeks). Helpful as well is the recognition of a depression of mood, a change in self-attitude, and a previous history of attacks of mania or depression. Treatment is discussed in Ch. 233 3.

Folstein, M., Folstein, S., and McHugh, P. R.: "Mini-mental state." A practical method for grading the cognitive state of patients for the clinician. J. Psychiat. Res., 12:189, 1975.
Wells, C. E. (ed.): Dementia. 2nd ed. Philadelphia, F. A. Davis Company, 1977.

227. ALZHEIMER'S DISEASE

Alzheimer's disease is a progressive degenerative process of the brain that produces a dementia in middle to late life. It is the most common specific pathologic entity provoking dementia in the United States. Autopsy diagnoses vary from 1 to 10 per cent in mental hospitals, the particular figure depending on whether the observers make a distinction between Alzheimer's disease and senile dementia. Its defining characteristics are its pathologic features.

The brain in Alzheimer's disease very gradually atrophies, nerve cells disappearing from the cortex. The major brunt of the atrophic process appears to be in the frontal and temporal regions of the brain, but microscopic examinations demonstrate pathologic changes throughout the cortex.

The atrophic cortex contains many "senile plaques," microscopic collections of granular argyrophilic particles which tend to form in a halo around an indefinite center containing sudanophilic fat and an amyloid-like substance. These plaques are collections of neuron particles, degenerative synaptic boutons, surrounding a central core of amyloid fibrils. In the cortex many of the neurons that remain show a peculiar alteration of their neurofibrils, which are thickened and twisted into distinctive "neurofibrillary tangles."

The dementia of Alzheimer's disease parallels the pathologic features. In fact the severity of the cognitive symptoms has been directly correlated with the quantity of plaques and tangles in a clinicopathologic study by Blessed et al. The dementia, as the pathology, is slowly but relentlessly progressive. The onset is insidious, and for a considerable period into the course only psychologic symptoms are found. Motor or sensory neurologic signs appear late, if at all.

A disturbance in memory for recent events is usually the first symptom. This amnesic difficulty is accompanied by some disorientation in time and place but may be otherwise the only symptom for some time. Usually within one or two years other cognitive difficulties, as in judgment, comprehension, or abstract reasoning, appear and gradually worsen.

With the development of these cognitive symptoms, emotional unrest can appear. This at first may take the form of anxiety and depression related to the patient's self-awareness of his difficulties. But usually after three or four years of illness, emotional reactions are prompted by delusionary false beliefs that develop in 30 to 40 per cent of these patients. Auditory and visual hallucinations are found in a smaller number of patients.

At approximately the same time in the progression of the illness, symptoms related to focal cortical injury such as aphasia, apraxia, and agnosia often become prominent. The aphasia begins as a naming problem, but quickly dysphasic jargon appears and severely disrupts communication.

By three or four years of the illness, when these intellectual and emotional disturbances are well advanced, neurologic functions begin to deteriorate. The first symptom of this sort is a disorder of gait. This takes the form of difficulty in starting the rhythmical movements of walking. A synchronous activation of agonists and antagonist muscles results in a locking of the legs and a hesitant shuffle. Focal or generalized seizures occur in approximately 15 per cent of patients in the far advanced stages of the illness. Within five to eight years of the onset of symptoms the patient reaches a terminal stage. Here there is a profound dementia and a decerebrate physical state with flexion contractures of all limbs. Death comes from an intercurrent infection or some other complication of the bedfast condition.

The age of onset varies. Because this disorder was first recognized among relatively young people, the term "presenile dementia" has been applied to Alzheimer's disease. But the cerebral pathology and the clinical course of patients who develop symptoms before or after age 65 are the same. Alzheimer's disease, defined as it is by the cerebral pathology of atrophy with senile plaques and neurofibrillary tangles, is a disorder appearing with increasing frequency as people age. A distinction between Alzheimer's disease and senile dementia is argued, but pathologically they are identical.

The cause of Alzheimer's disease is unknown. Most examples occur sporadically, but a few patients have a family history. It is not certain whether Alzheimer's disease is a specific response to one noxious biologic process or whether it is a more general response of the brain to many injurious processes. The latter possibility is suggested by the occasional appearance of Alzheimer pathology in such different situations as the punch-drunk syndrome of boxers, Down's syndrome (trisomy 21), and postencephalitic parkinsonism. Experimental neuropathology has produced intriguing results such as the occasional but far from regular production of a neuropathic condition in primate hosts following injections of tissue from Alzheimer patients, the recognition of a deficit in the cortical cholinergic system in Alzheimer's disease, and the discovery of an increase in aluminum in Alzheimer brains. But as yet no confirmation has been provided of what might constitute a primary cause and what the secondary effects.

Blessed, G., Tomlinson, B. E., and Roth, M.: The association between quantitative measures of dementia and senile changes in the cerebral grey matter of elderly subjects. Br. J. Psychiatry, 114:797, 1968.

Corsellis, J. A. N.: Mental illness and the Ageing Brain. London, Oxford University Press, 1962.

Sjogren, T., Sjogren, H., and Lindgren, A. G. H.: Morbus Alzheimer and morbus Pick: A genetic clinical and pathological study. Acta Psychiat. Scand. (Suppl. 82), 1952.

Wolstenholme, G. E. W., and O'Connor, M. (eds.): Alzheimer's Disease and Related Conditions. Ciba Foundation Symposium. London, Churchill, 1970.

228.   PICK'S DISEASE

Pick's disease is also a degenerative disorder of the cerebral cortex that produces dementia in middle and late life. It is distinguished from Alzheimer's disease by its morbid anatomy.

In contrast to Alzheimer's disease, in which the cerebral atrophy is diffuse, in Pick's disease, the relatively severe atrophy is confined to the frontal and temporal lobes. The microscopic pathology is distinctive and includes individually degenerating neurons characterized by the accumulation close to the nucleus of a globular argyrophilic mass that distends the cell body into a swollen ballooned form. This "Pick cell" is usually found widespread in the atrophying areas of cortex. There are usually neurofibrillary tangles and senile plaques as well in the atrophic parts of brain.

It is difficult to distinguish an example of Pick's disease from Alzheimer's disease on clinical grounds. Patients with Pick's disease may have less difficulty in gait than patients with Alzheimer's disease. Otherwise, the conditions seem clinically identical. Pick's disease is considerably less common than Alzheimer's disease, but, as in that condition, no definite cause has been identified. Some examples of Pick's disease appear to be transmitted by an autosomal dominant trait, but many examples lack a family history.

229. CREUTZFELDT-JAKOB DISEASE

The dementia in Creutzfeldt-Jakob disease is rapidly progressive, advancing noticeably day by day from its onset to a fatal termination, usually within a year. The dementia is accompanied by a variety of neurologic symptoms such as ataxia, aphasia, paralysis, and visual disturbances and by prominent myoclonic jerking of the limbs and body at some stage in the disorder. The EEG is abnormal early in the disturbance, its normal rhythms lost and replaced with a distinctive mixture of slow and sharp waves useful for diagnosis. The condition is the result of a degeneration of cerebral cortex thought to be caused by a transmissible agent of the latent or slow virus variety. It is more thoroughly discussed in Ch. 310.3.

230. HUNTINGTON'S CHOREA

Huntington's chorea is a distinctive disease entity in which a dementia associated with chorea appears usually in the fourth or fifth decade of life. Its neuropathology is characteristic, and the disease is transmitted as an autosomal dominant trait. The condition is discussed more fully in Ch. 277.3.

231. TREATMENT OF THE DEMENTED PATIENT

With the exception of the specific treatments for curable diseases, the issue of treatment for the demented patient is most often that of management of particular symptoms rather than reversal of a pathologic process. Often, a treatment based on some research finding is proposed for the degenerative disorders only to prove of little value when employed in a clinical trial. Thus the discovery that cerebral oxygen consumption is reduced in Alzheimer's disease led to treatments with both oxygen inhalation and hyperbaric chambers. But these treatments failed to produce significant improvement, almost certainly because the observed reduction in oxygen consumption is due to a reduction in the number of viable neurons rather than to an inadequate oxygen supply. Any treatment that is proposed for these distressing conditions is liable to be uncritically acclaimed, with eventual disappointment. The importance of the clinical trial with double-blind technique in assessing these treatments cannot be exaggerated.

Some general principles of management of the demented patient can be emphasized. First, complicating medical conditions such as congestive heart failure, dehydration, iron deficiency anemia, infections, and electrolyte imbalance can, even if not severe in themselves, make the mental condition of a patient with degenerative brain disease much worse and should be corrected. Second, much of the emotional unrest in demented patients is due to fear produced by their disorientation, misidentifications, and misinterpretations. Great relief of these symptoms can come from a willingness of nurses and doctors to explain repeatedly to the patient his situation and the proper interpretation of what is happening. Changes in surrounding and in nursing personnel should be minimized; well lighted rooms, preferably with familiar possessions, serve best, and an attitude that is accepting and supportive does much to assist the patient. Any situations that require effort beyond his capacity and so produce catastrophic reactions must be avoided. Third, considerable help for individual symptoms can be gained by the use of pharmacologic measures. Sleep disturbances in demented patients are best treated with chloral hydrate, up to 1.0 to 1.5 grams at night.

The agitated states associated with delusions, misinterpretations, and *catastrophic* reactions can be among the most disruptive features of these disorders. They can be considerably ameliorated by a combination of the supportive management described above and modest amounts of phenothiazine or butyrophenone medication. Thioridazine, in doses of 50 to 100 mg three to four times daily, or haloperidol, 2 to 5 mg three times daily, has proved helpful. Depressive symptoms respond to antidepressant medication (imipramine, 50 mg three to four times per day).

All these drugs should be used sparingly, as the patient with cerebral degeneration may demonstrate toxic signs at much lower doses than normal patients. Drug toxicity can worsen the condition severely.

In general, the management of the demented patient rests on an appreciation of the nature of his psychologic disabilities and the application of psychosocial medical and nursing principles. The response to this management is often gratifying.

Miller, E., and Pearce, J.: Clinical Aspects of Dementia. London, Bailliere Tindall, 1973, pp. 98–124.

Post, F.: Clinical Psychiatry of Late Life. New York, Pergamon Press, 1965.

Section Four PSYCHOLOGIC ILLNESS IN MEDICAL PRACTICE

Paul R. McHugh

232. THE CONCEPT OF DISEASE IN PSYCHIATRY

Any general hospital can provide an experience in psychiatry, because an example of every psychologic disorder will eventually appear among patients admitted to its services. However, many thoughtful physicians feel unsure of their ability to manage these disorders. They are apt to contrast their knowledge of somatic illness founded firmly in morbid anatomy and pathophysiology with their understanding of psychologic medicine in which classifications seem based on confusing mixtures of symptomatology and speculative theories, and the most effective treatments are empirical. Such physicians will continue uncertain until they grasp how the basic concept of disease can bring order to aspects of psychiatry as it does in all of medicine. This they must accomplish before they can profit from a review of the clinical facts of particular psychiatric conditions; hence this chapter.

The term "disease" is difficult to define, because it is a concept and not something concrete or given in nature. As a concept it focuses on patients as organisms and conveys the idea that among all the morbid changes in physical and mental health it is possible to recognize groups of abnormalities as distinct entities or syndromes separable from one another and from the normal and that these separations will prove to have some biologic explanation when the entities have been thoroughly investigated.

Abnormalities can as logically be viewed as quantitative changes merging imperceptibly into one another and into the normal, and can then be explained as consequences of disturbed interactions of a few vital processes. The Galenic concept of "humors" is just such a view. In fact the concept of disease based on qualitatively distinct syndromes is a convention championed by Sydenham, and remains but a convention today. However, this has been one of the most useful conventions in the natural sciences. It has become so indispensable in medical thinking that it is taken for granted in most discussions. Neglect of this convention explains much of the difficulty faced by students in psychiatry. Its logic thus needs review here.

The concept of any given disease passes through several stages as knowledge increases. At each stage attention focuses on certain features of the condition which are the "defining characteristics." At the first stage a "clinical disease entity" is recognized and defined as a constellation of symptoms and physical signs running a more or less predictable course or natural history. Dropsy, hemophilia, and epilepsy are typical clinical disease entities. But these entities are not pure species.

Each can be the expression of any one of several different pathologic conditions: glomerulonephritis, congestive heart failure, constrictive pericarditis. Thus the second stage is the division of the clinical disease entity into several "pathologic disease entities." When a disease can be conceived as a pathologic entity, the defining characteristics on which concept and diagnosis rest are results of laboratory tests that reveal pathologic function or morbid anatomy. Again, by way of example the demonstration of an elevated blood urea nitrogen and albumin and casts in the urine of a patient with dropsy leads to a presumptive opinion that the pathologic disease entity responsible for his condition is glomerulonephritis. This presumptive diagnosis is confirmed by studying the histopathology of the kidney. The third and final stage in the concept of a disease is the recognition of a particular etiologic agency. This recognition can derive from any aspect of biologic knowledge: genetics, microbiology, and biochemistry have all made their contributions. For glomerulonephritis the etiologic agency is the phenomenon of autoimmunity, and it will be from investigations of this phenomenon that physicians can expect to gain a complete understanding of glomerulonephritis as well as a treatment that can prevent and cure it.

For many medical diseases the mark of the twentieth century has been the discovery of etiologic agencies and their action. This is less so for psychiatry. For most psychiatric disorders knowledge has not passed the first stage on the traditional path, and for many even the hold on this stage is insecure. This insecurity arises in part from the difficulty of the subject matter, but also from a lack of consensus over the applicability of the disease concept in this field. It implies a distinction between those mental disturbances that arise in the mind of a subject coping with conflict and those that are a result of disease in the organism. This is a distinction some would deny, holding the opinon that *all* psychologic disturbances are to be viewed as emotional reactions to some form of environmental distress, and thus are quantitative abnormalities differing from normal in a continuous and smooth fashion rather than grouping into qualitatively distinct entities with separable pathologies and etiologies.

One objection to this view has to be the practical one that it discards for no obvious advantage a convention that has ordered other abnormalities successfully. Another is that it oversimplifies mental disturbances to make them all expressions of a few psychologic mechanisms. A consideration of the forms of disorder for which psychiatry assumes responsibility will demonstrate the utility found in the concept of disease for some of them.

Three groups of disturbances fall into manageable

psychiatric categories. *The first holds all those disturbances in mind and behavior that are a result of observable brain pathology.* Represented here are the clinical disease entities of delirium, dementia, and mental retardation. The conceptual and investigative approach to these conditions is indistinguishable from that for other somatic diseases. Such pathologic disease entities as Alzheimer's disease and such etiologic agencies as perinatal hypoxia, infections, and metabolic changes have been discerned.

The second group holds the two functional psychoses in which no obvious brain pathology is evident: schizophrenia and manic-depressive disorder. That these conditions are not unlike somatic disorders and should be conceived as clinical disease entities defined by symptoms and course is impossible to prove at this time. But this view was first prompted by the alien form of the psychologic symptoms such as hallucinations and delusions that appear in these disorders. It has been strengthened by the discovery of pharmacologic treatments specific to each entity and by the recognition of a few morbid conditions of the central nervous system leading to identical clinical conditions — amphetamine toxicity leading to a schizophrenia-like disorder, and the reserpine reaction that mimics a depressive disorder. It is now more conceivable that we are on the threshold of discoveries that will provide pathologic disease entities and etiologic agencies for these conditions than that they will be explained as quantitative exaggerations of emotional reactions.

The third group of disturbances in mind and behavior are the personality disorders and neurotic symptoms. The concept of disease with its logical extension from clinical entity through pathology to etiology does not fit these conditions. To seek, for example, a neuropathology provoking grief would seem an obvious category error — mistaking a subject's problem for an organism's disease. A different method is needed to explain problems. This method rests on the assumption that many expressions of distress in mood and behavior (neurotic reactions) can be understood from an appreciation of an individual's personality traits and his life experiences. His personality traits are the relatively stable features of temperament that distinguish him from others. They are quantitative distinctions and no more diseases than would be shortness of stature, plainness of face, or dullness of wit. Through an appreciation of his temperament, we can comprehend the meaning to him that links his past experiences, present events, mood, and behavior.

Psychiatry is the medical discipline that must consider both the subject and the organism in man. The concept of disease assists this consideration by organizing some clinical phenomena in a fashion similar to that of general medicine. In the following chapters the application of this concept to particular conditions as well as its distinction from methods for appreciating a subject's problems will be described.

Jaspers, K.: General Psychopathology. Translated by J. Hoenig and M. Hamilton. Manchester, Manchester University Press, 1963.

Scadding, J. G.: Diagnosis: The clinician and the computer. Lancet, 2:877, 1967.

Taylor, F. K.: Psychopathology. Its Causes and Symptoms. London, Butterworth and Co., Ltd., 1966.

Wightman, W. P. D.: The Emergence of Scientific Medicine. Edinburgh, Oliver and Boyd, 1971.

233. FUNCTIONAL PSYCHOSES

233.1. INTRODUCTION

The psychoses form a loose category that gathers together several different clinical entities. To be placed within the category an entity must produce disturbances in thinking and perception that are inexplicable solely as responses to experience and are severe enough to distort the patient's appreciation of the real world and the relationship of events within it. The category psychosis has no uniform foundation as in somatic pathology nor any more objective aspects of psychopathology to mark its distinction from other collections of psychiatric symptoms. It is thus a term difficult to use with precision. Sometimes psychosis is used as a euphemism for insanity, sometimes as a synonym for schizophrenia, one of the entities within the category, and sometimes to draw an elusive distinction as between neurotic and psychotic depression.

The unmodified term can be qualified by a differentiation into organic psychoses and functional psychoses. Here the term psychosis means only severe mental illness. The organic psychoses, delirium, dementia, and Korsakoff's syndrome, are produced by a variety of cerebral pathologies. The functional psychoses, schizophrenia and manic-depressive disorder, lack a recognizable neuropathology.

This differentiation is practical. It draws a distinction in kind that affects treatment and prognosis, and it indicates the character of the clinical problem. For the organic psychoses the central problem is the cause of the pathologic changes. For the functional psychoses the central problem is consistent diagnosis.

Schizophrenia and manic-depressive disorder are clinical disease entities. The criteria for their diagnosis are their symptoms alone. There are no objective tests verifying a diagnosis. Only the natural history or response to empirically discovered treatments can confirm a diagnostic opinion. Since they lack a recognized neuropathology and are by definition inexplicable as responses to experience, there are no comprehensive etiologic explanations for these disorders. Treatment therefore is symptomatic rather than fundamental. Both prevention and radical cure await a chance discovery or a major scientific advance in understanding the biologic foundations of human behavior.

233.2. SCHIZOPHRENIA

Schizophrenia is a most devastating mental illness. It is a disturbance of mind and personality appearing in clear consciousness and characterized by several distinctive alterations in mental experiences, modes of thinking, and mood that are seldom completely resolved. The most characteristic features occur during the active phases of the disturbance, and take the form of hallucinations, delusions, and altered behavior toward others. Specific intellectual and affective disabilities varying from minimal to severe can develop insidiously or remain after an attack. A crucial element of the definition is that all these symptoms occur in a patient free of any relevant and discernible pathologic change in his nervous system.

CLINICAL MANIFESTATIONS. The symptoms of schizophrenia can begin at almost any stage in life, but most commonly occur during adolescence and early adulthood and then either insidiously or as an acute attack followed by a series of attacks, each leaving behind personality defects of increasing severity.

In some patients it is possible to recognize a particular premorbid personality. They may have seemed more timid or seclusive than others. They may have been bookish, unsociable, and preoccupied with philosophic and religious ideas to the exclusion of friendships and community experiences. But this so-called *schizoid personality* is not found in most patients who develop schizophrenia. *At least half of schizophrenic patients had premorbid personalities indistinguishable from normal.*

Among the mental changes that mark the onset of a schizophrenic illness, only some are specific to this disorder. Emotional unrest, uncertainty, perplexity, and confusion can be found in many disorders other than schizophrenia, and therefore a diagnosis of schizophrenia cannot rest on them. There are, however, a number of mental changes that are more or less diagnostic. These can be usefully divided into abnormal mental experiences and disturbed modes of expression. The abnormal mental experiences are somewhat more reliable evidence of the illness simply because they are easier to elicit with confidence and less dependent upon interpretation than disturbances in expression.

Hallucinations and delusions are the outstanding schizophrenic mental experiences. Although hallucinations can occur in many disorders such as delirium, dementia, and occasionally manic-depressive disorder, certain forms of hallucinations are more specific for schizophrenia. Thus auditory hallucinations are the most common hallucinations in schizophrenia, and certain kinds of auditory hallucinations are almost diagnostic. Thus hearing one's thoughts aloud or hearing voices commenting about one's every action or several voices engaged in a conversation in which derogatory and praising remarks are passed with the patient discussed in the third person are the most typical schizophrenic hallucinations.

Although delusions, i.e., false beliefs that are incorrigible, idiosyncratic, and preoccupying, can be found in many disorders other than schizophrenia, in this illness delusional experiences are dramatic and well developed. They can begin as vague, fearful interpretations and "half-beliefs" and develop into firm incorrigible convictions. A delusion coming on suddenly, not prompted by any hallucination or previous delusion, nor related in any obvious way to the patient's mood, is called a "primary delusion" and is highly suggestive of schizophrenia. Many other schizophrenic experiences are of delusional form, but have such individual characteristics that they have been named for themselves.

Commonly schizophrenics have delusions about bodily control, the so-called passivity experiences. The patient feels as though he were under the control of some outside force or power making him behave as an automaton without a will of his own. He may feel hypnotized and feel forced to make particular movements, speak with a special voice, or walk to certain areas. The patient may believe these feelings come to him as penetrating waves from electronic or telephonic equipment.

The schizophrenic patient may experience changes in his thinking. Particularly he may feel that his thoughts are disrupted by some outside agency, that his thoughts are withdrawn from his mind, or that other thoughts are inserted into it. He may believe that people can hear his thoughts, which are leaving his mind as waves broadcast to others.

In contrast to these abnormalities of experience are the disturbances in the patient's mode of expression. Particularly noticeable is his abnormal language. Characteristically, he is difficult to understand. His thinking is expressed in a vague and awkward fashion with words poorly chosen and ideas poorly related to one another. Strikingly, the patient makes no effort to correct the vagueness of his thinking or to improve the clarity of his talk. Often, asking a question of the patient, the examiner receives a reply that is off the point and that goes into unnecessary details. Although the questions of the interview seem to start the patient toward a particular answer, it is never reached, but the patient takes up abstract and unnecessary ideas and must be redirected toward his goal. The examiner, laying the responsibility for the confusion on himself, may work to express himself more clearly, and only after considerable effort recognize that the difficulty in communication rests with the odd replies from the patient.

Another prominent disturbance is emotional expression of these patients. They seem distant, unresponsive, and cold. On some occasions the patient's emotional attitude seems incongruous, particularly for the thoughts he is expressing. Thus he may laugh while saying that he is in mortal danger. This cold or incongruous attitude and manner give the schizophrenic patient his most striking features, and even when at their mildest can be baffling and distressing symptoms to his family.

Other abnormal modes of expression of the schizophrenic patient are disturbances in stance and mobility called catatonic symptoms. Gestures may seem stiff, slow, and mannered. Some schizophrenic patients make repetitive movements or facial grimaces. Others may become totally immobile and mute. Still others may assume unnatural postures and hold them for long periods.

During the active phases of the schizophrenic illness the flamboyant subjective experiences are most prominent. During the chronic phase of schizophrenic illness expressive disturbances in thought and emotion are more evident, varying from mild to severe. Although at times some patients seem free of symptoms, whether a careful examination does reveal mild residual disturbances in thinking and emotional responsiveness is debated and difficult to disprove.

DIAGNOSIS. The diagnosis of schizophrenia rests on recognition of the distinctive clinical symptoms of this disorder and the exclusion of other conditions which may produce similar symptoms.

Many disorders of brain function can imitate schizophrenic symptoms; but with the exception of the three schizophrenia-like disorders to be discussed, patients with the other brain disturbances also manifest disturbed consciousness, disorientation, and disruption of cognitive abilities, particularly recent memory function, that are not found in schizophrenia.

Mania or depression can be confused with schizophrenia (to the considerable embarrassment of the diagnostician when the patient recovers completely on receiving treatment appropriate for these conditions). A source of difficulty is the occurrence of delusions, which are common enough in mania and depression but usually spring directly from the mood and the attitudes of self-confidence or self-blame that are so prominent in those disorders.

In schizophrenia disturbances in experience, including the auditory hallucinations and delusions just described, form the most secure basis for diagnosis. Thus, in a person free of brain disease or drug intoxication, recognition of auditory hallucinations with voices commenting on the patient in the third person, primary delusional experiences, passivity experiences, or disturbances in "thought control" permit the diagnosis of schizophrenia to be made with some confidence. In fact, Kurt Schneider has referred to these as "first rank symptoms" of schizophrenia because of the diagnostic confidence their discovery brings.

If these symptoms cannot be found, then diagnosis must rest upon recognition of manifest disturbances in thought and emotional expression. It should be pointed out, however, that opinion holding a person's thought to be illogical and vague, or his affective responses to be inadequate or incongruous, is an evaluative judgment and must be held with somewhat less confidence, if the difficulties are minimal or inconstant, than opinion resting on recognition of delusions and hallucinations.

Catatonic symptoms of immobility, posturing, and grimacing, along with the disturbances in behavior described as negativism or reluctance to cooperate, must be carefully interpreted. Only in those patients in whom no evidence of a prominent mood change can be found should a diagnosis of schizophrenia be made. Motility changes in the direction of psychomotor retardation are prominent features of depressive disorder, a condition as common as schizophrenia and more common than the catatonic variety of schizophrenia.

Symptoms of emotional unrest, anxiety, withdrawal, and hostility can be found in schizophrenic patients, but these are common to many other psychiatric disorders, and therefore can never form the basis for a secure diagnosis of schizophrenia. However, that diagnosis is rendered more likely if it can be established that the patient was developing normally without an apparently vulnerable personality, and if these symptoms appeared without a change in the patient's mood or the pattern of his life. Since these more general symptoms can be found in both schizophrenia and many other psychiatric disturbances, it is important to search carefully for the more basic symptoms of hallucinations and delusions from which emotional unrest and unpredictable behavior may stem. Often repeated efforts are required to gain cooperation of the patient so that he will divulge the existence of those basic symptoms that make a diagnosis of schizophrenia certain.

ETIOLOGY.   There is no neuropathology or consistent pathophysiology that can be observed to develop with progression of the disorder and that might give some hint of causation. An approach to a consideration of etiology has to be more circuitous and the opinions derived held with somewhat less assurance than is true of other clinical entities. Two aspects of etiology can be conveniently separated for the purpose of organizing the information we have. One aspect is "cause," that is, any prerequisite element needed to set in motion a train of events leading to the entity. The other is "mechanism," that is, the particular nature of the train of events, be they psychologic, neurologic, or biochemical, that produce the symptoms. For schizophrenia there is some information relating to "cause" and also to "mechanism," but it is far from conclusive.

"Cause" or Prerequisite Elements in Schizophrenia.   The genetic constitution has been decisively demonstrated to be one of the "causes" of schizophrenia. The risk of schizophrenia increases with the closeness of genetic relationship to a schizophrenic patient. Thus only 1 per cent of very distant relatives of a schizophrenic patient will themselves suffer from the disorder. This is no higher than the risk in the general population. But 5 to 6 per cent of siblings and 40 to 50 per cent of monozygotic twins of schizophrenic patients will have schizophrenia.

The possible objection that these data merely reflect the increasingly common environment of progressively closer relatives has been refuted by observations on monozygotic twins brought up apart who continue to show an identical high risk. Heston made the same point in a different fashion by studying a group of offspring of schizophrenic mothers. These particular children were raised from earliest infancy in foster homes by normal, nonschizophrenic mothers and fathers. The incidence of schizophrenia in these children was exactly the same as that reported for children raised by a schizophrenic parent. They thus resembled their biologic mother although reared apart from her.

It has nevertheless been impossible to fit schizophrenia into a clear mendelian pattern of dominant or recessive inheritance. Some students of the disease would describe the hereditary contribution to schizophrenia as polygenic, i.e., the sum of a number of contributions from the genes no one of which is solely responsible. The polygenic concept might permit environmental factors to play a larger role in causation. Thus a mild genetic vulnerability might express itself in a schizophrenic phenotype only in those who face stressful environments, whereas those carrying a more severe genetic vulnerability might show the disorder in any environment. It is difficult at the moment to propose a test that would exclude the polygenic hypothesis as a possibility.

Some studies that have established a genetic contribution to the etiology of schizophrenia have also given evidence of the inadequacy of genetics as a sufficient cause for the disorder. That 50 per cent of monozygotic twins of schizophrenic patients are free of this illness means one of the following: (1) Although the genetic constitution is necessary and sufficient to produce schizophrenia, the symptoms employed to define a case fail to provide an adequate means of recognizing all examples of the disorder, and 50 per cent are mistakenly called normal. (2) The defining symptoms encompass a mixed group of disorders, and in only 50 per cent of these disorders are genetic features necessary and sufficient causes for the symptoms. (3) A genetic vulnerability for schizophrenia is necessary but not sufficient. It must be combined with certain life experiences that need not be common for genetically identical individuals.

The present inadequacy of the genetic hypothesis to provide a complete description of the "cause" for schizophrenia reinforces a search for environmental and experiential causes. It has proved just as difficult to determine an environmental contribution as to define the genetic contribution. Thus the experiences of being raised by a cold and distant mother, or of receiving insistent, simultaneous, but incompatible directions from the parents, or of simply living in a disharmonious family incapable of providing a healthy environment for psychologic growth have all been considered causes of schizophrenia.

Such disturbed experiences have been found in the lives of some schizophrenic patients when viewed retrospectively after the onset of the illness. But none has proved to be a common experience in all schizophrenic people. Nor has it been possible to predict an increased incidence of schizophrenia among individuals living in comparably disturbed situations. Presently the most economical view of the role of life experiences in the "cause" of schizophrenia holds that *any* adversity, be it a psychologic shock, abnormality in critical relationships, or physical injury (particularly brain injury) may provide a partial contribution in causing schizophrenia, but that most of these adversities are exerting their causal effects upon a genetically vulnerable individual.

"Mechanism" of the Schizophrenic Syndrome. This is the other aspect of etiology. Given that some combination of genetic and environmental attributes is probably prerequisite for the illness, by what derangements are the symptoms produced? Are they produced by some change in a psychologic function that might have been learned or developed through experience, or are they produced by some morbid change in the nervous system that alters the normal capacity to perceive, integrate, and respond? There have been proposals for each of these "mechanisms."

It has been proposed that the mechanism of the disturbance has been through the production of a particular psychologic change fundamental to the whole syndrome and from which all the symptoms can be explained. Thus Federn has proposed a "loosening of ego boundaries" as the essential feature mediating this illness, whereas Bleuler proposed a basic disturbance in associational thinking. A crisis of identity has been proposed by exponents of existential psychiatry. These views have a ring of plausibility perhaps derived from their resemblance to experiences common to all men, part of which can seem to be reflected in the behavior of schizophrenic patients. But they depend on concepts that are difficult to define except in terms of what they purport to explain.

Other studies have attempted to demonstrate the possibility that the mechanism is a change in the central nervous system. No such change has been demonstrated in schizophrenia as yet, so supporters of this possibility have had to reason by analogy.

Three well documented conditions affecting the brain can give rise to a mental disturbance resembling schizophrenia. The most familiar is the syndrome found with *chronic amphetamine intoxication.* In this condition the patient is alert and oriented but preoccupied by auditory hallucinations and delusional ideas indistinguishable from those seen in schizophrenia. The disturbance may last from several days to a few weeks, but disappears eventually after the withdrawal of the stimulant.

Slater, Beard, and Glithero have demonstrated that among patients suffering from *psychomotor epilepsy,* caused by an irritative lesion in the limbic portions of the temporal lobe, a certain number develop a paranoid schizophrenia-like syndrome after 10 to 15 years of epilepsy. This condition displays all the classic delusional and hallucinatory symptoms of schizophrenia, but there is less tendency toward deterioration of thinking and personality.

Finally, certain patients, *withdrawing from excessive alcohol ingestion,* suffer from a period of auditory hallucinations. Although in most of these patients the hallucinatory experience clears within 24 to 48 hours, in a small proportion a chronic condition of persisting auditory hallucinations associated with delusional beliefs, incongruous affect, and disturbed thought develops. This chronic condition may be indistinguishable from the schizophrenic syndrome, and may persist for many years.

For all these schizophrenia-like conditions the possibility exists that the pertinent features might be the expression of a latent predisposition for schizophrenia in the affected individuals. But there is no evidence of a predisposition. The relatives of these patients do not have an increased incidence of schizophrenia, and the patients themselves do not have schizoid traits in their premorbid personalities.

The existence of these conditions demonstrates that the symptoms of schizophrenia are capacities of the damaged human brain. Yet we are ignorant of any common pathologic feature of these brain disorders that could by implication be the fundamental mechanism for schizophrenia. One possibility is that each of these disorders represents an extraexcitatory arousal of the brain, particularly of the reticular formation and limbic system, either directly via amphetamine or epileptic discharge or in rebound from long-continuing action of the depressant ethanol. It may be that the condition of schizophrenia itself is thus produced by some excessive activity in these or related brain regions evoked by the genetic-environmental "causes" discussed above. Mednick and Schulzinger have also found some evidence suggestive of hyperarousal in children of schizophrenic mothers who go on to develop the disease themselves.

Another proposed mechanism for producing schizophrenia is through some change in body metabolism or chemistry that could itself alter cerebral and psychologic functions. Many students have been prompted to consider this alternative because of the remarkable growth in biochemical methodology. In fact the difficulties in establishing a role for biochemistry in the etiology of schizophrenia rest not with the chemical methodology but with such issues as defining the group bing studied, avoiding chemical artifacts related to dietary habits or medications given chronically hospitalized people, and deciding what biochemical change to look for with little knowledge of what kinds of change might produce symptoms. The papers of Kety should be consulted for a more thorough discussion of these difficulties. A rare condition, periodic catatonia, has been documented by Gjessing to be associated with a phasic change in nitrogen balance, but no relationship between this disorder and schizophrenia in general has been found.

Snyder has proposed that a functional excess of cerebral dopamine may be the critical feature in schizophrenia. He based this suggestion mainly on the observation that the therapeutic potency of the phenothiazines parallels their relative capacities to block dopamine receptors. Although this evidence is indirect, the hypothesis has provided a specific focus to research efforts that seem close to providing some confirmatory evidence.

Thus our knowledge of "mechanism," as much as our knowledge of "cause," is still fragmentary and provisional. But on the bits of evidence at hand, the view that seems easiest to defend is that schizophrenia will prove to be due to some deranged neural mechanism that can occasionally be produced by coarse brain disease but more often is the outcome of an anomaly of the genetic constitution.

TREATMENT. The treatment for any schizophrenic patient is complex and should not be attempted by the inexperienced. A period of hospitalization will usually be required. There a program to include drug therapy, psychologic treatment, and social evaluation can be planned.

The sheet anchor of treatment now for schizophrenia is the *phenothiazine* drugs, discovered in the 1950's almost by accident. To date there is no secure explanation for their effectiveness. Clearly they are not simply acting by virtue of their sedative effect, since their remarkable action is not mimicked by other sedatives. They can remove the symptoms of schizophrenia, including the delusions, hallucinations, and disordered thought, and are not restricted to relieving excitement or anxiety as the term tranquilizer might imply.

The most versatile phenothiazine preparation is the original: chlorpromazine. The dose required to treat acute symptoms varies widely from patient to patient, and amounts from 200 to 2000 mg per day may be necessary. Maintenance dosage is similarly an individual matter, but 100 to 200 mg per day is usually an effective range. Since cessation of treatment results in the reappearance of symptoms in 60 to 70 per cent of patients within six months, drug therapy is often given over years. This practice, however, must be evaluated in light of a movement disorder (tardive dyskinesia) that may appear with prolonged use of phenothiazines. Tardive dyskinesia is a chronic choreoathetotic disorder affecting primarily the faciobulbar musculature but in some examples the extremities as well. It is resistant to most pharmacologic treatment with the exception of giving larger doses of the phenothiazines that provoked it originally. Since it is a particular danger of chronic high dose phenothiazine treatment, the attempt should be to employ as small a dose as possible in chronic administration. The report of Crane gives details.

The *psychotherapy* suitable for the schizophrenic patient has been a subject of intense controversy. The more radical approaches based on psychologic and particularly psychoanalytic views of the genesis of schizophrenia have not achieved their optimistic goals of curing the patient by relieving some basic psychologic conflict. More modest psychotherapy is indispensable when it is intended to help the patient in his everyday affairs, taking advantage of those personal assets that persist despite his illness, and establishing a relationship of friendly rapport in order to guide him in his management of personal and social issues, which, if mishandled, can lead to distress and further illness. A particularly pressing issue for the schizophrenic patient is the social situation into which he is placed after hospitalization. His psychiatrist, usually at first with the help of a psychiatric social worker, must strive to find a job that is regular and well within the patient's power but not excessively challenging, a domestic arrangement that is calm and supportive but not too emotionally demanding, and a daily routine that combats the tendency to withdraw from all social contacts into an isolated and perhaps fantasy-ridden existence. To accomplish these goals is one of the most challenging exercises in medical treatment. The growth of "halfway houses" as residences for previously hospitalized schizophrenic patients has been prompted by recognition of the need for stable and structured social environments for schizophrenic patients once they have improved enough to leave the hospital.

PROGNOSIS. Prognosis for any patient diagnosed as schizophrenic is always guarded. Certain features carry a good prognosis: high intelligence, a normal premorbid personality, an acute onset, catatonic features in the illness, and a family history of affective disorder. Other features carry a poor prognosis: low intelligence, schizoid premorbid personality, insidious onset of the illness, symptoms of thought disorder, affective blunting in the illness, and a family history of schizophrenia.

The use of phenothiazines has considerably improved the prognosis of schizophrenia, 30 to 50 per cent of patients having complete remissions on follow-up over five years. Another 30 to 40 per cent show some residual symptoms but are able to live in the community, and only 10 to 20 per cent require further hospitalization if phenothiazine treatment is begun and maintained after their first attack of the illness.

Connell, P. H.: Amphetamine Psychosis. Maudsley Monographs, No. 5. London, Chapman and Hall, Ltd., 1958.

Crane, G. E.: Persistent dyskinesia. Br. J. Psychiatry, 122:395, 1973.

Fish, F. J.: Schizophrenia. Bristol, John Wright & Sons, 1962.

Heston, L. L.: Psychiatric disorders in foster home reared children of schizophrenic mothers. Br. J. Psychiatry, 112:918, 1966.

Kety, S. S.: Biochemical theories of schizophrenia, I and II. Science, 129:1528, 1590, 1959, 1969.

Klein, D. F., and Davis, J. M.: Diagnosis and Drug Treatment of Psychiatric Disorders. Baltimore, Williams & Wilkins Company, 1969.

Mednick, S. A., and Schulzinger, F.: Some premorbid characteristics related to breakdown in children of schizophrenic mothers. J. Psychiat. Res., 6:267, 1968.

Schneider, K.: Clinical Psychopathology. Translated by M. W. Hamilton. New York, Grune & Stratton, Inc., 1959.

Shields, J.: The genetics of schizophrenia in historical context. *In* Coppen, A. J., and Walk, A. (eds.): Recent Developments in Schizophrenia. Brit. J. Psychiat., Special Publication No. 1, pp. 25–41, Ashford Kent, 1967.

Slater, E., Beard, A. W., and Glithero, E.: The schizophrenia-like psychoses of epilepsy. Br. J. Psychiatry, 109:95, 1963.

Snyder, S. N.: The dopamine hypothesis of schizophrenia: Focus on the dopamine receptor. Am. J. Psychiatry, 133:2, 1976.

233.3. MANIC-DEPRESSIVE PSYCHOSIS

The essential feature of this psychosis is an excessive disturbance of mood and self-appraisal from which its other mental symptoms seem to arise. This disturbance can be in the direction of elation and self-confidence or sadness and self-blame. The course tends to be episodic, even periodic, with attacks of elation (mania) or sadness (depression) interspersed with periods of apparent mental health varying in length from weeks to years. Individual patients may suffer attacks of only one kind throughout their lifetime. Single or repetitive attacks of depression seem to be the most common manifestation, but attacks alternately manic and then depressive or even repetitively manic are not unusual.

CLINICAL MANIFESTATIONS. Depression. During an

attack of depression the patient complains of feeling miserable and uncertain of himself. He may give evidence of his sadness by a dejected appearance and by restlessness and distractibility. Some patients are slowed in their activity, and this can progress to a psychomotor retardation of such severity that the patient seems totally unresponsive.

Mental examination of the depressed patient usually brings to light not only his feelings of sadness or misery but also a lowered self-esteem that can vary in intensity from feelings of inadequacy and incompetence to convictions of personal worthlessness, blameworthiness, and evil. This combination of depressed mood with self-blame is the diagnostic sign of this condition. It will also explain most of the other symptoms, modes of behavior, and dangers faced by the depressed patient.

Other symptoms include delusional extrapolations of the attitudes of self-blame. These can increase to a belief that the patient's guilt is notorious, that he is to be arrested, and that he will be condemned to die or to suffer some extraordinary punishment either in this world or the next. Suspiciousness and fear of mistreatment based on these delusional beliefs may be difficult to distinguish from similar attitudes in the paranoid schizophrenic patient. A useful if not cast-iron distinction is the depressive's belief that the suspected ill treatment comes as a justified punishment and not, as with the schizophrenic, as an undeserved persecution.

In some severely depressed patients delusional ideas can become bizarre and even grandiose in concept. Thus they come to believe that they have been the cause of cosmic disasters, that the sun is darkened by them, that whole cities have been deserted because of their presence, or that they and their progeny are accursed in the sight of the Divinity. Delusions of bodily change may take the form that their brains are rotting, their bowels totally blocked, or their bones fractured and dislocated.

Delusional ideas may concern the relationship of the patient to the world and to others. He may believe that he has lost all his money, that he has become a burden to others, that he is universally despised, or even that he gives off such a bad odor that people cannot stand his presence. Again, these beliefs are usually reflective of the patient's inner attitude of self-blame, self-contempt, and hopelessness.

The point about these opinions is that they are delusional and not just false. They are unshakable opinions held in the face of all contrary evidence. Only treatment of the depressive disorder will remove them.

The most worrisome symptom of the depressed patient is *inclination to suicide*. It is easily appreciated that attitudes of such hopelessness and despair as have been described could prompt self-destruction. But it is not necessary to have such exaggerated delusions for suicide to be a distinct risk. Vigilance for suicidal intentions must be maintained throughout the course of the depressive disturbance. The physician should ask any depressed patient about thoughts of self-injury. A series of questions useful in estimating suicidal risk is provided in Ch. 234.3. Often this simple action will reveal both the severity of the mood disturbance and the need to bring the patient into hospital for his own protection.

Homicide is also a possibility for the depressed patient, and is particularly likely in those who harbor be-liefs that their family shares in their guilt and accursed characteristics. Any suggestions by the patient that he might prefer death should be most seriously believed.

Along with these psychologic symptoms the depressed patient will often suffer from disturbances in his sleep, particularly waking early in the morning and being unable to return to sleep. Other physical disturbances include bodily aches and pains, loss of appetite, constipation, and weight loss. These features may combine with the retardation to give the appearance of chronic physical ill health. In fact, many depressed patients will first consult internists complaining of such physical symptoms. Helpful to the differentiation of the patient whose somatic symptoms are part of a depressive illness is a discovery of the features of depressed mood, and attitudes of self-blame or hopelessness when these features are combined with complaints of poorly localized pains, with loss of appetite or weight loss, or even with preoccupations about the state of the inner organs.

Mania.   Symptoms that are almost the exact opposite of those seen during an attack of depression appear during an attack of mania. Now the patient says that he is in excellent spirits, that he feels well, and in fact has never felt better. He is active and restless, and appears energetic, confident, and quick-witted. These characteristics tend to worsen, and it is in their more extreme form that they become recognized as symptoms. The restlessness and energy become overactivity, with the patient moving constantly and planning progressively less plausible projects. His speech becomes incessant, rapid, and disjointed, one idea following another with little connection between them. His attitude of confidence becomes grandiose self-satisfaction. He may be overbearing and pompous. He often will be irritated by his surroundings, easy to anger, and perhaps suspicious that the efforts being made to control him are unjust.

Although a manic patient can usually be recognized by his overactivity, ebullience, and great self-confidence, he can develop as well ideas of resentment and feelings that he is being in some way unfairly noticed or persecuted. These ideas, on investigation, are found to derive from his own delusional opinion that he is so important that he must be under scrutiny by forces such as foreign powers. Occasionally, these persecutory ideas are so prominent that a diagnosis of schizophrenia is entertained. It is, however, the direct connection of these ideas to the attitude of self-confidence that allows a diagnosis of mania to be made.

With the mental changes manic patients exhibit disturbed social behavior. They may have increased sexual interest and may become promiscuous. They tend to overspend and be reckless with money. They may insult their employers and so be fired from their jobs. In the first attack of mania and before the severe restlessness and disorganization of thought appear, these activities may not be recognized as the products of mental illness, but may be construed as actions for which the patient can be held accountable. Thus the patient can be subjected to severe losses, to legal actions, or to moral criticism that can hamper his life long after his manic attack is over. To protect him from these consequences hospitalization of the manic patient may be required.

ETIOLOGY.   "Cause" or Prerequisite Elements in Manic-Depressive Disorder.   As with schizophrenia, an important genetic contribution to the etiology of the manic-depressive disorder seems certain. There is a progressive frequency of incidence with increasing blood relatedness so that with monozygotic twins the concordance rate is over 50 per cent. It is likely that genetic constitution is a necessary but not sufficient cause for this disorder. Certain other features of the illness require consideration. First, the illness does appear in attacks interspersed with periods in which the person appears to be normal. Second, the attacks are somewhat seasonal, appearing more frequently in the spring and fall than in summer and winter. Third, although many attacks occur spontaneously, many seem to be precipitated by some disturbing event. Presumably some other elements must combine with the genetic vulnerability to explain these features. Again, the most easily defended position would hold that a necessary cause for manic-depressive disorder is the genetic constitution of the patient, but that any of a large number of environmental disturbances can bring out the disorder.

Mechanism in Manic-Depressive Disorder. As with schizophrenia, a pharmacologically induced disorder has enhanced confidence that, whatever the "cause," the mechanism for affective disorder is a neural one. Treatment with reserpine for hypertension produced depression in up to one of four patients, and this depression was accompanied by the typical delusional attitudes of the manic-depressive psychosis. The discovery that reserpine depleted brain neurons of biogenic amines, particularly norepinephrine and serotonin, has prompted a variety of hypotheses that propose some lack of norepinephrine, serotonin, or other biogenic amines at synaptic sites in the brain for emotional control. That many effective antidepressant agents also influence these same amines has been a further support to these hypotheses.

TREATMENT. The first rule in managing either manic or depressed patients is that most of them should be in a hospital. Their conditions can bring catastrophe to themselves and their families in the form of financial mismanagement in mania and suicide in depression. If these diagnoses are strongly suspected, then psychiatric opinion should be immediately sought so as to determine whether hospitalization should be imposed. It is critical to have expert help, because the patient can often hide the severity of the disorder in a mass of explanations which may appear quite plausible. In the hospital the suicidal patient must be closely supervised and definitive treatment should not be long deferred.

It is crucial to diagnose these patients and separate them from those with other conditions, because new drug treatments have proved effective for them and are specific to the affective disorders. Two classes of pharmacologic agents are effective in *depression.* Seemingly more effective are the so-called *tricyclic antidepressants,* the prototype of which is imipramine. This drug, given in doses of from 75 to 300 mg per day, will relieve a depressive attack in 50 per cent of patients. The recent development of the means for measuring plasma levels of tricyclic antidepressants has revealed a partial explanation for failures to respond. A narrow range (50 to 170 ng per milliliter) encloses therapeutic plasma nortriptyline levels. The failure to reach this level or the exceeding of it inhibits a full response. A rational pharmacology for these medications will soon require plasma measurements to be available as a routine. The

technologic advances to achieve this ideal seem near at hand. Maintenance therapy of 100 to 150 mg per day should be continued for six to eight months after recovery. If tricyclics are ineffective, the logical practice should be to switch to the other class, which includes the drugs that have as their primary action the capacity to inhibit the enzyme monoamine oxidase. These drugs, in doses of 45 to 75 mg per day, have also proved useful in depression.

If *monoamine oxidase inhibitors* are used, the patient must be warned to avoid foodstuffs such as cheese, broad beans, and some yeast extracts, which have pressor amines of the phenyl-ethyl-amine group that includes tyramine. If absorbed by patients whose monoamine oxidase enzyme is depleted, they can cause sudden elevation of blood pressure with headache, blurred vision, and even cerebrovascular hemorrhage.

The mainstay of treatment for severe depression is *electroconvulsive treatment* (ECT). In contrast to the drugs which relieve the symptoms of depression, ECT will terminate an attack of depression usually in four to eight treatments. This treatment can produce the most dramatic and quick recovery from the depths of a life-threatening depression, and should not be withheld from a delusional patient or any seriously depressed patient who has failed to respond to drug treatment after three to four weeks. Maintenance with imipramine, 100 to 150 mg per day for six months, is recommended after ECT for the avoidance of relapse shortly after successful treatment.

The *treatment of mania* is often very difficult, particularly if the patient is suspicious about medicines. Haloperidol in doses of 2 to 10 mg thrice daily taken orally has proved effective. This compound is liable to produce severe extrapyramidal side effects which can be combated with antiparkinsonian drugs and with Benadryl. Chlorpromazine in doses of 300 to 1000 mg per day can also be tried.

A recent and effective measure for controlling mania has been the use of lithium ion in the form of lithium carbonate. This compound is available in 300 mg tablets, and daily intake of 900 to 2400 mg per day can relieve manic excitement. It is, however, essential to follow plasma lithium concentration in these patients, because toxic signs of disorientation, tremor, anorexia, and diarrhea can appear if plasma lithium concentration rises above 2 mEq per liter. The therapeutic level and the toxic level of lithium are close, and therefore the medication must be started when the patient can be carefully supervised in a hospital. Maintenance lithium treatment can be recommended, because there is fair clinical evidence that in this fashion some further attacks of mania may be avoided.

PROGNOSIS. The prognosis for a single attack of mania or depression is excellent. Even without treatment patients tend to recover completely within six months. With antidepressant treatment the medication can be withdrawn after six to eight months with fair assurance that symptoms will not recur at this time.

The longer-range prognosis is not so favorable. Eighty per cent of people who have suffered one attack of affective disturbance will have another at some time in their lives, but this may not be for many years. Some patients, however, will have recurrent attacks of mania or depression interrupted by only brief intervals of normal behavior.

The best advice to give patients who have suffered from their first affective attack is that they will very likely be quite well for years, but that they and their family should be aware that their mood changes are to be considered seriously, and they should seek psychiatric attention promptly if such a mood change tends to persist or worsen. Prien's work indicates that individuals who suffer recurrent attacks of any form of manic-depressive disorder are best maintained on lithium for an extended, even an indefinite, period.

Astrup, C., Fossum, A., and Holmboe, R.: A follow-up study of 270 patients with acute affective psychoses. Acta Psychiat. Scand. (Suppl. 135), 1959.

Kragh-Sorensen, P., Hasen, C. E., and Asberg, M.: Plasma levels of nortriptyline in the treatment of endogenous depression. Acta Psychiat. Scand., 49:444, 1973.

Lewis, A.: Melancholia. J. Ment. Sci., 80:277, 1934.

Prien, R., and Caffey, E., Jr.: Relationship between dosage and response to lithium prophylaxis in recurrent depression. Am. J. Psychiatry, 133:567, 1976.

Prien, R., Klett, J., and Caffey, E., Jr.: Lithium prophylaxis in recurrent affective illness. Am. J. Psychiatry, 131:198, 1974.

Schildkraut, J. J.: The catecholamine hypothesis of affective disorders: A review of supporting evidence. Am. J. Psychiatry, 122:509, 1965.

234. PERSONALITY DISORDERS AND NEUROTIC SYMPTOMS

234.1. INTRODUCTION

GENERAL CONSIDERATIONS. The concept of disease entities that supports our understanding of the functional psychoses does not suit all psychologic disturbances and particularly those that are described as personality disorders or neurotic symptoms. There is uncertainty both in terms and in concept here. For example, the designation neurosis is ambiguous in that it seems a name for a clinical entity with some sharp distinction from normal, but a cardinal symptom of one neurosis, *anxiety*, is an experience of all people at some time and is an appropriate mood in certain circumstances. What then is abnormal in *anxiety neurosis*? Is this abnormality of a quantitative or a qualitative nature? To what kind of patient can the term anxiety neurosis be applied? Should we use it only for patients in the emotional "state" of anxiety, or is it suitable regardless of the present state if a patient has "traits" that make him prone to this emotion?

The term *personality* and particularly its extension, *personality disorder*, can be just as troublesome. Personality seems a word similar to such terms as character or temperament, words intended to describe aspects of human psychologic variation distributed in a smoothly graded fashion in the population. But if that is true, then the distinction personality disorder can seem an arbitrary, socially contrived, or judgmental decision, since no sharp dividing line is to be expected in smoothly graded characteristics. In Ch. 234.2 to 234.4, an attempt is made to dispel some of these ambiguities while considering several emotional disturbances often called neurotic that occur in a general medical setting.

Although many mental changes and emotional disturbances in patients can be ascribed to known or presumed pathologic changes in brain function, certain varieties of human psychologic constitution and certain life experiences can themselves provoke emotional disturbance and disrupted behavior. The terms personality disorder and neurotic symptoms are intended to describe the disturbances that result from variation in human constitution and experience by invoking the concepts of potential and response. Personality always means *potential*. It encompasses and describes the abiding and distinctive traits or tendencies of an individual to react to circumstances in a particular fashion. Thus by "optimistic personality" is meant an individual who can be expected to respond with cheerfulness and optimism in situations in which others are less likely to do so. An individual's personality is the sum of numerous traits, and a comparison with others is implicit in the description of each trait. Thus every trait can be conceived as a dimension of variation along which people can be dispersed in a fashion similar to their dispersal along the dimensions of height, weight, or intelligence. Any definition of an individual's personality is an attempt to place him in relationship to others in respect to one or more traits. An individual can be said to have a disorder of personality if he deviates to such an extreme along the range of variation for some trait that either he or others complain of its effects.

Whereas personality and personality disorder indicate potential, the neurotic symptoms are emotional *responses* displayed when the individual is troubled by circumstances. For anyone certain environments and life events are conducive to anxiety, others to depression, and still others to suspiciousness. People with a disorder of personality have an increased potential for these responses and are provoked to them by less extreme circumstances and less specific stimuli. Thus paranoid personality disorder is a term used to describe an individual who tends to show attitudes of suspiciousness and feelings of persecution (the neurotic symptoms) in settings so minimally threatening that they will seldom provoke such attitudes in others. If, however, his life is relatively free of threatening features, these feelings will be diminished and, despite his personality traits, symptoms may be avoided.

Before such concepts can be used in the evaluation and management of a particular patient, that patient must be well known to the doctor, and the possibility of other conditions that could produce similar symptoms must be excluded. For this a detailed psychiatric history, mental status, and physical examination are needed. The latter two can be obtained during the first interview, but historical information about the patient's family background, developmental milestones, sexual adjustment, scholastic and occupational achievement, habits, and medical problems may require several hours of examination. Observations from his relatives improve the accuracy of such information, and their descriptions of his personality are indispensable. All these data, combined with the knowledge of the patient's present condition, form the basis for diagnosis, treatment, and prognosis, and to embark on such matters without this information is to commit a capital error. The result is often failure of treatment, because the patient has been misunderstood and emphasis given to minor rather than major features of his problem.

As it becomes clear that a given patient's disturbance is the outcome of the kind of person he is and the situations that he faces, the data of the psychiatric history and the mental status examination can usually be divided into three categories which, although closely related, are usefully distinguished: (1) the predisposing factors for the disturbance, including personality traits and formative life experiences; (2) the precipitating factors; and (3) the symptoms themselves and their effect on the patient.

PREDISPOSING FACTORS. Predisposing factors are those features special to an individual that make him vulnerable to emotional disturbance. The most critical factor is personality, the traits of which are distinguished in the patient's temperament, attitudes, and predictable responses. But personality is the outcome of genetic constitution, intellectual endowment, and lifetime experiences, and each of these is a predisposing factor in itself. As intriguing examples of studies in these issues, the work of O'Connor on the role of intellectual subnormality in emotional instability and the study of Granville-Grossman on the relationship of parental loss to depression in adulthood can be recommended. Predisposing factors often overlooked are the patient's social status and cultural situation. The scholarly study of Dr. Beatrice Berle, *80 Puerto Rican Families in New York City*, and the recent work of the Dohrenwends in social psychiatry are excellent examples of empirical work in these areas.

Finally, the state of health is an important predisposing feature, because physical illness, through the distress it produces or by direct effects on the central nervous system, interferes with a person's capacity to cope with circumstances and thus leads to psychologic symptoms.

PRECIPITATING FACTORS. The precipitating factors are events or experiences that have disrupted emotional equilibrium and bear a close temporal relationship to the disturbance for which the patient seeks help. The common-sense expectations that personal illness, or conflict produced by changes in family or occupational circumstances, could precipitate psychologic distress have been confirmed in studies such as those of Brown and Birley. Holmes has attempted to grade life events in a hierarchy of emotional stressfulness, and many workers have found his scale useful for estimating the relative distress different patients have endured. Some psychologic precipitants are more recondite, because they depend on a special meaning an individual gives events, perhaps a symbolic meaning derived from the particular patient's early life experiences. Before emphasizing these more abstruse precipitants of a unique character, it is usually wise to consider the more immediate and obvious ones that may be present.

SYMPTOMS. In Ch. 234.2 to 234.4, the symptoms of anxiety, depression, and hysterical reaction are discussed, because they are common in the general practice of medicine.

All these neurotic symptoms emerge as complaints either of the patient himself or of others who must deal with him. They are symptoms in the sense that they disturb the patient's sense of well-being or they interfere with his behavior and his adaptability to circumstances. They can vary from mild to severe, and they can be acute or chronic.

In the assessment of these symptoms the patient should be encouraged to describe how he feels, how the symptoms developed, what seems to make them worse or better, what they are like when compared to previous emotional reactions, and how they disturb him now. *The aim is to come to appreciate these symptoms as understandable responses of this particular person to his particular circumstances.* The over-all principle is that we are considering here not classes of patients suffering from distinct disease entities, but individuals troubled by their special life circumstances and needing assistance tailored to their particular personal nature and situation. The specific symptoms, their characteristic predisposing and precipitating factors, their effects on behavior, and modes of treatment will be considered in the balance of this chapter.

Berle, B. B.: 80 Puerto Rican Families in New York City. New York, Columbia University Press, 1958.

Brown, G. W., and Birley, J. L. T.: Social precipitants of severe psychiatric disorders. *In* Hare, E. H., and Wing, J. K. (eds.): Psychiatric Epidemiology. New York, Oxford University Press, 1970.

Dohrenwend, B. P., and Dohrenwend, B. S.: Social Status and Psychological Disorder. A Causal Inquiry. New York, John Wiley & Sons, 1969.

Holmes, T. H., and Rahe, R. H.: The social readjustment score. J. Psychosom. Res. 11:213, 1967.

Jaspers, K.: General Psychopathology. Manchester, Manchester University Press. 1962.

O'Connor, N.: Psychology and intelligence. *In* Shepherd, M., and Davies, D. L. (eds.): Studies in Psychiatry. New York, Oxford University Press, 1968.

234.2. ANXIETY

DEFINITION. Anxiety is an unpleasant mood of tension and apprehension. It is fear's first cousin and, like fear, has prominent autonomic effects when severe. But fear is an emotion sharply focused on immediate dangers, whereas anxiety is usually imposed by the anticipation of future danger, distress, or difficulties. As an emotional response common to men, anxiety is useful. Activities that arouse it are avoided and those that diminish it are sustained. Although anxiety may spur people to perform difficult tasks skillfully and admirably, when excessive it is a hindrance, as some well prepared students demonstrate when facing a critical examination. *Anxiety is a medical problem when it is excessive, inappropriate, or without obvious cause.*

PREDISPOSING AND PRECIPITATING FACTORS. Anxiety is the psychologic response to anticipated troubles, real or imagined, dimly or accurately perceived. But men and troubles vary. Some persons, the timid, the inexperienced, the excessively conscientious, are frequently anxious in situations that seem not to affect others. Most people are at least mildly anxious whenever they seek medical advice, and when threatening dangers are intense or prolonged, as in chronic painful illness or in battle, even the most resistant individuals can develop incapacitating anxiety.

Resistance to anxiety varies with physical condition, and when tired, sick, or injured, people are more easily threatened. Also, they are more vulnerable to anxiety when their powers of analysis and discrimination are failing or underdeveloped. Thus, because of inadequate comprehension or imprecise perception, the immature, the elderly, or the person with brain damage may become anxious in situations in which a person with a healthy, mature brain is comfortable. In fact, one of the first indications of a dementia can be an attack of severe anxiety without obvious provocation.

Common precipitants of anxiety in daily life are circumstances of conflict in which an action is demanded but the correct action may be difficult to discern. Thus a person may be anxious over difficult decisions on which rest his economic and social success or because the decisions produce an unpredictable response in an inconsistent superior. Laboratory models for this kind of situation and its effects on the emotional state have been easy to produce. Pavlov trained dogs to respond to the picture of a circle by rewarding such responses with food. He did not reward responses to an ellipse. Then, by simply compressing the ellipse so that it gradually approached a circle in shape, he made the discrimination progressively more difficult. The emotional response of these dogs was remarkable. They became ferocious and violent when put into harness for the experiment. They tore at their restraints, barked uncontrollably, and refused to attempt the discrimination. In this state, not only did they make many mistakes, but they became unable to make discriminations that had previously been easy. It is not difficult to see analogies in both situation and behavior between Pavlov's dogs and men with emotional conflicts.

An emotional state of anxiety can be produced in other ways than as an understandable response to anticipated difficulties. A prolonged irritable anxiety state can follow a head injury as one of the symptoms of the so-called *postconcussional syndrome.* Gronwall and Wrightson demonstrate that it may be caused by a mild disturbance in cognitive capacity subjectively evident to the patient but demonstrable objectively only with difficulty. Similarly, a mood of tension and agitation with tremulousness can occur in the delirious states, such as those that follow withdrawal of alcohol or barbiturates and are sometimes produced by the hallucinogenic drugs such as LSD-25. In these situations, it may be disturbed perceptions and misinterpretations that arouse anxiety, but often the anxiety is independent of anything that the patient definitely experiences or understands. Roth describes a peculiar and chronic anxiety state that can follow a calamitous emotional experience. This condition, referred to as the *phobic anxiety syndrome,* occurs in mildly obsessional persons after a severe fright. The disturbance can last for many months. These patients are in a state of considerable anxiety, mostly unformulated, and, associated with this, they have an unwillingness to leave their homes because of vague fears. The peculiar psychologic response of *depersonalization,* which is a change in the awareness of self such that the person feels unreal, is present in many of these patients. In the phobic anxiety syndrome the mood of anxiety follows rather than precedes difficulty, demonstrating that anxiety, normally an anticipatory psychologic response, may take on a self-sustained activity after certain experiences such as severe frights or sudden disasters.

The role of learning and of conditioning has too often been neglected in considerations of anxiety. This probably derived from attempts to explain all anxiety in terms of basic instinctive drives. That a fear-provoking situation could train an individual to experience symptoms of anxiety in circumstances that resembled these situations is very likely, and is indicated by research on emotion in animals. The capacity to develop anxiety via conditioning mechanisms seems the probable explanation for certain cases of phobic anxiety focused on specific objects.

MANIFESTATIONS OF ANXIETY. The manifestations of anxiety are divisible into three groups. *First* are the inner feelings of tension, apprehension, and dread that form the anxious mood itself. *Second* are disturbances of the intellectual power of the anxious patient. He is unable to think clearly, to use proper judgment, to learn efficiently, or to remember accurately. *Third* are the autonomic, visceral, and endocrine changes that have been analyzed by Walter B. Cannon and his followers as the companions of emotional excitement and particularly of anxiety or fear. These include tremor, tachycardia, hypertension, increased perspiration, dilated pupils, and reduced salivation and gastric secretion. Increased activity of the sympathetic nervous system and of the adrenal medulla mediates the majority of these visceral responses to anxiety.

A model anxiety state is to be seen among front-line soldiers. The infantryman is a prepared subject for anxiety. He is always threatened with death or mutilation. He must go without sleep, remain exposed to the weather, and often be hungry. He is usually unable to understand what is happening around him. He is repeatedly frightened by gun fire and distressed by the death of comrades. If he is exposed long enough, he develops a severe and persisting anxiety state sometimes called "battle fatigue." He becomes tense and easily startled. His judgment is poor, and he cannot efficiently sustain a complex offensive action. Among other physical complaints, he suffers from headache, anorexia, and diarrhea. He is usually convinced that death is imminent. Almost all men develop this condition if exposed to battle long enough. Wolff reports that the average man in the army of the United States reached this point after 85 days of combat; 75 per cent could be expected to break down by combat day 140, and 90 per cent by combat day 210. These figures vary little among nations, although few are willing publish them. They make the point that, in his resistance to crippling anxiety, even the bravest man has a "breaking point." On reaching it, he does not betray his group or run from the enemy, but rather he becomes less efficient in protecting himself and runs a high risk of death.

The symptoms of anxiety that physicians see in patients are not different. The patients all have the same three groups of symptoms, but, depending in part on the cause, these symptoms can appear as a relatively brief attack or as a more prolonged, chronic disturbance of mood.

Anxiety attacks may be single episodes or may be periods of exacerbation in a chronic state of tension. They are short periods of tension, varying in severity from mild apprehension to severe panic. An anxiety attack can occur at any time. A favored time is when the patient is traveling in a plane, bus, or train. Most commonly, though, an attack develops at night when, with the disappearance of daytime distractions, a patient begins to ruminate on his troubles. The apprehensions grow to preoccupy his thoughts, and he develops visceral responses of fear. Clear thinking becomes impossible, as does sleep. The heart pounds. A common complaint in an anxiety attack is the sensation of tightness in the chest as though the lungs could not be adequately filled. The patient responds to this sensation by deep and sighing respirations. Sometimes he may produce in this way a respiratory alkalosis with feelings of giddiness and vertigo, tingling of his fingertips, and even tetany with carpopedal spasm. This is the *hyperventilation syndrome,* and the resulting symptoms may add to anxiety.

Full-blown anxiety attacks have an hysterical flavor and may, in part, depend on personal tendencies to self-dramatization and suggestibility. But they also can be the results of a psychic chain reaction, the initial apprehensions and anxiety stirring up cardiac and respiratory changes that are themselves frightening. Granville-Grossman and Turner have provided more evidence that visceral responses to anxiety can increase the subjective symptoms of anxiety by demonstrating that these latter symptoms are improved when an anxious patient is treated with propranolol, a drug that blocks the adrenergic beta-receptors of the sympathetic nervous system and slows the heart rate.

Chronic anxiety may be punctuated by or may begin with an acute attack, but it may be just a steady and distressingly prolonged disturbance of mood. The symptoms are less intense although not different in quality from those of acute anxiety. The patient is tense and "on edge." He may also report some feelings of sadness or hopelessness along with his anxiety. It can be difficult to differentiate his condition from an agitated depression. His intellectual powers are diminished, and he has considerable difficulty in concentration and in thinking. He will score poorly on intelligence tests, particularly on the performance subtests, just as does a patient with dementia. He will have a number of somatic complaints: frontal or occipital headache, anorexia, diarrhea, and weight loss, among other things. On examination, he may have the physical signs of tension, a fine tremor of the extended arms and brisk tendon reflexes, rapid heart beat, increased blood pressure, and pupillary dilatation. More extensive laboratory studies may reveal other visceral and endocrine disturbances, such as reduced gastric acid secretion or increased adrenocortical activity.

DIAGNOSIS. Usually diagnosis is not difficult. In both acute and chronic anxiety, the patient's major complaint is the distressing emotional state. Associated disturbances in thinking and autonomic function serve to confirm the diagnostic impression. For these patients, the major issue is not the diagnosis of anxiety, but rather the question of why they have become anxious now. This question must be answered from knowledge of the circumstances and personality of the patient.

An occasional patient focuses his complaints on his physical symptoms, such as irregularities in the beat of his heart, the change in bowel habits, weight loss, anorexia, or easy fatigability. From these symptoms a more severe illness such as a hidden malignancy, a chronic infection, or some endocrine disorder like hyperthyroidism of Addison's disease may be suspected. Although these conditions are usually seen to be only remote possibilities, laboratory studies may be required to exclude them. As with all psychologically disturbed patients, laboratory studies should not be delayed or protracted but should be decided upon, and this phase of the examination should be finished as promptly as possible.

TREATMENT. Treatment will vary with the cause and severity of anxiety. Many mildly anxious patients can be helped by a physician who is willing to listen carefully to their difficulties and offer some support and occasional advice. Most patients with anxiety have this mild type. Their disturbances are transient and are based on some particular problem or self-doubt that has developed acutely and is eventually resolved.

Those with more severe anxiety can be aided by a combination of pharmacologic treatment and repeated compassionate discussions of their troubles. Barbiturates have been the preferred agents for relief of anxiety in the past. However, barbiturates can be addictive, and there is the ever-present danger that they may be used in a suicide attempt by an anxious patient who is also depressed. In several double-blind clinical trials, chlordiazepoxide (Librium) has been found as effective as barbiturates for treating anxiety, and can be recommended. Dosage of 10 mg three to four times a day is usually effective. Up to 20 to 25 mg three times daily can be given to severely disturbed patients.

Patients with persisting anxiety can be referred with some confidence to specialists in psychotherapy. The effectiveness of psychotherapy seems to depend on the comfort provided by frequent sympathetic discussions and an increased recognition by the patient of the irrational aspects of his anxiety. The particular school of psychotherapeutic theory subscribed to by the therapist seems less important.

Only the most severely anxious patients need hospitalization and then usually only for an acute attack of anxiety. They are treated best with sedation; chlordiazepoxide in doses of 25 to 30 mg three times daily can be used. The somatic symptoms from the respiratory alkalosis of the hyperventilation syndrome can be treated by placing a bag over the nose and mouth that will retain the expired CO_2 for rebreathing.

Careful consideration should be given to any evidence that the anxious patient may be depressed. Agitated depression can be easily confused with simple anxiety. If depression is thought to be the diagnosis, then antidepressant medication, such as imipramine, 75 to 300 mg per day, should be given rather than sedatives.

For those individuals with restricted anxieties prompted by particular stimuli, i.e., phobias, there is growing evidence that deconditioning techniques based on learning theory may have an important place in therapy. Certainly some impressive controlled trials have been published indicating a faster response to this mode of management than to interpretive therapy for individuals suffering from a single phobia. This treatment, like any other, should not be attempted without experience and guidance.

Granville-Grossman, K. L., and Turner, P.: The effect of propranolol on anxiety. Lancet, 1:788, 1966.

Gronwall, D., and Wrightson, P.: Delayed recovery of intellectual function after minor head injury. Lancet, 2:605, 1974.

Roth, M.: The phobic anxiety-depersonalization syndrome and some general aetological problems in psychiatry. J. Neuropsychiatry, 1:293, 1960.

Wolff, H. G.: Every man has his "breaking point." Milit. Med., 125:85, 1960.

234.3. DEPRESSION

DEFINITION. Depression is a term for a mood of sadness and gloom. It can be a symptom of manic-depressive psychosis, and Ch. 233.3 should be consulted for a complete consideration of the subject. Here we are dealing with depression that occurs as a response to troubled life circumstances. Such depression can usually be given a more specific name, such as discouragement, demoralization, or grief — terms that carry specifically the connotation of an emotional reaction.

The troubled mood is usually not hard to recognize. The patient appears miserable, his face expressive of sadness and perhaps tension. He may move without confidence or purpose and report that his energy is decreased and his thinking slow and difficult. Appetite is usually lessened, often with weight loss, and sleep is restless and diminished. Sexual interest will be greatly reduced. The patient may also say that he is irritable and fearful. Depending on the severity of his depression, the patient will seem socially disorganized, proving inefficient in work, failing in duties, and neglectful of appearance. His acknowledged inadequacies in these respects may add to his sense of misery and may prompt thoughts of resigning from work, leaving his family, or even committing suicide.

Although various troubles can provoke depression, there is a specific response that illustrates features common to many depressive reactions. That response is *grief*, well studied by Dr. C. M. Parkes.

Grief is an experience in almost every lifetime and is the response that follows the loss, usually by death, of some relative or friend. The severity of the reaction and its duration depend upon many factors, but the most important is the closeness of the relationship and degree of dependence of the mourner on the lost individual.

Grief is a state that follows a pattern of development in which certain stages can be recognized even though the transition from one to the next is not possible to define exactly and features from one can persist in the others. *The first stage,* which lasts several days, begins upon learning of the death. The mourner feels stunned and appears bewildered, does not seem to grasp his loss fully or to relate its implications to his feelings coherently. He may appear irritable, tearful, or anxious, but can also seem calm and capable. Although his emotions and behavior may be unpredictable, they are often culturally modified as he carries out such customs as funeral rituals. He himself will usually report afterward that his emotions were blunted and his thinking uncertain, and that his depressed mood was not fully experienced. Parkes refers to this period as the stage of numbness, blunting, or shock.

This stage ends gradually but usually within one week of the bereavement, when there is an increase in the emotion of sadness and the appearance of an intense sense of loss that comes in waves, called pangs of yearning or pining by Parkes. In this *second stage,* between these surges of distressing feelings, which are so frequent at first as to be almost continuous, the patient is usually irritable and sad, with sleep and appetite diminished. Activity, which often takes the form of aimless moving about rather than productive work, may be increased, particularly so during a depressive surge, a point Parkes uses to support his analogy of this stage of grief to the searching behavior of animals separated from their mates. It is the phenomenon of *surges of misery,* however, that is most characteristic of grief and usually aids in its recognition. With time these occur less often, but it is common experience to have such a wave of depressive feelings sweep over a person following a reminder of the loss years after the bereavement.

The third period of grief appears with a diminution in the attacks of yearning and the anxious restlessness. This phase, usually entered into within several weeks of bereavement, customarily lasts the longest. It is a stage of depressed feelings with apathy and a disinclination to find purpose or interest in work. The patient is no longer restless, sleepless, or without appetite, but his emotional state is one of gloom and discouragement and his capacity for enjoyment or for physical or intellectual work is greatly reduced. Parkes refers to this as the stage of disorganization when the patient seems withdrawn, may complain of ill health, and fails to plan ahead. This state may last over a year and only gradually be replaced with more customary feelings. Recovery may be brought about in part by the natural but chance occurrence of new integrative activities and friendships, and can be facilitated by efforts of the mourner to expose himself to the opportunities for these restorative experiences.

Depressions that are responses to difficulties in life other than bereavement are very similar to this third stage. Symptoms like those in the first two stages of grief can appear briefly in distressing situations that have a sudden onset, such as being informed of an unexpected personal misfortune. But these are usually transient features and are soon replaced by a mood of sadness and discouragement very like that of the third stage.

PRECIPITATING FACTORS. In this form of depression it is usually not difficult to recognize the change as a response to some difficulty, for the patient is often preoccupied with the trouble itself and is ready to draw the link between it and his present mood. Precipitating situations can be of many kinds. They can be sudden and specific events in which something is lost, such as a relationship or a job. Other provocations are situations chronically thwarting to the sense of achievement and self-esteem, as in an education program in which students are confronted with their errors but given little effective teaching to overcome them. Moving away from home can provoke the very unpleasant depressive reaction, homesickness, especially in persons who depend a great deal on the support of friends and family. In general, circumstances that disturb a person's sense of stability, security, effectiveness, or worth provoke depressive responses.

The more such a precipitant is prolonged or accompanied by a growing realization of his difficulties, the more likely the person is to show a depressive response. A paradigm of these features for a precipitant is found in debilitating physical illnesses such as cancer. Here the protracted and continually worsening clinical situation provides constant reminders of losses suffered and brings more each day. That depression is a universal occurrence in such circumstances has been demonstrated by Hinton in his study of the dying.

For reasons not fully understood, there are some physiologic states and physical illnesses that commonly provoke depressive moods. Patients with hepatitis or any severe viral illness are particularly prone to report a depressive mood and to find reasons for it in trifles that did not trouble them when they were well. Endocrine alterations such as the postpartum state, Cushing's disease, or Addison's disease are also precipitants of depressive feelings that can be very distressing to the patient and of such profound degree as to occasionally promote a suicidal action. Certain brain diseases, particularly stroke, may also precipitate a prolonged and distressing depressive state. In all these circumstances the mood of depression may rest on some disturbed physiologic mechanism in the central nervous system as yet unknown. Their possible relationship to manic-depressive disorder is discussed in Ch. 233.3.

PREDISPOSING FACTORS. Given that situations of difficulty can lead to depression, there are features of personality that can make an individual more vulnerable to this response, perhaps by making him assess losses and difficulties more acutely and by inhibiting his power to resolve them. Especially vulnerable are those insecure and sensitive individuals who perceive criticism when none is intended and find a source of depressive feelings in their self-doubting.

Another depressive predisposition is that of the self-dramatizing and emotionally unstable and immature individual who tends to amplify emotional reactions of all sorts. When such an individual finds himself in situations of discomfort in which his feelings may be neglected, he seems more prone than others to develop a sense of dissatisfaction, distress, and depression. Slavney and McHugh present empirical evidence of this predisposition in their report of depressive symptoms in 80 per cent of patients hospitalized with the diagnosis of hysterical personality.

Finally, individuals limited in their capacity to cope with difficulties are predisposed to depressive responses. Particularly vulnerable for this reason are the mentally retarded. Even modest impairment in intellectual endowment will interfere with the person's ability to find solutions to situations that present him problems, and his failure and uncertainty tend to provoke a depressive mood. Borderline mental retardation is often overlooked in the search for predisposing factors, and a history of poor occupational and scholastic performance in a depressed patient warrants formal intelligence testing.

DIFFERENTIAL DIAGNOSIS. The differential diagnosis of depressive states can be difficult, particularly if it is not carried out methodically. The most important distinction to draw is that between depression as a response to troubled circumstances and depression as a symptom of manic-depressive disorder. This important discrimination rests on clinical grounds and cannot be made with certainty in all situations. Thus, although the depressions of the widow, the homesick, and the patient with a fatal illness can all be recognized as responses, the trap is in making this understandable connection with every depression and explaining it always as being due to some recent difficulty. If the family of the patient says he is more depressed than they would expect him to be under the circumstances, the diagnosis of a depressive response might be questioned. Also, the presence in the patient of remarkable changes in self-attitude such as the appearance of beliefs that he is a criminal or deserves punishment for minor transgressions, or that he is infectious and filled with physical corruption, are not seen in the usual depressive response and should lead to the consideration of manic-depressive psychosis. Finally, a previous history of mania or of depression, or a family history of affective disorder, should influence the interpretation of depression and sway the diagnosis away from the depressive response (see Ch. 233.3).

TREATMENT. Although the depressive response is characteristic enough to be recognized easily again and again, the particular predispositions, precipitants, and interactions are never the same from one patient to another. Treatment is based on these particulars and is thus unique to some extent to each occasion. It is therefore hard to describe the treatment of depression without some sense of dissatisfaction because, although the principles are simple, no list of them applies to every patient.

An important early decision in treatment is the need for hospitalization. This is usually determined by how severely the mood disturbance interferes with self-care, by the availability of a supportive and protective environment at home, and particularly by the presence of suicidal features. To assess the last, the patient must be asked if he has been considering self-injury. Although judgment is required in evaluating his answers, a sequence of questions probing for suicidal thoughts should be routine for every patient with depression. A proportion of the patients will deny all thought of self-

injury and can be assumed to be of lesser suicidal risk. Those who admit to such thoughts should be asked if they have any means in mind. To that question still more patients will reassure the doctor that their thoughts on suicide have not reached so severe an intensity. Those patients, however, who admit to having considered a means (pills, gas, shooting) must be considered of higher risk, and thought must be given to protecting them, perhaps by hospitalization or by guaranteeing that they are under the supervision of friends or relatives. Finally, the patients should be asked if they have acquired any means or done anything to try them out. Again a proportion of patients will say that they have not been that despondent, but those who say that they have done such things are at very high risk and should in most cases be hospitalized.

Once a decision is made about the site of treatment, in a hospital or on an outpatient basis, the act of reaching a secure diagnosis of a depressive reaction in a patient is the first step in its treatment, because this judgment requires that the doctor has come to understand the patient and his predicament. To gain this understanding the doctor's first meetings should be devoted to listening to the patient's description of his circumstances, of his emotional changes, and of the connections he draws between his experiences and his depressive mood. If appropriate, other informants such as relatives can amplify on the patient's statements and give details of his past modes of coping with trouble. All these efforts are intended to bring the doctor an appreciation of this particular individual and the circumstances that he faces. Such knowledge, combined with the relationships of trust, respect, and empathy that develop naturally in its acquisition, provides the resources for treatment.

The therapeutic efforts from this foundation are directed toward re-engaging the patient in life experiences in which success can be found, replacements for losses enjoyed, and a sense of integrity and control regained. Usually the first need of the patient is some help in simple tactics for the management of his current troubles and for the avoidance of their repetition in the future.

At this stage a sense of helplessness often prompts the patient to abandon many of his activities and efforts, but if at all possible he must be encouraged not to give in to these promptings, because doing so tends to perpetuate the disturbed mood by holding him from opportunities to reassess his situation and to try out solutions. His daily work, even when less efficiently performed, is often helpful in directing his attention to matters other than his troubles.

With assistance in simple matters of personal management, the patient can be helped to some success in his circumstances, bringing him encouragement and promoting a willingness to maintain his efforts and to plan for the future. Educating the patient in how certain circumstances strike his particular vulnerabilities and so provoke depressive responses can be helpful.

The most useful ingredient of the treatment is the support and interest of the doctor. This encourages the patient to express his feelings and discuss his circumstances. In this way not only is the physician provided with more information about assets and vulnerabilities of the patient, but often there is spontaneous recognition by the patient of causal features for his difficulties that brings both relief to his mood and self-perceived tactics for their resolution. If this supportive relationship can be maintained and developed, improvement of depression can be expected. For the occasional patient with whom such a relationship fails or who succumbs frequently to depressive reactions because of some intractable predisposition, more prolonged treatment by specialists in psychotherapy can be recommended.

Finally, treatment with pharmaceutical agents may help. Chlordiazepoxide, 10 mg three times daily, may relieve agitation somewhat in the bereaved or otherwise relatively depressed. A sleeping medication, flurazepam hydrochloride (Dalmane), is helpful for the sleeplessness. *The antidepressant medications,* although most useful in the manic-depressive psychoses, can be tried in some patients with a prolonged depressive response. Imipramine in a dose of 150 to 250 mg a day or the monoamine oxidase inhibitor phenelzine, 15 mg three times daily, has helped individual patients, but this symptomatic relief should be considered a minor part of the treatment plan in patients with this form of depression.

Granville-Grossman, K. L.: The early environment in affective disorder. *In* Coppen, A., and Walk, A. (eds.): Recent Developments in Affective Disorder. Br. J. Psychiatry, Special Publication No. 2, 1968.

Hinton, J. M.: Physical and mental distress of the dying. Quart. J. Med., 32:1, 1963.

Parkes, C. M.: The first year of bereavement. Psychiatry, 33:444, 1970.

234.4. HYSTERIA

DEFINITION.   Hysteria is a disturbance of behavior in which symptoms and signs of physical ill health are imitated more or less unconsciously for some personal advantage. As the phrase "more or less unconsciously" implies, hysteria may be hard to distinguish from "malingering," in which the imitation of illness is a well-appreciated fraud. Frank malingering is rare, though, because the power of human self-deception is usually adequate to persuade a person of the validity of his own symptoms. The only ones who can be called malingerers with any confidence are some self-mutilating patients and the remarkable pathologic liars, picturesquely called examples of the *Munchausen syndrome,* who travel from hospital to hospital gaining admission by means of dramatic acts of illness.

PREDISPOSING AND PRECIPITATING FACTORS.   Hysterical symptoms are to be seen as responses to distressing experiences. They can occur in almost any person facing danger or difficulty, especially if, as with soldiers in battle or prisoners, the distress is intense and prolonged and physical symptoms can provide a viable escape. Dull-witted or immature persons with inadequate powers of introspection and self-control may produce transparently hysterical symptoms in response to milder distress, such as school difficulties or family problems. Some of the exaggerations and elaborations of medical symptoms common in hospitalized patients may be similarly interpreted as responses to the distress of illness by persons whose capacity for self-control has been weakened by somatic illness. Hysterical symptoms can be the first manifestations of a dementing illness or of a depressive or schizophrenic psychosis, and these disorders must be considered when a previously well balanced adult develops a suspiciously hysterical symptom.

Commonly, though, hysteria is a disturbance in the be-havior of a person predisposed by an attention-seeking, emotionally unstable, and egocentric personality. In fact, these characteristics form what has become known as the "hysterical personality" even though hysteria can occur in other types of people, and these characteristics do not invariably produce hysterical symptoms. Most easily recognized in such people is their flair for the dramatic. They show this tendency in flamboyant dress and in exaggerated, even melodramatic, responses to questions about their symptoms. They are never so happy as when they are the center of attention. Karl Jaspers characterized the hysterical personalities as those who "crave to appear, both to themselves and others, as more than they are and to experience more than they are ever capable of." The zeal of these patients for exaggeration and drama renders them more liable to hysterical symptoms. But other kinds of people can have these symptoms. In all of them usually a discouraged, depressive mood has been prompted by difficulties in life, and the hysterical symptoms then emerge from this mood state.

SYMPTOMS AND SIGNS.   Many of the phenomena of somatic illness can be imitated by hysteria. The accuracy of the imitation depends on the medical sophistication of the patient. A doctor or nurse is more likely to produce a convincing imitation than is an unqualified person.

Common hysterical symptoms are vague subjective disorders, such as generalized weakness, dizziness, indigestion, or pain. Hysterical pain can occur in any part of the body, but the head and neck, the region over the heart, and the low back are particularly favored. Hysterical pain can be of any character, from dull aching to sharp and stabbing pain, but it is often described by the patient in vivid similes such as "like a bullet," "like a bolt of lightning," "aches like an abscessed tooth," or "sore as a hot boil." Usually, hysterical pain is not confined to a local area as around a pathologic lesion, nor is it referred into the distribution of a particular nerve or dermatome. Rather, hysterical pain is felt in a general region of the body and spreads, sometimes in bizarre ways, into contiguous areas without regard to neuroanatomic boundaries. Thus pain beginning in the face may spread along the side of the head and into the back, crossing from the region of the trigeminal nerve into the upper cervical nerve regions. Hysterical pain often varies in its character, intensity, and distribution, changing considerably with attention or suggestion. Occasionally it can be remarkably improved by a small amount of intravenous amobarbital sodium when analgesics do not help.

Although vague symptoms of a subjective kind such as pain or dizziness are the present vogue in hysteria, crude and gross symptoms are still seen. These may be psychologic, such as the amnesia or fugue states, in which memory is partially lost, often in situations in which the patient is depressed or anxious. Other psychologic symptoms shown occasionally include auditory and visual hallucinations and even flamboyant delusions. These must be carefully judged, but appear most commonly in young people who have read popular books on psychology and psychiatry and are apparently suggested into these symptoms by their reading at a time when they are distressed over other matters.

Motor disturbances in the form of abnormal movement, disturbed gaits, seizures, or paralyses are occasionally hysterical symptoms. Hysterical seizures can usually be distinguished from epileptic ones. The patients only rarely injure themselves, bite their tongues, or lose their urine. They do not have the typical tonic and then clonic phases of a seizure, but tend to show a dramatic flailing of the limbs. Consciousness is partially retained, and seizures hardly ever occur when the patient is alone. The EEG is normal.

Sensory disturbances are particularly favored hysterical symptoms. Thus, *blindness* or *deafness* is common, often developing dramatically at a time of emotional distress. Loss of sensation over one side of the body to pin prick or light touch is frequently found after a susceptible patient has been examined by a neurologist.

DIAGNOSIS. Diagnosis of hysteria is seldom easy and never popular. Ideally, it should rest on three supports: first, the *form* of the hysterical manifestation; second, the *personality* of the patient; and third, the *setting* in which the symptoms developed. Often it is not possible to find all three supports to a diagnosis, but all should be sought.

Commonly, hysterical symptoms are vague and variable. In fact, the more definite and consistent a patient's description of the onset, location, nature, and duration of his symptoms, the less likely the symptoms are to be hysterical. Hysterical symptoms and signs are also usually incompatible with what is known of anatomy and physiology. Thus sensory losses do not conform to patterns of nerve distribution; reflexes remain intact and unchanged in the palsies of arm and leg; seizures of the entire body do not disturb consciousness; total blindness appears without a disturbance of pupillary reflex or of opticokinetic nystagmus. The hysterically mute person can phonate on coughing. The hysterically deaf person speaks louder to be heard over increased ambient noises. Many other hysterical symptoms have been analyzed for such inconsistencies by Head.

Knowledge of the personality and past history of the patient is helpful to a diagnosis of hysteria. The recognition that the symptoms are occurring in an hysterical personality should prompt an observer to look very closely at the symptoms before embarking on extensive laboratory tests or upon surgery. Similarly, knowlege of a previous vague and poorly understood medical disturbance can lend weight to an opinion that a new symptom that has eluded diagnosis is occurring in an individual prone to hysteria. Conversely, hysteria can usually be eliminated as an explanation for symptoms in an emotionally stable, middle-aged person. People who have passed through adolescence and young adulthood without resorting to hysterical behavior are unlikely to employ it when older.

The setting in which the symptoms develop should be carefully scrutinized, and a search made for a distressing event that may have provoked an hysterical reaction or for any purpose that the hysterical symptoms may serve. Occasionally, a clear association between the symptoms chosen and a particular recent disturbance in the life of the subject can be found, such as an amnesia developing in a person who has done something shameful or criminal, or weakness and pain persisting in a person who is seeking financial compensation for an injury. Often, though, motivations behind hysterical symptoms are vague and uncertain. It is usual to find that the patient is unhappy or anxious about some aspect of his life circumstances and that the hysterical symptoms serve to call attention to his distress. Also, it may be possible to demonstrate that the development of particular symptoms has been prompted by suggestion: weakness of legs, for example, developing in a nurse caring for a paraplegic patient, or peculiar falling attacks after the patient has witnessed an epileptic seizure.

Guzé and his associates have pointed out a subgroup of patients with a chronic hysterical disorder who have had recurrent complaints of symptoms involving almost every bodily system. These patients, with what Guzé terms Briquet's syndrome, present diagnostic difficulties to many specialists as their complaints change, worsen, and improve in unpredictable ways. They usually have undergone multiple medical and surgical procedures. The same criteria that lead to the diagnosis of single hysterical symptoms can be applied to this group. Additionally they can be reliably differentiated from most medical patients by the sheer number of systems that have been involved in their past complaints. The role of particular personality traits in Briquet's syndrome has been explored by Kaminsky and Slavney.

A careful study of the symptoms, the personality, and the life setting of a patient usually allows a reasonably certain differentiation of hysterical symptoms from those of a medical illness. There are, however, certain medical problems that are notoriously easily confused with hysteria. These are the diseases that produce vague and changing symptoms that seem to vary with the patient's motivation and, at least in their early phases, lack convincing physical signs. If such an illness occurs in a patient who has features of the hysterical personality and who will therefore describe the symptoms in a dramatic and flamboyant fashion, physicians may be even more persuaded to believe that the illness is only deceptively physical. Examples of diseases frequently confused with hysteria because of their subtle clinical features are the first attack of multiple sclerosis, particularly if sensory changes alone are produced; the weakness of arms and legs seen early in acute idiopathic polyneuritis of the Guillain-Barré type; the difficulty in swallowing of bulbar myasthenia gravis; the attacks of muscular weakness in periodic paralysis; the tonic posturings and oculogyric crises of postencephalitic parkinsonism; the pain of a cauda equina tumor; and the abdominal pain of acute intermittent porphyria.

MANAGEMENT OF HYSTERIA. The management of hysterical patients is difficult. No one method can be recommended unqualifiedly. But there are certain principles that can be followed. To help hysterical patients it is essential to have sympathy for them. Many doctors find these patients irritating. It is just as possible to see them as individuals displaying an intriguing aspect of human behavior that has profound implications in their lives. It is pointless to argue with these patients about the validity of their symptoms. A useful approach is to agree that they have had an illness producing their symptoms, but that they are now improving even though total recovery has not arrived.

It is important to diagnose hysteria promptly. Hesitation in diagnosis leading to several hospital admissions for extensive laboratory investigations is a good way to solidify hysterical symptoms in a patient. Among other things, the uncertainty of doctors helps persuade a patient that the symptoms are real. Repeated examinations increase the consistency with which symtpoms are reported. Long hospitalization, mounting bills, and the inconvenience caused to others make it difficult for a patient to abandon symptoms without embarrassment. The gratifying attention given to the patient in the hospital, perhaps as an example of an intriguing diagnostic problem, can feed the self-dramatizing tendencies and so encourage the behavior.

There is always risk of error in any diagnosis, because diagnosis is only a weighing of probabilities. The diagnosis of hysteria, though, depends purely on a physician's judgment and, before relief of symptoms is accomplished, can be confirmed in the laboratory only by evidence of health. Physicians, for obvious reasons, fear more the error of calling a physically sick patient hysterical than the error of mishandling hysteria. They often prefer to exclude, by laboratory examination, progressively more unlikely diseases than to study carefully the symptoms and the individual who has produced them, even though this would lead more directly to a definite diagnosis as well as an understanding of the response. It may be unwise to counsel too strongly against this behavior because medical diagnosis is never easy. A compromise can be found in the admonition to perform immediately the laboratory tests that seem necessary for a patient, but when hysteria is suspected, to bring the period of investigation as quickly as possible to a close so that management of the specific symptom can be begun.

Treatment of the specific symptoms rests basically upon persuasion. The doctor is persuading the patient to perform the functions that the patient claims are disabled. Intravenous amobarbital sodium given to the point where the patient is mildly intoxicated and his speech slurred is particularly helpful in making and establishing a persuasion. Usually, some ingenuity is required for success. The hysterically blind person can, for example, be persuaded first that he can distinguish light from dark and then gradually to distinguish forms, to read large print, and, finally, small newspaper type. The person who claims he cannot walk can be encouraged first to move his legs in bed, and then to stand, to make a few tentative shuffles, and finally to stride out. The hysterically deaf person can be persuaded to hear through a stethoscope and then gradually that he can hear without it. A dramatic show of some kind is often helpful in removing these symptoms. If a physician has success in partially removing hysterical symptoms, he should persist in his treatment without interruption in order to bring about as much improvement as possible and even to restore full function. When there is recovery of function, the patient should perform his recovered skills in public — before his family, other patients, and several doctors — to prevent his relapsing immediately into his former state.

The fear that sudden removal of hysterical symptoms will result in a disastrous psychologic colllapse is exag-gerated. Rarely, a depressed patient with hysterical symptoms has an increase in depression, but it is clear that in those situations a depression was overlooked and the more secondary hysterical symptoms were emphasized.

Some hysterical disorders are refractory to treatment. Among these are the disorders assumed for some material gain, such as compensation. They usually are not improved until some settlement is made. Episodic disorders such as hysterical seizures can be hard to control. Sometimes, however, a statement to the patient that they will not recur, given with full authority by a physician whom the patient trusts and respects, may eliminate these symptoms. The longer the patient has hysterical symptoms, the harder they are to remove. This is a corollary to the aforementioned observation that hysterical symptoms produced for transparent reasons and bordering on malingering are more difficult to eliminate than are the ones produced by an attention-seeking personality in some emotional distress. Symptoms held for a long time cannot be easily abandoned without embarrassing the patient.

Simultaneously with treatment of the specific symptoms, the emotional state and present life of the patient should be studied to discover any distress that may have precipitated the hysterical symptoms. Then advice, social assistance, or guidance can be offered to aid the patient in resolving these difficulties. This aspect of their psychologic treatment depends on developing a relationship of friendship and mutual respect identical to that found necessary in treating an anxious or depressed person.

Long-term management of hysterical patients is much more difficult than treatment of individual symptoms. It is not wise to have the average hysterical patient embark on depth psychotherapy, because he tends to produce more symptoms and to recount involved sexual and other fantasies in order to maintain the interest of his doctor. If possible, these patients should be followed by one physician who understands them and the behavior that they are liable to produce and is also competent to recognize physical illness should it arise. This physician can save these patients from needless surgery and long hospitalization. He can remove hysterical symptoms promptly by being alert to the diagnosis and providing help for the difficulties that precipitate them.

Guzé, S.: The validity and significance of the clinical diagnosis of hysteria (Briquet's syndrome). Am. J. Psychiatry, 132:138, 1975.

Head, H. The diagnosis of hysteria. Br. Med. J., 1:827, 1922.

Kaminsky, M. J., and Slavney, P. R.: Methodology and personality in Briquet's syndrome: A reappraisal. Am. J. Psychiatry, 133:85, 1976.

Slavney, P. R., and McHugh, P. R.: The hysterical personality: A controlled study. Arch. Gen. Psychiatry, 30:325, 1974.

Walters, A.: Psychogenic regional pain, alias hysterical pain. Brain, 84:1, 1961.

Section Five PSYCHOLOGIC TESTING IN CLINICAL MEDICINE

Paul R. McHugh

235. INTRODUCTION

Psychologic tests are intended to assist clinical evaluation of behavioral disorders by bringing accurate measurement to the mental examination. Physicians are familiar with instruments, such as the thermometer or sphygmomanometer, that bring accurate measurement to observations in the physical examination. They are so easy to employ that knowledge of the normal readings in the human population and implications of deviations from normal have been established. Although psychologic tests are aimed at more abstract phenomena such as intelligence or personality, they similarly attempt to bring precision through numerical or graphic measurements and provide a means by which an individual can be compared in these features with others.

The mere provision of a numerical expression does not prove a test useful, as the numbers may not be meaningful. Often in our fascination with a new test and its intriguingly plausible scales for measurement, we overlook its failure to satisfy the criteria of *reliability* and *validity*.

The reliability of a measuring instrument, whether it be for a physical or a psychologic function, is an expression of the accuracy and reproducibility of its findings. No instrument is perfectly reliable, but the range within which it is unreliable must be a small fraction of the potential range of measurement if it is to be capable of detecting a genuine deviation in the variable under study. The validity of an instrument is an expression of its capacity to measure what it claims to measure.

How can we be sure that psychologic tests are actually measuring the psychologic variables that they claim to measure? How can we be sure that intelligence tests, for example, measure intelligence? The only proof that a psychologic test is valid is the demonstration that scores on it predict behavior in life thought to be the expression of the trait it claims to measure. For example, results on a valid intelligence test should correlate to some extent with scholastic performance.

The issues of reliability and validity are fundamental to all test evaluation. For more thorough consideration the reader is directed to Zubin's review and Messick's article.

236. INTELLIGENCE

The quantitative measurement of the mental attribute, intelligence, was first attempted by Binet at the turn of the century. His success and the Stanford-Binet battery of tests developed from his work brought such predictive power to the study of intelligence that they provide an impetus to the development of tests to examine other mental functions. But the tests of intelligence have through their revisions, particularly the *Wechsler Bellevue Intelligence Scale* published in 1939 and the *Wechsler Adult Intelligence Scale (WAIS)* of 1955,

remained the most secure and useful tests of mental function.

Intelligence is difficult to define. It is the abstract concept used to explain the observation that individuals vary in their mental capacities and in the effectiveness with which they employ them. Intelligence is more easily defined in practice by pointing to instances of its action. This way is in fact used in our daily life. We judge a man's intelligence by observing his bearing, his speech, his apparent grasp of situations, his judgments, and his emotional control. Then in the light of our past experience of watching other men, we call an individual bright or dull. We are doing nothing conceptually different when we estimate intelligence at the bedside or by means of psychologic tests. We organize the testing so that a series of observations can be made within a reasonable period of time. We add scope to our examination by asking for performance in several different kinds of mental activity. We bring accuracy to the observations by scoring the performance.

The questions on orientation, memory, attention and concentration, fund of knowledge, and capacity to reason abstractly that constitute the test of cognition routinely carried out at the bedside in the course of the physical and mental examination provide a doctor an estimate of his patient's intellectual functioning. In the light of knowledge of the patient's past life and demonstrated abilities, the doctor makes a judgment whether there has been damage to intellectual functioning. Psychologic tests are able to give a more accurate estimate of the intelligence of a patient at the moment of testing than do these bedside examinations, because these tests have proved both reliable and valid.

All these approaches, from the casual observations to the most refined test, are applications of a fundamentally identical method: an assessment of a performance thought on practical grounds to be a reflection of intelligence. However, any performance will be influenced by other factors, particularly the factors of education and experience. *Since these factors derive from opportunities and social heritage of the subject, every one of these assessments must be qualified and interpreted in the light of the subject's cultural and educational background.*

Subcultural differences that are obvious on bedside examination, being recognized as modifications in expression and in experience, *are allowed for almost automatically in that assessment but are sometimes forgotten when formal intelligence test scores are displayed.* Just as there is no culture-pure bedside examination, there is no culture-pure intelligence test. Test scores must be interpreted in relationship to all that is known about the patient. Particular care in the interpretation is demanded if he is a member of a subculture different from the standard criterion group employed in the development of the formal tests: urban, school-educated whites. The greater his divergence in this respect, the greater the allowance needed in interpreting the scores of his tests. Emotional disturbances or other preoccupations that interfere with the patient's concentration or cooperation will also obviously affect these performances. Allowances must be made for any of these features in assessing test scores, just as allowance is made for these features on bedside examination.

The *Wechsler Adult Intelligence Scale* is the most reliable and valid instrument we have for measuring the intellectual function of the adult. Its reliability has been demonstrated by the close correlation of test scores given on separate occasions to the same individuals and by the similarity of scores when one half of a test is compared with another half (split-half method). Its validity has been demonstrated by its correlation with life performances of individuals it scores as intelligent or dull.

In its present form the WAIS consist of 11 subtests of mental skill. Six of these subtests are "verbal tests." In these the patient is requested to define words, to recognize similarities between words, to do arithmetic, to remember numbers forward and backward, to answer questions on his fund of knowledge, and to judge and interpret proverbs. These tests are followed by five "performance tests," in which a patient is asked to work with rather unfamiliar material and solve problems set to him by that material. Tests here include the putting together of puzzles, work with symbols, the setting out of logical stories from pictures disorganized for the test, construction of patterns from multicolored blocks, and the recognition of things missing from drawings. The performance tests seem somewhat less related to the education of a person than are the verbal tests. All the subtests that have been chosen for the WAIS have a long history of investigation. They are combined together to produce a thorough and accurate instrument.

The scoring of the WAIS is in the form of the *Intelligence Quotient (I.Q.)*. In fact, the WAIS derives a verbal I.Q. from the verbal tests and a performance I.Q. from the performance tests. A full-scale I.Q. is derived from the combination of all 11 subtests.

The I.Q. compares an individual with others. Historically it was developed for children. I.Q. then was the ratio of mental age over chronologic age times 100 when mental age was defined in terms of a child's ability to succeed on tests which the average child of a given age could do. Thus a child solving problems which the average nine-year-old could solve had a mental age of nine. If he, himself, was nine years old at the time of the test, he had an average ability and an I.Q. of $9/9 \times 100$, or 100; if his chronologic age was six, he would be an advanced child with an I.Q. of $9/6 \times 100$, or 150. Terman demonstrated the constancy of I.Q. in the growing child.

But a ratio of mental to chronologic age is unlikely to be useful in adults because tested intelligence does not increase after the late teens. The WAIS and many other tests for adult intelligence continue to use the term I.Q. This is possible because of the fact that tests of intelligence appear to distribute individuals in a "normal" or gaussian fashion. This curve has a mean at I.Q. 100 and a standard deviation of ±15 I.Q. points. It is possible to divide the curve into percentiles of the population. The WAIS score of any person places him in the percentile of the population with similar scores, and his I.Q. can be extrapolated from percentile by means of the distribution curve. Thus an individual whose performance on the WAIS is equal to 50 per cent of the population is said to have an I.Q. of 100, whereas individuals whose test performances exceeded 98 per cent of the population will be said to have an I.Q. of 135 or above.

The WAIS has found its greatest clinical utility in the study of patients with brain disease. Any damage to the cerebral hemispheres will injure intellectual ability and disturb the scores on the WAIS. An intriguing observation is that early in the course of brain disease performance tests are disturbed before the verbal test scores change. This may indicate that verbal tests measure more what an indivdual has learned and practiced, whereas performance tests measure his capacity to meet new problems. The verbal and performance scores of normal individuals are usually comparable. The verbal I.Q. can be considered a fair estimate of the original intellectual endowment of an individual suffering from a brain injury. The decline of the performance I.Q. is a useful measure of the degree of injury to the cerebral tissue the patient has endured. With an advancing brain disease verbal I.Q. will fall eventually, but a patient will usually continue to demonstrate higher verbal than performance scores.

Emotional unrest such as anxiety or depression will also interfere with WAIS scores. Here, as with cerebral disease, the performance I.Q. will fall below the verbal I.Q., demonstrating that the capacity to work with unfamiliar material is disturbed more than tests of what has been well learned. But because these findings are identical to those in persons with brain disease, the differentiation of an emotional disturbance from dementia cannot come from WAIS results. It must rest on other information such as is derived from the history, physical examination, and mental status.

The WAIS is useful not only in demonstrating deterioration of intellectual function; when done serially, it can also document recovery of function with treatment. Since it is so simple to employ, its increasing utility in clinical research is assured.

237.   PERSONALITY

By personality is meant all the abiding traits of character that constitute an individual's potential to respond in particular ways to circumstances. All physicians are aware of how much information they must acquire through several interviews with the patient and from independent sources before they can have much confidence in their diagnostic opinion on personality. Tests that could elucidate personality more accurately and more rapidly would be useful. Two alternative approaches have been developed, "projective" tests and questionnaires, and each approach has raised particular problems.

In the so-called projective tests of personality ambiguous situations are set before the patient, and his responses are recorded. Thus he is presented with sentences to complete or a picture to interpret, or, in the most well known projective test, the Rorschach test, he is presented with a standardized set of ink blots and asked to describe the forms that he can recognize within them. Since there is nothing in the situations themselves that forces any particular response, the responses of the patient are thought to derive from his personal predilections and inner needs, drives, and conflicts. This seems logical. But logic is not the essential criterion for a test intended to aid the clinical examination. It must be demonstrated that the responses on projective tests provide measurements that are reliable and valid. This remains to be done.

Certain features of a patient can be expected to be seen in any set of his responses. For instance, overly conscientious persons will tend to be fixed on details, the schizophrenic patient with his disordered thought will demonstrate this feature in distorted expression, and the depressed patient will speak of unhappy themes as he discusses any matter. These features will appear whether the patient is being examined by his doctor or doing a projective test. Until the reliability and validity of projective tests can be demonstrated, it cannot be known whether they are superior to the clinical examination, and if they are not superior to the clinical examination, they are of doubtful utility to the physician. The question of their value is shrouded in controversy.

The other approach to personality measurement is the questionnaire. This was developed from the clinical examination. Since questions are used there to gain information from the patient, it seemed logical that a questionnaire including these and many other questions would improve on the clinical examination. It came as a surprise when tests developed in this fashion proved to be unreliable and invalid. This was demonstrated when different questionnaires intended to probe similar features of personality, such as introversion, did not correlate well with one another, and in fact could give quite opposite impressions of the same person. Questionnaires developed in this fashion proved so misleading that the method fell into disrepute. It was, however, eventually recognized that these early tests gratuitously assumed that questions would be accurately answered by patients. Consider the question, Do you lack self-confidence, yes or no? To presume that a person will understand this question exactly the same way as the examiner intends and that his criterion for a yes or nor answer is the same as that of all other people is to presume too much. Also these early tests failed to consider that many individuals might attempt to show themselves in some more favorable light and therefore not answer questions truthfully.

The most intriguing conceptual advance in the study of personality was the recognition that an objectively truthful answer to questions was not needed for a valid, useful test. In fact, more information can be obtained from observing the patient's replies to questions than from any belief that the statements they agree to or reject are in themselves accurate descriptions of their personality. The task of building questionnaires changed from finding questions that would display the inner feelings of people to finding questions that would be answered differently by different personality types.

To build such a questionnaire the first step was to gather together specific groups of people for study: normal people, anxious patients, hysterical patients, depressed patients, for as many groups as could be differentiated. These patients, the criterion groups, were asked a large number of questions, and the replies were compared from group to group. The questions which differentiated the groups best were then collected for the questionnaire. This questionnaire then given to an individual was interpreted not from the content of questions rejected or affirmed but from the number of questions replied to in the same fashion as in one or more of the criterion groups.

The most useful questionnaire that has been developed is the *Minnesota Multiphasic Personality Inventory (MMPI)*. The questions in that test have been carefully studied and chosen so that they differentiate the groups to the greatest degree possible with it. Because of the complexity of issues of personality, the numbers of questions needed to derive a profile with this test is 550. It was possible in the MMPI to fit in many questions that give an indication of the tendency of the patient to lie, exaggerate, or misunderstand questions.

The results of the MMPI are expressed as a series of ten scales or dimensions along each of which an individual is placed by means of his responses that correspond to responses of nine criterion groups. These scales were originally derived from clinical groups and given clinical names, i.e., hypochondriasis, depression, hysteria, psychopathic, masculine-feminine dimension, paranoid, psychaesthenic, schizophrenic, manic, and social introversion. Three so-called reliability scales are also scored for each test.

The MMPI is a reliable instrument, the accuracy and reproducibility of its readings having been demonstrated in repeated testing of individuals over many years. The validity of its scales varies. Some of the scales measure the personality characteristics for which they are titled. Scores on the psychopathic and manic scales do correlate with the clinical features intended by these terms. Scores on the schizophrenic and hysterical scales do not correlate well with these clinical disorders but with aspects of bizarreness and self-dramatization, respectively, features not specific to schizophrenia or hysteria. In an effort to avoid these invalid implications, the MMPI scales are no longer referred to by clinical titles, but by numbers of letters derived from the original names.

The tendency to look at specific scales for diagnostic impressions has been replaced by consideration of the "profile," or pattern of the several scales together, hoping to derive in this way a more global view of personality structure. This approach emphasizes the multidimensional character of personality. It takes advantage of the features of reliability found in this test. But, once again, the establishment of validity for these profiles must be accomplished. This is being attempted by matching the life course of individuals with predictions from the profiles, but work is still in progress.

Current practice is to find the MMPI useful as a screening and probing instrument that often suggests aspects of personality difficulty that might well be more carefully studied. However, its validity for the differentiation of clinical psychiatric entities or specific personality types is uncertain, and thus it must not be regarded as the arbiter in differential diagnosis.

Anastasia, A.: Psychological Testing. New York, Macmillan, 1976.

Butcher, H. J.: Human Intelligence, Its Nature and Assessment. London, Methuen & Co., Ltd., 1968.

Messick, S.: The standard problem — meaning and values in measurement and evaluation. Am. Psychol., 30:955, 1975.

Terman, L. M., and Oden, M.: The Gifted Group at Mid-Life. Genetic Studies of Genius, Vol. V. Stanford, California, Stanford University Press, 1959.

Welsh, G. S., and Dahlstrom, W. G.: Basic Readings on the MMPI. Minneapolis, University of Minnesota Press, 1956.

Zubin, J.: Classification of behavior disorders. Ann. Rev. Psychol., 18:373, 1967.

Section Six MEDICAL ASPECTS OF SEXUALITY

Harold I. Lief

238. THE PHYSICIAN'S ROLE

PREVENTION AS WELL AS THERAPY

In dealing with sexual problems, the physician has a splendid opportunity to practice preventive as well as therapeutic medicine. By aiding a young person to overcome sexual anxieties and inhibitions, he is helping to prepare that young person for satisfactory relationships and, eventually, marriage itself. By counseling a married couple, enabling them to obtain greater sexual pleasure and mutuality, the physician prevents increasing marital discord, perhaps even divorce itself, and the consequent emotional and physical sequelae for the couple and their children. Marital unhappiness and frustration have been implicated in a variety of illnesses, perhaps the most prominent of which is depression, which, in turn, is often a contributing factor to a variety of diseases. Helping patients with sexual problems is good medical care. It is more than the enrichment of life, important as that is, because sexual counseling reduces one of the most frequent sources of human suffering and thus aids in preventing individual illness, family uprooting, and resultant social disorganization.

Most sexual problems presented to physicians are in the context of a marital relationship, either as primary causes of marital dysfunction or as consequences of other areas of marital discord, but which nevertheless augment and maintain marital unhappiness. It seems reasonable then to make sex and marriage counseling a "package" in the training of the physician and in the delivery of medical care. Even in the case of the pediatrician, it is still logical, for he soon comes to recognize the direct connection between the marital relationship of the parents and the sexual problems of the child.

Although marriage counseling is important, it is not the only way the physician can practice effective preventive medicine. Early intervention can occur in a number of other clinical situations, e.g., premarital counseling, family-planning services during pregnancy, postpartum care, and family-life education for teenagers and young adults. The pediatrician and obstetrician have especially significant points of entrance into the system of health care, enabling these specialists to practice effective prevention.

PHYSICIAN COMFORT

Not only are marital and sexual problems frequent in medical practice, but they are often overlooked or avoided — either because of the physician's lack of training and his feeling of incompetence in this area, or because these problems impinge on his own marital and sexual conflicts or values and make him uncomfortable. Even if he consciously or unconsciously avoids the issue by failing to follow cues, changing the subject by responding with a trite and stereotyped form of reassurance, e.g., "this is just a phase — your problem will disappear in time," he is carrying out counseling of sorts. Vincent has stated it well: "The theoretical position that the physician cannot or should not engage in any marriage or sexual counseling becomes meaningless when the patients expect this role of their physician and when their illnesses have sexual and marital implications — if not origins. The majority of physicians literally have no choice; even to do and say nothing in response to the patient's questions and/or presentation of symptoms in the sexual and marital areas is, by default, one form of counseling."

To be competent in handling the therapeutic and preventive aspects of the sexual, marital, and family problems he sees almost daily in his practice, the physician must not only have a store of *information*, but must also develop a set of *skills* and *attitudes* that facilitate his making optimal use of his information. Surely the key factor in competent sex and marital counseling is the degree of comfort of the counselor. His skill in interviewing, in eliciting salient data about the most intimate, personal dimension of patients' lives, will depend directly on his capacity to react not with anxiety, anger, or self-righteousness, but with openness, ease, and a clear desire to achieve an atmosphere of genuine communication of feelings as well as thoughts. Lacking these skills and attitudes, his quantity of information, even if vast, is of little use.

LEVELS OF INTERVENTION

Four levels of intervention are possible for the physician treating patients with sexual dysfunctions, namely, (1) diagnostician, (2) educator, (3) counselor, or (4) therapist.

Diagnostician

Sexual problems fall into the following categories: overt, covert, associated with physical illness, associated with mental illness, and false or pseudosexual problems.

OVERT. Presenting complaints may be overtly sexual, e.g., impotence or anorgasmia. The physician has the task of discovering the meaning and importance of the symptom, whether it has been lifelong or acquired (following a period of adequate functioning prior to the onset of the symptom), generalized (with all partners in all situations), or situational (with one partner or in one situation). If it is situational, for example, limited to one partner, it will usually call for couple counseling rather than individual treatment.

COVERT. By contrast, with covert problems, the physician has to be on the lookout for the presence of sexual or marital problems that lie behind a host of physical symptoms — headache, backache, fatigue, menstrual irregularities, or dysmenorrhea. Osler said of syphilis that it was "the great imitator" of other disease states. Today it may be said more accurately that sexual dissatisfaction plays that role.

ASSOCIATED WITH PHYSICAL ILLNESS OR DRUG THERAPY. Although diabetes is the illness most often implicated in sexual dysfunction, other diseases, especially chronic ones not necessarily related to the neurologic or vascular pathways subsuming sexual responsivity, often have sexual connotations. Most physicians do not even discuss sex with their postcoronary patients, and when they do they may offer vague, uncertain advice such as "Take it easy." Patients who have a chronic illness or who have had an organ ablation such as hysterectomy *are* concerned about their sexual functions: How often? Under what circumstances? Am I still virile or attractive? Those are questions many patients are too embarrassed to ask. One study showed that only 10 per cent of women who had undergone mastectomy had discussed with their physicians their concerns about sexual behaviors, body-image, and the impact of the surgery on their husbands. The physician must be sensitive to when and how he can initiate such discussion with his patients. Antihypertensive drugs are frequently implicated in impotence, retrograde ejaculation, or diminished capacity for vaginal vasocongestion. Other medications, certainly the psychotropic drugs, may be similarly related to a decrease in sexual adequacy.

ASSOCIATED WITH MENTAL ILLNESS. Among the major mental illnesses, depression is the disorder most often found to have an adverse effect on sexual competence. The most frequent sexual consequence of depression is inhibition of sexual desire usually found in conjunction with a generalized anhedonia. This disturbance is found even more frequently than impotence; indeed, impotence often follows a decrease in sexual desire.

FALSE OR PSEUDOSEXUAL COMPLAINTS. Occasionally a patient will complain of a sexual problem as a primary reason for the consultation when, in fact, the primary difficulty may be a marital problem or depression. The sexual problem is used as a "calling-card" to gain entry into the health-care system, meanwhile avoiding some other problem that may be even more painful to face or to deal with.

Educator

As an educator, the physician can pass on to the patient correct information about sexual anatomy and physiology; he can discuss with the patient the range of sexual behaviors, including what is normative. He should always be mindful of the influence of society on what is judged "normal," for in today's changing sexual scene, yesterday's perversions and deviations are tomorrow's variations. Examples are masturbation, oral sex, premarital intercourse, and homosexuality. The physician has the opportunity to dispel sexual myths and misconceptions, e.g., anxiety about penis size, the effects of hysterectomy on sexual functioning, the frequency of coital orgasm in women, or the alleged effects of aging on sexual capacities. As an educator, a physician may point out to the patient the relations of the adverse or painful emotions ("emergency" emotions) — anxiety, anger, guilt — to the inhibition of sexual functioning. The physician-educator may convey appropriate information on psychosexual development to adolescents or to the parents of younger children.

Counselor

The educator role merges into the counselor role, and often there is more overlap than discontinuity. An example will illustrate this. The man recovering from a myocardial infarction can be told that the exertion in coitus is no more strenuous than climbing two flights of stairs; these comments constitute education. In the role of counselor, however, the physician would inquire into the patient's concerns about sexual capacity and, through the role of "inquirer" (expert listening is a crucial facet of counseling), would convey caring and understanding. In response to the patient's questions, the physician would be able to assume the role of educator more effectively, imparting more relevant information. The physician could counsel more precisely concerning resumption of sexual activity, the amount of activity, coital positions, and the like. By being precise, the physician will reduce the patient's anxiety and prevent the appearance of impotence or premature ejaculation. The physician-counselor may wish to discuss the situation with the patient's wife, elicit her cooperation, and reduce her fear that sexual activity will damage her husband. Anxiety is "contagious," and to reduce anxiety in one partner is not enough if the titer of anxiety is high in the other partner. In such a case, the anxiety of the spouse will spread to the patient, undermining the counseling efforts directed at the patient.

The physician who is too busy to set aside the time or who shies away from marital therapy may have to treat the couple by dealing with one patient only. Many situations can be handled in this fashion, e.g., the urologist who cures male dyspareunia by clearing up the patient's prostatitis, the internist who helps restore his patient's potency by reassuring him that sexual activity will not result in another coronary occlusion, the gynecologist who reassures his patient that she will suffer no loss of sexual drive after hysterectomy. *Yet sexual behavior involves a relationship; hence, in most instances therapy should also be directed toward the relationship.*

Therapist

The sex therapist is a specialty role requiring specialized training currently available in only a few first-rate training centers in the United States. The sex therapist should be competent in marital therapy and in individual psychotherapy and should be able to employ, as well, the specific behavioral techniques first set forth by Masters and Johnson. The sex therapist's greatest skill is in making an appropriate appraisal on the basis of which he can decide the form of treatment apt to be most effective in a given situation.

An encouraging sign is that more training centers in medical schools are being developed. A recent survey demonstrated that 39 per cent of United States medical schools now have separate sex therapy clinics; approximately 50 per cent carry out some form of sex therapy in their outpatient settings.

Of the four levels of intervention, most physicians will restrict their activities to the first three, namely,

TABLE 1. The Sexual System (Sexuality)

1. Biologic sex: chromosomes, hormones, primary and secondary sex characteristics
2. Core gender identity: sense of maleness and femaleness
3. Gender identity: sense of masculinity and femininity
4. Gender role behavior:
   a. Nonsexual gender role behavior: behavior that is often associated with masculinity and femininity
   b. Sexual behavior: behavior motivated by desire for sexual pleasure, ultimately orgasm (physical sex)
      (1) Proceptive behavior
      (2) Acceptive behavior
      (3) Conceptive behavior

diagnostician, educator, and counselor. A good rule of thumb for the physician-counselor is to arrange for his individual or couple patients to come in for six sessions. At the end of six sessions, if the physician feels that he is not making sufficient progress, he should refer patients to a sex therapist.

239. SEXUALITY

Sexuality refers to the totality of one's sexual being, of which physical sex is only one part. One's sense of being male and masculine, female and feminine, and the various roles these self-perceptions engender or affect are important ingredients of sexuality. Cognitive, emotional, and physical sex all contribute to the totality. In this sense, our sexuality is what we *are*, rather than what we *do*. Sexuality may be described in terms of a system somewhat analogous to the circulatory or respiratory system. The components of the sexual system are set forth in Table 1.

The brain is apparently programmed during fetal life for later sexual behavior. Fetal androgens during a critical period of fetal life (between the sixth and twelfth weeks) are necessary for an XY fetus to develop normally into a male. A deficiency of fetal androgens or androgen-insensitive tissues will interfere with normal male development. Similarly, excessive androgens in an XX fetus will bring about masculine changes. Chromosomal or hormonal abnormalities may create problems of intersexuality which may, if not corrected early in life, lead to conflicts in core gender or gender identity. The assigned sex is, with rare exceptions, more important in determining gender identity than is biologic sex. Sex-change procedures are usually unwise after the age of 18 months, when the sense of maleness and femaleness is far advanced. Some of the intersex patients and some without evident biologic defect have grave difficulties in developing a core gender identity of the same biologic sex. These are transsexuals. If they are biologic males, they think of themselves as "a female trapped in a male body." Transsexual biologic females consider themselves to be "a male trapped in a female body." With those relatively rare exceptions, development of sexuality leads to a secure sense of maleness or femaleness which is generally complete by the age of three. However, in our culture doubts and conflicts about masculinity and femininity are ubiquitous. Serious disturbances lead to paraphilias such as transvestism, fetishism, voyeurism, and exhibitionism.

SEXUAL SYSTEM AND PERSONALITY. Much more often the physician is called upon to deal with less overt conflicts about gender identity that create significant marital problems with sexual connotations; examples are the Don Juan who has to prove his masculinity by sexual conquests, the promiscuous housewife who tries to prove to herself her femininity by finding the elusive orgasm or by demonstrating her attractiveness, the woman who cannot respond sexually because she is afraid of being completely dominated or possessed by a male, and the husband who cannot have sexual intercourse with his wife on top because it seems unmanly. The "battle of the sexes" is carried out not only in bed but in every area of marital interaction, generally by people who are uncertain of their masculinity or femininity and who fight to gain self-respect by derogating the partner. Several generations ago these sexually related social roles were handed down or "assigned" by tradition; today, roles are negotiable, and problems become serious when negotiation is impossible to attain because of faulty communication, or when it breaks down because of disturbed perception or the fear of compromise. The sexual system develops as such an integral part of personality development that sexuality and personality are inseparably interwoven. The physician who wishes to be an effective sex counselor, therefore, must deal with sexual relations in the context of human, especially marital, relations.

GENDER ROLE BEHAVIOR. Gender role refers to the entire spectrum of roles for a particular sex, male or female, in a particular cultural system. The culture has orientations as to, for example, whether that sex should place primary emphasis on an occupational career or on a family; whether that sex should develop attributes of aggressiveness or of nurture; whether members of that sex should be leaders of a political party or of a religious group, or teach in a primary school or in a university system. The culture defines in sometimes clear and sometimes not so clear terms the expectations of society for males and females and the expectations of the males and females in each institution in society. There is a reciprocal relationship between gender identity and gender role behavior. How one feels about oneself as masculine or feminine affects one's behavior in institutional settings; conversely, one's behavior in a variety of institutional settings affects the way one feels about one's sex.

Sexual role behavior may be thought of as *proceptive, acceptive,* and *conceptive.* The proceptive is the phase of initial, erotic interaction between the couple — of attraction and attractiveness, solicitation and courtship. It may be initiated by either partner serially or by both reciprocally. In the absence of a partner, it may be initiated in imagery and fantasy. Whether alone or with a partner, the subjective experience includes anticipatory sexual drive, interest, or desire. The proceptive phase may be viewed in its longitudinal aspects, as part of psychosexual development, and it may be seen, as well, as part of a single sexual encounter, or of an ongoing relationship.

Proception is followed by acception, the phase of bodily interaction and potential genital union. This phase subdivides into stages of excitement, plateau, orgasm, and resolution. Excitement involves a subjective sense of sexual pleasure accompanying physiologic changes. The major change in a male consists of penile tumescence (erection). The major changes in the female consist of vasocongestion generalized in the pelvis with lubrication of the vagina and swelling of the external genitalia. Plateau consists of sustained sexual excitement and progressive physiologic changes. In the male there is the appearance of Cowper's gland secretion. In the female there is the development of the orgasmic platform, which is the swelling of the outer third of the vaginal vault, vasocongestion of the labia minora, breast tumescence, and ballooning of the inner two thirds of the vaginal vault. Orgasm consists of a subjective sense of ecstatic peaking of sexual pleasure with which sexual tension is resolved. The male has a sensation of ejaculatory inevitability preceding ejaculation of semen, propelled by spasmodic contractions of the prostate, seminal vesicles, and urethra. The female has spasmodic contractions of the outer third of the vaginal vault which may be subjectively experienced as either pulsatile or diffuse. Both male and female undergo generalized muscular contractions, usually including involuntary pelvic thrusting. Resolution consists of general muscular relaxation and a sense of well being and contentment. During this phase men are physiologically refractory to responding to additional sexual stimulation for a variable period of time. In women the refractory period may be very brief, depending on the intensity of the erotic stimulation and response.

Sexual inhibition may occur at the proceptive stage, leading to anxiety-ridden or neurotic forms of pair-bonding. Inhibition at this phase may also lead to inhibition of sexual desire. Inhibition in the acceptive phase may occur at any of the four subphases, although rarely is an inhibition of the resolution phase of primary clinical significance.

The conceptive phase is the phase of conception, pregnancy, childbirth and, eventually, parenthood. Pregnancy and parenthood usually have important repercussions on sexual behavior. The life-cycle changes often usher in sexual problems demanding the attention of the physician.

240. CLASSIFICATION OF SEXUAL DYSFUNCTIONS

The major sexual dysfunctions are listed in Table 2.

INHIBITED SEXUAL DESIRE

In most cases, a persistent inhibition of sexual desire is situational and acquired and is usually a result of marital conflicts and disappointments. If lifelong, it is a consequence of the early association of sexual pleasure with anxiety and/or guilt, occasionally resulting from sexual trauma such as rape or incest. Generalized inhibited sexual desire can occur as a defense against im-

TABLE 2. Types of Sexual Dysfunctions

Inhibited sexual desire
Inhibited sexual excitement (frigidity, impotence)
Inhibited female orgasm
Inhibited male orgasm
Premature ejaculation
Dyspareunia
Vaginismus
Other psychosexual dysfunctions

pulses (homosexual and sadomasochistic are the most common) that the patient is trying to ward off. Much more frequently it is caused by depression. Not uncommonly, one finds inhibited sexual desire as a consequence of chronic illness, even in the absence of depression. In men inhibition of desire may on rare occasions be associated with low levels of plasma testosterone, perhaps 250 nanograms per 100 ml, warranting a trial of replacement hormone; but usually there is no direct correlation between testosterone levels above 300 ng per 100 ml and sexual desire or capacity for erection. (In women there seems to be a more direct relationship between testosterone levels and sex drive and responsivity.) However, the relationship between the husband's sexual initiation and his wife's sexual responsivity, defined as the "sexual compatibility ratio," over a three-month period correlates significantly ($P < 0.05$) with the husband's average testosterone levels over the same period of time, indicating that biologic factors play a role in the frequency and responsivity of sustained sexual relationships.

INHIBITED SEXUAL EXCITEMENT

One of the most frequent sexual dysfunctions is the recurrent and persistent inhibition of sexual excitement during sexual activity with another person or alone. The inhibition is manifested by either (1) partial or complete failure to attain or maintain erection until completion of the sexual act (impotence), or (2) partial or complete failure to attain or maintain the lubrication-swelling response of sexual excitement until completion of the sexual act (frigidity). The term "frigidity" can be used if we narrow the definition to make it synonymous with "inhibited sexual excitement." In the past the term "frigidity" has been of little use, because it has been used to mean "inhibited sexual desire," "inhibited excitement," or "inhibited orgasm," or even the lack of pleasure in the presence of normal psychophysiologic responsivity. The diagnosis of "inhibited sexual excitement" should be made only if the clinician judges that the individual engages in sexual activity which is adequate in focus, intensity, and duration with the desired partner or means. Often, the failure to respond with adequate vasocongestion of either the penis or the vagina is a consequence of inadequate sexual stimulation due to either ignorance or selfishness.

IMPOTENCE. Impotence may be secondary to an inhibition of sexual desire. In the face of failure to attain or maintain an erection, the man's frustration is generally much more intense if there is adequate desire. The most common cause of impotence is anxiety with a particular partner, in which case marital-sexual therapy is the treatment of choice. If impotence is generalized and does not seem to be a consequence of marital conflict, the clinician should look for depression or some organic factor such as diabetes, and should also inquire about medication being used by the patient, e.g., antihypertensive drugs or psychotropic agents. Chronic alcoholism is often associated with impotence because testosterone metabolism seems to be adversely affected, with resultant low levels of plasma testosterone. This usually occurs in the presence of liver disease.

If the man gives a history of absent or infrequent morning or nighttime erections, or the inability to attain good erections with masturbation, rapid eye movement (REM) sleep studies are indicated, since the normal man has about 90 minutes of "erection time" associated with REM sleep during a nighttime of sleeping. It is possible to measure nocturnal penile tumescence (NPT) with special recording devices. If organic factors are present, there will be absent or inadequate erections during REM sleep.

FRIGIDITY (AS FORMERLY DEFINED). With either impotence or frigidity, lifelong inhibition of sexual excitement results from the association of adverse emotions, namely, anxiety, shame, and guilt, with sexual pleasure. In those cases, individual psychotherapy is often the treatment of choice, but only after a trial of conjoint couple therapy. However, most cases of inhibited sexual excitement in the female are acquired and are a consequence of the same negative emotions operating within the context of marriage. If the woman has been responsive earlier with her husband, or is now responsive with other partners, conjoint marital-sexual therapy is indicated, provided she is sufficiently committed to her marital relationship. This, in conjunction with specific behavioral techniques by which the woman is able to re-experience the sexual pleasure she has now lost, may be curative. However, if there is a great deal of hostility toward the spouse, marital therapy aimed at reducing anger and resentment must be carried out prior to specific sexual behavioral therapies. If frigidity is generalized, i.e., even with self-stimulation and/or with other partners, the clinician should search for organic causes. Here again, diabetes and medication are the most common causes of frigidity.

INHIBITED FEMALE ORGASM

This syndrome is characterized by the recurrent and persistent inhibition of the female orgasm, as manifested by delay or absence of orgasm following a normal sexual-excitement phase during sexual activity which is judged by the clinician to be adequate in focus, intensity, and duration. The majority of women are able to experience orgasm during clitoral stimulation but are not able to experience orgasm during coitus. There is evidence that suggests that in some instances this represents a symptomatic inhibition, justifying this diagnosis. In other women, failure to achieve orgasm during coitus represents a normal variation of the female sexual response. This is based on surveys which indicate that only approximately 30 per cent of women are able to achieve coital orgasm fairly frequently. If 70 per cent of women cannot achieve coital orgasm at all, or do so infrequently, it is probable that coital anorgasmia may be a normal variation, rather than a consequence of psychopathology. This difficult diagnosis can be made only by a thorough sexual evaluation, which may even require a trial of treatment. It is an important distinction clinically, since many women still ask for professional assistance because of this complaint.

The woman who is unable to achieve orgasm at all through *any* source of stimulation (about 10 per cent) can be helped in about 80 per cent of the cases by behavioral techniques. The use of sensate-focus as described by Masters and Johnson and the use of a vibrator have been helpful aids, at least in attaining noncoital orgasm. It is generally more difficult, even for the experienced sex therapist, to decrease a woman's inhibitions so that she is able to obtain coital orgasms fairly regularly. Referring back to the levels of intervention and the various roles of the physician, the physician-counselor is usually able to treat a woman who is completely anorgasmic, whereas it is generally necessary to refer a woman who wishes to achieve coital orgasm to a sex therapist.

INHIBITED MALE ORGASM

A relatively infrequent complaint compared with other types of sexual dysfunction is the recurrent and persistent inhibition of the male orgasm as manifested by a delay or absence of either the emission or ejaculation phases, or more usually both, following an adequate phase of sexual excitement. Although the vast majority of these cases are psychogenic, occasionally one finds this difficulty as a sequela of antihypertensive medication. Retarded ejaculation must be differentiated from retrograde ejaculation, which occurs most commonly after prostatectomy. Treatment of retarded ejaculation usually requires a combination of psychotherapy and couple-oriented behavioral techniques.

PREMATURE EJACULATION

It is impossible to use a normative length of time for the plateau phase of the sexual response cycle, i.e., the time between erection and ejaculation. Thus the diagnosis of premature ejaculation depends entirely on the man's distress over the recurrent and persistent absence of reasonable voluntary control of ejaculation and orgasm during sexual activity. Stated more simply, ejaculation occurs before the individual wants it. This dysfunction, with rare exceptions, is psychogenic and is a consequence of anxiety. The natural biologic sequence would be for rapid ejaculation after erection, and the male has to learn through experience to extend the plateau phase. Fortunately, there are excellent behavioral techniques for overcoming this frequent disorder. Use of the so-called "stop-and-start" technique during stimulation of the penis by his partner allows the male to recognize the sensations *prior* to ejaculatory inevitability. At the point when sensation will soon merge into ejaculatory inevitability, he signals his partner to cease stimulation for about 30 seconds, after which stimulation can be resumed. The same technique can be learned during copulatory pelvic thrusting. In this fashion over 95 per cent of men with premature ejaculation are reported to be cured of this distress. This technique is a simple one that can be easily taught to the patient; it thus comes under the province of the physician-counselor. The rare patient refractory to this method of therapy should be referred to a sex therapist.

"IMMEDIATE" CAUSES OF SEXUAL DYSFUNCTION

Every patient with inhibited excitement or orgasm or with premature ejaculation is adversely affected by "immediate" causes of sexual dysfunction. These are fear of failure, or anxiety over performance, which increases the underlying source of anxiety; the monitoring of one's own performance, called "spectatoring" by Masters and Johnson, that puts distance between the patient and his participation in the sex act; often an inordinate need to please the partner, providing another significant cause of increased anxiety; and the failure to talk about one's sources of anxiety, a reparative device which generally tends to accentuate anxiety. These dimensions of dysfunction can be dealt with by the physician-counselor, provided he is aware of them and is skillful enough to get his patient to discuss them. Reducing these immediate causes of sexual dysfunction is the first therapeutic task of any counselor or therapist. In many instances the immediate causes of sexual dysfunction turn out to be the only ones. For example, a man may lose his erection two or three times in the course of a week or two because of fatigue or preoccupation with business or because of some animosity toward his wife or because of too much drinking. This starts a vicious cycle of fear of failure or anxiety about performance, monitoring his own behavior, and being too exquisitely tuned to the reactions of his female partner. The anxiety increases into panic, and the inhibition becomes definite and pronounced. Indeed, anxiety can be differentiated from panic by the following quip: "*Anxiety* is the first time a man cannot get an erection twice, and *panic* is the second time he cannot get it once."

DYSPAREUNIA

Recurrent and persistent genital pain associated with coitus is not restricted to the female, although it is much more common in women than in men. Organic factors are frequent, so that adequate gynecologic and/or urologic examination is mandatory. Despite this, the most frequent cause of dyspareunia in the female is the relative absence of lubrication during the sexual response cycle. Coitus with a dry vagina often produces dyspareunia. A test of this can be made by having the woman use artificial lubrication. Dyspareunia may or may not be accompanied by vaginismus.

VAGINISMUS

Vaginismus can be diagnosed if there is a history of recurrent and persistent involuntary spasm of the musculature of the outer one third of the vagina that interferes with sexual activity. The diagnosis can be confirmed during a pelvic examination. If the vaginismus has been preceded by a history of dyspareunia, the underlying causes of dyspareunia must be discovered and treated first. If the vaginismus is psychogenic, the disorder can be readily overcome by a combination of psychotherapy and the use of graduated Hegar dilators. Very frequently the woman can be taught to dilate her own vagina in the so-called "sexological" examination. Techniques of doing this are demonstrated in the presence of her husband, as his cooperation is enlisted. Many but not all so-called "unconsummated" marriages are due to vaginismus. The treatment of the unconsummated marriage is then directed toward the treatment of vaginismus. (It should not be overlooked that a sig-nificant number of unconsummated marriages are due to either impotence on the part of the husband or to an inhibition of sexual desire in either or both husband and wife.)

OTHER SEXUAL DYSFUNCTIONS

In the absence of a specific sexual dysfunction, distress can come from a variety of other reasons. An individual may feel that he or she is not meeting some fantasied standard of sexual performance, or there may be feelings of inadequacy related to self-imposed standards of masculinity or femininity such as bodily habitus or size or shape of the sex organs. Sometimes a patient may express distress over the inability to respond sexually in certain specific situations in ways that are desired. Although the patient is desirous of sexual activity, there may be a marital conflict leading to avoidance of sexual activities, which in turn increases conflict. Sometimes the very intensity of sexual excitement can create anxiety and discomfort. Occasionally one finds a patient engaging in a variety of sexual behaviors, but who feels very little or no pleasure in the activity (sexual anhedonia). A very frequent couple conflict results when there are discrepant sexual desires for frequency, forms of foreplay, or coital positions, or when partner is exerting deliberate control of sexual expression over the other.

As has been discussed earlier, the physician-educator who is comfortable in dealing with sexual problems can clear up many sexual concerns by giving appropriate information. Sexual misunderstanding and misinformation are extensive; only a few examples are given here: the adolescent boy who thinks his penis is too small, or the teenage girl who thinks she is abnormal because of her sexual urges; the notion that oral-genital sex is a perverse activity; the frequent concept that coital orgasm is the only form of orgasm that is normal; that masturbation is abnormal and may even lead to mental illness; that direct clitoral stimulation must be continued until penetration occurs; that waxing and waning of sexual excitement is abnormal; that sexual activity during pregnancy or weeks after recovery from a coronary occlusion is dangerous; or that after the age of 50 or 60 or 70 a person is sexually "over the hill."

241. ADDITIONAL PROBLEM AREAS

When any of the specific sexual dysfunctions occur in a marital relationship, they may be the result of (1) sufficient psychopathology on the part of one or both spouses, (2) a poor relationship of "fit" between the spouses, or (3) relative ignorance of one or both partners. An example of the first category is the wife whose life experience taught her that sex is nasty and sinful and who cannot experience sexual pleasure, for the pleasure would increase her guilt inordinately. Patients in this category with longstanding sexual dysfunction are generally referred to psychiatrists. Patients whose difficulties stem largely from a poor marital relationship may be seen by the nonpsychiatric physician, who, unless he has had special training in sex and marriage counseling, must be mindful of his own capacities and limitations.

In evaluating any sexual problem, it is necessary to determine how much weight to attach to the three factors contributing to the problem. Often, all three are represented. The woman who has the concept of sex as a sinful activity and who inhibits her responsivity may have only a hazy idea of what pattern of stimulation is best suited to increase her sexual excitement, and may make all sorts of excuses to her husband ("I'm tired" or "I have a headache" or "It's my period") to avoid sex, or she may grant or withhold sex as a weapon to punish her husband or in bargaining for something she wants.

Although the sexual problems that arise in marriage constitute the most frequent and most important need for professional intervention, additional characteristic sexual problems arise during the life cycle. Including marital sexual problems, some of the more frequent problem areas are the following:

Helping children and their parents deal with problems of sexual development includes concerns about masturbation, sex play among children, menstruation, wet dreams, sexual fantasies, and coital activity among teenagers. "How do I, as a parent, talk to my children about sex?" is a question often asked of physicians.

Concerns of teenagers may include masturbation, penis size, how far to go during petting, the relation of sex to the relationships between sexes (how does sex relate to love?), erotic arousal for members of the same sex, contraception, and sexual performance. Unwanted pregnancy creates a need for abortion or "problem pregnancy" counseling. Venereal disease may occur at any age level, but it is increasing rapidly among teenagers.

Among young adults contemplating marriage, concerns include sexual performance and compatibility, as well as family planning.

Separation, such as occurs with divorce or death in the middle-aged or elderly, creates very special sexual problems. The loss of companionship and affection may be even more important than the decrease in sexual opportunities, although the interest in sex itself among the elderly is characteristically unrecognized or minimized by the physician.

Although *childhood sex play and masturbation* are now recognized as part of normal psychosexual development, parents are frequently concerned enough to ask their physicians about these behaviors. In most instances reassurance is all that is needed. If the sexual activity is "excessive" (and this is often subject to varying interpretation), it indicates a narrowing of the range of healthy social activities of the child rather than the abnormality of the sexual behavior per se. The basic points in talking to children or teenagers is to be as comfortable as possible, and to be brief, concise, and factual once the real concerns are elicited, by gently encouraging the child to talk and, above all, to avoid lecturing in a pontifical fashion. The physician is more apt to be "heard" if he discusses the pros and cons of sexual decision-making, rather than expressing his own value position in a forceful manner.

The problem of premarital coitus is characteristically presented by the unmarried girl who asks her physician for the "pill." If freedom of the physician is not restricted by his own set of values, this provides him with an opportunity to discuss with the young patient her feelings and expectations about her relationship with her actual or intended partner. Physicians are often concerned that prescribing contraception for the unmarried girl will be a license for sexual activity, and some still refuse to do so. Actually, the young girl usually asks for contraception *after,* rather than before, the initial coital experience. A study of over 500 unwed never-pregnant teenagers aged 13 to 17, who for the first time sought professional help to obtain contraception, showed that 96 per cent of those teenagers who asked for contraception were previously sexually active; most of them had been having intercourse for more than a year; few were using any contraceptives, and still fewer were using one of the most effective methods. It should be clear that if a minor requests contraception, she needs it. This study and others suggest that contraceptive information and educational programs directed at minors will not be a significant factor in their decision to become sexually active.

A special area of increasing concern to physicians is called *"problem pregnancy" counseling.* This is not restricted to teenagers, as the majority of abortions are performed on married women. The unmarried pregnant teenager, however, is in a highly vulnerable position, because pregnancy and childbearing may seriously interfere with her educational and economic status, while the negative social sanctions against abortion that still persist make her face difficult choices. The various options — e.g., continuing with the pregnancy and giving up the baby for adoption or keeping the baby, whether to marry or not, or whether to terminate pregnancy — must be discussed thoroughly, and outside pressures for decision-making should be separated from internal conflict. The availability of legal abortion for those who can afford it has greatly eased the situation. However, the decision for abortion should never be made lightly, because the physician should be fairly certain that the patient will not be in the small minority who suffer from depression or remorse after the abortion. This applies to married women as well as to the unmarried. Most patients (who are not harmed by the abortion procedure per se) would derive special benefits by more intensive contraceptive, sex, and family counseling than is ordinarily provided to women seeking abortion.

Family-planning counseling gives the physician an unparalleled opportunity for exploring the connections between sexual attitudes and behavior and contraceptive concerns. The choice of the appropriate method of contraception is influenced by the frequency of coitus, attitudes toward responsibility and decision-making, fears of bodily damage, and desires for greater sexual spontaneity, as well as religious and moral values. Contraceptive failures are related to risk-taking, to the failure to learn how or under what conditions conception occurs, or to the individual's being under stress so that "contraceptive vigilance" is reduced. Adequate communication with the partner about contraceptive planning is an important consequence of appropriate counseling. Family planning is much more than the prescription of a contraceptive method. It includes the timing of marriage, timing of the first child, child-spacing, the total number of children desired, and sex- and marriage-counseling, as well as counseling in contraception, problem-pregnancy, and sterilization methods. Genetic counseling may also be a significant dimension of family planning. In this sense, family-planning counseling is an essential feature of premarital counseling, but should be available throughout the childbearing years.

Patients frequently misperceive *the spouse's desired frequency of intercourse;* most often the wife overestimates her husband's desired frequency. In one sixth of the cases studied, there was a gross underestimation of the wife's desires. The perception of the problem is usually more significant than the reality. The physician can often help by asking each spouse separately how often each wants intercourse, and each one's perception of the spouse's desires. Better communication is the first step toward relieving this problem and, in many instances, may be all that is required. The physician also has to bear in mind that the sex drive in the male is at a peak between the ages of 15 and 25, whereas in the female it peaks a decade later.

242. HOMOSEXUALITY

The etiology of homosexuality — preferential or exclusive sexual activity with a member of the same sex — is not known. At present an intense debate among psychiatrists is raging whether to regard homosexuality as a normal sexual variant or as a psychopathologic development — in other words, a deviation. The American Psychiatric Association has removed homosexuality from its list of disorders (Diagnostic and Statistical Manual No. 2) and has established a category called "sexual orientation disorder" for those who are distressed by their homosexual desires or behavior and seek help to resolve this conflict.

Although homosexuality is found in virtually every society and culture around the world, there is no society in which it is the dominant or preferred mode of sexual activity. (If there were, it is clear that that particular society would eventually vanish.) It is also known that if, in a given society, repression of sexual behaviors — including homosexual play — is absent during prepubertal development, adult homosexuality is extremely rare. This implies, but is by no means a proven fact, that childhood repression of sexual behavior is the principal cause of adult homosexuality.

Sexual programming of the brain, principally the hypothalamus, during a critical period of fetal life prepares the individual for later sexual behavior. This occurs in every mammalian species studied, including man. It is conceivable but still highly conjectural that some as yet unknown mechanism interfering with this brain programming may be an important contributing factor in the etiology of homosexuality. It may take a combination of brain programming and certain types of social learning in childhood to bring about preferential same-sex behavior in the adults.

If called upon to give counsel to a homosexual, the physician's approach should in no way differ from the approach to a heterosexual. No attempt should be made to try to direct him into heterosexual behavior unless he specifically requests such help. If his motivation is high, if he still has heterosexual dreams or fantasies, if he has had one or more successful heterosexual encounters, and if his first homosexual experience occurred after the age of 16, the prognosis for changing to bisexuality or even preferential heterosexuality is reasonable. About one in three with these good prognostic indicators can be helped to become successfully heterosexual. This generally requires the skillful help of a competent and experienced psychotherapist.

LESBIANISM

The young woman who discovers that she is attracted to members of her own sex and who gradually develops an erotic interest in other females faces two major problems. One is the definition of her own gender identity; the other is a sense of isolation. Such women often remain uncertain of their sexual preferences for several years, and their resulting intense internal struggle is heightened by actual or anticipated parental and societal disapproval or rejection. Strong feelings of alienation accompany the self-condemnation of this internal conflict, and the affected woman may regard herself as unique with problems shared by few others, especially not by her friends or peers.

The physician or school counselor who is called upon to help these young women has to set a neutral, non-condemnatory, nonjudgmental course. Too quick an acceptance of the patient's lesbianism with facile reassurance may increase the young woman's anxiety, for she may be far from certain of her sexual preferences, whereas obviously a judgmental, censorious attitude will make her too uncomfortable to remain in treatment. The counselor's task is to help the patient reach some sort of closure (and this may take considerable time) about which direction she wishes to take, and then to help her with the social skills necessary to achieve a degree of intimacy, either heterosexually or homosexually. If the young woman decides that her preference is for lesbianism, the counselor also has to help the patient deal realistically with her parents and possibly with school authorities.

This is often a delicate matter, involving ethical decisions by the counselor, and tact, sensitivity, and good judgment are essential. Many schools have peer counseling adjuncts which, along with group counseling, may be useful in overcoming the woman's loneliness and feelings of inferiority. Although social condemnation for homosexual men and women is decreasing and "gay" groups are organized in many communities, most young people are afraid to identify themselves as being homosexual, and the adjustment to that special subculture, although ultimately helpful, is almost never without apprehension and even anguish.

SUMMARY

If the physician is interested in helping his patients with sexual problems, and if he is reasonably comfortable and tactful and has an appreciation of the role his own feelings and attitudes play in interviewing and treatment, he will be able to establish a feeling of confidence and hope in his patient. This empathic relationship, coupled with the physician's growing fund of information and skills in interviewing, makes possible the competent management of marital and sexual problems that heretofore have been either neglected or mishandled. In no other area of his practice can the physician derive greater reward and satisfaction from his efforts.

Abse, D. W., Nash, E. M. and Louden, L. M. R. (eds.): Marital and Sexual Counseling in Medical Practice. New York, Harper & Row, 1974.

Gadpaille, W. J.: The Cycles of Sex. New York, Scribners, 1975.
Kaplan, H. S.: The New Sex Therapy. New York, Bruner-Mazel, 1974.
Lief, H. I.: Sexual counseling. *In* Romney, S., Gray, M. J., Little, B., Merrill, J., Quilligan, T., and Stander, R. (eds.): Gynecology and Obstetrics: The Health Care of Women. New York, McGraw-Hill Book Company, 1975, Chap. 31, pp. 526–548.
Mandel, T., and Oline, P.: Counseling the lesbian. *In* Money, J., and Musaph, H. (eds.): Handbook of Sexology. Amsterdam, Excerpta Medica, 1977, Chap. 101, pp. 1279–1288.
Money, J., and Musaph, H.: Handbook of Sexology. Amsterdam, Excerpta Medica, 1977.
Vincent, C. E.: Sexual and Marital Health: The Physician as Consultant. New York, McGraw-Hill Book Company, 1973.

Section Seven   DRUG ABUSE, DEPENDENCE, AND INTOXICATION

243.   INTRODUCTION

Robert B. Millman

Drug abuse is behavior that results from the complex interaction of an individual, his social and cultural environment, and the pharmacology and availability of particular drugs. There is frequently no sharp line that distinguishes appropriate use from misuse of any drug. Drug abuse may therfore be defined as the use of any substance in a manner that deviates from the accepted medical, social, or legal patterns within a given society. This section will consider the abuse of drugs that are primarily used to induce alterations in mood, perception, and behavior. These may be grouped into six major classes: (1) opiates; (2) central nervous system depressants, including alcohol, hypnotics, and tranquilizers; (3) central nervous system stimulants, including the amphetamine group and cocaine; (4) cannabis; (5) psychedelics; and (6) miscellaneous inhalants.

Abuse of some drugs may be intermittent and lead to little physical, psychologic, or social deterioration. In other cases, the user may become dependent on the drug in order to function at what he perceives to be a satisfactory level. This *psychologic dependence,* or habituation, varies in intensity and may culminate in *compulsive drug abuse,* in which the supply and use of particular drugs become primary concerns of living. In addition, certain drugs have the capacity to produce *physical dependence.* This is an altered physiologic state induced by the repeated administration of a drug that requires the continued administration of the drug to prevent the appearance of a syndrome characteristic for each drug, the *withdrawal,* or *abstinence, syndrome.* The term "addiction" has been used in the literature to refer to either behavioral or pharmacologic events. As used herein, it refers to a pattern of compulsive drug use that includes both physical dependence and an overwhelming involvement with the supply and use of a drug. Neither a diabetic who is on insulin nor a well adjusted patient in methadone maintenance treatment is an addict in this sense of the term, although both are physically dependent on their medication.

ETIOLOGY AND PATTERNS OF ABUSE. No single factor is the basis of all drug-taking experience, and no person's drug taking has a single cause. Initially, drugs may be taken to satisfy curiosity, to reduce pain, to influence mood, to change activity levels, to reduce tension and anxiety, to decrease fatigue and boredom, to facilitate social interaction, to heighten sensation and awareness, and for many other reasons. If caffeine, nicotine, alcohol, and prescription and over-the-counter depressants and stimulants are included, few people in the United States would be found who take no psychoactive drugs. Patterns of abuse vary from the experimental or intermittent use of a particular drug or combination under defined circumstances, such as the use of marijuana and alcohol at a party, to a compulsive "polydrug-abuse" pattern, in which a variety of drugs are taken in a disorganized and dangerous manner on a daily basis.

SOCIOLOGIC FACTORS. Social and cultural factors determine which drug-abuse patterns are acceptable for a given group; and in some cases, groups derive their identity from particular drug-using behavior. The use of alcohol is condoned and even encouraged in many segments of society. Cannabis and psychedelic use are an integral part of membership in some white middle class groups. Heroin use, until recently, was considered an involving, exciting pursuit in inner-city ghetto areas. Given the limited opportunities to experience pleasure, satisfaction, or pride in certain underprivileged groups, moreover, the aggressive, goal-oriented life of a heroin addict may appear attractive to a young boy or girl. Social factors also determine the availability of particular drugs. Heroin is easily available in the inner city, whereas the suburban dweller may have to travel long distances to obtain the drug. The extent and patterns of abuse change rapidly in response to a variety of social and cultural factors. Accurate epidemiologic information is difficult to obtain because of the illegal or covert nature of the behavior and the necessarily indirect surveying methods. Currently (1978), the prevalence of heroin, alcohol, and polydrug abuse in this country appears to be increasing; amphetamine and psychedelic use are decreasing. Cocaine and marijuana appear to be more frequently used, and the patterns of abuse of these drugs have changed considerably over the last decade.

PSYCHOBIOLOGIC FACTORS. Personality and constitutional factors, in part, determine the psychoactive effects that drugs elicit in individual users and influence the choice of drugs and patterns of abuse. Amphetamines may produce tranquility in some people. Alcohol and barbiturates impair behavior control in others and may permit certain personality types to act in a hostile and violent manner. Genetic factors have been strongly implicated in the development of alcoholism.

Controversy exists as to whether drug abuse implies a personality disturbance that antedates drug use and that can be classified in distinct groups according to the drug and pattern of abuse. Some workers describe well defined addictive or alcoholic personality types, characterized by a mixture of neurotic traits and character disorders, although present evidence suggests that personality characteristics in drug-abusing populations vary considerably and that psychologic factors play a markedly variable role in the etiology of drug abuse. Although premorbid personality disturbances are crucial in the etiology of some cases of compulsive drug use, the psychopathology noted in other cases may be a reaction to the behavioral patterns of compulsive abuse in a society that condemns the drug-dependent life. *Moreover, no predictive test or system has been developed that will determine whether or not a person will become a compulsive user, nor which people will use which drugs.* It is generally agreed that the experimental or intermittent abuse of drugs is not necessarily an indication of psychopathology. Compulsive drug use *is* frequently associated with psychopathology. In some people the drug use may be an attempt at *self-medication* of painful feelings of anxiety, shame, inadequacy, loneliness, guilt, and depression. Others may be seeking to allay unacceptable aggressive or sexual drives or to control psychotic symptoms. At the same time, some severely disturbed people have experimented with alcohol, opiates, and other drugs and have not become compulsive users. The more aberrant an individual's drug-abuse behavior pattern is for his particular social or cultural milieu, the more likely there is a significant degree of psychopathology.

Conditioned learning is an integral part of the development and maintenance of compulsive drug-abuse patterns. The feelings of dysphoria that the drug-taking behavior allayed or some of the situations attendant to the behavior become, in time, the conditioned stimulus for the experience of drug craving and the persistence of drug-seeking behavior. This may occur in the presence or absence of physical dependence. The drug-craving and withdrawal syndrome that long abstinent ex-addicts experience when they return to a site of former drug use is, in part, a reflection of this conditioning process. Learning also influences the nature of the drug experience.

Various disease states are treated with psychoactive drugs for prolonged periods. The drug use of a small percentage of patients may come to exceed medically recommended dosages or indications and eventuate in drug dependence in some cases. Psychologic and sociologic factors should be considered in the etiology of these behavior patterns in addition to the physical and pharmacologic determinants.

PHARMACOLOGIC FACTORS. The nature of the psychic and physical effects of particular drugs is a determinant of their abuse potential. Considerations of physical dependence and tolerance influence the pattern of abuse. *Tolerance* refers to the decreased effect obtained from repeated administration of a given dose of a drug or to the need for increased amounts to obtain the effects that occurred from the first dose. Tolerance may be either *drug disposition* (metabolic) in type, in which there is more rapid inactivation or excretion of a drug, or *pharmacodynamic* (cellular), in which cells in the nervous system adapt to drug concentrations. Both may occur with the same drug. The physical dependence that develops concurrently with tolerance to opiates, barbiturates, and alcohol is poorly understood and may be related to pharmacodynamic tolerance mechanisms. *Cross-dependence* refers to the ability of one drug to suppress abstinence symptoms produced by withdrawal of another. Cross-dependence may be complete or partial, as with alcohol and the barbiturates.

DIAGNOSIS. To provide adequate treatment, it is necessary to characterize the specific problems of drug abuse and dependence in each patient as well as the psychologic set and the social situation attendant to the use of the psychoactive substances. The nature and degree of drug-induced psychoactive effects and any abstinence symptoms and signs should be assessed. This requires careful history taking when possible, including information on the type, amount, and pattern of chemical use, and a complete physical examination. Drug abusers are often poor historians and may minimize or exaggerate the extent of their drug use, depending on their perception of the situation, their needs, and the attitude of the examiner. It is likely that an opiate user will exaggerate the extent of his use so as to obtain more opiates during the detoxification process and perhaps suffer decreased abstinence symptoms. A college student may minimize his diazepam dependence, since the extent of his use might be considered evidence of weakness or serious psychopathology. Pressing social or legal needs should be identified with a view toward providing realistic, often necessarily short-term solutions.

Evaluation of the mode of administration and the adverse effects of the drugs of abuse is important in establishing a diagnosis. Signs of repeated intravenous injections ("tracks") suggest heroin, amphetamine, or cocaine abuse. These drugs are also "sniffed," whereby the material is inhaled and absorbed through the mucous membranes of the nasopharynx and respiratory tract. Chronic sinusitis or perforation of the nasal septum may suggest this mode of administration. Personal hygiene and patterns of behavior and dress may further define the clinical picture.

Routine qualitative procedures for the detection in urine of morphine (the major metabolite of heroin), methadone, amphetamines, cocaine, and the most frequently abused general depressants are currently available in many laboratories. Results will generally be positive if a dose sufficient to produce pharmacologic effects has been taken within 24 hours prior to the urine sample. Since results are not immediately available ordinarily and since false positives occur, these tests should be used to confirm the clinical impression. They are most useful as an adjunct to the long-term evaluation of patients already in treatment. In emergency situations, blood levels of suspected drugs can usually be obtained immediately.

TREATMENT AND PREVENTION. Treatment procedures should vary according to the individual and his social set, the pattern and extent of abuse, and the pharmacology of the abused drugs, as well as the goals of treatment. As distinct from most other patients, drug abusers frequently know more about the behavior and disability incident to drug taking than do their physicians. Serving to further complicate therapeutic efforts, drug abusers are often faced with prejudice and hostility on the part of treatment personnel, e.g., "They did it to themselves." Since many of their personality characteristics and behavior patterns occur in response to the attitudes of society, an inquiring, compassionate attitude is crucial in the treatment of this group of patients.

These patients commonly do not show consistent progress, often resuming the use of drugs after detoxification and varying periods of abstinence. This tends to frustrate the efforts of the physician or the treatment team, who may be provoked to give up on particular patients. The problem here may be a conceptual one;

physicians often regard substance abuse as an acute illness, not unlike pneumonia, and liable to complete cure after detoxification. This is an unrealistic assumption given the chronic nature of most psychologic and social difficulties. Then, too, the character of the pharmacologic dependence may be more protracted than previously imagined. Since the clinical course in some of these patients may be reminiscent of diabetes or schizophrenia, with remissions and exacerbations, treatment should be seen as consisting of both immediate and long-term measures. Patience and continuing enthusiasm are as essential as in most other branches of medicine.

Drug-abuse prevention programs have focused on educational efforts in which the risks of drug abuse are publicized, and on legal sanctions. Both approaches have serious deficiencies. Perhaps more important than either of these would be the provision of reasonably attractive vocational, recreational, and educational alternatives to drug abuse in those most at risk, namely, the young and psychosocially disadvantaged. Physicians must be extremely prudent in their prescribing practices with respect to potentially abusable drugs.

244. THE OPIATES

Robert B. Millman

Opiates or narcotic analgesics refer to natural or synthetic drugs that have pharmacologic actions similar to those of the derivatives of opium. Opium is obtained from the poppy plant *Papaver somniferum* and contains more than 20 alkaloids, of which morphine and codeine are relevant to this discussion. Heroin, the principal opiate of abuse in the United States, is converted from morphine by the addition of two acetyl groups (diacetyl-morphine). Meperidine and methadone are synthetic narcotic analgesics. Pentazocine is a synthetic analgesic compound that has actions similar to both the opiates and the narcotic antagonists.

INCIDENCE.   People have used opium for medical, religious, or recreational purposes since ancient times. Marked changes have occurred in the characteristics of the opiate-abusing population in the United States during the past 100 years. The use of patent medicines containing opiates was widespread in the middle class during the period from 1850 to 1906, when the labeling requirements of the Pure Food and Drug Act caused many preparations to be withdrawn. The Harrison Narcotics Act of 1914 and Supreme Court decisions in the 1920's made possession of narcotics without a prescription a crime and created a climate in which addicts were considered to be criminals and in which physicians could not prescribe narcotics to addicts. The number of oral opiate users declined, and the primary remaining group were those who injected heroin or morphine. Illegal dealers became the only source of opiates. Prices rose precipitously, and addicts frequently resorted to criminal activity to finance their addiction. The addict population from the 1930's to World War II predominantly consisted of white individuals involved in criminal activity or the entertainment professions who used intravenous heroin as well as morphine, cocaine, and other drugs. The growth of urban black ghettos and the development of efficient production and delivery systems ushered in the present era of extensive heroin use associated with a pervasive street culture that supports the heroin-dependent life.

Heroin use reached epidemic proportions in the United States in the mid- to late 1960's. The majority of users were members of ethnic minority groups and lived in major urban areas. Males predominated over females, and the population was quite young. In New York City in 1971, heroin was the major cause of death in males aged 15 to 35. Large numbers of affluent white suburban youths were also becoming addicted. During the early 1970's, the incidence of heroin addiction declined owing to a multiplicity of factors, including changing social and cultural styles, the proliferation of effective treatment programs, and decreased availability of heroin. More recently there appears to be a resurgence of the problem, with a shift in the highest rates of incidence to smaller cities and more rural areas. The total number of heroin addicts in this country in 1975 was estimated to be between 500,000 and 600,000.

PATTERNS OF ABUSE.   People initially experiment with heroin for many reasons, including a search for pleasure, curiosity, anxiety, immaturity, sexual problems, psychopathology, and peer pressure. In some urban ghetto areas, given the lack of attractive alternatives, using and selling heroin appears to be a rewarding, involving "career" that carries with it the illusion of wealth and significance. Users are generally introduced to the drug by a friend or acquaintance already using the drug. The majority of first-time users have already had drug-abuse experience, particularly alcohol and marijuana. The role of the nonaddicted drug dealer ("profiteer") is minimal in exposing new users to the drug. Street heroin ("smack," "scag," "junk," "dope") is adulterated ("cut") with quinine, lactose, mannitol, maltose, and other substances as it passes from the importer to the street user. The final amount of heroin in a street package costing from two to ten dollars may vary from 2 to 20 mg.

Initial street use is generally by "sniffing," in which the material is absorbed through the mucous membranes of the nasopharynx and respiratory tract. A user's first experience with the drug is often characterized as somewhat unpleasant because of nausea, vomiting, and anxiety; these symptoms abate with subsequent use. Effects may then be perceived as a sense of relaxation and peace with relief of worry and tension, a euphoric state in which all things are as they should be. At the outset, use may be intermittent and separated by weeks or months. It is not known how many people experiment with the drug and do not continue its use. Those who do continue to use heroin develop tolerance to its euphoric effects. In an attempt to maximize the euphoric effects of a given street amount, users will begin to inject the drug subcutaneously ("skin-popping") and eventually intravenously ("mainlining"). Intravenous injection produces a warm flushing of the skin and pleasurable sensations in the entire body, described as similar to sexual orgasm and called a "rush" or "kick." Many years of intravenous use of opiates and other drugs may result in obliteration of patent, available veins, necessitating a return to the subcutaneous mode of injection.

As tolerance increases and the awareness of physical dependence becomes manifest, more drug must be used more often. The urban street addict with little access to legitimate sources of money or drug must devote all his time and energy to the acquisition of heroin to support his addiction ("habit"). Involvement in the "junkie" subculture, with its own language and behavioral systems, ensures his supply of drug and provides for the transmission of skills, information, and ideology that make it possible to live as an addict. Any source of money is acceptable; males frequently engage in theft and forgery, whereas females will be prostitutes and shoplifters. Every user is a potential "dealer" of drugs, because this is the most efficient way of making money. Food, clothing, sexual desires, and dignity may become subordinate to the ever-present need for opiates. An unknown number of heroin addicts, particularly those in the entertainment professions, are able to maintain their employment and their families and do not become immersed in the behavior patterns of the street "junkie."

If heroin is not available or is in poor supply, addicts will use other opiates, particularly illicitly obtained ("street") methadone because of its long duration of action, to allay their withdrawal symptoms. Compulsive use of illicit methadone occurs, although usually after an initial period of heroin dependence. Primary methadone addiction is rare, because the drug is commonly available in oral form only and the intensity of its euphoric properties is less than that of heroin. Concurrent use of alcohol, sedatives, and marijuana occurs in up to 75 per cent of narcotic addicts, and mixed addictions in this group are frequently seen. Use of stimulants in association with narcotics is also quite common.

Opiate addicts are a heterogeneous group. They demonstrate a significant amount of psychopathology, including high levels of neurotic, personality, and psychotic characteristics, although no common pathologic pattern is apparent. Personality characteristics and behavior patterns frequently result from the interaction of the addict and the drug in the sociocultural environment of addiction. The incidence of premorbid psychopathology is controversial and depends in part on how deviant the behavior is relative to a given social milieu and how difficult it is to get the drugs. Inner-city minority-group addicts are often remarkably stable given their difficult living situations and the high degree of personality integration and intelligence required to survive as a street addict. Middle-class people are often more severely disturbed, and the drug use represents an attempt at self-medication for the symptomatology incident to borderline or psychotic personality disorders. The ability of the drugs to control severe symptomatology may derive from their anxiety-relieving qualities, direct antipsychotic effects, as well as the very structured existence street-heroin addiction often mandates. Some of these people are able to function effectively as street addicts but decompensate acutely or chronically when the heroin is withdrawn or when methadone is substituted. Under these circumstances, patients often will abuse other drugs, particularly those in the sedative-alcohol group.

PHARMACOLOGY. Opiates are absorbed from the gastrointestinal tract or the nasal mucosa, and after subcutaneous, intramuscular, or intravenous injection. Morphine and heroin lose much of their analgesic potency when taken orally, whereas codeine and meperidine remain quite active, and methadone retains most of its analgesic efficacy after oral administration. Heroin is hydrolyzed to morphine in the body and, except for its greater potency and more rapid onset of action, has pharmacologic properties similar to those of morphine. Morphine is concentrated in parenchymatous tissues, skeletal muscle, and, to a lesser extent, brain. It is conjugated with glucuronic acid and excreted primarily in the urine and secondarily in the feces. Traces of morphine can be found in urine for 48 hours, although 90 per cent or more is excreted within the first 24 hours.

Administered subcutaneously, methadone and morphine exert approximately equal analgesic effects; heroin is three times stronger, whereas meperidine and codeine are approximately one tenth as potent. Morphine or heroin taken intravenously is effective almost immediately; duration of action varies from three to six hours. Oral administration prolongs the action of all the opiates, particularly that of methadone, in which the onset of effect occurs within 30 minutes and the duration of action in nontolerant individuals is four to ten hours.

Morphine or heroin administered to a nontolerant individual induces analgesia through a reduction in the anxiety and tension that result from the perception of pain. Related to this is a positive feeling of well-being or euphoria. Somnolence, characterized by an inability to concentrate, sleepiness, or "nodding," also occurs. Opiates cause pupillary constriction, depression of respiration by decreasing the responsiveness of the brainstem to carbon dioxide, depression of body temperature, and stimulation of central nervous system centers to produce nausea and vomiting. Other acute effects include decreased motility of the stomach, diminished pancreatic and biliary secretions, decreased propulsive contractions of the small and large intestine, and increased tone of the anal sphincter, leading to constipation. Increased tone of the detrusor muscle leads to a sensation of urgency accompanied by increased tone of the vesical sphincter, resulting in urinary retention. An acute release of antidiuretic hormone is effected, as well as inhibition of release of ACTH, corticotropin-releasing factor, and gonadotropin. Peripheral vasodilatation occurs, resulting in pruritus and possibly causing the observed increase in perspiration. Histamine release occurs, frequently resulting in a wheal-and-flare reaction, or "hive," at the site of injection and in a "pins-and-needles" sensation.

ADDICTION AND WITHDRAWAL PROCESSES. Repeated use of narcotic analgesics produces tolerance to most of the acute narcotic effects, and the lethal dose is markedly increased. Whereas a 10-mg dose of morphine may produce euphoria in a nontolerant individual, the daily use of 5 grams has been reported in addicts. The rate at which this tolerance develops depends on the frequency and magnitude of use. Street addicts may spend from $20 to $200 or more daily on heroin and may inject themselves every three to six hours. Tolerance to all the opiate effects does not occur equally, because highly tolerant users will continue to demonstrate pupillary constriction and constipation. Cross-tolerance occurs with all narcotic analgesics. Tolerance to narcotics is primarily due to some form of cellular adaptation to the drug's action, with increased metabolism of lesser importance.

Physical dependence develops concurrently with tolerance and has been demonstrated after only a few exposures on succeeding days. It is marked by the development of an acute abstinence syndrome upon withdrawal of opiates, the "cold-turkey" process. This syndrome is quite variable in severity and characteristics and depends upon the particular drug, the dose, the interval between doses, and the duration of narcotic use, as well as on the personality and immediate environment of the narcotic addict. With heroin, the first withdrawal signs are generally seen shortly before the next scheduled dose. They are purposive in nature and include feelings of anxiety, restlessness, irritability, and drug craving. Lacrimation, rhinorrhea, yawning, and perspiration become apparent 8 to 15 hours after the last dose of narcotic. A restless sleep may intervene, the so-called "yen sleep," from which the addict awakens with more severe withdrawal symptoms and signs, including dilated pupils, sneezing, coryza, anorexia, nausea, vomiting, diarrhea, abdominal cramps, bone pains, myalgias, tremors, weakness, insomnia, goose flesh, and, very rarely, convulsions or cardiovascular collapse. With morphine and heroin, withdrawal symptoms peak at 36 to 48 hours, and most observable symptoms gradually subside over the next five to ten days. With methadone, the onset of withdrawal symptoms is more gradual, the peak is less pronounced and later, and the duration may be more than two or three weeks. The abstinence syndrome may be precipitated within minutes in opiate-dependent persons by administration of a narcotic antagonist such as nalorphine, levallorphan, or naloxone, although there are no medical indications for this diagnostic procedure.

Pentazocine (Talwin), a drug with weak opiate-antagonist effects and moderate opiate-agonist effects, elicits morphine-like subjective effects in nontolerant individuals. Higher doses produce dysphoric effects, including nervousness, anxiety, and, infrequently, bizarre alterations in perception and behavior. Tolerance and physical dependence occur, and cases of addiction to this drug are reported. Abrupt withdrawal of the drug from persons taking 500 to 700 mg daily results in an abstinence syndrome marked by irritability, abdominal cramps, nausea, vomiting, hyperthermia, lacrimation, and drug-seeking behavior. When pentazocine is administered to opiate-dependent patients, its antagonistic actions may precipitate withdrawal symptoms.

Subsequent to the termination of abstinence symptoms or after a course of detoxification with decreasing doses of opiates, most addicts experience recurrent urges for narcotics and generally resume their use of these drugs. The traditional psychologic theory of relapse presumes that, after withdrawal, the physiologic causes of drug taking have been removed, but that addicts have an "addictive personality" disorder that causes them to return to opiate addiction to escape reality. Psychologic factors play a role, although no predictive test has been developed to distinguish future addicts from future nonaddicts; nor are addicts able to be distinguished from nonaddicts by psychologic evaluation when they are observed under the same abstinent conditions. Evidence is accumulating that metabolic and neurophysiologic changes persist long after the detoxification process is completed, as does some tolerance. Protracted abstinence signs, as indicated by alterations in blood pressure, pulse rate, body temperature, respiratory rate, and pupillary size, and symptoms, including the depression and anxiety, have been documented for up to 30 weeks, and may relate to the chronic drug craving reported and the high incidence of relapse. The conditioned associations abstinent ex-addicts experience when they are exposed to their old neighborhoods and friends are also involved in the persistence of drug craving.

Narcotic addiction with its implicit relapses after periods of abstinence should be viewed as a disease of complex etiology in which *a persistent neurochemical disturbance*, as well as profound psychologic and social factors, contributes to the dominance of drug-seeking behavior.

MECHANISM OF OPIATE ACTION. The recent discovery of structurally and sterically specific receptors for the opiates in brain, spinal cord, and other nervous tissue in all vertebrates studied, including man, may shed light on the mode of action of the opiates and on the dependence-withdrawal cycle. These receptors seem to be localized in the areas of the nervous system associated with the integration of sensory information and emotion, particularly the limbic system. The presence of these receptors in species that have little or no contact with opiates led to the discovery of naturally occurring morphine-like peptides in the brain and gastrointestinal tract (enkephalins) and pituitary gland (endorphins) of many animal species. These endogenous morphine-like compounds elicit analgesia, produce tolerance and physical dependence, and compete with radioactive opiates for the receptor. It is of considerable interest that all the peptides so far identified except one have amino acid sequences present in the pituitary hormone, β-lipotropin. The function of these substances is not clear, but certain of them may be neurotransmitters and implicated in the control of pain, affective states, and appetitive drives. A model that includes a neurohumoral feedback mechanism has been postulated to play a part in the opiate addiction syndrome. If, under resting conditions, opiate receptors are exposed to a basal level of the morphine-like substances, when exogenous opiate is administered, the overloading of the opiate receptors might suppress the release of endogenous opioid. Termination of the exogenous opiate administration might produce a deficiency of the endogenous opioid at the receptor, which could be implicated in the immediate or protracted abstinence syndrome.

MEDICAL COMPLICATIONS. When a known dose of an opiate is administered under aseptic conditions, either occasionally or chronically, medical complications are almost unkown. There are well-documented cases of long-term opiate addiction in physicians and others in whom no adverse physical effects were found. The patterns of use, including life style, unknown and markedly variable opiate dose, lack of hygienic administration techniques, and the variety of adulterants used to dilute the opiate, are responsible for the extensive morbidity and mortality (estimated to be about 1 per cent per year) associated with opiate abuse and dependence.

Acute heroin reactions secondary to intravenous use of street drug are responsible for one half to three quarters of all fatalities from narcotics. Formerly thought of as true pharmacologic overdoses with respiratory depression, these reactions may also be due to opiate-induced cardiac arrhythmias or hypoxia by unexplained mechanisms. Acute reactions to adulterants, including quinine, allergic reactions, and synergistic effects from multiple-drug use, may also be implicated. The syndrome is marked clinically by the rapid development of cyanosis, pulmonary edema, respiratory distress, and varying levels of consciousness progressing to coma. Increased intracranial pressure and occasionally convulsive seizures are seen. Fever to 40° C may occur initially and may persist for 48 hours in association with leukocytosis. The pupils are usually pinpoint, although dilated, nonreactive pupils may occur in the presence of hypoxia or multiple-drug use. The pathologic picture includes pulmonary congestion and edema and frequently cerebral edema.

Skin abscesses, cellulitis, and *thrombophlebitis* are the most frequent complications of heroin addiction. Skin manifestations are particularly noted after the subcutaneous injection of heroin and its adulterants. Pentazocine injection causes characteristic chronic ulcers in areas of severe "woody" induration. *Septicemia* and *acute* and *subacute bacterial endocarditis* with involvement of either or both sides of the heart are seen. *Staphylococcus aureus* is frequently the causative organism in right-sided lesions. Peripheral and pulmonary embolic phenomena occur. Osteomyelitis occurs infrequently. Malaria was a frequent complication in the 1930's. The introduction of quinine as an adulterant and the eradication of malaria in this country have decreased the incidence of this complication.

Viral hepatitis transmitted by the communal use of contaminated needles is a frequent complication of intravenous drug use. Abnormal liver function tests, hypergammaglobulinemia, and increased serum immunoglobulins that persist for long periods of time after the acute episodes and that occur in addicts with no history of hepatitis are due in some cases to variants of chronic hepatitis, but may also be due to effects produced by alcohol, malnutrition, allergic phenomena, adulterants, and recurrent or chronic infections. False-positive serologic tests for syphilis are due to these factors, although there is a high incidence of syphilis and other venereal diseases in this population. The nephrotic syndrome has been seen in association with street heroin use as well.

Pulmonary complications include pneumonia, abscess, infarction, and tuberculosis. Disseminated extrapulmonary tuberculosis has been reported. Angiothrombotic pulmonary hypertension and granulomatosis result from the intravenous injection of foreign bodies, including talc or cotton. Vascular lesions include local arterial occlusion, phlebitis, mycotic aneurysms, and necrotizing angiitis.

Neurologic complications of street heroin use include transverse myelitis, peripheral nerve lesions, toxic amblyopia secondary to quinine, and muscle disorders, including acute rhabdomyolysis with myoglobinuria and a fibrosing chronic myopathy. Septic states may lead to bacterial meningitis and brain, subdural, and epidural abscesses. In this country, narcotism is a leading cause of tetanus, particularly when the drugs are injected by the intramuscular route. The course is generally more severe relative to a non-drug-using population, with mortality rates in the 50 to 75 per cent range.

Menstrual irregularities in addicted women have been described, although it is unknown whether these can be ascribed to narcotic-induced suppression of adrenocorticotropic hormone and gonadotropic release or to malnutrition, frequent infections, and the general life style of female addicts. There is a high incidence of toxemia and of prematurity in infants born to addicted mothers, probably because of these life-style factors and the lack of prenatal care. Withdrawal symptoms are noted in a variable percentage of these newborn. Sexual difficulties, including decreased libido, impotence, and delayed ejaculation, are frequent in male heroin addicts, although the etiology is unclear.

Homicide, suicide, and *accidents* account for between 20 and 40 per cent of all narcotic-related deaths. It is often difficult to distinguish these.

TREATMENT. Methods of treatment of narcotic dependence vary considerably, depending on the treatment goals, the factors that are thought to be most significant in the etiology of a patient's addiction, and the characteristics of individual patients. The magnitude of the addict's desire to stop using opiates is an important factor in the selection of the appropriate treatment modality as well as in the outcome. These motivational factors are difficult to assess, since, within one or two years after the onset of the addiction, most addicts express the wish to terminate it. Nevertheless, many continue the compulsive use of heroin for many years and suffer repeated treatment failures. Approaches are primarily psychosocial, pharmacologic, or combinations of these. Since addiction has physical, psychologic, and social determinants, treatment is best provided by a well-organized team approach. Individual practitioners should be prepared to make an accurate diagnosis, treat the acute and chronic sequelae of the drug use, and effect the appropriate referral.

WITHDRAWAL TECHNIQUES. Withdrawal of narcotics is most effectively accomplished by inpatient or outpatient substitution of oral methadone for any of the natural or synthetic narcotic analgesics (detoxification). Doses ranging from 20 to 40 mg daily are instituted, followed by a gradual reduction of dosage over the course of 10 to 14 days or more. Detoxification with decreasing doses of propoxyphene napsylate, a mild analgesic, has been effective, particularly when the degree of dependence is minimal or methadone is not available. In some cases, patients are withdrawn in a drug-free environment without opiate substitution, although this has proved less justifiable on medical and moral grounds. The chronic nature of this disease necessitates the provision of psychologic, legal, and vocational supportive services throughout the detoxification process and continuing into the drug-free period.

METHADONE MAINTENANCE

In this country, methadone maintenance has been the most widely used approach in the treatment of opiate dependence. This mode of therapy emphasizes social and emotional rehabilitation rather than abstinence. The treatment is based on the two major properties that distinguish methadone from other narcotics: good oral efficacy and long duration of action. After oral ingestion in tolerant individuals, the duration of action of methadone is extended to 24 to 36 hours owing to a reservoir of drug in tissues. Initially, oral methadone is administered daily in doses that will allay symptoms of abstinence. The dose is gradually increased until a stabilization level is reached at which patients will be tolerant to the euphoric effects of the drug and will experience no persistent craving for opiates. If the stabilization level is high enough (80 to 100 mg), there is a good degree of cross-tolerance to the effects of other narcotics, such that the effects of even large doses of intravenous opiates will not be felt ("narcotic blockade"). Approximately 65 per cent of patients in well-run programs remain in treatment. Improvement has been noted in the work and school records of patients retained in the program, and their criminal activity has declined markedly. Long-term methadone maintenance has been shown to be medically safe, with no toxicity when properly administered. Side effects include increased sweating, constipation, and some impairment of sexual function. Performance and learning are normal in methadone-maintained subjects. Medication should be dispensed in a clinic situation that provides medical care and extensive rehabilitative services so as to facilitate satisfactory re-entry into non-drug-dominated ("straight") society.

The effort to treat large numbers of people with limited budgets and space has produced overcrowded treatment programs that provide few ancillary services. A significant percentage of patients, although they may be heroin free, are unable to acquire the necessary skills and education to alter their life styles and continue to compulsively abuse alcohol and other drugs. Illicit diversion of methadone doses by clinic patients has led to the availability of the drug for the street-addict population.

Programs using methadone maintenance for varying periods of time followed by a slow-detoxification process are being evaluated, although the majority of adult patients with long-term addiction histories have been unable to remain drug free for extended periods of time. Clinical trials are presently under way with levo-alpha acetyl methadol (LAAM), a synthetic congener of methadone that extends opiate effects for 72 hours. Treatment might be rendered more efficiently if certain patients were required to attend clinics only three times weekly to ingest medication, and the risk of narcotic diversion would be minimized.

Various programs that would provide heroin under supervision are also being considered (heroin maintenance). The short-acting nature of the drug, the rapid development of tolerance, and the necessity to inject it render this form of treatment less potentially useful.

NARCOTIC ANTAGONISTS

Narcotic antagonists such as cyclazocine and naltrexone are being evaluated for the treatment of detoxified addicts. These agents block or attenuate the euphoriant effects of narcotics and prevent the development of physical dependence in patients who continue to use narcotics. Drug-seeking behavior might be extinguished insofar as it depends on conditioned associations to euphoric drug effects or abstinence symptoms. Prevention of the development of physical dependence might also minimize the continuation of narcotic use after a spree, and increase periods of abstinence. These drugs do not relieve the chronic opiate-drug hunger, and patients are prone to omit their dose of antagonist and relapse to heroin. A major advance would be the discovery of a medicine that relieves all symptoms of physical dependence, blocks the opiate-induced euphoria, does not itself produce physical dependence, and is not subject to abuse.

PSYCHOSOCIAL APPROACHES — ABSTINENCE PROGRAMS

A diverse array of programs exist that emphasize abstinence from opiates and other drugs as a primary component of treatment. These take the form of either voluntary groups or supervised institutionalization.

Voluntary groups are generally communities that are self-regulatory in nature and staffed predominantly by former drug users. The individual remains in the closed, drug-free environment for variable periods of time, frequently one to two years, and is encouraged to develop a new set of social and living skills that will enable him to remain drug free upon completion of the program. Outpatient programs are also under way. Intensive therapeutic techniques are utilized to eliminate the social and personality deficiencies of residents that led them to drug use. These facilities serve to reduce the sense of isolation felt by many drug users and attempt to provide role models for responsible behavior. Some of the well-known groups are Synanon, Daytop Village, and Phoenix House. Although sharing many common methods and doctrines, these communities vary considerably in the nature of the therapeutic milieu created and in the complex system of rewards and punishments provided residents. Therapeutic communities are valuable for many people, although only a small percentage of heroin addicts are motivated to enter a community, and follow-up studies of individuals who have returned to society are not presently available.

An alternative approach is programs which involve the nonpunitive incarceration of an addict for the purposes of rehabilitation (civil commitment). These programs generally include a period of enforced abstinence in a prison, hospital, or other locked facility, followed by a careful supervision of the individual in the community. If renewed drug abuse or other antisocial behavior is noted, the addict is reinstitutionalized. To date, these programs have met with meager success. If adequate rehabilitative services and facilities are made available in the future, the efficacy of these programs might be increased.

Results of traditional psychotherapeutic techniques, other than to enhance motivation, have been disappointing for the majority of compulsive opiate abusers. Specialized forms of group psychotherapy may be useful for some patients. After variable and sometimes prolonged periods of addiction, an unknown number of addicts spontaneously cease opiate use. This "maturing-out" process may be related to advanced age and the difficulty of obtaining drugs, a decline of internal psychologic conflicts, and the cumulative effect of various treatment programs.

245.   CENTRAL NERVOUS SYSTEM DEPRESSANTS

Robert B. Millman

All central nervous system depressants are subject to abuse. The most frequently abused drugs in this category are the short-acting barbiturates, particularly pentobarbital (Nembutal) and secobarbital (Seconal), assorted other hypnotics such as glutethimide (Doriden), methyprylon (Noludar), and methaqualone (Quāālude), and tranquilizers, particularly diazepam (Valium) and chlordiazepoxide (Librium), and amitriptyline (Elavil), an antidepressant with sedative properties. Bromide abuse has become rare. Since many of the characteristics of these drugs are similar, this discussion will center on the barbiturates, with other agents considered when relevant.

INCIDENCE AND PATTERNS OF ABUSE.   There is a continuum of depressant use that extends from appropriate use to compulsive abuse and addiction. Depressants in general and the benzodiazepines in particular have become the most widely prescribed drugs throughout the world. In 1971 alone, in the United States there were 50 million prescriptions for diazepam and 24 million for chlordiazepoxide. The medical indications are quite broad and include insomnia, depressive and anxiety states, convulsive disorders, and alcohol withdrawal. The pattern of use may begin as intermittent use at night to decrease anxiety and ensure sleep, progress to nightly use with increased doses, and culminate in prolonged daily use to maintain an adequate level of function. An individual may obtain drugs from several physicians at one time, none of whom are aware of the magnitude of their patient's depressant use. In this group there may be no illicit drug use, although alcohol is frequently used in association with the depressants.

Hypnotic and tranquilizer use is also present in urban drug subcultures. Heroin addicts use depressants ("downs") to supplement the poor quality of heroin available. Alcoholics will also use hypnotics when they are available, since the quality of the intoxications is similar. Although some people abuse depressants preferentially, concurrent physical dependence on alcohol or opiates is more common than pure depressant dependence in these groups. Illicit sources of drugs are most often employed, and a wealth of street names have evolved for the most popular hypnotics, including "reds" (secobarbital), "yellows" (pentobarbital), and "double trouble" (amobarbital and secobarbital). Most use is oral, although some individuals inject their drugs intravenously or intramuscularly. The amounts taken vary markedly, but some individuals have ingested as much as 30 hypnotic doses of the short-acting barbiturates or benzodiazepines daily over many months.

Recently, a marked increase in the use of illicitly obtained depressants has been noted in some adolescent and preadolescent populations. Patterns and extent of use vary markedly, but generally multiple-drug use occurs and is considered appropriate behavior within these groups. Intermittent users may take several times the therapeutic dose, possibly in addition to marijuana, alcohol, and amphetamines if they are available, to get "high" enough to enjoy a concert or party.

The "high" that obtains from abuse of depressant drugs has been characterized as the sense of tranquility or peace that occurs just prior to sleep in normal individuals. The world is seen as limited to the immediate. Inhibitions and anxiety are blunted, and there may be a feeling of aggressiveness, freedom, and pleasant numbness. Sexual pleasure and ability are said to be enhanced at low doses of these drugs; higher doses lead to a decreased ability to perform sexually. Violent and antisocial behavior occurs, frequently serving to isolate depressant abusers ("down heads") from other groups of drug abusers.

There appears to be a high incidence of serious psychopathology in compulsive abusers of the depressant drugs. Users may be seeking obtundation in attempts to cope with anxiety arising from a variety of sources.

PHARMACOLOGY. Barbiturates and related hypnotics are rapidly absorbed after oral administration and are distributed throughout the body. They are general depressants of nerves and of skeletal, smooth, and cardiac muscles, although at low doses the central nervous system is primarily affected. Central nervous system effects vary from mild sedation to coma, depending on the particular drug, the dose, the route of administration, the degree of excitability of the nervous system, and tolerance. In some individuals under certain circumstances, small doses produce an initial stimulation not unlike that produced by alcohol. Barbiturate-induced sleep is similar to physiologic sleep except for a reduction in the proportion of rapid eye movement (REM) sleeping time. Duration of action varies with the particular barbiturate. Aftereffects, including drowsiness, depression, impairment of judgment and performance, and occasionally hyperexcitability, may persist for many hours.

Both drug-disposition and pharmacodynamic tolerance to the barbiturates and related hypnotics develop rapidly with repeated administration. Drug-disposition tolerance in the short-acting barbiturates and some other depressants results from the activation of drug-metabolizing liver-enzyme systems and is characterized by the more rapid degradation of the drug and a decrease in sleeping time. The range of tolerance is narrow, and individuals tolerant to the sedating and intoxicating effects of 1 gram of pentobarbital may become intoxicated for prolonged periods upon the addition of 0.1 gram. Although the lethal dose of barbiturates varies in individuals, in distinction to the opiates, tolerance does not increase this dose significantly from that of nontolerant individuals. Severe poisoning is likely to occur when more than ten times the hypnotic dose is ingested at one time. Acute barbiturate poisoning may thus be superimposed on chronic intoxication at any time. The combination of sublethal doses of depressants with opiates or alcohol may also result in acute poisoning. Cross-tolerance develops to all barbiturates as well as to paraldehyde, meprobamate, and benzodiazepines. Partial cross-tolerance between alcohol and the depressants occurs.

CLINICAL MANIFESTATIONS. Acute depressant poisoning may occur either accidentally or incident to a suicide attempt. Accidental overdoses may be due in some cases to "drug automatism"; an individual may fail to fall asleep after several hypnotic doses, become confused, and ingest an overdose. Upon recovery, there may be no memory of the excessive drug ingestion. The clinical manifestations and treatment of poisoning are discussed in Ch. 251. The acute and chronic signs and symptoms of mild hypnotic intoxication resemble those of intoxication with alcohol. The individual shows general sluggishness, difficulty in thinking, slowness of speech and comprehension, poor memory, faulty judgment, emotional lability, and narrowed attention span. Neurologic signs of depressant intoxication include thick, slurred speech, nystagmus, diplopia, strabismus, vertigo, ataxic gait, positive Romberg sign, hypotonia, dysmetria, and decreased superficial reflexes. Sensation, deep-tendon reflexes, and pupillary responses are unaltered. Skin rashes have been reported. Unexplained seizures in adults should always prompt one to consider chronic depressant drug abuse.

With compulsive users, clothing may be unkempt and nutrition poor; needle marks and abscesses from intramuscular or intravenous use may be present. Adverse effects of chronic depressant use are poorly documented, but may be similar to those of alcohol on organ systems and the brain.

ABSTINENCE SYNDROME. Physical dependence, as indicated by abstinence signs and symptoms, develops to all the central nervous system general depressants. A characteristic *general depressant withdrawal syndrome* occurs and is similar to the symptoms of withdrawal from alcohol. It varies in severity, depending on the drug, dose, and frequency of use. *In contrast to the opiate withdrawal syndrome, that from depressants may be life-threatening.* The first manifestation of this syndrome might be considered the rebound increase in nightly rapid eye movement sleep, associated with nightmares and a sense of having slept badly, that occurs after discontinuation of use of only therapeutic doses of barbiturates for several nights. After a daily dose of 0.4 gram of pentobarbital for three months, abrupt withdrawal produces paroxysmal EEG changes without other significant symptoms. After 0.6 gram per day for one to two months, 50 per cent of patients experience insomnia, tremors, and anorexia. Sudden withdrawal from long-term daily use of only therapeutic doses of the benzodiazepines (45 mg of diazepam per day) will produce abstinence symptoms; withdrawal from higher doses may produce seizures and delirium. In general, the time required to produce physical dependence is shorter with the short-acting barbiturates and the withdrawal symptoms are more abrupt in onset and more severe than with the longer-acting sedatives.

When short-acting hypnotics are abruptly withdrawn, signs and symptoms of the intoxication clear over the initial 12 to 16 hours, and the patient appears to improve. Increases in restlessness, anxiety, tremulousness, and weakness then occur, which may be accompanied by cramps, nausea, vomiting, and orthostatic hypotension. These symptoms progress, and coarse hand tremors, muscle twitching, hyperactive deep reflexes, and increased blink reflex appear within 24 hours. Symptoms generally attain their peak during the second and third days, and convulsions may occur then or before. Some patients who have seizures may begin to show improvement, but 50 per cent develop a delirium that is marked by sensorial clouding, visual and auditory hallucinations, and disorientation to time and place. During the delirium, which usually occurs between the fourth and seventh days, hyperthermia, tachycardia, and agitation can lead to exhaustion and sometimes to fatal cardiovascular collapse. The abstinence syndrome generally clears by about the eighth day, and there is usually no residual physical damage. Clearing is frequently preceded by a period of prolonged sleep. With longer-acting barbiturates and benzodiazepines, seizures may not occur until the seventh or eighth day. Psychotic symptoms may persist for many months, but these may be related to pre-existing psychopathology.

TREATMENT. Treatment procedures include withdrawal and rehabilitative phases. Compulsive abusers of depressants are often considered more difficult to treat than any other class of drug abusers. Outreach and educational programs aimed at intermittent abusers of depressants before they become addicted may be important in this regard. The pattern of use and extent of physical dependence should be evaluated by means of a careful history and physical examination. Depressant abusers frequently distort or are unaware of the magnitude of their use, particularly those with a concurrent addiction to heroin.

If physical dependence is suspected, close observation or hospitalization is indicated. When the diagnosis is established, a suitable general depressant should be administered after the intoxication clears but before major withdrawal symptoms have begun. Phenobarbital orally is a suitable substitute for most of the general depressants. Its long duration of action provides for more constant blood levels and added protection against the development of either withdrawal symptoms or dangerous intoxication. Other barbiturates or benzodiazepines may be used as well if the pharmacology of both the drug of abuse and the withdrawal regimen are known. Patients who are taking large amounts of lesser known sedatives should probably be withdrawn from the original drug of abuse if it is known. If the patient will not tolerate the oral administration of phenobarbital or more rapid sedation is required, intramuscular injections of the same doses may be used. Patients may usually be switched to oral drugs after a few intramuscular injections. Sufficient phenobarbital should be given to produce a mild but manageable level of intoxication marked by inconstant slow nystagmus on lateral gaze, slight dysarthria, and ataxia. A rough approx-

imation of the dosage of phenobarbital to be given daily is calculated by substituting 30 mg of phenobarbital for each 100 mg of the short-acting barbiturate the patient reports using. Most patients will require between 100 and 300 mg daily for stabilization, to be given in four divided doses; a total of 600 mg daily should not be exceeded. This "stabilization dose" should be carefully controlled to prevent signs of increased intoxication, such as dysarthria, emotional lability, constant nystagmus, or gross ataxia. Patients should be maintained on this dose for 24 to 48 hours, after which the dose of phenobarbital should be reduced by 30 mg or less daily. The patient should be observed carefully for signs of insomnia, tremulousness, and orthostatic hypotension, at which time the withdrawal should be suspended for one to two days. If symptoms are severe, the patient should be given 100 mg of phenobarbital intramuscularly immediately, which will usually suppress them. Delirium, convulsions, or fever should be treated as emergencies with increased doses until the patient is able to sleep for 8 to 12 hours, after which the stabilization dose is determined, as described above. Once a withdrawal delirium develops, increased doses of phenobarbital may fail to restore equilibrium; agitation and disorientation may persist for several days.

Fluid and electrolyte losses must be replaced, and complicating medical and surgical conditions treated. Increasing fever without evidence of infection necessitates additional sedation, antipyretics, sponging, or cooling blankets. Phenothiazines, butyrophenones, and diphenylhydantoin are not indicated. In general, the use of the phenobarbital substitution technique may take from ten days to three weeks. It should not be hurried. During the process, patients should be encouraged to be as active as possible, eating regularly and taking part in group activities. Patients who are concurrently dependent on opiates should be withdrawn from the general depressant first, while being maintained on suitable doses of methadone. Opiate withdrawal procedures may then be effected.

After withdrawal is completed, provision must be made for high-frequency supportive counseling. Patients are frequently withdrawn and depressed, and the danger of relapse or suicide is great. The inclusion of patients in therapeutic programs, either on an inpatient or on an ambulatory basis, should be assured.

Physicians must be cautious when prescribing depressants for the relief of anxiety and insomnia. Attempts should be made to diagnose and treat the source of these symptoms without medication. If necessary, benzodiazepine tranquilizers may be used in low doses for well-defined, short periods or on an intermittent basis.

BROMIDES. Chronic bromide intoxication (bromism) has become rare, because bromide has been supplanted in modern medicine with more effective and less toxic sedative and analgesic compounds. The daily ingestion of small doses will result in an accumulation of this long-acting drug to toxic levels over a period of weeks. Central nervous system symptoms and signs are the most common features and include drowsiness, impaired thought and memory, dizziness, and irritability, leading in more severe cases to delirium, hallucinations, lethargy, and coma. Neurologic disturbances include tremors, thick speech, motor incoordination, and decreased superficial reflexes. The diagnosis of chronic bromide intoxication is established by serum bromide levels above 9 mEq per liter in association with the aforementioned clinical picture.

Treatment consists of the daily administration of 200 mEq of either sodium or ammonium choride, together with sufficient fluids to ensure a large urine output. This reduces the half-life of bromide to three or four days. Diuresis with chloruretic drugs may be useful if more rapid displacement of bromide is indicated. Hemodialysis rapidly clears bromides and may be indicated in treating comatose patients.

246. CENTRAL NERVOUS SYSTEM STIMULANTS

Robert B. Millman

Central nervous system stimulants or sympathomimetics that are subject to abuse include the *amphetamines, cocaine, methylphenidate* (Ritalin), *phenmetrazine* (Preludin), and *diethylpropion* (Tepanil). This discussion will consider the amphetamine group primarily, including amphetamine, dextroamphetamine, and methamphetamine, which are synthetic derivatives of ephedrine, and cocaine, an alkaloid of the coca plant which grows in the Andes in South America.

INCIDENCE AND PATTERNS OF ABUSE. *Amphetamine abuse* has been widespread in industrial societies, particularly in Japan, Sweden, Great Britain, and North America. Enormous quantities were prescribed by physicians for the treatment of a variety of conditions, including obesity, depressive syndromes, behavior disorders, narcolepsy, and the reduction of fatigue. Many patients, frequently middle-class women, became dependent on these drugs when they found that they had to continue to ingest the drug to prevent depression and to perform optimally. The advent of tolerance necessitated increased doses, occasionally five to ten times the original 5- or 10-mg amount prescribed. Amphetamine abuse by students, athletes, truck drivers, and others who want to increase their efficiency or productivity is common. In both these patterns, oral preparations are used. Hypnotics are often used by this group to ensure sleep, and concurrent dependence on both classes of drugs is not unusual. A decline in use and abuse has occurred recently as a result of federal and state regulations that severely limit prescribing and manufacturing practices with respect to the amphetamines.

Another category of amphetamine abuser is composed of multidrug users, primarily young, who use these drugs for their mood-elevating properties. Any amphetamine may be used, although methamphetamine ("speed," "crystal," or "meth") is preferred, because it has more pronounced central effects and less peripheral ones. The drugs are taken orally on occasion, although "sniffing" or intravenous use is common in drug-dominated groups. Most methamphetamine is manufactured in illegal laboratories, but commercially available oral preparations are also dissolved for intravenous use.

Upon "sniffing," or particularly after intravenous use, the user experiences a "flash" or "rush" that is described as a sense of increased mental capacity and physical strength, with little need for food or sleep, and a feeling of power and intensity that is quite distinct from the feeling of satiation induced by the opiates. Increased activity, planning, and talking occur. Dissipation of the drug effects after three to six hours is experienced as an unpleasant sense of fatigue and depression ("crashing"). Use may be intermittent and limited to special occasions such as a party or journey, or may be more regular. Rarely, chronic amphetamine abusers report that the daily, controlled use of these drugs decreases the anxiety and tension they experience normally, and enhances their ability to eat, sleep, and generally function.

Some individuals use the drug continuously, to maintain the "high" or stave off the "crash" for several days or even longer (a "run"). As tolerance develops, the dose is increased and the drug taken more frequently, such that 1 gram may be injected every two to four hours. At this stage, the compulsive user, or "speed freak," is usually nervous, irritable, and suspicious. There may be intense involvement in complicated and often unnecessary tasks such as disassembling a television set or reorganizing a room. When the supply of drug is depleted or the user becomes too disorganized or debilitated to continue, the "run" ends. Cessation of amphetamine use is usually followed by a prolonged deep sleep. Hypnotics or alcohol are often used to minimize the duration of the "crashing" phase and facilitate the induction of sleep. Upon awakening, although much of the paranoid ideation may be gone, a feeling of lassitude, apathy, and depression may be present. Intravenous users frequently inject other drugs alone or in combination with amphetamines. The combination of amphetamines or cocaine and heroin is known as a "speed ball."

Most of the psychoactive effects of *cocaine* are similar to those of the amphetamines with regard to elevation of mood, decreased need for food or sleep, and hyperactivity. Supply is always through illicit channels; it is more expensive than the amphetamines, with a variable "gram" costing between $60 and $100, and it is much shorter acting. After intravenous administration, the primary mode in this country until recently, effects last 5 to 15 minutes. Intravenous use is generally seen in the same population that abuses heroin. Psychologic dependence and compulsive use occur, such that during a "run" of varying druation, 1 to 10 grams may be used during the course of a day via injections every half hour. In contrast to the amphetamines, there has been a recent marked increase in cocaine abuse in all sectors, particularly by affluent and middle-class people in urban areas. Use in this group, by sniffing the much-adulterated white powder, is generally intermittent; it is regarded as luxurious punctuation for a variety of occasions, to be used in conjunction with alcohol, hypnotics, and marijuana.

PHARMACOLOGY. Systemic effects of amphetamines and cocaine include increased cardiac contraction, increased blood pressure and heart rate, relaxation of the bronchial musculature, increased contractility of the urinary bladder sphincter, increased venous pressure, pulmonary arterial pressure, and renal blood flow. Central effects include stimulation of the cerebrospinal axis and the medullary respiratory center. In low doses these drugs increase alertness and physical and cognitive ability, particularly when performance has been compromised by lack of sleep. The significant appetite depression seen is probably due to a combination of factors, including an inhibitory effect on the feeding center in the lateral hypothalamus as well as the improvement in mood that occurs. Cocaine is an effective topical local anesthetic and vasoconstrictor of mucous membranes.

Tolerance develops to both the peripheral and central effects of the amphetamines. Tolerance to cocaine is not thought to occur; there may be some degree of psychologic tolerance to the euphoric effects of this drug, although it apparently dissipates rapidly. Cross-tolerance exists between the amphetamines, but no cross-tolerance has been demonstrated between the amphetamines and cocaine.

Cessation of amphetamine or cocaine use does not generally produce major physiologic symptoms. The depression, anxiety, increased appetite, lassitude, and prolonged sleep that ensue might be considered an abstinence syndrome and evidence of some physical dependence. Moreover, during this sleep, a characteristic electroencephalographic pattern is produced that shows a marked increase in the percentage of REM sleep, and nightmares may occur. In some cases, withdrawal has been marked by headaches, profuse sweating, muscle cramps, disorientation, and confusion.

ADVERSE EFFECTS. Adverse physical effects in intermittent users of amphetamines or cocaine by the sniffing route may be limited to irritation of the nasal mucosa or perforation of the nasal septum. Chronic users may be markedly debilitated and subject to numerous infections as a result of lack of sleep and poor nutrition. A sensation of something crawling under the skin is described ("cocaine bugs"), such that chronic users will frequently have excoriations and open sores from constant scratching and pinching. The intravenous use of these drugs is fraught with the numerous complications that result from nonsterile conditions, which are detailed in Ch. 244. Reports of necrotizing angiitis and moderate-to-severe occlusion of cerebral vessels resulting from the direct toxic effect of chronic methamphetamine use require further clarification, but may be implicated in brain damage and cerebrovascular accidents in youthful populations. *Acute amphetamine toxicity* is marked by extensions of the sympathomimetic effects, including tachycardia, hypertension, and arrhythmias culminating in convulsions, cerebrovascular accidents, and coma. *Acute cocaine toxicity* is characterized by initial sympathomimetic effects followed by cortical depression and anesthetization of the midbrain and medulla, leading to respiratory failure and cardiovascular collapse. The incidence of sudden fatalities due to amphetamines or cocaine is unknown. The lethal dosage of amphetamines is variable, depending on the extent of tolerance; that of cocaine is estimated to be about 1.2 grams.

There is a high incidence of pre-existing psychopathology in compulsive amphetamine and cocaine abusers, and the abuse itself engenders severe psychologic complications. The most frequent complications of amphetamine and cocaine abuse are paranoid ideation and stereotyped compulsive behavior. Chronic users are frequently aware of these characteristics of the drugs and will not act on ideas of persecution. Antisocial or violent behavior may occur when this insight is lacking. Continued use frequently leads to a well described *amphetamine or cocaine psychosis* that is often indistinguishable from acute paranoid schizophrenia. These reactions appear to be inevitable if the dose and frequency of use of amphetamines and cocaine are continually increased or high doses maintained. Psychotic episodes have also been precipitated in some individuals after only one small dose. The syndrome is marked by paranoid ideation; stereotyped compulsive behavior; visual, auditory, and tactile hallucinations; and loosening of associations occurring in a setting of clear consciousness and correct orientation. The etiology of these disorders may be related to actions of amphetamines and cocaine in inhibiting the re-uptake inactivation of the catecholamines, dopamine, and norepinephrine, thus potentiating their synaptic effects. The psychotic episodes invariably appear while the patients are under the influence of the drug, and generally abate within a few days to several weeks after cessation of drug use. Prolonged psychotic episodes occur and may relate to the premorbid personality of the user.

TREATMENT. Amphetamine and cocaine abusers are a heterogeneous group who demonstrate markedly diverse patterns of drug use. Accordingly, treatment must be flexible. Treatment of the acute and chronic physical complications of abuse are considered in the appropriate chapters of this textbook. Treatment of sympathomimetic stimulation may be accomplished with diazepam or other depressant drug. Withdrawal from these drugs requires a safe, supportive atmosphere, much reassurance, and benzodiazepines when necessary for extreme anxiety. Detoxification with decreasing doses of the sympathomimetics is not generally indicated. Treatment of paranoid ideation or the overt psychotic episodes may necessitate short-term hospitalization. Phenothiazines or other major tranquilizers may be necessary for prolonged psychotic reactions.

After recovery, depressive symptoms should be sought and the possibility of suicide must be considered. The compulsive abuser may require long-term supportive care under close supervision, with provision for psychiatric and social rehabilitation.

Physicians would do well to prescribe amphetamines and related drugs with great caution. Some authorities suggest that the childhood hyperkinetic disorders and narcolepsy are the only indications for their use.

247. CANNABIS
(Marijuana and Hashish)
Robert B. Millman

Marijuana and hashish are derived from *Cannabis sativa,* the hemp plant, an herbaceous annual which grows readily in many parts of the world and reaches maturation in four to five months. All parts of both the male and female plants contain varying amounts of the major psychoactive principle, delta-9-tetra hydrocannibinol; its active isomer, delta-8-THC; and numerous other cannabinoids. The concentration of delta-9-THC in the flowering tops of these plants is a function of genetic and environmental factors and varies from less than 0.2 per cent in the fiber-type plants to more than 4 per cent in those plants grown for drug content. In the United States, *marijuana* refers to the dried mixture of crushed leaves and flowering tops with or without the inclusion of stems and seeds. The flowering tops of the plants secrete a clear, varnish-like resin, which when collected and compressed is called *hashish* and is thought to be four to eight times more potent than marijuana. Cannabis or its products are also called *kif, bhang, ganga, charas,* and *dagga* in various parts of the world.

INCIDENCE AND PATTERNS OF ABUSE. Cannabis has been used extensively in many societies since antiquity as a form of folk medicine, as a work adjunct, in association with religious practices, and for recreational purposes. The prevalence of cannabis use increased explosively in the United States and Western Europe during the past 20 years, in association with the changing styles of youth culture. Several recent surveys suggest that use continues to increase and that the number of people in the United States who have ever used cannabis is 36 million. Users fall heavily into the teenage and young adult group; more than 50 per cent of people from 18 to 25 are estimated to have used the drug. Increased use is being noted in older age groups as well. Whereas geographic, social, and cultural considerations are determinants of whether a person will use cannabis, personality characteristics are important in determining the frequency and pattern of use. Many people experiment with the drug and do not continue its use; over half are estimated to use the drug one or more times per month; about one in four who use it that often do so three times or more a week. The present trend toward the reduction or elimination of legal sanctions against cannabis possession and use may further broaden the demographic base of users and increase prevalence.

The drug is peripheral to the life of the occasional user, and frequently there is no other drug use. Others demonstrate a compulsive abuse pattern, in which their lives are dominated by the acquisition and use of cannabis and other drugs. Occasional users generally smoke in groups, where the ritual of preparation and sharing of the cigarette is an integral part of social interaction. Chronic smokers will also frequently smoke alone.

Marijuana is usually smoked in homemade cigarettes ("joints"). Hashish is smoked in a wide variety of small pipes. Both preparations may be ingested in combination with food or drink, although this is less common. The weight of a marijuana cigarette on the street may vary from 0.5 to 1 gram. The delta-9-THC content may vary from less than 1 per cent in domestic material to much more in imported varieties.

PHARMACOLOGY. Cannabis preparations are three to four times more potent when smoked than when taken orally. After inhalation, effects begin within minutes, peak within one hour, and are dissipated within three hours. After ingestion, effects begin in 30 minutes to two hours, peak at three hours, and persist for four to six hours. The effects of cannabis correlate with the appearance in plasma of active polar metabolites of delta-9-THC. Kinetic interactions have been described between several of the cannabinoids in marijuana, suggesting that, in accordance with popular belief, the pharmacologic and psychoactive effects of different strains may vary apart from the differences in delta-9-THC content.

The acute physiologic effects of cannabis are dose related and include an increase in heart rate, conjunctival vascular congestion, decreased intraocular pressure, bronchodilatation, increased airway conductance, and peripheral vasodilatation. Dryness of mouth and throat, fine tremors of fingers, ataxia, nystagmus, nausea, and vomiting have been noted. Orthostatic hypotension and loss of consciousness occur infrequently. Sleep patterns may be altered.

Psychoactive effects are highly variable and depend on the dose, the route of administration, the personality of the user, his prior experience with the drug, his personal expectations, and the environmental and social setting in which the drug is used. Enhanced perception of colors, sounds, patterns, textures, and taste is common. Mood changes are complex; a sense of increased well-being is frequently experienced, although anxiety and depression may be increased by the drug as well. Drowsiness or hyperactivity and hilarity may occur. Ideas may seem disconnected, rapid flowing, and associated with altered importance. Time seems to pass slowly, and short-term memory may be impaired. Motor performance is variably impaired, as is reaction time. Although attention can be maintained in certain situations, it is probable that alterations in attention are responsible for some of the reported decrements in performance and cognitive function. *Driving performance is significantly impaired by marijuana intoxication.*

Inexperienced users of cannabis report fewer subjective effects, but demonstrate more decrement in perceptual and psychomotor performance than experienced users. A learning process may be involved in the initial perception of psychoactive effects, although enzymatic induction with more rapid conversion of delta-9-THC to active metabolites is also possible. A varying degree of tolerance develops to some of the psychologic and

physiologic effects of the drug. Physical dependence on cannabis does not occur in man.

ADVERSE EFFECTS. There are no documented reports of human fatalities caused by an overdose of cannabis in any form. Decreased pulmonary function has been reported in chronic users, with an increased incidence of bronchitis, sinusitis, and nose and throat inflammations. The reported in vitro reduction in thymus-dependent lymphocytes and inhibition of DNA, RNA, and protein synthesis require clarification. Reduced testosterone levels and altered cellular characteristics of sperm in chronic cannabis users have been reported, but the functional significance of these findings is unclear.

Adverse reactions are generally psychologic in nature, infrequent, and dependent on dose, the personality of the user, and the setting. The most common adverse effects are simple depression, acute panic reactions, and paranoid ideation. These symptoms usually abate in several hours. An acute toxic psychosis, transient in nature, with confusion, disorientation, and auditory and visual hallucinations, occurs infrequently and is thought to be related to high doses of the drug. There is disagreement as to whether cannabis may precipitate a psychotic episode in a stable, well-structured personality. It is agreed that the drug may trigger a prolonged psychotic episode in people with borderline psychologic adjustments. Larger doses are associated with an increase in these reactions, though in a nonlinear way. "Flashback" phenomena similar to those seen with psychedelic use occur rarely.

There is no evidence that the chronic heavy use of marijuana causes diminished goal-directed activity, apathy, inability to master new problems, or poor social and work adjustment ("amotivational syndrome"), although it is possible that the drug may inhibit the output of workers who have complex tasks or for whom mental operations usually predominate. There is no evidence that cannabis use leads to criminal activity. Socially or psychologically predisposed individuals may experiment with other drugs as a result of positive experience with cannabis.

TREATMENT. Treatment of the frequently seen depressive and panic reactions should be personal, supportive, and reassuring. The patient must be continually reminded of the drug-induced nature of his difficulty. Tranquilizers are sometimes indicated in violent or aggressive states. Psychotherapy and hospitalization may be indicated in more severe or chronic disorders. The chronic use of marijuana may be associated with a subculture that rejects conventional mores and orientation. To be effective, treatment efforts should be sensitive to these value systems.

248. PSYCHEDELICS

Robert B. Millman

The distinguishing characteristics of the psychedelics is their ability to reliably produce distinctive alterations in perception, thought, feeling, and behavior. They are among the oldest known psychoactive drugs, having been used as an adjunct to religious practices in some societies. They are sometimes classified as hallucinogens, psychotogens, or psychotomimetics. In this country, the most frequently abused drugs in this category are related either to the indolealkylamines such as the synthetic *lysergic acid diethylamide (LSD, "acid")*, *psilocybin* ("magic mushrooms"), *psilocin, dimethyltryptamine (DMT)*, and *diethyltryptamine (DET)*, or to the phenylethylamines such as *mescaline*, which is derived from the peyote cactus, and the substituted amphetamines such as 2,5-dimethoxy-4-methylamphetamine *(DOM, "STP")*. Since the pattern of physiologic and psychologic effects produced by other agents is similar to that seen with LSD, this discussion will center on LSD. By virtue of their ability to produce bizarre alterations in behavior, anticholinergic compounds and *phencyclidine* ("angel dust," "PCP") a drug with anesthetic properties, will be considered in this chapter. Their psychoactive effects are distinct from the other psychedelics.

INCIDENCE AND PATTERNS OF ABUSE. LSD became available through illicit channels in 1960, and use apparently peaked in the 1967–1968 period, when the new styles of youth culture and its leaders were being popularized by the mass media. Estimates varied from 500,000 to 1 million users at that time, and have been lower since then.

Use has been primarily among middle-class, white, educated youth in this country who are seeking an enriching, ecstatic, mystical, or transcendental experience. A complex set of metaphysical and religious beliefs and social styles often distinguish the user.

Use is generally intermittent, frequently less than one "trip" monthly, separated by periods in which marijuana is used. Rarely, individuals may take the drug more often ("acid heads"), and some remain in intoxicated states for prolonged periods. Opiate and excessive alcohol use are not often seen in this population, although intermittent amphetamine and hypnotic use are not unusual in the intervening periods. The drug is generally taken in groups so that support is available in the event of a "bad trip." A naive user will frequently be attended by a guide who has previously had the psychedelic experience. As in the case of cannabis, a supportive, safe environment is sought for the experience to minimize the effects of unpleasant reactions.

LSD is generally synthesized in illegal laboratories and made available in a variety of forms, including impregnated paper or sugar cubes, capsules, and tablets. Users are often unaware of the dose they ingest or of whether the preparation is actually LSD or another of the psychedelics.

In contrast to LSD, abuse of illicitly produced phencyclidine has increased recently. It is available in a variety of forms and is used in a fashion similar to the other psychedelics.

PHARMACOLOGY. LSD is the most potent psychedelic known. It is more than 100 times more potent than psilocybin and 4000 times more potent than mescaline in producing psychologic effects. The usual illicit street dose is probably around 200 μg, but doses as low as 20 μg produce psychologic effects in susceptible individuals. It is generally taken orally, although it has been injected on occasion. Central sympathomimetic stimulation occurs within 20 minutes after ingestion, characterized by mydriasis, hyperthermia, tachycardia, elevated blood pressure, piloerection, increased alertness, and facilitation of monosynaptic reflexes. Nausea and occasionally vomiting occur.

Psychoactive effects are fully evident within one to two hours; these are quite variable from subject to subject and in the same subject under different conditions of dose, mood, expectation, setting, and time. Perceptions are heightened and may become overwhelming. Afterimages are prolonged and overlap with ongoing perceptions. Objects may seem to move in a wavelike fashion or melt. Illusions and synesthesias, the overflow of one sense modality to another, are common.

There may be a sense of unusual clarity, and one's thoughts may assume extraordinary importance. Time may seem to pass very slowly, and body distortions are commonly perceived. True hallucinations with loss of insight may occur in susceptible individuals. Mood is highly variable and labile, and may range from expansive reactions characterized by euphoria and self-confidence to a constricted reaction marked by depression and panic.

The syndrome begins to clear after 10 to 12 hours, and fatigue and tension may persist for an additional 24 hours. The duration of action of mescaline is about 12 hours, that of psilocybin is four to six hours, that of DOM is six to eight hours, and that of phencycline is two to four hours. DMT must be injected or sniffed, and effects last less than two hours.

Tolerance to LSD develops rapidly, repeated daily doses becoming ineffective in three to four days. Recovery is equally rapid, so weekly use of the same dose is possible. Cross-tolerance has been demonstrated between LSD, mescaline, psilocybin, and the amphetamine-based psychedelics, but not between LSD and amphetamine. Physical dependence does not occur with LSD or any of the psychedelic drugs.

Mechanisms of action of LSD are unknown, but may depend on a complex interaction of serotonin and norepinephrine systems in the central nervous system. LSD lowers the threshold for reticular arousal via sensory input and may influence the processes concerned with the filtration and integration of sensory information.

ADVERSE EFFECTS. Acute physiologic toxicity of the LSD-related psychedelic drugs is low at doses that produce marked psychologic effects. In man, no deaths directly attributable to the use of these drugs have been reported. Controversy exists as to whether the illicit use of LSD increases the rate of chromosome breakage in users and leads to an increased incidence of congenital defects in children born to parents who had taken this drug. Evidence suggests that pregnant women exposed to illicit LSD had an elevated rate of spontaneous abortions. LSD may inhibit antibody formation and disrupt the body's immune system. Additional study of these adverse effects are necessary because illicit users of LSD frequently take other drugs and may be malnourished and debilitated.

The acute panic reaction ("bad trip," "freak-out") is the most frequent complication of psychedelic use. These vary in intensity and have led to suicide attempts and accidents on rare occasions. Fear of death or insanity and sensations of breathlessness or paralysis are commonly reported. In most cases, this acute reaction subsides as drug effects are dissipated. Other complications include prolonged psychotic disorders, acute and chronic paranoid reactions, and depressive states. "Flashback" phenomena, the recurrence of some aspect of the drug experience when the individual is not under the influence of the drug, have been reported. The intensity, frequency, and duration of these episodes are quite variable. Adverse psychologic reactions are most frequent in emotionally disturbed individuals in crisis situations or insecure environments who take the drug in unsupervised settings. High doses of psychedelic drugs lead to an increased incidence of these complications. Whether the psychedelics cause prolonged adverse reactions in emotionally stable people is not clear.

Acute toxic effects of phencyclidine are frequent, and a

significant number of deaths have been reported. It may produce either depression or stimulation of the central nervous system, depending on the dose and the route of administration. Common features include emotional lability, excited intoxication, nystagmus, elevated blood pressure, and increased deep-tendon reflexes which may progress to a state of extreme muscular rigidity. High doses may lead to arrhythmias, convulsions, and coma. A chronic organic brain dysfunction has been described in phencyclidine abusers, marked by memory gaps, some disorientation, and visual and speech disturbances.

ANTICHOLINERGIC COMPOUNDS. Ingestion of the alkaloids *atropine, hyoscyamine,* and *scopolamine* in their natural plant forms is increasing incident to the ingestion of "herbal teas" or leaves, and several deaths have occurred. Excessive use of *antihistaminic* compounds with anticholinergic effects also occurs. Symptoms of the potent peripheral effects of intoxication with these drugs include dilated, fixed pupils, dry skin and mouth, flushing, hyperthermia, and tachycardia. Psychoactive effects are those of an acute toxic psychosis, with clouding of consciousness, delirium, and loss of memory for the period of intoxication. Vivid sensory phenomena are not prominent, although hallucinations may occur.

TREATMENT. Treatment of the acute panic reaction may usually be accomplished by ensuring a warm, supportive environment with someone in constant attendance and with a minimum of other external stimuli. The user should be reminded continually that the effects he is experiencing are due to the drug and will pass in time. In particularly agitated patients, phenothiazines or diazepam orally or intramuscularly may be used. In the event of precipitation of prolonged psychosis, hospitalization with supportive care may be required. Flashbacks are treated with reassurance and/or psychotherapy when these are severe. In general, the duration and severity of these decrease with time if psychedelic drug use ceases. Treatment of the acute intoxication caused by low doses of phencyclidine is similar to that for the other psychedelics, particularly with respect to reduction of external stimuli and tranquilization. Toxic reactions from higher doses may require hospitalization and intensive supportive care.

Treatment of anticholinergic poisoning is symptomatic and consists of protecting the patient from self-injury, providing fluids, and reducing the fever. Administration of cholinesterase inhibitors and suitable tranquilizers may be indicated, although phenothiazines are contraindicated because of their anticholinergic effects.

249. MISCELLANEOUS INHALANTS

Robert B. Millman

NITROUS OXIDE. Recreational inhalation of nitrous oxide alone or in combination with oxygen is a rarely reported phenomenon that occurs in some youthful populations. Psychoactive effects occur in 15 to 30 seconds and persist for less than five minutes. The experience is described as one of intoxication, euphoria, and hilarity. Adverse effects have not been reported.

ORGANIC SOLVENTS. The inhalation of a wide range of organic solvents, particularly the toluene in glue, has

received a good deal of attention from the mass media and law-enforcement agencies. It is likely that this publicity has contributed significantly to the incidence of this practice in the adolescent and preadolescent population. The material is usually squeezed into a plastic bag and the vapors inhaled. Prolonged exposure, as in the case of industrial workers, may have serious adverse effects on a variety of organ systems. As used recreationally, these solvents produce intoxication and dizziness not unlike that experienced with alcohol. Few side effects have been reported, although suffocation caused by the plastic bag has apparently occurred. A number of deaths have been reported secondary to the inhalation of the anesthetic agent halothane, a halogenated hydrocarbon. The inhalation of aerosol sprays containing fluorocarbon propellants is also occurring. The mechanism of toxicity and death may be the induction of cardiac arrhythmias or upper-airway obstruction and hypoxia.

AMYL NITRITE. Amyl nitrite ("amies," "poppers") inhalation occurs in some youthful drug-abusing populations, notably among homosexual men. A recent phenomenon is the similar use of other volatile nitrites that are marketed as deodorizers or "aromas" under a variety of exotic brand names. Use is intermittent and characterized by an instantaneous feeling ("rush") of flushing, dizziness, hilarity, and activity. Effects persist for minutes. Adverse effects include palpitations, postural hypotension occasionally proceeding to loss of consciousness, and headache. Chronic use is rare, and more severe adverse effects have not been reported.

Brecher, E. M., and the Editors of Consumer Reports: Licit and Illicit Drugs. The Consumers Union Report on Narcotics, Stimulants, Depressants, Inhalants, Hallucinogens, and Marijuana, Including Caffeine, Nicotine and Alcohol. Mount Vernon, N. Y., Consumers Union, 1972.

Dishotsky, N. I., Loughman, W. D., Mogar, R. E., and Lipscomb, W. R.: LSD and genetic damage. Science, 172:431, 1971.

Dole, V. P.: Narcotic addiction, physical dependence and relapse. N. Engl. J. Med., 286:988, 1972.

Dole, V. P., and Nyswander, M.: A medical treatment for diacetylmorphine (heroin) addiction. JAMA, 193:646, 1965.

Grinspoon, L., and Bakalar, J. B.: Cocaine: A Drug and Its Social Evolution. New York, Basic Books, 1976.

Isbell, H., Altschul, S., Kornetsky, C. H., et al.: Chronic barbiturate intoxication. An experimental study. Arch. Neurol. Psychiat., 64:1, 1950.

Jaffe, J.: Narcotic analgesics and drug addiction and drug abuse. *In* Goodman, L. S., and Gilman, A. (eds.): The Pharmacological Basis of Therapeutics. 5th ed. New York, Macmillan, 1975, p. 245.

Kales, A., Bixler, E. O., Tan, T-L., et al.: Chronic hypnotic-drug use: ineffectiveness, drug-withdrawal insomnia, and dependence. JAMA, 227:513, 1974.

Kreek, M. J.: Medical safety and side effects of methadone in tolerant individuals. JAMA, 223:665, 1973.

Peterson, R. C. (ed.): Marijuana Research 1976, NIDA Research Monograph No. 14. U. S. Department of Health, Education, and Welfare, July 1977.

Snyder, S. H.: The opiate receptor and morphine-like peptides in the brain. Am. J. Psychiat., 135:645, 1978.

Stimmel, B.: Heroin Dependency: Medical, Economic and Social Aspects. New York, Stratton Intercontinental Medical Book Corporation, 1975.

250. ALCOHOL ABUSE AND ALCOHOL-RELATED ILLNESS

Jack H. Mendelson

DEFINITION. The most widely accepted operational definition of alcohol abuse is excessive drinking which adversely affects an individual's health, impairs social function, or both. Although it is not difficult to assess the impact of alcohol abuse on biologic function, it is often impossible to quantify alcohol-related social impairment. Experts disagree about both the type and the severity of problem drinking which cause social dysfunction because of wide variations in societal norms for characterizing deviant drinking behavior. Attempts to establish criteria for normative drinking behavior based upon volume and consumption frequency indices have not been satisfactory because of conflicting social, cultural, religious, and even political perceptions of how individuals in various societies may consume alcohol.

The frequently used term "alcoholism" is ambiguous. "Alcoholism" is often not synonymous with alcohol abuse, but denotes a series of problems ranging from deviant drinking behavior (as defined by the society in which it occurs) to alcohol addiction. Some of the phenomena which are reported to occur during the progression of *alcohol abuse* to *alcohol addiction* include excessive drinking in normal social situations; drinking in isolation; drinking to reduce anxiety, apprehension, or anger; drinking to facilitate the induction of sleep during conditions of insomnia; early morning drinking; and alterations in memory function (blackout) during heavy episodic alcohol intake. All or none of these phenomena may be reported by individuals who demonstrate evidence of addiction to alcohol, and no specific pattern of events is pathognomonic of behavior attributes for transition of alcohol abuse to alcohol addiction.

Addiction to alcohol is characterized by both tolerance and physical dependence. Tolerance occurs when an individual consumes progressively larger quantities of alcohol over a period of time in order to induce changes in feeling states or behavior which previously were induced by smaller doses of alcohol. Physical dependence occurs when an individual develops subjective discomfort and/or overt withdrawal signs after partial or complete cessation of drinking. It is important to emphasize that withdrawal signs and symptoms may occur in alcohol addicts when they reduce drinking but do not completely cease all alcohol intake. Relatively small decrements in sustained high blood alcohol levels may be associated with precipitation of the withdrawal syndrome.

As with most behavior disorders, it is often impossible to establish a precise definition of clinical status, e.g., alcohol abuse versus alcohol addiction. The physician must make a judgment about the presence and severity of an alcohol-related problem on the basis of careful determination of physical and mental status, occupational performance, social interaction, and — not least important — the patient's own perception of how alcohol consumption enhances or compromises his or her health and well-being.

ETIOLOGY. No specific biologic, psychologic, or social variable has been shown to have high predictive value for determining which individuals are at high risk to develop and sustain problem drinking behavior. There are no known psychologic tests which can reliably differentiate alcohol abusers from normal drinkers. Many theories have purported to explain the causation of alcoholism in terms of psychodynamic factors, personality profiles, psychosocial developmental and growth characteristics, nutritional idiosyncrasies, allergic disorders, and specific and nonspecific metabolic derangements. To date, none of these theories of the causation of alcohol abuse or alcohol addiction have significant support from well-controlled laboratory and clinical investigations.

The contribution of specific genetic and environmental factors which may enhance the risk for development of alcohol-related problems has not been clarified. Many patients who develop alcohol-related problems have no family history of alcohol abuse or alcohol addiction. But it is also known that individuals with a family history of alcohol abuse, particularly those who report that both parents had alcohol problems, may be at very great risk for developing alcohol abuse themselves. It is likely that this enhanced risk occurs, in part, as a function of growing up in an environment where excessive drinking is employed for coping with or modifying social stress. Moreover, there are recent data which indicate that a genetic component may be associated with the causation of alcohol problems. Studies of adoptees in Denmark have demonstrated that these individuals are more likely to develop alcohol problems if their biologic parents were alcohol abusers than if the adopted parent had abused alcohol. Thus at present it appears reasonable to conclude that both genetic and developmental factors may contribute to the genesis of alcohol-related illness.

INCIDENCE AND PREVALENCE. Surveys of American drinking practices reveal that approximately two thirds of the adult population of the United States use alcohol at least occasionally. It is estimated that about 12 per cent of the American population are heavy drinkers, i.e., individuals who drink almost daily or who once a week consume five or more drinks per occasion. It is obvious that this definition of heavy drinking may be associated with a number of ambiguities, and it is difficult to rate relative degree of drinking (heavy versus light) from self-written reports about the volume and frequency of alcohol consumed. Thus, individuals may consume the same quantity of alcohol during a given interval of time, but variations in the spacing or the concentrating of the drinking may indicate vastly different drinking patterns. For example, alcohol addicts who are spree drinkers may consume enormous amounts of alcohol in a two- or three-day interval during a month and remain relatively abstinent the remainder of the time.

A recent survey of American drinking practices and problems revealed that the largest population of problem drinkers were city-dwellers of low socioeconomic status. The highest rates of alcohol-related problems were found in young (under 25) urban men; the number of heavy drinkers among white and black males was similar (22 and 19 per cent, respectively). However, black women reported a significantly higher rate of drinking (11 per cent) than white women (4 per cent). American Indians and Eskimos have high reported rates of alcohol abuse and addiction.

Repeated surveys have shown that alcohol problems can be found in anyone who drinks alcohol to excess and that individual variations obliterate the significance of any group, ethnic, or cultural qualities. Case finding in alcoholism is difficult because of the stigma associated with the disorder. However, most agree that alcoholism represents the major drug problem in America today. It has been estimated that about 5 million adults in the United States have significant alcohol-related problems. It is also estimated that an additional

4 million abuse alcohol to the extent that they are at high risk for the development of alcohol addiction. These figures imply that 7 per cent of the adult population have a significant alcohol-related problem.

PHARMACOLOGIC ASPECTS. After the consumption of alcohol, absorption occurs primarily from the small intestine, but gastric emptying and the rate of absorption from the intestine are influenced by a number of factors. The rate of absorption is accelerated with increasing concentrations of alcohol up to a maximum of 40 per cent. Concentrations of ingested alcohol above 40 per cent may be absorbed more slowly as a consequence of delayed gastric emptying. Similarly, high concentrations of congeners in beverage alcohol delay absorption because they impede gastric emptying by inducing pyloric spasm. The ingestion of food along with beverage alcohol also reduces the speed of absorption by delaying the emptying time of the stomach.

After absorption, ethanol is distributed to all portions of the body and achieves equilibrium with body water compartments. Blood alcohol levels are dependent upon the total body water concentration. No impermeable or semipermeable membranes impede the diffusion of alcohol into any body organ or tissue.

Alcohol is removed from the body primarily by metabolism in the liver, and only 2 to 10 per cent is excreted directly by the kidneys and the lungs. Alcohol is catabolized in the liver by well-known enzymatic mechanisms involving the enzyme alcohol dehydrogenase and the cofactor NAD. The rate of alcohol metabolism in normal drinkers and in abstinent alcohol addicts is not significantly different. However, the rate of ethanol metabolism may increase in alcohol addicts during the course of spree drinking, and it is believed that this increase is due to an ethanol-induced increase in rate of hepatic metabolism.

There are no known pharmacologic agents which may be utilized in clinical practice to enhance the rate of ethanol catabolism in man. Although it has been shown that high dosage administration of fructose may accelerate rates of ethanol metabolism, the clinical use of this is impractical.

Blood alcohol levels depend upon the amount of alcohol ingested and the weight of the individual. For the average man, it has been estimated that the consumption of 180 ml of distilled spirits on an empty stomach will produce a blood alcohol level of approximately 100 mg per 100 ml. Values around 100 mg per 100 ml have been established by most jurisdictions as the legal limit of sobriety for operating a motor vehicle. Blood alcohol levels achieved in usual social drinking situations average about 50 to 75 mg per 100 ml. At this blood level a subjective state of pleasant tranquility and a mild degree of sedation may occur. Overt signs of intoxication usually occur in social (nontolerant) drinkers between 100 and 200 mg per 100 ml. Severe intoxication is observed in social drinkers at levels above 200 mg per 100 ml, but alcohol addicts who are tolerant to the effects of ethanol may appear relatively intact and nonintoxicated with such blood alcohol levels. Regardless of the degree of tolerance, blood alcohol levels above 400 mg per 100 ml produce stupor and/or coma, and concentrations above 500 mg per 100 ml are frequently fatal.

ALCOHOL AND BEHAVIOR. Acute Intoxication. Although the concomitants of acute intoxication are well known and easily recognized (dysarthria, ataxia, and emotional lability), there is no simple correlation between the volume of alcohol consumed and an individual's ability to carry out cognitive and motor tasks successfully. Indeed, some individuals actually show improved performance on perceptual and psychomotor tasks with low to moderate doses of alcohol. This paradox obtains because small to moderate doses of ethanol may act in a manner similar to a minor tranquilizer, i.e., to reduce anxiety which may affect skill and performance. Individuals who demonstrate little impairment in performance of cognitive and motor tasks with high blood ethanol concentrations (150 to 200 mg per 100 ml) have probably developed tolerance for alcohol as a consequence of recurrent heavy drinking.

Moderate dosage of alcohol usually impairs visual-motor coordination in most social drinkers. In particular, brightness discrimination and visual adaptation after exposure to bright lights are often markedly reduced. Auditory and tactile sensation are usually unchanged. The integration and evaluation of sensory information, rather than the impairment of sensory input itself, are most severely compromised during acute intoxication. An individual's ability to initiate or maintain sustained attention to stimuli and to judge the qualities of stimuli is usually significantly diminished after moderate alcohol intake. Individuals under such conditions tend to underestimate the speed and distance of objects as well as to show impairment in making judgments regarding the passage of time.

Impairments of behavior associated with acute intoxication are also determined by factors related to the setting. If a person consumes alcohol in a situation in which drunkenness is both expected and tolerated, this anticipation may influence his behavior more than the dosage of alcohol ingested. Similarly, individuals who fear the consequences of intoxicated behavior may successfully mask the manifestations of acute inebriation even though they consume relatively large amounts of alcohol.

Alcohol, Aggression, and Accidents. Although it is well known that alcohol ingestion and acute intoxication are significant factors in accidents, the causal relationship is not a simple one. Alcohol intoxication may effect a number of patterns of behavior which combine to produce enhanced risk for an accident. These include compromised judgment, enhanced emotional lability, and inability to suppress expression of aggression. Acute alcohol intoxication also contributes to situations which result in death and injury as a function of violence and aggressive behavior. Homicide, armed robbery with aggravated assault, and other crimes of violence are frequent in perpetrators or victims who are acutely intoxicated.

Acute alcohol intoxication has been frequently implicated in fatal accidents. For example, over half of the nonhighway accident fatalities involve alcohol addicts or abusers. A recent survey carried out in a general hospital emergency room in which blood alcohol values were determined in accident victims showed that 30 per cent of the individuals involved in highway accidents, 22 per cent involved in home accidents, and 16 per cent involved in occupational accidents had elevated blood ethanol levels.

Alcohol abuse is a significant contributing factor to over 50 per cent of motor vehicle fatalities, and it was estimated during a recent 12-month period that 28,000 highway deaths were associated with alcohol intoxication. Increasing evidence suggests, however, that alcohol-related automobile fatalities may not be simply associated with episodic acute intoxication in social drinkers, but rather are phenomena related to chronic intoxication and alcohol addiction. Statistics obtained from studies of blood alcohol levels in individuals involved in single vehicle fatalities indicate that a majority had blood ethanol values above 150 mg per 100 ml. Such high blood levels are more characteristic of alcohol addicts than of social drinkers.

Alcohol and Sexual Function. The effect of acute intoxication on sexual behavior and function is poorly understood. The classic reference is Shakespeare's perception that intoxication increases desire but impairs sexual performance. Although the effects of acute alcohol intoxication on sexual behavior in moderate drinkers may be quite variable, sexual function and behavior are often markedly impaired in alcohol addicts. Male alcohol addicts often report sexual impotence and diminished heterosexual desire. A tendency to initiate or increase alcohol intake has been reported by female alcoholics during premenstrual periods. Gynecomastia and testicular atrophy have been reported in male alcohol addicts, particularly those who also show evidence of alcohol-related liver disease. Recent studies have demonstrated that alcohol administration to alcohol addicts is associated with suppression of plasma testosterone levels. Alcohol also suppresses plasma testosterone levels in normal males when blood ethanol levels are between 50 and 100 mg per 100 ml. Alcohol-induced suppression of testosterone is probably due to inhibition of testosterone biosynthesis in the testes. There is also evidence that chronic alcohol intake induces enzymes which enhance the rate of testosterone biotransformation in the liver.

The "Hangover." A well-known consequence of acute alcohol intoxication is a syndrome of generalized somatic discomfort, headache, nausea, agitation, and mild tremulousness which has been termed the "hangover." The physiologic mechanisms related to the hangover have not been determined. Current evidence indicates that the hangover may be the equivalent of a mild withdrawal syndrome. There is no evidence that any specific characteristic of beverage alcohol, such as its congener content, or any unique pattern of drinking, such as mixing different beverages, is the causal basis for the hangover. No specific form of pharmacotherapy is available for treatment of the problem, and there is little evidence that the plethora of popular remedies have any efficacy.

ADDICTION TO ALCOHOL. Addiction to alcohol is characterized by the presence of both tolerance and physical dependence. Although many individuals may frequently abuse alcohol, not all become physically dependent. Moreover, it is difficult to predict addiction liability on the basis of dosage of alcohol and frequency of consumption alone. There is no question, however, that physical dependence on alcohol is analogous to physical dependence induced by a number of other centrally acting drugs and is not caused by intercurrent illness or by vitamin or nutritional disorders. Withdrawal signs and symptoms have been observed in otherwise healthy alcohol addicts exclusively as a concomitant of cessation of drinking. Physical dependence has also been induced in a number of species of laboratory animals without producing derangements in nutritional or metabolic function.

Tolerance appears to develop more rapidly than physical dependence for alcohol and other drugs which affect the central nervous system (i.e., narcotics, barbiturates, and psychotropic drugs). Three forms of tolerance may be observed in the alcohol addict: behavioral tolerance, pharmacologic tolerance, and cross-tolerance to certain other drugs which have their primary effect on central nervous function.

Behavioral tolerance is manifest when the alcohol addict can consume relatively large amounts of ethanol without impairment in social behavior or psychomotor coordination. It has been observed clinically and demonstrated in research ward studies that some alcohol addicts can consume as much as 1 quart of beverage alcohol per day without evidence of gross intoxication. It has also been shown that many alcohol addicts can perform relatively complex tasks without error when their blood alcohol levels are twice the legal limit of intoxication for many state jurisdictions.

Pharmacologic tolerance reflects a metabolic adaptive change in the alcohol addict as a consequence of long-term drinking. Evidence of pharmacologic tolerance was originally inferred from the finding of low blood alcohol levels in alcohol addicts who had consumed large amounts of alcohol (up to 1 quart of bourbon per day for 20 consecutive days). Subsequent studies demonstrated an enhanced rate of ethanol metabolism in alcohol addicts during protracted episodes of drinking. The pharmacokinetics of alcohol-induced enhancement of ethanol metabolism have not been clarified, but they appear not to persist after long periods of sobriety. Pharmacologic tolerance may contribute to some small aspect of behavioral tolerance, but adaptive processes in the central nervous system are probably far more important for behavioral tolerance than alcohol-induced enhancement in rates of ethanol metabolism.

Clinical reports have stressed that alcohol addicts may show reduced sensitivity and responsivity to a number of other drugs: *cross-tolerance.* There are reports that alcohol addicts require significantly higher doses of both the barbiturate and volatile anesthetics for induction and maintenance of appropriate levels of surgical anesthesia. Alcohol addicts frequently show cross-tolerance for barbiturates, hypnotics, and psychotropic agents such as the minor tranquilizers. However, cross-tolerance and cross-dependence have not been demonstrated between alcohol and the opiates. It is important to point out that cross-tolerance occurs in alcohol addicts when they are temporarily abstaining from drinking. When alcohol addicts are intoxicated, both synergism and potentiation with narcotics, opiates and analgesics, barbiturates, and a variety of other psychotropic agents may occur. In fact, there is some evidence which indicates that the consumption of drugs such as barbiturates during heavy alcohol intake is associated with a decreased catabolic degradation of both agents.

Although tolerance for ethanol may appear to be very great for some alcohol addicts, the degree of tolerance which can be developed for ethanol is much smaller than that which can potentially occur in opiate or barbiturate addiction. Barbiturate addicts may ingest as much as 2 grams of secobarbital or pentobarbital daily without gross impairments of behavior. Heroin addicts may eventually employ a dosage 50 times larger than their initial intake. On the other hand, blood alcohol levels exceeding 450 mg per 100 ml for any drinker, social or addicted, are rarely observed, because this level is almost invariably associated with a comatose state. Moreover, the lethal level of 500 to 600 mg per 100 ml is no different for alcohol addicts as opposed to normal drinkers, because such blood alcohol levels cause severe and often irreversible respiratory depression.

Physical dependence upon alcohol is characterized by the appearance of withdrawal signs and symptoms after cessation of drinking. Tremulousness, delirium, and seizure disorders were first reported by Hippocrates to accompany alcohol abuse, and detailed descriptions of the abstinence syndrome are reported in the medical literature of the late eighteenth century. Systematic studies by Victor and Adams in 1953 are the basis for the classification of the withdrawal syndromes currently identified in clinical practice. Three types of withdrawal states have been differentiated: tremulous states, seizure disorders, and delirium tremens.

Tremulousness is the most frequent and benign type of abstinence syndrome. Although the onset of tremulousness usually occurs 12 to 48 hours after reduction of alcohol intake or initiation of abstinence, this sign may be observed as early as six hours after cessation of drinking. Tremor is usually mild with involvement of the hands, but in some instances it may be generalized with involvement of all extremities as well as the tongue and trunk. Tremor may be increased when the patient extends the arms with the palms upright and the fingers separated. Tremulousness usually remits or is significantly diminished by 72 hours after cessation of drinking, but in rare instances it may persist for five days.

Hallucinosis may be associated with a tremulous state or may occur independent of tremor. Hallucinations also may occur in alcohol addicts during conditions of severe intoxication as well as during conditions of complete or partial cessation of drinking.

Seizure disorders usually occur 12 to 24 hours after cessation or reduction of drinking. Seizures may be associated with tremulousness, but may be present without any other evidence of withdrawal signs. The seizure disorder is of the grand mal type, usually not preceded by auras but almost always followed by postictal stupor and even residual focal signs. Seizures may be observed in patients who have no overt evidence of a neurologic disorder and who have no abnormalities of the electroencephalogram. Victor and Adams have emphasized that approximately one third of all patients who have seizure disorders after cessation of drinking progress to develop delirium tremens.

Delirium tremens is the rarest form of the alcohol withdrawal syndrome. Delirium tremens is characterized by confusion, disorientation, delusions, hallucinations, psychomotor agitation, and autonomic dysfunction. The peak incidence of this syndrome is 72 to 96 hours after cessation of drinking. The severe confusional states and delirium which are the hallmark of delirium tremens are rarely observed in the more frequent instances of tremulousness after cessation of drinking. Patients who develop delirium tremens also often have profuse sweating, tachycardia, hypertension, and fever. Delirium tremens is a potentially lethal illness which requires hospitalization and intensive medical care.

Although the basic mechanisms underlying the alcohol withdrawal syndrome remain to be determined, a number of associated disorders affect the severity of the disorder. Significant disturbances in acid-base, water,

and electrolyte homeostasis may be associated with the abstinence syndrome. After cessation of alcohol intake, many alcohol addicts develop transient hyperventilation which may produce respiratory alkalosis and elevations in blood pH. This condition is usually associated with hypomagnesemia. The low serum magnesium levels observed in alcohol addicts during the withdrawal syndrome are probably caused both by poor dietary intake of magnesium during heavy drinking and by magnesium shifts from the intravascular to the intracellular fluid compartments associated with the pH shift of respiratory alkalosis. It is also important to remember that alcohol addicts who develop withdrawal syndromes may be not dehydrated, but in fact, overhydrated.

INTERCURRENT ILLNESS AND ASSOCIATED DISORDERS. Alcohol addicts are at high risk for developing a number of disorders which are observed frequently in general medical practice. These are discussed individually in other chapters of this text, but a few merit mention here.

Alcohol-related hepatic disease is a leading cause of morbidity and mortality in adult males. It has been demonstrated that alcohol intake alone without concomitant nutritional deficiency may induce hepatic disorders such as fatty metamorphosis, alcoholic hepatitis, and Laennec's cirrhosis (see Ch. 465.2). However, since many people consume large quantities of alcohol without developing these disorders, the crucial determinants of the interrelationships between heavy alcohol consumption and hepatic disease remain to be determined. Gastritis and pancreatitis (see Ch. 402 and Ch. 410.2 and 410.3) are also frequently seen in those who abuse alcohol. A variety of malabsorption syndromes may be associated with heavy alcohol intake (see Ch. 408).

The most severe neurologic disorders seen in alcohol addicts are peripheral neuropathies (see Ch. 335 to 337) which are characterized by motor and sensory impairments in the upper and lower extremities. Pain, paresthesia, motor weakness, and paralysis may occur as a consequence of poor dietary intake in conjunction with heavy ethanol intake.

Diseases of the central nervous system may also be associated with chronic alcohol abuse. Wernicke's disease and Korsakoff's psychosis (see Ch. 287) are characterized by derangements of memory function and disorders of thought processes. The genesis of many "organic brain diseases," which at present constitute the majority of first admissions to state mental hospitals, may be related to nutritional and metabolic derangements associated with alcohol abuse.

There is accumulating evidence that alcohol abuse may be a factor in the development of coronary artery disease and hypertension. Individuals who have a familial Type IV hyperlipidemia (see Ch. 532.5) are at high risk for developing elevations in blood triglyceride levels with even moderate alcohol intake. Studies carried out in the United States and France suggest that alcohol abusers are at higher risk for developing carcinoma of the oral cavity and esophagus. A number of cardiomyopathies have been found in alcohol addicts. Finally, it has been shown that chronic alcohol abuse may cause derangements in hematopoiesis, produce muscle wasting, and suppress immune mechanisms with consequence of higher risk for infection.

AFFECTIVE DISORDERS AND PSYCHOSIS. Some individuals with neurotic and psychotic affective disorders drink excessively, but many others with severe depression never abuse alcohol. In manic-depressive illness patients are more prone to drink excessively during the manic phase of their disorder than when they are depressed. There is also evidence to indicate that chronic alcohol abuse enhances rather than reduces feelings of depression.

Approximately 25 per cent of all suicide victims have detectable amounts of alcohol in body fluids on necropsy examination. It is estimated that one third of all suicides are associated with chronic alcohol abuse, but these findings may relate mainly to white middle-aged males. Suicide rates for black males over 35 are low, even though drinking problems may be high.

TREATMENT AND PREVENTION. Although there are occasional reports of children who die of respiratory failure associated with ethanol overdosage, death from *acute ethanol poisoning* is rare. Rapid ingestion of large amounts of ethanol usually induces vomiting. Those who consume large amounts of ethanol slowly usually become stuporous before they can ingest a dose necessary to produce significant respiratory depression. The rate of ethanol catabolism in man ranges from 15 to 22 mg per 100 ml per hour, and there are no clinically useful or efficacious methods for rapidly decreasing blood alcohol levels.

Acute ethanol intoxication may be complicated by concurrent intoxication with other centrally acting drugs. There appears to be an increasing degree of polydrug abuse in the United States, particularly drugs which act synergistically with or potentiate the actions of ethanol. Alcohol abusers also frequently abuse barbiturates and minor tranquilizers. The most commonly reported form of drug abuse in narcotic addicts maintained on methadone is with alcohol. In hospital practice it is advisable to obtain blood determinations for other possible central nervous system depressants when a severe depression of consciousness is noted in patients who appear only to be intoxicated with ethanol.

Many persons who seek a physician's aid during conditions of acute ethanol introxication have other medical disorders. These patients should receive the most careful physical examination and diagnostic workup. Most states have adopted legislation requiring that patients with alcohol-related illness, including acute intoxication, should not be denied admission to hospitals and medical facilities. In addition, the American Medical Association and the American Hospital Association have endorsed resolutions against discriminatory policies for patients with alcohol-related problems who seek admission to general medical facilities. Some patients may request hospital treatment for detoxification after chronic alcohol intake when there is no evidence of any significant intercurrent illness. If the patient's motivation for receiving medical assistance appears good, the physician should attempt to provide the best available hospital care. However, involuntary commitment of patients with alcohol problems is not legal in most jurisdictions if hospitalization is initiated only on the basis of a diagnosis of alcoholism without evidence of a serious psychotic disorder.

Treatment of the *alcohol withdrawal syndrome* has improved significantly during the past decade. Less than 15 years ago many hospitals reported a 15 per cent mortality in patients with delirium tremens. The current mortality rate associated with delirium tremens is less than 1 per cent. The major factor affecting reduction in both mortality and morbidity is the application of good general medical care. Patients requiring treatment for the withdrawal syndrome should have the following procedures carried out on a systematic basis: (1) a careful physical and roentgenologic examination to identify any traumatic injuries (especially trauma to the skull); (2) a search for infection of the pulmonary and genitourinary systems; (3) a search for hepatic, gastrointestinal, and cardiac disorders; and (4) an evaluation of the state of hydration, electrolyte, and acid-base status, with appropriate measures instituted to correct any derangements. It should not be assumed that patients exhibiting the withdrawal syndrome are dehydrated or have any particular derangement in electrolyte or acid-base balance status unless demonstrated by appropriate clinical and laboratory examinations.

Chlordiazepoxide is the best drug for reducing pyschomotor agitation in patients who have withdrawal syndromes, provided the agent is used judiciously. In general, the dosage employed should permit reduction of tremor and anxiety without compromising the patient's ability to tolerate fluid and foods orally. Patients exhibiting the withdrawal syndrome should not be sedated deeply simply to produce long periods of sleep. Whenever possible, medication should be given orally, although at the initial stages of the withdrawal syndrome it may be necessary to use the intramuscular route. The routine use of corticosteroids is contraindicated, and the efficacy of diphenylhydantoin (Dilantin) in controlling seizure disorders is questionable. Administration of multivitamins orally or intravenously should be based upon judgment of the patient's nutritional status.

The *treatment of chronic alcohol abuse* is often difficult because most patients with alcohol-related problems tend to deny the severity of their illness and to avoid or reject assistance by physicians and other health care professionals. It has been postulated that the patient's acceptance of treatment can be greatly improved if initial contacts with the physician and the hospital are sympathetic and positive. The point has often been made that treatment for the alcohol abuser and alcohol addict should have limited goals and that alcohol-related illness should be considered as a chronic disease analogous, in some ways, to chronic pulmonary and cardiac conditions. For the most part, physicians treating such illnesses strive to alleviate suffering and to induce compensation rather than achieve absolute cure. A reasonable treatment goal is to restore physical and behavioral status after decompensation in alcohol abusers, even if recidivism is expected. Multimodality therapy suited to the needs of the individual and his resources should be offered. However, the question of which treatment will maximally benefit the patient with alcohol problems remains unanswered.

At present there is no uniformly effective, specific treatment for alcohol abuse. A number of treatment techniques have been employed singly or in combinations which have proved effective for some patients. These include individual and group psychotherapy, Antabuse therapy, referral to self-help groups such as Alcoholics Anonymous, and a number of behavioral modification techniques. It is discouraging that the few relatively well controlled therapy evaluation studies have demonstrated a low rate of alcohol abstinence after therapy. But since these evaluations were carried out in specialized clinic treatment settings, it remains likely that the individual counseling and relationship offered by the family physician will offer a greater degree of success.

The spontaneous recovery rate for alcohol abusers has been estimated to be about 20 per cent over a three-year period. Thus physicians should not assume that alcohol-related disorders are intractable. Since all variants of alcohol abuse are multiply determined, alcohol problems present the treatment challenge of any complex behavioral disorder. Although there is no evidence to indicate that alcohol abuse is invariably associated with a predisposing psychiatric illness, the development of problem drinking rarely occurs in isolation from emotional, interpersonal, and job-related problems.

The physician should employ a multifaceted program of treatment which can be best determined from assessing the patient's motivation, resources, and ability to sustain treatment relationships. For some individuals, self-help groups such as Alcoholics Anonymous may be useful, but one must first explore whether any given patient can effectively utilize this form of assistance. The physician should familiarize himself with all available resources which exist in the patient's community for assistance with alcohol-related problems. It is often essential that the physician involve other members of the family in cooperating with some form of treatment program.

Adequate techniques for *prevention of alcohol-related disorders* have yet to be devised. Although significant emphasis has been placed upon public education and information concerning the responsible use of alcohol, the impact of such programs is difficult to evaluate. Since there are relatively poor incidence and prevalence data for alcohol abuse, it is impossible to argue that public education programs or attempts to shape attitudes have had any impact on alcohol abuse and alcohol addiction. Increased programs of public education and information may appear logical, but it should be remembered that problem drinking usually occurs in situations in which behavior is not determined by logical thinking but rather by internal and external stresses which are not highly amenable to rational persuasion.

Kalant, H.: Absorption, diffusion, distribution and elimination of ethanol: Effects on biological membranes. *In* Kissin, B., and Begleiter, H. (eds.): The Biology of Alcoholism, Vol. 1. New York, Plenum Press, 1971.

Mello, N. K.: Behavioral studies of alcoholism. *In* Kissin, B., and Begleiter, H. (eds.): The Biology of Alcoholism, Vol. 2 New York, Plenum Press, 1972.

Mendelson, J.H., and Mello, N. K.: Alcohol, aggression and androgens. Proc. Assn. Res. Nerv. Ment. Dis., 52:225, 1974.

Mendelson, J. H., and Mello, N. K.: Behavioral and biochemical interrelations in alcoholism. *In* Creger, W. P., Coggins, C. H., and Hancock, E. W. (eds.): Annual Review of Medicine. Palo Alto, Annual Reviews, Inc., 1976.

Wolfe, S., and Victor, M.: The physiological basis of the alcohol withdrawal syndrome. *In* Mello, N. K., and Mendelson, J. H. (eds.): Recent Advances in Studies of Alcoholism. Washington, D. C., U. S. Government Printing Office, Publ. No. (HSM) 71-9045, 1971.

251. ACUTE DRUG POISONING

Fred Plum

Almost any physician may be called upon to treat accidental or intentional drug overdose. Suicide produces a high death rate among all adolescent and adult age groups, and its incidence climbs steadily with age in single white males. Furthermore, psychologically engendered drug abuse plagues many countries, with fatal or near-fatal "accidents" often affecting youngsters of secondary school age as well as adults. No social stratum enjoys immunity. The physician's job is made harder by the fact that the mentally unbalanced or those just seeking new sensations have an ever-expanding roster of pharmaceutical or industrial chemicals to draw from. Nevertheless, changing fashions affect the minority, and the most frequent agents causing drug poisonings will undoubtedly continue to resemble those listed in Table 1.

Table 2 lists the most common drug poisonings presently encountered in the United States, gives their principal signs of toxicity, and outlines their treatment. Clinical appraisal still must be used to diagnose the agent causing several of these reaction patterns, specific chemical tests being either unavailable or impractically slow. Blood levels or size of the dose are generally unreliable guides to the potential danger with almost any of the drugs listed because tolerance develops to their chronic ingestion, making individuals react differently to similar doses. Also, the mixing of drugs with each other and with alcohol adds to the unreliability of blood levels as a guide to treatment or prognosis of the drugs listed in Table 2. Only the opiates and the sedatives create any appreciable risk of death; concurrent alcohol ingestion enhances both these risks. Opiate poisoning is discussed in more detail in Ch. 244. The rest of this chapter gives details of the management of sedative drug overdose. For the diagnosis and treatment of suspected drug or chemical poisonings not covered in these pages, physicians should consult the *Physicians' Desk Reference* or the Poison Control Center of a large city.

SEDATIVE OVERDOSE

PATHOGENESIS. All the sedative drugs depress the central nervous system, although not equally on a gram-molecular weight basis, and not to the same degree so far as different central structures are concerned. The duration of action varies widely and depends largely on how the particular drug is detoxified or eliminated. The short-acting barbiturates, pentobarbital, secobarbital, and amobarbital, are detoxified by the liver, as is methaqualone. They exert their maximal effects promptly after being absorbed and, even in huge doses, seldom cause neurologic depression lasting longer than three to five days. Barbital and phenobarbital are partially detoxified by the liver and partially excreted in the urine. Severe poisoning with the latter

TABLE 1. Drugs Used, in Order of Frequency, Among Severe Overdose Subjects, New York Hospital, 1969–1973

Alcohol	Lithium
Barbiturates, glutethimide	Salicylates
Heroin or methadone	Phenothiazines
Methaqualone	Diphenylhydantoin
Meprobamate	Bishydroxycoumarin, Coumadin
Scopolamine	Tolbutamide, phenformin
Amphetamine	Insulin
Imipramine	

TABLE 2. Common Drug Poisonings, Signs of Toxicity, and Treatment

Drug	Mild Toxic Signs	Tissue for Diagnosis	Treatment	Severe Overdose Signs	Treatment
Opiates: Heroin Morphine Demerol Methadone	"Nodding" drowsiness, small pupils, urinary retention, slow and shallow breathing; skin scars and subcutaneous abscesses; duration 4–6 hrs; with methadone, duration to 24 hrs	Urine	Levallorphan 1 mg IV, naloxone 0.4 mg IV or IM; repeat at 15-min intervals not more than twice; repeat in 3 hrs if necessary	Coma; pinpoint pupils, slow irregular respiration or apnea, hypotension, hypothermia, pulmonary edema	Levallorphan, nalorphine, naloxine; if no response by second dose, suspect another cause; treat shock; find and detect infection
Depressants: Alcohol Barbiturates Glutethimide (Doriden) Meprobamate (Equanil) Methaqualone (Quaalude, Sopor, Mandrax) Chlordiazepoxide (Librium) Diazepam (Valium)	Confusion, rousable drowsiness, delirium, ataxia, nystagmus, dysarthria, analgesia to stimuli Hallucinations, agitation, motor hyperactivity, myoclonus, tonic spasms Usually taken with another sedative if poisoning the attempt	Blood, urine, breath Blood Blood Blood Blood Blood	Alcohol excitement: diazepam or chlorpromazine None needed for acute toxicity; withdraw drug under supervision if patient is a chronic user	Stupor to coma; pupils reactive, usually constricted; oculovestibular response absent; motor tonus initially briefly hyperactive, then flaccid; respiration and blood pressure depressed; hypothermia; with glutethimide, pupils moderately dilated, can be fixed; with meprobamate, withdrawal seizures common; with methaqualone, coma, occasional convulsions, tachycardia, cardiac failure, bleeding tendency	Intubate, ventilate, gavage; drainage position; antimicrobials; keep mean blood pressure above 90 mm Hg and urine output 300 ml/hr; avoid analeptics; hemodialyze severe phenobarbital poisoning As above; diuresis of little help
Stimulants: Amphetamines Methylphenidate Cocaine Psychedelics (LSD, mescaline, psilocybin, STP) Atropine-scopolamine (Sominex)	Hyperactive, aggressive, sometimes paranoid, repetitive behavior; dilated pupils, tremor, hyperactive reflexes; hyperthermia, tachycardia, arrhythmia Acute torsion dystonia Similar but less prominent than above; less paranoid, often euphoric Confused, disoriented, perceptual distortions, distractable, withdrawn or eruptive, leading to accidents or violence; wide-eyed, dilated pupils; restless, hyperreflexic; less often, hypertension or tachycardia Agitated or confused, visual hallucinations, dilated pupils, flushed and dry skin	Blood None: clinical appraisal only	Reassurance if mild Chlorpromazine if intense Chlorpromazine Reassure Reassure; "talk down"; do not leave alone Reassure	Agitated, assaultive and paranoid excitement; occasionally convulsions; hypothermia; circulatory collapse Twitching, irregular breathing, tachycardia Panic Toxic disoriented delirium, visual hallucination; later, amnesia, fever, dilated fixed pupils, hot flushed dry skin, urinary retention	Chlorpromazine Sedation Reassure; diazepam satisfactory; avoid phenothiazines Reassure; sedate lightly; (1) avoid phenothiazines; (2) do not leave alone
Antidepressants: Imipramine (Tofranil), amitriptyline (Elavil) MAO inhibitors: tranylcypromine (Parnate), phenelzine (Nardil), pargyline (Eutonyl) Phenothiazines	Restlessness, drowsiness, tachycardia, ataxia, sweating Hypertensive crises, agitation, drowsiness, ataxia Acute dystonia, somnolence, hypotension	Clinical Clinical Clinical	Physostigmine for arrhythmias Withdrawal Benadryl 0.05 gram 3–4 times daily; withdrawal	Agitation, vomiting, hyperpyrexia, sweating, muscle dystonia, convulsions, tachycardia or arrhythmia Hypotension; headache; chest pain; agitation; coma, seizures and shock Coma; convulsions (rare); arrhythmias; hypotension	Symptomatic; gastric lavage Symptomatic; gastric lavage Symptomatic; gastric lavage

agent can cause coma lasting 10 to 14 days. Glutethimide has a short duration of action comparable to that of secobarbital, but it is poorly absorbed from the gut and may generate more long-lasting neurotoxic metabolites. Meprobamate has an intermediate duration of effect lasting for days. Bromide rarely causes full coma, but, once it reaches high levels, it replaces chloride in the blood and tissues, and persists for weeks to cause symptoms without further ingestion. Chemical autoanalyzers in hospital use do not differentiate these halide ions and report falsely high chloride levels in bromide poisoning.

Although the sedatives have few important effects outside the nervous system, glutethimide and meprobamate in toxic doses tend to produce hypotension. Also, glutethimide possesses anticholinergic properties and is the only sedative that predictably produces light-fixed pupils in toxic doses.

A withdrawal syndrome consisting of tremulousness, agitation, and sometimes delirium and convulsions can develop after prompt withdrawal of any of the hypnotic sedatives. Convulsions seem to be a particular problem after withdrawal from meprobamate and methaqualone.

CLINICAL MANIFESTATIONS. Stupor or coma caused by depressant drug poisoning presents the characteristic picture of severe metabolic brain disease. The depression of the central nervous system tends to be bilateral and symmetrical, and the drug affects simultaneously many levels, including the spinal cord. Respiratory and circulatory controlling mechanisms in the lower brainstem are affected only with very high doses or not at all, and, except with glutethimide, the pupillary light reflexes are preserved. Early in the course of poisoning, patients can demonstrate muscular hypertonus or even spasticity as the result of uneven depression of different neurologic levels. Within a short time, usually an hour or less, flaccidity supervenes, and the stretch reflexes tend to disappear. Even moderate degrees of drug depression depress or block the oculovestibular reflexes.

Four grades of coma have been described in order to aid in estimating the severity of poisoning and the effects of treatment. *Grade I* is light coma in which vigorous noxious stimulation evokes withdrawal or groaning. *Grade II* is deep coma in which only minimal grimacing or reflex responsiveness can be evoked by a noxious stimulus. In *grade III* subjects fail to respond in any way to a noxious stimulus. In *grade IV* unresponsive patients remain in deep coma for over 36 hours and, in addition, have serious respiratory or circulatory depression. As mentioned above, a relationship between the blood level of a sedative drug and the depth of coma is only approximate. Generally speaking, however, blood levels of short-acting barbiturates of more than 2.5 mg per 100 ml and phenobarbital blood levels of more than 12 mg per 100 ml are associated with grades III and IV coma.

DIAGNOSIS. The combination of unresponsiveness, preserved or sluggish pupillary reactions, absent oculovestibular reactions, motor areflexia, hypothermia, and depression of respiration and circulation is clinically diagnostic of sedative-anesthetic drug poisoning. Only pontine infarction resembles this clinical state, and with lesions of the pons the pupils are usually small or pinpoint, the stretch reflexes are generally preserved or hyperactive, and the plantar responses are extensor. Specific chemical tests will detect barbiturates, glutethi-

mide, meprobamate, methaqualone, and bromides in blood or urine, and are readily done as emergency measures.

MANAGEMENT OF COMA. There are no specific antidotes. Treatment consists of physiologic support and preventing complications until the drug is detoxified and is excreted. Proper management saves all but a very few patients if they survive to reach the hospital. Among the writer's very large series of patients with drug coma, fewer than 2 per cent have died. To achieve this low rate required meticulous attention to the airway and ventilation, to the circulation, and to the potential complications of the comatose state.

AIRWAY AND VENTILATION. Several mechanisms threaten to obstruct the airway of patients in coma from sedative drugs. If the subject lies on his back, the tongue and pooled secretions occlude the hypopharynx, with the result that secretions are aspirated into the lungs. The cough reflex and the ciliary action of the tracheobronchial mucosa are depressed. Many subjects aspirate stomach contents into the lungs, particularly if gastric lavage is attempted before tracheal intubation.

An oropharyngeal airway is sufficient to manage patients in light coma who cough when the larynx is stimulated. A cuffed endotracheal tube should be placed in more deeply anesthetized patients who lack a cough reflex. It is wise to precede intubation with atropine, 0.0008 gram intravenously, to reduce the danger of cardiac arrest. How long to leave the endotracheal tube in place in an unresponsive subject is often a difficult question. One practice is to deflate the cuff hourly for 5 minutes, to replace the tube at 24 hours, and to perform a tracheostomy at somewhere between 36 and 48 hours if the cough reflex has not returned or if no other signs indicate a lessening of coma.

To drain the lungs and improve oxygenation, patients should be placed in the prone position, as illustrated in the accompanying figure, and suctioned gently through the endotracheal tube every half hour, or more often if pulmonary secretions accumulate. It is desirable to administer low concentrations (25 per cent) of moistened oxygen, but not to occlude the tube with a large catheter. Tubes are removed when active coughing or bucking returns.

Hypoventilation should be treated with artificial respiration. Shallow breathing in a deeply comatose patient frequently reflects no more than the subject's depressed metabolism, but if the rate falls below 12 per minute or if the physician entertains serious doubts as to the adequacy of ventilation, artificial respiration is indicated. Ideally, arterial blood gases should be measured in deeply comatose patients and artificial respiration initiated if the arterial Pco_2 climbs above 45 mm of mercury. High concentration (>30 per cent) oxygen therapy should be avoided for patients not receiving artificial respiration, for its use increases the risk of hypoventilation and CO_2 retention.

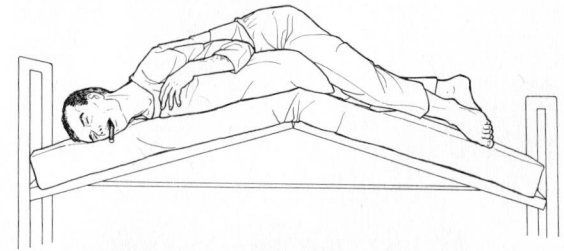

Circulation. Severe shock is rare with depressant drug poisoning unless the patient has been asphyxiated. However, moderate hypotension is common and significantly reduces glomerular filtration and renal clearance of the barbiturates. Fluids should be given liberally to restore blood volume and promote urine flow, and pressor agents, such as dopamine or isoproterenol, are indicated to keep the diastolic blood pressure above 60 mm of mercury and the systolic above 90 mm of mercury. Digitalis or similar compounds are useful only in patients with heart disease. Cardiac arrhythmias induced by tricyclic antidepressant ingestion should be treated with physostigmine. Corticosteroids are unnecessary.

Prevention of Complications. As long as he remains unconscious, the patient should be kept semiprone in the drainage position and changed from side to side in the semiprone position, but never placed on his back. Since the duration of unconsciousness is to be measured in days, the emergence of drug-resistant bacteria is of less concern than is pneumonia caused by already aspirated material. Thus it is useful to administer penicillin or tetracycline.

The blood pressure, pulse, and respiration should be recorded each half hour, and any abnormalities should be met appropriately. Body temperature elevations imply an infection if stimulants have not been given. Hypothermia above 32° C requires no special treatment. To evaluate the rate of urine flow, most physicians prefer to insert an indwelling catheter.

Other Measures. *Gastric lavage* is desirable for any patient who has ingested depressant drugs within the preceding few hours. A large Ewald tube must be used to remove capsular material. The procedure should be done gently to avoid producing pulmonary aspiration, and is best preceded by tracheal intubation with a cuffed tube in deeply comatose subjects. Subjects too lightly anesthetized to tolerate intubation should be turned prone before being lavaged. Care is required to avoid misplacing the tube and irrigating the lungs.

Forced diuresis and alkalinization of the urine have been recommended as adjuncts in treating barbiturate poisoning. Forced diuresis increases the renal clearance of both short- and long-acting barbiturates, and the quantity cleared increases proportionately to the volume of urine. Phenobarbital has a relatively high pK value, and raising the urine pH appears to increase its dissociation and excretion. Several programs have been employed to achieve diuresis. The first step is to assure an adequate blood pressure; the second, to infuse a hypotonic electrolyte solution. The infusions are given at hourly rates up to 600 ml, depending upon urine flow. Close attention must be given to hour-by-hour fluid balance and 12-hour electrolyte balance. If urine flow does not match the infusion rate by the second or third hour, infusions should be slowed and more attention given to raising the blood pressure. Chemical and osmotic diuretics are contraindicated. Hypokalemia is a greater risk than hyperkalemia.

For treating bromide intoxication, diuresis should be combined with a high intake of sodium chloride to displace bromide from blood and tissues.

Hemodialysis is not necessary to treat poisoning with the short-acting hypnotics. However, hemodialysis is indicated to shorten the duration of coma for patients who have ingested large amounts of long-acting barbiturates such as barbital or phenobarbital, or who are in grade IV coma from glutethimide overdose. Dialysis also is indicated for severe lithium or bromide poisoning.

Analeptics and pharmacologic stimulants are contraindicated for coma caused by depressant drug poisoning. Most carry the risk of overstimulating or producing convulsions in lightly poisoned patients.

RECOVERY AND PROGNOSIS. Patients recovering from coma require close medical supervision. Severe pneumonitis can develop as late as three to four days after recovery. If antimicrobial drugs were started during coma, they are best continued for at least 48 hours after it ends. Permanent physical sequelae to coma are rare. Among 356 cases, residual brain injury was observed only once (in a patient who suffered an acute cardiac arrest). Peripheral nerve injuries from pressure developed in 6 subjects, and 14 subjects had pressure skin lesions leaving scars. There were no other residua.

Later management varies according to the patient's underlying psychiatric disorder and his attitudes upon recovery. Serious suicide attempts are never accidents, and reports of near-fatal ingestion caused by misunderstanding the dose or forgetting previous doses carry little validity. The expert opinion of a psychiatrist should be sought before deciding whether to release a patient or to institutionalize him. The immediate prognosis is good, but there is a high incidence of recurrent attempts at self-destruction over the years.

Bourne, P. G.: Acute Drug Abuse Emergencies. New York, Academic Press, 1976.

Douglas, W. D., Rehder, K., Beyner, F. M., Sessler, A. D., and Marsh, H. M.: Improved oxygenation in patients with acute respiratory failure: The prone position. Am. Rev. Respir. Dis., 115:559, 1977.

Physicians' Desk Reference to Pharmaceutical Specialties and Biologicals. Published annually by Medical Economics Co., Oradell, N. J.

Section Eight THE HYPOTHALAMUS AND NEUROLOGIC DISORDERS

Fred Plum

252. INTRODUCTION

The hypothalamus links the emotional forebrain, the autonomic nervous system, and the endocrine system. Diseases involving this tiny spot not only produce protean symptoms but often develop insidiously and progress slowly, making early recognition difficult. Hypothalamic dysfunction must often be considered as a possible cause of emotional, autonomic, or endocrine disorders, and the following chapters should be read in conjunction with the description of the endocrine hypothalamus in Ch. 542.

253. FUNCTIONAL ANATOMY

The hypothalamus is made up of a diffuse reticulum of neurons richly traversed by fiber pathways. Only the paraventricular and supraoptic nuclei have sharp anatomic definition, other neuronal collections being defined better as regions or areas than as specific nuclei. Similarly, only a minority of the conduction pathways are collected into discretely identifiable tracts. This imprecise anatomy reflects itself in the localization of hypothalamic functions, many of which overlap several of the region's anatomic subdivisions (Table 1). Afferent connections come from the limbic forebrain, from the cerebral cortex of the frontal and temporal lobes, from the thalamus, and from the midbrain reticular formation. The hypothalamus, in turn, sends direct neural connections to the thalamus, the brainstem reticular formation, the brainstem autonomic nuclei, and the posterior lobe of the hypophysis.

From the standpoint of clinical medicine, ventromedian and posterior hypothalamic lesions tend to produce greater functional changes than ones elsewhere in the structure. Except for sympathetic activities, bilateral damage is required to produce discernible changes in hypothalamic function. Ventromedian lesions not only interfere bilaterally with hypothalamic functions localized in that area but commonly interrupt the flow of hypothalamus-to-pituitary neurosecretion as well. Posterior hypothalamic lesions both destroy local functions and interrupt descending common paths to the more caudal brainstem. Table 2 lists the most common causes of hypothalamic disease.

254. SLEEP AND AROUSAL

Sleep and arousal are active behavioral states influenced by nervous structures that extend from the anterior hypothalamus down to the mid pons. The hypothalamic components of this system appear to influence both sleeping and waking behavior more specifically than do the nuclei of the midbrain and pons. In animals, stimulation of the anterior hypothalamus produces a state that behaviorally and physiologically resembles true sleep; destruction of this region results in sustained insomnia. Conversely, posterior hypothalamic stimulation produces arousal, whereas its destruction results in sustained sleep-like unresponsiveness. In human beings, hypothalamic insomnia is rare, and has been observed only acutely with anterior hypothalamic injury. Posterior hypothalamic lesions, on the other hand, are a well established cause of lethargic behavior, hypersomnolence, or sleep-like coma and should be specifically searched for when these symptoms arise.

TABLE 1. Regional Functions of the Hypothalamus*

	Preoptic Anterior Hypothalamus	Tuberal and Ventromedian Hypothalamus	Posterior Hypothalamus
Receptor:	Thermal, osmotic	Caloric	Thermal set-point
Integrates:	Endocrine, thermal, autonomic	Cognition; endocrine; autonomic; caloric balance; fluid balance	Consciousness; cognition; complex endocrine; autonomic; thermal
Contains:	Sleep-inducing mechanism; forebrain parasympathetic paths	Thermoregulatory paths; final common endocrine paths	Reticular activating system; thermoregulatory effectors
Acute lesions:	Insomnia? diabetes insipidus; hyperthermia; diabetes insipidus; inappropriate ADH	Hyperthermia; diabetes insipidus; hypothalamic-endocrine disorders	Hypersomnia; emotional disorders; poikilothermia; autonomic storm
Chronic lesions:	Insominia; complex endocrine changes (e.g., precocious puberty); final common path endocrine changes; hypothermia; hypodipsia	Medial: memory loss; emotional disorders; hyperphagia and obesity; final common path endocrine disorders Lateral: emotional disorders; emaciation; loss of thirst	Memory loss; emotional disorders; poikilothermia; incoordination of autonomic reflexes; complex endocrine disorders (e.g., precocious puberty)

*As indicated in the text, functional localization is more precise for some activities than others.

TABLE 2. Principal Causes of Hypothalamic Diseases in Adolescents and Adults

Congenital midline brain defects, e.g., agenesis of corpus callosum
"Familial" disorders, e.g., diabetes insipidus
Chronic hydrocephalus or increased intracranial pressure
Tumors: craniopharyngiomas, glioma, hamartoma, dysgerminoma, dermoid, lipoma, lymphoma or leukemia, meningioma
Encephalitis: various viral encephalitides, exanthematous demyelinating encephalitides, disseminated encephalomyelitis
Granulomas: sarcoid, tuberculosis, histocytosis X
Trauma
Subarachnoid hemorrhage; aneurysms; arteriovenous malformation
Wernicke's polioencephalopathy (thiamin deficiency)
Progressive idiopathic degeneration

255. MEMORY AND EMOTION

The ventromedian hypothalamus stands in the pathway that links the limbic forebrain to the thalamus and the brainstem reticular formation. Damage to this region in man impairs recent and intermediate term memory, the severity of the defect roughly paralleling the anatomic extent of the damage. Present research leaves unsettled whether the critical anatomic structures include the mammillary bodies or the immediately more anterior hypothalamic region which contains projections from both the amygdala and fornix. Diseases that bilaterally invade or destroy this ventromedian area can produce a severe dementia, marked by memory loss, withdrawn and confused behavior, and, sometimes, aggressive outbursts. Loss of libido accompanies ventromedian hypothalamic disease but most probably reflects gonadal hypotrophism rather than a direct neural effect.

256. HEAT REGULATION

The question of hypothalamic dysfunction repeatedly arises in patients with cryptogenic fever. In fact, hypothalamic disease rarely or never produces subacute or chronic fever, although several kinds of hypothalamic damage reduce body temperature. Experimental evidence indicates that the preoptic anterior hypothalamus contains separate receptors for warmth and cold as well as for pyrogens. The hypothalamus integrates information generated by these receptors with stimuli arriving directly from peripheral thermoreceptors as well as from nonspecific sources, such as the subject's general level of arousal. Diurnal changes in central nervous system excitability and in the level of circulating ovarian hormones provide additional nonspecific stimuli. In turn, the hypothalamus activates varying combinations of behavioral, autonomic, and endocrine responses that conserve or dissipate the body heat.

Gross stimulation of the anterior hypothalamus activates mainly the more abundant warm receptors located in that region and leads to heat dissipation and a fall in body temperature. Conversely, acute anterior or lateral hypothalamic destruction causes transient hyperthermia that subsides gradually over several days to weeks as more caudally placed and peripheral thermoreceptors take charge.

The posterior hypothalamus integrates thermoregulation and generates the signals that initiate the physiologic, affective, and behavioral adjustments that guarantee the stability of body temperature. Selective stimulation of dorsomedial-caudal hypothalamic and rostral mesencephalic sites activates heat production mechanisms. In contrast, ventrolateral-caudal hypothalamic stimulation inhibits heat production and activates heat dissipation. Large posterior hypothalamic lesions destroy both heat loss and heat production mechanisms and result in poikilothermia.

HYPOTHERMIA. Relative Poikilothermia. Poikilothermia, defined as the fluctuation in body temperature of greater than 2° C with changes in ambient temperature, is the most common central abnormality of heat regulation in man. Most such cases are detected by a lowered body temperature. Poikilothermia results from degeneration or metabolic dysfunction of the final integrator and effector sites for thermoregulation located in the posterior hypothalamus and rostral mesencephalon. Lesions in this area impair not only autonomic heat regulating pathways but those that control thermal discomfort, and the behavioral regulation of body temperature as well. As a result, many patients with poikilothermia are unaware of their condition and do little to avoid it. At ordinary ambient temperatures of 20 to 25° C, the degree of hypothermia tends to be proportional to the degree of functional hypothalamic impairment. Relative poikilothermia resulting from impaired hypothalamic-autonomic function is frequent in the elderly, making them dangerously susceptible to lowered environmental temperatures. Chronic poikilothermia accompanies several degenerative disorders of the brain in children and adults. Metabolic causes of poikilothermia include acute or chronic sedative drug ingestion, hypoglycemia, and myxedema. Poikilothermia regularly accompanies extensive damage to the posterior hypothalamus or midbrain by stroke, trauma, or neoplasm.

Paroxysmal Hypothermia. *Sustained hypothermia* (as opposed to relative poikilothermia) is rare in man. Somewhat less uncommon is *paroxysmal hypothermia*, consisting of attacks of lowered body temperature that vary widely in frequency from daily to more than a decade apart. Such attacks usually begin abruptly, last from minutes to days, and are characterized by sweating, flushing of the skin, and a fall in body temperature, usually to 32° C or lower. Fatigue, decreased mental responsiveness, hypoventilation, hypotension, cardiac arrhythmias, ataxia, lacrimation, and asterixis may accompany the lowered body temperature. The attacks subside either slowly (hours to days) or rapidly with shivering and peripheral vasoconstriction. During hypothermia, mechanisms for both heat production and heat dissipation respond normally, but around a lower temperature set-point. Most of the patients have had direct evidence for hypothalamic disease; several have had agenesis of the corpus callosum.

HYPERTHERMIA. Hyperthermia resulting from central nervous system damage occurs only with acute pathologic processes, and rarely lasts for more than two weeks following the initial event. The most frequent causes include gross head injury, either surgical trauma or bleeding into the region of the anterior hypothalamus, or hemorrhage in the adjacent meninges or the third ventricle. With neurogenic hyperthermia, the body temperature can rise to potentially fatal levels of 42° C or higher as a result of active heat production unbalanced by heat dissipation. The cardiovascular changes that normally accompany fever are disproportionately lacking. Small (2 mg) doses of morphine can be useful in ameliorating dangerously high neurogenic fevers.

257. SYMPATHETIC AND PARASYMPATHETIC FUNCTIONS

Symptoms of sympathetic and parasympathetic dysfunction figure prominently in many medical and psychophysiologic illnesses. Nearly all these responses are mediated through hypothalamic pathways, and their presence repeatedly leads physicians to question whether these structures play a primary role.

Autonomic influences originating in the cerebral hemispheres converge on the hypothalamus and are integrated there to be transmitted down the neuraxis. Generally speaking, stimulation of the anterior hypothalamus evokes primarily parasympathetic responses, whereas posterior hypothalamic stimulation elicits sympathetic activity. Destructive lesions have the opposite effect. The evoked sympathetic responses occur mainly ipsilaterally and represent the only example of a unilateral localization and projection of a hypothalamic function.

Experiments of recent years have disclosed that the autonomic functions of the hypothalamus are specific to the degree that stimulation of an isolated fiber can engender a predictable response in specific peripheral organs. A similar precision applies to afferent pathways. Despite its capacity for individual autonomic responses, however, the predominant autonomic role of the hypothalamus is integrative. Without the hypothalamus, one can still obtain individually normal baseline autonomic activities, but the complex coordination of autonomic and behavioral responses that assures homeostasis is impaired or lost.

Central neurogenic autonomic abnormalities in man accompany acute disease of the hypothalamus and its efferent pathways. With the exception of partial sympathetic paralysis, however, chronic hypothalamic lesions rarely produce clinically detectable abnormalities in autonomic control systems.

CARDIOVASCULAR EFFECTS. An extensive clinical literature describes changes in cardiovascular function accompanying acute disease of the brainstem and hypothalamus. The abnormalities include hypertension, cardiac arrhythmias of various types, and a number of electrocardiographic abnormalities, some of which can simulate acute myocardial infarction. Many affected patients have no evidence of previous cardiovascular disease. Subarachnoid hemorrhage and acute diseases of the brainstem can induce multifocal myocardial necrosis, possibly due to coronary arteriolar vasoconstriction in response to the outpouring of catecholamines that accompanies the acute event. The specific relationship of such changes to hypothalamic damage has not been proved, and they may equally well reflect the effects of excitation of descending autonomic pathways.

Pulmonary edema and hemorrhage can be a sudden and striking accompaniment to acute hypothalamic injury in animals. Many observers believe that a similar process occurs in man, perhaps causing the wet lungs often observed after acute intracranial injury, infection, or hemorrhage. The response probably is nonspecific, however. Some patients develop pulmonary edema in association with anterior hypothalamic compression, intraventricular hemorrhage, or rupture of an anterior communicating arterial aneurysm. Others develop similar lung changes in association with lesions involving intracranial sites remote from the hypothalamus.

Theories of the pathogenesis of "neurogenic" pulmonary edema have centered on the excitation of an adrenergic cardiovascular mechanism producing acute hypertension and a shift of blood from the systemic to the pulmonary vascular beds. Direct studies in humans with acute neurogenic pulmonary edema, however, have failed to demonstrate either an elevated blood pressure or an elevated central venous pressure. Whatever its cause, acute pulmonary congestion accompanying acute central nervous system injury often requires urgent attention to minimize hypoxemia and the deleterious effects of overvigorous breathing efforts.

GASTROINTESTINAL FUNCTIONS. In laboratory animals, acute lesions placed anywhere from the level of the preoptic hypothalamus rostrally to the region of the vagal nuclei in the medulla caudally can result in gastrointestinal hemorrhage. Posterior hypothalamic lesions can result in ulceration, but anterior hypothalamic lesions generally confine their effects to producing hemorrhagic gastromalacia.

Hemorrhage and acute ulceration are the major gastrointestinal complications of central nervous system dysfunction in man, and they can affect the gastrointestinal tract anywhere from the lower esophagus to the large bowel. Intracranial surgery, head trauma, encephalitis, cerebral hemorrhage and infarction, acute multiple sclerosis, brain abscess, meningitis, and a variety of intracranial tumors all may precipitate acute gastrointestinal ulceration or hemorrhage. The common denominator of all these lesions is the acute nature of their onset. The most frequent specific gastrointestinal abnormality seems to be lower esophageal ulceration, an otherwise rare lesion. Gastric and duodenal ulcerations account for an even greater association, but much of this reflects their high non-neurogenic incidence. Neurogenic ulcers occur in all age groups from neonates to those over 80 years old. The ulcers themselves are morphologically identical to those that accompany the acute stresses of burns, pneumonia, and general body trauma. Acute gastrointestinal ulceration and hemorrhage in association with intracranial disease thus arises as a manifestation of nonspecific damage or an imbalance in descending central autonomic pathways rather than of any specific hypothalamic effect. Sympathetic hyperactivity elevating the systemic levels of catecholamines and parasympathetic hyperactivity producing elevated gastrin levels have been noted in affected patients. No one knows which of these is more important.

258. FEEDING BEHAVIOR AND CALORIC BALANCE

Forebrain and especially limbic system influences assume such an importance in feeding behavior in man that primary hypothalamic error accounts for no more than a tiny fraction of human obesity or emaciation.

In animals, stimulation of the ventromedian region inhibits feeding, whereas lesions destroying this region produce hyperphagia and a weight gain which later stabilizes at a new elevated set-point, after which time the hyperphagia subsides. The critical damage influencing feeding may be to the catecholaminergic pathways that lie in close proximity to the ventromedian nucleus as they traverse the hypothalamus toward the forebrain. Stimulation of the lateral hypothalamus in animals induces feeding behavior, whereas damage to the region results in a temporarily severe aphagia that slowly recovers to maintain a lowered body weight that represents a new set-point. The critical site affecting feeding behavior may be the paths traversing this lateral hypothalamic region, and not intrinsic hypothalamic neurons themselves.

HYPOTHALAMIC OBESITY. Most patients with hypothalamic obesity have shown at autopsy diffuse or large lesions involving the greater part of the structure, although frequently sparing the posterior hypothalamus. A few have had precisely placed abnormalities destroying the ventromedian hypothalamus with the size of the destructive lesion at least roughly corresponding with the degree of obesity. Occasional examples have been due to leukemic infiltration of the periventricular hypothalamus, with the most severe damage localized in the ventromedian region; others have been discrete tumors in this area.

These lesions in patients with hypothalamic obesity provide the most discrete localization of any disorder of the human hypothalamus. The patients have experienced remarkable combinations of food-seeking behavior, including hyperphagia, finickiness in food selections, decreased activity, and obesity, just as in the laboratory animal with medial tuberal damage.

The hypothalamus evidently contains a set-point mechanism that roughly regulates body weight. When one encounters a patient with hypothalamic obesity, the presence or absence of continued hyperphagia depends on whether or not the neurologic process is stable and the body weight set-point has been attained. Patients with obesity following upon surgical or blunt head trauma to the hypothalamus illustrate this principle. Characteristically, such individuals initially display a ravenous hyperphagia and gain weight quickly following the injury until they reach their new set-point, at which point they become normophagic and their weight stabilizes. After six months or so, many such patients then become hypophagic and their weight declines to reapproach the pretrauma level.

Emaciation sometimes accompanies hypothalamic disease in man, but in such instances the lesions usually have been large and their specificity uncertain. A causative association between hypothalamic disease and anorexia nervosa has not been established.

259. WATER BALANCE

Homeostatic control of body water and osmolality depends heavily on the hypothalamic coordination of affective thirst, drinking behavior, and antidiuretic hormone (ADH) release. Hypothalamic disease or dysfunction can produce four principal disorders of water balance. The syndromes of ADH deficiency (diabetes insipidus) and inappropriate ADH excess are dis-

cussed in Ch. 544.2 and 530, respectively. The syndromes of essential or central hypernatremia and of episodic hyperdipsia are often related to central nervous system dysfunction and are discussed in this chapter.

PHYSIOLOGY. The osmoreceptors that most influence thirst, water drinking behavior, and the osmotic control of ADH release lie within the preoptic anterior hypothalamic region. In laboratory animals, one can identify in this area cells that respond to both local sodium concentration and circulating levels of angiotensin, a polypeptide released during systemic dehydration. Osmoreceptors in other hypothalamic regions possess more limited functions.

Peripheral receptors influence water balance less strongly than do the hypothalamic receptors. Thirst is stimulated by osmoreceptors lying in the systemic interstitial fluids, as well as by receptors in the mouth responsible for the sensation of dryness. Excitation of volume receptors in the left atrium of the heart and in the large capacitance systemic veins tends to inhibit drinking behavior and ADH release. Baroceptor influences, ascending through the brainstem, exert a similar effect. Thermal stress, eating, psychic stress, and other influences all can activate drinking and ADH release so as to influence water balance.

The magnocellular neurons in the supraoptic and paraventricular nuclei of higher animals produce ADH and transport it to the median eminence and neurohypophysis, whence it passes into the blood. These neurosecretory cells maintain a low baseline firing rate that is increased by stimulation from excitatory osmoreceptors or decreased by stimuli from inhibitory volume receptors. All evidence indicates that the threshold for ADH release depends on the set-point of the associated osmoreceptor. Once above threshold, further changes in ADH release in response to changes of osmolarity appear to depend on the integrated sum of the various inputs. Under normal conditions, osmoreceptors are the most influential determinant of ADH release.

Most human disorders of water balance can be reproduced experimentally. Diabetes insipidus is the most easily obtained and requires a 90 per cent or greater loss of the magnocellular neurons of the supraoptic and paraventricular nuclei. Such a high percentage of cell loss requires direct hypothalamic damage, explaining why hypophysectomy (which spares the neurons secreting into median eminence vessels) usually causes only a temporary diabetes insipidus. Lesions that impinge on the supraoptic nucleus but do not destroy it result in an inappropriately high secretion of ADH, presumably by interrupting inhibitory pathways to the nucleus. Destruction of the receptor-containing preoptic region produces a permanent hypodipsia or adipsia accompanied by loss of the ADH response to osmotic stress.

Electrical stimulation of the lateral hypothalamus or nonspecific arousal in animals results in polydipsia, whereas destructive lateral lesions cause a temporary adipsia. Stimulation of higher limbic system structures tends most often to inhibit drinking and ADH release. Ventromedian hypothalamic stimulation inhibits drinking, whereas lesions of the ventromedian region may produce hyperdipsia.

THE SYNDROME OF ESSENTIAL HYPERNATREMIA. Four features characterize essential hypernatremia in man: (1) hypernatremia unaccompanied by a corresponding extracellular fluid deficiency, (2) a preserved renal tubular responsiveness to ADH, (3) an inadequate secretion of ADH in response to osmotic stimuli, and (4) the absence or deficiency of thirst with otherwise fully conscious behavior. True essential hypernatremia is rare; most cases of serum hyperosmolarity accompanying intracranial disease result from a nonspecific combination of dehydration and stupor.

Essential hypernatremia in its milder and more chronic forms often elevates the serum sodium only modestly, and such patients characteristically have no symptoms except for a remarkable lack of thirst. When sodium levels climb to the 160 to 170 mEq per deciliter range, however, most patients develop weakness and some, fever, as well as muscle tenderness and cramping that may progress to fatigue, ataxia, and even myoglobinuria. Mental symptoms include lethargy, anorexia, depression, and irritability. With elevations of serum sodium above 180 mEq per deciliter, most patients become confused or stuporous, and some will die. All patients with essential hypernatremia fail to demonstrate thirst, but many retain persistent habitual drinking, although at a volume insufficient to maintain a normal serum osmolality.

For poorly understood reasons, patients with essential hypernatremia lack clinical evidence of dehydration; only mild hypovolemia or even normovolemia can accompany serum sodium levels as high as 200 mEq per deciliter or more. An associated hypokalemia usually contributes to the muscular symptoms. Urine volumes may be low or normal but are always more dilute than appropriate for the serum hyperosmolality. The administration of exogenous ADH induces a much more concentrated urine. Further evidence of abnormal ADH release to naturally occurring stimuli comes from the observation that either an acute water load or a hypertonic saline load can produce an increase in free water clearance.

The hypothalamic defect producing essential hypernatremia in man is poorly localized. Almost all affected patients have associated neurologic abnormalities, but many have lacked radiographic evidence of morphologic central nervous system abnormalities. Others have had diffuse head trauma or space-occupying lesions destroying the entire hypothalamic region by the time of death. In a few affected patients restricted lesions have involved the preoptic and tuberal region. The mechanisms of essential hypernatremia remain unsettled and may not be the same in all instances. The absence of thirst is critical, and this, along with the lack of ADH response to changes in serum osmolality, indicates that osmo- and volume receptor function is uncoupled from the behavioral and hormonal control of water balance. Baroreceptor influences on ADH secretion may remain intact. The presence of normovolemia accompanying the hypernatremia remains difficult to explain.

Treatment consists of lowering the serum sodium and raising the potassium by manipulating the diet and conditioning the patient to drink several liters of water each day regardless of thirst. Spirolactone, chlorpropamide, and the thiazide diuretics contribute to achieving these ends. More vigorous treatment of hypernatremic crises must be initiated slowly. Becuse their intracellular osmolality has climbed to a new high steady state, patients with essential hypernatremia can develop symptoms of water intoxication if rapidly hydrated, even when the serum remains hyperosmolar compared to normal.

HYPERDIPSIA AND WATER INTOXICATION. Excessive water drinking in the absence of either hypovolemia or serum hyperosmolality is termed primary hyperdipsia and must be differentiated from the compensatory hyperdipsias of conditions such as diabetes insipidus, polyuric renal failure, or diabetes mellitus. In the absence of inappropriate ADH secretion, symptoms of severe hyperdipsia, i.e., hypervolemia, hyponatremia, and clinical water intoxication with stupor, delirium, and convulsions, are infrequent. These usually develop only in patients with renal dysfunction or those who imbibe greater than 15 liters per square meter per day of water, the quantity necessary to overcome the diluting capacity of the normal kidney. Because of the ability of the kidney to excrete large amounts of free water, almost all patients with water intoxication recover with fluid restriction and proper supportive care. Some, however, convulse, and a substantial proportion of these may suffer permanent brain damage.

Causes of primary hyperdipsia include habitual drinking and drinking in response to excessive thirst. Patients with *beer drinker's hyponatremia* drink up to 6 liters or more of beer per day, slowly developing chronic hyponatremia which predisposes them to symptoms from the acute water load associated with a binge. Other examples of habitual hyperdipsia produce their symptoms simply because of a tremendous ingestion of water over a brief period. Most such patients have acute psychiatric disorders and drink excessively to overcome delusional fears. Occasionally, acute water intoxication occurs in systematically healthy persons trying to quell the epigastric burning of gastritis or in youngsters drinking huge amounts of fluids on a dare, or during tea-party games.

Martin, J. B., Reichlin, S., and Brown G. M.: Clinical Neuroendocrinology. Philadelphia, F. A. Davis Company, 1977.
Plum, F., and Van Uitert, R.: Non-endocrine diseases and disorders of the hypothalamus. Res. Publ. Assoc. Res. Nerv. Ment. Dis., Vol. 56, 1977.

Section Nine   PROMINENT NEUROLOGIC SYMPTOMS AND THEIR MANAGEMENT

260.   PAIN

Jerome B. Posner

INTRODUCTION

Pain is the most common symptom for which patients seek medical assistance, and chronic pain is among the most vexing problems which physicians face. Pain can have no precise definition because only the individual suffering it, not the observer, perceives it. Sir Thomas Lewis described the situation exactly when he said pain is "known to us by experience and described by illustration." Pain always has two aspects: the first is an emotionally neutral perception of a stimulus which is usually sufficiently strong to produce tissue damage; the second is an affective response to the perception of that stimulus. Pain implies damage to the organism, either physical or psychologic, and chronic pain, if untreated, will itself damage the organism. It is the physician's twofold therapeutic task to discover and treat the cause of pain and also to treat the pain itself, whether or not the underlying cause is treatable. To meet this twofold task, the physician must know something of the anatomy, physiology, and biochemistry of pain pathways.

PAIN PATHWAYS

ANATOMY AND PHYSIOLOGY. The accompanying figure outlines schematically our current understanding of pain pathways. Pain receptors in the skin and other tissues (nociceptors) are believed to be the free nerve endings of small myelinated and unmyelinated fibers. "Free nerve endings" have never been identified microscopically, nor is there complete agreement on the adequate stimulus for discharging these receptors. Current studies suggest that nociceptors are stimulated either by strong mechanical deformation or by extremes of hot or cold. It is believed that tissue damage from mechanical or thermal injury liberates chemical substances which lower the firing threshold of the mechano- and thermonociceptors so that previously innocuous mechanical or thermal stimuli produce pain. Substances liberated by tissue damage which lower the threshold of pain receptors include potassium, acetylcholine, histamine, serotonin, prostaglandins, and bradykinin. There is some evidence that the lowering of nociceptor threshold is mediated by prostaglandins. Some investigators suggest that aspirin analgesia results from that drug's ability to inhibit prostaglandin synthesis.

The nociceptors are connected to two sets of peripheral fibers: small (6 μ), thinly myelinated, "A delta" fibers which conduct at about 35 meters per second, and unmyelinated "C" fibers (1 to 2 μ) which conduct at about 0.5 meter per second. This dual set of fibers explains the phenomenon of "double pain." A noxious stimulus elicits first a sharp, pricking, well-localized pain mediated by the more rapidly conducting

fibers, and the C fibers mediate a burning, poorly localized, exceedingly unpleasant "second pain." C fiber stimulation in man at a rate of 3 per second causes almost unbearable pain. Not all A delta and C fibers are "pain fibers"; a considerable number are low threshold mechanoreceptors which presumably subserve other sensory modalities.

All primary sensory afferents have their cell bodies in the dorsal root ganglion. Pain fibers enter the spinal cord via the dorsal root, lateral to the large myelinated (touch and proprioception) fibers. Experimental section of the lateral portion of the dorsal root decreases the perception of pain but leaves large fiber modalities intact. Nociceptive fibers enter the cord, and then ascend or descend for one or two segments in the medial portion of Lissauer's tract to enter the more ventrally placed dorsal horn. Lesions of the medial portion of Lissauer's tract contract the dermatomal field of a single root, indicating that it carries excitatory fibers from adjacent roots, and lesions in the lateral portion expand the dorsal root dermatome, indicating that it carries inhibitory fibers.

The dorsal horn consists of six laminae, with lamina 1 being the most dorsal. Laminae 2 and 3 taken together are often referred to as the substantia gelatinosa, but the functional boundaries of this area are not clearly defined. Fibers subserving pain probably end in all six laminae, with laminae 1 and 5

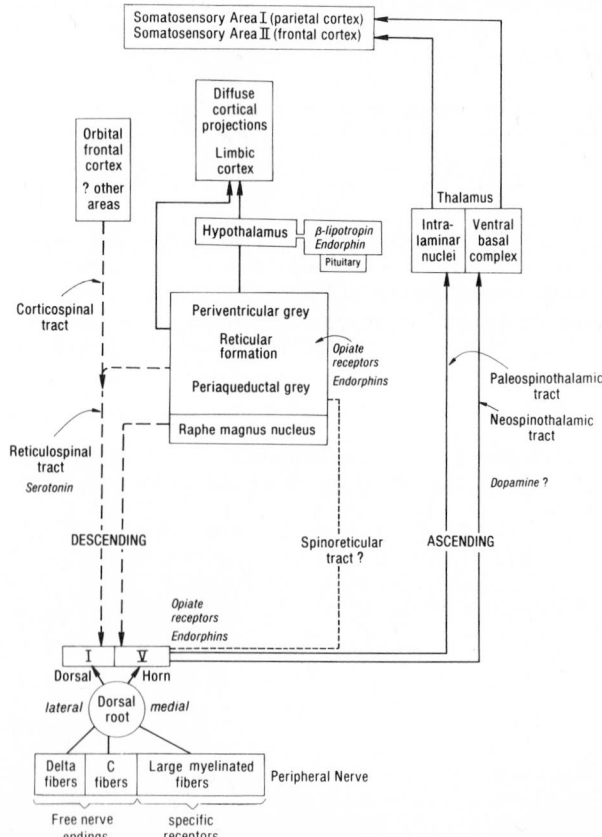

being most important. Interaction between neurons in the dorsal horn is an important site for modulating sensory input. These interactions in the substantia gelatinosa of the dorsal horn are the subject of the "gate control theory of pain," which, although highly controversial, has generated much experimentation. Melzack and Wall hypothesize that sensory fibers have two functions: (1) to carry patterned information, depending upon the specialized properties of each unit, and (2) to modulate the effectiveness of synaptic transmission between peripheral nerve and ascending spinal fibers. The first site of the putative modulating action is in the substantia gelatinosa of the spinal cord, where large fibers are presumed to activate an inhibitory system and small fibers stimulate an activating system. If large fiber stimulation is sufficient, synaptic transmission is inhibited and pain fiber activity which arrives later is less effective in exciting ascending spinal pathways. If the larger fiber stimulus is insufficient or absent, small fibers excite an action system and carry pain messages to higher centers. Descending fibers from cerebral cortex or lower structures also modulate this system.

The ascending pain pathways in the spinal cord are characteristically divided into two groups: the neospinothalamic tract, which is believed to subserve the perception of intensity and localization of pain, and the phylogenetically older paleospinothalamic tract, which is believed to subserve the arousal and emotional components of pain. The axons of the neospinothalamic tract arise from the dorsal horn (cell origin unknown), cross in the anterior commissure, and ascend in the anterolateral quadrant of the spinal cord. The axons terminate in the ventral basal complex of the thalamus, principally within the posterolateral ventral nucleus (VPL) ipsilateral to the side of their ascent. The thalamic terminations of these fibers coincide to a large extent with those of the dorsal column, and the pathway shows somatotopic localization at the thalamic level, the face and upper body being represented most medially. Third order neurons from the thalamus project to somatosensory area I (sensorimotor cortex), with the same somatotopic localization as other sensory modalities. Lesions made in the neospinothalamic pathway at either the thalamus or the cortex rarely relieve pain, and in fact lesions in this pathway at the thalamic level often lead to chronic so-called "thalamic pain." The paleospinothalamic tract, whose cells of origin in the dorsal horn receive C fiber input, also crosses in the anterior commissure and ascends in the spinal cord closely applied to but more ventral than the neospinothalamic tract. Many of the fibers of the paleospinothalamic tract give collaterals to the reticular formation of the brainstem, but some reach the thalamus, terminating in several nuclei, particularly the nucleus centralis lateralis and the intralaminar nuclei. None of these fibers project to center median despite the fact that lesions in this nucleus have been reported to relieve pain. The intralaminar nuclei of the thalamus project to somatosensory area II both ipsilaterally and contralaterally with some degree of somatotopic localization. The intralaminar nuclei also project diffusely, affecting large regions of both the frontal and parietal lobes. There is no somatotopic localization in projection. A third spinal ascending pathway which may play some role in nociception is the spinoreticular pathway, also referred to as the archispinal-lemniscal pathway, and phylogenetically the oldest of the nociceptive pathways. The pathway consists of projections from small myelinated and unmyelinated fibers. It originates in the dorsal horn and ascends via multiple synapses in the dorsal horn, mostly ipsilaterally, but to a lesser degree contralaterally, to terminate in the brainstem reticular formation, particularly that of the pons and medulla. The role this pathway plays in the conscious perception of pain in man is unclear, but it is unlikely to be major because spinal cord hemisection in humans usually completely eliminates pain contralaterally, thus ruling out a significant contribution by ipsilateral pathways. Such a multisynaptic ipsilateral pathway may explain, however, why some anterolateral cordotomies fail.

Fibers originating in the brainstem reticular formation receive input from several sources, including almost certainly the paleospinothalamic and spinoreticular pathways, and ascend in a polysynaptic projection to wide areas of the thalamus. The anatomy and physiology of the reticular formation is becoming increasingly important in our understanding of pain perception, because recent evidence (see below) suggests that electrical stimulation of this area produces analgesia and that the site of the action of narcotic drugs is here.

Descending pathways from fibers which originate in the orbital-frontal cortex and probably descend via corticospinal tracts, and fibers which originate in the midbrain reticular formation and raphe nucleus of the medulla and descend via polysynaptic pathways, both reach the dorsal horn to modulate input to all the laminae of the dorsal horn, particularly lamina 5. These descending fibers may influence activity at the dorsal horn level via either pre- or postsynaptic contacts and may be either facilitory or inhibitory. Electrical stimulation of the ventrolateral portion of a central gray substance of the mesencephalon and periventricular gray matter of the hypothalamus produces a profound analgesia in both animals and man, reversed by the opiate antagonist naloxone. There is no interference with motor function or the organism's responsiveness to other sensory stimuli. The anatomic substrate for these descending neural inhibitory systems is unclear, but their potency is striking.

BIOCHEMISTRY AND PHARMACOLOGY. A stereospecific receptor for narcotics has been identified in brain. This "opiate receptor" exists in highest concentrations in brainstem reticular formation, thalamus, and limbic system, the areas where narcotic analgesics are believed to act. The receptor binds both narcotic agonists and antagonists. In addition, several peptides called collectively the endorphins, which have morphine-like properties, have been isolated from brain. These analgesic peptides, enkephalin and β-endorphin, are smaller molecules of the pituitary hormone β-lipotropin and are believed to be neurotransmitters in pathways of pain or other behavior. The highest concentrations of both substances are in the same area as the opiate receptor. These substances bind to the opiate receptor, and can be displaced by opiate antagonists. They increase in concentration following electrical stimulation of the brainstem.

Another recent discovery has been the ability to dissociate biochemically opiate analgesia from opiate tolerance. Cyclohexamide, a protein synthesis inhibitor, blocks the development of tolerance to morphine in animals when given at doses that do not affect the acute response to morphine. Cyclic AMP and gamma-aminobutyric acid (GABA) accelerate the development of tolerance and physical dependence but at the same time decrease morphine analgesia. The ability to dissociate these two aspects of opiates biochemically suggests the possibility that a substance may be developed which will produce analgesia without the unwanted side effects of physical tolerance and dependency.

Other neurotransmitters, especially dopamine and serotonin, also appear to be important in pain biochemistry. Dopamine enhances the effect of both morphine analgesia and brainstem stimulation and may be the transmitter which subserves ascending inhibitory pathways to the brainstem reticular formation. Serotonin also has an inhibiting effect on pain perception and is probably the transmitter of descending inhibitory pathways which arise in the raphe nucleus of the medulla. GABA may be an inhibitory transmitter modulating pain at the level of the dorsal horn of the spinal cord.

DIAGNOSIS OF PAINFUL DISORDERS

Pain is either "acute" or "chronic." The point at which acute pain becomes chronic pain varies, but pain of over six months' duration is usually considered chronic. Several clinical features differentiate acute from chronic pain. In patients suffering severe acute pain, the autonomic nervous system is hyperactive, with tachycardia, hypertension, diaphoresis, mydriasis, and pallor. These autonomic signs serve as objective evidence of the patient's pain. In patients suffering from chronic pain, however, the autonomic nervous system adapts and the signs of autonomic hyperactivity disappear. The lack of such objective evidence forces the physician to rely upon the complaints of the patient and may lead the physician to believe that the patient's complaints are exaggerated. Since there are no reliable objective tests to assess chronic pain, the physician *must* believe the patient's report, taking into consideration his age, his cultural background, his environment, and other psychologic circumstances known to alter reaction to pain. *In general, the physician is wise to accept at face value the patient's report of the severity of his pain unless there is overwhelming evidence to the contrary.*

A thorough history, general physical examination, and careful neurologic examination are imperative in any patient complaining of pain. Often the description of the nature and distribution of the pain is so characteristic (e.g., trigeminal neuralgia or tabetic lightning pains) (see below) that it allows no other diagnosis. At times the history is so vague and bizarre and the distribution of pain so unanatomic as to suggest that the pain is a somatic delusion and not due to structural or even physiologic abnormality. Inquiry should be made concerning (1) the temporal pattern of pain, (2) its distribution, (3) exacerbating factors, and (4) relieving factors.

For example, headache beginning early in the morning before arising suggests increased intracranial pressure, whereas headache occurring late in the day is more suggestive of tension. Back pain and sciatica made worse by sitting or walking suggest disc disease, whereas back pain and sciatica which are worse while in bed suggest intraspinal tumor. Pain limited to a specific area is usually due to organ disease, whereas pain distributed in the distribution of a peripheral nerve or nerve root suggests that the nerve itself is diseased. Back pain and sciatica exacerbated by cough or sneeze suggest intraspinal disease, whereas similar pain not exacerbated by cough or sneeze suggests disease in the pelvis. Pain in the back or legs exacerbated by straight leg raising suggests disease of the nervous system, whereas a similar pain exacerbated by rotating the hips suggests pelvic or hip disease. Most pain caused by structural disease is relieved at least to some degree by analgesic drugs, whereas psychogenic pain often is not. Skeletal muscle relaxants or local heat may relieve pain of musculoskeletal origin. Both psychogenic and organic pain are relieved to some extent by distraction and a pleasurable environment. Both are exacerbated by anxiety or stress.

A careful psychiatric history, looking particularly for signs and symptoms of depression, should be elicited from all patients. Specifically, physicians should inquire about the degree to which pain has interfered with the patient's activities, whether he is having difficulty sleeping, and whether there is a change in appetite or bowel habits. Early morning awakening, anorexia, and constipation are somatic manifestations of depression, and either may be caused by chronic pain or may exacerbate the effects of the pain.

A general physical examination must be performed. Both the physical and laboratory examination should begin with the assumption that the site of pathologic change is at the site of pain. The painful areas should be examined for swelling and redness as well as for any obvious deformity. (The pain of herpes zoster usually precedes the rash, and occasionally on examination one may note only the faintest reddening of the skin in a dermatomal distribution.) The areas reported as painful should be palpated, the temperature estimated, and points of tenderness sought. (If the site of pain is in a soft tissue, bone, or joint, it should be tender to palpation as well as spontaneously painful.) Joints should be taken through a full range of motion and the effect of movement on the pain assessed. Nerve trunks going to the extremities should be palpated and stretched by movement of that extremity (e.g., straight leg raising; abduction and extension of the arm). Inflamed and compressed nerve roots and nerve plexuses are more painful when stretched. A careful neurologic examination must also be performed. If there are neurologic abnormalities (e.g., weakness, sensory loss, reflex changes) in the painful part, one can infer that nervous system disease is responsible for the pain. The absence of specific neurologic abnormalities on first examination does not guarantee, however, that the nervous system is free of disease, because the process may simply not have advanced beyond the stage of selectively involving pain pathways.

Finally, laboratory examinations are performed. If the site of disease appears to be in bones or joints, x-rays of those structures or radioisotope scans may localize it. First attention should be paid to the local site of pain but the physician should acquaint himself with the common referred patterns of pain (e.g., hip disease commonly causes knee pain, cardiac pain is frequently referred to the ulnar aspect of the arm and forearm, the pain of renal colic may be felt primarily in the groin and testicle, and pain resulting from disease of the throat may be referred to the ear).

Referred pain is pain perceived at a site remote from the source of the disturbance. Usually, referred pain is cutaneous and evoked by disease of deep structures innervated by the same dermatome. Referred pain may be associated with cutaneous hyperalgesia and even relieved by procaine injection into the area of referral. When pain is referred to the same dermatome or myotome as innervates the diseased structure (e.g., pain down the medial aspect of the arm [T1-T2] produced by myocardial infarction or angina pectoris), it is often helpful in diagnosis. However, pain is sometimes referred at a great distance from the primary site to segments not similarly innervated, and there the mechanism is perplexing (e.g., anginal pain referred to the jaw). Various theories have been suggested to account for referred pain. Such theories as division of the same nerve into deep and superficial branches, release of chemical mediators in the nervous system, and convergence of cutaneous and visceral nerves into common synaptic pools at the spinal cord all explain the dermatomal referral of pain but fail to explain pain at remote sites.

MANAGEMENT OF CHRONIC PAIN

In some patients, pain is best managed by treating the underlying disorder (e.g., steroids for giant cell arteritis relieve headache and muscle pain promptly; radiation therapy for bone pain caused by cancer is often helpful). In others, a particular kind of pain has a particular treatment (see Specific Pain Syndromes, below), but in many patients the pain is chronic and the physician is able neither to treat the underlying disturbances nor to offer specific therapy for that type of pain. In treating this type of chronic and severe pain, certain general principles should be followed:

1. The pain should be treated by the simplest means which will relieve it, but all efforts should be made to relieve it. Chronic pain is both physically debilitating and psychologically demoralizing. It should be treated by the physician as a serious symptom and all efforts made to relieve it to the extent that the patient is comfortable.

2. Pain should be treated early. There is both clinical and experimental evidence that if chronic pain goes untreated for an extended period of time, abnormal excitatory states arise in the central nervous system so that treatment directed toward peripheral structures which initially would have relieved the pain are no longer effective. In general, the earlier one undertakes to treat chronic pain, the more successful one is.

3. Pain should be treated promptly. Clinical evidence suggests that if analgesic drug doses are spaced so far apart that severe pain recurs, the analgesic becomes less effective. Thus patients should be encouraged to take analgesic agents when the pain first reappears rather than wait until it becomes unbearable.

4. Various treatments of pain are additive and should be used together rather than separately.

5. Narcotic drugs should be used with discrimination, but they should not be withheld if there is no alternative effective therapy. Long-term use of narcotics produces tolerance and physical dependence. These effects should not be confused with "addiction," which implies both a psychologic dependence and drug abuse for effects other than analgesia. The percentage of patients who actually become "addicted" to narcotics given for pain is unclear. Many physicians are impressed that narcotic "addiction" is unusual in patients treated for pain if the pain is later relieved by other means. The side effects of narcotic drugs include *tolerance*, which requires gradually increasing doses to maintain analgesia; *physical dependence*, which means that narcotics must be withdrawn gradually if they are to be discontinued after prolonged use; *constipation*, which requires careful attention to bowel function, including the use of stool softeners, laxatives and enemas; and at times *somnolence*. All narcotic drugs produce some degree of somnolence; in individual patients, if somnolence is a problem, lower doses should be given more frequently, amphetamines added, or several different narcotics tried, because the patient may tolerate a particular drug better than another in comparable doses. Other than those mentioned, the side effects of narcotic drugs are few. Methadone maintenance programs as well as other long-term studies have proved that patients can take narcotics in large doses over long periods of time without physical damage and continue to function usefully in society. Rarely, multifocal myoclonus and seizures may occur following repetitive doses of meperidine from accumulation of the metabolite normeperidine. Substitution of an alternative narcotic alleviates the seizures.

6. Psychogenic factors always play a role in chronic pain — the pain is more severe when the patient is anxious and stressed and less severe when he is relaxed. The physician must assess the psychologic factors in any patient with pain. However, no patient should be diagnosed as having psychogenic pain until an exhaustive examination has ruled out structural disease. Depression, whether endogenous or reactive, should be treated with antidepressant drugs. These may be effective in relieving pain by themselves, but more frequently are effective as analgesic adjuvants. Psychiatric consultation is necessary if psychogenic factors are causing the pain.

7. Placebo effects are important. In most clinical studies, about one third of patients report relief of pain when given a placebo, although the extent of relief is rarely equal to that achieved by analgesic drugs. The physician can utilize a patient's desire to be free of pain by approaching the therapy in an enthusiastic and reassuring manner. It is less important whether it is the placebo or the drug which was effective than that the patient be relieved of his pain.

8. Multidisciplinary pain clinics which diagnose and treat intractable pain exist in many centers and should be utilized to evaluate and treat severe problems.

Analgesic Agents

Analgesics are drugs which decrease pain without causing loss of consciousness. Analgesics (see accompanying table) can be divided clinically into those which are suitable for mild pain, generally non-narcotic agents; those suitable for moderate pain, usually narcotics or narcotic antagonists with low addiction potential; and those which are suitable for severe pain, generally narcotic agents except for methotrimeprazine. The mild analgesics appear to act peripherally by blocking the pain chemoreceptors and perhaps by relieving inflammation. There is also evidence for a central effect of some of these drugs as well.

The physician's strategy in treating chronic pain should begin with the mildest agents and add stronger agents or analgesic adjuvants only when mild agents fail to work. Drugs should always be given in sufficient amounts and at sufficiently short intervals to achieve relief of pain. Treatment should begin with aspirin or acetaminophen, 600 mg every three to four hours. If the pain is due to musculoskeletal spasm or if anxiety is prominent, one of the mild tranquilizers (diazepam or meprobamate) can be added. If the pain fails to respond to this mild regimen, one adds drugs used for the treatment of moderate pain (e.g., codeine or pentazocine). If the pain is still unrelieved and the physician satisfies himself that psychogenic factors are not responsible, the agents used for moderate pain should be discontinued, and agents used for severe pain should be added to the mild analgesic. Levorphanol, 2 mg, or methadone, 10 mg, every three to four hours is probably the agent of choice if oral drugs are to be used, and morphine, 10 mg every three to four hours, if a subcutaneous or intramuscular agent is necessary. If the pain continues as a chronic and unremitting problem not relieved by these drugs, or if anxiety and depression appear to be a major contributor to the pain, a major tranquilizer (phenothiazine) or antidepressant agent, or both, may be added to the mild analgesics and narcotic agents. At times a satisfactory resolution of an intractable problem may be achieved by the combined use of a narcotic and non-narcotic analgesic and a tranquilizer or an antidepressant. The physician must be careful to adjust the doses of each so as to produce maximal pain relief with minimal sedation and unpleasant side effects. The physician should be prepared to increase the dose of those particular drugs

Analgesic Agents

Type	Generic Name (Proprietary)	Usual Dose*		Comment
		Oral (mg)	Subcutaneous or Intramuscular (mg)	
Some agents used for mild to moderate pain	Aspirin	600 q 3–4 h		Side effects of dyspepsia and GI bleeding
	Acetaminophen (Tylenol)	650 q 3–4 h		Equal to aspirin but without GI side effects; less anti-inflammatory effect
	Phenacetin (aceto-phenetidin)	600 q 3–4 h		Probable renal toxicity with chronic use
	Dextropropoxyphene (Darvon)	65 q 3–4 h		Weak narcotic related to methadone, probably not superior to aspirin
	Indomethacin (Indocin)	25 qid		Useful only for pain associated with inflammation, probably not superior to aspirin
Some agents used for moderate to severe pain	Codeine	1 tab q 4–6 h	130 q 4–6 h	Narcotic with low addiction potential; additive effect if used with mild analgesics
	Oxycodone (with acetaminophen = Percocet)	5 q 4–6 h		Preferred over codeine by many patients
	Pentazocine (Talwin)	30–50 q 4–6 h	60 q 4 h	Narcotic antagonist (produces withdrawal in patients physically dependent on narcotics); low addiction potential; hallucinations and dysphoria in doses >80 mg IM or 200 mg PO
Some agents used for severe pain: narcotics and antagonists	Levorphanol (Levo-dromoran)	2 q 3–4 h	2 q 3–4 h	Long-acting oral narcotic
	Morphine		10 q 3–4 h	The standard narcotic agent for treatment of pain
	Meperidine (Demerol)	50–100 q 3–4 h	75 q 2–4 h	More rapid onset and shorter duration of action than morphine; possibly less spasmogenic and better for pain of biliary tree
	Methadone (Dolophine)	10–20 q 4 h	10–15 q 3–4 h	Long-acting oral narcotic; possibly less sedative effect than morphine
Non-narcotic	Methotrimeprazine (Levoprome)		20 q 4–6 h	Phenothiazine; no tolerance; produces sedation and postural hypotension
	Dextroamphetamine	10 q 6 h		Doubles narcotic effects and decreases somnolence in postoperative pain
Some agents used as analgesic adjuvants (probably little or no analgesic properties per se but used to relieve anxiety and/or depression)	Minor tranquilizers—muscle relaxants:			
	Diazepam (Valium)	5 qid		Useful with mild analgesics for acute or subacute pain associated with muscle spasm and/or anxiety
	Meprobamate (Miltown)	200–400 qid		
	Antidepressants:			
	Amitriptyline (Elavil)	75–100 hs		Reported useful in pain associated with depressive symptoms (esp. atypical facial pain); may be useful when combined with analgesic agents for chronic pain of many kinds; may cause oversedation or anticholinergic symptoms
	Phenelzine (Nardil)	15 tid		
	Imipramine (Tofranil)	25 qid		
	Phenothiazines:			
	Chlorpromazine (Thorazine)	25–50 qid		Reported useful in pain associated with anxiety or depression and in some specific pain syndromes (e.g., thalamic pain, postherpetic pain); these drugs may have analgesic properties or potentiate analgesics; fluphenazine and amitriptyline have been reported to relieve postherpetic pain; may cause oversedation, depression, Parkinson-like syndrome, hypotension, or urinary retention
	Promazine (Sparine)	50–100 qid		
	Promethazine (Phenergan)	25–50 hs		
	Fluphenazine (Prolixin)	1–3 qd		

*Intramuscular dose of narcotics is equivalent to 10 mg of morphine. Since tolerance develops to these drugs, doses must be increased with continued use. Oral doses are not equivalent to intramuscular doses but represent usual starting doses.

to which tolerance develops as is necessary to control pain. No tolerance develops to non-narcotic analgesics.

NON-NARCOTIC MILD ANALGESICS. Aspirin and acetaminophen (Tylenol, Tempra) are the most useful of the mild analgesics. Either aspirin or acetaminophen may be given in doses of 600 mg every three to four hours, either alone for relief of mild pain or in conjunction with more potent drugs for relief of severe pain. The degree of pain relief is linearly related to the logarithm of the dose of the drug, higher doses being not significantly more effective until doses are reached which produce unpleasant side effects. The side effects of aspirin (clotting disorders, dyspepsia, and gastrointestinal bleeding) make acetaminophen a safer drug and probably the drug of choice. There is no evidence that aspi-

rin and acetaminophen together are more effective than either one alone, but either aspirin or acetaminophen plus codeine is more effective than codeine alone. There is no evidence that the other mild, non-narcotic analgesics are superior in any way to the two most commonly used drugs.

NARCOTIC ANALGESICS. Tolerance develops to all narcotics. Thus there is no set dose of the drug, and with continued usage the dose must increase. *The physician is wise to learn to handle two or three of these drugs and use those consistently rather than using all the drugs occasionally.* He must be prepared to use more than one, because some patients find that side effects of the drugs make one preferable to another. Morphine, 10 mg intramuscularly, is the standard by which other narcotic analgesics are judged. Intramuscular morphine has its maximal effect in 60 to 90 minutes and lasts between three and six hours. It requires 60 mg or more of morphine orally to give the same analgesic effect as 10 mg intramuscularly. Levorphanol has a relatively high oral/parenteral ratio for analgesia; 2 mg given intramuscularly is equal to 10 mg of morphine intramuscularly, and 4 mg given orally is equal in total effect to 10 mg of morphine given intramuscularly. Methadone also has a relatively high oral/intramuscular potency ratio; 10 mg intramuscularly or 20 mg orally equals 10 mg of morphine intramuscularly. Codeine and dihydrocodeine are also effective orally and are generally used in doses of 50 to 60 mg as a mild analgesic. They often cannot be used to relieve severe pain, because side effects preclude high doses. Pentazocine can be used as a mild analgesic when given in doses of 30 mg and is equal to morphine if given in intramuscular doses of 60 mg. It is a weak narcotic antagonist with a high analgesic potential and has a dependence potential substantially less than that of morphine or meperidine (Demerol). Pentazocine is not included in the Federal Controlled Substances Act. However, hallucinatory effects and toxic psychoses have been noted in its users, and like the other narcotics it can produce respiratory depression. Dextropropoxyphene (Darvon) is structurally related to methadone and is a prescription drug not subject to the Controlled Substances Act of 1970. It is a weak narcotic with a low analgesic potential.

OTHER AGENTS. The phenothiazine methotrimeprazine (Levoprome) is a potent analgesic agent. Given intramuscularly in doses of 20 mg, it is equivalent to 10 mg of morphine intramuscularly. The drug is an effective antiemetic, and does not suppress cough or respiration but does produce sedation and postural hypotension, making it useful only for hospitalized patients.

Sedative and anticonvulsant drugs as well as other phenothiazines have been utilized by some physicians in the treatment of chronic pain, particularly that associated with depression or other psychologic symptoms. The antidepressant amitriptyline (Elavil), given orally in a single dose of 75 mg at night (when it helps counter insomnia) or orally in divided doses of 25 mg three to four times a day, has been effective in relieving some chronic pain or in decreasing the narcotic dose required. In conjunction with the phenothiazine, fluphenazine, the drug has been reported useful in the treatment of postherpetic neuralgia (see below).

Dextroamphetamine has been reported to enhance the effectiveness of narcotic agents in postoperative patients while counteracting the undesirable side effects of sedation and possibly respiratory depression. Whether the drug is also an effective adjuvant for chronic pain remains to be established.

Physical Methods of Pain Relief

There are a bewildering array of physical methods designed to relieve pain. These vary from simply rubbing a partially denervated area with a soft towel to placing radiofrequency lesions stereotactically in the thalamic and hypothalamic reticular formations. The simpler procedures can be carried out by the general physician or even by the patient; the more complicated ones, depending on their nature, demand the expertise of a skilled anesthesiologist or neurosurgeon.

The physician's approach to the use of physical methods for intractable pain should embody certain general principles:

1. Nondestructive procedures should be tried first. Cutaneous stimulation, either by hand or by battery-driven electrodes, or local anesthetic blocks in conjunction with analgesic drugs may be effective in relieving pain. If these simple procedures fail, the services of an anesthesiologist or neurosurgeon should be procured and a treatment plan embodying the use of analgesics and physical procedures outlined.

2. The least destructive procedure should be tried first. In general, the procedure should be directed first at the peripheral nervous system, and only if this fails, at the spinal cord, brainstem, or cerebrum. Quantitative data on the incidence of pain relief and its duration are sketchy for most of these procedures and seem to vary from center to center, depending on the skill and enthusiasm of the investigator reporting.

3. Thus the choice of a particular procedure often depends not only on the nature of the patient's disease but on the particular skills, experience, and bias of the physician.

4. If and only if a full trial of analgesic drugs has failed should destructive procedures for relieving pain be tried. These destructive procedures can and should be used in conjunction with analgesic drugs, because, even if the drugs have failed to relieve pain on their own, they may act synergistically with physical methods. Nerve blocks and surgical procedures often yield only temporary relief in patients with chronic pain. Thus many of the enthusiastic reports in the literature refer to patients followed for only a short period of time. When the patients are followed over months or years, the pain which was relieved shortly after the procedure often returns and is as bad as or worse than it was prior to the operation. For this reason, patients with cancer who are not expected to live a long time are often better candidates for surgical destructive procedures than are patients with pain originating from more benign conditions.

5. Patients with chronic pain being considered for destructive procedures must be thoroughly evaluated psychiatrically. If psychogenic factors play a major role in the genesis of pain, surgical procedures will not help, and often the pain will be exacerbated after surgical intervention.

CUTANEOUS STIMULATION. Cutaneous stimulation of a painful area, particularly one which has been partly denervated, is often effective in relieving pain. This procedure, which probably has its greatest use in the treatment of postherpetic neuralgia, consists of rubbing the painful area with a soft cloth or terrycloth towel, almost constantly at first but then with gradually lengthening intervals of rest between rubbing periods. Often a period of rubbing will yield relief which long outlasts the stimulus, and continued intermittent rubbings may totally relieve the pain. The "gate theory" offers an explanation of the rubbing phenomenon, i.e., rubbing stimulates large fiber afferents which may close the gate against incoming pain fibers. Whatever the explanation, the procedure is often useful in the treatment of painful phantom limbs and in chronic cutaneous or extremity pain after surgery. Recently, battery-powered electrical stimulators which give one control over the frequency and intensity of the cutaneous stimulation have become available. The electrodes of the stimulator may be placed over the painful area or over the peripheral nerve supplying the painful area, and stimulation using an intensity and frequency which produces a vibratory sensation is applied.

ACUPUNCTURE ANALGESIA. Acupuncture analgesia has become increasingly popular in the past few years, but no carefully controlled studies have reported on its usefulness. A needle is placed under the skin, often in a place remote from the painful site but at times into the painful site, and the area is stimulated either by twirling the needle or by electrically vibrating it. Recent experiments in animals and man suggest that the analgesic effect of acupuncture is reversed by naloxone, leading to the hypothesis that the mechanism of acupuncture analgesia is through enkephalin release. The usefulness of acupuncture in Western medicine is still not clear.

NERVE BLOCKS. Direct block of peripheral nerves, using either anesthetic agents (lidocaine) or neurolytic agents (phenol), has been popular in the treatment of thoracic and abdominal pain, particularly that pain which follows surgery. Blocks may be dangerous if used in the extremities, because they may paralyze as well as anesthetize; but in areas where they can be used, relief of pain sometimes long outlasts the period of anesthesia. The procedure is a simple one when performed by a skilled anesthesiologist.

Subarachnoid injection of anesthetics or neurolytics directed at nerve roots has been utilized in patients with widespread and intractable pain. Phenol can likewise be injected into the subarachnoid space and directed at particular nerve roots by positioning the patient. The mechanism of action is destruction of nerve fibers; if material spills into the cauda equina, bladder and bowel dysfunction are common. The relief of pain may only be transient.

OTHER PROCEDURES. Several nondestructive procedures directed at the affective component of pain are currently in use. These include not only psychotherapy and hypnotism but also more recently developed techniques of biofeedback and operant conditioning. The latter two methods have been gaining in popularity, but their role in the treatment of chronic pain is not yet certain. Neither psychotherapy nor hypnotism has been particularly useful in patients with chronic pain due to organic disease.

Each nonsurgical procedure directed at the *peripheral nervous system* has its surgical counterpart. In patients with chronic pain such as that which follows herpes zoster, the skin has been undercut in an attempt to totally denervate it. Postoperative infection is a complication at times and the pain relief is transient, thus contraindicating this procedure. Peripheral nerves can be cut, particularly in the thorax and abdomen, but this should not be done unless prior nerve blocks have indicated that it will be effective and sustained. The peripheral nerves regenerate after a time, and often the pain returns. Dorsal root ganglia in the thorax and abdomen can be removed for chronic pain or the dorsal roots themselves cut. This procedure also should not be done unless nerve blocks have indicated that it will be effective. Several roots must be cut off either side of the painful area if one is to achieve long-term pain relief.

SURGERY OF THE CENTRAL NERVOUS SYSTEM. There are three kinds of surgical procedures directed at the central nervous system for the relief of pain. *The first type,* a direct outgrowth of the gate control theory, involves the placement of electrodes to stimulate large fiber pathways, thus "closing the gate" against pain fibers. Electrodes have been placed on the skin, along peripheral nerves, and along spinal cord pathways. A few years ago there was some enthusiasm about electrodes surgically placed on the dorsal columns with a subcutaneous power pack which would allow the patient to control frequency and intensity of stimulation. Failure of this method to give prolonged relief and the morbidity of the procedure have led neurosurgeons to abandon it. More recently, electrodes have been placed stereotactically in the periventricular gray matter, again using a power source controlled by the patient. Total body analgesia with increase in pain threshold has been observed for three to eight hours following stimulation, but tolerance develops to the analgesic effect. This procedure is still an experimental one, and its effectiveness requires further evaluation.

The second type of procedure destroys pain pathways in the spinal cord, brainstem, or brain. Spinothalamic tracts can be destroyed either surgically, after a laminectomy (open cordotomy), or by the placement of a radiofrequency lesion through a needle (percutaneous cordotomy). These procedures are particularly effective in relieving pain in the lower extremities and have the advantage that, although pain and temperature sensations are lost, cutaneous sensation and motor power remain intact. At times the level of anesthesia approaches within one or two cord segments of the level at which the destruction lesion is placed, but often there is a drop to about five segments below the placement of the lesion. Thus the lesion must be placed considerably higher than the site of pain. If the lesion is placed unilaterally, pain often reappears on the other side of the body, necessitating another lesion. Bilateral lesions considerably enhance the risk of motor weakness and bladder and bowel dysfunction, but in skilled hands these risks are low. Occasional patients with bilateral percutaneous lesions in cervical cord suffer loss of automatic respiratory function (Ondine's curse). Percutaneous spinothalamic tract cordotomy, when done by a skilled technician, produces satisfactory pain relief in 70 to 90 per cent of patients, with a small mortality (1 to 5 per cent) and morbidity. The procedure is particularly useful in patients with terminal cancer, because the pain relief is usually sustained until death and the procedure does not require a major operation. An analogous lesion in the low brainstem placed in the descending tract of the trigeminal nerve has been reported useful in relieving facial pain. Pain and temperature sensation are lost, but cutaneous sensation remains intact. Lesions have been placed in the spinothalamic tract of the midbrain, so-called mesencephalic tractotomies. The dangers of this lesion are considerably greater than those of spinal cord lesions, and most centers have abandoned the procedure. Several neurosurgeons have placed lesions in the thalamus, both in the ventral-basal complex and in the interlaminar nuclei. Although good results are occasionally reported for both, the ventral-basal lesions appear only to produce transient relief of pain, whereas those placed in the intralaminar nuclei at the end-point of the paleospinothalamic tract appear to be more successful. There are rare reports of removal of sensory portions of the parietal lobe in relieving chronic pain, but the rarity of the reports implies the ineffectiveness of the treatment.

The third surgical method directed at pain relief is to place lesions in the frontal lobe, particularly the limbic projection to the frontal areas, in an attempt to alter the patient's psychologic response to pain rather than alter the pain pathways themselves. Several different surgical procedures, including frontal lobotomy, frontal leukotomy, and cingulotomy, have been tried with varied success. These procedures, which alter the patient's personality as well as his suffering, probably deserve trial only when all other procedures have failed.

Good statistical data comparing the various surgical procedures for pain are difficult to come by. The best extant data indicate that initial relief of pain occurs with almost all procedures in 50 to 80 per cent of patients, with spinothalamic tract cordotomies yielding the best results. Longer-term follow-up suggests that considerably less than 50 per cent of patients achieve lasting relief, in many series the figure being as low as 20 per cent. Patients with malignant disease seem to have greater pain relief even initially than those with more benign conditions, probably because selection of patients with benign conditions often includes many with psychogenic pain.

SOME SPECIFIC PAIN SYNDROMES

TRIGEMINAL NEURALGIA. Trigeminal neuralgia (tic douloureux) is a disease characterized by sudden, lightning-like paroxysms of pain in the distribution of one or more divisions of the trigeminal nerve. The pain is usually unassociated with identifiable structural disease of the nervous system (idiopathic trigeminal neuralgia) but occasionally may be a symptom of a gasserian ganglion tumor, of multiple sclerosis, or of a brainstem infarct involving the descending root of the trigeminal nerve (symptomatic trigeminal neuralgia).

The history is diagnostic. The pain occurs as brief, lightning-like stabs, frequently precipitated by touching a trigger zone around the lips or the buccal cavity. At times, talking, eating, or brushing the teeth serves as a trigger. The pains rarely last longer than seconds, and each burst is followed by a refractory period of several seconds to a minute in which no further pain can be precipitated. The pains, however, often occur in clusters so that the patient may report that each pain lasts for hours. The pain is limited to the distribution of the trigeminal nerve, usually affecting the second and third division or both. Spontaneous remissions and exacerbations are common, the exacerbations tending to occur in spring and fall. Between paroxysms of pain, the patient is asymptomatic. Tic pain rarely occurs at night. In idiopathic trigeminal neuralgia, the neurologic examination is entirely normal. In symptomatic trigeminal neuralgia, there may be sensory changes in the distribution of the trigeminal nerve, and such a finding should prompt a careful search for structural disease of the nervous system.

Carbamazepine is the drug of choice for the treatment of trigeminal neuralgia. This anticonvulsant drug is given in doses varying from 400 to 800 mg a day, but because of its sedative properties the initial dose is 100 mg twice daily, gradually increased to the required maintenance dose. No more than 1200 mg should be taken daily. The drug is not an analgesic and is only effective for specific kinds of pain such as trigeminal neuralgia, glossopharyngeal neuralgia, and the light-ning pains of tabes dorsalis. Rarely, aplastic anemia has been reported, and complete blood counts are procured prior to the initiation of therapy and at intervals thereafter. Other side effects include dizziness and sedation. Phenytoin in doses of 400 mg a day is also effective in trigeminal neuralgia but less so than carbamazepine. There is no evidence that the two drugs are synergistic. If medical treatment fails, section of the nerve root proximal to the ganglion affords permanent relief. Local anesthesia of the ganglion or the peripheral branches of the nerve at some time prior to surgery is desirable because some patients find the anesthesia produced by nerve section less tolerable than the pain itself.

GLOSSOPHARYNGEAL NEURALGIA. Glossopharyngeal neuralgia is characterized by pain similar to that of trigeminal neuralgia but in the distribution of the glossopharyngeal and vagus nerves. The trigger zone is usually in the tonsil or posterior pharynx, and the pain spreads toward the angle of the jaw and the ear. Occasional patients suffer cardiac slowing or arrest during these attacks as a result of the intense afferent discharge over the glossopharyngeal nerve. Carbamazepine is often effective, but if it fails, glossopharyngeal nerve roots are sectioned in the posterior fossa. Symptomatic glossopharyngeal neuralgia is occasionally the presenting complaint in a patient with a tonsillar tumor, and careful examination of the pharynx and tonsillar fossa for mass lesions must be carried out.

LIGHTNING PAINS OF TABES. The lightning pains of tabes are acute, short-lived pains in the trunk or lower extremities which occur with structural lesions of the dorsal roots and particularly with tabes dorsalis. Lightning pains are analogous to trigeminal and glossopharyngeal neuralgia. Like those two disorders, the pain usually responds to carbamazepine. There is no surgical therapy. (See Ch. 171.)

"REFLEX SYMPATHETIC DYSTROPHIES." This is a term which applies to pain, hyperalgesia, hyperesthesia, and autonomic changes, usually after injury to an extremity. If the injury has involved a peripheral nerve, particularly the sciatic or median nerve, the syndrome is called *causalgia* (hot pain). If the injury has not involved a peripheral nerve, such terms as post-traumatic painful osteoporosis, Sudeck's atrophy, post-traumatic spreading neuralgia, minor causalgia, shoulder-hand syndrome, and reflex dystrophy have been applied, the particular term depending on the outstanding symptom. Whatever the term, the pathophysiology of all these disorders appears to be the same, as do their clinical manifestations and response to therapy.

The disorder may follow either a major or minor injury to an extremity, after which severe pain, usually of a burning quality, develops in the extremity. The pain is continuous but exacerbated by emotional stress and is associated with severe hyperpathia, so that moving or touching the limb is often intolerable. At first the pain is localized to the site of the injury or the distribution of the nerve injured, but with time it spreads, often to involve the entire extremity. Along with the pain there are vasomotor changes, first of vasodilatation (warm and dry skin) but later a change to vasoconstriction (edema, cyanosis, cool skin). Other autonomic disturbances include either hyperhidrosis or hypohidrosis; trophic changes in the skin, subcutaneous tissue, and muscles; and osteoporosis. The entire symptom complex is rarely present in any one patient, and one sign or symptom usually predominates. Untreated, severe reflex sympathetic dystrophy leads to muscle atrophy, fixation of joints, osteoporosis, and a useless extremity. The exact mechanism of the pain and sympathetic changes is not understood.

Treatment should be undertaken as early as possible, because there is evidence that the earlier the treatment, the more effective it will be. Treatment begins with local anesthetic infiltration of the painful site, using 2 to 5 ml of 0.5 per cent lidocaine, repeated frequently enough to maintain relief of pain. When local measures fail, most patients are relieved by sympathetic block with lidocaine. This procedure often gives permanent relief, but if repeated local anesthetics produce only transient benefit, surgical sympathectomy should be performed.

POSTHERPETIC NEURALGIA. Postherpetic neuralgia refers to severe and prolonged burning pain with occasional lightning-like stabs in the involved dermatome after an attack of herpes zoster. Severe postherpetic neuralgia is usually a disease of elderly patients and, like most chronic pain, is exacerbated by emotional upset and relieved to some degree by distraction. Touching the involved area usually exacerbates the pain. Treatment of postherpetic neuralgia is not entirely satisfactory, but the initial treatment should be directed toward stimulating the painful area. Brisk rubbing for many hours a day with a terrycloth towel or stimulation of the dermatome with a cutaneous electrical stimulator often brings relief which long outlasts the stimulus. Initially, when therapy is undertaken, the hyperpathia may be so severe that the patient is unwilling to have the area stimulated. One can then spray the area with a local anesthetic (e.g., ethyl chloride) before stimulation is undertaken. During the first 48 to 72 hours, stimulation should be done as often as possible while the patient is awake and then decreased gradually. Care must be taken to keep the rubbing light so as not to excoriate friable skin. Relief of pain may take several weeks. Analgesic drugs are sometimes beneficial, and psychotropic drugs (amitriptyline, 75 mg daily, and fluphenazine, 1 to 3 mg daily) have been reported to be useful. The results of surgical therapy are usually poor. In many patients the disease runs its course, and after a year or two the pain disappears spontaneously. Thus mutilating surgical procedures are probably not indicated.

PHANTOM LIMB PAIN. Phantom limb pain is a chronic and severe pain appearing to be localized in an amputated or totally denervated limb. All patients suffer phantom sensations after amputation, but in only about 10 per cent is it painful, usually when there has been severe pain prior to operation. The pain is frequently similar to that suffered before amputation, or at times it may resemble muscle pain with the phantom seeming to be in a cramped or uncomfortable position. In most instances, the pain lessens and disappears with time, but in occasional patients it is a chronic and severe problem. Therapy is difficult. A search should be made for painful neuromas, but these are an uncommon cause of phantom pain, and even if small neuromas are found and removed, the pain is not usually relieved. Surgical procedures directed at the central nervous system are often not helpful. The pain may be triggered by touching the amputation stump, but over the passage of time healthy areas of the body when touched may also trigger pain in the phantom. Phantom pain is sometimes permanently abolished by cutaneous stimulation, either rubbing or electrical stimulation, or by repeated anesthetic blocks of peripheral nerves proximal to the stump. Narcotic analgesics may be helpful; other analgesic agents are usually not helpful. Sympathetic blocks have been reported to relieve pain in some patients for prolonged periods, but sympathectomy rarely produces relief as lasting as with causalgia. The mechanism of phantom pain is unknown.

MYOFASCIAL PAIN SYNDROMES. Pain arising from skeletal muscle is common. Unaccustomed exercise causes soreness and tenderness in the involved muscles but is rarely a source of patient complaint. Prolonged tonic contraction of skeletal muscles, however, has an underlying pathogenesis of psychologic tension, resentment, and anxiety, and may produce pain in which the cause is not immediately apparent to the patient. Examples are tension headache arising from chronic contraction of paraspinous muscles at the base of the skull, anterior chest pain from contraction of pectoralis major, posterior thoracic or lumbar pain from paraspinous muscle contraction, and abdominal pain from rectus muscle retraction. The pain is initially localized over the area of muscle contraction but may spread widely into a distribution characteristic for the muscles involved. The muscles are usually tender to palpation, and there is often a particular tender area somewhere in the muscle, called a trigger area, which, when palpated, reproduces the entire distribution of the spontaneous pain. When the pain is acute, it may be treated with rest, local heat, and mild analgesic drugs, along with muscle relaxant drugs such as diazepam or meprobamate. When the pain is chronic or severe, particularly when a trigger area is found, local anesthesia with ethyl chloride spray or local injection of 0.5 per cent lidocaine sometimes affords relief. At times, a single injection breaks the pain–muscle tension–pain cycle and permanent relief is achieved. At other times, repetitive injections with the addition of analgesic agents and muscle relaxants are required.

Bonica, J. J. (ed.): Symposium on pain. Arch. Surg., 112:749, 861, 1971.

Bonica, J. J.: Management of Pain. 2nd ed. Philadelphia, Lea & Febiger, 1974.

Bonica, J. J., and Albe-Fessard, D. (eds.): Advances in Pain Research and Therapy. New York, Raven Press, 1976.

Guillemin, R., Bloom, F., Rossier, J., Minick, S., Henriksen, S., Burgus, R., and Ling, N.: Recent physiological studies with the endorphins. In Goodman, M., and Meinhofer, J. (eds.): Peptides 1977, Proceedings 5th American Peptide Symposium. New York, John Wiley & Sons, 1977.

Mayer, D., and Price, D. D.: Central nervous system mechanisms of analgesia. Pain, 2:379, 1976.

Sternbach, R.: Pain Patients: Traits and Treatment. New York, Academic Press, 1974.

261. HEADACHE

Fred Plum

INTRODUCTION

Headache is man's most common pain, and in one form or another it affects some 90 per cent of the population. In any consideration of headache, two major points stand out: one is that *most* headaches come from structures *outside* the skull, and the other is that increased intracranial pressure, as such, does not necessarily cause headache. The following is an outline of the principal types:

A. Extracranial headaches have several causes and are listed roughly in declining order of frequency.

1. Vascular headaches. These are recurrent and vary widely in intensity, duration, and frequency. The following subtypes are recognized:

a. *Classic migraine*, with sharply defined, transient visual, other sensory and/or motor prodromes.

b. *Hemiplegic or ophthalmoplegic migraine*, featured by sensory and motor phenomena that persist during and after the headache.

c. *Common migraine*, without striking prodromes and less often unilateral than (a) and (d). Synonyms are "atypical migraine" and "sick headache."

d. *Cluster headache*, predominantly unilateral, associated with flushing, sweating, rhinorrhea, increased lacrimation and, often, Horner's syndrome. The headaches are usually brief in duration and occur in close-packed groups separated by long remissions.

e. *Lower half headache*, of possible vascular mechanism, centered primarily in the lower face. In this group are some instances of atypical facial neuralgia, sphenopalatine ganglion neuralgia (Sluder), and vidian neuralgia (Vail).

2. *Muscle-contraction headaches.* These present as occipito-frontal pains or sensations of tightness, pressure, or constriction associated with sustained skeletal muscle contraction and no permanent structural change. The ambiguous terms "tension," "psychogenic," and "nervous" headache refer largely to this group.

3. Combination of vascular headache of the migraine type and muscle contraction headache.

4. Anterior headache and nasal discomfort (nasal obstruction, rhinorrhea, tightness, or burning) can result from congestion, edema, and inflammation of nasal and paranasal mucous membranes. This is "sinus" headache.

5. Nonmigrainous vascular headaches associated with generally nonrecurrent dilatation of extracranial arteries. The category includes post-traumatic and hypertensive headaches.

6. Ocular headache due to increased intraocular pressure, excessive contraction of ocular muscles, trauma, new growth, or inflammation.

7. Aural headache due to trauma, new growth, or inflammation.

8. Dental headache.

9. Headache due to spread of pain from noxious stimulation of other structures of the cranium and neck (periosteum, joints, ligaments, and muscles or cervical nerve roots).

10. Cranial neuritides (caused by trauma, new growth, or infection).

11. Extracranial arteritis.

B. Intracranial headache:

1. Traction headache. Headache resulting from traction on intracranial structures, mainly vascular, by masses:

a. Primary or metastatic tumors of meninges, vessels, or brain.

b. Hematomas (epidural, subdural, or parenchymal).

c. Abscesses (epidural, subdural, or parenchymal).

d. Headache following puncture ("leakage" headache).

e. Pseudotumor cerebri and various causes of brain swelling.

2. Headache due to inflammation of cranial structures resulting from usually nonrecurrent inflammation, sterile or infectious. Examples include infectious, chemical, or allergic meningitis, subarachnoid hemorrhage, postpneumoencephalographic reaction, arteritis, and phlebitis.

C. Cranial neuralgias: trigeminal (tic douloureux) and glossopharyngeal (see Ch. 260).

D. Headaches of a delusional or conversion reaction, in which a somatic pain mechanism is nonexistent. The diagnosis is rare and must be made cautiously. Closely allied are hypochondriacal and depressive reactions in which tissue abnormalities relevant to headache are minimal.

PATHOGENESIS OF HEADACHE. Wolff and his colleagues identified the principal intracranial and extracranial pain-sensitive structures. Almost all the *extracranial* tissues are pain sensitive, the arteries especially so. Among intracranial structures, only a limited group of tissues can cause pain. These include the great venous sinuses and their venous tributaries from the surface of the brain, parts of the dura at the base, the dural arteries and the cerebral arteries at the base of the brain, the fifth, seventh, ninth, and tenth cranial nerves, and the upper three cervical nerves.

The cranium (including the diploic and emissary veins), the parenchyma of the brain, most of the dura, most of the pia-arachnoid, and the ependymal lining of the ventricles and the choroid plexuses are not sensitive to pain.

The fifth cranial nerve contains the pathways for pain from sensitive intracranial structures located on or above the superior surface of the tentorium cerebelli. Pain from these structures is experienced in various regions in front of a line drawn coronally joining the ears across the top of the head.

The ninth and tenth cranial nerves and the upper two or possibly three cervical nerves contain the pathways for pain from pain-sensitive structures on or below the inferior surface of the tentorium cerebelli. Pain from these structures is experienced in various parieto-occipital and upper cervical regions behind the line just described.

HEADACHE FROM INTRACRANIAL SOURCES

Headache from intracranial sources can result from the following mechanisms: (1) traction on and displacement of the great venous sinuses or of the veins that pass to them from the surface of the brain; (2) traction on and displacement of the middle meningeal arteries; (3) traction on and displacement of the large arteries at the base of the brain and their main branches; (4) dilatation and distention of intracranial arteries; (5) inflammation in or about any of the pain-sensitive structures of the head and portions of the pia and dura at the base of the skull; and (6) direct pressure by tumors on pain-sensitive cranial and cervical nerves. Intracranial diseases commonly cause headaches through more than one mechanism and may also cause secondary extracranial muscle-contraction headache, usually at the occiput, but often elsewhere.

The head pain associated with fever, bacteremia, sepsis, nitrite and foreign protein administration, carbon monoxide inhalation, hypoxia, and asphyxia is due principally to dilatation and distention of intracranial arterial structures. A similar mechanism probably causes the headaches that follow epileptic seizures (with or without convulsions) and certain "hangover headaches." Painful distention of intracranial arteries is responsible for the headaches that accompany sudden brisk rises in the arterial blood pressure, such as occurs with distention of the rectum or urinary bladder in paraplegics, rapid intravenous infusion of epinephrine, and the hypertensive crises occurring with pheochromocytoma or acute hypertensive encephalopathy.

The headache of meningitis is primarily related to the lowered pain threshold of inflamed tissues. The changes are usually most marked at the base of the brain. Under these circumstances, even the slight, usually painless arterial dilatation and distention during each cardiac systole become painful; hence, the characteristic throbbing headache.

Lumbar Puncture Headache

Dull, usually pulsating occipital headache develops in about one fifth of patients having lumbar puncture, particularly for the first time. For unexplained reasons, such headaches are less likely after repeated lumbar punctures. The headache usually begins 12 to 24 hours after the puncture, comes on in the erect position, and subsides if the subject lies flat. The headache usually disappears spontaneously in a day or so, and in most patients is made tolerable by routine analgesics. Occasionally, patients develop more prostrating symptoms that sometimes last as long as 10 to 14 days, accompanied by secondary muscle-contraction headache as well as nausea and vomiting.

The cause of postlumbar puncture headache is probably leakage of cerebrospinal fluid through the torn dural sac. The consequent loss of buoyance results in downward traction on unsupported, pain-sensitive posterior fossa tissues, particularly the veins. The headaches can often be avoided by accurate punctures, using No. 20 caliber sharp spinal needles, which minimize drainage through the dural needle wound.

Headache With Brain Tumor: With or Without Increased Intracranial Pressure

The headache with space-occupying lesions is deep, aching, steady, dull, and seldom rhythmic or throbbing. The pain is continuous in one tenth of the patients and is generally more intense in the morning. Aspirin, 0.3 gram, and local application of cold packs usually diminish the pain, and coughing or straining at stool may aggravate it. Some patients prefer the recumbent to the erect position. The headache is rarely as intense as that associated with migraine, ruptured cerebral aneurysm, or meningitis, and seldom interferes with sleep. Even when the tumor directly compresses and displaces pain-sensitive cranial nerves, headache may be absent or slight, and rarely is it as intense as the pain of tic douloureux, unless the tumor intermittently obstructs the cerebral ventricular system. In this instance, pain is excruciating and generalized, and may last 30 seconds to a half hour and then disappear as quickly as it commenced. During such an attack the sudden increases of intracranial pressure can be fatal.

Severe brain tumor headache is associated with nausea and vomiting. Vomiting caused by new growth also may occur with neither nausea nor headache, and is then usually the result of medullary compression. Being unexpected, such vomiting may be projectile.

When the headache is occipital or suboccipital, it is often associated with "stiffness" or aching of the muscles of the neck and tilting of the head toward the side of the lesion.

PATHOGENESIS. The initial headaches of brain tumor result from displacement of adjacent large arteries, veins, venous sinuses, and the cranial and somatic nerves, as mentioned. When the brain begins to shift away from the tumor, pain also can emanate form traction and displacement of structures remote from the space-occupying lesion. Increased intracranial pressure

per se need not cause headache, however. Indeed, in conditions such as benign intracranial hypertension, jugular venous obstruction or chronic communicating hydrocephalus, substantial elevations of intracranial pressure can occur with no headache.

(1) About one third of all headaches approximately overlie the tumor. (2) In the absence of increased intracranial pressure, two thirds of headaches are near or immediately over the tumor, and when unilateral are on the same side. (3) Occipital headache is almost always present and is the first symptom of posterior fossa tumors, except cerebellopontine angle tumors. When headache occurs with cerebellopontine angle tumors, it is frequently and sometimes solely postauricular. (4) Frontal headache is a first symptom in about one third of supratentorial tumors. Occipital headache rarely occurs with such growths unless associated with increased intracranial pressure or early tonsillar herniation. (5) A generalized headache with brain tumor signifies extensive displacement of the brain, usually with increased intracranial pressure, and has little localizing value.

MANAGEMENT. The most effective treatment for brain tumor headache is surgical removal of the mass. Transient decompression can be achieved by the intravenous infusion of either 500 ml of a 20 per cent sodium mannitol solution or 250 ml or a solution containing 30 per cent urea in 10 per cent invert sugar. Adrenal corticosteroids in high doses can also be employed to reduce brain edema and transiently decompress the mass. Lumbar drainage is contraindicated, nor does it predictably reduce headache of meningitis or subarachnoid hemorrhage.

If an inoperable tumor causes headache, ventricular drainage or shunting is sometimes employed.

Sometimes x-radiation or surgical procedures are justified in attempts to reduce headache caused by clearly defined metastatic disease. Headache resulting from craniopharyngioma or pituitary tumors does not in itself constitute an indication for surgical procedures, because removal provides no assurance that headache will be diminished or eliminated.

HEADACHES FROM EXTRACRANIAL STRUCTURES

Six main categories of head and face pain arise from extracranial tissues and related structures: (1) headaches due to painful dilatation and distention of cranial arteries; (2) headaches due to sustained contraction of skeletal muscle about the face, scalp, and neck; (3) headache from disease of the nose, paranasal spaces, eyes, ears, and teeth; (4) craniofacial pain of the major neuralgias and the postinfectious neuralgias and postinfectious neuritides; (5) headache due to nonspecific inflammation of cranial arteries ("cranial arteritis," "temporal arteritis"); and (6) head pain due to trauma, infection, or new growth involving extracranial tissues.

More than 90 per cent of all headaches are in the first two of these categories and occur or are intensified in a life setting that engenders frustration, resentment, anxiety, or depression.

Vascular Headaches

Vascular headaches are common; about 25 per cent of the population report having "migraine" or sick headaches, with about half this number suffering from unilateral headache. Such headaches are principally due to painful dilatation and distention of one or more of the extracranial and, probably, intracranial, i.e., dural, branches of the external carotid artery, with associated edema of adjacent tissues. The most common site of vascular headaches of the migraine type is the temple or the forehead, and one or both frontal, supraorbital, and superficial temporal arteries are most frequently involved, however. Many headaches at the back of the head and neck are associated with painful dilatation and distention of the postauricular and/or occipital arteries.

The lower half of the head and face and the upper jaw in the vicinity of the back teeth may all be the site of pain of vascular origin, with spread to the neck and even the shoulder. Such headaches may be accompanied by the awareness of unusually forceful throbbing in the neck. "Atypical facial neuralgia" is but one of the many designations applied to such headaches, which very probably result in good part from dilatation and distention of the extracranial portion of the middle meningeal artery, of the internal maxillary artery, and of the other branches and the trunks of the external and the common carotid arteries.

Migraine Syndrome

CLINICAL FEATURES. The migraine syndrome is a pattern of dysfunction integrated within the central nervous system and manifested as widespread bodily disturbances, both nonpainful and painful. The outstanding feature is periodic headache, usually unilateral in onset but at times becoming bilateral or generalized. The attacks may vary in duration from a few minutes to several days and, in severity, from trifling symptoms to prolonged disabling illness. The headaches are associated with "irritability," nausea, and often photophobia, vomiting, constipation, or diarrhea. Although most common in the temple, headaches may be experienced anywhere in the head, face, and neck. About 50 per cent of patients with classic migraine report a similar syndrome in a parent or grandparent.

Some patients experience vague symptoms for as much as several days before a migraine attack. These include a facial flushing or pallor and other transient cranial vasomotor phenomena such as vertigo. In the hour preceding the headache, a variety of visual and other neurologic abnormalities caused by transient local constriction of cerebral or retinal arteries occur in about 10 to 15 per cent of the instances. These prodromes may take the form of scintillating scotomas, visual field defects such as unilateral or homonymous hemianopsia, and, occasionally, hemiplegia. Rarely, more sustained neurologic defects and even cerebral infarction can occur. The risk of these cerebrovascular complications is higher in women than in men. The incidence of stroke reaches a fourfold increase over the control population in women with migraine who both smoke and take contraceptive pills. As the vasoconstriction phenomena recede, vasodilator headache commences, sometimes overlapping, sometimes beginning after a short symptom-free interval. The pain is throbbing and aching, is appreciably reduced by pressure on the common carotid and the affected superficial artery, and is characteristically eliminated or reduced by vasoconstrictor agents, particularly ergotamine tartrate. The walls of the dilated cranial arteries and the adjacent tissues become edematous and tender. With sustained vasodilata-

tion for several hours, the easily compressible arteries become rigid and relatively noncompressible, and the pulsatile pain becomes a steady ache. Redness and swelling of the eye with excessive tearing, and redness and swelling of the nasal mucosa with or without epistaxis, may occur. A secondary muscle contraction component of the headache may outlast the vascular pain and will not be modified by vasoconstrictor agents.

A variety of headache closely related to migraine is the *cluster headache.* This head pain is almost always unilateral, affects men more than women, and usually begins between the third and sixth decades. Attacks come on abruptly with intense throbbing pain arising high in the nostril and spreading to involve the region behind the homolateral eye and sometimes the forehead as well. During the attacks, which last up to two hours, the nose and eyes water. The skin reddens and a homolateral Horner's syndrome with pupillary constriction and ptosis may develop. The attacks tend to occur from once to several times daily, in clusters lasting weeks or, less often, months. Without apparent reason, the cluster subsides as suddenly as it began, and the patient commonly remains free of headache for weeks or months until another cluster begins. During a cluster period, but not between, alcohol is likely to induce attacks. When headaches recur in close succession, the Horner's syndrome may outlast the headache.

PATHOGENESIS. There is evidence of a general abnormality of vascular behavior in many migraine subjects, and the extracranial vessels of such subjects show more variability in their contractile patterns than those of normal subjects even during headache-free periods. Studies in man of the cerebral blood flow show that during the prodromal stages of the migraine attack the intracranial arteries are constricted, whereas during the headache itself the arteries become dilated. Humoral agents have long been sought as the basis of the migraine syndrome. Local fluid collected from sites of swelling at the point of maximal headache and tenderness during an attack contains a vasodilator polypeptide of the bradykinin type that lowers pain thresholds and may be a factor in a local sterile inflammation. However, kinins, histamine, or substances such as acetylcholine do not satisfactorily explain the generalized manifestations of the disorder. Several lines of evidence suggest that abnormalities in the metabolism of serotonin may play a role in the migraine syndrome. Reserpine, which induces a drop in serum serotonin levels, will often induce a migraine attack, and serum levels of serotonin have been found to drop spontaneously just before migraine attacks. During migraine attacks, an increased quantity of serotonin metabolites has been found in the urine. Evidence also indicates that a platelet abnormality may be connected with migraine. Transitory decreases in platelet monoamine oxidase activity have been recorded during migraine attacks. Increased platelet aggregability also has been noted; the full significance of these findings remains to be elucidated, however.

MANAGEMENT OF ACUTE HEADACHE. Traditionally, the vasoconstrictor effect of ergotamine tartrate taken orally, rectally, or by injection has provided the mainstay of treatment. Orally, two to eight Cafergot tablets (ergotamine tartrate, 1 mg; caffeine, 100 mg) may be given safely for any one headache attack. The intramuscular dose of ergotamine tartrate is 0.25 to 0.5 mg, and the rectal dose, by suppository, is 1 to 2 mg. Not more than 10 mg of ergotamine orally or 5 mg parenterally should be given in any week because of the hazards of arterial vasoconstriction. Recent evidence suggests that the combination of analgesics plus antiemetics sometimes may be superior to the use of ergotamine. Wilkinson reports that at the London Migraine Clinic most patients require for relief only an analgesic (aspirin, 0.6 to 0.9 gram, or acetaminophen, 0.5 to 1.0 gram) and an antiemetic (prochlorperazine, 5 mg). Codeine may be used judiciously, but using stronger narcotics threatens to produce addiction.

Cluster headaches are treated as above except that indomethacin almost specifically relieves some patients. Adrenocorticosteroids sometimes abort the clusters, but the effect is inconsistent. Methysergide has effects similar to its use in migraine.

PREVENTION. Prophylaxis against migraine is effective in perhaps 75 per cent of instances, and requires attention to both the medications and the personal problems of the patient.

Some patients relate recurrent headaches to the ingestion of chocolate, alcoholic beverages, or tyramine-containing foods such as cheese and wine. Such association deserves inquiry and appropriate restrictions. The most effective prophylactic drug is the serotonin antagonist methysergide, given as 2 mg three to four times daily. Methysergide must be used with caution, because it can cause a number of side effects, the serious ones including vascular insufficiency, retroperitoneal or pleural fibrosis, or fibrotic thickening of the heart valves. Side effects are minimized by enforcing drug-free periods of three to eight weeks' duration after every three-month treatment period. Less effective but sometimes successful agents used in prophylaxis include clonidine, cyproheptadine, and, occasionally, propranolol.

Patients with migraine often require considerable psychologic support and reassurance. Many such patients report becoming progressively more tense, resentful, and fatigued during periods of threat or conflict. Such feelings, along with a sense of anger or depression, often form the backdrop for a recurrence of headache. Treatment is best if it allows the patient free and repeated expression of his conflicts, resentments, and dissatisfactions; enables him to recognize the nature of his dilemma and its relationship to the physiologic basis of his pain; and guides him toward a more flexible attitude and personal adjustment.

Muscle-Contraction Headaches

The pain of a muscle-contraction headache is a steady, nonpulsatile, unilateral or bilateral ache located in the temporal, occipital, parietal, or frontal regions. Additional descriptive terms include tightness, bandlike or caplike sensations about the head, or sensations of weight, pressure, drawing, or soreness. Pain may be fleeting, with frequent changes in the site and intensity of recurrences, or localized in one region. The headache may last for weeks, months, or years.

PATHOGENESIS. The cause lies in long-sustained contraction of skeletal muscle about the face, scalp, and neck. Concurrent vasodilatation of the associated cranial arteries frequently contributes to the irritability of the involved muscles and the pain.

With prolonged sustained contraction, the muscles of the head, jaws, neck, and upper back become tender,

causing the patient to limit their motion. Palpation may reveal sharply localized painful areas or nodules. Commonly, it hurts to comb or brush the hair or to don a hat. Exposure to cold, with shivering, may precipitate or aggravate the headache. Pressure on the contracted, tender muscles may augment the intensity and may elicit tinnitus, dizziness, and lacrimation — features that also occur spontaneously.

Sustained muscle contraction giving rise to headache is often secondary to other head pains, including migraine or disease in the eye, ear, nose, paranasal spaces, teeth, or scalp, and to brain tumor. Painful, sustained muscle contraction is also the primary source of many headaches associated with emotional tension states, especially during periods of tension, anger, or depression.

MANAGEMENT. Reassurance, massage, manipulation, and manual stretching of the nuchal and occipital muscles, aspirin, and phenobarbital (30 mg three times a day) reduce or eliminate most such headaches. Diazepam is often used but enhances feelings of depression. Heat, warm baths, and the passage of time are important adjuvants. Particularly among patients susceptible to recurrent headache of this type, the antidepressant amitriptyline in doses of 25 to 75 mg daily may bring considerable relief.

Other Types of Extracranial Headache

RECURRENT ("CHRONIC") POST-TRAUMATIC HEADACHE. Head injury may rarely be followed by headaches that stem from intracranial sources such as subdural hematomas or subarachnoid hemorrhages. However, most post-traumatic headaches stem from nonintracranial sources, four types being most common: (1) pain or tenderness resulting from local tissue damage in a scar or at a site of impact, (2) muscle-contraction headache, (3) attacks of throbbing and aching vascular headache, and (4) infrequently, delusional headaches for which no tissue abnormality exists. The first two varieties are most common and are sometimes accompanied by fleeting vertigo with sudden movement or rotation of the head, nausea, irritability, and insomnia.

Many injured patients harbor resentment related to the circumstances of their accident or fear that they have sustained permanent brain injury. These reactions and attitudes are intimately related to the pathophysiology and "chronicity" of post-traumatic headaches, and the headache often fails to subside as long as compensation claims remain unsettled.

HEADACHES ASSOCIATED WITH ARTERIAL HYPERTENSION. When otherwise symptom-free and in the absence of hypertensive encephalopathy or pheochromocytoma, about 10 per cent of persons with arterial hypertension may experience severe, even disabling, headaches, particularly during the morning hours. Fluctuations in blood pressure correlate only poorly with the headaches, nor is the extent of the elevation directly related to the severity of the attacks. However, headache attacks tend to be less frequent when the blood pressure is least elevated.

The headache associated with arterial hypertension resembles the vascular headaches of migraine and muscle tension and often regresses spontaneously with reassurance and the effective treatment of the hypertension.

NASAL AND PARANASAL STRUCTURES AS SOURCES OF HEADACHE. Sinus headache is predominantly a short-lived problem, always associated with objective evidence of acute sinusitis. Most of the discomfort comes from the ostia, which are many times more sensitive than the relatively insensitive walls of the sinuses. Typically, "sinus" headache commences in the morning (frontal) or early afternoon (maxillary) and subsides in the early or late evening. The pain is dull and aching, is made worse by changing head position, and is seldom associated with nausea and vomiting. It is due to mucosal inflammation, so that engorged turbinates, ostia, nasofrontal ducts and superior nasal spaces should be visible. Most patients have sinus tenderness. Headache not associated with turbinate engorgement and inflammation is probably not due to sinus or nose disease. Sinus headache is best treated with decongestants and analgesics. Persistent purulent discharges should be cultured and appropriate antimicrobial drugs employed. Chronic suppurative disease in the frontal, ethmoid, and sphenoid sinuses, or in the mastoid air cells, may result in osteomyelitis and inflammation of adjacent cranial tissues. Headache persisting after surgical drainage of the diseased sinus is evidence for extradural and possibly subdural infection.

HEAD PAIN AND DISEASE OF THE TEETH. Noxious stimuli in a tooth usually evoke local toothache, but when severe, such pain can be extremely difficult to localize. Afferent fibers for sensation in the teeth are contained in the second and third divisions of the fifth cranial nerve. Headache in the areas supplied by the latter is, in rare instances, associated with prolonged, intense toothache, or follows a tooth extraction. More commonly, in association with toothache, tooth extraction or a tender, diseased tooth, distant tissues exhibit surface hyperalgesia, tenderness, and vasomotor reactions, such as tender eyeballs, reddening of the conjunctivae, and tenderness of the auricular and temporal tissues. Because of secondary muscle contraction, other sites of tenderness and pain may be noted behind the ears, behind the lower border of the mastoid process, and in the muscles of the occiput, neck, and shoulders.

The upper teeth frequently hurt in association with disease of the nasal and paranasal structures. Occasionally, in coronary insufficiency, pain is experienced in the lower jaw because of the close approximation of the fifth cranial and upper cervical neural segments in the cord. The teeth rarely cause craniofacial pains or "neuralgias" in the absence of toothache. Headache may not be attributed to a diseased tooth unless the injection of procaine into the tissues about the suspected tooth greatly reduces the intensity of, or eliminates, such headache.

HEAD PAIN AND DISEASE OF THE EAR. The fifth, seventh, ninth, and tenth cranial nerves contribute to the sensory innervation of the ear, and branches from the upper cervical roots supply the immediately adjacent scalp and muscles. Severe pain in the vicinity of the ear can be caused by disease of the teeth, acute tonsillitis, inflammatory and neoplastic disease of the larynx and nasopharynx, temporomandibular joint disorders, tumors, and inflammation in the posterior fossa and disease of the cervical spine and its soft tissues. Pain in the ear is also associated with vascular headaches and atypical facial neuralgias as well as herpes zoster of the fifth and seventh cranial nerves and, rarely, the glossopharyngeal nerve. True glossopharyngeal neuralgia causes severe pain radiating from the tonsil into the ear. It has the usual timing feature of "tic."

Primary ear disease is relatively infrequent — but important — as a source of headache, because it almost always indicates inflammation or destructive disease. Acute otitis media (purulent or nonpurulent), furunculosis of the ear canal, traumatic rupture of the tympanum, and fracture of the anterior wall of the bony canal all cause pain in the ear associated with sustained tender contraction of adjacent skeletal muscles. Osteomyelitis of the mastoid bone may be associated with inflammation of the nearby periosteum as well as dura and adjacent tissues (epidural abscess) — both sources of pain in or behind the ear. Pain in this region also accompanies tumors of the acoustic nerve and inflammation and thrombosis of the lateral sinus.

THE EYE AS A SOURCE OF HEADACHE. Errors of refraction (hypermetropia, astigmatism, anomalies of accommodation), disturbances of ocular muscle equilibrium, and glaucoma are universally described as causing headache. Refractive errors are also said to give origin to such other symptoms as aching of the eyes, "sandy" feeling in the eyes, pulling sensations in and about the orbit, and conjunctival congestion. Headache usually starts around and over the eyes and subsequently radiates to the occiput and back of the head.

The pain of increased intraocular pressure at first remains localized in the eyeball, then extends along the rim of the orbit and, finally, throughout most of the area supplied by the ophthalmic division of the trigeminal nerve. Nausea and vomiting sometimes accompany such headaches.

Headache accompanying various ocular disturbances is regarded as secondary to (1) sustained contraction of the intraocular muscles, which is associated with excessive accommodation effort, or (2) sustained contraction of the extraocular muscles, resulting from the effort to produced distinct retinal images, and single binocular vision with fusion. Simple myopia does not evoke headache because the myope, in attempting to improve his vision by the contraction of his eye muscles, actually makes his vision worse and soon abandons the attempt.

With inflammation of the iris and ciliary body, light may cause intense pain in the eye and adjacent areas when the light stimulus is accompanied by movement of the inflamed iris. When the iris is immobilized, pain is allayed.

Dalessio, D. J.: Wolff's Headache and Other Head Pain. 3rd ed. New York, Oxford University Press, 1972.

Harper, A. M., MacKenzie, E. T., McCulloch, J., and Pickard, J. D.: Migraine and the blood brain barrier. Lancet, 1:1034, 1977.

Norris, J. W., Hachinski, V. C., and Cooper, P. W.: Changes in cerebral blood flow during a migraine attack. Brit. Med. J., 3:676, 1975.

Vinken, P. J., and Bruyn, G. W. (eds.): Headaches and Cranial Neuralgias. Vol. 5. Handbook of Clinical Neurology. Amsterdam, North-Holland, 1968.

Waters, W. E., and O'Connor, P. J.: Prevalence of migraine. J. Neurol. Neurosurg. Psychiatry, 38:613, 1975.

Wilkinson, M.: The treatment of acute migraine attacks. Headache, 16:291, 1976.

262. HEARING LOSS

Robert W. Baloh

INTRODUCTION

Hearing loss is usually expressed in terms of the ability to hear pure tones which are defined by their frequency and intensity. In order to quantify the magnitude of hearing loss, normal hearing levels are defined by an international standard. These levels approximate the intensity of the faintest sound that can be heard by normal ears. A patient's hearing level is the difference in decibels (db) between the faintest pure tone that he can hear and the normal reference level given by the standard. The range of audible frequencies is approximately 20 to 20,000 Hz in young normal ears. The ear is most sensitive between 500 and 4000 Hz, which roughly corresponds to the frequency range most important for understanding speech. The hearing level in this range has several practical implications in terms of the degree of handicap and the potential for useful correction with amplification. A 30 to 40 db hearing level in the speech range would impair normal conversation, whereas an 80 db hearing level would make everyday auditory communication almost impossible (the social definition of deafness).

TYPES OF HEARING LOSS

Hearing disorders can be classified as conductive, sensorineural, and central, based on the anatomic site of pathology. *Conductive hearing loss* results from lesions involving the external or middle ear. The tympanic membrane and ossicles act as a transformer, amplifying airborne sound and efficiently transferring it to the inner ear fluid. If this normal pathway is obstructed, transmission can occur across the skin and through the bones of the skull (bone conduction) but at the cost of significant energy loss. For example, simple interruption of the ossicles results in a hearing level of approximately 25 db, whereas complete absence of the conduction system on a congenital basis results in a hearing level of about 60 db, i.e., the level of bone conduction. Patients with conductive hearing loss can hear speech in a noisy background better than in a quiet background because they can understand loud speech as well as anyone.

Sensorineural hearing loss results from lesions of the cochlea and/or the auditory division of the eighth cranial nerve. The sensory cells of the cochlea are force transducers converting sound energy in the inner ear fluid to action potentials in the auditory nerve. The spiral cochlea mechanically analyzes the frequency content of sound. For high frequency tones only sensory cells in the basilar turn are activated, whereas for low frequency tones all or nearly all sensory cells are activated. Therefore with lesions of the cochlea and its afferent nerve, the hearing levels for different frequencies are usually unequal and the phase relationship (timing) between different frequencies may be altered. Patients with sensorineural hearing loss often have difficulty hearing speech that is mixed with background noise and may be annoyed by loud speech.

Three important manifestations of sensorineural le-sions are diplacusis, recruitment, and tone decay. Diplacusis and recruitment are commonly seen with cochlear lesions; tone decay is usually seen with eighth nerve involvement. With diplacusis the tonal quality of a pure tone is distorted so that it may sound like a complex mixture of tones. Binaural diplacusis occurs when the two ears are affected unequally so that the same frequency has a different pitch in each ear, i.e., the patient hears double. Monaural diplacusis occurs when two tones or a tone and noise are heard simultaneously in one ear. With recruitment there is an abnormally rapid growth in the sensation of loudness as the intensity of a sound is increased so that faint or moderate sounds cannot be heard, whereas there is little or no change in the loudness of loud sounds. The inability to maintain perception of a continuous tone presented above auditory threshold is called tone decay. Patients with conductive or cochlear lesions can usually hear a continuous tone for at least 60 seconds, whereas the tone rapidly decays in patients with eighth nerve lesions.

Central hearing disorders result from lesions of the central auditory pathways. These consist of the cochlear and dorsal olivary nuclear complexes, inferior colliculi, medial geniculate bodies, auditory cortex in the temporal lobes, and interconnecting afferent and efferent fiber tracts. As a rule, patients with central lesions do not have impaired hearing levels for pure tones and they can understand speech as long as it is clearly spoken in a quiet environment. If the listener's task is made more difficult with the introduction of background noise or competing messages, performance deteriorates more markedly in patients with central lesions than in normal subjects. Lesions involving the eighth nerve root entry zone or cochlear nucleus, however, can result in unilateral hearing loss for pure tones. Since approximately 50 per cent of afferent nerve fibers cross central to the cochlear nucleus, this is the most central structure in which a lesion can result in a unilateral hearing loss.

EXAMINATION OF HEARING

BEDSIDE TESTS. A quick test for hearing loss in the speech range is to observe the response to spoken commands at different intensities (whisper, conversation, shouting). The examiner must be careful to prevent the patient from reading his lip movement. A high frequency stimulus such as a watch tick or coin click (approximately 4000 cps) should also be used, because sensorineural disorders often involve only the higher frequencies. Tuning fork tests permit a rough assessment of the hearing level for pure tones of known frequency. The clinician can use his own hearing level as a reference standard. The *Rinne test* compares the patient's hearing by air conduction with that by bone conduction. The fork (preferably 512 cps) is first held against the mastoid process until the sound fades. It is then placed one inch from the ear. Normal subjects can hear the fork about twice as long by air as by bone conduction. If bone conduction is greater than air conduction, a conductive hearing loss is suggested. The *Weber test* compares the patient's hearing by bone conduction in the two ears. The fork is placed at the center of the forehead or on a central incisor, and the patient is asked where he hears the tone. Normal subjects hear it in the center of the head, patients with unilateral conductive loss hear it on the affected side, and patients with unilateral sensorineural loss hear it on the side opposite the loss.

AUDIOMETRY. Tests Requiring Subjective Responses. *Pure tone* testing is the nucleus of most auditory examinations. Pure tones at selected frequencies are presented via either earphones (air conduction) or a vibrator pressed against the mastoid portion of the temporal bone (bone conduction). The minimal level that the subject can hear is determined for each frequency. Two *speech* tests are routinely used. The speech reception threshold (SRT) is the intensity at which the patient can correctly repeat 50 per cent of the words presented. The SRT is a test of hearing sensitivity for speech and should reflect the hearing level for pure tones in the speech range. The speech discrimination test is a measure of the patient's ability to understand speech when it is presented at a level that is easily heard. In patients with eighth nerve lesions, speech discrimination can be severely reduced even when pure tone thresholds are normal or nearly normal, whereas in patients with cochlear lesions discrimination tends to be proportional to the magnitude of hearing loss.

Recruitment is usually measured by the alternate binaural loudness balance (ABLB) test (if the hearing loss is unilateral). This test compares the loudness for tones of varying intensity as perceived by the pathologic ear and the normal ear. Recruitment is present if smaller increases in stimulus intensity are required in the poorer ear than in the better ear to maintain equal loudness. *Tone decay* is usually tested by presenting a tone at a prescribed suprathreshold level and asking the patient to respond as long as he hears the tone. Special tests for central auditory lesions assess the patient's ability to understand *distorted speech* or speech that is presented to one ear with a *competing message* in the other ear.

Tests Using Objective Measurements. By inserting a probe in the external canal that both presents and measures the sound pressure level of a tone, the acoustic impedance of the middle ear can be assessed. Two types of impedance measurements are routinely used: *tympanometry* and *stapedius reflex measurement*. Tympanometry, the measurement of impedance as a function of ear canal air pressure, is primarily useful for detection of middle ear disorders; stapedius reflex measurements are particularly useful for identifying lesions of the eighth nerve and/or brainstem. The stapedius muscle contracts and tightens the ossicular chain to protect the inner ear from excessively loud noises. The magnitude of the acoustic impedance change is an indirect measure of the strength of contraction of the stapedius muscle. The reflex arc consists of (1) auditory nerve, (2) brainstem interneurons, and (3) facial nerve. If the middle ear structures are intact, loss of the stapedius reflex suggests a lesion in this reflex arc.

Electrocochleography, a method for direct measurement of cochlear neural responses, and measurement of auditory evoked responses are two other promising objective tests of auditory function.

CAUSES OF HEARING LOSS

CONDUCTIVE HEARING LOSS. The most common cause of conductive hearing loss is *impacted cerumen* in the external canal. This benign condition is usually first noticed after bathing or swimming when a droplet of water closes the remaining tiny passageway. The most common serious cause of conductive hearing loss is inflammation of the middle ear, *otitis media*. Either infected (suppurative otitis) or noninfected (serous otitis) fluid accumulates in the middle ear, impairing the conduction of airborne sound. Since the air cavity of the middle ear is in direct connection with the mastoid air cells, infection can spread through the mastoid bone and occasionally into the intracranial cavity. Chronic otitis media with perforation of the tympanic membrane can result in an invasion of the middle ear and other pneumatized areas of the temporal bone by keratinizing squamous epithelium (cholesteatoma). Cholesteatomas can produce erosion of the ossicles and bony labyrinth, resulting in a mixed conductive-sensorineural hearing loss.

Otosclerosis commonly produces progressive conductive hearing loss by immobilizing the stapes with new bone growth in front of and below the oval window. Seventy per cent of patients with clinical otosclerosis notice hearing loss between the ages of 11 and 30, and there is a positive family history in approximately 50 per cent of cases. Initially, the hearing loss is purely conductive; but as the disease progresses, the cochlea may be invaded by foci of otosclerotic bone, producing an additional high frequency sensorineural hearing loss. Otosclerosis usually stabilizes when the hearing level reaches 50 to 60 db and rarely progresses to deafness. Other common causes of conductive hearing loss include trauma, congenital malformations of the external and middle ear, and glomus body tumors.

SENSORINEURAL HEARING LOSS. Congenital. Malformations of the inner ear can result from either abnormal genes or abnormal intrauterine factors. Genetically determined deafness may be present at birth, or it may become manifest years after birth as the normally developed inner ear structures deteriorate. In approximately one third of cases, there is a clearly defined syndrome, but in the majority of cases the diagnosis of *hereditary deafness* rests on the finding of a positive family history. In many instances the inheritance is through a recessive gene or a dominant gene with low penetrance, making it difficult to determine the genetic nature of the disorder.

Intrauterine factors resulting in congenital hearing loss include infection, toxic, metabolic, and endocrine disorders, and anoxia associated with Rh incompatibility and difficult deliveries. As many as 70 per cent of mothers who acquire *rubella* during the first trimester of pregnancy will produce a child with some degree of hearing loss. After conclusion of the first trimester, the risk is significantly less, but the infant's formed inner ear can still become infected from a maternal rubella infection. If the maternal infection occurs in the first six weeks of gestation, malformations of the eyes, cardiovascular system, and brain are also common. Since rubella rarely causes complete deafness, children with this type of congenital deafness may be helped with amplification. It is particularly important that children with congenital hearing loss of any variety be recognized, because they may be misdiagnosed as mentally retarded or brain damaged and appropriate educational opportunities not provided.

Acute. Infection of the inner ear (*labyrinthitis*) is the most common cause of sudden unilateral hearing loss.

Bacteria can enter the inner ear directly from the middle ear or from the cerebrospinal fluid via the cochlear aqueduct and internal auditory canal. In the former case, there is a history of recurrent or chronic otitis media; in the latter case, the patient has bacterial meningitis. In addition to the sudden hearing loss, the patient develops vertigo, nausea, and vomiting from involvement of the vestibular labyrinth. The end result is usually an irreversible unilateral deafness. In some instances there is not a direct bacterial invasion but rather an irritation of the labyrinth by bacterial toxins and endotoxins, producing biochemical damage to the membranes. This so-called toxic or serous labyrinthitis is associated with milder degrees of reversible hearing loss.

Viral labyrinthitis may be part of a systemic viral illness such as measles, mumps, and infectious mononucleosis or an isolated infection of the labyrinth without systemic symptoms. Mumps is a common cause of unilateral hearing loss in preschool and school-aged children, and there is serologic evidence that subclinical mumps infection may produce sudden unilateral hearing loss in adults. An infecting agent is rarely identified in adults with sudden unilateral hearing loss, but pathologic studies when obtained have suggested a viral cause in such patients.

Other common causes of sudden unilateral hearing loss include *head trauma* and *vascular occlusive disease.* Temporal bone fractures, particularly transverse fractures, are often associated with hearing loss. Sudden deafness that is either partially or completely reversible may also follow a blow to the head without skull fracture. This type of deafness is called inner ear concussion and is felt to be due to intense acoustic stimulation from pressure waves created by the blow. The role of vascular occlusion in the production of isolated sudden unilateral hearing loss is controversial, but this should be considered in patients with known vascular disease. Since the labyrinth is usually supplied by a branch of the anterior inferior cerebellar artery, transient hearing loss may be part of the basilar-vertebral insufficiency syndrome.

Subacute and Relapsing. *Menière's syndrome* is characterized by fluctuating hearing loss and tinnitus, episodic vertigo, and a sensation of fullness or pressure in the ear. In the early stages the hearing loss is completely reversible, but eventually severe permanent loss develops. In approximately 20 per cent of patients bilateral involvement will occur. The principal pathologic finding is an increase in the volume of endolymph associated with distention of the entire endolymphatic sac (endolymphatic hydrops). Viral and bacterial, including presumed syphilitic, labyrinthitis can lead to endolymphatic hydrops and must be considered in the differential diagnosis; but in the majority of cases, the cause is unknown. Multiple causes have been proposed for idiopathic Meniere's syndrome, including allergy, endocrine disturbance, focal infection, sympathetic vasomotor disturbance, and psychophysiologic reaction.

Ototoxic drugs are an important cause of bilateral subacute hearing loss. Salicylates in high doses, ethacrynic acid, and furosemide often cause a reversible hearing loss, whereas aminoglycoside antimicrobials usually produce a permanent hearing loss. The primary pathologic change with each of these drugs is loss of hair cells in the cochlea and vestibular end-organs. Commonly used aminoglycosides that cause hearing loss include neomycin, kanamycin, and gentamicin. Neomycin has the undesirable effect of producing hearing loss weeks to months after administration of the drug. Each of these drugs must be used cautiously in patients with impaired renal function, as small doses can create high blood levels and an increased incidence of ototoxic effects.

Chronic Progressive. The bilateral hearing loss commonly associated with advancing age is called *presbycusis.* Presbycusis is not a distinct disease entity but rather represents multiple effects of aging on the auditory system. Presbycusis may include conductive and central dysfunction, although the most consistent effect of aging is on the sensory cells and neurons of the cochlea. The typical audiogram of presbycusis is a symmetrical hearing loss gradually sloping downward with increasing frequency. The most consistent pathology associated with presbycusis is degeneration of sensory cells and nerve fibers at the base of the cochlea. *Noise-induced hearing loss* is extremely common in industrialized societies. The loss almost always begins at 4000 cps and does not affect speech discrimination until late in the disease process. With only a brief exposure to loud noise (hours to days) there may be only a temporary threshold shift, but with continued exposure permanent injury begins. The duration and intensity of exposure determine the degree of permanent injury. Damage to sensory cells is often confined to a small area at the base of the cochlea, centering around the area sensing 4000 cps.

Slowly progressive unilateral sensorineural hearing loss can be caused by a small benign tumor arising from the sheath of the vestibular division of the eighth nerve (*acoustic neuroma, neurilemmoma, vestibular schwannoma*). Acoustic neuromas initially compress the eighth nerve in the narrow confines of the internal auditory canal. As the tumor slowly enlarges, it protrudes through the internal auditory meatus, producing a funnel-shaped erosion of the bone surrounding the canal, stretching adjacent nerve roots over the surface of the mass and deforming the brainstem and cerebellum. The initial symptom is slowly progressive hearing loss in most cases, although rarely an acute hearing loss occurs from compression of the labyrinthine vasculature.

CENTRAL HEARING LOSS. Acute unilateral hearing loss is occasionally seen in patients with *multiple sclerosis* when a plaque involves the cochlear nerve root entry or cochlear nucleus. The hearing usually recovers in a period of days to weeks. *Infarction* in the lateral pontomedullary region can result in acute ipsilateral hearing loss along with multiple focal neurologic signs.

TREATMENT

Surgical treatment of hearing loss is limited to correcting abnormalities of the conduction system. *Hearing aids* amplify sound, usually with the goal of making speech intelligible. They are ideally suited for conductive hearing loss, but can also help sensorineural hearing loss if the inner ear is still able to discriminate speech. The most successful *medical treatment* of hearing loss is the use of appropriate drugs for microbial disease of the ear. The use of a low salt diet and diuretics may be effective in selected cases of Meniere's syndrome, particularly if episodes are precipitated by premenstrual water retention. There is little proof that vasodilator or anticoagulant drugs are effective in reversing sudden unilateral hearing loss of any cause. *Monitoring audiograms* in patients with noise or ototoxic drug exposure are critical for prevention of permanent hearing loss.

Davis, H., and Silverman, S. R. (eds.): Hearing and Deafness. 3rd ed. New York, Holt, Rinehart and Winston, 1970.

Dublin, W. B.: Fundamentals of Sensorineural Auditory Pathology. Springfield, Ill., Charles C Thomas, 1976.

Jerger, J. (ed.): Modern Developments in Audiology. New York, Academic Press, 1973.

Johnson, E. W.: Auditory test results in 500 cases of acoustic neuroma. Arch. Otolaryngol., 103:152, 1977.

Konigsmark, B. W.: Hereditary deafness in man. N. Engl. J. Med., 281:713, 1969.

Morrison, A. W.: Management of Sensorineural Deafness. Reading, Mass., Butterworth, 1975.

Schuknecht, H. E.: Pathology of the Ear. Boston, Harvard University Press, 1975.

263. DIZZINESS AND VERTIGO

David A. Drachman

THE COMPLAINT OF DIZZINESS

As a *complaint* rather than a *disease*, the term "dizziness" appropriately includes almost any sensation that a patient chooses to call by that name. By usage the term is applied to a number of uncommon sensations that are *not* part of daily experience. It is the thread of unfamiliar spatial disorientation that appears to bind these complaints together. When one listens carefully to a large number of "dizzy" patients, it is possible to sort their complaints into four types: a *rotational sensation*, *impending faint*, *dysequilibrium*, and *vague lightheadedness*.

Type I dizziness is a *definite rotational sensation* (vertigo) in which the patient feels that either he or the environment is spinning. Violent vertigo is often accompanied by nausea, vomiting, and a staggering gait. Oscillopsia — a visual hallucination of to-and-fro movement of the environment — may occur. The onset of vertigo is often instantaneous, and patients sometimes describe a sensation of being hurled to the ground. Although full-blown vertigo is unmistakable, with milder forms the patient may describe only a rocking sensation or vague lightheadedness. Recognition of mild vertiginous episodes is often aided by testing with the dizziness simulation battery described below.

Whenever the patient's dizziness is exclusively rotational, it is due to a disorder of the vestibular system: either the peripheral labyrinth or its central connections. Because of this close relationship, it is important to separate definite rotational vertigo accurately from other types of dizziness.

Type II dizziness is a *sensation of impending faint or loss of consciousness*. Pallor, dimness of vision, roaring in the ears, and diaphoresis, with recovery upon assuming the recumbent position, are common. Type II dizziness of cardiovascular origin is of abrupt onset and short duration. When faintness is gradual in onset or persists despite lying down, the relationship of the episodes to hypoglycemia or other disorders of cerebral metabolism should be sought.

The complaint of impending faint usually implies an inadequate supply of blood or nutrients to the entire brain, such as occurs in postural hypotension. It is not a feature of *focal* cerebral ischemia, although this mistaken impression is widely subscribed to by physicians. Other complaints of sudden alteration in the state of consciousness ("dreamy states") may be due to temporal lobe seizures, occurring in the absence of other, more obvious seizure phenomena.

Type III dizziness is *dysequilibrium*: the loss of balance *without* an abnormal sensation in the head. This experience occurs only when the patient is walking; it disappears as soon as he sits down. It is due to a disorder of motor system control.

Type IV dizziness is *vague lightheadedness* other than vertigo, faintness, or dysequilibrium. This designation includes dizziness that cannot be identified with certainty as any of the other types. When patients complain of lightheadedness, *fractional* or *poorly described* symptoms of vertigo, faintness, or dysequilibrium must first be looked for, e.g., a rocking sensation instead of spinning. Evidence of *hyperventilation* symptoms should next be sought, as well as symptoms pointing to a *psychiatric disorder*, particularly depression or anxiety. Finally, the evidence for *multiple sensory impairment* should be examined, especially a history of peripheral neuropathy, cervical spondylosis, or cataract surgery in an elderly or diabetic patient.

EVALUATING THE DIZZY PATIENT

The *history* must explore four major questions that critically distinguish the disorders producing dizziness: (1) the type of dizziness (I to IV) experienced by the patient; (2) the *abruptness* of attacks or *continuity* of symptoms; (3) the relation or independence of dizziness to *position or motion* (standing/sitting/lying; sudden change in position; walking); and (4) the *age* of the patient. The relation of these data to differential diagnosis will be discussed with specific entities.

A neurologic examination allows the distinction between central and peripheral causes of dizziness, and may reveal certain *patterns* of involvement that point to the diagnosis: e.g., brainstem syndrome (hemiplegia alternans), cerebellopontine angle syndrome, multiple sensory impairment.

The dizziness simulation battery is a series of eight bedside maneuvers that have proved valuable in distinguishing the various types of dizziness. Some produce dizziness in all patients, whereas others induce it only in patients with underlying disorders. After each maneuver the patient is questioned as to the similarity of the test-evoked sensation to his own dizziness. Identification of a provoked sensation as identical to the patient's dizziness is often more reliable than a verbal description, particularly if a single maneuver exclusively reproduces his symptoms.

1. *Orthostatic hypotension:* Blood pressure is measured supine, immediately on standing, and after three minutes.

2. *Potentiated Valsalva maneuver:* The patient squats for 30 seconds, then stands and blows into a mercury sphygmomanometer, raising the column to 40 mm Hg for 15 seconds.

3. *Carotid sinus stimulation:* The carotid sinus is unilaterally massaged for 15 seconds without continuous compression of the artery. ECG monitoring is required in the elderly, and the test should be omitted in patients with known cardiac disease.

TABLE 1. Positional Vertigo and Nystagmus

Benign	Central or Malignant
1. Latency of onset of vertigo and nystagmus	1. Immediate onset of vertigo and nystagmus
2. Adaptation and fatigue of vertigo and nystagmus	2. Persistence of nystagmus
3. Direction-fixed nystagmus	3. Direction-changing nystagmus
4. Severe vertigo and systemic symptoms	4. Mild vertigo; few systemic symptoms

4. *Neck-twist:* The patient rotates his head in each direction for 15 seconds as if watching an airplane fly past. Dizziness may result from "kinking" of a vertebral artery, cervicogenic dizziness, or a vestibular disorder.

5. *Walking and turning:* The patient walks in one direction and then quickly turns, reversing direction. This test reproduces dizziness occurring with multisensory deficits, gait apraxia, and disorders of balance.

6. *Hyperventilation:* The patient breathes deeply for three minutes.

7. *Nylen-Bárány maneuver:* The examiner carries the patient's head backward from a seated position, so that it is hanging 45 degrees below the horizontal and turned 45 degrees to one side. Vertigo *accompanied by nystagmus* indicates positional vertigo. The characteristics distinguishing a "benign" from a "malignant" form of this condition are listed in Table 1.

8. *Bárány rotation:* The patient is seated in a rotating chair, head tilted 30 degrees forward from the vertical. The examiner spins the patient in one direction ten times within 20 seconds, then abruptly stops the rotation.

LABORATORY TESTS (Table 2). *Electronystagmography* (ENG) may help to identify and distinguish disorders of the peripheral (labyrinth, eighth nerve) and central vestibular systems. Recording of the amplitude, speed, and duration of ocular movements is first made during a series of eye and head position maneuvers. In the *caloric test* the patient is positioned so that the horizontal semicircular canals are exactly vertical, and each ear is irrigated with cool and warm water (or air) to produce a convection flow of endolymph, which mimics rotational stimulation of each canal. Observations on the speed and duration of the nystagmus generated by this test provide information on the function of the vestibular apparatus.

Audiometric studies are used to evaluate lesions of the middle ear, labyrinth, and cochlear nerve, particularly in Menière's disorder and cerebellopontine angle tumors. Routine pure tone audiometry indicates the presence or absence of a hearing loss and may also distinguish banal causes (acoustic trauma, aging, otosclerosis) from specific cochlear and nerve disorders. More elaborate studies, such as the speech discrimination, alternate binaural loudness balance (ABLB), Békésy, threshold tone decay, and acoustic reflex tests, improve the accuracy of diagnosis. Recently, evoked re-

TABLE 2. Laboratory Tests in Dizziness

1. Electronystagmography (ENG) with caloric testing	6. Electrocardiogram with rhythm strip
2. Audiometry, ERA	7. Serum protein electrophoresis
3. Psychometric testing (MMPI)	8. Thyroid function studies
4. Skull x-rays with Stenvers' views	9. Electroencephalography
5. Cervical spine x-rays	10. Five-hour glucose tolerance test
	Optional: Petrous polytomography 24-hour cardiac monitoring

sponse audiometry (ERA), a signal averaging technique, has become a useful adjunct for distinguishing between brainstem and peripheral disorders.

SPECIFIC CONDITIONS PRODUCING DIZZINESS

It is not always simple to assemble the clinical and laboratory findings obtained from a dizzy patient into a specific diagnostic entity. A classification is provided here of the causes of dizziness, designed to parallel the four major complaints described earlier.

Vertigo and Other Vestibular Disorders

Vertigo accounts for only about a third of complaints of dizzy patients. When patients present with vestibular disorders, it is most important to distinguish between *peripheral* (labyrinthine) abnormalities and those involving *central* vestibular connections. The key to this distinction is the evidence for or against involvement of neighboring brainstem structures.

PERIPHERAL CAUSES OF VERTIGO. Benign Positional Vertigo. Benign positional vertigo is probably the most frequent cause of vertigo, accounting for about 25 per cent of patients with this complaint. The patient experiences a sensation of spinning when he rolls over in bed or makes other sudden head movements. Symptoms are greatest when he lies on his side with the affected ear underneath. The vertigo, sometimes accompanied by nausea and vomiting, lasts for less than five minutes, and between episodes the patient is free of symptoms. This condition, brought about *only* on change of position, differs from other vestibular disorders in which vertigo is increased by head motion but is present at other times as well. Benign positional vertigo occurs at any time during adult years; the cause is usually obscure, although it occasionally follows head trauma. The diagnosis is based on the typical history and on finding the "benign" type of vertigo and nystagmus on performing the Nylen-Bárány maneuver (Table 1). Caloric testing reveals depressed labyrinthine function in one ear in about half the patients. In the majority of cases symptoms persist for several weeks, although bouts may recur over a span of years with prolonged symptom-free intervals. This condition must be distinguished from so-called "central" or "malignant" positional vertigo and nystagmus (Table 1), which may occur with lesions (tumors, infarcts) involving posterior fossa structures; acute positional vertigo is uncommonly associated with such conditions.

Acute Peripheral Vestibulopathy ("Acute Labyrinthitis"; "Vestibular Neuronitis"). This condition is defined as a single bout of spontaneous vertigo, lasting for hours or days. Attacks occasionally follow a trivial respiratory or other infection, but the relation is not clear. Symptoms of vertigo, nausea, and vomiting usually improve within 48 hours, but may persist for 7 to 14 days. On examination the patient appears acutely ill, often pale and diaphoretic, resisting motion of the head. Nystagmus invariably accompanies the vertigo. As the patient recovers, he may feel "off balance" for weeks or months owing to unilateral impairment of vestibular function, present in about 50 per cent of patients. Hearing is not impaired in this condition.

Acute   and   Recurrent   Peripheral   Vestibulo-

pathy. Acute and recurrent peripheral vestibulopathy is clinically similar to the entity described above, but consists of *repeated* bouts of vertigo occurring over a period of months or years. This condition occurs in an older age group than acute peripheral vestibulopathy, and is associated with *less* severe vestibular impairment on caloric testing. Approximately half the patients presenting with a single attack of peripheral vestibulopathy experience a recurrence, linking this with the previous condition. The absence of auditory impairment distinguishes this condition from Menière's disorder.

Menière's Disorder. Menière's disorder is widely considered to be one of the most frequent causes of dizziness, but it actually accounts for only about 5 per cent of all dizziness and 10 to 15 per cent of vertigo. It usually occurs in adults and consists of recurring bouts of vertigo associated with *hearing loss* and *tinnitus* which may precede or follow the first bout of vertigo. Patients often complain of "fullness" in the ears, and are sometimes aware of *recruitment* as a sensation of auditory discomfort produced by loud noises. Bouts of vertigo last from hours to days, recurring as often as every week or as infrequently as every ten years. Hearing loss is unilateral in 80 to 90 per cent of patients, with a severe deficit in half the patients. Most patients develop chronic impairment of vestibular function, resulting in the syndrome of vestibular imbalance. In many patients the recurrent episodes of vertigo may "burn out" over the years.

Diagnosis depends on the characteristic history and the audiometric findings (low frequency pure tone impairment, poor speech discrimination comparable to the pure tone hearing loss, and recruitment). Caloric testing demonstrates abnormal vestibular function in 80 per cent of patients.

Pathologic studies have identified distention of the membranous labyrinth with endolymph as the immediate cause of this condition, but the explanation for the excess of endolymph remains obscure.

Toxic Damage to the Labyrinths. Drugs of the aminoglycoside groups (e.g., streptomycin, gentamicin) may produce toxic damage to the labyrinths. Although toxicity is generally dose related, some patients develop labyrinthine damage after brief treatment with ordinary doses of these drugs, particularly if renal function is impaired. Tinnitus, hearing loss, or vertigo may be the presenting symptom, along with severe impairment of balance, nausea, and vomiting. Vertigo continues for days or weeks. If the ototoxic drug is immediately discontinued, damage to the labyrinth is usually arrested. A characteristic loss of balance follows the acute stage of vertigo and may include blurring of vision on motion owing to loss of the vestibulo-ocular reflexes. With the loss of vestibular sensation, these patients are dependent on visual cues to maintain balance, and are unable to walk in the dark. After several months, adaptation to the loss of vestibular sensation develops, and many can lead fairly normal lives.

Diagnosis is based on the history of treatment with one of the ototoxic drugs, followed by the sequence described above. On examination the Romberg test is abnormal. Caloric tests demonstrate bilateral severe hypoactivity of the labyrinths. Bárány rotation may fail to elicit vertigo or nystagmus.

Other Peripheral Causes of Vertigo. Head trauma may be followed by persistent or positional vertigo. Dislocation of the otoliths from the macula of the utricle has been proposed as a cause of this condition. When vertigo immediately follows trauma, the etiologic relationship is clear, but in cases with medicolegal implications vertigo (and other forms of dizziness) may follow head trauma after a lengthy delay. It is often stated that the termination of pending litigation resolves such cases. *Cervicogenic vertigo,* although not vestibular in origin, may present with similar manifestations. Since the articulations and musculature of the cervical region provide extensive input to the brainstem vestibular system, cervical spondylosis or even painful muscular contraction may result in vertigo, nausea, and vomiting. *Dysproteinemias, hypothyroidism,* and *otitis media* are other occasional causes of vertigo.

TREATMENT. Management of vertigo resulting from most peripheral vestibular disorders is similar. When vertigo is severely disabling, the patient should be placed at bed rest or, in persistent cases, hospitalized. Meclizine, 25 mg four times daily, is of value in suppressing labyrinthine hyperactivity. Diazepam effectively suppresses central vestibular responses, and helps control the anxiety that often accompanies vertigo. Atropine tablets, 0.4 mg sublingually at the onset of attacks of vertigo, may abort the development of symptoms. Nausea and vomiting are controlled by trimethobenzamide hydrochloride (Tigan) suppositories, 200 mg every six hours, or in resistant cases by parenteral phenothiazines such as chlorpromazine (Thorazine), 25 mg every six hours.

Patients with benign positional vertigo may benefit from a soft foam rubber collar that limits cervical motion, thus preventing the stimulus for attacks.

Many patients with peripheral vestibular disorders have residual labyrinthine deficits after the acute vertiginous phase, and benefit from measures to improve their balance. A foam rubber collar is useful to limit neck motion, and methylphenidate (Ritalin) may enable them to react more quickly to the remaining sensory modalities. Balancing exercises help patients adapt to ambulation in the absence of normal vestibular function.

The treatment of acute attacks of Menière's disorder is similar to that for other vestibular disorders. A variety of medical and surgical treatments to prevent recurrences of vertigo and/or deterioration of hearing have been proposed; a discussion of their application and merits is beyond the scope of this chapter.

CENTRAL CAUSES OF VERTIGO. **Cerebrovascular Disease.** Cerebrovascular disease produces vertigo when basilar-vertebral artery ischemia damages the vestibular nuclei or their connections. In virtually all cases injury to adjacent brainstem structures occurs, and vertigo is unlikely to be due to a stroke when other neurologic symptoms or signs are absent. As with other patterns of cerebrovascular disease, elderly hypertensive patients with diabetes, heart disease, or hyperlipidemia are the most likely candidates. Caloric testing and evoked response audiometry (ERA) may help in the diagnosis by providing evidence of brainstem involvement of central vestibular and auditory pathways.

Transient ischemic attacks may be particularly difficult to diagnose, because at the time of examination the patient may have recovered completely. A reliable history of additional brainstem symptoms is necessary to establish the diagnosis. The treatment of cerebrovascular disease is discussed in Ch. 293 to 295.

Multiple Sclerosis. Multiple sclerosis may produce

vertigo in young patients, although this condition accounts for no more than 5 to 10 per cent of acute vertigo in those below age 40. Further, although multiple sclerosis may begin with vertigo, this is far less common than onset with optic neuritis or paresthesias. The diagnosis is discussed elsewhere; one must be aware that vertigo associated with ocular motor disorders that cannot be caused by purely peripheral vestibular disease (e.g., persistent diplopia, median longitudinal fasciculus syndrome, ophthalmoplegia) is strongly suggestive of this condition.

Treatment of the vertigo is similar to that for peripheral vestibulopathies; meclizine, diazepam, atropine, and Tigan are of value in controlling the vertigo and its associated nausea and vomiting.

Cerebellopontine Angle Tumors. Cerebellopontine angle tumors are a *rare* cause of vertigo, but must not be overlooked early in their growth when they are readily removable. The large majority are benign acoustic neuromas arising in the internal auditory meatus. These tumors develop in middle-aged patients who experience vague unsteadiness that progresses over a period of years. Vertigo when present may be of the "malignant" positional type (Table 1), and only rarely does acute spontaneous vertigo occur. Hearing loss, tinnitus, facial numbness or weakness, cerebellar ataxia, and occasional dementia complete the picture. Unilateral or bilateral acoustic neuromas are especially common in von Recklinghausen's disease (neurofibromatosis).

On caloric testing there is a markedly diminished response on the affected side. Audiometry demonstrates the findings of a "retrocochlear" lesion, including rapid tone decay, a diminished or absent acoustic reflex, and a Type III or IV curve on Békésy audiometry. Roentgenograms of the petrous bones are diagnostic and show erosion of the affected internal auditory meatus, a finding that is seen even earlier on polycyclic tomography.

Vertiginous Migraine. Vertiginous migraine may occur preceding the headache, during the headache phase, or as a "migraine equivalent" in place of the headache. Since both migraine and vertigo are common conditions, the occurrence of vertigo without a constant time relation to headache may represent only a coincidence in some unfortunate patients. Treatment is directed at prevention of the migraine attacks and control of the symptoms of vertigo, nausea, and vomiting as outlined above.

Viral Infections. Viral infections rarely cause vertigo except when herpes zoster affects the eighth nerve, often in conjunction with the Ramsay Hunt syndrome or geniculate herpes. Facial paralysis, vertigo, and hearing loss occur with herpetic vesicular lesions in the external auditory canal. Lymphocytes and polymorphonuclear leukocytes may be found in the cerebrospinal fluid. The diagnosis is established by demonstrating a rise of antibody titers to herpes zoster. Pathologically, lymphocytic infiltration of the sensory ganglia and nerve roots is seen. Treatment consists of the use of prednisone during the acute phase of the illness and the management of the vertigo, nausea, and vomiting as outlined above.

Cogan's syndrome is an uncommon vasculitis presenting in young adults with vertigo, deafness, and interstitial keratitis, as well as other systemic manifestations. Early in its course it may be mistaken for a minor vestibulopathy, although it may ultimately cause disability or death. Treatment with prednisone is of value and should be instituted promptly.

Deep-sea diving accidents may produce vertigo by a variety of mechanisms, including decompression sickness, air embolism, and rupture of the oval window. Investigation and treatment of these conditions should be carried out by physicians especially equipped to handle the problems of undersea medicine.

VESTIBULAR DISORDERS NOT PRODUCING VERTIGO. In some patients *hypoactivity* of the labyrinths may occur without antecedent episodes of vertigo. These patients describe lightheadedness on walking, turning, or changing position. The exact cause of the conditions producing these disorders is obscure. With *hyperactive* labyrinths, most often seen in anxious patients, instantaneous vertigo or loss of balance occurs on rapid turning. Caloric testing confirms the abnormal responsiveness of the labyrinths in either case. Patients with hypoactive or asymmetrical labyrinthine function benefit from methylphenidate (Ritalin), head restraint with a foam rubber collar, and a course of balancing exercises. Patients with hyperactive labyrinths are treated with meclizine, 25 mg three or four times daily, and diazepam, 5 mg three times daily.

Faintness: Syncopal and Seizure Disorders

SYNCOPAL DISORDERS (see also Ch. 264). **Orthostatic Hypotension.** In orthostatic hypotension the patient experiences faintness upon standing, resulting from a fall in blood pressure (at least 25/15 mm Hg). Acquired and idiopathic varieties are described. In the closely related Shy-Drager syndrome (see Ch. 278.6), manifestations of parkinsonism, peripheral neuropathy, dementia, and cerebellar abnormalities contribute to a multifactorial problem of dizziness. Recently, treatment with indomethacin, 50 mg three times daily, has been found to be effective in this condition.

Cardiac Arrhythmias. Patients with brief dizziness caused by episodic cardiac arrhythmias are often unaware of palpitations and complain only of faintness. When the arrhythmia is constantly present, it is easily recognized by observation of the jugular venous pulse, auscultation or electrocardiography. With infrequent runs of abnormal heart rhythm, the use of 12- or 24-hour ambulatory electrocardiographic monitoring is necessary. In young adults — especially women — mitral valve prolapse should be suspected as a cause of arrhythmia if a midsystolic click or late systolic murmur is heard on auscultation. Diagnosis and treatment are discussed in Ch. 364.

Carotid Sinus Hypersensitivity. Carotid sinus hypersensitivity resulting in bradycardia or temporary asystole may also present with Type II dizziness. The dizziness occurs abruptly and disappears rapidly, lasting no more than 15 seconds. The diagnosis is established by reproduction of symptoms with cautious carotid massage.

Vasovagal Syncope. Vasovagal syncope causes confusion with other forms of dizziness when the patient experiences faintness rather than actual loss of consciousness. The tendency to occur in young adults, the relation to precipitating emotional factors, the appearance of pallor at the onset, and the short duration are characteristic.

Cough, Micturition Syncope. Some patients experience faintness upon coughing or, with males, upon micturating while standing. The exact temporal relationship of faintness (or loss of consciousness) to these acts is diagnostic; the reproduction of symptoms by a potentiated Valsalva maneuver confirms the mechanism.

SEIZURE DISORDERS. Patients with temporal lobe seizures may describe feelings of "remoteness," "unreality," or, rarely, vertigo. When these events precede a typical psychomotor or generalized seizure, the cause is clearly *epileptic dizziness*. When the dizziness occurs as an isolated seizure phenomenon, it presents a diagnostic problem. Such patients *rarely* complain primarily of dizziness, however, because the epileptic phenomena dominate the picture.

Very rarely labyrinthine-induced vertigo may trigger "vestibulogenic epilepsy," a form of reflex seizure akin to reading epilepsy. If caloric testing is carried out while an electroencephalogram is taken, the observation of induced seizure activity establishes the diagnosis.

The reader is cautioned against diagnosing seizure disorders in patients whose dizziness is accompanied by mild abnormalities on electroencephalography without the other criteria mentioned.

Dysequilibrium: Impaired Balance

APRAXIA OF GAIT. This is a little-recognized but common disorder of the elderly. The patient walks with a broad-based gait, taking short steps and placing his feet flat on the ground, suggesting a person walking on ice. A tendency to retropulsion increases the danger of falling. On examination, motor power, coordination, and sensation are normal in the legs, although the gait is impaired and hopping on one foot is impossible. The finding of "frontal lobe" deficits, including dementia and grasp and suck reflexes, is confirmatory. Most cases of gait apraxia result from a degenerative process similar to Alzheimer's disease. Other causes include such conditions as subdural hematomas, tumors, normal pressure hydrocephalus, or a lacunar state.

When a specific disorder (e.g., a subdural hematoma) is found, treatment is directed appropriately. In the more common degenerative conditions treatment must be symptomatic. In some patients improvement may result from small doses of L-dopa (1.5 to 3.0 grams per day in divided doses). Mild stimulants (methylphenidate), balancing exercises, and a cane are of benefit, and patients should be encouraged to walk some distance *every day* to avoid total dependence.

PARKINSONISM. Patients with parkinsonism and a balance disturbance often complain of dysequilibrium. When tremor is minimal and impaired balance is prominent, it is difficult to distinguish between parkinsonism and gait apraxia. These patients often have a pronounced increase in axial tone, as well as frontal lobe signs and dementia.

CEREBELLAR LESIONS. Impairment of balance without other cerebellar signs may be seen in certain cerebellar lesions such as alcoholic cerebellar degeneration or tumors of the vermis. In addition some patients may develop "malignant" positional vertigo. Since a staggering gait and nystagmus are seen in peripheral vestibular disorders, the clinical distinction presents difficulties. Neurodiagnostic studies (radioisotope scan, computerized axial tomography, angiography) may be required to establish the diagnosis.

ASTASIA-ABASIA. Astasia-abasia is impairment of stance and gait on a psychogenic basis. In some patients the gait is quite bizarre, but in others it may resemble apraxia. The distinction depends on the absence of other frontal lobe signs and on the ability of the patient to walk *normally* under some circumstances, such as only indoors. Other evidence of a phobic or conversion reaction is often present.

Lightheadedness

Vague "lightheadedness" accounts for over 50 per cent of patients' complaints, and includes the largest spectrum of disorders.

Inevitably, some patients provide a *poor description of other types of dizziness* which more introspective or articulate patients would recognize as vertigo, faintness, or dysequilibrium. In addition, *fractional forms of other types of dizziness* are often described as "lightheadedness" even by observant patients. Almost half the patients who initially experience vertigo later complain of lightheadedness as their symptoms subside. The dizziness simulation battery helps to *identify* a sensation which the patient cannot easily *describe* verbally.

HYPERVENTILATION. This is the second most common cause of dizziness after vestibular disorders, and the most common under the age of 40. The disorder is discussed in detail in Ch. 265. In the acute form, young anxious patients present with brief episodes of shortness of breath, lightheadedness, paresthesias in the fingers and around the mouth, and feelings of panic. More difficult to identify is chronic hyperventilation, seen in patients who periodically sigh deeply.

The mechanism of hyperventilation-induced dizziness is presumed to be hypocapnia with secondary cerebral arterial contriction and diminished cerebral blood flow. Treatment of acute attacks with diazepam, 5 to 10 mg intramuscularly, is often effective. Rebreathing into a paper bag may abort the attack.

MULTISENSORY DIZZINESS. When several sensory modalities are impaired, perception of the environment becomes inadequate to maintain orientation, and the patient experiences dizziness when attempting to walk. The most common combinations of sensory impairment are peripheral neuropathy (with diminished touch, pressure, and proprioceptive sensation), visual loss from cataracts, and cervical spondylosis (with distortion of proprioception from cervical joints). Impaired vestibular and auditory function often add to the sensory disorientation. The aged and diabetic are especially prone to this condition. Patients with multisensory dizziness adopt a broad-based tentative gait, which may superficially resemble apraxia of gait, but the "frontal lobe" features are absent. Examination reveals the underlying neurosensory deficit — peripheral neuropathy, visual impairment, cervical arthritis, and hearing loss. Caloric testing may provide evidence of additional sensory impairment. When all five sensory modalities are severely impaired, patients may be unable to walk without assistance.

An important example of this condition is seen in the post-cataract-extraction patient who complains of disabling dizziness despite perfect restoration of visual acuity. Dizziness results from the distortion produced by the corrective lenses used after surgery. Patients who have no other sensory deficits are able to compensate for the visual distortions, but those with peripheral neuropathy cannot. Contact lenses eliminate these distortions, but unfortunately many elderly patients cannot manage them. Surgical replacement of opaque lenses wtih inert plastic implants promises to avoid this problem in suitable patients.

Treatment of multisensory dizziness includes balancing exercises and use of a foam rubber collar to eliminate extraneous head motion. A light cane should be used for balance. Methylphenidate (Ritalin) improves the speed of the patient's response to his perceived environment.

PSYCHIATRIC DISORDERS. In addition to patients with astasia-abasia or hyperventilation, some patients experience subjective dizziness on the basis of purely psychiatric disease. Some indicate that their dizziness consists of "difficulty concentrating"; others experience panic states when in crowded places; whereas some frankly psychotic patients describe the bizarre confusion of their perceived environments as "dizziness" for lack of a more explicit term.

In these patients, the diagnosis hinges on elimination of other causes of dizziness combined with evidence of significant psychiatric disease on interview or psychometric testing. It is often useful to demonstrate to such patients the negative findings on extensive tests for organic causes of dizziness, and to assure them that no cause has been overlooked.

Anxious patients complaining of lightheadedness may also manifest somatic symptoms, including tachycardia, palpitations, flushing, and tremulousness. In some cases the symptoms can be reproduced by the intravenous infusion of isoproterenol at a low rate (1 to 3 μg per minute), and have been attributed to "beta-adrenergic hyperactivity." Although the pathophysiology is obscure, such patients may derive benefit from treatment with propranolol hydrochloride, 10 to 40 mg four times daily.

Drachman, D. A.: Episodic vertigo. In Conn, H. (ed.): Current Therapy 1974. Philadelphia, W. B. Saunders Company, 1974, p. 684.

Drachman, D. A., and Hart, C. W.: An approach to the dizzy patient. Neurology, 22:323, 1972.

Fisher, C. M.: Vertigo in cerebrovascular disease. Arch. Otolaryngol. 85:529, 1967.

Harrison, M. S., and Ozsahinoglu, C.: Positional vertigo. Arch. Otolaryngol., 101:675, 1975.

Hart, C. W.: The evaluation of vestibular function in health and disease. In Otolaryngology. Vol. 1, Chap. 10. Hagerstown, Md., Harper & Row, 1972.

Naunton, R. F. (ed.): The Vestibular System. New York, Academic Press, 1975.

264. SYNCOPE

Albert Heyman

DEFINITION. Syncope is the cutting off or transient loss of consciousness. Although the term is usually applied to unconsciousness caused by a temporary decrease in cerebral blood flow, in this discussion a broader definition is employed that includes the brief disturbances in consciousness caused by changes in the chemical composition of the blood as in hyperventilation or hypoglycemia. Syncope has been found to occur in as many as 25 to 30 per cent of young, healthy adult males. It should be carefully differentiated from such disorders as epilepsy, vertigo, cataplexy, and strokes, all of which may produce transient disturbances in consciousness, generalized weakness, or inability to stand erect. The loss of consciousness in syncope may not be complete, but may consist of varying degrees of impaired sensorium with transient blurring of vision, weakness, and loss of postural tone. Such attacks may be described by the patient as dizziness, faintness, lightheadedness, or a "drunk feeling." These partial manifestations have the rapid onset, brief duration, and complete recovery characteristic of the fully developed faint.

PATHOGENESIS. Syncope is most frequently caused by a reduction in cerebral blood flow below a critical level and is usually associated with a sharp fall in blood pressure. This, in turn, is the result of either a loss of peripheral resistance, as seen in vasodepressor faint and in orthostatic hypotension, or a decrease in cardiac output, as in Adams-Stokes attacks. In many patients, however, loss of consciousness is not caused by reduction of blood pressure but by a decrease in such essential blood components as glucose, carbon dioxide, or oxygen. In other instances, as in micturition syncope and cough syncope, the faint seems to result from cerebral ischemia caused by extracardiac disturbances.

There are several features common to almost all types of syncope. Electroencephalographic changes usually appear, and consist of high voltage, 2- to 4-cycle per second slow waves that promptly return to normal after consciousness is regained. Brief convulsive movements, such as tonic or clonic contractions of the arms or turning of the head, can occur in all types of fainting, depending on the degree and duration of the cerebral ischemia. Fully developed seizures with tongue biting and urinary incontinence, however, are unusual. Recovery is usually hastened in the recumbent posture, which helps restore the normal cerebral circulation. The critical level of cerebral blood flow necessary to maintain consciousness has been estimated to be about 30 ml per 100 grams of brain per minute (normal value is 50 to 55 ml). The duration of asystole or the degree of hypotension necessary to produce critical levels of cerebral ischemia varies, depending upon the posture of the patient, the ability of the cerebral vessels to dilate, and other factors. In normal subjects in the erect posture, a mean arterial blood pressure as low as 20 to 30 mm of mercury or an asystole of four or five seconds' duration can produce syncope. In the recumbent position, longer periods of asystole may occur before loss of consciousness develops.

CLINICAL MANIFESTATIONS. Orthostatic Hypotension. Chronic orthostatic hypotension is a disorder of the autonomic nervous system in which syncope occurs when the patient assumes the upright posture. The condition is sometimes seen in diabetic neuropathy and in tabes dorsalis, but in many patients the site of the neurologic lesion is unknown. These people have an abnormality in the baroreceptor reflexes that ordinarily compensates for the pooling of blood in the lower extremities and viscera. When an attempt is made to stand upright, there is an inadequate degree of reflex arteriolar constriction, with a subsequent reduction in venous return. This is associated with an immediate and sharp fall in arterial blood pressure, followed by syncope. The pulse rate remains unchanged during the episode, and there are none of the usual prodromal symptoms of pallor, sweating, and nausea seen in vasodepressor faint. Orthostatic hypotension has also been associated with a Parkinson-like disorder sometimes referred to as the Shy-Drager syndrome (see Ch. 278.6).

A new syndrome of orthostatic hypotension known as hyperbradykininism has been reported, in which standing produces a fall in systolic blood pressure, an increase in diastolic pressure and heart rate, and purplish discoloration and ecchymoses over the legs. The disorder is characterized by high plasma levels of bradykinin, which may account for dilatation of the cutaneous venules and capillaries in the legs and reduction in venous return.

Failure of postural adaptation may appear after surgical sympathectomy for hypertension or the administration of vasodilating agents and antihypertensive drugs, especially the sodium-depleting diuretics and ganglionic blocking agents. Iatrogenic forms of syncope have also been noted in patients treated with tranquilizing agents such as phenothiazine derivatives or with L-dopa for Parkinson's disease. Commonly prescribed medications such as digitalis and quinidine may cause cardiac conduction disturbances resulting in arrhythmia and syncope. Patients recovering from chronic wasting illnesses associated with prolonged bed rest may experience syncope when they attempt to assume the upright position. Shorter periods of bed rest, particularly when associated with dehydration or electrolyte deficits, may also be associated with orthostatic hypotension.

Vasodepressor Syncope (the Common Faint). Vasodepressor syncope is by far the most frequent cause of transient loss of consciousness. The condition is characterized by a fall in blood pressure associated with the development of a variety of autonomic manifestations. In the early presyncopal period, there may be pallor, nausea, and sweating; in later stages pupillary dilatation, yawning, hyperpnea, and bradycardia appear. When the mean arterial pressure falls below critical levels, loss of consciousness and characteristic electroencephalographic changes occur. Bradycardia is often severe at the onset of unconsciousness, and pulse rates of 50 to 60 per minute may be observed even after recovery. The duration of syncope is brief, ranging from a few seconds to several minutes. In the postsyncopal period the patient may complain of headaches, weakness, nervousness, and slight confusion. Vasodepressor faint is most often evoked by sudden emotional stress associated with fear, anxiety, or pain. Hypodermic injections, trauma, minor surgery, and the sight of or withdrawal of blood are common precipitating events. Attacks usually occur in the standing or upright posture, and consciousness returns quickly once the patient is recumbent.

The initial event in this complex vascular and neurogenic reaction is dilatation of the vascular bed throughout the body, particularly in peripheral muscles. Vasodilatation in the limb muscles is a normal response to emotional stimuli, and is thought to represent preparation for "fight or flight." The absence of immediate muscle activity, however, and the fall in peripheral resistance are not compensated for by an increase in cardiac output, and as a result there is a reduction in cerebral blood flow.

Adams-Stokes Syndrome. In the early nineteenth century Morgagni, Adams, and Stokes separately observed and described fainting associated with a persistently slow pulse in the range of 40 per minute. Patients with this syndrome usually have a disordered atrioventricular conduction system. Syncope also occurs in patients with bilateral bundle branch disease, a condition which may precede complete heart block. The decision to insert a permanent pacemaker in such cases should be made only in patients with documented heart block or those with a clear-cut history of cardiac syncope. A rare form of syncope caused by ventricular fibrillation has been reported in children with hereditary prolonged Q-T intervals in the electrocardiogram, sometimes accompanied by congenital deaf mutism. Ventricular dysrhythmia and syncope caused by prolongation of Q-T intervals also has been described following drug intoxication and electrolyte imbalance. The clinical picture of syncope caused by cardiac arrhythmias is often characteristic. Loss of consciousness is abrupt; prodromal signs are not usually present. On regaining consciousness, the patient usually shows little confusion or postsyncopal residua. The attacks may occur several times a day and have no relation to posture or activity. Only a brief period of asystole of four or five seconds' duration will produce loss of consciousness in the erect position, but longer periods of asystole are not uncommon. In such instances, neurologic manifestations such as convulsive movements, pupillary dilatation, and prolonged confusion may be observed. Occasionally sudden death results from cardiac standstill. Syncope occurring for the first time in elderly patients should be suspected as being caused by heart block. Since these patients often have sinus rhythm with normal heart rate when seen by the physician, continuous tape-recorded electrocardiographic monitoring is often needed for diagnosis. Such monitoring can be carried out during the patient's routine activities; and by correlating the patient's symptoms with the appearance of an arrhythmia, a firm basis can be established for definitive treatment such as implantation of an intracardiac pacemaker.

Reflex Cardiac Standstill. Syncopal attacks may result from vagal reflex–induced cardiac standstill in persons without heart disease. A few authenticated cases of swallowing or deglutition syncope have been reported. Most such patients have been found to have diverticula or other disorders of the esophagus or underlying cardiac disease. Experimental distention of the esophagus with balloons can sometimes induce complete atrioventricular block and syncope. The alterations in consciousness and the electrocardiographic changes disappear when the pressure within the esophagus is relieved or after administration of atropine. The syncopal episode occasionally seen after drinking ice cold fizzy fluids, during digital prostatic examination (so-called prostatic prostration), or during thoracentesis or bronchoscopic examination may also be due to such reflex vagal mechanisms. Syncope caused by cardiac arrest has been observed in patients with paroxysmal pain in the throat due to glossopharyngeal neuralgia.

Carotid Sinus Syncope. In few patients is this the mechanism of actual syncope. Many persons, particularly those more than 60 years of age, show reflex slowing of the heart and fall of blood pressure during massage of one or both carotid sinuses. Such responses are frequent in patients with cardiac disorders, hypertension, or diseases of the carotid vessels such as atherosclerotic thrombosis or stenosis. The most common response to carotid sinus massage is either sinus bradycardia or sinoatrial block, both of which may be abolished by administration of atropine. Much less frequently, there may be a pure vasodepressor response without slowing of the heart. In a third but rare type of carotid response, fainting may appear in a few seconds without significant changes in either blood pressure or pulse; such instances probably occur only with vigorous pressure and when the opposite carotid is already thrombosed. Carotid sinus syncope is not accompanied by the prodromal symptoms seen in the common faint. It is more frequent in men, and usually occurs in the erect posture. It sometimes follows sudden head turning or pressure of a tight collar.

Very few of the patients who exhibit bradycardia or a reduction in blood pressure on carotid massage experience loss of consciousness. In eliciting carotid sinus responses, care should be taken to avoid obstructing blood flow to the brain by compression of the carotid vessels. Cerebral infarction and even death have been reported after carotid compression and massage. Massage of both carotid sinuses simultaneously may be hazardous. An increasing number of reports describe the use of a permanent demand pacemaker for relief of carotid sinus syncope. The rarity with which true syncope occurs with carotid sinus hypersensitivity, however, requires that such radical treatment be carefully evaluated.

Organic Heart Disease. Patients with myocardial infarction or valvular lesions may also have transient periods of unconsciousness. The mechanism of syncope in these disorders is not altogether clear, but may be related to a reduction in cardiac output with inadequate cerebral blood flow. In acute myocardial infarction, fainting probably results from decrease in stroke volume owing to a weakened myocardium. Transient arrhythmias, such as ventricular tachycardia, fibrillation, or heart block, may contribute to the syncopal reaction. Transient loss of consciousness may occur during attacks of angina pectoris, and is probably caused by ventricular fibrillation or various types of heart block associated with temporary periods of myocardial ischemia. Syncope also appears during paroxysmal tachycardia even in the absence of structural heart disease. In such cases the loss of consciousness usually occurs at the onset or at the end of the attack, at which time there may be a brief period of cardiac standstill.

Patients with aortic valvular or subvalvular stenosis often have syncope associated with physical exertion (effort syncope). The loss of consciousness in the early phases of such syncopal episodes may be due to shunting of blood to the peripheral muscles, but the later phases have been shown to be associated with transient ventricular asystole, tachycardia, or fibrillation, presumably caused by diminished coronary arterial blood flow. Sudden death may occur during these attacks. Effort syncope is also seen in patients with congenital heart disease such as patent ductus arteriosus or tetralogy of Fallot, as well as in those with pulmonary hypertension. Patients with atrial myxoma, on the right or left side, although rare, often present with recurrent syncope. In such cases, a pedunculated tumor intermittently obstructs the mitral or tricuspid valves.

Cough Syncope. Cough syncope usually follows a paroxysm of explosive and vigorous coughing. It is commonly observed in men but rarely in women. In adults, the condition is often seen in stocky, barrel-chested men with chronic lung disease or bronchitis; in children, it may occur during severe *pertussis*. The syncope is brief and there are no residua. The condition may recur in the recumbent patient or following hearty laughter. The loss of consciousness has been attributed to an increase in the intrathoracic and intra-abdominal pressure caused by vigorous coughing. This, in turn, is thought to produce a sudden sharp elevation in cerebrospinal fluid pressure, thereby "squeezing" blood from the intracranial and cerebral vessels. Other theories maintain that the condition is due to a Valsalva effect with reduction in cardiac output or to cerebral "concussive effect" caused by rapid rise in the cerebrospinal fluid pressure. There is clinical evidence to suggest that the presence of an intracerebral lesion such as brain tumor or stenosis of a major cerebral artery may produce increased susceptibility to syncope after paroxysms of cough. Such patients may have focal neurologic symptoms such as paresthesias or clonic movements of one limb prior to loss of consciousness. Therapy consists of the relief of the force, frequency, and duration of the cough by clearing of the bronchial secretions and suppression of cough reflex. In refractory cases, tracheostomy may be beneficial by reducing intrathoracic pressure during the paroxysms of cough.

Micturition Syncope. This form of syncope is most often seen during or immediately after micturition in men who rise in the middle of the night to urinate. The loss of consciousness is brief and there is no postsyncopal confusion or weakness. Many such people give a history of drinking large quantities of beer before retiring, and considerable bladder deflation may take place during micturition. A similar fainting may be observed after drainage of a distended bladder in urinary retention or after removal of a large quantity of ascitic fluid by abdominal paracentesis. It has been suggested that the loss of consciousness may be due to a reflex vasodilatation of the peripheral vascular system, a situation thought to be the converse of the paroxysmal hypertension seen in paraplegics during bladder distention. It is not likely to be due to a Valsalva maneuver during micturition but may be related to peripheral vasodilation associated with a warm bed and perhaps the recent consumption of alcohol.

Hysterical Fainting. Hysterical fainting is seen almost entirely in young women with emotional illness. It differs from the vasodepressor faint and the hyperventilation syndrome in that the patient is relatively free of anxiety and shows little concern regarding the fainting episodes. The attack usually occurs in the presence of others. The patient generally slumps to the floor gracefully, sometimes dramatically, without injury or awkwardness. It thus resembles the mid-Victorian drawing room swoon. A few decades ago, hysterical fainting often occurred in groups of young women during mass excitement, particularly that caused by the presence of screen or television idols. Although excited behavior is now often observed among young women attending "rock" concerts, swooning is seldom seen.

During the attack the patient may be motionless or may show bizarre resisting movements. The attack may last from several minutes to as long as an hour or more, with fluctuations of responsiveness. There are no abnormalities in pulse, blood pressure, or skin color. The electroencephalogram is normal during the attack, indicating that there may be no actual loss of consciousness. The diagnosis can usually be made without difficulty on the basis of the setting of the episode, the patient's underlying emotional disturbance, and the absence of physical abnormalities.

Cerebral Arterial Occlusive Disease. Patients with generalized atherosclerosis may have frequent episodes of loss of consciousness over a period of days or weeks.

In most instances the attack is accompanied by signs of focal neurologic deficits such as motor weakness, sensory loss, or cranial nerve disorders. In such cases the diagnosis of transient focal ischemia can be made without difficulty. Syncopal episodes in older persons, however, are often not associated with focal neurologic symptoms but consist only of transient giddiness and visual blurring and occur particularly on arising from bed in the morning or standing upright after stooping or bending over. Such patients with "blind staggers" frequently have evidence of hypertension, cardiac disease, or obstructive lesions in the extracranial cerebral vessels, but these conditions may not be responsible for their disturbing postural symptoms. It appears that the reflexes that normally compensate for sudden changes in posture are impaired in these individuals. Attempts to relieve such symptoms by surgical correction of extracranial arterial occlusive disease or by administration of various medications are often unsuccessful.

Hypoglycemia. Low levels of blood sugar often produce symptoms of weakness, trembling, sweating, tachycardia, hunger sensation, and confused behavior. Syncope is not a common occurrence, but prolonged hypoglycemia may result in seizures, coma, and serious brain damage. The majority of patients with these symptoms have anxiety reaction rather than hypoglycemia. The diagnosis of hypoglycemia must therefore be based on documented low levels of blood sugar at the time of the clinical manifestations which, in turn, can be relieved by ingestion of food or sugar. It is also important that the type of hypoglycemia be established. Reactive hypoglycemia is the most common type and may appear in thin, emotionally tense persons a few hours after ingestion of a high carbohydrate meal. It sometimes follows extensive gastric resection in association with the dumping syndrome and occurs in some people with mild diabetes. Hypoglycemia may also be due to islet cell adenoma of the pancreas. In this condition, nervousness, weakness, trembling, and sometimes convulsions occur after fasting and exercise. The fasting morning blood sugar level may be low, in contrast to that of patients with reactive hypoglycemia, in whom this determination is usually normal. Other conditions such as pituitary insufficiency, Addison's disease, hepatic failure, and large sarcomas may also produce hypoglycemia.

DIAGNOSIS. The diagnosis of syncope depends almost entirely upon a careful history of the attack and the setting in which it occurs. Differentiation of syncope from an akinetic epileptic seizure, such as petit mal or psychomotor attack, may be difficult. Careful evaluation of the electroencephalographic findings, the onset and duration of the attack, and the postsyncopal manifestations can usually distinguish these conditions. These factors are also helpful in differentiating the various types of syncope. In vasodepressor faint, the patient usually has prodromal signs of autonomic hyperactivity such as pallor, sweating, salivation, and bradycardia. In cardiac arrest, orthostatic hypotension, and carotid sinus syncope, loss of consciousness occurs abruptly, and prodromal symptoms are not usually present. Postsyncopal confusion, headache, and weakness often follow vasodepressor faint and the hyperventilation syndrome. In chronic orthostatic hypotension and Adams-Stokes attacks, recovery of consciousness is rapid and complete without postsyncopal symptoms.

Most types of fainting occur in the erect or upright position, but in cardiac arrest, syncope may appear while the patient is recumbent. The duration of syncope is brief in postural hypotension but prolonged in hyperventilation and hypoglycemia. Most of these differentiating manifestations can be determined by careful history, but specific procedures should be carried out during the physical examination. These consist of voluntary hyperventilation for approximately two minutes, careful massage of the carotid sinuses (preferably with electrocardiographic and electroencephalographic monitoring), auscultation for murmurs over the cervical vessels and base of the heart to exclude possible obstruction of blood flow through the extracranial cerebral vessels and aortic valves, and, finally, observations of pulse and blood pressure during change in posture from recumbency to erect position. If the blood pressure falls appreciably but the heart rate fails to accelerate, dysfunction of the autonomic nervous system should be suspected. If the patient with syncope has orthostatic hypotension with an appropriate rise in heart rate, hypovolemia caused by salt and water depletion or diuretic therapy may be present. An electroencephalogram is indicated whenever convulsive movements develop during the syncopal episode, or when focal neurologic manifestations are noted. In older persons, long strips of the electrocardiogram should be searched for episodes of arrhythmia, and prolonged ambulatory cardiac (Holter) monitoring should also be carried out whenever recurrent syncope is not otherwise explained. A glucose tolerance test should be made if there appears to be a relationship of syncope to meals, prolonged duration of altered consciousness, or recovery following ingestion of carbohydrates.

TREATMENT. Therapy in syncope consists primarily of treatment of the underlying disorder. In all types of fainting, recovery is usually aided by maintaining the patient in a recumbent position with elevation of the lower extremities. Application of cold water to the face and head and inhalation of spirits of ammonia or other pungent aromatics are time-honored and certainly do no harm.

Ad Hoc Committee on Hypoglycemia: Statement on hypoglycemia. Arch. Intern. Med., 131:591, 1973.

Dhingra, R. C., Denes, P., Wu, D., et al.: Syncope in patients with chronic bifascicular block. Ann. Intern. Med., 81:302, 1974.

Noble, R. J.: The patient with syncope. JAMA, 237:1372, 1977.

Shillingford, J. P.: Syncope. Am. J. Cardiol., 26:609, 1970.

Thomas, J. E.: Hyperactive carotid sinus reflex and carotid sinus syncope. Mayo Clin. Proc., 44:127, 1969.

Walter, P. F., Reid, S. D., and Wenger, N. K.: Transient cerebral ischemia due to arrhythmias. Ann. Intern. Med., 72:471, 1970.

Wright, K. E., Jr., and McIntosh, H. D.: Syncope: A review of pathophysiological mechanisms. Prog. Cardiovasc. Dis., 13:580, 1971.

265. HYPERVENTILATION

Albert Heyman

HYPERVENTILATION SYNDROME. The hyperventilation syndrome is one of the most frequent causes of impaired consciousness, usually producing "faintness" and "lightheadedness" without actual syncope. It is almost always a manifestation of acute anxiety. At the onset of an attack, the patient may complain of tightness of the chest and a feeling of suffocation. He may not be aware of overbreathing but usually recalls excessive deep sighing. Later, a sense of unreality develops, accompanied by feelings of apprehension and sometimes panic. Symptoms related to the heart and gastrointestinal tract consist of palpitations or pounding of the heart, precordial oppression, fullness in the throat, and epigastric discomfort. The syndrome may last for as long as a half hour or more and may recur several times a day. Sensations of "numbness" and "coldness" of the hands, feet, and perioral areas often develop. In prolonged attacks, tetany has been noted with the appearance of carpopedal spasm and Chvostek's sign, i.e., unilateral facial spasm following finger tapping of the facial musculature. Some patients develop chest pain.

The pathogenesis of the individual symptoms of this disorder is not altogether clear. With normal subjects, hyperventilation in the recumbent posture for as long as an hour will not produce loss of consciousness. They may, however, have sensations of decreased awareness, lightheadedness, and blurring of vision, but do not have the trembling, sweating, palpitations, or precordial distress frequently seen in patients with spontaneous overventilation. The serum calcium level remains normal, but there is often a decrease in serum phosphate. Within 15 minutes after onset of hyperventilation in voluntary subjects, arterial P_{CO_2} falls to levels of 20 to 30 mm Hg, where it may remain with only an occasional sighing respiration. The hypocapnia caused by overventilation results in cerebral vasoconstriction, which decreases oxygen delivery to the brain. Studies in laboratory animals have shown that prolonged hyperventilation produces an increase in lactic acid in the cerebrospinal fluid and brain due probably to ischemic cerebral hypoxia. A slight fall in blood pressure also occurs during hyperventilation caused by muscular vasodilatation. These factors alone are usually insufficient to produce syncope, and the occasional loss of consciousness with this syndrome is probably due to vasodepressor mechanisms as in the common faint.

The hyperventilation syndrome is often precipitated by acute emotional stress and is most common in nervous, anxious women who have other functional disturbances related to tension. The syndrome can often be reproduced by having the patient hyperventilate voluntarily for two or three minutes. Although the patient is often reassured by the fact that he can control the attack somewhat by breath-holding or breathing in a paper bag, therapy directed at the underlying emotional disturbance is usually necessary.

HYPERVENTILATION COMBINED WITH VALSALVA MANEUVER. The physiologic alterations produced by a combination of hyperventilation and increased intrathoracic pressure (secondary to variants of the Valsalva maneuver) account for several unique types of syncope. The "mess trick," a prank often indulged in by schoolboys, consists of sudden manual compression of the chest of the victim after he has been hyperventilating for about a minute. Loss of consciousness may also occur in the "fainting lark," in which the victim is instructed to hyperventilate in the squatting position, stand quickly, and immediately perform the Valsalva maneuver. The loss of consciousness observed in athletes lifting weights ("weightlifter's blackout") is due to similar mechanisms. During competition, these individuals often hyperventilate vigorously and then squat before grasping the weight. Lifting of the weight produces high levels of intrathoracic pressure which reduces venous return and causes decrease in cardiac output, stroke volume, and pulse pressure. These alterations, combined with the peripheral vasodilation caused by squatting and cerebral vasoconstriction caused by hyperventilation, result in a reduction in cerebral blood flow and loss of consciousness. Voluntary syncope has also been observed in muscular teenage boys who can maintain a prolonged Valsalva maneuver by vigorous stretching of the trunk and back muscles. Such instances of "stretch syncope" are often self-induced to provide a curiously satisfying experience.

Klein, L. J., Saltzman, H., and Heyman, A.: Syncope induced by the Valsalva maneuver: A study of the effects of arterial blood gas tensions, glucose concentration and blood pressure. Am. J. Med., 37:263, 1964.
Saltzman, H. A., Heyman, A., and Sieker, H. O.: Correlations of clinical and physiologic manifestations of sustained hyperventilation. N. Engl. J. Med., 268:1431, 1963.

Section Ten NEUROLOGIC DIAGNOSTIC PROCEDURES

Kathleen M. Foley

266. INTRODUCTION

Neurologic diagnostic tests supplement but do not substitute for a meticulous neurologic history and examination. The yield from diagnostic tests is directly related to the skill of the physician who must order the appropriate test suggested by the neurologic history and examination, and who must interpret the test based on the clinical findings.

The most valuable and commonly used of the neurologic diagnostic tests are described in the following chapters. Special attention is directed at those procedures which the general physician is likely to use in evaluating a patient with neurologic symptoms. These include the lumbar puncture, skull and spine x-rays, the electroencephalogram (EEG), the radionuclide brain scan, and computerized tomography (CT or CAT scan). It is imperative for the physician to familiarize himself with the indications and limitations of these studies to ensure appropriate interpretation. There is also a series of more selective neurodiagnostic procedures (i.e., arteriography, pneumoencephalography, myelography, cisternography, electromyography) which the physician may find useful and which are usually performed after consultation with a neurologist or neurosurgeon. In this presentation these procedures are considered in less detail. Many of the procedures are also discussed elsewhere in this text in the context of neurologic illnesses, and, when applicable, reference will be made to those chapters.

Certain general principles should govern the physician in his choice of any neurologic diagnostic procedure: (1) *No procedure should be considered routine.* The physician should order only those tests appropriate to answer specific questions posed by the neurologic history and examination. (2) *The procedure which yields the most information with the least risk to the patient should be performed first.* For example, if a brain tumor is suspected, computerized tomography is superior to either plain x-rays or radionuclide brain scans because it is much more informative, and is superior to arteriography and pneumoencephalography because it is much less of a risk and is less costly. (3) *The responsible physician should discuss the diagnostic problem with the specialist performing the procedure before it is done* to assure that the maximal information related to the patient's problem will be procured. The responsible physician should also review the completed study with the specialist to ensure an interpretation based on the clinical findings. (4) *The patient should be properly instructed in the nature of the procedure and in its potential risks, complications, and benefits.* Since patient cooperation is essential in these studies, adequate sedation should be employed when necessary.

267. COMPUTERIZED TRANSAXIAL TOMOGRAPHY
(CT Scan, CAT)

Computerized tomography has had a profound impact on the diagnostic evaluation of the patient with neurologic symptoms. It provides a simple, rapid x-ray procedure, applicable on an ambulatory basis, with diagnostic accuracy comparable to that of arteriography and pneumoencephalography. The procedure is unique in that it provides a direct two-dimensional view of the head with adequate visualization of bone, brain parenchyma, and cerebrospinal fluid spaces. The method computes differences in x-ray density of the many cranial and intracranial structures and draws a tomographic picture of the brain (usually 0.8 to 1.3 cm in thickness) such that the calvarium appears white, whereas less dense brain tissue is depicted in varying shades of gray. Cortical gray matter is more dense than central gray or white matter, and cerebrospinal fluid has an unusually low density and appears black against the brain parenchyma, allowing for delineation of cerebral and cerebellar sulci and fissures. Contrast enhancement by the intravenous administration of an iodinated x-ray contrast agent increases the absorption coefficient (density) of some normal and a number of abnormal intracranial structures, allowing for identification of lesions not seen on the unenhanced scan. The radiation exposure is approximately equal to that for a skull series (below 2 rads) and is well below the exposure of either the arteriogram or pneumoencephalogram.

The CT scan is the initial diagnostic procedure to assess and localize intracranial pathology. As an emergency procedure, it is particularly valuable in patients with head trauma to identify abnormal collections of blood, shifts in the ventricular system, or parenchymal injury, including cerebral edema and infarction. In the comatose patient with focal neurologic signs, it allows for rapid localization of a mass lesion and gives information as to its cause with characteristic appearances for hematoma, tumor, infarction, and abscess. In the patient with transient ischemic attacks and focal neurologic signs, it allows one to differentiate between infarction and hemorrhage before using anticoagulants. In the patient with metabolic encephalopathy and focal neurologic signs, it is used to exclude a focal cerebral lesion. As an elective procedure, it can be performed on an ambulatory basis to diagnose mass lesions, to evaluate ventricular size, and, in the patient with dementia, to diagnose cerebral atrophy or normal pressure hydrocephalus. Demyelinating disease can also be assessed. It is an important follow-up procedure in patients who have had treatment for intracranial tumors, either radiation therapy or neurosurgical intervention, to assess any remaining tumor or the reappearance of new tumor, as well as in patients who have had shunt procedures to evaluate ventricular size. The usefulness of the CT scan as an elective procedure eliminates the need of hospital admission for diagnostic work-up in numerous patients and facilitates the care of the patient with a neurologic emergency. The limitations include the fact that abnormalities must be greater than 5 mm in diameter to be visualized. There are certain areas, specifically the suprasellar region and the posterior fossa, which are not well visualized and may require other tests. Cerebral vessels are not well visualized, and although aneurysms and vascular malformations have been diagnosed by CT scan, it is not the procedure of choice to assess cerebral vessels and their abnormalities. Subdural hematomas, even of a clinically important size, may not show up well. The only major contraindication to CT scanning is allergy to iodinated contrast materials. In such cases, a no-contrast CT scan in conjunction with a brain scan may provide the necessary information.

NEWER TECHNIQUES. The use of coronal and sagittal slices as well as cisternal enhancement with radiopaque iodinated contrast agents will further increase the applicability of CT scanning by providing increased definition of the brain and cerebrospinal fluid spaces.

268. LUMBAR PUNCTURE

Cerebrospinal fluid (CSF) is sampled through a needle inserted between the lumbar vertebrae into the lumbar subarachnoid space. The procedure is simple and may be performed at the bedside or in the emergency room. Because it is so simple and commonly performed, special attention is required to consider both its indications and the amount of CSF required for complete assessment before starting the procedure. The indications are specific, nonspecific, or therapeutic. Lumbar puncture is the specific procedure to evaluate meningeal infection, subarachnoid bleeding, and meningeal carcinomatosis, and to directly measure intracranial pressure. In multiple sclerosis, the characteristic gamma globulin profile confirms the diagnosis. In the differential diagnosis of brain tumor, spinal cord block, and cerebrovascular disease, the lumbar puncture provides information about changes in the content of the CSF which are neither specific nor diagnostic. Therapeutically, it provides the route of administration for anesthetic agents in spinal anesthesia and for the treatment of central nervous system infection or malignancy by the administration of antimicrobial drugs. The major contraindications include clinical evidence of increased intracranial pressure caused by mass lesions (see Ch. 316) and infection at the lumbar puncture site. Other important contraindications include bleeding diathesis, thrombocytopenia with platelet counts below 30,000, and congenital malformations of the lumbar cord.

PROCEDURE.   Patient cooperation and proper positioning greatly facilitate the procedure. The patient should be placed in the lateral decubitus position with the knees flexed to allow for full extension of the space between the spinous processes. Under sterile conditions, local anesthesia should be administered. A 20-gauge stylet needle is then introduced slowly between the interspaces, most commonly L4-L5 or L3-L4 until it pierces the dura. The bevel should always be directed cephalad in order to pierce the dura in a vertical fashion. If the needle is advanced too far into the subarachnoid space, trauma to the ventrally located epidural venous plexus side will yield bloody fluid. Once the subarachnoid space is entered, a manometer should be attached to the lumbar needle and the opening pressure measured, with the patient as relaxed as possible, knees extended, and neck in a normal position. CSF should then be removed for study, and drugs or anesthetic agents administered. Lumbar puncture may also be performed in the sitting position but does not give reliable CSF pressure measurements. It does, however, allow for collection of CSF. In an unusually difficult situation, the procedure can be done under fluoroscopy to facilitate visualization of the normal bony landmarks. In special instances in which the lumbar route is not possible, CSF may be sampled from the cisterna magna. Although this is considered a routine method in other countries, the procedure should be done under fluoroscopy by a physician experienced in this technique. In patients with basilar meningitis from fungal or metastatic disease, a higher yield of positive cultures or of malignant cells may be found by this approach. The cisterna magna can also be the route of administration of radiopaque substances to outline the posterior fossa and the spinal cord above a spinal block. Once obtained, CSF samples are usually evaluated for cell count, glucose and protein content, and, if infection is suspected, Gram stain. Cell count and Gram stain are the responsibility of the physician performing the lumbar puncture (see Ch. 297). The sugar and protein content, bacterial, viral, and fungal cultures, and serologic and cytologic evaluation are customarily performed in hospital laboratories. More specialized studies to assess cerebrospinal fluid include viral cultures and titers, cryptococcal antigen, protein electrophoresis, and enzyme analysis. The normal values for CSF are found in Ch. 593. *Postspinal tap headache* is the most common complication of lumbar puncture and may be associated with bifrontal or occipital headache, neck stiffness, dizziness, and nausea. It resolves if the patient is placed in the prone or slightly head-down position, but may last up to ten days when the patient assumes the upright position. Although this is distressing for the patient, it does not produce any significant long-term effects. In rare instances transtentorial or cerebellar herniation may follow lumbar puncture, but if care is taken in the selection of patients, this complication should never occur.

269. CONVENTIONAL ROENTGENOGRAPHY

SKULL X-RAYS.   Plain films of the skull identify developmental anomalies (such as basilar impression), in-

tracranial calcifications, fractures of the skull vault, and longstanding increased intracranial pressure. In patients with head trauma, medicolegal considerations mandate skull x-rays unless CT scan is done. In fact, for serious head trauma, the CT scan provides much more direct information about the effects on brain parenchyma. Skull x-rays play a minor role in the evaluation of patients with brain tumors (see Ch. 316) and cerebrovascular disease (see Ch. 293 to 295). Specific radiographic projections are required to answer specific clinical questions. The anteroposterior and lateral views provide the general information about bony configuration and structure. Towne's view best identifies a calcified pineal, the base view shows the jugular foramen and other foramina of the base of skull, the inclined frontal view assesses superior orbital fissures and frontal sinuses, and Stenver's view assesses the mastoid and petrous pyramids.

SPINE X-RAYS.   Spine x-rays are the initial diagnostic procedure in patients with neck or back pain or dysfunction of the spinal cord. The spine films detect congenital anomalies, fracture or collapse of a vertebral body, inflammatory and degenerative diseases of the joint spaces, and spondylosis and spondylolisthesis of the spine. Prior to myelography they are required to assess the status of the lumbar spine. Three radiographic views provide the necessary information. These include the anteroposterior view, which provides information about the width of the spinal canal and integrity of the pedicles; the lateral view, which provides information about the status of the vertebral bodies, the disc spaces, and the size, shape, and alignment of the spinal canal; and the oblique view, which assesses the integrity of the joint and disc spaces, as well as the neural foramina. When necessary, specialized and coned-down views of the specific areas in question should be performed, particularly when one is concerned about areas which are poorly visualized on routine films, such as the C7-T1 region or the sacrum.

Plain radiographs of the skull and spine are limited by the fact that there must be 40 to 60 per cent change in bone density to detect changes on plain films. Alternative procedures include *the bone scan*, which provides a more sensitive method using specific radioisotopes, and which can demonstrate abnormalities three to four months before observable changes in plain x-rays; however, this procedure is nonspecific and cannot differentiate inflammatory diseases of bone from tumor. *Tomography* provides a more specialized radiographic technique to discern bony changes and is particularly useful in assessing areas of bony overlap such as the base of skull.

270. THE RADIONUCLIDE BRAIN SCAN

Radioisotope scans identify alterations of the blood-brain barrier and thus localize areas of intracranial pathology, especially tumor. Following intravenous injection of the radioisotope, most commonly technetium[99] pertechnetate, standard views of the brain are recorded on x-ray film, using a specialized scintillation camera, most commonly the gamma camera. This is a useful screening procedure to assess possible intracerebral mass lesions, infarction, subacute subdural hematomas, and abscess, because it provides a simple minimal-risk ambulatory procedure with a fair diagnostic accuracy. With the availability of the CT scan, however, its usefulness has diminished. At this time, radionuclide scanning is a second line procedure to futher clarify a normal or abnormal CT scan in the patient allergic to the contrast substances. The limitations of the procedure are significant: abnormalities must be 2 cm or greater to be visualized; changes in the skull vault may produce artifacts on the scan; and the diagnostic scope is restricted. Radionuclide scanning is not useful in assessing cerebral atrophy or ventricular enlargement, or in providing rapid diagnostic information in emergencies. Dynamic radionuclide brain scanning, available in some centers, employs a special camera attached to the scintillation camera which begins photographing the brain simultaneously with the injection of radioisotope. Cerebral blood flow, and particularly patency of the venous sinuses, can be estimated rapidly by this relatively low risk technique. In cerebrovascular disease, its diagnostic accuracy is less than that of arteriography. It is the initial procedure of choice to assess occlusion of the venous sinuses.

271. ELECTRO-ENCEPHALOGRAPHY

Electroencephalography (EEG) measures the electrical activity of the cortex, providing information about the functional status of the brain; it is considered in detail in Ch. 315. Because it is a simple and commonly available noninvasive procedure, it is often used by the general physician, but it provides limited diagnostic information except in certain types of epilepsy (petit mal), in patients with confusional states or unusual behavior who may display seizure activity on the EEG without motor or sensory component, and in patients with narcolepsy. The procedure provides nonspecific but, at times, important differential information in patients with metabolic encephalopathy (see Ch. 220). The EEG can help localize supratentorial brain tumors (see Ch. 316), but is not useful in the evaluation of posterior fossa tumors.

SPECIALIZED EEG TECHNIQUES. Specialized EEG techniques, used in some centers, include direct measurement of cortical activity with superficial and deep electrodes during ablative neurosurgical procedures for intractable epilepsy. Other techniques include computer analogues to assess sensory evoked responses of the visual, auditory, and sensory cortex in the evaluation of central visual and hearing loss, particularly in infants and children.

272. SELECTED NEURODIAGNOSTIC PROCEDURES

CEREBRAL ARTERIOGRAPHY. Cerebral arteriograms are performed by direct catheterization of the carotid artery in the neck or by catheterization of either the brachial or femoral artery and selective injection of the aortic arch and carotid and vertebral arteries, using a radiopaque contrast agent. Arteriography is the diagnostic procedure for assessing cervical or cerebrovascular occlusion, arteriosclerotic plaques, vasculitis, aneurysms, and other vascular malformations. Although it was formerly used as a diagnostic study in evaluating focal neurologic symptoms suggestive of brain tumor, the CT scan has replaced the arteriogram as the initial procedure.

PNEUMOENCEPHALOGRAPHY. This technique allows for visualization of the cerebrospinal fluid–filled ventricles, cisterns, and subarachnoid pathways, using air as the contrast agent. Special views and tomography are employed and selected by the radiologist during the examination. It is the specific diagnostic tool to assess the patency of the subarachnoid pathways, such as in patients with negative CT scans whose focal neurologic symptoms suggest pathology involving the parasellar area, the deep midline structures, or the posterior fossa. The major contraindications are those for lumbar puncture. The complications include transient fever, headache, and meningeal irritation, which usually clear within three to five days. In contrast to CT scans, this procedure is distressing for the patient, and in patients with normal pressure hydrocephalus it may produce transient worsening in their neurologic symptoms and signs.

MYELOGRAPHY. Myelography assesses abnormalities of the spinal cord, nerve roots, and meninges and is performed by the injection of a radiopaque contrast agent into the subarachnoid space, most commonly by the lumbar route. Although limited myelography is performed in some institutions, a full myelogram should be performed on every patient having the procedure. If a spinal block is suspected, a small amount of contrast is initially injected to assess the patency of the subarachnoid spaces. In cases of block, cisternal injection of contrast should also be performed to delineate the upper borders of the block and to assess the patency of the subarachnoid spaces above the block. This is particularly important prior to radiation treatment of patients with extradural metastatic disease and spinal cord compression who may have multiple blocks (see Ch. 332).

RADIOISOTOPE CISTERNOGRAPHY. Radioisotope cisternography involves the administration of a radioisotope into the subarachnoid space to study the dynamics of cerebrospinal fluid flow. Several radioisotope materials are currently used, and the basic principles of their dispersion involve both bulk flow and diffusion. The specific indications include the evaluation of patients with communicating hydrocephalus and cerebrospinal leaks, specifically CSF rhinorrhea.

ELECTROMYOGRAPHY. Electromyography is the investigative procedure which uses electrical activity of nerve and muscle to assess and localize disease involving the motor unit. Specifically, it provides the methods to differentiate lesions involving spinal motor neurons, roots, plexuses, entire nerves, branches of nerve, or muscle fibers. Its applicability is discussed in Ch. 338.

ECHOENCEPHALOGRAPHY. Echoencephalography uses pulses of ultrasound to detect shifts or alterations of structures within the cranial cavity, using the third ventricle as the reliable midline position. Although it is a simple, widely available procedure, it is nonspecific, and the patient requires further studies for a definitive diagnosis.

OTHER DIAGNOSTIC TESTS. The procedures outlined above, in conjunction with the neurologic history and examination, provide valuable information about the nature, site, and most likely pathologic process, but direct visualization of brain, nerve, and muscle provides the final diagnosis. *Brain biopsy* provides available tissue for neuropathologic evaluation and currently can be performed with minimal risk and discomfort to the patient. The specific indications are as follows: when the differential diagnosis is in question, e.g., benign vs. malignant disease; when knowledge of the pa-

thology will change or direct the therapy, e.g., brain abscess vs. tumor, toxoplasmosis encephalitis vs. herpes encephalitis; or when the pathology alone can provide the diagnosis and is necessary for genetic counseling, e.g., lipid storage diseases. *Muscle biopsy* is considered in Ch. 338.

Cohen, H. L., and Brumlik, J.: Manual of Electroneuromyography. New York, Harper & Row, 1976.

Gonzalez, C. F., Grossman, C. B., and Palacios, E.: Computed Brain and Orbital Tomography. New York, John Wiley & Sons, 1976.

Newton, T. H., and Potts, D. G. (eds.): Radiology of The Skull and Brain. St. Louis, C. V. Mosby Co., 1974.

Taveras, J. M., and Wood, E. H.: Diagnostic Neuroradiology. Baltimore, Williams & Wilkins Co., 1964.

Section Eleven   THE EXTRAPYRAMIDAL DISORDERS

273.   INTRODUCTION
Melvin D. Yahr

The basal ganglia or extrapyramidal diseases comprise a complex group of clinical disorders characterized by abnormal involuntary movements (dyskinesias), alterations in muscle tone, and disturbances in bodily posture. The major clinical states include parkinsonism, chorea, athetosis, dystonia, and hemiballism. These terms not only denote particular disease entities, but in a descriptive sense refer to a constellation of symptoms that may occur in a variety of central nervous system disorders involving the basal ganglia and/or their connections. They are recognizable, one from the other, by the degree, form, and combination of the triad of symptoms noted above and are distinguishable as disease entities by the age and mode of onset, the identification of particular etiologic and genetic factors, and the rate and manner of progression of symptoms.

The conventional anatomic concept of the basal ganglia as a group of nuclear masses in the forebrain has not proved adequate in explaining the clinical manifestations or what is known about the physiologic or pathologic aspects of these conditions. In consequence, neurologists have devised a functional anatomic approach that includes not only the basal ganglia nuclei, but also related structures in the brainstem as well as a neural network of connections with other parts of the nervous system. The structures of importance in this system are the caudate nucleus and putamen, which, because of their similarities in appearance, cellular structure, and phylogenetic development, are collectively known as the striatum; the globus pallidus or pallidum, an older structure but one in which many nonpyramidal pathways converge; the thalamus, another important way station and integrative region; and the subthalamic nucleus, red nucleus and substantia nigra, all brainstem centers with important connections to the basal ganglia. These nuclear masses, along with their connections with each other and with certain parts of the reticular formation, cerebellum, and cerebrum, make up an anatomic-physiologic unit that collectively has been

termed "the extrapyramidal system." The role of this system in maintaining normal motor activity in man is not definitely known, and has only been inferred from studies of animals, in which it is more highly developed and not dominated by the cerebral cortex. In submammalian forms, this system appears essential for maintaining normal locomotion, feeding, etc. In higher animals, except man, its integrity is necessary for the production of automatic movements and postural adjustments. Some believe that this same function is carried over to man and that coarse, gross automatic movements are mediated by the extrapyramidal system. Others have implied a more secondary role in which this system is incapable of initiating movements but provides a reinforcing and modulating influence on movements of cortical origin. The latter thesis seems more in keeping with present knowledge; hence it is best to view the pyramidal and extrapyramidal systems as operating in unison and constant balance. Movements having their origin in the cerebral cortex are mediated through the pyramidal tract but are influenced by reflex regulating mechanisms from various components of the extrapyramidal system. In this context, the prime role of the extrapyramidal system is automatic sensorimotor integration, which can be explained in terms of inhibition and facilitation of motor responses to appropriate stimuli. Hence dysfunction within this system results in motor responses that are delayed, slow, and incomplete and especially affect automatic or involuntary movements.

The manifestations of basal ganglia disorders fall into two general categories: those of a *positive* nature, such as abnormal movements, tremor, and chorea, and those of a *negative* nature, such as postural changes and loss of associated movements. Unfortunately, because of the nature of the disease processes affecting this region it has not been possible to correlate intimately the clinical symptoms with structural changes. Even the magnitude of the demonstrable morphologic changes often bears little relationship to the severity of the condition. During the past decade a growing body of evidence has related the underlying disturbance in these disorders to biochemical changes in the basal ganglia rather than to morphologic abnormalities.

The most prominent biochemical feature of the basal ganglia is their high content of putative neurotransmitter agents, notably acetylcholine (ACH), dopamine (DA), and gamma-aminobutyric acid (GABA). The substrates and enzymes necessary for their production and degradation are found within the cellular components of the basal ganglia. In some instances they are produced within the segment where they have their action, whereas in others cellular elements in one area produce the transmitters whence they are transported via connecting axons to another, where they are stored and then released to produce their effects. Experimental evidence is available indicating that dopamine, for example, is produced in the pars compacta of the substantia nigra and is transported via the nigrostriatal pathway to the caudate nucleus and putamen to exert its action. Normal function in the basal ganglia appears to depend on a balance among these various neurotransmitters. Neurophysiologically this balance may be viewed as existing between those whose action is inhibitory in nature (DA and GABA) versus those with excitatory properties (ACH). Disturbances of this balance result in symptoms. In general, dopamine deficiency allows for cholinergic hyperactivity and can be correlated with the akinetic rigid disorders such as parkinsonism. Dopamine hyperactivity and/or cholinergic hypoactivity results in the hyperkinetic phenomena encountered in Huntington's chorea. To a considerable extent present approaches to the etiogenesis and treatment of basal ganglia disorders are directed to a better understanding of the role of and re-establishing balance among these neurotransmitter agents.

In the clinical evaluation of extrapyramidal disorders it is essential to have a clear understanding of the many and varied symptoms encountered. Those of major significance are abnormal involuntary movements, alterations in muscle tone, and disturbances in bodily posture.

ABNORMAL INVOLUNTARY MOVEMENTS. *Tremor* is a rhythmic involuntary alternating contraction of opposing muscle groups, fairly uniform in frequency and amplitude. It may involve a limited segment such as fingers or lips, or may be widespread. Characteristically, tremor of extrapyramidal origin is augmented when the part is at rest and diminished or abolished during voluntary movements and sleep. It differs from that of anxiety, thyrotoxicosis, and those due to intoxications by being slower, of greater amplitude, and more rhythmic. Its occurrence at rest and suppression during voluntary movements and sleep distinguish it from the "action" tremor of cerebellar involvement. The anatomic and physiologic substrate of this type of tremor has not been defined with certainty. In Parkinson's disease in which such tremor is prominent, the substantia nigra invariably undergoes degeneration. However, not all such patients have tremor, and it remains controversial whether the pathologic changes are entirely limited to this structure. Discharges synchronous with the tremor have been recorded in certain thalamic nuclei, particularly lateralis posterior. These findings suggest derangement of a complex sensorimotor mechanism with possible multiple pathologic sites.

Athetosis denotes an involuntary movement that results from instability of posture combined with voluntary movement. The result is a slow, writhing, wormlike movement usually most prominent in the fingers and hand, but the face, neck, and feet may also be involved. Multiple areas of the extrapyramidal system, particularly the globus pallidus and striatum as well as the cerebral cortex, have shown pathologic changes.

Chorea refers to brief, distal, rapid, explosive movements which at first glance appear to be purposeful and coordinated but on closer inspection are aimless and uncoordinated. They involve upper and lower limbs, face, trunk, and head, and may occur with such rapidity that the individual appears in constant motion. Choreiform movements are accentuated by movement and environmental stimulation, and interfere with normal voluntary function. They are differentiated from tics by being unpatterned, unpredictable, and nonreproducible. Athetosis and chorea may coexist in such a pattern that they are indistinguishable from one another. Pathologic changes accompanying chorea have been found in many areas of the nervous system but especially in the striatum.

Dystonia is a term applied to an abnormally maintained posture resulting from a twisting, turning movement that usually involves the limbs, neck, or trunk. Although there is no specific pattern or posture that describes this disorder, the usual appearance is one of marked distortion of the affected part. The movements appear readily induced by ordinary stimuli, such as walking, talking, or light touch to the skin. The involved muscles appear to be alternately in a state of increased and decreased tone and, usually as the movement starts, the muscles involved appear to gradually build up tone. Patients with this type of movement cannot inhibit, modify, or terminate the posture, and voluntary movements become seriously impaired. In some instances the movements clear, but the abnormal postures become fixed with resultant torticollis, tortipelvis, and deformities of the limbs. Neither the pathologic nor physiologic substrate for this movement disorder has been defined.

Ballism is a violent dyskinesia consisting of forceful, flinging movements of the limbs. The muscles involved are in the shoulder and pelvic girdle, and usually only one side of the body or even one limb is affected. Ballism appears to be due to a discrete lesion, usually in the subthalamic nucleus of Luys or its immediate connections.

ALTERATIONS IN MUSCLE TONE. Although it is common to associate heightened muscle tonus (rigidity) with extrapyramidal disorders, some, such as chorea and athetosis, may show normal tone or hypotonus of the musculature. Rigidity, which is most commonly encountered in parkinsonism, must be differentiated from spasticity. The former is identifiable by passively flexing and extending the muscles of an extremity or rotating the hand on the wrist. The movement obtained is one of a series of interrupted jerks at regular intervals, the so called cog-wheel effect. Terms such as "plastic" or "lead pipe" are utilized to describe the homogeneous degree of rigidity. Rigidity may be limited to groups of muscles and may be evident only at some joints, or it may be generalized, affecting the entire musculature. The mechanism underlying the rigidity appears to be impairment of reciprocal inhibition of agonist and antagonistic muscle groups. Electromyographic analysis of these muscles shows continuing activity in both groups throughout a movement such as flexion of the forearm. Rigidity reduces muscle power and velocity of movement and also contributes to the production of deformities.

DISTURBANCES IN BODILY POSTURE. Patients with extrapyramidal disease, especially those with parkinsonism, have difficulty in preserving their equilibrium in the erect as well as the sitting position. They also have difficulty in changing from the horizontal to the upright position or in rolling over from back to front. Profound difficulties are noted in walking, when tendencies to propulsive or retropulsive gait are evident as well as shuffling and festination. Careful analysis of these defects has indicated that the subjects have loss of control of their center of gravity in both sagittal and coronal planes. These abnormalities are thought to be due to disturbances in righting reflexes, impairment of vestibular reflexes, and release of proprioceptor mechanisms subsequent to degeneration in the pallidum.

Carpenter, M. B.: Extrapyramidal pathways and interconnections. Pharmacol. Therap., 1:1, 1975.

Costa, E., Cote, L., and Yahr, M. D. (eds.): Biochemistry and Pharmacology of the Basal Ganglia. Hewlett, N. Y., Raven Press, 1966.

Duvoisin, R.: Clinical diagnosis of the dyskinesias. Med. Clin. North Am., 56:1321, 1972.

Lloyd, K. G.: Special chemistry of the basal ganglia 1. Monoamines. Pharmacol. Therap., 1:49, 1975.

Purpura, D. P.: Physiological organization of the basal ganglia. In Yahr, M. D. (ed.): The Basal Ganglia. New York, Raven Press, 1976, pp. 91–114.

Yahr, M. D.: Involuntary movements. In Scientific Foundations of Neurology. London, Heinemann, 1972, pp. 83–88.

274. THE PARKINSONIAN SYNDROME

(Paralysis Agitans, Shaking Palsy)

Melvin D. Yahr

274.1. INTRODUCTION

James Parkinson in 1817 first described the major manifestations of this syndrome, which is characterized by tremor, muscular rigidity, and loss of postural reflexes. Not only is it the most frequently encountered of the basal ganglia disorders, but parkinsonism is a prominent cause of disability. Its prevalence has been placed at close to one million patients in the United States, with the addition of 50,000 new cases each year. As a symptom complex its occurrence has been noted in a number of disease processes either as the sole manifestation or in association with other symptoms. However, in most cases no definable cause has yet been found; since the latter seem to have many features in common, particularly in regard to evolution, they have been designated as Parkinson's disease, paralysis agitans, or primary parkinsonism. The cases in which definable processes are found are best classified as secondary or symptomatic parkinsonism. This separation into clinical groups cannot be construed as indicative of a difference in pathophysiology or even pathogenic mechanisms for the production of symptoms, for all parkinsonism may well have a common origin. Indeed, from the standpoint of what is presently known about its chemical pathology, a deficiency of striatal dopamine is common to all types of parkinsonism. In most

instances of parkinsonism, regardless of cause, loss of pigmented neurons is found in the substantia nigra, locus ceruleus, and pigmented brainstem nuclei in association with other nonspecific changes diffusely distributed in the corpus striatum and cortex.

274.2. PARALYSIS AGITANS

(Parkinson's Disease)

The largest number of cases of parkinsonism fall into this category. The disease most frequently begins between the ages of 50 and 65 years. A rarely encountered juvenile form has been described. The disease affects both sexes and all races. There is no evidence to indicate a hereditary factor. Although the cause of Parkinson's disease is unknown, its appearance in the later years of life has suggested that it may relate to mechanisms involved in the aging process of neuronal cells, particularly in individuals in whom the nigral cells are highly vulnerable to such effects. One of the factors that has been given consideration and for which some evidence exists relates to the enzymes necessary for removing the oxidative products of catecholamine metabolism. Hydrogen peroxide is such a byproduct, and its removal depends on the enzymes peroxidase and catalase, both normally in high concentration in the substantia nigra and reduced with aging but more so in parkinsonian brains. Their reduction may allow for the accumulation of hydrogen peroxide and other toxic products which then leads to the destruction of nigral cells and the loss of tyrosine hydroxylase, the enzyme responsible for dopamine production.

The disease begins insidiously with any of its three cardinal manifestations either alone or in combination. Tremor usually in one or both hands, involving the fingers in a pill-rolling motion, is the most common initial symptom. This is often followed by stiffness in the limbs, general slowing of movements, and inability to carry out normal and routine daily functions with ease. As the disease progresses the face becomes "masklike," with a loss of eye blinking and failure to express emotional feeling; the body becomes stooped, and the gait becomes shuffling with loss of arm swing; and the patient is unable to readily gain and maintain an erect posture. Speech becomes slow and monotonous. There is a tendency to drool. The skin takes on an oily quality, and there is a tendency to seborrheic dermatitis. Although paralysis agitans is invariably progressive, the rate at which symptoms develop and disability ensues is extremely variable. Only rarely is the disease so rapidly progressive that the patient becomes disabled within five years of onset. In the majority, intervals of 10 to 20 years elapse before symptoms cause incapacity.

The major neurologic findings are as follows: (1) *Lack of facial expression,* with diminished eye blinking but ready induction of blepharospasm when the frontalis muscle is tapped (Myerson's sign). (2) *Tremor* of the distal segments of the limbs at rest, accentuated by suspension but decreased during active movements and eliminated in sleep. The tremor is rhythmical, alternatively affecting flexor and extensor muscles, and may involve upper or lower limbs, mouth, or head. (3) *Muscular rigidity,* readily evident on passive movement of a joint, and manifested by a series of interrupted jerks (cog-wheel phenomenon) rather than a smooth flowing, easy motion. (4) *Akinesia,* the tendency to slowness in the initiation of movement and sudden unexpected arrests of volitional movements while carrying out purposeful acts. The parkinsonian patient appears disinclined to move, and in the midst of performing a routine function suddenly finds himself "frozen" and unable to move through the sequence of motion necessary to complete the action. This is especially evident in writing or feeding and can be striking when, in attempting to walk, the patient finds that his feet are suddenly "frozen to the ground." (5) *Postural abnormalities,* most evident in the erect and sitting positions. The patient has a tendency to let his head fall forward on the trunk, and his body tends to fall forward or backward when seated on a stool unless supported; when pushed either from in front or behind in the erect position he falls, making no effort to catch himself either with a step or by movement of his arms. There is a tendency to deformities of the trunk, hands, and feet. Kyphotic deformity of the spine, causing a stooped posture, is a hallmark. There are ulnar deviations of the hand, flexion contractures of the fingers, and an equinovarus posture of the foot.

274.3. SECONDARY OR SYMPTOMATIC PARKINSONISM

In a long list of diseases and conditions of the nervous system parkinsonism has occurred as the predominant manifestation. Included are poisoning with carbon monoxide, manganese, and other heavy metals; brain tumors in the region of the basal ganglia; cerebral trauma; intoxication with neuroleptic agents; infectious processes such as encephalitis; multineuronal degenerative disorders of unknown cause; and association with cerebral arteriosclerosis as well as with endocrine dysfunction such as hypoparathyroidism. In most instances the presence of associated neurologic deficits, atypical features of the parkinsonian symptoms, and/or other systemic manifestations of the related disease process arouse suspicion that one is not dealing with primary parkinsonism. Of all the conditions noted, those most frequently encountered are postencephalitic and drug-induced parkinsonism and so-called arteriosclerotic pseudoparkinsonism.

POSTENCEPHALITIC PARKINSONISM

One of the most prominent sequelae of the epidemic of encephalitis lethargica (von Economo's disease) that occurred between 1919 and 1926 was the parkinsonian syndrome. The syndrome developed after mild as well as severe encephalitis lethargica, and, although in most instances it immediately followed the acute infectious process, in some patients prominent symptoms were not evident for intervals of up to ten years. The causative agent of encephalitis lethargica was never established. However, recent studies suggest that it was produced by a virus of the influenza A variety. Parkinsonism appears to have been a unique sequela of this form of encephalitis because it had rarely followed any other known viral encephalitides. There are still a significant number of survivors of encephalitis lethargica, and the evolution and consequences of this form of

parkinsonism differ from others, so its clinical recognition is of importance.

Postencephalitic parkinsonism has a number of distinctive features, including the following: (1) A history of encephalitis lethargica during the epidemic period 1918–1919. Since the pandemic of influenza occurred concurrently with encephalitis, it is essential that careful documentation be undertaken in differentiating these two infectious processes. (2) In addition to any or all of the parkinsonian symptoms indicated above, one or more of the following neurologic deficits may be found: hemiplegia, bulbar or ocular palsies, dystonic phenomena, tics, or behavioral disorders. (3) The parkinsonism itself is as a rule incompletely developed and has been static or slowly progressive over a period of years. (4) Episodes that have been termed oculogyric crises. These consist of attacks in which spasms of conjugate eye muscles occur so that the eyes are deviated upward, downward, or to one side for minutes or hours at a time.

DRUG-INDUCED PARKINSONISM

The use of neuroleptics as psychotherapeutic or antiemetic agents has resulted in the occurrence of a number of extrapyramidal syndromes. Parkinsonism indistinguishable from that previously described, dystonic movements involving the tongue and face, and akathisia, a restless fidgety state with a desire to be in constant motion, are those frequently encountered. Adults are more likely to develop parkinsonism and akathisia, whereas dystonic movements predominate in children. In some instances these reactions are dose dependent; in others they are related to individual susceptibility. The symptoms usually disappear within a few days when the drugs are withdrawn, but occasionally persist for months. In some subjects permanent remnants of parkinsonian symptoms have been found years after elimination of the drugs. Paradoxically, involuntary movements may make their initial appearance after withdrawal of neuroleptic agents. This condition, termed *tardive dyskinesia,* tends to occur in older patients who have been on phenothiazine drugs for extended periods of time, during which they have shown signs of parkinsonism. Stereotyped, repetitious movements of lips, tongue, and mouth and choreiform movements of limbs and trunk characterize this disorder. It may diminish in intensity or disappear spontaneously after weeks or months, but in some patients it has persisted indefinitely. Recently it has been shown that these abnormal movements may be controlled by the administration of large doses of choline chloride. In contrast, parkinsonism can be minimized by the simultaneous administration of one of the centrally active anticholinergic agents, such as benztropine (Cogentin) or trihexyphenidyl (Artane). In view of these potentially devastating side effects, physicians should employ neuroleptics cautiously with restricted doses. Drug holidays in those requiring long-term treatment should be routinely practiced and may be the best preventive measure.

ARTERIOSCLEROTIC PSEUDOPARKINSONISM

Atherosclerotic involvement of the cerebral vessels has been implicated by some as a cause of parkinsonism. Others have suggested that the nature of the symptoms warrants abandoning the term. Indeed, Critchley, who first proposed the term arteriosclerotic parkinsonism in 1929, has more recently re-emphasized the differing nature of the two disorders, and has recommended that when there is an underlying substrate of cerebrovascular disease, it be referred to as pseudoparkinsonism. Although the disorders superficially appear to resemble each other, there are distinctive differences as well as therapeutic implications. As a rule, the onset of symptoms is insidious, with most cases beginning in the seventh decade of life, although on occasion the occurrence has been noted in younger individuals as early as the fourth decade. Only rarely is there a history of a major stroke preceding onset, although symptoms referable to so-called minor strokes may be elicited. Early symptoms usually center around impaired mobility, with gait disturbance the most frequent complaint. Other presenting complaints may refer to pseudobulbar phenomena with dysarthria, some degree of dysphasia, and emotional incontinence. Some patients will present with progressive intellectual defects in association with poverty of movement. Tremor is rare, but alteration in muscle tone is common. It differs from the cog-wheel type, characteristic of Parkinson's disease, in that there is a stiffening of the limb in response to contact and a sense of resistance with attempted change of position. This type of alteration in muscle tone is known as gegenhalten. Hyperactive reflexes, abnormal plantar responses, and palmomental and snouting reflexes are all usually found. Pathologically, multiple small cerebral infarctions (lacunae) secondary to small vessel occlusion are found throughout the brain in these patients. The course of the disease is progressive, usually stepwise, and more rapid than that of Parkinson's disease. The usual antiparkinson drugs have little benefit.

274.4. MANAGEMENT OF THE PARKINSONIAN SYNDROME

GENERAL PRINCIPLES. Most patients will require life-long treatment, consisting of the administration of specific medications, supportive psychotherapeutic measures, physical therapy, and, in rare instances, surgical intervention.

SUPPORTIVE PSYCHOTHERAPY. The major symptoms of parkinsonism are markedly influenced by psychic factors, and a patient's outlook and motivation will affect the extent to which he can overcome disability. It is important for the physician to provide reassurance, encouragement, and sympathetic understanding to the patient and family so that they may meet the numerous difficulties to be encountered at various stages of the illness. To allay anxieties both should be counseled regarding the meaning of various symptoms, the nature of the disease in terms of its long and variable course, and the potential that most patients can lead active and productive lives for long periods after symptoms begin.

PHYSICAL THERAPY. Simple measures such as heat and massage will alleviate painful muscle cramps and the muscle contraction headache that often accompanies pronounced rigidity of the cervical musculature. Exercises help in preventing flexion contractures. Gait training, walking exercises, and minor rehabilitative measures may enable the patient to maintain his independence with regard to personal hygiene and daily living activities for many more years than his disabilities might allow. Physical therapy in parkinsonism need not be elaborate, but when indicated should be done frequently and for an indefinite period. The patient should be instructed in simple home exercises and encouraged to develop a program of physical activity. Most patients in the earlier stages like to take long walks and should be encouraged to continue this habit as long as reasonably possible. Every effort should be made to keep them gainfully employed and to adjust their occupations as indicated by their symptoms.

DRUG THERAPY. The drugs now employed in the treatment of parkinsonism are theoretically capable of restoring normal activity to the striatum. Thus any agent that crosses the blood-brain barrier and enhances the brain's dopaminergic function or that reduces cholinergic activity may be expected to influence parkinsonism favorably. As a general rule a combination of agents with such properties works best.

The dopaminergic system may be functionally enhanced by agents that increase the synthesis of dopamine (this is presumably the modus operandi of levodopa), delay the catabolism of dopamine (monoamine oxidase inhibitors), promote its release from presynaptic storage sites (amphetamine), simulate its action at receptors (apomorphine, bromocriptine), and block the reuptake of monoamines at the synaptic cleft (anticholinergics). Of the numerous means for improving dopaminergic function that have been tried to date, the most effective has been the administration of levodopa (3,4-dihydroxyphenyl-L-alanine). Given alone or in combination with a peripheral dopa decarboxylase inhibitor (benserazide, carbidopa), it is appreciably more effective and less toxic than any therapeutic agent previously available for the treatment of Parkinson's disease.

In the selection of patients for treatment with levodopa, the over-all severity of parkinsonism and the degree of functional impairment, as well as the existence of concomitant diseases of other organs, must be carefully considered. Patients with minimal signs and symptoms who are able to meet the demands of daily living need not involve themselves in a treatment program that may be rigorous and demanding and carries an implicit risk. The presence of occlusive vascular disease involving the heart or brain warrants careful assessment. Severe angina pectoris or transient cerebral ischemic attacks contraindicate the use of levodopa. A history of episodic cardiac arrhythmia presents an additional hazard. When the arrhythmia is associated with myocardial disease, the use of levodopa must be undertaken with extreme caution. Evidence of prior mental illness, particularly affective disorders or major "psychotic breaks," contravenes the use of levodopa. Although requiring careful monitoring, levodopa has been administered without adverse effects to patients with hepatic, renal, gastrointestinal, and hematopoietic disorders. The presence of hemolytic anemia and glucose-6-phosphate dehydrogenase (G-6-DP) deficiency contraindicates its use.

Clinical treatment with levodopa comprises two phases. The first or "introduction phase" extends over a period of weeks or months in which the dosage is slowly built up to the therapeutic range. During this phase, tolerance develops to many of the side effects of levodopa; and although improvement of symptoms occurs in most patients, the optimal therapeutic response may not be evident. A "maintenance phase" follows, in which the full benefits of treatment most often occur, and careful patient monitoring with readjustment of dosage and ancillary therapeutic measures may be required to maintain a stable therapeutic response. Each of these phases requires cooperation on the part of the patient and careful management by the physician to achieve the best therapeutic response.

Levodopa is an aromatic amino acid that is a relatively inert compound by itself, but several of its metabolites have profound pharmacologic effects. Levodopa is available in two main forms in the United States. One is as tablets or capsules of 100, 250, and 500 mg of levodopa alone. The other combines levodopa with an extracerebral decarboxylate inhibitor, carbidopa, in tablets marketed as Sinemet, containing 10 or 25 mg of carbidopa plus 100 or 250 mg of levodopa. Available in most countries in the world but not in the United States is a similar combination utilizing benserazide, 20 or 50 mg, as a peripheral decarboxylase inhibitor with levodopa, 100 or 200 mg (Madopar).

Levodopa can be given in slowly increasing dosages, starting with 250 mg three or four times daily after meals and slowly increasing by 125 to 250 mg every few days until maximal therapeutic effect or side reactions are encountered. The optimal dose for adults is 5.0 grams or even more. At this dose level, however, many patients experience side effects, including anorexia, nausea, feelings of nervous tension, or hypotension. Occasional transitory alterations in blood chemistry, including elevations of serum glutamic oxaloacetic transaminase (SGOT), alkaline phosphatase, and blood urea nitrogen (BUN), as well as depression of white blood cell count and development of a positive Coombs test, have occurred. To date, these have not been associated with symptoms of dysfunction in organ systems, nor has autopsy material shown structural alterations.

Many of the aforementioned side effects of levodopa may be avoided by the simultaneous administration of carbidopa or benserazide. These agents prevent the peripheral utilization of levodopa, making it more readily and rapidly available to brain and avoiding extracerebral dopaminergic action. Consequently, the induction phase is considerably shortened and one may obtain optimal therapeutic responses within a matter of days. Sinemet, the carbidopa-levodopa combination, is effective when administered in total daily doses of 50 to 100 mg of carbidopa with 500 to 1000 mg of levodopa. In general one starts with modest doses of Sinemet 10/100 (carbidopa 10 mg, levodopa 100 mg) given four times a day with increases at two-day intervals as required. Not available in the United States but in most other countries of the world is Madopar, a combination of benserazide, 25 or 50 mg, and levodopa, 100 or 200 mg. The average required daily dose of this combination has been benserazide, 200 mg, and levodopa, 800 mg, in four equally divided doses. Sinemet and Madopar appear to have an equivalent therapeutic effect.

Most patients on long-term or high-dose levodopa therapy sooner or later develop side effects attributable to the central nervous system action of the drug. Adventitious movements consist of choreiform movements of hands or feet. Grimacing may affect the face. Variability in therapeutic response may lead to a loss of dopa effect lasting for hours or even days. For all these reasons patients with parkinsonism need long-term supervision and drug adjustments to accomplish maximal benefits.

A number of other antiparkinsonian agents are useful as adjunctive drugs with levodopa; they are also indicated for those in whom levodopa is contraindicated and are preferred for patients with very mild symptoms in the very early stages of the disorder. Some are also the drug of choice in drug-induced parkinsonism. Most of these compounds possess central nervous system anticholinergic properties or augment striatal dopaminergic activity. Those most frequently used are trihexyphenidyl (Artane), available in 2 and 5 mg tablets; benztropine (Cogentin), as 1 and 2 mg tablets; cycrimine (Pagitane), as 1.25 and 2.5 mg tablets; and procyclidine (Kemadrin), 2 and 5 mg tablets. Treatment should be initiated with small doses such as trihexyphenidyl, 2 mg three times daily, and gradually increased until further increases yield no additional benefit or side effects reach an unacceptable degree of severity.

To obtain optimal results with anticholinergic drugs, careful titration of dosage against side effects is required. The goal is to find the dose that yields an optimal compromise between the limited symptomatic improvement of the parkinsonism and the disagreeable symptoms of cholinergic blockade of the central and peripheral nervous systems. Among the latter are blurring of vision, dryness of mouth and throat, anhidrosis, constipation, and urinary urgency or, sometimes, retention. The major symptoms of central anticholinergic intoxication are ataxia, dysarthria, hyperthermia, and a characteristic pattern of mental disturbances, including impairment of recent memory, confusion, delusional thinking, hallucinations, somnolence, and rarely coma.

A number of other agents, not primarily anticholinergics but with mild central anticholinergic properties, are useful. Diphenhydramine (Benadryl), orphenadrine (Disipal), and chlorphenoxamine (Phenoxene) are similar in pharmacologic action. In general, diphenhydramine has enjoyed the widest use and can be given in divided dosage up to 150 mg a day. It is particularly useful as an adjunct to levodopa, for in addition to benefiting symptoms of parkinsonism, it allays anxiety and tempers insomnia.

The antidepressants imipramine (Tofranil) and amitriptyline (Elavil) are minimally effective when used alone, but in combination with anticholinergic agents or levodopa they may be beneficial in relieving the depressive symptoms that so often accompany parkinsonism. With administration in limited dosage, one may avoid their adverse effects, which may resemble parkinsonism. Imipramine 10 to 15 mg given four times a day, or amitriptyline, 25 mg twice a day, can be safely administered for extended periods.

Introduced as an antiviral agent, amantadine HCl (Symmetrel) was accidentally found to have activity against parkinsonism. When used alone in doses of 100 mg twice a day, its therapeutic effects are evident within 48 to 72 hours, consisting of a mild reversal of symptoms of parkinsonism. More effective action can be achieved when it is added to an existing regimen of treatment consisting of anticholinergic agents or levodopa (or both). Its effects are short lived, tending to diminish after a month and rarely lasting for more than three months. Many of its side effects are similar to those of the anticholinergic agents, particularly the induction of confusional and delusional states. In some patients after long-term use, edema and a form of livedo reticularis develop over the limbs.

Recently clinical trials with a number of new agents designed to overcome the shortcomings of levodopa have been tried. In the main, they are directed toward patients who are unresponsive to levodopa, experience "on-off" response, or have an excessive degree of abnormal involuntary movements as a result of its use. Agents that have shown some promise are those having the property of directly activating postsynaptic dopamine receptors in brain — so-called dopaminergic receptor agonists. Some that have received particular attention are piribedil (Trivastal) and bromocriptine. Although piribedil has shown antiparkinson action, it has offered little advantage over levodopa administered with carbidopa (Sinemet). Indeed, its comparative efficacy is below that achieved with the latter combination. Bromocriptine in rather large doses, 100 to 200 mg a day, has produced beneficial effects in some patients who have been resistant to treatment. However, when added to an existing therapeutic regimen, in modest doses, it may add additional therapeutic benefit. Although the usual monoamine oxidase inhibitors have been avoided because of their potential for inducing hypertensive crises, when given with precursors of dopamine such reactions have not been encountered with the monoamine oxidase inhibitor deprenyl. Given in small doses, 10 mg a day, it has been possible to reduce the required dose of levodopa and produce a more efficacious therapeutic response. At the time of this writing, piribedil, bromocriptine, and deprenyl have not been approved by the Food and Drug Administration for general use in the United States.

At the time of this writing there is no doubt that levodopa given in combination with a decarboxylase inhibitor is the best available treatment for the large majority of parkinsonian patients. It is far from ideal, but its judicious use benefits a large proportion of those suffering from Parkinson's disease over an extended period of time.

SURGICAL MEASURES. Stereotaxic neurosurgical procedures, directed to the interruption of neural pathways in the brain responsible for producing symptoms of parkinsonism, were in considerable vogue before the advent of levodopa therapy. They have been almost entirely discontinued with the advent of the more successful medical therapy.

COURSE OF THE PARKINSON SYNDROME. All forms of parkinsonism reflect progressive disorders of the nervous system, leading over variable periods of time to a considerable degree of motor disability. The most progressive is the symptomatic form, in which, as part of a generalized disorder of the nervous system, marked disability and a fatal outcome can be expected within five years. Postencephalitic parkinsonism is unique in this regard, in that its evolution has been relatively slow and patients have remained functional for extended periods of time, in some instances for 30 years or more. Parkinson's disease, or what is now referred to as primary parkinsonism, prior to its treatment with levodopa, could be expected to produce severe disability or death in 25 per cent of patients within five years of onset, 65 per cent in the succeeding five years, and 80 per cent in those surviving for 15 years. Further, it had been estimated that those suffering from Parkinson's

disease had a mortality rate three times that of the general population matched for age, sex, and racial origin. Although there is no evidence to indicate that levodopa or any other therapeutic agent now in use alters the underlying pathologic process or stems the progressive nature of the disease, there are indications of a major impact on survival time and functional capacity. Recent studies show that the added risk of mortality from Parkinson's disease has been reduced by half and that longevity is extended by a number of years. More important, since the introduction of these newer therapeutic agents, the quality of life has been improved for parkinsonians in that they do not suffer the degree of incapacity and dependence which previously characterized this disease.

It must be emphasized, however, that the treatment of parkinsonism is still far from ideal. Long-term follow-up studies covering periods of up to eight years during which levodopa has been administered reveal a gradual loss of therapeutic efficacy. Optimal responses are obtained during the first three years of instituting treatment with levodopa regardless of duration of the disease, and then diminish. It is not known at this time whether this relates to intrinsic factors of the disease process itself or the loss of therapeutic efficacy of the drug.

Barbeau, A.: Parkinson's disease: Etiological considerations. *In* Yahr, M. D. (ed.): The Basal Ganglia. New York, Raven Press, 1976, pp. 281–289.

Cotzias, G. C., Papavasilou, P. S., and Gellene, R.: Modification of parkinsonism — chronic treatment with L-dopa. N. Engl. J. Med., 280:337, 1969.

Crane, G. E.: Persistence of neurological symptoms due to neuroleptic drugs. Am. J. Psychiatry, 127:1407, 1971.

Critchley, M.: Arteriosclerotic parkinsonism. Brain, 52:23, 1929.

Duvoisin, R. C., and Yahr, M. D.: Encephalitis and parkinsonism. Arch. Neurol., 12:227, 1965.

Gamboa, E. T., Wolf, A., Yahr, M. D., et al.: Influenza virus antigen in postencephalitic parkinsonism brain. Arch. Neurol., 31:228, 1974.

Hoehn, M. M., and Yahr, M. D.: Parkinsonism: Onset, progression and mortality. Neurology, 17:427, 1967.

Yahr, M. D. (ed.): Treatment of parkinsonism — the role of dopa decarboxylase inhibitors. Adv. Neurol., 2, 1973.

Yahr, M. D.: Evaluation of long-term therapy in Parkinson's disease: Mortality and therapeutic efficacy. *In* Birkmayer, W., and Hornykiewicz, O. (eds.): Advances in Parkinsonism. Basle, Editiones Roche, 1976, p. 435.

275. ESSENTIAL TREMOR

(Familial Tremor)

Melvin D. Yahr

This is a monosymptomatic condition in which tremor involves the hands and/or head and face. The tremor is usually more rapid than that encountered in parkinsonism, is accentuated by emotional factors, may be worsened by volitional movement, and is usually suppressed by the use of alcohol. The age of onset is variable, but in most cases the disorder begins prior to the age of 25 years and tends to persist throughout life. Some progression of the intensity of tremor and spread to other bodily parts usually occur over the years, which may result in significant physical and social disability. There is a strong familial incidence, with occurrence in several successive generations and members of the same family, but the genetic pattern of inheritance has not been determined. Some have suggested its transmission as an autosomal dominant trait. To date no specific pathologic lesion has been reported in the nervous system of people with this condition. It has been suggested that the condition is an abortive form of parkinsonism, but this concept does not appear justifiable at present. There is no specific effective therapy for controlling the tremor, although beta-adrenergic blocking agents, such as propranolol in dosage of 120 to 180 mg a day divided equally into three or four doses, have been useful in some patients. Responses, however, are variable and unpredictable, and cardiovascular alterations may limit the use of optimal dosage. Sedatives such as phenobarbital, in dosage of 15 mg three times a day, may reduce the intensity of the tremor. It is of utmost importance to differentiate essential tremor from parkinsonism. By and large, the distinguishing characteristics are earlier age of onset; lack of severe progression, akinesia, rigidity, or postural abnormalities; and the strong family history of tremor.

Baughman, F. A., Jr., Higgins, J. V., and Mann, J. D.: Sex chromosome anomalies and essential tremor. Neurology, 23:623, 1973.

Marshall, J.: Observations on essential tremor. J. Neurol. Neurosurg. Psychiatry, 25:122, 1962.

McAllister, R. G., Markesbery, W. R., Ware, R. W., and Howell, S. M.: Suppression of essential tremor by propranolol: Correlation of effect with drug plasma levels and intensity of beta-adrenergic blockade. Ann. Neurol., 1:160, 1977.

Scopa, J., Longley, B. P., and Foster, J. B.: Beta-adrenergic blockers in benign essential tremor. Curr. Ther. Res., 15:48, 1973.

276. SENILE TREMOR

Melvin D. Yahr

Tremor is a frequent finding in the elderly, most often involving the upper limbs and head. It differs from parkinsonian tremor in that it is finer and more rapid and at first occurs only with voluntary movements. As time goes on it becomes more constant and is also present while the limbs are at rest. There is no associated weakness or alteration in muscle tone. These features differentiate this form of tremor from parkinsonism. The cause is unknown. Since senile tremor has both cerebellar and extrapyramidal features, in that it occurs at rest and with movement, the assumption is that some critical pathway linking these systems has undergone degeneration. There is no effective treatment, although mild benefit may be derived from sedatives or the use of diphenhydramine (Benadryl) given in 25 mg doses three times a day. Most patients accept it as another of the many changes that come with advancing years. Occasional patients have to be reassured that they do not have parkinsonism or some other progressive neurologic disorder.

277. THE CHOREAS

Melvin D. Yahr

277.1. INTRODUCTION

There are a number of disease entities that, though wholly unrelated etiologically, have choreiform movements as their major manifestation. In some, intimate relationships with infectious processes have been found, whereas in others familial tendencies have pointed to a strong genetic component. In the light of newer concepts of inheritance, a common pathogenesis for all may be found. Although controversy exists as to the exact anatomic site from which movements of this type may derive, pathologic changes are commonly found in the striatum, particularly in the small cell components of the caudate nucleus and putamen. The classification of chorea into separate entities is at present somewhat arbitrary and is based on age of onset, association with identifiable disease processes or familial tendency, and occurrence of other neurologic abnormalities.

277.2. ACUTE CHOREA
(Sydenham's or Infectious Chorea, St. Vitus' Dance)

Acute chorea is a movement disorder encountered primarily during childhood and having its greatest incidence between the ages of 5 and 15 years. Occurrence beyond this age is uncommon, and then is usually in association with pregnancy or in persons who have had symptoms earlier in life. Females manifest these symptoms at least twice as often as males. Acute chorea has been reported in people of all races.

Considered as a symptom complex rather than as a specific disease entity, acute choreiform movements have been encountered as initial manifestations of a variety of conditions. They have been reported in epidemic encephalitis, in the encephalopathies occurring with exanthema, with pertussis and diphtheria, in idiopathic hypocalcemia, hyperthyroidism, systemic lupus erythematosus, carbon monoxide poisoning, vascular disease, tumors, and degenerative processes of the basal ganglia. These instances, however, account for only a small percentage of cases. The closest relationship appears to be with rheumatic fever. In more than half of the cases, rheumatic manifestations consisting of carditis, valvular heart disease, or arthritis occur prior to, coincident with, or following an attack of chorea.

There are no specific pathologic changes or anatomic sites of involvement that can be correlated with acute chorea. In fact, because acute uncomplicated chorea is rarely fatal, there has been a paucity of detailed pathologic studies. Cases that have come to autopsy have shown scattered changes in the cortex, basal ganglia, cerebellum, and brainstem. These have consisted of varying degrees of arteritis combined with cellular degeneration.

The outstanding clinical features of chorea are involuntary movements, incoordination, muscle weakness, and emotional lability. Although the onset of symptoms may be abrupt and obvious, it is more often insidious and subtle. The most frequent initial complaints include clumsiness of the limbs, evidenced by dropping objects from the hands or an awkward gait, particularly during emotionally tense situations. When these are coupled with irritability, poor performance in school, and generally fidgety behavior, frequently a hasty conclusion is reached, blaming the child or implying a psychiatric disorder. The typical choreatic movements may be noted in any part of the body, limbs, face, hands, tongue, or trunk. They may at first appear to be a part of the natural pattern of coordinated movements but are soon noted to be completely random, jerking, aimless, and purposeless. They occur at rest, are accentuated by any attempt at volitional movement, and disappear in sleep. They may be very mild and may minimally affect normal function or may be so forceful and frequent as to be totally disabling. Facial grimacing and difficulty in speech, chewing, and swallowing occur when the muscles subserving these functions are involved. Interruption of voluntary movements by involuntary ones leads to incoordination so that the person drops objects, walks in an awkward, ungainly fashion, and, in general, appears uncoordinated. Attempts to maintain forceful muscular contraction are similarly interrupted, and the resultant "waxing and waning" of motor power results in a relative degree of motor weakness. Although actual paralysis is rare, there is a disinclination to use a part of the body that is severely affected by involuntary movements of this type. Generalized reduction of muscle tone is an invariable feature of chorea and is readily demonstrable by hyperextensibility at finger, wrist, and ankle joints. In almost all choreatic children some degree of emotional lability is evident. It varies from total apathy to irritability, restlessness, and, infrequently, wild, inappropriate behavior.

Certain cardinal features can be found in almost all patients. These include (1) pronation of the forearm when the upper limbs are raised and extended; (2) inability to sustain muscle contraction when the examiner grasps the patient's hand or when the patient protrudes his tongue so that it darts rapidly in and out of the mouth; and (3) abnormal posturing of hands in which the wrist is noted to be sharply flexed and the fingers hyperextended at the metacarpophalangeal joints.

There are no specific laboratory tests for chorea. The cerebrospinal fluid is normal. The electroencephalogram may or may not show diffuse abnormalities correlated with the severity of the disease. Unless there are associated disease processes that manifest themselves in abnormalities of blood count, chemistry, or sedimentation rate, these studies are normal.

The age of onset and the distinctive involuntary movements readily differentiate acute chorea from other disorders of the basal ganglia. Tics and habit spasms may be confused with mild cases, but their movements are quite different, being stereotyped repetitive patterns localized to a single group of muscles. Huntington's chorea rarely begins in childhood and, in addition, there is a strong familial tendency with associated dementia. Movement disorders associated with cerebral palsy occur in infancy but have an athetoid element. The use of phenothiazines may induce abnormal movements, but the history of drug ingestion will differentiate these.

Acute chorea is a self-limited disease, recovery occurring in two to six months. Recurrence, with as many as two or three attacks over a period of years, appears in almost one third of the cases. There is no specific therapy. Bed rest and reduction of external stimuli to a minimum, combined with sedative drugs such as phenobarbital or chloral hydrate, are beneficial in controlling the severity of the movements. Paradoxically, the phenothiazines, such as thorazine and chlorpromazine, as well as reserpine in doses commensurate with individual tolerance, although capable of inducing chorea, have also been shown to be effective in its control. Because

of the high incidence of rheumatic valvular heart disease complicating acute chorea, prophylaxis with antimicrobial drugs over a long interval of time similar to that utilized in acute rheumatic fever is now recommended. If emotional symptoms are intense, psychotherapy may be in order. When specific abnormalities of calcium metabolism or thyroid dysfunction are found, their correction may completely ameliorate the symptoms. With recovery most patients show few or no neurologic sequelae.

Aron, A., Freeman, J., and Carter, S.: The natural history of Sydenham's chorea. Am. J. Med., 38:83, 1965.
Schwartzman, J.: Chorea minor. Review of 175 cases with reference to etiology, treatment and sequelae. Rheumatism, 6:89, 1950.

277.3. HEREDITARY CHOREA
(Chronic Progressive Chorea, Huntington's Disease)

Hereditary chorea is a progressive degenerative disease of the basal ganglia and cerebral cortex, beginning in adult life and characterized by choreiform movements and mental deterioration. The disease affects both sexes in equal numbers and is transmitted from parent to offspring in autosomal dominant fashion with full penetrance. Hence 50 per cent of children of sufferers will inevitably be affected. The disease is relatively rare, although its incidence may be high in geographic regions where affected families have resided for many generations.

Pathologically, widespread degenerative changes with cell loss and reactive gliosis are found, primarily in the cerebral cortex and caudate nucleus. Recently it has been demonstrated that glutamic acid decarboxylase and choline acetylase activity are reduced in the basal ganglia of patients with Huntington's chorea. This results in a deficiency of γ-aminobutyric acid, an inhibitory transmitter substance in brain, as well as depressed function of the excitatory transmitter acetylcholine. Disruption of the homeostatic relationship of these agents may underlie the choreatic manifestations of this disorder.

The clinical manifestations consist of choreatic movements, emotional disturbance, and intellectual deterioration in varying degrees, rate of appearance, and progression. The disease usually makes its appearance between the ages of 35 and 50 years, rather insidiously with any of the aforementioned symptoms, but as a rule with abnormal movements. The movements, though similar to acute chorea, are usually more jerky though less lightning-like and primarily involve the trunk and shoulder girdle and more often the lower limbs than the upper. This pattern of involvement tends to produce a dancing sort of gait, which is a prominent feature of the disease. In rare instances a Parkinson-like rigidity is encountered as the major manifestation rather than involuntary movements. The mental deterioration is similar to that of any organic dementia, with progressive impairment of memory and of intellectual capacity, and inattention to personal hygiene. Emotional disturbances include heightened irritability, bouts of depression, and fits of violent behavior.

With the typical triad of choreiform movements, dementia in adult life, and documentation of similar symptoms in family members, the diagnosis is readily evident. However, there is a tendency for families to deny the existence of mental disease, and it is sometimes difficult to obtain corroborative data even when the diagnosis is strongly suspected. Little difficulty occurs in differentiating hereditary chorea from acute chorea, but senile chorea may raise a problem. The latter, which comes on late in life, involves few mental changes, if any, lacks a familial history, and is usually benign in comparison. Other diseases such as the presenile psychoses, Alzheimer's and Pick's, because of their dementia and similarity in age of onset, may offer some difficulty, especially in instances in which choreiform movements are inconspicuous. Computerized axial tomography or pneumoencephalography demonstrating selective atrophy of the caudate nucleus may help to establish the correct diagnosis in such instances. There is a tendency to overdiagnose hereditary chorea, applying it to diverse neurologic disorders such as cerebellar degenerations and familial tremors. The dire implications of this form of chorea require strict adherence to the diagnostic criteria.

There is at present no known means of altering the underlying disease process or its progressive fatal outcome. Attempts to replace the defect in gamma-aminobutyric acid (GABA) metabolism by utilizing some of its precursors such as glutamic acid or to elevate its level by utilizing inhibitors of GABA catabolism such as dipropylacetic acid have been unsuccessful. Symptomatic control of the choreiform movements can be accomplished by the use of neuroleptic agents such as haloperidol and chlorpromazine. Recently it has been demonstrated that choline chloride given in dosages of up to 20 grams a day can ameliorate the choreiform movements to a considerable extent without the attendant rigidity occurring with the use of neuroleptic agents. Utilizing these drugs combined with supervision of the patient's daily activities allows for management at home during the early stages of the disorder. However, as the disease advances, confinement to a psychiatric facility becomes necessary. Of equal importance to treatment of the patient is appropriate genetic counseling of family members. They should be given a comprehensive understanding of the disease, their own risks as to inheritance as well as those of their children, and the value of predictive tests. In regard to such tests, none have been fully validated which permit detection of the disorder prior to development of symptoms.

Barbeau, A., Chase, T. N., and Paulson, G. W. (eds.): Huntington's chorea 1872–1972. Adv. Neurol., 1, 1973.
Bird, E. D., and Iversen, L. L.: Huntington's chorea: Post-mortem measurement of glutamic acid decarboxylase, choline acetyl transferase and dopamine in basal ganglia. Brain, 97:457, 1974.
Growdon, J. H., Cohen, E. L., and Wurtman, R. J.: Huntington's disease: Clinical and chemical effects of choline administration. Ann. Neurol., 1:418, 1977.
Paulson, G. W.: Predictive tests in Huntington's disease. *In* Yahr, M. D. (ed.): The Basal Ganglia. New York, Raven Press, 1976, pp. 317–329.

277.4.   SENILE CHOREA

Infrequently, choreiform movements are encountered as an isolated symptom in persons above 60 years of age. As a rule, the movements are mild and may involve the limbs on one side of the body or bilaterally.

Involuntary complex movements of the face, mouth, and tongue may occur, in association with limb movements or as the only manifestation of this disorder. No associated mental disturbance occurs in such patients, and no family history indicative of Huntington's chorea can be obtained. In many instances the symptoms come on abruptly, are unilateral, and show little or no progression. This has suggested an underlying vascular lesion, which may be found in an exceptional case. More often than not the pathologic findings are similar to those of Huntington's chorea insofar as involvement of the caudate nucleus is concerned, but the cerebral cortex is spared. This has led to the contrary consideration that these cases are a variant of Huntington's chorea occurring sporadically. Probably this form of chorea has several causes. As a rule, the symptoms are mild and the course benign so that therapeutic considerations are unimportant.

Martin, J. P.: Hemichorea resulting from local lesions of the brain. Brain, 50:637, 1927.
Weiner, W. J., and Klawans, H. L., Jr.: Lingual-facial-buccal movements in the elderly. II. Pathogenesis and relationship to senile chorea. J. Am. Geriat. Soc., 21:318, 1973.

278.   OTHER EXTRAPYRAMIDAL DISORDERS

278.1.   TICS
(Habit Spasms)
Melvin D. Yahr

A tic is a sudden, abrupt, rapid, purposeless, involuntary contraction of a muscle or group of functionally related muscles. Usually an irregular sequence of such contractions occurs that may result in eye blinking, head shaking, shrugging of the shoulder, or any sudden gesture of limbs or face. Tics may be voluntarily controlled for brief intervals, but such a conscious effort is usually followed by more intense and frequent contractions. Many persons experience minor transitory tic phenomena under periods of stress that are of no consequence. More persistent, sustained, and gross movements may be related to particular personality disturbances, and may be amenable to psychotherapy. In some instances tics have occurred during the acute phase of encephalitis; these are thought to be an expression of extrapyramidal dysfunction. Tics in younger patients must be differentiated from chorea. Their patterned, predictable, and stereotyped character makes this distinction.

An unusual form of generalized tic (*maladie des tics, Gilles de la Tourette's disease*) involving facial twitching, continuous gestures associated with echolalia, foul language, and obsessional ideas is occasionally encountered in childhood. Although at onset it may be difficult to differentiate simple tic phenomena from Tourette's disease, the progressive nature and development of associated symptoms make the diagnosis of the latter apparent. A number of reports have appeared indicating that haloperidol (Haldol) in divided dosage of 6 to 20 mg a day is effective both in reducing the movement disorder and in overcoming the unfortunate verbal outbursts.

Bruun, R. D., Shapiro, A. K., Shapiro, E., Sweet, R., Wayne, H., and Solomon, G. E.: A follow-up of 78 patients with Gilles de la Tourette's syndrome. Am. J. Psychiatry, 133:8, 1976.

Sweet, R. D., Solomon, G. E., Wayne, H., Shapiro, E., and Shapiro, A. K.: Neurological features of Gilles de la Tourette's syndrome. J. Neurol. Neurosurg. Psychiatry, 36:1, 1973.

278.2.   ATHETOSIS
(Mobile Spasms)
Melvin D. Yahr

This involuntary movement disorder is most frequently encountered in early infancy. Although in some respects it resembles chorea and although there are, in fact, transitional forms (so-called choreoathetosis), the athetotic movements are distinguishable by being slower, coarser, and more writhing. They occur when pathologic conditions involve the basal ganglia, primarily the pallidum, as well as additional motor pathways such as the corticospinal tract. Athetosis is most often found in the heterogeneous group of conditions now lumped together under the term "cerebral palsy" (CP). More often than not, patients with cerebral palsy have marked alteration in muscle tone consisting of a combination of spasticity and rigidity. Their extrapyramidal movements may be widespread or limited and encompass a wide variety of dyskinetic phenomena. Congenital defects, anoxia or trauma at birth, and other degenerative conditions have all been implicated. Some attempt has been made to identify specific entities based on clinicopathologic correlations. One such is athetosis simplex or status marmoratus. Cases of this disorder, which exemplifies all of the features of athetosis, show at autopsy a distinctive marbled appearance of the basal ganglia, the result of an abnormal overgrowth of myelin sheaths and increased numbers of glial cells. The cause of this morphologic abnormality is unknown. Other cases have been grouped together in which the prime pathologic change is cell loss and failure of myelin sheath formation in the region of the basal ganglia — so-called status dysmyelination. Still other cases have been encountered in which abnormal deposits of pigments occur or one of the lipoidoses or other storage diseases is found with the predominant clinical picture of athetotic movements. Athetosis is infrequently encountered in adult life, but when it is, tumors, vascular insufficiency, or malformations and the effects of toxic agents have been found in the region of the basal ganglia.

Typical athetosis possesses the following features in varying degrees. One or both sides of the body are involved. The movements involve the upper limbs to a greater extent than the lower and primarily in their distal segments. The muscles innervated by the cranial nerves are invariably involved so that facial grimacing, writhing movements of the tongue, and disturbances in articulation and swallowing are encountered. Abnormal postures of the limbs are assumed. In the upper extremities, these consist of adduction and internal rotation at the shoulder, semiflexion at the elbow, flexion of wrist and metacarpal phalangeal joints, and extension at interphalangeal joints. In the lower limbs the foot is maintained in internal rotation and plantar flexion with dorsiflexion of the toes. Superimposed on these abnormal postures are the athetotic movements described above. Muscle tone is increased during movement but is hypotonic during relaxation, and some degree of weakness is usually found. The reflexes may be hyperactive, with abnormal toe responses. In many instances some degree of intellectual impairment may be found.

The abnormal movements and postural abnormalities are distinctive enough to make this condition readily recognizable. The age at onset, the admixture of other neurologic abnormalities, and the manner in which the symptoms progress identify the disease. Since most instances of athetosis appear in early infancy, before one year of age, diseases of the perinatal period are considered primarily. Athetosis occurring in later childhood or adult life may be a part of other extrapyramidal disorders, such as dystonia, chorea, or hepatolenticular degeneration. Less frequently athetosis is a manifestation of a wide spectrum of neurologic disorders already mentioned in which the pallidum is coincidentally involved.

There is no specific therapy for the relief of athetosis. The use of anticholinergic agents as indicated in Ch. 274.4 may decrease the intensity of the movements. Thalamotomy has on occasion afforded some degree of relief, but one is hesitant to advocate this surgical procedure on a nervous system already extensively damaged by a variety of pathologic processes.

Courville, C. B.: Structural basis of athetosis in cerebral palsied children. Arch. Pediat., 78:461, 1961.

Mettler, F. A., and Stern, G.: On the patho-physiology of athetosis. J. Nerv. Ment. Dis., 135:138, 1962.

Narabayashi, H., and Nakamura, R.: Clinical picture of cerebral palsy in neurological understanding. Confin. Neurol., 34:7, 1972.

278.3.   DYSTONIA MUSCULORUM DEFORMANS
(Torsion Dystonia)
Melvin D. Yahr

The torsion dystonias comprise a group of movement disorders characterized by intense, irregular, sustained torsion spasms of the musculature, with resultant marked abnormalities of bodily posture. The dystonic movements may involve any or all of the musculature, but have a predilection for the trunk and shoulder and pelvic girdles. Although the site and underlying mechanisms by which symptoms are produced are unknown, sufficient evidence exists to indicate that they arise from dysfunction within the basal ganglia complex. In this regard a biochemical abnormality is suspected, because dystonic reactions may be induced by pharmacologic agents such as the phenothiazines and levodopa which affect striatal amine functions.

Based on genetic, clinical, and presumed causative factors, several forms may be recognized. In general, they fall into two categories: the symptomatic or acquired and the idiopathic or hereditary. The latter has a varied type of inheritance, being either autosomal recessive or autosomal dominant. Symptomatic dystonic movements occur with hepatolenticular degeneration, postencephalitic parkinsonism, tumors, or other diseases involving the basal ganglia. Morphologic changes indicative of these disease processes are found within one or another of the basal ganglia structures. In the idiopathic form no consistent morphologic abnormalities have been defined.

The autosomal recessive form is found most often in Ashkenazic Jews, beginning between the ages of 5 and 15 years. Its onset is variable but most frequently begins with intermittent spasmodic inversion of the foot, so that on walking the child finds difficulty in placing the heel on the ground. Bizarre stepping or a bowing gait may be noted when the dystonic movements affect the more proximal muscles of the leg or the spine. As the movements become more intense and the proximal musculature is more prominently involved, lordosis and tortipelvis appear. If the muscles of the neck and shoulder girdle are involved, torticollis is an early finding. Facial grimacing and difficulties in speech become evident as the muscles subserving these functions become involved. The continuous spasms over a period of time result in marked distortions of the body of a degree rarely seen in any other disease process. Although muscle tone and power appear to be normal, the involuntary movements interfere with function to such a degree as to make them useless. No changes in the deep tendon reflexes occur, and mentation remains normal.

The autosomal dominant form has its onset in early adult life and generally involves the axial musculature, with torticollis a frequent presenting symptom. In contrast to the recessive form, it remains more restricted in the regions of the body involved and is more slowly progressive. Recently it has been demonstrated that plasma dopamine beta hydroxylase activity is markedly elevated in the dominant form. This finding is strictly empiric, and although it is helpful in classification of the disease, neither the physiologic nor the biochemical significance of this finding has been elucidated.

In its early stages dystonia musculorum deformans must be differentiated from other movement disorders in which dystonic phenomena may occur. The history and physical findings exclude hepatolenticular degeneration and epidemic encephalitis. The age at onset and the involvement of proximal musculature in the movements are enough to differentiate it from athetosis. Chorea is characterized by movements more rapid and of shorter duration than those of dystonia. Hysteria is often a consideration; if it is not positively established by the personality characteristics of the patient, the course of the disease will soon suggest the correct diagnosis.

There is extreme variability in the rate of progression and eventual disability of both forms of the genetically determined disorder. In their early phases there may be complete remission of symptoms or lack of progression of initial symptoms for intervals of up to five years. Because the natural history is subject to wide variations, evaluation of the effects of treatment is difficult. Dystonic movements have been effectively controlled for varying periods of time by drugs and surgical intervention. Drugs which have proved useful are those which produce a degree of muscle relaxation, such as the benzodiazepines (diazepam [Valium], 15 to 30 mg per day, and clonazepam [Clonopin], 1.5 to 3 mg per day); and agents capable of inducing a degree of pseudoparkinsonism, such as the phenothiazines (chlorpromazine, 25 to 100 mg per day), butyrophenones (haloperidol, 6 to 10 mg per day), and carbamazepine (Tegretol,

800 to 1200 mg per day), which reputedly depresses neuronal activity in the thalamic nuclei. In mild cases a combination of these drugs with general supportive psychotherapeutic measures may be enough to control the patients' symptoms for years. Stereotactic thalamotomy has been reported to benefit patients for extended periods of time; however, it does require rather extensive bilateral lesions of the ventral lateral nuclei of the thalamus, which carries the risk of additional neurologic deficit, particularly speech disturbance. Attempts to utilize biofeedback mechanisms are of too recent origin to be assessed for value in this disorder.

Denny-Brown, D. E.: The nature of dystonia. Bull. N.Y. Acad. Med., 41:858, 1965.
Eldridge, R.: The torsion dystonias: Literature review and genetic and clinical studies. Neurology, 20(Part 2):1, 1970.
Marsden, C. D.: Dystonia: The spectrum of the disease. Res. Publ. Assoc. Res. Nerv. Ment. Dis., 55:351, 1976.

278.4.   SPASMODIC TORTICOLLIS
Melvin D. Yahr

The restriction of dyskinetic movements to neck muscles so that abnormal postures of the head result is the distinguishing characteristic of this symptom complex. Involuntary activity involves the sternocleidomastoids, trapezius, and scalenus muscles in sustained contractions that result in slow, twisting, turning movements of the head (torticollis) or less often forward flexion (anterocollis) or forceful extension (retrocollis). In most instances there is bilateral involvement, and the resultant postural deformity is maintained for varying lengths of time. The muscles of the neck appear under tension, and the continual muscular activity may lead to some degree of hypertrophy, especially evident in the sternocleidomastoid. Similar activity may spread to facial and brachial musculature. The amount of active motion or static postural deformity is extremely variable.

Spasmodic torticollis has variably been described as a psychogenic disorder, a fragment of dystonia musculorum deformans, or a compensatory postural defect in persons with congenital ocular muscle imbalance or defects of the cervical spine or musculature. In some instances it has occurred as part of a wide spectrum of extrapyramidal disorders that follow encephalitis lethargica. There is no information at present regarding either its pathophysiology or pathology.

The disorder has been encountered at all ages, but most frequently makes its appearance during the third to sixth decades of life. The course is extremely variable, being transitory and remitting after a few months in some patients and relentlessly progressive and leading to incapacity in others. Some cases reach a static phase in which movements cease or are minimal, and a minor postural deformity of the head persists.

The evaluation of this condition includes a search for ocular and vertebral signs, major psychiatric disturbances, and other neurologic conditions with which it may be associated. Definable conditions account for only a small percentage of cases. In most, no known cause is uncovered.

There is no specific therapy for torticollis except when an underlying correctable disease process is found. Many measures have been recommended to ameliorate the symptoms. Sensory biofeedback techniques have been utilized with some success. Of the number of pharmacologic agents used, the benzodiazepines, including diazepam (Valium), 15 to 30 mg per day, and clonazepam (Clonopin), 1.5 to 3 mg per day, as well as haloperidol (Haldol), 6 to 10 mg per day, have been reported effective in some patients. In those more severely affected, a variety of surgical measures have been attempted with inconsistent results. Denervation of the affected muscles by section of the anterior cervical root and/or the spinal accessory nerve has been utilized. Although the movements decrease on the operated side, they frequently recur in the contralateral group of muscles. Bilateral procedures may result in extensive disability. Although bilateral thalamotomy has been performed with reported improvement, one is hesitant to recommend a procedure of this magnitude except in extreme situations. A procedure involving iontophoresis of saline into the middle ear, which presumably suppresses labyrinthine function unilaterally, has produced encouraging results in one series.

Gilbert, G. J.: The medical treatment of spasmodic torticollis. Arch. Neurol., 27:503, 1972.

Herz, E., and Glaser, G. H.: Spasmodic torticollis. Clinical evaluation. Arch. Neurol. Psychiatry, 61:227, 1949.

Korein, J., and Brudny, J.: Integrated EMG feedback in the management of spasmodic torticollis and focal dystonia: A prospective study of 80 patients. In Yahr, M. D. (ed.): The Basal Ganglia. New York, Raven Press, 1976, pp. 385–426.

278.5. HEMIBALLISM

Melvin D. Yahr

This rather violent involuntary movement occurs when lesions involve the contralateral subthalamic nucleus, the corpus Luysii. Although a variety of pathologic processes such as tumor and infectious diseases have been found as underlying causes, most are a result of vascular lesions, either hemorrhagic or occlusive. In consequence, they are encountered in older patients, sometimes after a transitory hemiparesis. The event leading to the onset of this movement disorder often is an acute cerebrovascular accident with weakness and/or sensory deficit. As the neurologic signs clear or at a variable interval afterward, the ballistic movements begin. The movements do not occur during sleep, are localized to one side of the body, and involve the limbs in a forceful throwing movement, a result of almost continuous activity of the proximal musculature. Initially, their violence may exhaust and incapacitate the patient to such an extent that death may ensue. However, in most instances, the initial intensity decreases gradually so that they become tolerable, and in approximately six to eight weeks the movements stop spontaneously. Surgical measures, such as thalamotomy, are rarely needed for control. In this regard, it is interesting to note that hemiballism has followed attempted thalamotomy for other extrapyramidal disorders when poor localization for lesion placement has occurred. In such instances, the surgeon has inadvertently placed a lesion in the region of the corpus Luysii.

Carpenter, M. B.: Ballism associated with partial destruction of the subthalamic nucleus of Luys. Neurology, 5:479, 1955.

Hyland, H. H., and Forman, D. M.: Progress in hemiballismus. Neurology, 7:381, 1957.

Martin, P. J., and McCaul, I. R.: Acute hemiballism treated by ventrolateral thalamolysis. Brain, 82:104, 1959.

278.6. IDIOPATHIC AUTONOMIC INSUFFICIENCY

(Idiopathic Orthostatic Hypotension, Shy-Drager Syndrome)

Ira B. Black

DEFINITION. Idiopathic autonomic insufficiency is a rare degenerative disorder of unknown etiology which strikes during middle age, causing progressive autonomic dysfunction; severe debility or death may occur within 5 to 15 years of onset. Associated extrapyramidal abnormalities and lesions of pigmented brain nuclei may play a prominent role in the genesis of symptoms.

PATHOGENESIS AND PATHOLOGY. Histologic examination at autopsy has disclosed degenerative changes in autonomic ganglia in the periphery, and in the preganglionic, intermediolateral cell column in the spinal cord. In the brain, virtually all cranial nerve nuclei may undergo degeneration, and similar changes may occur in the hypothalamus, nigrostriatal system, pontine nuclei, and globus pallidus. Postmortem biochemical studies have revealed marked depression of catecholamine biosynthetic enzyme activities in sympathetic ganglia and in central noradrenergic neurons of the nucleus locus ceruleus; the substantia nigra may be similarly affected in patients with extrapyramidal symptoms. More specifically, dopamine-β-hydroxylase, which converts dopamine to norepinephrine, is decreased in sympathetic ganglia, whereas tyrosine hydroxylase, the rate-limiting enzyme in catecholamine biosynthesis, is decreased in locus ceruleus. In parkinsonian patients, tyrosine hydroxylase may be depressed in substantia nigra.

The pathogenesis of the disease is unclear. A number of observations suggest that preganglionic neuronal dysfunction may be an early, perhaps primary, event. First, degeneration of preganglionic neurons may be prominent in many patients. Second, although basal levels of plasma norepinephrine may be normal in some patients, suggesting that postsynaptic adrenergic neurons are functional, stress fails to cause the normal elevation of plasma norepinephrine, suggesting dysfunction of central autonomic pathways. Lastly, indirect-acting drugs such as tyramine, which cause sympathetic activation by releasing endogenous norepinephrine, may exert normal effects in patients with obvious sympathetic abnormalities. However, more recent studies indicate that preganglionic disease may not be *the* primary phenomenon in all cases. Thus the preganglionic intermediolateral column neurons may be histologically normal in the disease. The preganglionic cholinergic terminals in sympathetic ganglia may be biochemically normal with demonstrable postganglionic histologic and biochemical lesions. Finally, the pattern of enzyme deficits in adrenergic neurons of sympathetic ganglia is not entirely consistent with trans-synaptic dysfunction. It is possible that several different subpopulations are now included in this disease category, and that the respective pathogeneses differ.

Indeed, several observers have suggested that at least two entities may comprise idiopathic autonomic insufficiency. The first may consist of autonomic insufficiency alone, whereas the second may be characterized by autonomic insufficiency in association with a variety of neurologic signs, including movement disorders resembling Parkinson's disease. The great degree of clinical overlap between these groups, however, is also consistent with the existence of a broad continuum rather than distinct entities.

CLINICAL MANIFESTATIONS. Symptoms of autonomic dysfunction predominate early in the course. Characteristically, initial difficulties consist of sexual impotence, urinary hesitancy, urgency, or incontinence, and/or anhidrosis. These early symptoms are frequently unrecognized and undiagnosed. Within months to years, the hallmark of the disorder, postural hypotension, appears. This may be manifested as dizziness, giddiness, or frank syncope upon standing. Less frequently, patients complain of generalized weakness, cervico-occipital discomfort, or leg weakness upon standing. Attendant autonomic symptoms, including intermittent diplopia, dysphagia, and diarrhea, fecal incontinence, or constipation, may also occur. As the disease progresses, a variety of movement disorders may appear. A parkinsonian disorder, consisting of bradykinesia, coarse tremor, and rigidity, is common, and tends to progress inexorably. Myoclonus, gait disturbance, and signs of olivopontocerebellar dysfunction may also occur.

Physical signs parallel the aforementioned symptoms and include evidence of autonomic dysfunction. Orthostatic hypotension, greater than a 30/20 mm Hg fall in blood pressure upon assumption of the erect position, constitutes the hallmark sign. Other signs of possible autonomic-cardiovascular dysfunction include absence of sinus arrhythmia, absence of increased heart rate upon standing, and absence of the normal overshoot in diastolic pressure during phase IV of the Valsalva maneuver. In addition, autonomic dysfunction may manifest as Horner's syndrome or as anhidrosis even with elevated ambient temperature, as well as the bladder and bowel dysfunction described above. Neurologic examination may reveal signs indistinguishable from those of Parkinson's disease. Cerebellar ataxia, dysmetria, and dysdiadochokinesia may also be elicited. Muscle wasting, fasciculation, and extensor plantar responses have been observed.

A variety of clinical laboratory tests may be employed to evaluate autonomic function, and only the simplest will be delineated here. In addition to the bedside examinations described above, other observations may be helpful. *Miosis* in response to ocular administration of dilute solutions of methacholine, or *mydriasis* after instillation of dilute epinephrine, suggests respective parasympathetic or sympathetic denervation supersensitivity. On the other hand, absence of mydriasis after ocular instillation of cocaine or hydroxyamphetamine suggests that endogenous norepinephrine stores are defective. Absence of sweating with elevation of the ambient temperature and absence of the axon reflex after intradermal histamine suggest denervation of cutaneous structures. The presence of an abnormally accentuated blood pressure response to the intravenous infusion of norepinephrine is consistent with widespread denervation supersensitivity. Vagal dysfunction may be manifested by absence of sinus arrhythmia, absence of bradycardia after carotid sinus massage, absence of increased gastric acidity after insulin hypoglycemia, and altered gastrointestinal motility with retention of barium in the small bowel during x-ray studies.

DIFFERENTIAL DIAGNOSIS. Orthostatic hypotension itself may accompany intravascular hypovolemia (as with massive hemorrhage or adrenal insufficiency), vasodepressor syncope, acute cardiac failure from a variety of causes, familial hyperbradykininism, and intracranial posterior fossa mass or vascular lesions. However, in these conditions other signs of autonomic dysfunction are absent. On the other hand, autonomic insufficiency, including orthostatic hypotension, may occur with any disease that alters peripheral or central autonomic pathways. Many disorders conform to this description. A variety of peripheral neuropathies may be accompanied by dysautonomia, including the acute Guillain-Barré syndrome, the chronic neuropathies of diabetes mellitus, amyloidosis, Wernicke's disease and porphyria, and the congenital Riley-Day syndrome. Ganglion dysfunction may result from ingestion of ganglioplegic agents. Tabes dorsalis is commonly accompanied by autonomic signs. Autonomic dysfunction may result from interruption of descending pathways in the spinal cord, as observed with syringomyelia, trauma, or spinal tumor. Pontine hemorrhage may interrupt descending sympathetic pathways in the brainstem, thereby causing sympathetic dysfunction. However, differentiation from these diseases is easily accomplished with suitable history, examination, and laboratory tests. For example, peripheral neuropathies characteristically produce distal sensory, and often motor, impairment.

COURSE AND TREATMENT. Although treatment does not alter the underlying pathologic process, it may allow an otherwise bedridden invalid to lead a virtually normal life. Orthostatic hypotension may be treated with a variety of measures, dictated by the severity of the problem. The first line of defense consists of antigravity stockings, which prevent pooling of blood in the lower extremities upon standing. In moderately severe cases, intravascular volume expansion may be achieved by using the mineralocorticoid 9-α-fluorocortisone and sodium chloride, with potassium supplementation. In severe cases, oral sympathomimetic agents, including ephedrine or hydroxyamphetamine, may be added. Such combination therapy is effective in virtually all cases. Recent work suggests that indomethacin may be effective in selected patients for the treatment of orthostatic hypotension. The use of monoamine oxidase inhibitors may be potentially hazardous in those patients who are subject to denervation supersensitivity. Although the diet may be rigorously regulated in the hospital setting, this is rarely possible on an outpatient basis. For example, such foods as cheese, broad beans, Chianti, raisins, bananas, and aged or smoked meat contain significant quantities of vasoactive amines. Inadvertent ingestion of microgram quantities of vasoactive amines in the diet may result in alarming elevation of blood pressure in patients being treated with monoamine oxidase for widespread sympathetic denervation.

Parkinsonian signs and symptoms may be successfully treated with L-dopa and the customary anticholinergic agents.

Bannister, R., and Oppenheimer, D. R.: Degenerative diseases of the nervous system associated with autonomic failure. Brain, 95:457, 1972.

Black, I. B., and Petito, C. K.: Catecholamine enzymes in the degenerative neurological disease idiopathic orthostatic hypotension. Science, 192:910, 1976.

Bradbury, S., and Eggleston, C.: Postural hypotension: A report of three cases. Am. Heart J., 1:73, 1925.

Shy, G. M., and Drager, G. A.: A neurological syndrome associated with orthostatic hypotension. Arch. Neurol., 2:511, 1960.

Ziegler, M. G., Lake, C. R., and Kopin, I. J.: The sympathetic-nervous-system defect in primary orthostatic hypotension. N. Engl. J. Med., 296:293, 1977.

Section Twelve INHERITED DEGENERATIVE DISEASES OF THE NERVOUS SYSTEM

Roger N. Rosenberg

279. INTRODUCTION

The classic eponymic neurologic diseases discussed in this section produce characteristic pathologic changes in specific nuclei and fiber tracts in brain, spinal cord, and peripheral nerve. The disorders are usually progressive and symmetrical in their pathologic and clinical expression and often have a clear genetic basis of inheritance or suggestion of familial involvement. The disorders involve specific regions or systems of the nervous system such as cerebellar nuclei and fiber tracts or the corticospinal or extrapyramidal motor system, resulting in specific neurologic symptoms and signs referred to as system degenerations.

Gowers in 1902 referred to these inherited degenerative diseases as abiotrophies. This term implies the occurrence of neurologic disease resulting from an impairment in the metabolic state of the brain, spinal cord, or peripheral nerve. Recently, as discussed below, enzyme deficiencies, chromosomal breaks, specific immunologic defects, abnormalities in nerve growth factor, and slow latent viral-like infections of the brain have been identified as specific etiologic bases for some of these abiotrophies.

It is of great interest and importance that in most of the inherited degenerative disorders to be discussed the primary impact of disease involves the neuron, changes produced in astrocytes and oligodendrocytes being presumably of a reactive and secondary nature. Intensive research is currently underway in many laboratories concerning most of the disorders mentioned here. The past decade has witnessed an exponential increase in our knowledge concerning the basic enzyme defects and metabolic consequences of many autosomal recessive disorders in the categories of the gangliosidoses, leukodystrophies, mucopolysaccharidoses, glycogenoses, and heavy metal storage disorders; these will be discussed in greater detail in other chapters. Using these autosomal recessive diseases as models, it is hoped that the basic molecular defect in several autosomal dominant system degenerations discussed in the following chapters, such as Huntington's disease, olivopontocerebellar atrophy, striatonigral degeneration, nigrospinodentatal degeneration, tuberous sclerosis, and neurofibromatosis, will be clarified.

280. STRIATONIGRAL DEGENERATION

Striatonigral degeneration (Joseph's disease) is a rare disease of the nervous system inherited as an autoso-

mal dominant disorder in persons of Portuguese or Azorian ancestry. A nongenetic form of striatonigral degeneration also has been described by van der Eecken, Adams, and van Bogart. Patients with this form are diagnosed clinically as having Parkinson's disease, but the disease is different neuropathologically in that there is bilateral degeneration of the corpus striatum and substantia nigra, particularly the zona compacta portion. No cause has been found in any of the cases. Rosenberg, Nyhan, Bay, and Shore described a family of Portuguese ancestry with autosomal dominant striatonigral degeneration numbering 329 persons in eight generations, and Romanul et al. reported in another family of Portuguese-Azorian ancestry the presence of a striatonigral degeneration in a clinical setting of autosomal dominant disease with parkinsonism and polyneuropathy. No genetic link is present between these two families, who in fact come from separate and distant Azorian islands.

PATHOLOGY. The major pathologic findings in one deceased family member are a severe loss of neurons and glial replacement in the corpus striatum and a severe loss of neurons in the zona compacta portion of the substantia nigra. There is also a moderate loss of neurons in the dentate nucleus of the cerebellum and in the nucleus ruber of the midbrain. The cerebellum, cerebellar peduncles, inferior olives, corticospinal tracts in the brainstem, and basis pontis do not show gross atrophy. The cerebellar and frontal cerebral cortex appears normal histologically. There is no evidence of demyelination in the cerebellum, its peduncles, or the brainstem. Although the putamen shows significant neuronal loss, there is no increased pigmentation characteristic of the nongenetic forms of the striatonigral degenerations.

CLINICAL MANIFESTATIONS. The main neurologic findings include extremity weakness and spasticity of all extremities, especially the legs, often with associated dystonia of the face, neck, trunk, and extremities. Patellar and ankle clonus are common, as are extensor plantar responses. The gait is slow and stiff, with a slight increase in base and lurching from side to side due to spasticity. Affected persons have no truncal titubation. Pharyngeal weakness and spasticity cause difficulty with speech and swallowing. Of note are prominent horizontal and vertical nystagmus, the loss of the fast saccadic eye movements, hypermetric and hypometric saccades, and impairment of vertical gaze. Facial fasciculations, facial myokymia, and lingual fasciculations without atrophy are common and early manifestations.

The disorder is inherited as an autosomal dominant trait, the mean age of onset of symptoms in affected members examined being 25 years. Neurologic deficits increase progressively and result in death from debilitation within 15 years of onset. Patients retain full intellectual function, and the only significant involuntary movements are dystonia and tremor at rest in some affected members.

DIAGNOSIS. Autosomal dominant striatonigral degeneration should be considered in persons with an appropriate family history developing progressive dystonia, rigidity and spasticity of pharynx, trunk, and extremities, and associated hyperreflexia, clonus, and extensor plantar responses during the first or second decade. The entity is distinguished from Huntington's disease by the preservation of intellect and the absence of choreoathetosis. Dystonia musculorum deformans can be distinguished by the prominence of spasticity and the characteristic eye findings present in the striatonigral degenerations. The entity may be related to the nigrospinodentatal degeneration described by Woods and Schaumburg, which is also expressed as an autosomal dominant disorder producing rigidity and spasticity. However, the major pathology in their patients was in the dentate nuclei, the spinocerebellar tracts, and the middle cerebellar peduncle. Recent clinical and epidemiologic evidence indicates that this genetic disease can have a wide spectrum, and some patients in large families develop distal extremity atrophy, areflexia, distal sensory loss, hypotonia, and cerebellar truncal and extremity ataxia. Assays of the cerebrospinal fluid (CSF) for homovanillic acid are of value, as the mean concentration of this metabolite of dopamine in the CSF of five affected persons was 15.3 ng per milliliter as compared to a control value of 43.4 ng per milliliter.

281. MOTOR NEURON DISEASES

281.1. INTRODUCTION

The term motor neuron disease refers to a group of chronic neurologic disorders that selectively affect with varying combination and rapidity the anterior horn cells of the spinal cord and lower brainstem, plus, in some cases, those large motor neurons of the cerebral cortex that give rise to the corticospinal tract. Clinically significant sensory change or cerebellar dysfunction is absent in all instances. Cases in which upper motor neuron changes are prominent in addition to muscle fasciculation, atrophy, and weakness are called *amyotrophic lateral sclerosis* (ALS). *Progressive bulbar palsy* is a variant of ALS that produces relatively rapidly advancing upper and lower motor neuron involvement of the muscles of the jaw, pharynx, and tongue. Cases lacking signs of upper motor neuron disease and producing only a slow, progressive muscle wasting and weakness often are termed *progressive muscular atrophy* (PMA). A variety of clinical subtypes of PMA occur, some of which can produce restricted motor involvement that progresses extremely slowly over a period of many years. *Werdnig-Hoffmann disease* of infancy and young children and the *Wohlfart-Kugelberg-Welander disease* of older children and adolescents represent other variants of motor neuron disease. "Primary lateral sclerosis" is a nondisease. The ostensible condition included progressive spasticity but no lower motor neuron changes, and was at one time linked to the motor neuron diseases.

Subsequent studies have shown that such signs in fact always are attributable to other causes such as disseminated sclerosis, spinal cord compression, other degenerative disorders, or high spinal neoplasms.

281.2. AMYOTROPHIC LATERAL SCLEROSIS

Amyotrophic lateral sclerosis (ALS) can first affect bulbar muscles, a single limb, the extremities on one side of the body, the lower or upper extremities symmetrically, or all four limbs simultaneously, depending upon the individual case. The disorder occurs mainly in the fifth, sixth, and seventh decades of life and runs a progressive course lasting from as short as 18 to 24 months to as long as about seven years. The bulbar form runs a more malignant course. ALS usually occurs sporadically, but familial groupings of amyotrophic lateral sclerosis syndromes have occurred, indicating either a genetic predisposition for disease or common exposure to an unknown causative agent. Familial cases tend to come on younger and progress more rapidly than do cases in older adults. Recently Oldstone and associates have reported finding immune complexes associated with the mesangium of the renal glomerulus and basement membrane in patients with rapidly progressive but otherwise typical motor neuron disease. The implication in this instance is that motor neuron disease may be an autoimmune disorder. It also has been suggested that the disorder may be due to a slow latent viral infection such as a mutated poliovirus. Several reports cite the subsequent occurrence of motor neuron disease during late adulthood in patients having poliomyelitis in childhood. Despite these clues, the precise mechanism and cause of the motor neuron disorders is currently not known.

PATHOLOGY. The neuropathologic findings in ALS consist of degenerative changes and loss of the Betz cells in layers 3 and 5 of the precentral cerebral cortex, Brodmann's areas 4 and 6. These are absent in the more benign cases of progressive muscular atrophy. Neuronal loss also occurs in the motor cranial nuclei and the motor neurons in the anterior horns of the spinal cord. There are no characteristic features associated with the neuronal loss, and the musculature innervated by the affected motor cranial nuclei and anterior horn cells undergoes neurogenic atrophy as a result of denervation.

CLINICAL MANIFESTATIONS. ALS produces a variety of clinical patterns, all of which show muscle weakness and wasting but which vary in their rate of progression, the distribution of the major weakness, and the rapidity with which signs of upper motor neuron dysfunction occur. Patients develop a slowly progressive impairment of motor function affecting distal more than proximal structures, as evidenced by muscle atrophy involving the intrinsic muscles of the hand. Over a period of six months to a year, the process results in symmetrical muscle atrophy involving the hands, forearms, and shoulder girdle muscles. The disease may develop quite asymmetrically in some patients. Prominent and early in most patients is the occurrence of fasciculations due to acute and widespread denervation of entire motor units. The patient may have muscle cramps, as well as, rarely, mild distal paresthesias. The deep tendon reflexes are usually preserved in the upper extremities in the early phase of disease. Signs of upper motor neuron involvement may develop at any time but almost always by the time muscle involvement has lasted as long as a year. These include spasticity, particularly in the lower extremities with associated hyperreflexia, clonus, and extensor plantar responses on one or both sides. Characteristically, the superficial abdominal reflexes and the cremasteric reflexes as well as the bladder and anal sphincters remain normal. Generalized fasciculations and muscle atrophy in most instances involve the lower extremities later than the upper. These combinations of upper and lower motor neuron deficits are characteristic of ALS. Occasionally, spasticity predominantly involves the pharynx, larynx, and extremities, and signs of muscular atrophy and fasciculations are hard to detect; but they are always there, at least by electrical testing. The loss of the gag reflex, pharyngeal paralysis, lingual atrophy and fasciculations, and diffuse extremity atrophy and fasciculations with reduced myotatic reflexes would indicate a severe bulbospinal variant of ALS (progressive muscular atrophy almost always spares the cranial nerves). Musculature innervated by the fifth, seventh, tenth, eleventh, and twelfth cranial motor nuclei is involved in the bulbar form of ALS, but the disease spares the extraocular muscles. Patients may show signs of emotional lability, but intellectual functions are preserved, even in the terminal phases of the disorder. The cerebrospinal fluid is normal. The presence of fasciculations and other changes of acute muscle denervation can be confirmed by electromyography (EMG). The motor nerve conduction velocities remain normal, however, even in the presence of severe atrophy, a finding that separates this disorder from the peripheral motor neuropathies, in which conduction velocities are reduced.

DIFFERENTIAL DIAGNOSIS. Primary muscle disease, peripheral nerve disorders, spinal cord compression, or tumors and conditions damaging the corticospinal tracts so as to produce spasticity all can at least superficially resemble ALS. None of these conditions, however, are able to imitate the characteristic combination of painless, diffuse neurogenic muscle impairment plus spasticity and absent sensory change that marks severe motor neuron disease. Muscle disease can be separated by changes in serum enzymes, EMG, and biopsy. Peripheral nerve disorders mostly produce sensory impairment. They do not cause fasciculation, and they do cause slowing of nerve electrical conduction velocity. Cervical spinal cord compression from spondylosis or tumor often causes pain, and usually produces a destructive combination of weakness and atrophy restricted to the arms, plus spasticity and sensory changes in the legs.

Multiple sclerosis can result in spasticity, but not muscular atrophy or fasciculation, and sensory changes are usual. Intracranial disorders can produce bilateral spasticity, but other signs of brain involvement usually easily distinguish the condition.

TREATMENT. This must be symptomatic and supportive, as there is no specific therapy.

281.3. WERDNIG-HOFFMANN DISEASE

Werdnig-Hoffmann disease, occurring in infancy and early childhood, presents as a progressive impairment of the motor system. The lower motor neuron is exclusively involved, including musculature innervated by motor cranial mclei and anterior horn cells of the spinal cord. Infants and young children may present with this syndrome at birth or in the first few months of life with diffuse flaccidity, muscular atrophy, muscle fasciculations, and reduced to absent myotatic reflexes with associated respiratory and swallowing difficulties. There may be prominent lingual fasciculations and atrophy in the first few months of life. A muscle biopsy indicates neurogenic atrophy, and the cerebrospinal fluid is entirely normal. Electromyography shows acute denervation with normal peripheral nerve conduction velocities. The disorder usually appears either sporadically or as an autosomal recessive genetic disorder. The cause is not known.

281.4. WOHLFART-KUGELBERG-WELANDER DISEASE

Wohlfart-Kugelberg-Welander disease is an autosomal recessive disorder in which symptoms begin during late childhood, adolescence, or early adulthood and include progressive proximal muscle atrophy, weakness, and fasciculations. It is very slowly progressive and is usually compatible with a life span into the third or fourth decade. Typical examples have been described in families in which other children have Werdnig-Hoffmann disease. Thus varying penetrance of a single gene mutation inherited in an autosomal recessive manner may produce either an aggressive form of motor neuron disease in childhood (Werdnig-Hoffmann disease) or a more benign form of motor neuron disease in later childhood and early adulthood (Wohlfart-Kugelberg-Welander disease). The onset in the first and second decades of life of proximal weakness and atrophy with fasciculations but with a very slow progression without evidence of upper motor neuron involvement separates this disorder from amyotrophic lateral sclerosis. The presence of denervation without the insertional irritability characteristic of polymyositis can be determined by electromyography. Both Wohlfart-Kugelberg-Welander disease and polymyositis may present with progressive proximal weakness and atrophy; if fasciculations are not prominent, electromyography and muscle biopsy are of important differentiating value. Neurogenic denervation can be identified in biopsied muscle, thus separating it from the acquired or inherited myopathies. The cause of the disorder is unknown, and specific therapy is not available.

282. SPINOCEREBELLAR DEGENERATIONS

282.1. INTRODUCTION

This term applies to a group of progressive degenerative disorders in which ataxia and dysmetria resulting from predominant involvement of the cerebellum and its pathways are combined to greater or lesser degrees, with impairment of other sensory and motor systems. All represent system degenerations, and many of the specific entities have a well established genetic basis. Although clinical signs of cerebellar involvement predominate, the extension of the disorders to involve other regions of the nervous system can produce more complex neurologic symptoms. The important and common inherited spinocerebellar degenerations include (1) Friedreich's ataxia; (2) Roussey-Lévy syndrome; (3) Bassen-Kornzweig syndrome, (4) Refsum's syndrome; (5) olivopontocerebellar degeneration; (6) Marie's ataxia; and (7) dyssynergia cerebellaris myoclonica.

As classified by Greenfield, the spinocerebellar degenerations can be grouped into predominant spinal forms, spinocerebellar forms, and cerebellar forms. Further subclassification exists in the olivopontocerebellar degenerations, with at least five subtypes identified by Konigsmark and Weiner with both autosomal dominant and autosomal recessive forms of inheritance. The spinocerebellar degenerations have common neuropathologic features from the peripheral nerve through the spinal cord and up to the cerebellum with its attendant connections. Although these disorders are well described both clinically and pathologically, only in Friedreich's syndrome, Refsum's disease, and the Bassen-Kornzweig syndrome do molecular insights exist into the cause. The similarity of neuropathologic findings in the Bassen-Kornzweig syndrome and Friedreich's syndrome despite very different molecular defects indicates the vulnerability of the spinocerebellar system to different chemical abnormalities as well as its limited neuropathologic response.

282.2. FRIEDREICH'S ATAXIA

This form of spinocerebellar degeneration begins in childhood and is mainly inherited as an autosomal recessive or dominant disorder. Sporadic cases presumably represent spontaneous mutations. Friedreich's ataxia comprises a syndrome including several subtypes with common clinical features and pathologic changes. Causes of Friedreich's syndrome include several inborn errors of metabolism, including disorders of lipids (phytanic acid storage disease, abetalipoproteinemia, moderate beta-galactosidase deficiencies, and juvenile arylsulfatase deficiency), diseases of oxidative metabolism (neuromuscular disorders with "ragged red" fibers and abnormalities of cytochrome B or of NADH oxidation), aminoacidurias (intermittent maple syrup urine disease, gamma-glutamylcysteinyl transferase deficiencies, and Hartnup disease) and the partial deficiency of hypoxanthineguanine phosphoribosyltransferase (HGPRT).

Recently Blass et al. have described children in whom pyruvate oxidation was low in muscles from 4 of 7 patients with Friedreich's syndrome, in 4 of 12 patients with other ataxias, and in 8 of 19 patients with familial or idiopathic neuropathies. In those studies the degree of pyruvate dehydrogenase complex activity correlated with the severity and rapidity of the spinocerebellar disease process. For example, patients with less than 15 per cent of normal pyruvate dehydrogenase activity but with normal oxoglutarate dehydrogenase generally had severe neurologic disease and lactic acidosis beginning in infancy. Severe deficiencies of both complexes have been described in one infant with severe disease. Several patients with 20 to 30 per cent of normal pyruvate dehydrogenase activity had a milder illness in which ataxia was the most prominent sign. The patients with Friedreich's syndrome had the mildest defect, with 40 to 50 per cent of normal pyruvate dehydrogenase activity together with 50 per cent of normal oxoglutarate dehydrogenase activity. Thus a defect in pyruvate oxidation must be considered as a biochemical basis for one form of Friedreich's syndrome, and the evaluation of appropriate patients should include measurement of pyruvate oxidation.

PATHOLOGY. Demyelination with secondary gliosis affects the spinocerebellar tracts, the lateral corticospinal tracts, the posterior columns, and the peripheral nerves. Neuronal loss involves the primary sensory neurons in dorsal root ganglia as well as the cells of Clarke's column which give rise to the spinocerebellar tracts. Less often, neuronal loss affects the anterior horns of the spinal cord and cell layers in the cerebellar cortex and deep cerebellar nuclei. A diffuse and major loss of myocardial fibers with subsequent replacement by fibrosis may occur in some patients.

CLINICAL MANIFESTATIONS. Truncal ataxia appears first with impairment of gait, poor coordination, and frequent falling. Gait problems may be the only sign of disease for many years, but eventually dysarthria and ataxia of arm and hand emerge. By the midpart to end of the second decade of life most patients require assistance in walking. Nystagmus is an early and prominent feature, as is the loss of fast saccadic eye movements. A few patients develop optic atrophy during the later stages of the disease. Progressive skeletal deformities include kyphoscoliosis, pes cavus, and, less consistently, a deformed and high arched palate. Distal sensory deficits, especially in the legs, develop after several years and include impairment in position sense and vibratory sensation as well as, less prominently, a reduction in pain and temperature perceptions. Additional expressions of motor dysfunction include extensor plantar responses with normal or reduced tone in trunk and extremities and absent deep tendon reflexes. Moderate weakness and the occurrence of atrophy of the extremities and occasional fasciculations are late developments. About half the patients develop cardiomegaly, murmurs, bundle branch block, T wave inversions, and complete heart block on electrocardiograms. Cardiopulmonary arrest and congestive heart failure may occur. A small percentage of patients are mentally retarded.

DIAGNOSIS. The presence in childhood or young adolescence of insidiously beginning and slowly progressing truncal and extremity ataxia, with dysarthria and subsequent nystagmus, extensor plantar responses, and areflexia, is typical. When one adds the findings of scoliosis, pes cavus, and proprioceptive and vibratory loss in the lower extremities, hardly any other diagnosis is possible. Motor nerve conduction velocities are normal in the common neurogenic form of the disorder, but electromyography may detect denervation potentials, especially in the legs. In the hypertrophic neuropathic form of Friedreich's syndrome, the motor nerve conduction velocities are slowed and the peripheral nerves may be palpably enlarged with demyelination noted in peripheral nerve biopsies. The cerebrospinal fluid protein is normal. Muscle biopsies often show neurogenic atrophy but are unnecessary for diagnosis. The electrocardiogram may contain abnormalities as recorded above and the chest roentgenogram may show cardiomegaly.

DIFFERENTIAL DIAGNOSIS. Diagnosis of Friedreich's syndrome is not difficult if the case meets the aforementioned criteria. Multiple sclerosis and subacute combined degeneration of the spinal cord caused by vitamin B$_{12}$ deficiency differ in both age of onset and clinical characteristics. Cerebellar or spinal tumors produce a more rapid course and, usually, pain. The *Roussy-Lévy syndrome* is inherited as an autosomal recessive trait characterized by onset in childhood of ataxia, areflexia, pes cavus–clubfoot deformity, and kyphoscoliosis. It differs from Friedreich's ataxia in sparing position and vibratory sensation and by the absence of extensor plantar responses as well as of nystagmus and dysarthria. The Roussy-Lévy syndrome may be an intermediate disorder between Friedreich's ataxia and Charcot-Marie-Tooth disease. Patients with *Refsum's disease* caused by elevated serum phytanate as a result of a defect in lipid alpha-oxidase can have a Friedreich-like ataxia but suffer the additional defects of optic atrophy, pigmentary retinal degeneration, ichthyosis, and deafness. Patients with the *Bassen-Kornzweig syndrome* have spinocerebellar signs but also prominent steatorrhea, abetalipoproteinemia, and acanthocytosis.

Hereditary spastic paraplegia expresses an autosomal dominant, recessive, or sex-linked recessive trait by the occurrence of peroneal muscular atrophy, skeletal deformities, nystagmus, and prominent spastic paraplegia. The syndrome overlaps with other forms of spinocerebellar degeneration in some families.

282.3.   OLIVOPONTOCEREBELLAR DEGENERATIONS

The olivopontocerebellar atrophies represent a group of disorders manifested clinically by progressive involvement of cerebellar functions and pathologically by a reduction in neurons in the inferior olivary nuclei of the medulla, the basis pontis, the cerebellar cortex, and the deep cerebellar nuclei.

PATHOLOGY. Grossly, atrophy involves the cerebellum, cerebellar peduncles, and basis pontis. Microscopically, Purkinje cells, granule cells of the cerebellar cortex, and neurons from the dentate nucleus and other deep cerebellar nuclei all are severely reduced. Ultrastructurally, biopsies from the cerebellar cortex of patients at various stages of disease disclose a variety of nonspecific abnormalities but also reveal crystalloid inclusions resembling paramyxovirus-like tubular structures. These latter imply that infectious agents may participate in the pathogenesis of some autosomal dominant olivopontocerebellar degenerations.

CLINICAL MANIFESTATIONS. Olivopontocerebellar atrophy has several variants whose principal clinical manifestations vary with the phenotype. Sporadically arising cases outnumber those with clinically evident familial histories, but the pathologic changes are similar. Clinically, essential features include the development in mid-adult life of progressive ataxia, dysarthria, dysmetria, dysdiadochokinesia, nystagmus, and loss of fast saccadic eye movements. Subsequently, patients develop spasticity, optic nerve atrophy, distal sensory involvement, and late intellectual dysfunction.

In general, truncal ataxia develops initially in the second or third decades of life, and extremity ataxia and dysmetria and prominent dysarthria follow within a decade. After several years, perhaps a third of affected patients show spasticity with associated hyperreflexia, clonus, and extensor plantar responses. Nystagmus, optic nerve atrophy, and loss of fast saccadic eye movements occur frequently. A fraction of the patients display the late occurrence of muscle atrophy with fasciculations, including the facial muscles, muscles of mastication, and lingual musculature. Palatal myoclonus is an uncommon but almost pathognomonic accompaniment when it occurs. Variations in the illness include sensory deficits in a distal distribution, intellectual deterioration, signs of extrapyramidal dysfunction, external ophthalmoplegia, and early visual loss.

The olivopontocerebellar degenerations described by Holmes, Sanger-Brown, and Marie represent phenotypic variants of this general class of disease. The syndrome of *Ramsay Hunt's dyssynergia cerebellaris myoclonica* is another rare variant beginning in childhood and includes prominent, progressive ataxia and myoclonic seizures inherited as an autosomal dominant trait.

DIAGNOSIS. The olivopontocerebellar atrophies are readily characterized by the development early in adult life of progressive symmetrical involvement of cerebellar functions, followed in many instances by progressive and symmetrical development of spasticity in the legs. Abnormalities of eye movement, intellectual impairment, and muscle atrophy with sensory distal loss complete the clinical picture, sometimes with the addition of palatal myoclonus. Computerized tomography demonstrates cerebellar atrophy, pontine atrophy, and, late in the disease, cerebral atrophy and large lateral ventricles. Motor nerve conduction velocities may be slow, and muscle denervation may be detected by electromyography. The cerebrospinal fluid is normal. Neither specific diagnostic laboratory tests nor specific treatments exist. Progressive cerebellar deficits, which include truncal ataxia, nystagmus, and dysarthria, are also produced as a result of chronic malnutrition and as a remote effect of cancer, and these possibilities must be considered when a family history of cerebellar disease is lacking.

283.   SYRINGOMYELIA

Syringomyelia is derived from the Greek word syrinx, which means tube, and refers to the occurrence of a cavity within the spinal cord. Such cavities usually are located in the central region of the spinal cord at the cervical level; they often extend to higher levels in the medulla (syringobulbia) and may extend inferiorly into the thoracic and lumbosacral regions of the spinal cord. Acquired syringomyelia arises in association with approximately 25 per cent of intraspinal tumors. Syringomyelia in combination with spina bifida has been reported as a familial disorder.

PATHOLOGY. The syringomyelic cavity is usually associated with the central canal of the spinal cord but may be independent of it as well. The cavity may extend over many segments of the cervical cord and may be in direct anatomic communication with the fourth ventricle. The term hydromyelia is often used to describe those cavitary lesions of the spinal cord which do communicate with the fourth ventricle. The syringomyelic cavity dissects into and progressively replaces the gray matter of the posterior and anterior horns of the spinal cord, as well as disturbing the decussating fibers in the anterior commissure. The cavity wall is maintained by astrocytic glial and fibroblastic membranes and blood vessels. Most often, syringomyelia is associated with other congenital malformations at the cranial cervical junction, including the Arnold-Chiari malformation with herniation of the cerebellar tonsils, fusion of the cervical vertebrae (Klippel-Feil syndrome), or malformations at the lumbosacral region, including spina bifida and associated meningomyelocele. Hydrocephalus resulting from cranial cervical malformations or stenosis of the aqueduct of Sylvius occurs in some patients.

CLINICAL MANIFESTATIONS. Symptoms of syringomyelia most often begin in the second or third decade with a selective impairment in pain and temperature sensation with the preservation of the sense of touch. Earliest detected sensory changes are usually in the hands, but examination commonly discloses a similar dissociated sensory loss in the neck, shoulders, and upper chest and back. Sensory loss is accompanied by progressive atrophy of the musculature in the upper extremities with other skeletal malformations, principally kyphoscoliosis. These clinical manifestations are produced by the syrinx directly destroying the pain and temperature fibers in the anterior spinal commissure as well as the anterior horns to produce denervation of muscle. Progressive analgesia results in severe painless ulcers, burns, and Charcot joints. Atrophy of arm, forearm, and intrinsic hand musculature, fasciculations, and areflexia develop progressively. Later in the disease upper motor neuron signs arise in the legs owing to encroachment of the syringomyelic cavity into the lateral columns of the cord. Late involvement of vibratory and position sensations in the lower extremities and an associated Romberg sign indicate that the syrinx is extending into the posterior columns of the spinal cord. A preganglionic Horner syndrome may also develop due to dissection of the syrinx into the intermediolateral cell column of the lower cervical and first thoracic segment of the spinal cord containing sympathetic neurons. The kyphoscoliosis that sometimes heralds the disease results from the asymmetrical denervation and atrophy of paravertebral muscles. The disease process is progressive, usually symmetrical, and clearly evident in adult life.

Syringobulbia refers to the development of the syringomyelic cavity into the medulla with resultant destruction of the medullary structures in the lateral tegmentum. Dissociated impairment of pain and temperature over the face, nystagmus, pharyngeal and vocal cord paralysis, and lingual atrophy are most typical. Syringobulbia is always associated with syringomyelia and is not a separate process.

DIAGNOSIS. Lepromatous neuropathy, certain rare congenital and acquired peripheral neuropathies, and intramedullary destructive lesions of the spinal cord and brainstem are the only conditions causing insidiously developing and progressive, widespread, dissociated loss of pain and temperature sensation. Leprosy can be considered if the subject has grown up in an endemic area, but neither it nor other peripheral neuropathies produce signs of spinal cord involvement. When the dissociated sensory loss is coupled with signs of long tract disease in the lower extremities or is decidedly asymmetrical in distribution and dermatomal

in pattern, the principal differential consideration lies between congenital syrinx and intramedullary neoplasm. Pain is more frequent with tumors. Air or contrast myelography usually makes the necessary distinction, but even this may be difficult, especially when a secondary syrinx arises in association with a neoplasm. In such instances, surgical exploration may be necessary.

TREATMENT. Treatment generally is unsatisfactory. Surgical decompression of the distended syrinx by a laminectomy sometimes helps slow the disease progression. It has been claimed that dissection of the syringomyelic cavity also can be useful, but published results are few. Some surgeons claim that the placement of muscle tissue at the junction of the fourth ventricle and the upper cervical canal with or without a ventriculocardiac shunt has stabilized the neurologic status of patients. Syrinx associated with spinal tumor is treated by treating the tumor appropriately.

284. THE PHAKOMATOSES OR NEUROCUTANEOUS SYNDROMES

284.1. NEUROFIBROMATOSIS
(Von Recklinghausen's Disease)

Von Recklinghausen's disease or neurofibromatosis is a genetic disorder inherited as an autosomal dominant trait and characterized by the occurrence of pigmented skin lesions, multiple tumors of spinal or cranial nerves, tumors of the skin, and the associated occurrence of gliomas and intracranial meningiomas. There is an increased association with pheochromocytomas, cystic lung disease, renal vascular lesions causing hypertension, fibrous dysplasia of bone, gastrointestinal neurofibromas with chronic blood loss, and medullary thyroid carcinoma and other tumors of endocrine glands.

PATHOLOGY. The characteristic feature of the disease is the occurrence of multiple "neurofibromas" associated with nerves in their peripheral, intraspinal, or intracranial segments. Electron microscopic studies indicate that these tumors represent proliferation of fibroblasts or neurilemmal sheath cells (Schwann cells) in peripheral nerve. The tumors may become confluent in the region of the brachial or sacral plexus and produce large plexiform neuromas which can evolve into malignant sarcomas. Intracranial astrocytomas, ependymomas, glioblastomas, and meningiomas are also encountered with increased frequency, as are optic nerve gliomas in childhood. Stenosis of the aqueduct of Sylvius with noncommunicating hydrocephalus is also observed in this disease. The skin manifestations include pedunculated polyps, lightly colored pigmented lesions with sharp edges (referred to as café au lait spots), and depigmented lesions. Neoplasms of endocrine organs, including medullary thyroid carcinomas and pheochromocytoma with associated hypertension, have been reported in a number of patients.

Metabolic bone disease in some patients results in overgrowth of bone with the occluding of cranial foramina and rarefaction and cyst formation of bone due to replacement of normal bone with fibroblasts and fibrocytes in a pattern similar to that of fibrous dysplasia. The congenital absence of a portion of the sphenoid bone resulting in pulsating exophthalmos, congenital vertebral anomalies, bone cysts, pseudoarthrosis of the tibia, local gigantism of an extremity, and scoliosis are encountered in some patients. Histologic abnormalities of the cerebral cortex, ectopic islands of gray matter, and focal gliosis are described and may be the basis for the increased incidence of mental retardation.

Recently Schenkein et al. reported increases in nerve growth hormone–stimulating activity in serum from patients with neurofibromatosis. Nerve growth hormone or factor (NGF) is a protein which stimulates the proliferation and differentiation of spinal and sympathetic ganglia in vivo and induces differentiation of neurites from embryonic ganglion cells of the chick, mouse, and human neuroblastoma cells in culture. One can speculate that the high titer of the nerve growth factor during fetal life, when neurilemma sheath cells are most sensitive, induces a proliferation and transformation of sheath cells into benign tumor cells. Clinical manifestations of disease then result from the continued stimulation of these transformed tumor cells by the elevated levels of NGF. Possibly elevated NGF may serve as a useful marker in the future for individuals at risk for neurofibromatosis. Fialkow et al. studied tumor tissue from women with neurofibromatosis who also were heterozygous for the A and B genes at the X-linked glucose-6-phosphate dehydrogenase locus. The tissue contained both type A and type B isozymes. The implication is that hereditary neurofibromas have a multiple rather than a single cell origin.

CLINICAL MANIFESTATIONS. Neurofibromatosis, as is typical of diseases of dominant inheritance, can present in a variety of ways, but the presence of multiple cutaneous neurofibromas and café au lait pigmented skin lesions represent the hallmarks. The pigmented lesions are smooth with sharp, regular borders and occur most commonly over the trunk and in the axilla. Skin lesions greater than 3 cm in diameter and more than six in number are indicative of neurofibromatosis; smaller and fewer lesions can occur in persons who do not have this disorder. Nerve involvement can be solitary, involving individual nerves of the extremities, or multiple and diffuse. Multiple cranial nerves are affected as well, resulting in facial weakness, facial numbness, deafness, and visual loss with optic nerve atrophy. Multiple confluent tumors and fibrosis of the affected parts result in elephantiasis neuromatosa. A marked increase in the proliferation and overgrowth of skin and subcutaneous tissues of the skull, neck, and trunk can result in gross asymmetrical hypertrophy. Neurofibromas associated with the nerve root can invade the intervertebral foramen and result in compression of spinal cord or brainstem. Large neurofibromas of a cranial nerve can produce increased intracranial pressure due to hydrocephalus. Some such lesions present as a cerebellopontine angle mass lesion with ipsilateral cerebellar signs. The fifth, seventh, eighth, and tenth cranial nerves are commonly involved with neurofibromas, producing facial muscle weakness, facial numbness, weakness and atrophy of the muscles of mastication, deafness, and vertigo. Rarely, spontaneous fractures of vertebrae or long bones result because of fibrodysplasia or cystic bone formation.

The cerebrospinal fluid protein is elevated in patients having large tumors which result in cord compression. Roentgenograms of the skull and internal auditory meatus show erosion caused by adjacent tumors.

DIAGNOSIS. Neurofibromatosis is diagnosed readily by the occurrence of the characteristic neurofibromas and skin pigmented lesions. The tumors are often multiple and vary considerably in size. Most tumors are smooth, soft, and multilobulated, and can be palpated along the course of a peripheral nerve. Hypertensive patients must be evaluated for the possibility of renal artery stenosis as well as for pheochromocytoma with urinary determinations of catecholamines. Cranial nerve palsies and hydrocephalus signal the presence of an intracranial neoplasm and the need for computerized tomographic brain scans or angiography for precise definition. Cerebellopontine angle meningiomas and cranial nerve or spinal nerve tumors are usually resectable and must be considered in patients manifesting progressive brainstem or spinal cord deficits. There is no treatment for neurofibromatosis other than resection of symptomatic tumors and decompression of hydrocephalus.

284.2. TUBEROUS SCLEROSIS
(Bourneville's Disease)

Tuberous sclerosis (Bourneville's disease or epiloia) is a neurocutaneous disorder inherited as an autosomal dominant trait. Its triad of findings include facial nevi (adenoma sebaceum), epilepsy, and mental retardation. Although the clinical and neuropathologic features are well described, the basic biochemical defect remains unknown.

PATHOLOGY. The gross brain has many firm nodules which are apparent on the surface. These firm nodules are also present in the deep layers of the cortex, the underlying white matter, and the basal ganglia, and they also line the lateral ventricles as projections referred to as "candle gutterings." In addition these nodules are also encountered in the substance of the spinal cord, the brainstem, and the cerebellum. The histologic appearance of the nodules shows a proliferation of primitive glia with multinucleated giant cells. Vascular malformations, meningiomas, gliomas, and hamartomas of the brain also occur.

The cutaneous lesions include characteristic facial nevi and areas of fibrosis. These nevi are not true adenomas of the sebaceous glands but take their origin from terminal nerves in the subcutaneous region of the skin and include a hyperplasia of connective tissue and blood vessels. Funduscopic examination can disclose similar nodules or phakomas consisting of glial elements, fibroblasts, and ganglion cells arising from the retina. Rarely an optic nerve glioma develops. Rhabdomyomas of the heart can occur, as can renal tumors and neoplasms of endocrine organs, including testis, pancreas, ovary, and thyroid.

CLINICAL MANIFESTATIONS. The clinical appearance is characteristic. Patients develop mental retardation and epilepsy during the first decade of life. The first manifestation of disease is usually focal or generalized major motor seizures without other focal neurologic deficits. The occurrence of mental retardation is not evident until six years of age. Several years after the development of seizures the characteristic cutaneous facial lesions first develop. The facial nevi occur in a symmetrical distribution on the malar and nasal regions and appear to be yellow or orange-red, varying in size from several millimeters to 1 cm. The occurrence of areas of roughening of the skin (shagreen patches) in the shape of small spheres caused by fibrous hyperplasia, café au lait spots, areas of depigmented nevi, and, rarely, subungual neurofibromas are characteristic of tuberous sclerosis and link it genetically to von Recklinghausen's neurofibromatosis. The concurrent neoplasms in other organs rarely cause clinical complications. Papilledema and other focal neurologic deficits signal the occurrence of a large intracranial tumor.

DIAGNOSIS. The triad of facial nevi, epilepsy, and mental retardation is diagnostic. Examination of other family members may help make the diagnosis in an infant or child who presents with generalized seizures but may not yet have the characteristic cutaneous lesions. The characteristic periventricular phakomas are demonstrable by pneumoencephalography. Large periventricular calcifications seen on skull roentgenograms are diagnostic as well. There is no specific treatment. Seizures should be managed by appropriate anticonvulsant medication and development of brain tumors or increased intracranial pressure by surgical intervention and shunting procedures. Since a few affected patients may have normal intelligence, educational programs should be individualized accordingly.

284.3. STURGE-WEBER DISEASE

Sturge-Weber disease produces a port wine–colored capillary hemangioma on the face, accompanied by a similar vascular malformation of the underlying meninges and cerebral cortex. The cause is unknown, although the defect has been reported in more than one family member, indicating a genetic predisposition.

PATHOLOGY. The cutaneous hemangioma follows the distribution of one or more divisions of the trigeminal nerve. The underlying meninges contain a similar vascular lesion, and the capillaries of the cortex may show thickening and calcification, especially in the second and third cortical layers. The cerebral cortex may undergo atrophy with loss of nerve cells and a proliferation of glia. Cerebral calcification clearly outlines the cortical mantle in an undulating manner.

CLINICAL MANIFESTATIONS. The presence of a port wine facial nevus following the sensory dermatomal distribution of the first, second, or third portions of the trigeminal nerve is diagnostic. Generalized or focal motor seizures may occur with or without associated mental retardation. The patient can develop hemiplegic atrophy with shortening of the extremities contralateral to the calcified atrophic hemisphere. Exophthalmos, glaucoma, buphthalmos, optic atrophy, and other cutaneous port wine nevi and retinal angiomas can be present. There is no specific treatment; seizures are managed with anticonvulsant drugs.

284.4. HIPPEL-LINDAU DISEASE

Hippel-Lindau disease is a familial disorder inherited without a clear mendelian pattern, producing heman-

gioblastomas of the cerebellar hemispheres with associated angiomas of the retina and cystic change in the kidney and pancreas. It presents in the fourth to sixth decades of life, usually not associated with cutaneous vascular lesions. The disorder can present with signs of cerebellar mass lesion, cerebellar hemorrhage, brainstem vascular malformations, or hemangioma of the retina. A clinical association with pheochromocytomas and polycythemia has been noted, especially in the patients with cerebellar hemangioblastomas. The diagnosis should be suspected in any patient with cerebellar brain tumor or cerebellar hemorrhage, especially in association with an elevated hematocrit. Diagnosis and treatment are as for other such mass lesions.

284.5. ATAXIA TELANGIECTASIA

Ataxia telangiectasia is a neurocutaneous disorder that begins in the first decade of life with prominent telangiectatic lesions involving the bulbar conjunctivae, malar eminences, ear lobes, and occasionally upper neck regions, associated with cerebellar ataxia and nystagmus. The condition is usually sporadic in occurrence but occasionally presents in a pattern consistent with an autosomal recessive disorder. A chromosome translocation involving chromosome 14, increased chromosome breakage, and reduced lymphocyte response to phytohemagglutinin have been described and represent the only molecular clues to pathogenesis.

PATHOLOGY. The most prominent neuropathologic changes include loss of Purkinje, granule, and basket cells in the cerebellar cortex as well as of neurons in the deep nuclei of the cerebellum. Neuronal loss is also present in the inferior olives of the medulla. The posterior columns of the spinal cord undergo demyelination, and there is a loss of anterior horn cells in the spinal cord and ganglion cells of the spinal ganglia. The most consistent defect of the lymphoid system is a poorly developed or absent thymus.

CLINICAL MANIFESTATIONS. The onset of the telangiectatic lesions occurs in the first decade of life and is associated with progressive deficits in cerebellar functions with early onset nystagmus. Truncal ataxia, extremity ataxia, dysarthria, extensor plantar responses, myoclonic jerks, areflexia, and distal sensory deficits occur in a pattern somewhat resembling that of Friedreich's syndrome. The patients have a high incidence of recurrent pulmonary infections and neoplasms of the lymphoreticuloendothelial system.

DIAGNOSIS. Ataxia telangiectasia is diagnosed by the characteristic telangiectatic lesions in association with a truncal ataxia, other cerebellar deficits, and apractic eye movements. Serum protein electrophoresis documents the common occurrence of a deficiency of gamma globulins, especially IgA and IgE. Cellular immune abnormalities include lymphocytopenia, a reduced response to skin test antigens, and lack of sensitization to dinitrochlorobenzene (DNCB).

Barnett, H. J. M., Foster, J. B., and Hudgson, P.: Syringomyelia. London, W. B. Saunders Company, 1974.
Blass, J. P., Kark, R. A. P., and Menon, N. K.: Low activities of the pyruvate and oxoglutarate dehydrogenase complexes in five patients with Friedreich's ataxia. N. Engl. J. Med., 295:62, 1976.
Brady, R. O.: Inherited metabolic diseases of the nervous system. Science, 193:733, 1976.
Crowe, F. W., Schull, W. J., and Neel, J. V.: A Clinical Pathological

and Genetic Study of Multiple Neurofibromatosis. Springfield, Ill., Charles C Thomas, 1956.

Fialkow, P., Sagebiel, R., Gartler, S., and Rimoin, D.: Multiple cell origin of hereditary neurofibromas. N. Engl. J. Med., 284:298, 1971.

Hecht, F., McCaw, B., and Koler, R. D.: Ataxia-telangiectasia—clonal growth of translocation lymphocytes. N. Engl. J. Med., 289:286, 1973.

Horton, W. A., Eldridge, R., and Brody, J.: Familial motor neuron disease. Neurology, 26:460, 1976.

Konigsmark, B. W., and Weiner, L. P.: The olivopontocerebellar atrophies. Medicine, 49:227, 1970.

Kugelberg, E., and Welander, L.: Heredofamilial juvenile muscular atrophy simulating muscular dystrophy. Arch. Neurol. Psychiat., 75:500, 1956.

McFarlin, P. E., Strober, W., and Waldmann, T. A.: Ataxia-telangiectasia. Medicine, 51:281, 1972.

Meister, A.: The gamma-glutamyl cycle. Ann. Intern. Med., 81:247, 1974.

Oldstone, M. B. A., Perrin, L. H., Wilson, C. B., and Norris, F. H., Jr.: Evidence for immune-complex formation in patients with amyotrophic lateral sclerosis. Lancet, 2:169, 1976.

Refsum, S.: Heredopathia atactica polyneuritiformis: Phytanic acid storage disease (Refsum's disease). In Vinken, P. J., and Bruyn, G. W. (eds.): Handbook of Clinical Neurology, Chap. 10, Vol. 21, Part I. Amsterdam, North Holland Publishing Company, 1975, pp. 181, 229.

Rosenberg, R. N., Nyhan, W. L., Coutinho, P., and Bay, C.: Joseph's disease in California, Massachusetts, and the Azores. In Kark, P., Rosenberg, R., and Schut, L. (eds.): The Inherited Ataxias. Proceedings of an International Symposium, Nov. 1977, Los Angeles. New York, Raven Press, 1978.

Schenkein, I., Bueker, E., Helson, L., Axelrod, R., and Dancis, J.: Increased nerve-growth stimulating activity in disseminated neurofibromatosis. N. Engl. J. Med., 290:613, 1974.

Schwartz, J. F., Rowland, L. P., Eder, H., Marks, P. A., Osserman, E. F., Hirschberg, E., and Anderson, H.: Bassen-Kornzweig syndrome. Deficiency of serum beta-lipoprotein. Arch. Neurol., 8:438, 1963.

Section Thirteen NUTRITIONAL DISORDERS OF THE NERVOUS SYSTEM

Pierre M. Dreyfus

285. INTRODUCTION

Malnutrition, undernutrition, and the deficiency of specific nutrients such as vitamins are known to affect normal function of some parts of the central and/or the peripheral nervous system. It is well established that an isolated or combined deficiency of vitamins B_1, B_6, B_{12}, niacin, pantothenic acid, and perhaps riboflavin can be associated with a variety of neurologic disorders. However, despite increasing knowledge regarding the role of these vitamins in general metabolism, the specific mechanisms by which a deficiency state affects the normal development and function of the nervous system remain essentially unknown.

Most of the neurologic disorders discussed in this section, although commonly associated with chronic alcoholism, have also been described in malnourished, chronically debilitated, nonalcoholic patients. The inveterate drinker is frequently the victim of a primary nutritional deficiency which alters the normal metabolic activity of the nervous system. During periods of heavy drinking, the chronic alcoholic patient may change the composition of his diet, sharply decreasing vitamin and other essential nutrient intake, because of decreased appetite. Vitamin absorption, intestinal transport, tissue storage, utilization, and conversion to metabolically active forms may be curtailed while the need for many vitamins and essential nutrients increases. In addition to causing abnormal vitamin metabolism, the prolonged and abusive intake of alcohol leads to a somewhat unusual and extreme state of nutritional imbalance characterized by an excess of carbohydrate, fatty acid, cholesterol, glycerol, glycogen, and calories combined with a severe deficiency of B vitamins and other essential nutrients. The chronic alcoholic patient may also suffer from a secondary nutritional deficiency which may be the result of a chronic illness, such as infection, anemia, or blood loss, which increases his over-all metabolic demands.

The various nutritional syndromes described in this section may present separately in relatively pure form, but more frequently they occur together in varying combinations, some more prevalent than others. It is not known why, under seemingly identical circumstances, one nutritionally depleted patient develops one or several neurologic syndromes whereas another emerges essentially unscathed. Basic constitutional and genetic factors, such as aberrations in specific enzyme proteins, may underlie the individual response of patients to malnutrition and the chronic ingestion of alcohol.

Nutritional disorders of the nervous system are associated with one or more biochemical lesions which invariably antedate the appearance of symptoms and signs and histopathologic changes. These diseases all share the common neuropathologic attributes of other metabolic disorders of the nervous system by virtue of their predilection for specific areas or parts of the nervous system and because of the bilateral symmetry of the lesions.

286. NUTRITIONAL POLYNEUROPATHY

(Dry Beriberi, Alcoholic Neuropathy)

CLINICAL MANIFESTATIONS. Nutritional polyneuropathy, the most common of all the nutritional diseases of the nervous system, is characterized by progressive weakness and muscle wasting of varying degrees, involving, symmetrically, the legs more than the arms and the distal muscles more than the proximal ones. Weakness may be almost imperceptible or so severe that the legs are virtually paralyzed and the hands useless. Motor signs and sensory manifestations most frequently occur concomitantly. Abnormalities of sensation are usually striking. Patients complain of aching, coldness, hotness, deadness, numbness, prickliness, and tenderness, most commonly in the calves, on the plantar surfaces of the feet, and in the fingers. Deep pressure or light touch may be extremely unpleasant. In the most severe cases, the muscles become wasted, atrophic, flabby, and tender, and the skin may be dry, red, and shiny. Excessive perspiration of feet and hands is occasionally noted. The deep tendon reflexes, which may be exaggerated in some patients at the onset of the illness, are usually greatly diminished or totally abolished. The sensory loss is symmetrical, is most severe distally, and diminishes gradually over more proximal parts; all modalities are involved, some more than others. On rare occasions, severe burning, shooting, lightning, or "electric" types of pain can occur in the absence of clear-cut signs of neuropathy. The term "burning feet syndrome" has been applied to this variety of neuropathic disorder. This syndrome has been encountered in inmates of prison camps, chronic alcoholics, and patients undergoing dialysis for chronic renal failure. In rare instances, nutritional polyneuropathy may be accompanied by vertigo, deafness, hoarseness, dysphagia, and amblyopia.

The mode of evolution and the severity of nutritional polyneuropathy can be quite variable. Usually the onset is insidious, and the progression is slow. Sometimes the course is rapid and abrupt, crippling the patient in a matter of weeks. Recovery requires months and is sometimes incomplete. A temporary worsening of paresthesias and of weakness may follow the start of therapy. In early or mild cases, a prolonged nerve conduction velocity may be the only objective manifestation of the disease. Examination of the cerebrospinal fluid reveals a normal level or a very slight elevation of the protein content.

PATHOLOGY. The salient pathologic changes consist of demyelination and axonal destruction of peripheral nerves, involving distal parts to a greater degree than proximal ones. Occasionally dorsal root ganglia reveal a loss of nerve cells, and axonal reaction may be seen in some of the anterior horn cells of the spinal cord. In patients afflicted with hoarseness and dysphagia, degeneration of the vagus nerve and of the paravertebral sympathetic chain has been observed. It has been speculated that in nutritional polyneuropathy, primary axonal degeneration or a process of "dying back" results in destruction of both the axon and myelin sheaths in the periphery of the largest and longest nerve fibers.

PATHOGENESIS AND TREATMENT. Nutritional depletion probably alters the normal metabolism of peripheral nerves in several different ways. Both experimental and clinical studies support the view that a deficiency of several of the B vitamins can result in neuropathy. Certain neuropathies respond to the administration of thiamin alone. Recent studies have shown decreased levels of thiamin in the blood, urine, and muscles of patients afflicted with alcoholic neuropathy. Prior to nutritional replenishment, the activity of blood transketolase is usually reduced, and blood pyruvate levels, measured before and after the administration of glucose, may be elevated. The fact that biochemical evidence of thiamin deficiency in nutritional polyneuropathy cannot always be obtained is explained by the slow evolution of this disorder. Whereas the biochemical lesion antedates all clinical manifestations of neuropathy, the latter linger on for many months after the metabolic insult has been removed. A deficiency of pyridoxine has also been blamed for nutritional polyneuropathy. A neuropathic disorder has been observed in patients who were given desoxypyridoxine, a metabolic antagonist of vitamin B_6. The neuropathy that develops in the course of isoniazid (INH) therapy can be reversed by pyridoxine alone. Isoniazid causes a deficiency of the essential cofactor pyridoxal phosphate by interfering with phosphorylation of the vitamin. Pyridoxal phosphate is an essential cofactor for a number of enzymatic reactions known to participate in protein metabolism. The specific role of these enzymatic reactions in the metabolism of peripheral nerves remains to be defined. A deficiency of pyridoxal phosphate results in the inadequate synthesis of nicotinic acid from tryptophan. Reduced blood levels of nicotinic acid and nicotinamide have been measured in some patients with nutritional polyneuropathy. Pantothenic acid deficiency may also be involved in the production of some forms of nutritional polyneuropathy. It has been claimed that the administration of pantothenic acid relieves the burning feet syndrome, regardless of its cause.

287. WERNICKE-KORSAKOFF SYNDROME

Of all the disorders of the central nervous system associated with the protracted and abusive intake of alcohol and nutritional depletion, Wernicke's disease and Korsakoff's psychosis are the most frequent. The term "cerebral beriberi" has sometimes been applied to these conditions.

CLINICAL MANIFESTATIONS. *Wernicke's disease* is characterized by disturbed ocular motility, ataxia, impaired mentation, and, occasionally, polyneuropathy. The patient may complain of diplopia and unsteadiness of gait, but is usually unaware of his deficit. On examination, bilateral weakness or paralysis of the external recti muscles and paralysis of lateral conjugate gaze are common. Horizontal nystagmus is almost always present, although it sometimes cannot be elicited until abducens function has improved. Vertical nystagmus, particularly on upward gaze, is frequently present. Occasionally there are ptosis, complete paralysis of eye movements, miosis and, very rarely, unreactive pupils. The ataxia, which is almost always present, affects stance and gait primarily. It may be so slight that only special tests for cerebellar function betray its existence. When it is severe, the patient cannot stand or walk without help. Advanced polyneuropathy usually masks cerebellar ataxia. Intention tremor is less common and tends to affect the legs more than the arms. Scanning speech is a rarity. A mild to severe mixed sensory-motor polyneuropathy exists in at least 50 per cent of cases. When first seen, the patient with Wernicke's disease may display symptoms and signs attributable to alcohol withdrawal: i.e., delirium, tremulousness, confusion, agitation, hallucinosis, altered sense perception, and autonomic overactivity. More often, he lacks spontaneity, is apathetic, listless, indifferent, and disoriented in time and place, and tends to misidentify objects and people around him. Dull mentation, impaired retentive memory, and general lack of grasp are more common than drowsiness or unconsciousness. With improved nutrition and supplemental thiamin the patient becomes more alert, more attentive, and more readily testable. He may then display a characteristic amnestic syndrome known as *Korsakoff's psychosis*. In addition, the patient with Korsakoff's psychosis reveals a number of abnormalities of cognitive function. He may have a great deal of difficulty in forming visual and verbal abstractions. His capacity to shift from one mental set to another and his ability to learn are defective. Perceptual function and concept formation are affected. The most prominent and serious mental abnormality seen in Korsakoff's psychosis is the disordered memory function that renders some patients incapable of performing any but the simplest tasks. Recent retentive memory and the ability to learn newly presented material are strikingly impaired. An extensive retrograde amnesia covering a variable period of time is also common. Such patients may confabulate, i.e., fabricate fictitious or improperly sequenced stories. Confabulation is by no means unique to Korsakoff's psychosis and tends to disappear in the chronic stages of the illness.

Features of Wernicke's disease and Korsakoff's psychosis often coexist in the same patient. In many instances of Korsakoff's psychosis, slight, residual nystagmus and ataxia may be detected years later. The Wernicke-Korsakoff syndrome may be complicated by other stigmata of chronic malnutrition, including cirrhosis of the liver, anemia, and mucocutaneous lesions of various types. Many patients suffer from postural hypotension, dyspnea, and tachycardia, but full-blown beriberi heart disease is rare. The Wernicke-Korsakoff syndrome usually begins abruptly. Some degree of recovery is the rule, except in the most advanced cases and in those complicated by other illnesses. During the acute stage of the disease the mortality may be as high as 17 per cent. The ocular manifestations, except for nystagmus, respond promptly and dramatically to vitamin therapy. Ataxia improves more slowly, and incomplete recovery occurs in over half the patients; complete recovery from Korsakoff's psychosis occurs in less than one third of patients. The recovered patient usually shows permanent amnesia for the acute phase of the illness.

PATHOLOGY. The pathologic alterations that affect the cerebrum and the brainstem are remarkably constant. They almost always involve structures in a bilaterally symmetrical manner. Lesions are invariably seen in the mamillary bodies and the terminal fornices. Lesions in the periaqueductal region of the midbrain, in the floor of the fourth ventricle, in the vicinity of the dorsal motor nucleus of the vagus, and in the anterior superior parts of the cerebellar vermis probably account for the paralysis of gaze, nystagmus, and ataxia. The lesions involving thalamic nuclei (anteromedial, lateral dorsal, and pulvinar) and the hypothalamus and those seen in the mamillary bodies and fornices may underlie some of the psychologic abnormalities, particularly the amnestic syndrome. Microscopically, the lesions consist of necrosis of both nerve cells and myelinated structures. A striking glial reaction involves the center of the lesion. Both endothelial proliferation and hemorrhages are found, but the latter are usually fresh and may represent a nonspecific, terminal change. In the vermis of the cerebellum the principal changes consist of a loss of Purkinje cells and gliosis of the molecular layer of the cortex.

PATHOGENESIS. There is now an overwhelming body of evidence that favors a specific lack of vitamin B_1 as the main nutritional factor in the Wernicke-Korsakoff syndrome. Most patients give a history of inadequate nutrition and weight loss. Other stigmata of malnutrition, such as loss of subcutaneous fat and skin turgor, mucocutaneous manifestations, and an enlarged liver, are frequent. Clinical studies have shown that the continued intake of alcohol is not followed by aggravation of symptoms, provided adequate nutritional repletion is undertaken promptly. Thiamin alone, given orally or parenterally, can dramatically reverse some of the symptoms and signs. Victor and Adams maintained patients with Wernicke's disease on either glucose or a boiled rice diet containing no vitamins for brief periods, then gave them B vitamins selectively. Ophthalmoplegia, apathy, listlessness, and inattentiveness began to improve within a few hours and cleared completely within a few days after thiamin had been added to the regimen. Nystagmus and ataxia diminished, but Korsakoff's psychosis did not improve significantly. Other B vitamins were ineffective. The improvement of neurologic signs can be closely correlated with levels of blood transketolase activity, which are reduced prior to thiamin administration and increase toward normal with clinical improvement, sometimes within four to five hours after the injection of 25 to 50 mg of thiamin.

A recent study has suggested the existence of a genetic abnormality of transketolase (a thiamin-dependent enzyme) in serially cultured fibroblasts and red blood cells of some patients who have recovered from the disease. The aberrant enzyme binds the active cofactor of thiamin less tightly than does the normal enzyme. It is postulated that the presence of the aberrant enzyme predisposes the individual to clinically significant thiamin deficiency.

Although most commonly associated with chronic alcoholism, Wernicke-Korsakoff syndrome has been observed in clinical settings totally unrelated to abusive drinking. It has been described as a complication of chronic hemodialysis, pernicious vomiting of pregnancy, thyrotoxicosis, and gastric carcinoma, as well as after prolonged intravenous therapy.

288. NUTRITIONAL AMBLYOPIA

(Tobacco-Alcohol Amblyopia, Nutritional Retrobulbar Neuropathy)

CLINICAL MANIFESTATIONS. A remarkably uniform and stereotyped disorder of vision sometimes appears in chronically undernourished persons. Characteristically it evolves slowly and subacutely, the mode of onset of symptoms being much the same from patient to patient. Visual impairment usually starts insidiously and reaches a maximum in several weeks to months. Blurred or dim vision, difficulty in reading, photophobia, and retrobulbar discomfort on moving the eyes are the common presenting complaints. On examination, the patient has bilaterally symmetrical central, centrocecal, or paracentral scotomata. Ophthalmoscopic changes are restricted at first to slight redness of the temporal margins of the optic discs; minimal pallor is observed at a later stage. Often, no abnormality is visible. The peripheral visual fields are usually intact. The visual disorder is, to a large extent, reversible with improvement of nutrition.

PATHOLOGY. The pathologic change in nutritional amblyopia consists of bilaterally symmetrical loss of myelinated fibers in the central parts of the optic nerves, chiasm, and optic tracts, corresponding in location to the papillomacular bundle. In severe cases, the retina loses macular ganglion cells, probably secondary to the "zonal" destruction of medullated fibers in the retrobulbar parts of the optic nerve.

PATHOGENESIS. Nutritional amblyopia has been encountered in undernourished populations all over the world. It is commonly seen during famine, and among civilian and military prisoners of war. It is endemic in certain parts of Africa, Asia, and South America. Among the more privileged populations in the western world, the syndrome is seen in persons chronically addicted to alcohol or, occasionally, to tobacco, who neglect their nutrition. A similar syndrome also occurs as a complication of vitamin B_{12} deficiency and of diabetes mellitus. This visual disorder accompanies other neurologic syndromes believed to have a nutritional cause, such as *Strachan's syndrome*, in which amblyopia is combined with paresthesias of the feet, hands, trunk, and, occasionally, face, loss of reflexes, dizziness, deafness, hoarseness, spasticity, ataxia, and a variety of mucocutaneous lesions (genital dermatitis, corneal degeneration, glossitis, and stomatitis). In the chronic alcoholic patient, amblyopia may occur in conjunction with Wernicke's disease, cerebellar degeneration, Marchiafava-Bignami's disease, and peripheral neuropathy. The nutritional basis is well established, for if such patients are renourished their vision improves even if they smoke or drink alcohol. As yet, the metabolic aberration or specific vitamin deficiency responsible for the development of amblyopia has not been defined. A lack of vitamin B_{12}, thiamin, riboflavin, and pyridoxine or a failure in the detoxification of cyanide present in tobacco smoke has been implicated in the genesis of the syndrome. Except for isolated findings of reduced serum vitamin B_{12} levels, the abnormal urinary excretion of methylmalonic acid, and low levels of blood transketolase activity, no specific biochemical abnormalities have been reported.

TREATMENT. Treatment with oral or parenteral B vitamins and improved nutrition are usually followed by improvement, depending upon the severity of the amblyopia and its duration before therapy is instituted.

289. CEREBELLAR CORTICAL DEGENERATION

Cerebellar cortical degeneration, or parenchymatous cerebellar degeneration, has often been referred to as alcoholic cerebellar degeneration, although well documented instances of cerebellar cortical degeneration have occurred as a result of chronic nutritional depletion not attributable to alcohol. This disorder can be set apart from all other known forms of acquired or familial cerebellar degeneration because of the uniformity of the clinical and pathologic manifestations. The clinical and pathologic findings are discussed in Ch. 282.

A substantial body of evidence favors the contention that cerebellar degeneration is due to nutritional factors. The history of chronic alcoholic patients is admittedly unreliable, yet most admit improper eating habits. Many patients with cortical cerebellar degeneration give a history of progressive weight loss before the onset of their symptoms. Signs of malnutrition are common, and the cerebellar syndrome frequently occurs in conjunction with cirrhosis and other nutritional complications of alcoholism. Furthermore, a number of nonalcoholic patients develop cortical cerebellar degeneration in the setting of other diseases associated with nutritional depletion, such as pellagra, amebiasis, and protracted vomiting. In general, improved nutrition and supplementary B vitamins result in some degree of improvement of ataxia.

290. CENTRAL PONTINE MYELINOLYSIS

Central pontine myelinolysis is a relatively rare disease characterized by demyelination of the central portion of the pons. It was described originally in patients afflicted with chronic alcoholism and malnutrition but has since been encountered in nonalcoholic patients who were nutritionally deprived. The illness affects adults mainly, but has been reported in children; males and females are equally afflicted. Although the precise clinical course has not yet been defined, the principal neurologic abnormalities are progressive weakness of facial muscles and tongue, causing severe impairment of speech and deglutition. In a number of cases, pseudobulbar phenomena such as emotional lability and pathologic crying have been noted. Quadriparesis at the onset of the illness usually leads to a flaccid and areflexic quadriplegia with Babinski signs. Lack of response to painful stimuli and absence of corneal reflexes are said to be common. Urinary incontinence, decerebrate posture, and respiratory paralysis have been reported in isolated cases.

The illness evolves rapidly over a period of two to three weeks, usually ending in stupor, coma, and eventual death. Most patients succumb to medical complications, such as pneumonia, sepsis, or uremia. In rare instances, slow, gradual, and sometimes complete recovery occurs.

The clinical diagnosis of the disease is difficult to establish, but brainstem auditory evoked potential studies may help demonstrate impaired function of pontine pathways. Examination of the cerebrospinal fluid is unremarkable.

Pathologic examination reveals demyelination, variable in size and extent, involving the center of the basal portion of the mid and upper pons. In some cases the demyelination may also involve the midbrain, basal ganglia, and cerebral white matter. Axis cylinders, nerve cells, and blood vessels are relatively well preserved. An appropriate glial and phagocytic reaction is seen within the lesions. Vascular or inflammatory changes are absent. The clinical symptoms and signs depend upon the size and location of the lesions.

The pathogenesis is in some way related to malnutrition and its treatment. The lesion has been found at postmortem examination in patients suffering from alcoholism, other forms of chronic malnutrition, neoplasia, renal disease, hepatic insufficiency, and a variety of infectious processes. It has been suggested that the disease may be related to the treatment of dehydration and electrolyte imbalance rather than to malnutrition or alcoholism per se; in most instances, patients die after a period of intensive treatment. To date no biochemical data have been obtained.

291. MARCHIAFAVA-BIGNAMI DISEASE

Marchiafava-Bignami disease is a rare disorder occurring in the setting of severe malnutrition, usually with alcoholism. The disease affects males of middle age predominantly. The course is variable; it may evolve over a period of a few days or several months. Complete recovery is rare. The patients are agitated and confused, and have hallucinations (visual, auditory, and gustatory), disturbance of memory, negativism, impaired judgment, and progressive dementia. Neurologic symptoms and signs suggest bilateral involvement of frontal lobes and include disturbance of language, gait and motor skills, seizures, incontinence, rooting, grasping, sucking, and delayed initiation of action. Tremulousness of the hands and dysarthria have been reported.

Pathologically, symmetrical zones of demyelination affect the central parts of the corpus callosum, beginning in the most anterior parts and extending caudally. Similar changes affect the central parts of the anterior commissure, the optic chiasm and tracts, and, in severe cases, the central white matter of the frontal lobes. In zones of demyelination, axis cylinders tend to be preserved. Occasionally, there is extensive tissue destruction and cavitation. The degree of glial reaction in these areas depends on the chronicity of the process.

The disease originally was reported in males of Italian descent who consumed excessive amounts of crude red wine. The illness has since been encountered in patients of varied ancestry and with other alcoholic preferences. The characteristic pathologic changes of Marchiafava-Bignami disease have been encountered in conjunction with Wernicke's disease and nutritional amblyopia as well as in malnourished, nonalcoholic patients.

292. VITAMIN B₁₂ DEFICIENCY

DEFINITION. Insufficient absorption of vitamin B_{12} from the gastrointestinal tract can result in a subacute degeneration of the spinal cord, optic nerves, cerebral white matter, and peripheral nerves. Although the neurologic manifestations of vitamin B_{12} deficiency are frequently associated with a macrocytic anemia (pernicious anemia), the latter is not always present. Neurologic symptoms develop in approximately 80 per cent of patients between the ages of 25 and 75 years afflicted with pernicious anemia. They rarely occur as a result of secondary vitamin B_{12} deficiency complicating fish tapeworm (*Diphyllobothrium latum*) infestation, sprue, vegetarianism, or gastrointestinal surgery. (This subject is also dealt with in Ch. 479.)

CLINICAL MANIFESTATIONS. Symptoms and signs of spinal cord involvement (*combined system disease*) constitute the most common neurologic manifestations, and their mode of onset and progression is remarkably uniform. Symmetrical progressive paresthesias of the feet or hands in the form of numbness, tingling, burning, tightness and stiffness, and a feeling of generalized weakness constitute the most frequent initial symptoms. Vague asthenia and lameness progress to a measurable weakness and stiffness of the legs and an unsteadiness of gait that tends to be worse in the dark. The lower limbs may give way unexpectedly. The hands may be stiff and clumsy. When untreated, the illness progresses slowly and relentlessly. Spasticity, ataxia, and paraplegia ensue, often followed by bowel and bladder dysfunction. In the early stages of the disease, examination of the patient often reveals a few objective changes, but eventually signs of disturbed peripheral nerve and posterior and lateral column function become readily apparent. Diminution or loss of position and vibratory sense involves the legs, the hands, and, occasionally, the trunk, and tends to be pronounced. Pain, temperature, and tactile sensation are sometimes blunted over the distal parts of the legs in a pattern suggestive of peripheral nerve involvement. The motor examination reveals weak and, later, spastic legs and extensor plantar responses. The activity of the deep tendon reflexes is variable and appears to depend upon the severity of the illness. The knee jerks are often hyperactive and the ankle jerks absent. In advanced cases, all stretch reflexes may be diminished or absent, but may return when vitamin therapy has been promptly instituted. Psychologic symptoms range from apathy, irritability, and suspiciousness to confusion and dementia, and at times are the presenting neurologic abnormality. On rare occasions, failing vision caused by symmetrical centrocecal scotomata may be the presenting neurologic symptom of vitamin B_{12} deficiency.

PATHOLOGY. The lesions associated with subacute combined degeneration involve in sequence the posterior columns, the lateral columns, and the cerebral white matter. The earliest visible change consists of swelling of individual myelinated nerve fibers in small foci. These lesions subsequently coalesce into large, irregular, spongy, honeycomb-like zones of demyelination. Fibers with the largest diameter are predominantly affected. Axis cylinders tend to be spared. Myelin destruction frequently begins in the cervical and upper thoracic segments of the cord, spreading axially to involve other segments. The cerebral white matter is affected last. The large fibers of the peripheral nerves may show minimal loss of myelin.

DIAGNOSIS. A number of diseases other than vitamin B_{12} deficiency affect the posterior and lateral columns of the spinal cord, the most important being multiple sclerosis, tumors, cervical spondylosis, syphilitic meningomyelitis, and familial spastic paraplegia. These entities can usually be differentiated from one another clinically, but ancillary examinations such as myelography and special tests involving the cerebrospinal fluid may be necessary to establish a correct diagnosis. In B_{12} deficiency of the nervous system, the cerebrospinal fluid is usually normal. The electroencephalogram is often abnormal. The serum vitamin B_{12} content correlates well with the severity of the neurologic impairment and is invariably low in untreated cases. The Schilling test, using radioactive cyanocobalamin, is always positive, and gastric achlorhydria can be demonstrated in almost every instance. Blood and bone marrow examinations are of limited value, particularly when the patient has been treated with folic acid, which corrects the anemia but not the neurologic manifestations. The urinary excretion of methylmalonic acid, an intermediary metabolite in the conversion of propionic acid to succinic acid, is a sensitive indicator of vitamin B_{12} deficiency, but its relation to the lesions in the nervous system is as yet unknown.

PATHOGENESIS. The pathogenesis of the neurologic manifestations of vitamin B_{12} deficiency is unknown, although it probably differs from the biochemical lesion affecting the hematopoietic system, because the neurologic manifestations are independent of the anemia and may appear when folic acid corrects the anemia. The specific biochemical role of vitamin B_{12} in the nervous system has not yet been elucidated. It is an essential cofactor for at least two enzyme systems which exist in mammalian tissue, including brain: (1) methylmalonyl-CoA isomerase, which converts methylmalonyl-CoA to succinyl-CoA, a step in the utilization of propionic acid, and (2) N_5-methyltetrahydrofolate homocysteine methyltransferase, which is responsible for the synthesis of methionine from homocysteine. In experimentally induced vitamin B_{12} deficiency, the activity of both of these enzyme systems is reduced in brain. These enzymes may be essential to the maintenance of the myelin sheath. It has been shown that sural nerve specimens obtained from patients with pernicious anemia incorporate radioactively labeled propionate into abnormal fatty acids that have been identified as C_{15} branched-chain and C_{17} odd-chain acids. The presence of these abnormal fatty acids may explain, in part, the structural changes observed in central and peripheral myelin. An experimental approach to the study of the pathogenesis of the neurologic manifestations of vitamin B_{12} deficiency in animals has been greatly facilitated by the discovery of optic nerve and white matter lesions in monkeys maintained on a B_{12}-deficient diet for several years.

TREATMENT. Prompt initiation of therapy is of the utmost importance, because the early neurologic manifestations can be rapidly and completely reversed. The greatest degree of improvement is achieved in patients treated within three months of onset of symptoms, although variable degrees of amelioration can be attained after longer untreated periods (six to twelve months). In the first two weeks, daily intramuscular injections of 50 μg of cyanocobalamin, or an equivalent amount of liver USP, should be administered. During the next two months, 100 μg of cyanocobalamin should be injected twice a week. For the remainder of his life, the patient should receive a minimum of 100 μg intramuscularly every month to prevent a relapse. The administration of oral vitamin preparations containing folic acid must be avoided for patients with pernicious anemia, because folic acid may actually precipitate neurologic complications.

Agamanolis, D. P., Chester, E. M., Victor, M., Kark, J. A., Hines, J., and Harris, J. W.: Neuropathology of experimental vitamin B_{12} deficiency in monkeys. Neurology, 26:905, 1976.

Dreyfus, P. M., and Geel, S. E.: Vitamin and nutritional deficiencies. In Albers, R. W., Siegel, G. J., Katzman, R., and Agranoff, B. W. (eds.): Basic Neurochemistry. Boston, Little, Brown & Company, 1976, Chap. 29.

Gubler, C. J., Fujiwara, M., and Dreyfus, P. M.: Thiamine. New York, John Wiley & Sons, 1976.

Gyorgy, P., and Pearson, W. N.: The Vitamins. New York, Academic Press, 1967.

Kissin, B., and Begleiter, H.: The Biology of Alcoholism, Vol. 3, Clinical Pathology. New York, Plenum Press, 1974, Chaps. 7, 16.

Pant, S. S., Asbury, A. K., and Richardson, E. P., Jr.: The myelopathy of pernicious anemia — a neuropathological reappraisal. Acta Neurol. Scand., 44 (Suppl. 35), 1968.

Victor, M.: Polyneuropathy due to nutritional deficiency and alcoholism. In Dyck, P., Thomas, P. K., and Lambert, E. H. (eds.): Peripheral Neuropathy. Philadelphia, W. B. Saunders Company, 1975.

Victor, M., Adams, R. D., and Collins, G. H.: The Wernicke-Korsakoff Syndrome. Philadelphia, F. A. Davis Company, 1971.

Vinken, P. J., and Bruyn, G. W.: Handbook of Clinical Neurology. Vol. 28, Metabolic and Deficiency Diseases of the Nervous System. Amsterdam, North Holland Publishing Company, 1976, Chaps. 1–14.

Section Fourteen
CEREBROVASCULAR DISEASES

Fletcher H. McDowell

293. INTRODUCTION

It is estimated that there are 2 million persons alive today who have neurologic manifestations of cerebrovascular disease and that cerebrovascular disease of all varieties is annually responsible for approximately 200,000 deaths in the United States. Fully a half million Americans each year suffer a new, acute cerebrovascular attack. The over-all problem is even more imposing than the annual incidence and mortality figures. Recurrent vascular accidents are common in nearly all forms of cerebrovascular disease, each recurrence carrying a high risk of mortality. For the survivors, disability and dependency are the usual result. The need for medical care and hospital facilities for these patients is enormous and is an imposing challenge to medical and social service agencies alike.

In the following chapters, the cerebral vascular diseases are divided into two general groups, those producing ischemic *cerebral infarction* and those producing *intracranial hemorrhage.* Much of the material is derived from observations on 966 patients with clinically diagnosed cerebral vascular disease undergoing long-term study at the Cornell Division of Bellevue Hospital in New York City. As a rough index of the frequency of the different types of cerebral vascular accident or "stroke," 88 per cent of these patients had acute infarction or less severe cerebral ischemic attacks, and 12 per cent had intracranial hemorrhage. Of the infarctions, about one in eight was attributed to cerebral embolism.

294. CEREBRAL ISCHEMIA AND INFARCTION

DEFINITION AND ETIOLOGY

Cerebral thrombosis and cerebral emboli produce clinical symptoms by causing cerebral infarction, which means neural death from ischemia. Cerebral ischemia is the result of either a generalized or a localized prolonged reduction of blood flow to the brain. If ischemia is transient, less than 10 to 15 minutes, usually no discernible neurologic deficit remains. If it lasts longer than that, neural damage results, producing neurologic dysfunction, disability, and death.

The causes of cerebral infarction are numerous. The following are the most common ones:

1.   Atherosclerotic disease of the intra- and extracranial arteries.
2.   Cerebral emboli with (a) rheumatic heart disease, (b) myocardial infarction, (c) cardiac disease and atrial fibrillation, (d) subacute bacterial endocarditis, (e) nonbacterial thrombotic endocarditis.
3.   Reduced cerebral blood flow from severe hypotension or dysrhythmia of cardiac disease.
4.   Cerebral arterial spasm following subarachnoid hemorrhage.
5.   Generalized cerebral hypoxia from (a) cardiopulmonary insufficiency, (b) pulmonary emboli, (c) carbon monoxide poisoning.
6.   Cerebral thrombosis due to arteritis: (a) collagen vascular disease, (b) giant cell arteritis, (c) bacterial arteritis, including syphilis.
7.   Cerebral thrombosis due to polycythemia or ischemia caused by severe anemia.
8.   Cerebral thrombosis adjacent to intracerebral hemorrhage.
9.   Cerebral arterial vasoconstriction associated with migraine.
10.   Dissecting aneurysm of the aorta or great vessels in the neck.

INCIDENCE AND EPIDEMIOLOGY

Cerebral infarction is most commonly the result of cerebral atherosclerosis and cerebral emboli. In the Cornell-Bellevue series of 873 cases with nonhemorrhagic stroke, 92 per cent were clinically related to cerebral atherosclerosis and 8 per cent to cerebral emboli. In the group with cerebral emboli 20 per cent occurred in association with myocardial infarction, 26 per cent with rheumatic heart disease, most commonly with mitral stenosis, and atrial fibrillation, and the remainder in patients with atrial fibrillation associated with other varieties of heart disease.

Cerebral infarction is almost twice as frequent in males as in females. The peak age period is 60 to 69 years, but the incidence of stroke rises linearly with increasing age. In the Cornell-Bellevue study, stroke occurred earlier than the age of 50 in only 8 per cent of the patients.

NEUROPATHOLOGY

The brain is exquisitely dependent on its oxygen supply. There is no reserve of oxygen in cerebral tissue to sustain cerebral metabolism during periods of reduced or absent cerebral blood flow. When the brain is acutely and completely deprived of oxygen generally or locally, the electroencephalogram changes within 10 to 20 seconds, and irreversible and extensive neural damage occurs in the cerebral hemispheres after three to ten minutes. The determinants of brain ischemia are hypoxia and reduced general or local cerebral perfusion. The more important of the two is a decrease in perfusion. When ischemia is prolonged, the ischemic tissue softens, and the usually distinct margins between gray and white matter become unclear and occasionally hemorrhagic. Under the microscope, neurons are seen to be necrotic and shrunken, i.e., infarcted.

Cerebral infarctions that follow ischemia may be "pale" (nonhemorrhagic) or hemorrhagic. The extravasation of blood into tissues more commonly follows an embolic arterial obstruction, and pale infarcts more frequently follow atherosclerotic or thrombotic arterial obstruction. Often the two varieties of infarction blend together, and there is little advantage in extensively weighing the difference of causation.

A variable amount of *cerebral edema* accompanies cerebral infarction. With large infarctions the edema may be so extensive that portions of the swollen hemisphere shift under the falx or down through the tentorium cerebelli. This change in intracranial space relationships further impairs the flow of blood and cerebrospinal fluid, thus increasing the ischemia and neurologic deficit. This is often followed by secondary congestion and ischemia of the upper brainstem, which is almost invariably fatal.

It is common to find numerous old, small cerebral infarctions in patients dying from other causes, indicating that cerebral infarctions need not always give rise to symptoms. Old infarctions that have been hemorrhagic are identified at postmortem examination by the presence of hemosiderin in the wall of the infarct. As the infarct ages, the necrotic area breaks down, is absorbed, and eventually may be replaced by a fluid-filled cavity lined with glial and fibrovascular tissue.

MECHANISMS

Cerebral infarction is usually accompanied by abnormalities in the state of the arterial conducting system from the heart to the brain or the venous system draining the brain; the efficiency of the heart as a pump in producing a constant blood flow at a sufficient arterial

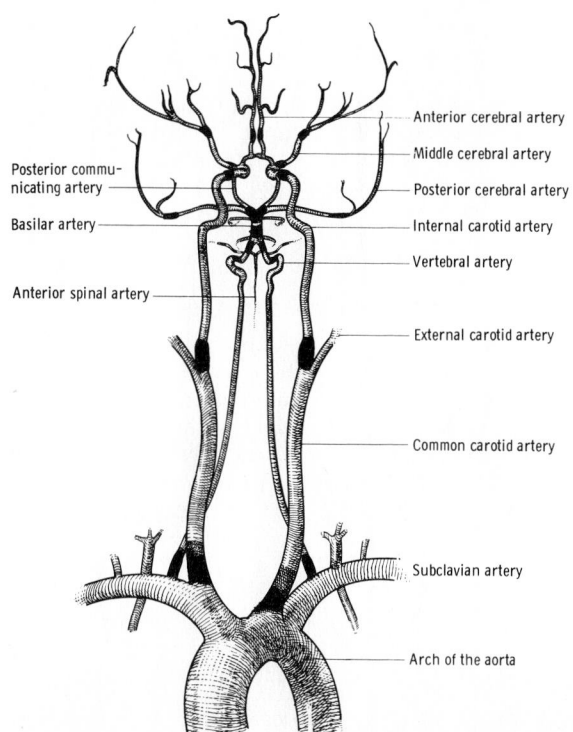

Figure 1. The darkened areas on the arterial diagram show the common sites of atherosclerosis and obstruction in the cerebral vessels.

Labels on figure:
- Posterior communicating artery
- Basilar artery
- Anterior spinal artery
- Anterior cerebral artery
- Middle cerebral artery
- Posterior cerebral artery
- Internal carotid artery
- Vertebral artery
- External carotid artery
- Common carotid artery
- Subclavian artery
- Arch of the aorta

pressure; and the character of the circulating medium (blood), its viscosity, its oxygen-carrying capacity, and its capacity to change from a colloidal suspension to a gel. Most cerebral infarctions are due to simultaneous changes in several of these factors.

The arterial conducting system is most often altered by atherosclerotic disease. In the third decade of life atherosclerosis is usually evident in the arteries leading to the brain, particularly in the larger cerebral arteries. Sites of predilection for plaques (Fig. 1) are the origins of the common carotid artery; just above the common carotid bifurcation; the internal carotid in its siphonous portion; the origin of the middle cerebral artery; and the vertebral arteries just after they enter the skull and the basilar artery. The atheromatous process in cerebral arteries is the same as that found elsewhere in the body, with lipid deposition in the intima, fibrous tissue overgrowth, hemorrhage into the plaques, ulceration of the plaques, and vessel obstruction.

Although atheromatous vascular disease begins early, it is a silent process for most of the life of the patient, and rarely produces symptoms until the middle years, when myocardial infarction, cerebral infarction, and lower extremity infarction occur. Most postmortem studies show that 80 to 90 per cent of all adult patients examined at autopsy have significant atheromatous disease. Since by no means all of these had experienced adverse clinical effects, the factors determining symptomatic complications assume major importance.

The first factor of importance is the degree and extent of atheromatous vascular disase, both in the arteries in the neck leading to the head and in the intracranial cerebral arteries. In general, persons who have cerebral **infarctions** have the most extensive cerebrovascular dis-

ease in the arteries in the neck and in the head. However, the pathogenesis of infarction depends on several mechanisms, and patients with only small or moderate amounts of vascular disease sometimes suffer serious cerebral infarcts. Conversely, extensive atheromatous disease can be found in large and small intracranial and extracranial cerebral arteries in patients without cerebral infarction.

Diabetes or *hypertension* can be detected in over two thirds of patients who have had cerebrovascular accidents. Patients with either diabetes or hypertension develop atherosclerosis at an earlier age, and the process develops more rapidly than in patients without these complicating illnesses. The atherosclerotic disease is extensive and is found in the smaller intracranial arteries.

The condition of the *cerebral collateral circulation* influences the development of cerebral infarction in persons with atherosclerosis. Most collateral circulation from one major intracerebral arterial system to another is through the circle of Willis via the posterior communicating arteries or the anterior communicating artery. Other sites of collateral circulation include the interconnections of the pial arteries on the cerebral surface between the anterior, middle, and posterior cerebral arteries. Sites of collateral circulation that become functional only when circulation through other routes is impaired are also found between the external and the internal carotid artery system, via the ophthalmic artery, and through muscular branches between the vertebral arteries and the external carotid artery in the neck.

Anomalies of the circle of Willis occur in nearly half the population. The most common is atresia of the posterior communicating artery, which tends to isolate the anterior (carotid system) circulation from the posterior (vertebral basilar) circulation. Anomalies in the circle of Willis are even more common in patients with cerebral infarction, and thus are believed to increase the chances of stroke in patients with cerebral atherosclerosis.

Inflammatory states involving the cerebral arteries are another cause of cerebral infarction. Inflammation produces edema and fibrosis of the vascular wall, which reduces the carrying capacity of the vessel and causes a decrease in cerebral blood flow distally. Collagen-vascular disease is the most common vascular inflammation causing cerebral infarction. Syphilis was formerly the most common inflammation of the cerebral arteries and a frequent cause of cerebral infarction, especially in young persons. Rarely, acute bacterial infections of the pharynx have been followed by vasculitis of the carotid arteries and cerebral infarction. Another uncommon illness is Takayasu's disease, which affects the origin of the cerebral arteries from the aortic arch and its branches, and often results in cerebral infarction, especially in young to middle-aged women.

Cerebral Emboli

Cerebral infarction can occur without intrinsic arterial disease when emboli block arteries and impair blood flow. The most common cause of cerebral emboli in patients under 50 is rheumatic heart disease with mitral stenosis and atrial fibrillation. Other conditions associated with embolus formation are myocardial infarction with mural thrombi, atrial fibrillation of unknown cause, subacute bacterial endocarditis, thyrotoxicosis with atrial fibrillation, and nonbacterial thrombotic endocarditis. Fat emboli are rare. Paradoxical emboli have been reported as a cause of cerebral infarction. These arise in distal veins, and are shunted through the heart to the brain through a patent foramen ovale.

The neuropathologic changes in the brain that follow embolic infarction are not different from those found with infarction from other causes except that hemorrhage into the infarct is found more often with emboli than with vascular occlusion from atherosclerotic disease. The actual embolic material is often not retrieved from the cerebral vessels at autopsy unless the embolus is large, presumably because most small emboli are lysed. This evanescence means that many instances of embolic cerebral infarction must be inferred by finding a source of emboli in other sites. Mutiple small areas of cerebral infarction are commonly found at autopsy in patients with embolic disease.

Cerebral emboli that originate from infected material with bacterial endocarditis or pulmonary infections may cause local inflammation as well as infarction. Infected emboli may produce cerebral abscess, local encephalitis, or mycotic aneurysm.

Recurrent emboli have been postulated as a cause for the transient attacks of neurologic dysfunction often seen in patients with cerebrovascular disease (see below). The surface of atheromatous plaques in the internal carotid artery is frequently ulcerated. A granular lipid debris is present on the ulcer, and the surface of some plaques has been noted to be covered with collections of platelets or organizing blood clot. It is believed that some of the granular or thrombotic material on the surface breaks off, is carried into and obstructs small cerebral vessels, and produces small areas of ischemia. Because only minute vessels are occluded, infarction usually does not occur. In support of this concept is the observation in the optic fundi of some patients having transient ischemic attacks of small white or yellow refractile bodies moving through or blocking the retinal arteries. These emboli have been identified as platelet collections or cholesterol crystals; it is believed that they represent atherosclerotic debris from plaques in proximal vessels and that similar emboli go to brain vessels, causing transient occlusions without necrosis. Embolic material from ulcerated atherosclerotic plaques can cause transient ischemic attacks in the absence of significant vascular obstruction.

Cerebral Venous Inflammation and Thrombosis

Cerebral infarction can result from thrombosis of one of the major venous sinuses, i.e., the superior sagittal sinus, the lateral sinus, or the cavernous sinus, or it can follow extensive thrombotic occlusion of cortical veins. The causes of cerebral venous thrombosis include dehydration, head injury, intracerebral hemorrhage, polycythemia vera, leukemia, infection, and the puerperal state. The most common cause is infection of the mastoid, the frontal sinus, or the subdural space. If the superior sagittal sinus is thrombosed anteriorly, both cerebral hemispheres become markedly congested, swollen, and hemorrhagic. The cerebral white matter may be involved, with small hemorrhages and edema. The surface veins become distended and filled with clot.

Thrombosis of surface veins is usually associated with cerebral or subdural abscess. The histologic picture is that of an acute inflammatory reaction with vascular congestion, edema, and neuronal loss.

Cavernous sinus thrombosis usually follows infection of the eye, face, or nose, and in many instances the thrombus extends through the perihypophyseal veins to involve the opposite cavernous sinus as well. Meningitis may follow spread of the infectious process through the sinus to the subarachnoid space.

Cardiac Disease

Hypotension and Hypertension

Cardiac disease contributes to infarction in patients with cerebral atherosclerosis as the result of periods of hypotension after myocardial infarction, congestive failure, and cardiac arrhythmia. In the Cornell-Bellevue series, clinical heart disease not only preceded cerebral infarction in half the patients, but was the actual cause of at least half the deaths after cerebral infarction.

HYPOTENSION. Both hypotension and hypertension have been implicated in the production of cerebral ischemia and infarction. Although cerebral blood flow in the normal person is relatively independent of the systemic blood pressure down to levels of 50 to 60 mm of mercury, it has been suggested that a lesser drop in blood pressure may produce cerebral ischemia when a significant obstruction is present in a vessel leading to the brain. A localized obstruction must reduce the vessel lumen by nearly 80 per cent to produce a significant distal drop in pressure, but luminal encroachment that extends over long distances theoretically could significantly decrease the distal arterial pressure with less severe grades of obstruction. However, the contribution to cerebral infarction of obstruction and distal decreases in blood pressure and flow is still an unsettled matter. Thus Marshall has reported that when patients with transient ischemic attacks were made briefly hypotensive with hexamethonium and tilting, nearly one half showed evidence of generalized cerebral ischemia only, and another one fourth developed evidence of generalized cerebral ischemia before any focal ischemia.

Failure to maintain the blood pressure may occur with cardiac arrhythmias and after myocardial infarction. The asystole that occurs in Stokes-Adams attacks, if prolonged, can reduce the cerebral blood flow so markedly that cerebral ischemia or infarction results.

HYPERTENSION. Longstanding hypertensive cardiovascular disease is probably the single biggest risk factor in stroke; the place of hypertension in the production of acute cerebral ischemia and infarction is less clear. Rapid elevations of blood pressure evoke an increase in cerebrovascular resistance, and model experiments have demonstrated that stenosis coupled with this increased resistance significantly reduces blood flow. In animal experiments, marked hypertension causes constriction in small cerebral vessels, leading, in turn, to areas of cerebral infarction. Transient marked increases in blood pressure may contribute to cerebral infarction.

Other physiologic changes in cerebral hemodynamics may contribute to cerebral ischemia. Osteoarthritis in the cervical spine may compress the vertebral arteries so that extension, flexion, or rotation of the head can reduce vertebral artery blood flow to the point that ischemic symptoms occur. Cerebral ischemia will be augmented in these instances if anomalies or extensive atherosclerotic deposits compromise the circle of Willis.

Changes in Blood: Clotting, Viscosity, and Anemia

A variety of blood changes have been linked to cerebral infarction. The most frequent is *thrombus formation,* although in many instances it is unclear whether this is primary or secondary to the ischemic process. Thus infarction is not invariably associated with clot-filled vessels, and when thrombi do occur, they arise most commonly in association with ulcerated atherosclerotic lesions or atherosclerotic plaques, which by themselves produce a marked degree of vessel obstruction. In vessels with greatly reduced or absent flow, clots form readily, and long, wormlike clots have been removed from the distal segment of a partially or completely obstructed internal carotid artery shortly after the development of symptoms and signs of cerebral ischemia. A plausible reconstruction of this sequence suggests that marked stenosis was present first and was suddenly increased by hemorrhage into the atherosclerotic plaque, after which clotting occurred distally to the occlusion.

Alterations in blood clotting suggesting hypercoagulability have been described in patients with cerebral infarctions. However, a state of altered clotting has not been observed before an infarction, and some evidence suggests that hypercoagulability is an epiphenomenon that follows, rather than precedes, infarction.

Other potentially deleterious changes in blood include *increased viscosity* with polycythemia and *decreased oxygen-carrying capacity* with anemia. About 15 per cent of patients with polycythemia die from thromboembolism in the brain. Transient ischemic attacks that occur in patients with polycythemia are believed to result from the increase in blood viscosity that occurs when the hematocrit rises above 55.

Severe *anemia* sometimes precipitates cerebral ischemia, particularly if the hematocrit falls below 20, i.e., if the oxygen-carrying capacity drops more than half. Any degree of anemia may supplement severe atherosclerosis, cardiac disease, or hypotension in causing cerebral ischemia.

Cerebral Infarction and Medication

Stroke occurring in young women of childbearing age is related to the use of oral contraceptive agents. The absolute risk of developing stroke in women of this age group is small (1 in 10,000), but with oral contraceptive agents it is increased five to six-fold. The risk is further increased in those women who have migraine or hypertension and who smoke. There is evidence relating the increased risk to the estrogen content of the medication, which is now known to alter blood clotting and intima of vessels. In patients with migraine and hypertension, when contraception is needed other means should be used.

THE PATHOGENESIS OF SYMPTOMS AND SIGNS IN CEREBROVASCULAR DISEASE

To make accurate clinical diagnoses in patients suspected of having cerebrovascular disease, the clinician requires an effective working knowledge of the structural and vascular anatomy of the brain. This is presented in the following paragraphs and diagrams, reference to which will explain why patterns of neurologic dysfunction after infarction or ischemia are related more to arterial territories than to specific neuroanatomic systems.

The brain is supplied by four large arteries, the two common carotids and the two vertebrals. One common carotid artery arises from the aortic arch and the other from the innominate artery in the upper thorax. The two vertebral arteries originate from the right and left subclavian artery. The common carotid artery bifurcates in the neck, forming the internal and external carotid arteries. Each internal carotid artery enters the skull through the homolateral foramen lacerum, passes through the cavernous sinus, and gives off branches in the following order: ophthalmic, anterior choroidal, and posterior communicating. It then bifurcates into the anterior and middle cerebral arteries.

The Anterior Cerebral Artery

As may be seen in Figures 2 and 3, the anterior cerebral artery supplies the medial and superior surfaces of the cerebral hemisphere and the whole of the most anterior portion of the frontal lobes. This area contains the motor and sensory cortex for the foot and leg and the supplementary motor cortex. The anterior cerebral artery also supplies several deep structures of impor-

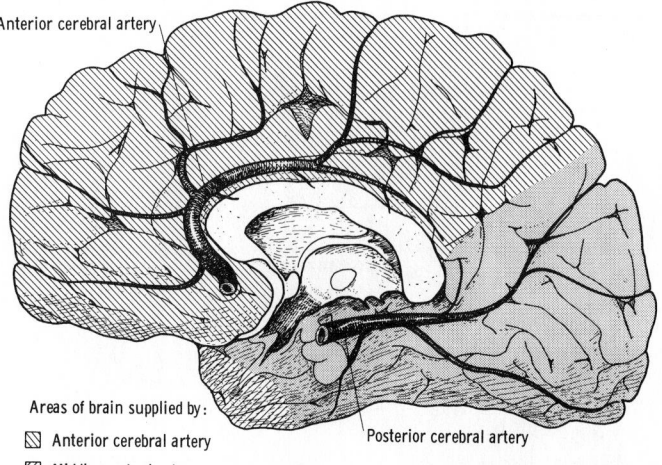

Figure 2. The medial surface of the cerebral hemisphere, showing the course of the anterior and posterior cerebral arteries and the area of brain supplied by each.

Anterior cerebral artery

Posterior cerebral artery

Areas of brain supplied by:

▨ Anterior cerebral artery
▧ Middle cerebral artery
▢ Posterior cerebral artery

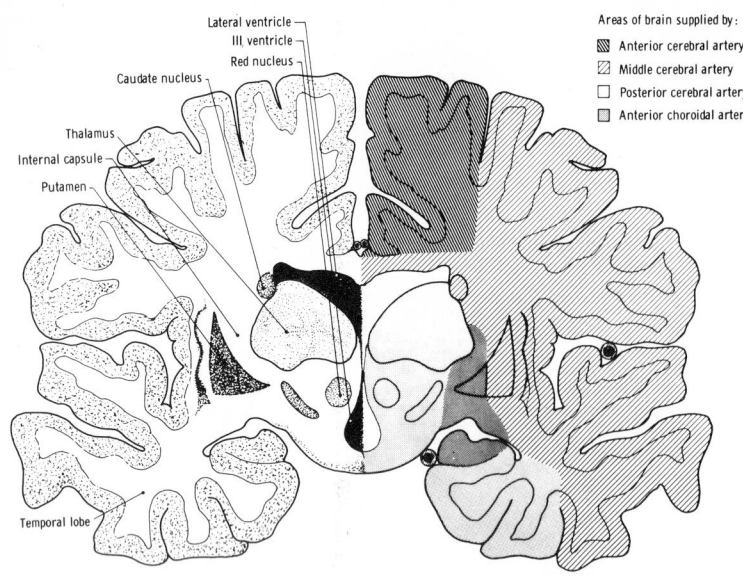

Figure 3. The cerebral hemispheres and the vascular supply, in coronal section.

tance, including the anterior nucleus of the thalamus and a portion of the anterior limb of the internal capsule.

The Middle Cerebral Artery

The middle cerebral artery (Figs. 3 and 4) supplies the lateral surface of the cerebral hemisphere with the exception of the occipital and frontal poles. The cortex supplied includes the primary motor and sensory area for the face, hand, and arm, the optic radiations, and, in the dominant hemisphere, the cortical areas for speech. The perforating branches of the middle cerebral artery reach the center of the cerebral hemisphere supplying the internal capsule and basal ganglia.

The Posterior Cerebral Artery

As shown in Figures 2 and 3, the posterior cerebral artery supplies the posterior pole of the lateral surface of the cerebral hemisphere and the posterior portion of the medial and inferior surfaces of the hemispheres. This area contains the calcarine cortex or the primary visual receptive area. The short perforating branches of the posterior cerebral artery supply the thalamus, part of the optic pathways, and other diencephalic structures including the midbrain.

The Vertebral and Basilar Arteries

The vertebral arteries reach the head via a bony canal in the transverse processes of the sixth through the second cervical vertebrae and enter the skull through the foramen magnum. Immediately after entering the skull each vertebral artery gives off a medial branch (these unite to form the anterior spinal artery) and, just distal to this, the posterior inferior cerebellar artery. At all levels along the brainstem, the ventral medial portion is supplied by short paramedian vessels. The ventrolateral portion of the brainstem is supplied by short circumferential branches from the vertebrals or basilar artery. The dorsal lateral portion and cerebellum are supplied by long circumferential branches: the posterior inferior, the anterior inferior, and the superior cerebellar arteries.

The vertebral artery lies on the ventral lateral surface

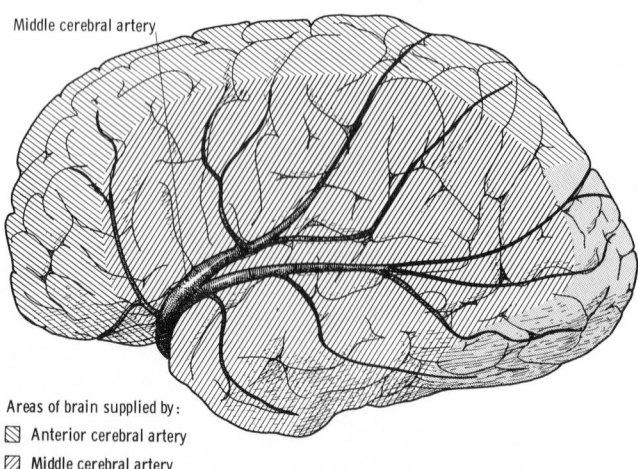

Figure 4. The lateral surface of the cerebral hemisphere and the course of the middle cerebral artery. The sylvian fissure has been opened to better illustrate the course of the vessel.

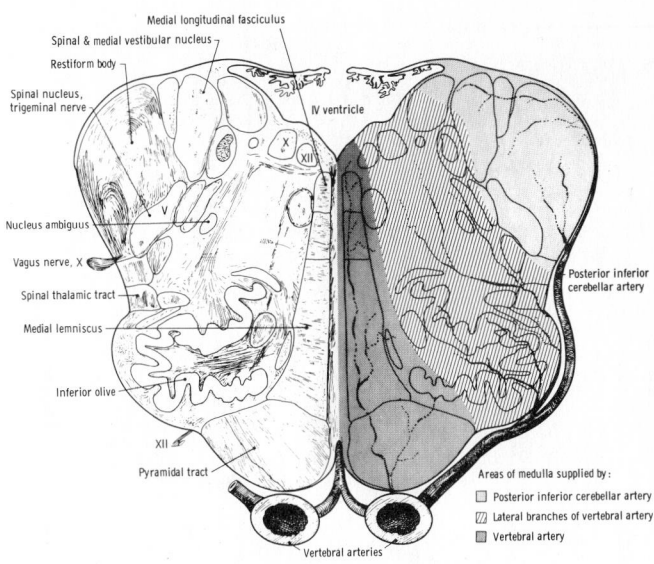

Figure 5. Cross section of the medulla oblongata seen from above at the level of the hypoglossal nuclei. The medial structures are supplied by short branches arising from the vertebral arteries and anterior spinal arteries. The lateral portions are supplied by longer branches and the dorsal and lateral areas by long circumferential branches, at this level called the posterior inferior cerebellar artery.

of the medulla oblongata, and from it and the anterior spinal artery short paramedian branches supply the pyramids, the inferior olives and medial lemniscus, the medial longitudinal fasciculus, and the emerging fibers of the hypoglossal nerve as shown in Figure 5.

The more dorsal portion of the medulla includes the spinothalamic tract, the vestibular nuclei, the sensory nucleus of the fifth cranial nerve, the restiform body, and the emerging fibers of the vagus and glossopharyngeal nerves, and is supplied by longer branches from the vertebral artery and branches from the posterior inferior cerebellar artery. The most cephalad and dorsal segment of the medulla includes the vestibular and cochlear nucei, and it and the posterior portion of the cerebellum are supplied by the posterior inferior cerebellar artery.

At the lower border of the pons, the two vertebral arteries unite to form the basilar artery. From this artery in the pons, short perpendicular branches enter the brainstem to supply paramedian structures, including the corticospinal tracts, the pontine nuclei, the medial lemniscus, the medial longitudinal fasciculus, and the pontine reticular nuclei (Fig. 6). Circumferential branches supply the lateral portion of the pons, which includes the emerging seventh and eighth cranial nerves, the trigeminal nerve root, the vestibular and cochlear nuclei, and the spinothalamic tracts. The anterior inferior cerebellar artery, the long circumferential branch at this level, also gives branches to the most dorsal and lateral of these structures as it runs dorsally to the cerebellum.

At the level of the midbrain the basilar artery lies in the interpeduncular fossa (Fig. 7). Short branches pass laterally and dorsally to both sides to supply the cerebral peduncles, the emerging third nerve roots, the medial portions of the red nuclei, the medial longitudinal fasciculus, the oculomotor nuclei, and the midbrain reticulum. Branches of the posterior cerebral artery supply the lateral portions of the peduncles, the red nuclei, and the medial lemnisci. The superior cerebellar arte-

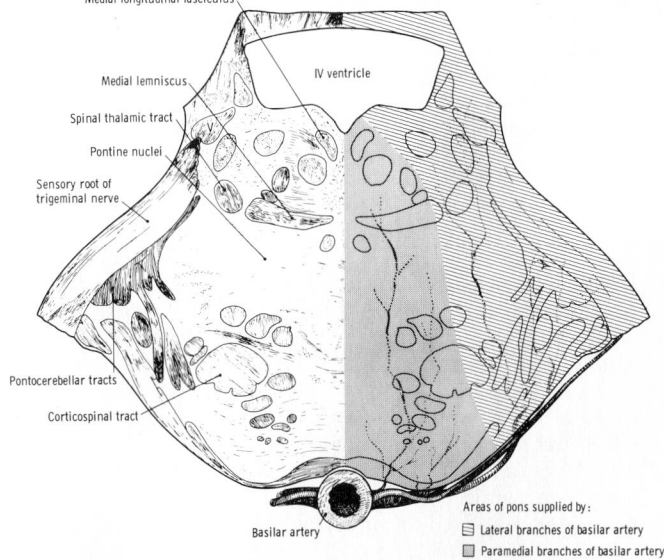

Figure 6. Cross section of the midpons. The most medial regions are supplied by short perforating branches from the basilar artery. The more lateral regions are supplied by lateral branches of the basilar artery. At this level, the more dorsal structures are supplied by the long circumferential branch, the anterior inferior cerebellar artery.

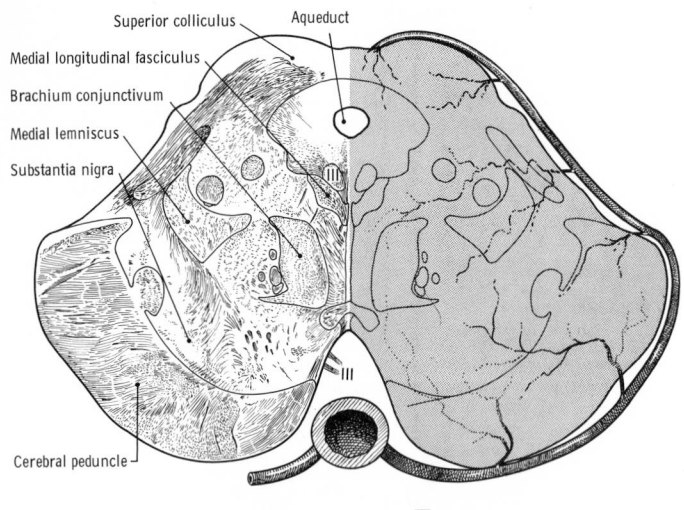

Superior colliculus
Aqueduct
Medial longitudinal fasciculus
Brachium conjunctivum
Medial lemniscus
Substantia nigra
Cerebral peduncle

Figure 7. Cross section of the midbrain seen from below. The medial, lateral, and dorsal regions are supplied by short branches from the posterior cerebral artery as it passes around the midbrain.

☐ Midbrain supplied by branches
of the posterior cerebral artery

ries supply some of the dorsal portions of the midbrain, including the colliculi and the anterior portion of the cerebellum on each side.

It will be clear from this review of neurologic and vascular anatomy that infarction can produce a large variety of clinical pictures, depending on the vessels involved. The pattern of most syndromes is helpful in localizing the area of the nervous system damaged by infarction, but only a few reliably indicate exactly which portion of the vascular tree is involved. As an example, diagnoses are often made of middle cerebral artery occlusion, but a review of the vascular anatomy of the brain quickly reveals why, with both anterior cerebral arteries filling from either side, an identical clinical picture can be associated with occlusion of the internal carotid artery at any point along its course.

SIGNS AND SYMPTOMS IN CEREBROVASCULAR DISEASE: STROKE SYNDROMES

An adequate exposition of the symptoms and signs of cerebrovascular disease requires a classification of the various clinical entities that make up the stroke syndrome.

Cerebrovascular accidents are classified on the basis of the anatomic site of ischemia or infarction, the cerebral vessels occluded or obstructed, and the temporal character of the entire clinical episode. The latter is clinically the most valuable in that the indicated therapy is often different for the three kinds of temporal profiles found. The three profiles have been defined as *transient ischemic attack, stroke-in-evolution* or *progressive stroke,* and *completed stroke.*

The term *transient ischemic attack* or incipient stroke refers to transient episodes of neurologic dysfunction caused by cerebrovascular disease. The attacks are believed to be caused by cerebral ischemia, and consist of fleeting, 5- to 30-minute disturbances in neurologic function that leave no permanent residue.

Stroke-in-evolution or progressive stroke refers to increasing neurologic dysfunction caused by cerebral ischemia over a period of minutes, hours, or, rarely, days.

Completed stroke refers to the clinical picture seen in patients who have ceased to show further progression in neurologic deficit or in those who have developed a slight to calamitous neurologic deficit earlier that is now stable or improving. *Cerebral embolism* is one cause of completed stroke in which the onset is an abrupt monophasic event, and there is clinically a demonstrable source of emboli.

Cerebral Transient Ischemic Attacks

The symptoms vary, depending upon which area of the brain is ischemic, but there are two main types: those associated with ischemia of parts or the whole of a cerebral hemisphere, and those associated with ischemia of the brainstem. The symptoms most often include transient contralateral weakness of the lower face, fingers, hand, arm, or leg, but such patients may also experience fleeting sensory symptoms such as tingling, "pin and needles," or numbness in parts of the body contralateral to the ischemia. Ischemia in the dominant hemisphere may cause dysphasia, with impairment in the context of speech and, at times, a transient lack of understanding.

Patients with ischemia in the portion of the brain supplied by the posterior cerebral artery may suffer blurred vision, or may notice transient hemianopic or altitudinal visual field defects or impairment of visual acuity.

Ischemia or insufficiency caused by internal carotid artery stenosis often produces transient retinal ischemia, resulting in monocular blindness or reduced acuity on the side of the stenosis, combined with contralateral weakness of the face, arm, or leg.

Ischemic attacks which result from involvement of the brain supplied by the vertebral and basilar arteries have an extremely wide range of symptoms. Common symptoms include vertigo, tinnitus, diplopia, dysarthria, dysphagia, and dysphonia. Patients may complain of unilateral or bilateral face, arm, and leg weakness and unilateral or bilateral sensations of numbness and tingling in the face, arms, or leg. There may be tinnitus, hearing loss, and ataxia. In addition, patients with brainstem ischemia may experience "drop attacks," in which they suddenly lose postural tone and fall to the ground without losing consciousness, then immediately regain postural control and rise quickly. The most common complaint with transient ischemic attacks from vertebrobasilar insufficiency is dizziness. However, dizziness is commonly associated with other physiologic disturbances and is rarely the only symptom of brainstem ischemia. When patients describe intermittent neurologic episodes with symptoms suggesting a generalized decrease in cerebral blood flow such as dizziness, lightheadedness, and generalized weakness, they should be carefully examined for cardiac dysrhythmia before being studied for the presence of extracranial arterial disease. Cardiac dysrhythmia, with a drop in cardiac output and subsequently in general cerebral blood flow, is a common cause of nonfocal transient ischemic attacks.

Symptoms of vertebral basilar artery ischemia, although variable, tend to occur in combinations that aid in their diagnosis. Vertigo, ataxia, dysarthria, paresthesia, diplopia, tinnitus, dysphagia, and focal weakness in the face, jaw, or pharynx tend to coexist, although not always in the same sequence or combination. Another grouping of symptoms is that of unilateral or bilateral weakness of the extremities with drop attacks and diplopia. The reason for these differences in symptom combinations can be found by referring to the diagrams of the blood supply to the brainstem. Ischemia of the dorsal and lateral portions of the brainstem supplied by the circumferential arteries produces the first group of symptoms. Ischemia of the more ventral portions supplied by the medial perforating arteries causes the second group.

Symptomatic vertebral basilar artery ischemia may occur with stenosis of the subclavian artery proximal to the origin of the vertebral artery. The arm on the side of the stenosis may be supplied by retrograde flow in the ipsilateral vertebral, and, during exercise, enough blood can be diverted from the vertebral system to the arm to cause symptoms of brainstem ischemia. This mechanism of producing brainstem ischemia has been called the *subclavian steal syndrome*. However, most instances of reversed vertebral artery flow with subclavian artery stenosis or occlusion are asymptomatic.

Ischemic attacks may occur many times a day or at weekly or monthly intervals. They may be intermittently present over several months or several years. Some patients with internal carotid artery occlusion have transient ischemic attacks for as long as two years before cerebral infarction occurs. Others have clusters of attacks lasting only a few hours or days before carotid occlusion becomes complete and causes infarction. *The major importance of transient ischemic attacks is that they signal the existence of significant cerebrovascular disease and clearly indicate the potential danger of cerebral infarction.* Studies of the natural history of transient ischemic attacks indicate that about one fourth to one third of patients afflicted will suffer a cerebral infarction within two to five years of onset of the attacks. It cannot always be predicted which patients with cerebral ischemia will develop cerebral infarction or even when it will occur. Transient ischemic attacks become more significant predictors of cerebral infarction if accompanied by extensive atherosclerosis as evidenced by abnormalities in the neurovascular examination, such as arterial bruit in the neck, absent temporal pulse, retinal embolization, and reduction of retinal artery pressure on

the appropriate side. Some varieties of cerebral ischemic attacks carry a better prognosis than others. Attacks suggesting ventral brainstem involvement, such as bilateral paresis or unilateral transient paresis or drop attacks, connote a poor prognosis. Carotid ischemic attacks that occur close together in clusters carry a poor prognosis, for in a large percentage of such patients cerebral infarction rapidly follows.

In the interval between transient ischemic attacks, the neurologic examination is usually entirely normal. During a transient ischemic attack, patients commonly have neurologic deficits corresponding to their symptoms. Thus with ischemia of a cerebral hemisphere, there may be a hemiparesis with reflex asymmetry and an extensor plantar response, or a mild hemisensory or visual field deficit. If the dominant hemisphere is affected, dysphasia may be noted: the patient has difficulty in naming and recognizing objects. Patients examined during a brainstem ischemic attack often exhibit nystagmus, complete facial weakness, palate and tongue weakness, and deviation, dysconjugate eye movements, sensory defects, and weakness on one side or on both sides of the body. The evaluation of patients with transient ischemic attacks must always include careful examination of the optic fundus through a dilated pupil, searching for cholesterol (bronze debris) or platelet emboli (white or invisible plugs) in the arterial tree. *The presence of such emboli in one eye is important evidence of an embolic source in the carotid artery.* Patients with such emboli should have cerebral angiography, and the presence of ulcerated atherosclerotic plaques should be determined.

Consciousness is usually unimpaired during transient ischemic attacks, although thinking is sometimes slowed. This lack of alteration of consciousness coupled with the absence of either aura or convulsive movements helps to distinguish these attacks from convulsive seizures. Other conditions that must be considered in the differential diagnosis are Menière's syndrome (which is rare in the elderly), migraine headache, cerebral emboli, or the progressive neurologic deficits caused by cerebral neoplasm.

Stroke-in-Evolution
(Progressive Stroke)

The evolving stroke is characterized by the gradual development of paralysis and sensory impairment over a period of several hours and, at times, one to two days. The symptoms and signs may develop as a series of steplike changes or as an unbroken continuum of worsening. When first examined, a patient may have mild weakness which, as the hours pass, is found to be more and more marked and to involve more and more of the body. The symptoms and signs found are identical to those of completed stroke; only the time course of onset is different. This course also occurs with subdural hematoma and brain tumor, but, for these disorders, the duration usually extends over several days or weeks.

Cerebral Infarction
(Completed Stroke)

Cerebral infarctions resulting from cerebral emboli or from cerebral atherosclerosis and thrombosis, respectively, cannot be distinguished by the neurologic disorders they produce. Differences between these two causes of infarction do exist, however, in the mode of onset of symptoms and in the general physical evaluation.

The pattern of onset of neurologic symptoms and signs in cerebral infarction often suggests the cause. Cerebral embolism causes an abrupt onset of symptoms, and headache often precedes other neurologic symptoms by several hours. Cerebral infarction caused by atherosclerotic vascular obstruction or occlusion often has a less sudden onset. There may be a distinct series of steplike increases in neurologic symptoms and signs, or infarction may be preceded by a series of transient ischemic attacks. A gradual onset with increasing neurologic deficit over several (one to five) hours is characteristic of the progressing stroke. A gradual onset of symptoms and signs over two days or, occasionally, one week, does occur but is uncommon. The frequency of these different patterns can be inferred from the experience of one large series of patients with ischemic infarction; about one third had a sudden onset of symptoms, about one fifth had symptoms that progressively increased over one to 12 hours, and only about one in 20 had symptoms that progressed for as long as 12 to 24 hours. One fifth of the patients with occlusive vascular disease and cerebral embolism had the onset of neurologic signs during sleep.

Headache is present in many patients with embolic or atherosclerotic infarction. The headache is usually mild and localized to the side of the infarction. Headache is believed to be caused by vasodilation of unoccluded vessels near the infarcted area, and is most common when vessels near the base of the brain are occluded.

Consciousness is usually not lost at the onset of infarction of the cerebral hemispheres, but may be reduced, particularly when large infarcts involve the dominant hemisphere. When unconsciousness is present from the onset or is the initial symptom, brainstem infarction is the most likely cause. When large hemispheric infarctions are complicated by rapidly developing and severe brain edema, loss of consciousness caused by diencephalic and upper brainstem compression may occur shortly after the onset of symptoms. This may give the false impression of loss of consciousness from the onset unless a careful history documents a lucid period at the very beginning of symptoms. Convulsive seizures are rare at the onset of cerebral infarction, but they occur in about 8 per cent of patients at some time in the course of the acute or convalescent phase of the illness. They are usually focal, but may be generalized.

When infarction is limited to the cerebral hemisphere, there is weakness or paralysis in the extremities contralateral to the infarction. Patients may also be aware that sensory perception on the side of weakness is impaired and may complain of heaviness or numbness in the arm or leg. They rarely have other sensory symptoms such as pain or paresthesias. Defects in visual fields are common but often escape the patient's notice. The defect is suspected when patients pay little attention to visual stimuli on one side of the body. At times, the eyes may be constantly deviated to the side away from the neurologic deficits.

The most serious consequence of infarction in the dominant hemisphere is dysphasia, which can range from a mild deficit of expression to aphonic mutism. The dysphasia is almost invariably a mixture of difficulty with expression (expressive dysphasia) and difficulty in understanding what is said, written, or indicated by gesture (receptive dysphasia); one or the other may predominate. In patients who have infarction in the nondominant hemisphere, lack of awareness or concern about paralysis of the contralateral side is often evident. Such subjects may, at times, be so completely unaware of their neurologic disabilities that they are hospitalized only after family or friends notice their disabilities. This phenomenon, *anosognosia*, is most common when a patient is obtunded and when there is a significant sensory deficit on the paretic side as a result of infarction of the parietal lobe. It accompanies nearly one fourth of all large strokes, but usually persists only if the patient remains obtunded or confused or has little return of sensation.

Infarctions in the brainstem produce a wide variety of symptoms. Among the most conspicuous are vertigo, diplopia, dysarthria, dysphagia, and ataxia. In addition, the patient may note unilateral or bilateral sensory impairment or weakness. Often patients note clumsiness and difficulty in performing skilled acts without paresis.

Specific Vascular Syndromes

Internal Carotid Artery Occlusion

Occlusion of the internal carotid artery at its origin from the common carotid or intracranially is the site of the major vascular lesion in nearly 20 per cent of strokes. The usual lesion is atherosclerotic with, at first, partial obstruction and, finally, occlusion with a thrombus. Occasionally the internal carotid artery is obstructed by a large embolus.

Symptoms and signs specific for internal carotid artery occlusion in the neck are intermittent visual impairment or blindness in the eye on the side of the occlusion (retinal artery insufficiency) combined with a contralateral hemiparesis and sensory loss (middle cerebral artery insufficiency). This clinical picture often begins with a series of transient ischemic attacks and only later causes permanent weakness and sensory loss. *Unless the history of intermittent blindness can be obtained*, it is difficult, on clinical grounds alone, to distinguish occlusion of the internal carotid artery from middle cerebral artery occlusion.

On neurologic examination, patients with cerebral infarction caused by internal carotid artery occlusion have paresis of voluntary movement, with weakness most noticeable in the contralateral face and upper extremity. Infarcts produce motility defects as their main manifestations, but there is usually some impairment of sensory perception and, at times, visual field impairment as well.

In the paretic extremities, deep tendon reflexes are hyperactive, and pathologic reflexes such as the Babinski sign (extensor plantar response) are found. Muscle tone becomes increased on the weakened side, and spasticity may be so marked that early contracture is evident. Sensory impairment is most evident in modalities such as position sense, vibration sense, two-point discrimination, and tactile perception of shape and texture. Touch and pain perception may be moderately impaired, and extinction of stimuli on the involved side may be evident on double simultaneous stimulation. The size of the cerebral infarction produced by internal carotid occlusion is extremely variable. When there is no collateral circulation through the anterior communicating, posterior communicating, ophthalmic, or surface collateral arteries, the infarct can involve nearly the whole cerebral hemisphere, both lateral and medial surfaces. With a richer collateral circulation, smaller infarcts and proportionately fewer neurologic defects result. Occasionally occlusion of the internal carotid is asymptomatic, and is discovered only as an incidental finding at autopsy or when cerebral angiograms are done.

Internal carotid artery occlusion or stenosis sometimes causes partial Horner's syndrome (slight ptosis and miosis) on the side opposite the paresis. The eye changes have been attributed to ischemia of the sympathetic fibers that lie in the adventitia of the arterial wall adjacent to the occlusion, but are more probably due to direct hypothalamic damage, for they can also be observed in patients with similar infarcts who do not have occlusion of the carotid arteries. An audible bruit in the neck at the angle of the mandible is a helpful indicator of stenosis of the internal carotid artery at that site. Occlusion of the internal carotid artery is also suggested when the retinal artery pressure on the affected side, as measured with an ophthalmodynamometer, decreases 25 per cent or more below the arterial pressure in the other eye. Study of blood flow in the supratrochlear artery, using a directional Doppler flowmeter, may show reversal of the usual direction of flow, which can be stopped by compression of the temporal artery. This finding is highly indicative of carotid artery occlusion with collateral circulation from the extracranial to the intracranial circulation via the ophthalmic artery.

Middle Cerebral Artery Occlusion

The cerebral tissue supplied by the middle cerebral artery is the most common area for infarction from emboli or vascular insufficiency, and the neurologic picture produced by either is the same.

When a middle cerebral artery is occluded, infarction occurs in the lateral portion of the hemisphere and produces varying degrees of contralateral paresis and sensory loss, mainly in the face, the upper extremities, and the hand, and often blindness in the contralateral, homonymous visual field. Occlusions at the origin of the middle cerebral artery produce extensive neurologic disturbance with profound contralateral hemiplegia and sensory loss. Occlusions in branches of the middle cerebral artery may produce a variable clinical picture. At times, only paresis is evident in the arm and face. In some patients, sensory impairment is the dominant and occasionally the only neurologic abnormality, and some patients have only dysphasia.

Anterior Cerebral Artery Occlusion

Anterior cerebral artery occlusion causes infarction in the cortical areas that control motor and sensory functions of the contralateral lower extremity, and impairs voluntary movement and sensory perception of that leg. The upper extremity and face are spared. Cerebral infaction caused by occlusion of the proximal portion of the anterior cerebral artery is uncommon because collateral circulation through the anterior communicating artery is usually adequate to supply both hemispheres.

Posterior Cerebral Artery Occlusion

Posterior cerebral artery occlusion causes infarction of the posterior lateral and posterior medial surfaces of the cerebral hemisphere, including the calcarine cortex. Proximal occlusions of the artery result in infarction of the thalamus and upper brainstem as well. Extensive infarctions in the occipital cortex cause homonymous hemianopic field defects, and those involving the dominant hemisphere may produce disturbances in reading, visual learning, visual recognition, and visual spatial orientation.

Infarction of both occipital poles can follow basilar artery stenosis or occlusion. The result is a double hemianopia and cortical blindness, a striking feature of which is that the patient is usually unaware that he is blind and may vigorously deny it (Anton's syndrome).

Brainstem Infarction

Brainstem infarction, although not as common as hemisphere infarction, produces several distinct clinical syndromes, best categorized by noting whether the clinical picture suggests involvement of ventral paramedian, ventrolateral, or dorsal brainstem structures. As noted in the discussion of neurovascular anatomy, these three areas receive blood supply through different groups of arteries.

Many of the particular groupings of symptoms and signs associated with various brainstem infarctions that have been given eponyms are believed to be common occurrences with brainstem infarction. However, in an analysis of 50 patients with brainstem infarction from the Cornell-Bellevue series, only two clearly fitted into these syndromes as originally described. The remaining 48 had an extensive mixture of symptoms and signs indicating an overlap in the areas believed to be infarcted with occlusions in specific arteries.

Midbrain Infarctions

Occlusion of the paramedian branches from the apex of the basilar artery or of the proximal posterior cerebral arteries causes infarction of portions of one or both cerebral peduncles, the oculomotor nerves, the oculomotor nuclei, the brachia conjunctivae, the red nuclei, and the midbrain reticular formation. The resulting symptoms and signs may be unilateral or bilateral, depending on the extent of the infarction. Unilateral signs include (1) ipsilateral oculomotor palsy and contralateral hemiparesis (Weber's syndrome), (2) ipsilateral oculomotor palsy, ipsilateral ataxia of gait, and poorly coordinated arm and hand movements (Nothnagel's syndrome). Bilateral signs include impaired consciousness, quadriparesis, divergent gaze, impaired vertical eye movements and midposition, or dilated pupils unresponsive to light. Purposeless, flail-like, involuntary movements (hemiballismus) may occur, and usually involve the upper extremity more than the lower. Patients in coma caused by infarction of the midbrain often have an unusual appearance, seeming to be almost awake although unable to communicate in any manner. This state has been called *coma vigil* or *akinetic mutism*. Such patients, although unresponsive, may exhibit a sleepwalking cycle.

When the dorsal area, supplied by the posterior cerebral artery, is ischemic or infarcted, the spinothalamic tract, the red nucleus, the descending sympathetic tracts, and the medial lemniscus are involved. The clinical picture consists of slight ptosis and miosis (Horner's syndrome), ipsilateral ataxia, and choreiform adventitious movements and contralateral impairment of all modalities of sensory perception of the entire body, including the face. This clinical picture is often called the superior cerebellar artery syndrome.

Pontine Infarction

Infarction in the pons is usually associated with basilar artery obstruction. Occlusion of the paramedian branches of the basilar artery causes necrosis of the corticospinal tracts, the pontine nuclei, the medial lemniscus, the medial longitudinal fasciculus, the abducens nucleus, the pontocerebellar tracts, and the pontine reticulum. Ipsilateral abducens palsy, facial weakness, and contralateral corticospinal tract dysfunction (Millard-Gubler syndrome) and the same findings with lateral conjugate gaze palsy (Foville's syndrome) are two unilateral syndromes that occur with occlusion in the paramedian arteries to the pons. Bilateral signs include quadriparesis, reduced reaction to noxious stimuli, and abducens paresis. Other signs include coma, hyperventilation, apneustic or ataxic breathing, small pupils, and internuclear ophthalmoplegia. If only the most ventral portion of the pons is damaged, awareness may be maintained even though the patient is quadriparetic.

With occlusion of arteries to the lateral pons, the signs and symptoms are unilateral and include tinnitus, deafness, nausea, vertigo, impairment of facial sensation, complete ipsilateral facial paralysis, nystagmus, miosis and ptosis (partial Horner's syndrome), and impaired conjugate gaze toward the side of the lesion. Impaired pain and temperature perception of half the contralateral body below the face is usually found. This clinical picture is often referred to as the syndrome of anterior inferior cerebellar artery occlusion.

Medullary Infarction

Occlusion of the paramedian branches of the vertebral artery in the medulla causes contralateral paresis of the arm and leg, contralateral impaired sensory perception to touch, position sense and vibration sense in the arm, trunk, and leg, and ipsilateral tongue paralysis. With occlusion of arterial branches to the lateral medulla, the clinical picture includes vertigo, nausea, vomiting, dysarthria, dysphagia, nystagmus, ipsilateral Horner's syndrome, ipsilateral vocal cord paralysis, and impaired ipsilateral facial sensory perception to pain with impairment of pain sensation on the contralateral half of the body below the face. This clinical picture is referred to as the syndrome of posterior inferior cerebellar artery occlusion or Wallenberg's syndrome. It results from occlusion of the vertebral artery itself as frequently as or more frequently than it does from occlusion of its branches.

Basilar Artery Occlusion

When the basilar artery is completely occluded, infarction is found mainly in the ventral pons, midbrain,

and occipital lobes. The clinical picture is like that seen with occlusion of the paramedian midbrain or pontine branches, but may include various defects in the visual fields and, at times, cortical blindness in addition. The brainstem tegmentum is almost invariably involved, causing major disturbances in consciousness.

Cerebral Embolism

The diagnosis of cerebral embolization is usually not difficult when it is remembered that the onset of neurologic symptoms and signs is abrupt, that they are often preceded by headache for a few hours before paresis is evident, and that a potential source for emboli is usually found on physical examination. Convulsive seizures occur at the onset, but they are uncommon. They are at first focal and later generalized in most patients. Loss of consciousness may occur and usually lasts for only a few minutes; but after onset, patients may be confused. The neurologic signs depend upon which artery is occluded; the most common clinical picture is that of middle cerebral artery occlusion. Cerebral emboli can lodge in any major cerebral artery, and emboli commonly recur often to the same artery. The cerebrospinal fluid is usually clear and without cells. When protein elevation and cells are found, subacute bacterial endocarditis should be suspected. Mitral stenosis with atrial fibrillation, myocardial infarction with mural thrombus, and subacute bacterial endocarditis are the cardiac disorders most commonly found. Normal sinus rhythm does not exclude the diagnosis of cerebral emboli, for it may be found in more than one third of such patients, particularly with a "tight" mitral stenosis or with past myocardial infarcts, respectively. Evidence of embolization to other sites strengthens the supposition that the cause of cerebral infarction is embolic.

Cerebral Venous Thrombosis

The symptoms of local cerebral venous thrombosis are headache, delirium, drowsiness, diplopia, and convulsions. The signs are usually those of increased intracranial pressure with papilledema and focal neurologic abnormalities. Focal fits are common, as are paresis and hemisensory loss. Such patients are restless, confused, and obtunded.

Superior sagittal sinus occlusion produces a somewhat similar clinical picture. At the New York Hospital, 21 patients with noninfective sagittal sinus thrombosis have been studied. Nine had terminal disease and marasmus, six had cyanotic congenital heart disease, and four had other, unexplained episodes of venous or arterial thromboses. Eleven of the 21 patients were children. Below the age of ten, cerebral infarction is more often due to venous than to arterial occlusion. Nearly all patients had fever, and their cerebrospinal fluids were under increased pressure, averaging 260 mm of fluid, and contained more than ten red blood cells. Neurologic symptoms appeared abruptly or progressed rapidly to a maximum, usually within 36 hours. Most patients were obtunded or confused and had headache. The white blood count was elevated in ten patients; in seven it was over 20,000. Nuchal rigidity was common, and papilledema, hemiparesis, and focal epileptic seizures occurred in about half the cases. Two patients presented later with signs of pseudotumor cerebri. The occurrence of hemiparesis or focal epilepsy was usually associated with cortical venous thromboses in addition to the sinus occlusion.

Cavernous sinus occlusion, usually a complication of sinus or paranasal skin infection, is characterized by proptosis, orbital chemosis, and edema, pain around the eye, papilledema, retinal hemorrhages, and fever. Extraocular palsy may be present. The disease carries a high risk of spread to the opposite cavernous sinus. Complications include meningitis and brain abscess.

Transverse or lateral sinus thrombosis, ususally secondary to mastoiditis, is now uncommon with the decline in the incidence of that disease. When it does occur, it is usually manifested by headache, tenderness over the mastoid process, and, occasionally, paresis of the structures supplied by the glossopharyngeal and accessory nerve, with dysphagia, dysphonia, and weakness of the ipsilateral sternomastoid and trapezius muscles.

In all varieties of cerebral venous thrombosis, there is usually some evidence of sepsis with fever, malaise, headache, and leukocytosis.

Although the condition is uncommon, a diagnosis of cerebral venous thrombosis should be kept in mind for patients with evidence of cerebral infarction who have focal seizures, increased intracranial pressure, or evidence of infection. Cerebral venous thrombosis is particularly likely as a cause of postpartum cerebral infarction.

PHYSICAL AND LABORATORY FINDINGS

The general evaluation of the patient with cerebral infarction usually reveals evidence of vascular disease at other sites as well as a variety of associated diseases. About one fifth of patients with atherosclerotic cerebral infarction in the Cornell-Bellevue series had had previous strokes, half of which had occurred in the preceding year. Another fifth had had myocardial infarction, usually within the previous year. Over one half of the patients were hypertensive, but the diastolic pressure was above 100 mm of mercury in only one third of the patients. Nearly one fifth of the patients had diabetes mellitus, and one in ten gave a history of peripheral vascular occlusive disease.

PHYSICAL EXAMINATION. The physical examination of most patients with cerebral infarction discloses a normal or slightly elevated body temperature. Careful examination of the heart should never be overlooked because the presence of cardiac enlargement, atrial fibrillation, and cardiac murmurs, suggesting rheumatic heart disease with mitral stenosis, aids in detecting the presence of cerebral emboli. Patients with cerebral infarction often have atherosclerotic cornary heart disease, and perhaps one fifth have had recent or associated myocardial infarcts.

Palpation may reveal absence of pulsation in easily felt peripheral arteries. In the lower extremities, this is indicative of atherosclerotic vascular disease in the aorta, iliac, femoral or popliteal arteries. In the upper extremities, it may indicate occlusions in the major branches of the aorta, such as the innominate or subclavian arteries. Absence of pulses in one or both upper extremities should alert the physician to such diagnoses as "pulseless disease" (Takayasu's syndrome) or the "subclavian steal syndrome."

Auscultation for bruit over the neck is helpful in identifying sites of extracranial stenosis. A bruit heard in the neck under the angle of the mandible suggests atherosclerotic disease of the carotid artery, and bruit heard just above the clavicles is associated with vertebral or subclavian artery stenosis. Bruit, when loud and localized, is associated with atherosclerotic obstruction at that site in more than three fourths of patients.

LABORATORY EXAMINATIONS. Laboratory tests are aimed at both confirming the diagnosis and identifying complications. Every patient suspected of stroke should have a lumbar puncture and skull roentgenograms, and, if there are any unusual features at all about the illness, computerized axial tomography (CAT scan) should be employed (see below).

The cerebrospinal fluid should be examined promptly to determine the presence of intracranial bleeding or an unsuspected infection. The lumbar puncture must be approached cautiously, however, when patients are in stupor or coma or when it is uncertain whether the illness is caused by stroke or by brain tumor, with increased intracranial pressure. In such instances, it is preferable to proceed with computerized axial tomography or an arteriogram, because lumbar puncture can inadvertently precipitate tentorial or foraminal herniation when there is an expanding intracranial mass.

The cerebrospinal fluid pressure is rarely over 200 mm of CSF in cerebral infarction. The fluid is usually clear and colorless, but bleeding and xanthochromia from hemorrhagic infarction may be found. The CSF protein level is usually normal, although slight elevations to 60 to 75 mg per 100 ml are found in perhaps one fifth of the patients. Elevations to 80 mg per 100 ml or above are found in less than 10 per cent, but particularly in those with basilar artery disease. With massive cerebral infarction, the protein may be raised to values of nearly 100 mg per 100 ml. Diabetes occasionally accounts for pronounced CSF protein elevations with stroke, probably by a leak of protein through damaged small vessels. Patients with high values should always be carefully reviewed for the possibility of brain tumor.

Skull roentgenograms should be examined for evidence of fracture, erosion of the posterior clinoids (suggesting chronically increased intracranial pressure), abnormal calcification, and pineal shift.

The general evaluation of patients with cerebral infarction should include an electrocardiogram (EKG) and a chest roentgenogram. The EKG may confirm the presence of an arrhythmia or may disclose a silent myocardial infarction. (A potentially confusing point is that the EKG may show minor T wave and S-T segment changes caused by cerebral infarction and not by primary cardiac disease.)

The development of computerized axial tomography (CAT scan) has added a major new dimension to the diagnosis and management of stroke and has replaced pneumoencephalography, electroencephalography, and echoencephalography in diagnosis. Its major use in cerebral infarction is in differential diagnosis, in which it is highly accurate in identifying or eliminating intracerebral hemorrhage and brain tumor as causes of neurologic deficit. It is the diagnostic means of choice to establish cerebral infarction as a cause of acute neurologic disability. It is further useful in defining the exact site and extent of an infarct. As the technique is based on the differential radiation absorption of tissue, during the first few days after infarction the CAT scan may not differentiate normal from infarcted brain, and small infarctions which are cystic may not alway be detected. On average the CAT scan will accurately detect cerebral infarction of 1 cm in diameter or larger in about 50 to 60 per cent of instances. Use of iodinated contrast media intravenously is useful in determining the degree of hemorrhage in an infarction. Computerized scans are helpful in delineating the degree of cerebral edema around an infarct and in following an infarct as it resolves.

Special Investigations

Arteriography

The technical quality and safety of arteriography has improved to the point that complications develop only in about 1 to 2 per cent of patients with cerebrovascular disease, and permanent worsening and death follow arteriography in less than 1 per cent of patients.

Cerebral angiography is indicated only for certain patients with cerebrovascular disease and has two main values. The first is in differential diagnosis for the patient with an atypical history and findings, or who is unable to give an accurate history because of dysphasia or depressed consciousness.

The second and more important value of cerebral angiograms is the accurate demonstration of the site, extent, and incidence of arterial obstructions and ulcerated atherosclerotic plaques that might be susceptible to surgical correction. Patients who need study include predominantly those who suffer transient ischemic attacks, very mild strokes, or strokes from which recovery has been substantial. In such cases, it is necessary to outline both the neck vessels and the nature and extent of the intracranial collateral circulation and the collateral channels from extracranial to intracranial vessels.

Rapid roentgenographic exposures have clarified some aspects of the physiology of cerebral blood flow in patients with cerebrovascular disease. Cerebral angiography may identify unusual patterns of blood flow in cerebral vessels, such as retrograde flow down one vertebral artery with proximal subclavian artery stenosis (subclavian steal). Ulceration of plaques can be demonstrated in about 41 per cent of patients with transient ischemic attacks coming to operation. The accuracy of the angiographic diagnosis when compared to findings at surgery is 90 per cent.

Brain scanning, using radiomercury-chlormerodrin or Tc^{99m} Pertechnetate, shows a high uptake of radioactive material in the area of a cerebral infarction. This technique may aid in accurate localization of the infarcted area, but an identical picture can result from brain tumor, thereby limiting its usefulness in differential diagnosis. A normal brain scan during the first few days after the onset of symptoms suggesting a stroke, followed by a positive brain scan, is highly suggestive of cerebral infarction.

DIFFERENTIAL DIAGNOSIS

The most common sources of error in the diagnosis of cerebral infarction are brain tumors, subdural hematomas, intracerebral hemorrhages, cerebral traumatic lesions, and cerebral infections.

When a clear history of the onset is available, cerebral infarction is seldom confused with other disorders. Stroke caused by cerebral emboli or cerebral thrombosis characteristically produces a maximal neurological deficit initially, with gradual improvement in function over days, weeks, or months. The first symptoms of brain tumor and subdural hematoma occasionally are mistaken for stroke, but the general tendency is for these two disorders to cause gradually progressive worsening, even though the first symptoms may seem to begin suddenly. In addition, both brain tumor and hematoma tend to produce disturbances in consciousness that are as prominent as or more prominent than focal neurologic defects, which helps in their differentiation from cerebrovascular disease. Often the problem in differential diagnosis is reversed in that the onset of stroke may include a gradual steady progression of symptoms and signs of focal neurologic defects, making the physician think first of tumor and only later of cerebral infarction. When doubt occurs about the diagnosis of infarction, subdural hematoma and neoplasm should be suspected, and cerebral angiograms and computerized axial tomography (CAT scanning) should be done.

Clinically, it is easier to confuse cerebral infarction with intracranial hemorrhage, for the onset is often similar. The cerebrospinal fluid examination usually helps, but blood can be found in both states —although considerably less often in cerebral infarction. Large amounts of blood in CSF under increased pressure is always caused by intracranial hemorrhage. Angiography or CAT scanning helps to settle the problem by demonstrating aneurysm, A-V anomaly, or intracerebral hematoma.

When it is not known where the patient could have suffered head trauma, it is often impossible to eliminate this as a cause of clinical states resembling cerebral infarction. Careful inspection for scalp lacerations and localized scalp edema and good quality skull roentgenograms identify most instances of trauma if it has been severe enough to cause neurologic injury. If trauma cannot be eliminated and the patient becomes progressively worse, CAT scanning or angiography must be done to eliminate consideration of subdural or epidural hematomas. CAT scanning is preferable, for it will not only indicate a hematoma but will also define other causes of illness such as tumor, or intracerebral hemorrhage.

Among the forms of intracranial sepsis only brain abscess is likely to be confused with cerebral infarction. The points that should alert the physician to the possibility of an abscess are a source of infection elsewhere in the body such as an ear, sinus, or chest infection; persistent headache; persistent low-grade fever; white cells, especially polymorphonuclear leukocytes, that persist more than 24 hours in the cerebrospinal fluid; a focal, highly abnormal EEG; and worsening of the clinical state. If abscess is suspected, angiograms performed on the side opposite the paresis will demonstrate the presence or absence of an intracerebral mass, which, if present, then must be surgically explored and drained to prove the diagnosis.

COURSE

Some improvement in function after the initial neurologic deficit can be expected after almost every cerebral infarction. During the first 72 hours, however, gradual worsening of neurologic deficits and increasing or beginning impairment of consciousness are frequent. This change may indicate extension of the cerebral infarction, but usually is associated with cerebral edema in and around the necrotic area. *Some degree of cerebral edema complicates every infarct.* It appears almost immediately, and with large infarctions may be so extensive as to shift the brain laterally and downward to produce herniation through the tentorium cerebelli and subsequent brainstem compression. This course of events, with its associated impairment of consciousness and other vital functions, is a common cause of death in patients with extensive infarction. The diagnosis of cerebral edema is especially likely when a patient shows a decline in awareness without a significant increase in focal neurologic deficits. Other causes of lethargy and stupor in patients with cerebral infarction are fever, electrolyte imbalance, the injudicious use of sedatives, tranquilizers or narcotics, and malnutrition.

In patients whose course is not complicated by severe cerebral edema, there is usually an early improvement in neurologic function. If some voluntary movement is preserved, there is a good chance for return of more. When function improves rapidly after the onset, the outlook for a good recovery is excellent. A slow return of function over weeks or months is associated with a less complete recovery. If flaccid paralysis is present from the onset with no return of voluntary movement over 30 to 60 days, the outlook for recovery is poor. Significant sensory loss impairs the chances of recovery of motor function. With brainstem infarction, the course is usually one of gradual improvement if the infarct is localized in the lateral medullary area. Symptoms of nausea, diplopia, and ataxia lessen and eventually disappear. Although some residual impairment of eye and extremity movement may be detected on examination, such patients often have little physical limitation. It is important to realize that recovery from cerebral infarction may continue for as long as one to two years.

PROGNOSIS

About one fourth to one fifth of patients with either thrombotic or embolic cerebral infarction die with their first attack. This figure varies somewhat with the cause of the infarction and especially with other factors such as age, cardiac status, and the degree of neurologic disability. The mortality rises sharply with increasing age; for patients over the age of 70 with cerebral infarction from atherosclerotic thrombosis or emboli the initial mortality is nearer 50 per cent. Patients with marked neurologic defects, coma, or extensive vascular disease elsewhere have an initial mortality of nearly 50 per cent. Infarction of the ventral portions of the brainstem after basilar artery occlusion, especially with quadriplegia, carries a poor outlook, although good medical and good nursing care may preserve a vegetative existence for long periods.

The prognosis for cerebral infarction is better in younger patients, in those with the least evidence of vascular disease at other sites, especially cardiovascular disease, and in those who do not have hypertension, diabetes, or severe neurologic defects.

About one fifth of patients who survive a cerebral infarction from atherosclerotic vascular disease suffer an-

other cerebrovascular accident within the next 12 to 24 months. However, the most significant limiting factor on survival is not recurrent stroke but cardiovascular disease. *Thus in the Cornell-Bellevue series, fully half of the patients who survived the initial cerebral infarction died at a later date from myocardial infarction or cardiac failure.*

Recurrence of cerebral infarction is common with cerebral emboli. In the New York Hospital series about 22 per cent of patients with cerebral emboli suffered recurrences, and nearly all the patients had more than one embolus if extracerebral sites were included. There is a strong chance that each cerebral recurrence will cause death or further neurologic disability.

TREATMENT

GENERAL. Treatment of cerebral infarction has four goals: to preserve life, to limit the amount of brain damage, to lessen disability and deformity, and to prevent recurrences.

The treatment program designed to preserve life is similar to that outlined for all seriously ill patients with neurologic illness. Efforts are directed toward maintaining a clear airway, an adequate fluid, electrolyte, and caloric intake, and an adequate urine output. Constant care is required to protect the skin from ischemia and necrosis resulting from pressure. Such a program is necessary for the obtunded or comatose patient, and must often be continued for the remainder of his life.

In patients with hemispheric infarction *cerebral edema* can impair consciousness and vital function early in the course of the illness. When cerebral edema subsides, the patient may again be able to cough, swallow, and voluntarily move paretic parts. A variety of measures can often temporarily reduce the brain swelling and carry the patient through a period of severe difficulty. Hypertonic urea solution, 1 to 1.5 grams per kilogram of body weight given intravenously, dehydrates normal brain, giving more space for edematous brain. The effect is transient, and a rebound effect has been reported. Hypertonic invert sugar, mannitol, has been used with similar results except that less rebound has been reported. One and one half to 2 grams per kilogram of body weight is given intravenously in a 20 per cent solution. In patients with cerebral infarction and brain edema this therapy is reserved until there is a serious threat to life with declining brainstem function, for the benefits are transient, and most patients can be carried through periods of depressed consciousness with careful nursing care alone. Although glucocorticoids such as methylprednisolone are often dramatically effective in improving patients with brain edema from primary and metastatic brain tumor, they have been found in carefully controlled studies to be ineffective in reducing cerebral edema after infarction.

Several agents have been utilized to increase cerebral blood flow in an effort to decrease the amount of ischemic tissue and limit the extent of cerebral infarction. Nearly all known agents that produce vasodilatation, including aminophylline, papaverine, tolazoline hydrochloride, nicotinic acid, and histamine, have been used without clear evidence of success in cerebrovascular disease. The only agent that produces effective vasodilatation in cerebral vessels is carbon dioxide. Although it has been used to treat acute stroke, there is no evidence that it reduces the neurologic defects.

Treatment for the late acute and convalescent phase of a

stroke is directed toward lessening deformity and disability, a goal that requires daily passive exercise of paretic parts to prevent joint fixation and to maintain normal muscle and tendon length. Some increase in muscle tone with spasticity invariably accompanies hemiplegia and tends to be most marked in the flexor muscles in the upper extremities and in the extensor muscles in the lower extremities. If this increase in tone in one muscle group over another persists and cannot be overcome by voluntary movement, daily passive movement of weakened or paralyzed parts through the full range of motion must be carried out by a nurse, physician, physiotherapist, or member of the family to prevent muscle and tendon contracture that may be nearly impossible to correct later on.

REHABILITATION. After cerebral infarction, *programs of retraining and rehabilitation should begin as soon as there is no longer evidence of increasing infarction.* Stabilization of the neurologic findings for 12 to 24 hours with some evidence of improvement is usually sufficient evidence to permit a start. Rehabilitation programs have as their goal the retraining of the remaining functions for maximal effectiveness. Although a few patients do require and benefit from special hospital facilities for rehabilitation, most such programs can be carried out on medical services without the aid of extensive equipment. An internist or general physician who is interested in rehabilitation can direct programs of activity and exercise, and can achieve results in rehabilitating hemiplegic patients that are nearly as effective as those of specialized centers.

An active program of rehabilitation begins by increasing the patient's tolerance to sitting and standing, which is impaired both by weakness and by changes in the sense of balance. Patients are allowed to sit up and then stand for increasingly long periods, beginning with five to ten minutes. During this period daily active and passive exercises of weakened extremities are carried out. When patients begin standing they need firm support and often splinting or bracing of the knee on the weakened side; marked quadriceps weakness may even demand a long leg brace. Ambulation is one of the main goals of rehabilitation. Gait training should begin when the patient can comfortably stand for 15 to 20 minutes without fatigue, and the support of parallel bars or a walker should be depended upon at first. After ambulation has started, it may be necessary to brace the foot to avoid the foot drop and supination that commonly occur after hemiplegia. At the same time that the patient is relearning to walk he should be trained in developing new skills with his unaffected arm and improving the strength and function in the paretic arm. This is done by an active program of exercise and by observing and retraining the patient in the activities of daily living such as eating, dressing and undressing, and personal hygiene. More complete details of programs of rehabilitation are outlined in other sources such as Covalt (1965) and can be followed by patients and their families under the direction of the physician. Usually, the maximal effect is gained in six to eight months, but some patients continue to show improvement over periods lasting as long as two years. Passive exercise must be continued indefinitely for severely paralyzed patients if contractures are to be avoided.

For patients with cerebral infarction who have mild to moderate dysphasia, speech therapy may be helpful. With severe dysphasia, therapy is rarely able to restore usable speech.

PREVENTION

The probability of an asymptomatic individual developing an atherosclerotic cerebral infarction has been analyzed by the Framingham study. The risk of developing stroke is increased in either sex and at any age by hypertension, diabetes, electrocardiographic evidence of heart enlargement, hypercholesterolemia, and cigarette smoking. The risk is higher with more than one of these factors operant and increases with the age of the individual. At the moment, the only factor which, if altered, is clearly related to a reduced risk of cerebral infarction is hypertension. In view of this, careful control of blood pressure in hypertensive individuals emerges as an important factor in prevention of signs and symptoms of cerebral ischemia. For management of hypertension, see Ch. 361.

Prevention of recurrent attacks and of cerebral infarction in patients with transient ischemic attacks and prevention of recurrent infarction in patients with cerebral atherosclerosis and cerebral emboli are the goals of much of the currently recommended treatment for stroke. Four methods to achieve this have been extensively evaluated: anticoagulation, drugs which alter platelet adherence, surgical correction of arterial obstructions, and removal of ulcerated atherosclerotic plaques.

ANTICOAGULANT DRUGS OR SURGERY IN TRANSIENT ISCHEMIC ATTACKS. *Anticoagulant therapy* was introduced to treat transient ischemic attacks after its use in myocardial infarction suggested a beneficial action. Reported studies of anticoagulants in transient ischemic attacks indicate that as long as patients receive anticoagulants and their prothrombin times are kept at two to two and a half times the normal value, they have fewer ischemic attacks and less chance of having a cerebral infarction. As a result, anticoagulants are accepted as effective in treating patients with transient ischemic attacks. The question is, which patients should receive the anticoagulants and for how long? The natural history of attacks is variable; attacks often stop spontaneously; some varieties carry a better prognosis than others. Even admitting these differences, anticoagulants should be given to the patients with transient ischemic attacks who do not have contraindications to their use. They should be continued for three to six months and then gradually discontinued. If transient ischemic attacks recur, they should be given again. The management of patients on anticoagulants is discussed in Ch. 357.

Drugs which inhibit platelet aggregation have been used to reduce platelet emboli as a cause of transient ischemic attacks. These agents include aspirin, dipyridamole, sulfinpyrazone, and cyproheptadine. Use of aspirin has been shown to reduce the frequency of transient ischemic attacks and to significantly reduce the occurrence of stroke in males with transient ischemic attacks. The required dose of aspirin is 0.3 gram four times a day.

Surgical correction of extracranial arterial obstruction with removal of ulcerated atherosclerotic plaques has been successfully used in the treatment of patients with transient ischemic attacks. Most carefully evaluated studies show that transient ischemic attacks stop after surgery and that the chances of future cerebral infarction are reduced. Arteriography of all precerebral vessels in the neck and the intracranial vessels should precede consideration of surgery, as the number and extent of sites of atherosclerosis are related to the success of operation. Isolated single obstruction or atherosclerotic plaques in accessible sites carry the best chance of successful treatment. Patients with multiple sites of extensive atherosclerosis, extra- and intracranially, should not be treated surgically and are best managed with anticoagulants or platelet aggregation inhibitors. If skillful, experienced surgeons are unavailable or referral to such surgeons is impossible for other reasons, anticoagulants or platelet aggregation inhibitors are the treatments of choice.

ANTICOAGULANT DRUGS OR SURGERY IN PROGRESSING STROKE OR STROKE-IN-EVOLUTION. Anticoagulants have been shown to significantly reduce mortality and morbidity among patients with stroke-in-evolution. Such situations are emergencies, and unless specifically contraindicated, anticoagulation must begin with heparin and must be continued with coumarin derivatives. Anticoagulants are usually given for four to six weeks. Surgical correction of an arterial obstruction for the patient with progressing stroke has sometimes been attempted as a means of reducing neurologic disability, but with poor results. Those patients in whom it can be demonstrated that showers of emboli from an ulcerated atherosclerotic plaque in the carotid artery are the cause of the progression, and who do not respond to anticoagulation or platelet antiaggregation agents, should have immediate surgical removal of the ulcerated plaque.

ANTICOAGULANT DRUGS OR SURGERY IN COMPLETED STROKE. For the patient with an already completed stroke, there is no clear treatment for preventing recurrences. Most series of patients with completed stroke studied by angiograms illustrate the widespread nature of atherosclerotic obstructive vascular disease. Intra- and extracranial vessels are commonly affected simultaneously and impose limiting factors on the successful outcome of surgical correction of extracranial arterial defects. A controlled evaluation of surgical therapy in this group of patients has been carried out and shows that surgical correction of an isolated carotid stenosis in patients with a mild neurologic defect is effective in reducing future mortality and morbidity. Surgical correction of arterial obstruction in patients with severe neurologic defects or with evidence of extensive atherosclerotic disease and occlusion does not change future mortality or morbidity.

Anticoagulants, given for one to four months, are useful during the acute and early convalescent period after a cerebrovascular accident to prevent pulmonary emboli in paralyzed, bedridden patients. The use of anticoagulants has also been recommended on a long-term basis for prevention of recurrent stroke. However, most studies of this problem indicate that there is no benefit from this form of treatment and that the complication rate is too high to warrant its use. Anticoagulation, therefore, can be recommended only for highly selected patients after cerebral infarction.

ANTICOAGULANT DRUGS IN CEREBRAL EMBOLIZATION. Anticoagulants greatly reduce the mortality and morbidity associated with recurrent embolization, and patients with a well established diagnosis of cerebral embolus should be placed on these drugs if there are no contraindications. If the source of emboli is rheumatic heart disease, anticoagulants are given continuously. When emboli follow myocardial infarction, treatment is usually given for one year. Coumarin anticoagulants are used and should be started immediately after the diagnosis has been made and the lumbar puncture has revealed bloodless cerebrospinal fluid.

Patients with cerebral emboli who have atrial fibrillation are often considered for conversion to normal sinus rhythm. This may be valuable in increasing cardiac output, but does not clearly reduce the chance of recurrent cerebral emboli.

General management of anticoagulant therapy is outlined in Ch. 357.

Hemorrhagic complications from anticoagulants are serious in about 2 to 4 per cent of patients and fatal in 2 per cent. Minor bleeding does not require that the medication be discontinued, but with serious bleeding it should be. Minor surgical procedures can be undertaken safely in most patients on anticoagulants if the prothrombin time is slightly lowered. Head injury, even of a minor nature, in patients on anticoagulants must be carefully evaluated and followed, as the chance of subdural hematoma in this group is high.

Heparin is the anticoagulant of choice for the initial treatment of patients with progressing stroke.

Patients with transient ischemic attacks, progressing strokes, or established strokes who also have hypertension should be treated with antihypertensive medication. Studies of patients with atherosclerotic cerebrovascular disease and hypertension show that when the blood pressure is returned to normal or nearly normal levels, the recurrence rate and mortality rate of stroke are reduced. Hypertension, depending on its severity, should be continuously treated with reserpine, chlorothiazide, or hexamethonium, and the blood pressure should be maintained as nearly normal as possible (see Ch. 361).

To sum up the prophylaxis of strokes: Patients with transient ischemic attacks should be treated with anticoagulants or platelet antiaggregation agents. If arteriography indicates significant extracranial vascular disease, especially ulceration of an atherosclerotic plaque, and experienced surgical care is available, the patient should be offered this form of treatment. Patients with completed strokes are not likely to benefit from any prophylactic treatment. If they are to remain bedridden for long periods, anticoagulants help to reduce the chances of pulmonary embolism.

HYPERTENSIVE ENCEPHALOPATHY

Hypertensive encephalopathy is an uncommon, acute neurologic syndrome characterized by headache, nausea and vomiting, convulsive seizures, transient focal neurologic defects, retinal artery spasm, papilledema, stupor, and coma. The cerebrospinal fluid pressure and protein content are commonly elevated. The syndrome is encountered in patients with longstanding hypertension. Its occurrence is associated with sudden marked increases in blood pressure from various causes, including malignant hypertension, eclampsia, and glomerulonephritis.

The mechanism by which hypertension causes neurologic dysfunction is believed to be acute cerebral vasospasm causing cerebral ischemia and edema.

Mild transient focal neurologic defects can be encountered in this syndrome. When neurologic defects are severe and sustained, the correct diagnosis is more likely to be cerebral ischemia or cerebral hemorrhage. When the blood urea nitrogen is above 100 mg per 100 ml, hypertensive encephalopathy can be difficult to distinguish from uremia, or can blend into that state.

The outlook for patients with hypertensive encephalopathy has been greatly improved with the use of antihypertensive medication, and temporary recovery is now frequent. The appearance of the syndrome, however, is usually associated with the end-state phases of advanced hypertensive vascular disease.

Hypertensive encephalopathy is a medical emergency, and treatment should be given to rapidly lower the blood pressure, for this is the only effective way to eliminate the symptoms. Initial treatment should be intramuscular reserpine, 2 to 5 mg per day. Blood pressure will begin to fall in two to three hours after administration of reserpine, and it can be maintained at desired levels with daily injections. Care must be exercised to avoid cerebral ischemia from hypotension. Permanent medical therapy must be instituted to maintain the blood pressure at more nearly normal levels, utilizing hydrochlorothiazide, reserpine, or alpha methyldopa (see Ch. 361).

PROGRESSIVE SUBCORTICAL ENCEPHALOPATHY

Progressive subcortical encephalopathy, described by Binswanger, is a rare disorder that occurs in patients with hypertension and atherosclerotic vascular disease. Progressive dementia, seizures, and focal neurologic signs characterize the clinical picture. The diagnosis is usually made at necropsy; the brain shows atrophy mainly in the temporal and occipital regions and patchy demyelination in the white matter of the hemispheres.

Barnett, H. J. M., et al.: The Canadian Cooperative Stroke Study Group: A randomized trial of aspirin and sulfinpyrazone in treatment of stroke. N. Engl. J. Med., 299:253, 1978.
Genton, E., Barnett, H. J. M., Fields, W. S., Gent, M., and Hoak, J. C.: Cerebral ischemia: The role of thrombosis and antithrombotic therapy. Stroke, 8:150, 1977.
Kannel, W. B., et al.: Risk factors in stroke due to cerebral infarction. Stroke, 2:423, 1971.
Katzman, R., Clasen, R., Klatzo, I., Meyer, J. S., Pappius, H. M., and Waltz, A. G.: Brain edema in stroke. Stroke, 8:512, 1977.
McDowell, F. H., and Brennen, R. W. (eds.): Cerebral Vascular Disease. Transactions of the Eighth Princeton Conference, 1972. New York, Grune & Stratton, 1973.
Millikan, C. H.: Reassessment of anticoagulant therapy in various types of occlusive cerebrovascular disease. Stroke, 2:201, 1971.
Scheinberg, P.: Cerebrovascular Diseases. Tenth Princeton Conference. New York, Grune & Stratton, 1976.
Vinken, P. J., and Bruyn, G. W.: Handbook of Clinical Neurology. Vols. 11 and 12: Vascular Diseases of the Nervous System. New York, American Elsevier Publishing Company, 1972.
Whisnant, J. P., and Sandok, B. A.: Cerebrovascular Diseases. Ninth Princeton Conference. New York, Grune & Stratton, 1975.

295. INTRACRANIAL HEMORRHAGE

DEFINITION

Intracranial hemorrhage, or apoplexy, comprises about one tenth of all acute cerebral vascular illness. Regardless of cause, intracranial hemorrhage is a serious illness with a high rate of mortality. At the bedside the physician can only suspect the diagnosis, which must be confirmed by finding blood in the cerebrospinal fluid or by the demonstration of a hematoma by computerized axial tomography, or angiography, or at surgery. The causes of intracranial hemorrhage are numerous, and the clinical pictures are similar regardless of the cause. It helps to understand the clinical problem better if one remembers that nontraumatic

bleeding within the cranium takes one of four separate anatomic courses and that these produce three relatively distinct clinical pictures:

1. Bleeding emanating from vessels on the surface of the brain and limited to the cerebrospinal fluid–filled space between the pial and arachnoid membranes is called *subarachnoid hemorrhage.*
2. *Subarachnoid hemorrhage with intracerebral extension* occurs when the sudden force of bleeding from a surface vessel also penetrates into the brain itself; signs and symptoms of both the subarachnoid and the parenchymal lesions result.
3. Bleeding from ruptured vessels within the substance of the brain is called *intracerebral hemorrhage.* This may remain isolated therein as a *cerebral hematoma.*
4. Intracerebral hemorrhage may extend through brain tissue to the ventricles or subarachnoid space, causing signs and symptoms of both the parenchymal and the subarachnoid lesions.

ETIOLOGY

Bleeding from ruptured arteries is the usual source of intracranial hemorrhage, although veins also may bleed. The accompanying table lists the common causes.

Arterial Aneurysms

BERRY ANEURYSMS. These are small, round, or saccular berry-shaped dilatations that form characteristically at arterial bifurcations at or near the circle of Willis. Their cause is uncertain, for aneurysms are not familial and they are rarely found in infants. They arise, however, from what are thought to be congenital defects in the media of cerebral vessels. The wall of an aneurysm is thin, composed usually only of intima and subintimal connective tissue. Muscle or elastic tissues may be evident at the origin of the aneurysmal sac from its parent vessel, but these tissues thin out and disappear as the sac enlarges. Most aneurysms are less than 1 cm in diameter; a few, however, dilate to as much as 2 to 5 cm. As the aneurysm enlarges, it may develop a narrow neck or may remain broadly attached to the vessel wall.

Most berry aneurysms, approximately 85 per cent, develop around the anterior portion of the circle of Willis, arising from the internal carotid, the posterior communicating, the middle cerebral, the anterior communicating, or the anterior cerebral artery, as shown in Figure 8. The most common site is the point of junction of the posterior communicating artery and the internal carotid. About 15 per cent of aneurysms arise from the vertebral-basilar artery system. Multiple aneurysms are found in about one of every six patients. Not all an-

Causes of Intracranial Hemorrhage

1. Arterial aneurysms
   a. *"Congenital" berry aneurysms*
   b. *Acquired arterial aneurysms*
      (1) Fusiform aneurysms
      (2) Mycotic aneurysms
2. Arteriovenous (A-V) anomalies
3. Hypertensive vascular disease
4. Vascular lesions associated with primary or metastatic brain tumors
5. Systemic bleeding diatheses
6. Undetermined and miscellaneous causes

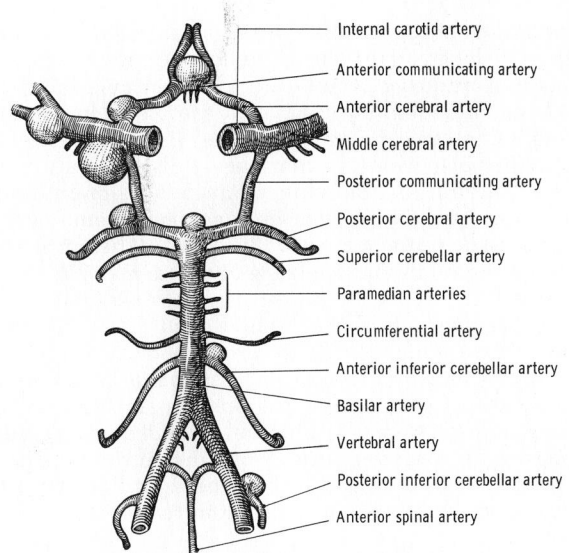

- Internal carotid artery
- Anterior communicating artery
- Anterior cerebral artery
- Middle cerebral artery
- Posterior communicating artery
- Posterior cerebral artery
- Superior cerebellar artery
- Paramedian arteries
- Circumferential artery
- Anterior inferior cerebellar artery
- Basilar artery
- Vertebral artery
- Posterior inferior cerebellar artery
- Anterior spinal artery

Figure 8. The more common sites of berry aneurysm. The size of the aneurysm at the various sites is directly proportional to the frequency at that site.

eurysms bleed, and some are found incidentally at postmortem examination. Occasionally, they become so large that they compress adjacent cerebral tissue or cranial nerves, and, rarely, they enlarge sufficiently to cause a clinical state that simulates brain tumor.

What makes an aneurysm rupture at any given instant is not clear, although several factors seem important. These lesions gradually enlarge with time under the stress of the arterial blood pressure. They are more frequent in patients who are hypertensive, and their incidence is high in subjects with coarctation of the aorta and polycystic renal disease, both of which cause early hypertension. Atheromatous plaques form in their walls, and clots line the aneurysms, but whether either of these conditions increases the chance of rupture is problematic. Probably a change in the blood pressure is the single final event that precipitates perforation of the sac.

FUSIFORM ANEURYSMS. These spindle-shaped dilatations along the course of an artery, usually the basilar, sometimes the carotid artery in the cavernous sinus, are due to atherosclerosis. The resulting elongated and tortuous dilatation may be large enough to compress adjacent cranial nerves or the brain itself. Hemorrhage from such an aneurysm is unusual, but characteristically damages the brain fatally when it does occur.

MYCOTIC ANEURYSMS. Mycotic aneurysms are produced by septic emboli associated with bacterial endocarditis. A local necrotic vasculitis occurs at the site where the embolus lodges and results in thinning and dilatation of the vessel wall, which may eventually rupture. Such lesions tend to be multiple, and they are the only aneurysms found distally in the smaller branches of the middle cerebral artery.

Arteriovenous Anomalies or Cavernous Angiomas

Arteriovenous (A-V) anomalies or cavernous angiomas are tangled, interconnected networks of vessels in which arterial blood passes directly to venous drainage without intervening capillaries. These lesions tend to

be supplied by more than one parent cerebral artery, and they range in size from the microscopic to a huge cavernous network large enough to cover most of one cerebral hemisphere or to occupy an entire lobe of the cerebellum. The vessels in an A-V anomaly are themselves malformed so that some structurally resemble arteries, others veins. Since these vessels are usually thin walled, circulating blood at arterial pressure distends and often eventually ruptures them, with a resultant subarachnoid hemorrhage, intracerebral hemorrhage, or both. Even without hemorrhage, large A-V malformations expand, and the neural tissue adjacent to the anomaly characteristically suffers an uneven pressure necrosis, causing progressively more abnormal neurologic signs and epilepsy. Hemorrhage can destroy all clinical evidence of a malformation of microscopic size and make postmortem diagnosis impossible.

Hypertensive Vascular Disease

Hypertension causes thickening and fibrinoid degeneration of the cerebral arterioles. Red cells can be found free in the perivascular spaces around many of the vessels, and microaneurysms have been described along the arteries since the time of Bouchard and Charcot in the nineteenth century. What part each of these abnormalities contributes to the eventual necrosis and rupture is still debated, although most contemporary pathologists view the fibrinoid degeneration as most important.

When hemorrhage occurs, it usually results from rupture of small arteries in the substance of the brain. This may occur anywhere; it is most common in the cerebrum and least common in the cerebellum and brainstem. In the cerebral hemispheres, small branches of the middle cerebral artery penetrating the region of the basal ganglia are most susceptible, and the lenticulostriate artery has even been termed "the artery of cerebral hemorrhage." In the brainstem, hemorrhages arise from paramedian perforating branches of the basilar more often than they do from the long circumferential branches of either the basilar or the vertebral arteries.

Hemorrhage in Brain Tumors

Hemorrhage may occur in either primary or metastatic lesions, usually in rapidly growing tumors with a large amount of vascular overgrowth. This complication is perhaps most common in glioblastoma multiforme and metastatic neoplasms from the lung. Among the more benign tumors pituitary adenomas have a tendency to cause apoplexy. Of the total number of cerebral hemorrhages, however, those from tumor contribute but a small fraction.

Bleeding Diatheses and Miscellaneous Causes

Leukemia, thrombocytopenia, and the ingestion of excessive amounts of anticoagulants all predispose to cerebral hemorrhage. In some patients it is difficult or impossible to establish what caused a cerebral hemorrhage. As mentioned, in some cases the hemorrhage may have erased the malformation. A hemorrhagic cerebral infarct can be so liquefied that it resembles a primary hemorrhage. However, with the increasing use of cerebral angiography and computerized axial tomography, more and more intracranial aneurysms and malformations are being demonstrated in all age groups as the cause of intracranial hemorrhage, and more strokes have been found to be small hemorrhages.

PATHOLOGY AND PATHOGENESIS

SUBARACHNOID HEMORRHAGE. Subarachnoid hemorrhage most commonly comes from rupture of a berry aneurysm, less commonly from an A-V anomaly or a mycotic or fusiform aneurysm. Blood suddenly released in this manner has several deleterious effects, each contributing to the seriousness of the disease. The sudden high pressure jet raises the intracranial pressure and sometimes acts like an acute concussion, causing sudden unconsciousness or, occasionally, rapid brain displacement and death. Blood is also a noxious agent, particularly as it hemolyzes and breaks down into its pigments. It irritates blood vessels, meninges, and the brain itself. Meningeal irritation causes the characteristic headache of subarachnoid hemorrhage, and later, within hours or days, the blood produces a sterile meningitis. This hemogenic meningitis itself becomes a source of considerable disability, for it not only causes subjective discomfort and systemic toxicity but leads to meningeal exudation, thickening, and scarring that can impair cerebrospinal fluid absorption and cause subacute or chronic communicating hydrocephalus. Moreover, the blood may irritate the underlying brain so as to evoke adverse descending autonomic discharges, causing hypertension and cardiac arrhythmias.

In addition to the brain destruction caused by the physical action of the hemorrhage, ischemic changes and infarction of brain tissue are found in as many as two thirds of patients dying from subarachnoid hemorrhage. The ischemia and infarction have been attributed to vascular spasm or vessel wall edema, and they are encountered most commonly in the area of the brain supplied by the artery with the ruptured aneurysm. Evidence for arterial spasm in subarachnoid hemorrhage comes from angiographic studies showing segmental vessel narrowing that correlates with a high incidence of clinical and pathologic evidence of cerebral infarction. The causative mechanism is believed to be a combination of the irritating effect of free blood and the production in the subarachnoid space of vasoactive substances, and of vessel injury. During surgery, mechanical stimulation of cerebral arteries causes significant and sustained vessel narrowing. Presumably, vascular spasm has a potentially protective action in reducing the amount of bleeding from a ruptured artery. Why in some instances it lasts long enough and is severe enough to reduce distal cerebral blood flow to the point of ischemia and neural death is unknown.

Extension of bleeding into the brain occurs in about half of all surface aneurysms and in nearly all A-V anomalies. The complication is particularly likely when the bleeding site lies close to cerebral tissue, as is true with aneurysms of the anterior communicating or anterior cerebral arteries, which are interposed between the frontal lobes, or of branches of the middle cerebral artery, which are buried within the sylvian fissure. Rupture from the anterior communicating vessel tends to damage one or both frontal lobes, and rupture of middle cerebral artery aneurysms tends to lacerate the temporoparietal or posterior frontal lobes.

INTRACEREBRAL HEMORRHAGE. Intracerebral hemorrhage is most often caused by hypertensive vascular disease or ruptured aneurysm, less often by a bleeding A-V malformation. The path that the blood takes with these lesions and the amount of bleeding are somewhat unpredictable. Some hemorrhages dissect the brain along fiber tracts, destroying relatively little brain tissue along the way. Others damage considerable amounts of neural tissue in the region of bleeding. All hemorrhages enlarge the brain and evoke cerebral edema. When the enlargement occurs rapidly, it displaces cerebral structures laterally across the midline under the falx and downward through the tentorium cerebelli, with resulting brainstem compression. Such a course of events is often fatal; at postmortem examination smaller areas of bleeding are found in the midbrain and pons in addition to the massive intracerebral hemorrhage. These secondary brainstem lesions have been attributed to venous obstruction and ischemia from transtentorial herniation.

Small intracerebral hemorrhages can remain entirely confined within the brain substance. Occasionally, the hematoma absorbs fluid, and this plus the surrounding edema can create the clinical picture of an expanding new growth. More often, however, the fluid is resorbed, and the remaining cavity shrinks almost to the point of disappearance.

Most large cerebral hemorrhages rupture into the subarachnoid space, the ventricular system, or both. Although serious consequences have been attributed to this course of events, it is likely that the large size of the hemorrhage causes the disastrous clinical effects rather than the fact that bleeding penetrated into the cerebrospinal fluid spaces.

CLINICAL MANIFESTATIONS OF INTRACRANIAL BLEEDING

SUBARACHNOID HEMORRHAGE. Subarachnoid hemorrhage has as its most common initial symptom a sudden violent headache. Initially the headache is usually described as an excruciating, intense, aching pain. Later it becomes dull and throbbing but remains severe, and most patients describe it as the most intense headache they have ever experienced. Even if it is at first localized, it soon becomes generalized, and frequently patients complain of severe neck and back pain. The initial localized headache is due to vascular distortion and injury. The later generalized headache is due to meningeal irritation from blood in the subarachnoid space.

Localization of headache at the onset is helpful in determining the site of the bleeding. Headache that begins in the back of the head suggests a posterior fossa origin of bleeding, and headache that begins in the anterior part of the head suggests a supratentorial bleeding source. If the initial headache is localized to one side, bleeding usually has occurred from a vessel on that side.

Other symptoms include dizziness, vertigo, vomiting, drowsiness, sweating and chills, stupor, and loss of consciousness.

Shortly after the onset of symptoms, the patient may lose consciousness for a few moments. With massive subarachnoid hemorrhage and intracerebral extension, the patient may lapse into and remain in coma until death. In some instances of subarachnoid hemorrhage death may be sudden and is related to intraventricular hemorrhage and sudden intense transtentorial herniation and brainstem compression. When hemorrhage is confined to the subarachnoid space or when intracerebral extension of bleeding is minor, consciousness is regained in a few minutes to a few hours. Delirium and lethargy often follow and may persist for as long as two weeks; severe mental clouding, delirium or coma usually indicates severe bleeding and brain damage.

Patients with subarachnoid hemorrhage usually complain of neck stiffness; this does not appear immediately in most patients but begins with the onset of the meningeal inflammatory reaction 6 to 12 hours later. When neck stiffness is evident shortly after the onset of symptoms, it is ominous and suggests that the meninges in the posterior fossa are stretched by beginning herniation of the cerebellar tonsils into the foramen magnum.

Although subarachnoid hemorrhage does occur during sleep, it most commonly occurs when patients are engaged in their usual activities. Many patients have reported that headache began during activity such as straining at stool, heavy lifting, or coitus.

Convulsions may occur, usually at onset, but sometimes during the acute phase of the illness. When present, they almost invariably indicate that the site of bleeding is in the anterior or middle fossa.

On examination the most conspicuous sign is marked neck rigidity and pain on attempting head movement. The most common localizing neurologic abnormality is pupillary inequality or paresis of vertical and medial movements of one eye that follows oculomotor nerve compression by aneurysms of the internal carotid artery.

Lateralizing neurologic signs, such as hemiparesis or hemiplegia, hemisensory defects or hemianopia, indicate either an intracerebral extension of bleeding or vascular spasm. The distribution of signs of neurologic dysfunction, particularly at onset, may be helpful in localizing the site of bleeding. Marked hemiparesis and severe hemisensory defects suggest bleeding from an aneurysm on the middle cerebral artery in the sylvian fissure. Unilateral oculomotor paresis with ptosis, diplopia, and mydriasis suggests that the bleeding source is from the region of the posterior communicating artery where it joins the internal carotid artery. This junction lies in close approximation to the oculomotor nerve as it passes from the posterior to the middle fossa. Bilateral paresis of the extremities suggests that the bleeding site is near the anterior cerebral–anterior communicating artery junction and suggests extension of bleeding into both frontal lobes. Paresis or sensory impairment present from onset is most likely to be caused by intracerebral extension of bleeding, whereas neurologic signs developing later are more often due to arterial spasm.

Examination of the optic fundi in patients with subarachnoid hemorrhage may reveal smooth rounded hemorrhages near the optic nerve head, "subhyaloid hemorrhages." They are often unilateral and, when present on one side, indicate the side of the bleeding. They are venous in origin and result from sudden increase in intracranial venous pressure at the time of the intracranial bleeding.

Fever caused by the hemogenic aseptic meningitis is common in patients with subarachnoid hemorrhage, appearing usually one to three days after onset and reaching 38 to 39° C. Greater elevations of body temperature usually suggest intraventricular or intracerebral extension of bleeding. Subsequent elevations of temperature during the course of the illness may suggest recurrent bleeding, but they are more often related to intercurrent infections.

RUPTURE OF AN ARTERIOVENOUS ANOMALY. The symptoms and signs of a subarachnoid hemorrhage from a ruptured A-V anomaly are identical to those from a ruptured aneurysm, because both bleed into the subarachnoid space or into the brain tissues. Bleeding into surrounding brain is common for a ruptured A-V anomaly, and symptoms and signs are like those of intracerebral hemorrhage from other causes. Seizures may occur at the onset of bleeding and are nearly always focal in pattern. The diagnosis of A-V anomaly is suggested by a history of pre-existing focal seizures or focal neurologic signs and of recurrent, always unilateral, vascular headache, each of which occurs in about a third of the patients. Rupture of A-V is more frequent at a younger age than is rupture of aneurysms, so that a history of focal seizures in a young patient with subarachnoid hemorrhage makes the diagnosis of arteriovenous anomaly particularly likely.

When the patient with an A-V malformation is examined, in addition to signs of meningeal irritation and focal neurologic defects, careful auscultation may disclose an audible bruit over the eyes or skull. Although bruits may be present with either A-V anomalies or aneurysms, they are more common with the former.

INTRACEREBRAL HEMORRHAGE. When intracranial hemorrhage occurs directly into the substance of the brain, the onset of symptoms is usually abrupt. Severe headache, nausea, and vomiting occur and sometimes precede other signs of a neurologic deficit or loss of consciousness by several hours. These early symptoms are the result of an acute increase in intracranial pressure. Focal neurologic dysfunction follows, with hemiplegia or hemisensory defects; this results from disruption or distortion of the main motor and sensory pathways in the cerebrum. Loss of consciousness within minutes after the onset occurs in more than one third of patients and indicates a large hemorrhage, intraventricular bleeding, or both. Among patients who are not initially in coma, half deteriorate with decline of awareness and eventually lapse into coma. With the progressive decline in consciousness, patients may show neurologic signs at first, indicating functional decortication and later indicating decerebration. This sequence follows herniation of the brain through the tentorial space with secondary brainstem compression.

In patients who retain consciousness but have motor or sensory deficits, it can be difficult to differentiate intracerebral hemorrhage from cerebral infarction until the cerebrospinal fluid is examined and found to be bloody. In about 20 per cent of patients, the intracerebral hemorrhage is circumscribed, and the fluid never becomes bloody. In these instances, except for the higher incidence of headache with intracerebral hemorrhage, it may be impossible to differentiate intracerebral hemorrhage from cerebral infarction.

The clinical picture produced by intracerebral hemorrhages at various sites is often characteristic and may enable an accurate localization of bleeding.

Capsular or Putamen Hemorrhage. Intracerebral bleeding into the region of the internal capsule causes abrupt flaccid hemiplegia, loss of sensory perception, and homonymous hemianopia. Capsular hemorrhages in the dominant hemisphere produce aphasia. When the hemorrhage is large, loss of consciousness promptly follows. With small hemorrhages changes are less severe. Paralysis is usually more prominent than sensory impairment, and paralysis of gaze to the side opposite the hemorrhage may be found.

Thalamic Hemorrhage. Hemorrhage into the thalamus also produces abrupt motor deficits, but in addition an impairment of all modalities of sensory perception is common and more prominent than deficits in motility or the visual fields. Consciousness is less likely to be lost with a thalamic than with a capsular hemorrhage. Thalamic hemorrhages are associated with distinct disturbances in eye movements. Patients commonly show paralysis of upward gaze. At rest, their eyes deviate downward and laterally and they are unable to look up on command or reflex. The pupils may be unequal and react poorly to light. There may be partial oculomotor palsy with ptosis and loss of convergence. The mechanism that causes the gaze palsy is compression of the region of the posterior commissure and the adjacent upper brainstem nuclei. Because the disturbances in gaze gradually clear, actual tissue destruction from extension of the hemorrhage into this area is probably not the cause of the defect.

Cerebellar and Brainstem Hemorrhage. Parenchymal hemorrhage in the posterior fossa can occur either in the cerebellar hemispheres or in the brainstem (usually pons). With intracerebellar hemorrhage, the patient may experience sudden severe occipital headache, diplopia, nystagmus, and ataxia. Examination reveals miosis, conjugate gaze palsy, and irregular respiration. In some subjects, these symptoms and signs may be present for several hours before any loss of consciousness; in others, loss of consciousness is immediate. When warning symptoms occur, the diagnosis can often be made from the clinical examination alone, and prompt evacuation of the hematoma can be lifesaving. Hemorrhage into the brainstem causes immediate impairment of consciousness, irregular breathing, pinpoint pupils, and quadriplegia followed by a rapid decline to death.

LABORATORY FINDINGS IN INTRACRANIAL BLEEDING

COMPUTERIZED TRANSAXIAL TOMOGRAPHY. Blood is more dense than brain tissue, and CAT scanning yields the diagnosis of most parenchymal hemorrhages greater than approximately 1 cm in diameter. Contrast enhancement with iodine accentuates the demarcation of such lesions.

CEREBROSPINAL FLUID EXAMINATION. Lumbar puncture can be safely carried out on most patients suspected of having intracranial hemorrhage, but should be done with caution when there is evidence of impaired consciousness or a progressive decline in awareness and focal neurologic defects. These signs indicate both extensive brain damage and the possibility of brainstem compression. With suspected intracerebral hemorrhages and hematoma, there is always the possibility of tentorial herniation, which may be precipitated or accentuated by changes in cerebrospinal fluid pressure

after puncture. In such instances lumbar puncture is best postponed until after CAT scanning has been carried out.

Examination of the cerebrospinal fluid shortly after the onset of intracranial bleeding (1 to 24 hours) reveals red cells with a constant red cell count in sequential samples. The supernatant fluid of a centrifuged specimen will have a pink color owing to the presence of oxyhemoglobin. The fluid reacts positively with benzidine. Cerebrospinal fluid examined after 24 hours will begin to show, in addition, a yellowish coloration (xanthochromia) caused by the degradation of oxyhemoglobin to bilirubin. This intensifies over a period of several days and usually reaches peak intensity at 36 to 48 hours after the onset of bleeding.

Bloody fluid caused by a traumatic lumbar puncture is indicated by the absence of pink or yellow discoloration of the centrifuged supernatant cerebrospinal fluid, i.e., not xanthochromic, by failure to obtain a positive benzidine test for hemoglobin in the supernatant fluid, and by a decreasing red cell count in sequential samples of the fluid. When there is still doubt about whether a traumatic lumbar puncture is the cause of bleeding, examination of the supernatant cerebrospinal fluid by spectrophotometry is helpful in proving that invisible amounts of hematin or bilirubin are not present and thus confirming the traumatic nature of the lumbar puncture.

The white cell count in the CSF, when determined shortly after bleeding, will be commensurate with the amount of bleeding — usually one white cell for every 1000 red cells. When the white cell count is made on specimens collected 12 hours or more after the onset of bleeding, it may be elevated. This increase in white cells is caused by the inflammatory reaction in the meninges and may reach levels as high as 500 per cubic millimeter. Early in the course of the inflammatory reaction, the cells may be polymorphonuclear leukocytes and lymphocytes; later, the cells are all lymphocytes.

An exudative reaction accompanies intracranial hemorrhage, and the cerebrospinal fluid protein is usually elevated to levels around 100 mg per 100 ml or more. During fresh bleeding, for each 10,000 red cells in the fluid, the protein is said to rise 15 mg per 100 ml. Protein elevations are maximal eight to ten days after bleeding and decline thereafter. The cerebrospinal fluid pressure is often elevated to levels of 200 to 300 mm (of CSF) with subarachnoid hemorrhage. Elevations may be much higher, 300 to 500 mm with large intracerebral hemorrhages. The white count in the peripheral blood can be elevated to levels up to 15,000, and some patients have a transient albuminuria and glycosuria.

ARTERIOGRAPHY. It is often impossible on clinical grounds alone to distinguish between a bleeding aneurysm, a bleeding A-V anomaly, or intracerebral bleeding of unknown cause. Cerebral arteriography is necessary to demonstrate the cause. Thus if the patient is a satisfactory operative risk, arteriography should be performed as soon as possible with the hope that specific treatment can be instituted.

Arteriography is most useful in demonstrating aneurysms and A-V anomalies. In patients with suspected ruptured aneurysm, cerebral angiograms will demonstrate the aneurysm in over 80 per cent of instances. They may also indicate whether the aneurysm can be approached surgically. In addition to the aneurysm, the angiogram may reveal distortion of the usual vessel patterns near the aneurysm, indicating a hematoma, and frequently there will be arterial narrowing. The technical details of arteriography are discussed elsewhere; however, the physician should see to it that the intracranial branches of both the right and left carotid arteries are visualized to determine whether more than one aneurysm is present. When more than one aneurysm is present, it is often difficult to determine which one ruptured. Points that are helpful are that the bleeding aneurysm is often irregular in outline and, in the surrounding area, there may be distortion of other vessels, suggesting a local hematoma, or the nearby vessels may show narrowing. Local hematoma is the most reliable evidence of bleeding. If an aneurysm is not seen in the carotid arterial tree, the vertebral and basilar arteries and their branches should be visualized. The demonstration of an aneurysm on the distal branches of the middle or anterior cerebral arteries is almost diagnostic of mycotic aneurysm.

A-V anomalies are readily demonstrated in cerebral angiograms, as the usually large flow of blood through these structures produces a characteristic picture of early arterial filling and venous drainage of the anomalous vessels.

Intracerebral hemorrhage often can be visualized on cerebral angiograms. Shift of midline vessels, widening of the space between the anterior and middle cerebral arteries, and downward or upward displacement of the middle cerebral branches are helpful evidence. However, roughly a quarter of small hematomas (20 to 30 per cent) escape detection by angiograms.

When hemorrhage has occurred into a cerebral neoplasm, angiograms help in demonstrating vascular changes suggestive of tumor. In addition to vessel distortion and shift of midline vessels, abnormal vessels in the tumor may fill with contrast media and produce a so-called "tumor stain."

PROGNOSIS

RUPTURED ANEURYSM. Subarachnoid bleeding from a ruptured aneurysm is extremely serious; the mortality rate is 45 per cent for each major attack, and there is a high risk of recurrence. Among those who succumb to bleeding, about one third do so within the first 48 hours, another one third within the next month, and the remainder from later major recurrences. Recurrence strikes about one patient in three, with the maximal danger during the first two weeks after the initial bleeding, when about 60 per cent of all rebleeding occurs. However, some patients bleed during the third and fourth weeks and about 20 per cent have late recurrences, most of which are within the first six months after leaving the hospital. Fatal recurrences have been reported as long as 20 years after the initial bleeding, and there is no way to predict which patient will have a recurrence of bleeding or when he or she is likely to have it. The high mortality and the frequency of recurrence make accurate statements of prognosis impossible for individual patients. In general, the longer a patient survives after the initial bleeding, the less are the chances of recurrence. Data submitted to the National Co-operative Study of Subarachnoid Hemorrhage indicate that if a patient with subarachnoid hemorrhage is alive one week after onset, the chance of surviving five more weeks is 65 per cent. Patients living two weeks without recurrence have a 76 per cent chance of living four more weeks. Patients 20 to 50 years of age have a better chance of survival than those over 60. As might be expected, patients with the least neural damage and the least impairment of consciousness have the best chance of survival. Long-term prognosis studied during a ten-year period of follow-up indicates that for patients with aneurysm who are alive six months after subarachnoid hemorrhage, rebleeding occurs at a rate of 3.5 per cent per year, with mortality from rebleeding of about two thirds.

RUPTURED ARTERIOVENOUS ANOMALY. The prognosis for bleeding from A-V anomalies is better than for aneurysm. The initial mortality is about 25 per cent and the possibility of recurrence less than that. Because of their location and the tendency to bleed into brain tissue, the neurologic disability among survivors of bleeding A-V anomalies tends to be high. Seizures with A-V anomalies are common before bleeding, and patients who do not have seizures often develop them after bleeding.

HYPERTENSIVE VASCULAR DISEASE. The prognosis for intracerebral hemorrhage from hypertensive vascular disease is poor; the over-all mortality is more than 50 per cent. Mortality is highest with hemorrhage into the ventricle or when severe brain edema causes temporal lobe herniation with resultant compression of the midbrain. The initial mortality rises with the age of the patient. It is about 40 per cent for patients in the 40 to 60 age range, 50 per cent in patients over 60 and 80 per cent in patients over 70. Patients who are in coma when first seen have a mortality rate of 70 to 100 per cent. Recurrence of intracerebral hemorrhage is uncommon, but tissue destruction and displacement at the time of bleeding cause serious neural damage and residual neurologic dysfunction. Patients with small intracerebral hemorrhages usually are left with only slight disability.

TREATMENT

The treatment of intracranial hemorrhage has three goals: preserving life, reducing disability, and preventing recurrence. Treatment directed toward preservation of life is similar for all causes of intracranial hemorrhage and for most other life-threatening neurologic illnesses. During the acute phase of intracranial hemorrhage, the patient should be in bed for as long as the symptoms of headache, stiff neck, and prostration require. Rebleeding is unlikely with ruptured A-V anomaly and hypertensive vascular disease, and a patient with one of these disorders need not be kept in bed for a long period once he feels well enough to get up. Just when to mobilize the patient with subarachnoid hemorrhage from intracranial aneurysm is a question more difficult to answer. Four to six weeks of bed rest is usually recommended, because this is the period of maximal danger from rebleeding. Recurrent hemorrhage has been noted to occur with straining at stool and with other activity, and rest in bed is believed to lessen the chances for potentially dangerous activity.

When the patient is in coma or has impaired consciousness after intracranial hemorrhage, meticulous care must be taken to maintain an adequate airway, blood pressure, and fluid and electrolyte balance. The skin and eyes must be protected from pressure and irritation. The urinary bladder should not be allowed to become distended from urinary retention. These are common problems for all patients with neurologic illness and depressed consciousness; they are discussed more fully elsewhere.

Patients with intracranial hemorrhage who are conscious usually complain of severe headache and stiff neck. They also frequently are restless and delirious. Analgesics such as codeine sulfate by mouth or codeine phosphate intramuscularly in doses of 60 mg may be needed as often as every two hours to relieve headache; in most instances this also relieves restlessness. Other narcotics for analgesia should be avoided because they depress respiration. *Delirium may persist for as long as two weeks.* No specific treatment is indicated, but having a member of the family present at all times and reducing examinations and procedures to a minimum greatly reduce the patient's anxiety and restlessness.

Protracted stupor or depression of consciousness following subarachnoid hemorrhage sometimes can be attributed to progressive communicating hydrocephalus. CAT scans demonstrating progressive cerebral ventricular enlargement in such instances can be a useful guide to instituting appropriate decompression measures.

Initially, patients with intracranial hemorrhage should not take fluid or food by mouth for 24 to 48 hours because of the danger of vomiting and aspiration. Subsequently, it is best to give clear fluids for another 24 to 48 hours and then a soft diet. During the period of restricted fluid and food intake, intravenous fluids should be given in the usual physiologic quantities.

Constipation must be avoided. When patients require codeine for relief of pain, mild laxatives or stool softeners should be given if the patient is able to take medication by mouth. Otherwise, small enemas should be given every other day.

When the blood pressure is elevated, it should be returned to nearly normal levels, particularly in patients with bleeding from intracranial aneurysms. This should not be done rapidly, however, because of the risk of precipitating a hypotension-induced cerebral ischemic infarct. Methyldopa or reserpine orally or parenterally is usually an effective antihypertensive.

RUPTURED ANEURYSM. Prevention of recurrent bleeding from aneurysms is the primary goal of treatment and, in view of the close approximation of recurrent bleeding to the initial hemorrhage, should be attempted as soon as possible. Thus angiograms to identify the source and site of bleeding should be made as soon as practicable, once the diagnosis of intracranial hemorrhage has been made. Similarly, if the aneurysm is believed to be amenable to surgical therapy, this is performed as soon as the patient's condition allows. Patients with no depression of consciousness, who are under 60 and normotensive, who have no evidence of arterial spasm on angiograms, and who have minimal neurologic deficits are considered good surgical risks and can be treated surgically immediately if this form of therapy is indicated for the particular aneurysm. Patients with depressed levels of consciousness or coma or with major neurologic deficits are very poor

candidates for surgery; operative mortality in this group is extremely high; operation, if indicated, should be postponed until improvement occurs. Patients over the age of 60 who are hypertensive and who have arterial spasm on angiograms also are poor operative risks, and surgery should be delayed until their condition improves.

The possibility that rebleeding is related to lysis of a clot plugging the aneurysmal sac has been suggested. Agents which inhibit the enhanced intrathecal fibrinolytic state that often follows subarachnoid hemorrhage have been evaluated to see if they decrease the chances of rebleeding. These agents include epsilon-aminocaproic acid and p-aminomethylbenzoic acid. Epsilon-aminocaproic acid must be given in large quantities, 20 to 30 grams per day intravenously, to be effective. Studies indicate that use of these agents reduces the chances of rebleeding and mortality. Complications related to altered blood clotting systemically are uncommon.

Surgical therapy is directed toward removal of the aneurysm or control of the bleeding by a direct surgical attack or toward decreasing the blood pressure in the feeding arterial tree by ligation of a proximal artery. Not all aneurysms can be treated surgically.

Some forms of surgical therapy are more suitable than others. In the past six years, several clinics and hospitals have worked together in a cooperative study to determine the type of surgery most suitable for a particular bleeding lesion. In the national cooperative study of ruptured aneurysm, surgical therapy has been found to reduce six-year mortality as compared to mortality in patients who did not have surgery. The reported mortality for patients with carotid artery aneurysm was 47 per cent; for middle cerebral artery aneurysm, 35 per cent; and for anterior cerebral artery aneurysm, 34 per cent. For those not surgically treated, mortality was 80 per cent. Carefully controlled studies in the United States and Britain have concluded that aneurysms arising from the internal carotid artery at the junction with the posterior communicating artery should be treated surgically, the procedure of choice being ligation of the common carotid artery in the neck or direct surgical attack on the aneurysm in good-risk patients.

The British controlled studies indicate that patients with anterior cerebral artery aneurysms probably do not benefit from surgery and may actually do worse. However, in properly selected patients, surgical correction of an aneurysm of the anterior cerebral or anterior communicating artery is beneficial.

The outcome of surgical treatment of middle cerebral artery aneurysms is more uncertain. In the British controlled treatment series, direct surgical attack provided better results in male patients, whereas women with middle cerebral aneurysms fared less well with surgery than when treated conservatively. The explanation of this difference appears to be that women are more prone to cerebral infarction after surgery than men. In addition, women have smaller, more fragile aneurysms that make surgery more difficult.

Aneurysms on the vertebral basilar vascular tree are difficult to reach surgically. The most successful surgery reported has been for aneurysms arising from the vertebral artery near the branching of the posterior inferior cerebellar artery.

Surgical treatment of ruptured intracranial aneurysm

is demanding, and should be performed using a surgical microscope. Surgical skill in this field is best maintained by frequent use. When physicians are considering surgery for their patients with aneurysm, these facts should be considered when selecting the surgeon.

If the patient is not suitable for surgical treatment or if surgery must be delayed, a program of medical treatment should be instituted as outlined above.

ARTERIOVENOUS ANOMALY. Surgery for A-V anomalies requires the tying of feeding vessels or the amputation of a portion of the brain containing the anomaly. The latter treatment is curative if the whole A-V malformation can be removed, but it is limited to those instances in which the anomaly lies entirely in or on the occipital pole or the frontal pole. The chance of neurologic disability associated with removal of A-V anomalies in other sites is usually too great to justify surgical therapy unless major disability had been present before bleeding.

Ligation of vessels feeding the anomaly has been recommended, but no carefully controlled evaluation of this form of surgical therapy has been done. Carotid ligation to reduce the blood pressure in the anomaly is also believed to reduce the chance of recurrent bleeding. Recently, artificial embolization with plastic spheres introduced into the feeding arteries has been reported to be successful in obliterating the anomaly.

Fortunately, the chance of recurrent bleeding with arteriovenous anomalies is less than with aneurysm. Also, bleeding carries a relatively low mortality, so that for most patients with A-V anomaly and intracranial hemorrhage, medical management identical to that described for ruptured aneurysm is the treatment of choice. The frequency of disability and mortality associated with surgical treatment is too high to justify its use except in highly special instances. Convulsive seizures are common with A-V anomalies and should be treated with anticonvulsants as outlined in Ch. 315.

INTRACEREBRAL HEMORRHAGE. Cerebral hemorrhage is a severe disease and one for which there is no satisfactory form of treatment. The immediate medical treatment was outlined earlier. It must include meticulous attention to the problems imposed by impaired consciousness and abrupt neurologic disability.

Whether and when to operate on cerebral hemorrhage is a recurrent question, and efforts have been made in this direction for years, although generally with poor results. Recently, McKissock and his colleagues in England carried out a carefully controlled evaluation of surgical treatment of acute cerebral hemorrhage caused by hypertensive disease, in which they showed that patients treated surgically fared less well than those treated conservatively. No matter what the treatment, patients in deep stupor or coma from intra-

cerebral hemorrhage rarely survive. For patients who survive the initial cerebral insult and become stable clinically, removal of a persistent encapsulated hematoma may lessen neurologic disability and hasten improvement.

Surgical removal of an intracerebral hematoma caused by bleeding from a ruptured aneurysm has been no more encouraging than when hypertensive vascular disease causes the hemorrhage. Patients with intracerebral hematoma from ruptured aneurysm are usually in coma and have severe neurologic dysfunction; survival in these circumstances is unlikely.

Removal of an intracerebral hematoma caused by bleeding from a ruptured A-V anomaly has been recommended for patients with neurologic disability. The results are difficult to appraise objectively, but surgical treatment has its best chance of offering relief if the patients have become stable clinically and have a well localized, encapsulated hematoma causing symptoms and signs of a mass lesion.

Patients who recover from intracerebral hemorrhage should begin programs of rehabilitation as soon as the effects of acute brain damage have subsided. Such a program begins with passive exercise of the paretic extremities to help avoid contractures and progresses to active exercises as voluntary movement returns. The program is as outlined under Treatment in Ch. 294.

Dinsdale, H. B.: Spontaneous hemorrhage in the posterior fossa. Arch. Neurol., 10:200, 1964.

Graf, C. J., and Nibbelink, D. W.: Cooperative study of intracranial aneurysms and subarachnoid hemorrhage. Report on a randomized treatment study, intracranial surgery. Stroke, 5:559, 1974.

McDowell, F. H., and Brennan, R. W.: Cerebral Vascular Diseases. Eighth Princeton Conference, 1972. New York, Grune & Stratton, 1973.

McKissock, W., Richardson, A., and Taylor, J.: Primary intracerebral hemorrhage. A controlled trial of surgical and conservative treatment in 180 selected cases. Lancet, 2:221, 1961.

McKissock, W., Richardson, A., and Walsh, L.: Anterior communicating aneurysms. A trial of conservative and surgical treatment. Lancet, 1:873, 1965.

McKissock, W., Richardson, A., and Walsh, L.: Middle-cerebral aneurysms. Further results in the controlled trial of conservative and surgical treatment of ruptured intracranial aneurysms. Lancet, 2:417, 1962.

Nibbelink, D. W., Torner, J. C., and Henderson, W. G.: Intracranial aneurysm and subarachnoid hemorrhage; antifibrinolytic therapy in recent onset subarachnoid hemorrhage. Stroke, 6:622, 1975.

Pool, J. L., and Potts, D. G.: Aneurysms and Arteriovenous Anomalies of the Brain: Diagnosis and Treatment. New York, Hoeber Medical Division, Harper & Row, 1965.

Sahs, A. L., Perret, G. E., Locksley, H. B., and Nishiotia, H.: Intracranial Aneurysms and Subarachnoid Hemorrhage. Philadelphia, J. B. Lippincott Company, 1969.

Whisnant, J. P., and Sandok, B. A.: Cerebrovascular Diseases. Ninth Princeton Conference, 1974. New York, Grune & Stratton, 1975.

Winn, H. R., Richardson, A. E. and Jane, J. A.: The long-term prognosis in untreated cerebral aneurysms: I. The incidence of late hemorrhage in cerebral aneurysm: A 10-year evaluation of 364 patients. Ann. Neurol., 1:358, 1977.

Section Fifteen INFECTIONS AND INFLAMMATORY DISEASES OF THE CENTRAL NERVOUS SYSTEM AND ITS COVERINGS

296. INTRODUCTION

Philip R. Dodge

The seriously ill patient with symptoms and signs of disease of the central nervous system and evidence of leptomeningeal inflammation presents a challenging diagnostic and therapeutic problem. Of crucial clinical significance is the determination of whether the involvement of meninges is primary, as in bacterial meningitis, or secondary, as in a variety of parenchymatous and parameningeal infections (e.g., encephalitis, brain abscess, subdural empyema). Central to this clinical problem is some degree of pleocytosis. Various bacteria, fungi, rickettsiae, viruses, and parasites may excite such a cerebrospinal fluid response. In addition, a similar reaction may be produced by a variety of noninfectious processes, including chemical irritation, hypersensitivity responses, and, occasionally, tumors. Elsewhere in this text many of the specific diseases that evoke an inflammatory response in the central nervous system and meninges are discussed. In this section emphasis will be placed on a systematic clinical approach to differential diagnosis and on the manner in which functions of the nervous system are deranged by such inflammatory processes.

297. AIDS TO DIAGNOSIS IN INTRACRANIAL AND INTRASPINAL INFLAMMATORY DISEASE

Philip R. Dodge

CEREBROSPINAL FLUID EXAMINATION

Because diagnosis rests in many instances on the cerebrospinal fluid (CSF) findings, the importance of a carefully performed lumbar puncture and of meticulous study of the CSF cannot be overstressed. The CSF findings characteristic of various inflammatory diseases of the central nervous system and meninges are outlined in Tables 1 and 2. Measurement of the initial pressure should be part of every CSF examination. In the presence of high pressure, just enough fluid should be removed slowly to allow for an adequate examination. Jugular compression (Queckenstedt's test) should be

avoided except in cases of suspected spinal cord compression. Deeply yellow (xanthochromic) fluid derives its color primarily from bilirubin pigment. In the absence of prior hemorrhage, this is most frequently associated with high concentrations of protein, and is often seen with impaired CSF circulation. Intense bilirubin staining of the CSF may also occur in jaundiced patients with meningitis (as in Weil's disease).

As few as 200 to 300 leukocytes per cubic millimeter will impart an opalescence to the fluid, and fluid containing thousands of cells will be turbid. The fluid should be examined promptly for cells in a counting chamber, and an accurate differential count should be performed on a stained smear of the sediment after centrifugation. In the event of a traumatic lumbar puncture, care must be exercised to ensure that an underlying pleocytosis is not missed. A gram-stained smear for bacteria should be studied. Recently, measurement of the concentration of bacterial antigens in CSF by countercurrent immunoelectrophoresis has proved highly reliable in the diagnosis of meningitis caused by *S. pneumoniae, N. meningitidis,* or *H. influenzae.* The test results can be provided within an hour. Whenever tuberculous meningitis is a consideration, a Ziehl-Neelsen or Kenyon stain should be performed on the sediment and on the protein coagulum or pellicle that frequently forms on standing. The India ink technique may outline *C. neoformans* in cases of cryptococcal meningitis (torulosis). The finding of budding forms of the yeast in CSF will help distinguish cryptococci from lymphocytes, with which they may be confused even by experienced observers; however, confirmation by culture is always necessary.

The CSF should be cultured whenever leukocytes are found or when an inflammatory process is suspected. A variety of media (blood agar, chocolate agar, thioglycollate broth) and various environmental conditions (reduced oxygen tension, increased CO_2 tension) are used routinely. Special media should be employed for the recovery of fungi or *M. tuberculosis.* The latter may also be injected into guinea pigs. Tissue culture techniques and inoculation of mice and embryonated eggs are used for virus isolation.

The concentration of protein in the CSF increases whenever there is interference with the blood-CSF barrier, as occurs with inflammation. In bacterial, tuberculous, mycotic, and carcinomatous meningitis the glucose concentration in the CSF is commonly reduced (hypoglycorrhachia). Although the mechanism of hypoglycorrhachia is incompletely understood, the high metabolic activity of rapidly growing cells, phagocyto-

TABLE 1. Initial Cerebrospinal Fluid Findings in Suppurative Diseases of the Central
Nervous System and Meninges

	Pressure (mm H$_2$O)	Leukocytes per cu mm	Protein (mg per 100 ml)	Sugar (mg per 100 ml)	Specific Findings
Acute bacterial meningitis	Usually elevated; average, 300	Several hundred to more than 60,000; usually few thousand; occasionally less than 100 (especially meningococcal or early in disease); polymorphonuclears predominate	Usually 100 to 500, occasionally more than 1000	Less than 40 in more than half the cases	Organism seen on smear usually; recovered on culture in more than 90% of cases
Subdural empyema	Usually elevated; average 300	Less than 100 to few thousand; polymorphonuclears predominate	Usually 100 to 500	Normal	No organisms on smear or by culture unless concurrent meningitis
Brain abscess	Usually elevated	Usually 10 to 200; rarely fluid is acellular; lymphocytes predominate	Usually 75 to 400	Normal	No organisms on smear or by culture
Ventricular empyema (rupture of brain abscess)	Considerably elevated	Several thousand to 100,000; usually more than 90% polymorphonuclears	Usually several hundred	Usually less than 40	Organism may be cultured or seen on smear
Cerebral epidural abscess	Slight to modest elevation	Few to several hundred or more cells; lymphocytes predominate	Usually 50 to 200	Normal	No organisms on smear or by culture
Spinal epidural abscess	Usually reduced with spinal block	Usually 10 to 100; lymphocytes predominate	Usually several hundred	Normal	No organisms on smear or by culture; may enter abscess on L.P. and get pus
Thrombophlebitis (often associated with subdural empyema)	Often elevated	Few to several hundred; polymorphonuclears and lymphocytes	Slightly to moderately elevated	Normal	No organisms on smear or by culture
Bacterial endocarditis (with embolism)	Normal or slightly elevated	Few to less than 100; lymphocytes and polymorphonuclears	Slightly elevated	Normal	No organisms on smear or by culture
Acute hemorrhagic encephalitis	Usually elevated	Few to more than 1000; polymorphonuclears predominate	Moderately elevated	Normal	No organisms on smear or by culture

TABLE 2. Comparative Cerebrospinal Fluid Findings in Nonsuppurative Meningitis

	Pressure (mm H$_2$O)	Leukocytes per cu mm	Protein (mg per 100 ml)	Sugar (mg per 100 ml)	Specific Findings
Tuberculous	Usually elevated; may be low with dynamic block in advanced stages	Usually 25 to 100, rarely more than 500; lymphoctyes predominate except in early stages when polymorphonuclears may account for 80% of cells	Nearly always elevated, usually 100 to 200; may be much higher if dynamic block	Usually reduced; less than 50 in ³/₄ of the cases	Acid-fast organisms may be seen on smear of protein coagulum (pellicle) or recovered from inoculated guinea pig or by culture
Cryptococcal	Usually elevated; average, 225	0 to 800; average, 50; lymphocytes predominate	Usually 20 to 500; average, 100	Reduced in more than half of cases; average, 30; often higher in patients with concomitant diabetes mellitus	Organisms may be seen in India ink preparation and on culture (Sabouraud's medium); will usually grow on blood agar; positive skin test
Syphilitic (acute)	Usually elevated	Average, 500; usually lymphocytes; rarely polymorphonuclears	Average, 100; gamma globulin often high	Normal (reduced rarely)	Positive reagin test for syphilis; spirochete not demonstrable by usual techniques of smear or by culture; positive countercurrent immunoelectrophoresis
Sarcoid	Normal to considerably elevated	0 to less than 100 mononuclear cells	Slight to moderate elevation	Normal	No specific findings
Tumor	Usually elevated; may be considerably so	0 to several hundred mononuclears	Elevated often to high levels	Normal or greatly reduced; (low in ³/₄ of carcinomatous meningitis cases)	Neoplastic cells may be identified on smear, by Millipore filter technique or by tissue block
Viral	Normal to moderately elevated	5 to few hundred; but may be more than 1000, particularly with mumps or echovirus 9; lymphocytes predominate but may be more than 80% polymorphonuclears in first few days	Frequently normal or slightly elevated; less than 100; may show greater elevation in recovering stages (particularly poliomyelitis)	Normal (reduced rarely)	Viral agent may be recovered in tissue culture, embryonated egg or animal inoculation

sis, and impaired glucose transport may all be involved. The gamma globulin concentration may be disproportionately increased in certain inflammatory disorders such as syphilis, subacute inclusion body encephalitis, and certain demyelinating disorders (postinfectious encephalomyelitis, multiple sclerosis). In addition to the time-honored tests for syphilis reagin, countercurrent immunoelectrophoresis is also useful here.

RELATIONSHIP OF CEREBROSPINAL FLUID FINDINGS TO ANCILLARY CLINICAL AND LABORATORY DATA

An immediate etiologic diagnosis is possible only when the responsible agent is identified. However, the clinical and CSF data can help to exclude certain clinical entities early in the diagnostic study. For example, when the symptoms and signs reflect involvement of the meninges and there is no evidence of cerebral or spinal cord disease, primary meningitis is probable. If, in addition, the CSF contains about 100 or so lymphocytes, a normal quantity of sugar, and an only slightly elevated protein concentration, then bacterial, including tuberculous, and cryptococcal meningitis are less likely, and some form of aseptic meningitis should be suspected. (However, it should be emphasized that the CSF sugar may be normal on initial examination of patients with tuberculous meningitis and may be reduced in samples obtained subsequently. It should also be appreciated that on occasion the CSF glucose may be reduced in aseptic meningitis.) A history of exposure to mumps and manifest parotitis make a diagnosis of mumps meningitis probable. On the other hand, the same findings in the CSF in a patient recovering from varicella, especially if there are symptoms and signs of cerebellar ataxia, suggest a diagnosis of postinfectious (varicella) encephalitis. In addition to primary meningeal disease, parameningeal infections can produce CSF abnormalities similar to those just described. The coexistence of a progressive dysphasia, superior quadrantanopsia, and hemiparesis on the right side and a history of a chronic draining left ear should immediately direct the physician's attention to the diagnosis of a left temporal lobe abscess. Unfortunately, however, a definite diagnosis cannot be made from either the initial clinical or CSF findings in many cases. Every attempt should be made to amplify the immediate and remote history, including epidemiologic data. One should search for foci of infection adjacent to or remote from the meninges. The extent of the dysfunction of the nervous system should be defined by repeated neurologic examinations and by laboratory studies. In addition to culturing the CSF, blood cultures should be obtained, because bacteremia is present in about half the cases of primary bacterial meningitis, and similar CSF changes may occur in bacterial endocarditis. Secretions of the upper and lower respiratory tracts also should be cultured for bacteria and fungi. Enteroviruses cause aseptic meningitis and encephalitis, and recovery of these agents from the stools of patients may aid in establishing the diagnosis. The development of specific neutralizing and complement-fixing antibodies will help confirm the diagnosis. Acute phase sera should be obtained on admission, and a convalescent serum sample obtained two to three weeks later. A four-fold rise

in complement-fixing or neutralizing antibody titer is usually evidence of a recent infection with that agent.

Roentgenograms of the skull, sinuses, chest, or spine may be helpful in establishing a diagnosis by disclosng a related focus of disease. An electroencephalogram or isotope scan may direct attention to a region of the brain that clinically is relatively silent. Computerized axial tomography (CAT), a noninvasive technique, is now established in the diagnosis of intracranial lesions and should be employed before resorting to invasive roentgenographic studies. Whether CAT will be equally reliable in the diagnosis of spinal lesions is now receiving study. Specialized contrast studies (myelography, pneumoencephalography, ventriculography, and angiography) are reserved for cases in which noninvasive studies are ambiguous or leave diagnosis in doubt. Occasionally the clinician must resort to a tissue biopsy; for example, the granulomatous lesions of sarcoidosis may be demonstrated in a lymph node or liver biopsy, and trichina, toxoplasma, or an unusual arteritis may be identified in microscopic sections of muscle tissue. Biopsy of the meninges or brain should be resorted to only rarely, but will at times help to establish the diagnosis in an obscure case. The pathologic findings in herpes, subacute sclerosing panencephalitis, and acute necrotizing hemorrhagic encephalitis are histologically specific enough to permit an exact diagnosis. Whenever tissue is obtained for routine histologic study, appropriate methods for the recovery of an infective agent should also be employed.

298.   PARAMENINGEAL INFECTIONS

Morton N. Swartz

The three major localized intracranial suppurative lesions are *brain abscess, subdural empyema,* and *cerebral extradural abscess.* Of paramount importance in their early recognition and subsequent management is an understanding of the nature of the predisposing suppurative conditions and of the portals by which infection has spread intracranially. Not only must these conditions be distinguished from one another but they must also, from a therapeutic viewpoint, be clearly distinguished from meningitis caused by bacteria or other infective agents.

BRAIN ABSCESS

DEFINITION. Brain abscess represents a poorly or sharply delineated suppurative process of brain substance, resulting from extension from adjacent foci or from hematogenous spread.

INCIDENCE. Despite the introduction of effective antimicrobial therapy, the over-all incidence of brain abscess has not changed significantly over the past two decades (about 7 per 1000 neurosurgical operations). It is seen approximately one sixth as frequently as bacterial meningitis in a large general hospital.

PREDISPOSING FACTORS. More than one third of intracerebral infections are a consequence of an adjacent primary focus of infection: middle ear, mastoid, paranasal sinuses, face or scalp and skull (osteomyelitis, compound fracture with wound contamination, or craniotomy wound infection). Another one third or so are a consequence of bronchiectasis, lung abscess, empyema, skin infections, acute bacterial endocarditis, or congenital heart disease with right-to-left shunt. In the remainder of brain abscesses an underlying cause cannot be determined.

Subacute and Chronic Middle Ear Infection and Mastoiditis. Over one third of all brain abscesses stem from ear and sinus infection. Infection usually spreads from the ear by either of two routes: direct extension to the roof of the tympanic cavity or mastoid bone (osteomyelitis) and then through the meningeal covering of the brain, or by extension along veins of the inner ear through diploic vessels of the skull and through intracranial venous channels into the substance of the brain. Thrombophlebitis of the pial vessels and dural sinuses, by impairing cerebral circulation, may cause infarction of brain tissue and facilitate development of local infection. The temporal lobe and cerebellum adjacent to the ear and mastoid are the most common sites of otogenic abscess.

Infections of the Paranasal Sinuses. Frontal and sphenoid sinuses are most frequently implicated in "rhinogenic" brain abscess of the frontal and temporal lobes, respectively. Infection may erode the sinus wall and invade the brain directly or, as with otogenic infection, may spread by way of veins communicating with the cavernous sinus and brain.

Infections of the Face and Skull. Intracranial spread of infection from the face or nose to the frontal lobe occurs by way of a septic thrombophlebitis. Compound fractures of the skull may result in brain abscess, particularly when dura and brain are lacerated, leaving a nidus of bone or foreign body in the devitalized tissue. Such abscesses may develop directly after the injury, or as long as 20 to 30 years later. Occasionally, the original trauma has seemed trivial and been overlooked. Brain abscess caused by a pencil point introduced through the orbit has occurred. Brain abscess may complicate stereotactic surgery and ventriculovascular shunts.

ETIOLOGY. A wide variety of microorganisms cause brain abscesses, and a careful attempt to establish a bacteriologic diagnosis should be made in every case. A gram-stained smear of purulent material should be studied at the time of surgery, and aerobic and anaerobic cultures, as well as cultures for fungi, should be obtained. In about 20 per cent of brain abscesses cultures are sterile. In about 25 per cent, most often when there is a contiguous extracerebral focus, two or more microbial species are isolated.

Various streptococci (either anaerobic or non-group A strains) and *Staphylococcus aureus* are the most frequently isolated organisms. *Streptococcus pneumoniae*, formerly a leading cause of brain abscess, is rarely incriminated today. Enterobacteriaceae (*E. coli, Proteus, Klebsiella*) are sometimes isolated. Anaerobic bacteria (streptococci, *Bacteroides* species, *Fusobacterium, Veillonella*) are isolated from 40 to 80 per cent of brain abscesses, particularly those of otogenic or rhinogenic origin. Rarely *Actinomyces* and *Nocardia* species may be recovered from an abscess cavity. Of interest is the frequent association of pulmonary alveolar proteinosis with pulmonary and occasionally cerebral nocardiosis. *Hemophilus aphrophilus* and the fungus *Cladosporium trichoides* rarely infect human beings, but when they do they show a curious affinity for the central nervous system.

When *Entamoeba histolytica* causes brain abscess, there are associated lesions of the liver or lung in virtually every case. In Central and South America and parts of Europe and Asia cerebral cysticercosis (usually solitary cysts containing the larval form of the pork tapeworm *Taenia solium*) should be considered in patients presenting with symptoms of brain tumor. In the racemose form of disease, obstructive hydrocephalus results from the growth of cysts in the third or fourth ventricle. The clinical picture may suggest a diagnosis of pseudotumor cerebri. Very rarely the brain is the site of echinococcal cysts and granulomas of schistosomiasis.

PATHOLOGY. Abscesses resulting from direct spread of infection are found in the brain adjacent to the primary extracerebral site; those resulting from retrograde venous propagation are often located at some distance from the primary focus in the distribution of the nearest venous sinus. Thus, for example, cerebellar abscess from otitis media is the result of spread of infection from the middle ear to its deep venous drainage into the transverse sinus, and thence medially into the veins draining the anterior superior portion of the ipsilateral cerebellar hemisphere. Metastatic abscesses are usually found in the distribution of the middle cerebral artery.

Initially, the site is edematous and infiltrated with polymorphonuclear leukocytes. The lesion is poorly demarcated at this stage and represents a local suppurative encephalitis. Usually within two weeks of onset the center undergoes liquefaction necrosis. The surrounding zone of fibroblasts becomes progressively thicker and contains more collagen; this constitutes the wall of the abscess, and astrocytes proliferate in the adjacent cerebral tissue. Multiple satellite abscesses may develop and frequently communicate with the principal cavity. Since abscess cavities usually spread through the central white matter, they often extend to and through the ventricular wall, producing the dire complications of ventricular empyema and meningitis. Brain abscess seldom or never results from primary bacterial meningitis. Coincidental occurrence of brain abscess and meningitis is usually related to intraventricular leakage of the abscess. In support of this view, the three most common organisms in primary pyogenic meningitis (*S. pneumoniae, H. influenzae,* and *N. meningitidis*) occur only rarely as the cause of brain abscess.

CLINICAL MANIFESTATIONS. Age Incidence. Brain abscesses are most common in the second to fifth decades, but may occur at any age. They are rare in infancy, even in patients with congenital heart disease.

General Features. The natural history of brain abscess consists either of a subacute to acute febrile illness with headache accompanied or followed by localizing neurologic symptoms, or of a "stroke-like" or tumor-like development of focal signs and symptoms in which evidence of infection is lacking. A history of fever at the time of invasion of the brain by the infective agent may be elicited; but a third of patients will lack a history of fever and remain afebrile under observation. Blood cultures are usually sterile except in those with an underlying acute bacterial endocarditis.

Headache, the most frequent initial symptom of brain abscess, may develop suddenly or insidiously while the attention of the patient and physician is directed toward the primary infection of ear, sinus, or lung. The development of unexplained headaches in a child with congenital cyanotic heart disease should be regarded as due to abscess until proved otherwise. The headache may be localized to the side of the abscess, but it is often generalized and increases in severity as the infection progresses. Heightened intracranial pressure, manifested by nausea, vomiting, drowsiness, bradycardia, confusion, and stupor, is common. Papilledema is a relatively late finding that is recognized in a minority of cases. The increased intracranial pressure may result in signs of sixth- and, less often, in those of third-nerve palsy. They are often false localizing signs, because the abscess may be remote from the cranial nerves. Although, pathologically, brain abscess progresses through several phases, there is no clear correlation with the clinical course of most patients. In some patients, usually those with metastatic brain abscesses, the illness runs a fulminating course, ending fatally in 5 to 15 days. In most, however, the course is considerably prolonged, and a diagnosis of cerebral neoplasm is often suspected.

Specific Neurologic Syndromes. TEMPORAL LOBE ABSCESS. The temporal lobes are the site of 30 per cent of brain abscesses; most are secondary to ear infection. Involvement of the dominant temporal lobe may produce a nominal (inability to name objects) or Wernicke's (inability to read, write, or understand spoken words) aphasia. Homonymous upper quadrantic or hemianopic field defects may occur. The only motor deficit may be a slight contralateral faciobrachial monoparesis. Herniation of the temporal lobe through the tentorium may develop precipitously and cause a homolateral third-nerve paralysis, coma, and bilateral pyramidal tract signs.

The presence of a second abscess should not be overlooked in a patient whose clinical state fails to improve or worsens after surgical treatment of a brain abscess. This is especially true in cases of temporal lobe abscess secondary to mastoiditis, in which cerebellar abscess may coexist.

CEREBELLAR ABSCESS. Cerebellar abscesses are almost exclusively otogenic and comprise 15 to 20 per cent of all brain abscesses. Increased intracranial pressure, suboccipital headache, and stiff neck may be the only manifestations. The patient may stagger and veer to the side of the lesion. Impaired coordination of extremities on the same side, with poor performance of rapid, alternating movements and with intention tremor, may be present. Nystagmus is frequent and usually coarser when the gaze is directed to the side of the abscess. Associated diseases of the inner ear may contribute to the unsteady gait and nystagmus, and may produce vertigo. Seizures do not occur with abscesses restricted to the cerebellum.

FRONTAL LOBE ABSCESS. Frontal lobe abscesses (30 per cent of brain abscesses) are most commonly associated with disease of the frontal or, less frequently, the ethmoid sinuses. Drowsiness, inattention, disturbed judgment, and impaired intellectual functions are common; the findings may suggest a psychiatric diagnosis. Mutism and increased grasp, suck, and snout reflexes are often present. In about a fourth of cases focal or generalized convulsions occur; deviation of the head and eyes to the side opposite the lesion is a common pattern of seizure. When the abscess is large or in the posterior frontal region, a contralateral hemiparesis usually develops. Rarely, dysphasia results from a lesion on the dominant side.

PARIETAL LOBE ABSCESS. Parietal lobe abscesses are usually hematogenous, but large otogenic temporal lobe abscesses may extend to the parietal lobe. Impaired position sense, two-point discrimination, and stereognosis are characteristic signs of an anterior parietal lobe abscess. Focal sensory and motor seizures occur. Homonymous hemianopia, visual inattention (often demonstrated by bilateral simultaneous stimulation of visual fields), and impaired opticokinetic nystagmus are encountered with more posterior and deep lesions. Dysphasia is a feature of inferior parietal lobe abscess on the dominant side. When the posterior parietotemporo-occipital region is affected, there may be impaired recognition of fingers, difficulty in differentiating left from right, acalculia, and agraphia (Gerstmann's syndrome).

BRAIN ABSCESS PRESENTING AS "ACUTE MENINGITIS." Occasionally patients with brain abscess present signs of meningitis, including fever, headache, stiff neck, and pleocytosis; focal neurologic signs are usually in evidence also. The syndrome is most often due to leaking of the abscess into the lateral ventricle. Massive rupture into the ventricle is a catastrophic event, with high fever, shock, and coma, and should be easily recognized. Pleocytosis with cell counts of more than 30,000 per cubic millimeter and reduced sugar concentrations are usual. Bacteria can often be seen on Gram stain and can be grown on culture.

In some patients with a similar clinical picture organisms are not found, and the syndrome may represent the phase of "bacterial encephalitis." The important point to be stressed is that one should be alert to the possibility of a brain abscess in any patients with chronic ear or sinus disease who develop "meningitis." These patients often improve on treatment of the meningitis only to develop evidence of an intracranial mass lesion one or two weeks later as encapsulation of the abscess progresses.

LABORATORY DIAGNOSIS. Modern neuroradiologic techniques presently provide the preferred and safest first step in laboratory diagnosis. When the diagnosis is suspected on clinical grounds, then skull films, supplemented as needed by x-rays of paranasal sinuses and mastoids, should be obtained. Brain scanning is the next step. The radionuclide scan will show increased uptake in almost all cases. Plain computerized tomography (CT) affords a similar high rate of detection of abnormality in cases of brain abscess and, in addition, provides much more detailed anatomic information, as well as increased accuracy in definition of multiple small lesions and loculi. Contrast enhancement may reveal an abscess capsule surrounding a central area of low absorption. (It should be recognized, however, that similar findings can be observed with cystic tumors, hematomas, or cerebral infarcts.) Angiography is generally less informative than the CT scan, but may provide further needed data (capsular staining, anatomic localization) when only the radionuclide scan is available. The EEG in brain abscess is localizing in the majority of cases, showing high voltage slow waves and, occasionally, sharp discharges over the margins of the abscess. However, it has little or no place if the CT scan is available.

The cerebrospinal fluid may require examination when meningitis is suspected, but lumbar puncture should be approached cautiously when clinical signs point to a mass lesion already being present. If the CT scan reveals no marked mass effect and that herniation is not occurring, lumbar puncture may be performed with less hazard. Cerebrospinal fluid pressure is commonly 200 to 300 mm H_2O, but may be considerably higher, particularly in the presence of intraventricular rupture. The cell count varies from a few to several hundred, with lymphocytes predominating. In cases of intraventricular rupture of the abscess, cell counts may be in excess of 50,000 (mainly neutrophils). Also, cell counts of several hundred to several thousand, with neutrophils predominating, may occur during the early phase of brain abscess ("bacterial encephalitis"). The glucose level is not reduced unless there is a simultaneous suppurative meningitis. The protein may be increased up to several hundred milligrams per 100 ml.

TREATMENT. Early diagnosis and prompt antimicrobial treatment are crucial. Intravenous mannitol is often employed to reduce brain edema. Parenteral corticosteroids have also been used for the same purpose during the perioperative period. Surgery is usually required once acute cerebral inflammation and edema are brought under control, and consists of initial aspiration of the abscess cavity, followed in some cases by excision at a later time, or primary total excision of the abscess. The method employed depends, to some extent, on the site of the lesion and the state of the patient, but whenever feasible, primary excision is probably preferable. The CT scan does provide a noninvasive means of following brain abscesses that have been drained rather than excised with an accuracy not previously possible.

Since in brain abscesses penicillin-susceptible organisms predominate, 10 million to 20 million units of penicillin per day intravenously should be started prior to operation. If there is reason to suspect an organism not susceptible to penicillin, e.g., gram-negative bacilli from a chronic ear infection, then chloramphenicol or similar drugs should be given concurrently. One of the semisynthetic penicillins, e.g., oxacillin, should be used if a penicillin-resistant *Staphylococcus* is suspected. The antimicrobial therapy should be modified as necessary at the time of operation, based on examination of a Gram-stained smear and culture of the abscess.

In selected cases it is possible that serial (plain or enhanced) CT scans will allow the delineation of the preabscess stage of acute bacterial encephalitis or cerebritis (previously not susceptible to definition except by invasive procedures), and the observation of its resolution or its evolution to abscess. However, it must be recognized that corticosteroid administration may significantly reduce contrast enhancement and obscure demonstration of an abscess capsule.

Mortality from brain abscess remains high despite antimicrobial and surgical treatment. Residual neurologic damage is frequent, and seizures are a significant sequela (up to 70 per cent) so that all patients should receive anticonvulsants for 24 months.

SUBDURAL EMPYEMA

DEFINITION. Subdural empyema refers to a collection of pus in the potential space between dura and arachnoid. It usually results from extension of infection from primary foci in the ears or sinuses. It is an infrequent complication of intracranial surgery, and may rarely represent a metastatic infection from a remote focus.

INCIDENCE. Subdural empyema is about one fifth as common as brain abscess. Its prevalence has not changed in the past two decades.

PREDISPOSING FACTORS AND PATHOLOGIC FEATURES. More than half the cases of subdural empyema develop in patients with chronic paranasal sinus infection, usually frontal. An acute exacerbation of the sinusitis just prior to the development of the subdural infection is common. Osteomyelitis of the frontal bone and an epidural abscess often accompany subdural empyema. Chronic otitis media and mastoiditis result in subdural empyema less often than formerly. Postoperative infection, penetrating wounds, infection in subdural hematomas, bacteremia, pulmonary infection, and (very rarely) bacterial meningitis are other sources of subdural empyema.

Infection spreads from the sinuses or mastoid by direct erosion of bone and dura or through infected veins. Thrombosis of cortical veins is observed in 90 per cent of fatal cases. Once pus forms in the subdural space it spreads widely over the convexity of the hemisphere and mesially along the falx. Rarely, the exudate extends beneath the falx to the opposite side. Purulent subarachnoid exudate is usually present immediately subjacent to the subdural exudate.

ETIOLOGY. Streptococci, often non-group A or anaerobic strains, are implicated most commonly, but a wide variety of gram-negative organisms are also found. Postoperative infections are usually due to *S. aureus*.

CLINICAL MANIFESTATIONS. The symptoms and signs of antecedent sinusitis, otitis, or osteomyelitis often blend into those of subdural empyema. Swelling and erythema of the tissues overlying the primary infection may be prominent, and percussion of the underlying bone may evoke considerable pain. In the early stages, pain or headache is mild and is limited to the area over the subdural infection. As the illness progresses, headache becomes generalized and severe; concomitantly high fever, chills, vomiting, and nuchal rigidity develop. Progressive obtundation, culminating in coma within 48 to 72 hours, occurs in untreated cases. Focal or generalized seizures and hemiparesis are common. Sensory deficits and visual field defects and dysphasia also occur. Although these signs are in part attributable to the compressive effects of a mass lesion, the associated thrombophlebitis of cortical veins and the consequent infarction of cerebral tissue are probably of equal importance. In the late stages, intracranial pressure is severely increased, but papilledema is rare except in chronic cases in which the clinical course has been modified by antimicrobial therapy. Without treatment, death usually occurs within a few days of onset of focal neurologic signs.

LABORATORY DIAGNOSIS. The cerebrospinal fluid pressure is elevated, and the fluid characteristically contains a few hundred to a thousand or more cells (either neutrophils or lymphocytes predominating), a normal glucose level, and no organisms. Roentgenograms of the skull may show destructive changes in the frontal or mastoid bones. In the past, carotid arteriography and/or burr hole examination have been diagnostic and distinguished subdural empyema from brain abscess. Although experience is as yet limited with the CT scan, it appears it can show up extracerebral collections of decreased density associated with a mass effect.

TREATMENT. The patient with a subdural empyema requires prompt and adequate surgical drainage by multiple burr holes or craniotomy. Surgical treatment of the accompanying sinusitis, frontal osteomyelitis, or mastoiditis is a secondary consideration and is usually postponed until the acute intracranial infection has subsided. Vigorous systemic therapy with penicillin (10 to 20 million units daily) and/or other antimicrobials, depending on the background of the case, is begun before surgery and continued until the infection has been completely controlled. The results of smear and culture of pus obtained at the time of operation may dictate changes in the antimicrobial regimen. Bacitracin or other antimicrobial drugs are commonly instilled into the subdural space at the time of operation and for a variable period thereafter.

CEREBRAL EPIDURAL ABSCESS

Epidural abscess is usually secondary to mastoiditis, sinus infection, osteomyelitis of the skull, skull fracture, or infection of an operative wound. Etiologic and pathogenetic considerations are identical to those described for subdural empyema. The close adherence of the dura to bone limits the size of the epidural abscess. It often represents granulations rather than a frankly purulent collection. Rarely, an extensive destructive osteomyelitis of the frontal bone ("Pott's puffy tumor") may be associated with an epidural abscess.

Diagnosis may be difficult. The patient is not as ill as with a subdural empyema, and the size of the collection is rarely sufficient to produce focal neurologic signs or increased intracranial pressure. Fever, pain, and tenderness over the affected area are the common manifestations. In most cases the cerebrospinal fluid is sterile, and contains few cells (lymphocytes predominating) and a normal concentration of glucose. Many times the diagnosis is made incidentally at the time of sinus or mastoid surgery or when intracranial surgery is performed for an associated subdural empyema or brain abscess. Some cases of epidural abscess are probably cured by antimicrobial therapy alone. Spread of infection from the mastoid along the ridge of the petrous bone may result in a small epidural granuloma or abscess that gives rise to a homolateral sixth-nerve palsy and temporoparietal pain from involvement of the sensory fibers of the fifth nerve (Gradenigo's syndrome).

THROMBOPHLEBITIS AND THROMBOSIS OF MAJOR VENOUS SINUSES

CORTICAL THROMBOPHLEBITIS. The syndrome of cortical thrombophlebitis characteristically appears some three to ten days after the onset of bacterial meningitis. The signs include a secondary rise in temperature, focal or generalized seizures, and focal neurologic deficits, such as a hemiparesis. In some instances at least, the underlying phlebitis has its inception earlier and is the basis for many of the seizures and signs of focal cortical disease encountered in the early stages of meningitis. Treatment includes continuation of the antimicrobial therapy and anticonvulsants. Anticoagulant drugs have no established place in therapy. In most cases the process is limited in extent and the patient recovers, but,

when the process is widespread, substantial neurologic deficits and death may result.

MAJOR DURAL SINUS THROMBOSIS

Thrombosis of the large dural sinuses may occur in meningitis, may complicate epidural or subdural abscesses, or may develop during the intracranial spread of infection from extracerebral veins. (For spontaneous sinus thrombosis, see Ch. 294.) The thrombotic process may spread to connecting sinuses and cortical veins. Abscess formation within the thrombosed vessel may result in septicemia and infected emboli that travel to distant sites. The cavernous, lateral, and superior sagittal sinuses are most frequently involved.

CAVERNOUS SINUS THROMBOSIS. Infection can spread to the cavernous sinus through venous channels by three routes: (1) from lesions of the upper half of the face through the facial veins communicating with the angular and superior ophthalmic veins, (2) from infections of the sphenoid and posterior ethmoid sinuses, inferiorly, and (3) from the ear, posteriorly. The initiating infection is usually a furuncle, acute sinusitis, or an ear infection. The use of antimicrobial drugs in the treatment of superficial infections has markedly reduced the incidence of this disease. The majority of infections are due to *S. aureus*.

Clinical Manifestations. The general clinical features are those of severe systemic infection: chills, fever, headache, nausea, lethargy, marked polymorphonuclear leukocytosis, and bacteremia. The specific findings are unilateral initially but become bilateral as the process extends to the opposite cavernous sinus via the connecting circular sinus. They include, in the case of infections about the face, unilateral edema of the forehead, eyelids, and base of the nose, as well as proptosis and chemosis — all caused by obstruction of the ophthalmic vein as it enters the cavernous sinus. The superficial veins over the forehead may be distended. The retinal veins become engorged or even thrombosed. Retinal hemorrhages and papilledema occur but may be late manifestations. Involvement of the ophthalmic branch of the fifth nerve produces pain in the eye, photophobia, and hyperesthesia of the forehead. Partial or even complete paralysis of the ocular muscles develops as a result of involvement of the third, fourth, and sixth cranial nerves as they pass through the sinus. The pupils are usually dilated but may be small; the pupillary reactions are often lost.

In infection spreading by the inferior route (e.g., sphenoid sinusitis) the process may be less acute initially. A meningeal reaction commonly occurs, usually without organisms in the cerebrospinal fluid, but pyogenic meningitis sometimes occurs. Rarely, infarction and abscess of the pituitary complicate septic cavernous sinus thrombosis.

Differential diagnosis includes other causes of proptosis, especially orbital cellulitis, abscess, or acute carotid-cavernous fistula. Retinal hemorrhages, papilledema, and palsies of cranial nerves innervating extraocular muscles rather than general restriction of ocular movement from the mechanical effects of orbital swelling are useful differential points.

LATERAL SINUS THROMBOSIS. Thrombosis of the lateral sinus is almost always a complication of acute or chronic otitis media, of mastoiditis, or of cholesteatoma formation. Rarely, infection may spread in a retrograde fashion from a focus in the neck or from a tonsillar abscess. Streptococci, predominantly group A, and staphylococci have been implicated most frequently. The clinical manifestations include chills, fever, and signs of increased intracranial pressure. Pain, venous engorgement, and edema behind the ear may result from associated involvement of the mastoid emissary vein and may extend into the neck over the jugular vein. Papilledema is common; it may be unilateral as a consequence of extension to the cavernous sinus on that side. A generalized increase in intracranial pressure is more frequent with occlusions of the right lateral sinus, which is commonly larger and more important for venous drainage than the left. Convulsive seizures and obtundation occur, but focal neurologic findings are rare except when the thrombophlebitis extends into cortical veins over the convexity of the hemisphere. Rarely, ninth-, tenth- and eleventh-nerve palsies develop, presumably owing to involvement of the jugular bulb and related venous channels.

Cerebrospinal fluid pressure is elevated, and the fluid contains several to many hundred leukocytes (lymphocytes predominating) but no bacteria.

SUPERIOR SAGITTAL SINUS THROMBOSIS. The superior sagittal sinus is less commonly involved in septic thrombosis than are the lateral and cavernous sinuses. Infection may spread from the lateral or cavernous sinuses, from the pelvis by way of the vertebral veins, from a primary meningitis, or from a contiguous osteomyelitis and peridural infection. If thrombosis is restricted to that portion of the sinus anterior to the rolandic veins, and there is no associated involvement of cortical veins, then the process is usually asymptomatic. Thrombosis of the posterior portion of the sinus results in increased intracranial pressure; at times there are engorgement of scalp veins and edema of the forehead. Extension of the inflammatory process into the cortical veins results in infarction of the underlying cortex. Focal seizures, which alternately involve one and then the other side of the body, are characteristic. Because the superior and mesial surfaces of the cerebral hemispheres are particularly liable to infarction, weakness and sensory changes are frequently more prominent in the legs. However, hemiparesis, homonymous hemianopia, aphasia, and paresis, or conjugate deviation of the eyes may occur.

The cerebrospinal fluid findings are similar to those in lateral sinus thrombosis. A suspected diagnosis of major venous sinus thrombosis can often be confirmed by angiographic study.

Treatment of Dural Sinus Thrombophlebitis. Appropriate antimicrobial drugs in high dosage and surgical drainage, with removal of infected bone and extradural or intrasinus abscess, constitute proper treatment for major sinus thromboses. Ligation of the jugular vein in lateral sinus thrombosis to prevent spread of infected emboli is usually not necessary. Because of the frequent involvement of penicillinase-producing staphylococci, the use of semisynthetic penicillins (nafcillin, oxacillin) is warranted until cultures are reported. Since infarction of cerebral tissue from venous thromboses tends to be hemorrhagic, anticoagulants are not employed. The prognosis for recovery is reasonably good when optimal treatment is given, although there are frequently residual neurologic symptoms and signs.

CEREBRAL MANIFESTATIONS OF BACTERIAL ENDOCARDITIS

Neurologic symptoms or signs occur in about 30 per cent of patients with bacterial endocarditis, and represent the major complaints in one half of these patients. The neuropathologic findings of subacute bacterial endocarditis (usually due to viridans streptococci) are distinct from those of acute bacterial endocarditis (see Ch. 131). Diffuse embolic infarctions, with a variable and usually limited inflammatory response about involved blood vessels and adjacent meninges, constitute the major neurologic findings in subacute bacterial endocarditis. Pyogenic brain abscess and purulent meningitis do not occur. The clinical picture can resemble that of diffuse encephalitis or toxic encephalopathy, or there may be focal signs such as hemiplegia and hemianopia. The cerebrospinal fluid contains modest numbers of polymorphonuclear leukocytes (sometimes red cells as well) and a normal concentration of glucose; bacteria are absent. Mycotic aneurysms, occurring in 2 to 10 per cent of patients with endocarditis, are generally small and located at the bifurcation of peripheral arteries. They are usually asymptomatic unless rupture occurs into brain or subarachnoid space. Clipping of superficial aneurysms may be possible; occasional mycotic aneurysms, demonstrated on angiogram, have been observed to disappear on subsequent study and following antimicrobial therapy.

In acute bacterial endocarditis caused by invasive pyogenic organisms (usually *Staphylococcus aureus*), brain abscess (usually small and multiple), acute purulent meningitis, and embolic infarction of cerebral tissue may occur.

Brain Abscess

Ballantine, H. T., Jr., and Shealy, C. N.: The role of radical surgery in the treatment of abscess of the brain. Surg. Gynecol. Obstet., 109:370, 1959.

Garfield, J.: Management of supratentorial intracranial abscess: A review of 200 cases. Br. Med. J., 2:7, 1969.

Gates, E. M., Kernohan, J. W., and Craig, W. M.: Metastatic brain abscess. Medicine, 29:71, 1950.

Heineman, H. S., and Braude, A. I.: Anaerobic infection of the brain. Am. J. Med., 35:682, 1963.

Matson, D. D., and Salam, M.: Brain abscess in congenital heart disease. Pediatrics, 27:772, 1961.

Samson, D. S., and Clark, K.: A current review of brain abscess. Am. J. Med., 54:201, 1973.

Swartz, M. N., and Karchmer, A. W.: Infections of the central nervous system. *In* Ballows, A., et al. (eds.): Anaerobic Bacteria. Role in Disease. Springfield, Ill., Charles C Thomas, 1974.

Zimmerman, R. A., Patel, S., and Bilaniuk, L. T.: Demonstration of purulent bacterial intracranial infections by computed tomography. Am. J. Roentgenol., 127:155, 1976.

Subdural Empyema

Conrood, D., and Dans, P. E.: Subdural empyema. Am. J. Med., 53:85, 1972.

Hitchcock, E., and Andreadis, A.: Subdural empyema: A review of 29 cases. J. Neurol. Neurosurg. Psychiatry, 27:422, 1964.

Kaufman, D. M., Miller, M. H., and Steigbigel, N. H.: Subdural empyema: Analysis of 17 recent cases and review of the literature. Medicine, 54:485, 1975.

Thrombophlebitis and Thrombosis of Major Venous Sinuses

Brown, P.: Septic cavernous sinus thrombosis. Bull. Hopkins Hosp., 109:68, 1961.

Kalbag, R. K., and Woolf, A. L.: Cerebral Venous Thrombosis. London, Oxford University Press, 1967.

Krayenbuhl, H.: Cerebral venous and sinus thrombosis. Clin. Neurosurg., 14:1, 1967.

Ray, B. S., and Dunbar, H. S.: Thrombosis of the superior sagittal sinus as a cause of pseudotumor cerebri: Methods of diagnosis and treatment. Trans. Am. Neurol. Assoc., 75:12, 1950.

Cerebral Manifestations of Bacterial Endocarditis

Jones, H. R., Siekert, R. E., and Geraci, J. E.: Neurologic manifestations of bacterial endocarditis. Ann. Intern. Med., 71:21, 1969.
Kerr, A., Jr.: Subacute Bacterial Endocarditis. Springfield, Ill., Charles C Thomas, 1955, Chap. V, p. 92.
Ziment, I.: Nervous system complications in bacterial endocarditis. Am. J. Med., 47:593, 1969.

299. SPINAL EPIDURAL INFECTIONS

Philip R. Dodge

DEFINITION. Spinal epidural infections consist of purulent or granulomatous collections contained within the spinal epidural space and overlying or encircling the spinal cord, roots, and nerves. Infection may be localized or may extend widely, at times involving the length of the spinal canal. In one large series an average extent of 4.3 bony segments was reported.

INCIDENCE. This is a rare type of infection in adults, being less than one twentieth — and in children one hundredth — as common as bacterial meningitis.

ETIOLOGY AND PATHOGENESIS. *Staphylococcus aureus* is involved in more than 90 per cent of cases, but group A streptococci, other streptococci, pneumococci, *Brucella, Salmonella,* and various other gram-negative organisms may be responsible. *M. tuberculosis* is an important cause of chronic epidural infections in areas where tuberculosis is prevalent; occasionally fungi and parasites may be recovered from epidural granulomas. There is a primary infective site remote from the spine in most cases. This usually involves the skin, and furuncles, boils, and cellulitis are the common underlying infections. Less often infections of the upper respiratory tract, genitourinary system, or bone may be responsible. Hematogenous or lymphatic spread of infection to the highly vascular epidural space is postulated. Occasionally the responsible organism may be cultured from the blood. Minor injury to the back frequently antedates the symptoms of epidural abscess, and trauma may in some way determine the site of infection. The lack of restraining fibrous tissue in the epidural fat allows the infection to spread caudally and rostrally, and epidural abscesses may extend into the extraspinal tissues; in contrast, the dura is rarely penetrated. In less than half the cases the spine and adjacent soft tissues are primarily affected, and the infection spreads secondarily to the epidural space. Only in tuberculous infections is primary osteomyelitis the rule. Epidural abscess may rarely complicate a lumbar puncture, myelogram, or spinal operation.

PATHOLOGY. The purulent material or granulomatous tissue is usually most abundant over the posterior aspect of the spinal cord. When the primary lesion is in a vertebral body, intervertebral disc, or some other anterior structure, the abscess may be predominantly ventral. Epidural abscess occurs most commonly in the thoracic region, but may develop at any level of the spinal axis. The lesion may be purulent or granulomatous.

The mechanism of neural dysfunction in spinal epidural abscess is uncertain. Since the lesion occupies space, direct compression of spinal cord, roots, and nerves is a prime consideration, but the small size of many epidural abscesses, in association with severe impairment of neural function, demands consideration of other possibilities. The most plausible of these and the one for which there are some supporting facts is a vasculitis with secondary venous and arterial occlusions resulting in infarction of neural tissues.

CLINICAL MANIFESTATIONS. Heusner has divided the clinical picture into four phases: spinal ache, root pain, weaknesses (voluntary muscles, sphincters, sensibilities), and paralyses.

Spinal Ache. The spinal ache, characteristically maximal at the level of the major pathologic process, soon spreads axially and may also include the paravertebral regions. Restricted movement of the spine, especially in the anteroposterior plane, is common. A functional or even a structural scoliosis may develop. The spines overlying the disease process are tender to percussion; pain so induced may be exquisite, particularly when there is vertebral caries. Signs of sepsis (fever, leukocytosis) are prominent, except in the more chronic cases. The diagnosis is rarely made at this stage.

Root Pain. Within two or three days (acute cases) nerve roots inevitably become encased by the purulent material, and radicular pains develop. Meningeal signs are present in most cases, and headache is a common symptom. At times reflex activity at the level of the involved segment may be depressed. An erroneous diagnosis of "neuritis" or "shingles" is frequently made, but at this stage of illness the combination of clinical symptoms and signs should permit an accurate diagnosis.

Weaknesses. The characteristic feature of this phase of the illness is progressive impairment of neural functions below the level of the lesion, the exact syndrome depending upon the site of maximal damage. If the abscess overlies the spinal cord, spastic weakness, heightened reflexes, and a sensory loss below the lesion are to be expected. There may be urinary urgency and incontinence. Abscesses in the lumbosacral region exert their effects on spinal roots and nerves, giving rise to dysesthesias in dermatomes supplied by the implicated nerves, along with appropriate pareses and depressed stretch reflexes. Pain is usually excruciating and nuchal rigidity extreme. The skin and soft tissues overlying the abscess may be swollen, warm, and red. High fever and signs of systemic toxicity are often present.

The diagnosis may be made as late as this with reasonable anticipation that prompt laminectomy and drainage of pus or removal of granulomatous tissue will effect considerable if not total recovery.

Paralyses. Within hours or at most a few days, severe or even total paralysis of nervous functions below the site of the lesion supervenes. Immediate surgical treatment is mandatory at this stage. Procrastination may vitiate the effect of any subsequent therapeutic measures, for *most patients who are paralyzed for more than a few hours remain so permanently*. When an epidural abscess remains unrecognized and untreated, death occurs in 25 to 33 per cent of cases.

It is axiomatic that the foregoing analysis of the clinical features of subdural abscess is arbitrary and somewhat artificial, because the various stages may merge one into the other. Yet, considered in this way the early stages are stressed and the importance of prompt diagnosis and treatment is underscored.

DIFFERENTIAL DIAGNOSIS. Spinal epidural abscess demands consideration in the patient with sepsis, back pain, and even minimal neurologic symptoms and signs. Confirmatory evidence may be obtained by tapping the epidural space with an ordinary spinal needle. This is most safely done in the lumbar area. Gentle suction is applied with a small (2 ml) syringe while slowly advancing the needle. If no purulent material is obtained, the stylet should be replaced in the needle and the subarachnoid space entered. The cerebrospinal fluid (CSF) is characteristically clear and xanthochromic. It may be acellular, but more often a few cells or a moderate pleocytosis (lymphocytes predominating) will be found. Normal sugar content and elevated CSF protein are the rule (several hundred to more than 2000 mg per 100 ml). A partial or complete manometric block below the lesion is found in most cases.

An acute viral, postinfectious, syphilitic, or necrotizing myelitis may produce a neurologic syndrome similar to that seen in stage 4 of a spinal epidural abscess, and may be associated with symptoms and signs of infection and CSF pleocytosis. There may be back pain in acute myelitis, but the duration of illness is compressed in time. Furthermore, xanthochromic CSF and manometric block are unusual in myelitis. They are seen, however, in progressive adhesive arachnoiditis, which may be confused with subacute or chronic epidural infections. Spinal caries, demonstrable by roentgenography in less than 20 per cent of cases of spinal epidural abscess, suggests the correct diagnosis. In questionable cases a myelographic study will confirm the presence of a space-occupying intraspinal lesion. Rarely, malignant tumors, especially lymphomas that lodge in the epidural space, may present with fever, backache, neurologic signs, and spinal block. Chronic epidural abscess in which evidence of an inflammatory disease is meager or wanting will, on occasion, be confused with the more benign intraspinal tumors.

TREATMENT. Prompt laminectomy with drainage of purulent material or removal of granulomatous tissue and the administration of appropriate antimicrobial drugs constitute proper therapy. The antimicrobials must be continued in high doses for a minimum of six weeks when pyogenic osteomyelitis is present.

Baker, A. S., Ojemann, R. G., Swartz, M. N., and Richardson, E. P., Jr.: Spinal epidural abscess. N. Engl. J. Med., 293:463, 1975.

Heusner, A. P: Nontuberculous spinal epidural infections. N. Engl. J. Med., 239:845, 1948.

Hulme, A., and Dott, N. M.: Spinal epidural abscess. Br. Med. J., 1:64, 1954.

300. TRANSVERSE MYELITIS OR MYELOPATHY

Philip R. Dodge

Transverse myelitis refers to a clinical syndrome in which there is evidence of complete or partial loss of neurologic functions below a lesion which pathologically usually has a limited longitudinal dimension in the spinal cord. Thoracic and cervical segments are most frequently involved. Although inflammation is implied, it should be appreciated that evidence for this is frequently lacking, and thus the term transverse myelopathy is preferred by many neurologists.

ETIOLOGY. As a syndrome rather than a disease, the spectrum of specific causes is broad (see accompanying table). However, the cause remains unknown in the majority of patients presenting with the typical clinical findings.

PREVALENCE. No precise epidemiologic data are available. Although rare in general medical practice, the syndrome is not uncommonly encountered in a neurologic setting. Sixty-seven cases (44 adults and 23 children) were encountered over a 25-year period at the Columbia Presbyterian Medical Center in New York. Males and females are affected about equally. Altrocchi, who reported on this experience, excluded compressive lesions, serious trauma, radiation myelopathy, those with evidence of concomitant cerebral involvement, and those thought to have multiple sclerosis.

PATHOLOGY. The pathology of myelitis or myelopathy includes varying degrees of destruction affecting either white or gray matter or often both, usually in an asymmetrical fashion with this irregular pattern of involvement present over the longitudinal extent of the lesion. Patchy destruction frequently involves several segments of the spinal cord but may be even more extensive. Demyelination, neuronal injury, and incomplete or complete necrosis of neural tissue have been described and may at times be associated with inflammatory cells, macrophages, or proliferation of astroglia. The form of the reaction is probably related to the du-

---

Diseases Which May Present as an Acute or Subacute Transverse Myelitis or Myelopathy

I. Myelitis due to viruses
   A. Poliomyelitis
   B. Coxsackievirus
   C. Herpes zoster
   D. Rabies
   E. B virus myelitis
   F. EB virus

II. Myelitis of unknown etiology
   A. Demyelination myelitis (acute multiple sclerosis)
   B. Postinfectious or postvaccinal myelitis
   C. Necrotizing myelitis (? myelopathy)

III. Myelitis secondary to inflammatory diseases of the meninges
   A. Syphilitic myelitis
      1. Acute meningitis
      2. Meningovascular spinal syphilis
      3. Tabes dorsalis
      4. Gummatous meningitis, including chronic spinal pachymeningitis
   B. Pyogenic or suppurative myelitis
      1. Subacute or chronic meningomyelitis
      2. Abscess of the spinal cord
      3. Subdural abscess
      4. Acute epidural spinal abscess or granuloma
   C. Tuberculous myelitis
      1. Pott's disease with spinal cord compression
      2. Tuberculous meningomyelitis
      3. Tuberculoma of the spinal cord
   D. Miscellaneous
      1. Parasitic and fungal infections producing an epidural granuloma, localized meningitis, or meningomyelitis
      2. Idiopathic meningomyelitis (chronic adhesive arachnoiditis)

IV. Myelopathies
   A. Vascular
      1. Anterior spinal artery occlusion
      2. Dissecting aneurysm with occlusion of major radicular arteries
      3. Arteritis, e.g., polyarteritis nodosa, lupus erythematosus
      4. Malformations
   B. Nutritional deficiencies

ration of the disease and its cause. Thickening of small arteries and veins within or adjacent to the parenchyma of spinal cord has been prominent in only a few of the recorded cases. Because death rarely occurs in the acute stage of the illness today, recent reports characteristically lack postmortem studies employing modern histochemical and cytologic techniques.

CLINICAL MANIFESTATIONS. The onset is usually abrupt, with the neurologic deficit evolving from the initial symptoms to maximal disability within hours to a few days or occasionally a few weeks. A premonitory history of an upper respiratory or other infection or minor trauma is reported in about 25 per cent of cases. The earliest symptoms are (1) muscle weakness, usually involving the lower limbs, (2) sensory aberrations, (3) back discomfort, or (4) root pain, all occurring with about equal frequency. Signs may be asymmetrical, but bilateral involvement of the spinal cord is invariable at some time in the course of disease. Bladder and bowel dysfunction are nearly universal as paresis of the limbs and sensory disturbances progress.

The degree of paraparesis is variable, but moderate to severe weakness of the legs obtains in about two thirds of patients. Weakness may affect the arms in as many as one quarter of patients. Sensory loss also is seen in approximately two thirds of reported cases, pain and temperature being more often affected than position and vibratory sensation. Segmental paresthesias and dysesthesias may occur. Stretch reflexes are often lost in the acute stage of the disease but become exaggerated later. Babinski signs are usual. Meningeal signs are encountered in up to one third of patients. There is fever in about one half of patients, although this may be referable to complicating infections of lung or urinary tract.

The cerebrospinal fluid (CSF) findings are extremely variable even during the acute stage of the disease. In some patients the CSF may be acellular with only a slight rise in the protein concentration, but there may be several hundred or a thousand or more leukocytes, often with a predominant polymorphonuclear reaction in the acute state. The protein concentration may be elevated to several hundred milligrams per 100 ml, and the percentage of gamma globulin can be increased significantly. The sugar content is typically normal. Spine radiographs are unrevealing, as is myelography, except in rare instances when spinal cord swelling is extreme, impeding the flow of dye. In such instances there also can be a manometric block.

DIAGNOSIS. Although the diagnosis of transverse myelitis or myelopathy can be suspected on clinical grounds, it is incumbent upon the physician to consider first those diseases which demand specific and prompt treatment. Spinal epidural abscess can mimic closely transverse myelitis, although the course of the latter condition is usually more rapid. Contrast myelography should be performed if there is any question about the diagnosis. (Spinal CAT myelography may eventually replace contrast myelograms, but this is not yet the case.) The risk of the myelography is minimal, and the danger of missing a compressive suppurative lesion which should be treated by surgery is of overriding concern. Intraspinal neoplasms and other compressive tumors will also be excluded by myelography except in those rare instances in which an acutely inflamed, swollen cord may mimic an intra-axial mass. Syphilis, especially the meningovascular form, may mimic nonspecific myelitis and deserves immediate treatment. The treatable nutritional myelopathies evolve more slowly and have a pattern of spinal cord involvement which is more diffuse. Other evidence of vitamin B_{12} deficiency or of pellagra should make exclusion of these disorders relatively easy. A vascular nevus at the segmental level of the spinal cord lesion should signal the possibility of an intraspinal vascular malformation which can be defined by selective spinal cord angiography. Every effort should be made to establish the diagnosis of specific viral infections by appropriate cultural and serologic means. A diagnosis of multiple sclerosis may become obvious only when lesions of the central nervous system disseminated in time and space appear.

TREATMENT. There is no specific treatment for transverse myelitis or myelopathy of unknown cause. The efficacy of pharmacologic doses of the glucocorticoids is unproved but might be considered, particularly if there is evidence of swelling of the spinal cord. Prevention or appropriate treatment for the complications of paraplegia is critical.

PROGNOSIS. Proper supportive care, including therapy for complicating infection, prevention of pressure sores, and attention to urinary tract function, renders the prognosis for survival excellent. According to Altrocchi, one third of patients make a good or complete recovery, one third do moderately well, and a poor recovery characterizes the course in the other third. Lipton and Teasdall found similar results. Recurrent neurologic problems are rare among the survivors.

Altrocchi, P. H.: Acute transverse myelopathy. Arch. Neurol., 9:112, 1963.
Greenfield, J. G., and Turner, J. W. A.: Acute and subacute necrotic myelitis. Brain, 62:227, 1939.
Hoffman, H. L.: Acute necrotic myelopathy. Brain, 78:377, 1955.
Lipton, H. L., and Teasdall, R. D.: Acute transverse myelopathy in adults. Arch. Neurol., 28:252, 1973.

301. SYPHILITIC INFECTIONS OF THE CENTRAL NERVOUS SYSTEM

Philip R. Dodge

A general exposition of *T. pallidum* infection is presented in Ch. 171. The following presentation is restricted to a discussion of neurosyphilis.

Although the spirochete invades the nervous system and its coverings during the early weeks of infection in nearly every case, neurosyphilis develops in less than 10 per cent of untreated cases.

PATHOLOGY. Involvement of the leptomeninges is an essential feature of all forms of neurosyphilis. A meningitis of varying severity and extent is present in every case of active neurosyphilis regardless of the neurologic syndrome. The cerebrospinal fluid (CSF) reflects this involvement. Even in cases of *asymptomatic neurosyphilis*, in which the presence of syphilis reagin constitutes the sole abnormality, rare postmortem examinations have disclosed definite meningeal inflammation and ependymal granulations. Similarly, in chronic tabes dorsalis with negative CSF examination, evidence of prior active meningeal disease will be revealed by pathologic study.

Postmortem study of a few cases of acute *syphilitic meningitis* has shown a meningeal inflammatory reaction in which lymphocytes and plasma cells predominate. Cellular aggregates collect about blood vessels, and evidence of early arteritis may be found, although cerebrovascular accidents are rare in this stage of the disease. Reactive fibrosis of the leptomeninges, especially about the base of the brain, is also seen. This accounts for the cranial nerve palsies and for impaired CSF circulation that can result in increased intracranial pressure. A granular ependymitis is commonly present, and, rarely, this may obstruct CSF flow through the aqueduct.

In so-called *meningovascular syphilis*, which is typically a more chronic disorder occurring months or a few years after the primary lesion, the inflammatory response is usually less acute and meningeal fibrosis more prominent. As the name suggests, there is an associated arteritis (usually small vessels) that predisposes to arterial occlusion and consequent infarction of neural tissue. When larger arteries become occluded, infarction of brain or spinal cord may be extensive. In some cases damage to regions of neural tissue adjacent to meninges occurs without obvious vascular occlusions.

In general paresis there is direct invasion of neural tissue by the spirochete, accompanied by meningeal involvement. In tabes dorsalis and primary optic atrophy, the pathogenesis is unclear. There is no convincing evidence that direct invasion by the spirochete plays a significant role; whether a reaction in the meningitis is important is uncertain. On gross inspection the dorsal roots appear gray and atrophic, and the dorsal aspect of the spinal cord appears wasted. Myelin sheaths are damaged as well, and demyelination of dorsal columns is easily demonstrated by appropriate stains. Involvement of anterior roots with resultant amyotrophy occurs also but is exceedingly rare. Why the syphilitic process shows a predilection for dorsal roots is unknown.

In general paresis one finds on gross examination meningeal thickening, atrophy of cerebral tissue (especially of frontal and temporal lobes), and enlargement of ventricles; a granularity of the ependymal surface is consistently present. Microscopically, diffuse destruction and loss of neurons, especially in the cortex, are found, and special stains may demonstrate a heavy infestation with *Treponema pallidum*. Reactive gliosis is often extreme, pleomorphic microglia being characteristically abundant. Inflammation of the meninges is prominent, and varying degrees of arteritis can be anticipated. Collections of subependymal astroglia account for the granularity noted grossly.

Focal *granulomatous accumulations* (gummas) are rare, but may occur in the meninges and extend into the parenchyma of the central nervous system. More diffuse granulomas of the dura (hypertrophic pachymeningitis) assume significance when they compress neural structures, especially the spinal cord.

CLINICAL SYNDROMES IN NEUROSYPHILIS

Asymptomatic Neurosyphilis

As the term suggests, the patient lacks symptoms or signs of neurologic disease, although pathologic involvement of the meninges and possibly of the nervous system parenchyma is implied. The diagnosis rests on the finding of cellular, chemical, or immunologic abnormalities of the CSF. This is the most common form of neurosyphilis and constituted about 30 per cent of cases in one large neurosyphilis clinic. With adequate treatment (see Treatment) the development of neurologic symptoms can be prevented in most cases.

Symptomatic Neurosyphilis

Meningitis

Symptoms and signs of an acute meningitis are encountered only rarely by physicians, an incidence of less than 2 per cent among syphilitic patients being reported from one general hospital series. It seems likely that some patients with mild or even moderate symptoms go unnoticed. Symptomatic syphilitic meningitis usually occurs during the early weeks or months of infection, often during the period of the secondary rash or concurrently with a mucocutaneous relapse in a patient previously but inadequately treated. The illness is usually of less than a month's duration, but symptoms may persist for longer periods. Headache, vomiting, malaise, and irritability are prominent symptoms. Kernig and Brudzinski signs develop. Occasionally, confusion, delirium, seizures, and cranial nerve palsies (seventh and eighth nerves most common) occur. Argyll Robertson pupils are not part of the constellation of findings in acute syphilitic meningitis. Acute syphilitic hydrocephalus with evidence of increased intracranial pressure, including papilledema, may lead to confusion with other inflammatory and neoplastic conditions. But the diagnosis should not be difficult if the physician considers the possibility of syphilis. The CSF will always contain an increased number of white blood cells (average about 500 per cubic millimeter — usually mononuclear, rarely polymorphonuclear), elevated total protein (average, about 100 mg per 100 ml), normal sugar concentrations (reduced rarely), and syphilitic reagins. An elevated gamma globulin concentration will be found in 70 per cent of cases. The serologic tests for syphilis are usually but not always positive.

The response to therapy is generally prompt and gratifying, although an occasional patient will subsequently develop some other form of neurosyphilis.

Meningovascular Syphilis

Although the incidence of this form of neurosyphilis is difficult to ascertain, a figure of 3 per cent of syphilitic patients has been recorded. As with the other forms of neurosyphilis, men are more often affected than women (3:1) Patients with meningovascular syphilis present most commonly from two to ten years after the primary lesion. Symptoms and signs of meningitis are lacking, although headache is a frequent complaint. The major neurologic abnormalities result from the arteritis and consequent arterial thromboses. The neurologic deficits may develop slowly as the circulation through small vessels becomes compromised, or there may be an abrupt loss of function consequent upon occlusion of a major vessel. The specific syndromes depend upon the distribution of infarction within the brain or spinal cord. The patient may develop hemiplegia, hemisensory defect, dysphasia, or homonymous hemianopia. Involvement of the cortex accounts for seizures in a small percentage of cases. Various spinal cord syndromes have been described. A transverse myelopathy can be expected to to produce varying degress of paraparesis, sensory loss, and impaired function of bladder and bowel. Infarction of the anterior two thirds of the cord, with resultant paraplegia and loss of pain sensation below the lesion, follows occlusion of the anterior spinal artery. Sensory functions subserved by the posterior columns are usually preserved. Asymmetric infarction of one half of the spinal cord will result in weakness and impairment of light touch and position sense on that side and diminished pain and temperature sensation on the opposite side below the anatomic lesion (Brown-Séquard's syndrome).

Some abnormality of the CSF is always found in meningovascular syphilis. A lymphocytic pleocytosis (few to 100 cells per cubic millimeter) and/or an elevated protein concentration is characteristic. The gamma globulin content is often elevated. Syphilitic reagins are nearly always present in the CSF as well as in the blood.

The progress of meningovascular syphilis can usually be halted by specific treatment, but the degree of functional recovery depends upon the extent and location of the infarcts and upon the many complex physiologic factors that condition recovery in cerebrovascular disease of any type.

General Paresis

(Dementia Paralytica, General Paralysis of the Insane)

This dread complication of syphilis makes its appearance from 2 to 30 (usually 10 to 25) years after the primary lesion. It occurs more often in men than in women (3:1), and 89 per cent of cases occur between the ages of 30 and 60 years. In one large series about 60 per cent of patients presented with simple dementia, and less than 20 per cent displayed manic symptoms and megalomania. Often faulty judgment, impaired memory (recent memory affected first), disturbed affect (depression or euphoria), or paranoia suggests the presence of a serious mental disturbance. This behavioral change will be especially noticeable when the afflicted individual has been a competitive member of society. Delusions and hallucinations occur less often but, when present, prompt a quick referral to the physician. The patient himself may complain of "nervousness," but characteristically lacks insight into the nature of his difficulty. Fine or coarse tremors, often affecting facial muscles and tongue, are present in about two thirds of the patients with fully developed general paresis. Abnormal pupillary responses, including Argyll Robertson pupil (see Tabes Dorsalis, below), impassive facies, slurred or dysarthric speech, exaggerated stretch reflexes, and extensor plantar responses are additional neurologic signs. Convulsions occur in 10 per cent of patients, and strokes secondary to vasculitis are also seen. When symptoms and signs of tabes dorsalis accompany those of paresis, the designation taboparesis is used.

The CSF is always abnormal, containing in excess of 5 white blood cells per cubic millimeter (mononuclear) in 85 per cent of untreated cases, and more than 30 cells per cubic millimeter in about a fourth of cases. An elevated total protein concentration (greater than 50 mg per 100 ml) of CSF can be anticipated in 75 per cent, and a level of 100 mg per 100 ml or higher in about 20 per cent of cases. An elevated gamma globulin level accounts for the first zone colloidal gold (Lange) curve, e.g., 5554433211, which is frequently found in general paresis. Nearly every patient will have a positive reagin test for syphilis in the CSF, and in more than 90 per cent of cases the blood serologic test will also be positive. Incomplete, prior treatment may modify but will not restore to normal the CSF.

General paresis, once established, evolves rapidly, and patients soon become disabled mentally, socially, and, in the late stage, physically. The term general paralysis of the insane derived from observations of patients helpless and bedridden in the terminal stages of the disease. Untreated general paresis is universally fatal, usually within three years.

If the disease is recognized early and treated vigorously, about 80 per cent of patients will return to some form of work, but only in about one half will complete recovery be achieved. There is little hope of a satisfactory result when treatment is delayed until the patient is demented, incontinent, and bedridden.

Tabes Dorsalis

(Locomotor Ataxia)

Tabes dorsalis develops in less than 5 per cent of patients with untreated syphilis, and symptoms usually become manifest 10 to 20 years after the primary infection. Rarely, there is a latent period of 30 or more years. Men are more often affected than women.

Dysfunction of affected posterior roots accrues slowly, and symptoms develop insidiously. Impaired joint position sense frequently results in stumbling and difficulty in walking, especially in the dark when visual compensation is imperfect. As the disease progresses, this sensory ataxia worsens, and a broad-based gait is assumed. Profound hypotonia, secondary to a lack of modulation of muscle tension by afferent fibers, is expressed frequently in a slapping gait. Paresthesias usually appear early in the disease but may be ignored by the patient until the appearance of lightning pains. These pains are characteristic of tabes dorsalis but are in no way specific, because they occur in other diseases affecting dorsal roots, e.g., diabetic neuropathy. Lightning pains develop in at least 75 per cent of patients and may appear in any area of the body, although they are most common in the lower extremities. Some patients insist that they are more troublesome when the barometric pressure is low. They may be described as sharp, burning, or aching. However, sharp jabs of pain are characteristic. These may be mild or excruciating, and frequently flit from one region to another. At times they are so transitory that by the time the patient has made the natural move to rub or massage the involved part, pain has disappeared. For a period of hours or days one spot will seem particularly vulnerable, but then the site of attack shifts to another place. Involvement of thoracoabdominal nerve roots gives rise to visceral pains (gastric or visceral crises), which may simulate intrinsic visceral disease and may lead to unnecessary surgery; in one series an estimated 25 per cent of tabetic patients had undergone operation for tabetic pain. The converse is also true: on rare occasions visceral pain has been ascribed to tabes dorsalis and suppurative appendicitis, or a ruptured peptic ulcer has gone undiagnosed. As the disease advances, pain sensation may be so dulled that recurrent trauma is unnoticed by the patient and indolent ulcers of the skin develop; the toes and balls of the feet are especially vulnerable. Weight-bearing joints and adjacent bone, deprived of pain sensation, are destroyed by the constant trauma of use in 5 to 10 per cent of tabetic patients (Charcot joints).

Unless general paresis coexists, as it does in a small percentage of cases *(taboparesis)*, tabetic patients are mentally normal. Optic atrophy complicates tabes dorsalis in about 10 per cent of cases or occurs as an isolated disorder. Pupillary abnormalities, including meiosis, irregularity, poor responsiveness to light and mydriatics, but retained reaction in accommodation (Argyll Robertson pupils), are present in most cases of tabes dorsalis. Involvement of other oculomotor functions is occasionally seen. Hypotonia, ataxia, and broad-based gait can usually be demonstrated. Affection of the sensory arc of the myotatic reflexes accounts for the greatly diminished or absent stretch reflexes. The Achilles reflex is affected more constantly. The plantar responses are normal in most cases of uncomplicated tabes dorsalis. Loss or diminution of position and vibratory sensation is found in every case. Increased swaying when the eyes are closed and the patient is standing with feet together (Romberg's sign) results from the impaired position sense. Variable degrees of hypesthesia and hypalgesia in a root distribution can be anticipated but may be difficult to plot. Isolated areas of hypalgesia (Hitzig zones) are sometimes found. Delayed perception of a pain stimulus (from one to several seconds) often can be demonstrated. Impaired deep pain sensation may account for a dramatic lack of responsiveness to squeezing of the Achilles tendon or testicles. Because of involvement of sacral nerve roots, functions of the urinary bladder and bowel are impaired in up to one third of cases; overflow incontinence and constipation develop. Impotence is a major complaint in the male. Characteristically a csytometrogram shows an absence of, or reduction in, the normal muscular contractions of the bladder in response to filling; the patient may be unaware of a volume in excess of 500 ml. Hydronephrosis and pyogenic infection are common complications of a hypotonic bladder.

Early in the course of tabes dorsalis, the serologic tests for syphilis are, as a rule, strongly positive. The CSF may reflect the meningeal inflammatory process with pleocytosis, an elevated total protein, and a positive reagin test. Late in the disease, especially after some antisyphilitic treatment, the serologic tests may be negative (in 25 to 50 per cent of cases), and even the CSF is negative in up to 20 per cent of cases.

The course of tabes dorsalis is unpredictable, and the response to antisyphilitic therapy is variable. In general, patients who have had symptoms for a few months or at the most a few years, with significant CSF abnormalities and no prior therapy, are most likely to improve with treatment. Patients with far-advanced disease and severe degeneration of dorsal roots and who suffer from the painful complications will not benefit significantly from antisyphilitic therapy. At least partial relief of pain may be achieved by analgesics, but when narcotics are used the risk of addiction is significant.

Recently, some benefit has been reported with diphenylhydantoin (Dilantin) treatment (200 mg per square meter per day). Recourse to spinal cordotomy and other surgical measures to relieve pain should be deferred until all medical measures have failed. Urologic assistance may be required to deal effectively with the tabetic uropathies, and surgery may be required for management of penetrating ulcers of the skin and Charcot joints.

Optic Atrophy

Visual impairment in syphilis may result from iritis, choreoretinitis, increased intracranial pressure (consecutive optic atrophy), or primary optic atrophy. Optic atrophy occurs in 1 per cent of patients with untreated syphilis and is five times more common in males than in females. It is stated that blacks are more prone than whites to optic atrophy, whereas the reverse is reported in other forms of neurosyphilis.

Because the outer portions of the optic nerve are first affected, the visual impairment tends to be peripheral in the early stages. Ultimately, however, the papillomacular bundle lying in the center of the nerve becomes involved, and impaired visual acuity and central and paracentral scotomas develop. It has been estimated that, without treatment, 50 per cent of patients will be blind in two years and 90 per cent in ten years. One eye is typically affected before the other. Optic pallor is usually present by the time symptoms appear, but in the early stages it is recognizable only by the reduced vascularity. A chalk-white disc with sharp margins and prominent lamina cribrosa constitute the fully developed appearance of optic atrophy. The optic atrophy of syphilis is indistinguishable from that caused by other diseases of the optic nerve in which there has been no antecedent papillitis or papilledema. The CSF is abnormal in most patients with active disease of the optic nerve. Intensive antisyphilitic therapy may arrest the disease process and preserve what vision remains, but return of vision already lost should not be anticipated.

Gumma

This rare complication of syphilis usually declares itself as an intracranial or intraspinal mass lesion and behaves in every way as a slowly growing neoplasm. The correct diagnosis may be suspected from a positive serologic test for syphilis or from CSF abnormalities. Frequently, however, the diagnosis is not made until the patient is operated upon, and histopathologic studies are made. Removal of the tumor mass, supplemented by antimicrobial therapy (see Treatment), should alleviate symptoms and prevent spread of the disease.

Congenital Neurosyphilis

Syphilis acquired by the fetus from an infected mother after the first trimester of pregnancy tends to be a fulminant disease. Miscarriages and stillbirths are common, and a wide spectrum of clinical manifestations may be recognized in the infant or child who survives. *Neurosyphilis* develops in an estimated 10 to 20 per cent of infants and children with congenital syphilis. *Asymptomatic neurosyphilis* may be diagnosed in the early months or years of life by doing routine CSF examinations on children of syphilitic mothers. But, as with acquired neurosyphilis, symptoms and signs develop only after a latent period that, in the case of *juvenile paresis*, may be as long as 20 years. More often symptoms first appear late in the first decade or during adolescence. Clinical syndromes and CSF findings mirror those found with the acquired disease except that *tabes dorsalis* is exceedingly rare and *choreoretinitis* more common. Hydrocephalus, cranial nerve palsies (eighth cranial nerve especially), and seizures may complicate congenital syphilitic meningitis, and syphilis should be remembered as a cause of cerebrovascular accidents in children. Previous studies emphasize that more than a third of all children presenting with juvenile paresis have been retarded mentally since early life. Although mental retardation is very likely due to other factors in some cases, such statistics emphasize the vulnerability of the developing nervous system to syphilitic infection.

Other non-neurologic stigmata of congenital syphilis include dental deformities (Hutchinson's teeth), saddle nose, frontal bossing of the skull, saber shins, and interstitial keratitis (usually developing during the second decade). These signs are not seen in acquired syphilis. Fortunately, the current practice of doing routine serologic tests on all pregnant women and on infants of syphilitic mothers has all but eliminated congenital neurosyphilis in many areas of the world. In this regard it should be remembered that the mother can acquire syphilis at any time during pregnancy and that negative serologic studies obtained early do not exclude the possibility that they might become positive later in the course of pregnancy. In some institutions blood from the umbilical cord is routinely tested for the reagin of syphilis.

Early and intensive treatment of infants with congenital syphilis materially reduces the morbidity (see Treatment) from neurologic complications. Unhappily, results from even optimal treatment of patients with juvenile paresis remain poor.

TREATMENT

Penicillin is the preferred drug for treating neurosyphilis. Reasonable therapy for adults with all forms of neurosyphilis, except general paresis, is a total dose of procaine penicillin G of 6 to 12 million units given over two to three weeks. A total dose if 18 to 24 million units administered over the same period of time is used to treat patients with general paresis. For children, approximately one half of the adult dose is employed, and one quarter of the adult dose is given to infants. We prefer to treat patients with active neurosyphilis in hospital (mandatory in general paresis), but this is not always feasible. When outpatient treatment is necessary, an initial dose of 3 million units of long-acting penicillin (benzathine penicillin G, Bicillin) should be given. The sole use of benzathine penicillin G at weekly intervals in doses equivalent to those presented above has been advocated by some in the treatment of neurosyphilis. It must be stressed that these therapeutic regimens are empirical. Nevertheless, they are reasonable and have stood the test of time. The author suspects that early diagnosis of syphilitic infection is far more critical than the precise dosage and the time course of therapy.

For a further discussion of treatment, the reader is referred to Ch. 171.

Clarke, E. G., and Danbolt, N.: The Oslo study of the natural history of untreated syphilis. J. Chronic Dis., 2:311, 1955.
Green, J. B.: Dilantin in the treatment of lightning pains. Neurology. 11:257, 1961.
Hahn, R. D., et al.: Penicillin treatment of general paresis (dementia paralytica) — Results of treatment in 1086 patients, the majority of whom were followed for more than 5 years. Arch. Neurol. Psychiat., 81:557, 1959.
Hooshmand, H., Escobar, M. R., and Kopf, S. W.: Neurosyphilis. A study of 241 patients. JAMA, 219:726, 1972.
Idsøe, O., Guthe, T., and Willcox, R. R.: Penicillin in the treatment of syphilis. Geneva, Bull. WHO, Supplement to Vol. 47, 1972.
Merritt, H. H., Adams, R. D., and Solomon, H.: Neurosyphilis. New York, Oxford University Press, 1946.
Montgomery, C. H., and Knox, J. M.: Antibiotics other than penicillin in the treatment of syphilis. N. Engl. J. Med., 261:277, 1961.

Section Sixteen   VIRAL INFECTIONS OF THE NERVOUS SYSTEM

302.   INTRODUCTION

Richard T. Johnson

Viral infections of the nervous system, in general, represent uncommon but important complications of systemic infections. With a few exceptions such as rabies or B virus (*herpes simiae*), nervous system infections are caused by agents which often infect man. Some of these viruses, such as polioviruses and arthropod-borne encephalitis viruses, cause clinically significant disease only on the rare occasion when the nervous system is involved. Others, such as herpes simplex and mumps virus, are frequent causes of mild disease that assumes a more serious form when the central nervous system is infected.

Experimentally, viruses have been shown to invade the nervous system by centripetal growth or movement in peripheral nerves, by penetration across the olfactory mucosa, or by a viremia. In man most viruses which infect the nervous system spread to the brain and meninges from blood, although neural spread appears to be important in rabies, B virus, and varicella-zoster virus infections. The infrequency of nervous system involvement can be attributed to a variety of host defense mechanisms, including cellular and humoral responses, interferon production, anatomic barriers of nonsusceptible cells, and the activity of the reticuloendothelial system which clears viruses from the blood. Youth, severe nutritional deficiency, and defects of cellular immunity have been shown to increase the risk of nervous system infection with some viruses, but in the majority of patients the factors which have permitted central nervous system invasion are not evident.

Viral infections of the nervous system can lead to diverse clinical signs and symptoms, varied clinical courses, and protean pathologic changes. This diversity can be explained by the following two principles: (1) the varied cell populations of the nervous system have different susceptibilities to different viruses; and (2) viral infections can have varied effects on susceptible cells. If infection is limited to the meninges covering the nervous system, then signs of headache, fever, stiff neck, and pleocytosis (i.e., meningitis) may be the only clinical manifestations. If the infection spreads to the parenchymal cells of the brain, in addition to signs of meningeal irritation, there may develop a depression of the state of consciousness, seizures, focal neurologic deficits, or increased intracranial pressure (i.e., encephalitis). Some viruses cause even more selective involvement of specific cell populations in the brain and spinal cord and thus evoke characteristic clinical symptoms and signs. For example, in poliovirus infections the selective vulnerability of anterior horn cells leads to a characteristic clinical finding of acute meningitis with lower motor neuron paralysis. On the other hand, rabies virus infections in animals tend to spare the cortical neurons involved in most types of encephalitis and infect neurons of the limbic system. Therefore, instead of obtundation, seizures, and motor or sensory deficits, the infected animal shows alertness, loss of timidity, aberrant sexual behavior, and aggressive activity. This selective infection of cells of the limbic system appears to be a diabolic adaptation of the rabies virus to specific cell populations, so that the clinical disease in animals can drive the host to transmit the virus to another host by biting. Glial cell populations may also be selectively involved, such as in progressive multifocal leukoencephalopathy in which virus infection and cell lysis appear limited to the oligodendrocytes, causing a slowly progressive demyelinating disease.

The virus-cell interaction may be quite varied. There may be *acute lysis* of the infected cell, transformation of the cell with production of neoplasm, or *chronic infection* causing cellular dysfunction, cellular degeneration, or no abnormality. In acute viral infections the clinical and pathologic abnormalities may result either from an acute viral destruction of cells, as in acute viral meningitis or encephalitis, or from the host's immunologic response to the infection, as has been postulated in postinfectious encephalomyelitis. A *latent infection* is a virus-host relationship in which the virus remains present in some form in the host without giving rise to any signs of infection, but which can, when some trigger mechanism comes into play, emerge as an acute infectious process. This appears to occur in herpes zoster and possibly in some cases of herpes simplex encephalitis. *Chronic viral infections* are those in which there is an ongoing active infection, which may give rise to a somewhat irregular or unpredictable course extending over many months or years. Chronic inflammatory disease of the central nervous system is seen with fetal infections by rubella and cytomegaloviruses. In these indolent infections virus can be recovered for long periods of time postnatally and may or may not cause continuing or evolving clinical signs of disease. *Slow infections* have a more predictable course than chronic infections. They are defined as infections with an incubation period lasting for months to years, followed by a protracted but predictable clinical course ending in death. Slow viral infections of the nervous system in man include kuru, Creutzfeldt-Jakob disease, subacute sclerosing panencephalitis, and progressive multifocal leukoencephalopathy (see Ch. 310).

303. VIRAL MENINGITIS AND ENCEPHALITIS

Richard T. Johnson

Viral meningitis is a benign, self-limited illness with clinical signs of headache, fever, and meningeal inflammation. *Viral encephalitis* is a more severe illness in which fever, headache, and meningeal inflammation are complicated by depression of the state of consciousness, seizures, and/or focal neurologic deficits suggesting inflammation within the parenchyma of the brain.

The clinical syndrome of viral meningitis is also called *aseptic meningitis* or *serous meningitis*, since some bacterial infections and chemical irritants can cause identical clinical symptoms and cerebrospinal fluid changes. Encephalitis is also called *meningoencephalitis* or *encephalomyelitis*, the latter indicating concurrent signs of spinal cord involvement.

ETIOLOGY. A variety of viruses have been associated with meningitis and encephalitis (Table 1). The two syndromes represent a clinical continuum and are caused by the same spectrum of viral agents. However, some viruses tend to cause predominantly benign disease such as the coxsackie- and echoviruses, which cause about half of all cases of viral meningitis but are only rarely associated with encephalitis. Other viruses tend to cause more severe disease such as arthropod-

TABLE 1. Viruses Associated with Acute Central Nervous System Infections in the United States

Enteroviruses
  Polioviruses
  Coxsackieviruses, groups A and B
  Echoviruses
Togaviruses (arboviruses)
  Eastern equine
  Western equine
  Venezuelan equine
  St. Louis
  Powassan
  California
Herpesviruses
  Herpes simplex, type 1 and type 2
  Varicella-zoster
  Epstein-Barr
  Cytomegalovirus
Myxoviruses and paramyxoviruses
  Influenza
  Parainfluenza
  Mumps
  Measles (rubeola)
Adenoviruses
Lymphocytic choriomeningitis virus
Rabies virus

*Data from Neutropic Viral Diseases Surveillance Reports, Center for Disease Control.

TABLE 2. Frequency of Association of Agents with Aseptic Meningitis and Encephalitis*

Etiologic Agent	Percentage of Cases of:	
	Aseptic Meningitis	Encephalitis†
Enteroviruses	30	8
Mumps	16	16
Lympocytic choriomeningitis	9	14
Leptospira	4	2
Herpes simplex	1	10
Arboviruses	1	14
Other‡	2	2

*Data from Meyer et al., 1960.

†Fatal cases in this study (eight of 139) associated only with herpes simplex and arbovirus infections.

‡Includes infectious mononucleosis, *Mycoplasma pneumoniae*, Rocky Mountain spotted fever, and fungal infections.

borne togaviruses (arboviruses) and herpes simplex virus, which are the major causes of fatal encephalitis (Table 2).

Enteroviruses are small, nonenveloped RNA viruses of the picornavirus family, and include polioviruses, group A and B coxsackieviruses, and echoviruses. The three serotypes of poliovirus are now largely controlled by immunization programs (see Ch. 307). Over 40 coxsackie- and echovirus serotypes have been associated with meningitis and encephalitis; the serotypes most frequently recovered from patients with viral meningitis are echoviruses 3, 4, 6, 9, 11, 18, and 30, coxsackievirus A9, and coxsackieviruses B1 through 5. Echovirus 9 has been associated with the largest epidemics.

Mumps virus is a large, enveloped RNA virus of the paramyxovirus group. Mumps is the single most common cause of viral meningitis and mild encephalitis. Lymphocytic choriomeningitis virus is a small, enveloped RNA virus of the arenavirus group, which also causes both meningitis and mild encephalitis.

Herpesvirus are large, structurally complex, enveloped DNA viruses which cause a variety of neurologic diseases. Type 1 herpes simplex virus is associated with severe encephalitis in adults and represents the most common cause of endemic fatal encephalitis. Type 2 herpes simplex virus, a major cause of fatal neonatal encephalitis, seldom causes severe encephalitis in adults but has been associated with cases of meningitis. Headache and pleocytosis often accompany herpes zoster infections, but it is not known whether meningitis without radicular pain or cutaneous eruptions can be a manifestation of recrudescences of latent varicella-zoster virus infections (see Ch. 305). The Epstein-Barr virus has been related to meningitis and encephalitis, complicating approximately 1 per cent of cases of infectious mononucleosis. Cytomegalovirus, like rubella virus, is associated primarily with chronic congenital infections. However, cytomegalovirus also causes encephalitis in immunocompromised adults, but such infections are usually asymptomatic and found incidentally at autopsy.

The acute neurologic disease associated with measles, vaccinia, and primary varicella (chickenpox) infections, in most cases, represents postinfectious encephalomyelitis (see Ch. 309.2). This may also be true of the encephalitis which has occasionally been reported with influenza and parainfluenza virus infections.

The arboviruses are small, enveloped RNA viruses of the togavirus family. Over 20 different arboviruses have been associated with encephalitis in varied geographic areas of the world; six cause encephalitis in the United States (Table 1). Over 100 cases of California virus encephalitis are reported annually over a wide geographic area. Eastern, Western, St. Louis, and Venezuelan equine encephalitis viruses cause localized epidemics; St. Louis virus has been the predominant cause of major epidemics in recent years.

Adenoviruses are respiratory viruses which only rarely cause meningitis or severe childhood encephalitis. Nonviral agents which cause clinical syndromes indistinguishable from viral meningitis or mild encephalitis include *Leptospira, Treponema pallidum, Mycoplasma pneumoniae,* and *Rickettsia.*

EPIDEMIOLOGY. Over 5000 cases of aseptic meningitis and over 2000 cases of encephalitis are reported to the Center for Disease Control annually, but this represents only a small fraction of the total number of cases per year in the United States. Both viral meningitis and encephalitis are reported with greater frequency during the later summer and early fall, and this increase results, in large part, from the seasonal dissemination of enteroviruses and arboviruses.

Epidemiologically the viruses causing meningitis and encephalitis in man fall into three categories: (1) Viruses that spread from man to man; these agents generally cause disease during a particular season of the year and often in epidemics. (2) Viruses acquired from infected animals (zoonoses); these agents may have distinct geographic distributions, and a history of animal contact in patients is often obtained. (3) Viruses spread by hematophagous arthropods and necessitating a cycle in the arthropod host; these viruses have very specific seasonal and geographic limitations.

The enteroviruses are spread from man to man by hand-to-mouth contact and to a lesser extent by respiratory spread or by fecal contamination of fomites or vectors. Virus growth is primarily in the intestinal tract. Although enteroviral infections occur throughout the year, the incidence of these infections increases dramatically in summer and early fall, often reaching epidemic proportions. Because of the mode of spread, family outbreaks are common, and the spread of virus is facilitated in families or communities with preschool children.

Mumps virus is spread by the respiratory route. Mumps occurs throughout the year, but there is a marked increase in incidence during the spring. Although the incidence of infection with mumps virus is equal between the sexes, males develop meningitis three times more frequently than females.

Lymphocytic choriomeningitis virus is the major zoonotic virus causing meningitis and encephalitis. The natural host of this virus is *Mus musculus,* the common house mouse, and the virus is present in its excreta. Man acquires the infection by contact with contaminated dust or food. Human disease is more common in winter, when the natural host tends to move indoors, increasing human exposure. Recently, lymphocytic choriomeningitis virus has also been found in hamsters, and human infections have been traced to laboratory and pet hamsters. Leptospiral infections are also acquired from both domestic and wild animals. These spirochetes are excreted in urine and contracted by man through contact with animal tissue, contaminated soil, or water polluted by animal urine.

Each of the arboviruses has a different epidemiologic cycle (see Ch. 101). In the United States, Eastern, Western, St. Louis, California, and Venezuelan equine encephalitis viruses are transmitted by mosquitoes. Powassan virus is transmitted by ticks. The seasonal occurrence of these infections is limited exclusively to seasons when the vectors are feeding. Eastern encephalitis virus is limited to the Atlantic and Gulf coasts and normally circulates between birds and salt marsh mosquitoes, which do not bite man. When ecologic changes alter the bird-mosquito balance, the virus can overflow into other arthropod vectors which feed on mammals. Regional deaths of horses or pheasants usually herald the rare human outbreaks. Western encephalitis virus is limited to the western two thirds of the country and normally circulates between mosquitoes and birds; horses and man become inadvertent hosts when bitten by infected mosquitoes. This virus causes many more human infections than does Eastern encephalitis virus, but only 1 in 100 of those infected develop encephalitis. St. Louis encephalitis virus causes both rural and urban disease over a large area of the United States. In the rural areas the virus has the same pattern as Western encephalitis virus, but in urban areas more explosive outbreaks can occur when the virus is introduced into urban breeding mosquitoes and urban birds and humans become the intermediate hosts. California virus has a different cycle involving woodland mosquitoes and small animals; birds are not involved. In recent years the virus has been related to encephalitis every year over a wide geographic area of the United States. Disease is confined almost entirely to children. Venezuelan equine encephalitis is transmitted from mosquitoes to animals, and the virus has recently spread into Florida and the southwestern states. Most people infected with the virus have an influenza-like illness, but about 3 per cent develop acute meningitis or encephalitis. Powassan virus has been found in ticks in Canada and along the northern border of the United States; it is a rare cause of encephalitis in man.

PATHOGENESIS AND PATHOLOGY. Viruses usually replicate in cells at the site of entry. For example, after oral ingestion enteroviruses grow in the gastrointestinal tract; after respiratory spread viruses grow in the respiratory tract; or after subcutaneous or intravenous inoculation arboviruses grow in local subcutaneous, vascular endothelial, or muscle cells. Following local replication, dissemination of virus usually occurs via the blood. Despite the longstanding belief that the blood-brain barrier was impervious to viruses, it is now evident that the majority of viruses invade the central nervous system from the blood. The cerebral capillary endothelium is nonfenestrated, has tight junctions, and is surrounded by a dense basement membrane with astrocytic processes apposed to the outer surface. These structures do constitute a relative barrier to virus invasion, but experimentally viruses are found to invade the nervous system both by infection of the vascular endothelial cells with subsequent infection of surrounding glia and neurons and by passage of virus through endothelial cells. Experimentally viruses have also been found to grow in the choroid plexus and to seed virus into the cerebrospinal fluid.

Since viral meningitis by definition is a benign disease, its histopathologic correlates are unknown. In fatal encephalitis an inflammatory reaction is usually prominent in the meninges and in a perivascular distribution within the brain. Although the perivascular inflammatory reaction is composed predominantly of mononuclear cells, polymorphonuclear cells may be evident. Neural cells may show degenerative changes, and apparent phagocytosis of neurons by macrophages or microglial cells (neuronophagia) is often found.

Pathologic changes in encephalitis cannot unequivocally distinguish the agent involved. Topographic localization of lesions is of little value except in distinguishing poliomyelitis, rabies, and herpes simplex virus infections. Intranuclear inclusions are seen in herpesvirus infections and in measles virus infections, and in the latter cytoplasmic inclusions may also be found. Cytomegalovirus infections produce a characteristic pathology with the induction of cytomegalic cells containing inclusion bodies. Although fatal cases of mumps virus encephalitis are rare, pathologic studies have shown both the acute inflammatory lesions usually seen in virus encephalitis and perivenular demyelination characteristic of postinfectious encephalomyelitis.

CLINICAL MANIFESTATIONS. Viral Meningitis. The major clinical manifestations of viral meningitis are headache, fever, and nuchal rigidity. Signs and symptoms are often abrupt in onset and may persist from three days to two weeks. Other symptoms may include general malaise, sore throat, nausea and vomiting, drowsiness, abdominal pain, and chills and fever. The headache is often frontal or retro-orbital and may be associated with photophobia. Fever is seldom elevated above 40° C. Nuchal rigidity may not be as severe as that seen in bacterial meningitis and may be detectable only with extreme flexion. Kernig and Brudzinski signs may or may not be positive.

Viral meningitis caused by several of the enteroviruses is often associated with rashes. The eruption usually appears at the same time as the fever and persists for four to ten days. In coxsackievirus A9 and 16 and echovirus 4, 6, 9, 16, and 30 infections the rash is typically maculopapular and nonpruritic, and may be confined to the face and trunk or may involve extremities, including the palms and soles. In echovirus 9 infections the rash may be petechial, causing confusion with meningococcal infections. In group A coxsackievirus infections herpangina may develop, characterized by grayish vesicular lesions on the tonsillar fossae, soft palate, and uvula. In coxsackievirus A5 and 16 infections a vesicular rash may involve hands, feet, and oropharynx (hand, foot, and mouth disease; see Ch. 95).

Mumps virus meningitis and encephalitis are associated with parotitis in approximately half the cases. However, the parotitis may precede or follow the meningitis by as much as a week. Oophoritis and pancreatitis may also be seen. Evidence of parotitis associated with meningitis is not diagnostic of mumps virus infection, because parotitis has also been reported with group B coxsackievirus and lymphocytic choriomeningitis virus infections.

Aseptic meningitis caused by the type 2 herpes simplex virus may coincide with the eruption of genital lesions. In some cases this meningitis has been associated with radicular pain simulating lumbar or sacral root compression.

Viral Encephalitis. In addition to headache, fever, and nuchal rigidity, alterations of consciousness characterize encephalitis; mild lethargy may progress to confusion, stupor, and coma. Focal neurologic signs usually develop, and seizures are common. Motor weakness, accentuated deep tendon reflexes, and extensor plantar responses may be observed. Abnormal movements are seen in some cases of encephalitis, and rarely a tremor characteristic of Parkinson's disease may develop. The hypothalamic-pituitary area may be involved, causing severe hyperthermia or poikilothermia, diabetes insipidus, and inappropriate antidiuretic hormone secretion. Involvement of the spinal cord can lead to flaccid paralysis, depression of tendon reflexes, and paralysis of bowel and bladder. Increased intracranial pressure can cause third and sixth cranial nerve palsies.

In herpes simplex virus encephalitis, signs often include bizarre behavior, hallucinations, and aphasia, suggesting the temporal lobe localization typical of that infection (see Ch. 304).

LABORATORY FINDINGS. Blood count may be normal, show moderate leukopenia, or show a moderate leukocytosis. Epstein-Barr virus infections are suggested by large numbers of atypical mononuclear cells, as well as by positive heterophil reactions. Serum amylase may be elevated with mumps virus infections. Lymphocyte choriomeningitis virus infections are frequently associated with pulmonary infiltrates.

Cerebrospinal fluid examination is essential to establish the diagnosis of aseptic meningitis and encephalitis, even though it is of little help in determining the specific virus involved. The cerebrospinal fluid may be under normal or moderately elevated pressure. The fluid is usually clear but may show xanthochromia if the protein content is over 100 mg per 100 milliliters. Cell counts are variable, but 10 to 1000 cells are usual with a predominance of mononuclear cells. If the fluid is examined early in the course of disease, there may be no cells or a preponderance of polymorphonuclear cells. Repeat examination in 24 hours will usually show the characteristic presence of mononuclear cells. Significant numbers of red cells are often present in herpes simplex virus encephalitis, but this finding is not a dependable point of differential diagnosis. The protein content is usually elevated. The glucose content in the cerebrospinal fluid is generally normal, although mild depressions are seen, particularly with mumps and lymphocytic choriomeningitis virus infections.

The electroencephalogram usually shows diffuse slowing, but shifting foci, marked asymmetry, and seizure activity may be evident in encephalitis. Diffuse slowing is not a grave sign in viral meningitis, because this abnormality can persist briefly even after the patient is asymptomatic.

Cerebral angiography, radioisotopic scans, and computerized axial tomography of the brain may show localization of lesions of the temporal lobes in herpes simplex virus encephalitis, but these studies are usually of no value in differentiating other forms of encephalitis.

DIAGNOSIS AND DIFFERENTIAL DIAGNOSIS. The most important aspect of differential diagnosis is to exclude those treatable diseases which may masquerade as viral infections. These include tuberculous and fungal meningitis, parameningeal infections, brain abscess, partially treated bacterial meningitis, subacute bacterial endocarditis, amebic encephalitis, and other illnesses which may present headache, fever, and nuchal rigidity. The differential diagnosis of encephalitis is important, as specific therapy is now recommended for herpes simplex virus encephalitis (see Ch. 304).

A definitive etiologic diagnosis can be determined only by appropriate virologic laboratory studies. However, an educated clinical guess regarding the cause can be based on public health information concerning agents currently being disseminated in the area; on knowledge of the agents endemic to the area and the season of the year; and on the patient's history, including past immunizations and illnesses, possible insect bites, place of residence, travel in areas where particular infections are prevalent, health of the family, and type of dwelling place.

The coxsackievirus and echovirus infections occur sporadically throughout the year but reach epidemic proportions in the late summer and fall. Furthermore, they cause family outbreaks and protean manifestations. Thus the patient with aseptic meningitis occurring in late summer or fall who gives a history of other family members with nonspecific illness, rash, pleurodynia, or other enterovirus-associated disease probably has meningitis due to a coxsackie- or echovirus. Transient lower motor paralysis reminiscent of poliomyelitis is also occasionally seen with these infections.

Mumps virus infections tend to occur in the spring, and a history of exposure is commonly obtained. Since there is no evidence that reinfection with mumps virus can occur, a clear-cut past history of parotitis during a mumps virus epidemic is good evidence against the patient's having mumps meningitis.

Patients with lymphocytic choriomeningitis virus infections often provide a history of living in mouse-infected houses or working in barns or other places frequented by mice. Alternatively, a history of exposure to or recent acquisition of a pet hamster should be sought. Lymphocytic choriomeningitis virus often causes a biphasic illness, with rather severe respiratory symptoms or pneumonitis preceding the abrupt onset of meningitis or encephalitis.

The mosquito-borne virus infections characteristically occur only in late summer and early fall before the frost. They vary in prevalence from year to year, depending on rainfall or other factors influencing mosquito, bird, and wildlife populations. Public health data regarding the dissemination of Eastern, Western, and St. Louis viruses in the population may be helpful in suggesting the diagnosis. California encephalitis virus shows little variation in frequency from year to year. Since this infection is usually acquired by children after exposure to woodland mosquitoes, a history of preceding recreational woodland exposure may be obtained.

Herpesvirus infections show no seasonal distribution. In type 1 herpes simplex virus infection, a past history of cold sores, exposure to herpes labialis, or presence of labial lesions at the time of encephalitis is of little help in ruling out or suggesting the diagnosis. The diagnosis is suggested by the severity of the encephalitis and signs of localization to the temporal lobes. In contrast, onset of type 2 herpes simplex virus meningitis may coincide with the appearance of genital lesions.

Obtaining a specific etiologic diagnosis in the laboratory necessitates obtaining acute and convalescent phase serum specimens. It is also useful to obtain specimens for isolation of virus (cerebrospinal fluid, stool, blood, and throat washings). Convalescent serum alone is of little value, as antibodies to most of the agents causing meningitis or encephalitis are widespread. Disease can be associated with a specific agent serologically only if a four-fold or greater increase in antibody is demonstrated between the early phase of disease and convalescence. Therefore blood should be drawn in the first few days of disease, and a subsequent serum specimen should be obtained two to six weeks later. The optimal specimens for viral isolation are dependent on the virus being sought. Arboviruses and enteroviruses can be isolated from the blood but are seldom recoverable at the time of clinical meningitis or encephalitis. During the acute disease coxsackie- and echoviruses are most readily isolated from stool or cerebrospinal fluid and, in some cases, throat washings. Lymphocytic choriomeningitis virus is most readily isolated from blood or cerebrospinal fluid. Mumps virus may be isolated from saliva, throat washings, or cerebrospinal fluid. Type 2 herpes simplex virus may also be isolated from the cerebrospinal fluid or blood. Unfortunately, type 1 herpes simplex virus can seldom be isolated from blood or cerebrospinal fluid, and serologic studies can be misleading. A definitive diagnosis of type 1 herpes simplex virus encephalitis at present still requires a brain biopsy.

TREATMENT. With the exception of adenine arabinoside, now recommended in treatment of herpes simplex encephalitis, specific antiviral therapy is not available for viral meningitis or other forms of encephalitis. Treatment consists of supportive therapy and the management of the complications of encephalitis, including coma, seizures, and increased intracranial pressure.

In both viral meningitis and encephalitis bed rest is indicated. Strict isolation procedures are not essential, as most of the viruses causing meningitis and encephalitis are common in our environment. If an enteroviral infection is suspected, precautions in handling of stools and handwashing should be instituted. If measles, chickenpox, rubella, or mumps virus infections are evident, the usual isolation from susceptibles is recommended.

The headache and fever of aseptic meningitis can usually be managed with judicious doses of aspirin. Severe hyperthermia may develop in encephalitis, necessitating use of more vigorous therapy, but it should be remembered that viruses are thermolabile. Therefore modest temperature elevations may serve as a natural defense mechanism, and attempts to reduce mild temperature elevations to normal or subnormal levels may be ill advised.

Patients with severe encephalitis are often in coma. Since these patients may make remarkable recoveries even after prolonged periods of coma, vigorous supportive therapy and avoidance of complications are essential. The airway must often be maintained by intubation or tracheostomy, and mechanical respiration may be necessary. Although intravenous fluids may suffice for brief periods, prolonged coma necessitates feeding with a nasogastric tube. Blood glucose and electrolytes should be checked frequently, because water, glucose, and salt control are not infrequently compromised during encephalitis. The respiratory tract, urinary tract, intravenous site, and skin are common sites of infection in comatose patients, and infections should be sought assiduously, treated vigorously, and avoided by skillful nursing, maintenance of bronchial drainage, frequent turning to avoid decubitus ulcers, and meticulous catheter care.

Although seizures frequently complicate encephalitis, prophylactic anticonvulsants are not usually recommended. If seizures develop, they can usually be managed with diphenylhydantoin and phenobarbital. If status epilepticus develops, more vigorous therapy should be instituted, remembering to treat the hypoxia and hyperthermia which complicate and aggravate status epilepticus.

Modest increases in intracranial pressure can be treated with glycerol given orally or by rectal tube. This osmotic agent is probably preferable to the use of urea or mannitol, because it can be given over a longer period of time. Steroids should generally be avoided in the treatment of encephalitis because of their inhibitory effects on host-immune responses and the potential of enhancement of viral invasion. However, when increased intracranial pressure is severe, the use of dexamethasone is probably indicated.

PROGNOSIS. Viral meningitis is a benign disease, and full recovery usually occurs within 5 to 14 days of onset, although some patients describe persistent fatigue, lightheadedness, and general asthenia which may persist for months.

The prognosis of encephalitis is dependent on the etiologic agent. The mortality rate of herpes simplex virus encephalitis is estimated at 50 per cent, with a high rate of sequelae in survivors. Encephalitis associated with arbovirus infections has variable mortality rates; the mortality rate with Eastern encephalitis is approximately 50 per cent; with St. Louis, 10 per cent; with Western, 10 per cent; with Venezuelan equine, 1 per cent; and with California, less than 0.5 per cent. The mortality rates for Western encephalitis are greater in children under one year of age, and for St. Louis encephalitis they are greater in the elderly. Nonfatal encephalitis caused by Eastern, Western, and St. Louis viruses leaves a relatively high rate of neurologic sequelae.

Encephalitis associated with mumps or lymphocytic choriomeningitis viruses is very rarely associated with death, and sequelae are infrequent. Recently, however, hydrocephalus has been reported as a late sequela of mumps meningitis and encephalitis in children.

Balfour, H. H., Siem, R. A., Bauer, H., and Quie, P. G.: California arbovirus (La Crosse) infections. I. Clinical and laboratory findings in 66 children with meningo-encephalitis. Pediatrics, 52:580, 1973.

Biggar, R. J., Woodall, J. P., Walter, P. D., and Haughie, G. E.: Lymphocytic choriomeningitis outbreak associated with pet hamsters. JAMA, 232:494, 1975.

Johnson, R. T., and Mims, C. A.: Pathogenesis of viral infection of the nervous system. N. Engl. J. Med., 278:23, 84, 1968.

Johnstone, J. A., Ross, C. A. C., and Dunn, M.: Meningitis and encephalitis associated with mumps infection. A 10-year survey. Arch. Dis. Child., 47:647, 1972.

McLean, D. M.: Arboviruses. *In* Rhodes, A. J., and Van Rooyen, C. E. (eds.): Textbook of Virology. 5th ed. Baltimore, Williams & Wilkins Company, 1968, p. 633.

Meyer, H. M., Jr., Johnson, R. T., Crawford, I. P., Dascomb, H. E., and Rogers, N. G.: Central nervous system syndromes of "viral" etiology. A study of 713 cases. Am. J. Med., 29:334, 1960.

304. HERPES SIMPLEX ENCEPHALITIS

J. Richard Baringer

DEFINITION. Adult encephalitis caused by herpes simplex virus is usually encountered as a sporadic illness, the consequence of infection by the antigenically distinct type 1 herpes simplex virus. Recently it has become apparent that most if not all of the cases previously designated as acute necrotizing encephalitis are related to infection by this virus. Electron microscopic examination of tissues from a number of these cases has revealed characteristic herpes simplex virus particles.

In newborn infants, herpes simplex virus encephalitis is seen as a result of maternal genital herpes infection. Usually the infection is due to type 2 herpes simplex virus, but some cases are related to infection by type 1 virus. The type 1 adult infection remains confined to the central nervous system, whereas in newborns the process is commonly disseminated in a variety of other organs, and the virus may be recovered from blood and cerebrospinal fluid. Type 2 virus may also occasionally produce a meningitis or polyradiculitis in adults, frequently in association with genital infection by the same strain.

Rarely the related B virus of monkeys has been incriminated as a cause of encephalitis in humans, usually as a result of accidental transmission of the virus to laboratory workers or attendants. This condition in humans is notable for its high mortality.

INCIDENCE.   Because of the difficulty in establishing the diagnosis of herpes simplex encephalitis by currently available means, the precise incidence of the condition is unknown. It has been estimated that 4000 cases may occur in the United States each year. Herpes simplex virus probably causes fewer cases than either mumps or the arthropod-borne viruses. However, the considerable mortality and morbidity resulting from herpes simplex virus infection rank it as the most common cause of sporadic viral encephalitis with severe sequelae. In view of the tendency for some infections to undergo spontaneous resolution and the difficulty in establishing the virologic diagnosis, it is possible that herpes simplex virus may be a more frequent cause of mild encephalitic illness than is currently recognized.

ETIOLOGY.   Herpes simplex virus is a large, 180 mμ diameter, enveloped, deoxyribonucleic acid–containing virus which is antigenically related to B virus of monkeys but antigenically distinct from the other herpesviruses. Herpes simplex virus has man as its natural host. It is known for its ability to cause recurrent cutaneous and oral or genital mucosal lesions. The virus commonly remains latent in trigeminal and sacral ganglion tissue of humans.

Early observations in man and laboratory animals suggested that various strains of herpes simplex virus behaved differently in regard to their ability to produce disease. Subsequent work has demonstrated that there are at least two distinct serotypes of herpes simplex virus (types 1 and 2) which differ not only antigenically but also in distribution. Type 1 is commonly isolated from oral and cutaneous lesions above the waist and from sporadic adult cases of herpes simplex encephalitis, whereas type 2 strains are commonly associated with genital infections and cutaneous lesions below the waist. Exceptions to these general rules are common. The two strains differ in several other respects. Type 1 has a slightly lower DNA density, produces smaller pocks on chick chorioallantoic membrane, produces a higher yield of virus in most tissue culture systems, possesses slightly less neurovirulence for mice and rabbits, and is slightly more sensitive to idoxuridine in tissue culture systems.

PATHOGENESIS.   Many aspects of the pathogenesis of herpes simplex encephalitis in adults caused by type 1

virus are poorly or incompletely understood. Although most such infections appear to have resulted from a primary infection with the virus, in a few cases a previous history of recurrent cutaneous or oral herpes simplex lesions has been obtained. Rare cases have been reported in patients whose immune systems were compromised by disease or immunosuppressive drugs, but most cases are encountered in previously normal adults.

In adults, there is usually no evidence of involvement of other viscera. Within the cerebrum the pathologic process has a characteristic bilateral distribution, necrotic and hemorrhagic lesions being most prominent in the hippocampus, amygdala and medial temporal lobe, orbital surface of the frontal lobe, insular cortex, and cingulum. The distribution is usually asymmetric. The posterior portions of the cerebrum, the cerebellum, the brainstem, and the spinal cord are usually spared. Histologically, the lesions are characterized by severe necrosis of all elements of the tissue. The presence of eosinophilic intranuclear inclusions in neurons, oligodendrocytes, and astrocytes is suggestive but not diagnostic of herpes simplex encephalitis. There is a brisk inflammatory reaction, consisting of mononuclear cells and lymphocytes and usually a mild to moderate meningeal exudate. Small hemorrhages within the lesions and on the pial surface are common.

The route by which the virus produces nervous system involvement has been the subject of much speculation. The consistent involvement of portions of the brain subserving olfactory functions has suggested that the virus may enter the nervous system by way of olfactory mucosa whence it may travel along the olfactory tract to reach the brain. The ability of herpes simplex virus to travel within nerves has long been recognized, but there is little evidence from human studies to indicate that the olfactory bulb or tract is uniformly or even commonly involved in cases of herpes simplex encephalitis. The possibility that the nervous system involvement might be the consequence of a viremia and a special affinity or susceptibility of neurons in the limbic system to hematogenous virus has also been considered, but there is little evidence from clinical or experimental data to support this hypothesis. Further information concerning the pathogenesis of the disease awaits careful studies of the distribution of lesions and virus in human cases of herpes simplex encephalitis.

CLINICAL MANIFESTATIONS.   Encephalitis caused by type I herpes simplex virus is a sporadic disease of the nervous system which often has devastating effects and a highly variable clinical course. It is uncertain whether or not the virus also causes a mild form of encephalitis, because the laboratory tests necessary to provide a definitive diagnosis are seldom feasible in patients with benign illness.

In contrast to other viral encephalitides in the United States, herpes simplex encephalitis is nonepidemic. In its severe form, the disease produces a combination of nonspecific signs and symptoms of an acute encephalitis plus focal manifestations of damage to the limbic system and frontal lobes. The onset in some patients is abrupt, with headache, fever, delirium, and, often, generalized or focal convulsions. Few illnesses can produce so much neurologic devastation in so short a time; within hours of the onset some patients may lose consciousness or undergo progressive dysphasia and/or unilateral or bilateral motor weaknesses.

Alternatively, the disease may have a subacute course. Behavioral changes are common early signs of disease and at times have prompted admission to psychiatric facilities. Some patients experience olfactory or gustatory hallucinations, presumably as a consequence of the focal involvement of temporal lobe structures. In others memory is impaired out of proportion to other cognitive functions, reflecting the bilateral involvement of the hippocampal system. Seizures may take the form of generalized, focal motor, temporal lobe, or occasionally myoclonic phenomena. Involvement of larger or deeper portions of the cerebrum is signaled by the appearance of hemiparesis, conjugate deviation of the eyes, or aphasia. The illness characteristically undergoes fluctuation in its intensity, and such fluctuation may help in distinguishing herpes simplex encephalitis from involvement of the cerebrum by tumor or abscess.

The type 2 herpes virus, which is the major cause of fatal disseminated herpes infections in the newborn, usually causes less severe neurologic disease in adults. This virus in adults has been associated with aseptic meningitis and with radicular pain, often over lower lumbar and sacral dermatomes. The pain may mimic symptoms of a herniated intravertebral disc but is often temporally associated with the eruptions of genital herpes.

DIAGNOSIS. The diagnosis of herpes simplex encephalitis rests upon clinical suspicion confirmed by laboratory data.

The cerebrospinal fluid (CSF) in most cases contains up to 500 cells per cubic millimeter, with lymphocytes or mononuclear cells predominating. Occasional cases, confirmed by isolation of the virus from the brain, have lacked cells in the CSF. Red cells in the CSF and/or xanthochromia frequently reflect the hemorrhagic nature of the lesions. The CSF protein concentration is commonly elevated, but this does not distinguish the process from a number of other affections. The CSF sugar is usually within the normal range, but occasionally is low.

Recent reports of the identification of herpesvirus antigen by fluorescent antibody study of cells in the CSF suggested a specific and convenient way of establishing the diagnosis, but further confirmatory experience is necessary. Attempts to isolate virus from the CSF have only rarely been successful.

Serologic tests for confirmation of the diagnosis have several inherent disadvantages. Comparison of acute and convalescent titers is of little practical value in the management of the acutely ill patient. Furthermore, fluctuations in the titer of antibody to herpes simplex virus are commonly encountered as a reaction to a variety of stimuli. Less than fourfold increases in titer do not necessarily signify recent herpes simplex virus infection; conversely in some confirmed cases of herpes simplex virus encephalitis, the titers have failed to rise. The utility of tests of complement requiring neutralizing antibody in serum or passive hemagglutinating antibodies in the CSF must await further experience from a variety of laboratories.

The electroencephalogram is virtually always abnormal, although the abnormality may not be specific. Diffuse slowing accentuated in one or both temporal lobes and the appearance of sharp waves or spikes in temporal areas are findings consistent with the diagnosis. Several cases have been associated with relatively specific, periodic sharp and slow wave complexes; such findings are highly suggestive of the disease, but their absence does not exclude it.

Brain scans reveal unilateral or bilateral uptake of the tracer substance, a reflection of the increased permeability of vessels in the lesions. Cerebral arteriography usually demonstrates an avascular mass in the temporal lobe with or without shift of midline structures. Computerized axial tomographic scans have frequently revealed bilateral low density temporal lobe lesions with positive uptake of contrast material.

A certain diagnosis of herpes simplex encephalitis requires the use of cerebral biopsy. This technique has several limitations and also some hazard, and it should be performed only in major medical centers possessing the necessary facilities for proper processing of the tissue. The limitations arise from the fact that the encephalitic process is often confined to the medial and undersurfaces of the temporal and frontal lobes, so that biopsy of the lateral or superior portions of temporal or frontal lobes or other portions of the brain may fail to demonstrate the process or identify the agent. The time at which the biopsy is performed is of additional importance. Herpes simplex virus disappears from neural tissue within a short time and cannot be recovered thereafter by ordinary techniques. Thus the biopsy should be performed as early as possible in the course of the illness, and the tissue should be subjected to histologic study, fluorescent antibody study, electron microscopy and viral culture. If the tissue is fixed in Bouin's solution for histology, intranuclear inclusions are stained to better advantage and can be more easily recognized than with formalin-fixed tissue. Fluorescent antibody study has the advantages of relatively great sensitivity for detection of viral antigen, and specificity for the virus when appropriate controls are included. The test may be completed within a few hours after the tissue is removed. Electron microscopy is less sensitive because of the inherent sampling problems. Viral culture offers the most sensitive method for demonstrating virus in nervous system tissue. The technique of inoculating trypsinized cells from the biopsy tissue onto indicator cultures may offer a better opportunity for recovery of virus than does inoculation of clarified suspension of homogenized brain.

Among conditions which must be distinguished from herpes simplex encephalitis, cerebral abscess presents the most difficult problem. Fever, headache, and seizures occur with cerebral abscess, and these features do not serve to differentiate abscess from herpes encephalitis. The presence of another site of pyogenic infection, especially in sinus or mastoid, should alert the clinician to the possibility of abscess. However, unusual psychiatric changes or an isolated disorder of memory are less common in cerebral abscess than in herpes, and abscesses usually produce more focal and fewer diffuse signs than herpes. CSF changes may be similar; there is some tendency for the protein to be higher and the cell count lower in cases of abscess than in encephalitis. In doubtful cases, the computerized axial tomographic scan, arteriogram, electroencephalogram, and brain scan are more apt to reflect the bilateral lesions in encephalitis, and periodic high voltage sharp waves which appear and disappear over a few days are characteristic of encephalitis but are not a feature of abscess. Rarely, proper diagnosis is not reached until craniotomy, but this is usually in patients in whom the diagnosis of encephalitis has not been given sufficient preoperative consideration.

The distinction between herpes encephalitis and a pyogenic or tuberculous meningitis is somewhat easier because of the prominence of meningeal signs, the more regular lowering of the CSF glucose, the presence of organisms, and the lesser frequency of focal signs in the latter conditions. Distinction between herpes simplex encephalitis and the postinfectious or other acute viral encephalitides may be difficult and rests with the history of one of the common viral exanthems or mumps in the weeks preceding the onset of the cerebral disorder. Cerebral neoplasm can usually be distinguished by its more slowly progressive course, by the absence of fever and of CSF findings suggestive of encephalitis, and by the appearance on scan and arteriographic studies.

TREATMENT. The difficulties in establishing the diagnosis of herpes simplex encephalitis, the infrequency with which cases are seen at any one medical center, and the great variation in course from one case to another have thwarted attempts to arrive at a reasonable evaluation of treatment. In any given case there is considerable uncertainty concerning the stage in the evolution of the disease at which treatment is instituted. In addition, recent improvements in supportive treatment may tend to invalidate comparisons between series of cases.

Individual reports involving single or small numbers of patients have appeared in which idoxuridine (IUDR) has been used to treat human encephalitis caused by herpes simplex virus. IUDR, a thymidine analogue, presumably exerts its antiviral effect by becoming incorporated into the viral DNA, thus producing a fraudulent molecule which cannot be replicated. However, controlled studies have shown it to lack effectiveness and to possess unacceptable toxicity.

Cytosine arabinoside (Ara-C), a pyrimidine nucleoside, has been shown to possess activity against herpes simplex virus both in tissue culture and with herpes simplex virus keratitis in animals. Although the drug has the practical advantages of being readily available and easily solubilized and there is more experience with its use, it retains some of the toxic effects of IUDR, including granulocytopenia and thrombocytopenia. Experience with Ara-C in treatment of herpes simplex encephalitis is limited to a few largely favorable reports. A controlled study of Ara-C in disseminated varicella-zoster infections revealed no therapeutic efficacy.

The purine nucleoside, adenine arabinoside (Ara-A), has been used in a small, placebo-controlled series of patients with biopsy-proved herpes simplex encephalitis. A reduction of mortality from 70 to 28 per cent was achieved with a daily dosage level of 15 mg per kilogram for 10 days. Toxicity appeared minimal. The material was effective only if given before loss of consciousness occurred. Further careful use of this compound in established cases of herpes encephalitis seems warranted on the basis of this information.

Some authors have recommended that corticosteroids be used in herpes simplex encephalitis to treat brain swelling and impending tentorial herniation. This effect must be weighed against the potential for corticosteroids to enhance the spread and delay the clearing of herpes and virus from lesions. Further data bearing upon this topic are necessary; in the meantime it would seem reasonable to use steroids only in situations in which brain swelling seems to be a critical factor threatening the patient's life, discontinuing their use as soon as possible.

PROGNOSIS. Because of the very great difficulty in establishing the diagnosis of herpes simplex encephalitis with certainty, as well as the tendencies for biopsy to be performed in more seriously ill patients and for cases to be reported only if they are confirmed by biopsy or autopsy, the outcome of herpes simplex encephalitis is quite difficult to predict. Published reports from many sources suggest that an over-all mortality of between 30 and 70 per cent is to be expected and that among survivors severe sequelae are common, including prominent impairment of memory. A few reports, however, emphasize that nearly complete recovery is possible even without any specific treatment.

Adams, H., and Miller, D.: Herpes simplex encephalitis: A clinical and pathological analysis of twenty-two cases. Postgrad. Med. J., 49:393, 1973.

Baringer, J. R.: Herpes simplex virus infection of nervous tissue in animals and man. Prog. Med. Virol., 20:1, 1975.

Boston Interhospital Virus Study Group and the NIAID-sponsored Cooperative Antiviral Clinical Study: Failure of high dose 5-iodo-2'-deoxyuridine in the therapy of herpes simplex virus encephalitis: Evidence of unacceptable toxicity. N. Engl. J. Med., 292:599, 1975.

Dayan, A. D., and Stokes, M. I.: Rapid diagnosis of encephalitis by immunofluorescent examination of cerebrospinal fluid cells. Lancet, 1:177, 1973.

Johnson, K. P., Rosenthal, M. S., and Lerner, P. I.: Herpes simplex encephalitis: The course of five virologically proven cases. Arch. Neurol., 27:103, 1972.

Sarubbi, F. A., Sparling, P. F., and Glezen, W. P.: Herpesvirus hominis encephalitis: Virus isolation from brain biopsy in seven patients and results of therapy. Arch. Neurol., 29:268, 1973.

Shope, T. C., Klein-Robbenhaar, J., and Miller, G.: Fatal encephalitis due to herpesvirus hominis: Use of intact brain cells for isolation of virus. J. Infect. Dis., 125:542, 1972.

Stevens, D. A., Jordan, G. W., Waddell, T. F., and Merigan, T. C.: Adverse effect of cytosine arabinoside on disseminated zoster in a controlled trial. N. Engl. J. Med., 289:873, 1973.

Thomson, J. L. G.: The computed axial tomograph in acute herpes simplex encephalitis. Br. J. Radiol., 49:86, 1976.

Whitley, R. J., Soong, S., Dolin, R., Galasso, G. J., Ch'ien, L. T., Alford, C. A., and the Collaborative Study Group: Adenine arabinoside therapy of biopsy proved herpes simplex encephalitis: NIAID Collaborative Antiviral Study Group. N. Engl. J. Med., 297:289, 1977.

305. HERPES ZOSTER

Richard T. Johnson

Herpes zoster is an acute viral infection of sensory ganglia and the corresponding cutaneous areas of innervation. The disease is characterized by localized pain along the distribution of the nerve and a vesicular skin eruption over a single or adjacent dermatomes. The disease is due to the same virus that causes chickenpox (varicella) and is thought to represent an acute localized recrudescent infection by the varicella virus that has remained latent in the sensory ganglia since the primary attack of chickenpox. (For a description of chickenpox, see Ch. 85.) Herpes zoster is also called shingles or zona.

ETIOLOGY. The varicella or varicella-zoster virus is a herpesvirus. The virus core measures 45 to 50 mμ and contains deoxyribonucleic acid. This is surrounded by a capsid with a diameter of 50 to 100 mμ and an outer envelope, giving a total diameter of the virion of 150 to 250 mμ. The virus is naturally pathogenic only for man, although chickenpox has been seen in anthropoid apes in zoos. There is some evidence of experimental transmission of the virus to several species of monkeys. The virus can be grown in a variety of cell cultures of human and primate origin but not in nonprimate cells. The virus is avidly cell-associated and can usually be transmitted in the laboratory only by the inoculation of infected cells, although the virus is stable in a cell-free form in the vesicular fluid. Morphologically, varicella virus resembles herpes simplex virus, with which it shares some common antigens, but it is markedly different from herpes simplex virus in its inability to infect nonprimates and nonprimate cell cultures and in its loss of infectivity in most cell-free preparations.

INCIDENCE. Herpes zoster occurs at a rate of three to five cases per thousand persons per year. The attack rate increases with age. The disease is rare in childhood and is most frequently seen in persons over the age of 50 years. It is estimated that half the people reaching 85 years of age have suffered from at least one attack of herpes zoster. Rates are higher in persons with malignancies or diabetes mellitus and in patients receiving immunosuppressant drugs or radiation therapy.

EPIDEMIOLOGY, PATHOGENESIS, AND PATHOLOGY. It has long been recognized that chickenpox may develop after exposure to a patient with herpes zoster, although this is less likely than development of chickenpox after exposure to chickenpox. In contrast, zoster rarely develops after exposure to chickenpox or other cases of zoster. These observations are supported by the epidemiologic findings that chickenpox is a seasonal disease occurring mainly in the winter and spring and occurs in epidemic proportions every two to four years. In contrast, zoster is not a seasonal disease, and there is no increase in incidence during the years of chickenpox epidemics. There is, in fact, some evidence that the incidence of zoster decreases slightly during years when there are large numbers of cases of chickenpox.

The precise pathogenesis of herpes zoster is unknown, but the following hypothesis is widely accepted. Chickenpox is transmitted from man to man by respiratory spread, and in the susceptible person the virus is probably disseminated throughout the body by a viremia. Infection of the skin occurs through the blood, and vesicles develop most prominently over the face and trunk. It is postulated that virus then spreads centripetally via sensory nerve fibers to the sensory ganglia, where it becomes latent in some form within the neurons or stellate cells. This latency of varicella virus in ganglia has not been documented in man or laboratory animals, but the recent demonstration of latency of herpes simplex virus in sensory ganglia has added credence to this hypothesis for varicella virus. Virus replication is later activated. In some cases activation is associated with the development of malignancy, local x-irradiation, immunosuppressive therapy, trauma, treatment with arsenicals, neurosyphilis, or tumor entrapment of the dorsal root ganglia or nerve root. Nevertheless, in most patients, there is no obvious exciting cause, and it is thought that the decline of immunity with age and the lack of exposure to children with chickenpox may promote reactivation. When virus multiplies in the ganglia, an active ganglionitis develops, causing pain along its sensory distribution. Virus is then thought to pass down the nerve and multiply again in the skin, causing characteristic clusters of vesicles. The localized zoster lesions are most common over

trigeminal or thoracic dermatomes corresponding to the areas of major eruption during the antecedent chickenpox infection. The more rapid secondary immune response may prevent hematogenous dissemination. Resolution and limitation of the rash of herpes zoster do not correlate well, however, with the development of antibody but appear to correlate with the collection of inflammatory cells and the presence of interferon in the vesicular fluid. This theory of pathogenesis is consistent with the occurrence of the disease with increasing age or development of malignancy, the lack of seasonal association with chickenpox, the observation that pain usually precedes the skin eruption, the dermatomal localization of the lesions of herpes zoster, and the pathology and patterns of distribution of herpes zoster.

Pathologic studies of herpes zoster have shown an acute ganglionitis with an intense inflammatory response, cell necrosis, and occasionally hemorrhages within the ganglia. In addition, there is inflammation in the adjacent segments of the cord or brainstem which is predominantly unilateral, more prominent in gray matter, and involves the posterior more than the anterior horns. A mild leptomeningitis is generally found which is most intense over the segments of involvement. Inflammation in the roots distal to the ganglia is also present, representing a true peripheral mononeuritis.

In the skin innervated by the nerve there is degeneration of the basal and deep prickle cell layers of the epidermis. Ballooning degeneration of these cells causes the formation of the intradermal vesicles. Giant cells and eosinophilic intranuclear inclusions are found in the base of the vesicles.

CLINICAL MANIFESTATIONS. The eruption of herpes zoster is often preceded by malaise and fever for two to four days. Pain or dysesthesia along the segmental dermatome also precedes the rash usually for four to five days. The pain is often a superficial tingling or burning sensation, but may vary from severe deep pain, suggesting appendicitis, cholecystitis, or pleurisy, to very mild itching. The pain may be intermittent or constant. Tenderness or hypesthesia may be detected along the dermatome on examination during this pre-eruptive stage. The cutaneous lesions present first as small, red macules which rapidly vesiculate, becoming tense, clear vesicles on an erythematous base. On about the third day, the vesicular fluid becomes turbid as inflammatory cells collect within the vesicles. Within five to ten days, the vesicles dry and crusts develop. However, in severe cases the vesicles may become confluent with a gangrenous appearance, and healing may be delayed for many weeks. During the course of the rash, there is usually enlargement of the regional lymph nodes, and there is often spread of a few vesicles to adjacent dermatomes but seldom to the other side of the body. The pain or dysesthesia usually persists for one to four weeks, but approximately 30 per cent of the patients over the age of 40 have pain that persists for months to years. This postherpetic neuralgia is more common in the elderly when there has been a prolonged period of pain prior to cutaneous eruption and a more severe rash.

Although herpes zoster may occur over any sensory nerve distribution, the thoracic dermatomes are the sites in over two thirds of cases. Cranial nerve involvement is next in frequency, and this tends to be more severe, with greater pain, frequent signs of meningeal irritation, paralysis, and sometimes involvement of the mucous membranes. The ophthalmic division of the trigeminal nerve is the most common site of cranial involvement, accounting for 10 to 15 per cent of all cases of herpes zoster. Fortunately, the eye is usually spared, but occasionally a keratoconjunctivitis develops. With ophthalmic zoster it is not uncommon to have involvement of oculomotor function, with extraocular muscle weakness, ptosis, and paralytic mydriasis. The fourth and sixth cranial nerves may also be involved, indicating that the infection is not confined to the trigeminal ganglia and its ophthalmic fibers, but may involve the brainstem and other nerve roots. The association of vesicles in the external ear and ipsilateral facial palsy (Ramsay Hunt's syndrome) was originally ascribed to infection of the geniculate ganglia. This localization of zoster may be accompanied by hearing loss, vertigo, loss of taste, or vesicles on the tongue, and probably represents involvement of multiple cranial ganglia and the associated localized encephalitis and neuronitis.

Since the primary lesion of herpes zoster is in the nervous system, the cerebrospinal fluid commonly shows a pleocytosis and elevation of protein, even when clinical signs of meningeal irritation or encephalomyelitis are absent. Not infrequently, the peripheral mononeuritis or local encephalomyelitis may cause muscle paralysis and atrophy in the area of the segmental rash. Acute urinary retention, urinary or fecal incontinence, and hemidiaphragmatic paralysis have also been seen. Signs of major central nervous system infections with herpes zoster are rare, but cases of acute transverse or ascending myelitis, disseminated encephalitis, and acute cerebellar ataxia have been described.

Zoster sine herpete is typical pain in an appropriate sensory area which is not followed by the development of the characteristic vesicles. Whether some of the common transient intercostal pains represent activation of varicella virus in ganglia without spread to the skin is a matter of speculation. An antibody response to varicella virus has been demonstrated in the absence of a rash in patients with transient facial pain resembling trigeminal neuralgia and in patients with facial palsy (Bell's palsy). However, these are rare occurrences, and the vast majority of cases of trigeminal neuralgia and Bell's palsy are not associated with serologic evidence of activation of the varicella or any other known viral infection.

Cutaneous dissemination is rare, occurring in less than 2 per cent of the cases. Dissemination is more common in patients with underlying malignancies, and about one quarter of the patients with Hodgkin's disease show a progressive spread of vesicles beyond the original one or two dermatomes of involvement. Such cutaneous dissemination, however, generally does not progress for more than six days, and spontaneous recovery occurs in most patients.

DIAGNOSIS. Characteristic development of pain and vesicular eruptions over single or adjacent dermatomes served by a segmental or cranial nerve branch usually presents no problem in differential diagnosis. However, similar zosteriform lesions can be caused by herpes simplex virus in infants.

Diagnosis can be confirmed by the demonstration of multinucleated giant epithelial cells with intranuclear inclusions in Giemsa-stained scrapings from the base of an early vesicle. Virions can also readily be found in

vesicular fluid by electron microscopic examination. However, neither of these tests differentiates zoster from herpes simplex virus infections, although they can be helpful in differentiating zoster or chickenpox from smallpox infections. Varicella and herpes simplex virus infections can be differentiated by fluorescent antibody staining of cells in scrapings from vesicles.

Virus can be isolated from vesicular fluid and, in some cases, from cerebrospinal fluid by inoculation of fluid onto cultures of human or primate cells. Serologic diagnosis can also be made, but in human sera some cross-reactions are found with herpes simplex virus, so that simultaneous serologic tests should be carried out against both viruses.

TREATMENT. Little can be done to treat the acute eruption of herpes zoster other than symptomatic application of powder or calamine lotion to the rash and the use of analgesics for the pain. A variety of previously advocated treatments such as protamide, vitamins, x-irradiation, vasodilators, antimicrobials, and gamma globulin have proved to be useless. In a controlled study corticosteroids have been shown not to affect the rate of healing of skin lesions but to shorten the period of the acute pain. This benefit must be weighed against the potential hazard that corticosteroids may promote dissemination.

Systemic cytosine arabinoside, a drug inhibitory against DNA virus replication in vitro, has been advocated for the control of severe and disseminated herpes zoster infections. However, in a placebo-controlled study, cytosine arabinoside was found to actually prolong the duration of dissemination in some patients compared to the placebo group. This adverse effect of cytosine arabinoside appeared to be related to its depression of antibody response, delay in vesicle interferon appearance, and possibly its effect on the cellular immune response. Preliminary results with adenine arabinoside and interferon have been encouraging, and definitive controlled studies are in progress to assess their value.

Postherpetic Neuralgia. The development of prolonged postherpetic neuralgia after recovery from herpes zoster presents a difficult problem in management. Although this pain usually abates over a period of months to years, it is very refractory to the usual analgesics. Application of cold to the area by use of an ethyl chloride spray may give some transient relief. Tranquilizers or sedatives can sometimes be of help, and tricyclic antidepressants (amitriptyline) in combination with substituted phenothiazines have been effective in relieving pain in some cases. Local injection or section of the nerve root is of no value, and narcotics should be avoided because of the problem of addiction. In the most severe cases when pain persists over long periods, the use of transcutaneous peripheral nerve stimulation or even cordotomy may be considered (see Ch. 260).

PROGNOSIS. There is a popular misconception that herpes zoster does not recur. However, zoster does not give immunity to further attacks, and the likelihood of a second attack is about the same as, if not slightly greater than, that of having suffered the first. Most patients recover uneventfully, although severe vesiculation may lead to permanent scarring. Scarring of the cornea after ophthalmic involvement may result in permanent visual impairment. Motor paralysis of the local nerves recovers to adequate function levels in over 75 per cent of cases. Even in patients with severe encephalomyelitis, the mortality rate appears to be less than 10 per cent, and permanent sequelae are rare. The prognosis, however, must be more guarded in those patients who have underlying neoplastic disease, in which both the disease and the chemotherapeutic agents used in the treatment of neoplasms may increase the possibility of cutaneous and visceral dissemination.

PREVENTION. No vaccine is available for varicella virus. Chickenpox can be modified if gamma globulin is given after exposure, and sera obtained from patients recuperating from herpes zoster can totally prevent chickenpox in children if given within 72 hours of the time of exposure. This zoster immune globulin is recommended for children on immunosuppressive therapy or with leukemia who have been exposed to chickenpox or herpes zoster. Similar measures are not recommended for disabled adults exposed to chickenpox or to zoster, although contact should be avoided in the adult patient with a compromised immune system, because it is in this group that occasional cases of zoster have been thought to be related to exposure to chickenpox or zoster.

Ch'ien, L. T., Whitley, R. J., Alford, C. A., Jr., Galasso, G. J., and the Collaborative Study Group: Adenine arabinoside for therapy of herpes zoster in immunosuppressed patients: Preliminary results of a collaborative study. J. Infect. Dis., 133 (Suppl):A184, 1976.
Hope-Simpson, R. E.: The nature of herpes zoster: A long-term study and a new hypothesis. Proc. R. Soc. Med., 58.9, 1965.
Jellinek, E. H., and Tulloch, W. S.: Herpes zoster with dysfunction of bladder and anus. Lancet, 2:1219, 1976.
Luby, J. P.: Varicella-zoster virus. J. Invest. Dermatol. 61:212, 1973.
McCormick, W. F., Rodnitzsky, R. L., Schochet, S. S., and McKee, A. P.: Varicella-zoster encephalomyelitis. Arch. Neurol., 21:559, 1969.
Stevens, D. A., Jordan, G. W., Waddell, T. F., and Merigan, T. C.: Adverse effect of cytosine arabinoside on disseminated zoster in a controlled trial. N. Engl. J. Med., 289:873, 1973.
Taub, A.: Relief of postherpetic neuralgia with psychotropic drugs. J. Neurosurg., 39:235, 1973.
Thomas, J. E., and Howard, F. M., Jr.: Segmental zoster paresis — a disease profile. Neurology, 22:459, 1972.

306. CYTOMEGALOVIRUS INFECTIONS

James B. Hanshaw

DEFINITION. Cytomegalic inclusion disease (CID), generalized salivary gland virus disease, cytomegaly, and inclusion disease are synonyms for an illness caused by cytomegalovirus infection. Although frequently an inapparent infection, it is a cause of fetal encephalitis with irreversible damage to the central nervous system. Disease also occurs in patients on immunosuppressive therapy and others subject to opportunistic infections. The virus has been associated with a mononucleosis-like illness in previously well patients and in individuals receiving transfusions of blood.

ETIOLOGY. Cytomegalovirus (CMV) infection is caused by a species-specific agent with the physiochemical and electron microscopic characteristics of a herpesvirus. It was isolated in human fibroblastic tissue culture in the mid-1950's from infants with CID as well as from the adenoid tissue of schoolage children. A cytopathic effect was noted in tissue culture which was characterized by large intranuclear inclusions. The propagation of the virus provided the basis for the development of specific serologic tests.

EPIDEMIOLOGY. Cytomegalovirus infection is worldwide in distribution. The prevalence of complement-fixing antibodies is especially high in communities where crowding and poor living conditions are extant. Although approximately 50 per cent of women in the child-bearing age group are seropositive, this may vary from 20 to 90 per cent. Approximately 4 per cent of pregnant women excrete the virus in the urine. In the several studies that have been done in this country and in the United Kingdom, 0.5 to 1.5 per cent of newborns are virus positive. Thus cytomegalovirus is the most common known fetal infection. In some countries infection occurs in the majority of infants at some time during the first year of life. In the United States complement-fixing antibody is present in approximately 5 to 15 per cent of infants from 6 to 24 months of age.

PATHOGENESIS AND PATHOLOGY. Cytomegalovirus does not induce a highly communicable infection. Thus a substantial number of individuals remain susceptible to the infection in adult life. The virus has been isolated from saliva, the upper respiratory tract, urine, milk, cervical secretions, semen, feces, and circulating leukocytes. Virus is probably transferred by intimate contact with an infected individual or by infusion of blood from an asymptomatic blood donor. Nursing personnel working on infant wards and newborn nurseries do not have a higher prevalence of complement-fixing antibody than women in the general population. There is evidence that the placenta itself is infected with the virus prior to transmission to the fetus.

The symptomatic newborn is rarely without neutralizing, complement-fixing, and immunofluorescent IgM antibodies in the cord serum. The presence of specific IgM antibody is of value in differentiating maternal from fetal antibody because of the failure of maternal macroglobulin to pass the placental barrier. Antibody in the serum of the congenitally infected infant does not prevent the persistence of virus excretion for years after birth. The precise mechanism of this remarkable persistence is not known.

Among adults undergoing immunosuppressive therapy after renal homotransplantation, over 90 per cent develop an active cytomegalovirus infection if they have cytomegalovirus antibody prior to surgery. Approximately half of the seronegative patients subsequently become infected on immunosuppressive therapy. Seronegative recipients receiving a kidney from a seropositive donor almost always develop a postoperative infection and are likely to develop symptoms.

CLINICAL MANIFESTATIONS. Congenital Infection. The most frequently encountered signs of the infection in symptomatic newborns are hepatosplenomegaly, jaundice, purpura, microcephaly, cerebral calcifications, and chorioretinitis—in approximate order of decreasing frequency. Any one of these signs may occur alone. A petechial rash on the first day of life is suggestive of CID. Occasionally there are no physical findings other than increased irritability or a general failure to thrive. Some infants have repeated respiratory infections. The incidence of various congenital abnormalities in infants with CID is increased. These include clubfoot, inguinal hernia, strabismus, high-arched palate, microcephaly, and deafness. There have been reports of associated congenital heart disease, but this coexistence may be coincidental.

The major complications of congenital cytomegalovirus infection relate to central nervous system sequelae. There is little evidence that extraneural involvement of viscera such as the liver, spleen, kidney, or lungs results in any permanent damage to these organs. Blindness is associated with macular chorioretinitis or optic atrophy. Deafness may be complete or limited to the higher frequencies. Spastic quadriplegia or hypotonia are common manifestations in severely affected infants. Psychomotor function may range from the vegetative state with no meaningful communication to milder abnormalities with minimal effect on speech, behavior, and motor coordination.

Acquired Infection. Cytomegalovirus acquired after birth is often inapparent but may also produce respiratory symptoms with pneumonia, paroxysmal cough, petechial rash, hepatomegaly, and splenomegaly. Central nervous system disease caused by infection acquired after birth has not been frequently demonstrated, although there are reports of associated myoclonic seizures in infants and infectious polyneuritis. Chorioretinitis has been documented after acquired infection.

Hepatomegaly and mildly abnormal liver function tests are found in well individuals excreting CMV in the urine as well as in patients with cytomegalovirus mononucleosis. The latter patients may experience malaise, fever, chills, myalgia, sore throat, headache, anorexia, and abdominal pain. On physical examination, pharyngeal edema without exudate, lymphadenopathy, and splenomegaly may be present. Atypical lymphocytosis is common. Some patients have maculopapular rashes, especially if ampicillin is administered, and abnormal serologic reactions, including cold agglutinins, antinuclear antibody, and cryoimmunoglobulins, have been described. An illness similar to cytomegalovirus infection has been described in patients who have received blood transfusions. This condition, referred to as post-transfusion mononucleosis, occurs two to four weeks after the administration of blood.

Acquired cytomegalovirus infection has also been associated with autoimmune hemolytic disease, ulcerative lesions of the gastrointestinal tract, post-transplantation pneumonia, and thrombocytopenic purpura.

There is equivocal evidence that the mild liver dysfunction associated with acquired CMV infection is capable of progressing to chronic hepatitis, granulomatous hepatitis, or cirrhosis of the liver. Children with chronic hepatitis or chronic liver disease may have a higher prevalence of active infection, but the relationship of this infection to the pathogenesis of chronic liver disease is uncertain. For the majority of CMV infections acquired *after* birth, recovery is without significant complications. Patients with CMV mononucleosis may experience recurrent or protracted periods of malaise, pharyngitis, and cervical adenopathy.

DIAGNOSIS. Congenital Infection. The diagnosis of congenital infection is usually not suspected at birth, because 90 per cent of infected infants are asymptomatic. The presence of infection (not necessarily disease) can be established by (1) virus isolation in human fibroblastic tissue culture from the urine, blood, upper respiratory tract, or biopsy material; (2) demonstration of cytomegalovirus IgM antibody in the cord or neonatal serum; (3) persistent cytomegalovirus complement-fixing or immunofluorescent antibody beyond the sixth month of life; or (4) demonstration of large nuclear inclusion-bearing cells in the urine sediment at birth.

Differential Diagnosis of Congenital Infec- **tion.** TOXOPLASMOSIS. Cytomegalovirus infection resembles toxoplasmosis in striking detail. Toxoplasmosis, however, is more likely to be associated with microphthalmia, *scattered* cerebral calcifications, hydrocephalus, and chorioretinitis. The demonstration of specific toxoplasma antibody titers persisting beyond six months of age or the presence of toxoplasma IgM antibody is tantamount to isolation of the organism.

RUBELLA. Congenital CMV and congenital rubella may be difficult to distinguish in the neonatal period. Both can be associated with a purpuric rash, jaundice, microcephaly, and deafness. The presence of central cataracts, however, is strong presumptive evidence for rubella. If these are associated with a congenital heart lesion, the probability of rubella is high. Specific laboratory tests for rubella virus or rubella IgM antibody or serial hemagglutination-inhibition antibody tests are required for a definitive diagnosis.

HERPES SIMPLEX. Herpes simplex infection is usually transmitted to the infant during labor and has its onset in the second week of life. The disease is often fulminant in character and may present as a meningoencephalitis, pneumonitis, or undiagnosed vesicular rash. The virus is readily isolated from vesicular lesions (see Ch. 304).

BACTERIAL SEPSIS. Infants with bacterial sepsis usually are more lethargic than infants with CID and rarely have a petechial rash. Although the diagnosis rests on a positive blood culture, the decision to treat with antimicrobial drugs must be made on the basis of the early clinical findings.

Acquired Infection. The diagnosis of cytomegalovirus infection in a patient with mononucleosis-like symptoms can be established by virus isolation as described above. Serologic determinations, such as the presence of specific immunofluorescent IgM antibody or a fourfold rise or decline in complement-fixing antibody, must be interpreted with more caution than in the newborn period because of cross-reactions with other cell-associated herpesviruses, and a tendency for CF antibody to fluctuate widely in normal subjects. Patients with cytomegalovirus mononucleosis are always heterophil antibody negative.

Cytomegalovirus mononucleosis may be difficult to distinguish from heterophil antibody-negative *infectious mononucleosis*, because both conditions occur in young adults and both have atypical lymphocytosis, pharyngeal symptoms, abnormal liver function tests, splenomegaly, and fever. In addition, the cytomegalovirus IgM (FA) test is positive in cytomegalovirus and infectious mononucleosis, presumably because Epstein-Barr virus (EB virus) and cytomegalovirus share common antigens. A patient with cytomegalovirus mononucleosis usually has virus in the urine, upper respiratory tract, and peripheral leukocytes. EB virus antibody can be measured by an indirect immunofluorescence technique. The complement-fixation tests for EB virus and CMV are specific for each agent.

A jaundiced patient with CMV mononucleosis may clinically resemble one with *hepatitis A or B* infection. A serum glutamic oxaloacetic transaminase level above 800 units is unusual for CMV infections at any age and common in icteric A and B hepatitis. Both conditions may be associated with mild atypical lymphocytosis. Jaundice in an adult is far more unusual in CMV infections than in infections with the hepatitis viruses. A history of recent contact with a jaundiced person is strong evidence in favor of hepatitis A. Hepatitis B antigen may be detected in the serum of many patients with serum hepatitis.

PROGNOSIS. Congenital. The prognosis is guarded for completely normal psychomotor development in an infant with symptoms of CID at birth. Approximately 75 per cent or more usually have some central nervous system sequelae. Although asymptomatic infants discovered on routine surveys have a more favorable outlook, there is evidence that approximately 50 per cent of infants with cytomegalovirus IgM in the cord serum have detectable CNS sequelae five years after birth. Bilateral deafness may become apparent after the second year of life. The absence of cytomegalovirus IgM antibody in the cord serum and a birth weight above 3000 grams are favorable prognostic signs.

Acquired. Although acquired cytomegalovirus infections are usually benign, they may be life-threatening in a patient subject to opportunistic infection. This usually is manifest as a progressive pneumonitis but may take the form of a hemolytic anemia, purpura, gastrointestinal ulceration, hepatitis, pericarditis, and rarely encephalitis.

TREATMENT. There is no satisfactory treatment for cytomegalovirus infections. The use of corticosteroids, gamma globulin, and antiviral drugs such as deoxyuridine, floxuridine, cytosine arabinoside, and adenine arabinoside have been reported with equivocal, beneficial, or no effect on the clinical course. These reports are difficult to evaluate because of the small numbers of individuals treated, the multiple factors operating simultaneously, and the variability of virus excretion in individuals tested at different times.

PREVENTION. It is not possible to prevent cytomegalovirus infection at present. Handwashing and gown technique should be used in working with patients with cytomegalovirus infection in a hospital setting. Usually this is ineffectual because of the difficulty the physician has in recognizing the infection. Almost everyone in a given population will acquire CMV at some decade in life. The infection cannot be prevented by a live or killed vaccine, although this approach is under active investigation.

Benyesh-Melnick, M.: Cytomegaloviruses. *In* Lennette, E. H., and Schmidt, N. J. (eds.): Diagnostic Procedures for Viral and Rickettsial Infections, 4th ed. New York, American Public Health Association, Inc., 1969, pp. 701–732.

Hanshaw, J. B., Scheiner, A. P., Moxley, A. W., Abel, V., and Scheiner, B.: School failure and deafness after "silent" congenital cytomegalovirus infection. N. Engl. J. Med., 295:468, 1976.

Jordan, M. C., Rousseau, W. E., Stewart, J. A., Nobel, G. R., and Chin, T. D. Y.: Spontaneous cytomegalovirus mononucleosis: Clinical and laboratory observations in nine cases. Ann. Intern. Med., 79:153, 1973.

Plummer, G.: Cytomegaloviruses in man and animals. *In* Melnick, J. L. (ed.): Progress in Medical Virology. Basel, S. Karger, 1973, pp. 92–125.

Weller, T. H.: The cytomegaloviruses: Ubiquitous agents with protean clinical manifestations. N. Engl. J. Med., 285:203, 267, 1971.

307. ACUTE ANTERIOR POLIOMYELITIS

Fred Plum

DEFINITION. Acute poliomyelitis is a highly contagious viral disease which ranges widely in severity. An *inapparent infection* consists of an invasion by polio-virus that produces an antibody response but no systemic symptoms. An *abortive infection* produces transient nonspecific symptoms of a minor illness without central nervous system involvement with a rise in antibody. In *nonparalytic poliomyelitis*, the major illness develops with signs and symptoms of central nervous system invasion and meningitis but no paralysis. *Paralytic poliomyelitis* consists of the major illness, often with a biphasic pattern, associated with flaccid weakness in one or more muscle groups, the result of the attack by the virus on the somatic motor and autonomic neurons of the spinal cord and lower brainstem.

Initially endemic in character, poliomyelitis became epidemic during the first half of this century in the highly developed countries of Western Europe and North America. Since the advent of effective vaccines in the 1950's, major epidemics have disappeared, but minor outbreaks have reappeared in groups of nonimmunized children and in specific areas such as the American-Mexican border.

ETIOLOGY. The polioviruses are small enteric viruses of the picornavirus group. The virus is naturally infectious only for selected primates, particularly man, and has no other known natural reservoir. Poliovirus can be classified immunologically into three distinct types. Infection with type 1, 2, or 3 confers immunity against subsequent infection with the same type, but cross-immunity from type to type is minimal, a fact reflected by well documented cases of second attacks of poliomyelitis. Occasionally cases of an acute paralytic illness clinically are caused by coxsackie- and echoviruses (see Ch. 90 to 98).

EPIDEMIOLOGY. The virus of poliomyelitis is worldwide, and the infection is spread largely if not entirely by human contact. In nonepidemic areas with poor sanitation and largely unvaccinated populations, the illness is mainly confined to infants and children who come in contact with fecal-borne virus during the early months of life. Such children have a high infection rate with all three types of virus. Presumably they get some protection from maternal antibody; there is little serious illness but an incidence of paralytic lameness in schoolchildren which is almost as high as the attack rate formerly reported from epidemics in the developed countries. Under the circumstances, a large percentage of the population develop antibodies early in life and, despite repeated exposures, become immune from epidemic spread. Once sanitation improves and infant mortality falls in a region, the average age incidence progressively rises, with a concomitant increase in the number of paralytic cases. Prior to the extensive use of preventive vaccines, as many as 35 per cent of affected patients in the northeastern United States were over 14 years old.

Individual epidemics are predominantly the result of a single virus type, although different types of virus may attack the same community in successive years. During epidemics, poliovirus can be recovered readily from the pharynx, nasopharyngeal secretions, and stools of both patients with clinical cases and those with inapparent infection. The ratio of inapparent infection to disease ranges from 50 to 1 to 500 to 1. Thus inapparent infections are by far the largest reservoir for transmission.

PATHOGENESIS AND PATHOLOGY. Naturally occurring poliomyelitis infection is transmitted by human contact. Poliovirus enters the body through the alimentary tract and multiplies in the oropharynx and lower intestinal tract. No symptoms accompany this early proliferative stage. From the alimentary canal, the virus disseminates to regional lymph nodes with subsequent viremia which corresponds to the early, nonspecific phase of the abortive illness. With inapparent and abortive attacks, although viremia occurs, the virus apparently fails to penetrate the barriers of the central nervous system.

Both virus and host factors influence whether poliomyelitis virus invades the central nervous system and the severity of CNS involvement. Different strains of the virus vary widely in virulence. Host factors are perhaps even more important. Both epidemiologic and tissue culture studies suggest that poliomyelitis in man is genetically determined. Age and excessive physical activity during the prodromal illness unfavorably influence the severity of paralysis. Pregnancy increases the risk of contracting paralytic poliomyelitis. Local injections received during the preceding six weeks appear to increase the risk of paralysis in the injected extremity, and previous tonsillectomy enhances the risk of bulbar poliomyelitis. Inapparent and abortive poliomyelitis infections presumably never invade the nervous system at all. In nonparalytic and paralytic cases, the distribution of lesions in the neural parenchyma is roughly similar, although the intensity of the changes increases proportionately to the degree of paralysis. No one knows just what factors govern the special susceptibility of the motor gray matter and the distribution of the virus along the neuraxis in any given patient. In paralytic cases, the spinal cord gray matter is diffusely reddened, swollen, and congested, particularly in the anterior horns; the involvement in fatal cases commonly extends rostrally to the hypothalamus and thalamus. Lesions in the cerebral cortex are confined to mild alterations of the motor area. Microscopically in regions of maximal damage there are marked perivascular cuffing and diffuse infiltrates of mononuclear cells. The anterior horn cells of the spinal cord and the motor nuclei of the lower brainstem show abnormalities ranging in severity from mild chromatolysis and pericellular infiltration to total destruction. Small areas of necrosis commonly dot regions of intense inflammation. Outside the anterior horns, the inflammatory reaction sometimes spreads into the intermediate horn of the spinal cord; posterior column demyelination and neuronolysis of dorsal root (sensory) ganglia are rare but well documented. In the brainstem, abnormalities can be found in the vestibular nuclei, the roof nuclei of the cerebellum, and that part of the reticular formation which regulates autonomic, respiratory, and circulatory functions.

Chronically active neural lesions do not follow poliomyelitis. In patients dying of motor neuron disease several years after poliomyelitis (see below), the pathologic changes have a degenerative rather than inflammatory character.

Outside the nervous system, pathologic changes of myocarditis may be found. Complications and secondary effects of the illness produce abnormalities in the lungs, gastrointestinal tract, urinary tract, bones, and muscles.

Cerebrospinal Fluid. The cerebrospinal fluid (CSF) in poliomyelitis is characterized by pleocytosis, a moderate increase in protein content, and normal values for sugar and electrolytes. The pressure is not significantly elevated. As many as 10 per cent of patients may have an initially normal fluid, but persistently negative findings are rare.

The white cell counts range from 5 to 10 to as many as 3000 per milliliter in acutely ill patients. Polymorphonuclear cells predominate at first but give way to a lymphocytosis within 72 hours. The initial protein content ranges between 30 and 100 mg per 100 ml, values over 150 mg per 100 ml being unusual. After the first week of the disease, however, the CSF protein rises to 100 to 150 mg per 100 ml or more, and by this time the cell count often has returned to normal.

CLINICAL FEATURES. One would not suspect that a systemic infection was caused by poliovirus unless the virus invaded the nervous system. Furthermore, once central nervous system invasion has taken place, the severity of the naturally occurring disease still has wide limits. Poliovirus can cause a relatively mild attack of aseptic meningitis in one patient but the most fulminating acute paralytic and encephalitic processes in another, all in the same epidemic. The illness often pursues a biphasic course. The early stage is the time of viremia and dissemination of virus in the tissues. The later phase reflects the effects of later damage to the cells of the nervous system. Nothing specific characterizes the early illness of poliomyelitis; vague malaise, low-grade fever, muscular aching, and sometimes headache are accompanied by coryza or moderate gastrointestinal difficulties with anorexia, sometimes nausea, and often diarrhea. This prodromal phase may subside in one to three days or can progress directly into the major illness. If it subsides, three to ten or more days of health may pass before the patient falls ill again.

Nonparalytic Poliomyelitis. The major illness progresses with more severity and intensity. Moderate nonspecific malaise develops first, often with a sense of muscular aching or stiffness that leads to unwise exercise to "work off" the discomfort. Generalized headache appears early. Children may have coryzal symptoms. Anorexia, nausea, diarrhea, constipation, and sometimes vomiting are frequent in adolescents and adults. Chilliness is frequent, but shaking chills are rare. Other visceral symptoms are also prominent; many patients have insomnia as well as excessive and localized sweating. Some report urinary hesitancy or retention even before paralysis develops elsewhere.

As the illness progresses, *muscle pain* becomes prominent, usually antedating paralysis. Patients also complain of a deep-seated low back discomfort that repeated changes in position fail to alleviate. Occasionally, frank muscle twitching and cramping develop in the early stages of the illness, and diffuse fasciculations can be seen.

Fever ranges between 38.5 and 40° C. The pulse is elevated commensurately, usually between 100 and 120 per minute. Most patients have mild hypertension. Patients with poliomyelitis usually look acutely ill. Their skin is flushed, and the lips of those with severe illness may show a dark cherry hue, bssociated with circumoral pallor. There is usually some facial sweating, and localized sweating in dermatomes or restricted bodily parts. Many patients are restless and anxious, even at a stage when paralysis has not set in. Along with the diffuse autonomic changes of the early stages of the illness, the psychologic symptoms may reflect the widespread involvement of the brainstem reticular formation or hypothalamus.

A stiff neck and back along with tight hamstring

muscles are usually prominent in the early stages of nonparalytic or preparalytic disease. The muscles may be tender, and cutaneous hyperesthesia is often a complaint. Early in the illness, muscle stretch reflexes are often hyperactive.

Paralytic Poliomyelitis. Paralysis in poliomyelitis may develop with overwhelming rapidity, proceeding from barely detectable weakness to tetraplegia in but a few hours, or it may pursue a more indolent course in which additional weaknesses appear over a four- or five-day period. Rarely this indolent progression may last for as long as 10 to 12 days. In general, the more rapid the early progression, the more severe the eventual involvement.

The virus has a predilection for large motor neurons, with weakness about large joints usually being noted first. Spread of the disease shows no consistent pattern; although there is a tendency for adjacent spinal and brainstem segments to be involved together paralysis is nearly always asymmetric and at times widely scattered in its distribution. The lower extremities and lower trunk are involved most frequently, whereas upper extremities and cranial nerves are seriously paralyzed less often. These general incidences are of no help in predicting how the individual case will progress.

Poliomyelitis causes flaccid paralysis with the involved part becoming toneless and inert. The stretch reflexes become reduced, and then disappear. Fasciculations are inconstant and transient, and the paralyzed part is initially painless. Sensory loss does occur in acute poliomyelitis, but it is extremely rare, and in most instances the finding of reduced sensation indicates some other illness.

Bulbar Poliomyelitis. Cranial nerve paralysis may develop at any time. When bulbar palsy initiates the paralytic disease, it is a dangerous sign, for the progress of paralysis seldom halts in less than four to five days. With bulbar poliomyelitis certain signs herald trouble. During the early hours, agitation and fear may become pronounced. Delirium is prone to occur at night. Fulminating bulbar polioencephalitis can produce stupor, acute excitement, or myoclonic twitches. Nystagmus on the extremes of gaze is frequent and carries no serious significance. More severe forms of ophthalmoplegia with opsoclonia or even total external ophthalmoplegia are usually limited to fulminating cases. The pupils, if they show any abnormality at all, tend to be constricted. Funduscopic abnormalities are absent during the acute stage of the disease.

Abnormalities in the rest of the motor cranial nerves are more common than those in the oculomotor nerves. Trismus may precede paralysis of the jaw. Facial paralysis is usually restricted to one or more muscles and rarely produces a total facial diplegia. Paralysis of swallowing is the most frequent abnormality in cranial nerve function. Many such patients later show little or no residual pharyngeal weakness, implying that the acute dysfunction results from involvement of the integrating center for swallowing in the reticular formation of the medulla.

In addition to impaired swallowing, involvement of other somatic motor functions of the vagus is frequent. Muscle paralysis of the larynx creates the danger of respiratory obstruction. Total aphonia is rare, but laryngeal involvement may be so severe that the voice sounds are limited to hoarse cries. Vagal autonomic disturbances occur commonly and include anorexia, vomiting, and constipation.

Autonomic Abnormalities. Many autonomic abnormalities complicate acute poliomyelitis. Hypertension and excessive sweating have already been mentioned. Over 50 per cent of adults suffer at least transient acute urinary retention. Sialorrhea and bronchorrhea are usually profuse in patients with severe bulbar disease. The autonomic involvement in such patients sometimes progresses into fulminating elevations of blood pressure, tachycardia, and fatal pulmonary edema. Cardiac arrhythmias are frequent with bulbar poliomyelitis and consist of partial heart blocks, wandering cardiac pacemakers, supraventricular tachycardias, or auricular flutter. Electrocardiographic tracings show abnormalities in the configuration of the T waves.

DIFFERENTIAL DIAGNOSIS. Poliomyelitis is singular in producing an acute febrile illness with headache, stiff neck, and asymmetric, flaccid, multifocal, and progressive muscle paralysis. However, unless poliomyelitis invades the nervous system, it cannot be differentiated clinically from many other viral diseases producing myalgia or influenza-like symptoms. Similarly, aseptic meningitis can be caused by mumps, coxsackieviruses and echoviruses that can be identified only by tissue culture or serologic studies. Bacterial or fungal meningitides can usually be separated from nonparalytic poliomyelitis by their characteristic cerebrospinal fluid alterations, including the reduction of glucose.

Diseases in which muscle pain is combined with weakness and fever provide the greatest difficulty in diagnosis. *Acute polyneuritis* can be differentiated by the presence of sensory changes in approximately 80 per cent of cases. Furthermore, patients with polyneuritis are seldom systemically ill or febrile, and the CSF rarely shows a persistent or significant pleocytosis. Protein elevations in the CSF above 100 mg per 100 ml are frequent in polyneuritis but unusual in polio. Paralysis in poliomyelitis usually lacks the symmetry which characterizes polyneuritis. *Epidemic neuromyasthenia* (benign myalgic encephalomyelitis, Iceland disease) has many clinical similarities to early poliomyelitis. It is characterized by insidious onset, headache, fever, diffusely aching and tender muscles, and the development of muscular weakness in approximatly one quarter of the cases. The disease comes in epidemics, predominantly affects adolescents and young adults, and produces emotional instability and lassitude. However, the cerebrospinal fluid is normal, and paresthesias as well as mild sensory loss are often prominent. Paresis fails to progress to severe paralysis, and stretch reflexes are preserved. Viral, bacterial, and serologic studies have thus far failed to identify a cause for this obscure illness.

The course of *acute viral encephalitis* usually differs from poliomyelitis. Although headache and some stiff neck are present in encephalitis, such patients usually have drowsiness, lethargy, convulsions, or mental changes. There may be pupillary changes, ophthalmoplegia, or spastic pareses, but lower motor neuron involvement is absent. The cerebrospinal fluid often is normal in acute encephalitis. Specific neutralizing antibodies can be detected in the blood within seven to nine days after attacks of equine or St. Louis encephalitis.

Less frequent diagnostic problems include acute porphyria, in which fever is lacking and the cerebrospinal fluid normal, and hysteria, which commonly arises during poliomyelitis epidemics.

TREATMENT. There is no specific treatment for the poliomyelitis viral infection. Patients with known or suspected acute poliomyelitis are best kept at bed rest and should be hospitalized if signs of nervous system involvement are detected. Patients with paralytic and nonparalytic poliomyelitis are most comfortable if placed on a firm bed with the back and head supported. A low head pillow helps relieve neck pain, and a thin pad placed beneath the small of the back minimizes lumbar discomfort. Footboards to support the weight of bedclothes help to prevent foot drop.

During the acute illness, aspirin and other non-narcotic analgesics should be used for pain relief. Narcotics and sedatives, with the exception of small doses of codeine, are dangerous and should be avoided. Hot packs provide comfort to painful muscles and should be gently laid on with minimal manipulations. More vigorous physical therapy should be deferred to the convalescent phase.

Patients should be on liquid or minimal diets until their appetite returns. If necessary, parenteral fluids totaling 2000 to 2500 ml should be given in order to maintain a high fluid intake and counteract the risks of immobilization. Either indwelling or intermittent catheterization can be employed to deal with urinary retention, parasympathomimetic drugs being of little help at this stage.

COMPLICATIONS. The acute complications of poliomyelitis result mainly from damage to motor neurons and autonomic centers in the upper spinal cord and the brainstem. *Swallowing paralysis* is common in bulbar poliomyelitis and is treated by a combination of withholding oral intake and postural drainage. If respiratory failure coexists, tracheostomy should be performed. *Respiratory failure* can result from either paralysis of the muscles of breathing (peripheral failure) or damage to the respiratory centers in the medulla oblongata (central failure). The treatment in either instance is the early and effective use of artificial respiration. The management of circulatory problems in poliomyelitis is similar to their management in other diseases.

During convalescence from acute poliomyelitis, almost all catheterized patients develop infections and many subsequently develop urinary calcium phosphate stones caused by the combination of skeletal demineralization and the alkaline, infected urine. Treatment should include effective antimicrobial therapy, and stones should be prevented by a high fluid intake and turning severely paralyzed subjects. Papilledema occurs in 5 to 10 per cent of patients during convalescence and has no serious significance. A few patients develop an unexplained but usually reversible increase in various muscle weakness as late as three to four weeks after the acute disease. A more severe complication is *late motor neuron disease after poliomyelitis.* This is the uncommon but well documented occurrence of clinically typical progressive muscular atrophy or amyotrophic lateral sclerosis developing 30 to 40 years after acute paralytic poliomyelitis. The frequency of the occurrence is several times that of spontaneous motor neuron disease and strongly suggests an association between the two illnesses. The pathogenesis is unknown.

PROGNOSIS. At the peak of the acute illness it is impossible to predict accurately how much recovery will take place. Less than 10 per cent of patients with paralytic poliomyelitis die when treated with modern methods. Only a few fail to recover significant strength during convalescence. It can generally be estimated that muscle groups which function partially at the end of the acute illness will recover considerably. Recovery or improvement in areas of total paralysis is less certain. Significant improvement in strength is unusual after the end of the first year, and improvement after this time is largely a matter of learning greater skill. Muscles that show no voluntary motion by three months after the illness rarely later develop functional usefulness.

Increased neuromuscular excitability with cramping on exercise or night cramps is sometimes a more or less permanent residuum of poliomyelitis. Many patients have fasciculations at least intermittently. These are sometimes so prominent and enduring as to suggest active motor neuron disease. In most instances such fascicular activity is benign and unaccompanied by any progression of weakness.

PREVENTION. Natural infection with any of the three types of poliovirus induces lifelong immunity to the specific infecting immunotype. Proper vaccination with either the inactivated poliovirus vaccine (IVP) or the live, attenuated oral poliovirus vaccine (OPV) appears to achieve a similar result and has largely eliminated epidemic poliomyelitis from the developed countries of the world. Nevertheless public apathy and failures of vaccine delivery in the United States have combined to produce a steady decline in immunization rates in both socioeconomically advantaged and disadvantaged groups as the menace of poliomyelitis has receded from public view. These unimmunized populations remain at risk of paralytic disease.

Although full courses of immunization with both IPV and OPV provide protective levels of serum antibodies in over 90 per cent of recipients, only OPV gives substantial immunity following a single dose. Moreover, OPV elicits secretory immunity of the alimentary tract, which prevents subsequent implantation of "wild" strains of poliovirus, thereby breaking the cycle of transmission. For these reasons OPV has almost completely replaced IPV in the United States. The chief disadvantage of OPV is the rare occurrence of vaccine-associated paralytic disease, estimated to be a risk of one case in a vaccine recipient for every 11.5 million persons vaccinated and one case in a household contact for every 3.9 million persons vaccinated. Two groups are at special risk: (1) young adult household contacts with normal immune status, and (2) immunodeficient children.

Immunization against poliomyelitis should be initiated in infancy, when a three-dose series of trivalent OPV should start at approximately two months of age. The second and third doses are given at eight-week intervals thereafter. A fourth dose should be given at 12 to 18 months of age. Additional doses are desirable on entrance to the first grade of school and the seventh grade. This last dose of OPV is designed to protect these young people in later years when they become parents, because it is then that they are at greater risk of paralytic poliomyelitis. Routine immunization is no longer recommended for adults residing in the United

States. If vaccination is required because of special occupational risk or travel to areas of high endemicity, the initial immunization of adults should be with IPV. IPV is also preferred for immunodeficient children and their siblings. In the event of an outbreak of poliomyelitis, the epidemic is best aborted by the use of either trivalent or homotypic monovalent OPV.

Grist, N. R., and Bell, E. J.: Enteroviral etiology of the paralytic poliomyelitis syndrome. Arch. Environ. Health, 21:382, 1972.

Horstmann, D. M.: Lagging immunity of our children. N. Engl. J. Med., 285:1432, 1971.

Mulder, D. W., Rosenbaum, R. A., and Layton, D. P.: Late progression of poliomyelitis or forme fruste amyotrophic lateral sclerosis? Mayo Clin. Proc., 47:756, 1972.

Nightingale, E. O.: Recommendations for a national policy on poliomyelitis vaccine. N. Engl. J. Med., 297:249, 1977.

Paul, J. R.: A History of Poliomyelitis. New Haven, Yale University Press, 1971.

Price, R. W., and Plum, F.: Poliomyelitis. In Vinken, P. J., and Bruyn, G. W. (eds.): Infections of the Nervous System. Part I, Vol. 000, Handbook of Clinical Neurology. Amsterdam, North Holland Publishing Company (in press).

308.   RABIES

(Hydrophobia, Lyssa)

Hilary Koprowski

DEFINITION. Rabies is an acute infectious disease of the central nervous system to which all warm-blooded animals and man are susceptible. The virus, frequently present in the saliva of an infected host, is usually transmitted by bites, by licks, and occasionally by the respiratory route. The disease is characterized by a profound dysfunction of the central nervous system and ends usually in death.

HISTORY. Rabies is one of the oldest diseases of man. First mention of it dates to the twenty-third century B.C., when it was referred to in the pre-Mosaic Eshunna Code. In the Americas, rabies as a bat-transmitted disease fatal to man was probably first described in the sixteenth century. Since 1753, when it was first recorded, its presence has been evidenced throughout the North and South American continents.

In 1975, 64 countries in the world reported rabies (26 countries reported the absence of rabies). In most countries, dogs were the main source of bite wounds or other human contact that required treatment. Cats were the second most frequent source of exposure to rabies, with rats, squirrels, foxes, jackals, cattle, and bats a main source in several countries. On the basis of species, the total number of rabid animals reported was as follows: dogs, 18,026; cats, 1529; foxes, wolves and jackals, 10,686; bats, 73; mongooses, 234; farm animals, 33,559; and others, 2180.

The total number of human deaths from rabies reported in 1975 was 352, as compared with 294 in 1974. Of these human deaths, 68 had received antirabies treatment and 284 were untreated. However, 288,333 were reported to have received antirabies treatment in 1975. In 1975, antirabies treatment resulted in 27 paralytic reactions.

ETIOLOGY, HOST RANGE, AND EXPERIMENTAL INFECTION. Virus recovered in nature, the so-called *street virus*, is characterized by extremely variable, usually long incubation periods and by its ability to invade salivary glands as well as central nervous tissue. The term *fixed virus* is used for strains of rabies that have been adapted to laboratory animals by means of serial intracerebral passages and are characterized by their neuro-

tropism and by causing disease after a shorter incubation period. Prolonged cultivation of some strains of rabies virus in the developing chick embryo or in tissue culture has resulted in modification to the point of complete loss of pathogenicity for animals injected extraneurally.

The physicochemical properties of the virus are shown in Table 1. In addition, the virus is readily inactivated by sunlight, ultraviolet irradiation, formalin, 50 to 70 per cent alcohol, and 0.1 to 1.0 per cent quaternary ammonium compounds, bichloride of mercury, and strong acids. It is relatively resistant to phenol. In aqueous solutions, its thermal death point is reached at 56° C after an exposure of one hour. It survives desiccation from the frozen state, and rabies-infected tissue may be stored successfully at 4° C in 50 per cent glycerol saline or kept frozen at temperatures below −20° C.

All warm-blooded animals are susceptible to rabies. It is principally a disease of mammals, including bats. The virus is also pathogenic for birds, but to a lesser degree than for mammals. As far as we know, the disease is not transmissible by insects or arthropods. It has been found in all parts of the world, in all climates and seasons. The virus apparently cannot invade the body through intact skin, but infection through unabraded mucosa seems possible. An airborne transmission of infection in caves inhabited by rabid bats, as well as by inhalation of aerosolized virus in a laboratory, has been described in several human cases.

Rabbits, guinea pigs, mice, and hamsters are most commonly employed for experimental infection. Hamsters are remarkably susceptible to intramuscular infection with street virus, but intracerebral injection of mice is usually employed for diagnostic purposes.

Epizootics of rabies occur in any climate during any

TABLE 1.   Specific Biologic Activities, Gross Chemical Composition, and Some Physical Properties of Purified Rabies Virus

Property	Observation
Specific infectivity	1×10^{10}–5×10^{10} PFU/mg protein
Specific hemagglutinating activity	10^4 HAU/mg protein
Specific complement-fixing activity	5×10^3 CFU/mg protein
Gross chemical composition	22% lipids 3% carbohydrates 1% RNA 74% protein
Virus structural proteins	Four major proteins, one of which is a glycoprotein and the other a phosphoprotein
Sedimentation coefficient	600 S
Buoyant density in sucrose solution	1.17 grams per cm³
Genome	Single-stranded RNA, 4.6×10^6 daltons molecular weight

PFU = Plaque-forming unit.
HAU = Hemagglutinating unit.
CFU = Complement-fixing unit.

season of the year. Wars and mass movements of men and animals favor the geographic spread of the disease. Man becomes an accidental host upon exposure to the infected saliva of the biting animal, and wild animals are often sources of human rabies. The attack rate in man, after exposure, depends to a certain extent on the location and on the severity of the inflicted wounds. Head and neck bites lead to a higher incidence of infection than bites on other parts of the body. The bites of rabid wolves are apparently very dangerous; an attack rate of 47 per cent was observed in 32 persons who were bitten by the same animal and did not receive antirabies treatment in time to be of any protective value.

PATHOLOGY. At autopsy, the brain is friable, edematous, and congested; the convolutions are broad and flattened. Severe vascular congestion of the white and gray matter may extend to the medulla and the spinal cord. Virus-infected salivary glands are usually soft and swollen. On microscopic examination of the central nervous system, the nonspecific findings consist of hyperemia, perivascular and perineuronal infiltration with mononuclear cells, and considerable neuronal degeneration. Mononuclear cell infiltration of periacinal interstitial tissue accompanied by degeneration of acinar cells may be observed in the parotid and sublingual and submaxillary salivary glands.

In the absence of Negri bodies (see below), the lesions are indistinguishable from those observed in some of the other viral encephalitides. The exact nature of the virus-host relationship is unknown.

INCUBATION. The incubation period in man varies from ten days to over twelve months. As minor and seemingly insignificant contacts with rabies virus in the saliva of an animal not obviously sick at the time of exposure are sometimes forgotten, claims of extended incubation periods (one to two years) have to be critically evaluated. In dogs, signs of rabies may appear after an incubation period of ten days to several months.

The length of the incubation period is related to the amount of virus introduced at the time of exposure and to the severity of the laceration. The *site* of the original exposure does not seem to affect the duration of the incubation period.

CLINICAL MANIFESTATIONS. Dogs. In dogs the prodromal phase of the disease lasts two to three days and consists of fever, anorexia, and, very frequently, a change in the tone of the bark. However, these signs are often so slight that only a trained observer may note them. The animal's disposition is altered, and symptoms give way to the excitation phase, usually lasting three to seven days, during which time the animal grows unnaturally restless and agitated. General tremor owing to stimulation of the muscular system appears frequently. In the furious type of the disease, agitation intensifies as the illness progresses. The animal, erratic and aggressive, growls and barks constantly. It will grab viciously at any object or animal encountered. At this stage, an unrestrained animal sometimes leaves home and travels great distances, inflicting damage on other animals and humans along the way. Convulsive seizures are often observed, and the animal may become completely paralyzed. In many cases, however, the excitation phase predominates until the time of death.

In the paralytic type of rabies, the excitation phase may be slight or totally absent, and the disease is characterized only by the paralytic syndrome. Paralysis of the lower jaw, accompanied by excessive salivation, appears as an early symptom, and the animal acts as though it were choking on a foreign body. Paralysis of the muscles of phonation may lead to loss of the bark. As the disease progresses, paralysis of the posterior extremities sets in, followed by general paralysis and death. The time from the onset of the disease to the death of the animal ranges from one to eleven days. On the other hand, dogs may die suddenly without noticeable signs of illness.

Man. In man, the prodromal phase is marked by fever, anorexia, headache, malaise, nausea, and sore throat. *Abnormal sensations around the site of infection*, such as intermittent pain, tingling, or burning, are of diagnostic significance. Extreme stimulation of the general sensory system is manifested by hyperesthesia of the skin to temperature changes and to drafts, and by acute sensitiveness to sound and light. Other symptoms include increased muscular tonus, prompt gag and corneal reflexes, dilation of pupils, and increased salivation.

As the disease progresses, spasmodic contractions of the muscles of the mouth, pharynx, and larynx on drinking — and later at the mere sight of fluid — are observed in the majority of cases. This dysfunction of deglutition gave the disease its common name, *hydrophobia*, or fear of water. Spasms of respiratory muscles and convulsive seizures leading to opisthotonos also may occur. The pulse is very rapid. Periods of irrational and often maniacal behavior are interspersed with those of alertness and responsiveness. Paralysis of the muscles of phonation may lead to hoarseness or loss of voice.

The excitation phase may remain predominant until the time of death. However, in many cases it gives way shortly before death to cessation of muscle spasms, to hyporeflexia or areflexia, and to general paralysis of the flaccid type.

In rabies in man *resulting from vampire bat infection*, the excitation phase is almost totally absent, and the disease is characterized by ascending paralysis without hydrophobia. Without an adequate history of exposure, clinical diagnosis of this type of infection may be difficult.

DIAGNOSIS. Profound dysfunction of the central nervous system, accompanied by impairment in deglutition, in persons who either were exposed to a bite or lick of any animal or may have recently visited caves harboring bats, facilitates the clinical diagnosis. Isolation of virus from saliva obtained in the course of the disease and from brain tissue obtained at autopsy, followed by proper identification of the agent by means of neutralization test, will confirm the diagnosis. Syrian hamsters, rabbits, guinea pigs, and, preferably, suckling mice are used for diagnostic purposes. Demonstration of rabies virus antigen in smears of brain tissue obtained from either patient or animal (preferably brainstem, cerebellum, or Ammon's horn) by means of specific staining with antibody coupled with fluorescein isothiocyanate is of diagnostic significance. The presence of intracytoplasmic inclusion bodies in the neuron (Negri bodies) is pathognomonic, but their absence does not exclude the diagnosis of rabies, as the presence of virus may be demonstrated by other means.

PROGNOSIS. Although inapparent infection with

street virus may be induced artificially in laboratory animals, and although animals have recovered completely after exhibiting signs of the disease, there are only two cases reported of the recovery of a human from rabies after showing signs of disease. In all other reported cases, the disease proved fatal to humans.

TREATMENT. General Considerations. Confinement and observation of the biting animal, preferably under the supervision of a veterinarian, for a period of not less than ten days for dogs and cats, is one of the most important steps in deciding whether an individual has been exposed to rabies. Biting wild animals should be sacrificed and their brain tissue examined properly by immunofluorescent staining. Treatment of severely exposed persons should be started without awaiting results of the laboratory diagnosis. If the absence of rabies infection in the biting animal is reported, treatment may be stopped.

Local Treatment of Wounds. Since the most effective available mechanism of protection against rabies is the elimination of the virus at the site of infection, all bite wounds, as well as scratches and other abrasions exposed to licks of animals, should be treated immediately by thorough cleansing and adequate mechanical flushing of the wound with soap solution followed by treatment with substances such as 40 to 70 per cent alcohol, tincture or aqueous solutions of iodine, or 0.1 per cent quaternary ammonium compounds, which are lethal to rabies virus. If debridement is necessary, infiltration with local anesthetics is not contraindicated. Bite wounds should *not* be sutured immediately. After determination of sensitivity to antirabies serum, the serum should be used in local application upon the wound.

Preliminary application of antimicrobial drugs is of no value as a prophylactic measure. However, antitetanus treatment and local application of antiseptics and antimicrobials should be instituted if indicated.

Indications for Specific Treatment. These are summarized in Table 2, prepared by the Expert Committee on Rabies of the World Health Organization. Emphasis

is placed on the condition of the biting animal at the time of exposure and during the ensuing ten days. It is assumed that the saliva of an animal that is not obviously ill at the time of exposure may be infectious during a maximal period of five days preceding the appearance of clinical signs of the disease.

New Human Vaccine. Plans have been well under way to have a new human rabies vaccine licensed in the United States. This human diploid cell vaccine, licensed in Europe and other countries, was used successfully in postexposure treatment of 45 Iranians who all survived after exposure to severe wolf and dog bites. This vaccine should be used preferentially for post- and pre-exposure immunization because it is more immunogenic than the currently available avian embryo vaccines and shows no side effects in contrast to the nervous tissue vaccines. The vaccine is administered either subcutaneously or intramuscularly in the upper arm. A single dose consists of 1 ml.

Administration of Postexposure Treatment. Passive-active immunization by the administration of antirabies serum of animal or human origin and immunogenically potent vaccine in repeated doses is the most effective protective specific treatment of the exposed persons. Experience indicates that vaccine alone is sufficient for minor exposures (see Table 2). Serum should be given in a single dose — 40 IU per kilogram of body weight for heterologous serum, and 20 IU for human antirabies gamma globulin; the first dose of vaccine is inoculated at the same time as the serum but at another site. Sensitivity to heterologous serum must be determined before its administration.

The human diploid cell vaccine (see above) is at present recommended to be given on days 0 (the day treatment begins), 3, 7, 14, 30, and 90. *All* other vaccines should be given daily for 14 consecutive days, with a booster inoculation given 10, 20, and 90 days after the regular course of vaccine. Treatments should be started as early as possible after exposure, but in no case should it be denied to exposed persons arriving late. In areas in which antirabies serum is not available, full

TABLE 2. Specific Systemic Treatment

| | Status of Biting Animal Irrespective of Previous Vaccination | | |
Nature of Exposure	At Time of Exposure	During 10 Days*	Recommended Treatment†
I. Contact, but no lesions; Indirect contact; no contact	Rabid	—	None
II. Licks of the skin; scratches or abrasions; minor bites (covered areas of arms, trunk, and legs)	(a) Suspected as rabid†	Healthy	Start vaccine; stop treatment if animal remains healthy for five days*‡
		Rabid	Start vaccine; administer serum upon positive diagnosis and complete the course of vaccine
	(b) Rabid; wild animal§ or animal unavailable for observation		Serum + vaccine
III. Licks of mucosa; major bites (multiple or on face, head, finger, or neck)	Suspect† or rabid domestic or wild animal,§ or animal unavailable for observation		Serum + vaccine; stop treatment if animal remains healthy for five days*‡

*Observation period in this chart applies only to dogs and cats.
†All unprovoked bites in endemic areas should be considered suspect unless proved negative by laboratory examination (brain FA).
‡Or if its brain is found negative by FA examination.
§In general, exposure to rodents and rabbits seldom if ever requires specific antirabies treatment.
FA = Fluorescent antigen.

vaccine therapy, including three booster inoculations, should be administered.

The administration of preventive treatment may give rise to local allergic reactions, to serum sickness (if combined serum-vaccine therapy is used), and to nervous system reactions (if vaccines containing nervous tissue are used). Treatment should then be either interrupted or continued with vaccines of non-nervous tissue origin. Many problems can be avoided if treatment is given only when specifically indicated (Table 2).

Treatment Once Clinical Signs Are Apparent. Although no specific therapeutic measures are available to save the life of a person exhibiting symptoms of the disease, the survival of two patients with human rabies indicates that all the tools of modern medicine should be used in the attempt to save the patient's life. These therapeutic measures should consist of (1) starting treatment immediately after signs of rabies appear; (2) placing the patient in the intensive medical care unit in a quiet environment, with constant monitoring to prevent cardiac failure; (3) using sedatives for the relief of anxiety and pain; (4) performing a tracheostomy and applying artificial breathing to maintain respiratory function; (5) using curare-like drugs to alleviate spastic muscular contractions if they occur; and (6) instituting intravenous perfusions and administering diuretics to assure proper hydration and diuresis. *Note:* Since rabies virus may be present in the saliva of the patient exhibiting signs of the disease, all attending personnel should be protected against contamination through the use of goggles, masks, and rubber gloves.

PRE-EXPOSURE IMMUNIZATION. Preferably, human diploid cell vaccine or, if that is not available, any other patent vaccine free from paralytic factors is recommended to be given at 1, 7, and 21 days to persons engaged in veterinary practice, experimental surgery involving handling of dogs and cats, spelunking, dog catching, or any other activity involving unusually high risk of exposure. The vaccinated person should be bled one month after the last vaccination to check the sera for the presence of antirabies antibodies. Such persons upon exposure may be given one booster dose of a *potent* vaccine. Persons without antibody should receive full treatment if re-exposed to rabies.

CONTROL MEASURES. Although the presence of rabies-infected bats in the Northern Hemisphere presents a difficult problem for rabies control, most human exposure can be prevented by the use of control measures that will rid an area of enzootics or epizootics of rabies.

The following measures should be applied in an efficiently organized rabies control program conducted by public health authorities: control of the canine population (registration, restraint, elimination of stray dogs), reduction in number of susceptible dogs by mass vaccination, reduction in number of wildlife species that are a reservoir of the virus, and continuous educational campaigns for the general public.

Baer, G. M. (ed.): The natural history of rabies, Vols. I and II. New York, Academic Press, 1973.

Bahmanyar, M., Fayaz, A., Nour-Salehi, S., Mohammadi, M., and Koprowski, H.: Successful protection of humans exposed to rabies infection. JAMA, 236:2751, 1976.

Expert Committee on Rabies: Sixth Report. WHO Techn. Rep. Ser., No. 523, 1973.

Hattwick, M. A. W., Weis, T. T., Stechschulte, C. J., Baer, G. M., and Gregg, M. B.: Recovery from rabies. A case report. Ann. Intern. Med., 76:931, 1972.

Hummeler, K., and Koprowski, H.: Investigating the rabies virus. Nature, 221:418, 1969.

Johnson, H. N.: Rabies. In Horsfall, F. L., Jr., and Tamm, I. (eds.): Viral and Rickettsial Infections of Man. 4th ed. Philadelphia, J. B. Lippincott Company, 1965.

Kaplan, M., and Koprowski, H. (eds.): Laboratory Techniques in Rabies. 3rd ed. Geneva, World Health Organization, 1973.

309. ENCEPHALITIC COMPLICATIONS OF VIRAL INFECTIONS AND VACCINES

Donald Silberberg

309.1. INTRODUCTION

Acute disseminated encephalomyelitis may be associated with banal viral diseases or may follow immunization. Neuroparalytic accidents following antirabies vaccination resemble acute disseminated encephalomyelitis, but specifically follow immunization against rabies. Reye's syndrome seems to be related to banal viral infections, but has distinctive features. Despite some points in common, these entities are best considered separately.

309.2. ACUTE DISSEMINATED ENCEPHALOMYELITIS

DEFINITION. Acute disseminated encephalomyelitis (postinfectious encephalomyelitis, postvaccinal encephalomyelitis, acute perivascular myelinoclasis, acute hemorrhagic leukoencephalitis) is an acute or subacute disease of the central nervous system which most commonly occurs after viral infections that do not normally affect the nervous system, or as a complication of immunization. Involvement of the brain and spinal cord may be widespread, or may be limited to discrete areas, such as optic nerves (optic neuritis, papillitis) or a single spinal cord level (transverse myelitis). Acute disseminated encephalomyelitis is characterized by varying degrees of perivenous mononuclear cellular infiltration and demyelination.

ETIOLOGY AND PATHOGENESIS. Predisposing factors include exposure to measles, mumps, varicella, rubella, influenza, infectious mononucleosis, smallpox, and banal upper respiratory infections. Similar disease has been associated with pertussis, tetanus, streptococcal infections, and mycoplasma pneumonia. Acute disseminated encephalomyelitis also follows immunization against smallpox, rabies, influenza, and tetanus. Disease occurring after immunization is often termed *postvaccination encephalomyelitis*, and the central nervous system disease which may follow immunization against smallpox with attenuated vaccinia virus is termed *postvaccinal encephalomyelitis*.

The neurologic complications of childhood viral diseases usually occur 4 to 18 days after the appearance of a skin rash or other systemic signs. However, encephalomyelitis can occur before, concomitant with, and even in the absence of systemic signs of viral infection.

The pathogenesis of acute disseminated encephalomyelitis may be viewed as the direct consequence of viral infection, as an immune disorder, or as the result of interaction of these two mechanisms. Historically an immune pathogenesis was considered first because of the histopathologic resemblance of acute disseminated encephalomyelitis to neuroparalytic accidents following antirabies vaccination and to experimental allergic encephalomyelitis (see Ch. 309.3).

There have been few attempts to recover an infectious agent from the central nervous system of patients with acute disseminated encephalomyelitis, using modern virologic techniques. Measles virus was isolated from the brain of a patient with postmeasles acute disseminated encephalomyelitis, using co-cultivation techniques. The patient's brain contained the typical histologic features of acute disseminated encephalomyelitis. Long after vaccination, vaccinia virus was isolated from the cerebrospinal fluid of a number of patients without neurologic symptoms, suggesting that persistent virus may play a role in postvaccinal encephalomyelitis. Mumps virus may be isolated from cerebrospinal fluid during the first few days of systemic illness in over half the patients.

At present no definite direct evidence exists for primary immune pathogenesis of human acute disseminated encephalomyelitis, except for the form that follows rabies immunization (see Ch. 308 and 309.3). However, several observations demonstrate that immune alterations occur in the course of the disorder. In the acute stages of disease, peripheral blood lymphocytes from patients show positive transformation on stimulation with homologous myelin basic protein. This may correlate with observations of lymphoblasts in the peripheral blood of similar patients. Cerebrospinal fluid lymphocytes from patients with acute disseminated encephalomyelitis also show an enhanced response to myelin basic protein, as do cerebrospinal fluid lymphocytes from patients with acute and progressive multiple sclerosis. These observations may relate to the liberation of myelin basic protein into cerebrospinal fluid, as has been shown in patients with multiple sclerosis.

INCIDENCE. Approximately 30 per cent of the reported cases of encephalitis in the United States are associated with childhood diseases. The incidence of neurologic complications may vary from epidemic to epidemic, but is approximately 1:1000 cases in measles, 1:5000 in rubella, and 1:8000 in scarlet fever, and probably exceeds these figures in pertussis. The fact that abnormalities in the electroencephalogram occur in approximately 50 per cent of neurologically uncomplicated cases of measles suggests that asymptomatic involvement of the nervous system is common. A variety of neurologic complications occur in approximately 1 per cent of patients with infectious mononucleosis, but acute disseminated encephalomyelitis is rare. In general, males are affected more frequently than females, approximating a ratio of 2:1 in some series. Infants younger than two years of age and the elderly are rarely affected; the age incidence reflects the age incidence of the precipitating disease.

Mumps resembles lymphocytic choriomeningitis in its central nervous system involvement. An increase of cells in cerebrospinal fluid is common in neurologically asymptomatic children with mumps. As many as 18 per cent of patients with mumps have convulsions, and

signs of meningeal irritation are frequent. Despite this, the incidence of acute disseminated encephalomyelitis associated with mumps remains low.

Postvaccinal encephalomyelitis, which is practically unknown in infants under two years of age, occurred in 17 of 800,000 people who were vaccinated during the 1962 epidemic of smallpox in South Wales, suggesting an over-all incidence of approximately 1 in 50,000 vaccinations. Several other series report similar figures. There is a greater incidence of postvaccinal complications after primary vaccination than after revaccination, with the highest incidence among children of school age (3 per 100,000). A long interval between primary vaccination and revaccination increases the incidence.

PATHOLOGY. The basic lesion in acute disseminated encephalomyelitis is the presence of mononuclear cells around small veins, chiefly in white matter, but to a lesser extent in gray matter as well. This is accompanied by varying degrees of perivenous demyelination. Individual lesions are scattered and rarely coalesce to give large lesions. Severe cases may include destruction of axons and nerve cell bodies, serous exudate, fibrin impregnation of vessel walls, polymorphonuclear infiltration, and hemorrhages. The inclusion of hemorrhages as well describes acute hemorrhagic leukoencephalitis.

CLINICAL MANIFESTATIONS AND COURSE. Acute disseminated encephalomyelitis usually begins with fever, headache, vomiting, and drowsiness. This is quickly followed by depressed consciousness and often coma. Irritability, behavior disturbances, and convulsions are common. Multifocal signs, including ataxia, involuntary movements, paralyses of one or more extremities, visual impairment, or other focal neurologic signs occur, often accompanied by signs of meningeal irritation. Lesions restricted to the optic nerves producing optic papillitis or retrobulbar neuritis occur. The duration of symptoms varies from a few days to weeks and sometimes months.

Myelitis predominates in approximately 10 per cent of instances. The lesion may affect only one cord level (transverse myelitis), or may progress to involve the entire spinal cord, producing successive backache, urinary retention, paraparesis, paraplegia, quadriplegia, and bulbar signs.

The cerebrospinal fluid may be normal or may show increased pressure and pleocytosis up to 1000 cells per cubic millimeter. The cell counts usually range from 15 to 250. Most cells are mononuclear, although polymorphonuclear cells may predominate during the first several days of illness. Approximately 60 to 70 per cent of patients with neurologic complications have pleocytosis, but over 10 per cent of patients with neurologically uncomplicated exanthemata also have pleocytosis. Cerebrospinal fluid protein may be normal and rarely exceeds 100 mg per 100 ml. The cerebrospinal fluid changes have no prognostic significance and no relation to the type or severity of neurologic disorder. The electroencephalogram is almost always diffusely abnormally slow.

Neurologic manifestations may precede signs of systemic infection by up to ten days or follow signs of systemic infection by up to 24 days. The average latent period is about five days. The occurrence and severity of neurologic symptoms appear to bear no relation to the severity of the systemic disease.

The immediate and long-term prognosis varies somewhat with the individual virus. Encephalitis associated with rubella, measles, and mumps has a higher mortality (20 to 50 per cent) than in scarlet fever (13 per cent) or varicella (10 per cent). Sequelae are most common in scarlet fever (45 per cent) and measles (35 per cent), and less so in varicella (20 per cent) and rubella (2 to 5 per cent). The clinical sign which correlates best with prognosis is the level of consciousness.

DIAGNOSIS. Identification of acute disseminated encephalomyelitis is not difficult when neurologic symptoms are preceded by a recognizable viral illness. Differential diagnosis includes acute infectious encephalitis and acute multiple sclerosis. Encephalitis caused by neurotropic viruses is almost always accompanied by increased cells and protein in the cerebrospinal fluid which are often lacking in acute disseminated encephalomyelitis. Fever and meningeal signs are rare in multiple sclerosis. Correct diagnosis in the absence of precipitating illness may depend entirely on direct virus isolation from all possible sites and by serum antibody determinations during the course of the illness in an attempt to detect evidence of a virus infection. Fatal cases provide the opportunity for attempts at direct recovery of virus.

TREATMENT. Corticosteroid therapy appears to produce improvement in some patients with acute disseminated encephalomyelitis. However, no controlled studies have been feasible because of the low frequency of cases, and there is no convincing evidence to support the use of steroids in the absence of increased intracranial pressure. Appropriate measures to reduce increased intracranial pressure, including intravenous mannitol, high doses of corticosteroids, and hyperventilation, may be required to sustain life during severe acute illness. Appropriate symptomatic support include reduction of fever with aspirin, the use of anticonvulsants and antimicrobial drugs when indicated (such as for pneumonia), and management of fluid and electrolyte balance.

PREVENTION. Initial smallpox vaccination during infancy reduces the danger of postvaccinal disease. The use of measles, mumps, and pertussis vaccines to induce active immunity to these diseases will reduce the frequency of acute disseminated encephalomyelitis.

Alvord, E. C.: Acute disseminated encephalomyelitis and "allergic" neuroencephalopathies. *In* Vinken, P. J., and Bruyn, G. W. (Eds.): Handbook of Clinical Neurology. New York, American Elsevier Publishing Company, 1970, Vol. 9, pp. 500–571.

Cohen, S. R., Herndon, R. M., and McKhann, G. M.: Radioimmunoassay of myelin basic protein in spinal fluid. N. Engl. J. Med., 295:1455, 1976.

Lisak, R. P., Behan, P. O., Zweiman, B., and Shetty, T.: Cell-mediated immunity to myelin basic protein in acute disseminated encephalomyelitis. Neurology, 24:560, 1974.

Lisak, R. P., and Zweiman, B.: In vitro cell-mediated immunity of cerebrospinal fluid lymphocytes to myelin basic protein in primary demyelinating diseases. N. Engl. J. Med. 297:1207, 1977.

ter Mullen, V., Kackell, Y., Muller, D., Katz, M., and Meyermann, R.: Isolation of infectious measles virus in measles encephalitis. Lancet, 2:1172, 1972.

309.3. NEUROPARALYTIC ACCIDENTS FOLLOWING ANTIRABIES VACCINATION

The production of neurologic disease is a dreaded complication of immunization against rabies. Neuro-

paralytic accidents following antirabies vaccination include a disease which resembles acute disseminated encephalomyelitis in its clinical manifestations and histology, and, less commonly, the Guillain-Barré syndrome. These complications are clearly related to the presence of brain tissue or other neural antigens in the vaccines. As vaccines produced in tissue cultures of human diploid cells replace the nervous tissue vaccines, the neurologic complications of antirabies vaccination described in this chapter should disappear (see Ch. 308).

The over-all incidence of postvaccinal encephalomyelitis varies from 1 in 2000 to 1 in 9000 of those receiving brain-containing vaccines. Practically no cases occur in young chidren, but as many as 1 per cent of young adults (20 to 40 years) developed encephalomyelitis after immunization with neural vaccines. The incidence after immunization against rabies with vaccines prepared in avian embryos is low, approximating 1 in 50,000.

With rare exceptions in which live rabies virus was accidentally introduced with vaccines, the pathogenesis of encephalomyelitis following antirabies vaccination seems to be immunologic. The low incidence and the age-related incidence strongly suggest that immune responsiveness plays a role in disease production. In addition, an experimental disease which is very similar histologically, experimental allergic encephalomyelitis (EAE), can be induced in a variety of animals by injection of homologous or heterologous brain tissue or myelin basic protein.

Encephalomyelitis following antirabies vaccination may be divided into encephalitic and myelitic forms. Both are distinguished by widely spread foci of demyelination and cellular infiltration throughout white and gray matter, but more pronounced in white matter. Brain lesions (encephalitic form) tend to be larger, and many are periventricular as well as perivenous. These lesions closely resemble plaques of multiple sclerosis. More acute lesions are distinguished by perivenous mononuclear cell invasion. Axis cylinders are spared in most instances. The myelitis form resembles acute disseminated encephalomyelitis, with smaller scattered areas of perivenous demyelination and cellular infiltration.

The interval from the last injection to the onset of symptoms averages 15 days with the myelitis form, and about 35 days with the encephalitic form. Headache, fatigue, and changes in mental function commonly precede the appearance of such focal neurologic signs as visual disturbance, hemiplegia, or paraplegia. Progression of neurologic signs and symptoms may proceed for days or weeks. Mortality is approximately 20 per cent, but most cases were reported before the availability of corticosteroids which may increase survival. Permanent sequelae occur, including changes in mentation or behavior.

If any signs of the possible development of encephalomyelitis develop during a course of immunization against rabies with a nervous tissue vaccine, immunization should be stopped. High doses of corticosteroids may be effective in reducing the morbidity of the acute process.

Immunization against rabies should be undertaken only when it is reasonably certain that there has been a bite by a rabid animal. Vaccines prepared in human diploid cells are unlikely to produce postvaccinal encephalomyelitis (see Ch. 308).

Shiraki, H.: The comparative study of rabies post-vaccinal encephalomyelitis and demyelinating encephalomyelitis of unknown origin with special reference to the Japanese cases. *In* Bailey, O. T., and Smith D. E. (eds.): The Central Nervous System: Some Experimental Models of Neurological Diseases. Baltimore, Williams & Wilkins Company, 1968, pp. 87–123.

309.4. REYE'S SYNDROME

DEFINITION. Reye's syndrome describes an acute and often fatal encephalopathy of childhood that is characterized by acute brain swelling associated with fatty infiltration and dysfunction of the liver. Reye's syndrome may follow a variety of common viral infections.

ETIOLOGY AND PATHOGENESIS. Reye's syndrome has been reported after infections with influenza B, varicella, adenovirus type 3, coxsackievirus A and B, reovirus, echovirus, herpes simplex, and parainfluenza. Viral infection is suggested as the initiating factor by recovery of virus from a few patients, by the frequency of varicella as the prodromal illness in sporadic cases, and by the reported increased incidence concurrently with outbreaks of influenza B infection in two epidemiologic studies. The pathogenic relationship between virus infection and the encephalopathy and hepatic injury is unknown.

It is possible that the encephalopathy is secondary to metabolic effects of the hepatic lesion. The combination of hypoglycemia and ammonia retention, together with other abnormalities of intermediary metabolism, may be sufficient to produce the coma and cerebral edema which occur. The early occurrence of mitochondrial abnormalities in liver and brain suggests that induction of a partially reversible mitochondrial injury may be instrumental.

INCIDENCE. Reye's syndrome occurs in children 6 months to 15 years of age. Approximatley 1000 cases have been reported. Large series have been described from Australia, Canada, Thailand, and the United States. It occurs both as a sporadic, rare disease, and in minor outbreaks in a particular area. It is a leading cause of death in children one to six years old in Thailand, where it is associated with ingestion of the fungal toxin, aflatoxin.

PATHOLOGY. Marked cerebral edema occurs, with astrocyte swelling, myelin bleb formation, and injury of neuronal mitochondria which resembles the concurrent mitochondrial changes seen in the liver. The liver is swollen and orange to pale yellow. Fatty infiltration occurs initially as diffuse small vacuoles in the periportal areas, and spreads to cause massive involvement in fatal cases. Electron microscopic examination of liver biopsy specimens shows swollen pleomorphic mitochondria and small droplets of triglycerides in hepatocytes. Fat deposition also occurs in the renal tubules and in the myocardium.

CLINICAL MANIFESTATIONS AND COURSE. Typically, Reye's syndrome starts with an upper respiratory infection or mild gastrointestinal disturbance. A symptom-free interval of hours to several days is followed by persistent vomiting and then by delirium and coma. Convulsions are common. Hyperpnea or irregular deep respiration is common. There are no meningeal or focal neurologic signs. Decerebrate posturing may occur as

increased intracranial pressure supervenes. Mild to moderate hepatomegaly is the only clinical suggestion of hepatic involvement, and even this is lacking in 50 per cent of cases.

Hypoglycemia is found less frequently now (5 per cent) than when the syndrome was first described. Cerebrospinal fluid protein is normal. Elevation of serum transaminases, hyperammonemia, and prolongation of the prothrombin time reflect hepatic damage. Bilirubin levels rise in a minority of patients. Hypocapnia, hyponatremia, and hypokalemia are common. Elevation of plasma free fatty acid levels reflects an initial impairment of fatty acid oxidation.

Deepening coma leading to death occurs in 25 to 50 per cent of patients. More recent reports indicate the lower mortality rates, both because of improved management and because milder cases are being diagnosed. Severe neurologic sequelae, such as mental impairment, seizures, or hemiplegia, occur in some survivors.

DIAGNOSIS. The diagnosis of Reye's syndrome is suggested by the clinical manifestations described above. Biopsy or autopsy demonstration of fatty infiltration of the liver is confirmatory but usually unnecessary.

TREATMENT. Treatment is empirical. Hypoglycemia and electrolyte disturbances should be corrected. Enemas, neomycin and low protein intake as employed in hepatic encephalopathy are commonly used. Peritoneal dialysis and exchange transfusions have been used to correct refractory metabolic abnormalities and to correct clotting factor deficiencies. Corticosteroids, mannitol, hyperventilation, and exchange transfusion may be used to reduce intracranial pressure.

Partin, J. C., Partin, J. S., Schubert, W. K., and McLaurin, W.: Brain ultrastructure in Reye's syndrome. J. Neuropathol. Exp. Neurol., 34:425, 1975.

Reye, R. D. K., Morgan, G., and Baral, J.: Encephalopathy and fatty degeneration of the viscera: A disease entity of childhood. Lancet, 2:749, 1963.

Schiff, G. M.: Reye's syndrome. Ann. Rev. Med., 27:447, 1976.

310. SLOW INFECTIONS OF THE NERVOUS SYSTEM

Richard T. Johnson

310.1. INTRODUCTION

Recently, slow viral infections have been related to several chronic and subacute neurologic diseases in which clinical signs of infection are lacking and in which the pathologic changes are those of degenerative or demyelinative processes. The term slow infection was originally coined in the veterinary literature to describe several transmissible diseases of sheep. Two of these sheep diseases, *scrapie* and *visna*, are the prototypes of slow infections of the nervous system. Both these diseases are transmissible. After inoculation of sheep with tissue from an affected sheep, there is a latent period of one to four years during which the sheep appear well. This is followed by the insidious onset of neurologic signs which progress without fever from one to six months and lead inevitably to death. Scrapie is clinically characterized primarily by ataxia and visna by progressive paralysis. Pathologically the diseases are very different. The lesions of scrapie are confined to the nervous system, where there is marked proliferation of astrocytes and the degeneration of neurons with vacuolization of their cytoplasms. By contrast, central nervous system lesions of visna are characterized by marked inflammation and demyelination. The agents responsible for these two slow infections of sheep are also very different. The scrapie agent has been transmitted to a variety of other animals, but the agent does not cause cytopathic changes in cell culture, and no virus-like particles have been found in infectious tissue by electron microscopy. The infectivity of this tissue remains remarkably stable on exposure to physicochemical treatments which inactivate classic viruses. Furthermore, animals naturally or experimentally infected with scrapie fail to develop any evidence of an immune response against the agent. In contrast, the visna virus is an enveloped RNA retrovirus. Although transmissible from sheep to sheep, it has not been transmitted to other animals but can be grown in a variety of tissue cultures. Of the four slow infections of the human central nervous system described below, kuru and Creutzfeldt-Jakob disease resemble scrapie pathologically, and the agents responsible for these diseases have properties similar to those described for the scrapie agent. Therefore scrapie, kuru, and Creutzfeldt-Jakob disease have been classified together as the subacute spongiform encephalopathies. Subacute sclerosing panencephalitis and progressive multifocal leukoencephalopathy, like visna, are due to classic viruses. These viruses have been visualized by electron microscopy, are antigenic in natural and experimental hosts, and can produce rapid cytolytic infection in some cell cultures even though they are capable of causing slow infections in man.

310.2.   KURU

Kuru is an endemic disease of Melanesian tribal people inhabiting a remote area of the Eastern Highlands of central New Guinea. The disease has been seen only among the Fore linguistic group and several neighboring groups with whom the Fore have intermarried. However, within this limited area, kuru, until recently, was the most common cause of death. The disease predominantly affected adult women, but children over age five were also affected but without sexual predilection. Adult males were least involved. The disease begins insidiously with unsteadiness of stance and gait. A progressive symmetrical cerebellar ataxia develops over a period of months and follows a relentless, afebrile course until the patient is unable to make the slightest movement without violent ataxic tremors. Late in the course of the disease, abnormalities of extraocular movement and mental changes develop. The disease invariably leads to death in three to six months. Extensive laboratory examinations have failed to show any abnormalities, and the cerebrospinal fluid remains normal. Pathologic changes are confined to the brain where there is a marked increase of astrocytes and degeneration of neurons with cytoplasmic vacuolization. The brain is diffusely affected, but the findings are most prominent in the cerebellum and pons and, to a

lesser degree, in the hypothalamus and basal ganglia. Inflammation is not found.

Because of the similarities between kuru and scrapie in terms of epidemiology, clinical progression, and pathologic changes, brain tissue from patients dying of kuru was inoculated into a variety of primates for long-term observations. After incubation periods of 18 months to 4 years, a similar disease developed in chimpanzees, and this disease has subsequently been transmitted from chimpanzee to chimpanzee and to several other species of primates. The agent can be transmitted with serial dilutions, proving that it replicates within the primate host. However, like scrapie, the agent of kuru has not been seen by electron microscopy, does not induce cytopathic changes in cell culture, is resistant to physical and chemical treatments that usually inactivate viruses, and fails to evoke a demonstrable immune response in man or experimentally infected primates.

In recent years, there has been a striking decline in the incidence of kuru, particularly among children, in whom the disease has disappeared. This decreasing incidence has coincided with the suppression of cannibalism is this primitive culture, and there is considerable circumstantial evidence indicating that kuru was transmitted during the practice of ritual cannibalism.

310.3.   CREUTZFELDT-JAKOB DISEASE

Creutzfeldt-Jakob disease is an uncommon form of rapidly progressive dementia accompanied by myoclonus and other neurologic signs. The disease usually develops between ages 40 and 65, is worldwide in distribution, and usually occurs sporadically, although a few familial cases have been reported. The dementia develops rapidly, so that deterioration from day to day or week to week is evident. Myoclonic jerks usually develop early in the disease, and often massive symmetrical myoclonic jerks of the limbs occur when the patient is startled by unexpected light or sounds. Pyramidal tract signs, cerebellar ataxia, visual disturbances, and muscle wasting with fasciculations are common but inconstant features. The disease is inexorably progressive, usually reducing the patient from good health to total helplessness or death in less than a year. The cerebrospinal fluid shows no abnormality; but the electroencephalogram becomes abnormal early in the disease, showing diffuse slowing with superimposed bursts of sharp waves.

Neuropathologic findings include diffuse loss of cortical neurons with a remarkable increase in fibrous astrocytes. Vacuoles are present in neurons and astrocytes, and this may give a spongiform appearance to the cerebral cortex. Inflammatory reactions and inclusion bodies are absent. Thus, despite clinical and epidemiologic differences, the pathologic findings in Creutzfeldt-Jakob disease are very similar to those of kuru and scrapie.

A similar disease develops in chimpanzees inoculated with brain tissue of most patients with Creutzfeldt-Jakob disease after an incubation period of 11 to 71 months. The chimpanzees developed somnolence, ataxia, tremor, fasciculations, and intermittent jerking of the extremities. The pathologic changes in the brains resembled those of Creutzfeldt-Jakob disease. The disease has also been transmitted from chimpanzee to chimpanzee, to Old and New World monkeys, to domestic cat, to guinea pig, and possibly to mouse. Little information is available on the agent of Creutzfeldt-Jakob disease, but the absence of virus-like particles on electron microscopic examination of infectious tissues, the failure to demonstrate cytopathic changes in cell cultures, and the absence of a demonstrable immune response suggest that the agent is similar to those causing kuru and scrapie.

The mode of spread is unknown, but the ability to transmit disease with tissues from familial cases suggests the importance of genetic factors or the possible vertical transmission of the agent. The failure to find increased incidences in medical personnel, laboratory investigations, or spouses of patients suggests a lack of significant communicability by respiratory, enteric, or sexual contact. Furthermore, the agent has not been detected in blood, sputum, or urine of patients, although it is present in extraneural tissue. On the other hand, apparent person-to-person transmission has been documented with the development of Creutzfeldt-Jakob disease in a patient 18 months after receiving a corneal transplant from another patient who proved to have the disease; by the occurrence of the disease in two young patients less than two years after cerebral corticography using the same implanted electrodes previously used in a patient with Creutzfeldt-Jakob disease; and by the occurrence of the disease in a number of patients within two years after undergoing intracranial surgery. In view of these observations, isolation of patients with Creutzfeldt-Jakob disease does not appear indicated, but careful disposal of needles and special sterilization of surgical instruments used on these patients appear mandatory. Medical personnel should avoid contamination of open sores or the conjuctiva with tissue, and no organs or corneas from patients with ill-defined neurologic diseases should be used for transplantation purposes.

No known treatment alters the relentless course of Creutzfeldt-Jakob disease.

310.4.   SUBACUTE SCLEROSING PANENCEPHALITIS
(Dawson's Encephalitis, Subacute Inclusion Body Encephalitis)

This is an uncommon, subacute encephalitis that usually occurs in children or young adults between the ages of 4 and 20 years. The onset is usually insidious and is characterized by deterioration in school work and behavioral disorders. This is followed in weeks or months by overt mental deterioration and neurologic signs, the most characteristic of which is myoclonus. The disease usually terminates after a third stage of stupor, blindness, dementia, and decorticate rigidity, which may last months to several years. Characteristically, the cerebrospinal fluid is under normal pressure and shows no pleocytosis but an increased concentration in gamma globulin, corresponding in large part to antibodies against measles virus. During the stage of active myoclonus, the electroencephalogram usually shows a typical pattern of general suppression of activity, with periodic (8 to 15 seconds) synchronous bursts of high-voltage slow and sharp waves. The clinical course is usually characterized by progressive deterioration, but occasionally an apparent arrest of the disease process or even transient clinical improvement is seen.

Although the disease follows a protracted afebrile course, a viral cause has long been suspected because of the pathologic changes. Perivascular infiltrates of mononuclear cells are characteristic, and eosinophilic intranuclear inclusion bodies are found in neurons and glial cells. Because of these inclusions, a herpesvirus was long suspected of being the etiologic agent. However, electron microscope studies of cerebral biopsies show virus-like particles resembling the nucleocapsids of paramyxoviruses. Astonishingly high levels of antibodies against measles virus can be demonstrated in the serums of most patients, and measles virus antigen is present in the brain. Nevertheless, the isolation of measles-like viruses from brains of patients with subacute sclerosing panencephalitis is difficult, requiring the establishment of cell cultures from brains of patients with the disease and subsequent cocultivation of these cultures with other cells. The measles virus associated with the disease is apparently defective.

The pathogenesis of subacute sclerosing panencephalitis is obscure. This disease bears little resemblance clinically or pathologically to the fulminating forms of measles virus infections, in which virus dissemination may lead to giant-cell pneumonia. Furthermore, it is quite distinct from parainfectious encephalomyelitis that occasionally complicates measles virus infections, in which acute neurologic disease occurs and perivascular demyelination is found in the brain and spinal cord. Epidemiologic studies have shown that subacute sclerosing panencephalitis is more common in males than females, in children of rural than of urban origin, and in patients with a history of measles during the first two years of life. These findings suggest that environmental factors and presence of residual transplacental passive immunity may play roles in inducing defective infection or precipitating disease.

Empirical treatments of patients with antiviral agents, interferon inducers, and immunosuppression and immunoenhancement therapies have provided no convincing evidence of beneficial effects. An apparent recent decline in numbers of cases suggests that the widespread use of measles vaccine may have some preventive effect.

In a small number of preadolescents with stigmata of congenital rubella virus infections, a progressive neurologic disease has developed which clinically resembles subacute sclerosing panencephalitis. In these patients antibodies to rubella virus have been elevated in serum and cerebrospinal fluid. Pathologic changes are similar to those of subacute sclerosing panencephalitis except that inclusion bodies are absent and mineralization, as seen in infantile congenital rubella encephalitis, is present. Rubella virus has been recovered from brain.

310.5.   PROGRESSIVE MULTIFOCAL LEUKOENCEPHALOPATHY

This is a rare demyelinating disease of the central nervous system. It usually develops in patients having preexisting disorders of the reticuloendothelial system such as leukemia, lymphoma, or sarcoidosis, but has also developed in patients immunosuppressed therapeutically or after organ transplantation. Although the underlying systemic disorder may be of long standing, the neurologic abnormalities develop rather suddenly and follow a subacute progressive course until death. The findings usually suggest multifocal disease. Abnormalities of motor function, sensation, vision, or speech are common, and dementia frequently develops. The cerebrospinal fluid shows little if any abnormality, and the electroencephalogram shows only nonspecific slowing. Pathologic lesions in the brain consist of multiple foci of demyelination in various stages of evolution. Oligodendrocytes are depleted within the foci, but surrounding the foci they are enlarged and contain eosinophilic intranuclear inclusions. The astrocytes within the demyelinated areas are often bizarre and contain mitotic figures. Inflammatory cells are usually not prominent.

The presence of the inclusion bodies and the occurrence against a background of disorders associated with impaired immunologic responses led to speculation that the disease might be caused by a viral infection. Electron microscopic examination in almost all cases has shown particles in the oligodendrocyte inclusions resembling small papovaviruses. Two small deoxyribonucleic acid viruses related to simian-virus 40 have been isolated from brain tissue of patients dying from progressive multifocal leukoencephalopathy. The JC virus, a new human papovavirus to which the majority of people have antibody since childhood, appears to be the causative agent in most cases. Viruses antigenically indistinguishable from simian-virus 40 have been related to two cases. Neither of these viruses has been associated with any disease in man except progressive multifocal leukoencephalopathy. Therefore progressive multifocal leukoencephalopathy apparently results from opportunistic infection of the brain by normally nonpathogenic agents. The viruses appear to selectively infect and lyse oligodendrocytes, the glial cells which maintain the myelin sheaths, and cause demyelination. The disease occurs in patients with impaired cellular immune responses, but it is not known whether this disease represents a primary infection of an immunologically incompetent patient or whether it represents a reactivation of a latent or persistent papovirus infection.

Evaluation of possible therapeutic agents has not been possible because of the rarity of cases and the infrequency of diagnosis during life.

310.6. OTHER NEUROLOGIC DISEASES

Since viruses can cause disease after a long incubation period, can produce disease with a subacute or relapsing course, and can give rise to noninflammatory pathologic changes, the possible role of slow or latent virus infection in a variety of neurologic diseases has been entertained.

In several chronic or relapsing inflammatory diseases of the nervous system, a viral cause has been suspected. *Chronic focal epilepsy* (epilepsia partialis continua, Kozhevnikov's epilepsy) is, in some cases, associated with a chronic focal inflammatory process in the brain. In the Soviet Union, this has been thought to represent a persistent focal infection with tick-borne viruses after acute encephalitis; and in several Soviet laboratories, tick-borne encephalitis virus has been isolated from surgically removed cerebral epileptogenic foci. No viruses have been isolated from similar cases in other countries. Chronic focal epilepsy can be a manifestation of focal disease processes such as neoplastic, vascular, or traumatic lesions, but chronic infection may play a role in some cases.

Recurrent acute meningitis or encephalitis occurs in three clinical syndromes of unknown cause in which latent viral infection has been suspected. *Mollaret's meningitis* is a rare, recurrent meningitis characterized by repeated attacks of headache, fever, and nuchal rigidity. Each attack is abrupt in onset and lasts for two to three days; the patient is entirely well between episodes. During attacks, the cerebrospinal fluid may contain large numbers of both polymorphonuclear and mononuclear cells and also large, poorly staining "epithelial cells," characteristic but not pathognomonic of this disease. More severe recurrent neurologic involvement can occur in *Behçet's syndrome* and in the *Vogt-Koyanagi-Harada syndrome*. Behçet's syndrome is a chronic disease characterized by recurrent oral and genital ulcers and inflammatory ocular lesions, usually taking the form of acute recurrent iritis. In about one quarter of the patients neurologic signs develop, consisting either of cranial nerve palsies, focal seizures, hemiparesis, or other focal signs or of severe depression of consciousness, coma, or meningeal signs, suggesting more diffuse neurologic involvement. Neurologic deficits usually remit and relapse but may be progressive. Neuropathologic findings include meningeal inflammatory reactions, perivascular inflammation, and focal areas of necrosis. The Vogt-Koyanagi-Harada or uveoencephalitic syndrome is characterized by depigmentation of skin and hair, inflammatory ocular lesions (usually consisting of iridocyclitis or exudative retinal detachment), and meningitis. Unlike Behçet's syndrome, neurologic involvement occurs in all cases, often precedes the ocular inflammation, and usually consists only of headache, nuchal rigidity, and a mononuclear cell pleocytosis. However, transient decrease in hearing and tinnitus may accompany the meningitis, or a severe encephalitis may develop, leaving permanent neurologic deficits. Neuropathologic findings have consisted only of a chronic arachnoiditis. Reports have been made of isolations of unidentified viruses from patients with Mollaret's, Behçet's, and Vogt-Koyanagi-Harada syndrome; but none of these claims have been entirely convincing. An allergic cause has also been postulated in each of these disorders, and consequently treatment with corticosteroids has been advocated.

Considerable interest in a possible viral cause of *multiple sclerosis* has been stimulated by epidemiologic data that indicate the role of a common exposure factor, serologic studies showing higher antibody levels against measles virus in patients with multiple sclerosis, observation of viral-like particles in brains, and unconfirmed claims of virus isolations. These data are still inconclusive. A notion that Parkinson's disease might have a viral cause has been entertained ever since the observation was made that a form of parkinsonism was a frequent sequela of encephalitis lethargica (von Economo's disease). Similarly, the possible role of a slow infection in amyotrophic lateral sclerosis and in a variety of other demyelinating and degenerative diseases has also been postulated. Although the spectrum of neurologic disease that can be potentially attributed to slow, latent, or chronic viral infections has greatly broadened in recent years, evidence is still scant for incriminating a transmissible agent in these chronic neurologic diseases.

Bernoulli, C., Siegfried, J., Baumgartner, G., Regli, F., Rabinowicz, T., Gajdusek, D. C., and Gibbs, C. J., Jr.: Danger of accidental person-to-person transmission of Creutzfeldt-Jakob disease by surgery. Lancet, 1:478, 1977.

Gajdusek, D. C.: Unconventional viruses and the origin and disappearance of kuru. Science, 197:943, 1977.

Johnson, R. T., and Herndon, R. M.: Virologic studies of multiple sclerosis and other chronic and relapsing neurological diseases. Prog. Med Virol., 18:229, 1974.

Johnson, R. T., and ter Meulen, V.: Slow infections of the nervous system. Adv. Intern. Med., 23:353, 1978.

Lampert, P. W., Gajdusek, D. C., and Gibbs, C. J., Jr.: Subacute spongiform virus encephalopathies. Scrapie, kuru, and Creutzfeldt-Jakob disease: A review. Am. J. Pathol., 68:626, 1972.

Narayan, O., Penney, J. B., Jr., Johnson, R. T., Herndon, R. M., and Weiner, L. P.: Etiology of progressive multifocal leukoencephalopathy: Identification of papovavirus. N. Engl. J. Med., 289:1278, 1973.

Padgett, B. L., Walker, D. L., ZuRhein, G. M., Hodach, A. E., and Chou, S. M.: JC papovavirus in progressive multifocal leukoencephalopathy. J. Infect. Dis., 133:686, 1976.

Roos, R., Gajdusek, D. C., and Gibbs, C. J., Jr.: The clinical characteristics of transmissible Creutzfeldt-Jakob disease. Brain, 96:1, 1973.

Section Seventeen   THE DEMYELINATING DISEASES

Labe C. Scheinberg

311.   INTRODUCTION

The term *demyelinating diseases* is applied to disorders that selectively damage or destroy central nervous system myelin but relatively spare the axis cylinders of the nerve cells. Traditionally, the term has been applied principally to multiple sclerosis and its variants. Several other inherited and acquired disorders also can affect central myelin rather selectively, however. Accordingly, Poser, in 1957, suggested assigning the term "demyelinating" to those relatively common disorders in which myelin is apparently normally formed but from some cause breaks down later in life. Multiple sclerosis is the most frequent of these diseases. The term "dysmyelinating" was employed, on the other hand, to designate a group of relatively rare disorders in which a known or presumed genetically determined enzyme deficiency results in defective myelin early in life. The term includes the leukodystrophies, other lipodystrophies, and some of the aminoacidurias. Table 1 lists these disorders of myelin.

BIOLOGY OF MYELIN. Myelin in the central nervous system appears to be formed mainly, if not entirely, by the oligodendrocytes. Astrocytes, in turn, may contribute to maintaining the nutrition and the ionic-metabolic homeostasis of the central tissue once it is formed. As the central nervous system develops, oligodendrocytes wrap their external plasma membrane concentrically around the axons of the larger nerve cells, producing a lamellar proteolipid sheet (myelin) that insulates the axon and guarantees its proper conduction of impulses. One oligodendrocyte may, by multiple extensions, form the myelin of many axons; as a result, destruction or disease of only a few oligodendrocytes may lead to a relatively large lesion of myelinated tracts. As the unit membrane of the oligodendrocyte forms myelin, the internal surfaces become apposed to form what one sees by electron microscopy as the dark major period line. The external surfaces give rise to the lighter intraperiod line, and the entire wrapping produces a structure composed of layers of concentric, tightly packed membranes of uniform thickness. The results of studies employing x-ray diffraction, electron

microscopy, and lipid analyses suggest that each layered unit membrane of myelin consists of a bimolecular lipid leaflet sandwiched between parallel layers of hydrated protein, in close contact with the polar groups of the lipids. The lipids that make up this leaflet appear to be interdigitated molecules of cerebroside, phospholipid, and cholesterol. Detailed chemical analyses of myelin indicate that protein (primarily proteolipid protein) makes up approximately 22 per cent of dry

TABLE 1.   Disorders Selectively Affecting Myelin

I. Demyelinating diseases (acquired breakdown of preformed normal myelin)
  A. Known or suspected disorders of the host's immune response to a foreign protein
    1. Postimmunization encephalomyelitis (smallpox, rabies, etc.)
    2. Parainfectious encephalomyelitis (postexanthematous, postinfectious, etc.)
    3. Acute disseminated encephalomyelitis without antecedent cause
  B. Multiple sclerosis and its presumed variants
    1. Optic and retrobulbar neuritis
    2. Neuromyelitis optica (Devic)
    3. Transverse myelitis
    4. Acute disseminated encephalomyelitis
  C. Disorders of known viral cause
    1. Progressive multifocal leukoencephalopathy
    2. Subacute sclerosing panencephalitis
  D. Disorders of presumed nutritional origin
    1. Combined systems disease (cyanocobalamin deficiency)
    2. Demyelination of the corpus callosum (Marchiafava-Bignami)
    3. Central pontine myelinolysis
  E. Disorders of anoxic-ischemic origin
    1. Delayed postanoxic cerebral demyelination
    2. Progressive subcortical ischemic encephalopathy (Binswanger)
II. Dysmyelinating disorders (genetic or developmental failure to form or maintain normally constituted myelin)
  A. The leukodystrophies
    1. Simple storage type; metachromatic leukodystrophy, glial insufficiency type of sulfatidosis
    2. Sudanophilic (Pelizaeus-Merzbacher)
    3. Globoid cell (Krabbe)
    4. Adrenoleukodystrophy (Schilder)
    5. Miscellaneous and mixed types (Seitelberger, Lowenberg-Hill, Alexander, Canavan, etc.)
    6. Lipidoses (Tay-Sachs, Gaucher, etc.)
  B. Aminoacidurias and developmental disorders
    1. Phenylketonuria, maple syrup urine disease, etc.
    2. Congenital thyroid deficiency, etc.

weight. The lipids contain approximately equal molar ratios of cholesterol and phospholipids with about one half as much galactolipid. These lipids in the myelin sheath are remarkably inert; once deposited at the time of myelin formation, they undergo little subsequent turnover. The biologic half-life of cholesterol in myelin is about one year, for example, compared to about ten days in other biologic membranes. Myelin should not be considered as metabolically inactive, however, because the components of white matter, and particularly the glial cells, account for about 30 per cent of the brain's total oxygen consumption.

The central myelin sheath is a compact, highly organized membrane extension of the oligodendrocyte which, though metabolically active, must be regarded as one of the more permanent tissue elements of the body.

The foregoing considerations indicate that primary central demyelination must be considered not just as a problem of myelin breakdown or dysgenesis but as the result of a basic disorder of the oligodendrocyte. In most primary demyelinating disorders, the precise cause remains unknown. The pathogenic agent may attack either the perikaryon (cell body) or the plasma membrane of the oligodendrocyte to produce demyelination.

PATHOGENESIS OF MULTIPLE SCLEROSIS. Multiple sclerosis is by far the most prevalent and clinically significant myelin disorder, affecting as many as 500,000 persons in the United States. Until a valid biochemical or immunologic test exists or until the etiologic agent is identified with certainty, we cannot say that the various symptoms and signs collected under the rubric multiple sclerosis are more than a syndrome. Clinical experience has shown, however, that if certain diagnostic criteria are met (see below), a group of central nervous system disorders in adults may be defined which are accompanied by consistent neuropathologic changes. Developments in the past few years suggest that multiple sclerosis results when an exogenous agent, presumably a viral infection, precipitates in the body an autoimmune response which, in turn, destroys central nervous system myelin.

The strongest stimulus for suspecting allergic factors in the pathogenesis of demyelinating diseases lies in the similarity of the neuropathologic abnormalities in multiple sclerosis to those of rabies postvaccinal encephalomyelitis. Rivers and coworkers in 1933 showed that multiple intramuscular injections of normal rabbit brain into monkey resulted in an encephalomyelitis with neuropathologic lesions similar to those of rabies postvaccinal encephalomyelitis. This line of investigation was accelerated by the extensive work of Kabat, Wolf, and coworkers in the 1940's, who showed that experimental allergic encephalomyelitis (EAE) could be produced by a single injection of adult autologous, homologous, or heterologous central myelin mixed with Freund's adjuvant (paraffin oil and killed mycobacteria).

The critical antigenic material in white matter to produce EAE appears to be a protein known as myelin basic protein (BP). This BP with Freund's complete adjuvant can initiate EAE, but if injected into animals with paraffin oil alone, later challenge of the animals with the usual encephalitogenic agent fails to produce EAE. Unfortunately, subsequent investigations in animals have shown variable and sometimes contradictory results in the role of BP as a therapeutic agent. BP has no current role in the treatment of prophylaxis of multiple sclerosis.

Other studies have shown that EAE is a delayed hypersensitivity reaction mediated by thymus-dependent lymphocytes (T cells) and may be transferred from one guinea pig to another by sensitized lymphocytes. Serum from EAE animals and from patients with multiple sclerosis can destroy myelin in tissue culture.

The strongest direct evidence for immunologic abnormalities in patients with multiple sclerosis is the presence of increased levels of gamma globulin (IgG) both in the cerebrospinal fluid (CSF) and surrounding the demyelinating lesions in the brain of most patients with multiple sclerosis. The highest incidence of the CSF abnormality is detected by visualizing specific "oligoclonal" bands in the gamma globulin region, and this abnormality may be detected even when the percentage of IgG is normal.

Widespread acceptance of multiple sclerosis as a disease incorporating abnormalities of cellular and humoral immunity has led to several efforts at using these changes to provide laboratory tests of diagnosis or disease activity. Thus far none of these measures have achieved a sufficient consistency or specificity to be clinically useful. Among these studies, one has demonstrated that leukocytes from patients with multiple sclerosis adhere to measles-infected epithelial cells to form rosettes. Such responses are much less pronounced with normal leukocytes or with those from patients with other neurologic disorders. Also, patients with multiple sclerosis often have elevated levels of measles antibody in blood and CSF, but the response is inconsistent and often includes other increased antibody levels as well. Other efforts to determine the activity of multiple sclerosis employ BP in a radioimmunoassay of myelin fragments present in the CSF. The test has correlated a high concentration of BP in the CSF during supposed active myelin destruction or exacerbation, but is not specific to multiple sclerosis.

The hypothesis that a viral agent could cause the chronic relapsing and remitting lesions of multiple sclerosis is based on three principal pieces of indirect evidence. One is the recently acquired knowledge that slow or chronic viral infections can produce chronic neurologic disorders in animals and man (see Ch. 310). The second is the evidence suggesting an excessive immunologic response to an exogenous agent in the tissues and CSF of patients with multiple sclerosis. The third is epidemiologic evidence that multiple sclerosis arises predominantly in individuals who have been exposed prior to a certain age to a (possibly infectious) environmental agent.

Multiple sclerosis (MS) is from three to over thirty times more prevalent in northern than in southern latitudes. Several epidemiologic investigations have shown that individuals who move from areas of higher to areas of lower MS prevalence after the age of about 15 years retain a risk of developing MS that is the same as in their original environment. Those who move before 15 years of age, however, develop the risk engendered by the new environment. A virus (e.g., measles) that differently affected adults and children and that infected individuals at an earlier age in southern than in northern latitudes could explain these observations. Poliomyelitis, for example, when it attacks at an early age, may cause mild illness yet afford lifelong immunity, but at a later age often produces paralytic disease. Factors of geography, economics, climate, and hygiene all seem to play significant roles in the prevalence of MS and are consistent with the theory of viral etiology.

Inconclusive or inconsistent results have attended efforts to identify a virus in the tissues of patients with MS. Reports of visualizing viral particles in the tissues by electron microscopy have not been confirmed. Parainfluenza viruses have reportedly been recovered from affected brains by co-cultivation techniques by some laboratories, but not others. Other laboratories have claimed that agents in the tissues of patients with MS will induce specific abnormalities in animals or cells in tissue culture, but this finding also stands as unconfirmed. Even the oligoclonal band in the CSF of patients with multiple sclerosis has thus far not been demonstrated to contain predominantly antibody to any specific virus.

Even if it turns out that MS results from infection by a virus, the epidemiologic data indicate that most of those infected do not get the disease. This implies a possible genetically determined susceptibility, and evidence supporting this speculation is gained from the fact that certain patterns of histocompatibility antigens are found more frequently in patients with MS than in normals. According to theory, an MS susceptibility gene occurs in close association with genes determining the body's immune response to viruses and modifies the response to such infection.

Since the HLA patterns associated with MS show differences in different parts of the world, however, the full significance of the association remains to be determined.

312. MULTIPLE SCLEROSIS

DEFINITION. Multiple or disseminated sclerosis (MS) is the most common demyelinating disorder. The disease characteristically is marked by recurrent attacks of demyelination (dissemination in time) distributed widely in the brain and spinal cord (dissemination in space). The disease includes a number of well recognized and readily diagnosed syndromes, but borderline cases may be difficult to categorize clinically and pathologically. The lack of comprehensive diagnostic laboratory tests adds to this difficulty. Generally, MS is chronic and relapsing, but fulminating attacks occur and as many as 30 per cent of the patients progress steadily from the onset. Most of the symptoms and signs reflect involvement of central myelin, but occasionally symptoms of neuronal or gray-matter involvement occur when the plaques extend into such areas.

PREVALENCE. The prevalence of MS in the United States varies from about 10 per 100,000 in the South to 60 per 100,000 in the North, with similar prevalence and distribution in Europe. The disease affects males and females about equally. About 67 per cent of cases begin between the ages of 20 and 40 years and 95 per cent between 10 and 50 years.

Populations residing between latitudes 40° N and 40° S (tropical and subtropical zones) have a low risk of MS, whereas populations residing north of this latitude in North America and Europe are at higher risk. Exceptions to these generalizations are found in other parts of the world; e.g., a low incidence is reported in the Union of South Africa and in Japan. Racial factors seem to play little part in the United States, because the incidence in blacks is almost the same as in whites. Reports of a greater family incidence than could be expected by chance fail to exclude the common effects of environmental factors. A purely hereditary basis seems to be excluded by a lack of concordance in identical twins.

PATHOLOGY. The external surface of the brain and cord generally shows no abnormality. Occasionally there is atrophy of the optic nerves, and rarely there is focal or generalized atrophy of the cerebral hemispheres. Acute large lesions may cause swelling of the cord. Rarely there may be sufficient focal swelling of the cerebrum to give the appearance of a neoplasm in roentgenologic contrast studies.

Cut sections of the brain or spinal cord reveal numerous scattered, grayish, well defined lesions that are slightly depressed and vary in diameter from a few millimeters to a few centimeters. These are found throughout the white matter of the brain, optic nerves, and spinal cord and occasionally extend into gray matter. The number of lesions is usually greater than would be expected from the clinical picture.

Microscopic abnormalities depend on the age of the lesion. Acute lesions show an infiltration of microglial phagocytes and mononuclear cells about vessels, as well as scattered in the lesion itself. The myelin sheaths are affected to varying degrees, from partial to complete destruction, with relative sparing of axons, glia, and other structures. In more severe lesions there may be total destruction of tissue and cyst formation. As the lesions become chronic, there is a proliferation of glial cells and fibers to give the typical "sclerotic plaque." The axons in these areas may be preserved or destroyed.

AGGRAVATING FACTORS. An *infective process* (upper respiratory infection, "influenza," urinary tract infection, gastroenteritis, etc.) is said to precede the initial attack or a relapse of MS in 10 to 40 per cent. *Immunizations* are without apparent effect on the course of the disease, and any exacerbations seen following these are probably coincidental.

Many workers have stated that *pregnancy* aggravates the disease, but this is open to question. The disease and pregnancy occur in the same age group, and although some studies show a higher incidence in married childbearing women, more attacks occur during the puerperium than during pregnancy itself. The physician must consider many nonmedical factors when advising on this problem. Pregnancy is generally considered nondeleterious to the course of MS in any patient who has had no attack in two years.

There seems to be no clear-cut association of attack or relapse with surgical procedures, and indications for *surgery* in patients with MS should be judged solely on their merit.

There is no statistical evidence to support a relationship between peripheral *trauma* and the onset or relapses of MS. There is a tendency for patients to associate trauma with the onset of an attack or relapse, but in many cases it is more likely that the trauma resulted from the disability of MS. *Emotional stress* has been incriminated as a precipitant of attacks or relapses of MS. This is difficult to substantiate, but it is reasonable to assume that cerebral changes in MS make it difficult for the patient to cope with emotional stress.

TABLE 2. Frequency of Occurrence of First Symptom of Multiple Sclerosis in Cases Proved by Clinical Study and Autopsy

Symptom	Autopsy (Carter et al.) (46 Cases)	Autopsy (Poser) (111 Cases)	Clinical Diagnosis (Carter et al.) (539 Cases)
	per cent	*per cent*	*per cent*
Weakness	42	39	54
Diplopia, impaired vision	35	32	21
Tremor, ataxia, incoordination	20	6	19
Paresthesias	13	16	32
Pain	11	1	—
Sphincter impairment	11	1	7
Dizziness or vertigo	7	1	8
Changes in muscle tone	7	—	—
Facial pain	2	—	—
Mental changes	2	2	—
Seizures	—	—	3

Certain diagnostic procedures such as lumbar puncture, pneumoencephalography, cerebral angiography, and myelography have been implicated in the worsening of symptoms in MS. However, these procedures are performed usually in patients whose disease is progressing or soon after an attack or relapse. They should be reserved for patients in whom one has serious questions whether a neoplasm exists in the nervous system, and not performed simply because "there's nothing else to be done."

CLINICAL MANIFESTATIONS. The clinical picture of MS is pleomorphic, but there are usually sufficient typical features to enable one to diagnose the disorder in the absence of a specific diagnostic test or without extensive "excluding" diagnostic procedures. The disease is chronic, often characterized by exacerbations and remissions, with evidence of multiple lesions in central white matter occurring in young adults without other systemic disorders. The symptoms of central white matter involvement are usually those of supranuclear weakness, incoordination, paresthesias, and visual complaints. Other symptoms and signs that are more characteristic of lesions in gray matter, e.g., aphasia, seizures, fasciculations, and neurogenic atrophy, are rare. Mental changes have an intermediate incidence and affect perhaps 30 per cent of patients.

The onset may be acute, with symptoms appearing within minutes to hours, or it may be insidious, with gradual, slow progression of symptoms over a period of months.

The frequency of occurrence of the first symptom of MS is given in Table 2.

The weakness usually begins or is most prominent in the lower extremities, but the upper extremities may be involved. When both lower extremities are involved, there are usually accompanying urinary complaints such as urgency or frequency. The weakness may be minimal, or there may be a total paralysis. There are usually upper motor neuron signs such as spasticity, hyperreflexia, and pathologic reflexes.

Visual complaints include blurring of vision with a central scotoma and decreased visual acuity or diplopia with extraocular paresis and nystagmus.

The incoordination is seen as ataxia or clumsiness and intention tremor of the upper extremities. Often a combination of spastic-ataxic gait is seen.

The paresthesias may involve any or all of the extremities. Usually there is impairment of vibratory sense and position sense in the lower extremities, whereas cutaneous sensation is relatively spared.

The typical clinical course of MS is one of exacerbations and remissions over a period of years, with increasing neurologic deficits caused by an increasing number of disseminated lesions. Less frequent are (1) an acute, severe course progressing to death in a few days or weeks; (2) a chronic, progressive course over a period of years; and (3) a benign form with relatively few presenting symptoms and signs and long-lasting remissions. In middle age the insidious onset of a progressive spastic paraparesis is often seen as the major clinical manifestation, particularly in women.

MS is sometimes divided into clinical types, depending upon which portion of the neuraxis is most involved, e.g., spinal, cerebral, brainstem-cerebellar, or mixed. The most common form is spinal with prominent features of spastic paraparesis, lower extremity paresthesias, and urinary complaints. The brainstem-cerebellar variety with prominent visual complaints, cranial nerve signs, nystagmus, vertigo, and incoordination is also common, but the cerebral form with mental changes and hemiparesis and hemisensory changes is uncommon.

Although most cases may be classified as one of these forms early in the course, almost all patients appear to have a mixed type of involvement after about 15 years.

In Table 3 may be noted the frequency of various symptoms and signs of MS in clinical and autopsy series reported by Carter et al. and by Poser.

Certain uncommon symptoms and signs such as nausea, vomiting, facial pain, seizures, dysphagia, atrophy, hearing loss, tinnitus, and changes in states of consciousness occur in 2 to 10 per cent of cases. Signs such as internuclear ophthalmoplegia are highly characteristic of multiple sclerosis; headache and aphasia are rare.

LABORATORY DATA. Abnormal findings in MS are usually confined to the cerebrospinal fluid (CSF). In the acute disease, there may be a mild mononuclear pleocytosis of as much as 200 to 300 cells per cubic millimeter, but usually less than 40. The protein content is usually normal or slightly elevated (50 to 100 mg per 100 ml); values higher than this are rare. The gamma globulin content is elevated in about two thirds of the cases and, correspondingly, there is often an abnormal colloidal gold curve (first or second zone), accompanied by a negative serologic test for syphilis. Closer examination of the gamma globulin region of the CSF by starch-gel or agar-gel electrophoresis shows specific oligoclonal bands of immunoglobulin in a majority of cases. These may be detected even when the percentage of gamma

TABLE 3. Frequency of Occurrence of Symptoms and Signs in Course of Multiple Sclerosis

	Carter et al. (46 Cases)	Poser (111 Cases)
	per cent	per cent
Weakness (symptom or sign)	89	96
Abnormal movements	67	
Abnormal reflexes (absent superficials, Babinski signs, or hyperreflexia)	99	95
Sphincter and genital difficulties	78	82
Visual disturbance (symptom or sign)	100	85
Nystagmus (any type)	85	70
Disc pallor, atrophy, decreased acuity	75	85
Third nerve impairment (and internuclear ophthalmoplegia)	67	
Tremor, ataxia	93	79
Impaired vibration and position sense	81	58
Impaired touch, pain, temperature sense	35	35
Mental changes (symptom or sign)	61	45
Paresthesias	44	65
Pain	42	19
Vertigo or dizziness	18	15

globulin is normal. Such oligoclonal bands also occur occasionally in neurosyphilis, subacute sclerosing panencephalitis, Guillain-Barré syndrome, brain tumor, and cerebrovascular disease, and are not of themselves diagnostic.

The electroencephalogram may be mildly abnormal in about two thirds of cases, but is not useful in diagnosis. Computerized tomography (CT) scans detect large confluent areas of cerebral demyelination but are not useful for diagnosis in most cases. Recently described blood immunologic tests require independent confirmation before they can be relied upon for diagnosis.

Visual evoked responses can extend the diagnostic examination in patients with suspected MS. The test involves the presentation of a patterned stimulus to the retina and recording the response at the occipital cortex by scalp electrodes. Abnormalities of the latency and/or configuration of the computer-averaged cortical response are readily detected and identify subclinical involvement of the visual pathways.

DIAGNOSIS. Because of the pleomorphic nature of the disease, it is often necessary to exclude many other neurologic disorders. Most often one must consider spinal cord, brainstem or cerebellar tumors, degenerative diseases such as the spinocerebellar degenerations, and combined system disease.

The fact that MS has a remitting nature in many instances and the dissemination of symptoms and signs should indicate that one is not dealing with an expanding lesion involving the nervous system. If all the symptoms and signs can be explained by a single lesion, then one should assume that the condition is not MS. If the patient complains of headache, seizures, or progressive focal neurologic signs, which are uncommon in MS, and if these are accompanied by abnormalities such as increased CSF pressure, roentgenographic changes in the skull or spine, and marked elevation of CSF protein, then one must proceed further to exclude a neoplasm. This can be done in most cases by a neuroroentgenologic procedure such as myelography, pneumoencephalography, cerebral angiography, or CT scan. Vascular disease, particularly that involving the brainstem, can be confused with MS in middle-aged patients. In some of these cases only prolonged follow-up reveals the true diagnosis.

Certain degenerative disorders of the nervous system can be confused with MS. However, the former tend to have a family history, to be slowly progressive without remission, and to confine themselves to systems, e.g., cerebellar, extrapyramidal, or motor system. In the differential diagnosis of spastic paraparesis of middle age, one should consider, respectively, motor neuron disease (amyotrophic lateral sclerosis), cervical spondylosis, or spinal cord tumor. The first has no sensory abnormalities, and the latter two both have characteristic roentgenologic abnormalities. Combined system disease can be excluded in most cases by hematologic studies and gastric analysis.

TREATMENT. There are several aspects to the management of MS. The first is to attempt to treat or affect the course of the disease itself. The second is to attempt to manage the painful and disabling complications of the disease, e.g., spasticity, tremor, decubiti, and urinary problems. The third aspect is the management of the patient with a chronic, unpredictable, and occasionally disabling disease.

Many authorities believe that adrenocorticosteroids favorably influence the onset or acute exacerbations of MS, and recommend the administration of ACTH, 40 to 80 units per day, or prednisone, 40 to 80 mg per day, over a period of three to four weeks, taking suitable precautions against complications. Controlled studies have suggested that such measures induce the more rapid clearing of acute symptoms and signs but leave the long-term outcome of the disease unaffected. Because of potential complications, long-term maintenance therapy with ACTH or corticosteroids is contraindicated. No evidence indicates that immunosuppressant agents have long-term benefit.

The greater gain in treatment lies in the management of some of the painful or disabling complications of the disease. Some are specifically neurologic and related to MS, whereas others are seen in any chronic disease. Three neurologic symptoms are responsible for most of the disability seen in MS: spasticity, incoordination, and urinary bladder problems. Spasticity with flexor spasms seems best controlled by use of baclofen, a substituted gamma-aminobutyric acid compound which inhibits central synaptic transmission. In doses of 30 to 100 mg per day* it is effective in most patients and causes few side effects or complications. Gait incoordination or truncal ataxia responds poorly to most measures, although intention tremor of the arm seems to respond to contralateral cryothalamotomy. Bilateral

*See p. vi, Dosage Notice, immediately following Preface.

thalamic surgery is not advised because of the occurrence of pseudobulbar symptoms. Pharmacologic agents such as propanolol, 40 to 320 mg per day, have been reported sometimes to relieve tremor. The management of the urinary bladder is of extreme importance regarding both the life expectancy of the patient and his or her self-esteem. Primarily the effort must be made to avoid a large residual urine with eventual infection of the bladder. Intermittent daily catheterization probably carries a lower risk of infection than prolonged use of an indwelling catheter, and many women can be taught self-catheterization. The prevention and management of decubiti, nutritional deficiency, contractures, infections, and psychologic problems are similar to those in other diseases. In MS, because of its often undeserved grim reputation, there is a frequent attempt to keep the diagnosis from the patients. This often results in unnecessary distress for the patients and family and loss of confidence in the physician. Usually, it is advisable to inform the patient when the diagnosis is established and to be supportive and optimistic. Statistics indicate an average survival of 35 years from onset of MS, with about two thirds of the patients remaining productive if not in physically demanding occupations.

The third aspect of the management of the patient with chronic, unpredictable, and occasionally disabling disease is the most important, rewarding, and neglected aspect. These patients are told often that there is no treatment — and indeed there is none for the MS itself — but this does not imply that one can do nothing for its complications. Medical neglect combines with disease progression in taking physical and psychologic toll on patient and family. In addition to disclosure and open discussion of the disease with the patient and family, one must be continuously supportive and even optimistic. Sexual problems, financial insecurity, and physical disability are reflected in a higher divorce and unemployment rate and should be met with counseling and judicious planning. Occupational therapy, with emphasis on activities of daily living, probably contributes more than physical therapy. Exhausting physical exertion and even exhausting physiotherapy may cause greater distress in patients already suffering lassitude. An increased body temperature may aggravate the symptoms of MS, and consequently swimming in a cool pool is a much advised form of therapy and general conditioning exercise. Splinting, tenotomy, and neurectomy may be necessary in the final stages to manage contractures and decubiti.

Pregnancy generally is best avoided within two years of an acute attack because of the associated fatigue and weakness. Pregnancy probably does not adversely influence the course of the disease over the years. The timing of elective surgery and other unnecessary stresses should be carefully weighed by patient and physician.

PROGNOSIS. In the early stages of the disease it is not possible accurately to predict the course, although certain symptoms seem to indicate a better prognosis. Monosymptomatic and acute symptoms lasting hours to weeks tend to give a better prognosis than polysymptomatic or slowly progressive manifestations. Cranial nerve, visual, and sensory symptoms carry a better prognosis for remission or a benign course than do motor or cerebellar symptoms. More than half the cases remit after an initial attack, but one cannot predict the next attack. The remission of certain symptoms, e.g.,

retrobulbar neuritis, may be so complete as to make the clinician doubt the history.

Within the first five years after onset, about 70 per cent of patients are able to be employed, although with occasional interruptions in some cases. By the end of ten years this drops off to 50 per cent. At the end of 20 years 35 per cent are still employed, with minor interruptions, and about 20 per cent of patients succumb to complications of the disease by this time. The major disabilities are spasticity, disturbances of coordination, and disturbance in bladder and bowel function.

Life expectancy varies considerably, ranging from a few weeks to over 50 years after the initial attack regardless of whether one considers hospitalized severe cases or the more benign forms. The average life expectancy in all patients is about 35 years after onset. This represents an increase of about 10 years in the last generation and is due to better management of intercurrent genitourinary or respiratory infections, the usual causes of death.

313. POSSIBLE MULTIPLE SCLEROSIS VARIANTS

OPTIC AND RETROBULBAR NEURITIS

Optic neuritis is a term used to describe involvement of the optic nerve as a result of inflammation, demyelination, or degeneration. When the site of the lesion is intraocular, ophthalmoscopy reveals papilledema and the terms *papillitis* or intraocular neuritis are employed. *Retrobulbar neuritis* indicates involvement of the orbital or intracranial optic nerve behind the eye. There is often a predilection for the papillomacular bundle, producing a characteristic central scotoma but usually with minimal or absent ophthalmoscopic abnormalities in the acute stage.

Optic neuritis has many known causes, such as nutritional deficiency, intoxications (tobacco, alcohol), local inflammatory conditions (sinusitis, meningitis, orbital infections), and metabolic diseases (diabetes mellitus, pernicious anemia, other vitamin deficiencies). Once these have been excluded, demyelinating disease must be considered as a likely cause. In several large series of patients who presented with retrobulbar neuritis and were followed for many years, 15 to 30 per cent later developed other manifestations of MS. Conversely, about 50 per cent of patients with MS exhibit symptoms of optic neuritis at some time during the course of the disease.

Both optic and retrobulbar neuritis are characterized by an abrupt or progressive loss of vision that is rarely total and is usually unilateral. Associated with the visual loss may be pain in and around the eye that is accentuated by ocular movement. There may be tenderness on palpation of the eyeball. Visual testing reveals decreased acuity and central or paracentral scotomas. In *intraocular neuritis* or *papillitis,* the optic disc appears inflamed, and there may be hyperemia, blurred margins, and even elevation. A few hemorrhages may be seen in the retina adjacent to the disc. In *retrobulbar neuritis* the ophthalmoscopic picture is normal, but the features are otherwise similar to those of optic neuritis.

It is essential to differentiate optic neuritis from papilledema associated with increased intracranial pressure or other conditions. Papilledema is almost always bilateral, and vision is usually well preserved until late in the course. The disc elevation is usually greater in papilledema, and the only visual field defect is an enlarged blind spot. In optic neuritis the cerebrospinal fluid pressure is almost always normal, and there may be other findings indicative of MS.

Optic and retrobulbar neuritis may be treated with ACTH or corticosteroids. However, almost complete spontaneous recovery often occurs, and the benefits of therapy are difficult to assess.

The prognosis in a single attack of optic or retrobulbar neuritis is usually good. There may be complete recovery, or there may be residual visual field defects, temporal pallor of the discs, or optic atrophy. The visual acuity may be further impaired with subsequent attacks, but complete visual loss is rare.

ACUTE TRANSVERSE MYELITIS

Acute transverse myelitis may appear as the initial event in a subsequently typical form of MS, or it may develop during the course of the disease. The findings include complete or partial paralysis of both legs or of all four limbs, variable sensory loss, and bladder and bowel involvement. The condition is described in detail in Ch. 300.

Subacute necrotizing myelopathy is often associated with vascular malformations of the spinal cord or thrombophlebitis (Foix-Alajouanine syndrome). In acute necrotizing myelopathy there is hemorrhagic necrosis of the spinal cord without any associated vascular malformation. Such cases, which are rare, show a rapidly ascending motor and sensory paralysis with polymorphonuclear cells in the cerebrospinal fluid, and death may occur in weeks or months.

NEUROMYELITIS OPTICA (DEVIC'S DISEASE)

This clinical syndrome is characterized by acute transverse myelitis and optic neuritis. It may be considered to be a variant of MS and may occur as the initial illness or later during the course of the disease. There may be sudden loss of vision in both eyes, with central scotoma or sudden onset of paraplegia with sensory loss. The ocular involvement may be due to optic or retrobulbar neuritis, and the transverse myelitis may be partial or complete. Days or weeks may elapse between the onsets of the two symptom complexes. In severe cases the motor symptoms tend to be permanent, but otherwise the course, laboratory data, and treatment are similar to those of MS.

TRANSITIONAL SCLEROSIS

Transitional sclerosis is probably a pathologic variant of MS in which the disseminated plaques tend to become confluent, creating large areas of myelin loss. Clinically these cases are indistinguishable from cases of typical MS. Transitional sclerosis probably represents an intermediate pathologic form between MS and Schilder's cerebral sclerosis.

ACUTE NECROTIZING HEMORRHAGIC ENCEPHALOMYELITIS

This is a rare and fulminant variant of demyelinating disease that often progresses to death in days or weeks. The disease is characterized by a rapid course, fever, headache, convulsions, progressive change in state of consciousness from drowsiness to coma, nuchal rigidity, and hemiplegia or quadriplegia. The cerebrospinal fluid examination reveals a pleocytosis up to several thousand white blood cells that are predominantly polymorphonuclear leukocytes, and an elevated protein content. On pathologic examination, there are large foci of hemorrhagic necrosis of white matter. Although most patients succumb within a few weeks, there are rare alleged reports of recovery. There appears to be an experimental allergic model of this disorder with similarities on histologic examination. The only therapy that can be offered is supportive, though ACTH and corticosteroids should be tried.

ACUTE DISSEMINATED ENCEPHALOMYELITIS

Occasionally acute neurologic symptoms may occur without apparent preceding infection. The clinical picture is dependent on the location of the lesions and may include the symptoms and signs of meningitis, encephalitis, myelitis, or any combination of the preceding. Some cases blend indistinguishably into chronic, typical MS and so may represent the initial acute attack of that disease. Other cases may be uniphasic, and the patient may recover with or without neurologic residua and have no further attacks. Only prolonged follow-up with a recurrence or progression of neurologic symptoms can enable one to diagnose acute MS and exclude acute disseminated encephalomyelitis.

DIFFUSE SCLEROSIS

There is a group of progressive neurologic disorders of young patients who manifest severe neurologic deficits of various types and progressive visual and mental deterioration. In three publications from 1912 to 1924, Schilder described three cases of diffuse disease of white matter that he proposed grouping under the name encephalitis periaxialis diffusa (called Schilder's disease). Additional publications by Schilder and others followed. It now seems likely that three separate conditions have been included under the rubric of Schilder's disease and that the eponymic designation should be discarded. Some of these cases represent the result of severe, confluent extensions of the myelinoclastic lesions of MS. Some represent leukoencephalitides of known viral origin, such as subacute sclerosing panencephalitis and progressive multifocal leukoencephalitis. A third group undoubtedly includes the leukodystrophies listed in Table 1. Among these, it is probable that adrenoleukodystrophy was the disorder that Schilder identified in one of his early cases. This condition only recently has been delineated fully. It is genetically transmitted, probably as a sex-linked recessive trait, and affects young boys, usually before the age of ten years.

The onset of adrenoleukodystrophy is usually insidious but may be acute. It is usually slowly progressive, but there may be successive bursts to simulate the course of MS. A typical presenting picture is of insidious mental deterioration with loss of recently acquired intellectual achievements, and this progresses slowly to dementia. Many patients develop aphasia, apraxia, and dysarthria. Visual loss with cortical blindness is characteristic, and auditory complaints with cortical deafness may follow involvement of the cortical radiations. Clinical signs of adrenal insufficiency occur in only a minority of the patients, but tests of adrenal function are almost always abnormal. Pathologic examination of the adrenal gland shows abnormalities predominantly in the zona fascicularis and zona reticularis. Neuropathologically, the changes in brain myelin resemble many of the abnormalities of MS, yet contain abnormal cytoplasmic inclusions. Since these ultrastructural abnormalities also occur in other tissues, adrenoleukodystrophy presently is regarded as an inherited metabolic disorder.

314. LEUKODYSTROPHIES

This group includes heredofamilial diseases in which normal myelin is probably not formed because of some genetically determined enzymatic defect. The classsification is not completely satisfactory; the group tends to merge with the lipidoses of the nervous system, so that authorities differ in their classifications. Only further elucidation of the enzymatic defects of myelin metabolism in these disorders will lead to a satisfactory classification.

METACHROMATIC LEUKOENCEPHALOPATHY

These are otherwise known as the glial insufficiency forms or the sulfatide lipidoses. This group includes those cases in which large amounts of metachromatic material accumulate in the central nervous system. The disease is inherited as an autosomal recessive and begins in the first ten years of life, usually with gait disturbances, convulsions of various types, hypotonia, ocular palsies, and dysarthria. There are coarse tremors of the extremities and, terminally, severe mental deterioration and spasticity or rigidity.

The cerebrospinal fluid protein is usually elevated (100 to 200 mg per 100 ml), and metachromatic material (staining red with toluidine blue) can be found in the urinary sediment. The metachromatic material also collects in the kidney, liver, gallbladder, spleen, or peripheral nerves, and biopsy confirms the diagnosis. Gallbladder function studies may be abnormal. The course is one of progressive neurologic deterioration leading to death in one to four years, although some patients have survived 10 to 20 years. Some cases may begin later in childhood and run a more protracted course. The disorder is one of the more common leukodystrophies and can often be diagnosed in life. There is no therapy.

SUDANOPHILIC LEUKODYSTROPHY
(Pelizaeus-Merzbacher Disease)

This is a very rare, familial leukodystrophy, predominantly of males. The pathologic changes consist of ex-

tensive diffuse demyelination in the cerebral hemispheres and cerebellum. The disease appears to be transmitted as a sex-linked recessive and begins in early life with a slowly progressive course. Disturbances of coordination such as intention tremor, gait disturbances, dysarthria, spasticity, abnormal movements, and mental deterioration occur. The illness lacks pathognomonic features, but the predominant progressive cerebellar symptoms in a male with a positive family history should make one suspect the entity. It runs a course of several years or more before fatal termination. There is no therapy.

GLOBOID CELL LEUKODYSTROPHY
(Krabbe's Disease)

This rare familial type of leukodystrophy begins in infancy and rapidly progresses to death. The typical pathologic feature is the deposition of cerebrosides in globoid cells of the brain. These may be glial or another type of macrophage. The cases described by Krabbe began at about four months of age with seizures, spastic quadriplegia, abnormal startle responses, cortical blindness, and optic atrophy, and progressed rapidly to death in one or two years. The protein in the cerebrospinal fluid is usually elevated. There is no therapy.

SPONGY DEGENERATION OF WHITE MATTER
(Canavan's Disease)

In this rare familial leukodystrophy there is widespread demyelination accompanied by microscopic vacuolation that gives rise to a spongy appearance. It appears to be transmitted as an autosomal recessive and seems to be most common among Jews. Usually it begins early in infancy with atonia of the neck muscles, spastic paraplegia, severe mental retardation, optic atrophy, abnormal reflexes, and enlargement of the head. Laboratory studies, except for skull roentgenograms showing enlargement, are usually normal. Death usually occurs at about 18 months of age. There is no therapy.

LIPIDOSES OF THE CENTRAL NERVOUS SYSTEM

These comprise disturbances of metabolism that result in an increase of lipids in the brain. Included are amaurotic idiocy, or Tay-Sachs disease (gangliosidoses) (see below); Niemann-Pick disease (sphingomyelin) (see Ch. 533.3); Gaucher's disease (cerebrosides) (see Ch. 533.2); and Hurler's disease (mucopolysaccharides) (see Ch. 538.1).

The dividing line is by no means sharp between the dysmyelinating diseases, characterized by faulty myelin formation, and the lipid storage diseases, characterized by the accumulation of lipid-staining materials within nerve cell bodies. The distinction is further blurred by the fact that demyelination also occurs in many of the lipidoses, particularly amaurotic idiocy.

Amaurotic idiocy, or cerebromacular degeneration, can have an infantile (Tay-Sachs), late infantile (Bielschowsky), or juvenile (Batten-Spielmeyer-Vogt) onset. The Tay-Sachs variety is found chiefly among children of Jewish descent and has a recessive genetic pattern. The incidence of the other forms is genetic recessive and nonracial. All three are characterized by a progressive decrease in vision leading to complete blindness within one to two years. Concomitantly, there is a progressive and usually severe dementia combined with convulsions and advancing weakness, leading eventually to the patient's being bedridden with paralysis. Diagnosis in all three forms depends upon the characteristic clinical combination of dementia and blindness plus, in the Tay-Sachs and Batten-Spielmeyer-Vogt varieties, either a cherry-red or red-purple discoloration, respectively, marking the area of macular degeneration in the retina. An adult form (Kufs') has also been recognized. This group of late onset neuronal storage disorders without organomegaly is characterized by seizures, pigmentary degeneration or cherry-red spot changes in the retina, pyramidal signs, basal ganglia signs, cerebellar signs, and dementia. The problem remains whether these disorders are examples of identical or different genetically determined enzymatic defects of the nervous system. Clinicopathologic changes are not diagnostic. Rectal biopsy disclosing fat-packed ganglion cells in Meissner's plexus provides morphologic confirmation of the diagnosis.

Carter, S., Sciarra, D., and Merritt, H. H.: The course of multiple sclerosis as determined by autopsy proven cases. Am. Res. Nerv. Ment. Dis. Proc., 28:471, 1950.

Davison, A. N., Humphrey, J. H., Liversedge, L. A., McDonald, W. I., and Porterfield, J. S. (eds.): Multiple Sclerosis Research. London, Her Majesty's Stationery Office, 1975.

McAlpine, D., Lumsden, C. E., and Acheson, E. D.: Multiple Sclerosis. A Reappraisal. London, E. & S. Livingstone Ltd., 1965.

Porterfield, J. S. (ed.): Multiple sclerosis. Br. Med. Bull., 33:1, 1977.

Poser, C. M.: Recent advances in multiple sclerosis. Med. Clin. North Am., 56:1343, 1972.

Prineas, J. W.: Paramyxovirus-like particles associated with acute demyelination in chronic relapsing multiple sclerosis. Science, 178:760, 1972.

Raine, C. S., Powers, J. M., and Suzuki, K.: Acute multiple sclerosis. Confirmation of "paramyxovirus-like" intranuclear inclusions. Arch. Neurol., 30:39, 1974.

Schaumberg, H. H., Powers, J. M., Raine, C. S., Suzuki, K., and Richardson, E. P.: Adrenoleukodystrophy. A clinical and pathological study of 17 cases. Arch. Neurol., 32:577, 1975.

Shein, H. M. (ed.): Interaction of brain cells and viruses. In Schmitt, F. O., and Worden, F. G. (eds. in chief): The Neurosciences: Third Study Program. Cambridge, Mass., M.I.T. Press, 1975.

Vinken, P. J., and Bruyn, G. W. (eds.): Multiple Sclerosis and Other Demyelinating Diseases. Handbook of Clinical Neurology, Vol. 9, Amsterdam, North-Holland Publishing Company, 1970.

Section Eighteen THE EPILEPSIES

315. THE EPILEPSIES

Gilbert H. Glaser

DEFINITION AND PREVALENCE. Epilepsy is derived from the Greek *epilepsia,* meaning a "taking hold of" or "a seizing." It refers to the many types of recurrent seizures produced by paroxysmal excessive neuronal discharges in different parts of the brain that can be due to a variety of cerebral and general bodily disorders. Designation of "the epilepsies" as symptom complexes, therefore, is more appropriate, and the term encompasses convulsions or convulsive disorders with loss of consciousness as well as nonconvulsive seizures with only slight changes in conscious awareness.

An accurate epidemiology of the epilepsies is difficult, but various studies indicate an over-all incidence of between 0.5 and 1.0 per cent in general populations involving all age groups. The experience of a single seizure is more common, especially in early childhood, but recurrence is necessary for the diagnosis of an epilepsy.

PATHOGENESIS. Basic Mechanisms of Epileptic Discharge. Given the sufficient and proper electrical and chemical stimuli, abnormal discharges and seizures can arise in even the normal brain. Certain regions of the brain are particularly sensitive to seizures, having a low threshold and a high susceptibility. These include particularly the motor cortex and the structures within the limbic system. The temporal lobe and its deeper nuclear aggregates, the amygdala and hippocampus, are especially susceptible; their vascularity is vulnerable to compression, and the tissues themselves are especially sensitive to biochemical disturbances. It sometimes is difficult to separate cause from effect in temporal lobe lesions, because morphologic abnormalities in these regions may result when a severe seizure produces secondary vascular insufficiency and hypoxia.

Factors related to age and development are important in the genesis of the epilepsies, and brain lesions acquired during the perinatal period often require many years to mature and produce clinical epileptic phenomena. Certain seizure types such as massive spasms are more common in infants; petit mal seizures appear in childhood rather than later in life. This is reflected by different electroencephalographic patterns associated with seizures in infancy and childhood, compared with those in older age groups. The immature brain also is more susceptible than that of the adult to biochemical disturbances such as hypoxia, hypocalcemia, hypoglycemia, and hyponatremia. The occurrence of seizures with high fever is almost confined to early childhood. The periodicity of epilepsy correlates with sleep or menstrual cycles in some patients.

Seizures may be *focal,* arising from an abnormal focus or a number of foci, or *generalized from the onset,* seemingly without focal origin. However, generalization throughout the brain of an initially focal paroxysmal discharge sometimes occurs so rapidly that the focal origin can be obscured. The attacks of many patients with fixed cerebral lesions and *secondary or symptomatic seizures* are in this category. It is still uncertain whether generalized seizures, such as idiopathic grand mal convulsions and the brief seizures of petit mal absence (see below), develop immediately as generalized cerebral discharges involving specific pathways or whether they are initiated by a localized discharge. Convulsions caused by metabolic disturbances such as water intoxication, hypocalcemia, or hypoglycemia may be considered examples of those generalized from the onset. In these instances, the initial detonation starting the seizure is believed to be in the subcortical mesodiencephalic nonspecific reticular systems with diffuse propagation bilaterally into the cerebral cortex. The rapid loss of consciousness that first occurs and the marked memory disturbance after the seizure can be related to this spread.

Hughlings Jackson concluded many years ago from clinical observations that most seizures develop from a focus or aggregate of abnormally excitable neurons, and many studies since his time have supported this hypothesis. It is postulated that the nerve cells of patients with epilepsy contain intrinsic intra- and extracellular metabolic disturbances which produce excessive and prolonged depolarization of the membrane, producing a defect in the recovery process after excitation. The cortical regions containing such cells generate shifts in slow or standing wave potentials as a result of abnormal electrical activity arising in the region of neuronal dendrites. The neurons in the abnormal, epileptic focus are a hyperexcitable aggregate, and they tend to discharge paroxysmally. Clinical seizures develop if the discharge propagates along neural pathways or if sufficient local recruitment occurs. The abnormal discharges, once initiated, spread through essentially normal brain; the manifestations of the particular seizure then depend upon both the focus of origin and the region of the brain subsequently involved in the propagated discharge. In certain cases, seizures may be provoked by various sensory stimuli ("reflex" or sensory-induced epilepsy), especially flickering light or visual patterns and sound. At other times, peripheral sensory stimulation can arrest the development of a seizure.

The metabolic environment of epileptogenic neurons is most important in the genesis of attacks, and many metabolic disturbances may be associated with seizures. For example, a balance of electrolytes is required to maintain the resting potential of the neuronal membrane. An alteration in membrane permeability with an increased, intraneuronal sodium content could be a significant change preceding seizure discharge. Initiation and maintenance of neuronal hyperexcitability have been related to increases in extraneuronal potassium. Depletion of available calcium ions upsets membrane stability and causes oscillations; conversely, an increase in calcium has a depressant, anticonvulsive effect. Both hypoxia and hypoglycemia deprive neurons of basic substrates, allowing insufficient energy for the maintenance of appropriate ionic gradients. However, if effects of excessive muscle metabolism and apnea during generalized convulsive seizure activity are eliminated, such seizures do not induce cerebral hypoxia; actually, cerebral blood flow increases to meet cerebral oxygen demands in this state.

The coenzyme function of pyridoxal phosphate is directly involved in the metabolic pathway of gamma-aminobutyric acid, which has neuronal inhibitory activity. Experimental alterations of this system can be produced by such substances as the antimetabolite methoxypyridoxine and the hydrazides, but pyridoxine deficiency seizures occur only rarely and in infants. The toxicity of isoniazid in high doses operates by this mechanism.

ETIOLOGY. It is customary to divide epilepsy into two categories, *idiopathic* and *symptomatic or acquired*. A diagnosis of idiopathic epilepsy is made when no specific cause is found; in acquired epilepsy the cause can be determined by available diagnostic procedures. Present techniques fail to uncover a specific structural or biochemical cause of epilepsy in up to 75 per cent of patients.

Idiopathic Epilepsy. Idiopathic epilepsy undoubtedly stems from a number of cryptic causes, in many instances accompanying a genetic predisposition to seizures. A family history of seizures exists in high incidence for some groups of seizures, particularly those beginning in early life. The relatives of patients with idiopathic epilepsy have a 3 to 5 per cent incidence of epilepsy, six to ten times that in the ordinary population. There is also an increased incidence of electroencephalographic abnormality in the relatives of seizure patients, particularly in monozygotic twins, in whom the incidence of concordant abnormalities may exceed 20 per cent. Since epilepsy may be but a symptom associated with other neurologic abnormalities, an inheritance pattern for a specific cerebral disease must be considered in some cases. There are also a number of indirect factors, such as cerebral birth trauma resulting from a narrow maternal pelvis, that tend to produce seizures in families.

Acquired Epilepsy. Most diseases or structural abnormalities of the brain may be associated with seizures. *Congenital malformations* induced chromosomally or otherwise, such as microgyria, porencephaly, and hemangiomas, have a varying incidence of associated epilepsy, depending upon the intensity of the abnormality and possibly on more general genetic factors. Maternal infection, as by rubella, can produce multiple cerebral abnormalities, and severe toxemia of pregnancy also can affect the fetus. Perinatal difficulties causing *birth trauma* and *asphyxia* are relatively common causes of cerebral damage and later epilepsy.

Acute, subacute, and chronic infections of the brain and its coverings, such as meningitis, encephalitis, and abscess, cause seizures, both during the active process and later as healing leaves cerebral scars. Acute viral encephalitis often causes seizures, and convulsions caused by cerebral tuberculomas (more often by tuberculous meningitis) remain common in certain countries such as India. Cysticercosis and schistosomiasis have specific geographic distributions and are frequent causes of seizures in highly endemic areas.

Febrile convulsions commonly accompany nonspecific infections in infants and young children and are to be distinguished from direct infection of the nervous system. The seizure usually accompanies a high rise in fever in an otherwise neurologically normal child. About 30 per cent of these children develop epilepsy later without fever. Sometimes febrile convulsions precipitate status epilepticus, which, in turn, causes permanent cerebral damage. The deep temporal lobe structures are particularly sensitive to the ill effects of prolonged seizures; the resulting lesions may later result in psychomotor seizures.

Head injury is a major cause of acquired epilepsy, the seizures occurring both in the acute phase and as a chronic residual. The incidence of late epilepsy after head injury is given differently in different accounts, but in Jennett's comprehensive series it was 5 per cent. Acute hematoma, seizures occurring immediately after the trauma, and depressed skull fracture all raise the risk. With severe head and depressed skull fracture or open penetration of brain in the sensorimotor area, the incidence of late epilepsy can rise to 50 per cent.

Brain tumors are an important cause of seizures, particularly in adults, but it has been difficult to ascertain the relative incidence of brain tumor with the large population of epileptics. Between 30 and 40 per cent of all patients with cerebral tumors have seizures especially if the tumor is supratentorial. The seizure is apt to be focal and, in 15 to 20 per cent of cases, is the first symptom. The brain tumors most likely to cause seizure are astrocytomas, meningiomas, and metastatic neoplasms, especially those from the lung.

Cerebral vascular disease is a relatively common cause of seizures, particularly in the older age groups. The attacks may result either from localized vascular insufficiency and secondary ischemic hypoxia or from a chronic residual scar, left after thrombosis, embolism, or hemorrhage. Episodes of loss of consciousness owing to diminished cerebral blood flow may progress into seizures, as in severe states of carotid sinus sensitivity and Adams-Stokes syndrome caused by heart block. Seizures appear in up to 20 per cent of patients with the various collagen disorders, e.g., systemic lupus erythematosus and periarteritis nodosa, and are the result of small vascular lesions involving the brain.

Various *allergic reactions* may be related to single seizures, but usually not recurrent epilepsy. Convulsions have been reported after immunizations in drug sensitivity reactions, and after insect bites.

Certain generalized *cerebral degenerative and demyelinating diseases* carry a significant incidence of seizures; in multiple sclerosis this is 5 per cent, and patients with Alzheimer-Pick dementia may experience generalized and myoclonic seizures. The complex cerebral lesions of tuberous sclerosis often produce seizures, including infantile massive spasms. The cerebral lipidoses, such as Tay-Sachs disease, may cause generalized and myoclonic seizures.

Toxic and metabolic disorders are an important cause of seizures since treatment may be directed quite specifically. Seizures are prominent during withdrawal from chronic drug intoxications, particularly from barbiturates (and other sedatives and tranquilizers), and from alcohol. Seizures developing in association with alcoholism usually appear within 48 hours after cessation of drinking and may precede delirium tremens. Carbon monoxide intoxication and other forms of hypoxia may cause seizures. Lead poisoning has been a common cause of convulsions in young children. Water intoxication or excessive hydration, with hemodilution, can produce seizures, again especially in the young. Other pertinent metabolic causes are pyridoxine deficiency, phenylketonuria, hypocalcemia (with or without hypoparathyroidism), porphyria, and hypoglycemia. Hypoglycemia may be a complication of the treatment of diabetes or may accompany islet cell tumors of the pancreas and other endocrine disturbances such as hypopituitarism. Seizures, especially myoclonic, are common in acute and chronic renal insufficiency but are relatively unusual in hepatic failure. Secondarily induced magnesium deficiency, such as follows severe gastrointestinal fluid loss, has been implicated in the production of seizures.

It is likely that, in many patients, several factors combine to produce attacks: a genetically determined predisposition, an increased cerebral excitability related to a general metabolic disturbance, the presence of a focal brain lesion or a tendency to vascular insufficiency, and a triggering disturbance such as emotional crisis or an excessively flickering light. Each patient, therefore, must be evaluated from many different aspects in order to establish full cause and develop appropriate total therapy.

CLINICAL MANIFESTATIONS. The classification of seizures employed here is based mainly on a combination of clinical manifestations and electroencephalographic correlates. Table 1 gives a recently adopted, more detailed international classification of the epilepsies.

Generalized Seizures (Grand Mal or Major Convulsions). The major tonic-clonic seizures have many causes and arise in all age groups. These seizures usually start with a *prodromal phase* that lasts minutes or even hours, with a change in emotional reactivity or affective responses, such as increasing anxiety or depression, often difficult to recognize. More commonly, the specific onset of the seizure is the *aura*, a brief experience directly related to the locus of origin of the seizure. Frequently experienced auras are a sense of fear, a peculiar epigastric sensation welling up into the throat, an unpleasant odor, various visual and auditory hallucinations, and strange sensations in an arm or leg. At times, localized movements of an extremity or portions of the face precede the onset of the general convulsion. The *convulsion* itself occurs with sudden vocalization (the "epileptic cry"), loss of consciousness, tonic extensor rigidity of the trunk and extremities, then clonic movements, a brief cessation of respiration, cyanosis, and then heavy, stertorous breathing. Incontinence of urine and feces can occur; subjects often bite the tongue and cheeks in the clonic phase. After some minutes, the excessive motor activity ceases, breathing becomes more normal, and consciousness gradually returns. Frequently a *postictal state* appears, characterized by confusion, general fatigue, headache, and, some-

---

TABLE 1.   A Classification of Seizures

I. Generalized seizures (bilaterally symmetrical and without local onset)
  1. Tonic-clonic seizures (grand mal)
  2. Tonic seizures
  3. Clonic seizures
  4. Absence seizures (petit mal); may be simple or complex (i.e., with brief automations)
  5. Bilateral epileptic myoclonus (myoclonic jerks)
  6. Infantile spasms
  7. Atonic seizures (often with myoclonic jerks)
  8. Akinetic seizures (loss of movement)
II. Partial seizures or seizures beginning locally (focal seizures)
  A. Elementary or simple (generally without impairment of consciousness)
    1. Motor (with march, as in jacksonian; or without; adversive, aphasic)
    2. Sensory (somatosensory, visual, auditory, vertiginous, olfactory, gustatory)
    3. Autonomic
  B. Complex (generally with some impairment of consciousness; may begin as simple)
    Includes symptoms of cognitive, affective, psychosensory, and psychomotor disturbance, i.e., the psychomotor–temporal lobe–limbic seizure complex
  C. Partial seizures with secondary generalization
III. Unilateral or predominantly unilateral seizures (mostly in childhood); these are mainly unilateral tonic, clonic, or tonic-clonic seizures
IV. Unclassifiable epileptic seizures (usually because of incomplete data)

times residual neurologic signs such as hemiparesis or monoparesis, sensory disturbances, and dysphasia. Automatic behavior may be present. As with the aura, these postictal phenomena can imply focal origins of the generalized seizure. The postictal paralysis, sometimes called "Todd's paralysis," ordinarily lasts for several minutes to hours after the seizure. In general, there is amnesia for a generalized seizure with the exception of possible recollections of the prodromal phase or the aura.

The designation *fragmentary seizure* is given to the occurrence of brief components of the generalized complex. For example, only auras may appear and may or may not be followed by abortive tonic movements or loss of consciousness. Such fragments occur particularly during therapy with anticonvulsant drugs and reflect incomplete control.

Grand mal seizures vary in their frequency from once or twice yearly to many times daily; 20 per cent of patients may have only nocturnal seizures. In women the seizures may appear cyclically with or immediately before the menstrual periods, and the incidence may increase or decrease with pregnancy, being increased by toxemia and water retention.

The *electroencephalographic (EEG) patterns associated with generalized seizures* are difficult to distinguish during the attack from movement artifact. Between attacks, the EEG often contains paroxysms of bilateral, synchronous, 4- to 7-cycle-per-second discharges from all areas, interspersed with nonspecific patterns of high amplitude spikes and slow waves. A paroxysmal or slow wave discharge localized to one region of the scalp suggests a focal cerebral lesion. Between seizures up to 25 per cent of patients have an electroencephalogram within the normal range.

Petit Mal (Absence Attack). The petit mal seizure is a specific form of minor epilepsy, consisting of a sudden brief lapse of consciousness, usually lasting no longer than 30 seconds, more commonly 5 to 10 seconds. Petit mal almost always appears in childhood, with onset usually between the ages of three and ten. The attacks diminish during postpuberty, and rarely persist into adult life after the age of 30. Usually, no specific cause is found. In rare instances a specific brain lesion such as a vascular calcified tumor of the frontal lobe or diffuse cerebral lipidosis has been reported with petit mal seizures, but the EEG was seldom entirely characteristic.

Clinically, the patient with petit mal has a sudden cessation of activity and stares blankly, making no movements, except at times a 3-per-second blinking of the eyelids, a slight deviation of the eyes and head, or brief minor movements of the lips and hands. The end of the spell is equally abrupt. More complex behavioral disturbances or postictal confusion or drowsiness suggest another type of minor seizure such as psychomotor automatism rather than petit mal. The attacks of petit mal can be as few as a flurry every several days to as many as 100 or more per day. As the frequency increases, the repeated absences sometimes produce difficulties in continuing motor tasks and in learning. The designation *petit mal status* or absence state refers to many attacks occurring close together for minutes to hours and producing confusion and disorientation.

The electroencephalographic correlate of the petit mal or absence seizure is a rhythmic 3-cycle-per-second spike and wave discharge appearing synchronously from all scalp regions both during and between seizures. Usually a discharge of more than a few seconds' duration is associated with a clinical absence. The characteristics of the seizure and the typical electroencephalographic discharge have led to these seizures being designated as "centrencephalic," implying an origin in the centrally placed, "integrating," mesodiencephalic regions of the brain. Experimentally, there is evidence to support this hypothesis, although direct confirmation in the human is inconclusive.

Akinetic Seizure. The term akinetic attack is applied to a generalized seizure associated with loss of consciousness and simple falling. It may be accompanied by an absence and minor movements, but generally there is a marked diminution of postural tone with falling and, often, self-injury. Afterward, the appearance of normal posture and mental clarity is common, although there may be a brief period of confusion. Electroencephalographically, there is a diffuse abnormality with slow wave discharges or atypical spike waves, often slower than 3 per second.

Myoclonic Seizures. These are characterized by sudden involuntary contractions involving an integrated response of a single muscle or several muscle groups, producing relatively simple arrhythmic jerking movements about a single joint or several joints, or of a segment of the body. The jerks may exist as an independent entity, as a phenomenon preceding and building up to a generalized grand mal convulsion, or as an accompaniment to petit mal absences in children. Myoclonic attacks are often sensitive to sensory stimulation and may be precipitated or accentuated by sound or light, by change in posture, by movement of an extremity, by drowsiness, or by an emotional upset. Myoclonic jerks occur as a normal phenomenon in normal subjects during drowsiness.

Myoclonus Epilepsy. The myoclonus epilepsy of Unverricht refers to generalized myoclonus and mental deterioration secondary to a diffuse degenerative metabolic disorder of undetermined origin. Other forms of myclonus appear in diseases of cerebral lipid metabolism, in subacute encephalitis, and with rare forms of cerebellar disease. A severe myoclonus appearing in the first 18 months of life and associated with general cerebral deterioration is called *infantile massive spasms* or jackknife seizures. In this condition, the infant develops severe flexion spasms of the head, neck, and trunk and extension of the legs and arms. Some known causes of this disorder are phenylketonuria, tuberous sclerosis, and Down's syndrome, but in most instances neither a biochemical nor an anatomic abnormality can be found.

The electroencephalographic correlates of the myoclonic seizure are variable depending on the severity of the seizure state; in mild instances, generalized, synchronous slow spike and wave complexes or sharp and slow wave elements occur intermittently with relatively normal electroencephalographic patterns between. Infantile massive spasms are commonly associated with *hypsarrhythmia*, which consists of more or less continuous, nonsynchronous, asymmetric discharges of spike and sharp wave elements along with slow waves from all regions.

Focal or Partial Seizures. Involvement by a lesion of a specific region of the brain may be manifested by characteristic seizures. They are typical of acquired epilepsy, although occasionally no anatomic abnormality is found. As indicated above, a focal onset seizure can occasionally spread extremely rapidly to become generalized, but in seizure states specifically classified as focal or partial, the attack usually remains limited. There often is a disturbance of consciousness or awareness with varying degrees of amnesia, but total loss of consciousness occurs only with general spread.

Lesions involving any of the motor regions of the brain, but particularly the so-called motor cortex, produce focal motor seizures. The classic *jacksonian motor seizure,* caused by a lesion sharply localized in a specific region of the motor cortex, begins as a repetitive movement of a distal portion of an extremity, such as the fingers or toes, and then spreads by a march of the clonic contractions up the extremity toward the trunk. Such a seizure usually remains limited to the extremity, but it may spread to the rest of the ipsilateral side, the face, and the contralateral side. Occasionally, these seizures begin at the corner of the mouth and are associated with masticatory movements and speech disturbances. Other focal motor seizures involve gross movements of the arms or legs without the classic jacksonian march. *Adversive seizures* produce turning movements of the head, eyes, and trunk toward the side opposite the cerebral lesion, which is usually in the profrontal cortex.

Focal seizures originating from the *supplementary motor area* of the mesial frontal supracingulate cortex are not common; they are characterized by gross body movements, especially raising of the contralateral arm with the head turning toward that arm, rhythmic bilateral arm and leg movements, and repetitive speech, usually of syllables, not words. Occasionally, speech is slowed or totally inhibited during such a seizure. Other experiences are peculiar sensations in the abdomen, generalized flushing, and palpitations.

Focal sensory seizures caused by a lesion involving the sensory cortex may be jacksonian with a march of abnormal sensations such as numbness and tingling spreading up an extremity. Other sensory areas of the cerebral cortex produce more complex seizures with paroxysmal visual, auditory, olfactory, gustatory, and vertiginous components in varying degrees of organization. As with other types of focal attacks, the pattern of onset is often the most accurate guide to the locus of an abnormal cerebral lesion.

Autonomic seizures are produced by focal lesions in the regions of the brain associated with autonomic representation, namely, the deep temporal, limbic, and diencephalic (hypothalamic) areas. Many autonomic symptoms are associated with other focal or generalized seizures, but they also appear in attacks more or less by themselves, as paroxysms of abdominal pain, sweating, piloerection, incontinence, salivation, and, rarely, fever.

Psychomotor (temporal lobe, limbic system) epilepsy is due to seizure activity involving the temporal lobe, its deeper nuclear masses (the amygdala and hippocampus), and their associated limbic system structures. Psychomotor epilepsy is common in both children and adults and occasionally coexists with grand mal seizures. Such patients often give a history of febrile seizures and status epilepticus in infancy. Evidence of an acquired lesion is found in more than half the patients, with a frequent history of trauma at birth or, later, encephalitis or neoplasm. Some patients with psychomotor seizures are found to have focal frontal or occipital lobe lesions, but even with these there is evidence that the discharges produce their eventual manifestations by propagation through temporal-limbic lobe structures.

Psychomotor-temporal-limbic seizures can take a number of forms, and several combinations can occur of the symptoms given in the following description. Many such attacks are manifested by an initial aura of anxiety and visceral symptoms, especially by a peculiar epigastric sensation welling up into the throat. An alteration in consciousness follows, associated with complex feeling and thinking states, as well as automatic somatic and autonomic motor behavior. Memory loss, disorientation, or a sense of re-experiencing the environment (déjà vu) may be prominent. Motor activity is first arrested or suspended, then simple movements can ensue, such as chewing, swallowing, sucking, lip smacking, and aimless twistings of the arms and legs. Automatisms of varying complexity can involve either partially purposeful or inappropriate and bizarre behavior. Usually, such automatisms are stereotyped, but, despite this, the movements usually interplay with the environment, and occasionally they appear to be determined in part by psychologic factors. The activities in this phase of the seizure may merge into normal behavior. The complex attack beginning with unpleasant olfactory hallucinations caused by lesions of the mesial portions of the temporal lobe, the uncus, was specifically called an uncinate seizure by Jackson, who also described the "dreamy" and confused state of the patient. Visceral manifestations are common in young patients, who experience hunger, nausea, vomiting, and abdominal pain as well as urinary incontinence. Destructive aggressive behavior occasionally occurs but usually is not goal-directed unless patients are forcibly restrained. Affective disturbances may include expressions of fear, anger, and depression. Occasionally, prolonged fuguelike states with running or wandering may last many minutes or even hours. During some psychomotor–temporal lobe seizures, patients experience hallucinations, visual or auditory as well as interpretive illusions involving their own bodies or the immediate environment. These symptoms frequently are associated with ideational blocking and forced thinking as well as peculiar feelings of familiarity called "déjà vu" and "déjà pensée." Amnesia is usually present.

ELECTROENCEPHALOGRAPHIC CONCOMITANTS OF FOCAL SEIZURES. These are represented by discharges of slow waves, spikes, and sharp and slow complexes localized over the particular cerebral region involved. Frequently, the abnormalities are bilateral but asynchronous, representing transmission and diffusion of the abnormal discharge from one hemisphere to its mirror point on the other. At times, deeply situated lesions produce only minimal or no significant alteration in the ordinary electroencephalogram recorded from the scalp.

Status Epilepticus. The rapid repetitive recurrence of any type of seizure without recovery between attacks is called status epilepticus. The term is usually applied to attacks of generalized epilepsy in which the patient remains unconscious and in continuous seizures, with tonic and clonic fluctuations, incontinence, severely disturbed breathing, high fever, excessive sweating, and elevation of blood pressure. Such status may last for hours, even days, and requires emergency medical treatment because of the possible dangers of cerebral damage, thought to be due to ischemic anoxia (or "consumptive" hypoxia) and cardiac and renal failure. Careful attention to ventilation and oxygen demands during such severe seizure activity reduces the associated risk of brain damage, but only stopping the seizures guarantees that no more damaging consequences will occur. Although status epilepticus sometimes begins spontaneously, most attacks follow sudden withdrawal from anticonvulsant medication or a too rapid shift of medication.

Focal motor seizures may recur in continuous fashion, lasting many hours; this state has been called *epilepsia partialis continua*.

Petit mal status is associated with sustained 3-cycle-per-second spike-wave discharges in the electroencephalogram. The patient is in a state of confusion, has a continuously dazed expression, and has minor movements around the lips or in the arms and legs. *Psychomotor* or *temporal lobe status* also occurs, but less frequently. Such patients are found in a confused state with persistent, inappropriate, bizarre complex behavior patterns lasting over many hours, occasionally associated with fluctuating visceral symptoms.

The Interseizure State.   A patient with a progressive cerebral degenerative disease, an extensive cerebral malformation, a severe encephalitis, or an expanding brain tumor may develop changes in behavior and intellectual functioning, primarily because of the underlying structural lesions and not directly because of any seizures that might be present. In the past much attention has been paid to the possibility of a specific personality distortion in epileptic patients. Most patients subject to seizures have normal behavior and intellectual functions between attacks and adjust appropriately to society, often excelling. In some instances, however, severe emotional problems do develop, usually in response to environmental restrictions. *Neurotic, maladjusted behavior* occurs with obsessional, particularly religious, preoccupations. Often, under these circumstances, the seizures increase and become more difficult to control.

An undetermined number of patients with frequent recurrent generalized seizures, especially status epilepticus, or with recurrent psychomotor temporal-limbic seizures, develop continuing defects in intellectual functions. Psychologic tests reveal persistent impairments of concentration and attention, memory lapses, word-finding distortions, subtle losses in the ability to associate, and perceptual difficulties. It is possible that prolonged subclinical seizure activity contributes to these disturbances.

More severe personality disturbances, ranging all the way to psychosis with schizophrenic manifestations, complicate the interseizure course of a few patients with either psychomotor or severe grand mal epilepsy. The psychotic reactions often have psychologic precipitating factors; occasionally, they follow control of the actual seizures by medication, and these instances may be related, in part, to a reaction to the drug. The symptoms include paranoid, depressive, and hallucinatory reactions, catatonic disorders, flattening of the affect, and severe obsessional states. The patients suffer marked difficulty in concentration and disorientation of time sequences. Defects in memory are present and are accompanied by abnormalities in perception as well as difficulties in word finding, in calculating, and in analyzing the thought content of written material. However, the patients usually attempt to maintain contacts

with reality, and major withdrawal is not present, in contrast to most examples of spontaneous schizophrenic illness. Diffuse electroencephalographic abnormality, with either bilateral temporal lobe involvement or diffuse spike wave paroxysms, accompanies some of these clinical phases, but with others the electroencephalogram remains normal.

DIAGNOSIS IN EPILEPSY.   The patient with epilepsy should receive a thorough diagnostic evaluation to determine causative factors and precipitating circumstances. This requires a thorough history, a detailed medical and neurologic physical examination, and selected laboratory investigations, with particular reference to blood chemistry tests, cerebrospinal fluid analysis, electroencephalography, and special roentgenologic studies. Every effort should be made to identify a specific medical illness or a focal cerebral lesion.

History.   The history must contain a detailed description of the attacks to help establish the fact of recurrent seizures. As much recollection as possible should be obtained from the patient, particularly of experiences of the aura and the onset of the seizure. The patterning or course of events during and after the seizure should be documented, especially by eyewitness accounts, with special attention to any phenomena that might possess localizing significance. Information should be sought as to the various circumstances under which seizures occur, such as the time of day or night, the frequency of attacks and how medication influences them, their relationship to the menstrual cycle, pregnancy, food intake, sound or light stimulation, intake of alcoholic drinks, or psychologic stresses. All symptoms of neurologic disturbances should be described, such as headache, hemiparesis, hemisensory disturbances, dysphasia, visual difficulties, or vertigo.

The *past medical and developmental history* is of great aid in establishing the cause. Information should be obtained concerning pregnancy, delivery, the neonatal period, the developmental neurologic milestones, head injuries, and reactions to immunizations and the various childhood illnesses such as measles, mumps, and chickenpox. The occurrence of any severe illness with delirium or coma that might be considered an encephalitis should be inquired about, as well as any exposure to toxic substances. Drug intake needs particular investigation, particularly with adults suspected of taking barbiturates or tranquilizer drugs. One must inquire into the patient's social development and behavior in and out of the family setting, his intellectual performance at school, and his vocational adjustments and performance. Any alteration in these phases of existence should be related to seizure occurrence, to the interseizure state, and to the possible effects of medication.

A *family history* of susceptibility to seizures may delineate a significant number with a history of febrile seizures in early childhood as well as of generalized and focal seizures extending into later life. The family history may reveal not only genetically determined cerebral disorders associated with seizures but also other neurologic abnormalities.

The *general medical history* can reveal evidence of pertinent cardiovascular disease, blood dyscrasias, and metabolic and endocrine disorders; a seizure may be the first manifestation of a cerebral metastasis or of a generalized vascular disease.

Clinical Examination. In most patients with seizures, physical examination fails to disclose significant physical or neurologic abnormalities. Nevertheless, a thorough general examination is warranted; careful examination of the skin, for example, may produce the diagnosis in cases of tuberous sclerosis, neurofibromatosis, or cerebral hemangioma. Examination of the lungs provides evidence for consideration of metastatic tumor or abscess; evaluation of the peripheral circulation and blood pressure gives an indication of the possibility of the various types of cerebral vascular lesions or aids in differentiating between syncope and seizure.

The *neurologic examination* serves two purposes: to elicit signs of any general neurologic disorder and to determine whether or not focal signs of a localized cerebral lesion are present. A neurologic examination is particularly valuable at the time of, or shortly after, a seizure if it reveals a transitory hemiparesis or related signs.

A battery of *psychologic tests* can aid the evaluation of both intellectual capabilities and psychologic adjustments. Simple tests of memory and perception are part of the regular neurologic examination. For more complete studies, the most useful tests include the Wechsler Intelligence Scale (especially the Kohs block test), the memory scales, the Bender-Gestalt, the Rorschach, and the Thematic Apperception tests. Attention should be paid to the patient's performance during these tests as well as to the actual scores.

Laboratory Investigations. Each patient with recurrent seizures, no matter the age, should be examined with certain laboratory investigations at least once and more often if changes develop in seizure patterns or neurologic signs. At different ages certain tests are more apt to produce results leading to specific etiologic diagnosis. Additional studies are necessary to evaluate the general health of the patient and follow the potentially toxic effects of medications.

There are no abnormal laboratory findings consistently associated directly with seizure activity except electroencephalographic discharges. Urinalysis is necessary to determine the state of kidney function; if abnormal, a specific renal disorder may be present, and certain drugs cannot be administered. Similarly, a complete blood count is necessary. Severe seizure states such as status epilepticus may be associated with proteinuria, leukocytosis, and fever as secondary manifestations. In certain instances, special blood chemistry studies are warranted, such as the blood sugar for the diagnosis of suspected hypoglycemia and in the evaluation of a diabetic with epilepsy, and the serum calcium determination for infants and young children with seizure states. Evaluation of fluctuations in serum electrolytes and acid-base balance is necessary to study both children and adults with disorders of the kidney, liver, heart, and lungs, or those suspected of water intoxication. Serologic tests help to diagnose past infections.

The *cerebrospinal fluid* is apt to be normal in all constituents and pressures, except in the minority of patients who have specific neurologic disease. After severe seizures, there may be a slight increase in the cerebrospinal fluid protein and white cell count. In structural neurologic disorders with seizures, the protein and/or pressure may be elevated persistently, and the specific diagnosis then depends on other tests, such as contrast roentgenologic studies. Chronic nervous system infection can be associated with an increase in the white cell count of the cerebrospinal fluid; occasionally, a cerebral tumor may be revealed by neoplastic cells in the fluid.

Roentgenograms of the skull and chest may be taken of all patients. The film of the skull may reveal asymmetry caused by early injury or maldevelopment, abnormal calcifications, shift of the calcified pineal, or signs of increased intracranial pressure. The chest film potentially detects pulmonary infection or tumor and aids in evaluating the cardiac status. Roentgenologic studies of the intracranial contents employing contrast media are extremely useful diagnostic procedures if employed at the proper time, but must be selected with care because of their morbid potential. Such procedures are considered when a focal intracranial lesion is suspected. In many countries, *computerized axial tomography* (CT scanning) of the brain has largely replaced ventriculography and pneumoencephalography in the diagnosis of suspected brain tumors or atrophic lesions. CT scanning with contrast material certainly is indicated in any epileptic in whom the least suspicion of a focal abnormality exists or in adults with seizures of recent onset. *Cerebral arteriography* is useful to demonstrate localized abnormal vascular patterns in neoplasms as well as intracranial hematomas, vascular malformations, and the location of vascular occlusions.

Radioactive isotopic brain scanning has largely been supplemented by CT scanning as a diagnostic tool in epilepsy.

Electroencephalography. The various electroencephalographic correlates of the different types of seizures have been described. The electroencephalogram is an indicator of a certain kind of cerebral activity determined by recording electrodes upon the scalp. This is important to realize, because electroencephalograms from up to 25 per cent of patients with seizures are normal; yet, abnormal discharges are disclosed in many of these same patients by depth electrodes recording from deeper cerebral structures such as the amygdala and hippocampus. The electroencephalogram, therefore, has limited diagnostic applications and must be correlated with other information from the various physical and neurologic examinations. It can be utilized to confirm the presence of a seizure disturbance, particularly if paroxysmal discharges are recorded during and correlated with a seizure. The use of television monitoring during electroencephalographic recording sometimes aids in establishing the specificity of the electroencephalographic pattern. An example of this specificity is that up to 85 per cent of children with petit mal will have the typical 3-cycle-per-second spike and wave discharges both during and between seizures, and in many instances these discharges can be precipitated during the recording by overventilation and light stimulation.

In other instances of epilepsy, the electroencephalogram contains generalized, nonspecific slow wave discharges that merely indicate the presence of cerebral dysfunction, but not a definite seizure disorder. Focal slow wave abnormalities in the electroencephalogram suggest a localized structural lesion and ordinarily lead to further investigations. In certain forms of focal epilepsy, the electroencephalogram may show focal discharges of spikes, sharp waves, and complex components indicative of the epileptogenic nature of the focus. Yet, in some of these instances, such an abnormality might be transmitted, the basic discharging focus being elsewhere.

In most laboratories of electroencephalography the test procedure involves recording in the waking state and during voluntary overventilation. Additional attempts are usually made to provoke generalized and focal paroxysmal discharges by means of sleep, sensory stimulation with light and occasionally sound, and sometimes by utilizing certain metabolic and pharmacologic adjuvants.

The recording of the electroencephalogram during sleep is useful in the attempt to demonstrate focal temporal lobe discharges in patients with psychomotor-temporal lobe epilepsy. In adults, such discharges are increased during sleep in up to 75 per cent of patients, but in children the increase occurs in only 30 per cent. In many patients, sleep produces increased bilateral appearance of abnormal temporal discharges. The use of sleep deprivation prior to a recording, then followed by sleep, may produce more abnormal discharges. The use of sphenoidal electrodes is occasionally of some help in lateralizing temporal lobe discharge, particularly when patients are being evaluated for surgical therapy. At times, barbiturate-induced fast wave activity is found to be diminished on the side of the involved temporal lobe. Photic stimulation identifies patients with light-sensitive epilepsy and, occasionally, produces lateralized discharges in patients with a sensitive focus. There have been many attempts to alter the electrical activity of the brain in susceptible patients by inducing metabolic changes, such as hydration after an injection of Pitressin. Various stimulant drugs have been used, such as pentylenetetrazole (Metrazol) and bemegride (Megimide). All these methods, particularly the use of the drugs, may produce paroxysmal discharges as well as clinical seizures, usually generalized. However many normal subjects respond with seizures to these procedures. Accordingly, these methods are not recommended for general use in the diagnosis of epilepsy. Occasionally, it may be important in the evaluation of a specific patient to study in detail the phenomena of the seizure and to determine focal components either in the electroencephalogram or clinically. In selected cases, this can be accomplished by the administration of a controlled dose of a seizure-producing drug, under very careful monitoring.

The use of the electroencephalogram in following patients with epilepsy is limited, because in many instances some degree of electroencephalographic abnormality persists even though seizures are controlled. This is most often the case in patients with psychomotor-temporal lobe epilepsy and least often in children with petit mal and myoclonic seizures.

DIFFERENTIAL DIAGNOSIS. The diagnosis of epilepsy has profound medical and psychologic implications as it affects the total life situation of the patient and his family. Consequently, careful attention must be given to make this diagnosis positively and specifically, and to differentiate it from nonepileptic disturbances that produce somewhat similar abnormalities of neurologic function.

Consciousness may be disturbed episodically by inadequate cerebral blood flow in attacks of *cerebrovascular insufficiency* or of *syncope* of various types, particularly the vasodepressor form. Disturbances of cerebral circulation affect older persons especially, and such pa-

tients generally suffer other evidence of hypertension and cerebral arteriosclerosis. Periodic blackouts and recurrent confusional states are manifestations of basilar artery insufficiency, as are other episodic signs of brainstem and cerebellar dysfunction. Patients with carotid arterial insufficiency characteristically experience transitory hemiparesis and hemisensory disturbances along with dysphasia, but the clonic movements of a paroxysmal disorder usually are absent. The electroencephalographic findings of paroxysmal discharge do not occur with cerebrovascular disease although, at times, bilateral rhythmic discharges are observed related to vascular lesions of the upper brainstem. The differential diagnosis is sometimes difficult and may require arteriographic confirmation of a vascular lesion as well as the usual evaluation of the history and general medical state of the patient.

Syncopal episodes may resemble akinetic or brief motor seizures; prolonged syncope can progress into a convulsion resulting from the persistence of cerebral ischemia and hypoxia. Girls and young women are more prone than boys to such severe syncopal attacks. The patient with syncope usually has indications of disturbed vasomotor reactivity with excessive sweating, pallor, and tachycardia. Specific precipitating factors often are present such as fear or other psychologic upset. The confusion, headache, and drowsiness that occur after a generalized seizure usually do not appear in syncope. The electroencephalogram during simple syncope consists of diffuse asynchronous slow waves without paroxysmal or focal discharges.

Certain *psychogenic disorders* resemble epileptic states and can be difficult to differentiate. Hysterical "seizures" not only occur as independent problems, but also complicate the course of a limited number of patients with known seizures, the combination being called "hysteroepilepsy." The clinical problem is difficult to unravel because of the interrelationships between the actual seizure and the reactive psychologic disturbance. The hysterical seizure is not associated with neurologic signs of reflex abnormality and, during it, the electroencephalogram contains no paroxysmal discharges. The pattern of hysterical seizures is often bizarre and not a stereotyped tonic-clonic movement sequence. During true seizures the pupils are fixed, and following grand mal convulsions caloric responses are briefly lost; neither change occurs with hysteria. Self-injury is an unusual result of hysterical seizures, and the postictal states of confusion, headache, and drowsiness are absent. Hysterical or psychotic fugue disturbances and dissociative reactions must be distinguished from psychomotor–temporal lobe seizures. The diagnosis of an hysterical seizure state requires careful psychiatric evaluation because of the severe neurotic process involved.

TREATMENT. Treatment of the epilepsies must take into account not only the patient and his disorder, but his family and general life situation. Much depends on the diagnostic evaluation and the finding of specific causes whenever possible that can be treated directly. This is clearly defined in instances in which metabolic disturbance is obvious, such as hypoglycemia and hypocalcemia, or when an operable cerebral tumor is found. However, in many cases of acquired epilepsy, the basic cause of the seizure cannot be treated directly. Seizures may continue in patients even after removal of a brain tumor because of scarring, or when the tumor

TABLE 2. Most Frequently Used Anticonvulsant Drugs: Dosage, Indications, and Toxic Effects

Acetazolamide (Diamox)

Dose:	250 mg tablets
Daily dosage:	Children: 0.75 to 1.0 gram; adults: 1.0 to 1.5 grams. Use intermittently; tolerance occurs
Indications:	As an adjuvant in all types of seizures, especially those in females related to menstrual cycles
Toxic effects:	Anorexia, acidosis, drowsiness, numbness of extremities; rarely, blood dyscrasias

Carbamazepine (Tegretol)

Dose:	0.2 gram tablets
Daily dosage:	Children: 20 mg per kg; adults: 0.2 to 0.8 gram
Indications:	Complex partial (psychomotor–temporal lobe) and other focal seizures, grand mal
Toxic effects:	Leukopenia, anorexia, "dizziness," drowsiness, rash

Clonazepam (Clonopin)

Dose:	0.5 mg, 1.0 mg, 2.0 mg tablets
Daily dosage:	Children: 1.5 to 4 mg; adults: 3 to 12 mg
Indications:	Myoclonic, minor motor, akinetic, petit mal, some complex partial seizures
Toxic effects:	Drowsiness, ataxia, behavioral problems, anorexia, hematologic (anemia, leukopenia)

Diphenylhydantoin (phenytoin, Dilantin)

Dose:	0.03 gram and 0.1 gram capsules; 0.05 gram tablets; 0.1 gram delayed action capsules; 0.025 gram per ml suspension; 0.1 gram in oil, capsules; 0.25 gram ampules for parenteral use
Daily dosage:	Children: 0.15 to 0.3 gram; adults: 0.3 to 0.6 gram. Effective blood level 10 to 20 μg/ml
Indications:	Grand mal, psychomotor and focal seizures; most useful in combination with phenobarbital or primidone
Toxic effects:	Rash, fever, gum hypertrophy, gastric distress, diplopia, ataxia, hirsutism (young females); drowsiness, uncommon; megaloblastic anemia (due to secondary folic acid deficiency); lymphadenopathy

Ethosuximide (Zarontin)

Dose:	0.25 gram capsules
Daily dosage:	Children: to 0.75 to 1.0 gram; adults: 1.5 grams. Effective blood level range 40 to 80 μg/ml
Indications:	Petit mal seizures (now the drug of choice); used with Dilantin in mixed seizure states
Toxic effects:	Blood dyscrasias (pancytopenia, leukopenia) unusual; dermatitis, anorexia, nausea, drowsiness, dizziness

Ethylphenylhydantoin (Peganone)

Dose:	0.25 gram, 0.5 gram tablets
Daily dosage:	Children: 0.5 gram to 1.5 grams; adults: 2.0 to 3.0 grams
Indications:	Grand mal, psychomotor and focal seizures
Toxic effects:	Similar to those of Dilantin but less frequent; may be substituted for Dilantin, but is generally less effective

Methylphenylethylhydantoin (Mesantoin)

Dose:	0.1 gram tablets
Daily dosage:	Children: 0.1 to 0.4 gram; adults: 0.4 to 0.8 gram
Indications:	Grand mal, psychomotor, and focal seizures
Toxic effects:	Rash, fever, drowsiness, ataxia, gum hypertrophy (less than Dilantin), neutropenia, agranulocytosis

Paramethadione (Paradione)

Dose:	0.15 gram, 0.3 gram capsules; 0.3 gram per ml solution
Daily dosage:	Children: up to six years of age, 0.3 to 0.9 gram; over six years of age, 0.6 to 1.8 grams; adults: 1.2 to 2.4 grams
Indications:	Peti mal, myoclonic, and akinetic seizures, massive spasms, occasionally psychomotor seizures (in children); often useful in combination with Dilantin and phenobarbital; somewhat less effective and less toxic than Tridione
Toxic effects:	Rash, gastric distress, visual symptoms (glare, photophobia), neutropenia, agranulocytosis

Phenacemide (Phenurone)

Dose:	0.5 gram tablets; 0.3 gram enteric-coated tablets
Daily dosage:	Children over five years of age, 0.5 gram to 2.0 grams; adults: 1.5 grams to 3.0 grams
Indications:	May be effective in all types of seizures, especially psychomotor-temporal lobe seizures; should be used only in very resistant cases
Toxic effects:	A highly toxic drug, producing liver damage, agranulocytosis, psychotic reactions, and rashes

Phenobarbital

Dose:	0.015 gram, 0.030 gram, 0.060 gram, 0.1 gram tablets; 4 mg per ml elixir
Daily dosage:	Children: 0.045 gram to 0.1 gram; adults: 0.1 gram to 0.3 gram. Effective blood level range 15 to 30 μg/ml
Indications:	All seizure states: grand mal, petit mal, psychomotor and other focal; most useful in limited dosage in combination with other drugs such as Dilantin
Toxic effects:	Drowsiness, dulling, rash, fever; irritability, and hyperactivity in some children

Primidone (Mysoline)

Dose:	0.05 gram, 0.25 gram tablets; 250 mg per 5 ml suspension
Daily dosage:	Children: 0.25 gram; adults: 0.75 to 2.0 grams. The daily dosage should be built up very slowly. Effective blood level range 5 to 15 μg/ml
Indications:	Grand mal, psychomotor and focal seizures; occasionally, petit mal; useful in combination with Dilantin
Toxic effects:	Drowsiness, ataxia, dizziness, rash, nausea, leukopenia (rare)

Trimethadione (Tridione)

Dose:	0.15 gram tablets; 0.3 gram capsules; 0.15 gram per 4 ml solution
Daily dosage:	Same as paramethadione, above. Effective blood level range 10 to 30 μg/ml
Indications:	Petit mal, myoclonic and akinetic seizures, massive spasms; often useful in combination with Dilantin and phenobarbital
Toxic effects:	Rash, gastric distress, visual symptoms (glare, photophobia) neutropenia, agranulocytosis, nephrosis

Valproic Acid (Depakene)

Dose:	0.25 gram capsules, 0.25 gram per ml syrup
Daily dosage:	15 mg/kg/day, increasing at one-week intervals by 5 to 10 mg/kg/day until seizures controlled or side effects preclude further increase; maximum daily dosage is 30 mg/kg/day; if daily dose exceeds 250 mg, it should be given in a divided regimen
Indications:	Petit mal (simple and complex absence seizures); adjunctive therapy in multiple seizure types
Toxic effects:	Nausea, vomiting, diarrhea, anorexia, sedation, ataxia, hair loss (rare, transient), rash, emotional reactions, altered bleeding time, leukopenia, hepatotoxicity (rare); may cause an increase in serum phenobarbital levels, and decrease or increase in serum phenytoin (diphenylhydantoin)

The following drugs may be used in the emergency treatment of status epilepticus:[*]

Diazepam (Valium):	2.5 to 10 mg intravenously
Sodium phenobarbital:	0.25 to 0.50 gram intravenously
Sodium amytal:	0.25 to 0.50 gram intravenously
Dilantin sodium (parenteral):	0.25 gram intravenously in patients previously receiving this drug or as much as 1.0 to 1.5 in previously untreated patients). *Caution:* Dilantin intravenously must be given slowly in 0.05 gram increments to avoid vasodepression

[*]General anesthetics such as ether, Avertin, and xylocaine have a limited usefulness in the treatment of status epilepticus. Careful nursing and attention to fluid and electrolyte balance, airway, cardiac and renal functions, and temperature control are essential in the over-all management of status epilepticus.

is found to be inoperable or incompletely removable. The diagnosis of an acquired epilepsy after head injury or encephalitis usually does not lead to specific therapy. Only a limited number of patients with post-traumatic epilepsy are satisfactory candidates for surgical removal of a localized meningocerebral scar. The administration of anticonvulsant drugs is necessary, therefore, for the majority of patients.

Medical Therapy. There are many available anticonvulsant drugs, but those listed in Table 2 are the main ones used by the general physician. No drug will achieve total seizure control in all patients, but careful selection and utilization in each case often leads to optimal results. Each physician should learn to use a number of these drugs well and to recognize disturbing side effects as early as possible. Periodic blood counts, urinalyses, and liver function tests are necessary with certain drugs.

The basic mechanisms of anticonvulsant drugs are not definitely known. Most of the drugs are neuronal depressants with certain variations in action. The hydantoin drugs reduce the synaptic activity of post-tetanic potentiation; the oxazolidine (methadone) drugs decrease nerve transmission during repetitive stimulation. The drugs are believed to increase the stability of excitable neuronal membranes by acting upon electrochemical characteristics involved in ion permeability and membrane polarization. Such stabilizing effects would decrease the activity of the hyperexcitable neuronal aggregates in an epileptogenic focus and prevent the spread of discharge through normal neuronal circuits.

The anticonvulsant drugs are administered to achieve the desired effect of seizure control and must be built up in dosage while not producing untoward toxic reactions. It is best to start with one drug of choice, but usually a single drug is not totally effective, and a second is necessary. Two drugs might be needed initially for patients with two different types of seizure such as grand mal and petit mal. This occurs in from 25 to 50 per cent of children with petit mal. The process may require weeks of adjustment, and during this time the patient's or parent's cooperation in reporting effects on seizure frequency or side reactions is most important. Determination of anticonvulsant blood levels, i.e., diphenylhydantoin, phenobarbital, primidone, may be helpful in identifying patients who are obtaining unsatisfactory control because they either fail to take the drug or metabolize it abnormally. Drugs should be started slowly and their doses changed gradually. Frequent and rapid shifting or replacement of drugs produces side effects and can precipitate seizures. Following blood levels in each individual patient and using the blood level to adjust medication dosage into the therapeutic range improves seizure control and reduces the risk of inducing toxicity.

Diphenylhydantoin metabolism is impaired in patients with acute and chronic liver disease, resulting in elevations of blood levels when standard doses of the drug are taken. By contrast, in the presence of uremia, the blood level of diphenylhydantoin is reduced; however, apparently adequate amounts of the drug unbound to plasma protein may be achieved with administered low dosage.

Other drugs can alter the rate of diphenylhydantoin metabolism induced in liver microsomal enzymes so as to lead to an increase in diphenylhydantoin blood levels even to toxicity. These drugs include isoniazid, bishydroxycoumarin, phenyramidol, disulfiram, methylphenidate, diazepam, chlordiazepoxide, phenylbutazone, chlorpromazine, prochlorperazine, and some estrogens. Carbamazepine and ethanol have been reported to lower diphenylhydantoin blood levels. On the other hand, diphenylhydantoin has been reported to lower blood levels of digitoxin, bishydroxycoumarin, metyrapone, and DDT. Diphenylhydantoin also has been found to stimulate enzymes which rapidly turn over endogenous or exogenously administered adrenocorticosteroids; this has resulted, in some instances, in increased adrenocorticotropic and cortisol production by negative feedback effects.

A specific anticonvulsant drug for each type of seizure is not available. However, there is one major therapeutic division; petit mal absences respond best to either succinimide or oxazolidines (methadiones). These drugs are not effective in the treatment of major generalized (grand mal) or focal cerebral seizures, nor are the hydantoins (used in grand mal and other seizures) effective in petit mal. It is stated that the drugs used in the therapy of petit mal may worsen a generalized seizure state, but this has not been proved.

Generalized grand mal and focal motor seizures are best treated by diphenylhydantoin sodium and phenobarbital. Initially, either drug may be administered to patients who have infrequent attacks, but generally the combination of diphenylhydantoin and phenobarbital produces the most effective seizure control. The average dose of diphenylhydantoin is 0.3 to 0.4 gram per day usually administered as 0.2 gram in the morning after breakfast and 0.2 gram after dinner. The dosage of phenobarbital is initially 60 mg at bedtime, with 30 mg increments over the day, up to three times daily, if necessary, limited by the unwanted sedative effect.

Patients with psychomotor–temporal lobe epilepsy are often more difficult to control. Many trials of different agents and different doses may be necessary in these cases; the best results are to be expected with diphenylhydantoin and either phenobarbital or primidone. Although in some clinics the two latter drugs are used together, primidone is partially converted to phenobarbital, and their sedative effects combine to make such administration difficult. It is most important with primidone to start therapy with small doses, such as 125 mg, increased at weekly intervals to reach a maximal dosage of 0.75 gram for children or 1.0 to 2.0 grams per day for adults.

Carbamazepine (Tegretol) is being administered more frequently to patients with psychomotor–temporal lobe seizures, often in combination with diphenylhydantoin, rather than the barbiturate-related drugs, as it is less sedative. The tendency for carbamazepine to produce leukopenia must be monitored carefully.

Acetazolamide is an adjuvant to the treatment of any type of seizure. It seems to have a general effect upon hyperexcitable cerebral neurons because of its properties of inhibition of carbonic anhydrase and production of acidosis. Because tolerance develops, the drug should be administered intermittently. It is occasionally useful, for example, in helping to control seizures appearing periodically in females at the time of menstruation. Under these circumstances, acetazolamide is administered for a week prior to and during menses.

Status epilepticus with major motor seizures is a medical emergency and requires immediately effective treatment to minimize the risk of brain damage. The first step is to establish an adequate airway and oxygenation. This requires insertion of an endotracheal tube if the subject remains unresponsive for more than 30 minutes or so. Anticonvulsants should be given intravenously, diazepam, 10 mg, being the initial drug of choice to stop convulsions. This can be repeated up to three times with 20-minute intervals, as it has a short duration of action. Maintenance anticonvulsants should follow immediately, injecting diphenylhydantoin slowly intravenously, 0.05 gram every one to two minutes to a total of 0.5 gram in patients previously receiving the drug and up to 1.0 or 1.2 grams in previously untreated patients. With the higher dosage, one should monitor pulse and blood pressure closely after each successive dose and stop the administration if any sign of bradycardia or hypotension develops. Additional anticonvulsants, including phenobarbital or diphenylhydantoin, can be given intramuscularly, as indicated.

The *results of drug therapy* are difficult to predict. With careful attention to individual details and general management, most patients with occasional generalized and psychomotor seizures achieve either complete or nearly complete reduction of seizures. Satisfactory or complete control can be achieved in most children with petit mal absences. However, each group of patients, especially those with grand mal and psychomotor epilepsy, contains a refractory number who suffer from troublesome side effects of drugs and from increasing psychologic and sociologic difficulties as the years go by.

In a relatively small number of patients under treatment with diphenylhydantoin and occasionally phenobarbital-related drugs, a paradoxical increase in seizures occurs, along with depressed mentation and increased electroencephalographic abnormalities. The blood levels of the drugs are usually in a "toxic" range, but not always, and other signs of "toxicity," such as nystagmus and ataxia, may not be present. Reduction of anticonvulsant drug dosage, in these instances, leads to a diminution of seizure activity and clearing of mental functions.

When to stop drugs for a patient whose seizures are completely controlled is a recurrent question. Some authorities recommend cautiously withdrawing anticonvulsants if patients have been free of attacks for two years. In relatively few cases, however, can drugs be withdrawn without seizures recurring even after symptom-free periods of three to five years. Thus continued treatment is indicated for most adults with grand mal and psychomotor epilepsy. The electroencephalogram may remain abnormal in clinically seizure-free patients, indicating persistent seizure potentiality, but even in patients with normal electroencephalograms drug withdrawal may be unsuccessful. Yet, in the management of some patients, it is understandable that a calculated risk of drug withdrawal be considered if this represents a psychologic achievement of great magnitude. Under these circumstances, the drug should be withdrawn carefully with some decrements over many weeks. Drug elimination may be carried out more successfully in children with controlled petit mal, particularly because there is a natural tendency for the absences to diminish with age and maturity.

Adrenocorticotropic hormone (ACTH) and adrenocortical steroids are now used in the treatment of massive spasms in infancy associated with the "hypsarrhythmic" electroencephalogram. Such therapy is administered after primary causes of massive spasms, such as phenylketonuria, have been excluded. Although initial improvements in the spasms and the electroencephalogram may occur, the prognosis is poor, particularly with regard to the mental deterioration accompanying this condition. Nothing is known about the mechanism of action of the hormones in this disorder; this is somewhat paradoxical because these hormones are known to raise cerebral excitability and precipitate seizures in older persons and in experimental situations.

Dietary Treatment. There are no dietary restrictions for the patient with epilepsy, nor is there a specific diet capable of aiding most patients. A diet high in fat content, the *ketogenic diet,* occasionally helps in treating young children with intractable petit mal and generalized motor seizures. Anticonvulsant drugs usually have to be continued, and the diet is difficult to maintain because it is unpleasant.

Psychologic Therapy and Sociologic Management. Many problems in the life adjustments of the patient need management even though drugs can achieve control of seizures. In many cases, the coexistence of seizures and personality problems requires a combination of medical therapy and psychologic management.

The sedative properties of anticonvulsant drugs usually are not used directly. The so-called tranquilizing drugs have limited usefulness in the management of seizure patients; chlordiazepoxide (Librium) and diazepam (Valium) may reduce disturbed behavior, particularly in children. The phenothiazine drugs have variable effects; an alerting phenothiazine, fluphenazine, is of some use in controlling abnormal behavior in certain patients with psychomotor seizures. However, other drugs in the chlorpromazine group are known to provoke seizures and paroxysmal discharges in the electroencephalogram.

Some patients in a state of psychologic turmoil experience increased seizures and require greater amounts of anticonvulsant drugs. The subsequent achievement of psychologic adjustment decreases the frequency of seizures and lessens the drug requirement. This needs to be developed in various ways, depending on the patient's age and his family and social circumstances. Family understanding is of primary importance, because the child with seizures has to live, insofar as possible, as a normal person within home and school settings. A great problem, still to be overcome, is the stigma attached by society to the diagnosis of epilepsy, and the lack of understanding that not only exists among people in general but is reflected by various restrictive legal practices. Most children with seizures are able to attend schools and vocational programs successfully; most adults with controlled seizures are capable of developing productive careers and engaging in the activities that are so much a part of our culture, such as marriage, childbearing, obtaining an education, driving an automobile, traveling from country to country, and working with appropriate safeguards, protected by insurance and worker's compensation programs. Only a relatively small number of patients require a protected environment, such as that in schools or colonies specifically developed for epileptic patients. Even these no longer should be institutions where many hundreds of epileptic patients are kept in essentially custodial care. "Colonies" with schools, homelike units, and small villages exist in Great Britain, Holland, and Denmark and take care of relatively small numbers of patients (up to a few hundred at most in each), involved in intensive programs of medical therapy, psychologic management, education, and vocational training. From these places increasing numbers of adequately controlled patients are sent out into the general community, where they live well adjusted and productive lives.

Only a few occupations are contraindicated for patients with seizures. These include activities of potential danger to either the patient or others, such as work requiring unprotected climbing to great heights and work utilizing heavy power equipment or dangerous chemical substances.

Informal and formal psychotherapeutic measures can be undertaken in order to reduce emotional disturbances. The role of the family physician is all-important in these considerations. Often he alone can judge the problems that exist in a family, school, or social setting. His understanding and guidance help both the patient and his family to overcome the feelings of despair, anxiety, fear, and self-consciousness that otherwise interfere with the normal adjustments of everyone involved. It is only when anxieties and depressive tendencies develop into more severe reactions, associated with paranoid states, increased withdrawal, and excessive obsessional tendencies, that more intensive psychiatric treatment becomes necessary. Occasionally, brief periods of hospitalization help in the evaluation of the intensity of the psychologic disturbance and any associated intellectual difficulties that may interefere with the patient's performance. Drug schedules may be revised at the same time, under controlled conditions.

Even the child with epilepsy and behavioral disorder can be cared for best if he attends a regular school in an understanding environment and is associated with a clinical outpatient service in which the physician and social service department work together with both the child and the family. It is becoming less necessary to arrange for either home tutoring or the placement of such children into schools or other facilities for the maladjusted.

Surgical Therapy. The patient with a potentially remediable lesion, such as a brain tumor, usually is considered for operation, whatever the state of the seizures. Surgical intervention for the removal of a focus of abnormal discharge is appropriate only for selected patients who have focal epilepsy that remains intractable after intensive medical therapy. A constant focally discharging area should be confirmed by serial electroencephalographic studies, and the region of brain considered for excision must be such that the patient will not be left afterward with a severe speech, memory, or other disabling neurologic deficit.

Patients so evaluated usually do not have gross space-occupying lesions, but the epileptogenic region eventually excised may contain an area of scarring (secondary to previous seizures, i.e., mesial temporal scle-

rosis), a hematoma, a small tumor, a vascular lesion, or a scar secondary to trauma or previous encephalitis. The surgical approach has been utilized particularly for patients with focal motor and psychomotor–temporal lobe seizures. Even though many patients are considered for surgical therapy, relatively few are chosen, and the numbers of patients so treated are still only in the hundreds the world over. In carefully selected series, about half the patients enjoy significantly improved control of seizures postoperatively, although this sometimes merely represents less anticonvulsant drug requirement. In some patients, generalized seizures appear instead of previous psychomotor–temporal lobe attacks. A small number experience relief from severe personality disturbances, particularly aggressive psychotic behavior, but this is an uncertain effect, and surgical intervention usually is not primarily directed toward this. Bilateral operations on the temporal lobe have been of limited success and have produced severe memory disturbances.

Cerebral hemispherectomy has been accomplished in a small number of carefully selected children with severe infantile hemiplegia, intractable convulsions, and behavior disturbances. Improvement in the seizures and behavior has occurred despite the persistence of motor and sensory neurologic disability.

Much more must be learned about the natural history of the epilepsies in order to evaluate thoroughly the different therapies. Adequate seizure control can be achieved now for most patients. The drugs involved are increasingly less toxic, but anticonvulsant medication remains essentially nonspecific and is directed against mechanisms of neuronal hyperexcitability that are little understood. A relatively small number of cases not responding to other management can be selected for surgical intervention. It is hoped that combined physiologic and biochemical studies of disturbed cerebral and bodily functions in the epilepsies will lead eventually to more rational and effective therapy.

Brazier, M. A. B. (ed.): Epilepsy. Its Phenomena in Man. New York, Academic Press, 1973.

Gastaut, H.: Clinical and electroencephalographic classification of epileptic seizures. Epilepsia, 11:102, 1970.

Glaser, G. H.: Limbic epilepsy in childhood. J. Nerv. Ment. Dis., 144:394, 1967.

Jasper, H. H., Ward, A. A., and Pope, A.: Basic Mechanisms of the Epilepsies. Boston, Little, Brown & Company, 1969.

Jennett, B.: Epilepsy After Non-missile Head Injuries. 2nd ed. Chicago, Heinemann–Year Book, 1975.

Laidlaw, J., and Richens, A.: A Textbook of Epilepsy. London, Churchill Livingstone, 1976.

Lennox-Buchthal, M. A.: Febrile Convulsions. A Reappraisal. Amsterdam, Elsevier Scientific Publishing Company, 1973.

Ounsted, C., Lindsay, J., and Norman, R.: Biological Factors in Temporal Lobe Epilepsy. London, Heinemann Medical Books Ltd., 1966.

Penfield, W. G., and Jasper, H. H.: Epilepsy and the Functional Anatomy of the Human Brain. Boston, Little, Brown & Company, 1954.

Solomon, G., and Plum, F.: Clinical Management of Seizures. Philadelphia, W. B. Saunders Company, 1976.

Woodbury, D. M., Penry, J. K., and Schmidt, R. P. (eds.): Antiepileptic Drugs. New York, Raven Press, 1972.

Section Nineteen INTRACRANIAL TUMORS AND STATES CAUSING INCREASED INTRACRANIAL PRESSURE

Robert A. Fishman

316. INTRACRANIAL TUMORS

Intracranial tumors include neoplasms, both benign and malignant, and other space-taking lesions of chronic inflammatory origin that develop in brain, meninges, or skull. Their clinical manifestations are diverse and vary according to tumor type and location. Errors in diagnosis are relatively common because the clinical manifestations of tumor may simulate a variety of neurologic disorders. Brain tumors occur at any age; they are common in children under ten, but have their peak incidence in the fifth and sixth decades of life. Race, occupation, and history of trauma have not been established as predisposing factors. Genetic factors are relevant to the occurrence of a few tumor types, e.g., hemangioblastomas, neurofibromas, and certain gliomas.

CLASSIFICATION AND PATHOLOGY. Most classifications include (1) primary tumors originating in brain, (2) meningeal tumors, (3) vascular tumors, (4) pituitary tumors, (5) congenital tumors, (6) adnexal tumors, (7) metastatic tumors, and (8) granulomas and parasitic cysts.

Primary Brain Tumors. The largest group of primary brain tumors are the gliomas, composed of malignant glial cells. These include the following:

GLIOBLASTOMA MULTIFORME. These most malignant gliomas are composed of very undifferentiated cells. Complete surgical removal is impossible. The average life expectancy varies from 6 to 36 months or so, according to location and treatment. They have a very rapid growth rate and are characterized by tissue necrosis and brain edema.

ASTROCYTOMA. Astrocytomas are composed of astrocytes that infiltrate the brain and are often associated with cysts of varying size. They are generally slow growing and may run a course of many years or even decades. They may infiltrate normal brain widely but with relatively little effect on brain function early in the illness. Complete surgical excision of cystic astrocytomas of the cerebellum may be possible, particularly in children, but in most other instances their invasiveness of brain prevents complete removal. Astrocytomas may undergo malignant change, and a highly malignant glioblastoma may develop within a relatively benign astrocytoma.

OLIGODENDROGLIOMA. Oligodendrogliomas, composed of oligodendroglial cells, are similar in behavior to astrocytomas and are distinguishable only on histologic study.

EPENDYMOMA. Ependymomas are derived from ependymal cells. They arise from the walls of the ventricular system, filling or obstructing the ventricles and invading adjacent tissues. They are malignant and cause death in about three years.

MEDULLOBLASTOMA. Medulloblastomas develop from a primitive cell within the cerebellum. They are chiefly tumors of childhood but can occur in older patients. They are highly malignant and frequently metastasize throughout the subarachnoid space to involve the cerebrum or spinal cord.

Meningeal Tumors. The most important tumor arising in the meninges is the *meningioma*, which may invade the adjacent bone as well as compressing and distorting the brain. It is slow growing, well circumscribed, often highly vascular, and may be calcified. It is benign, and complete removal is often possible unless the tumor involves critical structures.

Vascular Tumors. Tumors composed of vascular elements include the arteriovenous malformations (angiomas) and hemangioblastomas. The angiomas are congenital malformations composed of an abnormal collection of blood vessels of adult structure. They are present from birth but slowly enlarge and may not cause symptoms for many years. They may compress normal brain, may bleed intracerebrally or into the subarachnoid space, may be manifest only as a source of seizures, or may be an incidental finding at autopsy. Hemangioblastomas are true neoplasms composed of primitive vascular elements that may be quiescent for many years or may enlarge very slowly. They are most commonly found in the cerebellum but occur also in the cerebrum. Cerebellar hemangioblastoma may be associated with angiomatosis of the retina and cysts of the kidney and pancreas (the von Hippel–Lindau syndrome).

Pituitary Tumors. Pituitary tumors may arise from chromophobe, eosinophil, or basophil cells of the anterior pituitary. Of these, chromophobe adenomas are the most common. Chromophobe adenomas are nonfunctioning tumors that give symptoms by compression of the normal pituitary gland as well as the optic chiasm, the hypothalamus, and the adjacent brain with their suprasellar growth. Eosinophilic adenomas give rise to hyperpituitarism, acromegaly in adults, and gigantism in children, but do not generally compress suprasellar structures unless the tumor is mixed with chromophobe elements. Basophil adenomas are small and, although associated with Cushing's syndrome, are not responsible for symptoms by compression of adjacent tissues. *Craniopharyngiomas* derived from Rathke's pouch may be intrasellar or suprasellar in location, may compress the pituitary and optic chiasm, and are similar in effect to the chromophobe adenoma. They are frequently calcified and often contain cysts filled with thick, lipid-laden fluid. Endocrine aspects of pituitary tumors are discussed in Ch. 543.5.

Congenital Tumors. These tumors develop from congenital rests and include craniopharyngiomas of the pituitary, chordomas, dermoids, and teratomas. Chordomas are composed of cells derived from the embryonic notochord. They are midline and usually arise on the clivus, posterior to the sella. They grow slowly, but are highly invasive, and their total extirpation can seldom be accomplished. Dermoids and teratomas may occur anywhere in the central nervous system, particularly near the midline, adjacent to the ventricular system, or at the distal end of the cord. They tend to become symptomatic during the first decade of life, but may be silent for many years.

Adnexal Tumors. These tumors include those originating within the pineal body and those derived from the choroid plexus, the choroid papilloma. Pinealomas are rare tumors that cause symptoms by compressing the aqueduct, resulting in obstructive hydrocephalus and giving paralysis of vertical gaze by involvement of the pretectum of the midbrain. They may compress the hypothalamus and give rise to precocious puberty or diabetes insipidus. Choroid plexus papillomas are benign lesions that may cause intraventricular bleeding. They may cause increased intracranial pressure by obstructing the ventricular system or by excessive formation of cerebrospinal fluid.

Metastatic Tumors. Metastatic tumors constitute 10 to 25 per cent of brain tumors. They may originate from almost any primary tumor, most commonly those of breast and lung, but also from neoplasms of the gastrointestinal and genitourinary tracts, bone, thyroid, or nasal sinuses. They may be single or multiple, well encapsulated or diffuse, spread by extension from adjacent tissues or hematogenously. They may occur as a late manifestation in widespread carcinomatosis or as the first manifestation of an unrecognized primary visceral malignancy.

Granulomas and Parasitic Cysts. Granulomas affecting the nervous system include those associated with tuberculosis, mycotic infection, sarcoidosis, parasitic infestation, and syphilis. *Tuberculoma* may present as a solitary mass lesion within the brain; although rare in the United States, it is more common in Central and South America and in India. Tuberculoma usually develops without evidence of tuberculous meningitis, although evidence of pulmonary tuberculosis is common. Favorable results with surgical excision and antituberculosis therapy have been reported. *Toruloma* is the most common mycotic granuloma affecting brain. This is usually associated with evidence of meningeal involvement. The *granulomas of sarcoidosis* occur in the brain; there is usually evidence of meningeal or posterior pituitary involvement, although the evidence for systemic sarcoid may be minimal. *Cysticercosis,* caused by the larvae of *Taenia solium* or *Taenia saginata,* may be responsible for single or multiple cerebral masses. This is seen chiefly in South America and in the Middle East and India. *Syphilitic gummas* are extremely rare, presenting like slow-growing cerebral gliomas.

PATHOPHYSIOLOGY. Intracranial tumors give rise to focal disturbances in brain function and to increased intracranial pressure. Focal manifestations occur because brain is compressed or infiltrated by tumor, because the blood supply of the region is compromised, resulting in tissue necrosis, and because of cerebral edema. Tumors may be located either within or outside brain parenchyma, i.e., intra-axial or extra-axial in location. Brain dysfunction is generally greatest with rapidly growing, infiltrative intra-axial tumors, e.g., glioblastoma, because of marked infiltration, compression, and necrosis of brain. Cyst formation within tumors also compresses adjacent normal brain. Cerebral edema about tumors may greatly increase the neurologic deficit. It has the features of *vasogenic brain edema* with increased brain water and sodium and an expanded extracellular fluid volume. Extra-axial tumors, e.g., meningioma, which slowly compress brain, may reach great size with few, if any, clinical signs.

Tumors cause a generalized increase in intracranial pressure when they reach sufficient mass, because of the fixed volume of the intracranial cavity. Obstruction of the ventricular system also increases intracranial pressure and causes hydrocephalic dilatation of the proximal ventricles and thinning of the cerebral hemispheres. Tumors that obstruct the intracranial venous sinuses also cause increased intracranial pressure. Complete compensation with very little or even no rise in pressure can occur with slowly growing neoplasms, but with rapidly growing malignant tumors, increased intracranial pressure is an early sign. Increased intracranial pressure becomes life threatening when there is sufficient displacement of brain to cause herniation of the uncus or cerebellum. In *uncal herniation,* the most medial gyrus of the temporal lobe, the uncus, is displaced inferiorly by a hemispheric mass through the tentorial notch, thus causing compression of the midbrain. This results in depression of consciousness and ipsilateral or bilateral dilated and fixed pupils owing to compression of the third nerve. In *cerebellar herniation,* the tonsils are displaced downward through the foramen magnum by a posterior fossa mass, causing compression of the medulla and respiratory arrest. Characteristic vasomotor changes ensue with increased intracranial pressure when rapid or severe. These include *progressive bradycardia* caused by vagal slowing of the heart; *systemic hypertension,* which occurs as the intracranial pressure begins to approach arterial diastolic pressure, inducing medullary ischemia and compensatory systemic vasoconstriction; and, finally, *central respiratory failure.* Carbon dioxide retention will further increase intracranial pressure because of its cerebrovasodilator effects, and therefore adequate ventilation with maintenance of a clear airway is essential for the patient with increased intracranial pressure. (Drugs such as morphine, which depress respiration sufficiently to raise arterial carbon dioxide levels, are therefore contraindicated.)

CLINICAL MANIFESTATIONS. The natural history of intracranial tumor is characterized by insidious onset and progression of focal or general neurologic deficits, or both. Many tumors have rather characteristic manifestations that point to the diagnosis (see below). There is great variation, depending upon location and rate of growth. Occasionally symptoms may be explosive in onset, suggesting a vascular lesion, and there may also be variations in course, suggestive of a remission. The symptoms and signs of intracranial tumor are discussed below.

Headache. Headache is a major but not invariable symptom of intracranial tumor. Patients with extensive tumors may not complain of headache, particularly if they have slowly growing infiltrative tumors (astrocytoma) or slowly growing extra-axial tumors (such as meningiomas, acoustic neuromas, or pituitary tumors). Similarly, when tumors interfere with the higher intellectual functions, headache may not be reported. Tumors give rise to headache by displacing the pain-sensitive structures within the cranial cavity (see Ch. 261).

Mental Changes. Mental changes may occur either early or late in the history of brain tumor, depending upon tumor location. Subtle evidence of personality change may be the first manifestation of a mass in the cerebral hemispheres, particularly involving the frontal lobes. This may take several forms. The symptoms may be chiefly affective, simulating an involutional depression. Some patients develop confusional states, at times associated with episodes of bizarre behavior. The most common mental changes are progressive impairment of abstraction, recent memory and judgment, and a shortened attention span (see Ch. 226 to 231). However, some patients, particularly those with slowly growing neoplasms in the right (nondominant) hemisphere, may harbor huge tumors with only minimal impairment of intellect. Drowsiness progressing to stupor and coma accompanies severely increased intracranial pressure.

Disturbances of Speech. Various forms of aphasia occur with neoplastic involvement of the dominant hemisphere. The aphasic disorders are insidious in their development, and minor disturbances may be overlooked or erroneously attributed to psychologic factors. The various discrete forms of apraxia and agnosia may occur in evolution of the tumor syndrome, and may be the initial symptom in otherwise well persons.

Papilledema and Vision. The presence of the characteristic ophthalmoscopic appearance of papilledema suggests increased intracranial pressure; however, the funduscopic findings may be indistinguishable from those of optic neuritis or pseudopapilledema. Pseudopapilledema is a congenital change in the funduscopic appearance of the disc that simulates the swelling associated with increased intracranial pressure. Differential points include the late loss of visual acuity in increased intracranial pressure as opposed to early and more severe visual loss in optic neuritis. Visual acuity is generally unaffected in pseudopapilledema. Episodes of *amaurosis fugax*, fleeting moments of dimming vision, may be associated with a marked degree of papilledema and are a dangerous warning sign of potential loss of vision. The visual fields in true papilledema or pseudopapilledema may show enlargement of the blind spots. Disturbance of vision in patients with intracranial tumor also can be caused by extraocular muscle palsies, disturbances of the central visual pathways (see below), and disorders of visual interpretation, as in the alexias and visual agnosias. Uniocular papilledema with contralateral optic atrophy occurs characteristically, with subfrontal tumors that cause optic atrophy by direct involvement of the nerve and papilledema in the opposite eye owing to increased intracranial pressure. The fundi may not reveal papilledema despite very elevated intracranial pressure; this may be attributable to glaucoma when present, but may also occur for unexplained reasons.

Diplopia and Hemianopia. Diplopia with brain tumors is due to involvement of one or both sixth cranial nerves, either directly by the tumor or, more commonly, indirectly because of generalized increase in intracranial pressure (see False Localizing Signs, below). Third-nerve palsy may be due to involvement of the superior orbital fissure by meningioma, although the nerve may be involved by a variety of other lesions anywhere along its course. Hemianopias result from involvement of the visual pathways. Lesions affecting the optic chiasm, notably originating in or near the pituitary, give rise to bitemporal hemianopia. Lesions of the optic tract, optic radiation, or occipital cortex give rise to contralateral homonymous hemianopias. Lesions of the anterior temporal pole characteristically cause a contralateral homonymous, superior quadrantopsia.

Ataxia and Hemiplegia. Unsteadiness in walking may occur with tumor in various intracranial sites. Lesions affecting the midline cerebellum cause a characteristic truncal ataxia with lateralized ataxia of the extremities if the cerebellar hemispheres are also involved. Disease in the frontal lobes may give rise to unsteadiness in walking, an apraxia of gait, which may simulate cerebellar truncal ataxia. Drug intoxication caused by diphenylhydantoin or barbiturates may potentiate ataxia. Tumors of the hemisphere characteristically cause contralateral spastic hemiparesis; initially the signs may be so minimal as to be easily overlooked.

Sensory Disturbances. Hemisensory defects occur with intracranial tumors affecting the contralateral sensory pathways. The primary sensory modalities of touch, pain, temperature, and proprioception are impaired when the thalamus or the ascending spinothalamic pathways are involved. Tumors of the parietal sensory cortex cause loss of cortical sensory functions that results in impairment of sensory localization, two-point discrimination, graphesthesia, stereognosis, and position sense. Tumors of the thalamus may be manifested by episodes of pain affecting the contralateral side of the face or body. Tumors of the cortex may cause focal sensory seizures with a jacksonian march; these may be reported as an aura before a grand mal seizure. Pain in the face occurs with tumors affecting the base of the skull, particularly those arising in the nasopharynx and paranasal sinuses. Tumors affecting the trigeminal nerve may give rise to paroxysms of pain in the face simulating trigeminal neuralgia (tic douloureux), but unlike the latter there is also some loss of facial sensation.

Seizures. Seizures may serve as the first clinical manifestation of brain tumor, or may occur at any time in the course of the illness. The types include classic grand mal seizures and various forms of focal seizures. Typical petit mal is probably never due to neoplasm; minor seizures that at first may resemble petit mal generally are, in fact, either fragmentary grand mal seizures or a variety of psychomotor attack. With any cerebral seizure, it is extremely important to note its aura or the pattern of its onset, for this often provides a reliable indicator of the location of the neoplasm. Focal motor and sensory seizures may be limited to one region of the body or may progress (jacksonian seizures) to involve the entire body. Lesions in the temporal lobe characteristically give rise to psychomotor seizures. These may be associated with olfactory hallucinations (uncinate fits), disorders of visual or auditory perception, experiential attacks such as déjà vu, and various types of automatic behavior, for which the patient is generally amnesic (see Ch. 315). The onset of convulsions in an otherwise healthy subject over the age of 20 without history of convulsions raises the possibility of an expanding lesion.

Nausea and Vomiting. Nausea and vomiting occur as a result of direct or reflex stimulation of the emetic center of the medulla. This is most likely to occur in association with increased intracranial pressure, particularly with displacement of the brainstem owing to herniation or the presence of bleeding into the cerebrospinal fluid. The vomiting may occur without preceding nausea and may be projectile. Brain tumor is not suggested by the occurrence of nausea and vomiting alone, i.e., there are invariably other clinical manifestations of the tumor. Antiemetic drugs, e.g., the phenothiazines, inhibit this type of centrally induced vomiting.

Stiff Neck. Signs of meningeal irritation may occur in brain tumor, as a manifestation of cerebellar herniation through the foramen magnum, because of the effects of bleeding into the subarachnoid space, or with meningeal involvement. Cervical rigidity may be striking, but Kernig's sign is generally absent (see Tumors of the Cerebellum, below).

Vasomotor and Autonomic Changes. These occur as ominous late signs. They include bradycardia and hypertension, as described above. Apnea generally precedes cardiac arrest in fatal cases. Autonomic manifestations of brain tumor include gastric ulceration (Cushing's ulcer), which may present as a massive gastrointestinal hemorrhage. This may occur with mass lesions anywhere in the intracranial cavity. (The use of adrenocortical steroids in the management of patients with brain tumor may further increase this hazard.) Fever may also occur in patients with mass lesions in the absence of pulmonary, urinary, or other infection, because of a central disturbance, presumably of hypothalamic origin. Hyperthermia is not uncommon just prior to death, but hypothermia may also occur. Fever commonly accompanies the presence of blood in the subarachnoid space. This may occur with rapidly growing neoplasms or as a result of surgery. Disturbances of sweating may occur, lesions of hypothalamus and brainstem giving rise to contralateral signs of sympathectomy.

Metabolic Manifestations. The complex interrelationships between the hypothalamus and the anterior and posterior pituitary may be deranged with intracranial tumors, giving rise to various systemic metabolic disorders. These include diabetes insipidus, inappropriate secretion of antidiuretic hormone, hypopituitarism, and precocious puberty (see Ch. 544.2, 530, 543.6, and 548.3, respectively).

False Localizing Signs. These may occur with increased intracranial pressure or with shift of intracranial structures. The most common such sign is unilateral or bilateral lateral rectus palsy due to sixth-nerve compression. This need not imply neoplastic involvement of the nerve, for it frequently occurs as a pressure palsy of the nerve resulting from increased intracranial pressure itself. Signs of hemiplegia can occur ipsilateral to the tumor owing to compression of the opposite cerebral peduncle on the tentorium; i.e., hemiplegia need not be contralateral to the mass. There are relatively silent areas in brain, wherein tumors reach large size with relatively little clinical deficit; these are the right frontal and temporal lobes. This must be considered in evaluating patients with the syndrome of increased intracranial pressure without localizing signs (see below).

DIAGNOSIS. Patients suspected of having an intracranial tumor require complete medical evaluation to establish the relationship of the neurologic findings to possible coexisting systemic disease. Appropriate laboratory studies should be obtained to search for a primary systemic neoplasm, e.g., lung, breast, gastrointestinal, genitourinary, or thyroid malignancies. The major neurologic diagnostic techniques are described below.

Skull Roentgenograms. The films should be examined for the following: (1) changes suggestive of increased intracranial pressure, (2) bone destruction, (3) bony thickening or hyperostosis, (4) abnormal vascular channels, (5) abnormal calcifications, (6) the shape of the sella turcica, (7) the position of the pineal if calcified, and (8) the relationship of the skull to the cervical spine in suspected platybasia, basilar impression, and related disorders (see Ch. 321).

Characteristic roentgenographic changes may occur with chronically increased intracranial pressure as a result of pressure atrophy of bone, which produces a beaten-silver appearance in the cranial vault, decalcification of the clinoid processes, and separation of the sutures in children. Bone destruction is characteristic of metastatic neoplasms arising from distant organs and of directly invasive tumors that arise in the paranasal sinuses and nasopharynx. Focal hyperostosis of the skull, i.e., thickening of the inner or outer tables of the skull, or both, with increased calcification, is characteristic of meningioma. Generalized thickening of the skull occurs with Paget's disease. Hyperostosis frontalis interna, localized bilateral thickenings of the inner table of the skull, is generally considered an incidental finding without clinical significance. The vascular markings of the skull, which accompany arterial and venous channels, vary greatly in the normal subject. Focal enlargements of the markings occur characteristically with meningioma involving adjacent meninges and skull. Abnormal calcifications characteristically occur in very slowly growing primary neoplasms (astrocytoma, oligodendroglioma, craniopharyngioma, meningioma), in arteriovenous malformations, in aneurysmal walls, and in the glial nodules associated with tuberous sclerosis. Calcifications may also occur in the gliotic walls of old abscesses, in hemorrhagic cavities, and in granulomas of cerebral toxoplasmosis. Displacement of the pineal laterally more than 2 mm is pathologic, and this or a shift superiorly or inferiorly suggests the presence of a space-taking lesion.

Electroencephalography. The electroencephalogram can be used in screening for possible brain tumor when computerized tomography is not available. Focal changes, particularly slowing in frequency of the record, are common with tumors in the cerebral hemispheres. Rapidly growing tumors are more likely to evoke focal changes than are slowly progressive tumors with only minimal clinical manifestations, and with the latter the record may be normal. The electroencephalogram is often normal with posterior fossa neoplasms.

Cerebrospinal Fluid. Examination of the cerebrospinal fluid (CSF) for pressure, protein, sugar, cell count, cultures, serologic tests, and cytologic analysis is often helpful in the diagnosis of intracranial tumor. The incidence of abnormalities varies with the stage of the illness and the site and nature of the neoplasm. The fluid is crystal clear unless the protein exceeds about 150 mg per 100 ml or unless bleeding has occurred. With slowly growing neoplasms the intracranial pressure will remain normal, less than 200 mm, until late in the illness, whereas in rapidly growing tumors increased pressure may be an early manifestation. Jugular compression for the Queckenstedt test is contraindicated in patients who are suspected of having brain tumor. A protein content greater than 100 mg per 100 ml is frequently associated with rapidly growing tumors near the ventricles or subarachnoid space. With slowly growing tumors, the protein may be normal despite the presence of a huge mass. Of the posterior fossa neoplasms, acoustic neuroma commonly results in marked elevation of the protein, 100 to 500 mg per 100 ml. The fluid is normal in most patients with brainstem gliomas. The cell count is elevated from 5 to 100 white cells per cubic millimeter in about one third of the cases, and may exceed 1000 white cells, particularly when the tumor involves the ventricular wall and has undergone necrosis. Malignant cells may be detected with suitable techniques. The glucose content is normal with brain tumor, apart from patients with diffuse neoplastic involvement of the meninges, when it is characteristically reduced to levels below 40 mg per 100 ml; in some cases this may be the sole abnormality, although commonly 10 to 100 mononuclear cells are seen, and with special cytologic techniques malignant cells may be detected.

Lumbar puncture may be hazardous; it is *contraindicated* in critically ill patients with clinical signs of incipient herniation because the removal of fluid from the lumbar sac may increase the degree of *pre-existing* herniation of the temporal lobe or of the cerebellar tonsils.

Computerized Tomography. The increasing availability of computerized tomography has provided a great advance in diagnostic evaluation (see Ch. 267). As a relatively noninvasive test, and especially when used with contrast enhancement, it is very useful in screening patients suspected of having single or multiple brain tumors. Its excellent visualization of the ventricular system has reduced the need for pneumoencephalography or ventriculography as well as the frequency of hospitalization.

Roentgenographic Contrast Studies. *Pneumoencephalography* by the lumbar route, *ventriculography*, and *arteriography* are used in the diagnosis and localization of brain tumor. Lumbar pneumography delineates the ventricular system and the subarachnoid space and thus may reveal the presence of a mass lesion. In ventriculography, air is injected via burr holes in the skull directly into the lateral cerebral ventricles; this may prove necessary for patients with increased intracranial pressure, in whom the lumbar route is deemed hazardous, and for patients in whom there is nonfilling of the ventricular system by the lumbar route. Cerebral angiography may yield much information concerning the location and size of a tumor. The vascular patterns of the tumor, arterial, capillary, and venous, may give indications of its histology. The decision as to which contrast technique is most likely to give maximal information in any patient depends upon the specific circumstances of the diagnostic problem in question and must be resolved individually.

Isotope Encephalography. Various scanning techniques permit the recording of the radioactivity present over regions of the skull after intravenous administration of radioiodinated human serum albumin, technetium, and other gamma emitters. The isotope may enter more rapidly and in greater concentration into the tumor and its adjacent area of edema because of the greater permeability of the capillaries and adjacent cellular membranes. The isotope scan does not readily differentiate between focal changes caused by neoplasm, sepsis, or infarction, and is often negative with slowly growing tumors.

Ancillary Laboratory Tests. Audiometry and vestibular tests are necessary in evaluating patients with suspected tumor of the eighth nerve, and visual fields are valuable in assessing lesions of the visual system.

TUMOR SYNDROMES. Tumors of the Skull. Benign osteomas rarely reach a size sufficient to compress underlying brain; generally these can be extirpated. Malignant tumors arising in the paranasal sinuses or nasopharynx directly invade the base of the skull and cause chronic facial pain and multiple cranial nerve involvement. Tumors of the glomus jugulare (nonchromaffin paraganglioma) arise near the jugular bulb and often lead to progressive deafness and a bloody discharge in the external auditory canal. Other lesions that give roentgenographic evidence of bone destruction and that must be differentiated include Paget's disease, Hand-Schüller-Christian disease, eosinophilic granuloma, and cholesteatoma (epidermoids).

Diffuse Meningeal Neoplasia (Carcinomatous Meningitis). Carcinomas, gliomas, sarcomas, melanomas, and lymphomas may diffusely infiltrate the leptomeninges and subarachnoid space to produce a syndrome of chronic meningitis, which may simulate chronic meningitis caused by fungi, tuberculosis, sarcoidosis, and meningovascular syphilis. Common manifestations include headache, mental changes, cranial nerve palsies, areflexia, and minimal if any signs of meningeal irritation. The cerebrospinal fluid findings generally will establish the diagnosis. The pressure is usually normal; sugar content may be below 45 mg per 100 ml and as low as 10 mg per 100 ml; protein content is normal or elevated; cell count reveals from 5 to several hundred mononuclear cells; cultures are negative; cytologic studies usually reveal malignant cells. The diagnosis may not be apparent at autopsy because gross lesions are not seen, and microscopic sections are needed to verify the diagnosis.

Tumors of the Cerebral Hemispheres. Tumors affecting the cerebral hemispheres are characterized by progressive focal neurologic deficits and, commonly, by generalized or focal convulsive seizures. Hemispheric tumors involving any lobe may be associated with contralateral hemiplegia; when located in the parasagittal region the paralysis is greater in the leg than in the arm. Tumors of the frontal lobes are also characterized by early impairment of intellectual function. Tumors in the parietal region cause contralateral cortical (interpretive) sensory deficits, impairment of primary sensation, and homonymous hemianopia. Tumors in the occipital region also cause contralateral homonymous hemianopia plus disorders of visual interpretation. Tumors in the temporal lobe, in the nondominant hemisphere, are relatively silent apart from contralateral superior quadrantopsia. Tumors of regions adjacent to the sylvian fissure of the dominant hemisphere give rise to aphasic disorders; anterior lesions in the frontal lobe cause expressive aphasia, posterior lesions in the parietal region cause the receptive aphasias, and lesions in the superior temporal gyrus cause anomic aphasia.

Tumors of the Cerebellum. The common tumors of the cerebellum include medulloblastomas, which affect the midline vermis most commonly in childhood, and tumors of the cerebellar hemisphere, chiefly gliomas and metastatic tumors. Early manifestations of tumor of the midline vermis include truncal ataxia on tandem walking and symptoms of increased intracranial pressure. Tumors of the cerebellar hemisphere cause ipsilateral limb ataxia as an early manifestation. Tilting of the head to one side may be an early sign as well. Stiffness of the neck is often seen in posterior fossa neoplasms as an early sign of herniation.

Brainstem Tumors. These intrinsic tumors of midbrain, pons, and medulla are most commonly gliomas. The initial symptoms are those of cranial nerve dysfunction, most commonly affecting the extraocular muscles (nuclear or internuclear ophthalmoplegia), chewing and swallowing, as well as the long tracts, ascending and descending. Headache and other manifestations of increased intracranial pressure occur late in the course. The cerebrospinal fluid is often normal.

Pituitary Tumors. The earliest symptoms may be those of endocrine disturbances (see above) or may be due to effects on the visual system. Frontal headache may be an early symptom. Pituitary tumors may invade the sphenoid sinus and thus permit the development of bacterial meningitis. The cysts associated with craniopharyngioma may release lipid-laden fluid into the subarachnoid space, thus causing bouts of sterile meningitis.

Optic Nerve Glioma. Gliomas may develop in the intraorbital, retro-orbital, or chiasmatic region of the optic nerve, the first of these being the most common location. These tumors usually occur in early childhood with uniocular loss of vision as the most common presenting symptom. Proptosis is seen in about one third of cases. Uniocular optic atrophy or papilledema may be noted. Roentgenographic evidence of enlargement of the optic foramen is common. The tumor is most often a slowly growing astrocytoma and may be associated with neurofibromatosis.

Acoustic Neuroma (Cerebellopontine Angle Tumor). These neurofibromas (schwannomas) of the eighth nerve begin within the auditory canal or in the subarachnoid space. They are slowly growing and characteristically cause progressive tinnitus and nerve deafness. The vestibular portion is more seriously involved than the acoustic portion, and in patients who do not have a dead labyrinth on caloric testing, the diagnosis is suspect. There are few symptoms referable to loss of vestibular function. A mild sensation of giddiness or unsteadiness is common, but recurrent episodes of vertigo are very rare in acoustic tumors. Adjacent cranial nerves are also commonly involved, particularly the fifth, sixth, and seventh nerves. Large tumors cause ipsilateral cerebellar signs and manifestations of increased intracranial pressure. Meningiomas of the cerebellopontine angle may give a similar clinical picture without, however, enlargement of the auditory canal on roentgenograms of the skull.

Metastatic Tumors. The clinical pictures that result from metastatic neoplasms are very variable, depending on the site and number of metastases and their rate of growth. The diagnosis is readily made in patients with evidence of widespread metastatic disease who then develop focal neurologic signs. Frequently the metastatic tumor becomes symptomatic in brain with few if any manifestations of the primary tumor. Therefore patients with an apparently single intracranial mass lesion should be studied for a hidden neoplasm.

DIFFERENTIAL DIAGNOSIS. A wide variety of neurologic diseases may simulate brain tumor because they are also characterized by progressive focal neurologic signs or signs of increased intracranial pressure. Some of the more common problems in differential diagnosis are considered in the following paragraphs.

Syndrome of Increased Intracranial Pressure Without Localizing Signs. A major diagnostic problem is seen in the patient who presents with increased intracranial pressure manifested by headache and papilledema and who is otherwise apparently normal. The many diagnostic possibilities (see Ch. 318) include extra-axial neoplasms that obstruct the ventricular system, such as tentorial meningioma and pinealoma, and intraventricular tumors like ependymoma and glioma. Some patients have the syndrome of aqueduct stenosis, hydrocephalus, or chronic meningitis. Tumors of relatively silent areas like the right frontal and temporal lobes must be excluded. The diagnosis of idiopathic benign intracranial hypertension is made by exclusion of the many specific causes of the syndrome (see Ch. 318).

Tumor vs. Vascular Disease. The differential diagnosis between tumor and vascular disease is generally made on the basis of history; most tumors have an insidious onset and progress slowly, but most vascular lesions characteristically have an abrupt onset. However, some neoplasms such as glioblastoma or metastatic tumors may have a very abrupt onset, most often caused by bleeding into the tumor. Also, the stepwise progression ("stuttering onset") of hemiplegia in some patients with vascular disease of the extracranial portions of the internal carotid and vertebral arteries and, at times, of the intracranial arteries, may pose diagnostic uncertainty.

Tumor vs. Subdural Hematoma. The clinical picture in these patients simulates an expanding hemispheric mass: e.g., headache, drowsiness, papilledema, hemiparesis. About one third of patients with chronic subdural hematoma provide no significant history of head injury. The diagnosis can be made almost always with computerized tomography or arteriography.

Tumor vs. Demyelinating Diseases, Multifocal Leukoencephalopathy. The more common forms of multiple sclerosis do not usually simulate expanding intracranial lesions. Diagnostic difficulty may be encountered in patients with another disorder of white matter, multifocal leukoencephalopathy, which occurs in association with the lymphomas and malignant disease arising in lung and other organs. In this disorder, multiple foci of demyelination are associated with electron microscopic evidence of viral infection. Clinically, there are signs of multiple lesions in the brain that can simulate metastatic disease. However, despite clinical evidence of multiple lesions and rapid progression, signs of increased intracranial pressure are absent. Characteristic, confluent low density lesions in the white matter seen with computerized tomography assist the premortem diagnosis.

Tumor vs. Presenile Dementia. Progressive development of an organic dementia in middle age may be caused by many diseases, including frontal or bifrontal neoplasms. Tumors most likely to present with dementia include frontal and subfrontal tumors (olfactory groove meningioma and tumors of the corpus callosum, "butterfly glioma"). Roentgenographic contrast studies may be necessary to establish the diagnosis. A CSF protein greater than 100 mg per 100 ml favors tumor over the degenerative dementias.

Tumor vs. Abscess, Granuloma. Encapsulated brain abscess and the granulomas associated with cysticercosis may simulate brain tumor. Cysticercosis must be considered in any patient in an endemic area having signs of a cerebral mass lesion. An eosinophilic pleocytosis in the cerebrospinal fluid favors cysticercosis. Differentiation between tumor and abscess may be particularly difficult because patients with encapsulated brain abscess generally do not have systemic manifestations of infection (fever, leukocytosis), and the primary source of infection may be obscure. The cerebrospinal fluid may show little or no inflammatory change. The correct diagnosis of abscess or granuloma may not be made until surgery is performed.

Tumor vs. Epilepsy. The common occurrence of convulsive seizures with intracranial tumors requires consideration of this diagnosis when patients develop seizures (apart from true petit mal, which is never due to brain tumor). This is particularly true of patients in whom seizures first develop after the age of 20. The occurrence of transient focal neurologic signs in the postictal state (Todd's paralysis) favors the presence of a structural lesion as basis for the attacks. It is estimated that about 20 per cent of patients who develop seizures after the age of 20, who do not have post-traumatic seizures, will in time be shown to have intracranial tumors. The likelihood of a brain tumor diminishes with the passage of years if focal signs do not appear.

TREATMENT. Surgical Therapy. Total surgical removal without sacrifice of normal cerebral tissue is possible only with tumors that are extra-axial in location, such as some meningiomas, osteomas, neurofibromas, and pituitary tumors. Total surgical extirpation of the primary tumors of brain, glioblastomas, and the less malignant gliomas, is not possible, although there are rare exceptions, e.g., cystic astrocytomas of the cerebellar hemisphere. Complete surgical removal of angiomas may be possible. Therefore it is essential to establish the precise location and tumor type to allow optimal therapy. Surgical attack on primary brain tumors may be helpful as palliative therapy, e.g., internal decompression or partial removal of tumor and edematous brain may relieve headaches and prolong useful life, particularly if the tumor is cystic and in the nondominant frontal or temporal lobes. There is no absolute rule for the surgical treatment of metastatic tumors. In some patients with major symptoms caused by an apparent single brain tumor without widespread systemic disease, surgical excision may offer useful palliation.

Radiotherapy. The gliomas may have a high degree of sensitivity, and x-ray therapy is generally indicated for palliation. Although biopsy and tissue diagnosis are highly desirable prior to instituting radiotherapy, a specimen is not always obtainable, particularly when the tumor is located in an inaccessible area like the brainstem. In such cases, diagnosis must be made on clinical and roentgenographic grounds. Unfortunately, the response of the gliomas to radiation is often brief, and recurrent growth supervenes.

Supportive Measures. Anticonvulsant drugs are indicated for patients with a history of convulsive seizures and for patients who have had intracranial surgery. Diphenylhydantoin, 300 to 500 mg per day, and phenobarbital, 30 to 60 mg three times a day, are common dosages. Higher dosages of these and other anticonvulsant drugs may be necessary for seizure control (see Ch. 315). The use of hypertonic intravenous solutions such as 25 per cent mannitol to lower intracranial pressure has a limited place in management of patients

with increased intracranial pressure. This is chiefly for very acute situations while the patient awaits neurosurgical intervention. Adrenal corticosteriods, such as dexamethasone, in high dosages help to reduce cerebral edema associated with brain tumors, particularly in the postoperative period and during radiotherapy; gastrointestinal bleeding, however, is a potential complication. Dosages of dexamethasone of 22 mg in the first 24 hours and 16 mg per day thereafter have been recommended. The toxic effects of such high doses make such long-term use hazardous. The administration of parenteral fluids must be planned carefully when hydrating patients with increased intracranial pressure, because intravenous infusion of 5 per cent glucose in water can result in a significant increase in intracranial pressure. This danger can be avoided by use of normal saline, 5 per cent glucose in saline, or 5 per cent glucose in 0.42 per cent saline. The phenothiazines may be used as antiemetic agents for patients with severe vomiting. These drugs are depressants and must be used cautiously. A variety of chemotherapeutic agents for the treatment of brain tumor are under active study, but their value has not yet been established.

Dastur, H. M., and Desai, A. D.: A comparative study of brain tuberculomas and gliomas based upon 107 case records of each. Brain, 88:375, 1965.

Dixon, H. B. F., and Lipscomb, F. M.: Cysticercosis: An Analysis and Follow-up of 450 Cases. Medical Research Council Special Report, Series No. 299. London, Her Majesty's Stationery Office, 1961.

Fishman, R. A.: Brain edema. N. Engl. J. Med., 293:706, 1975.

Samson, D. S., and Clark, K.: A current review of brain abscess. Am. J. Med., 54:201, 1973.

Vinken, P. J., and Bruyn, G. W. (eds.): Tumors of the brain and skull. In Handbook of Clinical Neurology, Vols. 16, 17, and 18. New York, American Elsevier Publishing Company, 1974.

Walker, M. D., and Weiss, H. D.: Chemotherapy in the treatment of malignant brain tumors. In Friedlander, W. J. (ed.): Advances in Neurology, Vol. 13. New York, Raven Press, 1975.

317. RADIATION INJURY OF THE NERVOUS SYSTEM

Radiation injury of the nervous system occurs as a complication of x-ray therapy when tissue dosage has been excessive. Signs of injury may appear within hours or days of high-dosage irradiation in laboratory animals; in man, with the doses used therapeutically, the onset is delayed. Characteristically, a progressive neurologic deficit develops after a latent period of many months or years after the termination of radiotherapy. This complication occurs when irradiation has been directed at neoplasms of the brain or at other tumors in the head and neck. The spinal cord is also subject to injury from excessive radiation, whether directed at a primary cord tumor or at tumors overlying the spine and paraspinal regions, e.g., tumors of the thyroid or mediastinum. Peripheral nerves are relatively radioresistant but are injured also by high doses.

PATHOLOGY. The response of the central nervous system to ionizing radiation can be recognized in three phases: an acute phase of meningoencephalitis, a period of apparent normalcy, and a period of late nerve cell damage, demyelination, and vascular change. The lesions in the nervous system attributed to irradiation are extensive in both white and gray matter. There are hyaline thickenings in the walls of blood vessels that may partially or completely occlude the lumen. There is a variable degree of cellular necrosis and degeneration of myelin. Astrocytosis and thickening of the leptomeninges are common. The long latent period between the time of irradiation and the onset of progressive signs is poorly understood; it has been attributed to progressive ischemia caused by gradual narrowing of the vascular lumen. Latent radiation effects in skin are readily attributable to vascular and connective tissue damage; this lends weight to the primary importance of the vascular injury in the brain, although it is likely that neuronal degeneration is not due to progressive ischemia alone. It has been suggested that autoimmune mechanisms play a role in the tissue damage that develops after a latent period.

DOSAGES. The precise tissue dosage that will induce radiation injury is uncertain. The minimal dose in Lindgren's series of 71 cases that produced pathologic evidence of brain necrosis was 4500 to 5000 roentgens, with delivery through medium-sized fields over a period of 30 days. The spinal cord is vulnerable to somewhat lower doses; radiation myelopathy has been reported after 4000 r in 28 days directed toward the mediastinum. Boden has defined the tolerance of the brainstem and spinal cord from a review of his own material. With small treatment fields of 10 by 7 cm or less, tissue doses up to 4500 r in 17 days or their biologic equivalent seem to be tolerated by the cord and brainstem. With large fields, a tissue dose of 3500 r is considered as the maximal tolerance dose to the brainstem and cord. There is considerable biologic variation in susceptibility of normal tissue to radiation damage, and precise definition of the effects of various dosages on normal tissue is difficult.

CLINICAL MANIFESTATIONS. When radiotherapy has been administered to tumors close to, but sparing, the brain and spinal cord, the development of a focal neurologic deficit after a latent period raises the possibility of radiation injury. After radiotherapy to brain or spinal cord tumors, clinical improvement that persists for one to five years with subsequent regression suggests the possibility of late radiation damage to normal nervous tissue. A transient form of radiation myelopathy is not uncommon; its major manifestation is the occurrence of Lhermitte's sign 2 to 37 weeks after radiation. Symptoms most often appear about a year after irradiation. The onset is insidious, and the rate of subsequent progress is unpredictable. The process may become arrested or may progress to cause a major cerebral hemispheric deficit or complete functional spinal cord transection. The clinical differentiation between radiation injury and recurrent tumor growth may be very difficult and uncertain pending pathologic confirmation at autopsy, and both may be coexistent. A repeated roentgenographic contrast study may help in differentiation. There is no specific therapy for radiation injury of the nervous system.

Goodwin-Austen, R. R., Howell, D. A., and Worthington, B.: Observations on radiation myelopathy. Brain, 98:557, 1975.

Holdorff, B.: Radiation damage to the brain. In Vinken, P. J., and Bruyn, G. W. (eds.): Handbook of Clinical Neurology, Vol. 23. New York, American Elsevier Publishing Company, 1975, p. 639.

Lindgren, M.: On tolerance of brain tissue and sensitivity of brain tumours to irradiation. Acta Radiol. (Stockholm), (Suppl. 170):1, 1958.

Samaan, N. A., Bardash, M. M., Caderao, J. B., Cangir, A., Jesse, R. H., and Ballantyne, A. J.: Hypopituitarism after external irradiation. Evidence for both hypothalamic and pituitary origin. Ann. Intern. Med., 83:771, 1975.

318. BENIGN INTRACRANIAL HYPERTENSION

(Pseudotumor Cerebri)

DEFINITION. Benign intracranial hypertension (BIH) describes the syndrome of increased intracranial pressure in which intracranial mass lesions, obstruction of the cerebral ventricles, intracranial infection, and hypertensive encephalopathy have been *excluded*. It has also been termed pseudotumor cerebri, serous meningitis, and otitic hydrocephalus. BIH includes a heterogenous group of disorders in which a number of different etiologic factors have been identified, although in most cases the cause and pathogenesis of these syndromes are poorly understood. They are termed "benign" because spontaneous recovery generally occurs; however, serious threats to vision may occur.

CLINICAL MANIFESTATIONS. The presenting symptoms are headache and disturbance of vision. The headache is often worse on awakening and is aggravated by coughing and straining. It is often relatively mild and may be entirely absent. The most common ocular complaint is visual blurring, a manifestation of papilledema. Some patients complain of brief, fleeting movements of dimming or complete loss of vision, occurring many times during the day (amaurosis fugax), at times accentuated or precipitated by coughing and straining. This ominous symptom indicates that the patient's vision is in serious jeopardy. Visual loss may be minimal despite severe chronic papilledema, including retinal hemorrhages; however, blindness rarely may develop very rapidly — in less than 24 hours. Visual fields characteristically show enlargement of the blind spots, and may show constriction of the peripheral fields and central or paracentral scotoma. Diplopia caused by unilateral or bilateral sixth nerve palsy may develop as a result of increased intracranial pressure. The neurologic examination is otherwise normal. A major clinical point is that patients with BIH commonly look well; that is, their appearance and apparent well-being belie the ominous appearance of the papilledema. Although the disorder may last for months or perhaps even years, no serious sequels usually follow. In some patients, however, BIH may be responsible for the development of the *"empty sella syndrome,"* in which there is enlargement of the sella turcica on x-ray simulating a pituitary tumor. The enlarged sella is filled with CSF due to a defect of its diaphragm.

PATHOPHYSIOLOGY. The signs and symptoms of BIH are due to the effects of increased intracranial pressure; pressures between 300 and 600 mm are frequent. The intracranial pressure is normally between 50 and 180 to 200 mm of water as measured in the lumbar sac or ventricles with the patient in the lateral recumbent position. This pressure is dependent upon the pressure-volume relationships within the intracranial and spinal cavities. The intracranial cavity contains about 1400 ml of brain, 75 ml of blood, and 75 ml of CSF, and an additional 75 ml in the spinal subarachnoid space. The CSF pressure is directly dependent upon the intracranial venous pressure; changes in the latter pressure are readily transmitted to the CSF, and thus a sustained increase in intracranial venous pressure may result in the syndrome of chronically increased intracranial pressure. The intracranial pressure is largely independent of the systemic arterial pressure, and it is normal in essential hypertension; however, it falls with acute systemic hypotension and rises acutely with very acute increases in systemic blood pressure, e.g., with the administration of vasopressor drugs or in the syndrome of acute hypertensive encephalopathy. Increased intracranial pressure also accompanies increased cerebral blood flow resulting from CO_2 retention, as in acute asphyxia or with chronic pulmonary insufficiency. In patients with BIH apart from those with obstruction of the intracranial venous system and chronic pulmonary insufficiency, the mechanism of the increase in intracranial pressure is unknown.

The occurrence of a special form of "interstitial" brain edema has been suggested to occur in some forms of BIH associated with decreased CSF absorption at the arachnoid villi. This hypothetical mechanism has been invoked to explain the occurrence of BIH in patients with polyneuritis and spinal tumors; a similar defect in CSF absorption may occur in the more common forms of BIH in which there is no apparent explanation for the intracranial hypertension.

ETIOLOGIC FACTORS AND ASSOCIATED DISORDERS

(Table). **Intracranial Venous Sinus Thrombosis.** Increased intracranial pressure as a result of occlusion of the intracranial venous sinuses occurs as a consequence of otitis media with extension of the infection into the petrous bone and to the wall of the lateral sinus. This syndrome has been termed otitic hydrocephalus. It occurs as a complication of both acute and chronic infection; at times the evidence for otitis media is minimal and readily overlooked. The sixth cranial nerve may also be involved, giving rise to diplopia on lateral gaze. Thrombosis of the superior longitudinal sinus may occur as a consequence of relatively mild closed head injury and may give rise to a pseudotumor syndrome. (Occlusion of this sinus that drains both cerebral hemispheres is more likely to result in hemorrhagic infarction in the cerebrum as the thrombosis extends into the cerebral veins, giving rise to bilateral signs. In such cases, the course is frequently fulminant and the prognosis guarded, although occasionally complete recovery may occur.) Aseptic or primary thrombosis of the superior longitudinal sinus may also be responsible for a pseudotumor syndrome. This develops as a complication of pregnancy and has been reported to occur during the first two to three weeks post partum, at the end of the first trimester of pregnancy, and with the use of oral progestational drugs. A disorder of the blood clotting mechanism has been suggested as basis for these events during the postpartum period, although this has not been substantiated. Sinus thrombosis occurs as a complication of cachexia ("marantic" thrombosis), and in association with cryofibrinogenemia.

Endocrine and Metabolic Disorders. The most common association is the occurrence of BIH in women with a history of menstrual dysfunction. The women are frequently moderately to markedly overweight (without evidence of alveolar hypoventilation). Menstrual irregularity is common, often with amenorrhea.

Benign Intracranial Hypertension: Etiologic Factors and Associated Disorders

1. Intracranial venous sinus thrombosis
   a. Mastoiditis and lateral sinus thrombosis
   b. After head trauma
   c. Pregnancy and postpartum
   d. Oral progestational drugs
   e. "Marantic" sinus thrombosis
   f. Cryofibrinogenemia
2. Endocrine and metabolic disorders
   a. Obesity and menstrual irregularities
   b. Pregnancy and postpartum (without sinus thrombosis)
   c. Menarche
   d. Addison's disease
   e. Hypoparathyroidism
   f. Diabetic ketoacidosis
   g. Dialysis dysequilibrium syndrome
3. Drugs and toxins
   a. Adrenal steroids and steroid withdrawal
   b. Female sex hormone
   c. Vitamin A
   d. Tetracycline and nalidixic acid
4. Hematologic disorders
   a. Iron deficiency anemia
   b. Infectious mononucleosis
   c. Wiskott-Aldrich syndrome
   d. Polycythemia
5. Pulmonary encephalopathy
   a. Paralytic hypoventilation
   b. Pulmonary emphysema
   c. Pickwickian syndrome
6. High cerebrospinal fluid protein
   a. Spinal cord and cauda equina tumors
   b. Polyneuritis
7. Miscellaneous
   a. Roseola infantum
   b. Sydenham's chorea
   c. Familial
   d. Lupus erythematosus
   e. Empty sella syndrome
8. Idiopathic

Galactorrhea is a rare associated symptom. The histories usually emphasize excessive premenstrual weight gain. Endocrine studies thus far have not revealed any abnormalities of urinary gonadotropins or estrogens, and the pathogenesis is unknown. BIH has been reported as a complication of Addison's disease, improvement occurring with replacement therapy. The mechanism is obscure. Hypoparathyroidism may present with evidence of increased intracranial pressure. The presence of hypocalcemic seizures or cerebral calcifications roentgenographically may further complicate the clinical picture. Increased intracranial pressure disappears with replacement therapy.

Drugs and Toxins. BIH has been reported in patients treated with adrenal corticosteroids for prolonged periods. Many of the patients have been children with allergic skin disorders or asthma. The syndrome is more likely to occur when the steroid dosage is reduced, suggesting that relative adrenal insufficiency might have been present, but this has not been substantiated. BIH has been reported in women taking oral progestational drugs when angiography has excluded sinus thrombosis. BIH has been reported in otherwise healthy adolescents taking huge doses of vitamin A for the treatment of acne. Doses as low as 25,000 units per day orally have been noted to cause headache and papilledema; there is rapid improvement after cessation of the therapy. The syndrome is said to have occurred in Arctic explorers who consumed polar bear liver, a great source of the vitamin. A few cases of BIH, manifested by bulging fontanelle and papilledema, have been reported in children after the administration of tetracycline or nalidixic acid. The mechanisms involved are obscure. Spontaneous rapid recovery occurs when the drugs are stopped.

Hematologic Disorders. Papilledema and increased intracranial pressure have been attributed to severe iron deficiency anemia, with striking improvement after treatment of the anemia. The mechanism presumably is dependent upon the marked increase in cerebral blood flow that accompanies profound anemia. BIH occurs with infectious mononucleosis and the Wiskott-Aldrich syndrome, but its mechanism is not known.

Pulmonary Encephalopathy. BIH can be a major complication of chronic hypoxic hypercapnia caused by paralytic states such as muscular dystrophy and cervical myelopathy, as well as of obstructive pulmonary disease and the pickwickian syndrome. The mechanism is dependent upon the chronic increase in cerebral blood flow resulting from the anoxemia and carbon dioxide retention (see Ch. 344).

High Cerebrospinal Fluid Protein. BIH occurs rarely with tumors of the spinal cord or cauda equina as well as with polyneuritis. Papilledema and headache have disappeared with treatment of the spinal lesion or regression of the polyneuropathy. The mechanism may involve the effects of a very high CSF protein upon CSF absorption at the arachnoid villi, both in the cranial and spinal subarachnoid spaces.

Idiopathic. One of the more common forms of BIH is its occurrence in otherwise healthy subjects in the absence of any of the etiologic factors described above. Both sexes are involved, and the occurrence is most often between the ages of 10 and 50 years. These cases represent the idiopathic form of BIH; its pathogenesis is a mystery. There are rare case reports of BIH with roseola infantum, Sydenham's chorea, and lupus erythematosus in which the mechanism is unknown.

DIAGNOSIS. The patient with headache and papilledema without other neurologic signs must be considered to have an intracranial mass, ventricular obstruction, or intracranial infection until proved otherwise. Although the diagnosis of BIH may be suspected by the appearance of apparent well-being and by the history of some of the associated features listed above, the diagnosis is essentially one of exclusion dependent upon ruling out the more common causes of increased intracranial pressure. Brain tumor, particularly when located in relatively silent areas such as the frontal lobes or right temporal lobe or when obstructing the ventricular system, may be manifest only by headache and papilledema. Patients with chronic subdural hematoma, without history of significant trauma, may present in the same way. Diagnostic evaluation requires skull films, electroencephalography, and arteriography and/or air studies. Computerized tomography, when available, has negated the need for angiography or air studies in many cases. Lumbar puncture is necessary in these patients, but is generally deferred until arteriography or computerized tomography has revealed that the ventricular system is normal in size and location. Laboratory studies regarding possible hypoadrenalism or hypoparathyroidism may be rewarding in rare cases of these disorders that present with the pseudotumor syndrome. The cerebrospinal fluid pressure is elevated, between 250 and 600 mm, but the fluid is otherwise normal. The protein content is generally low normal, and lumbar CSF protein levels below 15 mg per 100 ml are common. The

electroencephalogram is normal in BIH. Pseudopapilledema may be a source of diagnostic confusion. It is a developmental anomaly of the fundus wherein the ophthalmologic appearance may be indistinguishable from that of the true papilledema; there is elevation of the optic disc, but exudates or hemorrhages are absent. The visual acuity is normal, although visual fields may show some enlargement of the blind spots. The unchanging appearance of the fundus in subsequent examinations favors the diagnosis of pseudopapilledema, as does the finding of normal CSF pressure on lumbar puncture.

TREATMENT. In patients with lateral sinus thrombosis caused by chronic infection in the petrous bone, surgical decompression is often indicated. When the pseudotumor syndrome is a manifestation of hypoadrenalism of hypoparathyroidism, replacement therapy is indicated. Vitamin A intoxication disappears when administration of the vitamin is stopped. Anticoagulation therapy has been recommended for patients with dural sinus thrombosis; however, for patients with extension of the clot into cerebral veins with infarction of tissue, anticoagulation is hazardous because it increases the likelihood of hemorrhagic infarction.

The idiopathic form of BIH and its occurrence in patients with menstrual disorders and obesity require individualized management. This syndrome is self-limited in most cases, and after some weeks or months spontaneous remissions occur, making evaluation of therapy difficult. Recurrent episodes have been noted in about 5 per cent of cases. In rare instances, the illness may last for years. In the very obese, weight reduction is recommended. The use of daily lumbar punctures has been advocated to lower pressure to normal levels by removing sufficient fluid; 15 to 50 ml of fluid may be required, but its value is dubious. Subtemporal decompression has been widely used in the past. This procedure may be necessary for patients with serious threat to vision caused by pressure, although its efficacy has been questioned in a number of reports. A CSF shunting procedure, such as a lumbar-peritoneal shunt, is probably the surgical procedure of choice in such cases. The use of dexamethasone has been advocated because it minimizes cerebral edema of diverse causes. Acetazolamide has been used because this carbonic anhydrase inhibitor has been shown to reduce CSF formation. Furosemide also reduces CSF formation and may be useful. Hypertonic intravenous solutions (25 per cent mannitol) to lower intracranial pressure can be used in acute situations when there is rapidly failing vision, while one awaits neurosurgical intervention; however, prolonged dehydration therapy is impossible because of its deleterious systemic effects. The use of oral glycerol has the disadvantage of high caloric intake for obese patients. Management of these patients is difficult and requires the attention of neurologists and neurosurgeons experienced in these problems.

Boddie, H. G., Banna, M., and Bradley W. G.: Benign intracranial hypertension: A survey of clinical and radiological features, and long-term prognosis. Brain, 97:313, 1974.

Johnston, I., and Patterson, A.: Benign intracranial hypertension: I. Diagnosis and prognosis, II. CSF pressure and circulation. Brain, 97:289, 1974.

Jordan, R. M., Kendall, J. W., and Kerber, C. W.: The primary empty sella syndrome. Am. J. Med., 62:569, 1977.

Lombaert, A., and Carton, H.: Benign intracranial hypertension due to A-hypervitaminosis in adults and adolescents. Eur. Neurol., 14:340, 1976.

Weisberg, L. A.: Benign intracranial hypertension. Medicine, 54:197, 1975.

319. INTRACRANIAL HYPOTENSION

The normal intracranial pressure is 70 to 200 mm water (or 5 to 15 mm Hg). Symptoms of intracranial hypotension occur with pressures of about 70 mm water or less; at times the CSF pressure is not measurable and the fluid can be obtained only by aspiration with a syringe. The symptoms of intracranial hypotension include severe headache precipitated by the erect position and relieved by the supine position. Symptoms are aggravated by cough or strain. There also may be nausea and vomiting precipitated by similar postural changes. A unilateral or bilateral sixth nerve palsy may accompany low pressure syndromes. The most common cause is previous lumbar puncture with persistent CSF leakage into the subdural or epidural spaces. Low pressure syndromes also occur owing to spontaneous or post-traumatic cerebrospinal fluid rhinorrhea, and with pituitary tumors. Bacterial meningitis may complicate such cases. Traumatic avulsions of spinal roots may also result in a CSF leak. Severe dehydration also results in intracranial hypotension. An erroneously low CSF pressure may be recorded in the presence of spinal block.

The management of post–lumbar puncture headache includes bed rest, preferably in the prone position, adequate hydration, and analgesics (see Ch. 261). In patients with persistent symptoms, the use of the "blood patch," in which 10 ml of the patient's blood is carefully injected into the *subdural* space, has proved valuable. Major CSF leaks, e.g., CSF rhinorrhea, require surgical closure.

Bell, W. E., Joynt, R. J., and Sahs, A. L.: Low spinal fluid pressure syndromes. Neurology, 10:512, 1960.

MacGee, E. E.: Cerebrospinal fluid fistula. *In* Vinken, P. J., and Bruyn, G. W. (eds.): Handbook of Clinical Neurology, Vol. 24. New York, American Elsevier Publishing Company, 1976.

Ostheimer, G. W., Palahniuk, R. J., and Shnider, S. M.: Epidural blood patch for post-lumbar-puncture headache. Anesthesiology, 41:307, 1974.

320. HYDROCEPHALUS

DEFINITIONS. Hydrocephalus is a pathologic state characterized by dilatation of the cerebral ventricles with an increase in volume of cerebrospinal fluid (CSF), almost always caused by an obstruction in the circulation of this fluid. In children, prior to fusion of the cranial sutures, there is enlargement of the skull. Hydrocephalus must be distinguished from other causes of macrocephaly in infancy, including subdural hematoma. In older subjects, cranial enlargement cannot occur. Hydrocephalus is termed "active," i.e., progressive and associated with increased intraventricular pressure, or "arrested," i.e., when the intraventricular pressure has returned to normal and is no longer a stimulus for ventricular enlargement. These forms of hydrocephalus are distinguished from hydrocephalus ex vacuo, which is characterized by an increase in the volume of CSF under normal pressure that is compensatory to a primary atrophy of the brain. Normal pressure occult hydrocephalus refers to the syndrome of ventricular dilatation associated with inadequacy of the subarachnoid spaces without evidence of increased intracranial pressure (see below).

ETIOLOGY AND PATHOPHYSIOLOGY. There are three possible mechanisms for the development of hydrocephalus: overproduction of CSF, defective absorption of CSF, and obstruction of the CSF pathways. *Overproduction* of the fluid has been documented to occur only with the rare papilloma of the choroid plexus. *Defective absorption* of the CSF at the arachnoid villi, where the fluid passes through these membranous structures to enter the venous sinuses, may occur with subarachnoid hemorrhage, with meningitis, and with a very high CSF protein. *Obstruction* of the CSF pathways, which results in dilatation of the channels proximal to the site of obstruction, is the most common underlying mechanism in both the hydrocephalus of infancy and of adults. When the block is within the ventricular system, the process is termed *noncommunicating hydrocephalus,* whereas *communicating hydrocephalus* describes ventricular dilatation in which there is free flow of fluid and air between the ventricular system and the spinal subarachnoid space. Communicating hydrocephalus is characterized by extraventricular obstruction of the CSF pathways, most commonly in the subarachnoid spaces about the brainstem at the incisura of the tentorium or in the subarachnoid spaces about the cerebral hemispheres, or both. Ventricular dilatation develops in hydrocephalus because the intraventricular pressures (both the mean pressure and the pulsatile pressures, synchronous with cardiac systole) are pathologically increased; these give rise to a transmural pressure gradient across the cerebral mantle sufficient to cause compression of the adjacent white matter that has a loss of protein and lipid but an increase in water and sodium content. The magnitude and duration of the transmural pressure gradient necessary to induce ventricular dilatation have not been well defined. These changes may be reversible if surgical therapy can successfully relieve the increased intraventricular pressure (see below).

The major causes of obstruction in the CSF pathways that produce hydrocephalus are neoplasms, congenital malformations, and post-traumatic and postinflammatory lesions.

Neoplasms most likely to give rise to hydrocephalus are those that arise within or adjacent to the ventricular system and obstruct the flow of CSF. These include gliomas and ependymomas of the third and fourth ventricles and of the aqueduct (see Ch. 316). Congenital stenosis of the aqueduct may give rise to symptoms early in life, or manifestations may be absent until adulthood. Congenital malformations of the craniovertebral junction also may be associated with hydrocephalus (see Arnold-Chiari Malformation in Ch. 321). Most frequently, hydrocephalus is related to postinflammatory or post-traumatic obstruction of the basilar cisterns, particularly in the region of the tentorium. In infancy, this follows intracranial bleeding at the time of birth, at times unrecognized, or episodes of bacterial meningitis or toxoplasmosis. These processes lead to progressive fibrosis of the subarachnoid pathways at the base of the brain, with subsequent obstruction. In adults, postinflammatory hydrocephalus may develop with or after purulent, tuberculous and mycotic meningitis or with cysticercosis, and also may follow subarachnoid hemorrhage caused by trauma or ruptured congenital aneurysm.

CLINICAL MANIFESTATIONS. The major signs and symptoms of hydrocephalus are those of increased intracranial pressure (see Ch. 316). In infancy, this is manifest by a greater than normal growth rate and size of the head and by distended scalp veins; in severe cases there is downward displacement of the eyes and mental retardation. Although the head size (occipitobregmatic circumference) in comparison with the chest circumference is of importance, repeated observations of the *rate* of head growth are more significant. Additional information can be obtained from measurements of the anterior fontanelle, as active hydrocephalus does not occur in conjunction with a closing fontanelle. On the other hand, a fontanelle enlarging from month to month is evidence for increased intracranial pressure, and further investigations are warranted.

In older children and adults, the major manifestations include headache, diplopia caused by sixth nerve palsy, papilledema, visual blurring, nausea, and vomiting. Thus occult hydrocephalus that is due to a benign process must be differentiated from intracranial mass lesions, including tumor without localizing signs and chronic subdural hematoma, as well as from the various forms of benign intracranial hypertension and the chronic meningitides, including fungal meningitis, sarcoidosis, and diffuse meningeal neoplasia (carcinomatous meningitis).

Occult "Normal Pressure" Hydrocephalus. In recent years, a new syndrome has been delineated as occult "normal pressure" hydrocephalus. Typically, there is a gradual development over weeks or months of a mild impairment of memory with mental and physical slowness which progresses insidiously to a severe dementia with unsteady gait and urinary incontinence. The patients are usually headache-free and have no signs of increased intracranial pressure e.g., they have normal fundi and normal CSF pressure at lumbar puncture. Computerized tomography reveals ventricular enlargement without cortical atrophy. Pneumoencephalography reveals enlarged ventricles and a lack of filling of the subarachnoid space over the hemispheres. Isotope cisternography (intraspinal injection of isotope with serial scanning of the skull) has revealed a pathologic reflux of the isotope into the ventricular system with delayed and inadequate visualization of the cortical subarachnoid space. Some patients have a previous history of head injury or subarachnoid bleeding; in others, the cause is obscure. Striking improvement in the mental state and gait has been noted to follow shunting procedures. Patients with short histories are more likely to respond to surgery. This treatable syndrome is uncommon but must be differentiated from the more frequent forms of organic dementia as discussed in Ch. 226 to 231.

DIAGNOSIS. Detailed neurologic study is necessary to determine the cause of increased intracranial pressure and ventricular dilatation. Skull films show characteristic signs of increased intracranial pressure in young children; the signs in adults are generally less striking and may be absent. Computerized tomography is valuable in demonstrating ventricular enlargement and the presence of obstructive lesions. Electroencephalograms may be normal or may demonstrate bilateral slowing of nonspecific nature. Carotid angiography will show displacement of the arteries and veins characteristic of ventricular enlargement. Air contrast studies will reveal the degree of ventricular enlargement, the presence of obstructive lesions in the cerebrospinal fluid pathways, and the adequacy of the subarachnoid spaces about the brainstem, base, and cerebrum. Precise neuroradiologic analysis is essential to establish the diagnosis. The cerebrospinal fluid pressure is characteristically, but not invariably, increased in the cerebral ventricles and lumbar sac. The protein content is generally normal; elevated protein levels favor an underlying neoplastic process in the absence of bleeding or chronic meningitis.

TREATMENT. The treatment of hydrocephalus is surgical; it is directed toward reducing the volume and pressure of cerebrospinal fluid by bypassing obstruction. A wide variety of shunting procedures have been used. The choice of procedure will depend upon technical factors and the skill and experience of the operating surgeon. If the block exists in the third ventricle, aqueduct, or fourth ventricle (as with intraventricular tumors or with "aqueduct stenosis"), the Torkildsen procedure is often employed (ventriculocisternal shunt), wherein a catheter is placed from one or both lateral ventricles over the occiput into the cisterna magna to enable normal CSF reabsorption into the intracranial venous sinuses. In patients with communicating hydrocephalus, direct shunting of the ventricular fluid into the venous system is generally used, particularly the ventriculoatrial shunt wherein the fluid exits from the ventricle through a valved tube, which extends into the superior vena cava and right atrium of the heart. There are many variations of these procedures in use, including shunting to other body cavities, e.g., ventriculopleural, ventriculoabdominal, and lumbar peritoneal shunts. Infections and recurrent obstruction of the shunt are common complications of the various shunting procedures, and the results of treatment particularly in young children are frequently discouraging. Acetazolamide, a carbonic anhydrase inhibitor, reduces the rate of formation of CSF; but there is no convincing evidence that it is useful in the management of the various forms of hydrocephalus. Some hydrocephalic children will have spontaneous arrest and may function within the normal range with only a prominent forehead and large hat size as residual defects. Shunting procedures have established occult "normal pressure" hydrocephalus as a treatable dementia.

Fisher, C. M.: The clinical picture in occult hydrocephalus. Clin. Neurosurg., 24:270, 1977.

Mathew, N. T., Meyer, J. S., Hartmann, A., and Ott, E. D.: Abnormal cerebrospinal fluid-blood flow dynamics. Implications in diagnosis, treatment and prognosis in normal pressure hydrocephalus. Arch. Neurol., 32:657, 1975.

Messert, B., and Wannamaker, B. B.: Reappraisal of the occult hydrocephalus syndrome. Neurology, 24:224, 1974.

Milhorat, T. H.: Hydrocephalus and Cerebrospinal Fluid. Baltimore, Williams & Wilkins Company, 1972.

321. ANOMALIES OF THE CRANIOVERTEBRAL JUNCTION, SPINE, AND MENINGES

A wide variety of neurologic syndromes are associated with morphologic anomalies in the region of the foramen magnum of the skull that are due to distortion of the brainstem, cervical cord, and cerebellum. The most common of these are (1) Arnold-Chiari malformation, (2) fusion of the cervical vertebrae (Klippel-Feil syndrome), (3) basilar impression and platybasia, and (4) spina bifida and meningocele. These defects may occur singly or together, with or without clinical symptoms. Symptoms result from compression, distortion, or malformation of adjacent neural structures. These are most often congenital lesions, but acquired defects caused by bone disease or neoplasms of this region may give rise to similar syndromes.

ARNOLD-CHIARI MALFORMATION

This congenital anomaly is characterized by downward displacement of the cerebellum through the foramen magnum of the skull and by similar caudal elongation of the medulla. These cases can be divided into two major types, the infantile and the adult.

INFANTILE FORM. The infantile form is commonly associated with other midline defects such as spina bifida and meningocele, hydrocephalus caused by aqueductal or fourth ventricular obstruction, and other congenital malformations of the brain and cord. The infantile form of the Arnold-Chiari malformation usually presents itself because of hydrocephalus in the early months of life, with evidence of spina bifida or frank paraparesis resulting from myelomeningocele. Therapy is directed toward surgical relief of the hydrocephalus with a ventricular shunting procedure and repair of the meningomyelocele. Prognosis is poor for patients with extensive defects.

ADULT FORM. The malformation may be asymptomatic until adult life, when there is the onset of symptoms and signs of damage to the cerebellum, lower cranial nerves, pyramidal tracts, and posterior columns. The presenting signs may be due to hydrocephalus secondary to obstruction of the cerebrospinal fluid pathways or to coexisting syringomyelia of the cervical spinal cord and medulla (see Ch. 320 and 334.3). Commonly, there is evidence, clinical or roentgenographic, of fusion of the cervical vertebrae, platybasia, or basilar impression. The Arnold-Chiari malformation in adults may simulate syndromes produced by tumors near the foramen magnum and by multiple sclerosis. Surgical enlargement of the foramen magnum and decompression of the cervicomedullary junction are beneficial in selected cases.

CONGENITAL FUSION OF CERVICAL VERTEBRAE
(Klippel-Feil Syndrome)

Fusion of one or more of the cervical vertebrae is a congenital malformation that may be an asymptomatic finding, detected only with roentgenograms of the cervical spine; malformation of the atlas and axis may coexist. Multiple fusions and condensaton of vertebrae result in shortening of the cervical spine, which produces a characteristic appearance of a short, thick neck, head set low on the shoulders, and limitation of neck movements.

Coexisting abnormalities are common, including undescended scapula (Sprengel's deformity), platybasia, basilar impression, Arnold-Chiari malformation, and other "dysrhaphic" disorders such as syringomyelia and meningomyelocele. Clinical evidence of spinal cord involvement is most likely to be due to coexisting syringomyelia. "Mirror movements" may occur with the Klippel-Feil syndrome and other anomalies of the craniovertebral junction and high cervical cord, in which voluntary movements of one upper extremity are involuntarily imitated by the other upper extremity. Surgical decompression may be indicated if there is evidence of spinal cord compression.

BASILAR IMPRESSION AND PLATYBASIA

Basilar impression refers to abnormal invagination of the cervical spine into the base of the posterior fossa of the skull. The diagnosis is made from lateral roentgenograms of the skull when there is excessive protrusion of the tip of the odontoid process of the axis above Chamberlain's line, that is, a line drawn from the back of the hard palate to the posterior margin of the foramen magnum. Other radiologic criteria are also useful. *Platybasia* refers to flattening of the base of the skull, wherein lateral roentgenograms of the skull reveal flattening of the angle between the orbital plates of the anterior fossa and the clivus, the sloping anterior floor of the posterior fossa. The angle is normally 135 degrees and becomes 145 degrees or more in platybasia. Platybasia alone is asymptomatic.

These malformations, which commonly coexist or may exist alone, are usually developmental in origin, and there may be hereditary transmission. Occasionally, these deformations of the base of the skull may result from metabolic bone diseases such as rickets, osteitis deformans, osteomalacia, or osteogenesis imperfecta. The congenital form may be associated with the Klippel-Feil syndrome, Arnold-Chiari malformation, and other congenital malformations of the atlas and axis, such as fusion of the atlas to the base of the skull, malpositioning of the odontoid process, or atlantoaxial subluxation. Minor degrees of deformity of the base of the skull give rise to no symptoms. The neck appears shortened, and its movements may be limited. With more severe invagination, there may be signs of impaired function of the cerebellum, lower cranial nerves, pyramidal tracts, and posterior columns. Syringomyelia and syringobulbia may also be present. Increased intracranial pressure may develop owing to obstruction of the foramina of the fourth ventricle and the basal cisterns. The clinical manifestations must be differentiated from those caused by neoplasms in the region of the foramen magnum and multiple sclerosis. When neurologic signs are progressive, surgical decompression of the posterior fossa and upper cervical cord may be indicated.

SPINA BIFIDA AND MENINGOCELE

Various malformations of the meninges and spinal cord result from developmental defects in the closure of the bony canal. Although many of these are obvious at birth, some may not be symptomatic until adult life. The classification of these defects would include the following: (1) *Complete rachischisis,* in which the bony vertebral arches are missing in the lumbar region, the cord is undeveloped or aplastic, and the nerve elements have no covering. (2) *Meningomyelocele,* an obvious soft tissue saccular mass which extends over the lumbosacral spine. The cerebrospinal fluid may leak from a defect which may be responsible for bacterial meningitis. (3) *Meningocele,* a bony defect in the spine associated with a meningeal diverticulum covered by atrophic skin. The spinal cord and roots are generally not involved and there may be no associated neurologic defect. (4) *Spina bifida occulta,* a defect in the bony arches in the lumbar region often discovered incidentally on roentgenographic examination. In most cases, neither cord nor roots are involved. The overlying skin may be the site of a tuft of hair, a pilonidal dimple, or a dermal sinus, which is continuous with the subarachnoid space. The latter may serve as a portal of entry for recurrent bouts of meningitis. It should be sought in all patients presenting with bacterial meningitis. These malformations may be associated with Arnold-Chiari malformation and with hydrocephalus. There may also be evidence of syringomyelia. The neurologic deficit varies with the degree of involvement of the spinal cord, conus medullaris, and cauda equina. In adults the chief manifestation may be a neurogenic bladder and defective anal sphincter. Asymptomatic spina bifida requires no therapy. Dermal sinuses, when responsible for bacterial meningitis, require surgical excision. In patients with neurologic deficits, attempts at surgical correction may be indicated.

Appleby, A., Foster, J. B., Hankinson, J., and Hudgson, P.: The diagnosis and management of the Chiari malformations in adult life. Brain, 91:131, 1968.

Embry, J. L., and MacKenzie, N.: Medullo-cervical dislocation deformity (Chiari II deformity) related to neurospinal dysraphism (meningomyelocele). Brain, 96:155, 1973.

Greenberg, A. D.: Atlanto-axial dislocations. Brain, 91:655, 1968.

Schmidt, H., Sartor, K., and Heckl, R. W.: Bone malformations of the craniocervical region. In Vinken, P. J., and Bruyn, G. W. (eds.): Handbook of Clinical Neurology, Vol. 32. New York, American Elsevier Publishing Company, 1978, p. 1.

Wilkinson, M.: The Klippel-Feil syndrome. In Vinken, P. J., and Bruyn, G. W. (eds.): Handbook of Clinical Neurology, Vol. 32. New York, American Elsevier Publishing Company, 1978, p. 111.

Section Twenty NONMETASTATIC EFFECTS OF CANCER ON THE NERVOUS SYSTEM

Jerome B. Posner

322. INTRODUCTION

When patients with systemic cancer develop nervous system dysfunction, metastasis is usually the cause. However, cancer also exerts deleterious effects on the nervous system in the absence of direct metastatic involvement. Recognition of these nonmetastatic neurologic complications can prevent inappropriate and perhaps harmful therapy directed at a nonexistent metastasis. Since at times the nervous system symptoms precede the discovery of the cancer, they can also lead the physician to the diagnosis of an otherwise occult neoplasm.

An almost bewildering variety of neurologic disorders have been ascribed to effects of systemic cancer, as shown in the accompanying table. Many of these bear only an indirect nutritional or metabolic (e.g., hepatic coma) relationship to cancer and are discussed elsewhere in this book. The term "remote effects of cancer on the nervous system" as used in this section applies to nervous system dysfunction of unknown cause occurring in association with cancer (see accompanying table). The classification is similar to that of Brain and Adams (see Brain and Norris), but progressive multifocal leukoencephalopathy is not included in the text, because its cause (a viral infection by a papovavirus) is known.

Remote effects of cancer on the nervous system are uncommon. Croft and Wilkinson found remote effects in 96 of 1465 patients, an incidence of 6.6. per cent, but a rather ill-defined weakness and wasting of proximal muscles associated with diminished deep tendon reflexes accounted for two thirds of their patients. The incidence varied according to the type of cancer, with ovary (16.4 per cent) and lung (14.2 per cent) leading the list. Rectal (0.5 per cent) and uterine (1.3 per cent) cancer rarely caused remote effects. Since carcinoma of the lung is much more common than ovarian carcinoma, about half of all their patients with remote effects had lung cancer, usually of the oat cell type. My experi-

ence is that "remote effects" are less common than the aforementioned series suggests, and the diagnosis should never be accepted until a thorough evaluation has excluded metastatic or other nonmetastatic (e.g., infection, vascular disease) causes of neurologic dysfunction. In particular, infiltration of nerve roots by tumor in the leptomeninges (meningeal carcinomatosis) may mimic a "remote" peripheral neuropathy.

The etiology and pathogenesis of these "remote effects" are unknown; suggestions for their cause have included autoimmune reactions, viral infections, toxins secreted by the tumor, and nutritional deprivation. It is possible that different mechanisms are responsible for the several types of remote effects. Although the neurologic disorders described below are separated into anatomic categories, there is often an overlap. This is particularly true of the dementias, which are often lumped together with brainstem, cerebellar, and spinal cord lesions as "carcinomatous encephalomyelitis," and of myopathy and peripheral neuropathy associated with cancer, often called "carcinomatous neuromyopathy." The latter term was also applied by Brain to all the remote effects of cancer on the nervous system.

323. BRAIN AND CRANIAL NERVES

CEREBRUM. About 40 per cent of patients suffering from remote effects of cancer on the nervous system are demented. The dementia may be the only neurologic abnormality or may be associated with other neurologic findings. The dementia is insidious in onset and progressive. There is usually a striking loss of recent memory and an alteration of the affect, either anxiety or depression. Generalized seizures are prominent in some patients, and others have a fluctuating confusional state mimicking metabolic encephalopathy. When other abnormal neurologic signs are present, they usually point

Nonmetastatic Effects of Systemic Cancer on the Nervous System

I. "Remote effects," cause unknown
  A. Brain and cranial nerves
    1. Dementia
    2. Bulbar encephalitis
    3. Subacute cerebellar degeneration–opsoclonus*
    4. Optic neuritis – retinal degeneration
  B. Spinal cord
    1. Gray matter myelopathy
      a. "Amyotrophic lateral sclerosis"
      b. Subacute motor neuropathy
      c. "Autonomic insufficiency"
    2. Subacute necrotic myelopathy
  C. Peripheral nerves and roots
    1. Dorsal root ganglionitis*
    2. Sensorimotor peripheral neuropathy
    3. Acute polyneuropathy, "Guillain-Barré" type
    4. Autonomic neuropathy
  D. Neuromuscular junction and muscle
    1. Polymyositis and dermatomyositis (dermatomyositis in older men*)
    2. "Myasthenic" syndrome*
    3. Myasthenia gravis (thymoma)
    4. Neuromyotonia
II. Metabolic encephalopathy
  A. Destruction of vital organs
    1. Liver (hepatic coma)
    2. Lung (pulmonary encephalopathy)
    3. Kidney (uremia)
    4. Bone (hypercalcemia)
  B. Elaboration of hormonal substances by tumor
    1. "Parathormone" (hypercalcemia)
    2. "Corticotropin" (Cushing's syndrome)
    3. Antidiuretic hormone (water intoxication)
  C. Competition between tumor and brain for essential substrates
    1. Hypoglycemia (large retroperitoneal tumors)
    2. Tryptophan (carcinoid)
  D. Malnutrition
III. Infections (usually associated with lymphomas)
  A. Parasites
    1. Toxoplasma cerebral abscess
  B. Fungi
    1. Meningitis (cryptococcosis)
    2. Encephalitis (aspergillus, mucormycosis)
  C. Bacteria
    1. Meningitis (*Listeria monocytogenes*)
  D. Viruses
    1. Herpes zoster (radiculitis, myelitis, encephalitis)
    2. Progressive multifocal leukoencephalopathy
IV. Vascular disease
  A. Intracranial hemorrhage (secondary to bleeding disorders)
    1. Subdural hematoma
    2. Subarachnoid hemorrhage
    3. Intracerebral hemorrhage
  B. Cerebral infarction
    1. Thrombotic (due to "disseminated intravascular coagulation")
    2. Embolic (tumor emboli, marantic endocarditis)
V. Effects of therapy
  A. Steroids
    1. Myopathy
    2. Psychosis
  B. Chemotherapy
    1. Central effects (asparaginase encephalopathy)
    2. Peripheral effects (vinca alkaloid neuropathy)
  C. Radiation
    1. Encephalopathy
    2. Myelopathy
    3. Neuropathy
    4. Radiation-induced neoplasms

*Neurologic disorders which may precede diagnosis of cancer but strongly suggest its presence.

to brainstem, cerebellar, or peripheral nerve involvement (see below). The electroencephalogram in the demented patients is diffusely slow, and there are sometimes 10 to 40 lymphocytes per cubic milliliter in the cerebrospinal fluid and a slight elevation of the protein content.

Pathologically, there are two main groups. In some patients, particularly those who also have subacute cerebellar degeneration, bulbar encephalitis, or carcinomatous neuropathy (q.v.), no significant pathologic changes can be found in the cerebrum despite clinical dementia. Other patients demonstrate widespread cerebral neuronal loss with perivascular collections of lymphocytes, particularly in the temporal lobes (limbic encephalitis) or the thalamus.

The etiology of the dementing illness is unknown, but the inflammatory changes have led some to propose that a virus is responsible. The differential diagnosis includes metastatic disease of the brain or meninges, fungal or parasitic infections of the brain, a metabolic encephalopathy, and multifocal leukoencephalopathy. In the first three, focal cerebral signs other than dementia are present, and appropriate contrast and cerebrospinal fluid studies support the diagnosis of infectious or metastatic disease of the brain. Metabolic encephalopathy can usually be diagnosed by appropriate laboratory tests, as indicated in Ch. 220. The presence of a progressive dementia in middle age accompanied by cerebellar, brainstem, or peripheral nerve dysfunction but no other focal cerebral signs suggests carcinomatous dementia. There is no treatment for the dementias associated with carcinoma.

BULBAR ENCEPHALITIS. Henson et al. have reported a few patients with brainstem dysfunction and usually dementia, which develops insidiously or subacutely and is progressive. The brainstem signs include vertigo, nystagmus, dysphagia, ophthalmoplegia, and at times ataxia and extensor plantar reflexes. The pathologic changes, predominantly in the lower pons and medulla, are those of neuronal loss and perivascular lymphocytic cuffing. The lymphocytic infiltration is responsible for the term encephalitis. The cause is unknown, and there is no effective treatment.

CEREBELLUM. Subacute cerebellar degeneration due to cancer has a clinical picture sufficiently characteristic to suggest strongly that cancer is present even if the neurologic symptoms predate the appearance of the tumor. There is a subacute onset of bilateral and symmetrical cerebellar dysfunction, the patient being equally ataxic in arms and legs. Severe dysarthria is usually present, but nystagmus is generally absent or mild. Many patients have neurologic signs pointing to disease outside the cerebellum: extensor plantar responses are common; tendon reflexes may be either diminished or exaggerated; and dementia occurs in about half. The cerebrospinal fluid is usually normal, but there may be as many as 40 lymphocytes per cubic milliliter and an elevated protein content. The disease, which is usually associated with either carcinoma of the lung or of the ovary, precedes the discovery of the neoplasm by periods of from weeks to three years in more than half the patients, and it tends to run a progressive course over six to eight weeks, rendering the patient severely disabled. Characteristic pathologic changes consist of diffuse loss of Purkinje cells in all areas of the cerebellum with lymphocytic cuffs around blood vessels. There is often additional neuronal degeneration of brainstem nuclei and subthalamic structures as well. This illness can be distinguished from cerebellar metastases by the symmetry of its signs and the absence of increased intracranial pressure, and from alcoholic-nutritional cerebellar degeneration because dysarthria and ataxia in the upper extremities are prominent in the carcinomatous cerebellar degenerations, and are usually mild or absent in the alcoholic variety. The hereditary cerebellar degenerations rarely run so rapid a course. There is no treatment for this disorder, and its cause is unknown. There is no evidence that treatment of the tumor reverses the neurologic disability.

Another, less common, cerebellar syndrome is that of opsoclonus (spontaneous, conjugate, chaotic eye movements most severe when voluntary eye movements are attempted). Opsoclonus is frequently associated with cerebellar ataxia and myoclonus of the trunk and extremities. It has been reported in adults as a remote effect of cancer, but is more common in children as a remote effect of neuroblastoma. In children, the neurologic symptoms respond to adrenocorticosteroid therapy and to removal of the tumor.

OPTIC NERVES.   Acute optic neuritis is a rare remote effect of cancer which may precede the discovery of the cancer by months or years. The disease is bilateral, acute or subacute in its onset, and associated with decreased vision, central scotomas, and papilledema. The cerebrospinal fluid is normal, and vision usually does not improve. Pathologically, there is widespread demyelination of the optic nerves with relative preservation of the axis cylinders and occasional perivascular cuffings with lymphocytes. The illness cannot be distinguished from the optic involvement which is a common accompaniment of meningeal carcinomatosis except by examination of the cerebrospinal fluid, which in meningeal tumor usually reveals increased protein and decreased glucose concentrations and the presence of malignant cells. Blindness from optic nerve or chiasm involvement has also been reported as an untoward effect of radiation therapy and chemotherapy in patients with leukemia, but in these instances the history is diagnostic. Treatment of the acute optic neuritis with corticosteroids is not helpful. Blinding caused by degeneration of retinal photoreceptors has recently been described as a remote effect of oat cell carcinoma.

324.   SPINAL CORD

Two rare but distinct myelopathies complicate cancer. The first, which involves spinal gray matter (particularly anterior horn cells), has clinical and pathologic findings at times indistinguishable from amyotrophic lateral sclerosis, except that the patients with cancer are usually older and suffer a more indolent course. Alternatively, the course may be subacute, more like poliomyelitis, but sometimes with sensory changes. In these patients, there are inflammatory changes in the spinal gray matter as well as neuronal loss. Rarely, gray matter myelopathies with clinical courses resembling syringomyelia or autonomic insufficiency (q.v.) complicate systemic cancer. The second myelopathy is that of a subacute necrotic destruction of the spinal cord in which both gray and white matter are affected to an equal degree. Clinically, there is a rapidly ascending sensory and motor loss, usually to midthoracic levels, the patient becoming paraplegic and incontinent within hours or days of the onset of symptoms. The neurologic symptoms often precede the discovery of the neoplasm, and the illness is clinically and pathologically indistinguishable from idiopathic subacute necrotic myelop-

athy. Since epidural spinal cord compression from metastatic tumor or arteriovenous spinal cord anomalies may present similar clinical signs, a myelogram is essential to the diagnosis. In addition to the two aforementioned entities, many patients with carcinomatous cerebellar degeneration develop extensor plantar responses, mild sensory changes, and reflex asymmetries and weakness associated with degenerations of long tracts and anterior horn cells of the spinal cord. However, spinal cord symptoms do not predominate in these patients.

325.   PERIPHERAL NERVES

Four types of peripheral nerve disorders occur in association with cancer. Characteristic of carcinoma is a subacute sensory neuropathy (dorsal root ganglionitis) marked by loss of proprioception and cutaneous sensory modalities with relative preservation of motor power. The illness sometimes precedes the appearance of the carcinoma and progresses over a few months, leaving the patient with a moderate or severe disability. The cerebrospinal fluid protein is usually elevated. Pathologically, there is destruction of posterior root ganglia with perivascular lymphocytic cuffing. There is wallerian degeneration of sensory nerves. Many of the patients have inflammatory and degenerative changes in brain and spinal cord as well. The entity is rare; in one series no examples were found on examination of 1476 patients with cancer. The illness is of interest, however, because it is almost pathognomonic of cancer. The pathogenesis is unknown. There is no treatment.

More common than sensory neuropathy is a distal sensorimotor polyneuropathy characterized by motor weakness, sensory loss, and reflex absence distally in the extremities. Croft et al. subdivided their 33 patients with cancer and sensorimotor polyneuropathy into three groups: (1) a mild neuropathy often occurring in terminal patients (10 patients), (2) a more severe subacute or acute neuropathy at times preceding discovery of the cancer (15 patients), and (3) a remitting or relapsing neuropathy (8 patients). The illness is pathologically characterized by both segmental demyelination and wallerian degeneration of sensory and motor peripheral nerves. Dorsal root ganglia are never involved to the same degree that they are in the purely sensory neuropathy. Pathologically and clinically, the sensorimotor neuropathy is indistinguishable from nutritional polyneuropathies as well as those associated with uremia and other metabolic defects. Indeed, some have suggested that the late or terminal polyneuropathy may be due to nutritional deprivation associated with cancer. Its etiology, however, is not clear, and it does not respond to treatment with vitamins and other nutritional supplements.

A polyneuritis clinically and pathologically indistinguishable from acute postinfectious polyneuropathy (Guillain-Barré syndrome) also complicates cancer, particularly Hodgkin's disease, in which it is probably related to impaired immunity. A few patients with neuropathy limited to the autonomic nervous system as a remote effect of cancer, usually oat cell carcinoma, have been reported.

326. NEUROMUSCULAR JUNCTION AND MUSCLES

NEUROMUSCULAR JUNCTION. *Myasthenia gravis* is associated with thymomas but not other systemic tumors. However, Lambert and Eaton described a *"myasthenic syndrome"* occurring predominantly in men over 40 and associated with intrathoracic tumors in 70 per cent of the patients (see Brain and Norris). The patients complain of weakness and fatigability of proximal muscles, particularly of the pelvic girdle and thighs. The cranial nerves and respiratory muscles are involved less. In addition, patients complain of dryness of the mouth, impotence, pain in the thighs, and peripheral paresthesias. On examination there is weakness of the proximal muscles, but strength increases over several seconds of a sustained contraction. The deep tendon reflexes are diminished or absent. The diagnosis is made by electromyographic studies in which repeated nerve stimulations at rates above ten per second cause a progressive increase in the size of the muscle action potential (exactly the opposite of the effect of myasthenia gravis). The neuromuscular defect in this illness is believed to be deficient release of acetylcholine. The illness responds poorly to anticholinesterase drugs, but does respond to guanidine hydrochloride given in doses of 15 to 40 mg per kilogram per day. There is no direct relationship between treatment of the tumor and change in the myasthenic syndrome.

MUSCLE. Typical *dermatomyositis* or *polymyositis* may appear as a remote effect of cancer. About 10 per cent of patients with this disorder have cancer, but this figure is higher in patients with dermatomyositis, particularly in men over 40. In at least 60 per cent of males over 40 with dermatomyositis, a cancer either can be found when the disease develops or will appear within a few months or years. The clinical picture is indistinguishable from that of dermatomyositis or polymyositis. Pathologically there may be two groups: one with the typical inflammatory lesions of polymyositis, and one with little inflammation but severe muscle necrosis. The latter group may suffer an explosive clinical course. The patients respond somewhat less well to corticosteroid therapy than do those with dermatomyositis unaccompanied by cancer, although improvement with steroid treatment does occur in some.

327. MUSCLE WEAKNESS

Some patients with cancer complain of weakness and fatigability which seems worse than can be accounted for by their cancer alone. Cachexia and weight loss alone do not usually cause measurable muscle weakness. The weakness is usually proximal and produces particular difficulty climbing stairs and getting out of low chairs. Ankle reflexes may be diminished or absent. Further neurologic evaluation does not yield findings diagnostic of one of the remote effects of cancer described above. Brain and his colleagues have labeled this entity a "neuromyopathy" because its exact anatomic locus is unclear, but Hildebrand and Coers have suggested that it is a nonspecific accompaniment of cachexia and systemic illness. Engle has demonstrated that specific (type II) muscle fiber atrophy develops early in patients with systemic cancer. The cause and treatment of the weakness are unknown, but Sloane and Truong suggest that some of the patients have mild neuromuscular transmission disorders of the "myasthenic syndrome" type and respond to guanidine HCl.

Brain, R., and Norris, F. H., Jr.: The Remote Effects of Cancer on the Nervous System. New York, Grune & Stratton, 1965.
Croft, P. B., and Wilkinson, M.: The course and prognosis in some types of carcinomatous neuromyopathy. Brain, 92:1, 1969.
Curries, S., Henson, R. A., Morgan, H. G., and Poole, A. J.: The incidence of the nonmetastatic neurological syndromes of obscure origin in the reticuloses. Brain, 93:629, 1970.
Thompson, R. A., and Green, J. R. (eds.): Neoplasia in the Central Nervous System. Advances in Neurology, Vol. 15. New York, Raven Press, 1976.

Section Twenty-One   INJURIES OF THE HEAD AND SPINE

Russel H. Patterson, Jr.

328. INJURIES OF THE HEAD

Trauma claims over 110,000 lives each year in the United States and ranks in frequency as a cause of death after heart disease, cancer, and stroke. Head injury accounts for death in 70 per cent of cases and surpasses all other causes in persons between the ages of 1 and 35. Good management can benefit many of these patients, but often responsibility for their care falls first on someone who lacks formal training in the field of cerebral trauma. This need not be a disadvantage if the physician follows a few simple principles of management based on an understanding of the pathophysiology of the injury. Properly prepared, he can recognize the indications for specialized diagnostic procedures and possible surgery.

PATHOPHYSIOLOGY. The scalp, hair, skull, and bones of the face protect the brain from trauma by absorbing energy from blows to the head. When struck by a blow of moderate velocity, the calvaria bends inward, but a few centimeters away the skull bends outward, and linear fractures radiate toward and away from the point of impact. A blow of higher kinetic energy may comminute or penetrate the skull to cause a depressed fracture.

Beneath the point of impact intracranial pressure may increase for a few milliseconds to as much as 5000 mm Hg, and low or even negative pressure can be recorded simultaneously in the brain at the opposite side of the skull. Cavitation occurs in the brain in regions of low pressure, which accounts for many contrecoup injuries. The pressure gradients distort the brain, which attempts to flow toward the foramen magnum, inducing shear stresses in the brainstem and upper cervical spinal cord. Other shearing forces, induced by rapid acceleration and deceleration of the head, tear axonal processes; this is manifest pathologically by chromatolysis in the cell body of the neuron and microglial proliferation in the white matter associated with abnormalities of the myelin sheath. These changes may not be visible macroscopically at autopsy but account for widespread dysfunction in the cerebral hemispheres, basal ganglia, and brainstem.

The brain and skull respond at different rates to forces of acceleration and deceleration produced by a blow which results in mass movements of the brain. Sharp and irregular surfaces inside the cranial cavity such as the orbital surface of the frontal fossa, the sphenoid ridge, the falx, and the tentorium lacerate and contuse the moving brain. Rotational forces shear nervous tissue around arterioles and result in parenchymal hemorrhages; fragile cerebral veins draining into the dural venous sinuses may tear and fill the subdural space with blood. Fractures that divide meningeal arteries or major venous sinuses commonly cause bleeding in the epidural space.

After brain injury cerebral blood flow may decrease in some areas owing to vasospasm, whereas in other areas the arterioles dilate and lose their capacity to regulate flow in response to change in arterial blood pressure. Loss of the normal autoregulatory mechanism accompanies many, but by no means all, severe head injuries. The resulting dilation of the vascular bed combines with cerebral edema and any hematoma that might be present to increase the intracranial pressure. The elevated intracranial pressure fluctuates rhythmically and, in cases of severe injury, periodically may rise further to levels of 25 to 100 mm Hg for several minutes at a time. These additional pressure elevations, known as *plateau waves*, are often associated with a transient deterioration in neurologic status.

Cerebral contusions and lacerations accompany 90 per cent of severe nonpenetrating injuries. Blood stains the cortical surface and subarachnoid space over both cerebral hemispheres, areas of hemorrhage are found in the brain parenchyma, and clots form in the subdural and epidural spaces. Edema further crowds the contents of an unyielding cranium. The swollen cerebrum displaces the uncus of the temporal lobe through the tentorial notch to compress the oculomotor nerve and the midbrain. Continued pressure obstructs the posterior cerebral artery and basilar vein, inducing ischemia and augmenting edema.

The supratentorial structures generally are most susceptible to damage from head trauma because a heavy layer of muscle protects the contents of the posterior fossa. But should the effects of an injury swell the cerebellum, the tonsils herniate downward through the foramen magnum to compress the medulla while the vermis pushes upward through the apex of the tentorial notch to squeeze the vein of Galen against the corpus callosum, which is backed by the rigid falx.

Increased intracranial pressure causes constriction of the peripheral vascular bed, bradycardia, and increased return of venous blood to the heart. The left ventricle of the heart may be unable to increase cardiac output suf-ficiently to prevent the development of high pressure in the left atrium and pulmonary edema. Even in the absence of pulmonary edema, pulmonary arteriovenous shunts may open in response to both the increased blood flow in the pulmonary artery and increased sympathetic tone in the pulmonary vascular bed. The consequence is frequently arterial hypoxemia even if the patient's ventilation is adequate to maintain normocapnia or hypocapnia. If the tongue or secretions obstruct the airway, hypoxia develops in association with hypercapnia. Hypercapnia augments cerebrovasodilatation and causes a further increase in intracranial pressure with the grave consequences outlined above. In addition, blood flow may be shunted to one area of the brain through a portion of the vascular bed that is dilated and of low resistance, thereby reducing circulation to other areas that become relatively ischemic.

Hemorrhages are found about the pituitary gland and hypophyseal stalk in about two thirds of patients dying of craniocerebral trauma. Necrosis of the anterior lobe is present in more than a fifth of cases and has been attributed to shock, swelling of the gland, and obstruction of the portal vessels. The consequence may be some combination of diabetes insipidus, absence of thirst, and hypoadrenalism producing a varied picture of abnormal fluid and electrolyte metabolism which can range from hypernatremia to water intoxication.

CONCUSSION

Concussion is a clinical term that may be defined as loss of consciousness after an injury to the head without macroscopic damage to nervous tissue. Recovery is usually prompt after less severe injuries, but long periods of unconsciousness or death may occur, and amnesia for events before and after the accident is common. Concussion implies that contusions and lacerations of the brain have not accounted for the symptoms, but the diagnosis must be presumptive except in occasional fatal cases studied at autopsy. Information about the pathophysiology of concussion therefore is derived largely from experiments with laboratory animals.

How an injury to the head causes unconsciousness is not entirely clear. Transmitted pressure gradients and rotational forces distort the brainstem, but bilateral injury to the cerebral hemispheres may be equally important. Changes in the brainstem probably account for the apnea and bradycardia that immediately follow the blow as well as for the unsteadiness and giddiness with change in position of which patients often complain for a time. Amnesia, forgetfulness, irritability, fatigue, and impaired memory are attributed to neuronal damage in the cerebrum, although long persistence of these vague symptoms after cerebral trauma may be hard to evaluate, particularly if a lawsuit is unsettled.

Microscopic changes in the brain after a concussive blow are observed in the neurons and glia within a few hours. Some cells may recover, but others do not, and thus permanent damage to the nervous system occurs. Psychologic tests and neurologic examination may not reveal evidence for the loss of a relatively few neurons, but the effects of repeated small injuries are cumulative as the dull, querulous behavior of the punchdrunk fighter testifies.

EVALUATION OF THE ACUTE HEAD INJURY

The initial examination of the head-injured patient is particularly important not only because it will guide immediate management but also because it serves as a baseline for subsequent observations. The physician must be able to assess neurologic improvement or deterioration in order to make decisions about the need for special diagnostic and therapeutic procedures.

Details of the accident suggest what parts of the brain may be injured, and the physician should remember that drugs, alcohol abuse, or underlying disease may contribute to the clinical picture. The duration of unconsciousness is a rough index to the severity of the injury; even brief unconsciousness is evidence of enough damage to merit hospitalization and careful observation. The neurologic examination is repeated at intervals to detect any change in consciousness, breathing, pupillary diameter, motor strength, speech, or vision, which may signal the presence of an expanding intracranial mass.

The blood pressure, pulse, respirations, and temperature should be recorded frequently after an injury to the head. However, the classic response to increasing intracranial pressure of bradycardia and arterial hypertension may not occur, and any instability of vital signs implies a change in intracranial homeostasis.

The head should be inspected carefully for evidence of trauma, remembering that a scalp laceration can be overlooked easily under a heavy growth of hair. If a scalp laceration is present, the underlying skull should be palpated under sterile precautions because sometimes a fracture will be discovered that is not obvious on subsequent roentgenograms. Likewise, ecchymosis around the mastoid or the leakage of blood or cerebrospinal fluid from the auditory canal may be the only evidence of a basilar skull fracture. If the patient is unconscious, the neck should be stabilized until roentgenograms and the clinical course show that the cervical spine is not fractured or dislocated.

As death after trauma is usually due to failure of the respiratory and circulatory centers, the physician must be particularly alert to the early signs of damage to the brainstem. Coma may result from extensive injury to both cerebral hemispheres, but stupor that progressively deepens usually results from distortion of the brainstem caused by an enlarging clot or progressively edematous brain. The evolution of these signs of dangerous rostral-caudal deterioration is emphasized later in this discussion. Grave signs, however, are fixed pupils, impaired oculovestibular responses, and decerebrate posturing.

If edema or a clot herniates the temporal lobe through the tentorial notch, the uncus compresses the ipsilateral third cranial nerve, and the pupil first dilates, then fixes to light. Occasionally the contralateral third nerve is first affected, but eventually both nerves are paralyzed, and both pupils dilate. Later, when sympathetic centers in the midbrain are damaged, the pupils may contract to become fixed in midposition. Treatment, to be fully effective, must reverse the process before this advanced stage.

Sometimes retinal hemorrhages follow intracranial bleeding, or an occluded venous sinus causes papilledema, but mydriatics alter pupillary responses and for this reason should not be used to obtain a better view of the ocular fundus.

DIAGNOSTIC PROCEDURES. Roentgenograms. Roentgenographic examination of the skull should be performed without undue delay in all cases of injury to the head. Fractures of the calvaria are generally visible, but most basilar fractures are obscured in the bony detail. The presence of skull fracture is reason enough to admit a patient to the hospital after an injury even if he appears to have sustained no brain damage. Roentgenograms perhaps will reveal an indriven fragment of bone, a displaced pineal gland, or intracranial air if a fracture through a paranasal sinus tears the dura and arachnoid. The patient is a likely candidate for an intracranial blood clot if fracture is found which crosses a venous sinus or meningeal artery.

Lumbar Puncture. Lumbar puncture is helpful in the differential diagnosis of coma because the cerebrospinal fluid is commonly xanthochromic after being centrifuged in cases of trauma. However, if a good history is available, lumbar puncture is better avoided because in a patient with an edematous brain or an intracranial clot the withdrawal of fluid can precipitate transtentorial or foramen magnum herniation.

Echoencephalography. A shift of the midline structures of the brain caused by edema or hematoma can be identified by a displaced pineal gland on roentgenograms of the skull or by echoencephalography if the gland is uncalcified. After evacuation of a clot, the displaced midline structures return to their normal position unless the clot reaccumulates. The absence of a shift does not necessarily mean that an intracranial clot is not present; bilateral subdural hematomas are common and may cause transtentorial herniation of the temporal lobes without shift of the midline structures.

Electroencephalography. The electroencephalogram is rarely helpful in the management of acute injury to the head. An abnormal tracing is common immediately after the trauma and tends to improve as recovery takes place. In cases of chronic subdural hematoma the electroencephalogram may be of value if low voltages and abnormal wave forms are recorded from the scalp overlying the hematoma.

Radioactive Scan. Chronic subdural hematomas are often well demonstrated by the radioactive scan technique. In acute injuries a scan is less helpful because the study does not differentiate space-occupying lesions from contused areas of brain.

Cerebral Angiography. Angiography is widely used in evaluating trauma to the head, and in some cases, such as subdural hematoma, the films are almost diagnostic. The procedure is not without danger, particularly when the circulation to a region of the brain is already impaired by an injury. Consequently, angiography is best reserved for patients in whom progressive deterioration or focal signs such as hemiparesis raise suspicion that a blood clot may be present.

Burr Holes. Burr holes placed in the skull can be used to diagnose and treat subdural and epidural hematoma. The advantages of the procedure lie in the speed with which the clot can be evacuated if the patient's condition is rapidly worsening. However, computed tomography (CT scanning) and angiography have many advantages over burr holes as diagnostic procedures. Consequently, burr holes are reserved for emergencies or occasions when the more complex studies are not available.

Air Encephalography. Air encephalography provides less information than angiography or CT scanning in patients with trauma and carries more risk because of the possibility that a change in pressure relationships in the head may precipitate an unfavorable shift in the brain with serious consequences. As a result, air studies are employed infrequently in the management of head injury.

Computed Tomography. CT scanning has proved of great value in the management of head injury. Acute intracranial hematomas are well identified and localized because of the high absorption of x-rays by freshly shed blood. In addition, the CT scan often can demonstrate areas of contused and edematous brain, displacement or hydrocephalic enlargement of the ventricles, the presence of pneumocephalus, and skull fractures.

Obtaining a CT scan in a restless patient may be difficult and require sedation with drugs such as diazepam. The airway must be preserved during the scanning procedure, so many patients will require tracheal intubation and perhaps supplemental oxygen. Roentgenograms of the cervical spine prior to the scan are also desirable to rule out a spine fracture, particularly in unconscious patients.

In managing acute head injury, enhancement with intravenous contrast agent is rarely necessary. However, contrast enhancement is appropriate in evaluating some of the subacute and chronic effects of injury, since the membranes and walls of hematomas and of abscesses may be made visible.

MANAGEMENT OF ACUTE HEAD INJURY

Although it sometimes accompanies a severe head injury, hypovolemic shock is rarely the consequence of moderate head trauma or a scalp laceration. Consequently, a patient with a head injury who is in shock deserves investigation for a source of an occult hemorrhage, such as a pelvic fracture with retroperitoneal bleeding. Scalp lacerations are best repaired in the emergency room before roentgenograms are obtained in order to control bleeding and to prevent infection. This is the time to initiate baseline observations of vital signs and neurologic status and to examine the patient for associated injuries of the skeleton, viscera, and soft tissues. Prophylaxis against tetanus is administered, as are antimicrobial agents if open fractures are present.

RESPIRATION. A number of steps may be taken to reduce edema in the brain after an injury. The most important is the establishment of an adequate airway. Hypoxia and hypocarbia have grave consequences on cerebral homeostasis as outlined earlier. If a stuporous patient is unable to clear his own airway, the trachea should be intubated.

Blood gases should be monitored even in patients who appear to be respiring adequately, because pulmonary edema and shunting in the lung, described above, may result in low values of arterial P_{O_2} that the administration of oxygen can correct. When spontaneous respirations cease, even if cardiac action continues, death is inevitable, and mechanical ventilation is unavailing.

Opiates and sedatives are avoided for patients with injuries to the head. These drugs further depress an already damaged nervous system, impair respirations, and increase stupor. Urinary retention often accounts for restlessness in drowsy patients and is readily treated by catheterization.

BLOOD AND FLUID REPLACEMENT. Motor vehicle accidents commonly result in multiple injuries. Hypovolemic shock occurs and is best treated by the ordinary measures except that the head-low position is avoided if the brain is damaged. Elevation of the extremities increases the return of blood to the heart without contributing to cerebral edema.

Cerebral swelling is increased when hypotonic fluids are administered. Five per cent dextrose in water becomes hypotonic as the sugar is metabolized, and therefore should not be given in large quantities. Isotonic saline or 5 per cent dextrose in one half isotonic saline is less hazardous, because sodium chloride passes the blood-brain barrier poorly. Consequently, fluids are mildly restricted for patients with brain injury, and more saline is employed than in ordinary practice.

Patients with head injury sometimes develop inappropriate secretions of antidiuretic hormone with consequent water intoxication, even if fluids are replaced with care. The resulting symptoms of stupor and seizures are often mistakenly attributed to extensive parenchymal damage. Water intoxication is confirmed by demonstrating a serum sodium of less than 120 mEq per liter associated with a serum osmolality of less than 280 mOsm per kilogram and a urinary sodium greater than 25 mEq per liter. The primary treatment consists of restricting water and perhaps giving small amounts of intravenous 5 per cent saline.

Occasionally trauma damages homeostatic centers in the hypothalamus so that diabetes insipidus results. A patient who is alert will ordinarily drink enough to prevent dehydration. However, if osmoreceptor mechanisms are also disturbed or the subject is in stupor with a lack of thirst, serum hyperosmolarity with high electrolyte levels occurs if adequate fluids are not administered. Replacement of water, restriction of salt, and administration of Pitressin (usually as Pitressin tannate in oil) are indicated until the condition corrects itself, as it usually does.

Severe injuries to the brain are sometimes associated with impaired renal function despite the absence of shock, or a reaction to blood transfusion, or other common causes of damage to the renal tubules. Characteristically the ouput of urine remains good, but the specific gravity is fixed at 1.010, albuminuria is present, and the sediment contains red cells, white cells, and casts. Death from renal failure may occur in spite of treatment. The mechanism of the renal damage is not entirely clear, but stimulation of certain cortical areas and destructive lesions in the hypothalamus cause similar renal lesions in laboratory animals.

OSMOTIC DIURETICS. By administering a hypertonic solution it is possible to establish an osmotic gradient across the blood-brain barrier that removes water from the brain and reduces cerebral edema. Drugs that penetrate the brain slowly are employed, such as a 30 per cent solution of urea in 10 per cent invert sugar or 20 per cent mannitol given intravenously or glycerin given by mouth.

The administration of an osmotic diuretic often stabilizes or improves the neurologic status of a patient who is deteriorating rapidly after a head injury. The beneficial effects, if observed, are only temporary, but respite even for an hour or two may be enough to obtain diagnostic studies. If the patient is sufficiently ill to warrant the use of osmotic diuretics, his state is serious enough to deserve prompt and vigorous management. Any temporary improvement that might follow their use should not lull the physician, because the patient's neurologic status once again may worsen rapidly when the drug effect wears off.

INTRACRANIAL PRESSURE MONITORING. In most cases of severe head injury the physician is faced with treating diffuse brain damage complicated by cerebral swelling and edema rather than intracranial hematomas that need surgical drainage. Changes in brain swelling are reflected by changes in intracranial pressure, which can be measured continuously by a variety of methods that employ an intraventricular cannula or devices positioned in the subdural or epidural space. As described earlier in this chapter, periodic elevations in intracranial pressure to greater than 25 mm Hg may be associated with neurologic deterioration. These increases in pressure can be aborted by the administration of an osmotic agent or perhaps a diuretic such as furosemide (Lasix). Sometimes the drugs must be given as often as every two to four hours, in which case the serum electrolytes need close monitoring.

The aggressive use of dehydrating agents to treat brain swelling is presently under study not only in cases of head injury but also in other conditions such as Reye's syndrome. Their ultimate value in head injury remains to be established. Possibly their use may improve the rate and quality of survival in certain cases, or they may prove unrewarding, as have surgical attempts at controlling brain swelling through extensive cranial decompression.

STEROIDS. The administration of steroids, which has been of great value in managing the edema associated with brain tumor, has proved disappointing in treating post-traumatic cerebral edema. Although steroids are widely used, various prospective studies have failed to show any benefit in patients treated with doses of up to 40 mg per day of dexamethasone. Some preliminary reports have suggested that higher doses (in the range of 100 mg per day) may be helpful, but this remains to be proved. The fact that the pituitary gland becomes necrotic in as many as 25 per cent of patients with severe head injury suggests that at least replacement doses of steroids may sometimes be necessary.

COMPLICATIONS OF HEAD INJURY

CRANIAL NERVE INJURY. Damage may occur to the cranial nerves as they exit from the skull. Among the more common complications, anosmia and blindness are often permanent in contrast to extraocular palsies and facial paralysis, which usually improve.

DEPRESSED FRACTURES. The incidence of epilepsy is 30 per cent or more after depressed fractures and penetrating wounds, but the risk is reduced if the fracture is elevated and fragments of bone and other foreign bodies are promptly removed. As seizures may occur even if the site of fracture is remote from the motor areas of the cerebral cortex, all depressed fractures should be elevated except possibly a small depression over a major venous sinus. If a laceration of the scalp overlies a depressed fracture, antimicrobial agents are administered to prevent the occurrence of osteomyelitis and intracranial infection.

Debridement of a depressed fracture or penetrating missile wound often leaves an unsightly cranial defect that a properly executed cranioplasty will correct. The current use of synthetic material such as tantalum, acrylic plastic, and stainless steel has simplified this operation and improved its cosmetic results. Some have thought that cranioplasty both ameliorates such subjective symptoms as headache and giddiness and reduces the frequency of convulsive seizures, but properly controlled studies do not bear this out.

BASILAR SKULL FRACTURE AND CEREBROSPINAL FLUID FISTULA. Because they are often not visible on skull roentgenograms, basilar fractures are usually diagnosed by clinical signs such as anosmia, Battle's sign, bilateral periorbital ecchymoses, and the drainage of blood or cerebrospinal fluid from the nose or ears. Cerebrospinal fluid can be distinguished from a mucoid nasal discharge by testing for sugar, which is best done by analysis rather than the use of paper test strips. Patients with cerebrospinal fluid fistulas should be treated prophylactically with antimicrobial agents to prevent meningitis until the leak stops, as it does in 75 per cent of cases of rhinorrhea and almost all cases of otorrhea. The ear or nose should not be probed or packed, and sealing of the leak may be hastened by repeated lumbar punctures in which 30 ml or more of cerebrospinal fluid is withdrawn. A fistula which persists more than 10 to 14 days demands surgical repair.

EPILEPSY. The incidence of epilepsy after head injury varies with the severity of the injury to the brain. Seizures occur in 40 per cent of patients who sustain penetrating missile wounds, but follow only 10 per cent of the blunt injuries characteristic of civilian life. Depressed skull fracture is associated with an increased incidence of epilepsy, which reaches 40 per cent if accompanied by evidence of severe brain damage such as traumatic amnesia lasting more than 24 hours. Elevation of the depressed fracture, debridement of the wound, prevention of infection, and the prophylactic use of anticonvulsant agents can reduce this toll.

The first convulsive seizure occurs within the first week after injury in 95 per cent of cases. These early seizures are typically focal motor in type and many do not recur. Late epilepsy, meaning seizures which occur after the first week, has a more ominous prognosis. It is treated by anticonvulsants. Fortunately in many patients the attacks decrease in frequency as the years pass and ultimately stop in half the cases. A persistent, debilitating convulsive disorder can sometimes be improved by surgical excision of the epileptogenic focus.

INTRACRANIAL HEMATOMAS. Both increasing edema and an enlarging hematoma cause neurologic signs that progress. As the two are difficult to distinguish, progressive signs are a justifiable reason in any patient to search for a clot by the diagnostic procedures outlined earlier in this chapter.

Epidural Hematoma. Although small amounts of blood are often found in extradural space after fracture of the skull, large hematomas are uncommon, occurring in only 1 or 2 per cent of injuries to the head. Despite their rarity, epidural hematomas are important because they are potentially fatal, yet proper treatment is followed by recovery with little or no neurologic deficit if the brain has not sustained other injuries.

Epidural hematomas most frequently occur in the temporal region from a tear in the middle meningeal artery but are sometimes found in the frontal parietal, occipital, and suboccipital areas. Typically, a patient receives a blow on the temple that results in transitory unconsciousness. After a lucid interval of a few minutes or hours the expanding clot causes headache, drowsiness, contralateral hemiparesis, and paralysis of the ipsilateral third cranial nerve. Signs of decompensation of the brainstem soon follow, and death results.

The classic case is easily recognized but not often encountered. The patient may relate that the blow was light and unconsciousness brief. His prompt recovery and normal roentgenograms apparently substantiate the unimportance of the injury. Yet an epidural hematoma may be present and may reach a critical size some hours later, and death may ensue if the patient has been sent home with inadequate observation.

Variations from the typical pattern are common. An associated serious brain injury may cause the patient to remain stuporous without the lucid interval, or symptoms may be delayed several days if the bleeding is slow or intermittent. Progressive coma without localizing signs is the rule with clots over the cerebellum, and occasionally occurs with supratentorial clots. At times a hematoma is missed at operation, especially in children in whom the dura adheres to the suture lines of the skull and restricts the spread of blood over the convexity.

About 40 per cent of patients with epidural hematoma die or are permanently incapacitated. Because the hematoma often occurs in patients with other severe injuries to the brain, some morbidity doubtless is inevitable. But the gratifying recovery that may follow surgery justifies a meticulous evaluation of every patient with severe head injury in a search for this infrequently occurring intracranial clot.

Subdural Hematoma. Subdural hematomas are conveniently divided into categories of acute, subacute, and chronic, which differ in both symptomatology and prognosis. A subdural hematoma is called acute when a rapid progression of symptoms leads to its discovery within hours or a day or two after the injury. Prospects for recovery depend on the severity of the associated brain damage. The fatality rate is 90 per cent in patients whose symptoms warrant operation within 12 hours of injury, but the outlook is much improved if the need for surgery is evident only after several days have passed.

Chronic Subdural Hematoma. Chronic subdural hematoma in adults usually occurs after the age of 50 and often in alcoholics because of their unsteadiness and frequent falls. With age the brain shrinks away from the dural lining of the skull and leaves a space that can fill with blood if a fragile vein should tear. The trauma that initiates the bleeding is often trivial and even forgotten when symptoms commence several weeks later. The clinical importance of such hematomas depends on their size, and many hematomas of 60 ml or less probably cause no symptoms. With larger clots, headache occurs in 90 per cent of cases. Even if a confused patient denies it, the family may testify to his earlier complaints of pain or to his increased consumption of aspirin. Fatigue and irritability are followed insidiously by drowsiness, urinary incontinence, and stupor, which may be attributed erroneously to a natural deterioration in senescence. Hemianopsia, hemiparesis, or pupillary abnormality is observed in less than half the cases. Lumbar puncture usually reveals normal pressure, but in 50 per cent of cases the fluid is xanthochromic. Bruises about the head are frequently present, but a fracture of the skull is identified in only one third of cases, and a calcified pineal is displaced in only one fifth.

The patient usually deteriorates at an irregular rate. Intervals of substantial improvement interrupt the gradual decline and give hope of recovery, but sudden decompensation and unexpected death may occur.

Small clots may be tolerated or occasionally resorbed, especially when treated with a course of corticosteroid agents. Persistent mass lesions cause edema and irreversible anoxic-ischemic demyelination of the underlying brain. Most subdural hematomas are therefore best treated by surgical drainage. The diagnosis is confirmed readily by angiography or trephination. CT scanning, even with contrast enhancement, may not demonstrate a hematoma when it is between two and six weeks of age because the hematoma is in an "isodense" stage. At this time, shift of the ventricles, if present, may provide the only evidence of hematoma. The results of treatment are good except that irreversible effects of pressure on the brain may leave a noticeable defect in mentation after recovery, particularly in elderly patients. If treatment is delayed until stupor signals dysfunction of the brainstem, evacuation of the clot and the administration of steroids and osmotic diuretics may be unable to reverse progressive transtentorial herniation that results in death.

Intracerebral Hematoma. Scattered petechial hemorrhages are commonly observed in fatal injuries to the brain, but large parenchymal hematomas occur in only 1 to 2 per cent of cases and are usually located in the frontal or temporal lobes or, less frequently, in the occipitoparietal region or cerebellum. The diagnosis is difficult because stupor from associated concussion or contusions may mask the focal neurologic signs produced by the hematoma. The mass is best demonstrated by CT scanning or angiography. The results of surgery are often disappointing because the hemorrhage has destroyed sufficient cerebral tissue to leave a substantial neurologic deficit.

VASCULAR COMPLICATIONS. A blow to the head may rupture the carotid artery within the cavernous sinus and establish a *carotid–cavernous sinus fistula*. The arterial pressure dilates the tributaries of the sinus such as the orbital veins, with the result that the eye protrudes and pulsates, a bruit is usually heard, and chemosis and extraocular palsies occur. Altered arterial circulation to the eye causes loss of vision and, eventually, blindness. If the fistula is small, the symptoms may progress slowly, but spontaneous cure is uncommon. Repair by a direct approach to the fistula through the cavernous sinus is possible but requires the complicated technique of profound hypothermia and circulatory arrest. Ligation of the carotid artery in the neck or trapping the fistula by ligating in addition the intracranial carotid artery is sometimes successful. Better results have been achieved by embolizing the fistula with bits of muscle, often after intracranial ligation of the carotid artery. A recent development is to pack the cavernous sinus with fine copper wire, which precipitates an asymptomatic thrombosis of the cavernous sinus, thereby eliminating the fistula.

Trauma about the head occasionally leads to *thrombosis of the internal carotid artery* in the neck, resulting in hemiplegia. Less frequently, *thrombosis of the middle cerebral artery* by a dissecting aneurysm accounts for an unexpected paralysis several days after the injury.

Depressed fractures may cause *occlusion of the superi-*

or longitudinal sinus, blocking venous drainage from the cerebral hemispheres and thereby raising intracranial pressure and causing the rapid appearance of papilledema and hemorrhages in the ocular fundus. Patients display paralysis of both lower limbs and often of one or both upper limbs.

INFECTION. Osteomyelitis of the skull, meningitis, and abscesses of the brain occasionally complicate open injuries of the head, and may recur for years after the injury. Antimicrobial therapy and proper debridement of the wound greatly reduce the incidence of these infectious complications.

CEREBRAL SWELLING. Enthusiasm for aggressive surgery to cope with cerebral edema in patients with serious head injury waxes and wanes. Experience has shown that extensive cranial decompression is rarely rewarded by survival with an acceptable degree of neurologic function.

CEREBRAL FAT EMBOLISM. Fat embolism is an infrequent complication observed after severe trauma in which a long bone is fractured, or occurs occasionally with just extensive soft tissue injury. Symptoms start between 12 and 48 hours after the accident; a frequent history is that a patient has remained comatose after general anesthesia to reduce a fractured extremity. Cerebral symptoms and signs consist of rapidly progressive stupor often associated with extensor plantar responses and decerebrate posturing but with preservation of pupillary responses. Petechiae may appear on the chest and in the conjunctivae; dyspnea, tachypnea, and cyanosis are evidence that the lungs are affected. The diagnosis is best made by bedside examination, but the finding of fat globules in urine and sputum can lend laboratory support to the clinical impression.

Although cerebral fat embolism has an ominous prognosis, some patients recover even after long periods of coma. Treatment consists of taking measures to prevent shock and hypovolemia, providing ventilatory support, and perhaps administering steroids to reduce cerebral edema. The value of intravenous ethanol or of anticoagulation with heparin, which have been suggested, remains to be seen.

PROGNOSIS IN SEVERE HEAD INJURIES. About 45 per cent of patients with severe head injury die of their illness. Among survivors, the young are more likely to make a good recovery than older patients. Signs indicating a relatively poor outcome include abnormal pupillary responses, abnormal oculovestibular responses, and extensor posturing of the extremities, either spontaneous or in response to noxious stimulation. Patients between 20 and 50 years old who remain in coma for as long as two weeks rarely make a good recovery, whereas patients less than age 20 sometimes recover from coma lasting several weeks. In patients over age 30, the combination of abnormal motor responses and coma makes recovery unlikely.

After head injury some patients remain in a *vegetative state*; in such a case the patient awakens but is unresponsive to his environment. At autopsy, multiple lesions are likely to be present throughout the brain, with the most consistent pathologic changes to be found in the periaqueductal gray matter of the rostral brainstem. Less severely damaged patients profit from intensive care in a rehabilitation center where their physical, emotional, and social disabilities receive appropriate attention. Recovery from the injury continues

for a long time, even several years. Ultimately 80 per cent can be returned to work, but others remain handicapped by permanent neurologic defects. Even some who appear to make a good recovery have subtle defects in memory, concentration, and comprehension which prevent their achieving their expected potential at work. Others manifest distressing psychopathology, ranging from mildly asocial behavior through psychosis or dementia.

329. INJURIES OF THE SPINE

GENERAL CONSIDERATIONS. The first morphologic changes in laboratory animals suffering experimental spinal cord injury appear in the microvasculature. Within minutes small hemorrhages appear in the gray matter, and in severe injuries the hemorrhages coalesce and blood flow to the region ceases for a long interval. Although blood flow is maintained for a few minutes in the white matter, axonal transmission is lost immediately, which suggests that mechanical trauma rather than hemorrhage or ischemia accounts for the acute loss of function following injury. In animals that recover from experimental trauma, blood flow in the white fiber tracts decreases transiently but tends to return toward normal by one hour. In contrast, impaired blood flow in the white matter lasts many hours if the paraplegia is to be permanent. Late changes seen in paraplegic animals include edema in the white fiber tracts and hemorrhagic necrosis in the central gray matter. The mechanism of these changes remains unclear. Experimental efforts at treatment have been attempted with reserpine, regional hypothermia, splitting of the cord to decompress swelling, and the administration of glucocorticoids and epsilon-aminocaproic acid. All have appeared helpful in certain circumstances, but their usefulness in the management of the spinal cord–injured patient remains to be established.

THE ATLAS AND AXIS. Most fractures of the atlas result from blows to the vertex. They are of two types: those of the posterior arch, and the less frequent burst fractures of the lateral masses (Jefferson's fracture). The former can be treated with a cervical collar, whereas the latter generally require traction with skull tongs.

One common fracture of the axis is known as the "hangman's fracture." It consists of a fracture through the lateral arch of the axis and may be associated with a dislocation between the axis and C3. These fractures are inherently stable and heal in traction. In contrast, fractures across the base of the odontoid process cause instability of the atlantoaxial joint that may lead to dislocation. For this reason they are often treated by spinal fusion.

THE MIDCERVICAL SPINE. Patients with hyperextension injuries of the cervical spine often can be identified clinically because of the presence of abrasions on the forehead. They may have cervical spine roentgenograms which are normal or show only a chip fracture of the anterior inferior corner of the vertebral body. However, the forced neck extension buckles the ligamentum flavum forward and pinches the spinal cord, especially in elderly patients, who often have arthritic spurs present anteriorly. A central cord syndrome is a common result.

The upper limbs are weaker than the lower, and a variable sensory loss occurs with relative sparing of touch, position, and vibration sense.

Flexion injuries may lead to unilateral or bilateral locking of the articular facet joints and a variety of vertebral body fractures. They have a propensity for blocking the circulation in the anterior spinal artery or for injuring the radicular arteries or the vertebral arteries in the intervertebral foramina. The resulting ischemic injury is most severe in the anterior portion of the spinal cord and often causes motor paralysis with relative preservation of position sense. Actual thrombosis of the anterior spinal artery is rare.

Patients with injury to the cervical spine must be handled carefully to prevent an unfavorable shift of the fracture-dislocation from further damaging the spinal cord. A conscious patient usually gives warning of his plight, but the possibility of an unstable spine is easily overlooked if the patient is unconscious. A gentle pull on the head in line with the spine is advisable to keep traction on the neck whenever the patient is moved. Spine boards to which the head and trunk can be strapped commonly are used to protect the spinal cord when removing a patient from a wrecked automobile. If one is not available, a bulky wrapping about the neck which supports the chin and occiput will help reduce motion that might be dangerous. A firm board or a door makes a better litter than a sagging canvas stretcher that flexes the neck. Roentgenograms are best obtained on the litter to avoid the manipulation of a transfer to the x-ray table.

The primary treatment of fracture-dislocation of the cervical spine is traction with tongs or wires inserted in the skull to achieve and maintain the reduction. The pull should be in the line of the spine, and weights exceeding 30 pounds should be used with care to prevent a sudden shift from causing further damage.

After reduction is obtained, traction can be continued for six weeks, after which the patient is ambulated in a collar that is worn for three months. An acceptable alternative that shortens the period of immobilization is to perform an operation at which loose fragments of bone and disc are removed and the vertebral bodies fused anteriorly. Atlantoaxial dislocations are characteristically unstable and are appropriately treated by early fusion of the first three cervical vertebrae.

THE THORACOLUMBAR SPINE. Fractures of the upper and mid-thoracic spine may range from the wedge fracture of the elderly to an injury in which a strong force applied to the dorsal surface of the spine shears the upper portion of the spine from the lower. The result of the latter injury is usually a stable fracture but accompanied by complete spinal paralysis. Injuries at the thoracolumbar junction result from a variable combination of flexion, rotation, and compression. This produces wedging of the vertebral body or sometimes a horizontal fracture through the vertebral body associated with facet fracture and vertebral dislocation.

Thoracolumbar fractures in the past have been treated by hyperextension in bed, plaster jackets, and decompression laminectomy. More recently it has proved possible to restore normal alignment to the spine in severe injuries by inserting metal rods at operation. Whether or not this will improve the final outcome remains to be established. Certainly, in most cases, the position of a stable fracture can be accepted and the patient treated by bed rest until the pain subsides, at which time progressive ambulation is begun.

SURGICAL DECOMPRESSION. Whether surgical decompression restores function to a traumatized spinal cord is a matter of controversy. Here the initial neurologic examination assumes importance because almost no patient with complete loss of motor power and sensation that persists more than 24 hours ever regains much useful function regardless of treatment. Examination should include the testing of perianal sensation, and current clinical research includes efforts to record electrical activity in the cerebral cortex when sensory nerves below the level of the lesion are stimulated. If either a trace of motor activity or persistent sensation confirms that the cord has been only partially interrupted, surprising improvement may take place and may continue as long as two years, even without surgery.

All agree that the rare patient who shows progression of the neurologic defect after an injury should have a decompressive operation. Surgical debridement and closure prevent a spinal fluid fistula in open fractures, and possibly damaged nerve roots of the cauda equina benefit from decompression. At present many patients with fracture-dislocation of the cervical spine are operated upon by the anterior approach to achieve decompression of the cord and fusion of the vertebral bodies. The results are difficult to assess because of the relatively good prognosis without surgery when the damage to the cord is incomplete, and a conservative approach is usually justified.

Babcock, J. L.: Cervical spine injuries. Diagnosis and classification. Arch. Surg., 111:646, 1976.
Becker, D. P., Miller, J. D., Ward, J. D., Greenberg, R. P., Young, H. F., and Sakalas, R.: The outcome from severe head injury with early diagnosis and intensive management. J. Neurosurg., 47:491, 1977.
Fell, D. A., Fitzgerald, S., Moiel, R. H., and Caram, P.: Acute subdural hematoma. Review of 144 cases. J. Neurosurg., 42:37, 1975.
Fuld, P. A., and Fisher, P.: Recovery of intellectual ability after closed head-injury. Dev. Med. Child Neurol., 19:495, 1977.
Gronwall, D., and Wrightson, P.: Cumulative effect of concussion. Lancet, 2:995, 1975.
Jennett, B., Teasdale, G., Braakman, R., Minderhoud, J., and Knill-Jones, R.: Predicting outcome in individual patients after severe head injury. Lancet,:1031, 1976.
Lepistö, P., and Alho, A.: Diagnostic features of the fat embolism syndrome. Acta Chir. Scand., 141:245, 1975.
Marar, B. C.: The pattern of neurological damage as an aid to the diagnosis of the mechanism in spinal cord injuries. J. Bone Joint Surg., 56-A:1648, 1974.
Miller, J. D., Becker, D. P., Ward, J. D., et al.: Significance of intracranial hypertension in severe head injury. J. Neurosurg., 47:503, 1977.
Norrell, H. A.: Fractures and dislocations of the spine. In Rothman, R. H., and Simeone, F. A. (eds.): The Spine. Philadelphia, W. B. Saunders Company, 1975, p. 922.
Rish, B. L., and Caveness, W. F.: Relation of prophylactic medication to the occurrence of early seizures following craniocerebral trauma. J. Neurosurg., 38:155, 1973.
Rutherford, W. H., Merrett, J. D., and McDonald, J. R.: Sequelae of concussion caused by minor head injuries. Lancet,:1, 1977.

330. SEVERE SPINAL CORD DYSFUNCTION AND PARAPLEGIA

Many disorders, including spinal trauma, neoplasms, acute myelitis, poliomyelitis, and multiple sclerosis, can result in extensive spinal paralysis and cause similar problems in care and in the management of complications.

Antimicrobial agents and improved medical care have greatly reduced the mortality among patients with paraplegia or other forms of extensive spinal paralysis. Life expectancy is related to the severity of the neurologic deficit. Patients who are partially paraplegic or tetraplegic have a mortality about twice that of the normal population, whereas complete paraplegia carries a mortality four times the normal, and complete tetraplegia twelve times the normal. The mortality stems from an increased incidence of renal disease, cardiovascular disease, and cancer, in that order.

PROGNOSIS. The degree of independence that a paraplegic achieves largely depends on how many muscle groups escape paralysis. The lower the spinal level of the injury or disease, the more skills a well motivated patient can develop if good care prevents the complications of muscle spasm, decubitus ulcers, and infection of the urinary tract.

An understanding of how much recovery is possible sets goals and supplies a yardstick with which to measure progress during rehabilitation. The patient with a complete or extensive lesion of the spinal cord just below C5 retains innervation of the neck musculature and some of the shoulder girdle. He is unable to move in bed, and becomes easily fatigued because of poor respiratory reserve, but he may be able to feed himself with special equipment. With lesions of the lower cervical cord, function of more muscles of the upper limb is preserved; thus the patient is able to roll over, sit up, propel a wheelchair, and possibly learn a job at home that does not require strength and dexterity of the hands. He depends upon an attendant for most of his needs.

High levels of thoracic spinal cord injury leave a functional upper limb, but the trunk is unstable, and intercostal breathing is not possible. The patient can transfer to and from a wheelchair, but even with bracing cannot develop a useful gait. Lower thoracic injuries, which leave a strong pectoral girdle and good respiratory reserve, permit the patient to be independent in all his daily activities. Bracing is still cumbersome, and ambulation is generally not practical.

Patients with lesions at T12 to L3 can usually walk in long leg braces and even negotiate stairs, but depend heavily on wheelchairs. Even with an injury below L3 a patient may sometimes use a wheelchair because such acts as arising from the sitting position, climbing steps, and standing for prolonged periods are difficult.

EMOTIONAL ASPECTS. Severe depression may accompany the realization that paralysis and partial dependency are permanent. Progress in rehabilitation is slowed, and recently learned skills may be temporarily lost, but emotional support from the hospital staff does much to reduce the depth and length of the depression. The environment of a center where others face and overcome similar hurdles also bolsters the morale of the paraplegic.

CARDIORESPIRATORY SYSTEM. Injuries in the cervical region paralyze the intercostal muscles and leave only diaphragmatic respiration. Exercise quickly results in dyspnea, so that the usefulness of a hand-driven wheelchair or braces for walking is limited.

Interruption of motor pathways in the cervical spinal cord isolates the thoracic sympathetic centers from higher control. Consequently, the patient cannot constrict peripheral arteries when he sits or stands. Blood pools in the limbs and viscera, thus reducing venous return to the heart, and even elastic supports cannot adequately compensate. Venostasis in the lower limbs also accounts for a higher incidence of pulmonary embolus in paraplegics who are confined to bed.

GASTROINTESTINAL SYSTEM AND NUTRITION. Paralytic ileus commonly follows spinal injury or acute poliomyelitis for a few days. In treatment oral feedings should be omitted until bowel activity returns. If abdominal distention occurs, a nasogastric tube is advisable to decompress the intestinal tract.

Most paraplegics eventually begin to defecate without an enema. However, fecal impactions are frequent in patients with acute spinal paralysis, so that stool softeners, gentle laxatives, or low enemas may be needed at first. As recovery progresses, a regular dietary schedule and adequate fluids are important to achieve spontaneous evacuation. Some patients initiate reflex evacuation by abdominal massage or digital stimulation of the rectum.

Adequate nutrition is imperative for recovery but is difficult to attain, particularly for patients confined to bed. A diet high in protein and calories helps repair injured tissue and prevent bedsores. A reasonable goal at first is 2000 to 2500 calories daily, although this may have to be lowered later to avoid obesity. During the early months the daily calcium intake should be kept below 0.5 gram to minimize the likelihood of urinary calculus. Transfusions to correct anemia and low blood volume in poorly nourished patients are often beneficial.

SKIN. Decubitus ulcers are a serious problem for paraplegics and can occur in any paralyzed, immobilized patient who is neglected. The danger of an anesthetic region is that it tolerates continuous pressure without the pain that ordinarily prompts a shift in position. After about two hours of immobility, ischemic changes begin in the subcutaneous tissue and are manifested by erythema of the overlying skin. Repeated ischemic insults are followed by ulceration.

Bedsores can be prevented by turning the patient at least every two hours, protecting reddened skin from further pressure, and maintaining adequate nutrition. Alternating air mattresses and rotating frame beds help to vary pressure points but are not by themselves guarantees against ulcers forming over the occiput, heels, trochanters, and sacrum. The weight of bedding is sometimes sufficient to erode the tips of the toes. Plaster casts over anesthetic areas may ulcerate the skin, and even supporting braces are dangerous.

Bedsores that heal with scar tissue remain particularly vulnerable to pressure. Therefore the most satisfactory coverage of a sizable decubitus ulcer is obtained by rotating pedicle tissue into the defect after trimming off any underlying bony prominence.

MUSCULOSKELETAL SYSTEM. Many operations and mechanical devices have been used to compensate for paralyzed muscles. Crutches, braces, or wheelchairs restore mobility. An automatic lift enables anyone to transfer a patient from bed to chair. Bracing or surgery can reconstruct the loss of pinch between the thumb and index finger and thus allow the patient to feed and shave himself.

Kyphosis or lordosis is a grave consequence of the unequal pull of partially paralyzed muscles that distorts the growing spine of a child. Spinal fusion halts progression of such deformity, and often can correct a moderate curvature. Good results have been reported with internal fixation of the spine to avoid the complications of plaster immobilization.

Although a certain amount of muscle spasm may help a paraplegic to support the trunk or to position an extremity, painful or recurrent spasms that forcibly flex or adduct the lower limbs interfere with sitting and ambulation and thus prevent rehabilitation. As flexor spasms are reflex responses, the first step is to remove sources of noxious, afferent stimuli such as infection of the bladder and bedsores. If these measures plus physical therapy fail, more drastic procedures may be required, such as myelotomy, excision of the distal end of the spinal cord, anterior rhizotomy, subthecal injections, peripheral neurotomy, or division of muscles and tendons. Any procedure that increases the neurologic deficit of an already paralyzed subject is undesirable. Accordingly, division of spastic muscles and tendons or a myelotomy that disconnects the afferent sensory input from the efferent limb of the spinal reflex is appropriate if motor or sensory function is present. Subthecal alcohol, anterior rhizotomy, or excision of the cord is suitable only for those who have no useful spinal cord function.

URINARY TRACT. Renal calculi, pyelonephritis, and hydronephrosis are the major causes of death in paraplegics and are sources of considerable disability in patients with lesser paralysis. These renal complications follow incomplete emptying of the bladder, which initially necessitates catheterization. Secondary infection and vesicoureteral reflux follow. These complications can be minimized by providing a low calcium diet, intermittently turning patients soon after the onset of paralysis, forcing fluids to achieve 1500 to 2000 ml of daily urine output, and treating culturally proved urinary tract infections promptly — but not prophylactically — with antimicrobial drugs. During recovery, nearly all patients with poliomyelitis and about 80 per cent of paraplegics become able to void without catheterization. Patients with poliomyelitis regain essentially normal bladder function. In paraplegics with high lesions of the spinal cord, reflex micturition occurs, mediated through the distal spinal segments. If an injury has destroyed sacral roots, suprapubic pressure may be necessary to empty the bladder.

Regaining spontaneous voiding after spinal injury is always difficult. In many patients a fluid intake of 3000 to 4000 ml daily and either intermittent catheterization or intermittent clamping of an indwelling catheter may establish spontaneous, automatic voiding. Intermittent catheterization using aseptic technique has given the best results as the urine remains sterile in three quarters of patients; if a catheter is left indwelling, one of the Gibbon type is preferred to the more irritating Foley. Some may need a transurethral resection of obstructing tissue at the bladder neck. If there is spastic hypertrophy of the bladder, especially with vesicoureteral reflux, satisfactory voiding usually cannot be obtained without partially interrupting the reflex arc. If there are no undesirable muscle spasms of the lower limbs, graded sacral rhizotomy is the most satisfactory procedure for enabling some patients to master bladder training. Myelotomy, as described earlier, is useful in managing patients with disabling spasticity of both the bladder and lower limbs. The more extensive procedures will also relieve autonomic hyperreflexia manifested by unpleasant episodes of sweating, hypertension, and headache triggered by contraction of bladder, bowel, or skeletal muscle. Recently, electrical stimulation of the conus medullaris to induce micturition has shown some promise, although the stimulus may also induce unwanted motion of lower limbs and penile erection.

Even patients who have apparently established satisfactory micturition may have slowly progressive hydronephrosis that, if unrecognized, will eventually cause death. Consequently, all patients should be evaluated periodically by intravenous pyelography. Progressive renal damage is an indication for urinary diversion, usually by implantation of the ureters into an ilial conduit.

Geisler, W. O., Jousse, A. T., and Wynne-Jones, M.: Survival in traumatic transverse myelitis. Paraplegia, 14:262, 1977.

Grimes, J. H., Nashold, B. S., and Currie, D. P.: Chronic electrical stimulation of the paraplegic bladder. J. Urol., 109:242, 1973.

Guttman, L.: Spinal Cord Injuries, Comprehensive Management and Research. Oxford, Blackwell Scientific Publications, 1976, p. 731.

Ivan, L. P., and Wiley, J. J.: Myelotomy in the management of spasticity. Clin. Orthop., 108:52, 1975.

Long, C., II, and Lawton, E. B.: Functional significance of spinal cord lesion level. Arch. Phys. Med. Rehabil., 6:249, 1965.

Wilcox, N. E., and Stauffer, E. S.: Follow-up of 423 consecutive patients admitted to the spinal cord centre, Rancho Los Amigos Hospital, 1st January to 31st December, 1967. Paraplegia, 10:115, 1972.

Section Twenty-Two
MECHANICAL LESIONS OF THE NERVE ROOTS AND SPINAL CORD

Albert J. Aguayo

331. SYMPTOMS OF NERVE ROOT AND SPINAL CORD COMPRESSION

Certain diseases result in compression of the nerve roots or spinal cord within the spinal canal. In general the symptoms and signs that accompany such intra-spinal lesions may be classified into two groups: radicular syndromes due to spinal root injury, and myelopathy caused by compression of the spinal cord; but a combination of both syndromes is common.

RADICULAR SYNDROMES

Compression of nerve roots causes pain, paresthesia, sensory loss, weakness, atrophy, and reflex changes which are confined to a radicular anatomic distribution. A single nerve root can be compressed, as in most cases of intervertebral disc protrusion, but several roots are often involved in arachnoiditis or when there is neoplastic invasion of the spinal canal.

The pain caused by root compression is experienced in the overlying spine, deep in certain muscles, or along the cutaneous distribution of the injured root (*dermatome*). This pain is often influenced by movement and increases with strain. Radicular pain is usually unilateral, but some intraspinal lesions, by compressing roots bilaterally, can give rise to pain in both limbs or on both sides of the thorax or abdomen. The most common sensory symptoms are hypesthesia and paresthesia, both of which may be described by patients as numbness. These sensory symptoms are usually accompanied by sensory impairment in the distribution of the compressed root or roots. Because of the more extensive overlapping of adjacent innervation for touch, this sensory loss is better outlined by testing responses to pinprick than to light touch.

Muscles supplied by roots that originate from the same spinal cord segment constitute a *myotome*. Because most muscles are supplied from more than one segmental level, compression of a single root causes different degrees of weakness and atrophy in different muscles. The effects of a root lesion on a muscle ultimately depend on the importance of the innervation provided by the injured root; weakness of certain muscles within a particular myotome may be difficult to elicit, whereas other muscles may be severely affected. For example, although fibers from the L5 root innervate approximately 30 different muscles in the lower limb, severe changes after compression of this root may be clearly apparent in only two: the extensor hallucis longus and extensor digitorum brevis muscles.

Muscle stretch reflexes are diminished or absent when reflex arcs are interrupted by root compression. At the level at which they can be clinically tested, reflex changes have an important localizing value (Table 1).

Differentiation between symptoms caused by nerve root and peripheral nerve lesions must follow anatomic guides (see figure and Table 2). In radiculopathy, as mentioned above, weakness and atrophy of muscles occur within a myotome. In a neuropathy weakness and reflex changes are confined to the anatomic distribution of the nerve, and sensory deficits do not fully

TABLE 1. Clinical Findings in the Four Most Common Radicular Syndromes

Root	Usual Distribution of Pain	Principally Affected Muscles	Sensory Loss	Muscle Stretch Reflexes Affected
C6	Neck, parascapular, lateral aspect of arm and forearm	Biceps, brachioradialis, wrist extensors and flexors	Radial border of forearm, thumb	Biceps and/or brachioradialis may be diminished
C7	Neck, parascapular, posterolateral arm, dorsum of forearm	Triceps, wrist, finger flexors and extensors	Dorsum of forearm; index and middle fingers	Triceps
L5	Low back, buttock, lateral thigh, dorsum of foot	Dorsiflexors of foot and toes	Anterolateral aspect of lower leg, dorsum of foot	Usually none, but ankle jerk may be diminished
S1	Low back, buttock, posterior thigh	Calf muscles, plantar flexors	Outer edge of foot and sole	Ankle jerk

TABLE 2.   Peripheral Nerve and Radicular
Innervation of Muscles

Upper Limb:

Nerves	Radicular Innervation					
	C-4	C-5	C-6	C-7	C-8	T-1
Suprascapular	– –Supraspinatus– –					
Axillary	– –Deltoid– – – – –					
Musculocutaneous		– –Biceps– – – – – – –				
Median			– –Flexor carpi radialis– –			
				– – – –Flexor pollicis longus– –		
				– –Flexor digitorum– –		
				– –Abductor pollicis longus– –		
					– –Opponens pollicis– – – –	
Ulnar				– –Flexor carpi ulnaris– – – –		
				– –Opponens digiti quinti– –		
					– –Abductor digiti quinti– – – –	
						– – –Interossei– – – – –
Radial			– –Triceps brachialis– – – – – – – – – –			
		– –Brachioradialis– –				
			– –Extensor carpi radialis– –			
				– –Extensor carpi ulnaris– –		
				– –Extensor digitorum longus– –		

Lower Limb:

Nerves	Radicular Innervation						
	L-1	L-2	L-3	L-4	L-5	S-1	S-2
	– –Iliopsoas– – – – –						
Gluteal					– –Gluteus maximus– – – – –		
Femoral			– –Quadriceps femoris– –				
Obturator		– –Adductors– – – – –					
Sciatic					– – – –Hamstrings– – – – –		
C. Peroneal				– –Tibialis anterior– –			
				– –Extensor digitorum brevis– –			
Tibial					– – – – –Gastrocnemius– –		
				– –Abductor hallucis			
					– –Abductor digiti quinti– –		

correspond to individual dermatomes. Differentiation is made easier when the affected muscles are supplied by different nerves (e.g., the deltoid and biceps may be weak in lesions of the C5 root; these muscles are supplied by different nerves: axillary and musculocutaneous nerves, respectively). Because of the proximity of roots and spinal cord within the spinal canal, both structures may be compressed together. Associated signs of spinal cord compression are not a feature in peripheral neuropathies except in rare disorders such as familial hypertrophic neuropathy, in which pathologically enlarged roots may encroach upon the spinal cord (Symonds and Blackwood).

SPINAL CORD COMPRESSION

The clinical symptomatology depends on the speed of compression, the transverse and longitudinal extent of the lesion, the functional role of the compressed level of the spinal cord, and the cause of compression.

The spinal cord accommodates to slow forms of compression such as occur with meningiomas and neurofibromas. As a result these tumors in their early stages may cause few symptoms and signs. However, an acute intervertebral disc protrusion or an epidural hematoma will result in rapid impairment of function with severe paralysis, sensory loss, and loss of bladder and bowel control.

The effects of compression may be limited to only a portion of the transverse area of the cord. When one half of the spinal cord is injured at levels higher than the tenth thoracic, the symptoms and signs that follow may be those of *Brown-Séquard's syndrome.* Such patients have spastic weakness, exaggerated muscle stretch reflexes, and an extensor plantar response (Babinski sign) all on the same side as the lesion. Joint position and vibration sense are decreased ipsilaterally, but pain and temperature are impaired on the opposite half of the body. The contralateral loss of pain and temperature sensation is due to crossing of spinothalamic fibers subserving these modalities. Spinothalamic fibers are somatotopically arranged within the ventrolateral columns of the spinal cord, with fibers originating at lower levels lying most laterally. Because of this anatomic organization, extrinsic compression tends to first produce symptoms below the site of the lesion, the level of sensory impairment gradually ascending as the compression affects deeper parts of the spinal cord. Conversely, because deep-seated lesions may spare superficially arranged fibers, sensation may be normal in the lower dermatomes in patients with intramedullary lesions (sacral sparing).

In addition, intramedullary lesions may give rise to sensory dissociation with loss of pain and temperature sensation and relative preservation of touch. This occurs when mainly crossed fibers are interrupted by a central cord lesion (*commissural or syringomyelia-like syndrome*). In addition, by predominantly disturbing postural sensibility, cord compression may cause ataxia.

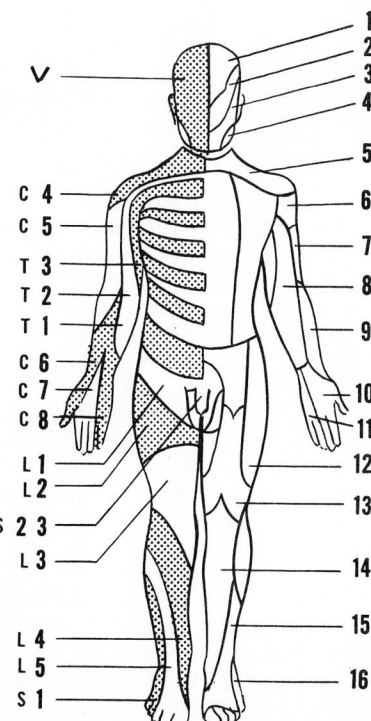

Schematic representation of dermatomes and peripheral nerve sensory areas:

1. Trigeminal 1st division
2. Trigeminal 2nd division
3. Trigeminal 3rd division
4. Greater auricular nerve
5. Branches from cervical plexus
6. Axillary nerve
7. Radial nerve
8. Medial brachial cutaneous nerve
9. Musculocutaneous nerve
10. Median nerve
11. Ulnar nerve
12. Lateral femoral cutaneous nerve
13. Femoral nerve
14. Saphenous nerve
15. Peroneal nerve
16. Sural nerve

LEVELS OF INTRASPINAL COMPRESSION

FORAMEN MAGNUM AND UPPER CERVICAL SPINE. Compression at this level may cause symptoms resulting from spinal cord, nerve root, or intracranial involvement. Pain in the neck and back of the head is the most common and earliest sign. The pain is made worse by head movement, particularly nodding. There may be weakness and atrophy of muscles of the neck and shoulder girdle with spasticity in the lower limbs. Paresthesia and sensory deficits may also occur in the occipital head region (C2 dermatome) and the neck (C3 dermatome). Motor and sensory signs may even extend to involve the hands (C6 to C8 segmental level); this extension to the mid- and lower cervical cord has been thought to be due to impaired circulation from compression of spinal vessels. Tumors of the formen magnum may also extend intracranially and cause increased intracranial pressure, cerebellar dysfunction, nystagmus, trigeminal sensory loss, and atrophy of the tongue.

The most common causes of compression at the craniocervical junction are bony abnormalities which result in basilar invagination, dislocation of the atlantoaxial and atlanto-occipital joints, and neoplasms, meningiomas in particular.

CERVICAL REGION. Compression at this level characteristically produces spinal and radicular signs in the upper limbs combined with long tract signs in the lower extremities.

There is loss of power and bulk in muscles of the shoulder girdle and arms. The biceps, brachioradialis, or triceps jerks mainly depend on the integrity of the C5, C6, or C7 reflex arcs, respectively, and may be diminished or absent. In addition, there can be "inversion" of the brachioradialis reflex; tapping the tendon of this muscle elicits a brisk reflex contraction of the hand and finger flexor muscles and not the usual flexion and supination of the forearm. This unusual response is due to efferent interruption of the segmental reflex arc; the spread of the response and hyperreflexia at lower spinal levels results from pyramidal tract involvement.

When sensory symptoms extend along the radial border of the forearm and thumb ("numb thumb"), they suggest involvement of the C6 cord segment or nerve root. Symptoms in the index and middle fingers point to C7, and sensory impairment in the ring and little fingers suggest C8. Lesions at the cervicothoracic junction can cause unilateral Horner's syndrome which can be associated with wasting of the small muscles of the hand and a sensory deficit on the ulnar border of the hand and forearm (C8, T1).

The most common causes of compression at this level are cervical spondylosis and protrusion of an intervertebral disc, but intramedullary and extramedullary tumors also occur.

THORACIC REGION. Compression is suggested by the finding of normal upper limbs and spasticity in the legs. When thoracic radicular symptoms are present, a more precise localization is possible. It is useful to remember that the projection of the thoracic segments coincides with that of the intercostal spaces. Important landmarks are the level of the nipples for the fourth thoracic, the xiphoid process for T7, and the umbilicus and groin for T10 and T12, respectively. Patients will often complain of a tight, bound feeling which usually coincides with the compressed root or segment. In addition, intercostal muscles may be wasted. In low thoracic lesions the umbilicus may elevate when the patient, in the supine position, raises his head against resistance (Beevor's sign).

Common causes of compression at the thoracic spine level are metastatic tumors, meningiomas, and neurofibromas. Intervertebral disc protusions are comparatively rare at this level.

LUMBOSACRAL REGION. Lower Spinal Cord. There is a close relation between the segments in the lower cord and the roots that form the cauda equina. As a result, pain, sensorimotor signs in the lower limbs, and loss of sphincter control can result from the involvement of either cord or roots. It is seldom that a discrete spinal cord segmental lesion can be clinically identified at this level.

Cauda Equina. In cauda equina compression, dull, aching pain may be experienced in the sacrum or perineum or can radiate to the legs in a sciatic distribution.

Symptoms depend on the level of compression and number of motor and sensory roots affected. Often there is atrophic, areflexic paralysis combined with asymmetrical bilateral radicular sensory impairment. Sensory dissociation does not occur. Progression of signs is usually slow, and loss of bladder and bowel control may occur late.

Presumably because of interference with blood supply to the roots of the cauda equina by compression, some patients with a narrowed lumbar spinal canal experience transient, radicular signs or pain in the calf muscles when walking or after prolonged standing. This syndrome has been named intermittent claudication of the cauda equina.

The most important cause of single or multiple root compression at the lower lumbar and sacral level is an intervertebral disc protrusion. Cauda equina compression occurs in congenital spinal stenosis and lumbar spondylosis, Paget's disease, and achondroplasia. Ependymomas, teratomas, and lipomas may constrict the lower segments of the cord and cauda equina. Tabes dorsalis, diabetic neuropathy, and other lesions affecting peripheral nerves to the lower limbs must be differentiated from lesions compressing the lumbosacral roots.

Aids to the Investigation of Peripheral Nerve Injuries. London, Her Majesty's Stationery Office, 1960.
Haymaker, W.: Bing's Local Diagnosis in Neurologic Diseases. 15th ed. St. Louis, C. V. Mosby Company, 1969.
Keegan, J. J., and Garett, F. D.: The segmental distribution of the cutaneous nerves in the limbs of man. Anat. Rec., 102:409, 1948.
Klenerman, L.: Cauda equina and spinal cord compression in Paget's disease. J. Bone Joint Surg., 48B:365, 1966.
Rewcastle, N. B., and Berry, K.: Neoplasms of the lower spinal canal. Neurology (Minneap.), 14:608, 1964.
Symonds, C. P., and Blackwood, W.: Spinal cord compression in hypertrophic neuritis. Brain, 85:251, 1962.

332. LABORATORY AIDS TO INVESTIGATION

To localize and establish the nature of lesions causing intraspinal compression, several diagnostic tests may be used. Roentgenographic investigations are the most important, but electrophysiologic techniques, radioisotope scanning, and cerebrospinal fluid examination are also helpful.

ROENTGENOGRAPHIC METHODS

Roentgenographic investigation should begin with plain films of the suspected site of spinal cord or root compression. Frontal, lateral, and oblique views are required for examination of the cervical spine; frontal and lateral views are generally satisfactory for visualization of the thoracic and lumbosacral spine. Lateral films of the cervical spine in flexion and extension are needed if recurrent subluxation is suspected. In certain situations, tomography may be necessary to define a bone lesion more precisely.

Plain films of the spine should be systematically examined, noting the number, shape, density, and alignment of the vertebrae and the contour of the pedicles, the size of the intervertebral foramen, the size and shape of the spinal canal, the width of the disc spaces,

and the presence of abnormal soft tissue shadows or calcifications. The anteroposterior depth of the spinal canal is a particularly important measurement. Sagittal diameters of less than 10 mm at any level of the cervical spine usually indicate spinal cord compression; bony compression of the cord is also possible with canals measuring 10 to 13 mm but improbable if measurements are greater than 13 mm. Increases in the transverse diameter of the spinal canal may be associated with thinning of the pedicles and are seen with syringomyelia or intramedullary tumors. Narrowing of the spinal canal with compression of the spinal cord or roots may occur in spondylosis, achondroplasia, and Paget's disease.

Plain x-rays of the vertebral column may suggest certain specific conditions. Dumbbell-shaped neurofibromas which enlarge the intervertebral foramen will become readily apparent in such x-rays. Congenital anomalies of the vertebral bodies are at times associated with intraspinal teratomas or lipomas. Bone caries suggests an infectious process such as tuberculosis, typhoidal infection, or brucellosis. Vertebral bone destruction by infection often involves the intervertebral discs; conversely, tumor metastases to the vertebral column spare the discs.

When surgical treatment is contemplated, radiopaque *oil myelography* by lumbar or cisternal injection is required for precise localization. In expert hands, *air myelography* is also a useful tool for the assessment of spinal cord size and for a diagnosis of small tumors. *Spinal angiography* is a specialized technique necessary for the detailed investigation of tumors and vascular malformations.

Computerized tomography using a body scanner is a new, yet to be fully evaluated tool for the investigation of lesions in the spinal canal and surrounding tissues.

SCANNING AND ELECTROMYOGRAPHY

Bone scanning after radioisotope injection may be helpful if metastases are suspected as cause of bone destruction. However, fractures, infection, and ankylosing spondylitis may also cause increased radioisotope uptake.

Electromyography is useful for the localization of intraspinal lesions affecting the motor unit at the anterior horn cell or the nerve root levels, as noted in Ch. 272.

CEREBROSPINAL FLUID EXAMINATION

Cerebrospinal fluid examination rarely provides specific diagnostic information about compressive spinal cord or root lesions. Therefore because satisfactory myelograms are difficult to obtain in patients who have had lumbar puncture in the preceding week, cerebrospinal fluid examinations are usually best performed at the time of myelography. In general, the examination of cerebrospinal fluid may suggest certain diagnostic possibilities. Xanthochromic fluid is seen with intraspinal hemorrhage or block of cerebrospinal fluid circulation. Intraspinal bleeding may originate from vascular malformations, ependymomas, or melanomas. Inflammatory cells indicate an infectious process or chemical meningitis caused by a ruptured teratoma or dermoid cyst. Tumor cells may be identified in the cerebrospinal fluid of patients with carcinomatous infiltration of the meninges.

In the absence of a block in the circulation of cerebrospinal fluid, elevations of CSF protein over 60 mg per 100 ml suggest other intraspinal lesions than an intervertebral disc protrusion or spondylosis. Spinal fluid blocks are best established by myelography; because irreparable damage to the spinal cord may result from displacement of an intraspinal mass after pressure changes resulting from jugular compression (Queckenstedt test), this procedure should not be done if spinal cord compression is suspected.

Aguilar, J. A., and Elvidge, A. R.: Intervertebral disc disease caused by the Brucella Organism. J. Neurosurg., 18:27, 1961.

Ambrose, G. B., Alpert, M., and Neer, C. S.: Vertebral osteomyelitis. A diagnostic problem. JAMA, 97:101, 1966.

Charkes, N. D., Sklaroff, D. M., and Young, I.: A critical analysis of strontium bone scanning for detection of metastatic cancer. Am. J. Roentgenol. Radium Ther. Nucl. Med., 96:647, 1966.

DiChiro, G., and Doppman, J. L.: Differential angiographic features of hemangioblastomas and arteriovenous malformations of the spinal cord. Radiology, 93:25, 1969.

Elsberg, C. A., and Dyke, C. G.: Diagnosis and localization of tumors of the spinal cord by means of measurements made on x-ray films of vertebrae and the correlation of clinical and x-ray findings. Bull. Neurol. Inst., 3:359, 1934.

Hammerschlag, S., Wolpert, S., and Carter, B.: Computer Tomography of the spinal canal. Radiology, 121:361, 1976.

333. MANAGEMENT OF PATIENTS WITH SUSPECTED NERVE ROOT OR SPINAL CORD COMPRESSION

The specific management of intraspinal compression of nerve roots or cord depends on the suspected diagnosis, the severity of the symptoms, and the extent of the neurologic signs.

CONSERVATIVE MANAGEMENT AIMED AT REDUCING PAIN AND PREVENTING FUTURE RECURRENCES. Patients in this category have acute localized pain in the spinal or paraspinal region with or without peripheral radicular radiation; they do not have neurologic deficits indicative of spinal cord or severe root compression. The most likely diagnosis is an acute intervertebral disc protrusion, and with time complete recovery can usually be anticipated. This approach is particularly justified when there is no history of similar previous episodes and when the pain follows minor trauma, effort, or strain.

Patients may stay at home and should rest on a firm bed and make no physical effort. Analgesics and muscle relaxants are given for symptomatic relief. When pain subsides, exercises aimed at strengthening the muscular support of the spinal column may help prevent recurrences.

Plain x-rays of the involved segment of the spine help ascertain changes in the vertebral bodies or discs. Initially, however, these investigations can be deferred if the patient is in considerable pain.

CONSERVATIVE MANAGEMENT AIMED AT DECIDING IF THE COURSE OF INTRASPINAL ROOT COMPRESSION IS PROGRESSIVE. Acute pain may be accompanied by signs of moderate sensory or motor deficit in a root dis-

tribution. Such signs are represented by some loss of strength, paresthesia, and mild sensory impairment or a loss of muscle stretch reflexes. If these signs worsen or do not subside after a trial of conservative treatment, admission to hospital should be arranged to assure immobilization and rest and to arrange further investigations.

MANAGEMENT AIMED AT POSSIBLE SURGICAL DECOMPRESSION. This approach is indicated for patients showing signs of spinal cord compression. It is also advisable for patients with nerve root compression if there is intractable or severe recurrent pain or if there are signs of severe neurologic deficit, particularly marked weakness and muscle atrophy. These patients should be admitted to hospital for investigation. If there are no contraindications to surgery, myelography should be performed to establish a diagnosis and determine the site and extent of compression. If indicated, operative treatment should soon follow.

PROMPT INVESTIGATION AND SURGICAL DECOMPRESSION. This approach is required for patients who rapidly develop spinal cord or cauda equina compression. A particular emergency is represented by impaired bladder or rectal control. Patients should be immediately admitted to hospital to undergo only those investigations which enable a localization of the lesion. Such investigations usually include plain films of the spine and an emergency myelogram. In the course of these investigations, patients should be kept fasting to allow for immediate anesthesia if surgical intervention is decided upon.

334. SPECIFIC DISORDERS THAT CAUSE NERVE ROOT OR SPINAL CORD COMPRESSION

334.1. INTERVERTEBRAL DISC PROTRUSION

Each intervertebral disc consists of fibrocartilage and has a soft center, the nucleus pulposus, surrounded by thicker fibrous tissue, the anulus fibrosus. The nucleus pulposus constitutes most of the disc substance in the young, but with age it loses volume and resilience. When, during effort or trauma, the disc is suddenly compressed and the nucleus pulposus is caused to protrude through the anulus, fragments of disc may be extruded into the spinal canal. The herniated disc is usually directed toward the spinal canal because the anulus and longitudinal ligament are thinner posteriorly. Disc disease is more common in the cervical and lumbar spine, where there is greater mobility; in the thoracic spine, where movement is limited, disc herniations are rare.

The signs and symptoms of disc herniation result from compression of pain-sensitive structures within the spinal canal, including nerve roots or the spinal cord itself. Posterolateral disc herniations tend to involve individual nerve roots at the intervertebral foramina, whereas central protrusions may compress the spinal cord or cauda equina. Commonly the compressed root approximately corresponds to the level of the protruded disc, but this may not be the case in the lumbosacral region where several roots can be compressed by a single disc. Furthermore, extruded disc material may move several centimeters along the dural sac and compress roots situated below the site of disc rupture.

CLINICAL MANIFESTATIONS. Pain is the main symptom of an intervertebral disc protrusion. It is usually severe and accompanied by local reflex contraction of paraspinal muscles. Other symptoms and signs depend upon the localization of the protruded disc.

Herniated Cervical Discs. Cervical disc herniations occur most frequently at the fifth and sixth interspaces with fewer protrusions at C4 and C7 interspaces. Symptoms are often precipitated by sudden twisting, hyperextension, or hyperflexion of the neck. The pain may radiate to the shoulder and parascapular region and usually has a boring, aching quality. If nerve roots are compressed below the midcervical level, pain may extend into the upper extremity. Movements of the neck, but particularly hyperextension and tilting toward the affected side, are limited by pain. Symptoms caused by compression of the C6 and C7 roots are summarized in Table 1, Ch. 331. More rarely cervical disc protrusion results in cord compression. In such patients, long tract signs which develop below the level of the lesion are mainly due to involvement of the corticospinal tract.

Herniated Lumbar Discs. The most common disc protrusions are in the lower lumbar region and affect the L5 and S1 roots (Table 1). There is often a poorly localized low backache (lumbago), and pain may radiate into the buttocks, thigh, and lower leg (sciatica). The pain is generally severe and follows effort, such as lifting. In some patients, however, the pain may be spontaneous; occasionally sensory and motor deficits caused by disc herniation occur in the absence of pain. In most patients, the radiation of pain is unilateral; when there is a central disc protrusion, however, pain may occur in both lower extremities.

On examination patients show straightening of the normal lumbar curvature, and the pelvis may be tilted away from the side of the protrusion. Paraspinal mucles and vertebral spinous processes are tender to palpation. Straight leg raising (Lasègue's maneuver) on the side of compression is limited by pain. In addition, the pain can occur with raising of the opposite leg ("crossover pain"). There may be tenderness on palpation of the sciatic notch.

Compression of several of the roots of the cauda equina may give rise to pain, asymmetric bilateral sensory and motor changes, and even to loss of sphincter control. Occasionally, bladder control may be lost in the absence of other symptoms.

DIAGNOSIS. The symptoms of an intervertebral disc protrusion must be differentiated from those caused by arthritis of the spine and other bone and joint diseases. Neuropathies caused by entrapment, neuralgic amyotrophy, and diabetic neuropathy may enter the differential diagnosis because they may present with localized pain, and with sensory and motor deficits.

Plain x-rays of the spine reveal narrowing of disc spaces in less than half the patients. In the cervical spine, oblique views are necessary to establish whether there is a reduction in the size of intervertebral fora-

mina. *Myelography should be performed only when the cause of compression is doubtful or when surgical treatment is contemplated.* Disc protrusions are evidenced by myelography as a filling defect at the level of the interspace. Obliteration of the root sleeve by a protruded disc may also be demonstrated by this procedure. The cerebrospinal fluid protein may be normal or increased; in the absence of complete block of cerebrospinal fluid circulation, protein values are usually below 60 mg per 100 ml.

TREATMENT. Patients presenting with acute pain should be treated with analgesics, muscle relaxants, rest, and immobility. A cervical collar or a lumbar brace may reduce mobility, and rest in bed on a hard mattress is often helpful. If improvement follows such measures, usually no investigations other than plain x-rays of the spine are necessary. If pain and other symptoms persist after a period of rest, hospitalization must be considered to ensure immobilization. Intractable pain, persistent disability, or development of progressive sensory or motor signs of radicular compression requires consideration of surgical treatment. Prompt operative treatment is mandatory when signs of progressive cord involvement or impairment of bladder or rectal sphincter control develop.

Recurrent symptoms after discoidectomy may be due to an incomplete removal of the disc, to disc herniation at an adjacent level, or to arachnoiditis. In addition the possibility that a herniated disc may have been associated with another type of intraspinal disease must be considered.

Fisher, R. G.: Protrusions of thoracic disc. The factor of herniation through the dura mater. J. Neurosurg., 22:591:1965.
Kessler, L. A., and Stein, W. Z.: Posterior migration of a herniated disc. Radiology, 76:104, 1961.
Love, J. G., and Schorn, V. G.: Thoracic disc protrusions. JAMA, 191:627, 1965.
Scott, P. J.: Bladder paralysis in cauda equina lesions from disc prolapse. J. Bone Joint Surg., 47B:224, 1965.
Spanos, N. C., and Andrew, J.: Intermittent claudication and lateral lumbar disc protrusions. J. Neurol. Neurosurg. Psychiatry, 29:273, 1966.
Spurling, R. G.: Lesions of the Lumbar Intervertebral Disc. Springfield, Ill., Charles C Thomas, 1953.
Spurling, R. G.: Lesions of the Cervical Invertebral Disc. Springfield, Ill., Charles C Thomas, 1956.

334.2. MYELOPATHY AND NERVE ROOT COMPRESSION DUE TO SPONDYLOSIS

Spondylosis refers to degenerative changes in the spine which may be neurologically asymptomatic or may cause symptoms by compression of nerve roots or spinal cord.

Spondylotic changes consist of intervertebral disc narrowing, osteophyte formation, and thickening of spinal ligaments. These changes most frequently involve the cervical or lumbar spine and are rare in the thoracic region. The term spondylosis is not generally used to describe acute protrusion of intervertebral discs, although the two conditions may be associated.

PATHOGENESIS. Spondylosis presumably results from the "wear and tear" of repeated spinal movement. Although more than one half of people older than 50 years of age have cervical spine osteophytes, associated neurologic symptoms and signs are much less frequent.

The single most important factor in the development of clinical manifestations caused by spondylosis is the size of the spinal canal. If the canal is congenitally narrow, the spinal cord may be compressed by relatively small osteophytes or ligamentous hypertrophy; on the other hand, a wide spinal canal may accommodate extensive spondylotic changes without causing appreciable neurologic signs of compression.

When the cervical spinal cord is compressed by osteophytes from the vertebral bodies or by thickening of the posterior longitudinal ligament and ligamentum flavum, symptoms and signs may follow trauma caused by neck movement or from impairment of spinal cord circulation. The cauda equina may also be injured in lumbar spondylosis. At both the cervical and lumbar levels, nerve roots are compressed by degenerative changes in bone and soft tissues adjacent to the intervertebral foramina.

CERVICAL SPONDYLOSIS

The most important symptoms and signs of cervical spondylosis are due to spinal cord (cervical myelopathy) and root (cervical radiculopathy) compression.

CERVICAL MYELOPATHY. Cervical myelopathy commonly develops insidiously, but symptoms may be precipitated by minor trauma. Sensory abnormalities are usually less striking than signs of disturbed motor function. Spastic paresis, clonus, and hyperreflexia in the legs as well as extensor plantar responses are the most common neurologic signs of this myelopathy.

In the upper limbs, there may be segmental muscle weakness and atrophy, as well as loss of muscle stretch reflexes, particularly if there is an associated radiculopathy. Vibration sense may be diminished in the lower limbs, but loss of joint position sense or pain and temperature sensation is uncommon. As a rule, bladder and bowel control are normal in patients with cervical myelopathy.

CERVICAL RADICULOPATHY. Cervical radiculopathy may occur in the absence of cervical myelopathy. Various radicular syndromes may develop, depending on the particular root affected. In the cervical spine the most common radiculopathies are those of the C6 and C7 root (Table 1, Ch. 331).

Pain and limitation of neck movements are common in cervical spondylosis, and some patients may present with occipital headaches.

DIAGNOSIS. X-rays of the cervical spine confirm the presence of cervical spondylosis. However, there is a high incidence of asymptomatic spondylotic changes, and careful clinical correlation is required for interpretation of such radiologic findings. To prove the diagnosis of cervical spondylotic myelopathy, the anteroposterior diameter of the cervical canal must be measured. If this measurement is less than 10 mm, there is almost certain cord compression. The extent of compression can best be determined by myelography which also shows soft tissue changes in spondylosis. Oblique x-ray views demonstrate narrowing of the intervertebral foramina.

PROGNOSIS AND TREATMENT. Because of wide variations in the natural course of cervical spondylotic myelopathy, it is difficult to assess the relative merits of conservative and surgical management. By and large, surgical treatment rarely is indicated for radiculopathy, but should be undertaken when clear evidence indicates progressive myelopathy. Most patients can usually be managed effectively with analgesics, muscle relaxants, and cervical immobilization.

LUMBAR SPONDYLOSIS AND SPINAL STENOSIS

In addition to compression of individual nerve roots by osteophytes encroaching upon intervertebral foramina, spondylosis of the lumbosacral spine may significantly reduce the size of the spinal canal. In such circumstances, spinal canal stenosis may cause injury to the cauda equina.

The pathogenesis of neurologic symptoms in patients with lumbar stenosis is similar to that in other bone diseases resulting in shallow lumbar canals, namely, congenital spinal stenosis, achondroplasia, and Paget's disease. In all these disorders, further narrowing by osteophytes, disc herniation, or ligamentous hypertrophy may give rise to compression of the cauda equina.

CLINICAL MANIFESTATIONS. The only symptom in patients with lumbar spinal stenosis may be backache after prolonged standing or effort. Signs of single or multiple root compression may develop gradually or have a sudden onset. These radicular symptoms are similar to those of intervertebral disc herniation and other causes of lumbosacral nerve root compression. Patients with lumbar spinal stenosis may suffer acute compression of the cauda equina after minor trauma or when subjected to prolonged hyperextension as during anesthesia for certain surgical procedures.

Intermittent Claudication of the Cauda Equina. Intermittent claudication of the cauda equina is a rare syndrome which may present in association with narrowing of the spinal canal. Typically, symptoms and signs are evoked or accentuated by walking and disappear soon after stopping. In other patients symptoms follow prolonged standing. In both varieties of intermittent claudication of the cauda equina, roots are compressed within a narrow spinal canal. The onset of symptoms has been explained by postulating that transient additional spinal narrowing is caused by the lordotic posture adopted during walking and standing. Patients usually present with pain in the low back and legs and may show weakness and sensory symptoms. During examination signs of motor and sensory deficit, as well as diminished reflexes, may be temporarily elicited by asking the patient to walk until symptoms reappear.

The absence of signs of vascular insufficiency in the iliofemoral and other arteries to the lower extremities helps differentiate claudication caused by compression from that which results from primary vascular disease.

DIAGNOSIS. The diagnosis of lumbar spinal stenosis requires radiologic demonstration of a narrow lumbar canal and myelographic confirmation of cauda equina compression.

TREATMENT. In advanced lumbar spinal stenosis, progressive signs of individual root or cauda equina compression can be relieved by surgical decompression.

Ehni, G., et al.: Significance of the small lumbar spinal canal: Cauda equina compression syndromes due to spondylosis: (Parts I to V). J. Neurosurg., 31:490, 1969.

Naylor, A.: Surgery in the treatment of cervical and thoracic disc protrusions. Br. Med. J., 1:821, 1977.

Stoltmann, H. F., and Blackwood, W.: The role of the ligamenta flava in the pathogenesis of myelopathy in cervical spondylosis. Brain, 87:45, 1964.

Turnbull, I. M. Microvasculature of the human spinal cord. J. Neurosurg., 35:141, 1971.

Waltz, T. A.: Physical factors in the myelopathy of cervical spondylosis. Brain, 90:395, 1967.

Wilkinson, M. (ed.): Cervical Spondylosis. Its Early Diagnosis and Treatment. Philadelphia, W. B. Saunders Company, 1971.

334.3. SPINAL CORD TUMORS

Depending upon their anatomic relation to the dura mater, tumors affecting the spinal cord may be classified as *extradural tumors*, which usually arise in the bone of the spinal column or within the extradural space; *intradural extramedullary tumors*, which lie between the dura mater and the spinal cord; and *intramedullary tumors*, which arise within the substance of the cord itself. The relative incidence in a general hospital population is approximately 50, 40, and 10 per cent, respectively.

EXTRADURAL TUMORS

Such tumors are usually manifested by symptoms and signs of spinal cord compression and are most often caused by extradural bone metastases. Common primary sources are carcinomas of the lung, breast, kidney, and prostate; less frequent sources are the gastrointestinal tract and thyroid gland. Spinal extradural compression may also occur in multiple myeloma, sarcomas, or lymphomas. Most metastases give rise to localized compression, but a few, particularly lymphomas and sarcomas, may extensively infiltrate the epidural space.

Pain resulting from bone destruction or root compression is the first symptom in the majority of patients with extradural tumors. It is usually dull, constant, and localized, is made worse by movements of the spine or pressure over the vertebral spinal processes, and is often exacerbated by bed rest. Radicular symptoms usually follow the local pain and are often bilateral. Pain alone is usually present for weeks or months before signs of spinal cord dysfunction develop; but once spinal cord signs appear, they usually progress rapidly over a few days or weeks to produce, if untreated, complete paralysis. More rarely, compression develops acutely, because of pathologic collapse of an infiltrated vertebral body or from hemorrhage within the metastasis. In either event, spastic weakness and loss of vibration and joint position sense below the level of the lesion are the first spinal cord signs to develop, whereas disturbances of bladder and/or bowel control generally occur late.

Radiologic changes are present on the plain x-ray films of most patients with malignant extradural metastases. Signs vary from osteoporosis to frank destruction of bone. When ordinary x-ray films of the spine are normal, evidence of bone involvement may be provided by radioisotope scanning. A definitive diagnosis of malignant extradural metastasis, however, can be made only by myelography, which must be carried out promptly if there is clinical suspicion of spinal cord compression, no matter what the plain radiograms reveal.

As a rule the cerebrospinal fluid protein is elevated, but there are no malignant cells. The CSF glucose is normal, in contrast to the decreased levels often seen in patients with carcinomatous invasion of the subarachnoid space.

Because metastatic tumors are a frequent cause of spinal cord compression in adults, this possibility should always be considered in patients with signs or symptoms of compression. In particular, the lungs and breasts should be carefully examined as sources of a possible primary malignancy. Anemia, bone pain, mediastinal enlargement, hepatomegaly, or splenomegaly all suggest metastatic disease or lymphomas. Bone x-rays, serum electrophoresis, testing for Bence Jones protein in the urine, and bone marrow examinations are all of help in diagnosing multiple myeloma.

Hormones, radiotherapy, and/or chemotherapy are used in the treatment of most of the extradural tumors involving the spine. The best results of medical therapy are usually obtained in patients with myeloma and lymphomas. Surgical decompression may be indicated when such therapy is ineffective, when there are signs of rapidly progressing compression of the cord, and when the etiologic diagnosis is unknown. Whatever form of treatment is chosen, it must be begun promptly and be vigorous, because if neurologic signs are mild, the chances of maintaining or improving neurologic function are better.

INTRADURAL EXTRAMEDULLARY TUMORS

The two most important tumors in this category are meningiomas and neurofibromas, which together account for almost two thirds of all primary intraspinal neoplasms. Less common tumors are teratomas, arachnoid cysts, some lipomas, and meningeal invasion by carcinoma.

Meningiomas show a high incidence among middle-aged women. They are usually single, relatively small, and located posterior or lateral to the spinal cord. Excluding those that occur in the region of the foramen magnum, approximately 90 per cent are found in the thoracic region. Signs of spinal cord compression develop insidiously so that an ataxic, spastic syndrome, which superficially resembles subacute combined degeneration of the spinal cord, may result. Moderate localized or segmental pain is presented in only 50 per cent of patients and is the central symptom in only 20 per cent. Tenderness on percussion of the vertebral spinous processes may be present. Tumors of the foramen magnum are particularly difficult to diagnose. Spastic ataxia and nystagmus can be early symptoms and may suggest multiple sclerosis rather than such a tumor. With foramen magnum tumor there may be pain or sensory loss in the C2 distribution, and the CSF protein is elevated.

X-ray may show bone erosion or calcification within a meningioma (4 per cent). Myelography is required for a precise localization of intraspinal meningiomas. In tumors of the foramen magnum a routine myelogram may be negative; therefore if such a tumor is suspected, myelography must be done in the supine as well as in the prone position to localize high, posteriorly placed tumors.

Neurofibromas arise from dorsal nerve roots, affect both sexes equally, occur at all ages, and may be present at any level of the spinal canal. Neurofibromas may extend extradurally but may also grow within the substance of the spinal cord. In some cases the tumors are part of a generalized neurofibromatosis. A small percentage of neurofibromas undergo sarcomatous changes and become invasive or metastasize.

Patients with intraspinal neurofibromas often give a history of longstanding radicular pain, and this symptom usually long precedes any sign of cord compression. When neurofibromas extend on either side of an intervertebral foramen, they may adopt a dumbbell or hourglass shape. X-rays, including oblique views of the spine, may show enlargement of a foramen and thinning of the adjacent pedicle. The degree of radiographic change may be out of proportion to the presenting symptoms. When the intraspinal portion of the tumor is small in comparison to the extraspinal, the latter may grow to such a large size that it is palpable externally even when there are few signs of cord compression.

As with meningiomas, the cerebrospinal fluid protein is almost always elevated. Myelography is essential for precise localization. A complete recovery usually follows the early surgical removal of both meningiomas and neurofibromas.

INTRAMEDULLARY TUMORS

Most of these tumors arise from constituent cells of the spinal cord. Ependymomas are the most common, followed by astrocytomas, glioblastomas, and oligodendrogliomas. In addition, vascular tumors (hemangioblastomas), lipomas, and even metastases may occur as intramedullary tumors.

Ependymomas arise at all levels of the spinal cord but have a preference for the caudal region. They represent more than two thirds of the tumors of the conus medullaris and are common causes of tumors of the filum terminale. Ependymomas may extend through several segments of the spinal cord; in rare instances the entire length of the cord is involved. Syringomyelia may develop in association with these and other intramedullary tumors. Spontaneous hemorrhages into ependymomas and hemangioblastomas occur and may give rise to sudden pain and neurologic deficit. Excluding glioblastomas and metastases, most intramedullary tumors have a slow progression. Dull, localized aching pain, muscle weakness or atrophy, impotence in males, and sphincter disturbances in both sexes are common early symptoms. Intramedullary tumors affecting the cervical or thoracic cord may cause sensory dissociation with predominant pain and temperature impairment. In such cases the sacral dermatomes are usually spared. In some patients, however, signs and symptoms may resemble Brown-Séquard's syndrome.

Longstanding intramedullary tumors may cause radiologically visible widening of the spinal canal and erosion of the pedicles. Contrast myelography usually demonstrates an enlarged spinal cord. In the lumbosacral region tumors may present as a pedunculated mass involving the cauda equina. Tumors of the filum terminale may be mobile and be a source of confusion for myelographic localization.

Successful surgical removal of intramedullary tumors is sometimes possible. Operative success is particularly high with ependymomas and hemangioblastomas, but recurrences may occur; gliomas respond poorly to any form of treatment, and lipomas are technically difficult to remove.

Davis, R. A., and Washburn, P. L.: Spinal cord meningiomas. Surg. Gynecol. Obstet., 131:15, 1970.
Harries, B.: Spinal cord compression. Br. Med. J., 1:611, 673, 1970.
Posner, J. B.: Neurological complications of systemic cancer. Med. Clin. North Am., 55:625, 1971.
Posner, J. B.: Management of central nervous system metastases. Semin. Oncol., 4:81, 1977.
Thomas, J. E., and Miller, R. E.: Lipomatous tumors of the spinal canal. Mayo Clin. Proc., 48:393, 1973.
White, W. A., Patterson, R. H., Jr., and Bergland, R. M.: Role of surgery in the treatment of spinal cord compression by metastatic neoplasm. Cancer, 27:558, 1971.

334.4. SPINAL ARACHNOIDITIS

Spinal arachnoiditis results from a low grade inflammation of the spinal meninges with formation of fibrous adhesions and loculation of cerebrospinal fluid. The changes extend throughout the length of the subarachnoid space or may be confined to a few segments. The adhesions may compress roots or the spinal cord itself.

Arachnoiditis may result from spinal surgery or spinal anesthesia and, more rarely, from myelography. It can be a late complication of subarachnoid hemorrhage, syphilis, tuberculosis, or other bacterial or parasitic spinal meningitides. In some cases no cause is found.

The development of symptoms and signs is insidious, the earliest symptoms usually reflecting multiple root involvement. This is particularly true if the adhesions extend into the lumbosacral spinal region, thereby involving the cauda equina. Pain is common and may be unrelated to movement; sensory symptoms usually exceed motor deficit. Signs of cord compression gradually develop and may progress to paraplegia; in other cases the disease process spontaneously arrests.

The diagnosis of spinal arachnoiditis depends upon the clinical course, as well as on examination of the cerebrospinal fluid and myelography. The CSF protein is elevated, and there may be pleocytosis. On myelography there are spotty, irregular collections of oil and an impairment of the flow of contrast material in the subarachnoid space.

When a specific infectious agent is identified, appropriate chemotherapy is indicated. Surgical exploration may provide histologic evidence as to the diagnosis, but laminectomy and removal of adhesions are not always beneficial for the relief of spinal and root compression.

Davidson, S.: Cryptococcal spinal arachnoiditis. J. Neurol. Neurosurg. Psychiatry, 31:76, 1968.
Guidetti, B., and LaTorre, E.: Hypertrophic spinal pachymeningitis. J. Neurosurg., 26:496, 1967.
Seaman, W. B., Marder, S. N., and Rosenbaum, H. E.: The myelographic appearance of adhesive spinal arachnoiditis. J. Neurosurg., 10:145, 1953.
Weiss, R. M., Sweeney, L., and Dreyfuss, M.: Circumscribed adhesive spinal arachnoiditis. J. Neurosurg., 19:435, 1962.
Wise, B. L., and Smith, M.: Spinal arachnoiditis ossificans. Arch. Neurol., 13:391, 1965.

334.5. ARTERIOVENOUS MALFORMATIONS AND OTHER VASCULAR LESIONS OF THE SPINAL CORD

Vascular malformations may be present on the surface of the spinal cord or within its substance. They may thus give rise to subarachnoid hemorrhage, intramedullary hemorrhage (hematomyelia), or both. Rarely, a spinal epidural hematoma results from such bleeding. The sudden development of partial or complete transverse myelopathy is the most common form of onset. This is manifested by paralysis, sensory impairment, and loss of sphincter control. If there is bleeding into the subarachnoid space, pain in the neck and back and other signs of meningeal irritation occur. Sudden headache, neck stiffness, and blood in the cerebrospinal fluid may be mistakenly attributed to hemorrhage of intracranial rather than intraspinal origin.

Arteriovenous malformations may also compress the spinal cord or give rise to hemodynamic changes that result in spinal ischemia. Distortion and compression of the cord by enlarged, abnormal vessels occur only gradually, and patients present with slowly progressive symptoms of spinal cord dysfunction. Transient exacerbation of symptoms may occur in association with menstrual periods or pregnancy.

Complete or partial recovery of function can follow episodes of spinal cord ischemia or even small hemorrhages. The unchanging localization of the attacks and the prominence of pain help to differentiate those symptoms caused by arteriovenous malformations from other recurrent neurologic disorders such as multiple sclerosis. In some patients a spinal bruit may be heard by auscultation over the site of the malformation.

Cavernous angiomas of the spinal cord are vascular hamartomas which may be associated with cysts and tumors in the organs or with hemangioblastomas of the cerebellum. Retinal vascular changes (von Hippel–Lindau syndrome) and cutaneous vascular nevi may be associated with spinal vascular malformations. The presence of these associated signs lends support to the assumption that, in a patient who presents them, spinal symptoms may be due to a vascular malformation.

Intraspinal bleeding caused by vascular malformation must be differentiated from bleeding that occurs as a complication of hemorrhagic diathesis, anticoagulant therapy, or collagen disease such as polyarteritis nodosa. In these conditions, however, there are usually signs of a more general disorder, cutaneous hematomas or other skin lesions, hematuria, or abnormal laboratory investigations.

In most patients with vascular malformations presenting with acute symptoms, examination of the cerebrospinal fluid reveals bloody or xanthochromic fluid, but, when there has been no recent bleeding, the only finding may be an elevated protein. Plain x-rays of the spine may show erosion, coexistent vertebral hemangiomas, or calcification within the spinal canal. On myelography, serpentine streaks within the column of oil may reveal the site of the vascular malformation. Angiography with regional catheterization of radicular vessels is a necessary preliminary to surgical treatment. Advances in microsurgery have increased considerably the chances for a satisfactory removal of spinal vascular malformations.

Antoni, N.: Spinal vascular malformations (angiomas) and myelomalacia, Neurology, 12:795, 1962.

Fine, R. D.: Angioma racemosum venosum of spinal cord with segmentally related angiomatous lesions of skin and forearm. J. Neurosurg., 18:546, 1961.

Henson, R. A., and Parsons, M.: Ischaemic lesions of the spinal cord: An illustrated review. Quart. J. Med., 36:205, 1967.

Houdart, R., Djindjian, R., Hurth, M., and Rey, A.: Treatment of angiomas of the spinal cord. Surg. Neurol., 2:186, 1974.

Matthews, W. B.: The spinal bruit. Lancet, 2:1117, 1959.

Taylor, J. R., and Van Allen M. W.: Vascular malformation of the cord with transient ischaemic attacks. J. Neurosurg., 31:576, 1969.

334.6.   SPINAL EPIDURAL HEMATOMA

Bleeding into the spinal epidural space may occur spontaneously but is more commonly associated with trauma, bleeding diathesis, or vascular malformations. It is a particular risk in patients receiving anticoagulants. The hemorrhage usually originates in the epidural venous plexus, and the hematomas tend to collect over the dorsum of the thoracic dura mater. Epidural hematomas vary in size, but the larger ones cause spinal cord compression. The clinical picture is characterized by the sudden onset of severe, localized back pain. Cord compression, when it occurs, results in the rapid development of flaccid paralysis, sensory loss, and impaired bladder and bowel control. The sudden onset of signs of cord compression in a patient on anticoagulants should allow few doubts as to the likelihood of a spinal epidural hematoma.

In epidural hematomas the cerebrospinal fluid may be clear or very slightly hemorrhagic.

Emergency surgical evacuation of the hematoma is essential. Although myelography is of great help in diagnosis and localization of epidural hematomas, this and other investigations should not take the place of prompt surgical intervention in order to avoid irreversible spinal cord damage.

Bidzinski, J.: Spontaneous spinal epidural hematoma during pregnancy. Case report. J. Neurosurg., 24:1017, 1966.

Jacobson, I., McCabe, J. J., Harris, P., and Dott, N. M.: Spontaneous spinal epidural hemorrhage during anticoagulant therapy. Br. Med. J., 1:522, 1966.

Markham, J. W., Lynge, H. N., and Stahlman, G. E. B.: The syndrome of spontaneous spinal epidural hematoma. Report of three cases. J. Neurosurg., 26:334, 1967.

Section Twenty-Three DISEASES OF THE PERIPHERAL NERVOUS SYSTEM

Peter James Dyck

335. DEFINITION OF PERIPHERAL NEUROPATHY

The term peripheral neuropathy includes any primary disorder of peripheral motor, sensory, and autonomic neurons. The clinical hallmarks are muscle weakness, with or without atrophy, sensory change, autonomic manifestations, or admixtures of these, from disease of peripheral neurons. The various clinical involvement patterns are of help in differential diagnosis and will be discussed in subsequent chapters.

The precise cause for many neuropathies is unknown, and the diagnosis of many neuropathies depends on their association with other diseases such as diabetes mellitus, carcinoma, or uremia.

Pathologic classifications are based on the nature of the fiber degeneration (wallerian, axonal degeneration, segmental demyelination) or the site of the pathologic changes, as well as on the specific histologic pattern (vasculitis, granulomatous reaction, hypertrophic repair, amyloidosis, and specific infective organism).

336. MONONEUROPATHIES AND PLEXUS NEUROPATHIES

336.1. CRANIAL NERVES

OLFACTORY NERVE. Anosmia is often the result of local disease of the nose, skull fracture, or brain tumor and may be reported by the patient as altered taste. Brief occurrences of stereotyped bad odors (or taste) not experienced by associates are from uncinate seizures — a condition not due to disease of the olfactory nerve but due to disease of the temporal lobe.

OPTIC NERVE. Altered vision is a symptom which may be due to refractive error, extra- and intraocular disease, developing diplopia or ptosis, optic nerve, optic tract, and optic radiation disease, and altered states of consciousness. Because of its serious implications and because treatment is available for many of its causes, this symptom should be investigated promptly by the appropriate medical specialist.

Disease of the optic nerve presents with loss of vision and a visual field defect. Temporary loss of visual activity followed by a pulsatile or sick headache is typical of migraine but may occasionally indicate cerebrovascular disease. Unilateral loss of vision accompanied by a central scotoma and an elevated optic disc is typical of papillitis. The appearance of the disc through the ophthalmoscope in papilledema may be no different from that of papillitis. Vision is not impaired in papilledema unless it is of long duration. In retrobulbar neuritis which not infrequently develops as a harbinger of more widespread multiple sclerosis, the patient has loss of vision (from a central scotoma) but no accompanying ophthalmoscopic abnormality. Intrinsic lesions of the optic nerve tend to produce scotomas, whereas untreated compressive lesions tend to produce monocular and binasal or bitemporal visual field defects. Such lesions include meningiomas, craniopharyngiomas, cholesteatomas, and chromophilic adenomas. Homonymous visual defects are usually the result of lesions of the optic pathways posterior to the chiasm from intrinsic brain disease.

OCULOMOTOR, TROCHLEAR, AND ABDUCENS. The motor nerves to the eyes may be damaged by a variety of diseases located anywhere in their long course from brainstem to orbit. In order of frequency the broad categories causing neurogenic extraocular palsies and pupillary disturbances are vascular disease (especially brainstem ischemia, hemorrhage and infarction, and aneurysm), neoplasm (both primary and secondary tumors), trauma, infections and postinfectious states, and congenital causes. The latter two causes are particularly common in the pediatric age group, whereas the vascular cause is especially common in old age, in hypertension, and in diabetes. The predominant symptom of dysfunction of these nerves is diplopia. Persons with a congenital palsy and those with disturbances of consciousness (especially in diseases affecting midbrain and pons) may be unaware of diplopia. Fluctuating diplopia, especially if improved with rest, suggests the diagnosis of myasthenia gravis.

The differential diagnosis of patients with an extraocular palsy and/or of a pupillary disturbance may not be easy. Congenital and traumatic causes are usually readily identified. In the former the deficit has been present since birth and is usually without symptoms. Trivial trauma does not as a rule produce extraocular palsy, and the maximal deficit is related in time to the trauma with usually slow improvement thereafter. An important cause of bilateral sixth cranial nerve palsy is increased intracranial pressure. Third cranial nerve palsy with pupillary enlargement and lid ptosis accompanying an ipsilateral cerebral hemisphere tumor is a sign of impending uncal herniation through the tentorium. Pontine gliomas, pituitary tumors, and nasopharyngeal and other tumors may directly displace the brainstem and cause damage of these cranial nerves. Episodic diplopia and pupillary disturbances may occur in transient cerebral ischemia (basilar artery), infrequently in migraine, and in berry aneurysm. Infectious and postinfectious states cause many of the transitory ocular palsies that affect children and young people. Extraocular palsies are especially common in chronic meningitis such as from tuberculosis, sarcoid, and cancer. They also may accompany presumptive viral meningitis and occur after trivial infections and exanthems. Short-lived extraocular palsy is not uncommon in acute inflammatory polyradiculoneuropathies. Third nerve palsy with sparing of pupillomotor function is associated with diabetes mellitus.

Abnormalities of pupillary size, shape, and reaction are not confined to third nerve injuries. The Argyll Robertson pupil is small, irregular, and usually bilateral, constricts to convergence accommodation but not to light, and responds poorly to mydriatics; it is common with neurosyphilis and rare with diabetes. The pupils of diabetics are often unequal, however, and may be nonreactive to light. Adie's myotonic pupil may cause confusion. It reacts only slowly to light or accommodation-convergence, but constricts to fresh 2.5 per cent methylcholine instilled into the conjunctival sac; a normal pupil lacks the latter reaction.

Bilateral external ophthalmoplegia of rapid or sudden onset occurs with four diseases, all of which are potentially serious and demand prompt treatment: acute myasthenia gravis, acute thiamin deficiency with Wernicke's encephalopathy, botulism, and acute inflammatory cranial polyneuropathy.

TRIGEMINAL. Generally speaking, disturbances of sensation of the face and anterior scalp are more likely to be due to brainstem lesions than to involvement of the gasserian ganglion, its roots, or its divisions. When they do occur, peripheral lesions are caused by tumor, infection, collagen disease, immunologic states, and intoxications. Herpes zoster and herpes simplex infections are discussed in Ch. 304 and 305. Painful states in the distribution of the trigeminal nerve include herpes zoster, trigeminal neuralgia (discussed in Ch. 260), and atypical face pain. Disturbed sensation in the face may accompany scleroderma. A hyperalgesic trigeminal neuropathy may be caused by stilbamidine and trichloroethylene.

FACIAL. Brain injury above the facial nucleus usually spares the innervation of the brow and forehead muscles because they are bilaterally represented at higher nervous levels; injury to the facial nerve at or peripheral to its nucleus paralyzes all the ipsilateral facial muscles. An intrapontine lesion causing facial weakness usually also affects abducens nerve function. As the facial nerve leaves the pons and enters the internal auditory meatus along with the acoustic nerve, it also carries fibers for lacrimation, salivation, and taste. As the nerve descends through the petrous bone, fibers to the lacrimal glands branch off first, and then salivary and taste fibers depart in the chorda tympani and cross the middle ear. Only motor fibers to the face emerge from the stylomastoid foramen. Thus the syndrome of seventh nerve damage varies according to the site of the injury. Acoustic neurinomas and other tumors of the cerebellopontine angle often involve the facial nerves, as do infections and neoplasms of the meninges.

Bell's palsy is a peripheral facial weakness of unknown cause and rapid onset, occasionally attended by aching pain about the angle of the jaw or behind the ear. Recent work has shown that the point of nerve conduction block is usually in the vicinity of the internal auditory meatus. Retraction of the angle of the mouth and eye closure are impaired, and the forehead is smooth on the affected side. Taste perception on the anterior part of the involved half of the tongue may be distorted. Rarely, hyperacusis results from paralysis of the stapedius muscle. Recovery usually begins within a week, and three of four patients fully recover over a period of several weeks. Occasionally, some permanent deficit remains after a protracted course. In such patients, asynchronous facial spasms may accompany voluntary facial movement. The use of adrenal corticosteroids begun near the onset of the illness and continued for seven to ten days is thought to speed recovery.

Herpes zoster affecting the geniculate ganglion produces a severe facial paralysis that is associated with a painful eruption within the external ear canal. This affection, often referred to as the Ramsay Hunt syndrome, may also involve the auditory nerve.

Chronic facial hemispasm affects middle-aged or older women somewhat more commonly than men, with spontaneous, unilateral, frequent, sudden, strong, brief contractions of part or all of the facial musculature. The condition usually begins in the orbicularis oculi muscle and, over many years, spreads to involve more of the face. In a few instances the disorder follows Bell's palsy. More often the cause is not known, but a slowly progressive, degenerative condition of the facial nucleus in the pons has been postulated, as has compression of the facial nerve by adjacent structures in the posterior fossa. Relief can be obtained by alcohol injection or section of the facial nerve, but it must be weighed against the facial paralysis necessarily produced. Relief has also been reported following intracranial surgical freeing of the facial nerve from adjacent structures.

Facial myokymia describes a condition of constant wormlike contractions of facial muscles. Such undulating, writhing, continuous movement is quite different from fasciculations, which are brief, synchronized contractions of muscle fibers. Myokymia is caused by intrapontine lesions such as tumors and multiple sclerosis.

AUDITORY. Disturbances of eighth nerve function are discussed in Ch. 262 and 263.

GLOSSOPHARYNGEAL. Glossopharyngeal neuralgia is described in Ch. 260.

HYPOGLOSSAL. This motor nerve to the tongue is uncommonly involved in its peripheral course, usually by neoplasms. Atrophy and fasciculation of the ipsilateral half of the tongue are seen, and the tongue deviates toward the affected side upon protrusion.

336.2. MONONEUROPATHY

PHYSICAL INJURY

Spinal nerves, plexuses, and peripheral nerve trunks may be injured by traction, compression, contusion, and laceration. Nerves may be damaged by electricity and radiation. Fractured bones may lacerate or compress nerves. Excessively tight casts or tourniquets may damage nerves by direct compression or by ischemia. Injection of penicillin or other medications into the sciatic nerve can cause serious injury, particularly if the vehicle for the medications is oil.

Recovery of nerve function is usually complete following acute compressive lesions and incomplete, faulty, or lacking in transected nerves. Recovery after contusion or section is greater in the young than in the old and in good than in poor fascicular apposition.

COMPRESSION AND ENTRAPMENT

The peripheral nerve trunks of the limbs are particularly prone to compression and entrapment, although any nerve passing over a rigid promontory or through a bony canal or tight fascial plane is vulnerable. The degree of compressive damage to nerves depends on the magnitude and duration of the force, on whether the force is repeated, on whether the nerve is anatomically situated next to soft or hard structures, on the physical habitus of the person, and on disease susceptibility. Malnutrition, diabetes mellitus, renal disease, and inflammatory neuropathy all are thought to predispose to compression damage. The tendency to compression damage is inherited in some families. For many years, investigators have differed as to whether ischemia or mechanical compression was the factor that produced nerve damage from compression. At an earlier time, the evidence favored ischemia; now it favors mechanical compression. Contusion and hemorrhage and later scarring may complicate some of the compressive lesions in man.

The term *entrapment* is given to the process by which nerves are damaged by repeated compression as they pass over a rigid structure or through a tight bony or fascial canal. Such injury occurs more readily when swelling, inflammation, or degeneration develops in adjacent joints and tendons (as may happen in pregnancy, rheumatoid arthritis, myxedema, and acromegaly). Suggestive evidence that multiple minor episodes of bruising of the nerve may contribute to the development of signs of entrapment comes from the common experience that excessive use of the wrist, in knitting or in gardening in the patient with the carpal tunnel syndrome, or in prolonged walking in patients with Morton's neuroma, will worsen symptoms. Sites of compression for the median nerve include the pronator teres muscle and the carpal tunnel ligament; for the ulnar nerve, the elbow wrist, pisohamate tunnel, palm, and metacarpal heads; for the radial nerve, the axilla, posterior aspect of the humerus, the supinator muscle, and radial aspect of distal forearm; for the lateral femoral cutaneous nerve, the pelvic brim; for the femoral nerve, the groin; for the saphenous nerve, the medial side of the knee; for the obturator nerve, the obturator canal; for the common peroneal nerve, the lateral aspect of the knee; for the superficial and deep peroneal nerves, muscle and fascial sheaths near their origin; for the posterior tibial nerve, the tarsal tunnel; and for plantar nerves, the sole of the feet.

The three most common entrapment neuropathies are the carpal tunnel syndrome, tardy ulnar palsy, and tardy peroneal nerve palsy.

CARPAL TUNNEL SYNDROME. In the carpal tunnel syndrome the median nerve is compressed as it passes through the canal made by the carpal bones and ligament. Some cases are idiopathic, and, in these, surgeons report a flattening of the median nerve just distal to the crease of the wrist and either thickening of the ligament or, more commonly, noninflammatory thickening of the synovia of the flexor tendons. The median nerve may be compressed within the carpal tunnel by a ganglion or by degenerative joint and synovial changes from rheumatoid arthritis, myxedema, and acromegaly.

This common disorder especially affects women. Pricking numbness and pain in the fingers and hands, coming on especially during the night and relieved by changing the position of the hands (shaking them), are characteristic. It is uncommon for patients to localize the numbness to the exact cutaneous distribution of the median nerve. Furthermore, the aching discomfort that may accompany the numbness may extend up the arm. Atrophy of the muscles innervated by the median nerve (for example, the thenar muscles) is not an early sign. In many cases it is possible to reproduce the painful numbness by holding the wrist in extreme flexion (Phalen's sign). Also, a burst of tingling may occur when the skin over the nerve at the wrist is percussed (Tinel's sign). There may be sensory loss in the distribution of the median nerve, although more frequently none is detected.

Measurement of Nerve Conduction. This provides an important confirmatory test and consists in determining the time from stimulation of the median nerve at a point above the carpal ligament to the appearance of the thenar muscle action potential. Similarly, one can determine the time from stimulation of digital fibers to the obtaining of an action potential in electrodes overlying the median nerve above the carpal ligament. In the carpal tunnel syndrome, the latency of both responses is usually prolonged.

Since the carpal tunnel syndrome may be brought on by an excess of gardening, ironing, sewing, crocheting, or similar activity, relief may follow the discontinuation of these activities. Immobilization of the wrist during the hours of sleep with a posterior splint of forearm and hand may give relief. Injections of corticosteroid preparations beneath the carpal ligament sometimes help. Treatment for an associated disease (myxedema, rheumatoid arthritis, acromegaly) may effect an improvement. However, in most instances the treatment of choice is surgical section of the carpal ligament, which usually provides almost immediate relief.

TARDY ULNAR NERVE PALSY. The ulnar nerve may be injured at the elbow, especially in persons with a shallow ulnar groove, those who rest their weight on their elbows excessively, and those who are cachectic and lie in bed.

Contrary to the findings in the carpal tunnel syndrome, muscle weakness and atrophy characteristically predominate over sensory symptoms and signs, possibly because the ulnar nerve at the elbow has relatively fewer sensory fibers than the median nerve at the wrist. Characteristically, the patient notices atrophy of the first dorsal interosseous muscle or difficulty in performing fine manipulations. There may be numbness of the small finger and contiguous half of the proximal and middle phalanges of the ring finger and ulnar border of the hand. Treatment consists of prevention of further injury. A doughnut cushion for the elbow may be helpful. Mobilizing and transplanting the nerve to a position in front of the medial epicondyle may prevent further progression of the disorder.

ACUTE RADIAL NERVE PALSY. The radial nerve may be compressed against a hard edge or surface in persons insensitized by an excess of alcohol or sedatives (Saturday night palsy) or may be compressed for excessive periods by the weight of a bed partner's head (bridegroom's palsy). Time usually provides complete recovery.

ACUTE AND TARDY PERONEAL NERVE PALSY. The common peroneal nerve is vulnerable where it crosses the head of the fibula, and can be injured when a person falls asleep in the sitting position with the knees crossed. A more chronic form occurs in cachectic patients who lie for prolonged periods with the legs externally rotated. In this disorder, dorsiflexion of the foot at the ankle and extension of the toes are weak, but usually little or no sensory loss is found over the lateral surface of the leg and on the dorsum of the foot.

TARSAL TUNNEL SYNDROME. Fractures of the ankle may compress the posterior tibial nerve, resulting in pain and numbness of the sole of the foot.

MERALGIA PARESTHETICA. Fat people wearing tight corsets, people wearing gun belts, and people with pendulous abdomens may develop superficial paresthesia and burning discomfort in the distribution of the lateral cutaneous nerve of the thigh. Presumably the trouble results from compression of this nerve as it passes beneath the inguinal ligament, but the condition sometimes arises without evident cause.

THORACIC OUTLET SYNDROME. Formerly, paresthesias of the fingers were frequently attributed to compression of the brachial plexus by a cervical rib or a tight scalene anterior muscle. Most such patients, however, prove to have either nerve root compression from a cervical disc or carpal tunnel syndrome.

336.3. MULTIPLE MONONEUROPATHY

Multiple mononeuropathy replaces the old term mononeuropathy multiplex. The term implies dysfunction that develops in the distribution of several individual nerve trunks at different times. At one time it was thought erroneously that this clinical pattern arose predominantly in association with vasculitis. It is now realized that the pattern may occur in leprosy (see Ch. 170), in necrotizing angiopathy, in inflammatory-immunologic disorders, in some metabolic diseases (some cases of uremia and diabetes mellitus), in familial disposition to pressure palsies, and in rare conditions involving blood and foreign body emboli to nerves and with iatrogenic nerve lesions.

A *necrotizing angiopathy* affects small arteries and arterioles within the epineurium of nerve trunks in periarteritis nodosa (see Ch. 53), in rheumatoid arthritis (see Ch. 56), and in other vasculitides. Such patients often have evidence of a multisystem disease affecting joints, skin, skeletal muscles, kidney, and other parenchymatous organs as well as evidence of a systemic illness with fever, cachexia, weight loss, and elevation of the sedimentation rate, and laboratory evidence suggesting a collagen-vascular involvement. Characteristically, the disorder begins with pain, paresthesias, or weakness in the distribution of a peripheral nerve which progresses to a maximal deficit within a few hours to several days. Other nerves become affected within days. The nerves of the lower extremities are affected more often than those of the upper, and neurologic signs are usually asymmetrical. After the initial involvement the disorder may improve,

relapse, or deteriorate. This type of neuropathy is a common manifestation of polyarteritis nodosa; it occurs less commonly with rheumatoid arthritis, Wegener's granulomatosis, Sjögren's syndrome, and Churg-Strauss syndrome.

The pathologic changes in most instances of necrotizing angiopathy affect the epineurial arteries of nerves. These may show degeneration of the media, fragmentation of the internal elastic lamina, thickening of the intima, and infiltration of the media and adventitia by mononuclear and polymorphonuclear cells (especially eosinophils). At necropsy segments of arterioles with occluded lumens may be widespread along the length of the nerve. Regions of nerve fiber degeneration do not coincide with these occluded vessels, but begin in isolated central regions of fascicles at watershed levels of poor blood perfusion. For the ulnar and median nerves this level is thought to be at mid-upper arm; for the peroneal and tibial nerves it is at midthigh. Because of separation and recombination of fascicles along the length of nerve, degenerating fibers arising from the focal areas of damage may be more randomly mixed with intact fibers in distal nerve.

336.4. PLEXUS NEUROPATHIES

BRACHIAL PLEXUS INJURY AND NEUROPATHY

The brachial plexus can be injured by traction, penetrating wounds, or compression. *Acute nontraumatic brachial plexus neuropathy* is a disorder of unknown cause. Antecedent needle injections into shoulder muscles, intercurrent infections, and an allergic basis have been suggested as possible etiologic factors. Factors causing it are also discussed in Ch. 337.3. Typically this disorder begins with aching pain in the lateral aspect of the shoulder or, less often, in the region of the elbow or arm. Muscle weakness develops within a few hours or days, and atrophy follows; sensory loss is usually minimal and is restricted to a small patch in the cutaneous distribution of the axillary nerve. The upper brachial plexus is affected more commonly than the lower, and therefore the weakness and atrophy are more often located in the region of the shoulder. In mild cases, improvement begins in a few weeks, and clinical recovery is complete within months. More characteristically, improvement does not begin for several months and may not be complete for years. Nevertheless, eventual complete or almost complete recovery is likely. Rarely, as one side improves, the other brachial plexus becomes affected. Careful examination by electromyography may reveal more extensive involvement of nerves than expected from the clinical examination. The cerebrospinal fluid is usually normal. There is no known treatment.

LUMBAR AND SACRAL PLEXUS AND ROOTS

Under the term *femoral neuropathy* (also called diabetic amyotrophy), a disorder has been described which in many cases involves lumbar roots and plexus. Many such cases occur in association with diabetes as described in Ch. 337.8, but sometimes no associated illness is found. Pain centered in the thigh and extending to the medial side of the leg may herald the onset of muscle weakness and atrophy, which usually develops rapidly over the next week. If the onset is abrupt and the neurologic signs are restricted to the distribution of the femoral nerve, an infarction of that nerve is a possibility. Careful examination and electromyography, however, often indicate that branches of multiple lumbar and sacral roots are affected with or without involvement of lumbar and sacral plexuses (in reality a lumbosacral radiculoplexus neuropathy). The cerebrospinal fluid protein may be elevated. Recovery may require months or years.

Occasionally, patients with lumbosacral plexus neuropathy present with the symptoms of sciatica, which differs from that caused by disc disease in the lack of a history of injury, the lack (usually) of marked back symptoms, and the clinical and electromyographic evidence of involvement of multiple roots and a negative myelogram. Although marked muscle weakness and wasting may occur, the outlook is usually favorable. The cause, pathology, and treatment are unknown.

337. POLYNEUROPATHY

337.1. DIFFERENTIAL DIAGNOSIS OF PERIPHERAL NEUROPATHY

SYMPTOMATOLOGY. Muscle weakness and atrophy are common in neuropathy. The first thing to decide is whether the weakness is myelopathic, neuropathic, neuromuscular, or myopathic. Spasticity, hyperreflexia, the Babinski sign, and a sensory level indicate a myelopathy. Muscle weakness associated with sensory symptoms, a reduction of tendon reflexes of a greater degree than accounted for by muscle atrophy, fasciculations, and a distal distribution of involvement favors neuropathy. In the absence of sensory changes, reliable differentiation of neuropathic from myopathic and from neuromuscular weakness depends heavily on the characteristics of nerve conduction and electromyographic examination. Reduction or absence of sensory nerve fiber action potentials, low nerve conduction of motor fibers, and the finding of fibrillation potentials with or without an increase in the size of motor unit potential favor a neuropathy. In myopathy motor unit potentials are small in amplitude and often polyphasic. Abnormalities of neuromuscular transmission in myasthenia gravis are recognized by a fall in amplitude of the muscle action potential when 3 per second supramaximal stimuli are given to the nerve. The abnormalities of neuromuscular transmission are different between the myasthenic syndrome, botulism, and drug-induced defects of neuromuscular transmission.

If it has been decided that the muscle weakness is neurogenic, one needs to know whether it is focal or diffuse and from what level along the length of the peripheral nerve it arises — roots, plexus, or nerve trunks. Proximal limb and axial involvement suggests proximal nerve involvement, raised cerebrospinal fluid protein suggests leptomeningeal (or root) involvement, and paraspinal denervation confirms this locus.

Sensory symptoms are typical of neuropathy and include two kinds. The first type occurs spontaneously and consists of symptoms of an "asleep feeling," "tightness," "coolness," "burning," "tingling," "aching," "tenderness," or other so-called "positive symptoms." These may be particularly bothersome during inactivity, as at night when they are characteristic of the "restless leg syndrome." In other patients "positive symptoms" of the feet are accentuated by walking and of the hands by their use in work or play. The second type of sensory symptom expresses the functional deficit from abnormal sensation, the so-called "negative symptoms." Unsteadiness, clumsiness, inability to recognize objects by feel, and mutilation without pain are examples of this group of symptoms.

Autonomic abnormalities are characteristic of some neuropathies. Postural hypotension is the most striking and usually implies involvement of the greater splanchnic nerves to the viscera. Impotence, incontinence of bladder and bowel, and anhidrosis are other important autonomic symptoms.

Peripheral neuropathy does not always present with the characteristic triad of distal limb muscle weakness and atrophy, absent tendon reflexes, and sensation loss. To illustrate, early in the course of neuropathy, loss of muscle stretch reflexes or reliable evidence of sensation loss may not be present. Several patterns of neuropathic symptomatology are useful in differential diagnosis.

PATTERNS OF NEUROPATHIC SYMPTOMS

HIGH ARCHES; CURLED UP TOES; AND PAINFUL CORNS AND CALLUSES. The recognition that a patient has a pes cavus foot deformity or other skeletal abnormality suggests an inherited neuromuscular disorder. If lower motor neurons are predominantly affected, such patients have a progressive muscular atrophy (hereditary motor neuropathy); if primary sensory neurons are predominantly affected, probably a hereditary sensory neuropathy; and if both lower motor and primary sensory neurons are affected, a hereditary motor and sensory neuropathy. Pes cavus is also common (probably because of the associated involvement of lower motor neurons) in spastic paraplegia and in spinocerebellar degenerations such as Friedreich's ataxia. Rarely, high arches are observed in longstanding myopathy.

CLAW HAND. This is the counterpart in the hand of pes cavus in the foot. Unlike pes cavus, however, which is usually due to neuromuscular disorders which begin in infancy or childhood, claw hand may come on at any age. If it occurs asymmetrically and without sensory abnormality, it may signal the onset of motor neuron disease or an unusual lower brachial plexus neuropathy. An associated sensory loss suggests the diagnosis of tardy ulnar palsy, cervical spondylosis, syringomyelia, intramedullary cervical tumor, or adult onset Tangier disease.

MUSCLE WEAKNESS OF LOWER LIMBS WITHOUT SENSORY SYMPTOMS. The absence of sensory signs is the important characteristic to look for. To confirm the lack of sensory involvement, recording of the latency and amplitude of afferent potentials over median, ulnar, and sural nerves should be obtained. Muscle weakness of lower limb muscles results in difficulties described as "unsteadiness," "stumbling," and "awkwardness in walking." Patients with bilateral foot drop tend to trip or stumble, and to walk with a steppage gait. Patients with weakness of plantar and dorsiflexion are unable to "stand still without holding onto something," or they may need to "brace their knees" against the cabinet of the sink when washing the face or shaving. Patients with quadriceps weakness may experience "collapsing" or "buckling" of the lower limb, to the point of falling down. They may not be able to arise from a seated position without the use of the hands or to climb stairs without a rail. A waddling gait reflects gluteal weakness.

The aforementioned symptoms suggest the possibility of a myopathy, a disorder of motoneurons, or, less often, a disorder of neuromuscular transmission. Reliable methods to distinguish myopathy and defects of neuromuscular transmission from neurogenic involvement are provided by the specialized techniques of electromyographic laboratories. Among neurogenic causes of weakness, poliomyelitis and motor neuron disease have mainly an asymmetrical distribution, whereas inflammatory polyradiculoneuropathy, porphyria, and hereditary motor neuropathy are mostly symmetrical.

BILATERAL DISTAL WEAKNESS OF THE HANDS, AND PROXIMAL WEAKNESS OF THE UPPER LIMBS WITHOUT SENSORY SYMPTOMS OR SIGNS. The list of conditions to be considered resembles that of the preceding category. Hyperreflexia, the Babinski sign, and long-tract sensory signs in the lower limb suggest possible cervical cord disease.

MUSCLE WEAKNESS OF LOWER LIMBS WITHOUT "POSITIVE" SENSORY SYMPTOMS BUT WITH SENSORY SIGNS. With a few exceptions, the lack of "positive" sensory symptoms in the presence of a testable abnormality of cutaneous sensation implies longstanding disease to which the patient has accommodated. The differential diagnosis includes inherited motor and sensory neuropathy, acute and chronic inflammatory polyradiculoneuropathy, and other rare conditions.

MUSCLE WEAKNESS OF LOWER LIMBS WITHOUT "POSITIVE" SENSORY SYMPTOMS. Sensory symptoms may be roughly divided into those found in patients with acute and subacute degeneration of large fibers, those associated with degeneration of small fibers, and those with mixtures of both.

Selective degeneration of large fibers of limb nerves results in abnormalities of touch-pressure, of vibration, and of joint position and motion sensations. Patients may describe their toes or feet as "asleep" or feeling as if a local anesthetic has been injected. The term pseudotabes has been applied when impairment of joint position is sufficient to result in locomotor ataxia. A similar involvement in the upper limbs may produce a disability to recognize the shape of objects by the sense of feel.

Selective degeneration of small myelinated and unmyelinated fibers often produces symptoms of hyperalgesia, described as "burning," "stinging," "prickling," or "aching." Tenderness and hypersensitivity are characteristic. The feet may have a raised threshold of sensation yet be hypersensitive once the threshold is exceeded, producing painfulness in walking.

Disorders which tend to affect large fibers selectively include inflammatory polyradiculoneuropathy, neuropathy associated with multiple myeloma, leukemia, and dysproteinemias, and neuropathy associated with hypothyroidism. Disorders which tend to involve predominantly small fibers include amyloidosis, inherited sensory neuropathy, Fabry's disease, and Tangier disease. A variety of toxins, drugs, and vitamin deficiencies (particularly thiamin deficiency associated with alcoholism and vitamin B_{12} deficiency in pernicious anemia), as well as less clear insults associated with uremia, amyloidosis, peripheral vascular disease, and malabsorption, may affect both large and small fibers. Diabetic neuropathy can affect large fibers, small fibers, or both.

SENSORY LOSS OF DISTAL LOWER LIMBS WITHOUT MUSCLE WEAKNESS. The differential diagnosis depends on whether large or small fibers are predominantly affected and on the chronicity of the disorder. Large fiber involvement is particularly seen in posterior inflammatory polyradiculoneuropathy and in spinocerebellar degeneration. Small fiber involvement with or without large fiber involvement occurs with herpes zoster, in hereditary sensory neuropathies, in carcinomatous sensory neuropathy, and in some cases of inflammatory sensory polyradiculoneuropathy. Mild neurogenic weakness in affected segments is common.

Patients with neuropathy involving small fibers often have autonomic symptoms, including postural hypotension, anhidrosis, impotence, and disturbances of gut motility. Whether these symptoms reflect preganglionic or postganglionic involvement or degeneration, or both, is not known for most disorders. The symptoms are characteristic of amyloidosis, hyperalgesic diabetic neuropathy, malabsorption syndromes, the Riley-Day syndrome, and the Shy-Drager syndrome.

DIFFERENTIAL DIAGNOSIS BY CHARACTERISTICS OF NERVE CONDUCTION AND ELECTROMYOGRAPHY

The determination of nerve conduction velocity and electromyography have assumed an increasingly important role in establishing the presence and type of neuropathic involvement. As described below, involvement of large, alpha motoneurons may be of at least three types: (1) rapid degeneration of the entire neuron (neuronal degeneration), (2) axonal degeneration of the distal axon (dying-back) with or without atrophy and with or without secondary segmental demyelination, and (3) primary segmental demyelination. In neuronal degeneration, nerve conduction velocity tends to remain within normal limits until marked muscle weakness occurs. Needle electromyography shows denervation and an increased size of motor unit potentials. In axonal degeneration, low conduction velocity occurs only when the majority of fibers show the features of axonal atrophy and secondary segmental demyelination and remyelination. The features of the electromyogram will be similar to those of anterior horn cell disorders. In primary segmental demyelination, Schwann cell function is altered because of an inborn error of metabolism, by toxin, or by immunologic mechanism. Nerve conduction velocity is reduced and muscle action potentials are reduced in size and dispersed. Special techniques can determine low conduction in both proximal and distal segments of nerve. Denervation, which often accompanies segmental demyelination, implies concomitant axonal degeneration.

The evaluation of abnormality of A alpha primary afferent neurons by clinical neurophysiologic techniques is less complete than for alpha motoneurons. A decrease in amplitude and increase in latency of ulnar, median, and sural nerve action potentials provide evidence of such an abnormality. Adequate clinical neurophysiologic evaluation of gamma motoneuron fibers, of A delta and somatic C fibers, and of sympathetic C fibers is not possible at this time. This lack is often not a serious limitation, as most neuropathic conditions also involve A alpha fibers.

DIFFERENTIAL DIAGNOSIS OF PERIPHERAL NEUROPATHY BY PATHOLOGY

Pathologic changes in peripheral nerve tissue can be divided broadly into interstitial and parenchymatous. Interstitial pathologic changes arise outside the nerve and Schwann cells and may damage these cells secondarily. Usually in interstitial neuropathies the initial change is in the supporting tissue of the nerve or in its blood vessels. Examples include amyloidosis, necrotizing angiopathy, and acute, chronic, and relapsing inflammatory polyradiculoneuropathy. In parenchymatous neuropathies, the nerve and Schwann cells are primarily affected from various causes such as inherited metabolic diseases, toxic substances, deficiency states, and other metabolic diseases. Examples of parenchymatous neuropathies are those caused by alcohol, lead, arsenic, diphtheria, and metachromatic leukodystrophy.

To help characterize the pathologic involvement it is helpful to ask the following questions: Which populations of neurons are affected? What is the level of damage within neurons? What is the type of fiber degeneration? How extensive? What kind of repair or regeneration has occurred?

A highly selective involvement by population of neurons may occur in neuropathic disease, e.g., in hereditary motor neuropathy, lower motor neurons; in Fabry's disease, A delta and somatic C neurons; and in Friedreich's ataxia, A alpha neurons.

The level of involvement within neurons may be characteristic for various neuropathies. To illustrate, in some neuropathies the entire neuron degenerates. This is seen in so-called anterior horn cell diseases, e.g., in poliomyelitis and in motor neuron disease. Such generalized neuronal degeneration may also affect primary afferent neurons, e.g., in herpes zoster and in Friedreich's ataxia. The degeneration of entire neurons is in contrast to diseases in which distal axons degenerate — dying-back neuropathies, e.g., in uremic neuropathy.

Several types of nerve fiber degeneration are recognized. In both wallerian and axonal degeneration, involvement of the axon is primary. In wallerian degeneration from crush or section of nerve, the distal axon inevitably degenerates by a series of rapid stereotyped histologic changes. In man wallerian degeneration occurs from compression, crush, or traction and from transection of fibers as, for example, in necrotizing angiopathic neuropathy. In axonal degeneration the course may be less rapid than in wallerian degeneration, axonal atrophy may precede degeneration, and electron microscopic abnormalities of axis cylinders may be present prior to dissolution of the myelinated fiber. Also, focal axonal abnormalities in some disorders may lead secondarily to wallerian degeneration of the distal axon.

At least two types of segmental demyelination are recognized. In primary segmental demyelination, the Schwann cells are affected first and predominantly. For example, in inflammatory polyradiculoneuropathy, involvement of interstitial mononuclear cells results in myelin damage, whereas in lead neuropathy a metabolic poisoning of Schwann cells probably is involved. A secondary segmental demyelination (secondary to axonal atrophy or disease) seems to characterize those neuropathies with axonal atrophy, e.g., in Friedreich's ataxia and in uremia.

The neurologic deficits from demyelinating lesions tend to be less severe and shorter lived than those from axonal degeneration. Nerve repair following a crush lesion is rapid and more complete than when the nerve trunk is transected. Nerve regeneration tends to be better in the young than in the old.

NERVE BIOPSY

Nerve biopsy can usually provide specific answers to the following questions: Is neuropathy present? What populations of fibers are affected? What type of fiber degeneration is occurring? How severe and how fast is it? Is regeneration or fiber repair occurring? Can specific diagnostic features be recognized? Cutaneous nerve biopsy (usually of the sural nerve) may provide diagnostic information in amyloidosis, in necrotizing angiopathic neuropathy, in leprosy, in sarcoidosis, and in various lipidoses such as metachromatic leukodystrophy and Fabry's disease. A presumptive diagnosis from nerve biopsy may be possible in inflammatory neuropathies, in lymphoproliferative disorders, and in myxedema. Despite its usefulness in diagnosis, however, nerve biopsy should be used sparingly because it may leave a longlasting, disagreeable, and sometimes painful numbness. Nerve biopsies should probably be performed only in centers which have specialized laboratories expert in dealing with this tissue.

337.2. NEUROPATHY ASSOCIATED WITH INFECTION

Diphtheria is commonly complicated by paralysis of the nasopharynx and oculomotor and ciliary muscles. More widespread cranial polyneuropathy is uncommon. A more generalized peripheral neuropathy may occur several weeks after the pharyngeal infection has subsided. The disease is discussed fully in Ch. 145.

Herpes zoster, with infection of the gasserian or spinal ganglia, produces a characteristic cutaneous lesion followed by a persistent hyperalgesic, anesthetic monoradiculopathy in the affected dermatome. The first division of the gasserian ganglion and intercostal dermatomes are most frequently affected. Although the painful state may persist for prolonged periods, it eventually remits in almost all instances (see Ch. 305).

Leprosy is one of the most common neuropathies on a worldwide scale. Diagnosis depends on recognizing the distinctive sites of predilection and the associated cutaneous involvement, and on histologic studies. New forms of treatment are completely changing the way these patients are being handled and their prognosis. This subject is discussed in Ch. 170.

337.3. NEUROPATHY ASSOCIATED WITH INFLAMMATION AND PRESUMED ALTERED IMMUNITY

Serum sickness neuropathy typically begins within seven to ten days of the injection of a foreign protein. The condition was more frequent when bacterial infections were treated with foreign antisera. A brachial plexus neuropathy occurs more frequently than does more diffuse peripheral neuropathy. One should consider serum sickness when the neuropathy is superimposed on a history of arthralgia, skin eruption, fever, albuminuria, and possible cerebral symptoms. Episodes of neuropathic involvement may recur over the course of several weeks. The pathogenesis is as follows: The introduction of foreign protein elicits an immune response. Initially because of an excess of antigen, the immune complexes are small and circulate freely. As antibodies build up, immune complexes become large and less soluble and are deposited between endothelial cells and basement membranes of blood vessels. Serum complement is bound and activated, and polymorphonuclear leukocytes release hydrolases which damage vessel walls. An acute inflammatory necrotizing vasculitis ensues.

337.4. ACUTE INFLAMMATORY POLYRADICULONEUROPATHIES

Acute inflammatory polyradiculoneuropathies are a group of disorders which probably have a similar pathologic and etiologic basis but can differ in their anatomic sites of predilection and their temporal profile. Understanding of etiologic and pathologic factors is incomplete, but investigators generally believe that infection, particularly by viruses, plays a role. Because a diverse group of viruses, bacterial agents, and foreign proteins may produce similar disorders, it seems unlikely that direct infection of nerve cells by these organisms is involved. Most likely, viruses produce an indirect effect through immunologic mechanisms. The pathologic hallmarks of the disorder are infiltrates of mononuclear cells around capillaries within nerve tissue, edema of the endoneurial compartment, and segmental demyelination and remyelination. Sensitized lymphocytes are thought to be involved in the myelin damage. The disorder may recur in some patients. Since the disorder may affect more than one family member, genetic factors may influence susceptibility. The pathologic lesions are patchy and tend to be widely distributed along the length of the nerves. In the motor variety, the predominant pathologic changes lie in the ventral spinal roots; in the sensory variety, in the posterior spinal roots; and in the autonomic variety, possibly in the sympathetic and autonomic ganglia of the abdomen. Four clinical syndromes are recognized: motor polyradiculoneuropathy, sensory polyradiculoneuropathy, autonomic neuropathy, and polyneuritis

cranialis. The clinical and pathogic features, at least of the motor and sensory syndromes, are sufficiently alike to seem to be explained by different anatomic sites of involvement rather than by different mechanisms. Pure syndromes of motor and of sensory involvement are uncommon. In mixed syndromes motor symptomatology predominates.

ACUTE INFLAMMATORY MOTOR POLYRADICULONEUROPATHY
(Landry-Guillain-Barré-Strohl Syndrome)

Approximately one half of patients give a history of a mild upper respiratory infection one to two weeks before the onset of muscle weakness. For the most part the specific virus or bacterial infection remains unknown, but the syndrome has been known to follow infection with measles, mumps, rubella, influenza A, influenza B, varicella-zoster, cytomegalovirus, infectious mononucleosis, vaccinia, variola, infectious hepatitis, coxsackievirus, and echoviruses. Cases have been described to follow the injection of a foreign protein, cat scratch, dog bite, blood transfusion or immunization, as was seen in the widespread influenza vaccine program of 1976 (see Ch. 82).

All the polyneuropathies tend to begin subacutely with relatively mild initiating symptoms and few or no systemic symptoms and signs. A small percentage of patients have unspecific malaise and headache, but chills, fever, stiff neck, and severe headaches are generally absent. Signs and symptoms of neurologic dysfunction usually appear first in a restricted part of the body, and are often relatively mild at onset. The rate of further progression varies widely. Some patients become severely paralyzed within no more than a few days, whereas in others the neuropathy worsens insidiously and slowly over a period of several days or even weeks.

In the syndrome originally described by Landry, there is an ascending paralysis which develops over the course of approximately one week, reaches a plateau for several weeks, and then improves. Most often, symptoms of acute polyneuropathy begin with some abnormality of walking, climbing stairs, or rising from a seated position. Muscle weakness tends to involve both proximal and distal limb muscles. The extent of paralysis varies widely from patient to patient. In the more severe cases, most of the cranial nerves except for the first, second, and eighth may be affected. Facial weakness and weakness of chewing and swallowing occur most frequently. Muscle weakness can affect all skeletal muscles of the limb and trunk.

Although muscle weakness and atrophy predominate in most patients, few fail to develop evidence of sensory involvement at some time during the course. Patients may report feelings of prickling numbness, bandlike tightness, altered sensation when the skin is touched, thermal sensations, and painful sensations. Typically these involve the feet but may extend upward to other parts of the lower limbs or the body. Sensory symptoms may accompany the onset of muscle weakness and then disappear, or may persist throughout the entire illness and be a major component of the disease. Some patients may have symptoms of unsteadiness in walking and severe loss of tactile sensation.

Involvement of the autonomic nervous system may

occur even in these predominantly motor polyradiculoneuropathies. Most commonly this is reflected by postural hypotension in the sitting or standing position after prolonged recumbency. Cramping abdominal pain may result from an atonic bowel. Bladder or bowel incontinence is rare.

The diagnosis is confirmed by the characteristic clinical course, the cerebrospinal fluid findings, the typical characteristics of the nerve conduction and electromyographic examination, and the lack of laboratory evidence of other disease. Characteristically the cerebrospinal fluid pressure is normal and the fluid is clear, contains less than 5 lymphocytes per cubic millimeter, and contains an elevated protein content. On occasion, however, either an increased number of lymphocytes or a normal protein level is found in otherwise typical cases. In approximately two thirds of cases, conduction velocity of motor fibers of distal limb nerves is less than 60 per cent of normal values. In such cases, the amplitude of the muscle action potential may be reasonably well preserved. When more proximal sites along the length of the limb nerves are stimulated, a reduction in muscle action potential may occur, implying a proximal block of motor fibers. In one third of cases, motor nerve conduction may be normal. In such instances, a proximal block or slowing of nerve fiber conduction would provide evidence of a segmentally demyelinating lesion in the proximal portion of nerves.

The differential diagnosis of acute inflammatory polyneuropathy includes acute intermittent porphyria and the neuropathy associated with leukemia, lymphoma, and multiple myeloma. Acute intermittent porphyria is recognized by the additional features of a delirium and by laboratory evidence of porphobilinogen excretion. The polyradiculoneuropathies associated with carcinoma and with lymphoma usually develop more insidiously and may be recognized by their radiographic and systemic alterations.

The first concern in the treatment of acute inflammatory motor polyradiculoneuropathy is to maintain an adequate airway and to provide ventilatory assistance as necessary. Fluid and food intake must be monitored so that supplementation may be begun either by tube feeding or by intravenous feeding. Corticosteroid hormones are reported to provide a small but significant improvement in the rate of recovery. The risk of complications is reduced by restricting such treatment to short periods of time. Convalescence may last for months or several years and should include physical therapy. Initially this should consist of passive exercises and later of active exercises. If at all possible the education of students should continue during this illness. Most patients make an almost complete improvement from this neuropathic disease.

ACUTE INFLAMMATORY SENSORY POLYRADICULONEUROPATHY

Involvement predominantly of the posterior root and spinal ganglion results in a sensory polyradiculoneuropathy which is probably the counterpart of the ventral spinal root involvement described above. As in the motor variety, a preceding infection may antedate the neurologic syndrome by several weeks. Typically the onset is marked by combinations of sensory dysfunction and pain. The sensory dysfunction is most commonly described as unsteadiness in gait or clumsiness in the use of the hands. Even more incapacitating are the painful dysesthesias which develop in some patients. Varying combinations of lancinating pain, prickling hyperesthesia, constricting band-like sensations, and burning or coldness of skin may be described. Most patients appreciate that the hyperesthetic skin is insensitive but that when the threshold for sensation is exceeded the discomfort is excessive. Any region of the body may be affected, and the disorder involves proximal as well as distal dermatomes. On clinical examination the lower extremities tend to be affected more than the upper, and the various modalities of sensation may be affected to different degrees. The patients often exhibit sensory ataxia, and, because of the severe impairment of joint position, the limbs may be held in distorted positions. Tendon reflexes are often diminished or absent.

Minor degrees of involvement of motor and autonomic neurons are not uncommon. In addition, patients have difficulty is sustaining muscle contraction in the presence of severe involvement of their afferent peripheral nervous system. The cerebrospinal fluid changes are similar to those in the motor variety. The motor nerve conduction velocity, the amplitude of the muscle action potential, and the distal latency may be within normal limits. By contrast, nerve action potentials cannot be elicited from stimulation of afferent nerve fibers either because the afferent fibers have degenerated or because the action potential is so dispersed.

Prognosis for recovery in sensory polyneuropathy is less good than in the motor variety, and symptoms of cutaneous hyperpathia often persist or recur for many years. The sensory ataxia usually improves but likewise often does not recover completely. This persistence of the neurologic deficit probably is explained by irreversible damage of spinal ganglion neurons. Affected craftsmen and professionals whose work depends on manual dexterity often require retraining in less skilled work.

ACUTE INFLAMMATORY AUTONOMIC NEUROPATHY
(Pandysautonomia)

Acute inflammatory autonomic neuropathy is a poorly understood, rare condition which may be the autonomic counterpart of the motor and sensory varieties described above. The onset and time course are similar to the motor and sensory neuropathies, but to date pathologic studies are unavailable. The principal symptoms include postural hypotension, cramping abdominal pain, and varying amounts of diarrhea and constipation. The hypotension may be so severe that the patient cannot sit up without losing consciousness. The cramping abdominal pain presumably is caused by regions of atonic bowel. Affected subjects reportedly improve with time, but few long-term follow-up studies are available. The use of fitted elastic stockings and oral fludrocortisone may hasten resumption of the erect position. The cramping abdominal pain may be modified by the use of frequent small bland feedings and antispasmodic agents.

337.5. CHRONIC INFLAMMATORY POLYRADICULONEUROPATHY

(Including Recurrent Polyradiculoneuropathy)

In chronic inflammatory polyradiculoneuropathy the neurologic deficit tends to develop slowly over months or years and persists for years. Some patients have a monophasic course over many years. Others have a stepwise progression to their maximal deficit and then slowly improve. Still others have a recurrent course with ultimate worsening or ultimate improvement. A few patients progress slowly to death several years later. As in the acute inflammatory polyradiculoneuropathies, the process tends to involve symmetrical proximal body structures and to affect motor, autonomic, and sensory peripheral neurons in varying proportions. The cerebrospinal fluid protein is usually elevated. The pathologic alterations initially resemble those of the acute variety, but with time hypertrophic neuropathy develops. Sural nerve biopsy may show features of the disease without cellular infiltrates. The characteristics of the nerve conduction and electromyographic examination are not unlike those of the acute variety, except that there probably are fewer cases with preserved normal nerve conduction. Over a period of years most patients eventually improve beyond their maximal deficit but continue to have a significant neurologic problem.

The use of prednisone often indicates a dramatic improvement. Regrettably, such effects soon wear off in most instances, and long-term steroid therapy should be avoided because of its complications.

337.6. SARCOID NEUROPATHY

Sarcoid neuropathy most commonly affects the facial nerve, and when it does it is indistinguishable from Bell's palsy. Occasionally other cranial nerves may be affected, or a more generalized neuropathy may be found (see Ch. 65).

337.7. NEUROPATHY ASSOCIATED WITH MESENCHYMAL DISEASE AND NECROTIZING ANGIOPATHY

Neuropathy is a relatively common complication of periarteritis nodosa, of Wegener's and other granulomas, and of rheumatoid arthritis. It is less commonly associated with Sjögren's syndrome and with cranial arteritis. Mononeuropathy may develop in any of these patients when nerves are compressed by immobilization, recumbency, or inflamed tissue within tight compartments. More often, these patients develop a characteristic and distinctive multiple mononeuropathy as a result of a necrotizing angiopathy. Usually such patients first develop a neurologic deficit in the distribution of a major limb nerve such as the peroneal or the ulnar. Characteristically, with peroneal nerve involvement, the patient becomes aware of his inability to dorsiflex the foot at the ankle. This is followed within hours or days by burning discomfort of the top of the foot and lateral side of the leg. In short succession other limb nerves may sequentially become affected. Pathologically, nerve fibers in regions of poor blood perfusion (usually at midthigh and mid-upper arm levels) become damaged only after occlusion of multiple epineurial arteries so that clinically one is seeing a late stage of the pathologic process. Corticosteroids are commonly used for treatment, usually with at least symptomatic improvement.

337.8. NEUROPATHY ASSOCIATED WITH DIABETES MELLITUS

FREQUENCY AND EPIDEMIOLOGY. The reported frequency of neuropathy among diabetic patients ranges widely, from 5 to 60 per cent. The difference is mainly due to differences of definition of what constitutes neuropathy and of the criteria and techniques used to diagnose it. If a mild reduction of nerve conduction velocity is used, neuropathy occurs in approximately 60 per cent of diabetics. The frequency of neuropathy increases with age and with the duration of diabetes.

ETIOLOGY. It seems unlikely that a single mechanism underlies the various types of diabetic neuropathy. Nerve damage from ischemia to distal lower limbs represents one variety, and compression may be another. The mechanism of nerve fiber damage in the more diffuse types of neuropathy is less well understood. A diffuse microangiopathy of endoneurial capillaries with alteration of blood nerve barrier seems a reasonable possibility. Alternative explanations include immunologic or biochemical derangements, insulin deficiency, or phospholipid deficiency. No explanation stands fully proved.

CLINICAL SYMPTOMATOLOGY AND CLASSIFICATION. The various types of diabetic neuropathy overlap each other, but the following classification illustrates the diverse types.

Asymptomatic Neuropathy. Although incompletely studied, asymptomatic low nerve conduction velocity is associated with morphologic abnormality of nerve fibers.

Neuropathy with Peripheral Vascular Disease. Diabetic patients with severe peripheral vascular disease affecting the distal lower limb may develop a distal, stocking-like ischemic neuropathy. Sensory and autonomic symptoms predominate. Only nerves in the territory of the ischemia are affected.

Ataxic Neuropathy (Pseudotabes Diabetica). A diffuse symmetrical distal neuropathy especially affecting the lower limbs is common in diabetics, particularly in longstanding disease and even in patients with mild diabetes mellitus. In most cases the neuropathy involves both large and small afferent fibers, as well as autonomic fibers and motor fibers. Mild cases produce nonpainful numbness of the toes and the front part of the foot. Varying degrees of sensory ataxia are found with more severe cases. The Achilles and, less frequently, the quadriceps reflex disappear. Touch-pressure, joint position, and vibration sensations are variably abnormal in the distal lower limb, less so in the upper. Pain and thermal discriminations tend to be spared.

Hyperalgesic Neuropathy. With hyperalgesic neuropathy the patients have burning painfulness of the skin of the toes, feet, and legs. In addition lancinating pain, tightness, hypersensitivity of the feet, and deep aching in the limbs may be present. Night pain in the legs, with the features of restless legs, can be improved only by movement such as getting out of bed and moving about. Autonomic involvement resulting in postural hypotension, anhidrosis, and impotence is more common in hyperalgesic than in ataxic neuropathy.

Autonomic Neuropathy. Autonomic symptoms of mild degree are common in diabetes, especially with neuropathy. In the variety called *autonomic neuropathy,* postural hypotension, impotence in the male, and bladder and bowel incontinence in both sexes are particularly troublesome. These patients tend to have hyperalgesic symptoms as well.

Diabetic Lumbosacral Plexus Neuropathy (Diabetic Amyotrophy and Femoral Neuropathy). The terms used to describe this type of diabetic neuropathy draw attention to different clinical presentations. So-called *femoral neuropathy* often begins suddenly with pain in the anterior aspect of the thigh, followed within a few days by marked weakness, and later atrophy, of the quadriceps muscle. The pattern of electromyographic denervation reveals that the disorder extends beyond the femoral nerve and involves either the lumbosacral plexus or the roots, or both. A rapid improvement in some cases speaks against the disorder's being due to vascular occlusion. If muscle weakness and atrophy predominate and the disorder affects both legs, the term *diabetic amyotrophy* has been applied.

TREATMENT. Only weak evidence indicates that close diabetic control prevents or ameliorates diabetic neuropathy. The pain in hyperalgesic diabetic neuropathy must be approached in several ways. One must allay anxiety and depression, encourage a normal sleep pattern, and find ways of dealing with the pain without addicting the patient. Cool soaks of the feet given for 15 minutes twice a day may help. Some patients find relief with phenytoin or carbamazepine. Aspirin with codeine may help others. Sedation should be reserved for night sleep. In the well adjusted male with impotence, an inflatable prosthesis may allow sexual function. Patients with insensitive feet should be instructed according to the direction given in Ch. 337.17.

337.9. NEUROPATHY ASSOCIATED WITH UREMIA

ETIOLOGY. The cause of uremic neuropathy is unknown. The lesion appears to be occurring less frequently than in the early days of hemodialysis, suggesting an effect from improved technique. Neuropathy generally disappears after renal transplantation.

PATHOLOGY. Abnormal nerve conduction is frequent in chronic uremics on hemodialysis. Pathologic studies in the diffuse symmetrical polyneuropathies show an axonal atrophy with secondary segmental demyelination that appears to precede a distal degeneration of nerve fibers.

CLASSIFICATION AND SYMPTOMATOLOGY. Subclinical neuropathies are common in patients with end-stage uremia on hemodialysis. Such patients may have slight weakness or dorsiflexion of the foot, absent ankle reflexes, and mild abnormalities of touch-pressure and vibration sensations. Patients with uremia are cachectic and prone to both compression and traumatic mononeuropathy. They also appear to be abnormally susceptible to acute inflammatory polyradiculoneuropathy. The most typical neuropathy seen in uremics, however, is a symmetrical, distal process in which variable severe sensory symptoms predominate, accompanied by mild motor and autonomic symptoms. Older men especially are predisposed. Uremic neuropathy develops earlier in patients with creatinine clearances below 5 ml per minute and more frequently when diabetes mellitus or polycystic kidneys are present. Treatment is difficult, and the benefit of hemodialysis in preventing or in improving the neuropathy is uncertain.

337.10. NEUROPATHY ASSOCIATED WITH HEPATIC DISEASE

Several kinds of peripheral neuropathy can accompany liver disease. These include those of nutritional deficiency as well as those associated with infectious mononucleosis, acute intermittent porphyria, various vasculitides, amyloidosis, celiac disease, and various intoxications. Acute inflammatory polyneuropathy can follow viral hepatitis. A sensory neuropathy may be associated with primary biliary cirrhosis.

337.11. NEUROPATHY ASSOCIATED WITH ENDOCRINE DISEASES

Hypothyroidism is associated with both a mononeuropathy and a diffuse peripheral neuropathy. Myxedematous changes of the connective tissues of the carpal tunnel often result in compression of the median nerve. Thyroid replacement may be curative. Diffuse peripheral neuropathy associated with myxedema tends to affect predominantly the lower limb. A sensory ataxia with or without hyperesthesia or hyperalgesia is characteristic. Motor and sensory nerve fiber conduction velocity is reduced, and the muscle action potential is dispersed. Thyroid replacement therapy results in clinical and electrophysiologic improvement.

Hyperthyroidism may also be associated with a neuropathy, but this may be a chance association.

Acromegaly commonly produces entrapment neuropathies at wrist and elbow. A diffuse and sometimes severe hypertrophic neuropathy may also occur. The neuropathy of acromegaly seldom improves with hormone replacement. The effects of hypophysectomy have not been well studied.

Inherited multiple endocrine neoplasia, commonly associated with thyroid and medullary adrenal carcinoma, is usually associated also with a peroneal muscular atrophy. The patients have pes cavus, peroneal muscular weakness, and sensory loss of the feet and legs. The facial features are distinctive, consisting of thickened lips and adenomas of the tongue, lips, and conjunctiva. Such patients and their relatives should be studied for the presence of endocrine neoplasms.

337.12. AMYLOIDOSIS

Inherited amyloidosis is frequent only in endemic regions such as Portugal and Japan. In the Portuguese variety, which is inherited as an autosomal dominant trait, the disorder usually begins in the third, fourth, and fifth decades and affects predominantly small sensory and autonomic fibers. Lumbosacral dermatomes show a syringomyelia-like loss of nociception and thermal discrimination with preservation of touch-pressure sensation. Loss of potency in the male, postural hypotension, and bladder and bowel incontinence are common in advanced stages. The disorder tends to progress over a decade or so. Biopsied sural nerves show a reduction in unmyelinated and small myelinated fibers with nodular deposits of amyloid along the nerve trunks.

In the Indiana type of inherited amyloidosis symptoms begin in the hands. Numbness of the thumb and first three fingers from compression of the median nerve at the carpal tunnel ligament is characteristic.

Noninherited amyloidosis may be divided into primary and secondary varieties. The peripheral neuropathy of primary amyloidosis also affects the distal aspects of the lower extremities more than the upper extremities and includes small fibers as much as or more than larger fibers. When typical symptoms of neuropathy are associated with heart enlargement, nephropathy, and enlargement of the tongue, the diagnosis of amyloidosis should be strongly suspected and can be confirmed by histologic examination of rectal mucosa, kidney, carpal ligament, muscle, gingivae, nerve, or bone marrow. No effective treatment for the neuropathy is available.

Some patients with multiple myeloma develop a symmetrical predominantly motor neuropathy with many of the clinical features of chronic inflammatory polyradiculoneuropathy. It is sometimes assumed that neuropathies associated with multiple myeloma are due to amyloidosis. Although amyloid deposition has sometimes been found in the nerves in myeloma, it is not clear that this causes the neuropathy. Multiple myeloma should be considered in chronic neuropathy of unknown cause.

Recently a new syndrome with peripheral neuropathy associated with solitary osteosclerotic myeloma has been reported from Japan. The patients had the additional features of skin hyperpigmentation and gynecomastia.

337.13. NEUROPATHY ASSOCIATED WITH CARCINOMA AND OTHER MALIGNANCY

Direct compression of nerves by metastatic tumors occurs within the spinal canal, within intervertebral foramina, and behind tight fascial sheaths, as in the retroperitoneal space of the pelvis. Bronchogenic, renal, prostatic, and breast carcinomas are especially prone to such metastases. The nonmetastatic neurologic effects of cancer are described in Ch. 322 to 327.

NEUROPATHY ASSOCIATED WITH NUTRITIONAL DEFICIENCY

See Ch. 286.

337.14. NEUROPATHY ASSOCIATED WITH THE USE OF DRUGS

Many drugs produce a peripheral neuropathy, some more frequently than others. When prescribing such agents, the risk-benefit ratio must always be considered.

The vinca alkaloids, particularly vincristine and vinblastine, are employed in the treatment of leukemias, lymphomas, and Hodgkin's disease. The drugs predictably produce a sensory neuropathy with sometimes painful paresthesias of the feet and a severity proportional to the dosage.

The use of clioquinol has been associated with a severe neurologic disorder, reported especially in Japan, called subacute myeloptical neuropathy (SMON). This disorder is characterized by loss of vision, ascending numbness, motor weakness, and autonomic involvement.

Nitrofurantoin commonly produces neuropathy when used for urologic infections in patients with impaired renal function who then develop high blood levels of the drug. Most common are paresthesias, but an ascending paralysis can occur.

Isoniazid used as an antituberculous agent interferes with pyridoxine metabolism. Paresthesias of the toes and feet associated with lower limb weakness can be prevented by pyridoxine supplementation.

Hydralazine occasionally produces a neuropathy, probably by producing pyridoxine deficiency.

The anticonvulsant phenytoin can produce a mild asymptomatic neuropathy with hyporeflexia.

Chloramphenicol occasionally produces mild peripheral neuropathy or optic neuritis.

Gold, used as sodium aurothiomalate for rheumatoid arthritis, can produce a peripheral neuropathy and cranial neuropathy as well as a confusional state.

Sodium cyanate is potentially useful in the management of sickle cell anemia but produces a distressing polyneuropathy in both man and laboratory animals.

Ethambutol, an otherwise promising antituberculous drug, produces optic neuritis and occasionally a peripheral neuropathy.

337.15. NEUROPATHY ASSOCIATED WITH HOUSEHOLD AND INDUSTRIAL POISONS

Large outbreaks of polyneuropathy can occur from inhalation of toxic substances in factories and from adulteration of food and drinking water. A variety of chemicals used as euphoriants or for suicidal purposes produce neuropathy.

Arsenic continues to cause a few cases of peripheral neuropathy each year in the United States. Often it is difficult even with intensive investigation to determine whether the intent of ingestion was homicidal or suicidal. A typical hyperalgesic neuropathy affects the feet and lower legs, and is accompanied by distal muscle weakness and a gastrointestinal upset. Cerebral and hepatic symptoms may occur. The skin may darken. Diagnosis depends on finding elevated arsenic levels in blood, in urine, in nail clippings, and in hair. Several months are required before one can reliably detect the diagnostic Mees lines on the fingernails.

Lead neuropathy is now rare. Abdominal colic, anemia, and wrist drop suggest the diagnosis.

Thallium neuropathy resembles arsenical neuropathy but with superimposed alopecia.

Methyl mercury, an industrial toxin, produces an encephalopathy with delirium and may be associated with loss of vision and a peripheral neuropathy. *Organophosphorus compounds* may produce an initial cholinergic block resulting in respiratory paralysis and at a later time a peripheral neuropathy. Of the organophosphorus compounds, tri-ortho-cresyl phosphate has resulted in the greatest number of cases of neuropathy in man owing to contamination of medicines and cooking oils.

Acrylamide, used for the waterproofing of underground tunnels and for various scientific purposes, when ingested results in a severe distal neuropathy.

Pesticides such as DDT and kepone (an ant insecticide) may be associated with a peripheral neuropathy.

A variety of organic solvents and plasticizers are associated with neuropathy. n-Hexane, used industrially in shoe factories and misused as a euphoriant agent, is known to produce neuropathy. Other toxic industrial chemicals producing neuropathy include methyl n-butyl ketone, hexachlorophene, carbon disulfide, and trichloroethylene.

337.16. INHERITED DISORDERS OF PERIPHERAL NEURONS

These represent a group of nonremitting, slowly progressive disorders probably caused by inborn errors of metabolism. Pathologically they are system atrophies which affect selective populations of neurons by type and size. In those with primary neuronal involvement, distal axonal atrophy and secondary segmental demyelination are characteristic.

The disorders are characterized by the type of inheritance, by their natural history by which population of neurons is involved, and by the nature of the pathologic involvement. Predominant involvement of lower motor neurons is called progressive muscular atrophy (inherited motor neuropathy); of sensory neruons, inherited sensory neuropathy; of both motor and sensory neurons, inherited motor and sensory neuropathy; and of autonomic neurons, dysautonomia. Predominant involvement of large sensory fibers and of corticospinal and spinocerebellar tracts constitutes spinocerebellar degeneration. Predominantly cerebellar involvement constitutes cerebellar ataxia. Predominant involvement of corticospinal tracts plus, as a rule, lower motor and sensory neurons constitutes spastic paraplegia.

The expression of clinical symptoms in inherited neuronal disorders varies widely from patient to patient and generation to generation. Usually functional disability is less than might be expected from the chronic neurologic signs. To confirm the presence of an inherit-

ed neuronal degeneration the patient's relatives often must be examined neurologically and by nerve conduction and electromyography.

DISORDERS OF PERIPHERAL MOTOR NEURONS
(Progressive Muscular Atrophies)

These are discussed fully in Ch. 281.

337.17. DISORDERS OF PERIPHERAL SENSORY NEURONS

Patients with disorders of peripheral sensory neurons characteristically suffer from pain, cutaneous injury from lack of sensation, unsteady movement from kinesthetic sensory loss, or combinations of these. Frequently they also have autonomic dysfunction. The nature of these symptoms and the associated sensory loss correspond reasonably well with the populations of fibers affected. Thus patients with loss of pain and temperature sensation and with autonomic impairment have degeneration, mostly of unmyelinated and small myelinated fibers, whereas patients with loss of touch-pressure sensation have degeneration of large myelinated fibers of cutaneous nerves. In advanced disease this selectivity of involvement by fiber size tends to be lost.

HEREDITARY SENSORY NEUROPATHY, TYPE I

Hereditary sensory neuropathy, Type I, is a dominantly inherited sensory radicular neuropathy. It has been variously described as perforating ulcers of the feet, mutilating acropathy, acrodystrophic neuropathy, and hereditary sensory radicular neuropathy. Variability in severity is commonplace. Sensory loss is usually much more severe over the feet and legs than in the hands and forearms, and some patients have lancinating pains. Pain and temperature sensation are affected more than touch-pressure sensation, and sensory ataxia is absent. Loss or decrease of sweating usually corresponds to the region of sensory loss. Nerve conduction of motor fibers is usually normal. Denervation may affect foot and leg muscles. The ankle tendon reflex may be absent. Life expectancy is normal in most cases. Late in the disorder, perforating ulcers of the foot may develop, especially when there has been poor foot care. In kinships, signs such as pes cavus, hammer toes, plantar calluses, inability to walk on heels, and sensation loss of acral parts of lower limbs point to an imcomplete expression of the affliction.

HEREDITARY SENSORY NEUROPATHY, TYPE II

This is a recessively inherited disorder, also called congenital sensory neuropathy, which usually manifests itself in infancy or childhood with a mutilating acropathy characterized by paronychia, whitlows, ulcers of the fingers and plantar surfaces of the feet, and, frequently, unrecognized fractures of the extremities. Sensory loss affects all types of cutaneous and sometimes kinesthetic sensation and is most marked distally in all four limbs. Tendon reflexes are usually absent. Sweating loss usually occurs over the distal limbs. Nerve action potentials of afferent fibers of cutaneous and limb nerves cannot be detected. Pathologically, there is an almost complete absence of myelinated fibers from the cutaneous nerves of the distal lower limb with preservation of decreased numbers of unmyelinated fibers.

HEREDITARY SENSORY NEOROPATHY, TYPE III
(Dysautonomia of Riley-Day)

Familial dysautonomia is a recessively inherited disorder of Jewish infants and children. It affects peripheral autonomic neurons, peripheral sensory neurons, peripheral motor neurons, and probably other central nervous system neurons. Characteristic are an onset in infancy, a history of poor feeding, repeated episodes of vomiting and pulmonary infections, autonomic disturbances, and premature death. Autonomic abnormalities include defective lacrimation, defective temperature control, skin blotching, excessive perspiration, hypertension, and postural hypotension. There are also insensitivity to pain, areflexia, corneal insensitivity, and absence of the fungiform papillae of the tongue. An abnormality of catecholamine metabolism has been demonstrated.

HEREDITARY SENSORY NEUROPATHY, TYPE IV

In this recessively inherited sensory neuropathy, insensitivity to pain, anhidrosis, and mental retardation are found. This disorder has been attributed to an abnormality of differentiation of the neural crest.

ANGIOKERATOMA CORPORIS DIFFUSUM
(Fabry's Syndrome)

This rare disorder is characterized by angiokeratomas, impaired renal function, and small purple to black spots distributed especially over the lower trunk and buttocks along segmental lines. Typically, patients have pain and numbness in the limbs but no motor symptoms. A deposition of glycolipids in the cell bodies of peripheral sensory neurons and a decrease in the number of small neurons of spinal ganglia and of unmyelinated and small myelinated fibers have been observed and may be important in explaining the painfulness of the disorder.

TREATMENT OF INSENSITIVE HANDS AND FEET

Persons with pain and temperature insensitivity of hands and feet are vulnerable to many injuries which potentially can cascade into ulceration, cellulitis, lymphangitis, osteomyelitis, and osteolysis. These events are seen particularly in the disorders of leprosy, inherited amyloidosis, and other inherited and acquired neuropathies with the aforementioned sensory loss. Congenital neuropathies with such sensory loss are particularly difficult to manage, because they occur at an age when it is difficult to obtain the cooperation of the patient. The goal in treatment is to prevent the onset of tissue damage or, when it has occurred, to promote healing and prevent further damage. Persons with loss of pain and temperature sensation should not engage in most forms of manual labor or perform repetitive tasks with hands and feet which can cause bruising. Repeated inspection of the feet and hands is necessary. Any bruise or ulcer on the foot should lead one to stop weight bearing until healing has occurred. Shoes should be wide and well constructed. The inside of the shoes must be inspected to remove retained objects or nails. The feet of such patients should be soaked in lukewarm water for 15 minutes twice a day and lightly covered with petrolatum lotion to retain moisture in the softened skin.

337.18.   INHERITED DISORDERS OF PERIPHERAL MOTOR, SENSORY, AND AUTONOMIC NEURONS

The disorders are usually inherited and progressive and have symmetrical signs. The pathologic features are nonfocal, and the nerve fibers show axonal atrophy and degeneration. The molecular cause is unknown.

HEREDITARY MOTOR AND SENSORY NEUROPATHY, TYPE I
(Dominantly Inherited Hypertrophic Neuropathy Type of Peroneal Muscular Atrophy)

This is a fairly common, mild, dominantly inherited variant of peroneal muscular atrophy. Affected persons may have no symptoms or signs, but may be identified by their position in a kinship and by low conduction velocities of all nerves.

Pathologically the disorder affects mainly myelinated fibers, producing segmental demyelination and remyelination and varying degrees of onion-bulb formation (the hallmark of hypertrophic neuropathy).

In involved kinships affected persons can be recognized by higher plantar arches, hammer toes (curled-up toes with convexity upward), frequent corns or calluses, and a high-stepping, awkward gait caused by paresis of the dorsiflexor muscles of the ankle and instability of the ankle joint. Persons with greater weakness may have weakness and wasting of the intrinsic hand muscles and weakness of the plantar flexor muscles. Ankle joint instability makes it difficult to stand still. The amount of muscle atrophy is usually not great. Typically, the tendon reflexes are reduced or absent, disappearing successively from the Achilles tendon, the quadriceps, and the upper extremity. Sensory loss is mild, affecting the modalities of touch-pressure, two-point discrimination, and joint position and motion in the distal parts of the extremities. Clinical enlargement of peripheral nerves may be detected in about one fourth of the cases. Some members of kinships have, in addition to the clinical features mentioned, a tremor of the head and outstretched hands which is indistinguishable from essential tremor (Roussy-Lévy syndrome). Foot ulcers occasionally occur. Corrective surgery should be reserved for patients who develop ulcers at pressure points owing to excessively high arches and for those with excessive inversion of the foot. Footdrop springs or braces may be used to elevate the toes in walking and to stabilize the ankle.

HEREDITARY MOTOR AND SENSORY NEUROPATHY, TYPE II
(Neuronal Type of Peroneal Muscular Atrophy; Charcot-Marie-Tooth Disease)

This dominantly inherited disorder usually begins in the second decade of life, occasionally as late as the fifth or sixth decade. Symmetrical muscle weakness with atrophy begins in small foot muscles, peroneal, long toe extensor, and ankle dorsiflexor muscles. Pes cavus and hammer toes may or may not be associated with the weakness. Initial symptoms include inability to pick up the toes in walking, instability of the ankle, difficulty in standing immobile, and visible atrophy of muscles. Later, weakness of small hand muscles develops. The muscle atrophy of the lower limbs may be typical of peroneal muscular atrophy, with a greater degree of atrophy in the distal aspect of thigh muscles and with much atrophy of leg muscles. Tendon reflexes are usually diminished or absent in the lower limbs. Touch-pressure, joint position, and vibration sensation are mildly decreased distally in lower limbs. Conduction velocities of motor fibers are normal in upper limbs and only slightly reduced in lower limbs. Sporadic cases occur. Leg braces that stabilize the ankle joint often permit these patients to stand still without losing balance.

HEREDITARY MOTOR AND SENSORY NEUROPATHY, TYPE III
(Recessively Inherited Hypertrophic Neuropathy)

This is a rare disorder transmitted as an autosomal recessive trait and beginning in infancy. Affected children learn to walk late, have great difficulty in walking even at their best point of neuromuscular development (ages 8 to 12), and are usually in wheelchairs by the age of 20 years. The patients are usually short, and most have a severe, symmetrical sensory motor neuropathy affecting predominantly the distal extremities with enlarged peripheral nerves. Some weakness of proximal muscles of the extremities usually is present also. Sometimes there are associated miosis and nystagmus. The conduction velocities of motor and sensory fibers of peripheral nerves are among the lowest determined in electromyographic laboratories. Pathologically, marked segmental demyelination and remyelination are found in myelinated fibers; unmyelinated fibers are not decreased in number but are probably affected also. A systemic biochemical abnormality involving ceramide hexoses and their sulfates has been found. No specific treatment is available.

HEREDITARY MOTOR AND SENSORY NEUROPATHY, TYPE IV
(Recessively Inherited Hypertrophic Neuropathy with Excess of Phytanic Acid; Refsum's Disease)

This rare progressive or relapsing disorder is inherited as an autosomal recessive trait and is due to the inability of affected subjects to alpha-oxidize ingested phytanic acid. Clinical manifestations usually begin in the second decade with night blindness and constriction of the visual fields owing to an atypical retinitis pigmentosa. Additionally, symptoms caused by a distal sensorimotor neuropathy develop, as well as an ataxia which is thought to be greater than that accounted for by kinesthetic loss. Ichthyosis, skeletal abnormalities, and death in the third or fourth decade from involvement of the heart all provide evidence of systemic extraneural involvement. The cerebrospinal fluid protein is usually markedly elevated. Pathologically, the peripheral nerves contain evidence of segmental demyelination and remyelination and onion-bulb formation. Pathognomonic is the occurrence of elevated levels of 3, 7,11,15-tetramethylhexadecenoic acid (phytanic acid) in the serum, red blood cells, liver, heart, kidneys, and skeletal muscles. Treatment consists of withholding dietary phytols (chlorophyll-free diet); if begun early, it can result in great improvement.

HEREDITARY MOTOR AND SENSORY NEUROPATHY WITH OPTIC ATROPHY, TYPE VI

In this very rare dominantly inherited disorder, there is optic atrophy in addition to peroneal muscular atrophy.

HEREDITARY MOTOR AND SENSORY NEUROPATHY WITH RETINITIS PIGMENTOSA, TYPE VII

This disorder has many of the features of Refsum's syndrome but without elevated plasma phytanic acid levels.

Asbury, A., Victor, M., and Adams, R.: Uremic polyneuropathy. Arch. Neurol., 8:413, 1963.

Austin, J.: Recurrent polyneuropathies and their corticosteroid treatment. Brain, 81:157, 1958.

Cooke, W., and Smith, W.: Neurological disorders associated with coeliac disease. Brain, 89:683, 1966.

Croft, P., Urich, H., and Wilkinson, M.: Peripheral neuropathy of sensorimotor type associated with malignant disease. Brain, 90:31, 1967.

Dyck, P. J., Lais, A. C., Ohta, M., Bastron, J. A., Okazaki, H., and Groover, R. V.: Chronic inflammatory polyradiculoneuropathy. Mayo Clin. Proc., 50:621, 1975.

Dyck, P., and Lambert, E.: Dissociated sensation in amyloidosis. Compound action potential, quantitative histologic and teased-fiber, and electron microscopic studies of sural nerve biopsies. Arch. Neurol., 20:490, 1969.

Dyck, P. J., Thomas, P. K., and Lambert, E. H.: Peripheral Neuropathy. Philadelphia, W. B. Saunders Company, 1975.

Iwashita, H., Ohnishi, A., Asada, M., Kanazawa, Y., and Kuroiwa, Y.: Polyneuropathy, skin hyperpigmentation, edema and hypertrichosis in localized osteosclerotic myeloma. Neurology, 27:675, 1977.

Raff, M., Sangalang, V., and Asbury, A.: Ischemic mononeuropathy multiplex associated with diabetes mellitus. Arch. Neurol., 18:497, 1968.

Sunderland, S.: Nerves and Nerve Injuries. Edinburgh and London, E. and S. Livingstone Ltd., 1968.

Thomas, P. K., and Lascelles, R.: The pathology of diabetic neuropathy. Quart. J. Med., 35:489, 1966.

Tyler, H.: Neurological complications of dialysis, transplantation and other forms of treatment in chronic uremia. Neurology, 15:1081, 1965.

Wiederholt, W., Mulder, D., and Lambert, E.: The Landry-Guillain-Barré-Strohl syndrome or polyradiculoneuropathy. Historical review, report on 97 patients, and present concepts. Mayo Clin. Proc., 39:427, 1964.

Section Twenty-Four DISEASES OF MUSCLE AND NEUROMUSCULAR JUNCTION

Lewis P. Rowland

338. INTRODUCTION

DEFINITIONS. Muscles can be weakened by many different disorders. When muscles become weak, they may waste away. Until recently it has been conventional to ascribe the varied causes of weakness and wasting to neurogenic and myopathic disorders, a fundamental pathologic distinction originally made a century ago. In the neurogenic disorders, the brunt of pathologic change was seen in the motor neuron or peripheral nerve; changes in muscle were less pronounced or could be attributed to secondary effects of denervation. In the myopathic disorders, the histopathologic changes in muscle were of different type and there was little abnormality in nerve cell or peripheral nerve.

Pathologic criteria, however, have limitations when one is dealing with living people. Muscle biopsy is possible, but there is no way of obtaining a sample of the spinal cord. Other criteria were therefore introduced to separate neurogenic and myopathic disorders: clinical and genetic characteristics, electromyography, nerve conduction velocity, and assay of serum activity of sarcoplasmic enzymes. Together, these criteria have provided a reasonably consistent basis for continued separation of those syndromes characterized by weakness into neurogenic and myopathic groups.

The concept, however, has been shaken in recent years. Denervation and cross-innervation studies of fast and slow muscles have shown that physiologic and biochemical characteristics of muscle are under neural control. A new kind of electrophysiologic evidence has been adduced to indicate a neurogenic cause for the muscular dystrophies, long held to be the prototype of myopathy. Unsurprisingly, there is confusion, perhaps more than necessary. Under the circumstances, the traditional separation of neurogenic and myopathic disease will be perpetuated in this section.

An air of vagueness pervades some of the language used to describe neuromuscular diseases, and the same words have different meanings to different authorities. Since the ideas are important, it is appropriate to define some of the more prevalent words. The word *atrophy* means, literally, "lack of nourishment." It has come to mean wasting of muscle, or loss of muscle bulk from any cause, and it is also used to denote single muscle fibers that are smaller than normal when viewed microscopically. But when used in the name of a disease, it always implies that the muscle wasting is secondary to a neural disorder, e.g., infantile spinal muscular atrophy, progressive spinal muscular atrophy, or peroneal muscular atrophy. To avoid ambiguity, it is therefore appropriate in examining patients to use "wasting" rather than "atrophy" to describe diminution in muscle bulk unless the cause is known to be neurogenic. *Myopathies* include disorders characterized by weakness or some other symptom of muscle dysfunction that is not due to emotional or neurogenic cause. Some authors speak of "primary" or "secondary" myopathies but there is little evidence that any muscle disease is really "primary," in the sense that there is an abnormality in muscle and nowhere else. In some myopathies, as in thyrotoxic myopathy, the fundamental disorder is elsewhere, and this could be true even in genetically determined diseases. The *dystrophies* are a subgroup of myopathy with three special characteristics: heritable transmission, progressive weakness, and histologic evidence of degeneration of muscle with no evidence of abnormally stored material or structural abnormality of the fibers. There are other genetic disorders of muscle in which the weakness seems to be stationary, and some in which progressive weakness is not the dominant symptom (transient attacks of weakness in periodic paralysis, cramps, and myoglobinuria in some glycogen diseases, or myotonia); other names are given to these conditions individually.

DIFFERENTIATION OF NEUROGENIC AND MYOPATHIC DISEASE

Sick muscles are usually weak. Few other symptoms result; sometimes muscles ache (myalgia); sometimes they relax with difficulty (myotonia); sometimes they shorten abruptly and painfully (cramp or contracture). Weakness is also the symptom that results from neurogenic diseases affecting corticospinal pathways, motor neurons, or peripheral nerves. The differential diagnosis of muscle disease is therefore a problem in distinguishing myopathic from neurogenic causes. Corticospinal disorders have characteristic signs that immediately identify them, and therefore they do not often enter into this differential diagnosis. Disorders of the lower motor neuron or peripheral nerve may be difficult and sometimes impossible to separate from muscle disease. In this kind of neurogenic disorder and in myopathies, weakness, wasting, and depression of myotatic reflexes are common to both groups. Neurogenic disorders are apt to affect distal muscles primarily, whereas myopathic disorders are more likely to affect proximal muscle, but there are so many exceptions that this is an unreliable guide. (Distal myopathy is rare but does occur; proximal weakness is not so rare in motor neuron disease or peripheral neuropathy.) Twitching of muscle is probably a reliable guide to motor neuron disease, but it is not yet definitely excluded as a myopathic sign. The combination of active reflexes in a limb with weak, wasted, and twitching muscles is almost pathognomonic of amyotrophic lateral sclerosis, especially if there are also Babinski signs. Sensory loss and an increased protein content of the cerebrospinal fluid are reliable guides to peripheral neuropathy, but once it is established that there is a peripheral neuropathy, it may be difficult or impossible to state whether there is also a concomitant myopathy. Because of these ambiguities in clinical diagnosis, increasing attention has been directed to three laboratory aids: serum enzymes, electromyography and nerve conduction velocities, and muscle biopsy. Some syndromes are virtually defined by electromyography: distal myopathy and "juvenile muscular atrophy simulating muscular dystrophy."

SERUM ENZYMES. Several different enzyme activities are increased in the serum of patients with X-linked dystrophies and polymyositis, whereas they are not increased in neurogenic diseases. It is often stated that determination of creatine phosphokinase (CPK) activity is the most sensitive. This enzyme is significantly increased in almost all muscle diseases, but it is, if anything, too sensitive; it picks up all the myopathic cases, but it is sometimes also increased in neurogenic disease. Other serum enzyme levels, e.g., SGOT or lactate dehydrogenase (LDH) and others, do not rise so much in myopathies, but neither do they give falsely positive reactions in neurogenic disorders. For this reason, it is useful to couple determinations of CPK with SGOT or LDH in evaluating individual cases. CPK has one other considerable advantage: it is not present in erythrocytes or liver and is therefore normal in serum contaminated by hemolysis or in patients with liver disease. Isoenzyme analysis has not improved diagnosis.

ELECTROMYOGRAPHY. Needle electromyography has been refined to a very useful technique. Normal muscle is electrically silent at rest, and patterns of potentials evoked by voluntary contraction have been analyzed in terms of frequency, duration, and amplitude of individual motor unit potentials. In denervated muscle, there is spontaneous activity (fibrillations from single muscle fibers or fasciculations from motor units), the number of potentials during a voluntary contraction is reduced, and the duration of potentials is increased. In myopathic disorders, there is usually no spontaneous activity, there is no reduction in the number of potentials under voluntary control, and the potentials are reduced in duration. These signs are usually reliable, but in some cases the results are equivocal, and there may be features of both a neurogenic and myopathic disorder.

NERVE CONDUCTION VELOCITIES. The speed of conduction along motor nerves can be recorded accurately, and slowing of conduction is a reliable guide to neuropathy. A normal conduction velocity, however, does not exclude a nerve lesion.

MUSCLE BIOPSY. The features of neurogenic and myopathic diseases can usually be differentiated in a muscle biopsy, especially with the new techniques of the rapid examination of frozen tissue and the application of histochemical methods. The electron microscope has opened new approaches that are still in the process of refinement. Only a few diseases can be definitively identified by muscle biopsy: periarteritis nodosa, trichinosis, sarcoidosis, and most (but not all) cases of lipid or glycogen storage disease. The congenital myopathies are best identified by histochemical and other special procedures.

In most cases, the results of all these special studies are consistent, one with the other. In some cases, however, the results are conflicting, and problems of classification remain.

Black, J. T., Bhatt, G. P., DeJesus, P. V., et al.: Diagnostic accuracy of clinical data, quantitative electromyography and histochemistry in neuromuscular disease. J. Neurol. Sci., 21:59, 1974.
Buchthal, F.: Electrophysiological signs of myopathy as related with muscle biopsy. Acta Neurol. Scand., 32:1, 1977.
Dubowitz, V., and Brooke, M. H.: Muscle Biopsy: A Modern Approach. Philadelphia, W. B. Saunders Company, 1973.
Lenman, J. A. P., and Ritchie, A. E.: Clinical Electromyography. Philadelphia, J. B. Lippincott Company, 1970.
McComas, A. J., Sica, A. E. P., and Campbell, M. J.: "Sick" motoneurones. A unifying concept of muscle disease. Lancet, 1:321, 1971.
Rowland, L. P.: Are the muscular dystrophies neurogenic? Ann. N. Y. Acad. Sci., 228:244, 1974.

339. INHERITED DISEASES

339.1. MUSCULAR DYSTROPHIES

DEFINITION. Muscular dystrophies are inherited myopathies, characterized primarily by progressively severe weakness. In the absence of known biochemical abnormality, they are distinguished from similar diseases by lack of histologic evidence of any metabolic storage material, or by changes other than those of degeneration and regeneration of muscle or tissue reactions to these processes.

ETIOLOGY. Although it is generally believed that inherited diseases must be due to a missing or structurally abnormal protein (either an enzyme or a structural protein), this abnormality has not been identified in any form of dystrophy. Increasing biochemical and ultrastructural evidence implicates the muscle surface membrane as the site of fundamental disorder. There is evidence of dysfunction of enzymes which are an integral part of the membrane, and there are gaps in the plasma membrane that permit the entry of large molecules such as horseradish peroxidase, a protein, or procion yellow, a dye. Membranes of erythrocytes from patients with Duchenne or myotonic dystrophy also exhibit biochemical and functional deviations from normal, although this is not reflected in any symptomatic disorder of red blood cells or anemia. Pathologic and biochemical abnormalities can be detected in muscle, and there is no clear evidence of neural abnormality in traditional terms. It is conceivable, however, that the fundamental abnormality is in another organ (such as the liver or bowel) and that the muscular abnormalities are secondary. There is still debate about the possible role of altered motor neurons, and some writers postulate a debatable vascular cause, functional ischemia of muscle.

CLASSIFICATION. No classification of the muscular dystrophies is entirely satisfactory, but clinical and genetic analysis provides the best approach at present. The classification in the accompanying table is based upon the clearly identifiable features of Duchenne dystrophy, facioscapulohumeral dystrophy, and myotonic muscular dystrophy. Limb-girdle dystrophy is probably not a single disease, but encompasses cases that do not fall into the other categories.

INCIDENCE. None of the muscular dystrophies are common. Incidence rates vary from 5 per million births for facioscapulohumeral dystrophy to about 250 per million births for Duchenne dystrophy. Many cases

Classification of Human Muscular Dystrophies

	Duchenne Dystrophy	Facioscapulohumeral Dystrophy	Limb-Girdle Dystrophy	Myotonic Dystrophy
Genetic pattern	X-linked, recessive	Autosomal, dominant	Autosomal, recessive	Autosomal, dominant
Age at onset	Before age 5	Adolescence	Adolescence	Early or late
First symptoms	Pelvic	Shoulders	Pelvic	Distal; hands or feet
Pseudohypertrophy	+	0	0	0
Predominant weakness, early	Proximal	Proximal	Proximal	Distal
Progression	Relatively rapid; incapacitated in adolescence	Slow	Variable	Slow
Facial weakness	0	+	0	Occasional
Ocular, oropharyngeal weakness	0	0	0	Occasional
Myotonia	0	0	0	+
Cardiomyopathy	0 or late	0	0	Arrhythmia, conduction block
Associated disorders	None (?mental retardation)	None	None	Cataracts; testicular atrophy and baldness in men
Serum enzymes	Very high	Slight or no increase	Slight or no increase	Slight or no increase
Prevalence (per million population)	38	5	20	25
Incidence (per million births)	251	5	47	—
Mutation rate	9×10^{-5}	5×10^{-7}	3×10^{-5}	10×10^{-6}

seen to be sporadic; the mutation rate of Duchenne dystrophy is high, 7×10^{-5}, and about two thirds of the cases appear sporadically, with no other affected individual in the family.

PATHOLOGY. Pathologic abnormalities are restricted to skeletal muscle, sometimes involving cardiac muscle. The brain, spinal cord, and peripheral nerves are devoid of histologic change, although some authors have implicated the brain because of a seemingly high incidence of mental retardation in children with Duchenne dystrophy. Terminal pneumonia may cause changes in the lungs, and there may be a variety of associated diseases not directly linked to the dystrophy. In myotonic muscular dystrophy, baldness and testicular atrophy are integral parts of the disease in men, and corneal opacities affect both sexes.

The abnormalities in muscle seem to involve all fibers in random fashion. Early, there is scattered evidence of necrosis and regeneration, with prominent variation in fiber size, including many fibers much larger than normal and many fibers that appear hyalinized. Later, fibers disappear, to be replaced by fibrous connective tissue and fat. "Pseudohypertrophy" is probably due to both "true" hypertrophy (large fibers) and increased accumulation of fat and connective tissue. In myotonic dystrophy, unusual figures form "ring fibers" (with one fiber running at right angles, encircling the other fibers in the same bundle) and "sarcoplasmic masses," or accumulations of sarcoplasm that are free of myofilaments. However, these abnormalities

occur occasionally in other diseases and are not pathognomonic of myotonic dystrophy. In Duchenne dystrophy, the myocardium may be affected by similar changes, but cardiac symptoms are rarely evident in life, a discrepancy that has been attributed to the sedentary life imposed upon the patients by advanced muscular weakness. Myopathic changes in the heart are common in myotonic dystrophy. There is no good evidence that smooth muscle is affected in any form of dystrophy. Ultrastructural investigations suggest an early, and perhaps primary, abnormality of the muscle surface membrane, but it is not clear how this might be related to the progressive degeneration of muscle. Disruption of myofibrillar structure, alterations of mitochondria, and degeneration of tubules and sarcoplasmic reticulum all seem to proceed together.

CLINICAL MANIFESTATIONS. The symptoms and signs of all forms of the muscular dystrophies are related to weakness alone, except that additional systems are involved in myotonic dystrophy. In other forms, the symptoms depend upon the distribution of weakness and the age at onset. In *Duchenne dystrophy* weakness is primarily proximal at onset, and symptoms begin early. By definition, girls are not affected. There are no symptoms in the first year of life, but walking may be somewhat delayed beyond 18 months. Once the child walks, some abnormality is usually evident to an experienced observer (either a parent with a previously affected child or a skilled physician). The boys tend to waddle when they walk, or walk on their toes, or fall frequently and have difficulty rising. They are probably never able to run, because they have difficulty raising their knees. These symptoms become more evident as the children grow older, and even the most unsuspecting parent becomes aware of some abnormality by age five. Teachers sometimes may detect the difficulty when the child starts school. Some cases are averred to start between ages five and ten, but these must be exceptional. It is difficult to examine individual muscles of a young child, but the waddling gait, the typical method of rising from the ground by "climbing up" himself (Gowers' sign), enlargement of calf or other muscles, and inability to run are characteristic. Myotatic reflexes may be normal at first, but by three years the knee jerks are usually lost, and later the ankle jerks disappear. As the child grows, increased growth and coordination may compensate temporarily for the concurrent progressive weakness and wasting, but the disease always prevails. There is increased difficulty walking. Going up grades or stairs first requires aid, then becomes impossible. Weakness of the trunk muscles leads to increased lordosis and a protuberant abdomen. Then the arms become weak. Finally, in early adolescence, the child becomes unable to walk. This may be accelerated by a period of inactivity after an injury or an orthopedic operation. Contractures appear, at first in the feet, as the gastrocnemius muscles tighten. When the child stops walking, flexion contractures limit motion of the knees, and scoliosis becomes more a problem with prolonged sitting. Ultimately respiration becomes shallow and the child is increasingly subject to pulmonary infection. Sooner or later, one of these infections is fatal, usually in the third decade. Although muscles are ravaged from the neck down, the cranial muscles are entirely spared. Congestive heart failure and abnormalities of cardiac rhythm are rare.

Becker dystrophy has manifestations similar to those of Duchenne dystrophy, but the onset is later in childhood or in adolescence, and the tempo is slower and more variable. This form may also be devastating, but some patients are able to function, albeit with limitations, well into adult life. The clinical similarities include pseudohypertrophy of calf muscles and increased serum content of creatine phosphokinase and other sarcoplasmic enzymes. However, although the two forms are similar, they are genetically separate; there are no mildly affected individuals in typical Duchenne families, nor are children affected severely in Becker families. In some families it is admittedly difficult to decide whether the disorder is Duchenne dystrophy of relatively late appearance or Becker dystrophy of relatively early appearance. The distinction awaits recognition of the biochemical abnormalities in the two or more forms.

The manifestations of *limb-girdle dystrophy* are also similar because weakness of muscles of the pelvic girdle usually initiates the syndrome, but symptoms start in late childhood or adolescence. Girls are affected as often as boys, and pseudohypertrophy is rare. Waddling gait, difficulty in walking and climbing, and frequent falls are common. Occasionally, symptoms begin in the shoulder girdle. In either case, there is usually weakness in all four limbs by the time the patient seeks medical attention. The severity, age at onset, and rate of progression vary considerably, suggesting that this category contains more than one disease.

Facioscapulohumeral dystrophy is distinct. Symptoms vary in severity so that some affected individuals never have any disability (but can be recognized by the signs), whereas others become incapacitated early; there are all grades in between. The first symptoms are apt to be related to difficulty in raising the arms or to prominence of the scapulae. Weakness of the legs may affect pelvic girdle muscles, or equally prominent weakness of the anterior tibial muscles may lead to a steppage gait. Truncal weakness may lead to prominent scoliosis. The face is always involved on examination; the perioral muscles may be more affected than those of the upper face, but ultimately patients develop difficulty in closing the eyes. The sternal head of the pectoral muscle is affected earlier than the clavicular head, a selectivity that can be detected on testing the individual muscles, and leads to a peculiar appearance of the axillary folds when the arms are dependent, because the anterior axillary fold of normal people is formed by the sternal portion of the pectoral muscle. Winging of the scapulae can be seen when the patient leans against a wall with the arms extended, and the weakness of shoulder girdle muscles leads to an unusual appearance because, viewed from the front, the superior margin of the scapula is higher than the clavicle.

Myotonic muscular dystrophy diverges from the preceding types in several respects. (1) The distribution of weakness differs in that cranial muscles are often affected and limb weakness is initially more marked in distal muscles. Thus weakness of the hands (as in twisting bottle caps or using tools) precedes shoulder weakness, and footdrop or steppage gait precedes symptoms of pelvic muscle weakness. *Ptosis, facial weakness,* and *dysarthria* are signs not seen in the other forms of dystrophy. Moreover, there is almost always selective weakness and smallness of the sternomastoids. The masticatory muscles either are poorly developed or waste early (even when not symptomatically weak), causing a characteristic long, lean facial facial appearance. (2) Myotonia, or difficulty in relaxation, may be symptomatic, and after a firm grip the patient may have difficulty letting go. Myotonia may cause other symptoms in patients with myotonia congenita (see below), but in the dystrophy only the hands are affected by this kind of stiffness. Myotonia of grip may be evident on examination, and can also be elicited by percussing the thenar eminence. In normal persons this evokes a rapid twitch, whereas in patients with myotonia, a sustained contraction of the adductor pollicis muscle persists for several seconds, only gradually relaxing. Similar responses to percussion may be elicited uncommonly in other limb muscles, but can often be seen in the tongue. Although myotonia is a dramatic sign and a symptom that can be relieved by drugs, it is not the symptom that causes the major disability in myotonic dystrophy; weakness is the problem. (3) Other systems are involved in this pleomorphic disorder; cataracts appear sooner or later in all patients, and are sometimes the only sign of the disease; most of the men (but not the women) have frontal baldness; testicular atrophy affects most of the men, but often after they have already sired children to perpetuate the disease (there is no definite evidence of gonadal insufficiency in affected women); the basal metabolic rate is often low, but other tests of thyroid function are normal (extrathyroidal hypometabolism). The incidence of diabetes mellitus may be increased. (4) Conduction defects are common in the electrocardiogram, and may lead to clinically significant arrhythmia or congestive heart failure.

Certain rare forms of muscular dystrophy are named after the prominent manifestations. *Ocular dystrophy* is a slowly progressive disorder in which ptosis of the eyelids and progressive immobility of the eyes are the cardinal features. The pupils are spared, and both eyes are usually affected symmetrically so that diplopia is uncommon. Other muscles of the head, neck, and limbs may also be affected, varying from family to family. This syndrome raises problems of definition; some cases probably are myopathic in origin, but this kind of ophthalmoplegia is often associated with other manifestations that are clearly neurogenic (such as spinocerebellar degeneration or peripheral neuropathy). The final distinction is often difficult or impossible to make because in the ocular muscles signs of myopathy in muscle biopsy or electromyography are not valid. In some patients with myopathic ophthalmoplegia, structural and biochemical abnormalities may be found in limb muscles. Abnormally large mitochondria are present in increased numbers; this can be seen dramatically in electron microscopy, and the numbers are sufficient to stain fibers red in the trichrome stain for light microscopy, leading to the appellation "ragged red fibers." In these cases there is apt to be an accumulation of glycogen, but the biochemical cause of this has not been ascertained.

Distal myopathy, as the name implies, affects distal leg and hand muscles first. It is probably the rarest form of dystrophy, and can be identified only by characteristic signs of myopathy in electromyography and muscle biopsy.

In the *scapuloperoneal syndrome* distal weakness in the legs resembles that of neurogenic peroneal muscular atrophy, but sensory loss is lacking, and there is proximal weakness in the shoulder girdle similar to that of facioscapulohumeral dystrophy. Some of these cases are myopathic and some neurogenic as distinguished by electromyography, muscle biopsy, and serum enzymes. In either case, autosomal dominant inheritance and a relatively slow progression seem characteristic.

DIAGNOSIS. The clinical picture of Duchenne dystrophy entails little diagnostic confusion. In its first stages, some children are merely regarded as clumsy, and some receive orthopedic care because of toe-walking; otherwise the diagnosis becomes obvious. As noted, the trait is transmitted as a sex-linked recessive, and once a case is recognized, members of the family rapidly detect the signs in subsequently affected youngsters. Once a family is known, affected individuals can be identified in the neonatal period because the serum enzymes are already markedly abnormal. Limb-girdle and facioscapulohumeral dystrophy must be differentiated from neurogenic diseases, from congenital myopathies, and from polymyositis, as will be discussed below. Myotonic dystrophy may be confused with endocrine disorders or, because of the distal weakness, with neuropathy or amyotrophy, or with hypothyroidism or gonadal disorders. Ocular myopathy must be differentiated from myasthenia gravis; there is no fluctuation of symptoms in the myopathy, and the weakness does not respond to cholinergic drugs.

These familial cases of progressive ophthalmoplegia (ocular muscular dystrophy) also have to be distinguished from an unusual syndrome that seems to be sporadic, not yet reported in more than one person in a family. This form is identified by progressive ophthalmoplegia, pigmentary degeneration of the retina, and onset before age 15. When these three features are identified, almost all the patients will be found to have evidence of heart block on the electrocardiogram and cerebrospinal protein content of more than 100 mg per deciliter. More than half of these patients also have short stature, hearing loss, and evidence of corticospinal tract or cerebellar disease. The constellation is sufficiently consistent to warrant designation as the Kearns-Sayre syndrome.

The differential diagnosis of the myopathies depends also upon the age of the patient. In childhood and adolescence, the major problems involve peroneal muscular atrophy (Charcot-Marie-Tooth) and "muscular atrophy simulating muscular dystrophy" (Wohlfart-Kugelberg-Welander). In adults, amyotrophic lateral sclerosis is the major problem. At all ages, polyneuritis must be considered.

TREATMENT. There is no specific treatment for the weakness of any form of dystrophy. Physical therapy exercises, splints, braces, and corrective orthopedic surgery are applied in different centers with varying degrees of enthusiasm. Some claim that walking can be prolonged into late adolescence in Duchenne dystrophy. The most poignant decisions concern the use of antimicrobial drugs or supported respiration for young men paralyzed from the neck down and with no hope of ultimate recovery. The myotonia of myotonic dystrophy can be relieved by diphenylhydantoin (0.3 to 0.6 gram daily), quinine (0.3 to 1.5 grams daily), or procainamide (4 to 6 grams daily), but this is rarely the problem, and nothing can be done for the weakness. Cataracts are treated surgically upon appropriate indication, and cardiac arrhythmias or congestive heart failure are managed accordingly.

PROPHYLAXIS. Genetic counseling offers the only possibility to control muscular dystrophy at present. Carriers of Duchenne dystrophy may often but not always be identified by abnormally increased serum enzyme activity (higher than normal, but not as high as in affected boys). In some centers, antenatal detection of sex allows selective prophylactic abortion. There is presently no way to determine whether a male fetus is affected, however. The development of methods to sample fetal blood has led to attempts to measure creatine phosphokinase. This technique may ultimately provide the way to identify the true biochemical abnormality in the fetus, assuming that it will be the same in both muscle and erythrocytes, an assumption that is not proved. Birth control ought to be effective in dominantly inherited diseases such as facioscapulohumeral and myotonic dystrophy, but since many cases are mild, few will accept continence. The high rates of mutation do not encourage optimism that genetic restriction can be the ultimate goal.

Berenberg, R. A., Pellock, J. M., DiMauro, S., et al.: Lumping or splitting? "Ophthalmoplegia plus" or Kearns-Sayre syndrome? Ann. Neurol., 1:37, 1977.

Mokri, B., and Engel, A. G.: Duchenne dystrophy: Electron microscopic findings pointing to a basic or early abnormality in the plasma membrane of the muscle fiber. Neurology, 25:1111, 1975.

Panayiotopoulos, C. P., and Scarpalezos, S.: Muscular dystrophies and motoneuron diseases. Neurology, 26:721, 1976.

Roses, A. D., Herbstreith, M., Metcalf, B., and Appell, S. H.: Increased phosphorylated components of erythrocyte membrane spectrin band II with reference to Duchenne dystrophy. J. Neurol. Sci., 30:167, 1976.

Rowland, L. P. (ed.): Pathogenesis of Human Muscular Dystrophies. Amsterdam, Excerpta Medica, 1977.

Walton, J. N.: Disorders of Voluntary Muscle. 3rd ed. Edinburgh, Churchill Livingstone, 1974.

Cornelio, F., DiDonato, S., Pelúchetti, D., et al.: Fatal cases of lipid storage myopathy with carnitine deficiency. J. Neurol. Neurosurg. Psychiat. 40:170, 1977.

DiMauro, S., and Eastwood, A. B.: Disorders of glycogen and lipid metabolism. Adv. Neurol., 17:123, 1977.

339.2. OTHER INHERITED BIOCHEMICAL DISORDERS

Although the glycogen storage diseases are discussed in more detail in Ch. 531.4, it is necessary to mention them here, because they enter into differential diagnosis and because they were the first inherited muscle diseases in which the biochemical defect was discerned. Of the several forms, the only ones that do not affect muscle are type 1 (lack of glucose-6-phosphate dehydrogenase) and type 6 (lack of liver phosphorylase).

Pompe's disease, the infantile form of glycogen storage disease Type 2, is associated with lack of acid maltase. It affects motor neurons and muscle, causing a clinical disorder that resembles Werdnig-Hoffmann disease, from which it is distinguished by glossomegaly and cardiomegaly with congestive heart failure. It is uniformly fatal by one year of age. In another group of disorders, the same enzyme is missing, but the disease starts later in childhood, or even in adult years. The syndrome is one of proximal limb weakness that resembles either limb-girdle dystrophy or polymyositis, and the only clinical clues to the nature of the disease are the prominence of respiratory failure and the presence of myotonic discharges in the electromyogram. Histologically, there is a vacuolar myopathy, which can be shown to be due to deposition of glycogen. Lack of acid maltase is demonstrated by biochemical assay of muscle homogenates or in the urine. Ketogenic diet and other dietary manipulations have been attempted, with little therapeutic effect.

Type 3 glycogen storage disease, caused by lack of the debrancher enzyme system, is usually manifest by hepatomegaly and hypoglycemia, but skeletal muscle may be involved with the liver, or even alone. This disorder may also resemble limb-girdle dystrophy or polymyositis. Again, diagnosis is suspected on the basis of histochemical study of muscle and proved by biochemical analysis. Types 5 and 7, resulting from lack of phosphorylase or phosphofructokinase, are causes of recurrent myoglobinuria.

Another group of diseases sometimes involves storage of glycogen, but the dominant biochemical abnormalities are lipid storage in muscle, sometimes with lactic acidosis, and often with proliferation of malformed mitochondria. These disorders may be manifest by a proximal myopathy alone, or in combination with mental retardation and seizures. One form of lipid storage disease is associated with abnormally low content of carnitine in muscle with no systemic abnormalities. Oral carnitine therapy may be beneficial. In another form, the liver is affected as well, with low tissue concentrations of carnitine in that organ and also in blood plasma, and the clinical disorder is punctuated by episodes of hepatic encephalopathy that may be fatal.

339.3. CONGENITAL MYOPATHIES

DEFINITION. These are rare diseases characterized by weakness that is usually mild but persists throughout life, either progressing slowly or remaining stationary.

ETIOLOGY. The cause is not known. A few of these disorders are familial and suspected of having a genetic basis, but so many cases are sporadic that other causes are not excluded, and there are no clear clues.

PATHOLOGY. These diseases are defined in terms of pathology, and most of them have been delineated within the past 15 years since the introduction of histochemical techniques to study muscle biopsy. The names of the diseases reflect the predominant anatomic disorder.

In *central core disease*, the central portion of the muscle fiber appears rather amorphous, in contrast to the fibrillar appearance of the surrounding normal portion. In cross-section, the central portion appears blue when stained with Gomori's trichrome, in striking contrast to the red periphery. The central areas lack all oxidative enzyme activity, and there are no mitochondria in this region. In *nemaline myopathy or rod myopathy*, small threadlike or rod bodies are scattered throughout the fiber. The rods are barely visible in conventional hematoxylin and eosin stains, but can be seen readily in phase contrast or with the trichrome stain. In electron microscopy the structures seem to originate in the Z-band, and circumstantial evidence suggests that they are composed of tropomyosin. *Myotubular myopathy* designates the appearance of myofibers that resemble a stage in the early development of fetal muscle, with nuclei located centrally rather than at the periphery and surrounded by a halo of apparently empty space. Because the pathogenesis of this appearance is uncertain, some investigators prefer the name *centronuclear myopathy*. In other disorders mitochondria have appeared abnormal, either in number (too many) or size (too large), often associated with accumulations of lipid droplets.

CLINICAL MANIFESTATIONS. Although designated "congenital," these disorders are only exceptionally symptomatic in the first year of life, except that the onset of walking may be delayed. Later, the symptoms of proximal limb weakness become evident: waddling gait, difficulty in climbing stairs, frequent falls, and scoliosis. Later, there may be weakness of the arms. There are few clinical clues to each specific histologic abnormality. Among the nemaline cases there have been skeletal abnormalities (kyphoscoliosis, pigeon breast, pes cavus, high palate, and an unusually elongated face). In two families with myotubular disease, ophthalmoplegia was present as well as limb weakness. Central core and mitochondrial disorders have not been associated with distinctive clinical signs other than proximal limb weakness. Abnormal mitochondria have been found in a variety of different clinical syndromes: euthyroid hypermetabolism (Luft's syndrome), proximal limb weakness with or without lactic acidosis or lipid storage, ocular myopathies, the Kearns-Sayre form of progressive ophthalmoplegia, variable limb weakness, cramps, and fatigue syndromes, among others. In none of the structurally defined congenital myopathies, therefore, is it possible to link the morphologic abnormality to a biochemical or physiologic cause of the weakness.

DIAGNOSIS. Proximal limb weakness in a young child is usually myopathic in origin, but must be distinguished from the neurogenic Wohlfart-Kugelberg-Welander syndrome and from polyneuritis. Myopathic abnormalities in the electromyogram, an abnormal family history, an incidence in girls, and especially the histologic abnormalities define the individual entities. The serum enzymes may be normal or slightly increased. In some clinics most cases of apparently congenital myopathy fail to meet the specific histologic criteria, showing only nonspecific myopathic changes in biopsy. There is no better designation for these cases than "congenital myopathy," but it is likely that there is more than one cause.

In infancy, the major cause of weakness is a form of motor neuron disease (Werdnig-Hoffmann disease). Among infants with multiple congenitally fixed joints (arthrogryposis multiplex), some prove to have myopathic disease as defined by muscle biopsy and electromyography. In some cases, neonatal difficulty in swallowing is followed by delayed onset of walking, possibly persistent weakness, obesity, childhood diabetes, mental retardation, and a characteristic facial appearance (Prader-Willi syndrome), but there is no abnormality on muscle biopsy or electromyogram.

TREATMENT AND PROGNOSIS. There is no specific treatment for any of these disorders. Physical therapy and orthopedic corrective measures are of value. There are too few cases to generalize about the course of these illnesses; most seem to be mild and nonprogressive, but occasional cases are more severe.

Afifi, A. K., Ibrahim, M. Z. M., Bergman, R. A., Haydar, N. A., Mire, J., Bahuth, N., and Kaylani, F.: Morphologic features of hypermetabolic mitochondrial disease. J. Neurol. Sci., 15:271, 1972.

Bharucha, E. P., Pandya, S. S., and Dastur, D. K.: Arthrogryposis multiplex congenita. J. Neurol. Neurosurg. Psychiatry, 35:425, 1972.

DiMauro, S., Schotland, D. L., Bonilla, E., et al: Mitochondrial myopathies. Which and how many? In Milhorat, A. T. (ed.): Exploratory Concepts in Muscular Dystrophy II. Amsterdam, Excerpta Medica, 1974, pp. 506–516.

Dubowitz, V.: The Floppy Infant. London, Spastics International Medical Publications, 1969.

Gordon, A. S., Rewcastle, N. B., Humphrey, J. G., and Stewart, B. M.: Chronic benign congenital myopathy; fingerprint body type. Can. J. Neurol. Sci., 1:106, 1974.

Hall, B. D., and Smith, D. W.: Prader-Willi syndrome: A résumé of 32 cases, J. Pediat., 81:286, 1972.

Kinoshita, M., Satoyashi, E., and Matsuo, N.: Myotubular myopathy and type 1 fiber atrophy in a family. J. Neurol. Sci., 26:575, 1975.

Kinoshita, M., Satoyashi, E., and Suzuki, Y.: Atypical myopathy with myofibrillar aggregates. Arch. Neurol., 32:417, 1975.

339.4.   MYOTONIA CONGENITA
(Thomsen's Disease)

DEFINITION. Myotonia congenita is a rare disorder characterized by difficulty in relaxation of skeletal muscle after forceful contraction, present from early childhood.

ETIOLOGY. There are occasional sporadic cases, but most are inherited in a pattern corresponding to an autosomal dominant trait. In a few families, the disease seems to be autosomal recessive. The biochemical fault is not known, but the muscle membrane is electrically unstable and tends to fire repetitively. The abnormality must be inherent within the muscle, because myotonic

phenomena may be elicited after all neural influences are abolished by spinal anesthesia, block of motor nerves by local anesthesia, or blockade of the neuromuscular junction by intra-arterial injection of d-tubocurarine. Myotonia is abolished, however, by the intramuscular administration of procaine. In human myotonia congenita, as in a genetic myotonia of goats, there seems to be an abnormality of chloride conductance in muscle, and this could account for the tendency to discharge repetitively. The disorder in myotonic muscular dystrophy seems to differ, and it is possible that the biochemical abnormality is different in each of the several forms of inherited human myotonia.

CLINICAL MANIFESTATIONS. The difficulty in relaxation is widespread. Difficulty in relaxing the grip may lead to prominent and sometimes embarrassing symptoms. Ocular muscles may be affected, so that the eyes seem momentarily "stuck" in one position, or the eyelids may remain closed after forceful closure. Sometimes oropharyngeal muscles are affected, with difficulty in speaking or swallowing. Startle reactions may induce stiffness of the legs, thwarting sudden attempts to catch a bus or run from home plate. There is no weakness, and one unexplained characteristic is the unusual muscular development of many patients, causing a Herculean appearance, perhaps related to involuntary and repeated isometric exercise. The myotonia can be elicited by tapping any muscle in severely affected cases. Reflexes are unaltered.

DIAGNOSIS. The major problem is in distinguishing the disorder from myotonic muscular dystrophy. Here the only symptoms and signs are related to myotonia. There is no weakness, cataract, baldness, or gonadal atrophy. So-called "transitional cases" are probably patients in families with myotonic muscular dystrophy who are only mildly affected and show only myotonia before the other manifestations. There may be some weakness in families with the rare autosomal recessive form of myotonia congenita. In general, families with myotonia congenita breed true.

TREATMENT. For many years, quinine was the staple treatment in doses of 0.3 to 1.5 grams daily. Recently, phenytoin has proved equally effective and less apt to cause disagreeable side effects in therapeutic doses of 0.3 to 0.6 gram daily. Should this fail, procainamide may also be used, in doses of 4 to 6 grams daily, but this drug is prone to induce lupus erythematosus.

Barchi, R. L.: Myotonia. An evaluation of the chloride hypothesis. Arch. Neurol., 32:1575, 1975.

Becker, F.: Myotonic syndromes. In Rowland, L. P. (ed.): Pathogenesis of Human Muscular Dystrophies. Amsterdam, Excerpta Medica, 1977.

339.5.   FAMILIAL MYOGLOBINURIA

Most cases of myoglobinuria are sporadic, and they will be described in Ch. 340.3. Some persons, however, have repeated attacks from early childhood, suggesting some genetic fault, and sometimes more than one individual in a family is affected. Some of these familial cases are due to lack of muscle phosphorylase or phosphofructokinase. They can be recognized by the ischemic work test in which contracture is induced and venous lactate fails to rise. (See Ch. 531.4.) In several families, recurrent myoglobinuria has been associated with lack of carnitine palmityl transferase, the enzyme necessary for the oxidation of long-chain fatty acids. In other cases, however, no abnormality has been found of either glycogen or lipid metabolism.

Bank, W. J., DiMauro, S., Bonilla, E., Capuzzi, D. M., and Rowland, L. P.: A disorder of lipid metabolism and myoglobinuria. Absence of carnitine palmityl transferase. N. Engl. J. Med., 292:443, 1975.

339.6.   FAMILIAL PERIODIC PARALYSIS

DEFINITION. Periodic paralysis is characterized by recurrent attacks of flaccid weakness usually associated with abnormally high or low serum potassium concentrations. Many cases are familial. In sporadic cases the abnormality may be secondary to aberrations of potassium metabolism.

ETIOLOGY AND PATHOGENESIS. Familial cases are distributed in a pattern consistent with autosomal dominant inheritance. Hypokalemia during attacks was the first metabolic abnormality to be recognized, with no loss of potassium in urine. It was presumed that potassium shifted from extracellular to intracellular compartments, especially muscle. This has been difficult to prove, and the anticipated hyperpolarization of the muscle membrane potential has not been substantiated by direct measurement with intracellular electrodes. Abnormalities of glucose metabolism have been suspected, because attacks can be precipitated by infusions of glucose and insulin, by eating a large meal, or by administration of epinephrine. However, biochemical studies have failed to pinpoint the abnormality.

During the past two decades it has been recognized that the serum potassium tends to rise in some patients, and attacks in these individuals are induced by the ingestion of potassium. This variety is therefore called "hyperkalemic periodic paralysis," and is generally considered to be the mirror image of the hypokalemic type, with potassium presumably shifting out of muscle and into blood during attacks. Why this should happen is not clear, but at least in the hyperkalemic type there are alterations of the intracellular potential in the direction required by theory. There are clinical differences between the two forms of periodic paralysis, but there are so many areas of overlap and so many common features that it is difficult to decide just how many genetically distinct forms there really are.

PATHOLOGY. In both forms of periodic paralysis there may be vacuoles within muscle fibers. These may be numerous or scanty, and it is not clear whether they are more frequent in paralyzed muscle. Most electron microscopists believe that the vacuoles are derived from the sarcoplasmic reticulum, but others think they originate in the T-system in areas of necrotic muscle. Glycogen seems to be increased in amount in ultrastructural studies, but the results of biochemical analysis have been inconsistent. There is no evidence that other organs are affected in either form of the disease. The heart is usually spared pathologically.

CLINICAL MANIFESTATIONS. There are clinical differences between the two forms. In the hypokalemic variety, attacks tend to start in late childhood or adolescence, frequently occur at night, are apt to be severe, and last for a day or more. In the hyperkalemic variety, attacks start at an early age, occur much more frequently, tend to be milder, and may last minutes or hours.

Moreover, patients with hyperkalemic periodic paralysis usually have some evidence of myotonia, often limited to percussion myotonia of the tongue. Lid-lag and Chvostek's sign are identified with the hyperkalemic type. These clinical distinctions may break down in application to individual cases and are only crude guides. Moreover, many features are common to both types: a dominant pattern of inheritance, a susceptibility to attacks during periods of rest after vigorous exercise, the ability to ward off attacks by mild exercise after a mild attack has begun, persistent weakness between attacks, vacuoles in muscle, a lack of clear relation between the serum potassium concentration and the severity of paresis, the induction of local weakness by cooling, and protection against attacks by acetazolamide. Some patients are affected by attacks in which the serum potassium may be either high or low.

Typical attacks start with weakness of the legs that ascends to the arms. Cranial muscles are affected in severe attacks only, and respiratory insufficiency is exceptional. The attacks may be mild and brief, or severe and prolonged, with all gradations in between. During severe attacks, the myotatic reflexes are lost, and the muscles are electrically inexcitable. Attacks are rarely apoplectic in onset and usually take an hour or more to develop, except that attacks beginning in sleep may be fully developed when the patient awakes. Paresthesias and myalgia may be prominent at the onset, or may be completely lacking. Some patients are aware of oliguria during the attack and of diuresis afterward.

The serum potassium is in the range of 2.5 to 3.5 mEq per liter in hypokalemic attacks, and 5.0 to 7.0 mEq per liter in the hyperkalemic type. Between attacks serum potassium values may be normal. The electrocardiogram is altered as would be predicted from the serum values, with low T waves in hypokalemia and peaked T waves in hyperkalemia.

Patients with hyperkalemic periodic paralysis may have mild myotonia, especially of the hands. When individuals in a family are studied, some may be found to have myotonia without any history of periodic paralysis.

In both types of the disease, there may be persistent weakness between attacks, most often proximal, sometimes distal. In the past this has been attributed to a permanent "myopathy," but experience with acetazolamide therapy indicates that even longlasting weakness may be reversible, regardless of pathologic changes in muscle. A few patients with intermittent normokalemic or hyperkalemic paralysis have had persistent cardiac arrhythmia, especially bigeminy, and bouts of ventricular tachycardia. The cardiac disorder is neither temporally related to attacks of limb weakness nor related to serum potassium content.

DIAGNOSIS. Periodic paralysis can be recognized by the history of typical attacks; no other disease causes this pattern of recurrent weakness. In myasthenia gravis, weakness may come and go, but less abruptly and with a duration of weeks rather than hours or days; remissions are less frequent so that it is less "periodic." Polymyositis may be transient, but episodes are rarely shorter than several weeks or months. Attacks of myoglobinuric weakness could conceivably be confusing if the pigmenturia were not recognized, but myalgia and malaise are so prominent that it is rarely mistaken for periodic paralysis. Hysterical attacks might be confusing.

If the patient is seen during the attack and the serum potassium is abnormal, other causes of hypo- or hyperkalemia must be considered. Low serum potassium concentrations with paralysis are also encountered in hyperaldosteronism; potassium-losing nephritis; potassium depletion caused by laxative abuse, diuretics, or diarrhea; and thyrotoxicosis. *Thiazide* and *thalidone diuretics* are in such widespread use nowadays that these drugs are likely to be an increasingly frequent cause of hypokalemic weakness; in one series, about 25 per cent of randomly chosen patients receiving these drugs had serum potassium contents below normal. Hyperkalemia is most often due to renal insufficiency, but may also occur in adrenal insufficiency, after administration of spironolactone, or as a manifestation of aldosterone deficiency.

Thyrotoxicosis can produce a variant of periodic hypokalemic paralysis closely resembling the familial variety. The condition especially occurs in young Chinese and Japanese men in their third or fourth decade, although other Asians and even women have occasionally been affected. The clinical manifestations of hyperthyroidism usually are not prominent, although tachycardia and even cardiac arrhythmias are frequent. Attacks commonly are precipitated by exercises or heavy carbohydrate meals. Serum potassium is low. Effective treatment of the thyrotoxicosis is curative.

A family history of periodic paralysis is useful in diagnosis, but sporadic cases may be indistinguishable from the familial disorder. If the patient is not having a spontaneous attack when studied, the only way to distinguish the two forms is to provoke an attack. The techniques to be described have been used in numerous centers with many patients, without serious complications. But induced attacks may be frightening to patient and physician, and should be left to experienced investigators. Facilities for supported respiration should be immediately available. Appropriately informed consent is mandatory. Because of the uncertainty of clinical distinction, it is advisable to start with glucose (100 grams) given intravenously in one hour with 20 units of regular insulin either in the infusion or given subcutaneously. Hypoglycemic symptoms should be anticipated, and the electrocardiogram should be monitored. Hypokalemia is induced as the blood sugar falls, usually within one hour after the infusion is completed. If an attack is induced, it can be terminated with administration of 7 to 10 grams of potassium chloride (KCl) by mouth. Whether or not an attack is induced by glucose and insulin, but especially if it is not, the patient should then be challenged with potassium. This poses problems because it is not clear how much potassium constitutes an adequate challenge. The writer starts with 3 grams of KCl by mouth. If this fails the dose is gradually increased on successive days to a maximum of 8 or 10 grams. Patients with hyperkalemic paralysis have attacks with serum potassium levels between 5 and 8 mEq per liter.

Other members of the family should be investigated clinically and electromyographically for evidence of myotonia.

TREATMENT. Acute attacks of hypokalemic paralysis are best treated with oral KCl, 5 to 10 grams. Relief of weakness usually commences within 30 minutes but may take several hours, and some attacks are peculiarly refractory. Hyperkalemia may be relieved by infusions of glucose and insulin. Chlorothiazide and calcium gluconate have also been reported to be effective. In severe attacks, weakness may persist even after the serum potassium has returned to normal concentrations.

The traditional method used to protect patients against hypokalemic paralysis was, until recently, a low-sodium diet supplemented by oral KCl, or perhaps by spironolactone or dexamethasone. Then, acetazolamide in small doses, sometimes only 250 per mg daily, sometimes more, was found to be effective prophylaxis in the hyperkalemic type. Subsequently, it was found that similar doses of acetazolamide were equally effective in the hypokalemic variety, so a single drug is beneficial in both forms. How it exerts this effect is not known. The best-known effects of this compound relate to its ability to inhibit carbonic anhydrase, but muscle lacks this enzyme, and no definite systemic effects of the drug have been recognized in the doses used, but respiratory acidosis may be responsible.

Gordon, R. M., Green, J. R., and Lagunoff, D.: Studies on a patient with hypokalemic familial periodic paralysis. Am. J. Med., 48:185, 1970.

Griggs, R. C., Engel, W. K., and Resnick, J. S.: Acetazolamide treatment of hypokalemic periodic paralysis: Prevention of attacks and improvement of persistent weakness. Ann. Intern. Med., 73:39, 1970.

Pearson, C. M., and Kalyanaraman, R.: Periodic paralyses. In Stanbury, J. B., Wyngaarden, J. B., and Fredrickson, D. S. (eds.): The Metabolic Basis of Inherited Disease. 3rd ed. New York, McGraw-Hill Book Company, 1972, pp. 1180–1203.

Ramsay, I.: Thyroid Disease and Muscle Dysfunction. Chicago, Year Book Medical Publishers, 1974.

Vroom F. Q., Jarrell, M. S., and Maren, T. H.: Acetazolamide treatment of hypokalemic periodic paralysis. Probable mechanism of action. Arch. Neurol., 32:385, 1975.

Zierler, K. L.: Speculations on hypokalemic periodic paralysis. Am. J. Med. Sci., 266:131, 1973.

339.7. MYOSITIS OSSIFICANS

This rare disorder is most dramatic in its consequences, producing the "stone man" of circus sideshows. Symptoms usually begin in early childhood, with transient and localized swellings of the neck and back. Ultimately there is progressive rigidity of the neck, trunk, and limbs. Palpable plates are discernible beneath the rigid parts. Severely affected patients may be able to stand and walk, and yet unable to bend so that they must be raised from bed with assistance. The bars beneath the skin are visible roentgenographically. Microscopically, muscle is replaced by bone and connective tissue. Whether the primary disorder is in the fibroblasts (leading to abnormal ossification) or in the muscle itself is not resolved. Muscle biopsy early in the disease may show widespread necrosis and inflammation, but serum enzymes are not always elevated, nor is the electromyogram always myopathic. Few cases are familial, but the disorder is believed to be inherited because digital abnormalities are almost always present in both the patients and other members of the family in a pattern suggesting an autosomal dominant inheritance. Microdactyly commonly affects the great toe, and clinodactyly (curved digits) may affect the hands. There is no detectable systemic abnormality of calcium and phosphate metabolism, and there has been no effective therapy, but recent reports suggest that administration of disphosphonates may prevent the deposition of bone. Once bone is formed, however, these drugs are ineffective.

Bassett, C. A. L., Donath, A., Macagno, F., Preisig, R., Fleisch, H., and Francis, M. D.: Diphosphonates in the treatment of myositis ossificans. Lancet, 2:845, 1969.

Lutwak, L.: Myositis ossificans progressiva. Am. J. Med., 37:269, 1964.

340. SPORADIC DISORDERS

340.1. THE PROBLEM PRESENTED BY DERMATOMYOSITIS AND POLYMYOSITIS

The main discussion of these conditions is found in Ch. 51. However, the concept of polymyositis is central to the analysis and concepts of acquired myopathies of adult life, and thus it is appropriate to review some of the problems here.

These conditions are usually considered together, but this practice may prove imprudent. *Dermatomyositis* is a recognizable syndrome, characterized by a rash and myopathy, both with distinctive features. The name is derived from the inflammatory cellular response that is usually found in skeletal muscle, but lymphocytic reaction is not present in all cases. This lack causes problems in defining *polymyositis,* a disorder presumably identical with dermatomyositis but without the rash.

There probably is such a disease as true dermatomyositis with scarcely detectable skin lesions. The rash of dermatomyositis may be so mild that it could be overlooked by parents or inexperienced clinicians, and there are patients with no history of rash who develop subcutaneous calcinosis, implying that the skin had been involved without visible dermatitis. But once the rash is taken away, an essential sign of dermatomyositis is withdrawn, and it becomes impossible to define polymyositis as the same condition. Polymyositis, therefore, is a syndrome, probably of diverse causes, and is identifiable by the following set of diagnostic criteria.

DIAGNOSIS. The diagnosis of dermatomyositis is a clinical diagnosis, depending upon the characteristic rash and limb weakness. In some patients, features of scleroderma may also be present, warranting the name "sclerodermatomyositis." However, there is no overlap with lupus erythematosus or periarteritis nodosa, and the visceral lesions of these conditions do not occur in dermatomyositis.

When there is no rash, the syndrome must be differentiated from the dystrophies by lack of family history, onset after age 35 (because no familial limb-girdle dystrophy starts so late), rapidity of onset in weeks or months rather than years, spontaneous improvement (which does not occur in dystrophy, by definition), distribution of weakness affecting cervical and cranial muscles, or systemic symptoms such as arthralgia or Raynaud's syndrome. Severe inflammation, when present, supports the diagnosis of polymyositis, but lack of leukocytic infiltration does not exclude the diagnosis. The electromyogram is helpful, but, again, not distinctive; there are the usual features of myopathy with the additional evidence of irritable muscle (increased insertional activity and some spontaneous activity). Serum enzymes tend to be high. There may also be an increased erythrocyte sedimentation rate, increased serum gamma globulin concentration, or a positive latex fixation test for rheumatoid factor. Evidence of lymphocytes sensitized to muscle may be demonstrable, but this has not yet attained diagnostic reliability.

The problem of diagnosis is best exemplified by a patient with limb weakness commencing at age 40 and evidence of myopathic disease in muscle biopsy and electromyogram. Search must be made for the known causes of muscle disease, to be discussed below. If none is found, the diagnosis of exclusion is polymyositis, no matter what the laboratory data show or do not show. That this residual group is all due to one disease seems unlikely, not only because there is clinical heterogeneity, but also because if there are so many known causes of the syndrome, others still remain to be recognized. Because inflammatory cells are not always seen in the muscle biopsy, some authorities eschew the word "polymyositis" and prefer "myopathy of unknown cause." This, at least, identifies the problem, but for the present "polymyositis" seems to be entrenched. Clinicians should recognize, however, that "polymyositis" is no more a specific diagnosis than "headache," "polyneuritis," or "convulsive disorder," terms that also imply inadequately defined syndromes of diverse etiology.

340.2. OTHER ACQUIRED MYOPATHIES

Proximal limb weakness in patients with no rash, with or without inflammatory lesions in muscle, and with or without increased serum enzyme activity, occurs in several disorders. These may be considered diseases associated with polymyositis, causing poliomyositis or simulating poliomyositis. To identify these disorders, appropriate diagnostic tools must be utilized.

CARCINOMATOUS MYOPATHY. Muscle weakness without rash may occur in patients with carcinoma of the lung or of any other primary site. Myeloma, macroglobulinemia, and other gammopathies may also be associated with myopathy. The tumor itself may or may not be symptomatic, and treatment of the tumor may or may not affect the muscular symptoms.

COLLAGEN DISEASES. Proximal limb weakness may occur in the course of systemic lupus erythematosus, progressive systemic sclerosis, rheumatoid arthritis, and, rarely, periarteritis nodosa or giant cell arteritis. In these circumstances, the myopathy is treated as part of the general disorder.

ENDOCRINE DISEASE. Thyrotoxic myopathy is a well-recognized syndrome. Usually there is clinical evidence of hyperthyroidism, but not always ("apathetic hyperthyroidism"). Signs of hypermetabolism are especially apt to be lacking in elderly patients. This myopathy inevitably disappears when the patient is rendered euthyroid by treatment. Similarly, weakness may complicate hypothyroidism. Another muscle syndrome of hypothyroidism is Hoffmann's syndrome, a peculiar difficulty in relaxing muscles that lack the characteristic electromyographic abnormalities of myotonia and is therefore called "pseudomyotonia," but may appear similar clinically. This, too, disappears with appropriate replacement therapy. Infants with cretinism may have unusually well developed muscles but not the disorder of relaxation.

Hyperparathyroidism and hyperadrenocorticism may also be responsible for weakness that looks like any other proximal myopathy. Surprisingly, because asthenia has so long been regarded as prominent, Addison's disease seems not to be a cause of this syndrome. Weakness may be part of hyperpituitarism, but acromegalic features always overshadow the myopathy. Myalgia, with or without weakness, may be a prominent symptom in patients with osteomalacia, and the muscular disorder may respond dramatically to administration of vitamin D.

INFECTIONS. Structures resembling viral particles have been seen with the electron microscope with polymyositis, and sometimes there are acute myopathic disorders in individuals with serologically proved influenza or other viral infections, or with encephalomyelitis assumed to be viral in origin. In one special form, children with congenital agammaglobulinemia develop dermatomyositis, and echovirus can be isolated from cerebrospinal fluid. Other infections or infestations that can be associated with clinical polymyositis are trichinosis, toxoplasmosis, cysticercosis, schistosomiasis, and trypanosomiasis.

SARCOIDOSIS. In muscle clinics, sarcoidosis is recognized as a significant cause of polymyositis. Usually there is other evidence of the disease, but sometimes the first symptoms are due to weakness, and in a few cases only muscle seems to be involved. Myalgia may be severe in these patients.

DRUGS. A variety of drugs used to treat more common disorders may themselves cause muscular weakness, especially triamcinolone and other fluorinated adrenal steroids (but probably all steroids), vincristine, chloroquine, bretylium, and guanethidine. Repeated injections of narcotics and other drugs may lead to fibrosis of muscle that simulates a diffuse myopathy.

ALCOHOLIC MYOPATHY. The clearest myopathic disorder in alcoholic persons is acute myoglobinuria. Some of these individuals, and some who never have an attack of pigmenturia, also suffer from proximal limb weakness, especially affecting the legs. The serum creatine phosphokinase is often elevated. The problem in some of these patients, however, is that they also suffer from the typical polyneuritis of alcoholism, and it then becomes difficult to prove that the muscular weakness is not also secondary to a neurogenic disorder. Too few patients have been evaluated to know whether abstinence and a good diet will reverse the persistent weakness. Chronic hypokalemia from any cause may be associated with the syndrome of polymyositis: weakness of relatively abrupt onset, muscle necrosis in biopsy, and high serum enzymes. This is most commonly seen in patients taking thiazide diuretics, but may also occur in hypokalemic states caused by chronic diarrhea. Hypokalemia may also contribute to some cases of alcoholic myopathy. (Other acquired disorders of potassium metabolism are discussed under Diagnosis in Ch. 339.6.)

Dietzman, D. E., Schaller, J. G., Ray, C. G., and Reed, M. E.: Acute myositis associated with influenza B infection. Pediatrics, 57:255, 1976.
Floyd, M., Ayar, D. R., Barwick, D. D., Hudgson, P., and Weightman, D.: Myopathy in chronic renal failure. Quart. J. Med., 43:509, 1974.
Frame, B., Heize, E. G., Block, M. A., and Manson, G. A.: Myopathy in primary hyperparathyroidism. Ann. Intern. Med., 68:1022, 1968.
Mastaglia, F. L., Gardner-Medwin, D., and Hudgson, P.: Muscle fibrosis and contractures in a pethidine addict. Br. Med. J., 4:532, 1971.
Perkoff, G. T.: Alocholic myopathy. Ann. Rev. Med., 22:125, 1971.
Rowland, L. P., Clark, C., and Olarte, M.: Therapy for dermatomyositis and polymyositis. Adv. Neurol., 17:63, 1977.
Scarpalezos, S., et al.: Neural and muscular manifestations of hypothyroidism. Arch. Neurol., 29:140, 1973.
Schott, G. D., and Wills, M. R.: Muscle weakness in osteomalacia. Lancet, 1:626, 1976.
Sharp, G. C., Irvin, W. S., Tan, E. S., Gould, R. G., and Holman, H. R.: Mixed connective tissue disease; an apparently distinct rheumatic disease syndrome associated with an antibody to extractable nuclear antigen. Am. J. Med., 52:148, 1972.
Silverstein, A., and Siltzbach, L. E.: Muscle involvement in sarcoidosis. Arch. Neurol., 21:235, 1969.

340.3. SPORADIC MYOGLOBINURIA

DEFINITION. Sporadic myoglobinuria comprises a group of disorders characterized by injury of muscle and excretion of myoglobin in the urine. *Rhabdomyolysis* has been proposed as a more precise term, but it is never used except when there is myoglobinuria and is therefore of dubious value.

PATHOGENESIS. Myoglobin may be released from muscle whenever there is extensive and rapid destruction. Sometimes the cause is evident, as in the *crush injuries* of World War II. Similar pressure injuries may occur in comatose persons who lie on one side without moving for prolonged periods. This kind of injury is perhaps more apt to occur when there are other causes of *metabolic depression;* for instance, in coma after suicidal ingestion of barbiturates or carbon monoxide intoxication, or prolonged unconsciousness in the snow. A similar effect may be induced by *arterial occlusion* by tourniquet or embolism, or even by prolonged knee-chest posture under anesthesia.

In other patients, the cause is less discernible. In every series of patients with myoglobinuria, a disproportionate number are *alcoholics,* but why this should occur is not known. Sometimes there has been exposure to a known *membrane toxin,* such as the bite of the Malayan sea snake. In some addicts, heroin itself seems to cause myoglobinuria. Or there may be *metabolic alterations* that do not ordinarily cause this kind of trouble, such as diarrhea with hypokalemia; potassium depletion caused by diuretics, amphotericin, or licorice; diabetic acidosis; or systemic infection with fever. In many attacks, however, not even these clues prevail.

The most common cause of myoglobinuria is probably unusually *vigorous exercise* by an otherwise normal person. Most cases have been reported by military physicians, and local designations include such titles as the "squat-jump syndrome." Some cases are attributed to "march hemoglobinuria." When large numbers of recruits endure these tortures, a certain number will have attacks of myalgia followed by pigmenturia. Why these individuals have attacks and others are spared is not clear, but this seems to be a "normal" variation. In civilians, cases have been caused by the excess muscular activity of an initiation rite into a club or fraternity, and isolated attacks have occurred after the vigorous muscular activity induced by succinylcholine before it achieves relaxation. In *malignant hyperthermia,* there is a rapid rise in temperature, widespread muscular rigidity, hyperkalemia, and metabolic acidosis, with a fatal outcome in about 75 per cent. The offending agents are usually halothane and succinylcholine. Increased serum activities of sarcoplasmic enzymes are the rule, and often there is myoglobinuria. The intense muscular contraction may be the proximate cause of myoglobinuria in this syndrome, but the widespread metabolic disorder probably contributes. Spontaneous convulsions and electroconvulsive therapy have also been followed by myoglobinuria. If an individual is subject to repeated attacks, it may be suspected that there is some kind of undiscovered genetic defect, although the only ones recognized now are deficiencies of phosphorylase, phosphofructokinase, or carnitine palmityl transferase.

CLINICAL MANIFESTATIONS. In attacks other than those caused by local crushing or arterial occlusion, the clinical picture is similar. Affected muscles are apt to be the ones subject to greatest physical strain (the legs in squat-thrusts, the arms after chinning or push-ups, the arms and legs after wrestling matches). The muscles ache, may be swollen, and are weak. Sometimes there is so much edema that local vascular abnormalities are suspected. There may be fever and considerable malaise. Symptoms persist for several days even though pigmenturia rarely lasts more than 48 hours. Recovery may be gradual. Cranial muscles are rarely involved, and although respiratory failure is uncommon it is a hazard. The most important threat to life is renal injury secondary to excretion of heme. There may be red cells or myoglobin in the urine as well as casts. Oliguria is followed by azotemia and hyperkalemia. This may be treated by appropriate measures.

DIAGNOSIS. The diagnosis of myoglobinuria can be made on clinical grounds and with relatively simple tests, but precise identification of the pigment depends upon biochemical analysis. The urine may appear red-brown because of hemoglobin, myoglobin, or porphyrins. The latter would not give a positive test with benzidine (or other heme-reacting reagents), and would give a positive Watson-Schwartz test for porphobilinogen. Besides, the neurologic disorder of porphyria is neuropathy, not an acute myopathy. If the urine gives a positive test for heme and contains no or few erythrocytes, the pigment is either myoglobin or hemoglobin. If it is hemoglobin, the serum would be pink (after a hemolytic reaction), whereas the color of the serum in myglobinuria is normal. (This distinction depends upon the affinity of serum haptoglobin for hemoglobin and not for myoglobin. Hemoglobin is not excreted until haptoglobin is saturated by visible amounts of the pigment, whereas myoglobin is excreted at much lower concentrations.) Furthermore, in attacks of myoglobinuria, the muscular weakness and myalgia are distinctive, and serum enzymes are greatly increased, whereas they are not in hemolysis. Positive identification of myoglobin can be achieved by several tests: absorption spectrophotometry is direct and simple, but in many laboratories the most convenient method is electrophoresis on starch gel or cellulose acetate. Immunochemical methods are gaining in favor.

Myoglobinuria should be considered a possible cause in cases of acute renal failure of uncertain etiology. If the serum content of sarcoplasmic enzymes is very high (e.g., creatine phosphokinase values to 10,000 to 50,000 units, with a method giving normal maximal values of 50 units), myoglobinuria is the likely cause.

TREATMENT. If there is no renal injury, myoglobinuria is not threatening. The hazards of renal injury are not directly correlated to the amount of pigment excreted, and other factors are probably involved. Once an attack starts, it is useful to encourage excretion of dilute urine, and some authorities favor alkalinizing agents although it has not been clearly demonstrated that these treatments protect the kidneys. Few patients are left with residual weakness, but in some the syndrome is characterized by prolonged weakness punctuated by attacks of myoglobinuria.

Demos, M. A., Gitlin, E. L., and Kagen, L. G.: Exercise myoglobinuria and acute exertional rhabdomyolysis. Arch. Intern. Med., 134:669, 1974.

Grossman, R. A., Hamilton, R. W., Morse, B. M., Penn, A. S., and Goldberg, M.: Nontraumatic rhabdomyolysis and acute renal failure. N. Engl. J. Med., 291:807, 1974.

Knochel, J. P.: Environmental heat illness. An eclectic review. Arch. Intern. Med., 133:841, 1974.

Moulds, R. G. W.: Biochemical basis of malignant hyperthermia. Br. Med. J., 2:241, 1974.

Rowland, L. P., and Penn, A. S.: Myoglobinuria. Med. Clin. North Am., 56:1233, 1972.

Ryan, J. F.: Procaine for malignant hyperthermia. N. Engl. J. Med., 291: 210, 1974.

340.4. MYASTHENIA GRAVIS

DEFINITION. Myasthenia gravis is a disease of unknown cause, due to circulating antibodies to acetylcholine receptors, and manifest by weakness that has special characteristics: predilection for ocular and other cranial muscles, tendency to fluctuate in severity, no signs of neural lesion, and amelioration of weakness by cholinergic drugs.

ETIOLOGY. Although the initiating event is not known, it seems clear that myasthenic weakness results from the presence of circulating antibodies to acetylcholine receptor (AChR). It has been found that rabbits and other species can be immunized with purified AChR. When antibodies appear in the blood, weakness results, and this weakness has all the essential physiologic and pharmacologic properties found in the human disease. Also, as in human myasthenia, there are morphologic changes at the neuromuscular junction, especially simplification of the postjunctional folds, and antibody can be demonstrated on the postjunctional membrane by immunocytochemical methods. As a result, the postjunctional membrane becomes less sensitive to the application of acetylcholine or other agonists.

When this experimental autoimmune myasthenia gravis was demonstrated and confirmed in other laboratories, similar antibodies to AChR were soon demonstrated in the blood of patients with myasthenia gravis. In a transient syndrome of infants born to myasthenic mothers, the symptoms disappeared when the antibodies disappeared. When purified IgG from patients was injected into mice, characteristics of myasthenia were induced in the animals, and if the plasma of patients was removed by plasmapheresis or thoracic duct drainage, the symptoms were ameliorated.

Some questions remain. Foremost is the nature of the events that initiate the formation of the antibodies. Also, it is not clear what role sensitized lymphocytes play, for there is evidence of altered cellular immunity, too. There are questions about the antibodies themselves, for they seem to be directed to antigenic sites on the AChR other than the combining site for acetylcholine. Simple blockade of AChR by steric hindrance is one possible mechanism, but the antibodies also seem to accelerate the loss of AChR, and other mechanisms of interference are possible. In intercostal muscle from patients with the disease, miniature end-plate potentials are reduced in amplitude and there is decreased sensitivity to cholinergic agonists.

Other evidence of an autoimmune disorder include abnormalities of the thymus gland in most patients, either germinal centers or thymoma; accumulation of lymphocytes in muscle and other organs; increased coincidence with other presumed autoimmune diseases; and increased frequency of nonspecific autoantibodies against nuclear antigens (ANA), striation-binding muscle antigens, and thyroid antigens.

NEUROMUSCULAR DISORDER. The symptoms of myasthenia gravis resemble those of curare intoxication. This observation led to the use of curare antagonists in the treatment of myasthenia gravis. All effective therapies have been derived from this initial observation, and all drugs currently in use are inhibitors of the enzyme cholinesterase. These drugs also partially repair a physiologic defect that can be detected in patients by relatively simple techniques. When the ulnar nerve of normal individuals is stimulated at rates of 15 per second or less, the action potential of the hypothenar muscles is sustained at a constant amplitude. In patients with myasthenia, however, there is a rapid decline in the height of the evoked potentials. If the patient is then given neostigmine, the amplitude of the evoked potentials is restored to normal. This abnormality has been regarded as characteristic and is consistent with the reduced amplitude of miniature end-plate potentials found in intercostal muscle. The use of repetitive stimulation for diagnostic purposes has disadvantages because it causes some discomfort to the patient and because decrementing responses can be encountered in diseases other than myasthenia gravis. Attention has therefore been given to single-fiber electromyography (SFEMG), which is less painful but has not yet been validated for specificity. In SFEMG, the intervals are measured between discharges of different fibers within the same motor unit. These intervals vary normally, a variation called "jitter," and the temporal limits have been defined. In myasthenia, jitter increases; when the intervals are very long, expected potentials do not appear, a phenomenon called "blocking," and the number of blockings increases in myasthenia. These abnormalities are attributed to slowing of and uncertainty of neuromuscular transmission.

INCIDENCE AND PREVALENCE. The prevalence of myasthenia gravis is about 33 per million population and the annual incidence about 2 to 5 million. Cases occur in all decades of life, most frequently at about age 40. Among young adults, the disease affects women about three times more frequently than men. Among children and older persons, however, men and women are affected equally. There are few familial cases, perhaps somewhat more than would be expected by chance, and there may be increased incidence of thyroid or other autoimmune disease in relatives of patients with myasthenia. Some genetic predisposition is suggested by a disproportionate frequency of particular transplantation antigen haplotypes in affected individuals, and these may differ in those with thymoma and in younger patients with no tumor.

PATHOLOGY. Pathologic changes in myasthenia gravis are limited to muscle and thymus. Skeletal muscles may appear completely normal, but there are often collections of lymphocytes around blood vessels. In some cases there is evidence of degeneration of muscle fibers, and the inflammatory cellular response may be more extensive. Rarely, similar lesions are encountered in the myocardium. The thymus gland is often abnormal. Encapsulated tumors (thymoma) occur in about 15 per cent of the cases, almost all after age 30. In about 25 per cent of these tumors there is evidence of local invasion, but distant metastases are virtually unknown and the local invasiveness is not a cause of symptoms. Lymphocytic proliferation, in the form of germinal centers, is seen in the thymus glands of almost all other patients, but sometimes the gland appears normal, and in some older individuals the gland is so involuted that it cannot be found. Patients dying of this disease usually have some pulmonary disorder (edema, atelectasis, infection) secondary to the terminal events. It has not been shown that myasthenia occurs more frequently in patients with cancer than might be expected on the basis of chance.

CLINICAL MANIFESTATIONS. The most common presenting symptoms relate to weakness of eye muscles, ptosis or diplopia. At the onset these symptoms may last only a few days, then disappear, only to return weeks or months later. Ptosis frequently varies even in the course of a single day. Diplopia may be noted in particular directions of gaze. Difficulty in chewing, dysarthria, and dysphagia are common. Limb weakness is more often proximal in accentuation, so that patients have difficulty climbing stairs or rising from chairs, or have difficulty lifting heavy objects or raising the arms overhead. However, distal weakness is not uncommon, and the initial symptoms may be related to the strength of the hands or fingers. Selective respiratory weakness is unusual. There is no alteration of consciousness, no pain, and, in untreated patients, no cramps or muscular twitching. Difficulty in chewing and swallowing may lead to considerable loss of weight, but there is no specific wasting of muscle except in patients with severe chronic weakness.

On examination, evidence of weakness of the appropriate muscle groups is found. If any sensory abnormality is found, there must be some other disorder, alone or in combination with myasthenia. Similarly, hyperactive reflexes and Babinski signs imply some other disorder, as does the complete loss of reflexes. Weakness is responsible for all the signs of myasthenia. Ptosis may be unilateral or bilateral. Most often, there is asymmetrical weakness of several ocular muscles in a pattern that cannot be explained by disorder of a particular ocular motor nerve. In addition, there is frequently weakness of eye closure because of paresis of the orbicularis oculi. Muscles of the lower face are involved later. Lingual and palatal weakness are evident in patients with dysarthria, producing a nasal twang and indistinct speech. In advanced cases, patients support the chin with one hand to help them talk, a maneuver almost pathognomonic of myasthenia. Neck weakness may be mild or severe enough to cause difficulty in holding the head erect. Limb weakness may be mild or so severe that the patient cannot walk or even turn in bed. Ventilatory insufficiency occurs only in severely affected patients and usually in generalized disease, but some patients with oropharyngeal weakness may be unable to breathe unassisted even though limb muscles are strong. Even though weakness fluctuates, a normal neurologic examination is inconsistent with the diagnosis of myasthenia gravis if the patient is symptomatic at the time.

COURSE. It is the experience of most clinicians that the nature of the disease in a given patient is established within weeks or months of onset, with fluctuations afterward. If after one year, or certainly after two years, myasthenia is still restricted to ocular muscles, it is most unlikely to become generalized; purely ocular myasthenia may account for 20 per cent of all cases.

SPECIAL FORMS OF MYASTHENIA. Neonatal Myasthenia. Infants born to myasthenic women may have a transient syndrome of weakness. The most prominent symptom is difficulty in sucking and swallowing. This may be the sole manifestation, or there may also be noticeable reduction in spontaneous movement and in the vigor of the baby's cry. Only rarely is there respiratory difficulty, but unrecognized neonatal myasthenia has been fatal in exceptional cases. The condition can be identified by the intramuscular injection of neostigmine (0.1 to 0.25 mg), followed by improved sucking, a louder cry, better response to the Moro reflex, and stronger spontaneous movements. Small doses of cholinergic drugs may be administered therapeutically, but more often all that is needed is a nasogastric tube to ensure adequate nutrition. Symptoms subside within a week or, at most, a month.

Congenital Myasthenia. Myasthenia gravis may commence at any age. But there are some children who seem to have had ophthalmoplegia from birth, with or without other signs of myasthenia. Although presumably congenital, this disorder rarely causes concern in the first year of life. It is only later, when the ophthalmoplegia is recognized, that the parents state the child's eyes have always been that way. There may be a disproportionate number of familial cases among children with congenital myasthenia; ophthalmoplegia occurs in almost all of them, and there may be somewhat less tendency for crisis and remission. Otherwise, there are no characteristics that distinguish this syndrome from myasthenia at any other age.

Thyrotoxicosis. About 5 per cent of patients with myasthenia have thyrotoxicosis at some time. Usually the two disorders occur simultaneously, but sometimes hyperthyroidism is evident for weeks or months before there are myasthenic symptoms. Only rarely does myasthenia come long before the thyrotoxicosis, and patients who appear euthyroid do not ordinarily have laboratory evidence of thyroid overactivity. Treatment of the two disorders is directed according to the usual indications for each.

DIAGNOSIS. In almost all cases the diagnosis of myasthenia is obvious from the history and examination. The diagnosis is immediately confirmed by the response to cholinergic drugs. For adults, 1 ml of edrophonium (10 mg) is given by vein intermittently; after injection of 2 to 3 mg, specific muscle groups are evaluated. If there is no response within 30 seconds, a second dose of 3.0 mg is given and the patient is evaluated once again. If there is still no response, the remainder is given, a total of 10 mg. This drug is preferred when cranial muscles are being tested because the response is prompt and dramatic. Cranial weakness cannot be simulated voluntarily, and placebo injections are therefore not necessary.

If it is desired to evaluate limb strength, the injection of neostigmine has advantages because the effect lasts longer, permitting more leisurely testing. The adult dose is 1.5 mg intramuscularly, and it is usually combined with atropine, 0.5 mg, to avoid the muscarinic symptoms of abdominal cramps and sweating. When limb strength is evaluated, it is sometimes advisable to evaluate placebo responses by giving the atropine 30 minutes before the neostigmine. In all cases of myasthenia gravis there is some response to these drugs, but the response is sometimes slight, and the test may have to be repeated on several occasions to provide convincing evidence.

To provide confirmatory evidence, the electromyographic response to ulnar nerve stimulation may be studied. The characteristic decline in amplitude of the evoked potential is usually seen in affected muscles, but the response may be normal when the disease is restricted to the eyes. As noted above, SFEMG is finding increasing use in diagnosis. Rarely, it is desirable to administer d-tubocurarine, a drug to which myasthenics are unusually sensitive. There are hazards in the administration of this drug, however, and its use should probably be left to research centers; d-tubocurarine should never be given without appropriate precautions to support respiration.

The most important diagnostic laboratory test is likely to be the demonstration of antibodies to AChR, as this seems to be present in virtually all these patients but not in the other diseases. The most sensitive and most specific assay system reported so far involves use of human AChR as antigen, and this is difficult to obtain. AChR from denervated rat muscle or from the electric organs of torpedo or eel may substitute, but seem less sensitive.

It is useful to perform a standard series of studies. Thymomas can almost always be identified in standard roentgenograms of the chest, supplemented by oblique views. Laminagrams may provide more information, but there is little need for thymic venography or mediastinal pneumography. Thyroid function should be tested, and it is useful to evaluate immunologic disorders by serum protein electrophoresis, LE cell preparation, latex fixation test for rheumatoid factor, and antinuclear antibodies. Tests for muscle antibodies or lymphocyte sensitivity are performed in special centers.

The differential diagnosis requires special consideration. Probably the most frequent error in diagnosis concerns patients with emotional fatigue states and hysterical weakness. There are no cranial muscle symptoms in these patients (except globus hystericus), whereas cranial muscles are involved in virtually all myasthenics. Their symptoms are not those of weakness but of exhaustion, and in tests of strength against resistance there is apt to be marked variation in effort, or dramatic giving way. The diagnosis of acute myasthenia may be mistakenly made in a patient with botulism. As the discovery of botulism calls for urgent action, for both patient and eating companions, the physician should be aware of this diagnostic pitfall (see Ch. 22.3). Amyotrophic lateral sclerosis and peripheral neuropathy may be confused with myasthenia when these disorders affect cranial muscles, but signs indicative of a neurogenic disorder distinguish them from myasthenia. Polymyositis may be confusing, but ocular muscle paresis is not found. There is some debate about the specificity of the therapeutic effect of cholinergic drugs, but for practical purposes it may be taken that an authentic (not placebo), convincing (not equivocal), and reproducible (not seen by one examiner only) effect is found only in myasthenia gravis.

TREATMENT. Therapeutic efforts fall into two categories: those which affect symptoms without influencing the course of the disease (cholinergic drugs), and those designed to induce remission of the disease itself (thymectomy, steroids, immunosuppressive drugs). Management starts as soon as the diagnosis is made, using cholinergic drugs. Then decisions are made regarding other forms of treatment.

Cholinergic Drug Therapy. The major drugs used to treat myasthenia gravis are inhibitors of cholinesterase, neostigmine and pyridostigmine. Another drug, ambenonium, is also used in some clinics, but has no special advantages. It is best to use only one drug; there is no benefit from combinations of two or more. Neostigmine is provided in 15 mg tablets, and pyridostigmine in 60 mg tablets; these are essentially interchangeable. The choice of drugs is arbitrary because there is no evidence that the maximal benefit achieved by one is more than that of the other. Most patients, but not all, prefer pyridostigmine because it is less apt to cause abdominal cramps and diarrhea, and it is less apt to cause noticeable peaks and valleys of strength. But these advantages have never been proved objectively, and some patients do very well with neostigmine. Pyridostigmine is also provided in a slow-release capsule (Timespan) of 180 mg, said to provide 60 mg immediately and the remainder in 8 to 12 hours. Some clinicians use the prolonged-action preparation throughout the day, but because of uncertainties of release, it seems advisable to use this only at bedtime for patients who would otherwise have to awaken at night or who are very weak on waking in the morning. (For patients who cannot swallow pills, both drugs may be administered parenterally, and pyridostigmine may be given as a syrup. The intramuscular dose is about one tenth of the oral dose, and the intravenous dose is one thirtieth of the oral dose.) Decisions about optimal dosage are sometimes difficult. Some authorities advocate the use of edrophonium to evaluate oral drug therapy; a test dose of 2 mg is given intravenously. If the patient improves, oral therapy has been too little. If there is aggravation of weakness, oral therapy has been too much. But other authorities find this an unreliable guide, and we do not use this technique. If edrophonium is not used, there is nothing but clinical observation to guide the therapist. For mild cases, two tablets of either neostigmine or pyridostigmine three times daily, with meals, is useful. If there is inadequate response, the dose may be increased, first by shortening the interval between doses, then by increasing the quantity of drug with each dose. Problems arise because these drugs never completely reverse symptoms. Therefore the dose should be increased only so long as there is clear-cut response, and it should not be increased beyond the amount giving some perceptible benefit.

Overtreatment itself can cause weakness; cholinesterase inhibitors may cause a depolarizing block at the neuromuscular junction. This probably does not occur often.

Drugs advocated as "adjuvants" include potassium chloride, ephedrine, and guanidine; they may have some effect in individual patients, but their true value is unproved.

Steroids and Immunosuppressive Drugs. Prednisone now enjoys widespread popularity in the treatment of myasthenia, but it has never been put to an adequately controlled prospective therapeutic trial. Some investigators report improvement in as many as 80 per cent of patients treated, with virtually no side effects. Others are less enthusiastic about beneficial effects and are more concerned about deleterious effects. Some treat virtually all patients; others restrict therapy to those with incapacitating disease. It is agreed that the minimal dose should be about 50 mg daily for an adult, often given as 100 mg on alternate days. For patients who are seriously ill, larger doses have been used. Alternatively, because worsening of myasthenia may attend initiation of therapy, some start with 25 mg on alternate days and gradually increase to the full dose. Some use prednisone in preparation for thymectomy; others reserve steroids until some interval after thymectomy. If there is no beneficial response, it is not clear how long prednisone should be continued before deeming the trial a failure; a minimum of three months at full dosage seems reasonable. No matter how used, steroid drugs should be initiated with close supervision and probably in hospital because of the danger of their temporarily increasing the weakness.

The mechanism of action of steroids in myasthenia is not known, but current theories favor an immunosuppressive role. More specific immunosuppressive drugs such as azathioprine, methotrexate, or cyclophosphamide have also been used. There is no indication that these drugs are any better than prednisone, and evaluation of them is probably best performed in research centers.

Surgical Treatment. A reasonable program for patients with myasthenia starts with thymectomy for those still disabled after cholinergic drug treatment. Thymectomy is followed by significant improvement in about two thirds of patients with myasthenia and no tumor. Patients with thymoma fare worse whether the tumor is excised or not. Chest surgeons, anesthesiologists, and respirator units for postoperative care are now so skillful that the risks of operation are almost negligible. Because it is difficult to predict which patients will benefit, however, there is still some uncertainty in the selection of patients. Some recommend the operation for all patients who are incapacitated in daily living for more than six months despite adequate drug therapy. In preparing patients for operation, their usual oral dosage is continued until the day of operation, then stopped. Endotracheal intubation is used for all patients with oropharyngeal weakness, and intermittent positive pressure breathing is used in the postoperative period. The endotracheal tube may have to be replaced by tracheostomy after a few days, but endotracheal intubation alone suffices in most cases. Specific cholinergic drug therapy is withheld for several days, until fever subsides, and then started again at a level of one half or less of the preoperative dose.

Crisis. Patients with myasthenia gravis may suddenly develop difficulty breathing, severe enough to require artificial ventilation. This may be induced by systemic infection or major surgical procedures, but often there is no apparent cause. Patients with oropharyngeal weakness are especially liable to this threat, perhaps because of aspiration. Whenever there is doubt about the adequacy of ventilation or the state of the airway, endotracheal intubation should be used for short periods of respiratory support, obviating the need for tracheostomy. The insertion of a cuffed tube makes intermittent positive pressure breathing feasible, and also reduces the hazard of aspiration. Patients are best transferred to a respiratory intensive care unit. Cholinergic drugs are stopped. After several days, usually after fever (an almost inevitable concomitant of crisis and tracheostomy) has started to subside, drugs may be started once again, at half the precrisis dosage. The cause of crisis is not clear, but it is usually transient, and will subside if the patient can be kept alive. The mortality rate of crisis was formerly about 50 per cent, but since the advent of intensive care units, only about 10 per cent die, and these are mostly elderly patients with complicating cardiac and renal disease.

Some patients require assisted ventilation for prolonged periods, some longer than one year. For these patients, trial programs of prednisone seem advisable.

PROGNOSIS. The course of myasthenia is variable. The disease may be restricted to ocular muscles for many years, with no threat of life. Other patients are disabled to a variable degree by oropharyngeal or limb weakness, and a few are crippled. Crisis occurs in about 25 per cent of the cases. The over-all mortality is probably about 15 per cent, and although myasthenia itself was formerly the main hazard, intercurrent and unrelated disease is now more often the cause of death.

Drachman, D. B.: Medical progress: Myasthenia gravis. N. Engl. J. Med., 298:136, 186, 1978.
Genkins, G., Papatestas, A. E., Horowitz, S. H., and Kornfeld, P.: Studies in myasthenia gravis. Early thymectomy. Am. J. Med., 58:517, 1975.
Harvey, A. M.: Myasthenia gravis: The first 100 years in perspective. Trans. Am. Clin. Climatol., 82:149, 1970.
Jaretski, A., III, Wolff, M., Olarte, M., et al.: A rational approach to total thymectomy in the treatment of myasthenia gravis. Ann. Thorac. Surg., 24:120, 1977.
Johns, T. R.: Treatment of myasthenia gravis. Long-term administration of corticosteroids with remarks on thymectomy. Adv. Neurol., 17:99, 1977.
Lindstrom, J. M., Einarson, B. L., Lennon, V. A., et al.: Antibody to acetylcholine receptor in myasthenia gravis; prevalence, clinical correlates, and diagnostic value. Neurology, 26:1054, 1976.
Lindstrom, J. M., and Lambert, E. H.: Content of acetylcholine receptor and antibodies bound to receptor in myasthenia gravis, experimental autoimmune myasthenia gravis and Eaton-Lambert syndrome. Neurology, 26:130, 1978.
Pinching, A. J., Peters, D. K., and Davis, J. N.: Remission of myasthenia gravis following plasma exchange. Lancet, 2:1373, 1976.

340.5. EATON-LAMBERT SYNDROME
(Myasthenic Syndrome)

DEFINITION. The Eaton-Lambert syndrome is defined essentially in terms of electromyography. It is a disorder with muscular weakness in which the amplitude of the first muscle action potential evoked by stimulation of the nerve is reduced, and with repetitive stimulation the amplitude of the action potential increases to more than three times the original height.

PATHOGENESIS. The first cases were associated with oat-cell carcinoma of the lung, but cases have been found with other tumors, other diseases, and sometimes with no complicating disorder. Microelectrode studies indicate that the defect is due to impaired release of acetylcholine at the nerve terminals.

CLINICAL MANIFESTATIONS. The first evidence of the Eaton-Lambert syndrome may be prolonged apnea after curarization for surgery. Formal testing with d-tubocurarine also indicates that patients are unduly

sensitive. Other patients may have symptoms of limb weakness, but cranial muscle weakness is never prominent. The response to cholinergic drugs is usually equivocal at best. Pain in the limbs may be prominent. Movements may be peculiarly slow. In tests of strength it may seem as though the patient gets stronger with continued effort. Myotatic reflexes are frequently depressed.

DIAGNOSIS. The signs listed above diverge sufficiently from myasthenia to avoid confusion; only limb weakness and curare sensitivity are similar. The remainder of the syndrome resembles polymyositis, and polyneuritis would also have to be considered. The diagnosis is made by the response to repetitive stimulation. Antibodies to AChR have not been found in typical cases.

TREATMENT. Guanidine promotes the release of acetylcholine, and the drug is effective in daily doses of 35 mg per kilogram of body weight, given orally. This drug may suppress bone marrow in many patients, however, and great caution must be taken. This effect limits treatment seriously, and the drug should probably not be used unless the neuromuscular disorder is disabling.

Eaton, L. M., and Lambert, E. H.: Electromyography and electric stimulation of nerves in diseases of motor unit: Observations in myasthenic syndrome associated with malignant tumors. JAMA, 163:1117, 1957.
Elmqvist, D., and Lambert, E. H.: Detailed analysis of neuromuscular transmission in a patient with myasthenic syndrome sometimes associated with brochogenic carcinoma. Mayo Clin. Proc., 43:689, 1968.
Oh, S. J., and Kim, K. W.: Guanidine hydrochloride in the Eaton-Lambert syndrome. Neurology, 23:1084, 1973.

340.6. UNUSUAL CAUSES OF NEUROMUSCULAR BLOCK

Botulism and *tick paralysis* are described in Ch. 22.3 and 33.12. Both cause a syndrome of flaccid quadriplegia with paresis of cranial muscles, and must be differentiated from polyneuritis, myasthenia gravis, and periodic paralysis. In neither is there a sensory disorder, but autonomic fibers may be affected in botulism, especially pupilloconstrictor fibers (resulting in a dilated, fixed pupil). The physiologic disorder in both syndromes is impaired release of acetylcholine from motor nerve terminals. The electromyogram in botulism may resemble that in the Eaton-Lambert syndrome, an observation that may be diagnostically important. Guanidine has been used with benefit to treat botulism and might also be effective in tick paralysis. Supportive therapy (tracheostomy and assisted respiration) is mandatory in severe cases. Tick paralysis is reversed by removal of the organism.

Several *aminoglycoside antimicrobial drugs* interfere with the release of acetylcholine, and may cause clinical syndromes in man. The offending drugs include neomycin, streptomycin, colistin, polymyxin, and kanamycin. The most common manifestation is postoperative apnea without other evidence of paralysis. This is most apt to occur in patients with renal failure, presumably with unusually high blood levels of the antimicrobial drug. In occasional cases, however, there may be flaccid quadriplegia. Administration of calcium and guanidine may be helpful, but the essence of management is supportive treatment and use of a safer antimicrobial.

Cherington, M., and Ryan, D. W.: Botulism and guanidine. N. Engl. J. Med., 278:931, 1968.
de Jesus, P. V., Slater, R., Spitz, L. K., and Penn, A. S.: Neuromuscular physiology of wound botulism. Arch. Neurol., 29:425, 1973.
McQuillen, M. P., Cantor, H. E., and O'Rourke, J. R.: Myasthenic syndrome associated with antibiotics. Arch. Neurol., 18:402, 1968.
Swift, T. R., and Ignacio, F. J.: Tick paralysis: Electrophysiologic studies. Neurology, 25:1130, 1975.

340.7. SYNDROMES OF MUSCULAR OVERACTIVITY: CRAMPS AND RELATED DISORDERS

Cramps, caused by painful, abrupt shortening of muscle, affect almost everyone at some time or other, Electromyographic investigation indicates that motor units fire at a rate of about 300 per second, much higher than the most vigorous voluntary contraction. It is presumably the high rate of discharge that causes the palpable muscle tautness and the pain. The pain can be relieved by stretching the affected muscle, or by massage. The stimulus responsible for cramps is not known; relief by stretching suggests that some central mechanism is involved, since this is the stimulus for receptors in muscle that inhibit discharge of the motor neuron to the same muscle. Certain conditions are associated with a propensity to cramps: denervation (especially amyotrophic lateral sclerosis), pregnancy, and electrolyte disorders (especially water intoxication and hyponatremia). Some people are more susceptible than others for unknown reasons. Sometimes cramps occur only at night, and can be prevented by quinine sulfate, 0.3 gram orally at bedtime. Sometimes cramps occur frequently during the day, occasionally so often that the individual is effectively crippled. Diphenylhydantoin, 0.3 to 0.6 gram daily, may be helpful to these patients, but some are resistant to this and to other drugs that may be tried, including diazepam and procainamide.

Tetany is a special form of cramp, identified by its predilection for flexor muscles of the hand and fingers, its association with laryngospasm, and its relationship to hypocalcemia. Tetany can be painful. It differs from other cramps electromyographically because of the characteristic rhythmic grouping of discharging potentials.

Contracture is the term reserved for the painful shortening of muscles in glycogen storage diseases, in which the muscles are electrically silent although maximally shortened.

Myokymia has been used to describe a variety of apparently different disorders characterized by cramps in association with spontaneous twitching of muscle. In some cases there are prolonged trains of spontaneous potentials, whereas in others there is grouping of potentials. Some of these patients have difficulty in relaxing grip, but, unlike myotonia, the muscular activity is abolished by neuromuscular blocking agents, indicating a neural rather than a muscular origin. Hyperhidrosis is prominent in some patients and is secondary to the increased muscular activity.

Continuous shortening of the muscle would lead to abnormal postures and abnormally increased resistance to passive movement. These abnormalities, of course, are often due to central neurologic disorders. In recent years, however, an increasing number of patients have been described because of fluctuating rigidity of axial and limb muscles. For want of a better name, and lacking understanding of the pathogenesis, this has been called the *stiff man syndrome*. The diagnosis requires that there be no signs of cerebral or spinal cord disease, and there must be continuous electromyographic activity despite authentic attempts to relax. Ordinary cramps may be superimposed upon the persistent stiffness. Diazepam, 30 to 60 mg daily, may bring dramatic relief.

A variety of other names have been applied to these syndromes, including *quantal squander, armadillo diease, neuromyotonia,* and *continuous muscle fiber activity.* Some cases of brief duration may be related to mild cases of tetanus. It will take some time to sort out the variety of causes. If these unusual forms can be analyzed, we may yet understand why an otherwise normal individual occasionally has a cramp.

Editorial: Writer's cramp. Br. Med. J., 1:67, 1972.
Garner-Medwin, D., and Walton, J. N.: Myokymia with impaired muscular relaxation. Lancet, 1:127, 1969.
Gordon, E. E., Januszko, D. M., and Kaufman, L.: A critical survey of stiff man syndrome, Am. J. Med. 42:582, 1967.
Isgreen, W. P.: Normocalcemic tetany. Neurology, 26:825, 1976.
Layzer, R. B., and Rowland, L. P.: Cramps. N. Engl. J. Med., 285:31, 1971.
Wallis, W. E., Van Poznak, A., and Plum, F.: Generalized muscular stiffness, fasciculations and myokymia of peripheral nerve origin. Arch. Neurol., 22:430, 1970.

PART XII
RESPIRATORY DISEASE

341. INTRODUCTION

John F. Murray

Normal respiration includes all of the processes concerned with O_2 uptake and CO_2 elimination. The lungs are the major organs of gas exchange, but the nose, oropharynx, extrapulmonary airways, brain, spinal cord, nerves, thoracic cage, respiratory muscles, and cardiovascular system are also involved. Thus respiratory diseases, literally interpreted, incorporate a large variety of abnormalities arising in all the different structures that contribute to gas exchange. In general, however, a more limited definition applies, and respiratory diseases are considered to include disturbances of the air passages, lungs, pleura, chest wall, muscles of respiration, and mediastinum (excluding the heart, systemic vessels, and esophagus).

Acute respiratory diseases are probably the most common affliction of mankind and are responsible for more absences from school and work than any other illness. Chronic respiratory diseases, particularly emphysema and bronchitis, are second only to cardiovascular diseases as causes of disability payments. Cancer of the lung kills more persons each year than any other kind of malignancy. Because of the remarkable incidence of these and other respiratory diseases, it is important that all physicians, not just internists and chest specialists, be well versed in the clinical manifestations and methods of diagnosis, treatment, and prevention of the most common disorders. The material concerned with respiratory diseases here and elsewhere in the book is intended as a primer of necessary knowledge with which to recognize and to treat the major respiratory diseases; additional information is available in the references cited at the end of each chapter.

Acute infections of the upper and lower respiratory tract caused by viruses, bacteria, fungi, protozoa, and helminths are discussed in appropriate chapters in Parts IX and X of the text. Although most infectious diseases of the air passages and lungs are viral in origin and prove to be relatively benign and self-limiting, the importance of other infections in the differential diagnosis of patients with respiratory disease cannot be overemphasized. These remain a major cause of morbidity and mortality that can largely be prevented by early diagnosis and use of appropriate chemotherapy. For example, tuberculosis, an eminently curable disease, is too often forgotten and tragically identified only at postmortem examination.

In view of their systemic manifestations, diseases that commonly involve the lungs such as sarcoidosis (see Ch. 65), Wegener's granulomatosis (see Ch. 68), eosinophilic syndromes (see Ch. 72), and the "collagen diseases" (see Ch. 49 to 53) are also discussed elsewhere. Another group of diseases that frequently involve the lungs both primarily and secondarily are disorders of the pulmonary circulation. Of these, pulmonary embolism and infarction (see Ch. 357.3) are by far the most important, but patients with primary pulmonary hypertension (see Ch. 358) and other vasculitic disorders are occasionally encountered. A major feature of many respiratory diseases, but not a disease itself, is pulmonary edema; this is discussed in part in Ch. 351 and in part in Ch. 355.

Part XII begins with a review of basic respiratory physiology (Ch. 342). Knowledge of physiologic principles provides the background for understanding how respiratory diseases affect the function of the lungs and for ordering and interpreting various pulmonary function tests. Next, Ch. 343 deals with the work-up of the patient with respiratory disease, including discussion of the indications for selecting particular diagnostic procedures among those traditional and newly available methods that have improved and often simplified the diagnosis of many diseases. These chapters are followed by those on categories of respiratory diseases: diseases associated with airways obstruction (Ch. 344); abnormalities of lung aeration (Ch. 345); diffuse infiltrative diseases (Ch. 346); lung abscess and bronchiectasis (Ch. 347); physical and chemical irritants (Ch. 348); neoplasms of the lung (Ch. 349); and diseases of the pleura, diaphragm, chest wall, and mediastinum (Ch. 350). Finally, because virtually all respiratory disorders can lead to disturbances of gas exchange, Ch. 351 discusses the diagnosis and treatment of respiratory failure. In this context the term respiratory is used in its broadest meaning to include abnormalities anywhere in the body that cause decreases in arterial P_{O_2} and increases in P_{CO_2}.

342. RESPIRATORY STRUCTURE AND FUNCTION

John F. Murray

342.1. INTRODUCTION

Knowledge of normal pulmonary physiology is a necessary background for understanding how abnormalities affect the function of the lungs. This information enables practicing physicians to order and to interpret results of the pulmonary function tests that have proved of considerable value in the diagnosis and management of patients with many types of lung disease.

Respiration can be defined as "those processes concerned with gas exchange between an organism and its environment." This definition, which emphasizes that the chief function of the respiratory system is *gas exchange*, is sufficiently comprehensive to apply to all animals, ranging from simple one-celled protozoa to infinitely more complex mammals. In human beings, the basic processes leading to gas exchange, or the uptake of O_2 and the elimination of CO_2, are usually separated into four functional subdivisions:

(1) *Ventilation* — the movement of air from outside to inside the body and the distribution of air within the tracheobronchial system to the gas exchange units of the lungs.

(2) *Diffusion* — the movement of O_2 and CO_2 across the alveolar-capillary membrane between the gas in alveolar spaces and the blood in pulmonary capillaries.

(3) *Perfusion* — the flow of mixed venous blood through the pulmonary arterial circulation, distribution of the blood to the capillaries of the gas exchange units, and removal of the blood from the lungs through pulmonary veins.

(4) *Control of breathing* — the regulation of ventilation, usually in accordance with changing metabolic demands.

342.2. VENTILATION

Air moves from outside the body into the gas exchange units of the lung because contraction of the muscles of respiration normally generates sufficient force to expand the lungs and chest wall and to overcome the resistance and inertia in the system. Accordingly, the volume of gas that reaches the individual gas exchange units is determined by the mechanical properties of the lung parenchyma, airways, and chest wall, and by the force provided by the muscles of respiration (or by a mechanical ventilator).

The amount of air that enters the lung with each breath is called the *tidal volume*. When the lungs are fully expanded, the amount of gas they contain is called the *total lung capacity*. The maximal volume of gas that a person can exhale from total lung capacity is called the *vital capacity*, and the amount of gas remaining in the lungs at the end of maximal expiration is called the *residual volume*. Another important static lung volume is the *functional residual capacity*, which is the volume of gas in the lungs at the end of a normal breath. The relationships among these different lung volumes, which vary in different disorders and which will be frequently referred to, are shown in Figure 1.

STATIC PROPERTIES

Both the lungs and chest wall are elastic structures. This means that they can distend and, when the distending force is removed, recoil back to their resting volumes. Although the lungs and chest wall are similar in this respect, they differ considerably in their respective resting volumes when there is no expanding force.

The elastic properties of isolated lungs are shown by the dashed line in Figure 1. The slope of the line, or the change in volume (ΔV) for a given change in pressure (ΔP), is known as the compliance of the lung. This curve demonstrates that (1) the lungs collapse almost completely when there is no distending pressure, (2) the slope of the volume-pressure curve is relatively steep at low lung volumes (i.e., as the lungs are beginning to inflate, their compliance is high), and (3) at high lung volumes, the curve flattens (compliance decreases) so that little increase in volume results from a large increase in pressure. The elastic forces of the lungs originate within the tissues that are being stretched, particularly those containing elastin and collagen, and from the surface tension of the film of *sur-*

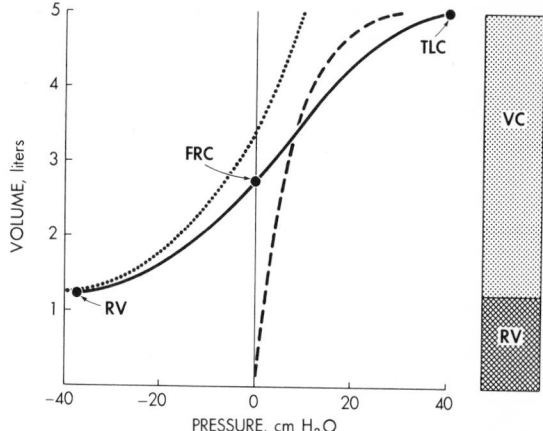

Figure 1. Schematic representation of the volume-pressure relationships of the chest wall (dotted line), lungs (dashed line), and chest wall and lungs combined (solid line). Total lung capacity (TLC) occurs when the lungs are fully expanded, and residual volume (RV) is the amount of gas remaining in the lungs at the end of a maximal expiration. Functional residual capacity (FRC) occurs at that volume at which the recoil pressures of the chest wall and lung are equal and opposite (i.e., the distending pressure = 0 cm H_2O). The bar graph on the right shows the vital capacity (VC) and RV subdivisions of TLC.

factant that lines the air-liquid interface of alveolar spaces. The static properties of the isolated chest wall (including the diaphragm and abdominal contents that must be displaced during breathing) are shown by the dotted line in Figure 1. The chest wall is a compressible and distensible structure that contains an appreciable volume in its resting state. To decrease the volume of the thorax, a force must be applied to overcome the tendency of the chest wall to resist compression and recoil back to its resting position. Conversely, to increase the volume of the thorax, the applied force must overcome the elastic forces in the chest wall that also cause it to recoil back to its resting position.

It is useful conceptually to consider the behavior of the lung and chest wall separately, but obviously they function together. Because their action is coupled by the pleural pressure that keeps the lung expanded against the chest wall, the lungs and chest wall ordinarily change their volumes by exactly the same amount. Thus the pressures required to inflate and deflate the respiratory system (or lung and chest wall combined) are obtained by simply adding the pressures necessary to achieve a given volume. The solid line in Figure 1 indicates the pressure that must be produced by contraction of the respiratory muscles, or by a mechanical ventilator, to inflate or deflate both the lungs and chest wall. Figure 1 also shows that functional residual capacity is the volume at which the inward recoil force of the lung is equal and opposite to the outward recoil force of the chest wall; in other words, functional residual capacity is that volume at which the net force of the respiratory system is zero.

During inspiration, the force developed by the contracting muscles of inspiration meets progressively increasing (inward) recoil forces from the combined expansion of the lung and chest wall. Furthermore, because shortening muscle fibers generate progressively less force, inspiration finally ceases at that volume (total lung capacity) at which the weakening inspiratory muscle forces can no longer overcome the increasing forces required to expand the lungs and chest wall. Similarly, during expiration, the net force developed by the contracting muscles of expiration meets progressively increasing (outward) recoil forces from the chest wall. In children and young adults, expiration ceases at that volume (residual volume) at which the decreasing expiratory muscle forces can no longer overcome the increasing forces required to compress the chest wall. In older persons, residual volume is governed mainly by factors that regulate the caliber and patency of peripheral airways; thus even though the expiratory muscles are capable of further compression, emptying is prevented by airway closure and trapping of gas in the lungs.

Vital capacity, or the volume between total lung capacity and residual volume, is determined by the factors that influence maximum inspiration and expiration, i.e., the balance of forces generated by the muscles of respiration and by the mechanical properties of the lungs and chest wall combined. Changes in these variables explain the characteristic changes in lung volumes that occur in patients with the respiratory disorders discussed in subsequent chapters.

Lung volumes also vary among healthy persons according to their age, sex, and physical structure (especially height). Because body build varies slightly from one ethnic group to another, it is important to have normal data that pertain to the population being studied. Measured volumes are usually expressed as both the observed value and the percentage of the predicted value for a normal subject of the same age, sex, and height.

$$\text{Per cent predicted} = \frac{\text{observed value}}{\text{predicted value}} \times 100$$

Measured values should not be considered abnormal unless thay are clearly outside the range of values likely to be found in normal persons (100 per cent ± 20 per cent for vital capacity and 100 per cent ± 25 per cent for total lung capacity, residual volume, and functional residual capacity).

Vital capacity is easily measured with a spirometer or one of a variety of commercially available recording systems. Most spirometers can also be used to determine airflow rates (see Dynamic Properties, below) but they do not measure total lung capacity, functional residual capacity, or residual volume.

To measure *all* the gas in the lungs at any of these volumes, one of two basically different methods must be used: either dilution or washout of an inert gas or whole body plethysmography. Functional residual capacity is usually determined because it is the normal end-expiratory lung volume and an easy volume for subjects to maintain during the breathing test. After measuring functional residual capacity, residual volume is derived by subtracting expiratory reserve volume, and total lung capacity is obtained by adding vital capacity to the residual volume.

Gas dilution or washout involves measurement of the volume and concentration of an inert gas such as nitrogen (N_2), neon (Ne), or helium (He). These methods measure the amount of gas that communicates freely with the airways during the breathing maneuver; dilution or washout techniques do not detect gas trapped beyond closed (or very narrowed) airways and in poorly communicating regions, like bullae.

Body plethysmography involves placing the subject in the plethysmograph, a large airtight box resembling a telephone booth, and having him breathe through a mouthpiece in which a shutter can be closed to stop the flow of air. When the subject attempts to pant against the closed shutter, the volume of the thorax and gas in the lungs expands and contracts, which changes the pressure measured inside the mouthpiece. Movement of the thorax also changes the pressure in the box by compressing and expanding the gas surrounding the subject. From application of Boyle's law, which states that the pressure times the volume of a gas is constant if temperature remains the same, the volume of gas in the thorax can be calculated. The body plethysmograph measures all the gas present during the breathing maneuver, including that in freely communicating airspaces and any that may be trapped behind poorly communicating airways or in closed spaces (pneumothorax).

In normal subjects, measurements of functional residual capacity by dilution (or washout) and plethysmographic techniques are virtually identical. In contrast, in patients with airways obstruction or bullous disease, the communicating volume may be considerably less than the plethysmographic volume and the difference is a measure of the noncommunicating (sometimes called trapped) volume.

DYNAMIC PROPERTIES

To cause air to flow from outside the body into the gas exchange units, a muscular (or other mechanical) force must be exerted to overcome not only the elastic recoil properties of the lungs and chest wall but also their resistive and inertial properties. In contrast to distensibility, which is not affected by the rate of movement, the forces required to offset resistance and inertia are markedly influenced by the velocity of airflow. Except in a few patients (e.g., those with severe obesity), inertial forces are normally small and usually ignored; thus only those factors affecting airways resistance need be considered in detail.

Resistance to airflow is affected chiefly by the caliber of the airways. Although the diameter of each successive generation of airways decreases, their combined total cross-sectional area increases steadily throughout the tracheobronchial tree from the main bronchi to the peripheral airways. This means that airways resistance progressively decreases and that most of the resistance of the human tracheobronchial tree resides in large airways: direct measurements reveal that about 80 per cent of total airway resistance originates in airways *greater than* 2 mm in diameter. A corollary of this observation is that changes can occur in the caliber of the small peripheral airways without having much effect on total airways resistance. Hence, small airways have been called the lung's "quiet zone," and because they are frequently involved early in the evolution of clinically important lung disease, new tests have been devised to examine their functional behavior.

Changes in the cross-sectional area of airways can also result from changes in lung volume and diseases of the lung parenchyma and airways. During inflation of the lungs from functional residual capacity, airways are

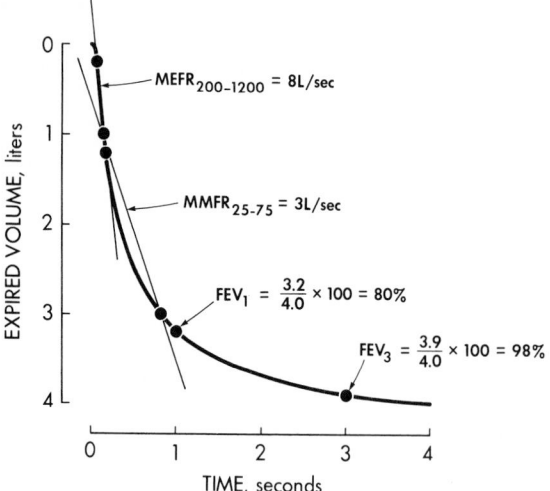

Figure 2. Schematic representation of a normal forced vital capacity (FVC) maneuver (expired volume against time, heavy line) and the derivation of several variables commonly used to evaluate airways obstruction. $MEFR_{200-1200}$ = maximal expiratory flow rate, measured between expired volumes of 200 and 1200 ml; $MMER_{25-75}$ = maximal mid-expiratory flow rate, measured between 25 and 75 per cent of the total FVC; FEV_1 = forced expiratory volume in one second, expressed as percentage of total FVC; FEV_3 = forced expiratory volume in three seconds, expressed as percentage of total FVC.

pulled open so that resistance to airflow decreases; during deflation, airways narrow and their resistance increases. Airway caliber changes during inflation and deflation because of the combined effects of the tethering action of the attachments between the lung parenchyma and small airways and the distending effect of pleural pressure on large airways. Elastic recoil of the lung, which governs the pull of the attachments and the magnitude of pleural pressure, affects the size of all airways. It follows that when elastic recoil is decreased, as in patients with emphysema, airways are narrowed and resistance is increased; this mechanism accounts for much of the airflow obstruction found in patients with emphysema.

Airway narrowing can also result from bronchospasm, edema of the mucosal lining, and secretions within the lumen. Also, changes in the viscosity and density of the inspired gas affect airways resistance, and gas mixtures of different densities are sometimes used to study the dynamic properties of the tracheobronchial system.

Airways resistance can be measured in a body plethysmograph; however, this procedure has limited clinical usefulness. Fortunately, the important dynamic properties of the respiratory system can be assessed by several readily available tests of airways function. The simplest and most widely used of these is the forced expiratory volume in one second (FEV_1), expressed as a ratio of the forced vital capacity (FVC), or FEV_1/FVC (Fig. 2). To perform the FVC maneuver, the subject inhales fully and then exhales as rapidly and completely as possible. In normal persons, the FVC equals the vital capacity from a slow or nonexpulsive maneuver, but in patients with airways obstruction, vigorous expiration may cause airways to narrow or close so that the FVC may be less than the vital capacity; the magnitude of

the difference between the two values is an indication of the amount of air trapped behind compressed airways. The FEV_1/FVC decreases with age in normal persons after reaching adulthood and is usually higher in women than in men at all ages.

Additional measurements of airways behavior besides the FEV_1 can be obtained from the tracing obtained during the FVC maneuver (Fig. 2): several derivatives of time such as the $FEV_{0.5}$ and FEV_3 (the subscript denoting the number of seconds after beginning expiration at which the expired volume is measured), the maximal expiratory flow rate (MEFR or often $MEFR_{200-1200\ ml}$, indicating that the flow rate was measured between expired volumes of 200 and 1200 ml), and the maximal mid-expiratory flow rate (MMFR or often $MMFR_{25-75\%}$, indicating that the rate was measured between expired volumes of 25 and 75 per cent of the FVC). None of these has any particular advantage over the FEV_1 except that the MMFR is less dependent on the effort exerted by the subject than the other variables and reflects the flow properties of small as well as large airways.

Another way of examining the events during an FVC maneuver is by recording flow against volume instead of volume against time, which provides a maximal expiratory flow–volume curve. From these records, maximal flow rates at any given fraction of the vital capacity, usually 50 per cent ($\dot{V}max_{50}$) or 25 per cent ($\dot{V}max_{25}$), can be determined and reported as the percentage of the predicted values for a subject of the same age, sex, and body size. The early portion of the maximal expiratory flow–volume curve, which includes peak flow, is determined by the effort exerted by the subject and is thus called the effort-*dependent* segment; the later portion is less influenced by effort and is called the effort-*independent* segment. Failure of increasing expiratory effort to augment the velocity of airflow (during the effort-independent portion of the curve) is explained by a fortuitous combination of circumstances through which increasing effort narrows airways by the phenomenon of dynamic compression, and increases airways resistance by just the right amount to offset the effect of the extra effort. Dynamic compression occurs mainly in large airways, from the trachea out to about the segmental bronchi. Compression is important during coughing because the increased lateral velocity of airflow in the narrowed airways produces a shearing effect that removes particles and other material deposited on the luminal surface.

Because events recorded in the effort-independent portion of the flow-volume curve require less cooperation and understanding by the subject, they are more reproducible than those in the effort-dependent portion. Once the effort-independent portion of the maximal expiratory flow–volume curve is reached, maximal flow is determined by only two factors: the elastic recoil of the lungs and the geometry (i.e., cross-sectional area) of the airways between the alveoli and the airways in which dynamic compression occurs. This concept means that tests of peak flow, MEFR, and even FEV_1 reflect mainly resistance to airflow offered by central "large" airways, whereas tests of MMFR and $\dot{V}max_{50}$ and $\dot{V}max_{25}$ reflect chiefly the characteristics of airflow in peripheral or "small" airways. Maximal expiratory flow-volume curves can also be recorded after a few breaths of 79 per cent He and 21 per cent O_2 ($He-O_2$) as well as after breathing room air (79 per cent N_2 and 21 per cent O_2). In normal persons, the two curves differ from each other because He is a less dense but more viscous gas than N_2. Thus higher flow rates are achieved with He-O_2 during the early and mid portions of expiration in which turbulence and convective acceleration (both density-dependent phenomena) occur; later, when slow laminar flow develops, viscous effects prevail and the He-O_2 curve is identical with or even lower than the room air curve. In general, in normal subjects, flow rates are higher with He-O_2 than with room air throughout most of expiration; appreciable differences in flows are evident at 50 per cent ($\Delta \dot{V}max_{50}$) and 25 per cent ($\Delta \dot{V}max_{25}$) of the vital capacity, and the volume at which the two curves intersect (Viso$_{\dot{V}}$) is close to residual volume.

In the presence of narrowing of peripheral airways, turbulence and convective acceleration are less prominent, so the He-O_2 curve is nearer to the room air curve than it should be; this means that $\Delta \dot{V}max_{50}$ and $\Delta \dot{V}max_{25}$ decrease and Viso$_{\dot{V}}$ increases. Comparison of maximal expiratory flow–volume curves obtained while breathing room air and He-O_2 may prove to be one of the most sensitive tests for demonstrating abnormalities that are presumably located in the small airways of the lungs; however, the value of these tests in detecting early bronchitis and emphysema remains to be proved.

DISTRIBUTION OF VENTILATION

During the movement of air from outside the body into the lungs during inhalation, the airstream is partitioned as it flows through the tracheobronchial to the terminal respiratory units where gas exchange takes place. Even in healthy persons ventilation is not distributed uniformly, and marked derangements may develop in patients with lung disease.

The unevenness of ventilation found in normal subjects results from the vertical gradient of pleural pressure between the uppermost and lowermost parts of the lungs. The origins of the vertical gradient are complex and include the weight of the lungs, their attachments at the hilum, and the shape and effects of the chest wall and abdominal contents. Because of the gradient in the pressure surrounding the lungs, alveoli are larger at the top than at the bottom, and the distribution of inspired ventilation differs from top to bottom.

When breathing normally from functional residual capacity, more inspired air is distributed to the dependent regions of the lungs than to the superior regions because the differences in pleural pressure cause the two regions to function on different segments of the same volume-pressure curve. Because the *change* in intrapleural pressure during quiet breathing is the same throughout the pleural space, the lower regions inflate more than the upper regions because they are operating on a steeper part of the curve and thus receive more volume for the same pressure change. When inspiration continues to total lung capacity, alveoli at the top and bottom of the lung inflate to nearly the same size because both regions are functioning on the flat portion of the volume-pressure curve even though the pleural pressure difference persists. During exhalation, the pleural pressure surrounding the most dependent portion of the lung becomes positive; this causes airways in that region to close. As expiration continues, airway closure progresses from the lowermost regions up the lungs involving more and more airways.

Regional differences in the distribution of ventilation can be examined by the test of closing volume, which is carried out by labeling alveolar gas during inspiration from residual volume to total lung capacity by one of two methods (bolus or resident gas techniques); in either case, the uppermost regions contain a higher concentration of the label than the lowermost regions. The gas concentration measured at the mouth during the subsequent exhalation varies according to the sequence of regional emptying and demonstrates that the first gas inhaled is the last gas exhaled. Phase 1 reflects the composition of gas from the tracheobronchial system and contains none of the label; the concentration rapidly rises during Phase 2 as alveoli containing the label begin to empty; a near-plateau is evident in Phase 3 as alveoli throughout the entire lung deflate; finally, the plateau terminates abruptly with a steep rise in concentration during Phase 4. Closing volume is the junction between Phases 3 and 4 and is that volume at which airways in the dependent regions of the lung begin to close; accordingly, the rising concentration of the label in the subsequent expirate indicates the progressively increasing contributions from the preferentially labeled alveoli in the upper regions of the lung.

Because an increase in closing volume reflects premature closure or narrowing of airways, an increase in closing volume occurs in patients with lung disorders in which the caliber of peripheral airways is decreased from either decreased elastic recoil (e.g., in emphysema) or abnormalities of the airways themselves (e.g., in bronchitis or asthma). Furthermore, increases in closing volume have been detected in asymptomatic patients, usually smokers, and may be an early manifestation of lung disease. In addition, the slope of Phase 3 is useful because it provides a sensitive measure of the adequacy of the distribution of ventilation. Well ventilated units fill and empty more completely and rapidly than poorly ventilated units; this means that the concentration of the label will be lower in the better ventilated regions that empty early during exhalation than in the poorly ventilated regions. Thus the more uneven the distribution of ventilation within the lung, the steeper the slope of Phase 3. The physiologic principles that govern the slope of Phase 3 in the closing volume test are the same as those in the single breath O_2 test for the distribution of ventilation designed by Comroe and Fowler many years ago.

Other tests of the distribution of ventilation utilize the gamma ray–emitting properties of certain radioactive gases, chiefly ^{133}Xe, which are nontoxic and can be detected after inhalation in low concentrations by external counters. The distribution of ventilation can be assessed during a breath hold at end-inspiration after a single breath of ^{133}Xe or at intervals during its elimination by normal breathing after the lung has been labeled uniformly by rebreathing ^{133}Xe from a closed system.

ABNORMALITIES OF VENTILATION

Lung diseases that cause abnormalities of ventilation are usually divided into two different categories: restrictive and obstructive ventilatory disorders. This classificaton is not completely satisfactory because it ignores the fact that disturbances of the distribution of ventilation are the earliest and by far the most common

TABLE 1. Characteristic Changes in Lung Volumes and Tests of Airways Resistance in Patients with Restrictive and Obstructive Ventilatory Disorders*

Test	Restrictive	Obstructive
Vital capacity	Decreased	Decreased or normal
Residual volume	Decreased	Increased
Total lung capacity	Decreased	Normal or increased
RV/TLC	Normal or slightly increased	Markedly increased
FEV_1/FVC	Normal or increased	Decreased
MMFR	Normal or decreased	Decreased
Single-breath O_2	Normal or increased	Increased

*Abbreviations: RV/TLC = residual volume to total lung capacity ratio; FEV_1/FVC = forced expiratory volume in one second to forced vital capacity ratio; MMFR = maximum mid-expiratory flow rate.

abnormality of ventilation and can occur in the absence of manifestations of coexisting obstructive or restrictive disorders.

DISTURBANCES OF DISTRIBUTION. Whenever a disease process involves the lung parenchyma or airways unevenly, abnormalities in the distribution of ventilation are likely to occur because more inspired gas will reach the normal regions of the lung compared with the regions distal to the site of bronchial narrowing, or the regions in which the distensibility is impaired. Whether these functional changes can be detected depends on the extent and severity of the disease and the sensitivity of the test being used. The single breath O_2 test, the slope of Phase 3 of the closing volume maneuver, and the washout of radioactive gases are all sensitive methods of detecting early abnormalities in the distribution of ventilation. Frequency dependence of compliance is also a sensitive test for distribution of ventilation but is seldom used owing to its technical complexities.

RESTRICTIVE VENTILATORY DISORDERS. The term *restrictive ventilatory disorder* denotes a pattern of abnormalities in lung function. The word "restrictive" is employed to indicate a restriction of or limitation to the amount of gas within the lungs. Thus restrictive ventilatory disorders are characterized by reductions in lung volumes (Table 1). The hallmark of restriction is a decreased vital capacity, but because this change also occurs in obstructive ventilatory disorders, it is important to exclude the presence of airways obstruction (see Obstructive Ventilatory Disorders, below) or demonstrate the presence of reductions in other lung volumes, particularly total lung capacity.

Many components of the lung, chest wall, and respiratory control system determine the amount of gas that can be breathed into the lungs. Accordingly, restrictive ventilatory disorders can develop in diseases that (1) affect the chest wall or respiratory muscles (pectus excavatum, myasthenia gravis), (2) cause infiltrations in the lung parenchyma or air spaces (diffuse interstitial fibrosis, pulmonary edema), (3) involve the pleura (pleural thickening), (4) occupy space within the thorax (tumors, effusions, cardiac enlargement), and (5) occur after lung resection (pneumonectomy).

OBSTRUCTIVE VENTILATORY DISORDERS. The term *obstructive ventilatory disorder* denotes the constellation of abnormalities that results from airways obstruction, regardless of its cause. Because the functional disturbances depend on the presence of increased resistance to

airflow, obstructive ventilatory disorders are detected mainly by tests of the behavior of the respiratory system under dynamic conditions (Table 1). The FEV_1/FVC test is the most widely used, but tests of maximal flow-volume relationships are being used increasingly and may prove superior to the FEV_1/FVC in the *early* diagnosis of airways obstruction, especially when the obstruction is situated in peripheral airways.

Obstructive ventilatory disorders are found in patients with asthma, bronchitis, emphysema, advanced bronchiectasis, or other diseases that cause narrowing of the tracheobronchial system. When the term "obstructive" was originally employed, it was not possible to differentiate among these various entities, so they were lumped together in the nonspecific category of chronic obstructive pulmonary disease. Now, however, it is possible by means of specialized tests of lung function to sort out the various diseases that cause airways obstruction, even when they coexist; the characteristic features of asthma, chronic bronchitis, and emphysema are described in subsequent chapters.

342.3. DIFFUSION

Diffusion can be defined as the movement of molecules from a region of higher to one of lower concentration; accordingly, diffusion tends to eliminate differences in concentration within the various regions accessible to the molecules. Diffusion is a passive process that results from the kinetic motion of the molecules and no extra energy is required. In the lung, O_2 moves by diffusion from alveolar gas into pulmonary capillary blood; similarly, in the tissues, O_2 moves by diffusion from capillary blood in peripheral tissues into neighboring cells. Carbon dioxide also moves by diffusion but usually in the direction opposite to that of O_2. Both O_2 and CO_2 undergo chemical reactions in the bloodstream at the start and finish of their journeys between the lungs and the peripheral tissues; O_2 reacts solely with hemoglobin, and CO_2 reacts in part with hemoglobin and in part to form bicarbonate.

DIFFUSING CAPACITY

The diffusing capacity of the lung for any gas (G) indicates the quantity of that gas that diffuses across the alveolar-capillary membrane per unit time ($\dot{V}_G$) in response to the difference in mean pressures of the gas within the alveolus (P_{A_G}) and pulmonary capillary ($P\bar{c}_G$). The diffusing capacity of the lung for any gas (DL_G) is expressed by the following general equation:

$$DL_G = V_G/P\bar{A}_G - P\bar{c}_G$$

Most inert gases (e.g., N_2) diffuse across the air-blood barrier so rapidly that the amount taken up by the lung is not detectably limited by the diffusibility of the gas and the properties of the lung and blood but is determined solely by the solubility of the gas and the volume of tissue and blood into which it can dissolve. This phenomenon enables use of highly soluble gases like acetylene, dimethyl ether, or nitrous oxide to measure lung tissue volume and pulmonary capillary blood flow.

The only two gases that measure the diffusing capacity of the lungs are O_2 and CO. Because of their unique ability to combine with hemoglobin, both have to diffuse across the alveolar-capillary membrane in large quantities to saturate the available hemoglobin at the gas pressure prevailing in the alveoli. Thus it may not be possible for complete equilibrium to occur before the hemoglobin-containing red blood cells leave the pulmonary capillaries and gas transfer ceases. Of the two gases, CO is much more widely used for the measurement of diffusing capacity than O_2 because of the ease and convenience of applying the various CO tests and because CO uptake is always diffusion limited. In contrast, O_2 uptake is not limited by diffusion (i.e., is not a test of diffusing capacity) in normal subjects except during heavy exercise or while breathing low concentrations of O_2.

The physical definition of the diffusing capacity of the lung and its mathematic definition are simple and straightforward. However, despite technical improvements in testing procedures, the interpretation of the results in normal subjects and especially in patients with lung disease is open to question. The chief problem lies in the difficulty of obtaining a true "mean" alveolar Pco. None of the several available methods of measuring diffusing capacity with CO yields a value for Pco that summarizes accurately the events taking place in the 100,000 gas exchange units of the lung, in each of which Pco varies according to the ventilation and blood flow to the unit. Despite this shortcoming, measurements of the diffusing capacity of the lung have provided useful empirical information concerning the function of the lung in healthy persons and patients with lung diseases.

Two general types of tests are available that involve either a breath-holding maneuver (single breath method) or continuous rebreathing (steady state methods). (1) The single breath test for the measurement of pulmonary diffusing capacity is noninvasive, easy for the subject to perform, rapid, and safe. Accordingly, it is widely used not only in pulmonary function laboratories but also in screening clinics for early detection of lung disease. However, some patients with severe dyspnea cannot hold their breath for ten seconds; similarly, the breath-holding requirement limits use of the single breath tests for CO-diffusing capacity during exercise. (2) All six steady state methods involve the continuous breathing or rebreathing of a gas mixture containing a small amount of CO, but each has a different approach to the derivation of mean alveolar CO pressure. Although steady state methods take longer to apply than the single breath method and nonuniformity of ventilation and blood flow probably affect the results of steady state methods more than those of the single breath technique, steady state methods are easier to use during exercise.

The quantity of CO that will diffuse in a known period of time from alveolar gas into capillary blood and combine with hemoglobin in response to a given pressure difference between gas and blood depends on (1) the solubility and diffusibility of CO in each layer of the air-blood barrier, (2) the surface area and thickness of the barrier, and (3) the rate of the chemical reaction between CO and hemoglobin within red blood cells. Because the solubility and diffusibility of CO are physical characteristics that presumably do not change under ordinary circumstances, the two chief components of diffusing capacity are the area and thickness of the alveolar-capillary membrane available for diffusion (DM) and the pulmonary capillary blood volume (Vc) (i.e., the reservoir of hemoglobin) with which the CO combines at a finite rate (θ).

It is now possible to derive the two components of overall diffusing capacity by performing several measurements of DL_{CO} with the subject breathing gas mixtures of different concentrations of CO and O_2. Because CO and O_2 compete with each other for available positions on the hemoglobin molecule, changing the O_2 concentration changes the rate with which CO reacts with hemoglobin, in other words θ, and thus affects DL_{CO}. The values from a series of tests can be plotted and solved graphically for DM and Vc according to the equation developed by Roughton and Forster that expresses the interrelationships among the various factors:

$$1/DL = 1/DM + 1/\theta Vc$$

Approximately half the total resistance to diffusion of CO from alveolar gas to capillary blood resides in the membrane compartment and the other half in the chemical reaction that takes place in the pulmonary capillary blood volume. Accordingly, changes in the hemoglobin concentration have a calculable effect on total CO diffusion that should be taken into account when establishing the predicted "normal" value for a patient with anemia or polycythemia.

Normal values for CO-diffusing capacity depend chiefly on the person's lung volume and therefore closely correlate with body size, especially height. Because single breath and steady state methods yield different results in the same subject, appropriate regression equations must be solved to obtain predicted normal values according to the test being used.

Diffusing capacity is normally higher in the supine than erect posture because position changes Vc. When blood flow to the lung increases, as in muscular exercise, Vc also increases owing to recruitment of previously nonperfused capillaries and dilatation of others; these phenomena account for the progressive increase in DL_{CO} during increasingly strenuous levels of exercise. Similarly, the elevated pulmonary arterial pressures encountered in persons who live at high altitudes also recruit capillaries, increase Vc, and cause an increase in "normal" DL_{CO}. For unexplained reasons (possibly genetic), natives of high altitudes have higher DL_{CO} values than sojourners fully acclimatized to the same altitude.

ABNORMALITIES OF CO-DIFFUSING CAPACITY

Based on the physiologic principles that govern the diffusion of CO, it can be inferred that DL_{CO} may increase or decrease in patients with various cardiopulmonary disorders that affect Vc, DM, or both. When tests of diffusing capacity were first used to study patients with various forms of lung disease, it was assumed that abnormalities of gas transfer would result from thickening of the air-blood barrier by a pathologic process that lengthened the pathway for diffusion of gases; this concept led to the formulation of what became widely known as the *alveolar-capillary block syndrome*. The "block" meant that the distance CO molecules had to travel from gas to blood was increased and, in turn, that extra time was required for diffusion to reach equilibrium across the air-blood barrier. This means that alveolar–end-capillary O_2 differences might occur during the period of time red blood cells normally spend in the pulmonary capillary. Now it is known that the importance of alveolar-capillary block has been greatly exaggerated because (1) arterial hypoxia in patients at rest with decreased diffusing capacities has been shown to be caused mainly by ventilation-perfusion inequalities and not by diffusion abnormalities and (2) decreases in D_L from changes in D_M, such as would occur with a "block," are rare, whereas decreases in D_L from changes in V_C are common.

Pulmonary vascular disorders, such as pulmonary emboli and pulmonary vasculitis, that affect (directly or indirectly) the pulmonary capillary bed decrease D_L through a decrease in V_C. Similarly, $D_{L_{CO}}$ is reduced because of decreases in V_C in patients with infiltrative disorders of the interalveolar septum that obliterate or destroy capillaries. This is the usual mechanism underlying reduction of $D_{L_{CO}}$ in patients with sarcoidosis, diffuse interstitial fibrosis, berylliosis, or collagen diseases of the lung.

Changes in D_M account for a decreased $D_{L_{CO}}$ in patients with diseases in which some form of intra-alveolar filling process has occurred and the air-to-blood diffusion pathway is actually lengthened: pneumonia, pulmonary edema, alveolar proteinosis. A decrease in both D_M and V_C produces a low $D_{L_{CO}}$ in patients with disorders associated with removal or destruction of lung tissue, such as resectional surgery and emphysema.

An increase in $D_{L_{CO}}$ results occasionally from an increase in V_C secondary to hemodynamic changes in the pulmonary circulation: an increase in pulmonary arterial or left atrial pressures or an increase in pulmonary blood flow. The $D_{L_{CO}}$ is sometimes increased in patients with bronchial asthma during an attack, but the cause of this change is not known.

342.4. PERFUSION

The pulmonary circulation delivers blood in a thin film to the gas exchange units so that O_2 uptake and CO_2 elimination can occur. The physiologic determinants of pulmonary blood flow are analogous to those of ventilation in that the total volumes of ventilation and blood flow must be adequate to meet metabolic needs, and the distribution of both must be such that proportionate amounts of inspired fresh air and incoming mixed venous blood are delivered to individual gas exchange units. Ventilatory volume is controlled by the factors that regulate breathing (see Ch. 342.5), whereas the volume of blood flowing through the lungs is determined mainly by the extrapulmonary mechanisms that govern cardiac output.

DISTRIBUTION OF PULMONARY BLOOD FLOW

Pulmonary blood flow is not distributed uniformly throughout the lung but is normally greatest in the dependent regions where pulmonary arterial pressure is highest and, conversely, is least in the superior regions where pulmonary arterial pressure is lowest. In the upright subject under resting conditions, the apices of the lungs are barely perfused and considerably more blood flows, even allowing for differences in the amount of lung tissue, to the basilar regions. The presence of nonuniform blood flow, which is not matched by comparable changes in ventilation, leads to important differences between regions of the lung in their defense capabilities and efficiency of gas exchange.

Distribution of pulmonary blood flow can readily be measured by injecting radioactive substances, such as ^{125}I-albumin aggregates or ^{133}Xe dissolved in saline, and then detecting their location in the lung with an external counter system. Abnormalities in the volume and distribution of pulmonary blood flow may result from diseases that involve the blood vessels themselves (emboli, vasculitis, emphysema), from compression of blood vessels (tumors, cysts), or from reactivity of blood vessels (vasoconstriction secondary to alveolar hypoxia).

OTHER FUNCTIONS

The pulmonary circulation has important functions besides providing blood flow for continuous gas exchange: (1) it acts as a filter of virtually the entire venous drainage; (2) it supplies substrates for the nutrition and metabolic needs of the lung, including the synthesis of surfactant; (3) it serves as a reservoir of blood for the left ventricle; (4) it affects endocrine function by modifying the pharmacologic properties of a variety of circulating substances; and (5) it provides a large surface area for the absorption and filtration of liquids and solutes.

342.5.   CONTROL OF BREATHING

The respiratory system must maintain gas exchange during periods of stress, such as exercise and other forms of increased metabolic needs. The O_2 consumption may increase more than tenfold from rest to strenuous exercise; over this range, arterial P_{O_2} remains remarkably constant. The correspondence between the volume of ventilation and the demands for O_2 uptake and CO_2 elimination results from the responsiveness of three reasonably well characterized receptor systems that interact to regulate breathing in normal subjects and patients with a variety of disease states: (1) receptors in the airways and lung parenchyma, (2) peripheral chemoreceptors, and (3) central chemoreceptors. Nerve impulse traffic from these receptors is integrated and modulated in the medulla with impulses arising from higher centers in the brain. The medulla can be viewed as the main headquarters for initiating, processing, and relaying messages concerning breathing to other parts of the body via nervous pathways. Some of the resulting medullary neural activity may reach the cerebral cortex and evoke conscious perception of breathing (i.e., the symptom of dyspnea); other impulses may travel through efferent pathways in the autonomic nervous system to the lungs and other organs; still other impulses may descend in the spinal cord to be processed with afferent impulses from peripheral nerves at different cord segments before finally being transmitted to the muscles of respiration and other effectors.

ABNORMALITIES OF CONTROL OF BREATHING

Variations, usually increases, in the rate and depth of breathing occur in patients with many common clinical disturbances such as fever, metabolic diseases, or psychiatric disorders. Several frequently used drugs (e.g., aspirin, antidepressants, and alcohol) also affect ventilation. *Hyperventilation* occurs when ventilation increases out of proportion to CO_2 production and arterial Pco_2 decreases; *hypoventilation* is the converse. *Hyperpnea* signifies an increase in the rate and depth of breathing, such as occurs during exercise, but carries no implication concerning arterial Pco_2 values. It should be emphasized that a decrease in the O_2 pressure (Po_2) of arterial blood has several causes. In contrast, the pressure of CO_2 (Pco_2) is governed simply by the relationship between CO_2 production ($\dot{V}co_2$) and CO_2 elimination by alveolar ventilation ($\dot{V}alv$):

$$Pco_2 = k\dot{V}co_2/\dot{V}alv$$

Because alveolar ventilation normally changes to keep pace with CO_2 production, for practical purposes abnormal arterial Pco_2 values can always be interpreted as indicating hyper- or hypoventilation.

Abnormalities of the control of breathing can result from excitation of intrapulmonary receptors (pulmonary embolism, pneumonia, asthma), depression of peripheral chemoreceptors (natives of high altitudes, sedative drugs, severe chronic bronchitis), stimulation of peripheral chemoreceptors (drugs such as doxapram), depression of central chemoreceptors (sedative drugs, obesity, myxedema, neurologic disorders), and stimulation of central chemoreceptors (drugs such as aspirin, irritative neurologic lesions). Special tests of the ventilatory response to breathing gas mixtures with increased CO_2 or decreased O_2 help in defining the physiologic derangements among these disorders.

342.6. GAS EXCHANGE

The end product of respiration is gas exchange, which in human beings consists of maintaining the values for Po_2 and Pco_2 in arterial blood within normal limits. As stated previously, respiration consists of ventilation, including the distribution of inspired air throughout the tracheobronchial system, diffusion, blood flow, including the distribution of mixed venous blood throughout pulmonary capillaries, and the control of breathing. Each of these contributes in a unique way to gas exchange such that an impairment in one process cannot be compensated for by improvement in another.

Normal values for the pressures of O_2, CO_2, N_2, and H_2O at sea level (barometric pressure 760 mm Hg) in ambient air, conducting airways (i.e., the dead space), gas exchange units, and arterial and mixed venous blood are given in Table 2. Ambient air consists primarily of N_2 and O_2 with varying amounts of water vapor. As air is inhaled, it is warmed to the subject's body temperature and fully saturated with water vapor (PH_2O 37° C = 47 mm Hg); the addition of water vapor has the effect of diluting the inspired mixture of N_2 and O_2 and reduces their respective pressures proportionately. During gas exchange in the alveoli, more O_2 is removed than CO_2 is added; this causes the volume of each respiratory unit to decrease slightly and raises the concentration and pressure of N_2 slightly.

The values given in Table 2 indicate that gas exchange in the healthy lung is not perfect because there is a small (5 mm Hg) difference between the Po_2 values in (mean) alveolar gas and arterial blood. The difference, known as the alveolar-arterial Po_2 difference, occurs because of the normal presence of a slight nonuniformity in the distribution of ventilation with respect to perfusion and a small right-to-left shunt. Note that the sum of the pressures of the individual gases in mixed venous blood is less than the total atmospheric pressure. Because the tissues and spaces of the body are in approximate equilibrium with venous blood, these structures are also subatmospheric. The "suction" serves to keep the lung expanded against the chest wall and to cause the reabsorption of gas from tissue spaces (e.g., a pneumothorax).

ABNORMAL GAS EXCHANGE

Measurements of arterial Po_2 and Pco_2 and calculations of the alveolar-arterial Po_2 difference are reliable guides to the over-all adequacy of respiration. In determining whether or not an abnormality is present, it must be remembered that normal values for Po_2, but not Pco_2, vary with age and that both Po_2 and Pco_2 are influenced by the altitude at which the subject is living. There are five physiologic mechanisms known to cause arterial hypoxia, defined as a decrease below normal of arterial Po_2: (1) hypoventilation, (2) decreased diffusion, (3) ventilation-perfusion imbalance, (4) right-to-left shunting of blood, and (5) breathing air (or a gas mixture) with a low Po_2. Except for a few uncommon clinical examples, such as breathing air with its Po_2 reduced by combustion of O_2 and addition of smoke or suffocation, item 5 can be ignored. Items 1 to 4 can be separated, at least for practical clinical purposes, by analyzing the values from a given blood specimen and a few easy tests.

TABLE 2. Normal Gas Pressures (in mm Hg) During Inspiration in Ambient Air, Conducting Airways, Terminal Respiratory Units (Alveoli), and Arterial and Mixed Venous Blood

Gas Pressure	Ambient Air	Conducting Airways	Terminal Respiratory Units	Arterial Blood	Mixed Venous Blood
Po_2	156	149	100	95	40
Pco_2	0	0	40	40	46
PH_2O	15*	47	47	47	47
PN_2	589	564	573	573	573
$PTOTAL$	760	760	760	755	706

*PH_2O varies according to humidity and has a proportionate effect on Po_2 and PN_2.

HYPOVENTILATION. The simplest disturbance of gas exchange occurs when not enough fresh air is breathed into alveolar spaces to raise pulmonary capillary Po_2 to normal levels and to allow CO_2 to leave the bloodstream. Although arterial Pco_2 may theoretically increase in patients with other disturbances of gas exchange (ventilation-perfusion abnormalities and right-to-left shunts), for clinical purposes an elevated value should be interpreted as indicating alveolar hypoventilation.

Pure hypoventilation is a relatively uncommon clinical event. When it is found, depression of the central nervous system resulting from anesthetic agents or other sedative drugs is the usual cause. More commonly, hypoventilation occurs in association with other disturbances of oxygenation. When these coexist, they can be recognized by the fact that the decrease in arterial Po_2 is more than can be accounted for by the increase in arterial Pco_2.

IMPAIRED DIFFUSION. Decreased diffusion, from either loss of pulmonary capillaries or thickening of the air-blood barrier, does not usually cause important alveolar-arterial Po_2 difficulties *at rest*. Thus abnormalities of diffusion can be ignored in patients with arterial hypoxia whose blood specimens are obtained while they are resting. In contrast, impaired diffusion is one of the two major causes of severely worsening hypoxia during exercise (right-to-left shunting of blood is the other). Regardless of the cause of the diffusing impairment, under resting conditions there is sufficient time to allow gas transfer to reach equilibrium between gas and blood. However, during exercise, cardiac output and the velocity of blood flow through pulmonary capillaries increase; thus the time for gas transfer is reduced and marked alveolar–end-capillary Po_2 differences occur.

VENTILATION-PERFUSION MISMATCHING. Because the distributions of inspired air and pulmonary blood flow in normal subjects are neither uniform nor proportionate to each other, a slight ventilation-perfusion imbalance exists in healthy persons. Moreover, increased (above normal) mismatching of ventilation and perfusion is by far the most common cause of arterial hypoxia encountered clinically. Virtually all forms of lung disease are associated with a detectable ventilation-perfusion abnormality.

When a unit is underventilated relative to its perfusion (i.e., has a low ventilation-perfusion ratio), O_2 uptake by that unit must decrease so that the Po_2 of its end-capillary blood is lower than normal; Pco_2 tends to increase but cannot rise above the value in mixed venous blood. Thus the process affects values for Po_2 more than Pco_2. Furthermore, in those units that are overventilated owing to a redistribution of inspired air, the high ventilation-perfusion ratio causes Po_2 to increase and Pco_2 to decrease. But there is an important difference in the effects of these changes in pressures on the actual quantities (contents) of O_2 and CO_2 in the capillary blood leaving units with high ventilation-perfusion ratios. Given the shapes of the respective dissociation curves, O_2 content is not appreciably increased but CO_2 content is decreased. Thus increasing ventilation with respect to perfusion in some regions corrects the tendency to CO_2 retention that would otherwise exist but does not correct the hypoxia caused by low ventilation-perfusion relationships in other units. Another invariable consequence of a ventilation-perfusion abnormality is an increase in the alveolar-arterial Po_2 difference.

RIGHT-TO-LEFT SHUNTING. A small right-to-left shunt of blood is found in normal persons, and shunts of considerable magnitude may occur in patients with pulmonary disease. A right-to-left shunt may be visualized as a pathway(s) through which mixed venous blood flows from the right to the left side of the heart without having contacted functioning gas exchange units along the way. Thus there is a continuous admixture of venous blood with arterialized blood that has come from normal pathways in the lungs. Arterial hypoxia and an increased alveolar-arterial Po_2 difference occur that vary in severity with the magnitude of the shunt and its O_2 content. Right-to-left shunts occur through intracardiac communications in patients with congenital heart disease. In patients with lung disease, although shunts may be extremely large, they seldom occur through abnormal vascular channels such as pulmonary arteriovenous fistulas; instead, they are caused by blood perfusing normal vessels in regions of lung that are atelectatic or in which alveoli are filled with edema fluid, pus, or blood; in either case, because gas transfer is impossible, a shunt occurs.

The consequences of a right-to-left shunt are similar to those of a ventilation-perfusion imbalance owing to basic similarities between the two disturbances. A shunt can be viewed as an extreme ventilation-perfusion abnormality in which there is perfusion but *no* ventilation at all. It is impossible to differentiate between a ventilation-perfusion disturbance and a right-to-left shunt while the subject is breathing ambient air; therefore the effects of both are combined and designated as venous admixture or a "shunt-like" effect. The two causes of hypoxia can be separated by giving the patient 100 per cent O_2 to breathe and measuring arterial Po_2 after all the N_2 has been washed out of the lungs. When a ventilation-perfusion abnormality exists, the N_2 is replaced by O_2 and all the blood perfusing the lungs equilibrates at a high Po_2 (approximately 600 mm Hg); in this way 100 per cent O_2 is said to "correct" a ventilation-perfusion disturbance. In contrast, in the presence of a right-to-left shunt, the admixture of mixed venous blood continues despite breathing 100 per cent O_2 and arterial hypoxia persists. In fact, the alveolar-arterial Po_2 difference in patients with a right-to-left shunt is higher during breathing of 100 per cent O_2 compared with room air, whereas the opposite occurs in patients with ventilation-perfusion inequalities.

SIGNIFICANCE OF ARTERIAL BLOOD GAS VALUES

The availability of accurate rapid analyzers for measuring Po_2, Pco_2, and pH has been one of the major clinical advances of the last 25 years. Virtually the entire therapeutic approach to patients with acute and chronic respiratory failure is dictated by the presence and magnitude of blood gas and pH abnormalities (see Ch. 351). Every physician should know the mechanisms of arterial hypoxia and how to differentiate them because it is important clinically whether a patient's hypoxia results from hypoventilation, impaired diffusion, ventilation-perfusion mismatching, or right-to-left shunting. Evaluating the course and prognosis of the lung disease, determining the need for and outcome of therapy, and assessing disability, operability, and the limits of resection in patients considered for pulmonary surgery all depend to some extent on the findings of blood gas analysis. Thus all physicians who care for patients must become familiar with the technique of arterial puncture and must know how to interpret the results of blood gas analysis.

Bates, D. V., Macklem, P. T., and Christie, R. V.: Respiratory Function in Disease; An Introduction to the Integrated Study of the Lung. 2nd ed. Philadelphia, W. B. Saunders Company, 1971.

Campbell, E. J. M., Agostoni, E., and Davis, J. N.: The Respiratory Muscles: Mechanics and Neural Control. 2nd ed. Philadelphia, W. B. Saunders Company, 1970.

Comroe, J. H., Jr., Forster, R. E., II, DuBois, A. B., Briscoe, W. A., and Carlsen, E.: The Lung; Clinical Physiology and Pulmonary Function Tests, 2nd ed. Chicago, Year Book Medical Publishers, 1962.

Comroe, J. H., Jr., and Nadel, J.: Screening tests of pulmonary function. N. Engl. J. Med., 282:1249, 1970.

Cotes, J. E.: Lung Function, 3rd ed. Philadelphia, J. B. Lippincott Company, 1975.

Jones, N. L. Campbell, E. J. M., Edward, R. H. T., and Robertson, D. G.: Clinical Exercise Testing. Philadelphia, W. B. Saunders Company, 1975.

Murray, J. F.: The Normal Lung: The Basis for Diagnosis and Treatment of Pulmonary Disease. Philadelphia, W. B. Saunders Company, 1976.

343. SPECIAL DIAGNOSTIC PROCEDURES IN PULMONARY DISEASE

Gordon L. Snider

Pulmonary disease comes to light because the patient has respiratory symptoms, because the physician finds abnormalities on physical examination, or because a chest roentgenogram has disclosed an abnormal shadow. With the data in hand from the history and physical examination, chest film (see below), and basic blood and urine laboratory tests, the physician must choose among a broad array of special procedures in order to establish a diagnosis and develop a plan of management. Clinical pulmonary function testing is discussed in Ch. 342. In the following chapters the special diagnostic procedures applicable to pulmonary disease will be reviewed, with comments on when they are to be used and on their limitations.

343.1. THE CHEST ROENTGENOGRAM

STANDARD VIEWS. As already noted, the chest roentgenogram can detect abnormalities in the asymptomatic patient with a normal physical examination of the chest. Even in the presence of respiratory symptoms, the chest roentgenogram may be abnormal when the physical examination is nonrevealing. On the other hand, the full inspiration chest roentgenogram provides no dynamic information, and rales denoting parenchymal disease or rhonchi indicating bronchial disease may be present when the lung fields appear normal in the roentgenogram. It follows that complete evaluation of the respiratory system in the individual who is symptomatic, or who is suspected on other grounds of having pulmonary disease, must include both a physical examination and a chest roentgenogram.

The standard projections are the posteroanterior (PA) and lateral views of the chest. The PA view is taken in full inspiration with the patient's anterior chest wall against the film and the scapulae rotated anterolaterally; the x-ray tube is about 2 meters from the patient so that divergence of the x-ray beam is minimal and the images of the heart and any pulmonary lesions are not magnified. The lower neck and upper abdomen should be included in the field of view. The lateral chest film is an essential part of the roentgenographic examination because it exposes to view portions of the lungs obscured in the PA view by the heart, the mediastinal structures, and the leaflets of the diaphragm. Precise localization of a lesion usually requires display in both the PA and lateral projections.

The normal chest roentgenogram is formed from images of the soft tissues, the bones, the air columns of the trachea and main bronchi, the heart and great vessels, pleural planes observed on end, and the pulmonary parenchyma. The last-named has two major components: (1) the respiratory tissues are strikingly radiolucent because they are more than 90 per cent air at total lung capacity; and (2) the pulmonary vessels present as a branching pattern of denser shadows gradually tapering from the hilum to the periphery but normally seen in a film of good quality to within 1 cm of the edge of the lung. The air columns in lobar and smaller bronchi are not usually seen except adjacent to the lung roots. Variations in density of the lung fields are caused not just by disease processes but also by differences in the depth of respiration and the technical factors of positioning the patient, x-ray exposure, and processing of the film.

Parenchymal abnormalities may be manifest by either an increase or a decrease in roentgenographic density. Diseases which cause an increase in density may be classified into predominant air-space disease, predominant interstitial disease, or shadows due to atelectasis. Air-space consolidation is characterized by poorly marginated densities, often patchy in distribution, and with a tendency to coalesce. Shadows of the air-filled bronchi may become visible in contrast to the consolidated lung tissue surrounding them, an appearance known as an air bronchogram. Densities abutting pleural surfaces are sharply marginated, a property which aids in their localization. The volume of affected lung is normal or even increased. Bacterial pneumonia and pulmonary edema are examples of air-space consolidation.

Processes which predominantly affect the parenchymal interstitium such as viral pneumonia and chemical injury of the lung tend to give rise to linear or lacy patterns of abnormal shadows. The processes are widespread but often uneven in intensity and may be accompanied by some degree of alveolar exudation. Fibrosis with incorporation of alveoli into the interstitium and loss of lung volume may occur.

Atelectasis is a state in which lung tissue is shrunken and airless. The process may be due to bronchial obstruction, to compression of lung by air or fluid in the pleural space, to pulmonary fibrosis, or to alveolar collapse from impaired surfactant activity. The volume of lung affected may vary from less than a segment to an entire lung. The shadows of atelectasis may be nonhomogeneous, but air bronchograms tend to be absent. Loss of volume is evidenced by shifts toward the lesions of the interlobar fissures, the chest wall, or mediastinal structures.

Dense, circumscribed shadows may result from neoplasms, inflammatory processes, or fluid-filled cysts. These shadows may be well or poorly marginated and single or multiple, and may range in size from less than 1 cm to densities which almost fill a hemithorax. It is common to refer to large solitary circumscribed shadows as mass lesions. Central radiolucencies representing necrosis and cavitation may be seen in circumscribed lesions.

There are a number of parenchymal processes which give rise to a decrease in roentgen density. In emphysema (see Ch. 344), the destruction of lung parenchyma results in increased transradiancy and attenuation of the vascular pattern. When the process is very severe locally, bullae may be evident as localized radiolucent zones partially or completely surrounded by arcuate hairline shadows. Increased transradiancy of lung parenchyma is also observed in conditions in which there is high-grade obstruction of the distal airways with pulmonary overdistention, as in severe asthma (see Ch. 344.1) and obliterative bronchiolitis (see Ch. 344.1). A decrease in the amount of blood in relation to tissue is also noted in congenital or acquired narrowing or obstruction of the pulmonary arteries. All the processes referred to above may be widespread or they may be confined to one lung, one lobe, or an even smaller moiety of lung tissue.

Some disease processes show predilections for particular zones of the lung. For example, postprimary tuberculosis occurs most frequently in the apical-posterior segments of the upper lobes; pulmonary embolism and infarction favor the lower lobes. These preferential localizations, although not always rationally explained, are often helpful in differential diagnosis.

Pleural fluid, whether serous, bloody, purulent, or chylous, causes an increase in roentgenographic density; the different types of fluid are not roentgenographically distinguishable. The fluid when free in the subcostal pleural space and small in amount presents as obliteration of the costophrenic angle; larger amounts of fluid present as homogeneous basilar densities with an upper border which is concave. Pleural fluid may occasionally present atypically with a border which is convex upward, mimicking an elevated hemidiaphragm — a so-called infrapulmonary effusion. Fluid may also be loculated in the interlobar fissures, in the subcostal pleura, or paramediastinally. Such shadows usually present as sharply marginated, homogeneous, ovoid densities. The pleura may also be the site of fibrous thickening, calcification, or neoplastic processes.

Pneumothorax is identified by the presence of a radiolucent zone without vascular markings which subtends part or all of the subcostal parietal pleura. In massive pneumothorax, the underlying lung may be completely collapsed and the mediastinum is shifted to the contralateral side. With lesser degrees of pneumothorax, the lung will be variably aerated and the sharp margin of the visceral pleural can be identified, separating the pneumothorax on one side and the slightly denser lung on the other. If fluid accompanies the pneumothorax, its upper border is horizontal, presenting as an air-fluid level.

FLUOROSCOPY. Fluoroscopy permits inspection of the chest during motion and is useful for establishing the diagnosis of diaphragmatic paralysis, for localizing circumscribed dense shadows in preparation for further roentgenographic study, or for guiding placement of a needle, a bronchial brush, or a biopsy forceps. The extent of diaphragmatic excursion during deep breathing is readily determined; paradoxical upward movement of the hemidiaphragm during an inspiratory sniff or downward movement during cough helps confirm the suspicion of paralysis. The anteroposterior placement of a shadow can be located by observing the lesion while the patient rotates on the vertical axis. The degree of motion is related to a structure of known anterior or posterior location such as a rib. The less relative motion there is between the lesion and the reference point, the closer they are together. Attempts to differentiate transmitted from intrinsic pulsation in studying a mediastinal or a paramediastinal mass are usually not helpful.

INSPIRATION-EXPIRATION VIEWS. Films taken a few moments apart in full inspiration and full expiration provide a record of the respiratory system at total lung capacity and at residual volume. The technique is useful for confirming the presence of a small pneumothorax. The air in the pleural space shows an apparent increase in size without change in radiographic density but air leaves the underlying lung, making it more dense and enhancing contrast with the pneumothorax. Inspiration-expiration films are also useful for the demonstration of unilateral or focal obstruction of airways, whether by foreign body or tumor in the large airways or by generalized disease of the small airways. In the expiratory film, the parenchyma beyond the involved airways will empty poorly and the mediastinum will shift away from the involved lung.

SPECIAL VIEWS AND TECHNIQUES. The lordotic projection throws the images of the clavicles and anterior ends of the first ribs upward, thus bringing the structures in the apical-posterior segments of the upper lobes into clear view. This projection demonstrates small nodular shadows due to granulomatous disease and may occasionally show a cavity which is not seen in the plain PA film; however, the lordotic view may conceal a lesion in the anterior segment of the upper lobe.

Overpenetrated PA and lateral views may be taken to more clearly see lesions which are concealed by overlapping structures such as the heart or thickened pleura. Portable films are views taken at the bedside in seriously ill patients using a portable x-ray machine. The views are anteroposterior (AP) in projection with the patient "upright" at an angle of 45 to 80 degrees. The tube-film distance is about 4 feet, resulting in magnification of the heart shadow. These films have more limitations in diagnostic potential than standard PA films but are frequently necessary. Some of these limitations may be overcome by ordering supine or upright AP films done with the patient lying or sitting on a litter in the x-ray department, but such films require the transporting of a seriously ill patient.

Lateral decubitus views are made with the patient lying on one side with the x-ray beam oriented in a horizontal plane. This technique is of great value in the identification of pleural effusions which are free in the major pleural space. Comparison of the lateral decubitus and PA films reveals the appearance in the former of a dense shadow along the lateral chest wall due to fluid which has flowed from above the diaphragm in response to the effects of gravity. Less than 100 ml of fluid may be identified, and the presence of fluid with an atypical presentation may be readily shown. The technique may also be used to confirm the presence of air-fluid levels in the thorax and for demonstrating whether a structure which appears within a cavity is really an intracavitary, freely moving body such as a mycetoma (fungus ball).

Comparison of current PA and lateral views with old films often yields information of signal importance. A solitary pulmonary nodule may be shown to have been present and unchanging for years or alternatively to have appeared in the recent past. The nature of a shadow may be made clear as with no other procedure, e.g., it may become obvious that an air-fluid level in the lung represents an infected bulla rather than a lung abscess. Few diagnostic procedures will as richly repay the physician's efforts as an assiduous search for old chest roentgenograms.

Special views for study of the bones are often helpful. Rib films in suspected fracture and spine films in the evaluation of chest pain are examples. Contrast studies of the esophagus and stomach are valuable in studying mediastinal masses and diaphragmatic hernias as well as in the detection of disorders of esophageal function such as achalasia or intrinsic disorders of these organs.

TOMOGRAPHY. Tomography is a technique in which films are exposed while the x-ray tube and the film move proportionally in opposite directions. The effect is to allow selective visualization of a predetermined layer of tissue to the exclusion of structures lying superficial or deep to this layer. In essence, the image is that of a thin "slice" of lung. The level of the slice which is in focus may be varied at will and is usually recorded as the number of centimeters from the roentgenograph table on which the patient is positioned.

The main indications for the procedure are providing more precise delineation of the morphology of lesions visible on plain films but obscured by overlying densities. Accurate diagnosis of the presence of cavitation within the lung is a good example of this application. Tomography is also capable of clearly demonstrating the presence of calcification within lesions, which is not readily seen in the plain films. The large airways are well shown, and pulmonary arteries and veins may also be more clearly delineated with this method, at times permitting their separation from other shadows such as lymph nodes or demonstrating the decrease in caliber characteristic of pulmonary emphysema. Tomograms may reveal shadows within the lung which are beyond the resolving power of the plain film. For example, small nodules of metastatic neoplasm not seen in the PA or lateral films may be detected tomographically.

BRONCHOGRAPHY. Bronchograms are made by taking a roentgenogram of the chest after the surface of the bronchial mucosa is coated by a contrast medium. The procedure is most often carried out after topical anesthesia of the bronchial tree but may be performed under general anesthesia. The contrast medium is usually oily propyliodone, although other contrast media have been used. Excellent films have been obtained with powdered tantalum, but this material has not yet been released for general use.

Bronchography is most useful for the diagnosis of bronchiectasis, although it is sometimes of value in investigating segmental bronchial obstruction when the nature of the obstructing process is not readily apparent from bronchoscopy or tomography. The procedure is used on occasion for the study of air-filled or solid densities within the thorax such as giant bullae or intralobar sequestration. The bronchogram also reveals dilation of submucosal mucous gland ducts in chronic bronchitis as well as impairment of filling of the smallest radicles of the bronchial tree in conditions such as chronic bronchitis, asthma, and obliterative bronchiolitis; filling of the microbullae of centrilobular emphysema presents a characteristic pattern known as the mimosa or lily-of-the-valley pattern; bronchography is virtually never justified for the sole purpose of displaying these abnormalities.

The performance of a bronchogram causes transient impairment of ventilatory and gas exchange function, with the amount of function loss dependent upon the amount of bronchographic medium used and the presence of a bronchoconstrictor response to the local anesthetic or bronchographic medium, as in asthma. Needless to say, in patients with pulmonary insufficiency, a bronchogram can precipitate acute respiratory failure. As with any diagnostic procedure, the risks must be weighed against the benefits, and in general the procedure should not be carried out unless its outcome is going to directly influence action taken by the physician.

ANGIOGRAPHY. Pulmonary Angiography. Pulmonary angiography is the making of a sequential series of chest roentgenograms, following the rapid injection of a contrast medium into the pulmonary arterial circulation. Although the bolus of contrast medium is sometimes injected into the inferior vena cava, better visualization is obtained if the injection is made through a catheter positioned in the pulmonary artery. More selective pulmonary angiograms may be made by injection into the right or left main pulmonary arteries or even into smaller branches. Although most information is obtained from a study of the opacified pulmonary arteries, the contrast medium is also usually followed as it passes through the capillary circulation of the lung into the pulmonary veins; the pulmonary angiogram also gives information about vascular transit times and the presence of anomalous vascular communications.

Pulmonary angiography is most frequently used for the diagnosis of pulmonary embolism and is the most accurate test for that entity. The presence of pulmonary emboli is revealed by the demonstration of areas of decreased perfusion or intravascular filling defects.

A less frequent but nevertheless important use of pulmonary angiography is the demonstration of oligemic areas in patients with unilateral hyperlucent lungs or in patients with giant bullous emphysema who are being considered for surgical therapy. In the latter group, pulmonary angiography usefully identifies lung which is being compressed by the giant bullae; the procedure is of less risk to the patient than bronchography. Pulmonary angiography is also useful for demonstrating congenital anomalies of the pulmonary vascular tree such as agenesis or hypoplasia of a pulmonary artery, stenosis of peripheral pulmonary vessels, idiopathic dilation of the pulmonary artery, and arteriovenous malformation of the lungs, including pulmonary venous varix. Rarely, pulmonary angiography may be the only way of settling whether an enlarged hilum is due to a dilated pulmonary artery or to lymphadenopathy.

In general, the procedure is well tolerated even by seriously ill patients. However, there is a decidedly increased risk of cardiopulmonary arrest when this test is performed in patients with severe pulmonary hypertension. If, in this circumstance, the physician decides that the procedure still must be done, the amount of contrast medium injected should be sharply decreased and consideration given to carrying out several small, selective injections.

Aortography. Aortography, best carried out by direct catheterization of the aorta by a percutaneously inserted catheter, is useful for the diagnosis of aneurysm of the aorta and the differentiation of dilations and distortions of the great vessels from other mediastinal masses. The procedure should also be performed prior to exploratory thoracotomy in a patient who may have intralobar sequestration of the lung in order to identify the anomalous aortic vessel which often supplies such a sequestration.

Superior Vena Cava Angiography. The superior vena cava is opacified by the injection of contrast medium into a catheter which has been passed into the vessel or into one of its large tributaries. The technique is useful in the investigation of obstruction of the superior vena cava, especially with incomplete manifestations of the superior vena cava syndrome. It is also used occasionally in preoperative staging of patients with carcinoma of the bronchus, especially when the primary lesion is in the right upper lobe, adjacent to the mediastinum.

Azygography. The azygos and hemiazygos veins can be outlined by injecting contrast medium directly into the intraosseous space of a lower rib or into a catheter which has been introduced percutaneously into the azygos vein. This technique has been used for evaluating the presence of mediastinal metastases in carcinoma of the lung and for studying enlargement of the azygos vein in obstruction of the superior vena cava, congestive heart failure, and severe cirrhosis of the liver. However, the technique has added little to other methods of study and is rarely used.

Bronchial Arteriography. The bronchial arterial circulation can be opacified by the injection of contrast medium through a catheter which has been passed through the aorta directly into one of the bronchial arteries. Bronchial arteriography carries the risk of spinal cord injury if contrast medium is injected into a vessel communicating with the anterior spinal artery. This technique has been useful in elucidating the hyperplasia of the bronchial circulation which occurs in such conditions as pulmonic stenosis and bronchiectasis, but has no proved value as a diagnostic tool. Bronchial arterial embolization is currently being explored as a means of controlling life-threatening hemoptysis.

COMPUTERIZED TOMOGRAPHIC SCANNING. Computerized tomographic (CT) scanning provides a 180 degree transverse image of a thin "slice" of the thorax. A thin beam or beams of x-rays passes through the thorax, and the change in the attenuation of the x-rays is measured by a series of detectors. A computer reconstructs a pictorial image which represents the differential absorption of the x-ray beam through the chest. Newer equipment performs two adjacent levels of scanning in approximately two to ten seconds, a time which permits breath-holding. The examination is usually performed in the supine position, but prone and lateral recumbent projections can also be utilized.

Experience with the method is still limited in the thorax, but preliminary studies show the equipment to be more accurate than conventional tomography in the evaluation of mediastinal mass lesions, especially those due to fat deposition, cystic lesions, and vascular enlargements. The method appears to be more sensitive than tomography in screening for the small nodular shadows of suspected metastatic neoplasm and is of unique value in differentiating pleural from peripheral pulmonary lesions. CT scanning is also extremely sensitive in detecting calcification and is therefore of value in studying solitary pulmonary nodules. The technique is also used for identifying pulmonary lesions in areas which are ordinarily poorly seen in conventional roentgenograms or laminograms such as the lung adjacent to mediastinal structures, including the paravertebral areas (especially at the thoracoabdominal junction) and the posterior costophrenic sulci. Lesions in the parenchyma which are obscured by complex pleural or parenchymal shadows are well shown.

Felson, B.: Chest Roentgenology. Philadelphia, W. B. Saunders Company, 1973.
Fraser, R. G., and Paré, J. A. P.: Diagnosis of Diseases of the Chest. Philadelphia, W. B. Saunders Company, 1970.
Heitzman, R. E.: The Lung; Radiologic-Pathologic Correlations. St. Louis, C. V. Mosby Company, 1973.

343.2.   RADIONUCLIDE IMAGING

In a relatively few years, radionuclide lung scanning has come into widespread use. The procedure is most often carried out with the gamma scintillation camera coupled to a digital computer system and cathode ray display; photographs of the display are made for permanent records. Lung scanning is most often used for the diagnosis of pulmonary embolism; however, the technique is also used clinically for the evaluation of regional lung function.

We will first consider the lung perfusion scan, which is based on the following considerations. There are billions of arterioles and capillaries in the lung which are less than 30 μm in diameter. Following the injection of about 50,000 microspheres of radioactive human serum albumin of 30 μm diameter, a small proportion of these vessels will be blocked temporarily by the particles. Because the density of the microspheres is comparable to that of red blood cells, their distribution throughout the lungs will be determined by the distribution of pulmonary arterial blood flow. External imaging of the radioactivity within the lung can be carried out in four projections: the anterior, posterior, and both lateral projections. Foci of the lung with impaired arteriolar and capillary perfusion will be disclosed as areas partially or completely devoid of radioactivity. Vessels occluded by emboli will thus be revealed as fairly sharply defined segmental or lobar defects. However, areas of parenchymal pulmonary infiltration caused by pneumonia, fibrosis, or tumor will also show as impaired zones of perfusion; the presence of such areas can, of course, be detected by a study of the plain chest roentgenogram. Emphysematous lung or areas where there is impaired perfusion due to focal increase in intra-alveolar pressure, as in asthma, will also appear as areas of impaired perfusion. Such perfusion defects are usually nonsegmental in nature and are vague in outline. It is apparent that this latter class of perfusion defects is not readily detectable from a study of the plain chest roentgenogram.

Regional ventilation can be determined by imaging with a scintillation camera the initial distribution and subsequent washout of air mixed with a radioactive gas, [133]xenon. Imaging after an initial period of breathing the gas to equilibration reveals "cold" areas of lung which may be aerated (as seen in the chest films) but not communicating with the bronchial tree. Study of images done at regular intervals during washout of the ^{133}Xe permits estimation of total and regional rates of ventilation. The normal lung is cleared of xenon at the end of about three minutes of breathing air. The perfusion scan, of course, gives information regarding regional perfusion. Regional ventilation and perfusion relations may be assessed visually or by processing of the information with the computer. The two lungs may be studied separately to give information comparable to that obtained by differential bronchospirometry but without the need for using an invasive technique. The computer may also be programmed to provide the ventilation-perfusion relationships of more limited zones of the lung such as the upper, middle, and lower lung zones of each of the lungs separately.

A negative perfusion lung scintigram of good technical quality excludes the diagnosis of angiographically detectable pulmonary embolism. In pulmonary embolism without infarction, perfusion of the embolized area is profoundly impaired, with minimal impairment of ventilation; in emphysema both regional perfusion and ventilation are impaired. Consequently, the combination of impaired perfusion with maintained ventilation permits improved accuracy in the diagnosis of pulmonary embolism.

Regional ventilation and perfusion relationships are also useful in preoperative evaluation of the risk of pulmonary surgery, in the evaluation of unilateral hyperlucent lung, and in more precise evaluation of the localized severity of emphysema than is possible in the plain chest roentgenogram. Impairment of perfusion with maintenance of ventilation has been demonstrated in patients with bronchogenic carcinoma who have involvement of their pulmonary arteries by tumor. Such patients have been shown to have a decreased rate of operability and of survival when resectional surgery is carried out.

[67]Gallium citrate, a radioisotope with a half-life of 78 hours which emits gamma rays, concentrates in rapidly dividing cells. Thus the radioisotope will appear in rapidly growing tumors and in inflammatory lesions. Although this technique is largely of research interest in pulmonary disease, it has been used to detect occult mediastinal metastases in patients with known bronchogenic carcinoma. Its use in establishing the activity of such diseases as idiopathic interstitial pulmonary fibrosis and sarcoidosis of the lungs is presently being explored.

Anderson, P. O., Rujanavech, N., Secker-Walker, R. H., and McNight, R. C.: Role of ^{133}Xe ventilation studies in scintigraphic detection of pulmonary embolism. Radiology, 120:633, 1976.

Bell, W. R., and Simon, T. L.: A comparative analysis of pulmonary perfusion scans with pulmonary angiograms. Am. Heart J., 92:700, 1976.

Gilday, D. L., and James, E., Jr.: Lung scan patterns in pulmonary embolism versus those in congestive heart failure and emphysema. Am. J. Roentgenol., 115:739, 1972.

Siemsen, J. K., Grebe, S. F., Sargent, E. N., and Wentz, D.: Gallium-67 scintigraphy of pulmonary diseases as a complement to radiography. Radiology, 118:371, 1976.

Wagner, H. N., Jr.: The use of radioisotope techniques for evaluation of patients with pulmonary disease. State of the art. Am. Rev. Respir. Dis., 113:203, 1976.

343.3. ULTRASONOGRAPHY

Ultrasound is the term applied to a class of mechanical pressure waves that can be propagated through liquids and solids and which, for medical use, have a frequency of oscillation between 1 and 20 MHz. A high frequency sound wave is emitted from a transducer which is applied to the patient's skin. A portion of the wave is reflected back to the transducer as it passes through the tissues being scanned. An image is produced on a cathode ray tube for immediate viewing or is photographed for producing permanent records. Ultrasonography can be applied in a variety of different modes which permit localization of the depth of visualized structures, show the rate of motion of structures such as the diaphragm and heart valves, or generate cross-sectional images which can show outlines of solid viscera such as the liver, large blood vessels, and solid or cystic masses.

Ultrasound waves do not penetrate far into the aerated lung, and the technique is therefore applicable only in pleural or juxtamediastinal disease. Ultrasonography has proved to be helpful in the evaluation of pleural opacities, especially in the localization and identification of loculated pleural effusions. Pleural effusion, whether serous, sanguineous, or purulent, presents as an echo-free space. Consolidated lung conducts sound but, unlike pleural fluid, produces numerous echoes. Pleural fibrosis behaves similarly to consolidated lung. Ultrasonography is useful for determining the site of thoracentesis and may be used to determine the depth to which the needle or a chest tube must be inserted in order to drain a pleural loculation. In most circumstances, ultrasonography is superior to fluoroscopy or chest roentgenography in assisting in the diagnosis and management of loculated pleural effusion. Its use is unnecessary in uncomplicated pleural effusion.

Doust, B. D., Baum, J. K., Maklid, N. F., and Doust, V. L.: Ultrasonic evaluation of pleural opacities. Radiology, 114:135, 1975.

Sandweis, D. A., Hanson, J. C., Gosink, B. B., and Moser, K. M.: Ultrasound in diagnosis, localization and treatment of loculated pleural empyema. Ann. Intern. Med., 82:50, 1975.

343.4. SKIN AND SEROLOGIC TESTS

Skin and serologic tests are of value in the investigation of many viral, bacterial, and fungal diseases of the lungs as well as in the investigation of hypersensitivity lung diseases. Skin tests may be divided into three broad categories: immediate or wheal-and-flare reactions, immune complex or Arthus-type reactions, and delayed or tuberculin-type reactions.

IMMEDIATE SKIN REACTIONS. Immediate, wheal-and-flare or Type I skin reactions result from the release of chemical mediators from IgE-sensitized basophils and mast cells which have contacted a specific antigen. Solutions for skin testing are made from extracts of material which are inhaled or ingested, and which may be causing symptoms, such as the pollens of trees, grasses and weeds, house dust, animal danders, mold spores, or foods. Dilutions may also be made from insect venoms and animal serums. These tests are most safely performed by applying the test solutions to scratches or pricks and demonstrating a wheal-and-flare reaction, which is usually obvious within 15 to 20 minutes after the test is performed and which is greater than the reaction produced by a simultaneously applied test diluent. Intradermal tests may be done with 0.02 ml amounts of solution when scratch tests have been negative. As with any laboratory test the results of skin tests must be interpreted in their clinical context.

The presence of antigen-specific serum IgE may also be detected by the radioallergosorbent test. In this test an insoluble polymer-antigen conjugate is mixed with the serum to be tested. IgE specific for the antigen present in the serum will attach to the conjugate. The quantity of antigen-specific IgE in the serum is quantified by adding[125] I-labeled anti-IgE antibody and measuring the amount of radioactivity taken up by the conjugate.

Bronchial inhalational challenge may be carried out by using graded doses of a highly dilute extract of the allergen to be tested. Development of airways obstruction is demonstrated by serial measurements of airways resistance or indices derived from the forced expiratory spirogram or flow volume loop. This method remains largely a research procedure.

IMMUNE COMPLEX SKIN REACTIONS. Skin test reactions manifest by an erythematous, edematous area developing about six hours after the intradermal injection of the test solution are known as Type III or immune complex reactions. They are believed to result from the deposition of a soluble circulating antigen-antibody (immune) complex in the vessels or tissues. Both wheal-and-flare and immune complex reactions may occur following the same skin test material, as with aspergillus antigen solutions. Except for aspergillosis, this type of skin test reaction has limited clinical use.

DELAYED SKIN REACTIONS. Delayed, tuberculin-type hypersensitivity or Type IV reactions are believed to be caused by activation of sensitized lymphocytes after contact with antigen. An inflammatory reaction results from direct cytotoxicity or from the release of lymphokines. A positive reaction is manifest by an area of induration occurring 48 hours or more after the injection of an appropriate test solution.

The intracutaneous or Mantoux test is the "gold standard" of delayed-type hypersensitivity testing in tuberculosis; 0.1 ml of stabilized solution of PPD-tuberculin containing 5 tuberculin units in injected intradermally into the skin of the forearm. The test is read on the second or third day after injection: 10 mm or more of induration is interpreted as a positive reaction indicating infection with *Mycobacterium tuberculosis*, with or without associated disease; induration of 5 to 9 mm diameter is interpreted as doubtful (such reactions can result from either infection with *M. tuberculosis* or one of the atypical mycobacteria), and the test must be interpreted in clinical context and may have to be repeated; 0 to 4 mm induration is interpreted as a negative reaction, representing either no evidence of infection with *M. tuberculosis* or low grade sensitivity caused by atypical mycobacterial infection.

Multiple puncture tests, such as the tine test, should be used only for screening, and positive reactions should be confirmed by an intradermal test. Skin tests with antigens produced from atypical mycobacteria may give larger reactions in patients with such infections than the tuberculin test done with standard PPD-tuberculin. Although these tests have proved useful in epidemiologic studies, they are rarely useful in establishing a diagnosis in the individual case, and skin testing materials are not available for general use.

Skin testing materials are available for studying patients who may have coccidioidomycosis (coccidioidin, spherulin) and histoplasmosis (histoplasmin); 0.1 ml of a 1:100 dilution is given intradermally, and induration of 5 mm or greater is interpreted as a positive reaction. As with the tuberculin reaction, the test may take several weeks after infection to become positive, is often negative in severe or disseminated disease, and may be falsely negative when there is cutaneous anergy as in advanced age or severe febrile illnesses, especially those due to viruses. The state of skin reactivity may be established by testing with a common antigen such as mumps or *Trichophyton*. Skin tests for blastomycosis, cryptococcosis, nocardiosis, and actinomycosis are not clinically useful. Many physicians believe that since, as noted below, the histoplasmin skin test often causes a rise in histoplasmin complement-fixing titer and is often negative in early or disseminated disease, this skin test is also of very limited clinical usefulness.

THE KVEIM TEST. The Kveim test for sarcoidosis is performed by intradermally injecting 0.1 to 0.2 ml of a crude saline suspension of tissue prepared from spleen or lymph node of a patient with active sarcoidosis. A positive reaction consists in the development of a sarcoid granuloma in tissue biopsied four to six weeks after the injection. The reaction is said to be positive in up to 80 per cent of patients; false-positive reactions are low with most but not all batches of the test material. Kveim antigen is not commercially available in the United States, and the test remains a research procedure.

SEROLOGIC TESTS. Serologic tests, which demonstrate the presence of specific antibodies in the patient's serum and which depend on agglutination, precipitating, complement-fixation, or other reactions, are useful in a variety of bacterial, viral, and mycotic infections. The specificity and sensitivity of these tests varies, and the experience of a particular laboratory with a particular test must generally be known to permit the most useful interpretation. The tests must always be interpreted in the light of the full clinical picture, and the results must often be considered confirmatory or supportive rather than diagnostic.

In acute viral, mycoplasmal, and rickettsial infections, the occurrence of recent infection must generally be documented by showing a rise in titer to the antigen occurring over time (10 to 21 days). A single positive test may indicate nothing more than infection in the distant past. Thus these tests are often of most value in identifying the nature of an epidemic in a community rather than being of help in the diagnosis and treatment of the acutely ill patient.

Nonspecific cold agglutination antibodies are found in about half the patients with *Mycoplasma pneumoniae* infections, and a rising titer of cold agglutinins in an appropriate clinical setting is strong evidence for the presence of this disease.

Precipitin reactions are positive during the early weeks of histoplasmosis and coccidioidomycosis and then wane. Complement-fixation (CF) tests then become positive. In coccidioidomycosis a rising CF titer, especially above 1:64, presages dissemination. In histoplasmosis, complement-fixing antibodies tend to disappear with dissemination. The coccidioidin skin test does not affect the coccidioidin CF test, but the histoplasmin skin test tends to cause a rise in histoplasmin CF titer. Serologic tests for blastomycosis are not useful.

Precipitin and CF tests for aspergillosis tend to be positive in patients with invasive aspergillosis and aspergilloma and in many patients with allergic bronchopulmonary aspergillosis. However, these tests are not highly specific and must be regarded as confirmatory rather than diagnostic.

Cryptococcal antigen in blood, or especially spinal fluid, is helpful in establishing the diagnosis of infection with *Cryptococcus neoformans* and in following the course of treatment; as the patient improves, antigen levels tend to fall and antibodies to the cryptococcus are detectable in increasing titer. These tests have little application in uncomplicated pulmonary cryptococcosis.

In autoimmune disorders, antibodies may develop to various components of the individual's own cells (see Ch. 38). These antibodies may be specific for components of the nucleus or of the cytoplasm of the cells. One of the most widely used of these is the antinuclear antibody test. The demonstration of the lupus erythematosus cell is also dependent upon this type of immune disorder.

Serologic tests have proved to be disappointing in the diagnosis of hypersensitivity lung disease. Although precipitin antibodies to the agent in question are often demonstrated in patients with these diseases, they are also frequently found in persons who have had inhalational exposure to the causative organic dusts but who have not developed any illness. The tests thus have a confirmatory rather than a pathognomonic role in diagnosis.

Emmons, C. W., Binford, C. H., and Utz, J. P.: Medical Mycology. Philadelphia, Lea & Febiger, 1970.
The Tuberculin Skin Test. Supplement to Diagnostic Standards and Classification of Tuberculosis and Other Mycobacterial Diseases. New York, American Lung Association, 1974.

343.5. EXAMINATION OF THE SPUTUM

COLLECTION OF THE SPECIMEN. It is estimated that the tracheobronchial glands and goblet cells produce about 100 ml of secretion per day. Virtually all this material is swallowed after being carried to the oropharynx by the mucociliary elevator. Expectoration of bronchial secretions represents an abnormal state, and much information can be garnered by a study of sputum using microscopic and cultural methods. In patients with acute or chronic pulmonary disease who are not expectorating sputum, a specimen may be obtained by passing a suction catheter through the nose into the trachea (the nasotracheal specimen), or sputum production may be induced by having the patient inhale an ultrasonically generated aerosol of physiologic saline for 15 minutes. An aerosol of a 10 to 15 per cent sodium chloride solution heated to near body temperature may also be used for this purpose. When cultural studies are to be carried out for organisms such as *M. tuberculosis* or pathogenic fungi, which can withstand an acid milieu, a specimen of lower respiratory secretions can generally be obtained by early morning aspiration of gastric contents. However, specimens obtained in this way do not have a higher yield than induced sputa.

Since expectorated sputum is always contaminated by mouth flora, anaerobic cultures can be performed only on specimens obtained by transtracheal aspiration. Transtracheal aspiration is performed under local anesthesia by inserting a thin-walled needle through the cricothyroid membrane into the lumen of the trachea. A sterile plastic catheter is threaded through the needle into the trachea, and secretions are aspirated after a few milliliters of sterile saline are instilled to provoke cough. Routinely obtained bronchoscopic specimens are invariably contaminated with mouth organisms.

INSPECTION. Inspection of sputum with the naked eye serves to distinguish mucoid from mucopurulent sputum and discloses the presence of blood, black pigment as in anthracosis, or stones and gravel as in broncholithiasis. The viscosity of the sputum and the presence of plugs or casts of the bronchi can be ascertained.

MICROSCOPIC EXAMINATION. A fleck of sputum, carefully chosen because it is opaque, is placed on a microscope slide. This is spread out under a coverslip and, after scanning with the low power lens, is examined with the oil-immersion lens with the condenser racked down and the diaphragm adjusted to give a quasi-darkfield effect. In such a preparation eosinophils can be recognized by their large, brightly refractile granules and a bilobed nucleus. The granules of neutrophils are smaller and often display brownian motion; these cells have multilobed nuclei. The numbers of cells present indicate whether grossly observed purulence of the sputum is due to eosinophils or neutrophils. The presence of more than 20 per cent eosinophils suggests the presence of atopic disease. Macrophages are larger, are rounded, and often contain granular and pigmented inclusions. These cells come only from the lower respiratory tract and are observed in large numbers in the quiescent phases of chronic bronchitis. In lipoid pneumonia, clear lipid droplets abound in their cytoplasm. Hemosiderin-laden macrophages are observed in chronic left ventricular failure and in idiopathic hemosiderosis.

Charcot-Leyden crystals, which are elongated, rhomboid, needle-like shapes varying from 10 to 400 μm in length, are derived from the granules of eosinophils and have the same significance. Fungi such as the budding forms of candida, sometimes with their pseudohyphae, the septate hyphae characteristic of aspergillus, and the endospore-filled spherules of coccidioidomycosis can be recognized. Detection of fungi may be improved by clearing the specimen with potassium hydroxide.

Epithelial cells are often seen. The presence of squamous epithelial cells identifies contamination with oral secretions, indicating that further microscopic and cultural examination should not be carried out on that portion of the specimen. Study of the morphologic variants of bronchial-epithelial cells by this method is of little clinical value.

The coverslip can be removed from the wet preparation and the smear may be stained with Gram's stain for evaluation of bacterial flora. Eosinophils and neutrophils cannot be distinguished in this preparation, but squamous epithelial cells are easily identified, and areas near such cells should be avoided or another smear made. The morphology and Gram-staining characteristics of organisms can be identified. The morphology of bacteria often permits tentative identification such as the flame-shaped, gram-positive diplococci that denote the pneumococcus or the clumped, rounded, gram-positive cocci of the staphylococcus; the fine gram-negative rod of *Hemophilus influenzae* can usually be differentiated from the plump, sometimes encapsulated gram-negative rod that is *Klebsiella pneumoniae*.

The predominance of large numbers of one organism suggests infection of the respiratory tract rather than colonization. Sheets of gram-negative rods, to the virtual exclusion of other organisms, suggest a gram-negative bacillary infection; a large number of gram-negative and gram-positive organisms of great morphologic variability suggests the possibility of a mixed anaerobic infection. Needless to say, the Gram stain is of little value by itself, but is often helpful in establishing a clinical diagnosis when its results are carefully integrated with all other clinical information. Although cultures of sputum provide the most accurate qualitative information, integration of the sputum Gram stain with cultural data provides the best easily available estimate of quantitative bacteriology of the respiratory tract.

Examination of a sputum smear stained by the acid-fast or Ziehl-Neelsen method (direct smear technique) provides the possibility of rapid discovery of acid-fast bacilli in the sputum and the diagnosis of a mycobacterial infection in the appropriate clinical setting. Concentration of sputum with low bacillary counts by smear of the sediment after solubilization of mucus by adding agents such as N-acetyl-cysteine increases the sensitivity of both the smear and cultural techniques and, when sputum is scanty, may be applied to sputum collected over a period of several days. Mycobacteria may be seen with even more sensitivity but somewhat less specificity in sputum smears stained with fluorochrome dyes and examined by ultraviolet microscopy.

SPUTUM CULTURES. Cultures of sputum may be made for pyogenic organisms, mycobacteria, and fungi; drug susceptibility testing can be carried out on the pyogens and mycobacteria. Reports on pyogens are usually available within 24 to 72 hours, but mycobacterial cultures take from three to eight weeks from time of planting and fungal cultures take about three weeks. As noted previously, mouth flora contaminates all expectorated sputum, and cultural studies must be interpreted in the context of a Gram stain and the clinical findings. Positive blood cultures in the appropriate clinical setting provide the most powerful evidence of the etiology of bacterial pneumonia.

When dealing with an exacerbation of a chronic bronchopulmonary process, it is appropriate to start antibiotic therapy for the most commonly found organisms (*D. pneumoniae* or *H. influenzae*) without doing a culture, provided that the Gram stain does not show predominance of some other organism.

Cultures for mycobacteria done on concentrated specimens are much more sensitive diagnostically than microscopic examination, and accuracy improves as multiple cultures, up to five in number, are performed. Cultures are also required for precise identification of mycobacteria.

SPUTUM CYTOLOGY. Smears are prepared for cytologic examination either by ethanol-ether fixation of a freshly expectorated specimen or by homogenization and concentration of a specimen previously expectorated into a fixative solution. Staining is carried out by the Papanicolaou method. Tumor cells can be identified in as high a proportion as 90 per cent of central tumors and a lower proportion of midzonal tumors. Cytologic study is of little value in diagnosing peripheral tumors. Diagnostic yield increases with the examination of multiple specimens, but there is little increase in the rate of return after five specimens have been examined. In many instances, the cytologist can accurately identify the histologic type of the tumor. It should be remembered that positive sputum cytology can result from neoplasms in the nasopharynx, larynx, mouth, and esophagus, a fact that is of special importance when the chest roentgenogram is negative.

Chodosh, S.: Examination of sputum cells. N. Engl. J. Med., 282:854, 1970.
Davies, D. F.: A review of detection methods for the early diagnosis of lung cancer. J. Chron. Dis., 19:819, 1966.
Epstein, R. L.: Constituents of sputum: A simple method. Ann. Intern. Med., 77:259, 1972.

343.6.   EXAMINATION OF PLEURAL FLUID

Inspection of pleural fluid, an inevitable part of every thoracentesis, provides useful information. The diagnosis of empyema is evident if pus is obtained. Hemorrhagic effusions are more frequent in carcinoma and pulmonary infarction than in infectious processes. The obtaining of milky white fluid establishes the diagnosis of chylous effusion, and the presence of shimmering reflections from the top of a test tube of pleural fluid suggests the presence of a cholesterol-containing pleural effusion.

Laboratory examinations of pleural fluid are definitive only if tumor cells are seen in cytologic examination of the specimen or when a specific agent is recovered which proves the etiology of an infectious process. However, the integration of relatively inexpensively obtained laboratory data with the clinical information often provides important clues to the diagnosis. Thus pleural fluid transudates, often a part of systemic edematous states, generally have a specific gravity of less than 1.015, total protein of less than 2.5 grams per 100 ml or a pleural fluid to serum protein ratio of less than 0.5, lactic dehydrogenase (LDH) levels of less than 200 IU, and pleural fluid to serum LDH ratios of less than 0.6. Pleural exudates, reflecting an inflammatory process, have a specific gravity greater than 1.018 and total protein of greater than 3 grams per 100 ml or a pleural fluid to serum protein ratio of greater than 0.5; the pleural fluid to serum LDH ratio is greater than 0.6.

In infectious effusions, glucose is often decreased to values of about half the serum value, but in rheumatoid pleural effusion, glucose is characteristically less than 10 mg per 100 ml.

Total and differential cell counts are helpful except when the pleural fluid is grossly purulent. A predominance of polymorphonuclear leukocytes (PMN's) suggests that bacterial infection is the cause, e.g., the pleural effusion accompanying a pneumonia. Such a fluid may be sterile, or microscopic examination of a pleural fluid smear stained with Gram's stain may reveal bacteria. A predominance of small lymphocytes, particularly with few mesothelial cells and total cell counts above 1000 per cubic millimeter, strongly suggests tuberculosis. Tubercle bacilli are rarely observed in acid-fast stains and are not commonly recovered on cultures. Lymphoma of the pleura is much less readily diagnosed on cytologic preparations than carcinoma. With pulmonary infarction, a mixture of PMN's, lymphocytes, and numerous mesothelial cells is often observed. Lupus erythematosus cells may be seen in the pleural fluid in systemic lupus erythematosus. Eosinophils in the pleural fluid have no diagnostic significance except to indicate chronicity of the process.

The pleural fluid complicating pancreatitis usually demonstrates an amylase concentration several times higher than that in serum. Pleural fluid pH of 7.2 or below tends to be associated with empyema or loculated effusions requiring drainage. In the cholesterol or pseudochylous effusion, cholesterol concentration is high but neutral and fatty acid concentrations are low. Such effusions are the result of longstanding chronic pleural disease, most commonly tuberculosis or rheumatoid disease. In chylothorax, the lipid content of the fluid is high as manifest by sudanophilic fatty droplets and a high concentration of neutral fat and fatty acids; the cholesterol content is low.

Black, L. F.: The pleural space and pleural fluid. Mayo Clin. Proc., 47:493, 1972.

Light, R. W., MacGregor, M. I., Luchsinger, P. C., and Ball, W. C.: Pleural effusions: The diagnostic separations of transudates and exudates. Ann. Intern. Med., 77:507, 1972.

343.7.   BRONCHOSCOPY

Bronchoscopy is the inspection of the lumen of the tracheobronchial tree with a lighted optical system or endoscope. Prior to 1967, all bronchoscopies were performed with the rigid bronchoscope, a hollow metal tube with a blunted tip, and a system for providing light at the end of the bronchoscope, either a minature electric light bulb or a fiberoptic light carrier. This instrument may be passed under either local or general anesthesia. The neck must be hyperextended and flexed to the right or left side to permit entry into the left or right bronchial trees, respectively. Visualization of the lobar and segmental orifices of both lower and the right middle lobes is readily possible. Visualization of the upper lobe bronchi bilaterally is usually possible but more difficult; segmental orifices can sometimes be seen using telescopes fitted with prisms which permit visualization at 45- or 90-degree angles to the axis of the telescope. These instruments permit ready appreciation of fixation of the bronchial tree owing to lymph node involvement by tumor; biopsy or surgical treatment of bronchoscopically visualized lesions and the removal of foreign bodies can be carried out.

During the last ten years the use of the rigid bronchoscope has been rapidly superseded by the flexible fiberoptic bronchoscope. In these instruments, light is carried to the tip of the device by fiberoptic light carrying bundles and the image is returned to the eye through an objective lens and fiberoptic bundle. Bronchoscopes for use in adults have a 5 to 5.2 mm tip and an aspiration channel which is approximately 2 mm in diameter. Aspiration may be carried out directly through this channel, or suction catheters, bronchial brushes, and various types of biopsy and grasping forceps can be passed through the channel. The distal end of the bronchoscope can be angulated to facilitate visualization and entry of various portions of the bronchial tree by moving a lever at the proximal end of the instrument.

The flexible fiberoptic bronchoscope can be passed through either the nose or the mouth with the neck in its normal position. Inspection of the tracheobronchial tree down to subsegmental bronchi or beyond is readily possible. Cytologic specimens can be collected on the bronchial brush, and fragments of bronchial wall can be readily removed with the biopsy forceps for histologic examination. Brush or biopsy forceps can be passed directly into solid lesions under fluoroscopic control. Small fragments of pulmonary parenchyma can be obtained with the biopsy forceps by grasping the walls of distal, thin-walled bronchi, a procedure known as transbronchoscopic lung biopsy. The small diameter of the bronchoscope permits ready bronchoscopy of patients who are receiving mechanically assisted ventilation. The instrument is passed through either the endotracheal or tracheostomy tube, and special adapters are used to maintain assisted ventilation during the procedure.

Bronchoscopy is a major tool in evaluating the patient with suspect bronchogenic carcinoma. Such patients present with hemoptysis or a shadow in the chest film which suggests bronchial obstruction or a mass lesion; the method is of greatest value in central and mid-zonal lesions. Although the flexible bronchoscope can be used for foreign body removal, the rigid bronchoscope is much more versatile for this purpose. Bronchoscopy can be used therapeutically for aspirating secretions, but since the method cannot be applied at frequent intervals, it is of limited value; the rigid bronchoscope accepts larger suction devices than can be passed through the flexible bronchoscope.

Although flexible fiberoptic bronchoscopy is much more widely applicable than rigid tube bronchoscopy, the procedure is not innocuous. Asthmatic patients may have an adverse reaction to the local anesthetic agent; mild hypoxemia is a regular accompaniment of the procedure and, although not troublesome in individuals with normal lung function, may be hazardous in patients with underlying lung disease. Life-threatening hemorrhage may complicate bronchial wall or transbronchoscopic lung biopsy. Fever may occur without a parenchymal pulmonary infiltration, and pneumonia may be a complication of bronchoscopy, especially in elderly individuals with obstructing bronchial lesions.

As with any diagnostic procedure, the risks of the procedure should be weighed against the benefits, and alternative methods for diagnosis should be considered. Thus, if precise anatomic information regarding the presence of an endobronchial tumor is not necessary, sputum cytology should be considered first for tumor diagnosis. In the elderly, seriously ill individual with a large peripheral tumor, cytologic examination of a specimen obtained by percutaneous fine-needle aspiration may entail a lower risk than bronchoscopy.

Khan, M. A., Whitcomb, M. E., and Snider, G. L.: Flexible fiberoptic bronchoscopy. Am. J. Med., 61:151, 1976.

Sackner, M. A.: Bronchofiberscopy. State of the art. Am. Rev. Respir. Dis., 111:62, 1975.

343.8.   BIOPSY TECHNIQUES

LYMPH NODE BIOPSY. Biopsy of palpable superficial lymph nodes is generally helpful in evaluating pulmonary disease that is part of a systemic process or when primary tumor of the lung has spread outside the confines of the thorax. When lymph nodes are not palpable, the scalene lymph node, situated on the anterior scalene muscle, may be biopsied through a small supraclavicular incision. Scalene lymph node involvement is much more likely when there is involvement of the paratracheal lymph nodes as observed in the chest roentgenogram. This procedure has a high yield in granulomatous disease such as sarcoidosis but a much lower yield in neoplastic disease.

MEDIASTINOSCOPY. Mediastinoscopy is performed under general anesthesia, using an endotracheal tube. An incision is made in the suprasternal notch, and the mediastinoscope, a metal tube with light carried to its beveled end, is inserted via the tissue planes adjacent to the trachea as far as the carina. Anterior mediastinal, right paratracheal, and even subcarinal lymph nodes may be seen and biopsied. The left paratracheal area is more difficult to approach because of the presence of the aortic arch. This procedure has almost 100 per cent yield in granulomatous disease such as sarcoidosis. The method is being widely used for staging patients with bronchogenic carcinoma, but the exact indications remain controversial.

PLEURAL BIOPSY. Biopsy of the parietal pleura using the side-cutting Cope or Abrams needles is of major importance in the diagnosis of pleural effusion. In patients who do not have an obvious explanation for pleural effusion, biopsy should be considered at the time of the initial thoracentesis. The Abrams needle has the advantage that large pieces of tissue can be obtained with a very low risk of inducing a pneumothorax, and several biopsies tangential to the needle puncture can be obtained with a single insertion of the needle. The Cope needle produces smaller pieces of tissue than the Abrams needle. An end-cutting core-biopsy needle, such as the Silverman needle, can be used when the pleura is very thick and adherent to the lung.

The major risk of pleural biopsy is bleeding due to injury of the intercostal artery, and biopsy should never be performed on the cephalad side of the intercostal puncture wound. The procedure should obviously not be performed on patients with a coagulopathy. Because of the focal nature of pleural disease, a second or third biopsy is often performed if the first biopsy has failed to yield diagnostic information. Consideration should always be given to culturing a piece of tissue as well as to histologic examination, because the yield of positive cultures for *M. tuberculosis* is much higher from tissue than from pleural fluid. Surgical or open pleural biopsy adds little to twice or thrice repeated needle biopsy of the pleura and is rarely used.

LUNG BIOPSY. In instances in which simpler diagnostic studies have not been fruitful, consideration should be given to obtaining lung tissue for laboratory diagnosis. The approach to sampling lung tissue for cytologic, histologic, or bacteriologic diagnosis varies, depending on whether the patient has a diffuse pulmonary lesion or has a circumscribed and presumably solid lesion.

The endoscopic approach to solid lesions by the means of the fluoroscopically guided biopsy forceps or brush has been referred to above. Material for cytologic examination can often be obtained by fine needle aspiration of the mass lesion carried out under fluoroscopic control. If the lesion is not adherent to the pleura, pneumothorax may result, requiring the insertion of a chest tube. When the lesion is adherent to the chest wall, core biopsy with a cutting needle, obtaining material for both cytologic and histologic examination, is probably a preferable procedure. Percutaneous methods

should be considered only when surgical therapy is contraindicated or the risk is so high that this form of treatment would not be undertaken without proof of diagnosis.

Diffuse pulmonary lesions may be approached by transbronchoscopic lung biopsy. This method should be particularly considered when the differential diagnosis includes lesions which can be readily diagnosed by the pathologist on small amounts of tissue. Included in this category are granulomatous and neoplastic lesions and the suspected presence of infectious agents readily identified histologically such as *Pneumocystis carinii*, aspergillus, or one of the obligatory pathogenic fungi. The procedure is less helpful in diagnosing lymphoma than carcinoma and is of limited value in the diagnosis of chronic interstitial fibrosis in which the histology of small amounts of tissue is nonspecific and there is a serious sampling problem. In the latter circumstance, open lung biopsy performed through a short intercostal incision permits biopsy of a larger portion of lung, often from two sites, and provides enough tissue for a variety of histologic, cultural, and immunopathologic examinations. Core biopsy, using the high speed air-powered biopsy drill or one of the core biopsy needles, has been applied to diffuse pulmonary lesions; but except in the hands of the most highly skilled and experienced operators, it carries more hazard than either transbronchoscopic or open lung biopsy.

Carr, D. T., Soule, E. H., and Ellis, F. H., Jr.: Management of pleural effusions. Med. Clin. N. Am, 48:961, 1964.

Gaensler, E. A., Moister, V. B., and Hamm, J.: Open lung biopsy in diffuse pulmonary disease. N. Engl. J. Med., 270:1319, 1964.

Gunstensen, J., and Wade, J. D.: Mediastinoscopy. An analysis of 320 consecutive cases. Br. J. Surg., 59:209, 1972.

Levine, H., and Cugell, D. W.: Blunt-end needle biopsy of pleura and rib. Arch. Intern. Med., 109:516, 1962.

Lillington, G. A., and Jamplis, R. W.: Scalene node biopsy. Ann. Intern. Med., 59:101, 1963.

Manfredi, F., and Krumholz, R.: Percutaneous needle biopsy of the lung in evaluation of pulmonary disorders. JAMA, 198:1198, 1966.

Niden, A. K., Burrows, B., Kasik, J. E., and Barclay, W. R.: Percutaneous pleural biopsy with a curetting needle. Special reference to biopsy without effusion. Am. Rev. Respir. Dis., 84:37, 1961.

Nordenstrom, B.: Transthoracic needle biopsy. N. Engl. J. Med., 276:1081, 1967.

Skinner, D. B.: Scalene-lymph node biopsy: Reappraisal of risks and indications. N. Engl. J. Med., 268:1324, 1963.

Steel, S. J., and Winstanley, D. P.: Lung biopsy with a high speed air drill. Thorax, 22:286, 1967.

Zavala, D. C.: Diagnostic fiberoptic bronchoscopy techniques and result of biopsy in 600 patients. Chest, 68:12, 1975.

343.9. MISCELLANEOUS PROCEDURES

THE ELECTROCARDIOGRAM. Electrocardiographic changes occur in only a small proportion of patients with pulmonary embolism, but the procedure is noninvasive and inexpensive and should therefore be regularly used when this diagnosis is suspected. The changes are transient so that serial examination is helpful; P pulmonale, right bundle branch block, right axis deviation, and supraventricular arrhythmias are most frequently seen (see Ch. 364). Electrocardiographic evidence of right ventricular hypertrophy correlates quite well with the degree of pulmonary hypertension and cor pulmonale in patients with disorders causing restriction of the vascular bed of the lung. The electrocardiogram is a less sensitive indicator of right ventricular enlargement in patients whose cor pulmonale is due to chronic bronchitis and emphysema (see Ch. 344). The changes of myocardial ischemia may be helpful in discerning the etiology of chest pain, and those of ischemia and left ventricular hypertrophy may be helpful in patients with acute cardiogenic pulmonary edema, especially when the presentation is atypical (see Ch. 356).

EXTRAPULMONARY RADIONUCLIDE IMAGING. Scintiscanning of the neck and mediastinum after administration of radioiodine is useful in the evaluation of an upper mediastinal mass which may be substernal goiter (see Ch. 546). Liver scans are useful in detecting bacterial or amebic abscess of the liver but are neither very sensitive nor specific in detecting metastatic bronchogenic carcinoma, and the technique should not be routinely used in the preoperative evaluation of patients with this neoplasm (see Ch. 349.2). Bone scans after ^{99m}technetium-labeled polyphosphate often can detect metastatic carcinoma before lesions are roentgenographically visible; however, focal injury to bone from any cause may cause increased concentration of radionuclide, and some highly lytic lesions may not be revealed by this method (see Part XXII).

TESTS OF MUSCLE FUNCTION. Disorders of the muscular system may involve the muscles of the respiratory system and be suspected because of loss of vital and total lung capacities. Brief reversal of the impaired vital capacity after administration of the short-acting anticholinesterase edrophonium supports the diagnosis of myasthenia gravis (see Ch. 340.4). Electromyography may be helpful in establishing this diagnosis as well as that of other neurologic or muscular disorders (see Ch. 272). Elevation of serum creatine phosphokinase and aldolase levels is helpful in the diagnosis of polymyositis or dermatomyositis (see Ch. 51).

SPECIAL TESTS. Sweat chloride concentrations above 60 mEq per liter in the absence of adrenal insufficiency or nephrogenic diabetes insipidus support the diagnosis of cystic fibrosis of the pancreas; 95 per cent of adult males with this disorder have azoospermia (see Ch. 412). Patients with Kartagener's syndrome (situs inversus, sinusitis, and bronchiectasis) have ultrastructurally identifiable abnormalities of their cilia which can be detected in nasal or bronchial mucosal biopsies. In homozygous alpha$_1$ antitrypsin deficiency, serum alpha$_1$ globulin and serum trypsin inhibitory capacity levels are markedly decreased.

344. DISEASES ASSOCIATED WITH AIRWAYS OBSTRUCTION

Benjamin Burrows

344.1. GENERALIZED AIRWAY DISEASES

The present discussion deals with chronic or recurrent generalized airways disorders which are not the direct result of an underlying "specific" bronchopulmonary disease. It includes asthma, the chronic bronchitis syndromes, emphysema, and chronic obstructive pulmonary disease.

INTRODUCTION

DEFINITIONS OF TERMS AND INTERRELATIONSHIPS OF DIAGNOSTIC ENTITIES. The bronchopulmonary system may respond in different ways when exposed to irritants or allergens. The type of response depends on the nature and severity of the exposure and on host susceptibility.

In subjects with hyperreactive or "twitchy" airways, exposure to a variety of provocative factors can lead to bronchospasm (i.e., constriction of bronchial smooth muscles, often accompanied by edema of bronchial walls and abnormal mucus production). Recurrent episodes of bronchospasm of sufficient severity to lead to symptoms are called *asthma*. Asthma is especially likely to develop in allergic individuals in whom exposure to inhaled allergens provokes recurrent Type I allergic bronchospasm. But it also occurs in nonallergic individuals who have hyperreactive airways, and, as used in this discussion, the term "asthma" has no specific etiologic implications.

The response is different when there is chronic, relatively low-grade exposure to bronchial irritants in a subject without hyperreactive airways. This results in stimulation of the mucus-secreting elements of the airway, reduction in bronchial ciliary activity, and impaired resistance to bronchial infection. In the present discussion, the resulting syndrome, characterized primarily by chronic productive cough, is called *simple chronic bronchitis*.

In a relatively small proportion of subjects, chronic exposure to bronchial irritants results in severe irreversible narrowing of airways, a condition called *chronic obstructive bronchitis*. Much of the obstruction is in airways less than 2 mm in diameter, including bronchioles as well as bronchi, and the term *"small airways disease"* has been introduced to emphasize this point. There would seem little use, however, in delineating this as a separate disease.

Finally, the lung may respond to noxious stimuli by developing *emphysema*, a condition characterized by dilatation of air spaces distal to the terminal bronchiole with destruction of their walls. As with chronic obstructive bronchitis, there appears to be considerable variability in susceptibility to the disorder. Emphysematous changes reduce the elastic recoil of the lung, allowing excessive airways collapse on expiration and leading to an irreversible obstructive problem.

The definitions of the aforementioned terms are in no way mutually exclusive. Indeed, in view of their common dependence on exposure to inhaled irritants, one would expect them to coexist frequently. Patients with chronic obstructive bronchitis may show superimposed recurrent bronchospasm, thereby fulfilling the criteria for asthma. Most patients with emphysema have a chronic productive cough at some stage of their illness, allowing a secondary diagnosis of simple chronic bronchitis. Some obliteration of small airways generally accompanies emphysema, and without elaborate tests it may be difficult to determine the relative importance of chronic obstructive bronchitis and emphysema in a severe irreversible airways obstructive disorder. This has led to the use of general terms such as *chronic obstruc-*

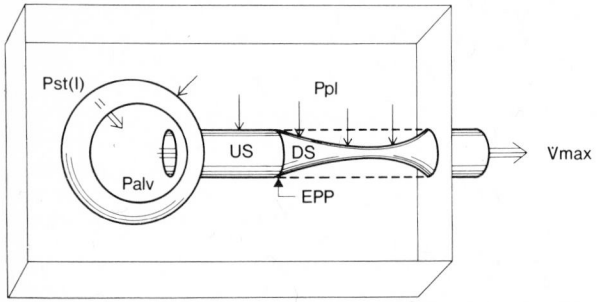

Figure 1. A schematic model of the respiratory system during forced expiration. The pleural pressure (Ppl) is applied to both alveoli and intrathoracic airways. The pressure driving air out of the system is the alveolar pressure (Palv), which is the sum of Ppl and the elastic recoil of the lung (Pst(l)). The pressure within the airway falls as one proceeds mouthward. At the equal pressure point (EPP), pressure within the airway just equals Ppl. In airways upstream (US) of this point, intraluminal pressure exceeds Ppl and airways remain dilated. Mouthward or downstream (DS) of this point, compression of intrathoracic airways occurs, and this acts as a governor on flow, causing a maximal flow (Vmax) to be achieved which is essentially independent of the Ppl generated by the expiratory muscles. (From Burrows, B., Knudson, R. J., and Kettel, L. J.: Respiratory Insufficiency. Copyright © 1975 by Year Book Medical Publishers, Inc., Chicago. Used by permission.)

tive pulmonary (or lung) disease (abbreviated COPD) to describe this clinical syndrome.

In practice, one generally applies the single diagnostic term which best describes the patient's major problem. But this must not limit one's therapeutic efforts. For example, a diagnosis of emphysema should not imply that measures directed at amelioration of bronchitis or prevention of bronchospasm are inappropriate. Therapy should be directed at all features of the patient's disease, not simply at those which determine the primary diagnosis.

The term *chronic bronchitis,* unqualified, has been used in various ways by different authors, sometimes referring to a simple smoker's cough and at other times (especially in the British literature) to severe COPD. In view of its ambiguity, it will be used in the present discussion only when qualified as "simple" or "obstructive."

PATHOPHYSIOLOGY OF AIRWAYS OBSTRUCTION. In clinical practice, airways obstruction is synonymous with slowing of forced expiration. To understand the determinants of the speed of forced expiration, one must consider the pressures which develop within the thorax during a maximum expiratory effort. These are depicted in Figure 1. The high intrapleural pressure (Ppl) developed by the expiratory muscles tends to drive air from the alveoli, but its effect on flow is limited by its tendency to compress intrathoracic airways. This "dynamic compression of airways" is resisted by the recoil of the lung (Pst) which causes the pressure within the alveoli and peripheral airways to exceed Ppl. Owing to flow resistance, however, the high pressure within the alveoli and peripheral airways is dissipated as air progresses mouthward, and during a forced exhalation there will be a point within the thorax where the pressure inside the airway just equals Ppl. Mouthward of this "equal pressure point," the pressure outside the airways exceeds that within, and airways compression occurs. This airways compression

acts as a governor on flow, and a maximum expiratory flow (Vmax) occurs which is essentially independent of the effort exerted by the subject. It depends only on the intrinsic resistance of the airways, the recoil of the lungs, and the compressibility of the airways mouthward of the equal pressure point. A high airways resistance, low lung recoil, or excessive collapsibility of airways will lead to a reduction in Vmax.

In determining whether Vmax is normal, its relationship to lung volume must be taken into account. When the lung volume is large, airways are maximally dilated and have a low resistance. Also, lung recoil is high. Thus Vmax is high when the lung is near full inflation. As lung volume decreases, airways resistance rises and lung recoil falls, leading to a reduction in Vmax. The relationship between lung volume and Vmax is readily seen in a maximum expiratory flow volume (MEFV) curve, depicted in Figure 2A. The same information is contained in a standard spirogram (Fig. 2B) in which volume is displayed against time; in this case, the rapidity of change in volume (the slope of the curve) reflects Vmax. The total volume exhaled during the test is called the "forced vital capacity" (FVC). Values for the volume exhaled during the first second of a forced exhalation (the FEV_1) or for the average flow during the middle half of the FVC (the MMEF or $FEF_{25-75\%}$) are readily determined from standard spirograms and are commonly used indicators of the speed of forced expiration. Instantaneous Vmax values are more readily measured from MEFV curves. They are most commonly

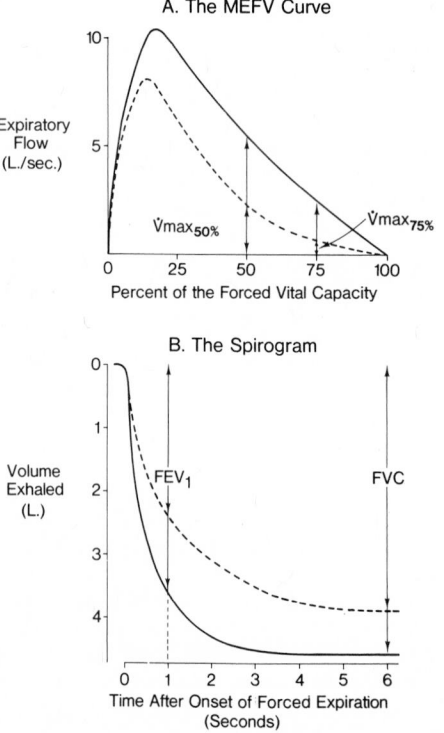

Figure 2. Solid lines are used to show a normal maximum expiratory flow-volume (MEFV) in *A* and a normal spirogram in *B*. Broken lines indicate typical curves for a patient with mild airways obstruction. Measurements of the forced vital capacity (FVC), the forced expiratory volume at one second (FEV_1), and forced flow rates at 50 per cent and 75 per cent of the FVC ($Vmax_{50\%}$ and $Vmax_{75\%}$) are depicted as vertical lines.

determined at 50 per cent or 75 per cent of the forced expired volume ($\dot{V}max_{50\%}$ or $\dot{V}max_{75\%}$, respectively*).

The $Vmax_{75\%}$ appears more sensitive than the FEV_1 for detecting subclinical airways dysfunction and has become popular in epidemiologic studies. However, since it is easily measured, is highly reproducible, has a relatively narrow normal range, and tends to reflect the clinical severity of disease, the FEV_1 is more widely used in clinical practice.

In order to determine that a low FEV_1 results from slowing of expiration rather than from a marked restriction in the total volume exhaled, the FEV_1/FVC ratio is examined. This ratio is regularly below 65 per cent in clinically significant airways obstructive diseases. Once the presence of airways obstruction has been confirmed by the presence of a low FEV_1/FVC ratio, the severity of the abnormality is best assessed from the degree of reduction in the FEV_1 itself.

Airways obstruction leads to an increased work of breathing. It also causes a diminished response to a ventilatory stimulus. The latter may lead to underventilation and hypercapnia if the disease is severe, if ventilatory drive is reduced (as with sedatives or narcotics), or if there is respiratory muscle weakness or fatigue.

Since the airways abnormalities and any accompanying parenchymal lesions are nonuniformly distributed throughout the lung, ventilation becomes uneven and may be poorly matched to blood flow. The nonuniformity of alveolar ventilation can be demonstrated by an increased "slope of phase III" on the single breath nitrogen test, by an abnormality in the nitrogen washout curve, or by prolongation of the helium equilibration time.

Continued perfusion of poorly ventilated regions of lung causes some alveoli to have very low ventilation/perfusion ($\dot{V}/\dot{Q}$) ratios. The blood traversing such areas does not become well oxygenated, an effect called "venous admixture," "physiologic shunting," or "relative shunt." This is the major cause of hypoxemia in airways obstructive diseases.

As a result of the mismatched ventilation and perfusion, other alveoli show very high $\dot{V}/\dot{Q}$ ratios. The ventilation which reaches these alveoli is largely wasted, resulting in an increased "physiologic dead space." This reduces the effective alveolar ventilation and necessitates an increase in overall ventilation if hypercapnia is to be avoided.

Obstructed airways tend to close prematurely during a maximum exhalation, leading to trapping of air and an increase in residual volume. In emphysema and during attacks of asthma, the total lung capacity is also increased. As might be expected, the pulmonary diffusing capacity measurement is almost always reduced in emphysema. It is usually within normal limits in asthma and gives variable results in chronic obstructive bronchitis.

The small airways have a very large total cross-sectional diameter, and extensive changes in this "quiet zone" of the lung are required to produce a discernible effect on measurements such as the FEV_1. More sensitive tests are needed to detect mild small airways ab-

normalities. Many new tests have been proposed, including measurements of $\dot{V}max$ late in forced expiration, "closing volume," and "frequency dependence of compliance." Although these tests may prove useful for detecting subclinical disease and in research studies, their specificity for small airways abnormalities is doubtful, and they have no proved clinical application. Recently, there has also been much interest in the helium responsiveness of the MEFV curve. In normal subjects, $\dot{V}max_{50\%}$ shows a marked increase after helium breathing. A smaller than normal increase in $\dot{V}max_{50\%}$ is considered evidence for small airways obstruction. The role of this test in clinical practice remains uncertain.

A report of the ACCP/ATS Joint Committee on Pulmonary Nomenclature: Pulmonary terms and symbols. Chest, 67:583, 1975.

Burrows, B., and Hasan, F. M.: Abnormalities in small airways. Disease-a-Month, Vol. 23, No. 10, July 1977, pp. 2–34.

Despas, P. J., Leroux, M., and Macklem, P. T.: Site of airway obstruction in asthma as determined by measuring maximal expiratory flow breathing air and a helium-oxygen mixture. J. Clin. Invest., 51:3235, 1972.

Knudson, R. J., and Burrows, B.: Early detection of obstructive lung diseases. Med. Clin. North Am., 57:681, 1973.

Macklem, P. T.: The pathophysiology of chronic bronchitis and emphysema. Med. Clin. North Am., 57:669, 1973.

Macklem, P. T., Thurlbeck, W. M., and Fraser, R. G.: Chronic obstructive disease of small airways. Ann. Intern. Med., 74:167, 1971.

Mead, J., Turner, J. M., Macklem, P. T., and Little, J. B.: Significance of the relationship between lung recoil and maximum expiratory flow. J. Appl. Physiol., 22:95, 1967.

Thurlbeck, W. M.: Chronic bronchitis and emphysema. Med. Clin. North Am., 57:651, 1973.

SIMPLE CHRONIC BRONCHITIS

PREVALENCE AND PATHOGENESIS. In epidemiologic studies, simple chronic bronchitis is diagnosed when productive cough is present on most days for at least three months of the year. Using this criterion, the diagnosis may be applied to a large proportion of heavy cigarette smokers, especially after age 45. Exposure to occupational or environmental air pollutants adds to the effects of smoking. Only a small fraction of subjects with this syndrome consult a physician. Most accept their "smoker's cough" as a penalty for their cigarette habit. Those who do see a physician are likely to have recurrent respiratory infections or some type of wheezing problem in addition to their cough.

The disorder results from three apparently direct effects of inhaling bronchial irritants: (1) stimulation of the mucus-secreting elements of the airway; (2) interference with ciliary activity with impaired mucus clearance; and (3) disturbance of alveolar macrophage function with reduced resistance to bronchopulmonary infection. Accumulation of secretions leads to cough. Bacterial colonization is common, the normally sterile bronchi now harboring organisms similar to those found in the nasopharynx.

PATHOLOGY. The most characteristic finding is hypertrophy of mucous glands and goblet cells. The "Reid index," representing the ratio of mucous gland to total bronchial wall thickness, exceeds its normal limit of 0.4. In addition, one finds retained bronchial secretions and variable degrees of inflammatory change in the bronchial walls. Even in the absence of clinically significant obstruction, careful studies may show narrowing or obliteration of some small airways and scattered centrilobular emphysema. Similar small airways and em-

---

*There is considerable confusion in use of these symbols. It has been recommended that $Vmax_{50\%}$ and $Vmax_{75\%}$ be expressed as $FEF_{50\%}$ and $FEF_{75\%}$, respectively. Also, the $Vmax_{75\%}$ as defined herein is sometimes reported as $\dot{V}max_{25\%}$, the 25% then referring to the portion of the FVC remaining when the flow measurement is made.

physematous changes are noted in asymptomatic smokers, however, and it is uncertain that they are related to simple chronic bronchitis except through their common association with cigarette use.

CLINICAL MANIFESTATIONS. In mild disease, cough is noted primarily on arising or after smoking the first cigarette of the day, is productive of a small quantity of mucoid sputum, and is present most regularly during the winter months. As the disorder becomes more severe, cough tends to recur throughout the day, symptoms persist throughout the year, larger volumes of sputum are raised, and increasingly severe paroxysms of cough are noted. Wheezing is common at the end of a severe coughing spell, probably representing cough-induced bronchospasm. Wheezing may also occur on reclining; this may first be noted by the patient's spouse. This type of wheeze is probably a direct result of retained secretions, as it is often relieved by cough.

Periodic exacerbations of symptoms occur, often accompanied by purulence of the sputum. Most such episodes appear to follow viral respiratory infections, and purulence of the sputum is regarded as evidence of bacterial overgrowth. Cultures generally show the normal nasopharyngeal flora, although *H. influenzae* and *S. pneumoniae* are often present as well. These organisms probably represent secondary invaders rather than primary causes of the exacerbations. Varying degrees of bronchospasm may occur during exacerbations, and there is no clear distinction between such episodes and asthma. Blood-streaked sputum occurs occasionally, but repeated or severe hemoptysis should lead one to suspect a more serious disease than simple chronic bronchitis.

With further progression of the disorder, the sputum may become chronically purulent. The term *mucopurulent bronchitis* is sometimes applied to this stage of illness. Sputum cultures may now reveal drug-resistant organisms such as *P. aeruginosa;* this is especially likely to occur if the patient has received a variety of antibiotics.

Physical examination may be entirely normal in mild disease. Later, scattered rhonchi and variable coarse rales are heard. These may clear or change location after cough. A wheeze or paroxysm of coughing is often induced by a forced expiratory effort.

LABORATORY FINDINGS. In uncomplicated cases, blood counts and differential smear are normal, as is the chest radiograph. Sputum examination shows variable numbers of leukocytes and a mixed flora of organisms, as already noted. Bronchograms reveal the enlarged ducts of hypertrophied mucous glands, mucus plugs which prevent filling of some medium-sized bronchi, and often mild diffuse dilatation of bronchi on inspiratory films. Bronchoscopy reveals retained secretions, diffuse hyperemia, and some mucosal edema. Spirometry may be within normal limits but often shows slight slowing of forced expiration.

COURSE AND PROGNOSIS. Patients with simple chronic bronchitis often show considerable fluctuation in symptoms. Cough and sputum production worsen with increased cigarette use, during inclement weather, and following acute respiratory infections. In mild cases, symptoms usually disappear completely with cessation of smoking. Although simple chronic bronchitis is often associated with slight reduction in ventilatory function, at least one prospective study has failed to show that smokers with chronic productive cough have a significantly greater rate of decline in lung function than asymptomatic smokers. This suggests that the effect of cigarette smoke on airways function is essentially independent of its effect on mucus secretion. It is clear, at least, that a diagnosis of simple chronic bronchitis does not imply that the patient will inevitably develop progressive disabling respiratory insufficiency.

DIFFERENTIAL DIAGNOSIS. The diagnosis is basically one of exclusion. It is justified when there is persistent cough which cannot be ascribed to a parenchymal lung disease, a disorder of the upper respiratory tract, a specific endobronchial disease, or an allergic reaction of the airway. Thus a chest radiograph is required to exclude a parenchymal lesion. A careful examination of the upper airway is indicated, and one must exclude physical findings which might indicate a localized airways disorder (such as a persistent localized wheeze). In children or in young adults with severe symptoms, mucoviscidosis also must be excluded.

One should be cautious in diagnosing simple chronic bronchitis in the absence of an obvious source of chronic bronchial irritation. In a nonsmoker, in a patient whose history suggests an association between symptoms and exposure to allergens, or in a patient with episodes of wheezing dyspnea, one should check for eosinophilia in the sputum and blood. High eosinophil levels suggest that the disorder is a variant of asthma. In any case, a secondary diagnosis of asthma is justified when recurrent reversible airways obstruction is an important feature of the disease.

Repeated or severe hemoptysis, or physical findings suggesting localized disease may call for bronchoscopy and even bronchography to rule out an endobronchial lesion or localized bronchiectasis, but these procedures are not indicated in the routine case. Some authorities recommend sputum cytology on all subjects with chronic bronchitis, especially over age 40. Spirometry should be carried out to determine the degree of associated ventilatory impairment.

There may be a problem in distinguishing severe mucopurulent bronchitis from bronchiectasis. Mild diffuse cylindrical dilatation of bronchi is noted in many severe bronchitics. Recurrent hemoptysis, repeated pneumonias in the same lung region, or areas of honeycombing on chest radiograph suggest that there may be areas of frank saccular bronchiectasis. Bronchography is required for accurate diagnosis but is usually indicated only if resection of the bronchiectatic areas would be considered. Otherwise, there is little difference in the therapy of mucopurulent bronchitis and bronchiectasis.

TREATMENT. Removal of the provocative factors (usually cigarettes) is of primary importance and may totally relieve the condition. When symptoms persist despite maximal efforts to avoid bronchial irritants or are severe enough to require more immediate relief, the following measures are employed:

Antibiotic Therapy. Noneosinophilic purulent sputum is regarded as evidence of infection and is treated with a seven- to ten-day course of tetracycline or ampicillin, 1 gram daily in divided doses. If the sputum fails to clear, further antibiotic therapy should be determined by sputum culture and sensitivity. Successive doses of different antibiotics should be avoided, however, because they tend to lead to a resistant flora. Failure of therapy is more often related to poor drainage of bronchial secretions than to inadequate antibacterial agents.

Recurrent infections may be treated with prophylactic tetracycline, prescribing 0.5 to 1.0 gram daily either continuously or for three weeks out of each month. Alternatively, the patient may be given a supply of tetracycline and advised to begin a seven- to ten-day course promptly if the sputum becomes purulent or if there are other signs of a lower respiratory tract infection. Prophylactic therapy appears to reduce the severity and duration of exacerbations but does not reduce their frequency.

Very severe exacerbations of disease generally respond better to ampicillin or cephalothin than to tetracycline, and it is reasonable to use these agents as initial therapy when the specific infecting organism is unknown. (Penicillin has proved inappropriate therapy for severe purulent exacerbations of bronchitis.) When resistant organisms are cultured from the sputum, the antibiotic regimen may have to be adjusted in accord with drug susceptibility studies.

Bronchodilator Agents. These are indicated on a regular basis for patients with mild reversible airways obstruction and for patients with prominent posttussic wheezing. Doses may have to be increased or medications first prescribed during exacerbations of disease. Inhaled bronchodilators are also useful adjuncts to bronchial hygiene treatments, as described below. Some degree of bronchospasm is generally present in patients with severe paroxysmal cough, and in them a trial of bronchodilators is justified even when frank expiratory slowing cannot be demonstrated. Bronchodilator therapy is discussed in more detail under the treatment of asthma.

Bronchial Hygiene Measures. The objective of these measures is to clear retained bronchial secretions. The most important steps are deep breathing followed by deliberate coughing. This may be made more effective by positioning the patient so that the most affected lung regions are in a superior position (postural drainage). In some subjects, chest percussion and vibration further increase sputum production.

Premedication with an inhaled bronchodilator may greatly improve the patient's tolerance of bronchial hygiene measures and increase their effectiveness. This may be followed by inhalation of bland mist in an attempt to loosen secretions. It has been difficult to show objective effects from bland mist therapy, but some patients are convinced of its beneficial effects. There is no evidence that use of complicated apparatus such as IPPB machines improves the effectiveness of therapy.

Thus for patients with troublesome cough or retained secretions, a bronchial hygiene treatment might consist of inhaling a bronchodilator medication followed by breathing of a bland mist, postural drainage, deep breathing with deliberate cough, and even chest percussion and vibration. Treatments are usually prescribed twice daily for ambulant patients and more often during exacerbations. It should be appreciated, however, that patients vary in their reactions to such therapy. Only those measures which prove effective for the individual patient should be continued, as the full program is time consuming, uncomfortable, and costly.

All patients should be encouraged to keep well hydrated to avoid inspissation of secretions. In acute exacerbations, this may require intravenous fluids. The usefulness of expectorant medications is questionable. Some authorities recommend 10 to 12 drops of a saturated solution of potassium iodide three times a day. This does seem to be effective in some patients, but it is associated with a high rate of side effects, some of which can be severe. Cough syrups and lozenges may help relieve a "tickle" in the throat but have little effect on the viscosity of bronchial secretions. Cough sedatives are generally contraindicated. They should be used only for acute episodes of severe nonproductive cough.

Burrows, B., and Lebowitz, M. D.: Characteristics of chronic bronchitis in a warm, dry region. Am. Rev. Respir. Dis., 112:365, 1975.

Burrows, B., and Nevin, W.: Antibiotic management in patients with chronic bronchitis and emphysema (editorial). Ann. Intern. Med., 77:993, 1972.

Ferris, B., Jr.: Chronic bronchitis and emphysema. Classification and epidemiology. Med. Clin. North Am., 57:637, 1973.

Fletcher, C. M., Elmes, P. C., Fairbairn, A. S., and Wood, C. H.: The significance of respiratory symptoms and the diagnosis of chronic bronchitis in a working population. Br. Med. J., 2:257, 1959.

Fletcher, C. M., and Peto, R.: The natural history of chronic airflow obstruction. Br. Med. J., 1:1645, 1977.

Proceedings of the Conference on Scientific Basis of Respiratory Therapy. Aerosol therapy. Physical therapy. Intermittent positive pressure breathing. Am. Rev. Respir. Dis., 110:85, 129, 169, 1974.

ASTHMA

PREVALENCE AND PATHOGENESIS. Approximately 3 per cent of the United States population are known to have asthma. In addition, there are many subjects in the population who have symptoms suggesting a subclinical form of the disease or who have features of asthma associated with a primary diagnosis of chronic bronchitis or chronic obstructive pulmonary disease. The disease often begins in childhood but may have its onset quite late in life. Childhood asthma is more common in boys.

The basic problem in asthma is hyperreactivity or "twitchiness" of the airways, causing the subject to develop bronchospasm in response to a variety of stimuli. Provocative factors include allergens; bronchial infections; irritant particles, fumes, and gases; mechanical irritation of the airways; certain pharmacologic agents; vigorous exercise; psychologic stresses; and irritation of the nasopharynx.

Bronchial Reactivity. The factors which lead to bronchial hyperreactivity are uncertain. They may include (1) the quantity, anatomic arrangement, or inherent contractility of bronchial smooth muscles; (2) the number of bronchial mast cells or their ability to produce and release mediators of bronchoconstriction; (3) the sensitivity of airways receptors and of vagally mediated bronchoconstrictor reflexes; and (4) the sensitivity of bronchial beta$_2$-adrenergic receptors. To some extent, bronchial reactivity is an inherited characteristic, but it is also susceptible to environmental influences. For example, increased reactivity may be noted for a prolonged period following an acute viral bronchitis. Also, postexercise bronchospasm is much more marked in young asthmatics who are still having attacks than after a prolonged remission. It appears that recurrent bronchospasm may cause the bronchi to become more irritable, hence the adage, "Asthma begets asthma."

Provocative Factors and Mechanisms of Their Effect. In children and young adults, inhaled allergens are usually important provocative factors. Typically, they produce immediate, "Type I," IgE-mediated, allergic reactions in the airway, although "Type III," IgG-mediated reactions may also occur in some individuals. The Type I reaction depends on release of chemical mediators of bronchoconstriction by bronchial mast cells. An inhaled allergen which traverses the bronchial mucosa bridges two antigen-specific IgE antibodies which are bound to a mast cell wall, leading to the formation of active mediators. Mediators include histamine, slow-reacting substance of anaphylaxis (SRS-A), eosinophilic chemotactic factor of anaphylaxis (ECF-A), prostaglandins, and a variety of other substances. The importance of each of these mediators remains to be determined, but histamine appears to be relatively less important in asthma than in some other allergic disorders. The ability of the mast cell to form mediators is moderated by intracellular levels of 3'5' cyclic AMP. Agents which increase 3'5' cyclic AMP, such as beta-adrenergic agonists and methylxanthines, tend to inhibit mediator production.

The parasympathetic nervous system also plays an important role in the asthmatic response. Cooling or cutting of the vagus nerve ameliorates experimental allergic bronchoconstriction. Cholinergic stimulation induces mediator production in the mast cell and causes contraction of bronchial smooth muscle. Parasympathetic reflexes apparently augment mucus secretion and may be responsible for the cough and hyperventilation associated with bronchospastic attacks. "Nasobronchial" reflexes are involved in the bronchoconstriction induced in some subjects by stimulating the upper airway with cold air or certain chemicals. The parasympathetic system also appears important in the bronchoconstriction induced by direct irritation or infection of the bronchial mucosa, and such reactions can be blocked with anticholinergic agents.

Vigorous exercise produces bronchoconstriction in some asthmatic subjects. The precise mechanism is uncertain, but release of mast cell mediators appears to be involved in many cases.

Asthmatic subjects are also unusually susceptible to bronchoconstrictor drugs, and responses to graded doses of inhaled histamine or methacholine have been used to assess the degree of bronchial reactivity. Therapeutically employed beta-adrenergic blockers (such as propranolol) may induce bronchospasm in asthmatic patients. By mechanisms which are less clear, aspirin, indomethacin, and certain yellow coloring agents used in foods and medications may also induce asthmatic attacks. This reaction to aspirin does not have an immunologic basis and usually occurs in nonatopic subjects.

Asthma-like reactions to inorganic chemicals and to organic dusts are described in Ch. 348.14.

The role of psychogenic factors is difficult to assess. Attacks can be precipitated by suggestion in some subjects, and many patients appear to have exacerbations of disease when subjected to emotional stress.

PATHOLOGY. In fatal cases, the lungs are hyperinflated and there is hypertrophy of bronchial smooth muscle. The bronchial walls are edematous and show eosinophilic infiltration as well as variable numbers of neutrophils, lymphocytes, and plasma cells. Extensive mucous plugging is noted in small and medium-sized bronchi.

CLINICAL MANIFESTATIONS. Several types of asthma have been described. There are atopic patients in

whom most attacks appear to be related to inhalation of allergens. These are generally younger subjects, and their disease is designated as "extrinsic," "atopic," or "allergic" in type. Hay fever is common in such subjects and often precedes the onset of asthma. Some patients give a past history of infantile eczema, and a family history of allergies is common. Attacks are likely to occur when environmental pollen counts are high (spring or fall) or in relationship to exposure to an obvious specific allergen, such as an animal dander. These subjects show other evidences of atopy, including multiple allergy skin test reactions and high levels of circulating IgE. Approximately 70 per cent of subjects with an onset of asthma before age 30 have this form of illness. Even in typical extrinsic asthma, attacks may be precipitated by nonallergic factors, including exercise, infections, nonspecific irritants, and even emotional factors.

A special form of allergic asthma is associated with *Aspergillus* organisms which grow in bronchial mucus plugs. The resulting syndrome, *allergic aspergillosis*, is characterized by relatively persistent asthma; recurrent pulmonary infiltrates, which may lead to lung fibrosis; localized bronchiectasis of relatively large airways; marked immediate hypersensitivity to *Aspergillus* (noted both by RAST and allergy skin tests); and very high circulating IgE. Findings suggesting a Type III allergy (modest levels of serum precipitins to *Aspergillus* and an Arthus reaction at the site of an intradermal allergy skin test) are common, and in some cases *Aspergillus* can be cultured from the sputum.

A second type of asthma, called "intrinsic" or "nonallergic," is characteristic of adult onset disease and is not associated with evidences of atopy. Attacks are generally precipitated by infections, exposure to nonspecific irritants, or emotional factors. Most patients deny a relationship to season, but some claim worsening during the winter months. Vasomotor rhinitis and nasal polyps are common. Many patients have some degree of chronic productive cough and are prone to recurrent respiratory infections. Approximately 70 per cent of asthma beginning after age 30 is of the "intrinsic" or "nonatopic" type. Aspirin intolerance is noted in some subjects, and the combination of persistent asthma, nasal polyps, and aspirin sensitivity has been called the "aspirin triad."

Another form of asthma is that which occurs in some patients with chronic obstructive lung disease. Even mild superimposed bronchospasm in such subjects may lead to a life-threatening exacerbation.

Regardless of the type of disease, the history is usually characteristic. After a period of relative well being, a sense of tightness or congestion is noted in the chest, usually accompanied by wheezing and slight cough. Over a period varying from minutes to days, symptoms increased in severity. Severe episodes culminate in an attack of incapacitating dyspnea. Although the attacks of dyspnea are often described as sudden in onset, the disease is usually more chronic than is appreciated by the patient. Serial spirometric measurements may show a gradual decline in FEV_1 long before the patient is aware of an attack. Symptoms then seem to develop suddenly when the airways obstruction reaches a level intolerable to the patient. Patients vary in the diurnal pattern of their attacks. In some, episodes are primarily nocturnal.

During a frank attack, physical examination reveals

obvious respiratory distress, hyperinflated chest, marked prolongation of forced expiration, frank wheezing, and, in severe cases, cyanosis. With increasing severity of the attack and marked diminution in expiratory flow rates, wheezing may become less pronounced, an ominous sign. As the episode is relieved, thick mucoid sputum may be raised. It often contains bronchial casts which illustrate the mucous plugging characteristic of the disease.

When symptoms persist despite bronchodilator therapy, *status asthmaticus* is said to exist. After many hours in "status," especially if the patient has been unable to sleep, respiratory muscle fatigue may develop, leading to hypoventilation and hypercapnia.

LABORATORY FINDINGS. During an attack, forced expiratory flow rates and the forced vital capacity are markedly reduced. Physiologic studies suggest that the obstruction is likely to involve the small airways to a greater extent in intrinsic than in extrinsic asthma. The residual volume and total lung capacity are increased, and the chest radiograph reveals hyperinflation. In some patients, recurrent pulmonary infiltrates accompany asthmatic episodes. These may result from subsegmental atelectasis behind a mucus plug. They may also result from an eosinophilic infiltrate in the lung, a characteristic finding in allergic aspergillosis.

During an acute episode, blood gases reveal variable degrees of hypoxemia. This may worsen temporarily after bronchodilator administration. Early in the episode, the arterial carbon dioxide tension is generally low, reflecting hyperventilation. With prolonged status asthmaticus the arterial carbon dioxide may return to normal or even become elevated, a grave prognostic sign.

In mild disease, spirometric tests generally return to normal between acute episodes, but more sensitive lung function studies often show subtle persisting abnormalities. In more severe disease, some slowing of forced expiration is likely to persist between attacks. This generally improves transiently following inhalation of a bronchodilator.

Sputum and blood eosinophilia are common and tend to reflect the activity of the disease. Eosinophilia occurs in both intrinsic and extrinsic forms of the disease.

In atopic subjects, serum IgE levels are elevated. The presence of IgE's specific for suspected antigens may be demonstrated directly by the RAST or indirectly by allergy skin tests.

COURSE AND PROGNOSIS. Asthma having an onset in childhood usually diminishes in severity during adolescence, and only 5 to 10 per cent of asthmatic children continue to have severe symptoms as adults. A history of infantile eczema is associated with a poorer prognosis. The prognosis is also less favorable for adult onset asthmatics. In them, symptoms tend to fluctuate in severity, but complete remission occurs in less than 25 per cent of cases. Persistence of frank spirometric abnormalities between symptomatic episodes and the presence of nasal polyps are poor prognostic signs.

Considering the high prevalence of the disease, death from asthma is relatively uncommon. Occasional sudden unexpected deaths do occur, however, even in young patients. Some of these may be the result of overuse of sympathomimetic drugs, leading to cardiac arrhythmias. Occasional deaths also occur in patients with status asthmaticus despite apparently optimal medical management.

A small number of subjects, especially those with late onset intrinsic asthma, appear to progress from typical paroxysmal asthma to persistent irreversible airways obstruction, but the actual relationship between asthma and COPD remains uncertain.

DIFFERENTIAL DIAGNOSIS. There is usually little difficulty in diagnosis. The recurrent episodes of wheezing dyspnea, often associated with known provocative factors, are quite characteristic. In patients with nocturnal episodes or with symptoms provoked by exertion, one must exclude congestive heart failure. Episodic dyspnea in the latter condition is almost always accompanied by cardiomegaly and other evidence of primary cardiac disease. Occasionally, however, a trial of diuretic therapy may be needed to distinguish nocturnal asthma from paroxysmal nocturnal dyspnea of cardiac origin.

It is also possible to mistake the hyperventilation syndrome for asthma on the basis of a casual history. In the hyperventilation syndrome, dyspnea is usually described as an inability to fill the chest sufficiently and is accompanied by a sighing rather than labored type of breathing. The conditions are readily distinguished if the patient is seen during an attack, because the hyperventilation syndrome is not associated with slowing of forced expiration.

Bronchospasm may be precipitated by aspiration, it may occur as part of the carcinoid syndrome, or it may represent a feature of a generalized immunologic disorder, particularly periarteritis nodosa.

In older subjects, it is sometimes difficult to distinguish asthma from COPD, and many patients show features of both disorders. In fact, the degree of reversibility of COPD (its "asthmatic component") can only be determined by a therepeutic trial. This is discussed further in the therapy of COPD.

THERAPY. Treatment of the Ambulent Patient. Asthma is a chronic disease characterized by hyperreactive airways. Regular management in an attempt to normalize function and prevent episodes of bronchospasm is essential, especially because the tendency to recurrent attacks appears to be reduced following a prolonged induced remission. The following measures are employed in the ambulant asthmatic patient:

AVOIDANCE OF PROVOCATIVE FACTORS. A careful history is required to identify factors which tend to aggravate symptoms. Nonspecific irritants, including smoking, should be eliminated or avoided. Dust suppression measures should be implemented in the home and work environment. Respiratory infections should be treated promptly and antibiotics prescribed if recurrent infections are a problem, as outlined in the treatment of simple chronic bronchitis. Aspirin and related compounds and beta-blocking agents should be used cautiously if at all in asthmatic subjects.

Allergens clearly related to attacks should be avoided. Unfortunately, identification of allergens responsible for attacks is often difficult. Atopic individuals usually have specific IgE's and positive skin tests to a wide variety of foreign proteins. Only a few are likely to be important in producing bronchospasm. Bronchial challenge tests with suspected allergens may be more specific, but these tests are difficult and time consuming, and their reliability in identifying clinically significant allergens remains uncertain. Immunologic tests are helpful in determining the general atopic predisposition of the patient, but they must be evaluated in conjunction with the clinical history in identifying agents of etiologic significance in the disease.

Severe asthmatics are often tempted to change their place of residence in order to avoid local allergens. For many, this does result in symptomatic improvement. Frequently, however they soon develop reactions to the aeroallergens in the new locale.

ANTIALLERGIC THERAPY. When it is clear that a few specific allergens cause a large fraction of the patient's symptoms, immunotherapy ("hyposensitization") is sometimes recommended. Such therapy, consisting of injections of increasing doses of antigen, induces the formation of IgG antibodies which block antigen binding with IgE. It may also lead to a reduction in specific IgE. Unfortunately, hyposensitization is prolonged, expensive, and only partially effective.

Antihistamines are generally ineffective except for controlling nasal symptoms. In fact, they should be used with caution in asthma, as they tend to lead to inspissation of secretions.

Immunosuppressive therapy of the type used in transplant patients has been attempted in very severe asthmatic subjects. Results are equivocal, and such therapy is rarely justified except in a research environment.

BRONCHODILATOR AGENTS. These are the mainstays of therapy for asthma, for control of any reversible component in COPD, and for management of bronchospasm associated with simple chronic bronchitis. Both the main classes of bronchodilators, beta-adrenergic agonists and methylxanthines, raise the level of 3'5' cyclic AMP in mast cells and bronchial smooth muscles, thereby inhibiting mediator production and reducing bronchial muscle contractility. Beta-adrenergic agents cause a conversion of ATP to 3'5' cyclic AMP by increasing adenylcyclase activity. Methylxanthines inhibit degradation of 3'5' cyclic AMP by interfering with phosphodiesterase activity. These agents may have additive or even synergistic effects. They are useful both to relieve existing bronchospasm and to prevent recurrent attacks.

Doses of beta-adrenergic drugs are limited by their side effects, and new drugs are continuously being introduced which have less alpha and $beta_1$ (cardiac) adrenergic effects while retaining $beta_2$ activity on bronchial mast cells and smooth muscles. Thus ephedrine, for many years the standard oral medication for asthma in doses of 25 mg three to four times daily, is being replaced by drugs such as metaproterenol, terbutaline, and salbutamol. (Salbutamol is not yet available in the United States but is considered the drug of choice in many other countries.) Oral medications are begun in small doses and gradually increased, depending on the patient's tolerance (e.g., terbutaline, 2.5 mg three times a day, increasing to 5 mg four times a day). The major side effects are tachycardia and tremulousness. Ephedrine may still have a role in some subjects, but it must be used with caution in older persons and should be not used in hypertensives or in men with prostatic disease, in whom it tends to cause urinary retention.

The newer beta-adrenergic drugs may also be used by aerosol and are replacing isoproterenol, long the standard inhaled bronchodilator. Metaproterenol, terbutaline, and salbutamol have longer durations of action as well as more specific $beta_2$ activity. Individual patients differ in their responses to these agents, however, and some still prefer isoproterenol (0.1 mg per inhalation) to newer aerosolized medications. Inhaled bronchodilators may be used regularly as preventive medication. They are especially useful as premedication for bronchial hygiene treatments, as described in the treatment of simple chronic bronchitis. In subjects with infrequent attacks, the aerosols may be used prior to exposure to known provocative factors or as therapy for episodes of dyspnea.

Inhaled bronchodilators are most conveniently administered from a pressurized container, but some authorities prefer a hand or powered nebulizer. One must limit use of aerosol medications to four or five times per day. Abuse of these is common and can lead to refractoriness or side effects such as cardiac arrhythmias. There is no evidence that complicated apparatus such as IPPB machines add significantly to the effectiveness of inhaled bronchodilator medications.

Methylxanthines are frequently given instead of, or in combination with, adrenergic agents. Oral therapy is begun with 100 to 200 mg of aminophylline three to four times daily and the dose increased gradually (up to 400 mg four times daily) until a satisfactory therapeutic effect is obtained or adverse side effects such as nausea occur. Aminophylline may also be administered rectally, using 250 to 500 mg of the drug in a suppository or rectal solution. Rectal aminophylline can be used at bedtime to prevent nocturnal attacks, but offers no real advantage over long-acting oral preparations.

Atropine and related drugs are effective in reversing bronchospasm in some subjects, but the place of anticholinergic agents in the management of asthma remains unclear.

DISODIUM CROMOGLYCATE (CROMOLYN). This unique type of therapy consists of inhalation of a powder containing 20 mg of cromolyn four times daily, using a special spinhaler. The only known effect of cromolyn is to stabilize mast cells, preventing mediator release. It is relatively effective preventive therapy for allergen- or exercise-induced attacks but is of no value for treatment of established bronchospasm as it is not a bronchodilator and must be used regularly to be effective prophylaxis. It has to be given for at least four weeks to determine its usefulness. It is generally ineffective, even as prophylaxis, in older intrinsic asthmatics. Cromolyn is irritating for some subjects, and the agent may be better tolerated if an aerosolized bronchodilator is used shortly before each cromolyn treatment. Cromolyn has no known side effects.

ADRENOCORTICAL HORMONES. The exact mechanism of action of adrenocortical steroids, the most potent antiasthmatic medications, remains unclear. They probably minimize inflammation by stabilizing lysosomes. Their use in asthma is justified when significant airways obstruction persists or recurs frequently despite maximal bronchodilator and cromolyn therapy. In the ambulant patient, drugs are given in moderate doses (e.g., 20 to 40 mg of prednisone per day) for a few days and rapidly tapered to the lowest level compatible with sustained improvement. In many cases, improvement is rapid and the medication may be discontinued totally within five to seven days. Occasional relapses are then treated by repeated short "bursts" of steroids. In some patients, however, symptoms recur when the steroid dose falls below a certain level. One must then taper slowly to the lowest dose compatible with patient comfort and reasonably normal ventilatory function. If possible, maintenance steroids should be administered as a single dose given on alternate days.

Once a maintenance dose has been reached, an attempt should be made to replace some or all of the oral corticosteroid with an inhaled nonabsorbed preparation such as beclomethasone. This agent is supplied in a pressurized container, and the standard dose is two inhalations (100 μg) four times a day. This generally replaces 7.5 to 10 mg per day of oral prednisone and produces no discernible systemic side effects. Some patients require premedication with an inhaled bronchodilator to ameliorate irritation from the beclomethasone aerosol.

Several problems may occur when inhaled steroids are substituted for oral medications. In the steroid-dependent patient who has received oral medication for many months or years, systemic medication must be discontinued very slowly (over several months) to avoid adrenal insufficiency. Nasal symptoms, previously suppressed with oral medications, may exacerbate, requiring reinstitution of oral medications. In some subjects (up to 30 per cent in some series) oropharyngeal candidiasis occurs. Fortunately, this responds promptly to specific therapy and rarely requires discontinuation of inhaled steroids.

OTHER MEASURES.   There are some asthmatic subjects in whom cough and sputum production are significant persistent problems. Such patients may be helped by the bronchial hygiene measures described in the therapy of simple chronic bronchitis.

Much has been written about a possible psychogenic basis for asthma. More often than not, however, emotional problems prove to be a result rather than a cause of the disease. Regardless, one must cope sympathetically with anxiety in both the patient and the family. Patients should be encouraged to lead as normal a life as possible. A full program of medications should be used to prevent attacks rather than severely limiting the patient's activities in an attempt to avoid provocative factors.

One must provide medications to use at home (e.g., an aerosol bronchodilator, rectal theophylline, or epinephrine for subcutaneous use) should a mild attack occur. One must also assure that the patient has emergency medical care readily available should home remedies fail to terminate an attack. Most importantly, one should encourage the patient to make regular office visits to be sure his disease remains in good control and to seek medical attention promptly if symptoms worsen.

Treatment of the Acute Attack.   Mild attacks in subjects not receiving regular bronchodilator management may respond promptly to an aerosol bronchodilator, rectal aminophylline, or even oral bronchodilator agents. In young subjects not already receiving adrenergic drugs, 0.1 to 0.2 ml of 1:1000 epinephrine subcutaneously is traditional therapy. In older subjects, 5.6 mg of aminophylline per kilogram of body weight given intravenously over 20 minutes may terminate an acute attack. (In patients already receiving aminophylline, the intravenous dose is lower and generally should not exceed 250 mg.) Since episodes tend to recur when effects of medications wear off, maintenance therapy should be prescribed until the patient returns for a regular office visit.

When patients fail to respond promptly to the aforementioned measures, *status asthmaticus* is said to exist and admission to hospital is generally required. Following the loading dose of intravenous aminophylline noted above, this medication is given as a continuous intravenous infusion in an attempt to maintain a therapeutic blood level, generally considered to lie between 10 and 20 mg per liter. A dose of 0.9 mg per kilogram of body weight per hour is commonly recommended, but patients vary in their aminophylline requirements, and the dose may have to be adjusted, depending on the patient's clinical response. Blood theophylline measurements can be helpful in regulating therapy.

In addition, patients should inhale beta-adrenergic agents, followed by bronchial hygiene measures, every four to six hours.

Supplemental oxygen is given in a dose sufficient to maintain the arterial oxygen tension in the range of 60 to 70 torr. Large doses of corticosteroids are indicated and should be begun early because their effect is delayed for several hours. An initial dose of 200 mg of hydrocortisone intravenously, followed by 100 mg every hour or two until symptomatic relief occurs, is conventional therapy. Even larger doses, up to 5 grams per day, have been used in refractory cases. When these measures fail to produce significant improvement over the first 12 to 24 hours, one should consider intravenous isoproterenol. Sedatives and narcotics should be avoided, as they may lead to underventilation. Should this occur, as evidenced by a rising arterial CO_2 tension, endotracheal intubation and mechanical ventilation are indicated. At this stage, sedatives and muscle relaxant agents may be used; they are sometimes required to allow the patient to coordinate with the ventilator.

Once bronchospasm is controlled, oral therapy is substituted for intravenous, and steroids are reduced slowly. Patients should remain in hospital until they have returned to their baseline state and should always be discharged on a full program of maintenance bronchodilators and steroids. Otherwise, return of severe symptoms is likely within 72 hours.

Antic, R., and Macklem, P. T.: The influence of clinical factors on site of airway obstruction in asthma. Am. Rev. Respir. Dis., 114:851, 1976.

Austen, K. F., and Orange, R. P.: Bronchial asthma: The possible role of the chemical mediators of immediate hypersensitivity in the pathogenesis of subacute chronic disease. Am. Rev. Respir. Dis., 112:423, 1975.

Brogden, R. N., Speight, T. M., and Avery, G. S.: Sodium cromoglycate (Cromolyn sodium): A review of its mode of action, pharmacology, therapeutic efficacy and use. Part I: Asthma. Drugs, 7:164, 1974.

Burrows, B., Lebowitz, M. D., and Barbee, R. A.: Respiratory disorders and allergy skin-test reactions. Ann. Intern. Med., 84:134, 1976.

Davies, G., Thomas, P., Broder, I., Mintz, S., Silverman, F., Leznoff, A., and Trotman, C.: Steroid-dependent asthma treated with inhaled beclomethasone dipropionate. Ann. Intern. Med., 86:549, 1977.

Godfrey, S., and König, P.: Exercise-induced bronchial lability in atopic children and their families. Ann. Allergy, 33:199, 1974.

Gold, W. M., Kessler, G.-F., and Yu, D. Y. C.: Role of vagus nerves in experimental asthma in allergic dogs. J. Appl. Physiol., 33:719, 1972.

Kaufman, J., and Wright, G. W.: The effect of nasal and nasopharyngeal irritation on airway resistance in man. Am. Rev. Respir. Dis., 100:626, 1969.

Klaustermeyer, W. B., DiBernardo, R. L., and Hale, F. C.: Intravenous isoproterenol: Rationale for bronchial asthma. J. Allerg. Clin. Immunol., 55:325, 1975.

Mitenko, P. A., and Ogilvie, R. I.: Rational intravenous doses of theophylline. N. Engl. J. Med., 289:600, 1973.

Pepys, J., and Hutchcroft, B. J.: Bronchial provocation tests in etiologic diagnosis and analysis of asthma. Am. Rev. Respir. Dis., 112:829, 1975.

Pepys, J., and Simon, G.: Asthma, pulmonary eosinophilia, and allergic alveolitis. Med. Clin. North Am., 57:573, 1973.
Woolcock, A. J.: Inhaled drugs in the prevention of asthma (editorial). Am. Rev. Respir. Dis., 115:191, 1977.

CHRONIC OBSTRUCTIVE PULMONARY DISEASE

PREVALENCE AND PATHOGENESIS.   Chronic obstructive pulmonary disease (COPD) is a major cause of disability in older subjects, ranking behind heart diseases and schizophrenia in United States Social Security statistics. It is also an increasingly important cause of mortality. Reported United States mortality rates, which are almost certainly underestimates, have increased several-fold over the last few decades, and the true mortality from COPD probably approaches that from lung cancer. The disease is usually first diagnosed between ages 55 and 65. It is much more common in men than in women, most series reporting a male:female ratio close to 9:1, but this may reflect only the different smoking habits of the sexes earlier in the century.

As already noted, COPD results from some combination of chronic obstructive bronchitis and pulmonary emphysema. Both disorders are closely related to cigarette smoking. The intrinsic airways disease is generally considered a direct consequence of bronchial irritation in a susceptible individual, but a possible role of chronic infection cannot be excluded. It is now generally believed that emphysema results from the effect of proteolytic enzymes on lung tissue. When there is a very severe congenital deficiency of serum antiproteolytic activity, emphysema is likely to develop by middle age even if the subject does not smoke. Without such a severe deficiency (which accounts for only 0.5 to 2 per cent of COPD), the development of emphysema depends on prolonged exposure to noxious irritants, usually cigarette smoke. Presumably, such exposure leads to reduction in lung defense mechanisms, low grade inflammatory changes in the lung parenchyma, and release of sufficient leukocytic proteases to overwhelm the body's antiproteolytic mechanisms.

Epidemiologic studies reveal a close relationship between cigarette smoking and slowing of forced exhalation. Whereas the average nonsmoking adult shows a rate of decline in FEV_1 of 20 to 25 ml per year of age, the average heavy smoker shows a decline of 40 to 45 ml per year. Thus an FEV_1 of 4.0 liters in a 25 year old would be expected to decline to approximately 3.1 liters by age 65 if he did not smoke but, on the average, would be close to 2.2 liters if he smoked one to two packs of cigarettes per day throughout adult life. The excess rate of decline appears to cease if smoking is discontinued. But this average effect of cigarettes is not sufficient to explain the much more severe impairment of FEV_1 noted in clinically significant COPD. Presumably, there are subjects who are especially susceptible to the effects of smoking.

There is great interest in identifying factors which cause a minority of smokers to develop clinically significant COPD. Respiratory disorders in childhood and intercurrent respiratory infections may be contributory factors. Genetic factors may also play a role. Certainly there are a few families in whom a deficiency of serum antiproteolytic activity is associated with a susceptibility to COPD. The serum's trypsin inhibitory capacity is determined by the *protease inhibitor* or "Pi" phenotype of the subject. A normal individual has two M genes (Pi phenotype MM). Severe deficiency of alpha$_1$ globulin, which contains most of the serum's antiproteolytic (antitrypsin) activity, occurs with a ZZ phenotype. This is found in approximately 1:4000 of the population. It is associated with hepatitis in infancy as well as emphysema in middle age. A heterozygotic state (phenotype MZ) is much more common, occurring in 3 to 5 per cent of the population. It is associated with moderate reduction in serum antiproteolytic activity. In some families, such an MZ phenotype appears to be associated with an increased tendency to COPD. On the other hand, general population studies have failed to show any over-all tendency for MZ subjects to develop an excess of respiratory disease or for respiratory disorders to be related to the level of serum trypsin inhibitory capacity except in ZZ subjects. A variety of other Pi genes have been identified (of which S is the most common), but only the Z gene is clearly associated with COPD.

The generally accepted concept of the early, preclinical history of COPD is that susceptible subjects who smoke show a very excessive rate of decline in lung function throughout adult life, a decline approximating 75 ml per year. According to this concept, the subject who will later develop COPD should be recognizable by age 40 because he will already show a mild ventilatory abnormality. This has led to some enthusiasm for screening of young to middle-aged adults in order to detect early COPD. There is no direct evidence, however, that the individual who will later develop severe disabling disease can be identified reliably by any physiologic test applied early in life. Indeed, it remains possible that the usual subject who develops COPD is indistinguishable from the average smoker until a relatively few years prior to the onset of symptoms when ventilatory function declines extremely rapidly.

PATHOLOGY.   The basic defect in emphysema is destruction of alveolar walls, leading to a reduced number of enlarged air spaces. This is often most severe in the central portion of the lobule (centrilobular emphysema) but it may occur uniformly throughout the acinus (panacinar emphysema). Both types of change may occur in the same lung, and severe centrilobular changes may progress to a point at which the process appears to involve the entire acinus. Centrilobular changes are closely related to chronic obstructive bronchitis, whereas panacinar changes, especially severe at the lung bases, are characteristic of homozygotic (ZZ) alpha$_1$-antitrypsin deficiency states.

Changes in the large airways characteristic of simple chronic bronchitis vary considerably in severity. But there are usually widespread abnormalities in small bronchi and bronchioles, including inflammation in and around air passages with narrowing of their lumens, mucous impaction, and obliterative changes. The extent of the abnormalities in small airways is not obvious on casual examination of the lung and can be quantified only by morphometric studies.

Small airways changes and emphysema may not be totally unrelated. Indeed, it is likely that one may induce the other. However, there is wide variability in the relative importance of intrinsic airways disease and emphysema among subjects with COPD, and these differences are reflected in the clinical and physiologic manifestations of the disease.

CLINICAL MANIFESTATIONS.   Dyspnea is the most common chief complaint, but some patients first see a physician because of cough, wheezing, recurrent respiratory infections, or even weakness or weight loss. The dyspnea is usually described as insidious in onset and progressive. Some patients, however, are aware of shortness of breath only during exacerbations of disease and give a history more suggestive of asthma than COPD. Others date their chronic symptoms from an acute respiratory infection.

Most patients admit to some cough and expectoration, but often this consists only of clearing a small quantity of mucus from the chest shortly after awakening. Other patients complain of more severe cough and more copious, sometimes purulent sputum.

Physical findings are extremely variable and depend to some extent on the stage of the disease. In relatively early illness (FEV₁ above 1.0 liter), the examination is often normal except for slowing of forced expiration. Rhonchi may be present or the chest may be unusually quiet on auscultation. Other physical findings occur with increasing frequency as the disease progresses. There may be gross overinflation with low diaphragms and a decreased area of cardiac dullness. Labored breathing, sometimes through pursed lips, may be present after slight exertion or even at rest. The patient may assume a stooped posture, tend to lean on his elbows when sitting, and use accessory muscles of respiration. Cyanosis may be present, and slight dependent edema is common.

Evidences of cor pulmonale generally appear only in advanced stages of illness when the FEV₁ is below 1 liter, but the severity of cardiac complications is quite variable. Pulmonary hypertension and cor pulmonale in COPD are more closely related to the severity of hypoxemia than to the degree of ventilatory impairment and are generally noted only when the resting arterial Po₂ is below 45 torr. Occasionally, patients first seek medical attention at this stage of illness, their major presenting features being those of heart failure secondary to cor pulmonale.

The variability in findings in patients with COPD is explained, at least in part, by differences in the severity of their emphysema and their intrinsic airway disease. Occasionally, relatively distinctive syndromes can be distinguished which relate to the underlying pathology. These have been called the emphysematous (Type A) and bronchial (Type B) types of COPD. Their features are summarized in the accompanying table. Since typical Type A patients often hyperventilate, thereby maintaining reasonably normal arterial oxygen tensions, they have been described as "pink puffers." Cyanosis and congestive heart failure are more common in Type B disease, and patients with these features have been called "blue bloaters." It should be recognized, however, that these clinical types represent extremes of a spectrum of presentations. Most patients display a mixture of findings, especially if followed over a period of time.

LABORATORY FINDINGS. Except for some erythrocytosis in severely hypoxemic patients, the routine blood count and differential are normal. The finding of eosinophilia should lead one to suspect that there is a reversible (asthmatic) component to the disease.

The chest radiograph may be entirely normal early in the disease, or it may reveal only the residua of previous inflammatory changes. With severe emphysema, marked overinflation is noted with flattening of the diaphragms, increased retrosternal space, and regional attenuation of vessels. In some cases, there are frank bullae demarcated by hairline margins. In homozygotic alpha₁-antitrypsin deficiency, emphysematous changes are usually most marked at the bases of the lungs.

The most characteristic feature of COPD is persistent reduction in forced expiratory flow rates. The residual volume is increased, as is the residual volume : total lung capacity ratio. Nonuniformity of ventilation and some mismatch of ventilation and perfusion are generally noted, but the severity of physiologic shunting and hypoxemia varies greatly from case to case. Most other pulmonary function abnormalities are also variable and depend to some extent on the relative severity of the emphysema and intrinsic airways disease, as indicated in the table.

Isotopic lung scans show the uneven ventilation and perfusion. Areas of diminished perfusion may even be mistaken for pulmonary emboli, and lung scans must be interpreted cautiously in patients with any chronic pulmonary disease.

The electrocardiogram is often normal, especially early

Features of the Bronchial and Emphysematous Types of COPD

	Emphysematous (Type A)	Bronchial (Type B)
Clinical features		
Dyspnea	Insidious onset, slowly progressive	Often noted first only during chest infections
Sputum	Usually scant and mucoid	Often copious and purulent
Weight loss	Often marked	Usually slight or absent
Chronic cor pulmonale with heart failure	Infrequent until terminal stages of the disease	Common
Chest examination	Quiet chest (except slight wheeze at end expiration), marked hyperinflation	Noisy chest, slight hyperinflation
Chest radiograph	Hyperlucent, overinflated lung; often regional attenuation of vessels	Often evidence of old inflammatory disease
Physiologic tests		
Total lung capacity	Increased	Normal or slightly decreased
Residual volume	Markedly increased	Moderately increased
Lung compliance, static	Increased	Near normal
Lung compliance, dynamic	Normal or slightly low	Very low
Lung recoil	Markedly reduced	Variable
Inspiratory airways resistance	Normal	Increased
Diffusing capacity	Markedly reduced	Variable
Arterial Po₂	Slight reduction at rest; usually falls with exertion	Often very low at rest; variable change with exertion
Arterial Pco₂	Usually normal or low	Often chronically elevated
Resting pulmonary artery pressure	Normal or slightly elevated at rest; increases with exertion	Often markedly elevated at rest
Cardiac output	Often low	Usually near normal

in the disease. Later, one may find some right axis shift and a delayed transition of the QRS complexes across the precordial leads. Peaked P waves ("P pulmonale") may be noted, especially during exacerbations of disease. These changes, although characteristic of severe COPD, are not well correlated with pulmonary hypertension or cor pulmonale. The most reliable indication of the latter condition is the presence of R waves over the right precordium.

COURSE AND PROGNOSIS. The initial response to therapy is variable and depends on the degree of bronchospasm associated with the disease. Some patients show considerable initial symptomatic and physiologic improvement. After this, the disease tends to progress slowly, with an average decline in FEV_1 between 50 and 75 ml per year. The rate of loss of function can be assessed only after several years of follow-up, however, because the variability in FEV_1 may exceed its true annual decline. Almost all symptoms also tend to worsen slowly. Cough and sputum production are exceptions. These often improve, especially if the patient stops smoking.

As a rule, patients note dyspnea on moderate exertion when the FEV_1 is between 1.2 and 1.5 liters, become limited to relatively sedentary activity when the FEV_1 is near 1 liter, and become invalided as the FEV_1 approaches 500 ml. Chronic hypercapnia, severe hypoxemia, and cor pulmonale are usually noted only when the FEV_1 is below 1 liter. Median survival is approximately ten years when the FEV_1 exceeds 1.2 liters, is near five years when the FEV_1 is 1.0, and approaches 2.0 years when the FEV_1 is less than 700 ml, but there is considerable variability around these median survivals, some patients living 12 to 15 years despite a very low initial FEV_1. Rapid heart rate at rest, severe blood gas abnormalities, or evidences of cor pulmonale are poor prognostic signs. Longevity is reduced in patients residing at altitudes in excess of 3500 feet.

Many patients show periodic exacerbations of their disease characterized by increased cough and dyspnea. These exacerbations often follow acute respiratory infections and are associated with variable degrees of bronchospasm. In patients with severe COPD, such exacerbations are life threatening, leading to acute respiratory failure and to heart failure secondary to cor pulmonale.

DIFFERENTIAL DIAGNOSIS. There are three criteria for the diagnosis of COPD: (1) there must be slowing of forced expiration, and the reduction of FEV_1 must be disproportionate to any reduction in FVC (i.e., both the per cent predicted FEV_1 and the FEV_1/FVC ratio must be reduced); (2) the expiratory slowing must persist despite prolonged and intensive medical therapy; and (3) specific bronchopulmonary diseases which might explain the physiologic abnormalities must be excluded. Failure to demonstrate extensive parenchymal disease on chest radiograph and an absence of any signs of upper airway obstruction (e.g., stridor, neck mass, or narrowing of the upper airway on chest radiogram) are generally considered sufficient for the last criterion. It is more difficult to exclude reversibility of the disease. This is discussed further under Treatment.

Determining the relative importance of intrinsic airways changes and emphysema may also present a challenge, but attenuation of vascular markings and increased transradiancy of the lung are usually noted on the chest radiograph if the emphysema is severe. A well-preserved diffusing capacity suggests that extensive emphysema is not present, whereas a relatively normal airways resistance measurement suggests that intrinsic airways abnor-

malities are limited in extent. The esophageal balloon measurements required to measure the elastic properties of the lung (the best guide to the severity of emphysema) are rarely justified for clinical evaluation.

In children and young adults, any syndrome resembling the bronchial type of COPD should suggest mucoviscidosis.

A homozygotic alpha$_1$-antitrypsin deficiency should be suspected when there is a family history of emphysema or when there is an early age of onset of an emphysematous type of COPD, especially if the patient is a nonsmoker or is female, or when the radiograph reveals a bilateral basilar distribution of the emphysematous changes. The diagnosis is confirmed by almost complete absence of alpha$_1$ globulin, by very low serum trypsin inhibitory capacity, and, most definitively, by demonstration of the pattern of a ZZ phenotype on crossed immunoelectrophoresis of the serum.

TREATMENT. The goals of therapy of COPD are as follows: (1) relief of any reversible component of the airways obstruction; (2) control of cough and bronchial secretions; (3) elimination and prevention of bronchopulmonary infection; (4) increase in exercise tolerance to the limits imposed by the patient's permanent physiologic impairment; (5) control of remediable complications of the disease, including cardiovascular problems and excessive hypoxemia; (6) avoidance of factors which may aggravate the disease such as inhaled irritants, sedatives and narcotics, or unnecessary surgery; and (7) relief of depression and anxiety which often accompany the disorder.

A comprehensive therapeutic program can ameliorate symptoms, reduce the frequency of hospital admission, prevent premature death, and allow patients to lead more active and more satisfying lives. Although it is true that most patients with severe COPD show a slow progression of ventilatory impairment despite treatment, this should not lead to therapeutic nihilism.

The usefulness of a team approach to therapy of COPD has been well demonstrated. There is no evidence, however, that equally satisfactory results cannot be obtained by a dedicated individual physician, perhaps assisted by an office nurse to help patients with bronchial hygiene and physical therapy measures.

Initial Treatment. One cannot predict accurately the degree of reversibility of the airways obstruction when the patient is first seen, and all patients should be regarded as having potentially reversible disease. Bronchodilators should be given to tolerance, as described in the therapy of asthma. Smoking should be eliminated or minimized and other sources of bronchial irritants avoided. Bronchial hygiene measures and, when appropriate, antibiotics should be used, as outlined in the therapy of simple chronic bronchitis. If signs of congestive heart failure are present, diuretics should be prescribed.

The appropriateness of this regimen should be evaluated after its effects on symptoms and ventilatory tests have been observed. Therapy may have to be adjusted to minimize side effects, and apparently useless measures (such as postural drainage which leads to no sputum production or symptomatic relief) should be discontinued. The physician must then decide if the possibility of further reversibility of the disease is sufficiently great to justify a three- to four-week trial of corticosteroids.

Although there are no hard and fast rules, the following features suggest potential reversibility of the disease and indicate that a trial of steroids is worthwhile in a patient with apparent COPD: (1) improvement in FEV_1 of greater than 20 per cent after inhalation of a bronchodilator; (2) similar degree of improvement in FEV_1 over several weeks of intensive bronchodilator therapy; (3) history of considerable fluctuation in severity of symptoms or of acute attacks of wheezing dyspnea not precipitated by exertion; (4) prominent wheeze or noisy chest on physical examination; (5) chest radiograph which appears normal except for hyperinflation; (6) eosinophilia of the blood or sputum; (7) evidences of atopy, such as a history of hay fever, positive allergy skin tests, or high serum IgE level; (8) associated vasomotor rhinitis or nasal polyps; or (9) normal pulmonary diffusing capacity measurement.

Corticosteroids are given in moderate doses (e.g., 20 to 40 mg per day of prednisone) for three to four weeks, and their effectiveness is assessed by changes in spirometric tests. Full doses of bronchodilators are maintained during this trial period. If significant improvement in FEV_1 is not observed, steroids should be discontinued gradually over one to two weeks. If improvement does occur, medications should be tapered to the smallest possible maintenance dose, as described in the therapy of asthma.

Maintenance Therapy. Even if no objective improvement is obtained with bronchodilator drugs, maintenance doses of theophyllines, perhaps in conjunction with beta-adrenergic drugs, are usually advised to prevent episodes of superimposed bronchospasm. Adrenergic aerosols may also be used prior to exposure to known bronchial irritants, for treatment of acute attacks of dyspnea, or as part of a bronchial hygiene program. In patients who show significant improvement with bronchodilators or with adrenocortical hormones, these drugs should be maintained as described in the therapy of asthma. Those measures described for the treatment of simple chronic bronchitis are fully applicable to patients with COPD who suffer from productive cough, recurrent bronchopulmonary infection, or retained secretions. Certain other types of treatment are more uniquely applicable to COPD.

PHYSICAL THERAPY. Unless contraindicated by a cardiac disorder, a program of gradually increasing exercise should be prescribed. This should have a specific goal which is important to the patient, such as walking a greater distance so the patient can go to a neighborhood store. Exercise does not improve lung function but it does train skeletal muscles to function more efficiently, thereby increasing exercise tolerance. For very severely disabled patients, exercise therapy may have to be initiated by a trained physical therapist, but in the usual case an appropriate program can be recommended directly to the patient by his physician. Patients with severe exertional hypoxemia may need supplemental oxygen during exercise, and it is advisable to obtain arterial blood gas at rest and after exercise before embarking on a vigorous exercise program in patients with an FEV_1 below 1 liter.

"Breathing exercises" are sometimes recommended. These generally consist of attempts to train the patient to breathe abdominally, in the hope of encouraging diaphragmatic activity. It is doubtful, however, that one can alter the patient's usual breathing pattern. More realistically, one can teach the patient that dyspnea per se is not harmful, that slow deep breathing relieves dyspnea more quickly than rapid shallow "panic breathing," and that breath holding during exertion is to be avoided. Mechanical devices, such as emphysema belts and IPPB machines, are of no proved value.

OXYGEN THERAPY. There are clear indications for home oxygen therapy in some patients with COPD. Low flow oxygen by nasal cannula may be employed during exercise in patients with severe exertional hypoxemia. Other patients require regular oxygen therapy to control severe pulmonary hypertension which has led to cor pulmonale and recurrent episodes of heart failure. In the latter instance, oxygen is generally administered during sleep, and there is a suggestion that it should be given for at least 15 hours per day to achieve maximum effects. The proper oxygen dose is one which achieves an arterial oxygen tension between 55 and 65 torr (usually 1 to 2 liters per minute by nasal prongs). In patients with resting arterial oxygen tensions consistently below 40 torr, continuous oxygen therapy may be needed to maintain ambulation and prevent congestive failure.

Oxygen should not be used to treat episodes of dyspnea. Patients become habituated to this form of therapy, adding to their invalidism.

ENVIRONMENTAL CONTROL. The possibility of a change in climate or locale is often considered for severely impaired patients. A move to a lower altitude is certainly justified for patients living at altitudes above 4000 feet. (All patients with severe COPD should be advised to avoid high altitudes, and those with severe hypoxemia may require supplemental oxygen when traveling by air.) A change in residence may also be indicated for patients residing in areas of very heavy air pollution.

Many patients consider moving to escape a cold winter climate. Some find relief in warm humid regions, whereas others prefer dry warm desert climates. There is no evidence that the overall course of the disease is altered by a move to either type of area. A decision to relocate in a more salubrious climate should be made only after weighing the possible symptomatic relief against the social and economic hardships of the move. The specific area is best chosen on the basis of a trial period to assess both symptomatic relief and the patient's fondness for the locale.

TREATMENT OF EDEMA AND COR PULMONALE. Pedal edema is common even in the absence of other evidences of congestive heart failure and is usually readily controlled with small doses of diuretics. Recurrent or chronic congestive failure secondary to cor pulmonale is a more difficult problem. In addition to the usual therapy for heart failure (using digitalis with great care), phlebotomies may be needed to maintain the hematocrit below 56, and all treatments may fail unless hypoxemia is controlled with oxygen therapy.

TREATMENT OF HYPERCAPNIA. Chronic hypercapnia is common in late stages of the disease. It requires no specific therapy but does indicate the need to monitor blood gases closely during exacerbations of the disease and to avoid totally the use of sedatives, tranquilizers, or narcotics. There is no justification for respiratory stimulants or mechanical assistance to ventilation in patients with chronic stable hypercapnia.

SURGICAL THERAPY. A few patients with very large bullae which compress relatively normal lung may be benefited by bullectomy. However, the selection of suitable operative candidates requires careful and detailed preoperative evaluation.

SUPPORTIVE MEASURES. It is essential that patients understand the nature of their disease, the significance of symptoms which may develop (e.g., purulent sputum), the possible side effects of medications, and the goals of therapy. Provision must be made for prompt treatment of exacerbations. Most importantly, patients must be encouraged to live active and interesting lives within the limits imposed by their respiratory impairment and within the constraints imposed by any therapeutic measures which are employed. Occupational therapy and vocational rehabilitation are useful for some patients.

Treatment of Exacerbations. Mild symptomatic exacerbations, often associated with infection, are treated with more vigorous application of the measures mentioned above. Antibiotics, increased bronchodilators, and even a course of steroids are often indicated. Blood gases should be monitored and cardiovascular status assessed. Severe hypoxemia, increasing arterial carbon dioxide tension, or evidence of congestive heart failure dictates immediate hospitalization. The management of acute respiratory failure and heart failure from cor pulmonale are discussed in Ch. 351.5 and 355. Patients with refractory bronchospasm superimposed on their COPD should receive the same type of management as patients with status asthmaticus, as described in the therapy of asthma.

Burrows, B., and Earle, R. H.: Course and prognosis of chronic obstructive lung disease. N. Engl. J. Med., 280:397, 1969.

Burrows, B., Fletcher, C. M., Heard, B. E., Jones, N. L., and Wootliff, J. S.: The emphysematous and bronchial types of chronic airways obstruction. Lancet, 1:830, 1966.

Burrows, B., Knudson, R. J., Cline, M. G., and Lebowitz, M. D.: Quantitative relationships between cigarette smoking and ventilatory function. Am. Rev. Respir. Dis., 115:195, 1977.

Burrows, B., Knudson, R. J., and Lebowitz, M. D.: The relationship of childhood respiratory illness to adult obstructive airway disease. Am. Rev. Respir. Dis., 115:751, 1977.

Filley, G. F., Beckwitt, H. J., Reeves, J. T., and Mitchell, R. S.: Chronic obstructive bronchopulmonary disease. II. Oxygen transport in two clinical types. Am. J. Med., 44:26, 1968.

Fletcher, C. M., and Peto, R.: The natural history of chronic airflow obstruction. Br. Med. J., 1:1645, 1977.

Hogg, J. C., Macklem, P. T., and Thurlbeck, W. M.: Site and nature of airway obstruction in chronic obstructive lung disease. N. Engl. J. Med., 278:1355, 1968.

Lertzman, M. M., and Cherniack, R. M.: Rehabilitation of patients with chronic obstructive pulmonary disease. Am. Rev. Respir. Dis., 114:1145, 1976.

Lieberman, J.: Alpha₁-antitrypsin deficiency. Med. Clin. North Am., 57:691, 1973.

Morse, J. O., Lebowitz, M. D., Knudson, R. J., and Burrows, B.: Relation of protease inhibitor phenotypes to obstructive lung diseases in a community. N. Engl. J. Med., 296:1190, 1977.

Proceedings of the Conference on the Scientific Basis of Respiratory Therapy: Oxygen therapy. Am. Rev. Respir. Dis., suppl. to Vol. 110, Dec. 1974, pp. 25–84.

344.2.　LOCALIZED AIRWAY OBSTRUCTION

Localized obstruction to airflow may result from extrinsic compression of airways, from diseases of the airways themselves, or from intraluminal obstructions. Signs and symptoms depend on whether the lesion is above or below the tracheal bifurcation, on whether the obstruction is complete or partial, and on the cause of the obstruction.

OBSTRUCTION ABOVE THE TRACHEAL BIFURCATION

PARTIAL OBSTRUCTION. The characteristic finding in partial obstruction above the tracheal carina is stridor, often accompanied by inspiratory retraction of the intercostal spaces. Slowing the air flow is noted on both forced inspiration and forced expiration, and the MEFV curve may have a characteristic appearance, showing a plateau which reflects a relatively constant forced expiratory flow over a large portion of the FVC. With severe obstruction,

adequate over-all ventilation may not be maintained, resulting in hypercapnia and hypoxemia.

Diseases intrinsic to the airways which may lead to partial obstruction include enlarged tonsils and adenoids (especially in young children); neoplasms of the hypopharynx, larynx, vocal cords, or trachea; stenosing lesions secondary to trauma; bilateral vocal cord paralysis; laryngeal edema or spasm; and inflammatory lesions of the pharynx (as in peritonsillar abscess), larynx (as in croup), or trachea (as in diphtheria). Extrinsic compression of the larynx or trachea may occur secondary to enlarged thyroid, paratracheal neoplasm, or, rarely, mediastinal infection. If the primary cause of the obstruction cannot be eliminated, an artificial airway, tracheostomy, or surgical repair is indicated.

COMPLETE OBSTRUCTION. Unless promptly relieved, complete obstruction above the tracheal carina leads to rapid asphyxiation. The presentation is pathognomonic with lack of air flow at the mouth despite inspiratory efforts and inspiratory retraction of the intercostal spaces. Acute obstruction is most commonly caused by aspiration of poorly chewed food. This emergency is treated by applying forceful pressure to the epigastrium, using the *Heimlich maneuver.*

Episodic complete obstruction of the upper airway occurs during sleep in a few very obese individuals owing to falling back of the glossopharyngeal structures. This form of sleep apnea causes frequent awakening, troubled sleep, and somnolence. The resulting clinical picture can be confused with the pickwickian syndrome.

Complete obstruction secondary to trauma, intractable laryngospasm, or chronic disease must be bypassed with an artificial airway or tracheostomy.

OBSTRUCTION BELOW THE TRACHEAL BIFURCATION

PARTIAL OBSTRUCTION. Characteristically, this results in a localized expiratory wheeze over the site of obstruction and hyperinflation of the distal lung. It is most commonly caused by a primary neoplasm which grows into or compresses an airway, but it may result from acute or chronic inflammatory lesions of the bronchi, aspiration of foreign bodies, compression of bronchi from enlarged hilar lymph nodes, or mucus plugs. Since airflow from the remaining lung is unimpaired, spirometry may be relatively normal, but other tests will reveal evidence of nonuniformity of ventilation. The area of diminished airflow may be detected by ventilation scans. Definitive diagnosis generally depends on bronchoscopy, and treatment is directed at the underlying disease.

Partial bronchial obstruction impairs clearance of secretions from the distal lung, leading to infection and even abscess formation. Recurrent infections in the same area of lung, slow clearing of pneumonia, or lung abscess should make one suspect partial obstruction of the bronchus leading to the affected region.

COMPLETE OBSTRUCTION. Air in the lung distal to a complete obstruction is absorbed into the bloodstream, leading to collapse of the affected region, a condition called "obstructive atelectasis." Its features are discussed under Atelectasis in Ch. 345. Any of the disorders mentioned above as causes of partial obstruction may progress to the point of complete occlusion of a bronchus and lead to obstructive atelectasis.

Ainger, L. E.: Large tonsils and adenoids in small children with cor pulmonale. Br. Heart J., 30:356, 1968.

Heimlich, H. J.: A life-saving maneuver to prevent food-choking. JAMA, 234:398, 1975.

Sackner, M. A., Landa, J., Forrest, T., and Greeneltch, D.: Periodic sleep apnea: Chronic sleep deprivation related to intermittent upper airway obstruction and central nervous system disturbance. Chest, 67:164, 1975.

Shim, C., Corro, P., Park, S. S., and Williams, M. H., Jr.: Pulmonary function studies in patients with upper airway obstruction. Am. Rev. Respir. Dis., 106:233, 1972.

345. ABNORMALITIES OF LUNG AERATION

Benjamin Burrows

LOCALIZED HYPOAERATION (ATELECTASIS)

Atelectasis refers to diminished aeration of the lung. It is a feature of many bronchopulmonary diseases, and several types of atelectasis have been described. When total airlessness of a portion of the lung occurs, blood traversing the region fails to participate in gas exchange and behaves as if it were being shunted directly from the right to the left side of the heart. Thus total atelectasis leads to an "anatomic-like" or "absolute" shunt. Unlike the "physiologic" or "relative" shunt noted in most bronchopulmonary diseases, the "absolute shunt" produced by atelectasis is not fully corrected by inhalation of 100 per cent oxygen.

TYPES OF ATELECTASIS AND THEIR PATHOGENESIS. When there is complete obstruction of an airway distal to the tracheal bifurcation, air in the lung behind the obstruction is gradually absorbed into the bloodstream, leading to complete collapse over a period of a few hours, a condition called *obstructive atelectasis*. The rate of collapse is limited by the poor solubility of nitrogen and is much more rapid in an oxygen-filled than in an air-filled lung. Thus high inspired oxygen tensions encourage the development of atelectasis behind obstructing mucus plugs.

Atelectasis may also occur when the recoil of a local area of the lung is greatly increased by fibrotic changes. This results in shrinkage of the involved region rather than total airlessness and is called *contraction atelectasis*.

When widespread alveolar instability occurs in the respiratory distress syndromes (in newborns owing to a surfactant abnormality), *patchy atelectasis* may develop throughout the lung.

A portion of the lung may be allowed to decrease in volume when the intrapleural pressure is elevated as a result of a large pneumothorax, pleural effusion, or other space-occupying lesion in the thorax. This has been called "compression atelectasis" but is more properly termed *relaxation atelectasis*, because it occurs as a result of the lungs' own tendency to recoil when distending forces are relaxed. With marked relaxation atelectasis, small airways in the affected region collapse, and any air remaining distally is removed by the bloodstream.

Finally, a condition called *plate-like atelectasis* may be noted on a chest radiograph. Its pathologic significance is uncertain. The horizontal radiopaque streaks which characterize the condition occur most often at the bases of the lung. They are associated with poor aeration of the lung and are commonly seen when the diaphragm is elevated or when the patient has been unable to breathe deeply for a prolonged period.

CLINICAL MANIFESTATIONS. The clinical and physiologic consequences of atelectasis depend on the extent and chronicity of the process. Sudden collapse of a large portion of the lung may cause severe dyspnea and profound hypoxemia. Over a period of hours, blood flow through the nonventilated lung diminishes, and both symptoms and hypoxemia become less severe. The acute picture is apt to be noted when obstructive atelectasis develops rapidly from retained secretions (as occurs occasionally in the postoperative period) or from aspiration of a foreign body. When the obstruction develops slowly, as is usually the case with bronchial neoplasms, there may be few or no symptoms and only minimal hypoxemia.

Physical findings depend on the type of atelectasis. With relaxation atelectasis, the findings are those of the underlying condition (e.g., pneumothorax or pleural effusion). In patchy atelectasis, findings are those of the respiratory distress syndrome, which is discussed in Ch. 351. Plate-like atelectasis is not associated with any distinctive physical findings and is basically a radiographic interpretation. With contraction or obstructive atelectasis, physical findings depend on the amount of lung involved. If the atelectatic area is sufficiently large, the trachea and mediastinum are deviated to the affected side, the diaphragm is raised, and the entire hemithorax may be smaller and show less respiratory motion than the unaffected side.

DIAGNOSIS AND TREATMENT. The presence of atelectasis is confirmed radiographically. If the appearance suggests an obstructive type of disease, bronchoscopy is needed to determine its specific etiology. Occasionally, it is possible to remove the occluding material through the bronchoscope. Obstructive atelectasis in a patient who is not severely ill always should raise the question of a bronchogenic neoplasm.

In nonobstructive types of atelectasis, treatment is directed at the underlying cause of the disorder.

THE RIGHT MIDDLE LOBE SYNDROME. In relaxation atelectasis, the lung is usually restored to normal when it is allowed to re-expand (as with relief of a large pneumothorax). With obstructive atelectasis, however, secondary infection is common, leading to fibrosis, abscess formation, and localized bronchiectasis. Thus after prolonged collapse, the affected lung may fail to re-expand normally when the obstruction is relieved. This is commonly noted when the right middle lobe bronchus has been compressed by large hilar lymph nodes in primary tuberculosis or other granulomatous lung diseases. When the lymph nodes finally decrease in size, the affected lung may fail to re-expand fully. It often shows bronchiectatic changes and becomes the site of recurrent or chronic infection. This has been called the *right middle lobe syndrome*. Less commonly, the same sequence of events occurs in other lung regions. When recurrent pneumonia, chronic suppuration, or hemoptysis occurs, the involved lung may have to be resected.

Albo, R. J., and Grimes, O. F.: The middle lobe syndrome; A clinical study. Dis. Chest, 50:509, 1966.

Wanner, A., Landa, J. F., Nieman, R. E., Jr., Vevaina, J., and Delgado, I.: Bedside bronchofiberscopy for atelectasis and lung abscess. JAMA, 224:1281, 1973.

LOCALIZED HYPERAERATION

A partial bronchial obstruction may lead to overinflation of the affected lung. Increased aeration is also seen in emphysematous lung regions, and pockets of air may be noted within cysts, abscesses, or cavities. Lung bullae and the so-called "unilateral hyperlucent lung" are discussed in Ch. 349.1.

346.   INFILTRATIVE DISEASES OF THE LUNG

Gareth M. Green

346.1.   INTRODUCTION

DEFINITION. Pulmonary infiltration is a radiologic term which connotes a variable but rather characteristic reticulonodular pattern on the chest radiograph. This radiographic pattern is nonspecific with regard to etiologic agent, pathologic entity, or mechanistic process, or as a guide to treatment or prognosis. It is seen as a terminal stage in lymphoma, leukemia, or carcinomatosis, in advanced metabolic derangement such as uremia, in acute viral infections, and in congestive failure, either acute or chronic; it can be found as the only manifestation of a chronic low level exposure to an occupational or environmental agent, such as silica dust or metals or exposure to an air pollutant or to a drug. However, since the radiograph is commonly the first point of recognition of an underlying disorder, these diverse diseases have been grouped by their generally similar radiographic appearance, a somewhat characteristic clinical presentation, and a set of common physiologic abnormalities.

In the past, the infiltrative diseases of the lungs have been classified chiefly according to pathologic reactions, and therefore diagnosis has depended either on examination of pulmonary tissue by lung biopsy or on strong historical evidence of exposure to an occupational or environmental agent known to be associated with the infiltrative or fibrotic process in the lung. Recent and current research has directed much more attention to biologic mechanisms in these diseases. As this new knowledge develops, a more organized and fruitful approach to diagnosis becomes possible and new classifications are introduced.

This chapter will commence with a discussion of features of the syndrome that are common to most of the group. Rather than explain each separate disease as a distinctive clinical entity — an unwarranted practice because of the great variation between and among the disorders — the different diseases will be distinguished by etiology, pathogenesis, or histopathology. Clinical features particularly characteristic of one specific disorder will be mentioned in the discussion of that disease, although it should be remembered that differentiation and diagnosis depend more on the meticulous collection and analysis of historical and laboratory data than on any clustering of clinical, physiologic, or radiologic findings.

The clinical presentation of diffuse infiltrative lung diseases (DILD) varies from asymptomatic to acute or chronically progressive dyspnea, tachypnea, and cyanosis. Commonly, an environmental or occupational exposure is not recognized, although it is the responsibility of the physician to ferret out this information from the history and recognize when an individual has been exposed to an agent that might account for the symptoms and pulmonary abnormalities. The chest film characteristically shows reticulonodular infiltrations diffusely throughout the lung, or localized to upper and lower lung fields or to one region, lobe, or segment. The syndrome, however, includes radiographs with a characteristic ground glass appearance and areas with localized consolidations and even cavitations. Although not characteristic, pleural effusions occur and enlargement of the hilar nodes is seen, particularly in infectious disorders, mineral dust exposures, and sarcoidosis. Cardiac enlargement of the right ventricular type reflects cor pulmonale in either acute or chronic form.

Abnormalities of respiratory physiology are variable, depending upon the chronicity and duration of the process. However, as a general statement, this group of diseases contrasts with obstructive pulmonary disorders by showing relatively little change in air flow dynamics, but, rather, reduction in pulmonary volumes, including vital capacity, functional residual capacity, and residual volume, and in pulmonary compliance and diffusing capacity. Minute ventilation is frequently elevated, distribution of ventilation is well maintained, and perfusion may be reduced and ventilation-perfusion ratios deranged by disease of the small airways. Reductions in both arterial P_{O_2} and P_{CO_2} are characteristic, with either a normal or elevated arterial pH. The symptoms of tachypnea and dyspnea are generally attributed to the changes in compliance and in the efficiency of gas transfer. The relatively stiffer lungs require greater respiratory effort, particularly on inspiration, a finding frequently reflected in augmented work of inspiration, the increased audibility of respiratory effort, and perceptible intercostal retractions. Additional findings on physical examination include tachypnea, increased tactile and vocal fremitus, coarsening of breath sounds with a tendency toward bronchovesicular and bronchial breathing, fine or crackling rales, particularly in the lower lung fields, normal percussion note unless there is consolidation or pleural effusion, accentuated S-2, prominent subxiphoid cardiac impulse, and peripheral cyanosis and clubbing of the digits in more severe cases.

ETIOLOGY. The infiltrative lung diseases are associated particularly with the inhalation of a wide variety of particulate agents, including minerals, metals, radioactive dusts, fungal spores and other allergenic substances, bacteria, viruses, and other microbial organisms. Infiltrative reactions also occur in response to the inhalation of irritant gases, such as nitrogen dioxide, ozone, and components of cigarette smoke; radioactive gases, such as radon; and a variety of other fumes produced principally as occupational exposures. Infiltrative reactions occur as the pulmonary component of disseminated vasculitis, systemic collagen vascular diseases, lymphatic carcinomatosis of the lung, or chronic congestive cardiac failure, particularly mitral stenosis; as a manifestation of pulmonary thromboembolic and venoocclusive disease; and as epithelial cell proliferation associated with certain drug reactions. The medical challenge is to discover by historical, epidemiologic, or laboratory analysis the specific agent producing the infiltrative response, to eliminate further exposure to that agent, and to suppress or control the infectious or inflammatory process by appropriate drug therapy. Since environmental and occupational agents loom large in the list of agents producing infiltrative responses in the lung, a detailed knowledge of such agents found both in the environment and as hazards of occupations is required for an astute diagnostic evaluation.

EPIDEMIOLOGY. As a group, the infiltrative lung diseases have not received the attention of the research and practicing medical profession warranted by the probable importance of this type of reaction in the lung. When studies have been made, it has become apparent that diffuse pulmonary infiltration and fibrosis are far more widespread than was previously suspected. The reason is that the medical profession has tended to rely on the chest radiograph for detection and diagnosis of these diseases. It is becoming increasingly apparent that the chest radiograph is considerably less sensitive to low-level chronic infiltrative and fibrotic processes in the lung than to the acute inflammatory variety. Thus an acute viral infection shows up well on the radiograph, whereas the diffuse early fibrosis associated with cigarette smoking and other environmental exposures can lead to considerable functional derangement before radiographic changes are apparent. Likewise, recent studies in the granite industry indicate that functional impairment may occur in advance of radiographic signs.

Thus epidemiologic studies relying principally on the chest radiograph do not indicate reliably the true prevalence of infiltrative lung disease in an exposed population. Recent advances in pulmonary physiologic and other laboratory techniques available for epidemiologic surveillance mandate extensive new studies of working and other populations before the true extent and significance of environmental and occupational exposure can be known.

PATHOGENESIS. As the name implies, infiltrative lung disease results from the infiltration of fluid, cells, fibrous tissue, inhaled particulates, or lipid substances into the interalveolar septa, the alveolar spaces, and the peribronchial and perivascular lymphatics. The pathology is widely variable, even with a fairly constant radiographic picture. Inhaled particles are phagocytized by alveolar macrophages and other alveolar phagocytic cells, which eradicate the inhaled particle in situ, exit up the bronchial ciliary escalator carrying the phagocytized burden, become immobilized in the interstitium of the lung with long-term retention of the particle, or trigger by release of chemotactic and other factors acute and/or chronic inflammatory processes.

Exposure to inert dust, such as coal, results in long-term passive accumulation of dust-laden cells which degenerate in time to leave coal dust deposits in the perivascular and peribronchial lymphatics. Exposure to highly irritant dusts such as silica or asbestos causes intracellular damage to phagolysosomal structures with release of proteolytic enzymes and stimulation of inflammatory processes and fibrosis. Inhalation of immunogenic particles leads to the influx of thymus-derived and/or bursa-equivalent lymphocytes which respond to the antigen by the synthesis of immune globulins or the transformation of sensitized lymphocytes. These cells in turn liberate additional mediators, with exacerbation or evolution of the inflammatory

process frequently associated with granuloma production, vasculitis, and fibrosis. The process seems to depend both on the physical, chemical, or immunogenic properties of the inhaled particle and gas and on poorly defined qualities in host defense mechanisms. In low grade fibrogenic exposures, such as to cigarette smoke, the response to exposure may not be associated with any inflammatory process. There appears to be a direct fibrinogenic relationship between the injured phagocytic cell on the one hand and the infiltrating fibroblast on the other. Although less dramatic than the more acute inflammatory processes, this form of silent fibrosis may be the most common cause of idiopathic progressive impairment and disability.

DIFFERENTIAL DIAGNOSIS. The differential diagnosis of infiltrative lung diseases is encyclopedic in terms of the specific agents which can produce a limited variety of histopathologic response in the lung. The classification used in this chapter is somewhat empiric but of clinical utility; it is based on the clustering of disease entities related by clinical or laboratory manifestations, association with systemic disorders, exposure to external agents such as drugs or occupational or environmental agents, or a variety of different agents producing disease by a common and defined pathogenic mechanism. Even with this type of classification, there is still a group of disorders simply classified as "other," without common agent, disease mechanism, histopathologic picture, or diagnostic or therapeutic approach.

Diseases associated with diverse immunologic mechanisms are the pulmonary infiltrates with eosinophilia, the pulmonary manifestations of systemic collagen vascular diseases, hypersensitivity pneumonitis or alveolitis, Wegener's granulomatosis and allergic granulomatosis, drug-induced infiltrative reactions in the lung, and Goodpasture's syndrome. Diseases caused by the inhalation of physically or chemically active agents include the pneumoconioses, pulmonary fibroses (caused by a variety of metallic fume and oxidant gas exposures), and fibrosis associated with exposure to ionizing radiation.

A group of diseases of unknown cause, but of rather characteristic clinical, radiologic, or pathologic presentation, includes sarcoidosis, eosinophilic granuloma, hemosiderosis, alveolar proteinosis, diffuse interstitial pneumonitis, desquamative interstitial pneumonitis, lymphoid interstitial pneumonitis, and usual interstitial pneumonitis (UIP) with fibrosis. Finally, diseases associated with lymphatic stasis include chronic passive congestion associated with mitral stenosis, lymphatic carcinomatosis, and thromboembolic disease of the lungs. A word should be said here about the *Hamman-Rich syndrome*, which is perhaps associated more with a characteristic tempo and intensity of inflammatory process in the lung than with any specific etiologic agent. It is a virulent form of infiltrative lung disease with active inflammatory and epithelial proliferative processes associated with acute shortness of breath and cyanosis, and an unrelenting course with death in three to six months. It is not yet clear that this is a specific etiologic entity or simply one end of a spectrum that is common to a variety of diffuse infiltrative lung disorders.

The diagnosis in this heterogeneous group of disorders is made by systematic analysis of the history for detection of etiologic or associated disease factors; by a study of respiratory tract cells and secretions for detection of characteristic cellular elements, such as eosinophils; by a detailed and specific immunologic evaluation of both the respiratory tract and the systemic immunologic system for evidence of immunization against specific environmental antigens; and by tissue biopsies of draining lymph nodes, of distant organs such as liver and bone marrow, or, most usually, of lung parenchymal tissue obtained by transbronchial or transthoracic needle.

TREATMENT. The selection of therapeutic agents to combat this group of pulmonary disorders is limited largely to the anti-inflammatory agents such as corticosteroids; immunosuppressive agents such as cyclophosphamide; specific antibiotics when appropriate; treatment of underlying diseases such as the collagen vascular diseases, neoplasias, and cardiovascular abnormalities; and removal and avoidance of any identified environmental or ingested causative agents (such as drugs). When the history fails to reveal a specific environmental agent known to produce a characteristic clinical picture, when the immunologic work-up is negative for the identification of a specific antigenic agent, and when examination of pulmonary secretions fails to reveal an etiologic agent, it is best to proceed to the analysis of a tissue specimen obtained either by transbronchial or transthoracic needle biopsy or by open lung biopsy. Although the needle biopsy procedures are capable of providing a diagnosis in more than 80 per cent of cases, the heterogeneity of the pulmonary reactions and the limited size of the biopsy obtained by the needle frequently do not provide a representative assessment of what is going on in the lungs. Under such circumstances, an open lung biopsy is required to fix the diagnosis.

There is growing research interest in the role of subsegmental bronchoalveolar lavage to obtain pulmonary cells and secretions for diagnostic purposes. This technique has become well established in the diagnosis of pulmonary alveolar proteinosis, has recently been found to be effective in the diagnosis of occult infectious processes, and is showing promise of giving useful information in the assessment of the nature of the inflammatory process in the lungs and possibly the state of activity of the disease in the lungs. It is too soon to know the full value of this procedure; but as more becomes known about the etiology and pathogenesis of diffuse infiltrative lung diseases, and as new technology, such as fiberoptic bronchoscopy and subsegmental lavage, becomes available, there will be less need to resort to invasive procedures such as open lung biopsy. Perhaps the two best examples of how developments in scientific knowledge and technology have virtually eliminated the role of open lung biopsy in diagnosis are in hypersensitivity alveolitis, in which diagnosis can frequently be made by immunologic assessment; and in occult infections of the lung in the immunosuppressed host, specifically *Pneumocystis carinii*, in which bronchopulmonary lavage may substitute for needle or open lung biopsy in identifying the causative agent.

PROGNOSIS. The prognosis in infiltrative lung disease is highly variable and difficult. In general, the acute actively inflammatory diseases respond more favorably to agents such as corticosteroids than do diseases of a chronic and slowly progressive variety that are discovered only late in their course. Acute inflammatory disorders more often give rise to symptoms

which bring the patient to the doctor, whereas chronic asymptomatic but progressive disorders are unlikely to do so until the late onset of symptoms of dyspnea and fatigue, when the pathologic process is well advanced and difficult to alter. When a specific agent can be identified and removed from the patient's surroundings, or from the therapeutic regimen, the disease process may subside completely. This is particularly true of diseases associated with drug ingestion and the immunologically produced diseases associated with inhalation of fungal spores or other antigenic material that can be identified and removed from the environment. On the other hand, when no agent can be identified and the pathologic process is obscure, as in the case of pulmonary manifestations of collagen vascular diseases or pulmonary fibrosis of unknown cause, the response to treatment may be minimal.

PREVENTION. A significant portion of the infiltrative lung diseases provides one of the best opportunities in medicine for prevention of disease. Infiltrative diseases associated with environmental exposures in the form of air pollutants, occupational exposures, or avocational exposures to materials around the home can be completely prevented if the disease process is recognized, if the susceptibility of the individual to the agent is identified, and if the offending agent is effectively removed. However, since many of these agents produce asymptomatic disease, it is not possible to rely on the symptomatic patient in order to control the disease. Instead, efforts must be developed to systematically and continuously monitor working and other populations exposed to a wide variety of environmental materials. This will require greatly increased skills and professional capability, but it is here that epidemiology and preventive medicine offer the greatest hope of long-term control of respiratory disease.

American College of Radiology Committee on Audio-visuals: Radiologic Diagnosis of Interstitial Disease of the Lung (videorecording). Chevy Chase, Md., 3M Company, 1975.

Baum, G. L.: Textbook of Pulmonary Diseases. 2nd ed. Boston, Little, Brown & Company, 1974.

Fraser, R. G., and Paré, J. A. P.: Diagnosis of Diseases of the Chest. Philadelphia, W. B. Saunders Company, 1977, p. 342.

Green, G. M., et al.: State of the art: Defense mechanisms of the respiratory membrane. Am. Rev. Respir. Dis., 115:479, 1977.

Petty, T. L.: Pulmonary Diagnostic Techniques. Philadelphia, Lea & Febiger, 1975, pp. 51, 171, 203, 243.

Schofield, N. C., et al.: Small airways in fibrosing alveolitis. Am. Rev. Respir. Dis., 113:729, 1976.

Spencer, H.: Pathology of the Lung: Excluding Tuberculosis. 3rd ed. Oxford and New York, Pergamon Press, 1976.

346.2. PULMONARY INFILTRATE WITH EOSINOPHILIA
(PIE)

Pulmonary infiltrate with eosinophilia (PIE) includes a variety of disease entities which have in common pulmonary infiltrations with local and/or systemic eosinophilia (Table 1). Although the diseases included under this term have little else in common, the grouping is useful as an easily recognized point of departure along the diagnostic pathway or for the identification of a specific entity. This clustering is also of interest because it illustrates that diseases of diverse etiology and clinical presentations have in common the attraction of a specific blood leukocyte, the eosinophil. This cell has

TABLE 1. Pulmonary Eosinophilia*

Classification	Clinical Data	Radiologic Features	Pathologic Findings
Simple pulmonary eosinophilia (Löffler's syndrome)	Minimal symptoms; peripheral blood eosinophilia; spontaneous resolution within one month	Migratory, patchy "infiltrates" with a predominantly peripheral distribution	Not well characterized
Prolonged pulmonary eosinophilia	Symptoms may be severe: fever, weight loss, cough, dyspnea; duration greater than one month or may be fatal; diminished pulmonary function; response to steroids, but relapse possible	Dense, progressive infiltrates primarily at periphery and nonsegmental	Variable, but may include eosinophilic and mononuclear cell collections in alveoli and interstitium; occasional granuloma formation and even microangiitis
Tropical eosinophilia	Persistent pulmonary symptoms, including cough, dyspnea, asthma; malaise, fever, weight loss; marked blood eosinophilia; high levels of antifilarial antibody and very high levels of serum IgE; improvement after antifilarial chemotherapy (e.g., diethylcarbamazine)	Diffuse finely nodular infiltrates; increased interstitial markings	Granulomatous nodules often surrounding degenerate microfilaria or with necrotic centers; alveolar and interstitial infiltrates composed of eosinophils and mononuclear cells
Pulmonary eosinophilia with asthma	Most commonly allergic bronchopulmonary aspergillosis, either as complication of longstanding asthma or as a cause of adult-onset asthma; elevations of both specific reaginic and precipitating antibodies	Nodular opacities of varying size; recurrent pneumonia; atelectasis; occasional bronchiectasis	Eosinophilic and mononuclear cell infiltrates of alveoli and interstitium; increased numbers of mast cells in walls of the air spaces
Pulmonary eosinophilia with periarteritis nodosa, and variants	Severe symptoms: pulmonary, systemic, and multisystem	Variable: interstitial markings, peripheral infiltrates, consolidations, nodules, and sometimes cavitations	Variable, but characterized by vasculitis and granuloma formation, both sometimes associated with eosinophils

*From Ottesen, E. A.: *In* Kirkpatrick, C. H., and Reynolds, H. Y. (eds.): Immunologic and Infectious Reactions in the Lung, Volume 1. New York, Marcel Dekker, Inc., 1976, p. 289.

long interested both clinicians and researchers, and it is only recently that significant information has accumulated to determine why it responds in such a wide variety of disease processes.

The eosinophil has long been associated with allergic and immunologic processes. Recently, a link between the eosinophil response and the lymphoid immune system has been determined through the identification of at least four distinct eosinophilotactic substances: eosinophil chemotactic factor of anaphylaxis (ECF-A), a product of the mast cell; eosinophil chemotactic factor produced by complement activation (ECF-C); eosinophil stimulation promoter (ESP); and a lymphocyte-derived eosinophil chemotactic factor (ECFP) requiring the presence of specific antigen-antibody complexes. These chemoatactic factors have been attributed to specific types (Type I through IV) of immunologic responses of the Coombs-Gell system, and this linkage has provided a rationale for the appearance of eosinophilia in immune responses of widely different pathogeneses. Individual rationales will be discussed further under the headings that follow.

SIMPLE PULMONARY EOSINOPHILIA
(Löffler's Syndrome)

Simple pulmonary eosinophilia is asymptomatic or minimally symptomatic in individuals who present with migratory pulmonary infiltrates which are generally patchy and peripheral or pleural based, most often in the upper lung fields, unilateral or bilateral, transient and migratory, and associated with peripheral blood eosinophilia. The condition is self-limited, with spontaneous resolution occurring usually within a month. These manifestations are attributed to an allergic response to a variety of causative agents, and the features

of this response are compatible with a Type I allergic reaction in which the allergen interacting with mast cell bound antibody, the reaginic (IgE) antibody, elicits the release of biologically active mediator substances, including SRS-A (slow reacting substance of anaphylaxis), histamine, and ECF-A (eosinophil chemotactic factor of anaphylaxis). These mediators act at local vessels to increase the concentration of cells and fluid giving rise to the characteristic pulmonary infiltrates. The most notable agents to elicit such responses are the tissue-invading parasitic helminths, including *Ascaris lumbricoides,* Strongyloides stercoralis, the dog and cat ascarids, *Toxocara canis* and *Toxocara cati,* and *Ancylostoma braziliense,* the dog hookworm. In addition, drugs, such as p-aminosalicylic acid, sulfonamides, and chlorpropamide, and chemicals, such as nickel carbonyl, also produce Löffler's pneumonia. There are, in addition, other unknown causes of this syndrome.

As the disease is self-limited and ordinarily results in no tissue damage, the importance of this syndrome is to differentiate it from infectious or other causes of pulmonary infiltration of more serious import. No specific treatment is indicated, except for the underlying parasite infestation if identified and for the removal of any offending drug that might be the cause of the reaction.

PROLONGED PULMONARY EOSINOPHILIA

This group of diseases is distinguished from simple pulmonary eosinophilia by the prolonged duration and more severe character of the clinical symptoms of fever, night sweats, weight loss, cough, and dyspnea. The specific causes for this syndrome are diverse, including parasitic, bacterial, and fungal infections, hypersensitivity pneumonitides, and drug allergies. The tissue reaction is more severe with accumulation of eosinophils, mononuclear cells, and occasionally multinucleate giant cells; with an edematous interstitium infiltrated with eosinophils and mononuclear and plasma cells; and with granulomas often showing necrosis and, on occasion, minimal microangiitis. The mechanism of disease appears to be a combination of immune complex (Type III) and cell-mediated immune (Type IV) responses, and responds dramatically to corticosteroid treatment. Recognition is important for this reason and to distinguish this form of pulmonary infiltration from pulmonary infections and other forms of pulmonary infiltration and fibrosis.

TROPICAL EOSINOPHILIA

Tropical eosinophilia bears a relationship to filarial infection and is characterized by persistent pulmonary symptoms of cough, paroxysmal nocturnal asthma, dyspnea, malaise, weight loss, fatigue, low-grade fever, peripheral blood eosinophilia greater than 2000 to 4000 cells per cubic millimeter, and high levels of antibody in all classes to filarial organisms. Duration is a few weeks to months, and clinical improvement occurs by treatment with antifilarial chemotherapy. For reasons that are not clear, the syndrome appears under certain circumstances in infection with the human filarial parasites *Wuchereria bancrofti* and *Brugia malayi*. In particular circumstances, it appears that the host localizes the larval infections to the pulmonary parenchyma, as there is no generalized microfilaremia and the pathologic lesions show microfilaria surrounded by necrotic tissue or eosinophilic leukocytes with granulomatous responses composed of epithelioid histiocytes, fibroblasts, and multinucleate giant cells. This granulomatous response is associated with interstitial infiltrates composed of eosinophils, lymphocytes, macrophages, and plasma cells. This pathologic response may represent immune injury from Type I and Type IV allergic responses mediated by ECF-A and ECF-C (the complement derived eosinophilic chemotactic factor) associated with antigen-antibody complex. Treatment is for the underlying filarial infection.

PULMONARY EOSINOPHILIA WITH ASTHMA

Eosinophilia may occur as a complication of longstanding asthma or in association with adult onset asthma. The disease is characterized by persistent wheezing, cough, fever, and tenacious sputum with rusty brown bronchial plugs. In addition to the pulmonary infiltrates, the syndrome is characterized by recurrent pneumonia, atelectasis, and proximal bronchiectasis. The finding of dilated proximal bronchi associated with pulmonary infiltrates, rubbery brownish bronchial casts, and eosinophilia is strong evidence for the diagnosis. The disease is most commonly caused by allergy to a noninvasive colonization of the bronchial airways by species of *Aspergillus* organisms. The fungal spores serve as potent immunogens, giving rise to both reaginic (IgE) and precipitating (IgG and IgM) antibodies in the patients. Stains of bronchial casts show masses of fungal filaments, and cultures yield the offending organism.

The Type I reaginic response appears to pave the way for the Type III antigen-antibody–mediated reaction, with asthma characterized by gradual onset, prolonged duration, greater severity, poor reversibility, fever, and leukocytosis. These responses are probably mediated by the activation of complement, with eosinophils responding to the complement-derived eosinophil chemotactic factor (ECF-C). Treatment with corticosteroids will interrupt this immunologic reaction, suppress the inflammatory response and lead to a reduction of secretions, fever, leukocytosis, and symptoms. Recurrence of the syndrome, however, is common, and control can be difficult.

PULMONARY EOSINOPHILIA WITH PERIARTERITIS NODOSA

This entity is included for completeness to distinguish the eosinophilias associated with vasculitis from those described above. However, it more logically belongs in the discussion of the collagen vascular diseases below. Pulmonary eosinophilia may also occur with a wide variety of other conditions, including infection, pulmonary infarction, neoplasia, and cardiac myopathies. However, in these conditions other aspects of the disease predominate and are likely to distinguish them from the aforementioned groupings of pulmonary infiltrates with eosinophilia. In all these disorders, the eosinophilia most likely results as a response to one of several eosinophil chemotactic factors, reflecting the immunologic mechanisms of the underlying disease.

Adickman, M., et al.: Pulmonary infiltrates and eosinophilia associated with drug reactions and parasitic infections. Postgrad. Med., 60:143, 1976.
Ottesen, E. A.: Eosinophilia and the lung. *In* Kirkpatrick, C. H., and Reynolds, H. Y. (eds.): Immunologic and Infectious Reactions in the Lung. Volume 1. New York, Marcel Dekker, Inc., 1976, p. 289.
Turner-Warwick, M., et al.: Cryptogenic pulmonary eosinophilia. Clin. Allergy, 6:135, 1976.

346.3.   HYPERSENSITIVITY PNEUMONITIS
(Extrinsic Allergic Alveolitis)

DEFINITION. Hypersensitivity pneumonitis, also known as extrinsic allergic alveolitis, is perhaps the most important immunologically mediated pulmonary disease to recognize because of the ubiquity of etiologic agents, the severity of acute symptoms, and the potential for permanent fibrotic damage to the lung, but, most importantly, because this disease is entirely preventable by removal of the etiologic environmental agent. Hypersensitivity pneumonitis is an inflammatory interstitial pneumonia that results from an Arthus-type immunologic reaction in response to a variety of inhaled organic dusts (Table 2). The reaction also involves the terminal and small airways and may present with an asthmatic component in addition to the symptoms and signs of pneumonitis. Precipitating antibody of the IgG class is generated in response to the inhalation of fungal spores of a variety of species frequently, although not always, associated with an occupational exposure. Recognition of the disease depends on knowledge of its clinical presentation, its timing with an environmental exposure, and the ability to identify one of the many possible etiologic agents.

ETIOLOGY. Hypersensitivity pneumonitis may result from the inhalation of small particle antigenic material

TABLE 2. Etiologic Agents in Hypersensitivity Pneumonitis*

Disease	Exposure	Antigen
Farmer's lung	Moldy vegetable compost	
Mushroom worker's lung	Moldy vegetable compost	*Micropolyspora faeni*
Bagassosis	Moldy vegetable compost	*Thermoactinomyces vulgaris*
Humidifier or air conditioner lung	Contaminated forced air system	*Thermoactinomyces saccharii*
Maple bark stripper's lung	Moldy bark	*Cryptostroma corticale*
	Moldy malt	*Aspergillus clavatus*
Sequoiosis	Moldy redwood dust	*Aureobasidium pullulans*
Paprika splitter's lung	Paprika dust	*Mucor stolonifer*
Wheat weevil disease	Wheat flour weevils	*Sitophilus granarius*
Cheese worker's lung	Cheese mold	*Penicillium caseii*
Suberosis	Moldy cork	*Penicillium* sp.
Bird breeder's lung	Pigeons, parakeets, etc.	Avian proteins
Pituitary snuff lung	Porcine, bovine pituitary	Porcine, bovine proteins

*From Fink, J. N.: *In* Kirkpatrick, C. N., and Reynolds, H. Y. (eds.): Immunologic and Infectious Reactions in the Lung, Volume 1. New York, Marcel Dekker, Inc., 1976, p. 229.

of biologic origin from animal or plant sources. The most common forms result from the inhalation of fungal spores, dried and fragmented fungal or insect particles, or particulate animal proteins, such as are found in pigeon or parakeet droppings or in pituitary powder originating from beef or pig serum proteins and used as snuff. The responsible fungal species are varied, but most belong to the thermophilic actinomycetes identified as *Micropolyspora faeni* or *Thermoactinomyces vulgaris* and *saccharii*. These fungi grow best at 45 to 60°C, usually in decaying vegetation as in molding hay, sugar cane, or other vegetable products. Fungi may also grow in heated water associated with air conditioning and may be disseminated to a rather large population through air conditioning or air heating systems in residential or commercial buildings. Other fungal materials, such as are found in wood dust or in association with tree bark, molding cheese, or brewery materials, may also be responsible agents. A partial list is shown in Table 2. The alert physician may discover new agents by careful study of the patient's environmental exposure, and by microbiologic characterization of discovered fungal species.

EPIDEMIOLOGY. Hypersensitivity pneumonitis most commonly occurs with an occupational exposure as in farmers, sugar cane workers, and bird handlers, or in the general population exposed to contaminated forced air systems, but the physician must be alert to the potential for this type of exposure in a wide variety of circumstances, e.g., snuff taking, moldy cellars, or molding wallpaper. Physicians who specialize in this area have patients with unique and unusual kinds of exposures that have been identified only after repeated hospitalizations and treatments for infectious or other pneumonias. In studies of air conditioning or forced air heating system exposure, it has been found that approximately 15 per cent of the individuals exposed to these particles will develop symptoms of hypersensitivity pneumonitis, and this may be taken as an index of the magnitude of the susceptible population in any given exposure. The development of hypersensitivity pneumonitis in housewives after inhalation of small particles of proteolytic enzymes in laundry detergents is perhaps the best example of how the right combination of susceptible population and conditions of exposure can lead to the disease in any epidemiologic setting.

PATHOGENESIS. The pathogenesis of hypersensitivity pneumonitis involves factors both in the environment and in the host. Vegetation decaying under conditions which give rise to temperatures between 45 and 60° C, such as in composting or when hay is baled wet, is favorable to the development of vast numbers of fungal spores of a particle size appropriate to reach the terminal airways of the lungs when the dust is released by breaking open the hay bale, turning the compost heap, starting up a forced air system in the fall, stripping off maple bark, or other such suitable conditions for exposure. The small respirable particles (between 2 and 5 microns) reach the depths of the lung where they are phagocytized by macrophages and other phagocytic cells of the alveolar surface. An immunologic response is characterized by development of precipitating IgG antibody to the antigen.

Only a fraction of those who develop antibodies exhibit symptoms and signs either acutely or chronically, depending on the nature of the exposure and other factors that are poorly understood. The precipitating antibody interacts with freshly inhaled or deposited antigen with the deposition of immune complexes. Their rephagocytosis by inflammatory cells and the release of inflammatory mediators, chemotactic agents, and lymphokines set up an acute or chronic inflammation. Although the disease is largely thought to be mediated by a Type III immune complex reaction in the pulmonary tissues, there is also evidence of granuloma production and the probable involvement of the Type IV cell-mediated immune response. Evidence of alveolar phagocyte involvement can be seen in histopathologic sections in which histiocytes contain foamy cytoplasm and are surrounded by large numbers of lymphocytes in the interstitium and in the alveolar space. Sarcoid-like granulomas may develop, and some may show foci of central necrosis. More severe cases, and particularly the chronic variety of disease, develop fibrosis in the interalveolar tissues with thickening of the walls of bronchioles and luminal obstruction by granulation tissue.

CLINICAL MANIFESTATIONS. Hypersensitivity pneumonitis is unified as a disease more by the character of the immunologic response than by etiology or by clinical manifestations. A wide variety of clinical presentations may occur, but in general the disease presents in either acute or chronic form. The *acute form* follows inhalation of the antigenic dust in patients previously sensitized to the agent at work or at home. Symptoms include dyspnea, fever, cough, chills, malaise, and myalgia, characteristically four to six hours after exposure. Symptoms persist for up to 12 hours, but spontaneous recovery is the rule. Patients may be treated repetitively for a mistaken diagnosis of acute respiratory infection until the immunologic nature is recognized and the etiologic agent identified.

On physical examination, patients may appear dyspneic, toxic, and acutely ill with bibasilar end-inspiratory moist rales. The chest x-ray most often shows diffuse and nodular reticulations throughout the lung fields, most marked in the lower lung fields, looking very much like an interstitial pneumonia. Pleural effusion is not part of the syndrome. A leukocytosis up to 25,000 cells may occur with a marked shift to the left and occasionally eosinophilia. Pulmonary function studies usually show an acute restrictive defect with a decrease in forced vital capacity and one second forced expiratory volume, but with little air flow obstruction. These signs appear four to six hours after exposure and may be accompanied by mild hypoxemia, hypocapnia, and decrease in pulmonary compliance.

Another type of response follows a two-stage course, with an immediate asthmatic type reaction with decrease in forced vital capacity and forced expiratory volume as well as expiratory flow rates. This pattern is then followed in four to six hours by the restrictive response described above.

The *chronic form* of disease is not accompanied by acute respiratory symptoms and presents with signs of respiratory failure, including dyspnea and cyanosis, fixed restrictive ventilatory impairment with decrease in total lung capacity and vital capacity, marked decline in diffusing capacity, and noncompliant lungs. However, in some of the chronic advanced forms of hypersensitivity pneumonitis, elevated residual volume and diminished respiratory flow rates with loss of pulmonary elasticity suggestive of emphysema are found.

DIAGNOSIS. The diagnosis of hypersensitivity pneumonitis used to depend on pathologic examination of lung tissue obtained by biopsy. However, recent advances in understanding the immunologic pathogenesis of the disease now make it possible to achieve the diagnosis in most cases on the basis of historical, radiographic, and immunologic features. A careful history reveals the relationship of the symptoms to the suspect exposure as part of an occupational or home environment. The radiograph reveals the characteristic reticulonodular interstitial infiltrations of either acute inflammatory disease or advanced fibrosis. Careful culture for environmental agents found in the suspect moldy vegetation, such as hay, or in dusts or contaminated liquids, such as in humidifiers, reveals the antigen. Subsequent exposure of the antigen to the serum from the patient may reveal the diagnostic precipitin lines. The diagnostic loop is completed on occasion by careful inhalation challenge of the patient with the suspect antigen in a laboratory setting, or to the suspect work or home environment such as barnyard or coop. After exposure the patient is carefully observed for 12 to 24 hours with blood pressure, temperature, white blood count, and pulmonary function studies. A characteristic decline in vital capacity and forced expiratory volume and sometimes an elevated temperature and leukocyte count occur at four to six hours following the exposure. These laboratory abnormalities, even in the absence of acute symptoms, in response to exposure to the agent and the finding of precipitins in the blood are considered diagnostic.

TREATMENT. Treatment with corticosteroids is indicated when acute symptoms fail to respond within 12 to 24 hours of observation, when symptoms are extreme and there is hypoxemia, or when an extensive exposure has occurred over a fairly long period of time. Corticosteroid treatment is provided to determine whether the fibrotic reaction is reversible. Steroid treatment should be followed with repeat studies of radiographic appearance and pulmonary function changes to determine the extent of response to treatment.

PREVENTION. Hypersensitivity pneumonitis is completely preventable by avoidance of exposure to the etiologic antigen. The principal deficiency in clinical management of this disease is failure to recognize the nature of the hypersensitivity process or to discern the etiologic antigen by careful historical assessment and by environmental analysis. The diagnosis made in the clinic or hospital should be the beginning of a systematic search of the patient's environment with either elimination of the offending agent, such as by the burning of moldy hay, or by engineering the work environment so that the patient no longer becomes exposed to an antigen, even when it is almost impossible to remove it from the work environment. For example, great advances have been made in the dairy industry in the designing of barns and the feeding process such that minimal or no exposure to the offending antigen takes place. At the very least, a person who is not sensitive to the antigen should substitute at the work step where exposure occurs. Careful attention to these aspects of the work environment rather than callously ordering the patient to give up his occupation will usually permit the patient to maintain his livelihood without undue hazard to his health.

PROGNOSIS. The prognosis for the acute disease is excellent provided that repetitive exposure to the offending antigen is avoided. Prognosis in the chronic fibrotic form is poor as far as reversal of pulmonary dysfunction is concerned, but good in terms of progression of the disease if further exposure is avoided. Corticosteroid treatment is generally not effective in improving pulmonary function in the chronic and fibrotic form of the disorder. Thus long-term prevention depends principally on alertness to the acute immunologic cause of diffuse infiltrative lung disease which might otherwise be mistaken for an acute pulmonary infection or, in a chronic form, for idiopathic pulmonary fibrosis.

Fink, J. N.: Hypersensitivity pneumonitis. *In* Kirkpatrick, C. H., and Reynolds, H. Y. (eds.): Immunologic and Infectious Reactions in the Lung, Volume 1. New York, Marcel Dekker, Inc., 1976, p. 229.

Kilburn, K. (ed.): International conference on pulmonary reactions to organic materials. Ann. N. Y. Acad. Sci., Vol. 221, 1972.

Richardson, H. B.: Allergic alveolar diseases. Problems in diagnosis and management. Postgrad. Med., 60:121, 1976.

346.4. PULMONARY VASCULITIS AND GRANULOMATOUS VASCULITIS (INCLUDING WEGENER'S GRANULOMATOSIS)

DEFINITION AND CLINICAL MANIFESTATIONS. Pulmonary vasculitis and granulomatous vasculitis are characteristic tissue reactions common to a broad group of systemic diseases that may also affect the lung and to a few diseases which primarily involve the lung. The pathologic entities usually require tissue diagnosis either by biopsy of the parenchymal lung tissue or by presumptive diagnosis through biopsy of other tissues, such as skin, muscle, or kidney, in the case of systemic disorders. Pulmonary vasculitis is associated with disseminated vasculitis in systemic lupus erythematosus and other collagen vascular diseases, in some of the drug-induced hypersensitivity states, in rheumatoid arthritis with vasculitis, in serum sickness, and potentially in any disorder in which disseminated vasculitis occurs. The pulmonary reaction may be an incidental or prominent part of this systemic disorder.

Pulmonary granulomatous vasculitis is characterized by granuloma formation in addition to the vascular inflammation. Diseases with this pathology primarily involve the lung, although reactions in other tissues, particularly the kidney, may be found. *Wegener's granulomatosis* is perhaps the best known of these diseases and is characterized by the triad of necrotizing granulomatous vasculitis of the upper and lower respiratory tracts, focal glomerulitis and glomerulonephritis, and a greater or lesser degree of disseminated vasculitis. Involvement of the upper respiratory tract may be manifested by mucosal ulcerations of the nose and by chronic and recurrent infections of the sinuses and middle ear. The renal involvement, when present, represents the most serious threat to life because of progressive renal failure (see Ch. 68 and 374.4). For this reason, the renal tract should always be carefully assessed and treatment modified accordingly. Carrington and Liebow have described a limited form of Wegener's granulomatosis which spares the kidney.

The pulmonary lesions may be asymptomatic, but more usually involve cough, hemoptysis, pleuritic pain, and sometimes neurologic symptoms associated with central nervous system involvement. The radiographs are frequently characteristic, showing solitary or multiple nodular densities resembling localized areas of pneumonia, with secondary cavitation in necrotic centers a common sequel. The nodules may be solitary or multiple, varying in size from 1 to several centimeters and may be unilateral or bilateral. The lack of mediastinal lymph node enlargement as well as the cavitation helps distinguish these lesions from acute sarcoidosis, although definitive diagnosis usually requires obtaining tissue by biopsy of the lung or, in the case of upper respiratory tract or renal involvement, tissue from those organs, respectively.

Less common forms of pulmonary granulomatous vasculitis are allergic granulomatosis with vascular necrosis involving the lungs, heart, skin, and nervous system in patients with an allergic background, and lymphomatoid granulomatosis in which a proliferative lymphoreticular disease is associated with necrotizing granulomatous vasculitis involving predominantly the lungs.

PATHOGENESIS. The mechanism of the vasculitis is thought to involve the deposition of circulating immune complexes (Type III allergic reaction) or the Type IV reaction caused by antigen reacting with sensitized lymphocytes, with the release of lymphokines and other mediators of inflammation in and around the blood vessels. Deposition of immune complex has been demonstrated in systemic lupus erythematosus, serum sickness, and rheumatoid arthritis, as well as in periarteritis nodosa. In these diseases, the predominant manifestations are those of the systemic disorder. Granulomatous arteritis and tissue and blood eosinophilia may follow a respiratory illness and lead to periarteritis nodosa, presumably because of a hypersensitivity state to

some agent initiating the respiratory illness. Asthma is usually not found in this type of periarteritis nodosa. Drugs such as sulfonamides, penicillin, busulfan, and others may induce vasculitis as part of a serum sickness–like syndrome, whereas the prolonged administration of hydralazine and procainamide has been associated with a lupus-like syndrome with small vessel periarteritis and vasculitis.

TREATMENT. Corticosteroid therapy is the treatment of choice for pulmonary vasculitis other than in Wegener's granulomatosis. When pulmonary vasculitis is associated with systemic disease, as in lupus erythematosus or rheumatoid arthritis, the treatment is generally governed by the systemic factors. In serum sickness and drug-induced hypersensitivity states, discontinuation of exposure to the agent will usually result in a clearing of the signs of the disease. However, a brief course of corticosteroid therapy is probably effective in reducing the inflammatory responses to the mediators released by the immunologic reactions and also in diminishing the release of proteolytic lysosomal enzymes by the stabilization of lysosomal membranes. Corticosteroids may also affect the immunologic process by suppressing the blastogenic lymphocyte response to mitogens.

Wegener's granulomatosis is the one disease in this group that has been determined to show an excellent response to the cytotoxic agents, particularly cyclophosphamide or azathioprine. Presumably these agents are effective through suppression of the production and proliferation of the lymphocytes which mediate the disease. Treatment with these agents is associated with lymphocytopenia, with a greater suppression of bursa-equivalent than of thymus-derived lymphocytes, a decrease of elevated serum immunoglobulin levels to normal, suppression of primary induction of delayed hypersensitivity in antibody responses to new foreign antigens, and decreased in vitro lymphocyte blastogenic response to certain antigens, but with intact mitogen-induced in vitro lymphocyte blastogenic response.

Fauci, A. S.: Pulmonary vasculitis. *In* Kirkpatrick, C. H., and Reynolds, H. Y. (eds.): Immunologic and Infectious Reactions in the Lung, Volume 1. New York, Marcel Dekker, Inc., 1976, p. 243.

346.5.   THE CONNECTIVE TISSUE DISORDERS

Although recognized and characterized primarily by their systemic manifestations, connective tissue diseases frequently show significant and often serious manifestations in the lungs. Indeed, pulmonary infiltration, pleuritis, and pleural effusion may be the earliest sign of the systemic connective tissue disorders. In addition to direct involvement in the connective tissue disease process, the lungs show increased susceptibility to pulmonary infection, so that a significant proportion of the pulmonary infiltrates call for treatment with antibiotic agents. Although the systemic connective tissue disorders may show nonspecific (or noncharacteristic) pathologic change such as vasculitis, the major diseases — systemic lupus erythematosus, rheumatoid arthritis, polymyositis-dermatomyositis, and scleroderma — can be recognized as distinct entities through their pulmonary manifestations. More general descriptions of these diseases are found in Ch. 50, 51, 52, and 56.

SYSTEMIC LUPUS ERYTHEMATOSUS

Pulmonary involvement in systemic lupus erythematosus (SLE) occurs in more than 50 per cent of patients. It is characterized radiographically by serosal as well as parenchymal changes. Serositis is manifested by cardiac enlargement, pericardial effusion, and pleuritis with or without effusion. The effusions are usually small, are frequently bilateral, are exudative in character, and may show LE cells. Pulmonary infiltrates most frequently involve the lung bases, are patchy, interstitial and migratory in nature, and are caused by infection, vasculitis, or interstitial pneumonitis. These parenchymal abnormalities produce the characteristic pulmonary functional abnormalities of volume restriction, impairment of diffusing capacity, and arterial hypoxemia, with the usual symptoms of cough and dyspnea.

Treatment should be governed by the systemic manifestations of the disease, and usually includes corticosteroids.

RHEUMATOID ARTHRITIS

Pulmonary involvement is a frequent and often unsuspected manifestation of rheumatoid arthritis, giving rise to pleuritis with or without effusion, diffuse interstitial pneumonitis, rheumatoid nodules often associated with dust exposure or pneumoconiosis as in *Caplan's syndrome,* and vasculitis with pulmonary hypertension. Pleural disease is probably the most common pulmonary manifestation of rheumatoid arthritis, occurs primarily in males, may precede or follow the onset of joint involvement, and may result in empyema and fibrothorax. The pleural fluid is an exudate, but its characteristically low glucose level (less than 30 mg per cent) is virtually diagnostic if tuberculous and malignant effusion can be excluded. This finding is useful in distinguishing rheumatoid from other causes of effusion and in indicating the likely cause of associated infiltrative or nodular disease in the lungs.

The fibrosing alveolitis found in rheumatoid arthritis is nondistinctive but may be diagnosed by the associated findings indicated above and by the serologic finding of rheumatoid factor. The pulmonary disease may precede or complicate joint manifestations. Whereas overt radiologic interstitial fibrosis is relatively uncommon in rheumatoid arthritis, evidence of parenchymal disease is more commonly found by pulmonary function studies, the characteristic findings being restrictive ventilatory impairment, reduced diffusing capacity, and hypoxemia.

The nodular form of rheumatoid pulmonary disease is more characteristic than the interstitial form. These nodules occur more frequently in men than in women and may be associated with occupational exposures such as coal mining, sandblasting, asbestos work, pottery, boiler scaling, and brass and iron work. Radiographically, the lesions are single or multiple, may develop rapidly, are characteristically rounded and sharply circumscribed, and may undergo cavitation. These radiographic changes may appear prior to the onset of joint disease and may be diagnosed clinically by lung biopsy and by association with high titers of rheumatoid factor. Patients with rheumatoid lung disease may show enhanced susceptibility to infection,

which should systematically be excluded when new symptoms and infiltrates appear.

DIFFUSE SYSTEMIC SCLEROSIS
(Scleroderma)

Scleroderma is a connective tissue disease primarily of females in the middle years, and is characterized by atrophic sclerosis of the skin, musculoskeletal system, heart, lungs, kidneys, and gastrointestinal tract. Involvement of the skin, esophagus, and lungs often presents a triad, and the presence of pulmonary fibrosis, vascular disease, or pleuritis occurs in over 80 per cent of the patients. Manifestations include cough and dyspnea, signs of hypoxemia, interstitial fibrosis, and, later, cor pulmonale. Progressive fibrosis with cystic changes, pulmonary calcifications, pleural effusion and pleural thickening, and enhanced pulmonary vascular markings and hypertension are other evidences of the progressive pulmonary disorder. Pulmonary function studies show reduction of pulmonary volumes, diffusing capacity, and lung compliance. Pathologic study of lung biopsy and postmortem material has shown the abnormality much more frequently than expected, with histopathologic findings focused principally in the blood vessels, which show marked intimal thickening with loose myxomatous connective tissue in the small pulmonary arteries and arterioles.

POLYMYOSITIS AND DERMATOMYOSITIS

Polymyositis and dermatomyositis, which are systemic diseases primarily affecting striated muscle, also affect the lungs, with interstitial pneumonitis and pneumonia. The pneumonia is a secondary complication of aspiration and hypostasis related to atrophy and weakening of chest wall muscles, with impairment of ventilation and cough. However, primary interstitial pneumonitis does occur in a small percentage of patients with these diseases, either in acute form or with gradual onset of dyspnea, cough, and diffuse pulmonary infiltrate. The histopathology is noncharacteristic, showing the changes of idiopathic fibrosing alveolitis with arteriolitis. There may be some improvement with corticosteroid therapy.

Matthay, R. A., et al.: Pulmonary manifestations of systemic lupus erythematosus: Review of twelve cases of acute lupus pneumonitis. Medicine, 54:397, 1975.

Matthay, R. A., Schwarz, M. I., and Petty, T. L.: Pleuro-pulmonary manifestations of connective tissue diseases. Clin. Notes Respir. Dis., 16:3, 1977.

346.6.   DRUG-INDUCED REACTIONS

DEFINITION. Among the many adverse reactions to drugs is allergy or hypersensitivity. This is thought to account for only 25 per cent of all drug-induced disease, and therefore other types of adverse reactions should be ruled out. Specific evidence of allergy or hypersensitivity, such as that established by laboratory immunologic investigation, should be obtained whenever possible to implicate that mechanism as responsible for the pathogenesis of the observed disease.

PATHOGENESIS. In order to induce immune response

TABLE 3.   Drugs that Produce Pulmonary Disease Possibly Through a Hypersensitivity Mechanism

Antibiotics
    Nitrofurantoin
    Sulfonamides
    Penicillin
Chemotherapeutic agents
    Busulfan, cyclophosphamide
    Methotrexate
    Bleomycin
    Procarbazine
    Melphalan
Analgesics, neuroactive and vasoactive agents
    Heroin
    Hexamethonium
    Methadone
    Methysergide
    Propoxyphene
Miscellaneous
    Blood
    Chlordiazepoxide
    Drugs that induce systemic lupus erythematosus
    Hydrochlorothiazide
    Pituitary snuff

and hypersensitivity reactions, a drug must first bind irreversibly to tissue macromolecules by covalent bonding. It thus serves as a hapten against which the antigenic determination is made. Hypersensitivity to drug reactions may occur as anaphylactic, cytotoxic, Arthus, or delayed hypersensitivity reactions. At least the last three, and probably all types, can be associated with acute or chronic diffuse pulmonary infiltration.

ETIOLOGY. A vast number of drugs are potentially associated with pulmonary hypersensitivity reactions, as listed in Table 3.

Nitrofurantoin. Probably the most commonly reported drug associated with diffuse infiltrative pulmonary disease is nitrofurantoin, a drug used over long periods of time as an antibacterial agent in the urine. The disease can occur in acute form with fever, cough, and pulmonary infiltrates, and it may be associated with pulmonary infiltration with eosinophilia; it is presumably of the Type II or Type III immune reaction. The reaction can begin within hours or days of beginning treatment, and a chest roentgenogram may have the appearance of noncardiac pulmonary edema. Eosinophilia and bronchospasm can occur, or even anaphylactic reaction, but remission occurs within 24 to 48 hours after the drug is discontinued. A positive response can be elicited by a small rechallenge dose.

Chronic disease associated with nitrofurantoin ingestion develops insidiously as cough and dyspnea over months to years after initiation of nitrofurantoin therapy. The disease is much like other forms of pulmonary fibrosis radiographically, functionally, and histopathologically. Diagnosis is made by history of drug ingestion and compatible histopathology by lung biopsy. Therapy is discontinuation of the drug and use of corticosteroids.

Busulfan, Cyclophosphamide, Methotrexate, and Methysergide. A very different histopathology is seen in the interstitial pneumonitis and fibrosis associated with busulfan and cyclophosphamide ingestion. Cough, dyspnea, and fever develop subacutely three to four years after starting the treatment. The pulmonary infiltrate may be interpreted as an opportunistic infection or a neoplastic infiltration. Lung biopsy shows a bizarre hyperplastic reaction of Type II alveolar cells

that appear almost neoplastic. Corticosteroids are of little benefit, and the patient usually dies even though the drug is discontinued. A similar disease without the atypical Type II cells can be produced by methotrexate. Methysergide, on the other hand, produces a fibrotic lung and pleural fibrosis.

Drug-Induced Systemic Lupus Erythematosus (SLE). A variety of drugs may be followed by diffuse pulmonary infiltration with pleuropulmonary reactions and laboratory findings of systemic lupus erythematosus. These drugs are listed in Table 4. Drug-induced SLE shows less renal and cutaneous reaction and more pleuropulmonary disease than spontaneous SLE. The reaction appears to be dose related and may simply represent an unmasking of a pre-existing propensity to SLE.

DIAGNOSIS. The x-ray and the laboratory offer little help in the diagnosis of diffuse infiltrative diseases of the lung induced by drug ingestion. In vitro detection of drug-induced antibodies is possible through physical, chemical, serologic, and in vitro live cell tests, but these are not generally available or useful clinically. The diagnosis depends almost entirely on physician awareness of the possibility of drug-induced diffuse infiltrative disease, careful elicitation of history, or, on occasion, the contribution of an alert pharmacist. Specific inquiry must be made into the drugs that may account for the clinical picture, for many individuals fail to recognize that a drug which they have taken routinely and for years, such as nitrofurantoin, is in fact a drug at all. Of course, all patients should be carefully questioned as to previous drug reactions, because the predisposition to drug reactions and hypersensitivity may indicate the possibility of cross-reactions, and such a patient is at a greater risk than one with no prior history. Rechallenge or provocative test is the most definitive method of diagnosing the drug-related nature of the patient's disease. This procedure, however, should be reserved for situations in which the drug is required as a therapeutic agent, because it is dangerous and may give rise to serious anaphylactic, inflammatory, or pancytopenic hypersensitivity reactions.

TREATMENT AND PREVENTION. Treatment consists of withdrawal of the drug, suppression of inflammatory or

TABLE 4.   Drugs Thought to Induce Systemic Lupus Erythematosus*

Definite	Reported
Chlorpromazine	Aminosalicylic acid
Diphenylhydantoin	Digitalis
Ethosuximide	Gold
Hydralazine	Griseofulvin
Isoniazid	Guanoxan
Mephenytoin	Isoquinazepon
Phenobarbital	Methyldopa
Primidone	Methylthiouracil
Procainamide	Oral contraceptives
Trimethadione	Penicillamine
	Penicillin
	Phenylbutazone
	Practolol
	Propylthiouracil
	Reserpine
	Streptomycin
	Sulfonamides
	Tetracycline
	Thiazides

*Adapted from Schwarz, J. A. Von: Arzneim-Forsch./Drug Res., 27:1856, 1977.

anaphylactic reactions with corticosteroids or sympath-omimetic amines, and other supportive measures as indicated. Preventive measures are most important, for legal as well as for medical reasons. Patient education as to the cause of illness and risks of re-exposure to the same or related drug and potential for cross-reactions with other drugs should be assiduously carried out. As always, thorough record keeping is mandatory, along with a mechanism available to alert others in the health care system to the risks of a patient's drug hypersensitivity. The use of Medic-Alert tags or bracelet or wallet cards and the availability of integrated computerized records, are recent and valuable approaches to prevention of recurrent episodes.

Bone, R. C., et al.: Desquamative interstitial pneumonia following chronic nitrofurantoin therapy. Chest, 69(2 Suppl.):286, 1976.

Gould, V. E., et al.: Sclerosing alveolitis induced by cyclophosphamide. Ultrastructural observations on alveolar injury and repair. Am. J. Pathol., 81:513, 1975.

Lundgren, R., et al.: Pulmonary lesions and autoimmune reactions after long-term nitrofurantoin treatment. Scand. J. Respir. Dis., 56:208, 1975.

Petty, T. L.: Editorial: What else can injure the lungs? N. Engl. J. Med., 294:954, 1976.

Rosenow, E. C., III: Drug-induced hypersensitivity disease of the lung. In Kirkpatrick, C. H., and Reynolds, H. Y. (eds.): Immunologic and Infectious Reactions in the Lung, Volume 1. New York, Marcel Dekker, Inc., 1976, p. 261.

346.7. INFILTRATIVE DISEASES ASSOCIATED WITH CAPILLARY BLEEDING

GOODPASTURE'S SYNDROME

Goodpasture's syndrome can now be considered a distinctive disease entity, characterized clinically by hemoptysis, pulmonary infiltrates, and hematuria. The glomerulonephritis and pulmonary hemorrhage are caused by complement-mediated damage to pulmonary and renal tissue produced when autoantibodies react with glomerular and alveolar basement membranes. Although the etiologic agent (or agents) is unknown, the immune reactions are probably triggered by an inhaled antigen or infectious agent. Progressive glomerulonephritis with proteinuria, hematuria, and renal insufficiency is punctuated with frequent episodes of hemoptysis, bilateral pulmonary infiltrates, and dyspnea. The clinical course is one of progressive renal failure, although cases of spontaneous resolution have been reported. Approaches to treatment have included corticosteroids, immunosuppressive therapy, and nephrectomy. The diagnosis is suspected by the clinical and laboratory findings, and substantiated by kidney or lung biopsies showing antglomerular or pulmonary capillary basement membrane antibody. This syndrome is also described in Ch. 374.4.

From the renal standpoint, the disease must be distinguished from Wegener's granulomatosis, acute glomerulonephritis, or other forms of glomerulonephritis or renal vein thrombosis. From the pulmonary standpoint, the disease must be distinguished from viral or bacterial pneumonia, allergic alveolitis, pulmonary edema, and other forms of pulmonary vasculitis. Goodpasture's disease is distinguished by the episodic nature of hemoptysis and dyspnea, the rapid resolution of the pulmonary infiltrates, the appearance of hemosiderin-laden macrophages in the sputum, hypochromic anemia and iron deficiency responding to iron therapy, the circulating anti-glomerular basement membrane antibody, the evidence of glomerulonephritis with microhematuria and red blood cell casts, and positive tissue immunofluorescence tests for anti-basement membrane IgG. Episodes of hemoptysis may vary from microscopic evidence only to massive hemoptysis with death from exsanguination or asphyxia. Treatment with prednisone is indicated because of the anti-inflammatory effect of this agent, with immunosuppressive agents such as cyclophosphamide to suppress immunoglobulin and cell-mediated immune reactions, and, in rare instances, with nephrectomy, presumably to remove the offending antigen.

IDIOPATHIC PULMONARY HEMOSIDEROSIS

Idiopathic pulmonary hemosiderosis is a disease entity of children and young adults characterized by cough, dyspnea, fatigue, pulmonary infiltrates, and microcytic hypochromic anemia with iron deficiency, progressing to pulmonary fibrosis. Although hemoptysis is occasionally manifested, the disease is characterized more by the symptoms of the anemia and the associated acute or chronic pulmonary infiltrates. Pathologic examination shows pulmonary inflammation and fibrosis with large numbers of hemosiderin-filled pulmonary macrophages with associated hematologic findings of hypochromia and deficiency of iron stores in the bone marrow. It appears that the cause of the disease is unknown. The pathogenesis is characterized by chronic and recurrent extravasation of blood into the pulmonary tissues, with subsequent low-grade inflammation and fibrosis and phagocytosis of blood elements, with permanent storage of the hemosiderin pigment isolated in the macrophages. The clinical characteristics, the nonspecificity of the pathology, and the absence of immunologic involvement are the keys to diagnosis.

The disease is distinguished from other forms of pulmonary interstitial disease by the evidence of the anemia and the large amounts of iron stored in the tissues. It is distinguished from Goodpasture's syndrome by absence of glomerulonephritis and anti-basement membrane autoantibodies. Suspicion of the disease should prompt examination of sputum with iron stains for hemosiderin; this finding indicates only that bleeding has occurred in the lung, but does not indicate the cause. The chronicity of the condition, the degree of pulmonary fibrosis, and the anemia without other apparent cause for blood loss should lead to a pulmonary biopsy to confirm the diagnosis. Also in the differential diagnosis is the chronic hemorrhage and pulmonary fibrosis associated with mitral stenosis, which may be similar pathologically to idiopathic pulmonary hemosiderosis. Other forms of chronic cardiac failure may produce a similar pathologic picture, although generally less severe, with clinical attention more appropriately focused on the cardiac disease. The disease must also be distinguished from other forms of pulmonary vasculitis and pulmonary manifestations of systemic connective tissue disease; again, these are more likely to show extrapulmonary manifestations with less predominance of blood loss anemia.

Benoit, F. L., et al.: Goodpasture's syndrome: A clinicopathologic entity. Am. J. Med., 37:424, 1964.

Dolan, C. J., Jr., et al.: Idiopathic pulmonary hemosiderosis. Electron microscopic, immunofluorescent, and iron kinetic studies. Chest, 68:577, 1975.

Donald, K. J., et al.: Alveolar capillary basement membrane lesions in Goodpasture's syndrome and idiopathic pulmonary hemosiderosis. Am. J. Med., 59:642, 1975.

Everett, D. E., et al.: Goodpasture's syndrome: Response to mercaptopurine and prednisone. JAMA, 214:1849, 1970.

Gonzalez-Crussi, F., et al.: Idiopathic pulmonary hemosiderosis: Evidence of capillary basement membrane abnormality. Am. Rev. Respir. Dis., 114:689, 1976.

Nowakowski, A., et al.: Goodpasture's syndrome: Recovery from severe pulmonary hemorrhage after bilateral nephrectomy. Ann. Intern. Med., 75:243, 1971.

Poskitt, T. R.: Immunologic and electron microscopic studies in Goodpasture's syndrome. Am. J. Med., 49:250, 1970.

Soergel, K. H., and Sommers, S. C.: Idiopathic pulmonary hemosiderosis and related syndromes. Am. J. Med., 32:499, 1962.

Wilson, C. B., and Smith, R. C.: Goodpasture's syndrome associated with influenza A2 virus infection. Ann. Intern. Med., 76:91, 1972.

346.8. SARCOIDOSIS

Sarcoidosis is "a disease characterized by the presence in all of several affected organs and tissues of noncaseating epithelioid cell granulomas proceeding either to resolution or to conversion into featureless hyaline connective tissue." The disease is usually systemic, affecting lungs, liver, spleen, eye, skin, and even heart. The systemic aspects of the disease are presented in Ch. 65; the disease is included here because it is commonly recognized first as a pulmonary disorder, characterized clinically by dyspnea, shortness of breath, and hypoxemia, and radiologically as a localized or diffuse pulmonary interstitial infiltration and/or characteristically enlarged "potato nodes" in the hilar regions.

DIAGNOSIS. The diagnosis of sarcoidosis depends on the accumulation of evidence that the symptoms and signs presented by the patient are related to a widespread noncaseating epithelioid cell granulomatosis with the clinical, immunologic, and pathologic characteristics associated with sarcoid. Diagnosis is strongly influenced by clinical and radiographic signs; by the age, sex, and race of the patient; by immunologic characteristics, including depressed cell-mediated immunity and reactivity to the Kveim antigen; and by characteristic histopathology. Lung biopsy is rarely needed, as histopathologic confirmation can be obtained by biopsy of lymph nodes, particularly of the mediastinum. Biopsy at the site of injection of the Kveim antigen in the presence of characteristic or concordant symptoms and signs and radiographic presentation is sufficient for diagnostic purposes.

In patients with pulmonary sarcoid, diagnostic workup should include stains and cultures of respiratory tract secretions or washings and biopsy material for acid-fast bacilli, mycobacterial organisms, and fungi. There will occasionally be some confusion between mycobacterial disease and sarcoid when characteristics of both are present, particularly when acid-fast bacilli may be seen on smear in a case that is otherwise characteristic of sarcoid. It is more appropriate to refer to both possibilities in the diagnostic categorization than to eliminate either one prematurely. Particular difficulty arises if the evidence of sarcoidosis is limited only to the lung without evidence of granulomas in other organs, and if the Kveim test is negative or inconclusive. In such cases, greater reliance must be placed on clinical analysis and observation and on the biopsy of lymph nodes or lung tissue. Diagnosis should also consider other findings associated with systemic sarcoidosis such as erythema nodosum, bilateral hilar adenopathy, uveitis, or other signs of systemic sarcoidosis, such as hypercalcemia and hypercalciuria.

TREATMENT. Treatment of sarcoidosis is nonspecific, as no etiologic agent has been identified against which therapy may be directed. The use of corticosteroids in pulmonary sarcoidosis is governed by evidence of active and progressive deterioration of pulmonary function rather than by the appearance of the chest x-ray. Indeed, the chest radiograph may look severely abnormal in acute inflammatory sarcoidosis, which may turn out to be self-limited with spontaneous resolution. Although clinical signs such as breathlessness may be used as guides, the best index is a measure of gas transfer such as the single breath diffusing capacity. Although measurements of arterial blood oxygen tension or pulmonary vital capacity will similarly reflect interference of pulmonary function, the single breath diffusing capacity, when measured serially, is a more useful guide to the activity of the disease and the response to corticosteroid therapy.

Initial treatment is with relatively large doses of corticosteroids (e.g., 40 to 60 mg of prednisone), continued until maximal improvement of pulmonary function is observed on sequential studies. At this point, the dose can be reduced slowly to the smallest dose that maintains the level of improvement. Treatment should be continued for six to twelve months, at which time there should be further gradual reduction of the dose, accompanied by careful observation of symptoms, radiographic appearance, and tests of pulmonary function. It is not uncommon for the inflammatory process to recur, even six to twelve months after initiation of corticosteroids, and indeed the flare-up may be more difficult to control than the original process. In the event of recrudescence, the steroid dose should be increased once again as in the original treatment schedule. It should be remembered that the majority of sarcoid cases require no treatment, even though radiographic findings may be substantial in the early phases. The tendency of the disease to recur when steroids are withdrawn, the limited evidence that steroid therapy of even long-term duration affects the fibrotic course of disease, the common finding that steroid treatment may require continuation for years, and the serious complications of long-term steroid therapy should temper the physician's decision to treat acute sarcoidosis automatically at the time of diagnosis. Indeed, it is better to follow the patient for several weeks or months to determine the natural course of the disease, whether self-limited or progressive, before commencing a long and potentially hazardous course of corticosteroid therapy.

Baum, G. L., Schwarz, J., and Barlow, P. B.: Sarcoidosis and specific etiologic agents: A continuing enigma. Chest, 63:488, 1973.

Editorial: Diagnosis of pulmonary sarcoidosis. Br. Med. J., 4:540, 1975.

Hirsch, J. G., Nelson, C. J., and Siltzbach, L. E.: The Kveim test. N. Engl. J. Med., 284:1327, 1971.

Israel, H. L.: Sarcoidosis. Postgrad. Med. J., 46:524, 1970.

Israel, H. L., Fouts, D. W., and Beggs, R. A.: A controlled trial of prednisone treatment of sarcoidosis. Am. Rev. Respir. Dis., 107:609, 1973.

Mitchell, D. N., and Scadding, J. G.: Sarcoidosis. In Murray, J. F. (ed.): Lung Diseases: State of the Art, 1974-75. New York, American Lung Association, 1976.

Siltzbach, L. E. (ed.): Seventh international conference on sarcoidosis. Ann. N. Y. Acad. Sci., Vol. 278, 1976.

346.9. MISCELLANEOUS INFILTRATIVE DISEASES

PULMONARY ALVEOLAR PROTEINOSIS

DEFINITION, ETIOLOGY, AND PATHOGENESIS. Pulmonary alveolar proteinosis, a disease of unknown cause and pathogenesis, is characterized by chronic and progressive filling of the alveoli with a proteinaceous, lipid-rich, granular material thought to represent surfactant and cellular debris. The disease is often found on a background of acute or chronic exposure to inhaled dusts or chemicals, and some have thought there to be an immunologic abnormality. Because of the diversity of preceding history, pulmonary alveolar proteinosis is thought to be a pattern of pulmonary response to a variety of environmental agents.

CLINICAL MANIFESTATIONS. The diagnosis may be suspected when there are progressive dyspnea and hypoxemia, with scanty sputum, x-ray infiltrates of a characteristic ground-glass appearance involving first the lower lung fields and later the upper lung fields, and pulmonary function tests showing ventilatory restriction, reduction in lung volumes, and hypoxemia. Arterial oxygen desaturation may be severe, with arterial blood oxygen tensions as low as 28 to 33 mm Hg in ambulatory patients with this disorder. Nevertheless, definitive diagnosis is usually made by lung biopsy. The histopathology shows essentially normal alveolar septal structure, with the alveolar spaces packed with eosinophilic, PAS-positive, proteinaceous, granular material rich in lipids. In the active phases of the disease, numerous macrophages may be seen, but few leukocytes or inflammatory cells are found. Recent electron microscopic studies of biopsies and bronchial washings in pulmonary alveolar proteinosis have demonstrated abundant annular inclusions in pulmonary alveolar macrophages, showing concentric layering of the bilamellar material characteristic of surfactant. The disease is thought to represent an accumulation of surfactant material due either to overproduction or decreased clearance, with secondary phagocytosis of the material by alveolar macrophages. Complicating infections may be a problem; for example, several cases have been reported in which nocardiosis developed.

DIAGNOSIS AND TREATMENT. Definitive diagnosis of the disease is important for two reasons: first, because blind steroid treatment renders the patient susceptible to secondary bacterial infection and produces no effect on the disease process; and second, because effective therapy can be rendered by the *technique of whole lung lavage* with massive volumes of balanced salt solution. The technique of large-volume lavage has been developed specifically for treatment of pulmonary alveolar proteinosis and involves careful volume-controlled inflow of fluid to minimize adverse effects on pulmonary blood flow. The course of the disease is highly variable; some patients show spontaneous resolution and some show resolution after lavage, but most patients will have a recurring accumulation of the material and a repeated need for lung lavage. Patients with an associated interstitial inflammatory process have in general a poorer prognosis than those in whom the alveolar septal structure is essentially normal. No preventive measures are known, except general measures to avoid inhaled dusts and chemical irritants.

EOSINOPHILIC GRANULOMA

Eosinophilic granuloma is a disease of unknown cause, found typically in young, adult, white males, either localized to the lung or presenting as a multifocal disease involving bone, brain, and endocrine organs as well as spleen, bone marrow, and lymph nodes. The pathologic lesion is one of granulomatous fibrosis, infiltration of histiocytes, macrophages, and eosinophils, and occasionally extensive endarteritis of the small blood vessels. The disease, when localized to the lung, presents with nonspecific symptoms of cough, shortness of breath, and weight loss, and x-ray findings of diffuse pulmonary infiltration or, in more severe cases, honeycomb lung. In multifocal disease symptoms of adrenal insufficiency, hypothyroidism, neurologic abnormalities, and diabetes insipidus may be found. The pulmonary disease is complicated by pneumothorax in about a quarter of the patients, and indeed some patients present with this complication.

The course is variable. In localized disease, it tends to be benign and may show spontaneous remission. Mortality is associated with extensive soft tissue involvement. In the progressive disease, treatment is not satisfactory and focuses on corticosteroids and immunosuppressive agents. Because of the granulomatous pathology and the response to corticosteroids and immunosuppressive agents, as well as abnormalities of delayed hypersensitivity and immunoglobulin levels, the disease is thought to have an immunologic mechanism and perhaps to reflect an immunologic response to an exogenous inhaled agent.

DESQUAMATIVE INTERSTITIAL PNEUMONITIS (DIP)

Desquamative interstitial pneumonitis, or DIP, is a disease of unknown cause but characteristic histopathology, consisting of the proliferation and desquamation into the alveolar spaces of Type II epithelial cells. The disease may be associated with a variety of environmental exposures to chemicals and dusts, and may be preceded by a history of respiratory infection, suggesting the possibility of viral involvement. Clinical, functional, and radiographic features do not distinguish it from other forms of diffuse infiltrative diseases of the lung, but diagnosis is important because the appropriate treatment is corticosteroids, to which this disease responds reasonably well. No other known therapy is available. Histopathology suggestive of DIP may be found simultaneously with areas that resemble pulmonary alveolar proteinosis and pulmonary fibrosis. These processes may be successive steps in the low grade inflammatory and fibrotic response of the lung to environmental agents. The factors that govern the appearance of one form or another are not understood.

USUAL INTERSTITIAL PNEUMONITIS (UIP)

Usual interstitial pneumonitis is a term coined to designate a fairly common and characteristic histopathologic picture in patients with clinical, functional, and radiographic evidence of diffuse infiltrative disease of the lung who have no identifiable environmental exposure, associated connective tissue disease, identifiable immunologic reaction, or other etiologic agent. Response to treatment with corticosteroids is variable.

LYMPHOID INTERSTITIAL PNEUMONITIS (LIP)

This disorder is similar to UIP, except that the histopathology is characterized by an extensive infiltration with lymphocytic cells and a tendency to be associated with the later appearance of diffuse lymphoma.

INFILTRATIVE DISEASE CAUSED BY PHYSICAL AND CHEMICAL AGENTS

Diffuse infiltrative and fibrotic diseases of the lung that are caused by identifiable physical or chemical agents such as inorganic dusts, industrial chemicals, or exposure to ionizing radiation are covered more extensively in Ch. 348, but are included here because of the importance of the differential diagnosis in considering the preceding diseases. Although some of these exposures produce a rather characteristic radiographic picture and histopathology, more frequently the x-ray is indistinguishable from those of other diseases in this group and the diagnosis is made by the historical association with an environmental or occupational exposure, or by a previous history of radiotherapy for lung cancer or pulmonary lymphoma. Diseases in this category do not usually call for lung biopsy when an adequate explanation for the changes can be found by historical evidence of exposure. For this reason, a careful and exhaustive occupational and environmental history is extremely important in all cases of diffuse infiltrative lung disease so that an agent can be implicated when present, the patient removed from exposure, and unnecessary lung biopsy avoided.

OTHER CAUSES OF INFILTRATIVE LUNG DISEASE

Diffuse infiltrative pulmonary disease can be a manifestation of a variety of other disorders: viral and bacterial infections; mycotic pneumonitis; rickettsial infection (psittacosis); gastric acid aspiration; cardiogenic pulmonary congestion and edema related to mitral stenosis or left ventricular failure, or to fluid overload; parasitic infestations; pneumonia caused by *Pneumocystis carinii;* diffuse pulmonary calcifications known as pulmonary alveolar microlithiasis; blood-borne anaerobic infection; septic emboli; the early stages of adult respiratory distress syndrome, occurring postoperatively or related to trauma and pulmonary contusion; kerosene or gasoline ingestion; and metabolic infiltrates associated with uremia, myxedema, and acute hypervolemia. This list is included to alert the physician to the wide range of agents and conditions which can induce diffuse interstitial pulmonary infiltrations and to encourage the student of disease to look more intensively to the lungs not only to recognize and resolve diseases of that organ, but to gain clues and insight into systemic disorders and diseases of other organs as well.

Costello, J. F., et al.: Diagnosis and management of pulmonary alveolar proteinosis: The role of electron microscopy. Thorax, 30:121, 1975.

Rogers, R. M., et al.: Hemodynamic response of the pulmonary circulation to bronchopulmonary lavage in man. N. Engl. J. Med., 286:1230, 1972.

Villar, T. G., Avila, R., and Marques, R. A.: Eosinophilic granuloma of the lung and the extrinsic pulmonary granulomatoses. Ann. N.Y. Acad. Sci., 278:612, 1976.

Zinkham, W. H.: Multifocal eosinophilic granuloma: Natural history, etiology, and management. Am. J. Med., 60:457, 1976.

347. LUNG ABSCESS AND BRONCHIECTASIS

Sydney M. Finegold

347.1. LUNG ABSCESS

DEFINITION. Lung abscess is a suppurative pulmonary infection producing destruction of lung parenchyma with the formation of a cavity with an air-fluid level. Some workers describe a similar process with multiple cavitations each less than 2 cm in diameter as necrotizing pneumonia. The distinction is arbitrary; they are different expressions of the same pathologic process.

ETIOLOGY. By far the most important background factor for abscess of the lung or necrotizing pneumonia is aspiration, usually related to altered consciousness. Common causes of altered consciousness in such patients are alcoholism, cerebral vascular accident, general anesthesia, drug overdose or addiction, seizure disorder, diabetic coma, shock, and other serious illness. Other factors in aspiration include dysphagia caused by either esophageal disease or neurologic disease, intestinal obstruction, and tonsillectomy or tooth extraction. Next to aspiration, the most important factor predisposing to lung abscess or necrotizing pneumonia is periodontal disease or gingivitis. Lung abscess is rare in an edentulous person and suggests the possibility of an associated bronchogenic carcinoma. Other underlying processes include bronchiectasis and secondary infection of a bland pulmonary embolus with infarction. Anaerobic bacteria are the primary organisms recovered. About 60 per cent of cases have only anaerobic bacteria as etiologic agents, with the majority of the balance having both anaerobes and facultative or aerobic forms recovered concurrently. There is generally an average of three organisms per case. The predominant anaerobes recovered are *Fusobacterium nucleatum, Bacteroides melaninogenicus, Peptostreptococcus, Peptococcus,* and microaerophilic streptococci. *Bacteroides fragilis* and *Fusobacterium necrophorum* may also be found. The predominant nonanaerobes recovered are streptococci of various types. Actually, the microaerophilic streptococci produce lactic acid as the major end-product of fermentation and therefore officially belong in the genus *Streptococcus.* However, anaerobic techniques are usually required for their isolation and characterization so that most workers continue to consider them along with the anaerobes.

Pneumonia, particularly that caused by *Staphylococcus aureus, Klebsiella pneumoniae,* and *Streptococcus pyogenes,* may be complicated by abscess formation. Pneumococcal pneumonia is rarely or never associated with abscess formation unless other organisms are involved in the infectious process with the pneumococci. *Pseudomonas aeruginosa* may cause necrotizing pneumonia but seldom causes lung abscess per se. Uncommon causes of lung abscess are actinomycosis, glanders, and melioidosis. Patients with impaired host defense mechanisms, particularly patients receiving high doses of corticosteroids or chemotherapy for malignancy, are predisposed to necrotizing pneumonia and lung abscess. An important cause in this group, although it may occur in the absence of such background factors as well, is *Nocardia asteroides.*

Bronchial obstruction may lead to lung abscess. Most often the obstructing lesion is a bronchogenic carcinoma, but it may be a foreign body or an enlarged mediastinal lymph node. Carcinoma of the esophagus may also be complicated by lung abscess, most often on an aspiration basis.

Metastatic lung abscess may occur, usually as a result of septic emboli from right-sided bacterial endocarditis (*Staphylococcus aureus* is the major pathogen in this setting) or from pelvic or other deep vein thrombophlebitis. Septicemia may result in lung abscess.

Occasionally, subphrenic abscess or other intra-abdominal infection will extend directly or indirectly to involve the lung. In this situation and with intestinal obstruction, *Bacteroides fragilis* is much more common than in the usual aspiration type of lung abscess.

Tuberculosis must always be a consideration in necrotizing pneumonia, and fungal infection (particularly histoplasmosis, coccidioidomycosis, and aspergillosis) may also produce this type of pathology. Bronchogenic cysts, which are lined with an epithelium containing secretory elements, commonly contain fluid which may constitute a good culture medium for various microorganisms. Factors which favor aspiration of oropharyngeal flora or which interfere with drainage may lead to infection of lung cysts. The bacteriology of these infected lung cysts is not unlike that of lung abscess.

Lung abscess is the primary manifestation of pleuropulmonary amebiasis, but pleural complications may occur as well.

INCIDENCE AND PREVALENCE. Although lung abscess was more common prior to the introduction of antimicrobial agents, large general hospitals still see at least ten cases each year; if necrotizing pneumonias are included, the figures are considerably higher.

EPIDEMIOLOGY. Lung abscess and necrotizing pneumonia are primarily of endogenous origin. Most of the bacteria involved are elements of the normal flora of the upper respiratory tract. Infections involving *Staphylococcus aureus, Klebsiella,* and occasionally other organisms may be of hospital origin.

PATHOGENESIS AND PATHOLOGY. The primary site of lung abscess is the posterior segment of the right upper lobe, with the same segment on the left less commonly affected. Next in frequency of involvement are the apical segments of the lower lobes. These segments are dependent, and the distribution relates to the fact that aspiration or inhalation is the primary background factor. Normally, aspirated material is handled effectively by ciliary action, cough, and alveolar macrophages; but if the protective mechanisms are not effective, infection may result. Thick or particulate matter and foreign bodies are not easily removed and thus may lead to bronchial obstruction and atelectasis. With aspiration, gastric acid and enzymes may be primary offending agents.

Subdiaphragmatic infection may extend to the lung or pleural space by way of lymphatics, directly through the diaphragm or defects in it, or by way of the bloodstream. Most amebic lung abscesses are located in the right lower lobe adjacent to the diaphragm, since they typically arise by direct extension of hepatic abscesses through the diaphragm. Infection may arise in or behind an obstructing neoplasm.

Although the virulence of the infecting organism(s) may be a factor determining the nature and extent of the infectious process, this is not usually important in the case of the anaerobes except for *Fusobacterium necrophorum.* However, the number of organisms aspirated may well be an important factor. With certain of the nonanaerobes, such as *Klebsiella, Staphylococcus,* and Group A streptococci, virulence may play an important role.

In the early stages of infection the pathology is that of an ordinary pneumonia. Later, necrosis supervenes upon the inflammation, and cavitation or abscess formation takes place. Subsequently, the abscess cavity may become partially lined with regenerated epithelium, and localized bronchiectasis and emphysema may develop. There is usually no significant vascular involvement in either necrotizing pneumonia or lung abscess. However, septic or bland pulmonary embolus may be the initial event. Once underway, the infection itself may give rise to pulmonary arteritis as in infection caused by *Pseudomonas aeruginosa.*

CLINICAL MANIFESTATIONS. The illness often begins as an acute pneumonic process with fever, malaise, cough, and often pleuritic pain. As a frank abscess is produced, the cough becomes productive of copious amounts of purulent sputum that is usually foul smelling. There may be hemoptysis. Symptoms have usually been present for two weeks or longer at the time of admission, and weight loss and anemia are common. When lung abscess complicates pneumonia caused by *Staphylococcus aureus* or *Klebsiella pneumoniae,* the symptoms are those of a severe pneumonia. There may be a history of unconsciousness, evidence of alcoholism, diseased gums, absence of the gag reflex, or other indications of the predisposing condition.

The physical findings are those of pneumonia, with or without pleural effusion, early in the course of the illness. Later there may be amphoric or cavernous breath sounds. Clubbing of the fingers is noted on occasion. In addition to the usual findings on roentgenograms (see Diagnosis, below), mediastinal lymphadenopathy may be seen on occasion. This may make the differential diagnosis more difficult.

The onset not uncommonly is more insidious than with acute pneumonia. There may be weeks or even months of malaise, low grade fever, productive cough, and significant weight loss before the patient seeks medical attention.

Approximately one third of lung abscesses are complicated by empyema. This may be seen with or without bronchopleural fistula. Brain abscess may also be a complication in patients not receiving appropriate therapy early.

In patients with amebic lung abscess, the symptoms of the associated liver abscess often have been present prior to the rupture through the diaphragm. Following perforation of the liver abscess into the lung, there is gradual development of cough and expectoration of a peculiar chocolate or anchovy sauce–like sputum. There is no odor to the sputum. The development of pulmonary amebic abscess varies from a very insidious phenomenon to a dramatic disease with sudden attack of severe cough productive of a large amount of brownish red sputum. There may be a history of diarrhea and appropriate travel. Complications of amebic abscess include spontaneous perforation to create a cutaneous sinus, hepatobronchial fistula, empyema, secondary bacterial infection, and amebic abscess of the brain.

In cases of secondary lung abscess, the basic process (bacteremia, endocarditis, or septic phlebitis) is usually evident in addition to the pulmonary process.

DIAGNOSIS. A typical lung abscess can be suspected on clinical grounds. Most diagnoses are made from the chest roentgenogram, specifically from the presence of a cavity with an air-fluid level. As indicated earlier, the majority of lung abscesses are located in dependent segments, most often the posterior segment of the right upper lobe, the posteroapical segment of the left upper lobe, and the superior segments of the lower lobes. The basilar segments of the lower lobes may also be involved. Diagnosis of the specific cause, as well as differentiation from similar lesions, depends on bacteriologic studies. Because of the universal presence of large numbers of anaerobes as indigenous flora in the mouth and the common presence, particularly in hospitalized individuals, of potential pathogens such as *Staphylococcus aureus* and *Klebsiella pneumoniae* as colonizers in the mouth and upper respiratory tract, it is necessary to obtain a specimen other than expectorated sputum for bacteriologic diagnosis. When empyema fluid is available, this provides an excellent source. On occasion, particularly in metastatic lung abscess, blood cultures may be positive and provide the specific etiologic diagnosis. However, in most cases of primary lung abscess or necrotizing pneumonia there is no accompanying bacteremia. In the absence of the aforementioned sources, percutaneous transtracheal aspiration is the easiest, safest, and most dependable way of establishing the specific etiology of lung abscess or necrotizing pneumonia. The procedure should not be used in individuals with a significant bleeding tendency or in those in whom it is difficult to provide adequate oxygenation. Percutaneous transthoracic aspiration has been used on occasion in adults but is more hazardous and, in the case of necrotizing pneumonia, provides a much smaller specimen than can be obtained by transtracheal aspiration. It is possible that specimens obtained through a fiberoptic bronchoscope, using special precautions to minimize contamination from normal upper airway flora, may be suitable when quantitative aerobic and anaerobic culture is employed. However, this remains to be established. The antibacterial activity of the topical anesthetic employed with bronchoscopy presents another problem with regard to that type of specimen. It is essential that material obtained for culture be placed under anaerobic conditions promptly before transport to the laboratory. It is usually desirable to aspirate the material to be cultured into a syringe, to expel all bubbles of air or gas from the syringe and needle, and to then transfer the specimen to a tube which has been gassed out with oxygen-free gas for transport to the laboratory.

Amebic lung abscess often provides distinctive clues, i.e., evidence of the disease in the liver. Although demonstration of underlying liver abscess is basic to the diagnosis of amebic involvement of the lung, one may be able to demonstrate motile trophozoites of *Entamoeba histolytica* in the patient's sputum. Presence of Charcot-Leyden crystals in the sputum is very suggestive of amebic infection. The usual procedures for diagnosis of intestinal or hepatic amebiasis should be undertaken. This would include stool examination, sigmoidoscopy, barium enema, and serologic tests. The vast majority of patients with extraintestinal amebiasis have high titers in hemagglutination or complement fixation tests.

Bronchogenic carcinoma can simulate lung abscess when a large tumor undergoes necrosis and cavitation. In addition, the two diseases may coexist. A true lung abscess may develop peripheral to a bronchus obstructed by tumor. In the case of a peripheral cavitating carcinoma, bronchoscopy may not provide the diagnosis. Factors which suggest a cavitating carcinoma rather than lung abscess include absence of predisposing factors for an aspiration abscess (including edentulous state), location of an abscess in a nondependent segment, irregular abscess wall, and failure to respond to antibacterial therapy. Tuberculosis may also simulate lung abscess or necrotizing pneumonia and should always be excluded in cases in which these diagnoses are considered. Cavitating fungal infection may also be confused with lung abscess but is usually distinguished without difficulty. Patients with infected lung cysts typically lack the systemic symptoms which may be seen in lung abscess, the cavity wall is thin, and there is no surrounding pneumonitis. Films taken prior to the illness may have shown an air-containing cyst. Other lesions which may occasionally simulate lung abscess include a cavitating bland pulmonary infarct, cystic bronchiectasis, and cavitating lesions of Wegener's granulomatosis.

TREATMENT. The primary therapy is administration of antimicrobial agents for prolonged periods of time. Treatment may have to be continued for two to four months in order to achieve cure without likelihood of relapse.

With the exception of the *Bacteroides fragilis* group and occasional strains of other anaerobes, the anaerobes involved in lung abscess or necrotizing pneumonia are susceptible to penicillin G. Penicillin V, ampicillin, and amoxicillin are roughly comparable in activity against the anaerobes. Carbenicillin and ticarcillin, in the high dosage usually employed, are active against 95 per cent of strains of the *Bacteroides fragilis* group. However, these agents would not ordinarily be the drugs of choice for this type of infection unless there was another indication for their use. Since some of the anaerobic cocci may require 8 units per milliliter or more of penicillin G for inhibition, one should use large doses of this agent (10 to 20 million units intravenously daily) in patients who are quite ill. The usual adult with anaerobic lung abscess is not seriously ill and usually responds satisfactorily to doses of 2 to 6 million units of penicillin G daily. After there has been a good clinical response, the regimen can usually be changed to 600,000 units of procaine penicillin G intramuscularly every 12 hours. Patients not very ill may be treated satisfactorily with one of the oral penicillins. It should be noted that penicillins other than those mentioned above are typically less active than penicillin G and often considerably less active.

Cephalosporins not uncommonly are less active against anaerobic bacteria than are the penicillins.

However, respiratory tract anaerobes are usually susceptible to cephalosporins (*Bacteroides fragilis* is a major exception), and oral cephalosporins such as cephalexin or cephradine may be used with good effect. Cefoxitin, an investigational beta-lactamase–resistant cephamycin, is much more active than the cephalosporins; 90 per cent of strains of the *Bacteroides fragilis* group are susceptible to this compound and virtually all other anaerobes, with the exception of some clostridia, are as well. Doxycycline and minocycline are more active than other tetracyclines against anaerobes, but a significant percentage of strains of most species are resistant. Accordingly, these compounds should be used only when susceptibility data are available or when the patient's illness is minor so that a therapeutic trial in the patient can be undertaken safely. Clindamycin is active against most anaerobes with the exception of some strains of *Peptococcus* and some strains of clostridia other than *C. perfringens*. It is almost always active against *Bacteroides fragilis*. Accordingly, it represents a good choice in individuals who have significant allergy to penicillins or cephalosporins and in seriously ill patients in whom the *Bacteroides fragilis* group may be present. It may be given intravenously or orally in a dose of 15 to 30 mg per kilogram of body weight per day in four equal doses every six hours. Chloramphenicol is active against nearly all anaerobes and represents another option in a seriously ill patient with necrotizing pneumonia or lung abscess in whom the *Bacteroides fragilis* group may be present. The succinate derivative may be given intravenously in a dosage of 30 to 60 mg per kilogram of body weight per day in adults, using four equal portions every six hours and giving the drug slowly, over a period of 30 minutes. Metronidazole, still investigational for treatment of anaerobic infections, has a broad spectrum of activity and is consistently bactericidal. All strains of *Bacteroides fragilis* are susceptible. However, some of the cocci, particularly those not obligately anaerobic, and *Actinomyces* are resistant.

For staphylococcal infections a penicillinase-resistant penicillin is preferable, but one of the parenteral cephalosporins or vancomycin may be used in the event of significant allergy. Penicillin G is the drug of choice for group A streptococcal infection. For infections caused by *Klebsiella pneumoniae* or other facultative or aerobic gram-negative bacilli which may be involved in the type of pulmonary infection under discussion, one of the aminoglycosides would represent the drug of choice. Gentamicin is ordinarily suitable, but in certain settings significant numbers of gram-negative bacilli are resistant to gentamicin, and then amikacin is the next choice. In seriously ill patients, particularly those who may be immunosuppressed, the use of carbenicillin or ticarcillin along with the aminoglycoside is desirable.

For nocardiosis, sulfonamides or co-trimoxazole, minocycline, and ampicillin all have significant activity. In seriously ill patients, a sulfonamide plus one of the antibiotics should be used. In amebiasis, drugs used for treatment of amebic liver abscess (in particular, metronidazole or emetine) constitute effective therapy, along with appropriate drainage. Treatment for the primary intestinal amebiasis should also be included.

Postural drainage is an important aspect of therapy of lung abscess. Bronchoscopy may be helpful in effecting good drainage at times and also permits removal of foreign bodies and biopsy diagnosis of tumors. Surgical resection of lung abscess is rarely required unless there is a coexisting malignant process. Indeed, surgery is contraindicated because of the hazard of uncontrollable spread of infection or asphyxiation from spillage of abscess contents during positioning of the patient on the table. Surgical drainage of lung abscess through the chest wall is almost never indicated. In the case of accompanying empyema, drainage is crucial and usually requires an open procedure with rib resection.

PROGNOSIS. The prognosis varies with the type of underlying or predisposing pathologic process, if any, and, in the case of acute severe necrotizing pneumonias, the speed with which appropriate therapy is instituted. The mortality in anaerobic lung abscess is 15 per cent or less. In anaerobic necrotizing pneumonia it is 25 per cent. The mortality may be significantly higher in acute pneumonias caused by *Staphylococcus aureus*, *Klebsiella pneumoniae*, and other facultative or aerobic gram-negative bacilli. Prognosis in amebic lung abscess is good when diagnosis and treatment are prompt. Nocardiosis often has a relatively poor prognosis, especially when it complicates a serious underlying disease.

PREVENTION. When possible, care should be taken to minimize the likelihood of aspiration. Thus nasogastric tube feedings should be employed with care. The head of the bed should be elevated for patients with achalasia or similar problems. If aspiration does occur, particulate material should be removed promptly. Proper treatment of periodontal disease and gingivitis will minimize pulmonary complications. Acute pneumonias and bacteremias should be treated promptly with appropriate drugs.

347.2.   BRONCHIECTASIS

DEFINITION. Bronchiectasis refers to abnormal dilatation of the bronchial tree. The distribution of the disease is patchy. There are usually no signs or symptoms directly related to the bronchial dilatation. The clinical picture is due to chronic or recurrent infection and hypersecretion of mucus.

ETIOLOGY. Various infections may cause peripheral bronchial obstruction and stasis which may then lead to bronchiectasis. At present, bronchopneumonia is the most common causative factor. Obstruction related to a foreign body or to tumor may also lead to chronic infection and development of bronchiectasis distal to the obstruction.

True congenital bronchiectasis may be seen in Kartagener's syndrome. This syndrome consists of dextrocardia, sinusitis, and bronchiectasis. In cystic fibrosis of the pancreas or mucoviscidosis, the thick secretions obstruct the lumen of the bronchi, resulting in distal atelectasis. Bronchiectasis commonly results from infection superimposed on the aforementioned process. Recurrent infection in individuals with congenital agammaglobulinemia also leads to bronchiectasis. Tuberculosis may cause it by distortion of bronchi in association with healing disease, obstructing lymph nodes, or destruction due to endobronchial disease.

PATHOGENESIS AND PATHOLOGY. Irreversible dilatation of the bronchi results from prolonged bronchial obstruction and infection. The infection may extend into the bronchial wall, disrupting smooth muscle and elastic tissue and, at times, invading adjacent peribronchial tissue. Ciliated columnar epithelium is replaced by nonciliated cuboidal epithelium and sometimes fibrous tissue, resulting in the formation of localized areas of dilatation or saccules. These anatomic changes lead to further stasis of infected secretions, and there may be traction as a result of peribronchial scarring. The posterior basal segments of the lower lobes are the areas most commonly affected by bronchiectasis. When the left lower lobe is involved, the lingular segment of the left upper lobe is also commonly involved. Upper lobe bronchiectasis tends to be in the posterior or apical segments and is commonly secondary to healed tuberculosis.

CLINICAL MANIFESTATIONS. As noted earlier, bronchiectasis is asymptomatic in the absence of superimposed infection. Some individuals with bronchiectasis may be asymptomatic for extended periods of time. The classic symptoms of bronchiectasis are cough productive of mucopurulent sputum, hemoptysis, and recurrent pneumonitis. The cough may be particularly bothersome when the patient lies down, thus emptying secretions from the dilated saccules of the dependent lower lobes into the larger bronchi. Large amounts of mucopurulent sputum are produced each morning. Classically, such sputum, when collected in a jar, will show three layers: a bottom layer consisting of pus cells and elastic tissue, a central watery layer, and a frothy top layer. The sputum is not uncommonly foul or putrid smelling but may have a sickening sweet odor. The hemoptysis may be massive on occasion. Recurrent pneumonitis involving the same segment or lobe repeatedly should raise suspicion of the possibility of underlying bronchiectasis, as well as of tumor or foreign body.

Many patients with bronchiectasis also have sinusitis and gingival or periodontal disease, but the relationship of the latter processes to bronchiectasis does not seem to be one of cause and effect.

Exertional dyspnea may be noted by patients with extensive disease. There may be pleuritic pain, usually mild in nature. Fatigue and malaise are common. Patients appear chronically ill. A significant number exhibit clubbing of the fingers and toes. The most characteristic finding is persistent moist, coarse rales over the area of involvement.

DIAGNOSIS. In overt cases the diagnosis is readily established clinically. Such cases are not nearly so common as in the preantimicrobial era. Roentgenograms of the chest may show increased coarse lung markings and even honeycombing. In extreme cases of saccular bronchiectasis there may be ring shadows and fluid levels. Ordinarily, bronchography is the most effective means of establishing the diagnosis. In the case of suspected endobronchial obstruction underlying the bronchiectasis, bronchoscopy is important.

TREATMENT. The treatment of choice, when it is feasible because of localized disease, is resection of the involved areas. Aside from this, treatment consists of use of antimicrobial agents in limited courses for complications such as pneumonitis or acute exacerbations of the disease. There is a paucity of good bacteriologic data as to cause of the infection in these patients, but what is known suggests that it is comparable to that observed in lung abscess and necrotizing pneumonia. Accordingly, penicillin G is ordinarily the drug of choice. Individuals who have had repeated and extended courses of antimicrobial therapy, patients with cystic fibrosis in particular, may have infection with more resistant organisms such as *Staphylococcus aureus* or *Pseudomonas aeruginosa*. For them, a penicillinase-resistant penicillin or aminoglycoside such as gentamicin or amikacin represents the drug of choice. A major aspect of therapy is postural drainage.

Before contemplating surgery for localized disease in a newly diagnosed case, the clinician should undertake conservative management and observation of the patient. It is important to realize that spontaneous reversion of the process may take place. Reversible bronchiectasis may follow pneumonia or expansion of a collapsed lobe. In some cases, it may take many months for the process to revert to normal.

PROGNOSIS. The disease is usually not progressive, and with judicious use of antimicrobial therapy the life expectancy can be normal.

Bartlett, J. G., and Finegold, S. M.: Anaerobic infections of the lung and pleural space. Am. Rev. Respir. Dis., 110:56, 1974.

Bartlett, J. G., Gorbach, S. L., Tally, F. P., and Finegold, S. M.: Bacteriology and treatment of primary lung abscess. Am. Rev. Respir. Dis., 109:510, 1974.

Brock, R. C.: Lung Abscess. Springfield, Ill., Charles C Thomas, 1952.

Finegold, S. M.: Anaerobic Bacteria in Human Disease. New York, Academic Press, 1977.

Ochsner, A., and DeBakey, M. E.: Pleuropulmonary complications of amebiasis: An analysis of 153 collected and 15 personal cases. J. Thorac. Surg., 5:225, 1936.

Wynn-Williaus, N.: Bronchiectasis: A study centered on Bedford and its environs. Br. Med. J., 1:1194, 1953.

348. PHYSICAL AND CHEMICAL IRRITANTS

Margaret R. Becklake

348.1. INTRODUCTION

Man, in taming his environment, in developing his complex industrial society, and, more recently, in pursuit of his hobbies, has become increasingly exposed to a wide variety of *inhaled agents, including particles, fumes, or vapors,* which are capable of affecting his lungs to the point of producing disease. Apart from community air pollution, most *such exposures occur in relation to occupations.* Although the title of this chapter implies that the harmful effects of all such agents can be attributed to *physical or chemical irritation,* it is in reality often difficult to characterize the mechanisms whereby they produce biologic effects, even though the physical and chemical properties of the environmental agents concerned can be precisely measured. Often when the precise nature of the agent is not known, the practical solution may be to *link the disease with the occupation concerned.*

The physician usually makes this link through *the occupational history.* An industrial physician is sensitized to the need for a detailed occupational history and the environmental hazards associated with different occupations. However, in many communities working men and women first seek medical advice from their personal physician who may easily fail to recognize an occupational exposure because it occurs in a small plant, using experimental materials, or in the processing as a secondary user of dangerous products whose hazards are neither recognized nor appreciated. Thus *a work history should always be exhaustive* and should cover every job ever held, even part-time or vacation jobs, together with the materials handled directly or indirectly, as well as safety measures recommended on the job and information about the health of co-workers. Furthermore in the past, the role of women in the workplace was often forgotten; thus the listing of a middle-aged or elderly woman's occupation as that of housewife may result in failure to recognize, for example, a link between pleural calcification and work in a talc factory when she was younger. In addition, place of residence is also important, as well as the occupation of other family members, because *neighborhood* and *"take-home"* risks are increasingly being identified, e.g., mesothelioma developing years later in someone whose childhood home was beside an asbestos plant, or in the wife or child of a previous asbestos worker.

Thus today *occupational lung disease* covers the reaction of the lung to *a variety of physical and chemical agents.* It includes those conditions originally described by the term *pneumoconioses,* which refers to lung disease consequent to the inhalation of dust, in keeping with its Greek derivation. The term has recently been redefined by the International Labor Organization (ILO) to mean *the accumulation of dust in the lungs and the tissue reactions to its presence.* For the purpose of this definition, "dust" means an aerosol of solid inanimate particles. The tissue reaction may be *noncollagenous,* i.e., alveolar architecture remains intact, stromal reaction is minimal and consists mainly of reticulin fibers, and the reaction is potentially reversible. By contrast, *collagenous* pneumoconioses are associated with permanent scarring of the lung. Although the term was originally applied only to inorganic (mineral) dusts, it has subsequently been extended to cover organic (biologic) "dusts" as well, because exposure to the latter is also frequently occupational. However, besides any nonspecific reaction these biologic "dusts" may evoke, especially if exposure is heavy, they may act as stimulants to the subject's immune mechanisms (see Ch. 346). In this chapter the ILO definition will be followed. A large number of variants of the term pneumoconiosis

Physical and Chemical Irritants: Working Classification of their Pulmonary Effects

Category of Agents	Effect on Lung	Agent	Circumstances of Exposure, Including Occupation(s) or Industry at Risk
Inorganic dusts	1. Pneumoconiosis (noncollagenous)	Carbon, tin, iron, coal, graphite	Mining, welding
	2. Acute silicolipoproteinosis	Free silica (uncombined SiO_2)	Tunnelling, sandblasting: exposure to high doses of fine particles
	3. Pneumoconiosis (collagenous)		
	a. Nodular	Free silica	Hardrock mining of any sort; quarrying, stonecutting and dressing; foundry, pottery, and enamel workers
	b. Diffuse	Asbestos (all fiber types)	Asbestos mining, milling and manufacturing; insulating
		Fume and other fine silica	Sandblasting
		Beryllium	Fluorescent light and space industry
	c. Complicated	An altered response to usually nonfibrogenic dust	Coal miners (progressive massive fibrosis)
	4. Neoplasia (lung) (see Ch. 349.2)	Asbestos (all fiber types)	Mining and industrial exposures
		Radioactive dusts	Mining operations
		Metal mining	Hematite, chrome
		Metal refining	Nickel, chrome
	5. Neoplasia (pleura) (see Ch. 350.1)	Asbestos (excluding anthophyllite)	Industrial exposure more at risk than mining exposures
	6. Chronic bronchitis	All dusts, given a high enough dose	Probably all types of exposure
Organic dusts	1. Asthma-like reactions (see Ch. 344.1)	Enzymes of *B. subtilis*	Manufacture of detergents
		Western red cedar dust	Wood workers
	2. Late onset airflow obstruction (eventually irreversible)	Cotton, hemp, flax, and jute	Processing of vegetable fiber, especially carding of cotton
	3. Hypersensitivity pneumonitis (see Ch. 346.3)	Fungal spores, especially *M. faeni*	Haymaking, grain handling, mushroom cultivating, sugar cane picking or processing the residue
	4. Chronic bronchitis	Organic material (nonspecific)	Grain handling
	5. Chronic interstitial pneumonia	Vaporized mineral oil	Smoking blackfat tobacco (Guyana); certain industrial exposures
Chemicals, including fumes and vapors	1. Acute pulmonary edema	Oxides of nitrogen	Silo filling, fire fighting
		Phosgene	Fire fighting
		Certain insecticides, e.g., paraquat	Accidental ingestion
	2. Asthma-like reactions (see Ch. 344.1)	Complex platinum salts	Platinum refining
		Aluminum solder flux	
		Toluene di-isocyanate (TDI)	Manufacture of polyurethane plastic
	3. Acute bronchitis	TDI (in heavier doses)	Manufacture of polyurethane plastic
		SO_2	Pulp and paper mills
		NH_3	Refrigeration industry
		Vanadium	
	4. Chronic bronchitis	All the aforementioned agents in lower dose	As above
	5. Pneumonitis	Cadmium, Hg, Mn	
Radiation	1. Pneumonitis	X-radiation	Medical treatment
	2. Neoplasia (see Ch. 349.2)	Radioactive dusts	Uranium and other mining

have been coined to describe specific occupations at risk or specific dust diseases, and these will be referred to where appropriate.

The accompanying table, although it implies more precise understanding of the mechanisms of lung response to the different agents than is justified by current knowledge, does, however, provide a working and essentially practical approach for diagnosis. Included also is reference to the recognized associations between these agents and neoplasia, although of course the mechanism of action is probably more complex than physical and/or chemical "irritation."

Pneumoconiosis redefined. Br. Med. J., 2:552, 1972.

348.2. INORGANIC DUSTS: DOSAGE, CLEARANCE, AND CELLULAR REACTION

The main biologic effects of inorganic dusts depend on their retention in the lungs of man for long periods of time, measured usually in years, not months. It has been suggested that any mineral dust, if relatively insoluble and not immediately toxic, can produce a pneumoconiosis when inhaled in sufficient quantities. The physician is probably better advised to adopt this over-suspicious attitude to mineral dusts than to fail in recognizing old as well as new pneumoconioses. In addition to effects attributable to retention of dust in lung tissue, less specific effects on airway function are being increasingly recognized, and will be discussed under the heading of occupational bronchitis (see Ch. 348.10).

Human lungs have been aptly called *"size-selective dust samplers."* Airborne dust, when inspired into the lung, undergoes a process of separation based on its aerodynamic behavior or falling rate, a function mainly of diameter, but also of size, shape, and density. Once particles make contact with any part of the airways or airspaces, they are not resuspended in the expiratory airstream. Other factors which influence penetration and deposition include breathing patterns, including the amount of time spent mouth breathing, as well as tidal volume and minute ventilation. There is also evidence to suggest that the state of the airways in smokers is such as to favor central deposition rather than deeper penetration of particles. Over 80 per cent of larger particles (6 μ and over) impact on the mucous lining of the larger airways to be removed, usually quite rapidly (i.e., within hours), by ciliary escalation; however, some particles of considerable length, e.g., asbestos fibers up to as much as 100 μ in length, may penetrate as far as terminal respiratory units. Small dust particles penetrate more deeply, fine particles (below 2 μ) constituting the majority of those which reach the alveolar spaces. The retention rate is about 40 per cent in the 2 to 1 μ size, and higher for those below 0.2 μ (see Fig. 1). It is ironic that in many industrial situations mechanization has resulted in an increase in the environmental risks, increasing not only the overall dust levels but in particular the fine particles with a higher retention rate.

Particles deposited in the major airways are removed rapidly (within hours) by the mucociliary escalator. However, since the respiratory bronchioles and alveoli are lined with surfactant, not mucus, dust particles set-

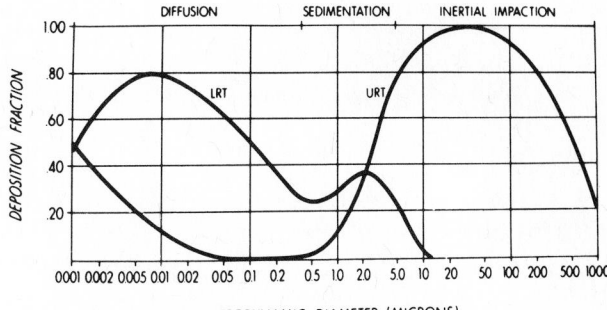

Figure 1. Deposition rate of particles in the human lung in the nose and supraglottic structures (URT) and in the tracheobronchial tree and lung parenchyma (LRT) in relation to aerodynamic diameter, a measurement which refers to the actual diameter in the presence of water vapor which may exceed the particle size in dry air. (Courtesy of Professor Paul Morrow, University of Rochester, N.Y. Reproduced from Lee, D. H. K. [ed.]: Environmental Factors in Respiratory Disease. New York, Academic Press, 1972.)

tling here are handled by other clearance mechanisms, which are slower, with half-clearance times of between 24 hours and 100 days. Important to them all is the process of alveolar phagocytosis; dust-laden phagocytes migrate toward the alveolar ducts and terminal bronchioles; if not extruded into the airways they may penetrate into lung interstitium and lymphatics. Furthermore, clearance mechanisms may be provoked, i.e., mucus and surfactant production, ciliary activity, and endocytosis may all increase, in response to the inhalation of irritants, particularly if exposure is intermittent. Heavy doses, on the other hand, tend to overwhelm the removal mechanisms, and their efficiency may also be reduced by associated pollutants, either industrial or personal (tobacco smoke).

The *lung tissue response to inorganic dust* has been likened to the color spectrum to emphasize the variety in the type of response and its intensity, ranging from noncollagenous tissue reactions in the presence of large amounts of retained dust, e.g., cotton and coal, to intense collagen fibrosis in association with relatively small amounts of retained dust. The nature of the tissue response is thought to depend on the physicochemical properties of the dust as well as on its antigenic properties. It is almost certainly dose related to *the amount of dust retained* (not to the exposure dose), which in turn is the consequence of the integrated personal exposure less the integrated clearance over the years, and probably also relates to how long the dust has been resident in the lung. Other factors which may influence the response are the presence or absence of infection, and possible synergistic or antagonistic effects of other respirable materials in the environment. Finally, although dust dose is probably the most important factor determining the lung response, there appear to be between-individual differences in susceptibility; it is not clear, however, whether this is a reflection of between-individual differences in clearance and therefore retention, or between-individual differences in tissue response.

The nodular pneumoconioses, either noncollagenous or collagenous, are caused by the relatively insoluble dusts, and the diffuse pneumoconioses by relatively soluble dusts.

Brain, J. D., and Valberg, P. A.: Models of lung retention based on the ICRP Task Group Report. Arch. Environ. Health, 28:1, 1974.

Seal, R. M. E., and Wagner, J. C.: Pathologic reactions of the lung to dust. *In* Morgan, W. K. C., and Seaton, A. (eds.): Occupational Lung Diseases. Philadelphia, W. B. Saunders Company, 1975, p. 39.

348.3.   INORGANIC DUST PNEUMOCONIOSES: DIAGNOSIS, LUNG FUNCTION, AND DISABILITY

The criteria for *diagnosis* of an inorganic dust pneumoconiosis depend on the purpose for which the diagnosis is to be used (e.g., working diagnosis, screening, or attributability for compensation), as well as the degree of certainty required. In general, it will be based on the characteristic changes in the chest roentgenogram, *provided that the subject in question has an appropriate exposure history*. Furthermore it is not unusual for there to be no physical signs and no impairment of physical performance, even in the presence of marked radiographic changes. In no other field therefore is the quality of the chest radiograph more important, and the technique used should be appropriate; e.g., low kv to define pleural calcification, high kv to define the pulmonary parenchyma and noncalcified pleural changes, oblique views often being necessary to demonstrate the latter. In addition, use of standard films in conjunction with the UICC/Cincinnati Classification of Radiographic Appearances of the Pneumoconioses (1970) will improve the accuracy of film interpretation. In this classification, which is descriptive rather than etiologic, parenchymal changes are classified according to *type* (round or irregular); *size* (p, q, and r for rounded opacities of <1.5, 1.5 to 3.0, and >3.00 mm diameter, respectively; s, t, and u for fine, medium, and coarse irregular opacities; A, B, and C for large opacities of <1.0, 1 to 5, and >5 cm in diameter, respectively); and *profusion* (from 0/- to 3/4 on a 12-point scale, with provision for indicating the zones involved). Provision is also made for recording pleural thickening (according to site, width, and extent, and whether the costophrenic angle is involved), ill-defined diaphragm and cardiac outline, and pleural calcification (according to its site, thickening and extent), as well as other changes in the hila, mediastinum, and heart. In the absence of an exposure history, or if the exposure is considered to be too short to account for the amount of radiologic change seen, it may be necessary to establish a *tissue diagnosis* by *mediastinal node biopsy or transbronchial* or *open lung biopsy*. However, the pathologic findings may also be inconclusive, because lung tissue has only a limited number of response patterns and a given response may be evoked by several stimuli, e.g., irritants and infections, and every attempt should therefore be made to identify the agent. This may require examination under the electron microscope, e.g., for asbestos fibers, as well as chemical analysis and mineralogic study with x-ray diffraction of adequate tissue samples (for which open biopsy is usually necessary). The electron microprobe may ultimately allow precise characterization of mineral in very small tissue samples, or even in the single ferruginous (asbestos) body. Since most pneumoconioses develop as a consequence of occupational exposure, *precise evaluation of disability* is fre-

quently called for, with a view to establishing compensation; hence, the many studies of pulmonary function in pneumoconiosis. However, the relationships between *organ malfunction* (as reflected in what might be called descriptive measurements of the lung, e.g., its size or volumes, and measurements reflecting its mechanical properties, including gas mixing and airway caliber), *organ failure* (generally considered to be present only when gas exchange function is impaired), and *disability* (diminution of performance as perceived by the subject himself) are not straightforward. Thus considerable organ malfunction (i.e., abnormality of lung function tests) can be present without organ failure (i.e., abnormal arterial blood gases) even under the stress of effort. It is generally believed that *dyspnea* is felt when the respiratory effort (either minute volume or muscular effort) for a given task is greater than the subject habitually experiences. In health there exists a tremendous reserve of cardiopulmonary function, indicated by the capacity to increase O_2 consumption (going from rest to maximal exercise) by a factor varying from 20 in the young athlete to perhaps 10 in the middle-aged man. In its early stages pneumoconiosis may produce only very minor measurable changes in organ function, affecting performance at high levels of exercise only, and this may well be interpreted by the subject as the natural consequence of aging. As the condition progresses, dyspnea may be more easily related to demonstrable changes in the lung function. In the following chapters, an attempt is made to describe the usual clinical picture and lung function findings in the different pneumoconioses in their different stages of development, and, because of the universal nature of the smoking habit, the effect that smoking will have in further modifying function. *In evaluating the individual case,* however, *there is no substitute for the detailed study of pulmonary function at rest and on effort*, with a view to determining performance at an average aerobic workload (such as many jobs demand) and possibly to determine maximal aerobic work capacity. This information can then be interpreted in the light of industrial history, the physical demands of the individual's job, dust exposure (quality and quantity), medical history (in particular, previous and present heart and lung disease), and appropriate laboratory investigations.

In a case of industrial lung disease, the physician's responsibility to his patient does not cease until he has assured himself that the case has been referred to the correct local authority in charge of industrial safety. This referral has social implications at two levels. In the first place, there is the question of attributability and compensation for the individual and for his dependents. In the second place, it is evident that the occurrence of a case of occupational disease represents failure of control measures, and it is essential that this point of failure be identified so that appropriate action can be taken to protect the future health of a new generation of workers, the younger colleagues and children of today's cases. The physician must ensure that these steps have been taken.

Bates, D. V. B., Macklem, P. T., and Christie, R. V.: Response to chemical and physical irritants. *In* Respiratory Function in Disease. Philadelphia, W. B. Saunders Company, 1971, p. 361.

Becklake, M. R.: Pneumoconioses. *In* Handbook of Physiology. Respiration. II. Baltimore, Williams & Wilkins Company, 1965, p. 1601.

ILO U/C International Classification of Radiographs of Pneumoconiosis. Geneva, International Labour Office, 1972.

348.4. NONCOLLAGENOUS PNEUMOCONIOSES

EXAMPLES. Examples include *coal workers' pneumoconiosis; siderosis* in welders; *pneumoconiosis* in hematite and magnetite miners; *stannosis* in tin miners; *baritosis* in barium miners; *pneumoconiosis* in *chromite* and *china clay* miners, and in *Fuller's earth* and *mica* workers. It should be noted that information on the noncollagenous pneumoconiosis is derived largely from coal workers' pneumoconiosis, which, because of the large numbers of men at risk in many countries and the resurgence of coal as a source of energy, has been under extensive study in recent years.

PATHOGENESIS AND MECHANISMS. The dusts mentioned above elicit a virtually noncollagenous response in the lung; hence the diseases associated with such exposure have been called the *"benign" pneumoconioses.* Thus particles which are phagocytosed by macrophages accumulate in these cells without killing them. Dust-laden macrophages then move toward the respiratory bronchioles, where they aggregate. Similar aggregations develop in pulmonary lymphoid tissue and round small vessels. As the bronchiolar aggregations enlarge, dust-laden macrophages collect upstream, resulting in the development of dust macules located in a centrilobular position, and visible to the naked eye on whole lung sections. At first the macules are little more than dust collections (see Fig. 2), but later reticulin fibers appear, with some collagen, usually distributed in a radial rather than a concentric fashion. Thus even in the presence of as much as 30 grams of coal dust per lung (autopsy measurements) the stromal reaction tends to remain for the most part noncollagenous; however, it is influenced by the other constituents of the dust, in particular mineral and silica content. This probably explains such regional differences as exist, for example, among the dust macule of the Welsh soft coal miner, the more fibrous macule of his counterpart in Belgium, and the *stellate "mixed dust" nodule* of the foundry worker. Indeed, if the silica content of lung dust exceeds 18 per cent, the associated lung lesions will almost certainly be collagenous, resembling those of classic silicosis. In addition, the radiodensity of the

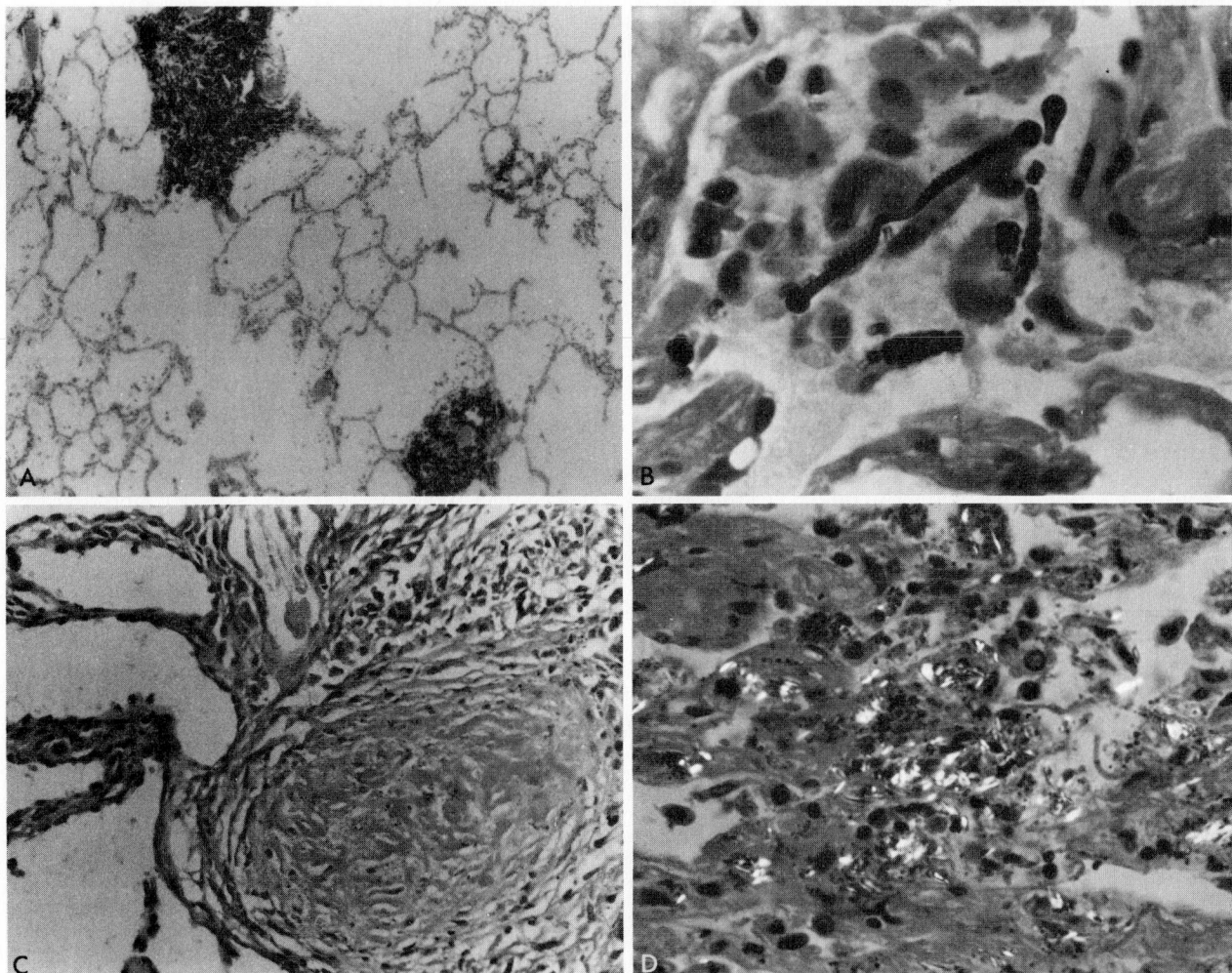

Figure 2. *A,* Coal macule located next to a distal airway; note the lack of collagenous response (× 30). *B,* Asbestos bodies in alveolar macrophages in an alveolus (× 500). *C,* Classic silicotic nodule showing a central core of dense hyalinized collagen fibers surrounded by loose fibers, arranged in a concentric manner; normal alveolar walls to one side (× 125). *D,* Classic silicotic nodule showing doubly refractile dust particles (× 300). (Courtesy of Dr. Nai-San Wang, Department of Pathology, McGill University, Montreal, Canada.)

nodules appears to be related to their iron content, endogenous iron accumulating around dust as it does around other foreign bodies. In time the respiratory bronchioles around the dust foci dilate, perhaps because of the local traction of the dust-encased bronchioles on the surrounding lung parenchyma, with bronchiolar dilatation and the development of *focal emphysema,* believed to be distinguishable from the more common centrilobular emphysema by the absence of an associated bronchiolitis. Indeed, it has been suggested that the dust sheathing accounts for this being a distention rather than a destruction emphysema.

The pathologic changes of generalized emphysema may also be seen in lungs which are affected by these nodular pneumoconioses, particularly when the nodulation is of the smaller variety (pinhead rather than micronodular). Such changes occur more frequently and to a more disabling degree (leading to pulmonary hypertension and right heart failure) in certain geographic areas, e.g., the iron mines of Lorraine and the coal mines of Belgium. Finally, pulmonary emphysema has been shown to occur more frequently in the lungs of miners than in the lungs of the nonmining population, even in the absence of pneumoconiosis, thus strengthening the evidence that dust exposure, particularly in the cigarette smoker, is a factor contributing to the development of chronic obstructive lung disease.

CLINICAL MANIFESTATIONS. The term "tattooing" of the chest roentgenogram has been applied to this group of *"benign" noncollagenous nodular pneumoconioses,* because even in the presence of diffuse radiologic nodular densities symptoms and signs of chest disease are rarely present. Thus the diagnosis is made on the basis of the presence of small rounded opacities on the chest roentgenogram characteristically distributed in the mid and upper zones; indeed, because of the close relationship between radiologic category and lung dust content, it has been suggested that the chest film remains "the only feasible method of determining and quantifying dust exposure in life." Likewise, most tests routinely used to evaluate pulmonary function, such as measurements of lung volume, flow rates, diffusing capacity at rest, and even the pulmonary mechanics, have been found to be within the normal limits in keeping with the histology of the dust macules. However, as the profusion of dust macules (reflected by advancing radiologic category) increases, detectable changes include an increase in residual volume, and a decrease in expiratory flow rates at the end of a forced expiration and in diffusing capacity (possibly related to the smaller type of nodulation), as well as abnormalities of gas distribution (reflected in dead space ventilation) and in gas exchange (reflected in A-a O_2 differences). Such changes, demonstrable at rest and exaggerated during effort, presumably reflect regional inequalities in ventilation vis-à-vis perfusion. However, they do not appear to affect function enough to cause symptoms or cause disability affecting performance; the latter, if present, is usually attributable to chronic obstructive airway disease.

EPIDEMIOLOGY AND PROGNOSIS. The prevalence rate of simple pneumoconiosis varies very much from operation to operation, even within the same industry; for example, in the 1970–71 National Coal Board survey in Britain, rates varied from 3.3 to 15.9 per cent of working miners, whereas in the 1969 Interagency study in the United States coal pits, rates varied from 4.6 to 46.0 per cent. In small uncontrolled operations prevalence may well be higher. These differences are thought to be related to the dust exposure levels, although differences in the reading of the chest roentgenogram, particularly for the lower categories of change, cannot be ignored. Prevalence usually falls dramatically as dust control becomes effective, e.g., in the Dutch coal miners rates fell from 270 to 160 per 1000 working miners over a seven-year period, but rates have leveled off in some countries, e.g., Britain — a trend attributed to increased mechanization and longer running times for coal machinery. An unfavorable influence of mechanization on prevalence has also been observed elsewhere, e.g., in the coal mines of central India. In addition, the British Coal Board study has shown that radiologic progression is related to mean mass concentration of airborne dust (not to particle counts), and occurs more rapidly in those men who develop radiologic change sooner.

In addition to the pathologic evidence quoted above, there is also epidemiologic evidence that the prevalence of symptoms of chronic bronchitis (e.g., sputum production) is increased in coal miners and that this is related to their occupation since dose relationships have been shown. However, other factors which influence its prevalence include environment (e.g., in some areas bronchitis appears to be as common among miners' wives as among the miners themselves) and cigarette smoking, since miners are frequently heavy smokers. Thus attributability is a taxing and difficult problem for compensation commissions, especially as the noncollagenous nodular pneumoconioses do not usually per se produce significant disability.

It is *unusual* for these noncollagenous pneumoconioses *to develop for the first time or to progress after exposure has ceased,* but this does occur. Likewise, the disappearance of radiologic changes after removal from exposure, though unusual, has been described, and is in keeping with animal experiments showing that dust nodules are not static structures but are the site of continuing phagocytic activity. Life expectancy does not appear to be affected by the presence of the noncollagenous pneumoconioses, provided that complicated pneumoconiosis, e.g., progressive massive fibrosis in coal miners, does not develop. This complication, by contrast, is associated with disability and premature death (see below).

Doig, A. T.: Baritosis: A benign pneumoconiosis. Thorax, 31:30, 1976.
Morgan, W. K. C., and Lapp, N. L.: Respiratory disease in coal miners. Am. Rev. Respir. Dis., 113:531, 1976.
Ryder, R., Lyons, J. P., Campbell, H., and Gough, J.: Emphysema of coal workers' pneumoconiosis. Br. Med. J., 3:481, 1970.

348.5. COLLAGENOUS PNEUMOCONIOSES (NODULAR)

EXAMPLES. Examples of these disorders include *classic silicosis of hardrock miners* (e.g., gold, tin, copper, uranium, chromite) and of *granite workers* and *cutters;* and silicosis in *iron and steel workers* and *sandblasters,* in the *pottery industry,* in industries using *silica flour,* and in those processing *bentonite* clays.

PATHOGENESIS AND MECHANISMS. If the dusts of carbon and coal represent those at the low end of the response spectrum, free crystalline silica dust represents the opposite end, with its almost unique biologic capacity to evoke a powerful fibrogenic tissue response. Silica particles are rapidly ingested by macrophages, but are only briefly retained within the phagosomes created by the invaginated cell wall before these rupture, owing to the action of lysosomal enzymes, thus freeing the particles now apparently in activated form, since cell death follows rapidly. This contrasts with the fate of the less fibrogenic dusts, which may be retained for long periods within the phagosomes of the macrophages without cell death. Other macrophages are recruited, perhaps by an autoimmune reaction, to reingest the particles with the same result. Released particles may penetrate lung tissue, with lymphatic clearance to the hilar lymph nodes, and preferential clearance from the lower lobes may explain why the subsequent tissue reaction appears more frequently in the mid and upper zones. Collagen formation follows, resulting from stimulation of fibroblasts, and finally hyalinization of the collagen to form the *characteristic fibrous silicotic nodule,* made up of whorled fibrous connective tissue like an onion. These appear first in the hilar nodes, and then in peribronchial, perilymphatic, or perivascular locations, presumably at the sites of accumulation of the activated dust particles, which, however, tend to remain on the periphery of the nodule and thus are capable of enlarging it or stimulating the formation of new nodules (see Fig. 2). Autoimmunity may play a role in recruiting macrophages to sustain the reaction and in altering the development of already established lesions, since diseases such as systemic sclerosis, which are thought also to be mediated through autoimmune mechanisms, occur with increased frequency in subjects with established silicosis and in some instances even in miners with dust exposure but no evident dust disease. An *unusual form of silicotic lung lesion* has recently been described in *Elliot Lake* (Ontario) *uranium miners,* in which the granulomas resemble those of sarcoid more than the classic silicotic nodule; the presence of radioactivity may account for this modified type of lung reaction. Extensive and marked fibrosis may be present in the lungs at autopsy with only relatively small amounts of dust (up to 10 grams, of which perhaps half is silica). Involvement of the hilar and mediastinal lymph nodes is common, occasionally with *egg-shell calcification,* but abdominal nodes are only occasionally affected. *Acute silicotic reactions* occur with heavy exposures to fine particles and may be associated with alveolar wall thickening and the accumulation of proteinaceous fluid in the alveolar spaces *(alveolar lipoproteinosis),* thought to be due in part to overloading of the clearance mechanisms and accumulation of surfactant. Sarcoid-like granulomas may also be seen, and complicating infection, particularly by mycobacteria, including atypical forms, is frequent. In nature, free crystalline silica occurs almost exclusively as quartz; however, other free crystalline silicas, e.g., crystobalite, tridymite, though rare in natural geologic formation, may be formed from quartz in steel-making and in other high-heat smelting processes, and probably have a more powerful silicosis-producing action than quartz.

Conglomerate silicosis is the result of the matting together by fibrosis of silicotic nodules, often with obliteration of bronchi and blood vessels, and frequently associated with caseous areas and cavitation, which often but by no means always show conclusive histologic evidence of tuberculosis. These changes account for the right heart strain, hypertrophy, and failure which may

develop subsequently, perhaps as a consequence of the pulmonary vascular bed's being reduced by the fibrosis and tissue loss and associated emphysematous changes in the adjacent lung. A reversible element in the pulmonary hypertension may also be present, related perhaps to hypoxia or hypercapnia or both.

CLINICAL MANIFESTATIONS. Nodular silicosis is essentially a chronic disease, and radiologic changes rarely appear before 20 years of exposure. However, even in this disease in which the radiologic lesions are fibrous nodules, not noncollagenous dust macules, there may be no clinical manifestations and no apparent impairment in pulmonary function, particularly for Category 1 radiologic disease. However, the proportion of cases without signs and symptoms is probably only about 20 per cent, in contrast to about 90 per cent in the noncollagenous pneumoconioses of equivalent radiologic category.

The first complaint in nodular silicosis is commonly *shortness of breath,* brought on by moderate, and then progressively less, exercise until it is present at rest. This symptom is probably due to the increased muscular work required to ventilate incompliant lungs and is aggravated by increased minute ventilation to offset impaired gas exchange. Lung volumes are reduced as the nodular disease becomes more widespread. Other changes may follow, including a reduction of diffusing capacity commensurate with the volume reduction, a further fall in compliance, impaired mixing, and disturbances of gas exchange (attributed to impairment of regional ventilation-perfusion balance), eventually with hypoxemia, first on exercise and then at rest. However, the over-all function profile is by no means always restrictive; in particular, miners who smoke may present with the symptoms, signs, and classic lung function pattern of chronic obstructive lung disease, even though the radiologic pattern is primarily that of diffuse nodular pneumoconiosis. Additional symptoms include *cough* and *sputum* (usually the consequence of cigarette smoking), *hemoptysis* and *chest pain* (usually associated with intercurrent infection), and, rarely, pressure effects of calcified hilar nodes on neighboring structures (superior vena cava, esophagus, phrenic nerves, and bronchus).

When *complicated pneumoconiosis* develops *on a background of classic silicosis,* the symptoms, signs, and clinical presentation usually represent a progression from an already symptomatic state, and the diagnosis is made from the chest radiograph which shows a conglomeration of existing lesions, usually in the upper mid-zones, often bilateral, with eventual progression to the characteristic bilateral "angels' wings" shadows. The lung function pattern may suggest restrictive disease but frequently shows a pattern characteristic of obstructive disease, or there may be a mixed picture. Infection with *M. tuberculosis* is more likely to be demonstrable in conglomerate silicosis than in the progressive massive fibrosis of coal workers, and is more likely to behave and progress as in the nonsilicotic lung with constitutional symptoms (see below). Right heart strain and failure may complicate the picture, particularly if chronic bronchitis and emphysema are present. *An accelerated form of silicosis* may develop with a shorter incubation period after first exposure (e.g., four to eight years) if exposure has been heavy. Its clinical features are similar to those of the chronic form, but the over-all course to death is rapid (approximately ten years), and complicating infection by mycobacteria is common (about 25 per cent of cases).

Acute silicolipoproteinosis, a variant of accelerated silicosis with characteristic histopathologic changes, runs an even more rapid course. Clinical features include weight loss, weakness, diffuse rales, and hypoxemia. Infection with mycobacteria (often atypical) is invariable, and the clinical course to death is usually only a matter of months.

In addition, the presence of silicosis appears to be associated with an *increased prevalence of autoimmune diseases*, such as rheumatoid arthritis, systemic sclerosis, and diffuse lupus erythematosus, which occurred, for example, in 10 per cent of New Orleans sandblasters who had developed an accelerated form of silicosis. An increased incidence of systemic sclerosis has also been reported in Witwatersrand gold miners.

EPIDEMIOLOGY AND PROGNOSIS. Prevalence rates vary between as well as within mines or other operations, the variations reflecting differences in airborne dust levels and, most important, its free silica content. Thus in the Witwatersrand gold mining industry, rates fell from 40 per 1000 underground miners in the 1920's to less than 10 per 1000 in the 1950's, and the average period of mining service prior to diagnosis rose from 10 to 23 years over this period. Comparable over-all prevalence figures for the United States metal mining industry for 1958 to 1961 were 34 per 1000. Complacency about exposures to dusts thought to be low in silica content, e.g., in bentonite mining in the United States or granite quarrying in the West country of the United Kingdom, has accounted for recent outbreaks and should alert the physician to exploring in full the occupational history even in industries not recognized to have a health risk. In addition, epidemiologic studies have now shown that *occupational exposure to most mining environments* is a risk factor in the *development of bronchitis*, the prevalence of which is dose related to estimated exposure (see Ch. 344.1) when the greater effect of cigarette smoking has been taken into account. This is not linked to the presence of pneumoconiosis. Thus it appears that exposure to the mining environment is associated with two types of tissue response: one specific (the fibrosis of pneumoconiosis), and one nonspecific (chronic mucus hypersecretion or chronic bronchitis) — both dose related to exposure, but not apparently related to each other. The simple silicosis of hardrock miners is undoubtedly a less benign disease than the simple pneumoconiosis of coal miners, despite the fact that it does not appear to affect life expectancy, and figures for Sweden indicate that, after withdrawal from exposure, x-ray changes never regress but progress in the majority of cases (Fig. 3).

Ziskind, M., Jones, R. N., and Weill, H.: Silicosis. Am. Rev. Respir. Dis., 113:643, 1976.

348.6. COLLAGENOUS PNEUMOCONIOSES (DIFFUSE)

EXAMPLES. These pneumoconioses include *asbestosis* in mining, milling, manufacturing, and all the secondary industrial uses of asbestos, including insulation workers, particularly those pulling out old insulation in ships and buildings; *aluminosis*, as in Shaver's disease; *talcosis* in miners and millers of talc in some industrial

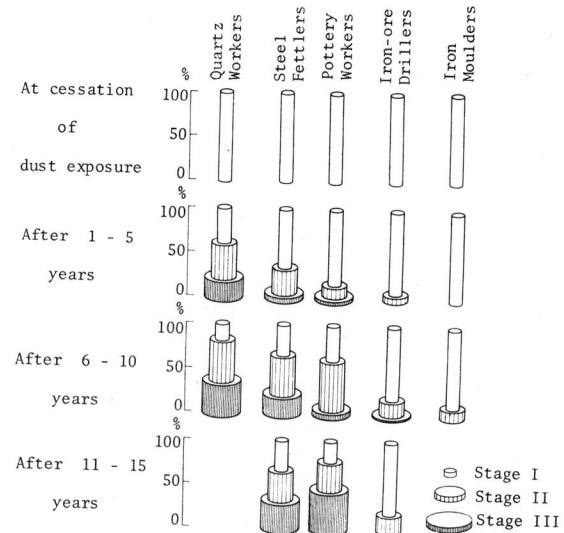

Figure 3. Rate of progression of different pneumoconioses after removal from dust exposure. The figures are based on five occupational groups of Swedish workers (each containing a minimum of ten cases) followed for 15 years after dust exposure ceased. (From Bruce, T., Nystrom, A., and Ahlmark, A. L.: Scand. J. Resp. Diseases, Supp. 63, 1968.)

processes, and also in its intravenous administration by drug users who inject solutions of talc-containing tablets; and *chronic beryllium disease of the lung*.

PATHOGENESIS AND MECHANISMS. Asbestos, the most important mineral in this group, occurs in several forms: *chrysotile* (a magnesium silicate, occurring as long, white, flexible fibers), the chief asbestos of commerce, mined primarily in Canada and the U.S.S.R. as well as in Italy and in Southern Africa; and the *amphiboles*, iron silicates (occurring as brittle fibers such as amosite, anthophyllite, and blue crocidolite) mined in South Africa, Australia, and Finland. Exposure occurs in mining and milling, and in the manufacture of a wide variety of the commodities used by modern man. *Asbestos cement products*, such as tiles and pipes, account for 70 per cent of production, and *insulation materials*, including floor tiles, for another 10 per cent; the rest is used in *paper*, *friction materials* (car brake and clutch linings), and *textiles* for use as protection against heat in industry and in homes.

The extent to which asbestos fibers penetrate the lung in all likelihood depends on their physical properties, the curly fibers of chrysotile being more likely to impinge on the mucus blanket than the short straight amphibole fibers. Some fibers appear to penetrate the interstitium directly and remain there, perhaps undergoing chemical and physical degeneration but nevertheless visible in much greater profusion than was ever suspected before the use of electron microscopy in their detection. Other fibers become engulfed by macrophages, and still others, but probably only a very small proportion of the longer fibers, become coated by a smooth protein film which becomes iron-impregnated, giving rise to the typical drumhead, golden-brown *asbestos bodies* (see Fig. 2), a process also attributed at least in part to macrophage action. There is some evidence that the coating of a fiber renders it nonfibrogenic. The pleura also appears to be a target organ, although it is not clear how the fibers gain access to the pleura, for pleural reactions may occur even in the absence of demonstrable fibers in the lung, and coated fibers are rarely seen in the pleura. It is possible that small fibers may be cleared to subpleural lymphatics and for some reason undergo dissolution here more readily than in other parts of the lung. *Pleural reactions* include *effusion* (often bloody); dense, fibrous, *adhesive pleurisy; plaques* and *calcification* involving parietal rather than visceral pleura; and malignancy in the form of *mesothelioma* (see below).

It is not known which fibers are, or become, fibrogenic; nor is their precise mode of action known. However, observed cytogenic effects include an interaction with the cell membrane, increasing permeability, and an interreaction of already ingested particles with the lysosomal membrane. Target cells include the macrophage, mesothelial cells, alveolar epithelial cells, and fibroblasts. Fibers deposited in alveolar structures elicit a cellular reaction similar to *desquamative alveolitis;* others at the level of the respiratory bronchiole produce an appearance of *bronchiolitis obliterans;* a third reaction is characterized by *interstitial edema* going on to *collagenization*. Nonspecific antinuclear antibodies may accelerate the fibrosis once it has started, and it eventually becomes confluent, obliterating air spaces and replacing them with cystic spaces lined by flattened epithelium ("honeycomb" lung). Other mineral dusts which produce this pattern of diffuse fibrosis are talc and diatomaceous earth.

Generalized pulmonary fibrosis may also be found in *chronic beryllium disease* of the lung, now thought to be the end result of a Type IV immune reaction to the inhalation of beryllium salts. The granulomas which characterize the earlier stage of the process are indistinguishable histologically from those of sarcoidosis, and may vary from loose collections of histiocytes to large circumscribed granulomas, often containing giant cells with various inclusion bodies. Although the lung is the organ most seriously affected, presumably because it is the portal of entry, granulomas are found throughout the body, involving hilar, mediastinal, and abdominal lymph nodes, liver, spleen, skin, and in fact all organs involved in sarcoidosis except the eye, parotid, and tonsil. Beryllium has been isolated, in varying amounts, from all these tissues (about 0.5 gram of tissue is necessary for this analysis), and the diagnosis can be made with certainty only by isolation of the element beryllium in tissues or body fluids. There is often a very long period of latency, up to 30 years, and initial exposure may have been only indirect, e.g., neighborhood exposure (residence close to a plant using beryllium), so that cases related to the manufacture of fluorescent light in the United States during World War II continue to be reported today, even though the use of beryllium in the fluorescent lamp industry ceased in 1949. Although its modern uses, particularly those concerned with space exploration, appear to be better controlled, physicians should remain vigilant because new cases continue to be added to the U.S. Beryllium Registry at the Massachusetts General Hospital.

CLINICAL MANIFESTATIONS. These are no different from those of diffuse pulmonary fibrosis, whatever the underlying cause. In some subjects *dyspnea* is the first symptom, brought on at first by considerable exertion and then by progressively less effort, until it is eventually present at rest. In other subjects, an *irritating dry cough* precedes the awareness of shortness of breath, often by many years. With the progress of the disease, the cough may become productive, and *spells of chest pain* may be associated with the coughing. When the condition is advanced, there are usually diffuse basal rales, but these may also occur early before radiologic evidence of lung changes. The lung signs may be modified by the presence of pleural thickening or calcification. Respiratory failure may only appear late in the course of the disease, with pulmonary hypertension, right heart strain, and right heart failure. Nor is the victim of these diffuse pneumoconioses immune from the attack by general atmospheric pollutants — in particular, cigarette smoking — which may encourage the development of chronic bronchitis and bronchiectasis and increase the risk of bronchial neoplasm.

The *radiologic changes* are also no different from those seen in all other forms of diffuse interstitial fibrosis except for the *prominence of the associated pleural changes;* in particular, calcification should direct attention to the possibility of exposure to asbestos or talc. Thus for the purpose of diagnosis of the individual case, the features to be evaluated are, in particular, prevalence, extent and character of *small irregular opacities in the parenchyma*, and the site, width, and extent of *pleural thickening or calcification*, as outlined in the ILO classification. Rounded opacities are more frequent when the exposure includes silica.

In certain parts of the world, e.g., Finland, *pleural calcification* may appear as the only manifestation of exposure to anthophyllite, asbestos, and less commonly talc and mica. It is rarely seen under 20 years of industrial exposure, and neighborhood cases are seen with diminishing frequency as the circumferential distance of the place of residence from the industry increases.

The *established case of asbestosis* is associated with changes in pulmonary function characteristic of restrictive lung disease, i.e., small volumes, reduced compliance, impaired gas exchange with reduced diffusing capacity, and hyperventilation on effort and eventually at rest. The earliest function changes in response to asbestos dust exposure appear to be reduced vital capacity and increased exercise ventilation, tests which may eventually prove useful in the longitudinal surveillance of exposed workers. In addition, the function changes of chronic obstructive lung disease are not infrequently seen, particularly in workers who smoke.

In addition, changes in lung function may be detected in the healthy worker before symptoms and sometimes before radiographic changes occur, changes which are thought to reflect the effects of asbestos exposure in the lung and which vary from subject to subject, presumably according to the particular location of the tissue responses in his lung, i.e., peribronchiolar, pleural, or interstitial. These include changes in tests thought to represent small airway status, as well as in vital capacity, exercise ventilation, and possibly diffusing capacity. Small changes in tests of this sort, particularly the vital capacity, although not likely to be useful in the diagnosis of the individual case, may, however, eventually prove useful in the *long-term surveillance of exposed workers*, particularly if followed over time from their recruitment into the industry.

EPIDEMIOLOGY AND PROGNOSIS. The *attack rate of asbestosis* varies in different industries from under 10 per cent of miners working in open pits, as in Quebec, up to over 70 per cent in men with long exposure in the insulation and construction industries. These differences are thought to reflect primarily differences in exposure levels to respirable dust, which is often higher in industrial operations with the progressive manipulation of the fiber and its fractionation into small particles, which penetrate the lung further with higher retention rates.

The epidemiology of *population exposure* to *asbestos* has been established from the search for asbestos bodies in lung scrapings or extruded lung fluid in routine autopsies. Positive results are reported in many parts of the world, ranging from 1 per cent in rural Italy to over 50 per cent in Finland, the site of the world's oldest known asbestos deposits; prevalence is also consistently higher in men than in women, increases with age, and shows within-city variation in relation to proximity of residence to industrial areas. Insofar as the lung is an accumulator over time, and the world's use of asbestos is increasing dramatically, it is not surprising that this percentage is increasing in adults in London; New York studies by contrast report between 50 and 60 per cent both in recent and in 1934 autopsy material. It must be emphasized that the presence of *ferruginous bodies* (as experts now urge that they be called) indicates exposure, not disease. Nor are they specific for asbestos, because other types of fibers, e.g., glass, wool, cotton, talc, may constitute their core, and the lung probably uses this method to "inactivate" a large variety of inhaled particles. However, their presence in the sputum or other biologic material should alert the physician to the strong possibility of an occupational exposure, past, even remote past, or present, which he should explore with vigor for its relationship to any current pulmonary disease.

Becklake, M. R.: Asbestos-related diseases of the lung and other organs: Their epidemiology and implications for clinical practice. Am. Rev. Respir. Dis., 114:187, 1976.

Hamilton, A., and Hardy, H. L.: Industrial Toxicology. 3rd ed. Acton, Mass., Publishing Sciences Group, Inc., 1974, p. 43.

348.7. COMPLICATED PNEUMOCONIOSIS

EXAMPLES. Examples of the complicated pneumoconioses include *progressive massive fibrosis of coal workers* and *Caplan's syndrome*.

PATHOGENESIS AND MECHANISMS. Progressive massive fibrosis (defined as a radiologic lesion greater than 1 cm in diameter) may develop as a complication of most inorganic dust pneumoconioses, including those which are noncollagenous, usually on the background of Category 2 or 3 disease, and this complication may occur even after exposure has ceased. Thus, although initially the response to dust exposure may be a macrophage reaction producing a noncollagenous response with little effect on the lung architecture, years later the same lung tissue may react to the same dust with severe fibrosis which obliterates and destroys all anatomic structure. On macroscopic examination the lesions of *progressive massive fibrosis in coal workers* (PMF) are amorphous, irregular, rubbery, and relatively homogeneous. Microscopic examination shows the central core of the lesion to be made up of an insoluble protein complex; its capsule consists of dust irregularly mixed with bundles of coarse, hyaline collagen fibers. Few blood vessels and air passages are seen, but the persis-

tence of internal elastic lamellae suggests that they have been obliterated by invading fibrous tissue. In addition, there is sclerosis of the vessel walls, often with invasion by dust-laden cells and evidence of endarteritis at the periphery of the lesion; *emphysema*, usually of an *irregular* nature, frequently develops in association with the lesions of PMF which often distort the major and medium-sized airways, and histologic or bacteriologic evidence of *Mycobacterium tuberculosis* is found in a high proportion of cases.

Several mechanisms may be operative in the development of complicated pneumoconiosis, of which infection by *M. tuberculosis* and/or atypical mycobacteria is probably the most frequent (the recovery rate of organisms both in life and at autopsy increases with increasing effort and has exceeded 50 per cent in some autopsy series). Clinical evidence includes the observation of an increased attack rate of PMF in miners who developed active tuberculosis after gastrectomy for peptic ulcer. However, the disease has been shown to develop in a substantial number of subjects with negative tuberculin skin tests (particularly in the United States), whereas in the Rhonda Fach in Wales a decline in attack rate of tuberculosis was not accompanied by a concomitant decline in the attack rate of PMF. Thus in some cases, other mechanisms may be important; these include the overwhelming of clearance mechanisms by lung dust; aseptic necrosis owing to interference with blood supply; significant silica contamination of the coal dust; and, finally, reaction on an immunologic basis, in which the coal dust acts as an absorptive surface for proteins. Immune mechanisms are also thought to play a role in the development of *Caplan's syndrome*. Caplan observed an association between rheumatoid arthritis and a particular radiologic picture in miners, characterized by well-defined opacities 0.5 to 5 cm in diameter, widely distributed and developing rather more suddenly than progressive massive fibrosis, often on a background of slight or no pneumoconiosis. Some lesions eventually cavitate, then shrink, perhaps with calcifications, and may later become incorporated into a mass radiologically indistinguishable from progressive massive fibrosis. Histologically, the rheumatoid nodule contains a central core of necrotic collagen separated by bands of dust, with a peripheral zone of active inflammation and a well-marked arteritis in the adjacent vessels. Caplan's syndrome, though first recognized and most frequently seen in coal miners, has been described in workers in foundries, asbestos, potteries, sandblasting, and boiler scaling. Most of the evidence supports the view that the lung lesions in Caplan's syndrome are a manifestation of *rheumatoid disease facilitated by the presence of dust*. Thus in Wales there is no evidence that coal mining predisposes to the development of rheumatoid arthritis, but the prevalence of PMF (and incidentally of tuberculosis) was increased in miners with this disease. Furthermore rheumatoid factor was positive with greater frequency in miners with Caplan's syndrome (approximately 70 per cent) than in those with PMF (30 to 40 per cent), whereas lower figures were observed in men with simple pneumoconiosis. By contrast in Appalachian coal miners, the prevalence of rheumatoid factor appeared to relate not to radiologic lesions suggesting Caplan's syndrome but to the type of coal mined, being highest in anthracite miners with PMF (74 per cent). Thus there remain aspects of the interrelationships of simple pneumoconiosis, PMF, and Caplan's syndrome which require clarification.

CLINICAL MANIFESTATIONS. In coal workers, the appearance of progressive massive fibrosis usually marks the onset of symptoms and signs of lung disease. The first symptom is commonly *dyspnea* on heavy effort, and subsequently at lesser work loads until it becomes evident at rest. The changes in function initially suggest loss of functioning volume, followed by a generalized restrictive lung disease. The symptom of cough does not appear to be more common in the earlier stages of complicated pneumoconiosis than in simple pneumoconiosis. *Melanoptysis* (sudden coughing up of a moderate amount of jet black fluid) is not uncommon, and frequently relates to cavitation. *Chest pain*, dull and aching, and diffusely located, is common, and there is an increasing tendency to *acute purulent bronchitis*. Pulmonary hypertension and right heart hypertrophy, leading ultimately to *right heart failure*, is present in many instances, with the usual symptoms and signs. When infection with *M. tuberculosis* appears to be the factor precipitating the development of the complicated pneumoconiosis, it is seldom accompanied by the usual systemic symptoms, i.e., fever, weight loss, and hemoptysis.

When the chest roentgenogram suggests Caplan's syndrome (see above), serum tests for rheumatoid factor are positive in over 70 per cent of cases, whereas arthritis, already present in about 50 per cent of cases, may develop in others only after a delay of several years.

EPIDEMIOLOGY AND PROGNOSIS. *Attack rates of PMF vary* within a region, chiefly in relation to the *background of radiologic category* (e.g., 0.7 and 4.3 per cent per year for Category 1 and 3, respectively, in South Wales), but they also decline steeply in relation to *age*. They tend to be higher in those whose chest radiographs show the *more rapid progression of disease*, but are apparently uninfluenced by smoking, energy expenditure, tuberculous infection, and even continued exposure. Considerable between-region differences (e.g., high in France and eastern Pennsylvania, low in Utah) may well be due to variations in some of the factors mentioned above. Rheumatoid pneumoconiosis occurs in 2 to 6 per cent of United Kingdom coal miners affected by pneumoconiosis, and should be suspected when PMF develops suddenly in an individual with minimal or no pneumoconiosis. By contrast with simple coal workers' pneumoconiosis, PMF does affect mortality, but it is of interest that this does not apply to lesions less than 20 sq cm in size on the chest radiograph.

Benedek, T.: Rheumatoid pneumoconiosis: Documentation of onset and pathogenic considerations. Am. J. Med., 55:515, 1973.
Morgan, W. K. C.: Coal workers' pneumoconiosis. *In* Morgan, W. K. C., and Seaton, A. (eds.): Occupational Lung Diseases. Philadelphia, W. B. Saunders Company, 1975, p. 149.

348.8. INORGANIC DUST PNEUMOCONIOSES: TREATMENT AND PREVENTION

TREATMENT. There is *no specific treatment for the simple nodular or diffuse inorganic dust pneumoconioses* once the diagnosis is established. Nor does it seem likely that any of the materials mentioned under Prophylactic Substances, below, will be effective, although so far aluminum is the only one to have received a careful clinical trial. Despite this, the physician has an extremely important role to play in management, both in support of and advice to an individual faced with a threat to his livelihood due to diagnosis of a disease related to the source of his livelihood. Advice depends primarily on evaluating *factors which influence outcome*, most important of which is diagnosis of whether the *pneumoconiosis is noncollagenous (and likely to affect health, function, or longevity)* or *collagenous (carrying threats to all of the above)*. Other factors include the *immune status* and *skin reactivity* to mycobacteria, *age*, and an *evaluation of the current as opposed to past risks* (including dust levels) in the *particular working environment* concerned. The physician must attempt to answer the following questions as accurately as he can: (1) *What is the likely outcome* in this particular case? (2) *Should he advise the patient to seek other employment?* These questions are easier to answer when the subject is a "patient" with complaints for which he seeks the physician's help, but much harder when the individual is working and believes himself to be in good health, but has an abnormality on the chest roentgenogram and/or a small loss of lung function. For the noncollagenous pneumoconioses, most physicians will permit continued employment given regular health surveillance measures. For the collagenous pneumoconioses, progression to complicated disease appears to depend as much on past as on subsequent exposure (see Fig. 2), and the decision is much more difficult. Although animal studies do suggest that withdrawal from exposure slows progression, extrapolation of these results to man must be done with caution, despite the intuitive reaction to act on them.

In *complicated pneumoconiosis*, the medical management of associated chronic obstructive lung disease and right heart failure and pulmonary heart disease is the same whether or not it coexists with pneumoconiosis (see Ch. 351). When active tuberculous infection with mycobacteria, including atypical types, can be demonstrated, and probably even when the only evidence is a positive skin test to PPD, appropriate chemotherapy should be instituted (see Ch. 167). The addition of rifampin to the treatment regimen has received favorable comment. Nevertheless, although treatment is usually successful in respect of sputum conversion, radiologic clearing is less impressive; and controlled clinical trials do not support the routine use of tuberculosis chemoprophylaxis in all cases of PMF irrespective of whether active tuberculous infection can be demonstrated. Neither antituberculous treatment nor steroids appear to influence the evolution of Caplan's syndrome. Since complicated pneumoconiosis is invariably accompanied by disability, often associated with right heart failure, most patients with complicated pneumoconiosis will have already left the industry concerned. Opinion is divided on the advisability of withdrawal from exposure if the patient is still so occupied.

In *acute silicosis*, progression to death is rapid and does not appear to be halted by any treatment measures, including steroids. Lung transplant has been carried out in two cases, one with survival up to ten months. The management of *alveolar lipoproteinosis* associated with silica exposure is no different on this account; however, if bronchial lavage is considered, the addition of PVNO (see below) to the lavage fluid might be considered on purely theoretical grounds, without as yet any published practical report.

DUST CONTROL. Inorganic dust pneumoconioses cannot be treated effectively, but they can be prevented, and *prevention* means, essentially, *dust control*. Attack rate increases with exposure, and there is a dust dose–disease relationship. Thus *control should be at an epidemiologic level*, aiming at controlling the exposure of the community at risk, not at a personal level with the use of masks or respirators, which should preferably be regarded as a measure for temporary use when circumstances force the suspension of other control measures. Indeed their use, often incorrectly, in the past has led to a false sense of security on the part of the worker and his employer; for instance, *inside* the hoods used, though not consistently, by Gulf sandblasters, respirable dust of high silica content reached average levels of three times, ranging up to 50 times, in excess of recommended standards. Dust can seldom be completely eliminated from industrial operations. However, disease could be controlled if the minimal exposure which produces health effects in a given industry were known, and increasing efforts are being made to translate available scientific information, in particular epidemiologic studies, into estimates of health risk. For instance, it has been estimated that the probability of a British coal worker developing Category 2 (or higher) pneumoconiosis is 3.4 per cent given a 35-year working exposure at an average dust concentration of 4.3 mg per cubic meter. Similarly, the risk of developing asbestosis has been estimated at under 1 per cent for a 50-year working exposure at an average fiber level of 2 per cubic centimeter. It is possible to envisage a future in which, using cumulative ongoing records of each worker's exposure, operations could be planned so that no worker would be likely to exceed the exposure known to produce disease within his working life. Such an ambitious scheme, already under way in the West German coal mining industry, is likely to be set up only in large industries able to mount extensive research programs. However, for smaller industries, it is quite valid to assert that *less dust means less disease*. Equally important aspects of environmental control are work practices, often best controlled not by directive but by worker education and worker participation in environmental monitoring with posting of information. Provision of laundry facilities at work to avoid the "take-home" hazards of the past—e.g., asbestos, beryllium—is equally important. *Threshold limit values* are annually revised by bodies such as the American Conference of Governmental Industrial Hygienists and provide general reference standards. However, it should be clear to the physician that these are only estimates of safe levels, based on the information presently available, and he should not be deterred from making the diagnosis of pneumoconiosis because the individual has worked in a controlled environment only; controls may fail and estimates may be inaccurate, and the physician must not automatically assume that his patient is "protected."

TUBERCULOSIS CONTROL IN WORKING POPULATIONS. Medical attention should be directed toward reducing the attack rates of complicated pneumoconiosis and silicotuberculosis. All subjects with pneumoconiosis are at a higher risk in terms of tuberculosis

than the general population; in addition the circumstances of employment may favor infection, e.g., recruitment of workers from populations in which infection with tubercle bacilli occurs relatively late in life. Case finding and control of tuberculosis should thus be of a particularly high standard in populations exposed to an inorganic dust hazard; at the very least this should include a pre-employment tuberculin skin test and chest roentgenogram, the latter to be repeated subsequently at appropriate intervals. Finally, gastrectomy for peptic ulcer should be avoided in subjects with pneumoconiosis (see above).

PROPHYLACTIC SUBSTANCES. Studies in laboratory animals have indicated that certain substances (ferric oxide, iron, coal, aluminum, and, more recently, poly-2-vinyl-pyridine-N-oxide or PVNO) depress or inhibit the biologic effects of silica dust. Of these materials only aluminum has received a trial in man as a prophylactic or preventive measure when it was introduced into the gold mines of Ontario in 1943; however, no conclusive evidence on its effectiveness has come out of this experience, and this type of prophylaxis is a sorry substitute for proper environmental dust control. PVNO has also received a limited trial in Europe.

Becklake, M. R.: Asbestos-related diseases of the lung and other organs: Their epidemiology and implications for clinical practice. Am. Rev. Respir. Dis., 114:187, 1976.

Dubois, P., Gyselen, A., and Prignot, J.: Rifampin-combined chemotherapy in coalworker's pneumoconiotuberculosis. Am. Rev. Respir. Dis., 115:221, 1977.

Kennedy, M. C. S.: Aluminum powder inhalations in the treatment of silicosis of pottery workers and pneumoconiosis of coalminers. Br. J. Industr. Med., 13:85, 1956.

Morgan, W. K. C., and Seaton, A.: Occupational Lung Diseases. Philadelphia, W. B. Saunders Company, 1975, pp. 108, 203.

348.9.   NEOPLASIA ASSOCIATED WITH DUST EXPOSURE

ASBESTOS. The carcinogenic potential of asbestos has been amply confirmed by animal experiments, and human exposure should also be regarded as always potentially carcinogenic. Thus in man it has been shown that exposure increases the attack rate (probably in a dose-related fashion) of *bronchial carcinoma*, and also of *laryngeal cancer*, particularly in smokers, suggesting a synergism between these carcinogens. It has been estimated that if smoking and asbestos exposure separately increase the risk of developing bronchogenic cancer about ten-fold, the two factors together increase the risk about 80-fold. In addition, the risk is increased by the presence of asbestosis, and some reports indicate that neoplasia will develop in 50 per cent of patients with already established asbestosis. However, the belief that all excess lung tumors are "scar cancers" (i.e., adenocarcinomas) is supported by only some of the studies examining cell types of cancer in asbestos-exposed victims of this disease. Exposure to asbestos dust is also associated with increased risk of *gastrointestinal neoplasia*, presumably because of dust swallowing. An unusual feature is the occurrence of multiple cancers, e.g., in lung and gut. Thus far, however, no link between nonoccupational exposure (e.g., to asbestos fibers in drinking water) and gastrointestinal neoplasia has been shown. Finally a rare tumor, *mesothelioma of the pleura and/or peritoneum*, occurs with greater frequency not only in industrially exposed populations, but also in association with indirect exposure, often after a long latent period, e.g., neighborhood exposure as a child 40 years before. This led to the supposition that this type of cancer was not dose related to exposure. However, careful fiber counts in affected lungs suggest that for this cancer, too, there is a dose relationship to fibers retained in the lung.

Although all types of asbestos fiber are implicated in the increased incidence of neoplasia, the order of increase varies, being on the whole higher for those engaged in processing and using than for those engaged in mining or milling. To what extent these differences are attributable to dust dose, fiber type, changes in physical and chemical properties with processing, and/or contamination by cocarcinogens remains to be determined. For mesothelioma, however, the evidence to date suggests that fiber type is important, the risk being greatest with exposure to crocidolite, less with amosite, and possibly even less with chrysotile.

AIRBORNE RADIOACTIVE PARTICLES. Knowledge of an excess mortality in the Schneeberg metal miners dates back to the sixteenth century, and is likely to have been due to lung cancer associated with the radioactivity of these mines. This risk has persisted into the twentieth century. In North America, an increased number of deaths from lung cancer have been observed in Colorado as well as Ontario uranium miners, the risk being related to the estimated radiation dose with a preponderance of small cell cancers. In these men also, smoking considerably increased the risk. Furthermore, regular sputum cytology examinations in this occupational group have shown progression from mild through moderate to marked atypia, over a time span of, on the average, up to ten years before the identification of a carcinoma in situ, information which permits a realistic evaluation of sputum cytology as a screening procedure. Increased deaths from lung cancer have also been observed in miners handling other materials, thought to be noncarcinogenic, in whom exposure has occurred to mine air contaminated by radon decay products from the ore-bearing rock or mine water, e.g., fluorspar miners of St. Lawrence, Newfoundland, and hematite miners in Cumberland, England.

OTHER OCCUPATIONS AT RISK. Increases in mortality from lung cancer have been reported in a number of other occupations which involve exposure to dusts and/or fumes and chemicals, without identification of the specific agent implicated. These include *chromate workers, workers in nickel refineries and in copper smelters, coke oven workers* in the United States, *gas workers* in the United Kingdom, and workers exposed to chlormethyl-ether. Indeed Doll has estimated that up to 50 per cent of cigarette-caused lung cancer may be dependent on the synergistic effect of an atmospheric pollutant, and the ever expanding number of occupations for which an increased risk has been demonstrated is in keeping with this belief.

Whether or not a neoplasm is occupation associated makes no difference to the outcome as far as the individual patient is concerned; *recognition of this association* on the part of the attending physician may, however, be important both from the patient's point of view (because of the question of compensation) and from the point of view of the patient's working colleagues, since index cases serve to direct attention to as yet unrecognized occupational hazards. It has been suggested as a rule of thumb that *for a working population of 1000 men, diagnosis of the second case of cancer of the lung* should arouse

suspicion in the mind of the occupational physician that there is an excess lung cancer risk requiring investigation.

Becklake, M. R.: Asbestos-related diseases of the lung and other organs: Their epidemiology and implications for clinical practice. Am. Rev. Respir. Dis., 114:187, 1976.

Seaton, A.: Occupational pulmonary neoplasms. *In* Morgan, W. K. C., and Seaton, A. (eds.): Occupational Lung Diseases. Philadelphia, W. B. Saunders Company, 1975, p. 357.

348.10. OCCUPATIONAL BRONCHITIS

Chronic bronchitis may be defined as a *clinical syndrome* characterized by *sputum production*, often with a *cough*, and frequently associated with *airflow obstruction*. A *relationship with exposure to cigarette smoke* was strongly suspected by clinicians, but was difficult to confirm by clinical observation alone for a number of reasons: a persistent cough is so frequently accepted as a "normal" phenomenon in a smoker, smoking is such a widespread habit, and few individuals consult a doctor for just a cough. It was through the study of its manifestations in the population at large, using the techniques of epidemiology, that the strength and importance of this relationship were revealed, a relationship which is now accepted as causal. By this the epidemiologist means that the relationship is consistent (i.e., has been found in almost all populations studied, in almost all circumstances, and in almost all countries), and is dose-related, including the influence of withdrawal (i.e., the manifestations occur more frequently in those who smoke more heavily, and tend to diminish in those who quit), as well as having a consistent time relationship (i.e., manifestations develop *after*, not *before*, the smoking habit is taken up). Additional *environmental risk factors* shown to be important are urban (as opposed to rural) living and social class (at least in Britain); *host factors* which influence its prevalence include sex, age, race, childhood health, and probably some genetic factors. In passing, it should be pointed out to the clinician who generally regards with scorn the epidemiologist's definition of bronchitis (positive answers to a standardized questionnaire indicating the presence of "cough with production of sputum occurring on most days for at least three months of the year during at least two years") that this definition, never intended for clinical diagnosis, was developed for use in population studies as an indicator of the presence of a clinical condition, and as such has proved a powerful tool in discerning the risk factors listed above.

Occupations which result in individuals being exposed to the *inhalation of dusts* (see above), *fumes, and vapors* (see below) have also been suspected by clinicians of contributing to the development of chronic bronchitis, but a problem has been to disentangle the relative importance of smoking (usually practiced by over 60 per cent of any particular occupation group). In addition, *in studies in which the population has also been at risk for developing other dust-related diseases*, in particular pneumoconiosis, *the two diseases (chronic bronchitis and pneumoconiosis) do not appear to be directly linked.* A likely explanation is that each represents the response to a different size range of dust particles, pneumoconiosis representing the lung tissue response to the smaller particles which penetrate deeply and are more likely to be retained, whereas chronic bronchitis is the consequence of the deposition of larger particles in major airways with perhaps irritation and stimulation of mucus glands and probably also goblet cells. When the possible responses to dust inhalation are considered separately in this way, and when smoking has been taken into account, an *increased prevalence of chronic bronchitis has been consistently found in mining populations*, and has invariably been shown to be dose related to estimated dust exposure. Occupations in which the prevalence of bronchitis appears to be increased include coal mining (in the United States, United Kingdom, Belgium, and Germany), gold mining (in South Africa), asbestos mining (in Canada), chemical workers (in the United Kingdom and Canada), and coke oven workers (in the United Kingdom), as well as cement workers, rubber workers, cotton workers, wool workers, and grain handlers. This list is not exhaustive.

A consistent finding, however, has been the *predominant influence of cigarette smoking compared to that of occupations* on the prevalence of bronchitis. Furthermore, some studies have shown the excess prevalence to be present in smokers only; others suggest synergism between the two factors, and yet others suggest the opposite. Nor is the association with airflow obstruction (reflected in pulmonary function tests) always clear. A next step is to re-evaluate the influence of dust exposure on symptoms (i.e., mucus hypersecretion) and airflow obstruction separately; it may be that these, too, are separate responses to dust exposure, in the same ways as they have recently been shown by Fletcher to be separate responses to cigarette exposure. Other unanswered questions include the relative importance of withdrawal from dust exposure and quitting smoking on symptoms and on airflow obstruction thought to be dust related, and the influence, if any, of both on morbidity and mortality.

There can be little doubt that *chronic bronchitis (either as diagnosed by the clinician or as detected by the epidemiologist) is a disease of multifactorial etiology, with risk factors attributable to both the host and the environment*, one of which is *exposure to different industrial environments in the pursuit of different occupations*. As in other conditions of multifactorial etiology, not only are difficulties encountered by the scientist attempting to study these factors and elucidate their relative importance in populations, but difficulties are also encountered by the physician attempting to translate this information into clinical practice, both in management of the individual case and in evaluation for compensation purposes. Society, through legislative action, is equally at a loss to know how to act, because it is as yet impossible to apportion relative importance of the different risk factors in an individual case. Should occupation be considered the only risk factor, and so compensated? Or should it be relegated to second place in the presence of the most important other risk factor, the cigarette? Neither seems just, and for the moment and until further evidence becomes available, a preferable way to proceed seems to be by clinical diagnosis, a procedure which, in scientific parlance, proposes the "best available hypothesis" to explain the known facts about the individual and all the occupations he has ever pursued, past and present.

Fletcher, C., and Peto, R.: The natural history of chronic airflow obstruction. Br. Med. J., 1:1645, 1977.

Higgins, I. T.: Epidemiology of Chronic Respiratory Disease: A Literature Review. Publication No. EPA-650/1–74–007. Washington, D.C., Office of Research and Development, Environmental Protection Agency, 1974.

Lapp, N. L.: Industrial bronchitis. *In* Morgan, W. K. C., and Seaton, A. (eds.): Occupational Lung Diseases. Philadelphia, W. B. Saunders Company, 1975, p. 265.

348.11. ACUTE AIRWAY REACTIONS TO ORGANIC PARTICLES

EXAMPLES. Examples include "asthma" in workers exposed to the enzymes of *B. subtilis* in the manufacture of detergents and asthma in workers with Western red cedar (*Thuja plicata*) and in grainhandlers.

PATHOGENESIS AND MECHANISMS. Inhalation of organic materials may provoke *airway reaction on a nonimmunologic basis*, the result of *stimulation of cough and irritant receptors* which cause *reflex constriction of the airways via vagal pathways*. These receptors are believed to be located in the complex network of nerve endings beneath and between the cells of the alveolar epithelium, cough receptors occurring in the major airways (especially in the larynx and carina), whereas irritant receptors, stimulation of which also results in hyperpnea, occur in the more peripheral airways. The trigger mechanism is likely to be *mechanical irritation* due to the deposition of inhaled particles. Of interest is the fact that *receptor reactivity may be enhanced in the presence of pathologic changes in the airways*, e.g., inflammation, and may account for epidemics of *acute febrile episodes associated with asthma* reported, for instance, by grain handlers, in association with the contamination of grain by bacterial toxins. Similar episodes have been described in cotton weavers.

In addition, inhaled organic materials may evoke *airway reactions on an immunologic basis*, and reactions may be immediate (within minutes), late (within the hour), delayed (within hours), nocturnal (following exposure), and even recurrent nocturnal (on subsequent nights without subsequent exposure) (see Ch. 344). *In the individual subject the mechanism underlying an airway response* will be determined not only by his *immunologic reactivity* (atopic status and probably also nonspecific airway reactivity), and *nature of the exposure* (in particular, whether there has been a previous sensitizing contact with the offending material), but also by the *dose of inhaled material* (heavy doses appear to be capable of provoking immune reaction in nonatopic individuals), as well as the *particle size distribution* (which will influence the site of deposition). More than one type of reaction may occur in the same individual so that it is not always possible clinically to determine the mechanism(s) responsible in a particular patient.

For a detailed discussion of the mechanisms, as well as the diagnosis, treatment, and management of the patient with airways reactions (asthma) of an immunologic nature attributed to the inhalation of organic material, the reader is referred to Ch. 344. Indeed, the list of respirable organic particles capable of producing asthma in the atopic individual is virtually limitless and includes not only those generated in daily living but also the wide variety of others generated by industrial and commercial enterprises. It is the relatively *heavy exposure* to the latter of *large numbers of individuals together in a workplace* that has directed attention to the often widespread occurrence of *asthma-like reactions in nonatopic individuals* and resulted in clarification of the nonimmunologic nature of their response, the subject for consideration here.

Two such exposures, recognized and studied over the last decade, are mentioned above under Examples. Reactions to these occupational exposures occur usually within months of first exposure in the case of the enzymes, but often only after years in the case of *Thuja plicata*. The nonatopic individual is as much at risk as the atopic individual, with up to 50 per cent of workers in some plants being affected. In the case of *detergent workers who are atopic*, bronchial provocation tests invariably elicit a dual response, i.e., immediate and late (within hours), attributed to Type I (IgE-mediated) and Type III (precipitin-mediated) hypersensitivity, respectively. In *nonatopic workers* (usually the majority of the factory personnel), the immediate effects appear to be on a nonimmunologic basis, but there is some evidence that the late effects are precipitin mediated and may involve the alveoli as well (see Ch. 344). Skin reactions are positive in about half the workers, but do not distinguish the symptomatic from the nonsymptomatic.

CLINICAL MANIFESTATIONS. In sensitized workers, symptoms follow exposure within minutes and include chest tightness, cough, and wheezing, with audible rhonchi. Without bronchodilators, the symptoms subside slowly over about four hours, to be followed by the development of *dyspnea, wheezing,* and *rhonchi,* and the general symptoms of headache, malaise, and muscle pains at about six hours. *Nocturnal exacerbations of wheezing* are also characteristic and have been attributed to inhibition of endogenous regulatory mechanisms, and their association with a daytime occupational exposure can easily be missed. There is no present evidence of serious and permanent lung damage, but the manufacture of these detergents is too recent to be certain that such effects may not occur, particularly because animal exposures, admittedly to much higher doses, have produced diffuse emphysema. The use (as opposed to the manufacture) of enzyme detergents may on occasion pose a risk, but probably only in the atopic individual, and the risk is probably less when the enzyme component is added in granular rather than powder form to the washing powder. A case of chronic granulomatous lung disease attributed to the inhalation of cedar sawdust has been reported.

TREATMENT AND PREVENTION. Sensitized individuals should be removed from exposure promptly once the diagnosis of an immunologically mediated airways reaction is established, but it may take several weeks for symptoms to disappear completely. However, since some 50 per cent of exposed workers appear to become reactive in many instances, control *must* be environmental. Improvements in plant housekeeping, including changes in production techniques and dust control measures, have successfully reduced the frequency of acute effects in a number of plants. In addition, coating the enzyme particles to increase their size (from 0.5 to 1.0 mm) reduces the chance that they will be inhaled into smaller airways. However, complacency is not justified in the detergent industry until more is known about long-term outcome of exposure, even to low levels.

Biological effects of proteolytic enzyme detergents (report of a symposium). Thorax, 31:621, 1977.

Nadel, J. A.: Parasympathetic nervous control of airway smooth muscle. Ann. N.Y. Acad. Sci., 221:99, 1974.

Seaton, A.: Occupational asthma. *In* Morgan, W. K. C., and Seaton, A. (eds.): Occupational Lung Diseases. Philadelphia, W. B. Saunders Company, 1975, p. 251.

348.12. AIRWAY OBSTRUCTION (EVENTUALLY CHRONIC) DUE TO ORGANIC PARTICLES

EXAMPLES. Examples include *byssinosis* in association with the processing of *cotton* (particularly spinning), *flax,*

and *soft hemp dusts; jute* may be implicated; *sisal* probably is not.

CLINICAL MANIFESTATIONS. An acute response to cotton dust may occur at first exposure. This type of response appears to occur in the atopic subject only, is almost certainly mediated through the subject's immune system, and may be very severe. However, this is not what is meant by *byssinosis,* a term reserved for the symptom complex described below which usually develops only after a number of years' exposure, and its appearance is unrelated to the subject's atopic status, with the nonatopic individual as much at risk as the atopic one. The diagnosis is made on the basis of a characteristic symptom pattern in a subject with *cough, tightness in the chest,* and *breathlessness,* occurring at first only occasionally on the first day of the working week (Grade ½), then regularly on Monday morning (Grade 1), then persisting beyond Monday (Grade 2), and finally, after several years, persisting throughout the week (Grade 3), when it is indistinguishable from nonindustrial chronic obstructive lung disease. There are no specific radiologic changes. Attack rates may reach over 90 per cent of exposed populations; a family history of atopy, with hypersensitivity to inhaled histamine, is unusual, and immediate skin reactions to cotton dust are infrequent — all observations in favor of a nonimmunologic mechanism to explain the airway reactions. The only host factor which appears important is cigarette smoking, which increases the risk and severity of the disease. The nonsymptomatic worker generally has normal pulmonary function; he may react to exposure with small shift decreases in tests reflecting major airway status such as FEV_1 and forced expiratory flow rates, or he may not (see Fig. 4). By contrast, the worker with the *Monday morning dyspnea of byssinosis* is likely to have lower spirometric values than his nonsymptomatic counterpart, and exposure usually results in more marked effects on FEV_1 and on the forced expiratory flow rates, particularly toward the end of expiration, as well as effects on residual volume and (less consistently) closing volumes, with, on occasion, arterial hypoxemia suggesting a response in peripheral as well as central airways. The airway effects can be improved by

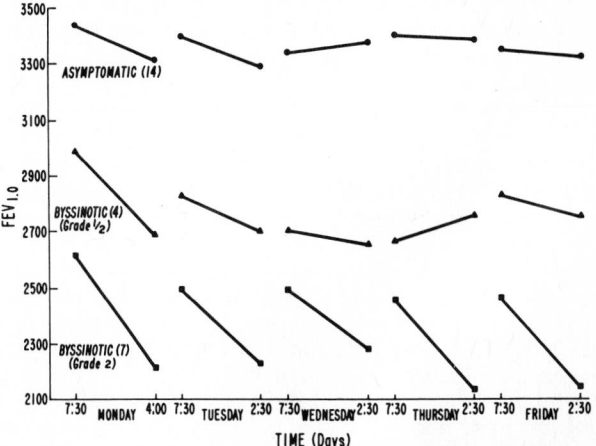

Figure 4. The pattern of physiologic response of exposure to cotton dust; $FEV_{1.0}$ during a five-day working week in 25 carders in a textile plant. (Courtesy of Dr. J. A. Merchant, Director, Appalachian Laboratory for Occupational Safety and Health, NIOSH, Morgantown, W. Va. Reproduced from Ann. N.Y. Acad. Sci., 221:39, 1974.)

isoproterenol inhalation. Antihistaminic drugs may also improve the flow rates in byssinosis without necessarily affording subjective relief, a finding pointing to the probable importance of small airway involvement. Pretreatment with orciprenaline, antihistamines, and ascorbic acid appears to diminish the biologic response to cotton dust.

PATHOGENESIS AND MECHANISMS. Despite the many studies and the variety of approaches used, the mechanism underlying the airway reactions in byssinosis is not fully understood. The hypothesis that the reactions are nonspecific, the result of stimulation of cough and/or irritant receptors, is no longer tenable. There is evidence to support the view that some fraction of the offending dusts (probably the protein fraction) causes the nonantigenic release of histamine and perhaps of other pharmacologically active substances; these reduce the caliber of large and/or small airways, the site of action perhaps being related to dust size and site of maximal deposition. Whether the histamine release is entirely nonantigenic, as originally proposed, or whether there is an antigenic component to the reaction (e.g., a Type III or Arthus reaction to a condensed polyphenol derived from the cotton plant), as recently proposed, has not been determined. Information on the long-term effects comes from published autopsy reports, the largest series being 43 patients compensated for byssinosis in the United Kingdom, in over half of whom no emphysema was noted. All lungs showed heavy dust pigmentation, but there was no excess fibrosis, granulomas were not noted, and vasculature was not remarkable. Mucous gland hyperplasia in the lobar bronchi suggests this as the site of major involvement rather than the smaller ones. In addition, occasional "ferruginous" bodies, more rounded than the usual asbestos body, were noted, containing what was assumed to be cotton fibers. There is a single report of extensive fibrosis with plasma cell infiltration, suggesting an immunologic background for the disease in that particular case, but this does not appear to be the rule.

EPIDEMIOLOGY AND PROGNOSIS. Attack rates of byssinosis vary widely, and are thought to relate to the *quality of the cotton* (being very low when high quality cotton is processed), to the *care with which it is picked* (there is some evidence that the active component is in the bracts), and usually, though not invariably, to the *environmental levels of cotton dust*. In addition, the jobs of carding and stripping carry a higher risk. In some instances plant modernization and air conditioning have even led to increased environmental dust. Reported rates for Egyptian workers vary from 0 to 90 per cent; for Swedish, Dutch, and British workers, about 50 per cent; and for American workers, up to 30 per cent (it has been estimated that at present there are 20,000 American workers with byssinosis, and this does not take into account those already retired). A study of retired rural Spanish workers shows a high prevalence of chronic disease. There are no data on the rate and inevitability of progression from Grade I (essentially reversible) to Grade III (essentially irreversible) disease. However, it is not insignificant and annual decrements of FEV_1 up to over 100 ml have been reported. Indeed, the recognition of byssinosis resulted from the observation of increased mortality and morbidity rates for cardiovascular and respiratory disease in certain Lancashire cotton workers.

PREVENTION. Present efforts to control byssinosis are directed toward dust control by means of environmental engineering, and its success depends on the accuracy with which it is possible to estimate the dust levels which constitute risk. *Reprocessing the cotton* by autoclaving has been found to diminish by ten-fold the incidence of the biologic response. Thus dust control of the future may well be a source intervention as envisaged many years ago by Schilling. Medical aspects of prevention include a *pre-employment examination* (to eliminate those with preexisting lung disease and those who show a marked response to dust) and *regular medical surveillance* to detect reactors and, if feasible, relocate them in a nonexposed job. Indeed, this may be one of the few industrial exposures in which progression to chronic disease may be halted by removal from exposure at any early clinical stage of the disease.

Bouhuys, A., Gilson, J. C., and Schilling, R. S. F.: Byssinosis in the textile industry. Arch. Environ. Health, 21:475, 1970.

Edwards, C., McCartney, J., Rooke, G., and Ward, F.: The pathology of the lungs in byssinotics. Thorax, 30:612, 1975.

Merchant, J. A., Lumsden, J. C., Kilburn, K. H., O'Fallon, W. M., Copeland, K., Germino, V. H., McKenzie, W. N., Baucom, D., Currin, P., and Stilman, J.: Intervention studies of cotton steaming to reduce biological effects of cotton dust. Br. J. Industr. Med., 31:261, 1974.

Morgan, W. K. C.: Byssinosis and related conditions. *In* Morgan, W. K. C., and Seaton, A. (eds.): Occupational Lung Diseases. Philadelphia, W. B. Saunders Company, 1975, p. 251.

348.13.   INTERSTITIAL (LIPOID) PNEUMONIA

EXAMPLES. Those affected have *inhaled vaporized mineral oil,* e.g., while oilspraying (usually *occupational exposures),* or while smoking tobacco (blackfat tobacco smokers' lung).

PATHOGENESIS AND MECHANISM. *Aspiration of oil in liquid form* into the lungs is associated with *acute reactions* such as hemorrhagic bronchopneumonia if the *oil is irritant* (usually the case if it contains animal fats), and with more *insidious reactions leading to chronic disease* in the case of the more *bland mineral oils.* Localization of such chronic disease to a zone or lobe is usual, and is attributed to the influence of gravity at the time of the aspiration. When chronic reactions result from *aspiration of mineral oil in vaporized form,* e.g., in association with its industrial use in cleaning aircraft parts, they tend to be more generalized in distribution, and may pose a much more series threat to health, as revealed by a recent investigation in Guyana. Here an unusually high prevalence of diffuse interstitial pulmonary fibrosis in older individuals, recognized for at least 25 to 30 years, has now been shown to be due to a chronic interstitial lipoid pneumonia, the consequence of many years of smoking blackfat tobacco. Blackfat tobacco is unusual in that certain oils are added to the leaf during processing, and smoking causes these to distil over into the lungs. The pathology (based on three postmortem lung biopsies) is in keeping with published reports on aspiration lipoid pneumonia. Thus in the early stages the lipid is present in the alveolar phagocytes, lying free in alveoli or in collections in the interstitium in a peribronchiolar or subpleural location where they evoke first a cellular and eventually (if the dose is large) a collagenous response, with lesions resembling those of liquid paraffin granulomas. The end result is a diffuse interstitial fibrosis and vasculitis, with deposits of lipid and black material in the walls of blood vessels and in the interstitium. The absence of any marked inflammatory reaction was in keeping with previous evidence that mineral oil is comparatively bland in its effect on lung tissue. It was possible to exclude hypersensitivity to the suspected agent, teichoic acid, and extrinsic allergic alveolitis as the background of the chronic interstitial fibrosis in the Guyana study.

CLINICAL MANIFESTATIONS. Localized disease may be asymptomatic and discovered by chance on a routine chest roentgenogram. When disease is diffuse, as in the Guyana series, symptoms include cough, dyspnea, and rather striking weight loss, with eventually pulmonary heart disease. Basal crepitations are characteristic, and wheezing is unusual except during superimposed infection. Radiologic and functional changes are those of diffuse interstitial fibrosis, except in the Guyana series, in which the function profile was obstructive rather than restrictive, perhaps because of the association with another inhaled pollutant, tobacco smoke. The finding of fat droplets in macrophages in the sputum is evidence of exposure, not disease.

TREATMENT, EPIDEMIOLOGY, AND PREVENTION. There is some evidence that x-ray changes associated with the aspiration of mineral oil of short duration (months, not years), are reversible on steroids. Presumably this occurs when the tissue reaction is primarily cellular rather than collagenous. Thus this form of treatment certainly merits consideration in the patient with recent occupational exposure to vaporized mineral oil. Once diffuse fibrosis has developed, however, treatment is essentially palliative, no different from that of other chronic interstitial lung diseases. In the Guyana series, giving up the smoking of blackfat tobacco was no guarantee that symptoms would not develop in the future. The steady decline in blackfat tobacco smoking in Guyana suggests that this local health problem is also on the decline. However, *recognition that inhaled additives to tobacco* can produce *long-term effects* of a *low-grade inflammatory type* on the lungs is of great importance to physicians the world over who are concerned with the health effects of tobacco smoking.

Fraser, R. G., and Paré, J. A. P.: Diagnosis of Diseases of the Chest, Vol. II. Philadelphia, W. B. Saunders Company, 1970, p. 964.
Miller, G. I., Ashcraft, M. T., Beadrell, H. M. S., Wagner, J. C., and Pepys, J.: The lipoid pneumonia of black fat tobacco smokers in Guyana. Quart. J. Med., 160:457, 1971.

348.14. ASTHMA-LIKE REACTIONS TO CHEMICAL AGENTS

EXAMPLES. Those affected include workers with *toluene di-isocyanate* (TDI) and *other isocyanates* (e.g., di-isocyanato diphenyl methane, [MDI]) used in the application of certain lacquers and resins and in the manufacture of polyurethane foams for cushioning, insulation, and soft toys; consumers using do-it-yourself polyurethane; and *cable jointers* using certain aluminum soldering flux. *Platinosis* (describing rhinorrhea, asthma, and urticaria) results from exposure to complex platinum salts in refineries.

PATHOGENESIS AND MECHANISMS. From carefully controlled occupational-type provocation tests monitored by measurements of forced expiratory volumes, it has been shown that immediate, late, and dual asthmatic reactions occur in workers sensitized to the chemical vapors, fumes, and dusts listed above. These reactions may be mechanically (due to irritation) or, less commonly, immunologically mediated. The presence of reaginic and

precipitating antibodies against *platinum salts* and against *soldering flux* in symptomatic subjects suggests an immunologic basis (Types I and III allergy) for reactions to these materials, and others may well come to light in the future. However, it has not been possible to date to show an allergic mechanism for *TDI sensitivity,* in keeping with the clinical observations that large numbers of those exposed have symptoms but are not atopic. Nor is skin reactivity to TDI correlated with respiratory responsiveness, which appears to be dose related. An alternative possibility is TDI interaction with specific IgE antibodies localized to the respiratory tract, with release of pharmacologic mediators. In addition, there is some evidence that TDI may increase bronchial reactivity. These reactions, which may follow exposure to very low doses, should be distinguished from the well recognized *irritant effects of the same chemicals in higher doses* and other chemicals discussed subsequently. Thus sensitization to isocyanate vapors may occur at very low exposure levels (0.002 parts per million) which is well below the present threshold limit value of 0.02 ppm, which is again below the level at which the irritant effects of isocyanates are seen. Even when measured environmental levels do not exceed 0.02 ppm, an excess fall in expiratory flow rates in the long term, linked to the occurrence of acute effects, has been shown in one study; however, this may be related to factors peculiar to that exposure and has not been shown in other studies.

CLINICAL MANIFESTATIONS. Symptoms (cough, chest pain, and tightness suggesting asthma which may be immediate and/or late and often nocturnal) develop after periods varying from one week to several months after first exposure and, if possible, should be distinguished from those of high dose irritation, of which eye, nose, and throat irritation are the most common. Decreases in forced expiratory volumes and flow rates, immediate, late, or delayed, accompany the symptoms. Symptoms subside after removal from exposure, and function may return to normal within days or weeks. However, reexposure regularly results in recurrence, often more violent. Most exposed persons show some reduction in expiratory flow rates during working hours, a change eliminated by the oral administration of an aminophylline compound.

DIAGNOSIS, TREATMENT, AND PREVENTION. Diagnosis depends on a high degree of suspicion, particularly when symptoms occur predominantly at night, and can be confirmed using carefully controlled occupational-type provocation tests as suggested by Pepys. These should be carried out only under hospital supervision with monitoring of forced expiratory flow tests, together with observation of the effects of isoproterenol and disodium cromoglycate on the reactions. Objective demonstration of sensitization is important, particularly for platinum salts and solder flux where an immunologic mechanism is likely, because it may be necessary to advise removal from exposure with potential financial and other hardships for the worker.

Since TDI sensitivity is rarely immunologically mediated, diagnosis in an individual exposed in a plant with other workers must be brought to the attention of the appropriate authority, because control should clearly be at the environmental and not the personal level. Thus the variation in the number of sensitized workers, ranging from 4 to 100 per cent, is most likely a reflection of plant housekeeping. Nor can satisfactory environmental control be assumed on the basis of area monitoring, which does not necessarily correlate directly with monitoring by personal sampler, and it should be supplemented by vigilant health surveillance of the working population with prompt action when cases are detected.

Butcher, B. T., Jones, R. N., O'Neil, C. E., Glindmeyer, H. W., Diem, J. E., Venkatram, D., Weill, H., and Salvaggio, J.: Longitudinal study of workers employed in the manufacture of toluene-diisocyanate. Am. Rev. Respir. Dis., 116:411, 1977.

Pepys, J., and Hutchcroft, B. J.: Bronchial provocation tests in etiologic diagnosis and analysis of asthma. Am. Rev. Respir. Dis., 112:829, 1975.

Peters, J. M., and Murphy, R. L. H.: Pulmonary toxicity of isocyanates. Ann. Intern. Med., 73:654, 1970.

348.15. ACUTE CHEMICAL BRONCHITIS AND/OR PNEUMONITIS

EXAMPLES. *Chemical agents with principal effects on airways,* with industries or occupations at risk for exposure, *include sulfur dioxide,* SO_2 (in the manufacture of pulp and refrigerators); *ammonia,* NH_3 (in the production of fertilizers, refrigerators, explosives, and plastics); *chlorine,* Cl_2 (in the production of alkalis, bleaches, and disinfectants); *phosgene,* Cl_2CO (in the chemical industry and in fire-fighting); and *hydrogen fluoride,* HF (in etching and metal refining).

Chemical agents with principal effects on both airways and pulmonary parenchyma, with occupations or industries at risk for exposure, *include osmium tetroxide,* OsO_4 (in alloy production); *vanadium pentoxide,* V_2O_5 (in the chemical industry); *cadmium oxide* (welding and ore smelting); *chromates* (in electroplating); *zinc chloride* (dry cell manufacture); and *trimellitic anhydride* (used to harden epoxy resins).

Neither of these lists is exhaustive, and they should be supplemented by consulting specialized texts.

PATHOGENESIS AND MECHANISMS. Reaction to chemical agents, usually inhaled in the form of fumes and/or vapors, tends to be primarily at the level of the airways for agents with a high solubility in biologic fluids, and further down the bronchial tree involving the parenchyma for agents with lower solubility. Thus when compared to CO_2, the most soluble of the physiologic gases (56.7 vols per cent in water at $37°C$ at 1 atmosphere), those whose effects are primarily on airways have a much greater solubility: equivalent values for SO_2, Cl_2 and NH_3 being 280, 257, and 139 vols per cent, respectively. Accidental inhalation of high concentrations results in rapid solution in the mucous membranes of the upper airways with the formation of irritant compounds, e.g., H_2SO_3 from SO_2, NH_4OH from NH_3, HCl from Cl_2. The initial irritation causing *bronchorrhea* is rapidly followed by sloughing and a *frank necrotizing bronchitis.* In fatal cases, the bronchial mucosa may be stripped down to the cartilage. If exposure is prolonged or unduly heavy, the lower respiratory tract becomes exposed, with the development of an *acute chemical pulmonary edema.* Recovery may be complete. However, residual mucosal scars and submucosal thickening are not uncommon, particularly if the mucosal sloughs were deep and secondary infection prominent. Acute chemical irritation may also result from the *aspiration of vomited or regurgitated material high in HCl content,* an event more common in the frail and elderly than is generally supposed, or in relation to blunting of the gag reflex as in anesthesia, head injuries, and alcohol-

ic or other intoxications. If the aspirate is chiefly water or saline in small amounts, absorption is quick and the consequences usually slight.

CLINICAL MANIFESTATIONS. When exposure to a chemical irritant is heavy, clinical manifestations are invariably immediate, the patient is alerted to his exposure, and he makes every effort to remove himself therefrom. *Conjunctivitis, irritation* and *burning* in the *mucosa* of the mouth and throat, *laryngitis, laryngospasm,* and *difficulty in breathing* are in keeping with the usual site of damage, i.e., upper respiratory tract, and coarse *rhonchi* are a characteristic physical finding, often with profound *mucorrhea,* which may be bloodstained. *Cough* is usually also a prominent symptom, although it is believed that the cough receptors are less responsive to chemical stimuli than are the irritant receptors. More profound *dyspnea* usually implies alveolar involvement resulting from either chemical edema or aspiration of bronchial sloughs. These complications can frequently be suspected from chest roentgenograms and may result in profound impairment of pulmonary blood-gas exchange with *severe arterial hypoxemia* and a low arterial CO_2 tension. Nausea, vomiting, and stupor may complicate the picture.

If the patient survives the acute event, complete recovery is usual. However, some patients may be left with chronic bronchitis or saccular bronchiectasis or both, sometimes of considerable severity, with residual effects on pulmonary function.

Chronic irritation from long-term exposure to low doses, e.g., SO_2, as in city air pollution, Cl_2, as in chlorine plants, may perhaps be more important in terms of community health, particularly in relation to the etiology of chronic obstructive lung disease.

TREATMENT. Recognition, the most important aspect of treatment, poses no difficulty for the acute accidental heavy exposure, but it seems likely that many exposures producing less dramatic effects go unrecognized in the complex modern industrial processes. These are more likely to be identified if a substantial number of individuals are affected, e.g., the outbreak of upper and lower respiratory tract disease in a Wisconsin rubber tire plant when a new thermosetting resin, containing resorcinol and a trimere of methylene aminoacetonitrile, was introduced into the tire formulation. Over 200 workers in all were affected, and lung biopsy revealed evidence of interstitial fibrosis as well as chronic peribronchiolar and perivascular inflammation. This shows that an exhaustive occupational history is an essential part of the investigation of all cases of idiopathic pulmonary fibrosis.

Acute chemical bronchitis and *acute chemical pulmonary edema* are *medical emergencies.* In the acute phase, survival depends on maintaining airway patency and adequate oxygenation. To aspirate sloughs, it may be necessary to employ intubation, lavage with saline, using modest amounts only (10 ml at a single flush), and even bronchoscopy. Controlled oxygen administration is usually necessary, and frequently must be supplemented with positive pressure respiration, assisted in mild cases, controlled in the severe ones. Corticosteroids, thought to modify the acute inflammatory reaction at the gas-exchange surface, should always be given in the presence of pulmonary edema and indeed are recommended by some in all cases of exposure on a prophylactic basis. Heavy initial doses should be reduced as the clinical picture improves. Infection should be controlled by the use of antimicrobial drugs.

DoPico, G. A., Rankin, R., Chosy, L. W., Reddan, W. O., Barbee, R. A., Gee, B., and Dickie, H. A.: Respiratory tract disease from thermosetting resins. Ann. Intern. Med., 83:177, 1975.

Fraser, R. F., and Paré, J. A. P.: Diagnosis of Diseases of the Chest, Vol. II. Philadelphia, W. B. Saunders Company, 1970, p. 948.

Hamilton, A., and Hardy, H. L.: Industrial Toxicology. Section Three: Chemical Compounds. Acton, Mass., Publishing Sciences Group, 1974, p. 203.

Walton, M.: Industrial ammonia gassing. Br. J. Industr. Med., 30:78, 1973.

348.16. CHEMICAL PULMONARY EDEMA

EXAMPLES. Chemical pulmonary edema can result from exposure to *oxides of nitrogen* in freshly filled silos *(silo-filler's disease);* welding in poorly ventilated spaces; misfires in blasting operations carried out in closed spaces (e.g., mines); burning of N_2-containing materials in closed spaces; *exposure to phosgene* after its liberation from many chlorinated substances, e.g., carbon tetrachloride in fire extinguishers; or *accidental ingestion of the herbicide paraquat.*

PATHOGENESIS AND MECHANISMS. The immediate clinical effects of exposure to the oxides of nitrogen and phosgene may be mild, but a severe, chemical pulmonary edema, often fatal, may develop after a *delay of several hours to several days.* The physicochemical processes underlying this delay are not fully understood, but changes in permeability and liquid transport appear to follow the direct injury to pulmonary alveolar and capillary cells by the inhaled agents, and the edema fluid is high in protein content. If the acute event is not immediately fatal, healing by fibrosis may lead to the development of *bronchiolitis fibrosa obliterans,* usually four to eight weeks after initial exposure, often with a fatal result. Autopsy studies show widespread organization of exudates, primarily located in the terminal bronchioles; atelectasis is not seen, however, presumably because of the collateral ventilation now recognized to be extensive in man.

Acute chemical pulmonary edema of delayed onset (one to three days) may also follow the *accidental ingestion of the herbicide paraquat* (1,1'-dimethyl-4,4'-dipyridilium), a common constituent of commercial weed-killers. Thus the acute effects of this poison, which also include acute oral, esophageal, hepatic, and renal damage, become evident only after a delay of several days, i.e., after the peak blood levels and at a time when most of the material has been excreted. These characteristics have earned it the name of the "hit and run" poison, and once the pulmonary damage starts, it invariably runs a relentless course to death within weeks from respiratory failure caused by a *diffuse progressive pulmonary fibrosis* and replacement of gas-exchanging tissue by cystic changes. Its mechanism of action is unknown, but it has been suggested that the primary action is to inactivate or depress formation of surfactant.

CLINICAL MANIFESTATIONS. Immediate effects of exposure to the oxides of nitrogen and phosgene, which may include cough, chest irritation, and sputum, are often so mild that the victim may even fail to report to the first-aid post, only to return from hours to several days later with the symptoms, signs, and chest roentgenogram of *acute, severe, pulmonary edema.* Hence it is reasonable to suggest observation in hospital for 48 hours after possible exposures (e.g., for firefighters who have been inside burning buildings), perhaps even giving steroid therapy if suspicion of exposure is strong. In the mild case of edema, symptoms may escape attention, changes on the chest film at the most may be equivocal, and the diagnosis depends on the finding of coarse rales, sometimes lasting over a short period only, with a transient hypoxemia. Clinical management has been discussed above; in cases of frank, severe edema, steroid therapy should probably be prolonged for six to eight weeks to cover the period when the subacute complication of bronchiolitis obliterans is likely to develop. This complication, probably avoidable if steroid therapy is given early, should be suspected when symptoms recur or appear at three to six weeks, and generally responds to steroid therapy.

Management of a patient known to have ingested paraquat should include heroic measures to prevent absorption. In laboratory animals bentylol and/or Fuller's earth by mouth has been shown to inactivate the material more effectively than charcoal. Forced diuresis and hemodialysis are recommended once blood levels have risen. There is some evidence that corticosteroids may be effective in the treatment of the pulmonary edema, and that O_2 therapy should be used with the utmost caution, experimental work indicating that it potentiates the action of the poison.

EPIDEMIOLOGY. Large-scale heavy exposure to, for instance, oxides of nitrogen occurs only in relation to mass disasters, e.g., in the Cleveland clinic fire in 1929 owing to the burning of stored x-ray film, and in the Cocoanut Grove fire in Boston in 1943 owing to the burning of nitrogen-containing plastics. Many modern plastics no longer contain nitrogen. However, in most fires involving domestic buildings in which wood is used, circumstances exist in which these fumes could be evolved, and three or four cases are seen annually in most city hospitals.

Fraser, R. F., and Paré, J. A. P.: Diagnosis of Diseases of the Chest, Vol. II. Philadelphia, W. B. Saunders Company, 1970, p. 948.

348.17. RADIATION

Increased use of x-irradiation in the treatment of cancer of the breast and of various intrathoracic organs led to the recognition that the lungs themselves may be affected by this procedure. *Acute changes* may come on within weeks of the onset of treatment up to six months after its cessation and possibly much longer, but rarely manifest themselves clinically while treatment is in progress. The initial damage is believed to occur in the capillary endothelium, which becomes necrotic and eventually collagenized; this is associated with an alveolar cellular reaction, followed by desquamation and exudation of protein-rich material, which itself is followed in some instances by hyaline membrane formation. Focal necrosis of the bronchial mucosa may develop as a result of damage to capillary endothelium with subsequent necrosis and vascular occlusion. These changes may resolve or go on to loss of lung volume, sometimes of marked degree, occurring rather suddenly, and usually ascribed to fibrosis, shrinkage, and hyalinization, particularly if there has been infection. Studies in animals, however, suggest that the loss of volume may, on occasion, be due to atrophy and that the hyalinization may be in part due to autohypersensitivity, the consequence of new cell antigens formed as a result of the ionizing radiation.

There may be no clinical manifestations of *radiation pneumonitis* even in the face of definite radiologic changes. Likewise, lung damage detectable by pulmonary function tests may occur in the absence of roentgenographic changes. The most common symptom is a persistent, hacking dry cough. Fever, some dyspnea, and weakness may be seen, and the symptoms of radiation esophagitis are common. On physical examination the effects of radiation on the skin of the thorax are usually evident; rales and a friction rub may be found. The chest film characteristically reveals regional or diffuse haziness usually corresponding to the area irradiated, and pulmonary function tests indicate a restrictive pattern. Spontaneous remission over weeks is frequent. Recommended therapy includes steroids (to lessen the chances of healing by fibrosis) and, less commonly, anticoagulants (which may lessen the ischemic effects of small-vessel thrombosis commonly seen at autopsy). When *radiation fibrosis* supervenes, clinical presentation will depend on how much functioning lung tissue is lost and on the function in the remaining lung. In severe cases the loss of lung volume is striking, with obliteration of all lung architecture and evidence of traction on the hilum and mediastinum. Respiratory failure, pulmonary hypertension, and right heart failure may all follow.

Some authors suggest that there is a parenchymal reaction to ionizing radiation of the thorax in 100 per cent of cases so exposed, that some degree of pneumonitis is common if not invariable, though symptoms occur in a smaller number (estimated at 10 per cent), and that progression to radiation fibrosis is rare. Factors thought to affect the attack rate include total dose (broadly speaking, there is a dose relationship but with considerable individual variation), the *time over which it is given* (the longer the time, the less likely an unfavorable reaction), and the technique of application. Clinically important reactions are unusual at total doses below 2000 rads and invariable above 6000 rads. The age of the patient, the chest wall thickness, the condition of the lung before treatment, and the presence of complicating disease may also be important. Individual factors remain to be identified, however, since identical doses can be harmless to one person and cause a severe reaction in another.

Gross, N. J.: Review: Pulmonary effect of radiation therapy. Ann. Intern. Med., 86:81, 1977.

349. CYSTS AND NEOPLASMS OF THE LUNG

Leo F. Black

349.1. CYSTIC LESIONS OF THE LUNG, BULLOUS DISEASE OF THE LUNG, AND UNILATERAL HYPERLUCENT LUNG

Classification of different types of cysts in the lungs is confusing because there is considerable variation in the definition of the terms cysts, blebs, bullae, and pneumatoceles. For this presentation, cysts will be considered to be abnormal air-containing spaces lined with bronchial epithelium. Blebs are collections of air within the layers of the visceral pleura. Blebs are formed by air that ruptures out of alveoli along the lobular septa and bronchovascular sheaths and dissects toward the pleura within the connective tissue framework. Bullae are emphysematous spaces at the pleural surface or within the lung parenchyma. Pneumatocele is a term sometimes used to describe a bullous lesion. At other times, this term is used more specifically to describe an intraparenchymal air collection caused by obstruction of small airways by an inflammatory process. This most commonly occurs with staphylococcal pneumonia in children. Infections in the lung parenchyma due to many bacteria, fungi, and parasites may be associated with abnormal air spaces, which are generally referred to as cavities rather than cysts, although they may have a similar appearance on the thoracic roentgenogram.

BRONCHOGENIC CYSTS

Bronchopulmonary foregut malformations are a group of developmental abnormalities that include bronchogenic cysts, enterogenous cysts, and bronchopulmonary sequestrations. Bronchogenic cysts may be located in the mediastinum or within the lung parenchyma. The cysts are thin walled, are lined with ciliated columnar epithelium, and usually are filled with mucus. They may contain all the elements normally found in the tracheobronchial tree such as cartilage, mucous glands, fibrous tissue, and smooth muscle. The respiratory epithelial lining may be destroyed when a cyst is infected, and in this instance it may be difficult to distinguish a congenital cyst from an acquired air-containing space.

In infants and young children, some authors describe congenital alveolar cysts that are considered to develop at the embryologic stage of alveolar formation. These cysts are usually peripheral and multiloculated. Both these and bronchogenic cysts may be asymptomatic, or they may produce coughing, wheezing, and respiratory distress by expanding and compressing the tracheobronchial tree and the surrounding lung parenchyma. They also may be associated with recurrent pulmonary infections. Treatment is surgical resection with conservation of as much normal pulmonary tissue as possible.

In adults, bronchogenic cysts are frequently asymptomatic and are discovered incidentally on the thoracic roentgenogram. They may, however, produce chest discomfort and be associated with recurrent pulmonary infections. The diagnosis of a bronchogenic cyst may be suspected on the basis of clinical findings and the findings on the thoracic roentgenogram. These cysts, when intrapulmonary, are most often in the lower lobes and present as solitary masses. If they have been infected and a bronchial communication has developed, then an air-fluid level may be visible. Bronchogenic cysts in the mediastinum may present as masses in the paratracheal, carinal, hilar, or paraesophageal regions on the thoracic roentgenogram. Definite diagnosis frequently cannot be made until thoracotomy. Treatment is surgical resection, with preservation of as much functioning lung tissue as possible.

Hutchin, P.: Congenital cystic disease of the lung. Rev. Surg., 28:79, 1971.

BRONCHOPULMONARY SEQUESTRATION

Bronchopulmonary sequestration is a congenital malformation that arises from accessory budding of the tracheobronchial tree early in its development. Sequestrations may present as masses separate from the lung (extralobar) or may occur within the visceral pleura of a lobe (intralobar).

Extralobar sequestrations represent maldeveloped pulmonary tissue that is enclosed in its own visceral pleura. The arterial supply is from the aorta or one of its branches. Venous drainage is into the systemic circulation. Approximately 90 per cent are on the left side and present as a mass between the lung and the diaphragm; the lesion may also be within the diaphragm or below it. It is frequently associated with an ipsilateral congenital diaphragmatic hernia. Because this type of sequestration has its own pleural covering, infection is unusual. This lesion is usually detected in infancy, and surgical excision is the treatment of choice.

Intralobar sequestration consists of a nonfunctioning portion of lung within the visceral pleura of a lobe. It has poorly developed respiratory structures and may be filled with mucus. The epithelium may be flat or ciliated columnar. The arterial supply is from the aorta or one of its branches, and the venous drainage is into the pulmonary veins. These sequestrations most commonly develop in the lower lobes, especially in the posterior basal segments. If infection has occurred and a bronchial communication has developed, cystic changes with air-fluid levels may be visible on the thoracic roentgenogram. Intralobar sequestrations are frequently not diagnosed until adulthood. They may be detected in asymptomatic patients when a routine thoracic roentgenogram reveals a solid or cystic lesion in the posterior portion of the lower lobes. In some patients, recurrent pulmonary infections are associated with the sequestration. Aortography may aid in diagnosis by demonstrating the abnormal arterial blood supply to the lesion. Treatment is surgical excision.

Heithoff, K. B., Sane, S. M., Williams, H. J., Jarvis, C. J., Carter, J., Kane, P., and Brennom, W.: Bronchopulmonary foregut malformations: A unifying etiological concept. Am. J. Roentgenol., 126:46, 1976.

HONEYCOMB LUNG

This term refers to the presence of multiple small cysts in the lung and is the end result of pulmonary involvement by many diseases, such as interstitial pneumonitis and fibrosis, histiocytosis X, rheumatoid lung, and scleroderma. The fibrotic lungs contain multiple cysts that are formed from dilated bronchi and bronchioles and are lined by columnar or cuboidal epithelium. They are associated with a grossly distorted pulmonary architecture. The cysts may have thickened fibrous walls. Occasionally, rupture into the pleural space produces pneumothorax. Treatment is directed at the underlying disease process responsible for the diffuse pulmonary changes.

BULLOUS DISEASE OF THE LUNG

DEFINITION. Bullous disease of the lung refers to the presence of bullae in the lung, and they may or may not be associated with obstructive airway disease.

PATHOLOGY. Bullae may result from any form of emphysema, including the panacinar, paraseptal, and irregular types. Reid has described several different types of bullae, based on their anatomic characteristics. Type 1 bullae are subpleural, are more common in the upper lobes, have a narrow neck, and represent small units of lung tissue that have become greatly expanded. These tend to occur independent of widespread emphysema and may represent examples of paraseptal or irregular emphysema. Type 2 bullae are subpleural, have a broad neck, and may be associated with panacinar or centrilobular emphysema as well as paraseptal and irregular emphysema. Type 3 bullae represent overdistention of relatively large areas of lung, may affect any lobe, and are located within the lung parenchyma.

CLINICAL MANIFESTATIONS. The symptoms produced by bullae vary greatly. In general, the presence of dyspnea depends on the size of the bullae and the functional status of the remainder of the lung. Bullae also may become infected and produce symptoms related to this. Pneumothorax is another possible complication.

Some patients have bullae in the apical areas of the lung and have no chronic symptoms. These may be discovered incidentally on a thoracic roentgenogram, or they may produce a pneumothorax, which results in acute pain and dyspnea. Another group of patients may have single or multiple bullae in one area of the lung and also have no symptoms unless pneumothorax develops.

Patients with multiple bullae may present with symptoms of chronic obstructive airway disease, such as cough and dyspnea. In them, it is not always easy to determine the relative contribution of the chronic airway disease and the bullae to the dyspnea. In many, the bullae represent emphysematous areas of the lung that are part of the basic problem of chronic obstructive airway disease. Some patients, however, have bilateral bullae demonstrable on the thoracic roentgenogram years before symptoms of chronic bronchitis develop. In such cases, bronchial obstruction secondary to bronchial compression by the bullae may have a role in the development of chronic bronchitis.

DIAGNOSIS. The diagnosis of bullae is usually established on the basis of the thoracic roentgenogram, which reveals single or multiple hyperlucent areas with a decreased vascular pattern. The hyperlucent areas may be bordered by hairline-curved densities representing the walls of the bullae and surrounding compressed lung. When bullae are infected, an air-fluid level may be detected.

Physical examination of the lungs may reveal suppression of breath sounds over the bullous areas if the bullae are large. If the patient has chronic obstructive airway disease, physical findings may include slowing of a forced expiration and generalized suppression of breath sounds.

Angiography and perfusion lung scanning may offer the best indications of the condition of the remaining lung in patients with obvious bullae. Pulmonary function tests reveal variable findings, depending on the size of the bullae and the presence or absence of chronic obstructive airway disease. In general, patients with bullae but no obstructive airway disease have relatively normal pulmonary function until the bullae become very large. The vital capacity may be reduced. The total lung capacity, measured by a gas dilution method, may be increased, normal, or decreased, depending on the degree to which the bullae communicate with the airways. Total lung capacity measured with the body plethysmograph will be increased in patients with large bullae. Expiratory flow rates, such as the one-second forced expiratory volume and the maximal mid-expiratory flow rate, are mildly reduced in the presence of large bullae. The diffusing capacity for carbon monoxide will be normal or decreased, depending on the extent of compression of the surrounding lung.

When chronic obstructive airway disease is present in addition to the bullae, pulmonary function tests may reveal a decreased vital capacity, increased total lung capacity, decreased expiratory flow rates, and a decreased diffusing capacity for carbon monoxide. Arterial blood gases may be abnormal depending on the extent of the disease.

TREATMENT. Treatment depends on the symptoms of the patient. Asymptomatic patients with bullae and no accompanying chronic obstructive airway disease require no specific therapy other than periodic follow-up to determine any progressive enlargement of the bullae. When the bullae are large (greater than one third the volume of one lung), resection may be considered when the patient is symptomatic. In the presence of chronic obstructive airway disease, the decision to resect the bullae is often very difficult. Occasionally, a patient will experience considerable benefit from resection of large bullae. Decisions regarding resection should be made only after the patient has been on a medical program for the airway disease and when the course of the disease has been determined by regular follow-up examinations.

When recurrent pneumothorax occurs owing to bullae, abrasion of the pleural space and resection of the bullae are indicated to prevent further recurrences.

Boushy, S. F., Kohen, R., Billig, D. M., and Heiman, M. J.: Bullous emphysema: Clinical, roentgenologic and physiologic study of 49 patients. Dis. Chest. 54:327, 1968.

Pride, N. B., Barter, C. E., and Hugh-Jones, P.: The ventilation of bullae and the effect of their removal on thoracic gas volumes and tests of over-all pulmonary function. Am. Rev. Respir. Dis., 107:83, 1973.

Reid, L.: The Pathology of Emphysema. Chicago, Year Book Medical Publishers, 1967, p. 211.

Thurlbeck, W. M.: Chronic Airflow Obstruction in Lung Disease. Philadelphia, W. B. Saunders Company, 1976.

UNILATERAL HYPERLUCENT LUNG

DEFINITION. Unilateral hyperlucent lung (Swyer-James syndrome, Macleod's syndrome) is characterized by the presence of a hyperlucent lung on the thoracic roentgenogram with a normal or smaller than normal lung volume.

PATHOLOGY AND PATHOGENESIS. The entire lung is characteristically abnormal, although not uniformly involved by the pathologic process. At times, only one lobe may be involved. Morphologically, there is evidence of bronchitis, bronchiolitis, and bronchiolitis obliterans. The patchy involvement allows some ventilation of the involved lung, and pathways of collateral ventilation prevent alveolar collapse. The lung parenchyma frequently shows panacinar emphysema, although sometimes there is minimal parenchymal destruction. The number of alveoli and finer branches of the pulmonary artery are reduced, thus suggesting that hypoplasia of these structures may be secondary to airway obstruction early in life, preventing the normal growth of these structures. Lower respiratory infections, especially viral, may be the cause of the widespread bronchial and bronchiolar disease. The pulmonary artery on the affected side, when examined at surgery, is larger than it appears on angiography but may be smaller than normal.

CLINICAL MANIFESTATIONS. Patients with this condition may be asymptomatic, and the abnormality is discovered on a routine thoracic roentgenogram. Some of them complain of cough and dyspnea on exertion, whereas others have histories of repeated lower respiratory tract infections.

DIAGNOSIS. Generally, the diagnosis can be established on the basis of the clinical findings and inspiratory and expiratory thoracic roentgenograms. Physical examination reveals decreased excursion of the affected hemithorax. Breath sounds are diminished over the involved lung, and occasionally scattered rales are heard.

The inspiratory thoracic roentgenogram reveals a hyperlucent lung of normal or smaller than normal overall lung volume. The hyperlucency is due to decreased vascular perfusion of the affected lung. The pulmonary artery to the involved lung may appear to be smaller than normal. The vascular markings of the contralateral lung may appear more prominent than normal because most of the pulmonary blood flow goes through the contralateral lung. The expiratory thoracic roentgenogram reveals air trapping in the involved lung and shifting of the mediastinum to the opposite side.

Bronchoscopy reveals the absence of an obstructing lesion in major airways on the affected side. Bronchograms show irregular dilated segmental bronchi that end abruptly or may terminate in small pools or dilations. The peripheral bronchi do not fill with the contrast material.

Radioisotope lung scans reveal decreased ventilation to the involved lung and delayed clearance of the isotope. Perfusion scans reveal reduced to absent pulmonary blood flow to the affected lung. Pulmonary angiograms reveal a small pulmonary artery on the affected side, the peripheral arterial tree is smaller than normal, and the vessels appear to be narrow and attenuated.

Pulmonary function studies reveal variable findings. The vital capacity may be reduced, as may be the expiratory flow rates. The diffusing capacity for carbon monoxide may be normal or reduced. Arterial blood gases may be normal or may reveal hypoxemia at rest or with exercise. Bronchospirometric measurements have shown decreased ventilation and oxygen uptake in the involved lung.

The presence of expiratory air trapping documented by expiratory thoracic roentgenograms differentiates this condition from agenesis of a pulmonary artery and embolic or thrombotic obstruction of a pulmonary artery. Hyperlucency of one lung secondary to partial bronchial obstruction generally is associated with increased lung volume on the affected side. Bronchoscopy is of diagnostic aid in ruling out a bronchial-obstructing lesion.

TREATMENT. Treatment of this condition consists of prompt therapy for respiratory infections. The prognosis is good.

Gottlieb, L. S., and Turner, A. F.: Swyer-James (Macleod's) syndrome: Variations in pulmonary-bronchial arterial blood flow. Chest, 69:62, 1976.

Macleod, W. M.: Abnormal transradiancy of one lung. Thorax, 9:147, 1954.

Swyer, P. R., and James, G. C. W.: A case of unilateral pulmonary emphysema. Thorax, 8:133, 1953.

Weg, J. G., Krumholz, R. A., and Hackleroad, L. E.: Unilateral hyperlucent lung: A physiologic syndrome. Ann. Intern. Med.·, 62:675, 1965.

349.2. NEOPLASMS OF THE LUNG

The lung may be the site of many types of neoplasms. Benign tumors such as hamartomas, lipomas, and papillomas occur infrequently compared with malignant tumors. Primary and metastatic malignancies involving the lung are common clinical problems. The classification of primary lung neoplasms by the World Health Organization is shown in Table 1. Groups I through V constitute approximately 90 per cent of the primary lung neoplasms and are commonly designated bronchogenic carcinomas.

BRONCHOGENIC CARCINOMA

DEFINITION. The frequency distribution of the different histologic types of bronchogenic carcinoma varies in several reported series, but in general the incidence is epidermoid carcinoma, 40 to 50 per cent; adenocarcinoma (bronchogenic and bronchiolo-alveolar), 15 to 20 per cent; large cell carcinoma, 15 to 20 per cent; and small cell anaplastic carcinoma, 15 to 20 per cent. Lung cancer is now the leading cause of cancer deaths in men and is the third leading cause of cancer deaths in women, after cancer of the breast and colon. Bronchogenic carcinoma occurs most frequently between the

TABLE 1.　World Health Organization Classification of Primary Lung Neoplasms

I. Epidermoid carcinomas
II. Small cell anaplastic carcinomas
　1. Fusiform cell type
　2. Polygonal cell type
　3. Lymphocyte-like ("oat-cell") type
　4. Others
III. Adenocarcinomas
　1. Bronchogenic
　　a. Acinar ⎤
　　b. Papillary ⎦ with or without mucin formation
　2. Bronchiolo-alveolar
IV. Large cell carcinomas
　1. Solid tumors with mucin-like content
　2. Solid tumors without mucin-like content
　3. Giant cell carcinomas
　4. "Clear" cell carcinomas
V. Combined epidermoid and adenocarcinomas
VI. Carcinoid tumors
VII. Bronchial gland tumors
　1. Cylindromas
　2. Mucoepidermoid tumors
　3. Others
VIII. Papillary tumors of the surface epithelium
　1. Epidermoid
　2. Epidermoid with goblet cells
　3. Others
IX. "Mixed" tumors and carcinosarcomas
X. Sarcomas
XI. Unclassified
XII. Mesotheliomas
　1. Localized
　2. Diffuse
XIII. Melanomas

ages of 45 and 75 years, and there is a male-to-female preponderance of about 7:1. However, in the United States, mortality rates from lung cancer are now increasing more rapidly for women than for men, and the sex ratio has started to decline.

ETIOLOGY AND PATHOGENESIS. The major factor in the development of bronchogenic carcinoma is the inhalation of carcinogenic pollutants, especially tobacco smoke, by susceptible hosts. Epidermoid and small cell anaplastic carcinomas have been most closely associated with cigarette smoking. The evolution of changes in the respiratory epithelium related to smoking has received detailed study. Three principal types of changes related to smoking have been described: a loss of cilia, an increase in the number of cell rows, and the presence of atypical cells. Each of these three changes increases with increased amounts of cigarette smoking. Epithelial lesions are much more frequent in cigarette smokers than in pipe and cigar smokers. Eventually, the columnar epithelial lining is replaced by metaplastic squamous epithelium. Subsequently, atypical proliferation, dysplasia, and carcinoma develop. When carcinomatous change is present and located above the basement membrane, the lesion is referred to as carcinoma in situ. Invasive epidermoid carcinoma is the end result of this progression. Studies have shown that ex-smokers have fewer hyperplastic epithelial cells than do current smokers. Ex-smokers also have fewer cells with atypical nuclei than do current smokers, and the number of such cells decreases progressively as the number of years of nonsmoking increases, although they do not reach the level seen in never-smokers. In agreement with these observations is the finding that the incidence of bronchogenic carcinoma decreases in ex-smokers compared with current smokers, although not reaching the incidence level in never-smokers.

Because many smokers do not develop lung cancer, host factors may be important in the development of this disease. Indeed, there is a significant excess mortality from lung cancer among relatives of lung cancer patients that cannot be accounted for by smoking. There appears to be a synergistic interaction between the familial and smoking factors. The nature of this familial influence has not been determined.

An increased incidence of lung cancer has been recognized in association with certain other environmental exposures. Higher mortality rates from lung cancer have been noted in heavily industrialized areas, where air pollution is characterized by elevated concentrations of benzo(a)pyrene and other polynuclear aromatic hydrocarbons. The increased incidence of lung cancer in asbestos workers is well documented. The frequency of lung cancer has been reported to be eight times the expected value in insulation workers employed in that industry for more than 20 years. It is of interest that lung cancer develops rarely in nonsmoking asbestos workers. The effects of smoking and asbestos exposure appear to be multiplicative rather than additive, thus resulting in the increased frequency of lung cancer in this group. The relative risk for the development of cancer also depends on the type of exposure and the type of asbestos fiber involved. Most, but not all, patients in whom lung cancer develops relative to asbestos exposure also have evidence of pulmonary fibrosis due to exposure to asbestos fibers.

Workers in uranium mines have an increased incidence of lung cancer which cannot be explained solely by smoking. The histologic types of these cancers are mainly epidermoid and small cell anaplastic carcinomas. The incidence of the lung cancers is related to cumulative radiation dosage. More recently, an increased incidence of lung cancer was reported in workers exposed to chloromethyl methyl ether. All these patients were males, and their ages ranged from 33 to 55 years. Most were smokers, but some had never smoked. The duration of exposure to this chemical varied from 3 to 14 years. These tumors were predominantly small cell anaplastic carcinomas. Other occupations in which an increased incidence of lung cancer has been reported include those in which workers are exposed to chromium, arsenic, nickel, and mustard gas.

Several reports have suggested that lung cancer, especially adenocarcinoma, may develop in areas of pulmonary fibrosis or scars. Such lesions may result from proliferating epithelial changes that are sometimes associated with chronic inflammation in the pulmonary parenchyma.

CLINICAL MANIFESTATIONS. The clinical manifestations of bronchogenic carcinoma depend on several factors related to the type and anatomic extent of the tumor. Symptoms may be related to the primary lesion, extension of the tumor beyond the lung parenchyma, distant metastasis, and syndromes produced by systemic nonmetastatic effects of the neoplasm. Many patients with lung cancer are asymptomatic when the pulmonary lesion is discovered.

Cough is a common symptom of lung cancer, and it may be a particularly troublesome symptom when the lesion is located near the carina. Because many lung cancers develop in smokers, a change in the character of a chronic cough may signal the development of the new lesion. *Sputum production* commonly accompanies the cough. The amount is generally small. Profuse expectoration may at times result from the presence of a diffuse bronchiolo-alveolar cell carcinoma, but even with this tumor large amounts of sputum are unusual. *Hemoptysis* occurs frequently owing to ulceration of the primary bronchial lesion. Usually, this is in the form of blood streaking of the sputum. Occasionally, the bleeding is more vigorous, as small blood vessels are eroded by the tumor. Massive hemoptysis leading to death occasionally occurs in advanced disease when the neoplasm erodes into a large blood vessel. *Dyspnea* is a frequent complaint. This may result from the primary tumor, an associated disease, or a combination of both. When lung function is otherwise normal, dyspnea may develop when the neoplasm involves a main bronchus and compromises ventilation to one lung or when it has spread extensively within the thorax.

Frequently, patients have associated chronic obstructive pulmonary disease, and this process is a factor in the development or worsening of dyspnea. The onset of dyspnea may be associated with the development of a pleural effusion due to the neoplasm, and at times, this occurs when the primary neoplasm is small but has spread extensively to the pleural space. Rarely, a primary lung neoplasm may be associated with the development of a pneumothorax, leading to an acute episode of dyspnea. *Fever and chills* resulting from pneumonitis may occur secondary to a bronchogenic carcinoma. The tumor may produce partial or complete bronchial obstruction, leading to an obstructive pneumonitis or atelectasis. Any patient with recurrent pneumonitis or an unresolved pneumonitis should be evaluated for the

possibility of a bronchial neoplasm. *Loss of weight* is a frequent symptom of bronchogenic carcinoma but generally occurs with more extensive disease beyond the time when the neoplasm is limited to the lung parenchyma. *Wheezing* occasionally may be the primary complaint of the patient when the primary bronchial lesion has narrowed a major airway to the degree that impaired air flow and secretion removal lead to the production of this symptom.

When the primary neoplasm has extended beyond the confines of the lung parenchyma, numerous additional symptoms may be present. *Chest pain* may be due to pleural involvement by the tumor or to direct involvement of the ribs and chest wall. The pain may have pleuritic qualities or may be dull and boring in character. *Dysphagia* may result from invasion or compression of the esophagus by a tumor that has spread into the mediastinum. *Hoarseness* is usually due to involvement of the recurrent laryngeal nerve owing to extension of a tumor from the left lung. *Superior vena caval compression or obstruction* results from mediastinal extension of a tumor. This produces edema of the face, neck, and upper extremities, along with a dilated superficial venous pattern in these areas. Some of these patients complain of headache and dizziness or vertigo. Neoplasms at the extreme apex of the lung may invade contiguous structures, producing the *Pancoast syndrome*. In this condition, pain is the most common initial complaint. This pain may be felt in the shoulder, scapular or interscapular area, upper anterior chest, arm, neck, or axilla. Other components of the syndrome include Horner's syndrome, muscle weakness of the upper extremity, and sensory disturbances in the upper extremity. The pain is due to neoplastic involvement of the pleura, ribs, spinal column, and brachial plexus. Horner's syndrome results from tumor extension into the inferior cervical sympathetic ganglion. The upper extremity weakness and sensory disturbances result from involvement of the inferior trunk of the brachial plexus or the eighth cervical and first and second thoracic nerves. Occasionally, such patients complain of hoarseness, which is due to tumor invasion of the right laryngeal nerve, which normally passes around the right subclavian artery in this area.

Distant metastasis is common with bronchogenic carcinoma and may result in a wide variety of symptoms. *Bone pain* may result from osseous metastasis, especially to the ribs, spinal column, and pelvis. *Headache, cranial nerve palsy, monoparalysis, hemiplegia*, and various other neurologic symptoms may result from metastasis to the central nervous system. *Lymphadenopathy*, especially in the supraclavicular and cervical areas, is common, and occasionally this finding is the first abnormality noted by the patient. *Anorexia, epigastric distress, and jaundice* may result from hepatic metastasis.

In recent years, a wide variety of syndromes have been noted in patients with lung cancer from the systemic effects of the neoplasm but not from metastasis. In some of these conditions, hormone or hormone-like secretion by the primary neoplasm has been demonstrated (see Ch. 525). In lung cancer the most commonly encountered endocrine syndromes are *inappropriate antidiuretic hormone secretion, Cushing's syndrome*, and *gynecomastia*. Small cell anaplastic carcinoma especially is associated with the development of these syndromes, suggesting hormone overproduction. Small cell anaplastic carcinoma may be derived from malignant change in the Kulchitsky or K-type cell in the basal layer of the bronchial epithelium. These cells may be of neural crest derivation and may have the potential for secreting many different chemical mediators.

Hypercalcemia associated with lung cancer may be due to metastatic destruction of bone, ectopic formation of parathyroid hormone, or formation by the tumor of an osteolytic substance other than parathyroid hormone. Hypercalcemia may be accompanied by such symptoms as nausea, vomiting, lethargy, polydipsia, polyuria, and mental confusion. The most common cell type of lung cancer associated with this finding is epidermoid carcinoma. Depending on the type of radioimmunoassay utilized, 20 to 70 per cent of tumors that cause hypercalcemia do so by producing ectopic parathyroid hormone. The serum phosphorus level varies, depending on the presence or absence of azotemia, but generally in nonazotemic patients the level is decreased. Removal of the primary lung tumor may lead to prompt return of the serum calcium and phosphorus levels to normal. Recurrence of the tumor may return the electrolyte abnormalities.

Hypertrophic pulmonary osteoarthropathy may be associated with various neoplasms, but it is most commonly associated with bronchogenic carcinoma. In one series, 41 per cent were epidermoid carcinomas, 22 per cent were adenocarcinomas, 16 per cent were large cell carcinomas, and 8 per cent were small cell carcinomas; the remainder included lymphomas, bronchial carcinoids, and other more infrequent tumors. This syndrome occurs frequently with large localized fibrous mesotheliomas of the pleura and may occur with metastatic tumors to the lung from the breast, uterus, and prostate. The syndrome consists of a symmetric proliferating subperiosteal osteitis with subperiosteal new bone formation. This process most commonly involves the distal long bones of the arms and legs. The ankles, knees, and wrists may show chronic synovitis, effusion, pannus formation, and cartilage erosion. This produces arthralgias, limitation of motion, and tenderness on palpation. The circumference of the limbs may be increased, and at times severe edema of the legs may be noted. Hypertrophic pulmonary osteoarthropathy is almost always associated with *digital clubbing*, but the latter frequently occurs alone. On pathologic examination, the subperiosteal new bone formation that takes place around the distal ends of the long bones of the extremities is characterized by a vascular, edematous osteoid matrix. The connective tissue overlying the periosteum undergoes proliferative changes and contains numerous thick-walled vascular channels, which appear to be arteriovenous anastomoses. Increased blood flow to the involved extremities has been demonstrated. In some way, a neural reflex appears to be involved also, because vagotomy decreases the abnormal blood flow in the extremities of patients with this syndrome. In animals with this syndrome, atropine does not produce the same effects as vagotomy, thus suggesting that the vagus may have a role as the afferent limb in a neurovascular reflex. The symptoms from this syndrome may precede, occur simultaneously with, or follow the development of symptoms related to the lung tumor. Removal of the lung tumor produces relief of symptoms, and in some cases vagotomy alone relieves symptoms. Bone changes may gradually revert to normal after resection of the tumor.

A number of *neurologic syndromes* that are not due to metastasis have been associated with lung cancer. The cause of these syndromes is unknown. These may be due to immunologic reaction, infection due to altered immunity, toxin production by the tumor, or utilization of an essential metabolite by the tumor. The neurologic symptoms may antedate discovery of the tumor by several years, may occur at the same time as symptoms from the tumor, or may develop after resection of the tumor. There is no correlation between the neurologic symptoms, the size of the tumor, and the presence or absence of metastasis. The neurologic symptoms may occur when the lung tumor is curable, but the neurologic manifestations generally do not change after resection of the tumor. The lung cancer is frequently of small cell anaplastic type, but the syndromes have been associated with all types of bronchogenic carcinoma. The neural and neuromuscular syndromes include *corticocerebellar degeneration, spinocerebellar degeneration, peripheral neuropathy, myasthenia,* and *myopathy* (see Ch. 322 to 327).

Thrombophlebitis, when it is recurrent or migratory and without apparent cause and when it is resistant to treatment with anticoagulants and involves unusual sites, suggests the possibility of an underlying lung neoplasm.

Nonbacterial thrombotic endocarditis may occur with lung neoplasms, especially with bronchiolo-alveolar cell carcinomas and adenocarcinomas. Vegetations occur most frequently on the mitral valve, but they may occur on the aortic valve alone or on both the aortic and mitral valves. These lesions may result in cerebral and myocardial embolization.

DIAGNOSIS. The diagnosis of bronchogenic carcinoma is generally established by some combination of clinical history, physical examination, thoracic roentgenogram, sputum cytologic examination, bronchoscopic examination, biopsy of involved structures, and thoracotomy. The many symptoms that bronchogenic carcinoma may produce have been described, and most of them are not specific for carcinoma. Physical examination of the chest may reveal a localized wheeze due to bronchial obstruction, dullness to percussion and decreased breath sounds due to presence of a pleural effusion, or other abnormalities such as rhonchi and expiratory slowing. However, in many patients, examination of the chest reveals no abnormalities. A complete physical examination is very important because it may reveal, for example, evidence of mediastinal spread of the tumor producing the signs of superior vena caval obstruction, as well as evidence of distant metastasis to supraclavicular or cervical lymph nodes or to the liver, with resultant hepatomegaly. Such findings are important in guiding the subsequent workup and evaluation of the patient.

The *thoracic roentgenogram* may reveal the presence of the neoplasm, give clues as to the histologic cell type of the neoplasm, and provide information on the extent of the neoplasm within the thorax. Epidermoid carcinomas most frequently present as hilar or perihilar masses, although they also may present as peripheral nodules. At times, the thoracic roentgenogram reveals obstructive hyperlucency, obstructive pneumonitis, or atelectasis that is secondary to the intrabronchial tumor. Cavitation has been reported to occur in about 7 per cent of patients with epidermoid carcinomas. The cavity may be thick walled and contain an air-fluid level, thereby resembling a lung abscess. The cavitation may be central or eccentric. Small cell anaplastic carcinoma generally presents as a hilar or perihilar mass, frequently with mediastinal widening. There may be associated obstructive pneumonitis or loss of lung volume. Large cell carcinoma appears most commonly as a peripheral mass. Cavitation may occur with this tumor, and the cavity usually appears to have a thick wall. Adenocarcinoma usually appears as a peripheral mass, and rarely it may also undergo cavity formation. Bronchiolo-alveolar cell carcinoma may present as single or multiple nodules or as diffuse lobar infiltrates. At times, one can recognize radiolucent spaces within the nodules. The margins of the nodules in alveolar cell carcinoma may be less sharply defined and less dense than nodules of metastatic tumor, and this may aid in the differential diagnosis of multiple pulmonary nodules.

In addition to these findings concerning the primary lung neoplasm, the thoracic roentgenogram also may demonstrate hilar and mediastinal lymph node involvement, pleural effusion due to the tumor, rib metastasis, elevation of a hemidiaphragm, tracheal compression or distortion, and pericardial effusion. Special roentgenographic studies may be helpful. Bilateral decubitus thoracic roentgenograms will demonstrate free pleural fluid and may demonstrate small amounts of pleural fluid that are not apparent on routine films. Tomograms of pulmonary nodules are helpful if they demonstrate central calcification suggestive of a granuloma or stippled calcification suggestive of a hamartoma. Eccentric calcification does not necessarily indicate a benign process because the calcium may have been engulfed by an enlarging neoplasm. Whole-lung tomograms may be helpful in differentiating a primary lung cancer and a metastatic lesion from a previously resected cancer elsewhere in the body. If these tomograms reveal multiple lesions, which may not be apparent on routine films, the diagnosis of metastatic disease is favored. Pulmonary nodules must be at least 1 cm in diameter before they can be detected on the routine thoracic roentgenogram. Lesions even larger than this may be hidden by overlying bone structures, the diaphragm, and the heart and great vessels.

Cytologic studies of the sputum are very helpful in establishing the diagnosis of bronchogenic carcinoma. The frequency of positive results in patients with lung cancer depends on the number and types of specimens examined and the location of the neoplasms. Centrally located lesions may be positive in about two thirds of cases, whereas peripheral lesions are positive in about one third of cases or less. Epidermoid and small cell anaplastic carcinomas that are central in location are most frequently associated with positive cytologic examinations. Bronchiolo-alveolar carcinoma, when present as a diffuse lesion rather than as a discrete nodule, can also be identified frequently by this means. Sputum for examination may be collected as a one-day spontaneous specimen, a three-day pooled spontaneous specimen, or an induced sputum specimen. Studies have shown that the three-day pooled specimen is superior to the one-day spontaneous specimen and has a similar percentage of positivity to induced sputum specimens. The induced sputum technique is of greatest value in patients who cannot expectorate spontaneously. Experienced cytologists can be very accurate in providing information regarding the cell type in epidermoid and small cell carcinomas and adenocarcinomas.

The sputum cytologic examination and the thoracic roentgenogram have been shown to be complementary in several studies. The thoracic roentgenogram is especially valuable in detecting early peripheral lesions, whereas sputum cytologic examination is more helpful in detecting early central lesions. False-positive sputum cytologic examinations are unusual, but can occur with such illnesses as acute pulmonary infections and pulmonary infarctions.

Bronchoscopic examination is an important technique in the diagnosis and localization of bronchogenic carcinoma. The recent introduction of the bronchofiberscope has increased the ability of this technique to establish a diagnosis, largely because this instrument enables close examination of the segmental and subsegmental bronchi in the upper lobes, which was not possible with previous instruments. A definitive diagnosis frequently can be established by direct visualization and biopsy of the lesion. Bronchial washings also may be obtained for cytologic examination. In addition, brushing of a peripheral lesion under fluoroscopic guidance may yield the diagnosis when direct biopsy is not possible.

Lung cancer may spread extensively within the thorax and metastasize widely throughout the body. The extent of local spread and distant metastases must be documented to determine prognosis and to plan therapy. *Biopsy of enlarged cervical and supraclavicular nodes* will establish the presence of extrathoracic metastasis. Liver metastasis is common, and when clinically suspected it may be detected by *liver function tests* and *isotope scans*. *Liver biopsy* may be indicated. *Bone roentgenograms* and *bone isotope scans* in patients with bone pain may demonstrate bone metastasis. Most metastatic lesions from lung cancer are osteolytic. The brain is a frequent site of metastatic disease, and when neurologic symptoms are present, this involvement can be documented by *neurologic examination, skull roentgenography, computerized tomographic studies*, and *angiography*. *Mediastinoscopy* may be needed to demonstrate metastasis to the mediastinal nodes and may preclude the need for thoracotomy. Some authorities employ this procedure almost routinely before deciding on surgery. Pleural effusion may be due either to direct tumor involvement of the pleura or to lymphatic obstruction by the tumor, or may be secondary to obstructive pneumonitis. Generally, the effusion is an exudate with a protein concentration that is greater than 3 grams per deciliter. Frequently, it is bloody or serosanguineous. *Cytologic examination of the pleural fluid or pathologic examination of material obtained by needle biopsy of the pleura* usually will establish the cause for the effusion. Some patients present with single nodules in the lung, and for various reasons they may not be suitable candidates for thoracotomy. The diagnosis of lung cancer in these patients frequently can be made by *cytologic examination of transthoracic needle aspirates*. The procedure is carried out under fluoroscopic guidance.

STAGING OF BRONCHOGENIC CARCINOMA. A method for staging lung cancer has been proposed that is helpful in determining prognosis and aids in the selection of proper therapy. This method, proposed by the American Joint Committee for Cancer Staging and End-Results Reporting (Table 2), is based on an estimate of the anatomic extent of the disease. In this system, the letter T describes the extent of the primary tumor, the letter N describes the presence or absence of regional lymph node involvement, and the letter M describes

TABLE 2.   Staging of Bronchogenic Carcinoma Proposed by the American Joint Committee for Cancer Staging and End-Results Reporting

TNM Classification
Primary tumor (T)
T0: No evidence of primary tumor
TX: Tumor proved by the presence of malignant cells in bronchopulmonary secretions but not visualized roentgenographically or bronchoscopically, or any tumor that cannot be assessed
TIS: Carcinoma in situ
T1: A tumor that is 3.0 cm or less in greatest diameter, surrounded by lung or visceral pleura, and without evidence of invasion proximal to a lobar bronchus at bronchoscopy
T2: A tumor more than 3.0 cm in greatest diameter, or a tumor of any size that either invades the visceral pleura or has associated atelectasis or obstructive pneumonitis extending to the hilar region; at bronchoscopy, the proximal extent of demonstrable tumor must be within a lobar bronchus or at least 2.0 cm distal to the carina; any associated atelectasis or obstructive pneumonitis must involve less than an entire lung, and there must be no pleural effusion
T3: A tumor of any size with direct extension into an adjacent structure as the parietal pleura or chest wall, the diaphragm, or the mediastinum and its contents; or a tumor demonstrable bronchoscopically to involve a main bronchus less than 2.0 cm distal to the carina; or any tumor associated with atelectasis or obstructive pneumonitis of an entire lung or pleural effusion
Regional lymph node involvement (N)
N0: No demonstrable metastasis to regional lymph node
N1: Metastasis to lymph nodes in the peribronchial or the ipsilateral hilar region, or both, including direct extension
N2: Metastasis to lymph nodes in the mediastinum
Distant metastasis (M)
MX: Not assessed
M0: No (known) distant metastasis
M1: Distant metastasis present in lymph nodes, brain, bones, liver, contralateral lung, bone marrow, pleura, skin, eye, or other areas

Stage Grouping

Occult carcinoma
TX N0 M0 — An occult carcinoma with bronchopulmonary secretions containing malignant cells but without other evidence of the primary tumor or evidence of metastasis to the regional lymph nodes or distant metastasis

Stage I
TIS N0 M0 — Carcinoma in situ
T1 N0 M0
T1 N1 M0
T2 N0 M0 — A tumor that can be classified T1 without any metastasis or with metastasis to the lymph nodes in the peribronchial and/or ipsilateral hilar region only, or a tumor that can be classified T2 without any metastasis to nodes or distant metastasis
NOTE: TX N1 M0 and T0 N1 M0 are also theoretically possible, but such a clinical diagnosis would be difficult if not impossible to make; if such a diagnosis is made, it would be included in stage I

Stage II
T2 N1 M0 — A tumor classified as T2 with metastasis to the lymph nodes in the peribronchial and/or ipsilateral hilar region only

Stage III
T3 with any N or M — Any tumor more extensive than T2, or any
N2 with any T or M — tumor with metastasis to the lymph nodes in
M1 with any T or N — the mediastinum, or any tumor with distant metastasis

the presence or absence of distant metastases. Utilizing this system, a clinical-diagnostic stage for all patients can be determined after the initial examination. If the patient undergoes thoracotomy, a surgical-evaluative stage or a postsurgical treatment–pathologic stage may be determined. A re-treatment stage may be assigned if the cancer recurs after treatment. Small cell anaplastic carcinoma has such a poor clinical course regardless of

the demonstrable extent of the disease that staging of it is not very helpful.

TREATMENT AND PROGNOSIS. *Surgery* remains the most effective therapy for bronchogenic carcinoma. One exception is in the patients with small cell anaplastic carcinoma. This tumor has an extremely poor prognosis, and for limited disease radiation therapy is superior to surgery. Many clinical trials utilizing polychemotherapy are now under way for this neoplasm. For stages I and II bronchogenic carcinomas, surgical resection is recommended. Some stage III carcinomas are resectable if the extent of the disease is such that all the cancer can be excised. This may be true for some peripheral lesions that directly involve the chest wall in which the entire disease can be removed en bloc. Overall, the prognosis for all patients with lung cancer is poor. The five-year survival rate for all stages of bronchogenic carcinoma has been about 9 per cent for the last 20 years. However, it is well recognized that the size and extent of the primary lesion are important determinants of survival. Relatively high five-year survival rates of about 70 per cent have been reported for patients with carcinoma in situ or minimally invasive carcinoma. Patients with peripheral lesions 4 cm or less in diameter also have been shown to have improved survival rates. In one study of 193 patients with peripheral lesions of this type, resection for cure was carried out in 182 patients or 94 per cent of the group. The operative mortality was 7 per cent. Of patients who survived surgery, the five-year survival rate was 51 per cent. The five-year survival rate for patients with lesions 2 cm or less in diameter was 68 per cent; for patients with lesions 2.1 to 3 cm in diameter, it was 46 per cent; and for patients with lesions 3.1 to 4 cm in diameter, it was 42 per cent. In this study, 49 per cent of the lesions were adenocarcinomas, 21 per cent were large cell carcinomas, 18 per cent were epidermoid carcinomas, 10 per cent were bronchiolo-alveolar cell carcinomas, and 2 per cent were small cell anaplastic carcinomas. The survival rates for patients with adenocarcinoma, epidermoid carcinoma, and large cell carcinoma were similar. The survival rate for those with bronchiolo-alveolar carcinoma was higher. Other studies have reported five-year survival rates of 50 to 80 per cent for patients with localized bronchiolo-alveolar cell carcinomas. Patients with the diffuse variety of bronchiolo-alveolar cell carcinoma have a uniformly poor prognosis. Further evidence of the importance of the extent of disease on survival can be noted in Table 3, in which two-year survival rates for various types of lung cancer are shown, based on the stage of the disease determined by the method previously discussed. Thus improvement in survival of patients with lung

TABLE 3.   Percentage of Two-Year Survivals in Carcinoma of the Lung*

Cell type	Stage of Disease		
	I	II	III
Epidermoid	46.6	39.8	11.5
Adenocarcinoma	45.9	14.3	7.9
Large cell	42.8	12.9	12.9
Small cell	6.0	5.0	3.8

*Adapted from Mountain, C. F., Carr, D. T., and Anderson, W. A. D.: Am. J. Roentgenol., 120:130, 1974.

cancer probably will come from earlier diagnosis of the neoplasm, at least until chemotherapy or other forms of treatment become more effective.

When a patient presents with a lesion that is compatible with a bronchogenic carcinoma, it is important to determine whether the patient is a surgical candidate. Surgery may not be feasible because of spread of the primary tumor or because of associated diseases. The patient is generally considered to be inoperable if there is widespread mediastinal lymph node metastasis, superior vena caval obstruction, neoplastic pleural involvement, or evidence of distant metastasis. Evaluation of general health is important, especially in relation to the presence of chronic obstructive pulmonary disease. When such disease is present, one must estimate the pulmonary function that the patient will have after the operation. In evaluating this, it is important to consider the extent of the contemplated surgery — lobectomy or pneumonectomy — and whether the tumor is significantly impairing pulmonary function preoperatively. For example, in a patient with a tumor occluding a mainstem bronchus, the results of pulmonary function tests before operation probably closely reflect what the patient will be able to do after the operation. However, a patient with a small peripheral lesion will undoubtedly lose functioning lung in the course of the operation. Patients with reduction of 50 per cent in the forced vital capacity, the one-second forced expiratory volume (expressed as a percentage of the forced vital capacity), maximal voluntary ventilation, and diffusing capacity for carbon monoxide are high-risk patients, but many can successfully undergo surgery. Additional studies, such as isotope perfusion scans, to evaluate the pulmonary capillary bed may help the clinician determine whether a patient can tolerate surgery in selected instances. With modern methods of intensive respiratory care, it is often surprising how well resectional surgery is tolerated.

Radiation therapy is recommended for stages I and II bronchogenic carcinoma only when surgical treatment is contraindicated. This form of therapy is indicated for stage III neoplasms when the disease is limited to the involved hemithorax and ipsilateral supraclavicular lymph nodes and when surgical treatment is not possible. Such therapy can eliminate evidence of cancer in as many as 30 per cent of such patients. Failure to cure such patients results from presence of metastatic lesions outside the field of therapy. Preoperative radiation to lung cancers has not increased survival rates in general. Preoperative radiotherapy to superior sulcus tumors has been advocated in some studies. Patients with advanced lung cancer frequently may receive palliation with radiotherapy. Bone pain, superior vena caval obstruction, pleural effusion, brachial plexus involvement, and hemoptysis may be controlled in as many as 75 per cent of the patients. When radiation therapy is considered for limited disease in patients with pulmonary insufficiency, it is important to realize that the radiation therapy will damage the adjacent lung tissue and thereby further impair lung function.

The poor over-all prognosis for lung cancer is related to the early and widespread dissemination of the cancer. *Chemotherapy* would seem to be a reasonable approach to this problem. At this time, many clinical trials are under way using chemotherapeutic agents, such as nitrogen mustard, cyclophosphamide, methotrexate, 5-fluorouracil, Adriamycin, and bleomycin. The responses to single drugs have been disappointing, but some combination-drug programs have produced encouraging results, particularly in patients with small cell anaplastic carcinoma.

Immunotherapy is currently being considered for bronchogenic carcinoma. This approach has been based on studies that suggest an impaired cellular immunity in patients with carcinoma. The cellular immune response has been evaluated by quantifying the number of circulating T cells and B cells, by skin testing with antigens such as purified protein derivative, mumps, *Candida*, and 2,4-dinitrochlorobenzene (DNCB), and by testing the ability of lymphocytes to undergo blast transformation in response to mitogens. At present, there is considerable uncertainty in regard to how and when the impaired cellular immunity develops in a patient with lung cancer and what the effect of this impaired immunity is on prognosis and survival. Animal experiments suggest that immunotherapy may be most effective when only a limited amount of tumor is present. Because immunotherapy is likely to be most effective when the tumor burden is minimal, clinical trials using nonspecific immunostimulating agents such as BCG vaccine as surgical adjuvants are under way. It is too early to know what the benefits will be.

In spite of the poor prognosis for most patients with advanced lung cancer, much can be done to alleviate their distress. Judicious use of analgesics and narcotics, together with appropriate radiotherapy, will control pain in many patients. Occasionally, neurosurgical procedures are necessary for symptomatic relief. Antibiotics for symptoms of obstructive pneumonitis, and bronchodilator therapy for dyspnea due to or aggravated by accompanying chronic obstructive pulmonary disease, are helpful. Occasionally, oxygen therapy at home aids in relieving dyspnea. Recurrent pleural effusion may be benefited by intercostal tube drainage with the instillation of sclerosing agents, such as nitrogen mustard or tetracycline.

Auerbach, O., Stout, A. P., Hammond, E. C., and Garfinkel, L.: Changes in bronchial epithelium in relation to cigarette smoking and in relation to lung cancer. N. Engl. J. Med., 265:253, 1961.

Auerbach, O., Stout, A. P., Hammond, E. C., and Garfinkel, L.: Changes in bronchial epithelium in relation to sex, age, residence, smoking and pneumonia. N. Engl. J. Med., 267:111, 1962.

Byrd, R. B., Carr, D. T., Miller, W. E., Payne, W. S., and Woolner, L. B.: Radiographic abnormalities in carcinoma of the lung as related to histological cell type. Thorax, 24:573, 1969.

Carbone, P. P., Frost, J. K., Feinstein, A. R., Higgins, G. A., Jr., and Selawry, O. S.: Lung cancer: Perspectives and prospects. Ann. Intern. Med., 73:1003, 1970.

Fontana, R. S., Sanderson, D. R., Woolner, L. B., Miller, W. E., Bernatz, P. E., Payne, W. S., and Taylor, W. F.: The Mayo Lung Project for early detection and localization of bronchogenic carcinoma: A status report. Chest, 67:511, 1975.

Holmes, E. C.: Immunology and lung cancer. Ann. Thorac. Surg., 21:250, 1976.

Jackman, R. J., Good, C. A., Clagett, O. T., and Woolner, L. B.: Survival rates in peripheral bronchogenic carcinomas up to four centimeters in diameter presenting as solitary pulmonary nodules. J. Thorac. Cardiovasc. Surg., 57:1, 1969.

Mountain, C. F., Carr, D. T., and Anderson, W. A. D.: A system for the clinical staging of lung cancer. Am. J. Roentgenol., 120:130, 1974.

Nathanson, L., and Hall, T. C.: Lung tumors: How they produce their syndromes. Ann. N.Y. Acad. Sci., 230:367, 1974.

Selawry, O. S.: The role of chemotherapy in the treatment of lung cancer. Semin. Oncol., 1:259, 1974.

Stenseth, J. H., Clagett, O. T., and Woolner, L. B.: Hypertrophic pulmonary osteoarthropathy. Dis. Chest, 52:62, 1967.

Tokuhata, G. K., and Lilienfeld, A. M.: Familial aggregation of lung cancer in humans. J. Natl. Cancer Inst., 30:289, 1963.

CARCINOID TUMORS

DEFINITION. The term "bronchial adenoma" has been used in the past to describe slow-growing intrabronchial lesions that subsequently have been subdivided into three distinct pathologic entities: bronchial carcinoids, cylindromas, and mucoepidermoid tumors. Because these tumors have different biologic courses, as well as different histologic features, they should be considered as separate entities rather than under the broad category of bronchial adenoma. True bronchial adenomas of bronchial gland origin are extremely rare. Carcinoid tumors arising elsewhere in the body are discussed in Ch. 551.

PATHOLOGY. Carcinoid tumors may develop from Kulchitsky's cells, which are found in the bronchial epithelium and in bronchial glands. These are of neural crest origin and contain neurosecretory granules. Also, small cell anaplastic carcinoma may be derived from them. At times, the pathologist may have difficulty in distinguishing, on a small biopsy specimen, a carcinoid tumor from a small cell anaplastic carcinoma. Carcinoids tend to grow into the bronchial lumen, but there is frequently considerable extension below the mucosa. Carcinoids may metastasize to the regional lymph nodes, liver, and bones. The bone metastatic lesions may be osteoblastic or osteolytic. About 10 per cent of these tumors may be pathologically classified as "atypical carcinoids." These have increased mitotic activity, pleomorphism, and irregularity of nuclei with prominent nucleoli, areas of increased cellularity with disorganization of the architecture, and areas of tumor necrosis. These tumors have a more aggressive clinical course.

CLINICAL MANIFESTATIONS. Carcinoid tumors have an equal sex distribution. The average age of the patient at diagnosis is about 48 years, with a range reported in one series to be from 15 to 73 years. As expected from this intrabronchial lesion, the most common symptoms are cough, hemoptysis, and recurrent pneumonitis.

Bronchial carcinoids may produce the carcinoid syndrome, with cutaneous flushes, diarrhea, bronchoconstriction, and cardiac valvular lesions (see Ch. 551).

DIAGNOSIS. The diagnosis may be suspected on the basis of the history, particularly if the clinical course has been prolonged, because the tumor is slow growing and many patients have cough or recurrent hemoptysis for several years. The findings on physical examination depend on the degree of bronchial obstruction produced by the tumor. There may be decreased breath sounds and dullness to percussion owing to atelectasis, or a localized wheeze may be audible because of partial bronchial obstruction.

The thoracic roentgenogram may reveal a peripheral nodule, a hilar mass, or secondary manifestations of the intrabronchial lesion such as loss of volume, atelectasis, obstructive hyperinflation, or obstructive pneumonitis. Results of sputum cytologic examination are generally negative. Bronchoscopic examination is the best procedure for diagnosis of lesions within the range of the bronchoscope. Care should be taken while these tumors are being biopsied, because excessive bleeding may ensue.

TREATMENT AND PROGNOSIS. The treatment of choice is surgical excision. The extent of the surgery depends on the findings at operation. Sleeve resection of a part of a bronchus, segmental resection, lobectomy, or pneumonectomy may be required. The over-all five-year survival rate for patients with typical bronchial carcinoids has been reported to be 94 per cent; if regional nodes are involved with metastasis, the five-year survival rate decreases to 71 per cent. Patients with "atypical" carcinoids, based on a more aggressive pathologic appearance of the tumor, have a poorer prognosis; metastasis develops in 70 per cent compared with 5 per cent for patients with typical carcinoids, and 57 per cent of patients with "atypical" carcinoids survive five years. Corticosteroids and the phenothiazine drugs have been reported useful in patients with the carcinoid syndrome due to bronchial carcinoids.

Melmon, K. L., Sjoerdsma, A., and Mason, D. T.: Distinctive clinical and therapeutic aspects of the syndrome associated with bronchial carcinoid tumors. Am. J. Med., 39:568, 1965.

Okike, N., Bernatz, P. E., and Woolner, L. B.: Carcinoid tumors of the lung. Ann. Thorac. Surg., 22:270, 1976.

PRIMARY LYMPHOMA OF THE LUNG

The major discussions of lymphomas are to be found in Ch. 500 to 503. The lung and intrathoracic lymph nodes may be the primary sites of Hodgkin's disease and non-Hodgkin's lymphoma. Pseudolymphoma and lymphocytic interstitial pneumonitis are additional entities that may lead to difficulties in establishing a diagnosis.

The clinical manifestations produced by Hodgkin's disease and non-Hodgkin's lymphoma are variable, depending on the extent of the disease. Fever, cough, dyspnea, pleuritic pain, and loss of weight are frequent.

With Hodgkin's disease, the thoracic roentgenogram may reveal a solitary mass that may cavitate, an area of parenchymal consolidation, pleural effusion, or obstructive pneumonitis or atelectasis due to bronchial occlusion. Mediastinal lymph node enlargement is common. The anterior mediastinal nodes are often involved, a finding that is rare in sarcoidosis, and may be helpful in the differential diagnosis of mediastinal adenopathy. Direct parenchymal invasion via the lymphatic vessels may occur and produce a pattern of diffuse linear infiltration on the thoracic roentgenogram. Non-Hodgkin's lymphoma may produce similar roentgenographic patterns. When this disease is primary in the lung, the most common pattern is that of a homogeneous mass within the lung parenchyma with or without hilar and mediastinal lymph node enlargement. Bronchial obstruction rarely occurs, and cavitation in the parenchymal mass is uncommon. Lesions caused by non-Hodgkin's lymphoma may seem to progress very slowly on serial thoracic roentgenograms.

Pseudolymphoma and lymphocytic interstitial pneumonitis are lymphoproliferative disorders that are incompletely understood at present. The pathologic changes are similar in both, with the pseudolymphoma presenting as a nodular lesion and lymphocytic interstitial pneumonitis presenting as a diffuse infiltrate. Pathologically, these lesions may be very difficult to distinguish from a well-differentiated malignant lymphoma of the lymphocytic type. In fact, some patients who were considered to have pseudolymphoma or lymphocytic interstitial pneumonitis initially have developed true malignant lymphoma. Involvement of the hilar or mediastinal lymph nodes in a patient in whom the differentiation is difficult points strongly toward the diagnosis of a malignant lymphoma.

Diagnosis of intrathoracic lymphoproliferative disease depends on obtaining tissue for pathologic examination. Bronchoscopy and cytologic studies of the sputum and bronchial washings are generally not helpful. Occasionally, bronchoscopic biopsy of an endobronchial lesion will be diagnostic in Hodgkin's disease. Transbronchoscopic lung biopsy, mediastinoscopy, mediastinotomy, and thoracotomy are employed to establish the diagnosis when the disease is limited to the thorax.

Hodgkin's disease and non-Hodgkin's lymphoma are treated with radiation therapy and chemotherapy. Surgical resection of non-Hodgkin's lymphoma localized to the lung parenchyma has been carried out at the time of thoracotomy for diagnosis, with radiotherapy given postoperatively in many patients. These studies report a five-year survival of about 45 per cent. Pseudolymphoma of the lung is generally resected when surgical exploration is carried out to obtain the diagnosis. The proper therapy for lymphocytic interstitial pneumonitis has not been established. Some clinicians have treated these patients with immunosuppressive drugs.

Greenberg, S. D., Heisler, J. G., Gyorkey, F., and Jenkins, D. E.: Pulmonary lymphoma versus pseudolymphoma: A perplexing problem. South. Med. J., 65:775, 1972.

Thiessen, P. N., and Couves, C. M.: Primary lymphosarcoma of the lung: A case report and review of the literature. Can. J. Surg., 17:117, 1974.

UNCOMMON PRIMARY LUNG MALIGNANCIES

Cylindromas or adenoid cystic carcinomas derive from the mucous glands of the bronchial epithelium. Most are located in the trachea or main bronchi. There is an equal sex incidence, and the age range at the time of diagnosis has been reported to be between 30 and 65 years. Cylindroma is the second most common tumor of the trachea (the most common being epidermoid carcinoma). It produces its symptoms by bronchial irritation and obstruction. Bronchoscopic examination reveals a polypoid infiltrative tumor that partially or completely obstructs the airway and may bleed easily. Treatment is surgical resection. The prognosis must be guarded because of the tendency for distant metastasis to develop ultimately.

Mucoepidermoid tumors are rare structures of mucous gland origin, occurring in the age range of 40 to 55 years. On bronchoscopic examination, they present as polypoid masses with a smooth surface. Treatment is surgical resection, and the prognosis is better with these than with adenoid cystic carcinomas.

Carcinosarcoma is a rare entity that has both malignant epithelial and sarcomatous elements. It may present as a peripheral parenchymal mass or as an endobronchial lesion with bronchial obstruction. Treatment is surgical resection.

Pulmonary blastoma probably is a malignancy of primitive mesodermal cells capable of producing both epithelial and stromal components. It tends to arise in the peripheral portion of the lung. Treatment is surgical resection, and the prognosis is poor.

Payne, W. S., Ellis, F. H., Jr., Woolner, L. B., and Moersch, H. J.: The surgical treatment of cylindroma (adenoid cystic carcinoma) and muco-epidermoid tumors of the bronchus. J. Thorac. Cardiovasc. Surg., 38:709, 1959.

METASTATIC NEOPLASMS OF THE LUNG

The lung is a frequent location of metastases from carcinomas and sarcomas. These lesions may have several different patterns on the thoracic roentgenogram, patterns which may provide clues to aid in the search for the primary lesion if it is not apparent. *Solitary metastatic lesions to the lung* commonly originate from carcinomas of the colon, rectum, breast, kidney, testis, and cervix and from melanomas. Osteogenic and synovial cell sarcomas may produce this pattern. *Diffuse hematogenous metastasis* may appear as multiple micronodular shadows or large masses on the thoracic roentgenogram. Nodules may be of one size, suggesting one shower of tumor emboli, or may vary in size, suggesting tumor embolization at different times. A fine micronodular pattern is suggestive of metastasis from thyroid, renal, or trophoblastic tumors or from bone sarcomas. Rarely, diffuse hematogenous metastasis may produce a clinical pattern of cor pulmonale, with the thoracic roentgenogram revealing large hilar vessels but no parenchymal infiltration or nodules. *Diffuse lymphatic metastasis* may develop owing to involvement of the bronchomediastinal lymph nodes, with retrograde spread through the pulmonary lymphatics, or to vascular metastasis, with invasion of the peripheral lymphatic vessel and spread toward the hilar regions. Tumors that frequently present these findings are carcinomas from the breast, stomach, pancreas, thyroid, larynx, and lung. The roentgenographic pattern is one of increased linear and reticulonodular markings throughout the lung. *Cavitation* in metastatic lesions is suggestive of an epidermoid carcinoma from the head and neck regions and female reproductive organs, of a carcinoma of the colon, or of a metastatic sarcoma. *Calcification* in metastatic lesions is suggestive of an osteogenic sarcoma or a chondrosarcoma. *Pleural effusions* may be produced by metastasis from almost any primary neoplasm. *Pneumothorax* may be due to metastatic lesions, especially from bone, or to synovial cell sarcomas.

Cytologic examination of the sputum may be positive in as many as 50 per cent of patients with lung metastasis, depending on the extent of the disease. Bronchoscopy with biopsy of endobronchial lesions due to metastasis is occasionally helpful in renal, pancreatic, and adrenal carcinomas and malignant melanoma.

Surgical resection should be considered for solitary metastases to the lung. Five-year survival rates of 30 per cent have been reported, with the rate for carcinomas being 32 per cent and for sarcomas, 23 per cent. The resection should be conservative, and the primary neoplasm should be controlled. There should be no other evidence of metastatic disease. It has been suggested that a patient with a presumed solitary metastasis should be observed three months to see if additional lesions develop before proceeding with surgery. In some situations (patients with metastatic osteogenic sarcomas), multiple lung resections have been performed, with good results. It is important to remember that a solitary nodule in a patient with a previous malignancy may be a new primary lung malignancy.

Thomford, N. R., Woolner, L. B., and Clagett, O. T.: The surgical treatment of metastatic tumors in the lungs. J. Thorac. Cardiovasc. Surg., 49:357, 1965.

BENIGN TUMORS OF THE LUNG

In comparison with malignant neoplasms of the lung, benign tumors are uncommon. They present as solitary nodules in asymptomatic persons or as endobronchial lesions. In the latter instance, they may produce cough, hemoptysis, dyspnea, and recurrent pneumonitis, depending on size and location. The *hamartoma*, the most common benign lung neoplasm, is composed of tissues normally present in the lung, but these elements are unorganized, and include fat, epithelial tissue, fibrous tissue, and cartilage. These tumors are usually not diagnosed until adulthood, and there is a 2:1 or 3:1 male predominance. Most of them are peripheral and present as a solitary lung nodule. There may be calcification in the lesion, and sometimes this has the characteristic stippled or "popcorn" appearance. About 10 per cent of hamartomas are endobronchial. Treatment is surgical excision, and the prognosis is excellent.

Papillomas are most often encountered as laryngeal tumors in children. They may involve the trachea and bronchi. Histologically, they are composed of vascular connective tissue covered by stratified squamous epithelium. They may be of viral cause. In an unusual situation in which multiple papillomas extend throughout many bronchi, the clinical course may be characterized by repeated pneumonitis, atelectasis, bronchiectasis, and chronic pulmonary infection. Management is difficult and includes repeated bronchoscopic removal of the tumors if possible. Malignant change has been reported.

Granular cell myoblastomas are rare benign tumors usually found in the walls of the large bronchi. They may present as a mass lesion on the thoracic roentgenogram or with symptoms suggestive of a bronchial obstructing lesion. Treatment is surgical resection. Other uncommon benign lung tumors include *lipomas, fibromas, leiomyomas, chondromas,* and *hemangiomas.*

Arrigoni, M. G., Woolner, L. B., Bernatz, P. E., Miller, W. E., and Fontana, R. S.: Benign tumors of the lung: A ten-year surgical experience. J. Thorac. Cardiovasc. Surg., 60:589, 1970.

350. DISEASES OF THE PLEURA, MEDIASTINUM, DIAPHRAGM, AND CHEST WALL

John H. McClement

350.1. THE PLEURA

INTRODUCTION

The pleura, a serous membrane of mesodermal origin, covers the lung, the chest wall, the diaphragm, and the mediastinum. It is a closed sac which encloses the pleural space and separates the lung from adjacent structures. The visceral pleura designates that portion of it which covers the lung; the remainder is the parietal pleura. The parietal pleura receives its blood supply from the systemic circulation, whereas the visceral is supplied by the pulmonary circulation. The normal pleural space contains no gas and only a small amount of serous fluid. During quiet breathing, the elastic recoil of the lung produces a subatmospheric pressure (-4 to -10 cm H_2O) in the pleural space.

Pleural pain and signs and symptoms secondary to collections of fluid and gas in the pleural space are principal indicators of pleural disease.

Pleural pain originates in the parietal pleura; stimulation of the visceral pleura does not cause pain. Typically, pleural pain is sharp, aggravated by respiration and thoracic motion, and relieved by splinting of the involved area. When it arises from the pleura of the chest wall, the pain is referred to the chest wall overlying the involved area; pain arising from the pleura of the central portion of the diaphragm is referred to the posterior part of the shoulder area; pain from the costal portions of the diaphragm is referred to adjacent parts of the chest wall and abdomen.

The formation and removal of pleural fluid are dependent on those forces which regulate the exchange of fluid into and out of capillary beds, and on lymphatic drainage. The hydrostatic pressure in the pleural capillaries (Pc), the hydrostatic pressure in the pleural space (Ppl), the oncotic pressures of the plasma (OPp) and the pleural fluid (OPpf), and the permeability of the pleural capillaries (K) are the factors which regulate the transport of fluid (F) into and out of the pleural capillaries. According to Starling's law of transcapillary exchange, this can be expressed as follows:

$$F = K(Pc - OPp) - (Ppl - OPpf)$$

The visceral pleura is supplied by arterioles from the low pressure pulmonary arterial system, whereas the parietal pleura is supplied by the higher pressure systemic arteries. There is evidence that the permeability (K) of the visceral capillaries is less than that of the parietal pleura. Normally a balance of these forces favors absorption of fluid by the visceral pleura at about the same rate it is formed. However, all these forces may be altered by disease, and the removal of fluid may be slowed or its formation increased. An increase in capillary permeability (K) from inflammation, a decrease in the oncotic pressure of the plasma proteins (OPp) from hypoalbuminemia, and an increase in the hydrostatic pressure in the pulmonary capillaries (Pc) are the common alterations that lead to pleural fluid collections. Uncommonly a decrease in the hydrostatic pressure in the pleura (Ppl) from a collapsed and nonexpandable lung will cause effusion. Protein, red blood cells, and particulate matter are removed from the pleural space by the pleural lymphatics. The absorption and transport of pleural fluid by way of the lymphatics is increased by diaphragmatic and intercostal activity. Decrease in this activity or obstruction of local or distant lymphatic channels may prolong or prevent reabsorption of pleural fluid.

METHODS OF EXAMINATION IN PLEURAL DISEASE

HISTORY AND PHYSICAL EXAMINATION. Pleural pain and shortness of breath are the symptoms which most often call attention to pleural disease. A dry, irritating, nonproductive cough may sometimes accompany the pleural pain. Shortness of breath may sometimes be caused by severe pleural pain, but usually indicates the presence of fairly large amounts of intrapleural fluid or gas. Early in the course of pleural inflammation a friction rub may be heard over the involved area. As fluid forms, the friction rub and the pain disappear, and dullness to percussion and diminished breath sounds on auscultation appear. At the upper limits of pleural fluid, egophony is sometimes elicited. Pleural disorders for the most part arise from derangements in cardiac, hepatic, or renal function which lead to increased collections of fluid, or by extension of disease from adjacent structures such as the lung, mediastinum, chest wall, esophagus, or the upper abdomen. Evidence of disease in these structures must be searched for in the history and physical examination.

RADIOLOGIC EXAMINATION. Up to 300 ml of fluid may be present in a pleural space and not be apparent on the usual upright chest x-ray film. Small amounts of fluid may sometimes be suspected, especially on the left side, from the presence of a density or apparent widening of the diaphragmatic shadow as it is seen between the gas-containing stomach and the lower limits of the lung. Decubitus films taken with the involved side dependent may also sometimes make small amounts of fluid apparent on the x-ray film. With larger amounts of fluid the characteristic density of pleural fluid with its curvilinear upper border appears. However, if pleural fluid occurs in a pleural space in which previous inflammatory disease has produced adhesions, the distribution of the fluid may produce varied shadows. The x-ray shadows of pleural fluid are characteristically adjacent to the chest wall; rarely fluid will collect in or become encapsulated in one of the interlobar fissures and produce a pattern similar to a parenchymal pulmonary tumor.

EXAMINATION OF PLEURAL FLUID. A detailed chemical, bacteriologic, and cytologic analysis of all pleural fluids aspirated is essential in patients in whom the diagnosis is not completely clear. Analysis for total protein and lactic acid dehydrogenase (LDH), a complete blood count with a differential count, cultures for bacteria including mycobacteria, a Gram-stained smear, and a search for malignant cells should be carried out initially on virtually all pleural fluids. Glucose, pH, amylase, fat, and cholesterol measurements may also sometimes be indicated. The specific gravity of pleural fluid was once recommended as a measurement that would help differentiate between exudates and transudates. Because the specific gravity depends almost entirely on the protein content of the pleural fluid, and because it is a measurement that is frequently inaccurate, it can usually be omitted if an accurate measure of protein content is available.

The differentiation of pleural transudates and exudates is most helpful diagnostically and can usually be accomplished from examination of pleural fluid. Transudates are those fluids which occur in response to a decrease in the oncotic pressure of plasma, an increase in hydrostatic pressures in the pleural capillaries, or a decrease in intrapleural pressure. Exudates result from infections or from inflammatory or neoplastic processes which alter the permeability of pleural capillaries. Characteristically, transudates have a low protein content, a low specific gravity, and few white blood cells, whereas exudates have a high protein, high specific

gravity, and increased numbers of white blood cells. Arbitrary limits have been chosen to separate transudates and exudates (e.g., total protein more than 3.0 ml per 100 ml and specific gravity greater than 1.015). Unfortunately, when these arbitrary limits are tested in patients who have pleural fluid in which the cause is certain, both transudates and exudates are sometimes misclassified. Light and his associates have examined the cellular and chemical characteristics of pleural fluid from patients in whom a definite diagnosis could be established. On this basis they were classified as transudates or exudates. The three measurements which they found most reliable in differentiating transudates and exudates were the pleural fluid to serum protein ratio (greater than 0.5 in exudates), the level of LDH (greater than 200 IU in exudates) and the ratio of pleural fluid to serum LDH (greater than 0.6 in exudates). Although white blood counts greater than 10,000 per cubic millimeter are usually found only in exudates and counts of greater than 2500 per cubic millimeter suggest that the fluid is an exudate, counts below 2500 per cubic millimeter do not distinguish transudates from exudates.

Chylothorax refers to the presence of chyle in the pleural space and results from trauma to or obstruction (most often by a neoplastic process) of the thoracic duct or some other major intrathoracic lymphatic. Chylous pleural effusions are characteristically milky in appearance and have a high fat content which can be identified both microscopically and chemically. The protein content is usually about half that of plasma.

Milky-appearing pleural collections may also occur late in the course of tuberculous pleural effusion, in the pleural effusions of rheumatoid lung disease, and in other chronic effusions from the accumulation of cholesterol and cholesterol crystals in these fluids. Chemical analysis of such fluids will show a high cholesterol content and a low fat content and distinguish them from chylous effusions.

PLEURAL BIOPSY. Biopsy of the pleura with a Cope or Abrams needle is indicated in nearly every patient in whom the diagnosis is not clear, and who has sufficient pleural fluid to make this a safe procedure. Material from the biopsy should be submitted not only for histologic examination, but also for culture for tubercle bacilli. Pleural biopsy has been particularly useful in establishing the diagnosis of tuberculous pleurisy and malignant neoplastic implants in the pleura.

SIMPLE HYDROTHORAX

Pleural fluid collections occur more often as a result of cardiac, hepatic, or renal disease than from inflammatory or malignant disease of the pleura. These fluid collections most often result either from increases in hydrostatic pressures in the pleural capillaries, from a decrease in the oncotic pressure of the plasma, or from a combination of these factors. There is some exchange of fluid between the peritoneum and the pleura through the diaphragmatic lymphatics, and in patients with ascites this mechanism may result in pleural collections. Clinically these fluid collections are usually identified by physical examination, from x-rays of the chest, or, if they are large, from the appearance of dyspnea. They occur much more frequently on the right side than on the left. Pleural fluid in patients with simple hydrothorax will have those characteristics of a transudate which have been described. Because the parietal pleura is thin and uninvolved, pleural biopsy often fails to yield any identifiable pleural tissue. The treatment of these pleural collections is the treatment of the underlying disease, and pleural aspiration should be used therapeutically only if these measures fail and dyspnea requires relief.

PULMONARY EMBOLISM AND PULMONARY INFARCTION

Pulmonary embolism frequently produces pleural manifestations. In patients with pulmonary embolism, confirmed by pulmonary angiography, more than half will have a clinically detectable pleural effusion. The pleural effusion does not appear immediately and is usually identified more than 24 hours after the embolic event. The pleural effusion is an exudate and sometimes has moderate numbers of red blood cells; however, it is usually a clear amber fluid. Unless repeated embolization occurs, the pleural fluid disappears as the pulmonary infarction resolves.

PLEURAL EFFUSIONS WITH PNEUMONIA: EMPYEMA

Inflammation of the adjacent pleura occurs in most patients with pneumonia whatever the cause. Bacterial pneumonia frequently has clinically significant pleural involvement; in most pneumonias caused by viruses and mycoplasma, pleural disease is not clinically prominent.

The extent of pleural inflammation in bacterial pneumonia varies widely from case to case. There may be minor inflammation which produces pleural pain with clinically undetectable amounts of fluid, and which leaves no clinical residue; or large collections of grossly purulent fluid containing large numbers of bacteria (empyema) resulting in marked pleural fibrosis and fibrothorax. In practice one encounters patients who produce a continuum between these two extremes. Treatment of these effusions depends largely on the severity and intensity of the pleural inflammation, but is primarily the treatment of the associated pneumonia with appropriate antimicrobial drugs. The less intense small serous effusions with relatively small numbers of white blood cells and few organisms will usually respond to drug treatment alone. With larger collections of fluid and more white blood cells, aspiration by means of closed drainage through an intercostal tube may speed resolution and lead to smaller pleural residues. The finding of a pH of lower than 7.30 in the pleural exudate correlates with a more protracted and complicated course and may be an indication for earlier surgical drainage. With grossly purulent fluid and larger numbers of bacteria, surgical rib resection and open dependent drainage may be necessary. Infrequently pleural inflammatory disease leads to persistent massive fibrous entrapment of the underlying lung even after the infection has been controlled. A so-called fibrothorax results; the affected lung has its volume greatly decreased; ventilation and perfusion are reduced; there is a shift in the mediastinum toward the entrapped lung, and overdistention of the contralateral lung occurs. In such cases surgical decortication may free the entrapped lung and restore pulmonary function.

TUBERCULOSIS OF THE PLEURA

DEFINITION. Localized tuberculosis of the pleura probably occurs in most patients with pulmonary tuberculosis. It is usually clinically inapparent, but does result in pleural adhesions over the involved area.

Tuberculosis of the pleura with pleural effusion and without apparent pulmonary tuberculosis is the principal or first clinical manifestation of tuberculous disease in a few patients. Characteristically it is a febrile illness, accompanied by a serous pleural effusion. Although the acute illness, even if untreated, usually subsides in a few weeks with resorption of the fluid, it is very frequently followed by pulmonary tuberculosis or some other form of tuberculosis. Roper and Waring found that 65 per cent of patients with serofibrinous pleurisy who did not receive antituberculous chemotherapy developed tuberculosis during the next five years. Thus recognition of the tuberculous cause is of great importance. Infrequently pleural effusions that are grossly purulent and contain large numbers of tubercle bacilli are encountered; such cases are designated as tuberculous empyema.

EPIDEMIOLOGY. Tuberculous pleurisy with effusion can occur at any age but occurs most often in older children and young adults. It usually occurs soon after tuberculous infection, and is uncommon in patients who are known to have had tuberculous infection for a long time.

PATHOLOGY AND PATHOGENESIS. Tuberculosis of the pleura in nearly all cases results from extension of disease from the lung. Extension from tuberculosis of adjacent bones or lymph nodes is rare. Usually this extension from the lungs results only in localized pleural disease, and pleural effusion is not significant. In an occasional patient there is a massive outpouring of pleural fluid, and tuberculous infection is generalized over the visceral and parietal pleura. Myriads of typical tubercles stud the pleural surfaces. The immunologic reasons why some patients have this acute, widespread disease whereas others have only insignificant localized disease are not known. In a few weeks the acute reaction subsides, the pleural fluid decreases and then disappears, and fibrous adhesions between the visceral and parietal pleura form. Infrequently the fluid persists, becomes more purulent, and has increased numbers of tubercle bacilli; a chronic tuberculous empyema is established, which may persist for many years. Perhaps because the adjacent subpleural area is richly supplied with lymphatics, there is easy access for the dissemination of tubercle bacilli. In any case the subsequent development of tuberculosis in the lung and in other organs is a common event after untreated tuberculous pleurisy with effusion.

CLINICAL MANIFESTATIONS. The onset of tuberculous pleurisy with effusion is usually fairly sudden and acute. Sharp, fairly severe pleural pain is the most common first symptom. It is usually unilateral, made worse by breathing, and relieved by splinting the affected area. It is sharpest and most painful for the first few days, and then with the outpouring of pleural fluid it becomes duller and gradually subsides. Shortness of breath which is sometimes severe results from large collections of pleural fluid. Fever, which is sometimes as high as 39 to 40° C, is usually present in the first two or three weeks, and gradually subsides. Physical examination and x-ray examinations will identify the presence of variable amounts of fluid. In the typical case the parenchymal focus in the lung from which the disease originated is not apparent radiologically.

DIAGNOSIS. The diagnosis of tuberculous pleurisy should be considered in every patient with a pleural effusion; should be strongly suspected if this is accompanied by skin reactivity to 0.0001 mg of PPD; and should be presumptively diagnosed if, in addition, the fluid has the characteristics of an exudate and another diagnosis cannot be firmly made. Fortunately, methods for making the diagnosis of pleural tuberculosis have improved to such an extent that, if they are all used in a concerted fashion before treatment is started, the number of cases in which only a presumptive diagnosis must be made is small. Tubercle bacilli can be cultured from pleural fluid in up to 20 per cent of cases, from the sputum in a similar number, and from pleural biopsy material in over 60 per cent of cases. Typical tuberculous granulation tissue is seen in over 60 per cent of pleural biopsies from cases of tuberculous pleurisy. Although none of these methods are diagnostic in all cases, if they are used together, bacteriologic or histologic evidence of tuberculosis will be found in most cases.

Congestive heart failure, metastatic carcinoma involving the pleura, pulmonary infarction, and the effusions of bacterial pneumonia are the most commonly encountered conditions from which tuberculous pleurisy with effusions must be differentiated. Pleural mesothelioma, subdiaphragmatic abscess with an associated pleural effusion, rheumatoid pleural disease, and disseminated lupus erythematosus are less common conditions that may resemble tuberculous pleurisy.

TREATMENT. The treatment of tuberculous pleurisy is the prolonged administration of isoniazid and at least one other antituberculous drug and is the same as that for pulmonary tuberculosis (see Ch. 167). Surgical decortication to free a lung trapped by pleural adhesions (fibrothorax) after chemotherapy has controlled the infection is rarely necessary. With prompt and adequate chemotherapy, pleural residues are usually minor and do not benefit from surgical correction.

NEOPLASMS OF THE PLEURA

METASTATIC CARCINOMA. Implants of metastatic carcinoma of the pleura are, especially in older age groups, a common cause of pleural effusions. Carcinomas of the lung and breast are the tumors that most commonly extend to the pleura, but almost any carcinoma can have this complication. If the primary tumor has already been identified, the diagnosis is usually quickly made. If the pleural effusion is the first indication of the tumor, the diagnosis may not be so apparent. Characteristically the pleural effusions of malignant implants in the pleura are not accompanied by fever, the fluid is an exudate and often contains a large number of red blood cells, and the course is marked by the continued outpouring of fluid. The diagnosis can be established by finding malignant cells in the pleural fluid, by the presence of tumor in the parietal pleura on

pleural biopsy, or by open surgical biopsy of the pleura.

Treatment is aimed at preventing the accumulation of fluid in the pleural space and eliminating the need for repeated thoracenteses for the relief of dyspnea. Obliteration of the pleural space may be produced by the instillation of various irritating substances (e.g., atabrine, nitrogen mustard, cyclophosphamide, tetracycline, radioactive gold), followed by aspiration of the fluid to assure that the visceral and parietal layers are opposed. The insertion of an intercostal tube attached to suction is sometimes used for continuous aspiration after the irritating material has stimulated an inflammatory response.

MESOTHELIOMA. Pleural mesotheliomas may be either localized or diffuse. The localized tumor, the so-called fibrous mesothelioma, is relatively benign, may grow to a very large size, is sometimes cured by surgical resection, but does have a tendency to recur. The diffuse mesothelioma is a highly malignant tumor which involves the pleura widely and produces massive encroachment on the pleural space with fluid and tumor. Formerly this was believed to be a very rare tumor. It is now being seen with increased frequency, and its association with exposure to asbestos has been established (see Ch. 348.9).

OTHER PLEURAL TUMORS. Benign tumors of the pleura include lipomas, fibromas, vascular tumors, and pleural cysts. Primary malignant tumors of the pleura other than mesotheliomas include various sarcomas. They are all very uncommon.

Pleural effusions from intrathoracic lymphoma are not uncommon and apparently can result either from direct involvement of the pleura or from intrathoracic lymphatic obstruction. Chylothorax is sometimes seen when there is lymphatic obstruction.

SPONTANEOUS PNEUMOTHORAX

The pleural space normally does not contain gas, and if gas is instilled into the pleural space, it is absorbed. The total pressure of dissolved gases in venous blood is 54 mm Hg less than the atmospheric pressure which is transmitted to the pleura. This negative gradient keeps the intact pleural space gas free. Air may enter the pleural space through either the chest wall or the lung. Trauma to the chest wall or lung, medical procedures that permit the entry of air through the chest wall or that puncture the lung, and the spontaneous entry of gas from a ruptured emphysematous bleb are the most common causes of pneumothorax. The rupture of lung abscesses and tuberculous cavities into the pleura are less common causes. Spontaneous pneumothorax occurs in at least two distinct populations: the young, tall, otherwise healthy male, and the older person with underlying and usually clinically apparent chronic obstructive pulmonary disease or some other disease that has produced pulmonary fibrosis and localized emphysema.

CLINICAL MANIFESTATIONS. Pleural pain and shortness of breath are the principal symptoms of spontaneous pneumothorax. The severity of the shortness of breath may vary from insignificant to very severe and depends on the amount of gas in the pleural space and the amount of underlying pulmonary disease which is present. Physical examination of the chest will sometimes show increased resonance to percussion over the affected side, but a decrease in the intensity of the breath sounds is a more definite and discernible sign. If the pneumothorax is large and there is a marked increase in intrapleural pressure, a shift in mediastinal structures away from the affected side may be detected. The chest x-ray will show air in the pleural space and the amount of collapse of the lung which has occurred.

DIAGNOSIS. The possibility of spontaneous pneumothorax should be considered whenever there is the sudden onset of shortness of breath and particularly when it is accompanied by chest pain. It is a diagnosis which is usually made easily when it occurs in an otherwise healthy person and when the clinical findings which have been enumerated are present. The diagnosis is occasionally missed when it occurs in an asthmatic, a patient with obstructive pulmonary disease, or in other patients who have some other disease that seems to explain their shortness of breath. Because it can be lethal in such patients if untreated, the possibility of its occurrence should be kept prominent.

If a vessel in the lung or chest wall is torn when a pneumothorax occurs, a hemopneumothorax may result. When the chest x-ray shows the presence of fluid as well as air, this possibility should be considered, and a thoracentesis should be performed. Massive intrapleural bleeding is uncommon, but if present it requires surgical correction.

TREATMENT. The treatment of pneumothorax is concerned with its immediate and acute management, and with the prevention of recurrences.

The methods used in the early management of spontaneous pneumothorax will depend on the size and cause of the pneumothorax, the presence or absence of complicating pulmonary disease, and whether the leak between the lung and the pleura is closed or continuing. If the pneumothorax has occurred in a young healthy person, is small (e.g., 10 to 15 per cent), is causing few or minimal symptoms, and does not increase during the first 12 hours of observation, it requires no treatment. However, the fact that it has indeed resorbed should be confirmed by chest x-ray about two weeks later. In a similar patient with a larger pneumothorax, and especially if there is significant shortness of breath, the gas may be removed by inserting a small venous catheter through a thoracentesis needle and aspirating the intrapleural gas. This simple method will usually succeed in patients who do not have underlying pulmonary disease and who do not have a continuing leak. If there is significant pulmonary disease, pleural adhesions, or evidence of a continuing bronchopleural fistula, a larger intercostal tube should be inserted and attached to an underwater seal. The relief of an increasing and positive pressure — a *tension pneumothorax* — by prompt decompression is occasionally lifesaving. If there is a significant continuing leakage of air or evidence of respiratory insufficiency, continuous suction is required. If the lung cannot be re-expanded or there is continued leakage for more than a few days, an open thoracotomy with resection and closure of the bronchopleural fistula may be required.

Recurrence. Spontaneous pneumothorax may recur once or many times over several years after the first episode. Recurrences may be on the same side or the opposite side. The possibility of recurrence can be greatly reduced or eliminated by surgical treatment. Surgical treatment includes the resection of blebs and bullae if they are sufficiently localized to permit this and the obliteration of the pleural space. The removal of the parietal pleura, the application of irritating substances to the pleura, and the scarification of the pleura followed by intrapleural suction are methods which are used to obliterate the pleural space.

MISCELLANEOUS PLEURAL DISEASES

The pleura is involved in a great variety of systemic diseases and in diseases of the lung and adjacent structures.

COLLAGEN VASCULAR DISEASES. Systemic lupus erythematosus and rheumatoid arthritis are the collagen vascular diseases in which pleural effusions are most often encountered. In rheumatoid arthritis pleural effusions are usually seen in older men in whom the arthritis is of long duration. The fluid is an exudate and characteristically has a very low glucose content.

PANCREATITIS. Pleural effusions secondary to acute and chronic pancreatitis are occasionally encountered. They may occur in either pleural space, but are more common on the left. There is often an associated pancreatic pseudocyst. The fluid is an exudate, may have extremely high amylase content (500 to 50,000 units per milliliter), and characteristically has a higher level of amylase than the serum.

ASBESTOSIS. Inhalation of asbestos dust commonly leads to pleural disease. Serous pleural effusion, pleural fibrosis, pleural calcification, and pleural mesothelioma are all complications of asbestos dust exposure.

The pleural effusion of asbestos exposure is commonly bilateral and frequently recurrent; the fluid is usually an exudate and is often serosanguineous. Pleural effusion is often accompanied by clinically apparent parenchymal fibrosis, but can occur in the absence of obvious asbestosis. Duration and intensity of exposure to asbestos can vary widely.

Pleural fibrosis is a common accompaniment of pulmonary asbestosis and has been identified in up to 14 per cent of cases of asbestosis. Like pleural effusion it may be seen in patients who do not have evident parenchymal fibrosis.

Pleural calcification is common among asbestos workers and has been found in more than 10 per cent of workers with prolonged exposure. It is often bilateral, predominantly involves the basilar portions, is primarily in the parietal pleura, and usually occurs only after lengthy exposures to asbestos.

Although pleural mesothelioma has been reported to follow these more benign forms of pleural disease from asbestos, it is an uncommon complication.

MEIGS' SYNDROME. Ascites, pleural effusion, a benign fibroma, or fibroma-like ovarian tumor, with cure of the ascites and pleural effusion by removal of the tumor, is a syndrome that Meigs called attention to in 1934. It is an uncommon cause of pleural effusion, but many cases of the syndrome have been reported. Most often the fluid is found in the right pleural space, but it can be present in either or both pleural spaces. The fluid is usually a clear transudate, but exudative fluids and serosanguineous collections have been reported. The amount of fluid in both the pleural and peritoneal spaces is variable, and in some cases the amount of ascites has been quite small. The mechanism for the formation of the pleural and peritoneal fluid has not been completely explained, but it is suggested that somehow the fibroma causes the ascites which is then transported to the pleural space by diaphragmatic lymphatics. Because this uncommon condition can be cured by pelvic surgery, it should be considered in women with pleural effusion of obscure origin, especially if there is evidence of concurrent ascites and pelvic disease.

SUBDIAPHRAGMATIC ABSCESS. Pleural effusion and pleurodiaphragmatic pain, particularly on the right side, are common manifestations of a subdiaphragmatic abscess, and are frequently the first indicators of the location of the infection. The pleural effusion is most often a serous exudate, and the organism in the subdiaphragmatic abscess is often not found in the pleural fluid. Amebic infection from the liver may also extend through the diaphragm and cause a pleural exudate, which is characteristically purulent and chocolate-colored and may contain amebae.

Berger, H. W., Rammohan, G., Neff, M. S., and Buhain, W. J.: Uremic pleural effusion. Ann. Intern. Med., 82:362, 1975.

Besson, L. N., Ferguson, T. B., and Burford, T. H.: Chylothorax. Ann. Thorac. Surg., 12:527, 1971.

Black, L. F.: The pleural space and pleural fluid. Mayo Clin. Proc., 47:493, 1972.

Gaensler, E. A., and Kaplan, A. I.: Asbestos pleural effusions. Ann. Intern. Med., 74:178, 1971.

Killen, D. A., and Gobbel, W. G., Jr.: Spontaneous Pneumothorax. Boston, Little, Brown & Company, 1968.

Light, R. W.: Management of parapneumonic effusions (editorial). Chest, 70:324, 1976.

Light, R. W., MacGregor, M. I., Luchsinger, P. C., and Ball, W. C., Jr.: Pleural effusions: The diagnostic separation of transudates and exudates. Ann. Intern. Med., 77:507, 1972.

Meigs, J. V.: Fibroma of the ovary with ascites and hydrothorax — Meigs' syndrome. Am. J. Obstet. Gynecol., 67:962, 1954.

Mellins, R. B., Levine, O. R., and Fishman, A. P.: Effects of systemic and pulmonary venous hypertension on pleural and pericardial fluid accumulation. J. Appl. Physiol., 29:564, 1970.

Potts, D. E., Levin, D. C., and Sahn, S. A.: Pleural fluid pH in parapneumonic effusions. Chest, 70:328, 1976.

Scharer, L., and McClement, J. H.: The isolation of tubercle bacilli from needle biopsy specimens of parietal pleura. Am. Rev. Respir. Dis., 97:466, 1968.

Szucs, M. M., Brooks, H. L., Grossman, W., Banas, J. S., Meister, S. G., Dexter, L., and Dalen, J. E.: Diagnostic sensitivity of laboratory findings in acute pulmonary embolism. Ann. Intern. Med., 74:161, 1971.

Wallach, H. W.: Intrapleural tetracycline for malignant pleural effusions. Chest, 68:510, 1975.

Yeoh, C. B., Hubaytar, R. T., Conklin, E. F., Simpson, D. G., and Ford, J. M.: Spontaneous pneumothorax: Treatment with small lumen polyethylene tube. New York State J. Med., 70:779, 1970.

350.2.   THE MEDIASTINUM

The mediastinum is that anatomic space which lies in the mid-thorax, separates the two pleural cavities, and is delineated by the diaphragm below and the suprasternal thoracic outlet above. It contains the heart, pericardium, esophagus, various great vessels, nerves, lymph nodes, and numerous other structures. Diseases of the mediastinum arise for the most part from infections, tumors, and other disorders of these contained structures. Because defining the principal anatomic locus of mediastinal disease may be helpful, the mediastinum has been arbitrarily divided into three or more zones: a superior area, above the heart, which contains the great vessels, thymus, and substernal extensions of the thyroid; a lower anterior area, which contains the heart, pericardium, and lymph nodes; and

a posterior area, which contains the esophagus, the descending aorta, and many different nerves.

INFECTIONS. Acute mediastinitis is fortunately rare and most often results from endoscopy, surgery, or trauma to the esophagus. Fever, widening of the mediastinal shadow by x-ray, and a history of surgery, perforation, trauma, or manipulation of the esophagus may suggest the diagnosis. X-ray studies with suitable contrast material may demonstrate esophageal perforation, or the development of a complicating pleural effusion may be observed. Repair of the esophageal perforation, if it is identified early, surgical drainage of mediastinal abscesses, and microbial treatment are the usual therapies.

Chronic mediastinitis from extension of tuberculosis or histoplasmosis of mediastinal lymph nodes is extremely rare but may cause organizing mediastinal fibrosis with venous obstruction (see Ch. 71).

MEDIASTINAL EMPHYSEMA. Mediastinal emphysema occurs when air enters the mediastinum from some adjacent air-containing organ. Although it may result from trauma to or rupture of the eosphagus or a large bronchus, in which case it has serious impact, it most often results from a dissection of air from the peripheral airways into the pulmonary interstitium either from a spontaneous tear or as a complication of positive pressure artificial ventilation. There then occurs a dissection of air along the peribronchial and perivascular structures into the mediastinum. Precordial pain or discomfort may be present, and on physical examination there may be a loud crunching sound over the precordium which is related to the heartbeat and not to respiration (*Hamman's sign*). Dissection of air out of the mediastinum and into the neck or even very extensively over much of the body may occur. The air in the mediastinum sometimes can be seen on the x-ray of the chest as x-ray translucencies that outline the pericardium, the heart, and other mediastinal structures. Mediastinal emphysema is usually a benign, self-limited condition that resolves without treatment and does not interfere with venous return or other mediastinal organ function. Surgical relief of intramediastinal pressure is rarely helpful or necessary.

TUMORS. Tumors of the mediastinum are the most common major disorder of this region. In young adults they are often primary in the mediastinum and benign; in older adults they are more often malignant and metastatic. Symptoms of mediastinal tumors may arise from pressure on or invasion of adjacent structures, and result in cough, shortness of breath, dysphagia, venous congestion, substernal pain, or phrenic or recurrent laryngeal nerve paralysis. Malignant tumors may cause constitutional symptoms. Many mediastinal tumors come to medical attention only because an asymptomatic mass is identified on an x-ray of the chest.

Tumors of the superior mediastinum are often of thymic origin and may be benign or malignant. Intrathoracic extensions of thyroid adenomas are also common causes of upper mediastinal tumors. Metastatic carcinoma from the lung or breast may involve the lymph nodes of the upper mediastinum. If there is extension to the superior vena cava, the so-called *superior vena caval syndrome* may result, with edema and swelling of the head, eyes, and upper extremity. Involvement of the various nerves in the upper mediastinum may result in vocal cord paralysis (especially on the left) or diaphragmatic paralysis.

Lymphoma may be a cause of upper anterior mediastinal tumor, but most often tumors of the anterior mediastinum are teratodermoids, usually benign. They may vary from a simple cyst to complex mixed tumors of ectodermal origin. Pericardial cysts arise from and are attached to the pericardium and must be differentiated from other tumors of this region. Congenital cysts that arise from the bronchi, bronchogenic cysts, usually are attached to the trachea or the large central bronchi and radiologically are seen as tumors of the central mediastinum. They are usually fluid filled and by x-ray present as solid spherical masses. Occasionally a bronchial communication is established, they contain air, and by x-ray they appear as cystic air-containing spaces.

In the posterior mediastinum the most common tumors are of neural origin; these, too, are usually benign. Neurofibromas may arise from the dorsal roots and the sympathetic chain.

Although many mediastinal tumors are benign and do not cause symptoms, the inability to establish a certain diagnosis, together with the possibility that they will undergo malignant degeneration, has usually resulted in their treatment by surgical removal.

Hamman, L.: Spontaneous mediastinal emphysema. Bull. Johns Hopkins Hosp., 64:1, 1939.

Sabiston, D. C., Jr., and Oldham, H. N., Jr.: The mediastinum. In Sabiston, D. C., Jr., and Spencer, F. C. (eds.): Gibbons' Surgery of the Chest. 3rd ed. Philadelphia, W. B. Saunders Company, 1976, pp. 406–424.

350.3. THE DIAPHRAGM

The diaphragm is the principal muscle of respiration. It separates the thorax and the abdomen, and it confines to the thorax the negative pressure of the pleura during inspiration. It arises from and is attached to the sternum, the lower ribs, the upper lumbar vertebrae, and from the fascia of the quadratus lumborum and the psoas muscles. It inserts into the central tendon of the diaphragm. Motor and sensory fibers reach the diaphragm by the phrenic nerves; some sensory fibers come from the lower intercostal nerves.

HERNIAS. Hernias of the diaphragm may be congenital, developmental, or traumatic.

Herniation of abdominal organs through the congenital and persistent foramina of Bochdalek and Morgagni is quite uncommon. Hernias of Bochdalek are more common than hernias of Morgagni; they occur in the posterolateral chest on either side, are predominantly a disease of infants and children, may result in massive herniation of small intestine or other abdominal viscera into the chest with collapse of the lung and intestinal obstruction, and often require emergent surgical correction.

Hernias of Morgagni are located anteriorly, in or close to the midline, and on either side, but more often on the right. Part of the liver or the omentum is the structure that most often protrudes through them; other abdominal viscera, e.g., colon, stomach, or small intestine, may be in the hernia. These hernias are often asymptomatic, found on a routine x-ray, and they present the diagnostic problem of an anterior mass connected to or adjacent to the diaphragm. Radioisotopic scans of the liver and x-rays of the gastrointestinal tract will often make the diagnosis. Diagnostic pneumoperitoneum with abdominal x-ray has sometimes been used.

Surgical exploration for diagnosis and repair is usually carried out.

The much more common herniation of the stomach through the esophageal hiatus is considered in Ch. 396.

Traumatic hernia of the diaphragm may result from direct injury to the diaphragm, e.g., knife or bullet wounds, or indirectly from severe abdominal trauma with compression. Because this complication may not be appreciated at the time the trauma occurs, it may come to attention later when abdominal viscera are found located in the thorax. Unfortunately the cause of the abnormalities is not always recognized, and the chest x-ray findings may be confused with a paralyzed diaphragm or a pneumothorax. These usually require surgical correction.

PARALYSIS. Paralysis of the diaphragm may result from interruption of the phrenic nerve anywhere in its course. It may be caused by trauma, infection (e.g., diphtheria), surgical interruption, or tumor, or it may be of unknown cause. Invasion of the phrenic nerve by a malignant tumor in the mediastinum is the most common cause. The paralyzed diaphragm is elevated and may move paradoxically in inspiration. If inspiration is performed swiftly, as with an inspiratory sniff, this paradoxical motion is accentuated and usually is very apparent.

Most of the physiologic studies in diaphragmatic paralysis were done on patients who had tuberculosis at a time when unilateral interruption of the phrenic nerve was a form of therapy. The physiologic changes were minor and consisted of some changes in the lung volumes.

EVENTRATION. Rarely, one of the diaphragms or part of one of the diaphragms is atrophic, and is replaced by a thin nonmuscular membranous structure. The cause is unknown, but is probably congenital. The involved portion of the diaphragm is high and moves paradoxically. It is often confused with a paralyzed diaphragm. The patient with an eventration is often asymptomatic, and the defect may be found on a routine x-ray examination. If it produces either thoracic or abdominal symptoms, surgical correction may be necessary.

HICCUP. Hiccup is an involuntary quick inspiration interrupted by a quick closure of the vocal cords. It is usually of unknown and benign cause and of short duration, and stops spontaneously or as a result of various self-administered respiratory maneuvers. Occasionally it is a symptom of serious disease, e.g., uremia. It occurs in various pulmonary, cardiac, pleural, and abdominal processes that irritate the diaphragm. In a rare case of persistent hiccup, if exhaustion becomes a problem, local anesthesia of a phrenic nerve has sometimes been successful. Fluoroscopy to determine if the process is unilateral should precede this therapy.

Agostoni, E., and Sant'Ambrogio, S.: The diaphragm. In Campbell, E. J. M., Agostoni, E., and Davis, J. N. (eds.): The Respiratory Muscles. Philadelphia, W. B. Saunders Company, 1970.

McCredie, M., Lovejoy, F. W., Jr., and Kaltreider, N. L.: Pulmonary function in diaphragmatic paralysis. Thorax, 17:213, 1962.

Paris, F., Tarazona, V., Casillas, M., Blosco, E., Conto, A., Pastor, J., and Acosta, A.: Hernia of Morgagni. Thorax, 28:631, 1973.

350.4. THE CHEST WALL

The chest wall may be disturbed in its structure and function by a variety of congenital, inflammatory, neuromuscular, pulmonary, pleural, and idiopathic diseases. The most common disturbances are from diseases of the spine that result in gross bony disarrangement (kyphoscoliosis), various congenital defects of the anterior thorax (pectus excavatum, pectus carinatum), and those that are secondary to pulmonary or pleural disease or its surgical treatment.

KYPHOSIS AND SCOLIOSIS

DEFINITION. Scoliosis is lateral curvature of the spine. It is almost always accompanied by some posterior curvature (kyphosis). It may occur in any part of the spine, but produces its greatest disturbance when it is in the thoracic region. In scoliosis there is usually a compensatory curve in the opposite direction in the spine below the primary curvature. Scoliosis is categorized as to the right or left according to the direction of the convexity of the primary curvature, and its degree is expressed as the angle which the converging limbs of the curvature form when measured on an x-ray of the spine. Kyphosis is described by the angle which the upper limb of the deformity forms with the vertical plane.

ETIOLOGY AND MECHANISMS. Most cases (70 to 80 per cent) of kyphoscoliosis are of *unknown cause* and are first recognized in childhood. A smaller and decreasing number are due to neuromuscular disease, especially poliomyelitis. Another relatively uncommon cause of kyphoscoliosis and scoliosis is intrinsic disease of the spine. Pulmonary and pleural disease, as well as chest surgical procedures, e.g., extensive thoracoplasty, may cause kyphoscoliosis.

CLINICAL MANIFESTATIONS. The most common disturbance which kyphoscoliosis or kyphosis causes is the psychologic effect of the skeletal deformity. Unless the scoliosis or kyphosis is severe, cardiorespiratory insufficiency usually does not appear. In the carefully studied group of patients observed by Bergofsky and his associates, this complication was seen only in those patients whose scoliosis exceeded 100 degrees or whose kyphosis exceeded 20 degrees. The effect of the kyphosis and scoliosis seemed to be additive.

Probably most patients with kyphoscoliosis have no pulmonary complaints. If their pulmonary function is measured, they will be found to have only minor decreases in lung volumes and ventilatory capacity without disturbances in gas exchange.

With more advanced skeletal deformity and especially with advancing age, some patients have first shortness of breath on exertion, hypoxia, and hypercapnia. Others will have extreme dyspnea on exertion, severe hypoxia and hypercapnia, even at rest, and cor pulmonale with profound right ventricular failure.

The mechanism for this cardiorespiratory failure was long thought to be due to complicating bronchitis and emphysema. It is now clear that this is usually not the case and that the skeletal and chest wall deformity leads to an increased work of breathing and eventually to decreased alveolar ventilation, hypoxia, hypercapnia, polycythemia, decreased carbon dioxide responsiveness, and increased pulmonary vascular resistance.

PROGNOSIS. Although it is known that cardiorespiratory failure occurs only with severe degrees of kyphoscoliosis, it is not certain how many individuals with severe deformities develop this complication.

Once cor pulmonale develops, the prognosis is poor; but vigorous treatment sometimes reverses many of the derangements, and with good care and medical supervision some patients have done well for many years after an episode of cardiorespiratory failure.

TREATMENT. Early prophylactic treatment of the skeletal deformity is primarily an orthopedic problem, but aggressive surgical treatment aimed at correcting and stabilizing the deformed spine in children and adolescents seems warranted and promising.

In older adults who are deformed but stable and asymptomatic, all measures which may prevent the development of complicating bronchitis should be taken, e.g., removal of bronchial irritants, prompt treatment of bronchial infection.

The treatment of severe cardiorespiratory insufficiency requires a multifactorial approach like that used in other forms of cardiopulmonary failure, in which one strives to identify reversible physiologic defects and correct them. Decreased alveolar ventilation may require assisted ventilation, although the chest deformity may make this difficult. Marked hypoxia may indicate the need for supplemental oxygen if ventilation can be maintained. Congestive failure should be treated with diuretics and digitalis. Sometimes with vigorous treatment, patients with severe cardiorespiratory failure recover, improve, and maintain this improvement for long periods. Nocturnal assisted ventilation with a Drinker respirator has been used chronically in some patients with decreased alveolar ventilation.

ANKYLOSING SPONDYLITIS

Ankylosing spondylitis of the thoracic spine produces a characteristic deformity of the chest with marked flexion of the thoracic spine, and rigidity from vertebral fusion (see Ch. 58.1). This disorder most commonly causes limitation in thoracic mobility and reduced vital capacity but little pulmonary disability. Recently it has been recognized that a small group of patients with ankylosing spondylitis also have pulmonary or pleural disease. Most commonly there is fibrobullous disease of the upper lobes; infrequently it is complicated by *Aspergillus* colonization or severe respiratory insufficiency. Pleural effusions or pleural fibrosis are also rare complications.

DEFORMITIES OF ANTERIOR CHEST WALL

PECTUS EXCAVATUM. This congenital defect is sometimes also called funnel chest. It consists of a shortening of the distance between the xiphoid and the vertebral bodies, backward displacement of the body of the sternum, and deformity of the costal cartilages to accommodate this displacement.

For most patients the only disability arises from the cosmetic effects and the psychologic symptoms it engenders. Extremely rarely the defect may be so severe that it causes cardiorespiratory symptoms. Surgical correction is possible but rarely necessary.

PECTUS CARINATUM. This defect has also been called pigeon breast. It is less common than pectus excavatum and consists of a swinging forward of the xiphoid and lower portion of the sternum and a lengthening of the costal cartilages. It causes cardiorespiratory symptoms even less frequently than pectus excavatum, and correction of the cosmetic defect is a rare indication for surgical correction.

Bergofsky, E. H., Turino, M., and Fishman, A. P.: Cardiorespiratory failure in kyphoscoliosis. Medicine, 38:263, 1959.

Gacad, G., and Hamosh, P.: The lung in ankylosing spondylitis. Am. Rev. Respir. Dis., 107:286, 1973.

Rosenow, E. C., Strimlam, C. V., Muhm, J. R., and Ferguson, R. H.: Pleuropulmonary manifestations of ankylosing spondylitis. Mayo Clin. Proc., 52:641, 1977.

Sinha, R. and Bergofsky, E. H.: Prolonged alteration of lung mechanics in kyphoscoliosis by positive pressure inflation. Am. Rev. Respir. Dis., 106:47, 1972.

351. RESPIRATORY FAILURE

John F. Murray

351.1. INTRODUCTION

Adequate respiration consists of the uptake of sufficient amounts of O_2 and the elimination of sufficient amounts of CO_2 to maintain Po_2 and Pco_2 in arterial blood at their respective normal values. It follows that *respiratory failure* is associated with disturbances in the exchange of O_2 and CO_2 between gas in alveoli and blood in pulmonary capillaries and that these abnormalities must be reflected by changes in the Po_2 and Pco_2 in arterial blood. Thus respiratory failure is defined as a condition in which arterial Po_2 is below the normal range (excluding hypoxemia from intracardiac right-to-left shunting of blood), or arterial Pco_2 is above the normal range (excluding respiratory compensation for metabolic alkalosis). This definition, which is physiologically precise as well as clinically applicable, implies that the diagnosis of respiratory failure depends chiefly on laboratory analysis of arterial blood and not on clinical findings.

Respiratory failure is not a disease but a disorder of function that can be caused by a variety of conditions that affect the lungs; in some instances, the lungs are completely normal (e.g., overdose of sedative drugs). Respiratory failure is analogous to heart failure and renal failure, both of which represent the consequences of impaired normal function resulting from numerous disparate diseases.

Respiratory failure is traditionally divided into acute and chronic varieties, depending on the time it takes for the abnormalities in gas exchange to occur. This arbitrary classification does not take into account the common clinical occurrence of an acute worsening of arterial Po_2 and Pco_2 in a patient who already has chronic respiratory failure as a result of some underlying disorder. However, the distinction between acute and chronic respiratory failure has important etiologic and therapeutic connotations and will be referred to frequently.

351.2. PATHOPHYSIOLOGY OF RESPIRATORY FAILURE

In human beings, respiration has been subdivided into four functional processes: ventilation, diffusion, perfusion, and control of breathing. Each of these contributes uniquely to the maintenance of normal values of Po_2 and Pco_2 in arterial blood. Therefore, abnormalities in any one of the four processes, if sufficiently severe, will cause respiratory failure; furthermore, in many common respiratory disorders, multiple abnormalities coexist.

NORMAL GAS EXCHANGE

The physiology of normal gas exchange is described in Ch. 342.6 and will not be reviewed here. However, understanding what is meant by normal is important, because arterial Po_2 varies with age and both arterial Po_2 and Pco_2 vary according to the altitude (i.e., the prevailing barometric pressure) at which the person happens to be when the blood specimen is obtained and to the extent of acclimatization. The normal range includes the biologic variabilities among individuals and the analytic variations inherent in the measurements. Because the diagnosis of respiratory failure should be made in the laboratory and not at the bedside, the physician's ability to establish the diagnosis depends on the accuracy of the laboratory tests used to measure Po_2 and Pco_2. Normal mean arterial Po_2 (Pa_{O_2}) values in subjects 20 years of age or older can be calculated from the regression equation $Pa_{O_2} = 100.1 - 0.323$ (age in years). The normal range of variation is ± 5 mm Hg from the mean value. Arterial Pco_2 does not vary with age and is normally within the range of 40 ± 5 mm Hg in healthy persons at sea level. Values of Po_2 *below* or Pco_2 *above* normal limits indicate the presence of respiratory failure.

ABNORMAL GAS EXCHANGE

The pathophsiology of abnormal gas exchange is also discussed in Ch. 342.6. Hypoventilation, impaired diffusion, ventilation-perfusion mismatching, right-to-left shunting of blood, and breathing air with a low Po_2 all cause arterial hypoxia (a decrease below normal of Po_2); in contrast, for practical purposes only hypoventilation causes arterial hypercapnia (an increase above normal of Pco_2). In view of the therapeutic importance of recognizing the abnormal mechanism(s) leading to a patient's respiratory failure, each will be reviewed briefly.

HYPOVENTILATION. As just mentioned, alveolar hypoventilation is present when the arterial Pco_2 is increased. Furthermore, as arterial Pco_2 increases, Po_2 decreases *except* when the patient is breathing gas with an enriched concentration of O_2. Because arterial Po_2 and Pco_2 change in opposite directions by nearly the same amount during hypoventilation, the contribution of hypoventilation to the patient's arterial hypoxia can be readily assessed. (In a 60-year-old person, for example, if $Po_2 = 50$ mm Hg and $Pco_2 = 70$ mm Hg, both have changed from their normal values by the same amount [30 mm Hg] and "pure" hypoventilation is present; in contrast, if $Po_2 = 30$ mm Hg and $Pco_2 = 70$ mm Hg, the change from normal of Pco_2 does not account for the entire change in Po_2; some other cause in addition to hypoxia from hypoventilation must be present.) Arterial hypoxia from alveolar hypoventilation is not associated with an increased alveolar-arterial Po_2 difference and is "corrected" by breathing 100 per cent O_2.

IMPAIRED DIFFUSION. Abnormalities of diffusion do not cause arterial hypoxia in persons at rest unless they are extremely severe. Although these occur in occasional patients with respiratory failure, for practical purposes the possible contribution of an abnormality of diffusion to a given patient's arterial hypoxia can be ignored except during exercise. This practice is permissible because diffusion disturbances can cause only relatively small increases in the patient's alveolar-arterial Po_2 difference, and this abnormality, if it exists, is readily corrected by adding small amounts of O_2 to the inspired air.

VENTILATION-PERFUSION IMBALANCE. When gas exchange units receive more blood flow than ventilation, arterial hypoxia results. Mismatching of ventilation-perfusion is by far the most common cause of arterial hypoxia and can be recognized by giving the patient 100 per cent O_2 to breathe; this causes the alveolar-arterial Po_2 difference from pure mismatching that is present while the patient breathes room air to decrease and arterial Po_2 to increase to normal values (>550 mm Hg). Although a "pure" ventilation-perfusion inequality can lead to CO_2 retention, this is an uncommon cause of hypercapnia because as arterial Pco_2 tends to increase, it stimulates peripheral and central chemoreceptors and increases ventilation; this, in turn, reduces Pco_2 back to normal values but, owing to the shape of the oxyhemoglobin dissociation curve, does not correct the hypoxia.

RIGHT-TO-LEFT SHUNTS. Shunts of blood from right to left may occur through abnormal anatomic communications in the lung (e.g., a pulmonary arteriovenous fistula) and frequently by perfusion of lung units that are completely unventilated because they are either collapsed (atelectasis) or filled with fluid (pulmonary edema, pneumonia, alveolar proteinosis). Regardless of the cause, an alveolar-arterial Po_2 difference results that increases when the patient breathes 100 per cent O_2 compared with the value obtained while breathing room air. For reasons similar to those occurring in patients with ventilation-perfusion imbalances, CO_2 retention seldom occurs in patients with right-to-left shunts.

HYPERCAPNIA. In contrast to arterial hypoxia, which may result from five different pathophysiologic derangements, arterial hypercapnia can always be interpreted as signifying alveolar hypoventilation. This is true because arterial Pco_2 (Pa_{CO_2}) is governed by the relationship between CO_2 production ($\dot{V}co_2$) and alveolar ventilation ($\dot{V}A$); $Pa_{CO_2} = k\dot{V}co_2/\dot{V}A$. Normally, however, even when CO_2 production increases markedly, alveolar ventilation increases proportionately and arterial Pco_2 is maintained within narrow limits. Thus an increase in arterial Pco_2 can always be viewed as respiratory failure in the sense that alveolar ventilation is inadequate to eliminate all the CO_2 being produced at that time. Severe ventilation-perfusion imbalances and right-to-left shunts can produce CO_2 retention, but this is uncommon because, as already emphasized, alveolar ventilation increases and corrects the disturbance.

An increase or decrease in Pco_2 in the blood has a direct effect on the amount of carbonic acid in the blood and a reciprocal effect on pH. Acute changes in Pco_2 have a more profound effect on pH than chronic changes owing to differences in plasma bicarbonate. With acute increases or decreases in Pco_2, there is little change in bicarbonate level and a considerable change in pH; after three to five days of sustained changes in

Pco_2, renal compensation has increased plasma bicarbonate in hypercapnia and decreased it in hypocapnia, both tending to restore pH toward normal. Many patients with respiratory failure have mixed respiratory and nonrespiratory acid-base disturbances. Knowledge of the time course of a patient's problem as well as the magnitude of changes in plasma bicarbonate is extremely useful in providing the necessary understanding for appropriate treatment of all components of the disorder.

RIGHT HEART FAILURE

Acute respiratory failure can cause acute right heart failure (acute cor pulmonale). The right ventricle cannot sustain sudden pressure loads over 40 to 50 mm Hg and fails. Thus acute right heart failure may develop in any condition in which pulmonary vascular resistance increases abruptly; this happens most commonly in patients with multiple pulmonary emboli with obstruction of much of the pulmonary vascular bed (usually >60 per cent). At times, acute cor pulmonale complicates the course of patients with severe bronchial asthma or other forms or marked airways obstruction.

Acute right heart failure may also occur in patients with chronic lung disease during an episode of acute respiratory failure. Most of these patients have right ventricular hypertrophy (chronic cor pulmonale) to begin with, and a subclinical or stable condition is worsened by the added effects of the superimposed acute lung disease (usually bronchitis or pneumonia). In these patients, resistance to blood flow through the lungs increases above its previous value for several reasons: (1) alveolar hypoxia and acidemia cause pulmonary arterial vasoconstriction; (2) certain lung diseases reduce the cross-sectional area available for perfusion; (3) hyperinflation of the lung increases pulmonary vascular resistance; and (4) arterial hypoxia may depress myocardial contractility. These factors are important to recognize because they are reversible and usually respond well to appropriate treatment of the intercurrent acute disorder.

351.3. CAUSES OF RESPIRATORY FAILURE

Because respiratory failure is defined as the presence of arterial hypoxia with or without hypercapnia, it is obvious that a large variety of disorders are capable of producing these abnormalities. For convenience, the multiple causes of respiratory failure can be classified (Table 1), depending on which component of the respiratory system is involved. Because most of these disorders characteristically cause either acute or chronic respiratory failure, they can be subdivided further into these categories.

DISEASES CAUSING AIRWAYS OBSTRUCTION

ACUTE. Obstruction may result from acute diseases that involve any portion of the upper and lower airways. The presence of respiratory failure depends on the magnitude and extent of the narrowing. Obstruc-

TABLE 1.   Classification of Common Disorders Associated
with Respiratory Failure

Diseases causing airways obstruction
  Acute
    Epiglottitis
    Laryngeal edema (croup)
    Foreign body
    Bronchiolitis
    Bronchial asthma
  Chronic
    Bronchitis
    Emphysema
    Bronchiectasis
Diseases causing parenchymal infiltration
  Acute
    Pneumonia
    Immunologic reactions
  Chronic
    Sarcoidosis
    Pneumoconioses
    Diffuse interstitial fibrosis
Diseases causing pulmonary edema
  Cardiogenic
    Myocardial infarction
    Mitral or aortic valve disease
    Left ventricular failure
  Noncardiogenic
    High altitude
    Shock from any cause
    Heroin
    Inhalation of chemical substances
    Sepsis
    Neurologic disorders
Pulmonary vascular diseases
  Acute
    Pulmonary emboli (blood clots)
    Fat emboli
  Chronic
    Pulmonary vasculitis
    Recurrent thromboembolism
Diseases of the chest wall and pleura
  Acute
    Flail chest
    Pneumothorax
  Chronic
    Kyphoscoliosis
    Obesity
    Massive pleural effusion(s)
Disorders of the neuromuscular system
  Brain disorders
    Sedative drugs, anesthesia
    Vascular diseases
    Infections
    Tumors
  Muscular disorders
    Muscular dystrophy
    Myasthenia gravis
  Peripheral nerve disorders
    Polyneuritis
    Poliomyelitis

tion of the *extra*thoracic airway (nasopharynx, larynx, extrathoracic portion of the trachea) usually causes stridor, a characteristic alteration of breathing that is associated with harsh, high-pitched respiratory noises that are louder and more pronounced during inspiration than expiration. In contrast, obstruction of the *intra*thoracic airways causes wheezing, an abnormality of breathing in which expiration is louder and longer than inspiration.

Obstruction of the upper airways can result from (1) inflammation-induced swelling of the mucosa secondary to infections, allergic reactions, and, less commonly, thermal or mechanical injuries, and (2) impaction of foreign bodies or, occasionally, tumors. Acute obstruction of the upper airways is particularly likely to devel-

op in infants and young children who have smaller and hence more vulnerable upper passages than older children and adults.

Acute obstruction of the lower airways is usually caused by swelling of the mucosa, secretions in the lumen, or bronchospasm. Accordingly, bronchial asthma, infections, bronchiolitis, and the inhalation of chemicals (such as nitrogen dioxide in silo-filler's disease) are important causes of acute respiratory failure.

CHRONIC. Diffuse obstruction may result from disorders originating in large bronchi (bronchiectasis), small bronchi (bronchitis), or the lung parenchyma (emphysema). These abnormalities characteristically progress gradually and lead to chronic respiratory failure. Of considerable importance are the intercurrent episodes of acute disease, usually pneumonia or bronchitis, that complicate the underlying disorder and often worsen the severity of existing respiratory failure.

DISEASES CAUSING PARENCHYMAL INFILTRATION

ACUTE. The most common cause of acute infiltration of the parenchyma is pneumonia, which may have a viral, bacterial, or occasionally chemical origin. Whether acute respiratory failure develops depends on the extent and severity of the disease. Immunologic reactions from drugs, migrating parasites, or leukoagglutinins are uncommon causes of acute respiratory failure but are important because of their special therapeutic requirements.

CHRONIC. There are over 100 different conditions that can cause chronic diffuse parenchymal infiltration. When severe, any of these can cause chronic respiratory failure. As in patients with chronic airways obstruction, patients with chronic infiltrative diseases may have intercurrent episodes of bronchopulmonary infection that cause acute worsening of their underlying respiratory status.

DISEASES CAUSING PULMONARY EDEMA

CARDIOGENIC. Pulmonary edema in patients with heart disease may be acute or chronic in onset; both varieties are caused by an increase in the hydrostatic pressure within pulmonary capillaries. Pulmonary edema may follow an acute myocardial infarction and acute left ventricular failure of any cause (hypertensive crisis, arrhythmias), or it may be precipitated in patients with valvular or other forms of chronic heart disease by sudden changes in their circulatory status (from arrhythmias, pulmonary emboli, or increased systemic blood pressure). Chronic pulmonary edema is found in patients with chronic, usually refractory, heart failure, but even in these patients the amount of edema increases and decreases according to changing hemodynamics and therapy.

NONCARDIOGENIC. It has long been recognized that acute pulmonary edema can accompany certain conditions that do not involve the heart. The basic pathophysiologic abnormality in most of these disorders appears to be an increased permeability of the pulmonary capillary endothelium, but other forms of pulmonary edema (high altitude pulmonary edema, re-expansion pulmonary edema) also occur. Pulmonary edema result-

TABLE 2. Partial List of Conditions That Have Been Associated with the Adult Respiratory Distress Syndrome

Shock of any etiology	Inhaled toxins
Infections	O_2 (high concentrations)
Gram-negative sepsis	Smoke
Viral pneumonia	Corrosive chemicals (NO_2, Cl_2,
Bacterial pneumonia	NH_3, phosgene, cadmium)
Trauma	Hematologic disorders
Fat emboli	Intravascular coagulation
Lung contusion	Massive blood transfusion
Nonthoracic trauma (including	Metabolic disorders
head injury)	Pancreatitis
Liquid aspiration	Uremia
Gastric juice	Paraquat ingestion
Fresh and salt water (drowning)	Miscellaneous
Hydrocarbon fluids	Increased intracranial pressure
Drug overdose	(including seizures)
Heroin	Eclampsia
Methadone	Postcardioversion
Propoxyphene	Radiation pneumonitis
Barbiturates	Postcardiopulmonary bypass
Colchicine	

ing from increased permeability is an important and apparently steadily increasing cause of acute respiratory failure, especially in patients who are hospitalized with serious medical or surgical illnesses that initially do not involve the lungs. After a latent period of 6 to 24 hours, these patients develop progressive arterial hypoxia, decreased compliance, and extensive roentgenographic infiltrations; in fatal cases, the lungs are found to be nearly airless, intensely congested, and filled with a proteinaceous edema fluid that also contains large numbers of red blood cells; occasionally, hyaline membranes are found. This constellation of clinical, physiologic, and pathologic events is now known as the *adult respiratory distress syndrome* and has been reported as a complication of many apparently unrelated conditions (Table 2). The feature common to all these disorders is the presence of diffuse injury to the alveolar-capillary membrane. Once damage has occurred, probably by many different pathways, and the permeability of the membrane is increased, pulmonary edema follows; thus the clinical, physiologic, and pathologic manifestations are similar, regardless of the cause of the injury.

PULMONARY VASCULAR DISEASES

ACUTE. Pulmonary embolism is usually accompanied by a decreased arterial Po_2 and Pco_2, the latter reflecting the hyperventilation that nearly always occurs. Pulmonary embolism is also an important cause of worsening respiratory failure in patients with underlying chronic lung disease. Fat emboli and emboli from platelet-fibrin aggregates can cause marked hypoxia by increasing the permeability of the alveolar-capillary membrane and producing severe pulmonary edema.

CHRONIC. Pulmonary vasculitis and recurrent thromboembolism are not common conditions and, when present, usually do not cause respiratory failure until the late stages of the disease. Recurrent thromboembolism occurs in intravenous drug abusers and in patients with chronic peripheral venous thrombi, sickle cell anemia, and schistosomiasis. Pulmonary vasculitis occurs in patients with scleroderma, other collagen diseases, and primary pulmonary hypertension.

DISEASES OF THE CHEST WALL AND PLEURA

ACUTE. The most important cause of sudden respiratory failure from acute disorders involving the thoracic cage is injury to the chest wall. Segmental fractures of several ribs or fractures of ribs on both sides of the sternum can result in a flail chest. Besides the impairment of ventilatory function that results from the unstable chest wall, gas exchange abnormalities are often compounded by contusion of the lung underneath the site of injury. Spontaneous or traumatic pneumothorax is an important cause of acute respiratory failure, which may be severe and which often afflicts otherwise healthy persons.

CHRONIC. Severe idiopathic or acquired kyphoscoliosis can cause chronic respiratory failure, which is often associated with cor pulmonale. Similarly, massive obesity is a well known cause of chronic respiratory failure. Patients with massive pleural effusion(s) or with thickened, constrictive pleural layer(s) may also have chronic respiratory failure.

DISORDERS OF THE NEUROMUSCULAR SYSTEM

Disorders of the neuromuscular system are classified into which part of the effector system is involved, i.e., the brain, neuronal pathways, or muscles of respiration, rather than into acute and chronic varieties. Patients with these disorders often have normal lungs; respiratory failure occurs from lack of ventilation.

BRAIN DISORDERS. Probably the most common cause of respiratory failure from impaired function of the central nervous system comes from the use of sedative drugs or anesthetic agents. Suppression of ventilatory drive from opiates, barbiturates, psychic depressants, alcohol, and a variety of sedative drugs results in hypoxia and hypercapnia that may be life threatening. Ventilatory stimuli can also be depressed by many diseases of the central nervous system, including vascular diseases, tumors, and infections.

SPINAL CORD AND PERIPHERAL NERVE DISORDERS. Injuries to the cervical or high thoracic spinal cord may produce immediate respiratory failure from paralysis of the muscles of respiration. Loss of anterior horn cell function in patients with poliomyelitis was an important cause of acute and chronic respiratory failure but is seldom encountered now because of the widespread use of vaccination. Polyneuritis, whether postinfectious (Guillain-Barré syndrome) or toxic, is an uncommon but important cause of respiratory failure in view of its inherent reversibility.

MUSCULAR DISORDERS. The final effectors in the system that controls breathing are the skeletal muscles of respiration. When these muscles are involved by generalized myopathies, such as muscular dystrophy or myasthenia gravis, respiratory failure results. Respiratory failure in patients with myasthenia gravis occurs during myasthenic or cholinergic crises. In contrast, respiratory failure in patients with muscular dystrophy is nearly always chronic and related to an advanced stage in the progression of the disease.

351.4. CLINICAL MANIFESTATIONS

Given the great variety of disorders that can cause respiratory failure (Table 1), it is obvious that the clinical manifestations in a given patient depend in large part on which underlying disease he has; these are dealt with elsewhere in this book. When respiratory failure ensues and if the blood gas disturbances are sufficiently severe, the signs and symptoms of hypoxia, and possible hypercapnia, become superimposed upon the signs and symptoms of the underlying disease. It should be emphasized that the clinical manifestations of hypoxia and hypercapnia are nonspecific and usually occur late in the evolution of the clinical problem. This statement underscores the earlier axiom that respiratory failure is a laboratory diagnosis and not a clinical diagnosis.

HYPOXIA

The signs and symptoms of acute hypoxia are chiefly caused by abnormalities in central nervous system and cardiovascular function. Characteristic features are impaired judgment and motor instability, a clinical picture closely resembling acute alcoholism. As hypoxia worsens, the brainstem is affected and death results from depression of the medullary respiratory centers. The initial cardiovascular effects of acute hypoxia are tachycardia and increased blood pressure; when hypoxia is very severe, bradycardia, myocardial depression, and shock ensue. Recognizable cyanosis of the lips, mucous membranes, and nail beds usually occurs when the concentration of reduced hemoglobin in the capillaries is >5 grams per 100 ml. Accordingly, cyanosis can result from decreases in either arterial Po_2 or blood flow. In patients with lung disease, cyanosis cannot be detected by most physicians until arterial Po_2 is <50 mm Hg; some observers cannot recognize cyanosis unless arterial Po_2 is <40 mm Hg!

In patients with chronic hypoxia, the central nervous system manifestations are drowsiness, inattentiveness, apathy, fatigue, and delayed reaction time. The chronic cardiovascular effects are often minimal, but pulmonary hypertension or even cor pulmonale with signs of right heart failure may be detected on clinical examination. One of the hallmarks of chronic hypoxia is erythrocytosis, which may cause noticeable plethora and changes in the hemoglobin concentration, hematocrit ratio, or red blood cell count. However, the increase in red blood cell mass in many patients with chronic hypoxia is masked by an almost proportionate increase in plasma volume; in these patients, the usual peripheral blood indexes of the red blood cell production (hemoglobin, hematocrit) do not reveal the full extent of the erythropoietic response.

HYPERCAPNIA

The physiologic consequences of hypercapnia depend not only on the amount of excess CO_2 in the body but also on the rate at which retention develops. Increases in Pco_2 from acute respiratory failure lead to a constellation of progressive disturbances of central nervous system function: apprehension, confusion, drowsiness, coma, and death. The vascular responses represent a mixture of vasoconstriction, from generalized sympathetic activity, and vasodilation, from local accumulation of CO_2; thus the cardiovascular abnormalities are variable and depend on whether vasoconstrictor or vasodilator influences predominate. There is usually tachycardia and sweating, but blood pressure may be high, low, or normal.

In contrast, if Pco_2 increases slowly, compensation takes place and the clinical consequences may be minimal at values of arterial Pco_2 that would cause death if reached suddenly. There are numerous patients with arterial Pco_2 values over 100 mm Hg who are ambulatory and at times living active lives, although most breathe supplementary O_2 to prevent life-threatening hypoxia. Patients with hypercapnia from chronic respiratory failure frequently complain of headaches and drowsiness; these symptoms are probably attributable to the potent cerebral vasodilating effect of excess CO_2. In addition, patients with chronic hypercapnia may have papilledema, muscular twitching, coarse myoclonic jerky motions, and asterixis. At times, the neurologic findings simulate those of a brain tumor.

351.5. TREATMENT OF ACUTE RESPIRATORY FAILURE

The time course of worsening abnormalities varies in patients with acute respiratory failure from almost instantaneous (flail chest, pulmonary embolism) to a gradual crescendo during a period of several hours or even days (respiratory tract infections, bronchial asthma). The demands for treatment and the speed with which it must be provided obviously differ from one patient to another. It is difficult to generalize about such an extremely variable clinical condition, but the principles of treatment of acute respiratory failure are as follows: *first*, establish an airway, administer O_2, and maintain adequate alveolar ventilation; *second*, identify and treat the underlying condition and monitor the patient's progress carefully.

ESTABLISH AN AIRWAY

The upper airway tends to be occluded in unconscious patients because of relaxation of the oropharyngeal muscles and tongue and the presence of saliva, vomitus, and other secretions. When respiratory arrest occurs away from medical facilities, clear all material from the oropharynx and place the victim on his or her back with the head tilted backward as far as possible and extend the jaw forward. Sometimes these simple maneuvers are all that is required to enable breathing to resume spontaneously. If it does not, start mouth-to-mouth breathing; after three or four quick full breaths without allowing time for deflation to occur, maintain deep breaths once every five seconds until the emergency is over.

An airway can be established by three different methods: an oropharyngeal tube, an endotracheal tube passed via the nose or mouth, and a tracheostomy. Selection of the procedure depends on available facilities and personnel and on the site and severity of the obstruction.

OROPHARYNGEAL AIRWAY. An oropharyngeal airway is valuable in unconscious patients who are breathing spontaneously (e.g., during recovery from general anesthesia, after a cerebrovascular accident). An oropharyngeal airway is also useful in patients who are apneic during emergency resuscitation but who are receiving some form of assisted ventilation (mouth-to-mouth respiration, bag-mask system) Although an oropharyngeal tube is commonly used in these clinical circumstances, its role must be viewed as temporary, either while the patient is waking up or until an endotracheal tube can be inserted.

ENDOTRACHEAL TUBE. The preferred method of establishing an airway in most emergencies is with an endotracheal tube. Once inserted, the tube is used to remove secretions and to provide ventilation. Endotracheal tubes can usually be passed quickly through the nose or, at times, through the mouth into the trachea by an experienced person; the airway is then sealed by inflating a balloon near the tip of the tube. Endotracheal tubes should be used in nearly all patients with acute respiratory failure severe enough to require control of their airways.

TRACHEOSTOMY. Emergency tracheostomy was formerly the only way of quickly establishing an airway in patients with acute respiratory failure. Now, emergency tracheostomy is contraindicated except in one clinical situation: acute obstruction of upper airways (e.g., from foreign bodies, trauma, or inflammation). Otherwise, intubation with an endotracheal tube is the treatment of choice for acute respiratory failure. Tracheostomy, if needed, can be performed at a later time in the operating room under ideal conditions. There is virtually no mortality and very little morbidity with an elective tracheostomy, in contrast to the high incidence of complications associated with emergency tracheostomy performed at the bedside.

The decision to convert a satisfactory endotracheal intubation to a tracheostomy is not an easy one and must be individualized in each case. The availability of tubes of inert plastic with low pressure cuffs permits endotracheal tubes to be used for weeks rather than days without prohibitive injury; the main mechanical difference between endotracheal and tracheostomy tubes is the trauma to the vocal cords from the former. The usual reasons for performing a tracheostomy in a patient with a satisfactory endotracheal tube are (1) failure to control secretions (sometimes it is difficult to suction the lungs adequately, especially the left side, through a long endotracheal tube) and (2) the need for prolonged (i.e., several weeks) intubation for assisted ventilation and/or removal of secretions (these circumstances are uncommon but occur particularly in patients with neuromuscular disease and chest wall injuries).

The presence of a tube and its cuff in the airway can cause necrosis of the mucosa of the trachea; at times the entire airway wall may be eroded with penetration of the esophagus (tracheoesophageal fistula) or a neighboring blood vessel (innominate artery), causing severe hemorrhage. Delayed complications after extubation are caused by damage to the trachea or larynx from the tube or cuff; injury to the vocal cords merely impairs phonation, but serious and life-threatening obstruction can result from stenosis or malacia of the tracheal wall. These complications should be considered and evaluated in any patient who complains of persisting hoarseness or who develops breathlessness or stridor at any time after endotracheal intubation.

HUMIDIFICATION. Insertion of an endotracheal or tracheostomy tube bypasses the normal source of humidification of the inspired air. When this occurs and unhumidified air or gas mixture is breathed, the result is drying of the mucosa and impairment of mucociliary clearance. Thus as long as the upper airway is bypassed, patients must receive air or a mixture of O_2 that is fully saturated with water vapor at their body temperature. This is easily accomplished if the patient is being ventilated with most commercial ventilators that have heated humidifiers in the circuit. If the patient is breathing spontaneously, humidified gas can be delivered through a T-piece connected to the endotracheal or tracheostomy tube. When proper humidification is carried out, remember that there is *no* insensible water loss through the respiratory tract when evaluating the patient's daily fluid balance.

ADMINISTER OXYGEN

Acute respiratory failure, by definition, includes decreased arterial Po_2. When respiratory failure is severe, death results from the central nervous system or cardiovascular consequences of hypoxia. During emergencies, supplementary O_2 is given without worrying about the concentration being used; in general, the higher the concentration of O_2, the better. After the patient's emergency condition has stabilized, attention is directed to administering O_2 in the lowest possible concentration required to correct the hypoxia. Any more O_2 than required to raise arterial Po_2 to a safe level exposes the patient to the direct toxicity of O_2 on the lung parenchyma and other undesirable effects: suppression of alveolar macrophage function and mucociliary clearance. Another possible complication of O_2 therapy that should be kept in mind is suppression of ventilatory drive; hypoventilation develops in patients with chronic CO_2 retention who are insensitive to hypercapnia and whose chief stimulus to breathe comes from the effect of hypoxia on the peripheral chemoreceptors. When these patients are given high concentrations of O_2, correction of their hypoxia removes the stimulus to breathe and further hypoventilation results. Deaths from severe hypercapnia and respiratory acidosis have resulted from this iatrogenic complication. However, the sequence occurs only in patients with chronic lung diseases, particularly airways obstruction, who are hypercapnic to begin with, and is one of the reasons for using "low-flow" O_2 therapy as in Ch. 351.6.

The usual goal of O_2 therapy in acute respiratory failure is to raise arterial Po_2 to between 60 and 80 mm Hg. Because these values lie on the flat portion of the oxyhemoglobin dissociation curve, most of the available hemoglobin is saturated with O_2; raising arterial Po_2 values even higher adds very little additional O_2 to the blood and may require increases in alveolar Po_2 concentrations to toxic levels. At times, especially when the mechanism of arterial hypoxia is right-to-left shunting of blood, arterial Po_2 may be considerably less than 60 mm Hg even with the patient breathing 100 per cent O_2. When this occurs, other maneuvers such as addition of end-expiratory pressure are required to raise arterial Po_2 and to allow a reduction in inspired O_2 concentration.

There are several ways of giving supplementary O_2 to a patient. Which method is chosen depends on the cause and severity of the arterial hypoxia and convenience to the patient. It is important to emphasize that no method can be relied upon to produce a certain increase in arterial Po_2; the response depends on which physiologic mechanism(s) is responsible for the hypoxia. Thus it is always advisable to monitor the effects of O_2 administration by serial analyses of arterial blood.

NASAL CANNULAS OR PRONGS. The concentration of O_2 in the inspired air can be enriched by nasal cannulas, catheters, or prongs. These devices work well even when patients breathe through their mouths. However, because of the drying effects of unhumidified O_2 on the nasal mucous membranes, if >3 to 5 liters per minute is needed to achieve satisfactory arterial oxygenation, other methods of administration are advisable.

VENTURI MASKS. These masks work on the principle of entrainment of a fixed proportion of air that mixes with the O_2 being supplied, and results in a constant inspired concentration: 24, 28, 35, or 40 per cent O_2. Although a properly used Venturi mask ensures that the inspired O_2 concentration is constant, the effects on arterial P_{O_2} vary considerably from one patient to another. The mask is somewhat uncomfortable and must be removed for eating and drinking. Because of these disadvantages and high cost, other simpler and cheaper methods usually suffice to deliver relatively low (21 to 41 per cent) concentrations of O_2.

RESERVOIR MASKS. When high concentrations of O_2 (40 to 80 per cent) are needed in patients who are not intubated, reservoir masks are used. To ensure optimal efficiency of operation, the masks must be tight fitting to avoid leaks; because this often causes discomfort, it is difficult to deliver high concentrations of O_2 by reservoir masks for long periods.

OTHER METHODS. Most of the recently developed mechanical ventilators have regulators that can be set to deliver an inspired O_2 concentration that ranges from 21 to 100 per cent. One of the best ways of ensuring that patients actually receive high concentrations of O_2 (60 to 100 per cent) is to use a mechanical ventilator connected to an endotracheal or tracheostomy tube.

MAINTAIN ALVEOLAR VENTILATION

Emergency resuscitation after respiratory arrest requires ventilation by mouth-to-mouth respiration or a bag and mask device. As soon as possible thereafter, if the patient does not resume spontaneous breathing, intubation and ventilation by a mechanical ventilator are required. Similar considerations apply to patients with acute respiratory failure whose breathing is insufficient to maintain adequate gas exchange. Because these patients are often receiving supplementary O_2, arterial P_{O_2} is not a good guide to the adequacy of their alveolar ventilation and reliance is placed on arterial P_{CO_2}. Intubation and mechanical ventilation are indicated in most patients with acute respiratory failure whose arterial blood gas studies reveal substantially elevated or increasing P_{CO_2} values.

MECHANICAL VENTILATION. Two types of mechanical ventilation can be used to provide assisted ventilation: pressure ventilators, in which a certain (adjustable) airway pressure is reached by the machine during each breathing cycle, or volume ventilators, in which a constant (adjustable) tidal volume is delivered to the patient with each breath. Most commercially available ventilators of both types can be set either to cycle automatically or to assist breathing once it is initiated by the patient. Most instruments also provide means of controlling inspiratory and expiratory flow rates. Pres-

sure ventilators were widely used for many years, but emphasis is now shifting from pressure to volume ventilators, which are more versatile and more reliable.

In general, pressure ventilators work best when the pressure required to deliver a satisfactory tidal volume does not exceed 30 to 40 cm H_2O — in other words, when the compliances of the lung and chest wall are normal or only slightly decreased and airways resistance is normal or only slightly increased. In contrast, volume ventilators deliver a preset tidal volume regardless of any respiratory mechanical abnormalities that might be present; these machines are particularly useful in patients with flail chests, massive obesity, or adult respiratory distress syndrome.

END-EXPIRATORY PRESSURE. Mechanical ventilators ordinarily raise airway pressure during inspiration and allow it to fall to zero (atmospheric) during expiration; this pattern of assisted ventilation is known as intermittent positive pressure ventilation, or IPPV. At times, it is desirable to add positive pressure to the airway during expiration as well as inspiration to hold the lung at a higher end-expiratory lung volume (functional residual capacity) than it would reach at zero end-expiratory pressure; this pattern of assisted ventilation is known as continuous positive pressure ventilation, or CPPV. Keeping the lung at a high functional residual capacity prevents closure of alveoli and airways during expiration and often improves arterial P_{O_2} considerably. Positive end-expiratory pressure (or PEEP) is most useful in patients with the conditions that cause the adult respiratory distress syndrome (Table 2).

Although end-expiratory pressure usually results in an improvement in arterial P_{O_2} and O_2 content, it may also decrease cardiac output by impairing myocardial contractility and increasing pulmonary vascular resistance. Accordingly, the actual delivery of O_2 to the tissues of the body may decrease. Thus it is important to monitor both the respiratory and circulatory responses to end-expiratory pressure to determine the optimal amount of pressure and the need for additional therapeutic interventions. Another common and serious hazard of end-expiratory pressure is its tendency to cause spontaneous pneumothorax and pneumomediastinum.

IDENTIFY AND TREAT THE UNDERLYING CONDITION

Acute respiratory failure always has a precipitating cause. Consequently, the cause of the condition should be identified as soon as possible after emergency measures have been started and the patient's condition has stabilized. Usually, the diagnosis can be established easily by a thorough history and physical examination, analysis of the blood and urine, and chest roentgenogram. Helpful auxiliary tests include those that evaluate central nervous system or cardiac function, those that determine the presence of drugs or poisons in the body, and bacteriologic study of secretions and blood.

Treatment obviously depends on the underlying cause, and the reader is referred to the appropriate chapters of this book for information about the therapy of specific pulmonary and other disorders that lead to acute respiratory failure. In all patients with acute respiratory failure, careful attention should be paid to fluid balance. Overhydration is a frequent and serious complication that can usually be avoided by careful attention to fluid replacement and monitoring of pulmonary capillary (wedge) pressure.

MONITOR THE PATIENT'S PROGRESS

The need for monitoring varies from patient to patient according to the response to initial treatment. If the disorder is readily reversible (e.g., bronchial asthma), the patient may respond sufficiently to go home shortly after being seen and treated. Other less rapidly responding conditions causing acute respiratory failure often require hospital care, and seriously ill patients are best treated in special acute care facilities (intensive care units) when available. Intensive care units provide an institutional focus of trained personnel and special equipment for the care of critically ill patients.

All seriously ill patients should have frequent measurements of blood pressure, constant monitoring of heart rate, careful recording of fluid intake and output, and determination of weight daily. Arterial blood gas analysis should be performed as often as needed but usually at least once daily. Special studies include measurement of cardiac output and placement of a Swan-Ganz catheter in the pulmonary artery for determination of pulmonary arterial and wedge pressures and sampling of mixed venous blood; this information is very helpful in guiding fluid replacement and ventilator adjustments, including levels of end-expiratory pressure. In general, wedge pressure values should be maintained in the normal range (5 to 10 mm Hg) and not allowed to increase above 10 mm Hg, especially in patients with the adult respiratory distress syndrome. Values of mixed venous O_2 saturation provide a rough guide, but the best presently available, to the balance between O_2 delivery to and utilization by all the organs of the body. Although satisfactory levels probably vary from one patient to another, saturations greater than 60 per cent or Po_2 values above 30 mm Hg should be maintained in mixed venous blood by various maneuvers that increase O_2 delivery: breathing supplementary O_2, increasing cardiac output, and increasing hemoglobin concentration. Per cent O_2 saturation of mixed venous blood is probably a better guide to the adequacy of O_2 transport than Po_2 because the affinity between O_2 and hemoglobin (i.e., the position of the oxyhemoglobin dissociation curve) may vary markedly in critically ill patients.

351.6. TREATMENT OF CHRONIC RESPIRATORY FAILURE

Patients with chronic lung disease often have sufficient alterations in their arterial Po_2 and Pco_2 values that they are said to be in chronic respiratory failure. Therapeutic regimens for these patients, whose disease is relatively stable, are delivered mainly on an outpatient basis and are designed to meet two objectives: (1) preventing or minimizing the number and severity of the intercurrent complications that would otherwise occur, and (2) treating maximally all reversible elements of the underlying disorder. Many of the specific remedies are used for both purposes, and the approaches to preventive and maintenance therapy for patients with the most common chronic lung diseases, asthma, bronchitis, and emphysema, are discussed in Ch. 344.

Despite emphasis on preventing intercurrent complications, these attacks continue to plague the lives of patients with chronic lung disease. Acute episodes of bronchopulmonary infection, pneumothorax, pulmonary embolism, surgical procedures, and misuse of sedatives all add their effects to those of the underlying lung disease and frequently produce serious disturbances of blood gases. These episodes are potentially life threatening, are usually associated with prolonged morbidity, and frequently require hospitalization. The principles of therapy are to maintain oxygenation while treating all new, presumably reversible, elements of the disease in an effort to restore the patient to his or her former state of health.

OXYGEN

Patients with chronic obstructive lung disease and superimposed episodes of acute respiratory failure nearly always have severe hypoxia from a combination of hypoventilation and ventilation-perfusion mismatching. Typical arterial blood values are Po_2 of approximately 30 mm Hg, Pco_2 of 70 mm Hg, and pH of 7.30. Neither the hypercapnia nor the acidemia is life threatening, but the hypoxia is potentially fatal. Thus treatment is directed mainly at alleviating the disturbance in oxygenation; the changes in Pco_2 and pH will return to baseline values as the acute condition improves. In view of the possibility that O_2 therapy may depress ventilation further by withdrawing the hypoxic stimulus to breathe, O_2 is given initially in low concentrations (1 to 3 liters per minute). The goal is to raise Po_2 to satisfactory levels (50 to 60 mm Hg) without depressing ventilation to the extent that unacceptable increases in Pco_2 and decreases in pH (particularly) occur.

The O_2 is usually started at 2 liters per minute, and an arterial blood specimen is analyzed 15 to 30 minutes later to determine the patient's response. Depending on the Po_2 value, the flow of O_2 can be adjusted. If hypoventilation and acidemia result from too much O_2 (e.g., Po_2 80 mm Hg, Pco_2 80 mm Hg, and pH 7.25), the supplementary O_2 should *not* be discontinued but the flow rate should be decreased. The Po_2 decreases much faster than the stimulus to breathe returns, and cardiac arrest or other serious complications of hypoxia may result.

INTUBATION-ASSISTED VENTILATION

Low-flow O_2 given in the manner described provides satisfactory relief of hypoxia in nearly all instances. Although the goal of low-flow O_2 is an arterial Po_2 of 50 to 60 mm Hg, at times one has to be satisfied with 40 to 50 mm Hg. When oxygenation cannot be achieved without intolerable hypercapnia and acidemia, the decision whether to intubate and ventilate the patient must be made. Experience with intubation and mechanical ventilation in this group of patients has been extremely unrewarding, particularly because of the prolonged need for assisted ventilation once intubation is performed and the poor prognosis for prolonged survival and return to useful life after recovery from the acute episode. Although each case must be considered individually, in general, patients with chronic obstructive pulmonary disease who develop superimposed acute respiratory failure should not be intubated. The major exception to this axiom is the need for ventilator support during the postoperative period. Doxapram (see Respiratory Stimulants, below) often allows administration of "extra" O_2 without depressing ventilatory drive.

BRONCHODILATORS

Most intercurrent episodes of acute respiratory failure in patients with chronic obstructive pulmonary disease are associated with increased airways resistance from the presence of secretions, edema of the mucosa, and bronchospasm. Because it is impossible to discriminate among these, bronchodilator drugs are always included in the treatment regimen to take advantage of the reversibility of whatever element of bronchospasm is present.

When patients seek medical attention for intercurrent attacks, they frequently have already tried — and failed to respond to — oral and aerosolized bronchodilators. In this circumstance, intravenous aminophylline is the initial drug of choice. Aminophylline can be injected slowly in 250-mg or 500-mg boluses, or, if the patient has been hospitalized and prolonged treatment is envisioned, by a loading dose (5.6 mg per kilogram of body weight) and constant sustaining infusion (0.9 mg per kilogram of body weight per hour). These dosages should be reduced in patients who have been receiving aminophylline, who are elderly, or, especially, who have liver disease or heart failure. It is advisable to determine the aminophylline plasma level 24 to 36 hours after the constant infusion regimen has been started to ensure that values are in the therapeutic range (10 to 20 mg per 100 ml) and to avoid toxicity.

Selective β-2 sympathomimetic drugs, administered either parenterally or by aerosol, are begun or continued at appropriate intervals. Aerosolized drugs that work topically should not be relied upon solely, because they fail to penetrate effectively throughout the tracheobronchial system in the presence of airways secretions and severe narrowing.

The indications for and dosage of corticosteroids in this clinical setting are controversial. Most patients who have typical attacks of intercurrent infectious bronchitis can be managed satisfactorily without corticosteroids. These drugs should be used in patients with either status asthmaticus or severe episodes of superimposed acute respiratory failure in which an important component of bronchospasm and airways inflammation is presumed to exist. Hydrocortisone, 100 mg intravenously every four hours or the equivalent dose by constant infusion, is indicated. Much higher doses of corticosteroids (e.g., methylprednisolone, 15 mg per kilogram of body weight per day in divided doses) have been recommended, but there is no evidence to suggest that these are more efficacious than the suggested dose of hydrocortisone.

ANTIMICROBIALS

Infections are the most frequent and important cause of acute respiratory failure in patients with chronic underlying lung disease. Intercurrent attacks usually begin as a typical cold, with rhinitis, pharyngitis, and headaches. Shortly afterward, lower respiratory involvement appears with increasing cough, sputum production, purulence, wheezing, and breathlessness. These episodes occur several times a year in most patients with chronic obstructive pulmonary disease. (It should be noted that fever, leukocytosis, and new roentgenographic infiltrations are uncommon in this setting.) When airway infection is present, the sputum is not only purulent but usually contains numerous microorganisms detectable by Gram stain of the secretions. Sputum cultures, however, often fail to reveal pathogenic bacteria, although at times *Diplococcus pneumoniae* and/or *Hemophilus influenzae* may be grown. Regardless of the presence or absence of identifiable pathogens, oral treatment with ampicillin (250 to 500 mg every six hours) or tetracycline (250 to 500 every six hours) frequently results in decreased volume of sputum, thinning of the secretions, change in sputum appearance from purulent to mucoid, and improvement in blood gases.

When pneumonia is present, signified by the presence of new infiltration(s) on the chest roentgenogram, Gram stain of the sputum is likely to show one bacterial species predominating, and the initial selection of antimicrobials should cover this organism. Therapy can be revised, if necessary, when the results of the sputum cultures are available.

CONTROL OF SECRETIONS

Many patients complain of thick tenacious sputum that is troublesome to clear. Although it seems desirable to attempt to alter the character of these secretions to facilitate their removal, there is no clear evidence that it is possible to do so by pharmacologic means. Iodides, enzymes, detergents, and acetylcysteine, administered orally or by aerosol, have been tried extensively, but none has been shown convincingly to be effective. Moreover, each has potential toxic side effects. Similarly, mist tents and ultrasonic nebulizers, once widely used, are seldom employed today. The best way to control secretions is to control infection with antimicrobials and to ensure adequate (but not excessive) hydration by the administration of intravenous fluids.

Patients with troublesome sputum retention may require intermittent nasotracheal suction to control the volume of secretions. Manual or mechanical percussion serves to loosen secretions and enhances their removal. Respiratory physical therapy, especially when carried out by a skilled therapist, often results in increase in arterial Po_2 related to the improvement in the distribution of ventilation from clearance of sputum.

TREATMENT OF HEART FAILURE

Cor pulmonale is an inevitable complication of severe chronic lung disease. Right-sided heart failure occurs secondary to the increased work load imposed on the right ventricle by the changes in the pulmonary circulation from the effects of lung disease. Resistance to blood flow through the lungs increases when pulmonary blood vessels are destroyed (as in emphysema), obstructed (as in pulmonary thromboembolism), narrowed (from vasoconstriction), or compressed (breathing at high lung volumes), or the blood is unusually viscous (polycythemia). Patients whose cor pulmonale is well compensated or even inapparent while their chronic lung disease is stable often develop acute right heart failure during intercurrent attacks of acute respiratory failure. Peripheral edema, increased venous pressure, and enlarged, painful liver are important clues to the presence of acute cardiac decompensation.

Most patients with right heart failure from cor pulmonale, even if severe, have a satisfactory diuresis when put to bed, given O_2, and treated appropriately for their underlying lung disease. Diuretics may make patients feel more comfortable by diminishing peripheral edema and hepatic and gastrointestinal congestion faster than spontaneous diuresis; but if used, the drugs should be administered orally in low doses. Intravenous ethacrynic acid or furosemide can cause excessive renal loss of Cl^- that worsens existing acid-base disturbances and depletes intravascular volume sufficiently to decrease cardiac output and blood pressure. A particularly dangerous situation occurs in patients who already have coexisting nonrespiratory (metabolic) alkalosis, often from Cl^--losing diuretics, in addition to their hypercapnia from chronic respiratory failure; when the measures designed to improve ventilation lower arterial Pco_2, the nonrespiratory alkalosis becomes "unmasked" and arterial pH becomes markedly alkaline. When this occurs, the patients can develop cardiac arrhythmias, become comatose, or manifest convulsive seizures or other focal neurologic abnormalities.

If an element of pulmonary edema or pulmonary vascular congestion is present from left heart failure, this may also respond to diuretics. Whether left heart failure can occur secondary to purely right-sided disease is controversial, but there is probably little or no relationship. Of greater importance are coexisting causes of left-sided involvement (e.g., valvular disease, coronary atherosclerosis); furthermore, chronic hypoxia and severe polycythemia may impair left ventricular as well as right ventricular function.

There is no clear evidence that digitalis or its derivatives are beneficial in patients with cor pulmonale; in fact, most of the recent evidence is to the contrary. Also, the use of digitalis is hazardous in patients with chronic respiratory failure owing to the sudden shifts in acid-base balance and electrolyte concentrations that may occur in these patients. Therefore digitalis should be used only in patients with digitalis-responsive arrhythmias or coexisting left heart failure.

RESPIRATORY STIMULANTS

With few exceptions, respiratory stimulants are obsolete. Nikethamide, picrotoxin, and ethamivan have been replaced by other less hazardous and more efficient methods of maintaining ventilation. Doxapram, a drug that works by stimulating carotid chemoreceptors rather than neurons in the brain, appears to be much safer than centrally acting stimulants. The chief use of doxapram is to minimize or prevent the depression of ventilation, with consequent increase in Pco_2 and decrease in pH, that occurs in some hypoxic patients with hypercapnia who are given O_2 to breathe.

SEDATION

All sedative drugs should be avoided in patients with chronic lung disease and intercurrent acute respiratory failure, including diazepam (Valium) and chlordiazepoxide (Librium), which can suppress ventilation. Exceptions to this cardinal rule are made from time to time, but usually only when the patient is being mechanically ventilated and sedation is required to enable breathing synchronous with the machine.

POSTOPERATIVE COMPLICATIONS

Patients with chronic respiratory failure are high risk operative candidates. Moreover, the closer the surgical incision to the thorax, the higher the incidence of postoperative complications. Despite this caveat, it is safe to say that virtually *all* patients who have respiratory failure can safely undergo *non*thoracic surgery. Postoperative complications can be anticipated and often prevented by attention to the general principles of care outlined in this chapter. Close observation and monitoring are usually required, and these can best be carried out in an intensive care unit.

Abraham, A. S., Cole, R. B., Green, I. D., Hedworth-Whitty, R. B., Clarke, S. W., and Bishop, J. M.: Factors contributing to the reversible pulmonary hypertension of patients with acute respiratory failure studied by serial observations during recovery. Circ. Res., 24:51, 1969.

Campbell, E. J. M.: The J. Burns Amberson Lecture. The management of acute respiratory failure in chronic bronchitis and emphysema. Am. Rev. Respir. Dis., 96:626, 1967.

Hopewell, P. C., and Murray, J. F.: The adult respiratory distress syndrome. Ann. Rev. Med., 27:343, 1976.

Moser, K. M., Shibel, E. M., and Beamon, A. J.: Acute respiratory failure in obstructive lung disease. Long-term survival after treatment in an intensive care unit. JAMA, 225:705, 1973.

Pontoppidan, H., Geffin, B., and Lowenstein, E.: Acute Respiratory Failure in the Adult. Boston, Little, Brown, & Company, 1973.

Sykes, M. K., McNicol, M. W., and Campbell, E. J. M.: Respiratory Failure. Oxford, Blackwell Scientific Publications, 1976.

Zwillich, C. W., Pierson, D. J., Creagh, C. E., Sutton, F. D., Schatz, E., and Petty, T. L.: Complications of assisted ventilation. A prospective study of 354 consecutive episodes. Am. J. Med., 57:161, 1974.

PART XIII
CRITICAL CARE MEDICINE

Byron D. McLees

352. THE MEDICAL INTENSIVE CARE UNIT

352.1. INTRODUCTION

Critical care medicine may be defined as the observation, diagnosis, treatment, and rehabilitation of patients with overt or potential failure of vital functions. Morbidity and mortality can be reduced by the concentration of these patients in special units where staff and equipment are oriented to special methods of care. In the following pages attention is focused on common problems of critically ill patients. Emphasis is placed on the distortions of physiology in patients hospitalized on intensive care units and the techniques and concepts of care integral to their treatment. Problems encountered in the critically ill are unique not only in their impact on all the vital systems but also in their time course of development and in the types of data required for adequate evaluation and treatment.

The most important requirement of an intensive care unit (ICU) is that there be an organization. The essential aspects for the organization of an ICU include the following points:

1. Formal educational programs for the nursing, technical, and medical staff.

2. Protocols for the management of commonly encountered problems to aid in the consistent application of a therapeutic approach to patient care by all members of the team.

3. Staffing patterns for nursing and technical personnel which are designed to meet the needs of each specific unit and not calculated from empirical formulas based on fixed ratios of patients to staff.

4. Patient selection criteria which are carefully developed and implemented.

5. Appropriate record-keeping to attempt to establish the effectiveness of the ICU.

Recognition, treatment, and rehabilitation are well recognized phases in the care of the critically ill patient. We must now emphasize *anticipation* as a critical stage in patient care, because early, appropriate management of the critically ill patient can frequently alter the natural history of the illness and perhaps obviate the need for major life support systems. The fact that intensive care units frequently treat patients presenting in extremis should not be interpreted as license to allow an illness to reach catastrophic proportions before transfer to an ICU.

GOALS AND LIMITATIONS OF INTENSIVE CARE: MEDICOLEGAL ASPECTS. Definition of therapeutic goals is an important requirement in the total care of a critically ill patient. Failure to define goals can lead to the application of maximal life support measures for the sake of appearances long after hope for survival has been abandoned. A prognostic classification system has been developed to aid in the assessment of patients, particularly with respect to deciding when a specific intervention (including cardiopulmonary resuscitation) is no longer advisable (Tagge et al.). This system establishes a process regularly exercised by the ICU staff to address the question of what is best for the whole patient and promises open communication regarding the elements of life and death decisions in the critical care setting.

Both the termination of life-supporting interventions and the failure to initiate therapy have substantial legal implications. The legal aspect of discontinuing life support is a controversial subject at present. Courts throughout the United States are concerned with this problem. Neurologic criteria are now frequently used as the basis for pronouncing the patient dead. The Harvard criteria for brain death have gained considerable medical acceptance: (1) absence of responsivity or receptiveness; (2) absence of spontaneous movement, breathing, or reflex activity; (3) presence of isoelectric EEG; and (4) all examinations repeated at two intervals 24 hours apart in the absence of hypothermia or drug ingestion.

These criteria provide the physician with a concrete means for determining clinical death and have been used to determine the time at which organs may be removed from transplantation donors. However, even these widely used criteria are not recognized by civil law in all states. The legal status of the termination of life-supporting therapy in patients who do not meet the criteria for brain death is not defined, and the medicolegal aspects of such action are far from clear. Both civil and criminal litigation could be involved. The law regarding failure to initiate therapy, thus permitting natural death from a fatal illness, is ambivalent; however, the practice has been upheld by the courts in cases in which the choice has been made by competent adults. There is no record of criminal action against a physician for neglecting to engage in the active treatment of a dying patient. The physician has the responsibility for the life of his patient but must also have an intelligent and sympathetic concern for the patient's death. It is incumbent upon the physician to formulate his ethical and medical decisions in the best interests of the patient and in recognition of the status of the law surrounding such action.

352.2. INSTRUMENTATION FOR THE INTENSIVE CARE UNIT

The purpose of this chapter is to discuss the instrumentation commonly used to facilitate care of the critically ill patient. The details of data collection and interpretation will be discussed in the chapters devoted to specific clinical problems.

AUTOMATED DATA MANAGEMENT. An intensive care unit has the potential to generate large amounts of data, and much effort is directed toward obtaining appropriate measurements to guide patient therapy. Unfortunately, less effort and thought may be given to the manner in which the data will be displayed and stored. It may be impossible to interpret very accurate cardiac output data because changes in fluid balance and medications relevant to the regulation of cardiac output were not recorded appropriately. Intelligent care of the patient frequently depends upon a knowledge of the patient's response to previous therapy. The most accurate and sophisticated data may become useless without detailed and accurate flow sheets, which should be tailored to each intensive care unit and to the individual patient.

The development of dedicated mini-computers designed specifically for critical care medicine permits the use of a computer-generated flow sheet. Some of the commercially available systems collect data directly from electronic transducers and conduct on-line processing and computation of the data. Data which cannot be collected directly, such as intake and output, body weight, and appearance, can be entered at a small bedside keyboard by the nursing staff. Computing systems complete with software (programs) are now commercially available; as the cost of these devices decreases, they may become more readily available to all intensive care units.

CARDIAC OUTPUT DEVICES. Contemporary care of the critically ill patient requires knowledge of the cardiac output. Serial determinations of cardiac output provide information essential to the cardiorespiratory and pharmacologic management of the patient. The development of bedside pulmonary artery catheterization permits the use of indicator dilution techniques for determination of cardiac output. Many substances have been used as indicators, but the two most commonly used are indocyanine green and cold saline or water. More recent thermodilution computers can use room temperature solutions.

Dye dilution is more cumbersome than the thermodilution technique, but will produce a more reliable value for cardiac output in the critically ill patient. A small volume of dye is injected into the pulmonary artery, and its appearance is measured spectrophotometrically at the arterial side of the circulation (brachial or femoral artery). Blood is withdrawn from the artery at a fixed rate by a mechanically powered syringe and passed through a densitometer, which records the dilution of dye with respect to time. Commercially available devices are available to calculate and digitally display the cardiac output in liters per minute immediately following injection of the indicator.

The thermodilution technique employs a bolus of cold indicator (10 ml of 5 per cent dextrose in water or normal saline) which is injected through a special purpose catheter. The bolus passes through a side hole located approximately 30 cm proximal to a thermistor, which is positioned near the tip of the catheter and senses the change in temperature as the indicator flows into the pulmonary artery. The thermodilution system does not require an arterial puncture; hence serial determinations may be performed without withdrawing blood samples. In some hands the thermodilution technique has been as reliable as the dye dilution technique, even in the critically ill patient.

FLUOROSCOPIC IMAGE INTENSIFIER. Intensive care medicine has been greatly facilitated by the availability of small, inexpensive image intensifiers which can be used at the bedside without special wiring or lead shielding. These devices can be used by the ICU staff, thus obviating the need to move critically ill patients for simple roentgenographic studies. Hydraulic, radiolucent beds simplify fluoroscopic interpretation but are not absolutely necessary. The effective and accurate use of vascular catheters and endotracheal and nasogastric tubes is greatly simplified by safe, rapid, and convenient fluoroscopy.

MASS SPECTROMETER. Stable low cost mass spectrometers have been developed to provide automated systems for monitoring respiratory gases on a practical clinical basis. These commercially available systems provide for the real time, simultaneous noninvasive measurement of inspired and expired gas concentrations on up to 12 patients. The partial pressures of oxygen, carbon dioxide, and nitrogen can be displayed and printed at preselected time intervals ranging from 10 to 60 minutes. Respiratory gas monitoring permits earlier detection of changes in respiratory function than blood gas determinations. Audible and visual alarms are activated if end-tidal gases exceed preset limits.

TRANSDUCERS. Pressure is quantified by strain gauges or transducers. Hydrodynamic pressure is transmitted to a diaphragm through a fluid-filled tube system attached to the catheter and is converted to an electrical signal. This signal is detected and amplified by an amplifier which displays the pressure on an oscilloscope or other suitable display device. The fluid-filled manometer has no role in the measurement of systemic or pulmonary artery pressures, and it is clearly a second choice even for measurement of venous pressures.

VENTILATORS. The function of a mechanical ventilator is to deliver an adequate volume of gas to the patient's airway. Many devices are available which fulfill this function; selection of a ventilator is principally a matter of preference, provided that the desired volume can be delivered at the desired rate. A mechanical ventilator should be simple and provide for the control of pressure, volume, flow rate, expiratory time, and oxygen concentration. The parameter used to regulate the quantity of gas delivered is frequently used to classify ventilators into pressure-, volume-, or time-cycled devices. *Pressure-cycled devices* terminate the inspiratory phase of ventilation when the airway pressure reaches a predetermined level regardless of the volume of gas delivered, and initiate the expiratory phase. These devices may be used for uncomplicated ventilation problems and are frequently successful in ventilating patients with respiratory failure accompanying chronic obstructive pulmonary disease. The tidal volume delivered is a function of chest wall and lung compliance (stiffness) and airway resistance; consequently, the expired volume must be measured frequently to ensure that the desired gas volume is being delivered. Patients with the syndrome of acute respiratory failure require large tidal volumes and may suffer frequent and rapid changes in pulmonary mechanics. Pressure-cycled devices are frequently inadequate and always inconvenient to use in this setting.

Volume-cycled ventilators deliver a predetermined gas volume regardless of the airway pressure. The simplicity, reliability, and reproducibility of the volume-cycled devices have made them popular ventilators for the management of patients with acute respiratory failure.

Time-cycled devices are also reliable and acceptable ventilators for the management of patients with acute respiratory failure; however, they have not been widely used in the United States, perhaps because of their expense and foreign manufacture. The cycling pattern in the time-cycled ventilators is determined by regulation of the length of the inspiratory and expiratory phases of the respiratory cycle. The tidal volume is determined by adjustment of the flow rate so that an appropriate volume is delivered during the time scheduled for inspiration.

Fluidic and pneumatic ventilators are commercially available as gas-powered, volume-cycled, and time-cycled devices. They require no electrical power and are especially useful for the transportation of critically ill patients requiring large tidal volumes, high oxygen concentrations, and end-expiratory pressures — conditions in which use of resuscitation bags is at best a tenuous means of respiratory support.

The performance of a ventilator is no better than its operator. If a machine is capable of delivering the required tidal volume at the desired rate and is appropriately adjusted, there is little to suggest any special therapeutic advantage for a particular ventilator over any other device capable of delivering the desired volumes and rates.

352.3. ACUTE RESPIRATORY FAILURE

The term acute respiratory failure includes pathologic states frequently labeled adult respiratory distress syndrome, post-traumatic pulmonary insufficiency, shock lung, or wet lung. Respiratory failure associated with decompensation of chronic lung disease is discussed separately in Ch. 351 because it is a different disease process in terms of etiology, pathophysiology, and therapy. It must be emphasized that the discussion to follow does not apply to decompensated obstructive bronchopulmonary disease, and the treatment outlined here for acute respiratory failure may result in substantial morbidity and possible mortality if applied to the patient with chronic obstructive lung disease as the *primary* illness.

Acute respiratory failure occurs in many clinical settings; Table 1 lists the etiologic factors frequently associated with this syndrome. The inclusion of so many diverse entities under the guise of a single syndrome is obviously unsatisfactory and should not be interpreted to suggest that etiology is irrelevant or unimportant. As our understanding of this syndrome increases, it may become unnecessary to lump undoubtedly separate entities into a single category termed acute respiratory failure. Unfortunately, the patient frequently presents to the intensive care unit with severe, progressive respiratory failure under conditions in which single etiolo-

TABLE 1. Etiologic Factors in Acute Respiratory Failure

Fat emboli
Fluid overload
Shock
Aspiration
Pulmonary infarction
Oxygen toxicity
Multiple transfusions
Disseminated intravascular coagulation
Sepsis
Pancreatitis
Septic abortion
Massive trauma and burns

gic factors cannot be defined. In each instance a detailed and diligent investigation should be conducted to define the etiologic factors which alone or in combination could be responsible for respiratory insufficiency. Frequently a number of factors, taken singly, seem insufficient to account for the onset of progressive respiratory failure; however, taken together they become sufficient to cause acute respiratory failure. If the search for an etiology is unrewarding, a pragmatic approach should be taken to management of the acute respiratory failure syndrome. Appropriate and effective therapy can usually be designed despite the inability to define an etiology, because the distortions of lung pathology and physiology are similar regardless of the initial insult.

CLINICAL FEATURES. Moore et al. have described the clinical features of acute respiratory failure and have outlined four phases which characterize progression of the syndrome.

Phase I: Injury and Resuscitation. This is the period immediately following the initial injury, hemorrhage, or infection. During this period the patient has almost invariably been resuscitated from a low flow state by infusion of large volumes of crystalloid or colloid and, perhaps, by cardiopulmonary resuscitation. Alkalosis is frequently present, but there is no evidence of respiratory distress and the chest x-ray is clear. It is important to recognize this setting as the milieu in which the syndrome of acute respiratory failure may appear so that appropriate plans can be made for careful observation of the patient.

Phase II: Circulatory Stabilization. Tissue perfusion, as reflected by mental status, renal function, and blood pressure, has returned to normal. This phase may last for five to seven days before the onset of pulmonary insufficiency becomes clinically apparent. The signs of acute respiratory failure frequently occur in an otherwise stable patient. *The most important and frequently the earliest sign of incipient respiratory failure is hyperventilation*, which may persist long after the initial injury and at a time when the chest x-ray and auscultatory findings are normal. The hyperventilation is frequently and erroneously attributed to anxiety, pain, or subclinical pulmonary congestion. The arterial oxygen tension is slightly decreased (60 to 70 mm Hg) on room air. However, measurement of the arterial oxygen tension following a 20-minute trial on 100 per cent oxygen will reveal a large alveolar-arterial oxygen tension difference ($Aa_{D_{O_2}}$) consistent with a large intrapulmonic shunt. These findings are frequently overlooked or dismissed because the patient looks and feels well and all are pleased with the results of a successful resuscitation; however, the presence of a large $Aa_{D_{O2}}$ points strongly to the incipient development of the acute respiratory failure syndrome. The intrapulmonic shunt (Qs/Qt) may be as high as 15 to 30 per cent at this phase of the patient's course. Aggressive therapeutic intervention promptly initiated may alter the natural course of the illness.

Phase III: Progressive Pulmonary Insufficiency. This phase is characterized by increasing respiratory difficulty manifested by tachypnea, progressive hypoxemia, and hypocarbia. Auscultation reveals scattered rales and rhonchi; the x-ray film shows spotty, diffuse infiltrates compatible with bronchopneumonia. Entities such as congestive heart failure, pulmonary emboli, bronchopneumonia, atelectasis, and aspiration pneumonitis are frequently invoked to explain this constellation of signs and symptoms. The assistance of a mechanical ventilator will frequently be required to support the patient's respiration. Sputum cultures may show growth of nosocomial organisms such as *Klebsiella, Pseudomonas,* or *Serratia* species. As time passes, the roentgenogram begins to show large areas of consolidation and the powerful respiratory drive begins to disappear; the patient becomes less alert. Hypoxemia is progressive, requiring increased oxygen concentrations to maintain satisfactory arterial oxygen tensions. The hypocapnia associated with the initial hyperventilation gradually disappears and may be replaced by hypercapnia in spite of mechanical ventilation with large minute volumes. Progressive hypercapnia precedes the terminal phase of illness; the mixed venous oxygen tension begins to fall, and the patient becomes comatose.

Phase IV: Terminal Hypoxia and Hemodynamic Decompensation. This phase of illness is usually brief, but with advanced life support techniques it may last several days. It is characterized by progressive coma, increasing intrapulmonary shunt, hypercapnia, and metabolic acidosis. The cardiac output finally begins to fall and requires pharmacologic support. Atrial and ventricular arrhythmias appear. Tissue perfusion deteriorates in spite of increasing hemodynamic support, and bradycardia and terminal asystole frequently mark the death of the patient.

The four phases of acute respiratory failure may be telescoped into a very short course of seven to ten days or may last up to several weeks. Unfortunately, the diagnosis of acute respiratory failure is frequently not entertained until the patient has progressed to the second phase of the illness; it is even more unfortunate when transfer to critical care facilities is delayed until the patient has progressed to the third or fourth phase of the syndrome. The importance of early recognition of the illness is again emphasized because early intervention with institution of appropriate therapy may be capable of modifying the natural history of the disease.

PATHOLOGIC CHANGES. Many types of injurious conditions which affect lung architecture produce similar reactions at the cellular level and cause a series of uniform morphologic responses to injury. The pulmonary capillaries are lined with endothelial cells which may be important in active transport and metabolism. The alveolar side of the capillary is lined with epithelial cells, termed Type I pneumocytes. Large, distinct cells, termed Type II or granular pneumocytes, are frequently located at junctions of the interalveolar septa. The Type II pneumocytes are progenitor cells and are thought to be capable of replacing the Type I pneumocytes. The capillary endothelial cells and the alveolar epithelial cells are separated by basement membrane and connective tissue components which compose the interstitium of the lung. The pulmonary capillaries course from arteriole to venule through the interstitial space of the interalveolar septum.

The pulmonary lymphatics represent a third circulating system for the lung and are of particular importance in the prevention of extravascular fluid accumulation. They are well designed to participate in the removal of fluid from the interstitial space and serve to protect the lung against increases in interstitial fluid.

The response of the lung to acute injury is characterized by the accumulation of fluid in the interstitial space; transudated fluid forms during oxygen toxicity, shock, and other acute injuries. A consideration of the determinants of capillary permeability in the absence of heart failure provides a convenient framework for the construction of a picture of acute respiratory failure. Swelling and disruption of the mitochondria in the endothelial cells of the pulmonary capillary are produced by many types of injuries. This process eventually leads to swelling of the capillary endothelial cells and causes the tight junctions between these cells to open, permitting the escape of fluid into the interstitial space. These junctions may become so distorted that cellular elements escape into the interstitium, followed ultimately by their deposition into the alveolus.

Extensive cellular damage involving the Type I and Type II pneumocytes is also observed. The Type I cells become detached from the basement membrane, leaving a completely denuded surface; Type II cells then line the alveoli as regeneration begins to take place. The Type II cells become vacuolated because of the destruction of the lamellar bodies. This may be an anatomic representation of the decrease in surfactant content found in the lungs of patients with acute respiratory failure. Many investigators feel that the common pathway for pulmonary injury is mediated through a decrease in surfactant production. The loss of surfactant tends to favor transudation of fluid from the vascular bed into the air spaces. The precise magnitude of the physical forces producing fluid movement at the alveolar-capillary junction is unknown, but it is likely that the sum of the Starling forces is normally slightly positive, producing a liquid layer which coats the air-tissue interface and is responsible, in part, for the normal pulmonary lymph flow. This normal flux of fluid into the lung may explain the genesis of severe pulmonary edema following capillary injury. Mechanical occlusion of the pulmonary capillary bed decreases its volume and may also produce pulmonary capillary hypertension with subsequent fluid transudation. Microaggregates containing erythrocytes, platelets, leukocytes and fibrin-containing thrombi are frequently found occluding the pulmonary arterioles and capillaries of patients dying from acute respiratory failure, but the extent of this microaggregation is generally thought to be insufficient to explain capillary hypertension on a purely mechanical basis. There is evidence, however, that these aggregates of cellular material may release intracellular substances which are capable of inducing capillary hypertension and directly altering capillary permeability. Prostaglandins, ADP, serotonin, and histamine all have the potential to produce pulmonary vasoconstriction and may play a role in the induction of pulmonary hypertension and pulmonary edema seen in acute respiratory failure. Thrombin produced by intravascular coag-

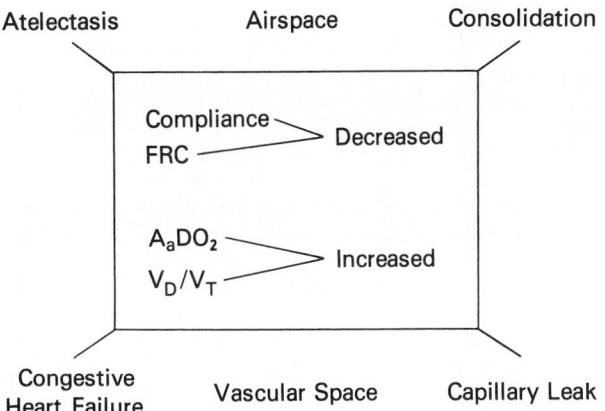

Figure 1. Interrelationship between primary pathologic changes in acute respiratory failure and alterations in pulmonary physiology. (From Wilson, R. F., and Pontoppidon, H.: Crit. Care Med., 2:293, 1974.)

ulation may directly cause an increase in pulmonary vascular resistance, in addition to its role in platelet aggregation and fibrin formation. The histologic features of pneumonitis may be produced in experimental animals following the release of vasoactive peptides, mediated perhaps through the action of lysosomal enzymes. When blood from septic dogs is perfused through an isolated canine pulmonary lobe, the pulmonary resistance is increased. A histologic picture of pneumonitis is produced only in the perfused lobe, and pretreatment of the septic animal with a protease inhibitor (Trasylol) prior to the perfusion will prevent the appearance of these lesions. In advanced stages of pulmonary injury the alveoli are filled with a hemorrhagic fibrinous exudate containing leukocytes, macrophages, and cellular debris. Fibrin covers many of the alveolar surfaces, alveolar ducts, and distal airways and may contribute to the formation of hyaline membranes.

In summary, the common morphologic and pathologic features of acute respiratory failure are (1) microaggregation of platelets and leukocytes within the pulmonary capillaries; (2) swelling and degeneration of the pulmonary capillary endothelium; (3) interstitial edema and hemorrhage; (4) marked reduction in capillary bed integrity; (5) extensive proliferation of granular pneumocytes, with the production of a cuboidal epithelial lining in the air spaces; (6) alveolar hemorrhage and edema; (7) hyaline membrane formation; (8) atelectasis; and (9) bronchopneumonia.

PHYSIOLOGY OF ACUTE RESPIRATORY FAILURE. The anatomic and morphologic changes discussed above produce the distortions of physiology seen in the clinical management of acute respiratory failure (Fig. 1). The functional residual capacity (FRC) equals the volume of gas in the lung at the end of tidal respiration; it is the equilibrium lung volume when the tendency of the lung to collapse is balanced by the tendency of the chest wall to "spring outward." The FRC serves two physiologic functions: (1) it buffers inspired gases to prevent large tidal swings in alveolar gas tension, and (2) it acts to keep airways open.

Reductions in the FRC may occur as a consequence of interstitial edema, hemorrhage, and pneumonitis; however, abdominal distention, pain, and body position also decrease FRC. Changes in lung volume affect pulmonary function primarily through changes in the distribution of ventilation. In large measure, the distribution of ventilation to the basilar or apical regions of the lungs depends upon the region of the pressure-volume curve over which ventilation is occurring. The effect of inspiration on the pressure-volume curve of the lung is illustrated in Figure 2. The degree of expansion manifested by any region of the lung depends upon its position on the pressure-volume curve. The base of the lung will undergo a larger change in volume than the apex because of its location on the steep part of the curve; it will, consequently, receive better ventilation than the apex in spite of the small resting volume.

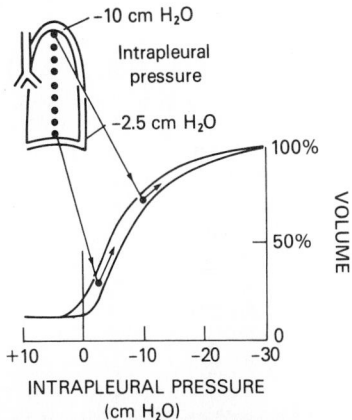
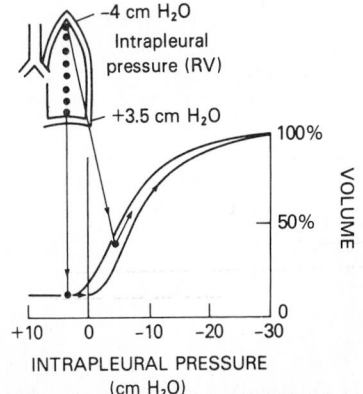

Figure 2.   Change in pressure-volume relationships in the lung with acute respiratory failure. In the normal upright lung (A), the transpulmonary pressure is less at the base than apex. During inspiration the change in transpulmonary pressure will be of equal magnitude at the base and apex of the lung; however, the alveoli at the base will expand more than those at the apex because of their position on a steeper portion of the curve. The slope of the curve for basal alveoli (compliance = volume/pressure) is greater for the basal alveoli; thus inspired air will preferentially move to the basal lung regions. If the lung volume is decreased by edema or atelectasis, as seen in acute respiratory failure (B), the alveoli at the base will remain closed with the initial change in transpulmonary pressure, causing the inspired gas to preferentially move to the apex. Once the critical opening pressure of the alveoli has been overcome, their volume will increase and proceed to move up the inspiratory limb of the curve. (From West, J. B.: Respiratory Physiology: The Essentials. Baltimore, Williams & Wilkins Company, 1974.)

Ventilation at low lung volumes can result in better ventilation of the apices because of airway closure in the poorly expanded basal portion of the lungs. The closing volume is operationally defined as the lung volume at which airway closure is detected. During expiration to very low lung volumes, the small airways, probably in the region of the respiratory bronchioles, functionally close or collapse. As long as the volume at which closure occurs is below the FRC, gas exchange will probably not be adversely affected; however, the reduction in FRC seen in acute respiratory failure may produce circumstances in which airways close prior to the end-expiratory position (FRC), resulting in impairment of gas exchange. If the volume required to open the airways (critical opening volume) is not achieved, the gas entrapped distal to the airway closure will be absorbed, resulting in atelectasis.

Compliance is defined as the change in volume per unit change in pressure and is determined by the slope of the pressure-volume curve (Fig. 2). A reduction in compliance signifies that the lungs are becoming stiffer and more difficult to ventilate, and reflects the decrease in FRC and the presence of edema, hemorrhage, and pneumonitis commonly seen in patients with acute respiratory failure. As the FRC decreases, more alveoli approach closing volume, producing atelectasis, impaired gas exchange, and further decrease in compliance. The fall in compliance, perhaps coupled with an increase in airway resistance secondary to airway edema and congestion, causes an increase in the work of breathing. The total work of breathing can be approximated by the following equation:

$$W = \frac{(V_T)^2}{2C} + 2R(V_T)^2 \, f \qquad \text{(Eq. 1)}$$

W = Work of breathing
R = Resistance to flow
V_T = Tidal volume
f = Respiratory frequency
C = Compliance

It can be seen that ventilation at small tidal volumes will minimize the work required for ventilation; the shallow, rapid respiration of the patient with acute respiratory failure typifies this pattern of breathing.

The volume of each breath which fails to reach functioning terminal respiratory units is termed wasted ventilation or physiologic dead space. Wasted ventilation may be calculated from a modification of the Bohr equation:

$$V_D = \frac{(Pa_{CO_2} - Pe_{CO_2})}{Pa_{CO_2}} \cdot V_T \qquad \text{(Eq. 2)}$$

V_D = Wasted ventilation (dead space)
Pa_{CO_2} = Partial pressure CO_2 in arterial blood
Pe_{CO_2} = Partial pressure CO_2 in mixed expired gas
V_T = Tidal volume

For bedside measurement a 10-liter Douglas bag may be used to collect the mixed expired gas sample over several breaths; a simultaneous sample of arterial blood should be obtained to permit calculation of the ratio of wasted ventilation, V_D, to tidal volume, V_T (V_D/V_T ratio). The $V_D V_T$ ratio is normally 0.3. An increase in the ratio implies that the efficiency of the lung for CO_2

removal is impaired and an increase in tidal volume will be required if the Pa_{CO_2} is to remain constant. During mechanical ventilation corrections should be made for mechanical dead space and gas volume compressed within the ventilator system (Caldwell and Moya). The most important factors influencing the V_D/V_T ratio are processes which deprive alveoli of perfusion, causing an increase in the ratio of ventilation to perfusion. In moderate respiratory failure the V_D/V_T ratio may assume values of 0.5 to 0.6, and occasionally values up to 0.8 may be present. Changes in the V_D/V_T ratio parallel alterations in compliance, FRC, and x-ray appearance and provide a simple means for evaluating pulmonary function in addition to the measurement of gas exchange.

BLOOD GAS EXCHANGE. The effectiveness of blood gas exchange is assessed by comparison of the gas tension in the arterial blood with that present in the alveoli. The mean alveolar gas tension can be calculated from a modification of the alveolar gas equation:

$$P_{A_{O_2}} = F_{I_{O_2}} (PB - 47) - \frac{Pa_{CO_2}}{RQ} \qquad \text{(Eq. 3)}$$

$P_{A_{O_2}}$ = Mean alveolar oxygen tension (mm Hg)
$F_{I_{O_2}}$ = Fractional concentration of O_2 in inspired gas
PB = Barometric pressure (mm Hg)
47 = Vapor pressure of water (mm Hg, 37° C)
Pa_{CO_2} = Arterial carbon dioxide tension (mm Hg)
RQ = Respiratory quotient (usually assumed to be 0.8)

This equation can be simplified for use at the bedside to:

$$P_{A_{O_2}} = 713 \cdot F_{I_{O_2}} - 1.25 \cdot Pa_{CO_2} \text{ (assume PB = 760 mm Hg)} \quad \text{(Eq. 4)}$$

An example is given for a patient with the following data:

$$F_{I_{O_2}} = 0.40 \; Pa_{O_2} = 150 \text{ mm Hg } Pa_{CO_2} = 35 \text{ mm Hg}$$

The mean alveolar oxygen tension can be calculated as shown:

$$P_{A_{O_2}} = (713)\,(0.40) - (1.25)\,(35) = 241 \text{ mm Hg}$$

The normal difference between the alveolar and arterial oxygen tensions is approximately 10 mm Hg; hence the predicted Pa_{O_2} would be 231 mm Hg. The alveolar-arterial oxygen tension difference ($Aa_{D_{O_2}}$) in this patient is 91 mm Hg and denotes a severe disorder of gas exchange in spite of what, superficially, appears to be an acceptable arterial oxygen tension (150 mm Hg).

The $Aa_{D_{O_2}}$ may be used to evaluate the etiology of arterial hypoxia (Table 2). It is characteristically increased in parenchymal pulmonary disease through one or more of the following mechanisms:

1. Impaired diffusion resulting principally from thickening of the alveolar capillary membrane, a reduction in pulmonary capillary blood volume, or both.

2. Nonuniform distribution of alveolar ventilation and blood flow to the gas exchange units, producing a ventilation-perfusion imbalance. A mismatch in ventilation and perfusion causes the ventilation-perfusion (Va/Q) ratio to deviate from the normal value of 0.8 and results in an abnormally wide $Aa_{D_{O_2}}$.

3. Physiologic or intrapulmonary (right to left) shunt

TABLE 2.   Causes of Arterial Hypoxia (a Reduction in Po_2) and Their Effect on Alveolar-Arterial Po_2 Differences (Aa_{DO_2})

Cause	Effect on Arterial Po_2	Effect on Aa_{DO_2}
Hypoventilation	Decreased	No change
Diffusion abnormality*	No change	No change
Ventilation-perfusion imbalance	Decreased	Increased
Right to left shunt	Decreased	Increased
Reduction in inspired Po_2	Decreased	No change

*Effects of diffusion abnormalities are infrequently encountered at rest and are more likely to be evident during exercise.

of blood past nonventilated alveoli to return mixed venous blood to the left atrium.

Intrapulmonary shunts are believed to be a major cause of arterial hypoxia in acute respiratory failure. The normal or physiologic shunt represents 3 to 5 per cent of the cardiac output and arises from bronchial and mediastinal veins, which anastomose with the pulmonary veins, and from the thebesian veins of the myocardium, which empty directly into the left ventricle. These physiologic shunts are responsible for an Aa_{DO_2} of approximately 8 mm Hg or less in normal subjects breathing room air; an Aa_{DO_2} of 20 to 40 mm Hg is found in normal subjects following exposure to 100 per cent oxygen. The pathologic changes of atelectasis, edema consolidation, and hemorrhage, discussed earlier, are associated with a decrease in FRC and compliance and result in the perfusion of nonventilated respiratory units. Shunting of blood past nonventilated alveoli provides a source of mixed venous blood which dramatically lowers the oxygen tension of normally arterialized blood at the level of the left atrium. This fall in oxygen tension is produced by the addition of blood containing unsaturated hemoglobin to fully oxygenated blood and explains why the arterial blood oxygen tension in patients with large intrapulmonic shunts (Qs/Qt) is refractory to the inhalation of increased oxygen concentrations. The Qs/Qt term represents the degree of venous admixture expressed as per cent of the total cardiac output and can be calculated from the following expression:

$$\frac{Qs}{Qt} = \frac{Cc_{O_2} - Ca_{O_2}}{Cc_{O_2} - Cv_{O_2}} \qquad \text{(Eq. 5)}$$

Where Cc_{O_2} = end-capillary blood oxygen content
Ca_{O_2} = arterial blood oxygen content
Cv_{O_2} = mixed venous blood oxygen content

The pulmonary-capillary oxygen tension cannot be measured but is assumed to be equal to that of the blood if it were allowed to equilibrate at mean alveolar oxygen tension. The value of the capillary oxygen content may be calculated from the following expression:

$$Cc_{O_2} = So_2 \times Hb \times 1.34 + (Pa_{O_2} \cdot 0.0031) \text{(Eq. 6)}$$
Where: Cc_{O_2} = end capillary blood oxygen content (vol per cent)
Hb = hemoglobin concentration (grams per 100 ml)
1.34 = ml oxygen combined with 1 gram hemoglobin

0.0031 = factor used to convert oxygen tension (mm Hg) to oxygen content (ml per 100 ml) in solution
So_2 = per cent saturation of hemoglobin

A similar expression can be applied to calculate the arterial oxygen content. Substitution of the expressions for arterial and end-capillary oxygen contents into Equation 5 gives the following expression in terms of oxygen tensions and is valid under conditions when the hemoglobin is *fully* saturated:

$$\frac{Qs}{Qt} = \frac{(0.0031)(Aa_{DO_2})}{(0.0031)(Aa_{DO_2}) + (Ca_{O_2} - Cv_{O_2})} \qquad \text{(Eq. 7)}$$

By assuming a value for the $(Ca_{O_2} - Cv_{O_2})$ term, this equation can be used to approximate the intrapulmonic shunt when only arterial blood gas data are available. This equation provides justification for using the Aa_{DO_2} as an index to the size of the right to left shunt during ventilation with 100 per cent oxygen. The Aa_{DO_2} is a practical, useful bedside tool for evaluation of a patient's status, but it is important to be aware of factors other than the shunt fraction which may affect the value of the Aa_{DO_2} (Table 3). The theoretical relationship between Qs/Qt, Pa_{O_2}, Pa_{O_2}, and mixed venous oxygen content is shown in Figure 3. At moderate values of Qs/Qt it is apparent (Fig. 3B) that small changes in the mixed venous oxygen content are reflected by large changes in the Pa_{O_2}. Failure to estimate the Aa_{DO_2} in a patient suspected of early acute respiratory failure may delay the initiation of therapy. The arterial Pa_{O_2} on room air may be abnormal, but this does not necessarily indicate that the patient is critically ill. However, if the Pa_{O_2} increases to only 100 mm Hg following ventilation with 100 per cent oxygen (Aa_{DO_2} = 560 mm Hg), then the presence of a large shunt is likely, and the patient should be considered to have acute respiratory failure and to be in the high risk category until proved otherwise. As a rule of thumb an approximation of an Aa_{DO_2} of 15 mm Hg (on 100 per cent oxygen) reflects a right to left shunt of approximately 1 per cent of the cardiac output, *provided that the cardiac output is close to normal.* In the example cited above, the Aa_{DO_2} of 560 mm Hg could be used to estimate the shunt to be 37 per cent. The development of balloon flotation catheters has permitted the safe and convenient sampling of pulmonary arterial blood for determination of the mixed venous oxygen content (Cv_{O_2}) and direct calculation of Qs/Qt (Eq. 5) to eliminate many of the uncertainties inherent in the use of the Aa_{DO_2} for estimation of the shunt fraction. The Cc_{O_2} term is calculated from Equation 6; the arterial and venous oxygen contents can be calculated from knowledge of the per cent saturation, hemoglobin concentration, and oxygen tension of the appropriate blood samples. A sample calculation of Qs/Qt, using the shunt equation (Eq. 5), is given on the following page.

TABLE 3.   Factors Affecting the Aa_{DO_2}

Fi_{O_2}
Impaired pulmonary function
Cardiac output
Oxygen consumption
Position of the oxyhemoglobin dissociation curve
Mixed venous oxygen content

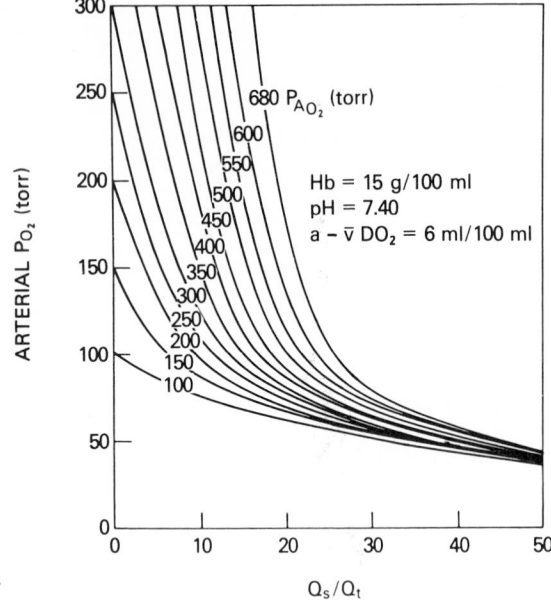

A

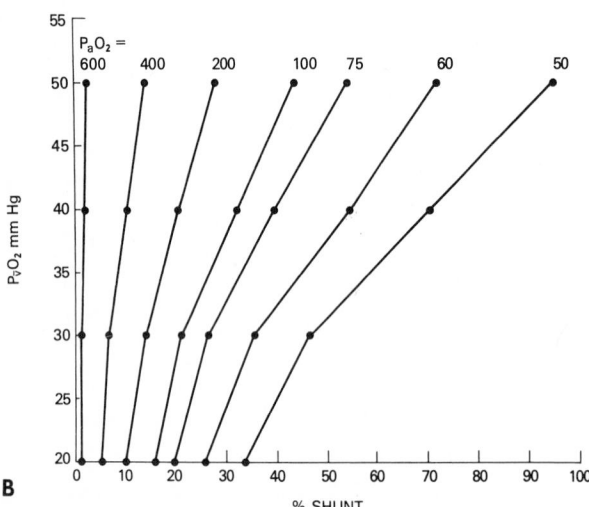

B

Figure 3. *A,* Relationship between arterial oxygen tension (P_{O_2}) and intrapulmonary right to left shunt at various levels of alveolar P_{O_2} ($P_{A_{O_2}}$). The $P_{A_{O_2}}$ varies with the inspired oxygen concentration. Note that the arterial P_{O_2} changes relatively slowly at shunt fractions exceeding 30 per cent. (From Pontoppidon, H., Laver, M. B., and Geffin, B., *In* Welch C. E. [ed.]: Advances in Surgery, Vol. 4. Chicago, Year Book Medical Publishers, 1970.) *B,* Effect of mixed venous oxygen tension ($P_{V_{O_2}}$) on shunt fractions Qs/Qt at constant arterial oxygen tensions ($P_{A_{O_2}}$) during inhalations of 100 per cent oxygen. For a given shunt fraction, the $P_{A_{O_2}}$ becomes dependent upon the mixed venous oxygen tension; this relationship becomes more marked at the higher shunt fractions. (From Moore, F. D., et al.: Post-Traumatic Pulmonary Insufficiency. Philadelphia, W. B. Saunders Company, 1969.)

T $= 38°$ C	pH $= 7.20$	$Sa_{O_2} = 98$ per cent
$Pa_{O_2} = 163$ mm Hg	$FI_{O_2} = 1.0$	$Sv_{O_2} = 35$ per cent
$Pa_{CO_2} = 40$ mm Hg		
$Pv_{O_2} = 25$ mm Hg		
Hb $= 13$ grams per 100 ml		

$P_{A_{O_2}} = (760-47)\ (1.0) - (1.25)\ (40) = 663$ mm Hg
$Ca_{O_2} = (0.98)\ (13.0)\ (1.34) + (163)\ (0.0031) = 17.58$ vol per cent

(Continued at top of next column)

$Cc_{O_2} = (1.0)\ (13.0)\ (1.34) + (663)\ (0.0031) = 19.47$ vol per cent
$Cv_{O_2} = (0.35)\ (13.0)\ (1.34) + 25)\ (0.0031) = 6.17$ vol per cent

$$Qs/Qt = \frac{(19.47 - 17.58)}{(19.47 - 6.17)}$$

$$= 14 \text{ per cent}$$

The patient has only a 14 per cent shunt; the large $Aa_{D_{O_2}}$ measured on 100 per cent oxygen is a consequence of the wide arterial-venous oxygen content difference (11.4 vol per cent), associated with a low cardiac output. In spite of the superficial appearance of a large Qs/Qt based on the $Aa_{D_{O_2}}$, direct calculation of the shunt fraction shows only a modest venous admixture and, in fact, represents the situation in a patient virtually moribund with septic shock and low cardiac output. Therapeutic efforts must be directed toward improvement of the cardiac output and decreasing the arterial-venous oxygen content difference.

HEMODYNAMIC RESPONSES. Myocardial function must be understood if the results of therapeutic interventions in acute respiratory failure are to be properly interpreted. In experienced hands it is relatively uncommon for death to occur because of failure of parenchymal lung function; survival in acute respiratory failure is frequently critically dependent upon myocardial function and pharmacologic support for a compromised circulation.

In the absence of tricuspid disease central venous or right atrial pressure measurements have frequently been used to evaluate ventricular function. Numerous studies have shown that the central venous pressure does not correlate with left ventricular function as determined by direct measurement of left atrial pressure. In view of this evidence, it is disturbing that central venous pressure is still widely used as a monitor of left ventricular function. Furthermore, disparate function of the right and left ventricles in the critically ill patient is now well recognized. This imbalance between right and left ventricular functions requires separate determination of both right and left ventricular filling pressures if myocardial function is to be critically evaluated.

The development of balloon-tipped flotation catheters now permits direct measurement of pulmonary artery and pulmonary capillary wedge pressures. The pulmonary capillary wedge pressure is the pressure value obtained when the tip of a catheter is wedged into a small, distal branch of the pulmonary vascular tree. This maneuver interrupts blood flow, and the value measured under these circumstances is an equilibrium pressure transmitted retrogradely from the left atrium through the pulmonary veins and capillaries to the catheter tip. The wedge pressure may also be obtained through the use of a balloon-tipped flotation catheter; use of this device is described in detail later in this chapter.

The pulmonary capillary wedge pressure is of major importance in the care of patients with acute respiratory failure. It is closely related to the left atrial pressure (± 1 mm Hg), which (in the absence of mitral valve disease) parallels the left ventricular end-diastolic pressure; hence the mean pulmonary capillary wedge pressure is of major importance in the assessment of left ventricular function. In the absence of pulmonary disease the pulmonary artery diastolic pressure is nearly identical to the pulmonary capillary wedge pressure; however, conditions which increase the vascular resis-

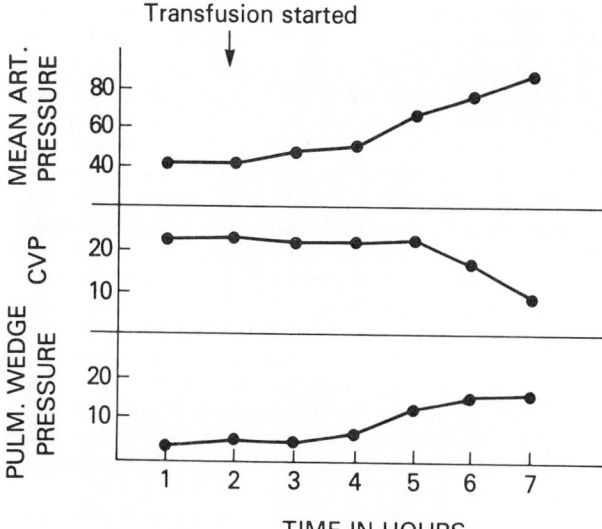

Figure 4. Relationship between CVP and pulmonary capillary wedge pressure (PCWP) in hemorrhagic shock. Prior to transfusion, the patient was severely hypotensive with an elevated CVP and low wedge pressure. Following successful volume replacement, CVP gradually fell to normal range and (PCWP) was increased to an acceptable level.

tance, such as hypoxemia, acidosis, or pulmonary fibrosis, convert the high capacitance pulmonary vascular bed to a low capacitance circuit, causing the diastolic pulmonary artery pressure to increase and exceed the capillary wedge pressure. Under these conditions the pulmonary artery diastolic pressure may be much higher than the capillary wedge pressure, and consequently the wedge pressure becomes a relatively useless guide to filling pressure and left ventricular function. The left atrial pressure is fundamentally related to pulmonary congestion; hence the capillary wedge pressure may be extremely useful in the evaluation of pulmonary congestion and establishing safe limits for volume expansion. Figure 4 illustrates the value of the capillary wedge pressure in patient care.

Measurement of the central venous pressure alone may have prompted therapeutic decisions to withhold the administration of plasma expanders and, perhaps, to administer a diuretic agent. Since the evaluation of ventricular function based on the measurement of filling pressures may be of limited value, it is frequently advisable to assess function of the myocardium through determination of ventricular function curves at the bedside. The effect of a carefully controlled volume challenge on the right atrial and capillary wedge pressures and cardiac output is determined over a 15- to 20-minute interval. If the cardiac output increases with only a small (2 to 3 mm Hg) increase in atrial or wedge pressure, the preload is again increased by rapid infusion of volume to obtain an optimal position on the function curve. The effects of pharmacologic support for the vascular system can be evaluated by the determination of function curves in a similar manner.

The importance of these measurements in the patient with acute respiratory failure cannot be overemphasized. The diagnosis of noncardiogenic pulmonary edema should not be considered unless left ventricular failure can be excluded unequivocally. Precise therapeutic manipulation of the cardiovascular system can

be accomplished only through measuring right and left atrial pressures and cardiac output and observing their response to volume expansion.

TREATMENT. The first problem in the management of acute respiratory failure centers on early recognition of the syndrome. It is important to be aware of the clinical settings which predispose the patient to the development of acute respiratory failure. Patients recovering from severe trauma, hemorrhage, or shock are, of course, at high risk; however, a number of other clinical settings have been recognized to contribute to the development of the syndrome (Table 1). If a trial on 100 per cent oxygen demonstrates the presence of a large Aa_{DO_2}, further studies should be conducted to help formulate the therapeutic plan.

Evaluation of Need for Mechanical Ventilation. The decision to institute mechanical ventilation requires clinical experience and judgment. A serious error frequently results when mechanical ventilation is postponed until the patient is in extremis. Such errors in judgment occasionally occur because of failure to appreciate the difference between the physiology of a patient with acute respiratory failure and that of a patient with decompensation of chronic obstructive bronchopulmonary disease. The patient with acute respiratory failure will be moribund if allowed to reach the stage of decompensation permitted in chronic obstructive bronchopulmonary disease prior to institution of mechanical ventilation. Pontoppidan and coworkers have formulated several useful guidelines in assessment of the need for mechanical ventilation (Table 4). These are only guidelines and should not be viewed as absolute criteria. Many patients who appear well but meet the criteria for mechanical ventilation will only deteriorate further if respiratory support is deferred on the basis of subjective clinical observations. In borderline or questionable situations the serial, frequent determination of the parameters listed in Table 4 will usually resolve the uncertainty.

Airway Control. Once the decision has been made to begin mechanical ventilation, attention must be directed toward airway control and endotracheal intubation. The choice between oral endotracheal or nasotracheal intubation is largely a matter of personal preference and skill of the intubationist, but patient comfort and maintenance of tube position and patency are frequently more satisfactory with nasotracheal tubes. Oral endotracheal intubation is the method of choice in emergency situations. It may frequently be necessary to paralyze the combative or disoriented patient with neuromuscular blocking agents prior to laryngoscopy and intubation when this route is utilized. The use of a fiberoptic bronchoscope as a guide to introduce either the oral endotracheal or nasotracheal

TABLE 4. Indications for Mechanical Ventilation

Pa_{O_2} (mm Hg)	<60 (on mask O_2)
Aa_{DO_2}	>400
($FI_{O_2} = 1.0$)	
Qs/Qt	30–40%
Respiratory rate	>35
Tidal volume (ml/kg)	<4
Vital capacity (ml/kg)	<15

These values suggest that mechanical ventilation should be considered; a downward trend from these values would make mechanical ventilation mandatory in the majority of patients.

tube decreases patient discomfort and increases the speed and safety of the procedure. The tube is passed over the tip of the bronchoscope, which is placed into the trachea under direct visualization. Supplemental oxygen can be administered through the suction channel of the bronchoscope during the procedure. This technique is especially valuable for intubation of the patient with cervical traction or limited neck motion. The recent introduction of low pressure, "floppy," large residual volume, highly compliant cuffs has resulted in the mechanical ventilation of patients for weeks without tracheal damage; however, inappropriate or careless management of even the best, most modern endotracheal tube for only a few hours can result in severe tracheal damage. The risk of cuff-induced tracheal damage is the same with either endotracheal or tracheostomy tubes. The use of endotracheal tubes subjects the patient to the uncommon complication of laryngeal destruction, with the resulting possibility of aphonia. The placement of a tracheostomy tube eliminates this complication and also improves patient comfort during long-term mechanical ventilation. Overinflation of the cuff by only 1 ml can result in unacceptable and dangerous pressures against the wall of the trachea and cause tracheal damage. Some general guidelines for the management of endotracheal tubes should be considered:

1. The minimal leak technique of ventilation should be utilized; the cuff should be inflated to allow an audible air leak at the end of inspiration. Such a leak will not be sufficient to affect the delivery of the desired volume or to interfere with the use of end-expiratory pressure. This technique will decrease the likelihood of cuff overinflation.

2. The volume of air necessary to achieve the minimal leak condition is recorded on a flow sheet for each nursing shift. If the volume of air begins to increase, a careful evaluation of the trachea should be conducted. Increasing cuff diameters may reflect the onset of tracheomalacia as the cuff begins to accommodate to a dilating tracheal wall.

The care of a tracheostomy tube should follow the same guidelines outlined for the endotracheal tube. It is important that the tracheostomy tube be connected to the respirator through a swivel connector and flexible tubing to minimize motion of the tip, which can produce trauma to the tracheal stoma and mucosa. The tracheostomy tube should be changed 72 hours after tracheostomy if the patient's condition is stable. The first postoperative tube change should be performed by a physician experienced in airway management. A tracheostomy tray should be immediately available, and the tube should be removed over a small catheter or guide wire placed into the trachea to facilitate placement of the new tube into position. Accidental extubation prior to maturation of the stoma is a potential emergency; it may be impossible to rapidly replace the tube because of the inability to identify the tracheostomy tract or stoma. If this situation should occur and the tube fails to be repositioned in a single try, the stoma should be sealed with a dressing and the patient ventilated by mask until an endotracheal tube can be positioned from above. Surgical assistance should be immediately obtained.

An uncommon complication of tracheostomy is massive hemorrhage from a tracheal innominate artery fistula, which may occur at any time following surgery. Hemorrhage occurring at the tracheostomy site which is not obviously superficial in origin should prompt immediate surgical consultation. The cuff should be tightly inflated and left in this position until surgical help arrives. If massive hemorrhage occurs following maximal cuff inflation, digital pressure should be applied against the anterior tracheal wall by insertion of a finger through the tracheal stoma. It is the physician's responsibility to see that appropriate equipment and personnel are always at hand for maintenance of airway control. Deaths have occurred because suction devices failed to function or because adapters needed to couple the endotracheal tube to a bag or ventilator could not be located. Such catastrophes reflect directly on the physician assuming responsibility for care of the patient and maintenance of airway control. These details cannot be delegated to the nursing staff, central supply, or other personnel.

Mechanical Ventilation. A description of ventilators suitable for use with the critically ill patient is presented in Ch. 352.2. A general approach to the selection of an optimal ventilation pattern is described below; the details of each pattern will of course vary, depending on the specific clinical condition. The optimal pattern is achieved through the use of large tidal volume ventilation. An initial tidal volume of 15 ml per kilogram should be selected; if the airway pressure at this volume exceeds 50 to 55 cm H_2O, the use of a smaller tidal volume should be considered in order to minimize the possibility of barotrauma (the airway pressure should be measured under no flow conditions). This can be easily achieved on the MA-I ventilator by reading the plateau pressure when the expiratory resistance knob is turned fully clockwise. (On other machines it may be necessary to occlude the expiration line momentarily at peak inspiration.) The use of periodic sighs or hyperinflations is superfluous with the large tidal volume ventilation, because each breath approaches a sigh in volume. A respiratory rate between 10 and 20 breaths per minute is desirable, and most patients will spontaneously assist at these rates as they become accustomed to the large tidal volume pattern. When the tidal volume and rate have been established, the ratio of inspired to expired time (I:E ratio) should be adjusted to provide a value between 1:2 and 1:3. On volume-cycled machines the ratio is adjusted by determining the length of the inspiratory phase with the flow control.

The ventilation pattern is selected and established without regard for the value of the Pa_{CO_2}. The pattern described above may be associated with a minute ventilation of 15 to 20 liters per minute (normal = 6 liters per minute) producing hypocapnia, frequently with Pa_{CO_2} values less than 30 mm Hg. Hypocapnia below 30 mm Hg should be corrected because it is deleterious and may be dangerous; it may cause an important decrease in oxygen delivery by changing the parameters listed in Table 5. Correction of severe hypocapnia can

TABLE 5. Effects of Hypocapnia

Decreased cardiac output
Decreased cerebral blood flow
Decreased seizure threshold
Sensitization of heart to arrhythmia
Hypoxemia secondary to ventilation-perfusion
Perfusion imbalance

frequently produce a substantial increase in the Pa_{O_2}. The Pa_{CO_2} should not be corrected through reductions in either tidal volume or respiratory rate. Normocapnia is best achieved by the addition of carbon dioxide to the inspired line of the ventilator or by the addition of dead space tubing to the breathing circuit. When possible, the ventilator should be operated in the assist mode, which allows the patient to receive a breath in response to a small inspiratory effort to trigger the machine. This mode of ventilation is often more acceptable to the patient, because a breath is delivered with each inspiratory effort. Occasionally the tachypneic, restless patient will trigger the machine at unacceptably high rates of respiration. In these circumstances the frequent use of reassurance and encouragement, coupled with the administration of morphine for relief of pain and diazepam to make the patient more comfortable, will usually result in the production of a more satisfactory respiratory rate. The rate should never be controlled by decreasing the ventilator sensitivity to a point at which the machine fails to respond to a few initial inspiratory efforts, but finally triggers in response to a desperate inspiratory gasp. This technique will undoubtedly decrease the respiratory rate, but it is antithetical to the primary goals of mechanical ventilation, which include the elimination of respiratory distress and a reduction in the work of breathing.

If the respiratory rate cannot be satisfactorily controlled by reassurance, sedation, and adequate oxygenation, it may rarely be necessary to eliminate the respiratory drive through muscular paralysis with a neuromuscular blocking agent such as pancuronium bromide or curare. The former has been especially safe and effective when used in the critically ill patient because of its lack of effect (except for tachycardia) on the cardiovascular system. Paralytic therapy not only represents another level of control from which the patient must be weaned, but also precludes neurologic evaluation of the patient, renders communication with the patient impossible, and totally obliterates the cough reflex with an attendant increase in the risk of infection. These agents greatly increase the danger associated with accidental disconnection of the electrical power and must not be used simply because the patient requires frequent emotional and pharmacologic support to synchronize respiration with the machine. The benefits of paralysis must be carefully weighed against these risks. If the patient is paralyzed, every attempt must be made to limit the duration of such treatment to the briefest possible period.

The syndrome of oxygen toxicity in the critically ill patient is poorly understood and does not develop in a predictable fashion. Prolonged exposure to high concentrations of oxygen can produce oxygen toxicity with pathologic changes similar to those described in acute respiratory failure, i.e., edema, hemorrhage, and hyaline membrane formation. The development of oxygen toxicity is considered to be both time and concentration dependent; oxygen concentrations of less than 40 per cent can be tolerated over long periods of time without apparent risks; concentrations of 60 per cent can certainly be tolerated in many patients for sustained periods of time without apparent damage, but this is generally considered to be an unsafe concentration for long-term ventilation. Attempts to avoid oxygen toxicity at the expense of hypoxemia will almost certainly result in unsatisfactory clinical results.

The patient should be ventilated at the lowest oxygen concentration capable of maintaining an arterial hemoglobin saturation of 90 per cent. If 100 per cent oxygen is required to maintain adequate oxygenation, it should be used until it is safe to reduce the inspired oxygen concentration. Patients ventilated on 100 per cent oxygen for two to three days or longer have survived. It must be remembered that most patients requiring oxygen concentrations greater than 60 per cent will have intrapulmonic shunts, with Qs/Qt exceeding 30 per cent, a range at which the Pa_{O_2} is not a sensitive function of the inspired oxygen concentration (Fig. 3A). Clinically, this means that a reduction in the $F_{I_{O_2}}$ from 1.0 to 0.7 will be associated with only a very small decrease in the Pa_{O_2}. However, a large fall in the Pa_{O_2} will occasionally accompany a modest decrease in the inspired gas concentration, so such trials should be conducted with caution.

Positive End-Expiratory Pressure. During conventional mechanical ventilation the airway pressure is returned to 0 at the end of expiration. If the expiratory limb of the breathing circuit is submerged under a column of water, the end-expiratory pressure will be positive and the magnitude of the pressure will depend upon the length of tubing below the water surface. The same effect has been more conveniently achieved by the design of the expiration valve so that a desired level of end-expiratory pressure can be obtained from a simple adjustment on the control panel. The reduction in lung volume and interstitial edema described in acute respiratory failure combine to produce airway closure during tidal breathing. These changes, collectively, are responsible for the physiologic intrapulmonic shunt and the increased $Aa_{D_{O_2}}$ difference described earlier. The goal of therapy with end-expiratory pressure is to increase the number of alveoli remaining open by raising the pressure at end-expiration above the critical opening pressure. The patient with acute respiratory failure usually has a marked reduction in FRC and may be expected to benefit from the application of end-expiratory pressure because the potential exists to "recruit" these collapsed alveoli. As more alveoli are recruited, the FRC increases and the shunt and $Aa_{D_{O_2}}$ decrease. Patients with a high or normal FRC are unlikely to respond to the application of end-expiratory pressure, because alveolar collapse is unlikely to be significant in the presence of a normal FRC. Excessive amounts of end-expiratory pressure may overdistend normal alveoli, decreasing perfusion to these units as the intra-alveolar pressure increases. This overdistention increases the dead space and may be associated with a rise in the Pa_{CO_2} and a decrease in the Pa_{O_2}; ultimately, overdistention may cause alveolar rupture and pneumothorax.

End-expiratory pressure will, of course, increase the mean airway pressure and may have a profound effect on the cardiac output because of the impedance to venous return reflected by changes in ventricular filling pressures. The importance of the increased airway pressure in producing changes in the circulation depends principally on the extent to which it is transmitted through the lung parenchyma to the pleural space. In the severely diseased noncompliant lung of acute respiratory failure the airway pressure may not be transmitted to the pleural space and, consequently, may have little effect on the filling pressures and cardiac output. In the more common situation in which airway pressure is transmitted to the pleural space, the pleural pressure will rise (become less negative) during inspiration, and the measured atrial and wedge pres-

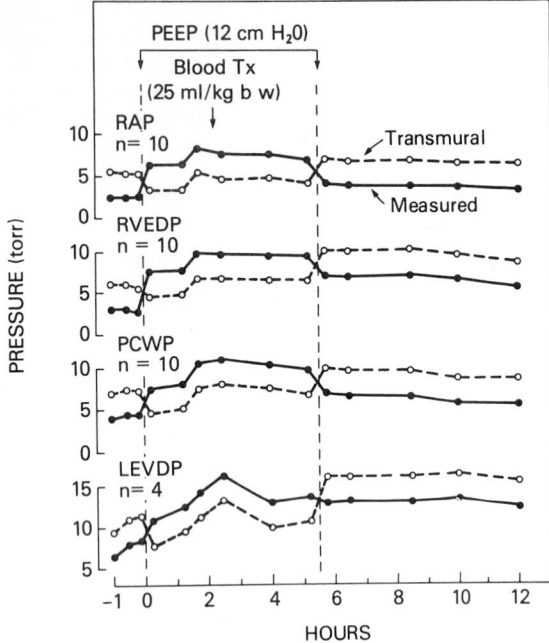

Figure 5. Pattern of response of right atrial pressure (RAP), right ventricular end-diastolic pressure (RVEDP), pulmonary capillary wedge pressure (PCWP), and left ventricular end-diastolic pressure (LVEDP) during 12 hours of positive end-expiratory pressure (PEEP). Note that the measured pressure (relative to the atmosphere) rose while the transmural pressures (measured pressure − pleural pressure) actually fell with application of PEEP. This pattern was reversed when PEEP was removed. (From Quist, J., et al.: Anesthesiology, 42:45, 1975.)

sures will increase secondary to the changes in pleural pressure. These pleural pressure changes will cause the measured values of the pulmonary artery, central venous, and capillary wedge pressures to increase as the end-expiratory pressure is increased. The measured pressure values, however, are determined with respect to atmospheric pressure and are not the correct values to be used in assessment of cardiovascular performance. The pressure across the vessel wall is the transmural pressure:

$$\text{Transmural pressure} = \text{measured pressure} - \text{pleural pressure}$$

The relationship between measured and transmural atrial pressure is shown in Figure 5. The transmural filling pressure actually decreases while the measured pressure increases following the application of end-expiratory pressure. Volume augmentation increases the ventricular preload and returns the transmural filling pressure and cardiac output to normal. Ventricular function curves have shown that these changes in cardiac output can be related solely to changes in filling pressure and not to changes in myocardial contractility. The sudden increase in venous return which occurs when end-expiratory pressure is suddenly discontinued may result in the appearance of pulmonary congestion. This paradoxical deterioration in cardiovascular function is most likely to occur in patients with underlying myocardial disease and physiologically may be considered analogous to the results of rapid volume expansion in the patient with pre-existing congestive heart failure. The appropriate use of end-expiratory pressure requires considerable thought. An increase in the

Pa_{O_2} may be negated by the decrease in cardiac output associated with the inappropriate use of end-expiratory pressure. The application of end-expiratory pressure solely to maximize the arterial oxygen tension is a potentially lethal maneuver; the cardiac output may be decreased by as much as 30 per cent with very little change in blood pressure. The enthusiasm associated with a dramatic initial increase in the Pa_{O_2} will subsequently be replaced by disappointment and frustration as the patient develops metabolic acidosis and hypotension and deteriorates in iatrogenic shock. Because pleural pressures are not routinely measured at the bedside and pulmonary capillary wedge pressures are probably unreliable at values of end-expiratory pressure exceeding 10 cm H_2O, it is advisable to examine other ways to assess the response of the cardiovascular system to the application of end-expiratory pressure. The mixed venous oxygen content and the arterial-venous oxygen content difference may be used along with cardiac output to measure the responses of the vascular system to the application of end-expiratory pressure. Careful examination of all parameters of cardiovascular function will usually provide sufficient data to resolve any doubts about the vascular response to end-expiratory pressure. If the response to volume augmentation is equivocal or uncertain, the fluid administration should be continued only with extreme caution. The administration of an inotropic agent will frequently provide sufficient hemodynamic support to permit the use of end-expiratory pressure under conditions in which its use would otherwise be impossible because of ventricular failure.

Suter and coworkers have shown that the end-expiratory pressure value associated with maximal oxygen transport (defined as cardiac output × the arterial oxygen content) is associated with maximal values of effective compliance as estimated from the tidal volume and plateau pressure registered by the airway pressure dial on the ventilator. The end-expiratory pressure corresponding to the maximal effective compliance has been termed the "best PEEP" value, because increases in the Pa_{O_2} obtained at end-expiratory pressures exceeding this value were negated by decreases in oxygen transport. It should be noted that the "best PEEP" values were determined in normovolemic patients who did not require changes in volume status during therapy. As a general rule the end-expiratory pressure should be increased by a maximum of 5 cm H_2O every 30 to 40 minutes. The response of the Pa_{O_2} is time dependent and may not reach the maximal value until 30 to 40 minutes after application of the end-expiratory pressure; when it is discontinued, the Pa_{O_2} may return to baseline values within three to five minutes. Concern is frequently expressed about the use of positive end-expiratory pressure during ventilation in the assist mode, because the inspiratory efforts may cause the airway pressure gauge to deflect in a negative direction, indicating that such efforts have caused a reduction of the positive end-expiratory pressure. The gradient of pressure across the lung (airway pressure to pleural pressure) will not be changed by the inspiratory efforts, and the effectiveness of the end-expiratory pressure is not lost under these conditions. The effectiveness of positive end-expiratory pressure depends upon this pressure gradient and not upon the absolute value of pressure indicated by the airway pressure gauge. Most important, there is no reason to sedate or paralyze the patient receiving end-expiratory pressure simply to eliminate the effects of respiratory efforts.

Use of the Swan-Ganz Catheter. Precise measurements of cardiac output, pulmonary capillary wedge pressure, and right atrial pressure are required to evaluate the nature and severity of pulmonary congestion and to direct therapeutic manipulations. These data also permit the need for hemodynamic support with inotropic agents to be assessed objectively. The development of the balloon-tipped flow-directed catheter has greatly facilitated bedside measurement of these parameters. A particularly useful version of the flow-directed catheter is a triple lumen device, which also contains a small thermistor for thermal dilution cardiac output determinations (see Ch. 352.2). One lumen is used to inflate the balloon with air or CO_2 (not saline or water). When the balloon is inflated to the volume denoted on the body of the catheter, it is carried by the blood flow through the right atrium and right ventricle into the pulmonary artery. A second lumen opens at the tip of the catheter and is used for recording pressures and for withdrawing pulmonary arterial blood samples for determining mixed venous oxygen content. A third lumen is positioned to open into the right atrium when the tip of the catheter is placed within the pulmonary artery. This permits the simultaneous determination of atrial and pulmonary capillary wedge pressure. A thermistor is located approximately 4 cm from the catheter tip and senses the temperature of the pulmonary artery blood to permit determination of the cardiac output, as described previously.

Catheterization of the pulmonary artery can be conducted at bedside with only pressure and electrocardiographic monitoring. A portable image intensifier (see Ch. 352.2) can greatly facilitate placement of the catheter but is not usually necessary. The catheter can be inserted percutaneously or through a small cutdown site at the antecubital fossa. Following insertion, the catheter is advanced into the thorax, denoted by the superimposition of respiratory variations upon the pressure tracing. The balloon is inflated and the catheter is rapidly advanced under continuous pressure monitoring (Fig. 6). The catheter is advanced until the wedge tracing is obtained. The balloon is deflated, and the pulmonary artery pressure waveform should immediately reappear. The validity of the wedge pressure tracing should be confirmed by the following points:

1. Balloon inflation should change the contour of the pulmonary artery pressure, and deflation of the balloon should cause immediate reappearance of the pulmonary artery waveform.

2. The wedge pressure should be less than or equal to the diastolic pulmonary artery pressure.

3. The trace should vary with respiration.

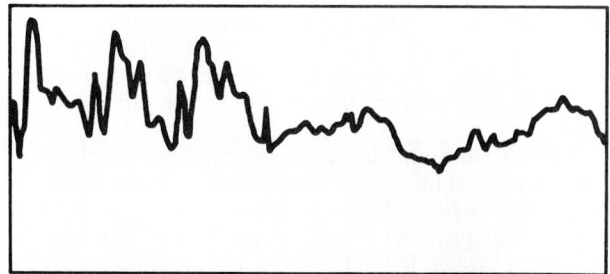

Figure 6. The change in pulmonary artery pressure to pulmonary capillary wedge pressure occurs when the balloon is inflated and the pulmonary artery is occluded proximal to the catheter tip.

4. A pressure trace which drifts up or down following balloon inflation is unsatisfactory.

5. The catheter tip is in the appropriate position if arterialized blood can be drawn through the distal lumen while the balloon is inflated.

The tip of the catheter should be positioned in a major branch of the pulmonary artery. After passage of the catheter into a wedge position, it is important to allow the catheter to assume a position independent of balloon inflation. The balloon should be reinflated to the volume at which the pulmonary artery trace changes to that of the wedge pattern. If this volume is significantly less than the balloon capacity, the catheter position should be readjusted so that balloon volumes approaching the capacity of the balloon are required to produce the wedge pressure trace.

The catheter frequently tends to migrate distally after insertion, causing the production of a continuous wedge pressure pattern with the balloon deflated. The pressure must be continually monitored so that the catheter may be repositioned immediately if such a fixed wedge tracing appears. Pulmonary infarction can result from such catheter migration. A digital display of the arterial pressure does not allow changes in the pressure waveform to be easily detected and, by itself, is not an adequate monitoring system for a Swan-Ganz catheter. The use of the Swan-Ganz catheter is not associated with a high risk to the patient; however, the complications of pulmonary infarction, pulmonary artery rupture, and air embolism are real, and the guidelines described above (Swan-Ganz) should be carefully followed if the values are to be reliable and disasters are to be avoided. Blood for the determination of mixed venous oxygen content can be aspirated from the distal lumen of the catheter with the balloon deflated. If the catheter is positioned as described above, the sample obtained should be representative of the mixed venous blood, provided that the withdrawal rate is 3 ml per minute or less. Large errors may occur if the blood is withdrawn rapidly or if the catheter is positioned peripherally within the pulmonary artery. These errors result from contamination of the mixed venous pulmonary blood with arterialized blood drawn from the pulmonary capillaries and veins.

General Considerations in the Treatment of Acute Respiratory Failure. Every attempt should be made to diagnose and treat the syndrome of acute respiratory failure as soon as possible after the onset of symptoms. Tachypnea, hypocapnia, and hypoxemia associated with intrapulmonary shunts have been discussed as early warning signs. Treatment must be initiated before the patient has developed obvious signs of respiratory distress.

Initial therapy should consist of administration of methylprednisolone sodium succinate (30 mg per kilogram intravenously every six hours for 48 hours). Corticosteroid therapy should be started as soon as the diagnosis of acute respiratory failure is entertained; following the appearance of overt respiratory failure, it is fruitless. The action of corticosteroids in this syndrome will undoubtedly depend upon the etiology and precise physiologic profile at the time therapy is started. There is impressive experimental evidence and suggestive clinical evidence for the efficacy of methylprednisolone in the prevention of the progressive pathologic features of pulmonary insufficiency. Pharmacologic doses of methylprednisolone have been reported to reduce the mortality from acute respiratory failure following shock and hypotension; however, there are no convincing clinical data to justify the use of corticosteroids in this syndrome. Wilson and colleagues have shown that the microcirculatory changes seen in the dog lung during shock can be almost totally prevented by the prior administration of corticosteroids. There are ample data to support the safety of pharmacologic doses of corticosteroids administered over a 48- to 72-hour period. Hyperglycemia is the only systemic side effect likely to be seen following the use of corticosteroids as outlined above. The fact that corticosteroids may alter the progression of respiratory failure while subjecting the patient to only a minimal risk suggests that their use may be prudent in a disorder associated with such a high mortality rate.

Intensive nursing care in the early phases of respiratory failure may do much to obviate the eventual need for mechanical ventilation. Frequent coughing and deep breathing should be coupled with position changes every 30 minutes without fail. Oxygen should be administered by mask to maintain an arterial hemoglobin saturation of 90 per cent. Ultrasonic nebulization may also be used to deliver medications to the airway and to augment humidification of the tracheobronchial tree. The incentive spirometer may be particularly useful for encouraging the cooperative patient to take deep breaths; the routine use of intermittent positive pressure breathing will probably be of little value unless carefully and expertly administered. The routine of mucolytic agents should be avoided; good nursing care and humidification should obviate the use of these agents, which may cause bronchoconstriction and bronchial irritation. Abdominal distention should be relieved and restlessness eased with gentle sedation. The use of salicylates to reduce fever may decrease the over-all energy expenditure of the patient. The over-all goals of therapy at this stage should be to obtain a well oxygenated, relaxed, comfortable patient and to encourage postural drainage, deep breathing, coughing, and frequent position changes.

Fluid Balance. The roentgenographic features of acute respiratory failure are frequently indistinguishable from those of acute pulmonary edema. Any questions regarding the presence or absence of congestive heart failure must be resolved, and it will frequently be necessary to measure vascular pressures to decide this question. Volume overload may cause profound hypoxemia and greatly prolong the course of the disease because of the inability to mobilize the extravascular lung water in this syndrome. Diuretic therapy and dehydration may be ineffective, perhaps because of changes in capillary permeability coupled with damage to the pulmonary lymphatics. As a first step the vascular volume should be adjusted to be as close to normal as possible; baseline values establishing the state of fluid and electrolyte balance should be collected. Perhaps because of the resemblance of the syndrome of acute respiratory failure to pulmonary edema, attempts are frequently initiated to dehydrate the patient by fluid restriction and diuretic therapy. Such therapy is potentially very dangerous; rapid diuresis can lead to reductions in cardiac output, with subsequent reductions in tissue perfusion leading to renal failure. There is no direct evidence that reduction of venous pressure improves pulmonary function; however, excessive lung water is present in acute respiratory failure, and it is probably desirable to initiate a carefully controlled, gradual reduction in the vascular volume. This reduction in volume should not

proceed unless it is unequivocally demonstrated that tissue perfusion is not compromised by this maneuver. A urine output of 1 ml per kilogram per hour will usually be sufficient to reflect adequate renal perfusion. The administration of furosemide (20 mg intravenously) once or twice daily will prevent the gradual accumulation of fluid frequently associated with mechanical ventilation. Failure to maintain adequate urine flow or to administer small amounts of a diuretic agent will almost invariably lead to the gradual accumulation of excess fluid. A critically ill patient receiving conventional intravenous fluid therapy can be expected to lose 0.5 kg per day; a stable body weight indicates that the patient is retaining fluid.

Patients receiving high levels of positive end-expiratory pressure may retain large quantities of fluid manifested as daily weight gain, but still require administration of fluid to maintain hemodynamic stability. Decisions regarding volume status should integrate all the clinical data, including input, output, osmolality, weight, and electrolyte concentrations. If uncertainty remains or if the patient fails to improve, the collection of hemodynamic data becomes essential. Pulmonary capillary wedge pressures greater than 16 mm Hg may contribute to pulmonary congestion, and, in general, myocardial performance should be optimized without exceeding this value of filling pressure. The use of colloids to increase the plasma oncotic pressure and assist in the mobilization of fluid from the interstitial space is controversial. Colloid may pass through the damaged capillary endothelium into the interstitial space and there act to potentiate interstitial edema. The administration of albumin should probably be limited to those patients with frank hypoalbuminemia (<2.0 grams per 100 ml). Hyperalimentation should be considered in all patients likely to require long-term mechanical ventilation. Parenteral hyperalimentation can be safely instituted as soon as hemodynamic stability has been achieved.

Hemodynamic Support. Signs of hemodynamic instability or deterioration are particularly ominous in the patient with acute respiratory failure. Deterioration of cardiopulmonary function is more frequently the immediate cause of death than failure to achieve adequate gas exchange. The use of inotropic agents should be considered for patients requiring high filling pressures (>16 mm Hg) to maintain an adequate cardiac output. A low cardiac output in the critically ill patient may represent a serious degree of hemodynamic decompensation, because the stress in these patients is virtually always associated with at least a high normal cardiac output in patients with normal cardiovascular responses. Isoproterenol and dopamine are useful inotropic agents; they can be easily titrated to the desired level and rapidly discontinued if necessary. They should not be reserved for the terminal, hypotensive patient, but should be used at the first sign of decreased perfusion to provide hemodynamic stability and to prevent further decompensation. The administration of these agents is discussed in more detail in Ch. 352.4.

Infection Control. Infection is a major cause of death in respiratory failure. The presence of infection may be particularly hard to establish in the critically ill patient with acute respiratory failure. The chest x-ray is frequently difficult or impossible to interpret; a leukocytosis may be present for other reasons or conversely may fail to appear in the seriously ill patient. Most patients have preexisting, intermittent low grade temperature elevations and may not become overtly febrile when infection develops. Cultures from the airway systems are always positive due to colonization of organisms. The physician is frequently presented with a picture of gradual deterioration in gas exchange coupled with slight changes in the chest x-ray. There is no simple answer to the management of this situation, but every attempt should be made to identify the presence of infection and the type of organism responsible prior to committing the patient to antimicrobial therapy. A positive sputum culture is not of itself sufficient indication for the initiation of antimicrobial therapy; however, if bacterial invasion occurs, it will frequently be caused by organisms colonizing the respiratory system. Daily Gram stains and sputum cultures are useful to monitor the changes and nature of the respiratory flora. If the patient fails to show a definite response to antimicrobial therapy, a more aggressive approach to the diagnosis of the problem should be entertained. Open lung biopsy can be performed on patients requiring mechanical ventilation with acceptable risks. Antimicrobial therapy for presumed infections will almost always give unacceptable clinical results if no signs of improvement are seen within 72 hours. This situation frequently leads to superinfection with resistant organisms, and the concern about infection turns into a self-fulfilling prophecy. Reactivation of tuberculosis can and does occur in the catabolic, critically ill patient, and this possibility should be considered in any patient developing a pneumonia on the intensive care unit.

Monitoring the Results of Therapy.   Arterial blood gas tensions are frequently used to follow the progress of a patient with acute respiratory failure; unfortunately, they provide little information about oxygen delivery. There is no satisfactory measurement of oxygen delivery at the tissue level, but the mixed venous oxygen tension (Pv_{O_2}) can provide additional insight into the delivery of oxygen throughout the body and is a valuable guide to the over-all changes in oxygen delivery. A mixed venous $Pv_{O_2} > 40$ mm Hg is normal and reflects good oxygenation, whereas values between 30 and 40 mm Hg reflect modest disturbances in oxygenation. Values of Pv_{O_2} between 20 and 30 mm Hg reflect severe disturbances in oxygen delivery and call for some intervention to improve the situation; values < 20 mm Hg are seldom compatible with life. In sepsis the Pv_{O_2} will occasionally be misleadingly high because of poor oxygen extraction by the peripheral tissues; the interpretation of this (and all) physiologic measurement must be considered in the total clinical context of the patient. Sequential changes are much more important than any single measurement. Metabolic acidosis caused by the accumulation of lactic acid is a late sign of circulatory failure. Any degree of acidosis in the critically ill patient should be assumed to be a consequence of hypoperfusion until proved otherwise. If the acidosis appears to be a consequence of poor oxygen delivery, every attempt should be made to improve the patient's status because of the very poor prognosis associated with metabolic acidosis, regardless of its severity. Cardiac output and arterial venous oxygen content difference can also be used to evaluate the hemodynamic status of the patient. These measurements are particularly valuable when it is necessary to optimize the hemodynamic status through the construction of ventricular function curves. They should also be obtained when changes in pH or mixed venous oxygen tensions suggest a deterioration in oxygen delivery. The delivery of oxygen is a function of the hemoglobin content, the cardiac output, and the level of hemoglobin

saturation. Each factor can be measured separately, and attempts can be made to improve oxygenation through the optimization of each value. In general, patients receiving adequate therapy with less than 40 per cent inspired oxygen concentration and less than 10 cm H_2O end-expiratory pressure will not require hemodynamic monitoring in the absence of other complicating factors. As long as the patient is hemodynamically stable, has normal renal function, and shows no evidence of hypoperfusion, careful sequential monitoring of the conventional clinical parameters will suffice. As treatment progresses, the patient should show a progressive improvement in effective compliance, $Aa_{D_{O_2}}$, and V_D/V_T.

Intermittent Mandatory Ventilation.   A system of mechanical ventilation has been developed which allows the patient to breathe spontaneously (Downs et al.) and still permits a mechanical ventilator to inflate the lungs at a predetermined rate. Figure 7 shows a schematic diagram of such a system (IMV). This technique of ventilation has been used primarily to facilitate weaning of patients from mechanical ventilators following long-term ventilation. It has also been reported to be effective in reducing the impedance to venous return caused by high levels of positive end-expiratory pressure. Used in these circumstances intermittent mandatory ventilation permits the use of levels of end-expiratory pressure which otherwise would be prohibited because of the deleterious effect on cardiac output related to decreased venous return.

352.4.   SHOCK

The definition, classification, and general features of the shock syndrome are discussed in Ch. 356. The purpose of this chapter is to discuss the problems of diagnosis and treatment of this syndrome as frequently encountered in the intensive care unit. Cardiogenic shock is discussed in Ch. 356.

DIAGNOSIS OF SHOCK.   The classic description of shock is well known: cold, clammy skin, restlessness, oliguria, diaphoresis, systolic hypotension (less than 90 mm Hg), and tachycardia associated with a metabolic acidosis. The patient with all or most of these signs would be dangerously, perhaps even irretrievably ill with irreversible

IMV CIRCUIT
(Respirator Off)

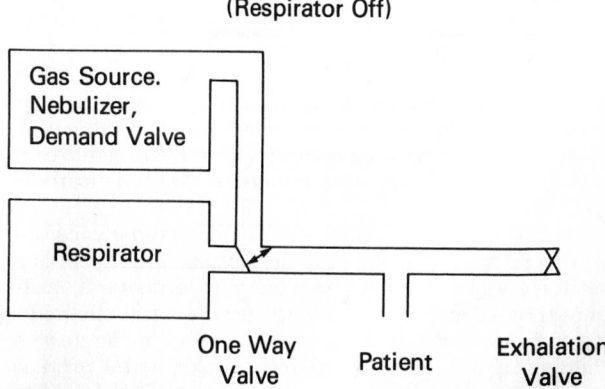

Figure 7.   Schematic diagram of intermittent mandatory ventilation (IMV) circuit. The patient's inspiratory effort opens the one-way valve, which permits delivery of fresh humidified gas. During ventilator-generated mandatory breath the one-way valve is closed.

shock. It should be remembered that hypotension is a relatively late sign in shock and appears only after the initial compensatory mechanisms are no longer able to conserve vascular volume. The diagnosis of frank overt shock should present little or no difficulty; however, the recognition of incipient, early shock presents a more challenging problem. Blood pressure is an important indicator of hemodynamic status but does not necessarily parallel cardiac output or blood flow.

The earliest manifestation of shock, particularly septic shock, is frequently hyperventilation, and the appearance of this sign should prompt immediate attention. Arterial blood gas analysis will show a respiratory alkalosis characterized by a low P_{CO_2}, an elevated pH, and a normal bicarbonate value. Determination of the Aa_{DO_2} following the administration of 100 per cent oxygen at this stage will generally fail to disclose a significant intrapulmonic shunt. If a shunt does exist, the situation is even more urgent. Restlessness, apprehension, and changes in mental status are particularly frequent manifestations of early shock, and their appearance should be assumed to represent an early stage of abnormal perfusion until further investigation can clearly resolve the problem. A cold, clammy skin frequently reflects the presence of increased systemic vascular resistance developed in compensation for a decrease in vascular volume. Inadequate renal perfusion may be indicated by a progressive decline in urine flow coupled with an increase in urine osmolality.

Metabolic acidosis can be considered an early sign of shock only in the sense that it may present prior to the onset of hypotension or oliguria; however, the presence of a metabolic acidosis resulting from abnormal perfusion always signifies a major derangement in the circulatory status and calls for immediate therapy.

ACID-BASE DISTURBANCES IN SHOCK. The metabolic (lactic) acidosis associated with shock is well recognized, but it is less well appreciated that the acid-base disturbances frequently progress as follows: normal → respiratory alkalosis → metabolic acidosis. The major significance of the respiratory alkalosis is to alert the physician to the incipient development of shock or respiratory failure. The recognition of metabolic acidosis is frequently delayed because of the presence of a mixed acid-base disturbance. A pH of 7.50 associated with a P_{CO_2} of 20 mm Hg will usually represent a mixed respiratory alkalosis and metabolic acidosis in spite of a pH value which indicates an alkalemia. This point is important, because an underlying acidosis suggests a serious and potentially catastrophic defect in perfusion. Nothing would be gained by delaying therapy until the development of frank acidemia. Valuable time will be lost if the situation is allowed to progress further, because the acidosis becomes more difficult to correct with the passage of time and will require the administration of very large amounts of sodium bicarbonate.

Lactate acidosis causes deleterious effects on myocardial contractility, cardiac rhythm, and serum electrolytes. Correction of the underlying circulatory or perfusion disturbance is the cornerstone of therapy for the metabolic acidosis of shock. If the acidosis is not corrected by aggressive therapy of the perfusion disturbance or if the pH falls below 7.30, the administration of bicarbonate should be instituted. Maintenance of the arterial pH above 7.30 may avoid the necessity for the rapid administration of large quantities of base. Sodium bicarbonate is the most convenient agent for the correction of acidosis. The amount of bicarbonate to be administered can be approximated from the following relationship: mEq HCO_3 = (base deficit) $\times$ 0.30 body weight (kilograms). The base deficit is approximated by subtraction of the carbon dioxide content from the normal bicarbonate value of 25 mEq per liter. The rapid administration of large quantities of base may cause severe disturbances in fluid and electrolyte balance. One half the calculated amount of bicarbonate should be administered at a rate not to exceed 5 mEq per minute. The remainder should be administered as indicated by pH determinations. In the presence of severe acidosis the volume of distribution of bicarbonate can be assumed to be 100 per cent of body weight. The approach to correction of metabolic (lactic) acidosis is considerably different from that applied in the management of diabetic ketoacidosis, in which treatment with bicarbonate is generally reserved for pH values of 7.1 or lower. The metabolic acidosis associated with shock may progress very rapidly and can be extremely difficult to correct under any conditions. It is prudent to correct the acidosis as early as possible, because lethal acidemia may develop even in the face of heavy bicarbonate therapy. The administration of base for the correction of acidosis substantially changes the serum potassium and ionized calcium levels; the consequences of these changes should be considered when treating metabolic acidosis.

Metabolic alkalosis is frequently encountered in the critically ill patient and is most often a consequence of diuretic administration or nasogastric suction; it may occur rarely as a consequence of poorly understood metabolic responses to shock. The first line of therapy for metabolic alkalosis is, naturally, to discontinue the administration of all alkalinizing agents. Antacids, bicarbonate, and diuretic agents are the most common offenders. Nasogastric suction should be discontinued and the serum potassium concentration maintained within normal limits. The administration of potassium chloride in addition to the measures above is frequently sufficient to correct the alkalosis. In severe alkalosis or in the face of hyperkalemia, the intravenous administration of hydrochloric acid (0.10 M) can safely correct the problem. This reagent should be administered into a central vein and the rate of flow adjusted by careful sequential measurements of the arterial pH.

In summary, acid-base disturbances should be diagnosed by frequent analysis of the appropriate electrolyte and blood gas data. Abnormalities should be corrected slowly after the perfusion and volume deficits have been treated. The correction of acid-base disturbances requires a knowledge of the interrelationship of pH, potassium, calcium, and magnesium levels.

ASSESSMENT OF THE PATIENT IN SHOCK. The patient in shock must be assessed and followed very carefully. Therapy will sometimes be necessary without the comfort of laboratory data and before vascular monitoring catheters can be placed for baseline values. All patients can be followed by observation and by recording the items listed in Table 6. The sequential measurement of these parameters will be sufficient to guide therapy when shock has been diagnosed early and the patient responds rapidly to initial treatment. This will frequently be the case for the younger patient without multisystem failure, but if the patient fails to respond to the initial administration of 1.5 to 2.0 liters of crystalloid for volume replacement or if multisystem failure is present, more sophisticated monitoring and treatment will generally be required.

TABLE 6. Critical Measurements for Patients in Shock

Arterial blood pressure
Pulse rate
Respiratory rate
Arterial pH
Arterial blood gases
Mental status
Urine flow and osmolality
Chest roentgenogram

The blood pressure can frequently be followed by sphygmomanometry, but this procedure may give falsely depressed values in the presence of severe vasoconstriction. In patients without obtainable blood pressures or with mean pressures calculated to be below 60 mm Hg, an arterial catheter should be placed for measurement of intravascular pressure. In the seriously ill or unstable patient the intravascular pressures provide a continually visible indication of vascular stability and allow the nursing personnel to spend time more profitably than by measuring cuff pressures. The radial artery pressure can be conveniently monitored by percutaneous insertion of a 20 gauge arterial cannula. The brachial artery should be avoided if possible because of the lack of collateral circulation around the elbow. In patients with severe vasoconstriction there may be substantial differences between the peripheral arterial pressure and that measured centrally in the aorta. In these circumstances a special catheter can be advanced from the brachial artery to the proximal aorta; alternatively a femoral cannula may be inserted to record pressures from the distal aorta. The use of these sites may be associated with substantial complications, and they should not be used without defined, specific reasons and unless the operator has previous experience in the placement of such devices.

The blood pressure should be monitored and maintained at a level sufficient to produce (1) a urine flow of at least 0.5 ml per kilogram per hour, (2) a normal mental status, and (3) a normal electrocardiogram. A mean systemic pressure of 55 to 60 mm Hg is usually sufficient to achieve these goals. It should be remembered that there is no obligatory relationship between blood flow and blood pressure, and that blood pressure values alone are not acceptable parameters in the management of a patient in shock. Urine flow is frequently correlated with renal blood flow and may also be used to reflect perfusion of other organs; however, urine flow alone may not be a valid reflection of renal function. The urine volume and specific gravity should be recorded systematically every 15 to 30 minutes. The use of simple laboratory tests can be of considerable value in the assessment of oliguria. The measurement of central venous pressure may be of some value as a guide to the replacement of volume in the patient with *simple* shock caused by hypovolemia; however, it is usually much more important to follow the urine flow, blood pressure, mental status, and indicators of peripheral perfusion. As with all clinical measurements, the change or trend of these values is worth more than any single measurement.

Careful chest auscultation is important during the rapid administration of large volumes of fluid. Pulmonary congestion may develop with surprising speed during volume replacement and may be a prelude to acute respiratory failure. The appearance of rales or an increase in the Aa_{DO_2} requires careful assessment of the clinical situation.

The use of the Swan-Ganz flotation catheter has been fully discussed in Ch. 352.3. Changes in the pulmonary capillary wedge pressure should also be interpreted very carefully in response to volume expansion. Extreme caution should be exercised at wedge pressures exceeding 18 mm Hg. The blind use of any physiologic measurement to the exclusion of careful clinical assessment of the patient, including auscultation and recording of urine flow, is a certain invitation to disaster.

Cardiac activity should be monitored to detect trends in the pulse rate and to identify arrhythmias. Tachycardia is the rule in shock; however, bradycardia may present in elderly patients with coronary artery disease and may contribute further to the abnormal perfusion state. Arrhythmias are important both in terms of electrical malfunction of the heart and because they may contribute substantially to deterioration in hemodynamic performance. Careful observation of the arterial blood gases will be rewarded by the detection of metabolic acidosis and deteriorating pulmonary function at a time when they may still be responsive to treatment.

Serum chemical concentrations should be followed frequently; the blood urea nitrogen, glucose, and serum electrolytes may have to be followed twice daily or even more frequently. The serum albumin, calcium, phosphorus, SGOT, LDH, bilirubin, and uric acid values should be followed at least every two to three days unless specific circumstances dictate the necessity for more frequent determinations. It is also important to follow daily determinations of the hemogram, including, during the acute phase of illness, prothrombin and partial thromboplastin times and platelet counts. The examination of each stool for occult blood is important, along with daily examination of the gastric aspirate for occult blood if a nasogastric tube is in place. Wound, tracheal, and urine cultures should be monitored frequently as long as endotracheal tubes and catheters are in position. Collection and analysis of data in a systematic manner will maximize the chance for early therapeutic intervention and recovery of critically ill patients.

FLUID REPLACEMENT. The appropriate replacement fluid for the patient in shock is controversial. Crystalloid solutions contain isotonic sodium chloride as the principal constituent. Colloid solutions contain osmotically active particles as the principal constituent. There is little objective evidence to dictate the selection of one crystalloid preparation over another. Comparison of patients resuscitated with either saline or Ringer's lactate solution showed no difference in survival or in electrolyte or acid-base balance. Comparison of resuscitation programs using blood plus colloid and blood plus saline suggested that the latter is a better combination for the resuscitation of combat casualties. The critically ill patient may sequester large amounts of fluid in areas of trauma or other third spaces such as the peritoneum or intestine. Alterations in cellular membrane potential may result in the movement of fluid from the extracellular to the intracellular space in addition to third space accumulation. The infusion of colloid contributes to expansion of the vascular space, but crystalloid infusion contributes expansion of the entire extracellular space and perhaps results in an improved chance for recovery. Blood is the only replacement fluid which can restore oxygen-carrying capacity; it also contains protein, which contributes to the maintenance of osmotic pressure. The principal disadvantage to the use of blood is its potential to transmit hepatitis; it can also cause serious transfusion reactions and is an expensive replacement fluid. Albumin is occasionally used in resuscitation from shock but principally to restore serum osmolality.

Resuscitation of the patient from shock may begin with the administration of 2 to 3 liters of crystalloid. If this results in hemodynamic stabilization with hematocrit above 30 per cent, the crystalloid administration should be continued at a maintenance level. If the patient is still unstable after the crystalloid administration and the hemoglobin concentration is adequate, at least one third to one half of the administered fluid should be in the form of colloid solution such as plasma or plasmanate. If the hematocrit falls below 30 per cent, the administration of packed red cells should be initiated. Sufficient albumin should be administered to maintain an albumin concentration greater than 2.0 to 2.5 grams per deciliter to maintain the serum colloid osmotic pressure.

The appropriate use of crystalloid has reduced the amount of blood required for the resuscitation of the patient from shock. Blood should not be considered to be the only replacement fluid for the patient in shock but one of the components which may be chosen for the individual patient. The replacement program described above permits the loss of 2 to 3 units of blood before replacement by transfusion is indicated. The use of blood for situations requiring massive blood transfusions is discussed in Ch. 352.6.

THE USE OF VASOACTIVE DRUGS IN SHOCK. Pharmacologic support of the vascular system is frequently required in the treatment of resistant or refractory shock. Replacement of volume deficits is the first priority in all forms of shock; patients failing to respond to volume augmentation have a poor prognosis and will frequently require the addition of a vasoactive drug to support their hemodynamic status. The use of such agents in hypovolemic shock has been popular because of their ability to produce an elevation in systemic blood pressure. The increase in blood pressure is usually produced through an increase in the systemic vascular resistance, which results in decreased tissue perfusion and serves to potentiate the abnormal perfusion pattern. The objective of treatment is to improve blood flow to the tissues, and the use of agents to raise the blood pressure by elevation of systemic resistance through vasoconstriction can be dangerous and should be undertaken only on good indication. For example, the elderly patient with clinical evidence of myocardial, cerebral, or renal ischemia is particularly susceptible to the effects of hypotension and may benefit from the judicious use of agents that increase peripheral vascular resistance to maintain a perfusion pressure to these vital organs.

The general use of specific vasoactive drugs and their combinations are discussed in Ch. 356. The use of dopamine, isoproterenol, and calcium in the critically ill patient deserves special consideration.

Dopamine produces vasodilation of the coronary, cerebral, renal, and mesenteric vascular beds. The administration of 1 to 5 μg per kilogram per minute (low dose) will frequently produce a dramatic increase in urine flow in the oliguric patient and cause little detectable change in cardiac output or blood pressure. The administration of dopamine at this dosage level may have value in the preservation of renal function in the critically ill patient, and its use for this purpose requires further investigation. Improvement in cardiac output and tissue perfusion is generally obtained by increasing the rate of administration to the range of 5 to 20 μg per kilogram per minute. Alpha-adrenergic stimulation begins to occur as the rate of administration is increased beyond this range and the function of the drug becomes similar to that of the conventional alpha agonists.

Isoproterenol is predominantly a beta stimulator. It decreases peripheral resistance as well as renal and coronary resistance to produce an increase in cardiac output and tissue perfusion. Isoproterenol frequently produces tachycardia and myocardial irritability; but if appropriate concentrations are used and the rate of administration is carefully controlled, these complications can be minimized. A concentration of 2.0 mg in 250 ml of diluent will facilitate the safe and convenient administration of this drug. The rate of administration should begin at 0.80 μg per minute and be increased slowly to obtain the desired hemodynamic response.

The use of alpha agonists such as norepinephrine is usually associated with a dramatic improvement in systemic blood pressure, but, unfortunately, the increase in blood pressure is frequently associated with a decrease in cardiac output, manifested by cold, cyanotic extremities and a decreased urine flow. These changes may also be accompanied by substantial increases in central venous and left atrial pressures. The use of alpha agonists alone will seldom contribute to improvement in the hemodynamic status of the patient. Their use when combined with vasodilators is discussed in Ch. 356.

Severe abnormalities in *calcium* metabolism occur in the critically ill patient. The administration of calcium is recommended following the transfusion of every 4 units of blood; however, there is little evidence that decreases in ionized calcium sufficient to cause coagulation abnormalities occur in association with blood transfusion. Patients receiving pharmacologic support of the circulation may undergo a marked depression of the serum ionized calcium levels. This depression of ionized calcium may occur in the absence of transfusions and while the total calcium level is normal. If facilities for the determination of ionized calcium are not available, every patient with persistent hypotension should receive a trial of intravenous calcium chloride. This may result in surprising improvement in cardiac output and tissue perfusion.

Many patients with refractory shock have impairment of myocardial function, but the use of digitalis preparations in patients with variable renal function and labile electrolyte and acid-base disorders can be particularly difficult. The safety, ease of administration, and ability to regulate the minute to minute dosage of agents such as dopamine and isoproterenol have led to the widespread use of these agents in place of digitalis in the unstable, critically ill patient. If digitalis is selected for use, digoxin is the agent of choice because of its relatively short half-life and rapid onset of action.

SEPTIC SHOCK. The terms sepsis and septicemia refer to a number of ill-defined clinical conditions in addition to bacteremia. The shock syndrome in sepsis is presumed to result from the effects of endotoxin. Organisms which are considered normal flora as well as highly virulent bacteria are capable of causing sepsis. Viruses, fungi, protozoa, and rickettsiae have all been implicated as etiologic agents in septic shock.

Gram-negative bacteria are a ready source of infection because of their prevalence in the hospital environment and their contribution to the patient's normal oropharyngeal, gastrointestinal, and dermal flora. The organisms are frequently resistant to all drying and chemical disinfectants; these properties are largely responsible for their role in the transmission of infection by contaminated medical devices.

Underlying host factors not only influence susceptibility of the patient to infection but also determine the likelihood of survival. The severity of the underlying disease is a more important determinant of survival than either the administration of an appropriate antimicrobial agent or the species of bacteria. In one study (Freid and Vosti), the mortality rate in patients with gram-negative bacteremia who were in otherwise good health was 16 per cent. If the underlying disease was anticipated to prove fatal in four to five years, the mortality was 46 per cent; the mortality rate was 90 per cent if the underlying disease was anticipated to prove fatal in less than one year.

Pathophysiology. The pathophysiology of septic shock is poorly understood and largely speculative, but the hemodynamic changes may result from a series of interactions occurring through activation of the complement system, which results in the production of chemotactic factors, histamine and bradykinin. The hemodynamic changes characteristic of gram-negative sepsis are illustrated in Table 7.

Diagnosis. Resuscitation from shock depends upon prompt recognition and treatment of sepsis. The classic description of shock, including tachycardia, cold, clammy skin, weak pulse, and hypotension, is discussed under Diagnosis of Shock, above, and applies in part to septic shock; however, some patients with sepsis present with a different clinical picture. The hallmark of this pattern is arterial vasodilation associated with an increased cardiac index and a hyperdynamic circulation. The blood pressure is usually lower than the patient's baseline pressure but not so low as the values associated with the classic picture of frank shock. The extremities may be warm and pink; occasionally the vasodilation may produce striking erythema. The mental status, electrocardiogram, and urine flow may be normal or may show only slight deterioraton. Hyperventilation is frequently present. In spite of the clinical appearance of apparently excellent perfusion, a metabolic acidosis may document the presence of an abnormal microcirculation. A mild hypoxemia may be present in spite of the hyperventilation. These hemodynamic findings reflect an increased blood flow associated with peripheral vasodilation and arteriovenous shunting. If this hyperdynamic circulatory state progresses or is unresponsive to therapy, the high output state gradually merges into the low output syndrome classically associated with shock.

Treatment. The best treatment of septic shock is prevention, especially because many patients develop this syndrome during hospitalization. Meticulous attention must be directed toward sterile techniques for the management of all catheters and cannulas placed into the patient. The use of prophylactic antimicrobials should be sharply curtailed and proper attention directed to nutritional support of the chronically ill, debilitated patient. These steps, coupled with restraint in the use of immunosuppressive drugs and an effective infectious disease committee, can do much to reduce the incidence of bacteremia and septic shock.

Shock associated with sepsis progresses rapidly. If sepsis is suspected on clinical grounds, a rapid examination of the patient for a source of infection should be conducted. Cultures and Gram stains should be performed on all appropriate specimens; at least three separate blood cultures should be obtained. All indwelling catheters should be removed and cultured; antimicrobials must be started as soon as cultures and smears are obtained. Definitive therapy for sepsis depends upon control of the infection with antimicrobials and surgical debridement and drainage when indicated. The institution of these steps should be considered an emergency and must not be postponed until supportive measures such as monitoring systems, fluid administration, and hemodynamic support can be established.

Surgical therapy, if indicated, should be performed as soon as the patient's condition is stabilized and may be required before the patient responds to therapy. If the infection cannot be controlled, the situation is hopeless and even the best supportive therapy will fail.

Antimicrobial selection and administration will be required before culture and sensitivity data are available. The choice of antimicrobial agent should be based on the most likely etiologic agent and the susceptibility pattern of bacteria applicable for each institution. Occasionally, in the presence of life-threatening infection, particularly in the compromised host, shotgun therapy with broad-spectrum antimicrobials may be appropriate, but the routine use of this practice is to be condemned because of the risk of superinfection with resistant organisms. Treatment of bacteremia with an appropriate antimicrobial will decrease the frequency of shock and subsequent fatal outcome; however, there is no difference in survival rates related to use of bactericidal or bacteriostatic antimicrobial agents.

The basic principles underlying fluid therapy have been discussed under Fluid Replacement, above. Patients with hypodynamic shock will have inadequate filling pressures and will respond to appropriate volume augmentation. If the hemoglobin concentration is adequate, the initial volume replacement should consist of a crystalloid solution. If hemodynamic stability has not been achieved following administration of 1000 to 1500 ml of fluid, a pulmonary artery catheter should be inserted to guide further therapy. The central venous pressure will frequently be high, but the pulmonary capillary wedge pressure will almost always be low (Fig. 4). The failure to initiate adequate volume augmentation is a serious error; however, it is

TABLE 7. Hemodynamic Changes in Sepsis

	Blood Pressure	Pulse	Cardiac Output	AVO$_2$D	Central Venous Pressure	Total Peripheral Resistance
Hypodynamic	↓	↑	↓	↑	↕	↑
Hyperdynamic	N ↓	↑	↑	↓	↕	↓ N

AVO$_2$D = Arterial-venous oxygen content difference.

equally important to avoid fluid overload and its disastrous pulmonary consequences.

The hemoglobin concentration should not be allowed to fall below 13 grams per 100 ml; blood transfusions will frequently be required to maintain the hemoglobin concentration in this range. Therapy for the hyperdynamic pattern of shock is not well established. One approach has been to optimize ventricular function through determination of wedge pressure and cardiac output values. It is important to ensure that these patients do not become volume depleted with resulting sudden deterioration manifested by the appearance of atypical hypodynamic shock. The hyperdynamic pattern of shock is frequently refractory to vasoactive drugs. The general principles underlying the use of these drugs in hypovolemic shock apply equally well to the treatment of septic shock. The administration of pharmacologic doses of steroids should be initiated as soon as sepsis is suspected and continued for 48 hours.

REFRACTORY SHOCK.   Resuscitation from shock can fail for a number of reasons, but failure is frequently related to myocardial, renal, pulmonary, or hepatic insufficiency. Myocardial dysfunction is an important element in refractory shock and may even be seen in young patients with no pre-existing heart disease. Subclinical coronary artery disease and the direct action of endotoxin have been suggested as causes of myocardial depression. A myocardial depressant factor (MDF) has been described in the plasma of animals following many forms of shock. If further studies document the authenticity of this factor, believed to be a small peptide, many episodes of myocardial failure associated with shock may be explained.

Renal failure accompanying shock is associated with a very high mortality. Dialysis does not alter the mortality associated with renal failure in this setting, and every therapeutic effort should be expended to prevent this catastrophic complication in the critically ill patient.

The pulmonary lesion in shock is discussed in detail in Ch. 352.3. Early and appropriate therapy of shock can do much to reduce the mortality associated with this disorder. Disseminated intravascular coagulation may be detected, but is not often a clinically important problem. When pathologic bleeding occurs in association with disseminated intravascular coagulation, the prognosis is extremely poor. The patient in shock with underlying hepatic disease has a particularly grave prognosis, perhaps attesting to the central role of the liver in maintaining metabolic homeostasis. Unless the patient responds rapidly to initial therapy, the mortality has been greater than 90 per cent. Advanced life support systems can maintain such patients for very long time periods but seldom with satisfactory results.

A number of reversible factors can be responsible for the lack of response to appropriate therapy: (1) inadequate or inappropriate fluid therapy; (2) sepsis, unrecognized or refractory to treatment; (3) pulmonary emboli; (4) pneumothorax; (5) occult adrenal insufficiency; or (6) malnutrition. A careful and systematic search for one or more of these factors should be conducted in every patient refractory to therapy for shock.

352.5. RENAL FUNCTION IN THE CRITICALLY ILL PATIENT

Acute renal failure is discussed in Ch. 372. The present discussion is limited to those aspects of renal failure relevant to the critically ill patient. Oliguria is defined as a urine flow less than 400 ml per day for a 70-kg patient and is the most common renal problem encountered in the seriously ill. The volume of urine excreted depends upon (1) the ability of the kidney to concentrate and (2) the solute load. A normal subject is capable of maximal urinary concentration to 1300 to 4000 mOsm per kilogram of water. This solute load will require a urine volume of 1 liter for excretion. A catabolic patient may require excretion of 1200 mOsm of solute per 24 hours; however, the seriously ill patient may be unable to concentrate urine to greater than 600 mOsm per liter. This set of conditions requires a large urine volume for the excretion of increased osmolar loads. The septic, catabolic patient may, in fact, be oliguric, with urine flows approaching 800 ml per day. A *minimal* output of 0.5 ml per kilogram per hour will usually provide a sufficient margin of safety to permit excretion of the increased solute loads in the presence of a decreased concentrating ability without the appearance of azotemia; however, urine flows of 0.8 to 1.0 ml per kilogram per hour provide a more acceptable margin of safety. Oliguria may be present if the hourly urine flow decreases below this level.

Oliguria is associated with a high incidence of renal failure. The need for immediate therapy requires oliguria to be characterized as prerenal, renal, or postrenal in origin. A rapid, thorough search must define the cause of oliguria in each case. Prerenal azotemia is caused by a decreased renal blood flow which is insufficient to cause intrinsic renal damage. Peripheral vasodilation, myocardial failure, and hypovolemia are all causes of prerenal oliguria. The kidney responds to minimize volume loss through secretion of aldosterone, antidiuretic hormone, and increased proximal tubular reabsorption of sodium. The increased reabsorption of sodium and water results in the production of urine characterized by a high solute concentration. The urine volume is decreased, whereas the concentration of sodium is low (<20 mEq per liter) and the potassium concentration is high. Tubular concentrating mechanisms function effectively in prerenal oliguria; the urine to plasma osmolality ratio is greater than 2:1, and the urine to plasma creatinine ratio is usually greater than 50. The use of the simple laboratory measurements in assessing the cause of oliguria is more fully discussed in Ch. 372. Postrenal failure must be considered if the patient remains oliguric following bladder drainage. Considerable judgment must be used in assessment of a patient for postrenal failure. Diagnostic aids include KUB films, intravenous pyelography, and retrograde pyelography. The hazard of infection associated with urinary tract instrumentation is real, and these procedures should be undertaken only in patients with specific indications pointing to bilateral ureteral obstruction.

If renal and postrenal uropathy are eliminated as causes of oliguria, the adequacy of vascular volume must be established. Oxygen delivery should be optimized through appropriate attention to cardiac output and hemoglobin concentration. If optimization of perfusion fails to produce an adequate urine flow, a trial of diuretics should be administered. The administration of large initial doses of furosemide to the hemodynamically unstable patient can produce severe hypotension unrelated to the diuretic effect of the drug. Large doses of loop diuretics are unlikely to alter the course of renal failure, and their use for this purpose is controversial; however, the administration of diuretics may convert oliguric renal failure to nonoliguric failure, which greatly simplifies the convenience and ease of patient management. The initial dose of furosemide should be 20 to 40 mg given intravenously, and this may be doubled every hour until a maximum single dose of 500 to 600 mg or a maximum cumulative dose of 1 gram in 24 hours has been administered. Dialysis should be instituted as soon as the diagnosis of acute renal failure is established. The patient should not be allowed to become uremic; frequent dialysis will also facilitate the administration of a high caloric intake. The hemodynamically unstable patient usually tolerates peritoneal dialysis well.

The preceding discussion has emphasized the importance of oliguria in assessment of the renal status. It is equally important to realize that a normal or high urine flow does not guarantee that renal function is normal. It may be used as an indicator of change in renal function, but other parameters such as BUN and creatinine should be used to monitor the renal status.

Patients with sepsis may have abnormally high urine flows; if these losses are not carefully replaced, oliguria may develop. The erroneous use of diuretics under these circumstances can be particularly hazardous because of the likelihood of volume depletion. The urine sodium concentration can be particularly useful in following such patients.

Polyuric syndromes have been described (1) following resuscitation from shock, (2) associated with sepsis, and (3) accompanying nonoliguric renal failure. The syndrome of acute nonoliguric renal failure is characterized by azotemia and a high urine flow. The urine sodium is less than 20 mEq per liter, and isosthenuria is usually present. Hyperkalemia is found less frequently than in the oliguric form of renal failure. The management of nonoliguric renal failure may be simplified because fluid restriction is not required, but the condition is by no means benign. The mortality is only slightly less than that reported for oliguric renal failure.

352.6. MASSIVE BLOOD TRANSFUSIONS

The principles underlying blood replacement are discussed in Ch. 352.4; however, special problems are encountered in massive blood transfusions. Massive blood loss requires replacement by typed, cross-matched blood. Blood should be transfused within 60 minutes of its removal from the blood bank unless proper storage facilities are available at the bedside. Patients requiring multiple blood transfusions over several days should have their serum tested for compatibility each day, because antibodies may develop to the transfused blood and react with future transfusions. Type-specific, cross-matched blood is always the first choice for replacement therapy, but under emergency circumstances blood may have to be administered under less than ideal conditions. The second choice is partially cross-matched, type-specific blood. Such blood should be available after a 15- to 20-minute delay; this blood is provided after the conventional cross-match procedure has been performed but before the Coombs test is completed. Type-specific ABO and Rh (D) noncross-matched blood may be administered if a five- to ten-minute delay is acceptable. In truly exsanguinating hemorrhage, type O Rh-negative blood may be administered while a cross-match is performed. Transfused antibodies may accumulate when a nongroup O patient receives type O blood. A substantial risk may be involved in returning

the patient to type-specific blood, and it may be necessary to continue administration of type O blood until this antibody titer decreases. Blood transfusions are frequently administered to improve the recipient's oxygen delivery. The hemoglobin-oxygen dissociation curve is shifted to the left during the first few days of blood storage, and this shift may remain for up to 24 hours following the transfusion of banked blood. Storage of blood in citrate-phosphate-dextrose (CPD) anticoagulant maintains the 2,3-diphosphoglycerate level, which increases the potential of transfused blood to deliver oxygen. Many blood banks are changing from the conventional acid-citrate-dextrose (ACD) solutions for this reason.

COMPLICATIONS OF MASSIVE BLOOD TRANSFUSIONS. The complications from transfusion of more than 5 units of blood are (1) pulmonary insufficiency, (2) leukocyte sensitization, (3) hypothermia, (4) acidosis, (5) hypocalcemia, (6) hyperkalemia, and (7) hemorrhage.

Banked blood stored in either acid-citrate-dextrose or citrate-phosphate-dextrose solution contains significant quantities of debris composed of platelets, leukocytes, and fibrin. This debris has been shown to produce changes in pulmonary hemodynamics; there is a substantial body of experimental evidence to implicate a contributory role for microaggregates of this debris in the pathogenesis of respiratory failure. Ultrafiltration of banked blood with small pore filters will remove the microaggregates. These filters are now commercially available and are capable of removing over 500 mg of microaggregated material per unit of stored blood. Most of these filters are manufactured of woven Dacron and can be used without causing substantial damage to the blood components or decreasing the flow rate. Failure to use these devices for administration of over 3 units of blood may place the patient at increased risk for the development of acute respiratory failure.

Sensitization of the recipient to leukocytes or platelets of the donor has been proposed as a cause of noncardiogenic pulmonary edema. The sudden appearance of pulmonary edema without evidence of circulatory overload following the administration of only 2 to 3 units of blood may be the only presenting sign of this phenomenon. Therapy for this rare syndrome has not been established, but the use of dextran and antihistaminic agents has been suggested.

The rapid administration of banked blood can quickly lower core temperature. A temperature decrease of only 0.5° C can induce shivering, which greatly increases oxygen consumption and cardiac output. These effects may be extremely deleterious in the patient with a marginal hemodynamic status. The incidence of cardiac arrest and ventricular arrhythmias during massive blood transfusion has been decreased by warming the blood prior to or during transfusion. A number of safe, inexpensive heat exchangers or blood warmers are now available and should be used for transfusions of more than 2 units.

The individual acid-base responses to blood transfusion are extremely variable; pH should be monitored during massive transfusion therapy to assess need for bicarbonate administration. The rapid administration of large quantities of ACD blood may contribute to the development of metabolic acidosis, in part because the pH of ACD blood may approach 6.5 following 14 days of storage.

Citrate intoxication may produce circulatory depression secondary to the binding of ionized calcium by citrate; there is little evidence to establish the clinical importance of hypocalcemia said to be associated with blood transfusions.

Hyperkalemia is frequently listed as a major complication of multiple blood transfusion; however, significant hyperkalemia does not frequenlty accompany administration of banked blood to patients with normal renal function. The patient with compromised renal function, hypovolemia, and massive trauma, however, is predisposed to hyperkalemia on other grounds unrelated to blood transfusion. It should be appreciated that the patient with normal renal function and not in frank shock may, in fact, become hypokalemic following massive transfusion and may actually require the administration of potassium to prevent the development of hypokalemia.

A hemorrhagic diathesis, manifested by bleeding from venipuncture sites, hematuria, or petechiae, may be seen following the administration of large amounts of stored blood. This bleeding tendency may be the result of dilutional thrombocytopenia, deficiency of factors V and VIII, or disseminated intravascular coagulation (DIC). Blood storage at 4° C may be capable of altering platelets sufficiently to cause their removal by the reticuloendothelial system soon after infusion. Infusion of ACD blood stored for more than 24 hours can produce dilution of the available platelet pool in patients losing large amounts of blood. This phenomenon is perhaps the most important cause of bleeding tendencies following massive blood transfusion. Factors V and VIII may decrease to values as low as 20 per cent of normal following three weeks of blood storage. This deficiency is rarely the cause of posttransfusion bleeding, but may act to intensify bleeding from other causes. The administration of fresh frozen plasma can correct this deficiency.

352.7. COAGULATION DISORDERS IN THE CRITICALLY ILL PATIENT

The most important coagulation disorders identified in the critically ill patient are those related to activation of the coagulation or fibrinolytic processes following shock or trauma and those related to therapy.

DISSEMINATED INTRAVASCULAR COAGULATION. The most important coagulopathy is termed disseminated intravascular coagulation. This syndrome is characterized by intravascular coagulation occurring within the peripheral vessels. This extensive coagulation process consumes normal clotting factors in the plasma to the point at which normal hemostasis is impossible and uncontrollable hemorrhage begins. Conditions frequently associated with intravascular coagulation are hypotension, shock, sepsis, burns, anaphylactoid reactions, hepatic disease, massive trauma, and cancer. Plasma factors I, II, V, and VIII and platelets are consumed through activation of both the intrinsic and extrinsic clotting systems. Activation proceeds through a final common pathway to the formation of thrombin which cleaves fibrinogen to form a fibrin clot. Thrombin also promotes the conversion of plasminogen to plasmin, which acts on fibrin to form fibrin split products. The hemorrhagic process is perpetuated by the split products which inhibit the action of thrombin on fibrinogen. The clinical manifestations of disseminated intravascular coagulation classically involve the skin. The petechiae, purpura, and hemorrhage at venipuncture sites are common clinical presentations of disseminated intravascular coagulation. Oral cyanosis and gangrene are also manifestations of disseminated intravascular coagulation. The diagnosis of this syndrome must be made from serial coagulation studies which include the partial thromboplastin time and prothrombin time, both of which are prolonged by consumption of clotting factors. The fibrinogen level and platelet count also decrease because of their consumption in the clotting process. The thrombin time is also frequenlty prolonged, but this may result from hypofibrinogenemia or the presence of even minute quantities of heparin. The use of these tests to diagnose disseminated intravascular coagulation and the special problems of their interpretation in the presence of hepatic disease are discussed more fully in Ch. 521.5.

The basic treatment of disseminated intravascular coagulation lies in the correction of the underlying disease process. In life-threatening hemorrhage the appearance of disseminated intravascular coagulation in the critically ill patient is associated with a grave prognosis, perhaps because of its frequent relationship to irreversible shock. In life-threatening hemorrhage a trial of heparin therapy may be initiated in an attempt to control the widespread coagulation process. The use of heparin in this condition is not established and is controversial, but in the face of life-threatening hemorrhage associated with disseminated intravascular coagulation its use can perhaps be justified. In any case, its use can, at best, only provide additional time for correction of the underlying disorder. The course of heparin therapy is best followed by its regulation to prolong the whole blood clotting time between two and three times normal. The partial thromboplastin time cannot be used, because depletion of the clotting factors and the presence of fibrin split products interfere with interpretation of the test. The administration of heparin should begin at 15 units per kilogram per hour. Several days may be required before the effects of heparin become apparent, and it may require even longer before improvement in the thrombocytopenia is noted. Heparin excretion depends both on renal and hepatic function; the dosage may require reduction in the presence of either hepatic or renal compromise. After the intitution of heparin therapy, the replacement of consumed factors may be considered. Fresh frozen plasma may be used to replace factors V and VIII; platelets may be given if necessary, and plasma may be administered if the fibrinogen level fails to respond to appropriate therapy. The role of fibrinolysis in disseminated intravascular coagulation is unclear, but primary fibrinolysis unrelated to disseminated intravascular coagulation is rare. The use of drugs to treat primary fibrinolysis can precipitate thrombotic complications if disseminated intravascular coagulation is present.

THROMBOCYTOPENIA. Thrombocytopenia is probably the most frequently encountered hematologic disorder in the critically ill patient. Its presence probably reflects increased platelet utilization caused by immune antibodies, drugs, or infections. Generalized marrow suppression may occur as a consequence of inanition or drug therapy. As a general rule platelet counts greater than 50,000 per cubic millimeter are not associated with an increased incidence of hemorrhage; however, if large numbers of inadequately functioning platelets are present, substantial hemorrhage may occur even in the presence of adequate numbers of platelets. A number of drugs interfere with platelet function, including aspirin, dipyridamole, phenylbutazone, indomethacin, glyceryl, guaiacolate, chlorpromazine, and diphenhydramine. Platelet dysfunction is also seen as part of the uremic syndrome and may be corrected by dialysis.

VITAMIN K DEPLETION. Factors II, VII, IX, and X are vitamin K dependent clotting factors. The prothrombin time and partial thromboplastin time are both prolonged by deficiencies of these factors. Biliary tract obstruction and malnutrition produce clotting disorders which are corrected by the administration of vitamin K. Unfortunately, malnutrition is still a problem in patients receiving long-term life support. It is hoped that the use of hyperalimentation techniques will reduce the incidence of this cause of clotting disorder. The vitamin K dependent clotting factors may be replaced by either infusion of fresh frozen plasma or a concentrate of factor IX.

Civetta, J. M.: The daily problems in the intensive care unit. Adv. Surg., 8:221, 1974.

Collins, J. A., and Ballinger, W. F.: The treatment of shock. *In* Ballinger, W. F., Rutherford, R. B., and Zuidema, G. D. (eds.): The Management of Trauma. 2nd ed. Philadelphia, W. B. Saunders Company, 1973.

Downs, J. B., Klein, E. F., Desautels, D., et al.: Intermittent mandatory ventilation, a new approach to weaning patients from mechanical ventilators. Chest, 64:331, 1973.

Freid, M. S., and Vosti, K. L.: The importance of underlying disease in patients with gram negative bacteremia. Arch. Intern. Med., 121:418, 1968.

Moore, F. D.: Post-traumatic pulmonary insufficiency. *In* Hardy, J. D. (ed.): Critical Surgical Illness. Philadelphia, W. B. Saunders Company, 1971.

Murray, J. F.: The Normal Lung. The Basis for Diagnosis and Treatment of Pulmonary Disease. Philadelphia, W. B. Saunders Company, 1976.

Pontoppidan, H.: Bedside pulmonary tools and their interpretation. *In* Caldwell, T. B., and Moya, F. (eds.): Advances in Respiratory Care and Physiology. Springfield, Ill., Charles C Thomas, 1973.

Pontoppidan, H., Geffin, B., and Lowenstein, E.: Acute Respiratory Failure in the Adult. Boston, Little, Brown & Company, 1973.

Rutherford, R. B.: The pathophysiology of trauma and shock. *In* Ballinger, W. F., Rutherford, R. B., and Zuidema, G. D. (eds.): The Management of Trauma. 2nd ed. Philadelphia, W. B. Saunders Company, 1973.

Suter, P. M., Fairley, H. B., and Isenberg, M. D.: Optimum end expiratory airway pressure in patients with acute pulmonary failure. N. Engl. J. Med., 292:284, 1975.

Tagge, G. F., Adler, D., Bryan-Brown, C., et al.: Relationship of therapy to prognosis in critically ill patients. Crit. Care Med., 2:61, 1974.

West, J. B.: Ventilation/Blood Flow and Gas Exchange. Oxford, Blackwell, 1970.

Wilson, R. F., Leblane, L. P., and Walt, A. J.: Shock due to trauma. *In* Walt, A. J., and Wilson, R. F. (eds.): Management of Trauma; Pitfalls and Practice. Philadelphia, Lea & Febiger, 1975.

353. CARDIOPULMONARY RESUSCITATION

DEFINITION. Cardiopulmonary arrest is a clinical syndrome characterized by apnea, pulselessness, unconsciousness, and a death-like appearance in a person not otherwise expected to die. Physiologically this syndrome is characterized by a sudden cessation of sufficient oxygen to maintain viability of the heart and brain.

SCOPE OF THE PROBLEM. In this chapter we will discuss the recognition of cardiopulmonary arrest and the application of resuscitation techniques necessary to maintain life until the patient recovers or until advanced life support measures become available. The causes of cardiopulmonary arrest in the hospital are legion. Virtually every diagnostic and therapeutic procedure performed has been complicated by cardiopulmonary arrest, which emphasizes the importance of a knowledge of the hazards and side effects of all medications and procedures administered by the hospital staff. The long-term survival following resuscitation from cardiopulmonary arrest occurring inside the hospital depends upon the environment in which the arrest occurs. Survival rates as high as 70 to 80 per cent have been reported for patients experiencing cardiopulmonary arrest following acute myocardial infarction. By contrast, survival rates of only 10 to 20 per cent have been reported for patients with chronic underlying disease who arrest on hospital wards. The survival of persons who arrest outside the hospital is even less, but is improved when there is widespread training in basic life support techniques, and when mobile coronary care units are available.

The most effective treatment for cardiopulmonary arrest is prevention; the identification of patients with specific risk factors at the time of hospitalization should permit the application of appropriate monitoring and treatment to decrease the over-all incidence of cardiopulmonary arrest. The relationship between etiology, prevention, and treatment of cardiopulmonary arrest can best be appreciated through an understanding of the underlying pathophysiology. Jude has defined four vectors which may interact to cause cardiac arrest: (1) decreased cardiac output, (2) decreased coronary perfusion, (3) decreased myocardial function, and (4) cardiac arrhythmias. These vectors may be considered to be the proximate cause(s) of cardiopulmonary arrest, producing a decreased delivery of oxygen and substrate to the tissues and resulting in cellular hypoxia. Each vector can be associated with anatomic, physiologic, or biochemical situations representing the etiologic factors leading to the arrest. The cardiac arrest circle (Fig. 8) facilitates treatment directed toward each vector and thus provides a logical basis for management of the appropriate pathophysiologic factor.

DEFINITION OF BASIC AND ADVANCED LIFE SUPPORT. The classic mechanistic approach toward cardiopulmonary arrest is a basic life support system designed to maintain the circulation of oxygenated blood to the tissue. This approach facilitates a reflex response by both medical and nonmedical personnel which suffices for all causes of cardiopulmonary arrest. It is a pragmatic approach of proven effectiveness, but it will not lead to an understanding of cause; nor will it direct attention to prevention of recurrence. Basic life support

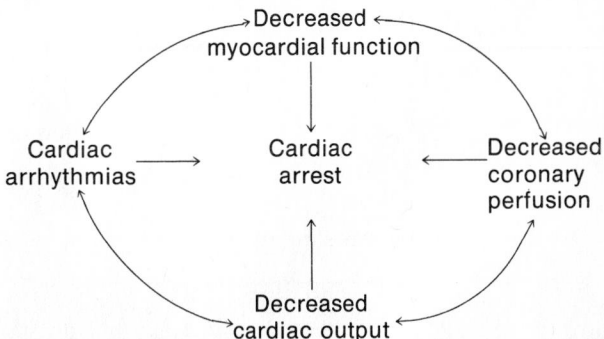

Figure 8. Cardiac arrest circle. The interaction of these four vectors may lead to the loss of effective circulation and cardiac arrest. Identification of factors giving rise to each vector facilitates a systematic approach to the causative factor(s). This permits a plan of treatment to be developed on a logical basis. (Modified from Jude.)

is emergency first aid designed for the management of cardiopulmonary arrest. It includes steps frequently recalled by the mnemonic *ABC*, which stands for *Airway*, *Breathing*, *Circulation*. These measures may be applied by medical or nonmedical personnel and do not require specialized equipment or the administration of drugs. Advanced life support includes monitoring, defibrillation, drug administration, and other therapies and equipment required to stabilize the patient; it requires the presence of highly trained personnel and the supervision of a physician (Fig. 9).

RECOGNITION OF CARDIOPULMONARY ARREST. Patients with unexpected collapse or loss of consciousness should be considered to have sustained cardiopulmonary arrest. Gasping respiration and absence of the cardiac impulse and major arterial pulses are important clinical criteria for recognition of cardiopulmonary arrest. The cessation of respirations may not occur for one to two minutes following circulatory failure, and dilatation of the pupils may take two to three minutes; hence these signs should not be required for the initiation of cardiopulmonary resuscitation. There must be a sense of emergency about initiating the basic life support steps in cardiopulmonary resuscitation. The initial seconds are critical. Chances of survival decrease rapidly with each minute of delay. The differential diagnosis can be considered after the institution of basic life support; the situation usually clarifies itself after beginning of the initial resuscitative efforts. Cardiopulmonary resuscitation should commence as soon as a cardiopulmonary arrest is suspected, and assistance should be summoned. All hospitals should have a well rehearsed plan for bringing personnel and equipment to the bedside in the shortest possible time.

ESTABLISHMENT OF AIRWAY. The first aspect of basic life support is the establishment and maintenance of airway control. The most frequent mistake is failure to open the airway prior to artificial ventilation. The airway is easily opened by placing the patient on his back and tilting his head backward as far as possible (unless there is a neck injury; see below). The rescuer places one hand beneath the patient's neck and the other hand on the forehead in order to tilt the head backward. This procedure (1) extends the neck and (2) moves the tongue from the posterior oropharynx. This decreases the possibility of airway obstruction by the tongue, opens the airway, and may even allow breathing to resume spontaneously. The head should be maintained in this position throughout resuscitation without fail.

If a neck injury is suspected, e.g., following an automobile or diving accident, the neck must not be hyperextended. In this case, the airway should be opened by using a modified jaw thrust, keeping the victim's head in a fixed, neutral position.

ASSISTED BREATHING. If the patient does not begin spontaneous respirations when the airway is opened, artificial ventilation must be started. The methods available for artificial ventilation are as follows: (1) expired air ventilation — mouth to mouth or mouth to nose; (2) bag-valve-mask system; (3) endotracheal intubation; and (4) esophageal obturator airway.

Mouth to Mouth. To perform mouth-to-mouth ventilation the patient's head is maintained in a position of maximal backward tilt while debris is removed from the patient's mouth. The patient's nostrils are closed; the resuscitator takes several deep breaths, makes a tight mouth-to-mouth seal, and exhales slowly into the patient's mouth. He then removes his mouth and allows the patient to exhale passively, while watching the chest fall. This cycle is repeated every five seconds (12 breaths per minute). The adequacy of ventilation can

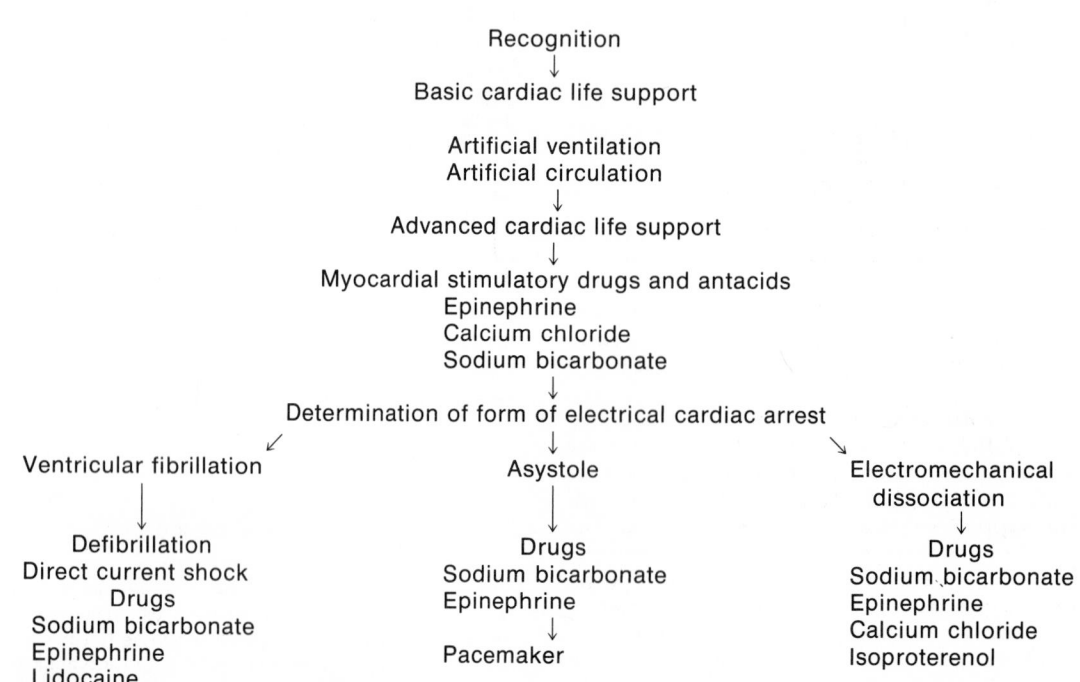

Figure 9. An approach to the management of cardiopulmonary arrest, incorporating elements of basic and advanced life support systems. (Modified from Jude.)

be assured by seeing the chest rise and fall with each breath and feeling the compliance and resistance of the patient's lungs as they expand. If difficulty is encountered in securing a tight seal about the patient's mouth, mouth-to-nose resuscitation can be used; with this technique the patient's lips are sealed by lifting the mandible during ventilation; subsequently it may be necessary to open the mouth slightly during expiration to allow the air to escape.

Bag-Valve-Mask Devices. The principal advantage of the manually operated, self-inflating bag-valve-mask units lies in their ability to deliver supplemental oxygen. With mouth-to-mouth or mouth-to-nose resuscitation the concentration of exhaled oxygen is approximately 18 per cent, which, under ideal conditions, will correspond to an alveolar tension of 80 mm Hg. This may result in marked hypoxemia because of substantial physiologic shunting and ventilation-perfusion imbalance which frequently accompany an arrest. The resuscitator bag devices usually provide tidal volumes less than are delivered by mouth-to-mouth ventilation, and it is very difficult to maintain a leakproof seal between the mask and face while assuring an adequate open airway. Considerable training and practice are required to ventilate a patient successfully with a resuscitator bag assembly; it is frequently more effective for the resuscitator to hold the mask and effect a seal to the patient's face while an assistant squeezes the bag. The resuscitator bag assembly should always be used with supplemental oxygen and should ideally have a reservoir assembly to permit administration of 100 per cent oxygen. Care must be taken to ensure that oxygen flows are not so high as to jam the valve system, rendering the bag useless and giving the impression that the valve malfunctions. Gas flow in the range of 8 to 10 liters per minute should be tolerated by a high quality bag assembly. If supplemental oxygen is not available, mouth-to-mouth resuscitation will provide more effective ventilation than use of the mask-bag-valve resuscitator bag assemblies.

Endotracheal Intubation. Cuffed endotracheal tubes undoubtedly provide ventilation superior to the methods discussed above. Mouth-to-mouth and bag-valve-mask ventilation promote gastric distention, posing the hazard of regurgitation and aspiration of gastric contents into the lungs. With a cuffed endotracheal tube the airway is patent, aspiration is prevented, and delivery of high concentrations of supplemental oxygen is ensured. In spite of these advantages, valuable time should not be wasted in attempts to intubate the patient during the first few minutes of resuscitation. This should be attempted only after the patient has been well oxygenated by mouth-to-mouth or bag-valve-mask ventilation. No more than ten seconds should be allowed for intubation. If the airway cannot be secured within this period of time, the patient should be ventilated with 100 per cent oxygen for a few minutes before the next attempt. Any interruption of ventilation and assisted circulation for longer periods of time will contribute to the irreversibility of the process. It is far better to use mouth-to-mouth resuscitation than to waste time while inexperienced personnel attempt to intubate the patient. If the airway cannot be established, an emergency cricothyroidotomy should be performed. The cricothyroid membrane should be incised and a 6 mm (OD) tube inserted into the tracheal lumen.

There is probably no role for a tracheostomy during cardiopulmonary resuscitation.

Esophageal Obturator Airway. Oxygenation of the lungs by exhaled air methods or by simple airway adjuncts often results in gastric distention, which may interfere with breathing or result in regurgitation. This can be avoided by endotracheal intubation; however, this technique requires special training, is often difficult in emergency situations, may cause delays and interruptions in administration of cardiopulmonary resuscitation, and may have serious complications. The esophageal obturator airway may be a useful alternative to endotracheal intubation. The airway may be introduced more easily and quickly than an endotracheal tube, and direct visualization is not required. Gastric distention and regurgitation are prevented by the soft plastic obturator, which blocks the distal orifice of the tube, and by the inflatable cuff, which completes the total occlusion of the esophagus. Multiple openings in the tube at the level of the pharynx provide adequate air flow in the trachea and ventilation of the lungs. This airway should be used only in patients who are not breathing or who are unconscious. Precautions must be taken to minimize or prevent regurgitation and aspiration of stomach contents during insertion and removal of the tube.

EXTERNAL CARDIAC COMPRESSION. The absence or questionable presence of a pulse is indication for starting artificial circulation by means of external cardiac compression. When cardiopulmonary arrest occurs, the airway must be controlled, artificial ventilation initiated, and external cardiac compression commenced in very rapid succession. The rescuer must (1) establish unresponsiveness of the patient and maintain the airway, (2) quickly ventilate the lungs four times, demonstrating good chest expansion, and (3) while maintaining an open airway, check for presence of the carotid pulse. The following procedure should be used in the application of external cardiac compression:

1. The patient remains supine in bed, or on the floor or ground, but is positioned on a firm surface such as a board or tray placed under the back.

2. Effective cardiac compression requires sufficient pressure to depress the lower sternum from 1½ to 2 inches. The heel of the hand should be palced on the lower portion of the sternum approximately 1 to 1½ inches from the xiphoid process toward the patient's head. The rescuer's fingers should not rest on the patient's ribs during compression, because lateral pressure increases the possibility of rib fractures. The heel of the hand should remain in constant contact with the chest wall during relaxation, but pressure on the sternum should be *completely* released so that it returns to its normal resting position between compressions. The compression should be smooth and regular, with the cycle equally divided between compression and relaxation time.

3. It is always preferable to have two rescuers, because artificial ventilation must be combined with artificial circulation. Under these conditions one rescuer positions himself at the patient's head *to maintain the airway* and to perform rescue breathing, while the other rescuer positions himself at the side of the patient to perform external cardiac compression. With two rescuers the compression rate is 60 per minute. This rate facilitates timing at 1 compression per second and per-

mits optimal coordination of ventilation and circulation by the rapid interposition on one breath after each five chest compressions *without* interruption of the mechanical compression (5:1 ratio). It is important to deliver the breath without a pause in external compression, because any interruption in cardiac compression results in a decrease in blood flow and blood pressure to zero. When there is only one rescuer, the compression rate is increased to 80 per minute, and two *quick* full lung inflations are delivered after each 15 compressions. This procedure produces a 15:2 ratio of compression to ventilation and results in an actual compression rate of 60 per minute. The two breaths must be delivered in rapid succession without allowing full exhalation to occur in order to maintain an adequate number of breaths and compressions per minute.

4. Palpation of the femoral and carotid pulses may be used to assess the effectiveness of circulatory support; however, there is often poor correlation between recorded intra-arterial pressures and the strength of the pulse to palpation.

It must be remembered that even under the best of conditions the cardiac output is less than 50 per cent of normal when external cardiac compression is applied. It is possible to achieve systolic pressures approaching 100 mm Hg (mean arterial pressure of 30 to 50 mm Hg); however, the average pressure obtained during resuscitation is frequently 40 to 60 mm Hg. External cardiac compressions must not be interrupted for longer than five seconds, even for insertion of intravenous lines or monitoring of cardiac rhythm, if a resuscitation is to be successful. Any interruption in cardiac compression results in a drop in blood flow and blood pressure to zero. The use of a stopwatch to time the interruptions of external massage is frequently useful to prevent additional hypoxic damage related to cessation of cardiac compression. Occasionally external cardiac compression will not provide adequate tissue perfusion. Progressive metabolic acidosis results, and the resuscitation is unsuccessful. Certain conditions preclude effective external massage; these include massive obesity and thoracic deformities such as kyphoscoliosis, pectus excavatum, and severe emphysema. In addition, hypovolemia, pneumothorax, and cardiac tamponade may produce poor ventricular filling and result in ineffective resuscitation. These three conditions are easily correctable and should come to mind when resuscitative efforts appear to be unsuccessful. Since the cardiac output during cardiopulmonary resuscitation is so dependent upon ventricular filling, it is frequently efficacious to elevate the legs during external cardiac compression to increase venous return and augment the cardiac output. If external cardiac massage is ineffective, open chest massage should be considered. This procedure is rarely performed outside the operating room and requires trained personnel, adequate equipment, and the presence of a thoracic surgeon. During prolonged resuscitation the efficiency of mechanical external compression decreases because of fatigue; rotation of individuals performing external compression should be considered at least every ten minutes. Mechanical devices are available to perform external cardiac compression, and they may be of great value in cases in which massage must be continued for more than an hour or the patient must be transported in a vehicle. They should not be used ini-

tially because of the time consumed at such a critical stage in the resuscitation.

FAILURE AND COMPLICATIONS. The most common causes for failure in cardiopulmonary resuscitation are excessive delay in initiating the resuscitative efforts, improper management of assisted ventilation and circulation, and extensive myocardial damage. Especially important in contributing to the failure of resuscitation efforts is the detrimental effect of discontinuing cardiac compression during endotracheal tube insertion or placement of intravenous lines.

Complications arising from cardiopulmonary resuscitation do occur and may be potentially lethal. The most frequent are fractures of the rib and sternum, which may be associated with laceration of the liver, esophagus, spleen, or kidney. Hemopericardium and pneumothorax may be related to rib fracture or intracardiac administration of drugs.

If the airway is patent and appropriate ventilation and perfusion are provided through basic cardiopulmonary resuscitation, definitive therapy can be formulated, based on an accurate diagnosis.

VENTRICULAR FIBRILLATION. Ventricular fibrillation is the most common cause of cardiac arrest and is treated by electrical defibrillation with a direct current defibrillator. If a defibrillator is not available and the patient is pulseless, a single thump should be delivered to the immediate mid-sternum–precordial area; if successful, this maneuver may restore the patient's circulation and obviate the need for cardiopulmonary resuscitation. If the single thump is unsuccessful, no harm will have resulted, provided that resuscitation has not been delayed unduly. If a defibrillator is available, the electrode paddles are placed at the cardiac apex and at the base of the heart at the right upper sternal portal. If electrocardiographic monitoring is not immediately available, a single 400 watt-second shock should be delivered prior to cardiopulmonary resuscitation. An unmonitored attempt at defibrillation will not adversely affect the patient with asystole or heart block. If a single countershock is unsuccessful, no further defibrillabion should be attempted until electrocardiographic monitoring is available; basic cardiopulmonary resuscitation must be continued. If ventricular fibrillation or asystole is shown to be present, basic resuscitation should be continued while an intravenous infusion route is established. A peripheral vein should be used if possible; the femoral or jugular veins provide acceptable alternative routes if a peripheral vein cannot be easily cannulated. The insertion of a subclavian intravenous cannula can be extremely difficult in the presence of *uninterrupted* cardiopulmonary resuscitation. Drug therapy with sodium bicarbonate (1 mEq per kilogram administered as a bolus) and epinephrine (0.5 mg, i.e., 5 ml of a 1:10,000 solution) should be initiated after the intravenous route is established. These drugs should not be mixed together, because epinephrine may be inactivated by the alkaline bicarbonate solution. External cardiac compression must be continued following injection to circulate the drugs. The cardiac rhythm may than be reassessed, and, if ventricular fibrillation is still present or rapidly returns after a brief episode of sinus rhythm, further administration of sodium bicarbonate and perhaps lidocaine is indicated. If the ventricular fibrillation presents a fine fibrillatory electrocardiographic pattern, epinephrine (5 ml of 1:10,000 solution) should be administered intravenously to produce a course pattern prior to further attempts at defibrillation. Continued failure to defibrillate the patient demands a reassessment of the perfusion, oxygenation, and pharmacologic management of the patient. Hypoxemia and acidosis are frequently responsible for the presence of ventricular fibrillation refractory to electrical conversion.

If reassessment of the cardiac rhythm shows the return of normal sinus rhythm, a bolus of lidocaine (1 mg per kilogram) should be administered, followed by a continuous infusion of 1 to 4 mg per minute. It may be necessary to repeat the bolus administration at three- to five-minute intervals, but extreme caution should be used in the administration of doses exceeding 300 mg because of the possibility of drug toxicity. Lidocaine toxicity is especially likely to occur in the presence of acute reductions in cardiac output, and this should be kept in mind with respect to individualizing the dosage for each patient.

If normal sinus rhythm returns, the pulse is checked and basic resuscitation discontinued if appropriate. If bradycardia is present *and associated with hypotension,* atropine (0.5 mg) may be administered intravenously and repeated every five minutes up to a total dose of 2.0 mg.

The presence of asystole or electromechanical dissociation (electrical myocardial activity without palpable pulse) indicates the need for further pharmacologic intervention and perhaps the use of a pacemaker.

Epinephrine (5 ml of 1:10,000 solution) given *intravenously* should be administered for the presence of asystole or electromechanical dissociation. This drug should not be administered by intracardiac injection if an intravenous route is present. The hazards of intracardiac administration include interruption of cardiac compression and ventilation, coronary artery laceration, pneumothorax, and intramyocardial injection, which may produce intractable ventricular fibrillation. If there is a delay in establishing the intravenous route, epinephrine may be given by intracardiac injection in the same dose. Calcium chloride (5 ml of a 10 per cent solution) may be especially useful in the presence of electromechanical dissociation and also in the restoration of an electrical rhythm during asystole. Isoproterenol (1 to 20 μg per minute) may be useful in the management of profound cardiovascular collapse associated with asystole or electromechanical dissociation; however, it must be used cautiously because it may result in the production of serious dysrhythmias.

DRUG THERAPY. The most important pharmacologic maneuvers in cardiopulmonary resuscitation are the administration of oxygen to combat hypoxemia and sodium bicarbonate to treat acidosis. All drugs are preferably administered through an intravenous line, followed by one to two minutes of external cardiac compression to ensure circulation of the agent. There is no indication for the intracardiac injection of any pharmacologic agent during cardiopulmonary resuscitation, provided that an intravenous route is present.

Ineffective perfusion and ventilation result in the appearance of metabolic and respiratory acidosis within minutes of the onset of cardiopulmonary arrest. Effective resuscitation critically depends upon the proper maintenance of acid-base balance. After the initial in-

jection of sodium bicarbonate (discussed above), further administration should be titrated on the basis of pH and arterial blood gas measurements determined every five to ten minutes during resuscitation. If laboratory facilities are not available, repeated doses of 1.0 mg per kilogram should be given every ten minutes until spontaneous circulation is restored.

If laboratory facilities are available, the dose of bicarbonate can be approximated as follows:

$$\text{mEq bicarbonate} = \frac{\text{base deficit (mEq per liter)} \times \text{patient weight (kg)}}{4}$$

The base deficit may be approximated as follows:

$$\text{pH change of 0.15} = \text{base change of 10 mEq per liter per liter}$$

The use of these two expressions allows one to approximate the amount of bicarbonate required from pH data alone. The respiratory component of acid-base balance can be assessed by correcting the measured pH appropriately for deviations of the P_{CO_2} from 40 mm Hg. Every 10 mm Hg change in P_{CO_2} is associated with a 0.08 unit change in pH. Using these guidelines, the measured pH can be corrected for the respiratory contribution; the corrected value can then be used to calculate the base deficit, which is then used in conjunction with the patient's weight to estimate the dose of bicarbonate. The full calculated dose of sodium bicarbonate should be administered during cardiopulmonary resuscitation. Correction of the acidemia will improve myocardial contractility and render the heart more sensitive to cardiovascular drugs; however, frank alkalemia is deleterious, because it sensitizes the myocardium to arrhythmias and results in a decreased release of oxygen because of the pH dependency of the oxyhemoglobin dissociation curve.

Vasopressor agents such as norepinephrine and epinephrine are frequently useful after the return of a regular cardiac rhythm to increase the peripheral vascular resistance, elevate central venous pressure, and improve coronary and cerebral blood flow. Their use should be limited to very brief time periods and discontinued as soon as the patient's status can be evaluated and adequate manipulations of the vascular volume and inotropic agents can be instituted to maintain cardiac output and peripheral perfusion. These powerful vasoconstrictor agents should not be needed for longer than a few minutes under most conditions.

PACEMAKERS. Persistent asystole or bradycardia resistant to therapy may require insertion of a pacemaker. Percutaneous insertion of a pacemaker into the left ventricle will usually provide sufficient myocardial contact to permit satisfactory pacing. Insertion of a transvenous pacemaker via the internal jugular vein will also usually provide for satisfactory pacing. Balloon-tipped flotation-directed catheters are difficult to place in emergency situations, because the blood flow is insufficient to provide a guiding force for the catheter. Electrical depolarization of the myocardium will be ineffective in the presence of acidemia and hypoxemia.

POSTARREST TREATMENT. After successful resuscitation, attention must be directed toward maintenance of the appropriate life support systems until the patient's primary disorder can be corrected. The maintenance of life support systems has been discussed in detail in Ch. 352.

Many patients experience recurrent cardiopulmonary arrest within minutes to hours of the initial episode. It is essential to provide continuous monitoring and evaluation of the patient during the first 24 to 48 hours following such an episode.

If central nervous system dysfunction persists following resuscitation, treatment should be administered to minimize adverse effects of the hypoxia-induced cerebral edema. Cerebral edema should be managed by (1) elevation of the head and chest, (2) mild hyperventilation (Pco_2 maintained between 25 and 35 mm Hg), (3) dexamethasone (6 mg every four hours), (4) diuretic administration (mannitol), and (5) mild hypothermia (temperature no lower than 32° C). If clinical absence of central nervous system function persists beyond 72 hours, an electroencephalogram should be obtained for further evaluation.

CONCLUSION. There is need for training in emergency cardiopulmonary resuscitation for all health professionals, especially physicians.

Committee on Emergency Cardiac Care, American Heart Association: Advanced Cardiac Life Support. Dallas, American Heart Association, 1975.

Committee on Emergency Medical Services, National Academy of Sciences, National Research Council: Standards for cardiopulmonary resuscitation and emergency cardiac care. J.A.M.A., 277:837, 1974.

Jude, J. R.: Classification of etiology, prevention and treatment of cardiac arrest. In Safar, P. (ed.): Advances in Cardiopulmonary Resuscitation. New York, Springer-Verlag, 1975.

PART XIV
CARDIOVASCULAR DISEASES

354. INTRODUCTION

354.1. PREVALENCE AND EPIDEMIOLOGY OF CARDIOVASCULAR DISEASE

Robert I. Levy

It is difficult to overemphasize the magnitude of the medical, social, and economic burden of cardiovascular diseases. An estimated 30 million Americans have some form of cardiovascular disease. Each year about 25,000 children are born with congenital heart disease, and of the 6000 of these children who die annually approximately half are less than one year of age. Over 100,000 children and 1.6 million adults have rheumatic heart disease, of whom almost 15,000 die each year. More than 4 million Americans have overt clinical signs of atherosclerosis, primarily of the coronary, cerebral, and peripheral blood vessels. Over 23 million adult Americans (15 per cent of the adult population of the United States) have hypertension as defined by a blood pressure of 160/95 or higher. Furthermore, the latter two major etiologic processes, atherosclerosis and hypertension, are interactive and result in an estimated 1.25 million heart attacks (of which 750,000 are first events) each year — a rate of 3400 per day or two per minute — and 500,000 strokes (of which 400,000 are first events) each year. In 1975, cardiovascular diseases accounted for 994,513 deaths or 52.5 per cent of all deaths in the United States, of which almost 650,000 were due to coronary artery disease (heart attack and sudden death) and 194,000 to cerebrovascular disease (stroke).

The age-adjusted death rate from rheumatic heart disease in the United States declined from 20.5 to 6.3 per 100,000 population between 1940 and 1970 and from 6.3 to 4.8 per 100,000 population between 1970 and 1975 (a 25.4 per cent decline). Although there are few reliable studies of the incidence of rheumatic fever, the data that are available indicate that a significant decrease in both severity and incidence of the disease has occurred in this country since 1940. It has been estimated that approximately 12,000 new cases of rheumatic fever occur at present in subjects between 5 and 14 years of age, based on a mean incidence rate of 11.0 per 100,000 population. Data on the prevalence of rheumatic heart disease are usually based on surveys of school children, with rates ranging between 0.5 and 3.7 per 1000.

The major risk factor for the development of rheumatic fever is the existence of a prior group A beta-hemolytic streptococcal throat infection; from 0.3 to 3.0 per cent of individuals so infected develop the disease. Environmental factors have been identified as signifi-cant additional risk factors, the most important being overcrowded living conditions. Other risk factors include low socioeconomic status, ethnic status, malnutrition, climate, and geography.

The onset of the downward trend in morbidity and mortality preceded the introduction of antibiotics, although the trend declined more precipitously following the introduction of effective treatment of streptococcal infections. Recurrent attacks of the disease have decreased dramatically following the institution of secondary prevention programs, in which effective drug therapy was utilized to prevent streptococcal infections in subjects who had previously experienced an episode of rheumatic fever. The additional impact of altered environmental factors, such as overcrowding, must be significant. Despite this decrease in morbidity and mortality, rheumatic fever and rheumatic heart disease continue to be the leading cause of death from heart disease in subjects between 5 and 24 years of age and second only to coronary heart disease as a reason for adults undergoing cardiovascular surgery.

The prevalence of coronary, cerebrovascular, and hypertensive diseases rises sharply with age. Although 8 per cent of adults under age 45 have hypertension, few have other manifestations of cardiovascular disease. Overt coronary heart disease is present in 6 per cent of males ages 45 to 64 and 11 per cent of males age 65 and over. For females the corresponding rates are 3 per cent and 7 per cent. Cerebrovascular disease, present in 1 per cent of persons ages 45 to 64, is present in 5 per cent age 65 and over. Hypertension is present in 44 per cent of women age 65 and over — compared to 37 per cent for men in that age group. In terms of mortality from these diseases, it is from coronary heart disease that mortality is highest. As in prevalence statistics, death rates rise steeply with age, especially after age 35, and for ages under 65 rates for coronary heart disease in men are more than double the rates in women. Death rates for cerebrovascular and hypertensive disease are large in number only after age 65.

Cardiovascular diseases rank second only to respiratory diseases in terms of days of bed disability. They rank first in terms of limitation of activity, Social Security disability, hospital discharges, and total hospital bed days (48 million per year). In terms of economic costs, cardiovascular diseases also rank first among all medical disorders. The estimated economic cost of cardiovascular diseases to the nation in 1976 totaled over $47 billion. Of this amount, $17 billion was related to the direct costs of illness and over $30 billion was due to indirect costs secondary to lost wages and productivity.

In America in 1900, infectious processes, such as pneumonia, influenza, and tuberculosis, reigned as our major health problems. As these disorders were brought under control, cardiovascular disease (especial-

TABLE 1.   Age-Adjusted Death Rates* for Major Cardiovascular-Renal Diseases and All Other Causes of Death Combined—United States, Decades 1900–1970 and 1975†

		All Causes Except Cardiovascular- Renal Diseases	Cardiovascular-Renal Disease				
Year	All Causes		Total	Heart Disease	Cerebro- vascular	Renal	All Other
1900	1778.5	1356.5	422.0	167.3	134.4	97.0	23.3
1910	1578.8	1101.6	477.2	201.7	126.4	107.0	42.1
1920	1423.6	952.2	471.4	203.6	122.6	105.9	39.3
1930	1246.1	754.9	491.2	252.7	106.5	102.5	29.5
1940	1076.1	590.3	485.8	292.7	91.0	79.0	23.1
1950	841.5	401.4	440.1	307.6	88.8	14.5	29.2
1960	760.9	361.6	399.3	286.2	79.7	5.7	27.7
1970	714.3	364.5	349.8	253.6	66.3	3.5	26.4
1975	638.3	338.4	299.9	220.5	54.5	2.8	22.1

*Rate per 100,000 population, age-adjusted to the United States population, 1940.
†Source: Vital Statistics of the United States, National Center for Health Statistics.

TABLE 2.   Age-Adjusted Death Rates* for Four Subgroups of Cardiovascular Disease—United States, 1940–1975†

Year	Coronary Heart Disease	Hypertensive Disease	Rheumatic Fever and Rheumatic Heart Disease	Congenital Heart Disease
1940	207.2	69.3	20.5	4.8
1945	208.2	59.7	17.1	4.9
1950	226.4	56.0	14.0	4.6
1955	226.0	41.2	11.2	4.3
1960	238.5	29.6	9.7	4.7
1965	237.7	22.4	7.5	4.3
1970‡	228.1	7.9	6.3	3.7
1975‡	196.1	5.1	4.8	3.1

*Rate per 100,000 population; age-adjusted to the United States population, 1940.
†Source: Vital Statistics of the United States, National Center for Health Statistics.
‡Rates since 1968 are not totally comparable with rates for previous years due to the change in the International Classification of Diseases.

TABLE 3.   Recent Mortality from Cardiovascular Diseases—United States, 1970–1976*

		Cardiovascular Diseases					Noncardiovascular Causes of Death
Year	Total	Coronary Heart Disease	Stroke	Hypertension	Rheumatic Heart Disease	Other Cardiovascular Disease†	
		Numbers of Deaths					
1970	1,032,500	666,500	207,000	23,500	15,000	120,500	888,500
1971	1,041,500	674,000	209,000	22,000	14,500	122,000	886,000
1972	1,060,000	684,500	213,500	21,500	14,000	126,500	904,000
1973	1,062,000	684,000	214,000	20,000	13,500	130,000	911,000
1974	1,035,000	665,000	207,500	19,000	13,500	130,000	899,000
1975	994,500§	642,500	194,000	17,500	13,000	127,500	898,500
1976‡	996,500	647,000	188,500	16,500	13,000	131,500	907,500
		Death Rate Per 100,000 Population (age-adjusted)¶					
1970	350.0	228.1	66.3	7.9	6.3	41.4	364.3
1971	344.4	225.1	65.2	7.2	6.0	40.9	355.5
1972	343.7	223.9	65.0	6.8	5.7	42.3	358.1
1973	336.6	218.9	63.7	6.3	5.4	42.3	356.3
1974	320.1	207.7	59.9	5.7	5.1	41.7	346.1
1975	300.3	196.1	54.5	5.1	4.8	39.8	338.0
1976	298.3	195.1	52.8	4.9	5.1	40.4	336.1

*Source: Vital Statistics of the United States, National Center for Health Statistics.
†Includes congenital heart disease.
‡Provisional.
§Below 1,000,000 for the first time since 1964.
¶Adjusted by age to the United States population, 1940.

TABLE 4. Percentage of All Deaths Due to Cardiovascular Diseases* by Age—United States, 1962, 1975†

Age	1962	1975
Total	55.1	52.5
Under 25	7.6	7.4
25–44	27.7	20.1
45–64	50.2	44.2
65–74	61.3	54.9
Over 74	71.3	67.5

*Includes congenital heart disease.
†Source: Vital Statistics of the United States, National Center for Health Statistics.

ly that of the coronary arteries) became more prevalent and virulent, raising the specter in the late 1940's and 1950's of an "epidemic" of cardiovascular disease and accounting for 55.1 per cent of all deaths in 1962. Over the last 30 years, however, this tide has gradually turned; age-adjusted cardiovascular death rates have been declining slowly since 1950 and then more sharply since 1963. In total, since 1950 age-adjusted cardiovascular death rates have decreased by more than 31 per cent. Most significantly, the decline in coronary and cerebrovascular disease mortality rates has been even more precipitous since 1970 (stroke deaths down 18 per cent and coronary deaths down 14 per cent between 1970 and 1975) and has continued through 1977. This decline in cardiovascular mortality rates has been observed in both sexes and all age decades from ages 20 to 29 to 70+ and has been so sharp that, despite a growing and aging United States population, cardiovascular disease accounted for fewer than 1 million deaths in 1975 and again in 1976 for the first time in a decade. This trend is generally not paralleled in the rest of the world, however. Between 1969 and 1973 the mortality from cardiovascular disease increased sharply in Sweden, Denmark, Norway, England, Scotland, and Hungary, with lesser increases documented in other countries. In spite of the encouraging trends in the United States, cardiovascular disease remains a problem of staggering proportions, causing over 50 per cent of all deaths in 1976. The gaps in our knowledge and management of cardiovascular disease thus continue to pose a formidable challenge.

It is hard to attribute the ebb and flow in cardiovascular morbidity and mortality to specific events. Clearly, the two major etiologic processes damaging both the heart and the blood vessels are hypertension and atherosclerosis. Both processes are silent but incessant. We now know that hypertension may be present for long periods, as measured by simple blood pressure measurement, without producing signs or symptoms and, similarly, that atherosclerosis develops secretly in focal areas in blood vessels beginning in the first and second decades of life. This secret process may then proceed for two to six decades with no overt signs or symptoms until after two thirds of a vessel's lumen is occluded or the lesion breaks off or hemorrhage occurs. Symptoms appear suddenly in the form of heart attack, sudden death, angina, claudication, or stroke. It is because of their silent nature that these processes did not receive more attention earlier. Because of their ultimately devastating effects on the cardiovascular system, they are now the major subject of cardiovascular disease investigation. As basic researchers seek the cause(s) of arteri-

osclerosis and hypertension, as well as a better understanding of their basic pathophysiologic effects on the heart and blood vessels, cardiovascular physiologists have sought to develop better invasive (angiography) and noninvasive methods (e.g., echocardiography, nuclear imagery, x-ray densitometry) to diagnose abnormalities of the blood vessels, heart muscle, and heart valves long before signs or symptoms appear. During the past 30 years, cardiovascular epidemiologists have also made important contributions by detecting risk factor traits or habits in individuals to identify those who are at increased risk for specific cardiovascular diseases.

Much of the epidemiologic evidence regarding the role of certain personal characteristics ("risk factors") in the occurrence of coronary heart disease derives from several long-term prospective studies of fairly large population samples. The Framingham Heart Study, conducted by the National Heart, Lung, and Blood Institute, is a prototype study in which a general population sample of 5209 residents of the town of Framingham, Massachusetts, has been followed. At their first examination in 1948–1950, these men and women were 30 to 62 years old. Every two years they are re-examined to assess their medical status and to measure the characteristics to be described below. In 1977–1979 the fifteenth biennial cycle of examinations is being conducted, yielding 28 years of follow-up experience on this group. The Tecumseh Study followed a similar design, using all the residents of Tecumseh, Michigan, of whom 8624 participated in the initial examination in 1959. Three subsequent examinations have been completed.

Similar epidemiologic studies included studies in Albany, using male civil servants aged 39 to 54 years; in Chicago, using male employees of the Chicago Peoples Gas Company aged 40 to 59 years, and another using male employees of Western Electric Company aged 40 to 55 years; and in Evans County, Georgia, using a total community in which one third of the population was black. The Tecumseh, Framingham, and Evans County studies included women as well as men.

A long list of major and minor cardiovascular risk factors have now been enumerated by these studies. They include as major factors *age, male sex, hypertension, cigarette smoking, plasma LDL and HDL cholesterol,* and *blood glucose,* and as lesser factors *overweight, sedentary way of life, hardness of water, family history of heart disease before age 65, personality type,* and *stress.*

Prospective epidemiologic studies in other areas have tended to confirm the findings of the aforementioned studies. Most of the other studies have used populations with lower over-all rates of heart disease such as Japanese men in Japan, Hawaii, and California, Puerto Rican men, urban and rural men in Yugoslavia, and male civil servants in Israel. The essential features of each of these studies were (1) an effort to obtain a large representative sample of the population, (2) careful assessment of a variety of measurements prior to the onset of clinically overt coronary disease, and (3) complete ascertainment of all cardiac events occurring during the subsequent years of follow-up.

As a result of studies such as those mentioned above, there is little doubt of the predictive power of the major cardiovascular risk factors (see accompanying figure). Estimates based on the Framingham Heart Study and

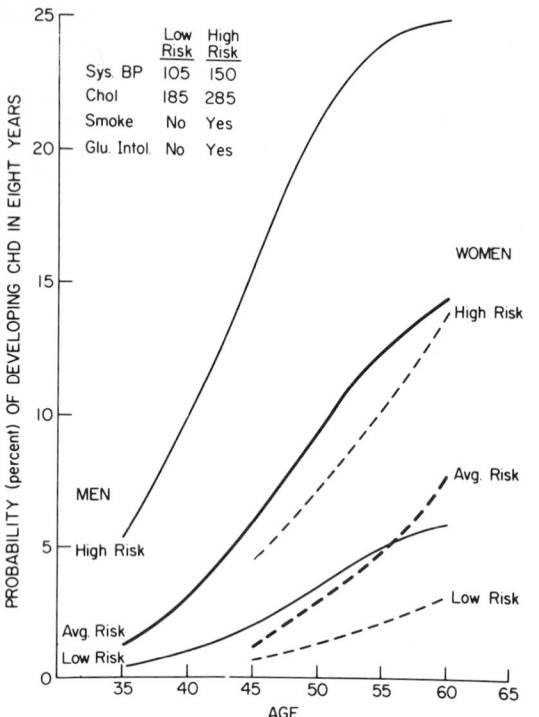

	Low Risk	High Risk
Sys. BP	105	150
Chol	185	285
Smoke	No	Yes
Glu. Intol.	No	Yes

Probability of developing coronary heart disease (CHD) in eight years by age, sex, and risk category. (From Feinleib, M.: Am. J. Epidemiol., 104:457, 1976.)

national vital statistics indicate that two out of every three coronary events (myocardial infarction, coronary death, or coronary insufficiency) occur in high risk subjects. As detailed in the basic prevalence figures, older age and male sex both are associated with increasing cardiovascular disease. Females seem to have a 15- to 20-year protective buffer before cardiovascular events begin to manifest themselves increasingly in the seventh and eighth decades of life.

Cigarette smoking has clearly been shown to be an independent, potent risk factor for coronary, cerebral, and peripheral vascular disease. Sudden cardiac death, heart attack, angina, claudication, and stroke incidence and prevalence can be related to the number of cigarettes one smokes. The heavier the cigarette smoking history, the higher the risk. Both the nicotine and carbon monoxide inhaled with cigarette smoking have been incriminated as causative factors, but definite understanding of cause and effect still eludes us. Cigar and pipe smoking are not associated with this heightened degree of cardiovascular risk. Furthermore, in contrast to the apparently cumulative relationship of cigarette smoking to lung cancer, a series of prospective and retrospective studies now indicates that if one stops smoking cigarettes, over 90 per cent of the increased cardiovascular risk disappears within 18 months.

Hypertension is not only a major direct cause of cardiovascular disease but also appears to greatly accelerate the atherosclerotic process, especially that of the coronary and cerebral vessels. Although we define blood pressures above 160/95 as hypertension, cardiovascular risk begins to increase at considerably lower levels. For example, in a 35-year-old man with a normal blood pressure of 120/80, the risk of mortality over the

next 20 years would increase almost two-fold if his pressure were 142/90. That risk increases 2.2 times with a pressure of 142/95, whereas a level of 152/95 raises the 20-year mortality risk 2.5 times.

An elevation of plasma cholesterol levels has long been associated with increased cardiovascular risk. Through second and third generation epidemiologic studies, our focus has become more specific. It is now clear that the cholesterol-rich low density lipoproteins (LDL), the major carriers of cholesterol in our blood, are directly and independently associated with cardiovascular risk. It has been observed recently that another plasma carrier of cholesterol, high density lipoprotein (HDL) (usually accounting for less than 25 per cent of the total plasma cholesterol) is independently but inversely related to cardiovascular risk. The higher the level of HDL, the lower the cardiovascular event rate. Although the biochemical basis of the apparently protective effect of HDL is still speculative, it is clear that the measurement of the plasma levels of HDL and LDL gives more information than the determination of total plasma cholesterol alone. LDL levels are in part genetically determined, although environmental factors, especially diet, appear to have major effects on the plasma levels of this lipoprotein. Diets high in cholesterol and saturated fats increase plasma LDL levels, whereas diets low in cholesterol and saturated fat and/or high in unsaturated fat decrease LDL levels. Plasma levels of HDL are much more stable in any given individual and appear to be under stronger genetic control. Exercise and modest ingestion of alcohol do appear to raise HDL levels, however. From the time of adolescence, males have levels of HDL that are 10 to 20 per cent lower than those of females, whereas LDL levels are 10 per cent higher. This sex difference may be explained by the direct inverse effects of estrogen and testosterone on plasma HDL and LDL levels.

Blood glucose is another independent cardiovascular risk factor, with higher levels directly related to the extent of vascular disease. This relationship is true for both the juvenile and adult onset diabetic, and in both groups premature macrovascular disease is the major cause of death. Of special interest is the observation that the female diabetic appears to lose all the protective cardiovascular effect usually attributed to the female sex.

Overweight, although associated with increased cardiovascular risk, does not appear to be an independent risk factor for cardiovascular disease. When other associated variables are factored out through multivariate analysis, obesity loses all its predictive risk power. It appears, rather, to exert its cardiovascular effect through other risk factors. Thus weight gain raises blood pressure, LDL cholesterol, and blood glucose levels and increases sedentary behavior, whereas weight loss has the opposite effect, lowering each of these variables.

The association of sedentary behavior, family history of premature heart disease, water hardness, and personality type with vascular disease risk seems clear cut. However, whether they represent primary or independent risk factors still must be clarified.

Although the existence of the risk factors enumerated above and their predictive value in assessing cardiovascular risk in an individual or group is now firmly established, evidence that modification of risk factors will alter cardiovascular risk is incomplete. Prospective and retrospective analysis leaves little doubt that cessation of cigarette smoking will decrease cardiovascular risk; in fact, it has been suggested that if all Americans stopped smoking, cardiovascular deaths would be reduced by 150,000 per year. Little doubt exists of the beneficial effects on many body functions of weight control and regular modest exercise. Therefore, although it has not been firmly established that weight reduction or exercise conditioning will decrease cardiovascular events, these measures are usually recommended. In the case of high blood pressure, there is little doubt that treatment of moderate and severe hypertension will decrease stroke, renal failure, and heart failure; hence we treat hypertension aggressively. However, whether treatment of high blood pressure will prevent heart attack has not been definitely proved in man. Similarly, it remains unclear whether treatment of mildly elevated blood pressure or elevated blood pressure in the elderly is efficacious. Furthermore, the potential preventive benefit of salt restriction and weight control in those at risk for hypertension remains to be definitely proved.

There is little doubt that dietary modifications in cholesterol and saturated fats will reduce levels of LDL cholesterol, and nonhuman primate studies suggest that cholesterol lowering through diet will actually lead to regression of existent atherosclerosis. However, we await the results of ongoing clinical trials in man to prove conclusively the benefit of lowering LDL. Similarly, the beneficial effect of lowering blood sugar levels is still being debated.

Conclusive demonstration of the benefit of risk factor modification is of central importance to our current approach to cardiovascular disease. It is increasingly apparent that the first clinical signs of cardiovascular disease may also be the last, because one fourth of first heart attacks manifest as sudden death. Epidemiologic evidence shows clearly that after a coronary event, the state of the heart and the degree of damage are more crucial than any of the aforementioned risk factors. There is little doubt therefore that the primary prevention of cardiovascular disease is important. If it can be demonstrated that the basic process of arteriosclerosis and hypertension can be delayed or prevented, either through risk factor modification or by other means, we will clearly have a very cost-effective remedy.

The striking association of the current waning cardiovascular "epidemic" with clear evidence of changing American life styles and habits is very hopeful. Since 1966, the number of cigarette smokers has declined in men by 25 per cent, in women by 10 per cent, and in physicians of both sexes by 33 per cent. Between 1963 and 1975, there has been a 22.4 per cent decline in per capita tobacco consumption, a 19.2 per cent decline in the consumption of fluid milk and cream, a 31.9 per cent decline in butter consumption, a 12.6 per cent decline in egg consumption, a 56.7 per cent decline in the ingestion of animal fats and oils, and a 44.1 per cent increase in the ingestion of vegetable fats and oils. These concomitant changes have been associated with evidence of a 4 to 8 per cent decline in plasma LDL cholesterol levels in the United States in the past ten years. Americans are more conscious of the need for exercise. Since 1972, a government-sponsored National High Blood Pressure Education Program has increased

by over 8 million the number of adult Americans aware of having hypertension, increased patient visits for hypertension by 50 per cent, and increased by an estimated 4 to 6 million the number of Americans under effective blood pressure control. These life style and habit changes coincide with a declining United States cardiovascular death rate (reinforced by the lack of evidence for a decline in either cardiovascular rates or risk factor status in Europe) and augur a potentially bright future for preventive cardiology.

Dawber, T. R.: Risk factors in young adults: The lessons from epidemiologic studies of cardiovascular disease — Framingham, Tecumseh, and Evans County. J. Am. College Health Assoc., 22:84, 1973.

Gordon, T., Garcia-Palmieri, M. R., Kagan, A., Kannel, W. B., and Schiffman, J.: Differences in coronary heart disease in Framingham, Honolulu and Puerto Rico. J. Chron. Dis., 27:329, 1974.

Kannel, W. B.: Prevention of cardiovascular disease. Cur. Prob. Cardiol., 1:1, July 1976.

National Center for Health Statistics, National Health Survey, 1972.

Stamler, J., and Epstein, F. H.: Coronary heart disease: Risk factors as guidelines to preventive action. Prev. Med., 1:27, 1972.

World Health Statistics Annual, 1972–1976. World Health Organization.

354.2. CIRCULATORY FUNCTION AND CONTROL

William W. Parmley

The normal cardiovascular system has a remarkable capacity to alter its performance. Such adjustments can increase cardiac output three to five times and heart rate two and a half times above basal values. The mechanisms responsible for this reserve capacity have been carefully studied over the years, resulting in a plethora of information about the circulatory system. The purpose of this chapter is not to detail these studies, but to provide a general overview of cardiovascular function. In particular, clinically important concepts will be stressed more than the details of data. Following a brief discussion of functional anatomy, the balance of the chapter will discuss the factors determining cardiac pump performance and overall circulatory function, and then discuss selected aspects of the response of the circulatory system to stress and heart failure.

FUNCTIONAL ANATOMY

The normal adult heart (weight approximately 300 grams) is about the size of a person's clenched fist — a gesture, interestingly enough, that the patient with angina pectoris frequently uses to describe the character of his cardiac discomfort. The atria are thin-walled shallow cups whose functional role is three-fold. When the atrioventricular (AV) valves are closed during ventricular systole, the atria serve a reservoir function by collecting blood from the systemic or pulmonary veins. In early diastole therefore there is rapid ventricular filling following opening of the AV valves. In mid-diastole, the AV valves remain open so that the atria serve as a conduit for the continuous flow of blood from the veins to the ventricles. Toward the end of diastole active atrial contraction ejects another increment of blood into the ventricle just prior to ventricular systole (about 20 per cent of stroke volume). The normal atria are thin walled, because they pump into the ventricles during diastole at low pressure.

The right ventricle is a thin-walled volume pump which has a low filling pressure (about 5 mm Hg) and ejects blood into the low pressure pulmonary artery (about 20 mm Hg). The right ventricle is formed by a concave free wall which opposes the convex septal wall, thus creating a crescent-shaped slit between them. Ejection of blood occurs by both shortening of the free wall and movement toward the interventricular septum, which compresses the chamber by a bellows action. This latter mechanism is extremely efficient in ejecting a large volume of blood with a minimum of muscle shortening, but can only function effectively at the low pressures normally found in the right-sided circulation.

The left ventricle is somewhat conical in shape, with its apex forming the apex of the heart. It can be considered as a thick-walled pressure pump whose medial wall is the thick interventricular septum. Ejection of blood from the left ventricle is primarily accomplished by a constriction of the muscular wall, although there is some shortening of the chamber.

The thickness of the ventricular wall is dependent on the relationship between wall stress, intraventricular pressure, and the radius of wall curvature as defined by the Laplace relation:

$$\sigma = \frac{PR}{2h}$$

(σ = wall stress [force/cross-sectional area], P = intraventricular pressure, R = radius of curvature of the wall, and h = wall thickness.) In general, wall stress is relatively constant throughout the heart. Thus the radius of curvature and wall thickness tend to be related. At the apex of the heart where the radius of curvature is short, the wall is thin. By contrast, the free wall of the left ventricle has a longer radius of curvature and a proportionally thicker wall.

Although emphasis is usually placed on a description of the systolic function of the heart, a greater appreciation of the importance of the diastolic properties of the heart has occurred over the past few years (Fig. 1). A thick hypertrophied ventricle with decreased compliance causes increased resistance to filling. This frequently leads to atrial dilatation and hypertrophy in order to maintain the atrial contribution to ventricular filling. The importance of this contribution is apparent in patients with severe hypertrophy due, for example, to aortic stenosis or idiopathic hypertrophic subaortic stenosis. Loss of an appropriately timed atrial contraction (as with atrial fibrillation) often results in marked exacerbation of left heart failure. In these patients during sinus rhythm, the left ventricular end-diastolic pressure is markedly elevated due to a large A wave, whereas mean diastolic pressure, which is reflected back through the pulmonary veins into the lungs, is maintained at a lower level. When atrial contribution and the A wave kick are lost, however, there is an increase in mean left atrial and pulmonary venous pressures in an attempt to maintain the same level of end-diastolic pressure and cardiac output. This frequently leads to disabling dyspnea.

Recent observations have also pointed out how the apparent compliance of the ventricles can be acutely altered by hemodynamic factors, such as raising and lowering arterial or right-sided pressures. Since the two ventricles are enclosed in a common pericardial sac,

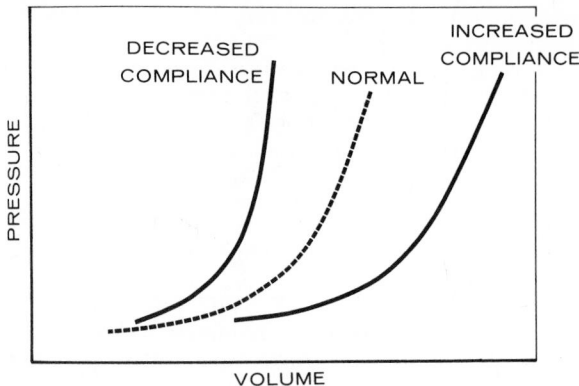

Figure 1. Representative passive pressure-volume relations of the left ventricle. The general exponential relationship between left ventricular diastolic pressure and volume is shown. At low pressures a small increase in pressure results in a large volume increment, whereas at higher pressures lesser volume increments occur with a rise in pressure. Chronic shifts in the passive pressure-volume relation can occur with various disease states. For example, with aortic stenosis and concentric hypertrophy, the left ventricular volume may be reduced at a given end-diastolic pressure (decreased compliance curve). On the other hand, with volume overload (e.g., mitral or aortic insufficiency) the curve may shift to the right with a larger volume at each end-diastolic pressure. In addition, recent evidence suggests that acute shifts in the left ventricular pressure volume relation may occur with changes in hemodynamics or ischemia. Vasodilator drugs which lower arterial pressure may produce a slight shift of the curve to the right (increased compliance).

which is quite stiff at high filling pressures, pressure or volume influences on one side of the ventricle can be transmitted to the other side of the heart. For example, administration of vasodilator drugs, such as nitroprusside or nitroglycerin, which reduce arterial and right-sided pressures in patients with heart failure, will tend to reduce left ventricular end-diastolic pressure at the same left ventricular end-diastolic volume. The presumed mechanism is a reduction in right ventricular volume (the more compliant chamber) and a reduction in the transpericardial pressure gradient, both of which result in an apparent increase in compliance of the left ventricle. Appreciation of the interaction of the right and left ventricles in a common intrapericardial space is important in any patient undergoing therapeutic maneuvers which rapidly alter right- and left-sided filling pressures.

CARDIAC PERFORMANCE

We will first consider the factors which alter the performance of the heart and then integrate these factors into the over-all function of the intact cardiovascular system. The four most important factors in determining the pump performance of the heart are preload, afterload, contractility, and heart rate.

Preload refers to the initial loading conditions of the heart. In isolated heart muscle, it is defined as the initial resting force stretching the muscle prior to contraction. In the intact heart, it is less easily defined. Estimates of preload include measurements of end-diastolic volume or end-diastolic pressure of the ventricle. In patients, it is often convenient to measure the filling pres-

INTERACTION OF PRELOAD (LVFP) AND AFTERLOAD ON STROKE VOLUME

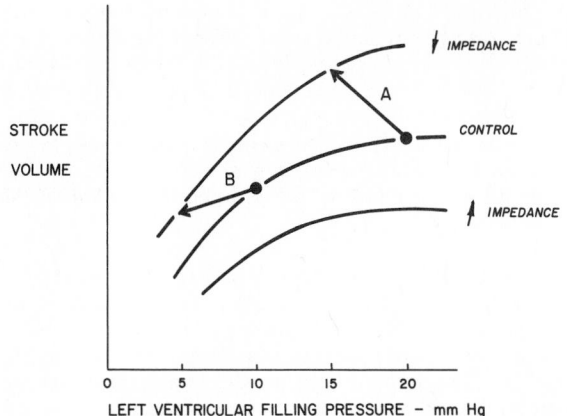

Figure 2.   Representative ventricular function curves following changes in afterload (impedance). Stroke volume is plotted as a function of left ventricular filling pressure (left atrial pressure). A vasodilator drug such as sodium nitroprusside, which decreases impedance, will shift the ventricular function curve up and to the left. Beginning at a high filling pressure, there will be a decrease in filling pressure and an increase in stroke volume (line A). Beginning at a low filling pressure, nitroprusside will also shift the patient to a new curve, but there may be a reduction in stroke volume (line B) because the patient moves down the ascending limb of the function curve. (From Chatterjee, K., and Parmley, W. W.: Prog. Cardiovasc. Dis., 29:305, 1977.)

sures (atrial pressures) of the ventricles as an index of preload. Within limits, as one increases the preload (end-diastolic pressure or volume of the heart), there is an increase in cardiac performance, manifested by an increase in the pressure developed or in the volume of blood ejected. This represents the ascending limb of the familiar Frank-Starling relationship (Fig. 2). The classic explanation of this phenomenon has been related on an ultrastructural basis to the degree of overlap of crossbridges between the thick myosin filaments and the thin actin filaments of each sarcomere. Newer evidence suggests that initial muscle length also has an effect on the amount of calcium available for contraction (length-dependent activation).

This over-all relationship is often referred to as a ventricular function curve (Fig. 2). Some measure of cardiac performance, such as stroke volume or stroke work (stroke volume × arterial pressure), is plotted as a function of some measure of preload, such as atrial filling pressure or end-diastolic pressure. The concept of the ventricular function curve is important for several reasons. First of all, it allows for a comparison between subjective signs and symptoms and objective measurements. Thus as the level of left atrial pressure rises, the symptoms and signs of pulmonary congestion and edema appear. The ensuing dyspnea is the most common symptom associated with heart failure. The second major symptom complex in heart failure is fatigue due to reduced cardiac output. This is related to the vertical axis of the ventricular function curve, because cardiac output is the product of stroke volume and heart rate. This correlation between subjective symptoms and objective measurements is an important conceptual one in evaluating patients with cardiovascular disease.

An important application of preload alteration is exemplified by the therapy of patients with severe acute power failure. In such hypotensive patients, optimization of left ventricular filling pressure will maximize stroke volume or stroke work. The normal left atrial pressure is about 10 mm Hg. The optimal left atrial pressure in critically ill patients appears to be approximately 15 to 20 mm Hg. At higher pressures, there is no further improvement or, in some cases, an actual decline in cardiac performance, whereas the symptoms of pulmonary congestion will increase. In patients who are hypotensive with a very low left ventricular filling pressure, volume administration is appropriate therapy to raise the filling pressure up to 15 to 20 mm Hg. This therapy is often sufficient to reverse the hypotension and low cardiac output state. An appreciation of preload therefore is of great practical importance in the characterization and management of patients with heart failure.

An important distinction must be made between the right atrial pressure, which represents the filling pressure of the right ventricle, and the left atrial pressure, which is the filling pressure of the left ventricle. Each atrial pressure is related to the functional status of its respective ventricle. In manipulating the volume status of the patients, however, it is far preferable to measure left ventricular filling pressure, because the left ventricle has a more important role in determining arterial pressure and forward cardiac output.

The term *afterload* refers to the load against which the heart must contract. In isolated heart muscle studies, it can be carefully defined as the load resisting shortening as the muscle is stimulated. In the intact heart, it is loosely approximated as the arterial pressure or impedance against which the heart has to work. The effect that afterload has on performance is relatively straightforward. As one increases arterial pressure, the stroke volume will go down because the ventricle has greater difficulty in ejecting blood against a higher load. Conversely, if one can reduce systemic vascular resistance and arterial pressure with vasodilator drugs, one can increase forward stroke volume and cardiac output. One must avoid severe hypotension, however, which will compromise coronary blood flow and therefore reduce cardiac performance. The principle of afterload manipulation is one of the most important new concepts in cardiac therapy within the past several years. Vasodilator therapy for both acute and chronic heart failure is emerging as one of the most important adjuncts to more standard forms of therapy.

It should also be pointed out that there is a close relationship between changes in preload and afterload. Thus as the arterial pressure is increased, the ventricle has greater difficulty in ejecting blood and tends to retain more end-diastolic volume, thus increasing its preload. The opposite sequence of events occurs when the afterload is reduced. Therefore when one monitors arterial pressure and left atrial pressures simultaneously, particularly in patients with heart failure, the two frequently undergo directionally similar changes.

In terms of a ventricular function curve, vasodilator drugs which reduce both preload and afterload may affect function differently, depending on the initial level of left ventricular filling pressure. As illustrated in Figure 2, a vasodilator drug such as sodium nitroprusside, which reduces the resistance (impedance) to aortic ejec-

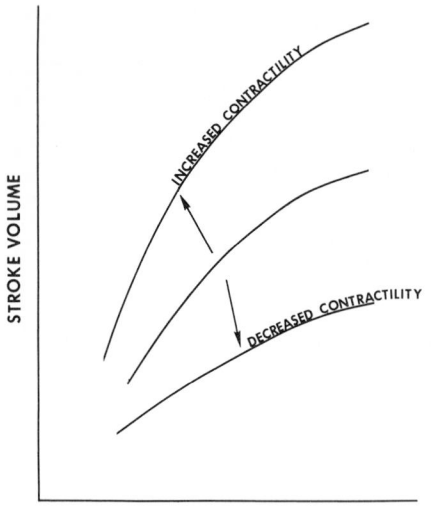

Figure 3. Representative shifts in ventricular function curves following changes in contractility. Left ventricular stroke volume is plotted as a function of left ventricular end-diastolic pressure. If the middle curve represents a baseline, drugs which increase contractility shift this curve upwards and to the left, while interventions which decrease contractility shift the curve down and to the right.

tion, will shift the ventricular function curve upward. Beginning at a high filling pressure (20 mm Hg), there will be both a reduction in filling pressure and an increase in stroke volume (line A, Fig. 2). At a normal filling pressure (10 mm Hg), however, the reduction in filling pressure will move the patient down the ascending limb of the ventricular function curve, and may reduce stroke volume (line B), even though the patient is on a higher curve.

Contractility refers to the vigor of contraction of heart muscle and is best defined in isolated heart muscle as an increased velocity of shortening at a given load. Drugs such as digitalis or the catecholamines increase contractility, whereas hypoxia, ischemia, acidosis, and certain antiarrhythmic drugs or beta-adrenergic blocking agents may reduce contractility. In terms of a ventricular function curve, drugs which increase contractility tend to increase stroke volume or stroke work at a given end-diastolic pressure. With a depression of contractility, the ventricular function curve shifts down and to the right with a reduction in stroke volume at a given left ventricular end-diastolic pressure (Fig. 3). Alterations of contractility may not always be beneficial. For example, in patients with coronary artery disease and limited coronary flow, a positive inotropic agent such as a catecholamine will markedly increase contractility and the need for myocardial oxygen. The partially obstructed coronary circulation may not be able to deliver the necessary increase in coronary blood flow. Under these circumstances, myocardial oxygen demand may outstrip supply and produce further ischemia and deleterious effects on the myocardium.

Heart rate is an obvious determinant of cardiac performance, and is one of the most important mechanisms available to the heart to increase cardiac output (cardiac output = stroke volume × heart rate). The magnitude of the heart rate may be an important indicator of the cardiovascular status of an individual patient. For example, in a patient with acute failure who

has a sinus tachycardia of 140, it is evident that the reduction in stroke volume (downward shift in ventricular function curve) is so great that a marked elevation of heart rate has resulted in an effort to maintain cardiac output at an acceptable level. Of course, stroke volume may be reduced because of low preload (hypovolemia) or because of severe failure with a high preload. It may be necessary to measure the preload to resolve this dilemma. Other factors which raise heart rate must also be considered, including fever, anemia, thyrotoxicosis, and others.

The effects of changes in heart rate on cardiac contractility are related to the interval strength relation. If one has a premature ventricular depolarization, that contraction is reduced, whereas the contraction following the pause is augmented (post-extrasystolic potentiation). This augmented contractility is apparently related to an increased availability of calcium during the subsequent beat. Although an increase in heart rate in and of itself causes a slight increase in the contractility of heart muscle, this is not a major effect when compared to interventions such as the catecholamines.

Although the importance of the ascending limb of the Frank-Starling curve is established, there is some question regarding the importance of a descending limb as preload is increased to extremely high levels. In general, studies in isolated heart muscle and whole heart preparations have shown that there is *not* a prominent descending limb. However, in patients with reduced cardiovascular reserve, it is possible to demonstrate a "descending limb" (reduction in cardiac performance and marked increase in preload) by provoking an exercise or afterload stress. For example, arterial pressure can be increased with drugs such as angiotensin or during isometric exercise, a potent mechanism for increasing arterial pressure. Under these circumstances, patients with reduced ventricular reserve may have a marked increase in left ventricular filling pressure and a decrease in stroke volume or stroke work index.

In response to an afterload stress, the heart utilizes the Frank-Starling mechanism and increased contractility to maintain compensation. When the limits of these compensatory factors are exceeded, a descending limb of the ventricular function curve will appear, predominantly related to the increase in afterload and not specifically to a descending limb of muscle function.

As quantitative indices of cardiac performance, cardiac pressures and volumes can be measured in the cardiac catheterization laboratory, or in patients in critical care units. For reference, normal pressures, volumes, cardiac output, and vascular resistance are listed in the accompanying table. Volume measurements are normalized for interpatient comparison by dividing by the body surface area (square meters). This latter value is obtained from a standard table, based on height and weight. One useful index of left ventricular function is the ejection fraction, which is defined as stroke volume per end-diastolic volume. A normal ejection fraction is 0.55 or greater. In severe heart failure, ejection fraction may be reduced to less than 0.20.

PERIPHERAL CIRCULATION

The arterial system represents the conduit system for delivery of blood to all parts of the body. Blood pressure remains relatively constant in this system until one

Pressures and Volumes in the Normal Heart

Pressures
  Left-sided
    1. Left atrial pressure (normal mean pressure $\leq$ 12 mm Hg)
    2. Left ventricular pressure
       a. Peak systolic pressure (wide normal range, usually 100–150 mm Hg in adults)
       b. Left ventricular end-diastolic pressure (normal $\leq$ 12 mm Hg)
    3. Aorta
       a. Systolic pressure (wide normal range, usually 100–150 mm Hg in adults)
       b. Diastolic pressure (wide normal range, usually 60–100 mm Hg in adults)
  Right-sided
    1. Right atrial pressure (normal mean pressure $\leq$ 6 mm Hg)
    2. Right ventricular pressure
       a. Peak systolic pressure (normal 15–30 mm Hg)
       b. Right ventricular end-diastolic pressure (normal $\leq$ 6 mm Hg)
    3. Pulmonary artery
       a. Systolic pressure (normal 15–30 mm Hg)
       b. Diastolic pressure (normal 4–12 mm Hg)
Volumes
  Left-sided (at rest)
    1. Left ventricular end-diastolic volume (normal 70–100 ml/m^2)
    2. Left ventricular end-systolic volume (normal 25–35 ml/m^2)
    3. Stroke volume (wide normal range, usually 40–70 ml/m^2)
    4. Ejection fraction (stroke volume divided by end-diastolic volume (normal 0.55–0.80)
Time-related measurements
    1. Heart rate (wide normal range, usually 60–100 beats/minute)
    2. Cardiac index (2.8–4.2 liters/minute/m^2)
Resistances
    1. Systemic vascular resistance (770–1500 dynes sec cm^{-5})
    2. Pulmonary vascular resistance (20–120 dynes sec cm^{-5})

reaches the level of the terminal arteries and arterioles. There is about an 80 per cent drop in pressure across this latter network, which is primarily responsible for regulating the peripheral vascular resistance. The subsequent cross-sectional area of the capillaries is enormous so that the relatively large velocity of blood in the aorta (40 to 50 cm per second) is reduced to about 0.07 cm per second in the capillaries.

The venous system is not only responsible for return of blood to the heart, but at one time contains about 75 to 80 per cent of the total blood volume. These larger thin-walled vessels therefore are extremely important in regulating shifts in blood volume between the central and peripheral circulation, depending on their relative constriction or dilatation. Various therapeutic agents can produce important volume shifts. For example, in patients with heart failure, a potent diuretic such as furosemide and sublingual nitroglycerin both produce prompt dilatation of systemic veins, resulting in a redistribution of blood away from the central circulation into the peripheral circulation. This is effective in reducing pulmonary venous and left atrial pressures, thus improving the symptoms of pulmonary congestion.

Cardiac output has an important regional distribution, which may be altered in various pathologic states. For example, the kidney accepts a high proportion of cardiac output (approximately 20 per cent), which is necessary for appropriate renal function. Abrupt reductions in cardiac output can compromise renal flow and markedly reduce urine output. Regional circulations, such as the cerebral and coronary circulations, have powerful autoregulatory capabilities so that blood flow can be maintained despite reductions in arterial pressure. Other regional circulations, including the skin and splanchnic bed, are often "sacrificed" during hypotension so that blood may be preferentially shunted to more vital organs.

The primary function of the heart is to pump nutrients and oxygen to all parts of the body. The amount of oxygen delivered to the body is the product of the cardiac output and the arterial-venous oxygen difference. During periods of reduced cardiac output, increased oxygen extraction by peripheral tissues can increase oxygen delivery to the body, although this is a minor compensatory mechanism. The kidneys receive a large share of cardiac output, but have relatively less demand for oxygen so that the arterial-venous oxygen difference across the kidneys is less than the rest of the body. At the other end of the spectrum, the heart itself tends to extract oxygen nearly maximally from the blood delivered through the coronary arteries. Thus an increase in oxygen delivery to the myocardium is accomplished primarily by an increase in coronary flow, rather than by an increase in oxygen extraction.

The capillary system has an enormous total surface area, which facilitates passage of substances into and out of the circulation. Lipid-soluble substances such as O_2 and CO_2 diffuse directly across the capillary walls. Blood flow in capillaries is not uniform and is dependent on the contractile state of the precapillary sphincters. True capillaries have no smooth muscle cells and therefore cannot actively change their cross-sectional area. Ions and small molecules move across the capillary walls at surprising rates, through pore sizes of 40 Å. The primary factor which restrains fluid from leaving the capillaries is the osmotic pressure of the plasma proteins, the most important of which is albumin. The Starling hypothesis states that hydrostatic forces are primarily responsible for fluid movement out of the capillaries, whereas oncotic pressure is primarily responsible for fluid movement back into capillaries. An example of imbalance between these forces is seen in pulmonary edema secondary to an increase in pulmonary venous pressure. Under these circumstances hydrostatic pressure exceeds oncotic pressure, resulting in movement of fluid into the interstitial space and eventually into the alveoli.

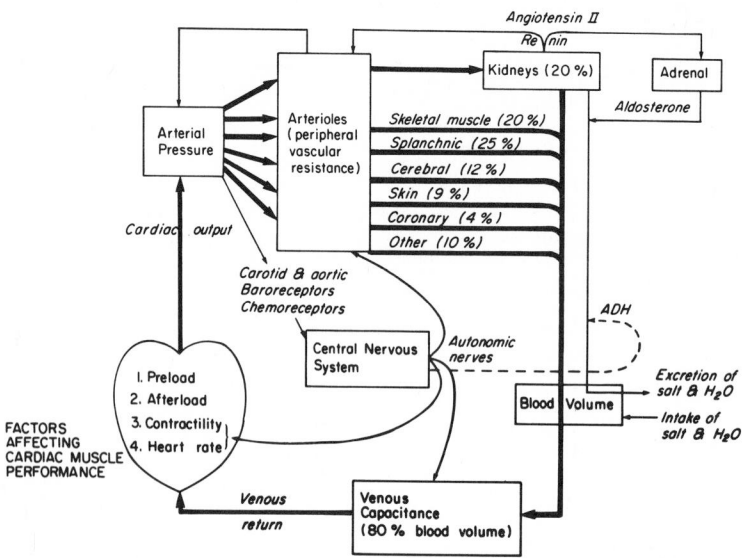

Figure 4.   Schematic representation of the circulatory system. See text for details.

INTEGRATED CARDIOVASCULAR FUNCTION

A simplified overview of the circulatory system is diagrammatically illustrated in Figure 4. The four factors directly affecting cardiac muscle performance have already been discussed in relation to left ventricular performance. Similar factors would apply to right ventricular performance and the pulmonary circulation, although they are not separately shown in Figure 4. The discussion to follow will summarize information related to these and other major factors listed in the diagram.

HEART RATE. The heart rate is determined by the frequency of the sinoatrial node impulses, which are related to the rate of depolarization of phase four of their action potential. Heart rate is also markedly affected by the autonomic nervous system. Branches of the sympathetic nerves increase heart rate via norepinephrine release, whereas branches of the vagus nerve decrease heart rate by release of acetylcholine. It appears that the parasympathetic system is the dominant factor in the normal control of heart rate. In individuals who have undergone exercise conditioning and have slow resting heart rates, the initial increase in heart rate during exercise is mediated by a gradual reduction in vagal tone. Only at higher levels of exercise are the sympathetic nerves active in increasing heart rate. On the other hand, in individuals who are not physically conditioned, the sympathetic influence is utilized much sooner in increasing heart rate. Emotional factors have an important influence on heart rate, as is evident during anxiety, fear, or anger. An increase in heart rate also occurs in anticipation of physical exertion before the exercise has been initiated.

Stretch receptors in both the carotid body and aortic arch exert important effects on heart rate. A change in arterial blood pressure alters the frequency of impulses from the baroreceptors to the central nervous system. In general, a drop in arterial pressure induces an acceleration of the heart, whereas an increase in arterial pressure tends to slow the heart. Similarly, externally applied digital pressure on a sensitive carotid body can promptly reduce heart rate. There are a number of other reflex effects mediated through the vagus nerve which may slow heart rate. These include stimulation of the respiratory tract as with intubation, nausea and vomiting, or painful stimuli of various kinds. On the other hand, an increase in heart rate accompanies any activity in which there is an increase in sympathetic tone or in circulating catecholamines.

CARDIAC OUTPUT AND VENOUS RETURN. In general, the cardiac output is normally determined by the peripheral needs of the body. Thus the heart is a relatively passive organ in the circulatory system. It merely pumps out all the blood that is returned to it, and cardiac output is determined by the venous return to the heart.

Changes in venous return and cardiac output are largely produced by the altered capacity of the peripheral vascular bed. Either an augmentation of blood volume or a reduction of venous capacitance will tend to augment venous return and thus raise cardiac output.

Any venoconstriction will improve cardiac filling by slightly elevating the pressure gradient for venous return, thereby displacing blood from the peripheral circulation toward the cardiopulmonary circulation. Since only about 20 per cent of the blood volume is in the arterial system, it is clear that there can be little or no displacement of blood by constriction of arteries or arterioles.

If one alters heart rate substantially under normal resting conditions, there is usually no change in cardiac output. As the heart rate goes up (as for example by artificial pacing), the stroke volume goes down in a reciprocal manner, and cardiac output remains constant. This further emphasizes the importance of peripheral factors in determining the normal cardiac output. The heart becomes the limiting factor in regulating cardiac output only when it begins to fail. When the diseased heart is unable to pump out all the blood that has returned to it and is unable to supply blood sufficient for the metabolic needs of the body, then a state of heart failure can be said to exist. Under these circumstances, the changes in cardiac output are extremely dependent on myocardial function, which then becomes the limiting factor. Under normal circumstances, however, the heart basically responds to the increased needs of the body and supplies the blood required by the organism at that particular time. Variations in venous return as produced by alteration in posture, activity, or intrathoracic pressure transiently influence cardiac output considerably. When one assumes the upright posture, gravitational forces tend to pool blood in the dependent parts of the body, which may transiently reduce venous return, central blood volume, and diastolic volumes of the heart. The normal changes in intrathoracic pressure which occur with breathing also influence the return of blood to the heart. During inspiration, the negative intrathoracic pressure enhances cardiac filling and stroke volume, whereas the reverse occurs during expiration. Changes in intrapericardial pressure may also markedly affect venous return to the heart in pathologic states. Pericardial effusion with tamponade, restrictive pericarditis, or endocardial fibrosis all markedly limit venous return and thereby limit forward cardiac output.

The most important factor in determining venous return and cardiac output is a change in peripheral metabolic needs such as might occur with exercise, fever, or thyrotoxicosis. The most common example of this increased need occurs during exercise in which the arterioles of the exercising muscle are dilated, resulting in a marked increase of blood flow to the exercising muscles. As catecholamine influence increases during exercise, there is also a constriction of the venous bed which markedly enhances the return of blood to the heart. Thus any activities associated with sympathetic stimulation would be expected to constrict the venous bed and augment venous return. Although elevation of venous pressure has some role in returning peripheral blood to the heart, the pressure difference between small veins and right atrium is too small to be an important factor. Furthermore, the venous bed is quite compliant so that even marked venoconstriction or venodilatation may result in only small changes of venous pressure relative to arteriolar pressure. Even though the pressure changes that occur may be relatively small, the displacement of volume and change in venous return may be quite substantial. Exercising leg muscles which compress veins with a one-way valve system are also quite important in returning venous blood to the heart during exercise.

ARTERIAL PRESSURE. In order for an individual to carry out a wide range of activities with a reasonably constant arterial pressure, it is clear that a stabilizing and regulatory system of some magnitude must exist. In this regard it is useful to consider the relation between blood pressure, cardiac output, and systemic vascular resistance. The formula relating them states that blood pressure = cardiac output × systemic vascular resistance. This equation assumes that central venous or right atrial pressure is small. Although a marked increase in cardiac output can lead to some elevation of blood pressure, the principal factor which regulates blood pressure is the peripheral vascular resistance, as primarily influenced by reflex neurogenic control.

Both extrinsic and intrinsic mechanisms influence systemic vascular resistance. Most important among the extrinsic mechanisms are neurogenic stimuli, although circulating hormones, including catecholamines and prostaglandins, have some minor role. The intrinsic mechanism for altering active tension of smooth muscle in arterioles has been termed autoregulation. Both the kidney and the heart have extraordinary abilities to autoregulate their arterioles and thus maintain blood flow at a needed level over a fairly wide range of perfusion pressures. This autoregulation is produced by two opposing mechanisms. Stretching of the vascular tissues increases the spontaneous activity of the smooth muscle and thus initiates progressive vasoconstriction. On the other hand, accumulation of tissue metabolites exerts a local vasodilator influence so that the opposing effects of pressure-induced vasoconstriction and metabolite-induced vasodilation tend to maintain flow at a level appropriate to the needs of the tissue. It is also possible that a decrease in oxygen in and of itself may be responsible for vasodilation. One clinically important vascular bed, however, that responds to hypoxia with vasoconstriction is the pulmonary bed, where pulmonary hypertension and pulmonary edema may occur at high altitudes with reduced oxygen content.

Although there are several pressure-sensitive receptors, the best studied baroreceptor involved in blood pressure control is the carotid body, which is located at the junction of the common carotid artery with its internal and external branches. Pressure-sensitive nerve endings in the wall of the receptor alter their discharge rate according to the pressure that is applied. At extremely high pressures the discharge rate is increased, whereas at low pressures the discharge rate from the carotid body is reduced. These impulses pass through the cardiovascular regulatory centers in the medulla, which then alter the relative magnitude of vagal and sympathetic tone. For example, as arterial pressure is increased, the impulses from the carotid body to the cardioregulatory center are also increased. These (1) stimulate the motor nucleus via the vagus to slow heart rate, and (2) inhibit the cardioaccelerator center, which reduces sympathetic tone and peripheral vascular resistance. This latter effect returns blood pressure toward the previous level. Alterations in the sympathetic vasoconstrictor outflow appear to be the most important mechanism for altering or producing changes in peripheral vascular resistance.

Chemoreceptors lying near the carotid bifurcation and in the aortic arch also respond to changes in pH, Pco_2 and Po_2. Reduced oxygen, increased CO_2, or lowered pH stimulates the chemoreceptors and leads to an elevation of systemic arterial pressure. A marked reduction in arterial pressure can also make the brainstem ischemic and result in severe peripheral vasoconstriction mediated through the sympathetic nerves. This is presumably an attempt to raise arterial pressure up to levels that would relieve the central nervous system ischemia. In general, these latter mechanisms are operative only under extreme conditions and probably are not involved in the normal regulation of arterial pressure.

There is considerable fluctuation in blood pressure around the clock, as influenced by all the factors of everyday life, including posture, emotion, exercise, stress, and sleep. For example, exercise generally causes an increase in both systolic and diastolic pressure which persists for some time after the termination of exercise. Sleep, on the other hand, usually results in a reduction in blood pressure, although intense dreaming may produce an elevation of both heart rate and blood pressure.

CARDIOVASCULAR RESPONSE TO STRESS. A major principle related to the evaluation of the cardiovascular system is the importance of its response to an imposed stress. Under certain circumstances, resting function may be normal, whereas the response to an imposed stress may be grossly abnormal, thus detecting the individual with reduced cardiovascular reserve. This principle is implicit in history taking when one inquires about shortness of breath, fatigue, chest pain, or other symptoms provoked by exercise and other activities.

The cardiac response to exercise involves the interrelated effect of increased heart rate, catecholamine stimulation, and the utilization of the Frank-Starling mechanism. A treadmill exercise test or other specialized tests are useful in quantitating cardiovascular reserve. Two different stresses which have been used are isotonic and isometric exercise, which represent the two major types of exercise conditioning. Isometric exercise implies little change in the length of exercising skeletal muscles. This would occur during weight lifting or any exertion in which there is little movement of muscles. The usual response to isometric exercise is some degree of peripheral vasoconstriction with an increase in arterial pressure. There is an increase in sympathetic outflow which increases the contractility of the heart and may result in a slight increase in cardiac output. There is also an increase in heart rate in response to the increased sympathetic tone. In patients with normal cardiovascular reserve, the ventricular function curve therefore shifts generally upward with little change in pulmonary capillary wedge pressure (Fig. 5). Patients with poor ventricular reserve, however, may

have an adverse response to the increased afterload produced by vasoconstriction. This is characterized by a substantial reduction in stroke volume or stroke work index, and a marked rise in left ventricular filling pressure (Fig. 5). The response to isometric exercise therefore can be useful in quantitating the cardiovascular reserve of individual patients.

Isotonic exercise implies considerable muscle movement against a constant but low load. This is characteristic of walking, jogging, or running. Those who engage regularly in isotonic exercise programs will "train" their cardiovascular system. This results in a lower resting heart rate with a far greater capacity to increase cardiac output during subsequent exercise. With isotonic exercise, there is a marked reduction in systemic vascular resistance, primarily in the exercising muscles. This improves forward flow and markedly increases cardiac output.

The normal distribution of cardiac output at rest is indicated in Figure 4. With exercise, there is a substantial increase in relative and absolute blood flow to the skeletal muscles and skin. There is also an increase in flow through the coronary circulation, but little absolute change in flow to the splanchnic, cerebral, or renal beds.

With the onset of heart failure and a reduced resting cardiac output, there is a reduction in the percentage flow to the renal bed and skin. Exercise during heart failure produces a marked reduction in relative flow to the renal and splanchnic beds, with a greater proportion of flow going to exercising muscles. The absolute increase of flow to skeletal muscle, however, is far less than that found in a normal person during exercise.

Initially, it was assumed that changes in preload (Frank-Starling mechanism) were responsible for the increased cardiac output during exercise. It is apparent, however, that most of the changes in cardiac output are mediated by an increase in heart rate. The adrenergic nervous system increases both heart rate and contractility, and leads to peripheral vasodilation. The tachycardia which occurs due to the increase in sympathetic tone tends to reduce the cardiac dimensions, and thus to counteract the changes which might occur if the heart were allowed to dilate via the Frank-Starling mechanism. During light or initial exercise, there may be a slight reduction in end-diastolic volume. Because of the increase in contractility of the heart, however, stroke volume tends to remain relatively constant, and the increase in cardiac output is produced primarily by the increase in heart rate. At more profound levels there may be a slight increase in heart size as the Frank-Starling mechanism is utilized.

BLOOD VOLUME. The magnitude of blood volume is another important factor affecting cardiovascular function. Some of the factors involved in the maintenance of extracellular fluid and blood volume are listed on the right-hand side of Figure 4.

An increase in blood volume as might occur by an increased intake of salt and water would increase cardiac output. This, in turn, would tend to increase arterial pressure and renal perfusion and thus increase urine output, which would decrease blood volume back toward normal. Atrial receptors sensitive to dilatation are also responsible for vasodilating reflexes to the kidneys, and reflexes to the central nervous system to diminish the secretion of ADH. Both these factors would tend to

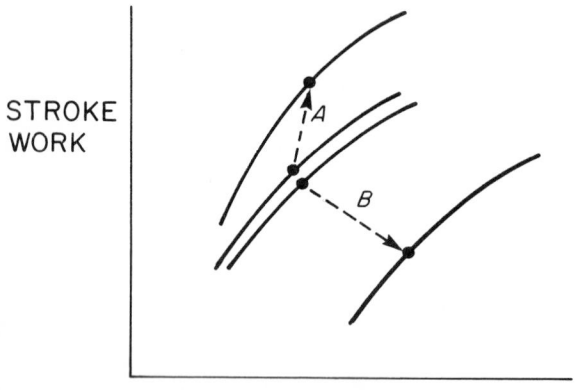

Figure 5. Altered ventricular function due to an elevation of arterial pressure produced by handgrip isometric exercise. A normal integrated response (patient A) shows an increase in stroke work with little change in left ventricular end-diastolic pressure (LVEDP). In this case, the increased contractile reserve has overcome the effects of the increased afterload (aortic pressure). The response of patient B indicates a substantial reduction in cardiovascular reserve. Under these circumstances, the marked increase in afterload has reduced the cardiovascular performance and produced a large rise in end-diastolic pressure.

increase the output of urine. These volume receptors, however, appear to have only transient effects and are not operative during heart failure with high atrial pressures.

Loss of fluid volume occurs primarily through the kidneys. Sweating, respiratory, and gastrointestinal losses are usually less important, except during extreme conditions. Since approximately 20 per cent of the resting cardiac output passes through the kidneys, they provide an ideal location for regulating salt and water balance. Since this subject is discussed in detail elsewhere, only some of the pertinent factors will be mentioned here.

Reduction in renal perfusion (reduced pressure and flow) is sensed by the juxtaglomerular apparatus, which releases renin. Other factors, such as ischemia and sodium depletion, have also been suggested as stimuli that affect renin release. Over-all, the phrase "effective blood volume" is a useful concept to keep in mind. Thus, decreased effective blood volume results in increased renin release, whereas increased effective blood volume turns off the stimulus for renin release. This concept forms the basis for alterations in sodium intake and volume as provocative tests for altering renin levels. Renin promotes the formation of angiotensin I from its precursor in the bloodstream. Angiotensin I is then converted to angiotensin II. Although angiotensin II is a powerful vasoconstrictor substance, this may not be its most important effect on blood pressure. Small suppressor doses of angiotensin II may increase aldosterone secretion, which may be one of its most important roles in regulating blood pressure. Angiotensin is also a potent stimulus for catecholamine release via the central nervous system vasomotor center and from the adrenal medulla.

Aldosterone promotes retention of salt and water. Under normal circumstances, salt and water intake are carefully balanced by their excretion. With congestive heart failure, there is an increased retention of salt and water which leads to edema formation and increased blood volume. There are usually increased aldosterone levels in severe heart failure secondary to reduced renal perfusion, and probably also due to decreased metabolism of aldosterone in the liver. It should be recalled that splanchnic flow is often reduced in heart failure, particularly during exercise.

In some patients with severe heart failure, free water excretion may also be severely impaired, and patients may be hyponatremic despite excess body sodium. Under such circumstances, restriction of fluid intake may be necessary to reduce fluid accumulation and reverse the hyponatremia. The potent diuretics available today are usually extremely effective in reversing the excess salt and water retention associated with heart failure. In some cases, excessive diuresis can lead to relative volume depletion and hypovolemia. Although uncommon, it is important to recognize this syndrome, because the associated hypotension and low cardiac output are effectively treated by liberalization of salt and water intake.

CIRCULATORY FAILURE. Heart failure is due to a number of causes, including mechanical or valvular defects, failure of the myocardium (cardiomyopathy), or loss of myocardium (myocardial infarction). In general, as myocardial failure occurs, there is reduction in heart muscle contractility, and the heart becomes the limiting factor in maintaining an appropriate level of cardiac output. In terms of the factors we have discussed, several characteristic alterations occur. First of all, cardiac output is decreased, and the preload of the heart is generally increased due to the reduced ability of the heart to eject blood (reduced ejection fraction) and to an increase in circulating blood volume. This may lead to elevated filling pressures on *both* the right and left sides of the heart. Second, there is evidence that the reduction in cardiac output which accompanies heart failure leads to a reflex increase in peripheral vascular resistance in an attempt to maintain arterial blood pressure. This increase in peripheral vascular resistance increases the resistance to ejection and may therefore further reduce cardiac output, resulting in a vicious cycle. The presumed existence of this cycle is supported by the fact that arteriolar dilating drugs such as hydralazine are extremely effective in increasing forward cardiac output in patients with severe heart failure, with no essential change in arterial pressure, heart rate, or pulmonary capillary wedge pressure. This suggests that systemic vascular resistance may be inappropriately high in heart failure for the level of cardiac output required. It should also be noted that the baroreceptor reflex mechanisms are markedly blunted in congestive heart failure. Thus interventions which reduce arterial pressure do not produce the same reflex increase in heart rate as in the normal individual.

In heart failure, there is a generally heightened sympathetic tone to the peripheral vasculature and to the myocardium, in an attempt to maintain cardiovascular compensation. This increased sympathetic tone causes more venoconstriction than in the normal individual, presumably in an attempt to maintain venous return and cardiac output. Heart rate may also be chronically elevated in heart failure in an attempt to maintain cardiac output. Arterial pressure often tends to be somewhat lower in heart failure as the ventricle loses the capacity to generate a normal or high blood pressure. In patients with hypertensive heart failure, however, blood pressure may remain at elevated levels for some time.

A consideration of the aforementioned factors suggests a rationale for the usual interventions employed in the treatment of chronic heart failure. Thus salt restriction and diuretics tend to reduce intravascular volume and therefore reduce preload below the level responsible for dyspnea. Digitalis stimulates the failing myocardium to increase its contractile state and thus improves the ability of the heart to eject blood. An inappropriately high systemic vascular resistance can be treated with arteriolar dilators to reduce the resistance to ejection and thus increase forward cardiac output. Venodilators, such as nitroglycerin, which predominantly dilate veins can redistribute blood away from the central circulation and also reduce pulmonary capillary wedge pressure.

In general, one does not attempt to control the sinus heart rate during heart failure, as this is the result of cardiac decompensation rather than a cause which has to be corrected. Of the four factors which affect cardiac performance therefore, therapy can be directed toward a correction of three of them (preload, afterload, and contractile state), and improved compensation will be reflected by a reduction in an elevated heart rate.

In summary, the cardiovascular system is a complex,

carefully regulated system which has extraordinary capabilities for altering its performance over wide ranges in response to the needs of the body. Usually the cardiac output is determined by the peripheral needs of the body as regulated by changes in venous return. Only when the heart is unable to meet these peripheral needs does a state of "heart failure" occur. At this point, the four factors affecting cardiac muscle performance become important considerations, and their regulation forms the basis of most of our therapeutic interventions in chronic heart failure.

Braunwald, E.: Control of cardiac performance. In Berne, R. (ed): Handbook on Circulation. Baltimore, Waverly Press, 1978, in press.

Chatterjee, K., and Parmley, W. W.: The role of vasodilator therapy in heart failure. Prog. Cardiovasc. Dis., 19:301, 1977.

Crexells, C., Chatterjee, K., Forrester, J. S., Dikshit, K., and Swan, H. J. C.: Optimal left heart filling pressure in acute myocardial infarction. N. Engl. J. Med., 289:1263, 1973.

Guyton, A. C.: Circulatory Physiology: Cardiac Output and Its Regulation. Philadelphia, W. B. Saunders Company, 1963.

Kivowitz, C., Parmley, W. W., Donoso, R., Marcus, H., Ganz, W., and Swan, H. J. C.: Effects of isometric exercise on cardiac performance: The grip test. Circulation, 44:994, 1971.

Parmley, W. W., and Talbot, L.: Heart as a pump. In Berne, R. (ed.): Handbook of Circulation. Baltimore, Waverly Press, 1978, in press.

Parmley, W. W., Tyberg, J. V., and Glantz, S. A.: Cardiac dynamics. Ann. Rev. Physiol., 39:277, 1977.

Rushmer, R. F.: Structure and Function of the Cardiovascular System. Philadelphia, W. B. Saunders Company, 1976, Chapters 3-7.

354.3.   APPROACH TO THE PATIENT WITH CARDIOVASCULAR DISEASE

Andrew G. Wallace

This chapter describes an approach to the collection of cardiovascular data, the principles behind certain laboratory tests used to obtain data, and strategies about data acquisition. The objective is to complement the following chapters, which emphasize the data in specific conditions and their use in management decisions.

A textbook of medicine is customarily organized by system. Diseases are presented for each system according to diagnostic categories, and for each category topics such as etiology, pathophysiology, symptoms, physical signs, laboratory data, and treatment are discussed. This approach provides the reader with an integrated picture of diseases that affect the system. The merits of the approach are numerous and outweigh shortcomings; however, there are shortcomings. One is that patients usually do not present to the doctor with an established diagnosis. Another is that textbooks frequently describe a composite of the manifestations of a disease; often patients fail to match this description, either because the description conveys inadequately the continuum of symptoms and signs produced by variable amounts of disease or because the evolution of symptoms and signs over time receives less than optimal attention. Establishing whether or not cardiovascular disease is present is the first objective of a complete evaluation. When disease is present, the diagnosis includes not only a definition of the structural abnormality it produces, but also its etiology and severity. The approach to the patient is at least as important as a knowledge of the clinical and laboratory characteristics which are expected in any given disease.

In an effort to exclude cardiovascular disease or to define more precisely structural changes and severity of diseases that are evident from clinical examination, the physician relies on laboratory methods. There are many laboratory methods available which give information about cardiovascular structure and function. Each method has particular conditions for which it is best suited, each has a predictable sensitivity and specificity with respect to particular questions, and among various methods there is an element of redundancy so that essentially the same information can be obtained in more than one way. Laboratory studies vary in cost and risk to the patient. They may give false or misleading information about a condition, especially if it is interpreted out of context with clinical data or other laboratory studies. The optimal approach to the patient requires a knowledge of changes in laboratory results produced by a disease, and also a strategy regarding which test and what sequence of studies will help in making the diagnosis and appropriately directing management of the patient.

Making a diagnosis is an important step in defining a clinical problem, but the diagnosis is not an end in itself. Patients within a given diagnostic category typically do not come to common end points within a predictable time. This is especially true in common chronic cardiovascular diagnoses such as hypertension, angina pectoris, and mitral stenosis. Prognosis is important to the patient because he or she wants to know what the future holds. Prognosis is important to the doctor because he or she needs to prescribe therapy and to select a therapeutic program. The number of descriptors which enable a physician to predict outcomes accurately is generally greater than the number needed to make a diagnosis. Large numbers of patients within a diagnostic category are needed to define which descriptors discriminate against certain outcomes. Finally, estimating prognosis is essentially an exercise in the application of probability statistics. The optimal approach to management decisions involves accurate collection of data which contribute to a definition of outcomes, the availability of information on many patients similar to the one being evaluated, and valid systems for assessing the impact of management choices.

COMPONENTS OF THE CARDIOVASCULAR DATA BASE

There are five components of the cardiovascular data base: the history, physical examination, electrocardiogram, chest x-rays, and laboratory studies. Patients with heart disease may or may not have symptoms, and they may be referred by one physician to another because of an abnormality or a suspected abnormality in any of the components of the data base. In practice, therefore, the starting point may be anywhere in this scheme. The sequence of acquiring data is less important than a thorough approach to each component. Indeed, it is instructive and useful to start purposefully with a different component of the scheme on different occasions, because it increases the likelihood of a thorough approach and skillful interpretation of each component.

THE HISTORY.   The cardinal symptoms of cardiovascular disease include chest pain, shortness of breath, hemoptysis, palpitations, swelling, faintness or syncope, and cyanosis. Chest pain is usually characterized by its location, quality, severity, duration, radiation, and factors which cause, aggravate, or alleviate the symptoms.

These features are sought in the history in an effort to distinguish between the common causes of chest pain: ischemic heart disease, pericardial disease, pulmonary infarction, aortic aneurysm, chest wall pain, and pain related to gastrointestinal disease. Shortness of breath may occur at rest, only with exertion, or only in certain positions. The history is designed to help distinguish between shortness of breath related to heart failure, pulmonary emboli, intrinsic lung disease, and anxiety. Hemoptysis is the production of bloody sputum during coughing. The quantity of blood, its color, and how it is mixed within the sputum (i.e., streaks, clumps, evenly mixed, or pure blood) all are important in distinguishing bronchitis, pulmonary infarction, pulmonary edema, and hemorrhage from a ruptured bronchial vein such as in mitral stenosis. Palpitation is an awareness of the heart beating in the chest. This sensation is not unusual in normal subjects when lying in bed or after vigorous exercise. On the other hand, when the sensation has an abrupt onset and termination, or is described as irregular or a skipping sensation, it usually signifies an arrhythmia. Swelling is edema in any part of the body. Edema implies retention of salt and water and is a common manifestation of heart failure. Local factors may cause or contribute to the site of edema formation. For example, edema of only one leg suggests venous disease. Dizziness or syncope may be a consequence of one of several mechanisms: arrhythmias, obstruction to blood flow, an orthostatic drop in blood pressure, loss of blood volume, or drugs. The history is particularly important in syncope, because abnormal signs are frequently absent. The relation to preceding incidents, associated symptoms such as pain and palpitations, and a history of blood loss or drug use are important to elicit. Other important causes of syncope include cerebrovascular disease, seizures, and hyperventilation.

To obtain a good cardiovascular history, remember these two principles: First, let the patient tell the story. Patients will frequently include information that would not come forth in response to a series of directed questions. Gestures used by the patient to describe symptoms and the situations in which they appear are often significant in subsequent management decisions. Second, after hearing the patient's story, ask direct questions to fill in any missing information and to determine the presence or absence of the cardinal symptoms of cardiovascular disease. Pursue each positive response in appropriate detail. Establish the chronology of the history, the severity of present symptoms, and whether the course is stable, progressive, or cyclic. Whenever possible, use the patient's words, not your own.

THE PHYSICAL EXAMINATION. There are five parts to the cardiovascular physical examination: physical appearance, venous pressure and pulse, arterial pressure and pulse, precordial movements, and auscultation.

Physical Appearance. The physical appearance of a patient is important for two reasons: it may give clues to a systemic disease that also affects the heart, and it may provide data relevant to the nature and severity of heart disease. Marfan's syndrome involves a typical body habitus and is sometimes associated with mitral and aortic insufficiency and aneurysms of the aorta. Mongolism (trisomy 21) is associated with endocardial cushion defects. Bony abnormalities of the upper extremity (especially a fingerized thumb) are associated with atrial septal defect and together constitute the Holt-Oram syndrome. Dis-

turbances of gait may suggest Friedreich's ataxia with associated cardiomyopathy. Acromegaly, disturbances of thyroid function, and rheumatoid arthritis are frequently associated with myocardial, pericardial, or valvular disease. Cyanosis and clubbing are clues to reversal of a shunt in congenital heart disease. A head bob and exaggerated arterial pulsations in the neck suggest increased diastolic run-off, as in aortic insufficiency. Edema and ascites suggest heart failure; when combined with obvious cachexia, they indicate longstanding and severe heart disease.

Venous Pressure and Pulse. There are two objectives to examination of the neck veins. The first is to estimate central venous pressure, and the second is to evaluate the wave form of the venous pressure pulse (Fig. 1). The examination is a visual one seeking a volume change in the veins. Because the venous system is a low pressure system, neck veins are nearly empty when the patient is sitting up, and they are distended when lying flat without a pillow. In either position a change in volume synchronous with the heartbeat is usually absent. To examine neck veins ideally, elevate the patient's head to an angle which maximizes the volume change in the veins throughout the cardiac cycle. The external jugular vein is a more reliable source to estimate venous pressure, but the internal jugular vein is a more reliable source to evaluate venous pulsations. Venous pressure is estimated by identifying the undulating meniscus in the jugular vein, measuring its height in centimeters above the sternal angle of Louis and adding 5 cm. The "A" wave results from atrial contraction and is exaggerated with right ventricular hypertrophy (reduced compliance), tricuspid stenosis, arrhythmias in which atrial contraction occurs against a closed tricuspid valve (i.e., cannon waves), and constrictive pericarditis. Obliteration of the "X" descent and a prominent "CV" wave are characteristic of tricuspid insufficiency. Elevated venous pressure with exaggerated "X" and "Y" descents is typical of pericardial constriction.

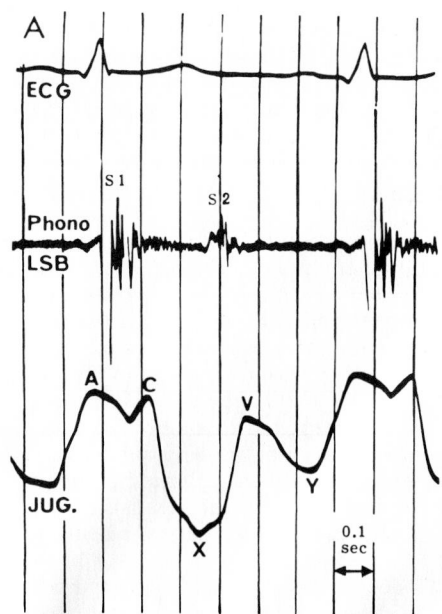

Figure 1.   Normal jugular venous pulse.

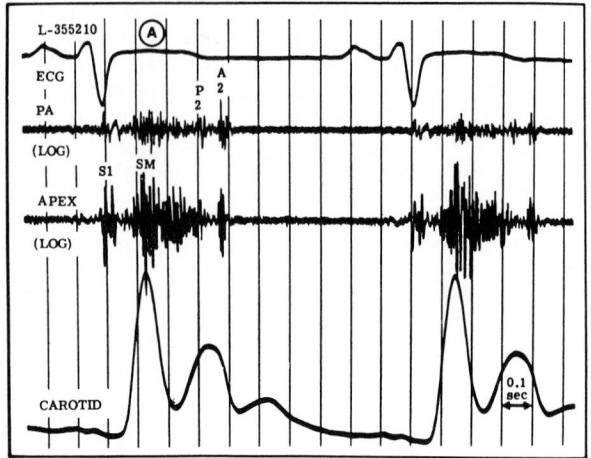

Figure 2. Bifid or bisferious carotid pulse in asymmetric septal hypertrophy with obstruction.

Arterial Pressure and Pulses. Arterial pulses are examined by palpation with the fingertips. The artery is compressed until it is displaced by the force of the arterial pressure pulse. This sensation of force on the fingertips is related to the amplitude of the pressure pulse, i.e., the difference between systolic and diastolic pressure, and not to pressure or flow per se. The carotid arteries are generally the most valid reflection of cardiac activity because they are centrally located and not influenced importantly by local factors which will affect the amplitude of the radial artery pulse independent of changes in cardiac activity. The amplitude of the carotid pulse is increased with anemia, thyrotoxicosis, and aortic insufficiency. In these conditions stroke volume and the rate of left ventricular ejection are enhanced. The carotid pulse is attenuated in myocardial failure, with rapid heart rates such as atrial fibrillation, and in aortic stenosis. These conditions are characterized by either a reduced stroke volume or a decreased rate of left ventricular ejection, or both. The arterial pulse becomes bifid in certain conditions in which left ventricular ejection is initially very rapid, producing a percussion wave, which is then followed by tidal wave which represents a reflected pulsation from the periphery (Fig. 2). A bifid or bisferious pulse is typically seen in asymmetric septal hypertrophy with obstruction (i.e., hypertrophic subaortic stenosis) and sometimes in aortic valve disease with predominate aortic insufficiency. In addition to examination of the carotid pulse, peripheral arterial pulses should be felt and compared. A diminished or delayed pulse at one site compared to another suggests arterial occlusion. If such a discrepancy is noted, it can be exaggerated by exercising the extremity supplied by the obstructed artery. In patients with claudication arterial pulses are frequently normal at rest, but they become reduced in the affected leg or foot with walking. This happens because at rest the distal arterial bed is constricted, flow in the leg is low, and as a consequence there is little or no gradient across the stenosis. With exercise the distal arterial bed opens up, flow into the leg is limited by the stenosis, and a gradient develops with a marked drop in pressure distal to the stenosis.

Arterial blood pressure should be measured with a cuff of appropriate size. If an elevated blood pressure is obtained in the arm, pressure in one leg should also be recorded. This procedure is used to exclude coarctation of the aorta in hypertensive patients. The arterial blood pressure should be recorded in both the supine and the standing positions. If the patient's blood pressure is elevated on the first measurement, several recordings should be obtained. Blood pressure is recorded to establish the presence or absence of hypertension. Discrepancies between pressure at two sites suggest obstruction or an arterial anomaly. A marked postural drop in arterial pressure suggests either hypovolemia or an inadequate sympathetic vasoconstrictor response. A change of systolic arterial pressure on alternate beats in sinus rhythm is referred to as pulsus alternans (observed in severe myocardial failure), and a change of systolic blood pressure of greater than 10 mm Hg with respiration is referred to as pulsus paradoxus (observed in pericardial tamponade).

Precordial Movements. Precordial movements should be evaluated by inspection and by palpation at the apex, in the left parasternal region, and in the right and left second intercostal spaces. The normal apical impulse is ascribed to left ventricular activity and is seen and felt as a tap of brief duration localized in the fourth or fifth interspace at the midclavicular line. Its distance from the midsternal line should be measured in centimeters and recorded. When the left ventricle is dilated, the impulse is displaced to the left and downward and occupies a larger area. With systolic overloads such as hypertension or aortic stenosis, the impulse is not displaced (in the absence of dilation) but is more forceful and sustained than normal (Fig. 3). Right ventricular enlargement typically produces an exaggerated left parasternal early systolic lift or thrust. A soft late systolic lift may be produced by mitral insufficiency. Dilation of the pulmonary artery or aorta (aneurysm) may produce a systolic pulse or tap in the second left or right intercostal spaces, respectively. In regional myocardial disease or in coronary disease with regional infarction, there is a paradoxical outward systolic movement felt in the third or fourth left intercostal space between the sternum and the nipple. Accentuated heart sounds are often palpable. Gallop sounds are usually palpable when they can be heard and reflect altered ventricular compliance. Palpation of the precordium is directed primarily at assessing ventricular size, ascertaining whether an increase in chamber size is due to dilation or concentric hypertrophy, assessing

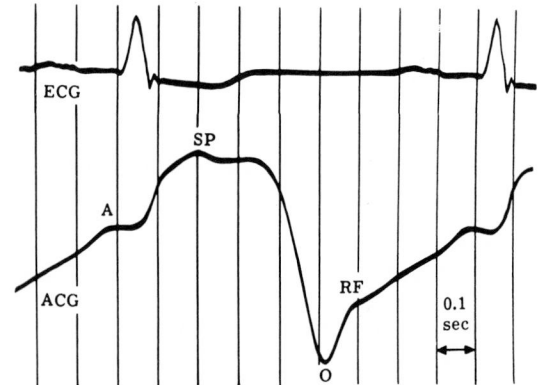

Figure 3. Apex cardiogram showing an exaggerated and prolonged outward systolic plateau (SP) due to left ventricular hypertrophy in a patient with aortic stenosis.

changes in compliance, and detecting asynchronous contraction of a region of the ventricle due to a regional disease process. For the experienced observer many cardiac diagnoses can be anticipated even before listening with a stethoscope.

Auscultation. The first principle of cardiac auscultation is to choose a stethoscope which fits the ears comfortably and which has tubing as short as possible. The second important principle is to carry out the examination in a room where the ambient noise level is as low as possible. Clinical experience and studies in hearing laboratories have shown that acoustic phenomena of diagnostic importance can be missed even by experienced observers if either of these principles is compromised.

The next important step in auscultation is to remember that you only hear what you listen for. A systematic approach in which you listen at specific locations and focus on specific sounds and parts of the cardiac cycle is essential. Devise a *mental check list* which you move through in stepwise fashion. For example, starting at the apex, ask yourself the following questions: (1) Which is the first and which the second heart sound? (2) What are their relative intensities, and is either accentuated? (3) Is there more than one component to either sound? (4) If there are two components to the first sound, is the extra component an S_4, an ejection click, or splitting? (5) Are there midsystolic or diastolic sounds? (6) Can a murmur be heard in either systole or diastole? Remember that high frequency sounds are best heard with the diaphragm, whereas low frequency sounds are best heard with the bell. Make it a standard part of your examination to listen with the patient supine, in the left lateral position, standing, and after exercise.

In chapters that follow this introduction, details of the physical examination in each of the major cardiac disorders will be presented. The point stressed here is the approach to the patient. The examination should be systematic. Abnormal physical findings may be so striking that they cannot be missed; more often, however, they are subtle. Therefore the most reliable approach is a mental check list. Progress through the list in an orderly fashion, and at each step optimize the conditions for eliciting the phenomenon which is sought.

It is rare for a cardiac condition to have only one manifestation on the physical examination. For example, when you see cyanosis you can anticipate certain findings on palpation or auscultation which will help explain it. When you feel an enlarged right ventricle, a palpable first heart sound, and a systolic pulse over the pulmonary artery in a middle-aged female, you can anticipate that auscultation may elicit an opening snap and diastolic rumble. Anticipating the next step is useful in examining a patient. For one thing, it is likely to increase the precision of the next step in the examination so that less will be missed. Absence of an anticipated finding may redirect tentative conclusions about the diagnosis. Finally, an anticipatory approach encourages synthesis of data as the examiner progresses through the check list. A diagnosis results from a synthesis of data; whether the history and physical examination yield a diagnosis or a definition of the problem which falls short of a diagnosis, synthesis helps to define what the next step should be and whether or not that step is necessary.

Laboratory studies play a central role in the diagnosis of cardiovascular diseases and, even more importantly, in quantifying the severity of these disorders. The paragraphs below are designed to highlight the role of commonly employed laboratory tests in cardiovascular diagnosis. It seems appropriate to discuss briefly the physical or physiologic principles behind these tests, because in some instances these techniques have been applied to cardiovascular studies only in the recent past, or because these principles help to clarify the uses and limitations of a particular test.

THE ELECTROCARDIOGRAM. Cardiac muscle is an excitable tissue. On each beat excitation begins at some site in the heart (normally the sinoatrial node), spreads from cell to cell initially over the atrium, then through the atrioventricular node, and finally to the ventricles. The form of the electrocardiogram at any point in time is determined by the location, size, and geometry of boundaries between excited and unexcited regions.

Whenever a boundary exists, the voltage difference across the boundary produces an electrical field at any point in the body. The positive side of this boundary can be viewed as a source of current, and the negative side of the boundary can be viewed as a sink. Regions on the body surface that face the current source will be on the positive side of the field, whereas those that face the current sink will be on the negative side of field. Because the location, spatial orientation, and size of the boundary change throughout excitation and recovery, the field changes in strength and orientation. On the body surface the amplitude and sign of the potential change with time. An electrocardiogram is a record of the voltage difference between two points on the body surface with respect to time.

The electrocardiogram is the most widely used and useful noninvasive cardiac diagnostic technique. Its diagnostic value has developed over the years of use through (1) correlations with clinical states and pathologic material, (2) physiologic studies designed to establish the relation between the electrocardiogram and normal and abnormal states, and (3) simulation. Analyses of the P wave and the QRS complex, their rate, and their temporal relation to each other provide a definitive approach for recognizing most disturbances of cardiac rhythm. The electrocardiogram gives diagnostic and localizing information about most myocardial infarctions. Criteria have been established for recognizing hypertrophy of the right or left atrium and the right or left ventricle. The electrocardiogram is an important diagnostic aid also in various forms of congenital heart disease. Because it can be obtained repeatedly in the same individual or monitored continuously over days, it is of particular value in assessing pathophysiologic phenomena that change over the interval between records (rhythm, hypertrophy, infarction or ischemia, electrolytes, and drug effects). The electrocardiogram is easily recorded during exercise.

THE X-RAY. Chest roentgenography is the oldest and one of the most useful techniques for imaging the heart. Radiographic examination utilizes x-rays which are a form of electromagnetic energy. X-rays are created by an energy conversion that occurs when rapidly moving electrons strike a metal target and atoms which comprise the target are converted from one energy state to another. This conversion is produced in an x-ray tube which is a modified vacuum diode tube. The cathode of an x-ray tube consists of a filament which is heated by electrical current. Electrons emitted from the cathode are accelerated by the voltage potential across the tube. These electrons strike the anode or target, which is usually made up of tungsten, and x-rays are emitted from the target. Useful x-rays emerge through a diaphragm at the base of the tube to form a beam which is directed at the patient. This beam consists of x-ray photons which are packets of electromagnetic energy. In passing through the chest a variable fraction of photons is absorbed by body tissues where absorption is determined by the composition of the tissues, their thickness, and the quality of the beam. The photons that emerge from the subject are used to expose a film. The picture created on the film is a superimposition of structures within the chest that absorb x-rays to a variable extent. The cardiovascular structures form silhouettes because of the marked difference between their x-ray absorptive characteristics and those of bone and lung.

The standard radiographic examination of the heart involves a posteroanterior view and a lateral view, usually supplemented by left and right oblique views with barium in the esophagus. Each view is designed to optimize conditions for visualizing various cardiac structures. With appropriate views one can assess the size of individual cardiac chambers, the size of the superior vena cava, the aorta, and the pulmonary artery. The pulmonary vessels can be seen on conventional x-rays, and typical patterns are produced by pulmonary venous engorgement, by increased or decreased pulmonary blood flow, and by pulmonary hypertension. Calcification of valves, the anuli of valves, coronary arteries, and pericardium can be observed, although conventional x-rays are less sensitive than fluoroscopy in detecting calcium. With fluoroscopy one also can visualize the motion of cardiovascular structures.

In many forms of congenital and acquired heart disease, a diagnosis can be made or strongly suspected on the basis of chest x-rays. In practice, however, x-rays are interpreted together with the history, physical examination, and electrocardiogram. In this context, the most useful role of the x-ray is to confirm structural changes suspected by physical examination, to identify structural changes not suspected by physical examination, and to assess on a semiquantitative basis the severity of anatomic and physiologic consequences of heart disease. One of the greatest values of the x-ray is to provide a method for determining the size of cardiovascular structures over time.

THE ECHOCARDIOGRAM. Echocardiography is a noninvasive technique in which high frequency sound waves are directed into the thoracic cavity and echoes reflected from moving cardiac structures are recorded (Fig. 4A). Echoes are produced at the interface between tissues of different acoustic impedance (i.e., at the epicardial surface, at the interface of endocardium and blood, and at the interface of structures such as septa and valves and the blood). The echoes produced by these structures vary in distance from the transducer throughout the heart cycle, and they vary in distance from each other with respect to time (Fig. 4B). With appropriate instrumentation and technique high quality echocardiograms can be obtained in approximately 75 per cent of individuals.

A complete examination should include visualization of the mitral, aortic, tricuspid, and pulmonary valves, and the left atrium, left ventricle, and right ventricle; a sweep from the left ventricle into the aortic root; and assessment of the presence or absence of pericardial fluid.

The importance of echocardiography can be inferred from several observations about its use and diagnostic valve. An echocardiogram is completely noninvasive, is without risk, and requires approximately 30 minutes. Mitral stenosis can be easily recognized, and the orifice of the stenotic valve can be measured. Aortic stenosis can be easily recognized, and although the orifice size is difficult to measure precisely, a demonstration of cusps which open to the periphery of the aortic root rules out significant aortic stenosis. A pulmonary artery diastolic pressure above 20 mm Hg produces a typical change in the diastolic contour of the pulmonary valve. Echocardiography is probably the most sensitive technique available for recognizing left atrial myxoma, mitral valve prolapse, and asymmetric septal hypertrophy with or without subaortic obstruction. It is the only available technique for visualizing vegetations on the valves in infectious endocarditis. The presence of small amounts of pericardial fluid can be detected, and the volume of fluid can be closely estimated. Although there are serious limitations to quantitation of ventricular volume and function from echo studies, chamber dimensions and a qualitative assessment of wall motion have proved to be reliable estimates of chamber size and left ventricular function. Images which are diagnostic of certain forms of congenital heart disease have also been reported. From this brief survey it can be concluded that echocardiography is capable of establishing the diagnosis in several important types of cardiac disease, and it provides important information about structure and function that is otherwise not available short of cardiac catheterization.

RADIONUCLIDE STUDIES. Radionuclide studies of the cardiovascular system involve the injection of an isotope into the circulation and subsequent detection of the energy emitted from the isotope by an appropriate external instrument. Isotopes vary in their mode of decay (for example, emission of electrons or positrons), in their half-life, and in the energy of photons that are liberated as a consequence of decay of the isotope. After variable absorption in body tissues, photons exit from the body and are available for detection. Most detection instruments rely on a thallium-activated sodium iodide crystal which has the property of giving off electrons (a photoelectric event) when struck by photons. The current generated by this event is then amplified many times by a photomultiplier tube and used to expose film or to modulate an oscilloscope beam, or, after conversion to a voltage, is stored in a computer. Imaging devices are of several types. The rectilinear scanner is a single small collimated probe that is moved over the area of interest. The Anger camera is a much larger crystal coupled to an array of 19 to 91 separate photomultiplier tubes which view a very large field. Multicrystal cameras consist of as many as 294 separate crystals. With appropriate collimation, scintillation cameras can be focused to produce tomographic images.

Decay of the positron-emitting isotope results in the emission of two photons per event, and the photons are directed at 180 degrees relative to each other. By placing detectors on opposite sides of the source and operating the detectors in a coincidence mode, events are recorded only if both detectors sense the annihilation photons simultaneously. This amounts to electronic collimation. By rotating the crystal array around the patient, positron cameras can be used to provide tomographic images; and

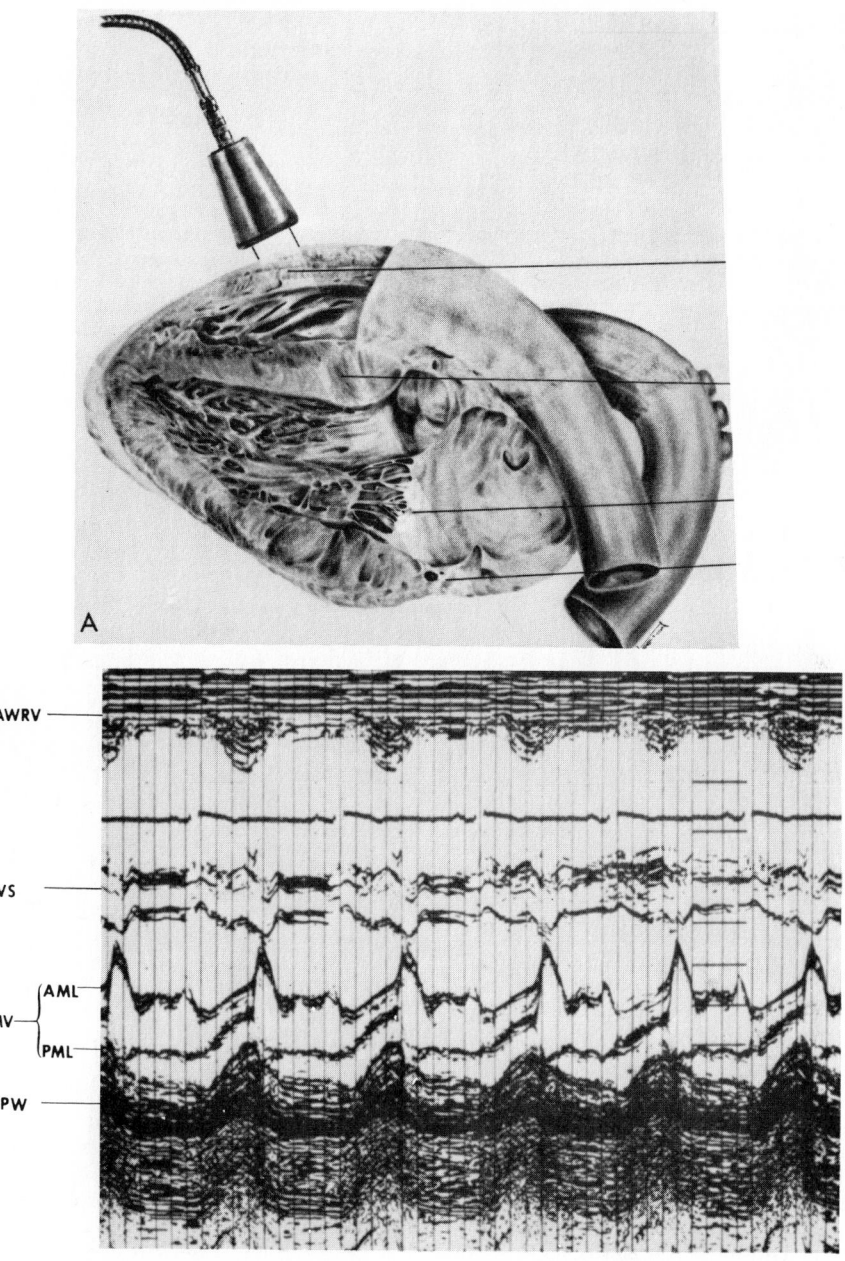

Figure 4. *A,* The ultrasound beam of an echocardiograph and its intersection with various cardiac structures. *B,* The echocardiogram, which shows the motion of various cardiac structures with respect to time and each other.

by an array of 48 crystals surrounding the patient, three-dimensional reconstruction or cross-sectional images can be produced.

Radionuclides can be used to label the blood pool and thus produce images of the cardiac chambers throughout the cardiac cycle to estimate chamber volume, ejection fraction, and wall motion (Fig. 5). A special application is the construction of time-activity plots over specific regions and the application of indicator dilution principles to locate and quantitate intracardiac shunts. Radionuclides such as potassium-43 and thallium-201 are extracted by normal muscle in proportion to blood flow and can be used to evaluate relative regional myocardial perfusion at rest and during exercise. Technetium-99m phos-

phate is localized to acutely necrotic myocardium and gives images that are diagnostic of acute infarction (positive images from 12 hours to three to five days after infarction). Theoretically, positron-emitting isotopes can be used for any of the aforementioned applications. A unique application of positron images results from the availability of isotopes of carbon, oxygen, and nitrogen which can be used to label natural metabolites and thus study regional metabolism of ischemic zones noninvasively and sequentially. It can be projected that noninvasive nuclear cardiology will replace the need for cardiac catheterization in some instances, complement catheterization in other situations, and provide unique data about cardiovascular function unattainable by other methods.

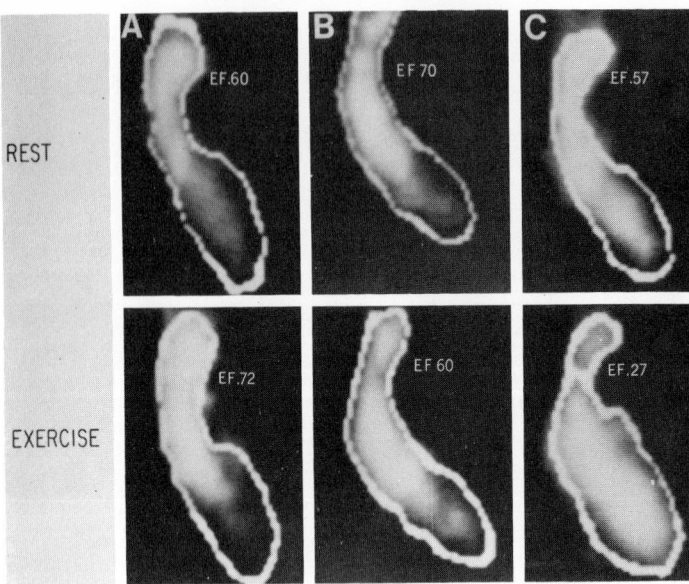

Figure 5. Radionuclide angiogram. Diastolic and systolic images at rest and during exercise are shown for three subjects: *(a)* a normal, *(b)* a patient with two vessel coronary artery disease, and *(c)* a patient with disease of the left main coronary artery. In the normal subject ejection fraction improves with exercise. In the patients with coronary artery disease, ejection fraction deteriorates with exercise.

CARDIAC CATHETERIZATION. Cardiac catheterization provides a method by which the pressure in any or all of the cardiac chambers can be measured with considerable accuracy. Gradients across stenotic valves can be measured, cardiac output and pulmonary blood flow can be estimated, and shunts between the systemic and pulmonary circulation can be localized and quantitated. Contrast agents can be injected to define radiographically the dimensions of the cardiac chambers, to estimate the volume of regurgitation through insufficient valves, and to visualize the anatomy of simple and complex congenital malformations. The aorta and most of its branches, including the coronary arteries, can be selectively catheterized, and deviations from normal anatomy can be defined. The contractile performance of heart muscle can be evaluated, and the adequacy of cardiac output and flow to many individual organs, including the heart, can be deduced from measurement of flow and the arteriovenous difference of several metabolites, including oxygen. Electrode catheters can be used to define the location of conduction delays within the heart, the sequence of excitation, and the mechanism of certain alterations of cardiac rhythm. Catheterization is a powerful diagnostic technique which provides definitive data about many cardiovascular disorders.

There are many cardiac conditions in which the diagnosis can be established by history, physical examination, and noninvasive tests. The severity of the condition can also be assessed with sufficient clarity to judge that the patient is a surgical candidate. Catheterization in these circumstances is performed primarily to provide the surgeon with anatomic and physiologic detail which will help direct his approach to the patient (e.g., an open or closed approach to mitral stenosis, or which coronary arteries should be bypassed in a patient with angina pectoris). Catheterization may also reveal conditions that are unsuspected on clinical grounds or that cannot be judged quantitatively with the accuracy needed to guide the surgical approach (e.g., the presence of associated anomalous pulmonary venous return in a patient with atrial septal defect or aortic insufficiency which was underestimated on clinical grounds in a patient with pre-

dominant mitral regurgitation). Catheterization provides information about myocardial function which may not be adequately assessed on clinical grounds and hence contributes to the evaluation of surgical risk and the likelihood that correction of a valvular, congenital, or coronary lesion will prolong survival and reduce symptoms.

Another role of cardiac catheterization in patients with known heart disease is to enhance our knowledge of the severity of the condition when there is a discrepancy between symptoms and data obtained from physical examination and noninvasive techniques. One of the most noteworthy examples of this situation is the question of whether or not significant mitral stenosis has persisted or recurred in a patient who had mitral commissurotomy with an initially favorable response. On the other hand, patients with hydraulically significant stenosis of the aortic or pulmonary valve or with atrial septal defect may present with clinical signs and EKG and x-ray findings which indicate the need for surgical correction, and yet there may be few symptoms or none at all.

In certain situations cardiac catheterization is performed as a diagnostic procedure in patients in whom a diagnosis can only be suspected on clinical grounds or to clarify the basis of symptoms or signs of unknown significance. Probably the most frequent example is the adult patient with recurrent chest pain compatible with angina in whom the electrocardiogram at rest and during exercise fails to provide evidence of myocardial ischemia. When other noncardiac causes of angina-like chest pain have been searched for and excluded, coronary artery disease cannot be confirmed or excluded as a basis for the symptoms without coronary arteriography. In this situation a normal arteriogram may be very useful in directing attention away from the heart. Similarly, the finding of significant coronary artery disease may lead to a course of therapy (medical or surgical) which is successful in relieving a symptom which was causing significant incapacity.

Despite the usefulness and necessity of cardiac catheterization for situations of the type described above and many others, most cardiac conditions can be recognized and their severity adequately assessed without resorting to catheterization. Catheterization requires hospitalization, it is an expensive test, it causes some discomfort to the patient, and there are risks of arterial injury, embolization, myocardial infarction, reactions to contrast agents, and even death. Fortunately, these occurrences are extremely rare. Cost and the incidence of untoward events are not sufficient reasons to defer or refrain from catheterization when a significant condition is present or suspected and the probability of obtaining data which will be useful to management of the patient is high. Conversely, catheterization should not be undertaken if significant heart disease can be reasonably excluded on the basis of history and physical examination with or without the use of noninvasive laboratory tests. Similarly, cardiac catheterization is not indicated even in the presence of heart disease if the data obtained will not contribute substantially to decisions about management. Furthermore, even when cardiac catheterization can contribute data which would be useful to management, it is not needed if the same or more definitive data can be acquired by a less invasive, less expensive, and lower risk procedure.

STRATEGIES

When the physician has obtained a thorough history and performed a complete physical examination of the cardiovascular system, the next question frequently is whether or not laboratory studies are indicated and, if so, what tests and in what sequence. The answer to this question is not as straightforward as it might seem. What is important is to have a general strategy and a willingness to adapt that strategy in a manner which is appropriate to the problem which led the patient to the doctor, or to the findings obtained from the clinical examination. In any situation it is appropriate to pursue studies until a potential problem has been reasonably excluded or until an actual problem has been defined at the level which is necessary to make a decision about the need for further tests or treatment.

The role of laboratory studies is influenced in part by the age of the patient and the reason for seeking the advice of a doctor. For example, when a teenager is evaluated prior to participating on a high school athletic team and the history and physical examination are normal, most doctors would agree that no laboratory studies are indicated. If the same individual is referred to a cardiologist because of a systolic murmur at the base which radiates to the carotid arteries, and the physical examination, x-ray, and electrocardiogram are otherwise normal, an echocardiogram may show a bicuspid aortic valve without evidence of stenosis. This additional information would provide a basis for encouraging athletic participation, and also advice about prophylactic antibiotics and follow-up over the years ahead.

Is there an age at which certain laboratory tests become routine even in the absence of a history of cardiovascular disease or abnormalities on the physical examination? Many physicians would respond to this question in the affirmative. One example is the physician who is oriented toward preventive cardiology and is interested not only in detecting the presence or absence of disease, but also in detecting conditions which may substantially increase the risk of disease in later life. This strategy is invoked by those who advocate measuring serum choles-

terol and its distribution between high and low density lipoproteins at least once in early adult life, particularly if there is a family history of premature atherosclerotic disease or hyperlipidemia.

There is another justification for obtaining selected tests on a routine basis in young adults. As patients grow older there is an increased probability that they will develop cardiovascular disease. There is also an increased probability that they will develop conditions which may require surgery (e.g., hernia repair, hip replacement). At that stage the consultation of an internist is frequently sought, particularly if the patient is over age 50, and an electrocardiogram and chest x-ray are obtained. If an abnormality is observed on one or both of these tests, it is useful to have a prior x-ray or electrocardiogram. It can be argued that the yield of abnormal electrocardiograms or chest x-rays does not justify obtaining them on a routine basis annually, especially prior to the age of 45 or 50. On the other hand, for the physician who is seeing patients over the age of 45, the availability of one electrocardiogram and chest x-ray at an earlier age when no disease was suspected can be of enormous value in evaluating later records.

When patients present with a history that indicates heart disease or with abnormal physical findings, laboratory tests take on a different role. At one level, certain tests are used to confirm or help interpret an abnormal physical finding. For example, the phonocardiogram can be used to confirm and document the presence and timing of abnormal sounds or murmurs, the apex cardiogram can confirm and document abnormal precordial movements, and external pulse recordings can confirm and document abnormal venous or arterial pulsations. These techniques are useful in teaching and they can be very important when a patient moves from the care of one doctor to another. Echocardiography is a new and exciting noninvasive cardiovascular diagnostic technique. It is probably the most sensitive available method to detect mitral valve prolapse, mitral stenosis, pericardial fluid, left atrial myxoma, and asymmetric septal hypertrophy. Not only is the method sensitive in these conditions, but it is probable that modern two-dimensional echocardiography will eliminate the need for cardiac catheterization to diagnose these conditions.

The most important point is that laboratory studies should be selected and pursued until the nature and severity of the disease can be established with reasonable certainty. If that can be accomplished with noninvasive methods, then tests of greater expense and potential risk are not necessary. On the other hand, when symptoms or signs suggest a severe disease potentially amenable to surgery, or if significant disease is suspected but cannot be clarified by noninvasive techniques, then catheterization is clearly indicated.

Most forms of heart disease are chronic. The approach of a physician whose focus is on prognosis, management, and follow-up requires more information than is required to make a diagnosis. Furthermore, accurate assessments of severity of disease and the response to management require quantifiable and reproducible descriptors. These considerations never justify the performance of costly unnecessary tests which subject the patient to a risk of complications. They emphasize, however, that a complete cardiac evaluation very often includes the use of laboratory procedures which exceed the minimal data base required to make a diagnosis.

355. HEART FAILURE

Alfred P. Fishman

The heart is part of an elaborate circulatory apparatus that is designed to serve two major functions: (1) to provide the tissues with sufficient blood (carrying oxygen, substrates, and nutrients) for their metabolic needs, both at rest and during activity; and (2) to reapportion the cardiac output according to the physiologic priorities of the moment, e.g., muscular exercise, heat loss, digestion. The same regulatory mechanisms that satisfy physiologic priorities in health also serve to protect vital organs, e.g., the heart and brain, when cardiac output is seriously compromised.

As a pump, the heart is remarkable not only for its capacity to adjust rapidly to metabolic need and to varying loads, but also for its durability. Unfortunately, it is also vulnerable to a wide array of congenital, metabolic, inflammatory, and degenerative disorders that affect its muscular walls, its linings, its valves, and particularly its nutrient vessels, i.e., the coronary arteries. Some cardiac disorders, such as arteriosclerosis of the small coronary arteries, progress slowly and insidiously, and their disease takes a lifetime to become clinically evident. Others, such as bacterial infection of the aortic valve, are often dramatic in onset and catastrophic in their consequences.

In general, signs and symptoms of heart disease are of two different kinds: those referable to the heart itself, such as pain and palpitation, and others that are extracardiac and originate in congested circulatory beds and hypoperfused organs. Considered out of context, each extracardiac manifestation may be disappointingly nonspecific. For example, breathlessness is a common symptom that is shared by disorders of the heart, the lungs, and the brain. Nonetheless, when breathlessness develops in a patient with left heart disease in association with other evidence of congested and edematous lungs, and grows worse when the patient lies flat, there is little question that the patient is suffering from left heart failure.

Subsequent chapters in Part XIV will deal with individual cardiac disorders. The present chapter will be concerned with heart failure, a final common pathway for many of the diverse etiologies and pathogenic mechanisms that will be discussed subsequently.

GENERAL ASPECTS

Heart failure may be considered in clinical, physiologic, or biochemical terms. *Clinically*, "heart failure" refers to a distinctive constellation of symptoms and physical signs that has emerged in a patient with an underlying cardiac disorder. *Physiologically*, heart failure is defined as the inability of the heart to match its output to the metabolic needs of the body (determined as O_2 consumption) even though filling pressures of the heart are adequate. The biochemical features are not as certain as the hemodynamic, but appear to involve defective conversion by the heart muscle of chemical energy to mechanical work.

No definition of heart failure is universally acceptable. However, experts generally use the term in one of two ways: (1) to indicate that inadequate performance

of some part of the heart, i.e., valves or myocardium, has evoked the florid clinical picture of pulmonary and systemic venous congestion, or (2) as a synonym for inadequacy of heart muscle secondary either to overloading or to intrinsic disease. In this chapter, the second alternative is chosen, and *heart failure* is used as a synonym for *myocardial failure*. This approach has some distinct advantages: the inept performance of the heart, and the clinical picture that ensues, can be related to physiologic and biochemical events in heart muscle and to the pathogenesis of the heart failure; it avoids confusion with nonmyocardial disorders, which often evoke the same clinical picture but which have different origins and require different therapeutic measures, e.g., valve replacement for aortic stenosis; and it requires that distinction always be maintained between left and right ventricular failure in tracing pathogenesis and with respect to applying therapeutic measures. This stipulation automatically excludes syndromes in which the seat of the difficulty is in abnormalities of the heart valves or pericardium or excessive heart rates — each of which can compromise the circulation even though the cardiac muscle is normal.

Disproportion between hemodynamic load and myocardial capacity to cope with it initiates the sequence that culminates in heart failure. In general, the heart tolerates volume overloads better than pressure overloads. For example, *volume* overload of the left ventricle produced by aortic insufficiency may exist for years without causing distress; in contrast, *pressure* overload from aortic stenosis generally elicits signs and symptoms of heart failure much earlier. Sustained overloads are also accommodated better than acute overloads. Thus chronic mitral regurgitation caused by rheumatic heart disease often lasts for years without signs of heart failure, whereas the acute mitral regurgitation produced by a ruptured chorda tendinea is apt to precipitate a disastrous syndrome of heart failure.

The myocardium responds differently to volume and pressure loads. Volume overloads generally elicit dilatation followed by hypertrophy; conversely, pressure overloads characteristically elicit hypertrophy until late in the natural history when dilatation supervenes. Primary myocardial disease generally elicits both dilatation and hypertrophy.

Categories of Heart Failure

In the clinic, the type of heart failure is generally identified by its duration (acute or chronic), initiating mechanisms, the ventricle that is primarily affected, the characteristic clinical syndrome, and the underlying physiologic derangements.

ACUTE VS. CHRONIC HEART FAILURE. The manifestations of heart failure usually begin insidiously, blurring at the outset with those of the underlying cardiac disorder and continuing gradually into a chronic state. However, the syndrome may also begin acutely, as after myocardial infarction. Between these extremes of acute and chronic heart failure are many instances of subclinical heart failure in which a successful cardiotonic program, coupled with self-restriction of activity by the patient, minimizes signs and symptoms even though cardiac performance remains seriously compromised. On the other hand, it is not uncommon for the course of chronic heart failure that is nicely controlled to be punctuated by bouts of acute heart failure that stem either from lapses in therapy or from progression of the underlying heart disease.

Both acute and chronic heart failure elicit compensatory adjustments. These include increase in peripheral vascular resistance, redistribution of blood flow, and increase in erythropoietic activity. But the adaptive mechanisms differ strikingly in type, degree, and intensity, and even in direction. For example, *acute* distention of the left atrium generally promotes a sodium-poor diuresis, whereas *chronic* distention of the left atrium elicits salt and water retention. This distinction between acute and chronic heart failure must be borne in mind when attempting to relate observations on experimental heart failure in animals to the clinical syndrome of chronic heart failure in man, because experimental heart failure is generally acute in onset, is fulminating in course, and is generally ended abruptly by the death of the animal.

INITIATING MECHANISMS. Each initiating mechanism generally imposes its own distinctive stamp upon the clinical syndrome. Thus rheumatic heart disease leads to a different constellation of symptoms and signs from that of hypertensive heart disease; in turn, both have a different natural history from cor pulmonale. Indeed, even a single etiology, arteriosclerosis, may have distinctly different consequences; progressive narrowing and gradual occlusion of *peripheral* branches of the coronary arteries may be so covert that the characteristic shortness of breath and undue fatigue of left ventricular failure may be misinterpreted as evidence of the general physical decline of advancing age. Conversely, abrupt closure of a major coronary artery, as a consequence of thrombosis superimposed on an arteriosclerotic plaque, may elicit massive myocardial necrosis, followed by extensive myocardial scarring and unremitting heart failure.

LEFT VS. RIGHT HEART FAILURE. With rare exception, one ventricle fails before the other. Because of the prevalence of cardiac disorders which overload or damage the left ventricle, e.g., coronary arteriosclerosis and hypertension, heart failure usually begins with the left ventricle. Breathlessness, the key clinical expression of pulmonary congestion and edema, is the most common initial complaint. Conversely, when the right ventricle fails, systemic venous congestion and peripheral edema generally predominate. Left ventricular failure is the most common cause of right ventricular failure, and breathlessness often improves as right ventricular output falls and pulmonary congestion diminishes.

The mechanism by which left ventricular failure causes the right ventricle to fail is not clear. The conventional explanation puts the blame on pulmonary hypertension secondary to left ventricular failure. But the degree of pulmonary hypertension in this circumstance is rarely enough to constitute a formidable burden on the right ventricle. Much more likely as a predominant mechanism is the continuity of heart muscle that envelops both ventricles. In contrast to the fact that left ventricular failure is the most common cause of right ventricular failure, how often right ventricular failure causes left ventricular failure is still a matter of debate. Resolution of this problem is difficult because of the frequency with which independent and unrelated left ventricular disease coexists with right ventricular failure.

The combination of left and right ventricular failure, in which evidences of systemic and pulmonary venous hypertension predominate, is traditionally referred to as "congestive heart failure." This is a colloquialism that conveys the image of severe physical incapacity, breathlessness, distended neck veins, hepatic engorgement, and troublesome peripheral edema. But it also highlights clinical features that can be measured at the bedside: a high venous pressure, a prolonged circulation time, and a diminished vital capacity, all of which improve as the patient gets better.

BACKWARD VS. FORWARD HEART FAILURE. Somewhat reminiscent of the fable about the blind men and the elephant is the vintage controversy about "backward" versus "forward" heart failure. "Backward failure" calls attention to the damming up of blood in the veins proximal to the failing ventricle and attributes to this venous congestion a critical role in the evolution of the syndrome of heart failure; "forward failure" assigns the same pivotal role to a decrease in cardiac output and underfilling of the arterial tree. In reality this distinction is meaningless, because it is inevitable in a closed circuit that the inability of the heart to sustain its output (forward failure) and the pooling of blood on the venous inflow side (backward failure) must go hand in hand.

LOW VS. HIGH OUTPUT FAILURE. Cardiac catheterization in man has made it possible to sort myocardial failure according to the level of the cardiac output. This practice has served at least three purposes: (1) to separate, on clinical and physiologic grounds, a type of myocardial failure ("high output failure") in which the circulation remains vigorous and the extremities remain warm despite venous congestion, edema, and a lower cardiac output than existed prior to the heart failure; (2) to emphasize that the level of the cardiac output and the circulatory adjustments during myocardial failure are, to large extent, a consequence of the cardiac output that existed prior to heart failure; and (3) to relate etiology and clinical evidences of heart failure to the state of the circulation: the more common causes of heart failure — arteriosclerosis, hypertension, myocardial disease, valvular disease, and pericardial disease — tend to be low output states; less common causes, such as hyperthyroidism, Paget's disease, anemia, beriberi, and arteriovenous fistula, tend to be high output states. But the hemodynamic hallmark of cardiac failure remains the same regardless of the level of cardiac output at rest: an inability of the heart to increase its output (or stroke volume or stroke work) as end-diastolic volume (as well as pressure) is increased (see Preload, below).

The separation into "high" and "low" output failure is concerned with the clinical manifestations, rather than the causes, of myocardial failure. But it is also a hemodynamic frame of reference to which the anatomist and the biochemist can relate the myocardial origins of heart failure. For example, "high output" failure probably has different biochemical bases from "low output" failure. Nor are all types of "low output" or "high output" failure apt to have the same biochemical origins. For example, it is unlikely that the "high output" failure of a peripheral arteriovenous fistula has the same anatomic or biochemical beginnings and evolution as the "high output" failure of severe anemia or malnutrition.

CONGESTIVE FAILURE VS. CONGESTED STATE. Overfilling of the circulation, without myocardial failure, is the hallmark of the "congested state." It may be induced by rapid infusions; it is common in severe anemia and in chronic renal insufficiency. Similar but less dramatic venous congestion may also complicate Paget's disease or beriberi. In each of these situations, venous hypertension arises from a combination of an expanded venous volume and heightened venomotor tone, rather than from heart failure.

It is true that persistence of a "hyperkinetic" congested state may, in time, cause the heart muscle to fail from overwork. The onset of myocardial failure may then be difficult to detect on clinical grounds, because the hyperkinetic circulation persists and the congestion may be only slightly increased during myocardial failure. Accordingly, the transition from the congested state to congestive heart failure may be difficult to detect on clinical grounds alone. But when heart failure does supervene, cardiac catheterization will disclose an inadequate increase in cardiac output during exercise as well as a considerable increase in cardiac output after digitalis. Fortunately, identification of the transition from a "congested state" to "congestive heart failure" is of greater theoretical than practical importance, because therapeutic measures, such as the administration of diuretics and the replacement of particular nutrients, e.g., thiamin in beriberi, are effective in both situations. However, digitalis will exert an important therapeutic effect once the myocardium has failed, whereas it is clinically useless when administered to a heart that is coping well with an overfilled circulation.

Subcellular Bases for Contraction

With each beat, the heart develops force and expends energy. Electrical activity at the cell surface activates the contractile machinery. Connecting the electrical activity at the surface and the contractile machinery within the muscle cell is the sarcoplasmic reticulum which plays a critical role in the release and uptake of calcium during contraction and relaxation.

For the development of the contractile force, heart muscle depends on interactions among contractile proteins, the hypothetical "elastic components" with which they are connected in series, and the constraining bounds within which the contractile elements function. The contractile proteins are contained within sarcomeres, repeating units that comprise the individual muscle fibers (myofibrils). Within the sarcomere, the contractile proteins are arranged in two orderly groups of myofilaments, one consisting of myosin, the other predominantly of actin. Holding the contractile apparatus at bay are two modulator proteins, troponin and tropomyosin. Delivery of calcium to troponin from the sarcoplasmic reticulum and sarcolemma sets the contractile process into motion.

To account for changes in the length of heart muscle during contraction and relaxation, the sliding filament hypothesis of Huxley is generally invoked: during contraction, the thin actin filaments slide past the thicker myosin filaments to shorten the sarcomere; the entire muscle cell follows suit. Conversely, during relaxation, the sarcomeres and the muscle cell resume their initial lengths as the original actin-myosin relationships are restored. Nearby mitochondria generate energy for the contractile machinery by oxidative phosphorylation of free fatty acids and glucose supplied by the circulation.

The tension that is developed in cardiac muscle during contraction depends on actin-myosin relationships. Projecting from the myosin filaments are cross-bridges. Before activation, these bridges are not attached to actin filaments. Upon activation, the cross-bridges on the myosin filaments lock into receptor sites on the actin filaments, thereby developing the force that leads to contraction. As the muscle shortens, the cross-bridges disengage and slide along the actin filament, like a pawl on a ratchet, to engage other sites. Depending on the number of cross-bridges that are interlocked at the same time, different tensions will be developed.

In addition to these subcellular elements that are directly involved in the contractile process, there appears to be a subcellular beta sympathomimetic system that can enhance the inotropic state. Although an increase in intracellular calcium is involved, the precise mechanism is unclear.

Evidence exists that for the sarcomere, as for the whole heart (see Preload, below), the tension developed during contraction is directly related to its initial length. This correspondence implies that, for the whole heart, stretching increases the ability of its individual contractile elements to develop force. Also, since stretching does not affect the rate of interaction of active sites, elongation of cardiac muscle fibers before contraction should not affect the velocity of the subsequent contraction. These considerations underlie many current notions about cardiac contractility. But it is still unclear whether the ultrastructural-physiologic correlations are real or simply models for eliciting a new kind of reflection about an exceedingly complicated problem.

PATHOPHYSIOLOGIC INTERPLAY

Each ventricle functions as a separate muscular pump supplied by its own booster pump (atrium). The two ventricles empty in unison, simultaneously dispatching their respective contents: the right ventricle sending blood to the lungs for arterialization, the left ventricle sending arterialized blood to the rest of the body for metabolic purposes. In the normal heart, at least 50 per cent of the end-diastolic volume is ejected with each beat. Much of the ejection force is the result of the inherent properties (fiber-length and inotropism) of the myocardium. But a wide range of adaptability to the ever-changing metabolic needs of daily life is provided by a superimposed series of extrinsic neurohumoral adjustments which, in daily life, modify and obscure the intrinsic inherent properties of the heart muscle.

Each ventricle, as with any man-made machine, is endowed with a finite capacity for stress, strain, and repair. The two ventricles also have somewhat different designs in keeping with their different long-range functions as pumps. The rate of obsolescence of each ventricle depends on the wear and tear to which it is subjected, its supply of nutriments and substrates, and its continuing state of good health. Before birth, both ventricles are taxed equally, because they bear the same pressure loads. After birth, as pulmonary arterial pressure falls, the right ventricular burden decreases and its walls thin. Consequently, other influences remaining equal, the durability of right ventricular performance is destined from birth to exceed that of the left ventricle. The brighter prospects of the right ventricle for longevity in performance are intensified by the greater vulnerability of the left side of the heart to disease and to disorders in its blood supply.

Assessment of Cardiac Performance

With respect to evaluating cardiac performance, the heart may be regarded from three points of view: as a pump; as a muscle; and as a component of the circulation. Hemodynamic measurements are used to characterize its behavior as a pump: cardiac output, stroke output, stroke work, stroke power, ventricular end-diastolic pressure, ejection fraction, and ventricular end-diastolic volume. To ascertain its behavior as a muscle, principles of muscle mechanics are applied. Its adequacy as a component of the circulation is reflected in the derangements that result from the low cardiac output, the redistribution of blood flow among tissues and organs, organ hypoperfusion, and venous congestion.

Heart as a Pump: Hemodynamics

By the time the heart fails, a variety of mechanisms are operating to bolster its flagging performance. In contrast to the inappropriately low cardiac output, the blood pressure generally remains normal or even increases.

CARDIAC OUTPUT. At each level of activity, in health and disease, a complicated interplay automatically adjusts the extent of shortening of myocardial fibers and, consequently, the stroke volume and the cardiac output. Four principal determinants set the stroke volume: preload (Table 1), afterload (ventricular emptying during

systole), the inotropic characteristics of the heart, and the coordinated pattern of contraction. A fifth determinant, the heart rate, sets the cardiac output (stroke volume times heart rate). For practical purposes, three of these five principal determinants of cardiac output — preload, afterload, heart rate — are quantifiable. Attempts are currently under way to depict quantitatively the fourth, i.e., the contribution of different regions of the ventricular myocardium to the ejection of blood from the heart. But the fifth, i.e., the inotropic state, remains difficult to assess (Fig. 1) except in the extreme, i.e., when the heart is large and evidence exists of venous congestion and organ hypoperfusion.

Relationships among these determinants are not fixed; they play greater or lesser roles, depending on the state of the heart. Thus when the inherent contractility (inotropic state) is impaired, stroke output and cardiac output may be maintained by ventricular dilatation (Frank-Starling mechanism). This flexible arrangement limits the value of cardiac output as a measure of cardiac contractility (inotropic state) to situations in which preload, afterload, and heart rate can be held constant. Unfortunately, this degree of control of loading conditions and heart rate is easier to achieve in the experimental laboratory than in clinical situations.

Indicator-dilution techniques are now widely used for the bedside determination of cardiac output. The normal range in adults at rest is between 2.5 and 3.6 liters per minute per square meter. A decrease in cardiac output at rest represents a late stage in abnormal cardiac performance. Failure to increase cardiac output during exercise occurs much earlier. Thus in normal subjects exercising in a supine position, the increase in cardiac output exceeds 600 ml per minute for each 100 ml increase in oxygen consumption. Lower values indicate abnormal cardiac performance. In heart failure, the arteriovenous difference for oxygen is abnormally wide,

---

TABLE 1.   Terms Used to Describe Mechanical Performance of the Heart

Term	Relation to Cardiac Function
Inotropic state	A measure of contractility.
Preload	Stretch of myocardial fibers at end-diastole.
Afterload (during ejection)	Force that the ventricle must develop during systole in order to eject the stroke volume. The two major determinants are aortic impedance and left ventricular volume. Afterload is usually expressed as wall stress or wall tension; also, as instantaneous force at some point during ventricular ejection or as mean wall force throughout systole.
Wall tension (during ejection)	Total force per unit of ventricular circumferential length. Determined as product of systolic pressure and radius of ventricle in accord with Laplace equation. Independent of wall thickness.
Wall stress (during ejection)	Force per unit of cross-sectional wall area. Determined as product of pressure and radius divided by wall thickness. Reduced by thickening of wall in ventricular hypertrophy.
Impedance (during ejection)	Instantaneous relationship between rate of change in aortic pressure and aortic blood flow. The aortic input impedance reflects the forces external to the heart that impose a load on the left ventricle, including stiffness of aortic wall. Determined primarily, but not exclusively, by total peripheral vascular resistance to run off from the arterial tree. Normal peripheral resistance is approximately 1500 dynes sec/cm^{-5} or 15 peripheral resistance units.
Energetics	Generally determined as myocardial oxygen consumption. For any contractile state, the force developed and maintained during contraction represents the major mechanical determinant of oxygen consumption. An increase in myocardial wall force (tension or stress) that accompanies an increase in filling pressure and radius (Laplace equation) in heart failure increases the energy cost of contraction.

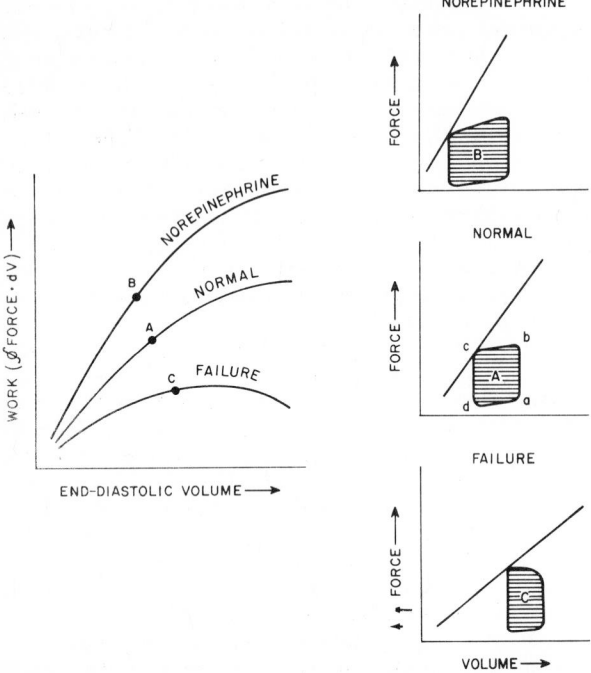

Figure 1. Schematic ventricular function (Frank-Starling) curves (left). By using work (instead of stroke output) on the ordinate, the work done per beat can be analyzed using force-volume curves (right). The three curves correspond to the normal (A), failing (C), and highly contractile (B) hearts on the Frank-Starling curves.

Left, The effects of preload and contractility on ventricular function curves. The normal left ventricle (A) increases its stroke output as preload (measured clinically as pulmonary wedge pressure) increases, moving up the ascending limb of the curve until preload reserve is exhausted. In severe heart failure, the ventricular function curve is displaced downward and to the right. The preload reserve is gone, and the heart is operating chronically on the descending limb of curve (C). An increase in contractility, as after administering norepinephrine, displaces the curve to the left, i.e., a large stroke output is accomplished at lower filling pressures (B).

Right, Work loops per beat corresponding to points B, A, and C on the ventricular function curves. The sloping line in each curve defines the contractility of the particular heart under consideration. On the perimeter of the work loop in the cardiac cycle are indicated the following landmarks: a = end diastole; b = opening of aortic valve; c = closure of aortic valve; d = start of filling of heart.

In comparison with the normal heart (center), the failing heart (lower) does just about as much work (total area under curve), at a high filling pressure, but ejects less per beat (d-a). Norepinephrine improves the contractility, so that the end-diastolic volume and pressure decrease whereas the stroke output (d-a) improves greatly. (Based on Weber and Janicki.)

resulting almost entirely from the low oxygen content of venous blood returning to the heart rather than from impaired oxygenation in the lungs.

During exercise, heart rate and cardiac output increase as linear functions of oxygen consumption. This is true during both supine and upright exercise, but for any level of exercise the cardiac output is appreciably lower in the upright position. These increases in cardiac output are accomplished principally by acceleration of the heart rate rather than by increase in the stroke volume. In heart failure, cardiac output is even more

dependent on heart rate, both at rest and during exercise.

VENTRICULAR END-DIASTOLIC PRESSURE. Inadequate ventricular emptying during systole leads to an increase in the residual volume of blood in the ventricle after systole, and thereby to an increase in end-diastolic ventricular volume. Since end-diastolic ventricular volumes are difficult to measure, end-diastolic ventricular pressures are generally substituted. This practice depends on the premise that a change in pressure is effected by a change in ventricular volume. However, exceptions to this rule do occur: structural changes in the myocardium (fibrosis, edema, hypertrophy, hemorrhage) and pericardial restriction cause end-diastolic pressure to increase without increment in volume, i.e., compliance is decreased. Conversely, in some states of chronic volume overloading of the ventricle, compliance decreases so that large volumes are accommodated at end-diastole without increasing pressure to abnormal levels.

An end-diastolic pressure in the *left* ventricle greater than 12 to 15 mm Hg is abnormal; for the right ventricle, the corresponding upper limit of normal is 10 mm Hg. It is rather simple to estimate the right ventricular end-diastolic pressure by measuring the central venous pressure; the left ventricular end-diastolic pressure is more difficult to estimate because of its inaccessibility. However, in the absence of mitral obstruction or of an increase in pulmonary vascular resistance, pulmonary arterial diastolic pressure provides a useful estimate of left ventricular end-diastolic pressure. Pulmonary wedge pressure is now widely used as a measure of left ventricular end-diastolic pressure.

The performance of the heart depends on two essential components: fiber length (Frank-Starling mechanism) and the inherent contractility (inotropic state) of the muscle. The normal heart is keyed to respond automatically to maintain the cardiac output. The factors that are involved are preload, afterload, contractility, and heart rate. In response to chronic overloading, the heart undergoes dilatation or hypertrophy or a combination of the two.

PRELOAD (THE FRANK-STARLING MECHANISM). According to this mechanism, an increase in end-diastolic volume (preload) is followed by a more forceful contraction that improves ventricular emptying. To assess the Frank-Starling mechanism, only preload should vary, i.e., afterload and heart rate are kept constant for each level of contractility. A distinctive "ventricular performance" curve exists for each state of contractility (Fig. 1). Thus the curve for a failing ventricle is depressed and flat so that small stroke volumes are delivered at abnormally high end-diastolic volumes. The high filling pressures are responsible for congestion and edema in the venous beds that lead to the ventricle that has failed.

In the normal heart, the Frank-Starling mechanism operates chiefly to match the stroke outputs of the two ventricles. But in heart failure, this mechanism plays an important part in sustaining the cardiac output.

AFTERLOAD. Afterload refers to the force that the ventricle must develop during systole in order to eject the stroke volume. In principle, it provides a measure of all factors that oppose active shortening of the ventricular fibers. In practice, because of the difficulties of estimating all these factors, impedance is estimated either from the arterial blood pressure or from a calculation of systemic vascular resistance (ratio of blood pressure to flow, expressed in dynes sec/cm^{-5} or in peripheral resistance units).

For clinical purposes, the relationship of blood pressure to cardiac output and peripheral resistance (P/Flow = R) is quite useful. For example, any intervention that causes a large increase in cardiac output without changing systemic blood pressure presumably causes vasodilation, thereby decreasing calculated peripheral vascular resistance, impedance, and afterload (wall force). Accompanying the improved emptying of the left ventricle is a decrease in its filling pressure (measured by pulmonary wedge pressure).

Increasing the afterload on the normal heart (while preload and contractility remain constant) decreases both the degree and speed of wall shortening; reduction in afterload has the opposite effect.

CONTRACTILITY. Increase in sympathetic nervous activity provides the major inotropic effect for the normal heart (in conjunction with increase in heart rate and venous tone). In contrast to the Frank-Starling mechanism, the increase in force and velocity of contraction is accomplished without corresponding increase in fiber length (end-diastolic ventricular volume). Contractility does not limit the performance of the normal heart. In contrast, the failing heart is limited in its myocardial performance as indicated by displacement of the ventricular function curve downward and to the right. An increase in afterload in severe heart failure moves the heart to the descending limb; conversely, improvement in contractility displaces the heart toward the normal curve.

Inotropic State. Clinicians would welcome an objective index of myocardial contractility in which the inotropic state (intrinsic contractility of the muscle) could be measured independent of change in the length of myocardial fibers (Frank-Starling relationship). This would be useful in three different ways: (1) to examine the effects on the myocardium of an acute intervention, such as the administration of digitalis, (2) to determine consecutive changes in the inotropic state of the myocardium in the same individual during the evolution of heart failure and in response to treatment; and (3) to compare the inotropic state in different individuals.

Unfortunately, distinction between the effects of fiber length and of intrinsic contractility is difficult to accomplish for the heart. The main obstacle stems from the strong influence of mechanical loading conditions on hemodynamic measurements. Thus a change in either the preload (length of ventricular fibers at end-diastole) or the afterload (force developed in ventricular muscle during systole) can modify ventricular performance greatly without affecting its intrinsic inotropic state. Another complication is the inability of conventional hemodynamic measurements to take heart size into account so that comparisons of contractility in hearts of different size are generally unreliable.

Because changes in mechanical loading conditions confuse determinations of inotropic state, attempts are being made (1) to make these determinations under constant conditions of mechanical loading (constant diastolic volume, aortic pressure) and heart rate, (2) to devise methods for determining inotropic state that are insensitive to loading conditions, or (3) to interpret hemodynamic values in terms of a change in inotropic state when loading conditions can be adequately dis-

counted. But when determinants of mechanical performance other than inotropic state cannot be discounted — which is usually the case — more independent indices of contractility have been sought, particularly the rate of rise in ventricular pressure in the pre-ejection phase of ventricular contraction and force-velocity relationships.

Rate of Increase in Intraventricular Pressure (dp/dt). Several indices of dp/dt are being used. In practice dp/dt is determined electronically as the first derivative of the ventricular pressure. For comparative purposes, measurements are generally made at some preselected point(s) in the cardiac cycle, e.g., at 40 mm Hg. Often the value for dp/dt is further standardized by reference to some common denominator; e.g., peak dp/dt may be divided by total pressure instead of being used as dp/dt, per se. At present, application in man of the dp/dt determinations is handicapped by the need for extraordinarily high fidelity recording systems and by the difficulty in reproducing loading conditions. Although it holds considerable promise for comparisons of contractile performance in a single patient before and after intervention, it has little prospect for comparing different hearts.

As in the case of pressure, the rate of development of wall tension is also decidedly abnormal in heart failure. Moreover, in contrast to the normal heart in which wall tension decreases during systole, wall tension in heart failure remains high throughout systole so that both the velocity and the degree of shortening are abnormal.

Velocity of Contraction. The use of the velocity of contraction as a measure of contractility became popular a few years ago. In principle, it was based on force-velocity relationships developed by A. V. Hill for skeletal muscle. However, the great promise that was envisaged for this approach has not materialized.

EJECTION FRACTION. The fraction of the end-diastolic volume that is ejected per beat is termed the "ejection fraction." It is widely used as a measure of contractility and is estimated angiographically or by echocardiography. The normal systolic ejection fraction ranges from 0.56 to 0.78. A reduction in ejection fraction suggests that the ventricle is excessively dilated as a result of a depressed inotropic state.

SYSTOLIC TIME INTERVALS. Simultaneous recording of the electrocardiogram, phonocardiogram, and carotid arterial pulse allows indirect bedside appraisal of cardiac function. By this combination of recordings, total electromechanical systole is subdivided into left ventricular ejection time and the pre-ejection period. In patients with abnormalities of myocardial contractility — even before overt congestive heart failure — pre-ejection time usually lengthens, whereas ejection time shortens (the normal ratio of pre-ejection time to left ventricular ejection time is 0.35 ± 0.04 SD). This noninvasive technique is most useful in chronic coronary artery disease, arterial hypertension, and the cardiomyopathies. It does not distinguish between inotropic state and other mechanical determinants of contractility, particularly loading of the ventricle. Disturbances in conduction, valvular disease, and other unanticipated disorders may invalidate the determinations.

Chronic Compensatory Mechanisms

In principle, the heart that is chronically in a state of failure has recourse to four compensatory mechanisms:

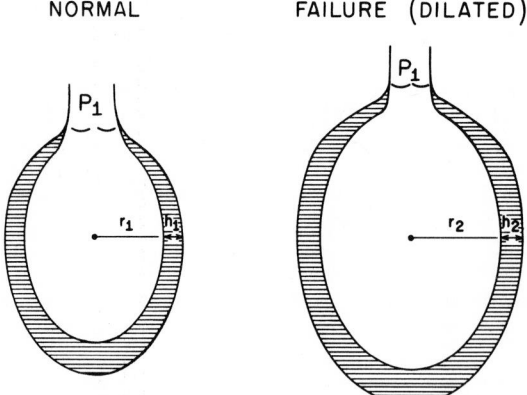

NORMAL   FAILURE (DILATED)

Figure 2. Laplace relationship applied to the dilated heart. The tension developed in the wall of the heart during systole (T) is a directional force that is proportional to the product of the mean pressure that the wall is supporting (P) and the mean radius (r). Dilatation of the heart ($r_2 > r_1$) at the same pressure ($P_1 = P_2$) increases wall tension ($T_2 > T_1$). Should the wall become thinner during dilatation, the wall stress would increase as the cross-sectional area of myocardium (h) decreased (equation 2). The use of wall force (equation 3) which is proportional to the pressure and volume of the chamber eliminates considerations of chamber size and shape and of the thickness of the myocardial wall.

Wall tension = Force per circumferential length of myocardium

$$= \frac{P \cdot \pi r^2}{2\pi r} \tag{1}$$

$$= \frac{P \cdot r}{2}$$

Wall stress = Force per cross-sectional area of myocardium

$$= \frac{P \cdot \pi r^2}{2\pi r h} \tag{2}$$

$$= \frac{P \cdot r}{2h}$$

Wall force = Pressure · cross-sectional area of chamber
$$= P \cdot \pi r^2 \tag{3}$$

increased contractility due to sympathetic nervous activity, tachycardia, hypertrophy, and dilatation. Of the four, the increase in sympathetic activity is more of a burden than a blessing, since it increases peripheral vascular resistance without contributing appreciably to the inotropic state of the faltering heart. Sympathetic activity does, however, contribute indirectly to support the cardiac output by reflexly increasing the heart rate.

HEART RATE. Chronic tachycardia is a feature of heart failure. Much of the increase in heart rate stems from cardiac reflexes that are stimulated by distention of the great veins at their junctions with the atria (Bainbridge reflex). However, in terms of energetics, tachycardia is a costly way to run the heart. Indeed, it is possible to produce, or to precipitate, heart failure by inducing tachycardia.

DILATATION. Progressive and persistent dilatation marks the transition between ventricular hypertrophy and failure. For a long while, dilatation may serve as a compensatory mechanism, increasing the contractile force of the heart by way of the Frank-Starling relationship. But dilatation gradually becomes inadequate to maintain stroke output.

Several different mechanisms seem to be involved in the ultimate inability of the dilated heart to maintain its output: (1) slippage and rearrangement of sarcomeres during progressive dilatation; as a result, they neither produce a coordinated contraction nor are properly stretched to enhance contractility as the heart dilates further; (2) high wall tension in accord with the

law of Laplace (Fig. 2); as the volume of the ventricle increases so that its wall tension for a given pressure in the ventricular cavity during contraction is greater than normal, the myocardial oxygen consumption increases accordingly; (3) protracted maintenance of high wall tension during contraction; in contrast to the normal heart, in which the wall tension decreases in the course of systole, wall tension remains high in the dilated heart; (4) high energy requirements coupled with an inefficient conversion of chemical to mechanical energy; despite the decrease in stroke output, the dilated heart does more internal work and has a higher myocardial oxygen consumption than does the normal heart. Because of these limitations, chronic enlargement is an inefficient and ill-fated mechanism for achieving sustained improvement in cardiac performance.

HYPERTROPHY. Chronic exposure to abnormal pressure and volume loads leads to hypertrophy, i.e., an increase in ventricular mass. This increase in muscle mass takes time to develop. It involves increased protein synthesis in response to mechanical overload or dilatation. The stimulus for hypertrophy may be an increase either in wall force (tension) in accord with the Laplace relationship (Fig. 2) or in the energy requirements of a heart that is chronically dilated or operating at high filling pressures.

The pattern of hypertrophy depends on the load. In response to chronic volume overloading, e.g., arteriovenous fistula, the total mass increases as the chamber size enlarges but thickness does not change. This pattern is known as "eccentric" hypertrophy. In contrast, in chronic exposure to increased afterload, e.g., systemic hypertension, the end-diastolic volume remains unchanged, whereas the wall thickens. This pattern is known as "concentric" hypertrophy.

Normal ventricular contraction is a smoothly coordinated process by which the ventricular wall moves inward during systole to eject its contents. Abnormal electrical conduction interferes with this smooth performance and with ventricular function. The coordinated mechanism is further disrupted by local disease that causes zones of fibrosis to alternate with normal zones. This disposition of normal and abnormal areas leads to hypertrophy of functioning muscle not only because the geometry of the abnormal ventricle causes it to operate at a mechanical disadvantage but also because normal muscle is obliged to do work, and to expend energy, in moving and stretching damaged muscle or scar upon which it abuts.

Early in hypertrophy, muscle mass and capillary vessels increase proportionately and the contractile properties of the myocardium are preserved. But later, the inotropic behavior becomes abnormal and the capacity of the myocardium to synthesize adrenergic transmitter decreases. Indeed, once hypertrophy begins, the myocardium has been eased on the road to failure.

In the depressed inotropic state associated with hypertrophy, circulatory function is maintained for a long while by the combination of the increase in muscle mass, the Frank-Starling mechanism (Fig. 2), and augmented sympathetic stimulation by way of circulating catecholamines. But as the myocardial inotropic state continues to deteriorate, perhaps after intrinsic catecholamine stores have been depleted, circulatory compensation can no longer be maintained. Resting cardiac output then fails and filling pressures increase, leading to the clinical and hemodynamic manifestations of congestive heart failure.

Heart As A Muscle

Most studies of ventricular performance during heart failure have centered around the contraction phase. Before embarking upon these considerations, it is pertinent to consider how events during diastole influence the subsequent contraction and how the energy for cardiac contraction is derived.

RELAXATION AND DISTENSIBILITY. Filling of the ventricle during diastole depends not only on the time available but also on the pattern of relaxation. Relaxation consists of two components: an active one, which promotes relaxation by way of intrinsic mechanisms; and a passive one, arising from extension of the fibers by the inflowing blood. Incomplete relaxation would be expected not only to increase the filling pressure of the heart but also to dissipate energy. In the normal heart, the active and passive components appear to work synergistically to minimize losses in chemical energy. But in heart failure the viscous and elastic properties of the heart muscle seem to change so that there is a diminished resistance to filling (decreased "impedance") and an increased extent of ventricular expansion on filling (increased "compliance"). Thus not only the velocity and duration of relaxation but also changes in the physical properties of the muscle seem involved in heart failure.

ENERGETICS. The heart does work and expends energy during each contraction. For its supply of energy, it depends on aerobic metabolism. Some energy is expended to satisfy its basic oxygen requirements and those of activation. But the bulk of the energy is spent during contraction.

Attempts have been made over the years to dissect physiologically the major determinants of oxygen consumption of the heart. The variables that have been examined are ventricular pressure, volume, work, wall force, and contractile state. The major determinant for any given contractile state has proved to be the force (calculated as the product of ventricular volume and pressure) that is developed in the myocardium at the start of ejection and that continues to the end of systole. At each instant during ejection this wall force is changing. It is the integral of systolic force that relates closely to myocardial oxygen consumption. Other important influences in addition to wall force are heart rate and contractility. In contrast, fiber shortening has negligible effect on myocardial oxygen consumption.

For its contraction, the heart depends on the conversion of the chemical energy of oxidizable substrates into the mechanical energy of muscular contraction. ATP participates in this process as the principal store of energy released by oxidation; its breakdown by myosin ATPase is the principal way by which chemical energy is transformed into mechanical energy. ATP resynthesis in the myocardium is accomplished chiefly through oxidative phosphorylation. The rate of ATP breakdown and the quantity of energy used by the myocardium depend chiefly on the tension that is developed in the myocardial fibers rather than on the degree of shortening or the work done; this developed tension causes the ventricular walls to contract and the blood to be ejected. From a biochemical point of view, the muscle of a ventricle has failed when its generation of free energy, or its utilization of that energy in the process of contraction, is insufficient for the circulatory load which it has to handle.

Unfortunately, the biochemical basis for heart failure is not yet settled. But it is now clear that there are no consistent defects in energy metabolism or in protein synthesis. The investigative focus at present is on excitation-coupling and the role of calcium in the contractile process.

Any physiologic change or pharmacologic intervention will increase myocardial oxygen requirements if it increases either preload or afterload, increases the contractile state of the myocardium, or increases the heart rate. The usual compensatory mechanisms in severe heart failure tend to increase myocardial oxygen requirements by increasing all these parameters: fluid retention increases preload; sympathetic mechanisms increase afterload, contractility, and heart rate. Similarly, the usual interventions employed in heart failure may or may not increase myocardial oxygen requirements further, depending on the balance of changes in the aforementioned determinants in each individual case.

Heart as Component of Circulation

As the overburdened ventricle fails, it elicits venous hypertension and slowed circulation, and sets into motion peripheral mechanisms to sustain blood pressure and cardiac output.

VENOUS HYPERTENSION. With the onset of failure, the ventricle fails to empty properly during systole so that the volume of blood left in the ventricle after contraction increases, i.e., ejection fraction decreases. An increase in diastolic pressure in the ventricles and in the atrium and veins that lead to the ventricle accompanies the increase in ventricular volume. Several other elements contribute to the venous hypertension: (1) heightened venomotor tone; (2) expansion of the blood volume as a consequence of sodium retention by the kidney; and, on occasion, (3) regurgitation of blood from ventricle to atrium as the atrioventricular valve becomes incompetent either from ventricular dilatation or from improper closure during an arrhythmia.

SLOWED CIRCULATION. The circulation time depends on the cardiac output and the volume of blood interposed between the sites of sampling and injection. Should either ventricle fail, the time for a tracer substance to pass from the site of intravenous injection to the site of detection will be prolonged. For example, in left heart failure, the arm-to-tongue circulation time, measured by using Decholin as a tracer, will be prolonged beyond the normal limits of 10 to 15 seconds; delay of the tracer in traversing the pulmonary circulation and dilated left heart, as well as excessive dilution of the tracer by the enlarged intervening blood volume, contributes to the delay. Similarly, the arm-to-breath circulation time measured after the intravenous injection of ether will be prolonged in right heart failure. By relating the circulation times to the central venous pressure, it may be possible to establish at the bedside which ventricle has failed. For example, in left heart failure, central venous pressure and ether circulation time will be normal, whereas Decholin time will be prolonged.

PERIPHERAL MECHANISMS TO SUSTAIN CARDIAC OUTPUT AND BLOOD PRESSURE. In order to sustain the cardiac output, to apportion it selectively, and to maintain the systemic arterial blood pressure, a variety of peripheral mechanisms are activated.

Autonomic Nervous System. Normally, a four- or fivefold increase in oxygen consumption elicits a doubling of the cardiac output. When the increase in cardiac output cannot keep pace with the level of activity, distribution of blood flow is altered to defend vital areas, e.g., brain and heart. The autonomic nervous system is deeply involved in this rearrangement of the circulation. It also contributes to activation of the mechanisms for retaining sodium and water.

Peripheral vasoconstriction and tachycardia are the hallmarks of the usual forms of heart failure. Paradoxically, despite a generalized increase in sympathetic nervous activity, norepinephrine stores in the heart muscle are depleted because of defective local synthesis. Consequently, the failing heart, denied local adrenergic support for its inotropic and chronotropic responses, is obliged to rely on norepinephrine delivered to it by the blood from the adrenal medulla and the peripheral vasculature. Pharmacologic agents, such as guanethidine, which further deplete the heart of its catecholamines, aggravate heart failure. In many respects, the performance of the human heart that has failed resembles that of both the "denervated" heart and the isolated heart-lung preparation that Starling used. The role that the parasympathetic nervous system plays in heart failure is ill defined, but evidence does exist to indicate that its contribution to the control of heart rate and baroreceptor activity is impaired.

PERIPHERAL VASOCONSTRICTION. Peripheral arteriolar and venoconstriction, mediated by heightened sympathetic nervous activity, are essential compensatory mechanisms in heart failure. The extent to which accumulation of sodium and water in the arteriolar wall contributes to increased arteriolar resistance is as yet unclear. Selective arteriolar vasoconstriction helps not only to sustain the blood pressure but also to preserve function in critical organs. The pattern of selective vasoconstriction, in turn, influences the cardiac output by determining the total peripheral resistance to cardiac emptying.

Selective venoconstriction promotes venous return by transfer of returning blood to the central veins. Although peripheral venoconstriction may contribute importantly to the increase in central venous pressure, the major determinant is myocardial incompetence in coping with the venous return.

REDISTRIBUTION. In order to maintain oxygen delivery to vital organs (brain and myocardium) during heart failure, blood flow is diverted by heightened sympathetic nervous activity from skin, kidneys, splanchnic viscera, and muscle. At first the redistribution of blood flow among organs occurs during activity or stress, i.e., as cardiac output fails to increase appropriately for the increment in metabolism; later it operates also at rest. The mechanism for diversion is the balance between sympathetic innervation and local metabolism: the circulations to skin, kidney, splanchnic organs, and skeletal muscle are richly innervated, and these viscera have low metabolic rates; sympathetic nervous vasoconstriction easily overrides local metabolites. In contrast, the circulations to brain and myocardium are poor in alpha-adrenergic receptors; these organs, with high oxygen consumption, produce ample metabolic dilators to counterbalance heightened sympathetic activity.

In the normal subject during exercise, as need for heat dissipation increases, cutaneous hyperemia develops. In contrast, the patient in heart failure fails to develop cutaneous hyperemia despite increasing need for heat dissipation. The net effect is that the patient in heart failure, suffering from a low cardiac output during exercise, preserves blood pressure and blood flow to vital organs by paying the penalty of impaired heat loss as well as inadequate blood flow to exercising muscles.

VALSALVA MANEUVER. An abnormal response to the Valsalva maneuver, in which intrathoracic pressure is maintained at approximately 40 mm Hg for 10 to 12 seconds, is a useful test for left heart failure. The autonomic nervous system, operating in conjunction with the expanded volume of blood in the left side of the heart and pulmonary venous system, contributes to the abnormal response. During strain, the normal subject manifests a characteristic decrease in blood pressure and pulse pressure and increase in heart rate; when straining stops, the blood pressure, pulse pressure, and bradycardia "overshoot." In contrast, the patient in left heart failure demonstrates a "square wave response" of blood pressure: at the start of straining, blood pressure increases abruptly, stays high during the maneuver, and drops precipitously to baseline after the maneuver, without overshoot. Throughout the procedure there is little or no change in pulse pressure and no tachycardia. The lack of reflex changes stems from the failure of stroke output or arterial pulse pressure to change during the straining phase, so that no reflex changes are elicited in peripheral vessels.

Salt and Water Retention. As the patient slips into heart failure, the reduction in cardiac output is associated with a decrease in renal blood flow and glomerular filtration rate, and with a redistribution of blood flow within the kidneys. These hemodynamic changes undoubtedly contribute to the sodium and water retention of heart failure, but in different ways and to different degrees according to the stage of heart failure. Early in heart failure, when filtration rate is decreased, much of the sodium retention is attributable to the decrease in the filtered load of sodium presented to the tubules for reabsorption. Later on, humoral factors, predominantly hyperaldosteronism and a group of extra-adrenal, sodium-retaining influences ("factor III") predominate.

There is little doubt that disturbed hemodynamics are importantly involved in the release of the humoral factors. Thus a large role is currently envisaged for diminished baroreceptor stimulation in the renal afferent arterioles or a decrease in the sodium load passing the macula densa, or both, in activating the renin-angiotensin-aldosterone mechanism. In addition, baroreceptor effects arising in the distended left atrium or underfilled arterial tree may affect renal hemodynamics and the renin-angiotensin-aldosterone system. Other reflexes engaged in the intense sympathetic activity of heart failure may also be involved. Clearly, the hemodynamic-neurohumoral interplay that results in sodium and water retention is complex and incompletely understood. On the other hand, awareness of the important role of hyperaldosteronism in the genesis of sodium and water retention has provided new approaches to the therapy of heart failure using aldosterone antagonists.

Not only urine but also sweat and saliva are sodium poor. But the underlying mechanisms are different. Antidiuretic hormone is not directly involved in the genesis of the edema of heart failure.

The expansion of the circulating blood volume contributes to sustaining the cardiac output and the perfusion of vital organs. Rarely is the expansion in blood volume marked, usually ranging from 10 to 20 per cent in moderately severe heart failure to 30 to 50 per cent in severe, refractory heart failure. But even modest expansion helps to augment the ventricular-end-diastolic volume, thereby improving ventricular performance by way of the Frank-Starling principle. Unfortunately, the high end-diastolic volume and pressures promote the formation of edema by raising capillary pressures in the circulation behind the failing ventricle. At a time when circulation blood volume may be increased by 20 per cent, the extravascular fluid volume may have doubled.

CLINICAL MANIFESTATIONS OF HEART FAILURE

The signs and symptoms of heart failure depend on the ventricle that has failed and the duration of the failure. The clinical syndrome of left ventricular failure is dominated by *symptoms* of pulmonary congestion and edema. In contrast, right ventricular failure is dominated by *signs* of systemic venous congestion and peripheral edema. Fatigue and weakness are common in both types of heart failure.

Left Ventricular Failure

Symptoms

Complaints of respiratory discomfort or distress dominate the symptoms of left ventricular failure. They vary with position, stress, and activity. They are often associated with physical signs of disturbances in the lungs or in respiratory control mechanisms.

DYSPNEA. Like pain or anxiety, dyspnea is subjective and difficult to quantify. Because breathing is ordinarily automatic and effortless except after strenuous exertion, the complaint of breathlessness may signify anything from awareness to distress. Dyspnea during modest exertion is usually the first symptom of left heart failure. Usually dyspnea is associated with increased rate of breathing (tachypnea).

The physiologic basis for the sensation of dyspnea remains unclear. Both lungs and the chest muscles may contribute. Thus interstitial edema in the vicinity of the pulmonary capillaries stimulates juxtacapillary receptors ("J-receptors"), thereby reflexly setting a pattern of rapid, shallow breathing; associated with this abnormal pattern is an increase in the work and oxygen cost of moving the stiff lungs. However, this increased amount of work on the lungs is done in the face of diminished blood flow to the respiratory muscles, a consequence of the diminished cardiac output and redistribution of blood flow. Consequently, the disproportion between work done by the respiratory muscles and the supply of blood delivered to them may contribute to fatigue of the respiratory muscles and to the sensation of dyspnea. Sensory elements within the respiratory muscles may also contribute to respiratory discomfort by registering the disproportion between the inordinate amount of energy that is being spent by muscles and the amount of ventilation that they produce.

Although precise mechanisms for dyspnea remain uncertain, its occurrence in left heart failure clearly depends on the increase in the blood and water content of the lungs at the expense of the air volume. Ventilation increases as the air volume is progressively encroached upon, and, as the minute ventilation approaches the maximal ventilatory capacity, the likelihood of dyspnea increases.

ORTHOPNEA. Progressive, and often urgent, dyspnea that occurs soon after lying flat is designated as orthopnea; it is relieved by sitting up. The physiologic basis for orthopnea is the augmented venous return from the lower extremities and splanchnic bed to the lungs that results from redistribution of gravitational forces in the supine position and the reabsorption of diurnal edema. In the patient with heart disease, orthopnea is reliable evidence of left ventricular failure. In contrast, the dyspnea of chronic lung disease or musculoskeletal disorders is rarely aggravated by lying flat.

The patient learns to avoid respiratory distress at night by supporting head and thorax by two or more pillows. In severe heart failure, orthopnea may force the patient to sleep upright in a chair rather than in bed. In some patients with extensive coronary artery disease and left ventricular failure, orthopnea occurs only in the left lateral position; the mechanism for this is unclear.

Cough and expectoration are common in left heart failure, presumably a consequence of reflexes from the congested lungs and bronchi. The patient may also manifest an orthopneic cough which has the same significance as orthopnea, and is presumably the consequence of venous congestion and edema of the tracheobronchial walls. In some patients, precordial distress may substitute for breathlessness in the supine position. This "nocturnal angina" is also somehow related to the mobilization of water from the tissues to the circulation when the patient goes to bed.

PAROXYSMAL NOCTURNAL DYSPNEA. A bout of urgent respiratory distress, verging on suffocation, may rouse the patient unexpectedly from sleep and cause him to seek relief desperately, either by sitting up or by rushing to the open window to breathe "fresh air." Respiration may be labored and wheezing, hence the designation "cardiac asthma." The episodes represent intolerable aggravation of pulmonary congestion and edema during sleep in the supine position. A combination of dulling of the respiratory center to sensory input from the lungs during sleep and increase in venous return to the lungs makes it possible for pulmonary venous congestion and edema to accumulate to the point of precipitating the frightening episode of breathlessness.

ACUTE PULMONARY EDEMA. In an acute episode of left ventricular failure, such as that which follows myocardial infarction, the inability of the left ventricular myocardium to handle the blood that the competent right ventricle is delivering to it may result in an abrupt increase in pulmonary venous and capillary pressure, followed by flooding of the interstitial spaces and alveoli. If the edema is confined to the interstitial spaces of the lungs, an increase in respiratory frequency because of stiff lungs would be expected to produce alveolar hyperventilation and respiratory alkalosis; conversely, once free fluid enters the terminal bronchioles and mounts the respiratory tree, respiratory acidosis may occur because of imbalances between alveolar ventilation and alveolar blood flow (ventilation-perfusion inhomogeneities).

Pulmonary edema may begin with a cough, with wheezing, or with breathlessness. Often there is a sense of oppression in the chest. At first, except for the abnormal breathing pattern and the evidences of heart disease, there may be few physical signs. In time, as free fluid enters the distal airways, rales become audible, most marked in the dependent parts of the lungs, but extending upward as the attack worsens. In a severe attack, the patient is pale, sweating, cyanotic, obviously gasping for breath, and usually producing frothy sputum which may be blood tinged.

HEMOPTYSIS. Rusty sputum, laden with heart failure cells (alveolar macrophages containing hemosiderin), occurs frequently in severe left heart failure. Frankly bloody sputum is generally a sign of pulmonary infarction. In severe pulmonary edema caused by left ventricular failure, the frothy fluid that pours from the bronchial tree is often pink, i.e., blood tinged, owing to the escape of red cells into the alveoli from the congested minute vessels of the lungs.

CHEYNE-STOKES RESPIRATION. Some patients with severe heart failure display periodic breathing characterized by alternate periods of apnea and hyperventilation. Cyclic changes in arterial blood gas tensions accompany this waxing and waning of the ventilation: during apnea, the arterial Po_2 reaches its peak, whereas the arterial Pco_2 reaches its nadir. At the same time, alveolar gas tensions are exactly opposite: the alveolar Po_2 reaches its peak during hyperpnea; the alveolar Pco_2 reaches its nadir during hyperpnea. This discrepancy between arterial and alveolar gas tensions has been attributed to the fact that changes in arterial blood gases *cause* the swings in ventilation, whereas the changes in alveolar gas tension are the *consequences* of the changes in ventilation. The critical role of the arterial blood gases stems from the prolonged circulation time between the lungs and the respiratory centers in the brain. This slowing of the circulation exposes the central respiratory control mechanisms to arterial blood that differs in gaseous composition from that in pulmonary venous blood. In essence, because of slowing of the circulation, negative feedback is delayed. As expected, the longer the circulation time, the longer the cycles of hyperventilation and apnea. The neurologic and cerebrovascular changes of old age predispose to Cheyne-Stokes breathing.

Physical Signs

In addition to being breathless, the patient is generally pale, a bit dusky, and sweaty. His handshake is cold because of peripheral vasoconstriction. The heart rate is rapid and the pulse pressure is narrow, with a modest increase in diastolic blood pressure. If only the left ventricle has failed, the neck veins are not distended.

THE HEART. Enlargement of the heart is usually evident to inspection and palpation of the apical impulse and is confirmed by roentgenologic and radiographic examination. Angina pectoris is not a manifestation of heart failure, nor is palpitation common unless overzealous administration of digitalis and diuretics has occasioned digitalis toxicity. As the left ventricle fails and pulmonary venous pressure increases, pulmonary arterial pressure also increases, and the heart sound attributable to pulmonary valve closure increases in intensity. Also, as the left ventricle dilates, the mitral valve leaflets fail to appose properly, resulting in mild mitral incompetence.

Gallop Rhythm. The advent of a third heart sound during diastole in an adult with heart disease signifies the advent of heart failure. The fixed sequence of the two normal sounds and the abnormal third sound, in conjunction with an increase in heart rate, is responsible for the characteristic cadence of a gallop rhythm. The third heart sound ("S-3 gallop") occurs early in diastole during the state of rapid ventricular filling. This ventricular gallop presumably originates in the vibrations of the ventricular walls as the rapidly inflowing blood is abruptly arrested; this extra sound, normal in young children and in young adults, is generally a reliable sign of ventricular failure in the middle-aged or elderly patient with heart disease.

A gallop rhythm may also originate in the atrial contribution to ventricular filling. This atrial or "S-4 gallop" is not unique for heart failure, because it may reflect diminished ventricular compliance resulting from hypertrophy or ischemia rather than myocardial failure. If a patient with a fourth heart sound develops heart failure, a third sound appears to cause a quadruple rhythm. If the heart rate is rapid or the P-R interval is prolonged, the atrial and ventricular gallop sounds summate ("summation gallop"). In the candidate for heart failure, summation gallop has the same implication as other diastolic gallop rhythms, particularly if it persists as the heart is slowed.

Pulsus Alternans. In patients with heart disease, particularly if the cause is hypertension, cardiomyopathy, or coronary arteriosclerosis, the appearance of alternating strong and weak beats, even though the fundamental rhythm remains regular, heralds the onset of heart failure. This pulsus alternans may be detected by palpation or by sphygmomanometry. It often follows an extrasystole. Rarely is this mechanical alternans associated with electrical alternans. The mechanism for pulsus alternans has been attributed to alternations in fiber length (ventricular end-diastolic volume) or to alternating increase and decrease in the number of contractile units, or to both.

THE LUNGS. A characteristic consequence of interstitial edema and pulmonary venous congestion is tachypnea. As left heart failure progresses, interstitial edema is succeeded by alveolar edema and fluid in the terminal bronchioles, particularly at the lung bases. Accordingly, bilateral basal rales are common in moderate failure of the left ventricle.

Electrocardiogram

Abnormalities in the electrocardiogram arise from the underlying cardiac disorder and from therapeutic agents, e.g., digitalis and diuretics, rather than from heart failure per se.

Radiologic Aspects

The x-ray can be exceedingly helpful in the diagnosis of left ventricular failure. Typically, the cardiac silhouette is enlarged, often assuming telltale configurations that are determined by the underlying disorder. In contrast to the normal, in which pulmonary *arteries* are prominent in the lower lung fields, pulmonary vasculature is prominent at the apices, reflecting pulmonary *venous* hypertension and redistribution of blood flow because of edema and fibrosis at the bases. Enlarged hilar shadows accompany the prominent pulmonary veins in the upper lung fields.

Prominent septal lines, particularly near the costophrenic angles (Kerley's lines), indicate the presence of interstitial edema. The advent of alveolar edema is signaled by a generalized clouding of the lung fields. Pleural effusion may occasionally occur in left heart failure, but is much more apt to occur in biventricular heart failure. Evidence of interstitial and alveolar edema often lessens or disappears when right ventricular failure supervenes. However, hydrothorax generally persists. A widened shadow of the superior vena cava may provide reliable evidence of right ventricular failure and systemic venous congestion.

Pulmonary Function Tests

Traditionally, the course of overt failure of the left ventricle, particularly the response to treatment, has been followed by consecutive determinations of vital capacity. This is an insensitive measure, usually associated with decrease in compliance and occasionally with increase in airway resistance. Recently it has been shown that earlier in the course of pulmonary edema — presumably when the excess fluid is still confined to the interstitial space around alveoli and terminal airways (less than 2 mm in diameter) — expiratory flow rates at *low lung volumes* are reduced and peripheral airways tend to close prematurely during expiration, trapping gas within the lungs and disturbing the distribution of alveolar gas with respect to pulmonary capillary blood. This has led to a variety of tests (e.g., "closing volumes") which are designed to detect premature closure and resultant maldistribution of air — presumably by interstitial edema — long before compliance falls and total resistance of airways increases. During recovery there is usually a delay before expiratory flow rates and closing volumes return to normal, even though left atrial pressure is again within normal limits. The basis for the persistent abnormalities is presumably the gradual removal of interstitial edema from the vicinity of the small airways and blood vessels.

Associated with the high closing volume is evidence of ventilation-perfusion abnormalities manifested by widening of the alveolar-arterial ΔP_{O_2} and a decrease in arterial P_{O_2} caused by "venous admixture." Nonetheless, arterial oxygen saturation is generally near normal unless independent lung disease is present. Along with the decrease in arterial P_{O_2} is a widening of the arterial venous difference in O_2 content owing to the increased extraction of oxygen in the tissues. Arterial CO_2 tension remains normal or low unless free fluid enters the terminal airways in the course of pulmonary edema. Abnormally high values for CO_2 tension indicate that considerable free fluid has made its way into the airways.

Right Ventricular Failure

Clinical Manifestations

Isolated failure of the right ventricle is uncommon, generally a consequence of cor pulmonale secondary to intrinsic lung disease. More often, right ventricular failure is a sequel to left ventricular failure. In right ventricular failure, neck veins are distended and fill from below; the engorged liver may be tender to gentle pressure, and compression causes a surge of blood into the neck veins (hepatojugular reflux). In time, when both ventricles have failed, evidence of right ventricular failure may dominate the scene; but continuing dyspnea and rales attest to the persistence of left ventricular failure, and the continuing low cardiac output is manifested by signs of increased sympathetic nervous activity and of organ hypoperfusion.

Weakness may be marked and is occasionally associated with anorexia, weight loss, and malnutrition ("cardiac cachexia"). Not only severe heart failure but also digitalis, diuretics, and electrolyte disturbances are generally involved in the genesis of this cachectic state.

CYANOSIS. Bluish discoloration of the skin and mucous membranes is designated as cyanosis. It is due to an abnormal concentration of reduced hemoglobin (more than 5 grams per 100 ml) in the subpapillary venous plexus of the skin. In right heart failure, the congested venules, containing blood from which considerable oxygen has been extracted because of the slow flow, account for the cyanosis. In left heart failure, cyanosis is usually caused by a complication, e.g., pneumonia, unless overt pulmonary edema is present.

ABNORMAL HEART AND LUNGS. Although the breathlessness of the left ventricular failure may be somewhat relieved by right heart failure, usually some dyspnea persists along with tachypnea and basal rales. Severe right heart failure (and dilatation) may produce tricuspid valvular insufficiency, thereby contributing to systemic venous engorgement. The murmur of tricuspid insufficiency is distinguished from that of mitral insufficiency by its location (lower left border of sternum) and by its tendency to increase during inspiration. Hydrothorax, generally unilateral, is more common than in isolated left ventricular failure.

SYSTEMIC VENOUS CONGESTION. Distention of systemic veins is a hallmark of right heart failure. Several different mechanisms contribute to its genesis: (1) the inability of the failing right ventricle to cope adequately with the venous return; (2) the increase in the quantity of blood contained in the large systemic veins; and (3) increased venomotor tone, resulting from heightened sympathetic nervous activity. The increase in systemic venous pressure underlies the hepatomegaly, splenomegaly, and peripheral edema that characterize right heart failure. Less apparent are the congestion and edema of the gastrointestinal tract that the systemic venous hypertension produces.

Pressure in the superficial jugular vein is a useful index of right atrial pressure and, with experience, may be reliably estimated from the height of the fluid column distending the cervical vein. Normally, the cervical veins are flat in the erect position, whereas in right heart failure they are prominent and distended, usually with a level that pulsates. Functional tricuspid insufficiency, complicating dilatation of the right heart, distorts the normal venous pulse by increasing its v wave. Usually superficial venous distention precedes the onset of hepatomegaly and peripheral edema. Occasionally, compression of the abdomen over the liver (hepatojugular reflux) is necessary to display the increased blood volume in the venous system.

LIVER. The liver is usually enlarged and palpable in right heart failure, often in association with mild abdominal discomfort, and generally somewhat tender to compression. In severe right heart failure, particularly if the onset is acute, constraint of the swollen liver by its tight capsule may cause right upper quadrant pain. Tricuspid insufficiency accompanying right ventricular dilatation may cause synchronous pulsations in neck veins and liver. Splenomegaly is uncommon except in prolonged congestion of the liver. Rarely is the enlarged spleen tender from congestion per se.

Early in hepatic congestion, sensitive liver function tests, such as the handling of Bromsulphalein, are apt to be abnormal, and modest increases in the concentrations of cellular enzymes in serum, such as glutamic oxaloacetic transaminase (SGOT) increases in serum bilirubin, are not uncommon. The hyperbilirubinemia consists of a combination of quick- and slow-reacting bilirubin, presumably a consequence of decreased oxygen delivery to the liver arising from hypoperfusion and venous hypertension. But jaundice is uncommon unless hepatic congestion is associated with longstanding pulmonary congestion and, often, with pulmonary infarction.

If cardiac output is severely curtailed and liver congestion is marked and protracted, hypoglycemia may occur, presumably owing to depletion of glycogen stores in the liver and increased formation of lactic acid from glucose because of hypoxia. During physical activity, hepatic blood flow in heart failure decreases further, resulting in a marked decrease in aldosterone breakdown, thereby furthering sodium retention.

Repeated bouts of right heart failure elicit atrophy and necrosis of liver cells in the vicinity of the central veins and stimulate extensive fibrosis ("cardiac cirrhosis"). Many months of reduced hepatic blood flow and high venous pressures are required for this reaction, which may result in a shrunken, fibrotic liver difficult to distinguish from posthepatitic cirrhosis. Hepatic coma is a rare, preterminal complication of severe hepatic congestion and fibrosis.

EXTRACELLULAR FLUID COMPARTMENTS. In normal subjects, the fluid compartments of the body are held remarkably constant as the result of an automatic interplay among *intake* (governed by thirst and appetite), *transcellular exchanges* of fluid and electrolytes (governed by passive and active mechanisms), and *excretion* (regulated mainly by the kidneys). In heart failure, this automatic balance tends to be upset mainly because of inordinate retention of salt and water by the kidneys. The result is an isosmotic expansion of the extracellular fluid in which the circulating blood volume shares. It is conceivable that early in heart failure the conservation of salt and water may serve a useful purpose by expanding the blood volume either to sustain venous return to the failing heart or to relieve the arterial baroreceptors from undue stimulation as the cardiac output fails. But this teleologic explanation does not apply when the myocardium can no longer respond to increased filling pressures and volumes, and the retention of salt and water only aggravates congestion and edema.

The distribution of the excess extracellular fluid varies from patient to patient. In the patient who is up and about, edema accumulates in the feet and ankles under the influence of gravity; in the bedridden patient, the fluid shifts to the sacral region. Low tissue pressure, as around the back of the ankle, predisposes to localization. The level of colloid osmotic pressure and the integrity of the lymphatic system also influence the distribution of the excess fluid.

Subcutaneous Edema. Dependent edema, manifested as swelling of feet or ankles, developing gradually during the day and subsiding by morning, is a characteristic feature of right heart failure. Invariably, it is anteceded by systemic venous congestion, but after diuresis subcutaneous edema may linger even though systemic venous hypertension has been relieved by the reduction in venous blood volume. Usually a gain in weight precedes clinical evidence of edema. If edema is allowed to persist, complications such as low-grade cellulitis may occur. The combination of edema and slowed venous flow predisposes to thrombosis and to pulmonary embolism. The massive pitting edema of the lower extremities that was commonly seen before the advent of potent diuretics is now rarely encountered except in instances of gross neglect.

Hydrothorax. It is so uncommon for hydrothorax to complicate isolated failure of the right ventricle, that the association of pleural effusion and cor pulmonale should lead to search for an independent mechanism for the pleural effusion, e.g., pulmonary infarction. On the other hand, as indicated previously, it is quite common in combined heart failure (right and left). The pathogenesis of hydrothorax involves impaired removal of water from the pleural space because of high venous pressures in both the pulmonary and systemic circulations, thereby not only compromising transcapillary exchange of water in the pleura but also impeding lymphatic drainage. Hydrothorax contributes to dyspnea not only by encroaching on the air volume but also reflexly, probably by stimuli from lungs and chest wall. Pulmonary infarction may cause pleural effusion in two ways: by direct contiguity of the infarcted area of the lung and the pleural space, or by aggravation of heart failure.

Ascites. Clinically evident excess of free fluid in the abdominal cavity is designated as ascites. It is a late manifestation of right heart failure, generally associated with marked systemic venous hypertension, severe peripheral edema, and hydrothorax. It occurs most frequently in patients with tricuspid valvular disease (or with constrictive pericarditis). Portal and hepatic venous hypertension, coupled with high pressure in the systemic veins draining the peritoneum, seem to be involved in the etiology of ascites; but retention of salt and water is a fundamental prerequisite for ascites to occur. Usually ascites is first noticed by the patient as a gradual increase in abdominal girth. But in severe right heart failure, it may cause anorexia, abdominal discomfort, or pain.

Pericardial Effusion. In severe and persistent heart failure, abnormal quantities of transudate may accumulate in the pericardial sac. Rarely does fluid accumulate to the level of tamponade.

Anasarca. Massive right heart failure may cause excess fluid to accumulate everywhere in the body, most conspicuously in subcutaneous tissues and abdominal and thoracic cavities. Because of the influence of gravity, face and arms are spared until preterminally.

GASTROINTESTINAL TRACT. The bowel wall shares in the systemic venous congestion and edema. These changes rarely interfere with absorption of drugs or foods unless heart failure is extreme. In severe congestive heart failure, anorexia, nausea, and vomiting may occur from reflex, central, or local causes. Occasionally, when right heart failure is severe, a protein-losing enteropathy may develop.

BRAIN. Neurasthenia, headache, and insomnia are common in heart failure. Usually these manifestations are attributed to a combination of a modest diminution of cerebral blood flow and triggering mechanisms, e.g., dyspnea contributing to insomnia. Cerebral manifestations are more frequent when the reduction in cerebral blood flow is superimposed on antecedent cerebrovascular disease, e.g., arteriosclerosis, or personality disorder. Severe heart failure is often associated with irritability, restlessness, and difficulty in fixing attention, particularly in older persons. Preterminally, stupor and coma may develop. The possibility exists that central nervous abnormalities may be enhanced by the delivery to the brain of abnormal products elaborated by remote organs (liver, endocrines, gastrointestinal tract) that suffer deranged metabolism during heart failure as a result of congestion and hypoperfusion.

KIDNEY. Oliguria occurs in both right and left heart failure but is much more striking in the latter. As the heart improves, urinary output increases. The urine is poor in sodium but has a high specific gravity (1.020 to 1.030). Azotemia is common but generally moderate except when intrinsic renal disease is present or after vigorous diuresis. The combination of azotemia and high specific gravity is distinctive for heart failure (and dehydration) and contrasts with the low specific gravity of intrinsic renal disease. Proteinuria is common but rarely severe — usually less than 1 gram per day. A variety of casts accompany the proteinuria. Renal function, as determined by clearance techniques, is only slightly depressed except in severe right failure of long standing.

OTHER MANIFESTATIONS. In severe congestive heart failure, the accumulation of edema may obscure the gradual loss of tissue mass. Often this tissue wasting is associated with *weakness*. In extreme instances, *cachexia* may

develop. At this late stage, the patient is usually suffering from anorexia, gastrointestinal upsets, anemia, and electrolyte upsets. Part of the picture undoubtedly stems from organ hypoperfusion and congestion, but often a large contribution has been made by overvigorous use of diuretics and digitalis.

Anxiety. It is not surprising that patients with organic heart disease become anxious. Indeed, anxiety is a regular feature by the time the heart fails. But not always is it an easy matter to distinguish between cardiac complaints as manifestations of anxiety or of the cardiac disorder. Part of the difficulty stems from the nonspecific nature of complaints, such as breathlessness, especially if the patient does have organic heart disease. The difficulty is compounded if the patient misinterprets or exaggerates his symptoms unconsciously. For example, the severely anxious patient may hyperventilate to the point of alkalosis, producing the characteristic lightheadedness, cold hands, and tingling fingers of hypocapnia, reduced cerebral blood flow, and peripheral vasoconstriction, thereby reinforcing his view of the organic nature of his breathlessness. Palpitation is also commonly misinterpreted by the patient suffering from anxiety as a telltale sign of organic heart disease.

The standard approach for the physician is the separate assessment of the organic versus the psychosomatic aspects of the heart disease. Particularly helpful in this regard are excessive or inconsistent complaints for the role of the cardiac disease. Not infrequently, hemodynamic measurements may be required to settle the role of organic heart disease in producing the clinical symptoms.

CLINICAL MANAGEMENT

General Measures

The aim of treatment in heart failure is to arrest and reverse the pathogenic sequence that led to the clinical signs and symptoms. The response to treatment of the more common types of heart failure, i.e., hypertensive and arteriosclerotic, is often dramatic. But each relapse marks another milestone on the road to refractory heart failure, not only by signaling progressive deterioration of the myocardium, but also because intensified and protracted treatment enhances the prospect for eliciting the toxic manifestations of the therapeutic agents.

INCREASING CARDIAC OUTPUT. In most forms of chronic heart failure, the cardiac output can be made to increase by decreasing the cardiac load, by improving myocardial contractility, or by a combination of the two. In the patient with severe bradycardia associated with heart failure, acceleration of the heart rate by cardiac pacing may cure heart failure that would otherwise be refractory. Conversely, severe tachycardia must be arrested if filling times of the ventricles are too greatly curtailed by the abbreviated diastole.

DECREASING THE WORK OF THE HEART. Lightening the cardiac load is prerequisite for the successful treatment of heart failure. The load is always assessed with respect to the state of the myocardium, i.e., a damaged heart may not be able to cope with a blood pressure or volume load that a normal heart handles easily. The aim of treatment is to promote ventricular emptying so that the stroke output of the heart will increase. If successful, the improved cardiac performance reverses the train of clinical manifestations that the low cardiac output had initiated.

The traditional mainstays of cardiotonic therapy are rest, digitalis to improve the inotropic state of the myocardium, and diuretics to reduce the filling pressure of the failing ventricle. Rest is sometimes overlooked as an effective instrument for decreasing the cardiac burden. It must be both physical and mental. For the patient in left ventricular failure, simply sitting upright and breathing more easily is conducive to mental ease. Reassurance is essential to decrease metabolic activity and tachycardia and to relax peripheral vasoconstriction. No amount of reassurance will suffice to relieve a patient experiencing the pangs of severe constipation or urinary retention. Oxygen by nasal catheter (4 to 6 liters per minute) often makes the patient more comfortable even though the degree of arterial hypoxemia is exceedingly modest, possibly by increasing oxygen delivery to the brain. After recovery from an acute bout of heart failure, a new life style of lessened activity may be required as part of the cardiotonic program. Should reassurance prove inadequate, sedatives or tranquilizers (such as chloral hydrate, 0.5 to 1.0 gram, phenobarbital, 15 to 30 mg, or diazepam, 2 to 10 mg, taken orally three times per day and at bedtime) may be needed to promote mental ease, particularly as the patient improves and grows restless. Narcotics are rarely needed in heart failure unless pulmonary edema has generated intolerable anxiety. Excessive sedation, to the point of immobilizing the patient, enhances the risk of venous thrombosis and embolism, particularly in the elderly.

It is remarkable how often the proper use of rest as the initial step in treatment will promote a vigorous diuresis, slow the heart rate, and relieve dyspnea, thereby allowing a more leisurely use of other cardiotonic agents, such as digitalis and diuretics. On the other hand, if metabolic demands remain high, as during undetected thyrotoxicosis or fever, heart failure may prove refractory to the conventional cardiotonic program until the thyroid overactivity is curtailed.

Acute Pulmonary Edema

Treatment of the acute pulmonary edema of left ventricular failure is begun with the patient in the sitting position, thereby draining the upper portions of his lungs of excess fluid. Meperidine, 50 mg, or morphine, 10 to 15 mg, is administered intravenously for restlessness or dyspnea. These agents seem to act primarily by relieving anxiety and agitation. Morphine is the traditional agent. How it works is still a matter of debate. Most clinicians credit its effectiveness to its role in relaxing the patient and in decreasing tachycardia. Evidence for a direct venodilating effect that would withhold blood from the overloaded ventricle is more convincing under experimental conditions than in human heart failure. Unfortunately, distressing side effects, such as nausea, vomiting, and urinary retention, are sometimes troublesome and force recourse to other sedatives. A rapid-acting diuretic, ethacrynic acid or furosemide, is administered intravenously. Even though arterial oxygenation may be near normal, high concentrations of humidified oxygen, 50 to 100 per cent, are frequently used empirically to relieve dyspnea, restlessness, and confusion.

Most initial or mild episodes of pulmonary edema respond quickly to the aforementioned program of rest, reassurance, morphine, and diuretic. When the prospect of severe and progressive pulmonary edema is likely, attempts are generally instituted to reduce preload or afterload, or both. The drugs that are used are considered subsequently under Unloading Agents. In addition to drugs, several other interventions are in common practice: rotating tourniquets on the extremities, phlebotomy (of the order of 200 to 300 ml of blood), or positive pressure breathing which impedes venous return. All three of these interventions have become less popular since the advent of vasodilator therapy. Systemic hypotension is a contraindication to phlebotomy or to positive pressure ventilation.

Digitalis is more essential for supporting the myocardium after the loads on the heart have been lessened than during the acute bout of pulmonary edema. However, a digitalis preparation is usually part of the first wave of therapy in the emergency room. Digitalis (digoxin or lanatoside C, 1.0 mg) may be administered intravenously if the patient has had none during the preceding two weeks. However, the urgency for intravenous injection of digitalis has decreased considerably since the advent of potent, rapid-acting diuretics. An exception to this generalization is the attack of pulmonary edema precipitated by a bout of tachycardia which can be slowed by digitalis, e.g., paroxysmal atrial fibrillation. In this instance, digitalis relieves the heart failure primarily because of its effect on slowing atrioventricular conduction and consequently the ventricular rate, rather than because of its inotropic effect on the heart. In ectopic tachycardias, it may be necessary to resort to DC electroshock in order to restore normal heart action and tolerable heart rates.

Face to face with a patient in pulmonary edema, the physician often feels compelled to apply a battery of strenuous measures in rapid succession or simultaneously. Especially for patients in poor condition, this treatment may be worse than the disorder, which is usually self-limited once the upright position has been assumed, mental rest accomplished, and a potent diuretic administered. As soon as the crisis is over, a more conventional cardiotonic program is begun, and a search is made for the cause of the left heart failure as well as for the mechanism that precipitated the episode.

The role of left heart failure in producing high-altitude pulmonary edema is not clear. Prompt recovery usually follows bed rest, descent to lower altitude, and the administration of oxygen.

Inotropic Agents: Digitalis

Although immediate therapeutic agents for coping with the acute episode of heart failure may not include digitalis, once the crisis is over, lasting improvement almost invariably requires the use of digitalis glycosides. Unfortunately, establishing the proper dose of digitalis is not always straightforward, because optimal doses vary somewhat from patient to patient and with associated clinical disorders. Moreover, unless standard brands of predictable potency are prescribed, tablets may vary considerably in effectiveness. Finally, the concomitant administration of other, apparently unrelated, medications may lead to drug interactions which interfere with the effect of the digitalis.

DRUG INTERACTIONS. Multiplicity of drugs is the rule in modern therapy. Some drugs are deliberately prescribed in combinations, either to reinforce a desirable therapeutic effect or to avoid an untoward side effect. A familiar example of this practice is the combination of digitalis, a potassium-losing diuretic, and potassium supplements for the treatment of heart failure; the dosage of each is individualized to achieve maximal inotropic effect on the heart and to relieve circulatory congestion. But other drugs, such as sleeping pills and anticoagulants that are administered concomitantly for subsidiary or unrelated purposes, may interact and decrease the effectiveness of the cardiotonic program.

There are several ways by which one therapeutic agent can influence the effects of another. Among these are (1) chemical interaction (cholestyramine, a cholesterol-lowering, ion-exchange resin, impedes absorption of digitoxin [and, to a much lesser extent, of digoxin] by binding in the intestine); (2) competition for binding sites on plasma proteins (digitoxin and ethacrynic acid compete for albumin); (3) induction of drug-metabolizing enzymes (phenobarbital and phenylbutazone enhance the metabolism of digitoxin by hepatic microsomal enzymes); and (4) enhanced excretion (polar metabolites of digitoxin are eliminated more rapidly in urine and bile than is digitoxin per se). In conventional dosages, few of these interactions seem to be clinically significant even though cholestyramine has been advocated in treating digitoxin intoxication. But they do introduce an element of unpredictability into standard therapeutic programs, and they do urge caution whenever medications are either added to or deleted from a stable therapeutic regimen.

Related to the concept of drug interaction is the broader concept of drug-biologic interaction which determines how drugs act. This broader concept includes reactions between the pharmacologic agent and some biologic aspect of the living subject. For example, digitalis effects depend heavily on ion fluxes at ultrastructural membranes; changes in ionic composition and behavior are known to modify the clinical influence of digitalis. Or the physiologic state of the patient may shape the response: acidosis blunts the effectiveness of norepinephrine; the administration of a conventional dose of a ganglionic blocking agent, when sympathetic vasomotor tone is high because of vigorous diuresis and depletion of blood volume, may precipitate circulatory collapse.

The concept of drug-biologic interaction is complicated by individual variability in responsiveness to drugs. Part of this variability is undoubtedly inherited; part is immunologic; most remains to be explained.

DIGITALIS: GENERAL ASPECTS. Digitalis improves the contractility of the failing myocardium regardless of the type of heart failure, the rate, or the rhythm. After digitalis has been given in effective doses and myocardial contractility has increased, the heart shrinks in size, cardiac output increases, end-diastolic volume and pressure decrease, venous pressure normalizes, and evidences of peripheral vasoconstriction, circulatory congestion, and organ hypoperfusion disappear. In the reordering of the circulation that follows relief of congestive heart failure, blood that had been sequestered in the splanchnic venous bed is redirected to the systemic veins by appropriate adjustments in vascular tone, thereby helping to sustain the improved cardiac output.

Molecular Bases. Although the full picture of how the digitalis glycosides improve cardiac contractility is not yet clear, they do seem to act by altering surface and intracellular (sarcoplasmic reticulum and mitochondria)

membranes so that they release calcium ions more readily. Another manifestation of a change in cellular membrane characteristics caused by the glycosides is inhibition of the Na^+-K^+-ATPase activity. However, it is unsettled whether this interference with ATPase, as well as the associated decrease of sodium pumping into the cell, is directly related to the inotropic effect of the glycosides.

Effect on Inotropic State. In low output heart failure, digitalis increases the cardiac output and restores the end-diastolic pressure in the left ventricle to normal. This is a consequence of increased myocardial contractility. A similar effect on contractility occurs in the normal myocardium, but the cardiac output does not increase because of a direct vasoconstricting effect of digitalis on the peripheral resistance vessels. But in low output heart failure in which sympathetic nervous activity is consistently high, restoration of the cardiac output by digitalis reflexly diminishes sympathetic tone, thereby overriding the direct vasoconstricting effects of digitalis on the vessels. These distinctions underscore the unique property of digitalis glycosides as inotropic agents because of their ability to improve myocardial contractility in heart failure without simultaneously eliciting antagonistic effects, such as peripheral vasoconstriction (or tachycardia).

Myocardial Oxygen Consumption. The increase in the strength of contraction produced by the digitalis glycosides increases the oxygen consumption of the myocardium in the normal heart. But this tendency is neutralized in the failing heart which responds to glycosides by shrinking in volume, thereby reducing wall tension and its associated oxygen consumption. Accordingly, the increase in contractility produced in the dilated failing heart is generally accomplished with no increase in myocardial oxygen consumption.

Catecholamine Depletion. Although reduction in cardiac catecholamines is a feature of chronic heart failure, this depletion leaves unaffected the positive inotropic effects of the digitalis glycosides.

Coronary Circulation. In the normal unanesthetized animal, ouabain elicits coronary vasoconstriction. Unfortunately, nothing is known about the behavior of the coronary circulation in response to digitalis during heart failure.

Systemic Circulation. Digitalis elicits an increase in cardiac output, thereby reducing the reflex vasoconstriction of the low output state. But because of the direct constrictor action of cardiac glycosides on vascular smooth muscle, there is apt to be a brief period of increase in systemic arterial pressure, particularly if large doses of cardiac glycosides are administered intravenously.

CHOICE OF DIGITALIS PREPARATION. Five digitalis preparations are in common use today in the United States: digitalis leaf, digoxin, digitoxin, deslanoside (Cedilanid-D), and ouabain. Their basic pharmacologic actions on the heart and their toxic-therapeutic ratios are quite similar. But they do differ considerably with respect to the rate and degree of absorption from the intestine and both the onset and duration of action.

Digoxin and digitoxin have replaced digitalis leaf for chronic oral administration; ouabain and deslanoside, as well as digoxin, are administered intravenously. Digitoxin is not as satisfactory an intravenous agent, because it is relatively slow in reaching its peak effect. Digitalis leaf is gradually disappearing from use, because it varies

TABLE 2. Administration of Common Cardiac Glycosides

| Preparation | Digitalization | | | Cardiotonic Effects | | Blood Levels | |
	Loading Dose* (mg/24 hrs)	Initial Dose† (mg)	Maintenance Dose (mg)	Onset of Activity (min)	Peak Effect (hrs)	Steady State Therapeutic Level/¶ (mg/ml)	Half-Life (hrs)
Digoxin (oral)	2.5	1.0	0.25	60–120	1–3	1.5	36
Digitoxin (oral)	1.2	0.75‡	0.1	30–120	4–6	17	96–144
Deslanoside (IV)	1.6	0.8§	—	10–30	1–2	—	33
Ouabain (IV)	0.25	0.25§	—	3–10	0.5–2	0.5	21

(These values are examples to illustrate orders of magnitude.)

*Total quantity to be administered in 24 hours for therapeutic effect.
†Assuming no prior digitalis during previous two weeks.
‡The same dose may be administered intravenously if urgent digitalization is required.
§When feasible, switch to oral maintenance doses of digoxin or digitoxin.
¶On conventional maintenance doses.

in potency, requires bioassay for standardization, and has no therapeutic advantage over digitoxin which is its principal constituent.

Traditional practice in digitalization has relied on a preliminary loading phase to achieve a therapeutic level, followed by maintenance dosage to sustain a balance between intake and elimination. Accordingly, the preset loading dose is administered over a period of one to three days (Table 2), providing enough digitalis to load body stores and to compensate for daily elimination. Unless a desperate situation — such as a life-threatening cardiac arrhythmia — calls for acute digitalization, slow digitalization is preferable. Indeed, if there is no hurry, continued administration of the maintenance dose, without a loading dose, has proved to be a practical way to achieve digitalization.

Dosages listed in Table 2 are intended to indicate orders of magnitude rather than precise schedules. Dosage is determined individually according to the nature and severity of the heart disease, the clinical setting, the use of other drugs such as potassium-losing diuretics, and continued observation of the patient's response.

Oral Preparations. Digoxin and digitoxin have replaced digitalis leaf for chronic oral administration.

DIGOXIN. The maintenance dosage of digoxin is determined by a balance between renal excretion, dose, and absorption. Ordinarily, between 75 and 90 per cent of an oral dose is absorbed. Digoxin is lipid soluble and absorbed from the small intestine by diffusion. Some variation in absorption may occur, depending on the solubility of digoxin molecules in the intestinal fluids. Variability in absorption may also result from different preparations of digoxin. Consequently, once a digoxin

preparation from one manufacturer has proved effective, changes should be avoided.

Digoxin is excreted primarily by the kidney, and most of the drug appears unchanged in the urine. When fully digitalized, the concentration of digoxin in serum is approximately 1 per cent or less of total body stores of digoxin. If renal function is normal, approximately one third of the body stores is eliminated per day; the maintenance dose replenishes this daily loss. The half-life of digoxin in serum is approximately the same in normal subjects and in patients with heart failure, averaging one and one half days. However, the half-life is prolonged in renal failure. The serum level of digoxin in renal insufficiency is directly related to the creatinine clearance and inversely to the concentration of urea nitrogen in the blood (BUN). Formulas have been devised to take these relationships into account, recognizing that, in contrast to the normal daily elimination of one third of body stores of digoxin, the anuric patient eliminates about one seventh. Accordingly, the anuric patient will require one half or less of the usual maintenance dose.

Only 5 per cent of digoxin in serum is bound to protein. Its polar structure accounts for the difference between its concentration and that of digitoxin (nonpolar) in the serum (Table 3).

Without an initial loading dose, patients receiving digoxin orally reach a steady state in the serum, reflecting equilibrium between body stores, intake, and elimination in about one week. The steady state level in serum is approximately 1 per cent or less of total body stores of digoxin. Body stores are related to lean body weight, because digoxin does not accumulate in fat or interstitial fluid. In an adult patient, body stores are generally of the

TABLE 3. Features of Cardiac Glycoside Preparations in Common Use

Preparation	Source	Usual Route of Administration*	Gastrointestinal Absorption	Protein Binding†	Principal Route of Elimination
Digoxin	*Digitalis lanata*	Oral	75–90%‡	23%‡	Kidneys
Digitoxin	*Digitalis purpurea*	Oral	90–100%	97%	Liver; kidney for metabolites
Deslanoside	*Digitalis lanata*	Intravenous	Erratic	—	Kidneys
Ouabain	*Strophanthus gratus*	Intravenous	Erratic	0	Kidneys

(These values are examples to illustrate orders of magnitude.)

*All can be administered intravenously.
†Affinity for protein (albumin) determines rate of urinary excretion and persistence in body.
‡Varies according to preparation. Different tablets differ in bioavailability of digoxin.

order of 0.01 mg per kilogram of body weight. Rarely are body stores required greater than 0.02 mg per kilogram of body weight. Therefore for a 70-kg patient, digitalization usually requires a minimal dose of approximately 0.7 mg. Should this digitalizing dose be exceeded in order to achieve better control of the clinical state, the prospects for toxicity will increase accordingly.

The essential features in using digoxin therapeutically are summarized in Table 2. Because of its short half-life, a single dose per day will cause a wide swing in serum concentration (and in body stores, including the heart) before the next dose is administered. In practice this swing is often unimportant; but, if desirable, its magnitude may be reduced (and therapeutic control improved) by administering one half the daily dose at 12-hour intervals. Many clinicians use digoxin for intravenous as well as oral administration, because its hemodynamic and biologic properties are comparatively well understood, and dosages are relatively easy to adjust.

DIGITOXIN. This agent is widely used for chronic administration. It differs importantly from digoxin in its metabolism and its slow rate of elimination; the main route of elimination is by metabolism in the liver, only a small fraction being eliminated by the kidney.

Digitoxin is completely absorbed after oral administration so that oral and intravenous dosages are identical. Body stores and digitalizing doses are approximately the same, but maintenance doses are quite different because of different rates of elimination. Approximately 12 per cent of body stores of digitoxin is eliminated per day in patients with normal renal function. The usual body store is estimated to be of the order of 0.8 mg in a 70-kg adult. Therefore the daily maintenance dose is generally 0.1 mg per day (0.12×0.8 mg). Because of its slow dissipation and elimination, serum levels of digitoxin vary less from hour to hour than do digoxin levels. But the drug accumulates insidiously so that maintenance doses established at the onset often prove to be toxic in time.

In contrast to digoxin, digitoxin has a strong avidity for albumin so that 97 per cent in plasma is nondialyzable. This combination is a critical factor in limiting glomerular filtration and excretion of digitoxin by the kidneys. After an oral dose of 1.0 mg, 50 per cent of the inotropic effect is reached in one hour; 85 to 100 per cent is achieved in four hours and sustained for the rest of the day. The average half-life is approximately five days. Digitoxin enters into an enterohepatic cycle. Between 30 and 60 per cent of the 1.0 mg dose is eliminated in the feces and urine, the larger fraction generally in the urine. The remainder is metabolized, primarily to digoxin, which is eliminated in the urine. Digoxin is preferable to digitoxin in renal or hepatic insufficiency.

Intravenous Preparations. As a rule, these are reserved for life-threatening situations. These include acute heart failure complicating a bout of atrial fibrillation with rapid ventricular rate, fulminating pulmonary edema as a complication of left ventricular failure, and the onset of heart failure or a serious arrhythmia during surgery. As a rule, the larger the dose of the glycoside, the more apt it is to create problems, particularly arrhythmias, of its own.

An intravenous bolus of a digitalis preparation may elicit a bout of hypertension, particularly if the dose is large, e.g., 1.0 mg of digoxin. The increase is generally of the order of 20/10, and the effect is generally short lived. But it may suffice to overburden the failing heart and to aggravate the situation until it subsides and is succeeded by the inotropic effect. Hypertension is rarely a problem if the intravenous dose is modest and administered slowly.

OUABAIN. This is the traditional digitalis preparation for intravenous use. It is a pure crystalline substance that is unsuitable for oral use because of erratic absorption from the gastrointestinal tract. Its latency after intravenous injection is exceedingly brief (less than five minutes); it is rapidly eliminated so that it is not suitable for maintenance of digitalization. The initial intravenous dose is 0.25 to 0.3 mg, administered slowly. An additional 0.15 or 0.3 mg may be repeated after 24 hours.

DESLANOSIDE. This preparation is identical with digoxin except for the addition of a glucose residue. It is gradually replacing ouabain in popularity for intravenous use. Its digitalizing effect appears in 10 to 30 minutes after intravenous injection, reaches peak effect in one to two hours, and regresses in 24 hours. For rapid intravenous digitalization, the full 1.6 mg may be given at once, or, preferably, 0.8 mg may be followed by another 0.8 mg, either in four hours or in divided doses, at two- to four-hour intervals for two to three additional doses. Maintenance of digitalization is preferably done by oral digoxin or digitoxin. But, if necessary, 0.4 mg may be given intravenously or intramuscularly at 8- to 12-hour intervals.

DIGOXIN. For rapid digitalization, 0.5 mg is given initially, followed by 0.25 mg every two to four hours as needed, but taking care to avoid exceeding a total dose of 2 mg in 12 hours. As soon as practical, the oral route is substituted for the intravenous route.

Diagnostic Preparations. ACETYLSTROPHANTHIDIN. This is a partial synthetic which, because of its exceedingly rapid onset of action and dissipation, has been advocated more as a diagnostic test for adequacy of digitalization than as a therapeutic agent for heart failure. In practice, repeated injections of the substance (0.25 mg in 5 ml of glucose and water) are made until toxic or therapeutic effects are observed. Because it is potentially dangerous, other diagnostic tests are being investigated.

GUIDES TO PROPER DOSAGE OF DIGITALIS. A major problem in using digitalis for its inotropic effect is the threat of inducing arrhythmias by virtue of its other effects on the heart (Fig. 3). On the other hand, if rapid atrial fibrillation coexists with heart failure, slowing of the ventricular rate, a consequence of slowed atrioventricular conduction, has proved to be a practical guide to digitalis dosage. Fortunately, slowing of the heart rate when atrial fibrillation coexists with heart failure also provides a rough measure of the inotropic effect (and of serum levels of the glycoside). On the other hand, when heart failure coexists with a normal sinus rhythm, slowing of the heart is a treacherous index of inotropic effect. Digitalis toxicity is common if large doses are administered in the attempt to slow the sinus tachycardia, particularly if a mechanism such as pulmonary emboli, infection, or hyperthyroidism is operating to sustain the rapid heart action.

The clinician now has available several different and effective digitalis preparations. Although none of these has any intrinsic advantage over the others with respect to myocardial contractility, they vary considerably with respect to speed of action, time course of effectiveness, and rates of elimination. Because of the ever-present prospect of digitalis toxicity, before starting to administer digitalis it is important to know whether digitalis, in any form, has been taken during the preceding week or two.

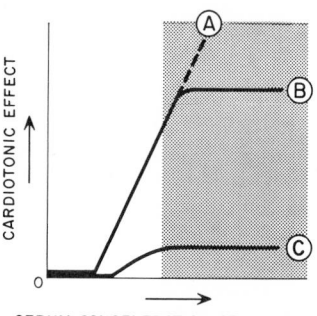

Figure 3. Hypothetical effects on contractility elicited by increasing doses (and serum concentrations) of digitalis. Once the inotropic effect of the digitalis preparation begins, it is unlikely that it will continue indefinitely as in A. Instead, it is likely that beyond a certain point the inotropic effects will taper to a plateau despite increasing serum concentration. When this plateau will occur depends on the capability of the heart to respond; a left ventricle that is suffering its first bout of failure is apt to manifest an excellent inotropic response for small increments in serum concentration before the plateau is reached (B). On the other hand, a spent heart that has suffered multiple myocardial infarctions may only manifest a sluggish inotropic response from the start and plateau early despite enormous increments in serum levels of glycoside (C). The shaded area is intended as a reminder of the increasing likelihood of serious arrhythmias as serum glycoside levels continue to increase.

Longer may be required if renal failure is present, particularly if digoxin was used. It cannot be overemphasized that the intravenous administration of a bolus of a digitalis preparation to a patient who has recently taken digitalis may precipitate ventricular tachycardia or fibrillation.

Clinical manifestations and the electrocardiogram are the key guides to dosage. As the circulation improves and signs and symptoms of heart failure abate, conventional dosage schedules are tailored to individual needs. The usual changes in the S-T segment and in the T waves produced by digitalis merely indicate that appreciable quantities of digitalis have been taken but provide no measure of dosage or efficacy. On the other hand, digitalis toxicity may first be manifested by electrocardiographic changes of abnormal conduction and of ectopic pacemakers.

Prophylactic. The perennial question of administering digitalis prophylactically, especially before surgical procedures, is again being discussed. This practice requires the administration of a preset dose without conventional criteria for distinguishing between adequacy and toxicity. Therefore uncertain guidelines for safe administration are coupled with questionable therapeutic benefits. Compounding this uncertainty is the prospect of hypoxia and electrolyte imbalance during surgery. Because of the availability of digitalis preparations that do act rapidly and effectively, there seems to be little basis at present for prophylactic digitalization.

DIGITALIS TOXICITY. Digitalis preparations are among the most dangerous, as well as the most useful, of current medications. The incidence of cardiotoxicity is staggering — of the order of 10 to 20 per cent in hospitalized patients receiving conventional doses of digitalis — and mortality from digitalis cardiotoxicity is estimated to run into the thousands per year.

Several different reasons account for much of this morbidity and mortality. (1) The narrow margin between therapeutic and toxic doses; this predisposes to digitalis toxicity during ordinary use but enhances its prospects when dosages are increased in the attempt to deal with increasing congestive heart failure. (2) The heavy reliance on slowing of heart rate and clearance of circulatory congestion as indices of improved contractility; this practice works well in atrial fibrillation but may be disastrous in normal sinus rhythm. (3) The ease with which changes in the clinical situation can derange stability of control; among the more common upsetting influences are electrolyte disturbances (particularly hypopotassemia), acute myocardial ischemia, upset acid-base balance, hypoxemia, renal impairment, autonomic nervous imbalances, other drugs, and infection. (4) Incomplete understanding by the physician of the distinctions in the clinical pharmacology of the various digitalis preparations; for example, differences in the renal handling of digoxin and digitoxin must be taken into account when choosing the proper glycoside in patients with renal insufficiency.

Recognition. The electrocardiogram is generally the final arbiter of digitalis cardiotoxicity. But three categories of clinical clues direct attention to the electrocardiogram: (1) the appearance of central nervous system evidence of digitalis toxicity, particularly anorexia and aversion to food; (2) a change in the arrhythmia, including unusual slowing or acceleration of the heart rate; and (3) regularization of the heart rate in the patient with atrial fibrillation while taking maintenance doses of digitalis.

Although serum levels are now quite popular as indices of digitalis toxicity, the lack of close correspondence between serum levels of glycosides and moderate cardiotoxicity in individual patients has kept alive interest in other tests to evaluate myocardial sensitivity to digitalis. These include the acetylstrophanthidin tolerance test, which is dangerous and should be reserved for experts. Among the more recent and innocuous is the salivary electrolyte test which relies on increases in the concentration of calcium and potassium in the saliva as an index of digitalis toxicity. This test is as yet empirical, because the mechanism for the increase in the concentration of these electrolytes is unknown. The practical value of this test remains to be established.

Digitalis cardiotoxicity is primarily a matter of arrhythmias. As might be expected from the diverse effects of digitalis on the heart, the arrhythmias are generally nonspecific. However, the coincidence of depressed atrioventricular conduction and stimulation of ectopic pacemakers is virtually unique for digitalis toxicity. This combination accounts for arrhythmias characterized by simultaneous rapid atrial rates and slow ventricular responses, for escape beats, and for nonparoxysmal junctional tachycardia. For example, atrial tachycardia with atrioventricular block, generally precipitated by overzealous administration of potassium-losing diuretics, is characteristic, although not specific, for digitalis toxicity. Even more distinctive is atrioventricular dissociation with junctional rhythm, in which two pacemakers operate independently above and below the intervening area of atrioventricular block. In atrial fibrillation, the advent of serious digitalis toxicity may be signaled by regularization of the ventricular rate because of acceleration of an ectopic focus below a high degree of atrioventricular block.

The usual cause of death in digitalis toxicity is ventricular fibrillation. Rarely does it appear unexpectedly. More often, it is presaged by multifocal premature contractions and runs of ventricular tachycardia. Consequently, premature ventricular beats that appear after digitalis has been started or during maintenance therapy have to be regarded as serious warnings of toxicity, particularly if they are multifocal in origin and if there is bigeminy involving premature beats that are bizarre in appearance. Rarely do ventricular arrhythmias occur without other evidence of digitalis intake, including the characteristic ST-T deformations, disturbances in atrial ventricular conduction, and atrial arrhythmias.

Treatment. The mainstay for treating digitalis cardiotoxicity is to stop the digitalis and to discontinue diuretics that contributed to hypokalemia. There is no specific antidote. Fortunately, most digitalis-induced arrhythmias are arrested by stopping digitalis. Thus junctional rhythms without excessive ventricular rates or evidence of ventricular irritability are generally treated without specific medication or intervention. But if the arrhythmia is characteristic of ventricular irritability or if it has caused hemodynamic upset in the form of hypotension, heart failure, and pulmonary edema, medical intervention is mandatory.

Potassium is the agent of choice for suppressing digitalis-induced automaticity. But because it slows conduction through the myocardium and specialized conduction tissues, thereby potentiating the depression produced by digitalis, it must be used with extreme caution when atrioventricular block is severe. In the latter case, the introduction of a temporary perivenous cardiac pacemaker may prove useful in tiding the patient over the period needed to eliminate the excess digitalis, particularly if antiarrhythmic drugs are to be used to suppress ectopic atrial or ventricular beats.

If the arrhythmia has produced no crisis, if renal function is adequate, and if there is no hyperkalemia, potassium salts (4 to 6 grams of potassium chloride per day) may be administered orally. On the other hand, if the situation is deteriorating rapidly because of ectopic beats or uncontrollable tachycardia, potassium salts may be administered intravenously. Continuous electrocardiographic monitoring is mandatory during intravenous administration. The combination of continuous monitoring and careful intravenous titration of the arrhythmia is generally safer than is oral administration. The usual preparation for intravenous use contains 40 mEq of potassium in a 500 ml solution of 5 per cent glucose in water; this is administered slowly, e.g., at a rate of 40 mEq per hour. This may be repeated, if necessary, for up to three doses. Hypotension may limit the amount of potassium that can be given by vein. The electrocardiogram is monitored throughout, recognizing that high plasma concentrations of potassium may per se cause death through cardiac depression, arrhythmias, or arrest. The characteristic changes in the EKG are disappearance of the P wave, widening of the QRS complexes, changes in the S-T segments, and tall, peaked T waves.

Antiarrhythmic drugs which decrease ventricular automaticity by slowing diastolic depolarization, such as procainamide, lidocaine, propranolol, and diphenylhydantoin, are effective but must be used cautiously. Procainamide is useful when potassium fails to control the arrhythmia or if potassium is contraindicated because of uremia or hyperkalemia. It also has the advantage of sustained action if digitalis toxicity should persist. But it runs the risk of hypotension, depression of contractility, and producing AV block.

Lidocaine (1 to 2 mg per kilogram in one to two minutes by intravenous injection or as continuous infusion) has been used to control premature ventricular beats and ventricular tachycardia resulting from digitalis. It produces an effect within 45 to 90 seconds which is dissipated within 20 minutes. It has the advantage over procainamide of not causing hypotension. Doses less than 750 mg per hour are rarely associated with significant toxic effects, i.e., neurologic disorders and convulsions.

Diphenylhydantoin has been advocated for the treatment of digitalis-induced arrhythmias because it does not depress atrioventricular conduction. It is administered intravenously at a rate of 5 to 10 mg per kilogram over a 5- to 15-minute period. Propranolol, quinidine, and chelating agents are also being used. Electroconversion by DC shock, which has proved to be remarkably effective in controlling many arrhythmias, is a desperate measure of last resort in digitalis-toxic arrhythmias because of the likelihood of producing uncontrollable paroxysmal ventricular arrhythmias.

BLOOD LEVELS. The pharmacologic effectiveness of most drugs depends on concentration at the site of action. Dosage may be a poor guide to this effective concentration because of biologic unpredictability with respect to absorption from the gastrointestinal tract, patterns of distribution throughout the body, and rates of metabolism and excretion. In general, it is anticipated that concentration of a drug in the blood (serum or plasma) will relate better to therapeutic consequences, including toxicity, than will dosage.

In recent years, as a result of advances in radioimmunoassay technology, determination of serum concentrations of some cardiac glycosides became practical and available as well as reliable, accurate, and specific. The application of these tests to patients taking digitalis preparations (digoxin, digitoxin) has shown that the frequency and severity of toxic effects increase progressively as serum concentrations exceed therapeutic levels.

But some overlap in concentrations does occur, particularly in the zone between toxic and therapeutic levels. Moreover, occasionally there is a complete disparity between serum concentration and clinical consequences. These divergences are not unexpected because of the multiplicity of physiologic, pathologic, and biochemical influences that can modify the response to a given concentration of glycoside in the serum (and at the site of action): e.g., hypokalemia, acid-base disturbances, hypoxemia, interaction with other drugs, hypoproteinemia, acquisition of tolerance. But the exceptions do emphasize that serum concentrations must be interpreted critically in the light of the clinical setting.

Currently, determination of serum concentration of a digitalis glycoside is most useful in patients who are suspected of digitalis toxicity but are unable to provide an accurate account of digitalis dosage. It also has a place in guiding dosage in candidates for digitalis toxicity, e.g., heart failure complicated by renal insufficiency or by violent biochemical and physiologic perturbations, as after cardiac surgery. At the other extreme, determination of serum concentration may indicate that refractory heart failure may simply be a consequence of inadequate dosage.

DIGITALIS IN ACUTE MYOCARDIAL INFARCTION. As a general rule, digitalis is the drug of choice for myocardial failure. Since some degree of left ventricular failure is characteristic of acute myocardial infarction, it might seem reasonable to afford high priority to digitalis in the therapeutic program. Although this generalization still applies to *severe* heart failure during acute myocardial infarction, particularly if the heart is enlarged, the value of digitalis in less urgent degrees of left ventricular failure during acute myocardial infarction is much less certain.

The dilemma stems from the noninfarcted myocardium. If the noninfarcted ventricle has failed, considerable improvement is to be expected from the inotropic effects of digitalis; conversely, if the noninfarcted ventricle is normal, the inotropic effect will be of little consequence, particularly when compared to the inotropic effects of circulating catecholamines that the acute crisis has promoted. The possibility also exists that, even if digitalis does enhance contractility of the noninfarcted area, the net effect on cardiac performance may not be impressive because of the paradoxical motion of the infarcted area during cardiac contraction.

In addition to these uncertainties concerning enhanced contractility, the threat exists that digitalis may promote ventricular irritability in the peri-infarcted, ischemic zone of the myocardium, thereby predisposing to ectopic foci and uncontrollable ventricular arrhythmias. This likelihood is accentuated by a variety of other concomitant influences that predispose to ventricular arrhythmias: increased sympathetic activity, hypokalemia, and hypoxemia (to which excess sedation may contribute).

These reservations, plus the availability of effective diuretics to clear pulmonary congestion and edema during the first few days of an acute myocardial infarction, encourage extraordinary circumspection in using digitalis during the acute episode. On the other hand, if heart failure persists after the acute crisis — because of either extensive scarring or unremitting hemodynamic overload — digitalis is clearly required because the myocardium has failed globally. Moreover, should atrial fibrillation with a rapid ventricular response complicate acute myocardial infarction early or late in its course, digitalis may be lifesaving. For other supraventricular arrhythmias, which generally require larger doses of digitalis and may even prove refractory, antiarrhythmic agents or electrical conversion are preferable during the phase of increased ventricular irritability.

OTHER INOTROPIC AGENTS: SYMPATHOMIMETIC AMINES. Although fashions in diuretics continue to change, no inotropic agent has as yet been found to compete with digitalis. Substitutes have been sought among the sympathomimetic amines which also stimulate the myocardium but differently from digitalis. The qualifications that have been sought include effectiveness after oral administration, improved contractility in conjunction with peripheral vasodilation, increased renal excretion of sodium, and a greater increase in coronary blood flow than in myocardial oxygen consumption. Three catecholamines have been singled out for close scrutiny because of their ability to stimulate the heart and to decrease peripheral resistance: epinephrine, isoproterenol, and dopamine. Unfortunately, none of these is on a clinical par with digitalis: all three provoke tachycardia; epinephrine decreases the elimination of sodium by the kidney, whereas isoproterenol usually has no effect on sodium excretion; dopamine has to be given intravenously, acts briefly, and causes undesirable increments in systemic arterial pressure.

Glucagon, a polypeptide hormone produced chiefly by the α cells of the pancreas, attracted considerable attention for a while as a possible adjunct for the patient in refracto-

ry heart failure who can tolerate no more digitalis. Like the catecholamines, glucagon presumably exerts its cardiotonic effects by activating adenyl cyclase. It has been given by continuous intravenous infusion (2 to 4 mg per hour for 10 to 13 days) and by injections of large single doses (10 to 25 mg). In these doses, the major side effect was nausea; abnormalities in blood sugar levels were uncommon. Unfortunately, enthusiasm for this agent has begun to wane because of recent evidence that the effects of glucagon on myocardial contractility are far less consistent in chronic heart failure than in the normal heart.

UNLOADING AGENTS (VASODILATOR THERAPY). The use of vasodilator agents began with refractory heart failure. Some patients with severe heart failure become unresponsive to increasing dosages of digitalis and diuretics and manifest toxicity. Because of their bleak outlook, the idea of improving the performance of the heart by administering vasodilators immediately caught hold. Its popularity was ensured by the availability of a wide assortment of agents for trial. At present, criteria have been liberalized so that the use of vasodilators is no longer restricted to refractory heart failure (Table 4). Indeed, questions are being raised about the feasibility of using these agents prophylactically.

Principles. The normal ventricle usually adjusts automatically to a change in afterload so that cardiac output and stroke volume remain virtually unchanged; if cardiac output does increase, it is because of an increase in heart rate. In contrast, the failing ventricle improves its emptying when afterload is reduced (Fig. 4), thereby increasing stroke volume and cardiac output without increasing heart rate. By this tactic, the failing heart responds to a decrease in afterload by shifting its ventricular function curve toward normal even though the inotropic state of the myocardium is unchanged. Thus by reducing afterload the failing heart can increase its output without increasing either preload or contractility. Since contractility, preload, and heart rate are major determinants of myocardial oxygen consumption, the use of agents that reduce afterload in heart failure includes the attractive prospect that better emptying of the ventricle will be achieved while decreasing myocardial oxygen requirements.

An early attempt at reducing afterload in severe heart failure was the use of arterial counterpulsation. This approach is still being used to treat patients who experience shock after myocardial infarction and involves the placement of an intra-aortic balloon device to reduce afterload and to raise diastolic aortic blood pressure. More recently, reduction in afterload has been approached using pharmacologic agents that induce systemic vasodilatation.

TABLE 4. Current Clinical Uses of Reduction in Afterload

Chronic myocardial failure
  Refractory heart failure in ambulatory patients
  Acute heart failure unresponsive to standard cardiotonic and
    diuretic program
Acute myocardial infarction
  Particularly with hypertension
  With severe heart failure
  With cardiogenic shock
Acute left ventricular failure due to cardiac overload
  Hypertensive crisis
  Acute aortic insufficiency
  Complications of acute myocardial infarction
    Ruptured chordae tendineae leading to mitral regurgitation
    Ventricular septal defect

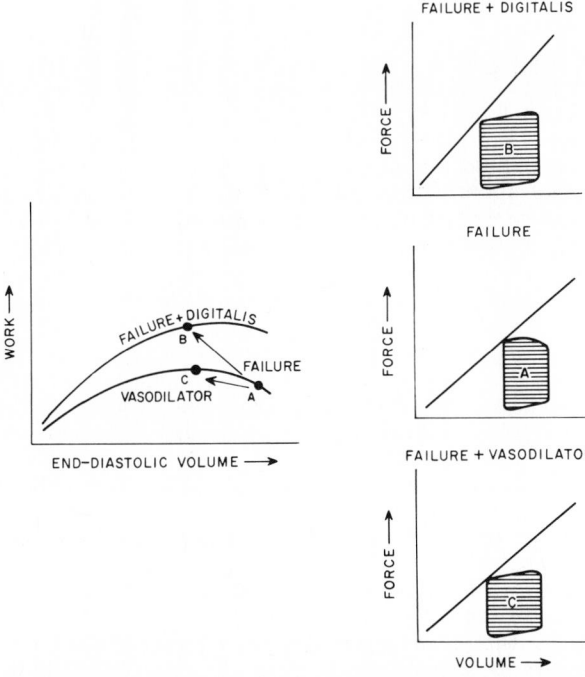

Figure 4. Schematic ventricular function curves comparing effects of vasodilator (reduction in afterload, per se) and vasodilator plus digitalis (inotropic effect) in heart failure. *Left,* The administration of a vasodilator in severe heart failure (A) moves the heart to an improved position on the lower curve of impaired contractility (B). Digitalis shifts the heart to a curve of improved contractility (C). *Right,* Analysis of work done per beat for points B, A, C shown on left. The landmarks on the work loops are the same as in Figure 2.

Three broad categories of vasodilators have been tried: arteriolar, venous, and a combination of the two (Table 5). The prototype is nitroprusside, which exerts its vasodilator effects directly on systemic arterioles and veins. Venodilation operates by pooling blood in peripheral veins, thereby decreasing venous return to the heart and decreas-

ing left ventricular end-diastolic volume and pressure (preload). Arteriolar dilatation decreases the impedance to left ventricular ejection (afterload). The over-all unloading effect of nitroprusside depends on the hemodynamic state of the heart. If the heart is not in failure so that output and filling pressures are normal, nitroprusside has little or no effect on stroke output; left ventricular end-diastolic pressure falls. The unchanged output and the concomitant decrease in filling pressure presumably reflect an equivalent reduction in preload and afterload by the nitroprusside. In contrast, if myocardial function is severely impaired, stroke output increases as left ventricular end-diastolic pressure falls because nitroprusside causes a greater decrease in afterload than in preload. In practical terms, the unloading effect of nitroprusside is most apt to be helpful when the left ventricular end-diastolic pressure is greater than 12 to 15 mm Hg and the cardiac output is low. Unloading of the heart by nitroprusside is not accompanied by a change in heart rate or in contractility. However, as systemic arterial pressure and end-diastolic volume fall, ventricular wall tension decreases and consequently the myocardial oxygen requirement falls. Thus in severe heart failure nitroprusside affords the prospect of achieving better emptying of the ventricle while decreasing myocardial oxygen requirements.

Phentolamine accomplishes vasodilation somewhat differently from nitroprusside. It is an alpha-adrenergic blocking agent as well as a direct dilator of systemic arterial and venous blood vessels. As in the case of nitroprusside, the effects of phentolamine on stroke output depend on the level of left ventricular filling pressure. However, phentolamine is less of a venodilator than an arteriolar dilator, so that it exerts a greater effect on impedance to ventricular emptying than on preload.

Nitroglycerin exerts its greatest effect directly by relaxing venous smooth muscle. As a result, venous return to the heart decreases. Therefore the predominant therapeutic effect of nitroglycerin is accomplished by reducing ventricular preload. Although nitroglycerin does have a vasodilator effect on systemic arterioles, the venodilator effect predominates.

Other vasodilator agents that are currently being tried are indicated in Table 5. Undoubtedly new agents will

---

TABLE 5. Representative Vasodilators Used to Reduce Afterload in Heart Failure

Agent	Route of Administration	Usual Dosage	Predominant Sites of Action	Predominant Hemodynamic Effects				Comment
				Blood Pressure	Cardiac Output	PA Wedge	Heart Rate	
Sodium nitroprusside	IV	Start with 15 µg/min and increase gradually;* maximum of 400 µg/min; usual, 65 µg/min	A, V†	+	++	++	0 or +	Hazard of thiocyanate or cyanide toxicity during prolonged therapy or high doses
Phentolamine	IV	Start with 0.1 mg/min;* maximum of 2 mg/min	A, V	+	++	++	+	Chief effect on arterioles; causes tachycardia
Nitroglycerin	IV Sublingual		V	+	+	+++	0	Transient (15-30 min); negligible effect on arterioles
Isosorbide dinitrate	Oral Sublingual	20-40 mg 2.5-10 mg	V	+	+	+++	0	Same as nitroglycerin but longer (1-4 hrs)
Hydralazine	Oral	50-75 mg q 6 hrs	A	0 or +	+++	0 or +	0	Sometimes used in conjunction with venodilator
Trimethaphan	IV	Start with 2-4 mg/min; decrease, maximum of 6 mg/min	A, V	+	++	++	0	No reflex increase in heart rate; adjust dose carefully to avoid marked hypotension

*Increase every 10 to 15 minutes, using arterial blood pressure and pulmonary wedge pressures as guides. Avoid large fall in systemic blood pressure while pulmonary wedge pressure is returning to about 15 mm Hg.
†A = Arterial bed. V = Venous bed.

continue to appear during the next few years. In applying any of these it is important to relate their predominant and side effects to the hemodynamic state of the patient.

Clinical application of agents that reduce afterload is not yet standardized. Vasodilators, such as hydralazine, trimethaphan, and diazoxide, have been successfully used to manage acute heart failure as a complication of hypertensive heart disease. This practice has been logically extended to the management of acute myocardial infarction and impaired ventricular performance in a patient with hypertensive heart disease. Vasodilators have also proved useful in managing heart failure that complicates acute myocardial infarction even though blood pressure is normal. At present, trials are being made of vasodilator agents in the management of chronic congestive heart failure in patients with chronic coronary heart disease.

Dramatic clinical improvement has followed the use of vasodilators in mitral regurgitation that follows papillary muscle dysfunction in acute or chronic coronary heart disease and in cardiomyopathies. Infusion of nitroprusside has increased the stroke output into the aorta while the regurgitant fraction decreases. Accompanying these changes is a decrease in left ventricular filling pressure and in systemic vascular resistance. In a similar fashion, nitroprusside decreases left-to-right shunting across a ventricular septal defect that occurs in the course of acute myocardial infarction; the drop in systemic arterial resistance that nitroprusside produces results in an increase in stroke output that decreases the left-to-right shunting and pulmonary congestion. Nitroprusside has also been of great value in improving cardiac function in the patient with severe aortic valvular insufficiency.

Diuretics

Inordinate retention of salt and water, followed by expansion of the plasma and the interstitial tissue compartments of the extracellular fluid volume, is a hallmark of congestive heart failure and is responsible for many of its symptoms. Consequently, elimination of the excess salt and water and contraction of the extravascular fluid volume by diuresis are essential for the successful treatment of heart failure.

"DRY" WEIGHT. The use of diuretics entails two separate problems: elimination of excess fluid, and the maintenance of edema-free ("dry") weight. In the hospital, where the patient is at rest and salt intake is precisely controlled, low dosages of diuretics may suffice to maintain dry weight. Out of the hospital, where the patient engages in various degrees of exercise, and salt intake is neither readily monitored nor controlled, larger doses may be needed. However, continued use of large doses of diuretics inevitably leads to serious derangements in electrolyte balance, often predisposing to digitalis toxicity by way of hypokalemia. Consequently, once the urgent need for brisk diuresis has passed — as during an episode of acute pulmonary edema — the optimal cardiotonic program relies heavily on digitalis and salt restriction and depends on diuretics as an ancillary measure.

SALT AND WATER RESTRICTION. Restriction of sodium intake should be directed not only at sodium chloride per se but also at sodium-containing medications, e.g., antacids. Restriction of water intake is rarely necessary except after the use of potent diuretics which predispose to hyponatremia and water intoxication. In mild heart failure, sodium intake is generally restricted to less than 3

grams per day; in severe congestive heart failure, intake of less than 0.5 gram per day is often needed to promote diuresis and to reduce the blood volume and venous pressure. Overzealous sodium restriction in conjunction with potent sodium-losing diuretics, particularly in the elderly or in others with impaired renal function, may lead to weakness, oliguria, and azotemia.

THE SODIUM CONTROL SYSTEM. The major diuretics increase the rate of sodium excretion by the renal tubule. As indicated previously, the tubule is the end organ of an elaborate control system that is influenced by hemodynamic and neurohumoral mechanisms. For some mysterious reason, the control system seems to be reset in heart failure so that an expanded extracellular fluid volume, usually a stimulus to diuresis, coexists with antidiuresis. Nonetheless, despite this reset, it is possible to modify the handling of sodium by intervening at several different sites in the control system.

The diuretics that will be considered interfere with the control system by modifying the reabsorption of sodium, with its accompanying anions and water, by the end organ, the renal tubule (Fig. 5). Five distinct categories of diuretics are in common use (Table 6). Each affects tubular reabsorption somewhat differently, and each produces its own characteristic abnormalities in electrolyte pattern, hydration, and acid-base balance. These abnormalities represent the pharmacologic consequences of effective drug action. When carried to extremes, or when effects interact, they are responsible for the toxicity of these different diuretics.

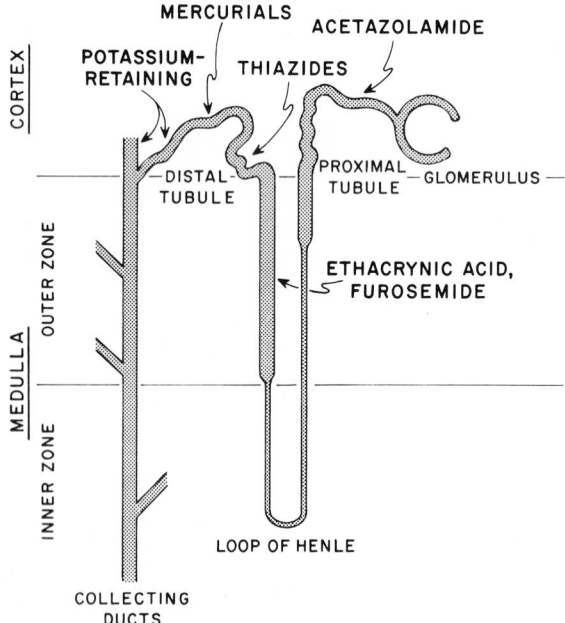

Figure 5. Schematic representation of a nephron, indicating predominant sites of action of the five groups of diuretics. Carbonic anhydrase inhibitors exert predominant effects on the proximal tubule. The potassium-retaining diuretics affect the distal nephron. The major diuretic effect of the thiazides is at a site of urine dilution in the cortical portion of the ascending limb of the loop of Henle. Ethacrynic acid, furosemide, and the organomercurials act chiefly on the loop of Henle, affecting both the diluting and concentrating segments to achieve potent diuretic effects.

TABLE 6. Diuretic Agents in Heart Failure

Type of Diuretic	Effect on Kidney		Effect on Electrolytes		Toxic Manifestations	Special Features
	Principal Site of Action	Mechanism	In Urine	In Blood		
Thiazides (chloruretic sulfonamides)	Ascending limb of loop of Henle; distal tubule	Interference with dilution of urine	Increased excretion of Na, Cl, K	Hypochloremic alkalosis; hypokalemia	Nausea; vomiting; skin rashes; hyperuricemia; hypercalcemia; hyperglycemia; azotemia	Loss of effectiveness and hypokalemia are common on continued administration
Ethacrynic acid*	Ascending limb of loop of Henle; distal tubule; probably proximal tubule	Interference with dilution and concentration of urine	Increased excretion of Na, Cl, HCO₃, K, H	Hypochloremic alkalosis; hypokalemia; hyponatremia	Hypotension; contraction alkalosis; hyperuricemia; hypercalcemia; azotemia; hyperglycemia; hearing loss	Causes renal vasodilatation; effective in renal insufficiency, systemic acidosis or alkalosis; potent diuresis often followed by rebound
Organomercurials	Proximal and/or distal tubule	Decrease of isosmotic reabsorption	Increased excretion of Na, Cl, H	Hypochloremic alkalosis	Mercury intoxication; sudden death (after IV injection); occasional agranulocytosis	Inactivated by hypochloremic alkalosis; hazardous in oliguria
Potassium-sparing†	Distal tubule	Aldosterone antagonism for Na-K exchange	Decreased excretion of K and H; slight increase in Na, Cl, HCO₃	Hyperkalemia	Generally nontoxic; GI upset; gynecomastia; rare agranulocytosis	Synergistic with thiazides and ethacrynic acid; avoid in renal insufficiency and in hyperkalemia
Carbonic anhydrase inhibitors	Proximal tubule	Inhibition of enzyme involved in acidification of urine	Increased excretion of Na, K, HCO₃; decrease in H	Hyperchloremic acidosis; hypokalemia	Generally nontoxic; mild GI and mental upsets; occasional sulfonamide idiosyncrasy	Not very potent and loses effectiveness in a few days

*Furosemide (Lasix), a nonthiazide sulfonamide, has practically the same indications and effects despite its different chemical structure.
†Spironolactone (Aldactone) operates as a competitive inhibitor of endogenous aldosterone; triamterene and amiloride are noncompetitive inhibitors and produce the characteristic effects on the urine even though aldosterone is absent.

THIAZIDES. Because of their effectiveness by mouth, their reliability, and their relative freedom from toxicity if administered circumspectly, the benzothiadiazine drugs are usually the diuretics of choice in cardiac edema. The prototypes of this group are chlorothiazide and hydrochlorothiazide (Table 7). *Acute* administration promotes the urinary excretion of sodium, chloride, and potassium without consistent change in urinary pH or bicarbonate excretion. The predominant diuretic effect (natriuresis and chloruresis) has been localized to inhibition of sodium absorption at a diluting site in the distal nephron (Fig. 5). Although there is also a carbonic anhydrase–inhibiting effect, it is generally insignificant until large daily doses are reached (of the order of 2000 mg per day). Kaliuresis depends on an increase in the quantity of sodium delivered to the distal nephron. Intravenous administration of chlorothiazide is uricosuric, whereas chronic administration results in hyperuricemia. The mechanisms responsible for the paradoxical uric acid effects are still unclear.

Hypokalemia is particularly apt to arise after intensive diuresis with thiazides or after prolonged thiazide therapy. Supplementary doses of potassium may then be required. Several generalizations have proved useful as practical guides to therapy. Acute hypokalemia that is modest in degree is managed by diet; if diet fails to correct the hypokalemia, supplementary doses of potassium may be required. Potassium chloride is generally the agent of choice for oral supplementation, because hypochloremic metabolic alkalosis usually accompanies diuretic-induced hypokalemia. For severe hypokalemia, intravenous infusions are used. To prevent hypokalemia during chronic administration of potassium-losing diuretics, aldosterone inhibitors are useful.

Certain precautions merit attention in applying these guides to therapy. Potassium salts administered orally in any form cause gastric irritation. This side effect is generally tolerable, especially in the hospital, where potassium chloride can be safely given in liquid form after meals.

Prolonged administration of potassium salts, particularly if enteric coated, is particularly hazardous because of the high incidence of intestinal ulceration, perforation, and peritonitis, often followed by intestinal stenosis and obstruction. No matter how administered, excessive doses of potassium are apt to lead to hyperkalemia. This likelihood is enhanced in older persons who often have slight renal impairment, especially if an aldosterone inhibitor is given concomitantly.

ETHACRYNIC ACID AND FUROSEMIDE. These are the most potent natriuretic agents currently available. Both are organic acids but otherwise are quite different chemically. Furosemide is a sulfonamide–anthranilic acid derivative related to the thiazide diuretics, whereas ethacrynic acid is a ketone derivative of aryloxyacetic acid (Table 7). Like the thiazides, they are effective orally and are rapid acting. They exert powerful diuretic effects by inhibiting both the renal diluting and concentrating mechanisms in the ascending limb of the loop of Henle (Fig. 5). Ethacrynic acid is without appreciable effect on carbonic anhydrase, whereas furosemide does elicit modest anti-carbonic anhydrase activity. Ethacrynic acid appears to relax vascular smooth muscle by a direct effect. Although this effect could contribute importantly to unloading the failing heart, it is exceedingly difficult to dissociate from the diuretic effect per se.

Ethacrynic acid, administered orally, exerts its effects in 30 minutes and continues to act for six to eight hours; administered intravenously, it acts within a few minutes, reaching its peak activity in one hour. Both agents elicit a marked increase in urine flow containing large quantities of sodium and chloride (of the order of 20 to 30 per cent of the filtered load). Kaliuresis is consistent and appreciable. In conventional doses, neither drug consistently increases bicarbonate secretion or modifies urine pH. But chronic administration of ethacrynic acid promotes hydrogen loss in a bicarbonate-free urine, i.e., produces metabolic alkalosis.

A cardinal virtue of these agents (in contrast with thia-

TABLE 7.   Administration of Diuretics

	Example	Relevant Chemical Structure	Preferred Route of Administration	Usual Range of Daily Dosage	Suggested Pattern of Administration
Thiazides	Chlorothiazide (Diuril)	Benzothiadiazine derivative	Oral	500 mg × 2–4	Standard type of diuretic to start treatment; few days on, few days off to avoid refractoriness and serious electrolyte disturbances
Ethacrynic acid*	Ethacrynic acid (Edecrin)	Ketone derivative of aryloxyacetic acid	Oral or IV*	50 mg × 2–3	Reserve for serious or refractory edema
Organomercurials	Mersalyl and theophylline	Theophylline plus organic mercurial	IM	2 ml	Adjunct diuretic or for moderately rapid response in hospital
Potassium-sparing†	Triamterene (Dyrenium)	Pteridine derivative	Oral	200 mg	Continuous administration in conjunction with more potent potassium-losing diuretics; do not use with potassium supplements
Carbonic anhydrase inhibitors	Acetazolamide (Diamox)	Sulfanilamide derivative	Oral	250 mg × 4–6	Episodic as booster diuretic; useful before injection of organomercurial for chloride-retaining effect

*Furosemide and ethacrynic acid may be given intravenously as well as by mouth. For ordinary use, however, furosemide is administered as a single oral dose in the morning. In an urgent situation (pulmonary edema), furosemide, as well as ethacrynic acid, may be administered intravenously (50 mg). Intravenous administration should not be administered at less than six-hour intervals.

†Spironolactone (Aldactone), 75 to 100 mg per day, is commonly used as a potassium-sparing diuretic. In refractory heart failure doses of 100 to 600 mg per day have proved helpful.

zides and carbonic anhydrase inhibitors) is their lack of effect on filtration rate or renal plasma flow unless sodium depletion occurs. This lack of direct hemodynamic effect is fortunate, because a decrease in filtration rate interferes with their action; conversely, increase in filtration rate, as by intravenous administration of mannitol or albumin, enhances their effects. At peak effect, both agents decrease renal vascular resistance.

Ethacrynic acid and furosemide remain effective despite gross electrolyte disturbances and hypoalbuminemia. If pushed, either may cause hyponatremia, volume depletion, fall in blood pressure, fall in urine volume, azotemia, and water retention. Because of the upsets in the electrolyte concentrations which they induce, other diuretics are preferred for maintenance treatment. They are most valuable in three situations: in acute pulmonary edema (25 to 50 mg intravenously), in severe or refractory heart failure, or when renal function is impaired (because they increase renal blood flow). Both agents produce "contraction alkalosis," i.e., an increase in plasma bicarbonate consequent to the decrease in extracellular fluid volume that follows excretion of a large volume of bicarbonate-poor urine. The metabolic alkalosis that follows hydrogen depletion and "contraction" predisposes to alveolar hypoventilation through its depressant effects on respiratory control mechanisms.

ORGANOMERCURIAL DIURETICS. Until the advent of potent oral diuretics, the organomercurials, generally a combination of an organic mercurial and theophylline, were the diuretic agents of choice in heart failure. Now they are generally reserved for parenteral administration in hospital. After administration of a maximally effective dose intravenously, large (and approximately equal) amounts of sodium and chloride are eliminated in the urine. The normal subject is apt to eliminate 10 per cent of the filtered load, whereas the individual who has been primed to the stage of hyperchloremic acidosis by prior administration of ammonium chloride may eliminate up to 20 per cent of the filtered load. Bicarbonate excretion does not increase, and urinary acidity persists during the diuresis. The effect on potassium excretion is variable and generally small, depending on prior rates of excretion. Generally they tend to decrease potassium.

Like ethacrynic acid and furosemide, the organomercurials exert an important inhibitory effect on sodium reabsorption in the loop of Henle, impairing both the diluting and concentrating mechanisms. In Figure 5, the organomercurials are shown as acting predominantly on the distal tubule, beyond the predominant sites of action of the thiazides, ethacrynic acid, and furosemide. However, these distinctions are far from absolute. Theophylline-containing mercurials usually elicit transient increases in filtration rate, but this effect is generally neutralized by volume concentration if diuresis is effective.

The organomercurials are almost invariably administered intramuscularly. After intramuscular injection, the onset of action is in one to two hours, reaching a peak in six hours, and lasting for 12 to 24 hours. Early in treatment, a brisk diuresis and natriuresis occur. But with continued use, refractoriness may result, generally for one of two reasons: (1) the onset of a hypochloremic hypokalemic alkalosis (with fairly normal sodium levels); responsiveness may then be restored by administering ammonium chloride; or (2) the advent of a low-salt syndrome in which sodium as well as chloride levels in the serum are severely depressed; this state responds to water restriction.

ALDOSTERONE ANTAGONISTS. A characteristic feature of chronic heart failure is high circulating levels of renin and aldosterone. Aldosterone, either by providing energy for active transport or by increasing permeability, enhances the movement of sodium through the distal tubular cell, from lumen to interstitium. Water follows passively. In addition to promoting sodium reabsorption, aldosterone also increases potassium excretion by a mechanism that is not entirely clear but is more than an ion-exchange mechanism. In heart failure the hyperaldosteronism causes continuing sodium retention, whereas potassium excretion remains normal, i.e., no hypokalemia. Aldosterone antagonists interfere with these actions, causing potassium retention and sodium excretion.

Three agents are available: spironolactone, triamterene, and amiloride (MK-870). Spironolactone is most popular; amiloride is not yet available for general use. Although all three act by competing for receptor sites in the distal tubule, the intimate mechanisms involved in electrolyte secretion may be quite different. The major site of action of spironolactone is in the distal tubule, in the region of the aldosterone-stimulated secretion of hydrogen and potassium. It is a specific competitive inhibitor of aldosterone and has no action if aldosterone is absent. It promotes natriuresis, water loss, and potassium retention by depressing aldosterone-dependent sodium-potassium exchange in the distal tubule. It is only effective in the presence of high levels of mineralocorticoid activity; it is devoid of effect after adrenalectomy. Conversely, triamterene (Table 7) and amiloride are noncompetitive inhibitors that inhibit potassium and hydrogen ion excretion even if aldosterone is absent. Their mechanism of action is unclear. Although these natriuretic agents are far less potent than the thiazides, ethacrynic acid, furosemides, and the organomercurials, they have the extraordinary advantage for prolonged use of continuing effectiveness, minor electrolyte derangements, and the virtual absence of toxicity as long as hyperkalemia is avoided. These agents are unique in that they are given without interruption, because, in contrast to the thiazides, ethacrynic acid, and furosemide, they do not lose effectiveness in a few days nor do they cause violent electrolyte upheavals.

Spironolactone is expensive but effective. Oral doses, ranging from 100 to 400 mg per day, are well tolerated for months. A few days may elapse before its action becomes apparent. It is currently being used primarily to potentiate the effects of the more powerful diuretics, particularly if potassium depletion is a serious consideration.

CARBONIC ANHYDRASE INHIBITORS. These agents are effective by mouth. They elicit an increase in excretion of bicarbonate, sodium, and potassium and an increase in urine pH. The most striking increments are in bicarbonate and potassium. By interfering with carbonic anhydrase activity in the kidney, they inhibit hydrogen ion secretion primarily in the proximal and distal portions of the nephron, exerting lesser effects on the loop of Henle, i.e., little effect on urinary diluting or concentrating mechanisms.

The prototype of this group is acetazolamide (Table 7). It is a weak diuretic and loses its effectiveness as hyperchloremic metabolic acidosis develops because of diminished hydrogen ion excretion (usually in 48 hours). Like ammonium chloride, this class of diuretics is particularly valuable in patients with high serum bicarbonate, as occurs in cor pulmonale or metabolic alkalosis. They are valuable in preparing for a mercurial diuresis because of the hyperchloremic acidosis that they produce. This group also enhances natriuresis produced by thiazides, ethacrynic acid, and furosemide. A contraindication for its use is severe acidosis, as from renal failure or hepatic insufficiency.

SPECIAL DIURETICS. This is a miscellaneous group of agents that are used with extreme caution and under special conditions. For example, osmotic diuretics such as mannitol and albumin, which expand the circulating blood volume, have the potential for increasing the renal blood flow and for blocking the reabsorption of sodium and water at the proximal tubule. However, in heart failure they entail the risk of circulatory overload and pulmonary edema.

COMBINATIONS. There are two main reasons for introducing a combination of diuretics into a cardiotonic program: to avoid serious electrolyte upsets that are bound to occur if the powerful primary diuretics are administered without pause, in large dosage, for long periods; and to stimulate diuresis when the prevailing cardiotonic program no longer suffices to prevent edema. In either case, the net diuretic effect of the combination will be determined by a wide variety of influences: the respective sites of action on the renal tubule of each agent, the extent of competitive inhibition at common receptor sites, the dose-response curves of the individual drugs, strategic timing of the administration of one agent with respect to the other, and the acid-base and electrolyte balances at the time that the agents are given.

A currently popular duo of diuretics is a potassium-sparing agent (triamterene or spironolactone) that is taken daily and a thiazide that is taken intermittently (e.g., for four days of each week). In time, the thiazide may be succeeded by ethacrynic acid or ethacrynic acid may be given sporadically as needed to sustain the edema-free state. On occasion, particularly in the hospital, a mercurial diuretic (after prior acidification) may prove helpful in overcoming a resistant state of edema. In contrast to the foregoing, other combinations hold little promise for success. Thus the combined use of acetazolamide and a mercurial diuretic is not apt to be exceedingly effective, because, by preventing acidification of the urine, the carbonic anhydrase inhibitor is apt to block, rather than to enhance, the diuretic effect of the mercurial.

The same general principles govern the use of combinations of diuretics in the treatment of refractory edema. This troublesome state is now relatively uncommon because of the advent of powerful primary diuretics, particularly furosemide and ethacrynic acid, coupled with a better understanding of the sites of action of the auxiliary diuretics. On the other hand, refractory edema may again become tractable by reversing electrolyte and acid-base imbalances that have been produced by unremitting administration of the primary diuretics for long periods. As a working principle, resistance to diuresis is overcome by deliberate selection of agents that act on different parts of the tubule. This approach presupposes that digitalis dosage is optimal. On occasion, aminophylline, by its inotropic effect, may reinforce the diuretic action of a thiazide or ethacrynic acid. Clearly, many opportunities exist for the physician to devise original sequences and combinations of diuretics. However, a restraining influence is imposed by the complicated interplay that is to be expected, not only between the diuretic agents per se, but also within the broad context of a deranged internal environment that generally is a feature of the state of refractory edema.

REFRACTORY EDEMA. This is a state of edema that resists conventional cardiotonic and diuretic measures. Before embarking on an endless train of drug combinations, the patient should be carefully re-evaluated for either a complication or an underlying disorder that has been overlooked: a surgically correctable disorder, such as mitral stenosis or constrictive pericarditis; a medical disorder, including hyperthyroidism, anemia, pulmonary emboli, bacterial endocarditis, persistent infection, and arrhythmias; inappropriate or excessive diuretic therapy that elicits serious disturbances in blood volume and electrolyte composition, digitalis toxicity, and water intoxication; physical overactivity; excessive salt intake and renal disease; sodium-containing medicaments, such as antacids, or agents such as reserpine, propranolol, and guanethidine which depress the myocardium to the point of failure.

COMPLICATIONS. A variety of disturbances may complicate effective diuretic therapy. These include hypotension and vascular collapse from rapid, massive diuresis; sodium depletion, usually the consequence of prolonged and effective diuretic therapy in conjunction with excessive water intake; hypokalemia from uninterrupted use of diuretics, predisposing to digitalis toxicity; hyperkalemia from injudicious administration of aldosterone antagonists and potassium supplements; metabolic alkalosis, either from a massive excretion of a bicarbonate-poor urine or from a combination of increased hydrogen ion excretion in the urine and alveolar hypoventilation as produced by ethacrynic acid or potassium depletion; and hyperuricemia after prolonged administration of small doses of the thiazides, ethacrynic acid, and furosemide, which share an inhibiting effect on uric acid excretion. In predisposed individuals, the hyperuricemia of prolonged diuretic therapy may precipitate an episode of gout. The thiazides, and occasionally furosemide, may precipitate diabetes which is rarely severe.

GENERAL COMMENTS. In treating heart failure, rarely is there a desperate need to restore everything to normal at once by vigorous diuresis. The temptation to restore the patient immediately to dry weight and to free him of breathlessness and congestion must be tempered by the penalty of dehydration and severe electrolyte disturbances. The more leisurely the diuretic therapy, the more durable and tolerable the relief.

The ability of these potent diuretics to elicit dramatic diuresis has led to their abuse. Thus without direct inotropic effect on the heart, a single injection of ethacrynic acid can effect a decrease in blood volume, a decrease in intracardiac filling pressures, an increase in cardiac output, and clear edema. But ethacrynic acid is rarely advisable as the mainstay of therapy unless edema is refractory and less drastic measures have proved ineffective. Only when coupled with a full cardiotonic program can judicious control of heart failure be maintained, particularly if the underlying heart disease is progressive and severe complications of diuretic therapy are to be avoided.

SURGICAL THERAPY OF REFRACTORY HEART FAILURE. Attempts are under way in several medical centers to provide temporary respite for the heart in acute refractory failure that is judged to be reversible, e.g., after myocardial infarction. The common feature of the different approaches is to unload the heart for hours to days while it is recuperating. The most popular devices are (1) venoarterial bypass, which assists the heart by diverting blood to a pump that returns it to the arterial tree, and (2) counterpulsation, which operates in synchrony with the heartbeat to adjust the aortic blood pressure by rhythmically changing either the volume of blood in the aorta (using an external pump) or the capacity of the aorta (using an internal balloon). All methods aim to reduce the external work of the heart and the tension that it develops during systole and to decrease myocardial oxygen consumption at the same time as coronary arterial perfusion is improved. Technical problems have restricted the use of these appliances in man to biding time in desperate situations, e.g., in cardiogenic shock. As yet, there are very few long-term survivors.

Cardiac replacement and the development of an artificial heart to assist or replace the failing heart are also being pursued as last measures for refractory heart failure. Experience with cardiac replacement began ten years ago, and approximately one fifth of the 346 heart transplant patients are still alive, the oldest nine years after transplantation. Because of great skill in surgery and in related techniques, expectations for one-year survival have improved to two out of three who undergo transplantation. However, the procedure is limited in applicability because of shortage of donor hearts and the burden of long-term immunosuppression and its complications.

The artificial heart program currently has the greatest promise as an assist device for the left ventricle. This modality is still experimental, has no long-term survivors, and is handicapped by incompatibilities between blood and artificial materials that comprise the synthetic heart.

Braunwald, E., Ross, J., Jr., and Sonnenblick, E. H.: Mechanisms of Contraction of the Normal and Failing Heart. Boston, Little, Brown & Company, 1976.
Cohn, J. N., and Franciosa, J. A.: Vasodilator therapy of heart failure. N. Engl. J. Med., 297:27, 254, 1977.
Dollery, C. T., George, C. F., and Orme, M. L. E.: Drug interaction in cardiovascular disease. Prog. Cardiol. 1:31, 1972.
Fishman, A. P. (ed.): Heart Failure. Washington, D.C., Hemisphere, 1978.
Fishman, A. P.: Pulmonary edema. The water-exchanging function of the lung. Circulation, 46:390, 1972.
Goldberg, M.: The renal physiology of diuretics. In Berliner, R. W., and Orloff, J. (eds.): Handbook of Physiology — Renal Physiology. Washington, D.C., American Physiological Society, 1973.
Mason, D. T.: Congestive Heart Failure. New York, Dun-Donnelley Publishing, 1977.
Weber, K. T., and Janicki, J. S.: Instantaneous force-velocity-length relations: Experimental findings and clinical correlates. Am. J. Cardiol., 40:740, 1977.

356. SHOCK

Francois M. Abboud

Shock is a complex clinical state which demands immediate care to avoid a fatal outcome. Few other clinical situations require such vigilant medical attention, careful hemodynamic monitoring, and thorough understanding of the basic principles of circulatory control and of the pharmacology of cardiac and vasoactive drugs. This chapter covers the basic principles of *circulatory control* as they relate to the shock syndrome, the *cellular mechanisms* involved in the pathogenesis of shock, and the *therapy* of shock.

DEFINITION. The common denominator in shock, regardless of cause, is a failure of the circulatory system to deliver the chemical substances necessary for cellular survival and to remove the waste products of cellular metabolism. In other words, the perfusion of tissues and cells with blood is restricted despite compensatory adjustments. This leads to cellular membrane dysfunc-

tion, abnormal cellular metabolism, and eventually cellular death. The goal is to recognize this state early and attempt to restore tissue perfusion.

The clinical picture is usually that of a patient who is hypotensive (with a systolic arterial pressure of 90 mm Hg or less); is hyperventilating; has cold, clammy, and cyanotic skin, constricted peripheral veins, a thready rapid pulse, and a dulled sensorium; may be confused or combative; and is oliguric, with a urinary output of less than 20 ml per hour. This basic clinical picture is present in addition to the signs and symptoms of the underlying precipitating disease, e.g., severe chest pain of acute myocardial infarction or dissecting aneurysm, visible bleeding, burn, peritonitis, sepsis.

STAGES OF SHOCK. The progress of this syndrome and its pathogenesis may be described in *three stages* which reflect the severity of the decline in tissue perfusion and intensity of cellular membrane damage. The basic elements in the pathogenesis of shock as they relate to the stages of the syndrome and the types of shock are portrayed in the accompanying figure. The causes and initiating mechanisms are listed in Table 1.

Stage I: Compensated Hypotension. Hypotension may be caused either by a fall in cardiac output or by vasodilatation. The initial event in a great majority of cases of shock is a fall in cardiac output rather than vasodilatation, except in septic shock in which peripheral vascular resistance is decreased significantly and cardiac output may be increased initially. The fall in cardiac output and hypotension trigger effective compensatory mechanisms mediated through the sympatho-adrenal and renin-angiotensin systems and other hormonal and local metabolic factors. These restore arterial pressure, and tend to restore blood flow to the more vital organs such as brain and heart. During this early stage the patients may not present with sufficient symptoms and signs to allow the clinician to suspect the possibility of impending shock. It is during this phase that intervention might be most effective in preventing further deterioration of the circulation and cellular death.

Stage II: Decreased Tissue Perfusion. Here the compensatory mechanisms to maintain perfusion of vital organs are maximal but insufficient. The evidence of decreased cerebral perfusion may be apparent from the mental status of the patient; decreased renal perfusion may reduce urinary output, and patients with coronary artery disease may begin to suffer from myocardial ischemia. The external appearance of the patient also reflects the excessive sympathetic discharge, with cyanosis and coldness and clamminess of the skin. The majority of patients are seen in this phase, and rapid aggressive intervention to restore cardiac output and perfusion of the tissues may reverse the shock syndrome.

Stage III: Microcirculatory Failure and Cellular Membrane Injury. Excessive and prolonged reduction of tissue perfusion leads to significant alterations in cellular membrane function, aggregation of blood corpuscles, and "sludging" in the capillaries. The vasoconstriction which has taken place in the less vital organs in order to maintain blood pressure is now excessive and has reduced flow to such an extent that cellular damage occurs.

Arterial pressure continues to fall progressively to a critical level at which even the perfusion of vital organs such as brain and heart is limited. Critical impairment

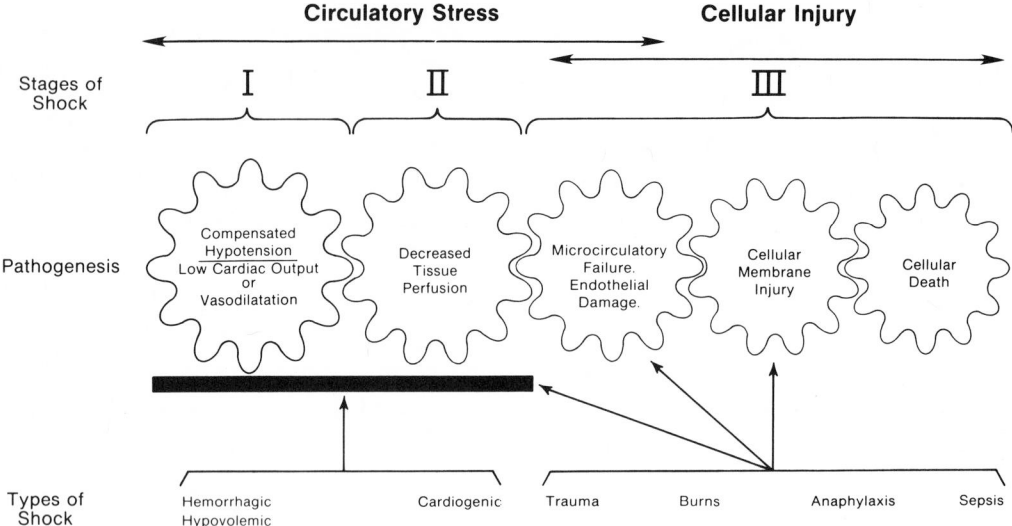

Pathophysiology of shock.

of renal perfusion leads to acute tubular necrosis as a result of ischemia of the cortical regions of the kidney. Ischemia of the gastrointestinal tract may lead to serious necrotic damage of the mucosa and the absorption into the circulation of bacteria and toxic bacterial products, which could have significant detrimental effects on other organs and might lead to a state of generalized endothelial damage with disseminated intravascular coagulation. Bacterial toxins react with neutrophils and cause the release of vasodilator poly-

peptides, which contribute to the fall in arterial pressure despite the excessive sympathoadrenal discharge and other vasoconstricting compensatory mechanisms. The severe acidosis resulting from anaerobic metabolism also contributes to vasodilatation. The decreased perfusion pressure of the coronary vessels, particularly in patients with coronary disease, results in reduction of myocardial perfusion, which in turn decreases myocardial contractility and creates a vicious cycle situation as the decreased contractility causes further decrements in arterial blood pressure. Similarly, reduction in perfusion pressure and ischemia of the central nervous system impair reflex neurogenic circulatory adjustments which help in maintaining arterial pressure. The loss of integrity of the capillary membranes leads to loss of fluid and proteins through the capillaries, with exacerbation of hypovolemia and hypotension. Damage to cellular membranes from ischemia leads to the leak of lysosomal enzymes and intracellular ions, to the progressive reduction in high energy phosphate reserves, and to cellular destruction.

CIRCULATORY CONTROL IN SHOCK

Major Determinants of Tissue Perfusion

The major determinants of hemodynamics and tissue perfusion are listed in Table 2. The perfusion of any organ is dependent upon the systemic arterial pressure (which is the driving force for blood to flow through all organs), the resistance offered by the vasculature of that organ, and the patency of nutritional capillaries. Systemic arterial pressure is in turn determined by the vigor of contraction of the heart (cardiac output) as well as the resistance of the total vascular tree. Vascular resistance is predominantly a function of the radius or caliber of blood vessels. Vascular caliber is influenced by neurogenic, humoral, and myogenic factors that regulate the tone of vascular smooth muscle. Thus blood flow to any one organ is dependent on cardiac function and on muscle tone and caliber of vessels in all the arterial tree as well as in the organ itself. The determin-

---

TABLE 1.   Causes of Shock and Initiating Mechanisms

I. Blood loss and decreased intravascular volume
  A. Acute hemorrhage: gastrointestinal bleeding, hemoptysis, hemoperitoneum, retroperitoneal bleeding, ruptured aneurysm
  B. Excessive fluid loss
    1. Vomiting (intestinal or pyloric obstruction)
    2. Severe diarrhea and dehydration
    3. Peritonitis, pancreatitis, splanchnic ischemia, intestinal obstruction and gangrene
    4. Fractures and extensive muscle injury
    5. Burns
  C. Relative hypovolemia
    1. Neurogenic vasodilatation: anesthesia (spinal), ganglionic and adrenergic blockers, spinal cord injury
    2. Metabolic, toxic, or humoral vasodilatation: septicemia (gram-negative endotoxemia or gram-positive bacteremia)
II. Cardiac
  A. Myocardial infarction, cardiac rupture
  B. Myocarditis and myocardial depression (hypoxia, acidosis, septic shock, myocardial depressant factors [MDF], drugs)
  C. Arrhythmias: severe bradycardia, tachycardia, and fibrillation
  D. Mechanical compression or obstruction
    1. Pericardial effusion or tamponade
    2. Positive pressure ventilation
    3. Pulmonary embolism
    4. Ball-valve thrombus or atrial myxoma
III. Microcirculatory endothelial injury and aggregation
  A. Anaphylaxis
  B. Disseminated intravascular coagulation
  C. Burns, septic shock, trauma
IV. Cellular membrane injury
  A. Septic shock
  B. Anaphylaxis
  C. Ischemia, prolonged hypoxia, pancreatitis, tissue injury

TABLE 2. Major Determinants of Hemodynamics and Tissue Perfusion

I. Systemic arterial pressure
  A. Total vascular resistance
     1. Total arteriolar resistance, vascular muscle tone
        a. Tissue metabolism
        b. Neurohumoral factors, toxins
     2. Viscosity of blood
  B. Cardiac output
     1. Heart rate
     2. Stroke volume
        a. Cardiac filling pressure
           i. Venous (vascular) tone
           ii. Blood volume
               Capillary hydrostatic pressure: post-precapillary resistance
               Capillary permeability
               Oncotic pressure, plasma proteins
        b. Myocardial contractility
           i. Arterial blood pH, Po_2
           ii. Myocardial O_2 supply
               Increase supply:
               ↑ Diastolic arterial pressure (norepinephrine, dopamine)
               Capillary diffusion
               Coronary dilatation (nitroglycerin, dopamine, metabolites)
               Decrease supply:
               ↓ Diastolic arterial pressure (isoproterenol, vasodilators)
               Coronary artery disease, myocardial infarction
               Hypoxia, anemia
           iii. Myocardial O_2 demand
               Increase demand:
               ↑ Cardiac size (pulmonary wedge pressure)
               ↑ Afterload (systolic arterial pressure, impedance)
               ↑ Contractility (norepinephrine, dopamine, isoproterenol) and heart rate
               Decrease demand:
               ↓ Cardiac size
               ⎧ Digitalis, ↑ ejection fraction
               ⎨ Venodilatation (nitroprusside, nitroglycerin, phentolamine)
               ⎩ Diuretics
               ↓ Afterload, impedance (vasodilators)
               ↓ Contractility and heart rate
           iv. Humoral factors
               Catecholamines
               Myocardial depressant factors
           v. Drugs
               Increase norepinephrine, dopamine, isoproterenol, digitalis
               Decrease propranolol, anesthetics
II. Organ vascular resistance
  A. Occlusive arterial disease
  B. Local arteriolar resistance
  C. Local venular resistance
  D. Viscosity of blood
III. Patency of nutritional capillaries
  A. Precapillary sphincter tone
  B. Intracapillary aggregation of corpuscles
  C. Capillary endothelial integrity

ant of exchange of substrates and metabolites with the tissues is the microcirculation. A patent nutritional capillary network is the critical interface between the circulation and the cell.

This discussion deals with cardiac, vascular, and microcirculatory factors.

CARDIAC FACTORS. Cardiac output is the product of heart rate and stroke volume. A rate of 70 beats per minute and a stroke volume of 70 ml per beat give a cardiac output of approximately 5 liters per minute, an amount more than sufficient to deliver 250 ml of oxygen per minute to all the tissues. This consumption of oxygen reflects metabolic needs at rest. A drop in cardiac output below 2 liters per minute per square meter is an indication of severe shock.

Heart Rate. Tachycardia usually increases cardiac output, but a marked increase in heart rate may limit cardiac filling time and result in a low cardiac output and arterial blood pressure. For example, ventricular tachycardia or rapid atrial fibrillation in a patient with recent myocardial infarction causes a reduction in cardiac output and arterial pressure which, if uncorrected, could result in cardiogenic shock. Immediate treatment to restore heart rate is essential. In considering the treatment of tachycardia in shock, one has to be cautious in avoiding treatment of a "compensatory tachycardia" often seen in patients with fever, anemia, sepsis, hemorrhage, or severe hypovolemia. Tachycardia is often an appropriate reflex circulatory adjustment to maintain cardiac output.

Extreme bradycardia may also cause a low output and hypotension. Sinus bradycardia and atrioventricular block are often seen immediately following myocardial infarction and should be reversed if they contribute to hypotension. Severe bradycardia is also seen in the "common faint" syndrome or vasovagal syncope; the patient usually falls to the horizontal position and recovers spontaneously. Rarely is it necessary to treat such patients with atropine.

Stroke Volume. A decrease in stroke volume may be caused by (1) a decrease in filling pressure, (2) a decrease in myocardial contractility, or (3) a mechanical obstruction to blood flow.

DECREASE IN FILLING PRESSURE. The amount of blood filling the ventricles at the end of diastole regulates the subsequent contraction and stroke volume (Starling's law of the heart). Although there are many factors that determine filling pressure such as the rate and duration of filling, ventricular compliance, and venous tone, a most important determinant is total blood volume. Reduction in blood volume may be either absolute or relative to the capacity of the vascular tree. Absolute reductions in blood volume are apparent when blood or fluids are lost, causing a hypovolemic state leading to hypovolemic shock. This is seen in hemorrhage (either external or internal bleeding), excessive vomiting, diarrhea, burns, renal loss of fluids such as in diabetes mellitus or diabetes insipidus, excessive diuresis, and excessive perspiration without fluid replacement. Internal losses of fluid occur in peritonitis, intestinal obstruction with extravasation of fluid, splanchnic ischemia with bowel necrosis and gangrene, fractures with extensive muscle trauma, hemothorax, and hemoperitoneum.

Relative decreases in blood volume occur when there is loss of vascular tone because of the administration of anesthetics or ganglion blockers, after spinal cord injury, and in patients with neuropathy or autonomic insufficiency. Pooling of blood thus results in a decrease in filling pressure. Compression of the heart may also prevent its filling, as is seen during pericardial tamponade, in tension pneumothorax, or in the superior vena caval syndrome.

DECREASE IN MYOCARDIAL CONTRACTILITY. Reduced contractility of the heart is the primary cause of shock after myocardial infarction, and it is a complicating factor in the late phases of any shock. There are many factors that contribute to it.

Hypoxia. Hypoxia resulting from ventilation-perfusion abnormalities of the lung occurs in the early phases of shock. In late shock malignant hypoxia accompanies the pathologic entity of shock lung. Hypoxia has several effects on the circulation. A direct, vascular effect tends to decrease vascular resistance and cause vasodilatation in organs such as the heart, brain, or contracting skeletal muscle, thus permitting the redistribution of blood to the organs with higher oxygen demand. Hypoxia also activates chemoreceptors, causing a sympathetic vasoconstrictor response in vessels of skeletal muscle, skin, and splanchnic bed, allowing for a redistribution of flow to the more vital organs. When the central nervous system is hypoxic and ischemic, a significant sympathetic discharge also takes place. Despite these and other compensatory adjustments, myocardial performance is impaired in the presence of decreased arterial Po_2. The severity of arterial hypoxia is often a reflection of the extent of myocardial damage following myocardial infarction. It is an important, potentially reversible cause of depression of myocardial contractility.

Acidosis. Acidosis results from anaerobic metabolism with release of lactate, from decreased renal perfusion with accumulation of organic acids, and possibly from hypoventilation of certain pulmonary segments, leading to respiratory acidosis. Acidosis reduces myocardial contractility and the vasoconstrictor response to various neurohumoral factors involved in the circulatory adjustment to the shock syndrome. This is another cause of myocardial depression which should be treated.

Myocardial Ischemia and Perfusion Pressure. Myocardial performance depends on perfusion of the ischemic myocardium, which is determined to a great extent by the level of arterial diastolic pressure. The fall in arterial pressure during hemorrhagic or hypovolemic shock in patients with coronary artery disease may complicate the syndrome by causing myocardial ischemia. Thus restoration of arterial pressure in any shock situation is critical to preservation of myocardial function. As stated above, the perfusion of any organ is dependent on arterial pressure and on the resistance to flow created by the vessels supplying that organ. In the presence of coronary artery disease, the resistance to flow is due to structural changes in the vessel wall, and the degree of reversible increase in vasomotor tone is minimal because of the excessive accumulation of metabolites downstream from the site of coronary narrowing and in the region of ischemia. Thus arterial pressure becomes the determinant of perfusion of the ischemic segment through collateral vessels or across a narrowing or a plaque.

Increased Myocardial Oxygen Demand Relative to Supply. Although oxygen supply to the ischemic myocardium is increased by increasing arterial pressure, hypertension is detrimental, as it increases myocardial work and oxygen demand. Conversely, hypotension decreases myocardial work and oxygen needs, but it also reduces myocardial perfusion as mentioned earlier. Thus judicious restoration of arterial pressure is necessary.

Increased cardiac size is associated with greater myocardial oxygen consumption as myocardial wall tension increases. Reductions in preload, cardiac size, and oxygen demand may be achieved with appropriate venodilator and diuretic therapy. Drugs such as isoproterenol might increase myocardial oxygen demand out of proportion to the associated increase in coronary flow and

would have a net detrimental effect. Conversely, propranolol decreases myocardial oxygen demand and could be protective, but its myocardial depressant action in patients with cardiogenic shock would be a hazardous complication.

Other Factors That Depress Contractility. Drugs may depress cardiac output by a direct effect on the myocardium such as might occur with the barbiturates or, more frequently, by suppression of the adrenergic drive to the myocardium such as is seen following the administration of propranolol, the administration of a ganglion-blocking drug, the use of catecholamine depleters such as reserpine or guanethidine, a high spinal anesthetic, spinal cord injury, or an intracranial lesion involving the medullary centers. These interventions not only depress myocardial contraction but also decrease peripheral tone and create a state of "relative hypovolemia" and a reduction in "effective blood volume."

Myocardial depressant factors (MDF) may be released from damaged cells in various organs during shock from burns, septicemia, or hemorrhage, and add an element of myocardial depression which compounds the syndrome.

MECHANICAL OBSTRUCTION TO BLOOD FLOW. Cardiac output may rapidly decline in situations in which there is a major obstruction to blood flow either in the heart or in the pulmonary circulation. In the heart, a ball-valve thrombus in the left atrium or an atrial myxoma might contribute to progressive hypotension and possibly shock. Similarly, extensive pulmonary embolism or acute occlusion of the large pulmonary vessels will result in severe shock. In these situations, early recognition and removal of the obstruction can be lifesaving.

VASCULAR FACTORS. These determine the resistance to blood flow and transcapillary exchange.

Arterial blood pressure is determined by cardiac output and total vascular resistance. The resistance to flow of blood to any organ is determined by the viscosity of blood and by the length and the cross-sectional area of the vessels. The cross-sectional area is the most important component, because the calculated resistance is inversely proportional to the fourth power of the radius of the vessels. The caliber of the vessels is in turn determined by the tone of vascular smooth muscle in the wall of the vessels. The vascular smooth muscle tone is modulated by neurogenic influences mediated primarily through the sympathoadrenal system and by circulating humoral and local metabolic factors.

Neurogenic Control. The sympathoadrenal discharge to the circulatory system is regulated by medullary neurons in the vasomotor center. The activity of these neurons is modulated by afferent neural impulses originating in various receptors located in strategic areas around the body. Some of these receptors trigger impulses which suppress the sympathoadrenal drive to the circulatory system, and others increase the activity of the sympathoadrenal system. Important among these receptors are the arterial and cardiac baroreceptors, the chemoreceptors, the somatic receptors in skeletal muscle, and the thermal receptors. Activity originating in various parts of the central nervous system (cerebellum, fastigial and vestibular nuclei, and hypothalamus) also impinges upon the vasomotor center to modulate its output. Activation of cardiac sensory afferent receptors, particularly those in the left ventricle during stretch of the myocardium, inhibits sympathoadrenal activity, causing hypotension and bradycardia. The severe bradycardia and hypotension often seen following myocardial infarction, especially the inferior-posterior wall infarction, could be ascribed to dyskinesis of the infarcted ventricle. Conversely, reduction in the stretch of these ventricular receptors during hypovolemia and hemorrhage releases the sympathoadrenal efferent activity to cause reflex tachycardia and vasoconstriction, to restore arterial blood pressure, and to release renin. The arterial baroreceptors, activated by a rise in blood pressure, suppress sympathoadrenal tone; conversely, during hypotension they increase sympathoadrenal drive and restore arterial pressure.

Severe hypoxia, often associated with shock from any cause, activates the chemoreceptor reflex and causes an increase in sympathoadrenal drive. Afferent impulses from baro- and chemoreceptors may be activated simultaneously during shock, and their interaction results in the ultimate response in the clinical situation. The reduction of central or cardiopulmonary blood volume and arterial pressure during hemorrhage activates the cardiopulmonary reflex and the arterial baroreceptor reflex simultaneously, and the two reflexes are synergistic with respect to the final sympathetic efferent activity. Similarly, the combined activation of the arterial baroreceptor reflex by hypotension and the chemoreceptor reflex by hypoxia results in a significant synergistic effect on the ventilatory response as well as the circulatory sympathetic drive. On the other hand, there may be situations in which the reflex responses have opposite effects. This may occur, for example, when cardiac receptors are activated following acute myocardial infarction by the dyskinetic bulge of the left ventricle, while the arterial baroreceptors are unloaded because of hypotension.

In the experimental preparation the inhibitory influence of the bulging left ventricular wall on the sympathetic outflow predominates and overrides the arterial baroreflex, preventing vasoconstriction and thus causing a decrease in cardiac afterload for the damaged left ventricle. Teleologically, this effect may be beneficial, as it will tend to decrease left ventricular work following its acute insult. There have been few studies of the effects of endotoxin on neurocirculatory reflexes. An increase in baroreceptor activity for any level of arterial blood pressure has been reported in endotoxemia, a situation which would tend to inhibit sympathoadrenal tone, and might explain in part, if confirmed, the decreased vascular resistance often seen in septic shock.

Humoral Factors. The release of hormones such as renin, vasopressin, steroids, prostaglandins, and kinins is partly mediated through the sympathoadrenal system and cardiovascular mechanoreceptors. In addition to their direct cardiovascular and renal effects these hormones have significant indirect effects by modulating central or peripheral adrenergic transmission and the release of the neurotransmitter (norepinephrine) at the adrenergic terminal.

RENIN-ANGIOTENSIN. Circulating levels of renin or angiotensin are too small to cause significant circulatory effects in physiologic states. However, angiotensin and renin may traverse the blood-brain barrier in the area postrema, where they influence medullary cardiovascular centers. A fall in arterial blood pressure or an increase in sympathoadrenal sympathetic discharge to the kidney causes the release of renin. The resulting formation of angiotensin causes peripheral vasoconstriction, maintains arterial pressure, stimulates the release of aldosterone to retain sodium and water, and has an intrarenal effect on tubular sodium reabsorption which permits greater sodium and water absorption and preservation of blood volume during hypotensive states.

VASOPRESSIN. This important constrictor hormone is released from the posterior pituitary primarily in response to changes in osmolality, and may also play a role in the circulatory control in shock. Its release may be significantly reduced by stretch of the left atrial receptors during hypervolemia or by stretch of the arterial baroreceptor during hypertension; conversely, during hemorrhage and systemic hypotension, or when patients are on cardiopulmonary bypass, the blood levels of vasopressin increase significantly. Recent observations suggest that thirst and the release of vasopressin may be induced by a central nervous system action of angiotensin.

KININS. A variety of potent vasodilator polypeptides are formed by the action of certain proteolytic enzymes on plasma protein precursors. The substance bradykinin serves as the prototype for this class of endogenous peptides. Their major physiologic role may be the local regulation of blood flow and function of such organs as the salivary gland and pancreas. In pathophysiologic states, kinins are believed to play a part in the hyperemia associated with inflammation and as vasodilators in hypotension produced by anaphylactic reactions and anaphylactic shock.

SEROTONIN AND HISTAMINE. Serotonin released from platelets and histamine released from mast cells during anaphylaxis or during complement activation in shock may play an important role in regulating local vascular tone and capillary permeability.

PROSTACYCLIN AND THROMBOXANE A_2. Prostaglandins are a family of endogenous acidic lipid-soluble materials with widespread distribution in the body and with diverse cardiovascular effects. They may be released in various organs during periods of ischemia and may therefore contribute to the reactive hyperemia and vasodilatation. The prostaglandin endoperoxides formed in platelets and in blood vessels from arachidonate are pivotal in the synthesis of two potent substances with opposing effects on the formation of thrombi. Prostacyclin, a powerful vasodilator and inhibitor of platelet aggregation, is synthesized in the vascular wall, mostly in the endothelial layers, from endoperoxides. In the platelets, however, endoperoxides are converted to thromboxane A_2, which causes vasoconstriction and platelet aggregation. In shock, damage to endothelial cells may inhibit synthesis of prostacyclin; in addition, platelets may release thromboxane A_2, causing intravascular platelet aggregation, clumping, and vasoconstriction.

Local Autoregulatory Adjustment of Blood Vessels. Blood vessels have an intrinsic ability to regulate vascular tone and thereby maintain blood flow to the organ over a wide range of perfusion pressures. This property has been referred to as the autoregulatory capacity for blood flow and is independent of systemic neurogenic influences or humoral factors. Different vascular beds vary with respect to their ability to maintain blood flow. The cerebral, coronary, and renal circulations are most potent. Thus during a fall in arterial pressure, vasodilatation of the cerebral, coronary, and renal vasculatures maintains blood flow and oxygen delivery to the brain and heart as well as sodium and water balance. Although a myogenic response intrinsic to the smooth muscle may explain the phenomenon, accumulation of tissue metabolites following a transient period of ischemia may also cause vasodilatation and restore blood flow. The specific mediator of metabolic vasodilatation is not known, but it is likely that a combination of changes in oxygen, carbon dioxide, hydrogen ion, and other cations, in osmolality, in the amount of adenosine compounds, and in Krebs cycle intermediates and other metabolites released in the immediate environment of blood vessels contributes to adjustments in vascular tone.

MICROCIRCULATION AND TRANSCAPILLARY EXCHANGE. Perhaps the most critical aspect of the pathogenesis of the shock syndrome takes place at the level of the microcirculation. The delivery of a significant amount of blood to an organ does not ascertain that all the segments of that organ and all capillaries are perfused appropriately.

Intraorgan Blood Flow Distribution. Adequate tissue perfusion depends on blood flow through vascular channels in which diffusion between the blood and tissues may occur. These are referred to as nutritional capillaries, as contrasted with non-nutritional vessels which do not permit capillary exchange. The latter are also referred to as arteriovenous shunts, although there may be little anatomic evidence for the existence of such shunts. An example of the importance of the intraorgan redistribution of blood flow is observed in myocardial infarction, in which an increase in coronary blood flow may not increase perfusion to the infarcted segment. Under some circumstances a coronary vasodilator might redistribute flow away from the ischemic into the nonischemic regions.

Similarly, intraorgan blood flow distribution may be critical in the kidney. Acute tubular necrosis associated with shock may reflect a reduction in glomerular filtration in the outer cortex because of a localized increase in vascular resistance in this region and a selective reduction in blood flow. Interventions that alter total renal blood flow can produce significant redistribution of flow within the kidney; for example, renal vasoconstriction following adrenergic discharge tends to shunt blood away from the outer cortex, whereas renal vasodilators such as furosemide shunt blood toward the outer cortical nephrons.

Pre- and Postcapillary Resistance. The *precapillary sphincters* regulate the patency of nutritional or "exchange" capillaries. The tone of those sphincters may be modulated by neurohumoral factors which contribute to the circulatory adjustments in shock. The metabolic products at the local tissue level are important determinants of the patency of these sphincters, which regulate the total capillary surface area and in turn determine the intravascular-extracellular fluid and solute exchange. The capillary hydrostatic force driving fluid out of the capillaries into the extracellular space is dependent on the ratio of the post- to the precapillary resistances. In hypovolemic or hemorrhagic shock, the fall in arterial pressure causes activation of the sympathoadrenal system, constriction of the precapillary resistance vessels, and a fall in capillary hydrostatic pressure, facilitating the movement of fluids from the extracellular into the intravascular space. This partially restores intravascular volume. Hematocrit and viscosity of blood and plasma oncotic pressure fall. The decline in plasma oncotic pressure may be partially corrected by rapid synthesis of new proteins; but as the hypotension persists and ischemia is prolonged, the vasoconstrictor response of the precapillary resistance vessels becomes less pronounced because of tissue acidosis but the resistance of *postcapillary* vessels (venules) increases, a situation in which more fluid is lost from the vascular to the interstitial space. Thus *venular resistance* and the reactivity of venules to the various vasoactive agents involved in the shock syndrome become important. The venules may even be *relatively* more reactive than the precapillary resistance vessels to catecholamines which activate constrictor alpha receptors. This differential effect in favor of postcapillary vasoconstriction also increases further hydrostatic pressure and intravascular fluid loss. The administration of alpha blockers in this situation might reverse this detrimental imbalance between post- and precapillary resistance. The ratio of post- to precapillary resistance and the consequent hydrostatic pressure may vary significantly from organ to organ as well as during the various stages of shock, and it is difficult to propose a specific uniform course of management directed at a reversal of that particular state, although one might consider the administration of a vasodilating drug in late stages of shock, in which the failure of the microcirculation is a predominant factor.

Capillary Permeability and Oncotic Pressure. The colloidal osmotic pressure (COP) is a major determinant of the intravascular volume. Albumin (molecular weight, 69,000) is the main osmotically active protein in plasma. The balance between the colloidal osmotic pressure and the capillary hydrostatic pressure determines the balance between the intravascular and extracellular fluid spaces. A significant degree of hypovolemia and hemoconcentration may take place either because of excessive capillary hydrostatic pressure from an increase in the ratio of post- to precapillary resistance or because of a reduction in plasma protein and consequently reduction of plasma oncotic pressure. Reduction of plasma protein and oncotic pressure might come about as the result of increased capillary permeability and loss of plasma protein from the intravascular to the extracellular space. The balance between oncotic and hydrostatic pressures is also an important determinant of the level of pulmonary edema and is critical in the management of shock and particularly of the shock lung syndrome with fluid replacement. Plasma oncotic pressure should be restored through careful selection of the type of fluid to be used in volume replacement. Fluids containing crystalloids may be undesirable, as these further decrease the oncotic pressure. On the other hand, administration of blood or colloids would be more appropriate, particularly to reduce pulmonary edema and accumulation of interstitial pulmonary fluid if pulmonary venous (or wedge) pressure is low.

Shock resulting from increased vascular permeability, such as anaphylactic shock or snake venom poisoning, is characterized by a dramatic reduction of plasma volume. Hematocrit rises sharply and oncotic pressure drops. This increase in capillary permeability may be partly related to the release of histamine from macrophages or the release of other metabolites or humoral factors which alter endothelial permeability.

Intravascular Hemagglutination and "Blood Sludging." The erythrocytes, leukocytes, and platelets undergo agglutination to a variable degree in association with the shock syndromes of thermal burn, sepsis, trauma, and perhaps even hemorrhagic shock. These aggregates may cause obstruction of capillaries as well as arterioles. The precipitating events are numerous. They may include platelet aggregation by catecholamines; damage to endothelial lining of small blood vessels and capillaries with subsequent fibrin deposition and accumulation of microthrombi; hypoxia increasing the rigidity of red cells; and release of vasoactive peptides and anaphylatoxins as a result of complement activation, which may in turn have an effect on permeability of endothelial cells and tone of precapillary sphincters, leading to further reduction in tissue perfusion and tissue damage.

Disseminated intravascular coagulation is a syndrome often seen in shock, particularly from gram-negative septicemia. The syndrome causes predominantly renal cortical necrosis and may contribute also to the pathogenesis of the shock lung.

Shock Lung. Pathologic studies of the lungs in patients dying from the shock syndrome may reveal marked capillary dilatation, pulmonary edema, alveolar hemorrhages, massive pulmonary vascular congestion and hyaline membrane formation, atelectasis, superimposed bronchial pneumonia, and, if the patient survives for weeks or months after the initial injury, pulmonary fibrosis. Shock affects the lung by producing endothelial damage in the vast capillary bed or precapillary arterioles. Microaggregates of platelets, polymorphonuclear leukocytes, and red cells block capillaries, destroy capillary endothelial cells by releasing hydrolytic enzymes, and eventually cause the increased capillary permeability that is responsible for the pulmonary interstitial edema seen in shock. In the balance of forces responsible for interstitial fluid in the lung, one must keep in mind the role of lymphatic drainage. Lymph flow is greatly increased in the very early stages of shock, and patients dying in hemorrhagic shock may have a widely distended pulmonary lymphatic system filled with proteinaceous material.

The decrease in pulmonary blood flow may also interfere with the production of surfactant. Lack of surfactant reduces the patency of alveoli and perpetuates leakage of fluid across pulmonary arterioles. Pulmonary venular constriction in response to tissue hypoxia may also contribute to pulmonary capillary congestion. It is also possible that with cerebral ischemia and hypoxia, neurogenic influences on the lung may cause a differential increase in venular resistance and increase capillary hydrostatic pressure and permeability. During *Pseudomonas* infusions in animals, there may be a direct effect of the endotoxin on capillary permeability, although sometimes a delayed response suggests an immune reaction with release of serotonin, contributing to the pulmonary edema. Regardless of its cause, the damage to the pulmonary capillary endothelium in shock perpetuates the resistance to blood flow, systemic hypoxia, and accelerates cellular death.

CELLULAR AND BIOCHEMICAL FACTORS IN SHOCK

OXYGEN-HB AFFINITY. Arterial blood with normal hemoglobin and oxygen saturation of 90 per cent at a P_{O_2} of 100 mm Hg carries close to 20 ml of O_2 per deciliter to the tissues. The mixed venous blood has an oxygen saturation of 75 per cent at a P_{O_2} of 40 mm Hg and contains 15 ml of O_2 per deciliter. The normal arteriovenous oxygen difference is 5 ml per deciliter. The extraction of oxygen from Hb by the tissues is not complete and depends to a large extent on the affinity of O_2 to Hb, i.e., the shape of the oxygen dissociation curve. Hydrogen ion (Bohr effect), carbon dioxide, and 2,3-diphosphoglyceric acid (2,3-DPG) cause greater dissociation of O_2 from Hb because of their preferential affinity for reduced hemoglobin. 2,3-DPG concentration in red cells results from a side reaction of glycolysis and increases during anemia, hypoxia, and acidosis. A drop in hemoglobin, hypoxia, and acidosis may thus be partly compensated for by a shift of the O_2 dissociation curve to the right, favoring greater delivery of O_2 to the tissues at the same P_{O_2}. This compensatory mechanism, in addition to the increase in cardiac output, provides for better oxygenation as extraction of O_2 from the O_2 reserve in venous blood increases. In certain tissues, however, such as the myocardium, extraction of O_2 at rest is already large, and any additional oxygen demand or a decrease in oxygen-Hb dissociation such as in alkalosis requires greater delivery of O_2, i.e., higher coronary blood flow.

In shock, the pH, carbon dioxide, and 2,3-DPG levels are changing, and one cannot calculate oxygen extraction from values of P_{O_2} because the shape of the O_2 dissociation curve cannot be predicted accurately. It is preferable to measure O_2 content or saturation of venous and arterial blood; if saturation is lower than predicted from values of P_{O_2}, one can deduce that there is a shift of the dissociation curve to the right, and vice versa. Overzealous correction of acidosis with bicarbonate may, through the Bohr effect on Hb affinity for O_2, actually reduce O_2 delivery to the tissues. Hypophosphatemia reported during hyperalimentation may decrease 2,3-DPG and O_2 delivery.

MITOCHONDRIAL FUNCTION. Survival of aerobic cells depends on the availability of substrates and oxygen to the mitochondria, which provide most of the high energy phosphate needs of the cell and utilize most of the available oxygen in the process. During oxidative phosphorylation, 36 moles of adenosine triphosphate (ATP) is produced per mole of glucose, whereas in the anaerobic state, glycolysis provides only two ATP molecules during the breakdown of one glucose molecule. Synthesis of the ATP from adenosine diphosphate (ADP) is associated with the most active state of respiration in mitochondria (state 3 respiration) and is determined by the cell energy demands. In addition to oxidative phosphorylation and ATP synthesis, the mitochondria bind and accumulate calcium. This function determines calcium availability for other intracellular organelles and thereby regulates biochemical processes or contractile events, as in cardiac or vascular muscle. Hypoxia may reduce the rate of ATP synthesis by mitochondria, but it does not cause significant damage to mitochondrial membrane functions unless it is severe, sustained, or associated with ischemia, which also reduces the availability of other substrates. In fact, an adaptation to hypoxia appears to take place such that when mitochondria are isolated from animal tissues after the animals have been exposed to brief periods of hypoxia (at P_{O_2} of 30 to 40 mm Hg), their capacity to respire and synthesize ATP in vitro is even enhanced. One of the earliest effects of hemorrhagic and endotoxin shock on mitochondrial function is the reduction in calcium transport by mitochondrial membranes, particularly in the organs that become ischemic. Effects on respiratory activity and ATP synthesis appear later, and finally mitochondrial damage ensues. The mechanism by which ischemia induces mitochondrial damage is not known. Whether such mitochondrial changes are the direct effects of deprivation of vital substrates during ischemia or are secondary to the release of lysosomal enzymes, changes in intracellular pH, or other changes in cellular ionic environment with accumulation of metabolites is not apparent.

Glucocorticoids may exert a protective effect on mitochondrial function in endotoxemia in rats. Very large doses of glucocorticoids completely protected the mitochondria when rats were given an LD 60 dose of endotoxin. The protective effect was not apparent, however, when a dose of LD 90 was given. One may summarize the mitochondrial effects by saying that hypoxia by itself triggers some adaptive mechanisms which tend to increase respiratory activity if oxygen and ADP become available, but ischemia during shock can induce significant mitochondrial damage which heralds cellular death.

CELLULAR STRUCTURE AND FUNCTION IN SHOCK. Several structural changes take place in cellular membranes in shock, and reversibility may occur at various stages. The earliest manifestation consists of swelling of the cell associated with an increase in intracellular sodium and clumping of nuclear chromatin, followed by dilatation of the endoplasmic reticulum. In this phase the cell membrane is unstable, and "blebs" may appear at the surface. The mitochondria will then begin to swell, and electron-dense clumps of flocculent material will appear within them. As the swelling of the mitochondria continues, Ca^{++} may or may not accumulate in them, depending on the type of cellular damage. The process of cell death becomes irreversible, lysosomes begin to disappear from the cell, and finally the cell is converted to a mass of debris, with large inclusions resembling myelin.

Two processes may lead to cellular death. One is a marked inhibition of the electron transport system caused by severe ischemia or anoxia or by the administration of cyanide or actinomycin A. This process leads to depletion of ATP, and the electron microscopic appearance of the cells undergoing that type of death does not show any calcium phosphate accumulation in the mitochondria. The other type of cell death is initiated by an injury to the cell membrane caused by activation of complement, by an antigen-antibody reaction, or by the administration of certain polyenes, such as amphotericin B, or certain bacterial or microbiologic products, such as the phospholipases or antitoxin. This type of cellular membrane damage is generally characterized by the precipitation of calcium phosphate in the mitochondria, presumably because active processes requiring ATP are preserved until late stages and calcium can be transported into the mitochondria.

One can relate the sequence of structural changes in the cellular membranes to specific biochemical changes. Initially there is probably an increase in cellular permeability for sodium and water causing cellular swelling, followed by increased sodium-potassium ATPase activity in an attempt to drive sodium out of the cell. Increased ATPase activity might eventually lead to the depletion of ATP and cyclic AMP, the latter leading to alteration of the cellular response to insulin, glucagon,

catecholamines, and other hormones. For example, the effect of insulin on glucose uptake in muscle of animals that have been subjected to hemorrhagic shock is reduced. The unresponsiveness to insulin in the peripheral tissues may be one of the reasons for hyperglycemia of injured individuals. There is also a marked decrease in ATP, particularly in the liver in early shock and in most other organs in late shock. It is difficult to determine the critical level of ATP that is necessary for cellular function, but it is believed that as long as there is ADP and oxygen, and substrate is provided, ATP generation can be resumed within minutes. The organs that are most seriously affected in the process of shock include, in descending order, the liver, kidneys, muscle, and lung.

THE LYSOSOMAL THEORY. Lysosomes are cytoplasmic granules which contain a variety of potent hydrolytic enzymes bound in a latent form in a relatively impermeable membrane. These enzymes are capable of hydrolyzing a wide variety of both natural and synthetic substances and can digest all intra- and extracellular macromolecules if they are released from their membranes. When released from the organelles, either inside or outside the cell, as a consequence of certain forms of cellular injury, they may contribute to the pathogenesis or the propagation and perpetuation of shock. They are most active at an acid pH, which would make them potentially more destructive in the setting of hypoxia and shock.

Numerous morphologic and biochemical observations implicate the lysosomal enzymes in the perpetuation of shock, but at this time the evidence for their primary involvement is not convincing. In organs such as liver, spleen, and intestine, the lysosomes enlarge and lose their granules during the early phases of shock. This is associated with a decrease in the total activity of lysosomal hydrolases in tissues and a corresponding increase in activity in the soluble fraction of the tissue homogenate. This has been interpreted to indicate a loss of lysosomal membrane integrity in vivo. When examined in vitro, the lysosomes obtained from animals in shock demonstrate an enhanced release of enzymes. A reduction in lysosomal membrane integrity has also been observed in animals after the administration of endotoxin. In several animal studies the levels of hydrolases found in blood, lymph, or serum seem to correlate with severity of shock.

The appearance of a *myocardial depressant factor* or factors (MDF) in shock, although still controversial, may be an indirect manifestation of the effect of lysosomal enzymes. In experimentally induced pancreatitis and in a variety of other shock states, plasma MDF activity closely parallels lysosomal hydrolases in the plasma. It has been suggested that pancreatic ischemia associated with shock results in the release of lysosomal and other enzymes within the pancreas, which act on an endogenous substrate to yield a peptide with low molecular weight and MDF activity, which is then released into the circulation. The resulting myocardial depression maintains the state of low cardiac output and sustains shock.

Another indication of the involvement of MDF has been the reproducibility of the shock syndrome with infusion of lysosomal hydrolases in animals. These animals demonstrate the hypotension, circulatory collapse, and pathologic changes in the tissues that are seen in experimental forms of shock.

Other suggestive evidence of the involvement of MDF has been the responsiveness of certain animals in shock to large amounts of corticosteroids. In vitro corticosteroids stabilize the lysosomal membranes and prevent their lysis. Treatment with steroids has been shown to suppress circulating serum levels of lysosomal hydrolases in a variety of shock states.

Endotoxemia is associated with increased levels of serum hydrolases, but in vitro the endotoxins do not increase the lysis of lysosome. It has been suggested that endotoxins may cause the formation of a lysosomal releasing factor, LRF, through activation of the alternative as well as the classic complement pathways. Activation of complement in fresh human serum has been found to generate a factor (LRF) which stimulates human polymorphonuclear leukocytes to release their lysosomal enzymes. This factor has many of the properties of human C5a, a complement component known to have chemotactic and anaphylatoxin activities.

COMPLEMENT ACTIVATION IN SHOCK. The complement system consists of a series of discrete plasma proteins which are present as inactive precursors until they are activated by highly specific biochemical reactions, some of which involve limited proteolytic cleavage. Nineteen components have been isolated and characterized. The activity of the immune system may depend on "complements" which may be the primary humoral mediators of antigen-antibody reactions. Not all antigen-antibody reactions depend on "complements." For example, the anaphylactic shock seen after penicillin or pollen antigens involving the IgE antibodies does not include complement. IgE immunoglobulins may act directly on cells to release histamine, slow reactive substance, and eosinophil chemotactic factor. In contrast, many other antigen-antibody reactions, particularly those involving the IgG and IgM immunoglobulins, which can also evoke an acute anaphylactic reaction, depend on complement as the primary humoral mediator of that reaction. The complement, when activated, can promote certain specialized functions by the cell, but could also eventually impair membrane function and cause cellular death. The various types of complements are designated numerically, and from a functional standpoint one could think of these various proteins as having a *recognition,* an *activation,* or a *cellular attack* function. The recognition function is carried out by three proteins forming a macromolecular complex in the plasma, which attaches itself to the membrane surface of a target cell with the appropriate antibody. The activation mechanism is triggered primarily by the antigen-antibody complex (classic pathway), but it may also be triggered by bacterial or fungal mucopolysaccharides without the participation of any immunoglobulins (alternative pathway). Regardless of pathways of activation, the results in terms of generation of various effectors, anaphylatoxins, or direct cellular damage are the same. Activation of complement causes the release of several low molecular weight vasoactive peptides from the complement molecules by cleavage, and these in turn have significant biologic effects. For example, during the activation of C2, a cleavage product occurs which has kinin-like activity, which then can significantly influence capillary permeability. Two other activation peptides, C3a and 5a, release histamine from mast cells, have chemotactic activity, and constrict vascular smooth muscle. Another fragment, C3b, acts as an opsonin and facilitates phagocytosis. Polymorphonuclear leukocytes may be attracted chemotactically through activation of esterases on their surface and may release their lysosomal enzymes if the concentration of the complement reaction product C5a is large enough. Platelets may have an increase in their procoagulant activity, and endothelial cells may contract. In addition to the direct and indirect effects of the fragments of activated complement on cells, their aggregation as decamolecular complexes on the surface of the cell membranes causes cellular destruction. The expressions of all these effects are increased capillary permeability; increased leukocyte accumulation and infiltration, such as is sometimes observed in glomerulitis; release of lysosomal enzymes, which could cause necrotizing vasculitis; and intravascular coagulation factors, which would induce the Shwartzman reaction, thrombocytopenia, and other manifestations of microcirculatory collapse and intravascular plugging seen in prolonged shock and in endotoxemia.

Although the side effects of complement activation in shock are detrimental, leading to cellular death, the fundamental biologic activities of the complement components are beneficial in enhancing phagocytosis and mediating the inflammatory response to local infection or irritation, in the vital neutralizing of viruses, and, finally, in modulating the immune response.

TREATMENT OF SHOCK

There are three main goals in the management of shock: (1) to restore or increase cardiac output to meet the demands of the tissues, (2) to distribute blood flow to vital organs if cardiac output cannot be increased effectively, and (3) to maintain arterial blood pressure in order to assure perfusion of the brain and of the ischemic myocardial segments in myocardial infarction, and to maintain glomerular filtration.

MYTHS IN THE TREATMENT OF SHOCK. *Myth 1: "All patients in shock die."* It is true that patients with extensive myocardial infarction, extensive burns, or overwhelming sepsis have a very meager chance for survival. On the other hand, a large number of patients with hypotension who are in the early phases of shock can be saved if an aggressive management is carried out to restore cardiac output and arterial blood pressure, particularly in situations in which reversible factors are contributing to the myocardial depression and hypotension.

Myth 2: "Norepinephrine (Levophed) is a lethal drug that should not be used in shock." This is another misconception which has emerged over the years from the assumption that all patients in shock have intense generalized vasoconstriction. Such is not the case in many shock syndromes, even after myocardial infarction, and particularly in septic shock. Furthermore, norepinephrine has a cardiotonic effect in addition to its vasoconstricting action, which will increase cardiac output and improve perfusion. Finally, it has a selective vasoconstrictor effect which spares the coronary and cerebral circulations and thus maintains perfusion of these vital organs and elevates arterial pressure for the perfusion of ischemic myocardial segments and glomerular filtration.

Myth 3: "Patients in cardiogenic shock should not receive intravenous fluid." This concern reflects the fact that patients in cardiogenic shock may have left ventricular failure and are bordering on pulmonary edema.

With careful monitoring of the pulmonary capillary wedge pressure (with a Swan-Ganz catheter), one can avoid fluid overload and yet administer sufficient fluid to compensate for hypovolemia and maintain a high left ventricular end-diastolic pressure necessary for an optimal stroke volume. It is also true that sometimes the shock lung syndrome associated with excessive transcapillary fluid loss into the lung may be reduced not by restricting fluid, but by giving fluids with high molecular weight colloids to increase oncotic pressure and reduce pulmonary edema.

Myth 4: "All patients in shock should be given a vasodilator." The assumption here is that the only way to improve tissue perfusion is to dilate blood vessels and decrease cardiac afterload. Drugs which produce vasodilatation may reduce arterial pressure, and thereby decrease perfusion of critically ischemic regions of the myocardium. For example, a vasodilator such as isoproterenol may increase blood flow to skeletal muscle, and a greater proportion of the cardiac output is diverted to that particular vascular bed, but the associated hypotension may reduce perfusion of the ischemic myocardium. Furthermore, unless vasodilatation includes the microcirculation, it might not necessarily be beneficial. This can be assessed by evaluating the metabolic changes in organs following the administration of a vasodilator. Isoproterenol, for instance, increases total myocardial blood flow; however, the distribution of flow within the microcirculation is such that perfusion of "exchange capillaries" is not increased and thereby the anaerobic state of that organ is not improved. In patients with myocardial infarction the intravenous administration of isoproterenol increases lactate production by the myocardium.

MONITORING PATIENTS IN SHOCK. Monitoring should include the following measures:

1. *The electrocardiogram.* Electrocardiographic monitoring promptly detects any premature ventricular contraction which could herald ventricular tachycardia and fibrillation or complete heart block, severe sinus bradycardia, or atrial arrhythmias, all of which should be treated if hypotension and low output are to be corrected.

2. *Arterial blood gases and pH.* These should also be monitored routinely. Correction of acidosis and hypoxia are essential elements in the management of the early phases of shock.

3. *Central venous and Swan-Ganz catheters.* The monitoring of central venous pressure provides an index of the status of absolute and relative blood volume and of the need for fluid replacement. The catheter should be inserted through the antecubital or external jugular vein; only if the physician is experienced should it be introduced through the subclavian or the internal jugular vein. Central venous pressure obtained with the catheter advanced to the superior vena cava is normally between 5 and 8 mm Hg, but it should be elevated to 10 mm Hg if one is to expect an adequate cardiac output in patients in shock. Central venous pressure reflects the filling pressure of the right ventricle.

The filling pressure of the left ventricle can be estimated from measurement of the "pulmonary capillary wedge" pressure with a Swan-Ganz balloon-tip catheter. A double lumen No. 7 F. catheter is introduced intravenously with or without fluoroscopy but with electrocardiographic monitoring. Its tip is advanced to the pulmonary artery; the balloon is inflated with air

and it can be floated to a wedge position in one of the pulmonary arteries. The recorded pressure downstream from the inflated balloon is the "pulmonary capillary wedge" pressure, and the appearance of the left atrial pressure wave form on the oscilloscope confirms the position of the catheter tip. The wedge pressure reflects left ventricular end-diastolic pressure, but a discrepancy between the two may occur if there is severe mitral stenosis or left atrial tumors. If for some reason one is unable to get the wedge pressure, the pulmonary artery diastolic pressure might be a useful index of the wedge pressure.

The double lumen Swan-Ganz catheter has been modified to include an extra lumen that allows measurement of right ventricular end-diastolic pressure simultaneously with the wedge pressure. Another modification includes a temperature sensor device at the tip that allows the detection of changes in temperature following injection of cold dextrose in the right atrium, and the temperature dilution curve obtained with the temperature sensor provides an estimate of cardiac output. A further modification of the Swan-Ganz catheter includes an electrical lead to allow the continuous monitoring of intracardiac electrocardiogram.

The Swan-Ganz catheter is expensive, and complications may accompany its use, such as arrhythmias, sepsis, or pulmonary infarction; nevertheless, it is a very important tool for monitoring patients with severe shock and for providing an important data base for judicious administration of fluids and sympathomimetic amines. One can suspect pulmonary infarction as a complication of Swan-Ganz catheterization if the pulmonary artery pressure rises, so occasional monitoring of the pulmonary artery pressure would be useful. The catheter should probably be removed within 48 hours after its insertion to avoid sepsis or pulmonary infarction, and should not be left continuously in the "wedged" position. The normal wedge pressure is 12 mm Hg, but it should be raised to 15 to 20 mm Hg in shock.

A discrepancy between right atrial and left atrial pressures may occur in patients with acute myocardial infarction, sepsis, or trauma when a high left atrial or pulmonary capillary wedge pressure may be accompanied by a low right atrial pressure, and under those circumstances monitoring right atrial pressure alone might lead to a dangerously aggressive replacement of blood volume. Conversely, patients with pulmonary disease, pulmonary embolism, pulmonary hypertension, and right ventricular infarction have relatively high levels of right atrial pressure compared to the pulmonary capillary wedge pressure, and the avoidance of fluids under those circumstances might deprive the patient of important therapy.

4. *Urinary catheter.* This allows the routine hourly measurement of urinary output. A decline in urinary output to less than 20 ml per hour is an indication of the inadequacy of arterial pressure and renal perfusion. It is a sensitive index of the progress of the shock syndrome and reflects the effectiveness of management. The most frequent cause of oliguria in shock is hypovolemia. Fluid deficits are often underestimated, particularly in the presence of sepsis. If oliguria persists despite adequate administration of fluid, diuretic therapy may be necessary to avoid acute renal tubular necrosis which complicates prolonged hypotension.

5. *Arterial catheterization for arterial pressure monitoring.* Patients with severe or persistent hypotension and

shock in whom it is difficult to measure blood pressure with the sphygmomanometer are candidates for intra-arterial pressure monitoring. There is often a discrepancy between the intra-arterial pressure measurements and the cuff pressure. There may be a low or even no recordable arterial pressure by the cuff technique when intra-arterial pressure by cannulation is normal or even at times slightly elevated. This discrepancy may result from severe peripheral vasoconstriction and low output and pulse pressure. Since the sphygmomanometric measurement of arterial pressure in shock may be erroneously low, it is advisable to palpate the femoral artery in the groin to get a better index of the strength of the pulse pressure in this more proximal large artery and to introduce an arterial cannula for monitoring arterial pressure before administration of vasopressors or resorting to counterpulsation. An arterial cannula also allows the frequent determination of blood gases and pH. The radial, brachial, or femoral arteries may be cannulated. We prefer to cannulate the femoral artery because of its size and the greater ease in identifying the pulse pressure in patients who are in shock.

6. *Cardiac output.* Measurement of cardiac output by thermal or dye dilution techniques is used for management of selected patients or for the evaluation of new therapeutic regimens. The mixed venous blood oxygen content may be used as an index of total body perfusion. Within certain limitations, one can estimate the effectiveness of total body perfusion and delivery of oxygen to the tissues by monitoring the oxygen content of mixed venous or pulmonary arterial blood. The assumptions are that the total body oxygen consumption is constant or does not change drastically and that the arterial oxygen content is high and does not vary significantly. An arteriovenous oxygen difference of 6 ml per deciliter or more indicates poor tissue perfusion.

MANAGEMENT. General Measures. Patients in shock may be in pain, apprehensive, and frightened. They should be reassured and put in a horizontal position with the legs slightly elevated, unless this position is uncomfortable or causes shortness of breath. In that case, they should be allowed to be in the most comfortable position. Pain should be relieved with morphine sulfate intravenously, preferably in small repeated doses of 2 to 5 mg; if side effects occur, such as hypotension, cold clammy skin, bradycardia, nausea, and vomiting, atropine may cause some relief. Another analgesic, meperidine, 50 to 100 mg, may be given intravenously. Intravenous fluid and monitoring of various functions should begin promptly to guide further therapy. Oxygen, norepinephrine, or dopamine may be initiated while the cause of shock is determined. Reversible factors which decrease cardiac output and cause hypotension should be corrected promptly.

CORRECTION OF HYPOVOLEMIA. Hypovolemia may occur in any type of shock whether or not it is associated with external signs of blood or fluid loss. If there is no evidence of actual fluid or blood loss, there may be a significant shift of fluid from the intravascular to the extracellular space because of increased capillary permeability and endothelial damage. This may occur in any vascular bed, but more specifically in the splanchnic and the pulmonary vasculature. Fluid may also shift intracellularly because of changes in cellular membrane permeability with increased intracellular sodium and water in any shock syndrome associated with decreased tissue perfusion. Fluid replacement is essential for the

restoration of cardiac output. Without an adequate filling pressure, there will not be an adequate cardiac output. The administration of potent cardiotonic drugs in the presence of hypovolemia and low cardiac filling pressure may be ineffective. On the other hand, these drugs increase cardiac output significantly if left ventricular end-diastolic pressure and volume are adequate.

If the patient has cardiogenic shock or if there are signs of pulmonary congestion or edema, one should insert a Swan-Ganz balloon catheter into the pulmonary artery or pulmonary arterial wedge position for measurements of the pulmonary artery diastolic pressure or the pulmonary capillary wedge pressure. If the pulmonary artery diastolic or pulmonary artery wedge pressure is less than 15 mm Hg, one should give 100 ml of Ringer's lactate, saline, or dextran every 10 to 15 minutes. If perfusion improves and wedge pressure remains less than 15 mm Hg, one should continue infusion at the same rate, trying to achieve a pressure between 15 and 20 mm Hg. If perfusion of the tissues is unchanged or worse, if wedge pressure increases above 20 mm Hg, or if there are signs of pulmonary congestion, one should stop volume expansion. Improvement in tissue perfusion is evaluated by examining the degree of cyanosis, clamminess of the skin, the level of arterial blood pressure, and urinary output, as well as the sensorium and alertness of the patient, blood gases, and pH.

In other types of shock, or if wedge pressure cannot be obtained the insertion of a central venous catheter is a helpful guide for administration of fluids. If the central venous pressure is less than 10 mm Hg, one should expand volume until arterial pressure and tissue perfusion return to satisfactory levels, central venous pressure is between 10 and 15 mm Hg, or pulmonary congestion develops. The central venous or pulmonary capillary wedge pressures should be measured with careful reference to a constant point marked on the chest at the level of the right atrium or the phlebostatic axis. Patients who are on respirators or are receiving positive pressure assistance or positive pressure ventilation will have an abnormally elevated pressure. Under those circumstances, the filling pressure should be recorded at the time the respirator is transiently disconnected.

Treatment for hemorrhagic hypotension is with blood replacement; but while waiting for typing and cross-matching, the patient should be given isotonic glucose or Ringer's lactate. The effects of these fluids are transient, because the crystalloids will rapidly leave the intravascular space. A more effective treatment might include colloids that stay longer in the circulation and increase oncotic pressure. This is particularly important when patients have manifestations of the shock lung syndrome, when extensive endothelial damage and interstitial edema are suspected, or when patients are chronically ill or malnourished and have hypoalbuminemia. Under those circumstances, dextran or mannitol, albumin or plasma would expand blood volume. The excretion of dextran or mannitol by the kidney will increase oncotic pressure in Bowman's capsule and create a favorable hydrostatic-oncotic pressure gradient across the glomerulus, facilitating filtration even at low arterial pressure. If arterial pressure is not rapidly restored or oliguria persists despite the administration of diuretics such as furosemide in conjunction with fluid replacement, then there might be danger of overexpansion of plasma volume and accentuation of the pulmonary edema. Dextran might not be indicated in the presence of hypofibrinogenemia and bleeding dyscrasias. The development of pulmonary edema is closely correlated with the gradient between plasma oncotic and pulmonary artery wedge pressure, which reflects the capillary hydrostatic pressure in the lung. Plasma oncotic pressure of normal adults is approximately 25 mm Hg, whereas pulmonary wedge pressure is 10 to 12 mm Hg. Capillary filtration takes place normally in the lung despite a low hydrostatic and a relatively high oncotic pressure, because of the equally high interstitial oncotic pressure in the lung. Plasma oncotic pressure may fluctuate. After 12 hours of bed rest, for example, it declines markedly. If oncotic pressure remains significantly higher (>8 mm Hg) than pulmonary capillary hydrostatic pressure, the risk of pulmonary edema is negligible; but if oncotic pressure is only 1 to 3 mm Hg higher than pulmonary wedge pressure, the patient is at high risk for pulmonary edema.

Types of Fluid. The isotonic saline solution contains 140 mEq of sodium and 140 mEq of chloride, whereas Ringer's lactate solution has 130 mEq of sodium, 4 mEq of potassium, 108 mEq of chloride, and 28 mEq of lactate. Lactate and acetate are converted to bicarbonate and maintain the alkalinity of the blood when large volumes of fluid are necessary. When large volumes of fluid are administered, isotonic saline causes a dilution acidosis, which can be avoided if Ringer's lactate is used.

Human serum albumin comes in two concentrations, 5 grams per deciliter, which is the usual dose used, or 25 grams per deciliter salt-poor albumin. The 25 grams per deciliter will be necessary only in the presence of severe hypoalbuminemia. An alternative is purified plasma protein, which is free of hepatitis virus contamination but has some contamination with vasoactive substances, causing the Food and Drug Administration to express concern about its use. Both albumin and purified plasma protein are expensive. They cost between $50 and $100 per 500 ml and represent a significant strain on blood donor programs. They should not be used indiscriminately.

There are two types of dextran: dextran 40 with 40,000 molecular weight, and dextran 70 with approximately 70,000 molecular weight. Dextran 70 comes in a 6 per cent solution, and dextran 40 comes in a 10 per cent solution. The dextran solutions maintain intravascular volume for several hours; but if given in amounts exceeding 1 liter, they may cause serious side effects, including platelet dysfunction and abnormalities in bleeding and coagulation, the nature of which is not clearly defined, and occasional anaphylactoid reactions. Approximately 5 per cent of patients receiving dextran have had such reactions, but very few of these are fatal.

With dextran 40 there is an incidence of acute renal failure, presumably because the rapid filtration of the low molecular weight dextran into the urine is accompanied by maximal reabsorption of the filtered salt and water, leading to a high intratubular concentration with an increase in intratubular viscosity and possibly physical occlusion of the renal tubule by dextran 40 precipitates. This does not seem to occur with dextran 70 because it is filtered at a much slower rate owing to its molecular size.

Another colloid is hydroxyethyl starch or hetastarch, which maintains volume expansion almost twice as long as dextran and has few of the side effects of dextran. It interferes minimally with coagulation, it has a very mild anaphylactoid effect, and its cost is one fifth that of albumin.

CORRECTION OF HYPOXIA. Often administration of 100 per cent oxygen by intranasal catheter may be sufficient to correct the hypoxia, although occasionally the use of positive pressure respirators to improve gas exchange has been necessary. Positive pressure ventilation may simultaneously decrease the venous return by increasing intrathoracic pressure, and thereby perpetuate and aggravate a low output state. Also, 100 per cent oxygen by mask may lead to toxic changes in the lung if continued more than a few hours. Thus when a respirator is required, the preferred approach is to select an F_{IO_2} of 50 per cent, and to increase the F_{IO_2} and employ positive pressure only if needed to achieve a P_{O_2} of about 70 mm Hg.

CORRECTION OF ACIDOSIS. If the arterial blood pH is less than 7.3 and respiratory acidosis has been ruled out, it is advisable to give 1 vial of sodium bicarbonate intravenously (44.6 mEq). On the other hand, if the arterial blood pH is less than 7.2, 2 vials intravenously may be administered and values repeated for further therapy in 15 to 30 minutes. Overcorrection of acidosis to alkalosis may decrease oxygen delivery to tissues by shifting the oxyhemoglobin dissociation curve.

TREATMENT OF ARRHYTHMIAS. Arrhythmias, particularly after myocardial infarction, may limit cardiac output and perpetuate shock.

Sustained ventricular tachycardia may be treated first with intravenous lidocaine in doses of 50 to 100 mg; if there is associated hypotension or any evidence of hemodynamic deterioration, electroshock should be used immediately. Ventricular fibrillation should be treated immediately with electroshock. If the first or second shock is unsuccessful, the patient must receive closed chest massage, mouth-to-mouth respiration, and possibly intravenous sodium bicarbonate before again attempting electrocardioversion.

Accelerated idioventricular rhythm is seen frequently in patients with myocardial infarction, particularly in those with diaphragmatic infarction. The rate is slightly faster than sinus rhythm, and a period of sinus bradycardia seems to favor the development of this arrhythmia. This benign condition can occasionally deteriorate into a fatal ventricular arrhythmia and should be treated with lidocaine or with atropine to increase the sinus rate.

Supraventricular arrhythmias (atrial tachycardias, flutter, fibrillation, or junctional rhythms) should generally be treated with digoxin; but if the rhythm persists or there is an associated hypotension or hemodynamic deterioration, electroshock therapy should be utilized immediately. Sinus bradycardia, if severe (less than 40 beats per minute), can contribute to hypotension. It is more commonly associated with inferior diaphragmatic infarction, and, if accompanied by frequent premature ventricular beats, restoration of a more rapid sinus rhythm can eliminate them. Atropine is most effective intravenously in doses of 0.4 mg up to 1 or even 2 mg. If bradycardia persists and hypotension or other signs of hypoperfusion are evident, electrical pacing should be instituted.

Conduction disturbances such as atrioventricular block carry a variable prognosis. The conduction disturbance which occurs with inferior diaphragmatic infarction has a better prognosis. It generally occurs early, is associated with sinus bradycardia, and may be caused by a temporary reflex increase in vagal tone to the conduction system or by atrioventricular nodal ischemia with only localized necrosis of this discrete structure. In anterior wall infarction, on the other hand, heart block is related to ischemic damage of the three fascicles of the conduction system, which results from a more extensive degree of necrosis and is associated with higher mortality. Patients with inferior infarction benefit from temporary electrical pacing if they do not respond to atropine, whereas those with anteroseptal infarction generally require a permanent pacemaker.

Treatment of Sepsis. Both gram-negative and gram-positive organisms have been associated with septic shock. In gram-negative septicemia, *E. coli* is the predominant organism, and infections with *Klebsiella-Aerobacter* (enterobacter) groups are not uncommon; endotoxin is an important factor in the pathogenesis of this syndrome. Gram-positive infections without endotoxemia, such as in pneumococcal pneumonia, *Staphylococcus aureus,* or streptococcal bacteremia, may cause shock. Chronic alcoholism is a common associated illness among these patients.

The characteristic hemodynamic abnormality in septic shock (whether gram-positive or gram-negative) is a marked decrease in peripheral vascular resistance; cardiac output may be increased, normal, or decreased. In contrast, in cardiogenic shock cardiac output is low and peripheral resistance is normal, increased, or occasionally decreased, and in hypovolemic shock cardiac output is low and peripheral resistance is increased. The treatment of septic shock includes the aggressive treatment of the infection with antibiotics and drainage of any abscesses. Although cardiac output may be normal or high, it may be insufficient to meet metabolic needs of the tissues, and an absolute or relative decrease in intravascular volume requires fluid administration. Therefore volume replacement with crystalloids or colloids is necessary to restore and raise central venous pressure to levels of 10 to 15 mm Hg or pulmonary wedge pressure to 20 mm Hg.

USE OF STEROIDS. The use of corticosteroids in septic shock has been adopted by most physicians and is used in very large doses early in the treatment of shock. Their beneficial effect appears to be related primarily to their action on cellular membranes. Steroids interact with biomembranes and probably become incorporated within their bilayer structures. The stabilizing effect of corticosteroids on biomembranes has been demonstrated in vitro in studies of lysosomes isolated from animals that have been treated with these agents. These lysosomes have a markedly increased resistance to lysis in vitro. Apparently this beneficial action of corticosteroids is not limited to their glucocorticoid properties. For example, testosterone is another potent membrane stabilizing agent. The reason for the continued question concerning the effectiveness of corticosteroids is that the consequences of membrane stabilization by corticosteroids in vivo are not really known. Experimental studies in animals subjected to septic, endotoxin, or hemorrhagic shock indicate improved survival with administration of corticosteroids. In shock, considerable damage to the microcirculation may be attributed to membrane interactions between platelets, polymorphonuclear leukocytes, and endothelium. Activation by the bacteria of the alternative complement pathway with the release of various peptides may favor platelet aggregation with endothelium and leukocytes, clot formation, and obstruction of the microcirculation. Corticosteroids may prevent these membrane interactions in vivo. Animals pretreated with cortisone exhibit an impressive resistance to endotoxin-mediated shock. On the other hand, it is not apparent whether corticosteroids are effective in the advanced shock state in which the physician often finds the patient. The use of corticosteroids in doses of 30 mg per kilogram of methylprednisolone as early as possible in patients with septicemia and hypotension might be justifiable, based on extensive work in vitro. The extension of the use of corticosteroids to patients with cardiogenic shock is unwise. There is evidence of malignant arrhythmias developing after the administration of corticosteroids to such patients, and the incidence of ventricular aneurysms may be increased because of interference with the inflammatory and healing processes of the myocardium.

It is claimed that corticosteroids have significant cardiovascular effects with possibly alpha receptor blocking activities, but pharmacologic studies indicate that the steroids have little if any significant direct cardiovascular action; they may augment the action of catecholamines, but they do not block alpha receptors.

Use of Sympathomimetic Amines. These drugs are used to increase cardiac output through their cardiotonic effect, and to redistribute blood flow to vital organs by their selective vasoconstricting action; by virtue of these two effects, they raise arterial pressure and allow the perfusion of ischemic regions, particularly in the myocardium, through collateral vessels. There are two potential problems with their use. If arterial pressure is elevated significantly, the hypertension may be detrimental, as it increases myocardial work and oxygen demand. Thus judicious elevation of arterial pressure to levels between 110 and 120 mm Hg systolic pressure would be reasonable. One cannot predict the optimal arterial pressure necessary to perfuse the coronaries in any particular patient because one does not know the severity of coronary disease and its extent, or the extent of myocardial reserves that would allow the heart to cope with a slight increase in afterload induced by the rising arterial pressure. Nevertheless, hypotension, particularly following myocardial infarction, should be corrected and arterial pressure maintained. The second potential problem with use of these drugs is their vasoconstricting effect; however, some vasoconstriction can be beneficial if it occurs in nonvital organs and if it is associated with increased cardiac output. This combination of effects raises arterial pressure and improves perfusion of vital organs. Therefore the proper use of sympathomimetic amines in shock requires a thorough knowledge of their cardiovascular effects. They have a structure similar to that of the natural adrenergic neurotransmitter norepinephrine and activate adrenergic receptors in various cells. Their action depends upon their affinity for various types of adrenergic receptors.

ADRENERGIC RECEPTORS. The adrenergic receptors may be classified as alpha or beta receptors with respect to their cardiovascular action. The alpha receptors are predominantly in blood vessels and mediate vasoconstriction. The beta receptors are present in the blood vessels as well as the myocardium. Activation of the beta-1 receptors in the myocardium causes an increase in myocardial contractility and in heart rate, whereas activation of beta-2 receptors in blood vessels causes vasodilatation. The same catecholamine may activate both alpha and beta receptors, depending on the dose and the organ in which it is acting.

NOREPINEPHRINE. Norepinephrine increases myocardial contractility by activating beta-1 receptors and thus may increase cardiac output. On the other hand, in blood vessels it activates primarily alpha or vasoconstricting receptors. The magnitude of its effect on alpha receptors varies from one organ to another. It is a very potent vasoconstrictor in skin, muscle, and splanchnic beds, whereas in the coronary vessels it activates the beta-2 receptors as well as the alpha receptors; and because there is a paucity of alpha receptors in the coronary vessels in contrast to other vascular beds, the drug causes vasodilatation of the coronaries.

It offers several distinct advantages in the treatment of shock. It increases cardiac output and redistributes blood flow away from the extremities and toward the heart and brain and increases arterial pressure, which in turn increases coronary flow to ischemic myocardium. It should be administered intravenously through an indwelling catheter to avoid the risk of extravasation, which results in necrosis of subcutaneous tissues. Two ampules of Levophed (4 mg base per ampule) may be dissolved in 500 ml glucose and water and an infusion rate started at a very low level to determine the smallest necessary dose to maintain arterial pressure between 100 and 120 mm Hg, which should provide adequate perfusion to the heart, brain, and kidney (unless the patient was hypertensive or has extensive arteriosclerotic disease). A dose of 4 μg per minute may occasionally be adequate; however, many patients require up to 40 μg per minute; and in general if such doses are necessary to maintain pressure, prognosis is poor. An average dose would be between 10 and 15 μg per minute. The lack of response to norepinephrine is probably an indication of significant myocardial damage if hypoxia, hypovolemia, and acidosis have been considered and corrected.

DOPAMINE. This is a naturally occurring catecholamine which is the precursor of norepinephrine. It has a different cardiovascular effect, depending on its dose level. When given in low concentrations, approximately 200 μg per minute, it has a vasodilator action in the renal and mesenteric vessels, with only slight dilatation of cerebral and coronary vessels. The dilator effect is mediated through beta-2 receptors and through specific dopaminergic receptors. In doses of 500 to 1000 μg per minute, it increases myocardial contractility and cardiac output through the activation of beta-1 receptors. In larger doses of 1500 to 3000 μg per minute, it causes vasoconstriction through activation of alpha-adrenergic receptors of arteries and veins in most vascular beds. Thus this drug may redistribute blood flow away from the extremities and toward the kidney, gut, heart, and brain; however, it may be necessary to give large doses to maintain arterial pressure and coronary blood flow, particularly following myocardial infarction, and these large doses will then tend to oppose to some degree the beneficial vasodilator effects seen in some vascular beds.

EPINEPHRINE. Epinephrine is released from the adrenal gland; it activates myocardial beta-1 receptors and vasoconstrictor alpha receptors in most vessels except in skeletal muscle and coronary vessels, where it activates beta-2 receptors when administered in low doses. It increases cardiac output, but redistributes flow away from the kidney and splanchnic circulations toward skeletal muscle. Given in a dose range from 2 to 30 μg per minute intravenously, its effect on the redistribution flow is not optimal, and its effect on arterial pressure is only modest because of its vasodilator effect in skeletal muscle.

ISOPROTERENOL. Isoproterenol is a synthetic sympathomimetic amine which activates primarily vascular beta-2 receptors, causing vasodilatation, and myocardial beta-1 receptors, increasing cardiac output. The magnitude of the vasodilator effect of isoproterenol varies in different vascular beds, depending on the density of beta-2 receptors and the affinity of the drug for them. The major vasodilator action of isoproterenol is in skeletal muscle beds.

This drug is not recommended in either cardiogenic or septic shock. In hemorrhagic shock, burns, or trauma the major line of treatment should be blood or fluid replacement. In cardiogenic shock, isoproterenol significantly increases myocardial oxygen requirement, and, despite the increase in coronary flow, there is evidence that the ischemic region of the myocardium may be hypoperfused as indicated by increased lactate production. In contrast, the administration of norepinephrine tends to decrease lactate production by the heart. Dopamine is also beneficial if arterial pressure is maintained. The use of isoproterenol should probably be limited to the treatment of complete heart block in an attempt to maintain an idioventricular rhythm until more definitive therapy can be carried out. The usual dose of isoproterenol is 0.5 to 4 μg per minute.

One can summarize the use of sympathomimetic amines by saying that the goal is to attain an arterial pressure sufficiently adequate to perfuse the kidney, the ischemic myocardial segment, and the brain without overloading the left ventricle. The drug used should redistribute blood flow toward the more vital organs and away from skin and muscle for the optimal utilization of the limited cardiac output in shock. Finally, the drug should also have an inotropic action, and drugs such as methoxamine and phenylephrine, which only cause arterial vasoconstriction by activating alpha receptors without stimulating the heart, should be avoided. With these goals in mind, norepinephrine and dopamine should be chosen in the management of shock, regardless of the initiating cause.

Vasodilator Therapy. The beneficial effects of vasodilator therapy are (1) to decrease myocardial oxygen demands by decreasing preload or cardiac filling pressure and cardiac size and decreasing afterload by decreasing arterial pressure and arterial impedance, and (2) to dilate microcirculatory vessels.

The effectiveness of vasodilators (nitroprusside, nitroglycerin, phentolamine, or hydralazine) is impressive in the acutely failing heart following myocardial infarction without shock and with an elevated left ventricular enddiastolic pressure or capillary wedge pressure above 20 or 25 mm Hg; but the presence of *hypotension* should be a contraindication to the use of this therapy alone. Under those circumstances one may have to use a vasodilator drug along with norepinephrine or dopamine.

REDUCTION IN PRELOAD. One can reduce oxygen demand of the myocardium by decreasing cardiac volume in patients who have a high filling pressure. Reduction in cardiac size decreases myocardial wall tension, which is a major determinant of myocardial oxygen requirements. It may be achieved by administration of diuretics or venodilator drugs, which reduce filling pressure by pooling blood in the peripheral veins. The goal of "venodilator therapy" is to decrease preload and cardiac size and not to decrease arterial blood pressure. This effect is desirable as long as cardiac filling pressure does not drop excessively, causing a drop in cardiac output. In some patients with severe pulmonary congestion and high cardiac filling pressure with systemic arterial hypotension, it might be necessary to combine the vasodilator therapy with another drug that will cause selective arteriolar vasoconstriction in certain organs and will increase peripheral vascular resistance and raise and maintain arterial pressure, such as dopamine or norepinephrine.

REDUCTION IN AFTERLOAD.   This is a beneficial effect of the vasodilators, because it will decrease the arterial impedance against which the left ventricle ejects its blood; thus ejection fraction may improve. This is desirable as long as it is not associated with a significant reduction in systemic arterial diastolic pressure, particularly in patients who are normotensive or have borderline hypotension. The dose of the vasodilator drug may be adjusted so that it would not cause a significant reduction in diastolic arterial pressure. Any drop in arterial pressure by more than 10 mm Hg should be avoided, and the diastolic pressure should certainly not be allowed to decrease below 65 mm Hg. Reduction in afterload is ideal in patients with chronic severe congestive failure with high filling pressure, pulmonary congestion, and low cardiac output, but without a significant reduction in arterial pressure. Patients with cardiomyopathy without coronary artery disease may be the best candidates for this therapy.

Neither a vasodilator alone nor propranolol, which also reduces myocardial oxygen demand, has a place in the management of cardiogenic hypotension following myocardial infarction. The elimination of the cardiotonic effect of the normal sympathetic drive by propranolol may significantly impair cardiac output and precipitate failure. If the patient has continuing pain and *a normal or elevated blood pressure,* despite the administration of narcotics, morphine or meperidine, and nitroglycerin, the administration of propranolol might then be considered.

MICROCIRCULATORY VASOCONSTRICTION AND ALPHA RECEPTOR BLOCKERS.   In some patients, despite prolonged administration of dopamine or norepinephrine, tissue perfusion is not improved. The reasons may be that the myocardial infarction or the cellular damage is extensive. It is also possible that constriction of microcirculatory vessels may be preventing the perfusion of exchange capillaries. The alpha receptor blocker phentolamine has a specific effect on the vasoconstricting α-receptors and does not block the beta receptors in the myocardium. Thus the cardiotonic effect of sympathomimetic amines would not be prevented, yet vasoconstricting effects at the microcirculatory level would be antagonized. Phentolamine has a preferential inhibitory effect on alpha receptors in venules and veins as opposed to arterioles, and its dilator action may therefore be greater in veins than in arterioles. This effect calls for a note of caution, because rapid relaxation of large veins may abruptly lower cardiac filling pressure if the patient is hypovolemic. For this reason, it is essential to ascertain that the patient has received adequate amounts of fluid before giving phentolamine.

In this setting of shock with high circulating catecholamines and after prolonged infusions of high concentrations of norepinephrine and dopamine and with persisting evidence of decreased tissue perfusion, the use of the alpha receptor blocker phentolamine offers several theoretical advantages over other vasodilators based on animal work. It dilates venules to decrease capillary hydrostatic pressure and opens up precapillary sphincters, which allow perfusion of nutritional capillaries. Other vasodilators may have a negligible effect on veins and venules, and although they increase blood flow, they do not necessarily increase perfusion of the microcirculation. Unfortunately there are no clinical studies which would confirm the

beneficial effects of phentolamine* in that stage of shock, which in general carries a poor prognosis. An initial dose of 2 mg given intravenously, followed by 5 mg, should be attempted, with careful monitoring of the intra-arterial and central venous pressures to ascertain that the patient is not hypovolemic and does not have a decreased effective blood volume. If hypotension results from this small dose, more rapid fluid replacement will be necessary before adding phentolamine. Generally phentolamine may be added to the intravenous fluid containing norepinephrine. One or 2 ampules of phentolamine (5 mg per ampule) may be added for each ampule of norepinephrine in the intravenous fluid. If given alone, 4 ampules in 500 ml or 40 μg per milliliter is a reasonable concentration, and the usual dose is between 20 and 80 μg per minute.

NITROPRUSSIDE.   This is a very effective vasodilator drug that causes relaxation of veins to decrease preload and some relaxation of arterioles to decrease arterial impedance. It may be started intravenously at a dose of 16 μg per minute and increased to 200 μg per minute with constant monitoring of arterial pressure. Occasionally larger doses have been necessary.

Other vasodilator drugs, such as hydralazine, which primarily exert an action on the arterioles, would not be very effective in reducing cardiac size and myocardial oxygen demand, and may be detrimental in causing a significant reduction in arterial blood pressure.

Digitalis.   One should consider the administration of digoxin to patients with cardiogenic shock only if there is evidence of pulmonary congestion and an elevated pulmonary artery wedge pressure. The initial loading dose of digoxin may be reduced because in the setting of myocardial infarction hypoxia may predispose to myocardial irritability, and the renal excretion of digoxin may be impaired because of decreased renal perfusion and arterial blood pressure.

Surgical Treatment in Cardiogenic Shock.   In cardiogenic shock, experience has been obtained with the use of intra-aortic balloon counterpulsation. The balloon is introduced into the aorta at the end of a catheter inserted through the femoral artery. It is inflated during early diastole and is collapsed during systole. This sequence increases the pressure during diastole and reduces it during systole, thus decreasing afterload during ejection and increasing diastolic coronary perfusion pressure and coronary flow during diastole. Improvement of the hemodynamic status has been observed, but because a large number of patients with myocardial infarction and shock have extensive coronary artery disease, the long-term survival is still disappointing. The balloon counterpulsation appears to be of greatest potential benefit in the support of patients who have seriously compromised hemodynamics after myocardial infarction and who are candidates for a surgical procedure. This mechanical assistance sustains the hemodynamics during cardiac catheterization and coronary arteriography in preparation for surgery. Emergency revascularization surgery or infarctectomy, which has been carried out on occasion, has not been encouraging. Two complications of myocardial infarction require surgical intervention and carry a reasonable prognosis; these are ruptured papillary muscle and interventricular septal perforation. In both, there is decreased ejection from the left ventricle and a fall in arterial pressure. Attempts to increase systemic arterial pressure with drugs exaggerate the regurgitation or the left to right shunt. In these circumstances, the selective

---

*Experimental drug for this purpose.

lowering of arterial systolic pressure with intra-aortic balloon counterpulsation is ideal, as it will facilitate ejection and reduce mitral regurgitation or left to right shunt. A significant reduction in afterload and vasodilatation may also be achieved with drugs such as nitroprusside or nitroglycerin, but the associated fall in diastolic pressure may extend the myocardial ischemia. Surgical management, as soon as it is feasible and safe, should be the course to pursue. Severe papillary muscle dysfunction or papillary muscle rupture (the posterior more frequently than the anterior) may cause significant left ventricular failure, and the surgical replacement of the mitral valve has been satisfactory, particularly in patients with good myocardial function. Patients with a perforation of the ventricular septum have congestive failure in association with the sudden appearance of a pansystolic murmur, often accompanied by a thrill. Clinically, it is often impossible to differentiate this condition from a ruptured papillary muscle. The demonstration of a left to right shunt by cardiac catheterization confirms the diagnosis. Rupture of the septum should be treated surgically, preferably six to eight weeks after infarction, so that the margins of the defect can have sufficient scar tissue to permit surgical closure with relative ease.

Abboud, F. M., et al: Reflex control of the peripheral circulation. Prog. Cardiovasc. Dis., 18:371, 1976.

Braunwald, E.: Protection of the ischemic myocardium. Circulation, 53 (Suppl. 1):1, 1976.

Braunwald, E.: The Myocardium: Failure and Infarction. New York, H. P. Publishing Company, 1975.

Goldberg, L. I.: Dopamine — clinical uses of an endogenous catecholamine. N. Engl. J. Med., 291:707, 1974.

The Cell in Shock. Proceedings of a Symposium on Recent Research Developments and Current Clinical Practice in Shock. The Upjohn Company, April 1976, pp. 16–29, 30–34, 35–38.

The Organ in Shock. Proceedings of the Second Symposium on Recent Research Developments and Current Clinical Practice in Shock. The Upjohn Company, April 1977, pp. 8–15, 24–31, 38–49.

Weil, M. H., et al.: Treatment of circulatory shock. JAMA, 231:1280, 1975.

Winslow, E. J., et al.: Hemodynamic studies and results of therapy in 50 patients with bacteremic shock. Am. J. Med., 54:421, 1973.

357. THROMBOEMBOLIC DISEASES

357.1. THROMBOSIS

Patrick A. McKee

A *thrombus,* as defined by Welch in 1899, is "a solid mass or plug, formed in the living heart or vessels from constituents of the blood." This definition remains valid, and thrombosis, which is the formation of a thrombus, can be contrasted with the term blood clotting or blood coagulation, which refers to the conversion of blood from a liquid to a solid outside the circulatory system. The primary difference between the two terms has to do with the mode of initiation and the in vivo contribution of flowing blood to the microanatomy of the thrombus. The term *embolus* refers to the dislodgment, in total or in part, of a thrombus from its site of origin and its movement by the flow of blood to a more distant site within the circulatory system. The general topic of *thromboembolism* refers to all those diseases which have as part of their pathogenesis, course, or outcome the occlusion of some part of the vascular system by a mass formed from blood constituents. Al-

though the exact mortality and morbidity attributable to thromboembolic diseases are not known precisely, it is known that the incidence of thromboembolic diseases has increased appreciably in proportion to man's longevity. As an index of the over-all importance of this condition, it is estimated that diseases either complicated or caused by thromboembolism occur approximately three times more frequently than cancer in general. Despite extensive research, the precise mechanisms involved in the pathogenesis of thrombosis have not been defined, and the general circumstances which predispose to thrombi remain the sharpest features of our understanding about their pathogenesis. These situations are defined by the presence of one or more features of Virchow's triad of abnormalities of blood flow, the vessel lining surface, and the blood constituents. To date our ability to measure meaningful changes in any one of these three descriptors remains elusive.

The consensus is that all thrombi, whether developing in arteries or veins, are initiated by platelets adhering to the endothelial surface of the vessel. For many years it has been known that venous thrombi are mostly influenced by marked slowing in the flow of blood, i.e., "stasis," and that this somehow leads to the activation of certain serine protease clotting factors with the formation of thrombin and then the conversion of fibrinogen to fibrin. This type of thrombus has been termed a "red thrombus" because it contains a fairly even distribution of red and white blood cells and platelets in a network of fibrin. More recent data, however, strongly suggest that, even in veins, platelets comprise the initial nidus of thrombi and that such an aggregate of platelets is analogous to the head of an arterial thrombus, which is referred to classically as a "white thrombus." The latter has long been recognized as being initiated and attached to the arterial endothelium by a large mass of platelets that grossly has a whitish appearance in contrast to the rest of the thrombus. Pathologic examinations have shown that deep venous thrombi usually begin in the concavity formed by the juncture of a venous valve leaflet with the vein wall. At this site, layers or aggregates of platelets can be seen, and it is believed by many that these platelet clumps trigger the events which culminate in the conversion of fibrinogen to fibrin and hence the formation of a thrombus. In the arterial vasculature overt stasis is not very important as a predisposing factor to thrombosis; however, relative stasis, such as might occur in areas of nonlaminar blood flow, may contribute significantly to the development and progression of a thrombus. Since arterial thrombi occur mostly in diseases characterized by atherosclerotic lesions, and on or in close proximity to such lesions, it is commonly believed that this attests to the importance of both disrupted laminar flow and an abnormal endothelial surface predisposing to thrombosis. The mechanism by which platelets adhere to a damaged endothelial surface is presumably due to the exposure of collagen fibrils in the subendothelial area. Although this can be shown to occur in vitro, it is not unequivocally established that the same phenomenon occurs in life. As platelets adhere to a surface, adenosine diphosphate (ADP) is released, which causes additional platelet aggregation. Other substances are also recognized as important in platelet-surface and platelet-platelet interactions; for example, the soluble plasma protein, von Willebrand factor, is known to be required for certain platelet adhesion and aggregation reactions. In addition, arachidonic acid, precursor to prostaglandin synthesis, and prostaglandin G_2 and thromboxane A_2, which are formed and released by the metabolically active platelet during platelet aggregation, promote further platelet aggregation. As platelets aggregate, other important components are also released which participate in reactions occurring at the blood-platelet membrane interface. This leads to the activation of certain plasma clotting factors, particularly those of the intrinsic system, thereby initiating a cascade of reactions which generates thrombin and culminates in the conversion of fibrinogen into fibrin (see Ch. 519 for blood clotting scheme).

Despite numerous studies, it is still unknown whether measurable changes in the levels of various blood clotting factor activities predispose to thrombosis. There are a number of nonspecific and not very sensitive differences in the levels of various clotting factors which have been found statistically significant when large populations of patients with certain thromboembolic disorders have been compared to those without such problems. For example, a shortened whole blood clotting time, a shortened partial thromboplastin time, increased levels of fibrinogen, circulating fibrin multimers, excess levels of activity of factors V, VII, and VIII, the presence of fibrin degradation products, increased platelet number or stickiness, decrease in the concentration of normal plasma serine protease inhibitors (antithrombins and antiplasmins), and reduction of the normal fibrinolytic activity have each been taken to signify a tendency to form thrombi. The results of such tests, however, have been ambiguous, and in general they are not very useful measurements for the diagnosis or management of thromboembolic disorders. In actuality, the presence of certain risk factors or the presence of certain diseases correlates better with the ability to predict or suspect thromboembolic disease than any laboratory assessment currently in use. Although in most instances local atherosclerotic changes are a prerequisite for arterial thrombosis, and venous stasis is recognized as the major predisposing factor to deep vein thrombosis, the question of whether "hypercoagulable" blood changes are also required in either situation remains debatable. Clearly, many of the reports that indicate such changes are necessary may have quantitated the result rather than the cause of thrombosis. The most important evidence to suggest that blood constituents may themselves trigger thrombosis is derived from observations that show thrombi do form in situations in which no obvious disturbance of flow has occurred and on endothelial surfaces which, as closely as one can detect, appear normal.

Recently it has become apparent that there are normally occurring plasma proteins which inhibit certain of the blood clotting factor enzymes, particularly those which are serine proteases. Since their inhibitory effects are relative with respect to specificity, rate, and completeness, these inhibitors can be viewed as modulators of the over-all activity of the blood clotting system. The more important inhibitors are thought to be antithrombin III, α_2-macroglobulin, and antiplasmin. The best evidence of their biologic importance is the well established observation that congenital deficiencies of antithrombin III predispose to venous thromboses in otherwise normal, healthy young people. Whether transient, acquired deficiencies of these inhibitors truly predispose to thromboses remains unknown. Of interest, however, is the fact that probably the most frequently reported and reproducible abnormality of the blood clotting system in women taking oral contraceptives is a decrease in antithrombin III concentration. Lastly, diminished fibrinolytic activity has also been offered as an explanation for the propensity to develop and sustain a thrombus. Most data supporting this notion are derived from epidemiologic studies, particularly those conducted in Africa, which show an increased fibrinolytic state to be associated with an absence of vascular disease. Studies in other countries have frequently not confirmed this. Isolated reports of patients who have reduced fibrinolytic activity and a predisposition to thromboses have also been used to marshal support for this theory.

Included among the more common thromboembolic diseases are deep venous thrombosis, pulmonary embolism, ischemic heart disease, cerebral vascular disease, thromboembolism as a complication of prosthetic heart valves, and thromboses confined to the microcirculatory system (e.g., diffuse intravascular coagulation, thrombotic thrombocytopenic purpura). Thromboembolism causes a reduction or cessation of blood flow to an organ or area of the body with attendant impairment or loss of function. When such blockage occurs in the microcirculation, microangiopathic hemolytic anemia may develop if red cell damage occurs when blood is forced through a vessel lumen partially obstructed by fibrin strands; paradoxically, a bleeding disorder due to utilization of coagulation factors and platelets in the microthrombi may also develop. Thromboembolism frequently complicates the course of malignancies, possibly by the release into the circulation of thromboplastin, which then interacts with certain of the clotting factors. Similarly, thromboplastin or analogous substances may enter the circulatory system, which becomes open during certain complications of pregnancy. Finally, in women receiving oral contraceptive agents, the problems of spontaneously occurring thromboses, particularly in the deep leg veins with subsequent pulmonary embolism or cerebral arterial thrombosis, have also received considerable attention.

Besides the more or less acute type of thromboembolic disorders, it has also been postulated that the blood coagulation system is involved in the pathogenesis of the initial atherosclerotic lesion. The initial stimulus is thought to be endothelial damage, probably due to shear stresses exerted on its surface by hypertensive blood pressure levels. This is believed to be followed by the formation of a nonocclusive, platelet-rich thrombus that becomes adherent to the arterial endothelial surface and then over time becomes organized, infiltrated with lipid, and partially endothelialized. During the attachment of platelets to subendothelial structures, the platelets are believed to release substances which stimulate smooth muscle cells to proliferate and migrate toward the lumen. Gradually a multiple-layered lesion composed of smooth muscle cells develops and protrudes into the lumen of the vessel; this lesion is thought eventually to become infiltrated with lipid and, ultimately, to become an atherosclerotic plaque. It is important to emphasize that, although currently very popular, this is only one theory of atherogenesis.

The therapy of thromboembolism continues to be aimed at altering the coagulability of the blood or the ability of platelets to stick to surfaces or each other. Because some epidemiologic studies have indicated that acetylsalicylic acid may be useful in preventing the development of thrombosis, it has received considerable attention; however, it is still not clear whether it prevents thromboses associated with any disease or predisposing situation. Biochemical data indicate that aspirin acetylates, and thereby inhibits, cyclo-oxygenase, which is an enzyme important in forming prostaglandin G_2 from arachidonic acid; as a consequence, the stimulant effect on platelet aggregation of prostaglandin G_2 and the subsequent metabolite, thromboxane A_2, is greatly diminished. Very low levels of aspirin are required to do this, and the effect seems to be irreversible during the life span of the platelet. *Coumarin* derivatives continue to be the mainstays in the long-term management of thromboembolism, particularly in situations such as deep vein thrombosis or recurrent pulmonary embolism. Recent analyses of older studies and results of new studies suggest that their use may decrease both morbidity and mortality in the acute and chronic stages of myocardial infarction. Coumarins serve as vitamin K antagonists in reactions which, although poorly understood, lead to the attachment of an additional carboxyl group on certain glutamic acid residues to form the dicarboxylic amino acid, γ-carboxyglutamic acid, in the vitamin K dependent clotting factors. It is thought that the dicarboxylic acid groups are important in binding calcium and lipid during the conversion of the zymogen forms of these clotting factors to active serine proteases. When a coumarin is administered, the clotting factor is synthesized without the addition of the extra carboxyl group to the specific glutamic acids, and as a result the conversion of the precursive form of the clotting factor to the active enzyme is greatly impaired. The levels of the zymogen protein, however, are normal. The other commonly used anticoagulant, *heparin,* is usually employed in a hospital setting where it is given subcutaneously or intravenously. The introduction of low-dose heparin therapy, i.e., doses administered subcutaneously in the range of 5000 units two or three times daily, has effected a dramatic reduction in the incidence of fatal thromboembolism following major thoracoabdominal surgery. This level of heparin does not ordinarily prolong the whole glass clotting time or the partial thromboplastin time. It is to be emphasized that low-dose heparin has only been found effective for the prevention of thromboses; much higher heparin levels are recommended for the treatment of established thromboembolism. To date no oral form of heparin has been found useful. For heparin to be effective as an anticoagulant, it requires a protein cofactor in plasma, antithrombin III. Evidence suggests that heparin temporarily binds and alters the shape of antithrombin III, thereby greatly accelerating the rate of covalent bond formation between an amino acid in its sequence and the active site serine amino acid residue in several of the clotting factor proteases. This mode of inhibition occurs rapidly at fairly low levels of heparin and is believed to be permanent.

Obviously advances have occurred in our understanding of the diseases and situations which predispose to thromboses, the biochemistry of blood clotting, and the therapy of thromboembolic disorders. Of concern, however, is our lack of knowledge about the precise mechanisms which trigger and perpetuate thromboses. It is probable that these must be defined if thromboembolism is to be prevented.

Chalmers, T. C., Matta, R. J., Smith, H. J., and Kunzler, A-M.: Evidence favoring the use of anticoagulants in the hospital phase of acute myocardial infarction. N. Engl. J. Med., 297:1091, 1977.
Davie, E. W., and Hanahan, D. J.: Blood coagulation proteins. *In* Putnam, F. W. (ed.): The Plasma Proteins. 2nd ed. New York, Academic Press, 1977, pp. 422–544.
Majerus, P. W.: Why aspirin? Circulation, 54:375, 1976.
Rosenberg, R. D.: Actions and interactions of antithrombin and heparin. N. Engl. J. Med., 292:146, 1975.
Ross, R., and Glomset, J. A.: The pathogenesis of arteriosclerosis. N. Engl. J. Med., 295:369, 420, 1976.
Salzman, E. W., Deykin, D., Shapiro, R. M., and Rosenberg, R.: Management of heparin therapy. N. Engl. J. Med., 292:1046, 1975.
Sherry, S.: Low-dose heparin prophylaxis for post-operative venous thromboembolism. N. Engl. J. Med., 293:300, 1975.
Sherry, S., Brinkhous, K. M., Genton, E., and Stengle, J. M. (eds.): Thrombosis. Washington, D.C., National Academy of Sciences, 1969.

357.2.   THROMBOPHLEBITIS AND PHLEBOTHROMBOSIS

Sol Sherry

The presence of a thrombus in a vein is referred to clinically as thrombophlebitis or phlebothrombosis. Adherence to the vein wall incites an inflammatory reaction with local symptoms, and because of the associated phlebitis the process is referred to as thrombophlebitis. When the thrombus is poorly adherent and extends primarily into the free-flowing circulation, local symptoms of phlebitis may be minimal or absent, and the process may be referred to as phlebothrombosis. Since the two states are, for the most part, identical and subject to the same complications, little virtue attaches to such a clinical differentiation; hereafter only the term thrombophlebitis will be used.

ETIOLOGY, RISK FACTORS, PATHOGENESIS, AND PREVALENCE. Multiple causes probably initiate venous thrombosis. Injury to the vessel wall by mechanical trauma, infection, chemical irritants, or the process of thromboangiitis obliterans is responsible for some cases, particularly the superficial variety.

In most instances, stasis with slowing of blood flow and venous distention appears to be the major predisposing factor, e.g., in the venous thrombi which frequently complicate the use of constricting garments, and in such clinical conditions or states as the hyperviscosity syndromes (including polycythemia vera), severe obesity, varicose veins, postoperative and postpartum states, trauma (particularly when extensive or involving fractures of the pelvis or femur), acute myocardial infarction, heart failure, hemiplegia, debility, and cachexia. Long periods of cramped sitting, e.g., in travel or watching television, or in fact any state involving partial or complete immobilization, particularly in the older age group, because of the loss of the normal pumping action of the leg muscles, is subject to an increased incidence of venous thrombosis. The risk of stasis-mediated as well as other forms of venous thrombosis is increased when there has been a previous episode of thrombophlebitis or pulmonary embolism.

Alterations in blood components have received much attention, but a "hypercoagulable state," i.e., one predisposing to thrombus formation, has defied simple description. Rather, it is recognized that many disorders of the blood may be associated with predisposition to venous thrombosis. These include thrombocythemia as well as certain thrombocytopathies, particularly those involving shortened survival and increased platelet functional activities (adhesion, aggregation, and coagulant properties), dysfibrinogenemias, accelerated thromboplastin generation, constitutionally elevated levels of plasma factors V and VIII, heightened antifibrinolytic activity, and decreased antithrombin III activity.

Finally, many other clinical conditions are associated with an increased incidence of thrombophlebitis, but the responsible factors have not been adequately elucidated. These include ulcerative colitis, malignancies of all types (possibly more so of the pancreas), homocystinuria, and prolonged administration of large doses of estrogens or estrogen-containing oral contraceptive agents. The presence of a "migratory thrombophlebitis" should cause suspicion of an underlying malignancy, collagen disease, thromboangiitis obliterans, or polycythemia vera. When thrombosis occurs without evidence of a known predisposing factor or associated clinical condition, the term *idiopathic* thrombophlebitis may be used.

Thrombosis in veins occurs most commonly in the deep and superficial veins of the lower extremities. Deep leg vein thrombi usually begin in the soleal arcade of the calf muscles where they may resolve, organize, extend, or trigger additional thrombi at independent sites. As long as the thrombus remains limited to the soleal veins, no significant clinical problem is posed. However, once extension into the major deep vessels of the leg occurs, or additional thrombi appear at other sites in the major deep veins, the patient is at significant risk for one or more complications (circulatory obstruction, valve damage, postphlebitic insufficiency syndrome, pulmonary embolism). When extension occurs from the soleal vessels, the thrombus extends proximally into larger vessels, frequently progressing to involve the popliteal, superficial femoral, common femoral, and iliac veins. More rarely the inferior vena cava is also affected. Thrombi originating in the major deep veins usually begin at the base of valve pockets and then extend either up along the vein wall or into the flowing circulation, or they may completely obstruct the entire vascular lumen. When the latter occurs, retrograde thrombosis as well as continued proximal growth is likely.

Next in frequency to thrombi in the deep leg veins are thrombi in the pelvic venous network, the right cardiac chambers, and the veins of the upper extremities. However, thrombi may occur in any veins (retinal, cerebral, renal, hepatic, portal, mesenteric) and contribute significantly to disease of the organ system involved.

Until recently, data on the incidence and frequency of leg vein thrombi were inadequate, because most of these are inapparent clinically. In studies in which leg vein dissections were carried out post mortem, the incidence was shown to be very high, varying from 27 to 80 per cent, depending on the nature of the series and the extent of the dissection; in most, the incidence ranged from 44 to 65 per cent. This incidence did not appear to depend on sex or clinical diagnosis, for the likelihood of thrombosis was similar in patients dying of medical, surgical, and traumatic causes. The most important factors influencing the frequency of leg vein thrombosis appeared to be the duration of bed rest and advancing age, although other factors undoubtedly contributed to those incidence figures.

With the advent of the ^{125}I-labeled fibrinogen leg-scanning technique, important epidemiologic and prevalence data are being obtained on leg vein thrombi appearing during life and in nonfatal situations. For example, in Kakkar's study of 469 consecutive patients aged 40 or over, undergoing elective surgery, 28 per cent developed deep vein thrombosis; older patients undergoing major operations had an incidence of over 50 per cent. Half the thrombi developed within the first 24 hours postoperatively, and the remainder occurred three to seven days after surgery; in one third of the patients, the thrombi were bilateral. The incidence in other conditions was as follows: fractured hips, 75 per cent of pertrochanteric and 34 per cent of subcapital femoral neck fractures; retropubic prostatectomy, 50 per cent; acute myocardial infarction, 38 per cent; stroke, 60 per cent in the hemiplegic lower extremity; gynecologic patients over 30 years of age and undergoing major abdominal or vaginal surgery, 18 per cent; and obstetric patients during the puerperium, 4 per cent. Probably the highest risk is in patients undergoing reconstructive or total hip replacement.

In over 90 per cent of the patients undergoing thrombosis, leg vein thrombi appear first in the veins of the calf; one fifth of these soleal thrombi extend proximally into the major deep vessels of the leg and thigh; of the latter, half embolize. In acute myocardial infarction, in which the over-all incidence of leg vein thrombosis is approximatley 20 to 25 per cent, 5 per cent of patients may be expected to develop thrombi in the major deep vessels of the leg or thigh, and in 2 to 3 per cent the illness will be complicated by an acute pulmonary embolism; the risk of leg vein thrombosis, extension, and embolization, however, is doubled in patients in the older age group who develop shock or congestive heart failure with their infarction.

CLINICAL MANIFESTATIONS AND DIAGNOSIS. Thrombophlebitis occurs suddenly or gradually. Superficial thrombophlebitis is not difficult to diagnose, because the thrombosed vessel can usually be felt beneath the skin as a tender cord, and the lesion may be accompanied by a surrounding area of localized inflammation. With more extensive use of the venous route for both therapy and drug abuse, the incidence of this form of thrombophlebitis has increased sharply. Although it is usually benign, a significant number of patients may become infected, e.g., after the use of contaminated equipment or when intravenous catheters have been left in situ for periods of more than 48 hours, and this may lead to a serious septic state.

Deep vein thrombophlebitis is much more difficult to diagnose, because it may or may not be accompanied by local (pain and tenderness) and systemic (fever) symptoms; these occur in only 20 to 30 per cent of patients. In the absence of local findings, the diagnosis should be suspected when there is a "doughy" feeling or an unexplained increase in the circumference of the limb and the presence of *Homan's sign* (pain in the calf and/or popliteal space on dorsiflexion of the foot). The *sphygmomanometer cuff pain test of Lowenberg* may also prove useful, particularly when carried out during ambulation. A blood pressure cuff around the involved part of the extremity is slowly inflated to 200 mm Hg and then deflated. During inflation, discomfort is normally experienced at or above 160 mm Hg. In venous obstructive disease, discomfort or tenderness is evident at a lower level (60 to 150 mm Hg). The test may often be positive when other symptoms and signs are absent, but it is not sufficiently specific to be considered diagnostic. The most useful noninvasive diagnostic techniques are the *augmented Doppler ultrasound examination* and *electrical impedance phlebography* with a thigh cuff; with experience, the results of these latter tests will correlate well with venography. However, these tests are positive only when the major deep veins are obstructed; they do not detect thrombi limited to the soleal veins. *Venography* is the most specific for diagnostic purposes, but it has limitations; it is expensive, may require a cut-down, and cannot be interpreted properly unless all the deep veins, including the soleal vessels, are filled adequately; there is also the possibility (still unresolved) that the large amounts of dye used in the procedure will aggravate an underlying thrombophlebitis.

Unless the patient has local complaints, the signs of venous thrombosis are often overlooked until the occurrence of pulmonary embolism calls attention to the limbs. Therefore special attention should be paid to the possibility of venous thrombi in all patients who are predisposed, and frequent observations should be made in older patients immobilized for any period of time.

Local tenderness in the calf and pain on forced dorsiflexion of the foot should suggest involvement of the deeper branches of the popliteal vein. Edema and mottled cyanosis will be present when the superficial femoral vein is affected; these findings are absent when adequate collateral channels exist. When the disease extends to involve the common femoral and iliac veins, edema and cyanosis of the leg may develop rapidly, often with diminished pulsation of the femoral artery. When associated perivenous inflammation and pelvic lymphatic involvement accompany thrombosis of the iliac vein, the swelling can be massive and result in a "milk leg" or *phlegmasia alba dolens*. In a particularly serious from of deep vein thrombosis called *phlegmasia cerulea dolens,* cyanosis and swelling of the extremity are associated with a disappearance of the arterial pulses; the leg becomes cold; gangrene appears imminent and may follow. This is associated with massive venous occlusion involving the deep, superficial, and intercommunicating veins so that there is almost total outflow obstruction; the rapid rise in tissue pressure compromises the arterial inflow and produces the picture of combined arterial and venous occlusive disease.

Damage to the venous valves resulting from an extensive episode or repeated attacks of deep vein thrombophlebitis may cause venous stasis and insufficiency; this leads to chronic edema, fibrosis, pigmentation, and trophic ulceration in the limb. The eventual deformity in this *postphlebitic syndrome* may be extreme and disabling. However, the most frequent and serious complication of thrombophlebitis is pulmonary embolism, a subject discussed in Ch. 357.3.

PROPHYLAXIS. Stasis should be eliminated whenever possible, particularly in the older patient. This includes the wearing of elastic or supportive hose in the presence of varicose veins; avoidance of long periods of cramped sitting and of constricting garments about the abdomen and lower extremities; and the use of appropriate measures during periods of immobilization or illness or after surgery, trauma, or fracture. The value of elastic hose during periods of immobilization is very limited, as are foot and leg exercises, even when carried out frequently and in the elevated position. More effective are physical devices which ensure repeated

calf muscle contraction or intermittent pulsation of the leg veins. Early but active ambulation is to be encouraged after illness, surgery, or trauma.

Iatrogenic thrombophlebitis can be minimized by avoiding prolonged use of intravenous catheters or administration of hypertonic or chemically irritating solutions.

Prophylactic therapy with anticoagulants is to be considered in high risk groups, i.e., those most likely to develop venous thrombi and pulmonary embolism. Included in this category are patients over the age of 50 who will be bedridden or immobilized for long periods of time as a result of extensive fractures, particularly of the femur, or other forms of trauma, debilitating disease, cardiac failure, myocardial infarction, or surgery, particularly hip arthroplasty. The pharmacologic basis for the use of anticoagulation in the prevention of venous thrombotic disease is sound, and its effectiveness in reducing thromboembolic complications after fractured hips or extensive trauma, during the postoperative state, and after acute myocardial infarction has been established in several series of observations. When indicated, anticoagulant therapy should be instituted immediately; it can be carried out solely with *oral agents (coumarin or indandione compounds),* for although these agents take several days to induce an appropriate antithrombotic state, the danger period for pulmonary embolism usually begins somewhat later. Anticoagulation should be continued until full mobilization is completed, because the risk of thrombosis remains as long as stasis exists. Such anticoagulation is not a contraindication to surgery or other procedures. Surgery can be performed without much danger either before or shortly after the institution of anticoagulant treatment, because hemostasis is not impaired for several days; later, in the more chronically anticoagulated patient, surgery can be undertaken after reduction of the level of anticoagulation with careful attention to wound hemostasis. Nevertheless, despite its proved value, physicians have been reluctant to use such prophylactic anticoagulant therapy except in cases of recurrent thrombophlebitis or pulmonary embolism; cited are the hazard of bleeding and the difficulties in maintaining adequate anticoagulation in older patients. Some of these difficulties can be avoided by elimination of a loading dose and recognition of the various factors which influence drug responsiveness (see below).

Infusion of *dextran* 40 or 75 (500 to 1000 ml on day of surgery, 500 ml daily for next five days)* can also be used to prevent postoperative thrombophlebitis, presumably by increasing blood flow and preventing surface interactions. However, although effective, it provides little advantage over anticoagulants, because it also enhances the risk of bleeding and is tolerated poorly in individuals with impaired cardiac reserve.

The most important advance in the prevention of deep vein thrombi in immobilized patients is administration of small doses of *heparin,* i.e., 5000 units twice a day subcutaneously into the abdominal wall during periods of high risk. This regimen maintains circulating heparin blood levels at a fraction of that ordinarily achieved with conventional therapeutic doses as used in the treatment of established thrombosis (see below), and does not significantly affect the Lee-White clotting time and activated partial thromboplastin time; nor

---

*Experimental drug for this purpose.

does it enhance the risk of bleeding. However, there is sufficient circulating heparin to activate enough heparin cofactor (antithrombin III) to block the action of earlier activated enzymes of the clotting reaction (notably Xa and IXa). In several trials, prophylactic therapy with low dose heparin has strikingly reduced the incidence of venous thrombosis occurring postoperatively (except after femoral fractures and hip arthroplasty) and after acute myocardial infarction as measured by ^{125}I-labeled fibrinogen scanning. A large multicenter, multinational study also has revealed that this mode of prophylaxis results in a significant reduction in pulmonary embolism in older patients following major abdominothoracic surgery.

The use of *platelet function inhibitors*, e.g., *aspirin*, *dipyridamole*, and *sulfinpyrazone*, for the prevention of deep vein thrombosis remains unclear; aspirin (600 mg twice daily) has been claimed to be effective in preventing deep vein thrombosis following reconstructive hip surgery, and sulfinpyrazone (600 to 800 mg daily) has been found useful in reducing the incidence of arteriovenous shunt thrombosis in patients undergoing chronic renal dialysis, and in decreasing the frequency of attacks in patients with recurrent thrombophlebitis who are refractory to coumarin therapy. When sulfinpyrazone is used with coumarin, the dose of the latter should be lowered because of occupation by sulfinpyrazone of coumarin-binding sites.

TREATMENT. General Measures. Acute superficial thrombophlebitis is most often self-limited, unless infected, and usually responds promptly to analgesics, bed rest, warm moist packs, and elevation of the affected limb. Pulmonary embolism is a rare complication unless there is also involvement of the deep venous system. Antimicrobial drugs are not indicated except in septic phlebitis, in which the choice of agent depends on the organism responsible for the infection.

Acute deep vein thrombophlebitis must be managed more aggressively because of the tendency of these thrombi to extend, embolize, and produce serious venous obstruction and damage to venous valves (a postphlebitic insufficiency syndrome occurs in about 5 per cent of those with an ascending thrombophlebitis). In addition to the local measures described above, the objectives of treatment are to prevent further disease and, if indicated, to remove the obstructing thrombus.

Anticoagulants. Currently the principal therapeutic agents for the prevention of further extension and embolization are the anticoagulants, and with their use alone most cases can be managed successfully and without complication. In the absence of contraindications (bleeding diathesis, hemorrhagic lesions, malignant hypertension, known allergy to heparin) anticoagulation should be instituted immediately with heparin, for it is the most effective of the agents available and induces an immediate antithrombotic state.

Heparin can be administered intravenously or by the intramuscular and subcutaneous routes. Based on control of antithrombotic effects, the intravenous route is most often recommended, particularly for the first several days of therapy. Because of local pain and frequent hematomas, intramuscular injections are the least desirable. Even with the intravenous route, dosages and regimens vary. Continuous intravenous infusions of heparin, although requiring special care in administration, are becoming the preferred mode of therapy; control of dosage is easier and, more important, evidence

is accumulating that bleeding complications can be reduced significantly. A suggested procedure is to begin with a loading dose of 75 IU per pound of body weight, followed by a sustaining infusion of 10 IU per pound per hour through an indwelling plastic catheter placed above the antecubital fossa. Subsequent dosage is adjusted to maintain the activated partial thromboplastin time at twice normal (range 1½ to 2½); with Lee-White clotting times, the range is 2 to 2½ times normal. If the intermittent injection technique is employed, it is suggested that 60,000 IU be given during the first day (e.g., 10,000 units every four hours) and that, beginning on the second day, dosage be regulated by coagulation determinations; one hour before the next injection, the activated partial thromboplastin time or Lee-White clotting time should be at the level recommended above for sustaining infusions.

Once the dose requirement has been established, the clotting time may be checked once daily at an appropriate time to exclude possible increase or decrease in the anticoagulant effect and to allow for variations in heparin requirement during the course of therapy. Not infrequently, patients in whom thrombosis is occurring require more heparin in the first 24 to 48 hours of treatment than several days after the institution of therapy. Heparin therapy is recommended for periods of seven to ten days before relying solely on oral anticoagulation with coumarin drugs; this will ensure the most potent antithrombotic state and allow the underlying thrombus to become firmly fixed to the vessel wall.

"Burning fingers" and an occasional allergic reaction may be seen with heparin (osteoporosis and alopecia are additional adverse effects associated with long-term administration), but the primary risk in heparin therapy is bleeding. In one series it was as high as 50 per cent in women over the age of 60; usually the incidence is of the order of 5 to 8 per cent. This risk can be reduced by better control of the anticoagulant state, eliminating aspirin and aspirin-containing compounds, and avoiding intramuscular injections and invasive procedures. It should be remembered that patients whose hemostatic mechanism is impaired before heparin is instituted are predisposed to bleed. When significant bleeding occurs, heparin in the circulation can be immediately neutralized with protamine sulfate; the latter reacts with heparin stoichiometrically and on a milligram per milligram basis. Protamine is administered slowly intravenously after dilution in physiologic saline in an amount equivalent to half the last dose of heparin but not in excess of 100 mg.* For this calculation 100 units of heparin can be taken to represent 1 mg.

Oral anticoagulation with *coumarin* (or, less popularly, *indandione*) compounds should be instituted several days before the discontinuation of heparin therapy. It should be continued for six weeks to six months, unless the phlebitis is associated with immobilization, in which case the drug should be continued until full physical activity is resumed. If thrombi recur when anticoagulants are discontinued, the treatment should be resumed, and long-term therapy may be necessary. Patients with known recurrent episodes of phlebitis may require prophylactic anticoagulant therapy extending over years.

The action of coumarin compounds is indirect, i.e., the induction of a hypocoagulable state, in contrast to

---

*See p. vi, Dosage Notice, immediately following Preface.

the action of heparin as an immediate activator of antithrombin III. At present, the aim of therapy is to reduce the level of the prothrombin complex factors (factors II, VII, IX, and X) to approximately 20 per cent of normal and sustain it there. (Antithrombin III levels are increased during coumarin administration and may contribute to the antithrombotic effect.) This is achieved by regulating dosage so as to prolong the one-stage prothrombin time test to one and a half to two times the control time by the Quick test. Levels of two and a half times or greater are associated with an increased incidence of bleeding, and levels of less than one and a half times the control may not be effective.

There is little difference in the onset of effect or smoothness of control among the various coumarin derivatives, and vitamin K_1 is equally effective in counteracting their action. Because factor VII of the various vitamin K dependent factors (II, VII, IX, and X) has the shortest half-life, it is depressed most quickly by coumarin therapy. However, the rapid depression of factor VII does not provide good antithrombotic protection but does enhance the risk of bleeding. Accordingly, previous regimens involving the use of a loading dose are being employed less frequently. A suggested regimen is to give warfarin, 10 to 15 mg daily, until the desired effect on the prothrombin time is achieved and the dose adjusted to maintain that level. Individualization of dosage is essential, because a variety of drug interactions, other pharmacologic considerations, and metabolic factors influence the sensitivity and response to the coumarin compounds. *Drugs to be avoided during warfarin therapy* include aspirin, phenylbutazone, oxyphenbutazone, and indomethacin, and the following have been shown to potentiate its effect: anabolic steroids, certain antimicrobials (particularly chloramphenicol and those which affect the intestinal bacterial flora), chloral hydrate, clofibrate, disulfiram, ethacrynic acid, glucagon, mefenamic acid, methylphenidate, quinidine, quinine, and sulfinpyrazone. Those agents which inhibit the prothrombinopenic effect of warfarin include barbiturates, corticosteroids, cholestyramine, ethchlorvynol, glutethimide, griseofulvin, haloperidol, meprobamate, and oral contraceptives. Also, older patients, particularly women, are more sensitive to warfarin, as are individuals suffering from febrile illnesses, malnutrition, steatorrhea, and hepatic or pancreatic disease, as well as those in the immediate postoperative state. Increased resistance to warfarin is associated with hyperlipidemia and hyperuricemia. Warfarin also interferes with the metabolism of other drugs; it enhances the action of diphenylhydantoin, chlorpropamide, and tolbutamide.

In patients being switched from heparin to warfarin therapy, a period of overlap is necessary because of the delay in the antithrombotic effect of the coumarin. A suggested procedure is to give warfarin, 10 to 15 mg daily for two to three days, until the desired therapeutic range for the prothrombin time is achieved; then, while continuing maintenance warfarin therapy, heparin dosage is progressively reduced over another three- to four-day period before discontinuation. Since prothrombin times are influenced by the presence of heparin, such assays should be carried out on blood specimens with a normal or near normal activated partial thromboplastin time; otherwise, the in vitro addition of protamine may be necessary.

Bleeding is a significant hazard with oral anticoagula-

tion, occurring in 3 per cent or more of patients on long-term therapy; vitamin K_1 in doses of 5 to 10 mg is usually corrective. Long-term therapy should not be undertaken unless a reliable laboratory is available and the patient's cooperation can be assured. Individuals on such therapy should avoid contact exercise, aspirin, and aspirin-containing compounds, and should be observed carefully even after slight trauma (subdural hematoma in the aged is often an unsuspected complication of coumarin therapy). Invasive procedures, including needle biopsies and spinal taps, are to be avoided unless the prothrombin time is first restored to or near the normal range. Other adverse effects are minimal; probably of most interest is the occasional appearance of skin necrosis and the rare "purple toe syndrome." Contraindications to coumarin therapy are similar to those previously mentioned for heparin and, in addition, pregnancy. Not only has coumarin administration been shown to increase teratogenicity in animals during the first trimester but, unlike heparin, it crosses the placental barrier and can produce fetal hemorrhage. The use of coumarins also should be avoided, when possible, for patients with severe liver disease or advanced renal insufficiency.

Other Antithrombotic Agents. Low molecular weight *dextran* infusions, based on their ability to improve flow rates by expanding plasma volume and to inhibit platelet adherence and aggregation, have been recommended by some as a useful adjunct in the management of acute thrombophlebitis. In contrast to its proved value in prevention, the efficacy of such therapy for thrombophlebitis remains to be established; at present there is little justification to have dextran infusions replace anticoagulant therapy. Also, there is considerable interest in the use of defibrinating agents; the most promising agents in this respect are the highly purified fraction (*Arvin*) obtained from the venom of the Malayan pit viper, and *Defibrase*. It remains to be established whether these agents will have advantages over heparin.

Surgical Therapy. Surgical procedures may be helpful in the management of some cases of thrombophlebitis; *proximal interruption of venous flow* can be employed to prevent embolization, and thrombectomy to relieve obstruction. The surgical procedures of choice to protect adequately against pulmonary embolization from the lower extremities and pelvis are inferior vena caval ligation, plication, or the insertion of an appropriate filter or umbrella. The last-named can be accomplished transvenously and does not require abdominal surgery. Each procedure has its adherents, and all but the first obviate the difficulty of sudden acute fluid sequestration with hypovolemia and impaired venous return, an event which may be tolerated poorly by people with underlying heart disease. Since all these procedures are usually followed by retrograde thrombosis, and consequently carry a significant incidence of distressing sequelae, both immediate and late, and do not permanently protect (large collaterals develop in several months and may provide a new route for embolization), they are not given consideration except in the presence of pulmonary embolism, or when pulmonary embolism has been known to occur in the past and there is a contraindication to the use of anticoagulant therapy.

Thrombectomy, including the use of Fogarty and similar types of catheters, has been employed successfully in the management of occasional cases of phlegmasia cerulea dolens. However, since this procedure is often followed by venous rethrombosis as well as complicating the subsequent use of anticoagulation, it is currently indicated only for those patients in whom acute fluid sequestration and high tissue tension sufficiently jeopardize the arterial circulation as to threaten the survival of the limb.

Thrombolytic Therapy. Clot-dissolving agents are useful in selected cases as adjuncts in the management of deep vein thrombophlebitis, for they provide the only medical means for directly lysing a thrombus already formed. The most useful agents for thrombolytic therapy are *streptokinase* and *urokinase*, activators of the naturally occurring human fibrinolytic enzyme system. Streptokinase is a secretory product of the hemolytic *Streptococcus* and can be produced readily in large quantities and relatively inexpensively for therapeutic purposes. Its major disadvantage is its antigenicity; this poses problems in dosage and, more important, in retreatment should thrombosis recur. Urokinase, a normal constituent of human urine, is nonantigenic and simpler to use therapeutically, but more expensive. Although originally prepared from urine, currently it is being processed from the culture medium of fetal kidney tissue cells. Both agents are given intravenously; for thrombophlebitis, a suggested procedure for streptokinase is to give 250,000 units as a loading dose over a 20- to 30-minute period, followed by a sustaining infusion of 100,000 units per hour for 48 to 72 hours; with urokinase, 2000 units per pound of body weight is given as a loading dose, followed by a sustaining infusion of the same amount per hour for 24 to 48 hours. Heparin therapy is instituted at the termination of the fibrinolytic therapy so as to prevent rethrombosis. Although both agents when used in appropriate dosage age capable of lysing large thrombi in the deep leg veins, the intense fibrinolytic state has a propensity to induce bleeding. Consequently, current recommendations are to limit their use to those patients with extensive occlusions of the major deep veins of the extremity or with a rapidly ascending thrombophlebitis or pulmonary embolism.

Follow-up Therapy. When the systemic symptoms and signs of thrombophlebitis have subsided and the involved limb is pain free and nontender, the patient can begin walking with the leg supported by elastic stockings, unless such activity is followed by return of symptoms. After walking has been resumed, the patient should be advised to elevate the extremity above heart level for several half-hour periods a day. Elastic stockings should be worn until measurement of the extremity reveals no accumulation of edema fluid. Early and persistent therapy is important to prevent development of the postphlebitic syndrome. Once the brawny swelling and induration of the postphlebitic limb have occurred, they may be relieved somewhat by long periods of elevation, elastic compressions, vigorous massage, special exercises and mechanical devices, providing that there has been no recent recurrence of phlebitis. Gross deformities, ulcerations, and persistent or repeated infections may ultimately require one or more surgical procedures.

Basu, D., Gallus, A., Hirsh, J., and Cade, J.: A prospective study of the value of monitoring heparin treatment with the activated partial thromboplastin time. N. Engl. J. Med., 287:324, 1972.

Coon, W. W., Willis, P. W., III, and Keller, J. B.: Venous thromboem-
bolism and other venous disease in the Tecumseh Community Health Study. Circulation, 48:239, 1973.

Foster, C. S., Genton, E., Henderson, M., Sherry, S., and Wessler, S. (eds.): The epidemiology of venous thrombosis. Milbank Memorial Fund Quarterly, 50(1), Part 2:9, 1972.

Gallus, A. S., Hirsh, J., Tuttle, R. J., et al.: Small subcutaneous doses of heparin in prevention of venous thrombosis. N. Engl. J. Med., 288:545, 1973.

Genton, E.: Guidelines for heparin therapy. Ann. Intern. Med., 80:77, 1974.

Harris, W. H. Salzman, E. W., Athanasoulis, C. A., et al.: Aspirin prophylaxis of venous thromboembolism after total hip replacement. N. Engl. J. Med., 297:1246, 1977.

Koch-Weser, J., and Sellers, E. M.: Drug interaction with coumarin anticoagulants. N. Engl. J. Med., 285:547, 1971.

O'Reilly, R. A., and Aggeler, P. M.: Studies on coumarin anticoagulant drugs. Institution of warfarin therapy without a loading dose. Circulation, 38:169, 1968.

357.3. PULMONARY EMBOLISM AND INFARCTION

Sol Sherry

DEFINITION. Pulmonary embolism is the impaction in the pulmonary vascular bed of a previously detached thrombus or foreign matter. Its major complication, pulmonary infarction, is the necrosis of lung parenchyma resulting from interference with blood supply. Since pulmonary embolism is the more common event, is not invariably accompanied by infarction, and has distinguishing features of its own, this chapter will be devoted primarily to pulmonary embolism; however, discussion of pulmonary infarction will be included as indicated.

ETIOLOGY. Pulmonary embolism is a complication, not a primary disease; therefore its etiology is considered in terms of the nature and source of the offending embolus. Almost all pulmonary emboli originate as thrombi; on occasion nonthrombotic materials such as amniotic fluid, fat, air, bone marrow, or tumor may embolize to the lung.

Venous thrombi in the deep veins of the lower extremities are the most common source for pulmonary emboli, accounting for 80 to 90 per cent. Another important source for pulmonary embolization is thrombi in the pelvic veins and prostatic plexus. Prostatic vein thrombosis may accompany malignant disease of the prostate but more frequently follows prostatic surgery. In the female, thrombosis in the pelvic veins may follow parturition or surgery; a particularly severe form, with frequent and protracted embolization, may complicate septic abortion. Pulmonary emboli may also arise from the right heart and are seen in association with cardiac failure, atrial fibrillation, myocardial infarction, the primary cardiomyopathies, and bacterial endocarditis (involving the tricuspid or pulmonic valves). Thrombi in the right heart frequently embolize and are said to account for approximately 25 per cent of pulmonary emboli among cardiac patients.

The factors controlling detachment of the whole or part of a venous thrombus into the general circulation are even less well understood than thrombus formation itself; frequently such thrombi will break away without apparent cause. It was formerly believed that embolization occurred more frequently with phlebothrombosis, but evidence to support this concept is lacking, and symptomatic thrombophlebitis is often complicated by embolization. Of more importance are the location of the vessel (embolism is rare from a superficial vein but very frequent from the iliofemoral vein), the presence of a free floating tail, and factors which acutely change pressure relationships in veins or suddenly increase venous blood flow; these include straining at stool, exertion, and ambulation after a long period of immobilization.

Once a thrombus is released into the venous circulation, it is usually carried rapidly through the great veins and right heart into the pulmonary arteries, except under those circumstances in which the embolus is shunted, through a patent foramen ovale or other defect, into the heart and systemic circulation *(paradoxical embolization)*. However, even this latter condition tends to occur most frequently after a bout of pulmonary embolism, for the associated pulmonary hypertension predisposes to paradoxical embolization.

INCIDENCE AND PREVALENCE. Pulmonary embolism with or without infarction is a common disorder and a most important cause of morbidity and mortality. It is frequently misdiagnosed. Next to pneumonia, it is the most common acute pulmonary lesion seen in hospitalized patients today. Thirty per cent of pulmonary emboli occur in cardiac patients, another 30 per cent occur among medical noncardiac patients (particularly among the aged), and most of the remainder occur postoperatively. Immobilization, venous disease, and prior cardiopulmonary disease are the factors most frequently predisposing to pulmonary embolism. The over-all incidence of pulmonary embolism in general autopsy series ranges from 5 to 14 per cent, but the incidence is considerably higher (25 per cent) in institutions for the care of the aged, and highest (30 to 45 per cent) among cardiac patients. The incidence of pulmonary embolism appears to have increased progressively over the past several decades.

Embolism to the main pulmonary artery or its primary branches so as to occlude acutely the major portion of the circulation through the lungs, although less frequent than embolism of smaller vessels, is the third most common cause of sudden death (5 per cent) among hospitalized patients. It occurs in about 3 per cent of general autopsy series, but with antemortem diagnosis of only one in eight.

Embolism to medium-sized vessels, i.e., lobar and segmental vessels, is observed approximately three to five times more frequently in autopsy series than is embolism of the major vessels; but since the former is commonly not fatal and is often recurrent, the actual incidence of acute episodes is relatively much greater. Furthermore, in contrast to embolism of the major vessels, the presence of medium-sized emboli at autopsy can be considered only incidental in two thirds of the cases; in the other third, the clinical features are such as to suggest some relation to the fatal termination. Pulmonary infarction complicates embolism of medium-sized arteries in less than 25 per cent of cases. In cardiac patients, the incidence of infarction after such embolism is considerably increased; in one autopsy series, more than 90 per cent of the lungs of cardiac patients with emboli were found to have areas of infarction.

Embolism to small-sized vessels, i.e., subsegmental arteries and their branches, probably occurs with great frequency, but the incidence is difficult to assess. As an isolated and focal lesion, such embolization has little clinical significance, for it usually is not large enough to produce a macroinfarction, and in routine autopsies the lesion is likely to be overlooked unless there are associated emboli in the larger vessels. However, multiple small emboli scattered throughout the lungs are frequently observed in association with embolic occlusions of larger vessels; under these circumstances they contribute significantly to the impairment of pulmonary circulation and associated morbidity. Miliary small vessel occlusion is also the major cause of morbidity when nonthrombotic emboli, such as fat, amniotic fluid, air, or nitrogen, are involved.

PATHOLOGY. Pulmonary emboli may be single or multiple and vary in size from microscopic particles to large saddle emboli that completely occlude the pulmonary artery and its major branches. In addition a large embolus may break up during passage through the heart or upon impaction and not only obstruct a major vessel but further embolize into one or more smaller branches in both lung fields. Also, there is evidence that, subsequent to impaction, emboli may shift or further fragment into previously unobstructed pulmonary vessels.

With occlusion of the main pulmonary artery or of both its primary branches, or when there is extensive involvement of medium-sized vessels so as to cut off the major portion of the pulmonary arterial circulation, there is acute mechanical obstruction to pulmonary blood flow; the pulmonary artery is distended by the presence of both clot and blood, the right ventricle is acutely dilated, the peripheral veins are engorged, and the liver is congested. Acute infarction rarely occurs; either the lung parenchyma is fairly normal or there is moderate atelectasis, usually explained by the loss of surfactant, and edema. Although the low incidence of acute infarction is possibly attributable to the rapidity with which death occurs (90 per cent of the deaths from acute pulmonary embolism occur within the first two hours), other factors are probably responsible for this phenomenon. In 40 per cent of the cases there is evidence of previous embolization and infarction.

Emboli which pass beyond the pulmonary artery and its major branches tend to impact the arteries of the lower lobes, more often the right than the left. Embolism to other lobes is much less frequent; combined, they account for only 25 per cent of cases. The more frequent involvement of the lower lobes is believed to be due to the fact that these areas lie in the more direct stream of the pulmonary arteries.

When *infarction* occurs, its spreads to involve a pleural surface, either peripheral or interlobar. The infarcted area is airless and hemorrhagic; the hemorrhage is both interstitial and alveolar. Because of the associated pleuritis, hypoventilation, and pre-existing disease, there may be surrounding atelectasis and edema as well. Although occlusion of the larger medium vessels, e.g., interlobar arteries, tends to be associated with infarcts of larger size, the relation between size of vessel occlusion and infarction is a poor one; other factors appear to be more critical in determining the presence and size of the infarct. By roentgenography, infarcts are poorly visualized on the first day. Thereafter they usually appear as humped, wedge-shaped, or, less commonly, rounded shadows. When they occur near the bases, considerable diaphragmatic elevation and restriction of motion may be observed. In 30 to 40 per cent of cases, infarcts are associated with a variable amount of *pleural effusion* that may be serous, serosanguineous, or frankly hemorrhagic; usually the specific gravity is in the range of 1.014 to 1.017 (protein, 3 to 3.5 grams per 100 ml) and there is mild to moderate increase in cell content.

Some shadows clear rapidly (two to three days) on roentgenographic examination and have been referred to as "incomplete" infarcts; however, it is likely that this clearing represents reventilation of an atelectatic or congested area occasioned by the embolic occlusion rather than true resolution of an infarct. "Complete" infarcts clear slowly over a two- to three-week period, ending as an area of linear fibrosis.

MECHANISMS OF DISEASE, INCLUDING PULMONARY IN-FARCTION. Emboli lodging in the pulmonary arterial tree acutely reduce the circulation distal to the site of obstruction. Potentially, the effects are four-fold: (1) less blood proceeds through the pulmonary circuit to the left heart and systemic circulation; (2) there is a damming back of blood behind the mechanical obstruction; (3) hemorrhagic necrosis of the ischemic area may occur; and (4) pulmonary function is impaired (pulmonary capillary perfusion and diffusion; later, ventilation may be compromised as well).

Except for the occurrence of infarction, which must be considered as a localized or focal disorder, the average person is believed capable of withstanding considerable obstruction of the pulmonary arterial bed without serious consequences to the vascular dynamics; in normal animals, a 60 to 70 per cent obstruction is usually well tolerated. Nevertheless, exceptions occur, particularly in the presence of underlying heart disease, when less extensive occlusions may elevate pulmonary arterial pressure or significantly reduce pulmonary venous outflow and when pulmonary circulation has been previously impaired by disease or prior embolization.

With a large occlusion of the main pulmonary artery or its primary branches, the effects are acute and primarily mechanical: rapidly rising pulmonary artery pressure, failure of the right ventricle, cyanosis, venous engorgement, and hepatic congestion. The consequences of impaired pulmonary venous return are sharp reduction in left ventricular filling, diminished cardiac output, reduced coronary and cerebral blood flow, hypoxia (also caused by pulmonary blood shunting), dyspnea, pallor, tachycardia, and hypotension, often progressing quickly to shock and death. Sudden dyspnea and retrosternal pain are frequently the most prominent initial complaints; the dyspnea is believed to be due to anoxia, apprehension, and stimulation of Hering-Breuer and other reflexes; the angina is usually attributed to acute coronary insufficiency, but direct stimulation of sensory nerves in the wall of a rapidly distending pulmonary artery may also play a significant role.

The effects of embolization to medium-sized vessels depend on the number, size, and distribution of the emboli and the prior state of the lung and circulation. Several patterns may be observed. (1) There may be no observable effects; a transient episode of dyspnea may be the only clue to its occurrence. (2) The picture may be predominantly one of pulmonary infarction with hemoptysis, pleuritic chest pain, friction rub, and abnormal roentgenographic shadows. Often, however, some elements of this pattern may be absent, notably the hemoptysis or the evidence of pleural involvement. (3) There may be an acute picture similar to, but frequently not as severe as, that seen with embolization of the main pulmonary artery or its primary branches, in which pattern the primary difficulty is one of extensive and sudden compromise of the pulmonary arterial circulation but here by multiple emboli or recurrent embolization; it may or may not be complicated by infarction. (4) There may be a chronic and

insidiously developing syndrome of cor pulmonale from progressive pulmonary hypertension that has evolved slowly after repeated episodes of embolization with or without infarction. This is often superimposed and obscured by the presence of other underlying chronic disease.

Controversy exists concerning the factors that acutely compromise the pulmonary circulation when emboli impact in medium-sized or smaller vessels. Some hold that vasoconstriction (pulmonary and perhaps coronary), mediated through reflexes from occluded arterioles or by the local release of serotonin, prostaglandins, or other vasoactive substances, plays an important role. It seems probable, however, that the continuing effects of most pulmonary emboli are primarily mechanical; when a major segment of the circulation is organically occluded, pulmonary hypertension and decreased venous outflow result. The suggestion has been made, and experimental studies have been cited to support the concept, that idiopathic pulmonary hypertension and pulmonary arteriosclerosis may result from repeated small pulmonary emboli.

The mechanism of pulmonary infarction is poorly understood. It does not result from ligation of pulmonary vessels and is unusual after embolization in animals with normal lungs; however, it does occur with great frequency in the congested, infected, or hypoventilated lung. Currently the best working hypothesis is that when medium-sized embolization occurs, enhancement of the circulation through the bronchial artery collaterals and bronchopulmonary vascular anastomoses distal to the embolus ordinarily serves to sustain the lung. However, in the presence of congestion or other conditions that predispose to local intrapulmonic circulatory stasis, augmentation of the collateral circulation is delayed or its benefits voided, and infarction occurs.

Hemorrhagic necrosis of the lung tissue and the overlying pleural inflammation are responsible for the characteristic clinical features of pulmonary infarction. The former accounts for the hemoptysis, cough, and fever; the latter for the pleural friction rub and pain. Since both lung tissue and the visceral pleura are devoid of sensory nerves, infarcts that do not extend to the outer surface of the lung to involve the parietal pleura do not cause pleural pain. When pain is present, it usually occurs over the ribs in the axillary region, but occasionally it may appear in the abdomen along the costal margin, or, when there is involvement of the parietal diaphragmatic pleura, in the shoulder or neck. The mechanism of the pain has usually been attributed to friction over an inflamed pleura, but an alternative explanation that may better explain its features (accentuation only on inspiration) is tension exerted during inspiration on those sensitized nerve ends of the parietal pleura that are attached to the intercostal muscles.

CLINICAL MANIFESTATIONS. The manifestations of *massive pulmonary embolism* (defined for clinical purposes as occlusion of 50 per cent or more of the pulmonary arterial circulation and representing approximately one third to one half of the suspected cases) may include sudden dyspnea; tachypnea; cyanosis; precordial or substernal oppressive pain, occasionally with radiation to shoulders and neck; evidence of right-sided cardiac dilatation and failure; tachycardia; restlessness; anxiety; syncope, occasionally with convulsions; and hypotension.

With massive embolism, death may be sudden or may occur over a period of several hours. In the latter instance, shock with vascular collapse becomes prominent. In an additional 2 to 3 per cent of patients, death may be delayed from one to several days; but when blood pressure spontaneously returns to normal, recovery is likely (unless the course is complicated by recurrence or an underlying disease). The physical signs noted include pulsation in the second left interspace, accentuation of P_2, a pseudo- or pleuropericardial friction rub, systolic or diastolic murmurs in the second left interspace, an interscapular bruit, S_3 or S_4 gallop rhythm, increased cardiac dullness to the right, distended neck veins, increased venous pressure with an hepatojugular reflex, and enlarged liver. Dislodgment of a large obstructing embolus may be associated with the dramatic transient appearance of a "red arterial wave" suddenly passing over a pallid cyanotic face.

Serial *electrocardiograms* reveal transient changes in most patients (85 per cent), but the pattern is extremely variable. The most frequent initial finding is T wave inversion (40 per cent). The electrocardiographic signs of acute cor pulmonale ($S_1Q_3T_3$, complete right bundle branch block, P pulmonale, or right axis deviation) are present in only 25 per cent of patients; left axis deviation is observed more frequently than right axis deviation. Rhythm disturbances (most commonly, premature ventricular beats) are observed in 10 per cent, as is a pseudoinfarction pattern. Patients with prior cardiopulmonary disease have a greater frequency of arrhythmias, conduction disturbances, and QRS changes; patients with extensive embolization demonstrate more QRS, RST, and T wave changes. In general, little change occurs during the first 24 hours, but after five to six days the QRS, primary RST segment, and T wave abnormalities begin to disappear. Roentgenographically, massive pulmonary embolism may result in the appearance of a large pulmonary arterial shadow that terminates abruptly; in some cases the ischemia may produce radiolucency of portions of the lung field (Westermark's sign).

With *submassive embolism*, i.e., occlusion of less than 50 per cent of the pulmonary circulation and usually involving the medium-sized or smaller vessels, the clinical manifestations may vary from a transient episode of dyspnea or the sudden or insidious worsening of an underlying pulmonary or cardiac disease, to the full-blown picture described for massive embolism (submassive embolism in patients with prior embolism or severe underlying cardiopulmonary disease frequently presents with the findings usually attributable to massive embolism); however, when pulmonary infarction occurs, its manifestations may also be superimposed.

The manifestations of *pulmonary infarction* are usually less dramatic. They vary in intensity from silent to those characterized by pleuritic chest pain, hemoptysis, cough, moderate dyspnea, fever, tachycardia, pleural friction rub, areas of dullness or flatness on percussion, and diminished breath sounds, occasionally with tubular breathing and rales. The leukocyte count is usually elevated, the sedimentation rate is accelerated, and, subsequently, the serum bilirubin and serum lactic dehydrogenase levels rise. Roentgenographic examination may show typical humped or wedge-shaped shadows; on occasions the lesions are rounded or indistinguishable from pneumonic infiltrates. At other times, a pleural effusion may be the only clue to an underlying infarct. The average patient with pulmonary infarction runs a moderately febrile course for a few days, which is followed by clearing of roentgenographic and physical signs in one to three weeks.

DIAGNOSIS. Despite the introduction of such diagnostic aids as pulmonary isotopic and ventilation photoscanning and selective pulmonary angiography, the diagnosis of pulmonary embolism with or without infarction is accurately made in no more than 50 per cent of cases when compared to autopsy findings. Frequently the diagnosis is overlooked because the disorder appears in the guise of congestive heart failure or pneumonia rather than as a distinctive syndrome; furthermore, the cardinal features do not occur with any great regularity. In half the patients subsequently proved to have recurrent infarction, no evidence of phlebitis, pleural pain, pleural friction rub, or hemoptysis is present, and in any one episode the incidence of each of these is less than 20 per cent. Thus in the absence of classic features, the diagnosis must be made on the basis of a high index of suspicion followed by confirmatory laboratory findings.

Pulmonary embolism with or without infarction should be suspected in all cases of chest pain of unknown cause, atypical pleural effusion, or bronchopneumonia. The possibility of this complication should also be considered in any patient who has a proved or suggestive history of a previous episode (present in 25 per cent of cases), in groups at high risk for deep vein thrombosis, and, most carefully, in critically ill patients with congestive heart failure; the incidence among the last-named group approaches 50 per cent and is much higher among those who exhibit unexplained fever or the *triad of tachycardia, digitalis toxicity, and edema unresponsive to diuretic therapy*.

Actually, the presence of one or more of the following symptoms, signs, or laboratory findings should raise the possibility of pulmonary embolism for consideration: sudden or increased dyspnea, tachypnea, cough, or cyanosis; substernal or pleuritic chest pain; hemoptysis; phlebitis; acute right-sided failure or sudden worsening of congestive heart failure; shock; pulmonary consolidation; pleural friction rub; roentgenographic evidence of pulmonary infiltration, elevated diaphragm, large areas of increased radiolucency, or pleural effusion; unexplained arrhythmias or electrocardiographic changes, particularly when the latter is indicative of acute right heart strain or dilatation; pulmonary function studies indicating an increased ventilatory dead space, i.e., reduction in the mean alveolar carbon dioxide tension in the presence of a normal or nearly normal arterial carbon dioxide tension; or unexplained fever, leukocytosis, elevated erythrocyte sedimentation rate, serum bilirubin, lactic dehydrogenase, and fibrinogen/fibrin split products (normal levels of fibrinogen/fibrin split products and fibrin monomer are rare in pulmonary embolism).

The most reliable *screening procedures* for excluding an acute pulmonary embolism are pulmonary isotopic photoscanning with technetium-labeled microspheres or macroaggregates of human serum albumin, and an arterial P_{O_2} determination; a negative four-positional (anterior, posterior, and both laterals) lung scan virtually eliminates acute embolism, and it is rare when the arterial P_{O_2} is 90 mm Hg or above.

Confirmation of the diagnosis can often be achieved through the use of either selective pulmonary angiography or pulmonary isotopic photoscanning; on occasion, both techniques will be necessary. Since selective *pulmonary angiography* provides direct visualization of the vascular tree, it is the more definitive of the two procedures, and is the choice for establishing the diagnosis of pulmonary embolism. However, there are limitations to its usefulness. It is expensive and requires a skilled team; catheterization of the pulmonary artery is associated with some morbidity; the technique does not distinguish between new and old emboli; the subsegmental and smaller vessels are not visualized adequately; and there may be errors in interpretation unless the angiographer is experienced and strict criteria are used.

Pulmonary isotopic photoscanning has the advantages of convenience and lack of significant morbidity, and allows for repeated observation in following the course of the patient. However, unlike pulmonary arteriography, photoscanning does not visualize the pulmonary arterial tree; rather, it is a measure of the distribution of blood flow or pulmonary capillary perfusion, and defects in perfusion may be misinterpreted as to cause, especially in the presence of any underlying pulmonary lesion, e.g., infiltrates, blebs, cysts, emphysema, an acute asthmatic attack, or alterations in perfusion as a result of previous or associated disease. Since the scan is not specific for pulmonary embolism, perfusion defects should be characterized as to whether they are segmental or not and only interpreted as having a high, medium, or low probability of being due to an embolism. Although emphysema may also be responsible for high probability perfusion defects, the differential diagnosis can usually be resolved by a radioactively labeled xenon ventilation scan, because such a scan is unaffected by pulmonary embolism, at least for a period of five days. Pulmonary isotopic photoscanning is most useful for demonstration and quantitating the perfusion defect of a pulmonary embolism when the chest roentgenogram is normal; it may also be diagnostic by revealing multiple perfusion defects (indicative of multiple pulmonary embolism) when only an isolated infiltrate or lesion is present roentgenographically. Resolution of the perfusion defect after an embolism occurs progressively (50 per cent in two weeks), and this, too, may be useful diagnostically. It is noteworthy that patients with underlying cardiac disease have an impaired resolution rate.

Acute pulmonary embolism may be most readily confused with acute myocardial infarction, pulmonary edema, acute asthma, atelectasis, pericarditis, spontaneous pneumothorax, ball-valve thrombus in the left atrium, dissecting aneurysm, and pulmonary artery thrombosis. The last-named condition occurs rarely as a primary form of obscure cause or as a complication of a partially obstructing embolus, invading tumor, narrowed vascular lumen, or atherosclerotic plaque; it is also seen in sickle cell disease and the mixed sickle cell hemoglobinopathies.

The differential diagnosis of pulmonary infarction includes pneumonia, pleurisy, other forms of pleural effusion, neoplasm, acute upper abdominal conditions, and the various causes of pulmonary hemorrhage. During resolution, an occasional infarct may slough out, leaving a thin-walled cavity which may be confused with an abscess.

To distinguish between an infarct and pneumonia may be difficult, yet this question arises frequently. Findings that are helpful in pointing to the diagnosis of infarct are a history or the presence of one of the preconditions of infarct, e.g., recent surgery, trauma, cardiac disease, previous venous disease, or pulmonary embolism; an extremely rapid appearance of roentgenographic abnormalities from the time of the first respiratory symptom; illness that seems disproportionately mild in relation to the extent of the pulmonary involvement or leukocytosis; and relative lack of cough or lack of preceding respiratory disease.

A spontaneous form of pulmonary infarction occurs in sickle cell disease, in the mixed sickle cell hemoglobinopathies, or in persons with sickle cell trait who are exposed to high altitude.

TREATMENT. General Measures. Supportive treatment for the usual acute embolism should include bed rest, an analgesic or narcotic (preferably meperidine hydrochloride [Demerol]) for pain and apprehension, and oxygen as indicated. The administration of antimicrobial drugs to prevent bacterial disease of the lungs is not indicated unless a septic infarct is suspected. All sudden effort should be avoided, especially straining at stool. Stool softeners and colonic lavages may prove useful. Pleural effusions may require aspiration, particularly if dyspnea is progressive. Digitalization is indicated if cardiac failure appears or worsens, but usually is of little benefit.

In more severe cases, continuous oxygen therapy should be employed, and positive pressure oxygen may prove particularly useful when pulmonary edema is present. Cardiac arrhythmias, which occur in 10 per cent of cases, should be treated appropriately. If shock occurs, fluids and isoproterenol should be given. Intravenous fluids should be monitored by central venous pressure measurements but maintained below 150 mm saline to prevent pulmonary edema. For hypotension, isoproterenol, because of its inotropic effect on the heart, is the agent of choice. It should be given intravenously slowly, usually at a rate of 2 μg per minute to sustain the systolic blood pressure at about 100 mm Hg (preferably at 120 mm Hg in previously hypertensive patients). Aminophylline, 250 to 500 mg (by suppository, intramuscularly, or by slow intravenous administration), may prove useful, particularly when dyspnea is prominent or pulmonary edema is present. Venesection may be dangerous, however, because of impaired left ventricular filling. The value of pulmonary vasodilators, e.g., papaverine, and bronchodilators, e.g., atropine, is still highly controversial.

Anticoagulants. In the absence of contraindications, heparin therapy should be instituted immediately in all patients with pulmonary embolism to lessen the danger of a recurrent and frequently fatal embolic accident (when heparin allergy is present, anticoagulation should be instituted immediately with coumarin compounds). Hemoptysis from pulmonary infarction is not a contraindication to anticoagulant therapy. The regimen for heparin therapy and subsequent oral coumarin anticoagulation is as described under the treatment of thrombophlebitis (Ch. 357.2). Aspirin and aspirin-containing compounds should be avoided because of the increased risk of bleeding. Coumarin therapy is continued for six weeks unless there is a chronic disease, e.g., cardiac failure, that predisposes to repeated venous thrombus formation; under these circumstances anticoagulant therapy should be continued for prolonged periods.

Thrombolytic Agents. These provide an important adjunct to the management of the more seriously ill patient with pulmonary embolism. Clinical trials have demonstrated that urokinase and streptokinase lyse pulmonary emboli extensively, reduce the hemodynamic abnormalities, improve pulmonary capillary perfusion, and increase gas exchange. These effects are observed fairly rapidly and are most striking in patients with massive embolism. Regimens as described previously for thrombophlebitis also will reduce significantly the need for surgical embolectomy, particularly when the therapy is combined with temporary cardiac bypass to tide the patient over the most critical period. Whether local perfusion of the agent directly into the pulmonary artery has any advantage over intravenous administration remains to be established. At present, thrombolytic agents are not indicated for the treatment of submassive embolism when stable vital signs are present; in the absence of complications, the patient is destined to recover and there is little need to increase the risk of bleeding; however, they are indicated in massive embolism with or without shock and in submassive embolism with shock. *Arvin,* the defibrinating agent, may also prove to be of benefit in the management of acute pulmonary embolism, but its advantage over heparin remains to be established.

Surgical Therapy. Inferior vena caval ligation, plication, or the insertion of a filter or umbrella should be reserved for those patients in whom anticoagulants are contraindicated, must be discontinued, or whose disease for one reason or another cannot be successfully managed with this form of therapy. Since these procedures carry a significant incidence of sequelae, they are not indicated unless there has been massive embolism or there is evidence of recurrent embolization (a minor recurrence of symptoms, due either to further small emboli or a shift in the position of a previous embolus, is observed in about 10 per cent of patients during the first few days of heparin therapy, and should not be considered as a failure of anticoagulant therapy unless the episode is significant clinically or continues to recur during adequate levels of anticoagulation).

Surgical embolectomy may be lifesaving in critically ill patients. However, this procedure requires cardiac bypass, and because of the condition of the patients, the mortality in patients treated with surgical embolectomy is still very high. At present, the indication for embolectomy is limited to patients who are in extremis or are deteriorating with angiographic evidence of massive embolism of the main pulmonary artery or its primary branches and with sustained peripheral hypotension despite the use of appropriate supportive measures, including thrombolytic therapy. Pulmonary embolectomy may also be considered for patients who have survived a massive embolism but in whom pulmonary hypertension resulting from the presence of an accessible embolus is leading to the development of cor pulmonale.

PROGNOSIS. The prognosis of pulmonary embolism is difficult to establish because the clinical diagnosis is frequently obscure. Of those who succumb, approximately 90 per cent die immediately or within the first two hours. Another 2 to 3 per cent die of protracted shock during the next 48 hours. Once stable vital signs are established, subsequent mortality approximates 7 per cent and is usually attributable to recurrent embolism or adverse effects on an underlying cardiopulmonary disease. The likelihood of a fatal episode is increased with succeeding embolic attacks and, most important, in the presence of a significant impairment of cardiopulmonary reserve. The greatest hope for the management of this problem is prevention.

Unfortunately, such measures as the use of elastic stockings or bandages, leg exercises for immobilized patients, and early ambulation postoperatively have not greatly affected the high incidence of pulmonary embolism; nevertheless, the intelligent use of such measures, and particularly of the more recently developed mechanical devices which enhance blood flow, is to be encouraged. In addition, serious consideration should be given to the use of anticoagulants for all patients predisposed to thrombus formation. When used carefully, anticoagulants have significantly reduced the incidence of pulmonary embolism after fracture of the femur and in cases of congestive heart failure. This form of therapy should not be undertaken lightly, because the hazards, in any specific case, may outweigh the benefits to be derived. Low-dose heparin should obviate this problem.

Anticoagulation also has an important role to play in the *prevention of arterial embolism.* Coumarin therapy is useful in avoiding systemic embolization from endocardial mural thrombi in the left ventricle, e.g., after acute transmural infarction, and in the left atrium, e.g., in rheumatic mitral disease or during an electrical conversion of an arrhythmia. For acute myocardial infarction, coumarin therapy should be administered to those at high risk for such embolic episodes; the high risk factors include age over 60, previous myocardial infarction, shock, congestive heart failure, and evidence of large transmural infarction as judged by the levels of serum enzymes, fever, leukocytosis, sedimentation rate, and the extent of the electrocardiographic abnormalities. Therapy should be initiated at the onset of the illness and continued for a period of four weeks. Patients with rheumatic mitral disease with a nonseptic embolus (anticoagulants are contraindicated in subacute bacterial endocarditis) should be maintained on long-term anticoagulation or until surgical correction of the lesion. For individuals undergoing electrical conversion of an arrhythmia, coumarin therapy should be initiated two to three weeks prior to attempting reversion to a sinus rhythm in all patients with previous emboli or evidence of mitral stenosis; in other situations the need for anticoagulation should be considered and evaluated on an individual basis.

Coumarin anticoagulation is less effective for the prevention of platelet emboli such as may occur from prosthetic heart valves and in the transient ischemic attack syndrome. Better results are being obtained for the former condition when coumarin anticoagulation is combined with antiplatelet agents, e.g., sulfinpyrazone* (800 mg daily) or dipyridamole* (400 mg daily). For the transient ischemic attack syndrome, aspirin (1.2 grams daily) appears to be the antiplatelet agent of choice.

Medical therapy of an acute embolic event with antithrombotic agents is as described under the management of thrombophlebitis and pulmonary embolism.

Anticoagulants in acute myocardial infarction. Results of a cooperative clinical trial. JAMA, 225:724, 1973.

Kakkar, V. V., Corrigan, T. P., and Fossard, D. P.: Prevention of fatal postoperative pulmonary embolism by low doses of heparin: An international multicentre trial. Lancet, 1:45, 1975.

Kakkar, V. V., Howe, C. T., Flanc, C., and Clarke, M. B.: Natural history of postoperative deep vein thrombosis. Lancet, 2:230, 1969.

McIntyre, K. M., and Sasahara, A. A.: The hemodynamic response to pulmonary embolism in patients without prior cardiopulmonary disease. Am. J. Cardiol., 28:288, 1971.

Miller, G. A. H., Hall, R. J. C., and Paneth, M.: Pulmonary embolectomy, heparin and streptokinase: Their place in the treatment of acute massive pulmonary embolism. Am. Heart J., 93:568, 1977.

Paraskos, J. A., Adelstein, S. J., Smith, R. E., et al.: Late prognosis of acute pulmonary embolism. N. Engl. J. Med., 289:55, 1973.

Sasahara, A., Hyers, T. M., Cole, C., et al. (eds.): The urokinase pulmonary embolism trial. Circulation, 47 (Suppl. II):II–5, 1973.

Stein, M., and Moser, K. M. (eds.): Pulmonary Thromboembolism. Chicago, Year Book Medical Publishers, 1973.

---

*Experimental drug for this purpose.

358. PULMONARY HYPERTENSION

Daniel S. Lukas

358.1. INTRODUCTION

Morphologically and physiologically, the circulation of the lungs differs from that of all other organs. Although the entire cardiac output passes through the lungs, a mean pressure in the pulmonary artery only one ninth of the pressure in the aorta is needed to sustain this flow. Under a wide variety of physiologic circumstances, simple adjustments of the pulmonary vascular bed minimize increases of pulmonary arterial pressure. Because many diseases of the heart and lungs can seriously compromise this regulatory capacity, pulmonary hypertension is a common clinical phenomenon. In some disorders elevations of pulmonary arterial pressure are acute and episodic, whereas in others the pulmonary hypertension is chronic and progressive.

The mechanisms producing pulmonary arterial hypertension in the major categories of disease are sufficiently different to warrant separate consideration and are best appreciated in the context of the normal structure and funciton of the pulmonary circulation.

THE NORMAL PULMONARY CIRCULATION

STRUCTURE. The pulmonary arterial tree consists of three distinct types of arteries that differ from each other in the composition of their walls and in size. The elastic arteries include the main pulmonary artery, its major branches, and arteries with external diameters greater than 1.0 mm. The muscular pulmonary arteries range in diameter from 0.1 to 1.0 mm. The smallest pulmonary arteries, the arterioles, have diameters less than 0.1 mm. The walls of all three types of arteries are much thinner than those of systemic arteries, and aside from the main pulmonary artery and its branches, these vessels have no strict anatomic counterparts in the systemic vascular bed.

The media of the main pulmonary artery and the elastic arteries contains a small amount of smooth muscle, collagen, and elastic fibers that are short, irregularly branching, and fragmented in appearance. The media of the aorta, in contrast, is 1.5 to more than 2 times thicker, and its elastic fibers are long, unbranching, and distributed in parallel fashion.

The muscular pulmonary arteries are closely apposed to the bronchioles and alveolar ducts. They have a large lumen and a thin wall that is composed of an intima and a thin media of concentrically oriented smooth muscle fibers bounded by internal and external elastic laminae.

The arterioles differ vastly from those of the systemic circuit, because they contain no muscle except at their point of origin. They consist of an endothelium, a single elastic lamina, and a scanty adventitia.

The pulmonary capillaries are the most prominent structural component of the alveolar walls, in which they form an extensive, interlacing network that is separated from the alveolar air by the lining cells of the alveoli and their basement membrane. The total surface of the capillaries that is available for gas exchange in adults has been estimated to comprise 60 to 70 square meters.

The pulmonary venules are thin-walled structures histologically indistinguishable from the arterioles. The structure of the veins is less ordered than that of the muscular arteries. The media, which is not bounded by well-defined elastic laminae, blends indistinguishably with the adventitia, and both contain smooth muscle and fragmented elastic fibers. The main venous trunks acquire a layer of cardiac muscle before they enter the left atrium. The venules and veins, unlike the arteries, do not course with the bronchial tree but are lodged in the septa that separate lobules and segments of the lung.

The bronchial arteries wind in spiral fashion around the bronchi and anastomose extensively with each other in and around the walls of the airways. They also form vasa vasorum in the adventitia of the elastic and larger muscular pulmonary arteries. Evidence that the two arterial systems intercommunicate in the normal lung is inconclusive. The bronchial veins, however, normally form numerous, small anastomotic channels with the pulmonary veins.

It is of considerable significance that the pulmonary arteries in the fetus and newborn differ structurally from those of the adult and do not attain their final form until the sixth to twelfth month of postnatal life. In the newborn, the media of the main pulmonary artery is as thick as that of the aorta and contains numerous, tightly packed, long, elastic fibers that are fairly uniform in thickness and are arranged in parallel fashion as in the aorta. Progressively after birth, the media diminishes in thickness, and the elastic fibers become fragmented, irregularly shaped, randomly distributed, and less densely packed, until they assume the full adult appearance. The muscular pulmonary arteries in the newborn resemble small systemic arteries. Typically, the wall contains a wide media composed of circularly oriented smooth muscle, and its thickness exceeds the diameter of the lumen. Rapid increase in luminal and external diameters and thinning of the media occur during the first sixth months of life. The arterioles at birth are surrounded by dense connective tissue and their lumina are barely patent. Their wall:lumen ratio likewise rapidly diminishes in the first few months of life.

During the early days of the postnatal period, the mean pulmonary arterial pressure is two or more times greater than that of the adult and may be high enough to reverse flow through the ductus arteriosus. The pulmonary arterial pressure declines to normal adult values within the first month, well before the metamorphosis of the pulmonary vasculature has been completed.

HEMODYNAMICS. The average normal pressure in the pulmonary artery at rest is 19/6 mm Hg (systolic/diastolic) with a mean pressure of 11 mm Hg. Normally at rest, the systolic pressure does not exceed 25 mm Hg, and the mean pressure is not greater than 15 mm Hg. Mean pressures in the large pulmonary veins and left atrium are essentially identical, ranging from 3 to 8 mm Hg, with an average of 5 mm Hg. Thus a pressure gradient from the pulmonary artery to the large pulmonary veins of only 6 mm Hg is sufficient to sustain a blood flow in the normal adult at rest of approximately 6.0 liter per minute. These values are eloquent testimony to the low resistance offered to the flow of blood by the thin-walled and capacious pulmonary vessels. Calculated in the conventional manner as the mean pressure gradient divided by flow, the normal pulmonary vascular resistance is 1.0 mm Hg per liter per minute, or 80 dyne sec cm^{-5}, a value only 7 per cent of the normal systemic vascular resistance. The linear distribution of resistance in the pulmonary vascular bed is uncertain, but measurements in dogs indicate that the pulmonary arteries are responsible for approximately half the total resistance, the pulmonary capillaries for 30 per cent, and the veins for 20 per cent.

Several observations testify to the capacity of the pulmonary vascular bed to accommodate increases in blood flow with disproportionately small increases in pressure. During exercise, two- to three-fold increases in cardiac output are associated with increments of only 25 to 50 per cent in mean pulmonary arterial pressure, but the pressure doubles when the output rises to four to five times the resting value. Large left-right shunts through an atrial septal defect that commonly triple the pulmonary blood flow are tolerated for many years with no more than slight elevations of pulmonary arterial pressure. After pneumonectomy or occlusion of either main branch of the pulmonary artery by a balloon catheter and in patients with congenital absence of a main branch of the pulmonary artery, the pulmonary arterial pressures remain within the normal range at rest if the perfused lung is normal.

Augmentation of pulmonary blood flow is facilitated and concomitant changes in pressure are minimized by several mechanisms that combine to expand the net cross-sectional area of the pulmonary vessels and thereby decrease the resistance they offer to the flow of blood. One of these mechanisms relates to the effect of changes in intravascular pressures on the caliber of the vessels. It has been demonstrated that increases in pulmonary arterial pressure well within the normal operational range are associated with large decreases in pulmonary vascular resistance and that the resistance declines further with the addition of a 2 to 3 mm Hg rise in left atrial pressure. The vessels are also subjected to the deforming effects of the pressures that surround them. The total pressure that acts on the vascular wall is the transmural pressure, or the difference between the intravascular and perivascular pressures. Some uncertainties exist regarding perivascular pressures in the lungs, but for vessels that are not intrinsic components of the alveolar structure, perivascular pressure is considered to approximate pleural pressure; for intra-alveolar vessels, the alveolar pressure has been regarded as the extravascular pressure. Since the vessels that account for the major fraction of the pulmonary vascular resistance are exposed to the normally negative pleural pressure, their transmural pressures exceed the hydrostatic pressures within them.

During exercise, the more negative pleural pressures generated to augment tidal volume increase the transmural pressure gradients acting on the extra-alveolar vessels, thereby stretching them open further and decreasing their resistance to flow. Pressure changes within the pleura and the lungs can profoundly affect the pulmonary vasculature. For example, when intrapleural and alveolar pressures are greatly increased, as during a Valsalva maneuver, pulmonary vascular transmural pressures fall, some vessels collapse, and the resistance rises markedly.

Primarily because of gravitational effects on regional intravascular pressures, the lungs are not evenly perfused. In the erect position, the height of the blood column from the apices of the lungs to the midpoint of the left atrium is sufficient to reduce pressures within the pulmonary arteries at the apices almost to zero and to decrease the transmural pressures of the pulmonary capillaries and veins in these regions to less than zero. Consequently, the vascular bed in the apices is not open, whereas at the bases of the lungs the vessels are subjected to the distending effects of the overlying column of blood and all are patent. These regional differences in vascular resistance produce a progressive decrease in regional blood flow within the lungs from base to apex, and in the upright position blood flow per unit volume of lung is eight times greater at the base than at the apex. At some point below the apices of the lungs, the transmural pressures of the arteries and the arterial limbs of the alveolar capillaries are high enough to maintain patency of the vessels, but the pressure within the venous segment of the capillaries or the venules is less than or just equals the perivascular pressure. The collapsible vascular segments in this region behave like sluices; they are either barely open or closed, and flow of blood through them no longer depends on the pressure gradient between the arterial and venous limbs but varies directly with the pressure difference between the arterial end of the segment and the pressure surrounding the collapsed segment. These hemodynamic conditions have been compared to those of a waterfall.

With increases in pulmonary flow, small changes in intravascular pressures open previously closed or partially collapsed vessels, thus expanding the size of the vascular bed and further lowering resistance to flow. This recruitment of small vessels and capillaries partly explains the increase of pulmonary diffusing capacity that occurs during exercise.

The volume of blood contained by the pulmonary vessels of an average size adult is approximately 400 to 500 ml, 70 to 100 ml of which is in the pulmonary capillaries. Because of its geometric complexity and the probably nonuniform dimensional rearrangements that the pulmonary vascular bed undergoes with changes in volume, the interrelationships among resistance, pressures, flow, and blood volume in the vessels of the lungs are far from simple. It is clear that the distensibility of the pulmonary arterial tree is much greater than that of the systemic arteries, and that this partially accounts for its lower resistance to flow. The large pulmonary veins, however, are less compliant than the major systemic venous segments. Also, the compliance of the small pulmonary vessels is not uniform; the capillaries are less distensible than the arteries and veins. In one study of normal subjects during an exercise that evoked an almost two-fold increase in cardiac output, the pulmonary blood volume increased by only 27 per cent, mean pulmonary arterial pressure increased slightly, and pulmonary vascular resistance fell. The pulmonary vasoconstriction produced by hypoxia is associated with a decrease in pulmonary blood volume, despite the increase of pressure in the elastic pulmonary arteries.

The compliance of the pulmonary vessels is finite, and changes in the volume of blood in the lungs do produce changes in vascular pressures. For example, the intense constriction of the systemic vessels that sometimes occurs after injury to the brain (*Cushing reflex*) results in systemic hypertension, displacement of blood from the systemic circuit into the lungs, and marked pulmonary venous and pulmonary arterial hypertension.

Whereas the systemic vessels are closely regulated by the autonomic nervous system and respond to a wide variety of endogenous compounds and drugs, adjustments of the pulmonary vascular bed appear to result almost entirely in response to physical forces. The pulmonary arteries are supplied with autonomic nerves, and there is experimental evidence in animals that the larger pulmonary arteries can be reflexly induced to stiffen, but reflex control of the pulmonary circulation has not been convincingly demonstrated in man. Similarly, many pharmacologic agents considered on the basis of experiments in animals to exert a vasoconstrictor action on the pulmonary arteries (norepinephrine, epinephrine, and serotonin) or a vasodilator effect (bradykinin, isoproterenol, and acetylcholine) have been shown to have either little or no direct action on the normal human pulmonary vascular bed. Because these compounds profoundly affect the systemic circulation and may alter pulmonary mechanics, the changes in pulmonary vascular pressures and resistance that are observed after they are administered are mainly secondary consequences of their actions elsewhere.

HYPOXIA. Ample evidence of several types indicates that hypoxia directly constricts the pulmonary bed and elevates the pulmonary vascular resistance by direct action on the muscular pulmonary arteries, which are separated from the inner surface of the small airways by only 0.1 mm. Extensive investigations in the past have failed to disclose the mechanism of this effect, but some studies have shown that in contrast to its action on systemic arterial smooth muscle, hypoxia may stimulate production of adenosine triphosphate and facilitate membrane depolarization in pulmonary arterial smooth muscle. Evidences that the actions of hypoxia on the pulmonary vessels are mediated by catecholamines, histamine, prostaglandins, angiotensin II, or serotonin generated or released by the lung either are inconclusive or have been convincingly refuted.

The vasoconstrictor response to hypoxia is greatly potentiated by increases in blood hydrogen ion and is almost abolished by alkalosis. The hypoxic reflex serves a useful local regulatory function by limiting blood flow to underventilated pulmonary segments and thereby restores the regional ventilation-perfusion ratio to normal, but when the hypoxia is generalized, the response is far from beneficial. Inhalation of 12 per cent oxygen at sea level (Po_2: 91 mm Hg) promptly results in twofold increases of pulmonary vascular resistance and pulmonary arterial mean pressure, with no increase in cardiac output or left atrial pressure.

PULMONARY ARTERIAL PRESSURE AT HIGH ALTITUDE. Chronic exposure to the hypoxia of high altitude produces a sustained increase in pulmonary arterial pressure. The average values of pulmonary arterial pressure in natives of Morococho, Peru, which is at 14,900 feet above sea level (Po_2: 80 mm Hg), are 41/15 mm Hg (systolic/diastolic), with a mean pressure of 28 mm Hg at rest and 77/40 (mean: 60 mm Hg) during exercise. Their right ventricles are hypertrophied, and their small pulmonary arteries are thicker and contain increased amounts of smooth muscle, which extends farther down into the smallest vessels than normally. After two years of residing at sea level, the pulmonary

arterial pressures of these people fall to normal values at rest but still rise to abnormal values with exercise.

Studies of the pulmonary circulation in residents of Leadville, Colorado (altitude: 10,200 feet; Po_2: 100 mm Hg), have emphasized the considerable individual variation in the reactivity of the pulmonary vasculature to chronic hypoxia. The average mean pulmonary arterial pressure at rest in one group of subjects was increased to 25 mm Hg, but it varied from 10 to 45 mm Hg, and in one 15-year-old woman the pressure rose to 105 mm Hg during exercise. This subject's pressure became normal after she had resided at sea level for 11 months.

The individuality of the response to hypoxia is further emphasized by the occurrence of acute pulmonary edema at high altitudes in susceptible persons who are otherwise normal. The pathogenesis of the pulmonary edema, which responds promptly to inhalation of oxygen, has not been fully elucidated, but it is not due to left ventricular failure, and pulmonary venous constriction has not been proved to be the cause. It occurs at altitudes greater than 9000 feet in persons who have not previously been exposed to altitude as well as in residents at high altitude within 12 to 36 hours after returning from even a brief sojourn at a lower level. Such persons are liable to recurrence of pulmonary edema with each transition from low to high altitude. Studies of susceptible subjects have revealed hyperreactivity of their pulmonary vessels to hypoxia. Their pulmonary hemodynamics and pulmonary function are normal at sea level, but at 10,000 feet after a day of exposure to the altitude and a period of vigorous activity at higher altitude, despite the maintenance of normal pulmonary wedge pressures and no evidence of pulmonary edema, their pulmonary arterial pressures were two to three times greater than those of normal subjects at the same altitude.

In many disease states affecting the pulmonary circulation, including those not producing alveolar hypoxia, individual variations in pulmonary vascular reactivity are common, and the spectrum of physiologic and structural abnormalities of the pulmonary vessels in each condition is usually wide.

358.2. PRIMARY PULMONARY HYPERTENSION

Primary pulmonary hypertension is a disease of unknown cause characterized by marked increase in the pulmonary vascular resistance and pulmonary arterial pressure. Despite exhaustive search while the patient is alive, or at autopsy, no evidence can be found of underlying diseases known to produce pulmonary arterial hypertension, such as congenital or acquired heart disease, pulmonary disease, disorders of respiration, and systemic diseases that affect the pulmonary vessels.

INCIDENCE. Primary pulmonary hypertension is uncommon. In one series of 10,000 patients with heart disease, it was found in only 17. Among reported cases, the patients ranged in age from 1 to 68 years, but most were 20 to 40 years old. There were three times as many women as men; most of the women were in their early thirties and had borne children. The disease is known to occur in a familial form. Among 20 families reported, the ratio of males to females in the 47 members with the disease was approximately 2 to 1. In six families, apparent parent-to-offspring transmission was documented, and in one kindred five members of three generations manifested the disease. The mode of genetic transmission is uncertain. In five families, the mother and either a daughter or a son were affected; in the other family, the father and his son and daughter died of the disease.

PATHOLOGY. In all patients, the pulmonary arteries show structural abnormalities characteristic of hypertensive pulmonary vascular disease usually of the most advanced degree (Grades 4 to 6 of Heath and Edwards). The walls of the muscular arteries and arterioles are greatly thickened, and their lumina are markedly narrowed and even obliterated. The smooth muscle in the media of the muscular arteries is hypertrophied and extends well down into the arterioles, which normally do not have a distinct media. In the arterioles and extending back to the smaller muscular pulmonary arteries less than 0.3 mm and occasionally those as large as 0.5 mm, marked cellular proliferation and fibrosis of the intima are seen. In some of the vessels, the intimal proliferation is concentric, shows an onion-layering appearance, and encroaches evenly on the lumen; in others, the masses of protruding fibrous tissue are unevenly distributed and create an eccentric, irregularly shaped lumen. The fibrous tissue contains elastic fibrils and eventually assumes a hyaline appearance.

Although the media attains a thickness equivalent to 30 per cent of the external diameter of the small arteries in some areas, in other areas the media is atrophied and the vessels dilated. Such generalized dilatations of the arterial wall are often found at and downstream from an occluded segment of a small muscular artery or arteriole and upstream from occlusions in the medium-sized arteries.

In addition to the generalized dilatations, localized dilatations that form morphologically complex, saccular structures develop from the walls of the smallest muscular arteries and arterioles. One of these structures, known as a plexiform lesion, is characterized by a thin-walled sac protruding from the wall of the vessel. The sac frequently contains a thrombus, over which an area of cellular intimal tissue has proliferated to form a complex, plexiform pattern. An overlying layer of fibrous tissue is continuous with the intimal proliferative layer of the artery. In other dilatation lesions, groups of thin-walled, cavernous vessels arise from thin-walled branches of muscular arteries, or occluded arteries give rise to veinlike branches that have been misinterpreted as arteriovenous anastomoses. Because of their thin walls, the vessels of dilatation lesions are subject to rupture and are associated with focal collections of hemosiderin-laden macrophages in the pulmonary tissue.

In the most advanced stage of hypertensive pulmonary vascular disease (Grade 6), fibrinoid necrosis occurs in the media of some of the muscular arteries. The necrotic muscle produces an inflammatory reaction consisting of polymorphonuclear leukocytes and some eosinophils that may invade all layers of the vessel. The necrotizing arteritis may destroy the entire vessel or only a segment of it, and thrombi are found in the lumina of some of the affected arteries.

The elastic pulmonary arteries, especially the main trunk and its branches, are greatly dilated, but the walls are thick. The media shows an increase in muscle mass that in the main pulmonary artery causes the thickness of the media to approximate or exceed that of the aortic media. The elastic fibers in the media are fragmented, irregularly shaped, and arranged in a loose network characteristic of the adult pulmonary artery. This configuration of the elastic tissue is evidence that the pulmonary hypertension was acquired rather than present at birth, because in patients with congenital heart diseases that produce pulmonary arterial hypertension from birth, the elastic fibers of the main pulmonary artery retain their fetal form and appear like those in the aorta. In a few reported cases of primary pulmonary hypertension, an orderly array of elastic fibers in the media signified that the hypertension existed in the neonatal period. In all cases, the media contains an excess of acid mucopolysaccharides that can accumulate in cystic fashion. A few atheromas are often found in the intima of the main pulmonary arteries; in occasional patients, they are numerous and scattered throughout the intima of all the elastic arteries.

The capillaries, veins, and parenchyma of the lungs are normal.

The right ventricle is extensively hypertrophied and dilated, and the ring of the tricuspid valve is often dilated. The right atrium is also dilated, and in a few patients, the foramen ovale is patent. The systemic arteries are usually free of significant abnormalities, although James has reported the occurrence of fibrous lesions in the intima of the small arteries of the sinus node in patients with primary pulmonary hypertension.

ETIOLOGY AND PATHOGENESIS. None of the several theories proposed for the pathogenesis of primary pulmonary hypertension has been verified. Amniotic fluid embolization of the pulmonary arteries has been suggested as a cause because of the preponderance of young women among patients with the disease, some of whom experienced their first symptoms after pregnancy. Congenital defects in the pulmonary arteries, such as medial aplasia or failure of the pulmonary arteries to undergo normal transformation from their fetal form, have been suggested; however, with only a few exceptions, the appearance of the elastic fibers in the media of the main pulmonary artery of patients with primary pulmonary hypertension indicates that the hypertension was not present from birth, as would be expected if the pulmonary arteries maintained their thick-walled, fetal form. The theory of medial aplasia holds that the areas of dilatation and thinning of the media observed in the muscular arteries represent congenital defects of the media and that the intima over these areas is subject to the development of intimal proliferation that then acts as the primary obstructive lesion. This explanation neglects the fact that all patients with primary pulmonary hypertension do not manifest dilatation lesions or defects of the media other than hypertrophy.

The occurrence of Raynaud's disease in some patients with primary pulmonary hypertension has prompted the speculation that the hypertension is due to vasospasm or to involvement of the pulmonary arteries by a systemic disease of a collagen, autoimmune, or allergic variety. Pulmonary vascular lesions and marked pulmonary hypertension are the predominant abnormalities in rare patients with lupus erythematosus, scleroderma, or sarcoidosis, but other stigmata of these diseases are evident during life or at autopsy. Neurogenically or humorally induced spasm of the pulmonary arteries is an attractive possibility, especially because these vessels in a few patients manifest medial hypertrophy with only slight abnormalities of the intima, but the hypothesis lacks support. Alveolar hypoxia, a potent pulmonary vasoconstrictor, is not present in these patients, and there is no history of residence at altitude, although an occasional patient may first experience symptoms during an excursion to a region several thousand feet above sea level.

The possibility that primary pulmonary hypertension is the consequence of multiple pulmonary emboli is most difficult to deny. Recurrent, small emboli to the lungs are often "silent" and can eventually produce marked increase in pulmonary arterial pressure and a clinical and physiologic syndrome identical to that of primary pulmonary hypertension. It is often difficult to distinguish between the two conditions by examination of the vasculature of the lungs, because the small pulmonary arteries in widespread pulmonary embolization often exhibit the medial hypertrophy and intimal proliferation of hypertensive pulmonary vascular disease, and recanalized, fibrotic emboli in the small arteries can resemble occlusive intimal lesions. Differentiation of the two conditions depends on identification in the embolic disease of intraluminal thrombi, recent or old, throughout the pulmonary arteries, especially in the larger elastic arteries, and absence of plexiform and dilatation lesions and necrotizing arteritis, which do not occur in the embolic disorder.

The practical difficulty in discriminating between pulmonary hypertension of the primary type and that caused by recurrent pulmonary embolization can be illustrated by the author's experience with 14 patients who after extensive study were considered to have primary pulmonary hypertension. Nine of these came to autopsy, and no cause for the hypertension other than the pulmonary vascular lesions of primary pulmonary hypertension was found in five. All five were women 32 to 33 years of age, except for one who was 44. In the other four patients, multiple thromboemboli were present in the pulmonary arteries. Two of these were men age 37 and 60 years, and two were women, 48 and 53 years of age. This and other reported experiences suggest the likelihood of an embolic cause of unexplained pulmonary hypertension in patients older than 40 years, especially if they are men. These data were collected before the widespread use of oral contraceptives, and it is conceivable that the proportion of young women with thromboembolism among patients with cryptic pulmonary hypertension may be modified in the future. Predisposition to pulmonary thromboembolism in one reported family with pulmonary hypertension was suggested by elevated plasma and serum antiplasmin activity in seven of its members.

An apparent increase in the frequency of pulmonary hypertension followed the introduction in a few countries of aminorex (2-amino-5-phenyl-2-oxazoline), an appetite depressant with pharmacologic actions similar to those of amphetamine. Although many of the patients had taken the drug, its role in the production of the "epidemic" of pulmonary hypertension was not established, and even after prolonged administration of large doses the compound does not cause pulmonary hypertension or pulmonary vascular lesions in laboratory animals. An association, probably also coincidental, of pulmonary hypertension with use of phentormin has been reported.

Whatever the cause, it appears that once pulmonary hypertension is established, the media of the pulmonary arteries reacts by progressive hypertrophy of its smooth muscle mass, probably as a consequence of increased arterial wall tension and work. The intima subsequently responds to the elevated pressure by proliferation, perhaps as the arterioles do in systemic hypertension. Thus each structural response of the pulmonary arterial tree leads to further compromise of its patency, further elevation of pressure, and the eventual development of the highest grades of hypertensive pulmonary vascular disease.

PATHOLOGIC PHYSIOLOGY. The cardinal hemodynamic abnormality is marked increase in the pulmonary vascular resistance with no evident physiologic cause. The resistance is usually 12 to 18 times normal and in the range of the systemic vascular resistance, and in an occasional patient it exceeds the systemic resistance. In one series, the average pulmonary arterial systolic pressure was approximately 110 mm Hg and the mean pressure approximately six times normal. During exercise the pulmonary vascular resistance remains fixed, and the pulmonary arterial pressures rise further. At rest and during exercise, the pulmonary wedge and left atrial pressures are normal. In contrast, the right ventricular end-diastolic and right atrial pressures are usually greatly increased. In some patients, the cardiac output is normal at rest, but more often it is only 50 to 60 per cent of normal and fails to increase appropriately with exercise. As the function of the right ventricle declines under its enormous afterload, cardiac output dwindles further, and evidences of tricuspid regurgitation may appear. Because of the small stroke volume, systemic arterial systolic and pulse pressures are frequently low.

The arterial oxyhemoglobin saturation is usually normal at rest and during exercise, but a few patients display mildly (91 to 92 per cent) and rarely substantially diminished (less than 90 per cent) saturation. Slight reduction in arterial carbon dioxide tension reflects the hyperventilation that commonly exists.

Infusion of tolazoline or acetylcholine into the pulmonary artery has been observed to produce slight to moderate decrease of pulmonary vascular resistance and pulmonary arterial pressure in some patients. Inhalation of oxygen has little effect.

CLINICAL MANIFESTATIONS. These are the direct result of the physiologic and anatomic disturbances produced by the disease. Dyspnea during exertion, closely intertwined with fatigue and weakness, is a universal symptom. An oppressive substernal sensation and even frank angina are commonly experienced during effort, although this symptom, which is most likely the result of right ventricular ischemia, can occur in some patients in the form of recurrent and exceedingly disturbing episodes at rest. Syncope on exertion is an ominous sign because patients with primary pulmonary hypertension are subject to sudden death. There is evidence that an abrupt fall in cardiac output secondary to acute right ventricular failure or arrhythmia is the essential mechanism producing the syncopal attacks. Rupture of the flimsy walls of localized arterial dilatation lesions probably accounts for the intermittent minor hemoptyses experienced by some patients. An occasional patient may experience hoarseness related to compression of the left recurrent laryngeal nerve by the enlarged left pulmonary artery.

Overt signs of right ventricular failure develop in many patients before death and initially respond to digitalis and diuretics, but within a short period of time become increasingly more difficult to control. Because of the marked and fixed obstruction to flow in the pulmonary vessels and severe impairment of right ventricular function, the cardiac output is not only low but does not increase on demand to meet peripheral needs. Consequently, systemic arterial pressure can fall precipitously and fatally during anesthesia; after vaso-depressor drugs, such as barbiturates; with physiologic stresses, such as fever and hemorrhage; and during diagnostic procedures, such as cardiac catheterization and angiocardiography. Because of the enormous obstruction to blood flow in the lungs, resuscitation from cardiopulmonary arrest is usually unsuccessful.

The patient usually appears normally developed and in good nutritional state. Occasionally the nail beds are slightly cyanotic, but the peripheral origin of the cyanosis is demonstrated by its disappearance after rubbing the digits. Clubbing is absent. Its presence should promptly suggest other causes of the pulmonary hypertension. Depending on the state of right ventricular function, the jugular veins may be distended; almost invariably, they show a prominent and sustained atrial contraction wave ("a" wave). If right ventricular failure and dilatation are advanced, the systolic wave of tricuspid regurgitation can also appear. The carotid arterial pulse is usually small.

The heart may be of normal size or considerably enlarged to the left and right. In contrast to the localized and unimpressive apical impulse, the heave associated with vigorous contraction of the hypertrophied right ventricle can be seen and felt along the left sternal border. Especially in patients with thin-walled and long chests, the prominent systolic pulsation of the enlarged main pulmonary can be seen and palpated for several centimeters to the left of the sternal border in the second left intercostal space. In almost every patient, a loud, sharp, pulmonic ejection sound can be heard and often felt. The second sound is usually closely split (0.02 to 0.03 sec), but in some patients the splitting may be wider (0.04 to 0.05 sec) and may vary relatively little during the respiratory cycle. The sound of pulmonic valvular closure is invariably accentuated in intensity, sharp or ringing in quality, and often palpable. Murmurs may be absent, but in many patients a systolic ejection murmur that is rarely harsh is heard in the third left interspace and extends well up along the left sternal border over the pulmonary artery. The diminuendo, medium-high-pitched murmur of pulmonic valvular regurgitation is audible in the third and fourth left interspaces in patients whose main pulmonary artery is very large, and is most easily detected with the patient erect and his chest held in full expiration. Either an atrial gallop sound (fourth sound) or an early diastolic gallop sound (third sound) or both are often heard over the lower right ventricle; increase in their intensity with inspiration signifies that they are generated in the right heart. When both gallop sounds are present, they can create the auditory illusion of a mitral diastolic rumble, an illusion that is enhanced by the early ejection sound, which may be misidentified as the loud closure sound of a stenotic mitral valve. A systolic murmur of tricuspid regurgitation that increases with inspiration may be heard in the fourth and fifth intercostal spaces along the left sternal border; it occasionally radiates well toward the apex if the tricuspid valve has been displaced to the left by a very enlarged right atrium and right ventricle. The usual signs of right ventricular failure and systemic venous congestion may be present.

Early in the course of the disease, the only abnormality in radiograms of the chest is enlargement of the main pulmonary artery and its major branches. Hypertrophy of the right ventricle is first manifested by its encroachment on the retrosternal space in lateral films and by a globular appearance of the heart in the posteroanterior projection. The heart is seldom massively enlarged, but the right ventricle may be sufficiently hypertrophied and dilated to displace the heart posteriorly, thereby creating some difficulty in assessing the size of the left ventricle. The right atrium usually appears rounded in frontal view, and eventually it and the superior vena cava dilate well into the right chest. The lung fields appear normal or slightly avascular, and the normal size of the small pulmonary arteries contrasts sharply with the dilated central arteries, which can attain considerable size. The pulmonary veins and left atrium are normal in size.

The electrocardiogram invariably reveals evidences of right ventricular hypertrophy, usually of the type associated with a systemic arterial systolic pressure in the ventricle. The mean QRS axis is at 90 degrees or more to the right. Lead V_1 shows an R wave of 1.0 to 1.5 mV with a small S wave, and the T waves in leads V_1 and V_2 are inverted. The P waves are tall (greater than 0.25 mV) and peaked in leads II, III, and aV_f; in V_1 the P wave is upright, peaked, narrow, and associated with a long PR segment. Higher grades of right ventricular hypertrophy are reflected by increasing amplitude of the R wave in V_1 and V_2, prominent S waves in the left precordial leads, and depression of the S-T segment and increasingly negative and coved T waves in V_1 and V_2 and even V_3.

Polycythemia occurs in some patients late in the course of the disease despite a normal or only slightly decreased arterial oxyhemoglobin saturation.

DIAGNOSIS. Although the diagnosis of primary pulmonary hypertension can be made on the basis of the clinical, radiographic, and electrocardiographic manifestations, it is very difficult in some patients to be certain on these grounds alone that an underlying lesion of the heart, such as septal defect, cor triatriatum, or silent mitral stenosis, does not exist. It is especially difficult to exclude multiple pulmonary emboli or a systemic disease as the fundamental disorder.

In the rare patient with marked pulmonary arterial hypertension and auscultatorily silent mitral stenosis, enlargement of the left atrium and calcification of the mitral valve may be the only clinical clues to the presence of the valvular lesion and should be assiduously sought by radiographic and electrocardiographic means. Echocardiography is exceptionally effective in identifying stenosis and other abnormalities of the mitral valve (see Ch. 360.2 to 360.4) and in measuring the dimensions of the left atrium and ventricle. Since it can also detect a left atrial myxoma, cor triatriatum, and septal defects, all patients suspected of having primary pulmonary hypertension should be carefully studied by this noninvasive method before submitting them to cardiac catheterization.

Cardiac catheterization should be performed to establish the diagnosis, to assess the severity of the hemodynamic derangements, and to demonstrate conclusively that the pulmonary arterial hypertension is not secondary to a congenital defect, mitral stenosis, or other lesion that produces left atrial or pulmonary venous hypertension. In pulmonary angiograms, filling defects or occlusions of the larger elastic pulmonary arteries are certain signs of pulmonary thromboemboli that are not found in primary pulmonary hypertension. Large areas lacking radioactivity in the lung fields in radioisotopic perfusion scans of the lungs constitute further evidence of the presence of embolic obstruction of large pulmonary arteries.

Because death of patients with primary pulmonary hypertension has been reported to occur during or immediately after cardiac catheterization and angiocardiography, considerable judgment and care must be exercised in performing these studies and determining how extensive they should be. The general state of the patient, the blood pressure, and the electrocardiogram should be meticulously monitored throughout the procedure and for some time afterward. Arrhythmias and frequent ectopic beats should be promptly suppressed; significant falls in blood pressure should be immediately corrected with an infusion of norepinephrine to maintain perfusion of the right ventricular myocardium. Many patients with primary pulmonary hypertension have undergone these essential diagnostic studies without complication.

The appropriate laboratory tests, including skin biopsy to exclude scleroderma and lupus erythematosus, should be performed in all patients with primary pulmonary hypertension, especially those who manifest Raynaud's phenomenon. Sarcoidosis involving the pulmonary arteries almost exclusively and producing pulmonary hypertension is exceedingly rare and has only recently been reported. The author has also observed one such case in which the cause was uncovered only at autopsy. The possibility of reversing the pulmonary hypertension by the administration of corticosteroids should prompt a search for signs of this disease.

Lung biopsy should not be performed because of the great risk and because the vessels in the tissue obtained may not manifest representative lesions of the pulmonary hypertensive vascular disease, which typically vary widely in type and severity throughout the lungs. A small pneumothorax in a patient with primary pulmonary hypertension was reported to precipitate an alarming increase in pulmonary arterial pressure and death.

Pulmonary function studies in patients with primary pulmonary hypertension usually reveal no major abnormalities aside from slight arterial hypoxemia and hyperventilation. If the patient does not have a right-left shunt through a patent foramen ovale, substantial hypoxemia at rest or during exercise owing to intrapulmonary arteriovenous shunting greatly increases the probability that thromboemboli are the cause of the pulmonary hypertension.

TREATMENT. No effective method for producing a sustained decrease in the pulmonary arterial pressure has been found. Chronic treatment with tolazoline or prolonged infusions of this drug or acetylcholine into the pulmonary artery have proved to be ineffective. Nor is there evidence that long-term administration of oxygen decreases the pulmonary arterial pressure or in any way modifies the course of the disease. Transplantation of a single lung is an appealing therapeutic maneuver but is impractical because of the currently short viability of pulmonary homotransplants. Because of the difficulty in excluding recurrent pulmonary emboli and because in situ thrombosis can occur in pulmonary arteries affected by hypertensive pulmonary vascular disease, chronic anticoagulation therapy has been widely advocated. Such therapy should be closely monitored in view of the deleterious consequences of hemorrhage in these patients. The usual cardiac glycosides, diuretic agents, and restriction of sodium intake should be used to control cardiac failure. The patient should not travel to altitudes above sea level.

PROGNOSIS. The patient usually dies during a syncopal spell, or after an acute, short-lived, shock-like episode, or of intractable right heart failure within three to four years after the onset of symptoms. Rarely, dissection of the main pulmonary artery is the lethal event. An occasional patient may survive for 12 or more years, but with progressively disabling dyspnea, angina, and syncope with exertion.

358.3.   OTHER CAUSES OF PULMONARY VASCULAR DISEASE

CONGENITAL HEART DISEASE

These remarks are intended to supplement the discussion of congenital heart disease in Ch. 359.

Pulmonary arterial hypertension is exceedingly common in patients with congenital defects that produce left-right shunting of blood within the heart or between the great vessels. The hypertension is usually the result of augmentation of pulmonary blood flow by the left-right shunt, structural abnormalities within the pulmonary arterial tree, or most commonly both. There are distinct differences in the frequency and severity of the pulmonary vascular abnormalities associated with these congenital lesions.

In patients with left-right shunts that traverse the left ventricle, such as those produced by ventricular septal defect, patent ductus arteriosus, aortic septal defect, and ostium atrioventricularis with a large ventricular septal defect, hypertensive pulmonary vascular disease is very frequent. The severity of the arterial lesions varies among patients, depending on the size of the defect, the magnitude of the left-right shunt it is capable of conducting, and individual susceptibility. If the communication is small and produces a pulmonary blood flow that exceeds systemic blood by 50 per cent or less, the pulmonary arteries are usually normal or show minimal changes and the pulmonary vascular resistance and pulmonary arterial pressure are also normal or only slightly elevated.

With larger defects, hypertensive pulmonary vascular disease of the type described in Ch. 358.2 is almost universally present. Most commonly, the small pulmonary arteries and arterioles simply manifest thickening of their walls owing to hypertrophy of the smooth muscle of the media (Grade 1 hypertensive pulmonary vascular disease, according to the classification of Heath and Edwards), but other obstructive lesions may be superimposed on this basic abnormality to produce increasingly advanced vascular disease. An early additional change is cellular proliferation of the intima of the arteries (Grade 2), which may subsequently undergo fibrosis and fibroelastic organization (Grade 3). The development of generalized and focal dilatations of the arterial wall with the formation of complex vascular structures occurs in Grade 4 disease, and in Grade 5 the dilatations are scattered throughout the lung and associated with hemosiderosis. Necrotizing arteritis occurs in the most severe form of the disease (Grade 6).

The development of the vascular disease is initiated shortly after birth by failure of the pulmonary arteries to undergo normal transformation from their fetal form. Instead of regressing, the increased mass of smooth muscle in the arterial walls persists, hypertrophies, and extends distally into the arterioles. The elastic fibers in the media of the main pulmonary artery and its major branches also fail to develop their adult form. They persist as dense, thick structures in parallel array, closely resembling their appearance in the media of the aorta. This important histologic sign indicates that the pulmonary vascular disease began in the neonatal period; it is not found in patients who acquired their pulmonary hypertension later in life.

The size of the communication determines the subsequent development of arterial lesions. Ventricular septal defects larger than 1 sq cm and patent ducti that approximate 1 cm in diameter are usually associated with more advanced grades of pulmonary vascular disease. Progression of the vascular lesions appears to occur early in life, but the most advanced abnormalities are found in patients older than 15 to 20 years. The pulmonary vascular resistance, however, in patients with only moderate pulmonary arterial hypertension (systolic pressure of 50 to 60 mm Hg) does not appear to increase significantly during the course of many years.

Why pulmonary vascular lesions develop in patients with post-tricuspid valvular shunts is uncertain. One possible factor is that these shunts early in life load the left ventricle and consequently produce higher left ventricular diastolic, left atrial, and pulmonary venous pressures than would normally exist, thus from the outset exhausting the distensibility of the pulmonary arteries and subjecting them thereby to higher pressures. Another theory holds that the transmission directly into the pulmonary arteries of part of the kinetic energy that is generated in the left venticle is the responsible factor.

The height of the pulmonary arterial pressure in patients with ventricular septal defect or patent ductus arteriosus is determined by the pulmonary vascular resistance, the size of the left-right shunt, and consequently the magnitude of the pulmonary blood flow. If the resistance is only slightly increased, large shunts and pulmonary flows as large as twice the systemic blood flow can occur with pulmonary arterial mean pressures three times normal and systolic pressures of 60 to 70 mm Hg. With increasing resistance, the pulmonary arterial pressures rise and the left-right shunt diminishes. Evidence of right-left shunting at first appears only during exercise when pulmonary arterial and right ventricular

pressures increase further or under circumstances when the systemic vascular resistance falls. Eventually, the pulmonary arterial systolic pressure attains systemic arterial levels at rest and the right-left shunt becomes larger and more sustained. Despite persistence of bidirectional shunting, the pulmonary blood flow declines to values usually less than normal. As a consequence of the right-left shunt and the diminished pulmonary blood flow, chronic arterial hypoxemia that is accentuated by exertion appears. In patients with patent ductus arteriosus, because the right-left shunt is directed into the descending segment of the aortic arch, the arterial unsaturation is more pronounced or even confined to the lower body and, occasionally, may also appear in the left arm and left side of the head. It is possible that the polycythemia and consequent increase in blood viscosity contribute to the resistance to flow in the pulmonary vessels.

Aside from cyanosis, which is usually accompanied by clubbing of the fingers and toes, the clinical signs and symptoms of patients with marked pulmonary hypertension and right-left shunts are similar to those of patients with primary pulmonary hypertension, but the course is usually considerably longer, and survival to an age of 30 to 40 years occurs frequently. The cyanosis is especially striking when polycythemia is marked. In patent ductus arteriosus with bidirectional shunting, the toes are cyanotic and clubbed, whereas the fingers are not or are much less so. Some signs of the underlying cardiac lesion are often evident. A precordial bulge is usually present. In some patients, the characteristic murmurs are intermittently audible, but in most, the murmurs are greatly modified. A pulmonic ejection sound is almost always present; the sound of pulmonic valvular closure is loud and sharp in quality, and a diastolic murmur of pulmonic regurgitation is frequent. Persistent enlargement of the left ventricle may be manifested by a forceful, diffuse apical thrust. Suggestive evidences of left ventricular enlargement may also be present in radiograms of the heart and in the electrocardiogram, but these and the radiographic signs of increased pulmonary blood flow tend to disappear as the pulmonary vascular disease advances.

In patients with a left-right shunt that does not traverse the left ventricle, structural abnormalities in the pulmonary arteries are slight, and the pulmonary arterial pressure remains normal or only slightly increased until late in the course of the disease. An atrial septal defect of the secundum type is the most common lesion producing such a shunt; other causes are partial or complete anomalous drainage of the pulmonary veins into the right atrium or its main venous trunks. Only in occasional patients with enormous shunts, caused by complete anomalous pulmonary venous drainage or an atrial septal defect of such size that the atria are converted into a common chamber, are pulmonary vascular disease and significant pulmonary hypertension established early in life. In most patients, despite pulmonary blood flows consistently 2.5 to 3 times greater than normal, the pulmonary arterial pressure remains at the upper limits of normal for 20 to 30 years and even longer. Thereafter, however, pulmonary vascular lesions begin to appear and the pulmonary arterial pressure rises. The earliest structural abnormality is fibrosis of the pulmonary veins followed by cellular proliferation of the endothelium of the widely dilated arterioles and small muscular arteries. At this stage, the pulmonary vascular resistance may no longer be less than normal as it must be to maintain a normal pulmonary arterial pressure in the presence of the large blood flow. The resistance is also fixed, and even though its value is within the limits of normal, the persistently augmented flow produces a proportionate increase in pulmonary arterial pressure.

The pulmonary venous pressure remains normal in atrial septal defect until the onset of myocardial failure, manifested by elevation of the diastolic pressures of both ventricles. As a consequence of the increased left ventricular diastolic pressure, the pressures in the left atrium and pulmonary veins rise to three to four times their usual values. A substantial left-right shunt nevertheless persists, and pulmonary arterial systolic pressure commonly attains values of 60 to 70 mm Hg.

Episodes of pulmonary embolization, which are common in patients with atrial septal defect, and progression of the hypertensive pulmonary arterial lesions eventually produce seven-fold or greater increases of pulmonary vascular resistance that throttle the pulmonary flow and promote right-left shunting through the defect.

The classic clinical, radiographic, and electrocardiographic features of atrial septal defect (see Ch. 359.2) usually persist throughout the patient's course, and provide for ready recognition of the lesion. The diagnosis is less evident in the occasional patient who has developed high-grade pulmonary vascular disease and pulmonary hypertension early in life and shows little evidence of increased pulmonary blood flow and a hypertrophied but not very large right ventricle.

TREATMENT.   The response of the pulmonary arterial pressure to closure of a septal defect or patent ductus arteriosus is governed by the relative roles of the left-right shunt and the pulmonary vascular resistance in elevating the pressure. If the pulmonary vascular resistance is normal preoperatively, the pulmonary arterial pressure declines to normal values postoperatively. When the shunt constitutes 50 per cent or more of the pulmonary blood flow and the resistance is only moderately increased, a substantial decrease can be expected. When the left-right shunt is small and the pulmonary vascular resistance and pressures approximate those in the systemic circuit, and especially if a significant right-left shunt exists, the pressure does not decrease and the risk of death during or shortly after the surgical procedure is great. Decision as to advisability of surgical correction of the lesion should be made on an individual basis after consideration of all physiologic and clinical data. Some have advocated preoperative measurements of the response of the pulmonary arterial pressure and pulmonary vascular resistance to infusion of tolazoline or inhalation of oxygen as a means of identifying a vasospastic component of an increased resistance.

Except in occasional infants with lower grades of hypertensive pulmonary vascular disease, the pulmonary vascular resistance does not usually fall after closure of an atrial or ventricular septal defect, and although the patient may be greatly benefited by the procedure, some degree of pulmonary hypertension persists.

STENOSIS OF PULMONARY ARTERIAL BRANCHES.   Although multiple coarctation-like, congenital stenoses of the large branches of the pulmonary artery produce an increase in pressure only in the pulmonary arterial segments upstream from the stenotic regions, the malformation in some patients raises the systolic pressure in the

main pulmonary artery and right ventricle to 70 to 80 mm Hg and can create difficulty in diagnosis. The lesions can occur in isolated form, but they often coexist with supravalvular aortic stenosis or an atrial septal defect. The total obstructive effect is usually slight, and the systolic pulmonary arterial pressure is increased to only 35 to 40 mm Hg at rest. The stenoses generate a continuous murmur or simply a systolic murmur that can be heard over the upper right or left precordial region. The diagnosis is conclusively established by an angiogram of the pulmonary arteries. An acquired form of pulmonary arterial branch stenosis can be produced by mediastinal fibrosis.

PULMONARY EMBOLI

Thrombi, globules of fat, and particulate matter of amniotic fluid can embolize the pulmonary arteries and produce acute pulmonary hypertension. The pathophysiologic basis for the hypertension is described in Ch. 357. Repeated embolization of the pulmonary arteries by thrombi (see Ch. 357 and 358.2), schistosomal ova (see Ch. 210), tumors, and cotton fibers and foreign matter contained in some drugs illicitly administered by vein cause chronic, progressive pulmonary hypertension by their primary obstructive effects and by the subsequent development of hypertensive pulmonary vascular lesions. In addition, schistosomal ova and particulate foreign matter evoke a granulomatous inflammatory reaction in the intima and walls of the arteries.

Although fragments of several types of cancer can embolize the pulmonary arteries after the tumor has invaded the liver or the inferior vena cava, the propensity of choriocarcinoma (chorioepithelioma) to metastasize in this manner deserves special consideration. Choriocarcinoma may remain undetected for several years after pregnancy, but soon after it originates it can invade the inferior vena cava and repeatedly discharge fragments of tissue into the pulmonary circulation. These embolic episodes may give rise to symptoms and signs of acute pulmonary embolization, or they can be clinically silent. The consequent obstruction of the larger pulmonary arteries can be extensive and give rise to marked pulmonary hypertension before the tumor invades the walls of the pulmonary arteries and appears in the lung fields.

Choriocarcinoma should be suspected in a woman who has had a recent pregnancy or even one a few years previously and has repeated bouts of pulmonary embolization or unexplained pulmonary hypertension. An increased concentration of human chorionic gonadotropin in the urine and the demonstration of multiple occlusions of the pulmonary arteries by angiography confirm the diagnosis. The tumor is exquisitely sensitive to methotrexate, actinomycin D, and 6-mercaptopurine, and complete cure has been achieved in 50 per cent or more of patients by administration of these agents.

COLLAGEN AND MULTIPLE SYSTEM DISEASES

Pulmonary hypertension caused by the pulmonary arterial lesions of scleroderma, lupus erythematosus, and sarcoidosis has been discussed in Ch. 358.2. The clinical features and diagnosis of these diseases are presented in Ch. 50, 52, and 65, respectively. It is worth emphasizing that the pulmonary hypertension and its secondary effects may rarely be the only clinically apparent manifestations of these disorders. Hemodynamic studies of patients with scleroderma have demonstrated the high frequency of increases in pulmonary vascular resistance and slight pulmonary hypertension without involvement of the pulmonary parenchyma by the disease.

HEPATIC CIRRHOSIS AND PORTAL HYPERTENSION: THE PORTOPULMONARY HYPERTENSION SYNDROME

The development of marked pulmonary hypertension has been observed in a number of patients with portal hypertension secondary to longstanding hepatic cirrhosis or obstruction of the portal vein by a congenital malformation or thrombus. Collateral vessels joining the portal and systemic veins were present in all patients and were often extensive. In some patients, the manifestations of pulmonary hypertension appeared only after a portacaval or equivalent shunt had been surgically created to alleviate bleeding from esophageal varices.

Except for the presence of portal hypertension in all the patients and hepatic cirrhosis in most of them, the clinical features, course, and hemodynamic disturbances were identical with those of primary pulmonary hypertension and are readily distinguishable from those of the high cardiac output state, which is a far more common circulatory complication of alcoholic or postnecrotic cirrhosis. The hyperkinetic state affects both cardiac ventricles and can produce mild to moderate pulmonary arterial hypertension when the pulmonary venous pressure rises as the result of faltering left ventricular function. In the portopulmonary hypertension syndrome, the pulmonary arterial pressure and vascular resistance are usually strikingly elevated, the right ventricle reacts to this burden and often fails, pulmonary venous pressure is normal, and left ventricular function appears unimpaired.

Morphologic studies of the pulmonary vessels at autopsy of patients with the syndrome have revealed the typical lesions of advanced pulmonary hypertensive disease, including plexiform lesions in all and necrotizing arteritis in a few. In almost 75 per cent of the cases, thromboemboli in various stages of organization were widespread throughout the muscular pulmonary arteries. The portal veins of a few patients contained large thrombi, and clots were also present in the eosphageal and gastric varices of one patient.

Naeye attributed the pulmonary vascular disease to the effects of multiple small pulmonary emboli that originated in the portal venous bed and entered the right heart via the copious portal systemic venous collateral vessels, thereby escaping entrapment in the liver. He was the first to propose that thrombogenic materials which are released into or generated in the portal venous blood and normally inactivated in the liver could in similar fashion gain access to the pulmonary circulation and incite the formation of thrombi therein. Others have proposed that vasoconstrictive or vasculotoxic substances which arise from the gut and normally undergo hepatic transformation to inactive compounds might serve as the pathogenetic agents. In searching for models of the syndrome, attention has been focused on the capacity of *Crotalaria spectabilis* (a leguminous annual plant used as a cover-crop) and monocrotaline, a complex alkaloid contained by the plant, to produce hepatic damage, pulmonary vascular disease, and marked pulmonary hypertension in animals. In man, however, ingestion of the plant leads to liver injury without evidences of pulmonary hypertension.

In reconstructing the pathogenesis of the hypertensive pulmonary vascular disease, it is difficult to exclude a primary role for pre-existing hyperkinemia. In 50 per cent of patients with portal cirrhosis, the cardiac output at rest is increased and is generally higher in those with a surgically created portacaval shunt. Outputs that are twice and even three times normal have been measured, and augmentation of output during exercise is greater than normal. Such marked increases in pulmonary blood flow, especially when they are of long standing, may in some patients promote the development of structural abnormalities in the pulmonary arteries as they do in patients with intracardiac left-right shunts. The few available hemodynamic studies of the syndrome have shown that the cardiac output is usually low to normal, but in occasional patients the output exceeded normal values, thereby enhancing the severity of the pulmonary hypertension.

The frequency of the portopulmonary hypertension syndrome is unknown, but it appears to be rare. Nevertheless, patients with portal hypertension and naturally occurring or surgically produced portacaval anastomoses should be periodically and carefully monitored for signs of pulmonary hypertension. Treatment for the condition is like that for primary pulmonary hypertension. It is difficult to advance a blanket recommendation concerning anticoagulant therapy in the syndrome because of the enormous risks of such therapy in these patients.

358.4. LEFT ATRIAL AND PULMONARY VENOUS HYPERTENSION

Elevation of pulmonary venous pressure is the most common cause of pulmonary arterial hypertension. Most frequently, left atrial and pulmonary venous hypertension are the result of dysfunction of the left ventricle characterized by impairment of its contractile state, decrease in its compliance, or both. Even in the absence of clinical signs of left ventricular failure, left ventricular end-diastolic pressure can be elevated, at first only with physical exertion or stress; later, as ventricular function becomes more impaired, it is chronically increased even at rest. Two-fold increases in left atrial, pulmonary venous, and pulmonary arterial pressures are common. During episodes of acute left ventricular failure, pressures in the pulmonary veins and capillaries rise to levels exceeding 25 mm Hg.

The state of left atrial function is a significant determinant of the degree of left atrial and pulmonary venous hypertension. A properly timed, vigorous atrial contraction will generate a considerably increased left ventricular end-diastolic pressure without the need for much increase in left atrial pressure during the rest of diastole, but when the pumping function of the left atrium is lost because of atrial arrhythmia or left atrial failure, its pressure throughout diastole becomes greater. Thus for a given level of ventricular end-diastolic pressure, mean pressures in the atrium and the entire pulmonary vascular circuit are higher in the presence of left atrial failure or arrhythmia, such as atrial fibrillation, than in the presence of normal atrial function.

Disorders of the mitral valvular apparatus are another frequent cause of left atrial hypertension. In general, stenosis of the mitral valve and stenosis combined with regurgitation produce more severe degrees of left atrial hypertension than does mitral regurgitation alone. Nevertheless, in certain patients with chronic, marked mitral regurgitation caused by rheumatic valvular disease or rupture of the chordae tendineae, high-grade hypertension can occur in the left atrium, pulmonary veins, and pulmonary artery.

Less common causes of obstruction at the mitral valve are left atrial myxoma and left atrial ball-valve thrombus. A ball-valve thrombus almost invariably occurs with preexisting mitral stenosis. A myxoma which is tethered by a stalk attached to the atrial septum in the region of the fossa ovalis, produces left atrial hypertension by obstructing blood flow through the mitral orifice in diastole, but it can also pass through the mitral valve and obstruct left ventricular outflow. Other tumors of the left atrium can obstruct the mitral valve and may also grow into and obstruct the main pulmonary veins.

Cor triatriatum, a congenital anomaly in which an abnormal diaphragm with one or more small perforations partitions the pulmonary venous outflow region from the main left atrial chamber, mimics mitral stenosis in its effects on the pulmonary circulation. However, it is often not associated with a diastolic murmur and can thus escape clinical detection. Although cor triatriatum and left atrial myxoma are rare, their recognition is of great importance because they can be completely corrected by appropriate surgical procedures.

Mediastinal collagenosis with constriction of the extra-pulmonary veins and diffuse pulmonary veno-occlusive disease are rare causes of pulmonary venous hypertension. The etiology of the latter disease, which occurs predominantly in women, is unknown. The small and medium-sized pulmonary veins are narrowed and occluded by thrombi and fibrous tissue without evidence of inflammation in the venous walls. The clinical picture resembles that of primary pulmonary arterial hypertension; however, because of increased pressure in the pulmonary capillaries, radiographic evidence of pulmonary congestion and edema is present. The disease leads relentlessly to death in a few weeks to five years after the onset of symptoms.

PULMONARY CIRCULATION IN MITRAL STENOSIS

The physiologic and anatomic modifications of the pulmonary circulation induced by various degrees of chronic pulmonary venous hypertension are well illustrated by the extensive observations that have been made in patients with mitral stenosis. When the mitral orifice is only slightly restricted, left atrial pressure and intravascular pressures throughout the pulmonary circuit may be normal when the patient is at rest, but they exceed normal values with exercise or during other states accompanied by augmentation of cardiac output, such as fever, anemia, pregnancy, thyrotoxicosis, and hypermetabolism of other causes. Tachycardia alone, by abbreviating diastole, requires the generation of a higher left atrial pressure to maintain cardiac output through the stenotic valve. At this stage, as in animals with acutely produced mitral stenosis not severe enough to cause pulmonary edema, the modest vascular hypertension dilates the small pulmonary vessels and produces a decrease in their resistance to flow. In these circumstances, the increase in pulmonary arterial pressure is less pronounced than the increase in pulmonary venous and left atrial pressures.

In moderate and severe mitral stenosis with valvular orifice areas less than 1.5 sq cm, left atrial mean pressure at rest is often in the range of 25 to 30 mm Hg and rises with slight exercise to values of 40 to 55 mm Hg, especially if cardiac output increases substantially. Even if the pulmonary vascular resistance is normal, the pronounced pulmonary venous hypertension causes the mean pressure in the pulmonary artery to exceed normal values by three- to six-fold. In most patients, however, pulmonary vascular resistance is greater than normal, resulting in an increase of pulmonary arterial pressure that is disproportionately greater than that caused by the left atrial hypertension alone.

The range of abnormality of pulmonary vascular resistance in mitral stenosis is wide. In a series of 180 patients studied by the author, the resistance was two or more times greater than normal in 67 per cent of the patients. In 11 per cent, the resistance and consequently the pulmonary arterial pressure equaled or exceeded systemic arterial values. Patients with such advanced disturbances usually have very severe mitral stenosis and appear also to have a predisposition to advanced alterations in the pulmonary arteries in response to hypertension in the pulmonary veins and arteries that is not shared by other patients whose mitral obstruction and left atrial hypertension are equally pronounced. The clinical features of such patients resemble in many respects those of patients with primary pulmonary hypertension. A mitral diastolic murmur may not be audible, mainly because the cardiac output is greatly diminished as the result of the pulmonary vascular restriction and marked right ventricular dysfunction. Normal sinus rhythm persists in many of them despite the advanced mitral stenosis. Unlike patients with primary pulmonary hypertension, however, they do not experience frequent syncope.

In mitral stenosis, structural lesions are present in all segments of the pulmonary vascular bed. The pulmonary veins are dilated, and their walls are greatly thickened by medial hypertrophy and proliferation of the intima. In some patients, numerous anastomoses develop between the pulmonary and bronchial veins. These anastomotic channels form submucosal varicosities in the bronchi that can rupture and produce brisk hemoptysis when the left atrial pressure rises acutely.

The basic anatomic expression of increased hydrostatic pressure in the pulmonary capillaries is dilatation and engorgement of these vessels with edema of the alveolar walls and leakage of edema fluid into the alveolar spaces. Measurements made by the simultaneous injection of isotopically labeled water and a nondiffusible indicator into the pulmonary artery of patients with mitral stenosis and with pulmonary venous hypertension of other causes have demonstrated expansion of the interstitial pulmonary water volume directly related to the increase in left atrial pressure. At left atrial pressures of 25 to 30 mm Hg, the extravascular water volume is three or more times normal. Increased transport by the lymphatics is reflected by dilatation of these vessels. When the pulmonary capillary pressure exceeds values of 20 mm Hg, which is on the threshold of plasma protein osmotic pressure, the lymphatic vessels and the edematous interlobular septa at the bases of the lungs become sufficiently radiopaque to appear as short lines extending horizontally to the pleura (Kerley B lines) in radiograms of the chest.

Rupture of alveolar capillaries and pulmonary venules leads to scattered microhemorrhages and subsequent hemosiderosis. When the edema is of long standing, it promotes the development of interstitial fibrosis in the alveolar walls and the surrounding parenchyma that is most marked in the bases of the lower lobes and the lower segments of all lobes. These regional differences attest to the gravitational augmentation of capillary pressure and the consequently greater and more persistent edema in the dependent regions of the lungs. In these regions, the alveolar septa are markedly thickened and the pulmonary capillaries are compressed or obliterated. Rarely, the fibrotic regions become ossified and appear as small calcified nodules scattered throughout the lower lung fields.

The small pulmonary arteries manifest the medial hypertrophy, proliferation and fibrosis of the intima, increased wall thickness, and diminished internal diameter characteristic of hypertensive pulmonary vascular disease; however, dilatation lesions and necrotizing arteritis that are the hallmarks of the most advanced grades of pulmonary vascular disease are very rarely found. Also, in contrast to the hypertensive pulmonary vascular disease associated with congenital heart disease and primary pulmonary hypertension, the distribution of the arterial lesions conforms to a regional pattern. The arteries in the lower lobes are most affected and show the greatest restriction of their lumina; even in the upper lobes, in which the larger arteries are dilated and the small arteries are relatively spared, the vascular lesions are more prominent in the lower segments. As a consequence of the pattern of distribution of the vascular abnormalities and probably because of the more pronounced interstitial fibrosis in the lower lobes, blood flow is preferentially directed to the upper zones of the lung and away from the lower zones, resulting in reversal of the normal ratio of perfusion between the two zones. The ratio of upper zone perfusion to lower zone perfusion can be as large as 4:1 in contrast to the normal ratio of 1:8. The degree to which perfusion of the upper zones exceeds that of the lower regions is directly related to the height of the pulmonary venous pressure. The ratio also increases directly with the pulmonary vascular resistance, but when the resistance attains values in the range of the systemic vessels, the ratio decreases toward normal, probably because of more widespread distribution of the vascular abnormalities.

Pulmonary embolization and infarction are exceedingly frequent in mitral stenosis and in one series were found at autopsy in approximately one third of the patients who had manifested moderate to severe pulmonary arterial hypertension during life. These occlusions and the secondary effects on the parenchyma of the lung undoubtedly contribute to the restriction of the pulmonary vascular bed.

The main pulmonary artery and its central branches are dilated, and their intima often contains atherosclerotic plaques. The cross-sectional diameter of these vessels increases directly with the pulmonary arterial pressure. When the internal diameter of the main pulmonary artery is 4.0 cm or more, the murmur of pulmonic regurgitation (Graham Steell murmur) commonly appears.

Some insight into the mechanisms producing the pulmonary arterial hypertension and the relative roles of the various vascular disturbances in the genesis of the increased pulmonary vascular resistance is offered by observations of the hemodynamic changes that occur after successful mitral valvotomy or replacement of the mitral valve by a prosthetic valve with a functionally adequate orifice. In almost all patients whose left atrial pressure is lowered by the surgical procedure, the pulmonary vascular resistance decreases and the decline in pulmonary arterial pressure is consequently even greater than that of the pulmonary venous pressure. Substantial decreases in pulmonary vascular resistance have been observed as early as two days after surgery and have been attributed to dilatation of muscular pulmonary arteries that had been reflexly induced to constrict by the left atrial and pulmonary venous hypertension. However, failure of the resistance to fall immediately after the surgical procedure despite the decrease in left atrial pressure has been interpreted as indicating that interstitial and perivascular edema exert a cardinal role in the pathogenesis of the increased resistance and that resolution of the edema lags behind the fall of pulmonary venous pressure. In the ensuing weeks and months, the pulmonary vascular resistance often decreases further; even in patients whose preoperative values exceeded systemic vascular resistance, the arterial pressure and vascular resistance in the lungs can eventually attain values only slightly in excess of normal. The most striking changes occur in patients whose left atrial pressures postoperatively at rest and during exercise are normal or only slightly greater than normal. Evidence is now available that regression of the medial hypertrophy and intimal proliferation in the small pulmonary arteries is responsible for the progressive decline of the vascular resistance, but the way in which the pulmonary venous hypertension initiated the development of the structural abnormalities in the pulmonary arteries remains uncertain.

358.5. PULMONARY DISEASES AND DISORDERS OF RESPIRATION

Constriction of the pulmonary arteries by hypoxia and destruction or restriction of the pulmonary vascular bed are the two basic mechanisms that operate to increase the pulmonary arterial pressure in diseases of the lungs and disorders of the respiratory system. Primary alveolar hypoventilation is an example of a condition in which the disturbances in gas exchange alone initiate the pulmonary hypertension; but in most diseases of the lungs, anatomic restriction of the pulmonary vessels alone in the early stages of these diseases usually increases pulmonary arterial pressure only slightly because of the enormous reserve capacity of the pulmonary vasculature. By the time that the disease process has obliterated enough of the vessels to produce high-grade pulmonary hypertension, structural damage of the pulmonary parenchyma is sufficiently advanced to result in marked disturbances in gas exchange. In most pulmonary diseases therefore both mechanisms are operative.

Since diseases of the lungs and respiratory system are described in Part XII, only those features of significance in the production of pulmonary hypertension, its consequences, manifestations, and treatment are considered here.

PATHOLOGIC PHYSIOLOGY. In *chronic obstructive pulmonary disease*, loss of pulmonary capillaries accompanies the loss of alveoli. Some muscular arteries adjacent to terminal bronchioles may show intimal fibroelastosis of sufficient extent to obliterate their lumina. The media of the muscular arteries is slightly thickened, but these vessels and the arterioles show few of the changes characteristic of hypertensive pulmonary vascular disease.

The loss of pulmonary vessels is tolerated with little or

no increase of pulmonary arterial pressure at rest, although the pressure does rise to abnormal levels when pulmonary blood flow is augmented by exercise. In such patients, defects in distribution of ventilation and perfusion within the lungs and reduction in diffusing capacity exist but are not severe enough to cause hypercapnia and more than slight hypoxemia. With increase in the extent of hypoventilated but perfused pulmonary segments, marked hypoxemia develops and the pulmonary arterial pressure rises in direct proportion to the degree of oxygen unsaturation of systemic arterial blood. The hypercapnia that accompanies more widespread alveolar hypoventilation does not appear to affect the pulmonary arteries directly, and its effect on blood pH is minimized by concomitant increase in plasma bicarbonate concentration. Acidosis, arising as the consequence of sudden increase in carbon dioxide tension or failure of the buffering capacity to keep pace with the hypercapnia, potentiates the pulmonary vasoconstrictor response to the hypoxia and further raises the pulmonary arterial pressure.

The greater afterload to ejection of blood created by the increased pulmonary vascular resistance and pulmonary hypertension is met by hypertrophy of the right ventricle. Since the pulmonary arterial mean pressure at this stage is usually no more than twice normal, the right ventricle does not fail until a bronchopulmonary infection or some other event aggravates the bronchial obstruction and the disturbances in gas exchange and produces marked, generalized alveolar hypoventilation. Under such circumstances, as much 80 per cent of the cardiac output perfuses underventilated alveoli, and the arterial oxyhemoglobin saturation falls to values of 40 to 80 per cent; the arterial carbon dioxide tension rises to 60 to 80 mm Hg, and the arterial pH falls to values as low as 7.20. Renal blood flow and glomerular filtration decrease; the excretion of sodium and water diminishes, and the extracellular volume expands. The consequent increase in blood volume is augmented by hypoxia-induced polycythemia of variable degree. The end-diastolic pressure of the right ventricle increases and raises the pressure in the right atrium and systemic veins. The contractile function of the right ventricular myocardium is progressively depressed, and the right ventricle dilates and fails. Several studies have demonstrated that left ventricular function, if it was previously normal, is not disturbed by these events, and that left atrial and pulmonary venous pressures remain within the range of normal.

The relative pathogenic role of each physiologic disturbance in producing the sudden increase in pulmonary arterial pressure in this complex state has been difficult to assess. Correction of the hypoxemia or the acidosis while the failure persists reduces the pulmonary arterial pressure, but it remains considerably elevated. Phlebotomy does not promptly lower the pulmonary arterial pressure. In some patients, because of infection and hypermetabolism, the cardiac output is higher than in the prefailure period, but in many patients the cardiac output is subnormal.

It is striking that as the manifestations of acute respiratory insufficiency and congestive right ventricular failure resolve with appropriate treatment, the pulmonary arterial pressure gradually falls and, together with the systemic arterial oxyhemoglobin saturation, finally returns to its prefailure values. It is difficult to avoid assigning a cardinal role to hypoxia in the pathogenesis of the marked pulmonary hypertension and the overt cor pulmonale.

During recurrent acute exacerbations of respiratory failure, and occasionally as the result of pulmonary thromboembolism to which these patients are prone, signs of increased pulmonary hypertension and right ventricular failure reappear. Eventually these manifestations and the disturbances in gas exchange do not respond fully to treatment, and the cor pulmonale becomes chronic.

In *fibroproliferative and chronic inflammatory diseases of the lungs,* the pulmonary vascular bed is compromised in many ways. In the diffuse interstitial disorders that affect the alveolar walls, such as *sarcoidosis* and other granulomatous diseases, the *Hamman-Rich syndrome, scleroderma, polymyositis, berylliosis, asbestosis, lymphangitic carcinomatosis, radiation fibrosis,* and *idiopathic pulmonary hemosiderosis,* the alveolar capillaries are compressed or obliterated. In massive pulmonary fibrosis caused by *silicosis* or coal miner's *pneumoconiosis,* the fibrotic nodules develop in proximity to muscular and small elastic arteries, and as they enlarge, they engulf and obliterate these vessels.

In all these disorders, increasing disruption of parenchymal structures and fibrosis cause progressive distortion, obstruction, and obliteration of pulmonary vessels. With the development of pulmonary hypertension, the medial hypertrophy and intimal proliferation of hypertensive pulmonary vascular disease are superimposed.

Early in the course of the pulmonary disease, as for example in the interstitial disorders of the lung, pulmonary hypertension may be only slight at rest despite marked restriction of lung volume, but the pressure usually rises steeply with exercise. Similarly, hypoxemia is only mild at rest, but the arterial oxygen saturation usually falls during exercise. With diminution of pulmonary diffusion capacity, the development of marked maldistribution of alveolar ventilation and perfusion, and increase in the extent of intrapulmonary arteriovenous shunting, oxygenation of arterial blood is progressively impaired, pulmonary arterial pressure rises further, and the right ventricle fails. Episodic exacerbations of failure are often precipitated by respiratory infections as in obstructive pulmonary disease, but reduction of pulmonary arterial pressure with treatment is less impressive, and once right ventricular failure occurs, it usually becomes chronic. The highest grades of chronic pulmonary hypertension secondary to pulmonary disease are found in fibrotic diseases of the lungs.

In bronchiectasis, tuberculosis, and other chronic inflammatory diseases of the lungs, extensive intercommunications can develop between the bronchial and pulmonary arteries; occasionally, the mammary and intercostal arteries participate in the formation of the anastomoses. The bronchial collateral flow through these channels is usually small, but in a rare patient it is large enough to constitute a significant left-right shunt that increases the pulmonary blood flow, further elevates the pulmonary arterial pressure, and taxes the left ventricle.

Alveolar hypoventilation pronounced enough to produce hypoxemia and hypercapnia, secondary constriction and hypertension in the pulmonary arteries, and right ventricular failure is encountered in a group of disorders characterized by a *defective ventilatory apparatus.* The fundamental defect exists in the chest bellows, as in *kyphoscoliosis, marked obesity* and *neuromuscular diseases* that affect the respiratory muscles, or in the respiratory control centers, as in hypoventilation of central nervous origin (*Ondine's curse*). The lungs and pulmonary vessels are intrinsically normal except in patients with severe kyphoscoliosis, whose pulmonary vascular bed is restricted by the inordinately small dimensions of the lungs and in whom concomitant bronchiectasis, areas of atelectasis, and bronchopulmonary infections are common.

Regardless of the nature of the basic defect in this group of diseases, alveolar ventilation not only is diminished at rest, but also fails to increase normally with exercise and increased metabolic demand, which consequently accentuates the hypoxemia and hypercapnia. In patients with these disorders, as well as in those with primary lung diseases who have had bouts of hypercapnia, the sensitivity of the chemoreceptors to both carbon dioxide and hypoxemia is progressively impaired, and the loss of ventilatory response to these stimuli enhances the propensity to the development of cor pulmonale. A respiratory infection commonly precipitates the development of marked pulmonary hypertension and right ventricular failure.

CLINICAL MANIFESTATIONS AND DIAGNOSIS. Pulmonary disease is usually readily identified by the history, the physical findings, and radiograms of the chest, but clues to the presence and severity of pulmonary hypertension may be masked by the pulmonary disease. In some patients, the classic signs of pulmonary hypertension described in Ch. 358.2 may be present, but in others, especially those with chronic obstructive disease, the cardiac sounds are barely audible or are obscured by adventitious pulmonary sounds, and enlargement of the right ventricle and main pulmonary artery cannot be detected with certainty. Despite considerable pulmonary hypertension, the sound of pulmonic valvular closure may not be audibly accentuated.

The patient with right ventricular failure typically presents a history of a recent respiratory infection followed by exacerbation of his usual respiratory symptoms and progressive dyspnea. He presents the appearance and physical signs of a patient with acute pulmonary insufficiency. Cyanosis is usually marked, especially in the presence of polycythemia, but often it is not impressive despite pronounced decrease in the arterial oxyhemoglobin saturation. If hypercapnia exists, drowsiness and the other central nervous system manifestations of hypercapnia may be evident. The jugular veins are distended and are further engorged by applying pressure over the enlarged, usually tender liver. Edema of the lower extremities may be present. The cardiac rate is rapid, and an early diastolic gallop sound may be audible over the mid-left precordium.

Radiograms usually reveal a prominent main pulmonary artery and enlargement of its main branches; but if the pulmonary hypertension is not marked or has not been sustained for a prolonged period of time, these vessels may appear normal in size. Especially in patients who have manifested chronic cardiac failure, the right ventricle and the right atrium are grossly enlarged. In other patients with obvious failure, the cardiac dimensions seem surprisingly normal, but serial films will often show diminution in the size of the right ventricle and right atrium with recovery from the failure.

The electrocardiographic manifestations of right ventricular hypertrophy are also modified by lung disease; even in patients with considerable pulmonary hypertension and right ventricular hypertrophy, the usual criteria considered diagnostic of hypertrophy and enlargement of the right ventricle are often not present. Large S waves in the precordial leads as far to the left as V_5 or V_6, a small rS or rSR' complex in V_1, negative T waves in the right precordial leads, a vertical or slight rightward displacement of the mean QRS axis in the frontal plane, and peaked P waves in the limb leads (P pulmonale) may be the only signs that the right ventricle is hypertrophied. These electrocardiographic alterations may not be present if the pulmonary arterial pressure is not two or more times greater than normal at rest. Regression of these electrocardiographic features in the course of recovery from an episode of respiratory failure often permits a retrospective appreciation of their significance. Atrial arrhythmias, especially flutter and fibrillation, and ventricular premature contractions are common in patients with acute respiratory insufficiency and cor pulmonale. Although it appears most commonly in such patients, chaotic atrial rhythm is an infrequent complication and bears a poor prognosis.

The findings of a reduced oxyhemoglobin saturation, diminished oxygen tension and pH and elevated carbon dioxide tension in the arterial blood, increase in plasma bicarbonate, and polycythemia support the diagnosis of pulmonary hypertension caused by pulmonary disease or respiratory disorder. Studies of pulmonary function are useful in defining the disorder, monitoring the effects of treatment, and assessing the probability that cor pulmonale will develop. Primary alveolar hypoventilation of central origin as the cause of pulmonary hypertension and congestive cardiac failure may go undetected without measurements of arterial blood gases and studies of the ventilatory response to carbon dioxide. In some patients with cardiac murmurs or evidence of left ventricular enlargement, the issue of whether the pulmonary hypertension is primarily due to the pulmonary disease or is secondary to an intracardiac lesion or left ventricular dysfunction may sometimes be resolved only by hemodynamic and angiographic studies. Pulmonary disease does not protect the patient from the development of coronary arteriosclerosis or systemic hypertension, which may compromise left ventricular function. The left ventricle may also be directly affected by scleroderma, polymyositis, sarcoidosis, certain forms of muscular dystrophy, and obesity. The features of the cardiopulmonary syndrome of obesity, in which marked pulmonary hypertension can occur, are described in Ch. 474.

TREATMENT. Treatment must be simultaneously directed at improving the function of both the lungs and the heart. The specific measures to be used are described in Part XII. When cardiac failure appears, a cardiac glycoside and a diuretic, such as hydrochlorothiazide or furosemide, should be administered. Losses of body potassium during diuresis should be replaced, but because of pre-existing disturbances in potassium balance and impairment of renal function, serum potassium should be closely monitored as a guide to such replacement. The hypoxemia, hypercapnia, acidosis, and electrolyte imbalances appear to predispose the heart of patients with cor pulmonale to arrhythmias and to the toxic effects of cardiac glycosides. Daily maintenance doses larger than 0.1 mg of digitoxin or 0.25 mg of digoxin should be used with caution, and manifestations of digitalis intoxication should be watched for. Correction of hypoxemia by inhalation of oxygen in concentrations that do not depress alveolar ventilation is a cardinal feature of therapy during an acute episode of failure, and chronic administration of oxygen may be indicated to control pulmonary hypertension in patients with marked chronic hypoxemia. Because polycythemia enhances the tendency to develop thromboemboli and increases viscosity of the blood and consequently the resistance to its flow, periodic phlebotomy is indicated to maintain the hematocrit at 50 per cent in patients with marked polycythemia.

PROGNOSIS. The development of pulmonary arterial hypertension and right ventricular failure in patients with pulmonary disease is a serious complication, but its prognostic significance depends on the underlying disorder. With appropriate treatment, the patient with chronic obstructive pulmonary disease may survive repeated bouts of cardiac and pulmonary failure over the course of many years. In patients with pulmonary fibrosis, the course after the onset of cardiac failure is variable but generally much shorter.

Blount, S. G., Jr., and Grover, R. F.: Pulmonary hypertension. *In* Hurst, J. W., and Logue, R. B. (eds.): The Heart, Arteries and Veins. 2nd ed. New York, McGraw-Hill Book Company, 1970, p. 1126.

Fishman, A. P.: Hypoxia on the pulmonary circulation. How and where it acts. Cir. Res., 38:221, 1977.

Harris, P., and Heath, D.: The Human Pulmonary Circulation. Its Form and Function in Health and Disease. Baltimore, Williams & Wilkins Company, 1962.

Heath, D., and Edwards, J. E.: The pathology of hypertensive pulmonary vascular disease. A description of structural changes in the pulmonary arteries with special reference to congenital cardiac septal defects. Circulation, 18:533, 1958.

Levine, O. R., Harris, R. C., Blanc, W. A., and Mellins, R. B.: Progressive pulmonary hypertension in children with portal hypertension. J. Pediat., 83:964, 1973.

Naeye, R. L.: "Primary" pulmonary hypertension with coexisting portal hypertension. A retrospective study of six cases. Circulation, 22:376, 1960.

Wagenvoort, C. A., and Wagenvoort, N.: Primary pulmonary hypertension. A pathologic study of the lung vessels in 156 clinically diagnosed cases. Circulation, 42:1163, 1970.

Yu, P. N.: Pulmonary Blood Volume in Health and Disease. Philadelphia, Lea & Febiger, 1969.

359.   CONGENITAL HEART DISEASE

Joseph K. Perloff

359.1.   INTRODUCTION

DEFINITION. "Congenital" is a Latin derivative from *con*, together, and *genitus*, born. However, the simple implication that congenital heart disease merely means "present at birth" requires qualification. The natural history begins before delivery, because most anomalies compatible with six months of intrauterine life permit live offspring at term. A congenital anomaly originating in the developing fetus is often considerably modified, at least physiologically, by the dramatic circulatory adjustments at birth. Weeks, months, or even years may elapse before the anomaly evolves into the "typical" clinical picture. Both physiologic and structural changes subsequently continue. The ductus in a premature infant sometimes remains widely patent for months, finally closing spontaneously, leaving the baby with a normal heart. A ventricular septal defect that delivers a large left to right shunt in infancy may gradually develop progressive infundibular pulmonic stenosis, so that years later the physiologic and the clinical picture resembles cyanotic Fallot's tetralogy. A congenital bicuspid aortic valve that is functionally normal at birth can take two, three, or more decades to stiffen, calcify, and

present as overt aortic stenosis. Accordingly, congenital heart disease should not be viewed narrowly as a fixed group of anatomic defects present at birth, but as dynamic anomalies that originate in fetal life and alter during postnatal development. Certain defects that are not "anatomic" in the gross morphologic sense are nevertheless considered congenital, such as congenital complete heart block, whereas others that are anatomic, such as the aortic root disease of Marfan's syndrome, are, by convention, not classified as congenital.

INCIDENCE, CHANGING POPULATION, AND ROLE OF THE INTERNIST AND MEDICAL CARDIOLOGIST. The prevalence of congenital heart disease has little meaning unless certain preconditions are met. An impression of over-all prevalence can be derived from population figures at the beginning of this decade when 3,718,000 live births were registered in the United States. An estimated 28,000 infants were born with congenital heart disease, i.e., 0.8 per cent. About half died within the first year, leaving 14,000 survivors. Both over-all incidence and incidence of specific defects vary according to patient age (neonate, infant, child, adolescent, young adult, older adult) and according to whether figures are derived from living subjects or necropsy material. A further distinction must be made between incidence based upon *natural* history and the incidence modified by *palliative* or *corrective* surgery. It is now possible to perform palliative or corrective surgery on almost all congenital cardiacs, even the most complex. Survival patterns are affected, often profoundly. We are therefore confronted with a changing population of congenital heart disease. Recent decades of intense diagnostic and therapeutic effort have resulted in survival of increasing numbers of adolescents, postadolescents, and adults with congenital defects of the heart or circulation. Accordingly, postpediatric congenital heart disease is represented not only by anomalies with a natural tendency for long survival, but also by those in which palliative or corrective surgery has been successfully employed. Operation not only increases life expectancy in anomalies with a natural tendency for long survival, but may also permit larger numbers of patients with disorders hiterto fatal in infancy or childhood to reach postadolescence or even adulthood. Appropriate long-term management requires an understanding of both the preoperative anomaly and the effects of surgical repair. *Thus congenital heart disease from the point of view of patient care should be considered not only in terms of age of onset, but also in terms of the age range that potential survival now permits.* Such patients require specialty care, be it by a pediatric cardiologist who extends an interest to older subjects or by a medical cardiologist who has a satisfactory comprehension of congenital cardiac disease. By the same token, just as it is necessary for the pediatrician to provide primary general pediatric care for the infant or child with congenital heart disease, the internist must provide primary general medical care for the late teenager and adult with these malformations.

ETIOLOGY. Congenital heart disease is etiologically multifactorial, the result of a complex interplay between genetic and environmental factors. These determinants in part include heredity, chromosomal defects, teratogens, prematurity, altitude at birth, sex, and maternal age.

Some tendency exists for congenital heart disease to

run in families. There is an increased incidence of defects in the offspring of propositi. Distribution and incidence are difficult to ascertain, because survival into the reproductive age is a requirement for transmission. Atrial septal defect commonly permits adult survival, and can be both familial and recurrent through a number of generations. Parents who in childhood experienced spontaneous closure of ventricular septal defects may live to adulthood and produce offspring with ventricular septal defects. There is also the prospect that increasing numbers of *operated* congenital cardiacs will reach childbearing age and produce a higher incidence of offspring with congenital defects of the heart or circulation. About 2 per cent of siblings of propositi have congenital heart disease. If one of a nonidentical twin pair has a congenital cardiac anomaly, the incidence in the co-twin is about the same as for sibs in general, but about 25 per cent of identical twins with congenital heart disease have affected co-twins with a high probability of identical defects.

Certain abnormal chromosome patterns are associated with predictable types of congenital cardiac disease, although chromosomal abnormalities per se are uncommon in the general population of congenital cardiacs. Down's syndrome (trisomy 21) has a high incidence of endocardial cushion defects, and about 50 per cent of patients with complete endocardial cushion defects have trisomy 21. Typical Turner's syndrome (phenotypic female with XO) occurs with coarctation of the aorta; trisomy 18 occurs with right ventricular origin of both great arteries; the Holt-Oram syndrome heightens suspicion of ostium secundum atrial septal defect, and the Ellis–van Creveld syndrome predicts common atrium.

The role of *teratogens* at critical times in fetal development is epitomized by the effects of thalidomide taken by the pregnant mother. Maternal rubella (German measles) during the first trimester increases the risk of offspring with patent ductus arteriosus and stenosis of the pulmonary artery and its branches.

Ventricular septal defect and patent ductus arteriosus are relatively common in *premature infants*. It has been postulated that the expected intrauterine time of ventricular septal closure is not limited to early fetal life but sometimes continues through gestation into the postpartum period. Delayed closure of the ductus arteriosus is more likely to occur in premature infants, and the duct may remain patent for as long as four to six months after birth. Incompletely developed cholinergic innervation and reduced constrictor response to oxygen of the premature ductus may in part account for this.

The *altitude at birth* is another factor that influences the occurrence of congenital heart disease. Patency of the ductus arteriosus is six times as frequent in people born at high altitudes as in those born at sea level. Reduced oxygen tension in ambient air at high altitudes may provide inadequate stimulus for ductal constriction even if cholinergic innervation of the ductal wall is well developed.

Parental age has been considered an etiologic factor. There is no evidence that paternal age plays a role, but *maternal age* has been called into question. Late maternal age (immediate premenopausal) seems to increase the risk of Fallot's tetralogy.

Sex distribution has been a point of interest in congenital diseases of the heart and circulation. The bicuspid aortic valve is predominantly a male disease. In fact, aortic valve disease in general has a strong male prevalence. The male-to-female ratio in ventricular septal defect with aortic regurgitation is twice as high as in uncomplicated ventricular septal defect. Aortic atresia is almost exclusively a disease of male infants. On the other hand, patent ductus arteriosus predominates in females (sex ratio of 2 or 3:1). Female predominance in ostium secundum atrial septal defect is estimated to be as high as 3.5:1, and females predominate in partial endocardial cushion defects. Congenital aneurysms of sinuses of Valsalva carry a male-to-female ratio of 4:1. A similar male-to-female ratio occurs in complete transposition of the great arteries, with a range of 2 to 4:1.

PHYSIOLOGIC ADAPTATION AFTER BIRTH. The concept has been underscored that congenital heart diseases are not static in time, but change anatomically and functionally during the course of their natural histories. A given congenital cardiac defect may exist in harmony with the fetal circulation, but is confronted with dramatic circulatory changes at birth that alter this harmony to widely varying degrees. It is therefore appropriate to examine briefly the principal immediate and delayed circulatory alterations at birth and in the neonatal period. The immediate changes consist of (1) a colossal fall in pulmonary vascular resistance associated with expansion of the lungs; (2) a pronounced rise in systemic vascular resistance associated with elimination of the low resistance placental circulation; (3) a fall in blood flow to the right atrium owing to abolition of umbilical venous return; (4) an abrupt rise — as much as tenfold — in pulmonary blood flow, which is promptly translated into a rise in left atrial volume and pressure; (5) functional closure of the valve of the foramen ovale caused by the rise in left atrial and the fall in right atrial pressure; and (6) constriction of the ductus arteriosus at about 12 hours after birth in response to an increase in systemic arterial Po_2. Several important delayed changes complete the picture. The thick-walled fetal pulmonary arterioles are designed to meet the full force of systemic right ventricular pressure the instant the lungs expand. After this need has been met, the fetal arterioles involute during the first few months of life. As respiration is established at birth, there is a marked rise in alveolar and systemic arterial oxygen tension to which pulmonary arterioles are exquisitely sensitive, setting the stage for dilatation and anatomic involution. In addition, the larger pulmonary arteries may also play a role — though much less — in determining the total drop in pressure across the lungs after birth. Maturational changes may affect the neonatal disparity in size between the main and branch pulmonary arteries as well as the angulation at the origins of the right and left branches; both these factors have been held responsible for a physiologic drop in pressure distal to the pulmonary trunk. The third important delayed change relates to the fetal right ventricle, which slowly loses its relative thickness during the first year of life. Adaptive hypertrophy is an expected feature of the fetal right ventricle, which ejects at systemic pressure via the ductus arteriosus. After birth, with the stimulus of right ventricular afterload eliminated, there is a gradual reduction in its thickness relative to septum and left ventricle. The thick neonatal right ventricular wall does not undergo regression; it merely does not increase its thickness as rapidly as the left in the growing infant.

These physiologic adaptations of the normal heart to the events at birth are remarkable in their own right. It is no surprise that congenital defects of the heart or circulation will, to varying degrees, interact with or be modified by adaptations to extrauterine life. A few examples suffice. At one end of the spectrum is the ductus arteriosus, which is a normal part of the fetal circulation. However, when the fetal ductus remains widely patent after birth, the neonatal fall in pulmonary vascular resistance establishes a left to right shunt; pulmonary blood flow increases; the left ventricle is volume overloaded and may fail under the burden. Thus a normal structure in the fetus becomes a potentially hazardous congenital defect after birth. At the other end of the spectrum, aortic atresia is an example. This anomaly is characterized by an atretic aortic valve, a rudimentary left ventricular cavity, and a rudimentary or atretic mitral valve. The left atrium has no effective exit, but in the fetus this is not a handicap, because flow into the left atrium via the lungs is negligible and right to left flow across the foramen ovale is not vital. Accordingly, survival to term is the rule, because systemic venous blood received by the fetal right heart is pumped into the systemic circulation via the ductus, bypassing the left heart. However, at birth, the lungs expand and pulmonary blood flow suddenly and dramatically increases, abruptly delivering a large volume into a left atrium that has no effective outlet because forward flow through the left ventricle is totally obstructed by the atretic mitral and/or aortic valves. Temporary survival depends upon decompression of the left atrium via a herniated valve of the foramen ovale. Death follows shortly. An intermediate case in point is large ventricular septal defect which, although abnormal, does not disturb the fetal circulation because it allows right ventricular blood to enter the aorta in a fashion analogous to the fetal ductus. However, after birth, a fall in pulmonary vascular resistance establishes a left to right shunt which may significantly disturb the postnatal circulation. Subsequently, the pulmonary vascular resistance may rise again and, in a decade or more, reverse the shunt (Eisenmenger's complex), re-establishing a circulatory state similar to the intrauterine presence of the ventricular septal defect.

The principle to be extracted from these examples is clear. The anatomy and physiology of the heart and circulation in congenital heart disease change with the passage of time from the fetus, to the dramatic changes at birth, to further changes in the infant, child, adolescent, and adult survivor. Some of these changes result in neonatal death; others express themselves gradually over weeks, months, years, or decades. A satisfactory comprehension of the clinical manifestations of congenital heart disease requires that these patterns be taken into account.

DIAGNOSIS. The clinical diagnosis of congenital heart disease can represent the epitome of applied medical logic. When sound inferences are drawn from accurate observations, correct diagnoses can be made with gratifying frequency. The clinical expressions of congenital cardiac disease are best dealt with in terms of the anatomic and physiologic mechanisms responsible for their production. Logical thought should be encouraged and memorization minimized. The pathologic anatomy must first be clarified in order to shed light on the resulting physiologic derangements. The question can then be asked: "What clinical manifestations result from these anatomic and physiologic derangements?" The stage is now set for the clinical diagnosis, which depends upon a synthesis of information derived from the history, the physical signs, the electrocardiogram, the x-ray, and the noninvasive and cardiac catheterization laboratories. Similarly, the physical diagnosis consists of a synthesis of information from its own five sources, namely, physical appearance, the arterial pulse, the jugular venous pulse, precordial movements and palpation, and auscultation. It is axiomatic that emphasis is placed on the *relationship of the parts to the whole*, a relationship that ideally results in a complete, harmonious picture devoid of internal contradictions, and *not* a loose confederation of unrelated observations. Maximum data should be extracted from each clinical source while relating information from one source to another. A simple principle emerges — on the one hand, depth; on the other, synthesis. Each step should advance our thinking and narrow the diagnostic possibilities. By the end of the clinical appraisal, untenable considerations should have been abandoned, diagnostic possibilities retained for due consideration, and high priority probabilities brought into sharp focus. Conclusions should become more and more refined as the clinical evaluation progresses step by step. The essence of this thesis stems from Herophilus' adage that the best physician is one who is able to distinguish between the possible and the impossible. A single additional word gives this comment modern relevance — distinguish between the *probable*, the possible, and the impossible.

Diagnostic thinking benefits from the devices of anticipation and supposition. Anticipate what the next step might reveal, and less will be missed. Having drawn tentative conclusions from the history, it is useful to pause momentarily and ask, "If these assumptions are correct, what can I expect the physical examination to reveal? What specific points might I anticipate in the electrocardiogram or x-ray in order to support or refute the conclusions based on the history?" The device of *anticipation* not only helps achieve a synthesis of each step with the next but also serves to heighten interest and suspense as the clinical assessment progresses. The device of *supposition* lends itself to the clinical classification of congenital heart disease in Table 1. Clinical information can be directly related to this classification so that orderly thinking begins apace. For example, we can ask, "*Suppose* this were a *congenital* cardiac defect in an *acyanotic* patient with a *left to right shunt;* which if any of the malformations in this category are appropriate to the information thus far at hand?" By simply asking, "Suppose this were so, what is likely to follow?" one is permitted the dual advantages of thoughtful consideration without inflexible commitment.

Diagnostic information is best handled within the framework of an orderly classification (Table 1) selected because it is practical, is clinical, and can be used effectively irrespective of which of the five sources of information one is dealing with. There are shortcomings in any classification, but these shortcomings, provided they are recognized and minimized, should not obscure the value of a practical, orderly grouping. *The fact that a number of defects are listed in more than one category simply emphasizes the variability of their clinical expressions.* The classification, first proposed by Paul Wood over two decades ago, is based upon the answers to the

TABLE 1.   A Clinical Classification of Congenital Heart Disease*

General

Innocent or normal murmurs
Congenitally corrected transposition of the great arteries
Congenital positional anomalies of the heart—cardiac malpositions
Congenital complete heart block

Acyanotic without a Shunt

Malformations originating in the left heart
1. Aortic stenosis
   a. Valvular
   b. Discrete subvalvular
   c. Supravalvular
2. Congenital aortic regurgitation
3. Coarctation of the aorta
4. Congenital mitral regurgitation
   a. Endocardial cushion defect
   b. Congenitally corrected transposition of the great arteries
   c. Primary endocardial fibroelastosis (dilated)
   d. Anomalous origin of the left coronary artery from the pulmonary trunk
   e. Miscellaneous (e.g., double orifice mitral valve, congenital perforations, accessory commissures with anomalous chordal insertion, congenitally short or absent chordae, cleft posterior leaflet, parachute mitral valve)
5. Primary endocardial fibroelastosis
6. Congenital obstruction to left atrial flow
   a. Cor triatriatum
   b. Mitral stenosis
   c. Pulmonary vein stenosis
Malformations originating in the right heart
1. Pulmonic stenosis
   a. Valvular
   b. Infundibular
   c. Supravalvular (stenosis of the pulmonary artery and its branches)
   d. Subinfundibular
2. Idiopathic dilatation of the pulmonary trunk
3. Congenital pulmonary valve regurgitation
4. Primary pulmonary hypertension
5. Ebstein's anomaly of the tricuspid valve

Acyanotic with a Shunt (Left to Right)

Shunt at atrial level
1. Atrial septal defect (isolated)
   a. Ostium secundum
   b. Ostium primum
   c. Sinus venosus
2. Atrial septal defect with mild pulmonic stenosis
3. Total anomalous pulmonary venous connection with low pulmonary vascular resistance
4. Partial anomalous pulmonary venous connection with intact atrial septum
5. Atrial septal defect with mitral stenosis (Lutembacher's syndrome)
Shunt at ventricular level
1. Ventricular septal defect (isolated)
   a. Infracristal
   b. Supracristal
   c. Muscular
   d. Endocardial cushion location
2. Ventricular septal defect with mild pulmonic stenosis
3. Ventricular septal defect with right ventricular origin of both great arteries
4. Ventricular septal defect (infracristal) with congenitally corrected transposition of the great arteries
5. Ventricular septal defect with aortic regurgitation
6. Ventricular septal defect with left ventricular to right atrial shunt
Shunt between aortic root and right heart
1. Coronary arteriovenous fistula
2. Ruptured sinus of Valsalva aneurysm

3. Anomalous origin of the left coronary artery from the pulmonary trunk
Shunt at aorticopulmonary level
1. Patent ductus arteriosus
2. Aorticopulmonary septal defect
3. Truncus arteriosus with large pulmonary arteries and low pulmonary vascular resistance
Shunts at more than one level
1. Complete endocardial cushion defect (complete persistent common atrioventricular canal)
2. Ventricular septal defect with patent ductus arteriosus
3. Ventricular septal defect with atrial septal defect

Cyanotic

Increased pulmonary blood flow
1. Complete transposition of the great arteries
2. The Taussig-Bing anomaly (right ventricular origin of both great arteries with supracristal ventricular septal defect or right ventricular aorta with biventricular pulmonary trunk)
3. Truncus arteriosus with large pulmonary arteries
4. Total anomalous pulmonary venous connection
5. Single ventricle with low pulmonary resistance and absent or mild pulmonic stenosis
6. Common atrium
7. Fallot's tetralogy with pulmonary atresia and increased collateral arterial flow
8. Tricuspid atresia with large ventricular septal defect and no pulmonic stenosis
9. Atrial septal defect with caval connection to left atrium
Normal or decreased pulmonary blood flow
1. Dominant left ventricle
   a. Tricuspid atresia
   b. Ebstein's anomaly with right to left interatrial shunt (mechanical dominance)
   c. Pulmonary atresia with intact ventricular septum and diminutive right ventricle
   d. Congenital vena caval to left atrial communication
   e. Single ventricle with pulmonic stenosis and non-inversion of the infundibulum
   f. Large pulmonary arteriovenous fistula in infancy
2. Dominant right ventricle
   Normal or low pulmonary arterial pressure
   a. Pulmonic stenosis or atresia with ventricular septal defect and right to left shunt (cyanotic Fallot's tetralogy)
   b. Pulmonic stenosis with right to left interatrial shunt
   c. Complete transposition of the great arteries with severe pulmonic stenosis
   d. Pulmonic stenosis with right ventricular origin of both great arteries
   e. Pulmonic stenosis with single ventricle and inversion of the infundibulum (electrical dominance)
   f. Truncus arteriosus with hypoplastic or absent pulmonary arteries
   Elevated pulmonary arterial pressure (pulmonary hypertension)
   a. Atrial septal defect with reversed shunt
   b. Ventricular septal defect with reversed shunt (Eisenmenger's complex)
   c. Patent ductus arteriosus or aorticopulmonary septal defect with reversed shunt
   d. Right ventricular origin of both great arteries with high pulmonary vascular resistance
   e. Hypoplastic left heart (aortic atresia, mitral atresia, complete interruption of the aortic arch)
   f. Complete transposition of the great arteries with high pulmonary vascular resistance
   g. Single ventricle with high pulmonary vascular resistance
   h. Total anomalous pulmonary venous connection with high pulmonary vascular resistance
3. Normal or nearly normal ventricles
   a. Pulmonary arteriovenous fistula
   b. Congenital vena caval to left atrial communication

---

*From Perloff, J. K.: The Clinical Recognition of Congenital Heart Disease. 2nd ed. Philadelphia, W. B. Saunders Company, 1978.

TABLE 2. Five Basic Questions

1. Is the patient acyanotic or cyanotic?
2. Is pulmonary arterial flow increased or not?
3. Does the malformation originate in the left or right heart?
4. Which is the dominant ventricle?
5. Is pulmonary hypertension present or absent?

TABLE 6

Acyanotic with a shunt. Where is the left to right communication, i.e., where does it originate and what chamber or vessel receives the shunt? Start proximally and end distally:

1. Atrial level
2. Ventricular level
3. Great artery level (aortic root, aortic arch)

TABLE 3

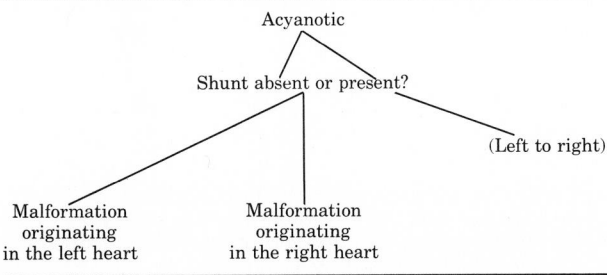

TABLE 7

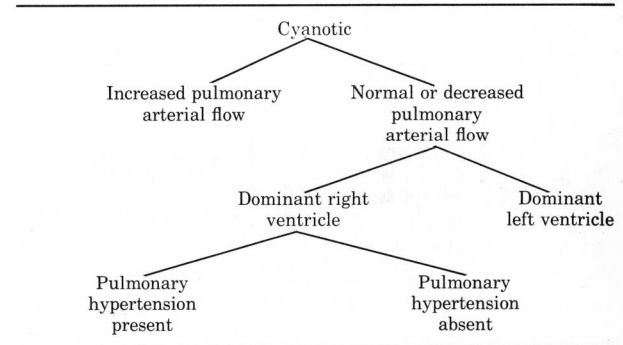

TABLE 4

Acyanotic without a shunt, malformation originating in the right heart. Start proximally (venae cavae) and end distally (pulmonary arteries):

1. Venae cavae
2. Right atrium
3. Tricuspid valve
4. Right ventricular inflow
5. Right ventricular outflow
6. Pulmonary artery and branches
7. Pulmonary arterioles

TABLE 8

Cyanotic with normal or decreased pulmonary arterial flow, dominant right ventricle, and pulmonary hypertension. Where is the right to left shunt? Start proximally and end distally.

1. Atrial level
2. Ventricular level
3. Great artery level

TABLE 5

Acyanotic without a shunt, malformation originating in the left heart. Start proximally (pulmonary veins) and end distally (aorta):

1. Pulmonary veins
2. Left atrium
3. Mitral valve
4. Left ventricular inflow
5. Left ventricular outflow
6. Thoracic aorta

TABLE 9

Cyanotic with normal or decreased pulmonary arterial flow, dominant right ventricle, and no pulmonary hypertension.

1. Pulmonic stenosis or atresia with right to left shunt at ventricular level.
2. Pulmonic stenosis or atresia with right to left shunt at atrial level.

five questions in Table 2. It is not even necessary to ask all five questions for each patient, although the first two questions are obligatory. If the answer to question 1 is "acyanotic," only two additional questions need be posed, first: "Is pulmonary arterial flow increased or not?" (i.e., is a shunt absent or present?), and second, if a shunt is absent: "Does the malformation originate in the left or right heart?"

Let us illustrate by dealing first with an acyanotic patient (Table 3). If the patient is *acyanotic* and the answer to question 2 is negative (acyanotic without shunt), we must then ask question 3: "Does the malformation originate in the left or right heart?" Now move step by step in the direction of blood flow. If the malformation originates in the right heart (Table 4), is it at the level of the venae cavae (persistent left superior vena cava) tricuspid valve—right ventricular inflow (Ebstein's anomaly), right ventricular outflow (stenosis or regurgitation, the former infundibular, valvular, or supravalvular), or the pulmonary arterioles (primary pulmonary hypertension)? Similarly, if the malformation originates in the left heart (Table 5), is it at the level of the pulmonary veins (congenital pulmonary vein stenosis), left atrium (cor triatriatum), mitral valve (stenosis or regurgitation), left ventricular inflow (endocardial fibroelastosis), left ventricular outflow (stenosis or regurgitation, the former subvalvular, valvular, or supravalvular), or the thoracic aorta (coarctation)? If the answer to question 2 (Table 2) is that pulmonary arterial blood flow is *increased* in an acyanotic patient, then the shunt by definition is left to right because cyanosis is absent. We can then consider methodically the origin of the shunt and the chamber or vessel that receives it. Again, move step by step through the heart in the direction of blood flow (Table 6), i.e., shunts at atrial level (atrial septal defect), ventricular level (ventricular septal defect), from the aortic root to right heart (e.g., coronary arteriovenous fistula), or from aortic arch to pulmonary artery (patent ductus).

Now, let us deal with *cyanotic* patients (Table 7; see accompanying figure). If pulmonary arterial blood flow is *increased*, there are, for all practical purposes, about eight or nine possibilities (Table 1, Cyanotic with Increased Pulmonary Blood Flow), only three of which are relatively common — namely, complete transposition of the great arteries, truncus arteriosus, and total anomalous pulmonary venous connection. If pulmonary arterial flow is *normal or decreased* (Table 7), and the *left* ventricle is dominant (question 4), there are six possibilities, only two of which are likely — namely, tricuspid atresia and Ebstein's anomaly of the tricuspid valve. If the *right* ventricle is dominant, question 5 must be asked: "Is pulmonary hypertension present or absent?" If pulmonary hypertension is *present,* again move step by step through the heart in the direction of blood flow (Table 8). Is one dealing with a pulmonary hypertensive right to left shunt at atrial, ventricular, or great artery level, i.e., reversed shunt through a pulmonary hypertensive atrial septal defect, ventricular septal defect, or patent ductus arteriosus? *Absence of pulmonary hypertension* (Table 9) necessarily implies obstruction to outflow into the pulmonary bed, i.e., normal or low pulmonary arterial pressure with high right ventricular pressure. In practical terms, the probabilities are two: pulmonic stenosis with right to left shunt at atrial or ventricular level, i.e., pulmonic stenosis with reversed flow through a foramen ovale or atrial septal defect, or through a ventricular septal defect (Fallot's tetralogy).

In dealing with the history, physical examination, electrocardiogram, x-ray, and diagnostic laboratories, it is worthwhile briefly to call attention to a few points especially appropriate to congenital heart disease. In the history, questions should include the pregnancy, for example, maternal exposure to teratogens such as rubella in the first trimester, or the altitude at which the patient was born. Maternal age may be important. Details of a cardiac murmur — the detection of which often heralds the diagnosis of congenital heart disease — should be precise regarding

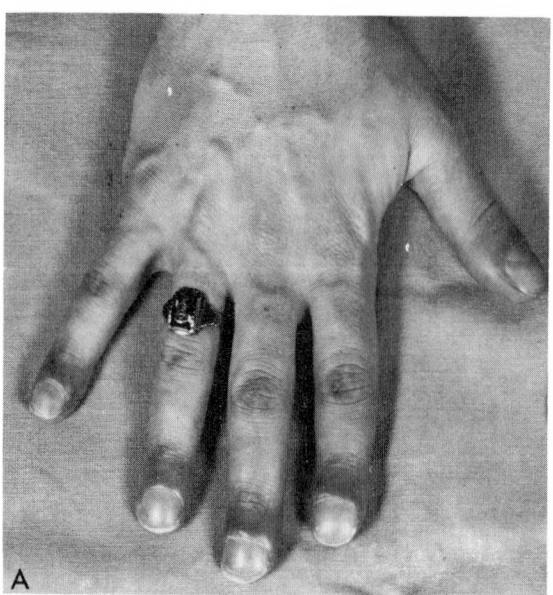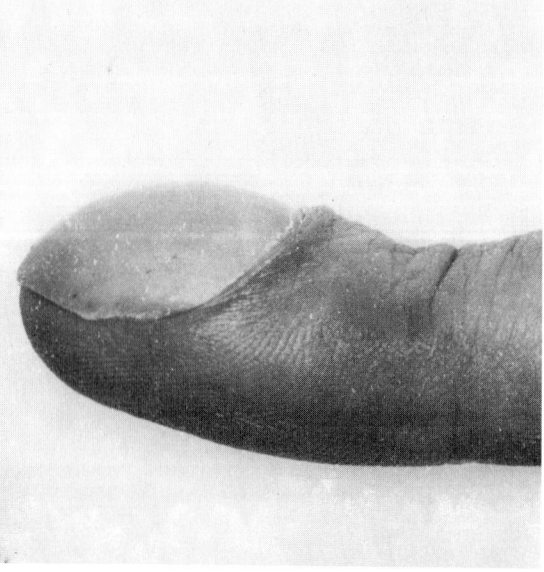

A, Hand of a cyanotic adult, showing the change in skin color of the distal phalanges. *B,* Profile of the index finger of another cyanotic adult, showing both a change in skin color and dramatic clubbing. (From Perloff, J. K.: The Clinical Recognition of Congenital Heart Disease. 2nd ed. Philadelphia, W. B. Saunders Company, 1978.)

onset and intensity. Was the murmur present at birth (newborn nursery), or was it first detected in early infancy, adolescence, or young adulthood? Was the murmur consistently and readily heard irrespective of patient cooperation (conspicuous murmur), or was it absent at times, difficult to hear, or believed to be unimportant? Was a new murmur ever commented upon (ventricular septal defect with subsequent aortic regurgitation)? Cyanosis should similarly be defined precisely according to time of onset, degree, and distribution. A history of squatting in a cyanotic patient typically applies to Fallot's tetralogy. Patterns of growth and development should be established. It is worth recalling that the clinical manifestations of congestive heart failure differ in infants, older children, and adults. Family history of congenital cardiac disease may shed light on the defect in the patient, especially if kinship is close. Susceptibility to lower respiratory infections suggests large left to right shunts. Neck pulsations (arterial or venous) may provide useful clues. A history of infective endocarditis calls attention to a relatively limited number of susceptible defects.

Physical appearance should apply to the presence of certain *somatic* congenital defects that are associated with specific types of congenital *cardiac* anomalies, such as *mongolism* (endocardial cushion defect), *Turner's syndrome* (coarctation of the aorta), *peculiar facies and dentition* associated with supravalvular aortic stenosis and pulmonary artery stenosis, the *Holt–Oram syndrome* (defects in the atrial septum), the *Ellis–van Creveld syndrome* (common atrium), or trisomy 18 (double outlet right ventricle).

The arterial pulses should be compared in the upper and lower extremities (coarctation of the aorta), but the brachials should also be palpated (cyanotic male infant with absent brachials and present femorals may mean aortic atresia). Right and left systemic arterial pulses should be compared (increased pulse pressure in the right carotid and brachial arteries in supravalvular aortic stenosis). The jugular venous pulse deserves special attention as soon as the patient is old enough to permit such observation (the short neck of the infant usually makes examination difficult or impossible). Percussion is useful in establishing visceral positions (cardiac and hepatic dullness and gastric tympany) to avoid missing a congenital positional anomaly. Palpation should carefully define each precordial movement according to chamber or great artery of origin, avoiding vague, meaningless terms such as "point of maximum impulse." During auscultation, designations such as "pulmonary area, aortic area, or mitral area" should be avoided, because they assume normal topographical anatomy of the heart, i.e., situs solitus without transposition of the great arteries and without ventricular inversion, assumptions which cannot be made, especially in the context of congenital heart disease. Simple descriptive terms should be used, such as apex, left or right lower, mid or upper sternal border, and the like. Murmurs should be precisely characterized, especially their timing in the cardiac cycle, with systolic murmurs classified as early, mid, late or holosystolic; diastolic murmurs as early diastolic, mid-diastolic or presystolic; and the continuous murmur defined as one that begins in systole and continues without interruption through the second heart sound into all or part of diastole.

The 12-lead surface electrocardiogram should be supplemented by leads V_3R and V_4R, and a vectorcardiogram is often necessary to clarify complex electrocardiograms.

Technically satisfactory plain films of the chest in the posteroanterior, lateral, right and left oblique positions have for all practical purposes replaced cardiac fluoroscopy except for the detection of intracardiac calcium. *Echocardiography* is a valuable source of diagnostic information and can be repeated without discomfort or risk. Cardiac catheterization and angiocardiography should be an extension of clinical judgment, a judgment which should decide not only when and which patients should be selected for study, but also which type of investigation is most appropriate for a given subject. Accurate diagnosis depends upon synthesis of the broad range of clinical data with the results of carefully planned and well-executed laboratory studies.

SCOPE OF THESE CHAPTERS. Survival in congenital heart disease results from natural selection or from surgical intervention. Ch. 359.2 to 359.5 will emphasize defects with a natural tendency to survive beyond the pediatric age group. Such emphasis is appropriate for a textbook of medicine. It must be stated, however, that congenital cardiac disease is a continuum from birth to adult life and that the only way to understand the patterns of postpediatric survival is to have dealt at some point with the same disorders in the infant and young child. The following categories will be considered: (1) *common* congenital cardiac defects in which postpediatric survival is expected; (2) *uncommon* congenital cardiac defects in which postpediatric survival is expected; (3) *common* congenital cardiac defects in which postpediatric survival is exceptional; and (4) *uncommon* congenital cardiac defects in which postpediatric survival is exceptional. Congenital cardiac anomalies (common or uncommon) in which postpediatric survival is unknown will not be considered. Chief emphasis will be placed on the common or uncommon anomalies with *expected* postpediatric survival. The common or uncommon defects with exceptional postpediatric survival will be touched upon more briefly to provide necessary perspective. It should be borne in mind, however, that as time goes on more and more congenital cardiacs beyond the pediatric age group will be postoperative; this is only as it should be.

359.2. COMMON CONGENITAL CARDIAC DEFECTS IN WHICH POSTPEDIATRIC SURVIVAL IS EXPECTED

FUNCTIONALLY NORMAL BICUSPID AORTIC VALVE

The frequency of congenitally bicuspid aortic valves — functionally normal, stenotic, and/or incompetent — may approach 2 per cent of the population. If this figure is correct, it means that the bicuspid aortic valve is not only the most frequent congenital anomaly of the heart or great vessels, but that the most common congenital cardiac defect in man manifests itself in the *postpediatric population*. The typical bicuspid aortic valve consists of two commissures and two cusps. One cusp, generally the larger, contains a low ridge or raphe ("false commissure"), adjacent to the aortic wall but not reaching the edge of the leaflet. If the free edges of a congenital bicuspid aortic valve are sufficiently redundant to permit unimpeded forward flow (no systolic gradient) yet not redundant enough to cause malapposition in diastole (little or no aortic regurgitation), then the bicuspid aortic valve is said to be "functionally normal." The natural history of such a valve is variable. A bicuspid aortic valve that functions normally at birth may continue to do so throughout life and be found incidentally at necropsy in late adult life. However, the same valve may take three unfavorable courses. The first is the tendency to become thickened, fibrotic, calcified, and stenotic during early or mid-adulthood. Second, infective endocarditis may convert a functionally benign lesion into the catastrophic mechanical fault of acute severe aortic regurgitation. Third, the larger of the two cusps may progressively evert or prolapse, causing progressive aortic regurgitation that ultimately can be severe. It is not yet known what determines which of these courses a given functionally normal congenitally bicuspid valve will take.

A functionally normal bicuspid aortic valve can be suspected clinically especially in teenagers and young adults. Innocent systolic murmurs in this age group, except for infraclavicular radiation of the innocent brachiocephalic systolic murmur, are not maximally heard at the right base. Accordingly, a short, somewhat impure Grade I to II midsystolic murmur loudest at the right base in a child, adolescent, or young adult is suspect. If that murmur is introduced by an ejection sound and if careful auscultation detects the soft murmur of aortic regurgitation, the clinical diagnosis reaches a high degree of probability. Physical interventions that increase aortic pressure (squatting, isometric exercise with clenched fists) increase audibility of faint murmurs of aortic regurgitation. Suspicion is always greater in males, because the congenital bicuspid aortic valve, whether functionally normal or not, is predominantly a male disease. If clinical suspicion is high, an argument can be made for verification by thoracic aortography, because the bicuspid aortic valve is highly susceptible to infective endocarditis and appropriate antimicrobial prophylaxis must be recommended. However, the simplest means of verification is echocardiography.

CONGENITAL VALVULAR AORTIC STENOSIS

Congenital obstruction to left ventricular outflow can be *valvular*, *subvalvular*, or *supravalvular*. The most common type is valvular and, in the adult, is usually characterized by narrowing of a bicuspid valve which can be intrinsically stenotic from birth or, more typically, becomes stenotic after progressive thickening and calcification (see above). Unicommissural unicuspid aortic valves are relatively frequent causes of intrinsically stenotic aortic valves at birth but, like the congenital bicuspid valve, sometimes exhibit delayed obstruction owing to thickening and rigidity.

Congenital valvular aortic stenosis is much more prevalent in males, with a sex ratio approximating 4 or 5:1. If the obstruction is present at birth, the murmur is likely to date from the newborn nursery. On the other hand, the functionally normal congenital bicuspid aortic valve is usually undetected in infancy or childhood, but may subsequently generate the prominent murmur of aortic stenosis in the second, third, or fourth decade. Angina and effort syncope arouse suspicion of aortic stenosis in acyanotic young patients with a history of

dyspnea, fatigue, and a prominent cardiac murmur dating from infancy or a murmur appearing in the second, third, or fourth decade. Cerebral symptoms can be subtle, consisting of nothing more than mild giddiness or lightheadedness, especially with effort. On the other hand, recurrent syncope is dangerous and heralds sudden death even in childhood or adolescence. Inappropriate sweating sometimes occurs and increases with the advent of cardiac failure. Infective endocarditis is a serious complication of congenital valvular aortic stenosis; all varieties are susceptible. The pulse pressure is small, and is accompanied by a slow rate of rise, a sustained peak, and a gentle collapse when obstruction is severe.

Precordial palpation reveals a left ventricular impulse that varies from normal (mild stenosis) to the strong, sustained heaving movement characterizing the hypertrophied left ventricle of severe obstruction. Presystolic distention of the left ventricle implies increased force of left atrial contraction, and is good evidence in young adults that the obstruction is significant. The thrill of aortic stenosis may be trivial or absent with mild obstruction, or with severe obstruction and advanced heart failure. The typical aortic stenotic thrill radiates upward and to the right, is maximal in the second right interspace, and is readily detected in the suprasternal notch and over both carotids. In some patients the thrill is confined to the apex or, if the heart is small, to the lower left sternal edge where the atypical location can be misleading. In addition to the thrill, the sharp impact of an ejection sound can often be palpated at the apex in congenital valvular aortic stenosis.

An ejection sound is a characteristic although not invariable feature. The sound is caused by abrupt upward movement of the dome-shaped or truncated congenitally stenotic valve and implies good valve motion. In adults calcification may impair valve mobility so that the ejection sound diminishes or vanishes. The aortic stenotic murmur begins after the first sound (or with the ejection sound), rises in a crescendo to a systolic peak, and declines in a decresendo to end before the aortic component of the second sound. The quality at the right base is harsh, rough, and grunting, especially when loud. Although configuration, length, and loudness do not necessarily relate to the degree of stenosis, the longer and louder the murmur and the later its systolic peak, the greater the likelihood of severe obstruction. However, an unimpressive midsystolic murmur — or none at all — may occur in severe aortic stenosis with advanced heart failure or in adults with increased anteroposterior chest dimensions. The right basal location and radiation of the murmur of valvular aortic stenosis are related to the upward and rightward direction of the high velocity jet within the ascending aorta. The second heart sound should be judged with regard to the intensity of the aortic component and the presence, degree, and type of splitting. In congenital valvular aortic stenosis with mobile valve, the aortic component of the second sound is well preserved even in the presence of appreciable obstruction. Prominent inspiratory splitting usually (but not invariably) means mild obstruction, because the duration of left ventricular ejection is not prolonged. *Paradoxical* splitting is a sign of severe obstruction and generally indicates that the duration of left ventricular ejection is appreciably prolonged. However, the majority of patients with aortic stenosis exhibit a second sound that is single or closely split through a wide range of severity.

A soft murmur of aortic regurgitation may be heard with congenital valvular aortic stenosis but is more common with discrete subvalvular obstruction because of cusp distortion (see below). A fourth heart sound in aortic stenosis is the acoustic counterpart of presystolic distention of the left ventricle and is likely to mean appreciable obstruction. However, after age 40, the fourth heart sound is not a reliable sign of severity, because there is an age-related incidence.

Electrocardiographic estimates of severity should be made with caution; mild valvular aortic stenosis sometimes occurs with left ventricular hypertrophy, and severe obstruction occasionally exists with a normal electrocardiogram. Sudden death may occur in patients with severe congenital aortic stenosis and normal electrocardiograms. Although these points must be borne in mind, they should not obscure the value of the scalar tracing. The best electrocardiographic index of appreciable obstruction is the combination of both voltage and repolarization criteria for left ventricular hypertrophy, especially in preadolescent patients. In congenital valvular aortic stenosis the x-ray features are poststenotic dilatation of the aorta with a relatively convex, globular left ventricular contour. In adults, aortic calcification is presumptive evidence of valvular obstruction and must be sought with the aid of echocardiography and an image intensifier.

Despite considerable clinical sophistication, cardiac catheterization and angiocardiography are generally required to be precise about the morphologic type and severity of congenital valvular aortic stenosis. If clinical evidence strongly points to mild obstruction, diagnostic intervention may be deferred, the risk of postoperative endocarditis far exceeding the benefits of operation. When clinical findings point to severe obstruction, diagnostic investigation should precede selection for surgery. If valvular obstruction is severe and the patient is *asymptomatic*, surgical intervention depends in large part upon the morphologic type of obstruction. Direct repair may provide excellent results at low risk. Severe valvular aortic stenosis in the *symptomatic* patient — especially with angina or syncope but without significant congestive heart failure — requires surgical intervention even if this means valve replacement. In severe obstruction, the greater the left ventricular dysfunction, the smaller the gradient, the smaller the ejection fraction, the higher the surgical risk, and the poorer the results.

COARCTATION OF THE AORTA

The basic anatomic fault is a localized deformity of the media manifested by a curtain-like infolding that eccentrically narrows the aortic lumen. The zone of coarctation is characteristically located distal to the origin of the left subclavian artery at or just beyond the insertion of the ligamentum arteriosum. Occasionally coarctation is situated at or just proximal to the left subclavian artery so that the orifice of that vessel is in the low pressure zone.

Nearly 25 per cent of patients with coarctation of the aorta have bicuspid aortic valves which may be functionally normal or may take one of the courses described above. The most important noncardiac anomaly is an aneurysm of the circle of Willis which may remain clinically silent or may announce itself by rupture.

Aortic coarctation predominates in males. After early infancy, patients are usually asymptomatic when the malformation is diagnosed. Serious symptoms are relatively uncommon before age 15 years, but it is uncommon for symptoms to be absent after age 30. The majority of patients live to adult life, but only a minority reach age 40, and only 10 per cent live beyond age 50. The longest survival was recorded in 1828 by Reynaud in his account of coarctation in a 92-year-old man. Discovery of systemic hypertension provides the initial suspicion unless the brachial and femoral pulses are palpated. A number of minor symptoms such as headache, spontaneous epistaxes, and leg fatigue sometimes occur. Major symptoms are related to four complications: congestive heart failure, rupture of the aorta or dissecting aneurysm, infective endocarditis or endarteritis, and cerebral hemorrhage. The incidence of cardiac failure is highest in early infancy or after the third decade and can develop in adults previously devoid of symptoms related to the malformation. Rupture of the aorta or dissecting aneurysm occurs most frequently in the 20's and 30's. The rupture originates either in the proximal ascending aorta or in a postcoarctation aneurysm. Infective endocarditis or endarteritis is most frequently implanted on the peculiarly susceptible bicuspid aortic valve; endarteritis at the site of coarctation occurs less frequently. Cerebral hemorrhage, the fourth major complication, is usually due to rupture of an aneurysm of the circle of Willis. In the pregnant female with coarctation, blood pressure fluctuations are similar in direction to those of uncomplicated pregnancy. The incidence of toxemia is lower in women with coarctation than in pregnant women with other forms of hypertension; intracranial hemorrhage is not more likely to occur, and cardiac failure seldom develops. However, pregnancy does increase the risk of rupture of the aorta, especially at the end of the third trimester. Furthermore, the bacteremia that may accompany labor and delivery can cause endocarditis or endarteritis.

The physique in coarctation is at times impressive; an athletic appearance of the chest and shoulders contrasts with narrow hips and thin legs. Coarctation of the aorta is sometimes suspected because of the characteristic physical appearance of *Turner's syndrome*, namely, a female with short stature, webbing of the neck, absent or scanty pubic and axillary hair, wide-set nipples, low hairline, small chin, and wide carrying angle of the arms.

Abnormal differences in upper and lower extremity arterial pulses are the clinical hallmarks of coarctation of the aorta. Diagnostic differences in arm and leg blood pressures should be based upon systolic and not diastolic levels. These pressure differences between arm and leg are exaggerated by exercise, which can therefore be a useful adjunct in confirming mild coarctation. The level of upper extremity blood pressure must be interpreted according to the patient's age. A blood pressure that is normal in an adult may be hypertensive in a child. As patients with coarctation grow older, the systolic pressure rises relatively more than the diastolic, so the pulse pressure increases. Such patients exhibit conspicuous, forceful carotid and suprasternal pulsations resembling aortic regurgitation, which may coexist. In addition, the subclavian arteries can sometimes be seen pulsating below the clavicles. Collateral arteries, even when abundant, are seldom obvious and must be specifically sought by having the patient stand and bend forward with the arms hanging at the sides. The examiner inspects the back, particularly around and between the scapulae, using a tangential light source to expose the subcutaneous collaterals in shadowed relief. The retinal arteries may be tortuous and narrowed, but hypertensive retinopathy is rare.

The right and left brachial arteries should be simultaneously compared by palpation and blood pressure determination. An absent or relatively small left brachial pulse means that the coarctation is at or just proximal to the left subclavian artery. In aortic stenosis with coarctation, the brachial arterial pulse (and pressure) may be relatively normal rather than hypertensive, whereas the femoral pulses are diminished or absent. Conversely, aortic regurgitation increases the femoral pulse, especially in mild coarctation, so the clinical diagnosis of the combined defects may be obscured.

Precordial palpation detects a left ventricular impulse that varies from normal to the sustained heaving impulse of ventricular hypertrophy. A dilated ascending aorta can cause a visible and palpable systolic impulse at the right base. Suprasternal thrills are relatively frequent in uncomplicated coarctation, but precordial thrills are seldom present without coexisting aortic stenosis.

An aortic ejection sound increases suspicion of coexisting bicuspid aortic valve, although the sound may arise in the dilated aortic root. Coarctation of the aorta is associated with systolic, diastolic, or continuous murmurs. Systolic murmurs originate from arterial collaterals, the coarctation itself, and the bicuspid aortic valve. Collateral systolic murmurs are distributed widely over the thorax. There is a tendency for these murmurs to be especially conspicuous along the left sternal border (the left internal mammary artery). Collateral murmurs are crescendo-decrescendo in shape and delayed in onset because of origin in arteries distant from the heart. The coarctation itself is responsible for a localized midline posterior murmur, the level of which is related to the site of aortic constriction. With mild coarctation, the posterior systolic murmur is relatively short; as the degree of obstruction increases, the murmur gets longer and may extend well into diastole, becoming "continuous." The most common *diastolic* murmur is aortic regurgitation, a useful sign of bicuspid aortic valve.

Isolated *right* ventricular hypertrophy is for all practical purposes confined to infants in the first six months of life with heart failure and reactive pulmonary hypertension. In uncomplicated coarctation, left ventricular hypertrophy is manifested by both voltage and repolarization criteria. However, prominent S-T segment depressions with deeply inverted T waves seldom occur with uncomplicated coarctation and suggest coexisting aortic stenosis.

The x-ray provides considerable information regarding both the diagnosis and the anatomic variations of coarctation of the aorta. Notching of the ribs results from collateral flow through dilated, tortuous, pulsatile *posterior* intercostal arteries. The notches typically appear as irregular, scalloped areas on the undersurfaces of the posterior ribs. The *anterior* ribs are spared be-

cause the anterior intercostal arteries do not run in costal grooves. Notching seldom appears before six or seven years. When the coarctation is located *proximal* to the left subclavian artery, collateral circulation fails to develop on the left side; *unilateral* notching appears in the *right* posterior ribs. In older children or adults, the lateral x-ray may show *retrosternal* scalloping caused by dilated tortuous internal mammary arteries. In classic coarctation of the aortic isthmus, the hypertensive ascending aorta is dilated. Aortic dilatation *distal* to the zone of coarctation (poststenotic enlargement) produces a recognizable leftward convexity of the descending thoracic aorta. When this sign is accompanied by the convex shadow of a dilated left subclavian artery, the two convexities form a typical "figure 3" in the frontal projection.

Cardiac catheterization and angiocardiography define the anatomic features of coarctation, including the collateral circulation, but as a rule they are not necessary for a secure clinical diagnosis upon which a therapeutic decision can be based. If there is clinical suspicion of coexisting bicuspid aortic valve, the inclination to perform thoracic aortography is increased, because confirmation gives insight into the postoperative natural course and the need for continued prophylaxis for infective endocarditis. The presence of all but mild coarctation warrants consideration for surgical repair. It is still the consensus that optimal age for correction awaits the seventh year. On the other hand, selection of patients for elective repair at earlier ages has been liberalized, because subsequent recurrence of coarctation has been shown to be negligible even when correction is done in early childhood. In fact primary repair in small infants with persistent heart failure is now selectively and successfully accomplished. In older patients, risk of technical complications during surgery increases. Irrespective of the quality of the repair, the risk of infective endocarditis on a coexisting bicuspid aortic valve is not diminished, and we do not know whether the risk of intracranial hemorrhage (berry aneurysm) is affected. Although the incidence of heart failure continues to rise during the fourth decade in unoperated coarctation, after age 40 there appears to be an even chance of death from incidental causes. In those surviving to this age, the efficacy of correction becomes debatable. Furthermore, long-term analyses of patients after surgical correction of coarctation of the aorta have revealed a high incidence of premature cardiovascular disease despite adequate operation. Particularly disturbing in this regard are the data on unexplained late postoperative hypertension.

PULMONIC STENOSIS

Congenital obstruction to right ventricular outflow can be valvular, subvalvular, or supravalvular. *Valvular* pulmonic stenosis, the most common variety, is characterized by a conical or dome-shaped valve with a narrow outlet at its apex. Three raphes extend from the small central opening to the wall of the pulmonary artery, although separate leaflets cannot be identified. Males and females are equally affected. Rarely, valvular pulmonic stenosis is caused by myxomatous dysplasia of the valve.

The functional consequences of valvular pulmonic

stenosis are related to the resistance to right ventricular outflow. Early discovery of the murmur is the rule, because the anatomic and physiologic conditions necessary for its production are present at birth. Survival into adulthood is relatively common. The tendency for the valve to grow in proportion to body size may in part account for this. However, with advancing age fibrous thickening and even calcification may reduce valve mobility and increase the degree of obstruction.

Familial occurrence is not a feature of ordinary valvular pulmonic stenosis. However, in congenital pulmonic stenosis caused by dysplasia of the valve, some relatives may have pulmonary valve dysplasia and others typical dome-shaped valvular pulmonic stenosis.

Subjective complaints tend to increase with age, although equivalent degrees of stenosis may handicap one patient in childhood yet leave another relatively unlimited in the fourth decade. An appreciable number of patients with moderate to severe stenosis are virtually symptom free well into the postpediatric age group. Dyspnea and fatigue are the most common symptoms. These complaints tend to remain absent as long as the right ventricle can maintain a normal stroke volume at rest and augment its output with effort. Right ventricular failure is the single most common natural cause of death. Patients with valvular pulmonic stenosis sometimes experience giddiness, lightheadedness, or frank syncope, especially with effort. Children as well as adults occasionally have chest pain resembling myocardial ischemia. Some patients with severe pulmonic stenosis are subjectively aware of giant A waves in the jugular venous pulse, especially during effort or excitement. The stenotic valve is susceptible to infective endocarditis.

Infants with typical valvular pulmonic stenosis may appear remarkably healthy, with good fat deposits and chubby round faces. Even older patients may have faces that are wide, full, or even bloated, with highly colored cheeks. Males or females with many of the phenotypic features of Turner's syndrome but normal chromosomal complements (46XX or XY) tend to have valvular pulmonic stenosis. *Myxomatous dysplasia* of the pulmonic valve may be associated with slow body growth and abnormal facies (triangular face with hypertelorism, ptosis of the eyelids, and low-set ears).

The jugular venous pulse exhibits an A wave that gets progressively larger as the degree of obstruction increases. Exercise and excitement augment these A waves. In addition, powerful right atrial contraction may be associated with presystolic pulsation of the liver. An increase in the height of the V wave occurs with the advent of right ventricular failure and tricuspid regurgitation.

Thrills mirror the location and intensity of accompanying murmurs (see below). In valvular pulmonic stenosis, the thrill is maximal in the second or occasionally third left interspace, radiating upward and toward the left, because the intrapulmonary jet is directed toward the left pulmonary artery. A right ventricular systolic impulse is an important physical sign of pulmonic stenosis and, when absent, casts doubt on the diagnosis. The location of the parasternal right ventricular impulse can sometimes be related to the level of obstruction, because the transmitted systolic movements originate in the high-pressure zone proximal to the level of stenosis. Presystolic distention of the right ventricle is caused by forceful contraction of the right atrium and is typically accompanied by a large jugular venous A wave.

An ejection sound is a characteristic feature of valvular pulmonic stenosis and is important in identifying this form of obstruction. The pulmonic ejection sound is high pitched, sharp or clicking, and maximal in the second left interspace, often selectively decreasing during inspiration. An ejection sound is not present in valvular pulmonic stenosis caused by myxomatous dysplasia or in the rare adult with a calcified pulmonic valve.

The systolic murmur of typical valvular pulmonic stenosis is maximal in the second left interspace, although it may be just as loud in the third. The lower location may be related to secondary subvalvular hypertrophy. The murmur, like the thrill, radiates upward and to the left, and when loud may be heard in the suprasternal notch and at the base of the neck, especially on the left. Loudness per se is not necessarily an index of severity, although as a rule intensity tends to vary directly with the degree of obstruction. However, the magnitude of stenosis is the major determinant of the *duration* of right ventricular ejection which, in turn, determines the *length* of the systolic murmur. A soft, symmetrical murmur, peaking in midsystole, is a feature of mild pulmonic stenosis; whereas a loud murmur, peaking late in systole and extending well beyond aortic closure, is a feature of severe obstruction.

The intensity of the pulmonic component of the second sound varies from normal to inaudible as severity increases. However, the *timing* of the pulmonic component is more important than intensity in assessing severity. A relatively slight increase in expiratory splitting, with normal intensity of the pulmonic component, is evidence of mild stenosis, whereas a marked increase in splitting with a faint or absent pulmonic component is evidence of severe obstruction.

The electrocardiogram commonly shows tall, peaked P waves. The QRS axis in the frontal plane shifts to the right, the degree of right axis deviation tending to vary directly with right ventricular pressure. The severity of pulmonic stenosis corresponds fairly well to the R/S ratios in V_1 and V_6 and to the height of the R wave in V_1. In mild pulmonic stenosis an rSr' pattern in V_1 is sometimes difficult to distinguish from normal. In severe pulmonic stenosis, leads V_1 and V_3R exhibit tall monophasic R waves, and lead V_6 shows an rS pattern. Between these extremes all gradations exist. In severe pulmonic stenosis, deeply inverted T waves that curve upward on the downstroke and that extend beyond V_2 are typical and assume greater significance when accompanied by ST segment depressions. Upright T waves occur with increased right ventricular pressure in young children, and upright T waves in the right precordium are the only electrocardiographic signs of right ventricular hypertension in some children with mild pulmonic stenosis.

The x-ray evaluation of valvular pulmonic stenosis should concentrate on (1) the peripheral intrapulmonary) vascular pattern, (2) the main pulmonary artery and its branches, and (3) the size and contour of the right ventricle and right atrium. The peripheral pulmonary vascular pattern is normal even in severe valvular stenosis until the output of the right ventricle falls. Poststenotic dilatation of the pulmonary trunk is characteristic and is often accompanied by conspicuous enlargement of the left branch. Calcification of the congenitally stenosed pulmonary valve is rare and confined to adult survivors. The left anterior oblique view is best for defining the right ventricular contour, whereas a prominent right atrial sweep may be seen in the posteroanterior projection. A conspicuous increase in right heart size is almost always a sign of severity, especially at an early age. Cardiac catheterization and angiocardiography permit definitive diagnosis of the level, morphologic type, and severity of obstruction to right ventricular outflow. However, patients with mild valvular pulmonic stenosis can be identified with such clinical confidence that invasive diagnostic investigation is generally not required. But in this group, clinical distinction from idiopathic dilatation of the pulmonary trunk may be difficult or impossible.

In typical valvular pulmonic stenosis, surgical repair is probably indicated for patients with resting gradients of 50 mm Hg or more, although a single determination may be misleading, because gradients vary considerably with cardiac output (transvalvular flow). The risk of operative repair in valvular pulmonic stenosis is low, and results are excellent. Postoperative pulmonary regurgitation often occurs, but as a rule it is mild and functionally unimportant. In severe valvular pulmonic stenosis, secondary hypertrophic subpulmonic stenosis may require resection. This intervention should not be taken lightly, because right ventriculotomy is necessary, although repair via the tricuspid valve is feasible.

ATRIAL SEPTAL DEFECT

Atrial defects are designated according to their sites in the septum: (1) in the region of the fossa ovalis (ostium secundum), (2) between the fossa and the inferior vena cava, (3) in the upper part of the septum (sinus venosus), (4) in the lower part of the septum (ostium primum), and (5) in the position normally occupied by the coronary sinus. The most common variety that will be dealt with here is referred to as *ostium secundum defect*.

The physiologic consequences of an atrial septal defect depend chiefly upon the magnitude and duration of the shunt, the adaptive response of the volume-loaded right ventricle, and the behavior of the pulmonary vascular bed. Two mechanisms have been proposed to explain left to right shunting. First, in infancy the right and left ventricles have similar distensibility characteristics and hence should have similar end-diastolic volumes. As pulmonary vascular resistance falls in the neonatal period, the right ventricle ejects into a low resistance bed and would be expected to have a larger ejection fraction than the left. During the subsequent diastole the volume received by the right ventricle would increase, and a left to right shunt would therefore be established. Second, as the pulmonary arterioles involute, the relatively thick-walled neonatal right ventricle becomes thinner and offers less resistance to filling than the left. Conditions become appropriate for augmenting flow from left atrium across the defect. The left to right shunt occurs in the presence of low pulmonary vascular resistance *and* normal pulmonary arterial pressure. This may in part explain the relative infrequency of subsequent pulmonary hypertension in young people with atrial septal defect. Pul-

monary hypertension is rare in infants and children with uncomplicated atrial septal defects and does not reach its peak incidence of about 14 per cent until early adult life.

In ostium secundum atrial septal defect the female-to-male ratio ranges from 2 to 3.5:1. Family history is important, because these defects not only can be familial, but also may recur through a number of generations.

Atrial septal defects often go unrecognized for years, because symptoms may be trivial or absent and physical signs subtle. The relatively soft pulmonic midsystolic murmur is easily overlooked in restless or crying children and may be mistaken for an innocent murmur in both children and young adults. In apparently healthy normal adults, atrial septal defect is often first suspected because of a routine chest x-ray. Life expectancy is shortened, although adult survival is the rule, and some patients live to an advanced age. Survival is more limited in young adults who develop pulmonary hypertension, but even in them the span of life generally averages more than 40 years. It is not rare to find atrial septal defects beyond age 70 years. Death may be unrelated to the defect, but when a relationship exists, cardiac failure is the most common natural cause. Since the natural history of uncomplicated ostium secundum atrial septal defect spans the childbearing age and since the majority of such patients are female, it is noteworthy that pregnancy is usually well tolerated. After the third or fouth decade, complications arise, and practically all patients who survive to the sixth decade are symptomatic. Effort dyspnea and fatigue are most frequent. Older patients with large left to right shunt atrial septal defects may experience not only effort dyspnea but also orthopnea. In the presence of decreased lung compliance caused by longstanding large left to right shunts, the work of breathing is greater in the supine than in the sitting position.

Infective endocarditis is rare in isolated ostium secundum atrial septal defect, a rarity attributed to the absence of jet lesions or turbulence because of the low velocity diastolic shunt.

Older patients with ostium secundum atrial septal defects deteriorate chiefly on three accounts. First, degenerative diseases such as coronary artery disease or systemic hypertension cause the left ventricle to become less distensible, so a larger volume of left atrial blood preferentially flows across the defect, adding to the work of an already overloaded right ventricle. The second problem is a rise in pulmonary arterial pressure in the face of a persistent large left to right shunt. The third concern is the advent of atrial arrhythmias — fibrillation, flutter, or paroxysmal atrial tachycardia. After the fourth decade atrial arrhythmias increase in frequency and represent one of the most serious complications.

Physical appearance of adults with ostium secundum atrial septal defect is generally normal, but children often exhibit a delicate, frail, or gracile habitus, with weight affected more than height. A left precordial bulge is common and is often associated with Harrison's grooves. A distinctive appearance that heightens suspicion of an ostium secundum atrial septal defect is the *Holt-Oram syndrome*. The thumb is hypoplastic, with an accessory phalanx that gives it a "crooked" appearance. Apposition of the thumb with other digits is difficult, and in some cases the thumb is rudimentary or absent.

The jugular venous pulse in ostium secundum atrial septal defect may show A and V waves of equal heights, because the two atria are in free communication. Pulmonary hypertension results in an increased force of right atrial contraction and a dominant A wave which may reach giant proportions.

Precordial movement and palpation characteristically detect a right ventricular impulse that is hyperdynamic, even tumultuous, and relatively brief in duration. This pattern occurs because the left to right shunt distends the right ventricle in diastole, and the chamber then contracts vigorously into a low resistance pulmonary bed. The dilated pulmonary trunk is often palpated in the second left interspace. A systolic thrill at that site indicates either a very large shunt or coexisting valvular pulmonic stenosis. In the presence of pulmonary hypertension, the right ventricular impulse becomes sustained and less dynamic, and presystolic distention may result from an increased force of right atrial contraction.

The "first heart sound" at the left sternal edge and apex may be split and the *second component* relatively loud. It has been variously proposed that the loud second component originates from the tricuspid valve or represents a pulmonic ejection sound. The location and lack of selective attenuation with inspiration favor the former, although the two mechanisms may coexist. The typical murmur accompanying atrial septal defect results from rapid ejection of a large right ventricular stroke volume into a dilated pulmonary trunk. The murmur is usually Grade 3 or less, maximal in the second left intercostal space, beginning after the first heart sound, crescendo-decresendo in shape, peaking in early or midsystole, and ending well before both components of the second heart sound. The septal defect itself is, with rare exception, acoustically silent. A murmur exceeding Grade 3 is likely to mean an unusually large shunt or associated valvular pulmonic stenosis. In slightly built patients, widely distributed thoracic systolic murmurs can sometimes be heard in the right chest, axilla, and back because of rapid flow through peripheral pulmonary arteries in low resistance, high-flow atrial septal defects.

A hallmark of atrial septal defect is the behavior of the second heart sound. The aortic and pulmonic components are widely and persistently split and exhibit little or no change in the degree of splitting with respiration or Valsalva maneuver. The relative loudness of the two components is usually normal, although at times the second component is increased despite little or no pulmonary hypertension. Proximity of the dilated pulmonary trunk to the chest wall and the brisk elastic recoil of the distended pulmonary trunk may account for this.

Two types of diastolic murmurs occur in atrial septal defect with left to right shunt. One is mid-diastolic and is caused by torrential flow across the tricuspid valve, indicating a sizable left to right shunt. The second diastolic murmur is rare and is due to pulmonary regurgitation in the absence of pulmonary hypertension; a very large pulmonary trunk is probably responsible.

Auscultatory signs in atrial septal defect with pulmonary hypertension differ from the foregoing. The pulmonic midsystolic flow murmur is replaced by a softer, shorter midsystolic murmur caused by ejection of a normal stroke volume into a dilated pulmonary trunk. Tricuspid flow murmurs vanish. Typical pulmonic ejec-

tion sounds appear, especially in the second left interspace, and exhibit characteristic respiratory variation (selective decrease with inspiration). The pulmonic component of the second heart sound becomes progressively louder, although fixed splitting persists as long as a significant left to right shunt exists. With abolition or reversal of the shunt, the pulmonic component becomes very loud, and the wide fixed split disappears. A *Graham Steell murmur* may develop. The holosystolic murmur of tricuspid regurgitation appears when the pressure load of pulmonary hypertension results in right ventricular failure. Since the right ventricle occupies the cardiac apex in atrial septal defect, the tricuspid murmur is heard at that site and can be mistaken for the murmur of mitral regurgitation.

After the third decade *atrial arrhythmias* increase, especially atrial fibrillation, but atrial flutter and paroxysmal atrial tachycardia also occur. When right atrial P waves are present, they generally manifest themselves by peaking in lead II rather than by an increase in amplitude. The QRS duration is usually upper limits of normal with a tendency to prolong with age. As QRS duration increases, the pattern resembles complete right bundle branch block, but this rarely develops before the fourth decade. Depolarization is typically clockwise, with q waves in inferior leads and a vertical QRS axis. These electrical directions are important, because they distinguish ostium secundum from ostium primum defects in which the axis is directed upward and to the left and depolarization is counterclockwise (see below).

An electrocardiographic sign of atrial septal defect is the rSr' complex in right precordial leads. This feature is believed to stem from delayed activation of the crista supraventricularis, depolarization of which causes the terminal electrical forces to be directed superiorly, to the right, and anteriorly. These terminal force patterns do not result from interference of electrical impulses through the proximal right bundle branch. In fact, the sequence of ventricular activation is normal, so the term "incomplete right bundle branch block" is inappropriate. With the advent of pulmonary hypertension, the right ventricular free wall thickens and lead V_1 exhibits an increase in the amplitude of the R' wave together with a gradual decrease in the depth of the S wave.

The *chest x-ray*, especially in postadolescents and adults, is often distinctive. The lung fields show increased pulmonary arterial vascularity that generally extends to the periphery. The combination of a small aorta and a markedly dilated pulmonary trunk with disproportionate enlargement of the right branch can be striking. With the advent of pulmonary hypertension, peripheral pulmonary vascularity is replaced by relatively clear lung fields, the pulmonary trunk and its proximal branches get still larger, and the right branch presents as a huge inverted comma with an abrupt cutoff that makes the contrast between large central vessels and clear lung field stand out in bold relief. In an occasional older subject, the main pulmonary artery and its branches dilate aneurysmally and calcify.

Right atrial enlargement is ordinarily seen as a rightward convexity in the posteroanterior projection. Although radiographic signs of left atrial enlargement are occasionally found in adults, this is rarely so in children. Dilatation of the right ventricle is an expected feature, resulting in a convex lifted apex that usually forms an acute angle with the diaphragm. Dilatation of the outflow tract sometimes causes relatively smooth continuity or even a hump-shaped appearance below the enlarged pulmonary trunk. In the left oblique projection the right ventricle casts a rather typical convex anterior shadow.

Although uncomplicated ostium secundum atrial septal defect in the young is among the most easily diagnosed congenital malformations of the heart, the same anomaly may be misleading in some adults. Mitral stenosis with pulmonary hypertension comes under suspicion because of dyspnea, orthopnea, atrial fibrillation, an increased V wave in the jugular venous pulse, a right ventricular impulse, a loud first heart sound, a delayed pulmonic component of the second sound that is mistaken for an opening snap, a tricuspid flow murmur mistaken for a mitral diastolic murmur, vascular peripheral lung fields believed to represent pulmonary venous congestion, and a cardiac silhouette that exhibits dilatation of the pulmonary trunk and occasionally of both right and left atria. Similarly, mitral regurgitation may be suspected because the holosystolic murmur of tricuspid regurgitation is heard at the apex which is occupied by the right ventricle. A delayed pulmonic component of the second sound followed by a tricuspid flow murmur may be mistaken for the opening snap and the mid-diastolic murmur of coexisting mitral stenosis. In older subjects, coronary artery disease, systemic hypertension, atrial arrhythmias, or inverted left precordial T waves may cloud the issue. A catalogue of these misleading clinical points makes impressive reading, but it is rare to be confronted with all of them at once. However, even when the entire clinical picture is considered, the correct diagnosis may remain uncertain, although clues generally emerge to provide the background for an intelligently planned laboratory study.

Echocardiography has been a major step forward in the noninvasive diagnosis of atrial septal defect, defining not only the expected large right ventricular dimensions but also paradoxical motion of the interventricular septum. Normally, the interventricular septum moves *away* from the anterior chest wall during systole, behaving as part of the left ventricle. In ostium secundum atrial septal defect (volume overload of the right ventricle), the septum moves *toward* the anterior chest wall in systole.

Cardiac catheterization is generally employed even in patients in whom the clinical diagnosis is not in doubt. Such an intervention provides precise preoperative quantitative data that set the stage for comparative postoperative assessment. In addition to quantification of the shunt and confirmation of intracardiac pressures, there are a number of other reasons why cardiac catheterization is undertaken. An attempt should be made to separate ostium secundum from sinus venosus atrial septal defects which clinically can be indistinguishable. Patients with pure ostium secundum atrial septal defects sometimes exhibit mitral leaflet prolapse. This movement can be detected by left ventricular angiography and echocardiography and need not be accompanied by auscultatory signs.

Patients with high flow, low resistance uncomplicated ostium secundum atrial septal defects (pulmonary to systemic flow ratios of 2:1 or more) should be electively repaired, optimally in childhood. At this age, surgical risk is minimal, and delay gives rise to concern over postoperative residua, especially regression of dilatation and hypertrophy of the right ventricle. There has been debate regarding surgical correction in older patients (beyond age 40), but current experience has shown that patients in the fifth, sixth, or even seventh decades with relatively low resistance–high flow ostium secundum atrial septal defects benefit from surgical repair which can be undertaken at comparatively low risk. What is still more encouraging is that older patients can be operated upon at an acceptable risk despite moderate pulmonary hypertension and cardiac failure, provided there is still a sizable left to right shunt. In patients of any age in whom pulmonary resistance has reached or exceeded systemic so that the left to right shunt has been abolished, operative repair is contraindicated.

PATENT DUCTUS ARTERIOSUS

Patent ductus arteriosus represents persistence of a normal fetal vascular channel between the pulmonary artery and the aorta. The pulmonary orifice of the ductus is located immediately to the left of the bifurcation of the pulmonary trunk. The aortic end of the duct usually arises just beyond the origin of the left subclavian artery. A patent ductus is apt to be largest at its aortic insertion, exhibiting the shape of a truncated cone, because the tendency to close begins at the pulmonary arterial end. The ductus arteriosus in full-term infants normally undergoes an initial stage of *functional* closure, followed by a later stage of *anatomic* closure. At the end of a week the ductus is generally no more than probe patent, and by four to eight weeks anatomic closure is usually established.

The physiologic consequences of persistent patency of the ductus arteriosus depend upon the size of the communication and the level of pulmonary vascular resistance. When the ductus is small, the pulmonary arterial pressure remains normal; the left to right shunt and hemodynamic burden are negligible despite continuous aortic to pulmonary flow. When the duct is large, aortic pressure is transmitted directly into the pulmonary trunk, so pulmonary hypertension exists with pressure overload of the right ventricle. Under these circumstances the direction of flow through the ductus depends upon the relative resistances in the pulmonary and systemic beds. If pulmonary resistance is appreciably lower than systemic, a sizable left to right shunt exists, with volume overload of the left heart and pressure overload of the right. If pulmonary resistance is appreciably higher than systemic, left to right flow through the ductus is abolished, leaving a pure right to left shunt and pure pressure overload of the right ventricle. The vast majority of patients with isolated patent ductus arteriosus, literally 95 per cent, have left to right shunts with pulmonary arterial pressures considerably below systemic. Only 5 to 7 per cent have very high pulmonary vascular resistances with exclusive right to left shunts.

For all practical purposes the history in patent ductus arteriosus does not begin at birth, because the diagnosis is usually not entertained in the newborn. The mother is likely to report that her infant was examined and pronounced normal. As the neonatal pulmonary vascular resistance falls, a left to right shunt is established, the ductus murmur emerges, and the diagnosis becomes apparent. Patent ductus arteriosus predominates in females, with a sex ratio as high as 3:1. The female preponderance is even greater in older patients with this anomaly. Family history is important, because patent ductus tends to recur in siblings. The prenatal history also deserves comment, especially regarding maternal rubella in the first trimester. Patent ductus arteriosus (together with pulmonary artery stenosis) is the most common congenital cardiac defect in the offspring of mothers who have had rubella in the first trimester. Birth weight in uncomplicated patent ductus is normal but in the rubella syndrome low birth rate is the rule, and there is failure to thrive even when the shunt is small and cardiac failure absent. Another interesting point in the history is the *altitude* at which the patient is born. It has been estimated that persistence of the ductus arteriosus is six times as frequent in patients born at high altitudes as in those born at sea level, and there is a tendency for such patients to develop pulmonary hypertension. The physical appearance in patent ductus may be characterized by underdevelopment owing to a large shunt, cardiac failure, and recurrent respiratory infections. In addition, maternal rubella results not only in patent ductus and low birth weights, but also in poor growth irrespective of the size of the duct. Differential cyanosis and clubbing occur when pulmonary vascular resistance exceeds systemic so that unoxygenated pulmonary arterial blood flows through the ductus and enters the aorta distal to the left subclavian artery; this unoxygenated blood goes to the lower extremities so that the toes are cyanotic and often clubbed.

A wide pulse pressure is an important physical sign of patent ductus with large left to right shunt. Diastolic flow from aortic root into pulmonary artery lowers the aortic diastolic pressure, whereas the large left ventricular stroke volume caused by the left to right shunt results in elevation of aortic systolic pressure.

Precordial impulses are normal with small patent ductus. A moderately large ductus causes isolated volume overload of the left heart; the left ventricular impulse is somewhat dynamic, the right ventricular impulse is unimpressive, and a continuous thrill with systolic accentuation is present in the first or second left intercostal space. A large ductus with appreciable left to right shunt results in marked volume overload of the left ventricle with pulmonary hypertension; the left ventricular impulse is hyperdynamic, and a heaving right ventricular impulse appears. If a thrill is present, it is more likely to be systolic. When flow through the ductus is reversed, pulmonary hypertension exists without volume overload of the left ventricle. Palpation detects right ventricular and pulmonary arterial impulses and a loud pulmonic component of the second sound, but the ductus thrill is absent and a left ventricular impulse is trivial or absent.

Auscultation is virtually diagnostic when the classic murmur of uncomplicated patent ductus arteriosus rises to a peak in latter systole, continues without interruption through the second sound, and declines in intensity during the course of diastole. High velocity flow through a small duct results in a relatively soft high-frequency continuous murmur. The larger ductus is likely to cause a loud, noisy "machinery" murmur, accentuated in latter systole and punctuated with "eddy" sounds. The ductus

murmur is typically loudest in the first or second intercostal space or just beneath the left clavicle. With progressive elevations in pulmonary vascular resistance, the classic murmur is shortened, always beginning with the diastolic portion, and is finally abolished, to be replaced by auscultatory signs of pulmonary hypertension per se. Such patients present with pulmonic ejection sounds, short pulmonic midsystolic murmurs, a single or closely split second heart sound, and a loud pulmonic component of the second sound followed by the Graham Steell murmur of pulmonary regurgitation. Under these circumstances the diagnosis of patent ductus arteriosus cannot be made on auscultatory grounds. Differential cyanosis (cyanotic toes, acyanotic fingers) may be the key.

The electrocardiogram is normal when the ductus is small. Variations depend upon the degree and duration of volume overload of the left heart and pressure overload of the right.

In the x-ray, the ductus can sometimes be seen in the frontal projection as a separate convexity between the aortic knuckle and the pulmonary trunk. In older patients calcium is occasionally identified in the ductus; this should be sought in the frontal, left oblique, and lateral projections. A large left to right shunt *without* appreciable pulmonary hypertension results in varying degrees of pulmonary plethora while the pulmonary trunk and its branches increase in size. The ascending aorta is normal in infants but tends to enlarge in older children or adults because shunt flow traverses the aortic root. Volume overload of the left heart results in left ventricular dilatation and left atrial enlargement. The increase in left atrial size is usually mild to moderate but can occasionally be marked. In infants and young children, a sizable patent ductus arteriosus with left to right shunt and pulmonary hypertension is often associated with congestive heart failure and appreciable cardiomegaly; all four chambers contribute to the cardiac silhouette.

When flow through the ductus is reversed (suprasystemic pulmonary vascular resistance), a different radiologic picture emerges. The left ventricle and the left atrium are normal in size, and the right ventricle is hypertrophied but not conspicuously dilated. The pulmonary trunk and its main branches enlarge, but the ascending aorta tends to be normal, and the peripheral pulmonary vasculature is normal or reduced.

The typical patient with uncomplicated patent ductus in childhood, adolescence, or early adult life can be confidently diagnosed clinically. However, the sick infant with congestive heart failure and large left to right shunt should be investigated preoperatively, not only to confirm the clinical suspicion of patent ductus but also to determine the presence or absence of coexisting anomalies, especially ventricular septal defect. Also requiring diagnostic investigation are patients (generally postadolescent) with increased pulmonary vascular resistance, in whom the degree of left to right shunt must be firmly established before division of the ductus is recommended.

Typical patent ductus presenting in childhood is corrected by surgical division. A number of variations in therapeutic judgment are required, however. Since patency of the ductus with *delayed* spontaneous closure is frequent in premature infants, there is a tendency to delay surgery in such patients because of the prospect of spontaneous closure within months. On the other hand, large patent ductus is a relatively common cause of congestive heart failure in acyanotic infants, and generally requires operative intervention which may take the form of ligation rather than division. After the first year of life most patients with patent ductus are asymptomatic. Division of the ductus in such patients not only carries a low risk but also results in complete anatomic and physiologic correction. The adult poses a more complex problem. The simplest decision is in the adult with a large left to right shunt, relatively low resistance patent ductus, and no ductal calcification. Operation should be advised once the diagnosis is established. Calcification of the patent ductus increases the risk, but, if the shunt is large, operation is still advisable. When pulmonary resistance has exceeded systemic, abolishing the left to right shunt, patients are inoperable. A difficult decision occurs in the occasional adult with a small hemodynamically insignificant patent ductus. The answer hinges on a comparison of the risk of infective endocarditis as opposed to the risk of surgery. Each case requires individual judgment. If there has been a previous episode of infective endocarditis and the patient expresses concern regarding recurrence, surgical correction should be advised. If there has been no previous episode of infective endocarditis and the patient is reluctant to undergo thoracotomy, operation should be deferred.

VENTRICULAR SEPTAL DEFECT WITH PULMONIC STENOSIS

(Fallot's Tetralogy)

This combination encompasses a wide anatomic, physiologic, and clinical spectrum. Two elements of the tetralogy are of prime importance, namely, pulmonic stenosis and a nonrestrictive ventricular septal defect (right ventricular pressure at systemic levels). Large ventricular septal defect with mild to moderate pulmonic stenosis is looked upon as *acyanotic* Fallot's tetralogy; large ventricular septal defect with severe pulmonic stenosis and right to left shunt as *classic cyanotic Fallot's tetralogy;* and large ventricular septal defect with complete obstruction to right ventricular outflow as *Fallot's tetralogy with pulmonary atresia.* It is wise to remain flexible, however, and use appropriate *anatomic* designations instead of, or coupled with, the eponym, to serve the cause of clarity.

In classic cyanotic Fallot's tetralogy, the aorta may be left ventricular in origin, or biventricular to varying degrees, but the posterior aortic wall maintains anatomic continuity with the anterior mitral leaflet. Pulmonic stenosis can be located in the pulmonary trunk, pulmonary valve, infundibulum, or subinfundibular zone, although typically the obstruction is infundibular. Pulmonary atresia can be viewed as the ultimate expression of pulmonic stenosis and therefore the most severe form of Fallot's tetralogy. With pulmonary atresia, the pulmonary circulation is supplied chiefly by large collateral arteries, especially bronchial.

The degree of obstruction to right ventricular outflow may progress with the passage of time. When life expectancy is prolonged by an anastomotic operation, the patient may develop progressive narrowing of the zone of stenosis culminating in complete closure (atresia). Furthermore, infundibular stenosis in acyanotic patients with sizable left to right shunting can progress

sufficiently to reverse the interventricular shunt. Accordingly, a single patient may exhibit a broad spectrum of severity ranging from mild stenosis with large left to right shunt to marked obstruction with reversed shunt.

A number of *additional congenital cardiac malformations* have a tendency to occur with Fallot's tetralogy: (1) right aortic arch, (2) persistent left superior vena cava, (3) hypoplasia, stenosis, or absence of a pulmonary artery, (4) absence of the pulmonary valve, (5) incompetence of the aortic valve, and (6) a coronary arterial anomaly consisting of origin of the left anterior descending coronary artery from the right coronary artery.

The *physiologic consequences* depend upon three variables, namely, the degree of pulmonic stenosis, the size of the interventricular communication, and, to a lesser extent, the systemic vascular resistance. These variables can best be understood by beginning with a large ventricular septal defect upon which increasing degrees of pulmonic stenosis are imposed. When the stenosis is mild, the shunt is entirely left to right, and the condition closely resembles large isolated ventricular septal defect with increased pulmonary blood flow and volume overload of the left heart. As the degree of obstruction increases, the left to right shunt diminishes. When the resistance offered by the obstruction equals systemic resistance, the shunt is balanced. As the stenosis increases still further, a right to left shunt is established because it becomes easier for the right ventricle to eject into the aorta than into the pulmonary trunk. Since right ventricular blood under these circumstances preferentially enters the aorta, circulation to the lungs is reduced and the left heart is underfilled. When the stenosis is complete (pulmonary atresia), the entire right ventricular output is ejected through the ventricular septal defect into the aorta. No matter how severe the pulmonic stenosis, the right ventricle decompresses into the aorta via the large ventricular septal defect, so right ventricular systolic pressure does not exceed systemic. The magnitude of right ventricular systolic overload is then determined by *aortic* pressure.

The *history in typical Fallot's tetralogy* generally dates from the neonatal period because of detection of a murmur or cyanosis. Arterial unsaturation is usually obvious by three to six months. When an infant is born with very severe pulmonic stenosis or atresia, cyanosis dates from birth, and the murmur is relatively inconspicuous. A history of *squatting for relief of dyspnea* has long been a hallmark of Fallot's tetralogy. In addition, Taussig clearly described the preference for certain other postures, such as the knee-chest position, sitting with the legs drawn underneath, or lying down. A history of right ventricular failure is rare in classic Fallot's tetralogy. The neonatal right ventricle is well equipped to pump at systemic pressures, and is seldom called upon to do more, because the ventricular septal defect permits direct decompression into the aorta. A number of other complications occur in the natural history, such as recurrent cerebral hypoxia that can lead to brain damage and mental retardation, cerebral venous sinus thromboses, cerebral embolism, or brain abscess. Death from brain abscess is twice as frequent in cyanotic Fallot's tetralogy as in any other form of congenital cardiac disease. Infective endocarditis sometimes occurs on the zone of pulmonic stenosis. There are two chief determinants of long survival: a degree of pulmonic stenosis that permits adequate but not excessive pulmonary blood flow with little or no cyanosis, and pulmonary stenosis that evolves gradually enough to permit the formation of a well developed collateral circulation.

After age four, most cyanotic children with congenital heart disease have Fallot's tetralogy. This malformation is also present in the largest number of *cyanotic adults* with congenital heart disease.

The physical appearance of the majority of patients with cyanotic Fallot's tetralogy is characterized by small size and physical underdevelopment. When Fallot's tetralogy occurs with little or no cyanosis, the physical appearance is generally normal.

Knowledge of the brachial arterial systolic pressure allows an accurate bedside estimate of the gradient. Since right ventricular systolic pressure is the same as systemic, the gradient across the zone of stenosis is simply the difference between the brachial arterial systolic pressure and the estimated pulmonary arterial systolic pressure (15 to 25 mm Hg).

The jugular venous pulse in classic cyanotic Fallot's tetralogy is seldom elevated; the A wave is normal or nearly so, because the right ventricle maintains its neonatal capability of ejecting at systemic pressures without extra help from its atrium.

Precordial movement and palpation in classic Fallot's tetralogy detect a relatively inconspicuous right ventricular systolic impulse that is usually located inferior to the third left intercostal space because of the stenosed infundibulum. The right ventricle ejects at systemic pressures without an appreciable increase in the vigor of contraction and without dilating. In cyanotic Fallot's tetralogy, especially in the presence of pulmonary atresia, a right aortic arch is relatively frequent, and can sometimes be suspected because of movement imparted to the right sternoclavicular junction.

The auscultatory signs mirror the pathologic physiology. The incidence of aortic ejection sounds varies inversely with the degree of obstruction; the more hypoplastic the pulmonary trunk, the larger the aortic root, and the more likely an aortic ejection sound. The systolic murmur in cyanotic Fallot's tetralogy originates at the zone of stenosis and not across the ventricular septal defect. The murmur tends to be maximal in the third left interspace, because obstruction is usually infundibular. The length and loudness of the murmur (and accompanying thrill) are of considerable importance in estimating the severity of obstruction. A loud, long murmur extending up to the aortic component of the second sound means that an appreciable amount of blood is being ejected into the pulmonary trunk. As resistance at the zone of stenosis arises, there is an increase in the right to left shunt and reciprocal fall in pulmonary blood flow; the murmur gets shorter and softer. When obstruction is complete (pulmonary atresia), the pulmonic stenotic murmur vanishes altogether and is replaced by a soft midsystolic murmur caused by ejection into the dilated aorta. A continuous murmur is an auscultatory sign of pulmonary atresia because of flow through collateral arterial circulation. The pulmonic component of the second heart sound is inaudible in cyanotic Fallot's tetralogy and pulmonary atresia, but when cyanosis is mild or absent a soft delayed sound can sometimes be detected. When a large ventricular septal defect is associated with mild pulmonic stenosis, the auscultatory signs resemble those of uncomplicated ven-

tricular septal defect, although the murmur tends to have midsystolic accentuation (a combination of the ventricular septal defect and pulmonic stenotic murmurs) and there is likely to be moderately wide splitting of the second heart sound.

The *electrocardiogram* is another useful index of the physiologic spectrum encompassed by ventricular septal defect with pulmonic stenosis. Since the force of right atrial contraction is not appreciably increased, P waves of right atrial enlargement are absent about half the time. The mean QRS axis in the frontal plane is rarely to the right of 150 degrees so that right axis deviation takes the form of a dominant S wave in lead I but dominant R waves in leads II and III. In the precordial leads, a tall monophasic R wave is usually confined to lead V_1 with rS complexes in the remaining chest leads. In left precordial leads, q waves are conspicuous by their absence in cyanotic Fallot's tetralogy, because the left ventricle is underfilled. When the shunt is balanced, right ventricular pressure remains at systemic levels, so the electrocardiogram continues to exhibit right ventricular hypertrophy as described. However, the left heart is no longer underfilled, so left precordial leads exhibit well developed R waves and small q waves. When a large ventricular septal defect exists with mild pulmonic stenosis, the electrocardiogram resembles that of isolated ventricular septal defect with right ventricular hypertension.

The *x-ray* in ventricular septal defect with pulmonic stenosis shows vascular markings that are normal or increased when a large defect exists with a balanced or left to right shunt. Severe obstruction to right ventricular outflow diverts more right ventricular blood into the aorta, so that pulmonary blood flow falls and lung vascularity diminishes. In adults, these oligemic lungs may have an emphysematous appearance. In cyanotic Fallot's tetralogy the pulmonary artery segment is characteristically represented by a *concavity*. The aortic arch size varies inversely with the pulmonary trunk. In pulmonary atresia the aorta receives the entire output from both ventricles, so the rightward sweep and knuckle are especially prominent. A right aortic arch occurs in 20 to 30 per cent of patients with cyanotic Fallot's tetralogy, the incidence increasing with the severity of pulmonic stenosis, so that a right arch is most frequent with pulmonary atresia. In cyanotic Fallot's tetralogy the left atrium and left ventricle are normal or small because the left heart is underfilled; the right atrium and right ventricle cope with systemic pressure without dilating, so the cardiac size is normal or nearly so. In pulmonary atresia, however, the cardiac silhouette tends to be larger, especially in older subjects. The configuration of the heart has long been a subject of interest in cyanotic Fallot's tetralogy because of the distinctive boot-shaped appearance caused by a combination of concentric hypertrophy of the right ventricle, an abnormally small left ventricle, a relatively horizontal ventricular septum, and a concave pulmonary artery segment. In Fallot's tetralogy with little or no cyanosis (balanced or bidirectional shunt), the right ventricle remains concentrically hypertrophied, but the left ventricle is not underfilled. The cardiac apex is more likely to be smooth and rounded. When a large ventricular septal defect exists with mild pulmonic stenosis, the x-ray in many ways resembles that of large isolated ventricular septal defect except that the size of the pulmonary trunk may be comparatively small.

The *echocardiogram* serves a useful purpose in identifying biventricular origin of the aorta and continuity between posterior aortic wall and anterior mitral leaflet. Cardiac catheterization and angiocardiography are important in characterizing the morphology of the right ventricular outflow tract, in identifying the location of the ventricular septal defect, and in ruling out right ventricular origin of both great arteries. Intracardiac repair is technically a lesser problem in the patient with large ventricular septal defect, left ventricular aorta, and acquired pulmonic stenosis, even if the stenosis is severe enough to have reversed the shunt. Large ventricular septal defect with biventricular aorta and hypoplastic right ventricular outflow tract is far more difficult to repair (classic cyanotic Fallot's tetralogy). Primary intracardiac repair (total correction) is the treatment of choice and can be accomplished even in infancy. Nevertheless, shunt operations (Waterston or Blalock) are still applied in cyanotic symptomatic infants, especially those less than one year old. A previous shunt operation adds to the risk of complete repair. Postoperative "complete right bundle branch" is expected after right ventriculotomy. The long-term effects of ventriculotomy per se and of a patch for relief of outflow obstruction are still to be assessed.

359.3. UNCOMMON CONGENITAL CARDIAC DEFECTS IN WHICH POSTPEDIATRIC SURVIVAL IS EXPECTED

SITUS INVERSUS. The term "situs inversus" refers to an organ arrangement the reverse of normal (mirror image dextrocardia). Situs inversus is often accidentally discovered on a routine chest x-ray or physical examination, because the malposition is likely to occur with an otherwise normal heart. Such patients experience normal longevity and hence fall into age groups that are susceptible to acquired cardiac disease. Pain of myocardial infarction may be referred to the *right* chest and pain of acute appendicitis to the *left* lower quadrant. Palpation and percussion identify the cardiac apex and stomach on the right and the liver on the left; the left ventricular impulse forms the apex. The heart sounds are louder in the right chest, and splitting of the second sound is detected in the second right intercostal space. The electrocardiogram shows negative P, QRS, and T waves in lead I; the complexes in lead aVR and aVL are the reverse of normal, and right precordial leads resemble those normally recorded from the left chest. The x-rays are the exact mirror image of normal, so that the viewer must identify the symbols on the film that designate left and right. The aortic arch and stomach bubble are on the right, together with the cardiac apex.

DEXTROVERSION OF THE HEART. This term applies when thoracic and abdominal viscera are in normal position but the cardiac *apex* is on the *right* (right thoracic heart). In early fetal life the cardiac apex begins on the side opposite to that which it ultimately occupies. When the apex remains on the right while the aortic arch, left atrium, and stomach are in their normal left-sided positions, the term "dextroversion" is used. Dextroversion of the heart is likely to be detected because of other congenital cardiac anomalies which almost invariably coexist. The most common of these are congenitally corrected transposition of the great arteries (see below), pulmonic stenosis, and ventricular or atrial septal defect. Palpation and percussion identify the cardiac apex and liver on the right with the stomach on the left (normal abdominal situs with right

thoracic heart). Heart sounds and murmurs are louder on the right. The electrocardiogram shows upright P waves in lead I, because the atrial situs is normal. Prominent R waves or RS complexes are recorded from the right chest, whereas the left chest leads exhibit small septal q waves and small r waves. The x-ray shows the aortic arch and stomach bubble on the left but the apex on the right; the heart retains its peculiar silhouette whether or not the film is reversed.

CONGENITAL COMPLETE HEART BLOCK. This is a straightforward diagnosis by electrocardiogram. The AV block is identified as congenital if the slow heart rate existed from infancy (or in utero) and if the QRS configuration exhibits a "supraventricular configuration," i.e., a normal sequence of ventricular excitation. If liberal use were made of the electrocardiogram in infants and children with inappropriately slow heart rates, few cases of congenital heart block would be missed. The conduction defect is generally discovered accidentally in otherwise healthy asymptomatic children, or an alert obstetrician may detect a slow fetal heart rate. The arterial pulse is inappropriately slow for age, the upstroke brisk, the pulse pressure wide, and the rhythm regular. The jugular venous pulse shows intermittent "cannon waves" (right atrial contraction against a closed tricuspid valve), with independent A waves occurring at rates faster than the carotid pulse. The left ventricular impulse is dynamic (large stroke volume). The first heart sound varies in intensity from booming to soft, and there are short midsystolic basal flow murmurs, soft intermittent fourth heart sounds, and intermittent summation sounds. The x-ray may show mild cardiac enlargement related to increased diastolic filling (slow heart rate). The slow rate, regular rhythm, intermittent cannon waves, and variation in intensity in the first heart sound constitute a diagnostic combination.

CONGENITALLY CORRECTED TRANSPOSITION OF THE GREAT ARTERIES. In this anomaly there is a right to left interchange of the ventricles and their respective AV valves. Right atrial blood flows across an AV valve that is morphologically mitral into a venous ventricle that is morphologically left, and then into the pulmonary trunk. Left atrial blood flows across an AV valve that is morphologically tricuspid into an arterial ventricle that is morphologically right, and then into the aorta. Since the pulmonary trunk springs from an anatomic left ventricle and the aorta from an anatomic right ventricle (ventriculo–great artery discordance), the term "transposition of the great arteries" is appropriate. Since right atrial blood finds its way into the pulmonary trunk (albeit across a mitral valve and through an anatomic left ventricle) and since left atrial blood finds its way into the aorta (across an anatomic tricuspid valve and through an anatomic right ventricle), the "transposition" can be considered "congenitally corrected." Hemodynamic consequences of congenitally corrected transposition depend chiefly upon the presence of *associated defects*, the most common of which are (1) incompetence of the left AV valve which is tricuspid and deformed by Ebstein's anomaly (see below), (2) ventricular septal defect, and (3) disturbances in AV conduction. Theoretically, *uncomplicated* congenitally corrected transposition (a rarity) should cause little or no physiologic disturbance. However, even when the malformation is uncomplicated, "spontaneous" failure of the systemic ventricle tends to occur before the fourth decade, although some patients live longer. The unanswered question is the durability of an anatomic right ventricle as a systemic pump, i.e., whether a right ventricle subjected to systemic work loads will fail for that reason alone.

IDIOPATHIC DILATATION OF THE PULMONARY TRUNK. This malformation is characterized by congenital dilatation of the main pulmonary artery and occasionally its branches in the absence of anatomic or physiologic cause. Patients are asymptomatic, and physical appearance, arterial pulse, and jugular venous pulse are entirely normal. Palpation of the precordium may detect a pulmonary arterial impulse but no right ventricular impulse. Auscultation discloses a characteristic pulmonic ejection sound that introduces a soft, short pulmonic midsystolic murmur and normal or exaggerated splitting of the second heart sound. The electrocardiogram is normal. The chest x-ray is also normal except for a conspicuous convexity caused by the dilated pulmonary trunk.

DISCRETE SUBVALVULAR AORTIC STENOSIS. There are two relatively common forms of discrete congenital subaortic stenosis — the tunnel, tubular or fibromuscular, and the localized fibromembranous. "Tunnel" subaortic stenosis is represented by a long narrow fibromuscular channel; the lesion is typically severe at its onset, is usually associated with hypoplasia of the aortic ring, and is seldom seen beyond childhood. Somewhat more appropriate to this discussion is the fibromembranous variety, which is characterized by a thin (1 to 2 mm), crescent-shaped fibrous membrane 2 cm or less below the aortic valve. The membrane extends across the anterior portion of the left ventricular outflow tract, each end inserting onto the anterior mitral leaflet. Fibrous thickening and mild incompetence of the aortic valve commonly coexist and are believed to result from impact of the high velocity jet from the zone of subaortic obstruction. Accordingly, this anomaly is susceptible to infective endocarditis. Fibromembranous subaortic stenosis has a relatively high incidence in the young (11 per cent of left ventricular outflow obstruction below age 15 years), but survival into or beyond the fifth decade is a rarity. Progression in severity and perhaps later transformation into fibromuscular (tunnel) and/or asymmetric septal hypertrophy apparently conspire to shorten life span, accounting for the age-related difference in prevalence in children and adults. The arterial pulse is similar to that of valvular aortic stenosis. The systolic thrill is maximal in the first or second right interspace with radiation into the neck. The left ventricular impulse is sustained, and presystolic distention with an accompanying fourth heart sound may be present. *An aortic ejection sound is typically absent.* The midsystolic stenotic *murmur* is rough and noisy, and its location and radiation correspond to the thrill. The aortic component of the second heart sound is normal or reduced; a soft early diastolic murmur of aortic regurgitation is relatively common (see above). The electrocardiogram is indistinguishable from other forms of discrete aortic stenosis. In the x-ray, the ascending aorta is usually normal, although slight to moderate poststenotic dilatation may occur.

Precise characterization of the level and degree of obstruction requires cardiac catheterization and angiocardiography. The echocardiogram is characterized by abnormal echoes within the left ventricular outflow tract, abnormal systolic movement of the aortic valve (spike plateau contour caused by rapid opening followed almost immediately by partial closure for the rest of systole), and concentric hypertrophy of the left ventricle. Discrete fibromembranous subvalvular aortic stenosis is amenable

to direct surgical repair, although it should be remembered that the aortic leaflets are often distorted and that care must be taken not to damage the anterior mitral leaflet to which the subvalvular fibrous collar is attached.

SUPRAVALVULAR AORTIC STENOSIS. This malformation is typically characterized by a segmental hourglass-shaped narrowing immediately above the aortic sinuses. Occasionally there is tubular hypoplasia of the ascending aorta. Associated mental retardation is presumptive evidence that the aortic stenosis is supravalvular. Under these circumstances stenosis of the pulmonary artery and its branches almost always coexists. Physical appearance is sometimes sufficiently typical to permit these diagnoses to be entertained at a glance: small chin, large mouth, malformed teeth, abnormal bite, and retarded growth. The brachial and carotid arterial pulses may be asymmetrical, with the pulse pressure and rate of rise conspicuously greater on the right. The left ventricular impulse is similar to other forms of discrete aortic stenosis. An aortic ejection sound is absent, and the midsystolic stenotic murmur tends to be more conspicuous in the *first* right intercostal space with disproportionate radiation to the right neck. The aortic component of the second sound is normal or soft, and the murmur of aortic regurgitation is rare. The electrocardiogram is similar to that of valvular or discrete subvalvular aortic stenosis. The x-rays are distinguished by one chief feature — not only is poststenotic dilatation of the aorta absent but the ascending aorta is usually undersized. Precise diagnosis of morphology and severity requires cardiac catheterization and angiocardiography. Surgical repair, although possible, is difficult and at times untenable, as with tubular hypoplasia of the ascending aorta.

SUBVALVULAR PULMONIC STENOSIS. The location can be either infundibular or, rarely, subinfundibular. Discrete infundibular stenosis generally results from localized narrowing of the entrance to the outflow tract, beyond which the infundibulum may be somewhat dilated. Subinfundibular stenosis, a rare variety of right ventricular outflow obstruction, may be caused by hypertrophy of either abnormal muscle groups or normal bulbar muscle. Subvalvular pulmonic stenosis is uncommon as an isolated anomaly and is generally associated with ventricular septal defect. Isolated infundibular pulmonic stenosis can be suspected if the right ventricular impulse does not reach the third left interspace, if the murmur and thrill are maximal in the fourth interspace, if an ejection sound is absent, and if the x-ray shows a nondilated pulmonary trunk, a right aortic arch, and a local indentation at the site of the ostium of the infundibulum. Cardiac catheterization and angiocardiography delineate the level of obstruction, its morphologic type, and the degree of severity. It must be borne in mind that surgical correction may require right ventriculotomy, so operative risk is greater than with valvular pulmonic stenosis.

SUPRAVALVULAR PULMONIC STENOSIS (STENOSIS OF THE PULMONARY ARTERY AND ITS BRANCHES). This defect results from narrowing of the pulmonary trunk, its bifurcation, or its primary or peripheral branches; it may be unilateral or bilateral, single or multiple. Stenosis of the pulmonary artery and its branches causes hypertension in the proximal pulmonary trunk, whereas the converse is true with valvular or subvalvular obstruction. Isolated stenosis of the pulmonary artery and its branches exhibits the following features: murmurs, which may be discovered in early life but are sometimes inconspicuous or even absent in infants and young children; an occasional history of maternal rubella with low birth weight, physical and mental underdevelopment, cataracts, and deafness; familial occurrence; rarely hemoptysis from rupture of thinwalled poststenotic aneurysms; or the distinctive appearance associated with supravalvular aortic stenosis (see above). Auscultatory signs include absence of an ejection sound, normal intensity and splitting of the second heart sound, and left basal midsystolic murmurs with peripheral murmurs of nearly equal intensity in the axillae and back. X-rays show little or no dilatation of the pulmonary trunk but may reveal clusters of poststenotic dilatation of intrapulmonary vessels. Cardiac catheterization and angiocardiography establish the severity and define the anatomic pattern and distribution. Stenosis of the pulmonary artery and its branches is not currently amenable to surgical repair except in the occasional patient with isolated segmental obstruction confined to a zone within the pulmonary trunk.

CONGENITAL PULMONARY VALVE REGURGITATION. Healthy, asymptomatic individuals may be found to have cardiac murmurs and dilatation of the pulmonary trunk on routine chest x-rays. When congenital pulmonary regurgitation accompanies *idiopathic dilatation of the pulmonary trunk*, the clinical features are those of idiopathic dilatation (see above) plus the characteristic diastolic murmur described below. Regurgitation caused by *structural abnormalities of the valve itself* results in the following picture. Palpation detects a right ventricular impulse that becomes progressively more dynamic as the degree of incompetence increases. Systolic expansion of the pulmonary trunk may cause an additional impulse in the second left intercostal space. Auscultation reveals a characteristic diastolic murmur maximal in the second or third left interspace, medium to low in frequency, crescendo-decrescendo in shape, delayed in onset, short in duration, and louder during inspiration. A midsystolic pulmonic flow murmur may also be heard; the second sound can be normal or widely split and the pulmonic component soft or inaudible. The electrocardiogram is generally normal or exhibits volume overload of the right ventricle with an rSr′ pattern in lead V_1. The echocardiogram should display systolic anterior motion of the ventricular septum (paradoxic septal motion due to right ventricular volume overload). The x-ray shows moderate dilatation of the pulmonary trunk and occasionally of the right ventricle.

EBSTEIN'S ANOMALY OF THE TRICUSPID VALVE. Displaced, fused, malformed portions of tricuspid valvular tissue project into the right ventricular cavity. The portion of the right ventricle underlying adherent tricuspid valvular tissue is thin and functions as a receiving chamber analogous to the right atrium (*"atrialized right ventricle"*). Abnormal function of the right heart is related to three derangements: the malformed tricuspid valve, the "atrialized" portion of right ventricle, and the reduced capacity of the pumping portion of the right ventricle. Ineffective emptying of the right atrium may result in an appreciable increase in right atrial volume and a right to left shunt through a foramen ovale or an atrial septal defect, although most patients are acyanotic. Tricuspid regurgitation caused by the malformed leaflets adds to the hemodynamic burden. However, Ebstein's anomaly is compatible with a relatively long and active life, because there is a considerable range of severity. The majority of patients survive into the second, third, or fourth decade, but fewer than 5 per cent live beyond age 50.

Ebstein's anomaly can generally be diagnosed clinically. Bouts of paroxysmal rapid heart action — especially in cyanotic subjects — raise the index of suspicion. A key to the clinical recognition of Ebstein's malformation with right to left shunt is the combination of cyanosis with normal or diminished pulmonary blood flow and a functionally dominant *left* ventricle (see Table 1). A right ventricular impulse is conspicuously lacking, although the infundibulum may be palpable. A large jugular venous V wave is lacking despite tricuspid regurgitation because of decompression in the large right atrium. The murmur of tricuspid regurgitation is either absent or early systolic, because tricuspid regurgitation occurs with normal or low right ventricular systolic pressure. The murmur is of medium frequency, tending to be maximal over the region of the displaced tricuspid valve, i.e., further toward the cardiac apex. Third and fourth heart sounds commonly cause triple or quadruple rhythms. Short mid-diastolic or presystolic murmurs occur, especially when the P-R interval is prolonged, which is often the case. Type B Wolff-Parkinson-White electrocardiograms are noteworthy, and, in the context of cyanotic congenital heart disease, are likely to mean Ebstein's anomaly. The electrocardiogram otherwise shows prominent right atrial P waves and generally right bundle branch block but no right ventricular hypertrophy. The chest x-ray may have a relatively characteristic appearance with normal or clear lung fields, small vascular pedicle, and globular cardiac silhouette caused by rightward convexity of the enlarged right atrium and leftward convexity of the infundibulum. On echocardiography, recordings are readily obtained from the large mobile anterior tricuspid leaflet. These echoes are consistently abnormal, showing marked delay in tricuspid leaflet closure as well as increased amplitude of motion and an abnormally anterior position of the leaflet throughout diastole.

CONGENITAL PULMONARY ARTERIOVENOUS FISTULA. The fistula consists either of one or more relatively large vascular trunks or of a thin aneurysmal sac or a tangle of distended tortuous vascular channels. The arterial supply is derived from one or more abnormal branches of the pulmonary artery. Drainage is almost always through anatomically recognizable dilated pulmonary veins. Such connections are truly *pulmonary* arteriovenous. The physiologic consequences depend chiefly on the amount of unoxygenated blood delivered through the right to left shunt. As a rule the shunt is sufficient to cause cyanosis but not large enough to impose a hemodynamic burden. These fistulas are usually discovered in healthy young adults who are found to have abnormal densities in routine chest x-rays or who exhibit cyanosis or hereditary hemorrhagic telangiectasia. Dyspnea and fatigue are mild even in the presence of conspicuous cyanosis. Intermittent hemoptysis may punctuate the history. Recurrent bleeding also occurs from nose, mouth, or lips (telangiectasia), and members of the family may have similar complaints. Cerebral symptoms include dizziness, vertigo, paresthesias, faintness, visual aberrations, speech disturbances, headache, extremity weakness, mental confusion, and convulsions, although the mechanisms are unclear. Physical appearance is characterized by cyanosis and clubbing, together with small ruby patches (telangiectasia) on the face, tongue, lips, skin and nail beds, and nasal or oral mucous membranes. Thoracic auscultation detects delayed systolic murmurs (or none at all), or occasionally continuous murmurs with systolic accentuation, usually located over the lower lobes or the right middle lobe. The murmurs are generally less than Grade 3 and may get louder with inspiration or Müller's maneuver and softer with expiration or Valsalva's maneuver. The lung fields show densities that are single or multiple, unilateral or bilateral, small or large, typically located in the lower lobes or right middle lobe. The opacities are homogeneous, rounded or lobulated, fairly well demarcated, and attached to the hilus by bandlike shadows that represent dilated vessels entering and leaving the fistula. The size of a mass tends to decrease with Valsalva's maneuver and to increase with Müller's maneuver. In simple terms, pulmonary arteriovenous fistula is a cause of cyanosis with normal ventricles (see Table 1). The combination of cyanosis and telangiectasia with normal electrocardiogram and normal cardiac silhouette is distinctive in its own right, and conclusive when the fistulas cause shadows in the films.

LUTEMBACHER'S SYNDROME.   The eponym generally refers to a congenital atrial septal defect upon which acquired mitral stenosis is superimposed. A large atrial septal defect has an ameliorating effect upon mitral stenosis, which in turn aggravates the hemodynamic effects of the interatrial communication. Left atrial pressure is relatively low, and symptoms of pulmonary venous congestion are attenuated. Atrial fibrillation is relatively common, and the systemic arterial pulse may be small owing to a decrease in left ventricular stroke volume. The jugular venous pulse can exhibit a prominent A wave in the absence of pulmonary hypertension, because the left atrial pressure pulse is transmitted into the right atrium. The right ventricular impulse tends to be especially dynamic. Auscultation does not readily detect the telltale signs of mitral stenosis which as a rule are incomplete or absent altogether. The pulmonary flow murmur is prominent, because an especially large right ventricular stroke volume is ejected into a dilated pulmonary trunk. The electrocardiogram shows P waves of combined atrial enlargement, although left atrial P waves need not be present; evidence of right ventricular hypertrophy is common. The x-ray exhibits pulmonary plethora without pulmonary venous congestion; the right atrium and right ventricle are conspicuously dilated, and the pulmonary trunk may reach a remarkable size. Lutembacher's syndrome is more common in females, because the sex predilection exists for both isolated atrial septal defect and isolated mitral stenosis. The echocardiogram is useful in identifying both volume overload of the right ventricle (systolic anterior motion of the ventricular septum *and* mitral stenosis (slow EF slope and diastolic anterior motion of the posterior mitral leaflet). Lutembacher's syndrome is amenable to complete intracardiac repair.

COMMON ATRIUM.   This relatively rare variety of interatrial communication is the result of complete or virtual absence of the atrial septum. The right-sided portion of the common chamber has anatomic features of a *right* atrium and receives both venae cavae and the coronary sinus. The left-sided portion has anatomic features of a *left* atrium and receives the pulmonary veins. Absence of the septum means that the septum primum is deficient, so that elements of the endocardial cushion malformation coexist, especially a cleft anterior mitral leaflet with or without regurgitation. The physical appearance of the Ellis–van Creveld syndrome heightens suspicion. The clinical picture resembles large atrial septal defect, with the following exceptions: (1) symptoms begin earlier and are generally

more severe; (2) cyanosis exists without sufficient pulmonary hypertension to account for its presence; (3) the physical signs are those of atrial septal defect in which a large left to right shunt persists despite the presence of cyanosis (cyanosis with shunt vascularity; see Table 1); (4) the P wave axis tends to shift leftward, because there is absence of the upper or sinus venosus portion of the atrial septum with absence of a right sinus node); the QRS shows left axis deviation resembling endocardial cushion defect; and (5) the chest x-ray resembles a large atrial septal defect in which pulmonary arterial blood flow is increased even though cyanosis is present. Common atrium can be surgically corrected, more readily if mitral regurgitation is trivial or absent.

CONGENITAL CORONARY ARTERIOVENOUS FISTULA. Both coronary arteries arise from the aorta, but a fistulous branch of one communicates directly with a cardiac chamber or the pulmonary trunk. The right coronary artery is more frequently involved than the left. However, the *drainage* site is of greater clinical importance than the vessel of origin. Ninety per cent of coronary arterial fistulas drain into the right heart (arteriovenous). Most of these enter the right atrium, coronary sinus, or right ventricle, whereas relatively few enter the pulmonary trunk. Congenital coronary arteriovenous fistula should be considered when an asymptomatic acyanotic child or young adult is found to have an atypically located precordial continuous murmur that is relatively soft and "superficial"; the suspicion is heightened when the murmur does not peak around the second heart sound but instead is louder in either systole or diastole. The precordial location is determined by the chamber or vessel that receives the fistula and not by the vessel of origin. In young patients with small fistulas, an "atypical" continuous murmur is likely to be the only clinical abnormality. Larger flows acting over longer periods of time can result in the following pictures. When the fistula enters the *right atrium* or *coronary sinus*, precordial palpation detects both left and right ventricular impulses; the continuous murmur tends to be louder in systole and maximal along the right sternal border, over the lower sternum, or close to the lower left sternal edge; volume overload of both ventricles may be seen in the electrocardiograms; the x-ray shows increased pulmonary arterial flow. When the communication drains into the body of the *right ventricle*, palpation detects right and left ventricular impulses; the continuous murmur is louder in either systole or diastole and is maximal along the mid to lower left sternal border or subxiphoid area; volume overload of both ventricles may be seen in the electrocardiogram; the x-rays exhibit increased pulmonary arterial flow. When the pulmonary artery receives the fistula, palpation detects only a left ventricular impulse; the continuous murmur is usually indistinguishable from patent ductus arteriosus in both configuration and location; volume overload of the left ventricle may appear in the electrocardiogram; the x-ray may show increased pulmonary arterial flow. Coronary AV fistulas should be surgically ablated to abolish the left to right shunt, to eliminate the risk of infective endocarditis, and to channel coronary blood flow into the capillary circulation.

CONGENITAL ANEURYSMS OF THE SINUSES OF VALSALVA. Sinuses of Valsalva are three small dilatations in the wall of the aorta immediately above the attachments of each aortic cusp. More than 90 per cent of congenital aneurysms originate in the right or noncoronary sinus and project into the right ventricle or right atrium. The typical aneurysm begins as a blind pouch or diverticulum; the entire sinus is not dilated, but instead the aneurysm projects as a finger-like or nipple-like extension with a perforation at its tip. Acute rupture of a large aneurysm creates a dramatic clinical picture; a previously healthy young adult, generally male, develops sudden chest pain, dyspnea, a loud continuous murmur, bounding arterial pulse, and relentless cardiac failure that follows a period of temporary improvement. The arterial pulse resembles that of aortic regurgitation; the jugular venous pulse is elevated, and dynamic biventricular impulses are palpable. The continuous murmur is maximal below the third intercostal space along the right or left sternal border or over the lower sternum. The murmur is usually louder in either systole or diastole and does not peak around the second heart sound as in patent ductus. The electrocardiogram is likely to show biatrial P waves and left ventricular or combined ventricular hypertrophy. The chest x-ray displays increased pulmonary arterial flow which may be obscured by pulmonary venous congestion, dilatation of both ventricles, and enlargement of the right and occasionally the left atrium. Small perforations sometimes progress slowly and at first go unnoticed. Such patients come to attention because continuous murmurs are detected. Occasionally, unruptured aneurysms announce themselves by to-and-fro or diastolic murmurs, or because of heart block or myocardial ischemia resulting from coronary arterial compression by the aneurysm.

Cardiac catheterization and angiocardiography are usually definitive. Ruptured congenital aneurysms of the sinuses of Valsalva are amenable to complete correction by relatively simple intracardiac repair.

VENA CAVAL TO LEFT ATRIAL CONNECTION. Isolated drainage of a vena cava into the left atrium is a rare anomaly, but its presence can be suspected with a high degree of accuracy. The malformation is a form of *cyanotic* congenital heart disease *without* right ventricular hypertrophy (see Table 1). Cyanosis dates from early life, but cardiac symptoms are absent or nearly so. A right ventricular impulse is absent, whereas the left ventricle is normal or slightly thrusting. There are no significant murmurs. The electrocardiogram is usually normal but occasionally exhibits left ventricular hypertrophy. The x-ray reveals a normal cardiac silhouette, normal or diminished pulmonary blood flow, and perhaps the shadow of a persistent left superior vena cava.

359.4. COMMON CONGENITAL CARDIAC DEFECTS IN WHICH POSTPEDIATRIC SURVIVAL IS EXCEPTIONAL

VENTRICULAR SEPTAL DEFECT. The most common variety of ventricular septal defect lies below and posterior to the crista supraventricularis in the region of the membranous septum. Variations in both location and size of ventricular septal defects deserve special comment. The normal growth of the heart is most rapid in the first two years of life, during which the defect remains about the same in size or enlarges less rapidly than the rest of the heart. Accordingly, there is a tendency for the *relative* size of the defect to diminish. This tendency ideally results in complete spontaneous closure. Ventricular septal defects are

seldom seen after the fourth decade, not because patients have succumbed but probably because their communications have spontaneously closed or diminished to the point that they are clinically unrecognizable. The physiologic consequences of an isolated ventricular septal defect depend chiefly upon its size and the pulmonary vascular resistance. Both variables may change with time, and the physiologic and clinical manifestations will vary accordingly. A small defect causes little or no functional disturbance, because the shunt is negligible and the pressures in the right heart are normal. With moderately large defects, the left to right shunt increases and, up to a point, occurs with little or no elevation in pulmonary arterial pressure. In such patients the physiologic derangements are essentially due to volume overload of the left heart. A large defect (nonrestrictive) results in equalization of systolic pressures in the two ventricles. The amount of flow into the pulmonary and systemic beds then depends upon their relative vascular resistances. Three regulatory mechanisms affect the volume and direction of the interventricular shunt and the level of pulmonary arterial pressure in infants born with large ventricular septal defects: first, the pattern taken by the pulmonary vascular resistance; second, the relative decrease in size that the defect undergoes, especially in the first two years of life; and third, the development of obstruction to right ventricular outflow, i.e., acquired infundibular pulmonic stenosis.

A *small ventricular septal defect* is ordinarily suspected because of a prominent holosystolic parasternal murmur in a patient in whom cardiac evaluation is otherwise normal. The murmur is generally absent at birth but is readily detected at the first well-baby examination. With passage of time, if the size of the defect decreases, the holosystolic murmur becomes shorter, softer, and higher pitched and is early systolic prior to complete closure. Similarly, *very small defects* are associated with soft, localized high frequency early systolic murmurs. *Large ventricular septal defects* with appreciable left to right shunts cause congestive heart failure in infancy, with retarded growth and development (failure to thrive), diaphoresis, poor feeding, and recurrent lower respiratory infections. Physical examination reveals hyperdynamic biventricular impulses, a harsh holosystolic left parasternal murmur accompanied by a thrill, an apical mid-diastolic flow murmur, and normal or wide splitting of the second heart sound with a relatively prominent pulmonic component. The electrocardiogram exhibits biatrial and biventricular hypertrophy with volume overload of the left ventricle. The x-ray shows pulmonary plethora, a large pulmonary trunk, a normal ascending aorta, dilatation of both ventricles, and often dilatation of the left and right atria as well. Spontaneous improvement is related to a reduction in left to right shunt caused by a decrease in the size of the defect, especially in the first year, by an increase in pulmonary vascular resistance, or by acquired infundibular stenosis (see above).

In *large ventricular septal defect with reversed shunt (Eisenmenger's complex)*, cyanosis ordinarily dates from childhood but not from birth. Effort dyspnea occurs without left ventricular failure. The jugular venous pulse is usually normal and the precordium quiet, with moderate right ventricular and pulmonary arterial impulses. There are auscultatory signs of pulmonary hypertension but *no murmur of ventricular septal defect*. The electrocardiogram shows right ventricular hypertrophy with little or no evidence of volume overload of the left heart. The x-ray exhibits normal or decreased pulmonary vasculature, a relatively normal cardiac silhouette, moderate dilatation of the pulmonary trunk, and normal aortic arch (see Table 1).

In patients with typical small ventricular septal defects, the clinical diagnosis is so evident and the physiologic consequences so benign that cardiac catheterization and angiocardiography are not necessary; such patients should be followed expectantly. They are, however, at risk of infective endocarditis. Patients with *large* ventricular septal defects and pulmonary hypertension (nonrestrictive defects) require investigation to establish the magnitude of left to right shunt and pulmonary vascular resistance, the location of the defect or defects, and the absence or presence of coexisting anomalies.

Large ventricular septal defect with congestive heart failure in infancy is a special problem that will not be dealt with here. Beyond infancy, patients with ventricular septal defects and pulmonary to systemic flow ratios in excess of 1.7:1 should have elective correction. If the pulmonary to systemic flow ratio is less than 1.5:1 because the defect is small, the benign functional consequences do not warrant the risk of operative repair. If a similar flow ratio is the result of *high pulmonary resistance* with *large* ventricular septal defect, operative risk is high and results are poor, because little or no beneficial effect on the pulmonary resistance follows elimination of such a small shunt.

VENTRICULAR SEPTAL DEFECT WITH AORTIC REGURGITATION. The murmur of the ventricular defect is usually known from infancy. Between the ages of three and eight years a *new* murmur appears, together with the gradual development of bounding arterial pulses and a dynamic left ventricular impulse. The combined murmurs are *not* continuous but are holosystolic and early diastolic. The electrocardiogram and x-ray show left ventricular hypertrophy and enlargement out of proportion to the estimated size of the left to right shunt. As time goes on, the ventricular septal defect may decrease in size while the aortic regurgitation progressively worsens. Survival to adult life occurs, although cardiac failure eventually develops because of the volume of regurgitation.

ENDOCARDIAL CUSHION DEFECT. The endocardial cushions of the embryo contribute to the development of the mitral and tricuspid valves and to the growth and convergence of the atrial and ventricular septa. Defects therefore include varying combinations of anomalies in these four contiguous parts of the heart. Three general categories are recognized, namely, complete endocardial cushion defect, partial or incomplete endocardial cushion defect, and transitional forms. In the complete variety, separate atrioventricular valves do not exist as such. There is a common AV valve lying in a canal formed by an atrial septal defect above and a ventricular septal defect below. The partial or incomplete form is represented by an ostium primum atrial septal defect and a cleft mitral valve. Transitional forms represent intermediates between complete and partial endocardial cushion defects. Less commonly, any one of the four component lesions occurs as a clinically isolated anomaly. The physiologic consequences depend upon the presence and degree of the various combinations of the four anatomic components. The following remarks will relate to partial endocardial cushion defects in which postpediatric survival is possible.

An ostium primum atrial septal defect with cleft mitral valve occurs more frequently in females than males. The physical signs resemble ostium secundum atrial septal defect except that the left ventricle occupies the apex and is accompanied by the holosystolic murmur of mitral regurgitation. Congestive heart failure may begin in childhood, especially when marked mitral regurgitation exists with a large left to right shunt. Growth and development are poor and lower respiratory infections frequent. If mitral regurgitation is relatively mild and the left to right shunt moderate, symptoms may be delayed for one or two decades. The incompetent left atrioventricular valve is susceptible to infective endocarditis. Mongolism occurs, but not so frequently as with transitional or complete endocardial cushion defects. The electrocardiogram is important, because the frontal plane exhibits counterclockwise depolarization with left axis deviation; precordial leads show the rSr' pattern of expected volume overload of the right ventricle. In persistent ostium primum with cleft but competent mitral valve, this electrocardiogram is the only distinguishing clinical feature from ostium secundum defect.

The most important laboratory study in identifying endocardial cushion defect is a left ventricular angiocardiogram in the frontal projection which shows a characteristic "goose neck" deformity of the outflow tract caused by the cleft anterior mitral cusp and its abnormal chordal arrangements. The echocardiogram is likely to show displacement of the anterior mitral leaflet into the left ventricular outflow tract with prolonged diastolic apposition to the left side of the ventricular septum. Surgical repair in partial endocardial cushion defect is complicated chiefly by the degree of mitral regurgitation rather than the presence of the atrial septal defect.

TRICUSPID ATRESIA. In this disorder tricuspid valvular tissue cannot be identified. A small imperforate dimple is found on the floor of the right atrium, but no direct connection exists between right atrium and right ventricle. The only outlet for the right atrium is an interatrial communication which can take the form of a fossa ovale or an atrial septal defect. Variations beyond the mitral valve form the basis of Edwards' anatomic classification from which physiologic inferences can be drawn and clinical manifestations of tricuspid atresia understood. According to this classification, tricuspid atresia occurs either with or without transposition of the great arteries and, in each of these two categories with no pulmonic stenosis, with pulmonic stenosis, or with pulmonary atresia. Given an adequate interatrial communication, pulmonary blood flow is the chief determinant of longevity. Life expectancy is greatest when pulmonic stenosis of just the right degree exists so that blood flow to the lungs is favorably regulated. When the great arteries are normally related, the subpulmonic obstruction is generally marked, and most patients die in the first year. Nevertheless, occasional examples of survival have been recorded from the second through the fifth decade, with one exceptional survival to age 57. When the great arteries are *transposed*, pulmonic stenosis is more likely to permit longer survival. Sporadic patients in this category have lived into the second, third, and fourth decades, and one died at age 56. The key to the clinical diagnosis of tricuspid atresia is the presence of cyanosis, normal or diminished pulmonary blood flow, and a dominant left ventricle (see Table 1). The electrocardiogram shows right atrial P waves with left axis deviation and adult progression of the QRS in the precordial leads. Definitive diagnosis is achieved by angiocardiography. Palliative surgery is possible through (1) creation of an atrial septal defect in those patients with a foramen ovale, or (2) a shunt operation to improve pulmonary blood flow.

In addition, blood from the right atrium has been directed through a conduit to the pulmonary artery, permitting the right atrium to act as a pumping chamber for the pulmonary circulation.

COMPLETE TRANSPOSITION OF THE GREAT ARTERIES.

According to Elliott and Edwards: "In complete transposition, there are two ventricles. . . . The aorta, with the coronary arteries arising from it, takes origin from the right ventricle, while the pulmonary trunk takes origin exclusively from the left ventricle. Both atrioventricular valves are patent and have the corresponding structure of the right and left sided atrioventricular valves of the normal heart. The connections of the systemic, pulmonary and coronary veins are normal." Survival in complete transposition requires the presence of some means of blood exchange between the pulmonary and systemic circulations which exist in parallel rather than in series. The term "transposition" is best applied to hearts exhibiting ventriculo–great artery discordance, i.e., each great artery arises separately from an anatomically inappropriate ventricle (pulmonary artery–left ventricle; aorta–right ventricle). Connections between the greater and lesser circulations may take the form of an interatrial communication, ventricular septal defect, or patent ductus arteriosus. As a general rule, complete transposition of the great arteries is a congenital cardiac anomaly that exists with *cyanosis* and *increased* pulmonary blood flow (see Table 1). The large majority of patients die within the first year, often within the first months. Isolated examples of unusual longevity have been recorded into the second, third, or fourth decade; one patient aged 56 years at autopsy was believed to have complete transposition. Definitive diagnosis is by angiocardiography. Two physiologic corrective operations are currently applied. The Mustard operation redirects venous inflows, whereas the Rastelli operation achieves redirection of ventricular outflows.

359.5. UNCOMMON CONGENITAL CARDIAC DEFECTS IN WHICH POSTPEDIATRIC SURVIVAL IS EXCEPTIONAL

Anomalous origin of the left coronary artery from the pulmonary trunk is characterized by normal origin of the right coronary artery from the aorta and anomalous origin of the left coronary artery (LCA) from the pulmonary trunk. The aberrant left coronary artery is relatively small and thin walled, resembling a venous channel, whereas the right coronary artery is dilated and tortuous, especially in patients who survive childhood. Myocardial ischemia is a serious problem. The ischemic derangement is not due to the fact that only *one* coronary artery originates from the aorta, but is due instead to direct flow from the right coronary artery to the LCA through intercoronary anastomoses which bypass the capillary bed. Thus the anomalous left coronary artery distributes blood *into* the pulmonary trunk but does not receive blood from it.

In the natural history of this anomaly, three general patterns emerge: serious symptoms in early infancy with death before one year; early illness followed by improvement so that by childhood symptoms may be absent or nearly so; and absence or virtual absence of early symptoms with survival into adulthood. About 15 to 20 per cent of individuals with anomalous origin of the LCA reach adulthood; relatively few survive through the fourth decade, although one of the first known patients with this anomaly was a 50-year-old woman. The intercoronary anastomoses often result in a continuous murmur, and the myocardial ischemia results in papillary muscle dysfunction with mitral regurgitation. The electrocardiogram is important, because at a relatively early age deep Q waves appear in leads I and aVL. Definitive diagnosis is by cardiac catheterization and aortography or selective right coronary arteriography. A left to right shunt from right coronary through intercoronary anastomoses to anomalous LCA into the pulmonary trunk is identified. Selective coronary arteriography (injection into the right coronary) traces this pathway and provides specific anatomic diagnosis. Two surgical interventions have been applied. In infancy, ligation of the anomalous left coronary artery interrupts retrograde flow and improves capillary circulation. In older children or adults, the left subclavian artery or the internal mammary artery or a saphenous vein graft can be directly anastomosed to the left coronary artery, which is then ligated at its origin from the pulmonary trunk.

Cor triatriatum is characterized by drainage of the pulmonary veins into an accessory left atrial chamber that lies proximal to the true left atrium. The distal compartment communicates with the mitral valve and contains the left atrial appendage and the fossa ovalis. The fibrous or fibromuscular diaphragm that partitions the left atrium harbors one or more openings, the size of which determines the degree of left atrial obstruction. Cor triatriatum is therefore a congenital anomaly that is acyanotic without a shunt, with the malformation originating in the left heart (see Table 1). Severe cor triatriatum is ordinarily detected in infants or young children, but symptoms may not begin until adolescence or adulthood. Patients with mild obstruction may be entirely asymptomatic. The functional consequences are analogous to mitral stenosis with elevated pulmonary venous and pulmonary arterial pressures. However, the auscultatory signs of mitral stenosis are lacking, and enlargement of the left atrial appendage is absent, because that structure is in the distal low pressure compartment. It is wise to consider cor triatriatum in postadolescents with clinical signs of obstruction to left atrial flow but without signs of mitral stenosis. The diagnosis is materially assisted by echocardiography that detects a nonstenotic mitral valve, and by angiocardiography which, with pulmonary arterial injection of contrast material, defines the zone of obstruction as dye opacifies the left heart. Surgical intervention can completely remove the partition and relieve the left atrial obstruction.

Total anomalous pulmonary venous connection (TAPVC) is a condition in which all venous blood from both lungs enters the right atrium directly or through one of its tributary veins. The four anomalously connecting pulmonary veins emerge individually from the lungs and either enter the right atrium directly or, more often, unite in the mediastinum to form a confluence which joins the right atrium via (1) the coronary sinus, (2) an anomalous vertical vein or left superior vena cava, that connects the left innominate vein to the right superior vena cava, or (3) the right superior vena cava directly or via the azygos vein. In the right atrium, there is mixing of systemic and pulmonary venous blood, part of which enters the left heart via an atrial septal defect and most of which enters the right ventricle and low-resistance pulmonary bed. Accordingly,

TAPVC is classified as a cyanotic congenital anomaly with increased pulmonary arterial blood flow (see Table 1). The clinical picture in many ways resembles isolated atrial septal defect with large left to right shunt except for cyanosis which varies from subtle to marked. However, the patient is likely to be male, and symptoms generally begin in early childhood, although some individuals reach adult life with surprisingly little disability. The jugular venous pulse may exhibit a large A wave because of pulmonary hypertension. Palpation and auscultation are similar to atrial septal defect with large left to right shunt, but signs of pulmonary hypertension are more likely to coexist. Similarly, the electrocardiogram shows right atrial and right ventricular hypertrophy. The x-ray resembles atrial septal defect with large left to right shunt, but there is one distinctive picture. When the pulmonary veins communicate with the left innominate vein via a left vertical vein, the heart may exhibit a "figure of 8" appearance. The upper part of the figure of 8 is the left vertical vein on the left and the dilated right superior vena cava on the right. The lower part is the cardiac silhouette itself, i.e., dilated right atrium and right ventricle.

Diagnosis is established by cardiac catheterization and angiocardiography; the latter defines the specific connecting pathways. Echocardiography is similar to a large shunt ostium secundum atrial septal defect. Surgical correction is achieved, especially when the confluence of pulmonary veins can be anastomosed directly to the left atrium and the vascular channel to the systemic venous bed divided.

Right ventricular origin of both great arteries and "double outlet right ventricle" are synonymous terms for a congenital malformation in which the pulmonary artery arises in its normal position but the aorta arises wholly from the right ventricle. A ventricular septal defect provides the left ventricle with its only outlet. Pulmonary stenosis may or may not coexist. Right ventricular origin of both great arteries can exist with a ventricular septal defect above or below the crista supraventricularis. In double outlet right ventricle with infracristal ventricular septal defect and no pulmonic stenosis, two steps help in clinical diagnosis. The first step involves recognition of large ventricular septal defect with left to right shunt and pulmonary hypertension. Since both great arteries originate from the right ventricle, pulmonary arterial pressure is by definition systemic. It is a good rule to consider double outlet right ventricle in all patients who present with the picture of large left to right shunt pulmonary hypertensive ventricular septal defect. The second step in the clinical diagnosis consists of recognizing a QRS that exhibits left axis deviation and counterclockwise depolarization. The clinical diagnosis depends chiefly on left axis deviation in the presence of a pulmonary hypertensive ventricular septal defect with a large left to right shunt. Favorable adjustments in pulmonary vascular resistance sometimes regulate pulmonary blood flow so that, even though increased, it is not excessive. Under these circumstances longevity is improved; patients occasionally survive into young adulthood, and one underwent successful surgical correction at 53 years of age.

In right ventricular origin of both great arteries with supracristal ventricular septal defect, the defect lies just beneath the pulmonary valve (subpulmonic). This anomaly, called *Taussig-Bing complex*, is a diagnostic consideration in patients with *increased* pulmonary blood flow and *cyanosis* from birth or early infancy. Radiologic, electrocar-

diographic, and physical signs of pulmonary hypertension are obligatory. In the presence of patent ductus arteriosus (which often coexists) and high pulmonary vascular resistance, a distinctive type of reversed differential cyanosis occurs in which the toes are less cyanotic than the fingers, because oxygenated blood from the left ventricle is ejected into the pulmonary trunk and then through the ductus into the descending aorta, whereas unsaturated right ventricular blood is ejected into the aortic root and brachiocephalic vessels. It is a good rule to consider the Taussig-Bing anomaly in patients who appear to have Eisenmenger's complex but in whom cyanosis dates from birth or early infancy.

Right ventricular origin of both great arteries occurs with all grades of pulmonic stenosis (mild to severe to complete, i.e., pulmonary atresia). The ventricular septal defect is usually infracristal if pulmonic stenosis coexists. Double outlet right ventricle with mild to moderate pulmonic stenosis resembles ordinary large ventricular septal defect with equivalent pulmonic stenosis except for the electrocardiogram, which may exhibit counterclockwise depolarization with left axis deviation (see above).

Right ventricular origin of both great arteries with severe pulmonic stenosis closely resembles cyanotic Fallot's tetralogy and should be considered whenever the clinical diagnosis of cyanotic Fallot's tetralogy is entertained. Clinical distinction between the two is difficult, although some points favor double outlet right ventricle: (1) auscultatory evidence of a holosystolic murmur at the lower left sternal edge despite the presence of cyanosis (obligatory left to right shunt through the ventricular septal defect); (2) palpable left ventricular impulse in this context; and (3) electrocardiogram showing small q waves in leads I and aVL and relatively broad slurred S waves in leads I, aVL, and V_{5-6}. The echocardiogram may assist by identifying lack of continuity between the posterior aortic wall and anterior mitral leaflet, because in double outlet right ventricle there is no continuity between the anterior mitral leaflet and the wall of *either* artery. Definitive diagnosis is angiographic. Corrective surgery is technically feasible, although complex.

Truncus arteriosus is a congenital anomaly in which a single great artery leaves the base of the heart through a single semilunar valve. The truncus is situated just above a ventricular septal defect, receives blood from both ventricles, and gives rise to the coronary arteries and to the pulmonary and systemic circulations. No remnant of a second semilunar valve is present. Truncus arteriosus with large pulmonary arteries occurs with cyanosis and pulmonary plethora (see Table 1). Both pulmonary branches may arise from a common short pulmonary artery that emerges from the truncus, or the two branches may arise directly from the truncus.

The outlook is better when the pulmonary arteries are moderately stenotic at their truncal origins, advantageously controlling pulmonary blood flow and delaying death from cardiac failure. Occasional patients with favorably regulated pulmonary circulations have survived into the third or fourth decade, and one died at the age of 43 years. However, postpediatric survival is rare, especially with truncus arteriosus and large unobstructed pulmonary arteries.

Definitive diagnosis of truncus arteriosus is by angiocardiography. Physiologic correction is feasible, employing an operation which joins the two pulmonary arteries to the outflow of the right ventricle with a conduit.

Single ventricle refers to a congenital anomaly in which there are two atria but only one anatomic ventricular chamber that receives both the mitral and tricuspid valves. The usual type is a morphologic left ventricle or primitive ventricle with a small outlet chamber that represents the infundibular portion of the right ventricle. The infundibulum is a subdivision of the single ventricle, not a separate ventricular chamber. The great arteries are almost always transposed. If the infundibulum is situated at the right basal aspect of the heart, this arrangement is called "noninversion"; if the infundibulum is situated at the left basal aspect of the heart (corresponding to its expected location with congenitally corrected transposition), this arrangement is termed "inversion." Pulmonic stenosis may or may not coexist. Single ventricle without pulmonic stenosis occurs with increased pulmonary blood flow, and hence is an anomaly exhibiting cyanosis with pulmonary plethora (see Table 1). In single ventricle with high pulmonary vascular resistance, cyanosis is conspicuous and pulmonary blood flow normal or diminished (see Table 1). Single ventricle with pulmonic stenosis is an anomaly exhibiting cyanosis with normal or diminished pulmonary blood flow (see Table 1).

Survival depends chiefly upon a favorable balance between resistances to flow into the pulmonary trunk and aorta. Although the average patient dies in childhood, survival into adolescence or early adult life is not rare. The natural history occasionally extends into the third, fourth, or even fifth decade, with one survival to age 56 years. Moderate pulmonic stenosis without aortic obstruction favors longevity. Definitive diagnosis depends upon cardiac catheterization and angiocardiography, although precatheterization diagnoses are accomplished with a high degree of accuracy. On echocardiography, separate AV valves (tricuspid and mitral) are simultaneously recorded *without* an intervening septal echo. On a base to apex scan, there is absence of the ventricular septal echo in any of its expected locations. Surgical intervention is palliative, and consists of either banding the pulmonary trunk to limit pulmonary plethora or providing a shunt operation to improve pulmonary blood flow in patients with critical pulmonic stenosis or atresia.

de la Cruz, M. Z., Anselmi, G., Romero, A., and Monroy, G.: A quantitative and qualitative study of the ventricles and great vessels of normal children. Am. Heart J., 60:675, 1960.

Edwards, J. E., Carey, L. S., Neufeld, H. N., and Lester, R. G.: Congenital Heart Disease. Philadelphia, W. B. Saunders Company, 1965.

Feigenbaum, H.: Echocardiography. 2nd ed. Philadelphia, Lea & Febiger, 1976.

Gault, J. H., Morrow, A. G., Gay, W. A., and Ross, J., Jr.: Atrial septal defect in patients over age 40 years. Clinical and hemodynamic studies and the effects of operation. Circulation, 37:261, 1968.

Higgins, C. B., and Mulder, D. G.: Tetralogy of Fallot in the adult. Am. J. Cardiol., 29:837, 1972.

Higgins, I. T.: The epidemiology of congenital heart disease. J. Chronic Dis., 18:699, 1965.

Maron, B. J., Humphries, J. O., Rowe, R. D., and Mellits, E. D.: Prognosis of surgically corrected coarctation of the aorta. A 20-year postoperative followup. Circulation, 47:119, 1973.

Mitchell, S. C., Korones, S. B., and Berends, H. W.: Congenital heart disease in 56,109 births. Circulation, 43:323, 1971.

Morganroth, J., Perloff, J. K., Zeldes, S. M., and Dunkman, W. B.: Acute severe aortic regurgitation. Ann. Intern. Med., 87:223, 1977.

Nadas, A. S., and Flyer, D. C.: Pediatric Cardiology. 3rd ed. Philadelphia, W. B. Saunders Company, 1972.

Nora, J. J.: Multifactorial inheritance hypothesis for the etiology of congenital heart disease. Circulation, 38:604, 1968.

Perloff, J. K.: Pediatric congenital cardiac becomes a postoperative adult. The changing population of congenital heart disease. Circulation, 47:606, 1973.

Perloff, J. K.: The Clinical Recognition of Congenital Heart Disease. 2nd ed. Philadelphia. W. B. Saunders Company, 1978.

Perloff, J. K.: Postpediatric congenital heart disease: Natural survival patterns. Cardiovasc. Clin., in press.

Polani, P. E., and Campbell, M.: An aetiological study of congenital heart disease. Ann. Hum. Genet., 19:209, 1955.

Roberts, W. C.: The congenitally bicuspid aortic valve. Am. J. Cardiol., 26:72, 1970.

Rudolph, A. B.: Changes in the circulation after birth. Their importance in congenital heart disease. Circulation, 41:343, 1970.

360.   ACQUIRED VALVULAR HEART DISEASE

John Ross, Jr.

360.1.   INTRODUCTION

Before considering the characteristic features and treatment of each acquired valvular heart lesion, it will be useful to consider broad differences in the physiologic effects of these lesions and to suggest a general diagnostic approach to the patient with valvular heart disease. It will also be worthwhile to discuss the indications for cardiac catheterization, as well as the general considerations that enter into a decision to recommend surgical treatment.

GENERAL PHYSIOLOGIC EFFECTS OF VALVULAR HEART DISEASE

The consequences of stenosis or regurgitation of the heart valves may be considered in relation to their direct effects on the cardiac chamber that must compensate for the valvular lesion by undergoing hypertrophy or dilatation, and their secondary effects on intravascular pressures and blood flow in the aorta, pulmonary vascular bed, and systemic veins. When a semilunar valve of the heart (aortic or pulmonic) is stenotic or regurgitant, or when an atrioventricular valve (mitral or tricuspid) is regurgitant, the primary burden is placed upon the adjacent *ventricle*. With aortic stenosis and regurgitation, important secondary effects occur in the aortic pressure pulses, and with mitral regurgitation there are major secondary effects on the pulmonary venous bed. When an atrioventricular valve is stenotic, the primary burden is placed on the *atrium*, and secondary effects are prominent on the adjacent venous bed; in tricuspid stenosis, for example, there are right atrial overload and secondary elevation of pressure in the systemic veins. These general consequences of stenotic and regurgitant valvular lesions are summarized in Figure 1.

Aortic stenosis places an overload on the left ventricle during systole, a pressure gradient being developed to overcome the obstruction at the aortic valve (see Fig. 1). This leads to progressive hypertrophy of the left ventricular wall without an increase in chamber volume. Aortic regurgitation, in contrast, places a volume overload on the left ventricle during diastole. This leads to an augmented forward stroke volume into the aorta which, in turn, causes a substantial increase in the systolic pressure in the aorta and left ventricle, an increase

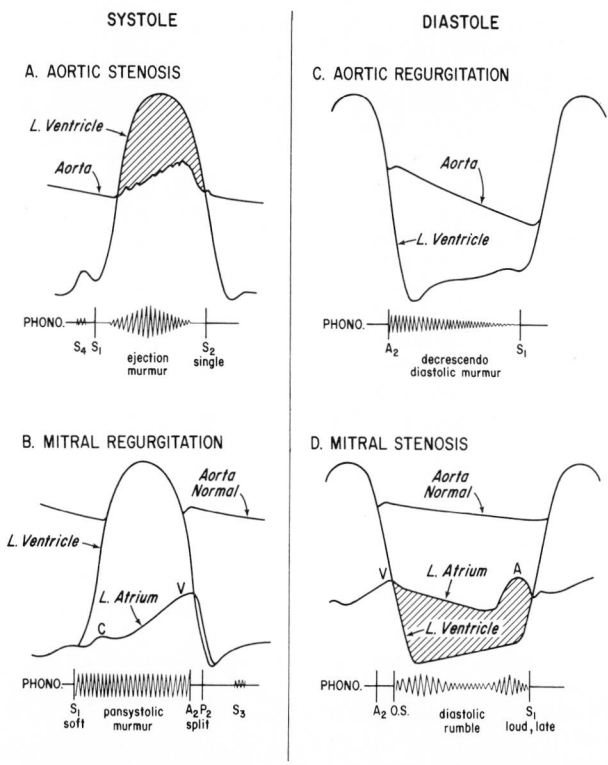

Figure 1. Diagrams of pressure tracings and phonocardiograms in valvular heart disease. The left-hand panels illustrate systole; the right-hand panels, diastole.

A, Pressure tracings in the aorta and left ventricle in aortic stenosis. The shaded area indicates the pressure gradient between left ventricle and aorta. The presystolic (A wave) in the left ventricle is shown, which correlates with the atrial diastolic gallop (S_4) on the phonocardiogram (Phono.). The murmur follows the time course of the pressure gradient during ventricular ejection, and the prolonged left ventricular ejection time results in a single second heart sound (S_2).

B, Pressure tracings in the aorta, left ventricle, and left atrium in mitral regurgitation. (Similar events occur in the right atrium, jugular venous pulse, and right ventricle in tricuspid regurgitation.) A prominent V wave is visible in the left atrium, and the pansystolic murmur on the phonocardiogram persists as long as there is a pressure gradient from left ventricle to left atrium across the leaking mitral valve. The A_2P_2 interval is more widely split than normal because of a shortened left ventricular ejection time in severe mitral regurgitation. The rapid filling wave in the left ventricle and left atrium is illustrated, which is often accompanied by a ventricular diastolic gallop (S_3).

C, Pressure tracings in the aorta and left ventricle in aortic regurgitation. There is a widened arterial pulse pressure with a rapidly falling aortic diastolic pressure. On the phonocardiogram the decrescendo diastolic murmur can be seen to follow the time course of the diminishing diastolic pressure gradient from the aorta to the left ventricle across the leaking aortic valve.

D, Pressure tracings in the aorta, left ventricle, and left atrium in mitral stenosis. (Similar events occur in the right atrium, jugular venous pulse, and right ventricle in tricuspid stenosis.) The left atrial pressure is elevated and the pressure gradient between left atrium and left ventricle during diastole is indicated by the shaded area. The slow fall in left atrial pressure after the V wave (slow Y descent) indicates obstruction to left atrial emptying, and the prominent A wave of left atrial contraction is not transmitted to the ventricle. The dumbbell-shaped diastolic rumble of mitral stenosis in the presence of normal sinus rhythm follows the time course of the pressure gradient, which is greatest early and again late in diastole. It can be seen how an increase or a decrease in the height of the left atrial pressure will move the mitral opening snap (O.S.) closer to or farther from, respectively, the aortic closure sound (A_2); similarly a higher left atrial pressure will result in a later and louder first heart sound (S_1).

in left ventricular volume, and moderate hypertrophy of the left ventricular wall. An excessive oxygen consumption by the left ventricle occurs in aortic stenosis because of the hypertrophy and increased pressure required to drive blood across the narrowed valve, and myocardial oxygen consumption also is increased to some degree in aortic regurgitation because of the large stroke volume and the increased systolic pressure in the aorta. In addition, there is a low diastolic aortic pressure available for coronary artery perfusion in aortic regurgitation and a low aortic pressure relative to left ventricular pressure in severe aortic stenosis (see Fig. 1), which can lead to imbalances between coronary

blood flow and myocardial oxygen demands. Angina pectoris is therefore common in both these conditions. Both aortic stenosis and regurgitation, in time, lead to left ventricular myocardial dysfunction.

Mitral regurgitation also places a diastolic volume overload on the left ventricle, but it differs importantly from aortic regurgitation in that the regurgitant leak occurs during ventricular systole and takes place into a relatively low pressure chamber, the left atrium (see Fig. 1). The ventricular chamber dilates to allow the increased total stoke volume (forward plus backward flow), but the ventricular systolic pressure is not elevated, wall hypertrophy is only moderate, oxygen demands are not greatly augmented, and coronary artery perfusion pressure is normal. Therefore this lesion, when it develops slowly, tends to be well tolerated, and left ventricular myocardial dysfunction develops late in the course of the disease. Mitral stenosis does not place an overload on the left ventricle; rather, obstruction at the mitral valve overwhelms the capacity of the atrial booster pump to maintain forward blood flow, and progressive elevation of left atrial pressure ensues (see Fig. 1).

The secondary effects of these valvular lesions on the arterial and venous beds are many. As mentioned above, the reduced aortic pulse in aortic stenosis and the wide aortic pulse pressure with low diastolic pressure in aortic regurgitation have important effects on coronary artery perfusion. In addition, when valvular lesions are sufficiently severe, or when left ventricular myocardial failure supervenes, the forward cardiac output becomes reduced, the arterial pulse weakens, and there is reflex systemic vasoconstriction with cool extremities and peripheral cyanosis. Such signs constitute evidence of *"forward" cardiac failure.* The effects of *"backward" cardiac failure* in the presence of left-sided valvular lesions are due to left atrial and pulmonary venous hypertension, and they are reflected in the lungs and the right heart. In mitral stenosis, obstruction to left atrial emptying leads to left atrial hypertension, distention of the pulmonary veins, interstitial edema of the lung, reactive pulmonary arteriolar constriction, and eventually pulmonary arterial hypertension. However, the same sequence of effects can also occur when aortic stenosis becomes extremely severe, or when left ventricular myocardial dysfunction becomes significant in the presence of aortic valve disease or mitral regurgitation. The common denominator under these conditions is marked elevation of the left ventricular diastolic pressure, and late in the course of each of these left-sided valvular lesions left atrial and pulmonary venous hypertension, lung congestion, and pulmonary arterial hypertension can also occur, as in mitral stenosis.

Once severe pulmonary hypertension develops, the resulting pressure overload on the right ventricle may then result in secondary right ventricular failure, tricuspid regurgitation, and right atrial hypertension. This, in turn, leads to congestion of the systemic venous bed and the peripheral tissues (liver, abdomen, and extremities). Tricuspid stenosis alone can produce such effects, the right atrial hypertension being caused by mechanical obstruction at the tricuspid valve.

APPROACH TO THE PATIENT WITH VALVULAR HEART DISEASE

Five basic steps in the evaluation of a patient with acquired valvular heart disease should be taken in a logical sequence: (1) the history, (2) the physical examination, (3) the chest roentgenogram (usually with multiple views and barium swallow), (4) the electrocardiogram, and (5) other special tests (phonocardiogram, echocardiogram, cardiac catheterization). The patient is often seen initially, of course, because of an abnormal finding in one of these areas (cardiac murmur, abnormal electrocardiogram, unusual chest x-ray).

HISTORY. The clinical course of patients with each major type of acquired valvular lesion tends to be rather characteristic, and often the findings to be encountered on physical examination can be predicted on the basis of a careful history alone. Thus in mitral stenosis the earliest symptoms are those due to episodic left atrial hypertension and pulmonary congestion, occurring particularly when the heart rate is rapid during exercise, and during intermittent atrial fibrillation or tachycardia. Such symptoms often begin in early adult life, and the dyspnea increases as the mitral valve narrowing progresses and reaches a critical degree. In contrast, patients with aortic stenosis or regurgitation, or mitral regurgitation, tend to develop dyspnea in relation to the duration and severity of the overload on the left ventricle. In acquired isolated aortic stenosis, there is often a long period without symptoms while the stenosis progresses and left ventricular hypertrophy increases; this is followed by a rather abrupt downhill course over four or five years, beginning at age 55 or 60, as the compensatory mechanisms are exhausted. The average downhill course in patients with chronic rheumatic aortic regurgitation tends to be less precipitous than that of aortic stenosis after symptoms begin, taking place over seven or eight years, but it usually begins somewhat earlier in life. On the other hand, in chronic mitral regurgitation the onset of symptoms is gradual and deterioration tends to be slow owing to the relatively favorable loading conditions on the left ventricle, discussed above.

These average clinical courses represent those of patients who experienced rheumatic fever in childhood, or who develop progressive stenosis of a congenitally bicuspid aortic valve. Departures from the typical patterns occur when, for example, coronary artery disease leads to angina pectoris in the presence of mild aortic stenosis, or when mitral regurgitation occurs acutely as a consequence of chordal rupture or papillary muscle dysfunction associated with coronary heart disease. Such deviations from the usual history should arouse the suspicion of a nonrheumatic etiology of valve dysfunction, or of other associated disease.

PHYSICAL EXAMINATION. In examining the heart, it is well to develop an ordered approach, commencing with careful inspection of the neck veins, palpation of the carotid arteries, and inspection and palpation of the precordium. Palpation of the carotid arteries may be highly useful, for example, in differentiating aortic stenosis caused by valvular obstruction from that caused by hypertrophic subaortic stenosis. Estimation of the jugular venous pressure (which, with practice, can be done reliably within 1 or 2 cm H_2O) and examination of the contour of the jugular venous pulse waves carry great importance, because these veins provide direct clues to events occurring in the right atrium. The jugular veins therefore serve as an "external manometer," and the characteristically slow downslope of the jugular venous pulse (Y descent) associated with tricuspid stenosis (see Fig. 1) or the dominant V wave of tricuspid regurgitation, may suggest organic tricuspid valve involvement. The jugular venous pulse waves often disclose atrial arrhythmias, or provide a clue to the presence of pulmonary hypertension and right ventricular hypertrophy, evidenced by a prominent venous A wave.

Auscultation of the heart is of course the key to an accurate diagnosis in valvular heart disease. An orderly sequence for listening should be developed, each area being examined first for normal or abnormal heart sounds and then for cardiac murmurs. Simultaneous palpation of the carotid artery and observation of the neck veins should be used as aids in the proper timing of the heart sounds and murmurs. By listening first at the aortic area, the aortic component of the second heart sound can be readily identified; the intensity of the pulmonic closure sound and its movement with respiration can then be assessed at the pulmonic area. As one moves down the left sternal border with the diaphragm of the stethoscope, the opening snap of mitral stenosis may be revealed even before the murmur is heard at the apex, or the high-pitched blowing murmur of aortic regurgitation may be audible. The tricuspid and mitral areas should then be examined for the characteristics of the first heart sound. Sometimes a very loud first heart sound alerts the examiner to the possibility of mitral stenosis, whereas mitral regurgitation leads to a reduction in the intensity of the first heart sound at the apex (see Fig. 1).

The duration and intensity of the murmurs of valvular heart disease occur with, and tend to follow, the time course of the pressure gradients between two adjacent cardiac chambers or between a chamber and its great vessel. Thus the diamond-shaped systolic murmur ("ejection" murmur) of aortic stenosis increases and decreases with the pressure gradient, and the velocity at which blood is forced across the narrowed aortic orifice rises and falls (see Fig. 1); this type of murmur does not occur during isovolumetric ventricular contraction and relaxation, and therefore begins well after the first heart sound and ends before the second sound. The decrescendo murmur of aortic regurgitation occurs as the diastolic pressure gradient between the aorta and the left ventricle gradually falls during left ventricular filling (see Fig. 1). The holosystolic (pansystolic) murmur of mitral or tricuspid regurgitation begins with the first heart sound and persists as long as active ventricular contraction maintains a positive pressure gradient from the ventricle to the passively filling atrium (see Fig. 1). The duration and intensity of the diastolic rumbling murmurs of mitral or tricuspid stenosis closely follow the diastolic pressure gradient across the valve from atrium to ventricle (see Fig. 1). Presystolic accentuation of the murmur during the A wave of atrial systole tends to disappear when atrial fibrillation occurs; and if the stenosis is mild, the pressure gradient and the mumur may disappear midway during diastole. It also can be seen from Figure 1 why the first heart sound is both late and loud in mitral stenosis, the left ventricle contracting rapidly and forcefully by the time it has built up sufficient pressure to close the mitral valve, and why the interval between the aortic closure sound and the mitral opening snap becomes progressively shorter as left atrial pressure rises.

Finally, it is important that changes in body position and certain other maneuvers become a regular part of the complete physical examination in a patient with valvular heart disease. The murmur of mitral stenosis may not be heard until the patient is placed in the left lateral decubitus position; the same position may be required to move the left ventricle sufficiently close to the chest wall to allow a ventricular diastolic gallop to be appreciated. The diagnosis of mitral stenosis should also not be excluded until a brief period of muscular exercise, or an isometric handgrip, has been performed

to accentuate the murmur by increasing the heart rate and cardiac output, thereby augmenting the pressure gradient across the mitral valve. The handgrip maneuver tends to increase aortic pressure as well, and it is useful for augmenting a left ventricular gallop, or for accentuating the murmur of aortic regurgitation. The faint murmur of mild aortic regurgitation may also be detected only when the patient leans forward and breathes out completely. Sometimes the standing position is required to bring out the murmur of hypertrophic subaortic stenosis; the Valsalva maneuver is also useful for accentuating this murmur and for diminishing the murmur of valvular aortic stenosis. Other maneuvers, such as amyl nitrite inhalation, sometimes are used to produce characteristic changes in murmurs; for example, the murmur of rheumatic mitral regurgitation is diminished, whereas that of mitral valve prolapse is prolonged by this agent, and the murmur of aortic stenosis is increased.

CHEST ROENTGENOGRAM. As mentioned above, the jugular venous pulse provides a "direct access" route to the right atrium and allows estimation of the right atrial or systemic venous pressure. The pulmonary veins, of course, are inaccessible to physical examination, and therefore the chest roentgenogram is relied upon heavily to aid in detecting left atrial and pulmonary venous hypertension. Often, when there is left atrial hypertension, enlargement of the upper lobe pulmonary veins reflects redistribution of pulmonary blood flow, with reduced perfusion of the lung bases relative to the upper lobes (reversing the normal pattern in the upright posture), and there are signs of interstitial pulmonary edema (such as the Kerley B line) which usually precede the development of pulmonary (intra-alveolar) edema.

Oblique, overpenetrated views of the heart with barium swallow provide valuable information in evaluating valvular heart disease. Left atrial enlargement may be disclosed in the frontal view by a round "double density" or by elevation of the left mainstem bronchus in the frontal view, but it also may be detected only in the right anterior oblique view as a discrete, posterior displacement of the barium-filled esophagus. This view is also useful for identifying right ventricular enlargement in patients suspected of having pulmonary hypertension. The left anterior oblique projection is the most reliable for detecting enlargement of the left ventricle. Other clues to the location of valvular heart lesions include poststenotic dilatation of the aorta in valvular aortic stenosis or calcification in a heart valve. Sometimes the latter is detected only by image intensification fluoroscopy.

THE ELECTROCARDIOGRAM. In acquired valvular heart disease, the electrocardiogram should be carefully scrutinized for signs of chamber enlargement. Left atrial enlargement may be the only electrocardiographic sign of isolated mitral stenosis in the patient with sinus rhythm, and this single sign disappears when atrial fibrillation occurs. The presence or absence of left ventricular hypertrophy is of importance in considering the hemodynamic severity of aortic stenosis and in assessing the degree of mitral regurgitation; in the patient with mitral stenosis who has an apical systolic murmur, the presence of left ventricular hypertrophy may indicate that associated mitral regurgitation is of significance. The suspicion of associated coronary heart disease or myocardial disease may be raised by a bundle branch block pattern or by evidence of a previous myocardial infarction. Prominent (septal) Q waves associated with left ventricular hypertrophy can also occur with hypertrophic subaortic stenosis. Right axis deviation or right ventricular hypertrophy suggests significant pulmonary hypertension. Sometimes the vectorcardiogram is employed to confirm the presence or absence of myocardial infarction or ventricular hypertrophy.

SPECIAL LABORATORY TESTS. Short of cardiac catheterization (discussed below), two other noninvasive tests are highly useful in the precise diagnosis of acquired valvular heart disease: the *phonocardiogram* and the *echocardiogram*.

The *phonocardiogram* is of value particularly for ascertaining the timing of normal and abnormal heart sounds. Recorded with the heart sounds are the indirect carotid pulse wave, which substitutes for the arterial pressure tracing; the indirect jugular venous tracing, which resembles the atrial pressure pulse; and the apex cardiogram, which corresponds roughly to the diastolic left ventricular pressure pulse. For example, a mitral opening snap can be identified by its close relation to the onset of left ventricular filling on the apex-cardiogram, and its precise timing in relation to the aortic closure sound can be determined from the carotid pulse wave (see Fig. 1). A prolonged left ventricular ejection time and a single second heart sound are often associated with the abnormal carotid pulse wave of severe aortic stenosis (see Fig. 1). The phonocardiogram is not particularly useful for detecting soft cardiac murmur; these are better identified by careful auscultation at various locations and by the several maneuvers described above.

The *echocardiogram* can aid considerably in reaching an accurate clinical diagnosis (Fig. 2). Thus the characteristically abnormal pattern of anterior mitral valve leaflet motion can be demonstrated in mitral stenosis (see Fig. 2), or the fluttering movement of this leaflet associated with a diastolic Austin-Flint murmur can be identified. The echocardiogram may show posterior mitral leaflet prolapse when mitral regurgitation is associated with the click-murmur syndrome or with papillary muscle dysfunction (see Fig. 2). The characteristic anterior movement of the mitral leaflet during systole (see Fig. 2) and echocardiographic identification of septal hypertrophy have simplified the diagnosis of hypertrophic subaortic stenosis (hypertrophic cardiomyopathy with obstruction). In this condition, there is also asymmetric septal hypertrophy (ASH) (see Ch. 366.2). The applications of echocardiography are many, and the technique is finding increasing application in the study of cardiac diseases of all types.

DECISIONS CONSIDERING CARDIAC CATHETERIZATION AND OPERATION

Cardiac catheterization is rarely necessary for the *diagnosis* of valvular heart disease. An accurate diagnosis can usually be accomplished by careful application of the approaches described above, including the use of special noninvasive techniques such as echocardiography when necessary. Therefore cardiac catheterization and angiography are generally reserved until the patient is considered a potential candidate for a corrective operation. Of course there are some occasions when

cardiac catheterization is used to make a definitive diagnosis, such as in differentiating angina pectoris caused by aortic stenosis from that resulting from associated coronary atherosclerosis, or in the differential diagnosis of pulmonary hypertension. In the latter situation, it is clearly important not to make a diagnosis of primary pulmonary hypertension until valve obstruction has been carefully excluded by hemodynamic studies.

Prior to considering a surgical procedure, cardiac catheterization is usually undertaken for several purposes: (1) To determine whether the valve lesion (stenosis or regurgitation) is sufficiently severe to make it likely that surgical correction will relieve symptoms. (2) To assess carefully the degree of left ventricular myocardial dysfunction or failure associated with aortic valve lesions and mitral regurgitation. (3) To detect significant associated lesions, such as unexpectedly severe mitral regurgitation or aortic stenosis in a patient with mitral stenosis. (4) To study the coronary circulation, particularly in older subjects or in patients with aortic valve disease in whom symptoms may be due primarily to coronary heart disease rather than the valvular lesion. (5) To assess the relative significance of myocardial and valvular disease in patients with recurrent symptoms after previous cardiac surgery.

Once appropriate information has been assembled concerning the mechanical severity of the valve defect, the degree of involvement of the left ventricular myocardium, the severity of any associated coronary artery disease, and possible complicating illnesses (such as diabetes mellitus, liver disease, anemia, or thyroid disease), a decision concerning the advisability of a cardiac operation can be undertaken. Such a decision must also be based upon knowledge in several other important areas:

1. The risk to the patient's life of the proposed operation versus the risk of medical management alone. Operative risk is related to the nature of the surgical intervention required. Must a valve prosthesis be inserted, or is a commissurotomy possible? Is more than one valve involved? Is there associated coronary artery disease that will require a myocardial revascularization procedure? The patient's age and the presence of associated noncardiac illness also influence the operative risk.

2. The usual natural course of the valve lesion and the long-range outlook after operation. Knowledge of the natural history as well as the likely course after operation is important. For example, once significant symptoms begin in patients with aortic stenosis, the downhill course is usually rapid and the risk of *not* operating outweighs that of the surgical procedure. The average downhill course is somewhat slower after the onset of symptoms in patients with aortic regurgitation, but the degree of secondary left ventricular myocardial dysfunction must be considered, and operation should be undertaken before myocardial disease becomes irreversible. A similar consideration applies in patients with chronic mitral regurgitation, but their more gradual downhill course allows a more leisurely decision concerning the proper time for surgical intervention. The probable finite limitations in the life span of the various valvular prostheses should be taken into account before recommending operation in a young patient who has only moderate limitation of activity.

3. The social setting. This must be considered care-

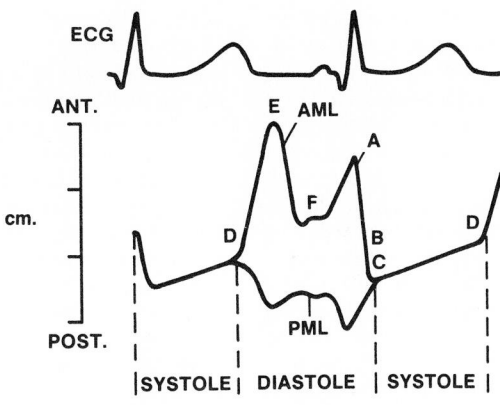

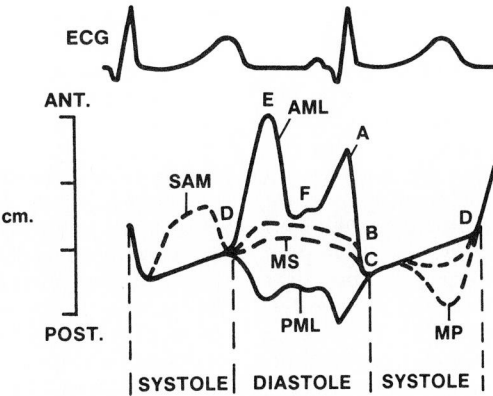

Figure 2. Characteristic normal and abnormal motions of the mitral valve.

Upper panel, Simplified diagrammatic echocardiogram of the motions of normal mitral valve as obtained by M-mode echocardiography. AML = Anterior mitral leaflet; PML = posterior mitral leaflet. ECG = simultaneously recorded electrocardiogram. The scale is in centimeters from anterior (ANT) to posterior (POST). During left ventricular systole the two leaflets are normally closed and there is a gradual anterior motion, as the whole heart moves forward during ventricular ejection. With the onset of diastole (D) the leaflets open rapidly in opposite directions, and during early rapid ventricular filling the anterior leaflet rapidly reaches its most forward position (E). The anterior leaflet then moves back to a partially closed position as rapid filling diminishes (E to F slope), and a brief period of slow filling or diastasis is shown, followed by another rapid opening of both leaflets due to late rapid filling during atrial contraction which reaches a peak at point A. With atrial relaxation the leaflets again close. The onset of mechanical ventricular contraction sometimes causes a notch (not shown) at point B, and is then followed by closure of the mitral valve at point C.

Lower panel, Abnormal mitral valve motions indicated by dashed lines.

In the typical patient with severe mitral stenosis (MS), the abnormalities are represented by the dashed lines during diastole. *Both* the anterior and posterior mitral leaflets move anteriorly during diastole; the forward excursion of the anterior leaflet to the E point is much reduced, and its E to F slope is greatly diminished.

In the patient with hypertrophic subaortic stenosis, during systole (on the left) the dashed line illustrates marked systolic anterior movement (SAM) of the anterior mitral leaflet. In some instances this motion may cause the anterior leaflet to touch the hypertrophied interventricular septum during systole, thereby leading to obstruction in the left ventricular outflow tract.

Mitral valve prolapse (MP) occurs during left ventricular systole, as illustrated in the right-hand systolic period. Typically, the leaflets move posteriorly during the latter half of systole, the motion often being most marked in the posterior leaflet, as shown. Occasionally, the posterior movement is holosystolic.

fully, for in the final analysis the expected benefits of the operation must be judged in relation to the patient's age, occupational needs, family responsibilities, and expectation of substantially improved longevity and functional capacity.

360.2. MITRAL STENOSIS

ETIOLOGY AND PATHOLOGY. Mitral stenosis in the adult usually develops as a sequel to rheumatic fever;

only rarely is obstruction caused by such malformations as congenital cor triatriatum (see Ch. 359.5) or left atrial myxoma. It is the most common single valvular lesion to follow acute rheumatic fever, accounting for over half the patients with chronic rheumatic heart disease. About two thirds of the subjects are female.

The rheumatic mitral valve shows fibrosis and thickening of the cusps, with partial fusion of the commissures; in patients with longstanding disease, leaflet fusion may produce restriction of the mitral orifice to as little as 0.5 sq cm. There are thickening and shortening of the chordae tendineae, and there may be heavy calcium deposits in the valve. The left ventricle is generally normal in size and weight unless there is associated mitral regurgitation or disease of the aortic valve, but the left atrium is enlarged and thick walled. Microscopic examination of the myocardium often shows evidence of old rheumatic myocarditis (Aschoff bodies). In the lungs, there is thickening of the muscular walls of the pulmonary arterioles and venules with intimal proliferation, and in the late stages of mitral stenosis there is diffuse hemosiderosis (primarily disintegrated hemoglobin within alveoli), and there may be interstitial fibrosis and pulmonary infarction.

PATHOLOGIC PHYSIOLOGY. The primary physiologic abnormality in mitral stenosis is mechanical obstruction to emptying of the left atrium produced by the narrowed valve orifice. Left ventricular function is usually normal, and therefore the defect in mitral stenosis stands in marked contrast to that of mitral regurgitation, or of aortic valve disease, in each of which a chronic overload is placed in the left ventricle.

When the mitral valve orifice is only mildly reduced, the mean left atrial pressure and filling of the left ventricle remain normal at rest. However, the rate of blood flow across the mitral valve is dependent not only on the orifice area of the valve and the driving pressure gradient (from left atrium to left ventricle), but also on the *time* available for flow across the mitral valve during diastole. With an increase in heart rate, the duration of left ventricular systole shortens only slightly, and tachycardia therefore occurs mainly at the expense of diastolic filling time per minute. Hence patients with mild mitral stenosis generally experience their earliest symptoms only during severe exertion, or with the onset of rapid atrial fibrillation. With exertion, both the normal tachycardia of exercise and the increased cardiac output lead to an increased left atrial pressure, whereas with atrial fibrillation and an uncontrolled ventricular rate the increased rate alone leads to a left atrial pressure elevation because of compromised filling time per minute.

With increased narrowing of the mitral orifice, the mean left atrial pressure becomes somewhat elevated at rest (over 12 mm Hg), but as the mitral orifice is reduced to below 1 sq cm the resting cardiac output can be maintained only at the expense of a markedly elevated left atrial pressure (often in excess of 20 mm Hg), in which the high pressure gradient forces blood across the narrowed orifice at high velocity. In this stage of the disease, the increased left atrial pressure and critically narrowed mitral valve often lead to pulmonary edema. Although pulmonary edema theoretically should occur when the pulmonary venous pressure exceeds about 30 mm Hg, higher levels have occasionally been recorded without its occurrence. This may be related to thickening of the alveolar-capillary membrane, which has been noted in the lungs of patients with mitral stenosis.

As the disease progresses, the elevated pressure in the pulmonary veins leads to pulmonary artery hypertension (see also Ch. 358.4). When pulmonary hypertension becomes persistent at rest, it reflects two major factors: first, the elevated left atrial pressure is transmitted retrogradely and requires an increased pressure head in the pulmonary artery to drive blood forward; and second, pulmonary arteriolar vasoconstriction

occurs. This vasoconstriction is accompanied in time by organic changes, mainly intimal proliferation and medial thickening in the walls of the small pulmonary arteries. At this stage, the pulmonary vascular resistance becomes elevated, which in turn leads to a reduction in the resting cardiac output. This sequence tends to limit any further increase in the left atrial pressure, which may even fall somewhat as the cardiac output becomes diminished. Symptoms of pulmonary venous congestion and pulmonary edema often diminish at this stage. In late mitral stenosis, pulmonary hypertension may become extreme, with the systolic pressure in the pulmonary artery equal to or exceeding that in the systemic arterial bed. Even with less marked elevations in pulmonary arterial pressure, the right ventricular end-diastolic volume and pressure become elevated, and this may lead to functional tricuspid regurgitation. Finally, signs of right ventricular failure appear with peripheral venous congestion.

CLINICAL MANIFESTATIONS. Symptoms and Clinical Course. After one or more attacks of rheumatic fever in childhood, there is a latent period averaging about 12 years before mitral stenosis becomes clinically manifest, symptoms and signs usually first becoming apparent in young adulthood. There is commonly then a relatively long period (five to eight years) of mild to moderate symptoms as the scarring and obstruction at the valve gradually progress.

The earliest manifestation of mild to moderate mitral stenosis is dyspnea caused primarily by the increased cardiac output and tachycardia of exercise, leading to transient elevation of left atrial pressure, as discussed above. Elevation of the left atrial pressure causes pulmonary venous hypertension, increasing lung stiffness and the work of breathing, and thereby leads to the subjective sensation of dyspnea. As the disease progresses, orthopnea at night commences as a result of redistribution of the peripheral blood volume into the central circulation and of peripheral resorption of fluid caused by the supine posture. Coughing, particularly at night, may also be a troublesome symptom. Dyspnea eventually becomes extreme with minimal activity, and hemoptysis may occur owing to rupture of dilated endobronchial vessels, which appear to form collateral channels between the pulmonary and bronchial venous systems. The hemoptysis, consisting of bright red blood which can accumulate in sufficient quantities to cause atelectasis, usually subsides with bed rest and sedation with opiates; most commonly it occurs in patients who do not have severe elevation of the pulmonary vascular resistance. An increased number of pulmonary infections may occur, perhaps related to the interstitial pulmonary edema present in this stage of the disease, and other factors such as severe emotional stress, sexual activity, and fever with tachycardia may acutely worsen the patient's symptoms.

Significant left atrial enlargement develops as the left atrial hypertension becomes persistent, and atrial premature beats, paroxysmal atrial tachycardia, or atrial fibrillation commonly occur. The sudden onset of atrial fibrillation with rapid ventricular rate may precipitate acute pulmonary edema when the obstruction at the mitral orifice is of sufficient severity. Eventually, sustained atrial fibrillation supervenes, requiring control of the ventricular response with digitalis. Intermittent atrial fibrillation, in particular, may be associated with peripheral embolic phenomena, and the incidence of emboli in patients with chronic atrial fibrillation is substantial. As the left atrium enlarges and stasis occurs, thrombus formation is most frequent within the left atrial appendage, and adherent clots have been found at operation in this location in about 30 per cent of patients. Small emboli may break loose to become lodged in the renal, splenic, or cerebral circulations, and the effects of such emboli, causing a convulsion or perhaps a renal infarction, sometimes provide the initial symptom in a patient with mitral stenosis. Coronary artery embolization with myocardial infarction has also been reported. Sometimes a large embolus to the brain results in serious and permanent sequelae, and saddle embolus in the aorta has been encountered on a number of occasions. Infrequently a thrombus within the left atrium may become sufficiently large to obstruct a pulmonary vein, leading to localized unilateral pulmonary edema, and rarely a pedunculated "ball-valve thrombus" can be formed which mimics the findings of left atrial myxoma (see below).

As mitral stenosis progresses further, the pulmonary vascular resistance rises, tending to limit flow across the pulmonary bed; with the associated diminution of pulmonary venous hypertension, hemoptysis and pulmonary interstitial edema diminish. Thus in patients with longstanding, severe mitral stenosis, dyspnea on exertion and orthopnea often become less prominent and fatigue now predominates. The development of functional tricuspid regurgitation may result in a further drop in the cardiac output and some reduction in the pulmonary artery pressure. In this stage of the disease weakness and signs of right heart failure become extreme, and abdominal discomfort with hepatomegaly, ascites, and peripheral edema dominate the clinical picture. Pulmonary embolus with pulmonary infarction is a common late complication.

Physical Findings. The patient (usually a female) with severe mitral stenosis may exhibit peripheral cyanosis and a "mitral facies" (blue-tinged with malar flush), and often there is some degree of emaciation. In such advanced cases, peripheral edema and ascites may also be evident.

The peripheral arterial pulses are typically small, and the blood pressure is normal or low. The jugular venous pulse is initially normal in the presence of moderate mitral stenosis, but as pulmonary hypertension develops, the mean venous pressure is increased and the A wave becomes prominent owing to right ventricular hypertrophy and elevation of the right ventricular end-diastolic pressure. In the presence of atrial fibrillation, there is a dominant V wave in the jugular veins.

In patients with mitral stenosis without pulmonary hypertension, palpation of the precordium may be unremarkable except for the presence of a diastolic thrill localized just inside the left ventricular apex. The accentuated first heart sound and sometimes an opening snap may be palpable. The apical impulse is otherwise normal, and the heart is not enlarged. In patients with pulmonary hypertension, there is a right ventricular lift in the left parasternal area, and the bulging pulmonary artery segment and pulmonic closure may be palpable at the upper left base if the mean pulmonary arterial pressure is in excess of 50 mm Hg.

On auscultation, the first heart sound is generally loud, snapping in quality, and somewhat delayed (see Fig. 1, Ch. 360.1). These features occur because the left atrial pressure is elevated, and additional time is required for the left ventricle to build up sufficient pressure to close the mitral valve; the rate of change of left ventricular pressure (dP/dt) is rapid by that time, which results in the more forceful than normal mitral valve closure. The aortic closure sound is normal, but a mitral opening snap follows the second sound, the snap being audible at the lower left sternal border and the apex. A general correlation exists between the severity of mitral stenosis and the timing of the opening snap, necessitating careful evaluation of the interval between aortic closure and the opening snap on the phonocardiogram. As the left ventricular pressure declines during the isovolumetric relaxation period after aortic valve closure, eventually it falls below the left atrial pressure and the stenotic mitral valve then snaps open. The higher the left atrial pressure, the closer this event must occur in relation to aortic closure (A_2). This time interval (the so-called A_2-OS interval) tends to be long (0.10 second or more) in patients with mild mitral stenosis and mean left atrial pressures below 15 mm Hg, whereas in patients with severe mitral stenosis and mean left atrial pressures of 20 mm Hg or more, the interval is usually shorter (less than 0.09 second). As might be expected, however, the interval will vary considerably with the heart rate. If the heart rate is below 100 and the interval 0.07 second or less, the mitral stenosis is usually of significant degree.

The opening snap is followed immediately by a low-pitched *diastolic rumble* resulting from turbulent flow across the stenotic mitral orifice. The murmur is usually localized to an area about 2 cm in diameter near or just inside the left ventricular apex in the fourth or fifth left intercostal space, and it is best brought out by positioning the patient in the lateral decubitus position. The mitral rumble is loudest in early diastole; it diminishes somewhat as the pressure gradient between left atrium and left ventricle falls, and, in patients with sinus rhythm, it then becomes loud (presystolic accentuation) as the left atrium contracts to again raise the pressure gradient (see Fig. 1, Ch. 360.1). When the stenosis is mild, the diastolic murmur may not be audible until the patient is placed in the lateral decubitus position *after* performing mild exercise or during a handgrip maneuver, when the cardiac output and heart rate are increased, thereby augmenting the pressure gradient across the valve. In the presence of atrial fibrillation, presystolic accentuation disappears; when the ventricular rate is slow, the murmur may occur only in the early and middle phases of long diastolic periods, because given sufficient time the left atrial and left ventricular pressure will come into equilibrium. In patients with severe mitral stenosis and a very low cardiac output, the murmur may be unusually difficult to appreciate. It is most important therefore to position the patient properly and to listen carefully over a wide area of the left chest for the well localized murmur, as well as to carry out the aforementioned exercise maneuvers. When such precautions are taken, "silent" mitral stenosis will be encountered rarely. Occasionally the murmur is inaudible when massive right ventricular enlargement places the left ventricle far posteriorly from the chest wall.

Individuals with "pure" mitral stenosis have a small fixed orifice, and it is not uncommon to hear a soft systolic murmur at the cardiac apex, which presents a trivial mitral regurgitant leak. When a louder pansystolic murmur at the left ventricular apex is accompanied by a third heart sound, by left ventricular enlargement on physical examination, or by electrocardiographic signs of left ventricular hypertrophy, the associated mitral regurgitation is undoubtedly of significance. In the patient with severe pulmonary hypertension, when a very large right ventricle fills the anterior chest and displaces the left ventricle posteriorly, the murmur of tricuspid regurgitation can mimic that of mitral regurgitation. The systolic murmur of tricuspid regurgitation is ordinarily heard best at the lower left sternal border; it increases with inspiration, and is not heard in the axilla or over the spine posteriorly, features which serve to distinguish it from the murmur of mitral regurgitation. With severe pulmonary hypertension the high-pitched, early diastolic blowing murmur of pulmonic regurgitation (the Graham Steell murmur) may also be audible. This murmur, heard best at the left sternal border, is usually indistinguishable from that of mild aortic regurgitation.

DIAGNOSIS. Electrocardiogram. In patients with moderate mitral stenosis and sinus rhythm, the electrocardiogram may be normal, or it may show only left atrial enlargement, with a notched and prolonged P wave in the limb leads and an increased negative component of the P wave in lead V_1. When there is atrial fibrillation, patients with rheumatic heart disease tend to show coarse fibrillation waves, presumably owing to the thickened atrial wall and enlarged chamber volume, a finding which contrasts with the fine fibrillatory waves often found in patients with coronary heart disease.

The right ventricle is the next chamber to be affected as mitral stenosis progresses, and in severe mitral stenosis with pulmonary hypertension the electrocardiogram often shows right axis deviation. Usually, if the QRS axis is 100 degrees or more or the R/S ratio in V_1 exceeds unity, the mean pulmonary artery pressure is over 35 mm Hg. Evidence of left ventricular hypertrophy in a patient with mitral stenosis generally indicates accompanying aortic valve disease or significant associated mitral regurgitation.

Roentgenographic Features. Minimal enlargement of the left atrium may be the only radiographic abnormality in patients with moderate mitral stenosis. It may be apparent only with barium swallow, the right anterior oblique view showing best the localized, posterior displacement of the barium-filled esophagus. As the disease progresses, left atrial enlargement becomes distinct, and this chamber is visible as a large round "double density" in the center of the cardiac shadow on the frontal view. The left mainstem bronchus is elevated by the enlarged left atrium (the angle formed by the bronchus with a central, vertical line increasing to more than 45 degrees), and enlargement of the left atrial appendage results in straightening of the left heart border.

As left atrial and pulmonary venous hypertension develop, there is a redistribution of the pulmonary vascularity in the lung fields. Initially, in the upright posture the normal, relative avascularity of the upper lobes is lost, and the pulmonary vascular pattern appears equal in the upper and lower lungs. In later stages of the disease, vascularity in the upper lobe vessels is increased.

Redistribution of the pulmonary vascular pattern generally occurs when left atrial pressure exceeds 15 mm Hg, and evidence of interstitial pulmonary edema commonly appears when the mean left atrial pressure at rest exceeds 20 mm Hg. Interstitial edema may be evidenced by *Kerley's B lines*, transverse linear densities about 1 cm in length and located at the lung bases laterally above the diaphragm, representing engorged septal lymphatic vessels. Acute pulmonary edema is reflected by typical butterfly densities in the hilar regions.

As pulmonary hypertension develops, the pulmonary artery segment becomes enlarged, the peripheral pulmonary arteries become dilated, and enlargement of the right ventricle and right atrium is evident. With long-standing pulmonary hypertension a diffuse reticular pattern in the lung fields may result from pulmonary hemosiderosis. Calcification in the mitral valve should be searched for, using image intensification fluoroscopy. The presence of calcification makes it less likely that the valve will prove amenable to valvuloplasty.

Phonocardiography. The phonocardiogram is particularly useful for timing the A_2-OS interval (see Physical Findings). Also, the configuration of the apexcardiogram, as it reflects diastolic events in the left ventricle (see Fig. 1, Ch. 360.1), may show loss of a rapid early filling wave and absence of a presystolic (A) wave in patients with significant mitral stenosis.

Echocardiography. Reflected ultrasound to confirm the presence of mitral stenosis and to estimate its severity has found widespread application. The echo recorded from the mitral leaflets exhibits characteristic features in the presence of significant mitral stenosis, the degree of the abnormality correlating in general with the severity of stenosis. Thickening of the anterior and posterior leaflets can often be identified, and there is a reduced anterior excursion of the leaflet during diastole (see Fig. 2, Ch. 360.1). Also, the degree of separation of the anterior and posterior leaflets during diastole is reduced in the presence of mitral stenosis. Both the anterior and posterior leaflets move forward with diastole as the domed, stenotic valve opens (in a normal valve, the posterior leaflet opens in an opposite direction to the anterior leaflet). Because of the persistent pressure gradient from left atrium to left ventricle, the normal posterior floating motion of the anterior mitral leaflet during mid-diastole does not occur; the leaflet is held open in an anterior position and moves only slowly posteriorly (see Fig. 2, Ch. 360.1). This posterior motion (the so-called E to F slope) is reduced to less than 15 mm per second when mitral stenosis is severe and is usually less than 25 mm per second when it is moderate. Although a general relation exists between the hemodynamic severity of mitral stenosis and the degree of reduction of the E to F slope, the slope by itself has not proved to be a reliable measure of the severity of stenosis; thus other factors such as the cardiac output and the left ventricular diastolic compliance also affect this measurement. Cross-sectional echocardiography, as with a mechanical sector scanner, offers the promise of direct estimates of the mitral valve orifice area, but this approach remains to be further validated.

The detection of characteristic moving echoes from behind the mitral valve can indicate the presence of left atrial myxoma or a ball-valve thrombus.

Pulmonary Function Tests. Patients with longstanding mitral stenosis generally have a reduced pulmonary compliance owing to elevation of the left atrial pressure and interstitial pulmonary edema. The vital capacity, total lung capacity, maximal breathing capacity, and oxygen uptake per unit of ventilation may be reduced, and abnormalities of ventilation-perfusion relations are often seen as well.

Cardiac Catheterization. In the young patient with obvious features of pure mitral stenosis and marked symptoms, cardiac catheterization is not performed in some centers prior to operation. On the other hand, when there is uncertainty about the severity of the stenosis in relation to the level of symptoms, cardiac catheterization should be performed to document objectively the degree of valve narrowing, and to calculate the orifice area. At cardiac catheterization, the typical patient with significant mitral stenosis will exhibit an elevated mean pulmonary artery wedge pressure. If a satisfactory wedge pressure tracing cannot be obtained, transseptal left atrial puncture is often performed. If the patient is in sinus rhythm, the forceful left atrial contraction produces a dominant A wave in the tracing, and there is a slow fall in the pressure after the V wave (reduced rate of the Y descent), reflecting obstruction to left atrial emptying during diastole. The left ventricular end-diastolic pressure is usually normal (below 12 mm Hg). The pressure gradient from left atrium to left ventricle is high early in diastole, falling progressively as left ventricular filling occurs, but the gradient is again increased late in diastole by left atrial contraction (see Fig. 1, Ch. 360.1). In patients with atrial fibrillation, the V wave is dominant and left atrial pressure continues to fall throughout diastole until the onset of ventricular systole.

The *mitral valve orifice area* can be calculated if both the cardiac output and the pressure gradient are known. By the Gorlin formula, the valve orifice area is directly proportional to the flow across the valve per second of diastole and is inversely proportional to the square root of the pressure gradient. In simple terms, this means that if the flow doubles, the pressure gradient will quadruple. Because of this nonlinear relation, measurement of the left atrial or wedge pressure alone can be misleading in assessing the severity of the mitral stenosis. Thus if the cardiac output is unusually high, an elevated left atrial mean pressure may give a false picture of the severity of the stenotic lesion; if it is low, a moderate left atrial pressure elevation may belie the presence of severe stenosis. Also, if the heart rate is abnormally rapid or slow and a shorter or longer diastolic filling time is available, the left atrial mean pressure may not reflect accurately the size of the mitral orifice. The area of the normal mitral valve is about 4 sq cm. Mitral stenosis is generally considered mild when the calculated orifice area is over 1.2 sq cm, moderate when it is between 1.2 and 0.9 sq cm, and severe when it is below 0.8 sq cm. Thus an area of 1.1 sq cm or less is usually considered to represent stenosis of sufficient severity to warrant operation.

Left ventriculography usually shows the left ventricle to contract normally, with a normal end-diastolic volume. It also provides information concerning the degree of thickening and fusion of the chordal attachments of the mitral valve, the pliability of its leaflets, and the degree of associated mitral regurgitation. All these factors, together with the presence or absence of valve calcification, weigh in the decision of whether to perform mitral valvuloplasty, or whether to recommend replacement of the valve with a prosthesis.

In older patients, selective coronary arteriography is indicated to search for significant coronary vascular disease. Cardiac catheterization will also document the severity of any associated aortic valvular disease; in patients with recurrent systemic emboli, a pulmonary angiogram may verify the presence of a left atrial thrombus.

DIFFERENTIAL DIAGNOSIS. Clinical findings of pulmonary hypertension should raise the suspicion of mitral stenosis. *Primary pulmonary hypertension* usually occurs in young females; it is associated with hyperventilation, chest pain, fatigue and dyspnea, and effort syncope, but with a relative paucity of objective physical findings. Whenever this diagnosis is considered, mitral stenosis and left atrial myxoma, treatable causes of left atrial and pulmonary hypertension, should be excluded by measurement of left atrial pressure directly or from an adequate pulmonary arterial wedge pressure. *Pulmonary hypertension caused by severe chronic lung disease* usually presents no diagnostic difficulty; but sometimes patients are given a diagnosis of ordinary bronchial asthma, when in fact their wheezing is due to mitral stenosis with left atrial hypertension ("cardiac asthma").

The murmur of rheumatic mitral stenosis may be mimicked by that resulting from a *left atrial myxoma*. However, with the latter lesion there may be other abnormal diastolic sounds, and the murmur may disappear when the patient's position is altered. In addition, symptoms can vary with changes in body position, syncope may occur, and there is usually an elevated sedimentation rate, anemia, fever, or other evidence of systemic disease. Echocardiography may detect the left atrial myxoma. In the young patient, *congenital cor triatriatum* (a rare malformation consisting of a fibrous partition within the left atrium above the mitral valve) may be considered.

The diastolic rumble which occurs in the presence of severe aortic regurgitation, the *Austin Flint murmur*, may be attributed to organic mitral stenosis. This murmur is typically ushered in by a ventricular diastolic gallop (S_3) rather than an opening snap, and it is loudest in mid-diastole. Amyl nitrite inhalation decreases this murmur by lowering diastolic aortic pressure, but the reflex tachycardia and increased cardiac output increase the murmur of mitral stenosis. Echocardiography is particularly helpful in differentiating the Austin Flint murmur from that of mitral stenosis by detecting a characteristic fluttering motion of the anterior leaflet during diastole as its motion is affected by the regurgitant jet.

In the older patient, *atrial septal defect* is occasionally mistaken for mitral stenosis. In atrial septal defect, the tricuspid closure sound is loud, the widely split second heart may mimic the opening snap of mitral stenosis, and the rumble of excessive flow across the tricuspid valve may be confused with the murmur of mitral stenosis. The murmur of mitral stenosis diminishes with inspiration, in contrast to this murmur and the murmur of tricuspid stenosis, which increase.

TREATMENT. Medical Management. In the patient with mild mitral stenosis and few symptoms, restriction of strenuous activity may result in many years of comfortable existence. If the patient is under 40 years of age, monthly Bicillin injections or oral penicillin (sulfonamides may be used in the allergic patient) are advisable to prevent infection with the beta-hemolytic *Streptococcus* and recurrence of acute rheumatic fever (see Ch. 130). In addition, antimicrobial drugs in therapeutic doses should be recommended prior to and after dental procedures or surgical manipulations, particularly those on the genitourinary tract, to prevent infective endocarditis (see Ch. 131).

In patients with moderate symptoms, limitation of activity should be combined with *sodium restriction* and/or administration of a *diuretic* agent. There is little rationale for the use of digitalis in patients with sinus rhythm, because left ventricular function is normal and this agent has no effect on exercise-induced tachycardia. *When atrial fibrillation occurs* for the first time, one or more attempts at *electrical reversion of the rhythm*, followed by maintenance with oral quinidine, are generally indicated. When mitral stenosis is significant, however, permanent atrial fibrillation will generally supervene in time, despite such therapy. In the presence of chronic atrial fibrillation, *digitalis* should be administered to maintain the ventricular rate at an acceptable level both at rest and during moderate exertion. In patients in whom the ventricular rate is difficult to control even with high doses of digitalis, the addition of a *beta-adrenergic blocking agent* (such as propranolol) in small doses may result in very effective control of the ventricular response. Moreover, during acute stress, such as a pneumonia, patients with atrial fibrillation may develop a rapid ventricular response caused by enhanced atrioventricular conduction consequent to excessive sympathetic nervous discharge; under these circumstances the addition of a beta-adrenergic blocking agent to digitalis may allow effective reduction of the ventricular rate in a safer manner than with high doses of digitalis alone. When the ventricular rate is refractory to digitalis in the absence of acute stress, or when signs of heart failure are out of proportion to the degree of mitral stenosis, hyperthyroidism should be suspected. Obvious signs of thyrotoxicosis may be masked in the presence of cardiac disease; but if such hyperthyroidism is detected and treated, symptoms caused by mild mitral stenosis may disappear.

In patients who have suffered a systemic embolus originating from the left atrium, long-term *anticoagulation* with Coumadin derivatives has been shown to be effective in preventing recurrence. The risk of recurrent embolization is greatly increased by atrial fibrillation and may occur even with mild mitral stenosis accompanied by atrial fibrillation. Minor neurologic episodes, or a frank convulsion, often provide the earliest sign of systemic embolization. Emboli also may occur to the legs, to the spleen, or to the mesenteric artery (causing abdominal pain and bowel necrosis), and prompt surgical treatment with embolectomy is required. Coronary artery embolization also occurs occasionally. If systemic embolization recurs while the patient is on adequate anticoagulant therapy, a mitral valve operation with removal of left atrial clot may be recommended for the patient with somewhat milder mitral stenosis, or with less marked symptoms than are usually required for an elective operation.

When pregnancy occurs in a patient with mitral stenosis, symptoms frequently develop for the first time or intensify. Such symptoms become most severe during the second trimester, when increased cardiac output and blood volume are maximal, and a substantial period of hospital treatment may be required. Generally, such symptoms diminish during the third trimester, and only rarely is a mitral commissurotomy necessary during pregnancy.

Once severe symptoms begin in the patient with tight mitral stenosis (New York Heart Association [N.Y.H.A.] Class III), the average mortality in patients treated medically approaches 30 per cent at five years. In severely limited patients (Class IV), the outlook without operation is extremely poor, less than 20 per cent of patients being alive after five years if data gathered prior to the cardiac surgical era are considered. Surgical treatment has greatly altered this outlook.

Surgical Treatment. In the typical younger patient with symptoms on normal activity (N.Y.H.A. Class II) and findings of pure mitral stenosis, the decision of whether to recommend operation is usually reached by considering the individual in his desired activity setting. In the patient with significant mitral stenosis who has had a complication such as a systemic embolus and who develops symptoms on ordinary exertion, operation is usually recommended. In the older patient in functional Class II who has evidence of mitral valve calcification on x-ray and physical findings suggesting a thickened and immobile mitral leaflet (soft first heart sound and reduced or absent opening snap), or in whom significant associated mitral regurgitation is suspected, a waiting period until symptoms are more severe is justified, because mitral valve replacement with a prosthesis will undoubtedly be necessary. Other features which indicate that valve replacement will probably be required are evidence of left ventricular hypertrophy, previous valvotomy, and a markedly thickened, immobile anterior leaflet on echocardiography. In patients with symptoms on less than normal activity (N.Y.H.A. Class III) or at rest (Class IV), the outlook without surgical treatment is poor and the indication for operation is clear.

The presence of severe pulmonary hypertension was considered at one time to represent a relative contraindication to operation, but more recent studies have indicated that even marked elevations of the pulmonary vascular resistance invariably regress postoperatively. Some reduction in the pulmonary vascular resistance occurs within a few hours postoperatively. In most patients studied by cardiac catheterization six months to one year after operation, the pulmonary artery pressure and pulmonary vascular resistance have returned to normal or near normal levels, provided the left atrial pressure is normal.

Surgical practices differ somewhat as to the type of procedure performed in the patient with mitral stenosis. Closed mitral valvulotomy by opening the valve commissures with the finger, inserted through the left atrial appendage, sometimes combined with the use of a mechanical dilator passed through the left ventricular apex, is still employed by some surgeons without the use of cardiopulmonary bypass (heart-lung machine). In many centers, open mitral commissurotomy is now carried out even in the uncomplicated patient, the left atrium being opened with the patient on cardiopulmonary bypass and the mitral stenosis relieved by blunt and sharp dissection under direct vision. The operative risk of such a mitral valvuloplasty is now about equal to that of cardiopulmonary bypass alone (under 2 per cent). This approach also allows removal of any clot that may be present within the left atrium. If significant mitral regurgitation is produced by the attempted valvuloplasty, it is then possible to proceed readily with replacement of the mitral valve by a ball-valve or other prosthesis.

The late results of valvuloplasty have been poor when there is significant mitral regurgitation, or if there is calcification with severe shortening and thickening of the chordae tendineae and immobilization of the mitral valve leaflets. When the valve exhibits such unfavorable anatomic signs, it is replaced with a prosthetic device, the caged ball-valve (Starr-Edwards) and, more recently, the glutaraldehyde-preserved porcine aortic valve xenograft being employed in many centers.

After a valvuloplasty, the average patient experiences 8 to 12 years of symptomatic relief, but a second operation is often necessary (usually mitral valve replacement). The average age at the time of mitral valve replacement is between 50 and 53 years, and about 30 per cent of patients have had a previous mitral commissurotomy. Most experience has been obtained with the caged ball-valve (Starr-Edwards) type of prosthesis. Operative mortality currently averages between 3 and 7 per cent, but it is higher in patients who are in N.Y.H.A. Class IV (average 20 per cent) and in patients who have objective findings of a very large left atrium and right ventricular hypertrophy. Mitral valve replacement usually results in marked alleviation of symptoms and appears to offer substantial prolongation of average life expectancy, when compared to earlier studies on the natural history of medically treated patients with mitral valve disease who were in Classes III and IV. At five years postoperatively, about 75 to 80 per cent of the patients who survive mitral valve replacement are alive, and about two thirds are still alive at the end of a ten-year follow-up. The long-term outlook is poorer for Class IV patients, however, with only about 50 per cent surviving at the end of six years. Thus results appear to support the desirability of operating on patients with mitral valve disease before Class IV symptoms appear, and before great left atrial enlargement with right ventricular overload are present. Thromboembolism is a significant complication with the ball-valve prosthesis, and continuous anticoagulation with sodium warfarin is customarily employed. Embolism occurs at rates of from 3 to 8 per cent per year, depending upon the adequacy of anticoagulation, the type of valve (cloth-covered versus non-cloth-covered), and the size of the left atrium. There also is some risk of a major complication, or death, from bleeding complications associated with the anticoagulation, and about one quarter of late deaths are related to the ball-valve prosthesis (e.g., thrombotic occlusion of the valve, bacterial endocarditis, embolism, or bleeding).

The follow-up after replacement of the mitral valve with the porcine xenograft valve is shorter and involves fewer patients. However, the incidence of thromboembolism has been lower (approximately 1 to 3 per cent per year), and generally patients have not been maintained on anticoagulants after the first three postoperative months. Anticoagulation may be continued, however, in those patients with left atrial enlargement and atrial fibrillation. Some centers have reported lower operative mortalities after xenograft mitral valve replacement than with the ball-valve prosthesis, and late deaths related to the xenograft so far have been rare. Long-term valve durability beyond five years is still an unresolved question with this type of valve substitute.

360.3. MITRAL REGURGITATION

ETIOLOGY AND PATHOLOGY. A wide spectrum of disease processes can result in mitral regurgitation, although rheumatic involvement is easily the most common cause. Rheumatic mitral regurgitation occurs more commonly in males, in contrast to mitral stenosis, and the murmur is commonly heard during or soon after the acute rheumatic episode, again in contrast to the relatively late development of the murmur of mitral stenosis. In chronic rheumatic disease, the left ventricle is generally dilated and the wall thickened, there is left atrial enlargement, and the mitral valve exhibits mild, diffuse scarring of the leaflets associated with some thickening of the chordae tendineae. The finding of associated aortic valve disease favors a rheumatic cause.

Other forms of mitral regurgitation include rupture of one or more chordae tendineae, most commonly resulting from bacterial endocarditis, but also sometimes attributed to rheumatic disease, trauma, or unknown causes. Papillary muscle dysfunction is usually secondary to necrosis or fibrosis of one or both papillary muscles owing to coronary artery disease, mitral regurgitation resulting from poor contraction of the muscles, and systolic eversion of the mitral leaflets. In acute myocardial infarction, rupture of a papillary muscle causes sudden, severe mitral regurgitation (see Ch. 363.3). Congenital mitral regurgitation can occur as an isolated condition, but more commonly it accompanies such lesions as ostium primum atrial septal defect or Marfan's syndrome in which the valve may resemble that found in the floppy valve syndrome, but is associated with other stigmata.

Mitral regurgitation also occurs as a secondary phenomenon in patients with obstructive hypertrophic cardiomyopathy, as discussed subsequently. In primary myocardial disease, mitral regurgitation may be secondary to massive dilatation of the left ventricle and the mitral anulus. Acquired, heavy calcification of the mitral anulus, which typically occurs in elderly women, is sometimes associated with significant mitral regurgitation. The mitral valve prolapse syndrome has been recognized with increased frequency and is considered in Ch. 360.4.

PATHOLOGIC PHYSIOLOGY. With insufficiency of the mitral valve of the type found in chronic rheumatic heart disease, regurgitation of blood from the left ventricle into the left atrium commences as soon as the left ventricular pressure during early systole exceeds that in the left atrium, and persists until the left ventricular pressure falls below the left atrial pressure. Therefore the regurgitation is pansystolic, commencing with the first heart sound and often ending with or just after the second heart sound, and at the peak of the atrial V wave. The prominent V wave in the left atrial pressure pulse is due to the normal inflow of blood from the pulmonary veins (when the mitral valve is ordinarily closed) which is augmented by the regurgitant leak.

An important physiologic characteristic of mitral regurgitation relative to the function of the left ventricle is that this lesion provides a relatively low impedance pathway for blood to exit from the left ventricle, pressure in the left atrium being lower than that in the aorta. The pressure in the left ventricle tends to fall more abruptly than normal late in ventricular systole because of the leak, and the average afterload or active tension in the wall of the left ventricle is thereby reduced. This effect favors increased shortening of the myocardial wall because of the inverse relation between force and fiber shortening (and velocity), and the ratio of stroke volume to end-diastolic volume (ejection fraction) may therefore be normal or even high in mitral regurgitation. In addition, although myocardial oxygen consumption is greatly enhanced by lesions which cause increased systolic pressure work or augmented wall tension, it is little affected by the increased volume load imposed by mitral regurgitation. These favorable mechanical loading conditions and the minimal effect of this lesion on oxygen consumption help to explain the prolonged clinical course observed in many patients with chronic mitral regurgitation.

In chronic mitral regurgitation the diastolic volume of the left ventricular chamber becomes increased because of ventricular dilatation and increased muscle mass. The increased diastolic ventricular size allows delivery of a much larger than normal *total* stroke volume during systole (forward stroke volume plus the regurgitant volume), but with a normal extent of shortening of each unit of the enlarged left ventricular circumference. When left ventricular myocardial function is not impaired, the left ventricular end-diastolic pressure is normal or only slightly elevated, and the forward cardiac output is well maintained. Under these conditions, the *mean* left atrial pressure may be minimally elevated, because the exaggerated V wave occurs only briefly during the cardiac cycle. There is no impairment of left atrial emptying into the left ventricle and hence little or no rise in mean left atrial pressure during exercise.

With longstanding, severe mitral regurgitation, left ventricular myocardial contractility is eventually depressed. When this happens, the extent of shortening of the left ventricular wall becomes reduced, the residual volume in the left ventricle at the end of ejection increases, the ejection fraction falls, and the end-diastolic volume and left ventricular end-diastolic pressure rise. The latter, in turn, leads to elevation of the mean left atrial pressure and subsequently to pulmonary hypertension. Left atrial hypertension also occurs when there is some associated narrowing of the mitral valve. The mechanism of pulmonary hypertension in mitral regurgitation resembles that in mitral stenosis, and in later stages elevations of the pulmonary vascular resistance as severe as those seen with mitral stenosis have been encountered.

The aforementioned description encompasses most patients with chronic rheumatic mitral regurgitation, but there are unusual physiologic manifestations seen late in the course of chronic disease or with acute mitral regurgitation, such as that caused by ruptured chordae tendineae. In the former category is the finding of giant left atrium with low mean left atrial pressure and greatly reduced cardiac output. This syndrome appears to be due to a combination of poor left ventricular function with reduced forward cardiac output and diminished regurgitant volume, as well as to a capacious and compliant left atrium, which absorbs the regurgitant leak with little change in the pressure. At the other extreme is the situation in sudden, severe mitral regurgitation. In this setting, the left atrium is small, distended, and noncompliant, and the large regurgitant leak produces a giant V wave which can reach 70 to 80 mm Hg (so-called "ventricularization" of the left atrial pressure pulse). Severe pulmonary hypertension and reduced forward cardiac output accompany such marked, acute regurgitation.

CLINICAL MANIFESTATIONS. Symptoms and Clinical Course. As mentioned earlier, the mean left atrial pressure may not be significantly elevated at rest in patients with mitral regurgitation in whom the left ventricle is compensated, and, unlike mitral stenosis, there is little increase in left atrial pressure during exercise or with tachycardia. Therefore the earliest symptom in mitral regurgitation is often exertional fatigue, which reflects inability to maintain a normal forward cardiac output to supply the exercising skeletal muscles. Mild symptoms of this type may persist for many years without significant dyspnea or pulmonary congestion.

Later in the course of severe chronic mitral regurgitation, with the onset of early left ventricular failure, the ventricular end-diastolic pressure increases, left atrial hypertension develops, and dyspnea on exertion and orthopnea occur. However, paroxysmal nocturnal dyspnea and acute pulmonary edema are distinctly unusual in this condition. With the onset of pulmonary hypertension, right heart failure accompanied by venous distention and peripheral edema may occur. Atrial fibrillation is a common complication, but left atrial thrombi are relatively unusual, and systemic emboli occur much less commonly than with mitral stenosis.

Chronic mitral regurgitation is the best tolerated of the lesions involving the left side of the heart. Frequently, patients remain relatively asymptomatic for 10 or 20 years, even in the presence of severe regurgitation, and it is not uncommon for patients to respond well to medical therapy for an additional 10 years or more before progressive left ventricular failure causes serious progressive difficulty and death. This long clinical course undoubtedly reflects in part the favorable loading conditions of this lesion on the left ventricle, as discussed earlier. It seems likely that a sizable number of patients with only moderate mitral regurgitation never experience serious difficulty and may have a normal life expectancy.

Physical Findings. When mitral regurgitation is severe, the peripheral pulse is sharp and abbreviated, owing to lack of sustained forward stroke volume in the face of the regurgitant leak. The jugular venous pulse is normal unless there is pulmonary hypertension or tricuspid valve disease. Atrial fibrillation is frequently present.

On palpation of the precordium, the left ventricle is enlarged, the apex beat is hyperactive and displaced laterally, and frequently there is a systolic thrill at the apex. In the lateral decubitus position, a rapid outward movement in early diastole (rapid filling wave) may be palpable. If pulmonary hypertension is present, there is a right ventricular lift. When the left atrium is markedly enlarged and the mitral regurgitation is severe, expansion of this chamber during systole may push the right ventricle and pulmonary artery out against the chest wall in the third and fourth left interspaces during late systole, a finding which may be confused with right ventricular enlargement.

The characteristic feature of mitral regurgitation in chronic rheumatic disease is a high-pitched *pansystolic murmur* at the cardiac apex which is transmitted to the left axilla (see Fig. 1, Ch. 360.1). If the lesion is severe, it is accompanied by four other findings: (1) soft first heart sound, (2) loud ventricular diastolic gallop (third heart sound), (3) short early diastolic rumble, which accompanies the rapid inflow of blood to the left ventricle, and (4) wide splitting of the second heart sound caused by early closure of the aortic valve. The last-named finding is caused by shortening of the left ventricular ejection time consequent to the regurgitant leak.

Although the murmur of mitral regurgitation is usually pansystolic, variations may be heard. When mitral regurgitation is due to papillary muscle dysfunction, the murmur begins well after the first heart sound and may have a crescendo-decrescendo quality. These characteristics result from posterior herniation of the mitral leaflet as the papillary muscles fail to contract normally late during ventricular systole. In the *click-murmur* or mitral valve prolapse syndrome, late ballooning of the mitral leaflets into the left atrium also occurs, but caused by intrinsic mitral valve disease. In this condition the late systolic murmur may be ushered in by one or more midsystolic clicks. In sudden, severe mitral regurgitation, sinus rhythm is often preserved and there may be a loud fourth heart sound, a most uncommon finding in chronic mitral regurgitation. When a giant left atrial V wave accompanies acute mitral regurgitation, the murmur may occur early in systole; but it is short and terminates before the end of systole, because the left ventricular pressure and massive left atrial V wave equalize near or even before the time of aortic valve closure.

DIAGNOSIS. **Electrocardiogram.** In patients with mild to moderate mitral regurgitation the electrocardiogram may be normal; but with longstanding moderate disease or with severe regurgitation the electrocardiogram usually shows left ventricular hypertrophy and atrial fibrillation. Typically, there is evidence of a so-called diastolic overload pattern, with upright T waves and voltage criteria for left ventricular hypertrophy. Right ventricular hypertrophy may develop in the late stages of the disease when there is pulmonary hypertension. If sinus rhythm is present, left atrial enlargement may be evident.

In the "click-murmur syndrome" S-T segment and T wave abnormalities may be observed and evidence of old or recent myocardial infarction may be seen with papillary muscle dysfunction caused by coronary heart disease.

Roentgenographic Features. The left ventricle and left atrium are usually enlarged. Occasionally, the left atrium is of giant size and can extend well into the right chest. The left ventricle is observed to contract vigorously on fluoroscopy, and systolic expansion of the left atrium may be striking. The presence of calcium in the mitral valve suggests some degree of associated mitral stenosis. If left atrial hypertension is marked, the findings in the lung fields resemble those of mitral stenosis.

Echocardiography. The echo from the mitral valve leaflets can be particularly useful in detecting abnormal posterior prolapse of one or both mitral leaflets into the left atrium during systole (see Ch. 360.4). A flail mitral leaflet may be identified in the presence of a ruptured chorda.

Cardiac Catheterization. Cardiac catheterization is indicated prior to considering cardiac surgery in order to confirm the presence of severe regurgitation, assess the degree of left ventricular myocardial dysfunction, exclude associated coronary artery disease, and assess the severity of any associated valvular lesions.

The severity of mitral regurgitation can be estimated by cineangiography, with injection of contrast medium into the left ventricle. The backward regurgitation of contrast medium into the left atrium during ventricular systole is readily apparent, and it is also possible to calculate the diastolic volume of the left ventricle, the total stroke volume, and the ejection fraction. If the forward cardiac output and forward stroke volume are calculated by the Fick method, when the regurgitation is severe the regurgitant volume per beat may be well in excess of the forward stroke volume.

An elevated V wave in the left atrium (peak of the V wave over 20 mm Hg) may be detected on the pulmonary artery wedge pressure tracing, or from direct measurement by transseptal puncture, with relatively normal mean left atrial pressure. The increased V wave is followed by a rapid pressure fall (the Y descent) as the ventricle

relaxes, the mitral valve opens, and an excessively rapid inflow of blood (forward plus regurgitant volume) crosses the mitral valve in early diastole (see Fig. 1, Ch. 360.1). Even with pure mitral regurgitation, there is often a pressure gradient across the mitral valve in early diastole, reflecting functional mitral stenosis in the presence of increased flow. A normal, simultaneous rise in left atrial and left ventricular pressures then ensues later in diastole, with no pressure gradient.

With the onset of left ventricular dysfunction, the ventricular end-diastolic pressure increases, the ratio of stroke volume to ventricular end-diastolic volume (ejection fraction) falls to less than 55 per cent, and the forward cardiac output diminishes. At this stage of the disease, pulmonary hypertension of moderate degree is generally present.

Mitral regurgitation due to ruptured chordae tendineae may result from bacterial endocarditis or may occur spontaneously with rheumatic or other types of degenerative valve disease, such as Marfan's syndrome or the click-murmur syndrome. In some patients the onset is insidious, but in others it is acute and characterized by a small left atrium, a murmur that is not prominent, sinus rhythm with S_3 and S_4 gallops, and severe congestive heart failure.

DIFFERENTIAL DIAGNOSIS. Several conditions may produce a systolic murmur resembling that of mitral regurgitation. The thrill and murmur of *ventricular septal defect* are pansystolic, but their location at the lower left sternal border is characteristic. The murmur of *tricuspid regurgitation* may be heard well to the left of the sternum whenever the right atrium and right ventricle are markedly enlarged, but the prominent V waves in the jugular venous pulse and the characteristic increase in intensity of the murmur with inspiration should help differentiate this lesion from mitral regurgitation.

When the jet of mitral regurgitation caused by a leak through the posterior mitral leaflet strikes the interatrial septum, the murmur is heard well in the aortic area, and it may be confused with the murmur of *aortic stenosis.* However, the murmur of mitral regurgitation increases when systemic arterial pressure is raised (as with the handgrip maneuver), and it decreases when the systemic arterial pressure is lowered (as with amyl nitrite inhalation), whereas opposite responses tend to occur in aortic stenosis.

The ejection type of murmur associated with *idiopathic hypertrophic subaortic stenosis* may be well heard at the apex, as well as at the left sternal border. The characteristic increase of this murmur with the Valsalva maneuver should provide a point of differentiation.

TREATMENT. **Medical Management.** In the absence of significant symptoms, the only therapeutic measures necessary are *antimicrobial prophylaxis* against streptococcal infections in the younger patient with a history of rheumatic fever and antimicrobial prophylaxis against bacterial endocarditis with dental or surgical procedures. With the onset of fatigue, dyspnea, or atrial fibrillation, the use of *digitalis* is indicated both to control the ventricular rate and to improve the contractile function of the left ventricle. Frequently, even in patients with severe mitral regurgitation, the use of an oral diuretic and digitalis, together with reduced sodium intake, will serve to maintain the patient in a comfortable status for a number of years.

In patients with sudden, severe mitral regurgitation, as with ruptured chordae tendineae, the use of a peripheral vasodilating agent such as sodium nitroprusside, to reduce the afterload on the left ventricle, often will improve the cardiac output and decrease left ventricular failure until replacement of the mitral valve can be carried out.

Surgical Treatment. Surgical treatment is generally indicated when symptoms of severe fatigue or dyspnea occur on less than normal activity (N.Y.H.A. Class III or IV), despite appropriate medical management. Such symptoms generally indicate the onset of significant left ventricular myocardial disease. Obviously, in reaching the decision to recommend operation, the prolonged natural course of this disease should be kept in mind, and the low incidence of serious complications such as acute pulmonary edema, systemic emboli, and sudden death should be considered. Nevertheless, it is desirable to recommend operation prior to the development of irreversible left ventricular myocardial disease, and the persistence of significant symptoms while the patient is maintained on adequate medical therapy is generally considered to presage the onset of this process.

Occasionally, the surgical repair of a ruptured chorda or of a deficient posterior leaflet is possible. Almost always, however, in rheumatic and other forms of mitral regurgitation, replacement of the valve with a prosthesis is necessary. Sudden, severe mitral regurgitation is not well tolerated and generally requires early surgical intervention. Different types of prostheses, complications, and late results of mitral valve replacement are discussed in Ch. 360.2.

360.4. THE MITRAL VALVE PROLAPSE SYNDROME

This syndrome, initially recognized by its auscultatory features, has received a variety of names, including the "floppy mitral valve" syndrome and the mid-systolic click–late systolic murmur or "click-murmur" syndrome. It has been recognized with increasing frequency in recent years as a result of the enhanced diagnostic accuracy available through echocardiography. It now seems likely that this common disorder, with some exceptions, is generally associated with a benign clinical course.

ETIOLOGY AND PATHOLOGY. Pathologic findings in the mitral valve prolapse syndrome include myxomatous degeneration of the mitral valve, often associated with redundant valve tissue and with elongation and other abnormalities of the chordae tendineae. Sometimes degenerative changes in the valve are associated with deposition of acid mucopolysaccharide material. The cause of these pathologic abnormalities is unknown, although the disorder has been associated with the Marfan syndrome (in its complete or incomplete forms), osteogenesis imperfecta, and other connective tissue diseases, as well as occasionally with coronary artery disease. It has been reported in up to 15 per cent of patients with ostium secundum atrial septal defect. The syndrome is seen more frequently in women than in men, and it occurs quite commonly in several members of the same family.

PATHOLOGIC PHYSIOLOGY. The abnormal mitral valve structure involves both the anterior and posterior leaflets, but effects often are most prominent on the posterior leaflet. With the onset of left ventricular contraction normal closure of the mitral valve initially takes place, but during ventricular ejection, as cardiac volume decreases, there is abrupt movement of the valve leaflets toward the left atrium; this rapid posterior motion is followed by

tensing of the chordae and other valve structures, leading to the mid-systolic click. The subsequent prolapse or herniation of the leaflets into the left atrium is associated with the late systolic murmur of mitral regurgitation. In some patients, the posterior prolapse of the leaflets starts more gradually early in systole and is not associated with a click. Mitral regurgitation can be absent, mild, or severe, and occasionally it is progressive over several years. Also, rupture of a mitral valve chorda with acute mitral regurgitation (sometimes associated with infectious endocarditis) occurs with increased frequency in patients with this syndrome.

Localized regional contraction disorders of the left ventricle have been described in many patients studied by angiocardiography, but whether or not they are causally related to the prolapse is not clear. In some patients, infusion of a pressor agent has reproduced their symptom of chest pain, suggesting the possibility of subendocardial ischemia, and it has also been suggested (without direct evidence) that small vessel coronary artery disease may play a role. Generally the major coronary arteries are normal, and there is no clear pathologic explanation for the chest pain or the frequent dysrhythmias that are observed in patients with this disorder.

CLINICAL MANIFESTATIONS. Symptoms and Clinical Course. The spectrum of symptoms is broad, but most commonly they include chest pain, weakness, fatigue, palpitations, lightheadedness, and dyspnea. The chest pain usually is not typical of angina pectoris; commonly it is nonexertional, and it may be prolonged. Sometimes symptoms are vague in nature, and there is an increased incidence of abnormal psychologic tests in patients with this disorder. Symptoms of lightheadedness or palpitations ordinarily are not associated with simultaneous cardiac rhythm abnormalities. Complaints of dyspnea usually are not progressive, nor are they accompanied by signs of cardiac failure.

The natural history of the mitral valve prolapse syndrome has not yet been defined clearly. However, its relatively high frequency in the general population (probably well over 1 per cent) suggests that symptoms never occur in many individuals. In one retrospective follow-up study of over 50 patients identified an average of 14 years earlier, there was an over-all incidence of serious complications of 15 per cent. These included progressive mitral regurgitation (9 per cent), bacterial endocarditis (6 per cent) (one patient died after rupture of a chorda), and nonfatal ventricular fibrillation (one patient); one patient died suddenly following institution of quinidine therapy for frequent ventricular premature beats. A late systolic murmur, rather than an isolated systolic click, was present in the patients with complications. Prospective studies are needed to define whether or not the few patients at risk of complications can be identified early in their course.

Physical Findings. The hallmark of this syndrome is the occurrence of one or more mid-systolic clicks, which generally occur 0.14 second or more after the first heart sound. Sometimes this finding is present alone, but more commonly the click is followed by a crescendo-decrescendo late systolic murmur; occasionally, patients with the echocardiographic features of mitral prolapse exhibit a holosystolic murmur without a click. Alterations in the characteristics of the click and murmur produced by certain maneuvers aid in the identification of the syndrome. Maneuvers which decrease cardiac volume tend to increase mitral valve prolapse, thereby causing the click and murmur to occur earlier during systole (prolonging the murmur), whereas those that increase cardiac volume tend to move the click and the murmur later in systole. The standing position and the Valsalva maneuver decrease the left ventricular volume, moving the click closer to the first heart sound and prolonging the murmur. Inhalation of amyl nitrite typically produces a biphasic response, initially only decreasing the intensity of the murmur, but later moving the click and murmur closer to the first heart sound. The squatting position (or production of bradycardia with agents such as propranolol) increases cardiac volume and moves the click later in systole while shortening the murmur. It is usually possible to document clearly the effects of these interventions by the use of phonocardiography.

DIAGNOSIS. Electrocardiogram. The electrocardiogram is abnormal in a relatively large proportion of patients, the most common finding being T wave inversions in leads II, III, and aVF and occasionally in leads V_5 and V_6; ST segment changes and Q waves are rather uncommon. Prominent U waves and prolongation of the QT interval have also been reported, particularly in patients with a positive family history. ST segment abnormalities are sometimes seen on the exercise ECG, but do not consistently correlate with the occurrence of chest pain. A variety of rhythm disturbances are common, and some surveys have shown frequent ventricular ectopic beats in 40 to 50 per cent of nonselected patients during 24-hour ECG monitoring; in a significant proportion of patients with frequent ventricular ectopic beats, brief or even prolonged bouts of ventricular tachycardia have been reported. Atrial premature contractions and supraventricular tachycardia also are quite common. As mentioned earlier, subjective complaints of palpitations and dizziness usually do not correlate well in time with dysrhythmias recorded on the ECG. In many patients, arrhythmias can be brought out by exercise stress testing, although 24-hour ECG monitoring appears to be the most sensitive method of detection.

Echocardiography. Two types of echocardiographic abnormalities have been described. In the more common variety, an initially normal closure of the anterior and posterior leaflets is followed by a horizontal or slightly posterior motion during early ventricular ejection and then by abrupt posterior motion of the valve during the latter half of left ventricular systole (a pattern said to resemble a "question mark placed on its side") (see Fig. 2, Ch. 360.1). Often, multiple echoes are recorded from the redundant valve tissue. The second type of abnormality consists of posterior motion of the mitral valve leaflets early after the onset of systole, reaching the most posterior position during mid-ejection, followed by a gradual motion anteriorly (yielding a "hammock" configuration). The first echocardiographic pattern tends to be associated with the click and late systolic murmur; the second, with a holosystolic murmur alone. These findings on the echocardiogram have also occasionally been reported to occur without associated physical findings, and rarely the echocardiogram is normal despite typical findings on physical examination.

Cardiac Catheterization. Left ventriculography has shown abnormalities in almost all patients studied. Usually, the intracardiac pressures and cardiac output are normal, except in those uncommon patients with associated hypertrophic cardiomyopathy or severe mitral regurgitation. The frontal and lateral plane angiocardiograms generally show markedly enlarged, scalloped mitral valve leaflets that prolapse into the left atrium during systole; often, scalloping and prolapse of the posterior leaflet are most prominent. Left ventricular contraction abnormalities, including hypokinesis of the posterior wall, systolic cavity obliteration, and the so-called "systolic contraction ring," are often observed. Some patients have been found to have angiographic evidence of associated prolapse of the tricuspid valve as well. An accompanying atrial septal defect may be detected in some patients.

DIFFERENTIAL DIAGNOSIS. The murmur closely resembles that associated with papillary muscle dysfunction and mitral regurgitation due to coronary heart disease. In its physical findings the mitral valve prolapse syndrome also closely resembles hypertrophic subaortic stenosis (hypertrophic cardiomyopathy, asymmetric septal hypertrophy), although many other features and the ECG differ (see Ch. 366.2). The murmur of hypertrophic subaortic stenosis has a crescendo-decrescendo character and responds in a qualitatively similar manner to that of mitral valve prolapse during the maneuvers described above, but it is greatly intensified during the Valsalva maneuver, whereas that of the prolapse syndrome tends instead to become more prolonged. Moreover, the murmur of hypertrophic subaortic stenosis is not initially decreased with amyl nitrite inhalation intensity, but is increased throughout the inhalation; if ectopic beats are present, the murmur of hypertrophic subaortic stenosis increases during the postextrasystolic beat, whereas that of mitral valve prolapse diminishes.

Systolic anterior motion of the anterior mitral leaflet in hypertrophic subaortic stenosis is followed by posterior motion ("SAM"; see Fig. 2, Ch. 360.1), but this event occurs anterior to the C point of the echocardiogram, whereas with mitral valve prolapse the posterior motion occurs posterior to the C point (see Fig. 2). Amyl nitrite administration during echocardiography enhances systolic anterior motion in hypertrophic subaortic stenosis but increases posterior motion in the mitral prolapse syndrome.

TREATMENT. In some patients with significant symptoms, beta-adrenergic blockade with propranolol (up to 320 mg per day in divided doses) has been found to relieve chest pain, whereas nitroglycerin often is ineffective. Propranolol may, however, increase symptoms of fatigue or dyspnea. Although dysrhythmias are common, treatment with antiarrhythmic drugs usually is reserved for patients with severe symptoms or life-threatening arrhythmias. In patients with significant symptoms, 24-hour ECG monitoring is recommended. Sudden death has been reported rarely, usually in association with a positive family history, and ventricular fibrillation has been reported in individuals with a prolonged Q-T interval. Therefore antiarrhythmic therapy appears warranted in patients with either of these features, as well as in patients with a history of ventricular fibrillation or syncope. In some patients, palpitations may respond to propranolol. Often, however, the control of arrhythmias with propranolol or other antiarrhythmic medications is difficult.

The true incidence of infectious endocarditis is not known, but there have been several reports of this complication, usually associated with viridans streptococci. Therefore prophylaxis against endocarditis at the time of dental or surgical procedures should be recommended in all patients with the mitral valve prolapse syndrome.

Rarely, mitral regurgitation appears to be progressive, and, if unresponsive to medical management, mitral valve replacement may be required. Also, following rupture of a chorda tendinea, some patients may require valve replacement for acute, severe mitral regurgitation.

It should be re-emphasized, however, that in most patients the clinical course of this disorder is benign. Thus reassurance of the patient usually is in order, and specific therapy should be reserved for patients with disabling symptoms or serious dysrhythmias.

360.5. AORTIC STENOSIS

ETIOLOGY AND PATHOLOGY. There is evidence that a congenitally bicuspid aortic valve is present in more than one half of adult patients with isolated aortic stenosis, most of the remainder being of rheumatic cause. Although the bicuspid valve is frequently not stenotic in early life, this malformation sets up abnormal stresses within the valve, leading to progressive fibrosis and thickening, with eventual immobility of the leaflets and calcification. This sequence may take many years, and the typical patient presents with findings of significant stenosis in the sixth decade of life. Three quarters of patients with isolated valvular aortic stenosis in adult life are male. The varieties of congenital aortic stenosis as they present in childhood and adolescence are discussed in Ch. 359.2. When aortic stenosis is due to rheumatic heart disease, the sex distribution is relatively equal, and frequently there is evidence of associated mitral valve involvement. With rheumatic disease, the aortic valve is tricuspid and shows fusion of one or more commissures and scarring and thickening of the leaflets; calcification may also be present. Acquired aortic stenosis may also occur in elderly subjects as a degenerative process without fusion of the commissures, stenosis resulting from heavy deposition of calcium within the valve leaflets. When calcification of the aortic valve is marked, the calcium may extend into the anulus and even into the upper portion of the ventricular septum, leading to involvement of the bundle of His or the left bundle branch.

When aortic stenosis is significant, the left ventricle shows concentric hypertrophy with marked thickening of the left ventricular wall, and there is poststenotic dilatation of the ascending aorta. The left atrium is usually normal unless there has been left ventricular failure.

PATHOLOGIC PHYSIOLOGY. The earliest physiologic response to obstruction at the aortic valve, as in acute experimental constriction of the ascending aorta, is an increased left ventricular diastolic volume and pressure and compensatory use of the Frank-Starling mechanism. Consequent to the more forceful contraction, the systolic left ventricular pressure is elevated and a pressure gradient is created across the aortic valve, forcing blood across the narrowed orifice at high velocity. The chronic effect of longstanding systolic pressure overload on the left ventricle is to induce hypertrophy of the ventricular wall, a compensatory process which tends to maintain the force or tension in the wall relatively normal, without substantial enlargement of the left ventricular cavity. (Wall tension, or stress, is directly related to systolic pressure but inversely proportional to wall thickness, and in concentric hypertrophy the increased pressure load is distributed over a larger number of muscle fibers.) The stroke volume is generally well maintained by these mechanisms until very late in the disease. Even when the pressure gradient across the aortic valve

is quite large, the compensatory left ventricular hypertrophy, coupled with a forceful left atrial contraction, serves to maintain the cardiac output at a normal level. This strong left atrial "booster pump" generates a prominent presystolic wave in the pressure tracings, leading to an elevated end-diastolic pressure in the hypertrophied and noncompliant ventricle (often near 20 mm Hg). However, elevation of the end-diastolic pressure by this mechanism does not indicate left ventricular failure, and the mean left atrial pressure is maintained relatively normal.

It should be recognized that a significant gradient is not produced across the aortic valve until the valve orifice is narrowed substantially, by more than 60 per cent of its normal area. A murmur may be created by turbulent flow in the absence of a pressure gradient; but as the stenosis progresses beyond this critical point, an increasing systolic pressure gradient develops between the left ventricle and aorta.

With the increased heart rate which accompanies muscular exercise, diastole is primarily abbreviated, and therefore more time is available per minute for systolic ejection. Hence the aortic valve gradient does *not* tend to increase during exercise, despite an augmented cardiac output, and the left ventricular end-diastolic pressure and mean left atrial pressure may also remain unchanged. This finding is in marked contrast to the situation in mitral stenosis, when filling occurs during diastole and less time is available for flow during exercise.

The arterial pulse pressure is usually narrow when there is significant aortic stenosis, and an important accompanying effect is a tendency toward reduction of the diastolic aortic pressure. The perfusion pressure available to the coronary circulation is therefore diminished. In addition, the oxygen demands of the left ventricle are increased because of the hypertrophy and the need to maintain an elevated systolic pressure in the ventricle (often well over 200 mm Hg in severe aortic stenosis). Heart rate, as well as pressure development, is an important determinant of myocardial oxygen consumption, and the increased heart rate during exertion, together with a limitation of coronary perfusion pressure, can lead to an imbalance between oxygen supply and demand in the left ventricle. Thus *angina pectoris* is common in aortic stenosis in the absence of coronary artery disease. Transient myocardial ischemia in the hypertrophied heart may also explain, at least in part, the tendency toward *sudden serious arrhythmia* which can lead to sudden death. Likewise, this mechanism, perhaps coupled with transient hypotension caused by momentary inability to maintain cardiac output (such as may occur with sudden assumption of the upright posture), may have a role in the *syncopal attacks* which sometimes mark the clinical course of patients with aortic stenosis.

Longstanding pressure overwork by the hypertrophied left ventricle in aortic stenosis eventually leads to evidence of myocardial disease with inability of the heart muscle to maintain normal basal contractile processes, often associated with some degree of myocardial fibrosis. With the onset of left ventricular dysfunction, the degree of emptying becomes reduced. This, in turn, leads to an increased residual ventricular volume and elevation of the end-diastolic volume, with a further increase in the end-diastolic pressure. Elevation of the left atrial mean pressure then ensues, with the onset of orthopnea and exertional dyspnea through the same mechanisms discussed in Ch. 360.2. In the late phases of myocardial failure, pulmonary hypertension develops and cardiac output falls.

CLINICAL MANIFESTATIONS. Symptoms and Clinical Course. Usually there is a latent period of many years, during which aortic stenosis is present and progressing in severity but symptoms are absent. When congenital aortic stenosis is severe, symptoms may occur in childhood, but typically they begin in middle or late life. If there is associated mitral valve disease in patients with rheumatic aortic stenosis, particularly mitral stenosis, the onset of symptoms may be much earlier and may lead to earlier detection of the associated aortic lesion. The three cardinal symptoms of aortic stenosis are (1) angina pectoris, (2) syncope, and (3) symptoms caused by left ventricular failure.

The pathophysiology of *angina pectoris* in aortic stenosis, an imbalance between oxygen supply and demand, is discussed above. It may mimic in every way the exertional chest pain which occurs in patients with coronary artery disease. In the older patient, the *coexistence* of coronary heart disease should be considered. Thus even when the aortic stenosis is moderate, or when stenotic lesions in the coronary vessels are moderate, increased oxygen utilization by the myocardium may lead to angina pectoris. Angina pectoris is often the first symptom in patients with aortic stenosis, and in the young patient it usually indicates severe obstruction to left ventricular ejection.

Syncope is sometimes the initial symptom in patients with aortic stenosis. This may be due to a transient arrhythmia such as atrial or ventricular tachycardia. The tendency of the hypertrophied ventricle to develop transient ischemia undoubtedly makes it more susceptible to ventricular fibrillation or ventricular tachycardia. Other mechanisms for syncope may consist of a transient fall in blood pressure during or immediately after exercise, or upon abruptly assuming the upright posture; such mechanisms are related to transient inability of the left ventricle to maintain a normal forward cardiac output, as discussed earlier, or are perhaps associated with metabolic or reflex peripheral vasodilatation. So-called presyncope may also occur, in which the patient experiences a transient graying out or loss of vision.

One of the major problems in the patient with hemodynamically significant aortic stenosis is the occurrence of *sudden death*, which is occasionally the first sign of the disease. In postmortem studies of patients who have died from aortic stenosis, death was sudden in about 15 per cent. It should be recognized, however, that most of these patients had significant symptoms, and that only 3 to 4 per cent of the patients who die do so without prior symptoms. The mechanism of sudden death is unclear, but it may be due to serious arrhythmia or mechanisms similar to those occurring with syncope.

With longstanding pressure overload, and increasing obstruction at the aortic valve, *left ventricular myocardial dysfunction* eventually develops. The earliest symptom of left ventricular dysfunction is usually orthopnea, caused by elevation of the left atrial mean pressure. Mild dyspnea on exertion may then ensue, which progresses to dyspnea on minimal exertion. In the late stages of aortic stenosis, pulmonary edema or evidence of pulmonary hypertension with right ventricular failure and peripheral edema may occur.

The onset of *atrial fibrillation* in patients with aortic stenosis is uncommon, but when it occurs in the absence of mitral valve disease it is ominous. Usually it indicates an elevated mean left atrial pressure with left atrial distention. Because of the loss of left atrial contribution to ventricular filling, further elevation of the mean left atrial pressure, fall in the cardiac output, and severe cardiac failure may ensue.

The onset of symptoms in a patient with significant aortic stenosis has real importance, because the subsequent course is generally downhill. Although earlier mortality figures based on retrospective clinical analyses of patients with aortic stenosis may be modified somewhat by the advent of modern diuretic, antiarrhythmic, and antimicrobial therapy, the typical course after symptoms begin remains relatively short. Thus the average life expectancy in an adult patient after the onset of congestive heart failure is 18 months to 2 years; after the onset of angina pectoris it is about 5 years; and when syncope begins it is about 6 years, although survivals as long as 18 to 20 years after onset of syncope have been reported. The natural history in the patient with severe stenosis who has few or no symptoms has not been clearly established.

Complications of aortic stenosis include *infective endocarditis*, which has been estimated to occur in as many as 25 per cent of patients during their lifetime. Rarely, hemolytic anemia has been seen in patients with severe calcific aortic stenosis, presumably owing to local blood trauma at the valve, and perhaps also to intrinsic red blood cell abnormalities. Systemic emboli have been reported as a result of calcium or fibrin particles breaking loose from the aortic valve.

Physical Findings. The primary findings on physical examination can be related to three features: abnormal ejection of blood into the arterial bed, turbulent flow and prolonged ejection across the stenotic aortic orifice, and left ventricular hypertrophy. Physical findings reflecting all three phenomena can generally be detected in hemodynamically significant aortic valve obstruction; but despite their helpfulness, such signs do not always predict accurately the degree of stenosis in the individual patient.

The patient with aortic stenosis is typically not debilitated or wasted, the cardiac output being well maintained until late in the course of the disease. The mean jugular venous pressure is generally normal, although the A wave may be prominent in patients with hemodynamically significant aortic stenosis, presumably because of septal hypertrophy with decreased right ventricular compliance. The carotid pulse is small, the upstroke is delayed, and a systolic thrill may be felt in the carotid vessels. The blood pressure is usually low-normal, with narrowing of the pulse pressure, but in elderly patients having reduced compliance (increased stiffness) of the aortic wall and arteries it is not unusual to find an elevated *systolic* blood pressure, even in the presence of significant aortic stenosis. However, marked systemic hypertension with a substantial diastolic pressure elevation is not encountered in the presence of severe aortic stenosis.

On palpation of the precordium, there is a systolic thrill at the aortic area, the apex beat is enlarged, and there is a sustained apical impulse. A presystolic atrial impulse may be palpable at the apex in the lateral decubitus position. The first heart sound is usually normal, and the aortic component of the second heart sound is diminished. Often, the second heart sound is single owing to a prolonged left ventricular ejection time; or aortic valve closure may even follow pulmonic valve closure, leading to paradoxical splitting of the second heart sound (decreased splitting during inspiration) (see Fig. 1, Ch. 360.1). The *systolic murmur* of aortic stenosis is crescendo-decrescendo in quality, is loudest at the aortic area, is transmitted to the carotid arteries, and is also audible at the apex. Being ejection in type, the murmur begins well after the first heart sound and ends well before the second heart sound. In the presence of severe aortic stenosis, the murmur is long and peaks in mid- or late systole. Frequently there is an atrial diastolic gallop (fourth heart sound), which reflects both reduced compliance of the thickened left ventricular wall and forceful left atrial contraction. This gallop is best heard in the left lateral decubitus position.

When aortic stenosis is mild, there tends to be less delay of the carotid upstroke, the duration of ventricular ejection may be normal, and the second heart sound splits normally with respiration. The systolic murmur tends to be less intense and shorter, peaking early in systole. It should be appreciated, however, that in the late stages of aortic stenosis, when cardiac failure and low cardiac output supervene, the murmur of aortic stenosis may also become markedly diminished in intensity. Under these circumstances, the left ventricle is generally substantially enlarged, and there are symptoms and signs of cardiac failure.

It is not uncommon to hear a soft, early diastolic blowing murmur at the left sternal border caused by mild aortic regurgitation, even in patients with severe aortic stenosis. This small leak occurs because of the small, fixed orifice. The murmur of associated mitral stenosis should be searched for carefully, particularly in female patients with aortic stenosis, because the association of these two obstructive lesions serves to diminish the physical findings of each. When mitral and aortic stenosis coexist, the cardiac output tends to be reduced, the severity of aortic stenosis may be underestimated, and the murmur of mitral stenosis may be difficult to appreciate.

DIAGNOSIS (see table). **Electrocardiogram.** In both children and adults, a normal electrocardiogram is rarely found in the presence of significant aortic stenosis. In children under 10 or 12 years of age, the degree of left ventricular hypertrophy on the electrocardiogram tends to relate to the degree of obstruction, but in adults relatively marked degrees of left ventricular hypertrophy are sometimes seen in mild or moderate obstruction. Typically, the electrocardiogram shows voltage criteria for left ventricular hypertrophy, with associated S-T segment and T wave changes and left atrial enlargement. Occasionally, intraventricular conduction delay or left bundle branch block is seen, particularly late in the course of the disease, and atrial fibrillation is a late and relatively uncommon problem. Complete heart block has been reported in some patients resulting from extension of aortic calcification into the conduction system.

Roentgenographic Features. There may be little or no over-all cardiac enlargement, but when aortic stenosis is significant some degree of left ventricular enlargement is usually discernible, with straightening of the left heart border, downward displacement of the left ventricular apex, and overlapping of the spine by the left ventricular shadow at 60 degrees of rotation in the left anterior oblique view. In the presence of left ventricular failure, the chamber is enlarged and the left atrium is also usually dilated, causing posterior displacement of the barium-filled esophagus. When significant left atrial

Differential Diagnosis in Aortic Stenosis

	Valvular Aortic Stenosis	Idiopathic Hypertrophic Subaortic Stenosis
Carotid pulse	Delayed	Rapid and bifid
Systolic murmur, location	Second right ICS, neck and apex	LLSB and apex
Effect of Valsalva maneuver	Murmur decreased	Murmur increased
Aortic closure sound	Soft	Normal
Systolic ejection click	Common when valve not calcified	Rare
Diastolic murmur of aortic regurgitation	Common	Rare
Electrocardiogram	LVH	Marked LVH; deep Q waves (septal in origin); left atrial enlargement
Chest roentgenogram	Normal heart size	Cardiomegaly (left ventricular); left atrial enlargement
Poststenotic dilatation of aorta	Present	Absent
Calcium in aortic valve	Present	Absent

LLSB = Lower left sternal border; ICS = intercostal space; LVH = left ventricular hypertrophy.

enlargement is seen, however, it should always raise the suspicion of associated mitral stenosis. Poststenotic dilatation of the ascending aorta is common in the frontal view, and calcification of the aortic valve should be searched for on the plain roentgenogram. However, image intensification fluoroscopy may be necessary for detection of mild valve calcification. In the presence of left ventricular failure, there is evidence of pulmonary venous engorgement and interstitial pulmonary edema.

Phonocardiography. Recording of heart sounds and the external carotid pulse wave may help in assessing the severity of aortic stenosis by documenting the presence or absence of a single second heart sound, paradoxical splitting, or a prolonged ejection time. A slow rising carotid pulse wave and the characteristics of the ejection murmur can also be documented. Usually, the carotid wave has an anacrotic notch or shudder and continues to slowly rise throughout the duration of the murmur (see Fig. 1, Ch. 360.1).

Echocardiography. In the presence of valvular aortic stenosis the echocardiogram will usually detect thickening of the aortic leaflets; if the opening of the leaflets is less than 1.5 cm during left ventricular systole, the diagnosis of aortic stenosis may be suspected. However, because of multiple echoes and difficulty in assuring that the echocardiographic beam is precisely traversing the aortic orifice, this sign is difficult to quantify and often unreliable. Sometimes because of eccentric placement of the aortic orifice relative to the aortic wall, it is possible to ascertain that a bicuspid valve is present. Hypertrophy of the left ventricular wall (posterior wall thickness over 1.1 cm) may further support the diagnosis of aortic stenosis. Cross-sectional echocardiography of the aortic valve may allow, in the future, a more quantitative assessment of aortic valve orifice size.

Cardiac Catheterization. In patients who have symptoms, cardiac catheterization is carried out to determine whether the degree of mechanical obstruction at the aortic valve is sufficient to warrant surgical treatment. It is important to measure both the systolic pressure gradient between left ventricle and aorta (see Fig. 1, Ch. 360.1) and the cardiac output at the time of left heart catheterization because of the nonlinear relation between the pressure and flow across the stenotic orifice, the orifice area being directly related to flow and inversely proportional to the square root of the pressure gradient (see Ch. 360.2). Thus if the cardiac output is reduced by 30 per cent, the pressure gradient will fall by about 50 per cent and the severity of the stenosis will be underestimated if the pressure gradient alone is relied upon. For example, when myocardial failure is responsible for a reduced resting cardiac output, the peak gradient from left ventricle to aorta may be below 50 mm Hg, even in the presence of marked aortic valve narrowing.

When the cardiac output is normal, with relatively mild aortic stenosis the aortic valve orifice area is between 0.75 and 1.5 sq cm in the adult (normal area 2.5 sq cm), and the systolic pressure gradient across the aortic valve is small. When aortic stenosis is moderate, the orifice area is 0.5 to 0.75 sq cm and the peak pressure gradient usually exceeds 50 mm Hg. With very severe or "tight" aortic stenosis, the orifice area is 0.5 sq cm or less, there may be a left ventricular systolic pressure in excess of 250 mm Hg, and the transvalvular pressure gradient is often over 100 mm Hg. The right heart pressures are normal, unless there is left ventricular failure which can produce pulmonary hypertension. Simultaneous measurements should be made of the pulmonary artery wedge pressure and the left ventricular pressure to exclude associated mitral stenosis.

It is important that selective left ventricular angiography be carried out to document the functional status of the left ventricle. Such a study will indicate whether or not the left ventricular end-diastolic volume is elevated and the ejection fracton reduced to below 55 per cent, factors which bear on the operative risk in the individual patient. In older patients, it is also important that selective coronary arteriography be performed. Lack of appreciation of significant coronary artery lesions can lead to difficulty during surgical treatment, and coronary revascularization procedures are sometimes carried out at the time of the aortic valve replacement.

DIFFERENTIAL DIAGNOSIS. An ejection murmur at the aortic area and lower left sternal border can be heard in the patient with *hypertrophic subaortic stenosis* (hypertrophic cardiomyopathy, asymmetric septal hypertrophy), although the murmur is generally poorly transmitted to the carotid vessels and has other special features. The key differentiating points between this lesion and valvular aortic stenosis are shown in the table. The echocardiographic features of each are also distinctive (see Ch. 360.1).

In the younger patient who has a murmur suggesting congenital aortic stenosis, other locations for the lesion (supravalvular, subvalvular membrane) should be considered. Occasionally the murmur of papillary muscle dysfunction or ruptured chordae tendineae, caused by mitral regurgitation through the posterior leaflet, can mimic the murmur of aortic stenosis. The mitral regurgitant jet impinges on the interatrial septum, which is directly contiguous to the posterior wall of the aorta, leading to transmission of the murmur to the aortic area; however, this murmur tends to transmit poorly to the carotid arteries; it increases with isometric handgrip and diminishes with amyl nitrite inhalation, whereas the murmur of aortic stenosis will behave in an opposite manner with these two maneuvers.

TREATMENT. Medical Management. The adult patient with findings suggestive of moderate aortic stenosis and no symptoms may be followed carefully, although cardiac catheterization is sometimes done to be certain of the severity of obstruction. In such patients, very strenuous physical exertion, such as competitive athletics, should be prohibited in order to minimize risk of sudden death. Antimicrobial prophylaxis for dental or surgical procedures is advised to prevent the development of bacterial endocarditis. In children or adolescents with congenital aortic stenosis who are suspected of having obstruction, cardiac catheterization is generally advised even when they are without symptoms.

Early symptoms of orthopnea or mild dyspnea may respond temporarily to digitalis, sodium restriction, and diuresis. However, as soon as significant symptoms appear (angina, syncope, or symptoms of left ventricular failure), the adult patient should usually be sent for cardiac catheterization and coronary arteriography, and consideration should be given to early operation.

Surgical Treatment. In children or young adult patients with congenital aortic stenosis, surgical treatment is generally advocated even in the absence of significant symptoms if the obstruction is severe, because the risk of operation appears to be lower than the risk of sudden death. The bicuspid valve in the young patient is generally favorable for a valvuloplasty, and clinical improvement may be experienced for a number of years.

In the adult patient with symptoms and significant narrowing of the aortic orifice (less than 0.75 sq cm) or peak systolic pressure gradient over 50 mm Hg with normal cardiac output, aortic valve replacement, using a prosthesis or a graft, is carried out, using cardiopulmonary bypass. Without operation, the outlook for such patients is poor. The average age at which such operations are performed is about 56 to 58 years. Associated coronary artery disease is often found in older patients, and insertion of one or more coronary artery bypass grafts sometimes is combined with replacement of the aortic valve. Sometimes mitral valve replacement also is necessary if an associated mitral valve lesion is sufficiently severe. Most experience has been obtained with the caged ball-valve (Starr-Edwards) prosthesis. The average operative mortality currently is between 5 and 10 per cent, but patients who are in NYHA Class IV exhibit a higher risk (approximately 15 per cent). Great improvement in symptoms generally occurs after the operation. Also, life expectancy is prolonged in survivors of the operation, 75 to 80 per cent being alive at five years and about 60 per cent of patients surviving after ten years. These late survival figures appear to be modified by the size of the left ventricle; thus if the ventricle is small, five-year survival is 95 per cent; whereas if it is greatly enlarged, five-year survival is approximately 60 per cent. The incidence of thromboembolism is significant after ball-valve replacement, averaging 2 to 3 per cent per year if the patient is continuously anticoagulated with sodium warfarin, although the use of certain types of cloth-covered ball-valves may improve this figure somewhat. If anticoagulation is inadequately maintained, the embolic rate is up to 8 per cent per year. Also, with long-term anticoagulant therapy, the incidence of important complications from bleeding (such as intracranial hemorrhage) averages about 1.5 per cent per year. Figures are comparable for prostheses such as the tilting disc (Björk-Shiley) device.

There is relatively less experience with application of porcine xenograft valves for aortic valve replacement. Operative mortalities and survival rates appear to be comparable to those reported with ball-valve devices, but the rate of embolization appears to be significantly lower with the xenograft, and long-term anticoagulation has not been employed. However, unless a large valve size can be inserted, blood flow characteristics through xenograft valves in the aortic position have been less favorable than with ball-valves of comparable ring size, and significant pressure gradients across this valve have sometimes been found postoperatively. The question of the durability of xenograft valves beyond five years also remains to be settled, although early results have been promising.

The question of whether the adult patient with documented, hemodynamically severe aortic stenosis but with few symptoms should be operated upon is not settled at present. The risk of aortic valve replacement is now relatively low in many centers, but whether the risk of sudden death in asymptomatic patients over a period of several years approaches this figure is unknown. Therefore older patients are referred for operation only if they have significant symptoms.

360.6. AORTIC REGURGITATION

ETIOLOGY AND PATHOLOGY. Aortic regurgitation is usually the result of rheumatic fever, but it has been described as a complication of an increasing number of systemic diseases (see below). A careful history may be of substantial help in ascertaining etiology. In chronic aortic regurgitation of rheumatic etiology, the aortic valve leaflets are scarred, thickened, and retracted and do not close during diastole. With longstanding disease, marked dilatation of the ascending aorta and the aortic anulus may add further to the insufficiency. Combined aortic stenosis and regurgitation are most frequently associated with rheumatic disease, but can also be seen in the late stages of a congenitally bicuspid valve. Aortic regurgitation may be associated with the most marked enlargement and hypertrophy of the left ventricle encountered in valvular heart disease. Approximately 70 per cent of patients with predominant aortic regurgitation are male.

Isolated congenital aortic regurgitation has rarely been reported as a consequence of a bicuspid aortic valve, but congenital aortic regurgitation can occur as a complication of discrete subvalvular stenosis which produces secondary thickening and insufficiency of the aortic leaflets. In younger children, ventricular septal defect may be complicated by prolapse of an aortic valve leaflet, thereby causing aortic regurgitation.

Acquired aortic regurgitation occurs in association with the following conditions: (1) *Syphilis*, which causes scarring and degeneration of the media and intima of the ascending aorta, resulting in part from disease of the vasa vasorum. There can be an aneurysm in the ascending aorta and dilatation of the aortic anulus, with thickening of the aortic leaflets, as well as narrowing of the coronary ostia caused by syphilitic involvement of the aortic intima. (2) *Ankylosing spondylitis*, in which associated medial disease of the aorta results in significant aortic regurgitation. (3)

Rheumatoid arthritis; degeneration of the aortic valve leaflets and the ascending aorta have been described. (4) *Marfan's syndrome,* in which loss of elastic tissue and connective tissue degenerative changes can lead to marked dilatation of the aorta and aortic anulus with severe aortic regurgitation. (5) *Hurler's syndrome,* or mucopolysaccharidosis, which may be accompanied by significant aortic regurgitation. (6) *Relapsing polychondritis,* which can exhibit associated aortic root involvement with aortic regurgitation. (7) *Severe systemic hypertension,* which can be associated with aortic dilatation and relative aortic insufficiency; other complications associated with hypertension, such as ascending aortic aneurysm or dissecting aneurysm, may also cause aortic regurgitation. (8) *Infective endocarditis,* which usually occurs on a deformed valve, and can lead to rapid progression of aortic regurgitation or to fenestration of the leaflets.

PATHOLOGIC PHYSIOLOGY. The physiologic defect in aortic regurgitation is retrograde leakage of blood from the aorta into the left ventricle during diastole. This results in low diastolic aortic pressure and increase in the end-diastolic volume of the left ventricle. The amount of blood ejected during systole is abnormally large, because it consists of the normal stroke volume plus blood regurgitated during the previous diastolic period. In severe aortic regurgitation the amount of blood regurgitated per beat may equal or even exceed the forward stroke volume. The initial compensation to this volume overload on the left ventricle is by the Frank-Starling mechanism (increased end-diastolic volume), and in mild aortic regurgitation there is increased systolic emptying as well, with little chronic dilatation of the ventricle. As regurgitation becomes more severe, the left ventricle slowly dilates, and new sarcomeres are laid down both in parallel and in series in the left ventricular wall during the process of dilatation and hypertrophy. This compensatory mechanism allows the enlarged left ventricle to deliver a greater stroke volume, but with normal shortening of each unit of the enlarged circumference.

The pathophysiology of aortic regurgitation somewhat resembles the volume overload of mitral regurgitation, but there are two important differences. (1) The increased foward stroke volume is delivered into a high impedance system (the aorta), and because the total forward stroke volume is increased, the left ventricular and aortic systolic pressures are elevated (sometimes to 160 mm Hg or higher). This, together with the increased size of the left ventricular chamber, leads to pressure as well as volume overloading and a somewhat elevated myocardial oxygen consumption. (2) The lowered diastolic aortic pressure tends to impair coronary artery perfusion. Normally the coronary blood flow occurs during diastole; with the reduced diastolic pressure which accompanies aortic regurgitation, coronary blood flow may become inadequate either during exercise or when heart rate and hence the diastolic pressure become very low, as during sleep. The increased myocardial oxygen consumption coupled with relative underperfusion of the coronary bed may lead to an imbalance between oxygen supply and demand. Thus unlike patients with mitral regurgitation, patients with severe aortic regurgitation commonly develop *angina pectoris* in the absence of coronary artery disease.

With adequate left ventricular myocardial contractility the ejection fraction of the left ventricle (ratio of stroke volume to end-diastolic volume) is maintained at normal (over 55 per cent), the forward cardiac output is normal, and left ventricular end-diastolic pressure may remain nearly normal despite ventricular dilatation. However, because longstanding overload leads to myocardial damage and depression of contractility, the extent of wall shortening during ejection tends to diminish, the residual volume in the left ventricle rises, and the end-diastolic pressure in the left ventricle becomes elevated. Indeed, in the late stages of severe aortic regurgitation the diastolic pressure in the aorta and that in the left ventricle may reach equilibration near the end of diastole, leading to an abbreviation of the murmur. Occasionally, "preclosure" of the mitral valve even occurs, leading to a dissociation between the rising left ventricular pressure and the left atrial pressure, which remains at a lower level. This situation may occur in sudden severe aortic regurgitation, such as with bacterial endocarditis, when sufficient time has not elapsed for ventricular dilatation and hypertrophy to occur. Such mitral valve preclosure may be audible as a snapping sound in mid- to late diastole.

In the late stages of aortic regurgitation the cardiac output decreases, and the left ventricular end-diastolic pressure becomes further elevated because of myocardial failure. The mean left atrial pressure then rises, leading to decreased pulmonary compliance and interstitial edema, and acute pulmonary edema occasionally occurs.

CLINICAL MANIFESTATIONS. Symptoms and Clinical Course. The typical patient with rheumatic aortic regurgitation has experienced acute rheumatic fever in childhood, and a period of about ten years then follows during which the severity of the regurgitant lesion progresses. Marked aortic regurgitation may become apparent by age 18 or 20, and there often follows a period of compensation during which the patient is asymptomatic, despite the presence of severe regurgitation. Occasionally during this stage of the disease, palpitations caused by transient atrial arrhythmias, headache caused by the high systolic blood pressure during exercise, or subjective sensations resulting from cardiac hyperactivity may be noted. Studies in children followed for many years after developing severe aortic regurgitation indicate that even after 20 years about 25 per cent of the individuals with this lesion remained asymptomatic. However, the average duration of the latent or asymptomatic period in severe aortic regurgitation is about ten years.

The earliest symptoms are usually due to the onset of left ventricular dysfunction or to coronary insufficiency. Mild dyspnea on exertion is noted as a result of elevation of the left ventricular end-diastolic and mean left atrial pressures during exercise. The length of time between onset of this symptom and death of the patient averages seven to ten years, although it should be recognized that many of these data were derived before the advent of modern diuretic therapy and rheumatic fever prophylaxis. Angina pectoris usually begins somewhat later, postdating the onset of dyspnea by two to three years. It may occur during exertion, and may or may not respond to nitroglycerin. Angina pectoris can also be atypical and occur at rest or at night, presumably caused by low heart rate which can lead to very low diastolic aortic pressure and inadequate coronary perfusion during long diastolic periods. The onset of severe nocturnal angina associated with profuse sweating, particularly in young patients, can portend a poor prognosis. Also, in young patients with rheumatic aortic regurgitation without significant symptoms who were followed prospectively, it has been reported that a triad of findings portends the occurrence of angina, heart failure, or death within six years in nearly 90 per cent of patients; these included marked left ventricular hypertrophy in the electrocardiogram, roentgenographic evidence of moderate or marked left ventricular enlargement, and a systolic arterial pressure over 140 mm Hg and/or a diastolic pressure below 40 mm Hg.

Once left ventricular decompensation begins, patients with severe aortic regurgitation usually tolerate infections poorly. They may experience severe congestive heart failure, and they are also at some risk of unexpected death. There are no clear-cut figures on the incidence of sudden death in patients with severe aortic regurgitation; although not as common as in aortic stenosis, it is by no means rare and probably results from sudden ventricular arrhythmia. In the late stages of severe aortic regurgitation, orthopnea and paroxysmal nocturnal dyspnea occur, and eventually symptoms and signs of right ventricular failure may supervene.

The natural history in the other forms of aortic regurgitation depends largely on the rapidity with which the lesion develops and on its severity. Patients with aortic regurgitation caused by syphilis may exhibit a course resembling that of rheumatic disease, although it usually begins later in life. With acute regurgitation such as that in bacterial endocarditis, there is insufficient time for chronic compensation to occur, and the clinical course may be fulminating. Under these circumstances, severe intractable left ventricular failure may develop.

Physical Findings. The diastolic pressure determined by sphygmomanometry correlates generally with the severity of the regurgitant leak, although in some patients there is severe regurgitation with diastolic pressure as high as 60 mm Hg. A diastolic sound over the artery is usually audible down to 0 mm Hg when regurgitation is severe, but the level at which the diastolic sound muffles corresponds reasonably well to the directly measured aortic pressure at the end of diastole, determined by a needle within the artery. The systolic arterial pressure is elevated. Characteristic clinical features caused by the large stroke volume and rapid runoff of blood from the aorta consist of *head bobbing* (a nodding motion of the head with each systole, which may be visible from a considerable distance), *visible pulsations of the carotid arteries*, a *Corrigan or water-hammer pulse* (sharp upstroke with collapsing quality), *Quincke's sign* (on light compression of the fingernail, alternate blushing and blanching are visible in the nailbed with each cardiac cycle), *pistol shot sounds* on auscultation with a stethoscope over the femoral arteries, and *Duroziez' murmur* (a to-and-fro bruit over the femoral artery, using slight compression with stethoscope diaphragm). Palpation of the carotid arteries may reveal a bisferious or bifid pulse, particularly if there is some associated aortic stenosis.

On palpation of the precordium, a diastolic thrill may be felt at the lower left sternal border, and a systolic thrill is palpable at the aortic area, the jugular notch, and the carotid arteries. The left ventricle is enlarged, the apex is displaced laterally, and the apex beat is hyperkinetic with marked retraction during systole.

The first heart sound may be normal or slightly reduced; the aortic component of the second heart sound is diminished or inaudible in the presence of severe regurgitation. Frequently, a loud third heart sound is audible at the apex, and there may also be a fourth heart sound. The most characteristic feature of the lesion is a decrescendo, blowing *diastolic murmur* at the left sternal border in the third and fourth intercostal spaces (see Fig. 1, Ch. 360.1). In the presence of mild aortic regurgitation, this murmur is high pitched, soft, and heard only in early diastole; it may be appreciated only with the patient in an upright position, leaning forward, and with held expiration. With a more severe regurgitant leak, the murmur may have a somewhat rougher quality and may last throughout diastole. Late in the course of severe aortic regurgitation, or with acute aortic regurgitation, the diastolic murmur may be shortened by equilibration of aortic pressure with a markedly elevated left ventricular end-diastolic pressure before the end of diastole; occasionally, a snapping sound caused by mitral valve "preclosure" is audible (see above). In patients in whom the aortic regurgitation is due primarily to aneurysmal dilatation of the ascending aorta or to enlargement of the aortic anulus, as in Marfan's syndrome, the diastolic murmur may be loudest to the *right* of the sternum, thereby providing a clue to the cause.

Invariably, when aortic regurgitation is severe, there is a systolic ejection murmur at the aortic area which is transmitted to the jugular notch and carotid arteries. This may be very loud even in the presence of pure aortic regurgitation, reflecting the extremely large stroke volume delivered across a deformed aortic valve, but usually there is little or no pressure gradient from left ventricle to aorta during systole. Frequently in the presence of severe aortic regurgitation, an *Austin Flint diastolic rumble* is audible at the apex. Although true mitral stenosis may accompany aortic regurgitation of rheumatic origin, the Austin Flint rumble is characterized by its onset with a third heart sound; it is loudest in mid-diastole and often exhibits some presystolic accentuation. The Austin Fint murmur is probably due not only to interference with opening of the anterior mitral leaflet by the regurgitant jet, but also to a more rapid rise in the left ventricular than the left atrial diastolic pressure. The effect is to prevent full opening of the normal mitral leaflets during diastole, leading to turbulent flow across the mitral orifice (see Differential Diagnosis in Ch. 360.2).

Sometimes, in the late stages of aortic regurgitation when left ventricular dilatation and failure are present, a holosystolic murmur of relative mitral regurgitation may be audible at the cardiac apex. Signs of pulmonary hypertension and right ventricular enlargement may also be encountered in the late stages of the disease.

DIAGNOSIS. Electrocardiogram. The electrocardiogram usually shows left ventricular hypertrophy, sometimes of marked degree, with associated S-T segment and T wave changes. Left atrial enlargement may also be present, particularly when the left ventricular end-diastolic pressure becomes elevated. When myocardial disease develops, left axis deviation, intraventricular conduction defects, or left bundle branch block may occur. Atrial fibrillation is a late and relatively uncommon complication.

Roentgenographic Features. The major findings are enlargement of the left ventricle and aorta with vigorous pulsations of the ascending aorta on fluoroscopy. The left ventricular enlargment is characterized by a downward and lateral displacement of the left ventricular apex, the left ventricle being particularly prominent and overlying the spine in the left anterior oblique view. With severe aortic regurgitation, left atrial enlargement may be apparent on the right anterior oblique view with barium in the esophagus. When aortic regurgitation is associated with aortic root disease, the ascending aorta may be markedly dilated or aneurysmal, although sometimes the major dilatation takes place posteriorly and may not be visible on the plain chest films. Occasionally, calcium is seen in the aortic valve, and calcification in the ascending aortic wall is characteristic of syphilitic involvement.

Echocardiography. By the use of ultrasound, calculation of the diameter of the aortic root and of left ventricular chamber size may be feasible. In addition, in the presence of an Austin Flint rumble there is a characteristic fluttering motion of the anterior mitral leaflet during diastole caused by the impinging aortic regurgitant jet. This finding, together with absence of mitral valve thickening and normal excursion of the posterior leaflet, provides evidence against organic mitral stenosis. However, such diastolic fluttering has not proved to be a reliable sign of the severity of the leakage. Often the echocardiogram will reveal left ventricular dilatation or hypertrophy when aortic regurgitation is severe, and there may also be left atrial enlargement. In severe aortic regurgitation, particularly of the acute variety, the echocardiogram may detect early closure of the mitral valve in mid-diastole. Such premature mitral valve closure appears to be due to massive aortic regurgitation associated with rapid elevation of the left ventricular diastolic pressure until it exceeds the more slowly rising left atrial pressure, whereupon the mitral valve closes. Sometimes, a group of multiple eccentric echoes from the aortic valve will signify the presence of vegetations due to infectious endocarditis.

Cardiac Catheterization. It is generally desirable to perform cardiac catheterization prior to undertaking cardiac surgery in order to characterize the status of left ventricular myocardial function and to exclude associated lesions. Supravalvular injection of contrast medium into the aortic root often provides adequate radiographic visualization of the left ventricle and the anatomy of the ascending aorta, and also allows assessment of the severity of the aortic regurgitation. The systolic, left ventricular, and aortic pressures are moderately elevated; there may be a slight systolic pressure gradient across the aortic valve and a low diastolic aortic pressure (see Fig. 1, Ch. 360.1). A normal or moderately elevated left ventricular end-diastolic pressure (less than 20 mm Hg) is encountered when left ventricular myocardial function is maintained, and the forward cardiac output is normal. There may be an early diastolic gradient across the mitral valve from the pulmonary artery wedge or left atrial pressure tracing to the left ventricle; this is probably related to the rapid early rise of left ventricular diastolic pressure and impaired opening motion of the anterior mitral leaflet consequent to the aortic regurgitation. Simultaneous recordings of this nature should exclude the presence of associated organic mitral stenosis, in which there is usually a pressure gradient throughout diastole. In longstanding aortic regurgitation there is elevation of the calculated left ventricular end-diastolic volume (in excess of 90 ml per square meter), with or without an elevation of the left ventricular end-diastolic pressure.

A reduced ejection fraction, an impaired forward cardiac output, and marked elevation of the left ventricular end-diastolic pressure all indicate depressed left ventricular myocardial function, which may increase the operative risk. Under these conditions, the left ventricular and aortic diastolic pressures may become equal late in diastole at a pressure of 35 to 40 mm Hg, or even higher. It is under the latter circumstances that early closure of the mitral valve can occur (see above), leading to a higher pressure in the left ventricle than in the left atrium in the last portion of diastole. Finally, selective coronary arteriography should be carried out in older patients to search for significant coronary artery disease.

DIFFERENTIAL DIAGNOSIS. When mild aortic regurgitation is associated with mitral valve disease, the aortic pulse pressure may be normal and the early diastolic blowing murmur may be confused with that of pulmonic regurgitation (Graham Steell murmur). If severe mitral valve disease with pulmonary hypertension is present, it may not be possible to make this differentiation on physical examination; but when aortography is performed, such a murmur has been shown to be due most commonly to aortic regurgitation. Handgrip, which increases aortic pressure, augments the murmur of aortic regurgitation but usually does not affect that of pulmonic regurgitation.

TREATMENT.   Medical Management.   In marked aortic regurgitation, some restriction of physical exertion is advisable to reduce the likelihood of sudden arrhythmia. In the younger patient with a history of rheumatic fever, prophylaxis against streptococcal infection is indicated, and the use of antimicrobial drugs to prevent bacterial endocarditis during and after dental or surgical procedures is important at all ages. Patients with syphilitic aortic regurgitation should receive a full course of treatment with penicillin. When acute aortic regurgitation occurs, as in patients with infective endocarditis, the use of a vasodilator such as sodium nitroprusside can, by reducing the afterload, relieve acute left ventricular failure until operation can be undertaken.

In the patient with angina pectoris, nitroglycerin is not always effective, but it may be worth a cautious trial; it should be recalled, however, that nitroglycerin causes peripheral arterial vasodilatation and may lower the aortic diastolic pressure even further. With the onset of dyspnea or orthopnea (symptoms of early left ventricular failure), the use of digitalis, sodium restriction, and diuretics when necessary can result in substantial improvement, and consideration for operation can sometimes be postponed.

Surgical Treatment.   Once signs of left ventricular failure become significant, the course of the disease tends to be downhill. Although the natural course is not as abrupt as that in aortic stenosis, the life expectancy averages only about seven years after onset of significant symptoms. When dyspnea or angina becomes troublesome on less than ordinary activity (N.Y.H.A. Class III) despite optimal medical management, surgical treatment should clearly be considered. In younger patients with the triad of severe left ventricular enlargement, marked electrocardiographic changes, and systolic arterial pressure over 140 mm Hg or diastolic arterial pressure below 40 mm Hg, it appears that a large percentage of such patients will develop symptoms or die within a few years, and operation may therefore be recommended even in the absence of significant symptoms.

An additional factor in selecting the appropriate time for operation is the finding that in some patients, despite hemodynamic improvement after aortic valve replacement, left ventricular dilatation and myocardial dysfunction may persist. Therefore it is desirable that surgical treatment be undertaken prior to the onset of such irreversible left ventricular disease. It may be hoped that improved noninvasive methods eventually allow detection of this potential problem before permanent changes occur.

Sudden, severe aortic regurgitation is poorly tolerated, and the average life expectancy is short. Therefore surgical treatment should usually be undertaken promptly.

In the great majority of patients, replacement of the diseased aortic valve with a prosthesis is necessary. The average age at the time of aortic valve replacement for aortic regurgitation is between 45 and 47 years. In some patients with marked dilatation of the aortic root and aneurysm formation, aortic valve replacement is combined with replacement of a portion of the ascending aorta. The various types of prosthetic aortic valves employed, the complications, and the results of operation are discussed in Ch. 360.5.

360.7.   TRICUSPID VALVE DISEASE

TRICUSPID STENOSIS

Tricuspid stenosis is rare as an isolated lesion. Almost always it accompanies rheumatic involvement of other cardiac valves, and it is of clinical significance in only about 5 per cent of patients with rheumatic heart disease. Seventy to 80 per cent of patients with tricuspid stenosis are female, and most often they have accompanying disease of both the mitral and aortic valves. *Rare causes* of tricuspid stenosis include *carcinoid heart disease, endomyocardial fibroelastosis, congenital malformations,* and obstruction from a *right atrial myxoma.*

The primary abnormality in tricuspid stenosis, like that in mitral stenosis, is mechanical obstruction to atrial emptying. This results in an elevated right atrial pressure and a pressure gradient across the tricuspid valve during diastole. It is important to measure simultaneous pressures in the right atrium and right ventricle at cardiac catheterization, because signs of peripheral venous congestion may occur with substantially lower pressure gradients (less than 10 mm Hg; often only 3 or 4 mm Hg) than are observed with mitral stenosis. Generally, the cardiac index is reduced substantially.

Tricuspid stenosis should be suspected particularly in the patient who has signs of multivalve disease and severe right-sided venous congestion but no evidence of marked pulmonary hypertension. The patient may also be relatively free of signs and symptoms of pulmonary venous congestion, despite the presence of mitral valve stenosis. This feature may be due to a limiting effect of this lesion on the cardiac output (a protective effect of the tricuspid stenosis) which may prevent sudden augmentation of blood flow into the pulmonary vascular bed. Such an effect would help explain the unusually prolonged clinical course seen in some patients with tricuspid stenosis.

On physical examination, the mean jugular venous pressure is elevated, and in patients with sinus rhythm there is a very sharp, prominent A wave which reflects right atrial contraction against the stenotic valve. There is a characteristic slow fall in the jugular V wave (delayed Y descent), caused by the obstruction to right atrial emptying and the resulting slow fall in right atrial pressure during diastole (see Fig. 1, Ch. 360.1).

On palpation of the precordium, the right ventricle is not enlarged, and a diastolic thrill may be palpable at the lower left sternal border. The diastolic murmur of tricuspid stenosis will often be missed unless specifically searched for at that location. It resembles that of mitral stenosis, having a low-pitched rumbling quality often beginning with a tricuspid valve opening snap (somewhat later than a mitral opening snap), and an early diastolic decrescendo murmur is followed by presystolic accentuation if sinus rhythm is present. A characteristic feature in differentiating the murmur from that of mitral stenosis is augmentation in the intensity of the tricuspid rumble during *inspiration,* or during the *Müller maneuver* (attempted inspiration against a closed glottis). This augmentation is due to the transitory increase in right atrial filling and tricuspid valve flow, which results from the negative intrathoracic pressure. Both these maneuvers diminish the murmur of mitral stenosis. There may be an associated abnormal increase in the venous pressure during such inspiration in tricuspid stenosis. When atrial fibrillation is present, the murmur is even more difficult to detect, because it may occur only in early diastole and can be confused with the murmur of pulmonic regurgitation.

The electrocardiogram, if sinus rhythm is present, exhibits peaked P waves in leads II and V_1, evidence of right atrial enlargement, but atrial fibrillation is often present. There is no evidence of right ventricular hypertrophy. On the chest roentgenogram, in addition to the findings caused by associated valvular lesions, there is enlargement of the right atrium. Echocardiography may detect a reduced posterior diastolic motion (low E to F slope) of the anterior leaflet of the tricuspid valve similar to that observed in mitral stenosis, although here also it should be recognized that this slope is influenced by tricuspid valve flow as well as by right ventricular diastolic compliance.

Surgical treatment is not indicated for mild tricuspid stenosis, but if it is severe or if the patient must undergo operation for a mitral valve lesion, surgical treatment may be undertaken. The tricuspid valve is usually not favorable for valvuloplasty, and most often a tricuspid valve prosthesis is inserted. Sometimes the tricuspid stenosis is not detected prior to a mitral valve operation, and is recognized only when unexpected signs of right-sided congestion develop postoperatively.

TRICUSPID REGURGITATION

Tricuspid regurgitation, like tricuspid stenosis, is usually associated with rheumatic disease of other cardiac valves, particularly the mitral. It may occur as an organic lesion, or more commonly it is a functional lesion secondary to right ventricular dilatation with severe pulmonary hypertension. Such functional tricuspid regurgitation usually occurs late in the course of mitral valve disease. Other forms of severe pulmonary hypertension, such as the Eisenmenger reaction in congenital heart disease or pulmonary hypertension caused by chronic lung disease, can also cause functional tricuspid regurgitation. Rheumatic involvement of the tricuspid valve can result in tricuspid regurgitation when the right ventricular systolic pressure is normal, although most frequently such organic lesions are of mixed variety, with both stenosis and regurgitation. Isolated tricuspid regurgitation can occur congenitally (as in Ebstein's malformation), and progressive tricuspid regurgitation caused by traumatic damage to the valve has been reported after crush injuries of the chest. The normal tricuspid valve can serve as a focus for bacterial endocarditis, particularly in drug addicts.

Tricuspid regurgitation constitutes a leakage of blood retrograde into the right atrium during right ventricular systole, which places an augmented volume load on the right ventricle. The pathophysiology resembles that of mitral regurgitation but involves the right heart. In mild tricuspid regurgitation, when the right ventricular end-diastolic pressure is not elevated, the right atrial mean pressure is normal and the V wave may not be particularly prominent. As the right ventricular and mean right atrial pressures rise in the presence of more severe regurgitation, the V wave becomes increased. If the right ventricle fails, the right ventricular diastolic and mean right atrial pressure rise, and the V wave becomes markedly enlarged.

Examination in severe tricuspid regurgitation may show the V wave in the jugular venous pulse high in the neck, with the patient in the upright position. Sometimes the height of the venous pressure may be difficult to discern, because the mean pressure may exceed 20 cm of water, and the top of the column may not be visible even in the sitting position. Systolic hepatic pulsations may be present, and there may be marked hepatomegaly, ascites, and peripheral edema. In tricuspid regurgitation secondary to severe pulmonary hypertension, there is a palpable pulmonary artery segment in the second left interspace, and a markedly accentuated pulmonic closure sound is evident. With severe tricuspid regurgitation, there is a thrill over the lower left sternal border and lower sternum, and an enlarged right ventricle is palpable along the left sternal edge and in the subxiphoid region. A pansystolic murmur is heard near the lower left sternal border and lower sternum, transmitted to the right sternal edge or the subxiphoid region. An early diastolic rumble caused by increased blood flow across the tricuspid valve may be audible; when there is organic involvement of the tricuspid valve by rheumatic disease, a longer diastolic murmur caused by associated tricuspid stenosis may be present. A characteristic feature of the murmur of tricuspid regurgitation is its augmentation during inspiration *(Carvallo's sign),* and the murmur can also be increased by the Müller maneuver (see Tricuspid Stenosis, above). These maneuvers lead to decreased intensity of a mitral regurgitant murmur.

There is electrocardiographic evidence of right ventricular hypertrophy, and atrial fibrillation is usually present in severe tricuspid regurgitation. Enlargement of both the right atrium and the right ventricle is evident on the chest roentgenogram. Infectious vegetations on the tricuspid valve may be detected by echocardiography, particularly when there is infective endocarditis secondary to intravenous drug use.

The *treatment* of tricuspid regurgitation, if moderate and secondary to severe pulmonary hypertension, is conservative. Generally, the patient will respond to medical measures aimed at the left-sided valvular disease (sodium restriction, diuresis, digitalis). When aortic or mitral valve surgery is undertaken, such functional tricuspid regurgitation generally disappears gradually after relief of the left-sided lesion, as the pulmonary hypertension regresses. Occasionally, plication of the tricuspid valve anulus is done in patients with functional tricuspid regurgitation who are undergoing operation on other cardiac valves. If the functional tricuspid regurgitation is very severe, or if organic disease of the tricuspid valve is present in the absence of severe pulmonary hypertension, replacement with a prosthesis is necessary.

360.8. PULMONIC VALVE DISEASE

PULMONIC REGURGITATION

Regurgitation at the pulmonic valve most commonly accompanies severe pulmonary hypertension caused by left-sided valvular heart disease. The murmur is high pitched, decrescendo in quality, and best heard at the lower left sternal border. It may be indistinguishable from the murmur of mild aortic regurgitation; however, it should be noted that by far the most common cause of such a murmur in the patient with rheumatic valvular heart disease is aortic regurgitation. Isolated congenital pulmonic regurgitation with a normal pulmonary arterial pressure occurs rarely, and in this situation the murmur occurs later in diastole, is lower in pitch, and may be confused with the murmur of tricuspid stenosis. Pulmonic regurgitation with a normal pulmonary artery pressure can also occur in association with bacterial endocarditis on a normal pulmonic valve, particularly in drug users. Occasionally, if antimicrobial therapy is unsuccessful in this condition, excision of the pulmonic valve has been used to eradicate the source of infection, and this procedure does not appear to result in serious hemodynamic difficulties.

PULMONIC STENOSIS

Pulmonic stenosis usually occurs as a congenital malformation and is discussed in Ch. 359.2. Occasionally, acquired subpulmonic stenosis occurs in association with hypertrophic subaortic stenosis, owing to bulging of the interventricular septum into the right ventricular chamber. Rarely an intrapericardial tumor can compress the main pulmonary artery or right ventricular outflow tract, resulting in a pressure gradient between the right ventricle and the pulmonary artery.

Barnhorst, D. A., Oxman, H. A., Connolly, D. C., Pluth, J. R., Danielson, G. K., Wallace, R. B., and Mcgoon, D. C.: Long-term follow-up of isolated replacement of the aortic or mitral valve with the Starr-Edwards prosthesis. Am. J. Cardiol., 35:228, 1975.

Braunwald, E., Lambrew, C. T., Rockoff, S. D., Ross, J., Jr., and Morrow, A. G.: Idiopathic hypertrophic subaortic stenosis. I. A description of the disease based upon an analysis of 64 patients. Circulation (Suppl. 4), 30:3, 1964.

Cohen, L. S., Gault, J. H., and Ross, J., Jr.: Mitral regurgitation. In Barondess, J. A. (ed.): Diagnostic Approaches to Presenting Syndromes. Baltimore, Williams & Wilkins Company, 1971, p. 1.

Feigenbaum, H.: Echocardiography. 2nd ed. Philadelphia, Lea & Febiger, 1976.

Hancock, E. W., and Fleming, P. R.: Aortic stenosis. Quart. J. Med., 29:209, 1960.

Mills, P., Rose, J., Hollingsworth, J., Amara, I., and Craige, E.: Long-term prognosis of mitral valve prolapse. N. Engl. J. Med., 297:13, 1977.

O'Rourke, R. A., Crawford, M. H., Johnson, A. D., Davidson, R. M., LeWinter, M. M., and Karliner, J. S.: Prolapsing mitral valve leaflet syndrome. West. J. Med., 122:217, 1975.

Rees, J. R., Epstein, E. J., Criley, J. M., and Ross, R. S.: Haemodynamic effects of severe aortic regurgitation. Br. Heart J., 26:412, 1964.

Ross, J., Jr., and Braunwald, E.: Aortic stenosis. Circulation (Suppl. 5), 37:61, 1968.

Ross, J., Jr., Braunwald, E., Gault, J. H., Mason, D. T., and Morrow, A. G.: On the mechanism of the intraventricular pressure gradient in idiopathic hypertrophic subaortic stenosis. Circulation, 34:558, 1966.

Salazar, E., and Levine, H. D.: Rheumatic tricuspid regurgitation, the clinical spectrum. Am. J. Med., 33:111, 1962.

Salomon, N. W., Stinson, E. B., Griepp, R. B., and Shumway, N. E.: Mitral valve replacement: Long-term evaluation of prosthesis-related mortality and morbidity. Circulation (Suppl. 2), 56:11, 1977.

Sanders, C. A., Harthorne, J. W., DeSanctis, R. W., and Austen, W. G.: Tricuspid stenosis: A difficult diagnosis in the presence of atrial fibrillation. Circulation, 33:26, 1966.

Segal, J., Harvey, W. P., and Hufnagel, C.: A clinical study of one hundred cases of severe aortic insufficiency. Am. J. Med., 21:200, 1956.

Spagnuolo, M., Kloth, H., Taranta, A., Doyle, E., and Pasternack, B.: Natural history of rheumatic aortic regurgitation. Criteria predictive of death, congestive heart failure, and angina in young patients. Circulation, 44:368, 1971.

Wood, P.: An appreciation of mitral stenosis. Parts I and II. Br. Med. J., 1:1051, 1113, 1954.

361. ARTERIAL HYPERTENSION

C. T. Dollery

DEFINITION. A wide range of blood pressure values is found among human populations. The values are not normally distributed, and there is a skew toward higher ones. The distribution of blood pressure readings (Fig. 1) has no natural break separating normality from abnormality, so the definition of what constitutes hypertension is empirical. Much effort has been expended, probably needlessly, in trying to define hypertension. Several different operational definitions are possible. Very high values of blood pressure — say, above 230 systolic and 130 diastolic mm Hg — are associated with a high probability that the individual will develop left ventricular failure or accelerated hypertension and thus present with a clinical illness which can be termed hypertension. Below this level of pressure most patients are not ill, but there is an increasing incidence of some symptoms such as morning headache with pressure from approximately 170 systolic and 110 diastolic mm Hg upward. However, the real problem for the individual with a blood pressure in the upper part of the distribution range is not the development of

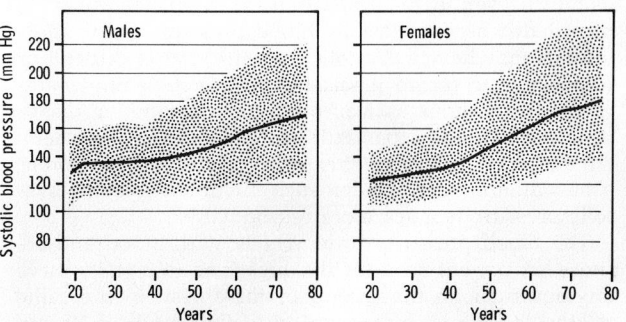

Figure 1. Median systolic blood pressure with 5 per cent and 95 per cent limits in male and female inhabitants of Bergen, Norway, over the whole span of age found in an adult population sample. (From Boe et al.: Acta Med. Scand., Suppl. 321, 157:1–252, 1957.)

symptoms due to the blood pressure but the sudden and apparently unpredictable catastrophe of a myocardial infarction or a cerebrovascular accident. Several prospective epidemiologic studies of human populations have shown that the risk of such a catastrophe is graded with the level of blood pressure throughout the range of pressures found. Normality in the sense of freedom from risk has no meaning in relation to blood pressure.

Thus the main clinical importance of hypertension is not that it is a disease in the usual sense but that it is the most important single factor that enables a physician to make a prediction about the future risk of vascular disease, and that furthermore it is a risk that can be controlled by lowering the blood pressure.

MEASUREMENT OF BLOOD PRESSURE. The sphygmomanometer column is calibrated in 10- and 2-mm divisions. Most physicians show a strong preference for numbers ending in zero and record the blood pressure only to the nearest 10 mm Hg. As decisions about patient management may be altered by differences in diastolic pressure of this magnitude, it is much preferable to read the instrument to the nearest 1 or 2 mm. It is also important to deflate the cuff slowly when taking blood pressure. Rapid deflation may bring about a considerable difference in the pressure in the cuff and that indicated by the column because of the inertia of the mercury. Furthermore, it is almost impossible to read the column accurately if the meniscus is rushing past the calibration points.

It is useful to make a rough check of the systolic pressure by palpation during inflation and to start deflation from 20 mm Hg above the systolic value. This avoids the problem of errors caused by "silent zones" during deflation which can cause the observer to fail to record the true (and much higher) level of systolic pressure. As the column falls, the silence is broken by a faint but distinctive tapping sound in time with the pulse. This is phase 1 of the sounds described by Korotkoff and corresponds with the systolic pressure. Less skilled observers usually record this value more accurately than the diastolic pressure, which has a less clear-cut endpoint. During further deflation the quality of the sound changes. At first it grows louder and has a roaring quality and then it becomes abruptly muffled. The point of muffling is the fourth phase, and the disappearance of sound, which usually occurs soon afterward, is the fifth phase. The true diastolic pressure lies between the fourth and fifth phase sounds, but as it is usually closer to the fifth, it is now official policy to record this as the diastolic blood pressure. Some individuals may have a diastolic pressure that is difficult or impossible to record precisely because the sound fades gradually without a clear point of muffling or disappearance. This is a particular problem if the peripheral circulation is dilated after exercise or under the action of a vasodilator drug. Under such circumstances the systolic pressure is much more reproducible.

The blood pressure varies widely with mood and activity. A patient seen for the first time is usually more anxious than on the second or third visit to the same doctor and clinic. It is common to find a fall of 10 mm Hg in systolic pressure from the first visit to the second, and about 4 mm Hg from the second to the third. A blood pressure taken at the beginning of a consultation is almost always higher than one taken near its end. There has been much debate as to which, if any,

of these is the most representative. The blood pressure taken on the first visit without any special preparation is often termed "casual" blood pressure. It probably corresponds most nearly to those used in epidemiologic surveys. The blood pressure recorded under conditions of rest, tranquillity, and even sedation is sometimes referred to as the "basal" blood pressure. As there is no generally agreed preparation for recording a "basal" reading, it cannot be precisely defined. There is evidence that a series of readings taken over the waking day provides a better prediction of prognosis than a single casual one, but portable equipment to provide such readings is expensive and not generally used.

Reading the mercury column of the sphygmomanometer is prone to systematic bias as well as digit preference and boundary avoidance. For exact work such as therapeutic trials and epidemiologic surveys, it is usual to employ an instrument that has provision for concealing the mercury columns, which are stopped by pressing a switch, or for incorporating a device to offset the zero by up to 80 mm Hg, so that the observer cannot anticipate any particular pressure level. The zero offset can only be read after the systolic and diastolic pressures have been recorded.

EPIDEMIOLOGY. Many factors affect the blood pressure of an individual within a population or may cause differences between two populations. Study of these factors may yield information about pathogenesis and suggest possible preventive measures.

Age and Sex. Blood pressure tends to rise throughout life, although the rate of rise varies at different ages. There is a relatively rapid rise from the low values of the neonate to the higher values of a child and young adult. The upward trend is slower between the ages of 20 and 45 years in both men and women; it then resumes an upward march, rising at an average rate of 0.5 to 1.0 mm Hg of systolic pressure each year until the seventh decade is reached. Values in older people are affected by differential mortality of those with higher pressures, and population means tend to level out or even fall in extreme old age. Women have slightly lower pressures than men in the third and fourth decades and slightly higher ones thereafter. The rate of rise of pressure is not uniform within a population, and the range of pressures found widens as age advances. There is some evidence that this occurs because those in the higher part of the range have a pressure that increases more rapidly than those in the lower part of the range. Recent work has suggested that individuals who ultimately develop pressure levels requiring treatment may lie in the upper part of the distribution as young as the age of one year.

Race and Environment. Studies of the distribution of blood pressure values have been carried out in many countries of the world, and almost all populations show a progressive rise in pressure with age and a distribution of values resembling in varying degrees that found in Western Europe and the United States. Although the pattern is similar, the proportion falling into higher pressure categories shows some interesting geographical and racial variations. Black people in West and East Africa, the West Indies, and the United States have a similar proportion of higher values to those found in whites, and in some samples significantly more. The proportion of individuals with higher values appears to be somewhat lower in population samples from the Indian subcontinent. Some communities have been found in which the blood pressure shows little increase with age and the distribution curve lacks the upward skew of higher values found in Caucasians. Such communities include nomads in East Africa, bushmen in Southern Africa, and the inhabitants of some Pacific islands such as Pukapuka in the Northern Cook Islands.

There is conclusive evidence that blood pressure is heritable, but wide divergencies of opinion exist concerning the proportion of the blood pressure variability in populations which is genetically controlled. Estimates of the genetic contribution to variation in systolic blood pressure range from as high as 82 per cent to as low as 30 per cent. The evidence of a major genetic contribution comes from several sources. Blood pressures of parents and their natural children are highly significantly correlated (r 0.3), whereas those of adopted children are not. There is a much lower correlation of spouse blood pressures than of family members who are genetically related. The correlation of blood pressures in monozygotic twins (0.55) is higher than that in dizygotic twins (0.25). It was once contended that blood pressure distribution in populations was bimodal and controlled by a single gene. The error arose because of digit preference for blood pressures ending in zero and boundary avoidance of pressures around 150 mm Hg systolic. It is now generally agreed that blood pressure is unimodally distributed and must be controlled by several genes. How many genes are important and what they control are still in doubt.

Extremes of body weight and salt intake can alter blood pressure, so that differences in body weight and salt intake found between races probably exercise some influence on the range of blood pressures that prevail among them. There is also the question of how much urban and social pressures may contribute to the elevation of arterial pressure. The evidence here is conflicting. Some studies of rural populations have demonstrated pressures as high as, or even higher than, those of genetically similar people living in crowded conditions in cities. A group with one of the highest proportions of high blood pressure values ever reported is black people living in rural Georgia in the United States. Yet studies of Pacific islanders have suggested that groups in closer contact with modern society have higher pressure values than those found in communities from which they migrated. The practical implication of these results is that, with the possible exception of obesity, no factor has yet been identified that can be utilized in a program to prevent high blood pressure.

Body Weight. Many epidemiologic studies have demonstrated a positive correlation between body weight and both systolic and diastolic blood pressure. The correlation is strongest among young and middle-aged adults. Prospective studies suggest that weight gain is associated with a significant rise in blood pressure in those initially normotensive, and, conversely, that weight loss lessens the chance of developing hypertension in those who were normotensive at the outset. There is also epidemiologic evidence that loss of weight among individuals who are hypertensive lowers blood pressure. Clinical studies have been conflicting in that loss of weight does not always lower blood pressure, and it has been argued that when it does so reduced sodium intake may be as important as reduced total calorie intake and body mass.

The improved nutrition of many countries that has resulted from improvements in agriculture and food

distribution may increase the number of individuals who are both overweight and hypertensive as well as increasing the number with glucose intolerance. The prevention of obesity is a worthwhile objective in relation to several other health problems besides hypertension, but practical ways of reducing the food intake of whole populations, short of famine or war, have not been identified.

Salt Intake. One of the earliest effective methods of lowering the blood pressure was the rice diet introduced by Kempner which owed its efficacy to its very low content of sodium chloride. Unfortunately, few patients were willing to persist with this tasteless and monotonous regimen, and such an extreme reduction of salt intake would be impractical as a preventive measure. Even the word salary is a reminder that the Roman legionaries were partly paid in salt, and the craving for this substance is deep seated in man and animals. Several studies have been made both within and between communities to establish how far variability in blood pressure is due to salt intake. Variations between communities are difficult to interpret because of genetic differences, but it has been established that the range of salt intake found in western populations does not appear to be an important influence upon levels of blood pressure. It appears unlikely that any practical degree of reduction of salt intake would lower blood pressure. Interesting selective breeding experiments have been carried out in a rat colony at Brookhaven, in which it has proved possible to breed a strain of animal that readily develops severe hypertension when given a high salt intake. Another strain was bred from the same original stock that was highly resistant to the blood pressure–elevating effect of a high salt intake. If there is a human counterpart to this experiment, it would probably involve extremes of salt intake that are rarely encountered in the population.

RISK FACTORS FOR PREDICTING VASCULAR DISEASE. Physicians are accustomed to making predictions about the likely future course of an illness to recovery or death. The use of risk factors to predict the future likelihood of developing an illness is no more than an extension of the same principle. The first to make extensive use of this concept were the life insurance companies, who recognized that factors such as high blood pressure, overweight, and proteinuria increased the probability of their having to pay out the proceeds of a policy, and they learned to adjust their premiums accordingly. It is instructive to reflect that life insurance companies were loading premiums for individuals with moderately elevated blood pressures at a time when their physicians were still patting them on the back and telling them that there was nothing to worry about. As a result of prospective epidemiologic studies such as those carried out in Framingham, Massachusetts, by the National Institutes of Health, it has been possible to study whole populations and to calculate correlation coefficients for many factors that have predictive power in relation to the risk of developing vascular disease. The concept is a most important one to grasp, because it alters radically the clinical management of a patient with a given level of pressure, depending upon the burden of associated factors of risk. It is also important to grasp the difference between absolute risk and relative risk. A young man with a systolic blood pressure of 160 mm Hg has two and one half times the chance of dying compared with a stand-

TABLE 1. Effect of Associated Risk Factors upon Outcome in Hypertension*

	Case I	Case II
Age	45 years	45 years
Sex	Male	Male
Systolic blood pressure	170 mm Hg	170 mm Hg
Cigarette smoker	Yes	No
Serum cholesterol	260 mg/100 ml	185 mg/100 ml
Glucose intolerance	Yes	No
Left ventricular hypertrophy on the ECG	Yes	No
Relative risk compared with age/sex average	7.15	0.78
Patient's risk of developing cardiovascular disease over eight years	54.1	6.33
Average risk for this age and sex group over eight years	8.0	8.0

*Based upon data from the Framingham Survey (program by courtesy of Dr. R. H. Roberts, Ciba-Geigy, Summit, N.J.).

ard risk. In an older man, the ratio is slightly lower. But as older men who are not hypertensive have a much higher chance of suffering a stroke or myocardial infarction, the absolute risk for the older man is much greater than for the younger one.

The three most important risk factors for predicting the future risk of myocardial infarction are level of blood pressure, level of blood lipids, and cigarette smoking habit. Other important factors include the presence of both voltage and T wave signs of left ventricular hypertrophy, glucose intolerance, and obesity. In absolute terms age and sex are most important, because the incidence of morbidity and mortality from vascular disease increases sharply as age advances, but the incidence at younger ages is less in women than in men. Simple computer programs have been constructed that make it possible to calculate the relative risk by providing information about these risk factors, and their importance is illustrated by two case histories for a man of 45 years who has a systolic pressure of 170

mm Hg with and without a high risk category in other respects (Table 1).

A further illustration is given in Figure 2, which shows histograms of risk of developing coronary disease at various levels of systolic pressure from 105 to 195 mm Hg as the burden of other risk factors increases. It can be seen that the risk of the lower pressure category in someone with a full load of other factors is greater than that of someone in the highest pressure category who is free of other risk factors.

The concept of risk factors is very important, but it has certain limitations. The demonstration of a correlation with predictive power does not by any means prove that there is a cause-and-effect relationship. It cannot be assumed that reduction of a risk factor will automatically bring about a proportional, or indeed any, reduction in risk. However, if a risk factor can be diminished without any obvious countervailing disadvantage, it is a matter of common sense to try to reduce it while awaiting the scientific evidence. This argument

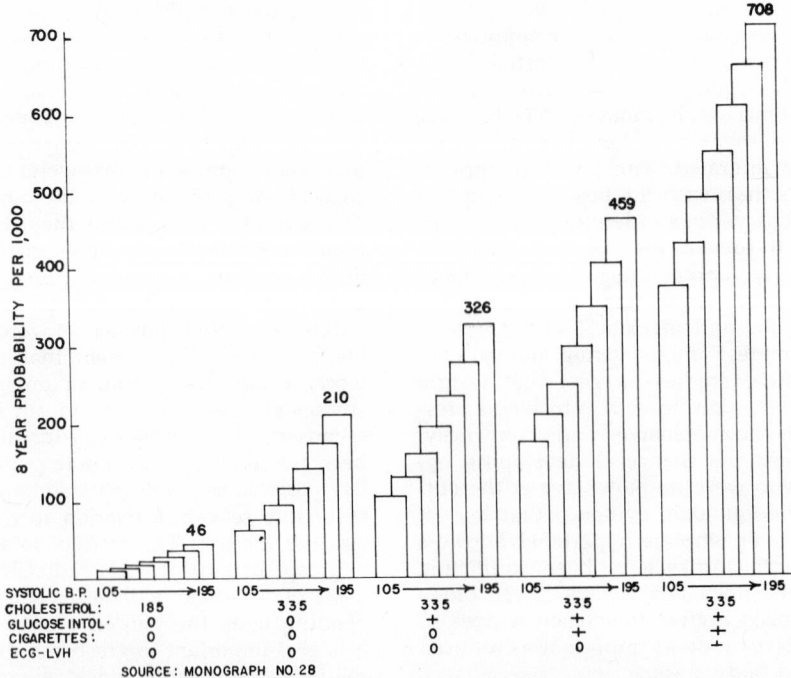

Figure 2. Risk of cardiovascular death according to systolic blood pressure at specified levels of other risk factors in 40-year-old men in Framingham, Mass. (By permission of Dr. W. B. Kannel.)

applies especially strongly to reduction of cigarette intake and body weight. The value of reducing lipids is a matter that has caused great controversy. There is evidence that lipid fractions such as the low and very low density lipoproteins may be more important than the total cholesterol or triglycerides. Measures that reduce blood lipids may not automatically reduce the amount of lipid in atheromatous lesions of the arterial wall. Drugs used for this purpose have not been entirely free of unwanted effects, and thus far there is no evidence of benefit in secondary prevention trials, i.e., when they have been used in individuals who have already suffered a myocardial infarction. The results of primary prevention trials are awaited.

CAUSES OF DEATH IN HYPERTENSION. The main causes of death in hypertensive individuals are from damage to blood vessels in vital organs causing myocardial infarction, stroke, peripheral vascular disease, and renal failure. The only causes of death that relate directly to the level of pressure at the time are accelerated hypertension, cerebral hemorrhage, heart failure, and (possibly) dissecting aneurysms. Myocardial infarction is by far the most important and accounts for over half the deaths.

A number of prospective studies, such as that carried out at Framingham, have demonstrated the steep gradient of risk with levels of blood pressure for each of these causes of death. Comparing normotensive individuals with those having a pressure exceeding 160 systolic and 95 diastolic mm Hg, the gradients were three-fold for coronary disease and peripheral vascular disease, four-fold for congestive heart failure, and seven-fold for stroke. The increase in risk with level of blood pressure is most striking for stroke deaths. In the age group 40 to 49 years the risk of stroke is ten times higher in individuals with a diastolic pressure exceeding 104 mm Hg than in those in whom it is below 85 mm Hg.

These data also highlight a problem when the control of blood pressure is used as a public health measure to decrease the incidence of stroke and coronary disease. The risk is much greater at high pressure levels, but the number of individuals involved is relatively small. Individuals with modest elevations of blood pressure are so much more numerous that they account for a large fraction of the hypertension-related morbidity and mortality, although at present many of them would probably not be considered for treatment.

CLINICAL MANIFESTATIONS. The assessment of the patient with hypertension has three main objectives: to ascertain the extent of organ damage that has already resulted from the high pressure, to detect any treatable cause, and to define and, when possible, to reduce the factors that determine a high risk of cardiovascular disease. Information relevant to these three factors can be obtained from the history, physical examination, and laboratory investigations.

The Extent of Organ Damage. Patients with severe hypertension may present to the physician with symptoms, although most patients with mild to moderate hypertension have no symptoms directly referable to the disease. Common symptoms include headache, dyspnea, giddiness, and blurred vision. The relationship of headache to hypertension has caused much confusion. Most headaches, including those in the majority of patients with a high blood pressure, bear no rela-

tionship to the level of blood pressure. However, patients with diastolic pressures exceeding about 110 mm Hg, especially younger patients, often complain of morning headaches similar to those seen in patients with other causes of raised intracranial pressure. These headaches are related to the level of blood pressure. Breathlessness and/or a slow walking pace are also common symptoms at higher pressure levels, but many patients with these complaints also have ischemic heart disease. The complaint of giddiness or unsteadiness is common in patients with untreated hypertension, although rather similar complaints may arise as a result of reducing the pressure to a point where cerebral perfusion is impaired. Blurred vision usually indicates the presence of cotton wool spots and/or macular edema, but also arises as a result of a branch retinal vein occlusion, which is more common in hypertensives than in normotensive people. There is a change in the normal diurnal rhythm of urine flow in many patients with hypertension, and they may complain of nocturia even though there is little other evidence of impaired renal function. Hypertension also commonly presents as a result of local ischemia which has resulted from atheromatous narrowing or occlusion of an artery in the brain, heart, or lower limbs. Unfortunately, some patients with hypertension have already suffered such severe damage to the function of the brain or myocardium as to make the value of treatment debatable.

Clinical examination is mainly focused upon the cardiovascular system and the brain. Patients with severe hypertension usually have an apex beat which is displaced to the left and which has a forceful sustained character. They frequently also have an atrial sound. In some patients there may also be signs of left ventricular failure, basal crepitations in the lungs, a third heart sound, pulsus alternans, or congestive heart failure with a raised jugular venous pressure and peripheral edema. Patients with mild to moderate hypertension often have a normal heart on clinical examination. It is important to feel the main arterial pulses, including the femoral, posterior tibial, and dorsalis pedis, and to time the femoral against the brachial artery pulse. The carotid artery should be auscultated at the angle of the jaw, the renal artery just above and about 2 inches lateral to the umbilicus, and the femoral artery at the inguinal ligament.

Careful retinal examination is essential, and this should be done in a darkened room, if possible, with the pupils dilated. The disc margin and the disc color should be carefully inspected, and the presence of the normal optic cup confirmed. The four main vessel groups should be followed for at least three diameters from the disc, taking note of the caliber of the artery, the uniformity of its diameter, the color of the blood column, and the shape of the crossings. The blood vessel wall is not visualized in the normal retina. The red lines of the "vessels" are the column of red cells within them. The cells are surrounded by a shell of plasma and a transparent vessel wall, neither of which is visible with the ophthalmoscope. When the wall becomes thickened and fibrosed, it begins to obscure the red cells column and may ultimately become an opaque white sheath. Cotton wool spots usually occur within three diameters of the optic disc and close to the main vessel groups. Flame-shaped hemorrhages have a similar distribution. Hard exudates are usually best seen close to the macula as radial spokes.

The most important investigations designed to assess organ involvement are the ECG, the chest radiograph, and tests of renal function, particularly the serum creatinine concentration. The ECG should be carefully examined. Common findings are an increased voltage and flattening or inversion of the T waves in leads 1, aVL, and V_{4-6}. The chest radiograph may confirm the clinical assessment of left ventricular enlargement. There is frequently some evidence of aortic disease such as dilatation or tortuosity with unfolding of the thoracic aorta. The degree of renal impairment varies, but some reduction of glomerular filtration rate is present in most patients with severe hypertension, although usually only to about 65 ml per minute if the patient is not in the accelerated phase. Mild and moderate hypertension usually leave renal function unimpaired.

Detection of Treatable Causes. There has been much controversy about the extent to which it is desirable to investigate patients for etiologic factors which may be treatable by surgery. The three main classes of treatable causes are excess catecholamine production from a tumor of the chromaffin tissue; excess mineralocorticoid production from the adrenal, e.g., Cushing's syndrome or hyperaldosteronism; and vascular obstruction such as coarctation of the aorta or renal artery stenosis. Causes of renal disease other than arterial disease are less important, because they less commonly lead to cure of hypertension.

The basic screening investigation for pheochromocytoma is the urinary vanillylmandelic acid (VMA), which some clinics measure in all hypertensive patients. It should certainly be measured in patients with a suggestive history or severe hypertension. The simplest screen for mineralocorticoid excess is measurement of serum potassium and sodium concentrations. There is debate about the extent to which it is necessary to search for renal artery disease if there are no suggestive features such as resistance to treatment or rapid onset of a high pressure level.

Evaluation of Risk. Much of the basic data for evaluating risk will have been derived from the patient's history. This includes date of birth, sex, previous vascular episodes, family history of hypertension and vascular disease, and history of renal disease or diabetes. These findings will be reinforced by the clinical examination and in particular by the blood pressure, body weight and height, and urinalysis for protein and sugar. The only information of value in prediction of risk to be derived from investigations is the ECG for evidence of left ventricular hypertrophy and/or ischemia.

Case Finding. As most patients with elevated levels of blood pressure are symptomless, the only practical way of detecting them before a catastrophe occurs is to conduct an active case-finding program. This means that every physician ought to take the blood pressure of every patient he sees, whatever the primary reason for the consultation. Several attempts have been made to develop rules about the frequency of rescreening if the pressure has been taken in the past. Based upon epidemiologic data, it seems reasonable to rescreen after ten years if the initial diastolic pressure is less than 80 mm Hg, after five years if it lies in the range of 80 to 89 mm Hg, and every year if it is in the range of 90 to 104 mm Hg. Higher pressures than this would normally be treated as would some in the range of 90 to 104 mm Hg.

CLINICAL SYNDROMES OF HYPERTENSION. High blood pressure can present clinically in a wide variety of ways. Before treatment of mild to moderate hypertension became widespread, patients frequently presented with accelerated hypertension, left ventricular failure, or cerebral hemorrhage. A few patients still slip through the net of case-finding programs and suffer these catastrophes prior to initiation of antihypertensive therapy, but these are less common than they used to be. The clinical presentation of hypertension is now most commonly as part of the spectrum of risk factors in a patient who has suffered a stroke or a myocardial infarction, or as a chance finding during clinical examination for another purpose.

Malignant or Accelerated Hypertension. The patient with malignant hypertension is almost always ill with symptoms such as morning headaches, blurred vision, dyspnea, and/or symptoms of uremia. Such patients are commonly in their fourth, fifth, or sixth decade of life, and about half have underlying chronic renal disease. Their blood pressure is almost always above 110 mm Hg diastolic in adults and frequently much higher, with diastolic pressures in the range of 130 to 170 mm Hg being commonplace. Clinical examination usually reveals an enlarged left ventricle and early signs of pulmonary edema such as persistent rales at the lung base. The retinal finding of cotton wool spots and papilledema is essential to make the diagnosis. Investigation usually shows some degree of renal impairment with raised blood urea and serum creatinine values. The serum potassium concentration is often reduced. The blood film may show evidence of intravascular coagulation of "microangiopathic hemolytic anemia" with circulating red cell fragments and fibrin degradation products. The platelet count may be reduced. Irrespective of whether the underlying cause is renal, there is likely to be proteinuria and microscopic hematuria. The characteristic pathologic change of accelerated hypertension is fibrinoid necrosis of small arterioles. Evidence will be presented later that the insudation of plasma and deposition of fibrin follow sudden dilatation of small arterioles whose smooth muscle cells have been unable to generate sufficient tension to withstand the intravascular pressure. This process can be termed high pressure autoregulatory failure, as it represents the upper limit of pressure at which tissue perfusion can be held approximately normal by progressive constriction of arterioles in the face of a rising systemic arterial pressure. High pressure autoregulatory failure is particularly likely to occur if the pressure has risen rapidly or if there are associated factors such as anemia which may impair autoregulation. If the rate of rise of pressure is slow, both smooth muscle hypertrophy and replacement of muscle by fibrous tissue increase the strength of the vessel wall and render it better able to stand the bursting strain of the high intravascular pressure. This probably explains the infrequency of accelerated hypertension in the elderly even though high pressure levels are very common among them. Conversely, younger patients, especially children, may develop the retinal features of accelerated hypertension at lower levels of pressure than is the case in older people.

Accelerated hypertension is a medical emergency because this condition is causing progressive damage to the blood vessels in vital organs, particularly the kidney. Such a patient is also in severe danger of suffering cerebral hemorrhage. When the diagnosis is made, a patient should be admitted to hospital at once for blood pressure reduction.

RETINOPATHY IN ACCELERATED HYPERTENSION. The diagnosis of malignant or accelerated hypertension is based clinically upon the retinal finding of cotton wool spots, linear hemorrhages, and papilledema, and its pathologic hallmark is the presence of fibrinoid necrosis in the arterioles of many organs, particularly the kidney. The retinal changes in accelerated hypertension are all direct consequences of the pressure elevation. As the pressure rises, the arterioles constrict and thus maintain an approximately normal pressure in the distal arterioles and the capillaries. If the pressure rises to a very high level, particularly if it does so quickly, the arterioles may not be able to withstand the high level pressure and begin to give way. The result is that a much higher pressure than usual is applied to the proximal ends of capillaries. In the retina the high pressure capillaries fed directly from the arterioles lie amid the nerve fibers; when hemorrhage takes place from these capillaries, its spread is confined by the nerve fibers so that it has a linear or flame-shaped appearance. A general transudation of fluid as a result of the disturbed Starling pressure equilibrium in the capillary leads to the formation of a grayish retinal edema. The walls of some arterioles which have given way in the face of the high pressure become disrupted, allowing the insudation of plasma through the endothelial cells into the wall. The plasma penetration is often accompanied by cellular elements such as platelets and red cells. This stage can be recognized on a fluorescence angiogram of the retina by the presence of multiple leaking points on small arterioles. The swelling and disruption of the arteriolar wall as a result of the penetration of plasma may obstruct the lumen and lead to a small retinal infarct downstream. This infarct is the cotton wool spot. Pathologic examination of the wall of the arteriole at this stage shows necrosis of myofibrillae in smooth muscle cells, penetration of plasma, and precipitation of fibrin. This is the appearance which pathologists term fibrinoid necrosis. The term is exactly descriptive of the appearances but misleading in the terms of the pathophysiology, because the deposition of fibrin has little or nothing to do with the causation of the lesion. Autoregulatory failure in the vessels of the nerve head causes swelling, engorgement of the capillaries, transudation of fluid, and sometimes also formation of cotton wool spots on the nerve head itself. Keith, Wagener, and Barker (1939) described the presence of hemorrhages and exudates as the third grade of retinopathy, and papilledema as the fourth. As they have the same basic pathogenetic mechanisms, it seems best to describe both as accelerated hypertension. Hard exudates are not present in the earlier stage of the development of hypertensive retinopathy, but they appear soon after cotton wool spots and papilledema are established and are often arranged in radial spokes from the macula, giving the appearance of a star or fan. Hard exudates are fine, punctate, shiny deposits of lipid in the deep layers of the retina and are readily distinguished with the ophthalmoscope from the larger, more diffuse white cotton wool spot with blurred edges which lies in the nerve fiber layer. The cotton wool spot is made up of swollen ischemic axons. The ischemia leads to an interruption of both anterograde and retrograde axoplasmic flow, so that organelles and other materials which are normally moving up and down the axon come to rest in the area of ischemia. These lead to swelling of the axon and its cloudy white appearance. Eventually some of these materials aggregate into dense masses within the neuron, where they have the superficial appearance of a cell nucleus. The swollen axon containing its pseudonucleus is sometimes referred to as a cytoid body. As cotton wool spots clear, they can take on a punctate appearance which may be confused with hard exudates. The punctate white areas are the cytoid bodies.

Hypertensive Encephalopathy. This term tends to be misused to describe any transient neurologic deficit in a patient with severe hypertension. True hypertensive encephalopathy is the cerebral counterpart of the retinal pathology of accelerated hypertension. It is caused by cerebral autoregulatory failure, which brings about generalized cerebral edema and patchy damage to arterioles with leakage of plasma constituents into their walls. Hypertensive encephalopathy often occurs in patients who also have the retinal features of accelerated hypertension, but these are not always present.

The patients usually present clinically with a very high level of pressure and increasingly severe headaches. These progress to general impairment of higher functions and eventually to stupor. Focal and usually transient neurologic signs may develop in the course of the illness. Investigation shows generalized swelling of the brain substance, and animal studies have demonstrated leakage of plasma from arterioles. The diagnosis is a most important one to make accurately, because the patient's condition will improve rapidly if the blood pressure is reduced to a level at which cerebrovascular autoregulation is once again possible.

There is a resemblance between hypertensive encephalopathy and other syndromes in brain autoregulatory failure such as high altitude cerebral edema or carbon dioxide narcosis, although these less commonly manifest focal neurologic signs.

Hypertension in Pregnancy. A raised arterial pressure during pregnancy usually leads to impaired placental function and a small baby. There is an increased risk of intrauterine death and increased neonatal mortality because of prematurity. Toxemia of pregnancy is characterized by a rise in blood pressure from 28 weeks' gestation onward, with edema and proteinuria. The most feared complication is progression to severe hypertension with fits and coma. Eclamptic convulsions are essentially hypertensive encephalopathic attacks occurring in a previously normotensive young woman who has suffered a rapid rise in blood pressure. They should never occur in women who have received proper antenatal care and control of blood pressure. Toxemia is hypertension provoked by pregnancy, but many women who have mild hypertension become pregnant or may be first found to be hypertensive when they consult a physician at about 8 to 12 weeks of pregnancy for antenatal care. Because of the separation that exists between medical specialties, there was in the past a different approach to treatment in a pregnant hypertensive than in the nonpregnant female with high blood pressure. This view is now changing, and most physicians and obstetricians use the same methods of management in pregnancy as at other times but aim to achieve particularly accurate control of pressure during the pregnancy. There is evidence that effective antihypertensive therapy reduces fetal loss during pregnancy, and the aim should be to keep the pressure below 140 systolic and 90 diastolic mm Hg if possible. The main drug used to control blood pressure is methyldopa. There has been concern that antihypertensive drugs might damage the development of the fetal nervous system by interfering with catecholamine pathways, but studies of babies whose mothers have been treated for hypertension with these drugs are reassuring. Some obstetricians are concerned about the use of beta-adrenergic blocking drugs because it obscures the interpretation of fetal bradycardia, an important clinical sign of both fetal and neonatal hypoxia.

Hitherto, pregnant hypertensives often had to spend many weeks resting in hospital to keep the blood pressure down. This is sometimes still necessary, but in many cases the blood pressure can be controlled with drugs and the patient can remain ambulatory.

Cerebral Hemorrhage. Abrupt onset of major neurologic signs, sometimes accompanied by severe headache and progressing rapidly to loss of consciousness, usually signifies the onset of intracranial bleeding in a hypertensive patient. The bleeding may occur into the subarachnoid space from a berry aneurysm, but the common source in hypertensive patients appears to be the minute arterial aneurysms on the striate arteries on the base of the brain, first described by Charcot and Bouchard in France over 100 years ago. These aneurysms are rare in individuals who have a normal blood pressure. Their pathogenesis has not been completely elucidated, but there may be areas of high pressure autoregulatory failure on the thin-walled cerebral vessels. The hemorrhage usually begins in the substance of the brain but may rupture into the ventricular system. Once intracranial bleeding has reached the subarachnoid space, the prognosis is very poor. Small hemorrhages have a better prognosis and can be difficult to differentiate clinically from the cerebral infarction caused by vascular occlusion. If there is any question of using anticoagulants, this differentiation can be important, and in such cases further investigation by lumbar puncture and computerized axial tomography is indicated. Carotid arteriography is indicated if there is clinical suspicion of a berry aneurysm and if the patient's condition improves sufficiently to warrant consideration of neurosurgical intervention.

Hypertensive Left Ventricular Failure. The presence of a high systemic arterial pressure increases the afterload of the left ventricle, and in consequence the ventricle hypertrophies. As the pressure rises to a very high level, the ventricles dilate and eventually fail, and the patient then presents with pulmonary edema. This may range in severity from a patient who is asphyxiating with airways full of white or pink froth to mild dyspnea on exertion or occasional attacks of nocturnal dyspnea. In older people with hypertension the clinical presentation of pulmonary edema is frequently precipitated by the onset of atrial fibrillation or by ischemic heart disease. If pulmonary edema is caused by high pressure, the clinical improvement as a result of pressure reduction can be almost miraculous in its rapidity.

"Benign Essential" Hypertension. Patients with an elevated pressure who are not in the accelerated phase are often described as having benign essential hypertension. The term benign is inappropriate, as an elevated blood pressure always carries some risk. Although no cause can be identified in most individuals with high pressure, the use of the word essential to describe it adds nothing, and it, too, is probably better avoided.

What then are the clinical features of hypertension which is not in the accelerated phase? They are rarely dramatic. The elevated level of pressure is often the only clinical finding of note. A mild degree of left ventricular hypertrophy may be identified clinically, or by means of the electrocardiogram or chest x-ray. Vascular damage may be evident either from its consequences on the heart or brain or by loss of pulses or arterial bruits.

RETINOPATHY IN "BENIGN" HYPERTENSION. Keith, Wagener, and Barker applied the terms grade I and grade II retinopathy to the retinal changes found in hypertensive patients who are not in the accelerated phase. The main features which they described included narrowing of the arterioles, often with caliber irregularity, and nicking of the veins at the crossing. The appearance of the arteriole wall changed so that it became shinier and more irregular, whereas the color of the underlying blood columns was partly concealed so that it took on a coppery or silvery hue. Narrowing of the retinal vessels is due to vasoconstriction. All the other changes represent thickening of the vessel wall as a result of muscle hypertrophy and fibrous replacement. The problem with these features is that none of them is by itself characteristic of hypertension. Elderly people who are normotensive may show all of them. They are still of clinical value if the patient is young but of little use in drawing conclusions about the severity of hypertension in the elderly. Recording of these features is very prone to observer error, and attempts to standardize the recording of the diameter of the arteries by comparing them with the nearby veins have foundered on the variability of the branching pattern of the retinal vessels. The presence of these features does not add much to knowledge of the patient in most cases.

MECHANISMS. The systemic arterial pressure must be maintained at a level which permits the brain and eye to function and allows pressure filtration in the kidneys and perfusion of the coronary arteries. It is not surprising that this most vital function is defended by several different control systems which prevent its falling too low. The blood pressure must also be prevented from rising too high, because vascular damage might result. Four control systems play the major part in maintaining the blood pressure between these limits. These are the arterial baroreflex, the regulation of body fluid volume, the renin-angiotensin system, and vascular autoregulation. All these mechanisms participate in blood pressure regulation in normotension and in hypertension. It is uncertain how far derangement of any one of them plays a role in the pathogenesis of hypertension.

The Arterial Baroreflex. The main concentration of pressure sensors lies in the carotid sinus, although there are others in the aorta and the wall of the left ventricle. These sensors continually monitor the level of arterial pressure, and their rate of firing changes between systole and diastole. They form the afferent limb of the fastest responding blood pressure regulating system. Sensory impulses from the baroreceptors are relayed and processed in the brainstem. Norepinephrine and epinephrine containing fibers around the nucleus of the solitary tract play an important part in regulating the gain of the baroreflex. The efferent fibers proceed through sympathetic adrenergic nerves to the heart and blood vessels and through vagal cholinergic fibers. A sudden rise in pressure causes baroreflex discharge, which results in vagally mediated cardiac slowing and vasodilatation with decreased sympathetic tone. The result is to lower the blood pressure, although not all the way to the prestimulus level. A sudden fall in pressure diminishes the rate of firing and causes sympathetic stimulation of the rate and force of cardiac contraction and constriction of peripheral arterioles and veins. The result is partly to restore the level of blood pressure. Denervation of the carotid sinus in animals causes extreme lability of blood pressure, which is sometimes termed neurogenic hypertension. However, the rise in arterial pressure is not usually very great except when the animal is stimulated, and the characteristic is more of extreme instability than sustained elevation of pressure.

It is important to realize that the baroreflex arc is not simply a fixed feedback loop such as might be found in an amplifier. Depending upon the physiologic circumstances, the response to the same level of blood pressure can be quite different. A blood pressure of 85 systolic and 55 diastolic mm Hg caused by bleeding would cause an intense sympathetic discharge and tachycardia. The same level of pressure during deep sleep would be accompanied by the normal bradycardia of the sleeping subject. A pressure of 200 systolic and 100 diastolic mm Hg is readily achieved during heavy exercise and is accompanied by tachycardia. The same pressure brought about by infusion of norepinephrine would cause severe cardiac slowing mediated by the baroreflex. The pressure is the same, but the interpretation at CNS level is completely different.

If the pressure remains elevated, the baroreflex begins to regulate at the new level within 24 to 48 hours. The ability of the baroreflex to reset so quickly argues against its playing an important role in long-term pressure regulation. Baroreflex function in patients with hypertension appears to be intact and not to differ qualitatively from that found in normotensives.

The effector side of the baroreflex is chiefly the sympathetic nervous system through its ability to constrict arteries and veins and to stimulate cardiac contractility and rate. The importance of this side of the reflex is seen in the postural hypotension suffered by many patients in whom it is inhibited by ganglion-blocking or adrenergic neuron–blocking drugs. The baroreflex is not the only control system that uses the adrenergic nerves to raise blood pressure. The rise in pressure that occurs with fear, anxiety, pain, or mental activity is also mediated by increasing cardiac output or peripheral resistance through these pathways. One possible mechanism for long-term elevation of blood pressure would be excessive central nervous system–mediated stimulation of adrenergic nerves. Evidence for this possibility has been sought by comparing the level of blood pressure at rest with the plasma concentration of the adrenergic neurotransmitter norepinephrine. Some research workers have found a very close relationship between blood pressure and plasma norepinephrine; others have not. It has not proved possible to devise any method of measuring the basic level of sympathetic impulses other than the plasma and urinary catecholamines that represent the totality of these processes and not just the vascular ones. There is evidence for a wider spread of norepinephrine levels in plasma in hypertensives, about 40 per cent of them lying above the normal range, but not yet sufficient to conclude that hypertension in some individuals is caused by the brain.

Fluid Volume. If the body is severely depleted of salt and water, the blood pressure falls; if it is overloaded, the pressure rises. The mechanisms involved are complex and have been discussed cogently by Guyton. Changes in fluid volume alter the distention of the venous system and change the venous return to the heart. If the cardiac filling pressure rises, so does the cardiac output; if it falls, the output also falls. The short-term effects of cardiac output changes upon blood pressure are buffered by the baroreflex, but in the longer term changes in tissue perfusion which are inappropriate to metabolic requirements lead to autoregulatory changes in the peripheral resistance and thus to changes in the blood pressure. If the kidneys are intact, a rise in pressure leads to a diuresis and a fall in pressure to conservation of salt and water. Thus the feedback loop is closed, and Guyton has claimed that this system, unlike the baroreflex, has infinite gain so that it can exactly restore the previous level of pressure.

Pathologic changes that alter the pressure threshold at which the kidneys excrete salt and water will alter the level of systemic arterial pressure. At one extreme a complete lack of kidneys should lead to a great sensitivity to changes in volume, and this has proved to be the case. Relatively small increases in salt and water intake in nephrectomized individuals cause a large increase in blood pressure. This type of hypertension is sometimes termed "renoprival." Other mechanisms such as the lack of a renal depressor substance may also play a part in the abnormal pressure regulation. If excretory function is diminished, the blood pressure will become responsive to an abnormally high sodium load. Mineralocorticoid excess will cause the kidney to retain salt at a pressure level at which it would normally be excreted and thereby raise the arterial pressure. Anything that increases the pressure gradient between the aorta and the glomeruli will tend to raise the systemic arterial pressure as renal retention of salt and water endeavors to restore the preobstruction renal perfusion pressure. This will apply to obstruction of the main renal arteries and of the arterial branches within the kidney. An experimental analogy is the one-kidney Goldblatt model. Here one kidney has been removed and the other has an arterial clip upon it. The renin levels are low, and the pressure gradient across the renal artery appears to be the important factor in causing the hypertension through the salt and water retention that results from diminished perfusion pressure applied to the clipped kidney.

Renin and Angiotensin. Renin is an enzyme released from the kidney which splits a decapeptide from a plasma globulin substrate. This decapeptide, angiotensin I, has little pharmacologic activity, but a dipeptide residue is removed by a converting enzyme in the lung to form an octapeptide, angiotensin II. Until the discovery of the thromboxanes, this was the most potent vasoconstrictor agent known. Angiotensin II has a direct action upon blood vessels, but it is also an important physiologic stimulant of aldosterone secretion from the adrenal gland.

Renin and angiotensin levels in the blood respond in the direction anticipated if they were participating in physiologic blood pressure regulation. Standing or salt depletion raises renin, and recumbency and salt loading reduce it. In conditions of primary mineralocorticoid excess the renin falls to a low value. Four control mechanisms have been identified that control the release of renin from the kidney. The first mechanism is the renal barostat, which senses changes in renal perfusion pressure and releases renin when the pressure falls; the second mechanism is the short feedback loop of plasma angiotensin II levels upon renin release. If angiotensin effects are blocked with its competitive antagonist saralasin, renin levels rise rapidly. The third mechanism is mediated by beta-adrenergic receptors in the kidney which release renin when they are stimulated, and the fourth mechanism depends upon sensing the tubular concentrations of sodium.

The importance of angiotensin II in maintaining blood pressure at any particular time depends upon the level of sodium intake. In a sodium replete individual inhibition of angiotensin II has little effect upon blood pressure; but if the same person is salt depleted, the result of inhibition may be a substantial fall. There is good evidence that angiotensin II is the cause of the blood pressure elevation in the experimental two-kidney Goldblatt hypertension and in human hypertension caused by renal artery stenosis. In the two-kidney Goldblatt model one kidney is clipped and the other is not. Thus the unclipped kidney should be able to prevent a rise in pressure due to salt and water retention resulting from the pressure gradient across the clipped artery. In the first phase of this form of hypertension the blood pressure rises and so do the plasma renin and angiotensin. Infusion of the competitive angiotensin II antagonist saralasin causes a prompt fall to a normal level of pressure. However, in experimental hypertension and probably also in human hypertension the pressure continues to rise in the second phase, whereas the renin subsides almost to normal. Short-term infusion of saralasin will not lower the blood pressure, which appears to be no longer angiotensin dependent. However, a 12-hour infusion of saralasin or a converting enzyme inhibitor gradually lowers the pressure to normal in animals and may do so in man. Thus the hypertension in phase II is still angiotensin dependent but apparently by a different mechanism.

The role of angiotensin II in other forms of human hypertension remains to be elucidated in full, but it seems very unlikely that it plays a central role in the majority of patients. In malignant hypertension the renin levels are usually high because of the multiple small areas of ischemia within the kidney. Angiotensin II plays some part in the maintenance of blood pressure and is undoubtedly responsible for the secondary hyperaldosteronism that frequently causes mild potassium depletion in these patients.

Vascular Autoregulation. In many tissues, of which the brain is the best example, a change in perfusion pressure does not cause a corresponding change in tissue perfusion. Instead, the vascular resistance is adjusted by local mechanisms to keep perfusion roughly constant over a wide range of arterial pressures. This phenomenon is known as "vascular autoregulation." If flow changes rather than pressure, autoregulation will diminish the vascular resistance in response to a reduction in flow and raise it in response to an increase. Thus changes in cardiac output which are inappropriate to metabolic demand should produce corresponding changes in blood pressure. It seems likely that this is an important mechanism in the causation of the hyper-

tension that accompanies salt and water overload, but it is uncertain how significant it is in other circumstances. It has been suggested that some patients with essential hypertension may go through a phase of increased cardiac output before hypertension becomes established, but this has not been proved beyond doubt. Reduction of cardiac output may be the main mode of action of beta-adrenergic blocking drugs in lowering the blood pressure, but this, too, remains to be established.

Circulatory Dynamics. In broad terms the level of the systemic arterial pressure is set by the match between cardiac output and peripheral vascular resistance. Elevation of blood pressure could result from either or both. In the early stages of hypertension some patients have a raised cardiac output and some a raised peripheral resistance, but in the majority of patients with established hypertension the cardiac output is normal and peripheral resistance is raised. In the later stages of severe hypertension the cardiac output is often less than normal and the peripheral resistance is greatly increased. Thus in looking for new factors that may cause hypertension, it seems most profitable to concentrate upon those which raise the peripheral resistance.

Elevation of the arterial pressure causes many other changes in the cardiovascular system. A high level of pressure stimulates hypertrophy of the vessel wall and increases the thickness of the smooth muscle coat. These changes probably account for the enhanced sensitivity to pressor stimuli in patients with established or early hypertension. Such stimuli include exposure to cold, fear, mental arithmetic, and so forth. A greater thickness of muscle means that the change in vessel caliber for a given degree of fiber shortening will be greater. Hypertrophy of the vessel wall also raises the minimum vascular resistance of tissues such as the human forearm under conditions of maximal vasodilatation.

Besides the hypertrophic changes, other structural changes take place in the arteries. Some of the muscle in the thickened wall is replaced by fibrous tissue. The most important vascular change is that the deposition of atheroma is increased by the presence of hypertension. The reason is not known, but it is a change manifest in pulmonary hypertension as well as systemic hypertension. As the predominant causes of death in hypertensive patients are stroke and myocardial infarction, the significance of accelerated formation of atheroma cannot be denied, but the mechanism is uncertain.

The cardiac muscle also hypertrophies, and, if pressure elevation is extreme, the cavity of the ventricle dilates. Local imbalance between metabolic demand and perfusion within the increased muscle mass may lead to relative ischemia and areas of fibrosis. These may lead to ineffective contraction which, combined with the dilated chamber and the afterload of the high pressure, will eventually bring about heart failure.

The regulation of plasma volume is altered in hypertension. Some patients have a relatively contracted plasma volume with a high hematocrit, probably because of the increased capillary pressure. There is a marked diurnal variation of plasma volume, with the value almost 10 per cent lower in the morning than in the evening in hypertensive subjects. An infused sodium load is excreted more rapidly by hypertensive patients than by normotensive controls.

ETIOLOGY. In most diseases the need to establish a diagnosis is paramount because the prognosis and the treatment given may be entirely different, depending upon which of the possible alternatives is the cause of the illness. The position with hypertension is somewhat different. There are very few causes of hypertension which are life threatening other than by their effect upon the blood pressure. The most important condition in this category is renal failure, but this is usually readily detected clinically, or by the use of a biochemical screen at presentation. Only coarctation of the aorta and a pheochromocytoma are sufficiently serious in themselves as well as through the pressure elevation they cause to make it essential that they should be diagnosed at once. Although it is desirable to make a diagnosis of renal artery stenosis or primary hyperaldosteronism, if present, some delay will not usually cause harm to the patient if the pressure has been controlled with drugs in the meantime. Thus the diagnostic problem in a patient with hypertension is how to detect as large a proportion as possible of the rare treatable causes without exposing millions of patients without such factors to unnecessary and uncomfortable investigations. The answer is to use screening tests and to be willing to reconsider the diagnosis in treated patients if the clinical course is atypical.

Obstruction or Loss of Elasticity in the Large Arteries. COARCTATION OF AORTA (see Ch. 359.2). Routine palpation of the femoral pulses with simultaneous timing against the radial is part of the basic clinical examination of a patient with hypertension. Other clinical features, such as a wide pulse pressure in the arteries fed by the aorta proximal to the coarctation, palpable or visible collaterals, or tortuous retinal arteries, help to confirm the diagnosis that has been made. Occasionally the diagnosis is first made radiologically by direct visualization of the coarctation or of rib notching on a routine chest radiograph. Operative treatment is indicated if it is technically feasible.

SYSTOLIC HYPERTENSION. Many elderly patients and some younger ones present with considerable elevation of the systolic pressure while having a relatively normal diastolic pressure. A typical pressure might be 200 systolic and 80 diastolic mm Hg in such an individual. The principal factors governing the magnitude of the pulse pressure are the stroke volume and acceleration of the blood from the left ventricle and the elasticity of the large arteries, particularly the aorta. Factors that increase the stroke volume such as bradycardia, aortic incompetence, anemia, and anxiety may all lead to an increase in systolic pressure with a normal or low diastolic pressure. In the elderly the most common cause is not an increase in stroke volume but a loss of elastic compliance of the large arteries. Epidemiologic studies have shown that such patients have an increased risk of cardiovascular morbidity and mortality even if their diastolic pressure is relatively low. However, it is not clear whether this cardiovascular disease is a cause or consequence of the systolic hypertension. It may be that the presence of a systolic hypertension is itself a marker of arterial disease and the level of systolic pressure has no other significance. There is no evidence as to whether reduction of systolic hypertension with a normal diastolic pressure conveys any advantage to the patient.

Hypertension Associated with Catecholamine Excess. PHEOCHROMOCYTOMA (see Ch. 550). Pheochro-mocytoma is a very rare cause of hypertension. It can be suspected clinically in half to two thirds of the patients. Pounding palpitations and/or headaches, paroxysmal skin color changes, tremor, sweating, agitation, glycosuria, and hypermetabolism may all point to the likelihood of this diagnosis.

Some patients are aware that pressure over the tumor area can provoke an attack. A very rare but striking example is the precipitation of a paroxysm by micturition in a patient with pheochromocytoma of the bladder. In some patients there are only occasional spikes of hypertension, or even of hypotension, whereas in others there may be a sustained elevation in the blood pressure. There is sometimes quite marked orthostatic hypotension in the absence of the use of drugs with a postural effect.

It is common practice to measure the urinary VMA as a screening test to detect pheochromocytoma in all hypertensive patients irrespective of clinical suspicions. A single estimate is about 80 per cent reliable in detecting a pheochromocytoma, but many slightly elevated values occur as false positives. Once firmly suspected, the diagnosis should be confirmed by further measurements of the urinary VMA and of metanephrines or catecholamines. Other causes of increased sympathetic activity such as left ventricular failure and myocardial infarction should be ruled out. Increasingly the measurements of plasma norepinephrine are being used to make and confirm the diagnosis of pheochromocytoma. These, combined with segmental venous sampling, may supplement radiologic methods of localizing the tumor.

MONOAMINE OXIDASE INHIBITORS: INTERACTION WITH TYRAMINE. Patients taking drugs which inhibit the monoamine oxidase in the gut wall and in the body at large may develop paroxysmal hypertension if they consume food or drink containing tyramine or medicines such as cold cures which contain indirectly pressor amines such as phenylpropanolamine. Tyramine and phenylpropanolamine are both capable of releasing norepinephrine from adrenergic nerve endings. Normally the amounts of these releasing agents that penetrate into the body are small because of metabolism by monoamine oxidase in the gut wall. If this enzyme is inhibited, larger amounts reach the systemic circulation where the adrenergic nerve endings contain an excessive amount of norepinephrine because of the local inhibition of monoamine oxidase. The result can be a catastrophic increase in circulating norepinephrine, causing a very high blood pressure with a risk of cerebral hemorrhage or paroxysmal cardiac arrhythmia.

CLONIDINE WITHDRAWAL. The imidazoline clonidine is an effective antihypertensive agent. It acts centrally as an alpha-adrenoceptor agonist and causes a decrease in the sympathetic outflow. If treatment with the drug is suddenly withdrawn, patients may develop a syndrome of catecholamine excess 16 to 48 hours later which closely resembles a pheochromocytoma. Patients complain of anxiety, tremor, palpitations, and insomnia with severe headache. Both plasma and urinary catecholamines can reach levels found in patients with pheochromocytoma. The precise mechanism underlying this reaction has not yet been determined, but sympathetic efferent activity is greatly increased. The blood pressure can be controlled by restarting clonidine or by use of alpha-adrenergic blocking agents.

CATECHOLAMINE EXCESS IN ESSENTIAL HYPERTENSION. A wide range of values of both plasma norepinephrine and urinary metabolites of catecholamines are found in both normotensive and hypertensive individuals. Some studies have found a fairly close correlation between the height of the blood pressure and the concentration of norepinephrine in the plasma, but this has been denied by others. The plasma norepinephrine rises slightly as age advances, and this may account for some of the reported differences between values in hypertensives and normotensive laboratory controls. It is still an open question whether prolonged chronic sympathetic overactivity is one of the causes of essential hypertension.

MANAGEMENT OF CATECHOLAMINE EXCESS HYPERTENSION. The long-term treatment of hypertension associated with gross excess of circulating catecholamines is to treat the cause. However, in the short term the blood pressure and cardiac rhythm disturbances, if present, must be controlled. Alpha-adrenergic blocking drugs such as injections of phentolamine should be used to control the immediate rise in pressure; oral agents such as phenoxybenzamine which alkylate the alpha receptor can be used in longer-term treatment. Tachycardia or tachyarrhythmias can be controlled by use of beta receptor blocking agents, such as propranolol. Patients with a pheochromocytoma should always be prepared for surgery by pharmacologic control of hypertension and cardiac arrhythmias.

Renal Hypertension. All forms of chronic renal disease may be associated with an increased incidence of hypertension. This is true of chronic glomerulonephritis due to immune complex deposition, chronic pyelonephritis due to infection, vascular lesions such as occur in polyarteritis nodosa and lupus erythematosus and in the main renal arteries due to congenital bands, intimal fibroplasia, and atheroma. Renal carcinoma can cause hypertension as can polycystic disease, although isolated renal cysts rarely do so. Obstructive uropathies, analgesic abuse, and renal calculi can also cause hypertension. Acute renal failure resulting from glomerulonephritis or tubular necrosis can cause rapid elevation of blood pressure, especially in fluid-overloaded patients.

There are two main reasons for making an accurate diagnosis of renal hypertension. The first is that the renal or urologic condition which has caused the hypertension may itself require treatment, e.g., infection, stone, obstruction, tumor. Of the conditions that fall into this category, infection is the most important. Pyelonephritis is an important cause of renal damage and hypertension, especially in children. Its numerical importance in relation to adult hypertension is difficult to establish because of the difficulty of proving a diagnosis of chronic pyelonephritis.

The relationship between bacilluria and hypertension is disputed, but there is an increased incidence of hypertension in patients whose urograms show "pyelonephritic scars." There are vascular lesions in the vicinity of these scars, and there seems little doubt that the scars are ischemic in origin. Such lesions can be caused by hypertensive changes in the vessels without any infection, and it is not clear how far infection of the renal parenchyma can cause vascular lesions and initiate the ischemia that leads to scar formation and hypertension in a previously normotensive individual. But in children with vesicoureteral reflux, urinary infection, renal scars, and hypertension, there seems little doubt that reflux and infection start the whole process.

If there are renal symptoms or a history of urinary infection, the urine should be cultured; if the culture is positive, an appropriate antimicrobial should be given.

There is no evidence that this will modify the course of the hypertension, but it may prevent further loss of renal parenchyma due to infection. Investigation of urologic causes of recurrent infection such as stone should proceed as it would in a normotensive patient.

The second reason for investigating a patient to determine if hypertension has a renal cause is the possibility of surgical cure of renovascular disease or unilateral renal disease. Cure of hypertension has resulted from nephrectomy in several types of unilateral renal disease, including pyelonephritis, hydro- and pyonephrosis, and tumor. One of the best pieces of direct evidence that pyelonephritis can cause hypertension is the cases of surgical cure when the disease was predominantly unilateral. Unfortunately, pyelonephritis is rarely completely unilateral; and as cure rates are only 30 to 40 per cent even in carefully selected patients, modern policy is to conserve functioning renal tissue when possible. Attempts at cure are focused on renovascular disease.

SALT AND WATER OVERLOAD HYPERTENSION. Patients without kidneys or those in terminal renal failure with very low values of glomerular filtration are extremely sensitive to changes in salt and water balance. The plasma renin and angiotensin II levels are usually low unless the patient has entered the accelerated phase of hypertension. This form of hypertension can usually be managed successfully by restriction of salt and water intake and elimination of excess by dialysis. The body weight is often a better guide to progress than the sphygmomanometer. The experimental counterpart to this form of hypertension is salt-loading animals that have had one kidney and part of another removed or else have had one kidney removed and an arterial clip applied to the other.

RENIN-DEPENDENT HYPERTENSION. The extent to which renin contributes to elevation of blood pressure in the majority of patients with hypertension is controversial, but most studies suggest that the proportion is quite small. The spread of renin values is wider among hypertensives than normotensives, and those above and below the normal range, related to sodium intake, are often called "high renin" and "low renin" hypertensives. It was suggested that renin might be itself a factor causing damage to blood vessels and that high renin hypertensives had a much increased incidence of stroke and myocardial infarction. That view has found little support from further studies. As plasma renin falls with age and the risk of vascular disease increases, a negative association has been proposed based upon epidemiologic studies. Renin contributes to the elevation of blood pressure in accelerated hypertension and causes it in renal disease associated with ischemia. Many types of renal disease can be associated with localized areas of ischemia, but the most important is renal artery obstruction caused by medial fibroplasia or atheromatous disease. The detection of these conditions has given rise to much controversy on the grounds of prevalence, costs, and results of surgery.

RENAL ARTERY STENOSIS. There are no reliable figures for the incidence of renal artery stenosis in the community. It may cause 3 to 5 per cent of severe hypertension treated in hospital but probably less than 1 per cent of the mild hypertension now being treated in the community.

There are few clinical features that help in making a diagnosis. Suspicion should be aroused by severe hypertension in a patient under 35 years old, or sudden increase in severity in an older patient. Rarely an attack of flank pain may point to a renal artery embolus, and a bruit above and radiating laterally from the umbilicus may be helpful. Unfortunately the majority of bruits heard over the abdominal aorta do not originate in the renal arteries. The most common means of diagnosis is an intravenous urogram. Typical features include one kidney more than 1.5 cm shorter than the other, delay in appearance of contrast on the ischemic side on a two-minute film, and delay in emptying on that side later in the urogram because of the low flow of concentrated urine. The most reliable means of confirming the diagnosis is an angiogram of the abdominal aorta and renal arteries. At one time a high proportion of patients with hypertension were subjected to abdominal aortography, but the yield of cases was low and appreciable discomfort and cost were involved. Routine aortography has now been abandoned almost everywhere. Some have argued against the value of the urogram in hypertension, especially when there is no indication other than the level of pressure itself. The cost of the investigative procedures per patient eventually cured of hypertension is rather high.

When the diagnosis of renal artery stenosis has been confirmed anatomically, it is still necessary to try to establish whether the elevation of blood pressure is due to it. The methods used currently include measurement of renin concentration in blood drawn from both renal veins. The difference should exceed 1.5 to 2 times, and the unprotected kidney has its production of renin suppressed. Antagonism of the effect of circulating renin is another promising method of establishing the diagnosis. This can be done by infusing the angiotensin II antagonist Sar-1-Ala-8-angiotensin II (saralasin) or a converting enzyme inhibitor such as the nonapeptide SQ 20881. The predictive power of these tests for results of surgery is good but not perfect.

At present the usual method of managing renin-dependent hypertension is to seek a treatable cause such as renal artery obstruction and to repair it by surgical means. Results depend upon the skill of the surgeon, but normotension has been achieved in half to two thirds of patients in some centers. In patients in whom operation is not technically feasible or whose general health does not permit, the blood pressure can be lowered by antihypertensive drugs, and the long-term survival of operated and medically managed patients is similar. Mortality tends to be high in both groups, because patients with atheromatous stenosis of the renal artery usually have extensive atheroma elsewhere. A special situation may arise in patients with renal failure and bilateral renal artery obstruction, in whom surgery can sometimes improve overall renal function. Drugs that reduce the sympathetically mediated release of renin are indicated if medical management is to be used, and a beta-adrenergic receptor blocking agent such as propranolol would be the first choice. As propranolol only inhibits sympathetically mediated renin release, it is not completely effective in reducing the plasma renin. Inhibitors of the converting enzyme active by the oral route hold out more promise but are still at an early stage of clinical trial.

MINERALOCORTICOID EXCESS HYPERTENSION. Mineralocorticoids, both natural and synthetic, can cause retention of salt and water and resultant hypertension. Thus hypertension is a common complication of Cushing's syndrome, both natural and iatrogenic. The contraceptive pill is capable of causing elevation of blood pressure, and there are worrying indications that this may be progressive over several years. The elevation each year is a trivial 1 or 1.5 mm rise in diastolic pressure, but the cumulative effect over several years can begin to be significant in epidemiologic terms in relation to the incidence of stroke and myocardial infarction. Blood pressure elevation may also result from the salt-retaining effects of carbenoxolone sodium given to treat gastric ulcer.

Among these factors the contraceptive pill gives rise to by far the greatest difficulty because of the extent of its use. Severe hypertension in users of the pill is very uncommon, although accelerated hypertension has been reported. More commonly a woman who has used the pill for several years develops a pressure level which is on the threshold of an indication for treatment. There is no certain method of establishing whether the pill is responsible short of stopping it for six weeks. Some women taking the pill are unwilling to stop taking it for fear of unwanted pregnancy, and it may be necessary to treat their hypertension without establishing beyond doubt that the contraceptive pill is its cause.

Endogenous mineralocorticoid excess can also pose difficult problems of detection and treatment. Cushing's syndrome or congenital adrenal hyperplasia as a cause of hypertension can usually be diagnosed clinically, although patients with an ACTH-producing malignant tumor may present with hypertension and severe hypokalemia without much other evidence of Cushing's syndrome. The main problem is the diagnosis of primary hyperaldosteronism. Some patients will give a history that suggests potassium depletion with muscle weakness and edema, but most do not. The presence of hypokalemia is a useful guide if the patient has not received a thiazide diuretic, but most patients have been treated with these agents before they get to a hospital clinic. If potassium depletion is severe and the serum sodium is high, the diagnosis is very likely to be hyperaldosteronism, and it can be confirmed by measuring plasma or urinary aldosterone and plasma renin. A patient with primary hyperaldosteronism has an increased production of aldosterone with a suppressed plasma renin. A trial of treatment with the aldosterone antagonist spironolactone predicts fairly accurately the eventual response of both blood pressure and serum potassium concentration to operative removal of an adrenal tumor. Primary hyperaldosteronism can be caused by an adrenal adenoma or by diffuse "micronodular" hyperplasia. A few patients have been described with hypertension due to primary hyperaldosteronism who had a normal serum potassium level some or all of the time. These patients are impossible to diagnose without full investigation of aldosterone and renin, and this does not appear justified as a routine procedure for the very low yield of treatable cases likely to result.

TREATMENT. The intellectual challenge of diagnosis often attracts more interest than the time-consuming persistent effort required for effective long-term drug treatment. The problem is evident in the management of hypertension, in which surgically treatable patients have tended to attract more attention than those requiring drug therapy. Although it is important for the patient with a surgically treatable cause to be detected, this must not be done at the expense of the great majority of patients who do not require elaborate clinical investigation but do need careful blood pressure control by use of drugs to diminish the risk of cardiovascular disease. The proportion of hypertensive patients in the community who might benefit from pressure reduction and who have a surgically remediable cause is very small, probably only 1 to 2 per cent of those requiring treatment.

Reduction of Risk. The aim of patient management in hypertension is to reduce the likelihood of cardiovascular complications, and the approach adopted depends upon the level of blood pressure and the burden of associated risk factors. If the blood pressure is very high, this is the dominant consideration, and other considerations can be deferred until the pressure has been reduced. However, in many patients with only moderate elevation of pressure, other factors such as cigarette smoking, serum lipids, glucose intolerance, and obesity may be of comparable significance to the blood pressure. Careful assessment is required to decide which factors should receive the most attention. A patient who is told to stop smoking, to lose 20 pounds in weight, and to take pills to lower blood pressure is likely to find the task so difficult that he will end up doing none of them. Failure to comply with the physician's advice is the most common cause of treatment failure, and strategies must be developed to try to improve it. A close relationship between the patient and a single physician is a significant factor. A patient who knows, likes, and trusts his physician is more likely to take his advice irrespective of its quality. That advice should be simple and unequivocal. A general advice to lose weight rarely has much impact, but a specific instruction to lose 1 pound per week for 20 weeks backed up by regular weighing and scrutiny of the results may succeed.

The drug regimen should consist of as few different drugs and tablets as possible, and regimens that require doses to be taken during the working day should be avoided. The patient should know the name and purpose of each tablet, and when and how many to take. The very fact that the doctor takes an interest in the drugs reinforces their importance in the eyes of a patient. A hastily written prescription handed over without an explanation may have the contrary effect. Patients often find it helpful to purchase a small metal pillbox and to count their tablets for the next day into it just before they go to bed. If the box is empty again by the next evening, the patient will know he has taken exactly the right amount. If the patient is elderly or confused, a family member can be enlisted to help count out the tablets and make sure they have been consumed. A wife or husband often seems more concerned about the outcome of therapy than the patient does.

Despite these measures to improve compliance with advice, some patients will drop out from treatment and attendance at follow-up. Few will do so by deliberate rejection of therapy, which is their right. In most cases it is more a matter of oversight. A well-run clinic should have a system to detect nonattendance and to issue reminders. A special register for hypertensive patients is the best arrangement.

Antihypertensive Drugs. In most countries there are many different antihypertensive drugs available, and the range of choice may seem bewildering. If the drugs are categorized in terms of their main pharmacologic action, much of this confusion disappears, and the choice of a particular drug within a group is of less importance than the correct choice of the main action. The main groups of drugs used to lower blood pressure are diuretics, beta receptor–blocking drugs, vasodilators, and centrally acting sympathetic inhibitors (Table 2). Drugs that blockade autonomic ganglia and adrenergic neurons are used less often than formerly. There has been increased interest in drugs that blockade alpha-adrenergic receptors, and in the combination of more than one property in a single molecule, e.g., alpha- and beta-adrenergic blockade.

DIURETICS. Most of the diuretics used to treat hypertension are based upon the molecular structure of chlorothiazide and, despite differences in activity per unit weight and duration of action, are of similar efficacy. It is more convenient for the patient to use a diuretic with a long duration of action for hypertension, because a sudden diuresis is an inconvenience. All diuretics of this type cause depletion of salt and water with a loss of extracellular and plasma fluid volume. During long-term treatment these changes in volume are less marked but the blood pressure reduction is maintained. There is a reduction of peripheral vascular resistance without alteration in the cardiac output. The dose response curve is relatively flat, which is an advantage, as it permits use of a single fixed dose in most patients. The precise mechanism of action in reducing peripheral resistance is not well defined, but probably depends upon changes in the fluid and ionic content of the blood vessel wall. The main advantage of the thiazides and related diuretics is that they cause few symptoms in most patients, and in this respect they approach the ideal more closely than any other antihypertensive drug. Serious toxicity is rare. The main long-term

TABLE 2. Drugs and Doses Used to Treat High Blood Pressure

Type of Action	Drug Name	Dose Range in General Use (mg per Day)
Diuretic	Bendrofluazide	5–10
	Hydrochlorothiazide	50–100
	Chlorthalidone	25–50
	Polythiazide	1–2
Beta-adrenergic blocker	Propranolol	40–640
	Oxprenolol	40–640
	Atenolol	50–100
	Metoprolol	200–600
Centrally acting alpha agonist	Methyldopa	500–3000
	Clonidine	0.3–1.0
Vasodilator	Hydralazine	50–300
	Minoxidil*	5–40
Alpha receptor antagonist	Prazosin†	0.5–15
Norepinephrine-depleting agents	Reserpine	0.1–0.25
Adrenergic neuron–blocking drug	Guanethidine†	10–100

*Investigational drug.
†Special care is needed to avoid postural hypotension. Start with a low dose.
See manufacturers' data sheets for full prescribing information and contraindications.

concern with thiazide diuretics has been in respect of their metabolic effects such as potassium depletion, hyperuricemia, glucose intolerance, and reduction of urinary calcium excretion. Some reduction of serum potassium value, averaging about 0.6 mEq per liter, almost always occurs, but this rarely causes any problem unless the patient is on a digitalis glycoside. The serum potassium concentration can be increased by eating a diet rich in high potassium foods (e.g., fruit, meat), and by taking oral potassium supplements or a potassium-retaining diuretic (amiloride, triamterene, or spironolactone). It is questionable whether routine use of potassium supplements or potassium-retaining diuretics is necessary.

Reduction of urate clearance and elevation of serum urate values are also almost invariable accompaniments of treatment with thiazide diuretics. Use of a diuretic occasionally precipitates an acute attack of gout, but it is not clear whether the mild hyperuricemia of prolonged diuretic therapy increases the incidence of acute gouty arthritis. Routine use of allopurinol or probenecid does not appear to be necessary.

A potentially more serious problem is a slow deterioration of glucose tolerance among patients treated with thiazides. Decreased glucose tolerance is much more likely if it is already abnormal, such as in patients with obesity. At present there is not sufficient evidence to seek to restrict the use of thiazides, but administration for very long periods should be accompanied by occasional urine testing for sugar. There is also a moderate increase in serum lipid concentrations during treatment with the thiazides, but the significance of this in relation to cardiovascular risk factors is still open.

Thiazide diuretics also reduce the urine calcium concentration and cause a small increase in the serum concentration, averaging about 0.15 mEq per liter. This is probably not of significance unless there is an additional cause of hypercalcemia such as sarcoidosis.

BETA-ADRENERGIC RECEPTOR BLOCKING DRUGS. Beta-adrenergic receptors are widely distributed in the heart, lungs, blood vessels, and metabolic and endocrine systems. Beta-adrenergic receptor blocking drugs cause competitive blockade of the action of norepinephrine and other beta receptor agonists. Their main cardiovascular action is to reduce the rate and force of cardiac contraction and thus lower the cardiac output. They also blockade bronchial beta receptors and may precipitate asthma in susceptible individuals. Among the many other consequences of beta receptor blockade are inhibition of sympathetically mediated renin release from the kidney and inhibition of sympathetically mediated mobilization of muscle glycogen. Some beta receptor–blocking drugs readily penetrate the central nervous system, and central sites of action have been postulated.

The mechanism of the hypotensive action of beta receptor–blocking drugs is still disputed among four main hypotheses. These are reduction of cardiac output, inhibition of renin release, a central action upon sympathetic receptors, and a peripheral action upon a beta receptor on the presynaptic surface of the adrenergic nerve endings. Reduction of cardiac output with loss of the full baroreflex-mediated compensatory increase in peripheral resistance seems the most likely of these explanations. Low concentrations of propranolol will cause maximal inhibition of renin release, but higher concentrations are required for an optimal effect upon blood pressure.

Beta-adrenergic blocking drugs do not cause a large and immediate fall in blood pressure such as can be seen with a drug that blocks sympathetic transmission elsewhere, at the alpha receptor or the sympathetic nerve ending, for example. However, the blood pressure begins to fall in two to four hours after a large dose, and most of the hypotensive effect is manifest within two or three days. In mild hypertension the fall in pressure achieved is comparable to that obtained with diuretics, but in more severe hypertension results comparable to those with methyldopa and guanethidine have been obtained. The reduction in pressure is similar in the lying and standing positions, and the normal rise in pressure on exercise is much reduced. A wide range of doses of propranolol has been used to treat hypertension, and the dose response curve appears to be steeper than it is for the diuretics. Other beta-blocking drugs such as atenolol have a flatter dose response curve.

The main contraindications to the use of beta-blocking drugs are a history of asthma or wheezing and the presence of cardiac conduction defects. The risk of precipitating an attack of asthma is greatest in patients with a history of this disease and is less in patients with a history of chronic bronchitis and emphysema. It is very rare for an asthmatic attack to be precipitated in a patient with no previous history of wheezing. The main concern about cardiac conduction defects has been that a patient who develops complete heart block while on beta-blocking drugs may have a dangerously slow ventricular rate. Opinions differ about the wisdom of using these drugs in patients with bundle branch or fascicular block, but they are probably best avoided in any situation in which a serious conduction disturbance is particularly likely to occur, such as the sick sinus syndrome and atrioventricular or intraventricular block. Less categorical contraindications include heart failure and diabetes requiring hypoglycemic agents. A failing heart depends upon sympathetic drive to maintain its contractility and beta receptor blockade may worsen heart failure. It would be most unwise to use beta receptor–blocking drugs in the early stages of treatment of a patient with severe heart failure, but once the blood pressure has been reduced these drugs can be used with little hazard. In patients with an enlarged left ventricle who are not in failure, the use of beta-blocking drugs in combination with diuretics is often effective and is rarely attended by evidence of impaired cardiac function. Recovery from hypoglycemia depends chiefly upon the mobilization of liver glycogen which is alpha-adrenergic receptor mediated in man. If the liver glycogen is depleted by starvation or ketosis, mobilization of muscle glycogen by beta-adrenergic receptor stimulation becomes important, and this cannot be achieved if the patient is beta blocked. Beta-blocking drugs should be used with great care, if at all, in unstable diabetics on insulin or sulfonylureas.

Beta-adrenergic blocking drugs cause many symptoms, but few of them are disabling. The reduction of cardiac output may cause cold extremities in cold weather and may worsen intermittent claudication in patients with obstructive disease of their leg arteries. Central nervous system side effects include a feeling of "muzziness," an exactly descriptive English word that appears to have no American equivalent, vivid dreams, and insomnia. Some patients may suffer daytime visual hallucinations. Serious toxicity has been very rare, but one beta-adrenergic blocking drug, practolol, had to be withdrawn from use because it caused a dry eye, progressing in some cases to perforation of the anterior chamber, a psoriasiform skin rash, and peritoneal fibrosis. It appears that this toxicity was unique to practolol, but some concern about the safety of new beta-adrenergic blocking drugs is bound to remain until much longer experience has accumulated.

Besides competitive beta receptor blockade, these drugs may possess in varying degree three other pharmacologic properties. These are cardioselectivity, membrane effects, and partial agonist activity. Cardioselective agents appear to be just as effective in lowering the blood pressure as nonselective ones. Their main advantage is a lesser degree of blockade of bronchial beta receptors and thus a lesser likelihood of precipitating asthma and a greater ease of treating it with beta receptor agonists if it occurs. Unfortunately the degree of selectivity for the cardiac, or beta-1, receptors is insufficient to avoid a substantial amount of bronchial beta blockade, especially at higher doses. Membrane activity such as is seen with the local anesthetic lidocaine is demonstrated by some beta-blocking drugs such as propranolol, but it is insignificant at the concentrations achieved by the usual dosage schedules in hypertension. Partial agonist activity means the ability to stimulate as well as blockade the beta receptors; it is sometimes referred to as "intrinsic sympathomimetic activity" or ISA. The consequence of partial agonist activity is less slowing of the resting heart rate. Claims have been made that drugs with partial agonist activity are less likely to precipitate heart failure of asthma and cause a lower incidence of cold extremities. The evidence to support these claims, particularly the first two, is slender, and it seems unlikely that the comparatively minor stimulation of beta receptors makes much difference to the therapeutic use of the drug.

Beta receptor–blocking drugs also vary in their lipid solubility and thus in the readiness with which they enter the central nervous system. The more hydrophilic drugs may have less tendency to cause vivid dreams and sleep disturbance than the lipid-soluble ones that enter the brain in high concentration.

CENTRALLY ACTING DRUGS. The level of efferent sympathetic activity is controlled by the brain. Drugs such as methyldopa and clonidine diminish the flow of impulses in peripheral sympathetic nerves as a result of a direct action upon alpha receptors in the brainstem. Methyldopa must be transformed into methylnorepinephrine to exert this effect, but clonidine is an alpha receptor agonist in its own right. Stimulation of alpha receptors in the brain potentiates the effect of the vasodepressor baroreflex, and this is one reason why the action of these drugs is accompanied by slowing of the heart rate. The reduction of sympathetic activity is manifest by a lowering of the plasma norepinephrine concentration and reduced amounts of catecholamine metabolites in the urine. As the baroreflex remains intact, postural adjustments of pressure can still be made, although there is sometimes a degree of fall in pressure on standing. The main problem of this type of action is that stimulation of brain alpha receptors also causes sedation and reduction in the flow of saliva. These are troublesome side effects for some patients, especially in the early days of therapy or after an increase in dose. In other respects, there are important differences between methyldopa and clonidine.

Methyldopa must be decarboxylated in the brain before it can exert its effect, and there is a delay of three to six hours after an oral dose before the full hypotensive effect is seen. In part the delay is caused by slow absorption from the gut, and in part by the need for metabolic transformation to the active form. Methyldopa modifies the rise in pressure on exercise but to a much lesser extent than beta receptor–blocking drugs. Apart from its central nervous system side effects, the main concern with methyldopa has been with its toxicity. Ten to 30 per cent of patients given the drug develop a direct antiglobulin test on their red cells, depending upon the dose used. A very small proportion of these will go on to develop an autoimmune hemolytic anemia. Mild diarrhea is a common symptom. A less common problem is the development of a maculopapular skin rash. Rarer forms of toxicity include a drug-induced fever, usually manifest in the first 14 days of therapy, and a hepatitic type of liver damage. However, the drug has been very widely used and is effective, and problems with toxicity have necessitated withdrawal in only a small proportion of patients.

Clonidine has a similar action to methyldopa, but the sedation and dry mouth it causes are marginally more prominent than with the equiactive doses of methyldopa. Clonidine causes constipation rather than diarrhea and is free of other types of toxicity. The main concern with the drug has been a syndrome of sympathetic hyperactivity with tachycardia, high blood pressure, tremor, sweating, and insomnia that occurs if the drug is stopped suddenly. Pressure begins to rise within 16 to 24 hours of cessation of therapy.

NOREPINEPHRINE-DEPLETING AGENTS. A number of hypotensive agents deplete neuronal stores of norepinephrine, but only the reserpine alkaloids appear to do this as their main pharmacologic action. The substances available include rauwolfia (whole root), reserpine, alseroxylon, deserpidine, rescinnamine, and syrosingopine. The differences among the action of these drugs are small, and reserpine itself is the most widely used. In high doses reserpine is an effective hypotensive agent and at one time injections of 1 to 5 mg parenterally were used to treat hypertensive crises. Chronic oral dosing at this level produces an unacceptable incidence of severe depression, and only low doses are now used. At these low doses reserpine is not of much use as single drug but is a valuable agent in combination with diuretics and vasodilators. Unfortunately, even in low doses reserpine increases the incidence of depression. There have also been several reports of increased incidence of breast cancer in middle-aged women treated with reserpine. Other studies have not supported this contention, although the argument has not been completely settled. Perhaps in consequence of these problems and also because of their greater efficacy, there has been a change to the use of beta-adrenergic blocking drugs in circumstances in which reserpine was used in the past. Reserpine has the virtue of cheapness, and it is worth recalling that the Veterans Administration trials, which still provide the best evidence of the efficacy of hypotensive therapy, used a triple combination of reserpine, hydralazine, and a diuretic.

VASODILATORS. As the main hemodynamic abnormality in hypertension is an increased peripheral vascular resistance, it would appear that use of a drug that directly dilates the blood vessels might be the most logical approach to treatment. Hydralazine is the most widely used drug of this class, although minoxidil and diazoxide are also important. Vasodilators share many properties in common. Acute administration leads to dilatation of arteriolar beds, with flushing of the skin, a fall in pressure, stimulation of the baroreflex, and a reflex increase in heart rate and force. If the patient has ischemic heart disease, the resultant increase in left ventricular work can precipitate angina or even myocardial infarction. Concurrent use of a beta-adrenergic blocking drug prevents most of the increase in heart rate caused by vasodilators, and as a result there has been a great increase in the use of this combination.

Hydralazine, the most widely used vasodilator, becomes tightly bound to the smooth muscle of blood vessel walls and in consequence has a much longer duration of action than its plasma half-life would suggest. The duration of action is such that twice or even once daily dosing will give effective control of pressure through the day and night. The main problem with hydralazine is its toxicity if the dose is increased above 200 mg daily. A proportion of patients develop a drug-induced lupus syndrome with arthralgia, muscle pains, fever, and skin rashes. As in other drug-induced lupus syndromes, the DNA binding is normal.

Hydralazine is a hydrazine, and like other hydrazines such as isoniazid it is metabolized by acetylation. In Caucasian populations there are roughly equal numbers of slow and fast acetylators, and it is the slow acetylators who develop the lupus syndrome. If the acetylator phenotype is known to be fast, it is possible to increase the hydralazine dose to 300 mg daily without undue risk of drug-induced lupus. Because of the limitation on dosage imposed by its toxicity, hydralazine is only a moderately effective hypotensive agent and is usually combined with both a beta-adrenergic blocking drug and a diuretic.

Several other vasodilators are under investigation, and two that have been studied extensively are diazoxide and minoxidil. Diazoxide is little used by the oral route because it causes diabetes in a high proportion of patients, but minoxidil is as effective as high doses of hydralazine but without the problems of lupus syndrome. The main problems associated with minoxidil therapy are fluid retention, which requires high doses of a loop diuretic in some cases, and increased growth of lanugo hair on the face, body, and limbs. The drug has shown considerable promise in controlling the pressure of patients with very severe hypertension otherwise difficult to control with existing drugs.

ADRENERGIC NEURON–BLOCKING DRUGS. These drugs — examples include guanethidine, bethanidine,* and debrisoquine* — are concentrated in adrenergic nerve endings by the amine pump and, once they achieve a high enough concentration, blockade transmission by preventing norepinephrine release. The result is to inhibit both alpha and beta adrenoceptor–mediated responses. The drugs are effective hypotensive agents, but interfere more severely than other agents with normal blood pressure regulation. There is often a substantial fall in blood pressure on standing and after exercise. Ejaculation during

*Investigational drug.

sexual intercourse in the male may be inhibited. Because of these problems these drugs are less widely used, although they are still an effective alternative when other measures fail or are contraindicated. Tricyclic antidepressants, which blockade the amine pump in adrenergic nerve endings, interfere with the hypotensive effect of adrenergic neuron–blocking drugs.

ALPHA-ADRENERGIC RECEPTOR–BLOCKING DRUGS. The alpha-adrenergic receptor–blocking drugs phentolamine and phenoxybenzamine have been known for some years and are used to treat hypertension due to excess circulating catecholamines. They are not very effective hypotensive agents in patients without excess catecholamines in the circulation. This in itself is surprising, because drugs that prevent stimulation of alpha receptors by diminishing catecholamine release are effective. The explanation may be that there are alpha receptors on both sides of the synaptic cleft, on the innervated structure and on the neuron. Inhibition of the neuronal presynaptic receptors causes increased release of norepinephrine, which partly negates the effect of postsynaptic receptor blockade. Prazosin, a new hypotensive agent, has an alpha receptor–blocking action which is almost entirely upon the postjunctional alpha receptor. It is a powerful hypotensive agent, although prone to cause postural hypotension, especially with the first dose, unless this is very small. It appears that some degree of postural hypotension is an unavoidable consequence of alpha receptor blockade, although the extent varies, and only a minority of patients have sufficient fall in blood pressure on standing to cause symptoms of faintness and weakness.

COMBINED DRUG TREATMENT OF HYPERTENSION. The main groups of antihypertensive drugs lower the blood pressure by somewhat different mechanisms; if more than one type of action is used at the same time, the result is often an additive effect. As unwanted drug effects are often dose related, this opens the possibility that drug combinations could be used to achieve the same or greater fall in pressure without so many side effects. A second possibility is that the effect of the use of two drugs might be greater than the addition of the two individual actions because of a synergistic action of the combination. The most widely used combination is that of a vasodilator with a beta-adrenergic blocker with the aim of minimizing the reflex rise in cardiac output caused by the vasodilator and the fall in cardiac output caused by beta-adrenergic blockade. This appears to be because other reflex adjustments such as a sympathetically mediated vasoconstriction are not completely inhibited. However, even if there is no synergy, there may be a useful additive effect such as has been demonstrated with the components of the vasodilator–beta blocker–diuretic combination and for combinations of diuretics with all other types of hypotensive agents (Table 3).

EMERGENCY REDUCTION OF BLOOD PRESSURE. There are only a few circumstances in which it is necessary to reduce

TABLE 3. Blood Pressure Response to Combined Drug Therapy*

Regimen	Fall in Pressure from Placebo (mm Hg)
Diuretic alone	21/11
Beta-adrenergic blocker alone	26/16
Diuretic + beta-adrenergic blocker	34/20
Diuretic + beta-adrenergic blocker + vasodilator	46/26

*Figures taken from Wilcox and Mitchell: Br. Med. J., 2:547, 1977.

the blood pressure rapidly. These include hypertensive left ventricular failure, hypertensive encephalopathy, including eclampsia, and accelerated hypertension. Other situations such as intracranial bleeding and dissecting aneurysm need careful evaluation before a decision is reached. Sudden reduction of blood pressure may be dangerous, and it is rarely necessary to reduce the level abruptly to 120 systolic and 80 diastolic mm Hg or below. Reduction to a level which relieves the immediate crisis is all that is necessary; fine adjustment can more safely be done later with oral therapy.

There are many methods of lowering the blood pressure quickly. If an immediate action is needed, an intravenous bolus injection of 300 mg of diazoxide or an infusion pump–controlled administration of sodium nitroprusside is effective in most cases. The patient must be carefully monitored with frequent readings of blood pressure, and baseline investigations such as an ECG and plasma electrolytes should be taken, if possible, before lowering the pressure. If reduction within a few hours is the objective, an oral loading dose of 1000 mg of methyldopa is effective, but the sedation that accompanies the fall in pressure may be diagnostically confusing in some circumstances. Diuretics and beta-adrenergic blocking drugs are not usually suitable for rapid reduction of pressure. Hydralazine is useful, but given alone it causes flushing and tachycardia and may precipitate angina. Pretreatment with a beta-adrenergic blocking agent will obviate this problem but may cause delay.

STOPPING HYPOTENSIVE THERAPY. Once drug treatment of hypertension has begun, it can rarely be stopped. Both patient and doctor should understand the long-term nature of the decision they have taken. If the drugs are stopped, the subsequent course of the blood pressure is highly variable. It may return to pretreatment levels within a few days, but more commonly it slowly rises over a few weeks or months. At one stage it was hoped that reversal of cardiovascular hypertrophy and a downward resetting of the pressure control mechanisms might make it possible to withdraw treatment after several years of blood pressure control. Results in the small number of patients in whom it was tried were disappointing, but the amount of hard data available on this point is small. Withdrawal of treatment is usually brought up in three circumstances: extreme old age, intercurrent illness, and surgery. If the main reason for treating hypertension is to prevent a late risk of myocardial infarction or stroke, there is little point in continuing it in a patient who is terminally ill. Old age of itself is not a reason for stopping therapy, but extreme senility would be. There is usually no need to interrupt therapy for a surgical operation, but it is essential that the anesthesiologist should be aware of current therapy.

THERAPEUTIC CHOICES. Three main considerations govern the choice of antihypertensive drugs for a particular patient: simplicity, tolerability, and efficacy. Absent from this list is one important consideration, the prediction of individual drug response.

As some patients do not respond well to one drug but do to another, it would be advantageous if an accurate prediction could be made to avoid the delays of trial and error. Some progress has been made in making predictions. There is evidence that the small proportion of hypertensives who have a low plasma renin respond less well than other patients to beta-adrenergic blocking drugs such as propranolol. However, a response to propranolol can be obtained even in low renin patients by using higher doses of propranolol (greater than 240 mg daily), although the response is never as great as in normal or high renin patients. There is also some evidence that patients with a urinary VMA in the higher part of the normal range respond better to a centrally acting hypotensive agent such as methyldopa than do patients with a urinary VMA in the lower part of the normal range. Patients with a low renin respond particularly well to diuretics, and, surprisingly, high VMA patients also respond well to diuretics. It has been suggested, largely on theoretical grounds, that patients with a raised cardiac output would respond particularly well to beta-adrenergic blocking agents, but this does not seem to be borne out in practice, and it is possible that the converse may be true.

It is too early to translate these findings into a flow chart to predict the optimal drug for a particular patient, although that stage may be reached in the medium-term future. One difficulty is that the unresponsive groups, low renin and low VMA, are a relatively small fraction of the total number of patients. A more substantial difficulty lies in the general use of drug combinations. There is no evidence about the predictability of response to drug combinations, and it may be that the "catch-all" philosophy of two- or three-drug combination therapy largely obviates the need to find the optimal single drug.

The ideal treatment for hypertension would be a once for all intervention that permanently lowered blood pressure. Surgical thoracolumbar sympathectomy at one time promised that this might be possible, but the effects waned as the nerves regenerated. In animals central administration of 6-hydroxydopamine, which destroys adrenergic nerve endings in the brain, seems to produce a long-lasting fall in blood pressure, but this agent is too damaging to contemplate using in man. Long-term daily administration of hypotensive agents — effective but inconvenient — is all that we have to offer at present.

Two measures are possible to simplify the patient's regimen. The first is to use drugs with a long duration of action to avoid the necessity of a midday drug dose, and, when possible, to give the drugs only once a day. The second is to be prepared to use combined drug preparations when the mutual efficacy of the components has been well proved. Thus combinations of diuretic, beta-adrenergic blocker, and vasodilator in a single tablet are useful, just as similar combinations in which reserpine replaced the beta blocker were in the past.

Making a regimen tolerable for a patient is chiefly the ability to predict the acceptability of drug side effects. Drugs which interfere with male sexual function, such as the adrenergic neuron–blocking drugs and, to a lesser extent, the centrally acting drugs, are unsuitable for younger men. Fatigue on exertion and cold extremities or a past history of Raynaud's phenomenon would be a contraindication to the use of beta blockade in a patient who had to do heavy muscular work and/or work out of doors in cold weather. Sedation and dry mouth are tiresome side effects for patients who have to do intellectual work or speak in public. Some patients who speak in public find a positive virtue in the lessening of palpitations and shaking hands brought about by beta-adrenergic blockade. Younger women do not relish the hirsute face and limbs brought about by minoxidil. A patient troubled by insomnia may find his problem worse while taking propranolol, but better on methyldopa. A depressed patient is always much more troubled by drug side effects than one with a normal mood, and drugs with prominent side effects should be avoided in such a patient.

It may seem a strange inversion to deal with efficacy last, but the truth is that there are a number of equally effective regimens available, and no drug is effective if the patient will not take it. A simple step care approach should prove adequate in all but the most severely hypertensive patients.

Because of freedom from side effects and a flat dose response curve, it is wise to use a thiazide diuretic as the first choice in patients with diastolic pressures up to 114 mm Hg. A fixed dose can be used. The second step is a beta-adrenergic blocking drug. In most cases the dose should be started low and titrated upward. If the patient has a diastolic pressure of 115 mm Hg or higher, it would be sensible to begin treatment with both a thiazide diuretic and a beta-adrenergic blocking agent. The alternative to the beta-blocking drug is to use a centrally acting drug or reserpine. The third step would be to add a vasodilator such as hydralazine to the existing two-drug combinations, beginning with a low dose and increasing quickly to the practical maximum. If these three steps are inadequate and minoxidil is available, this should be substituted for the hydralazine. Alternatively an adrenergic neuron–blocking drug or a combination of alpha- and beta-adrenergic blockade should be tried. Never accept poor pressure control too readily. It can always be improved, provided that sufficient time and care are spent. Depending upon the type of patient, it is reasonable to anticipate that about half the patients can be controlled with one drug, and another 30 per cent with two; the remaining 20 per cent will require three or more.

Blood pressure should be reduced as close to normal as symptoms will allow. The target of reducing the diastolic blood pressure below 100 mm Hg, which many clinics set when treating severe hypertension in the 1960's, is quite inadequate today. A diastolic of 90 mm Hg might be acceptable, but one of 80 to 85 mm Hg would be even better.

PROGNOSIS. In patients with accelerated hypertension and left ventricular failure the results of treatment are so dramatically beneficial that a controlled clinical trial was never considered necessary to establish them. Improvement in pulmonary edema is often evident within seconds of lowering the blood pressure, although full resolution may take much longer. The retinopathy of accelerated hypertension ceases to progress within two or three days of pressure reduction, and those lesions that appear after pressure reduction were probably already in process of formation at the time treatment began. All the features of accelerated hypertensive retinopathy will eventually regress in periods varying from 6 to 12 weeks for the cotton wool spots, linear hemorrhages, and papilledema, to up to a year or more for the macular star figure of hard exudate. Renal function ceases to deteriorate at a rapid rate, and in patients with an abrupt onset of accelerated hypertension there may be some improvement in glomerular filtration. The survival of patients with accelerated hypertension is greatly improved by treatment, although still dominated by the extent of deterioration of renal function at the time of diagnosis. Patients with severe impairment of renal function tend to continue to deteriorate despite pressure control. The availability of renal dialysis and transplant programs has become the main consideration in the long-term survival of these patients. However, the five-year survival of patients with accelerated hypertension under treatment is now 35 to 50 per cent without the help of renal support, which compares with only 1 to 5 per cent prior to the introduction of antihypertensive therapy. Accelerated hypertension should be looked upon as a preventable condition, and the widespread introduction of treatment for mild to moderate hypertension is leading to a progressive decrease in the number of patients with accelerated hypertension who are being diagnosed.

The great majority of patients with elevated blood pressure are not in the accelerated phase, and the benefits of treatment are less obvious in the short term. Some symptoms such as headache in the mornings are relieved by blood pressure reduction, but the loss of some symptoms is often roughly balanced by the gain of others which are due to the drugs. The only objective signs of improvement may be a reduction in the size of the heart and a reduction in the voltage and improvement in repolarization abnormalities in the electrocardiogram. Retinal vascular changes such as caliber irregularity and crossing changes rarely show much change when the pressure is lowered. However, if the rise in pressure has been recent and rapid and the retina shows a uniform narrowing of the retinal arteries, there may be some dilatation when the pressure is lowered.

The benefits of treatment of this type of hypertension had to be established by controlled clinical trials. Considering the very large numbers of patients who might potentially be treated, proof of the benefit of treatment rests upon a very small number of properly controlled trials. Of these the largest and best known are those conducted by the Veterans Administration in the United States. Only men were included in these trials, and the incidence of complications among the control groups was rather high, probably because the patients were drawn from those referred to hospitals rather than from a community sample. The pressure levels quoted in the trial are those after six weeks on placebo, a point to bear in mind when relating them to first visit casual pressures. In individuals with diastolic pressures of about 115 mm Hg, the benefits of treatment were so striking that the trial was stopped on ethical grounds. Deaths and major complications such as stroke, heart failure, and progression to accelerated hypertension appeared entirely in the placebo-treated group. For patients with diastolic pressures of between 105 and 114 mm Hg, there was a statistically significant benefit with treatment, with fewer deaths and many fewer hypertensive complications than in the control group, although the difference was less dramatic than in the patients with a diastolic of 115 mm Hg and higher. For the group with diastolic pressures of between 90 and 104 mm Hg there were fewer incidents in the treated group than in their controls, but this difference did not reach statistical significance. Based upon these results, most physicians have concluded that patients with diastolic pressures above 105 mm Hg on the first visit would benefit from treatment, and no further placebo-controlled trials among patients with this level of pressure are being undertaken. It should be noted that there is no direct proof that this is the case in women, as almost all of the clinical trial evidence was derived from men. Women with untreated hypertension have fewer complications over a given time than men.

Two major areas of doubt remain concerning the efficacy of hypotensive therapy. The first concerns the benefit of treatment in the great majority of hypertensive patients whose casual pressure lies in the range 90 to 104 mm Hg. Trials are in progress in the United Kingdom, the United

States, and Australia to try and answer this question. Until the results are available in the early to mid-1980's, it seems reasonable to treat those patients with a particularly high burden of risk factors but not to treat those who lie in a relatively low risk group. The second question concerns the effects of treatment upon different types of cardiovascular pathology. The vascular pathology of accelerated hypertension does not rise in patients whose blood pressure has been well controlled throughout. If a patient already has accelerated hypertension, the progression of the vascular changes is halted but tissue damage, had it already taken place, remains. The onion skin proliferative changes of the intima of renal arteries is still present in patients many years after their accelerated hypertension has been brought under control. The risk of death from cerebral hemorrhage is also very greatly reduced by lowering the blood pressure, and this probably indicates that the Charcot-Bouchard aneurysms are remodeled or obliterated after a period of pressure control. The effect of hypotensive therapy upon atheromatous disease and particularly myocardial infarction is much more difficult to answer, yet is of central importance. The majority of deaths in patients with mild to moderate hypertension occur as a result of myocardial infarction. None of the individual clinical trials thus far carried out has shown a significant reduction in morbidity or mortality from myocardial infarction, although the pooled results of several trials suggests that there may have been a reduction of as much as 50 per cent. There is room for modest optimism about the prospect of achieving a worthwhile reduction of the incidence of myocardial infarction by hypotensive therapy, but full proof is still necessary. The widespread use of beta-adrenergic blocking drugs may alter the picture, as two of these, alprenolol and practolol, have been shown to reduce the risk of sudden death in the first three years after a myocardial infarction.

Berglund, G., Hansson, L., and Werkoe, L. (eds.): Conference on Pathophysiology and Management of Arterial Hypertension. Moelndal, Sweden, Lindgren & Soner, 1975.

Dollery, C. T.: Adrenergic drugs in the treatment of hypertension. Br. Med. Bull., 29:158, 1973.

Genest, J., Koiw, E., and Kuchel, O. (eds.): Hypertension. New York, McGraw-Hill Book Company, 1977.

Pickering, G. W.: High Blood Pressure. 2nd ed. London, J. & A. Churchill, 1968.

Sackett, D. L., and Haynes, R. B. (eds.): Compliance with Therapeutic Regimens. Baltimore, Johns Hopkins University Press, 1976.

Stamler, R., and Pullman, T. N.: The Epidemiology of Hypertension. New York, Grune & Stratton, 1967.

Veterans Administration Cooperative Study Group on antihypertensive agents. JAMA, 202:1028, 1957, and 213:1143, 1970.

362. ATHEROSCLEROSIS

Harvey Wolinsky

HISTORY. The antiquity of atherosclerosis has been established from studies of Egyptian mummies. Attempts to relate pathologic changes in the coronary vessels to clinical symptoms, particularly angina pectoris, followed upon early descriptions of sclerotic vessels by Leonardo da Vinci in the sixteenth century. The term *atheroma*, derived from the Greek word meaning porridge, was not used in the context of arterial disease until 1904, when Marchand coined the term *atherosclerosis*. This disease is lipid rich, as contrasted with *arteriosclerosis*, an older and more general term for thickening and stiffening of the vessel wall. Another important distinction still made today is that arteriosclerotic involvement of a blood vessel wall tends to be concentric and diffuse, whereas atherosclerotic le-

sions are more eccentric and focal. The interrelation among coronary disease, myocardial damage, and clinical syndromes was not appreciated before the emergence of pathology as a separate discipline in the latter part of the nineteenth century. It was not until 1918 that the proposal by Herrick of a connection between clinically detected nonlethal heart damage and atherosclerotic coronary disease gained acceptance.

OCCURRENCE AND EPIDEMIOLOGY. Atherosclerosis tends to involve large and medium-sized arteries. Most commonly affected are the aorta and the iliac, femoral, coronary, and cerebral arteries. Clinical symptoms occur because the mass of the atherosclerotic plaque reduces blood flow through the involved artery and thereby compromises tissue or organ function distal to it.

Ischemia or necrosis of the perfused tissue results in characteristic clinical syndromes, and myocardial infarction and sudden death are common fatal outcomes. In terms of public health, cardiovascular diseases, particularly myocardial infarction and stroke, are the most common lethal diseases in the United States and other industrialized societies, accounting for more than 50 per cent of all deaths. For example, well over 500,000 deaths per year in the United States are attributable to acute myocardial infarction. The risks of developing clinical evidence of a cardiovascular disease by age 65 are 37 per cent for a man and 18 per cent for a woman. A downward trend in death rates from myocardial infarction of approximately 20 per cent has been documented since 1970. The precise reasons for this are not yet clear.

PATHOLOGY. By the time it is large enough to cause clinical events, the atherosclerotic plaque is a complicated mixture of three components: (1) cells, mostly smooth muscle in origin, (2) connective tissue (elastin, collagen, glycosaminoglycans), often concentrated as a "cap" on the lesion, and (3) lipid deposits, both intra- and extracellular, representing complex aggregates of cholesteryl ester, cholesterol, triglyceride, and phospholipids. Cell necrosis is a prominent feature which contributes to the gruel-like nature of the lesion. Calcification is often present in advanced lesions, and hemorrhage from small ingrowing vessels frequently occurs. A slowly progressive increase in the plaque mass is usually responsible for its clinical sequelae. Other events in the blood vessel wall which can provoke acute symptoms include transient or progressive deposition of platelet clumps or thrombus on the irregular luminal surface, rupture of the plaque and release of its components, hemorrhage into a plaque, or dissection of blood into the wall.

Basic knowledge of the progressive stages of atherosclerosis is essential to the physician who cares for patients with vascular disease and who attempts to influence its progression. Clinical events in middle age which are associated with the advanced plaque represent the culmination of decades of slow growth of the lesion beginning in childhood. In the first decade of life, blood vessels undergo structural remodeling, which mainly involves the intima. This takes the form of concentric fibromuscular intimal thickening and development of intimal cushions at branch sites. In all human populations studied (even all mammals), this thickening develops progressively throughout life. However, in those populations which have a predilection for development of later atherosclerosis, this arteriosclerotic thickening is especially well developed long before lipid deposition is prominent. Enhanced intimal thickening of certain artery segments, especially in the male, also predicts patterns of subsequent atherosclerotic lesions. In those human societies not vulnerable to atherosclerosis, this concentric intimal thickening, even when prominent, does not in itself seem to seriously compromise blood flow.

Upon this matrix, lipid accumulates in the form of *fatty streaks* in all populations. These yellow, soft, raised lesions may be transient, but their prevalence increases with age to a peak in the third decade of life. Microscopically, these consist largely of smooth muscle cells in the intimal layer which are filled with lipid deposits, mainly cholesterol and cholesteryl ester. In populations prone to atherosclerotic vascular disease, *plaques*, as described above, begin to be seen in the third decade and become more numerous with time in common disease sites, such as the proximal coronary vessels. The *fibrous plaque* is grayish white, focal, and raised and microscopically consists of a prominent extracellular matrix, with less prominence of visible lipid (although by biochemical analysis the lipid content is high). It is thought that these lesions may arise de novo at times, but that they usually develop from fatty streaks. The forces required for this transformation in susceptible populations are not well understood, but hypertension seems to be one such stimulus. The further accumulation of cells, connective tissue, and fat over decades results in the severe or *complicated lesions* which are so often found at autopsy to provide the "explanation" for a clinical event.

LOCALIZATION. Although tending to occur in large elastic and muscular arteries, the distribution of atherosclerosis is far from uniform. The aorta is heavily involved, particularly its abdominal portion. The large caliber of this distributing vessel makes it an uncommon site for occlusive symptoms, although it may be a source of embolic clot or plaque material to peripheral branches. Atheromas are most common in the proximal coronary tree, although lesions occur peripherally as well. Curiously, lesions occur in the extramural portions of the coronary blood vessels and not in those segments which are intramural and surrounded by muscle. It is also of interest to those who stress the role of hemodynamic factors in localization that the renal arteries, arising from the heavily diseased abdominal aorta, are remarkably spared of disease despite having a caliber similar to that of the main coronary arteries.

Arteries of the lower extremities have much more atherosclerosis than those of the upper limbs. The distribution patterns may be focal and proximal or more diffuse. Clinical symptoms rarely arise from isolated lesions because of the rich collateral blood supply. The major hazard to those having peripheral vascular disease, even when symptomatic, stems from the likelihood of concurrent coronary artery disease in the same individuals.

The vertebral or carotid vessels may develop patchy lesions which present clinically with neurologic deficits. Particularly likely sites are the proximal portions of these arteries or the carotid bifurcation. Intracranial predisposed sites are the basilar artery, the middle cerebral artery, and the carotid artery as it angulates in the region of the carotid siphon.

Atherosclerosis of the smaller muscular arteries is especially common in individuals who use cigarettes or have glucose intolerance. Since basement membrane abnormalities also frequently occur in small blood vessels of diabetics, it is not certain that atherosclerotic involvement alone explains the notable symptoms of vascular insufficiency in these individuals.

Again of special interest to the proponents of hemodynamic factors in atherogenesis is the observation that the low-pressure venous system and pulmonary arteries are infrequent sites of atherosclerosis except under circumstances of increased intravascular pressure, as occurs in pulmonary hypertension.

RISK FACTORS. The concept of risk factors for atherosclerosis derives from epidemiologic studies. A profile of risk can be obtained from evaluation of the frequency with which specific characteristics and chemical measurements are associated with occurrence of certain clinical events in a given population. It should be stressed that the epidemiologist can only point out associations; he can neither determine mechanism nor even be certain of a direct interaction between a particular characteristic and the presence of disease. The value of these constructs, however, is that they identify high-risk populations in which "reduction" of risk factors can be attempted, and they suggest to the experimentalist potentially fruitful areas of investigation to elucidate mechanisms of pathogenesis. Possible links between known risk factors and aspects of cellular involvement in atherogenesis are summarized under Pathogenesis, below.

Finally, it is important to stress that for virtually every risk factor, the risk is a continuous gradient throughout the entire range of observed values, habits, or characteristics. For example, an increasing risk of occurrence of a cerebrovascular event is seen with increasing blood pressure, even within the "normotensive" range of blood pressures. It is only within the "hypertensive" range, however, that the growing gradient of risk is generally felt to justify intervention.

Age. The risk of myocardial infarction increases with age regardless of sex. Little is known about this factor, although it is assumed that it simply represents duration of exposure to other factors. For example, recent epidemiologic studies of children have shown the appearance of significant subgroups in the teenage years with blood pressures and serum lipids at levels of the general adult population.

Sex. A 10- to 15-year lag in extent of atherosclerosis of the coronary, cerebral, and peripheral vasculature and its sequelae is seen in women compared to men until approximately 50 years of age. After that point, which roughly corresponds to the menopause, the rates of disease in both sexes are more similar. This may represent increased risk in women or decreased risk in men due to early elimination of high-risk males. The acceleration of vascular disease in younger individuals with diabetes mellitus blurs the usual sex differences.

Blood Pressure. Experimental and clinical evidence has convincingly shown the importance of blood pressure as an accelerator of atherosclerosis. A systolic blood pressure of greater than 160 mm Hg or a diastolic of greater than 95 mm Hg carries a five-fold increased risk of coronary heart disease compared to normotensive individuals. Hypertension is the strongest risk factor over-all for clinical disease in individuals older than 45 years; it is especially predictive of atherosclerotic brain infarction. (In the absence of uniform autopsy reporting, this designation may include pure hemorrhagic stroke as well as atherosclerotic sequelae.) Recent studies have shown a clear-cut effect of blood pressure reduction on the incidence of stroke, when hypertension is defined as a diastolic pressure of 105 to 115 mm Hg, but, disappointingly, no reduction in myocardial infarction was found after a three-year period of treatment. This difference might reflect the major contribution of pressure to stroke, whereas the coronary lesion reflects the chronic, degenerative aspects of atherosclerosis which, once established, may be more difficult to reverse.

Hyperlipidemia. Another major risk factor is the presence of elevated circulating blood lipids — cholesterol and triglyceride. The problem may be broken down into two components: (1) the generally elevated lipid levels in industrialized populations compared to agricultural societies, and (2) identification of high-risk individuals with high lipid levels within a given population range. The increased levels found in entire populations seem largely due to diet, although genetic factors may play a role. The increased intake of saturated fat, refined sugar, and total calories by a sedentary population seems of major importance.

Using ultracentrifugal and electrophoretic techniques, four major lipoprotein classes have been identified as carriers of lipid in plasma (see Ch. 532.3). For the purposes here, it is necessary only to summarize briefly the major constituents of these lipoprotein classes. Chylomicrons are the largest particles, contain the most lipid (mainly triglyceride) and least protein (1 to 2 per cent by weight), and are normally found in the circulation only shortly after meals. In the fasting state, very low density lipoproteins (VLDL) carry most circulating triglycerides as well as lesser amounts of cholesterol and cholesteryl ester. Low-density lipoproteins (LDL) are derived from metabolism of VLDL and carry most of the serum cholesterol and cholesteryl ester. High density lipoproteins (HDL), the smallest particles, contain the most protein (50 per cent by weight); phospholipid and cholesterol account for about 45 per cent and 35 per cent, respectively, of the lipid. HDL are involved in the esterification of free cholesterol released into plasma from the tissues. It has been shown that whole plasma triglyceride accurately reflects VLDL levels and that total plasma cholesterol generally reflects LDL-cholesterol levels in man, although this latter relationship is not as consistent (see below).

The three most common electrophoretic patterns of serum lipoproteins in individuals with premature atherosclerotic vascular disease are increased LDL or Type IIa (elevated cholesterol, normal triglyceride), increased VLDL and LDL or Type IIb (elevated cholesterol, elevated triglyceride), and increased VLDL or Type IV (normal or slightly increased cholesterol, elevated triglyceride). These three patterns appear with about equal frequency in survivors of an acute myocardial infarction below age 60. Approximately one third of all such individuals will have one of these patterns, and familial distributions of each have been demonstrated. Whereas Types IIa and IV show autosomal dominant inheritance and are clearly monogenic, the inheritance of Type IIb is not yet completely defined. What is important, however, is that when Type IIb is found in a proband, familial expressions may include elevations mainly of

cholesterol or triglyceride or both. To screen for the most common disorders, therefore, measurement of total plasma cholesterol and triglyceride provides the same detection of risk as do the more complicated lipoprotein pattern analyses. In adults under age 55, a value of plasma cholesterol greater than 250 mg per deciliter or fasting triglyceride greater than 150 mg per deciliter indicates the need for further investigation (see Ch. 532.3).

Current knowledge about lipoprotein metabolism does not permit a clear-cut assessment of the precise roles of various lipoproteins in the clinical definition of risk for unselected populations. However, prospective epidemiologic studies do show a positive correlation between plasma cholesterol levels (particularly LDL) and risk of clinical atherosclerotic events. This relationship is evident under age 50, but is not detectable in older age groups. Increasing plasma VLDL (triglyceride) levels seem to add risk to a given plasma LDL (cholesterol) level. Triglyceride levels alone, however, are less strongly related to clinical atherosclerotic events. The risk associated with triglyceride, seen more clearly in women, is eliminated when obesity or glucose intolerance is taken into account and may therefore not be an independent variable. More recently, the emergence of HDL as an important protective factor has complicated the use of total plasma cholesterol to assess risk. That is, the risk of coronary heart disease is inversely related to the level of HDL cholesterol. Since this can only be detected by examining isolated HDL and LDL, the total cholesterol level alone is less informative. HDL levels are significantly higher in women than in men at all age levels, are reduced by the presence of diabetes mellitus, are increased by regular exercise (e.g., jogging), and are not predictably related to levels of LDL in the same individual. Therefore a plasma lipid profile of total cholesterol, HDL cholesterol, and fasting triglyceride may be the best predictor of coronary disease.

Cigarette Smoking. Increased risk of atherosclerotic vascular disease manifested by stroke, myocardial infarction, and intermittent claudication is seen in male smokers compared to nonsmokers; in female smokers, the occurrence of intermittent claudication is increased. By age 45, the excess risk in males approaches 70 per cent. The increased incidence of atherosclerosis found in smokers at autopsy correlates with the degree of previous smoking activity. In addition to atheromatous changes in larger coronary blood vessels, small intramyocardial arteries show increased diffuse fibromuscular intimal thickening. Not only are these changes related in degree to numbers of cigarettes smoked, but cigar and pipe smokers have impressive increases over nonsmokers as well.

Sudden death is the most frequent clinical event associated with cigarette smoking. Cessation of smoking promptly and sharply reduces the risk of this event. Levels of carboxyhemoglobin are significantly increased in smokers, of whom about 15 per cent regularly achieve levels of carboxyhemoglobin of 5 per cent or more. Men in the age group of 30 to 69 years who achieve this level of carboxyhemoglobin show a 20-fold increased prevalence of atherosclerotic vascular disease events (myocardial infarction, angina pectoris, intermittent claudication) compared to nonsmokers or smokers with levels of 3 per cent or less. A narrowed coronary artery may be unable to deliver the 20 per cent increase in blood flow required to offset the decreased availability of oxygen from blood containing 5 per cent carboxyhemoglobin and thereby prevent ischemia. Indeed, a lower threshold for angina pectoris occurs in cardiac patients in whom comparable levels of carboxyhemoglobin have been experimentally achieved. Nicotine, once considered a culprit, has not been implicated in recent studies. Glycoprotein components of tobacco leaf and tar, which contain rutin moieties, appear to promote thrombosis in normal animals and cardiac arrhythmias in sensitized experimental animals, and have also been shown to be allergenic in man.

Glucose Intolerance. Glucose intolerance, defined as a casual blood glucose of 120 mg per deciliter or more or the presence of glucose in the urine, acts independently of other commonly associated risk factors, namely, triglyceride elevation, obesity, and hypertension. It is somewhat more important in women than in men. The excess risk associated with glucose intolerance may be 100 per cent. Intermittent claudication is the cardiovascular symptom most associated with glucose intolerance. When present in combination with a fasting plasma triglyceride level of greater than 150 mg per deciliter, a marked synergistic effect of diabetes mellitus on development of angiographically demonstrable, diffuse coronary artery disease is found. The contribution to this process of basement membrane abnormalities found in the small coronary branches in diabetics is not known.

Obesity. Obesity, particularly at 20 per cent or more above ideal weight, carries significantly increased risk. However, when associated variables, including hypertension, hyperlipidemia, and diabetes mellitus, are removed, obesity per se makes no clear contribution. The salutary effect of weight reduction on the other variables, however, makes it a prime focus of intervention.

Physical Activity. It is difficult to separate the risk of this variable from other confounding factors. Sedentary individuals have many other risk factors operating as well. Epidemiologic studies show that only heavy physical work, of the type done in rural communities or by the most active dockworkers, is associated with decreased risk of myocardial infarction and sudden death. The remarkably striking decrease in sudden death in these groups suggests that exercised myocardium may be less vulnerable to a fatal ischemic event. Exercise tolerance can be improved in individuals with coronary artery disease through a program of regular, moderate exercise.

Personality Factors. A strong suspicion has long been held that angina pectoris and sudden death are strongly associated with emotional stress or anxiety. The Type A pattern of behavior (enhanced aggressiveness, ambitiousness, competitive drive, and chronic sense of time urgency) is frequently associated with many other risk factors, and the converse Type B is less closely associated. A prospective study by the Western Collaborative Group showed that even after removal of associated risk components, Type A behavior, determined from interviews, had a residual two-fold risk of clinical coronary heart disease over the Type B personality type. The possible metabolic, genetic, and other components of this behavior pattern have not been identified, nor has behavior modification been convincingly shown to be feasible or effective in modifying risk.

Genetic Factors. Familial inheritance patterns of hyperlipidemia, hypertension, and diabetes mellitus are well known. Segregation of behavioral factors within families, including tobacco smoking, obesity, and perhaps physical activity, is also seen. These associations may provide the physician his best opportunities to detect clusters of risk factors and to attempt preventive measures.

Other. A host of other variables associated with cardiac risk have been enumerated, but in sum they appear to contribute only a minor portion of risk. Included among many others are lung vital capacity, blood uric acid level, blood group type, and mineral salt content of local drinking water. Moderate alcohol consumption seems to be associated with decreased risk of myocardial infarction, perhaps through a positive effect on HDL:LDL ratios. Electrocardiographic evidence for left ventricular hypertrophy carries about a three-fold risk for new coronary artery disease, independent of other variables, including blood pressure.

Unknown. All known risk factors taken together account for approximately 50 per cent of the risk of an individual's developing coronary heart disease in the United States. It is clear that important risk determinants remain to be discovered. For example, little has been said about the contribution made by inherent properties of vascular tissue, genetic or otherwise, to cardiovascular disease. Each risk factor must ultimately be expressed at the tissue or cellular level if it is in fact related to the development of the manifest vascular disease we call atherosclerosis. Therefore further identification of specific cellular and tissue metabolic patterns under well defined conditions of risk may provide additional risk factors.

PATHOGENESIS. Atherosclerosis is undoubtedly multifactorial in origin and progression. The sharp contrast between the frequent suddenness of clinical events and the slow progressiveness of vascular lesions suggests that different factors are responsible for each and that different strategies might be needed for intervention. Pioneering studies of quite advanced lesions generated the classic theories which invoked processes such as vascular injury, lipid infiltration, thrombosis, and hemorrhage. Although still useful in a descriptive pathologic sense, these terms are being incorporated into concepts more consonant with newer knowledge of cell biology. Vascular tissue is increasingly appreciated to be a dynamic responsive organ system of great complexity, rather than a conduit arrangement with rather limited responses. The normal blood vessel is a tightly organized, highly regulated, and closely integrated fibrocellular system. The two major cell types found in blood vessel walls are smooth muscle cells and endothelial cells. Each has been shown experimentally to have characteristic, far-ranging metabolic capabilities. Endothelium seems to be important in determining the rate of entrance of circulating materials, including lipoproteins, into the blood vessel wall and in maintaining the nonthrombogenicity of the vascular surface. Smooth muscle cells elaborate the extensive connective tissue matrix of the arterial wall and metabolize those circulating plasma components which gain entrance to the vessel wall. When atherosclerosis occurs, the same basic wall components are present, but the picture is a distorted one of smooth muscle cell proliferation, connective tissue deposition, and lipid accumulation.

Alteration in the functional or structural barrier presented by the endothelial cell-lining layer is thought to be an early event in the pathogenesis of atherosclerosis. Local turbulence or shear force generated by blood flowing at high pressure could determine the special susceptibility of certain sites to disruption of the surface layer. Two major consequences of endothelial loss would be increased thrombogenicity of the denuded sites and increased entrance of circulating lipoproteins and other plasma components into the blood vessel wall. Platelet adhesion and aggregation quickly occur on the exposed region; platelets contain a mitogen which can stimulate smooth muscle cell proliferation in vitro. Other evidence obtained in vitro suggests that LDL itself might stimulate proliferation of these cells. The recent evidence that cells in each human atherosclerotic plaque tend to be monoclonal raises the possibility that selective growth advantage or even neoplastic transformation of certain cells could contribute to this aspect of plaque growth. Experimentally produced atherosclerotic lesions are polyclonal, so that this issue is far from resolved.

Increased connective tissue synthesis is closely linked to cell proliferation whether studied in the intact blood vessels or in isolated cell systems. Specific stimuli at the cellular level for increased synthesis of connective tissue proteins have not been identified, although hypertension in particular seems to promote fibrosis and estradiol given experimentally seems to retard it. Circulating lipoprotein, particularly LDL, can be immunologically detected in very low concentrations in normal human blood vessels. With loss of endothelial integrity, it is presumed that an increased influx of this lipoprotein occurs which may result in progressive accumulation of lipid by two mechanisms. First, binding to excessive extracellular matrix in more advanced lesions might occur. Perhaps a more important determinant in early lesions, however, is the metabolic capacity of the vascular smooth muscle cell to cope with the incoming lipid. The ability of the cell to maintain balance among internalization and catabolism of complex lipoproteins (including hydrolysis of cholesteryl ester to free cholesterol and fatty acid) and synthesis of lipid may determine its susceptibility to intracellular lipid accumulation. In the sense that ingress of substrate may exceed egress of product, the lipid accumulation can be thought of as a subtle form of storage disease in the muscle cell, which becomes a repository of slowly permeant cholesteryl ester and other lipids. Based on available information, it seems plausible that many "risk factors" exert an influence on this influx-efflux balance. For example, the relationships among LDL and HDL levels and risk of disease may derive at least in part from the putative role attributed to LDL of carrying cholesterol to the cell and to HDL of carrying cholesterol away from the cell. The influence of sex, age, and exercise as risk factors might stem, at least in part, from associated changes in levels of these lipoproteins. The increased vascular permeability seen with hypertension could lead to increased influx of lipoprotein into the cell, and, based on recent experimental evidence, diabetes mellitus might act to reduce efflux from the cell.

Plasma membrane receptors, endocytosis, lysosomal function and intracellular lipoprotein metabolism by this cell, and the nature of lipid transfer between isolated lipoprotein fractions and the cell are therefore active areas of inquiry in current research. Perhaps the best evidence for the appropriateness of the recent emphasis on the cellular biology of vascular tissue comes from the observation that a phenotypic hypercholesterolemia with monogenic inheritance is associated with a specific deficiency of surface receptors for LDL molecules in cultured cells obtained from afflicted individuals. Absence of the normal function of these receptors in regulating intracellular cholesterol synthesis results in hypercholesterolemia. The mechanisms by which this deficiency is translated into a marked predisposition to lipid accumulation by these cells and by which other "risk factors" exert their effects at the cellular level are yet to be identified.

TREATMENT, REGRESSION, AND PREVENTION. Current treatment of clinical atherosclerotic complications revolves around highly sophisticated coronary care units, replacement of diseased vascular segments with prosthetic or natural grafts, the use of antiarrhythmic agents, anticoagulants and plasma lipid lowering agents, and even heart transplantation. Although these approaches are remarkable accomplishments, they are addressed to the late stages of a disease process for which prevention is clearly the best goal. Significant regression of modest lesions in nonhuman primates follows extreme manipulation of diets from cholesterol-rich to cholesterol-poor content. However, the great reductions in serum lipid levels after this maneuver are not usually possible in man. Although an occasional study suggests that progression of atherosclerotic lesions may be slowed or arrested by stringent risk factor control in man, conclusions about real benefit are premature. Despite these uncertainties about the ultimate effects of available preventive measures on the atherosclerotic process, the clinician might adopt an approach which emphasizes a "prudent" course for his patients. Moderation of intake of total calories and saturated fat, reduction of elevated blood pressure and cigarette use, and control when possible of the other risk factors at the very least carry real benefits of improved general well-being and decreased likelihood of other serious diseases.

Benditt, E. P., and Benditt, J. M.: Evidence for a monoclonal origin of human atherosclerotic plaques. Proc. Natl. Acad. Sci. USA, 70:1753, 1973.

Fowler, S., and Wolinsky, H.: Lysosomes in vascular smooth muscle cells. In Bohr, D., Somlyo, A. P., and Sparks, H. V. (eds.): Vascular Smooth Muscle. Handbooks on Circulation. Washington, D.C., American Physiological Society, 1979.

Fry, D. L.: Responses of the arterial wall to certain physical factors. In Porter, R., and Knight, J. (eds.): Atherogenesis: Initiating Factors. Proceedings, Ciba Foundation Symposium No. 12. Amsterdam, Elsevier, 1973, pp. 93–120.

Geer, J. C., and Haust, M. D.: Smooth muscle cells in atherosclerosis. In Pollak, O. J., Simms, H. S., and Kirk, J. E. (eds.): Monographs on Atherosclerosis. New York, S. Karger, 1972, Volume 2.

Goldstein, J. L., and Brown, M. S.: The low-density lipoprotein pathway and its relation to atherosclerosis. Ann. Rev. Biochem., 46:897, 1977.

Goldstein, J. L., Hazzard, W. R., Schrott, H. G., Bierman, E. L., and Motulsky, A. G.: Hyperlipidemia in coronary heart disease. J. Clin. Invest., 52:1533, 1544, 1569, 1973.

Gordon, T., Castelli, W. P., Hjortland, M. C., Kannel, W. B., and Dawber, T. R.: High density lipoprotein as a protective factor against coronary heart disease. The Framingham Study. Am. J. Med., 62:707, 1977.

Kannel, W. B., Castelli, W. P., Gordon, T., and McNamara, P. M.: Serum cholesterol, lipoproteins, and the risk of coronary heart disease. The Framingham Study. Ann. Intern. Med., 74:1, 1971.

McGill, H. C., Jr. (ed.): The Geographic Pathology of Atherosclerosis.

Baltimore, Williams & Wilkins Company, 1968. (Reprinted from Lab. Invest., 18:463, 1968.)

Ross, R., and Glomset, J. A.: Atherosclerosis and the arterial smooth muscle cell. Science, 180:1332, 1973.

Wissler, R. W., Vesselinovitch, D., and Getz, G. S.: Abnormalities of the arterial wall and its metabolism in atherogenesis. Prog. Cardiovasc. Dis., 18:341, 1976.

363. DISORDERS OF THE CORONARY ARTERIES

363.1. INTRODUCTION

Desmond G. Julian

Disorders of the coronary arteries are the most common causes of death in developed countries and are responsible for much disability. The most frequent disease process involved is coronary atherosclerosis; other abnormalities include embolism, luetic aortitis, spasm, and, rarely, arteritis.

Coronary arterial disease usually exists for many years before it has any adverse effects upon the myocardium. Ischemic heart disease develops when the coronary circulation is insufficient to supply myocardial oxygen demands. The development of ischemia depends upon the location and severity of the stenosis or stenoses, the presence or absence of collateral vessels, and the demands of the myocardium.

Ischemic heart disease has three major manifestations: angina pectoris, myocardial infarction, and sudden death. Angina pectoris is a clinical syndrome resulting from transient and reversible myocardial hypoxia. Myocardial infarction is the term used to describe acute necrotic changes in the myocardium which are usually secondary to coronary occlusion.

It is important to recognize the differences in concept between the two syndromes. One — angina pectoris — is essentially a symptom complex; the other — myocardial infarction — by definition is a pathologic entity. The borderline between them is by no means always clinically distinct, and there are patients who exhibit features characteristic of both conditions. Some such patients, suffering from the "intermediate syndrome," may have symptoms suggesting myocardial infarction but no evidence of necrosis; others may have typical features of angina pectoris when, in fact, necrosis has taken place.

The initial presentation and course of ischemic heart disease vary strikingly from one patient to another. In about 25 per cent of cases, the first manifestation of ischemic heart disease is sudden death. In others, sudden death complicates acute myocardial infarction, whereas in still others it follows a prolonged period of angina pectoris. Myocardial infarction may be the first presentation, although it is frequently preceded by new or worsening attacks of angina pectoris. The patient who has recovered from myocardial infarction may be symptom free but often experiences angina pectoris and is liable to sudden death. The patient with angina pectoris may retain this symptom without any complications for years or decades. However, at any time other manifestations of ischemic heart disease may supervene.

The prognosis in ischemic heart disease is determined to a large extent by the location and severity of coronary arterial stenosis and the state of the myocardium, although other factors such as coexistent hypertension and cigarette smoking play a role.

363.2. ANGINA PECTORIS

Desmond G. Julian

DEFINITION. Angina pectoris describes a syndrome of discomfort in the chest and adjacent areas resulting from transient and reversible myocardial hypoxia.

The term was originally coined by William Heberden, whose description in 1768 has not been bettered:

"There is a disorder of the breast marked with strong and peculiar symptoms, considerable for the kind of danger belonging to it, and not extremely rare which deserves to be mentioned more at length. The seat of it, and the sense of strangling and anxiety with which it is attended, may make it not improperly be called angina pectoris.

"They who are afflicted with it, are seized while they are walking (more especially if it be uphill, and soon after eating) with a painful and most disagreeable sensation in the breast, which seems as if it were to extinguish life, if it were to increase or continue; but the moment they stand still, all this uneasiness vanishes.

"In all other respects the patients are, at the beginning of this disorder, perfectly well, and in particular have no shortness of breath, from which it is totally different. The pain is sometimes situated in the upper part, sometimes in the middle, sometimes at the bottom of the os sterni, and often more inclined to the left than to the right side. It likewise very frequently extends from the breast to the middle of the left arm."

ETIOLOGY. Coronary atherosclerosis is responsible for angina pectoris in about 90 per cent of cases. Coronary angiographic and postmortem studies have demonstrated that it is usual for at least one of the three major coronary arteries to be stenosed by 80 per cent or more before angina develops. In most cases, two or three of the major vessels are involved.

Another important cause of the syndrome is aortic stenosis; angina occurs less often in aortic regurgitation if this is isolated, but it is common in combined lesions. It is also a feature of syphilitic aortitis, although this is now a rare cause.

Coronary arterial spasm is being increasingly recognized as a mechanism of angina pectoris, but its frequency has not yet been established.

Rarer causes of angina pectoris include congenital anomalies of the coronary arteries, cardiomyopathies, mitral valve disease (particularly mitral valve prolapse), and diseases affecting small coronary arteries, including the connective tissue disorders such as systemic lupus erythematosus and polyarteritis nodosa.

Angina may also occur with marked right ventricular hypertrophy associated with pulmonary stenosis and pulmonary hypertension.

Conditions which may aggravate angina pectoris, although seldom responsible for it in the absence of other forms of disease, include hypotension, thyrotoxicosis, anemia, and polycythemia.

PATHOPHYSIOLOGY. Angina pectoris occurs when

there is an inadequate supply of oxygen for the needs of the myocardium. The quantity of oxygen available to the heart depends upon the coronary blood flow and the arteriovenous oxygen difference. In the normal heart under basal conditions, the heart extracts a very high percentage of the oxygen in the coronary arterial blood. The reserve available for increased demands is therefore very limited, and these can only be met by an increase in coronary blood flow. Coronary blood flow is determined by aortic pressure and coronary vascular resistance. Only a modest increase in coronary blood flow can be obtained by increasing arterial pressure; in the normal heart augmentation of flow in response to increased demands is mainly achieved by coronary vascular dilatation. Dilatation of the coronary vessels seems to be activated by oxygen lack, although the mechanism by which this occurs is not yet clearly identified.

The increase in coronary vascular resistance which is present in coronary arterial disease cannot be readily compensated for by an increase in arterial pressure or by increased oxygen extraction. However, as the disease process often affects only one or two of the major proximal vessels, the development of a collateral circulation may compensate. The degree of narrowing necessary to produce symptoms is variable, but in general a reduction in coronary blood flow in the basal state will be seen only when at least one vessel is obstructed 80 per cent or more, although there may be a limitation of coronary flow on exercise in the presence of only 50 per cent reduction. In patients with critically narrowed arteries, the coronary vessels beyond the obstructions are maximally dilated and are therefore unable to respond by further dilatation to increased demand.

The main determinants of myocardial oxygen demand are the contractile state of the myocardium, the heart rate, and the tension in the ventricular wall. Exercise, the chief provoking agent of angina, increases all three of these factors. In the presence of coronary arterial stenosis, it is usual for there to be segmental inadequacy of coronary blood flow, in spite of the presence of any collaterals. Furthermore, subendocardial blood flow suffers disproportionately.

During an attack of angina pectoris it is usual for there to be a moderate tachycardia, a rise in systemic blood pressure, and an increase in the end-diastolic pressure in the left ventricle. It seems probable that the last of these is due to decreased compliance (increased stiffness) in the ventricular wall. The contractility of the affected region of myocardium is impaired; contraction may cease completely and the ischemic area may move paradoxically.

Regional hypoxia also leads to metabolic changes, including loss of potassium and excessive lactate production as a result of anaerobic glycolysis. The actual cause of anginal pain is undetermined, although it seems probable that some as yet unidentified chemical stimulates the nerve endings. Many substances — acetylcholine, adenosine, histamine, and the kinins — have been thought to be possibly involved, but in no case has this been proved.

CLINICAL MANIFESTATIONS. Angina pectoris is by definition a symptom complex, and the diagnosis can usually be made readily from the patient's description. Sometimes, however, the features may be atypical or the individual's powers of expression inadequate. Observations which suggest or prove myocardial hypoxia at the time of the discomfort are of value, although they cannot prove the diagnosis.

Symptoms. There are four cardinal features of the angina syndrome: its site, its character, its relationship to exertion, and its duration. In the most typical case, all these features are present in their characteristic form, but one or more of them may be atypical.

SITE. Angina pectoris is most commonly located in the region of the middle or upper third of the sternum. However, it is quite frequently most severe in other areas or radiates to or from them. Such areas include the lower sternal region, the xiphisternal region, one or both sides of the chest (particularly the left), the arms (particularly the left), and the neck or lower jaw. More rarely, the pain is epigastric, interscapular, or over one scapula.

In milder attacks the discomfort may be located at only one site, but as it becomes more severe it may spread to the other areas. Similarly, when angina first occurs it is often localized, but with advancing severity it becomes more diffuse.

In its most typical form, the discomfort starts in the sternal region and radiates to the left shoulder and upper arm. It frequently extends further down one or both arms to the elbow, wrists, or fingers. In many cases, areas are "skipped" so that some patients complain of pain in the left shoulder and hand with the rest of the arm being uninvolved. In a few patients, the discomfort arises first in a peripheral area such as the jaw or wrists, and only with increasing severity is the sternal region involved. It is important to emphasize that the left submammary region is seldom involved in angina, and only very rarely is it the only site.

CHARACTER. The discomfort of angina pectoris is usually of mild to moderate severity and can be controlled by slowing down or stopping. Many patients emphatically deny that the discomfort in their chest is a pain. The sensation may be described as one of oppression, heaviness, or tightness. Other descriptions include "bandlike" or "viselike"; it is not knifelike or stabbing.

The discomfort in the arms is usually described as a heaviness or sense of uselessness or ache, but in the fingers there is often the sensation of numbness or tingling. In the neck, the feeling is one of choking, whereas in the jaw it is an ache, sometimes similar to toothache.

EXERCISE, EMOTION, AND OTHER PROVOKING FACTORS. The most common provoking factor of angina pectoris is physical exercise, and it is usual for the subject to be first aware of discomfort when walking uphill or in a hurry. Many patients manage to continue at their occupations even if they involve physical labor but find travel to or from work difficult. The syndrome is more likely to occur in the cold or after a meal. There is a marked variation in the amount of exercise that may be required to provoke the pain from time to time, and symptoms may disappear in warm weather only to return in the winter. In general, there is a tendency to progressive worsening over a period of several years.

Although less common, anginal pain may be readily provoked by arm movements, and for a given amount of work, it would seem that arm movements are more likely to produce angina than is walking. In the most severe cases, such activities as rubbing oneself after a shower or shaving may provoke angina.

Emotion is almost as important as exercise as a precipitating factor. Anger and anxiety are obvious causes, and the watching of competitive sport is frequently responsible. Car driving and public speaking are other common provokers of angina. Angina on sexual intercourse is particularly common, but frequently is not spontaneously mentioned by the patient.

Many patients complain of angina when first getting into bed, and others are troubled by being awakened by it, sometimes being aware that the syndrome is preceded by dreams which may be exciting or involving physical exercise. Angina which occurs whenever a patient lies down — "angina decubitus" — is rare and usually indicates advanced disease.

In most cases of angina, there is a clear precipitating factor. However, in a proportion of patients attacks of angina occur quite unexpectedly and in relation to no evident cause. Such patients often exhibit S-T elevation in the ECG, in contrast with the usual S-T depression which is a feature of exercise- or emotion-induced angina pectoris. Such cases, often classed as "Prinzmetal's angina" or "variant angina," will be discussed at the end of this chapter.

The ways in which angina may be relieved are almost as specific as its provoking factors. When it is provoked by exertion, rest usually produces relief of symptoms within a short time. Similarly, the pain subsides with the relief of emotion. Carotid sinus pressure may abbreviate an attack, provided that bradycardia can be induced. This test should be carried out with the patient recumbent and should not be undertaken if there is any evidence of carotid artery stenosis. Nitroglycerin can usually terminate an attack of angina pectoris in less than three minutes; an inability to achieve this relief should then cause one to question the diagnosis. In particular, when pain is more prolonged and is unresponsive, myocardial infarction should be suspected.

DURATION. Most attacks of angina pectoris last for about two or three minutes. It is rare for them to last less than a minute or for more than 15 minutes, although, particularly in emotion-induced angina, longer attacks may occur. However, too much emphasis must not be placed on the patient's estimation of duration, as most people find it difficult to know precisely how long an attack has lasted.

"NONVERBAL" DESCRIPTIONS OF ANGINA. It is always difficult to describe a pain and to know how long it has lasted. This appears to be particularly so in the case of angina pectoris, but there are some "nonverbal" ways in which the patient conveys valuable information about his discomfort. Patients may lay their hands across the chest or sweep them from side to side, a gripping motion may be made in front of the sternum, one hand may be placed on each side of the chest with the fingers touching over the sternum, or both hands may be placed laterally in this way. All these gestures are suggestive of angina, whereas the diagnosis is exceedingly unlikely if the patient points to the location of the pain with the tip of a finger, particularly if he points to the left submammary region.

ACCOMPANYING SYMPTOMS. Although Heberden pointed out the difference between dyspnea and angina, the two symptoms commonly coexist. Specific questions may have to be asked to elicit a history of one in the presence of other.

Palpitation is uncommon, except in those cases in which paroxysmal arrhythmias are responsible for the syndrome. Nausea and sweating sometimes occur, and some patients experience "angor animi" — a sense of impending dissolution. Dizziness occurs occasionally, but loss of consciousness is very unusual except when bradycardia, resulting from either sinus slowing or atrioventricular block, is responsible for both the chest discomfort and syncope.

Physical Examination. Physical examination plays a relatively small role in the diagnosis of angina pectoris, except in those patients in whom such disorders as aortic stenosis or cardiomyopathy are responsible. On the other hand, it may reveal important abnormalities which must be taken into account in the assessment of the patient and which may require correction. Such factors include overweight, hypertension, and anemia.

Apart perhaps from detecting high blood pressure, examination of the cardiovascular system is relatively unhelpful in most patients between attacks. There may, however, be features of myocardial malfunction due to old myocardial infarction or hypertension. Thus there may be cardiomegaly or left ventricular hypertrophy; a fourth heart sound is not uncommon. A third heart sound is much rarer, as is the murmur of mitral regurgitation secondary to papillary muscle malfunction. Occasionally, the paradoxical pulsation of a ventricular aneurysm may be detected.

During an actual attack of angina pectoris, the pulse rate is usually moderately increased and the blood pressure higher than prior to the attack. Other features which are occasionally noted are a fourth heart sound, paradoxical splitting of the second heart sound, and pulsus alternans. More rarely, an apical systolic murmur resulting from transient mitral regurgitation can be heard.

DIAGNOSIS. As angina pectoris is a symptom complex, the diagnosis depends upon an accurately taken and interpreted history. Because it is essentially a subjective phenomenon, no test can prove or disprove the diagnosis, but investigations are valuable in confirming the presence of concomitant myocardial ischemia and for demonstrating the pathologic processes which are responsible for it or are the consequences of it.

Electrocardiography. The ECG is normal in some 50 to 75 per cent of patients with angina pectoris. Changes which may be found in the remainder include evidence of old myocardial infarction, particularly Q waves and, less often, persistent S-T segment elevation or T wave inversion. The changes of left ventricular hypertrophy secondary to hypertension may be present. In many patients there are minor ECG abnormalities, such as flattening or inversion of the T waves; in others there may be arrhythmias.

Attacks of angina pectoris at rest are seldom witnessed, and ECG recordings are therefore not often obtained in this situation. However, if such attacks are observed, particularly in the context of an intensive care unit or by Holter monitoring, it is most usual to see depression of the S-T segments. However, in cases of so-called Prinzmetal's angina, S-T segment elevation develops.

Because the ECG is so often normal at rest and because angina is characteristically a symptom evoked by exercise, stress tests provide valuable evidence in its diagnosis. The longest established method of doing this is the so-called Master two-step test, which involves the performance of 15 to 25 trips up and down two steps each 9 inches high in a period of 1½ minutes. The number of trips is varied, depending on the age, weight, and sex of the patient. The test is discontinued if the pain is experienced, but is repeated if the patient remains symptom free and the ECG remains normal. ECG records are recorded immediately and for up to ten minutes after the conclusion of the test. S-T segment depression of 0.5 mm is suggestive of myocardial ischemia, provided that it is horizontal or downward sloping, but more severe degrees of S-T depression provide more definite evidence of ischemia. This test is rather unsatisfactory, as few patients can exercise themselves sufficiently to produce chest pain or the tachycardia which usually precedes it. An additional major disadvantage of the Master two-step test is the inability to monitor the ECG during the exercise.

Most cardiac centers now carry out exercise tests using either a treadmill or bicycle ergometer. These may be either "submaximal" or "symptom-limited" tests. In submaximal tests, the patient is exercised to a target heart rate which is related to the maximum anticipated heart rate for an individual of a given age and sex. Increasingly, symptom-limited maximal exercise tests are being undertaken, because it is common for patients with heart disease to reach symptom-limited work capacity before they achieve the expected target heart rate. Several different techniques are used, but all should include the recording of at least three chest leads during exercise and the recording of leads I, II, and III and three chest leads immediately after exercise and several times over the succeeding ten minutes. During the test, the workload is progressively increased at three-minute intervals until fatigue, chest pain, dyspnea, or other symptoms limit it. Blood pressure is recorded each three minutes, and the ECG is continuously monitored. The test should be discontinued if marked S-T changes develop, if the blood pressure falls, or if there are any other untoward signs. It may be regarded as positive if there is a 1-mm depression of the S-T segment persisting until 0.08 second after the J point, and it is most diagnostic if this is downward sloping. The heart rate and blood pressure response is extremely important, and it is essential to note at what level angina or S-T segment changes develop and at what work load the test has to be discontinued. Failure to raise the blood pressure significantly during the test or discontinuance of the test at low heart rates is suggestive of severe disease of the proximal parts of the coronary arteries.

Exercise ECG stress tests must be interpreted with considerable caution, as there are many false-positive and false-negative results. These tests are of little value when the patient is receiving digitalis or has certain ECG abnormalities such as bundle branch block.

There is almost no risk in a carefully conducted exercise test, provided that the precautions mentioned are observed. Very rarely, ventricular tachycardia or fibrillation may ensue, and it is essential to have a defibrillator and other apparatus available for cardiopulmonary resuscitation.

An alternative method of stress testing is by pacing of the atrium during cardiac catheterization. The tachycardia so induced increases oxygen demand, although not to the same extent as an equivalent degree of tachycardia produced by exercise. The heart rate is accelerated to 160 to 180 beats per minute or until chest pain or S-T changes develop. Although not as satisfactory a test of myocardial ischemia as the exercise test, it is valuable in assessing patients who are unable to perform satisfactorily on a bicycle or treadmill.

The demonstration of lactate production by coronary sinus sampling during stress testing provides further evidence of myocardial ischemia.

Chest Roentgenogram. This is of little value in the diagnosis of angina except when calcification of a coronary artery can be seen, but the demonstration of cardiomegaly or of a ventricular aneurysm may be important in assessing prognosis or planning treatment.

Coronary Arteriography. Coronary arteriography enables one to visualize the major coronary arteries and their branches and to demonstrate areas of narrowing in these vessels. It is the only method of proving the diagnosis of atherosclerotic disease, and is essential in patients being considered for coronary artery surgery. It also provides valuable information on prognosis. Notwithstanding the advantages of this technique, its dangers and its limitations must be borne in mind, and it should not be undertaken unless one or more of a number of indications are present.

The investigation is carried out either by means of a brachial arteriotomy (Sones technique) or by a percutaneous femoral approach, using special preformed catheters (Judkins technique). The method in experienced hands should have a mortality of less than 0.5 per cent. It should only be undertaken in laboratories in which at least 100 such investigations are undertaken annually and in which there is a highly trained team. Risks include ventricular fibrillation, bradycardia and hypotension, provocation of myocardial infarction, and dissection of a coronary artery, as well as local disorders in the intubated artery. All these complications are very unusual in competent hands. The risks are particularly low in those with little or no coronary arterial disease and are highest in patients with disease of the left main coronary artery. Measurement of the left ventricular pressure and left ventriculography are carried out at the same procedure. It has been shown that prognosis is closely related to the number of coronary vessels involved and to the nature and extent of ventricular malfunction.

Coronary arteriography is a quite sensitive test for coronary atherosclerosis, but one cannot assume that the presence of this pathologic process proves the presence of angina or ischemia, for such changes are common in symptom-free populations.

Coronary arteriography is indicated when the possibility of surgery on the coronary arteries is under consideration. The major group of patients is that for whom medical treatment has failed to control the symptoms. It is also of value in the diagnosis of coronary arterial disease and is particularly useful when it is desired to rule out coronary atherosclerosis in younger patients, in whom such a diagnosis would have adverse effects on their careers and future plans.

Nuclear Imaging. Imaging techniques are rapidly coming into widespread use in spite of their expense and the restricted availability of appropriate gamma cameras. The techniques used in angina are of two main kinds.

One of these is "cold spot scanning," in which an

isotope is injected which is taken up uniformly by well-perfused myocardium but poorly in ischemic areas. The most commonly used indicator at present is thallium-201. If this isotope is injected during exercise-induced angina, the isotope is not taken up in the ischemic area; when this area recovers, the "cold spot" disappears.

A different technique involves the use of gated blood pool scanning in the ventricles, using a label such as technetium-labeled albumin, to permit visualization of the ventricle in systole and diastole and, with more sophisticated techniques, throughout both periods. This allows an assessment both of over-all left ventricular function and of regional abnormalities.

DIFFERENTIAL DIAGNOSIS. A positive diagnosis of angina pectoris can usually be made on the basis of history, buttressed if necessary by the exercise ECG, but difficulties may arise when the pain is atypical.

Musculoskeletal pains are frequent in the chest wall, and often no cause can be found. Such pains may be aggravated by exertion, but the areas affected are often tender and seldom in the midline. The pain is most likely to be provoked by such factors as lifting, rotating the trunk, and pulling, which produce tension in the muscles attached to the ribs. Among more specific musculoskeletal conditions are Tietze's syndrome (in which there is inflammation of one or more costochondral junctions), metastatic lesions in the ribs, and fractured ribs. The pain of cervical spondylosis may be most severe in the upper chest region and is accompanied by discomfort in the shoulders and arms. However, such pains are not so clearly related to walking or emotion and are most likely to be provoked by movements of the neck.

Patients with anxiety neuroses are prone to chest pains and frequently think that these are due to cardiac disease. Most often they take the form of a persistent aching over the left breast region, but stabbing pains may also occur in the same area. If there is a relationship to exercise, this is usually after rather than during the effort. Chest pain in these patients forms a part of a group of symptoms which include breathlessness on little or no exertion, sweating, and faintness. On examination, the physical signs of anxiety are present, with cold moist hands and sighing respiration. Patients with these symptoms and signs have been designated in the past as suffering from "neurocirculatory asthenia," "effort syndrome," or "soldier's heart." Although it is possible to differentiate these features from those of angina pectoris, particularly if there is a clear-cut psychologic cause, angina and an anxiety state may coexist.

Rarely, the pains of pericarditis or pleurisy may be confused with that of angina, particularly as these may be aggravated by exercise. However, a carefully elicited history will show that the pain is aggravated on taking a deep breath or, perhaps, by lying flat.

One of the conditions most difficult to differentiate from angina pectoris is that of an esophageal reflux, which may be associated with hiatus hernia. The pain is usually central in the lower sternal region; it may radiate up toward the neck, but rarely to the shoulders or arms. It may be provoked by exercise, but is more commonly related to stooping or lying flat. It may be associated with flatulence or heartburn and be relieved by alkalis. The mere presence of a hiatus hernia does not prove the diagnosis, but the demonstration of esopha-

gitis by esophagoscopy and the provocation of pain by an acid perfusion test are virtually diagnostic.

The pain of peptic ulceration may radiate from its usual site in the epigastric region to the chest. There is usually associated epigastric tenderness, and the pain is related to food rather than exertion. It is usually relieved by alkali or milk and not by nitroglycerin. Cholecystitis and cholelithiasis may also give rise to pain in the lower sternal region, but it is usual for there to be tenderness in the right hypochondrium.

The pain of angina pectoris has, of course, to be differentiated from that of myocardial infarction. The pain of infarction is usually more prolonged and severe but is not necessarily either. However, the lack of relationship to exercise, the greater systemic upset, and the eventual ECG and enzyme abnormalities permit the establishment of the diagnosis of myocardial infarction, although 24 to 48 hours may elapse before one can be certain.

PROGNOSIS. Although in the lay mind angina pectoris is a diagnosis with sinister connotations, the majority of patients with this condition live for many years, and perhaps one half survive at least ten years. However, the risk of sudden death and myocardial infarction exists even in those apparently doing well. The severity of symptoms is, indeed, a poor guide to prognosis, and those with severe symptoms may live for many years, whereas those with mild angina may die suddenly. Clinical features which carry a bad prognosis include cardiomegaly, a third heart sound, and electrocardiographic abnormalities at rest. Hypertension is an unfavorable feature, as is marked S-T depression on the exercise test. Cardiac failure is particularly sinister.

More accurate prognosis may be obtained from coronary angiography and left ventriculography. If only one of the main coronary arteries is involved, the annual mortality is 2 to 4 per cent; if two are involved, it is 6 to 8 per cent; and if three are involved, it is 10 to 12 per cent. If the left main coronary artery is involved, the mortality is even higher. Malfunction of the left ventricle is also important. Those with apparently normal left ventricular function have an excellent prognosis in contrast to those whose ventricles contrast very poorly, whose mortality is very high.

TREATMENT. The aims of treatment are (1) to alleviate the patient's symptoms, (2) to educate him to live as rewarding a life as possible within his limitations, and (3) to improve prognosis.

General Management. The general management of a patient with angina is of paramount importance. Whether or not his symptoms can be controlled with medical or surgical measures, the patient will have to reappraise his life style in the light of the disorder. First of all the physician must reassure him that the diagnosis of angina pectoris is not a sentence of death. The relatively good prognosis should be stressed, but the long-term benefits of general health measures such as the avoidance of overweight and the stopping of smoking must be emphasized.

Moderate exercise, provided that this does not provoke angina, should be encouraged, and, if possible, a program of increasing activity should be prescribed. On the other hand, the patient should be cautioned against strenuous exercise, particularly if it involves heavy lifting or walking uphill against a wind.

The known risk factors for coronary arterial disease

should be controlled, particularly in the younger patient. Hyperlipidemia should be corrected by appropriate dietetic and, if necessary, drug measures. Coexistent hypertension should be treated. Often the most appropriate therapy for this is a beta-adrenergic blocking drug, which is also of value in the management of the chest pain. Smoking must be stopped.

Drugs. Attention to such factors as obesity and modifications of life style can often completely abolish angina pectoris, if only for some months. If symptoms can be controlled in this way, there seems no special point in prescribing drugs, but many patients do indeed require pain relief.

For more than 100 years, nitrates have been used to control angina. Their mode of action is still not entirely understood. They can be shown to have a dilator effect on the coronary arteries, but this is probably not the reason for their effectiveness except in patients who have coronary arterial spasm. They also dilate the peripheral arteries and veins and thereby reduce both the afterload and the preload on the myocardium. This in turn leads not only to a reduction in oxygen demand but also to a fall in left ventricular end-diastolic pressure, which allows a relative increase in endocardial blood flow.

Glyceryl trinitrate (nitroglycerin) is the drug in most common use. It must be administered sublingually and acts within about two minutes, its duration of action lasting for about 45 minutes. Patients should be encouraged to use it both prophylactically and therapeutically. Long-acting nitrates are also in common use, but are probably best reserved for those whose angina is proving troublesome or for those who find unacceptable the headache which may be produced by nitroglycerin. Isosorbide dinitrate, 2.5 to 5 mg sublingually, may give relief for one to two hours.

The beta-adrenergic blocking drugs have achieved an importance almost equal to that of the nitrates in the management of angina. Several double-blind studies have proved their efficacy, provided that they are given in adequate doses. Beta-adrenergic blocking drugs reduce the oxygen demand on the myocardium. They slow the heart rate, reduce the rise of blood pressure that occurs on exercise, and diminish the velocity of cardiac contraction. Propranolol is the most commonly used drug in this group and the only one currently available in the United States. It is classified as a "nonselective" drug in that it blocks both the beta receptors in the heart (beta-1) and those in bronchial smooth muscle and in the peripheral arterioles (beta-2). As a consequence, it may lead to bronchoconstriction in patients with obstructive airways disease and may cause cold extremities, particularly in those with peripheral atherosclerosis or poor peripheral circulation. Selective beta blockers, such as metoprolol and atenolol, which are available in most other countries, effectively block only the cardiac receptors. They reduce the risks of bronchoconstriction and also seem less liable to produce cardiac failure, which may occur with propranolol therapy.

Because of the risks of provoking cardiac failure and bronchospasm, it is wise to start propranolol in a relatively small dose of 10 mg four times daily. If this is well tolerated, there is usually little problem with larger amounts, and the daily dose may be rapidly increased to 160 mg, 240 mg, or higher as necessary. Bradycardia

at rest may be produced by quite small doses, but full beta blockade has not been achieved until the tachycardia of exercise has been largely abolished.

The major side effects of propranolol are cardiac failure and bronchospasm, but these are uncommon if patient selection is careful. Minor side effects are more common but are frequently overlooked. They include fatigue and depression, nightmares, cold extremities, and the aggravation of intermittent claudication. Propranolol should not be withdrawn abruptly, as this may lead to the sudden worsening of angina or even the precipitation of myocardial infarction.

Several new drugs, not yet available in the United States, are of value in patients who respond inadequately to beta-adrenergic blocking drugs.

Perhexilene, 100 to 200 mg twice daily, effectively relieves pain in many otherwise resistant patients. Its toxic effects include dizziness, ataxia, and, rarely, peripheral neuritis. Liver function test results are sometimes disturbed, but no untoward effects seem to ensue.

Prenylamine, 60 mg four times daily, is effective in a few patients but can cause repetitive ventricular arrhythmias.

Verapamil, 60 mg thrice daily, is particularly effective in coronary arterial spasm (Prinzmetal's angina). It has few side effects but may produce atrioventricular block.

Surgery. Surgery plays a major role in the management of angina pectoris (see Ch. 363.5). The discomfort can be relieved in nearly all subjects and abolished in most. The effect on mortality for coronary disease is still uncertain, except in the case of severe disease of the left main coronary artery, in which there appears to be undoubted benefit. The benefits and risks of coronary artery bypass operations should be considered when the patient with angina is first seen and should be regularly reappraised from time to time.

Surgery is clearly called for when anginal symptoms cannot be adequately controlled by medical measures. However, there is as yet insufficient evidence to recommend surgery for the improvement of prognosis.

UNSTABLE ANGINA. The term unstable angina is used to describe an increase in the severity of angina for which there is no obvious explanation. Although it has been applied to the first appearance of the symptom, it is better reserved for those patients in whom there is a progressive deterioration, with the pain becoming more prolonged or occurring on minimal exertion or at rest. It has been long recognized that patients with this condition are at a relatively high risk of proceeding to myocardial infarction, and the syndrome has been described as "impending infarction" or "preinfarction angina." This situation has also been described as "acute coronary insufficiency." It is likely that a variety of circumstances can be responsible. Thus in some cases a small myocardial infarction may have occurred, in others coronary arterial spasm may be responsible, and in yet others such factors as arrhythmias, anemia, or increased catecholamine drive following acute stress may be involved. Most commonly, however, it is likely that unstable angina develops because the natural progression of the disease has reached a critical stage.

During the attacks of pain, the S-T segments become depressed or the T waves inverted, although in a few cases the S-T segments may become elevated. By definition, no diagnostic enzyme changes occur, nor do the

Q waves of infarction appear. Some 10 to 20 per cent of affected patients proceed to myocardial infarction within the succeeding days or weeks; a small number die suddenly from ventricular fibrillation.

In the majority of patients, the situation can be stabilized by putting the patient to bed and treating with nitroglycerin, long-acting nitrates, and beta-adrenergic blocking drugs. In a few, symptoms continue to be severe in spite of these measures; coronary artery surgery should then be considered.

PRINZMETAL'S (VARIANT) ANGINA. A relatively uncommon but important variant of angina pectoris is characterized by recurrent attacks of angina, usually at rest, accompanied by S-T elevation and, sometimes, by ventricular arrhythmias. Coronary arteriography during the spells of pain has shown that there is usually spasm affecting one of the major coronary arteries. This may occur in an otherwise normal artery or in one affected by coronary atherosclerosis. The pain usually responds to nitroglycerin. Long-acting nitrates are helpful in prevention. Beta-adrenergic blocking drugs may either help or provoke the syndrome. Coronary arterial surgery is indicated only if there is severe concomitant coronary atherosclerotic disease.

Braunwald, E.: Control of myocardial oxygen consumption: Physiological and clinical considerations. Am. J. Cardiol., 27:416, 1971.

Bristow, J. D., Burchell, H. B., Campbell, R. W., Ebert, P. A., Hall, R. J., Leonard, J. J., and Reeves, T. J.: Report of the ad hoc committee on the indications for coronary arteriography. Circulation, 55:969a, 1977.

Dunkman, W. B., Perloff, J. K., Kastor, J. A., and Shelbourne, J. C.: Medical perspectives in coronary artery surgery — a caveat. Ann. Intern. Med., 81:817, 1974.

Gorlin, R.: Pathophysiology of cardiac pain. Circulation, 32:138, 1965.

Julian, D. G. (ed.): Angina Pectoris. Edinburgh, Churchill Livingstone, 1977.

Ross, R. S.: Ischemic heart disease: An overview. Am. J. Cardiol., 36:496, 1975.

Sheldon, W. C., Rincon, G., Pichard, A. D., Razari, M., Cheanvechai, C., and Loop, F. D.: Surgical treatment of coronary artery disease — "pure" graft operation. Prog. Cardiovasc. Dis., 18:237, 1976.

Vlodaver, A., and Edwards, J. E.: Pathology of coronary atherosclerosis. Prog. Cardiovasc. Dis., 14:256, 1971.

363.3. MYOCARDIAL INFARCTION

Desmond G. Julian

DEFINITION. Myocardial infarction is the term used to describe acute necrotic changes in the myocardium due to a sudden and catastrophic diminution in coronary blood supply.

ETIOLOGY AND PATHOLOGY. Atherosclerosis of the major coronary arteries is responsible for nearly all cases of acute myocardial infarction. Infarction may also result from such conditions as coronary embolism complicating rheumatic heart disease or the use of prosthetic valves, or from the occlusion of a coronary artery from syphilitic aortitis.

Infarction usually follows acute coronary arterial occlusion from thrombosis, subintimal hemorrhage, or rupture of an atheromatous plaque. However, a coronary artery may occlude without causing infarction if collateral blood flow is adequate. Infarction can also occur without total occlusion and without thrombosis.

Many patients dying during acute heart attacks do so within two hours of the onset of acute symptoms. In such cases, it is unusual to be able to demonstrate the classic features of acute myocardial necrosis. This may be due to the fact that no such necrosis has taken place and death has been due to an arrhythmia. On the other hand, changes may not be found because currently available pathologic techniques are unable to detect the earliest changes of infarction. When a patient dies several hours or days after the onset of the attack, necrotic changes can nearly always be seen.

The role of thrombosis in infarction remains a controversial issue. Thrombosis appears to be relatively uncommon in those who die suddenly or with a subendocardial infarction. It is nearly always present in patients dying with full thickness infarctions, particularly if there has been left ventricular failure or shock.

PATHOPHYSIOLOGY. The most important factor determining the hemodynamic response to myocardial infarction is the amount of myocardium involved. The size of the infarct depends on the location of the coronary arterial lesion responsible for it and the state of the other coronary artery vessels, but it is important to appreciate that the area of myocardium which is eventually infarcted is affected by influences operating after the onset of the heart attack. These include factors which increase or decrease the preload and afterload on the heart.

In the early stages after infarction, particularly if it is located inferiorly, there may be a strong vagal discharge with sinus bradycardia and hypotension. Many patients have a sympathetic response which leads to vasoconstriction, hypertension, and tachycardia unless a coexistent vagal effect is more powerful. Inadequate preload resulting from hypovolemia may lead to a lowered arterial pressure, which, although it diminishes afterload, may reduce the coronary perfusion below a critical level. Drugs which increase myocardial oxygen demand by increasing either contractility or afterload may have deleterious effects. Such drugs include digitalis, isoproterenol, and norepinephrine. The arrhythmias also may impair myocardial function by causing excessive bradycardia or tachycardia. In severe cases, arterial acidosis and hypoxia develop, and these may further damage the myocardium.

Other complications include papillary muscle malfunction or rupture leading to mitral regurgitation, rupture of the ventricular septum, and asynergy caused by left ventricular aneurysm.

In patients with mild attacks, the cardiac output is maintained or slightly abnormal; in those who proceed to heart failure or shock, it is profoundly depressed. In such patients, there may be elevation of left ventricular end-diastolic, left atrial, and pulmonary arterial pressures. The right atrial pressure may rise, especially when the infarction affects the right ventricle, as it may in inferior infarction.

Generally speaking, the severity of the hemodynamic disturbance parallels the seriousness of the clinical condition; but when pump failure supervenes, it may be difficult to determine the mechanisms responsible. Careful monitoring of the patient with intracardiac pressure recordings may be necessary to delineate the factors involved.

CLINICAL FEATURES. Symptoms. The most common presentation is with the onset of pain which may either develop abruptly or build up gradually over a period of minutes or hours. Sometimes it occurs in a stuttering fashion with short episodes lasting ten minutes or more. Although often severe, there may be only a slight discomfort. The sensation may be described as "heavy," "tight," or "vise-like." It may also be choking, aching, or bursting. The pain usually persists for half an hour to several hours, but sometimes lasts for only a few minutes. It is usually located in the region of the middle or upper sternum but may be lower down. It frequently radiates to one or both sides of the chest, to the neck and lower jaw, and to one or both arms. In some patients, more particularly the elderly, chest pain is either absent or overshadowed by other symptoms such as dyspnea or syncope. Other common complaints include sweating, giddiness, nausea, and vomiting.

Some two thirds of the patients have experienced an exacerbation of pre-existing angina or the onset of new angina in the month prior to the attack itself.

Physical Examination. At the start of the attack, the patient who is experiencing severe pain appears distressed, sweating, pale, and cold. Either bradycardia or tachycardia may occur at this time; similarly, blood pressure may be either raised or abnormally low. The patient may look "shocked," but this appearance is usually related to the severity of the pain and disappears rapidly when this is relieved. These features may be the consequence of increased vagal tone or sympathetic activity. Many patients look surprisingly normal within an hour or two.

Hypotension may occur transiently with the pain in the initial stages but may in this case be quickly reversed. However, there is usually a gradual fall in the blood pressure over the next few hours or days, followed by a slow rise which may or may not reach the preinfarction level. In 10 to 20 per cent of patients, blood pressure falls progressively until cardiogenic shock develops; such patients frequently die.

The venous pressure is often slightly raised in the first hours after infarction but usually subsides toward normal again. Persistent venous engorgement caused by right-sided heart failure is a feature of severe myocardial damage and usually takes some days to develop.

The apex beat is often impalpable but may be displaced to the left and downward, particularly if there is left ventricular enlargement secondary to longstanding hypertension or previous myocardial infarction. If the infarction has affected the anterior wall of the heart, it is common for a systolic pulsation to be felt in an area internal to and above the apex beat.

On auscultation, first and second heart sounds are often abnormally soft. A fourth heart sound can frequently be heard; a third heart sound or gallop rhythm is less common and indicates left ventricular failure. A soft systolic murmur at or internal to the apex, resulting from functional mitral regurgitation, is common; rarely, a loud systolic murmur can be heard due to rupture of the ventricular septum or of a papillary muscle. A pericardial rub can be heard in about 10 to 20 per cent of patients; it usually lasts for only a few hours and occurs on the second or third day. Crepitations are frequently audible at the lung bases. If they are widespread and persist after coughing, they suggest the presence of left ventricular failure but can occur in its absence in the recumbent patient. Most patients with myocardial infarction sustain a mild pyrexia which develops within 12 to 24 hours, reaches its peak by the second day, and gradually subsides over the next few days.

Most of the abnormal physical signs disappear over the succeeding two or three days. In patients with left ventricular failure, sinus tachycardia and a third heart sound may persist.

CLINICAL COURSE. The mortality of acute coronary heart attacks in the first four weeks is about 40 per cent. About half of these deaths occur within the first two hours of the onset of symptoms. Patients who survive to reach hospital have, without special care, a 20 to 30 per cent risk of dying. The most common mechanism of death is ventricular fibrillation, which is responsible for the majority of early deaths. Shock and left ventricular failure are responsible for most of the deaths after the first day.

Some 50 to 70 per cent of patients have a relatively uncomplicated course and escape severe arrhythmias, hypotension, or pulmonary congestion.

Early Complications. ARRHYTHMIAS AND DEFECTS OF CONDUCTION. Some disorder of rate, rhythm, or conduction is almost invariable. In about half the patients, they are severe enough to be of clinical importance.

Sinus tachycardia is common. When encountered soon after the onset, it may be the result of apprehension or pain; but when it is persistent, it usually indicates severe myocardial damage and is a feature of cardiac failure and shock. Sinus bradycardia is common during the first three hours and is particularly associated with inferior infarction. It can also result from therapy with drugs such as morphine and digitalis. In the early stages it may be dangerous because of hypotension or may be responsible for ventricular ectopic rhythms, but when seen later on during the course it is usually a good prognostic feature.

Atrial tachycardia and flutter are rare, but atrial fibrillation occurs in about 10 to 15 per cent of patients, mostly developing on the second or third day. It is often brief and self-limiting; but if the ventricular rate is fast, cardiac failure may be induced or aggravated.

Ventricular ectopic beats can be detected in most patients. Although they have been regarded as harbingers of ventricular fibrillation, this is probably not the case except when they are of the R-on-T variety or in prolonged runs, constituting ventricular tachycardia. Ventricular tachycardia is dangerous not only because of its association with ventricular fibrillation but because it can lead to cardiac failure and hypotension. Ventricular fibrillation is seen in 5 to 10 per cent of patients with myocardial infarction treated in hospital. It is responsible for most of the many deaths that occur in the first two hours, usually developing at home or at work.

Minor degrees of heart block are common in the first few hours and are usually vagal in origin. More persistent and severe atrioventricular conduction disturbances usually complicate inferior myocardial infarction. This association is a result of the right coronary artery supplying both the atrioventricular nodal tissue and the diaphragmatic surface of the heart. This form of block may be well tolerated but can cause hypotension or episodes of asystole. It usually resolves spontaneously within hours or days. A less common but more sinister type of atrioventricular block occurs in anterior myocardial infarction; it results from interruption of conduction in the right bundle and both fascicles of the left bundle. Widespread myocardial damage is usually present, and the prognosis is poor.

THE SHOCK SYNDROME. Between 5 and 15 per cent of

patients admitted to hospital with myocardial infarction develop shock; in the majority of cases this leads to a fatal outcome. The features of the shock syndrome include hypotension associated with a cold and clammy skin, pallor, mental dulling, and oliguria. Characteristically, the systolic blood pressure is less than 90 mm Hg, but may be higher than this in patients who were previously hypertensive. The most important factor in shock is probably the amount of contracting myocardium that is lost. Apart from the initial pathologic cause of the myocardial infarction, during the early hours additional factors come into play which, if they are not corrected, may augment the size of the eventual infarct. These include arterial hypotension, excess catecholamine drive, arrhythmias, and hypovolemia. It is probable that severe pain may be a factor in the early stages, associated as it is with sinus tachycardia and hypotension.

LEFT VENTRICULAR FAILURE.   In most patients, there is no evidence of left ventricular failure on admission to hospital, although in a few this is the presenting feature. However, the majority of patients develop some evidence of pulmonary congestion within the first 48 hours. Signs of left ventricular failure include tachycardia, a third heart sound, and widespread pulmonary rales. On the chest roentgenogram the features of pulmonary venous congestion or edema may be demonstrated.

THROMBOEMBOLISM.   Thromboembolic episodes in myocardial infarction may be either pulmonary or systemic.

Pulmonary embolism was common in former years when patients were confined to bed for several weeks in the management of myocardial infarction. Anticoagulants were found beneficial in reducing the many deaths which used to occur from this cause. With earlier ambulation, pulmonary embolism is much less common and is largely confined to patients with severe complications such as cardiac failure, in which prolonged recumbency is the rule.

Massive pulmonary embolism may cause sudden breathlessness, hypotension, or syncope. Any of these features accompanied by raised venous pressure, cyanosis, and the ECG patterns of right heart strain or right bundle branch block suggest the diagnosis. More commonly, pulmonary embolism is manifested by pulmonary infarction, which may produce pleuritic pain or hemoptysis and which can be detected on a chest roentgenogram.

Systemic emboli usually arise from thrombus originating in the left ventricle on the endocardial surface of a myocardial infarction. In some cases, however, they can arise in the atrium, particularly when there is atrial fibrillation.

PERICARDITIS.   Pericarditis develops in 15 to 20 per cent of patients, usually on the second or third day. It often produces the recurrence of chest pain, but one that is typically aggravated by deep breathing, lying flat, or swallowing. A pericardial rub may be heard, but it is frequently transient, lasting only for minutes or hours. Usually, the only treatment required is the relief of pain. If the patient is on anticoagulants, these should be discontinued unless there is a strong reason for their continuation, as hemorrhagic pericarditis leading to tamponade may occur.

CARDIAC RUPTURE.   Rupture of the myocardium is most likely to occur several days after the onset of symptoms. Rupture through the free wall of the left ventricle usually causes sudden collapse with loss of blood pressure and pulse but with the electrocardiogram demonstrating persistence of sinus rhythm. In a few cases, classic cardiac tamponade ensues over a period of minutes or hours; in such cases it may be possible to correct the defect surgically. Rupture through the interventricular septum occurs in approximately 0.5 per cent of patients with myocardial infarction, mainly those who have anteroseptal infarcts with bundle branch block. The usual clinical picture is of the sudden onset of severe heart failure, with a systolic thrill and loud murmur developing in the region of the left sternal edge. In most cases, the patient deteriorates rapidly and dies within a few days; in a small proportion of cases there may be survival for several weeks. The diagnosis may be confirmed by floating a Swan-Ganz catheter into the right side of the heart and demonstrating a left-to-right shunt at the ventricular level. If the patient is too ill to withstand corrective surgery at the time of the acute event, he may be kept alive by intra-aortic balloon counterpulsation for one or two weeks until surgery can be more safely undertaken.

PAPILLARY MUSCLE RUPTURE AND MALFUNCTION.   Mitral systolic murmurs caused by papillary muscle malfunction are common during the first few days after myocardial infarction but usually disappear subsequently. In a small proportion of patients a papillary muscle ruptures and leads to severe cardiac failure, accompanied by a loud systolic murmur with thrill internal to the apex. Death may occur within the next few hours or days; as with interventricular septal rupture, the patient may be kept alive with intra-aortic balloon counterpulsation until mitral valve surgery can be undertaken.

DIAGNOSIS.   In most cases, the presence of myocardial infarction is suspected because of the severe, prolonged nature of the chest pain with its typical heavy or gripping character and its radiation to the arms and throat. The patient's extreme distress and the changes in heart rate and blood pressure also help to suggest the diagnosis. However, this can never be regarded as proved unless there are ECG abnormalities, preferably supported by enzyme changes.

The Electrocardiogram (see also Ch. 364.2).   The electrocardiogram in myocardial infarction is associated with changes in three different features of the ventricular complexes. The most specific of these is the appearance of Q waves, indicating myocardial necrosis. Highly suggestive, but less diagnostic, are elevation and alteration in configuration of the S-T segment, indicating myocardial injury. Least specific are the T wave changes of myocardial ischemia.

The earliest changes are usually those of the S-T segment, which develop within minutes or hours of the onset of the attack. The raised S-T segment may initially retain its normal upward concavity, but within a short time it usually becomes convex upward. The S-T elevation develops in relation to the area of the infarct; other leads may show "reciprocal" S-T depression. Usually, the S-T segment returns to the isoelectric line within a few days. Persistence of the S-T segment elevation suggests an aneurysmal or akinetic segment. The S-T changes described, although nearly always due to myocardial infarction, are not specific. Similar changes may be seen in Prinzmetal's angina. However, when the characteristic pattern develops over a period of days and is supported by enzyme abnormalities, a confident diagnosis of infarction may be made.

Q waves, which usually develop between the first and

sixth hour after the onset of symptoms, are much more specific. Indeed, the development of pathologic Q waves (i.e., 0.03 sec or more) in appropriate leads in association with a typical history can be regarded as diagnostic of infarction even though enzyme abnormalities have not been demonstrated. However, Q waves, because they indicate necrosis, may persist indefinitely. The mere presence of Q waves therefore does not prove recent infarction; the changes may be old. When Q waves are present, the infarction is often called transmural, although in such cases the whole ventricular wall is not necessarily involved. When no Q waves can be seen, the infarction may be described as subendocardial or nontransmural.

T wave changes usually occur late in the first day or subsequently and become more pronounced as the S-T segment returns to the isoelectric line. These changes are quite nonspecific and may be seen in a number of different conditions. One should therefore be hesitant to make the diagnosis of infarction when the only ECG abnormalities detected are those of T waves.

The electrocardiogram is of great value in demonstrating the location of the infarct. Anteroseptal infarctions lead to changes in leads V_2 to V_4; anterolateral infarctions, in V_3 to V_6. Inferior or diaphragmatic infarctions produce abnormalities in leads II, III, and aVF. The electrocardiogram is less satisfactory in demonstrating infarctions affecting the posterior surface of the left ventricle; in this situation, none of the conventional leads overlies the infarct, but the loss of posterior left ventricular forces leads to apparent right ventricular preponderance, with a tall R wave appearing in V_1 and V_2. Right bundle branch block does not obscure the changes of myocardial infarction, a common variety being the appearance of an initial Q wave in V_1 to V_4, as opposed to the initial R wave expected in right bundle branch block. On the other hand, left bundle branch block usually obscures the changes of myocardial infarction because of the abnormal initial QRS vector.

Serum Enzyme Concentrations. The myocardium contains many enzymes which are released into the circulation by necrosis. The different enzymes vary from one another in the rate at which they are released; the pattern of enzyme rises in the serum is of diagnostic importance.

Creatine phosphokinase (CPK) occurs in heart, skeletal muscle, and brain. The CPK activity in serum rises within six hours of the onset of infarction and reaches its peak in 18 to 24 hours. It may become normal by 72 hours. Apart form myocardial infarction, high levels of CPK are seen in muscle diseases and cerebrovascular damage. Unfortunately, intramuscular injections can give rise to high CPK levels; as these are often given in the early phases of infarction, they may reduce the value of the enzyme level as a diagnostic test. Three CPK isoenzymes can be identified by electrophoresis. These have been designated BB, characteristic of brain; MM, found in skeletal and heart muscle; and MB, found only in myocardium. Changes in MB isoenzyme activity are virtually specific for myocardium and highly suggestive of myocardial infarction. Unfortunately, the assay is relatively expensive and is not in universal use. Glutamic oxaloacetic transaminase (GOT) is found particularly in the heart, skeletal muscle, brain, liver, and kidney. Normal values vary somewhat from laboratory to laboratory, but in most normal serum activity is 20 to 40 Frank-Karmen units or 30 to 60 international units. After myocardial infarction, the serum activity rises in about 12 hours, reaching its peak in 36 to 72 hours and

gradually falling to normal by about the fifth day. As with other enzymes, repeated estimation on a daily basis is desirable in establishing the diagnosis. Caution must be exercised in the presence of liver disease. In general, the height of the GOT reflects the severity of acute myocardial infarction. Sometimes, extremely high levels are encountered in myocardial infarction, e.g., 2000 or 3000 units; when this occurs, it suggests acute hepatic necrosis due to a severe reduction in the splanchnic blood flow associated with shock.

Lactate dehydrogenase (LDH) is also found in the heart. There are five LDH isoenzymes, of which the rapidly migrating isoenzyme LDH I predominates in the heart. The same isoenzyme is found in red cells. The rise in lactate dehydrogenase occurs later than the other enzymes mentioned, reaching its peak 48 hours or more after the onset of infarction; it may remain abnormal for one to three weeks. LDH is less specific than the other enzymes, but is valuable when it is suspected that the infarct has occurred some days prior to sampling or when concomitant diseases diminish the significance of CPK or GOT findings.

It has been shown that the release into the serum of enzymes from the myocardium reflects the severity of myocardial damage. This observation has been used to quantitate the severity of infarct by analyzing the area under the CPK curve. The validity of such estimates remains to be determined.

Nuclear Imaging. Certain chemical substances, such as pyrophosphate and diphosphonate, accumulate in the mitochondria of ischemic or infarcted myocardial cells. Technetium-labeled pyrophosphate and diphosphonate have been used for "hot-spot" scanning for the diagnosis of myocardial infarction. This has proved to be a quite sensitive method of detecting myocardial infarction, but its specificity remains undetermined.

Other Laboratory Abnormalities. A polymorphonuclear leukocytosis occurs in most cases, starting on the first day and persisting for five to seven days. The increase is usually to 12,000 to 15,000 leukocytes per cubic millimeter. In general, the extent of the leukocytosis reflects the severity of the infarction, but levels beyond 15,000 should suggest some other complication. The erythrocyte sedimentation rate rises more slowly and may remain elevated for several weeks.

DIFFERENTIAL DIAGNOSIS. The most common diagnostic problem is the differentiation of myocardial infarction from *angina*, particularly of the "unstable" type. The pain of myocardial infarction is usually more severe and prolonged and is more likely to be accompanied by breathlessness, syncope, nausea, and vomiting, as well as by evidence of hypotension and cardiac failure. None of these features is diagnostic, however, and the distinction between these disorders depends essentially on the finding of the characteristic ECG and enzyme abnormalities of myocardial infarction.

Massive pulmonary embolus may present great diagnostic difficulty, particularly in the patient recovering from surgery or trauma. Massive pulmonary embolism often presents with acute dyspnea, tachypnea, and cyanosis, rather than severe chest pain, although this can be present. Syncope is sometimes the only major manifestation. Additional diagnostic evidence is provided by the features of deep vein thrombosis. Many of the physical signs occur in both conditions, including tachycardia, hypotension, and gallop rhythm.

Many patients with pulmonary embolism have a persistently normal ECG, but Q waves and T wave inversion may appear in lead III; in these cases there is commonly an S wave in lead I. Other ECG abnormalities include P pulmonale, partial or complete right bundle branch block, and transient T wave inversion in the right chest leads. The S-T depression of myocardial ischemia is sometimes seen, but S-T elevation is not a feature. Enzyme abnormalities, including elevation of GOT, CPK, and LDH, may occur in pulmonary embolism, although not to the same extent as is found in myocardial infarction. The MB isoenzyme of CPK remains normal in pulmonary embolism. A lung scan may demonstrate unperfused areas of lung, which is highly suggestive, particularly if the chest roentgenogram is normal. The diagnosis may be established firmly by carrying out a pulmonary angiogram.

Acute pericarditis may produce a pain similar to that of an acute myocardial infarction, although it is usually made worse by lying flat, by breathing, or by swallowing. It is often sharper in character than the pain of myocardial infarction and seldom radiates to the arms, although it may reach the shoulders, neck, and upper abdomen. Acute pericarditis is commonly a complication of a viral infection, in which case pyrexia usually precedes rather than follows the onset of the pain, as in myocardial infarction. In pericarditis Q waves do not appear, but there is usually S-T elevation, which usually remains concave upward but is followed by T wave inversion. The ECG abnormalities tend to be more widespread than they are in myocardial infarction, and reciprocal S-T depression is not characteristically seen. Enzyme abnormalities are either absent or slight.

Dissecting aneurysm of the aorta may be difficult to diagnose. As with infarction, the pain is central and severe. However, it is often described as "tearing" in character and frequently starts in the back rather than in the front of the chest. Furthermore, it tends to move to the front of the chest and sometimes to the abdomen. The patient often has the appearance of shock with pallor and diaphoresis, but the blood pressure is frequently in the hypertensive or normal range, having previously been raised. Features which suggest the diagnosis of dissecting aneurysm include weakness or transient paralysis of the limbs, hemiplegia, hemothorax and aortic regurgitation, and differences in the pulses in the peripheral arteries. Roentgenographic features include a left pleural effusion and widening of the mediastinum. The ECG usually either is normal or shows the features of left ventricular hypertrophy. Transient elevations of serum enzyme activities may occur, although they are usually not great. Aortography can demonstrate the presence of the aneurysm, but is potentially hazardous.

Spontaneous pneumothorax may sometimes produce central chest pain, but usually it is pleural in character. The physical signs and roentgenographic features are diagnostic.

Perforation of a peptic ulcer is usually associated with severe abdominal pain accompanied by tenderness and rigidity. A roentgenogram taken in the upright position will usually demonstrate air under the diaphragm.

Rupture of the esophagus may simulate myocardial infarction, but is usually precipitated by violent vomiting. The chest roentgenogram may show air in the mediastinum.

Pancreatitis may also simulate myocardial infarction, although the pain is usually predominantly in the abdomen. It may radiate into the lower chest, and the picture is made more confusing by the quite frequent occurrence of S-T and T wave abnormalities in the electrocardiogram. Transaminase levels may be raised, but in pancreatitis the serum and urinary amylase levels are usually markedly elevated.

Biliary colic may mimic myocardial infarction, particularly when it is due to a gallstone wedged in the cystic duct. The pain may radiate to the chest and right shoulder region but not to the arms. Vomiting is frequent, and there is virtually always tenderness or rigidity in the right hypochondrium or epigastrium. The diagnosis may be established by appropriate roentgenographic examinations.

PROGNOSIS. The mortality of acute heart attacks is approximately 40 per cent within one month of the onset. A substantial proportion of these deaths are instantaneous or nearly so. The fatality rate in the remainder is in the order of 30 per cent, but this varies considerably with the age of the patient as well as other factors such as a previous history of coronary disease, the presence or absence of other diseases, and the complications of infarction. The mortality below 50 years of age is little more than 10 per cent, but it rises to more than 50 per cent in the elderly. Quite apart from the very early deaths, mortality is highest during the first day and progressively decreases thereafter. Death on the first day is usually due to ventricular fibrillation, although shock and failure may be fatal at this time. These latter complications are responsible for most of the deaths on the second and third days, but they become less common causes subsequently. Later, death may be due to cardiac rupture, pulmonary embolism, or recurrent myocardial infarction.

Unfavorable prognostic features include cardiogenic shock, persistent tachycardia, gallop rhythm, and the development of right-sided heart failure. Bundle branch block, high serum enzyme levels, and persistent arrhythmias are also sinister observations.

There is a high mortality in the first six months after myocardial infarction, but it progressively decreases over the first year and in succeeding years. Over-all, some 85 per cent of patients surviving one month after infarction live for one year, and about 70 per cent live for five years.

In those who survive an acute infarction, the most important correlate with early death is the severity of left ventricular malfunction. Indices of this include cardiomegaly, persistent tachycardia, a third heart sound, and signs of pulmonary congestion or edema. Ventricular arrhythmias are also associated with a bad prognosis, although this may be because they reflect the severity of left ventricular damage rather than being independent risk factors.

TREATMENT. The aims of treatment are (1) to relieve the patient's discomfort, (2) to minimize the oxygen demands of the myocardium in the hope of limiting the extent of the infarction, and (3) to prevent or correct complications.

Relief of Symptoms. The most urgent measure in most cases is the relief of pain. This usually requires the use of morphine sulfate in a dose of 5 to 15 mg given intravenously or intramuscularly. This may have to be repeated. Morphine may produce respiratory depression, hypotension, or bradycardia. It should not be given if possible in those with known obstructive airways disease. Bradycardia can be avoided by simultaneously administering atropine. Alternatively, morphine may be given with an antihistamine drug which diminishes the risk of vomiting and hypotension. It is probably unwise to use meperidine, as this may also cause hypotension and can increase the ventricular rate undesirably. In patients with less severe pain, pentazocine, 15 to 30 mg intravenously, may be helpful. When these powerful pain-relieving drugs are not available, the inhalation of nitrous oxide, 50 per cent, and oxygen, 50 per cent, is useful and can be administered by paramedical personnel.

Most patients respond well to these drugs and the pain is relieved within a short period of time. Furthermore, apprehension, a common feature of myocardial infarction, will usually be alleviated. If it is not, chlordiazepoxide (Librium) or diazepam (Valium) may be used.

General Management. PLACE OF CARE. The initial care of a patient with myocardial infarction will usually be in his home or at his place of work. Ideally, appropriately trained personnel will attend him where he develops the attack and treat his symptoms and complications immediately. This is best achieved by a mobile coronary care unit (see below). In most cases, and as soon as the patient has been made comfortable and any complications corrected, he should be transferred to hospital and admitted to a coronary care unit.

Although hospital admission is the almost invariable practice in the United States, the wisdom of transferring a patient from his home has been questioned in some European countries, notably the United Kingdom. Some controlled studies have suggested that patients do as well at home as they do in hospital, and it has been claimed that the physical and emotional stress of an ambulance journey and admission to an unfamiliar environment may evoke unfavorable responses, including dangerous arrhythmias. These studies are not scientifically satisfactory, and the high risk of unexpected sudden death within the first few hours suggests strongly that it is advisable for patients to be under intensive care during this period. This applies particularly to the younger patient, but it is not unreasonable to treat those patients at home who are seen there many hours after the onset of symptoms, particularly if they are in good general condition or if they are elderly.

BED REST. The obvious need to restrict demands on the myocardium has led many physicians in the past to insist on bed rest for a period of some weeks. The apparent advantages of such strict rest are outweighed, however, by the disadvantages that immobility imposes. The risks of deep vein thrombosis and subsequent pulmonary embolism are well known, but there is also a danger of "deconditioning" so that, when the patient becomes ambulatory, there is a tendency to orthostatic hypotension and undue increases in heart rate. Furthermore, the psychologic effects of the disorder are enhanced, and the patient is more liable to anxiety and depression.

It certainly seems wise to keep the patient in bed for at least 48 hours, although a bedside commode may be used except for those who have severe hypotension. If the patient's initial condition appears satisfactory, he may be allowed to feed himself and should be encouraged to exercise his legs gently. Within a few days, he may be allowed to sit out of bed although still resting in a comfortable armchair. Patients with mild cases may be permitted to walk a few steps after four to five days and be ready for hospital discharge in one to two weeks.

On the other hand, if the infarction has been more severe, being complicated by dangerous arrhythmias, cardiac failure, or shock, a more prolonged period of strict bed rest may be required until the complication has been brought under control. Affected patients need careful observation over the next two to three weeks and may require three to six weeks in hospital.

REASSURANCE. Rehabilitation is often impeded by undue anxiety on the part of the patient and his relatives. This anxiety is frequently engendered by inappropriate remarks made by doctors and nurses. By the time a patient is admitted to a coronary care unit, the most dangerous phase of the illness has already passed and the major complications which may yet develop can usually be controlled. The patient and his relatives can therefore be reassured that there is an excellent chance of survival and that there will be a probability of return to work within the subsequent two or three months. An optimistic attitude must be conveyed to the patient from the moment of his admission and constantly reinforced by his medical attendants. There is often a period of enhanced anxiety when the patient leaves the protective atmosphere of a coronary care unit for progressive care; it must be emphasized to the patient that he has done so well that careful monitoring is no longer necessary. Similarly, a sense of dependence on the hospital must be avoided so that at the time of discharge there is not another period of worry.

DIET. As the acutely ill patient usually has little appetite in the first few days, it is desirable to provide an attractively prepared, low calorie diet with moderate sodium restriction. When the acute phase is over, a normal diet may be given except for the overweight patient, for whom the calorie content should remain low.

SMOKING. Smoking should be absolutely prohibited during the phase of acute infarction and allowed subsequently only with the greatest reluctance.

BOWEL AND BLADDER FUNCTION. Patients are often constipated during the first few days in hospital, partly because of bed rest, partly because of inhibitions imposed by the unfamiliar surroundings, and partly because of the use of narcotics. Bedpans should be used only if they are essential, and in most cases patients should be allowed to use a bedside commode. Many will benefit from the use of a stool softener such as dioctyl sodium sulfosuccinate (Colace), 100 mg twice daily.

Some patients, particularly those with mild prostatic obstruction, develop urinary retention in the first few days. This may be aggravated by such drugs as atropine and disopyramide. If there is evidence of urinary retention, and particularly if there is hypotension, a knowledge of the urinary output is of great importance in management, and an indwelling catheter should be inserted with aseptic technique.

OXYGEN THERAPY. Nearly all patients with myocardial infarction have arterial hypoxemia; in many this is so mild that the additional discomfort of oxygen administration does not seem worthwhile. However, any patient who is breathless, or who has other features of cardiac failure or of shock, should receive oxygen, which is best given by nasal cannula or Venturi mask. High oxygen concentrations should be given except to patients suspected of having obstructive airways disease, in which case the concentration of oxygen should be limited to 28 per cent.

ANTICOAGULANT THERAPY. In the days when patients were confined to bed for long periods of time, it was shown that anticoagulant therapy reduced the risk of deep vein thrombosis and serious pulmonary embolism. With early ambulation and the encouragement of limb movements in bed, these risks have been substantially reduced and are largely confined to those with more severe reactions to the infarction. There is no evidence that anticoagulant therapy has any effect upon coronary thrombosis or the development of the myocardial infarction, although it may have a beneficial effect in reducing the risk of systemic embolism. It seems appropriate to confine anticoagulant treatment to those patients who have evidence of a severe course, including left- or right-sided cardiac failure, shock, and prolonged arrhythmias, particularly atrial fibrillation. They should be given to patients with a previous history of deep vein thrombosis or pulmonary embolism, but avoided if possible in those with known history of ulcer or hemorrhagic tendency, and in the presence of pericarditis.

Disorders of Rate and Rhythm. Sinus bradycardia is usually well tolerated and requires no treatment. However, particularly in the early stages, it may lead to hypotension, cardiac failure, or ventricular ectopic rhythms. The heart rate may be accelerated if the venous return is increased by raising the patient's legs. If this maneuver fails, atropine should be given, starting with not more than 0.5 mg but repeating it if necessary. The action of this drug usually lasts two to four hours. Larger doses may give rise to an undesirable degree of tachycardia, which may rarely lead to ventricular arrhythmias, including ventricular fibrillation. The drug should not be repeated many times, as it may provoke mental confusion and urinary retention and aggravate pre-existing glaucoma. Sinus bradycardia usually disappears after a few hours; but even if it persists, it seldom gives rise to serious hemodynamic disturbances. If it should do so, temporary pacing can be established with the electrode tip placed in the right ventricle. This procedure is particularly helpful when the "sick sinus syndrome" is present, as it permits the use of digitalis or other drugs required to control the concomitant atrial arrhythmias.

ATRIAL ARRHYTHMIAS. Frequent atrial premature beats require no treatment, although they may presage other atrial arrhythmias. Atrial tachycardia may respond to carotid sinus pressure. If it does not do so, therapy should depend upon the hemodynamic disturbance which it has caused. If the patient is in good condition, treatment with digoxin is adequate. However, if the patient is distressed and the blood pressure has fallen precipitately, synchronized direct current shock should be administered. If paroxysmal atrial tachycardia with block occurs, one should first check whether digitalis could have been responsible; if it has not, digitalis is called for if the heart rate is fast. Atrial flutter may be treated as atrial tachycardia.

When atrial fibrillation occurs, the ventricular rate may not be very fast. If this is the case, no treatment may be necessary. However, if the ventricular rate is sufficient to cause hemodynamic disturbance, it may be treated with digoxin in the first place. If this does not produce an adequate fall in heart rate, direct current shock may be necessary. Following a reversion to sinus rhythm, digitalis should be administered for several days because there is a risk of recurrence.

VENTRICULAR ECTOPIC BEATS. In recent years, ventricular ectopic beats and short runs of ventricular tachycardia have been regarded as harbingers of ventricular fibrillation, and therefore great efforts have been expended on detecting and treating them promptly. Certain types of ventricular ectopic beat have been regarded as particularly sinister: those which occur in pairs or are multiform, or those of the R-on-T variety. The most effective drug in this situation is lidocaine. Therapy should be started with an intravenous injection of 50 to 100 mg given over a period of one to two minutes (*not* rapidly as a "push," as this may produce neurotoxic effects). Subsequently, an intravenous infusion of this drug should be given, starting with 3 to 4 mg a minute for the first half hour and then gradually reducing to 2 mg a minute and 1 mg a minute over the next 12 to 24 hours. Further injections of 75 to 100 mg may be required to suppress recurrences of ventricular ectopic beats.

There is increasing dissatisfaction with this method of trying to prevent ventricular fibrillation. In the first place, many episodes of ventricular fibrillation occur without "warning" arrhythmias. Secondly, conventional monitoring techniques often fail to detect "warning" ventricular arrhythmias. It seems more logical therefore to use lidocaine prophylactically in all cases in which it is not contraindicated. However, the drug has important side effects if given in excessive doses. Mild confusion is common; more serious effects include convulsions and coma. It is preferable to give the drug by an infusion pump.

Several alternative drugs are available if lidocaine fails. These include procainamide and quinidine sulfate. Diphenylhydantoin is less effective but occasionally of value when the other drugs are unsuccessful. The adrenergic blocking drug bretylium tosylate* may also be valuable in difficult cases. An alternative method of treatment is by overdrive suppression, using a temporary pacing electrode.

VENTRICULAR TACHYCARDIA. The management of ventricular tachycardia is similar to that of ventricular ectopic beats, except that the treatment is more urgent. If drug therapy is not immediately successful, consideration should be given to direct current shock therapy.

VENTRICULAR FIBRILLATION. This should be corrected immediately by direct current shock. Usually 200 wattseconds is sufficient; but if this fails, larger shocks should be administered. If the first shock is not successful, the usual techniques of cardiopulmonary resuscitation, including ventilation and closed chest cardiac compression, should be undertaken (see Ch. 353). Acidosis usually ensues and should be corrected by intravenous sodium bicarbonate; recurrence of ventricular fibrillation should be prevented by intravenous lidocaine, or by other drugs used for suppressing ventricular ectopic beats.

Disorders of Conduction. First-degree heart block (prolonged P-R interval) requires no treatment, but monitoring for more advanced degrees of block should be undertaken. The Wenckebach type of second degree block is a common complication of inferior infarction, usually requires no treatment, and, in the first few hours, can often be corrected by atropine administration. It generally carries a good prognosis but may progress to complete heart block. Mobitz type II heart block, in which there are unexpected dropped beats or 2:1 heart block, occurs with a slow ventricular rate, is usually due to extensive myocardial damage to the bundle branches, and is liable to lead to an extremely slow heart rate or asystole. Such patients should have an electrode inserted with the tip in the right ventricle. Pacing should be instituted if the heart rate is slow enough to cause hypotension or if episodes of asystole have occurred. Therapy of complete heart block depends on the anatomic location of the block

---

*Investigational drug.

and the heart rate. When complete heart block is due to inferior myocardial infarction, the ventricular rate is often adequate and the hemodynamic status satisfactory. When heart block complicates anterior infarction, the block is usually in the bundle branches and the idioventricular rate is slow. Transvenous pacing is called for when the bradycardia leads to hypotension or cardiac failure or to episodes of asystole or ventricular fibrillation. If electrical pacing is not immediately available, isoproterenol may be administered as intravenous infusion of 2 to 5 mg in 500 ml dextrose. The rate of infusion should be adjusted to keep the heart rate between 70 and 100 per minute. Atrioventricular conduction defects in acute infarction nearly always resolve spontaneously within hours or days. Only very rarely is long-term pacemaking required, although there is a risk of late recurrence of heart block and sudden death in those with anterior infarction. Some physicians consider that long-term pacemaker therapy should be instituted in such patients even though normal conduction appears to have been restored.

BUNDLE BRANCH BLOCK. When infarction leads to block in two or more of the fascicles, such as the right bundle and the left anterior or left posterior fascicle, there is a risk of the sudden onset of complete heart block or asystole. Many physicians think it wise to insert a pacing electrode with its tip in the right ventricle as a prophylactic measure and to remove it when the danger of heart block appears to have passed.

Shock. When the shock syndrome has developed, the mortality is high whatever treatment is given. Prevention is therefore of great importance, and this depends upon the avoidance of hypotension, if possible, in the early phase, the relief of pain, and the correction of such unfavorable factors as arrhythmias and hypovolemia.

Once the features of the shock syndrome have developed, it is desirable to monitor the patient's hemodynamic status carefully, preferably with a Swan-Ganz catheter positioned in the pulmonary artery. If there is severe hypotension and the other features of shock, but left ventricular filling pressure is in the normal range, one may infuse fluid provided that the pulmonary capillary wedge pressure does not exceed 20 mm Hg. It is important not to rely on the right atrial (central venous) pressure in this context, as this may be within normal limits when the pulmonary wedge pressure is high.

Controversy persists as to the value of vasopressors in the management of shock syndrome. Norepinephrine and isoproterenol have been used in the past in this context, but both these drugs potentially may increase the size of the myocardial infarction and, in the case of isoproterenol, may produce peripheral vasodilatation. Myocardial oxygen consumption may be increased, which leads to an increase in the size of myocardial infarction. Dopamine and dobutamine may be of greater value in this context.

The most effective way of counteracting shock is by the use of intra-aortic balloon counterpulsation (see Ch. 356). With this technique, aortic systolic pressure is lowered and diastolic pressure is augmented, thus increasing coronary perfusion and reducing the work of the left ventricle.

Cardiac Failure. Mild degrees of pulmonary congestion may require no treatment; but when dyspnea or pulmonary edema is present, it is wise to give a diuretic such as furosemide intravenously or orally. The role of digitalis remains controversial. There is evidence that it may, by increasing myocardial contractility, lead to a disproportionate myocardial oxygen demand and thus increase the size of the infarct. Furthermore, the drug is particularly likely to induce arrhythmias in the context of myocardial infarction. On the other hand, when there is cardiomegaly, the drug, by reducing cardiac size, may improve cardiac efficiency. It may be wise therefore to reserve cardiac glycosides for patients with cardiomegaly and, of course, for those with atrial arrhythmias.

Substances which reduce cardiac afterload, e.g., nitroglycerin and sodium nitroprusside, may be effective in improving left ventricular performance; the combination of one of these drugs with an inotropic drug such as dopamine may be particularly beneficial.

Coronary Care Unit. The natural mortality in the first two or three days after the onset of myocardial infarction is very high. Some of the major causes of death, notably ventricular fibrillation, can be prevented if the patient is under close observation and if appropriate therapy, including cardiopulmonary resuscitation, can be applied without delay. In order for this to be done, the patient himself and his electrocardiographic and hemodynamic status must be under continuous observation. This can best be achieved by concentrating patients at maximal risk in specially designed areas, by ensuring that they are cared for by nurses and doctors with appropriate training, and by having apparatus for monitoring and resuscitation immediately available. The patients are best accommodated in a quiet environment, preferably in single rooms but under direct visual inspection by nurses at a central monitoring station. The nurses require training in the recognition of arrhythmias, in the administration of the main antiarrhythmic drugs, and in the techniques of cardiopulmonary resuscitation, including the application of direct current countershock. The patient's electrocardiograms are under continuous scrutiny so that any important arrhythmias are detected and treated without delay. In many coronary care units, not only are the electrocardiographic features observed but continuous hemodynamic monitoring is carried out in patients with suspected pump failure.

It is believed that coronary care units have substantially reduced mortality from acute myocardial infarction in hospitals, mainly by the prevention of death from ventricular fibrillation, but also by the more skillful care of the patient with pump failure. However, because many patients die before reaching the coronary care unit, the concept of mobile coronary care has been developed. The mobile coronary care unit is a facility for bringing the principles and practices of coronary care units to patients wherever they may be, at home, in the street, or in the factory. The patients who probably benefit most from this are those who "drop dead" away from hospital and are kept alive initially by cardiopulmonary resuscitation until the mobile unit can arrive and give appropriate therapy. These units are usually staffed by highly trained paramedical personnel, who are authorized to give antiarrhythmic drugs and to carry out defibrillation, as necessary.

PREVENTION OF RECURRENT HEART ATTACKS. Several approaches have been made to the prevention of recurrent heart attacks. The earliest of these involved the use of anticoagulant drugs such as warfarin. Although in some studies, there appeared to be a reduction in recurrent infarction, the risks of this form of therapy and the difficulty of controlling treatment have meant that the earlier enthusiasm for long-term anticoagulant therapy has dissipated. Recently, the use of sulfinpyrazone as a form of antithrombotic therapy appears to have reduced the incidence of recurrent heart attacks in patients who have recovered from myocardial infarction. Further information is needed before this form of therapy can be widely recommended.

As discussed in Ch. 363.4, there is evidence that certain beta-adrenergic blocking drugs, e.g., alprenolol, may reduce the incidence of death and, particularly, of sudden death in the months following an acute myocardial infarction. Whether these observations are applicable to propranolol is not yet known.

LATE COMPLICATIONS. Ventricular Aneurysm. A ventricular aneurysm has been defined as a protrusion of a localized portion of the external aspect of the ventricle accompanied by a corresponding protrusion of a ventricular cavity. Such aneurysms occur in 10 to 20 per cent of patients following acute myocardial infarction. They occur when the infarction affects the full thickness of the ventricular wall, which becomes extremely thinned and replaced by fibrosis. The asynergy adds to the load on an already impaired ventricle and may lead to cardiac failure. It is rare for aneurysms to rupture, and although they almost invariably contain organized clot, embolism is not common. They may be suspected clinically in any patient who, following a myocardial infarction, has persistent cardiac failure, a systemic embolism, or persistent arrhythmias. The characteristic physical sign is the presence of a palpable and visible systolic expansion in the anterior chest wall, giving rise to a double apical impulse. Third and fourth heart sounds are often present. The ECG usually shows evidence of old myocardial infarction, and in many cases there are large Q waves associated with persistent S-T segment elevation in the affected leads. The S-T elevation may become more pronounced on exercise. An abnormal rounded bulge may be seen on chest roentgenogram, but this is often absent. The diagnosis is best established by left cineventriculography, which shows the paradoxical movement of the affected area. If symptoms are troublesome, it should be removed surgically.

Postmyocardial Infarction Syndrome (Dressler's Syndrome). This syndrome occurs in 1 to 5 per cent of patients and usually begins one to six weeks after the onset of myocardial infarction. It is thought to be due to an autoimmune reaction to cardiac muscle damage and affects particularly the pericardium, pleura, and lungs. Pleural or pericardial pain is accompanied by malaise and pyrexia. Large effusions and tamponade are unusual, but anticoagulants should be discontinued because of the risk of hemopericardium. Many minor cases resolve spontaneously; but if severe symptoms persist, they can be brought under control quickly by corticosteroids or indomethacin.

Shoulder-Hand Syndrome. A small number of patients develop limitation of movement in the shoulder joint, especially the left, associated with pain and stiffness in the arm. There may also be swelling of the associated hand, the skin of which may become tense and shiny. It is less common than it used to be and is probably a consequence of prolonged immobility. It usually responds to physiotherapy.

Bigger, J. T., Jr., Dresdale, R. J., Heissenbuttel, R. H., Weld, F. M., and Wit, A. L.: Ventricular arrhythmias in ischemic heart disease: Mechanism, prevalence, significance, and management. Prog. Cardiovasc. Dis., 19:255, 1977.

Chatterjee, K., and Swan, H. J. C.: Hemodynamic profile of acute myocardial infarction. *In* Corday, E., and Swan, H. J. C. (eds.): Myocardial Infarction. Baltimore, Williams & Wilkins Company, 1973, Chap. 6.

Coronary Drug Project Research Group: Factors influencing long-term prognosis after recovery from myocardial infarction: Three-year figures of the coronary drug project. J. Chron. Dis., 27:267, 1974.

Fowler, N. O. (ed.): Treatment of acute myocardial infarction. *In* Cardiac Diagnosis and Treatment. 2nd ed. New York, Harper and Row, 1976, Chap. 35.

Meltzer, L. E., and Dunning, A. J. (eds.): Textbook of Coronary Care. Amsterdam, Excerpta Medica, 1972.

Multicentre International Study: Improvement in prognosis of myocardial infarction by long-term beta-adrenoreceptor blockade using practolol. Br. Med. J., 3:735, 1975.

Pantridge, J. F., Adgey, A. A. J., Geddes, J. S., and Webb, S. W.: The Acute Coronary Attack. London, Pitman Medical, 1975.

363.4. SUDDEN DEATH

Desmond G. Julian

Death is often sudden and unexpected. Every year almost half a million inhabitants of the United States die instantaneously or within 24 hours of the onset of fresh signs or symptoms. A high proportion of these succumb within less than half an hour of the onset of the final disorder. Nearly all these very rapid deaths are due to cardiovascular causes, predominantly coronary atherosclerosis. Other cardiac causes include aortic stenosis, cardiomyopathies, and various rare types of rhythm disorder, including Wolff-Parkinson-White syndrome and the prolonged Q-T syndromes. Noncardiac causes include cerebral hemorrhage; drug overdose, toxicity, or idiosyncrasy; pulmonary thromboembolism; and chronic obstructive pulmonary disease. Patients with chronic alcoholism may also die within a few hours of the onset of an acute illness.

MECHANISM OF SUDDEN CARDIOVASCULAR DEATH. Most cases of sudden death take place in circumstances in which the determination of the mechanism is impossible. However, a sufficient number of cases have been observed to occur under close observation and electrocardiographic monitoring to assert that the majority of sudden deaths are due to ventricular fibrillation. It is particularly common in patients dying with severe coronary atherosclerosis, either with or without an accompanying acute myocardial infarction. Ventricular asystole or extreme bradycardia may be responsible for death in some cases. This is relatively rare as a consequence of atherosclerosis but is more common in those with chronic heart block or the sick sinus syndrome. Death may also occur from a sudden reduction in cardiac output, as in acute massive pulmonary embolism, or from cardiac tamponade from such causes as acute pericarditis and cardiac rupture. Death often occurs suddenly in cases of severe aortic stenosis; the mechanism is not known in many cases, although arrhythmias are responsible for some. In others, it would appear to be due to sudden ventricular failure, and this may also be the cause of death in some patients with acute myocardial infarction. Acute vasodepressor reflexes may be responsible for some deaths, including those of the so-called "voodoo" type. In such cases, there may be a sudden reduction in arterial pressure and heart rate. Organic causes include pulmonary thromboembolism, carotid sinus syndrome, and primary pulmonary hypertension.

PREDICTION OF SUDDEN DEATH. The identification of

the person liable to sudden death is clearly important, as it is only by instituting prophylactic therapy in such individuals that the mortality of acute coronary disease can be substantially reduced. In general, it is true that the risk factors for sudden death are essentially the same as those for myocardial infarction, although heavy cigarette smokers may be at particular risk. The situation is different in those who have already sustained a myocardial infarction. The risk of sudden death in the months after infarction is particularly high in those who have evidence of serious left ventricular malfunction, such as cardiomegaly and persistent sinus tachycardia, in the convalescent phase; those who additionally show ventricular arrhythmias are especially vulnerable.

PREVENTION OF SUDDEN DEATH. Many people can be saved from sudden death by the prompt treatment of ventricular fibrillation. This is relatively easy in the emergency room or in the coronary care unit, but most sudden deaths take place away from hospital. Success in such cases depends on the rapid initiation of artificial ventilation and closed chest cardiac massage by lay or paramedical personnel until a defibrillator can be made available. There are now many areas where mobile coronary care is provided so that a defibrillator can be brought to the patient wherever cardiac arrest takes place. The value of such a scheme has been demonstrated particularly clearly in Seattle, where more than 50 patients each year are resuscitated successfully from ventricular fibrillation. This has required the organization of a very rapid response system operated by fire department paramedical personnel and, importantly, the training of a quarter of the whole population of the area in the techniques of cardiopulmonary resuscitation. Notwithstanding the impressive results, the consequent reduction in mortality from acute coronary heart attacks is probably of the order of only 5 to 8 per cent. More substantial reduction in sudden death must depend on preventive measures, either of coronary atherosclerosis or, more particularly, of ventricular fibrillation.

There is good evidence that one important factor in sudden death is the habit of smoking cigarettes. Stopping smoking appears to lead to a reduction in the risk of sudden death, certainly in those who have recovered from an infarction. There is also highly suggestive evidence that certain beta-adrenergic blocking drugs, e.g., alprenolol, can prevent sudden death in postinfarction patients. Whether this also applies to patients who have not had an infarction and whether other beta blockers are so effective have yet to be established. As yet, there is no definite evidence that coronary arterial surgery or the long-term use of antiarrhythmic drugs prevents sudden death.

Cobb, L. A., Baum, R. S., Alvarez, H., and Schaffer, W. A.: Resuscitation from out-of-hospital ventricular fibrillation: Four years' follow-up. Circulation (Suppl. 3), 51–52:223, 1975.

Goldstein, S.: Sudden Death and Coronary Heart Disease. Mount Kisco, N.Y., Futura Publishing Company, 1974.

Kannel, W. B., Doyle, J. T., McNamara, P. M., Quickenton, P., and Gordon, T.: Precursors of sudden coronary death. Circulation, 51:606, 1975.

Kuller, L., Cooper, M., and Perper, J.: Epidemiology of sudden death. Arch. Intern. Med., 129:714, 1972.

363.5. SURGICAL TREATMENT OF CORONARY ARTERY DISEASE

David C. Sabiston, Jr.

Although a number of surgical procedures have been devised to revascularize the myocardium, the development of the aortocoronary bypass graft during the past decade has made a remarkable impact on the management of ischemic heart disease. For the first time, significant numbers of patients with symptomatic coronary disease have undergone a direct surgical attack, and this procedure is currently the most common operation performed in the field of cardiac surgery. Although aortocoronary bypass grafts (CABG) have been supported by both cardiologists and surgeons with encouraging results, a cautious attitude nevertheless remains appropriate until a final assessment based upon long-term evaluation is available. Controversy continues concerning the effect of the CABG procedure on extending the life span of patients with symptomatic coronary disease, but there is general agreement that complete relief of anginal pain is achieved in the majority of patients. For specific anatomic lesions, such as significant stenosis of the left main coronary artery, it is also clear that patients managed surgically survive longer than those treated by medical means, as demonstrated in randomized studies.

A knowledge of the natural history of coronary atherosclerosis is of considerable importance in selecting the appropriate therapeutic approach, and a number of factors are of significance in evaluating the prognosis of a patient with angina pectoris. These factors include the number of coronary arteries involved, the severity and extent of the atherosclerotic lesions, the status of left ventricular performance, and the presence of associated conditions such as a valvular lesion or ventricular aneurysm. The prognosis in these patients is known to be adversely affected by several other factors, including a familial history of coronary disease, hypertension, diabetes, and a history of cigarette smoking.

Studies of the natural history of angina pectoris indicate that significant stenosis (greater than 70 per cent) of a *single* coronary artery is associated with a relatively low threat to life, the mortality in this group being in the range of 2 to 4 per cent each year. As the extent of the disease increases, the risk of death becomes greater such that with significant lesions in *two* main vessels the death rate increases to 7 to 8 per cent annually. For *three*-vessel disease, the annual mortality is even greater, being 10 to 15 per cent. Finally, for patients with *left main* coronary lesions, the death rate is even higher, leading to the position that nearly all patients with this condition are candidates for surgery.

SELECTION OF PATIENTS FOR SURGICAL THERAPY. It is difficult to state precisely the number of patients who are appropriate candidates for myocardial revascularization. However, it is generally estimated that some 20 per cent of those with angina do not obtain satisfactory pain relief by pharmacologic means alone. In some patients, drug intolerance becomes a problem, whereas in others the anginal pain is refractory to medication, especially in those with severe and diffuse coronary lesions. The most common indication for CABG is *relief of anginal pain,* and the majority of patients obtain complete relief, and all but a few of the remainder are considerably improved. In appropriate circumstances, CABG is also indicated for other manifestations of myocardial ischemia, including refractory cardiac dysrhythmias, preinfarction angina, and congestive heart failure in the presence of a ventricular aneurysm.

In selection of patients for myocardial revascularization, selective coronary arteriography is essential. The diseased vessels which are to be potentially grafted should have a reasonable lumen, and whenever possible the distal runoff should indicate a patent peripheral coronary bed. A coronary artery suitable for anastomosis should have a diameter of at least 1 mm. If extensive intrinsic disease is present in the distal coronary arteries, the postoperative result is apt to be unsatisfactory. Experience has shown that in 80 to 90 per cent of patients with symptomatic coronary disease the anatomy *is* appropriate for direct aortocoronary grafts. The majority of surgical candidates have several significant lesions in the proximal portions of the major coronary arteries, which are potentially correctable by a graft. It should be emphasized that in patients with *complete* occlusion of a proximal coronary artery the collateral circulation at the time of arteriography may be inadequate to opacify the vessel distally despite the fact that a lumen is present, as studies have demonstrated that a significant number of distal vessels which do not opacify can be shown to be patent at the time of operation or autopsy.

In addition to selective coronary arteriography, cardiac catheterization frequently adds many data of importance for an understanding of the total hemodynamic status. Such studies are not only helpful but often essential in objectively documenting left ventricular function. Cardiac catheterization reveals the status of left ventricular wall motion and also provides an assessment of the aortic and mitral valves. Certain features are associated with an *increased* surgical risk; these include cardiomegaly, a low ejection fraction (below 25 per cent), an increased left ventricular volume, a large arteriovenous oxygen difference (greater than 6 volumes per cent), and, to a lesser extent, an elevated left ventricular end-diastolic pressure. It should be emphasized, however, that the presence of any of these abnormalities does not necessarily represent a contraindication to operation or to a successful result.

The use of noninvasive radionuclide angiography has simplified the diagnostic approach, and with this technique it is possible to obtain objective values for ventricular volume, ejection fraction, cardiac output, and left ventricular wall motion not only at rest but during exercise. Thallium injections, which demonstrate ischemia during exertion, and ventricular function studies, which demonstrate a deterioration of ejection fraction and local abnormalities of wall motion, enhance ability to recognize ischemia by noninvasive techniques and to assess the significance of coronary arterial lesions demonstrated by angiography. With the use of a bicycle ergometer, the cardiodynamic status can be assessed both at rest and — of more importance — during graded exercise. Such data provide very helpful information in the total assessment of myocardial function and of the potential role of myocardial revascularization.

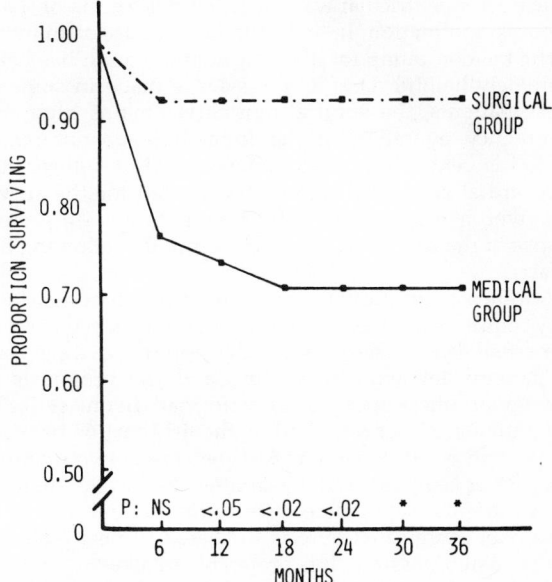

Accumulative survival rates of 83 patients with significant lesions of the left main coronary artery, who were randomly allocated into medical or surgical treatment groups in 1972, 1973, and 1974. There were 41 patients in the medical group and 42 patients in the surgical group. (From Takaro, T., Hultgren, H. N., Lipton, M. J., and Detre, K. M., and Participants in the Study Group: Circulation [Suppl. 3], 54:107, 1976.)

Significant stenosis of the *left main* coronary artery is known to be associated with considerable risk, and several studies have confirmed the fact that the death rate ranges up to 50 per cent in the two-year period following diagnosis by arteriography (Cohen et al.). In another study of 30 patients with left main arterial lesions, among those in whom operation was not performed the mortality was 33 per cent, with all deaths occurring within a month after arteriography. In an important and frequently cited cooperative study conducted by Veterans Administration Hospitals, 83 patients with critical stenosis of the left main coronary artery were randomized into surgical and medical groups for a three-year period. In the 41 patients in the medical group, 70 per cent survived, whereas among the 42 patients managed surgically, the survival was 93 per cent (see accompanying figure).

Left ventricular *aneurysms* may follow myocardial infarction and are hazardous both for the paradoxical dilatation which occurs during systole, producing cardiac inefficiency, and also as a source of systemic arterial embolism. These aneurysms may also be the site of electrical instability and cause refractory dysrhythmias.

Urgent or emergency aortocoronary bypass grafts have been recommended for patients with impending myocardial infarction (preinfarction or unstable angina) with good results. Nevertheless, others prefer to withhold operation for these patients until a procedure can be done electively.

Several groups have made an intensive effort to reduce the mortality of *acute* myocardial infarction associated with intractable *shock* with modest success. An immediate CABG procedure is performed, often combined with resection of ventricular wall for either dyskinesia or frank aneurysm formation. In this situation, the use of an intra-aortic balloon pump for diastolic augmentation has been extremely helpful. Despite the salvage made in some of these patients, the surgical mortality remains high and emergency operation in the immediate postinfarction period is generally not recommended. Most believe that myocardial revascularization is indicated for the survivors who have persistent refractory angina, with performance of the procedure three to six months following the infarct.

Another complication of myocardial infarction, which may require surgical intervention, is an acquired *ventricular septal defect*. These lesions develop in 1 to 2 per cent of patients following infarction, and the prognosis is quite poor unless operation is performed. In one series of 157 patients, 24 per cent died on the first day, 65 per cent by the end of two weeks, and 81 per cent at two months. Only 7 per cent survived a year after the development of the ventricular septal defect. Since the natural history is very poor, surgical closure is indicated in nearly all patients. When possible, it is preferable to allow the infarct to heal to permit the edges of the defect to become fibrotic and permit a better repair. Intractable heart failure often ensues following the development of these defects, and earlier or even urgent operation may be necessary. *Multiple* ventricular defects are present in approximately a third of patients and should be carefully sought at operation. The defect is generally closed with the use of a plastic prosthesis, and coronary bypass procedures may also be necessary in order to provide adequate ventricular function. If early operation is mandatory, the results are less favorable than for those who are able to survive for several weeks with elective scheduling of the operative procedures.

SURGICAL PROCEDURES. For most patients undergoing a CABG procedure, an *autologous vein* is anastomosed between the ascending aorta and the coronary artery distal to the obstruction. The saphenous vein is usually chosen, and the vessel is reversed to permit blood flow in the direction of open valves. Extracorporeal circulation is used to assure a quiet heart and to permit a careful coronary arterial anastomosis to be performed. It is well recognized that meticulous attention to detail is essential in making the anastomosis if a good postoperative result is to be obtained. The use of a very fine monofilament suture, often placed with the use of magnifying lenses, has been quite helpful in achieving long-term patency in these small vessels. It has also been shown that all major coronary arteries with significant stenoses should be grafted if the best results are to be obtained. Moderate total body hypothermia is usually employed, and the temperature of the heart may be further lowered by infusion of a potassium solution at 4° C to produce cardioplegia. During the procedure, the heart can also be continuously surrounded by cold saline or ice slush. The cardioplegia produces a flaccid heart, and the hypothermia simultaneously reduces the oxygen consumption to a very low level, preventing ischemic cellular changes within the myocardium. After placement of the coronary grafts, intraoperative electromagnetic flowmeter determinations have shown that significant volumes of blood flow through the anastomoses. Average flows for right coronary grafts are approximately 60 ml per minute (range of 28 to 150 ml), for the anterior descending coronary artery 80 ml per minute (range of 20 to 160 ml), and for the circumflex artery 75 ml per minute (range of 60 to 90 ml). In some patients with severe lesions and with borderline ventricular performance, the use of an intra-aortic balloon from the beginning of the operative procedure has been found helpful. This device is also of considerable importance in weaning difficult patients from cardiopulmonary bypass following the revascularization procedure. In those with extensive disease, the heart may be unable to assume a normal cardiac output immediately, and an intra-aortic balloon pump may be necessary for a period of several hours or days, during which time cardiac function improves sufficiently to maintain the circulation. Its use under these circumstances has clearly led to improved survival. In extenuating circumstances, this device has been used up to several weeks with successful results.

In the recent past there has been an increasing awareness of the association of severe coronary artery disease in patients who present primarily with disorders of the aortic and mitral valves. In these individuals, a surgical attack on the valve alone may be inadequate, and a simultaneous CABG for coronary lesions may be necessary. Similarly, patients with infarction of the papillary muscle and resulting mitral insufficiency often require a CABG procedure in addition to replacement of the mitral valve.

While autologous veins are chosen for the bypass graft in most patients, the internal mammary artery may be used in appropriate circumstances. In some reports, long-term patency has been greater in this vessel than with venous grafts.

POSTOPERATIVE MANAGEMENT. A number of postoperative problems may arise in patients following myocardial revascularization, and prompt diagnosis and immediate therapy are of prime importance. Adequate oxygenation is essential, and the endotracheal tube is generally left in place for the first day to assure adequate ventilation by a respirator. The effectiveness of the ventilatory support should be assessed by blood gas measurements, including Po_2, Pco_2, and pH. The cardiac output should be maintained at a normal level by continuous monitoring of central venous pressure, systemic arterial pressure, the electrocardiogram, and urinary output. Determinations of cardiac output are also important, especially if doubt exists concerning the circulatory status. Should a *low cardiac output syndrome* develop postoperatively, isoproterenol, dopamine, nitroprusside, and other agents should be employed as necessary with careful and continuous monitoring, including pulmonary artery diastolic and left atrial pressures. Cardiac dysrhythmias are common and may require the use of appropriate drugs or electrical cardioversion.

Myocardial infarction following CABG is usually reported in the range of 5 to 15 per cent, and in some series has been higher. The incidence of perioperative myocardial infarction is largely dependent upon the sensitivity of the diagnostic tests employed. For example, when CPK-MB isoenzyme activity is determined, the incidence of intraoperative and perioperative myocardial infarction is generally 30 per cent or more, as this determination is quite sensitive. This contrasts with an incidence of 15 per cent or less in studies in which new Q wave development is the primary criterion upon which the infarction is based. It is interesting that the presence of a perioperative myocardial infarction is generally not dependent upon whether or not the segment of myocardium involved received a graft or, indeed, if the graft was patent postoperatively. Moreover, in most patients in whom perioperative infarction occurs, the clinical manifestations are minimal and the diagnosis is made primarily upon electrocardiographic and enzymatic changes. It is relatively unusual for such patients to experience the signs and symptoms of a clinical myocardial infarction in the characteristic sense. In other words, in the majority of these patients, the infarction might well be unrecognized were it not for the electrocardiographic alterations and changes in serum enzymes.

RESULTS. Although the surgical *mortality* in early reports following CABG ranged up to 12 per cent or more, the figure has fallen considerably in the last several years and is currently in the range of 1 to 2 per cent for patients with *uncomplicated* angina pectoris. The mortality is correspondingly higher in those with severe left ventricular dysfunction, ventricular aneurysms, or associated valvular disease.

Relief of Pain. In nearly all series, an excellent symptomatic response is obtained. In approximately 65 per cent of patients the angina is *completely* relieved with no further medication being required, and much improvement occurs in an additional 25 per cent. With the passage of time pathologic changes may occur in some of the vessels, both in the native coronary arteries and in the inserted grafts. Such changes may be responsible for reappearance of symptoms. When these are present, further clinical evaluation, including coronary arteriography, is indicated.

Graft Patency. The patency rate of venous grafts during the first year following operation approximates 90 per cent. Later, intimal fibrosis may occur in the vein graft and reduce its caliber or produce complete obstruction. The graft may also thrombose, and this is generally the cause of *early* graft failure. In addition, technical features at the site of the anastomosis such as kinking of the graft can produce obstruction. Nevertheless, the distinctive fibrous proliferation which occurs in these grafts is the most common cause of failure and has been described in detail. Of additional interest is the continuation of the basic atherosclerotic process which progresses in the coronary arteries. In one series of patients followed one to four years postoperatively with repeat arteriography, 55 per cent of the original lesions *proximal* to the graft had progressed, whereas only 7 per cent of lesions *distal* to the anastomosis progressed. In this series, 14 per cent of the ungrafted vessels showed progression of atherosclerosis (McLaughlin et al.).

Reoperation. If symptoms recur following myocardial revascularization, reoperation may be indicated. However, the technical problems of the procedure are appreciable, due primarily to epicardial scarring and fibrosis, which make difficult the dissection and anastomosis of the coronary arteries. In one group of 21 patients undergoing reoperation, 33 per cent obtained complete relief of angina, 29 per cent obtained partial relief, and in 38 per cent there was no change. It is therefore apparent that the results following reoperation are less satisfactory than for the original procedure. For this reason, careful consideration should be given the indication when a second CABG procedure is planned.

RESULTS OF MEDICAL VERSUS SURGICAL MANAGEMENT IN RANDOMIZED STUDIES. The preferred method for resolving a problem concerning a controversial form of therapy is its evaluation by a double-blind, randomized study. For surgical forms of therapy, the double-blind feature is generally not feasible, but a randomized study of medical versus surgical treatment can be appropriately undertaken. With this objective, a group of cardiologists and surgeons in a group of Veterans Administration Hospitals combined to perform a cooperative study of patients with ischemic heart disease (Murphy et al.). The patients were randomized to medical and surgical management in an effort to determine the effect upon survival. In a series of 596 patients, 310 were managed by medical means and 286 were randomized to the surgical group. In the latter group a CABG procedure was performed, and the operative mortality at 30 days was 5.6 per cent. At an average of one year following operation, 69 per cent of the grafts were patent and 88 per cent had at least one patent graft. At 36 months, 87 per cent of the medical group and 88 per cent of the surgical group were alive.

This study has been the subject of much interest and considerable controversy, because the results suggest that the CABG procedure does not increase the life span when compared randomly with patients managed medically. Supporters and critics of this study have been numerous, and the principal points of view have been concisely summarized. Controversies of this type frequently arise when the goal of therapy is not *cure*, but rather *improved quality of life*. It has been difficult to define objective criteria to assess the results of either medical or surgical therapy for this group of patients as a whole. Critics of the VA study call attention to the high operative mortality in the series (5.6 per cent) and of the low rate of graft patency (69 per cent at one year), especially when these figures are compared to those which currently prevail. Another criticism is that selectivity was involved in the VA study, with exclusion of patients with unstable angina, left main coronary disease, ventricular aneurysms, and generalized poor ventricular contraction, as well as patients with markedly increased end-diastolic pressure and a large left ventricle with a poor ejection fraction. By exclusion of such patients, the series may have been artificially weighted.

In summary, for those patients who fail to achieve relief of anginal pain despite adequate medical therapy, myocardial revascularization is indicated and can be performed with expectation of very favorable clinical results and a low mortality. In addition, patients known to have a poor prognosis with medical management alone, such as those with significant lesions of the left main coronary artery, are also candidates for revascularization and have been shown in randomized studies to have an improved life expectancy when compared with similar patients managed medically. In a consideration of the total group of patients with symptomatic myocardial ischemia, questions remain concerning the ultimate effect of revascularization upon the life span, and further long-term evaluation will be required before this problem is finally clarified.

Cohen, M. V., Cohn, P. F., Herman, M. V., and Gorlin, R.: Diagnosis and prognosis of main left coronary obstruction. Circulation (Suppl. 1), 45–46:57, 1972.

Daggett, W. M., Guyton, R. A., Mundth, E. D., Buckley, M. J., McEnany, T., Gold, H. K., Leinbach, R. C., and Austen, W. G.: Surgery for postmyocardial infarct ventricular septal defect. Ann. Surg., 186:260, 1977.

Humphries, J. O.: Survival after myocardial infarction. Prognosis and management. Modern Concepts Cardiovasc. Dis., 46:51, 1977.

Kaiser, G. C., Marco, J. D., Barner, H. B., Codd, J. E., Laks, H., and Willman, V. L.: Intraaortic balloon assistance. Ann. Thorac. Surg., 21:487, 1976.

McLaughlin, P. R., Berman, N. D., Morton, B. C., McLoughlin, M. J., Aldridge, H. E., Adelman, A. G., Goldman, B. S., Trimble, A. S., and Morch, J. E.: Saphenous vein bypass grafting. Changes in native circulation and collaterals. Circulation (Suppl. 1), 51–52:66, 1975.

Murphy, M. L., Hultgren, H. N., Detre, K., Thomsen, J., Takaro, T., and participants of the Veterans Administration Cooperative Study: Treatment of chronic stable angina. A preliminary report of survival data of the randomized Veterans Administration Cooperative Study. N. Engl. J. Med., 297:621, 1977.

Rerych, S. K., Scholz, P. M., Newman, G. E., Sabiston, D. C., Jr., and Jones R. H.: Cardiac function at rest and during exercise in normals and in patients with coronary heart disease. Evaluation by radionuclide angiocardiography. Ann. Surg., 187:423, 1978.

Sabiston, D. C., Jr.: The coronary circulation. The William F. Rienhoff, Jr., Lecture. Johns Hopkins Med. J., 134:314, 1974.

364. CARDIAC ARRHYTHMIA

Anthony N. Damato

364.1. INTRODUCTION

Normally, the pacemaker of the heart is the sinoatrial (SA) node, which is an elongated structure (1.5 cm in length) located at the junction of the superior vena cava and the lateral border of the right atrium. In 55 per cent of cases the SA node receives its blood supply from the right coronary artery, and in 45 per cent of the cases, from the left circumflex artery. Cells of the SA node possess the property of automaticity which is responsible for the spontaneous rhythmicity of the heartbeat. Automatic or pacemaker cells undergo spontaneous diastolic depolarization (phase 4 depolarization) in contrast to nonautomatic or working myocardial cells which maintain a steady diastolic or resting potential. When an automatic cell achieves threshold potential, it undergoes depolarization and serves as the excitatory or depolarizing stimulus for adjacent cells. Increasing the rate of diastolic depolarization of sinoatrial nodal pacemaker cells increases the heart rate and vice versa. The property of spontaneous diastolic depolarization can also be found in certain cells of the atrium, atrioventricular (AV) junction, bundle branches, and Purkinje network, but not in ordinary working myocardial cells. These specialized cells serve as latent or potential pacemakers of the heart, and their rate of spontaneous diastolic depolarization is normally less than that of the sinoatrial node. However, if sinus node function is depressed, latent pacemaker activity can emerge and establish an escape rhythm. At other times, certain stimuli such as digitalis excess, ischemia, or hypoxia can enhance the rate of spontaneous diastolic depolarization of latent pacemakers beyond that of normal sinus node automaticity, which then results in an ectopic rhythm.

The transmission of impulses from the sinus node to the ventricles occurs along specialized conducting tissue which includes the AV node, the bundle of His (also called the common AV bundle), the right bundle branch, the left bundle branch, including its fascicular divisions, and the subendocardial Purkinje network. The bundle of His, bundle branches, and Purkinje network are commonly referred to as the His-Purkinje system or the ventricular specialized conducting system. In addition, three internodal connecting pathways (anterior, middle, and posterior internodal tracts) have been described which originate from the sinus node region and insert into different parts of the AV node.

Fibers from these internodal pathways also spread in various degrees from the right to the left atrium. It has been suggested by some investigators that transmission of the sinus node impulse to the AV node and between the atria is along these specialized and preferential pathways and not by radial spread alone. Internodal pathways have also been invoked to explain some cases of short P-R interval in which it is suspected that an atrial impulse either partially or completely bypasses the AV node during its conduction to the ventricles.

The AV node lies beneath the right atrial endocardium, anterior to the os of the coronary sinus, and above the insertion of the septal leaflet of the tricuspid valve. The human adult AV node measures between 5 and 7 mm in length, and its deep surface abuts the central fibrous body of the heart. Anteriorly, the AV node is directly continuous with the bundle of His. Most of the fibers of the internodal tracts, mentioned above, enter the superior and posterior margins of the AV node, and a smaller number of fibers enter along its lateral margin. Conduction velocity within the AV node is slow (0.05 meter per second), which accounts in part for the normal physiologic AV delay that is reflected in the P-R interval. In most human hearts, the AV node receives its blood supply from the right coronary artery, which explains the association of AV nodal conduction abnormalities seen in some cases of inferior or diaphragmatic myocardial infarctions.

The anterior and deep part of the AV node becomes the common AV bundle or bundle of His in which the muscle fibers are arranged in parallel. The bundle of His penetrates the collagenous central fibrous body and lies on the upper margin of the muscular interventricular septum. At the posterior margin of the membranous interventricular septum the common bundle gives off a relatively wide left bundle branch which courses over the left side of the interventricular septum. The left bundle branch divides into anterior and posterior fascicles which enter the anterior and posterior papillary muscles, respectively. In addition, fibers from the left bundle insert directly into the interventricular septum. On the right side of the heart, the common bundle continues as a slender right bundle branch which courses over the interventricular septum and enters the anterior papillary muscle. Peripheral arborization of the right and left bundle branches constitutes the Purkinje network. In contrast to the AV node, the velocity of conduction throughout the His-Purkinje system is more rapid, being within the order of 1.0 to 3.5 meters per second.

The AV node and the proximal portion of the bundle of HIs are in close anatomic relationship to the tricuspid and mitral valve rings. In addition, the distal part of the bundle of His and the proximal portions of the bundle branches lie in close proximity to the noncoronary artery aortic cusp. These anatomic relationships of the AV conducting system are important to bear in mind, because inflammation, fibrosis, or calcification of the valve rings or central fibrous body may cause different types of AV block.

The P-R interval represents a combination of intra-arterial, AV nodal, and His-Purkinje conduction times. Unfortunately, the electrical activities of the sinus node, AV node, bundle of His, bundle branches, and subendocardial Purkinje network are not recorded by the surface electrocardiogram. Figure 1 presents in a schematic way the electrical events occurring during the P-R in-

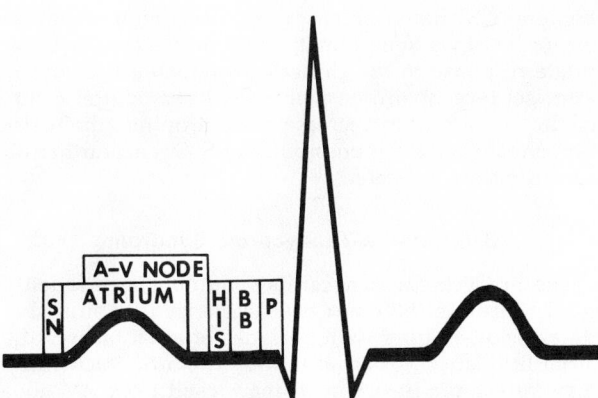

Figure 1. Schematic representation of the sequence of AV conduction in relationship to the P wave, P-R segment and QRS complex. SN = sinus node impulse; AV node = atrioventricular node; HIS = His bundle; BB = bundle branches; P = subendocardial Purkinje system. (Modified from Hoffman, B. F., and Singer, D. H.: Prog. Cardiovasc. Dis., 7:226, 1964.)

terval. The sinus node generates an impulse prior to the inscription of the P wave. As the atrial muscle is being depolarized (P wave), the sinus node impulse enters the AV node. Conduction within the bundle of His, bundle branches, and subendocardial Purkinje network occurs during the P-R segment. The QRS complex represents depolarization of the ventricular muscle.

It has become possible to record electrical activity of the bundle of His in man, using an electrode catheter which is fluoroscopically positioned in the region of the tricuspid valve. The electrode catheter records a low atrial electrogram (A), a His bundle deflection (H) which appears as a bi- or triphasic deflection within the P-R segment, and a ventricular electrogram (V) (Fig. 2). His bundle recordings permit division of the P-R interval into two subintervals, namely the A-H and H-V intervals. The A-H interval represents an approximation of AV nodal conduction time, and the H-V interval represents conduction time within the His-Purkinje system. Normal values for A-H and H-V inter-

vals have varied slightly as reported by different investigators, but in general are 60 to 140 msec and 30 to 55 msec, respectively. Bundle of His recordings provide a more precise method of localizing sites of AV conduction delay and block which may occur proximal to, within, or distal to the bundle of His. In addition, bundle of His recordings provide an accurate method for determining whether beats are of supraventricular or ventricular origin. Beats of supraventricular origin are preceded by His deflections with H-V intervals which are normal or greater than normal. In general, beats of ventricular origin are not preceded by His deflections.

364.2. ARRHYTHMIAS

SINUS ARRHYTHMIA

Sinus arrhythmia is characterized by irregular changes in the sinus rate which most often occur in relationship to the phases of respiration. The sinus rate increases at end inspiration and decreases at end expiration. The respiratory changes in sinus rate are believed to result from changes in vagal tone. Sinus arrhythmia is a normal phenomenon seen more frequently in children and young adults and tends to become less pronounced with increasing age. Electrocardiographically the P wave configuration is normal but may show slight changes in shape. The P-P intervals show cyclical increases and decreases in relation to the phase of respiration, whereas the P-R intervals remain fairly constant. Sinus arrhythmia requires no treatment.

SINUS BRADYCARDIA

Sinus bradycardia has been arbitrarily defined as a sinus rate of less than 60 per minute. It is a normal finding in a significant number of young healthy adults and is the expected finding in well trained athletes. Sinus bradycardia may result from administration of drugs such as digitalis, propranolol, morphine, reserpine, and prostigmine. Normal sinus rates return when these drugs are withdrawn. A temporary sinus bradycardia may occur during acute diaphragmatic myocardial infarction. Usually, sinus bradycardia is associated with normal AV conduction (1:1 AV response with a normal P-R interval). In older patients sinus bradycardia and AV block may coexist. Sinus bradycardia at rates of 40 per minute or less should raise the possibility of a 2:1 sinus node exit block, which is a rare phenomenon (see Fig. 4).

In general, sinus bradycardia requires no treatment. In most cases, the sinus rate shows a normal acceleration in response to exercise, atropine, or other appropriate stimuli. An inappropriate response to such stimuli raises the possibility of the sick sinus syndrome. If symptoms such as lightheadedness, syncope, congestive heart failure, or angina pectoris are the result of a low resting heart rate or inappropriate acceleration of the heart rate during stressful situations, a permanent ventricular pacemaker should be inserted.

SINUS TACHYCARDIA

For adults, sinus tachycardia is defined as a sinus rate in excess of 100 per minute. Most often, sinus ta-

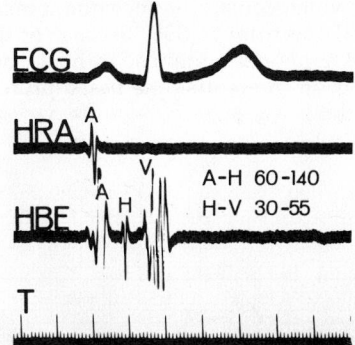

Figure 2. Tracings from top to bottom are as follows: surface ECG; a recording from the high right atrium (HRA); His bundle electrogram recording (HBE); and time lines (T) at 10 and 100 msec. A = Low atrial electrogram; H = His bundle electrogram; V = ventricular electrogram. During sinus rhythm the sequence of activation is from the high to low atrium. During retrograde conduction across the AV node, the sequence of atrial activation is reversed; the low atrial electrogram precedes the high atrial electrogram.

chycardia represents a normal physiologic response to stressful situations such as exercise, fright, emotional upset, fever, congestive heart failure, and hypotension. Under these conditions, the increase in sinus rate is generally associated with a normal or less than normal P-R interval, because the sympathetic stimuli causing sinus node acceleration also enhance AV nodal conduction. Vagolytic drugs, such as atropine, can also produce a sinus tachycardia. The treatment for sinus tachycardia is that of the underlying condition. Carotid sinus pressure will produce a temporary and incomplete slowing of the sinus rate which quickly returns to original levels. If sinus tachycardia is the result of congestive heart failure, digitalis will slow the sinus rate as the failure improves. However, digitalis will be ineffective in sinus tachycardia from other causes such as fever or thyrotoxicosis.

SICK SINUS SYNDROME

The sick sinus syndrome (SSS) refers to a variety of electrocardiographic abnormalities which result from dysfunction of the sinoatrial node. Included in SSS are the following:

1. Persistent, severe, or unexpected sinus bradycardia. At times, sinus bradycardia may alternate with episodes of supraventricular tachyarrhythmias, and this combination has been termed the bradycardia-tachycardia syndrome.

2. Sinoatrial block or exit block not related to drug therapy.

3. Sinus arrest (cessation of sinus rhythm) for short or long intervals, during which time either no escape rhythm arises or an atrial, junctional, or ventricular rhythm emerges.

These electrocardiographic abnormalities result because (1) the sinus node fails as an impulse generator, or (2) the sinus node impulse is delayed or blocked in its conduction out to the atrial muscle. Often, patients with SSS have an associated AV block or intraventricular conduction abnormality. The most commonly encountered symptoms in SSS are lightheadedness, dizziness, syncope, convulsions, dyspnea, fatigue, and angina pectoris.

Sinus Bradycardia

Sinus bradycardia may be the initial manifestation of SSS, and consequently not all sinus bradycardias are benign. SSS should be suspected when sinus bradycardia occurs in a symptomatic patient or is an inappropriate response to the clinical environs, such as during exercise, fever, pain, or congestive heart failure. Failure of the sinus rate to increase after atropine administration should raise the possibility of SSS, and further observations are indicated.

Bradycardia-Tachycardia Syndrome

The bradycardia-tachycardia syndrome is included in the spectrum of SSS and is characterized by sinus bradycardia alternating with episodes of atrial tachycardia, atrial fibrillation, or atrial flutter. The atrial tachycardia may be ectopic in origin or may result from AV nodal re-entry (Fig. 3). Symptoms may be related to either slow or rapid heart rates or both.

TREATMENT. Sinus bradycardia as a manifestation of SSS is generally, although not always, unresponsive to pharmacologic treatment. If belladonna alkaloids, atropine, or sympathomimetic amines are ineffectual in speeding up the sinus rate and the patient is symptomatic from the slow heart rate, a permanent ventricular pacemaker should be inserted. In the bradycardia-tachycardia syndrome the therapeutic problem is compounded by the fact that not only are agents such as procainamide and quinidine often ineffectual in controlling the atrial tachyarrhythmias, but these drugs may aggravate the sinus bradycardia. Likewise, digitalis, which can effectively slow the ventricular response during a period of supraventricular tachycardia, may also worsen the bradycardia. The most effective therapy to date has been the insertion of a permanent ventricular pacemaker by which the ventricular rate can be controlled and pharmacologic agents more safely administered to control the atrial arrhythmia.

SINOATRIAL BLOCK

The tissue surrounding the sinoatrial node normally imposes a conduction delay between the sinus node impulse and depolarization of the atrial myocardium. Disturbances in conduction of the sinus node impulse can take the form of first, second, or third degree SA block, all of which constitute uncommon manifestations of the clinical spectrum of SSS. Because of the inability to record the sinus node impulse in man, the diagnosis of SA block is an inferential one based primarily on the behavior of the P waves.

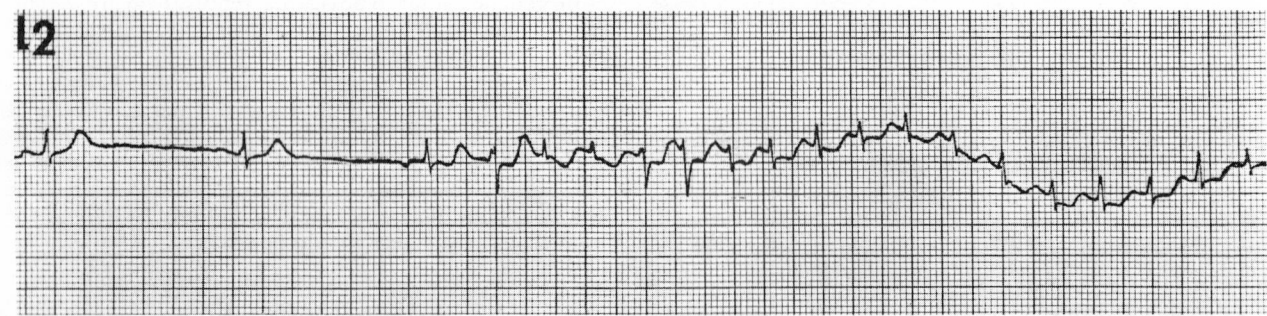

Figure 3. Bradycardia-tachycardia syndrome. After two sinus beats (rate, 45 per minute), two ectopic atrial beats occur, the second of which initiates an AV nodal re-entrant tachycardia. The initial part of the tachycardia shows aberrant ventricular conduction.

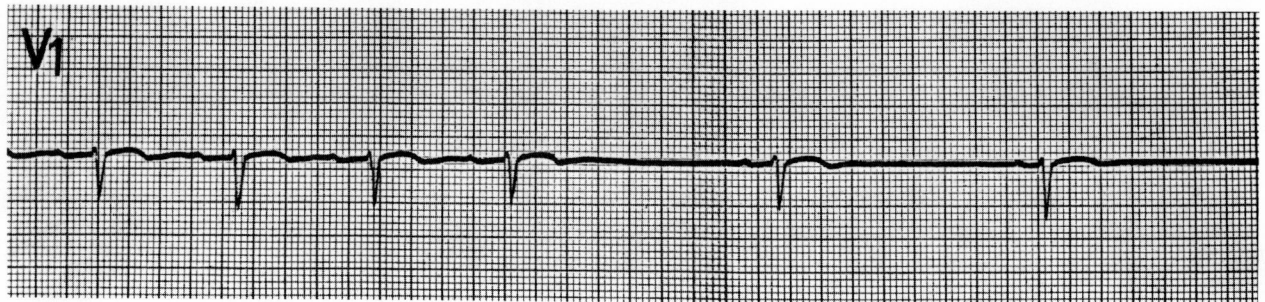

Figure 4. 2:1 SA exit block. The sinus rate is suddenly halved.

First Degree SA Block

In the first degree SA block the sinus node impulse is conducted more slowly out to the atrial myocardium. However, the clinical diagnosis of uncomplicated first-degree SA block cannot be made, because each sinus impulse elicits a P wave and the degree of delay is not reflected in the EKG recording.

Second Degree SA Block

Second degree SA block, like second degree AV block, has been classified into types I and II.

Type I Second Degree SA Block

In type I second degree SA block, sinoatrial conduction is of a Wenckebach type in which there is progressive conduction delay until a sinus node impulse fails to elicit a P wave. Like AV nodal Wenckebach cycles, the increment of SA conduction delay increases throughout the cycle so that the P-P intervals progressively shorten prior to the dropped wave. The P-P interval encompassing the dropped P wave is less than twice the P-P interval preceding the absent P wave.

Type II Second Degree SA Block

In type II second degree SA block, a sinus P wave is intermittently and unexpectedly dropped. The resultant pause is equal to twice the normal P-P interval. Atrial extrasystoles, which are hidden in the T wave and followed by a near compensatory pause, may simulate a type II SA block. In 2:1 SA block the normal sinus rate is halved. The resultant bradycardia is indistinguishable from the usual variety of sinus bradycardia unless an abrupt spontaneous doubling of the heart rate occurs (Fig. 4). Atrial bigeminy in which the ectopic P waves are masked by the T wave may simulate 2:1 SA block.

Third Degree SA Block

In third degree SA block, all the sinus impulses are blocked and there is absence of P waves. After a period of arrest, a subsidiary pacemaker located in the atrium, AV junction, or ventricles usually emerges as an escape rhythm. Third degree SA block is indistinguishable from sinus node arrest in which the pacemaker cells fail to generate impulses (Fig. 5).

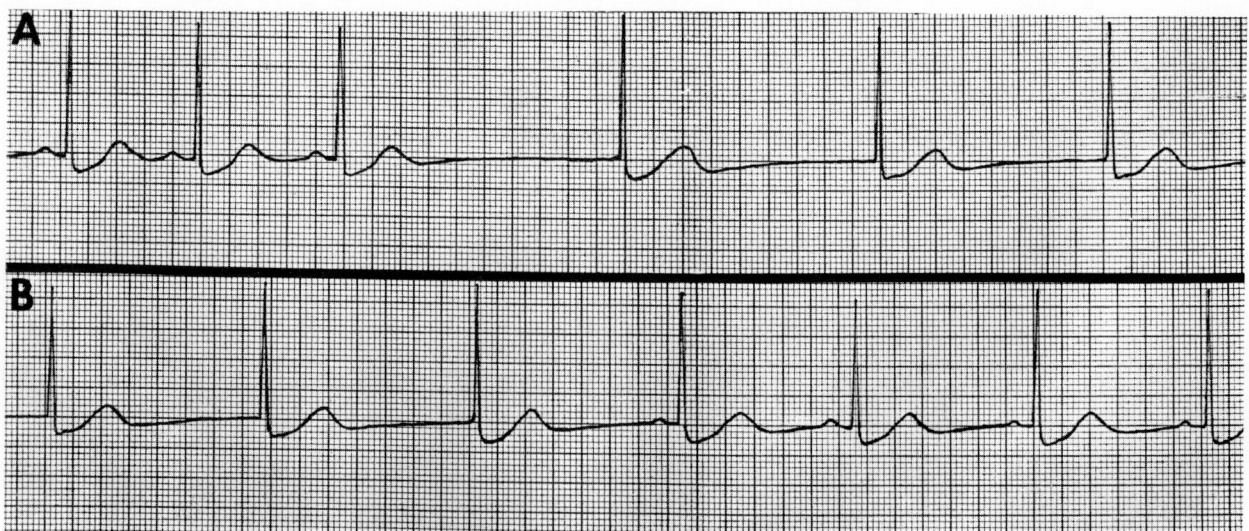

Figure 5. Third degree SA block. After three sinus beats, the sinus node impulse either fails to be generated or to exit from the sinus node. An AV junctional pacemaker emerges, followed by resumption of sinus rhythm. During the AV junctional rhythm, the QRS complexes are similar to those of sinus origin.

ABERRATION

Ventricular aberration is defined as an alteration in the sequence of ventricular activation which results whenever an impulse of supraventricular origin is asynchronously conducted within the His-Purkinje system. Aberration results because a supraventricular impulse enters the His-Purkinje system during its refractory period. For atrial impulses the determinants of aberration include (1) the degree of prematurity of the atrial impulse; (2) the cycle length (R-R interval) preceding the premature atrial impulse; (3) the speed of AV nodal conduction; and (4) the state of recovery of excitability of the His-Purkinje system. In general, the more premature an atrial impulse, the greater the tendency for aberration to occur. Fast or relatively rapid AV nodal conduction enhances the possibility of aberration, because the premature atrial impulse can be delivered to the His-Purkinje system during its refractory period. However, at very close coupling intervals, aberrant ventricular activation may disappear if the premature atrial impulse encounters sufficient AV nodal delay that its arrival time within the His-Purkinje system is delayed and the latter is no longer refractory.

A direct relationship exists between cycle length (R-R interval) and refractoriness within the His-Purkinje system. Refractoriness of the His-Purkinje system increases with longer R-R intervals and decreases as the R-R interval shortens. A long R-R interval preceding a sufficiently premature atrial beat favors aberration, whereas decreasing the preceding cycle length may abolish aberration.

Aberrant conduction involving the right bundle branch is seen more commonly than aberration involving the left bundle branch. Given the right conditions, aberrant ventricular activation can occur in normal or abnormal hearts and therefore is not a sign of heart disease. Aberrant conduction of consecutive beats during a surpaventricular tachycardia can mimic a ventricular tachycardia. Examples of aberrant conduction of supraventricular impulses are shown in Figures 3, 6, and 8.

ATRIAL EXTRASYSTOLES

Atrial extrasystoles are premature depolarizations of the atria resulting from impulses which originate in ectopic foci located anywhere within the atria. Atrial extrasystoles are also referred to as premature atrial beats, premature atrial contractions, or premature atrial systoles.

Atrial extrasystoles result in P waves (P') which are different from sinus P waves. These differences, which may be marked or subtle, are due to an altered sequence of atrial activation resulting from an ectopic origin of the depolarizing impulse.

Atrial extrasystoles may have a constant or inconstant coupling interval to the preceding sinus beat and can occur in a bigeminal or trigeminal sequence. Three or more consecutive atrial extrasystoles occurring at a rate of 100 per minute or greater constitute an ectopic atrial tachycardia.

Atrial extrasystoles occurring late in the diastolic period may be associated with little or no AV conduction delay, in which case the P-R interval will be the same as or close to that of the sinus beats. Extrasystoles of greater prematurity are almost always associated with an increased P-R interval (relative to sinus beats), which may be due to conduction delay within the AV node, His-Purkinje system, or both.

Atrial extrasystoles may result in normal or aberrant ventricular activation, the determinants of which are discussed above. Aberrant ventricular activation may mimic premature ventricular extrasystoles if the premature atrial P' wave is not recognized or is obscured within the T wave of the preceding QRS complex (Fig. 6). Atrial extrasystoles which are not conducted to the ventricles may block within the AV node or His-Purkinje system. A nonconducted atrial extrasystole may result in prolongation of the P-R interval of one or more subsequent sinus beats — a phenomenon which is called concealed conduction.

Atrial extrasystoles generally invade and prematurely depolarize the sinus node pacemaker, causing a reset of the sinus cycle which is reflected in the pause that follows the atrial extrasystole. If the delay in the appearance of the postextrasystolic sinus beat equals the prematurity of the atrial extrasystole, the pause is said to be compensatory. In a fully compensatory pause, the sum of the pre- and postextrasystolic R-R intervals equals two sinus cycle lengths. Complete compensatory pauses are uncommonly associated with atrial extrasystoles. More often, one sees postextrasystolic pauses which are incompletely compensatory; that is, the sum of the pre- and postextrasystolic pauses is less than two sinus cycles. Occasionally, one may see significant suppression of sinus node automaticity after an extrasystole.

Atrial extrasystoles are common and may occur in completely normal individuals or may be associated with various types of organic heart disease. They may presage atrial fibrillation, atrial flutter, ectopic atrial ta-

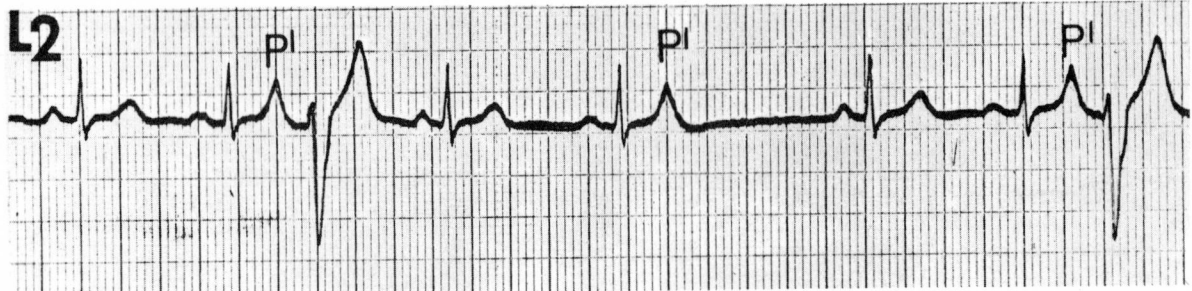

Figure 6. The third, sixth, and ninth P waves (P') are atrial extrasystoles which occur with trigeminal regularity. The first and third atrial extrasystoles are aberrantly conducted to the ventricles. The second atrial extrasystole is blocked.

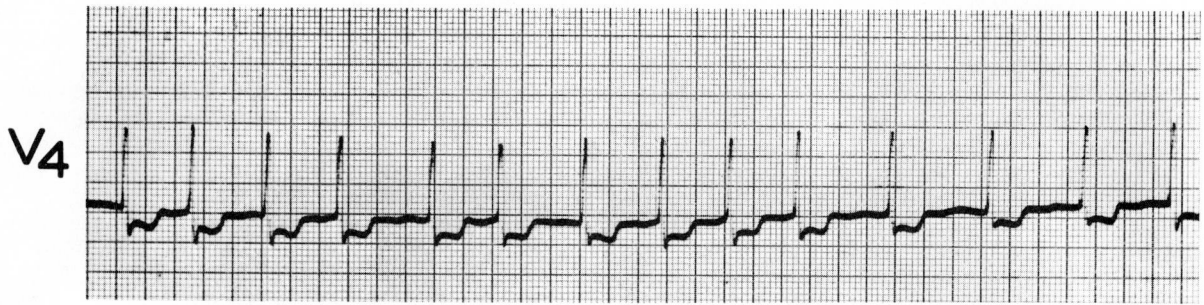

Figure 7. Untreated atrial fibrillation. There is absence of P waves with an irregular ventricular rate.

chycardias, or AV nodal re-entrant tachycardias. Very often, patients are unaware of the presence of infrequent atrial extrasystoles, and no special treatment is required. The patient may complain of "skipped beats" and "palpitations" which are the result of the pause and forceful ventricular contraction that follow the extrasystole. Mild sedation and abstinence from alcohol, tobacco, or caffeine may be all that is required to treat occasional extrasystoles which produce mild symptoms. Quinidine sulfate is used to treat atrial extrasystoles which cause disturbing symptoms, foreshadow other atrial arrhythmias, or are unabated by conservative measures.

ATRIAL FIBRILLATION

Atrial fibrillation is a frequently encountered cardiac arrhythmia which commonly occurs in association with some form of organic heart disease. Most cases of atrial fibrillation are associated with arteriosclerotic heart disease, followed in frequency by rheumatic and hypertensive heart disease. A high incidence of this rhythm disorder is seen in patients with thryotoxicosis. The greater tendency for enlarged atria to fibrillate may explain the frequent occurrence of atrial fibrillation in patients with congestive heart failure and mitral valvular disease. Atrial fibrillation, usually paroxysmal in nature, can occur in apparently healthy individuals who have no detectable evidence of associated heart disease.

The exact mechanism(s) underlying the development of atrial fibrillation is uncertain. Many of its characteristics are compatible with re-entry of multiple activation fronts. However, the fact that atrial fibrillation is frequently induced by premature atrial extrasystoles suggests that alterations in automaticity also play a role in the mechanism of this arrhythmia. Factors which favor the development and perpetuation of atrial fibrillation include frequent atrial extrasystoles, increased vagal tone, and an increase in atrial muscle mass wherein significant differences in conduction and refractoriness exist in adjacent fibers. Atrial fibrillation can be precipitated by a single atrial extrasystole which occurs in the so-called vulnerable period of the atrial cycle. At sinus cycle lengths the atrial vulnerable period has been estimated to be between 180 and 300 msec after a sinus P wave.

ELECTROCARDIOGRAPHIC FEATURES. Atrial fibrillation is characterized by absence of P waves and an irregular ventricular response. Normal sinus P waves are replaced by irregular chaotic and rapid atrial impulses occurring in excess of 400 per minute. The presence or absence of P waves is best observed in leads II and V_1. Atrial fibrillation has been described as "coarse" when the baseline of the electrocardiogram presents rapid, irregular fibrillatory (f) waves of varying amplitude, and "fine" when practically no atrial activity is detected. In untreated and uncomplicated atrial fibrillation, the irregular and rapid ventricular response is generally between 110 and 160 per minute, and most or all of the QRS complexes are of normal configuration for that patient (Fig. 7).

Concealed conduction within the AV node is the major determinant of the irregular R-R cycles during atrial fibrillation. The inherent capacity of the AV node to accept and transmit impulses to the ventricles is exceeded by the rapid, irregular atrial rate in atrial fibrillation. Consequently, many atrial impulses are blocked or concealed within the AV node, thereby altering its state of refractoriness which in turn affects the conduction of subsequent impulses. Impulses which exit from the AV node and enter the His-Purkinje system almost invariably result in a ventricular response. Uncommonly is the His-Purkinje system the site of concealment. Digitalis, propranolol, or increased vagal tone increases the degree of concealment or block within the AV node and thereby slows the ventricular response. The irregular R-R intervals during atrial fibrillation predispose to the occurrence of aberrant intraventricular conduction. In atrial fibrillation the distinction between aberrant conduction and ventricular ectopy is an important one which unfortunately is made more difficult because of the absence of P waves. The diagnosis of aberrant conduction is favored (80 per cent of the time) if the beat in question (1) has a right bundle branch block pattern, (2) terminates a short cycle which is preceded by a long cycle, and (3) has initial vector forces which are the same as known supraventricular beats. No single criterion or combination of criteria provides absolute evidence for the origin of any beat. The distinction can be made with bundle of His recordings. In atrial fibrillation with a rapid ventricular response, aberration may persist for many consecutive cycles and may simulate ventricular tachycardia. The occurrence of aberrant conduction during digitalis administration for atrial fibrillation is not a contraindication to continued use of the drug. In fact aberration usually disappears when the desired effect of ventricular slowing is achieved with digitalis. On the other hand, ventricular ectopy may signify digitalis toxicity or the presence of an additional dysrhythmic problem.

TREATMENT. Treatment of atrial fibrillation depends upon the urgency of the situation. If the irregular rapid ventricular response is causing severe dyspnea, hypotension, congestive heart failure, or severe anginal pain, conversion to normal sinus rhythm by DC countershock is the treatment of choice. DC countershock is contraindicated if it is suspected that digitalis intoxication is the cause of atrial fibrillation, which is uncommon. In less urgent situations, ventricular slowing is achieved with digitalis. Digoxin, 0.5 mg, is given intravenously and followed by a second dose in one half to one hour. If the ventricular rate is slowed (80 to 100 per minute), maintenance therapy of 0.25 mg digoxin per day is started. If the ventricular rate is not slowed within two hours of the initial dose, 0.25 mg digoxin is given every three to four hours until the desired effect is obtained. Infrequently, digitalis may convert atrial fibrillation to sinus rhythm. Propranolol may be used in conjunction with digitalis for those patients requiring excessive amounts of digitalis to slow the ventricular rate.

Once the ventricular rate is under control, consideration is given as to whether conversion to sinus rhythm is indicated. Conversion should not be attempted in those patients who have longstanding chronic atrial fibrillation, or in whom previous conversions have been unsuccessfully maintained. In some patients with severe heart disease, the loss of atrial contribution to the cardiac output may be significant, and conversion to sinus rhythm is necessary in order to avoid intractable heart failure. Patients with atrial fibrillation of recent onset should be converted to sinus rhythm, using either DC countershock or quinidine sulfate. The maintenance dose of digitalis should be withheld for one to two days prior to DC countershock.

ATRIAL FLUTTER

Atrial flutter is characterized by a rapid, regular atrial rate between 220 and 350 beats per minute. However, there is no universal agreement about which range of atrial rates specifically defines atrial flutter and separates it from an ectopic atrial tachycardia. There can be an overlap in the lower ranges of atrial rate; some ectopic atrial tachycardias may achieve trial rates of 220 beats per minute, whereas some cases of atrial flutter may be associated with rates of less than 220 beats per minute. Atrial flutter is almost always associated with some form of organic heart disease (coronary artery disease, cor pulmonale, rheumatic valvular disease), and rarely does it occur in normal healthy individuals. Digitalis is rarely a cause

of atrial flutter. Clinical symptoms associated with atrial flutter are related primarily to the ventricular response. Atrial flutter with a 3:1 or 4:1 AV conduction ratio may result in no symptoms, and the patient may be unaware of any dysrhythmia. On the other hand, during a 2:1 or a varying AV conduction ratio, the patient may experience palpitations, shortness of breath, anginal symptoms, or congestive heart failure.

ELECTROCARDIOGRAPHIC FEATURES. The following are the commonly found electrocardiographic features associated with atrial flutter: (1) the atrial rate is between 220 and 350 beats per minute; (2) the P waves are broad, bizarre atrial deflections which have been termed F waves; (3) leads II, III, and AVF show a "sawtooth effect with absence of an isoelectric period between flutter waves." One flutter wave appears to be merging directly with the next. The "sawtooth" effect may be absent in lead I and left-sided chest leads (v_5, V_6); (4) in most cases of atrial flutter, atrial activation is in a caudocranial direction; and (5) some degree of AV block exists which may be fixed, alternating, or variable. Many of the characteristic features associated with atrial flutter are presented in Figure 8.

A 1:1 AV response in atrial flutter is very uncommon, because atrial rates of 220 or greater generally exceed the inherent transmission capacity of the AV node. The presence of atrial flutter with a suspected 1:1 AV response should raise the possibility of an accessory or anomalous AV pathway such as exists in the Wolff-Parkinson-White syndrome. Conduction ratios of 2:1 or 4:1 are more commonly observed. Effective vagotonic maneuvers such as carotid sinus pressure temporarily increase the degree of AV block, permit a more positive identification of the atrial flutter waves, and do not significantly affect the atrial flutter rate. At times an increase in vagal tone which causes a shortening of atrial refractory period may convert atrial flutter to atrial fibrillation. By a similar mechanism, digitalis may convert atrial flutter to fibrillation.

TREATMENT. Direct current countershock is very effective in converting atrial flutter to sinus rhythm and is often the treatment of choice. Conversion can be achieved with low energy discharges. Direct current countershock is certainly the treatment of choice when the ventricular response is rapid and the patient is symptomatic.

Atrial pacing by means of an electrode catheter at rates slightly or greatly in excess of the inherent flutter rate has been used in the treatment of atrial flutter. Cessation of pacing may result in normal sinus rhythm or atrial fi-

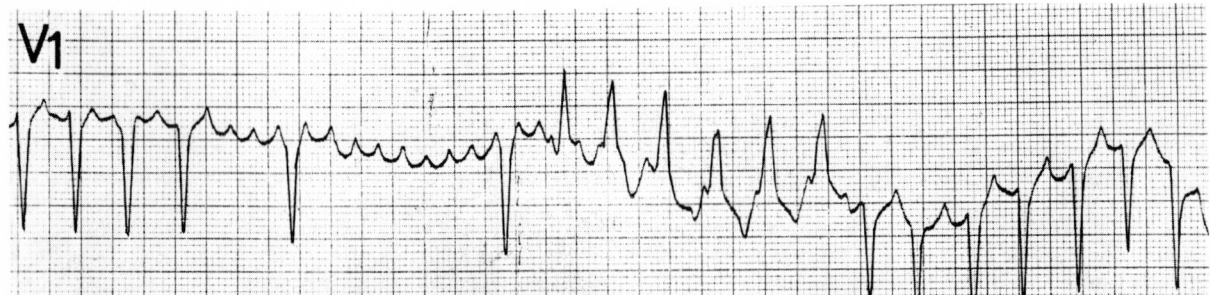

Figure 8. Atrial flutter with varying degrees of AV block. In the middle of the tracing, a period of high degree AV block occurs, during which time the atrial flutter waves are more easily identified. The second to the sixth beats after the long pause are aberrantly conducted with a right bundle branch block pattern.

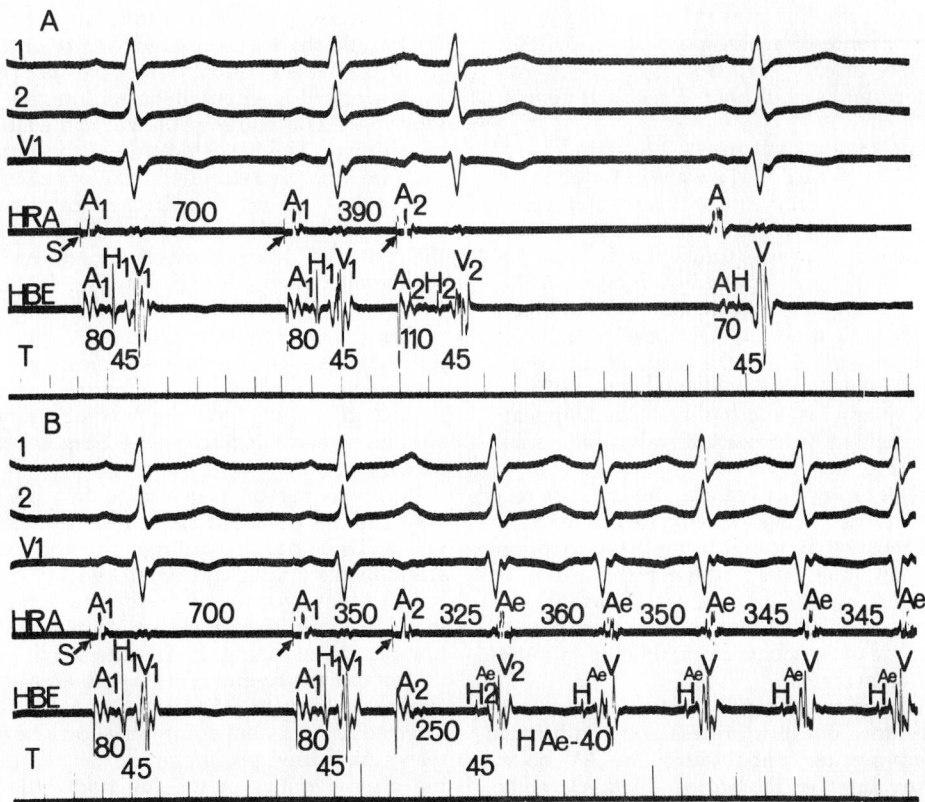

Figure 9. Re-entry within the AV node resulting in paroxysmal atrial tachycardia. In panels *A* and *B*, the tracings from top to bottom are electrocardiographic leads 1, 2, and V_1, a high right atrial electrogram (HRA), His bundle electrogram (HBE), and time lines (T) at 10 and 100 msec. In each panel, the first two beats are the last in a series of paced atrial beats at a constant cycle of 700 msec (A_1-A_1). The A-H and H-V intervals are 80 and 45 msec, respectively. Note that the sequence of atrial activation for paced atrial beats and sinus beats (fourth beat in Panel *A*) is from the high to low, right atrium. In Panel *A*, a premature atrial depolarization (A_2) is induced 390 msec after A_1. A_2 conducts with some AV nodal delay (A-H 110 msec), after which sinus rhythm resumes. In Panel *B*, A_2 is introduced 350 msec after A_1 and conducts more slowly through the AV node (A-H 250 msec). For this patient an AV nodal conduction time of 250 msec was apparently sufficient to induce an AV nodal re-entrant tachycardia at a cycle length of 345 msec. Note that during re-entry, atrial activation (Ae) occurs within the QRS complex and from the low to high right atrium.

brillation. Usually atrial fibrillation is not sustained and may convert to normal sinus rhythm in a matter of seconds or hours. The atrial pacing technique is useful when repeated DC shocks are required because of recurrent or persistent atrial flutter.

Digitalis and quinidine sulfate are the primary drugs used in the treatment of atrial flutter. Depending upon the urgency of the situation, digitalis may be given intravenously or orally. Its main function is to increase the degree of AV nodal block and to slow the ventricular rate. Rarely does digitalis convert atrial flutter directly to sinus rhythm; it may, however, convert flutter to atrial fibrillation, whereupon withdrawal of digitalis may re-establish sinus rhythm or atrial flutter may resume. Once the ventricular rate is controlled with digitalis, quinidine sulfate is given orally to convert the atrial flutter to sinus rhythm. It is preferred not to give quinidine initially without first digitalizing the patient, because quinidine may slow the atrial flutter rate, enhance AV nodal conduction, and precipitate dangerously rapid ventricular rates. If digitalis and quinidine are the primary therapies and prove to be unsuccessful, cardioversion by direct current countershock can be used but only after digitalis has been withheld for several days, because countershock and excessive amounts of digitalis may precipitate more serious ventricular dysrhythmias.

PAROXYSMAL ATRIAL TACHYCARDIA

Paroxysmal atrial tachycardia (PAT) is a relatively common arrhythmia. Several types of PAT are recognized which differ in etiology, underlying mechanism, and therapeutic approach. PAT may result from sustained re-entry within the AV junction or may be ectopic in origin. Three types of AV junctional re-entry have been reasonably well defined; these include AV nodal re-entry, re-entry utilizing a VA accessory pathway, and the Wolff-Parkinson-White syndrome (considered below). Undoubtedly, there are other types of junctional re-entries, but these appear less common and less well defined.

PAT Due to Sustained Reciprocation or Re-entry Within the AV Node

PAT that is due to AV nodal re-entry is seen in all age groups and frequently occurs in the absence of any clinically detectable heart disease. Characteristically, these tachycardias begin and terminate abruptly. During the tachycardia the patient may be keenly aware of a rapid heart rate and may complain of a fluttering within the chest or palpitations. Other associated symptoms include dyspnea, lightheadedness, or diaphoresis. Syncope may occur upon termination of the tachycardia if a sufficiently long pause follows prior to re-establishment of sinus rhythm or the occurrence of an escape beat. In patients with coronary artery disease, episodes of PAT may produce angina pectoris and significant S-T segment depression.

ELECTROCARDIOGRAPHIC FEATURES. Sustained re-entry within the AV node is almost always initiated by an atrial extrasystole. It is uncommon for this type of tachycardia to be precipitated by a ventricular extrasystole. If an atrial extrasystole encounters sufficient antegrade delay within the AV node (as indicated by a prolonged P-R or A-H interval), the impulse may at some point enter a nonrefractory pathway within the AV node and may be retrogradely transmitted back to the atria. If the retrogradely conducted impulse finds the antegrade pathway recovered, it may re-enter it, and the sequence is repeated, resulting in sustained reciprocation and a paroxysmal atrial tachycardia (Fig. 9).

During the reciprocating tachycardia, the atria are retrogradely activated. The P waves are inverted in leads II, III, and AVF and most often occur during the inscription of the QRS complex. The rate of these tachycardias is generally between 150 and 250 per minute. Aberrant conduction may occur for the first few beats or may persist for the entire episode of the tachycardia, thereby mimicking a ventricular tachycardia.

Perpetuation of a re-entrant tachycardia depends primarily upon a balance of refractoriness and conduction between the reciprocating limbs within the AV node. Consequently, any intervention which alters AV nodal conduction or refractoriness can terminate these tachycardias. Abrupt termination of these tachycardias can be achieved by increasing vagal tone with carotid sinus massage, gagging, Valsalva maneuvers, or raising the blood pressure. Propranolol and digitalis, both of which increase AV nodal conduction time and refractoriness, have been used successfully to treat AV nodal re-entrant tachycardias.

Prophylactic therapy could be directed toward eliminating atrial extrasystoles, which are the most frequent initiating cause, or toward altering refractoriness and conduction within the AV node. Quinidine can be used to eliminate atrial extrasystoles, whereas digitalis alone or in combination with propranolol can be used to affect the AV node.

PAT Due to Re-entry via a V-A Accessory Pathway

Evidence has accumulated supporting the idea that there exist within the AV junction accessory pathways which conduct unidirectionally, i.e., from ventricles to atria. These VA accessory pathways, located at the base of the heart, may be right or left sided; they differ (at least functionally) from the classic Kent bundles of the Wolff-Parkinson-White syndrome in that there is no antegrade conduction and hence no telltale sign of a delta wave. It is estimated that approximately 20 per cent of patients previously thought to have PAT due to AV nodal re-entry represent re-entry due to a V-A accessory pathway.

It is thought that during sinus rhythm, atrial impulses block at or within the atrial end of the accessory pathway, leaving it refractory even for retrograde conduction after the ventricles are activated. However, if a properly timed atrial extrasystole encounters sufficient AV delay, the accessory pathway may recover after the ventricles are activated and permit retrograde conduction back to the

atria. Recovery of the AV node for anterograde conduction would then set the stage for a re-entrant tachycardia to occur. The AV conduction delay may be within the AV node (long P-R interval) or within the bundle branch (aberrant conduction) ipsilateral to the site of the accessory pathway. The basal location of these pathways means that the atria are retrogradely activated after the inscription of the QRS complex. Thus re-entry via a VA accessory pathway should be suspected in any patient in whom the inverted P waves (leads II, III, and AVF) during a PAT appear after the QRS complex (Fig. 10). In most cases of PAT due to AV nodal re-entry, the retrograde P waves are within the QRS complex (compare Figs. 9 and 10). Properly timed ventricular extrasystoles may also initiate re-entrant tachycardias if the impulse is retrogradely conducted to the atria via the VA accessory pathway and simultaneously blocked in the bundle branch AV nodal pathways.

Evidence that one is dealing with a VA accessory pathway can be obtained from electrophysiologic studies, using His bundle recordings and the ventricular extrastimulus technique. In patients with VA accessory pathways, a closely coupled premature ventricular extrasystole will result in atrial activation prior to the ventricular impulse depolarizing the bundle of His.

Therapy for re-entry via a VA accessory pathway is similar to that for AV nodal re-entry. Therapy may be directed toward abolishing atrial or ventricular extrasystoles (quinidine, procainamide) or altering the conducting characteristics of the AV node (digitalis, propranolol).

Ectopic Atrial Tachycardia

Areas within the atria but outside the sinus node can serve as the pacemaker of the heart. Depolarization of the atria by an ectopic atrial pacemaker in excess of 100 beats per minute constitutes an ectopic atrial tachycardia. The atrial rates of most ectopic tachycardias are between 150 and 220 per minute. The tachycardias may be sustained for long periods of time or occur in paroxysms lasting seconds to hours. Ectopic atrial tachycardias can occur in all forms of heart disease. They may occur in association with digitalis toxicity, chronic obstructive lung disease, or enlarged diseased atria, or may be associated with no apparent heart disease.

ELECTROCARDIOGRAPHIC FEATURES. In ectopic atrial tachycardias the configuration of the P waves is different from that of sinus beats. If all the ectopic P waves are of the same size and shape, it is called unifocal ectopic atrial tachycardia. A multifocal ectopic tachycardia is one in which the ectopic atrial impulses arise from different parts of the atria, and consequently the configuration of P waves varies.

Depending upon the atrial rate and the capacity of the AV node to transmit impulses to the ventricle, ectopic atrial tachycardias may be associated with 1:1 AV conduction with normal or prolonged AV conduction times, AV nodal Wenckebach cycles, or 2:1 AV block. Digitalis toxicity is a frequent cause of rapid unifocal ectopic atrial tachycardias with 2:1 AV block (Fig. 11). Multifocal ectopic atrial tachycardias are frequently associated with chronic obstructive lung disease or marked atrial disease and may precipitate atrial fibrillation.

The differentiation between paroxysmal atrial tachycardias caused by AV nodal re-entry from a unifocal ectopic tachycardia may at times be difficult. Tachycardias

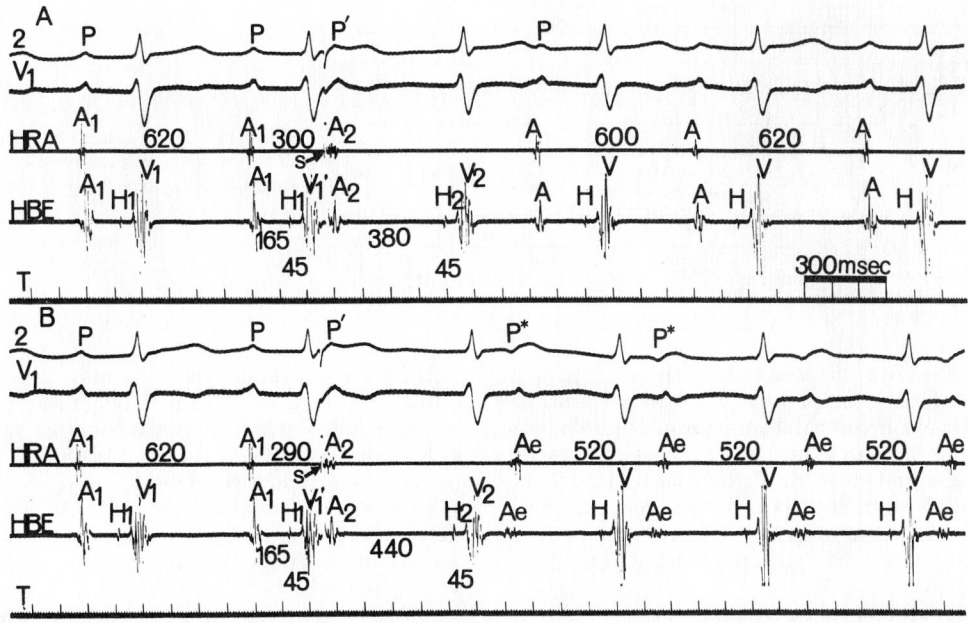

Figure 10. PAT in a patient with a VA accessory pathway. In panels *A* and *B,* the tracings from top to bottom are as follows: electrocardiographic leads 2 and V₁, a high right atrial electrogram (HRA), His bundle electrogram (HBE), and time lines at 10 and 100 msec. In each panel the first two beats are of sinus node origin with upright P waves in lead 2, a high to low sequence of atrial activation, AV nodal conduction time of 165 msec, and His-Purkinje conduction time of 45 msec. In panel *A*, a premature atrial depolarization (P′ or A₂) introduced 300 msec after the sinus beat (A₁) is conducted with an AV nodal delay of 380 msec. After activation of the ventricles sinus rhythm resumes. In panel *B,* a slightly earlier atrial extrasystole (P′ or A₂) encounters greater AV nodal delay as indicated by an A-H interval of 440 msec, which for this patient was sufficient to initiate a re-entrant tachycardia at a cycle length of 520 msec. Note that atrial activation occurs after the inscription of the QRS complex and is from the low to high right atrium, and that the P waves are inverted in lead 2. Atrial activation during the tachycardia is indicated by a P* on the surface ECG and by Ae on the intracardiac recordings.

associated with inverted P waves in leads II, III, and AVF favor re-entry within the AV node as the mechanism but do not exclude a rhythm of ectopic origin. Upright P waves in these same leads strongly suggest an ectopic tachycardia. If the configuration of the P waves during the tachycardia is the same as the initiating atrial extrasystole, ectopy is favored, especially if the P waves are upright in leads II, III, and AVF. If the initiating atrial extrasystole is upright in II, III, and AVF and inverted in these same leads during the tachycardia, re-entry is likely. Abrupt termination of the atrial tachycardia by carotid sinus massage or an electrically induced atrial extrasystole favors a mechanism of AV nodal re-entry. These maneuvers generally produce a temporary slowing or pause in the ectopic atrial tachycardia, followed by resumption of its inherent firing rate.

TREATMENT. The treatment of digitalis-induced ectopic atrial tachycardias is withdrawal of the cardiac gly-coside and administration of potassium supplements. Treatment of ectopic tachycardias in patients with chronic obstructive lung disease should first be directed toward correcting hypoxemia, hypercapnia, acid-base imbalance, or other metabolic imbalances, which frequently are present and are the initiating cause of these rhythm disturbances. Ectopic atrial tachycardias or other causes should be treated with either quinidine or procainamide.

VENTRICULAR EXTRASYSTOLES

Ventricular extrasystoles (ventricular premature beats, contractions, or systoles) are a common occurrence in patients with and without heart disease. In young healthy individuals, the incidence varies between 0.5 and 2.0 per cent. They may be caused by emotional stress, tobacco, alcohol, caffeine, anoxia, sympathomimetic

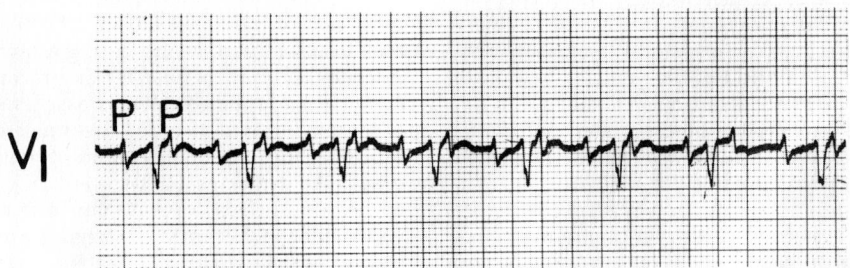

Figure 11.   Digitalis-induced atrial tachycardia with 2:1 AV block.

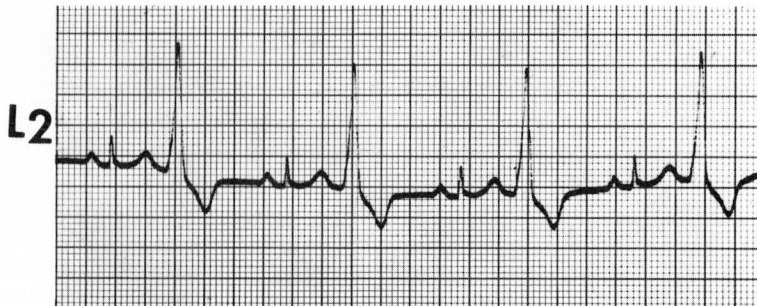

Figure 12. Ventricular bigeminy. A single premature ventricular extrasystole is coupled at a constant interval to each sinus beat.

drugs, or exercise. They are associated with all forms of heart disease and occur frequently (up to 80 per cent) in patients with acute myocardial infarction. Digitalis excess is a common cause of ventricular extrasystoles, especially if hypokalemia is present. Patients with occasional or even frequent ventricular extrasystoles may be completely unaware of their presence. On the other hand, some patients complain of "pauses," "palpitations," or "thumping" in the chest.

ELECTROCARDIOGRAPHIC FEATURES. Ventricular extrasystoles are characterized by wide QRS complexes (0.12 sec) with S-T and T wave changes. They may occur early or late in the cardiac cycle and very often have a constant coupling interval to the preceding sinus beat. The coupling interval is considered constant if the variation is within 0.08 sec (80 msec). A single ventricular extrasystole occurring after each sinus beat is referred to as ventricular bigeminy (Fig. 12). The term trigeminy refers to repeat cycles of either two sinus beats followed by a single extrasystole or one sinus beat followed by two consecutive ventricular extrasystoles.

Recurrent ventricular extrasystoles which always exhibit the same QRS morphology are referred to as unifocal in origin (arising from the same ectopic focus), whereas recurrent extrasystoles of different morphologies are termed multifocal in origin. Ventricular extrasystoles can arise anywhere within the bundle branch–Purkinje network. Extrasystoles arising from the left side of the conduction system result in QRS complexes which resemble right bundle branch block patterns, and those arising from the right side result in QRS complexes resembling a left bundle branch block pattern. Infrequently, extrasystolic impulses may arise high in one of the bundle branches, close to the bundle of His, and conduct with slight asynchrony down both bundle branches, resulting in narrow QRS complexes.

Most ventricular extrasystoles occur late in the cardiac cycle, i.e., after completion of the T wave of the preceding sinus beat, and are frequently coupled to the preceding sinus beat by a fairly constant interval. Less commonly, ventricular extrasystoles occur in early diastole, near the peak of the T wave or on its descending limb. This has been called the R on T phenomenon; it may reflect a very serious situation, because extrasystoles occurring near the so-called vulnerable period of the ventricle may lead to ventricular tachycardia or ventricular fibrillation.

Ventricular extrasystoles may be associated with various types of retrograde conduction patterns. The more common of these patterns include the following:

1. Complete retrograde conduction may occur across the AV conducting system, resulting in premature retrograde depolarization of the atria with inverted P waves in leads II, III, and AVF.

2. The extrasystolic impulse may retrogradely block within the AV node. This may result in the phenomenon of retrograde concealed conduction in which the next sinus impulse either is blocked or conducts with a P-R interval longer than sinus beats.

3. During prolonged retrograde AV nodal conduction delay, the extrasystolic impulse may reciprocate within the AV node and return to the ventricles, producing a ventricular echo beat.

4. Very premature extrasystolic impulses may retrogradely block within the His-Purkinje system. This type of retrograde conduction pattern cannot be determined from the electrocardiogram.

TREATMENT. The treatment of ventricular extrasystoles depends upon their cause, the underlying cardiac condition, severity of symptoms, their frequency, the coupling interval, and whether they are unifocal or multifocal in origin.

Ventricular extrasystoles which are related to emotional upsets, tobacco, alcohol, or sympathomimetic drugs may require only reassurance, mild sedation, or abstinence. Withholding of digitalis therapy for one or more days, in conjunction with oral potassium supplements, may be all that is necessary to treat extrasystoles caused by excess digitalis.

Ventricular extrasystoles occurring during an acute myocardial infarction require antiarrhythmic therapy. Therapy is urgently indicated if the extrasystoles have a close coupling interval, occur at a rate of five or more per minute, or are multifocal in origin. Irrespective of the underlying cardiac condition, antiarrhythmic therapy is indicated for ventricular extrasystoles which demonstrate the R on T phenomenon, are multifocal in origin, or occur consecutively in pairs.

VENTRICULAR TACHYCARDIA

Three or more consecutive beats occurring at rates greater than 100 per minute and arising from a focus located below the bundle of His constitute an episode of ventricular tachycardia. Most ventricular tachycardias occur at rates between 120 and 180 beats per minute; they may occur in paroxysms lasting a few seconds to several minutes or may persist for hours or days. Ventricular tachycardia is almost always associated with some form of organic heart disease, the most common being arteriosclerotic, rheumatic, and hypertensive heart diseases. As many as 50 per cent of patients with acute myocardial infarction may have one or more episodes of ventricular tachycardia of varying duration. Toxic doses of digitalis are a common cause of ventricular tachycardia. Other precipitating causes of paroxysmal ventricular tachycardia include hypoxia, hypokalemia, exercise, drugs (such as epinephrine, quinidine, and procainamide), cardiac catheterization of either the right or left heart, and anesthetic agents (cyclopropane, chloroform). Ventricular aneurysms may be the cause of recurrent or drug-resistant ventricular tachycardias.

Paroxysmal ventricular tachycardia has been reported to occur in young patients (less than 30 years old) in whom no evidence of heart disease could be detected. In this group, some attacks have been demonstrated to occur during exercise or emotional stress, implying a relationship between increased sympathetic tone and the ventricular dysrhythmia. In other patients, no precipitating factor could be demonstrated.

ELECTROCARDIOGRAPHIC FEATURES. In ventricular tachycardia, the QRS complexes are wide (0.12 sec or greater) and bizarre, recurring regularly at rates over 100 per minute (usually 120 to 180). Since the pacemaker is located below the bundle of His (i.e., within the bundle branches or Purkinje network), ventricular tachycardia is characterized electrophysiologically by the absence of a His bundle electrogram preceding the onset of ventricular activation. The bundle of His is retrogradely activated, and although in most cases it is not discernible, it is located within the ventricular electrogram. Initiation of the tachycardia may begin with a premature ventricular beat occurring close in time to the peak of the T wave of a preceding sinus beat; at other times, the initiating beat is located at the end of or after inscription of the T wave. Once initiated, ventricular tachycardia may be continuous for long periods of time or intermittent with one or more sinus beats interspersed (Fig. 13).

Often, it is extremely difficult to define the pattern of atrial activity during episodes of ventricular tachycardia from standard electrocardiographic tracings. Esophageal or intra-atrial recordings can be quite helpful in defining the frequency of atrial activity and its relationship to the QRS complexes.

During ventricular tachycardia, the atria may be dissociated from the ventricles, in which case independent P waves will be observed. At other times, various degrees of retrograde capture of the atria will occur (1:1, 2:1 retrograde Wenckebach cycles). If discernible, the P waves would be inverted in leads II, III, and AVF during retrograde activation of the atria.

An important and sometimes difficult clinical problem is the differentiation of supraventricular tachycardia with aberration from ventricular tachycardia. In aberrant conduction a His deflection with a normal or greater than normal H-V interval precedes ventricular activation, whereas in ventricular tachycardia there is absence of a His bundle electrogram preceding ventricular activation.

From the electrocardiographic point of view the presence of fusion beats during a sustained tachycardia provides strong supportive evidence that the rhythm in question is of ventricular origin. Fusion beats refer to partial activation of the ventricles by both supraventricular and ventricular impulses. During ventricular tachycardia, fusion beats may result because the atria are dissociated from the ventricles, and a sinus impulse occurring at an appropriate time in the cardiac cycle penetrates the AV conducting system and partially activates the ventricles; or during retrograde Wenckebach cycles, the impulse may reciprocate within the AV node and return to the ventricles, resulting in partial activation of that chamber. Complete activation or capture of the ventricles by either of the aforementioned mechanisms may terminate the tachycardia for one or more cycles, during which time sinus beats may appear, after which the tachycardia usually resumes.

A diagnosis of ventricular tachycardia is favored if one can discern independent atrial activity at a rate slower than the ventricular rate. On the other hand, supraventricular tachycardia with aberration is favored if carotid sinus pressure or other vagal maneuvers abruptly terminate the tachycardia.

TREATMENT. The choice and urgency of treatment for ventricular tachycardia depends on a number of factors, including its cause, the age and general condition of the patient, the severity and type of the underlying heart disease, blood pressure, and the state of consciousness. Causative factors such as hypoxia, hypokalemia, or other metabolic imbalances must be recognized and corrected.

DC countershock and drug therapy are the two commonly used methods for treating ventricular tachycardia. DC countershock is generally reserved for emergent situations in which the ventricular dysrhythmia is continuous or causes profound hemodynamic disturbances, or when drug therapy is ineffective. DC countershock is not the preferred treatment for ventricular tachycardias caused by digitalis toxicity.

Lidocaine is the most commonly used drug for the conversion of ventricular tachycardia to sinus rhythm. It is administered intravenously as a 50 to 100 mg bolus which can be repeated in two to three minutes if the initial injection is totally or partially ineffective. After suppression of the arrhythmia, lidocaine may be given as a continuous intravenous drip of 1 to 4 mg per minute. Ap-

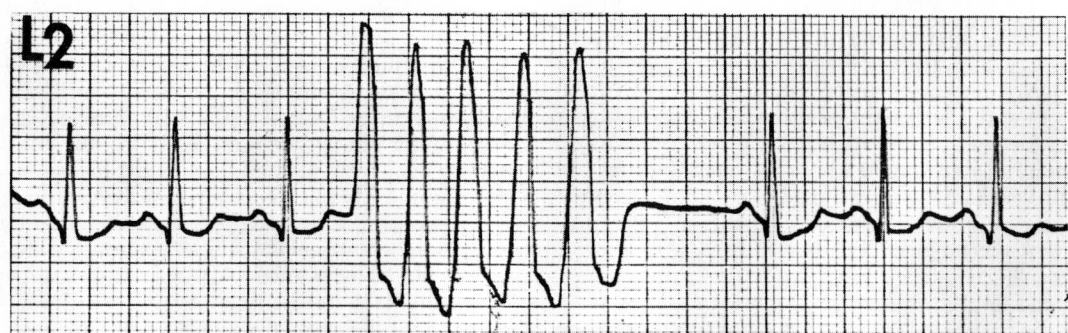

Figure 13. A short episode of a unifocal ventricular tachycardia interspersed between periods of sinus rhythm.

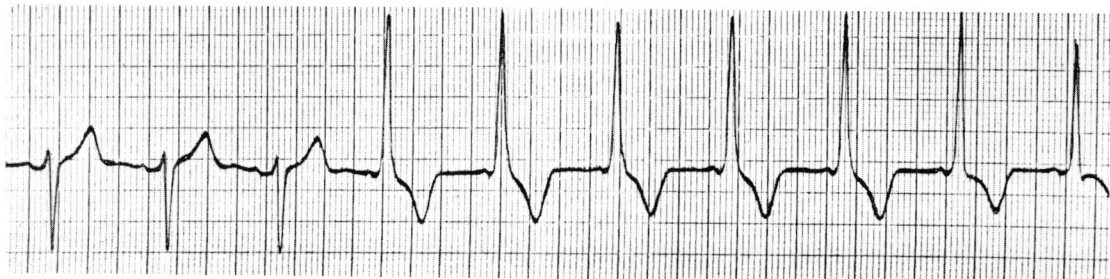

Figure 14. Accelerated idioventricular rhythm which begins just prior to the fourth sinus P wave. The rates of the sinus node and idioventricular pacemakers are nearly identical, thereby resulting in a period of isorhythmic AV dissociation.

proximately 90 per cent of ventricular tachycardias can be suppressed at lidocaine blood levels of 2 to 4 μg per milliliter. The more common side effects of lidocaine include drowsiness, paresthesias, decrease in auditory acuity, agitation, and convulsions. Since lidocaine is metabolized by the liver, lower doses of the drug may cause side effects in patients with hepatic dysfunction.

Intravenous procainamide is also highly effective in the treatment of ventricular tachycardia. The drug can be administered at a rate of 25 to 50 mg per minute until either the tachycardia is terminated or 1000 mg has been administered. Most ventricular tachycardias are suppressed at blood concentrations of 4 to 8 μg per milliliter. Occasionally, higher concentrations are required. Continued suppression of the tachycardia can be achieved by a continuous intravenous drip at a rate of 2.5 mg per minute. Procainamide, like most antiarrhythmic drugs, may cause significant hypotension after intravenous administration, especially if the underlying myocardial dysfunction is severe. At other times the arrhythmia is the cause of a lowered blood pressure which improves when normal sinus rhythm is restored.

If lidocaine and procainamide are ineffective in controlling the arrhythmia, one can use diphenylhydantoin, propranolol, or quinidine sulfate. On occasion, a combination of drugs is required.

If ventricular tachycardia is associated with an underlying complete or high degree of AV block, an electrode catheter should be positioned within the right ventricular cavity and endocardial pacing initiated immediately upon terminating the ventricular tachycardia with drug therapy. This is required because effective drug therapy may suppress all idioventricular pacemaker activity and ventricular asystole may ensue.

ACCELERATED IDIOVENTRICULAR RHYTHMS

Accelerated idioventricular rhythms (AIVR) is a term applied to ectopic ventricular rhythms with rates intermediate between idioventricular escape rhythms (30 to 40 per minute) and ventricular tachycardia (120 to 180 per minute). Most frequently the rates are between 75 and 100 per minute. Accelerated idioventricular rhythms are commonly associated with myocardial infarction or digitalis toxicity. Current thinking holds that AIVR represents an enhancement of the normal escape rhythm of latent ventricular pacemakers. Like other ventricular rhythms, the QRS complexes are bizarre and wide (0.12 sec). The rate of the AIVR is usually close to that of the sinus rate, and consequently it becomes manifest when

sinus rhythm is slowed by an increasing vagal tone (carotid sinus massage) or premature atrial extrasystoles, or when some degree of AV block develops. AIVR usually begins late in the cardiac cycle, and it may start with a fusion beat (Fig. 14). AIVR may also begin early in the cardiac cycle. If dissociation between the atria and ventricles is present, fusion beats may occur frequently. If 1:1 retrograde conduction occurs, the AIVR may persist for long periods of time. Some patients manifest, at different times, episodes of AIVR and ventricular tachycardia in which the QRS morphology during both rhythm disturbances is the same. The AIVR may represent ventricular tachycardia with a degree of exit block from the ventricular focus. Acceleration of the sinus rate by atropine or atrial pacing usually suppresses the AIVR. AIVR can also be suppressed with lidocaine or procainamide. Treatment of AIVR is the same as that of ventricular tachycardia. Also, acceleration of the sinus rate by atropine or atrial pacing can and usually does suppress AIVR.

BIDIRECTIONAL TACHYCARDIA

Bidirectional tachycardia is an infrequently encountered arrhythmia which is characterized by (1) rapid regular rate of 140 to 180 beats per minute, (2) alternating rightward and leftward axis shifts in the frontal plane, and (3) a constant right bundle branch block pattern in lead V_1. Most bidirectional tachycardias occur in the presence of severe myocardial disease or digitalis toxicity and are associated with a poor prognosis. Hypokalemia has also been implicated as a cause of bidirectional ventricular tachycardia. Two different mechanisms have been proposed to explain the electrocardiographic pattern of bidirectional tachycardia. One suggested mechanism is that bidirectional tachycardia originates from a supraventricular tachycardia in which there is permanent aberrant conduction within the right bundle branch along with alternating aberrant conduction in the two divisions (anterior and posterior fascicles) of the left bundle branch. The other mechanism, confirmed by His bundle recordings, indicates that bidirectional tachycardia results from an ectopic focus located in the left ventricle, which would account for the permanent right bundle branch block pattern observed (Fig. 15). It is as yet unclear whether the alternating rightward and leftward axis shift is the result of alternating routes of ventricular activation by a single ectopic left ventricular focus of alternating discharge of two separate left ventricular foci. The treatment of bidirectional tachycardia is withdrawal of digitalis and administration of potassium and an antiarrhythmic agent such as lidocaine or diphenylhydantoin.

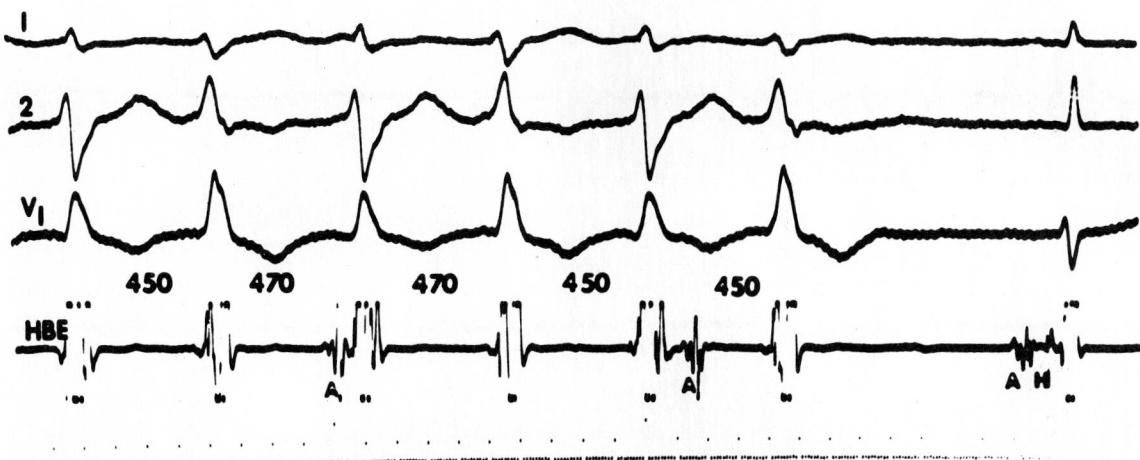

Figure 15. Bidirectional ventricular tachycardia. The first six QRS complexes show a persistent RBBB pattern in lead V_1 and alternating left and right axis deviation in lead 2. The ventricular origin of these beats is indicated by absence of a His deflection preceding the QRS complex. Ventricular activity is dissociated from atrial activity. The last beat shows a normally conducted atrial impulse with normal A-H and H-V intervals. (From Kastor, J. A., and Goldreyer, B. N.: Circulation, 48:897, 1973. Copyright 1973, American Medical Association.)

VENTRICULAR FIBRILLATION

Ventricular fibrillation consists of rapid, disorganized, multifocal depolarizations of the ventricular myocardium. The absence of rhythmic coordinated muscular contractions produces a loss of the pumping action of the heart and causes a precipitous fall of the blood pressure to zero levels and unconsciousness. Ventricular fibrillation is most often seen in patients with significant underlying cardiac disease, especially ischemic heart disease. It may also occur in patients without clinical or pathologic evidence of heart disease. It may accompany digitalis toxicity, especially if hypokalemia or other metabolic imbalances are present. Quinidine sensitivity or toxicity may also be the cause of ventricular fibrillation. Ventricular extrasystoles occurring within the so-called vulnerable period of the ventricles (R on T phenomenon) may initiate ventricular fibrillation (Fig. 16).

The treatment of ventricular fibrillation must be prompt and decisive. The patient must be ventilated and defibrillated, using DC countershock at 400 watt-seconds.

AV DISSOCIATION

AV dissociation is a general term which describes any rhythm in which the atria and ventricles are independently activated by different pacemakers discharging at similar or dissimilar rates. The atria may be activated by either the sinus node or an ectopic atrial pacemaker,

whereas the ventricles may be under the control of either a junctional or an idioventricular pacemaker. AV dissociation may occur with an essentially intact AV conduction system and may be of short duration, lasting for one or a few cardiac cycles, or it may persist for much longer periods. AV dissociation may be caused by (1) acceleration of a junctional or idioventricular pacemaker (Fig. 14), (2) slowing of an atrial pacemaker accompanied by an escape rhythm located in either the AV junction or ventricles, or (3) SA or AV block accompanied by an escape rhythm (Fig. 5).

Isorhythmic AV dissociation is one type of dissociated rhythm in which (1) the atria and ventricles are controlled by independent pacemakers discharging at equal or nearly equal rates, and (2) the P waves remain in close proximity to the QRS complexes; they may precede, occur simultaneously with, or follow the QRS complex. An example of isorhythmic AV dissociation in which the ventricles come under control of a junctional pacemaker is shown in Figure 17. As the atrial cycle length increases, the ventricles come under control of a junctional pacemaker, and the P waves which remain under control of the sinus node appear to be "marching" into the QRS complex and maintain a fixed R-P relationship, during which time the atria may remain under control of the sinus node or be retrogradely activated by the junctional pacemaker. After a variable period of time, acceleration of the sinus rate occurs, the P waves reappear in front of the QRS complex, and sinus rhythm is re-established. Sinus acceleration results from changes in baroreceptor activity, consequent to changes in arterial pressure or the

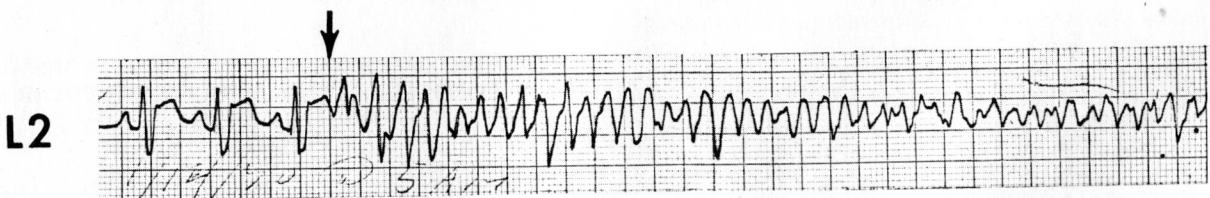

Figure 16. Ventricular fibrillation initiated by a rapid burst of ventricular activity (arrow).

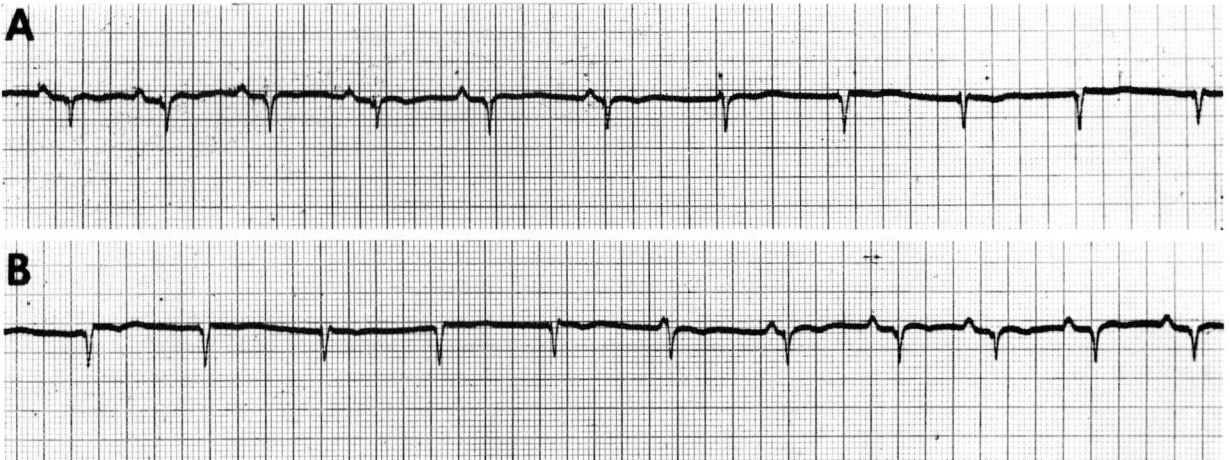

Figure 17. Isorhythmic AV dissociation. After the first five sinus beats, the sinus rate slows and an AV junctional pacemaker emerges, starting with the sixth QRS complex. The atria continue to be activated by the sinus node, and the P waves are obscured within the QRS complex. In the bottom strip, accelerating forces cause an increase in the sinus node rate and sinus rhythm is reestablished.

effect of right atrial stretch, or both. Acceleration of the sinus rate is dependent upon the magnitude of these accelerating influences and the responsiveness of the sinus node.

JUNCTIONAL RHYTHMS

Traditionally, AV nodal rhythms have been described as arising from the upper, middle, or lower portions of the AV node. This classification has been based primarily on the relationship of inverted P waves (leads II, III, AVF) to the QRS complex. In upper AV nodal rhythms the inverted P wave precedes the QRS complex, whereas in middle or lower AV nodal rhythms the P wave occurs simultaneously with or follows the QRS complex, respectively. It has been recommended that the terms "junctional" or "AV junctional rhythms" replace that of "AV nodal rhythms," because (1) experimentally it has been difficult to consistently and convincingly demonstrate pacemaker activity (phase 4 depolarization) in all three regions of the AV node and (2) pacemaker activity in other areas of the heart (coronary sinus, left atrium, and bundle of His) can result in electrocardiographic patterns similar to those ascribed to AV nodal rhythms.

AV junctional rhythms are primarily escape rhythms with rates usually in the range 40 to 70 per minute. They become manifest if there is (1) significant sinus slowing, (2) AV block, or (3) SA block. If the discharge rate of the sinus node falls below that of a subsidiary junctional pacemaker, as may occur during sinus bradycardia or after premature discharge of the sinus node by an extrasystolic impulse, an area within the AV junction can take over as the pacemaker of the heart. In similar fashion, an escape junctional rhythm can emerge when sinus node impulses fail to conduct to surrounding atrial myocardium such as occurs in SA block (Fig. 5). Escape junctional rhythms also occur during AV block in which supraventricular impulses block in the AV node and proximal to the site of a junctional pacemaker (see Fig. 27). In complete AV block in which the nonconducted atrial impulses block below the bundle of His, the escape rhythms are located below the AV junction (idioventric-

ular pacemaker). AV junctional rhythms result in QRS complexes which are similar to those of sinus rhythm.

JUNCTIONAL EXTRASYSTOLES

Extrasystolic impulses arising from the AV node or bundle of His are referred to as junctional extrasystoles. Their occurrence late in the cardiac cycle results in normal QRS complexes which are not preceded by P waves. More premature extrasystolic impulses may result in aberrant ventricular conduction, producing a wide QRS complex which mimics a ventricular extrasystole. Closely coupled extrasystolic impulses may encounter anterograde refractoriness within the bundle branches (no QRS complex) and retrogradely block in the AV node. Retrograde concealment in the AV node may affect conduction of subsequent sinus impulses. A variety of AV conduction patterns may result, depending upon frequency, regularity, and coupling interval of these concealed junctional extrasystoles. These include (1) sudden and expected prolongation of a P-R interval, (2) type I second degree AV block, (3) type II second degree AV block, (4) 2:1 AV block, and (5) alternation of the P-R interval. Patients exhibiting type II second degree AV block produced by a concealed junctional extrasystolic impulse do not require pacemaker therapy. Concealed junctional extrasystoles may disappear spontaneously, or may be suppressed during exercise or administration of atropine. When they occur in patients receiving digitalis, withholding the glycoside for a few days may be all that is necessary. Lidocaine and procainamide are also effective treatment. Diagnosis of concealed junctional extrasystoles can be made when the aforementioned conduction abnormalities occur in ECG tracings along with junctional extrasystoles, which are conducted to the ventricles.

SYNDROME OF SHORT P-R INTERVAL, NORMAL QRS COMPLEXES, AND SUPRAVENTRICULAR TACHYCARDIAS
(Lown-Ganong-Levine Syndrome)

The syndrome of short P-R interval (0.12 sec or less), normal QRS complexes (0.10 sec), and paroxysmal supraventricular tachycardias is known as the Lown-Ganong-Levine syndrome. The mechanisms responsible for both the short P-R interval and the tachycardias have remained obscure. Several theories, based primarily on anatomic considerations, have been proposed to explain the short P-R interval. The most popular theory centers on the presence of specialized internodal pathways by which atrial impulses can partially or completely bypass the AV node. Recent electrophysiologic studies, using His bundle recordings and atrial pacing techniques, have shown that most cases of short P-R interval are associated with AV nodal conduction times which are at the lower range of normal values. The A-H intervals were 60 to 80 msec, whereas H-V intervals were between 30 and 55 msec. In addition, in most patients when the right atrium was stimulated at progressively increasing rates, the expected A-H interval increases were qualitatively similar to, but quantitatively less than, that observed for subjects with normal P-R intervals. In only an occasional patient with a short P-R interval was the A-H interval found to be less than 60 msec or did the A-H interval not increase as the paced atrial rate was increased. These limited data suggest that most cases of short P-R interval are due to an abbreviated AV nodal conduction time which could be due to (1) atrial impulses partially bypassing the AV node (? specialized internodal tracts), (2) an anatomically small AV node, (3) preferential intranodal pathways, or (4) a combination of these. In only occasional patients are the electrophysiologic data compatible with a complete bypass of the AV node, accounting for the short P-R interval. It should be pointed out that prolonged periods of isorhythmic AV dissociation can mimic a short P-R interval with normal QRS complexes. Studies to date have shown that AV nodal re-entry is a common mechanism for the paroxysmal supraventricular tachycardias in this syndrome.

WOLFF-PARKINSON-WHITE SYNDROME

The electrocardiographic pattern of the Wolff-Parkinson-White syndrome is characterized by a short P-R interval (less than 0.12 sec) and a widened QRS complex, starting with an initial delta wave. This abnormal electrocardiographic pattern occurs in approximately 0.1 to 0.4 per cent of routine tracings. A significant number of patients exhibiting this pattern have episodes of supraventricular tachycardia. The Wolff-Parkinson-White syndrome may be associated with Ebstein's anomaly of the tricuspid valve and idiopathic hypertrophic subaortic stenosis (IHSS). Other terms used to describe this phenomenon include anomalous AV excitation, ventricular pre-excitation, and accessory AV conduction.

Over the years, many hypotheses have been put forth to explain the electrocardiographic findings in this syndrome. Currently, there is anatomic as well as electrophysiologic evidence indicating that atrial impulses pre-excite the ventricles via accessory bypass tracts composed of myocardial fibers which connect the atria and ventricles. These bypass tracts are referred to as bundles of Kent. Atrial impulses are simultaneously conducted to the ventricles via the normal AV nodal His-Purkinje conducting system and the accessory pathway. AV conduction via the latter results in shortening of the P-R interval, and pre-excitation of the ventricle produces the delta wave. In most cases, the QRS complex in the Wolff-Parkinson-White syndrome represents fusion activation, the delta wave being an expression of ventricular excitation via the accessory pathway, and the remaining portion of the QRS the result of excitation via the normal AV nodal His-Purkinje conducting system. If significant delay or block exists within the AV nodal His-Purkinje pathway, the QRS complex may represent one of total pre-excitation. Alternatively,

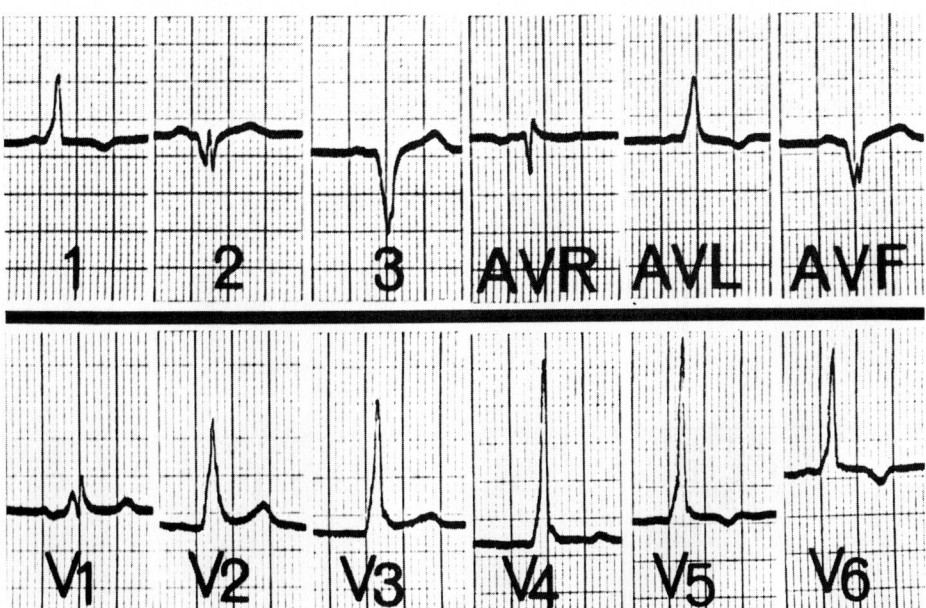

Figure 18. Wolff-Parkinson-White syndrome, showing Type A QRS complexes. The delta wave can be seen in almost all leads. The precordial leads resemble a right bundle branch block pattern. In leads 2, 3, and AVF the delta wave produces a Q wave which mimics a diaphragmatic myocardial infarction.

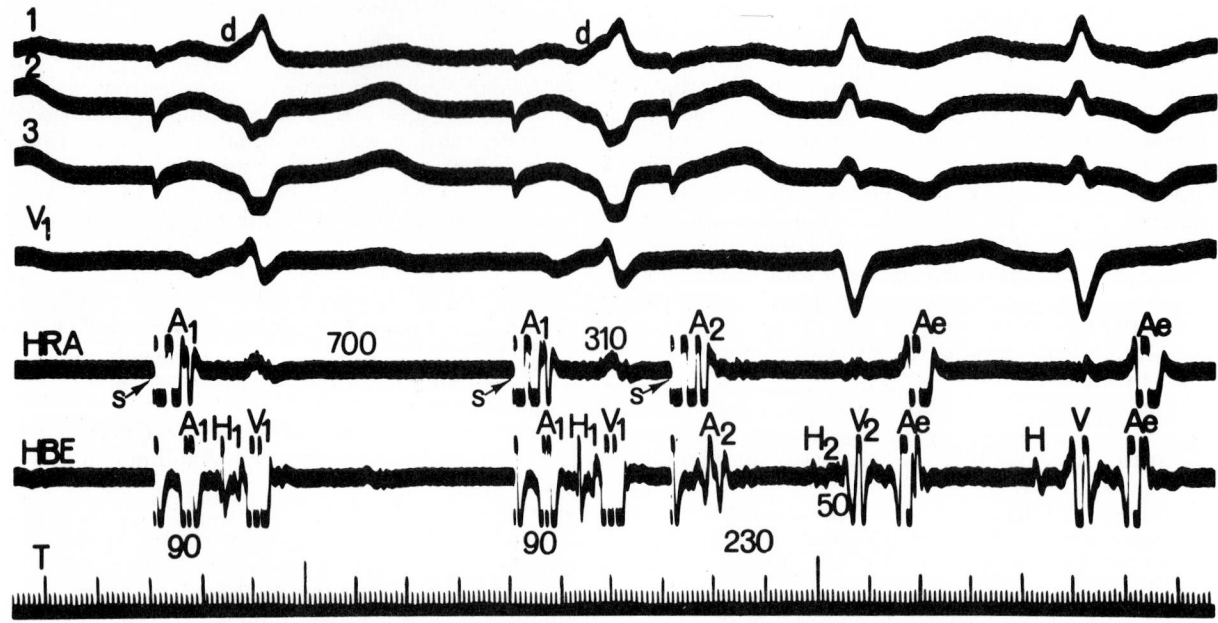

Figure 19. The first two QRS complexes show a Wolff-Parkinson-White type of ventricular excitation in which the delta wave (d) in leads II and III mimics a diaphragmatic myocardial infarction. Atrial impulses are also conducted along the AV nodal His-Purkinje system; bundle of His activation occurs at about the time of the onset of the delta wave. The third P wave (A$_2$) is premature and finds the accessory pathway refractory. Exclusive conduction along the AV nodal His-Purkinje system results in normal ventricular activation, followed by a re-entrant supraventricular tachycardia. Note the absence of electrocardiographic evidence of myocardial infarction.

if AV nodal conduction time is shortened, as may occur with increased sympathetic tone or during an isoproterenol infusion, activation of the ventricles by the AV nodal His-Purkinje system is increased and the QRS tends toward normalization. Anomalous AV excitation may be always present during sinus rhythm, or it may intermittently alternate with periods of normal activation. At times, anomalous AV excitation may mimic the electrocardiographic pattern of a myocardial infarction (Fig. 18). Bundle of His recordings in conjunction with atrial pacing techniques can establish the correct diagnosis (Fig. 19).

For a long time, the Wolff-Parkinson-White syndrome was divided into types A and B. In type A the

accessory bundle crosses the AV sulcus on the left side, causing pre-excitation of the base of the left ventricle. The vector of the delta wave is directed anteriorly in all precordial leads (upright in V$_1$ V$_6$), and the QRS pattern resembles right bundle branch block pattern (Fig. 18). In type B, the accessory bundle pre-excites the lateral margin of the right ventricle and the initial delta forces are directed leftward and posteriorly, producing a biphasic or negative delta wave in V$_1$ and QRS complexes resembling the left bundle branch block pattern.

It is now known from intraoperative epicardial mapping studies that accessory pathways may be located at a variety of sites within the tricuspid and mitral annuli. Accessory pathways have been located in the anterior,

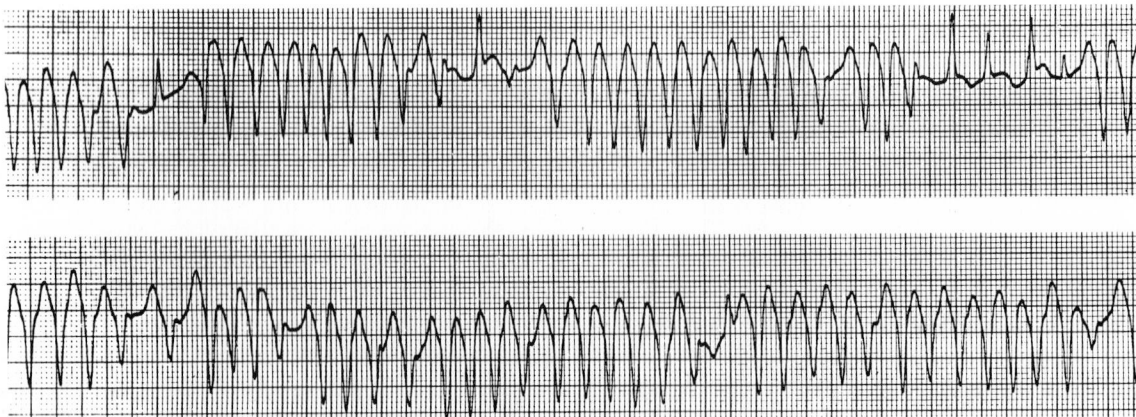

Figure 20. Patient with known Wolff-Parkinson-White syndrome who develops atrial fibrillation with rapid conduction over the accessory pathway (wide, negative QRS complexes). Intermittently, activation of the ventricles occurs over the normal AV nodal His-Purkinje system, producing upright QRS complexes of normal duration.

lateral, posterior (paraseptal), and medial aspects of the tricuspid annulus, as well as the anterior, lateral, and posterior (paraseptal) regions of the mitral annulus. On standard ECG tracings, pre-excitation of the ventricles from these various sites produces different delta wave vector forces which can be used to approximate the earliest site of epicardial excitation.

Supraventricular Tachycardias in Wolff-Parkinson-White Syndrome

Between 25 and 70 per cent of patients with Wolff-Parkinson-White type QRS complexes have episodes of supraventricular tachycardia, and most of these appear to be re-entrant in nature. However, it should be noted that atrial tachycardias which are ectopic in origin may also occur in these patients. Most re-entrant tachycardias occurring in the patients with the Wolf-Parkinson-White syndrome have normal QRS complexes with long P-R intervals and are initiated by premature atrial beats. Less commonly are re-entrant tachycardias associated with pre-excitation type QRS complexes.

There are two possible mechanisms to explain re-entrant supraventricular tachycardias with normal QRS complexes in patients with the Wolff-Parkinson-White syndrome. If a closely coupled premature atrial beat finds the accessory pathway refractory to antegrade conduction, it may traverse the AV nodal His-Purkinje conducting system (usually with some delay) and activate the ventricles, producing a normal QRS complex. If sufficient time has elapsed to permit recovery of excitability of the accessory pathway, retrograde conduction back to the atria will occur via the accessory pathway. If, after atrial activation, the AV nodal His-Purkinje conducting system has recovered, activation of the ventricles will follow and a self-sustaining re-entrant tachycardia will result (Fig. 19). Alternatively, a re-entrant supraventricular tachycardia with normal QRS complexes could be initiated by a premature ventricular beat which was retrogradely blocked within the His-Purkinje AV nodal conducting system but which retrogradely activated the atria via the accessory pathway. Recovery of excitability of the AV nodal His-Purkinje conducting system would allow antegrade conduction to ventricles to follow retrograde activation of the atria; if the process is repetitive, a sustained tachycardia with normal QRS complexes will result.

The second mechanism involved in producing re-entrant supraventricular tachycardias with normal QRS complexes is one in which reciprocation or re-entry occurs only within the AV node; the accessory pathway, although present, is not utilized in the re-entrant process. This type of re-entry is the same as that occurring in patients who have paroxysmal atrial tachycardia without Wolff-Parkinson-White complexes.

Re-entrant supraventricular tachycardias with pre-excitation type QRS complexes result when antegrade conduction occurs via the accessory pathway and the impulse is retrogradely returned to the atria via the AV nodal His-Purkinje pathway.

A potentially life-threatening situation may occur in patients with the Wolff-Parkinson-White syndrome who develop atria fibrillation (Fig. 20). Rapid irregular activation of the ventricles via the accessory pathway exclusively or both pathways simultaneously may lead to ventricular fibrillation. DC countershock is the treatment of choice in this situation.

TREATMENT. Most re-entrant tachycardias associated with the Wolff-Parkinson-White syndrome respond to vagotonic maneuvers such as carotid sinus stimulation, the Valsalva maneuver, or elevation of blood pressure (Fig. 21). Increased parasympathetic tone alters the re-entrant pathway by increasing refractoriness and delaying conduction within the AV node. Similarly, digitalis and propranolol can terminate re-entrant tachycardias by the same mechanism. DC countershock is reserved (1) for those tachycardias which are resistant to vagotonic maneuvers and require excessive amounts of drug therapy, (2) for those associated with very rapid ventricular responses and hemodynamic compromise, and (3) for atrial fibrillation with anterograde conduction over the accessory pathway.

Prophylactic drug therapy can be directed at (1) suppressing the atrial extrasystoles which are a common initiating cause of re-entrant tachycardias in the Wolff-Parkinson-White syndrome; quinidine sulfate may be used for this purpose; (2) altering refractoriness and conduction in the AV node so that re-entry cannot be sustained; digitalis and propranolol alone, or in combination, have been successfully used; or (3) altering conduction and refractoriness of the accessory pathway; procainamide or quinidine may be tried to accomplish this end. We have found digitalis, given daily with or

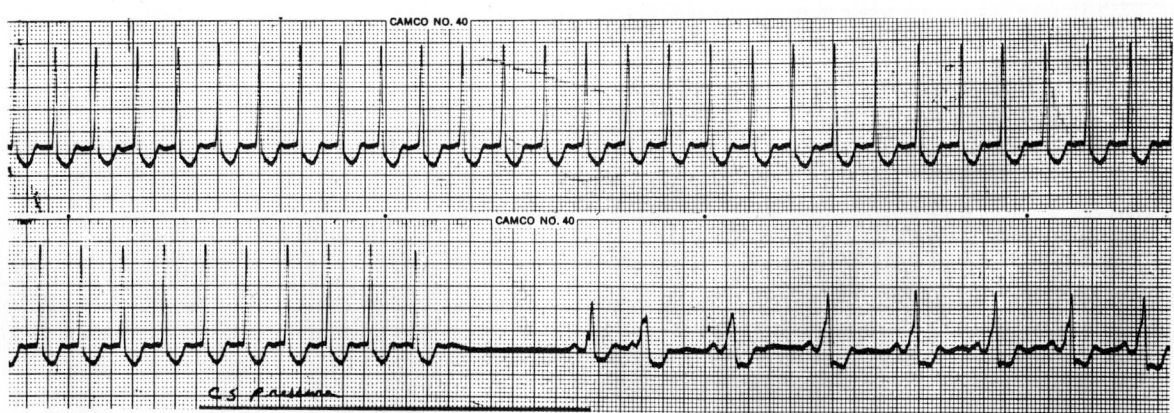

Figure 21. Paroxysmal atrial tachycardia in a patient with type A Wolff-Parkinson-White syndrome. Top tracing shows PAT with normal QRS complexes. Retrograde P waves are buried within the S-T segment. Bottom tracing depicts termination of the tachycardia by carotid sinus pressure with the characteristic QRS complexes of pre-excitation during the subsequent sinus rhythm.

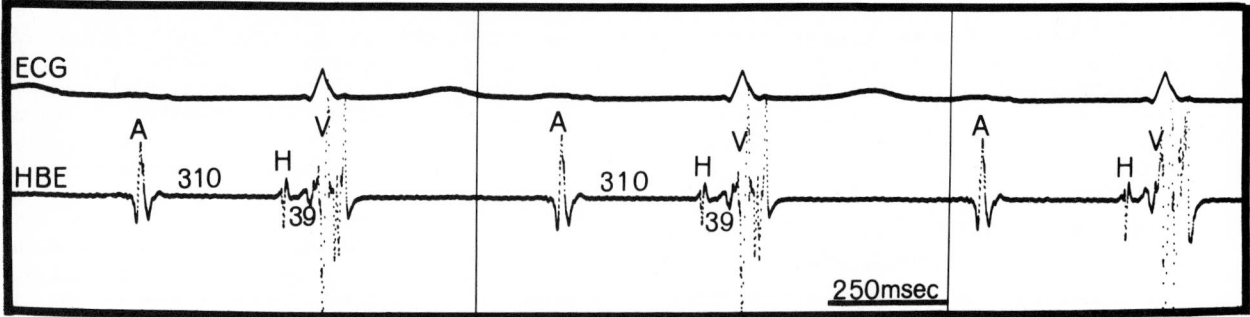

Figure 22. First degree heart block due to AV nodal delay.

without propranolol, an effective form of therapy for most of our patients. Arrhythmias are either not sustained or more easily terminated by carotid sinus massage or Valsalva maneuvers.

A small percentage of patients with the Wolff-Parkinson-White syndrome have frequent severe episodes of supraventricular tachycardia which, in addition to causing disabling and life-threatening symptoms, are resistant to control by drug therapy alone. An operative procedure has been devised for surgically interrupting the anomalous atrioventricular bypass tract which can effectively prevent or significantly modify recurrences of tachycardias. Surgical therapy in these selective patients requires that the region of the anomalous bypass tract be localized by epicardial mapping studies.

Preoperative evaluation in these patients should be directed toward (1) documenting that the patients' symptoms are related to arrhythmias caused by the presence of a bypass tract; (2) documenting that the arrhythmias are resistant to single and combination drugs (blood levels of drugs should be obtained and side effects noted); and (3) determining whether any associated cardiac anomalies exist, such as Ebstein's anomaly of the tricuspid valve or IHSS. A preoperative electrophysiologic study should be performed with the following goals in mind: (1) Confirming the presence of an accessory pathway and presumptively localizing its site. Some patients may have more than one accessory pathway. (2) Identifying the nature of the arrhythmias which the patient is experiencing and the participation of the accessory pathway in those arrhythmias. (3) Characterizing the functional characteristics of both the accessory pathway and the normal AV nodal–His–Purkinje systems. Examining the effect of drugs on both the normal and accessory pathways. A postoperative electrophysiologic study should also be performed to determine the effectiveness of surgical interruption of the accessory pathway.

DISORDERS OF AV CONDUCTION

First Degree Heart Block

In adults a P-R interval of more than 0.20 sec constitutes electrocardiographic evidence of first degree heart block which most commonly (90 per cent or more) is due to conduction delay occurring within the AV node. First degree heart block in the presence of normal QRS complexes is almost always due to AV nodal conduction delay, an example of which is presented in Figure 22. Bundle of His recordings reveal that the A-H interval was

prolonged at 310 msec and His-Purkinje conduction time was within normal limits at 39 msec.

Drugs such as digitalis and propranolol cause P-R prolongation by delaying conduction within the AV node. Neither drug affects conduction within the His-Purkinje system to any significant degree. The A-H interval returns to normal when these drugs are discontinued. At times, first degree AV nodal block may alternate with periods of type I second degree AV block or 2:1 AV block. In general, no specific treatment for first degree AV block is required. In most patients an increase in sympathetic tone, such as occurs during exercise or vagal blockade by atropine (0.5 to 1.0 mg intravenously), causes a decrease in the A-H interval concomitant with an increase in sinus rate so that 1:1 AV conduction is maintained.

His-Purkinje Delay

Less commonly, first degree heart block is due solely to conduction delay within the His-Purkinje system. Figure 23 is an example of P-R prolongation and right bundle branch block in which AV nodal conduction (A-H interval) is within normal limits and His-Purkinje conduction time (H-V interval) is markedly prolonged at 90 msec. The presence of a prolonged H-V interval is almost always associated with a bundle branch block pattern or widened QRS complex. However, not all patients with a bundle branch block pattern have prolonged H-V intervals. A prolonged H-V interval (greater than 60 msec) in the presence of a bundle branch block pattern usually indicates that there is conduction delay within the contralateral bundle. In asymptomatic patients, no specific treatment is required.

AV Nodal Plus His-Purkinje Conduction Delay

First degree AV block may be due to conduction delays in both the AV node and His-Purkinje system.

Intra-His Bundle Delay

Conduction delay occurring within the bundle of His itself can cause a prolongation of the P-R interval. However, this is an uncommon cause of first degree heart block.

Second Degree AV Block

Second degree heart block has been classified into two types. Type I second degree heart block (Wenckebach phenomenon, Mobitz type I AV block) is electrocardio-

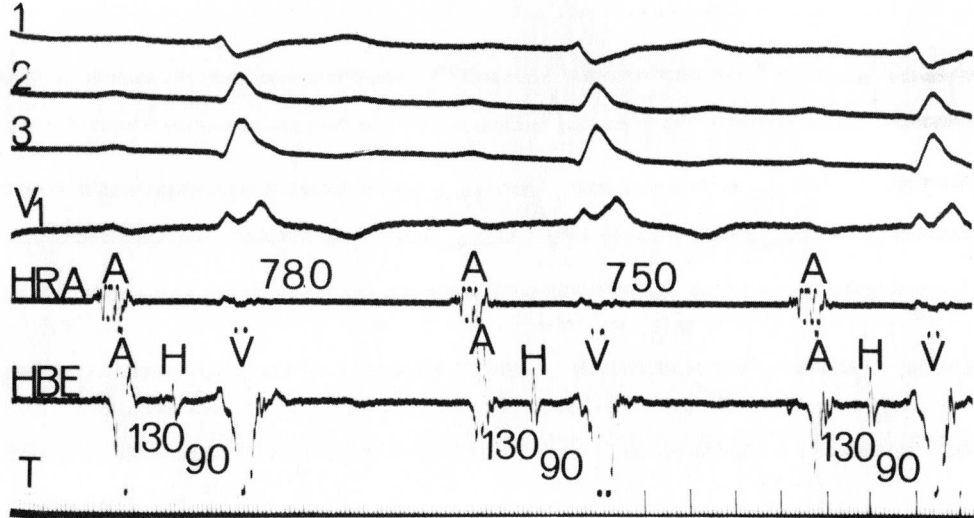

Figure 23.   First degree heart block due to a prolonged H-V interval (90 msec) in a patient with right bundle branch block.

graphically characterized by a progressive prolongation in the P-R interval preceding a nonconducted atrial beat. After the nonconducted P wave, the P-R interval is shorter. Type II second degree AV block (Mobitz II) is electrocardiographically characterized by a constant P-R interval preceding an unexpected nonconducted atrial impulse.

Type I Second Degree AV Block

The electrocardiographic pattern of type I second degree AV block can result from Wenckebach type conduction occurring within (1) the AV node, (2) the bundle of His itself, or (3) the bundle branch–Purkinje system. Delay in the AV node is by far the most common cause (more than 90 per cent) of type I AV block. The next most common site is the bundle branch–Purkinje system, and the least common is the bundle of His itself.

Classically the AV nodal Wenckebach phenomenon is depicted as one in which the greatest increment in P-R interval occurs with the second beat of the Wenckebach cycle and thereafter progressively diminishes. This results in a decreasing R-R interval in the presence of increasing P-R intervals. Some AV nodal Wenckebach cycles do not follow this classic pattern, and the greatest increment in P-R interval may occur with the last conducted beat. Also, one may observe little or no change in the P-R interval for several beats throughout the cycle.

Figure 24 is an example of type I second degree AV block resulting from progressive conduction delay and block within the AV node. Type I AV block in the presence of normal QRS complexes is almost always AV nodal in origin. At times, the second beat of the Wenckebach

cycle may be aberrantly conducted to the ventricles. Aberrant conduction is favored by the fact that the nonconducted atrial impulse of the preceding Wenckebach cycle results in a long R-R interval. In a 3:2 AV nodal Wenckebach cycle, aberrant conduction of every second beat may simulate a ventricular bigeminy, especially if the P wave of the aberrant beat is obscured by the T wave of the preceding QRS complex.

Type I AV block occurring within the AV node may be associated with inferior wall myocardial infarctions or excessive digitalis administration, and in both of these situations the block is generally reversible. Small doses of atropine, which enhances AV nodal conduction, usually re-establish 1:1 AV conduction. However, in some cases atropine may increase the sinus rate without appreciably affecting AV nodal conduction, and higher degrees of AV block (2:1, 3:1) may result. In type I AV block of AV nodal origin, the ventricular rate is seldom slow enough to warrant aggressive drug therapy or temporary right ventricular endocardial pacing.

The electrocardiographic pattern of type I second degree AV block can also result from Wenckebach type conduction occurring within the His-Purkinje system, as illustrated in Figure 25. During 3:2 AV conduction in the presence of a fixed right bundle branch block pattern, a small increase in the P-R interval precedes a nonconducted P wave. The H-V interval increases from an initially abnormal value of 60 msec to 100 msec, indicating progressive conduction delay within the left bundle branch and the third P wave blocks within the His-Purkinje system. Patients exhibiting the findings illustrated in Figure 25 will also have intermittent periods of high degree (e.g., 2:1, 3:1) AV block within the His-Purkinje

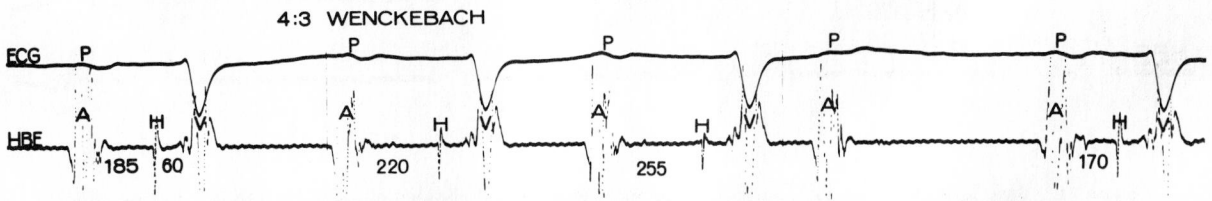

Figure 24.   Type I second degree AV block due to progressive conduction delay and block within the AV node.

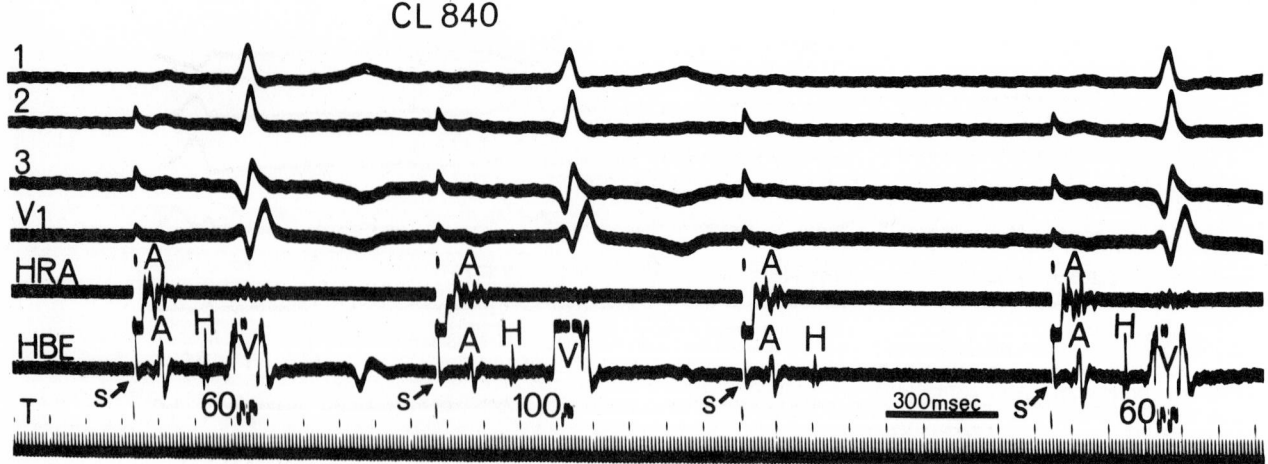

Figure 25.   Type I second degree AV block within the His-Purkinje system.

system, which accounts in part for their symptoms of fatigue, dizziness, and even syncope. Also, these patients almost invariably go on to develop complete AV block within the His-Purkinje system.

In the presence of a fixed bundle branch block pattern, the distinction, based solely on the ECG tracings, between type I second degree AV block occurring within the AV node and that of His-Purkinje origin may be quite difficult. In general, although not always, the increase in P-R interval from the first to the last of the conducted beats is significantly less in a His-Purkinje Wenckebach cycle than in an AV nodal Wenckebach cycle. However, when AV nodal Wenckebach type conduction is superimposed on a pre-existing first degree AV nodal block, the difference in P-R interval changes from the first to the last of the conducted beats may be of the magnitude seen with His-Purkinje Wenckebach cycles.

The least common site for the occurrence of Wenckebach type conduction is within the bundle of His itself. This phenomenon is characterized by the recording of two His deflections (H and H'), which signifies intra-His bundle conduction delay. As the P-R interval increases, the H-H' interval increases, and the nonconducted atrial impulse of the Wenckebach cycle is followed by only a single His deflection (H).

Type II Second Degree AV Block (Mobitz II)

Type II second degree AV block occurs less commonly than type I; it is almost always associated with a bundle branch block pattern and is a forerunner to complete AV block. The AV conduction ratio may be 3:2, 4:3, 5:4, and

so forth, and the P-R intervals preceding the nonconducted atrial beat are constant. His bundle recordings have consistently demonstrated that the site of block is within the His-Purkinje system. Figure 26 is a typical example of type II second degree AV block; a left bundle branch block pattern is present, and 3:2 AV conduction progresses to 2:1 AV block. The third P wave, which is unexpectedly blocked within the His-Purkinje system, is preceded by constant P-R intervals. A prolonged H-V interval of 76 msec in the presence of left bundle branch block indicates that a significant conduction delay also existed in the right bundle branch system.

In patients with type II second degree AV block, acceleration of the atrial rate by atropine, exercise, or atrial pacing generally leads to an increase in the degree of AV block within the His-Purkinje system. Lightheadedness, dizziness, fatigue, syncope, convulsions, and congestive heart failure are common symptoms and signs associated with type II AV block. The demonstration of type II AV block requires that a permanent ventricular pacemaker be inserted, because this form of block almost always progresses to complete AV block within a relatively short period of time.

During complete AV block, atrial impulses continue to block within the His-Purkinje system, and the ventricles come under the control of an idioventricular pacemaker discharging at a rate of 35 to 50 per minute (see Fig. 29). It is not unusual for patients with type II AV block which progresses to complete AV block to demonstrate 1:1 retrograde conduction during ventricular pacing at a rate faster than the sinus rate. This is called unidirectional block.

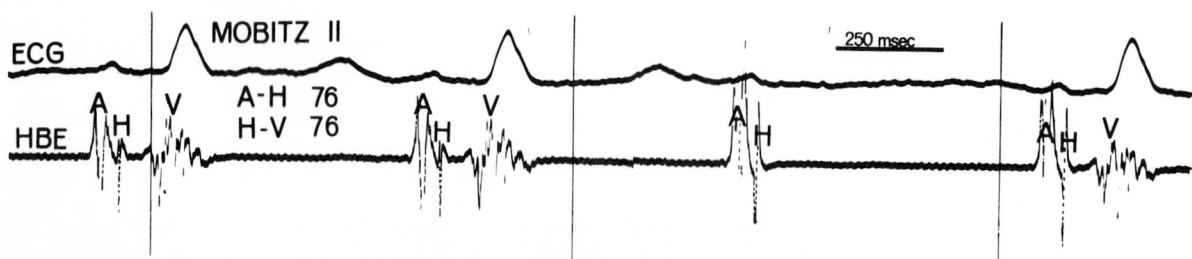

Figure 26.   Type II second degree AV block in a patient with left bundle branch block and 3:2 AV conduction which progressed to 2:1 AV block. The third P wave is blocked within the His-Purkinje system.

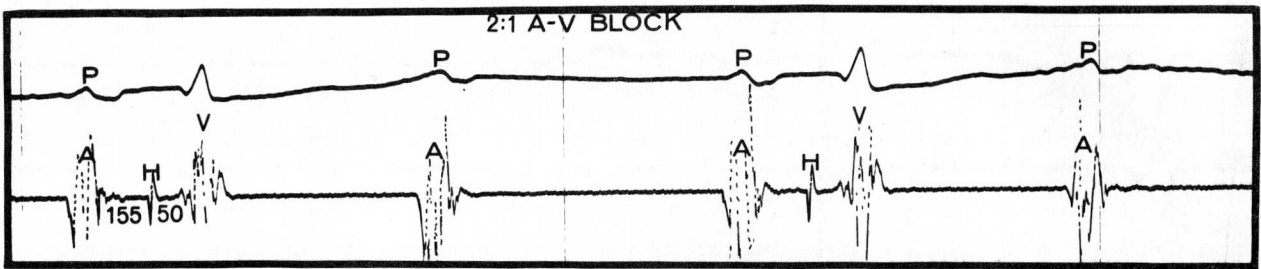

Figure 27. 2:1 AV nodal block in a patient with normal QRS complexes.

2:1 AV Block

Like all other forms of AV block, 2:1 AV block may result from lesions in the AV node, bundle of His, or bundle branch–Purkinje system.

A fixed 2:1 AV block in the presence of normal QRS complexes is almost always due to AV nodal block, and the nonconducted P waves are not followed by bundle of His deflections (Fig. 27). The P-R interval of the conducted atrial impulses may be normal or prolonged. Uncommonly, 2:1 AV block with normal QRS complexes is due to block within the bundle of His itself. Each of the nonconducted atrial impulses is associated with a bundle of His deflection, and the P-R intervals of the conducted beats are normal.

In 2:1 AV block with a bundle branch block pattern, the localization of block by electrocardiographic recordings alone is difficult. In our experience, block within the His-Purkinje system is slightly more common than AV nodal block.

Third Degree AV Block

Third degree AV block (also referred to as complete AV block) may result from lesions located in the AV node, bundle of His, or bundle branch–Purkinje system.

In third degree AV nodal block (Fig. 28), atrial impulses are blocked within the AV node. The bundle of His usually emerges as the subsidiary or escape pacemaker, activating the ventricles at a rate of 40 to 60 per minute. Each QRS complex is preceded by a single His bundle deflection, and in general both the QRS complex and H-V intervals are the same as prior to the occurrence of AV block. Patients with complete AV nodal block and a junctional pacemaker (bundle of His) may remain asymptomatic for relatively longer periods of time, and therefore the mere presence of complete AV block is not an indication for pacemaker therapy. Junctional pacemakers generally increase their discharge rate in response to exercise or after administration of atropine.

Complete AV block within the bundle of His itself is characterized by nonconducted atrial impulses which are followed by a His bundle deflection (H) and QRS complexes which are preceded by His bundle deflections (H'). The QRS complexes may be normal or abnormal and the H'-V intervals normal (30 to 55 msec) or greater than normal. It is believed that the junctional pacemaker is located within the bundle of His but distal to the site of block. These patients may not demonstrate acceleration of their ventricular rates in response to exercise or atropine. This would not be surprising if the process which caused the intra-His bundle block also affected the autonomic innervation of the common bundle . In these cases the need for pacemaker therapy depends upon the patients' symptoms.

Complete AV block distal to the bundle of His is characterized by nonconducted atrial impulses which are followed by His bundle deflections and abnormal QRS complexes which are not preceded by His bundle deflections (Fig. 29). The subsidiary pacemaker is located somewhere within the bundle branch–Purkinje system, and its discharge rate is generally between 35 and 50 per minute. These patients are almost always symptomatic (fatigue, dyspnea, dizziness, syncope, congestive heart failure) and require permanent ventricular pacemaker therapy.

Functional or Physiologic AV Block

At sinus rates of 60 to 100 per minute, the spontaneous occurrence of various types of AV block usually represents an abnormal response of the AV conducting system. On the other hand, acceleration of the atrial rate in resting subjects, such as may occur with atrial flutter, with an ectopic atrial rhythm, or during electrical stimulation of the atrium, can result in various degrees of AV block which may be considered physiologic or functional in nature. Normally, the autonomic nervous system mediates a fine balance between atrial rate and AV nodal conduction. During exercise or other stressful situations, sympathetic stimulation simultaneously increases sinus

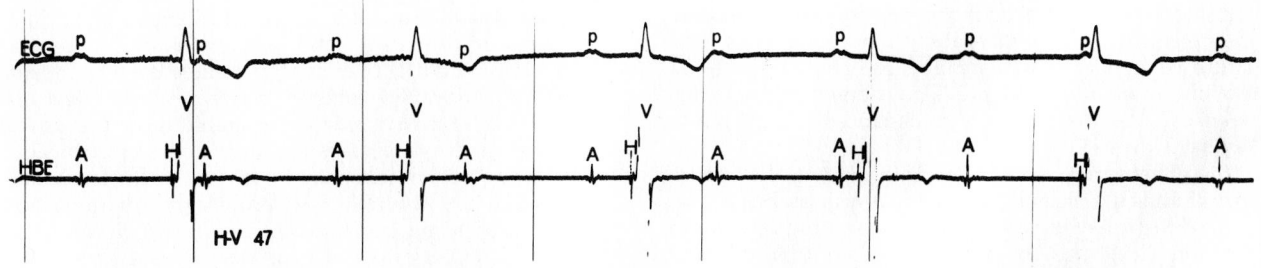

Figure 28. Third degree AV block. Atrial impulses are blocked within the AV node and dissociated from the ventricles. The latter come under control of a bundle of His pacemaker. H-V interval of 47 msec is within the normal range.

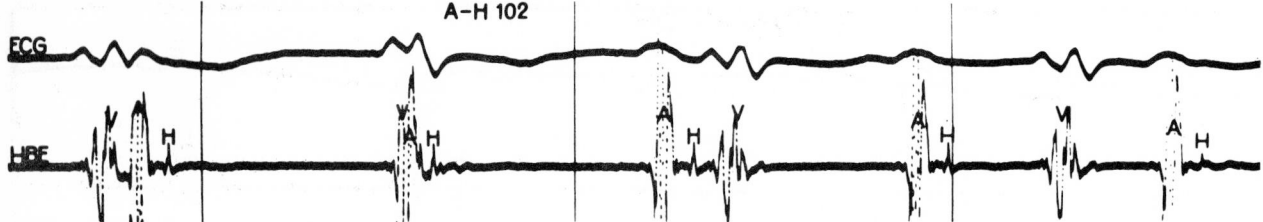

Figure 29. Third degree AV block within the His-Purkinje system. Nonconducted atrial impulses are followed by His bundle deflections. The wide QRS complexes come under control of a subjunctional pacemaker and are not preceded by bundle of His deflections.

rates and enhances AV nodal conduction so that there occurs little or no change in the P-R interval. During nonsympathetically mediated increases in atrial rate, the capacity of the AV node to transmit impulses to the ventricles is exceeded and a functional AV nodal block ensues.

Caracta, A. R., and Damato, A. N.: Significance of His bundle electrocardiography. *In* Fowler, N. O. (ed.): Cardiac Diagnosis and Treatment. New York, Harper & Row, 1976, pp. 979–1008.

Damato, A. N., Lau, S. H., and Bobb, G. A.: Cardiac arrhythmias simulated by concealed bundle of His extrasystoles in the dog. Circ. Res., 38:316, 1971.

Gallagher, J. J., Gilbert, M., Svensen, R. H., Sealy, W. C., Kassell, J., and Wallace, A. G.: Wolff-Parkinson-White syndrome. The problem, evaluation and surgical correction. Circulation, 51:767, 1975.

Gallagher, J. J., Svensen, R. H., Sealy, W. C., and Wallace, A. G.: The Wolff-Parkinson-White syndrome and the pre-excitation dysrhythmias. Medical and surgical management. Med. Clin. N. Am., 60:101, 1976.

Hoffman, B. F., and Cranefield, P. F.: Electrophysiology of the Heart. Mount Kisco, N. Y., Futura Publishing Company, 1976.

Narula, O. S.: His Bundle Electrocardiography and Clinical Electrophysiology. Philadelphia, F. A. Davis Company, 1975.

Rosen, K. M., Rahimtoola, S. H., and Gunnar, R.: Pseudo A-V block secondary to premature nonpropagated His bundle depolarizations. Documentation by His bundle recordings. Circulation, 42:367, 1970.

Wellens, H. J. J., Lie, K. I., and Janse, M. J.: The Conduction System of the Heart. Structure, Function and Clinical Implications. Philadelphia, Lea & Febiger, 1976.

364.3.   ANTIARRHYTHMIC DRUGS

Several drugs, which may be administered singly or in combination, are available for the treatment of a variety of cardiac rhythm disturbances. Proper management of cardiac arrhythmias begins with a precise electrocardiographic diagnosis of the arrhythmia at hand. Equally important is knowledge of the clinical setting in which the rhythm disturbance is occurring. Prior to initiating therapy one should obtain the following information: Does the patient have heart disease, and, if so, to what extent? Are there initiating or contributing factors present which, if corrected, will either preclude the use of antiarrhythmic drugs or enhance their effectiveness (e.g., hypokalemia, hypoxia, acidosis, thyrotoxicosis, caffeine, amphetamines)? Does the patient have congestive heart failure or hypotension? Is this a recurrent arrhythmia, and, if so, what was the previous therapy and its effectiveness? Are there known intolerances to any antiarrhythmic drugs?

The effectiveness of a given drug regimen in treating arrhythmias will be enhanced if the physician has knowledge of the following aspects of a given drug: (1) sites(s) of action, (2) dosage, route, and rate of administration, (3) site of metabolism and route of excretion, (4) range of therapeutic plasma concentration, and (5) clinical and electrocardiographic manifestations of side effects or toxicity.

LIDOCAINE

This drug finds its greatest utility in the coronary care unit for the treatment of ventricular extrasystoles and ventricular tachycardia. It is ineffective in the treatment of atrial arrhythmias. Lidocaine is given initially as an intravenous bolus injection of 50 to 150 mg over a one- to two-minute period, followed by a constant infusion of 1 to 4 mg per minute. The pharmokinetics of lidocaine are such that following a single bolus injection there occurs within a few minutes a rapid decline in blood concentration to subtherapeutic levels. A constant infusion is used to maintain therapeutic blood levels between 0.5 and 5.0 μg per milliliter. As soon as it is established that the ventricular arrhythmia is under control, the infusion rate of lidocaine should be decreased to the minimal amount which will maintain control. Lidocaine is metabolized in the liver, and therefore patients who have liver dysfunction or decreased hepatic blood flow should receive lesser amounts of the drug and be more carefully observed for toxic effects.

Toxicity to lidocaine is not uncommon and is most frequently expressed as central nervous system effects. There include dizziness, paresthesias, confusion, agitation, muscle tremors, and seizures. Although toxic effects are most commonly seen when blood levels exceed 5.0 μg per milliliter, they may also be observed when blood levels are within the therapeutic range. This latter effect may be due to the accumulation of pharmacologically active metabolites of the drug.

PROCAINAMIDE

Procainamide is a very effective agent in the treatment of ventricular arrhythmias. When given intravenously, it is administered at a rate of 20 to 25 mg per minute until either the arrhythmia is abolished or a total of 1000 mg has been given. The width of the QRS complex should be monitored and the drug cautiously given after there is a 25 per cent widening over control values. If a 50 per cent widening of the QRS complex occurs without effect on the ventricular arrhythmia, one should stop the drug. After the acute intravenous therapy, a constant infusion of 1 to 5 mg per minute may be given. Most ventricular arrhythmias are controlled at serum concentrations between 4 and 8 mg per liter. Within this concentration range, toxic effects are minimal. Major toxicity begins to occur at serum concentrations above 8 mg per liter.

Procainamide can also be given orally on a long-term

basis for control of ventricular arrhythmias. In most clinical situations the drug is well absorbed from the gastrointestinal tract, with peak plasma concentrations occurring after one hour. In patients without significant cardiac, renal, or hepatic dysfunction, the serum half-life varies between 2 and 4 hours (mean, three hours). It has been demonstrated that dosing at an interval of every six hours produces wide fluctuations in plasma concentration, and therefore it is recommended that oral procainamide be given at intervals close to its half-life, i.e., every three to four hours. Some patients may need dosing at the shorter interval, whereas others demonstrate good control at a dosing schedule of every six or eight hours. N-acetylprocainamide (NAPA) is one of the metabolites of procainamide which has been reported to approximate the antiarrhythmic activity of the parent compound.

In urgent clinical situations, a priming dose of procainamide may be given in order to achieve adequate serum concentrations as quickly as possible. The loading dose is twice the three- to four-hour maintenance dose (i.e., load, 500 to 1000 mg). Forty to 70 per cent of the drug is excreted unchanged by the kidney, and therefore the dose may have to be modified in patients with renal disease. Side effects of procainamide include nausea, vomiting, fever, and skin rashes. The most troublesome side effect is the development of a lupus-like syndrome. Various reports indicate that between 20 and 75 per cent of patients taking procainamide develop positive ANA titers but only 5 to 30 per cent develop clinical symptoms. Symptoms usually remit with discontinuance of the drug. An ANA titer should be determined for each patient who is to receive prolonged procainamide therapy. If a positive titer develops, the drug should be stopped and a substitute drug given.

QUINIDINE

The electrophysiologic properties of quinidine are similar to those of procainamide. Quinidine appears to be more effective than procainamide against atrial arrhythmias but is equally effective against ventricular arrhythmias. Quinidine is primarily used as an oral agent; it may be administered intramuscularly and is rarely given parenterally. The primary indications for quinidine are (1) for the pharmacologic conversion of atrial flutter or fibrillation to sinus rhythm, (2) as prophylaxis in patients with paroxysmal atrial flutter, atrial fibrillation, or junctional re-entrant tachycardia, and (3) for suppression of ventricular arrhythmias.

Quinidine is rapidly and almost completely absorbed from the gastrointestinal tract. Absorption is better on an empty stomach. The drug is metabolized in the liver. Unchanged quinidine (25 to 50 per cent) and its metabolic products are excreted in the urine. The dosage of quinidine should be adjusted downward in patients who have liver dysfunction or renal disease. With short-acting preparations of quinidine, peak blood levels are achieved in one to three hours; long-acting preparations achieve peak levels in approximately four hours. Therapeutic blood levels range from 2 to 7 mg per liter. An average oral dose of quinidine is 400 mg every six to eight hours (range, 100 to 600 mg).

The electrocardiographic alterations resulting from quinidine are a prolongation of the QRS and Q-T intervals. These occur because quinidine increases conduction and refractoriness in the His-Purkinje system. Quinidine can be given to patients who have a pre-existing bundle branch block pattern.

Quinidine is vagolytic and as such can cause an increase in the sinus rate and enhance AV nodal conduction. It is this latter effect which requires that patients with atrial fibrillation or flutter be given digitalis prior to being given quinidine, lest the ventricular response increase to an undesirable level. In atrial flutter, the ventricular response may increase because quinidine both slows the atrial rate and enhances AV nodal conduction. Quinidine can cause hypotension by decreasing myocardial contractility and causing vasodilatation.

So-called quinidine syncope is a major but fortunately uncommon complication of therapy. Self-limiting episodes of ventricular tachycardia or ventricular fibrillation have been demonstrated to be a cause of quinidine syncope.

Gastrointestinal toxicity includes anorexia, nausea, and vomiting. Diarrhea is the most common adverse effect. High blood levels may cause tinnitus, vertigo, and nausea (cinchonism). In a fair number of cases, quinidine causes thrombocytopenia.

PROPRANOLOL

Propranolol is a beta-adrenergic receptor blocking drug which has as its major electrophysiologic effects slowing of the sinus rate and AV nodal conduction time. As an antiarrhythmic agent the drug has its greatest usefulness in the following situations: (1) in cases of atrial fibrillation and atrial flutter in which the ventricular response cannot be controlled by digitalis alone or when digitalis is contraindicated, (2) as acute or prophylactic therapy in cases of AV junctional re-entrant tachycardias, and (3) for suppression of ventricular extrasystoles and ventricular tachycardia, especially those suspected of being due to excessive catecholamines or increased sympathetic tone. In most cases of ventricular arrhythmias, propranolol is not the first drug of choice.

Propranolol may be given orally or parenterally. It is almost completely absorbed form the gastrointestinal tract, with peak effect occurring in one to one and a half hours. Oral therapy is given every four to six hours. Since sympathetic tone varies considerably among individuals, the clinically effective dose varies from patient to patient (usual range, 20 to 80 mg four times per day). When given intravenously, the drug is administered at a rate of 1 mg per minute up to a maximum of 10 mg.* As with any intravenous therapy for cardiac arrhythmias, ECG and blood pressure monitoring should be performed.

Propranolol has a negative inotropic effect and may aggravate or precipitate heart failure in patients with borderline cardiac function. It may cause significant sinus bradycardia or hypotension or may intensify AV block. Beta-adrenergic blockade causes bronchial constriction, and therefore the drug is contraindicated in patients with bronchial asthma and chronic obstructive lung disease. Propranolol may mask the premonitory signs of hypoglycemia in patients with diabetes mellitus.

DIPHENYLHYDANTOIN†
(Phenytoin)

Diphenylhydantoin (DPH) is an anticonvulsant drug which has been shown to have cardiac antiarrhythmic

---

*See p. vi, Dosage Notice, immediately following Preface.
†Experimental drug for this purpose.

effects. Its effects on the electrophysiologic properties of the heart are similar to those of lidocaine and appear to be opposite to those of procainamide and quinidine. DPH has been shown to be effective against ventricular extrasystoles and tachycardia caused by digitalis and other agents. It is ineffective in converting atrial flutter or fibrillation to sinus rhythm. Effectiveness has been demonstrated in the treatment of atrial arrhythmias resulting from digitalis excess. DPH is not a first line drug; it is primarily used when other drugs have failed or when combination therapy is required. DPH may be given intravenously or orally. Intravenous administration should be at a rate of 20 mg per minute until (1) the arrhythmia is abolished, (2) 1000 mg has been given, or (3) serious side effects occur. Oral administration may be rapid or slow. To attain therapeutic blood levels rapidly by the oral route, 1000 mg is given within 24 hours, followed by 500 to 600 mg per day for two days. Thereafter, maintenance doses of 300 to 500 mg are given daily. If one starts by giving 300 to 500 mg per day, therapeutic blood levels will be attained in five to seven days. Therapeutic plasma levels are between 10 and 18 μg per milliliter. Toxic effects are generally seen at >20 μg per milliliter.

DPH is metabolized in the liver, and the dosage should be adjusted downward in patients who have liver dysfunction or decreased hepatic blood flow. The administration of usual doses of DPH in combination with isoniazid and aminosalicylic acid has resulted in toxic levels of DPH. Barbiturates increase microsomal enzyme activity, which accelerates the rate of DPH metabolism, causing diminished pharmacologic activity. Parenteral DPH may cause drowsiness, nystagmus, circumoral tingling, vertigo, nausea, and vomiting. Too rapid injection of DPH (>50 mg per minute) may cause cardiovascular collapse.

DISOPYRAMIDE

Disopyramide phosphate (Norpace) is an antiarrhythmic agent which has recently been approved for oral use. Its electrophysiologic actions appear to be similar to those of quinidine sulfate. Disopyramide is reported to be effective in the treatment of unifocal and multifocal ventricular extrasystoles and ventricular tachycardia. The usual adult dosage is 400 to 800 mg per day given in divided doses four times daily. Disopyramide is rapidly and almost completely absorbed from the gastrointestinal tract. Peak plasma levels are achieved within two hours of dosing. Therapeutic plasma levels are 2 to 4 μg per milliliter. Fifty per cent of the drug is excreted in the urine unchanged, and dosage should be lowered in patients with renal or hepatic impairment. The more common adverse effects are associated with the anticholinergic properties of the drug, which include dry mouth, urinary hesitancy or retention, constipation, and blurred vision. The drug should not be used in patients with glaucoma unless miotics are first given. Disopyramide may cause QRS widening and Q-T prolongation.

Benowitz, N. L.: Clinical applications of the pharmokinetics of lidocaine. Cardiovasc. Clin., 6:77, 1974.
Bigger, J. T., and Giardina, E. G. V.: Rational use of antiarrhythmic drugs alone and in combination. Cardiovasc. Clin., 6:103, 1974.
Koch-Weser, J.: Clinical application of the pharmokinetics of procaine amide. Cardiovasc. Clin., 6:63, 1974.

364.4. CARDIOVERSION OF ARRHYTHMIAS BY DC ELECTROSHOCK

DC shock applied externally to the chest wall is an effective method of converting several types of cardiac arrhythmias to sinus rhythm; these include atrial fibrillation, atrial flutter, paroxysmal atrial tachycardia, ventricular tachycardia, and ventricular fibrillation. AC cardioverters were originally used clinically but have been replaced by DC cardioverters. The advantages of DC cardioverters or defibrillators are as follows: (1) they are lighter in weight and more effective than AC defibrillators, (2) they can be made independent of line current and portable, and (3) the short duration of the electrical discharge (a few milliseconds) allows it to be delivered at a preset time within the QRS complex. This is called synchronized cardioversion. AC cardioverters produce sinusoidal pulses which deliver their energy over a period of 150 to 250 msec. Thus with AC cardioverters the ability to deliver a shock during the so-called vulnerable period of ventricles, and thereby to induce ventricular fibrillation, is greater than with DC cardioverters.

Cardioversion of supraventricular rhythms and ventricular tachycardia should always be performed in the synchronized mode. Input of an ECG signal into the defibrillator automatically programs it to discharge within the terminal portion of the QRS complex, thus avoiding the ventricular vulnerable period. It is extremely important to be sure that the synchronizer circuit is not activated when the defibrillator is used for the treatment of ventricular fibrillation. Since there are no QRS complexes generated during ventricular fibrillation, the activated synchronizer circuit will prevent the defibrillator from discharging.

Prior to cardioversion, patients should receive either thiopental or diazepam to create an amnesic state. Skin resistance must be decreased by the application of a suitable electrode paste or saline-soaked pads. Alcohol-soaked pads should never be used because passage of an electric current may cause them to burst into flames. Application of electrode paste should be limited to the diameter of the electrode paddles (3½ inches). One must avoid contact between the two areas of conductive material (bridging), as this will cause the electrical current to travel along the skin, causing burns and ineffectual cardioversion.

ATRIAL FLUTTER. Synchronized DC shock is considered by many to be the treatment of choice for atrial flutter. Sinus rhythm can be established in more than 90 per cent of patients. It is certainly the treatment of choice in those uncommon situations in which atrial flutter exists with 1:1 AV conduction. If a patient is receiving digitalis to slow the ventricular rate, it should be omitted for one or two days prior to electrical cardioversion. An oral dose of quinidine may be given one to three hours prior to cardioversion. Treatment of atrial flutter may begin with energy levels of 25 watt-sec (joules) and progressively increased until conversion occurs. The decision as to whether patients should receive long-term quinidine therapy to prevent future occurrences will depend upon the frequency of the episodes of atrial flutter and tolerance to the drug. In chronic or recurrent atrial flutter which is not prevented by quinidine, one may have to accept the persistence of the arrhythmia and maintain a suitable ventricular rate with the use of digitalis.

ATRIAL FIBRILLATION. Although most cases of atrial fibrillation can be converted to sinus rhythm, not all remain in sinus rhythm; nor should conversion be attempted in all cases of atrial fibrillation. Conversion by DC shock should be done immediately for those patients with the Wolff-Parkinson-White syndrome who have developed atrial fibrillation with rapid ventricular rates caused by conduction over the accessory pathway. Immediate conversion by DC shock should also be considered in the patient with atrial fibrillation with a rapid ventricular rate (>180 per minute) in whom significant hypotension, heart failure, or angina pectoris develops. Most other patients with atrial fibrillation can be treated with digitalis and/or propranolol for control of the ventricular rate, after which a decision for conversion to sinus rhythm can be made.

Conversion should not be attempted in the following: (1) Patients who have had established atrial fibrillation of several years' duration. (2) Patients in whom previous attempts to maintain sinus rhythm have been unsuccessful despite adequate prophylactic therapy with quinidine. (3) Patients with known sensitivity or idiosyncratic reactions to quinidine. (4) Patients with the bradycardia-tachycardia syndrome (sick sinus syndrome), in whom conversion of atrial fibrillation results in an inadequate sinus rate. (5) Patients with very large left atria. (6) Elderly patients (65 to 70 years of age).

Patients who are maintained in atrial fibrillation should be considered for anticoagulant therapy for the prevention of systemic embolization.

VENTRICULAR TACHYCARDIA. Drug therapy (e.g., lidocaine, procainamide) is the preferred method for treating ventricular tachycardia. Synchronized DC shock should be used for those patients who are resistant to conversion by drugs or in whom significant hypotension or shock is present. DC shock should be avoided in ventricular tachycardia due to digitalis toxicity. However, if DC shock must be used, one should begin with the lowest energy levels, i.e., 25 watt-sec. A lidocaine drip should be started and maintained during the postcardioversion period to prevent recurrences of ventricular tachycardia.

VENTRICULAR FIBRILLATION. Ventricular fibrillation should be immediately treated with 400 watt-sec energy levels. If anoxia and acidosis are present, it is more difficult to convert ventricular fibrillation and therefore these abnormalities must be corrected by adequate ventilation and $NaHCO_3$. If the initial one or two attempts at defibrillation are unsuccessful, basic life support measures should be applied while ventilatory and metabolic abnormalities are being corrected.

Ewy, G.: Cardiac arrest and resuscitation: Defibrillators and defibrillation. *In* Harvey, P. (ed.): Current Problems in Cardiology, Vol. II, no. 11. Chicago, Year Book Medical Publishers, 1978.

364.5. PACEMAKERS

The sick sinus syndrome and symptomatic AV block constitute the major reasons for insertion of cardiac pacemakers today. Much less frequently pacemakers are used in (1) control of drug-resistant ventricular tachycardia and (2) drug-resistant paroxysmal supraventricular tachycardia in which abrupt termination of the tachycardia is associated with a significant pause and symptoms prior to resumption of a sinus or escape rhythm.

Cardiac pacing may be performed by the transvenous method or by electrodes implanted directly onto the ventricular epicardium. Transvenous pacing may be temporary or permanent. In temporary transvenous pacing an electrode catheter is introduced into a peripheral vein and fluoroscopically positioned against the endocardium of the right ventricle. The proximal electrodes are connected to an external cardiac pacemaker which has an adjustable rate and milliamperage control. Temporary transvenous pacing is utilized (1) prior to the insertion of a permanent pacing system and (2) in situations in which the indication for pacing is judged to be reversible (drug-induced AV block or bradycardia) or possibly irreversible and progressive (AV and bundle branch blocks associated with myocardial infarction). Permanent transvenous pacing is performed under sterile surgical conditions. An electrode catheter is positioned in the right ventricle through a subclavian vein, and the proximal electrode terminals are attached to a pacemaker which is implanted subcutaneously.

Electrodes may be unipolar or bipolar. A unipolar lead-electrode system contains a single electrode in direct contact with the myocardium which is connected to the negative terminal of the pacemaker. The positive terminal functions as the indifferent electrode of the pacing system. In a bipolar lead electrode system, the electrodes are in close proximity to each other and are situated within or on the heart. Unipolar leads produce larger stimulus potentials on ECG tracings than do bipolar leads. In addition, unipolar leads are more sensitive to extraneous sig-

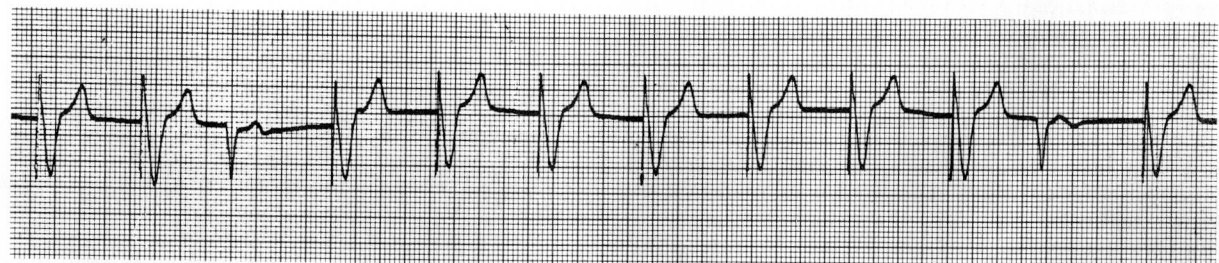

Figure 30. QRS-inhibited demand pacemaker functioning in both the pacing and sensing modes. Each paced QRS complex is preceded by a stimulus artifact. The stimulus interval is approximately 840 msec. The first two QRS complexes are paced beats. Following the second paced beat a single spontaneous QRS complex occurs approximately 720 msec after the last pacemaker discharge. The inherent beat is sensed by the pacemaker, which inhibits itself from firing. Absence of subsequent spontaneous activity results in the pacemaker functioning in a fixed mode. Sensing, inhibition, and subsequent pacing are repeated with the last two beats.

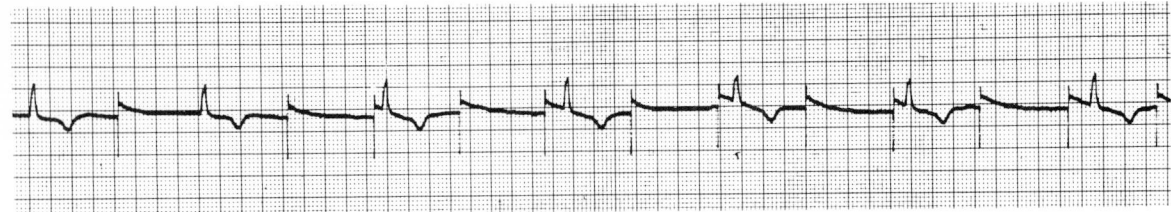

Figure 31. Sample tracing from a patient with a QRS-inhibited demand pacemaker. There is complete failure to capture, and only intermittent sensing. All QRS complexes are generated by the inherent heart rate, which varies between 1600 and 1720 msec. The stimulus interval of the pacemaker is 840 msec. The second spontaneous QRS complex, which occurs 40 msec before the expected discharge of the pacemaker, is sensed and inhibits the pacemaker. Thereafter, none of the QRS complexes are sensed and the pacemaker discharges at a fixed rate, but none of the stimuli capture the ventricles.

nals than are bipolar leads. In the event of a wire breakage, a bipolar lead system can be converted to a unipolar lead.

Cardiac pacing can be performed in the fixed or demand modes. In fixed rate cardiac pacing, the pacemaker is preset to discharge at a constant rate, irrespective of the inherent cardiac rate. The ability of fixed rate pacemakers to induce competitive rhythms which may cause tachycardia or fibrillation has discouraged their general use. Demand pacemakers may be QRS inhibited or QRS triggered. Both types of demand pacemakers are programmed to sense the inherent R-R interval (heart rate). In a QRS-inhibited demand pacemaker, the pacemaker will be inhibited from discharging a pacing stimulus if the inherent R-R interval is less than the preset firing rate of the pacemaker (stimulus to stimulus interval). It will also be inhibited if the interval from a paced or stimulated beat to a subsequent spontaneous beat is less than the preset firing interval (Fig. 30). If spontaneous ventricular activity is absent or consistently less than the preset firing rate, the demand pacemaker will essentially function as a fixed rate pacemaker (Fig. 31). QRS-triggered demand pacemakers are also programmed to sense the inherent R-R interval. However, when the R-R interval is less than the preset firing rate, these pacemakers discharge their stimulus within the spontaneously generated QRS complex. The pacemaker-generated stimulus is ineffectual because it occurs during the absolute refractory period of the ventricular myocardium. When the inherent R-R interval is greater than the preset firing rate of the pacemaker, the stimulus will be effective in eliciting a ventricular depolarization.

Temporary pacing as described above is usually not performed with the same catheter in place for more than five days, especially if phlebitis or local skin infection develops. If additional temporary pacing time is required, another vein with a new catheter will have to be used.

When failure to reliably pace occurs with the use of an external pacemaker, the physician should embark upon a systematic check of the pacing system: (1) Check to see that the proximal electrodes of the pacing catheter are secured within the positive and negative terminals of the external pacemaker. (2) Raise the milliampere level to ensure that it is above the minimum threshold for pacing. (3) Check for wire breaks on the externalized portion of the electrode catheter. (4) Check that the pacemaker batteries are not depleted. (5) Obtain appropriate x-rays of the chest to confirm location of the catheter.

A not infrequent complication of transvenous right ventricular pacing is dislodgment of the cardiac catheter from its endocardial pacing site. The design of newer

electrode catheters has helped to overcome this problem. Dislodgment results in failure to reliably capture or sense, or both. Perforation of the electrode catheter through the myocardium into the pericardial space is another cause for intermittent capture and sensing. Right ventricular apical pacing produces the electrocardiographic pattern of left bundle branch block with left axis deviation. A change from this pattern to one of right bundle branch block should suggest perforation of the electrode catheter and pacing of the left ventricle. Less commonly, failure to sense or capture is due to a wire break in the electrode catheter.

The development of newer battery energy sources has extended the functioning period of pacemaker power packs from two to five years before replacement is required. Nuclear-powered pacemakers are purported to last 20 years. After implantation of a permanent pacemaker, patients should be followed at monthly intervals for a few months, and thereafter the frequency of follow-up should be extended. The frequency of visits should be increased as the end of the expected life of the power source is approached. Transtelephonic monitoring has also been used for pacemaker surveillance.

Patients with cardiac pacemakers are subject to a wide variety of potential electrical dangers both in and outside the hospital. Patients with temporary transvenous electrode catheters are especially vulnerable to random current leakage, which, when bypassing the normally high skin resistance and delivered directly to the heart, may cause life-threatening ventricular arrhythmias. Malfunction of pacemakers may also occur from electromagnetic currents generated by electrocautery, diathermy, microwave ovens, television transmitting stations, or automobile ignitions. Skeletal muscle potentials have been reported to trigger the QRS sensing circuit of QRS-inhibited pacemakers and temporally suppress their function.

365. DISORDERS OF THE PERICARDIUM

Robert E. Whalen

365.1. INTRODUCTION

Claudius Galen first noted and named the pericardium in the second century A.D. He also recognized that the pericardium could be the site of inflammation in animals, that pericardial effusions had a deleterious

Etiology of Disorders of the Pericardium

I. Inflammatory
  A. Acute pericarditis
    1. Nonspecific "benign" or idiopathic
    2. Infections
      a. Viral
      b. Bacterial
      c. Tuberculous
      d. Fungal
      e. Others
    3. Myocardial infarction
      a. Acute myocardial infarction
      b. Postmyocardial infarction
    4. Postpericardiotomy or thoracotomy
    5. Post-traumatic
    6. Connective tissue disorders
    7. Allergic and hypersensitivity disorders
    8. Metabolic disorders
    9. Physical or chemical agents
  B. Chronic pericarditis (virtually all of the above)
II. Neoplastic disease
  A. Benign
  B. Malignant
    1. Primary
    2. Secondary
III. Congenital lesions of the pericardium
  A. Pericardial cysts and diverticula
  B. Partial or complete absence of the pericardium
IV. Disease of diverse or unknown etiology

effect on cardiac motion, and that the pericardium could be the site of tumor formation. Diseases of the pericardium typically present in one or more of three clinical forms: acute pericarditis, pericardial effusion, and pericardial constriction. Pericardial involvement may progress from inflammation to effusion and then constriction, or it may present as effusion or constriction without clinical evidence of preceding inflammation.

The pericardium may be the site of a variety of inflammatory, neoplastic, and congenital disorders. The incidence of such disorders, which are listed in the accompanying table, has changed markedly over the past several decades. This change stems from four major factors: the introduction of antibiotics, which has significantly decreased the incidence of bacterial involvement of the pericardium; the increasing clinical awareness of the involvement of the pericardium in various connective tissue diseases; the marked increase in the postpericardiotomy syndrome accompanying the advent of modern cardiac surgery; and the growing recognition of acute and delayed signs of pericardial involvement associated with myocardial infarction.

365.2. ACUTE PERICARDITIS

By far the most common initial manifestation of pericardial disease is acute pericarditis. This condition may be due to diverse causes. In many cases the same etiologic factors may persist over long periods of time and thus produce a recurrent, subacute, or chronic disorder.

ETIOLOGY. Nonspecific "Benign" or Idiopathic Pericarditis. This is perhaps the most common type of acute pericarditis in adults. The term benign should probably not be applied to this entity, because the symptomatology is certainly not benign and the disease can be accompanied by acute pericardial effusion and tamponade. The syndrome's designation is actually a reflection of our inability to determine an etiologic factor. For many years this syndrome has been attributed to either a viral agent or a hypersensitivity reaction, but there has been no effective proof of this. As detection and isolation techniques for viral diseases have been perfected and the skill of detecting other underlying diseases, such as connective tissue diseases and myocardial infarction, has improved, more and more cases of so-called idiopathic or nonspecific pericarditis have been removed from this category; but the cause of the rest remains unknown. Typically the syndrome occurs in late adolescence and early adulthood. It is often preceded by an upper respiratory infection days to several weeks before fever and precordial pain bring the patient to medical attention. The syndrome usually lasts one to several weeks, during which time the patient is mildly febrile and has varying degrees of precordial pain. Occasionally pericardial effusion may appear early, and sometimes it is the first sign of the syndrome. Although the acute symptoms may subside after a brief time, the patient may be left with easy fatigability for several months. This may reflect the fact that in virtually all cases of acute pericarditis there is some inflammatory response in the subepicardial myocardium, and there may be a greater degree of myocarditis than is recognized clinically. Exacerbations of the syndrome, particularly of precordial pain, are not rare and may occur sporadically for several months to years after the initial attack. The development of constrictive pericarditis is extremely rare. There are no classic differentiating laboratory studies, although the majority of patients have a mild leukocytosis. The electrocardiogram is almost always abnormal and shows the changes discussed under Laboratory Findings. Chest x-ray may show slight increase in cardiac size as compared to previous baseline x-rays; this may be due to either a small pericardial effusion or thickening of the inflamed pericardium. Pulmonary infiltrates are frequently noted, and pleural effusion may occur in one fourth of patients. In most cases bed rest and analgesics will produce relief of symptoms in one to two weeks. If these measures fail to produce relief of pain, various nonsteroidal anti-inflammatory agents, such as aspirin and indomethacin, have been effective. In patients with unusually severe and prolonged pain, adrenal corticosteroid hormone therapy may be indicated, but this should be undertaken only if bacterial infection can be excluded.

Infectious Pericarditis. Infections of proved etiology account for a significant number of cases of pericarditis. Various *viral agents* have long been suspected as causes for "idiopathic nonspecific" pericarditis. However, even with careful viral isolation studies, only a small percentage of cases have been demonstrated to be associated with viral infection of the pericardium or myocardium. The most common viral agent is coxsackievirus Type B; rarely, coxsackievirus Type A is the agent. Pericarditis has also been reported to be due to Type A echovirus, mumps, and infectious mononucleosis. The clinical course, physical findings, and method of treatment in proved cases of viral pericarditis are not significantly different from those discussed under Nonspecific "Benign" or Idiopathic Pericarditis. Although it has been suggested that diffuse myalgias, rubelliform rashes, and lymphadenopathy are more common in viral pericarditis than in idiopathic pericarditis, there have been insufficient viral studies in patients labeled as having idiopathic pericarditis to warrant this as being a diagnostic feature for separating the two entities, if indeed they are truly separate.

Bacterial infections of the pericardium may arise by direct extension of infection from foci in the thorax such as pneumonia or empyema. Less frequently bacterial pericarditis is caused by a septicemia which is initiated from a distant site of infection. The emergence of antibiotic-resistant strains of staphylococci, particularly in the hospital, has served to increase the frequency of this organism as a causative agent in relation to other previously classic bacterial causes for pericarditis. The unique susceptibility of the pneumococcus to penicillin has almost completely eliminated this as a cause for bacterial pericarditis, and cases are seldom seen unless treatment has been long delayed and the patient has empyema. A large number of other types of organisms have been implicated in the development of pericarditis, including the meningococcus, gonococcus, *Hemophilus influenzae,* and streptococcal organisms. Although gram-negative organisms are a relatively rare cause for acute pericarditis, their frequency has increased because of the development of antibiotic-resistant strains, particularly in patients having complications after cardiac surgery and in patients on immunosuppressive therapy for malignancies. *Pseudomonas, Proteus, E. coli* and *Klebsiella* have produced increasingly more difficult to treat pericardial infections in such patients. When typhoid fever was a scourge in earlier generations, involvement of the pericardium was recognized as a complication of this disease. Nontyphoidal *Salmonella* organisms are a very rare cause for pericarditis. Bacterial pericarditis rarely is the initial sign of infection and often appears only as a late complication of either untreated or poorly controlled bacterial infection. When it does appear, it may present with the classic signs of acute pericarditis and may eventuate in a pericardial effusion or constriction. However, it is important to recognize that the classic signs of acute pericarditis are present in probably less than half of patients with bacterial pericarditis, and therefore the diagnosis should not be discarded because of the absence of clinical signs of acute pericarditis. Laboratory signs are not significantly different from those seen in other forms of pericarditis except for the expected leukocytosis. Once the diagnosis is suspected, diagnostic studies must be initiated immediately, for time is of the essence if the infection is to be successfully treated. If suspicion is sufficient and diagnostic pericardial fluid cannot be obtained by pericardiocentesis, an exploratory thoracotomy should be performed promptly. If the diagnosis is not established either by pericardiocentesis or exploratory thoracotomy, a pericardiectomy, if feasible, or a pleuropericardial window procedure should be performed.

Although *tuberculous* involvement of the pericardium might justifiably be considered with the bacterial forms of pericarditis, it has earned a place of its own because of its prevalence in earlier decades and its propensity to produce constrictive pericarditis. Tuberculous pericarditis occurs predominantly in males, particularly in blacks, who have approximately ten times the incidence of the disease found in whites. Although tuberculous pericarditis may be the only evidence of the infection, it probably arises as a secondary manifestation of the disease rather than as a primary focus. Approximately half the patients with tuberculous pericarditis have evidence of previous or concurrent infection of the lung. In the acute phase it cannot be differentiated from other forms of infectious pericarditis. In the chronic phase it may have an insidious onset characterized more by systemic symptoms such as low grade fever and weakness. In the chronic form the progressive constrictive process may be its predominant manifestation. The disease must be considered in any patient presenting with acute pericarditis, pericardial effusion, or constriction. The diagnosis may sometimes be made by examination and culture of the pericardial fluid, although this is extremely difficult unless large volumes of pericardial fluid can be obtained. The diagnosis is more likely to be made by suitable pathologic examination and culture of pericardial tissue obtained at surgery.

TREATMENT. Evidence of old or active tuberculosis by chest x-ray or the presence of a positive tuberculin skin test in a patient who had a previous negative skin test not only heightens the likelihood of the diagnosis but should raise the question that antituberculous therapy should be started on clinical grounds alone. The effects of progressive tuberculous involvement of the pericardium are so devastating and the institution of antituberculous therapy is of such relatively low morbidity that on some occasions the clinician will feel forced to treat pericarditis of unknown etiology as though it might be tuberculous. When the diagnosis is likely on clinical grounds but cannot be proved by culture or pathologic studies, a more conservative approach with a combination of isoniazid and rifampin or ethambutol for 18 months, along with continued follow-up to be certain that there is no progression, may be indicated. If the index of suspicion is great and pericardiocentesis has not demonstrated an organism, a pericardiectomy, both to establish a diagnosis and to prevent future constriction, is frequently employed. When the diagnosis is established, triple therapy with isoniazid, streptomycin, and rifampin or ethambutol is indicated for 18 to 24 months. If the diagnosis has been made and antituberculous therapy has not eliminated signs of effusion or constriction in several months, a pericardiectomy should be performed.

Various *fungal disorders*, including histoplasmosis, coccidioidomycosis, actinomycosis, and nocardiosis, have been reported as etiologic agents in the development of pericarditis. Although these represent an extremely small number of cases, the possibility should be considered in patients who are uniquely susceptible to fungal infections, particularly those with lymphomas and leukemia and those who are undergoing immunosuppressant therapy for other systemic diseases. *Parasites* represent a very small but definite class of etiologic agents in the development of pericarditis. Infection with *Entamoeba histolytica* has been reported to produce pericarditis by hematogenous spread to the pericardium or by rupture of a hepatic cyst into the pericardial space. Although *Echinococcus* is a rare cause of pericarditis, over 100 cases of such involvement have been reported in the literature. Pericardial infection almost inevitably stems from initial invasion and cyst formation of the myocardium with rupture into the pericardial space.

Myocardial Infarction. Pericarditis associated with myocardial infarction may take two forms, and on occasion it may be difficult to be certain whether one is dealing with a late-appearing *acute pericarditis* or an early appearance of *postmyocardial infarction pericarditis.*

Acute inflammation of the pericardium frequently accompanies acute myocardial infarction, particularly if it is transmural. The clinical recognition of this, such as the development of consistent typical pericardial pain and a pericardial friction rub, is directly related to the frequency with which the patient is examined. With repetitive examination, signs may be recognized in at least two thirds of patients rather than the 20 per cent previously reported. The symptoms usually occur between the second and fifth days and rarely after the tenth day. The syndrome is thought to be due to an inflammatory response in the subepicardial region of the infarcted myocardium with some extension of inflammation to contiguous areas of the epicardium. It is almost inevitably a self-limited process and requires only analgesics or a nonsteroidal anti-inflammatory agent to control the symptoms. A pericardial effusion rarely presents a problem unless the patient has been anticoagulated. A second form of pericardial involvement occurs at any time from several weeks to several months after an acute myocardial infarction. This so-called *postmyocardial infarction pericarditis,* or *Dressler's syndrome,* is characterized by the onset of typical pericardial pain, particularly precipitated by changes in position or cough. It may be accompanied by fever and significant pericardial effusion. There may be a friction rub and systemic symptoms such as malaise and myalgias. Pericardial effusion may occur in such patients, particularly if they have received anticoagulants. The major differential diagnosis in such patients is the possibility of a recurrence of myocardial infarction, but the almost constant complaint of accentuation of symptoms by changes in body position, coughing, and inspiration, along with the presence of a pericardial rub without further evidence of infarction by ECG, serves to alert the clinician to the correct diagnosis.

TREATMENT. The syndrome is usually self-limited and can be treated with analgesics or nonsteroidal anti-inflammatory agents, but on occasion the syndrome may become so repetitive that it is necessary to rely on corticosteroid hormone therapy.

The Postpericardiotomy Syndrome. This has become a commonly recognized form of pericarditis. Although the incidence of the syndrome is reported to be approximately 10 per cent among patients undergoing cardiac surgery, it is undoubtedly higher than this, particularly if minor manifestations of the syndrome are taken into account. The exact cause of the syndrome is not understood. It has been suggested that a common denominator which ties together the pericarditis following myocardial infarction, cardiac surgery, and trauma to the pericardium is blood in the pericardium which produces an inflammatory response. However, it is clear that the presence of blood in the pericardium is not mandatory for the development of the syndrome, and there has been recent evidence to suggest that there may be a viral agent involved, perhaps arising from infection carried in the multiple transfusions often associated with cardiac surgery. The syndrome may occur as early as a week postoperatively, but frequently will not manifest itself until several weeks or months after surgery. Although the typical findings of acute pericarditis, such as fever, substernal chest pain, and a pericardial rub, usually are associated with the syndrome, it may appear with only one of these manifestations. Fever, typical ECG changes, and even an elevation of sedimentation rate may not accompany the

syndrome, and thus the absence of these abnormalities should not be used as evidence against the diagnosis of the postpericardiotomy syndrome. Actual entrance into the pericardium at surgery is not a necessity for the development of the syndrome, because it has been reported after thoracic surgery for pulmonary resection and repair of a hiatus hernia. It is frequently accompanied by a diffuse pleural reaction and associated small pleural effusions. Although the development of pericarditis several weeks postoperatively always raises the specter of a complicating postoperative bacterial pericarditis, the syndrome is almost invariably due to the postpericardiotomy syndrome rather than actual bacterial infection. However, it is important to keep in mind the possibility of a bacterial infection, particularly if the patient does not respond promptly to a brief course of anti-inflammatory agents.

Post-traumatic Pericarditis. Pericarditis may develop after both penetrating and nonpenetrating injury to the chest. The syndrome may appear early after a penetrating wound, and under these circumstances there is always concern that it may be due to bacterial infection of the pericardial space. The syndrome tends to occur weeks or even months after blunt trauma to the chest such as a steering wheel injury. Under these circumstances the concern about bacterial infection is less and one can move quickly with anti-inflammatory agents to suppress the symptoms.

Connective Tissue Disorders. These have become commonly recognized causes of pericarditis. In childhood the most common cause may be acute rheumatic fever. However, in the adult pericarditis is a relatively rare manifestation of acute rheumatic fever. In adults connective tissue disorders, such as systemic lupus erythematosus, rheumatoid arthritis, periarteritis, and, less likely, scleroderma, are much more frequent causes of pericarditis. Pericarditis may be the first sign of systemic lupus erythematosus and may precede other manifestations by months. It may be associated with a rapidly accumulating effusion which may present such a predominant and life-threatening clinical picture that other signs of the disease do not gain attention until the symptoms of pericarditis and effusion are controlled. Pericardial involvement has been noted in up to 40 per cent of documented cases of systemic lupus erythematosus. The diagnosis can be reasonably inferred when LE cells and anti-DNA antibodies are detectable in the blood. Steroid therapy is almost invariably necessary to control the symptoms of pericarditis. Clinical signs of typical acute pericarditis may be seen in approximately 3 per cent of patients with rheumatoid arthritis, even though autopsy series indicate that at least 10 per cent of patients with rheumatoid arthritis have an inflammatory response in the pericardium. Pericarditis is most commonly seen in patients with active rheumatoid disease, particularly those with rheumatoid nodules and markedly elevated titers of rheumatoid factor in serum. The pericarditis is seldom severe, but on rare occasions it can be accompanied by significant effusion. Examination of the pericardial fluid reveals a characteristic marked decrease in the concentration of glucose and elevated LDH enzyme levels as well as increased globulins and decreased complement values. Large round or oval multinucleated cells have been noted in the fluid and are thought by some to be pathognomonic of the disease. These ''RA'' cells contain cytoplasmic inclusion bodies thought to represent phagocytized rheumatoid factor complex. Other connective tissue disorders, such as periarteritis nodosa and scleroderma, as well as giant cell arteritis, have been reported to be associated with pericarditis less commonly. In particular, scleroderma more frequently involves the myocardium and is a rare cause of pericarditis.

Allergic and Hypersensitivity Disorders. Serum sickness, giant urticaria, and allergic responses to penicillin have been associated with pericarditis. In addition to penicillin, other drugs, including diphenylhydantoin, hydralazine, and procainamide, have been implicated in the development of pericarditis. With the renewed emphasis on prevention of cardiac arrhythmias following myocardial infarction and the consequent increased use of procainamide, a lupus-like syndrome involving the pericardium has been more frequently recognized after prolonged use of this drug.

Metabolic Disorders. Uremia and myxedema may provoke pericardial reactions. It has long been recognized that pericarditis, frequently with hemorrhagic pericardial effusions, may occur in the terminal phase of uremia; but before the advent of dialysis programs the incidence of this complication was relatively low, because the patient usually succumbed to renal failure before signs of pericarditis could develop. As many as 15 per cent of patients on dialysis programs may develop pericarditis. Indeed, one of the serious complications that must be watched for during long-term dialysis is the sudden development of a life-threatening pericardial effusion. The etiology of uremic pericarditis is not well understood. It has been seen to develop in patients well controlled with dialysis, but it has been noted that more frequent dialysis may lead to a remission in the pericarditis and pericardial effusion.

Cardiomegaly is not uncommon in hypothyroidism. In the majority of cases this cardiomegaly is due primarily to pericardial effusion. Effusions usually develop slowly and may become quite large with a minimum of symptoms. Hemodynamic embarrassment is rare. The condition responds promptly to thyroid replacement therapy.

Physical or Chemical Agents. The recent popularization of high dose radiation therapy for lymphomatous disease in the mediastinum has disclosed that the pericardium is more susceptible to radiation injury than had previously been thought. Acute pericarditis, pericardial effusion, and constriction have all been reported to follow high dose radiation to the mediastinum. This entity now is recognized as an uncommon but definite complication of radiation therapy, and congestive heart failure may result from either pericardial effusion or constriction, even as a late complication of therapy. Pericarditis is a rare complication of asbestosis and may be associated with a granulomatous thickening of the pericardium. It has also been suggested that irritation of the pericardium by urate crystals in patients with gout may on very rare occasions provoke pericarditis.

CLINICAL MANIFESTATIONS. The hallmark of acute pericarditis is the development of substernal chest pain, which is usually sharp and knife-like but may be a dull or oppressive sensation. The pain frequently is referred or radiates to other areas of the chest, particularly the left supraclavicular region. It may also be referred to the neck and shoulders, which may lead to an initial false impression that the symptom is primarily musculoskeletal in origin rather than due to acute pericarditis. Deep inspiration, rotation of the trunk, and coughing usually will precipitate the pain. Many patients find that it is accentuated and virtually intolerable when they lie on the back or the left side, but the pain can be partially alleviated by sitting up and leaning forward. Fever usually accompanies or initiates the pain and is often associated with other systemic symptoms, such as malaise, fatigue, and myalgias.

A characteristic physical finding in acute pericarditis is a pericardial friction rub. This leathery or scratchy sound may be heard over any portion of the anterior precordium, but it is most frequently heard low along the left sternal border. It may consist of one, two, or three components, presumably depending upon the extent of inflammatory involvement of the pericardium. When there is only a single component to the rub, it is confined to systole and may mimic a systolic cardiac murmur. Changes in the intensity and quality of the isolated systolic rub produced by variations in respiration and positions during auscultation will help differentiate a rub from a cardiac murmur. More commonly the pericardial rub has two or three components. When two components are heard, they occur during systole and diastole and are due to the rubbing of the inflamed epicardial surface against the parietal pericardial surface during systole and diastole. The presence of a third component to the rub, which is common, will eliminate any confusion as to whether the rub is due to an intracardiac murmur or pericardial inflammation. The third component of the rub is due to atrial contraction and occurs in the presystolic phase of the cardiac cycle. Frequently a rub may have a variable number of components, depending upon the position in which the patient is examined. Acute pericarditis is often accompanied by cardiac arrhythmias, which may be intermittent. The vast majority of arrhythmias are supraventricular arrhythmias, including frequent premature atrial contractions, paroxysmal atrial tachycardia, fibrillation, and flutter. This has been attributed to irritation and involvement of the sinus node, which lies close to the epicardial surface of the heart.

LABORATORY FINDINGS. Acute pericarditis is usually accompanied by a leukocytosis and an elevation in sedimentation rate, but these are by no means invariable. Chest x-ray may show a slight increase in cardiac size owing to either inflammatory thickening of the pericardium or a small pericardial effusion. In addition, there may be evidence of pleural involvement characterized by small pleural effusions. Pulmonary infiltrates also are common accompaniments. These changes reflect the fact that the inflammatory process involving the pericardium frequently will also involve the pleura. The electrocardiogram usually shows a typical pattern of S-T segment elevation without changes in the QRS morphology. The S-T segment elevation may last for weeks at a time, and frequently the elevation will show evolutionary changes with T wave inversion several days to weeks after the onset of the S-T segment changes. These electrocardiographic changes may be isolated to only several leads and are due to involvement of the subepicardial myocardium rather than involvement of the pericardium itself, because the pericardium is electrically silent. Serum levels of enzymes such as glutamic-oxaloacetic transaminase (SGOT) and lactic dehydrogenase (LDH) may be moderately elevated because there is inflammatory involvement of the subepicardial portion of the myocardium. Cardiac isoenzyme changes, including the presence of CPK-MB and LDH-1 greater than LDH-2 configurations, are less frequent but have been noted. The echocardiogram may show thickening of the pericardium and will often show a variable amount of pericardial effusion, as there is an almost inevitable increase in fluid in the pericardial space above the 25 to 35 ml normally present in the cavity.

DIFFERENTIAL DIAGNOSIS. When acute pericarditis presents in a young patient with sudden onset of sharp or grating substernal pain accentuated by changes in position and partially relieved by sitting up, plus a characteristic multicomponent rub and S-T segment elevation, the diagnosis is relatively simple. However, frequently the condition does not present in such a classic fashion; in such cases it is necessary to entertain other diagnoses, including acute myocardial infarction, pleurisy with or without pneumonia, pulmonary embolization, dissection of the aorta, pneumothorax, mediastinal emphysema, or an abdominal source for the complaint. Examination of serial electrocardiograms and serum cardiac isoenzyme levels will usually establish whether the primary process is due to myocardial infarction or pericarditis alone. The rub accompanying pleurisy which may raise the possibility of pericarditis is clearly related to and accentuated by the respiratory cycle and is usually heard diffusely over the chest or frequently in the lateral portions of the chest rather than in the precordial area. Pulmonary embolization may mimic pericarditis; but when further studies, such as serial chest x-rays, lung scans, and, if necessary, pulmonary arteriograms, are obtained, the differentiation becomes clear. Dissecting aortic aneurysm may simulate pericarditis and on occasion may actually be a cause for pericarditis owing to rupture of the base of the aorta, with a leak of blood into the pericardium which provokes a pericardial inflammatory reaction. However, the pain of dissection is usually more severe and unremitting than that of pericarditis and is usually noted in the infrascapular area, which is uncommon in pericarditis. Pneumothorax can be differentiated from pericarditis by physical examination which indicates absent breath sounds on the affected side if it is a large pneumothorax and by chest x-ray if it is not discernible by physical examination. Intra-abdominal events may produce pain which suggests acute pericarditis. Acute cholecystitis with referral of pain to the supraclavicular area must be considered. Pancreatitis can also produce a confusing picture suggestive of pericarditis. When there is inflammatory involvement of the diaphragm, there may be an associated small pleural effusion as well as nonspecific T wave changes. Splenic infarction may also provoke an inflammatory response in the diaphragm, and the pain may be referred to the left supraclavicular area, a favorite site for the referral of the pain of acute pericarditis.

365.3. PERICARDIAL EFFUSION

PATHOPHYSIOLOGY. Pericardial effusion, the accumulation of serous or serosanguineous fluid in excess of the normal 25 to 35 ml of lymphatic fluid in the pericardial space, may present in either acute or chronic form. It may be the first sign of acute pericarditis, and its severe hemodynamic consequences may actually obscure the classic signs of the underlying pericarditis. Although chronic pericardial effusion may be accompanied by a pericardial rub, the insidious development of this condition without other evidence of pericardial involvement may simulate progressive heart failure and, unless readily recognized, may lead to death, even though it is a readily treatable condition. An understanding of the pathophysiology of pericardial effusion makes the physical findings of this disorder more obvious and understandable. The circulatory effects of pericardial effusion are directly related to the rate at which the effusion develops. The sudden development of a pericardial effusion of several hundred milliliters of fluid may provoke profound hemodynamic changes, whereas the slower, more gradual development of pericardial effusion may be almost asymptomatic despite accumulations of several liters of fluid. The primary cause for the clinical and hemodynamic signs of pericardial effusion is the accumulation of fluid in the pericardium sufficient to prevent adequate filling of the cardiac chambers. Since venous inflow to the heart is markedly decreased, there is accumulation of blood in the venous system that is reflected in marked jugular venous distention and hepatic engorgement. If the process is chronic, there is usually peripheral edema as well. Jugular venous distention may be increased or at least unchanged by deep inspiration, a maneuver which usually decreases jugular venous pressure caused by increased venous return to the heart if no restriction to filling is present. In pericardial effusion deep inspiration may actually decrease venous filling of the ventricles and thus increase the volume of residual blood in the jugular veins, producing what has been called Kussmaul's sign. Since venous return to the heart is markedly diminished, cardiac output also falls, leading to a narrow pulse pressure and usually a reflex tachycardia.

CARDIAC TAMPONADE. The most severe complication of a pericardial effusion, no matter what its cause, is the development of cardiac tamponade. Cardiac tamponade is a classic example of the vicious cycle process in medicine. Accumulation of fluid in the relatively nondistensible pericardium initially limits cardiac filling and therefore cardiac output. As cardiac output declines, arterial pressure and coronary artery filling decrease. Coronary flow and thus myocardial function are further compromised by external pressure on the superficially lying coronary arteries. Eventually this decline in cardiac filling, decrease in cardiac output, fall in arterial and coronary artery filling pressure, and decreased coronary flow lead to severe myocardial ischemia, which initiates an even greater decline in myocardial function. Unless this cycle of events is contravened by elimination of the effusion, a fatal outcome is certain.

CLINICAL MANIFESTATIONS. A characteristic of a pericardial effusion is the presence of an abnormal paradoxical pulse. The paradoxical pulse is actually an exaggeration of a normal physiologic response. It is detected by determining the systolic blood pressure during inspiration and expiration. During normal inspiration the capacitance of the lung to accept blood volume is increased, and there is a decrease in venous return and a decreased filling pressure in the left heart. Thus left ventricular stroke volume falls, as does systolic blood pressure. The normal variation in systolic blood pressure between inspiration and expiration is in the range of 8 to 10 mm Hg. In the case of a pericardial effusion the systolic pressure may decline during inspiration to a point at which it is undetectable. In severe cases of pericardial effusion, this can be observed by simply palpating the peripheral pulse and noting a decrease in volume or complete absence of the pulse during inspiration. Although this finding is a prominent one in pericardial effusion, it is also a frequent accompaniment of chronic obstructive lung disease and cannot be used as a pathognomonic sign of pericardial effusion alone.

Dyspnea, tachycardia, distended jugular veins which do not decrease in size with inspiration, cyanosis, varying degrees of consciousness, and a rapid thready pulse with a frequently palpable decrease in the force of the peripheral pulse during inspiration warn of the presence of pericardial effusion. Examination of the lung fields may elicit Ewart's or Pins' sign, characterized by increased dullness, increased fremitus, and bronchial breath sounds at the base of the lung below the angle of the left scapula. These findings are believed to be due to compression of the lower lobe of the left lung by the distended pericardial sac. In large pericardial effusions percussion over the lower half of the sternum will reveal dullness caused by the underlying fluid in the pericardial sac, whereas under normal circumstances percussion over this region produces a resonant note. This sign may be obscured when there is obvious deformity of the anterior chest wall or emphysema, and it may be falsely present when there is marked obesity or right ventricular hypertrophy. Examination of the heart may reveal a quiet precordium with no palpable cardiac activity, but this is by no means the rule, and frequently significant pericardial effusions may be present with quite a distinct cardiac apex impulse. On auscultation the heart sounds may be normal or muffled, and there is frequently a pericardial rub even though the effusion may be a chronic one.

LABORATORY FINDINGS. The electrocardiogram may appear entirely normal, show generalized low voltage, reveal S-T segment elevation with or without T wave inversion, or demonstrate complete electrical alternans, which is characterized by a decrease in the size of the P, QRS, and T waves with alternate beats. Chest x-ray may show a normal-sized heart if the pericardial effusion is acute; but even in this situation, if previous chest x-rays are available, it will be apparent that there has been an increase in cardiac size.

In less acute situations the cardiac shadow may slowly enlarge and assume a pear shape. The normal contour of the left heart border may become straightened, and there may be a convex bulging of the right cardiophrenic junction. Signs of pulmonary congestion are variable. Cardiac fluoroscopy is suggestive but not definitive for the diagnosis if there is markedly decreased or no discernible cardiac pulsation and the epicardial fat line lies significantly inside the border of the presumed cardiac shadow. Further radiographic evidence of a pericardial effusion can be sought by placing a catheter in the right atrium and noting that the catheter tip cannot be passed to the lateral border of the right atrium, indicating that there is either a significant effusion or pericardial thickening between the lateral border of the right atrium and the lateral border of the cardiac shadow. This can be further confirmed by injection of contrast media, which will outline the chamber size in relation to the total cardiac shadow.

Similar conclusions can be drawn when carbon dioxide is injected into the right atrium while the patient is lying in the left lateral position and a lateral decubitus chest x-ray is obtained. Under these circumstances the radiolucent collection of carbon dioxide will be noted beneath the superiorly positioned lateral wall of the right atrium, and there will be a difference of greater than 10 mm between the superior dome of the carbon dioxide level and the border of the cardiac shadow. Since the development of echocardiography these invasive catheterization techniques are seldom warranted, because even small pericardial effusions can be detected with a high degree of accuracy with the echocardiogram. However, in rare cases in which the pericardial effusion is loculated, particularly in the space anterior to the heart, echocardiographic study may not be definitive and angiographic studies may be necessary.

TREATMENT: PERICARDIOCENTESIS. The ultimate proof of the diagnosis of pericardial effusion and also an often mandatory procedure to provide relief from cardiac tamponade is pericardiocentesis. This is accomplished by inserting a medium-sized needle high in the epigastrium in the angle formed between the left border of the xiphoid process and the lower left rib cage. After suitable local anesthesia, the exploring metal needle is connected by an insulated wire to the V lead electrode of the ECG. The needle is slowly advanced upward and slightly posterior in a line toward the medial third of the right clavicle. While the needle is being advanced, the electrocardiogram should be continuously monitored. Contact with the epicardium will be signaled by the development of marked S-T segment elevation on the electrocardiographic record. This procedure not only helps prevent puncture of the heart but also provides confidence that one has not perforated the heart if a frankly bloody pericardial effusion is encountered. In acute cases of tamponade such as can occur with aortic dissection or cardiac trauma, it may be impossible to ascertain whether one is draining the pericardial space or actually removing blood directly from a cardiac chamber. This quandary can usually be eliminated by making certain that there has been no evidence of a current of injury on the recorded V lead of the ECG. Once fluid is obtained by aspiration, it should be examined microscopically for the number and type of cells present and the presence of bacteria. The fluid should also undergo cytologic examination, be submitted for bacterial and tuberculous culture, and be analyzed for sugar and protein content, as well as LDH enzyme and rheumatoid factor if clinically indicated.

365.4. PERICARDIAL CONSTRICTION

PATHOPHYSIOLOGY. Constrictive pericarditis may be the last step in the process initiated by acute pericarditis and followed by a pericardial effusion. However, in many cases it develops insidiously without any previous evidence of pericardial disease, and its first manifestations are those suggestive of heart failure. The pericardium can become thickened, fibrosed, and eventually calcified in a remarkably short time. There are well documented cases of this whole process occurring in less than six months after the onset of bacterial or tuberculous disease involving the pericardium. The fundamental anatomic derangement which leads to the ultimate symptomatology of constrictive pericarditis is obstruction or constriction of either the cardiac chambers or the orifices of the great veins entering the heart. The constrictive process can be localized to isolated chambers of the heart and even small areas of the pericardium surrounding these chambers. Cases of localized constriction in the region of the outflow tract of the right ventricle have simulated subpulmonic stenosis. Isolated adhesions and constriction of the posterior portion of the epicardium have led to severe left ventricular dysfunction. The fundamental pathophysiologic process is one of inexorable decrease in cardiac filling, with consequent venous pooling in the periphery and decline in cardiac output. The process may be so slow that the onset of new symptoms is almost unrecognized by the patient and his physician. If the constriction is prolonged and generalized enough, there may be necrosis of myocardial tissue, and even eventual relief of the constriction will still not eliminate symptoms of heart failure because of residual myocardial damage.

CLINICAL MANIFESTATIONS. The classic clinical picture of constrictive pericarditis is the patient who appears emaciated with obvious venous distention in the neck, a potbellied appearance caused by ascites, and spindly, wasted, and often edematous extremities. The patient may be overtly dyspneic at rest or may complain only of dyspnea on exertion. Careful examination of the neck veins will demonstrate a prominent "Y" descent which corresponds with sudden brief right ventricular filling. Examination of the heart may reveal a quiet precordium with no palpable apical impulse, although this is by no means the rule. The heart sounds may be muffled, and frequently there is a prominent third heart sound occurring 0.09 to 0.12 second after the aortic closure sound. This so-called "pericardial knock" can easily be confused with the S_3 gallop associated with congestive heart failure. Atrial fibrillation is frequently encountered in the late stages of the disease. Hemodynamic deterioration of a patient with atrial fibrillation who has been given digitalis on the presumption that he has congestive heart failure should alert the clinician to the possibility of constrictive pericarditis. Administration of digitalis to the patient with rapid atrial fibrillation and heart failure should relieve signs of failure. However, the patient with constrictive pericarditis may be dependent for an effective cardiac output on a relatively rapid ventricular rate. When this ventricular rate is lowered by digitalis in a patient with atrial fibrillation, the patient is unable to increase ventricular filling and generate a greater stroke volume to maintain a normal cardiac output. Thus hemodynamic deterioration rather than improvement ensues.

LABORATORY FINDINGS. The electrocardiogram is almost invariably abnormal, with a decrease in QRS voltage, nonspecific S-T and T wave changes, and an irregular contour to the P waves. Chest x-ray will usually show a heart of smaller than expected or even normal size in view of the evidence of severe hemodynamic derangement. However, this is not invariable, and the diagnosis should not be discarded if the cardiac size is large, because much of this enlargement may be due to a markedly thickened pericardium. A characteristic of pericardial constriction is the presence of calcium in the pericardium, but this may not be seen on the standard chest x-ray because of technical factors. Thus if it is suspected, overpenetrated x-rays of the heart in different views should be obtained. Careful fluoroscopy with image intensification will demonstrate calcification in over 75 per cent of cases of constrictive pericarditis. Echocardiography may play an important role in alerting the unsuspecting clinician that he is dealing with constrictive pericarditis rather than advanced heart failure. An echocardiogram which demonstrates a thickened pericardium, small ventricular chamber size, and increased atrial chamber size should raise the possibility of constrictive pericarditis. Cardiac catheterization provides a series of typical findings, but they are not absolutely diagnostic of constrictive pericarditis. The right atrial pressure may be seen to rise with inspiration, which is analogous to Kussmaul's sign seen in the jugular veins; the right atrial pressure tracing shows a typical "M or W" shape; and the right ventricular pressure demonstrates a so-called early diastolic dip and a late diastolic shoulder. The early diastolic dip conforms to the early rapid filling of the ventricle and is coincident with the sharp "Y" descent seen in the jugular venous pulse. There is a generalized equalization of all end-diastolic pressures in the chambers of the heart as well as in the pulmonary artery. Although these findings are typical, it should be noted that exactly the same findings can be observed in patients with cardiomyopathies, and thus their presence or absence should not be the sole determining factor as to whether a patient should undergo an exploratory thoracotomy or not. In occasional patients with subclinical constriction, these hemodynamic findings become evident only after they have received a rapid infusion of saline.

Angiography is frequently helpful in demonstrating that the cardiac chamber is markedly smaller than might be surmised from the total cardiac contour. Furthermore, an unusual downward tugging of the bifurcation of the opacified main pulmonary artery during systole has been noted and is presumably due to the flexible uninvolved pulmonary artery actually being tugged back toward the heart by the contracting ventricles that are encased in an immobile pericardial sac. Results of liver function studies are almost inevitably abnormal, and there may be hypoalbuminemia on the basis of both hepatic disease and a protein-losing enteropathy.

TREATMENT. The definitive treatment for constrictive pericarditis is a pericardiectomy. If delayed too long, the constrictive process may be so advanced that adequate stripping, particularly of the epicardial portion of the pericardium, cannot be accomplished, or there may have been such advanced degeneration of myocardial muscle that postoperative results are less than satisfactory. It should be noted that there are well documented cases of isolated epicardial constriction which is not apparent until the epicardium is actually dissected away from the myocardium itself. The prognosis for recovery from constrictive pericarditis is a function of the age of the patient, the severity of the fibrotic process, and the degree to which the patient's general medical condition has deteriorated before the pericardiectomy is performed. With the lowering of the operative mortality for pericardiectomy to the range of 5 per cent, particularly if done early, there is a general tendency now to operate at the first suggestion of constriction, particularly if the patient is known to have had a bacterial or tuberculous pericardial infection in the past.

365.5. NEOPLASTIC DISEASES

The pericardium may be the site of primary or metastatic tumors. Primary tumors are rare and may be generally classified into mesotheliomas, which encompass tumors that have previously been classified as fibromas and sarcomas, vascular tumors such as hemangiomas and lymphangiomas, pericardial cysts, lipomas, and tumors of heterotopic tissue such as bronchial cysts, teratomas, and dermoids. The pericardium is not a rare location for metastatic tumors. Metastatic tumors from the lung in men and the breast in women are the most common types encountered in the pericardium. Lymphomatous disease, particularly Hodgkin's disease, also may involve the pericardium. Occasionally involvement of the pericardium and its attendant restriction, either by tumor mass or effusion, may be the first sign of a malignancy. Pericardial effusion, which is often bloody, can be found with even small sized tumors and a small number of metastases.

365.6. CONGENITAL LESIONS OF THE PERICARDIUM

Congenital true pericardial cysts may be celomic, lymphangiomatous, bronchial, or teratomatous. These seldom produce significant clinical symptoms and usually come to light when a routine chest x-ray is obtained. The major problem they present is that of differentiation from a mediastinal tumor. They may gradually increase in size and necessitate an exploratory thoracotomy to rule out malignant disease. In addition to true congenital pericardial cysts, a diverticulum of the pericardium may occur. The diverticulum appears as a sharply outlined semicircular or oval area protruding from the cardiac silhouette, usually in the region of the right lower portion of the cardiac shadow. Such diverticula cannot be differentiated from a pericardial cyst without exploratory thoracotomy.

There may be a congenital complete or, less frequently, partial absence of the pericardium. When the defect is a partial one, it occurs on the left side of the pericardium in two thirds of the cases and is seen most frequently in males. Herniation of the heart, particularly the left atrial appendage through the defect, has been associated with recurrent syncope and, rarely, sudden death. The defect should be suspected when the left atrial appendage appears disproportionately prominent on chest x-ray. The diagnosis can be confirmed by inducing a pneumothorax which demonstrates a pneumopericardium in addition to the pneumothorax.

365.7. DISEASES OF DIVERSE UNKNOWN CAUSE

In addition to all the conditions discussed previously, the pericardium may be the site of involvement in a variety of other diseases. *Familial Mediterranean fever*, which involves various serous membranes, may also involve the pericardium. Although *sarcoidosis* more frequently involves the myocardium, granulomas can be found in the pericardium and on rare occasions may lead to signs of constrictive pericarditis. *Hydropericar-*

dium, which is an excessive accumulation of transudate in the pericardial cavity, may occur in conjunction with advanced cardiac or renal failure, as well as in association with inflammatory or malignant diseases which may obstruct lymphatic drainage from the pericardium. A *chylous pericardial effusion* may develop following traumatic rupture of the thoracic duct or in association with primary or metastatic malignant diseases which obstruct the thoracic duct. The pericardial fluid is milky white or brownish yellow, contains fat globules which can be visualized under the light microscope, and has markedly elevated triglyceride levels. *Cholesterol pericarditis*, which is characterized by an elevated level of cholesterol in the pericardial effusion and frequently by the appearance of a shiny or scintillating gold paint quality to the effusion, has been thought to be a separate clinical entity in the past. However, cholesterol pericarditis has been associated with a variety of disease states. Approximately one fourth of the cases reported have been associated with hypothyroidism. It is now thought that it is a manifestation of prolonged pericardial effusion with impairment of absorption of cholesterol from the chronically inflamed or scarred pericardium. There is subsequent gradual accumulation of large amounts of cholesterol crystals which give the effusion its unique appearance. Early treatment of hypothyroidism may produce a prompt elimination of the syndrome if the primary cause is hypothyroidism. However, if treatment is delayed in the case of hypothyroidism or if the condition is due to other causes, a pericardiectomy is the treatment of choice.

Bush, C. A., Stang, J. M., Wooley, C. F., and Kilman, J. W.: Occult constrictive pericardial disease: Diagnosis by rapid volume expansion and correction by pericardiectomy. Circulation, 56:924, 1977.
Cortes, F. M. (ed.): The Pericardium and Its Disorders. Springfield, Ill., Charles C Thomas, 1970.
Dressler, W.: The postmyocardial infarction syndrome. A report on forty-four cases. Arch. Intern. Med., 103:28, 1959.
Feigenbaum, H.: Echocardiography. In Pericardial Disease. Philadelphia, Lea & Febiger, 1976, p. 419.
Holt, J. P.: The normal pericardium. Am. J. Cardiol., 26:455, 1970.
Koontz, C. H., and Ray, C. G.: The role of coxsackie Group B virus infection in sporadic myopericarditis. Am. Heart J., 82:750, 1971.
Shabetai, R., Fowler, N. O., and Guntheroth, W. G.: The hemodynamics of cardiac tamponade and constrictive pericarditis. Am. J. Cardiol., 26:480, 1970.
Spodick, D. H.: Diagnostic electrocardiographic sequences in acute pericarditis. Circulation, 48:575, 1973.

366. DISEASES OF THE MYOCARDIUM

366.1. INTRODUCTION

Victor S. Behar

Myocardial failure may occur as the result of primary myocardial disease or secondary to hyperkinetic states or valvular or ischemic heart disease. The following chapters will deal with the primary myocardial diseases in which the basic pathology specifically involves the myocardium, thereby differentiating them from those caused by abnormalities of other cardiac structures. Much of the ambiguity surrounding the generalized term of cardiomyopathy stems from the inability of our predecessors to arrive at an etiologic diagnosis in patients with ill-defined heart disease. This frequently led them to the use of such terms as chronic myocarditis, myocardial degeneration, idiopathic myocardial hypertrophy, idiopathic cardiomyopathy, and noncoronary myocardial degeneration, to name a few. In many of the underdeveloped parts of the world, primary myocardial disease may account for 15 per cent or more of the patients with clinical heart disease. It has been estimated that in the United States, however, fewer than 1 per cent of cardiac deaths are due to primary myocardial disease. This may be a gross underestimate because of the difficulty in recognizing the disease as well as the tendency to attribute its etiology to a more common process such as coronary atherosclerosis.

The presentation and clinical course of patients with a cardiomyopathy are variable. The onset may frequently be silent and accompany an infectious disease with the development of a myocarditis manifest only by nonspecific electrocardiographic changes. These patients usually do not suffer any cardiac disability, and the persistence of the electrocardiographic abnormalities is variable. Although complete recovery is common with this type of presentation, patients may develop asymptomatic cardiomegaly, frequent bouts of congestive heart failure, systemic or pulmonary emboli, or rapid deterioration and sudden death.

The symptoms of a cardiomyopathy are not unlike those of other forms of heart disease. Weakness, fatigue, and dyspnea on exertion are the most frequent manifestations and are due to a low cardiac output. The signs and symptoms of right ventricular failure may occur soon after the development of left ventricular failure, and the combination appears to be more common than in other forms of heart disease. The low cardiac output may also produce peripheral cyanosis, falsely suggesting congenital heart disease. Although uncommon, chest pain may be suggestive of angina in character or due to an associated pericarditis. Right upper quadrant pain caused by congestive hepatomegaly is much more likely to occur and can be especially distressing during acute right ventricular decompensation. Palpitations are frequent and may be due to extrasystoles or arrhythmias, especially in acute myocarditis, alcoholic cardiomyopathy, or the familial cardiomyopathies.

The diagnosis of primary myocardial disease should be suspected in the young, normotensive individual with cardiomegaly or congestive heart failure in the absence of a prior history of congenital, valvular, or ischemic heart disease. The electrocardiogram characteristically demonstrates left ventricular hypertrophy, arrhythmias, or conduction defects. Because of the lack of etiologic information in the majority of these patients, it has proved useful to classify them by their pathophysiology into congestive, hypertrophic, and restrictive types.

In the congestive cardiomyopathies, there is systolic pump failure and dilatation of the left ventricle. These patients may remain asymptomatic for years, however, before developing congestive heart failure. On physical examination, there is frequently sinus tachycardia, pulsus alternans, and an enlarged apex beat with both atrial and ventricular gallop sounds. In addition, a murmur of mitral regurgitation is common, as is tricuspid regurgitation in the presence of right ventricular failure. The presence of Q waves on the electrocardiogram may falsely suggest myocardial infarction, making it difficult to differentiate these patients from those with ischemic heart disease. In addition, conduction defects, including bundle branch block, bifascicular block, and sinoatrial node abnormalities, may be present. The chest x-ray demonstrates cardiomegaly and pulmonary congestion. The congestive type of cardiomyopathy may have the following causes: (1) infective, i.e., viral, bacterial; (2) metabolic, i.e., puerperal, endocrine, hemochromatosis, beriberi, amyloid; (3) heredofamilial neuromuscular diseases; (4) systemic diseases, i.e., collagen, sarcoid; (5) toxic, i.e., alcohol, heavy metals, drugs; (6) hypersensitivity reactions, i.e., serum sickness, postvaccinal; and (7) irradiation.

In hypertrophic cardiomyopathy, the pump function of the heart is usually maintained until late in the disease. The abnormal muscle reduces ventricular compliance and produces diastolic failure of the left ventricle with impaired diastolic filling. Outflow tract obstruction is common but not invariable. Although the majority of patients with this form of cardiomyopathy may be asymptomatic, others may complain of angina, dyspnea, syncope, or congestive heart failure. On physical examination, the classic findings include bisferious pulse, a bifid or trifid apical impulse, systolic ejection murmur, atrial gallop, and ventricular gallop in the presence of significant mitral regurgitation. This type of cardiomyopathy is most often familial and transmitted as an autosomal dominant trait. The clinical genetic marker is asymmetric septal hypertrophy (see Ch. 366.2).

Restrictive cardiomyopathies are rare and are most often due to an infiltrative process which frequently involves the endocardium. Pump function may be maintained and heart size normal, with symptoms being produced by restriction to ventricular filling. Although chest pain may be a presenting complaint, the majority of patients are asymptomatic and are referred because of an abnormal electrocardiogram or physical examination. Reduced ventricular compliance, secondary to the myopathic process, can simulate constrictive pericarditis because of the high venous pressure, rapid "y" descent, and loud early diastolic filling sound. In addition, at cardiac catheterization there may be an early diastolic dip in the right ventricular pressure recording, followed by a late diastolic plateau compatible with both restrictive and constrictive heart disease. When the restrictive process is disproportionately more severe on the left side of the heart, however, left ventricular end-diastolic, left atrial, and pulmonary artery pressures will be increased. Under these circumstances, the symptoms of pulmonary congestion may predominate. In constrictive pericarditis, there is equalization of diastolic pressures in all four chambers and normal pulmonary systolic pressure. This restrictive type of pathophysiology occurs in amyloidosis and less commonly in endomyocardial fibrosis of the African type and Löffler's fibroplastic eosinophilic endocarditis.

Goodwin, J. F.: Clarification of the cardiomyopathies. Mod. Concepts Cardiovasc. Dis., 41:41, 1972.

Mattingly, T. W.: Clinical features and diagnosis of primary myocardial disease. Mod. Concepts Cardiovasc. Dis., 30:677, 683, 1961.

Oakley, C. M.: Clinical recognition of the cardiomyopathies. Circ. Res., 35 (Suppl. II):II-152, 1974.

Perloff, J. K.: The cardiomyopathies — current perspectives. Circulation, 44:942, 1971.

Stapleton, J. F., Segal, J. P., and Harvey, W. P.: Clinical pathways of cardiomyopathy. Circ. Res., 35 (Suppl. II):II-168, 1974.

366.2.   ASYMMETRIC SEPTAL HYPERTROPHY

Victor S. Behar

In recent years, asymmetric septal hypertrophy (ASH) has been identified as the unifying characteristic of the elusive disease which has been called idiopathic hypertrophic subaortic stenosis (IHSS), hypertrophic obstructive cardiomyopathy (HOCM), and muscular subaortic stenosis (MSS). Early accounts of this abnormality described marked hypertrophy of the left ventricular outflow tract with obstruction to ventricular ejection, leading ultimately to generalized ventricular hypertrophy. Our understanding of this disease progressed most rapidly with the advent of cardiac catheterization and echocardiography as diagnostic and research tools. These techniques have provided documentation of the unique clinical, physiologic, and pathologic characteristics of ASH. It was soon appreciated that patients with similar symptoms and physical findings may fall along a spectrum of hemodynamic abnormalities, ranging from severe resting gradients to gradients only with provocative maneuvers or to total absence of outflow tract obstruction. The confusion in this dynamic entity was greatly alleviated by the observation that the asymmetric septal hypertrophy, so readily seen at autopsy, can be visualized noninvasively during life through the use of echocardiography. The echocardiographic demonstration of a septal to posterior free wall ratio of 1.3 or greater provides a clinical marker for identifying patients with ASH independent of the existence of outflow tract obstruction (see accompanying figure). Although IHSS was originally felt to exist in both sporadic and familial forms, documentation of the latter was possible in only about 30 per cent of cases. The presence of asymmetric septal hypertrophy by echocardiogram throughout the entire spectrum of the disease provides a unique opportunity to study its pattern of inheritance. Such studies in first degree relatives of propositi illustrated that ASH is a genetic disease in almost all patients and is inherited as an autosomal dominant trait with a high degree of penetrance.

The most common clinical manifestations in symptomatic patients include dyspnea, angina, presyncope, syncope, paroxysmal nocturnal dyspnea, and palpitations. These symptoms bear a striking resemblance to those occurring in valvular aortic stenosis. However, in valvular aortic stenosis, syncope is associated with severe aortic valvular gradients, whereas patients with ASH and syncope frequently have little or no outflow tract gradients at rest. In addition, syncope in ASH is often postural in nature or produced after the cessation of exercise, whereas in valvular aortic stenosis syncope usually occurs during the actual performance of exercise.

On physical examination, a large "A" wave may be seen in the jugular venous pulse due to reduced distensibility of the right ventricle. The carotid arterial pulse is brisk and bifid in contour with a rapid initial rise followed by a mid-systolic dip and late systolic rise. This bisferious character of the pulse is most prominent in the presence of outflow tract obstruction. The heart is usually enlarged with a double apical impulse owing to presystolic expansion during atrial contraction. On auscultation, there is usually a loud atrial gallop. A parasternal thrill is frequently palpable and accompanies a holosystolic or systolic ejection murmur of variable intensity best heard at the left sternal border and apex. The second heart sound is usually normal but may be single or paradoxically split. A diastolic murmur is uncommon. A ventricular gallop may also be present at the apex. The variable intensity of the outflow tract murmur is due to its dependence upon the dimensions of the outflow tract and consequently the degree of obstruction during ventricular systole. Widening of the outflow tract with reduced obstruction occurs with an increase in end-diastolic volume, an increase in distending pressure during systole, or a decrease in the inotropic state of the myocardium. Increased obstruction occurs with opposite hemodynamic conditions. Because of these effects, the murmur classically increases in intensity during the Valsalva maneuver or upon assumption of the upright position; the murmur will decrease in intensity during leg raising and may completely disappear during squatting. Inhalation of amyl nitrite markedly increases the intensity of the murmur and outflow tract obstruction by its ability to decrease blood pressure and increase heart rate, as well as to increase the level of myocardial contractility. Other provocative maneuvers which increase outflow obstruction include postextrasystolic potentiation of the beat following a premature ventricular contraction, digitalis, nitroglycerin, isoproterenol, and exercise. Methoxamine or phenylephrine infusion and hypervolemia increase the dimensions of the outflow tract, thereby reducing or obliterating the gradient.

The electrocardiogram usually shows normal sinus

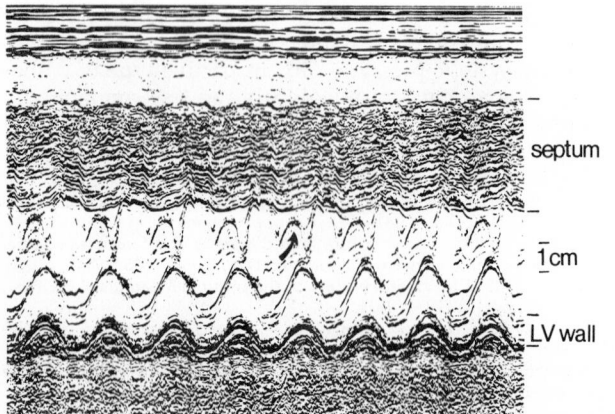

septum

1cm

LV wall

Time motion echocardiogram of the left ventricle in idiopathic hypertrophic subaortic stenosis. The septal thickness is markedly increased, and the septal to posterior free wall ratio is abnormal at 3.5. In addition, the arrow identifies anterior motion of the anterior leaflet of the mitral valve during ventricular systole. The apposition of the septum and anterior mitral leaflet is responsible for the outflow tract obstruction.

rhythm and left ventricular hypertrophy. The occurrence of atrial fibrillation is an ominous sign because of the dependence of diastolic filling on atrial contraction. A short P-R interval, either with or without a delta wave and QRS prolongation characteristic of the Wolff-Parkinson-White syndrome, is not uncommon. Large Q waves may occur in more than half the patients, simulating a previous myocardial infarction. This has been attributed to abnormal septal depolarization.

The chest x-ray shows left ventricular enlargement, which is frequently manifest by a prominent "bump" along the anterolateral wall of the left ventricle as viewed in the frontal projection. Left atrial enlargement is less common. The aorta is usually not dilated, and the absence of aortic valvular calcification is helpful in excluding fixed valvular stenosis.

At cardiac catheterization, a resting gradient is frequently present within the left ventricular outflow tract or can be elicited with provocative maneuvers as described above. The gradient is labile and may vary on a beat-to-beat basis as well as during serial observations. Elevation of the left ventricular end-diastolic pressure is common. The angiocardiogram demonstrates marked thickening of the ventricular septum and left ventricular free wall. The papillary muscles are large and distort the shape of the ventricle, producing an hourglass configuration. Mitral regurgitation is common and is probably related to the altered geometry of the ventricle rather than deformity of the leaflets themselves. Systolic anterior motion of the anterior mitral leaflet is common and is thought to produce the outflow tract obstruction by its apposition to the hypertrophied septum. Systolic anterior motion of the anterior mitral leaflet may also be demonstrated by echocardiography (see figure) and correlates well with the presence of obstruction, on a beat-to-beat basis as well as during longitudinal studies and following surgery.

In patients with obstruction, the basic pathologic abnormality is felt to reside only in the asymmetric septum. The ventricular free wall is thickened but has a similar configuration to the chamber in patients with valvular aortic stenosis, suggesting that free wall hypertrophy is secondary to obstruction. Ultrastructural studies show bizarre cell-to-cell and intracellular abnormalities in the septum, with only rare cellular changes in the free wall. In nonobstructive patients, however, there are similar septal changes but a nonuniform distribution of free wall thickening associated with many disorganized and bizarre cells. This is interpreted as evidence that unlike obstructive ASH, in which the genetic defect is localized to the septum, the functional impairment in nonobstructive ASH is due to a diffuse expression of the genetic defect.

Although the echocardiographic finding of asymmetric septal hypertrophy and the histologic observations of myocardial fiber disarray are important morphologic features of this cardiomyopathy, recent studies have shown that they are not pathognomonic. ASH has been demonstrated in the normally developing heart and in the newborn. In addition, an abnormal septal to free wall ratio has been observed in approximately 20 per cent of patients with congenital heart disease primarily involving the right heart. Although a minor degree of ASH has been found in adult hearts with acquired right ventricular hypertrophy as well as in patients with coronary artery disease, the septal to free wall

ratio on the echocardiogram generally does not exceed 1.3. The absence of ASH in first degree relatives of these patients indicates that this disproportionate septal hypertrophy does not represent genetically transmitted ASH. Focal zones of myocardial fiber disarray have also been observed in the normal heart and occur at the junction of the septum and free wall, as well as in the right ventricular infundibulum. Severe fiber disorganization has been found in congenital defects, characterized by hypertrophied ventricles, obliterated cavities, and outflow tract atresia, such as pulmonic atresia or the tetralogy of Fallot. These severe histologic abnormalities have not been found in acquired heart disease with right, left, or biventricular hypertrophy.

Relatively few patients with ASH are symptomatic. In the presence of symptoms the echocardiogram can be used to substantiate the diagnosis, and a trial of propranolol should then be attempted. Drugs such as nitroglycerin, digitalis, and diuretics should be avoided except for control of atrial fibrillation or the symptoms of congestive heart failure. As an important adjunct to therapy, patients should be taught to avoid the rapid assumption of the upright position, the Valsalva maneuver, and paroxysms of coughing. Approximately 10 to 15 per cent of symptomatic patients will not respond to medical therapy and will require surgery. Cardiac catheterization should be performed prior to surgery to document the severity of the resting or inducible gradient. The surgical procedure receiving greatest acclaim is that of left ventriculomyotomy and myectomy, which is performed through a vertical aortotomy while the patient is on cardiopulmonary bypass. Excellent symptomatic improvement has been reported in these patients with respect to dyspnea, angina, and syncope, but the amelioration of congestive heart failure has been somewhat disappointing. Postoperative hemodynamic studies in patients with obstruction at rest preoperatively have demonstrated complete abolition of the resting gradient in 90 per cent of patients, with the remainder having residual gradients of 25 mm Hg or less. Although mitral valve replacement has been advocated for the treatment of IHSS at some medical centers, the consensus suggests that valve replacement is not necessary even in the presence of significant mitral regurgitation, which has been found to regress clinically following left ventriculomyotomy and myectomy.

Braunwald, E., Lambrew, C. T., Rockoff, S. D., Ross, J., Jr., and Morrow, A. G.: Idiopathic hypertrophic subaortic stenosis. Circulation, 30 (Suppl. IV):IV-3, 1964.

Bulkley, B. H., Weisfeldt, M. L., and Hutchings, G. M.: Asymmetric septal hypertrophy and myocardial fiber disarray. Features of normal, developing, and malformed hearts. Circulation, 56:292, 1977.

Clark, C. E., Henry, W. L., and Epstein, S. E.: Familial prevalence and genetic transmission of idiopathic hypertrophic subaortic stenosis. N. Engl. J. Med., 289:709, 1973.

Henry, W. L., Clark, C. E., and Epstein, S. E.: Asymmetric septal hypertrophy. Circulation, 47:225, 1973.

Henry, W. L., Clark, C. E., Roberts, W. C., Morrow, A. G., and Epstein, S. E.: Differences in distribution of myocardial abnormalities in patients with obstructive and nonobstructive asymmetric septal hypertrophy (echo and gross anatomic findings). Circulation, 50:447, 1974.

Maron, B. J., Ferrans, V. J., Henry, W. L., Clark, C. E., Redwood, D. R., Roberts, W. C., Morrow, A. G., and Epstein, S. E.: Differences in distribution of myocardial abnormalities in patients with obstructive and nonobstructive asymmetric septal hypertrophy. Circulation, 50:436, 1974.

Morrow, A. G., Reitz, B. A., Epstein, S. E., Henry, W. L., Conkle, D. M., Itscoitz, S. B., and Redwood, D. R.: Operative treatment in hypertrophic subaortic stenosis. Circulation, 52:88, 1975.

366.3. FAMILIAL CARDIOMYOPATHY

Victor S. Behar

Although the term familial cardiomyopathy suggests a single disease entity, it more likely encompasses a variety of clinical and pathologic conditions. Included in this broad category are familial cardiomyopathy, asymmetric septal hypertrophy with or without obstruction, endocardial fibroelastosis, glycogen storage disease, Hunter's and Hurler's syndromes, and the heredofamilial neuromyopathic diseases.

FAMILIAL CARDIOMYOPATHY. Evans proposed the term familial cardiomyopathy in 1949 when he described three cases of heart disease in a single family. Clinically, the patients had palpitations, presyncope, congestive heart failure, or sudden death. Physical examination showed cardiomegaly and signs of left ventricular failure. The electrocardiogram showed extrasystoles, arrhythmias, and conduction abnormalities. At autopsy, there was generalized myocardial fibrosis and hypertrophy of the remaining myocardium. In addition, mural thrombi were present. The prognosis in young patients was worse than in adults, and death occurred from progressive congestive heart failure or was sudden. In recent years, the most frequent form of familial cardiomyopathy seen clinically is *asymmetric septal hypertrophy (ASH)*, either with or without left ventricular outflow tract obstruction. As described in Ch. 366.2, the unifying link in this disease is the demonstration of asymmetric septal hypertrophy either at autopsy or by echocardiography. Although it was originally felt that the disease could occur in either the sporadic or the familial form, echocardiographic studies in first degree relatives of patients with ASH demonstrate genetic transmission as an autosomal dominant trait. Most patients are asymptomatic, although angina, presyncope, syncope, and congestive heart failure may occur either with or without outflow tract obstruction.

ENDOCARDIAL FIBROELASTOSIS. Endocardial fibroelastosis is an obscure disease of unknown cause which may occur as an isolated lesion or in association with other cardiac anomalies. The occurrence of the isolated form in twins as well as siblings has suggested genetic transmission as an autosomal recessive trait. Endocardial fibroelastosis occurs in infancy and has no predilection for sex or race. The symptoms are usually dyspnea, orthopnea, wheezing, cyanosis, and failure to thrive. The course may be acute with rapid deterioration due to heart failure and death in several weeks, or chronic with remissions and exacerbations. Ninety per cent of patients are dead within one year because of heart failure, emboli, arrhythmias, or infection. The electrocardiogram shows left ventricular hypertrophy and, to a lesser extent, low voltage and conduction abnormalities. At autopsy, there is cardiomegaly with endocardial fibroelastosis involving all chambers, especially the left side of the heart. Grossly, the endocardium appears thickened, smooth, and porcelain white. The heart valves may be thickened and sclerotic in half the cases. The microscopic findings show increased amounts of endocardial ground substance with dense accumulation of elastic tissue and collagen at the junction with the subendocardium. Signs of inflammation and fibrous scarring of the myocardium are conspicuously absent. In addition, there is a periarterial adventitial hyperelastosis. The group of patients with

associated cardiac anomalies may have aortic stenosis, mitral stenosis, coarctation of the aorta, ventricular septal defect, or the hypoplastic left heart syndrome. Although a genetic cause has been proposed, other suggested causes include maternal infection, fetal endocarditis, anoxia, or mechanical factors resulting from pressure or volume overload. Attention should be directed toward excluding associated cardiac anomalies and providing supportive therapy.

POMPE'S DISEASE. This severe form of glycogen storage disease, also known as Type II glycogenosis, is characterized by the generalized deposition of normal glycogen in the tissues and severe cardiomegaly. The defect is a deficiency of α-1,4-glucosidase and is transmitted as a single autosomal recessive gene. Clinically, the infant appears cretinoid with an enlarged tongue and has marked muscular hypotonicity and cardiomegaly. Hypoglycemia, ketosis, and hyperlipidemia do not occur, as in other types of glycogen storage disease. Tissue damage is thought to be due to progressive replacement by glycogen. The electrocardiogram shows left ventricular hypertrophy, and pathologically the interventricular septum is particularly involved and may produce outflow tract obstruction. Microscopic examination reveals glycogen-filled vacuoles, thought to be lysosomes.

HURLER'S SYNDROME AND HUNTER'S SYNDROME. Both these mucopolysaccharidoses may be associated with a cardiomyopathy. Hurler's syndrome is transmitted as an autosomal recessive trait and Hunter's syndrome by an X-linked gene. Hurler's syndrome is differentiated from Hunter's syndrome by its more severe clinical manifestations. They are characterized by the deposition of dermatan sulfate and heparan sulfate within cells and connective tissues. The cardiomegaly is generalized with involvement of the heart valves as well as the endocardium. In addition, there is intimal proliferation of the coronary arteries. Death is primarily due to congestive heart failure.

FABRY'S DISEASE. This is a sex-linked disorder characterized by deficient activity of α-galactosidase A. Males are primarily affected by this disorder, which results in the deposition of glycosphingolipids (chiefly globotriaosylceramide) in the walls of blood vessels, myocardium, and nerves. There is progressive cardiomegaly and death from left ventricular failure.

HEREDOFAMILIAL NEUROMYOPATHIC DISEASES. The nonmyotonic muscular dystrophies are frequently complicated by a cardiomyopathy. It is most common in the classic, rapidly progressive, sex-linked Duchenne's pseudohypertrophic form, which affects males in the first five years of life. The cardiomyopathy occurs in as many as 50 per cent of patients. The symptoms of heart failure are unusual in these patients because of their markedly diminished activity. On physical examination, it is common to hear atrial and ventricular gallop sounds as well as the murmur of mitral regurgitation. Cardiac chamber abnormalities are difficult to interpret by chest x-ray because of the severe thoracic abnormalities which are present. Cardiac involvement is most readily detected by the electrocardiogram. These changes include tall R waves in leads V_1 and V_3R, with an increased R/S ratio in V_1 together with deep Q waves in the standard limb leads and lateral precordial leads. Identical changes have been observed in female carriers of the dystrophy, who have also been demonstrated to have creatine phosphokinase abnormalities.

In addition, the electrocardiogram shows labile sinus tachycardia, premature atrial and ventricular extrasystoles, and atrial or ventricular tachycardia. Postmortem studies show selective scarring of the posterobasal left ventricle and the posteromedial papillary muscle. Noninflammatory degenerative changes have also been described in the arteries supplying the sinoatrial and atrioventricular nodes with sparing of the larger epicardial vessels.

Slowly progressive Duchenne's dystrophy (sex-linked recessive), limb-girdle dystrophy of Erb (autosomal recessive), and fascioscapulohumeral dystrophy of Dejerine and Landouzy (autosomal dominant) may also be associated with a cardiomyopathy, in decreasing order of frequency.

Myotonic muscular dystrophy is a heredofamilial multisystem disease which produces myotonia, muscle atrophy, myopathic facies, cataracts, frontal baldness, testicular atrophy, and a cardiomyopathy. The electrocardiogram is the most sensitive indicator of cardiac involvement and is abnormal in over half the patients. The electrocardiographic changes include sinus bradycardia, intraventricular and atrioventricular conduction disturbances, left axis deviation, low voltage, and supraventricular tachycardias. The conduction abnormalities may progress to complete heart block with Stokes-Adams attacks and sudden death. At autopsy, there is myocardial fibrosis and fatty infiltration.

Friedreich's ataxia is a neurologic heredofamilial disease characterized by ataxic gait, areflexia in the lower extremities, Babinski reflexes, sensory loss, scanning dysarthria, and skeletal deformities of the thorax. The cardiac symptoms include congestive heart failure and, less commonly, chest pain. The heart is clinically involved in 30 to 50 per cent of patients, although electrocardiographic changes may be present in as many as 90 per cent. These changes include sinus tachycardia, supraventricular tachycardias, and T wave inversion primarily involving leads I, II, AVF, and V_3 to V_6. In addition, left and right ventricular hypertrophy have been observed. Family members with the disease often show similar electrocardiographic changes. At autopsy, the heart demonstrates myocardial fiber hypertrophy, interstitial fibrosis, focal degeneration, and occasionally active necrosis. The coronary arteries may show atheromatous changes, and there is frequently medial degeneration and intimal hyperplasia in the small intramural vessels. Death is due to congestive heart failure or cor pulmonale secondary to the severe thoracic deformities.

Evans, W.: Familial cardiomegaly. Br. Heart J., 11:68, 1949.
Griggs, R. C.: Hypertrophy and cardiomyopathy in the neuromuscular diseases. Circ. Res., 35 (Suppl. II):II-145, 1974.
Perloff, J. K.: Cardiomyopathy associated with heredofamilial neuromyopathic diseases. Mod. Concepts Cardiovasc. Dis., 40:23, 1971.
Rosahn, P. D.: Endocardial fibroelastosis: Old and new concepts. Bull. N.Y. Acad. Med., 31:453, 1955.
Still, W. J. S.: Endocardial fibroelastosis. Am. Heart J., 61:579, 1961.

366.4. INFLAMMATORY OR INFECTIVE CARDIOMYOPATHY
(Myocarditis)
Victor S. Behar

The ubiquitous nature of myocarditis in a variety of infectious diseases makes it important to recognize.

Myocarditis may be associated with viral, bacterial, rickettsial, parasitic, fungal, or spirochetal disease, although with varying degrees of documentation. Myocarditis also may occur secondary to a systemic process such as a hypersensitivity reaction or connective tissue disease. The true incidence of myocarditis in the population is impossible to ascertain. Focal or diffuse myocarditis has been found to be relatively common in routine autopsy cases, ranging from 3.4 to 9.3 per cent. In addition, as many as one third of patients with common infectious diseases may have electrocardiographic abnormalities suggesting myocardial involvement. From these observations, it appears that myocarditis is most often silent and not accompanied by overt ventricular dysfunction. It has been postulated, however, that chronic cardiomyopathy may be a late manifestation of an acute myocarditis. It is well documented, for example, that such diseases as acute rheumatic carditis, Chagas' disease, and toxoplasmosis may progress to a stage of chronic fibrosis. Further credence is given to this postulate from observations that the incidence and severity of experimental myocarditis are increased by hypoxia, exercise, or concomitant exposure to bacterial toxins. In addition, treatment of experimental myocarditis with steroids may lead to diffuse myocardial abnormalities rather than focal lesions. One may speculate that factors such as these may select out patients with "silent" myocarditis to develop more extensive disease over time, leading ultimately to an "idiopathic" cardiomyopathy.

Myocarditis is frequently unrecognized either because of its subclinical nature or because of the severity of associated conditions. When symptomatic, the patient may complain of fever, palpitations, pleuropericardial pain, dyspnea, edema, or fatigue, or may die suddenly. The physical examination shows biventricular failure, including elevated venous pressure, cardiomegaly, soft first heart sound, ventricular gallop, mitral and tricuspid regurgitation, pulmonary rales, and congestive hepatomegaly. A pericardial friction rub is heard in the presence of an associated pericarditis. The electrocardiogram may show atrial and ventricular extrasystoles, arrhythmias, conduction disturbances, and ST-T wave abnormalities. Measurement of cardiac isoenzyme activities may be helpful in differentiating cardiac involvement from passive hepatic congestion.

Specific treatment is indicated for such conditions as rickettsial or *Mycoplasma pneumoniae* infections. The management of congestive heart failure includes digitalis, diuretics, and salt restriction. Short-acting digitalis preparations are recommended because of the propensity of these patients to develop digitalis toxicity. In addition, patients should be placed at bed rest and administered oxygen, if hypoxic, to reduce the deleterious effects of activity and hypoxia observed in experimental myocarditis. Lidocaine, quinidine, or procainamide may be necessary to control arrhythmias, but propranolol should be used with caution because of its negative inotropic effect. Although steroids may be of great benefit in acute rheumatic carditis, they should be used only as a last resort for infectious myocarditis because of the potential of more widespread myocardial disease as shown in the experimental model.

VIRAL MYOCARDITIS. Myocarditis without pericarditis is frequently caused by Group B coxsackieviruses. Group A coxsackieviruses are implicated much less often, as are echoviruses, measles, mumps, and poliomyelitis, as well as many others. Human infection with Group B coxsackievirus was first documented in neonatal infants and later in nursery epidemics, with the virus being recovered from the myocardium itself. Since then, coxsackievirus B heart disease has been identified in adults and is frequently associated with pericarditis. The only clinical manifestation may be electrocardiographic changes. Less commonly, cardiac enlargement and decreased exercise tolerance may occur. Idiopathic benign pericarditis, which is frequently associated with a myocarditis, is increasingly felt to represent coxsackievirus B disease.

Myocardial damage by a virus may result from its myocytolytic effect, through direct cellular invasion and multiplication, or by an autoimmune process. Microscopically, interstitial edema, round cell infiltration, loss of striations, and areas of necrosis are found. The newborn infant is particularly susceptible to viral myocarditis, which may be rapidly progressive, leading to congestive heart failure and death. In the adult, complete healing usually occurs, but chronic fibrosis may ensue. Although it has not been possible to isolate a virus in the chronic stage of the disease, studies in mice have shown continued inflammation and fibrosis well after disappearance of the virus from the myocardium. Through fluorescent antibody techniques, viral antigens have been identified in human cardiomyopathies, suggesting the possibility of a chronic, active process. Appropriate laboratory studies must be carried out during the acute or subacute stages in order to define the specific offending agent. These include viral isolation from pharynx and feces by tissue culture, and analysis of paired sera for type-specific IgM neutralizing or hemagglutination-inhibiting antibodies.

Poliomyelitis is frequently accompanied by myocarditis as manifest by conduction abnormalities and ST-T wave changes on the electrocardiogram. The significance of these changes is difficult to ascertain, however, as they may be due to concomitant brainstem disease, metabolic imbalance, or hypoxia. Cardiovascular collapse is a frequent cause of death in patients with bulbar poliomyelitis. The myocarditis is significantly more severe in these patients than in those dying of other polio-related causes. The myocardial lesions range from perivascular inflammation to diffuse myocardial involvement with edema, loss of striations, and fragmentation of myocardial cells. In addition, these patients appear to have more extensive involvement of the reticular substance in the medulla. A combination of vasoconstriction, mediated by the medullary lesion in bulbar poliomyelitis, and the extensive myocarditis may be responsible for the acute heart failure with pulmonary edema and cardiogenic shock.

Many other viruses in addition to coxsackievirus and poliomyelitis have been implicated in the production of myocarditis. These include measles, mumps, *Mycoplasma pneumoniae*, influenza, rabies, varicella, choriomeningitis, and infectious mononucleosis. Treatment of viral myocarditis is largely supportive and symptomatic. Since it appears that steroids may be responsible for more widespread inflammation during the early intracellular viral infection, they should be withheld initially and added later to inhibit the chronic inflammatory process. The efficacy of steroids in limiting chronic inflammation and subsequent fibrosis is still controversial.

BACTERIAL MYOCARDITIS.   Primary bacterial invasion of the myocardium is rare. It remains a grave complication, however, of bacterial endocarditis and may account for ventricular dysfunction because of myocardial microabscess formation. Later, during the reparative stage, ventricular dysfunction may result from chronic myocardial damage. The organisms most commonly involved are streptococci and staphylococci.

DIPHTHERITIC MYOCARDITIS.   Myocarditis is an ominous complication of *Corynebacterium diphtheriae* infection and accounts for the majority of deaths. The protein exotoxin responsible for many of the clinical manifestations of the disease is thought to interfere with the synthesis of polypeptide chains by inhibiting the transfer of amino acids from soluble RNA. In the myocardium, the oxidation of long-chain fatty acids is inhibited with resultant accumulation of triglycerides.

In a large compilation of patients with diphtheria, the over-all mortality rate has been reported as 11 per cent, whereas in those with an associated myocarditis the mortality rate may be as high as 60 per cent. The electrocardiogram is a sensitive histotoxic indicator of myocardial involvement and is abnormal in 20 to 40 per cent of patients by the second week of the disease. Clinically evident myocarditis, however, occurs in less than 10 per cent of cases. The prognosis for patients with P-R interval prolongation and T wave changes is excellent. Conduction disturbances which occur later in the illness have a poor prognosis, with reported mortality rates of 50 per cent for bundle branch block and 100 per cent for patients with complete heart block. Causes of death include congestive heart failure and arrhythmias. At autopsy, the hearts are dilated and flabby. Histologic examination reveals interstitial edema, fibrinoid degeneration and necrosis, and focal infiltrates of inflammatory cells. The treatment for diphtheria is prevention by immunization, antitoxin, and symptomatic therapy for the complications caused by myocarditis.

TOXOPLASMA MYOCARDITIS.   *Toxoplasma gondii* is a protozoan which infects humans as both a congenital and an acquired disease. The prevalence of *Toxoplasma* infection is highest in women of childbearing age and approaches 90 per cent in some areas of the world. The congenital form is thought to arise by transmission in utero and frequently results in abortion, premature birth, or neonatal death. Maternal infection in the first trimester of pregnancy is most likely to cause fetal infection with resultant central nervous system damage. Myocarditis is not prominent in congenital toxoplasmosis. The mode of transmission is unclear for the acquired form, and both domestic and wild animals have been implicated. In the adult, the disease is usually subclinical or mild and self-limiting. It is common for several members of the same family to be infected. Lethal disseminated toxoplasmosis may occur, however, and myocarditis or pericarditis is frequent in this situation. The disseminated form usually occurs in debilitated patients receiving cancer chemotherapy, irradiation, or steroids. The myocarditis is characterized pathologically by scattered areas of focal necrosis and inflammation. Intracellular organisms without surrounding inflammation are frequently observed in the myocardium, whereas other areas show severe inflammatory foci in the absence of the protozoan. The antemortem diagnosis is difficult and depends on the demonstration of the organism in tissue by animal inoculation or positive serologic tests. The latter include the Sabin-Feldman methylene blue dye test, hemagglutination, and fluorescent antibody tests. Although treatment is frequently unsatisfactory, the treatment of choice is combined pyrimethamine and sulfonamides, which act synergistically against the organism.

TRICHINOSIS. Although trichinosis is thought to be the most common helminthic infestation in man, the majority of patients are asymptomatic. Neurologic and myocardial involvement account for the fatalities. Symptoms of encephalitis begin during the stage of larval dissemination during the second week; more localizing neurologic signs begin during the encystment stage in the third week. Myocardial involvement, characterized by retrosternal chest pain, tachycardia, dyspnea, and congestive failure, usually begins after the third week. The electrocardiogram reveals nonspecific ST-T wave changes, conduction abnormalities, and extrasystoles. The majority of patients recover, but when death occurs it is usually between the fourth and eighth week. At autopsy, cardiomegaly, scattered areas of myocardial necrosis, and inflammatory infiltrates are found. Steroids appear to be beneficial for both the neurologic and cardiac complications.

TRYPANOSOMIASIS. Chagas' disease is produced by a protozoan, *Trypanosoma cruzi*, which is harbored by hematophagous insects more common in South and Central America. Although less than 1 per cent of infected individuals develop the acute form of Chagas' disease, approximately 30 per cent will develop chronic chagasic myocarditis 20 years after the initial infection. Acute Chagas' disease has a mortality rate of 1 per cent, largely resulting from myocarditis or meningoencephalitis, whereas approximately 20 per cent of those with the chronic myocarditis die within two years of diagnosis. Most cases of acute chagasic myocarditis are self-limited, and most patients recover with only transient cardiomegaly and minor electrocardiographic abnormalities. In patients with fatal cases, however, there is rapid deterioration due to congestive heart failure secondary to a panmyocarditis. Parasites are present in variable numbers within myocardial fibers, and there is extensive interstitial inflammation, necrosis, and hyaline degeneration. Toxic as well as immunoallergic mechanisms have been postulated. Chronic chagasic myocarditis manifests itself most commonly as a congestive cardiomyopathy and less often with restrictive signs and symptoms simulating constrictive pericarditis. The electrocardiogram classically shows right bundle branch block and S-T segment changes compatible with acute infarction. Right bundle branch block occurs in as many as 60 per cent of patients and is frequently associated with left anterior hemiblock, whereas left bundle branch block is rare. Premature ventricular contractions are common, as are ST-T wave changes and Q waves mimicking myocardial infarction. The diagnosis is made by demonstrating the organism in the patient's blood, culture, complement fixation test, or xenodiagnosis. Treatment is directed toward control of the arrhythmias and congestive heart failure.

GIANT CELL MYOCARDITIS. Idiopathic giant cell myocarditis is an uncommon disease of unknown cause that may present clinically as congestive heart failure, arrhythmias, or sudden death. All ages may be affected, and there is no predominance of either sex. Proposed causes include viral infection, autoimmune disease, and sarcoidosis. Histologically, there is interstitial edema with scattered areas of granulomatous lesions associat-ed with fibrosis, multinucleated giant cells, plasma cells, lymphocytes, histiocytes, and fragments of degenerating myocardial fibers. In areas of myocardial necrosis, multinucleated giant cells are rare and polymorphonuclear cells are common. No other organs are involved. These observations by light microscopy and electron microscopy suggest that the process involves an unusual form of myocardial degeneration in which the multinucleated giant cells are myogenic in origin. The initiating cause of this degeneration is unknown, but of interest is the association with other diseases, including thymoma, myositis, thyroiditis, and systemic lupus erythematosus. There is no specific therapy, and the reports of results with steroids are conflicting.

Abelmann, W. H.: Myocarditis. N. Engl. J. Med., 275:832, 944, 1966.
Gleason, T. H., and Hamlin, W. B.: Disseminated toxoplasmosis in the compromised host. Arch. Intern. Med., 134:1059, 1974.
Gray, D. F., Morse, B. S., and Phillips, W. F.: Trichinosis with neurologic and cardiac involvement. Ann. Intern. Med., 57:230, 1962.
Hildes, J. A., Schaberg, A., and Alcock, A. J. W.: Cardiovascular collapse in acute poliomyelitis. Circulation, 12:986, 1955.
Hirschman, S. Z., and Hammer, G. S.: Coxsackie virus myopericarditis. Am. J. Cardiol., 34:224, 1974.
Ledbetter, M. K., Cannon, A. B., and Costa, A. F.: The electrocardiogram in diphtheritic myocarditis. Am. Heart J., 68:599, 1964.
Pyun, K. S., Kim, Y. H., Katzenstein, R. E., and Kikkawa, Y.: Giant cell myocarditis. Arch. Path., 90:181, 1970.
Rosenbaum, M. B.: Chagasic myocardiopathy. Prog. Cardiovasc. Dis., 7:199, 1964.

366.5.   NUTRITIONAL CARDIOMYOPATHY

Victor S. Behar

Nutritional deficiencies have been known to produce as well as contribute to heart disease in virtually all parts of the world, although most commonly in the underdeveloped countries. In most instances, the precise cause remains unknown, and multiple factors no doubt exist.

Two identifiable forms of nutritional heart disease have been described in Africans. *Bantu hypokinetic heart disease* occurs in the adult Bantu with a poor nutritional background. The diet of those afflicted is primarily composed of carbohydrate and lacks protein and essential amino acids. No single food factor or vitamin has been identified. The patient has cardiomegaly and recurrent episodes of congestive heart failure. The circulation is described as "hypokinetic," and the cardiac output is usually between 1 and 2 liters per minute. In the early stages, the disease is reversible by the intake of a balanced diet. Without dietary therapy, the heart failure becomes intractable to conventional therapy and death is frequently sudden. At autopsy, there is cirrhosis of the liver with histologic features of hemochromatosis or cytosiderosis. The heart is dilated and hypertrophied, with mural thrombi seen on gross examination. Microscopically, there is interstitial edema and scattered areas of fibrosis, which at times may be extensive. Hemosiderin is not seen in the heart.

The second form of nutritional African heart disease is *kwashiorkor*, which is produced by a protein deficiency in infancy. The infant appears markedly cachectic with hepatomegaly and edema. With cardiovascular involvement, venous distention, decreased pulse pressure, cold extremities, and peripheral cyanosis occur. The heart is characteristically small both on chest x-ray and at autopsy. The histologic appearance is nonspecific. The electrocardiogram shows low voltage, and arrhythmias are uncommon. The Q-T interval is prolonged, and there are broad, deep ST-T wave changes. The severity of these findings is of prognostic value; they frequently revert to normal following adequate protein intake. Death is often sudden and unexplained.

Beriberi is responsible for the most common cause of nutritional heart disease in the world. The criteria for beriberi heart disease have been broadened since its first description in the Orient. The classic description was that of a hyperkinetic circulation with bounding and pistol shot pulses, predominant right heart failure with venous engorgement, flushing of the skin with peripheral vasodilation, and syncope or shock. In the Occidental form, there is usually biventricular failure, and the hyperkinetic aspects are masked or absent. The common denominator, however, is the low nutritional intake of vitamin B$_1$ (thiamin) and a high carbohydrate diet. The polished rice diet in the Orient accounts for this combination, whereas in the Western countries the disease occurs primarily in chronic alcoholics. It is an uncommon form of heart disease in alcoholics, however, but it may complicate the course and treatment of other organic types of heart disease. The electrocardiogram shows low voltage, nonspecific ST-T wave changes and prolongation of the Q-T interval. Conduction disturbances and arrhythmias are uncommon. Pathologically, the heart is markedly dilated, especially the right ventricle, and hypertrophied. Mural thrombi are not uncommon and may result in emboli. The histologic changes are nonspecific and include interstitial edema and hydropic degeneration, especially in the subendocardial myocardium.

The clinical diagnosis can be made in the presence of cardiomegaly, edema, increased venous pressure, peripheral neuritis or pellagra, and dietary deficiency of three months or greater, with improvement following thiamin therapy. The hemodynamic abnormalities of high cardiac output, low arteriovenous oxygen difference, and low peripheral vascular resistance return toward normal both acutely and chronically following the administration of thiamin. Digitalis and diuretics have also proved useful for the control of congestive heart failure.

Potassium deficiency produces characteristic abnormalities on the electrocardiogram. These include prolongation of the Q-T interval, depressed S-T segments, flattening of the T wave, and the appearance of large U waves. Prolonged hypokalemia in animals fed a diet deficient in potassium or made hypokalemic by the administration of desoxycorticosterone acetate has been shown to produce typical histologic changes in the kidneys as well as the heart. Similar histologic changes have been observed in humans with chronic steatorrhea following prolonged periods of hypokalemia. The myocarditis of potassium deficiency is characterized by an early focal infiltration of polymorphonuclear neutrophils surrounding normal myocardial fibers, and later by loss of muscle striations, necrosis, influx of inflammatory cells, and bands of fibrosis. Treatment is, of course, early potassium replacement in order to prevent the development of permanent changes and fibrosis.

ALCOHOLIC CARDIOMYOPATHY. This is a well known clinical entity characterized by congestive heart failure in the absence of a known cause for heart disease other than the presence of alcoholism. The dietary state of these patients is usually adequate, and there is no deficiency of thiamin or other essential nutrients. Chronic alcoholism may be defined as the daily intake of eight ounces of whiskey, one quart of wine, or two quarts of beer for five years or more. The clinical recognition of cardiomyopathy in patients with chronic alcoholism is usually not difficult and can be documented by hemodynamic abnormalities of ventricular function both invasively and noninvasively. With these techniques, it has been shown that patients with an alcoholic fatty liver in the absence of clinical evidence of cardiac involvement may also have significant depression of ventricular function. Studies in noncardiac chronic alcoholics reveal that the depressed resting level of ventricular function may be further depressed by the acute ingestion of ethanol in a moderate dose, but not following a low dose. However, normal subjects receiving a similar low dose, which produces nonintoxicating ethanol blood levels, showed significant transient depression of ventricular performance. These findings suggest that there is a myocardial adaptation to chronic alcohol use in which the threshold for myocardial depression is increased. Metabolic studies in animals and man during acute ingestion of ethanol in intoxicating amounts show a rise in the myocardial respiratory quotient followed by a return to control levels in 90 minutes. This is accompanied by a decrease in myocardial free fatty acid extraction and an increase in triglyceride uptake. Transient myocardial injury following ethanol administration has been demonstrated by an efflux of ions and transaminase in coronary sinus blood. It is therefore apparent that chronic ingestion of alcohol adversely affects the heart and that these changes are reversible prior to development of the overt cardiomyopathy of alcoholism.

The clinical manifestations are palpitations, secondary to extrasystoles and arrhythmias, followed by the symptoms of congestive heart failure and thromboembolic episodes. On physical examination, a resting tachycardia, cardiomegaly, atrial and ventricular gallop sounds, and the murmurs of mitral or tricuspid regurgitation are found. Other common signs of heart failure include venous distention, hepatomegaly, and edema. These signs of a hypokinetic circulation are readily differentiated from the hyperkinetic circulation of beriberi. The electrocardiogram shows distinctive T wave changes described as spinous (peaked), dimpled (shallow notch in Q-T segment), and cloven (cleft at summit of low T wave). The T waves may later become inverted, falsely suggesting coronary disease. In addition, there may be left ventricular hypertrophy, conduction disturbances, S-T segment depression, pathologic Q waves, and arrhythmias, including premature atrial and ventricular systoles as well as atrial fibrillation. The chest x-ray reveals cardiomegaly and pulmonary congestion.

At autopsy, there is marked cardiomegaly with both dilatation and hypertrophy. Mural thrombi are common. Histologic study shows hypertrophy of the myocardial fibers, increased glycogen and neutral lipid, interstitial edema, necrosis, and fibrosis. Electron microscopic studies of tissue obtained by endomyocardial biopsy following acute infusion of ethanol show severe alterations of myocardial cellular organelles. These changes include mitochondrial swelling with loss of its cristae and swelling of the sarcoplasmic reticulum.

In the natural course of alcoholic cardiomyopathy the three-year mortality rate exceeds 40 per cent after the development of symptoms. The prognosis is significantly better in those patients with a shorter duration of symptoms and those who are able to abstain from further alcohol ingestion. Prolonged bed rest has not substantially improved the long-term response to conventional therapy, which is largely supportive and symptomatic.

COBALT-BEER CARDIOMYOPATHY. In August, 1965, a bizarre cardiomyopathy became manifest in Quebec City, affecting heavy beer drinkers who were primarily males over the age of 25. The illness was fulminating with biventricular failure associated with polycythemia, low cardiac output, cyanosis, cardiomegaly, gallop rhythm, pericardial effusion, cardiogenic shock, and severe lactic acidosis. A similar disease occurred in Minneapolis and Omaha, as well as in several other cities throughout the world. The electrocardiogram in these patients showed sinus tachycardia, whereas arrhythmias were rare. A rightward shift of the P wave and QRS complex was observed, as were large Q waves simulating anterior myocardial infarction. The chest x-ray revealed cardiomegaly and signs of pericardial effusion. Serum glutamic oxaloacetic transaminase, lactic dehydrogenase, and creatine phosphokinase were markedly elevated. The mortality rate ranged from 40 to 45 per cent. At autopsy, electron microscopic studies of the heart showed dissolution of myofibrils, with loss of myofibrillar proteins and replacement by glycogen; abnormal and shrunken mitochondria, which contained large intramitochondrial vacuoles; and dilatation of the sarcoplasmic reticulum, with formation of large vesicles. The sarcolemma appeared to be intact. The thyroid gland demonstrated follicular hyperplasia and little or no colloid. These changes in the thyroid gland were an important clue in the final identification of cobalt as the toxic agent. Because of the extensive use of detergents in washing glassware, beer poured into glasses with residual detergent was unable to maintain its foam. Cobalt chloride was therefore added to the beer in order to stabilize the foam. The metabolic action of cobalt is to block the oxidation of pyruvate to acetyl-CoA and α-ketoglutarate to succinyl-CoA without affecting the synthesis of glycogen and triglyceride. The relative toxicity of cobalt on the heart is complicated by other factors such as duration of ethanol intake, dietary protein, thiamin deficiency, and pre-existing heart disease. Although the majority of survivors had a satisfactory recovery, residual electrocardiographic changes and chronic heart failure were not unusual. Since the removal of cobalt from beer, no additional cases have been reported.

Ahmed, S. S., Levinson, G. E., and Regan, T. J.: Depression of myocardial contractility with low doses of ethanol in normal man. Circulation, 48:378, 1973.

Akbarian, M., Yankopoulos, N. A., and Abelmann, W. H.: Hemodynamic studies in beriberi heart disease. Am. J. Med., 41:197, 1966.

Demakis, J. G., Proskey, A., Rahimtoola, S. H., Jamil, M., Sutton, G. C., Rosen, K. M., Gunnar, R. M., and Tobin, J. R.: The natural course of alcoholic cardiomyopathy. Ann. Intern. Med., 80:293, 1974.

Higginson, J., Gillanders, A. D., and Murray, J. F.: The heart in chronic malnutrition. Br. Heart J., 14:213, 1952.

McAllen, P. M.: Myocardial changes occurring in potassium deficiency. Br. Heart J., 17:5, 1955.

Morin, Y. C., Foley, A. R., Martineau, G., and Roussel, J.: Quebec beer-drinkers' cardiomyopathy: 48 cases. Can. Med. Assoc. J., 97:881, 1967.

Regan, T. J., Levinson, G. E., Oldewurtel, H. A., Frank, M. J., Weisse,
A. B., and Moschos, C. B.: Ventricular function in noncardiacs with alcoholic fatty liver: Role of ethanol in the production of cardiomyopathy. J. Clin. Invest., 48:397, 1969.

Smythe, P. M., and Swanepoel, A.: The heart in kwashiorkor. Br. Med. J., 1:67, 1962.

366.6. CARDIAC AMYLOIDOSIS

Victor S. Behar

Cardiac amyloidosis is a disease of unknown cause characterized by the widespread tissue deposition of an amorphous hyaline-like substance. The disease is uncommon under age 40 and affects the sexes equally. The prevalence of amyloidosis in the general population is not known. Although patients with multiple myeloma may have an incidence of amyloidosis as high as 15 per cent, it occurs in less than 1 per cent of unselected cases at autopsy. The relationship of amyloidosis to the aging process is of particular interest, as it has been found in as many as 90 per cent of patients dying of senile dementia when specifically looked for in brain, heart, or pancreas.

There have been many attempts to classify amyloidosis; it appears most useful to divide them into the following groups: (1) primary amyloidosis (no coexisting disease), (2) myeloma associated amyloidosis, (3) secondary amyloidosis (coexisting, chronic inflammatory disease), (4) localized amyloidosis (single organ involvement), and (5) familial amyloidosis. Amyloidosis presents clinically most often with renal involvement, especially the nephrotic syndrome, congestive heart failure, carpal tunnel syndrome, sprue, peripheral neuropathy, or orthostatic hypotension. The most common symptoms are fatigue, weight loss, edema, dyspnea, and, to a lesser extent, hoarseness, paresthesias, or the carpal tunnel syndrome. Although the edema may be produced by either the nephrotic syndrome or congestive heart failure, the presence of dizziness, syncope, and orthostatic hypotension should suggest cardiac amyloidosis.

On physical examination, hepatomegaly, splenomegaly and macroglossia are usually found, the last being more common in patients with multiple myeloma. In addition, there may be lymphadenopathy, especially in the submandibular region, purpura, and skin lesions. The cardiac manifestations may simulate constrictive pericarditis because of impaired ventricular filling during diastole and include an elevated jugular venous pressure with a rapid "y" descent and an early diastolic filling sound. However, if the left heart is more severely involved, the signs of left heart failure may predominate.

The electrocardiogram shows low voltage, which may falsely suggest constrictive pericarditis, as well as Q wave abnormalities, which may be misinterpreted as old myocardial infarction. Supraventricular arrhythmias are frequently seen, as well as the entire spectrum of conduction abnormalities. Many investigators have made the observation that patients with cardiac amyloidosis are particularly susceptible to digitalis-induced arrhythmias, possibly because of the infiltration of amyloid in the perivascular region of the sinoatrial node.

Pathologically, the heart is increased in size and firm in consistency. Nodular lesions may be seen in the endocardium, valves, and pericardium. Histologic examination reveals diffuse interstitial infiltration of amyloid within the myocardium and in the blood vessels. Amyloid is identified by its distinctive green birefringence when stained with Congo red and examined under a polarizing microscope. In the electron microscope, the amyloid is seen to consist of rigid, nonbranching fibrils. In systemic primary amyloidosis these fibrils are identical to the variable portion of monoclonal Bence Jones protein. When Bence Jones proteins are subjected to pepsin digestion, amyloid fibrils are produced. This has led to the speculation that light chains produced by the plasma cells are precursors of the amyloid fibril, either being produced within the cell and secreted or being secreted to form the fibrils in the surrounding tissue. The association of Bence Jones protein and amyloidosis has been further substantiated by a report from the Mayo Clinic in which 50 per cent of their patients with primary amyloidosis were found to have a monoclonal protein in either the serum or urine. Similar monoclonal abnormalities were present in 89 per cent of patients with multiple myeloma–associated amyloidosis. The clinical diagnosis is proved by tissue biopsy from the rectum in over 80 per cent of patients, and in more than 90 per cent when tissue is obtained from the kidney, carpal tunnel, or liver. Two-year survival for patients with primary amyloidosis is 35 per cent, but only 10 per cent for those with amyloidosis associated with multiple myeloma. Congestive heart failure is the most common cause of death, and sudden death, presumably from arrhythmias, is also frequent.

Brigden, W.: Cardiac amyloidosis. Prog. Cardiovasc. Dis., 7:142, 1964.
Buerger, L., and Braunstein, H.: Senile cardiac amyloidosis. Am. J. Med., 28:357, 1960.
Cohen, A. S.: Amyloidosis. N. Engl. J. Med., 277:522, 1967.
James, T. N.: Pathology of the cardiac conduction system in amyloidosis. Ann. Intern. Med., 65:28, 1966.
Kyle, R. A., and Bayrd, E. D.: Amyloidosis: Review of 236 cases. Medicine, 54:271, 1975.

366.7. OTHER CARDIOMYOPATHIES

Victor S. Behar

ENDOMYOCARDIAL FIBROSIS. Endomyocardial fibrosis has been reported to be responsible for approximately 15 per cent of the cardiac deaths from heart failure in Uganda. The disease has also been reported in Celon and Sudan. No known cause has been defined, although increased consumption of African plantain, which is rich in serotonin, has been implicated, as well as persistence of the infantile form of fibroelastosis, hypersensitivity reactions, and inflammation caused by viral or parasitic disease. Both sexes and all age groups are affected. The manifestations are progressive biventricular failure with dyspnea, edema, ascites, and pain from hepatic congestion. Mitral regurgitation is common, and tricuspid regurgitation may occur in the presence of right ventricular failure. The signs of a restrictive cardiomyopathy are usually dominant both on physical examination and at cardiac catheterization, falsely suggesting constrictive pericarditis. The frequent occurrence of pulmonary hypertension, however, is strong evidence against constriction.

At autopsy, all chambers may show the endocardial and myocardial changes, but the ventricles are more severely involved. Microscopically, the endocardium demonstrates the presence of an acellular, hyalinized, fibrous tissue. These changes, together with granula-

tion tissue, extend into the inner one third of the myocardium. Mural thrombi are common despite the infrequent history of systemic emboli. There is no specific treatment for endomyocardial fibrosis other than the symptomatic management of congestive heart failure.

LÖFFLER'S FIBROPLASTIC ENDOCARDITIS. In 1936, Löffler reported a series of patients with progressive and refractory heart failure who had a febrile illness associated with a persistent eosinophilia and multiple systemic emboli. The mode of onset may be either acute, with abdominal, cerebral, or respiratory symptoms, or insidious, with a gradual decrease in exercise tolerance and a clinical picture simulating constrictive pericarditis. Mitral regurgitation is common, but murmurs of mitral stenosis and tricuspid regurgitation may also be heard. The electrocardiogram demonstrates low voltage with nonspecific S-T segment and T wave abnormalities. The chest x-ray shows pulmonary congestion and infiltrates as well as pleural effusions.

The acute phase of the disease is characterized by an eosinophilic arteritis involving the heart and other organs. In the late stages of the disease, the heart is enlarged and there is a leathery, grayish-white thickening of the endocardium which involves all chambers. The fibrosis extends into the myocardium as well as the papillary muscles and chordae tendineae, with resultant mitral and tricuspid valvular incompetence. The disease is inevitably fatal, and there is no specific form of therapy, although steroids have produced some improvement during the acute stage.

SARCOIDOSIS. Although clinical manifestations of cardiac involvement are unusual in sarcoidosis, postmortem studies have demonstrated parenchymal cardiac involvement in 20 per cent of cases. The patients with cardiac symptoms are frequently young or middle aged, with equal prevalence in males and females. There is almost always a known history of sarcoidosis. The clinical manifestations are most often palpitations, presyncope, or syncope; chest pain and congestive heart failure occur less often. Congestive heart failure is primarily due to cor pulmonale and not to direct myocardial involvement. The electrocardiogram demonstrates a high incidence of atrioventricular block, bundle branch block, ventricular ectopic beats, and ventricular tachycardia and fibrillation. Worsening of the arrhythmias has been noted during exercise testing. Death frequently occurs within six months of the onset of cardiac symptoms, and 75 per cent of patients are dead within two years. The cause of death is unexplained and sudden in approximately two thirds of patients. Arrhythmias and complete heart block, which occur in 30 per cent of patients, must, of course, be implicated. At autopsy, the typical lesion is a noncaseating granulomatous follicle composed of epithelioid cells and giant cells of the Langerhans type surrounded by a narrow zone of lymphocytes. Although many organs are involved, the lungs are frequently most severely affected, with progressive fibrosis leading to cor pulmonale. The myocardial lesions most often involve the left ventricle and the upper posterior part of the interventricular septum. The histologic lesions are variable but may be categorized as exudative, granulomatous, granulomatous plus fibrotic, and predominantly fibrotic. Although treatment is frequently disappointing, improvement in the recurrent arrhythmias has been observed with prednisone alone or in various combinations with procainamide, quinidine, and propranolol.

PERIPARTUM CARDIOMYOPATHY (PUERPERAL MYOCARDITIS). Peripartum cardiomyopathy is characterized by congestive heart failure in the last month of pregnancy or within five months of delivery in the absence of any pre-existing form of heart disease. The incidence is highest in multiparous blacks and is more common with increasing age, poor nutrition and prenatal care, toxemia, and multiple births. The onset of left ventricular failure occurs most often within the first three months post partum. The electrocardiogram may show left ventricular hypertrophy with inverted T waves, low voltage, and nonspecific ST-T wave abnormalities. The chest x-ray demonstrates cardiomegaly and pulmonary venous congestion.

Although the early prognosis is good, significant cardiac disability and death may ensue. The patients seggregate into low risk and high risk groups, according to changes in heart size. In as many as 50 per cent of patients, heart size may return to normal within six months. In these patients, the persistence of gallop sounds, recurrence of heart failure, or recurrence of postpartum failure following subsequent pregnancies is rare. In the patients with persistent cardiomegaly, however, chronic heart failure and pulmonary or systemic emboli are common. Furthermore, in this poor risk group, subsequent pregnancies frequently result in worsening of symptoms and death. Long-term survival for these patients is approximately 15 per cent in five years.

Myocardial biopsy obtained within three months of the onset of heart failure shows myocardial hypertrophy and varying degrees of fibrosis. At autopsy, the heart is dilated and appears hypertrophied. Mural thrombi are common and frequently result in emboli. Histologically, there is myocardial hypertrophy, fibrosis, interstitial edema, and focal accumulation of lymphocytes.

No specific form of therapy is indicated other than the management of congestive heart failure. The risk of subsequent pregnancies is substantial, and the likelihood of carrying the pregnancy to term is reduced.

RADIATION MYOCARDITIS. In recent years, the goal of radiation therapy has increasingly been complete eradication of the malignancy. Cardiac injury is clinically apparent in approximately 5 per cent of patients receiving 4000 rads or more in the form of either orthovoltage or supervoltage. Patients receiving larger amounts of radiation, as in those undergoing retreatment therapy for Hodgkin's disease, have a much higher incidence of carditis. In the large series of patients treated at Stanford, 50 per cent of those receiving more than 6000 rads developed carditis, which in some cases was a severe pancarditis. Radiation heart disease is most commonly manifest in the form of pericardial disease, including acute pericarditis, chronic effusion, or chronic constrictive pericarditis. Less commonly, myocardial fibrosis may accompany pericarditis and has been observed to produce conduction disturbances, including bundle branch block and varying degrees of heart block, as well as ventricular dysfunction and mitral regurgitation. Of particular interest is the controversy that radiation injury produces premature coronary atherosclerosis. Indeed, there are many autopsy reports of patients dying in the second or third decade with extensive coronary artery disease and myocardial infarctions following radiation therapy. In addition to these clinical observations, there are experimental data that the changes induced in the dog aorta by radiation are very similar to those which occur during the normal aging process. Other studies in atherogenic animal models further substantiate the clinical observation in that more severe atheromatous lesions occur following exposure to high dose radiation. The microcirculation has also been shown to participate in the process of myocardial damage from radiation. Immediately following exposure, there is an acute and transient inflammatory exudate in all cardiac tissues. After a latent period, however, a focal cytoplasmic degeneration occurs in the endothelial cells of myocardial capillaries, followed by a proliferation of these cells in an apparent attempt to form new capillaries. Ischemia and diffuse myocardial fibrosis result from this gradual loss of the microcirculation.

With the advent of megavoltage therapy and innovative rotational techniques, more effective tumor doses can now be delivered and survival significantly prolonged. As a byproduct of this, however, the treatment of thoracic malignancy also results in more radiation to the heart, and because of the longer survival there is greater opportunity for the delayed effects of myocardial damage to occur. It is important to acknowledge the fact that although acute pericarditis may occur during the period of radiation treatment itself, it is more likely that the signs and symptoms of cardiac damage will occur after a variable latent period, frequently years. Thus the development of cardiac symptoms following a course of radiation therapy does not necessarily indicate recurrence of tumor in the myocardium but may be a manifestation of radiation disease of the heart.

DRUG-INDUCED MYOCARDITIS. Adriamycin, which closely resembles its parent compound daunorubicin, has been observed to produce cardiotoxicity during the treatment of far-advanced cancer. The cardiotoxicity is manifest as electrocardiographic changes or congestive heart failure. The electrocardiographic abnormalities occur in 10 per cent of patients and include sinus tachycardia, ST-T wave changes, and premature ventricular contractions. These are reversible upon discontinuance of the drug. An additional 10 per cent of patients develop intractable biventricular heart failure, with death within three weeks of the onset of symptoms. This appears to be dose related, with virtually all affected patients receiving more than 500 mg per square meter of Adriamycin. Impaired left ventricular function has been observed by noninvasive studies in patients receiving as little as 300 mg per square meter, and this technique should be useful in detecting subclinical cases of cardiotoxicity. These early changes are reversible, but the recovery time is directly related to the cumulative dose. The toxicity appears to be due to the aglycone metabolite of the drug.

Other drugs which may produce electrocardiographic changes or toxicity include the tricyclic antidepressants, phenothiazines, and emetine.

Cohn, K. E., Stewart, J. R., Fajardo, L. F., and Hancock, E. W.: Heart disease following radiation. Medicine, 46:281, 1967.
Davies, J. N. P.: Some considerations regarding obscure diseases affecting the mural endocardium. Am. Heart J., 59:600, 1960.
Demakis, J. G., Rahimtoola, S. H., Sutton, G. C., Meadows, W. R., Szanto, P. B., Tobin, J. R., and Gunnar, R. M.: Natural course of peripartum cardiomyopathy. Circulation, 44:1053, 1971.

Fajardo, L. F., and Stewart, J. R.: Pathogenesis of radiation-induced myocardial fibrosis. Lab. Invest., 29:244, 1973.

Lefrak, E. A., Pitha, J., Rosenheim, S., and Gottlieb, J. A.: A clinico-pathologic analysis of Adriamycin cardiotoxicity. Cancer, 32:302, 1973.

Matsui, Y., Iwai, K., Tachibana, T., Fruie, T., Shigematsu, N., Izumi, T., Homma, A. H., Mikami, R., Hongo, O., Hiraga, Y., and Yama-moto, M.: Clinicopathologic study on fatal myocardial sarcoidosis. Ann. N.Y. Acad. Sci., 278:455, 1976.

Rinehart, J. J., Lewis, R. P., and Balcerzak, S. P.: Adriamycin cardio-toxicity in man. Ann. Intern. Med., 81:475, 1974.

Stein, E., Stimmel, B., and Siltzbach, L. E.: Clinical course of cardiac saroidosis. Ann. N.Y. Acad. Sci., 278:470, 1976.

366.8.   TUMORS OF THE HEART

Robert E. Whalen

The heart itself can be the site of a host of primary as well as metastatic tumors. Almost every type of malignant tumor has been found in metastatic form in the heart, but by far the most frequent metastatic tumors include malignant melanomas, leukemia, and malignant lymphomas. Although metastatic tumors of the heart are more frequent than previously realized, they seldom play a significant role in the course of the patient. A large variety of primary tumors of the heart itself have been described, including myxomas, lipomas, fibromas, hemangiomas, lymphangiomas, mesotheliomas, and sarcomas.

The cardiac myxoma is the most frequent and also clinically the most significant primary tumor of the heart, for its discovery and treatment can be lifesaving, whereas its continued presence can be fatal. Myxomas can arise from the endocardial surface of any of the cardiac chambers, but 95 per cent of them arise in the atria, with at least 75 per cent of these arising in the left atrium. The classic location for a myxoma is the region of the fossa ovalis in the left atrium. Bilateral atrial myxomas have been reported. Myxomas have been reported from youth to old age, but most frequently they occur in the middle years. In most series there is a higher incidence among females. They usually present in one or more of three typical ways. The most frequent presentation, which is due to progressive enlargement of the tumor within the cardiac chamber, involves progressive decrease in exercise tolerance, increased dyspnea on exertion, and pulmonary or peripheral edema. Next, the first sign of a myxoma may be produced by occlusion of a major artery with fragments of the myxoma or thrombus previously lodged on the surface of the intracardiac myxoma. Cerebrovascular accidents and sudden ischemia to limbs from this mechanism often herald the presence of a myxoma. The last and least frequent manifestation of a myxoma is the development of systemic symptoms which may simulate acute rheumatic fever, bacterial endocarditis, systemic lupus erythematosus, or a fever of unknown etiology.

Myxomas are almost always accompanied by a regurgitant heart murmur, usually due to incompetence of either the tricuspid or the mitral valve produced by distortion of the valve leaflets. Less frequently the murmur of tricuspid or mitral stenosis may be the most prominent feature due to obstruction of either one of these orifices. The hallmark of the myxoma, frequently detected by auscultation, is a third heart sound which varies in time after the second heart sound. This "tumor plop" is due to the acceleration of the tumor mass through the atrioventricu-lar valve and its impact against the ventricular wall. The presence of any of the aforementioned manifestations in the setting of a normal cardiothoracic ratio, particularly with atrial prominence by chest x-ray, should raise suspicion of a myxoma. The electrocardiogram may show atrial hypertrophy. The presence of a variable third heart sound by phonocardiography, the presence of either an elevated sedimentation rate or increased gamma globulin level, and the variable indentation of the barium-filled esophagus during systole under fluoroscopic observation should enhance suspicion.

The diagnosis of a myxoma is best confirmed by echocardiography, which provides a characteristic picture of the tumor mass as it moves from the atrium to the ventricle during diastole. Angiocardiography, formally the sine qua non for making the diagnosis, is seldom necessary. The life-threatening nature of a cardiac myxoma, the ease with which the diagnosis can be made by echocardiography, and the success of open heart surgery in eliminating the condition emphasize the importance of having a high index of suspicion when seeing a patient with symptoms suggestive of heart failure but with a normal heart size.

Fine, G.: Neoplasms of the pericardium and heart. *In* Gould, S. E. (ed.): Pathology of the Heart and Blood Vessels. Springfield, Ill., Charles C Thomas, 1968, p. 851.

Hardin, N. J., Wilson, J. M., Gray, G. F., and Gay, W. A.: Experience with primary tumors of the heart: Clinical and pathological study of seventeen cases. Johns Hopkins Med. J., 134:141, 1974.

Johnson, M. L., Sieker, H. O., Behar, V. S., and Whalen, R. E.: Echocardiographic diagnosis of a left atrial myxoma found attached to the free left atrial wall. J. Clin. Ultrasound, 1:75, 1973.

Peters, M. N., Hall, R. J., Cooley, D. A., Leachman, R. D., and Garcia, E.: The clinical syndrome of atrial myxoma. JAMA, 230:695, 1974.

Selzer, A., Sakai, F. J., and Popper, R. W.: Protean clinical manifestations of primary tumors of the heart. Am. J. Med., 52:9, 1972.

367.   DISEASES OF THE AORTA

Noble O. Fowler

367.1.   INTRODUCTION

The aorta begins just superior to the aortic valve and ends at the aortic bifurcation opposite the fourth lumbar vertebra. Diseases of the aorta cannot be entirely separated from diseases of the aortic branches. A pathologic process which involves both the aorta and its branches may provoke obstruction or occlusion of these branches and thereby call attention to the existence of aortic disease. For example, in the aortic root, obstruction of a coronary artery at its origin may be caused by aortic intimal disease, thus causing the pain of myocardial ischemia (angina pectoris). Takayasu's arteritis and syphilitic aortitis may represent examples of this mechanism. In a like manner, involvement of the aortic arch can lead to a constellation of symptoms known as the aortic arch syndrome. In this syndrome, obstruction of the orifice of the innominate or left common carotid artery can cause symptoms of cerebral ischemia or visual disturbance. Narrowing of the orifice of the innominate artery or left subclavian artery may cause ischemia of the upper extremities or syncope because of the "subclavian steal" syndrome. Thus patients with aortic atherosclerosis or Takayasu's arteritis may have attacks of syncope, transient pain or syncope with use of the arm with impaired blood supply, or transient monocular blindness. In the abdominal aorta, occlusion of the mesenteric arteries may lead to bowel ischemia with postprandial abdominal angina, or even to infarction of the bowel. Occlusion of a renal artery may lead to systemic hypertension through the Goldblatt mechanism, with increased renin production by the affected kidney causing activation of an alpha$_2$ globulin in plasma to angiotensin. Obstructive disease of the aorta may lead to absence or diminution of pulse in one or more areas; these include the carotid arteries, the subclavian or brachial arteries, and the femoral arteries. Extensive aortic intimal atherosclerosis may lead to cholesterol emboli or atheroembolism, which may cause transient cerebral ischemic attacks (TIA), renal insufficiency, pancreatitis, or cyanosis of one or more toes. Cholesterol emboli to the retinal arteries may be visualized by ophthalmoscopy.

There are other ways in which aortic disease may come to attention. When the aortic lumen is narrowed by disease, murmurs may be produced. Supravalvular aortic stenosis, aortic coarctation, and dissecting hematoma of the aorta each may produce a systolic murmur which is loudest downstream to the site of narrowing. On the other hand, when the aortic lumen is enlarged by aneurysm formation, the aneurysm may occasionally be appreciated on the chest wall or by physical examination of the abdomen; but more often it is detected because it produces pain, because it compresses other vital structures, or because it begins to leak, thereby causing bleeding and shock.

Many times aortic disease is discovered or evaluated more precisely by roentgenograms. Much of the length of the thoracic aorta can be studied by posteroanterior, oblique, and lateral roentgenograms of the chest without the use of contrast media. Although the sinuses of Valsalva are usually lost within the cardiac shadow, when the walls of an aneurysm are calcified, it may be possible to identify and evaluate the aneurysm precisely by plain radiograms, even though it is in the aortic sinuses. The employment of contrast medium increases the accuracy of evaluation of both the thoracic aorta and the abdominal aorta. Areas of narrowing of the lumen, irregularity of the lumen, and dilation of the aorta are thereby more accurately evaluated. Newer noninvasive methods of studying the aorta include echocardiography and dynamic radioisotope scanning (radioisotope aortogram). At present only the ascending thoracic aorta and the abdominal aorta can be studied accurately by echocardiography. In adults the remainder of the thoracic aorta lies too deep within the chest for good echocardiographic evaluation.

Moldveen-Geronimus, M., and Merriam, J. C., Jr.: Cholesterol embolization: From pathologic curiosity to clinical entity. Circulation, 35:946, 1967.

367.2. CONGENITAL DISEASES OF THE AORTA

Congenital diseases of the aorta are not rare in children. They are rather uncommon problems in adult life and will be considered briefly here.

SUPRAVALVULAR AORTIC STENOSIS. Eliot and Ed-

wards classify supravalvular aortic stenosis into three types: an hourglass form, a tubular form, and a fibrous diaphragm-like form. Supravalvular aortic stenosis may be associated with aortic intimal proliferation which may compromise the origin of the innominate artery or the left common carotid or subclavian artery. Thus blood pressure is often different in the two arms. The intimal process often involves the aortic valve as well, so that aortic insufficiency may occur. Coronary arterial stenosis also may occur. Supravalvular aortic stenosis is of two major etiologic backgrounds. One is the familial variety. In this variety mental deficiency and the characteristic facies are absent as a rule. The other variety is that associated with a characteristic facies, which consists of widely spaced teeth, dental malocclusion, full cheeks, elfin face, pug nose, and a wide mouth with pouting lips. Mental deficiency is usually present, and there is often a history of infantile hypercalcemia. In both varieties pulmonary arterial branch stenosis is a common associated disorder. Supravalvular aortic stenosis is diagnosed by left ventricular and aortic catheterization, which demonstrate the obstruction by showing a higher systolic pressure in the left ventricle and proximal ascending aorta than is found in the distal ascending aorta and aortic arch. The nature of the obstruction is shown more clearly by aortography. When the obstruction is sufficiently severe, it may be relieved by surgical operation.

COARCTATION OF THE AORTA AT THE AORTIC ISTHMUS. The most common variety of aortic coarctation consists of a narrowing of the isthmus of the aorta just distal to the left subclavian artery. This is a congenital disorder and is several times more common in males than in females. Occasionally the narrowing is proximal to the origin of the left subclavian artery. The ductus or ligamentum arteriosum may be inserted proximal or distal to the coarctation. The coarctation may be associated with patent ductus arteriosus. In some instances there is pulmonary hypertension and reversed flow of pulmonary arterial blood through the ductus arteriosus into the distal aorta beyond the coarctation, causing cyanosis of the lower extremities but not of the upper extremities. With aortic coarctation, the degree of aortic luminal narrowing varies greatly. At times the opening between the aortic arch and the ascending aorta is completely obliterated or only a few millimeters in diameter; in other instances the opening is 1 cm or more. The characteristic physical finding in this condition is hypertension in the upper extremities and low blood pressure and delayed pulse in the femoral arteries. The condition will rarely be overlooked if the blood pressure and pulse in the upper and lower extremities are compared in every patient with hypertension. Hypertension in these patients is usually not severe, and the blood pressure is usually of the order of 170/100 mm Hg. This is one variety of hypertension in which malignant hypertension is said not to occur.

The mechanism of hypertension in aortic coarctation is not clearly understood. The two principal theories are (1) that it is caused by mechanical blockage in the aorta and (2) that it is caused by impairment of renal blood flow. Studies of a limited number of patients have failed to show elevation of renal venous blood renin, thus failing to support the theory of restricted renal arterial blood flow as the cause of the hypertension.

Patients with aortic coarctation have collateral circulation between the aortic arch and the lower aorta. This is carried by three main routes: (1) the internal mammary arteries, which communicate through their anterior intercostal arteries with the posterior aortic intercostal arteries; (2) the internal mammary artery continuation, the superior epigastric artery, and anastomoses with the inferior epigastric branch of the external iliac artery; and (3) the anastomoses between subclavian artery branches and posterior aortic intercostal arteries around the scapula. In addition to the blood pressure differences between the upper and lower extremities, patients with aortic coarctation may have a murmur over the back caused either by the collateral circulation or by the obstruction in the aorta itself. The murmur caused by the narrowed aorta tends to be a systolic murmur when the opening is more than 3 mm in diameter; it may be continuous when the opening in the aorta is smaller than this. The collateral intercostal vessels may be seen or palpated over the posterior thorax. Approximately 50 per cent of patients with coarctation have a bicuspid aortic valve, and about 10 per cent have aortic insufficiency. Ventricular septal defect, subaortic stenosis, and congenital mitral stenosis are also found at times in patients with aortic coarctation. When the obstruction lies between the origins of the left common carotid and left subclavian arteries, the blood pressure is higher in the right than in the left arm. This is an uncommon occurrence. Ordinary radiologic examination of the chest tends to show bilateral notching of the inferior margins of the ribs between the third and tenth ribs. This notching is produced by dilation of the enlarged intercostal arteries which carry increased collateral flow. The aortic knob or arch is invisible on plain chest radiogram in approximately half the patients. A barium esophagram may show a so-called figure E or "reversed 3" sign. The upper esophageal compression is produced by prestenotic dilation of the aorta by the enlarged left subclavian artery and carotid arteries, and compression of the lower esophagus is produced by the poststenotic dilation of the aorta. The aortic coarctation can be best diagnosed and quantified by aortography.

Because of their associated difficulties and later complications, only a few patients with aortic coarctation have a normal life span, although many survive to adult life. Approximately 60 to 70 per cent of untreated patients die before 40 years of age. The common complications of this condition are congestive heart failure, bacterial endarteritis, aortic rupture or dissection, and bleeding intracranial berry aneurysms. The treatment ordinarily consists of surgical removal of the obstruction, except when there is severe pulmonary hypertension with reversal of blood flow through the patent ductus arteriosus.

PSEUDOCOARCTATION OF THE AORTA. This is probably a poor term. The aortic arch is elongated by hypertension or arteriosclerosis and is kinked downward in the region of the ligamentum arteriosum. This abnormality can resemble a mediastinal tumor or can be associated with a true aneurysm in this area. As a rule there is no true obstruction, and there is no blood pressure difference between the proximal aorta and the descending aorta. Subclinical true coarctation may exist in some instances.

COARCTATION OF THE ABDOMINAL AORTA. In addition to coarctation of the aorta at the usual site just distal to the left subclavian artery, coarctation may occur in the abdominal aorta. This lesion may be congenital, or it may be associated with Takayasu's syndrome (see Ch. 367.9). Coarctation of the abdominal aorta may involve the celiac axis, the mesenteric arteries, and the renal arteries. There may be associated hypertension because of the renal arterial involvement. Abdominal aortic coarctation is more common in women, whereas thoracic coarctation is more common in men.

Surgical Treatment. Ordinarily the diagnosis of coarctation of the aorta is in itself considered an indication for surgical correction. The preferable age for repair is between 8 and 12 years. However, when infants with coarctation have congestive heart failure which does not respond to medical management, surgical repair may be needed at that time. Surgical repair is generally not advisable in patients over the age of 50 years, because the operative risks are increased and the potential gain is less. In most patients repair can be done by resection of the coarctate area and end-to-end aortic anastomosis. In some, the coarctate area must be resected and a tubular prosthesis of Dacron inserted.

Results. In patients treated by experts in the field, the in-hospital mortality rate is low and should not exceed 2 per cent in uncomplicated cases. It is important, however, that the repair be done by an expert and not by an occasional cardiac surgeon. The early postoperative period may be complicated by abdominal pain and mesenteric arteritis. There is increasing evidence, from studies of James and Kaplan at the Cincinnati Children's Hospital, that hypertension is not completely relieved in many patients. These investigators found residual hypertension in 11 of 14 patients who were 9 to 22 years of age at the time of surgical repair. The failure to relieve hypertension is usually not due to an inadequate relief of the aortic narrowing. The mechanism of persistent postoperative hypertension is at present unknown.

ABSENCE OF THE AORTIC ARCH. The aortic arch may be absent or atretic. In this case the descending aorta is supplied with blood from the pulmonary artery through a patent ductus arteriosus. Thus there is unoxygenated blood entering the descending aorta, and there tends to be cyanosis and clubbing of the toes but usually not the hands — although the left hand may be involved. This is called differential cyanosis and clubbing. Whether or not the left hand is cyanotic depends upon the origin of the left subclavian artery. Associated defects are common. Among these are ventricular septal defect and aortic stenosis.

RIGHT-SIDED AORTIC ARCH. There are two basic types of right-sided aortic arch. In one, the aorta passes behind the esophagus and descends on the left. In this variety, associated congenital heart disease is less common (Knight and Edwards). When the arch remains on the right and descends to the right of the esophagus, additional congenital heart disease is usually present. The most common variety is tetralogy of Fallot; others include pulmonary atresia, tricuspid atresia, and truncus arteriosus. The right-sided aortic arch with a right-sided descending aorta is a common complication of tetralogy of Fallot and is found in approximately 25 per cent of patients with this disorder. It is also common in patients with truncus arteriosus. When right-sided aortic arch occurs as an isolated phenomenon, it may be mistaken for a mediastinal tumor. Right-sided aortic arch is a normal component of mirror-image dextrocardia. Isolated right-sided aortic arch is usually asymptomatic and can be recognized on plain roentgenogram or by demonstration of compression of the right side of the barium-filled esophagus. Knight and Edwards found that the right aortic arch was part of a double aortic arch pattern in 4 of 78 instances. Each arch gives rise to the common carotid artery on its side and then passes behind the esophagus to join the other arch, thus forming a vascular ring about the trachea and esophagus. Three of the four cases had an additional congenital cardiac anomaly. Dysphagia may be associated with double aortic arch or with right-sided aortic arch crossing behind the esophagus to descend on the left of the esophagus.

AORTIC ATRESIA. Aortic atresia may be associated with atresia of the aortic valve and, at times, with mitral atresia. This is part of the hypoplastic left heart syndrome and is not compatible with long survival. In this disorder the blood entering the left atrium through the pulmonary veins escapes into the right heart through the foramen ovale and then into the descending aorta through the patent ductus arteriosus from the right ventricle. The ascending aorta is extremely small, and carries blood in retrograde fashion from the patent ductus arteriosus to supply the coronary arteries. In patients with mitral atresia, blood enters the left ventricle and aorta from the right ventricle through a ventricular septal defect. In aortic atresia pulmonary venous pressure is high, tending to cause pulmonary edema. Death often occurs before the age of one week.

CONGENITAL AORTIC ANEURYSM. There may be a congenital aortic aneurysm of the sinus of Valsalva. These aneurysms involve either the right or noncoronary sinus in 90 per cent of instances. Those of the right aortic sinus usually project into the right ventricle, and those of the noncoronary sinus, into the right atrium. Aortic sinus aneurysms are difficult to see on plain roentgenogram of the chest unless they are calcified. They are recognizable, however, by echocardiography and by aortography. These aneurysms tend to rupture eventually, usually into the right atrium or ventricle where they produce a continuous shunt. The continuous shunt is associated with a continuous systolic and diastolic murmur, widening of the systemic arterial pulse pressure, and a tendency to heart failure. These conditions may be corrected surgically. The murmur of an aortic sinus aneurysm which has ruptured into the right heart resembles that of a patent ductus arteriosus except that, rather than being louder in the first and second left intercostal spaces like that of a patent ductus, it tends to be louder in the fourth and fifth left intercostal spaces near the sternum. As in other communications between the systemic circulation and the lesser circulation, the systemic arterial pulse pressure tends to be increased. It is said that these congenital aortic sinus aneurysms tend to rupture into the heart, whereas acquired syphilitic aneurysms in the same location tend to rupture into the pericardial sac. A similar condition is that of aortico–left ventricular tunnel in which there is a long tubular communication between the aortic sinus and the left ventricle. The unperforated aortic sinus aneurysm is usually asymptomatic but may cause cardiac conduction disturbances, myocardial ischemia due to coronary occlusion, or pulmonary stenosis or tricuspid insufficiency (Bulkley et al.).

Another congenital condition is that of aberrant right subclavian artery. It is said to occur in one of 200 individuals. In this condition the right subclavian artery is the last major branch of the aortic arch, rather than arising from the innominate artery as it does normally. It then passes behind the esophagus to reach the right arm. As a result the blood pressure may be lower in the right arm than the left; the pulse may be absent in the right upper extremity. These patients may have dysphagia produced by the pressure of the aberrant artery on the esophagus. The condition can be demonstrated by barium esophagram, which shows an oblique compression of the posterior esophagus. Aortography, of course, shows the condition more clearly. Rarely the aberrant right subclavian artery may be associated with coarctation of the aorta proximal to the left subclavian artery. In this condition arterial pulses tend to be feeble or absent in both upper and lower extremities.

Bulkley, B. H., Hutchins, G. M., and Ross, R. S.: Aortic sinus of Valsalva aneurysms simulating primary right-sided valvular disease. Circulation, 52:696, 1975.
Eliot, R. S., and Edwards, J. E.: Pathology of congenital heart disease. In Hurst, J. W., and Logue, R. B. (eds.): The Heart. Arteries and Veins. New York, McGraw-Hill Book Company, 1974, pp. 627–667.
James, F. W., and Kaplan, S.: Systolic hypertension during submaximal exercise after correction of coarctation of the aorta. Circulation, 49–50 (Suppl. II):27, 1974.
Knight, L., and Edwards, J. E.: Right aortic arch. Types and associated cardiac anomalies. Circulation 50:1047, 1974.

367.3. HEREDOFAMILIAL DISEASES OF THE AORTA

There are a number of heredofamilial disorders of connective tissue which may be associated with diseases of the aorta and its branches (McKusick). These conditions most commonly cause weakening of the aortic wall which may cause aneurysms, but at times there is occlusive aortic disease owing to thrombosis.

MARFAN'S SYNDROME. Marfan's syndrome, also known as arachnodactyly, is a heredofamilial disorder of connective tissue which may be associated with hydroxyprolinuria. Hydroxyprolinuria is neither a specific nor a constant finding, according to McKusick. The aortic lesion is characteristically that of cystic medial necrosis. The disease affects the blood vessels, the osseous skeleton, and the ligaments. Typically, arachnodactyly, increased height, ectopia lentis, and hypermobile joints are found. Abdominal hernia, pectus excavatum, and kyphoscoliosis are common. The principal cardiovascular manifestations are in the ascending aorta. The second most common cardiovascular abnormality involves the mitral valve. Occasionally, the tricuspid valve or the pulmonary artery is affected. Smaller arteries are usually not involved. The aortic lesion characteristically produces either sinus of Valsalva aneurysm or dilation of aneurysm in the ascending aorta above the sinuses. Its principal complications are dissecting aneurysm of the aorta, rupture of the aorta, and aortic insufficiency. Rarely, there is abdominal aortic aneurysm. The mitral valve involvement may cause mitral prolapse and mitral insufficiency.

EHLERS-DANLOS SYNDROME. This disorder is also known as cutis hyperelastica. Dissecting aortic aneurysm is a recognized complication. Also, there may be spontaneous rupture of the aorta or aortic rupture following slight trauma.

HOMOCYSTINURIA. Homocystinuria is a disorder which has some features in common with Marfan's syndrome. Ectopia lentis and disease of the aorta may occur in either condition. In homocystinuria more commonly there is occlusive disease of systemic arteries and veins. The coronary arteries may be occluded. Thrombosis of the terminal aorta may occur in this disorder. The elastica pattern of the aortic media is abnormal. It is uncertain whether aortic aneurysm is an essential part of this disease. In this disorder the enzyme cystathionine synthetase is lacking. Mental deficiency is common, whereas the patient with Marfan's syndrome usually has normal mental development.

OSTEOGENESIS IMPERFECTA. With osteogenesis imperfecta, deafness, fragilitas ossium, and blue sclerae are the common features. These patients often have a dilated aortic root and may suffer from aortic insufficiency. Mitral insufficiency is also a common cardiovascular manifestation.

MUCOPOLYSACCHARIDOSES. In these disorders, including Hurler's syndrome, Hunter's syndrome, and others, there may be gargoyle cells in the aorta. The principal involvement is of the aortic valve and coronary arteries. Aortic dilation and the aortic arch syndrome (see Ch. 367.9) have been described.

PSEUDOXANTHOMA ELASTICUM. Thrombosis of the terminal aorta has been described in this disorder, but its relationship to pseudoxanthoma elasticum is uncertain. Thrombotic occlusion involving coronary arteries and those of the extremities is a recognized complication. The iliac and femoral arteries may be smaller than normal, leading to impaired pulsations in the lower extremities and thus to confusion with coarctation of the aorta.

McKusick, V. A.: Heritable Disorders of Connective Tissue. 4th ed. St. Louis, C. V. Mosby Company, 1972.

367.4.   EFFECTS OF AGING UPON THE AORTA

Arteriosclerosis affects the aorta more commonly in our civilization than in more primitive societies. The process tends to be progressively more severe as one proceeds down the descending aorta, in contrast to syphilitic aortitis, which is more pronounced in the ascending aorta just superior to the aortic valve. The process may lead to elongation or dilation of the aorta, producing an irregularity observed on chest radiogram. Commonly, in older patients one sees a calcific deposit in the aortic knob (arch). Roentgen evidence of aortic atherosclerosis includes calcification of the knob, increase in the width of the aorta, and unusual tortuosity or uncoiling. These changes are not seen in normal persons under the age of 30 years and in only 2.5 per cent of individuals under the age of 40 years (Felson). Extensive atherosclerosis involving the aortic intima may lead to ulcerative lesions with cholesterol deposits and to emboli. These emboli may consist of cholesterol or may arise from thrombi. There may be cholesterol emboli to the retinal arteries; emboli in the renal arteries may cause hypertension; peripheral emboli may cause impairment of femoral blood flow. Arteriosclerosis is believed to be the common cause of aortic aneurysm. Aortic aneurysms caused by arteriosclerosis are most common in the abdominal aorta just inferior to the renal arteries but may occur also in the thoracic aorta and in the abdominal aorta above the origin of the

renal arteries. Aortic arteriosclerosis causes loss of elasticity with decreased compliance during left ventricular ejection. Thus left ventricular work may rise with aging, contributing to a decrease of circulatory reserve with age.

Felson, B.: Chest Roentgenology. Philadelphia, W. B. Saunders Company, 1973.

367.5.   INCREASED AORTIC DIMENSIONS

The enlarged aorta may increase in length or diameter or both. Increase in length usually reflects arteriosclerotic changes with aging. Increase in length may lead to an irregular margin, to apparent widening, or to kinking, tortuosity, or buckling. Increased diameter of the aorta may be generalized, as occurs in hypertensive disease, or localized. Localized increase of dimension may be called *ectasia* when of minor degree but more commonly is called *aneurysm*. Aneurysms of the aorta may be saccular or fusiform.

Aortic aneurysms are discussed in detail under the headings of the individual causative diseases. However, it is useful to summarize the relation of the location of an aneurysm to its etiology. Aortic aneurysms may be classified by etiology into congenital and acquired groups (DeBakey and Noon). By location, they are classified as follows: (1) ascending aorta, (2) aortic arch, (3) descending thoracic aorta, and (4) thoracoabdominal. Aortic sinus aneurysms are most commonly of congenital origin or due to Marfan's syndrome, syphilis, or infective endocarditis. Ascending aortic aneurysms are most commonly due to syphilis, Marfan's syndrome, aortic dissection, or cystic medial necrosis without the other features of Marfan's syndrome. Aortic arch aneurysms are most often due to syphilis, dissection, or Marfan's syndrome. An aneurysm of the descending thoracic aorta may be caused by syphilis, arteriosclerosis, or dissection. An aneurysm at the beginning of the descending aorta may be caused by trauma. Aneurysms of the abdominal aorta are most often caused by arteriosclerosis but may be the result of syphilis or the extension of aortic dissection from the thoracic aorta.

A number of other diseases may cause aortic aneurysms, which are usually smaller than those enumerated above and in varying sites. Among these is septicemia, which may cause mycotic aneurysms. Mycotic aneurysms may be caused by tuberculosis as well. Relapsing polychondritis may lead to aneurysm of either the thoracic or abdominal aorta. Localized aortic aneurysms often occur with Takayasu's aortitis and with giant cell aortitis.

ARTERIOSCLEROTIC AORTIC ANEURYSM. Arteriosclerotic aneurysms of the aorta, most common in the abdominal aorta, usually originate below the renal arteries. Arteriosclerotic aneurysms are most common in men over the age of 50 years. One study reported an autopsy incidence of 1.8 per cent of such aneurysms. Probably more than 95 per cent of abdominal aortic aneurysms are of arteriosclerotic origin. These aneurysms are most often discovered by roentgen examination of an asymptomatic patient. However, they may be discovered for the first time when the patient has pain — the pain may be in the back or the epigastrium, or may radiate to the flanks. Unfortunately, the first evidence of aneurysm may be that of rupture attended by the onset of severe and persistent pain and shock. Persistent abdominal pain of lesser severity may precede the more severe pain of aortic rupture.

ABDOMINAL AORTIC ANEURYSMS. Abdominal aortic aneurysms may be diagnosed by physical examination, but there are many possible errors. In obese or muscular patients or in those with small aneurysms, physical examination is unlikely to reveal the problem. On the other hand, abdominal aneurysm may be diagnosed in error. It is important to determine that there is actual increase in the width of the aorta and not merely a prominent aortic pulsation. Prominent pulsation of the abdominal aorta is common as a normal finding, especially in thin women with lax abdominal walls and lumbar lordosis. This often leads to the diagnosis of aneurysm by physical examination where none exists — "students' aneurysm." A prominent aortic pulsation may be due to an uncoiling of the aorta resulting from atherosclerosis or to aortic insufficiency or to a high output state producing an increased pulse pressure in the absence of aneurysm. Another pitfall in diagnosis is that a tumor overlying the aorta, such as pancreatic neoplasm, may appear to have an intrinsic pulsation and thus be mistaken for an aneurysm. Abdominal aneurysms may lead to ureteral obstruction with hydronephrosis. These aneurysms may also lead to consumption coagulopathy with diminished circulating platelets, reduced serum fibrinogen, and prolonged prothrombin time. A clue to the presence of aortic abdominal aneurysm may be that of cholesterol emboli to the smaller arteries of the feet and toes, leading to digital cyanosis and coldness.

Diagnosis. Roentgenograms of the abdomen may be helpful by showing calcification in the walls of the aneurysm. It is important to have lateral and oblique views in addition to anteroposterior views. Aortic wall calcification per se does not signify an aneurysm unless there is definite increase in the diameter of the aorta. The psoas shadow may be obliterated when rupture has occurred. Ultrasound scanning and radionuclide angiography may be useful in the diagnosis of abdominal aortic aneurysms. Aortography with radiopaque contrast medium is usually the diagnostic method of choice.

Prognosis. The prognosis of patients with abdominal arteriosclerotic aneurysms is generally considered poor, with only a small percentage of patients surviving for five years or more. The outlook is considered to be better when the lesion is less than 7.5 cm in diameter. However, it is difficult to know the true prognosis. Most patients who are operated upon and most patients who have been followed without operation were originally discovered because they had symptoms. The prognosis might conceivably be more favorable in patients who are symptomatic. Many unoperated patients had a poor prognosis because operation was considered inadvisable owing to an associated severe illness.

Surgical Treatment. Once the diagnosis of abdominal aortic aneurysm is made, one should in general recommend surgical replacement of the aneurysm even though the patient is asymptomatic. If the patient is having pain in relation to the aneurysm, replacement should be considered as an emergency. Surgical removal with insertion of a synthetic aortic graft of woven Dacron is the usual operative procedure. Aortic homo-grafts are no longer used because they tend to rupture at the line of anastomosis. However, late rupture at the suture line may be a problem even with synthetic grafts (Thompson et al.). There are two groups of patients in whom surgical resection might not be recommended. One is composed of those who are asymptomatic with aneurysms under 6 cm in diameter; the other group is patients who have some other life-threatening disease or who are extremely elderly and debilitated. Among the conditions which would be contraindications to resection are intractable heart failure, advanced renal failure, metastatic neoplasm, severe coronary artery disease with unstable angina pectoris or recent infarction, advanced cerebrovascular disease, and severe pulmonary insufficiency. In recent years the reported in-hospital mortality rate of abdominal aneurysm resection in several large series ranged from 5.3 to 9.5 per cent. It is greatly increased when there is severe cardiorenal disease or advanced age. The signs, symptoms, and treatment of thoracic aortic aneurysms are discussed in Ch. 367.7.

Bergan, J. J., and Yao, J. S. T.: Modern management of abdominal aortic aneurysms. Surg. Clin. N. Am., 54:175, 1974.

DeBakey, M. E., Beall, M. C., and Mattox, K. L.: Surgical treatment of diseases of the aorta and major arteries. In Hurst, J. W. (ed.): The Heart. 4th ed. New York, McGraw-Hill Book Company, 1978, Chap. 103.

DeBakey, M. E., and Noon, G. P.: Aneurysms of the thoracic aorta. Mod. Concepts Cardiovasc. Dis., 44:53, 1975.

Thompson, W. M., Johnsrude, I. S., Jackson, D. C., et al.: Late complications of abdominal aortic reconstructive surgery; roentgen evaluation. Ann. Surg., 185:326, 1977.

367.6. TRAUMATIC AORTIC DISEASE

The aorta may be damaged by nonpenetrating as well as penetrating trauma. The portion of the aorta most likely damaged by trauma is that lying just beyond the origin of the left subclavian artery. When the body is moving rapidly, followed by a sudden deceleration as in a fall or auto accident, differential rates of acceleration are greatest in this area because the aortic arch is relatively fixed by the root vessels. The second most common site of injury is the ascending aorta. The aorta may be lacerated or may rupture with either complete or almost complete transection. There may be a false aneurysm with extravasation of blood tamponaded by the mediastinal structure. Patients with nonpenetrating aortic trauma may have little or no external evidence of chest injury. In an acute setting, following decelerative-type injury, the patient may be in shock with evidence of a rapidly developing hemothorax — most commonly on the left side. Anuria and paraplegia, with absence of pulse in the femoral arteries and cold, pale lower extremities, are common. The initial findings thus simulate those of coarctation of the aorta. Arterial hypertension may be present as well. A routine chest radiogram may show widening of the mediastinum. A possible sequel is chronic traumatic aortic aneurysm, which may rupture during a period of days or years after the original injury. The characteristic location of an aortic traumatic aneurysm is distal to the origin of the subclavian artery (Fig. 1). The definitive diagnosis is made by aortography, and the treatment is that of surgical removal. Usually a graft replacement is employed in order to preserve aortic continuity.

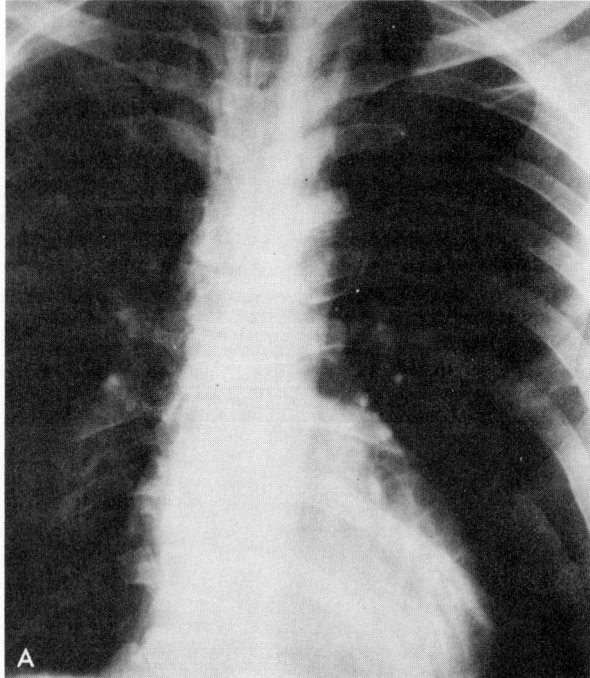 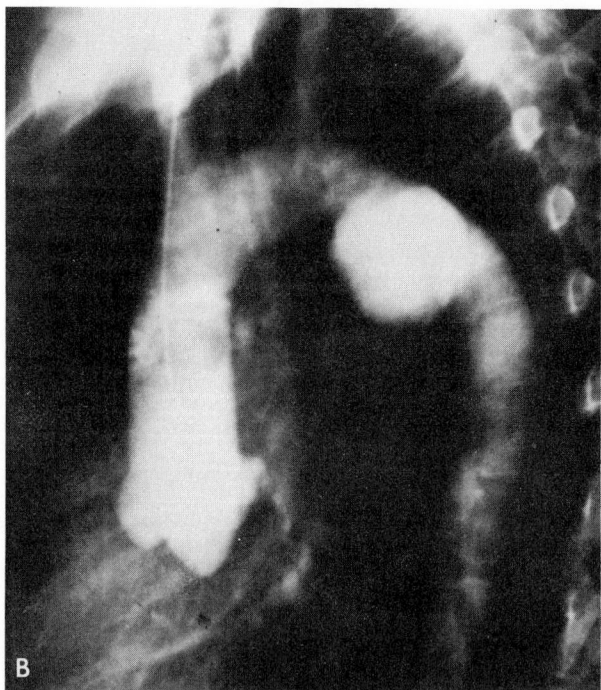

Figure 1. Traumatic aortic aneurysm just distal to the subclavian artery. A, This posteroanterior roentgenogram demonstrates calcification in the aneurysm, which appears in the region of the aortic knob. B, Aortogram demonstrating opacification of the aneurysm, which lies just beyond the subclavian artery. (From Fowler, N. O.: Cardiac Diagnosis and Treatment, 2nd ed., 1977. With permission of Harper & Row, Publishers, Inc.)

367.7. SYPHILITIC AORTITIS AND SYPHILITIC HEART DISEASE

Syphilitic aortitis is the principal cardiovascular manifestation of syphilis. Syphilis does not ordinarily affect the cardiac valves, although the aortic valve commissures may be separated. Rarely, it may affect the myocardium. It may affect the coronary arteries more often, but usually only the proximal few centimeters of these vessels are involved. Thus the principal cardiovascular effect of syphilitic disease is aortitis with its complications of aortic insufficiency, angina pectoris, and aortic aneurysm. Syphilitic aortitis, as a rule, is a late lesion of acquired syphilis and is usually recognized 10 to 30 years after the initial primary chancre, but occasionally it occurs as early as a few years after the original infection. The disease characteristically produces aortic medial destruction with necrosis of smooth muscle and elastic tissue and periarterial inflammation with lymphocyte cuffing of the vasa vasorum. There is also intimal wrinkling with treebark formation and a tendency to narrow the lumen of the orifice of the coronary arteries, as well as to produce the dilation of the aortic root that leads to aortic insufficiency or aneurysm. At times, innominate artery aneurysm may occur, but more distal arterial aneurysms are unusual. The syphilitic process, in distinction to that of arteriosclerosis, is usually most intense in the aortic root and becomes less intense as one examines the more distal aorta. Congenital syphilis seldom produces aortitis. Because of the delay in clinical manifestations, patients with syphilitic aortitis are ordinarily more than 30 years of age when recognized clinically and are usually over 50 years of age when

syphilitic aneurysms are recognized. Uncomplicated syphilitic aortitis ordinarily produces no symptoms and may be recognized only at the autopsy table. It produces dilation of the aorta and perhaps calcification in the ascending aorta. The latter may be detected radiologically (Fig. 2).

SYPHILITIC AORTIC ANEURYSM. This lesion occurs most often in the ascending aorta. Aneurysms occur in 10 to 40 per cent of patients with syphilitic aortitis. Syphilitic aneurysms, once the most common cause of thoracic aneurysms, are much less commonly seen now than a few decades ago. Nearly half occur in the ascending aorta; 30 to 40 per cent of syphilitic aneurysms are found in the arch and 15 per cent in the descending thoracic aorta. Syphilitic aortic aneurysms may occur in the abdominal aorta but are distinctly uncommon in this location and especially so if there is no syphilitic aneurysm in the thoracic aorta. If the aneurysm involves the ascending aorta, aortic insufficiency is often present; rarely there is a visible pulsatile mass in the first and second right intercostal spaces with exaggerated pulsations of the right sternoclavicular joint or in the episternal notch. Chest pain, the most common symptom, may occur owing to rib, sternal, or vertebral erosion. The pain is usually substernal, in the dorsal spine, or at the side of the chest. It may extend to the neck, shoulders, lower back, or abdomen. Increasing intensity of pain is usually an ominous sign associated with impending rupture. A chest radiogram may demonstrate erosion of ribs and sternum by the aneurysm. Respiratory difficulty may indicate that the aneurysm is in the arch of the aorta; there may be a tracheal tug with hoarseness and a brassy cough because of recurrent laryngeal nerve paralysis. There may be Horner's

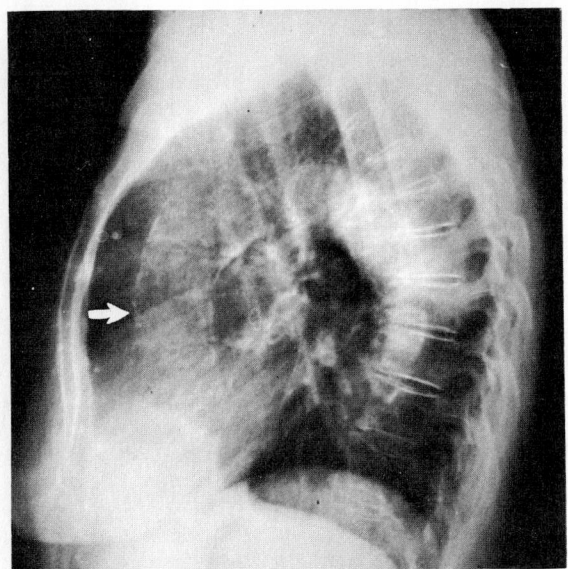

Figure 2. Calcification of the ascending aorta in syphilitic aortitis.

syndrome with ptosis, miosis, and decreased sweating on the left side of the face. There may be superior vena caval obstruction with distended nonpulsatile jugular veins, dyspnea, and collateral venous circulation over the thorax. Aneurysm in the aortic arch may produce compression of the left mainstem bronchus, with atelectasis of the left lung or of the left lower lobe. Hemoptysis may occur because of tracheal or bronchial ulceration. Hematemesis may indicate rupture into the esophagus. In the descending thoracic aorta, rarely the aneurysm may present as a pulsatile mass medial to, or inferior to, the angle of the left scapula. In these cases, vertebral erosion may occur. Cardiac enlargement does not occur because of aneurysm alone.

Radiologic studies are helpful in diagnosing thoracic aneurysm of any cause. When there is calcification in the ascending aorta, syphilitic aortitis is strongly suggested. A mass continuous with the aorta with calcification in its wall is very likely an aneurysm. When there is no calcification, then aortic aneurysm must be distinguished from other mediastinal masses, especially tumors of lymph nodes, dermoid cysts, thymic tumor, and substernal thyroid gland. Evaluation of pulsations of a mass by fluoroscopy is virtually worthless, because pulsatory movements transmitted into contiguous tumors are indistinguishable from those of intrinsic pulsations of the aorta. Conversely, aneurysms which are lined with thrombus may fail to show visible pulsations. Contrast or radionuclide aortography is the precise way of settling the diagnosis.

Course and Prognosis. Syphilitic aneurysms tend to rupture eventually. The rupture may take place into the right or left pleural space, into the trachea or esophagus, or into the pulmonary artery, where it produces a continuous murmur like that of patent ductus arteriosus. The aneurysm may rupture into the right heart, producing a continuous murmur like that described in Ch. 367.2. Laplace's law states that tension in walls of a cylinder is equal to the product of pressure times radius. Hence the tension in the wall of an aortic aneurysm is greater than that in the adjacent aorta. Because of its

tendency to expand according to Laplace's law and eventually to rupture, surgical resection of syphilitic aneurysms is recommended when feasible and when the patient does not suffer from some other disease which materially limits life expectancy.

Serologic studies of patients suspected of syphilitic aortitis may be misleading. The Kahn serologic test may be negative in as many as 23 per cent of patients with syphilitic aortitis. The VDRL test is said to be positive in 98 to 99 per cent of such patients but may be negative in patients over 65 years of age. The *Treponema pallidum* immobilization test may be positive when the VDRL test is negative and is especially useful when the patient is over 65 years of age or has had antisyphilitic therapy.

Antisyphilitic Treatment.   For the patients who have cardiovascular syphilis, the Venereal Disease Control Advisory Committee has recommended that the patient receive benzathine penicillin, 2.4 million units intramuscularly weekly for three successive weeks, or aqueous procaine penicillin, 600,000 units intramuscularly daily for 15 days. There is no assurance that such therapy will allay the progression of syphilitic aortitis or aneurysm, as the weakened aortic wall continues to expand despite the absence of active infection.

Syphilis: Recommended Treatment Schedules, 1976. Center for Disease Control, Atlanta, Georgia. Ann. Intern. Med., 85:94, 1976.

367.8. DISSECTING ANEURYSM OF THE AORTA

Dissecting aneurysm of the aorta is also called dissecting hematoma of the aorta. The disease tends to occur in certain settings. It is most common in men of middle age with a background of hypertension, but is also found in the setting of Marfan's syndrome, cystic medial necrosis, or coarctation of the aorta and seems to be more common in pregnancy. Dissecting aneurysm may also occur in certain heritable disorders of connective tissue, including Ehlers-Danlos syndrome, and has been described as a complication of relapsing polychondritis. Its relationship to arteriosclerosis of the aorta is questionable. It probably bears no relationship to syphilitic aortitis, which may, in fact, offer some protection against the process because of the fibrosis of the aortic media which occurs in syphilis.

Ordinarily the dissection begins with an aortic intimal tear, followed by a dissecting channel in the media, followed in turn by a point of re-entry from the intima back into the aortic lumen or, occasionally, rupture through the adventitia. Thus a double-barreled aorta may be produced. Approximately 50 per cent of aortic dissections begin in the ascending aorta, 30 per cent in the aortic arch, and 20 per cent in the descending aorta. Dissecting aneurysm may be related to trauma, especially that produced by an angiographic catheter or aortic balloon catheter (Alpert et al.) striking an arteriosclerotic plaque in the aorta. A dissecting aneurysm may extend proximally to involve the aortic valve area, thus causing aortic valvular insufficiency; it may surround the coronary arteries, producing myocardial infarction; it may extend along the carotid sheath to cause hemiplegia. It may involve the blood supply to the spinal cord, leading to paraplegia and anesthesia below the level of involvement. It may involve the renal artery, thus aggravating pre-existing arterial hypertension. Hypertension may also be aggravated by a carotid artery involvement when it interferes with the carotid sinus baroreceptor response. Rupture into the pericardium may lead to cardiac tamponade and rapid demise.

HISTORY. Most dissecting aneurysms are associated with chest pain, which may radiate into the abdomen or into the back. The pain of aortic dissection must be distinguished from that of myocardial ischemia. The pain of ischemic heart disease seldom radiates to the back and infrequently extends below the diaphragm, so that those features should suggest the possibility of aortic dissection. In some patients, however, there is complicating myocardial infarction when a proximal aortic dissection involves the coronary arteries, and then the condition may masquerade as a case of myocardial infarction. When the patient with aortic dissection suffers from rupture into the pericardium, he may develop cardiac tamponade; on the other hand, when there is a gradual leak into the pericardial sac, the patient may appear to have unexplained pericarditis. Approximately 25 per cent of patients with aortic dissection are believed to develop aortic insufficiency. The sudden appearance of aortic insufficiency should raise the possibility of dissecting aneurysm even when pain is absent. Hemiplegia, paraplegia, or syncope may be the presenting features, as may the aortic arch syndrome (see Ch. 367.9). The prevalence of pain is believed to be about 70 per cent. Occasional patients appear with aortic insufficiency, a large heart, and heart failure without a history of an acute episode of aortic dissection.

PHYSICAL FINDINGS. The patient is often hypertensive and often complains of chest pain. The patient is most often a man between the ages of 40 and 60 years. When the process extends to involve the orifices of the femoral arteries or arteries to the head and neck, asymmetrical arterial pulses may be found. Although abnormal peripheral arterial pulses were found in 13 of 18 cases in one series of patients with aortic dissection, most series show that it is the minority of patients who have significant differences of pulse and blood pressure in the arms, legs, or carotid arteries. Possibly 25 per cent of patients develop aortic insufficiency. Either sternoclavicular joint may transmit an abnormal pulsation. Unilateral distention of the left external jugular vein results from pressure of the expanded aorta upon the left innominate vein. This sign suggests the possibility of aneurysm of the aorta. It is not specific for dissecting aneurysm, however, and may occur in a patient with an elongated and kinked arteriosclerotic or hypertensive aorta in the absence of aneurysm.

LABORATORY STUDIES. The electrocardiogram may be normal or may show left ventricular hypertrophy. It may show evidence of acute pericarditis. In approximately one case in six of one series, the electrocardiogram showed changes of myocardial infarction. The chest roentgenogram is very important in the study of patients, especially if there are serial studies. A change in the width of the aorta, especially involving the aortic arch, is very suggestive of dissection or of mediastinal bleeding. At times, the chest radiogram may show changes virtually specific for dissection by demonstrating a separation of more than a few millimeters between a calcified intimal plaque and the external border of the aorta. However, the majority of patients cannot be diagnosed from plain roentgenogram; aortography is usually required to make the diagnosis (Fig. 3). The

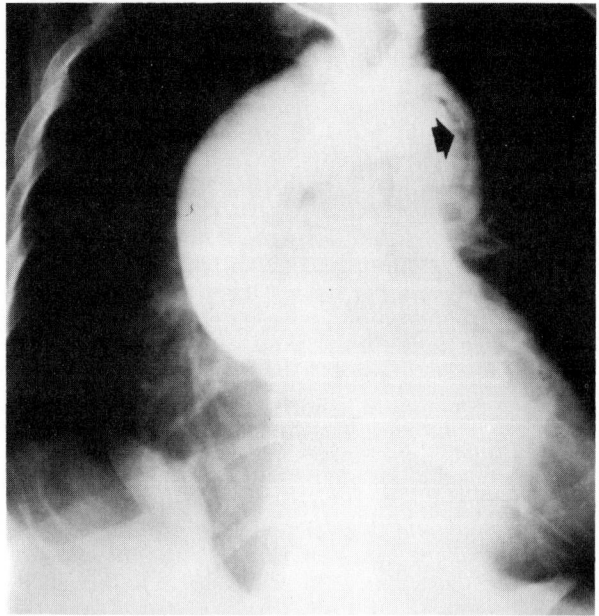

Figure 3. Aortogram: dissecting aneurysm. The arrow indicates line of separation between true and false channels. (Courtesy of Dr. Harold Spitz.)

aortographic features of dissecting hematoma are evidence of intimal tear, opacification of a false channel, and the indirect evidence of a false channel produced by narrowing of the original lumen. When the process involves the ascending aorta, echocardiography may be of value in showing thickening of the aortic wall.

The diagnosis requires a high index of suspicion. A patient thought to have myocardial infarction should be suspected of dissecting aortic aneurysm if the pain radiates to the back or into the abdomen, if the electrocardiogram shows no change or changes of pericarditis, and if the serum enzyme test results (especially the MB fraction of creatine phosphokinase) remain normal. Aortic dissection should also be considered when there is aortic insufficiency of recent onset or if there are impaired arterial pulses in the neck or extremities. Changes in aortic contour demonstrated by serial roentgenograms are highly suggestive. Once the suspicion of aortic dissection arises, the diagnosis may be proved in most cases by aortography. Uncommonly, when the dissection is entirely intramural, without either an entry or an exit channel, the aortogram does not show specific changes and the diagnosis can only be suspected from the unusual thickening of the aortic wall.

In one series described from Massachusetts General Hospital (Slater and DeSanctis), syncope with aortic dissection was usually caused by cardiac tamponade. There were differences between dissection involving the proximal ascending aorta and the distal dissection group when the descending thoracic aorta was involved. In 53 patients with proximal dissection, the patients tended to be younger and to have a significantly higher incidence of Marfan's syndrome or cystic medial necrosis. Anterior chest pain, pulse deficit, neurologic compromise, aortic insufficiency, and congestive heart failure were more common. With distal dissection, back pain was more common; hypertension and atherosclerosis were also more common. Chest radiograms almost always showed an abnormal aortic contour, although aortography was necessary to be certain of the diagnosis.

PROGNOSIS. The prognosis is poor in aortic dissecting aneurysm. If untreated, approximately 20 per cent of patients die within 24 hours and 27 per cent in 48 hours. A small percentage of patients with aortic dissection, probably less than 10 per cent, live for a year and may survive with chronic or even severe aortic insufficiency. With surgical resection of the diseased segment and aortic graft replacement, as many as 75 per cent may survive. The prognosis is better for either medical or surgical treatment when the dissection begins distal to the aortic arch. In this group, 50 per cent may survive the first three weeks even without modern therapy.

TREATMENT. Treatment may be either surgical or medical. Surgical management consists of resection of the involved segment and replacement with a prosthetic graft. Operative management is especially to be considered in the following circumstances: (1) when there is leaking from the dissection, which most commonly takes place into the left hemithorax or pericardium; (2) when the process is in the ascending aorta or arch; (3) when the cerebral circulation is compromised but not to a degree incompatible with recovery; (4) with severe heart failure caused by aortic regurgitation; (5) when there is evidence of continued dissection; (6) when pain and blood pressure cannot be controlled; and (7) when hypertension is absent.

Medical Management. Medical management involves control of hypertension and administration of drugs to lessen the systolic ejection force of the heart. Hypertension is controlled by such agents as trimethaphan (Arfonad) or, alternatively, intramuscular reserpine, 0.5 to 2 mg every six hours. One may also use oral or intravenous alpha methyldopa. The systolic blood pressure is reduced to 100 to 120 mm Hg. Along with these antihypertensive agents, oral propranolol is begun in a dosage of 10 to 40 mg four times daily so as to reduce the velocity of left ventricular ejection. In one series, 17 of 33 patients treated medically survived, and in another, 10 of 12. In the Peter Bent Brigham Hospital series, 26 of 31 patients with aortic dissection had contraindications to medical therapy; 17 of 22 did well after surgical correction. When dissection was limited to the descending aorta, none of 14 patients had contraindications to medical therapy, which was successful in each instance.

Medical management may be considered when the process is more than two weeks old. Resection of the dissected area, followed by grafting, may be carried out later when the condition of the patient is stabilized. Progressive enlargement of the aneurysm is an indication for surgical repair in patients who have received medical therapy. The majority can be brought through the acute phase of the illness alive. However, the long-term outlook in medically treated patients is questionable, and undoubtedly many of them will do better with surgical treatment once the condition has stabilized. Long-term antihypertensive therapy should be considered if indicated. This might include single drugs or combinations of methyldopa, propranolol, guanethidine, and diuretics as required.

Alpert, J., Bakhtan, E. K., Gielchinsky, I., et al.: Vascular complications of intra-aortic balloon pumping. Discussion. Arch. Surg., 111:1190, 1976.

Slater, E. E., and DeSanctis, R. W.: The clinical recognition of dissecting aortic aneurysm. Am. J. Med., 60:625, 1976.

367.9.   MISCELLANEOUS FORMS OF AORTITIS AND THE AORTIC ARCH SYNDROME

The aorta may be affected by a number of inflammatory processes in addition to those previously described. In some instances the aortic involvement is caused by septicemia; in others, by inflammation of contiguous structures. In still others, the aortic disease is a part of the generalized disorder of connective tissue. The process may encroach upon the origin of the aortic arch vessels. Symptoms may arise owing to impairment of the blood supply to the areas supplied by these vessels, namely, the innominate artery, the left common carotid artery, and the left subclavian artery. This syndrome is called the aortic arch syndrome. Thus one may find cerebral ischemia, syncope, visual difficulties, claudication during exercise of the upper extremities, impairment of the pulse in the upper extremities, or intermittent claudication of the jaw muscles with chewing. The aortic arch syndrome may be produced by Takayasu's syndrome, by syphilis, by arteriosclerosis, or by dissecting aneurysm. The aorta may be involved by tuberculosis, usually as a result of inflammation of continuous tuberculous lymph nodes. Septicemia may lead to mycotic aneurysm of the aorta. This may be a complication of infectious endocarditis. Relapsing polychondritis may lead to aortic involvement, and aortic aneurysms occur fairly frequently in this condition. The aneurysms may involve both the thoracic and abdominal aorta. The aorta may be involved by idiopathic aortitis, a process which resembles syphilis anatomically but occurs in the absence of serologic or bacteriologic evidence of syphilis. This process may lead to calcification of the ascending aorta and even to calcification of the aortic and mitral valves. The aorta may be involved in rheumatic fever and in rheumatoid disease (Heggtveit et al.). Giant cell aortitis may occur. This syndrome is closely allied to temporal arteritis and polymyalgia rheumatica. It may lead to the aortic arch syndrome. In ankylosing spondylitis, 5 to 10 per cent of patients develop a proximal aortitis closely resembling syphilitic aortitis. Aortic regurgitation often occurs. The disease affects men nine times as often as women.

TAKAYASU'S SYNDROME. Takayasu's arteritis is a form of aortic involvement which appears to be much more common in females and in Japan, although increasing numbers of patients are being recognized in the United States. This syndrome has also been called "pulseless disease," but since there are other diseases which affect the arterial pulses similarly, this term should be either discarded or qualified. Nakao and associates reviewed 84 patients. They divided the patients into three types. One was the *aortic arch type* (they usually had stenosis or occlusion of branches of the aortic arch). Forty-seven patients, of whom 41 were women, were in this group. The second type was the *extensive type*, which involved the entire aorta and its branches. There were 27 cases in this group. The third type was the *descending thoracic and abdominal type*, of which there were ten patients, seven of them female. The first symptoms usually appeared between the ages of 11 and 48 years. In 66 of the 84 patients the first symptoms appeared between the ages of 11 and 29 years. Eleven patients had angina pectoris, presumably from coronary artery involvement. In the early stages of the disease dyspnea, cough, and edema may be present, only to disappear later. Twenty-seven patients had localized pain over the affected arteries, but only two had loss of arterial pulse. Fever was present in 17. Dizziness, syncope, headache, and impaired vision with claudication in the upper or lower extremities were commonly described. Thirty-four of 75 had slight anemia, and 46 of 76 had an increased erythrocyte sedimentation rate. C-reactive protein was present in 30 of 68. Aortographic studies were essential in confirming the diagnosis. In some, aortography showed localized aneurysms in each of the three types. In the aortic arch variety, extensive stenosis or occlusion of the proximal part of the aorta or aortic arch branches was found. This was present in all of 28 of the arch type and in most of the extensive type. Acquired coarctation of the aorta occurred occasionally. Six of 15 of the *extensive type* who were studied showed coarctation of the abdominal aorta, and eight of nine of the *descending thoracic and abdominal aortic type* showed abdominal aortic coarctation. Both the extensive and the descending aorta type frequently showed encroachment upon, and narrowing of, the lumen of the renal or mesenteric arteries (Fig. 4), and some showed femoral artery occlusion.

The patients commonly complained of arthralgia; carditis and high fever were not present. Five had erythema nodosum. Six of the patients in this report died; three died of left-sided heart failure, one had angina and pericarditis, and two died suddenly. Two died in less than a year from the onset of symptoms; two, in one to four years; and two, 20 to 29 years after the onset of symptoms.

Pathologic Lesions. Takayasu's disease is a segmental panaortitis, or panarteritis, characterized by cicatrization of all layers of involved arteries and dense bands of medial inflammatory cells. In advanced stages, the arteries become thick walled, rigid tubes, followed by luminal obliteration caused by superimposed thrombosis. There may be occlusive narrowing of the coronary ostia. The fibrous mural thickening exceeds that usually seen in other forms of aortic disease.

Treatment. Twenty-nine of the patients received adrenal corticosteroids; of these 29, 18 had remissions and 11 had no suppression of the inflammatory findings. Anticoagulants were used but were thought helpful in only one of 12 patients in whom they were used. Although a few of the patients had increased antistreptolysin "O" serologic titers or positive rheumatoid factor tests, none met the clinical criteria for either rheumatoid arthritis or acute rheumatic fever.

Heggtveit, H. S., Hennigar, G. R., and Morrione, T. G.: Panaortitis. Am. J. Path., 42:151, 1963.
Nakao, K., Ikeda, M., Kimata, S., et al.: Takayasu's arteritis. Clinical report of eighty-four cases and immunological studies of seven cases. Circulation, 35:1141, 1967.

367.10. AORTIC OCCLUSION SYNDROMES

Occlusion of the terminal aorta at its bifurcation may be produced by traumatic severance, by arteriosclerotic thrombosis, or suddenly by embolism. The predisposing causes of emboli are most commonly atrial fibrillation, infective endocarditis, myocardial infarction, cardiomyopathy, prosthetic heart valves, ventricular or aortic aneurysm, and rheumatic mitral disease. Gradual occlusion of the terminal aorta is often well tolerated

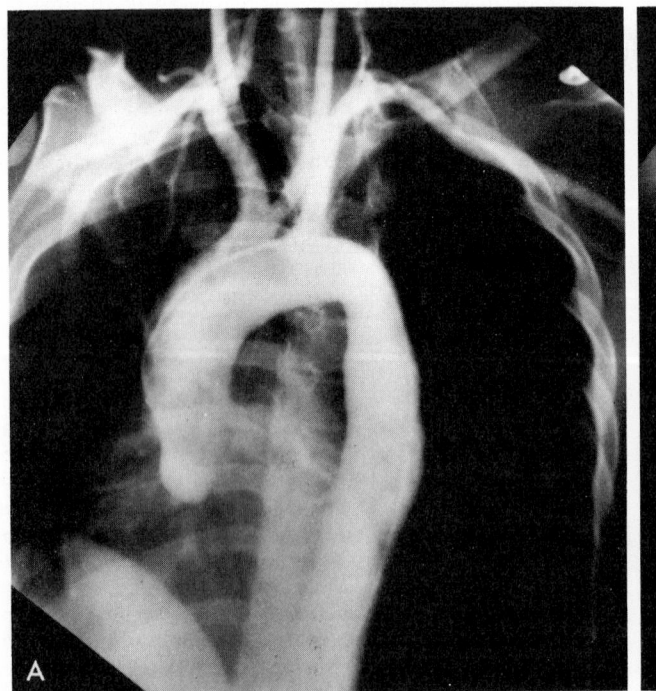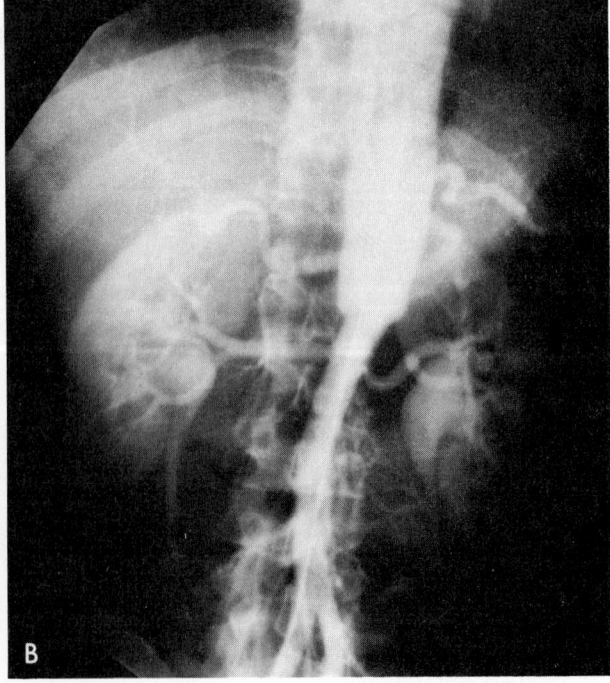

Figure 4. Takayasu's aortitis in a 26-year-old black man. Thoracic (*A*) and abdominal (*B*) aortograms show dilation, irregularity, and wall thickening extending from proximal descending thoracic aorta to the abdominal aorta a few centimeters above the renal arteries. *A*, The cervical branches of the aortic arch are normal. *B*, There is a 30 per cent narrowing of the left main renal artery. The picture is consistent with Takayasu's arteritis. (Courtesy of Dr. Harold Spitz.)

without gangrene of the lower extremities, although the patient may have pain and claudication in the hips and thighs with exercise, and the male may suffer from impotence (Leriche's syndrome). Sudden occlusion of the aorta at its bifurcation is poorly tolerated, and immediate embolectomy is needed. Patients with this condition suffer from pain (but pain may be absent in as many as 50 per cent of instances), loss of the femoral pulses, coldness, pallor, and often ensuing gangrene of the lower extremities. Weakness or paralysis of the lower limbs, loss of deep tendon reflexes, and impairment or loss of sensation are usually present. Two instances seen within the last two years at the Cincinnati General Hospital were referred to neurologists because of sudden paraplegia. The diagnosis was originally overlooked because of failure to examine the femoral pulses. The superficial veins of the lower extremities are usually collapsed. The diagnosis is made clinically and confirmed by aortography. Without embolectomy, massive fatal gangrene of the lower extremities and pelvis is likely. With chronic aortic thrombotic occlusion at the bifurcation, a synthetic bypass graft is used to bridge the obstructed area, provided that the iliac and femoral arterial vascular beds are adequate. Endarterectomy may be employed alone when the process is quite localized, or combined with bypass grafting when the process is more extensive.

Fairbairn, J. R., II, Juergens, J. L., and Spittell, J. A., Jr.: Peripheral Vascular Diseases. 4th ed. Philadelphia, W. B. Saunders Company, 1972.

368. DISEASES OF THE PERIPHERAL VESSELS

Jay D. Coffman

368.1. PERIPHERAL VASCULAR DISEASES DUE TO ORGANIC ARTERIAL OBSTRUCTION

ARTERIOSCLEROSIS OBLITERANS

DEFINITION. Arteriosclerosis obliterans is caused by arteriosclerotic narrowing or obstruction of large and medium-sized arteries supplying the extremities; symptoms and signs are produced by ischemia.

ETIOLOGY. The etiology of arteriosclerosis is discussed in Ch. 474.

INCIDENCE. Arteriosclerosis obliterans is the leading cause of obstructive arterial disease of the extremities after age 30. The lower extremities are involved most commonly; the superficial femoral artery is affected by stenosis or obstruction in approximately 90 per cent of patients. The aortoiliac and popliteal areas are the next most common sites. The greatest incidence of superficial femoral and more distal arterial disease occurs in the seventh decade, but aortoiliac disease has its peak a decade earlier. The disease is more common in males than in females, especially before the menopause (about 9:1). Patients with diabetes mellitus develop arteriosclerosis obliterans more frequently and at an earli-

er age than nondiabetics. Diabetics have the same incidence of femoropopliteal disease but a greater frequency of vessel involvement between the knee and ankle than nondiabetics. In patients with isolated aortoiliac disease, high plasma cholesterol and total lipid concentrations are frequent findings, but diabetes mellitus is not.

PATHOLOGY. The stenotic or occlusive process is usually segmental, and surgical therapy depends on this characteristic; however, the intima also displays widespread arteriosclerotic changes proximal and distal to the segmental lesion. Although the occlusive or stenotic lesions causing symptoms are usually proximal to the knee, the incidence of concomitant lower leg arterial occlusions is high (45 per cent in some surveys) and rises steeply with increasing age. Of the vessels in the calf, the posterior tibial artery is most often affected. A specific lesion of arteriolar and capillary endothelial proliferation has been described in diabetes by some investigators but has not been found by others. In patients with diabetes the development of indolent ulcers in the presence of adequate pulses may be due to diabetic neuropathy and not to small vessel disease.

PATHOPHYSIOLOGY. Symptoms and signs are produced by inadequate oxygenation of the tissues distal to the arterial lesion, secondary to the decrease in blood flow or pressure at rest or during exercise. Large and medium-sized arteries must have a decrease in cross-sectional area of 70 to 90 per cent before a decrease in blood flow or pressure occurs at rest; during exercise a 60 per cent decrease may suffice. The critical stenosis diameter which decreases flow or pressure is dependent on the velocity of flow and therefore the peripheral resistance; the length of the stenotic segment has a lesser effect. Factors affecting peripheral resistance are discussed below. In patients who develop ischemic symptoms only during exercise, the calf blood flow may be normal at rest; however, during exercise the blood flow may stop or be abnormally slow. The decreased blood pressure in the arterial vasculature distal to the obstructing lesion allows the contracting muscle to obstruct arterial flow partially or completely during exercise. Also, if full vasodilatation (reactive hyperemia) is produced in an involved limb, the total blood flow is usually much less than in the normal limb.

Although all the vessels of a system contribute to its total resistance, the arterioles and precapillary sphincters are of greatest importance. Peripheral resistance is regulated reflexly by the sympathetic nervous system and locally by the formation of vasodilator metabolites. Activity of the sympathetic nervous system usually causes cutaneous vasoconstriction, thereby increasing peripheral resistance. This normal activity, i.e., reflex vasoconstriction when exposed to cold, can be harmful to an ischemic extremity. Removal of vasoconstrictor activity in an extremity results in vasodilatation. Blood vessels in skeletal muscle also are affected by sympathetic activity but only to a very limited extent during exercise when vasodilator metabolites are active.

Blood supply to the limb distal to an obstructing or stenotic arterial lesion is via collateral blood vessels. Most of these collaterals are present in the normal limb but unused until an obstruction occurs; many appear almost immediately after an acute arterial occlusion, but others form more gradually over a period of months. Little is known concerning the reactivity of the collateral vessels in man; in animals, exercise and systemic blood pressure elevation decrease collateral vessel resistance, whereas a decrease in systemic blood pressure increases collateral vascular resistance. Blood flow can be increased through collateral vessels in man by raising the systemic blood pressure.

CLINICAL MANIFESTATIONS. The most common symptom of arteriosclerosis obliterans is *intermittent claudication* (intermittent limping). The patient experiences cramping pain, tightness, numbness, or severe fatigue in the muscle group being exercised. The amount of exercise producing the pain is relatively constant in each patient, and the pain is relieved promptly by rest. In a few patients, pain may disappear on further walking, perhaps because of an unconscious slowing of gait. Intermittent claudication is most frequent in the calf muscles because femoral artery disease is so common. However, even in more proximal lesions (aortoiliac disease) the calf is the most common site of claudication because these muscles do the most work in walking. Low back, buttock, thigh, and foot claudication may also occur; the site of the symptoms localizes the obstructing lesion proximally.

Rest pain is the other important symptom of obstructive arterial disease. Rest pain is a grave sign indicating that the blood supply is not sufficient even for the small nutritional requirements of the skin. It may be localized to one or more toes but often has a stocking distribution. The latter distribution means that ischemic neuritis is not usually the cause of rest pain. Rest pain is worse at night and is relieved somewhat by dependency and by cooling.

Other symptoms of arteriosclerosis obliterans include coldness, numbness, paresthesias, and color changes in the involved extremity.

Examination of the patient with intermittent claudication reveals diminished or absent pulses distal to the site of obstruction. Although the dorsalis pedis pulse may be absent congenitally in more than 10 per cent of people, the posterior tibial pulse is absent in only 2 per cent, and both pulses in approximately 0.5 per cent. If pulses are palpable in the presence of an obstructive lesion, exercise will make the pulses disappear; this is often a valuable diagnostic test. The second important part of the examination is to listen with the stethoscope over the aorta and peripheral arteries. The presence of a systolic or continuous bruit usually indicates a proximal obstructive or stenotic lesion; a continuous bruit denotes a very low diastolic pressure distal to the obstruction and therefore an inadequate collateral blood flow.

Examination may also reveal signs of ischemia. Distal to an arterial obstruction, the limb is often cool when compared with the proximal part of the same extremity or the symmetrical part of the opposite extremity. Skin temperature may vary widely in health, and even profound coldness, if present in all extremities, particularly in a cool environment, may be physiologic. Severe coldness that persists in a warm environment is usually abnormal, and, if unilateral, definitely abnormal. A warm extremity with normal color but absent pulses means collateral blood flow is adequate. The involved extremity may also show color changes: pallor, owing to a markedly decreased blood flow; cyanosis, caused by a diminution in blood flow not sufficient to cause blanching of the skin; rubor, a persistent red or reddish-blue discoloration owing to injury from anoxemia of the cutaneous capillaries and venules. Trophic

changes may develop: the subcutaneous tissue becomes puffy and thickened; the skin becomes dry, atrophic, shiny, and tightly drawn with an absence of hair; and the toenails become hard, brittle, thickened, ridged, and deformed. Indolent ulceration and gangrene indicate severe local ischemia. Ischemic ulcers on the toes, and sometimes over the anterior and lateral lower calf, are usually quite painful and sensitive.

Isolated aortoiliac disease (Leriche's syndrome) produces a characteristic picture. Intermittent claudication of the low back, buttock, thighs, or calves may be present. Global atrophy of the limbs and pallor of the legs and feet are frequent findings. Other trophic changes are usually absent; if present, concomitant femoropopliteal disease is often found. Hypertension may be present in the upper extremities; impotence has been emphasized as a symptom but it is not frequent. All pulses are usually absent in the legs, but weak femorals may be felt if the collateral circulation is well developed or if the occlusive process is only partial. A systolic murmur is often heard over both femoral arteries and lower abdomen.

DIAGNOSIS. By careful palpation of pulses and auscultation for bruits, the diagnosis and site of obstruction or stenosis are easily determined in most patients. The presence of coldness, discoloration, and trophic changes indicates the degree of ischemia. A triad of tests can be used to evaluate the degree of ischemia and collateral circulation. With the patient supine, the involved limb is raised to a 45 degree angle. Normally the plantar surface remains pink; pallor indicates a deficient blood supply. If pallor occurs only after ankle exercise, the circulation is not as compromised. Then the patient sits up quickly, allowing the extremities to assume a dependent position, and flushing and filling of the veins of the feet are timed. Flushing should occur immediately; veins should fill in about 10 seconds. Flushing and venous filling times of greater than 20 and 30 seconds, respectively, denote a severely ischemic limb with inadequate collateral circulation. These tests should be performed in a warm room to rule out vasospasm; varicosities invalidate the venous filling time. The use of a Doppler velocitometer to measure systolic blood pressure in the dorsalis pedis and posterior tibial arteries with the pneumatic cuff on the thigh and then at the ankle is especially helpful in diagnosing obstructive disease (the pedal pressures should be equal to or higher than the brachial artery pressure) and its site. A pressure less than 30 mm Hg indicates very severe ischemia and often presages gangrene. In doubtful cases, the most sensitive test is the measurement of pedal arterial systolic blood pressure before and after exercise by use of a Doppler velocitometer. In patients with a pedal pressure similar to the brachial artery pressure, the pedal pressure below an obstructive lesion will fall to low levels for more than 30 seconds after exercise. Other tests include measurement of blood flow during exercise by the disappearance of a radioisotope (^{131}I, ^{133}Xe) from the involved muscle. During exercise the disappearance rate either falls to zero or is abnormally slow in claudicators compared with that in normal subjects. The postexercise disappearance rates are also usually abnormal in obstructive arterial disease. Postexercise or postischemic flow can also be measured with a plethysmograph, but there is some overlap of values between claudicators and normal persons.

The presence or absence of calcification by x-ray of

the extremities is usually meaningless. *Arteriography* is always performed if surgery is being considered to reveal the exact location and extent of the obstructive lesion and the collateral circulation.

Intermittent claudication may occur in *severe anemia* and in *McArdle's syndrome;* both are easily distinguished from arteriosclerosis obliterans by the presence of normal pulses. The pain of *arthritis* may radiate to the thighs or calves, but is present at rest and not usually worse with exercise. *Arterial embolism* pain does not develop as insidiously as arteriosclerotic ischemic symptoms. In occasional patients with *lumbar disc, spinal canal, or cauda equina disease,* pain may occur only with exercise; also vasospasm may be intense so that distal pulses cannot be felt. Usually neurologic signs are present or appear with exercise. Even large vessel pulsations may disappear in patients taking *vasoconstrictive drugs* (see Ergotism and Methysergide Toxicity in Ch. 368.2.); patients should be carefully questioned concerning the use of these drugs.

Ischemic ulcers resulting from arteriosclerosis obliterans must be differentiated from ulcers that occur in patients with hypertension *(Hines' ulcers).* In hypertensive ischemic ulcers, pulses in the leg and foot are normal, and signs of ischemia are absent elsewhere in the extremity. The hypertensive ulcer is most commonly located on the lateral aspect of the leg or ankle, but arteriosclerotic ulcers are usually on the toes. Hypertensive ulcers are more common in females and are extremely painful. They begin as a purplish plaque which develops into a hemorrhagic bleb; the bleb then ulcerates, leaving a lesion with purplish red margins.

PROGNOSIS. Often intermittent claudication is the first symptom of generalized arteriosclerotic vascular disease, and most patients die eventually from myocardial infarctions or cerebrovascular accidents. Seventy to 90 per cent of patients with femoral artery disease remain stable in their symptoms or improve over a nine-year follow-up period. If diabetes mellitus is present, the prognosis is grave, for progression of the disease almost always occurs. The prognosis after surgical revascularization appears good in large vessel (aortic or femoral artery) disease.

TREATMENT. If the patient has only intermittent claudication with a normal-appearing limb, he should be treated conservatively. He will be able to walk farther without pain if he slows his gait and loses excess weight. Tobacco should never be used in any form, for it causes cutaneous vasoconstriction via the sympathetic nervous system. The patient is advised to exercise frequently to the development of pain but to rest until the pain totally disappears. It is hoped that exercise will stimulate further growth of collateral blood vessels, but proof is lacking for this point. Recent studies indicate that treatment of hyperlipoproteinemias may prevent or improve arteriosclerotic lesions; they may be a contributing factor and should be sought and treated if present (see Ch. 532.7). Patients should protect their limbs from cold or trauma; careful attention to keep the skin scrupulously clean, dry, and soft is important. Even minor infections such as the dermatophytoses may produce problems. Toenail trimming should be done regularly and with care.

If the claudication is found to be progressively worse over a six-month to two-year observation period, if it interferes seriously with the patient's daily activity, or if even minor ischemic symptoms such as numbness or

paresthesias are present, *surgery* should be considered. Since the lesion is often localized and segmental, restoration of circulation beyond segmental stenotic or obstructive areas by graft bypass is the treatment of choice. Currently autogenous saphenous vein grafts are used most frequently because the incidence of thrombosis is less than with grafts made of synthetic materials. Often patch grafts are used on one portion of the vessel. Bypass grafts are favored over excision and graft replacement, because collateral circulation is not destroyed with the bypass method. Before a grafting procedure can be performed, arteriography must be done to determine that there are patent vessels below the obstruction ("good runoff"). However, connection of a graft to an "isolated" popliteal segment (no calf vessels patent) may produce good results with healing of trophic lesions. Vein grafts have been connected to distal arteries in the lower calf and foot with success in saving ischemic, even gangrenous, feet. In patients with aortoiliac disease who cannot undergo major surgery, subcutaneous axillofemoral or, if one femoral is patent, femorofemoral grafts have been a very successful innovation. In patients with more than one obstructing lesion in the vessels supplying an extremity, correction of the most proximal obstruction often produces relief of symptoms. Endarterectomy of an obstructed deep femoral artery in a limb with superficial femoral artery obstruction may supply enough collateral blood flow to allow a limb to survive. The success of a surgical attack on involved vessels is proportional to the size of the vessel involved; aortoiliac operations have a 90 per cent or better success rate; femoropopliteal, 70 to 80 per cent; and posterior tibial artery, 50 per cent.

If surgery cannot be performed because of poor runoff or other serious disease, and rest pain or gangrene is present, rest in bed is essential. The affected extremity should be kept 20 to 30 degrees below the horizontal, for the dependent position increases blood flow and pressure and occasionally is the only position the patient can tolerate. If edema is present, the extremity should be kept horizontal but never elevated. External local warmth, if used at all, is best applied by means of a thermoregulated cradle kept at a temperature below 38° C. Direct application of external heat should never be used, because ischemic tissue blisters and burns at much lower temperatures than normal tissue. Rest pain may require the use of sedatives and analgesics, even narcotics. Ulcers caused by ischemia are treated the same as rest pain; warm saline soaks should be used to keep the ulcer open, moist, and clean. Enzymatic debridement is not advised because of possible local allergic reactions. If infection is present, the appropriate systemic and local antimicrobial drug should be used as determined by culture and sensitivity tests.

Preganglionic lumbar sympathectomy may be performed to increased skin blood flow when rest pain or small areas of ulceration or gangrene are present. Before surgery, it must be demonstrated that the sympathetic nervous system is intact in the extremity, especially in diabetics in whom peripheral neuropathy sometimes produces an autosympathectomy. To assess sympathetic activity in an extremity, plethysmographic foot blood flow, toe pulse, or skin temperature may be measured before and after a procedure to remove sympathetic activity. Methods used to remove sympathetic activity are (1) a warm environment, (2) local anesthesia of sympathetic ganglia, (3) local anesthesia of appropriate mixed nerves, (4) spinal anesthesia, or (5) autonomic blocking agents. An increase in the parameter being measured after one of these procedures indicates that a sympathectomy may be beneficial. Sweating of the involved extremity is also an indication of sympathetic activity. Although superficial ulcers often heal after the operation, sympathectomy alone rarely improves intermittent claudication.

Arteriosclerotic *gangrene* often necessitates *amputation* of the limb. In the presence of gangrene with ascending infection (advancing lymphangitis, fever, and leukocytosis), antimicrobial chemotherapy is indicated. Prompt amputation must be considered, because the efficacy of the antimicrobial agents may be limited by the ischemia of the affected tissues and by local necrosis. The level of amputation is determined by palpable pulses and the presence of warm viable tissue of good color. The percentage of patients who become ambulatory after amputation is much higher with below-the-knee than above-the-knee operations.

Vasodilator drugs and agents are widely advertised but have little, if any, place in the treatment of arteriosclerosis obliterans. They are consistently ineffective in relieving intermittent claudication but may increase muscle or skin blood flow at rest in some patients. The efficacy of drugs with prolonged vasodilator action depends upon the degree to which structural disease has rendered the peripheral arteries rigid and incapable of dilatation; it has yet to be shown that they are active on the collateral vessels. Vasodilator drugs often lower systemic blood pressure so that flow to the ischemic limb may be decreased; even intra-arterial administration has been shown to decrease foot flow in some patients.

Long-term anticoagulation has also been recommended for treatment of arteriosclerosis obliterans, but conflicting results have been reported. Fibrinolytic therapy with intravenous streptokinase has been evaluated for chronic arterial occlusive disease, and a few patients, especially those with a recent onset of symptoms, have benefited.

Barndt, R., Jr., Blankenhorn, D. H., Crawford, D. W., and Brooks, S. H.: Regression and progression of early femoral atherosclerosis in treated hyperlipoproteinemic patients. Ann. Intern. Med., 86:139, 1977.

Coffman, J. D.: Peripheral collateral blood flow and vascular reactivity in the dog. J. Clin. Invest., 45:923, 1966.

Coffman, J. D., and Mannick, J. A.: An objective test to demonstrate the circulatory abnormality in intermittent claudication. Circulation, 33:177, 1966.

Coffman, J. D., and Mannick, J. A.: Failure of vasodilator drugs in arteriosclerosis obliterans. Ann. Intern. Med., 76:35, 1972.

Mannick, J. A., and Coffman, J. D.: Ischemic Limbs. New York, Grune & Stratton, 1973.

Schadt, D. C., Hines, E. A., Jr., Juergens, J. L., and Barker, N. W.: Chronic atherosclerotic occlusion of the femoral artery. JAMA, 175:937, 1961.

Verta, M. J., Jr., Gross, W. S., van Bellen, B., Yao, J. S. T., and Bergan, J. J.: Forefoot perfusion pressure and minor amputation for gangrene. Surgery, 80:729, 1976.

Young, D. F., Cholvin, N. R., Kirkeeide, R. L., and Roth, A. D.: Hemodynamics of arterial stenoses at elevated flow rates. Circ. Res., 41:99, 1977.

THROMBOANGIITIS OBLITERANS
(Buerger's Disease)

DEFINITION. Thromboangiitis obliterans is an obliterative vascular disease or syndrome, probably inflammatory in type, affecting chiefly the peripheral arteries and veins. Identified first as endarteritis obliterans (von Winiwarter, 1879), it was described more fully and given its present name by Buerger (1908).

INCIDENCE. All races are subject to thromboangiitis obliterans, but the greatest incidence is in the Ashkenazic Jews, of whom 20 in 100,000 develop the disease compared with 7 or 8 per 100,000 in the general population. The disease is also common in the Orient. The incidence of the disease in the United States has decreased markedly. Men are affected far more frequently than women, in a ratio of about 75 to 1. Thromboangiitis obliterans has been observed at all ages but occurs most frequently between 20 and 45.

ETIOLOGY. Although many agents, toxic and infectious, have been suggested, no etiology has received general acceptance. Cigarettes are used moderately or excessively by many, but not all, patients with thromboangiitis obliterans and have been thoroughly investigated as a causative agent, for smoking aggravates the disease. An increased skin sensitivity to tobacco has been reported by some investigators but not found by others. The higher carboxyhemoglobin levels observed in smokers have been proposed as an etiologic factor by increasing the affinity of hemoglobin for oxygen. A thrombotic etiology is supported by the reports of abnormal thromboplastin generation tests and higher levels of heparin precipitable fraction of fibrinogen in plasma in patients with thromboangiitis obliterans than in normal persons or patients with arteriosclerosis obliterans. A rise in adhesive platelet counts has also been described in the disease and apparently correlates with tobacco smoking.

Considerable skepticism has been expressed that this disease is an entity different from arteriosclerosis occurring in young people. Evidence has been presented that its clinical and pathologic pictures are specific; however, it may be a syndrome with more than one cause.

PATHOLOGY. The lesions are segmental in that diseased sections of arteries or veins are separated by normal areas. In the acute stage cellular proliferation of the intima is accompanied by the formation of red thrombi in small and medium-sized vessels, but the internal elastic lamina usually remains intact. Polymorphonuclear leukocytes, lymphocytes, and giant cells infiltrate all coats of the artery and extend into the thrombus. The formation of sterile microabscesses within the thrombi is a specific finding in this disease. Additional segments of artery or vein are involved acutely at intervals from days to years; hence, a single long artery may exhibit many stages, ranging from the acute picture to dense scar formation. Late stages cannot be distinguished pathologically from arteriosclerosis obliterans.

PATHOPHYSIOLOGY. The disease is characterized by alternating periods of activity and quiescence. Depending upon the time relation between the developing occlusion and compensation by collateral circulation, the onset and course vary from insidious to fulminant. Usually occlusion gradually outstrips the developing collateral circulation, and definite peripheral ischemia brings the patient under medical care within one to four years after the first mild symptoms appear. The disease often has an initially more active course of six to twelve years, and then advances much less rapidly; at this stage it is very difficult to differentiate from arteriosclerosis obliterans.

CLINICAL MANIFESTATIONS. The typical patient with thromboangiitis obliterans is a young male who smokes cigarettes, presents symptoms of peripheral vascular ischemia, and may have a history of thrombophlebitis. The lower extremities are affected most commonly, and the most frequent presenting complaint is persistent coldness of the limbs. The upper extremities are involved in more than 70 per cent of patients (sometimes without symptoms), the digital arteries being affected more frequently than the ulnar or radial. Raynaud's phenomenon, hyperhidrosis, and ulcers of the digits are common. In comparison with other vascular diseases, the pain is often excruciating. Migratory thrombophlebitis may precede or accompany arterial involvement and occurs in approximately 40 per cent of patients. Tender, red, elevated areas about 1 cm in diameter appear suddenly in the skin near the valves of small, superficial veins, and gradually disappear during two to three weeks, to be followed after irregular intervals by new lesions. Other symptoms and signs (intermittent claudication, rest pain, ulcers, gangrene) are the same as in arteriosclerosis obliterans except that femoral artery disease is less frequent and aortoiliac, rare. Thromboses of the mesenteric, coronary, cerebral, and renal arteries have been described but are uncommon.

DIAGNOSIS. The diagnosis may be suspected when a young male presents with peripheral vascular insufficiency and thrombophlebitis, but it can be definitely proved only by biopsy of an active lesion. The age group, sex, thrombophlebitis, frequent involvement of upper extremities, Raynaud's phenomenon, and normal blood cholesterol concentration and glucose tolerance test result help differentiate the disease from arteriosclerosis obliterans. Arteriography can be helpful in demonstrating normality of vessels between lesions, absence of atheroma, a characteristic tree root configuration of the collateral vessels around the point of abrupt occlusion, and asymptomatic involvement of the upper extremities. Since Raynaud's disease is rare in men, affects the upper extremities more severely, and usually does not obliterate arterial pulsation at the wrist or ankle, it should not be confused with Raynaud's phenomenon in thromboangiitis obliterans. Migratory thrombophlebitis without symptoms or signs of arterial involvement cannot be diagnosed as thromboangiitis obliterans unless histologic proof is obtained.

PROGNOSIS. The prognosis for life is good, but amputation of extremities is common, especially in the fulminant form. In the late stages, the prognosis and course are similar to arteriosclerosis obliterans.

TREATMENT. The treatment is the same as that outlined for arteriosclerosis obliterans, but it is imperative that tobacco never be used in any form. Nicotine produces transient vasoconstriction and probably favors extension of the disease. Bilateral preganglionic sympathectomy has been advocated for established, gradually advancing thromboangiitis obliterans, especially if vasospasm is prominent. This major operation is not indicated in mild cases responding well to medical treatment or in advanced cases with massive gangrene. Opinion is still divided concerning the usefulness of sympathectomy in this disease. In thromboangiitis obliterans resistance to infection is fairly high and collateral circulation usually good, so that minor amputations may be performed more safely than in arteriosclerotic gangrene.

Astrup, P., Hellung-Larsen, P., Kjeldsen, K., and Mellemgaard, K.: The effect of tobacco smoking on the dissociation curve of oxygen hemoglobin. Scand. J. Clin. Lab. Invest., 18:450, 1966.
Barker, N. W.: Diagnosis and treatment of thromboangiitis obliterans (Buerger's disease). Minn. Med., 39:303, 1956.
Craven, J. L., and Cotton, R. C.: Haematological differences between thromboangiitis obliterans and atherosclerosis. Br. J. Surg., 54:862, 1967.
Goodman, R. M., Elian, B., Mozes, M., and Deutsch, V.: Buerger's disease in Israel. Am. J. Med., 39:601, 1965.
McKusick, V. A., Harris, W. S., Ottesen, O. E., Goodman, R. M., Shelley, W. M., and Bloodwell, R. D.: Buerger's disease: A distinct clinical and pathologic entity. JAMA, 181:5, 1962.
Wessler, S., Ming, S. C., Gurewich, V., and Freiman, D. G.: A critical evaluation of thromboangiitis obliterans. N. Engl. J. Med., 262:1149, 1960.
Williams, G.: Recent views on Buerger's disease. J. Clin. Pathol., 22:573, 1969.

ARTERIAL EMBOLISM

DEFINITION. Fragments of centrally located thrombi or atheromatous material may embolize and occlude large or small peripheral blood vessels.

ETIOLOGY. Emboli usually originate from mural or valvular thrombi in the left side of the heart (atrium or ventricle), less commonly from an atheromatous ulcer in the aorta or a more peripheral artery, and from thrombi in aneurysms. Paradoxical emboli originate from venous thromboses, travel to the right side of the heart, and pass through a patent foramen ovale. Most emboli occur in association with myocardial infarction, atrial fibrillation associated with mitral valve disease, chronic congestive heart failure, cardiomyopathies, or endocarditis. With the advent of surgical replacement of heart valves, prostheses have become a common source of emboli. Emboli in the upper extremities often originate from a compressed subclavian artery in the thoracic outlet syndromes.

PATHOPHYSIOLOGY. Emboli lodge at bifurcations of arteries and at narrowed arteriosclerotic areas. The most common site is at the junction of the femoral artery with the profunda femoris; emboli at the origin of the iliac arteries from the aorta (*saddle emboli*) are also frequent. The embolus stops blood flow through the artery and is followed within a few hours by secondary progressive arterial thrombosis below and sometimes above the point of obstruction. Secondary vasospasm has been assumed to be an important factor causing ischemia of the affected extremity, but convincing experimental evidence has not been presented to support this theory. The amount of muscle and skin ischemia that occurs depends on the degree of collateral circulation development.

PATHOLOGY. Emboli from the heart or aneurysms show the same pathology as the parent thrombi. Emboli lodged in arteries usually organize by the ingrowth of connective tissue, and later recanalization may occur. However, fragmentation of the embolus before organization is not uncommon with fragments lodging in more distal vessels. Emboli that originate from friable, ulcerated atheromatous lesions produce either large vessel obstruction by amorphous debris or arteriolar and capillary blockage by a variable combination of cholesterol crystals and lipoid material. The cholesterol crystals incite an inflammatory response which leads to fibrosis and complete vessel obstruction.

CLINICAL MANIFESTATIONS. In approximately half of patients, there is the sudden onset of severe pain in the extremity distal to the site of embolization. The other cases have an insidious beginning over one to several hours; numbness and paresthesias may precede the pain. Pain is present in 80 per cent of patients and may become excruciating within one or two hours, particularly if the patient exercises the limb. Paresthesias occur in about 60 per cent of cases, and 20 per cent develop muscular weakness or actual paralysis. With an aortoiliac embolus, fainting, nausea, vomiting, and abdominal pain may precede a shocklike state.

Examination of the involved extremity reveals pallor and coldness, sharply demarcated distal to the site of embolization, viz., at the inguinal ligaments or sometimes as high as the umbilicus in saddle embolus, at the lower third of the thigh in femoral artery embolus, and at midcalf in popliteal artery embolus. Arterial pulses are absent below the embolus by palpation or oscillometry. In the arms, because of the easy palpability of the brachial artery, the site of embolus lodgment can be determined by the disappearance of the pulse. Occasionally there is tenderness directly over the embolus in an artery. The extremity may also show collapsed veins, decreased to absent reflexes and sensation, and weakness and paralysis. Later the initial pallor changes to a blotchy cyanosis. If collateral circulation is good, the extremity soon shows signs of improvement in color and temperature, but muscle tenderness and pitting edema may develop. If the collateral circulation is inadequate, massive gangrene follows with bleb formation, spotty vermilion discoloration of the skin, and mummification.

Large emboli from thrombi or amorphous atherosclerotic debris show the aforementioned picture. Smaller emboli may produce only local digital cyanosis with or without pain. Atheromatous microemboli (cholesterol crystals and lipoid material) may produce sudden leg pain, tender muscles, cool legs with pulses, petechiae, livedo reticularis, and plaquelike reddened elevations of the skin. Pedal pulses may disappear later in this syndrome. The spontaneous appearance of painful dusky discoloration of a toe or toes in the presence of pulses should suggest atheromatous microembolism.

DIAGNOSIS. The diagnosis of embolization is not difficult in the patient with the acute onset of a painful, ischemic extremity who demonstrates a source for embolus formation. Acute arterial thrombosis can be distinguished from an embolus only by the presence or absence of underlying etiologies; absent or decreased arterial pulsations in the opposite limb support a diagnosis of acute thrombosis. Patients with acute iliofemoral thrombophlebitis sometimes have no palpable pulses in the affected extremity and may show signs resembling those of arterial embolus. Detection of a feeble pulse by oscillometry, distended veins, and massive edema of the extremity helps rule out embolus. In patients with symptoms and signs of embolization or microembolization and normal pulses, angiography must be performed to look for ulcerative atherosclerotic lesions, aneurysms, or fibromuscular dysplasia in the proximal large vessels. Microembolization is often confused with polymyositis or polyarteritis nodosa; muscle biopsy may be necessary to demonstrate the cholesterol crystals.

PROGNOSIS. The prognosis in acute arterial embolization depends on several factors, including size of vessel affected, age of patient, collateral blood supply, and speed of treatment. The larger the artery involved, the worse the prognosis without surgical treatment. Gangrene is much more common after the age of 60 years, probably because of concomitant arteriosclerotic involvement of the blood vessels and collaterals. The development of collateral circulation is very important, for sufficient collaterals may save a limb without surgical

treatment. The presence of patent companion vessels, e.g., around the elbow, gives a favorable outlook. The earlier an embolus can be removed surgically, the better the prognosis for survival of the severely ischemic limb.

With any method of treatment, the mortality in most studies is usually greater than 20 per cent, owing to the underlying disease and recurrent embolization to vital areas. The incidence of embolus recurrence is very high. After either medical or surgical treatment, limb incapacity from muscle fibrosis with tendon shortening or intermittent claudication is common.

TREATMENT. Although embolectomy should restore the normal physiology and is strongly recommended in the surgical literature, conservative medical management often gives as good end results. The exception is emboli at the aortic bifurcation, when surgery is the optimal treatment. When the patient is first seen, treatment should be instituted to improve blood flow to the extremity, and a vascular surgeon should be immediately called in consultation. Anticoagulation with heparin should be started at once to prevent thrombus formation below and above the embolus, and further embolization (long-term anticoagulation is usually indicated to prevent recurrent emboli). Thrombolytic therapy with streptokinase may be valuable in acute embolization in about one third of patients; such therapy is given intravenously and must be followed by adequate anticoagulation (see Ch. 357.3). The limb should be positioned in 15 degree dependency and adequate analgesics given to relieve the pain. The affected limb should be kept comfortably warm, as in a thermoregulated (30 to 34° C) cradle, and the body and uninvolved extremities warmed in an effort to produce reflex vasodilatation in the involved limb. Every precaution should be taken to prevent burning during heat application; ischemic limbs burn at much lower temperatures than normal limbs. Lumbar sympathetic block by paravertebral injection of procaine or xylocaine has been recommended to relieve vasoconstrictor tone and vasospasm if present; if used, it should be performed before anticoagulation.

If conservative medical therapy is not effective in greatly improving the extremity in two to four hours and the underlying condition of the patient will allow surgery, embolectomy is indicated. Early diagnosis is essential, as the greatest success with embolectomy is within eight to ten hours of the incident. Embolectomy has been performed longer than 48 hours after the acute insult with some success, although less than with earlier operations. Muscle tenderness and edema often occur after embolectomy and may be mistakenly diagnosed as thrombophlebitis. In cases presenting with gangrene, amputation is usually necessary. In atheromatous embolization or emboli from aneurysmal thrombi, surgical attack on the proximal lesion may be successful in preventing further emboli; the use of anticoagulants in this situation has not been shown to be of value.

Amery, A., Deloof, W., Vermylen, J., and Verstraete, M.: Outcome of recent thromboembolic occlusions of limb arteries treated with streptokinase. Br. Med. J., 4:639, 1970.

Eliot, R. S., Kanjuh, V. I., and Edwards, J. E.: Atheromatous embolism. Circulation, 30:611, 1964.

Freund, U., Romanoff, H., and Floman, Y.: Mortality rate following lower limb arterial embolectomy: Causative factors. Surgery, 77:201, 1975.

Jacobs, A. L.: Arterial embolism in the limbs. Edinburgh, E. & S. Livingstone, Ltd., 1959.

Karmody, A. M., Powers, S. R., Monaco, V. J., and Leather, R. P.: "Blue toe" syndrome. Arch. Surg., 111:1263, 1976.

Silverblatt, C. W., Wasserman, F., and Wolcott, M. W.: Pulmonary artery embolism and paradoxical embolization. Arch. Intern. Med., 107:105, 1961.
Szekely, P.: Systemic embolism and anticoagulant prophylaxis in rheumatic heart disease. Br. Med. J., 1:1209, 1964.
Wessler, S., Sheps, S. G., Gilbert, M., and Sheps, M. C.: Studies in peripheral arterial occlusive disease. III. Acute arterial occlusion. Circulation, 17:512, 1958.

PERIPHERAL ARTERITIS AND GANGRENE IN SYSTEMIC INFECTIONS

Symptoms and signs of peripheral vascular disease, mild or severe, appear occasionally as complications in bacterial, viral, rickettsial, and fungal infections. Bacterial arteritis and abscess of the wall of an artery are uncommon complications of bacterial endocarditis and septicemias and may lead to hemorrhagic lesions or aneurysm formation. The rickettsial diseases, especially typhus and Rocky Mountain spotted fever, may cause endothelial proliferation of the arterioles, capillaries, and venules followed by degeneration and necrosis of the media; thrombosis of larger arteries may occur rarely. In infectious arteritis with direct vascular involvement, signs of subacute or acute arrest of peripheral blood flow occur with necrosis of skin and sometimes massive gangrene. However, peripheral ischemia may be transitory and, in large part, vasospastic. Gangrene of the extremities may follow acute infectious conditions, such as pneumonia and gastroenteritis, especially in children; the cause is unknown.

Tuberculosis of the peripheral arteries is rare, but occasionally metastatic infection or embolism produces panarteritis or endarteritis with fully developed tubercles in thrombosed vessels. Direct involvement by extension from adjacent tuberculous lesions, although common in centrally located vessels, is rare in the extremities.

Syphilis may diminish peripheral circulation by producing periarteritis, obliterative intimal hyperplasia, or panarteritis, but the media is much less affected than in the large arteries. True gummas have been found in the vessels of gangrenous limbs. Peripheral vascular complications of syphilis are more common in men than in women. Peripheral ischemia, vasospastic or organic, appears insidiously or suddenly, but gangrene is rare. Active antisyphilitic therapy usually arrests the acute progress of the disease and relieves vasospasm, but organic occlusion remains.

Collins, R. N., and Nadel, M. S.: Gangrene due to the hemolytic *Streptococcus* — a rare but treatable disease. N. Engl. J. Med., 272:578, 1965.
Derick, C. L., and Hass, G. M.: Diffuse arteritis of syphilitic origin. Am. J. Path., 11:291, 1935.
Koten, J. W.: Peripheral gangrene in infancy and childhood. Br. Med. J., 3:798, 1967.
Learmouth, G. E.: Gangrene of the lower extremities complicating scarlet fever. Can. Med. Assoc. J., 15:69, 1925.
Slaughter, W. H.: Symmetrical gangrene of malarial origin. JAMA, 86:1607, 1926.

SHIN SPLINTS AND ANTERIOR TIBIAL COMPARTMENT SYNDROMES

The anterior tibial compartment is a closed space in which the muscles and blood vessels are surrounded by nonexpanding fascia and bone. Swelling of the tissues in this compartment can cause mild to severe complications.

Shin splints is a frequently encountered syndrome of pain and discomfort in the lower anterior part of the leg after repetitive, unusual exertion. The syndrome is presumably a result of ischemia from an abnormally high tissue pressure compressing the blood vessels. It often occurs in athletes or dancers early in the season. The pain in the front of the legs occurs during or after exercise and is only slowly relieved by rest. Tenderness is most frequent at periosteal attachments of the muscles to the tibia or interosseous membrane. Mild swelling and a slight rise in local skin temperature may be present. When the pain is reproduced by repeated dorsiflexion of the foot against resistance, the anterior tibial muscles become very hard and bulge prominently; a pulsation may become visible over the front of the legs. Arterial pulses are normal. Treatment consists of rest of the muscles, supportive strapping, and a program of graduated exercise.

The *acute anterior tibial compartment syndrome* is a rare condition caused by the rapid onset of ischemic necrosis of muscles in the anterior tibial space. Swelling of the muscles compresses muscles, nerves, and blood vessels. The cause is usually unknown, but there is often a history of excessive exertion. The syndrome may occur after fractures of the tibia or fibula or restoration of blood flow to an acutely ischemic extremity. A dull, aching pain which becomes progressively severe is the major symptom; it is unrelieved by rest and sometimes by analgesics. Extreme tenderness is present over the entire anterior tibial compartment, and the fascia rapidly becomes tense and boardlike. The skin becomes glossy, erythematous, and edematous as muscle necrosis occurs; a slight fever and leukocytosis may be present. Loss of dorsiflexion of the great toe and foot then occurs, and sensation may be lost between the first and second toes (deep peroneal nerve compression). The dorsalis pedis pulse may be present or absent. Treatment must be immediate and involves surgical decompression of the anterior tibial compartment by fasciotomy. If treatment is delayed, complete necrosis of the muscles occurs with a resultant permanent footdrop.

A *chronic anterior tibial compartment syndrome* also has been described with pain similar to intermittent claudication in the front of the lower leg on severe exertion but not with ordinary walking. The discomfort disappears with rest. Tenderness is present over the entire compartment when the pain occurs; arterial pulses are normal. The syndrome is thought to be due to an abnormally small compartment. Treatment is usually unnecessary, but a fasciotomy will relieve the symptoms.

French, E. B., and Price, W. H.: Anterior tibial pain. Br. Med. J., 2:1290, 1962.
Reneman, R. S.: The anterior and the lateral compartmental syndrome of the leg due to intensive use of muscles. Clin. Orthop., 113:69, 1975.
Rorabeck, C. H., and MacNab, I.: The pathophysiology of the anterior tibial compartmental syndrome. Clin. Orthop., 113:52, 1975.
Slocum, D. B.: The shin syndrome. Am. J. Surg., 114:875, 1967.

368.2. PERIPHERAL VASCULAR DISEASE DUE TO ABNORMAL VASOCONSTRICTION OR VASODILATATION

RAYNAUD'S PHENOMENON AND DISEASE

DEFINITION. Raynaud's phenomenon is a syndrome characterized by paroxysmal, bilateral ischemia of the digits induced by cold or emotional stimuli and relieved by heat.

ETIOLOGY. Raynaud's phenomenon may be secondary to an underlying disease or anatomic abnormality, but the most common cause is *Raynaud's disease*, which is of unknown etiology. It is less common before puberty and after age 40 but may occur at any age. Women are affected more frequently than men (5:1). Raynaud concluded from his early studies (1862, 1874) that excessive sympathetic activity was responsible for the attacks, but Lewis found that the digital vessels were abnormally reactive to local cold. Since ischemic attacks can still be induced after sympathectomy, it may be concluded that there is a local fault in the blood vessels in Raynaud's disease which is aggravated by the normal degree of reflex sympathetic nervous activity. However, about a dozen cases of Raynaud's phenomenon associated with pulmonary hypertension have been reported, suggesting that a neurohumoral mechanism may be operative in causing both syndromes.

Raynaud's phenomenon may occur in occlusive arterial disease (thromboangiitis obliterans, arteriosclerosis obliterans, arterial emboli), collagen disease (especially scleroderma), after trauma (pneumatic hammer disease, injuries to pianists or typists), after gangrene from any cause, drug intoxication (ergot, methysergide), blood dyscrasias (cryopathies, cold hemagglutinins), and neurogenic lesions (thoracic outlet compression syndromes, carpal tunnel syndrome, poliomyelitis, syringomyelia, causalgia). In Raynaud's phenomenon from secondary causes, the syndrome is caused usually by irritation of the sympathetic nerves, pathologic alterations in the small blood vessels, or sludging and agglutination of red blood cells.

PATHOLOGIC PHYSIOLOGY. The paroxysmal ischemia of the digits is due to constriction of the digital and palmar or plantar arteries; initial pallor indicates that vasoconstriction involves the small cutaneous vessels. Later the digital capillaries and venules become dilated, and the slowed blood flow allows the hemoglobin to release more of its oxygen, producing cyanotic, cold digits. When the vasconstriction is relieved, blood flow increases greatly (reactive hyperemia), imparting a red color to the previously ischemic digits. Total and capillary fingertip blood flow are smaller in patients with Raynaud's phenomenon and disease than in normal subjects. With a cooling stimulus, patients show a significant decrease in fingertip capillary flow not seen in normal subjects.

PATHOLOGY. In the early stages of the disease, the blood vessels are histologically normal. Later, in progressive cases, the intima is thickened and the muscular coats of the arteries are hypertrophied. Eventually thrombosis of small arteries may occur and focal gangrene of the digital tips may form, although elsewhere the arteries are still histologically normal or show only slight hypertrophy.

CLINICAL MANIFESTATIONS. In typical Raynaud's phenomenon, the fingers of both hands show well demarcated blanching on exposure to cold and then may turn cyanotic; sometimes only cyanosis occurs. During recovery, a bright red color (reactive hyperemia) replaces the cyanosis. During the ischemic phase, the digits are cold and numb. In the reactive hyperemia phase, throbbing pain, tingling, swelling, and a rise in skin temperature are found. The digits are affected to different levels in each patient (sometimes extending to the wrist), but the terminal phalanges are always most severely involved. Initially, attacks may be unilateral and involve only one or two digits, but they soon become bilateral and may be induced by emotional upsets as well as by cold exposure.

In Raynaud's disease, the onset is usually gradual with attacks only in the winter. Attacks may be rare, or they may occur several times a day; they may last a few minutes in mild cases to two hours or more in severe cases. They end spontaneously or can be terminated by immersing the hands in warm water. Between episodes, the digits are normal or, in severe cases, mildly cyanotic.

The hands alone are affected in half the cases, hands and feet in the remainder; nose, cheeks, ears, and chin are affected much more rarely. The course of the disease varies; after onset it may persist indefinitely in mild form, improve spontaneously, or become more severe. In the small number of cases that are progressive, the attacks become more frequent, persist during the summer, and last longer; finally, mild cyanosis may be present constantly.

Trophic changes appear in progressive cases, usually one to four years after onset. The fingers become thin and tapering and their skin smooth, shiny, less mobile, and eventually tightly stretched (sclerodactyly). The nails grow slowly and are ridged or curved. Recurrent infections, blisters, and small areas of local cutaneous gangrene appear on the fingertips, but gangrene of a whole digit is rare. The gangrenous areas are extremely painful and, on healing, leave tiny depressed scars.

DIAGNOSIS. Criteria which should be present in patients with Raynaud's phenomenon in order to diagnose Raynaud's disease include (1) absence of any disease or anatomic abnormality to which paroxysmal digital ischemia might be secondary; (2) well demarcated digital pallor or cyanosis occurring in intermittent attacks, induced by cold or emotion; (3) symmetrical or bilateral involvement of digits; and (4) gangrene, if present, usually limited to small areas of skin. Previously, presence of symptoms for two years with no evidence of an underlying cause had been considered a fifth diagnostic point; however, Raynaud's phenomenon may precede the diagnosis of scleroderma by many years. It is probably unsafe to diagnose the idiopathic disease in the presence of an elevated sedimentation rate or minor symptoms or signs suggestive of an underlying disease (arthralgias, telangiectasis). Raynaud's phenomenon is diagnosed by discovering an underlying disease or condition known to cause attacks.

Raynaud's disease and phenomenon are distinguished from acrocyanosis by the intermittency of attacks. The cyanotic, cold, and edematous limb affected by poliomyelitis or other diseases causing paralysis is also persistent in nature. The cause of sudden "bilateral gangrene of the digits" (Lewis), which appears rarely in children or young adults without previous attacks of discoloration and without cold exposure, is unknown. The fingers, toes, nose, and ears become permanently cyanotic, and within a few days gangrene develops in the distal phalanges of one or more fingers, often symmetrically and bilaterally. The gangrene is extensive and is due to sudden thrombotic occlusion of the final end branches of the digital arteries. The relationship of this syndrome to Raynaud's disease is uncertain, although typical cyclic color changes may appear during the healing stage.

PROGNOSIS. Mild cases of Raynaud's disease improve slowly or remain stationary for years, and the attacks, being few and avoidable, are merely an inconvenience. In a large series of cases, the disease caused no deaths and very little disability; amputations of terminal phalanges were necessary in only 0.4 per cent, and the phenomenon improved or disappeared in 46 per cent. The progressive form, with recurring infection and local gangrene, becomes increasingly painful and disabling, usually despite treatment, but only rarely results in the loss of more than the distal phalanges. The prognosis for secondary Raynaud's phenomenon depends on the underlying cause. Generalized scleroderma and rheumatoid arthritis, which are frequently associated with Raynaud's phenomenon, may produce extreme deformity and disability.

TREATMENT. Mild cases of Raynaud's disease with infrequent attacks limited to cold exposure, and without trophic changes or gangrene, may be relieved by reassurance, sedatives or tranquilizers, and protection from cold exposure. Smoking has been shown to produce cutaneous vasoconstriction, and the use of tobacco should therefore be avoided. Rauwolfia* products in continued small oral doses (reserpine, 0.25 to 0.5 mg daily) will often decrease the severity and frequency of attacks. Guanethidine* (10 to 40 mg daily) and alpha methyldopa* (1.5 to 2.0 grams daily) are also effective in treatment. If necessary, a vasodilator drug (tolazoline long-acting tablets, 80 mg every 12 hours) can be added to the therapeutic regimen. The addition of thyroid substances and androgens has been recommended but helps little, if any.

Vasoconstrictor tone caused by sympathetic nervous system activity is an important factor in bringing on and maintaining attacks of digital ischemia, whether or not the local arteries are abnormally reactive to cold. Removal of vasoconstrictor impulses by regional sympathectomy may be of benefit for the progressive type of Raynaud's disease with indolent ulcers or local gangrene. The success of the sympathectomy depends upon the extent to which the normal capacity for vasodilatation is preserved, as shown by the vasodilator response to body warming or sympathetic ganglion nerve block with lidocaine. In early Raynaud's disease of the lower extremities, lumbar sympathetic ganglionectomy gives complete relief of symptoms. For the upper extremity, preganglionic cervicodorsal sympathectomy is the operation of choice but usually is of temporary (six months to two years) benefit.

The treatment of Raynaud's phenomenon secondary to an underlying disease or anatomic abnormality is directed at the secondary cause. Sympathectomy is of little or no benefit in scleroderma or arthritis but may be helpful in Raynaud's phenomenon secondary to pneumatic hammer disease or causalgia (reflex sympathetic dystrophy).

Coffman, J. D., and Davies, E. T.: Vasospastic diseases: A review. Prog. Cardiovasc. Dis., 18:123, 1975.
Coffman, J. D., and Cohen, A. S.: Total and capillary fingertip blood flow in Raynaud's phenomenon. N. Engl. J. Med., 285:259, 1971.
Cosgriff, T. M., and Arnold, W. J.: Digital vasospasm and infarction associated with hepatitis B antigenemia. JAMA, 235:1362, 1976.
Farmer, R. G., Gifford, R. W., Jr., and Hines, E. A., Jr.: Raynaud's disease with sclerodactylia: A follow-up of seventy-one patients. Circulation, 22:13, 1961.
Gifford, R. W., Jr., and Hines, E. A., Jr.: Raynaud's disease among women and girls. Circulation, 16:1012, 1957.
Lewis, T., and Pickering, G. W.: Observations upon maladies in which the blood supply to digits ceases intermittently or permanently, and upon bilateral gangrene of digits; observations relevant to so-called "Raynaud's disase." Clin. Sci., 1:327, 1934.
McGrath, M. A., and Penney, R.: The mechanisms of Raynaud's phenomenon. Parts 1 and 2. Med. J. Aust., 2:328, 1974.
Tsur, N., Adar, R., Bechor, I., Bogokowsky, H., and Mozes, M.: Upper thoracic sympathectomy. Israel J. Med Sci., 9:53, 1973.

ACROCYANOSIS

Acrocyanosis (Croq, 1896; chronic acro-asphyxia, Cassirer, 1900) is a symmetrical cyanosis of the hands and, less commonly, the feet with few or no symptoms and no complications.

ETIOLOGY AND PATHOLOGY. It is primarily a vasospastic disturbance of the smaller arterioles of the skin of unknown cause, but is probably due to local cold sensitivity. When compared with normal digits, acrocyanotic digits have a heightened arteriolar tone at average room temperature. Secondary dilatation of the capillaries and the subpapillary venous plexus occurs, and the slower blood flow allows the hemoglobin to release a greater part of its oxygen content, accounting for the blue color. Acrocyanosis occurs without special age or sex incidence, and may be associated with various endocrine disorders or asthenias as well as with certain anxiety states. No specific pathology has been described.

CLINICAL MANIFESTATIONS. Patients usually present with an unevenly blue and red discoloration of the skin which may extend from the digits to the wrists and ankles but is most intense distally. The digits are also persistently cold and sweat profusely. Puffiness of the digits and mild hypesthesia may be present, but other trophic changes are rare. The cyanosis is intensified by cold or emotional upsets and is relieved by warmth.

DIAGNOSIS. Acrocyanosis can be distinguished from Raynaud's disease by the persistent nature of the discoloration. The presence of normal arterial pulses rules out obstructive arterial disease. Since the discoloration is limited to the hands and feet and disappears when the extremities are warmed, it should not be confused with various types of generalized cyanosis.

TREATMENT. Except for reassurance, treatment is usually unnecessary. Possible endocrine abnormalities should be investigated. To prevent reflex sympathetic vasoconstriction, general body protection from cold, as well as local measures, helps to decrease the intensity of the discoloration. For cosmetic reasons, vasodilator drugs (reserpine, 0.25 to 0.5 mg daily, or tolazoline long-acting tablets, 80 mg every 12 hours) may be used. Sympathectomy is helpful but seldom warranted.

Elliot, A. H., Evans, R. D., and Stone, C. S.: Acrocyanosis: A study of the circulatory fault. Am. Heart J., 11:431, 1936.
Larsson, Y.: The vasoconstrictor tone of the cutaneous arterioles in acroasphyxia, hypertension, and in the cold pressor test. Acta Med. Scand. (Supp. 206), 130:146, 1948.

---

*Experimental drug for this purpose.

Lewis, T., and Landis, E. M.: Observations upon the vascular mechanism in acrocyanosis. Heart, 15:229, 1930.
Lottenbach, K.: Vascular response to cold in acrocyanosis. Helv. Med. Acta, 33:437, 1966.

ERGOTISM AND METHYSERGIDE TOXICITY

DEFINITION. Intense vasoconstriction of small and large blood vessels, producing symptoms and signs of peripheral vascular ischemia, may result from the ingestion of ergot or methysergide.

ETIOLOGY. Ergotism results from the use of ergot-containing drugs or the ingestion of bread made from rye or wheat infected with the ergot fungus (*Claviceps purpurea*). It formerly occurred in epidemic form, but is now seen only sporadically (due to the fungus), or after the repeated administration of ergotamine (Gynergen, Cafergot) for migraine or pruritus or of ergot in abortion. Methysergide is a synthetic serotonin antagonist useful in the treatment of migraine headaches. Approximately 7 per cent of patients develop peripheral vascular symptoms or signs with methysergide ingestion, usually after large doses, although as little as 1 mg has caused symptoms in some patients.

PATHOPHYSIOLOGY AND PATHOLOGY. Both drugs induce large and small blood vessel vasoconstriction. Ergot induces vasoconstriction mainly by stimulation of the alpha adrenoceptors of vascular smooth muscle and can lead to thickening and fibrosis of the arterial wall resembling fibromuscular dysplasia. Secondary intimal hyperplasia and thrombosis may occur, resulting in gangrene. In methysergide toxicity, the arterial adventitia is markedly thickened by circular fibrous apposition. Its mode of action is unknown, but it does potentiate the effect of catecholamines on blood vessels.

CLINICAL MANIFESTATIONS. *Acute ergotism* produces diarrhea, colic, and vomiting, followed by headache, vertigo, paresthesias, convulsive seizures, and occasionally gangrene of the digits, nose and ears. It is rarely seen with the drug ingestion. In *chronic intoxications*, intermittent claudication, muscle pains, numbness, coldness and pallor of the digits, and even Raynaud's phenomenon may occur. Examination reveals only cool, pale digits or mottling of the skin with normal or decreased arterial pulsations; however, complete absence of medium- and large-vessel pulsations in the extremities may occur. Gangrene may develop in the severe cases. A similar picture of peripheral vascular ischemia may follow methysergide ingestion. Abdominal angina, angina pectoris, and cerebral ischemic symptoms have also been caused by these drugs. Methysergide has been implicated as an etiologic agent in periureteral or retroperitoneal fibrosis which can extrinsically obstruct arteries and veins.

DIAGNOSIS. The diagnosis is made from the history of drug ingestion associated with symptoms and signs of peripheral ischemia. Arteriography characteristically shows diffuse or segmental narrowing of large arteries and often very constricted distal vessels with collateral vessels present. Arteriosclerosis obliterans, Raynaud's disease, and acrocyanosis are differentiated from ergotism and methysergide toxicity by the history of drug ingestion and, if necessary, by arteriography.

PROGNOSIS. The prognosis is excellent if gangrene has not appeared before treatment and if drug administration is stopped.

TREATMENT. Treatment involves anticoagulation to prevent thromboses and the use of vasodilators, e.g., sodium nitroprusside, 50 μg per minute or more intravenously or intra-arterially,* to counteract the vasocontriction. Body warming is recommended to produce reflex vasodilatation in the involved extremities, but is often unsuccessful as is vasodilator drug therapy. With avoidance of the offending drug, the vasoconstriction usually subsides in one to three days. Sympathetic nerve block or sympathectomy may be necessary in pregangrenous or gangrenous cases.

Carliner, N. H., Denune, D. P., Finch, C. S., Jr., and Goldberg, L. I.: Sodium nitroprusside treatment of ergotamine-induced peripheral ischemia. JAMA, 227:308, 1974.
Graham, J. R.: Methysergide for prevention of headache. N. Eng. J. Med., 270:67, 1964.
Müller-Schweinitzer, E., and Stürmer, E.: Investigations on the mode of action of ergotamine in the isolated femoral vein of the dog. Br. J. Pharmacol., 51:441, 1974.
Rackley, C. E., Mengel, C. E., Pomerantz, M., and McIntosh, H. D.: Vascular complications with use of methysergide. Arch. Intern. Med., 117:265, 1966.
Regan, J. F., and Poletti, B. J.: Vascular adventitial fibrosis in a patient taking methysergide maleate. JAMA, 203:1069, 1968.

ERYTHROMELALGIA
(Erythermalgia)

DEFINITION. Erythromelalgia (Mitchell, 1878) is a rare syndrome of paroxysmal, bilateral vasodilatation of the feet and, less often, the hands, associated with burning pain, increased skin temperature, and redness of the skin.

ETIOLOGY AND PATHOLOGY. The cause is unknown. It has occurred as a hereditary affliction. Increased blood flow is usually present, but symptoms may occur in a limb in which the arteries are occluded by a blood pressure cuff. Therefore it is thought that there is a hypersensitivity of the skin to heat or tension. No uniform pathologic condition has been found, but data are scarce. The syndrome occurs without special age or sex incidence.

CLINICAL MANIFESTATIONS. The patient with erythromelalgia complains of attacks of bilateral burning pain, superficial or deep, involving circumscribed areas on the soles or palms, the entire foot or hand, or even the whole extremity. The attacks follow stimuli that normally induce only physiologic peripheral vasodilatation or engorgement such as local heat, a warm environment, exercise, standing, or simple dependency of the extremity. The onset is gradual, and symptoms may remain mild for years or may become so severe and continuous that total disability results. Examination during an attack (which may be produced by exposure to a 32 to 36° C environment) usually reveals that the affected skin is hot and red and often sweats profusely; arterial pulsations are normal. Trophic changes, gangrene, and ulceration do not occur, but swelling may be present.

The syndrome may be either idiopathic or secondary to polycythemia vera, hypertension, myeloproliferative diseases, or lupus erythematosus. The condition may precede the polycythemia by as long as 12 years. Secondary erythromelalgia occurs more commonly in an older age group, is more often unilateral, and produces pain of lesser intensity than idiopathic erythromelalgia.

---

*See p. vi, Dosage Notice, immediately following Preface.

DIAGNOSIS. Arteriosclerosis obliterans may produce localized and often unilateral burning pain and redness but, unlike erythromelalgia, is not associated with normal pulses or a rise in skin temperature. Neuritis, infectious ganglionitis, and poisoning by thallium, lead, or arsenic may produce painful peripheral hyperemia. Chronic inflammatory states produce in the skin a "susceptible state" with diminished capillary and arteriolar tone. Burning pain (erythralgia, Lewis) is then induced by mild grades of heat, cold, friction, and congestion that leave normal skin unaffected. A temporary reactive vasodilatation of the cutaneous vessels also normally occurs after prolonged exposure to cold in response to a histamine-like substance liberated by local tissue damage (Lewis). This is easily distinguished from erythromelalgia by the history.

TREATMENT. Attacks can be avoided or aborted by rest, elevation of the extremity, and cold application. Aspirin (0.6 gram orally) quickly relieves pain in some cases, and the remarkable response is of diagnostic value. Vasoconstrictor agents such as ephedrine (25 mg orally) may be useful; methysergide* (1 to 4 mg orally) has also produced relief. Even vasodilator agents (isoproterenol, nitroglycerin) have been reported to be helpful. Contrast baths, using heat below the threshold for pain, often afford considerable but temporary relief. Severe attacks require liberal doses of sedatives, and the therapy is generally unsatisfactory. Occasionally section or alcohol injection of peripheral nerve is required; sympathectomy has been successful in the treatment of three cases.

PROGNOSIS. The prognosis in idiopathic erythromelalgia is guarded, because the severe pain may become disabling. Prognosis of secondary cases depends on the underlying disease; treatment of the disease often relieves the symptoms.

Alarcon-Segovia, D., and Diaz-Jouanen, E.: Erythermalgia in systemic lupus erythematosus. Am. J. Med. Sci., 266:149, 1973.
Babb, R. R., Alarcon-Segovia, D., and Fairbairn, J. F., II: Erythermalgia. Review of 51 cases. Circulation, 29:136, 1964.
Catchpole, B. N.: Erythromelalgia. Lancet, 1:909, 1964.
Cross, E. G.: The familial occurrence of erythromelalgia and nephritis. Can. Med. Assoc. J., 87:1, 1962.
Lewis, T.: Clinical observations and experiments relating to burning pain in extremities and to so-called "erythromelalgia" in particular. Clin. Sci., 1:175, 1933.

368.3. PERIPHERAL VASCULAR DISEASES DUE TO EXPOSURE TO COLD

Exposure to cold induces vasoconstriction by a direct action on blood vessels and also by reflex sympathetic nervous system activity. Cold application to the forehead or to one extremity stimulates vasoconstriction in all extremities. The decreased blood flow and local anoxia may lead to tissue damage, depending on the degree and duration of exposure and the susceptibility of the patient.

Even brief exposure to nonfreezing cold is followed in sensitive persons by an exaggerated and prolonged type of reactive vasodilatation, low-grade edema, and tingling pain. Similar exposure in more susceptible patients produces pronounced edema of the angioneurotic or urticarial type on exposed areas; even mucous membranes may be involved on ingesting cold substances. A systemic reaction with increased pulse rate, decreased blood pressure, flushing of the face, and even syncope may accompany the edema. After swimming in cool water, this reaction has proved fatal in some instances. Familial cases of cold urticaria have been described; this is a milder condition not affecting mucous membranes. Histamine has been shown to be released and measurable in the blood and urine in the nonfamilial cases. The passive transfer of cold urticaria has been demonstrated with both IgE and IgM fractions of patients' serum. Diagnosis is made by exposure of a hand or arm to 12 to 14° C water; edema will develop during or after exposure. Antihistamines or cyproheptadine (Periactin, 4 mg three times a day) or repeated short episodes of cold exposure may be of use in the treatment of cold sensitivity, but protection of the patient from cold exposure is most important.

Bentley-Phillips, C. B., Black, A. K., and Greaves, M. W.: Induced tolerance in cold urticaria caused by cold-evoked histamine release. Lancet, 2:63, 1976.
Tindall, J. P.: Cold urticaria. Postgrad. Med., 50:133, 1971.
Wanderer, A. A., and Ellis, E. F.: Treatment of cold urticaria with cyproheptadine. J. Allergy Clin. Immunol., 48:366, 1971.
Wanderer, A. A., Maselli, R., Ellis, E. F., and Ishizaka, K.: Immunologic characterization of serum factors responsible for cold urticaria. J. Allergy Clin. Immunol., 48:13, 1971.

IMMERSION FOOT
(Trench Foot)

DEFINITION. Immersion foot is due to prolonged exposure of the extremities to water; syndromes characterized only by painful, swollen feet or hands to the more serious manifestations of muscle necrosis, ulceration, and gangrene may result.

ETIOLOGY. Although prolonged exposure (greater than 48 hours) to dampness or water is the important factor in the production of immersion foot, immobility and dependency of the lower extremities, constricting garments, chilling of the body, trauma, exhaustion, or dehydration, and, in some instances, semistarvation with deficient intake of protein and vitamins are often contributing causes. Two types, cold water and warm water immersion foot, exist and present different clinical pictures. The combination of wetness plus cold (not necessarily freezing) temperatures produces the most serious condition. Warm water injuries have been divided into warm water immersion foot and the more severe tropical immersion foot (paddy-field foot).

PATHOPHYSIOLOGY. The factors causing cold water immersion foot tend to decrease blood flow to the extremities. Vasoconstriction is caused by direct and reflex cold stimulation; actual cellular damage and the ensuing hyperemia are important in producing the clinical and pathologic picture. Persistent local anoxia leads to tissue necrosis and injures the capillary walls. Capillary filtration increases remarkably, and plasma and protein pass freely into the interstitial tissue, producing a tense edema. The resultant increased viscosity of the blood leads to stasis and occlusion of small vessels. The local anoxia may also produce wallerian degeneration of the nerves in the affected area.

---

*See p. vi, Dosage Notice, immediately following Preface.

Warm water immersion foot is thought to be caused by waterlogging and swelling of the stratum corneum together with abrasion from footwear. *Pseudomonas aeruginosa* can usually be cultured from the affected areas and may contribute by digesting human callus with its proteolytic enzymes. Tropical immersion foot may be caused by water entering the dermis through water-damaged stratum corneum.

PATHOLOGY. The early pathologic picture of the cold type has not been studied. In late stages, a nonspecific picture of vascular occlusion, desquamation of the skin, deep fibrosis, and superficial gangrene is seen. The nerves may be embedded in contracting fibrous tissue, and fibrosis of the media of arterioles and venules is present. Hyperhydration of the plantar stratum corneum is the only finding reported in warm water immersion foot. The pathologic features of tropical immersion foot are a lymphocytic infiltration, diapedesis of red blood cells, and swelling and proliferation of the endothelial lining of capillaries in the upper dermis.

INCIDENCE. Immersion foot is common in most wars. Non-Caucasians are thought to be more susceptible to the cold water type, perhaps on the basis of acclimatization.

CLINICAL MANIFESTATIONS. At the time of rescue from sea, or when first seen in trench warfare, cold water immersion foot often presents as pulseless, cold, red feet with a sock distribution of hypesthesia or anesthesia. The condition may develop insidiously with only numbness, paresthesias, and slight swelling as long as the tissues are supported by boots or shoes. As soon as the support is removed, edema, tingling, itching, and severe pain occur. The skin later becomes mottled yellow, blue or black. This is called the prehyperemic stage and lasts a few hours to a few days. A hyperemic stage follows, characterized by red, hot, dry feet, burning paresthesias, and intense pains, shooting or stabbing in nature. Pulses are now bounding. Edema increases with formation of blisters, which may weep serous fluid and then slowly heal. In severe cases, muscle weakness and wasting, ulcerations, and gangrenous patches develop. Gangrene is often superficial, and the necrotic skin sometimes sheds in large pieces, leaving healthy skin beneath. Even in the absence of gangrene, extensive exfoliation is common. This stage lasts one to ten weeks, depending on the grade of initial injury.

The recovery stage (posthyperemic) blends indistinguishably with the hyperemic stage; there is a return of vascular tone with restoration of normal skin color and temperature. Recovery may be complete in mild cases within two to five weeks, but severe cases often require three to twelve months. A few patients show late sequelae such as sensitivity to cold with Raynaud's phenomenon; general or marginal hyperhidrosis; paresthesias that are increased by warmth, dependency, or exertion; rigid toes caused by fibrosis of muscles; contracted joints in the feet and toes; or painful, indolent ulcers of the digits or their stumps.

Warm water immersion foot presents with painful and extremely tender feet, especially over pressure areas. Wrinkled, white, convoluted plantar surfaces and even maceration are seen on examination in the mild syndrome. In the more severe cases, called tropical immersion foot, pronounced erythema and edema of the ankles and dorsal aspects of the feet (boot area), fever, and femoral lymphadenopathy may occur. During healing, these patients develop diffuse ecchymoses, vesicles, and a maculopapular rash. Symptoms and signs subside within a week, usually leaving no residua.

PROPHYLAXIS. Drying of the feet overnight is the best method to prevent immersion foot. Avoidance of constricting clothing, prolonged dependency, or immobility; frequent rest periods; and several changes of clothes and boots will also help. If these conditions are impractical, application of silicone grease once a day may reduce the incidence of the affliction.

TREATMENT. In the prehyperemic stage of cold water immersion foot, bed rest and body warming are important. It is probably best to keep the extremities at heart level until pulses are present. Treatment of the hyperemic stage consists of complete bed rest, cooling of the hyperemic tissues to control pain and edema, keeping the body warm, elevation of the extremities above heart level, and correction of dietary deficiencies. If cleansing is necessary, light washing with dilute hexachlorophene solution may be used. Infected tissue and epidermophytosis should be treated with appropriate agents. For cooling, it may be sufficient to expose the extremities to room air, but sometimes electric fans with water sprays or ice bags are needed. With cooling, pain is usually relieved in a few hours, but in some instances it is necessary to discover an optimal temperature, because too low a temperature may again produce pain. Analgesics must be used. Tobacco smoking is prohibited. The patient is ready to walk when edema does not occur on dependency.

Sympathectomy has been helpful in the hyperemic stage but appears to improve late sequelae such as chronic painful ulcers, persistent vasospasm, and hyperhidrosis.

The treatment of warm water and tropical immersion foot involves bed rest with extremity elevation until edema and pain entirely disappear. Other measures are usually unnecessary; the symptoms and signs disappear in one to seven days.

Akers, W. A.: Paddy foot: A warm water immersion foot syndrome variant. Parts I and II. Milit. Med., 139:605, 1974.
Allen, A. M., and Taplin, D.: Tropical immersion foot. Lancet, 2:1185, 1973.
Lange, K., Weiner, D., and Boyd, L. J.: The functional pathology of experimental immersion foot. Am. Heart J., 35:238, 1948.
Montgomery, H.: Experimental immersion foot; review of physiopathology. Physiol. Rev., 34:127, 1954.
White, J. C.: Vascular and neurologic lesions in survivors of shipwreck. I. Immersion foot syndrome following exposure to cold. II. Painful swollen feet secondary to prolonged dehydration and malnutrition. N. Engl. J. Med., 228:211, 1943.

CHILBLAIN AND PERNIO

Chilblain and pernio (*erythrocyanosis*) occur commonly in patients, especially females, with a history of cool limbs in summer as well as winter. The etiologic and pathogenic factors are unknown, but the disease is seen only in cold, damp climates. However, it is much more frequent in England than in areas of the United States with comparable climates.

Acute chilblain occurs on the dorsum of the digits, hands, or feet as localized, warm, red, intensely pruritic swelling that may disappear spontaneously in a few days. Pernio is probably the same disease but involves the lower parts of the legs, especially in women who, because of their mode of dress, do not adequately protect their legs from cold weather. Rarely, indolent lesions, dull red or violaceous, proceed to painful bleb formation. The blebs contain blood-stained serous fluid and often lead to ulcer formation.

In some patients exposed repeatedly to cold, recurrent and chronic lesions, often appearing in crops, may develop. The lesions are erythematous and ulcerative and may leave residual scarring, fibrosis, and atrophy of the skin and subcutaneous tissues. The disease is more active during the cooler months and subsides in warm weather. Bilateral and symmetrical parts of the extremities are involved. This state is called chronic chilblain or pernio (erythrocyanosis frigida crurum).

Treatment is nonspecific. Corticosteroid creams may be used for itching and inflammation, antimicrobials for sepsis. Reserpine (0.25 mg orally daily)* has been reported to ameliorate the disease.

Eskell, J.: Reserpine in the treatment of chilblains. Practitioner, 189:792, 1962.

Lewis, T.: Observations on some normal and injurious effects of cold upon the skin and underlying tissues. II. Chilblains and allied conditions. Br. Med. J., 2:837, 1941.

McGovern, T., Wright, I. S., and Kruger, E.: Pernio: A vascular disease. Am. Heart J., 22:583, 1941.

Thomas, E. W. P.: Chapping and chilblains. Practitioner, 193:755, 1964.

FROSTBITE

DEFINITION. Frostbite is due to freezing of tissues which may result in damage to skin, muscle, blood vessels, and nerves.

ETIOLOGY. Superficial freezing of tissues evidently begins when the temperature of deeper tissues reaches about 10° C. During the Korean War, most cases of frostbite occurred at –6.5° C or below, after 7 to 18 hours' exposure. High winds, dampness, and general chilling of the body make frostbite more likely at above-freezing temperatures. Predisposing factors include any type of peripheral vascular insufficiency, improper clothing, exhaustion, and previous cold injury. Lack of acclimatization and geographic origin have also been implicated; the black race is more susceptible to frostbite. Most frostbite is of the slow freezing type, but a rapid frostbite (occurring in a few minutes) takes place at high altitudes with extremely low temperatures and has a predilection for the extremities rather than the face and ears.

PATHOPHYSIOLOGY. Whether actual tissue freezing or decreased blood flow from vasoconstriction is most important in producing cell injury is unknown. Damage is probably due to a combination of direct freezing with the formation of extracellular ice crystals, inducing dehydration of cells, and intense vasoconstriction. The vasoconstriction is due to direct cold exposure of the tissues but may also involve reflex vasoconstriction from chilling of other body areas. The reduced blood flow leads to capillary stasis and arteriolar and capillary thromboses. Capillary permeability is increased and results in edema formation.

PATHOLOGY. The pathologic findings vary with the stage of the disease and the depth of tissue affected. In early stages, low-grade vasculitis and inflammation are seen in all tissues. Later the skin is atrophied and may be keratinized, muscle is necrosed and shows waxy degeneration, arterioles and capillaries are thrombosed, and nerves demonstrate fibroblastic proliferation and neurolysis.

CLINICAL MANIFESTATIONS. The first indication of frostbite is often a sharp, pricking sensation that draws attention to a yellowish-white, numb area of hardened skin. However, cold itself produces numbness and anesthesia that may allow freezing of tissue without warning. When the freezing is superficial, thawing leads to local reddening and wheal and flare formation. When freezing involves deep tissues, subcutaneous edema occurs with thawing, followed by formation of vesicles and bullae. A hyperemic, reddish zone may be apparent between frozen and normal tissue. As the edema subsides in a day or two, necrosis and gangrene may become evident. However, it may take two to three months before final demarcation between viable and dead tissue can be ascertained. In the healing phase, a black eschar usually covers the area.

The traditional classification of frostbite has been from first to fourth degree, depending of the depth of tissue injury. Since the true extent of tissue damage cannot be judged on initial examination, a simpler classification of superficial and deep frostbite is more practical. The prognosis depends on the depth of freezing, as superficial cases usually have no sequelae, whereas deep freezing may end in amputation.

PROPHYLAXIS. Frostbite is preventable and occurs rarely among those who have been instructed how to protect themselves. Prophylactic measures include observance of each other for signs of frostbite; wearing adequate, loose fitting, dry clothing and mittens; exposure for only brief periods when exercise is not possible; and avoidance of smoking before and during exposure. Feet and socks should be kept dry.

TREATMENT. Superficial frostbite can be treated immediately by rewarming; affected areas on the face and ears can be warmed with the hands, hands can be placed in the axillae, or frostbitten parts can be warmed on the torso of a partner. Frostbitten areas should not be rubbed with snow or exercised.

Treatment of deep frostbite should be delayed until adequate facilities for rewarming are available. Therapy should always be very conservative, because the depth of tissue damage is difficult to ascertain, sometimes for months. It is best to rewarm the tissue as rapidly as possible in 40 to 44° C water. Massage, exposure to too high temperatures, and reactive hyperemia should be avoided because they tend to increase pain and edema. Analgesics usually are needed during rewarming. After rewarming, which usually requires about 20 minutes, the frostbitten area is exposed to room air (21 to 26° C). Although pressure dressings may be used, the open method with sterile surroundings is usually preferred. Vesicles, bullae, and eschars are left untouched. Antimicrobial drugs are indicated if infection is present. Tobacco smoking should be prohibited. Regional sympathectomy has been reported as beneficial, both clinically and experimentally, if performed at an optimal time of 24 to 48 hours after frostbite occurs. Sympathectomy may conserve tissue and lead to earlier demarcation, cessation of pain, and healing of tissue.

Eventual recovery is usually surprisingly good, the black eschar peeling off to leave normal tissue beneath.

---

*See p. vi, Dosage Notice, immediately following Preface.

Sensitivity to cold, paresthesias, and a predilection to repeated frostbite often persist. In severe frostbite, fibrosis of tissue may lead to disability, and gangrenous extremities may require amputation.

Golding, M. R., Martinez, A., DeJong, P., Mendosa, M., Fries, C. C., Sawyer, P. N., Hennigar, G. R., and Wesolowski, S. A.: The role of sympathectomy in frostbite, with review of 68 cases. Surgery, 57:774, 1965.

Lapp, N. L., and Juergens, J. L.: Frostbite. Mayo Clin. Proc., 40:932, 1965.

Meryman, H. T.: Tissue freezing and local cold injury. Physiol. Rev., 37:233, 1957.

Washburn, B.: Frostbite. What it is, how to prevent it, emergency treatment. N. Engl. J. Med., 266:974, 1962.

368.4. PERIPHERAL VASCULAR DISEASES DUE TO ABNORMAL COMMUNICATIONS BETWEEN ARTERIES AND VEINS

ARTERIOVENOUS FISTULA

DEFINITION. Arteriovenous fistulas are abnormal communications, single or multiple, between arteries and veins by which arterial blood enters the veins directly without transversing a capillary network.

ETIOLOGY. Arteriovenous fistulas created to facilitate renal dialysis are the most common fistulas. Acquired arteriovenous fistulas, usually single and saccular, may develop after a bullet or stab wound involving an artery and a contiguous vein, after vessel puncture (especially the vertebral artery), or after biopsy (especially the kidney). Fistulas of the iliac vessel may occur after surgery for intervertebral disc disease. Congenital fistulas are present from birth and are usually multiple; they result from defects in differentiation of the common embryologic anlage into artery and vein. There is no special sex incidence, and any part of the body may be involved. There is an association between large vessel congenital fistulas of the extremities and small cutaneous fistulas resembling angiomatoses.

PATHOPHYSIOLOGY. Arterial blood, following the path of least resistance, flows directly into the vein, bypassing the corresponding capillary bed. The arterial pressure is transmitted to the venous side of the fistula; the distal vein pressure is increased, but the proximal vein pressure may actually be negative during systole owing to the high velocity of blood flow. The elevated venous pressure leads to the development of varicose veins and venous stasis changes in the limb. Increased blood flow makes the tissues near the fistula abnormally warm, and diminished flow distal to the fistula may produce peripheral coldness and trophic changes. Large fistulas impose a burden on the heart; the cardiac output must be increased above normal by an amount proportional to the size of the fistula in order to maintain the general circulation. Total blood volume may be increased. The low peripheral resistance of the involved area tends to decrease diastolic and increase systolic and pulse pressures systemically. Large fistulas may lead to cardiac decompensation. Even the small fistulas created for renal dialysis induce a small increase in cardiac output and heart rate and occasionally have led to

heart failure. These fistulas have also led to ischemia or venous stasis and varicosities in the hand.

PATHOLOGY. In the region of the fistula, the intima and media of the involved veins become thickened, and newly developed elastic fibers appear. The arteries show a thinning of their walls with loss of elastic tissue and muscular fibers in the media.

CLINICAL MANIFESTATIONS. Patients complain of aching pain, edema, varicosities, or hypertrophied extremities. Occasionally, cardiac symptoms such as palpitation, substernal pain, and dyspnea on exertion are present. Examination reveals tortuous, dilated superficial veins in the extremity, and venous pulsation can be felt unless the fistula is small and deeply placed. In congenital fistulas, the skin temperature is usually elevated locally but decreased distal to the fistulas, although in acquired lesions, the temperature of the digits may be greater than in the opposite normal limb. A bruit and thrill are common over acquired fistulas; the bruit lasts throughout systole and diastole and has a coarse, machinery-like quality. The tissues near the fistula may be tender, edematous, and either red or slightly cyanotic. The circumference of the extremity is increased by edema or true hypertrophy, but bony structures are hypertrophied only if the fistula was present before epiphyseal closure. Stasis pigmentation and chronic indurative cellulitis with or without indolent ulceration may be present distal to the fistula. In contrast to the postphlebitic limb in which ulcers form around the medial malleolus, the ulceration of fistulas may affect the distal parts of the foot. Rarefaction of bone in the extremity may also occur. Temporary compression of the artery supplying a large fistula diminishes the heart rate (*Branham's sign*) and may be a helpful diagnostic sign.

DIAGNOSIS. If the diagnosis cannot be made from the clinical manifestations, other examinations may be helpful. The oxygen saturation of blood removed from proximal veins of an extremity with a fistula will be found to be greater than that of blood removed from corresponding veins in the opposite extremity. Arteriography will reveal the lesion, its location, and the number and size of communications. Edema of one or both extremities after surgery for intervertebral disc disease should suggest the possibility of a fistula. Thrombophlebitis and the postphlebitic extremity can be distinguished from fistulas by the oxygen studies and arteriography.

PROGNOSIS. The prognosis of acquired and single congenital fistulas is good after surgical repair. In acquired iliac vessel fistulas, congestive heart failure develops in two thirds of patients, and immediate repair is important. Without surgical repair, which is often not possible in multiple fistulas, the outlook is for a chronically swollen limb with varicosities, stasis pigmentation, and ulceration. Bacterial infection of acquired fistulas occurs but is rare.

TREATMENT. Single fistulas can be repaired surgically by re-establishing the continuity of the involved artery and vein walls by a variety of procedures (arteriorrhaphy, end-to-end suture, grafting). Ligation of the involved artery and vein leads to a high incidence of arterial and venous insufficiency of the extremity and should be avoided if possible. If the arterial supply depends upon a large anomalous artery, ligation of this vessel, followed by sclerosing injections of the dilated veins, may be effective. Multiple fistulas are much less amenable to surgery. Ulcers, edema, and pain may be relieved by wearing elastic bandages or stockings; pressure on the veins encourages blood flow to follow the arterial pathway. Amputation is required for large inoperable fistulas producing cardiac decompensation or gross deformity.

Binak, K., Regan, T. J., Christensen, R. C., and Hellems, H. K.: Arteriovenous fistula: Hemodynamic effects of occlusion and exercise. Am. Heart J., 60:495, 1960.

Johnson, G., Jr., and Blythe, W. B.: Hemodynamic effects of arteriovenous shunts used for hemodialysis. Ann. Surg., 17:715, 1970.

Lawton, R. L., Tidrick, R. T., and Brintnall, E. S.: A clinicopathologic study of multiple congenital arteriovenous fistulae of the lower extremities. Angiology, 8:161, 1957.

Nickerson, J. L., Elkin, D. C., and Warren J. V.: The effect of temporary occlusion of arteriovenous fistulas on heart rate, stroke volume, and cardiac output. J. Clin. Invest., 30:215, 1951.

Rossi, P., Carillo, F. J., Alfidi, R. J., and Ruzicka, F. F.: Iatrogenic arteriovenous fistulas. Radiology, 111:47, 1974.

Rusin, L. J., and Harrell, E. R.: Arteriovenous fistula: Cutaneous manifestations. Arch. Dermatol., 112:1135, 1976.

Wakim, K. G., and Janes, J. M.: Influence of arteriovenous fistula on the distal circulation in the involved extremity. Arch. Phys. Med. Rehabil., 39:431, 1958.

GLOMANGIOMA OR GLOMUS TUMOR

DEFINITION. Glomangioma or glomus tumor designates painful enlargement of a glomus body.

PATHOLOGY. The pathology consists of hypertrophy of the glomus body which contains an arteriovenous anastomosis with its associated smooth muscle coat, nonmyelinated nerve fibers, and connective tissue. Histologically, the lesion is encapsulated, occasionally diffuse but never invasive, and contains numerous epithelioid cells with no inflammatory cells.

CLINICAL MANIFESTATIONS. Glomus tumors are extremely tender but inconspicuous subcutaneous nodules which develop slowly during adult life. Pain may be present before the nodule becomes visible. They are found in various parts of the upper and lower extremities, but most frequently (30 per cent) beneath the fingernail. The diameter of the tumor is usually only a few millimeters. The nodule has a flat or slightly raised surface with reddish-blue to purplish discoloration. Excruciating burning or shooting pain, both local and referred up the extremity, occurs spontaneously or is produced by the slightest pressure. Hyperhidrosis, abnormal vasomotor activity, increased skin temperature, and tissue atrophy in the involved limb may be present. Heat, cold, and even contact with clothing may become intolerable so that protection is required continuously day and night. In glomus tumors beneath nails, a small excavation of the phalanx from erosion by the tumor can often be seen by roentgenography.

TREATMENT. Surgical excision leads to complete and immediate relief without recurrence.

Bailey, O. T.: The cutaneous glomus and its tumors — glomangiomas. Am. J. Path., 11:915, 1935.

Cooke, S. A. R.: Misleading features in the clinical diagnosis of the peripheral glomus tumor. Br. J. Surg., 58:602, 1971.

Horton, C., Maguire, C., Georgiade, N., and Pickrell, K.: Glomus tumors: An analysis of 25 cases. Arch. Surg., 71:712, 1955.

368.5. DISEASES OF THE PERIPHERAL VEINS

THROMBOPHLEBITIS

This subject is discussed in Ch. 357.2.

VARICOSE VEINS AND THE POSTPHLEBITIC SYNDROME

DEFINITION. Varicose veins are distended, tortuous veins with imcompetent valves. The postphlebitic syndrome denotes the chronically swollen extremity with trophic changes secondary to chronic venous stasis; despite the name, a previous history of thrombophlebitis is often not obtainable.

ETIOLOGY. Varicose veins are considered to be caused either by congenitally defective valves or by a condition that deforms valves or obstructs venous outflow over long periods of time. Varicosities resulting from congenital defects may develop early in life. Thrombophlebitis may lead to the formation of varicosities by deformation or destruction of venous valves and venous obstruction. Pregnancy, ascites, abdominal tumor, excessive weight or height, and prolonged weight bearing are all considered accelerating factors which cause increased venous pressures in the legs, distention of veins, and finally incompetency of valves. A generalized abnormality of the veins has been suggested as a predisposing factor. An increased forearm vein distensibility and a decreased amount of collagen and hexosamine in uninvolved veins have been demonstrated in patients with lower extremity varicosities; however, genetic evidence is not substantial. Since the majority of patients do not have obvious causes and varicose veins are an affliction of Western civilization, other factors in our society have been sought. The constipation associated with the Western countries' low-residue diet has been proposed as a frequent etiologic factor in varicosities. Emphasis is placed on the association of varicosities with hemorrhoids and diverticulosis, as a result of either increased intra-abdominal pressure during bowel movements or local pressure exerted by the bowel on intra-abdominal structures.

INCIDENCE. Varicose veins are very common, appearing in approximately 40 per cent of women; the incidence is less in men. The saphenous veins in the lower extremities are most frequently affected.

CLINICAL MANIFESTATIONS. The dilated, tortuous, sacculated varices are easily visible. Some patients with extensive superficial varicosities have no other symptoms or signs, but others have aching pain or easy fatigability of the calf muscles and edema after weight bearing. The edema usually disappears with bed rest overnight. Rarely the varicosities are so large that postural hypotension may result from pooling of blood in the lower extremities. When the communicating or deep veins are incompetent, symptoms and signs are more common. Chronic venous insufficiency is manifested by edema, which may later become fibrosed to produce a brawny induration. Extravasation of blood locally may cause a brownish pigmentation; an itchy, eczematoid rash may appear in the area. Finally the skin may ulcerate, producing an indolent, nonpainful lesion, usually above the medial malleolus near a palpable, incompetent communicating vein. This picture of chronic swelling and stasis dermatitis is called the postphlebitic syndrome. Arterial pulses are normal. When the deep venous system is blocked, pain similar to intermittent claudication may rarely occur.

DIAGNOSIS. The diagnosis can be made from the clinical picture. Retrograde flow of blood past incompetent valves can be demonstrated by the Trendelenburg test and its variations. The leg of the recumbent patient is elevated to empty the veins, and then a tourniquet is applied to occlude the superficial veins. The patient quickly assumes a standing position, the tourniquet is released, and the veins will become distended immediately if back flow is present. If two tourniquets are applied and left in place when the patient stands, filling of the saphenous veins between the tourniquets indicates an incompetent communicating vein. Application of the tourniquets to different levels on the limb can delineate exactly the sites of vein pathology. Venography may be used in doubtful cases or to be certain the deep venous system is patent. In a patient with varicosities and edema, other causes of edema, e.g., cardiovascular and renal disease, should be investigated.

PROGNOSIS. The prognosis for simple superficial varicose veins is good with treatment. Once the postphlebitic syndrome has developed, progressive disability usually can be expected despite treatment.

TREATMENT. Uncomplicated varicose veins respond well to support with elastic stockings or bandages to prevent progression. Panty girdles should never be worn. Frequent periods of elevation of the extremity above heart level, high ligation with stripping of the saphenous veins, and injection of sclerosing solutions may become necessary to prevent or treat the postphlebitic syndrome. However, since saphenous veins may be needed for arterial (coronary or peripheral) surgery, stripping should be performed only when absolutely unavoidable. Venous stasis ulcers are treated with sponge rubber pressure dressings or gelatin boots; local or systemic antimicrobials are indicated if infection is present. Sometimes the entire fibrosed area must be removed and a skin graft applied to heal an indolent ulcer.

Alexander, C. J.: The theoretical basis of varicose vein formation. Med. J. Aust., 1:258, 1972.
Burkitt, D. P.: Hemorrhoids, varicose veins and deep vein thrombosis: Epidemiologic features and suggested causative factors. Can. J. Surg., 18:483, 1975.
Fegan, W. G.: Conservative treatment of varicose veins. Prog. Surg., 11:37, 1973.
Hobbs, J. T.: The Treatment of Venous Disorders: A Comprehensive Review of Current Practice in the Management of Varicose Veins and the Post-thrombotic Syndrome. Philadelphia, J. B. Lippincott Company, 1977.
Mullarky, R. E.: The Anatomy of Varicose Veins. Springfield, Ill., Charles C Thomas, 1975.
Thurston, O. G., and Williams, H. T. G.: Chronic venous insufficiency of the lower extremity, Arch. Surg., 106:537, 1973.
Wood, J. E.: The Veins. Boston, Little, Brown & Company, 1965.

368.6. DISEASES OF THE PERIPHERAL LYMPHATIC VESSELS

Lymph is formed by the transudation of plasma through capillary walls into tissue spaces. The plasma that is not reabsorbed into the venular end of the capillaries is collected by a rich intercellular network of tiny lymphatic vessels. These vessels possess semilunar valves and become larger as they convey lymph to the regional lymph nodes; then the lymph travels through trunk lymphatics to the thoracic duct and finally to the left internal jugular vein. In the extremities, there are superficial and deep lymphatic systems which probably are joined by communicating vessels. The flow of lymph depends on intrinsic, rhythmic contractions of the lymph vessels, muscular contraction, respiratory movements, and, to a certain extent, gravity. The lymphatic vessels are responsive to sympathetic nerve stimulation, but the functional significance of this is not known.

LYMPHEDEMA

DEFINITION. Lymphedema is a form of chronic unilateral or bilateral edema of the extremities caused by the accumulation of lymph secondary to abnormalities or blockage of the lymph vessels or pathologic conditions of the lymph nodes.

ETIOLOGY. Primary lymphedema may be a hereditary disease or may occur sporadically. Various classifications exist according to whether the lymphedema is present at birth (*congenital*), appears at or near puberty (*praecox*), occurs after age 35 (*tarda*), or is familial and congenital (*Milroy's disease*). The mode of inheritance is probably dominant but has not been thoroughly investigated. An increased incidence occurs in ovarian dysgenesis syndromes. Primary lymphedema affects females predominantly (about 8:1); the onset of the disease occurs before age 40 in more than 90 per cent of cases.

Secondary lymphedema is most commonly caused by inflammation and follows recurrent lymphangitis (see below). In tropical and subtropical regions, filariasis often leads to lymphedema. Neoplasms are the second most common cause either by invasion or compression of lymph vessels or nodes. Surgical removal of lymph nodes and the fibrosis that follows irradiation may also cause lymphedema. Secondary cases have no special sex incidence and are uncommon before age 40.

PATHOLOGY. Examination of primary lymphedematous limbs by lymphangiography has revealed aplasia, hypoplasia, or hyperplasia (varicosities) of the lymphatic vessels. The lymph nodes may also be aplastic or hypoplastic, producing an obstructive type of lymphedema. No specific pathologic picture has been correlated with the current classification system but the few cases of Milroy's disease examined have revealed aplasia (or absence) of the lymphatic vessels. There is some indication that lymphedema may be part of a generalized defect in lymphatic vessels. Patients with lymphedema have been reported to have chylous pleural effusions, chylous ascites, and even intestinal lymphangiectasis. A syndrome of yellow nails, recurrent pleural effusion, and lymphedema occurs and is believed to be secondary to lymphatic abnormalities in each area. Another familial syndrome of recurrent intrahepatic cholestasis and lymphedema exists, the cholestasis probably being caused by defective hepatic lymphatic vessels. In secondary lymphedema, innumerable small, irregular lymphatics are usually seen beside normal or tortuous, sometimes varicose, vessels.

CLINICAL MANIFESTATIONS. Primary lymphedema is usually gradual in onset and asymptomatic; the distal portion of the extremity or whole extremity, or even a portion of the trunk, may increase in size. The edema is soft and pitting at first and disappears with treatment but later becomes firm and nonpitting, and cannot be relieved completely by treatment. At this stage, the skin becomes thickened and resists wrinkling; hair follicles are prominent. The lower extremities are involved most often; about half the patients develop bilateral swelling. The edematous tissue is especially susceptible to episodes of lymphangitis and cellulitis, which add to the deformity.

Secondary lymphedema is seldom bilateral. Lymphedema of the inflammatory type follows recurrent episodes of lymphangitis. Each attack leaves more residual edema after the inflammation subsides. The skin finally becomes thick, coarse, folded, and hard so that the eventual deformity may be extreme (elephantiasis). Secondary lymphedema resuting from neoplasm and other noninflammatory causes produces painless swelling of an extremity. Painless swelling of an extremity in an elderly male must be considered secondary to carcinoma of the prostate until proved otherwise.

DIAGNOSIS. Painless chronic swelling of an extremity suggests the diagnosis of lymphedema. Differentiation from venous insufficiency may be made by the lack of prominent veins, stasis dermatitis, and ulceration; lymphangiography and venography may be necessary. Mixed lymphangiomatous and hemangiomatous malformations that cause enlarged limbs can be diagnosed by the obvious tumor mass. In lipodystrophy, lymphangiography is necessary to delineate the normal lymphatics displaced by the lipomatous masses.

PROGNOSIS. Primary lymphedema usually progresses inexorably to a chronically swollen limb or limbs despite treatment. However, the lymphedema associated with gonadal dysgenesis may disappear spontaneously in months to years. Secondary lymphedema caused by infection may be controlled with adequate treatment. The prognosis is that of the underlying disease in other causes.

TREATMENT. In primary lymphedema, the most important aim of therapy is to keep the involved extremities free of edema in order to prevent fibrosis and recurrent infection. Frequent elevation of the extremity (including sleeping with the extremity above the heart level), elastic support applying graded pressure from the foot or hand proximally, external pneumatic compression, low sodium diet, and diuretics are usually necessary. Recently, a group of drugs containing benzopyrones has been reported in uncontrolled studies to be useful in treating lymphedema; their main action may be to increase the lysis of accumulated proteins in the lymphedematous tissue. Local infection and obvious lesions, such as epidermophytosis, should be eradicated. Surgical attack in advanced cases with fibrosis and resistant edema (Kondoleon operation and its modifications) has produced some relief but is usually disappointing.

Dilley, J. J., Kierland, R. R., Randall, R. V., and Shick, R. M.: Primary lymphedema associated with yellow nails and pleural effusions, JAMA, 204:670, 1968.

Gough, M. H.: Primary lymphedema: Clinical and lymphangiographic studies. Br. J. Surg., 53:918, 1966.

Hall, J. G.: The flow of lymph. N. Engl. J. Med., 281:720, 1969.

Kinmonth, J. B.: The Lymphatics: Diseases, Lymphography and Surgery. Baltimore, Williams & Wilkins Company, 1972.

Piller, N. B., and Cloduis, L.: The use of a tissue tonometer as a diagnostic aid in extremity lymphedema; a determination of its conservative treatment with benzopyrones. Lymphology, 9:127, 1976.

Sigstad, H., Aagenaes, Ø., Bjorn-Hansen, R. W., and Rootwelt, K.: Primary lymphoedema combined with hereditary recurrent intrahepatic cholestasis. Acta Med. Scand., 188:213, 1970.

Smith, R. D., Spittell, J. A., Jr., and Schirger, A.: Secondary lymphedema of the leg: Its characteristics and diagnostic implications. JAMA, 185:80, 1963.

LYMPHANGITIS

DEFINITION. Lymphangitis is an acute or chronic inflammation, usually pyogenic, of the lymphatic vessels.

ETIOLOGY. In the majority of cases of lymphangitis the hemolytic *Streptococcus* is the infecting agent; second most common is the coagulase-positive *Staphylococcus*. The bacteria enter the skin via areas of local trauma, trichophytosis, or arterial ischemic or venous stasis ulcers, although a portal of entry cannot always be discovered. Infection then spreads by the lymphatic vessels to the local lymph nodes; an accompanying diffuse cellulitis of the extremity is often present. An immune response to previously present bacteria or their products has been postulated as a cause of lymphangitis when an organism cannot be isolated, but proof of this is lacking.

PATHOLOGY. Acute, subacute, or chronic inflammation is found in the subcutaneous tissues and regional lymph nodes.

CLINICAL MANIFESTATIONS. Attacks of lymphangitis may be ushered in by malaise, headache, nausea, vomiting, and shaking chills followed by fever. Systemic symptoms, however, may not be present. Red streaks appear in the affected extremity, originating at the portal of entry and following the pathway of lymphatic vessels. Regional lymph nodes are usually enlarged and tender. There may be a surrounding area of cellulitis with tenderness and red discoloration in the lower part of the extremity, which is usually swollen with a soft, pitting edema.

DIAGNOSIS. The clinical picture is usually typical and allows the diagnosis to be made easily. A leukocytosis is often present. The inciting organism should be sought by culturing the portal of entry if obvious or by needle puncture of the subcutaneous tissues. A difficult diagnosis to rule out is acute thrombophlebitis, especially when a diffuse cellulitis is present, for symptoms and signs are similar; it is often wise to administer therapy for both diseases simultaneously.

PROGNOSIS. For an initial attack in a limb without underlying disease, the prognosis with treatment is excellent. However, some patients have recurrent attacks, often mild, which can lead to the development of lymphedema. In recurrent cases, the limb may remain somewhat larger after each attack.

TREATMENT. Systemic antimicrobial drugs should be administered as indicated by culture (and sensitivity studies if necessary). If no organism is cultured, penicillin should be given because the *Streptococcus* is so commonly the etiologic agent. Drainage of any focus of origin is also extremely important. Adjunctive measures include rest, elevation of the extremity above heart level, and warm wet dressings. Possible fungal infections in the feet and causes of secondary lymphedema should be sought. When attacks subside, elastic support should be worn on the extremity for three months to prevent residual swelling. In recurrent cases, either with or without underlying lymphedema, prophylactic long-term antimicrobial therapy should be instituted. Lymphangitis is especially dangerous in the ischemic tissues of patients with obstructive arterial disease; only under these unfavorable conditions is prompt amputation sometimes required.

Babb, R. R., Spittell, J. A., Jr., Martin, W. J., and Schirger, A.: Prophylaxis of recurrent lymphangitis complicating lymphedema. JAMA, 195:871, 1966.

Edwards, E. A.: Recurrent febrile episodes and lymphedema. JAMA, 184:858, 1963.

INDEX

Note: In this index the expression "vs." has been used to denote "differential diagnosis." Thus "Amebiasis, vs. malaria" is the equivalent of "Amebiasis, differential diagnosis from malaria." **Boldface entries and folios** in the index indicate main discussions in the text. *Italic folios* indicate illustrations and tables.

Dipetalonema perstans, 605, 632, **635**
Dipetalonema streptocerca, 632, 637
Diphenhydramine
in anaphylactic reaction complicating
therapy of serum sickness, 154
in angioedema, 163
in drug allergy, 157
in insect stings, 163
in parkinsonism, 755
in senile tremor, 757
Diphenoxylate
in diarrhea, 1480
in diarrhea of carcinoid syndrome,
2213
Diphenoxylate hydrochloride
in diarrhea after extensive small
intestinal resection, 1544
in malabsorption syndrome, *1536*
Diphenylhydantoin, 1265–1266
as nephrotoxin, 1432
hypocalcemia induced by, 2241
in cramps, 930
in digitalis toxicity, 1099
in epilepsy, *859,* 860
in intracranial tumors, 869
in myotonia congenita, 920
in myotonic dystrophy, 918
in status epilepticus, 861
in tabes dorsalis, 815
rickets or osteomalacia induced by,
2253
2,3-Diphosphoglycerate, in oxygen
dissociation, 1771
2,3-Diphosphoglyceric acid, levels of, in
shock, 1113
Diphtheria, 429–433
cutaneous, 431
vs. tropical phagedenic ulcer, 530
peripheral neuropathy with, 905
vs. infectious mononucleosis, 266
vs. streptococcal pharyngitis, 372
Diphtheria antitoxin, 432
Diphtheritic myocarditis, 431, 432, 1282
Diphyllobothrium latum, 559, 605, 606,
607
Diphyllobothrium mansonoides, 607
Diphyllobothrium pacificum, 607
Diplacusis, in sensorineural hearing
loss, 734
Diplopia, 899
in brain tumors, 865
in myasthenia gravis, 926
in thyroid eye disease, 2333
Dipylidium caninum, 611
Dirofilaria conjunctivae, 637
Dirofilaria immitis, 637
Dirofilaria repens, 637
Dirofilaria tenuis, 637
Dirofilariasis, 637
Disaccharidase deficiency, 1529, **1539**
Disc(s)
cervical, herniated, 894
intervertebral, protrusion of, 893–894
staphylococcal infections of, 402
lumbar, diseases of, vs.
arteriosclerosis obliterans, 1301
herniated, 894
Discoid lupus erythematosus, 176
Disease. See names of specific diseases.
Disequilibrium, linkage, 39
Disequilibrium syndrome
after dialysis in chronic renal failure,
1366
complicating maintenance
hemodialysis, 1381

Disodium cromoglycate, in asthma,
958
Disodium ethane-1-hydroxy-1,1-diphos-
phonate, in Paget's disease, 2259
Disopyramide, 1266
Dissecting aortic aneurysm, 1295–1297,
1296
vs. acute pericarditis, 1273
vs. myocardial infarction, 1233
**Disseminated encephalomyelitis, acute,
836–838, 849**
Disseminated infection, "atypical"
mycobacteria causing, 500
Disseminated intravascular coagulation
hypofibrinogenemic syndromes
associated with, 1893–1894
in cancer patient, 1906
in critically ill patient, 1052
in shock, 1113
without hypofibrinogenemia,
1894–1895
Disseminated listeriosis in infants, 472
Disseminated tuberculosis, vs. glanders,
469
**Dissociation, atrioventricular,
1255–1256,** *1256*
Distal myopathy, 918
Disuse osteopenia, 2236, 2237
"Disuse" osteoporosis, 2244, 2245
Diuresis, forced, in acute drug
poisoning, 714
Diuretics. See also names of specific
agents.
as nephrotoxins, 1432
hypercalcemia and, 2237
hypokalemia from, 1957, 1958
in arterial hypertension, 1212, *1212,*
1213
in heart failure, 1102–1106, *1102, 1103,
1104*
in nephrotic syndrome, 1389
metabolic alkalosis from, 1966
osmotic, in accidental poisoning, 74
in head injury, 882
Diuril. See *Chlorothiazide.*
Diverticulitis, 1582–1584
Meckel's, 1500, 1501
sigmoid, vs. Crohn's disease of colon,
1578
vs. ulcerative colitis, 1572
vs. acute appendicitis, 1581
vs. amebiasis, 592
Diverticulosis
colonic, 1501–1502
gallbladder, 1634
vs. diverticulitis, 1583
Diverticulum(a)
cecal, solitary, 1502
colonic, 1501–1502
angiography in, 1471, *1471*
gastrointestinal bleeding in,
1522
duodenal, 1500
bile duct obstruction by, 1632
epiphrenic, 1500
esophageal, 1499–1500
gastric, 1500
hypopharyngeal, 1499
ileal, 1500–1501
jejunal, 1500–1501
malabsorption in, 1537
Meckel's, 1500–1501
radionuclide imaging in, 1470
mid-esophageal, 1499
pericardial, 1276

Diverticulum(a) (*Continued*)
urethral, 1458
Zenker's 1499
Diving
atmospheric pressure changes with,
98, *98*
deep-sea, accidents during, vertigo
caused by, 740
hazards of, 98, 99, 102, 103
scuba, air travel after, 96
Dizziness, 737–742
conditions producing, 738–742
epileptic, 741
evaluation of, 737–738, *738*
hyperventilation-induced, 741
in cerebral transient ischemic attacks,
785
multisensory, 741, 742
psychiatric disease producing, 742
types of, 737
Dizziness simulation battery, 737, 738
DNA, 31
replication of, 31
synthesis of, slowed, megaloblastic
anemia from, 1723, 1724
Watson-Crick model for, 31
DNA–anti-DNA complexes, in systemic
lupus erythematosus, 134
Dog tapeworm, 611
Dolichostenomelia, 2053–2054
Dolophine. See *Methadone.*
DOM, 704
Dominance, functional, 656
Donovan body, in granuloma inguinale,
429
Donovania granulomatis, 429
L-Dopa, in assessment of growth hormone, 2092
Dopamine, 751, 2199, 2200
cerebral, functional excess of, schizo-
phrenia and, 668
in shock, 1048, 1120
Doriden. See *Glutethimide.*
Dorsal root ganglionitis, in cancer, 878
Double outlet right ventricle, 1173
Downey cells, in infectious
mononucleosis, 266
Down's syndrome
acute leukemia in, 1814
clinical and cytogenetic characteristics
of, *52*
frequency and sex ratio of, *48*
heterozygote detection in, *58*
intrauterine diagnosis of, *59*
Doxinate. See *Dioctyl sodium sulfosuccinate.*
Doxorubicin. See also *Adriamycin.*
in oncologic treatment, 1936, 1937
Doxycycline, 557, 562
in epidemic louse-borne typhus, 319
in louse-borne relapsing fever, 528
in rickettsial diseases, 316
in trachoma and inclusion conjunctivitis, 334
dp/dt, indices of, 1085
Dracontiasis, 633
Dracunculus medinensis, 605, 633
Dramamine. See *Dimenhydrinate.*
Dressings, wet, in dermatologic therapy, 2275, *2275,* 2276
Dressler's syndrome, 1237, 1271
Drop attacks, in brainstem ischemia,
784, 785
Droplet nuclei, tuberculosis infection
by, 480

Opsonins, in pneumococcal pneumonia, 349

Optic atrophy, 813, **815**
  hereditary motor and sensory neuropathy with, 913

Optic nerve
  disorders of, 899, **2327–2329**
  glioma of, 868
  in sarcoidosis, 2329
  in sickle cell diseases, 2331

Optic neuritis, 848–849
  acute, in cancer, 878
  complicating ethambutol therapy of pulmonary tuberculosis, 488

Optic neuropathy, ischemic, in giant cell arteritis, 2319

Oral cholecystography, 1622, *1623*
  in chronic cholecystitis, 1625

Oral contraceptives, 2195–2197
  cerebral infarction and, 781
  contraindications to, 2197
  hypertension and, 1211
  side effects of, 2195, 2196

Oral hypoglycemic agents, in diabetes mellitus, 1986, *1986*

Oral-facial-digital-syndrome, *2300*

Orbit, pseudotumor of, 224

Orbital cellulitis
  vs. cavernous sinus thrombosis, 808
  vs. Romaña's sign in Chagas' disease, 582

Orbital mucormycosis, in diabetes mellitus, 2320

Orchitis, 2174
  in epidemic pleurodynia, 272
  in mumps, 262

Organic particles
  acute airway reactions to, 996–997
  airways obstruction due to, 997–998, *997*
  pulmonary effects of, *984*

Organic solvents
  as nephrotoxins, 1434
  inhalation of, 705

Organomercurial diuretics, in heart failure, *1103, 1104,* 1105

Organophosphorus compounds, neuropathy from, 911

Orgasm, 687
  female, dysfunction of, 688, 2198, 2199
  male, dysfunction of, 688, 2198

Oriental cholangiohepatitis, 1633

Oriental sore, 587–589, *588*

Oriental tussock moth, dermatitis caused by, 119

Ornithine transcarbamylase deficiency, *2018,* 2022, 2044

Ornithinemia, 2022

Ornithodoros erraticus, 529

Ornithodoros hermsi, 529

Ornithodoros moubata, 526, 529

Ornithodoros tholozani, 529

Ornithodoros turicata, 529

Ornithosis, 336–338

Oropharyngeal tube, in acute respiratory failure, 1025, 1026

Orotic aciduria, *42,* 2044
  prevention and management of, 55

Oroya fever, 331–332

Orthopedic surgery
  in degenerative joint disease, 205
  in rheumatoid arthritis, 193

Orthopnea, in left ventricular failure, 1089

Orthostatic hypotension, 742, 743
  faintness in, 740
  idiopathic, 762–763
  in diabetes mellitus, 1980

Oscillopsia, in vertigo, 737

Osler's nodes, in infective endocarditis, 389

Osler-Weber-Rendu syndrome, 1880, *2298, 2301*

Osmium tetroxide, exposure to, respiratory effects of, 1000

Osmotic agents, in constipation, 1482

Osmotic diarrhea, 1479

Osmotic diuretics
  in accidental poisoning, 74
  in head injury, 882

Osseous hydatid, 609, 610

Osteitis deformans, 2257–2259

Osteitis fibrosa, in chronic renal failure, 1359, 1360

Osteitis fibrosa cystica, in hyperparathyroidism, 2215, *2216,* 2217

Osteoarthritis, 202–205, *203*
  erosive, 204
  hypertrophic, primary generalized, 204
  vs. rheumatoid arthritis, 190

Osteoarthropathy, hypertrophic, 201, 2263
  in bronchogenic carcinoma, 1007

Osteochondritis dissecans, 2260

Osteodystrophy, renal, 1360, **2254–2257**

Osteogenesis imperfecta, 2245
  aorta in, 1292
  vs. Ehlers-Danlos syndrome, 2055
  vs. juvenile osteoporosis, 2246

Osteoid seams, 2247

Osteolysis, in Paget's disease, 2258

Osteomalacia, 2247–2254
  anticonvulsant, 2253
  axial, 2254
  in cadmium poisoning, 82
  in chronic renal failure, 1360, 2254
  in malabsorption syndrome, 1528
  vs. hyperparathyroidism, 2217

Osteomyelitis, 2260–2261
  due to contiguous infection, 2261
  in blastomycosis, 540
  in subdural empyema, 807
  pyogenic, subacute, 2260
  refractory, hyperbaric oxygen therapy in, 105
  Salmonella causing, 2260
    in sickle cell anemia, 451
  staphylococcal, 402–403, 2260
    vs. sporotrichosis, 545
    vs. actinomycosis, 474

Osteonecrosis, 2259–2260
  dysbaric, of divers and caisson workers, 102

Osteopenia, disuse, 2236, 2237

Osteopetrosis, 2263

Osteopoikilosis, 2264

Osteoporosis, 2242–2246
  endocrine, 2244
  in adrenocorticosteroid therapy of rheumatoid arthritis, 192
  in homocystinuria, 2028
  in malabsorption syndrome, 1528
  in multiple myeloma, 1858, *1859*
  in rheumatoid arthritis, 189
  juvenile, 2246
    vs. osteogenesis imperfecta, 2245
  painful, post-traumatic, 727

Osteoporosis (*Continued*)
  postmenopausal, 2190, 2191, 2243, 2244
  primary, 2243–2244
  senile, 2243, 2244
  treatment of, 2246
  vs. hyperparathyroidism, 2217

Osteoporosis circumscripta, in Paget's disease, 2258

Osteoradionecrosis, hyperbaric oxygen therapy in, 104, 105

Osteosclerosis
  in agnogenic myeloid metaplasia, 1828
  in chronic renal failure, 1360

Ostium primum atrial septal defect, 1171

Ostium secundum atrial septal defect, 1160, 1161, 1162

Otitic hydrocephalus, 871

Otitis media
  air travel and, 96
  hearing loss from, 735
  Hemophilus influenzae in, 425
  in measles, 248
  in streptococcal pharyngitis, 373

Otomycosis, 547

Otosclerosis, hearing loss from, 735

Ototoxic drugs
  hearing loss from, 736
  vertigo from, 739

Ouabain, in heart failure, *1096,* 1097

"Ouch-ouch" disease, 82, 1429

Ovale malaria, 567
  clinical manifestations of, 571
  relapse of, 574

Ovarian steroid biosynthesis, pathways of, 2178, *2178*

Ovary(ies), 2175–2199
  cyst of, twisted, vs. acute appendicitis, 1581
  disorders of, 2179–2199
    amenorrhea due to, 2185–2186
    ascites in, 1593
  function of, 2175–2179
    status of, breast cancer and, 1918
    tests of, 2179, 2180, *2180,* 2181, *2181*
    hormones of, function of, 2176, *2177,* 2177–2178
    hyperfunction of, organic precocious pseudopuberty due to, 2182, 2183
  polycystic, 2188–2190
    resistant, syndrome of, 2186
    sclerocystic, 2189
  structure of, 2175–2179
    tuberculosis of, 496
    tumors of, carcinoid features of, 2212

Oversuppression syndrome, prolactin levels in, 2092

Oxacillin, *557,* 559
  in bacterial meningitis, 415
  in infective endocarditis, 393
  in infective endocarditis prophylaxis, 396
  in osteomyelitis, 2261
  in staphylococcal meningitis, 404
  in staphylococcal pneumonia, 402

Oxamniquine, in schistosomiasis, 616

Oxazolidinediones, as nephrotoxins, 1432

Oxprenolol
  in arterial hypertension, *1212*
  in hypertension of chronic renal failure, 1362

Oxycodone, in pain, 724

Peptic ulcer (*Continued*)
roentgenography in, 1509, 1510, *1510,*
1511, 1511, 1512, *1512*
stress causing, 1504
surgical treatment of, 1518–1520, *1519*
chronic postoperative morbidity in,
1520
symptoms of, 1507
vs. acute appendicitis, 1580
vs. angina pectoris, 1227
vs. chronic cholecystitis, 1625
Peptidergic neuron systems, central,
2077, *2078*
Peptococcus asaccharolyticus, 441
Peptococcus magnus, 441
Peptococcus prevotii, 441
Peptostreptococcus anaerobius, 441
Peptostreptococcus intermedius, 441
Peptostreptococcus micros, 441
Peptostreptococcus species, 367
Perchlorate discharge test, 2118, *2119*
Percutaneous antegrade pyelography, in
obstructive nephropathy, 1449
Percutaneous transhepatic
cholangiography, 1473–1474, *1473,*
1474
Percutaneous transtracheal aspiration,
microbiologic diagnosis by, 342
Perennial allergic rhinitis, 157
Perforation
colonic, in amebiasis, 591
in ulcerative colitis, 1575
gallbladder, in acute cholecystitis,
1626, 1628
gastrointestinal, in cancer patient,
1906
ileal, in regional enteritis, 1564
intestinal, in typhoid fever, 447, 448
of peptic ulcer, 1518
vs. acute cholecystitis, 1627
vs. myocardial infarction, 1233
Perfusion, 932, **938**
impaired, radionuclide imaging in,
944, 945
in airways obstruction, 953
Perhexilene, in angina pectoris, 1228
Periactin. See *Cyproheptadine.*
Periampullary neoplasms, vs.
choledocholithiasis, 1630
Perianal abscess, 1617
Periarteritis nodosa, 165, **180–183,** *2298*
cutaneous signs in, *2301*
drugs causing, 156
eyes in, 2317
malabsorption in, 1543
neuropathy in, 908
renal involvement in, 181, 1400
vs. toxocariasis, 628
vs. trichinosis, 631
Pericardial constriction, 1274–1275
Pericardial effusion, 1273–1274
chylous, 1276
in right ventricular failure, 1093
Pericardial friction rub, in acute
pericarditis, 1272
Pericardiectomy, in constrictive
pericarditis, 1275
Pericardiocentesis
in pericardial effusion, 1274
in tuberculous pericarditis, 494
Pericarditis
acute, 1269–1273
vs. myocardial infarction, 1233

Pericarditis (*Continued*)
allergic disorders associated with,
1272
amebic, 592
cholesterol, 1276
complicating maintenance
hemodialysis, 1382
connective tissue disorders causing,
1271, 1272
constrictive, 1274–1275
protein-losing enteropathy and,
1549
enteroviruses causing, 272–273
idiopathic, 1269
benign, vs. rheumatic fever, 383
in bacterial meningitis, 414
in chronic renal failure, 1365
in pneumococcal pneumonia, 353, 354
treatment of, 356
in systemic lupus erythematosus, 180
in tularemia, 467
infectious, 1269–1270
metabolic disorders causing, 1272
nonspecific, 1269
physical or chemical agents causing,
1272
postmyocardial infarction, 1231, 1270,
1271
postsurgical, 1271
post-traumatic, 1271
staphylococcal, 404
tuberculous, 494–495, 1270
vs. acute appendicitis, 1581
vs. angina pectoris, 1227
vs. peptic ulcer, 1507
vs. pulmonary embolism, 1133
Pericardium
bacterial infections of, 1270
congenital absence of, 1276
congenital lesions of, 1276
disorders of, 1268–1276
etiology of, *1269*
diverticula of, 1276
in pneumococcal pneumonia, 349
tumors of, 1276
viral infections of, 1269
Perifolliculitis of ascorbic acid
deficiency, 1675
Perihepatitis, gonococcal, 408, 409
vs. acute cholecystitis, 1627
Perinatal polycystic kidney disease,
1453
Perinephric abscess, 1410
Periodic catatonia, 668
Periodic fever, 2055–2057
Periodic paralysis
familial, 921–922
hyperkalemic, 921, 1959
vs. hysteria, 679
Periosteal nodules, in rheumatoid
arthritis, 187, 188
Periostitis
in blastomycosis, 540
in syphilis, 510
in yaws, *520,* 521
Peripartum cardiomyopathy, 1287
Peripheral arteries, in diabetes mellitus,
1981
Peripheral arteritis, in systemic
infections, 1305
Peripheral circulation, 1066–1067
Peripheral lymphatic vessels, diseases
of, 1314–1315

Peripheral nerves
in rheumatoid arthritis, 187, 189
nonmetastatic effects of cancer on,
878
Peripheral nervous system
diseases of, 899–913
in periarteritis nodosa, 182
Peripheral neuritis
drugs causing, 156
in diphtheria, 432
vs. polymyositis, 173
Peripheral neurons, inherited disorders
of, 911
Peripheral neuropathy(ies), 899–913
alcohol-related, 709
diabetes mellitus and, 908–909, 1979,
1980. See also *Neuropathy(ies),*
diabetic.
differential diagnosis of, 903–905
glossitis and, in malabsorption
syndrome, 1529
in bronchogenic carcinoma, 1007
in chronic renal failure, 1365
in multiple myeloma, 910, 1860
respiratory failure in, *1023,* 1024
symptoms of, 903, 904
vs. amyotrophic lateral sclerosis, 766
vs. idiopathic autonomic
insufficiency, 763
vs. myasthenia gravis, 927
vs. radiculopathy, 889, *890, 891*
with carcinoma, 910
with drug use, 910
with endocrine diseases, 909
with hepatic disease, 909
with household and industrial
poisons, 910
with infection, 905–906
with inflammation and presumed
altered immunity, 906
with mesenchymal disease and
necrotizing angiopathy, 908
with uremia, 909
Peripheral sensory neurons, disorders
of, 911–912
Peripheral vascular diseases, 1299–1315
diabetes mellitus and, neuropathy in,
908
due to abnormal communications
between arteries and veins,
1312–1313
due to abnormal vasoconstriction or
vasodilatation, 1305–1309
due to exposure to cold, 1309–1312
due to organic arterial obstruction,
1299–1305
Peripheral vasoconstriction, in heart
failure, 1088
Peripheral veins, diseases of, 1313–1314
Peripheral vestibulopathy
acute, 738
acute and recurrent, 738, 739
Periphlebitis, retinal, in sarcoidosis,
2329
Perirectal abscess(es)
enteric bacteria causing, 455
tuberculous, 492
Perirectal fistula, in regional enteritis,
1562
Peristalsis, esophageal, 1478
Peritoneal dialysis, 1377–1378
in accidental poisoning, 74
Peritoneoscopy, 1592